Success in the Classroom, in Clinicals, and on the NCLEX-RN®

Classroom

- Detailed lecture notes organized by learning outcome
- Suggestions for classroom activities
- Guide to relevant additional resources
- Comprehensive PowerPoint™ presentations integrating lecture, images, animations, and videos
- Classroom Response questions
- Image Gallery
- Video and Animation Gallery
- Online course management systems complete with instructor tools and student activities available in a variety of formats

---

PEARSON **mynursinglab**®

- Saves instructors time by providing quality feedback, ongoing formative assessments and customized remediation for students
- Provides easy, one-stop access to a wealth of teaching resources, such as test item files, PowerPoint™ slides, and video suggestions
- A built-in electronic gradebook tracks students' progress on assessment and remediation activities

Clinical

- Suggestions for Clinical Activities and other clinical resources organized by learning outcome

---

Real Nursing Simulations Facilitator's Guide: Institutional Edition

- 25 simulation scenarios that span the nursing curriculum
- Consistent format includes learning objectives, case flow, instructions for set up, student debriefing questions and more
- Companion online course cartridge with student exercises, activities, videos, skill checklists, and reflective questions also available for adoption

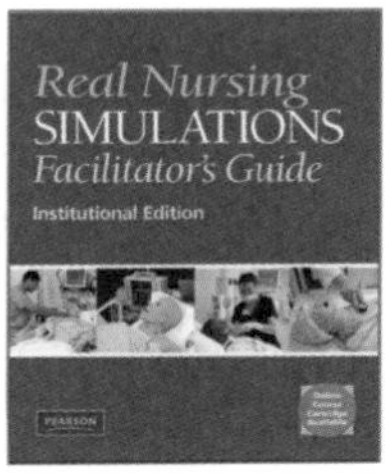

NCLEX-RN®

- Test Item Files with NCLEX®-style questions and complete rationales for correct and incorrect answers mapped to learning outcomes–*available in TestGen, Par Test, and MS Word*

Instructor Resources

***More** information and instructor resources*
***visit** www.mynursingkit.com*

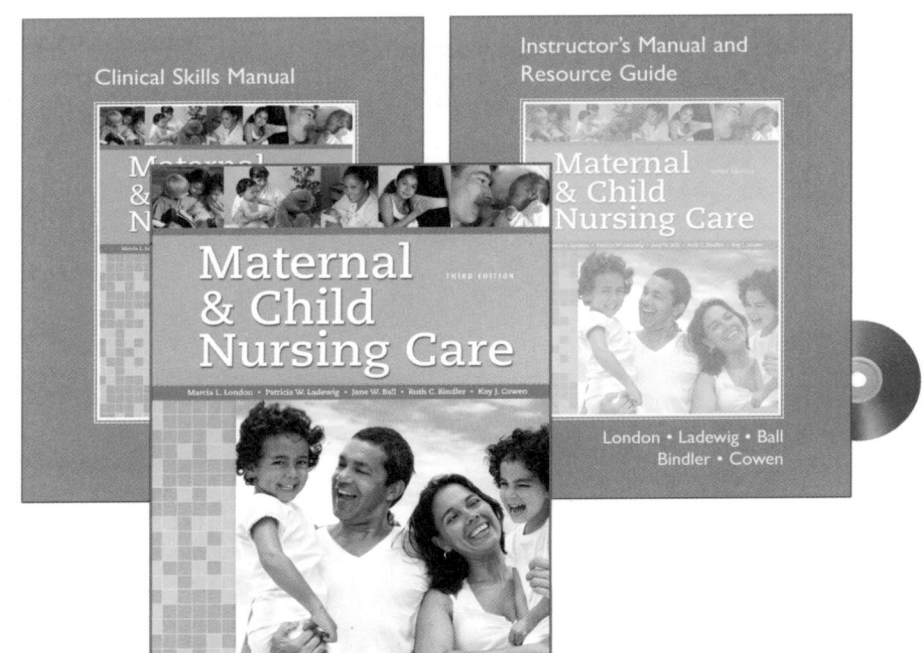

Brief Contents

EXPLORE PEARSON mynursingkit™

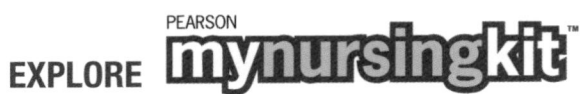

STEP 1: Register

All you need to get started is a valid email address and the access code below. To register, simply:

1. Go to **www.mynursingkit.com**. Click on the appropriate book cover.
2. In the "First-Time User" column, click "**Register**."
3. Read the **License Agreement** and **Privacy Policy**. If you accept, click "**I Accept**."
4. Under "**Do you have a Pearson account**?" select:
   - "**Yes**" if you have a Pearson account and know your Login Name and Password.
   - "**Not Sure**" if you do not know if you already have an account or do not recall your Login Name and Password.
   - "**No**" if you are sure you do not have a Pearson account.
5. Using a coin, scratch off the silver coating below to reveal your access code. Do not use a knife or other sharp object, which can damage the code.
6. Enter your access code in lowercase or uppercase, without the dashes, then click "**Next**."
7. Follow the on-screen instructions to complete registration.

After completing registration, you will be sent a confirmation email that contains your Login Name and Password. Be sure to save this email for future reference.

Your Access Code is:

Note: If there is no silver foil covering the access code, it may already have been redeemed, and therefore may no longer be valid. In that case, you can purchase access online using a major credit card. To do so, go to www.mynursingkit.com. Find and click on the cover of your textbook, then click "Get Access," and follow the on-screen instructions.

STEP 2: Log in

1. Go to **www.mynursingkit.com**.
2. Find and click on the appropriate book cover. Cover must match the textbook edition used for your class.
3. Enter the Login Name and Password that you created during registration. If unsure of this information, refer to your registration confirmation email.
4. Click "**Login**."

Got technical questions?

Customer Technical Support: To obtain support, please visit us online anytime at http://247pearsoned.custhelp.com where you can search our knowledgebase for common solutions, view product alerts, and review all options for additional assistance.

SITE REQUIREMENTS
For the latest updates on Site Requirements, go to www.mynursingkit.com. Find and click on the cover of the book you are using. Click on "**Needs help?**" link at bottom of page. Under "**Technical Problems**" select the link "**What do I need on my computer to use this site?**"

Important: Please read the Subscription and End-User License agreement, accessible from the book website's login page, before using the *mynursingkit* website. By using the website, you indicate that you have read, understood, and accepted the terms of this agreement.

0135078466

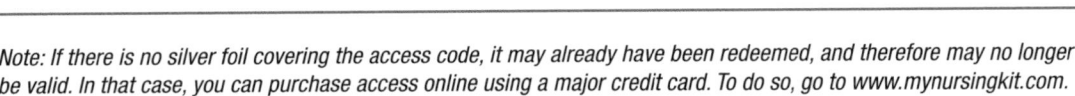

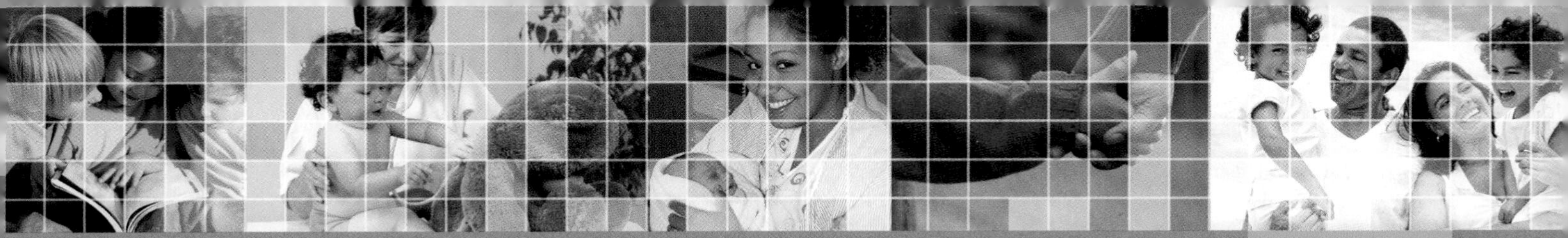

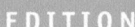

EDITION 3

Maternal & Child Nursing Care

Marcia L. London, RN, MSN, APRN, CNS, NNP-BC
Senior Clinical Instructor and Ret. Director of Neonatal Nurse Practitioner Program
Beth-El College of Nursing and Health Sciences
University of Colorado, Colorado Springs, Colorado
Staff Clinical Nurse
Urgent Care and After Hours Clinic
Colorado Springs, Colorado

Patricia A. Wieland Ladewig, PhD, RN
Professor and Academic Dean
Rueckert-Hartman College for Health Professions
Regis University
Denver, Colorado

Jane W. Ball, RN, CPNP, DrPH
Consultant
American College of Surgeons
Gaithersburg, Maryland

Ruth C. Bindler, RNC, PhD
Professor
Washington State University
College of Nursing
Spokane, Washington

Kay J. Cowen, RNC, MSN
Clinical Associate Professor
University of North Carolina at Greensboro
Greensboro, North Carolina

Pearson

New York Boston San Francisco
London Toronto Sydney Tokyo Singapore Madrid
Mexico City Munich Paris Cape Town Hong Kong Montreal

Library of Congress Cataloging-in-Publication Data
Maternal & child nursing care / Marcia L. London . . . [et al.]. — 3rd ed.
p. ; cm.
Includes bibliographical references and index.
ISBN-13: 978-0-13-507846-4
ISBN-10: 0-13-507846-6
1. Maternity nursing. 2. Pediatric nursing. I. London, Marcia L. II. Title: Maternal and child nursing care.
[DNLM: 1. Maternal-Child Nursing—methods. 2. Pediatric Nursing—methods. WY 157.3 M42525 2011]
RG951.M3145 2011
618.2'0231—dc22

2009052407

Publisher: Julie Levin Alexander
Assistant to Publisher: Regina Bruno
Editor-in-Chief: Maura Connor
Editorial Assistant: Marion Gottlieb
Editorial Assistant: Luz Costa
Executive Acquisitions Editor: Kim Mortimer
Assistant Editor: Sarah Wrocklage
Director of Marketing: Karen Allman
Marketing Specialist: Michael Sirinides
Development Editor: Dana Knighten
Development Project Manager: Molly Mullen Ward
Managing Editor, Production: Patrick Walsh
Production Editor: Lynn Steines, S4Carlisle Publishing Services
Production Liaison: Anne Garcia
Media Project Manager: Rachel Collett
Manufacturing Manager: Ilene Sanford
Senior Design Coordinator: Maria Guglielmo-Walsh
Interior Design: Wanda España
Cover Design: Wanda España
Composition: S4Carlisle Publishing Services
Manager, Visual Rights and Permissions: Zina Arabia
Manager, Visual Research: Beth Brenzel
Manager, Cover Visual Research & Permissions: Karen Sanatar
Image Permission Coordinator: Vickie Menanteaux
Printer/Binder: Courier Kendallville
Cover Printer: Lehigh-Phoenix Color/Hagerstown

PEARSON

www.pearsonhighered.com

10 9 8 7 6 5 4 3 2 1
ISBN-13: 978-0-13-507846-4
ISBN-10: 0-13-507846-6

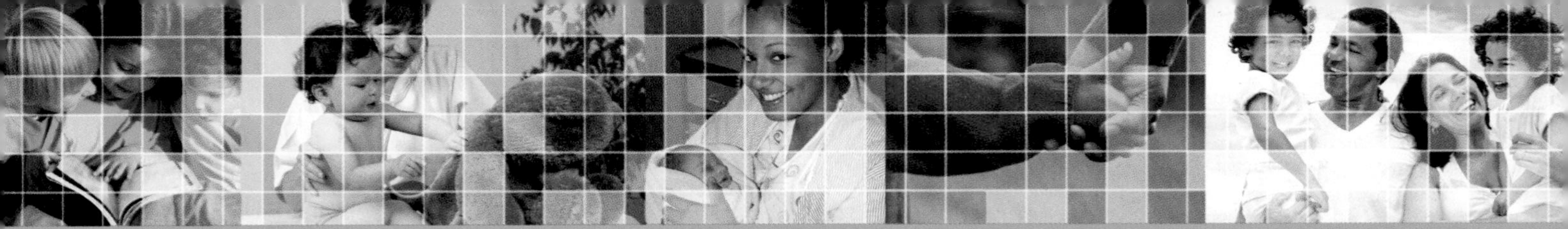

About the Authors

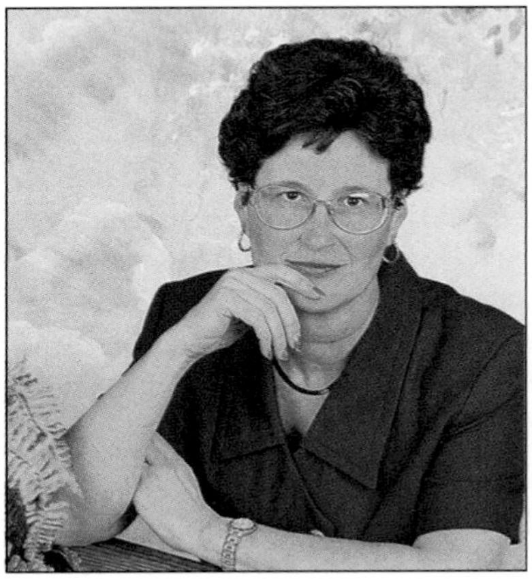

MARCIA L. LONDON Marcia L. London has been able to combine her two greatest passions by being both a nurse caring for children and families, and a teacher for almost 39 years. She received her BSN and School Nurse Certificate from Plattsburgh State University in Plattsburgh, New York, and her MSN in pediatrics as a clinical nurse specialist from the University of Pittsburgh in Pennsylvania. She began her nursing career as a pediatric nurse at St. Luke's Hospital in New York City and began her teaching career at Pittsburgh Children's Hospital Affiliate Program. Mrs. London began teaching at Beth-El School of Nursing and Health Science in 1974 (now part of the University of Colorado, Colorado Springs) after opening the first intensive care nursery at Memorial Hospital of Colorado Springs. She has served in many faculty and administrative positions at Beth-El, including assistant director of the School of Nursing and coordinator of undergraduate nursing care of children. Mrs. London maintains her clinical skills by working in an urgent care and after-hours clinic and doing undergraduate pediatric clinical supervision. She obtained her postmaster's neonatal nurse practitioner certificate in 1983 and subsequently developed the neonatal nurse practitioner (NNP) program and the master's NNP program at Beth-El. She is active nationally in neonatal nursing and was involved in the development of the Neonatal Nurse Practitioner Educational Program Guidelines. She has contributed five chapters to various neonatal nursing texts. Mrs. London is active in nurse practitioner education in general. She was involved in the revision of the Core Competency for Nurse Practitioners and Curriculum Guidelines for Nurse Practitioner Education, as a member of the Education Committee of the National Organization of Nurse Practitioner Faculties, and she also participated as part of the Core Competency Validation Expert Panel. Mrs. London has also pursued her interest in college student learning by taking doctoral classes in higher education administration and adult learning at the University of Denver in Colorado. She feels fortunate to be involved in the education of her future colleagues. Her teaching philosophy is that, with support, students can achieve more than they may initially believe they are capable of achieving. Mrs. London and her husband, David, enjoy reading, travel, and hockey games. They have two sons: Craig, who lives in Florida, works with Internet companies; and Matthew works in computer teleresearch. Both are more than willing to give Mom helpful hints about computers.

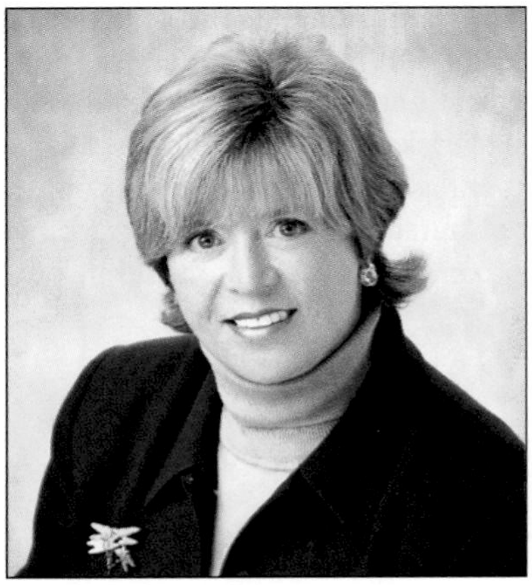

PATRICIA A. WIELAND LADEWIG Patricia A. Wieland Ladewig received her BS from the College of Saint Teresa in Winona, Minnesota. After graduation, she worked as a pediatric nurse before joining the U.S. Air Force. After completing her tour of duty, she relocated to Florida, where she accepted a faculty position at Florida State University. There she embraced teaching as her calling. Over the years, she taught at several schools of nursing while earning her MSN in maternal-newborn nursing from Catholic University of America in Washington, DC, and her PhD in higher education administration from the University of Denver in Colorado. In addition, she became a women's health nurse practitioner and maintained a part-time clinical practice. In 1988 Dr. Ladewig became the first director of the nursing program at Regis College in Denver and, in 1991, when the college became Regis University, she became dean of the Rueckert-Hartman College for Health Professions. Under her guidance, the School of Nursing has added a graduate program. In addition, the college has added a School of Physical Therapy, a School of Pharmacy, and two departments: the Department of Health Services Administration and Management and the Department of Health Care Ethics. When not at work or writing textbooks, Pat and her husband, Tim, enjoy skiing, baseball games, and traveling. However, their greatest pleasure comes from their family: son Ryan, his wife, Amanda, and grandchildren Reed and Addison, and son Erik, his wife, Kedri, and granddaughter Emma.

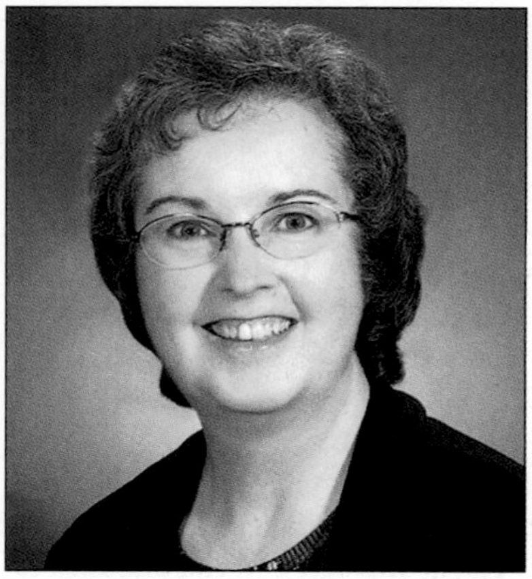

JANE W. BALL Jane W. Ball graduated from The Johns Hopkins Hospital School of Nursing, and subsequently received a BS from The Johns Hopkins University. She worked in the surgical, emergency, and outpatient units of the Johns Hopkins Children's Medical and Surgical Center, first as a staff nurse and then as a pediatric nurse practitioner. Thus began her career as a pediatric nurse and advocate for children's health needs. Jane obtained both a master of public health and doctor of public health degree from the Johns Hopkins University Bloomberg School of Public Health with a focus on maternal and child health. After graduation she became the chief of child health services for the Commonwealth of Pennsylvania Department of Health. In this capacity she oversaw the state-funded well-child clinics and explored ways to improve education for the state's community health nurses. After relocating to Texas, she joined the faculty at the University of Texas at Arlington School of Nursing to teach community pediatrics to registered nurses returning to school for a BSN. During this time she became involved in writing her first textbook, *Mosby's Guide to Physical Examination,* which is currently in its seventh edition. After relocating to the Washington, DC, area, she joined Children's National Medical Center to manage a federal project to teach instructors of emergency medical technicians from all states about the special care children need during an emergency. Exposure to the shortcomings of the emergency medical services system in the late 1980s with regard to pediatric care was a career-changing event. With federal funding, she developed educational curricula for emergency medical technicians and emergency nurses to help them provide improved care for children. A textbook entitled *Pediatric Emergencies, A Manual for Prehospital Providers* was developed from these educational ventures. For the past 16 years, she was the executive director of the federally funded Emergency Medical Services for Children National Resource Center, providing consultation and resource development for state health agencies, health professionals, families, and advocates to improve the emergency healthcare system for children. Dr. Ball currently serves as a consultant to the American College of Surgeons assisting states to develop and enhance their trauma systems.

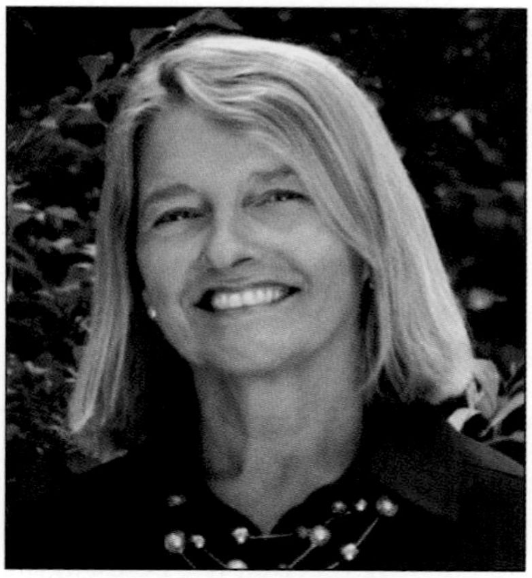

RUTH C. MCGILLIS BINDLER Ruth Bindler received her BSN from Cornell University–New York Hospital School of Nursing in New York. She worked in oncology nursing at Memorial–Sloan Kettering Cancer Center in New York, and then moved to Wisconsin and became a public health nurse in Dane County. Thus began her commitment to work with children as she visited children and their families at home, and served as a school nurse for several elementary, middle, and high schools. As a result of this interest in child healthcare needs, she earned her MS in child development from the University of Wisconsin. A move to Washington State was accompanied by a new job as a faculty member at the Intercollegiate Center for Nursing Education in Spokane, Washington, now the WSU College of Nursing. Dr. Bindler has been fortunate to be involved for 35 years in the growth of this nursing education consortium, which is a combination of public and private universities and offers undergraduate, masters, and doctoral nursing degrees. She has taught theory and clinical courses in child health nursing, cultural diversity, graduate research, pharmacology, and assessment, served as lead faculty for child health nursing, and is presently director of the PhD Program. Her first professional book, *Pediatric Medications,* was published in 1981, and she has continued to publish articles and books in the areas of pediatric medications and pediatric health. Her research efforts are focused in the area of childhood obesity, type 2 diabetes, and cardiovascular risk factors in children. Ethnic diversity has been another theme in her work. Dr. Bindler believes that her role as a faculty member has enabled her to learn continually, to foster the development of students in nursing, and to participate fully in the profession of nursing. In addition to teaching, research, publication, and leadership, she enhances her life by service in several professional and community activities, and by outdoor activities with her family.

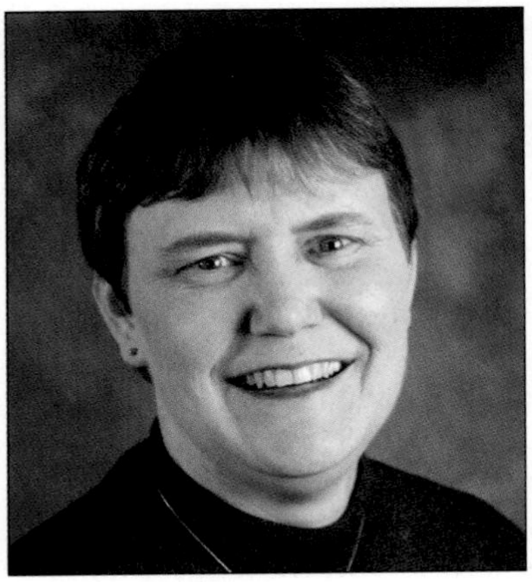

KAY J. COWEN Kay Cowen received her BSN degree from East Carolina University in Greenville, North Carolina, and began her career as a staff nurse on the pediatric unit of North Carolina Baptist Hospital in Winston Salem. She developed a special interest in the psychosocial needs of hospitalized children and preparing them for hospitalization. This led to the focus of her master's thesis at the University of North Carolina at Greensboro (UNCG) where she received a Master of Science in Nursing Education degree with a focus in maternal child nursing. Mrs. Cowen began her teaching career in 1984 at UNCG, where she continues today as Clinical Associate Professor in the Parent Child Department. Her primary responsibilities include coordination of the pediatric nursing course, teaching classroom content and supervising a clinical group of students. Mrs. Cowen shared her passion for the psychosocial care of children and the needs of their families through her first experience as an author in the chapter "Hospital Care for Children" in *Child Health Nursing: A Comprehensive Approach to the Care of Children and Their Families* published in 1993. In the classroom Mrs. Cowen realized that students learn through a variety of teaching strategies, and she became especially interested in the strategy of gaming. She led a research study to evaluate the effectiveness of gaming in the classroom and subsequently continues to incorporate gaming in her teaching. In the clinical setting Mrs. Cowen teaches her students the skills needed to care for patients and the importance of family-centered care, focusing on not only the physical needs of the child but also the psychosocial needs of the child and family. During her teaching career, Mrs. Cowen has continued to work part time as a staff nurse, first on the pediatric unit of Moses Cone Hospital in Greensboro and then at Brenner Children's Hospital in Winston Salem. In 2006 she became the part-time pediatric nurse educator in Brenner's Family Resource Center. Through this role she is able to extend her love of teaching to children and families. Through her role as an author, Mrs. Cowen is able to extend her dedication to pediatric nursing and nursing education. She is married and the mother of two college-age sons.

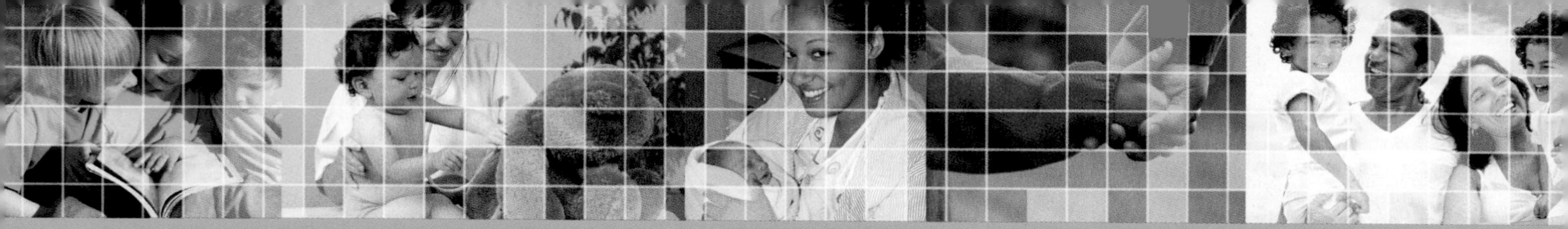

Thank You!

We are grateful to all the nurses, both clinicians and educators, who reviewed the manuscript of this text. Their insights, suggestions, and eye for detail helped us prepare a more relevant and useful book, one that focuses on the essential components of learning in the fields of maternal, newborn, and child health nursing.

Susan Beggs, RN, MSN, CPN
Austin Community College
Austin, Texas

Constance Bobik, RN, BSN, MSN
Brevard Community College
Cocoa, Florida

Pam Bowden, RN, MS, PNP
North Hennepin Community College
Brooklyn Park, Minnesota

Pamela Cleveland, MSN, RN, FNP
South Texas College
McAllen, Texas

Cheryl DeGraw, RN MSN, CRNP, CNE
Florence-Darlington Technical College
Florence, South Carolina

Cherste K. Eidman, BS, BSN
Metropolitan State University
St. Paul, Minnesota

Renee Zubay Fife, RN, MSN, CPN
Purdue Calumet School of Nursing
Hammond, Indiana

Pamela Fowler, MS, RN
Rogers State University
Claremore, Oklahoma

Mary Ann Helms, RN, MSN, MRE, EdD
Tennessee State University
Nashville, Tennessee

Rita Horgos, MSN, RN, CPN
Community College of Allegheny County, South Campus
West Mifflin, Pennsylvania

Kathy Jo Keever, RNC-OB, CNM, MS
Anne Arundel Community College
Arnold, Maryland

Lori Keough, APRN-BC, MSN, MEd
University of Massachusetts
North Dartmouth, Massachusetts

Carmen Kiraly, RN, BSN, MSN, C-WHNP
Suffolk Community College
Brentwood, New York

Kathleen Kleefisch, RN, MSN, FNP, BC
Purdue Calumet University
Hammond, Indiana

Kelli D. Lewis, RN, MSN
Rend Lake College
Ina, Illinois

Karen Lincoln, RNC, MSN
Montcalm Community College
Sidney, Michigan

Kathy Martin, MNSc, WHNP, RNC
Cox College
Springfield, Missouri

Linda L. Miedema, RN, BNS, MSA, PhD
Brevard Community College
Titusville, Florida

Carol Ann Moseley, PhD, MS, BAN, BA, RN
Blessing-Rieman College of Nursing
Quincy, Illinois

Deborah Naccarini, RN, MSN
Carroll Community College
Westminster, Maryland

Jeanette Nodorft, RNC, BSN, MSN
Southwest Wisconsin Technical College
Fennimore, Wisconsin

Janet Pinkelman, MSN, RNC
Owens Community College
Toledo, Ohio

Leslie S. Reifel
Sentara School of Health Professions
Chesapeake, Virginia

Katherine Roberts, MSN, RN
Lamar University
Beaumont, Texas

Nancy Rogers, RN, MA, BSN
Carroll Community College
Westminster, Maryland

Martha C. Ruder
Gulf Coast Community College
Panama City, Florida

Nora F. Steele, DNS, APRN
Delgado Community College
New Orleans, Louisiana

Marilyn L. Weitzel, PhD, RN
Cleveland State University
Cleveland, Ohio

Donna Wilsker
Lamar University
Beaumont, Texas

Marianne M. Wollyung, RN, MSN
Pottsville Hospital School of Nursing
Pottsville, Pennsylvania

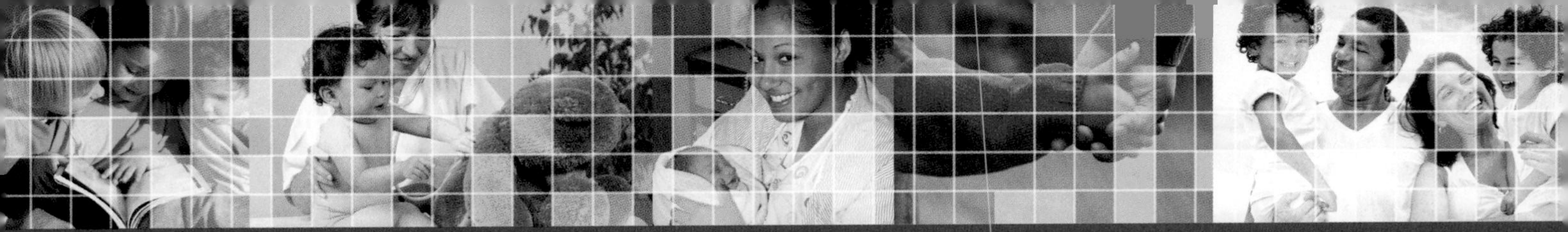

Dedication

Throughout the ages, nurses have cared for families, fathers, mothers, and their children—treating, healing, soothing, educating, and advocating.

And so we dedicate this book to nurses—

For their wisdom, expertise, and compassion
For their willingness to challenge the system when necessary
For their ability to remain strong during times of difficulty and stress
And for their unfailing commitment to the families they assist.

And to nursing students everywhere—

For seeking to serve others when so many have become self-serving
For committing their minds and talents to a proud profession
For accepting the challenges posed by the changes in health care
And for daring to envision a brighter tomorrow.

Then, too, as always, we honor our beloved families—

David London, Craig and Matthew
Timothy Ladewig, Ryan, Amanda, Reed and Addison, and Erik, Kedri, and Emma
Ronald Ball
Julian Bindler, Dana and her husband Brady, and Ross
Fred Cowen III, Benjamin and Michael

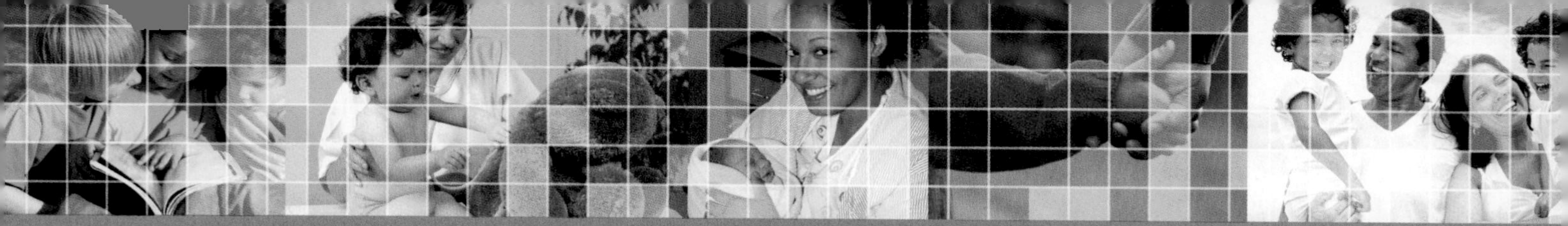

Preface

Faculty and students in today's maternity and pediatric nursing courses face a wide variety of issues and challenges. Courses are growing increasingly shorter, clinical experiences are more limited, and patients in hospitals are often more seriously ill. Time is precious for both students and faculty, and competence in nursing practice is essential. The primary goal in this edition is to present key content in an accurate, readable format that helps students and faculty focus on what is important. This textbook helps students develop the skills and abilities they need now and in the future in an ever-changing healthcare environment. This is done through the Learning Outcomes and the Critical Concept Review feature at the end of each chapter, through the illustrations and photographs that clarify concepts more efficiently than words can do, and through the electronic resources in MyNursingKit, which depicts clinical situations and requires students to engage in critical thinking. In its structure, format, and delivery, this text provides a concise look at maternal-newborn, women's health, and pediatric nursing.

ORGANIZATION

The organization of the text also reflects a time-saving approach. As educators and nurses, we know how difficult it is to teach everything that students need to learn in so little time. Consequently, we sought to reduce duplication in the text by carefully integrating maternity and pediatric nursing topics. For example, two introductory chapters address concepts important for maternal, newborn, and child nursing. Chapter 1 discusses introductory concepts of family-centered care, health promotion, community and home care, evidence-based practice, legal issues, as well as the complex ethical considerations related to reproductive decisions, cord blood banking, stem cell research, terminating life-sustaining treatment, and organ transplantation issues. Chapter 2 addresses concepts that are important for culturally appropriate care for the entire family, such as cultural norms related to childbearing and childrearing, cultural assessment, and complementary and alternative therapies. Throughout the text we cross-reference to other chapters to avoid the duplication of content, and we have worked to eliminate potentially conflicting information.

Subsequent chapters focus on reproductive issues and women's health, pregnancy, birth processes, postpartum care, and newborn management, and then transition into the pediatric care chapters. The pediatric chapters begin with introductory concepts, such as growth and development, assessment, nutrition, health promotion for children ranging from newborn to adolescents, and care of the child in the community and hospital settings. Chapters 46 through 59 cover the nursing care of children with various disorders, organized by body system.

IMPORTANT THEMES IN THIS EDITION

Central to this edition are several key themes that are increasingly evident in nursing care of childbearing and childrearing families.

FAMILY-CENTERED NURSING CARE

Nursing care for pregnant women and children is a family-centered process, and it is essential to providing culturally competent care. The underlying philosophy of *Maternal & Child Nursing Care* is simple: We believe that family members are co-participants in care during pregnancy and childbirth. Parents must be integrated into the care of an infant or child at any stage of development, as they are the central influence on the child's life. Families experience the excitement and exhilaration of welcoming a healthy infant into their home, but they also experience sorrow and concern when a health problem occurs. Nurses play a pivotal role in helping families celebrate the normal life processes associated with birth, in promoting the health of the family and child, in fostering the child's growth and development from infancy through adolescence, and in caring for the child with any health condition. We are committed to providing a text that integrates the needs of families across the continuum from conception through adolescence.

HEALTH PROMOTION

In this textbook, we subscribe to the paradigm that all childbearing and childrearing families and children need health promotion and health maintenance interventions, no matter where they seek health care or what health conditions they may be experiencing. Families may visit offices or other community settings specifically to obtain health supervision care. Nurses may also integrate health promotion and health maintenance into the care for childbearing and childrearing families and for children with acute and chronic illness in a variety of inpatient and outpatient settings. This textbook integrates health promotion and health maintenance content throughout, most visibly in four chapters: Chapter 5, "Health Promotion for Women," Chapter 36, "Health Promotion and Maintenance: General Concepts, the Newborn, and the Infant," Chapter 37, "Health Promotion and Maintenance: The Toddler, the Preschooler, and the School-Age Child," and Chapter 38, "Health Promotion and Maintenance: The Adolescent."

HEALTH PROMOTION

In addition, a feature entitled **Health Promotion** summarizes the needs of children with specific chronic conditions, such as asthma or diabetes. These overviews teach the student to look at the child with a chronic illness like any other child, with health maintenance needs for prevention, education, and basic care.

NURSING CARE IN THE COMMUNITY

Most maternity and pediatric nursing care occurs in the community setting, especially since most children and pregnant women are healthy and have only episodic acute health conditions. Even women with high-risk pregnancies and children with serious chronic health conditions are receiving more care in their homes and in the community. This textbook integrates community and home care throughout, including information on long-term management of complex health conditions, which are especially challenging to manage in community settings.

Five chapters provide a theoretical perspective and important tools in caring for childbearing and childrearing families in the community setting: Chapter 10, "Antepartal Nursing Assessment," Chapter 11, "The Expectant Family: Needs and Care," Chapter 31, "The Postpartal Family: Needs and Care," Chapter 39, "Family Assessment and Concepts of Nursing Care," and Chapter 40, "Nursing Considerations for the Child and Family with a Chronic Condition." In addition, Nursing Care in the Community is a special heading used throughout this text.

CLIENT EDUCATION

Client education remains a critical element of effective nursing care, one that we emphasize in this text. Nurses teach their clients during all stages of pregnancy and the childbearing process during the child's health visits, and while providing care for specific conditions. Throughout the book, we include Teaching Highlights that pre-sent a special healthcare issue or problem and the related key teaching points for care by the family.

THINKING CRITICALLY

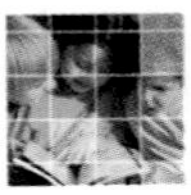

Nurses are faced with the responsibility to manage care for multiple families with diverse healthcare needs, and to work collaboratively with other health professionals to enhance care. Thus, nurses must be able to think critically, communicate well, and problem solve effectively.

To promote the development of critical thinking skills that will support nurses in challenging situations, **Thinking Critically** boxes provide brief scenarios that ask students to determine the appropriate response. Students can test their own decision-making skills by submitting answers to these questions on the MyNursingKit website, where the feature also appears. The instructor can then grade their answers using the suggested answers provided in the Instructor's Manual, which is replicated online in MyNursingKit and MyNursingLab. Students can access a variety of critical thinking exercises and case studies in MyNursingKit on the textbook's website at www.mynursingkit.com.

Another feature that emphasizes these skills is the **Critical Thinking in Action** feature. This case study introduces a client situation at the end of each chapter with questions to enable the student to decide which nursing actions are appropriate. Answers appear in MyNursingKit. The Instructor's Resource Manual has more suggestions for critical thinking exercises for both the classroom and clinicals.

EVIDENCE-BASED NURSING PRACTICE

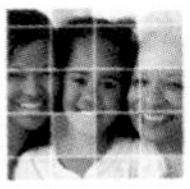

Healthcare professionals are increasingly aware of the importance of using evidence-based approaches as the foundation for planning and providing effective care. The approach of evidence-based practice draws on information from a variety of sources, including nursing research. To help nurses become more comfortable integrating new knowledge into their nursing practice, a brief discussion of evidence-based practice is included in Chapter 1.

A feature entitled **Evidence-Based Nursing** further enhances the approach of using research to determine nursing actions. It describes a particular problem or clinical question and investigates the evidence that suggests solutions to the problem. In these features, we provide an interpretation explaining the implications of the studies and then invite the student to apply critical thinking skills to further identify nursing care approaches.

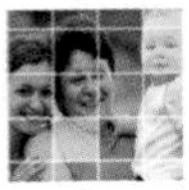

A new feature entitled **Evidence in Action** presents evidence from a variety of sources, including systematic reviews of research literature, recent research findings, and national organization policy that have direct application to nursing practice.

DEVELOPING CULTURAL COMPETENCE

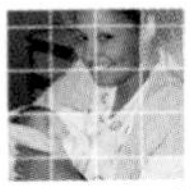

The influence of a family's culture on health beliefs and healthcare practices cannot be underestimated. Chapter 1 briefly introduces cultural issues relevant to maternity and child nursing care. Additionally, we include Chapter 2, "Culture and the Family."

We also emphasize cultural competence throughout the text. We highlight specific cultural issues and their application to nursing care in the **Developing Cultural Competence** features.

OTHER NEW OR EXPANDED CONCEPTS IN THIS EDITION

Many other important concepts are emphasized throughout this text:

- **Assessment** is an essential and core role in the nursing process. Several chapters are dedicated to helping the student perform an assessment at each stage along the pregnancy continuum, initially of the fetus and newborn, and later through the stages of childhood. In addition, body system assessment guidelines are provided in many of the pediatric chapters.

- **Communication** is one of the most important skills that students need to learn. Effective communication is the very fiber of nursing practice. This book integrates communication skills in an applied manner where students can most benefit. It is an essential part of the **Nursing Process** and **Teaching Highlights** boxes.
- **Ensuring appropriate nutrition** during pregnancy, infancy, and childhood is important to promote growth, development, and health. A growing national focus on healthy nutrition patterns underscores the importance of this information. Chapters 12, 30, and 34 address nutrition for pregnant women, newborns, and children.
- **Pain** is now considered the fifth vital sign, and pain management is a priority in healthcare settings. All of the chapters in Part 4, "Birth and the Family," address pain assessment and management, and it is the primary focus in Chapter 20, "Pharmacologic Pain Management." Pain assessment and management is also a focus in six chapters (23, 24, 26, 28, 31, and 32) of Part 5, "The Postpartal Family and the Newborn." In Part 6, Chapter 41 addresses pain assessment and management in the nursing care plan, and it is the primary subject in Chapter 42, "Pain Assessment and Management in Children." We discuss applicable pain management when appropriate in other chapters, including each of the chapters in Part 7, "Caring for Children with Alterations in Health Status."
- **End-of-life care** has gained greater national prominence. Expanded focus on the care of the family and the child who is dying has been added to Chapter 43, "The Child with a Life-Threatening Condition and End-of-Life Care." Grief and loss associated with miscarriage is addressed in Chapter 16, "Pregnancy at Risk: Gestational Problems." Care of the family experiencing perinatal loss is presented in Chapter 22, "Childbirth at Risk: Labor-Related Complications."

TOOLS THAT FOCUS STUDENT REVIEW TO MAXIMIZE TIME

Both instructors and students value learning aids that unify the objectives and concepts of a chapter as well as reinforce the overall themes in a text. In keeping with our theme of family-centered care, each chapter begins with a **Family Quote** that helps set the stage for content that follows from the family's perspective. This is followed by a list of **Learning Outcomes** and **Key Terms** with page numbers to identify the place where the term first appears in the chapter. An **Audio Glossary** of these terms commonly used in the field of maternal-newborn and child nursing can be found on MyNursingLab, the book's companion website, with audio pronunciations of the terms as well as printed definitions.

CRITICAL CONCEPT REVIEW

This feature is a direct response to instructors' and students' requests that the text provide more opportunities for review. Each chapter ends with a Critical Concept Review, a feature designed to help students retain the most important concepts from a chapter in a short period of time. This visual tool isolates the essential content in a chapter by means of a flowchart that links **Learning Outcomes** to their corresponding **Concepts**. Students save time by having the important concepts identified for them, allowing them to use more of their study time for reviewing the concepts themselves.

EXPLORE MYNURSINGKIT

The review section ends with a list of references and a section entitled EXPLORE mynursingkit. This last section encourages students to use the additional chapter-specific NCLEX-RN® review questions and other interactive exercises that appear on MyNursingKit and MyNursing Lab. These online offerings will further enhance the student's learning experience, build upon knowledge gained from this textbook, prepare students for the NCLEX-RN®, and foster critical thinking. In addition, throughout the chapters themselves, thumbtabs appear along the edges of the pages that point the reader to supplements on MyNursingKit that relate to a topic discussed near the thumbtab. The thumbtabs cross-reference specific animations, case studies, activities, and other materials that will assist students in understanding key concepts.

APPLICATION OF THE NURSING PROCESS

NURSING MANAGEMENT

The nursing process is emphasized throughout the nursing care chapters. The heading **Nursing Management** highlights nursing actions. In chapters with frequently seen or high-risk health issues or conditions, the expanded section on nursing management helps students understand and apply the nursing process more completely. The expanded section includes the headings Nursing Assessment and Diagnosis, Planning and Implementation, and Evaluation.

In keeping with changing approaches to nursing care management, we feature **Nursing Care Plans** and **Clinical Pathways** throughout the text.

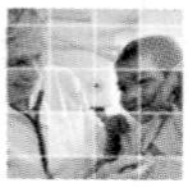

The **Nursing Care Plans** address nursing care for clients who have complications, such as a woman with preeclampsia or a child with otitis media. We designed this feature to help students approach care from the nursing process perspective. Care Plans integrate Nursing Diagnosis, Nursing Intervention Classifications (NIC), and Nursing Outcome Classifications (NOC).

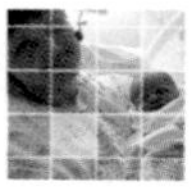

The **Clinical Pathways** describe nursing actions to help students plan and manage care within normally anticipated time frames as the patient's health status improves. The nursing care plans and clinical pathways help students become familiar with two approaches to managing care so that they are better equipped for variations in clinical settings.

VISUALS THAT TEACH

The conviction that art can teach is evident throughout the book. There are hundreds of contemporary photographs of childbearing and childrearing families and children in healthcare and related settings throughout the textbook, as well as illustrations, all of which serve to display conditions, compare developmental stages, and depict concepts.

PATHOPHYSIOLOGY ILLUSTRATED

In particular, **Pathophysiology Illustrated** figures allow the student to see into the body and to visualize the causes and effects of conditions on childbearing women, newborns, and children. Each Pathophysiology Illustrated feature box begins with a tab like the one shown here.

AS CHILDREN GROW

As Children Grow illustrations help the student visualize the important anatomic and physiologic differences between a child and an adult. These features illustrate how the child progresses through developmental stages and the important ways in which a child's development influences healthcare needs and how the child progresses through developmental stages. Each As Children Grow feature box begins with a tab like the one shown here.

Nursing is facing many new challenges: an ongoing nursing shortage, dramatic advances in healthcare knowledge, and natural and humanmade disasters that create a critical need for skilled nurses. We believe that nursing is becoming reenergized and is facing these issues and challenges with enthusiasm and commitment. Many people feel a strong desire to choose professions that make a difference—professions such as nursing. We, like you, know that expert nurses can have a tremendous impact on the lives of childbearing and childrearing families. Our goal in writing this text is to help prepare nurses with the skills and knowledge to make a difference—one family at a time.

Marcia L. London
Patricia W. Ladewig
Jane W. Ball
Ruth C. Bindler
Kay J. Cowen

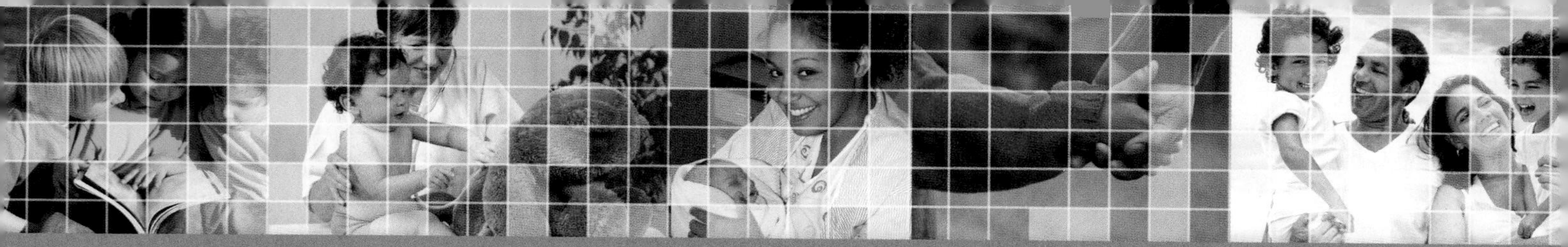

Features That Help You Use This Textbook Successfully

Instructors and students alike value the in-text learning aids that we include in our textbooks. The following guide will help you use the features and resources from *Maternal & Child Nursing Care*, Third Edition, to be successful in the classroom, in the clinical setting, on the NCLEX-RN® examination, and in nursing practice.

Each chapter begins with **Learning Outcomes** and a chapter opening **Vignette.** These personal stories illustrate the diversity of cultures, parental concerns, and family situations that nurses will encounter throughout the course of their careers.

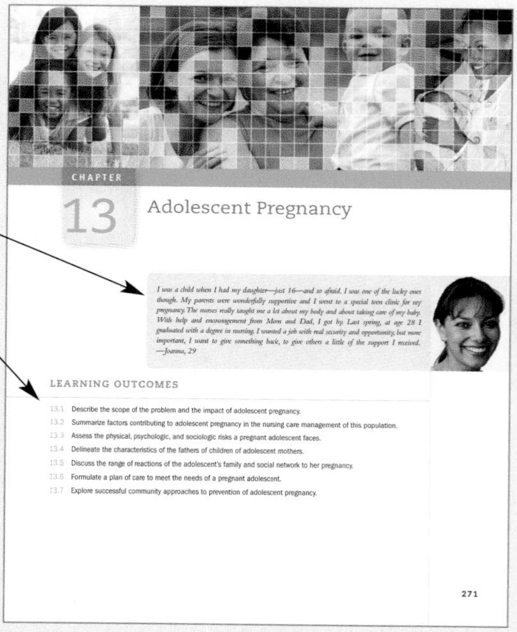

CHAPTER

13 Adolescent Pregnancy

I was a child when I had my daughter—just 16—and so afraid. I was one of the lucky ones though. My parents were wonderfully supportive and I went to a special teen clinic for my pregnancy. The nurses really taught me a lot about my body and about taking care of my baby. With help and encouragement from Mom and Dad, I got by. Last spring, at age 28 I graduated with a degree in nursing. I wanted a job with real security and opportunity, but more important, I want to give something back, to give others a little of the support I received. —Joanna, 29

LEARNING OUTCOMES

13.1 Describe the scope of the problem and the impact of adolescent pregnancy.
13.2 Summarize factors contributing to adolescent pregnancy in the nursing care management of this population.
13.3 Assess the physical, psychologic, and sociologic risks a pregnant adolescent faces.
13.4 Delineate the characteristics of the fathers of children of adolescent mothers.
13.5 Discuss the range of reactions of the adolescent's family and social network to her pregnancy.
13.6 Formulate a plan of care to meet the needs of a pregnant adolescent.
13.7 Explore successful community approaches to prevention of adolescent pregnancy.

271

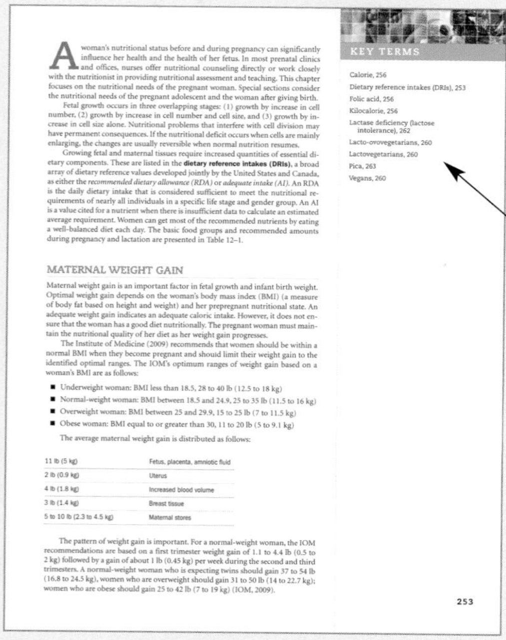

A woman's nutritional status before and during pregnancy can significantly influence her health and the health of her fetus. In most prenatal clinics and offices, nurses offer nutritional counseling directly or work closely with the nutritionist in providing nutritional assessment and teaching. This chapter focuses on the nutritional needs of the pregnant woman. Special sections consider the nutritional needs of the pregnant adolescent and the woman after giving birth.

Fetal growth occurs in three overlapping stages: (1) growth by increase in cell number, (2) growth by increase in cell number and cell size, and (3) growth by increase in cell size alone. Nutritional problems that interfere with cell division may have permanent consequences. If the nutritional deficit occurs when cells are mainly enlarging, the changes are usually reversible when normal nutrition resumes.

Growing fetal and maternal tissues require increased quantities of essential dietary components. These are listed in the **dietary reference intakes (DRIs)**, a broad array of dietary reference values developed jointly by the United States and Canada, as either the *recommended dietary allowance (RDA)* or *adequate intake (AI)*. An RDA is the daily dietary intake that is considered sufficient to meet the nutritional requirements of nearly all individuals in a specific life stage and gender group. An AI is a value cited for a nutrient when there is insufficient data to calculate an estimated average requirement. Women can get most of the recommended nutrients by eating a well-balanced diet each day. The basic food groups and recommended amounts during pregnancy and lactation are presented in Table 12–1.

KEY TERMS

Calorie, 256
Dietary reference intakes (DRIs), 253
Folic acid, 256
Kilocalorie, 256
Lactase deficiency (lactose intolerance), 262
Lacto-ovovegetarians, 260
Lactovegetarians, 260
Pica, 263
Vegans, 260

MATERNAL WEIGHT GAIN

Maternal weight gain is an important factor in fetal growth and infant birth weight. Optimal weight gain depends on the woman's body mass index (BMI) (a measure of body fat based on height and weight) and her prepregnant nutritional state. An adequate weight gain indicates an adequate caloric intake. However, it does not ensure that the woman has a good diet nutritionally. The pregnant woman must maintain the nutritional quality of her diet as her weight gain progresses.

The Institute of Medicine (2009) recommends that women should be within a normal BMI when they become pregnant and should limit their weight gain to the identified optimal ranges. The IOM's optimum ranges of weight gain based on a woman's BMI are as follows:

- Underweight woman: BMI less than 18.5, 28 to 40 lb (12.5 to 18 kg)
- Normal-weight woman: BMI between 18.5 and 24.9, 25 to 35 lb (11.5 to 16 kg)
- Overweight woman: BMI between 25 and 29.9, 15 to 25 lb (7 to 11.5 kg)
- Obese woman: BMI equal to or greater than 30, 11 to 20 lb (5 to 9.1 kg)

The average maternal weight gain is distributed as follows:

11 lb (5 kg)	Fetus, placenta, amniotic fluid
2 lb (0.9 kg)	Uterus
4 lb (1.8 kg)	Increased blood volume
3 lb (1.4 kg)	Breast tissue
5 to 10 lb (2.3 to 4.5 kg)	Maternal stores

The pattern of weight gain is important. For a normal-weight woman, the IOM recommendations are based on a first trimester weight gain of 1.1 to 4.4 lb (0.5 to 2 kg) followed by a gain of about 1 lb (0.45 kg) per week during the second and third trimesters. A normal-weight woman who is expecting twins should gain 37 to 54 lb (16.8 to 24.5 kg), women who are overweight should gain 31 to 50 lb (14 to 22.7 kg); women who are obese should gain 25 to 42 lb (7 to 19 kg) (IOM, 2009).

253

Opposite the chapter title page is a list of **Key Terms** that will be introduced in the chapter. Page numbers are included with each key term to identify the place where the term first appears in the chapter.

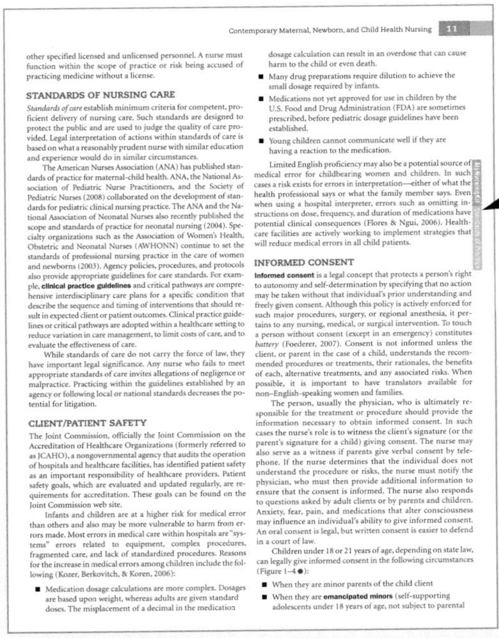

Contemporary Maternal, Newborn, and Child Health Nursing 11

other specified licensed and unlicensed personnel. A nurse must function within the scope of practice or risk being accused of practicing medicine without a license.

STANDARDS OF NURSING CARE

Standards of care establish minimum criteria for competent, proficient delivery of nursing care. Such standards are designed to protect the public and are used to judge the quality of care provided. Legal interpretation of actions within standards of care is based on what a reasonably prudent nurse with similar education and experience would do in similar circumstances.

The American Nurses Association (ANA) has published standards of practice for maternal-child health. ANA, the National Association of Pediatric Nurse Practitioners, and the Society of Pediatric Nurses (2008) collaborated on the development of standards for pediatric clinical nursing practice. The ANA and the National Association of Neonatal Nurses also recently published the scope and standards of practice for neonatal nursing (2004). Specialty organizations such as the Association of Women's Health, Obstetric and Neonatal Nurses (AWHONN) continue to set the standards of professional nursing practice in the care of women and newborns (2003). Agency policies, procedures, and protocols also provide appropriate guidelines for care standards. For example, **clinical practice guidelines** and critical pathways are comprehensive interdisciplinary care plans for a specific condition that describe the sequence and timing of interventions that should result in expected client or patient outcomes. Clinical practice guidelines or critical pathways are adopted within a healthcare setting to reduce variation in care management, to limit costs of care, and to evaluate the effectiveness of care.

While standards of care do not carry the force of law, they have important legal significance. Any nurse who fails to meet appropriate standards of care invites allegations of negligence or malpractice. Practicing within the guidelines established by an agency or following local or national standards decreases the potential for litigation.

CLIENT/PATIENT SAFETY

The Joint Commission, officially the Joint Commission on the Accreditation of Healthcare Organizations (formerly referred to as JCAHO), a nongovernmental agency that audits the operation of hospitals and healthcare facilities, has identified patient safety as an important responsibility of healthcare providers. Patient safety goals, which are evaluated and updated regularly, are requirements for accreditation. These goals can be found on the Joint Commission web site.

Infants and children are at a higher risk for medical error than others and also may be more vulnerable to harm from errors made. Most errors in medical care within hospitals are "systems" errors related to equipment, complex procedures, fragmented care, and lack of standardized procedures. Reasons for the increase in medical errors among children include the following (Kozer, Berkovitch, & Koren, 2006):

- Medication dosage calculations are more complex. Dosages are based upon weight, whereas adults are given standard doses. The misplacement of a decimal in the medication dosage calculation can result in an overdose that can cause harm to the child or even death.
- Many drug preparations require dilution to achieve the small dosage required by infants.
- Medications not yet approved for use in children by the U.S. Food and Drug Administration (FDA) are sometimes prescribed, before pediatric dosage guidelines have been established.
- Young children cannot communicate well if they are having a reaction to the medication.

Limited English proficiency may also be a potential source of medical error for childbearing women and children. In such cases a risk exists for errors in interpretation—either of what the health professional says or what the family member says. Even when using a hospital interpreter, errors such as omitting instructions on dose, frequency, and duration of medications have potential clinical consequences (Flores & Ngui, 2006). Healthcare facilities are actively working to implement strategies that will reduce medical errors in all child patients.

INFORMED CONSENT

Informed consent is a legal concept that protects a person's right to autonomy and self-determination by specifying that no action may be taken without that individual's prior understanding and freely given consent. Although this policy is actively enforced for such major procedures, surgery, or regional anesthesia, it pertains to any nursing, medical, or surgical intervention. To touch a person without consent (except in an emergency) constitutes *battery* (Foederer, 2007). Consent is not informed unless the client, or parent in the case of a child, understands the recommended procedures or treatments, their rationales, the benefits of each, alternative treatments, and any associated risks. When possible, it is important to have translators available for non–English-speaking women and families.

The person, usually the physician, who is ultimately responsible for the treatment or procedure should provide the information necessary to obtain informed consent. In such cases the nurse's role is to witness the client's signature (or the parent's signature for a child) giving consent. The nurse may also serve as a witness if parents give verbal consent by telephone. If the nurse determines that the individual does not understand the procedure or risks, the nurse must notify the physician, who must then provide additional information to ensure that the consent is informed. The nurse also responds to questions asked by adult clients or by parents and children. Anxiety, fear, pain, and medications that alter consciousness may influence an individual's ability to give informed consent. An oral consent is legal, but written consent is easier to defend in a court of law.

Children under 18 or 21 years of age, depending on state law, can legally give informed consent in the following circumstances (Figure 1–4 ●):

- When they are minor parents of the child client
- When they are **emancipated minors** (self-supporting adolescents under 18 years of age, not subject to parental

MyNursingKit thumbtabs in each chapter remind you to use the accompanying supplemental materials found on the text's companion website, MyNursingKit. These thumbtabs cross-reference additional information or specific activities related to the concepts introduced on that page in the textbook. These resources enhance learning and provide an application beyond the textbook experience. For example, you can see an animation of placenta formation in Chapter 4.

As Children Grow boxes illustrate the anatomic and physiologic differences between children and adults. These features illustrate how the child progresses through developmental stages and the important ways in which a child's development influences healthcare needs.

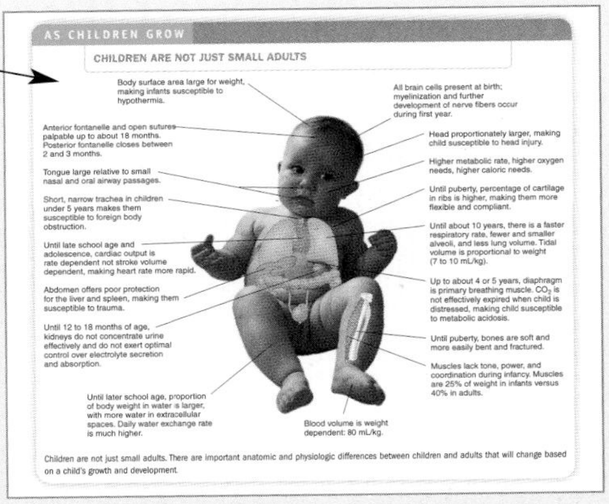
AS CHILDREN GROW
CHILDREN ARE NOT JUST SMALL ADULTS
Body surface area large for weight, making infants susceptible to hypothermia.
All brain cells present at birth; myelinization and further development of nerve fibers occur during first year.
Anterior fontanelle and open sutures palpable up to about 18 months. Posterior fontanelle closes between 2 and 3 months.
Head proportionately larger, making child susceptible to head injury.
Tongue large relative to small nasal and oral airway passages.
Higher metabolic rate, higher oxygen needs, higher caloric needs.
Short, narrow trachea in children under 5 years makes them susceptible to foreign body obstruction.
Until puberty, percentage of cartilage in ribs is higher, making them more flexible and compliant.
Until late school age and adolescence, cardiac output is rate dependent not stroke volume dependent, making heart rate more rapid.
Until about 10 years, there is a faster respiratory rate, fewer and smaller alveoli, and less lung volume. Tidal volume is proportional to weight (7 to 10 mL/kg).
Abdomen offers poor protection for the liver and spleen, making them susceptible to trauma.
Up to about 4 or 5 years, diaphragm is primary breathing muscle. CO_2 is not effectively expired when child is distressed, making child susceptible to metabolic acidosis.
Until 12 to 18 months of age, kidneys do not concentrate urine effectively and do not exert optimal control over electrolyte secretion and absorption.
Until puberty, bones are soft and more easily bent and fractured.
Muscles lack tone, power, and coordination during infancy. Muscles are 25% of weight in infants versus 40% in adults.
Until later school age, proportion of body weight in water is larger, with more water in extracellular spaces. Daily water exchange rate is much higher.
Blood volume is weight dependent: 80 mL/kg.
Children are not just small adults. There are important anatomic and physiologic differences between children and adults that will change based on a child's growth and development.

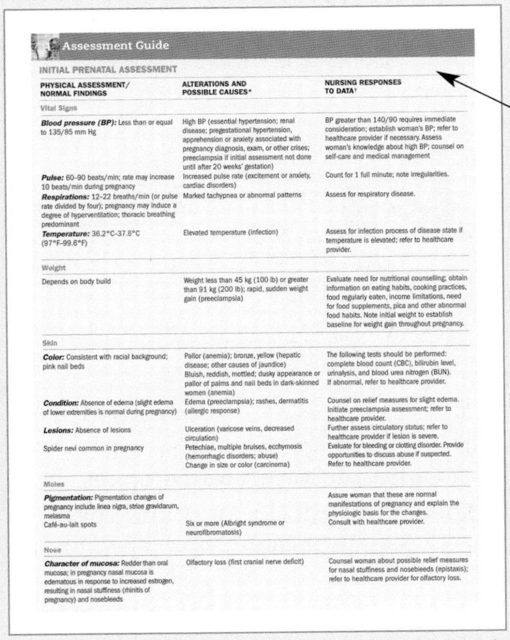

Assessment Guide

INITIAL PRENATAL ASSESSMENT

PHYSICAL ASSESSMENT/ NORMAL FINDINGS	ALTERATIONS AND POSSIBLE CAUSES*	NURSING RESPONSES TO DATA†
Vital Signs		
Blood pressure (BP): Less than or equal to 135/85 mm Hg	High BP (essential hypertension; renal disease; pregestational hypertension, apprehension or anxiety associated with pregnancy diagnosis, exam, or other crises; preeclampsia if initial assessment not done until after 20 weeks' gestation)	BP greater than 140/90 requires immediate consideration; establish woman's BP; refer to healthcare provider if necessary. Assess woman's knowledge about high BP; counsel on self-care and medical management
Pulse: 60–90 beats/min; rate may increase 10 beats/min during pregnancy	Increased pulse rate (excitement or anxiety, cardiac disorders)	Count for 1 full minute; note irregularities.
Respirations: 12–22 breaths/min (or pulse rate divided by four); pregnancy may induce a degree of hyperventilation; thoracic breathing predominant	Marked tachypnea or abnormal patterns	Assess for respiratory disease.
Temperature: 36.2°C–37.6°C (97°F–99.6°F)	Elevated temperature (infection)	Assess for infection process of disease state if temperature is elevated; refer to healthcare provider.
Weight		
Depends on body build	Weight less than 45 kg (100 lb) or greater than 91 kg (200 lb); rapid, sudden weight gain (preeclampsia)	Evaluate need for nutritional counselling; obtain information on eating habits, cooking practices, food regularly eaten, income limitations, need for food supplements, pica and other abnormal food habits. Note initial weight to establish baseline for weight gain throughout pregnancy.
Skin		
Color: Consistent with racial background; pink nail beds	Pallor (anemia); bronze, yellow (hepatic disease; other causes of jaundice) Bluish, reddish, mottled; dusky appearance or pallor of palms and nail beds in dark-skinned women (anemia)	The following tests should be performed: complete blood count (CBC), bilirubin level, urinalysis, and blood urea nitrogen (BUN). If abnormal, refer to healthcare provider.
Condition: Absence of edema (slight edema of lower extremities is normal during pregnancy)	Edema (preeclampsia); rashes, dermatitis (allergic response)	Counsel on relief measures for slight edema. Initiate preeclampsia assessment; refer to healthcare provider.
Lesions: Absence of lesions	Ulceration (varicose veins, decreased circulation)	Further assess circulatory status; refer to healthcare provider if lesion is severe.
Spider nevi common in pregnancy	Petechiae, multiple bruises, ecchymosis (hemorrhagic disorders; abuse) Change in size or color (carcinoma)	Evaluate for bleeding or clotting disorder. Provide opportunities to discuss abuse if suspected. Refer to healthcare provider.
Moles		
Pigmentation: Pigmentation changes of pregnancy include linea nigra, striae gravidarum, melasma		Assure woman that these are normal manifestations of pregnancy and explain the physiologic basis for the changes.
Café-au-lait spots	Six or more (Albright syndrome or neurofibromatosis)	Consult with healthcare provider.
Nose		
Character of mucosa: Redder than oral mucosa; in pregnancy nasal mucosa is edematous in response to increased estrogen, resulting in nasal stuffiness (rhinitis of pregnancy) and nosebleeds	Olfactory loss (first cranial nerve deficit)	Counsel woman about possible relief measures for nasal stuffiness and nosebleeds (epistaxis); refer to healthcare provider for olfactory loss.

Assessment Guides, found in the maternal-newborn chapters, assist you with diagnoses by incorporating physical assessment and normal findings, alterations and possible causes, and guidelines for nursing interventions. Assessment guides within several chapters of Part 7, "Caring for Children with Alterations in Health Status," provide a system-oriented approach to assessing the child's health condition.

Clinical Manifestations charts help you understand the association between the pathophysiology and the signs and symptoms of a particular condition. In some cases, these tables present several similar conditions so that you can visually differentiate the conditions. In others, the tables include treatment for the clinical manifestations and conditions.

Clinical Manifestations

NEWBORN WITHDRAWAL

CENTRAL NERVOUS SYSTEM SIGNS
- Hyperactivity
- Hyperirritability (persistent shrill cry)
- Increased muscle tone
- Exaggerated reflexes
- Tremors and myoclonic jerks
- Sneezing, hiccups, yawning
- Short, unquiet sleep
- Fever (accompanies the increased neuromuscular activities)

RESPIRATORY SIGNS
- Tachypnea (greater than 60 breaths per minute when quiet)
- Excessive secretions

GASTROINTESTINAL SIGNS
- Disorganized, vigorous suck
- Vomiting
- Drooling
- Sensitive gag reflex
- Hyperphagia
- Diarrhea
- Poor feeding (less than 15 mL on first day of life; takes longer than 30 minutes per feeding)

VASOMOTOR SIGNS
- Stuffy nose, yawning, sneezing
- Flushing
- Sweating
- Sudden, circumoral pallor

Cutaneous signs
- Excoriated buttocks, knees, elbows
- Facial scratches
- Pressure-point abrasions

In keeping with the changing approaches to nursing care management, **Clinical Pathways** are designed to help you plan and manage care within normally anticipated time frames.

Clinical Pathway

THE POSTPARTAL PERIOD

CATEGORY	FIRST 4 HOURS	4 TO 8 HOURS PAST BIRTH	8 TO 24 HOURS PAST BIRTH
Referral	Report from labor nurse if not continuing in an LDR room	Lactation consultation as needed	Home nursing, WIC referral if indicated **EXPECTED OUTCOMES** Referrals made
Assessments	Postpartum assessments q30min × 2, q1h × 2, then q4h. Includes: ■ Fundus firm, midline, at or below umbilicus ■ Lochia rubra less than 1 pad/h; no free flow or passage of clots with massage ■ Bladder: voids large amounts of urine spontaneously; bladder not palpable following voiding ■ Perineum: sutures intact; no bulging or marked swelling; no c/o severe pain. Minimal bruising may be present. If hemorrhoids present, no tenseness or marked engorgement; less than 2 cm diameter ■ Breasts: soft, colostrum present Vital Signs: ■ BP WNL; no hypotension; not > 30 mm systolic or 15 mm diastolic over baseline ■ Temperature: less than 38°C (100.4°F) ■ Pulse: bradycardia normal, consistent with baseline ■ Respirations: 16 to 24/min; quiet, easy Comfort level: less than 3 on scale of 1 to 10	Continue postpartum assessment q4h × 2, then q8h Breast: evaluate nipple status; should be no evidence of cracks or bruising Observe feeding technique with newborn Vital signs assessment q8h; all WNL; report temperature greater than 38°C (100.4°F) Assess Homans' sign q8h Continue assessment of comfort level	Continue postpartum assessment q8h Breasts: nipples should remain free of cracks, fissures, bruising Feeding technique with newborn: should be good or improving Vital signs assessment q8h; all WNL; report temperature greater than 38°C (100.4°F) Continue assessment of comfort level **EXPECTED OUTCOMES** Vital signs medically acceptable, voids qs, postpartum assessment WNL; comfort level: less than 3 on 1 to 10 scale, involution of uterus in process, demonstrates and verbalizes appropriate newborn feeding techniques

Information is included for both vaginal birth (VB) and cesarean birth (CB). However, because many of the nursing care interventions are the same for either, specific interventions or suggestions related to vaginal birth are designated VB, and those specific to cesarean are designated CB.

ADL, activities of daily living; BP, blood pressure; CB, cesarean birth; CNM, certified nurse-midwife; c/o, complaints of; D/C, discharge; DC, discontinue; LDR, labor, delivery, and recovery; LOC, level of consciousness; LOS, level of sensation; OOB, out of bed; OR, operating room; PCA, patient-controlled analgesia; PO, per oral; PP, postpartum; PRN, as needed; qs, quantity sufficient; s/s, signs and symptoms; TC & DB, turn-cough and deep breathe; VB, vaginal birth; VS, vital signs; WNL, within normal limits.

(continued)

Complementary Care

COMMON TREATMENTS FOR INFERTILITY

Couples experiencing infertility may seek out alternative treatments. Some common treatments include acupuncture and herbs.

Acupuncture: Acupuncture is a therapy used in traditional Chinese medicine (TCM), and has become a popular complementary treatment. Acupuncture involves inserting sterile needles into specific points on the body to control the flow of chi, or life energy. Acupuncture treatment would focus on balancing the flow of chi in the kidneys and adrenal glands. Several clinical studies have shown acupuncture to be effective in treating infertility in both men and women (Cheong, Hung Yu Ng, & Ledger, 2008).

Herbal Treatments: Herbs frequently recommended to treat infertility include ginseng and astragalus. Herbalists cite the healing and hormone-balancing effects of these herbs. Ginseng has historically been used in TCM to enhance male virility and fertility. Several studies also cite ginseng, as well as astragalus, in enhancing in vitro sperm motility (Skidmore-Roth, 2006).

The nurse should be alert for signs that the couple is pursuing complementary therapies out of desperation. A sensitive, nonjudgmental approach will go a long way toward comforting a couple and assuring them that many complementary therapies used are helpful and not harmful.

Complementary Care boxes present information about commonly used alternative and complementary measures to treat or provide comfort for various conditions.

Critical Thinking in Action proposes a real-life scenario and a series of critical thinking questions so that you can apply to the clinical setting what you learned in class.

CRITICAL THINKING IN ACTION

You are working in the OB/GYN clinic when Sally Smith, a 17-year-old teenager, comes in complaining of irregular menses. She believes her periods are really "messed up" and interfering with her active schedule. She wants them to be more regular and asks you for birth control. She tells you that she is a member of the swimming team and is a senior in high school. She says she is planning to start community college next year to obtain an associate degree in computer technology. You assess Sally's history as follows: menarche began at age 12; periods occur every 28 to 32 days. She usually experiences cramping in the first 2 days and the flow lasts 4 to 5 days. She uses an average of 4 to 5 tampons a day during her period. She has never been hospitalized, has no prior medical problems, and is up to date on her immunizations except for meningitis.

1. Based on your knowledge of menstruation, how would you describe Sally's menstrual cycle?
2. What is your primary goal in discussing Sally's menstrual cycle with her?
3. What information would you give Sally relating to her menstrual cycle?
4. What important request does Sally have?
5. Sally expresses problems dealing with the cramping she experiences with the first 2 days of her menses. What would you suggest to Sally to cope with the discomfort?

See MyNursingKit for possible responses.

Developing Cultural Competence

RACIAL DISPARITY IN STIs

Racial disparities exist in all STIs, with the highest rates found among African Americans. Although African Americans comprise 12% of the population, they account for 70% of gonorrhea cases and almost half the cases of chlamydia and gonorrhea. Though less marked, disparities also exist among Hispanics. These disparities may result, in part, because people from minority populations are more likely to seek care in public health clinics, which report STIs more accurately than private providers do. However, socioeconomic barriers to high-quality health care and to STI prevention and treatment play a role. It is essential that these barriers be addressed if such disparities are to be eliminated (CDC, 2009).

Developing Cultural Competence boxes highlight specific cultural issues and their application to nursing care.

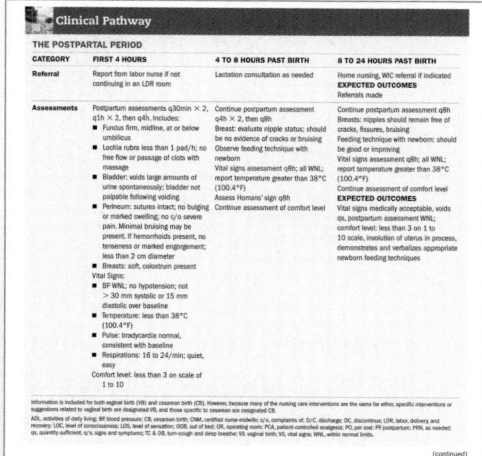

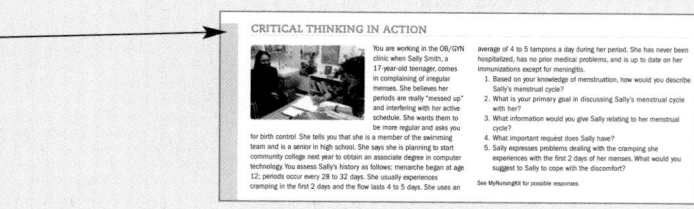

Drug Guides for selected medications commonly used in maternal-newborn and child nursing aid you in correctly administering the medications and evaluating their actions. Some Drug Guides are provided in tabular format to provide an overview of the types of medications that can be used for a specific condition and nursing considerations associated with their use.

Drug Guide

METRONIDAZOLE (FLAGYL)

Overview of Action

Metronidazole is an antiprotozoal and antibacterial agent. It possesses direct trichomonacidal and amebicidal activity against *T. vaginalis* and *E. histolytica*. Metronidazole is active in vitro against most obligate anaerobes but does not appear to possess any clinically relevant activity against facultative anaerobes or obligate aerobes. It is used in the treatment of various infections caused by organisms that are sensitive to this drug. It is used predominantly to treat the following infections in women: *T. vaginalis*, bacterial vaginosis, endometritis, endomyometritis, tubo-ovarian abscess, and postsurgical vaginal cuff infection.

Route, Dosage, Frequency

Trichomoniasis–1-day treatment: 2 g orally in a single dose; 7-day treatment: 500 mg orally twice a day for 7 consecutive days (CDC, 2006).

Amebiasis–Adults: 750 mg orally three times a day for 5–10 days; children: 35–50 mg/kg/24 hours orally divided into three doses for 10 days.

Bacterial vaginosis–500 mg orally twice a day for 7 consecutive days or one full applicator of metronidazole gel 0.75% intravaginally, once daily for 5 days (CDC, 2006).

Contraindications

Blood dyscrasias
Breastfeeding women (drug secreted in breast milk)
Impaired kidney or liver function
Active CNS disease

Side Effects

Convulsive seizures
Peripheral neuropathy
Nausea/vomiting
Weakness
Insomnia
Cystitis
Headache
Anorexia
Diarrhea
Epigastric distress
Abdominal cramping
Constipation
Metallic taste in mouth
Dizziness
Vertigo
Uncoordination
Ataxia
Confusion
Irritability
Dysuria
Reversible neutropenia and thrombocytopenia
Flattening of the T wave on ECG
Polyuria
Incontinence
Pelvic pressure
Proliferation of *Candida* in the vagina and mouth
Joint pains
Decreased libido
Dryness in the mouth, vulva, and vagina
Dyspareunia
Depression

Nursing Considerations

1. Inform woman about potential side effects.
2. Stress the importance of contraceptive compliance during course of treatment.
3. Obtain baseline renal and liver function tests as ordered.
4. Teach woman about the signs, symptoms, and treatment of vulvovaginal candidiasis.
5. Counsel the woman to avoid alcoholic beverages while taking the medication.
6. If the woman is taking oral contraceptives, a backup nonhormonal contraceptive method is recommended during treatment.
7. Take thorough history to rule out the woman's exposure to this medication within the last 6 weeks.
8. Teach woman to monitor the signs and symptoms of her infection.
9. Encourage cooperation with the entire course of treatment.

Evidence-Based Nursing

ACUPUNCTURE AND ASSISTED CONCEPTION

Clinical Question

Is acupuncture effective in helping women conceive?

The Evidence

Families who have difficulty conceiving are often interested in any measures that may increase their chance of successful pregnancy and birth. Acupuncture has been studied as a potential adjunct to assisted reproductive treatment. Cheong, Hung, & Ledger (2008) appraised 13 randomized controlled trials of adjunct acupuncture during assisted reproductive treatments. A meta-analysis was conducted, which allows the authors to draw conclusions about the magnitude of effect that may be produced by the intervention. While these trials each had small samples, in aggregate they represent a strong level of evidence.

Best Practice

The data from this meta-analysis suggest that acupuncture may increase the live birth rate when combined with assisted reproductive treatment, but only when it is performed on the day of the embryo transfer. The live birth rate of those receiving acupuncture on the day of embryo transfer was 35% compared with 22% for those without acupuncture. However, the authors caution that it is difficult to control the placebo effect in studies of acupuncture, and so these numbers may be inflated. There is no benefit to performing acupuncture at the time of oocyte retrieval or in repeating the acupuncture 2 to 3 days after the transfer. No single acupuncture point or procedure was found to be the most effective. Acupuncture after conception and in early pregnancy should be avoided until evidence is generated that demonstrates no harm to mother or baby.

Critical Thinking

1. What is the best acupuncture procedure to assure optimal results?
2. What are potential complications of acupuncture in early pregnancy?

Reference

Cheong, Y. C., Hung, Yu Ng E., Ledger, W. L. (2008). Acupuncture and assisted conception. *Cochrane Database of Systematic Reviews*, Issue 4. Art. No. CD006920.

Evidence-Based Nursing boxes present recent nursing research, discuss implications, and challenge you to incorporate this information into your nursing practice through activities.

Evidence in Action boxes present evidence from a variety of sources including systematic reviews of research literature, recent research findings, and national organization policy that have direct application to nursing practice.

Evidence in Action

Acupuncture in conjunction with embryo transfer improves the rate of pregnancy and live birth in women undergoing in vitro fertilization (Systematic review and meta-analysis) (Manheimer, Zhang, Udoff, et al., 2008).

Growth and Development

VEGETARIANISM AND THE PREGNANT ADOLESCENT

When a pregnant teen follows a vegetarian diet, she needs additional help to encourage adequate nutrition (Johnston & Sabate, 2006). A 24-hour or 2-day diet diary helps identify nutritional needs. Consider additional pregnancy needs for energy, protein, omega 3 fatty acids, iron, vitamin D, and calcium; note that Vitamin B_{12} is recommended as a supplement. Use the vegetarian Food Guide Pyramid available through the American Dietetic Association.

Growth and Development boxes, found exclusively in the pediatric chapters, provide information about the different responses of children at various ages to health conditions.

A feature entitled **Health Promotion** summarizes the needs of children with specific chronic conditions, such as asthma or diabetes. These overviews teach you to look at the child with a chronic illness like any other child, with health maintenance needs for prevention, education, and basic care.

HEALTH PROMOTION

COUPLES WHO MAY BENEFIT FROM PRENATAL DIAGNOSIS

- Women age 35 or over at time of birth
- Couples with a balanced translocation (chromosomal abnormality)
- Family history of known or suspected Mendelian genetic disorder (e.g., cystic fibrosis, hemophilia A and B, Duchenne muscular dystrophy)
- Couples with a previous child with chromosomal abnormality
- Couples in which either partner or a previous child is affected with, or in which both partners are carriers for, a diagnosable metabolic disorder
- Family history of birth defects and/or mental retardation (e.g., neural tube defects, congenital heart disease, cleft lip and/or palate)
- Ethnic groups at increased risk for specific disorders (see "Cultural Perspectives: Genetic Screening Recommendations for Various Ethnic and Age Groups" on page 162)
- Couples with history of two or more first trimester spontaneous abortions
- Women with an abnormal maternal serum alpha-fetoprotein (MSAFP or AFP) test
- Women with a teratogenic risk secondary to an exposure or maternal health condition (e.g., diabetes)

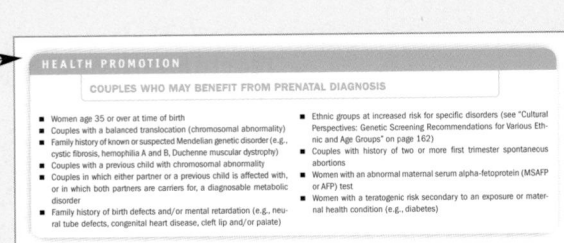

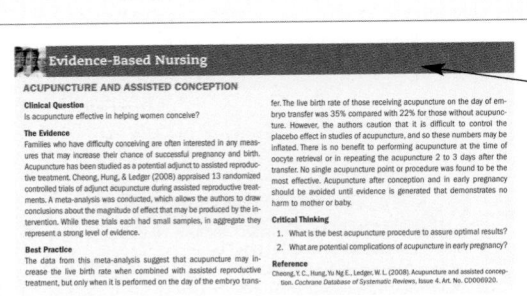

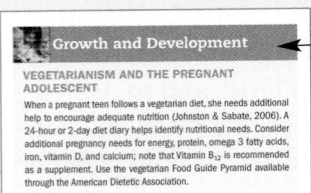

Nursing Care Plan

LANGUAGE BARRIERS AT FIRST PRENATAL VISIT

INTERVENTION	RATIONALE	EXPECTED OUTCOME
1. Nursing Diagnosis: Ineffective Health Maintenance related to alteration in verbal and written communication skills		
NIC Intervention: Effective communication: Developing and providing prenatal instruction for a non-English-speaking client.		**NOC Outcome:** Effective communication occurs. The client will gain an understanding of basic prenatal information as evidenced by using hand gestures, by pointing to pictures on posters and translated phrases on handouts, and through an interpreter, if one is available.
Goal: Client will demonstrate understanding of health information received during prenatal visits.		
■ If no interpreter is available, refer to posters with pictures to explain routine care and procedures during the prenatal examination.	■ Posters put words into verbal images and are helpful in communicating information.	
■ Provide handouts and brochures about prenatal care in the woman's native language.	■ Translated handouts provide information that the client can refer to at home. This reinforces information discussed during the visit and helps the family understand what the woman will experience during the pregnancy and at each visit.	
■ Use teaching models to demonstrate procedures. Teaching models may include plastic pelvis, knitted uterus, fetal model, breast model, birth control devices, ultrasound equipment, and so forth.	■ Visual aids help to communicate information during the examination.	
■ Schedule an interpreter for subsequent prenatal visits.	■ If a family member cannot translate the health information to the client, an independent translator is essential to ensure that information is accurately provided. When an interpreter is used (especially a family member), the nurse should be sure that the interpreter is translating information received from the woman and not simply answering the questions for her.	
■ Refer the woman to prenatal classes taught in her own language, if available.	■ Prenatal classes taught in the woman's language enable her to receive health information that is easily understood, which will provide a better understanding of what she should expect during pregnancy, birth, and postpartum. Prenatal classes may also provide a social outlet for clients.	
■ Involve other members of the healthcare team in planning and providing care.	■ Cultures vary in language, nonverbal expression, dietary habits, use of time, spatial expectations, and so forth. Use of medication and blood products may also be influenced by cultural beliefs. Social workers who are familiar with the client's cultural beliefs, for example, may help the client adjust to different healthcare practices while providing suggestions to ensure prenatal care that is more in line with the woman's cultural beliefs. Dietitians may help the woman plan meals that are aligned with her cultural practices while meeting the nutritional needs of pregnancy.	

Also provided are **Nursing Care Plans** that address nursing care for women who have complications such as preeclampsia or diabetes mellitus, as well as for high-risk newborns and children. We designed this information to enhance your preparation for the clinical setting.

Nursing Practice features offer hands-on suggestions and clinical tips. These are placed at locations in the text that will help you apply them. They include topics such as legal and ethical considerations, nursing alerts, and home and community care considerations.

Nursing Practice

Nursing responsibilities in Genetic Counseling include:

- Identify families at risk for genetic problems.
- Determine how the genetic problem is perceived and what information is desired before proceeding.
- Assist families in acquiring accurate information about the specific problem.
- Act as a liaison between the family and genetic counselor.
- Assist the family in understanding and dealing with information received.
- Provide information on support groups.
- Aid families in coping with this crisis.
- Provide information about known genetic factors.
- Assure continuity of nursing care to the family.

PATHOPHYSIOLOGY ILLUSTRATED

PREECLAMPSIA

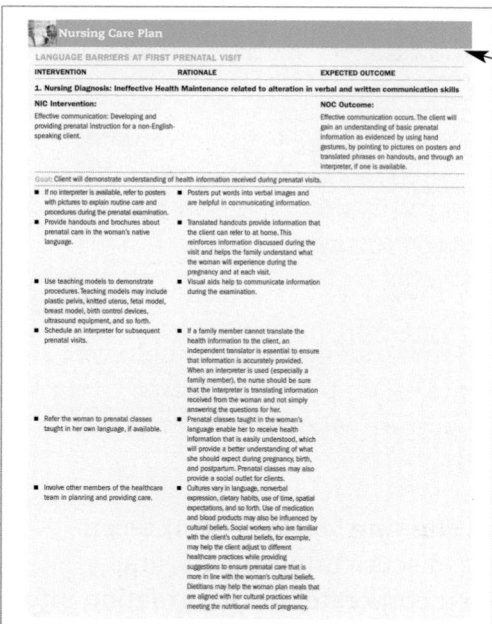

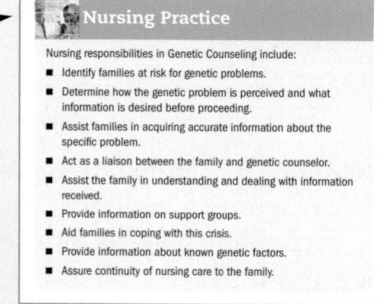

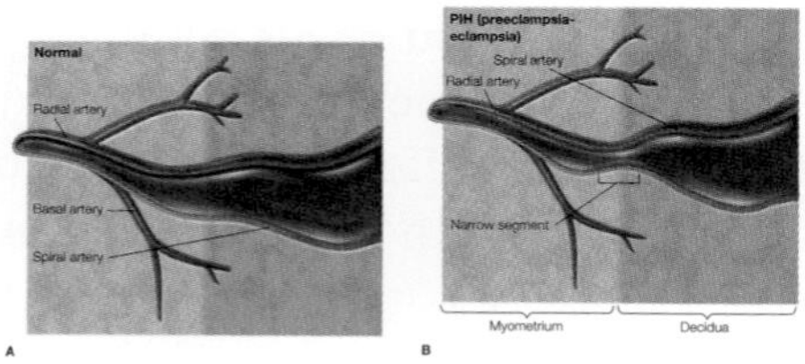

A, In a normal pregnancy, the passive quality of the spiral arteries permits increased blood flow to the placenta.
B, In preeclampsia, vasoconstriction of the myometrial segment of the spiral arteries occurs.

Pathophysiology Illustrated boxes feature unique drawings that illustrate conditions on a cellular or organ level, and may also portray the step-by-step process of a disease. These images visually explain the pathophysiology of certain conditions to increase your understanding of the condition and its treatment.

Teaching Highlights present special healthcare issues or problems and the related key teaching points for care by the family.

Teaching Highlights

INCLUDING GRANDPARENTS AND CULTURAL HEALTH PRACTICES IN THE TEACHING PLAN

When you care for a family in which the grandparents play a key role in decision making, be sure that they are present if you are teaching something that is important for the family to understand and act upon if necessary. This might include, for example, signs of illness in the newborn that need immediate follow-up.

If a specific cultural health practice is important to the family and will not cause harm, such as prayer, chanting, or specific foods, respect the family's beliefs and develop a teaching plan that includes those practices. Respecting their values improves the likelihood that the newly recommended healthcare actions will be accepted.

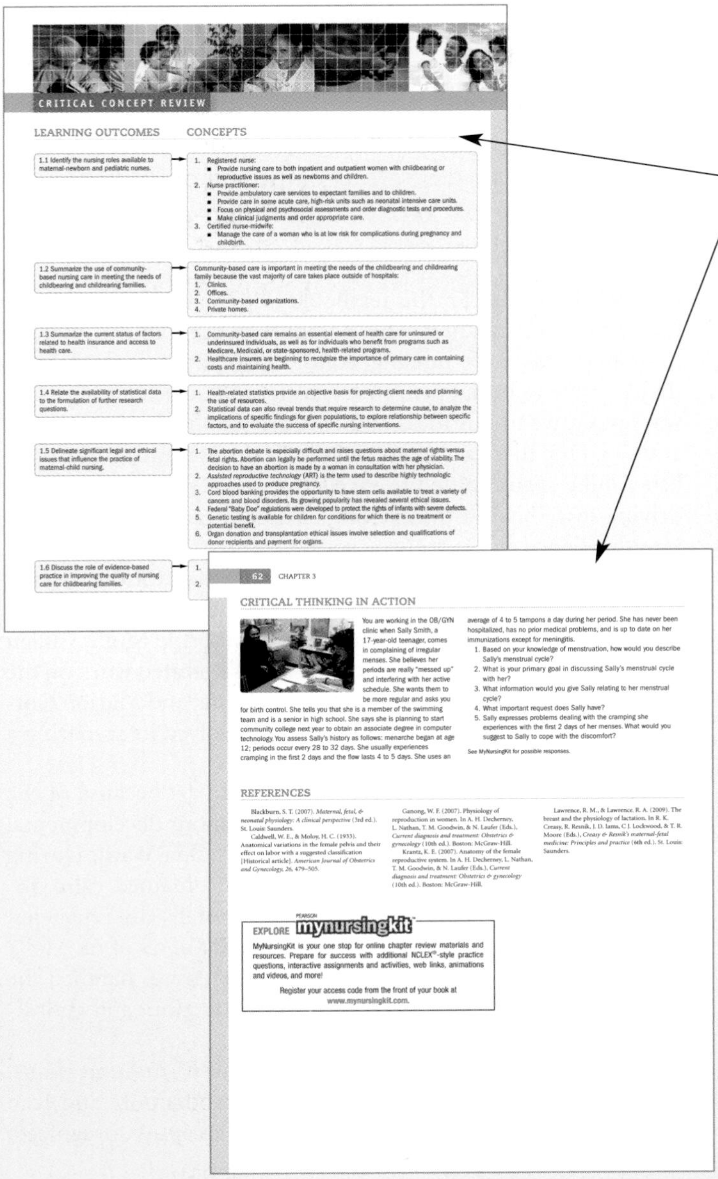

CRITICAL CONCEPT REVIEW

LEARNING OUTCOMES	CONCEPTS
1.1 Identify the nursing roles available to maternal-newborn and pediatric nurses.	1. Registered nurse: ▪ Provide nursing care to both inpatient and outpatient women with childbearing or reproductive issues as well as newborns and children. 2. Nurse practitioner: ▪ Provide ambulatory care services to expectant families and to children. ▪ Provide care in some acute care, high-risk units such as neonatal intensive care units. ▪ Focus on physical and psychosocial assessments and order diagnostic tests and procedures. ▪ Make clinical judgments and order appropriate care. 3. Certified nurse-midwife: ▪ Manage the care of a woman who is at low risk for complications during pregnancy and childbirth.
1.2 Summarize the use of community-based nursing care in meeting the needs of childbearing and childrearing families.	Community-based care is important in meeting the needs of the childbearing and childrearing family because the vast majority of care takes place outside of hospitals: 1. Clinics. 2. Offices. 3. Community-based organizations. 4. Private homes.
1.3 Summarize the current status of factors related to health insurance and access to health care.	1. Community-based care remains an essential element of health care for uninsured or underinsured individuals, as well as for individuals who benefit from programs such as Medicare, Medicaid, or state-sponsored, health-related programs. 2. Healthcare insurers are beginning to recognize the importance of primary care in containing costs and maintaining health.
1.4 Relate the availability of statistical data to the formulation of further research questions.	1. Health-related statistics provide an objective basis for projecting client needs and planning the use of resources. 2. Statistical data can also reveal trends that require research to determine cause, to analyze the implications of specific findings for given populations, to explore relationship between specific factors, and to evaluate the success of specific nursing interventions.
1.5 Delineate significant legal and ethical issues that influence the practice of maternal-child nursing.	1. The abortion debate is especially difficult and raises questions about maternal rights versus fetal rights. Abortion can legally be performed until the fetus reaches the age of viability. The decision to have an abortion is made by a woman in consultation with her physician. 2. *Assisted reproductive technology* (ART) is the term used to describe highly technologic approaches used to produce pregnancy. 3. Cord blood banking provides the opportunity to have stem cells available to treat a variety of cancers and blood disorders. Its growing popularity has revealed several ethical issues. 4. Federal "Baby Doe" regulations were developed to protect the rights of infants with severe defects. 5. Genetic testing is available for children for conditions for which there is no treatment or potential benefit. 6. Organ donation and transplantation ethical issues involve selection and qualifications of donor recipients and payment for organs.
1.6 Discuss the role of evidence-based practice in improving the quality of nursing care for childbearing families.	1. 2.

62 CHAPTER 3

CRITICAL THINKING IN ACTION

You are working in the OB/GYN clinic when Sally Smith, a 17-year-old teenager, comes in complaining of irregular menses. She believes her periods are really "messed up" and interfering with her active schedule. She wants them to be more regular and asks you for birth control. She tells you that she is a member of the swimming team and is a senior in high school. She says she is planning to start community college next year to obtain an associate degree in computer technology. You assess Sally's history as follows: menarche began at age 12; periods occur every 28 to 32 days. She usually experiences cramping in the first 2 days and the flow lasts 4 to 5 days. She uses an average of 4 to 5 tampons a day during her period. She has never been hospitalized, has no prior medical problems, and is up to date on her immunizations except for meningitis.

1. Based on your knowledge of menstruation, how would you describe Sally's menstrual cycle?
2. What is your primary goal in discussing Sally's menstrual cycle with her?
3. What information would you give Sally relating to her menstrual cycle?
4. What important request does Sally have?
5. Sally expresses problems dealing with the cramping she experiences with the first 2 days of her menses. What would you suggest to Sally to cope with the discomfort?

See MyNursingKit for possible responses.

REFERENCES

Blackburn, S. T. (2007). *Maternal, fetal, & neonatal physiology: A clinical perspective* (3rd ed.). St. Louis: Saunders.

Caldwell, W. E., & Moloy, H. C. (1933). Anatomical variations in the female pelvis and their effect on labor with a suggested classification [Historical article]. *American Journal of Obstetrics and Gynecology, 26*, 479–505.

Ganong, W. F. (2007). Physiology of reproduction in women. In A. H. Decherney, L. Nathan, T. M. Goodwin, & N. Laufer (Eds.), *Current diagnosis and treatment: Obstetrics & gynecology* (10th ed.). Boston: McGraw-Hill.

Krantz, K. E. (2007). Anatomy of the female reproductive system. In A. H. Decherney, L. Nathan, T. M. Goodwin, & N. Laufer (Eds.), *Current diagnosis and treatment: Obstetrics & gynecology* (10th ed.). Boston: McGraw-Hill.

Lawrence, R. M., & Lawrence, R. A. (2009). The breast and the physiology of lactation. In R. K. Creasy, R. Resnik, J. D. Iams, C J. Lockwood, & T. R. Moore (Eds.), *Creasy & Resnik's maternal-fetal medicine: Principles and practice* (6th ed.). St. Louis: Saunders.

EXPLORE PEARSON mynursingkit

MyNursingKit is your one stop for online chapter review materials and resources. Prepare for success with additional NCLEX®-style practice questions, interactive assignments and activities, web links, animations and videos, and more!

Register your access code from the front of your book at www.mynursingkit.com.

Each chapter ends with a **Critical Concept Review** that outlines the main points of the chapter as they relate to each Learning Outcome, a list of **References**, and directions to link to **MyNursingKit** for additional resources.

In addition, **cross-reference** icons help you to easily locate related information in other chapters. Important **laboratory values** are highlighted in a different color as a tool for you to assess your patients' conditions. Where relevant, SKILLS found in the companion book, *Clinical Skills Manual for Maternal and Child Nursing Care* (ISBN 0135097231), are cited.

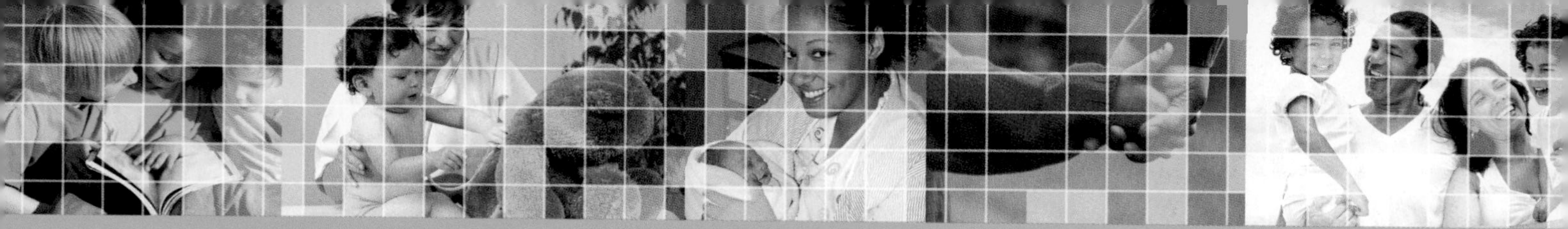

Acknowledgments

Nursing is a dynamic, exciting healthcare profession. As curricula develop, many nursing programs have begun to teach nursing of childbearing families and nursing of children together in a single course. This combined format requires that faculty approach these two fields with a similar framework and philosophy, and with similar teaching methods, so that students can maximize learning. With this third edition, we have created a tool that will enable students to master these two critical areas of nursing—the care of childbearing families and the care of children. Creating a dynamic and integrated text would not be possible without the skill and dedication of a host of people.

We wish to acknowledge the contributions to the MyNursingKit and MyNursingLab companion websites. These individuals brought their specialized knowledge to the project:

Melissa Black, RN, MSN, FNP
Mary C. Carrico, MS, RN
Amy M. Corbitt, MSN, RN
Laurie Gasperi Kaudewitz, RN, RNC-OB, BSN, MSN
Kathleen L. Peterson-Sweeney, PhD, RN, PNP-BC
Jacquelyn Reid, MSN, EdD, CNE
Cheryl Shaffer, RN, MS, PNP
Lisa South, RN, DSN
Jane K. Walker, BBA, PhD(c), RN, ASLNC-C, CNE

We also wish to acknowledge the authors of the Instructor's Resource Manual:

Michael D. Aldridge, MSN, RN, CCRN, CNS
University of Texas at Austin

Jenny C. Clapp, RN, MSN
University of North Carolina Greensboro School of Nursing

Bernadette Dragich, PhD, APRN, BC
Bluefield State College, West Virginia

We are also grateful to Janet Houser, PhD, RN, for developing the Evidence-Based Practice boxes and to Barbara Cheuvront, PhD-c, RN, for developing the Evidence in Action boxes that are presented in the women's health and maternal-newborn sections of this textbook.

We would personally like to thank several people. At Pearson Education, Maura Connor, editor-in-chief, first envisioned and supported the need for this textbook. Her creative, visionary enthusiasm is outstanding. This edition has been guided by Kim Mortimer, our new nursing editor, who merits our deepest thanks. She has been open, enthusiastic, and dedicated; she is always receptive to our ideas and encourages our development as authors. Our thanks also go to Julie Levin Alexander, our publisher. Julie is committed to excellence and creativity. She is the driving force behind the exciting changes occurring at Pearson Health Science and is truly a creative futurist in publishing. We also wish to thank Maria Guglielmo, art director, for the striking design of the text; Anne Garcia, production editor, for her calm coordination of the production of the manuscript; Molly Mullen Ward, freelance editor, for her carefully orchestrated work on the supplements; and Sarah Wrocklage, Luz Costa, and Marion Gottlieb for helping with the myriad details involved in preparing a manuscript of this size.

Operationally, this book exists in large part because of the tremendous dedication, patience, and skill of our developmental editing team, Dana Knighten and Molly Mullen Ward. During the long months of hard work, they both remained calm, focused, organized, and creative. Dana noted discrepancies, worked for continuity, and earned the respect of all of us. Molly managed communication within the author team, handled the many details of readying the book for production, and coordinated all of our efforts.

Special thanks to the people of S4Carlisle Communications, especially Lynn Steines, for coordinating production, and Jean Ives, for her work as copyeditor. They are perceptive, organized, and skillful in all of the tasks of publishing.

Finally we all wish to thank our other co-authors. As five individuals, but two teams, we came together with our own ideas, writing styles, and vision for this book. Over three editions we have grown closer in our collaboration, with productive discussions of important issues that have ultimately resulted in a new and different text for maternal, newborn, and child health nursing. We hope that this book and associated learning aids will be a useful tool for legions of nursing students to come.

Marcia L. London
Patricia W. Ladewig
Jane W. Ball
Ruth C. Bindler
Kay J. Cowen

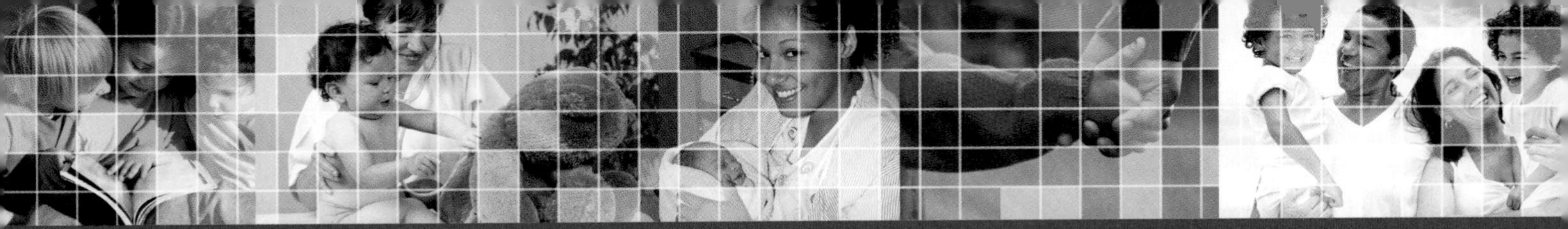

Contents

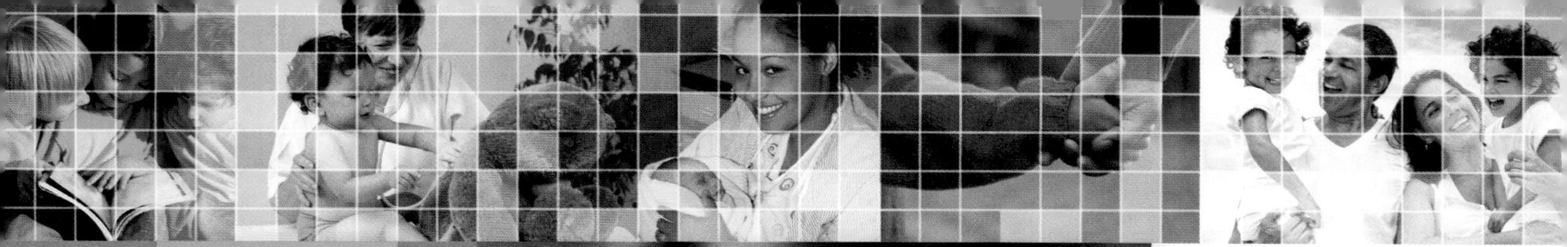

PART

1

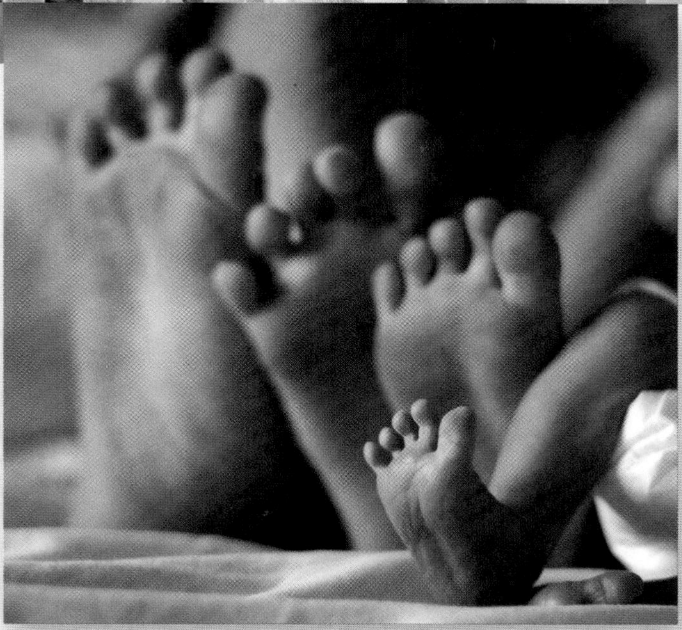

Introduction to Family-Centered Care

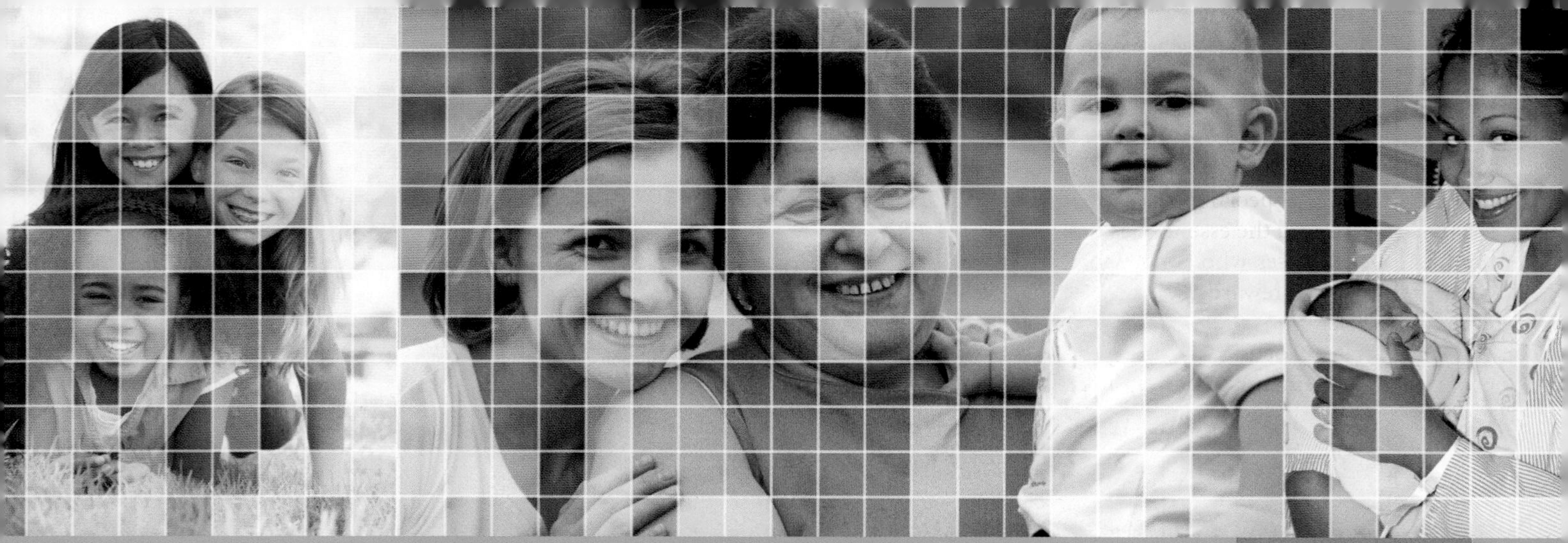

CHAPTER 1

Contemporary Maternal, Newborn, and Child Health Nursing

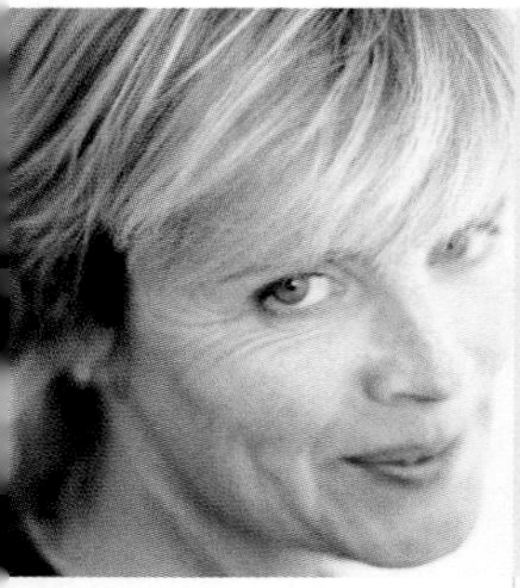

My younger son turned 21 today—officially a man now. I remember so well the night he was born in a birthing room at our local hospital. I watched my husband rock our baby and talk to him just minutes after his birth. Over the years we sought emergency health care for our son several times—when he was diagnosed with asthma as a high school freshman, when he fell skateboarding and needed surgery to put three pins in his wrist, when he fell snowboarding and dislocated his shoulder. Active kids do get their share of bumps! It is easy to take good health care for granted, but we shouldn't. It can make all the difference. —Marjorie, 47

LEARNING OUTCOMES

1.1 Identify the nursing roles available to maternal-newborn and pediatric nurses.

1.2 Summarize the use of community-based nursing care in meeting the needs of childbearing and childrearing families.

1.3 Summarize the current status of factors related to health insurance and access to health care.

1.4 Relate the availability of statistical data to the formulation of further research questions.

1.5 Delineate significant legal and ethical issues that influence the practice of maternal-child nursing.

1.6 Discuss the role of evidence-based practice in improving the quality of nursing care for childbearing families.

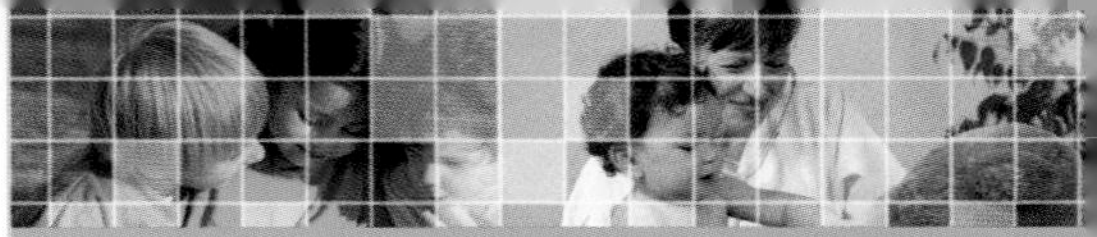

KEY TERMS

Advance directives, 13
Assisted reproductive technology (ART), 14
Birth rate, 8
Case management, 4
Certified nurse-midwife (CNM), 4
Clinical nurse specialist (CNS), 4
Clinical practice guidelines, 11
Emancipated minors, 11
Evidence-based practice, 16
Infant mortality rate, 9
Informed consent, 11
Intrauterine fetal surgery, 14
Maternal-child nursing, 3
Maternal mortality rate, 9
Mature minors, 12
Nurse practitioner (NP), 4
Nurse researcher, 4

Skilled nurses care for people, care about people, and use their expertise to help people care for themselves. This is the essence of nursing. Most nurses experience special moments professionally, times in which they know that they have practiced the essence of nursing and, in doing so, have touched the lives of others. For nurses who work with childbearing families or with children and their families, the rewards that come from skilled nursing practice can be especially rich.

This chapter focuses on introductory concepts related to the nurse and childbearing families, infants, children, and adolescents.

NURSING ROLES IN MATERNAL-CHILD NURSING

Traditionally, **maternal-child nursing** refers to the care of women during pregnancy, birth, and postpartum, as well as the care of infants, children, and adolescents. However, this label is somewhat misleading because it fails to acknowledge clearly the consideration due to fathers, partners, and family members. As nurses who work with families quickly learn, a holistic, inclusive approach is crucial to effective nursing care.

The nursing process provides the framework for delivery of direct nursing care. The nurse assesses the client—whether childbearing woman, infant, child, or adolescent—and identifies the nursing diagnoses that describe the responses of the individual and family to the condition or area of needed knowledge. The nurse then implements and evaluates nursing care. This care is designed to meet specific physical and psychosocial needs. For children the care is tailored to the individual developmental stage, giving the child additional responsibility for self-care with increasing age.

Nurses play a major role in minimizing the psychologic and physical stress experienced by childbearing families and by children and their families. This often involves listening to concerns, being present during stressful or emotional experiences, and implementing strategies to help the individual and family members cope. Nurses can help families by suggesting ways to support their loved one in the hospital, in community settings, and in the home. Nurses also suggest ways to support families with informational resources, family support groups, referral for healthcare services, and, in some cases, respite care.

Client education is a major component of maternal-child nursing. During pregnancy, nurses provide anticipatory guidance to prepare the woman and her partner, if he or she is involved, for the changes that each month brings. For example, the woman is taught self-care measures to relieve discomforts and learns to identify the warning signs that she should report. Both partners receive information on the psychologic changes of pregnancy that they may experience. Education for the laboring woman focuses on activities that help her deal successfully with a challenging experience—childbirth—whereas postpartum teaching addresses the needs of the woman and her newborn to prepare them for discharge.

In pediatric nursing, education is especially challenging because nurses must be prepared to work with children at various levels of understanding and to include family members in all aspects of care. As client educators, nurses help children adapt to the hospital setting and prepare them for procedures.

When a child is ill, most hospitals encourage a parent to stay with the child and to provide much of the direct and the supportive care under the guidance of a nurse. Nurses teach parents to watch for important signs and responses to therapies, to increase the child's comfort, and even to provide advanced care. Taking an active role during hospitalization helps prepare the parent to assume total responsibility for care after the child leaves the hospital.

Developing Cultural Competence

LOWERING THE READING LEVEL OF CLIENT EDUCATION MATERIALS

Approximately 36% (75 million) of the adult population in the United States cannot read and understand basic health information needed to make appropriate decisions regarding their health (Jones, 2007). The materials need to be provided in the appropriate language and at an appropriate reading level. Printed materials to educate children and families about a health condition might be readily available, but they often are written at too high a reading level. The recommended reading level for educational materials is fifth grade equivalency (Bauman, Massicotte, Ray, et al., 2007). Just because printed material may be available in the primary language of the client and family, do not assume that the family has reading skills in that language.

In developing client education materials with a lower reading level:

- Use short, familiar words with one or two syllables and short sentences.
- Substitute simple language for a medical term.
- Use arrows, white space, or bold type to point out the key message.
- Use action words and simple art or photos.
- Describe or show in art only the correct behavior.

Nurses also serve as advocates, acting to safeguard and advance the interests of families. To be an effective advocate, the nurse must be aware of the individual's needs, the family's needs and resources, and the healthcare services available in the hospital and the community. The nurse can then assist the family to make informed choices about these services and to act in their best interests. Nurses must also ensure that the policies and resources of healthcare agencies meet the psychosocial needs of childbearing women and of children and their families.

Collaborative practice is a comprehensive model of health care that uses a multidisciplinary team of health professionals to provide high-quality, cost-effective care. In maternal-newborn settings the team generally includes certified nurse-midwives (see later discussion), physicians, nurse practitioners, nurses, and other health specialists such as pharmacists, lactation consultants, or childbirth educators. Similarly, the multidisciplinary team assembled when a child has a significant health problem or handicapping condition may include physicians, nurses, social workers, physical and occupational therapists, and other specialists. Their goal is to create an interdisciplinary plan designed to meet the child's medical, nursing, developmental, educational, and psychosocial needs. Because nurses spend large amounts of time providing nursing care for the client and family, they often are better informed than other healthcare professionals about the family's wishes and resources. As a member of the team, the nurse serves as an advocate to ensure that the plan of care considers the family's wishes and contains appropriate services.

Case management is a process of coordinating the delivery of healthcare services in a manner that focuses on both quality and cost outcomes. This is often a collaborative practice with other healthcare providers designed to promote continuity of care. The nurse case manager has control over the use of healthcare resources that are considered appropriate for the client's condition and links the client and family to these services. The goal is to help the individual and family have the best healthcare outcome and decrease fragmentation of care, while controlling the cost of healthcare services. In maternal-child nursing, case management is often used for a complicated high-risk pregnancy and for long-term care of children with chronic conditions.

Discharge planning is a form of case management. Effective discharge planning promotes a smooth, rapid, and safe transition into the community and improves the results of treatment begun in the hospital. To be a discharge planner, the nurse needs to know about community medical resources, appropriate home care agencies, educational interventions, and services reimbursed by the individual's health plan or other financial resources.

In addition, several advanced-practice roles are available to maternal-child nurses with additional education. A **nurse practitioner (NP)**, who has specialized education in a Doctor of Nursing Practice (DNP) program or a master's degree program often provides ambulatory care services to pregnant women, newborns, children, adolescents, and families. (Note: Early nurse practitioner programs were sometimes certificate programs.) The area of specialization determines the NP's title, so that there are family nurse practitioners, neonatal nurse practitioners, pediatric nurse practitioners, women's health nurse practitioners and so forth. NPs focus on physical and psychosocial assessments, including history, physical examination, and certain diagnostic tests and procedures. They make clinical judgments and begin appropriate treatments, seeking physician consultation when necessary. **Clinical nurse specialists (CNSs)** have a master's degree and specialized knowledge and competence in a specific clinical area. They often are found on mother-baby units, on pediatric units, and in intensive care units assisting staff to provide excellent, evidence-based care. The **certified nurse-midwife (CNM)** is educated in the two disciplines of nursing and midwifery and is certified by the American College of Nurse-Midwives. The CNM is prepared to manage independently the care of women at low risk for complications during pregnancy, birth, and the postpartum period, as well as the care of healthy newborns (Figure 1–1 ●).

The **nurse researcher** has an advanced doctoral degree, typically a Ph.D., and assumes a leadership role in generating new research. Nurse researchers are typically found in university settings although more and more hospitals are employing them to conduct research relevant to patient care, administrative issues, and the like.

FAMILY-CENTERED MATERNAL-CHILD CARE

Contemporary childbirth is family centered—that is, characterized by an emphasis on the family and the family's choices about their birth experience. Consequently, today the concept of family-centered childbirth is accepted and encouraged. Fathers

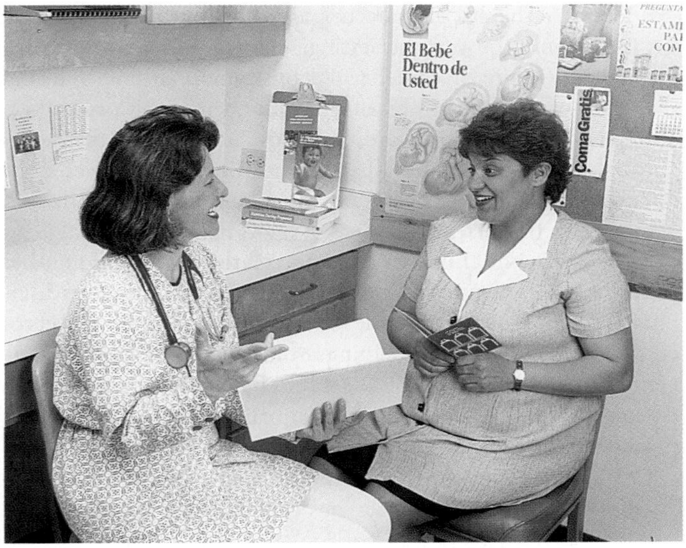

● **Figure 1–1** A certified nurse-midwife confers with her client.

and partners are active participants, not simply bystanders; siblings are encouraged to visit and meet the newest family member, and they may even attend the birth.

New definitions of family are evolving. For example, the family of a single mother may include her mother, her sister, another relative, a close friend, a lesbian partner, or the father of the child. Many cultures also recognize the importance of extended families, and several family members may provide care and support. See Chapter 2∞.

The family can make choices about the place of birth (hospital, birthing center, or home), the primary caregiver (physician, CNM, or even lay midwife), the approaches to childbirth (Lamaze, Bradley, and so forth), and birth-related experiences (position for birth, use of analgesia and anesthesia, and methods of childbirth preparation, for example) as well as breastfeeding and childcare choices.

In pediatric settings, *family-centered care* is designed to meet the emotional, social, and developmental needs of children and families seeking health care. Families have important knowledge to share about their child, their child's health condition, and how their child responds to various actions and events. Families are important in helping the child recover from illnesses and injuries. As partners in the child's care, families need to learn about the child's condition and participate in decisions regarding the child's care. The family and healthcare team collaborative relationship should address cultural values and respect diversity (Gance-Cleveland, 2006). The Society of Pediatric Nurses and the American Nurses Association nursing practice guidelines for family-centered care are provided in Table 1–1.

CONTEMPORARY CHILDBIRTH

In the early 1990s, women who gave birth vaginally remained in the hospital for about 3 days. This provided time for nurses to complete essential teaching. In the late 1990s, in an effort to control costs, discharge within 12 to 24 hours after birth became the

Table 1–1 Elements of Family-Centered Care

Elements
The family at the center: Incorporate into policy and practice the recognition that the family is the constant in a child's life, while the service systems and support personnel within those systems fluctuate, and that the illness or injury of a child affects all members of the family system.
Family-professional collaboration: Facilitate family-professional collaboration at all levels of hospital, home, and community care for: care of the individual child; program development, implementation, evaluation, and evolution; and policy formation.
Family-professional communication: Exchange complete and unbiased information between families and professionals in a supportive manner at all times.
Cultural diversity of families: Recognize and honor cultural diversity, strengths, and individuality within and across all families, including ethnic, racial, spiritual, social, economic, educational, and geographic diversity, and ensure this is reflected in policy and practice.
Coping differences and support: Recognize and respect different methods of coping and implementing comprehensive policies and programs that provide families with the developmental, educational, emotional, spiritual, environmental, and financial supports needed to meet their diverse needs.
Family-centered peer support: Encourage and facilitate family-to-family support and networking.
Specialized service and support systems: Ensure that hospital, home, and community service and support systems for children needing specialized health and developmental care and their families are flexible, accessible, and comprehensive for diverse family-identified needs.
Holistic perspective of family-centered care: Appreciate families as families, and children as children, recognizing that they possess a wide range of strengths, concerns, emotions, and aspirations beyond their need for specialized health and developmental services and support.

Adapted from: Lewandowski, L. A., & Tesler, M. D. (Eds.). (2003). Family-centered care: Putting it into action. *The SPN/ANA Guide to Family-Centered Care.* Washington, DC: American Nurses Association.

norm. This practice did not necessarily cause problems for women with supportive families, thorough prenatal preparation, and adequate resources. However, because there was less time available for client teaching, women with little knowledge, experience, or support were often inadequately prepared to care for themselves and their newborn. Fortunately, the negative impact of this practice gained recognition nationwide and resulted in legislation that provides for a postpartum stay of up to 48 hours following a vaginal birth and up to 96 hours following a cesarean birth at the discretion of the mother and her healthcare provider.

The place of birth is an important decision. As discussed in Chapter 8∞, birthing centers and special "homelike" labor-delivery-recovery-postpartum (LDRP) rooms in hospitals have become increasingly popular. Some women choose to give birth at home, although healthcare professionals do not generally recommend this approach. Most professionals are concerned that, in the event of an unanticipated complication, delay in receiving emergency care might jeopardize the well-being or even the life of the mother or her infant. Consequently, the majority of home births are attended by direct-entry midwives who are not RNs. Today's direct-entry midwives often complete a direct-entry midwifery education program and seek certification through either the American College of Nurse-Midwives or the North American Registry of Midwives (NARM).

In many areas there is a movement from normal to high-tech birthing. This movement is influenced in part by childbearing families, sometimes called generation Y or the iGeneration, who have grown up with technology and know no other way. They may view elective induction and mother-requested caesarean birth as accepted options, for example. This movement is often reinforced by caregivers who, aware of legal liability issues, practice defensive medicine. Furthermore, many hospitals now support a high-tech model of maternity care because it is "easier" to manage more women if their pain is controlled by epidurals and their contractions are monitored by electronic fetal monitors (Zwelling, 2008). Maternal-child nurses are beginning to analyze their personal attitudes and beliefs about childbirth and the impact of this approach to birthing. Additional research is also indicated to determine the long-term impact on the family and on caregivers.

CONTEMPORARY CARE OF CHILDREN

More than 82.1 million children age 19 years or younger live in the United States. They account for 27.4% of the population (U.S. Census Bureau, 2008). In today's society, children have special value, but they are also considered to be vulnerable and to need protection.

Pediatric nursing is a specialized area of nursing that focuses on caring for children in many different settings within the hospital and the community. These settings include the following:

- Various hospital units, such as pediatric units, intensive care units, emergency department, radiology, rehabilitation units, and specialty care clinics
- Physician offices, healthcare centers, clinics
- Schools, childcare centers, homeless shelters
- The child's home

Pediatric health care occurs along a continuum that reflects not only the various settings of care, but also the complexity and range of care needed by individual children and their families. For example, all children need health promotion and health maintenance care, but some children need care for chronic conditions, acute illnesses and injuries, and even end-of-life care. See Figure 1–2 ● for the model of pediatric health care used in this textbook.

Managing the child's transition from the hospital to another setting involves planning the discharge, implementing interdisciplinary plans, ensuring that the family understands the aspects of care they need to provide, helping the family to develop an emergency care plan in the event their child has an unexpected health care crisis, and collaborating with a broad range of healthcare professionals.

● **Figure 1–2** The Bindler-Ball Continuum of Pediatric Health Care for Children and Their Families. The outer bars represent the family, cultural, and community influence on the care that the child receives, either through the services sought by the family or the services provided in the community. Cultural influences include the family's values and beliefs, and the cultural competence of the nurse in caring for a child and family.

The inner categories represent the range of health care needed by children. All children need health promotion and health maintenance services, represented by the base of the triangle. Notice the arrows representing the upward and downward movement between the levels of care as the child's condition changes.

Children may be healthy with episodic acute illnesses and injuries. Some children develop a chronic condition for which specialized health care is needed. A child's chronic condition may be well controlled, but acute episodes (such as with asthma) or other illnesses and injuries may occur, and the child also needs health promotion and health maintenance services. Some children develop a life-threatening illness and ultimately need end-of-life care. A healthy child may also experience a catastrophic injury leading to death and the family needs supportive end-of-life care.

Source: Bindler & Ball, 2007.

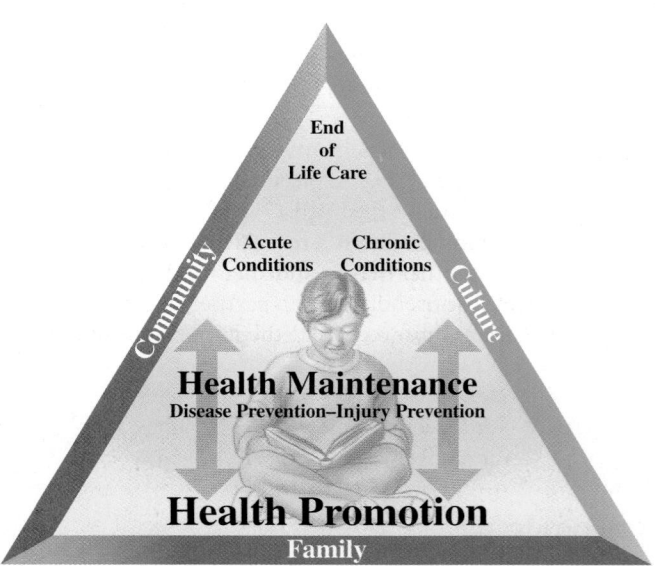

MATERNAL-CHILD CARE IN THE COMMUNITY

Primary care is the focus of much attention as caregivers search for a new, more effective direction for health care. Primary care includes a focus on health promotion, illness prevention, and individual responsibility for one's own health. These services are best provided in community-based settings. Third-party payers are beginning to recognize the importance of primary care in containing costs and maintaining health. Community-based healthcare systems providing primary care and some secondary care are becoming available in schools, workplaces, homes, churches, clinics, transitional care programs, and other ambulatory settings.

The growth and diversity of health payer plans offer both opportunities and challenges for women's and children's health care. Opportunities for improved delivery of screening and preventive services exist in community-based models of coordinated and comprehensive well-woman and well-child care. A challenge that health payer plans face is how to relate to essential community providers of care, such as family-planning clinics, women's health centers, and well-child centers that offer a unique service or serve groups of women and children with special needs (adolescents, women and children with disabilities, and ethnic or racial minorities).

Community-based care remains an essential element of healthcare for uninsured or underinsured individuals, as well as for individuals who benefit from programs such as Medicare, Medicaid, or the State Child Health Insurance Program (now referred to as CHIP [not SCHIP]). Some of these programs are broad based, such as those offered through public health departments, while others, such as parenting classes for adolescents, are geared to the needs of a specific population.

Maternal-child nurses are especially sensitive to these changes in healthcare delivery because the vast majority of health care provided to childbearing and childrearing families takes place outside of hospitals in clinics, offices, and community-based organizations. In addition, maternal-child nurses offer specialized services such as childbirth preparation classes, sibling classes, and parenting classes.

Home Care

Providing health care in the home is an especially important dimension of community-based nursing care. Shorter hospital stays end in the discharge of individuals who still require support, assistance, and teaching. Home care helps fill this gap. Home care also enables infants, children, and women to remain at home with conditions that formerly would have required hospitalization.

Nurses are major providers of home care services. Home care nurses perform direct nursing care and also supervise unlicensed assistive personnel who provide less skilled levels of service. In a home setting, nurses use their skills in assessment, intervention, communication, teaching, problem solving, and organization to meet the needs of childbearing and childrearing families. They also play a major role in coordinating services from other providers, such as physical therapists or lactation consultants.

Postpartum and newborn home visits help ensure a satisfactory transition from the birthing center to the home. This trend is a positive method of meeting the needs of childbearing families and hopefully will become standard practice. See Chapter 32∞ for discussion of home care and guidance about making a home visit. Information on home care is also provided as appropriate throughout this text.

Many children with serious chronic conditions and disabilities assisted by technology are now cared for at home by families rather than by long-term hospitalization. After studies in the 1980s found that home health care was substantially less expensive than hospital care, Congress amended laws to permit payment of home care services with federal funds, such as through Medicaid. Approximately 21% of children with special healthcare needs under 6 years of age use durable medical equipment, and 8% require home care services (Health Resources and Services Administration, Maternal and Child Health Bureau, 2008). Children with conditions considered fatal 15 years ago are thriving with home care and are participating in family, community, and school life. See Chapter 40∞.

COMPLEMENTARY THERAPIES

Interest in complementary care, previously termed complementary and alternative therapies (CAM), continues to grow nationwide and affects the care of childbearing and childrearing families. Complementary care includes a wide array of therapies, such as acupuncture, acupressure, therapeutic touch, biofeedback, massage therapy, meditation, herbal therapies, and homeopathic remedies. Concepts related to the use of complementary care by families are presented in more detail in Chapter 2∞ and in special boxed features throughout the text.

ACCESS TO HEALTH CARE

In 2006, healthcare expenditures in the United States were $2.1 trillion, a 6.7% increase over the previous year. The healthcare share of the gross domestic product (GDP) was 16% (National Center for Health Statistics [NCHS], 2009). Despite this increase in spending, however, not all pregnant women and children in the United States have access to health care. In 2006, 17% of the population (43.9 million people) were without health insurance. For people living in poverty, Medicaid is the most prevalent form of insurance, covering 14% of people (36.2 million), including pregnant women who fall into specified income categories (NCHS, 2009).

For women who become pregnant, early prenatal care is one of the most important approaches available to reduce adverse pregnancy outcomes. In 2005, 83.9% of pregnant women in the United States began prenatal care in the first trimester. However, these percentages vary significantly among groups, with black or African American, Hispanic or Latina, and Native American women less likely to receive early and adequate prenatal care than white and Asian women (NCHS, 2009).

In 2007, 8.1 million children, 11.1% of all those below 18 years of age, had no health insurance (Families USA, 2008). Nearly 27.4% of children are covered by public insurance programs such as Medicaid, Medicare, and the State Children's Health Insurance Program (CHIP) (Inglehart, 2007). More than two-thirds of the nation's 8.9 million uninsured children come from families with incomes at or below two times the federal poverty rate (Kaiser Commission on Medicaid and the Uninsured, 2008). Most of these children have difficulty obtaining the most basic preventive health care, including immunizations.

Efforts to provide universal access to health care for children continue to grow. Congress passed initial legislation to create CHIP in 1997 and reauthorized it in 2007. In 2009, the Children's Health Insurance Program Reauthorization Act (CHIPRA) was passed. It extends and expands CHIP and is projected to provide coverage for 4.1 million children in CHIP and Medicaid who would have been uninsured by 2013 (Kaiser Commission, 2009).

In a given month about 48.1 million people are enrolled in Medicaid. Of these, 23.5 million, or 48.9%, are children (Centers for Medicare and Medicaid Services [CMS], 2007). CHIP is a complement to Medicaid and enables more children to obtain access to essential healthcare services. States are allocated federal funds to encourage enrollment of children living with families whose income is above Medicaid eligibility levels (Kaiser Commission, 2008). Children enrolled must be provided with health benefits coverage that is substantially equal to the benefits coverage in the federal or state employee benefits plan or the plan of the largest health maintenance organization in the state. In 2007, 7.1 million children were enrolled in CHIP at some time during the year (CMS, 2008). Many pregnant adolescents are also served in these state programs.

CULTURALLY COMPETENT CARE

The population of the United States daily becomes more diverse. Approximately 42% of all children less than 18 years of age are from families of minority populations (Forum on Child and Family Statistics, 2007). Thus, it is vitally important that a nurse who cares for women and for children recognizes the importance of a family's cultural values and beliefs, which may be quite different from those of the nurse.

Specific elements that contribute to a family's value system include the following:

- Religion and social beliefs
- Presence and influence of the extended family, as well as socialization within the ethnic group

Developing Cultural Competence

CULTURAL CONFLICTS

Conflicts can occur within a family when traditional rituals and practices of the family do not conform with current healthcare practices. Nurses need to be sensitive to the potential implications for the child's health care, especially after the child is discharged from the hospital. When cultural values are not part of the nursing care plan, parents may be forced to decide whether the family's beliefs should take priority over the healthcare professional's guidance.

- Communication patterns
- Beliefs and understanding about the concepts of health and illness
- Permissible physical contact with strangers
- Education

When the family's cultural values are incorporated into the care plan, the family is more likely to accept and comply with the needed care, especially in the home care setting. It is important for nurses to avoid imposing personal cultural values on the families and children in their care. By learning about the values of the different ethnic groups in the community nurses can develop an individualized nursing care plan for each child and family.

Because of the importance of culturally competent care, this topic is discussed in more depth in Chapter 2 and throughout the book.

STATISTICAL DATA AND MATERNAL-CHILD CARE

Health-related statistics provide an objective basis for projecting client needs, planning the use of resources, and determining the effectiveness of specific treatments. The use of statistics helps identify certain healthcare trends and high-risk target groups. The following sections discuss descriptive statistics that are particularly important to maternal-child health care.

BIRTH RATE

Birth rate refers to the number of live births per 1000 people in a given population. Worldwide, birth rates vary dramatically as Table 1–2 indicates. In the United States in 2007, the preliminary birth rate rose by nearly 1%, to 14.3 per 1000. Increases in birth rate were seen in most age groups except among the youngest (aged 10 to 14) and the oldest (aged 45 to 49), which were unchanged. The birth rate for teenagers aged 15 to 19 increased for the second straight year (Hamilton, Martin, & Ventura, 2009). This increase and its implications for teenage pregnancy prevention efforts have sparked considerable discussion among healthcare professionals (see Chapter 13). In addition, childbearing by unmarried women reached record high levels. Specifically, in every age group 15 years and older, increases in nonmarital births dramatically outpaced increases in total births (Hamilton et al., 2009).

Statistics also indicate that the caesarean birth rate rose 2% in 2007, reaching a record high at 31.8% of all births. Over the last decade this rate has increased by more than 50% from 20.7 in 1996 (Hamilton et al., 2009).

The statistics do raise questions. For example: What is the impact of cultural differences and changing societal values on birth rates? Do birth rates change when access to information on contraception increases? What role does government policy, such as China's legislation limiting births to one child per family, play?

Table 1–2 Live Birth Rates and Infant Mortality Rates for Selected Countries (2007)

Country	Birth Rate	Infant Mortality Rate
Afghanistan	46.2	157.4
Argentina	16.5	14.3
Australia	12.0	4.6
Cambodia	25.5	58.5
Canada	10.8	4.6
China	13.5	22.1
Egypt	22.5	29.5
Germany	8.2	4.1
Ghana	29.9	53.6
India	22.7	34.6
Iraq	31.4	47.0
Japan	8.1	2.8
Mexico	20.4	19.6
Russia	10.9	11.1
United Kingdom	10.7	5.0
United States	14.2	6.4

Source: Data from *The World Fact Book 2008.* Washington, DC: The Central Intelligence Agency.

MATERNAL MORTALITY

The **maternal mortality rate** is the number of deaths from causes related to or aggravated by pregnancy or the management of pregnancy during the pregnancy cycle (including the 42-day postpartum period) per 100,000 live births. It does not include deaths of pregnant women due to external causes such as accidents, homicides, and suicides. The maternal mortality rate in the United States in 2005 was 15.1 deaths per 100,000 live births. However, black women have a significantly higher risk of maternal death than white women have. The maternal mortality rate for black women was 36.5 deaths per 100,000 live births as compared to 11.1 deaths for white women. The maternal mortality rate for Hispanic women is cited as 9.6, but inconsistencies in reporting Hispanic origin on death certificates and on censuses and surveys make this number less precise (Kung, Hoyert, Xu, et al., 2008).

Factors influencing the long-term decrease in maternal mortality include the increased use of hospitals and specialized healthcare personnel by maternity clients, the establishment of care centers for high-risk mothers and infants, the prevention and control of infection with antibiotics and improved techniques, the availability of blood products for transfusions, and the lowered rates of anesthesia-related deaths. Additional factors may be identified by asking the following research questions: Is there a correlation between maternal mortality and age? Is there a correlation between maternal mortality and availability of health care? Economic status?

INFANT MORTALITY

The **infant mortality rate** is the number of deaths of infants under 1 year of age per 1000 live births in a given population. In 2005, the infant mortality rate in the United States was 6.86 per 1000 live births. This rate is not significantly different from the 2000 rate of 6.89 and represents an unwelcome plateau in the decline in infant mortality rates that had occurred over the last 60 years (MacDorman & Mathewes, 2008). Figure 1–3 ● reflects infant mortality rates from 1950 through 2005. *Neonatal mortality rate* refers to deaths of infants less than 28 days old per 1000 live births while the *postneonatal mortality rate* refers to deaths of infants from 28 days through 11 months per 1000 live births.

However, the infant mortality rate varied widely by the race of the mother. Infant mortality rates were highest among non-Hispanic black women (13.63 per 1000 live births). This compares with 5.76 among non-Hispanic white women. Not surprisingly, infant mortality rates are higher among infants born in multiple births, infants born prematurely, and those born to unmarried mothers (MacDorman & Mathews, 2008).

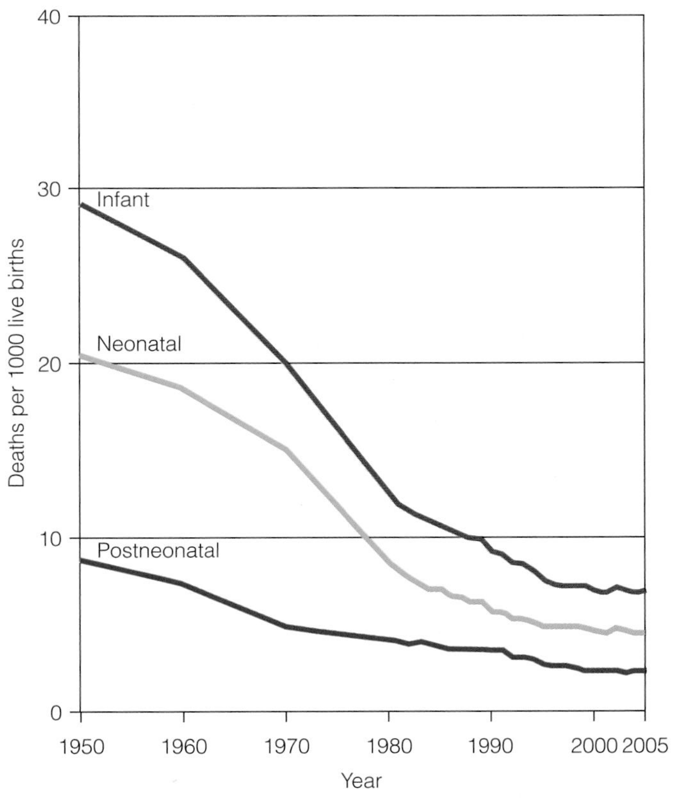

● **Figure 1–3** Infant, Neonatal, and Postneonatal Mortality Rates, United States, 1950–2005.

Source: Health, United States, 2008.

In 2005, 36.5% of all infant deaths were related to preterm birth. Not surprisingly, although very preterm infants account for only 2% of births, they account for over half of all infant deaths (MacDorman & Mathews, 2008). Overall, the five leading causes of infant death in order of frequency were congenital malformations and chromosomal abnormalities, disorders related to prematurity and low birth weight, sudden infant death syndrome (SIDS), maternal complications of pregnancy, and complications of the placenta, cord, and membranes (Kung et al., 2007).

The U.S. infant mortality rate continues to be an area of concern because the United States has fallen to 29th place in the world in infant mortality, tied with Slovakia and Poland (MacDorman & Mathews, 2008). Healthcare professionals, policy makers, and the public continue to stress the need for better prenatal care, coordination of health services, and provision of comprehensive maternal-child services in the United States.

Table 1–2 identifies infant mortality rates for selected countries. As the data indicate, the range is dramatic among the countries listed. Information about birth rates and mortality rates is limited for some countries because of a lack of organized reporting mechanisms.

The information raises questions about access to health care during pregnancy and after birth and about standards of living, nutrition, and sociocultural factors. Additional factors affecting the infant mortality rate may be identified by considering the following research questions: What are the leading causes of infant mortality in each country? Why do mortality rates differ among racial groups?

PEDIATRIC MORTALITY

Surprisingly, mortality rates for children between 1 and 19 years of age are higher in the United States than in Canada, Australia, and the United Kingdom, and the United States' mortality rate for children between 1 and 14 years ranks 20th among 26 economically developed countries (Duderstadt, 2007). The most common cause of death in 2005 for U.S. children between 1 and 19 years of age was unintentional injury. For children ages 1 to 4 years the next leading causes of death were congenital anomalies, cancer, homicide, and diseases of the heart while for children ages 5 to 14 the next leading causes of death were cancer, congenital anomalies, homicide, and suicide (National Center for Health Statistics, 2009).

Between 2000–2005, motor vehicle traffic-related accidents were the major cause of unintentional injury in all children ages 5 to 19. In children 1 to 4, the leading cause of unintentional injury was drowning, followed by pedestrian-related injuries, fires and burns, and motor vehicle accidents. In children 5 to 9 and 10 to 14, pedestrian accidents followed motor vehicle transportation-related injuries as the most common cause of unintentional death. However, for youths ages 15 to 19 years, poisoning was the next most common cause of unintentional injury (Borse, Gilchrist, Dellinger, et al., 2008).

PEDIATRIC MORBIDITY

Morbidity—an illness or injury that limits activity, requires medical attention or hospitalization, or results in a chronic condition—also varies according to the age of the child. In 2005 there were 3.5 million hospital discharges for children in the United States between 1 and 21 years of age, an average of 4 discharges per 100 children. This represents a 33% decrease in overall hospitalizations for children between 1 and 14 years of age between 1985 and 2003 (Health Resources and Services Administration, 2006). Respiratory diseases are the leading cause of hospitalization in children between 1 and 9 years of age. Although injury is a leading cause of death in children 1 to 19 years of age, it accounted for only a small number of hospitalizations. Mental disorders were the leading cause of hospitalization in children between 10 and 19 years of age. Pregnancy and childbirth was the leading cause of hospitalization for female adolescents between 15 and 21 years of age.

IMPLICATIONS FOR NURSING PRACTICE

Nurses can use statistics in a number of ways. For example, they can use statistical data to:

- Determine populations at risk.
- Assess the relationship between specific factors.
- Help establish databases for specific client populations.
- Determine the levels of care needed by particular client populations.
- Evaluate the success of specific nursing interventions.
- Determine priorities in caseloads.
- Estimate staffing and equipment needs of hospital units and clinics.
- Apply for funding to support health needs.

Nurses who use this information are better prepared to promote the health needs of maternal-newborn clients and their families.

In the report *Healthy People 2010,* the U.S. government established updated objectives to improve pregnancy outcome and the health of women, infants, children, and young adults. Many of these objectives focus on improving pregnancy outcomes and reducing the incidence of death and disability from the major causes of death. Federal funding is available to healthcare organizations for the development of programs aimed at reducing the number of deaths from these factors in specific high-risk groups. A midcourse review identified progress in achieving these objectives (U.S. Department of Health and Human Services, 2006).

LEGAL CONSIDERATIONS IN MATERNAL-CHILD NURSING

SCOPE OF PRACTICE

The *scope of practice* is defined as the limits of nursing practice set forth in state statutes. Although some state practice acts continue to limit nursing practice to the traditional responsibilities of providing client care related to health maintenance and disease prevention, most state practice acts cover expanded practice roles that include collaboration with other health professionals in planning and providing care, physician-delegated diagnosis and prescriptive privilege, and the delegation of direct care tasks to other specified licensed and unlicensed personnel. A nurse must function within the scope of practice or risk being accused of practicing medicine without a license.

STANDARDS OF NURSING CARE

Standards of care establish minimum criteria for competent, proficient delivery of nursing care. Such standards are designed to protect the public and are used to judge the quality of care provided. Legal interpretation of actions within standards of care is based on what a reasonably prudent nurse with similar education and experience would do in similar circumstances.

The American Nurses Association (ANA) has published standards of practice for maternal-child health. ANA, the National Association of Pediatric Nurse Practitioners, and the Society of Pediatric Nurses (2008) collaborated on the development of standards for pediatric clinical nursing practice. The ANA and the National Association of Neonatal Nurses also recently published the scope and standards of practice for neonatal nursing (2004). Specialty organizations such as the Association of Women's Health, Obstetric and Neonatal Nurses (AWHONN) continue to set the standards of professional nursing practice in the care of women and newborns (2003). Agency policies, procedures, and protocols also provide appropriate guidelines for care standards. For example, **clinical practice guidelines** and critical pathways are comprehensive interdisciplinary care plans for a specific condition that describe the sequence and timing of interventions that should result in expected client or patient outcomes. Clinical practice guidelines or critical pathways are adopted within a healthcare setting to reduce variation in care management, to limit costs of care, and to evaluate the effectiveness of care.

While standards of care do not carry the force of law, they have important legal significance. Any nurse who fails to meet appropriate standards of care invites allegations of negligence or malpractice. Practicing within the guidelines established by an agency or following local or national standards decreases the potential for litigation.

CLIENT/PATIENT SAFETY

The Joint Commission, officially the Joint Commission on the Accreditation of Healthcare Organizations (formerly referred to as JCAHO), a nongovernmental agency that audits the operation of hospitals and healthcare facilities, has identified patient safety as an important responsibility of healthcare providers. Patient safety goals, which are evaluated and updated regularly, are requirements for accreditation. These goals can be found on the Joint Commission web site.

Infants and children are at a higher risk for medical error than others and also may be more vulnerable to harm from errors made. Most errors in medical care within hospitals are "systems" errors related to equipment, complex procedures, fragmented care, and lack of standardized procedures. Reasons for the increase in medical errors among children include the following (Kozer, Berkovitch, & Koren, 2006):

- Medication dosage calculations are more complex. Dosages are based upon weight, whereas adults are given standard doses. The misplacement of a decimal in the medication dosage calculation can result in an overdose that can cause harm to the child or even death.
- Many drug preparations require dilution to achieve the small dosage required by infants.
- Medications not yet approved for use in children by the U.S. Food and Drug Administration (FDA) are sometimes prescribed, before pediatric dosage guidelines have been established.
- Young children cannot communicate well if they are having a reaction to the medication.

Limited English proficiency may also be a potential source of medical error for childbearing women and children. In such cases a risk exists for errors in interpretation—either of what the health professional says or what the family member says. Even when using a hospital interpreter, errors such as omitting instructions on dose, frequency, and duration of medications have potential clinical consequences (Flores & Ngui, 2006). Healthcare facilities are actively working to implement strategies that will reduce medical errors in all child patients.

MyNursingKit Standards of Practice

INFORMED CONSENT

Informed consent is a legal concept that protects a person's right to autonomy and self-determination by specifying that no action may be taken without that individual's prior understanding and freely given consent. Although this policy is actively enforced for such major procedures, surgery, or regional anesthesia, it pertains to any nursing, medical, or surgical intervention. To touch a person without consent (except in an emergency) constitutes *battery* (Foederer, 2007). Consent is not informed unless the client, or parent in the case of a child, understands the recommended procedures or treatments, their rationales, the benefits of each, alternative treatments, and any associated risks. When possible, it is important to have translators available for non–English-speaking women and families.

The person, usually the physician, who is ultimately responsible for the treatment or procedure should provide the information necessary to obtain informed consent. In such cases the nurse's role is to witness the client's signature (or the parent's signature for a child) giving consent. The nurse may also serve as a witness if parents give verbal consent by telephone. If the nurse determines that the individual does not understand the procedure or risks, the nurse must notify the physician, who must then provide additional information to ensure that the consent is informed. The nurse also responds to questions asked by adult clients or by parents and children. Anxiety, fear, pain, and medications that alter consciousness may influence an individual's ability to give informed consent. An oral consent is legal, but written consent is easier to defend in a court of law.

Children under 18 or 21 years of age, depending on state law, can legally give informed consent in the following circumstances (Figure 1–4 ●):

- When they are minor parents of the child client
- When they are **emancipated minors** (self-supporting adolescents under 18 years of age, not subject to parental

● **Figure 1–4** Marvin, a 15-year-old boy with acute nonlymphocytic leukemia, has definite opinions about his treatment. His parents have a difficult time accepting his opinions when they differ from their own. At what age can children make an informed decision about whether to accept or refuse treatment?

control). In most states, a pregnant teen is considered emancipated.

- When they are adolescents between 16 and 18 years of age seeking birth control, mental health counseling, or substance abuse treatment (Anderson, Schaechter, & Brosco, 2005)

Mature minors (14- and 15-year-old adolescents who are able to understand treatment risks) can give consent for treatment or refuse treatment in some states.

Refusal of a treatment, medication, or procedure after appropriate information is provided also requires that the individual sign a form releasing the doctor and clinical facility from liability resulting from the effects of such a refusal. Jehovah's Witnesses' refusal of blood transfusions is an example of such refusal.

Nurses are responsible for educating clients about any nursing care. Before each nursing intervention, the maternal-child nurse lets the individual and/or family know what to expect, thus ensuring cooperation and obtaining consent. Afterward the nurse documents the teaching and the learning outcomes in the person's record. The importance of clear, concise, and complete nursing records cannot be overemphasized. These records are evidence that the nurse obtained consent, performed prescribed treatments, reported important observations to the appropriate staff, and adhered to acceptable standards of care.

Because children are not considered competent to make healthcare decisions, parents, as the legal custodians of minor children, are customarily requested to give informed consent on behalf of a child. Both children and parents must understand that they have the right to refuse treatment at any time. In an emergency, consent for treatment to preserve life or limb is not required. When parents are divorced, some states limit the parental rights to give informed consent to the parent with custody. When parents have joint custody, in most cases either may give consent. Obtain legal advice from the agency's designated legal experts for complex family issues related to guardianship, divorced parents disagreeing over care, or a caregiver who is not the legal guardian.

Growth and Development

By 7 or 8 years of age, a child is able to understand concrete explanations about informed consent for research participation. By age 11, a child's abstract reasoning and logic abilities are advanced. By age 14, an adolescent can weigh options and make decisions regarding consent as capably as an adult.

Parents or guardians have absolute authority to make choices about their child's health care except in certain cases. Specifically:

- When the child and parents do not agree on major treatment options
- When the parents' choice of treatment does not permit lifesaving treatment for the child
- When there is a potential conflict of interest between the child and parents, such as with suspected child abuse or neglect

In some cases the court may be requested to appoint a proxy decision maker for the child or to determine that the child is capable of making a major treatment decision.

Children should become more actively involved in decision making about treatment procedures as their reasoning skills develop. Children too young to give informed consent can be given age-appropriate information about their condition and asked about their care preferences. Their parents, however, make ultimate decisions about their care.

With regard to children's participation in research, federal guidelines state that children 7 years of age and older must receive information about a research project and give assent (the voluntary agreement to participate in a research project or to accept treatment) before they are enrolled. Children should be given adequate time to ask questions and be told that they have the right to refuse to participate in the study. If children choose not to participate, they dissent to the proposed treatment or research participation. The child's refusal to participate in research should be respected (Hoehn & Nelson, 2004).

RIGHT TO PRIVACY

The *right to privacy* is the right of a person to keep his or her person and property free from public scrutiny. To protect this right for clients and families, only those responsible for their care should conduct an examination or discuss their case.

The right to privacy is protected by state constitutions, statutes, and common law. The ANA, the National League for Nursing (NLN), and the Joint Commission have adopted professional standards protecting the privacy of clients. Healthcare agencies should also have written policies dealing with client privacy. The Health Insurance Portability and Accountability Act of 1996 (HIPAA), which was fully implemented in 2002,

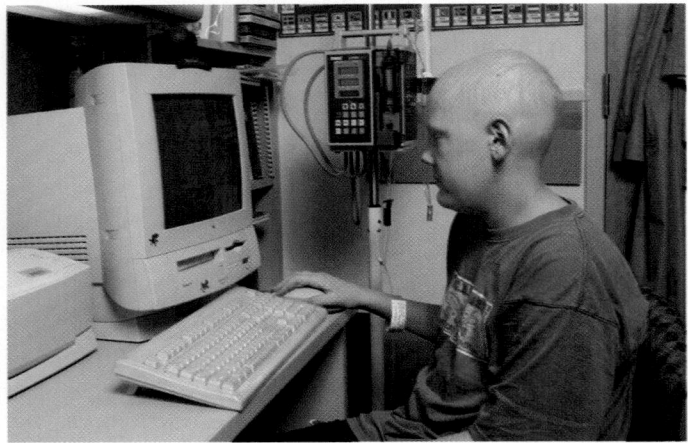

Nursing Practice

Breaching confidentiality is a potential problem for adolescents, who are just learning whom they can trust in the healthcare system. Make sure you openly discuss the limits of confidentiality for such things as mandatory reporting requirements with the client and family. Inadvertent disclosure of personal information may lead to psychologic, social, or physical harm in some clients.

also has a provision to guarantee the security and privacy of health information.

Laws, standards, and policies about privacy specify that information about clients' treatment, condition, and prognosis can be shared only by health professionals responsible for their care. Information considered vital statistics (name, age, occupation, and so on) may be revealed legally, but is often withheld because of ethical considerations. The client should be consulted as to what information may be released and to whom.

Children and Confidentiality

Concerns about privacy and the fear of disclosure of sensitive information to parents is a major reason why adolescents do not seek health care (Campbell, 2006). When the child is an emancipated or mature minor, many states permit healthcare providers to provide birth control and treatment for sexually transmitted infections, including HIV/AIDS, pregnancy, and substance abuse, without informing the child's parents (Anderson, Schaechter, & Brosco, 2005).

PATIENT SELF-DETERMINATION ACT

The federal Patient Self-Determination Act directs healthcare institutions to inform hospitalized patients about their rights, which include expressing a preference for treatment options and making **advance directives** (writing a living will or authorizing a durable power of attorney for healthcare decisions on the individual's behalf). Nurses often discuss these issues with clients and their families. Minor children and their parents should also be informed of their rights. Adolescents with serious acute or chronic conditions with a higher risk of death should be encouraged to talk with their parents about their healthcare wishes and to prepare advance directives jointly (Fletcher, 2004).

Do not resuscitate (DNR) or *allow natural death* orders have become more common for children with terminal illnesses in which no further treatments are possible or desired. In many cases these children are cared for at home or in a hospice program. Implementation of DNR orders for such children then becomes a community issue, to ensure that resuscitation measures are not initiated by any emergency care provider when the child has a life-threatening event. State health policies must be developed so children with these signed orders are easily identified and appropriate documentation of the orders is on file.

ETHICAL ISSUES IN MATERNAL-CHILD NURSING

Although ethical dilemmas confront nurses in all areas of practice, those related to pregnancy, birth, newborns, and children seem especially difficult to resolve.

MATERNAL-FETAL CONFLICT

Until fairly recently the fetus was viewed legally as a nonperson. Mother and fetus were viewed as one complex client—the pregnant woman—of which the fetus was an essential part. However, advances in technology have permitted the physician to treat the fetus and monitor fetal development. The fetus is increasingly viewed as a client separate from the mother. This focus on the fetus intensified in 2002 when President George W. Bush announced that "unborn children" would qualify for government healthcare benefits. This move was designed to promote prenatal care, but it represented the first time that any U.S. federal policy had defined childhood as starting at conception.

Most women are strongly motivated to protect the health and well-being of their fetus. In some instances, however, women have refused interventions on behalf of the fetus, and forced interventions have occurred. These include forced cesarean birth, coercion of mothers who practice high-risk behaviors such as substance abuse to enter treatment, and, perhaps most controversial, mandated experimental in utero therapy or surgery in an attempt to correct a specific birth defect. These interventions infringe on the autonomy of the mother. They may also be detrimental to the baby if, as a result, maternal bonding is hindered, the mother is afraid to seek prenatal care, or the mother is herself harmed by the actions taken. Attempts have also been made to criminalize the behavior of women who fail to follow a physician's advice or who engage in behaviors (such as substance abuse) that are considered harmful to the fetus. This raises two thorny questions: (1) What practices should be monitored? and (2) Who will determine when the behaviors pose such a risk to the fetus that the courts should intervene?

The American College of Obstetricians and Gynecologists (ACOG) Committee on Ethics (2004) has affirmed the fundamental right of pregnant women to make informed, uncoerced decisions about medical interventions and in 2005 took a direct stand against coercive and punitive approaches to the maternal-fetal relationship (ACOG, 2005).

Cases of maternal-fetal conflict involve two clients, both of whom deserve respect and treatment. Such cases are best resolved by using internal hospital mechanisms, including counseling, the intervention of specialists, and consultation with an institutional ethics committee. Court intervention should be considered a last resort, appropriate only in extraordinary circumstances.

ABORTION

Since the 1973 Supreme Court decision in *Roe v. Wade,* elective abortion has been legal in the United States. Abortion can be performed until the period of viability. After that time, abortion is permissible only when the life or health of the mother is threatened. Before viability, the rights of the mother are paramount; after viability, the rights of the fetus take precedence.

Personal beliefs, cultural norms, life experiences, and religious convictions shape people's attitudes about abortion. Ethicists have thoughtfully and thoroughly argued positions supporting both sides of the question. Nevertheless, few issues spark the intensity of response seen when the issue of abortion is raised.

At present the decision about abortion is to be made by the woman and her physician. Nurses (and other caregivers) have the right to refuse to assist with the procedure if abortion is contrary to their moral and ethical beliefs. However, if a nurse works in an institution where abortions may be performed, the nurse may be dismissed for refusing to assist. To avoid being placed in a situation contrary to personal ethical values and beliefs, it is important to identify the practices of an institution before going to work there. A nurse who refuses to participate in an abortion because of moral or ethical beliefs has a responsibility to ensure that someone with similar qualifications is available to provide appropriate care for the client. Clients must never be abandoned, regardless of a nurse's beliefs.

INTRAUTERINE FETAL SURGERY

Intrauterine fetal surgery, an example of therapeutic research, is a therapy for anatomic lesions that can be corrected surgically and are incompatible with life if not treated. The procedure involves opening the uterus during the second trimester (before viability), performing the planned surgery, and replacing the fetus in the uterus. The risks to the fetus are substantial, and the mother is committed to cesarean births for this and subsequent pregnancies (because the upper, active segment of the uterus is entered). The parents must be informed of the experimental nature of the treatment, the risks of the surgery, the commitment to cesarean birth, and alternatives to the treatment.

As in other aspects of maternity care, caregivers must respect the pregnant woman's autonomy. The procedure involves health risks to the woman, and she retains the right to refuse any surgical procedure. Healthcare providers must be careful that their zeal for new technology does not lead them to focus unilaterally on the fetus at the expense of the mother.

REPRODUCTIVE ASSISTANCE

Assisted reproductive technology (ART) is the term used to describe highly technologic approaches used to produce pregnancy. *In vitro fertilization* and *embryo transfer (IVF-ET),* a therapy offered to selected infertile couples, is perhaps the best known ART technique.

Some legislative efforts have been made to address consumer concerns about ART. In the United States, the federal Fertility Clinic Success Rate and Certification Act (FCSRCA) of 1992 requires standardized reporting of pregnancy success rates associated with ART programs and addresses issues related to laboratory quality. To help ensure data accuracy, a validation process, which includes site visits to a portion of reporting clinics, is completed.

More than one third of pregnancies that result from ART are multifetal pregnancies (March of Dimes, 2006). Multifetal pregnancy occurs because the use of ovulation-inducing medications typically triggers the release of multiple eggs, which, when fertilized, produce multiple embryos, which are then implanted. Multifetal pregnancy increases the risk of miscarriage, preterm birth, and neonatal morbidity and mortality. It also increases the mother's risk of complications, including cesarean birth. To help prevent a high-level multifetal pregnancy, the American Society for Reproductive Medicine (ASRM) has issued guidelines to limit the number of embryos transferred. These guidelines are designed to decrease risk while allowing for individualized care (ASRM, 2006). This practice raises ethical considerations about the handling of the unused embryos. However, when a multifetal pregnancy does occur, the physician may suggest that the woman consider fetal reduction, in which some of the embryos are aborted to give the remaining ones a better chance for survival. Clearly this procedure raises ethical concerns about the sacrifice of some so that the remainder can survive.

Prevention should be the first approach to the problem of multifetal pregnancy. It begins with careful counseling about the risks of multiple gestation and the ethical issues that relate to fetal reduction. No physician who is morally opposed to fetal reduction should be expected to perform the procedure; however, physicians should be aware of the ethical and medical issues involved and be prepared to respond to families in a professional and ethical manner (ACOG, 2007).

Surrogate childbearing is another approach to infertility. Surrogate childbearing occurs when a woman agrees to become pregnant for a childless couple. She may be artificially inseminated with the male partner's sperm or a donor's sperm or may receive a gamete transfer, depending on the infertile couple's needs. If fertilization occurs, the woman carries the fetus to term and releases the infant to the couple after birth.

These methods of resolving infertility raise ethical issues about candidate selection, responsibility for a child born with a congenital defect, and religious objections to artificial conception. Other ethical questions include the following: What should be done with surplus fertilized oocytes? To whom do frozen embryos belong? Who is liable if a woman or her offspring contracts HIV from donated sperm? Should children be told about their conception?

EMBRYONIC STEM CELL RESEARCH

Human stem cells can be found in embryonic tissue and in the primordial germ cells of a fetus. Research has demonstrated that in tissue cultures these cells can be made to differentiate into other types of cells such as blood, nerve, or heart cells, which might then be used to treat problems such as diabetes, Parkinson and Alzheimer diseases, spinal cord injury, or metabolic disorders. The availability of specialized tissue or even organs grown from stem cells might also decrease society's dependence on donated organs for organ transplants.

Positions about embryonic stem cell research vary dramatically, from the view that any use of human embryos for research is wrong to the view that any form of embryonic stem cell research is acceptable, with a variety of other positions that fall somewhere in between these extremes. Other questions also arise: What sources of embryonic tissue are acceptable for research? Is it ever ethical to clone embryos solely for stem cell research? Is there justification for using embryos remaining after fertility treatments?

The question of how an embryo should be viewed—with status in some way as a person or in some sense as property (and, if property, whose?)—is a key question in the debate. Ethicists recognize that it is not necessary to advocate full moral status or personhood for an embryo to have significant moral qualms about the instrumental use of a human embryo in the "interests" of society. The issue of consent, which links directly to an embryo's status, also merits consideration. In truth, the ethical questions and dilemmas associated with embryonic stem cell research are staggeringly complex and require careful analysis and thoughtful dialogue.

CORD BLOOD BANKING

Cord blood, taken from a newborn's umbilical cord at birth and stored or "banked," may play a role in combating leukemia, certain other cancers, and immune and blood system disorders. This is possible because cord blood, like bone marrow and embryonic tissue, contains hematopoietic stem cells, which can replace diseased cells in the affected individual.

Cord blood banks that store cord blood have been established in the United States. Public banks receive cord blood given on a volunteer basis and are designed to support unrelated-donor transplant programs. Private banks are for-profit entities designed primarily for families who plan to use the cord blood for the infant who provided the blood or for another family member who might need transplantation therapy in the future because of a genetic blood condition, cancer, bone marrow failure, or inborn error of metabolism, for example (ACOG, 2008).

Ethical concerns focus on the issue of confidentiality for the mother and family throughout the process; the question of ownership of the blood (donor, parents, the blood bank, or society); the concern about fair distribution of the harvested blood; and obligations to the family that may arise if testing of the blood reveals genetic disorders or infectious diseases.

Both ACOG and the American Academy of Pediatrics (AAP) have issued statements about umbilical cord blood banking. ACOG (2008) stresses the importance of providing balanced information about the advantages and disadvantages of public versus private banking and the need for healthcare professionals to disclose any financial interests they have in private cord blood banks.

The AAP (Lubin & Shearer, 2007) recommendations support the ACOG opinion and address other clinical considerations too. Key recommendations include the following:

- Parents are encouraged to bank their newborn's cord blood privately if they have an older child who has a condition that could benefit from a cord blood transfusion.
- In general, parents are encouraged to donate their newborn's cord blood to a public bank because it might help treat someone in need.
- Private cord blood banking as "insurance" against possible future personal or family need is discouraged because often the genetic traits associated with the condition that develops are present in the cord blood.
- Collection centers should test all donated cord blood for infectious and genetic disorders and should have a protocol developed for notifying families of abnormal results.
- Written consent for cord blood donation should be obtained before labor begins.

MAKING TREATMENT DECISIONS FOR CHILDREN

Technology makes it possible to sustain the lives of children who previously would have died, thus creating many ethical issues. Conflict often arises between health professionals and parents when parents choose to withhold therapy or to request aggressive therapy on behalf of their child and the health professionals have a different opinion about treatment. Nurses often face ethical dilemmas when providing care to such a child, especially as they witness parents struggling to decide among treatment options.

When making treatment decisions in pediatrics, healthcare professionals need to determine whether their responsibility is limited to the child or includes the interests of the parents. The healthcare institution's ethics committee often plays a role in resolving conflicts about treatment decisions. Courts should make ethical decisions only when healthcare professionals and parents are unable to agree about providing or withholding treatment.

MyNursingKit Case Study: Cord Blood Banking

TERMINATING LIFE-SUSTAINING TREATMENT

Federal "Baby Doe" regulations were developed to protect the rights of infants with severe defects. The federal regulations made child neglect a relevant factor in treatment decisions for neonates (Annas, 2004). Parents of such infants are usually the ultimate decision makers about the child's care. Factors important to parents in making their decision include the child's quality of life, degree of pain and suffering, likelihood for improvement, and physician recommendations (Sharman, Meert, & Sarnaik, 2005). Physicians may believe treatment will help the child and improve the quality of life (sometimes defined as a meaningful existence or an ability to develop human relationships). Physicians are not obligated to offer interventions that cause extreme pain and suffering when there is limited or no potential benefit. Treatments that only prolong life represent a misuse of expensive healthcare resources. Federal regulations require a formalized ethical decision-making process before physicians accept or reject a parent's wishes.

The ethics committee members consider all the options according to their individual beliefs and their perceptions of the value of specific interventions for an individual child, using ethical theory to guide decision making. When treatment has a reasonable chance of success and the infant will likely survive and be able to interact with the environment, even if burdened by a serious disability, the best interest of the infant is treatment (Silber & Batshaw, 2004). There may be no right or wrong answer; and a plan of action may result that is a compromise about which neither the health professionals nor family is totally happy (Tripp & McGregor, 2006).

ORGAN TRANSPLANTATION ISSUES

The death of a child can benefit another child through organ transplantation. The National Organ Transplant Act (PL 98-507) generated laws, regulations, and guidelines for organ collection and transplantation. For example, the healthcare facility has specific requirements to approach family members when brain death is suspected or confirmed to request organ donation. The limited supply of organs has created numerous ethical issues: Which individuals on a waiting list should receive the organs available? Should a child with multiple congenital anomalies or abnormal chromosomes be eligible for a transplant? Should families be permitted to pay donor families for organs? Should the family's ability to pay for an organ transplant give a child higher priority for an organ?

GENETIC TESTING OF CHILDREN

Genetic testing and screening of children is now possible for the presence of carrier status or to the presymptomatic detection for a specific condition, such as Duchenne muscular dystrophy. Testing may also be available for some conditions for which there is no definitive treatment or prevention of the condition. When genetic testing is considered, both the risks and benefits of receiving the genetic test information should be discussed when seeking informed consent process. Current recommendations are that children should be tested only if it is in the child's best interest, such as by getting appropriate interventions if the test for a condition is positive (Williams, Skirton, & Masny, 2006). See Chapter 6∞ for more information on genetic testing.

IMPLICATIONS FOR NURSING PRACTICE

The complex ethical issues facing maternal-child nurses have many social, cultural, legal, and professional ramifications. Ethical decisions in maternal-child nursing are often complicated by moral obligations to more than one client. Straightforward solutions to the ethical dilemmas encountered in caring for children and childbearing families are often, quite simply, not available.

Nurses must learn to anticipate ethical dilemmas, clarify their own positions related to the issues, understand the legal implications of the issues, and develop appropriate strategies for ethical decision making. To accomplish these tasks, they can read about bioethical issues, participate in discussion groups, attend courses and workshops on ethical topics pertinent to their areas of practice, and serve on ethics committees.

EVIDENCE-BASED PRACTICE IN MATERNAL-CHILD NURSING

Evidence-based practice—that is, nursing care in which all interventions are supported by current, valid research evidence—is emerging as a force in health care. It provides a useful approach to problem solving and decision making and to self-directed, client-centered, lifelong learning. Evidence-based practice builds on the actions necessary to transform research findings into clinical practice by also considering other forms of evidence that can be useful in making clinical practice decisions. These other forms of evidence may include statistical data, quality measurements, risk management measures, and information from support services such as infection control.

As practicing clinicians, nurses need to meet two basic competencies related to evidence-based practice. Nurses need to:

1. recognize which clinical practices are supported by good evidence, which practices have conflicting findings as to their effect on client outcomes, and which practices have no evidence to support their use; and
2. use data in their clinical work. In truth, market pressures are also a force in the use of evidence-based practice because they are forcing nurses and other healthcare providers to evaluate routines to improve efficiencies and provide better outcomes for clients.

Nurses need to know what data are being tracked where they work and how care practices and outcomes are improved as a result of quality improvement initiatives. However, there is more to evidence-based practice—competent, effective nurses learn to question the very basis of their clinical work.

Throughout this text we have provided *snapshots* of evidence-based practice related to childbearing women and families, such as the one on page 215. We believe that these snapshots will help you understand the concept more clearly. We also expect that these examples may challenge you to question the usefulness of some of the routine care you observe in clinical practice. That is the impact of evidence-based practice—it moves clinicians beyond practices of "habit and opinion" to practices based on high-quality, current science.

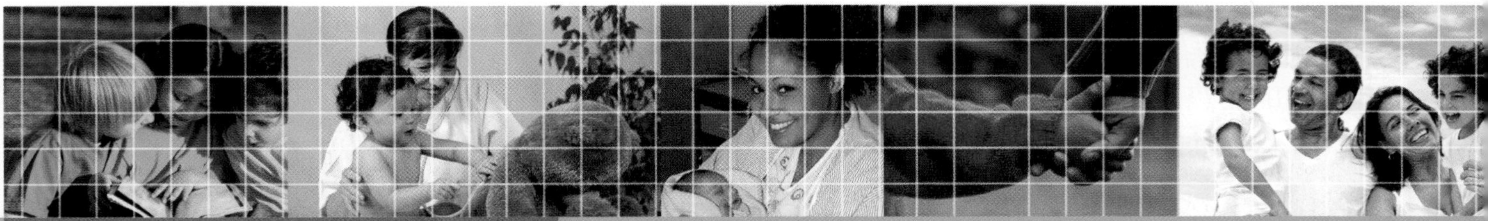

CRITICAL CONCEPT REVIEW

LEARNING OUTCOMES / CONCEPTS

1.1 Identify the nursing roles available to maternal-newborn and pediatric nurses.

1. Registered nurse:
   - Provide nursing care to both inpatient and outpatient women with childbearing or reproductive issues as well as newborns and children.
2. Nurse practitioner:
   - Provide ambulatory care services to expectant families and to children.
   - Provide care in some acute care, high-risk units such as neonatal intensive care units.
   - Focus on physical and psychosocial assessments and order diagnostic tests and procedures.
   - Make clinical judgments and order appropriate care.
3. Certified nurse-midwife:
   - Manage the care of a woman who is at low risk for complications during pregnancy and childbirth.

1.2 Summarize the use of community-based nursing care in meeting the needs of childbearing and childrearing families.

Community-based care is important in meeting the needs of the childbearing and childrearing family because the vast majority of care takes place outside of hospitals:

1. Clinics.
2. Offices.
3. Community-based organizations.
4. Private homes.

1.3 Summarize the current status of factors related to health insurance and access to health care.

1. Community-based care remains an essential element of health care for uninsured or underinsured individuals, as well as for individuals who benefit from programs such as Medicare, Medicaid, or state-sponsored, health-related programs.
2. Healthcare insurers are beginning to recognize the importance of primary care in containing costs and maintaining health.

1.4 Relate the availability of statistical data to the formulation of further research questions.

1. Health-related statistics provide an objective basis for projecting client needs and planning the use of resources.
2. Statistical data can also reveal trends that require research to determine cause, to analyze the implications of specific findings for given populations, to explore relationship between specific factors, and to evaluate the success of specific nursing interventions.

1.5 Delineate significant legal and ethical issues that influence the practice of maternal-child nursing.

1. The abortion debate is especially difficult and raises questions about maternal rights versus fetal rights. Abortion can legally be performed until the fetus reaches the age of viability. The decision to have an abortion is made by a woman in consultation with her physician.
2. *Assisted reproductive technology* (ART) is the term used to describe highly technologic approaches used to produce pregnancy.
3. Cord blood banking provides the opportunity to have stem cells available to treat a variety of cancers and blood disorders. Its growing popularity has revealed several ethical issues.
4. Federal "Baby Doe" regulations were developed to protect the rights of infants with severe defects.
5. Genetic testing is available for children for conditions for which there is no treatment or potential benefit.
6. Organ donation and transplantation ethical issues involve selection and qualifications of donor recipients and payment for organs.

1.6 Discuss the role of evidence-based practice in improving the quality of nursing care for childbearing families.

1. Evidence-based practice refers to clinical practice based on research findings and other available data.
2. Evidence-based practice increases nurses' accountability to integrate current knowledge and research into practice and results in better client outcomes.

CRITICAL THINKING IN ACTION

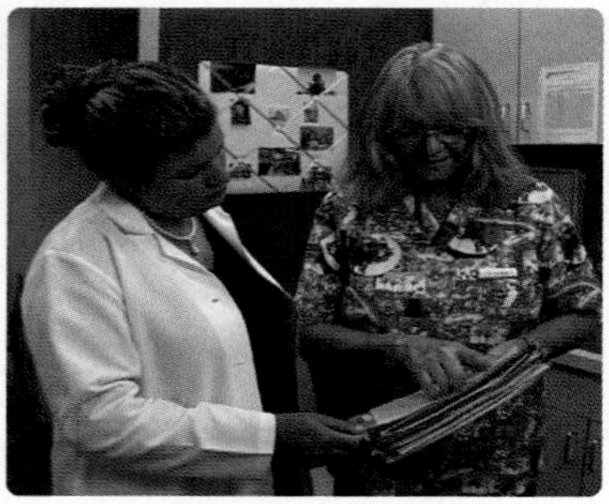

You are working as a prenatal nurse in a local clinic. Before entering a client's room, you review the chart for pertinent information such as cultural background, significant family members, weeks of gestation, test results, birth plan, and education for health promotion. You greet each client and family members by name and ask how they are coping with the pregnancy. Depending on the trimester of the pregnancy, you review the discomforts or concerns of the mother/family and what they may expect. You examine the mother, including fundal height, fetal heart rate and fetal position if appropriate, maternal blood pressure, weight gain, and urine analysis. With each client, you discuss the community resources available such as prenatal classes, lactation consultants, and prenatal exercise/yoga classes. Based upon the information you obtain, you might refer the mother to social services or the WIC program as appropriate. At the end of the clinic session, you review the clients with the collaborating physician.

1. How would you define the terms *family* and *family-centered care*?
2. Describe how the nursing process provides the framework for the delivery of direct nursing care.
3. How would you describe the concept of community-based care?
4. How would you describe culturally competent care?

See MyNursingKit for possible responses.

REFERENCES

American College of Obstetricians and Gynecologists (ACOG). (2004). *Parent choice: Maternal–fetal relationship.* (Committee Opinion No. 214). Washington, DC: Author.

American College of Obstetricians and Gynecologists (ACOG). (2005). *Maternal decision making, ethics, and the law.* (Committee Opinion No. 321). Washington, DC: Author.

American College of Obstetricians and Gynecologists (ACOG). (2007). *Multifetal pregnancy reduction.* (Committee Opinion No. 369). Washington, DC: Author.

American College of Obstetricians and Gynecologists (ACOG). (2008). *Umbilical cord blood banking.* (Committee Opinion No. 399). Washington, DC: Author.

American Nurses Association and the National Association of Neonatal Nurses. (2004). *Neonatal nursing: Scope and standards of practice.* Washington, DC: American Nurses Association.

American Nurses Association, National Association of Pediatric Nurse Practitioners, and the Society of Pediatric Nurses. (2008). *Pediatric Nursing: Scope and standards of practice.* Silver Spring, MD: Nursesbooks.org

American Society for Reproductive Medicine and the Society for Assisted Reproductive Technology. (2006). Guidelines on number of embryos transferred. *Fertility and Sterility, 86* (suppl. 5), S51–52.

Anderson, S. L., Schaechter, J., & Brosco, J. P. (2005). Adolescent patients and their confidentiality: Staying within legal bounds. *Contemporary Pediatrics, 22*(7), 54–64.

Annas, G. J. (2004). Extremely preterm birth and parental authority to refuse treatment—the case of Sidney Miller. *New England Journal of Medicine, 351*(20), 2118–2123.

Association of Women's Health, Obstetric and Neonatal Nurses. (2003). *Standards for professional nursing practice in the care of women and newborns* (6th ed.). Washington, DC: Author.

Bauman, M. E., Massicotte, M. P., Ray, L., & Newburn-Cook, C. (2007). Developing educational materials to facilitate adherence: Pediatric thrombosis as a case illustration. *Journal of Pediatric Health Care, 21*(3), 198–206.

Bindler, R. C., & Ball, J. W. (2007). The Bindler-Ball healthcare model: A new paradigm for health promotion. *Pediatric Nursing, 33*(2), 121–126.

Borse, N. N., Gilchrist, J., Dellinger, A. M., Rudd, R. A., Ballesteros, M. F., & Sleet, D. A. (2008). CDC Injury Report: Patterns of unintentional injuries among 0–19 year olds in the United States, 2000–2006. Retrieved June 12, 2009 from www.cdc.gov/safechild/images/CDC-ChildhoodInjury.pdf

Campbell, A. T. (2006). Consent, competence, and confidentiality related to psychiatric conditions in adolescent medicine practice. *Adolescent Medicine Clinics, 17,* 25–47.

Centers for Medicare and Medicaid Services (CMS). (2007). 2007 CMS Statistics. Retrieved March 21, 2009, from www.cms.hhs.gov

Centers for Medicare and Medicaid Services (CMS). (2008). FY 2007 SCHIP Annual Enrollment Report. Retrieved March 21, 2009, from www.cms.hhs.gov

Duderstadt, K. G. (2007). Health of U.S. children from the global view. *Journal of Pediatric Health Care, 21*(6), 403–406.

Families USA. (2008). Still too many uninsured children. Retrieved September 16, 2008, from http://familiesusa.org/assets/pdfs/still-too-many-uninsured-kids-2008.pdf

Fletcher, J. (2004). Adolescents and the Patient Self-Determination Act. *Pediatric Ethicscope,* 15(1). Washington, DC: Children's National Medical Center.

Flores, G., & Ngui, E. (2006). Racial/ethnic disparities and patient safety. *Pediatric Clinics of North America, 53,* 1197–1215.

Foederer, A. A. (2007). Appropriately navigating through treacherous medicine: Health care decision-making panels for vulnerable minors. *Journal of Nursing Law, 11*(2), 108–117.

Forum on Child and Family Statistics. (2007). *America's children: Key indicators of well-being, 2007.* Retrieved July 28, 2007, from www.childstats.gov/americaschildren

Gance-Cleveland, B. (2006). Decreasing health disparities. *Journal for Specialists in Pediatric Nursing, 11*(1), 72–76.

Hamilton, B. E., Martin, J. A., & Ventura, S. J. (2009). Births: Preliminary data for 2007. *National Vital Statistics Reports, 57*(12), 1–23.

Health Resources and Services Administration, Maternal and Child Health. (2006). *Child Health USA, 2006.* Rockville, MD: U.S. Department of Health and Human Services. Retrieved September 16, 2008, from http://www.mchb.hrsa.gov/chusa_06/healthstat/children/0313hdt.htm

Health Resources and Services Administration, Maternal and Child Health Bureau. (2008). *The national survey of children with special healthcare needs chartbook 2005–2006.* Retrieved May 12, 2008, from http://mchb.hrsa.gov/cshcn05

Hoehn, G. L., & Nelson, R. M. (2004). Advising parents about children's participation in clinical research. *Pediatric Annals, 33*(11), 779–781.

Inglehart, J. K. (2007). Insuring all children—the new political imperative. *New England Journal of Medicine, 357*(1), 70–76.

Jones, J. H. (2007). Patient illiteracy. *American Operating Room Nurse Journal, 85*(5), 951–955.

Kaiser Commission on Medicaid and the Uninsured. (2008). *Health coverage of children: The role of Medicaid and SCHIP.* Washington, D.C.: The Henry J. Kaiser Family Foundation.

Kaiser Commission on Medicaid and the Uninsured. (2009). *Children's health insurance program reauthorization Act of 2009 (CHIPRA).* Washington, D.C.: The Henry J. Kaiser Family Foundation.

Kozer, E., Berkovitch, M., & Koren, G. (2006). Medication errors in children. *Pediatric Clinics of North America, 53,* 1155–1168.

Kung, H. C., Hoyert, D. L., Xu, J. Q., & Murphy, S. L. (2007). QuickStats: Infant mortality rates for 10 leading causes of infant death—United States, 2005. *MMWR, 56*(42), 1115.

Kung, H. C., Hoyert, D. L., Xu, J. Q., & Murphy, S. L. (2008). Deaths: Final data for 2005. *National Vital Statistics Reports, 56*(10), 1–9.

Lubin, B. H., & Shearer, W. T. (2007). Cord blood banking for potential future transplantation. *Pediatrics, 119*(1), 165–170.

MacDorman, M. F., & Mathews, T. J. (2008). Recent trends in infant mortality in the United States. *NCHS Data Brief,* (9), 1–8.

March of Dimes. (2006). Multiple pregnancy and birth: Considering fertility options. Retrieved July 17, 2007, from www.modimes.com

National Center for Health Statistics (NCHS). (2009). *Health, United States, 2008. With Chartbook on Trends in the Health of Americans.* Hyattsville, MD: Author.

Sharman, M., Meert, K. L., & Sarnaik, A. P. (2005). What influences parents' decisions to limit or withdraw life support? *Pediatric Critical Care Medicine, 6*(5), 513–518.

Silber, T., & Batshaw, M. L. (2004). Ethical dilemmas in the treatment of children with disabilities. *Pediatric Annals, 33*(11), 752–761.

Tripp, J., & McGregor, D. (2006). Withholding and withdrawing of life sustaining treatment in the newborn. *Archives of Diseases in Childhood, Fetal and Neonatal Edition, 91,* F67–F71.

U.S. Census Bureau. (2008). *Statistical Abstract of the United States: 2008.* Retrieved September 15, 2008, from www.census.gov/prod/2007pubs/08statab/pop.pdf

U.S. Department of Health and Human Services, Office of Disease Prevention and Promotion. (2006). *Healthy People 2010 Midcourse Review.* Washington, DC: Author, Retrieved April 24, 2007, from www.healthypeople.gov/data/midcourse/pdf/FA14.pdf

Williams, J. K., Skirton, H., & Masny, A. (2006). Ethics, policy, and educational issues in genetic testing. *Journal of Nursing Scholarship, 38*(2), 119–125.

Zwelling, E. (2008). The emergence of high-tech birthing. *Journal of Obstetric, Gynecologic, and Neonatal Nursing, 37*(1), 85–93.

PEARSON

EXPLORE mynursingkit™

MyNursingKit is your one stop for online chapter review materials and resources. Prepare for success with additional NCLEX®-style practice questions, interactive assignments and activities, web links, animations and videos, and more!

Register your access code from the front of your book at
www.mynursingkit.com

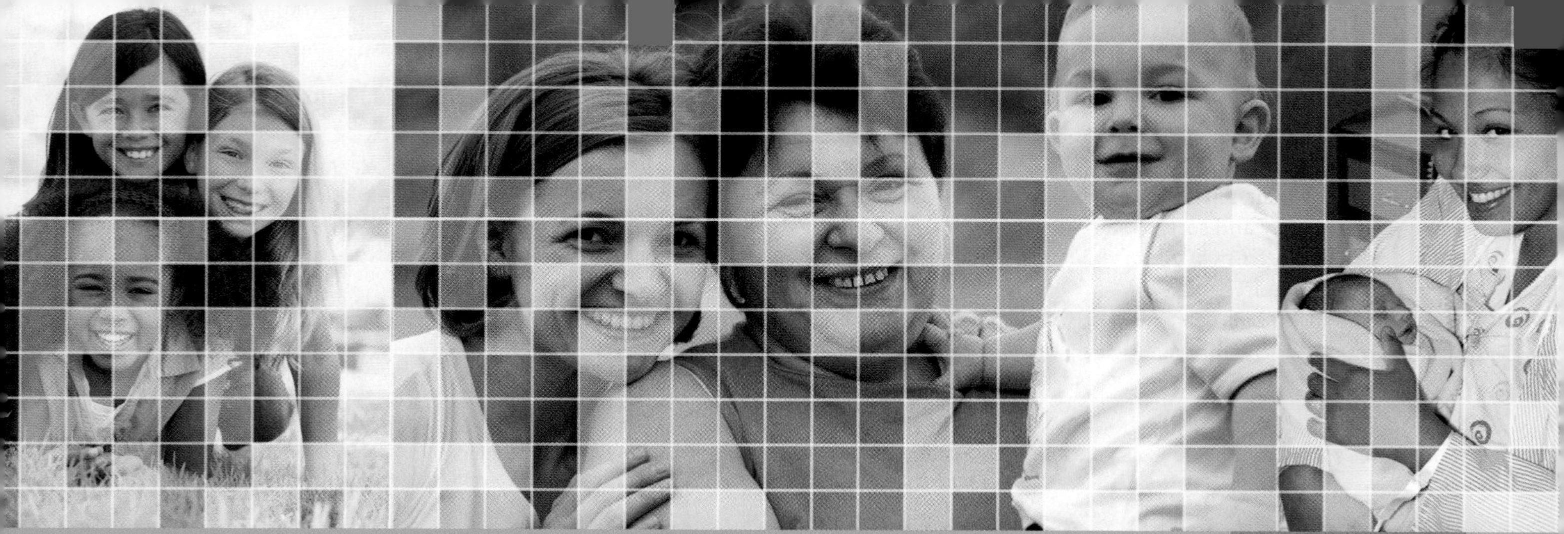

CHAPTER 2

Culture and the Family

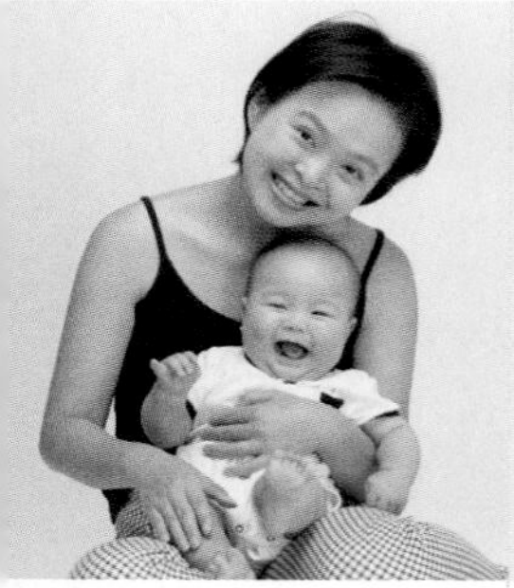

My parents came here from China when I was three. They wanted the chance to make a better life and they wanted another child. Needless to say, although I have always felt loved and cherished, I know how thrilled they were when my brother was born. Sometimes I feel as though I am walking a line between their ways and the ways I have learned growing up in this country. My husband is Chinese but he, too, grew up here. We are expecting our second baby in a few months. We talk often about which Chinese ways we want to retain and which new ways make more sense. I am not sure that my parents will understand, however. To them the old ways are always best. —Li Wei, 29

LEARNING OUTCOMES

2.1 Distinguish among several different types of families.

2.2 Identify the stages of a family life cycle.

2.3 Identify prevalent cultural norms related to childbearing and childrearing.

2.4 Summarize the importance of cultural competency in providing nursing care.

2.5 Discuss the use of a cultural assessment tool as a means of providing culturally sensitive care.

2.6 Identify key considerations in providing spiritually sensitive care.

2.7 Distinguish between *complementary* and *alternative therapies.*

2.8 Identify the benefits and risks of complementary and alternative therapies.

2.9 Discuss complementary therapies appropriate for the nurse to use with childbearing and childrearing families.

Individuals do not live in isolation. Their values, beliefs, behaviors, decisions, attitudes, and biases are shaped by many factors, including their families, their culture, and their religious beliefs. Nurses who provide effective, holistic care recognize this reality and seek to learn about and care for the entire family.

This chapter begins with a brief discussion of family types, functioning, and assessment. It then addresses the impact of culture on the family and concludes with a brief examination of some of the complementary and alternative therapies a family might use.

THE FAMILY

The U.S. Census Bureau defines a **family** as two or more individuals who are joined together by marriage, birth, or adoption and live together in the same household (U.S. Census Bureau, 2008). More broadly, however, a family may be a self-identified group of two or more persons joined together by sharing resources and emotional closeness.

Families are guided by a common set of values or beliefs about the worth and importance of certain ideas and traditions. These values often bind family members together, and these values are greatly influenced by external factors including cultural background, social norms, education, environmental influences, socioeconomic status, and beliefs held by peers, coworkers, political and community leaders, and other individuals outside the family unit. Because of the influence of these external factors, a family's values may change considerably over the years.

TYPES OF FAMILIES

Families are diverse in structure, roles, and relationships. Various types of families—both those considered traditional and nontraditional—exist in contemporary American society. This section identifies common types of family structure.

- In the *nuclear family,* children live in a household with both biological parents, and no other relatives or persons. One parent may stay home to rear the children while one parent works, but more commonly, both parents are employed by choice or necessity. Two-income families must address important issues such as childcare arrangements, household chores, and how to assure quality family time. Dual-career/dual-earner families are now considered the norm in modern society.
- In an *extended family,* a couple shares household and childrearing responsibilities with parents, siblings, or other relatives. Families may reside together to share housing expenses and childcare. However, in many cases, the child may be residing with the grandparent and one parent because of issues associated with unemployment, parental separation, parental death, or parental substance abuse. Grandparents may raise children due to the inability of parents to care for their own children.
- An *extended kin network family* is a specific form of an extended family in which two nuclear families of primary or unmarried kin live in close proximity to each other. The family shares a social support network, chores, goods, and services. This type of family model is common in the Latino community.
- Although rare in the past, the *single-parent family* is becoming increasingly common. In the traditional single-parent family, the head of the household is widowed, divorced, abandoned, or separated. Some single-parent families are established by choice and have good support. Other single-parent families face difficulties because the sole parent may lack social and emotional support, need assistance with childrearing issues, and face financial strain. Single-parent families experience higher rates of poverty, which has important implications for the children (Denham, 2005) (Figure 2–1 ●).

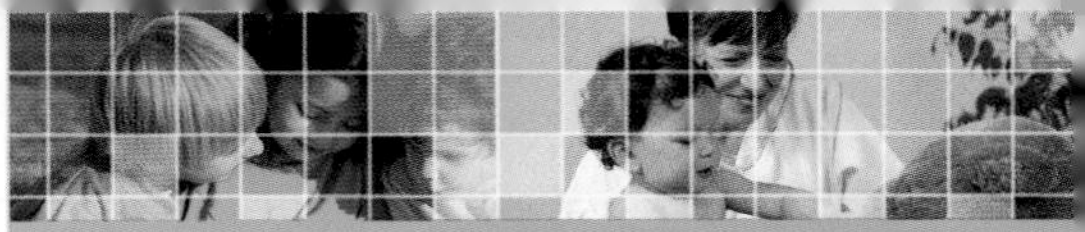

KEY TERMS

Acculturation, 24
Alternative therapy, 32
Assimilation, 24
Complementary therapy, 32
Cultural competence, 29
Culture, 23
Ethnicity, 24
Ethnocentrism, 28
Family, 21
Race, 24
Shaman, 26
Spirituality, 26
Stereotyping, 24
Taboo, 27

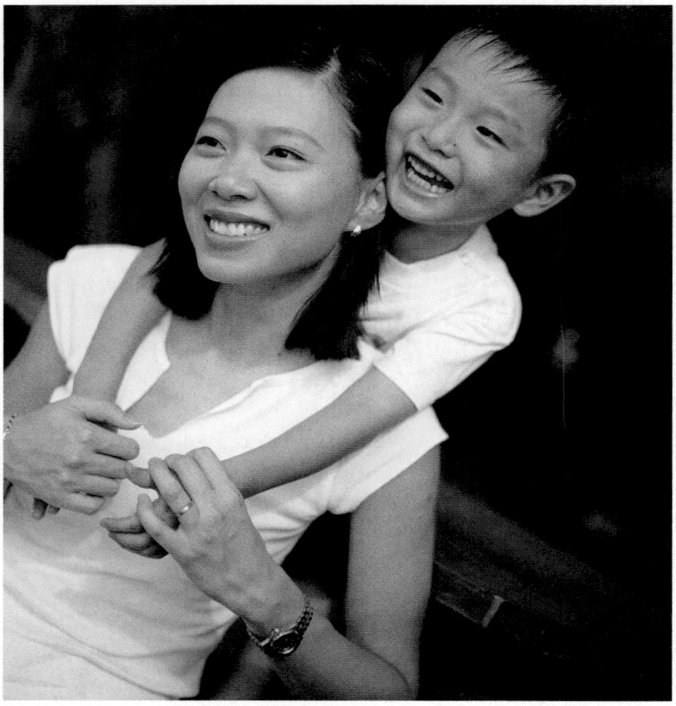

● **Figure 2–1** Single-parent families account for nearly one third of all U.S. families. What types of challenges do single-parent families face?
Used with permission from Joyce Choo/CORBIS.

- The *blended or reconstituted nuclear family* includes two parents with biologic children from a previous marriage or relationship who marry or cohabitate. This family structure has become increasingingly common due to high rates of divorce and remarriage. Potential advantages to the children may include better financial support and a new supportive role model. Stresses can include lack of a clear role for the stepparent, lack of acceptance of the stepparent, financial stresses when two families must be supported by stepparents, and communication problems.
- A *binuclear family* is a postdivorce family in which the biologic children are members of two nuclear households, with co-parenting by the father and the mother. The children alternate between the two homes, spending varying amounts of time with each parent in a situation called co-parenting, usually involving joint custody. Joint custody is a legal situation in which both parents have equal responsibility and legal rights, regardless of where the children live. The binuclear family is a model for effective communication. It enables both biologic parents to be involved in a child's upbringing and provides additional support and role models from extended family members.
- A *nonmarital heterosexual cohabitating family* describes a heterosexual couple who may or may not have children and who live together outside of marriage. This may include never-married individuals as well as divorced or widowed persons. While some individuals choose this model for personal reasons, others do so for financial reasons or to seek companionship.

Nursing Practice

It is important to establish which parent has legal custody, current visitation policies, and other variables (restraining orders, supervised visitation, etc.) when communicating information to parents about their children. Certain legal issues may prohibit the nurse from sharing some information with the noncustodial parent.

- *Gay and lesbian families* include those in which two or more people who share a same-sex orientation live together as domestic partners with or without children, and those in which a gay or lesbian single parent rears a child. Small studies that have evaluated children reared by same-sex couples found no significant differences in childrearing or in the children's adjustment from children reared in other types of families. These children have been found to do as well as those born into heterosexual families (Pawelski, Perrin, Foy, et al., 2006). Lesbian and gay parents are believed to be as effective as heterosexual couples in providing healthy and supportive environments for their children (American Psychological Association, 2004).

FAMILY DEVELOPMENT FRAMEWORKS

Family development theories use a framework to categorize a family's progression over time according to specific, typical stages in family life. These are predictable stages in the life cycle of every family, but they follow no rigid pattern. Duvall's (1977) eight stages in the family life cycle of a traditional nuclear family have been used as the foundation for contemporary models of the family life cycle that describe the developmental processes and role expectations for different family types. Table 2–1 lists Duvall's eight stages to illustrate important developmental transitions that occur at some point in most families.

Other family development models have been developed to address the stages and developmental tasks facing the unattached young adult, the gay and lesbian family, those who divorce, and those who remarry. Textbooks on families and developmental psychology provide further information on this topic.

FAMILY ASSESSMENT

The nurse's understanding of a family's structure helps provide insight into the family's support system and needs. A *family assessment* is a collection of data about the family's type and structure, current level of functioning, support system, sociocultural background, environment, and needs.

To obtain an accurate and concise family assessment, the nurse needs to establish a trusting relationship with the woman or child, and the family. Data are best collected in a comfortable, private environment, free from interruptions.

Basic information should include the following:

- Name, age, sex, and family relationship of all people residing in the household.
- Family type, structure, roles, and values.

Table 2–1 Eight-Stage Family Life Cycle

Stages	Characteristics
Stage I	Beginning family, newly married couples*
Stage II	Childbearing family (oldest child is an infant through 30 months of age)
Stage III	Families with preschool children (oldest child is between 2.5 and 6 years of age)
Stage IV	Families with school children (oldest child is between 6 and 13 years of age)
Stage V	Families with teenagers (oldest child is between 13 and 20 years of age)
Stage VI	Families launching young adults (all children leave home)
Stage VII	Middle-aged parents (empty nest through retirement)
Stage VIII	Family in retirement and old age (retirement to death of both spouses)

Adapted from: Duvall, E. M. (1977). *Marriage and family development* (5th ed.). Philadelphia: Lippincott; Duvall, E. M., & Miller, B. C. (1985). *Marriage and family development* (6th ed.), New York: Harper Row; Friedman, M. M., Bowden, V. R., & Jones, E. G. (2003). *Family nursing: Research, theory, and practice* (5th ed.). Upper Saddle River, NJ: Prentice Hall; Gedaly-Duff, V. Heims, M. L., & Nielsen, A. E. (2005). Family Child Health Nursing. In S. M. H. Hanson, V. Gedaly-Duff, & J. R. Kaakinen, *Family health care nursing* (3rd ed., pp. 291–321). Philadelphia: F. A. Davis.
*Keep in mind that this was the norm at the time the model was developed, but today families form through many different types of relationships.

- Cultural associations, including cultural norms and customs related to childbearing, childrearing, and infant feeding.
- Religious affiliations, including specific religious beliefs and practices related to child bearing.
- Support network, including extended family, friends, and religious and community associations.
- Communication patterns, including language barriers.

The nurse also gathers information about the health of individual family members because health status can have a major impact on family functioning. When possible, it is helpful to have information about the family's home environment as well. In many cases this information is gathered during client interviews. However, a home visit provides far more data about family relationships, roles, needs, and preparation for a new baby. See Chapter 39∞ for more information about family assessment.

CULTURAL INFLUENCES AFFECTING THE FAMILY

When caring for families, it is critical to consider the influence of culture, which may affect how a family responds to health-related issues. **Culture** has many definitions and is currently described as "the thoughts, communication, actions, customs, beliefs, values, and institutions of racial, ethnic, religious, or social groups" (U.S. Department of Health and Human Services: Office of Minority Health, 2005). Culture is characterized by certain key elements, including the following:

- *Culture is based upon shared values and beliefs, and expected behaviors.* Each culture identifies and articulates its shared values and beliefs. Expected behaviors and roles emerge that are consistent with those values and beliefs. This belief system suggests what preventive health measures and treatment for diseases are sought and accepted. It may also state the importance of children, of the family, of other individuals, and of the collective group, all of which can influence the choices people in the culture make regarding health.
- *Culture is learned and dynamic.* A child is born into a culture and starts learning the beliefs and practices of the group from birth. Children who are members of two cultural groups, such as African and immigrant, learn about both groups as they grow and develop. Immigrants may face challenges when integrating the rules of the dominant culture. Children who have family members from two or more cultural groups integrate parts of the worldview from each group. Therefore, although culture is connected with groups, each individual's manifestation of his or her own cultural background will be unique. Culture evolves and adapts as new members are born into or join the group, and as the surrounding social and physical environments change. For example, as first-generation immigrants enter a new country, they generally closely follow the cultural patterns of their native lands. As their children grow, the youth maintain some of the family cultural patterns but begin to incorporate some of the new culture (Figure 2–2 ●).
- *Culture is integrated into life and uses symbols.* Culture is integrated through social institutions such as schools, churches, mosques or synagogues, friendships, families, and occupation. This provides a variety of opportunities for learning about one's culture. The sense of integration may be disrupted or harder to maintain as individuals

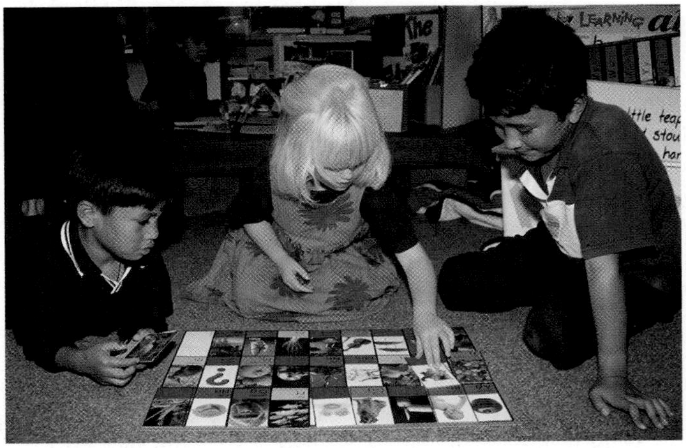

● **Figure 2–2** Preschoolers from various cultural backgrounds play together. How can nurses partner with families to assist children to understand and respect cultural differences?

move frequently and as cultures intertwine with each other. Symbols are an important way that many cultures communicate with each other and with the outside world. Language, dress, music, tools, and nonverbal gestures are symbols a culture uses to display and transmit the culture.

Race refers to a group of people who share biologic similarities such as skin color, bone structure, and genetic traits. Examples of races include white (sometimes called Caucasian or European American), black (sometimes called African American in the United States), Hispanic, Natives (such as Native Americans, Alaskan Native, Hawaiian Native, and First Nation people of Canada), and Asian.

Ethnicity describes a "cultural group's sense of identification associated with the group's common social and cultural heritage" (Spector, 2009, p. 349). Examples of ethnic groups include Hmong, Jews, and Irish Americans. Even the mainstream or majority of groups usually identify with an ethnic group. Some beliefs and practices are common among certain ethnic groups, but it is important to avoid **stereotyping** individuals, assuming that all members of a group have the same characteristics. The nurse should assess the woman or child and family to see which characteristics common to a group are possessed by the client rather than assume that because individuals identify themselves as a specific ethnicity they must practice certain customs.

Acculturation refers to the process of modifying one's culture to fit within the new or dominant culture. **Assimilation** is related to acculturation and is described as adopting and incorporating traits of the new culture within one's practice (Spector, 2009). Acculturation frequently occurs when people leave their country of origin and immigrate to a new country. Often acculturation is associated with improved health status and health behaviors, especially if the immigration is associated with improved socioeconomic status, which leads to better nutrition and access to health care. This is frequently true for people who immigrate to the United States from a developing country. On the other hand, health sometimes declines with acculturation. For example, obesity is a problem that is growing rapidly within the United States and particularly among immigrant populations.

FAMILY ROLES AND STRUCTURE

A family's organization and the roles played by individual family members are largely dependent upon cultural influence. The family structure defines acceptable roles and behavior of family members. For example, culture may determine who has authority (head of household) and is the primary decision maker for other members of the family. Additionally, the role of decision maker may change according to specific decisions. In some cultures, decisions regarding the family's health care are primarily the responsibility of the female, while other decisions are male dominated. Family dominance patterns may be *patriarchal,* as may be seen in Appalachian cultures; *matriarchal,* as may be seen in African American cultures; or more *egalitarian,* as may be seen in European American cultures. Nurses need to be alert for roles and functions in families since teaching may need to be directed to those responsible for decision making in order to promote health for all family members.

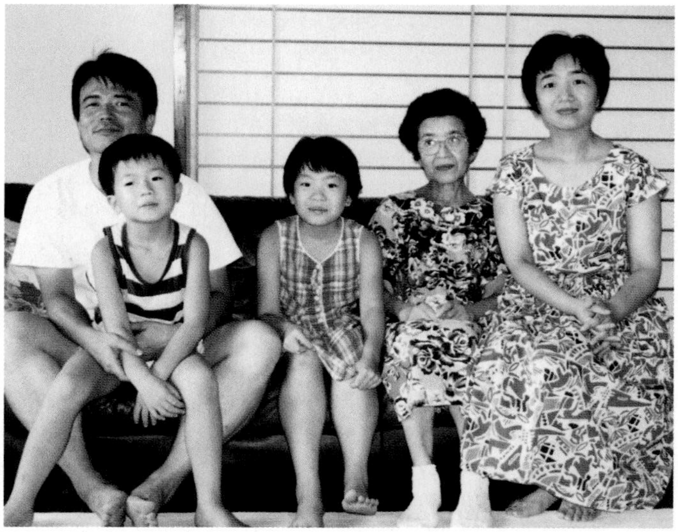

● **Figure 2–3** Many cultures value the input of grandparents and other elders in the family or group. In this multigenerational family, the grandmother's guidance is highly valued and significantly influences the family's childrearing practices.

Culture also defines gender roles, the role of the elderly, and the role of the extended family. For example, Native Americans may consult tribal elders (considered part of the extended family) before agreeing to medical care for a pregnant woman or for a child. In some cultures, major decisions for the family, including a child's health care, include input from grandparents and other extended family members (Figure 2–3 ●). Grandparents may even assume responsibility for care of the children in the family. In these cases, nurses must direct teaching for health promotion and demonstration for treatment procedures to the grandparent.

Family goals are also determined by cultural values and practices, as are family member roles and childbearing and childrearing practices and beliefs.

Teaching Highlights

INCLUDING GRANDPARENTS AND CULTURAL HEALTH PRACTICES IN THE TEACHING PLAN

When you care for a family in which the grandparents play a key role in decision making, be sure that they are present if you are teaching something that is important for the family to understand and act upon if necessary. This might include, for example, signs of illness in the newborn that need immediate follow-up.

If a specific cultural health practice is important to the family and will not cause harm, such as prayer, chanting, or specific foods, respect the family's beliefs and develop a teaching plan that includes those practices. Respecting their values improves the likelihood that the newly recommended healthcare actions will be accepted.

HEALTH BELIEFS, APPROACHES, AND PRACTICES

Three views of health described by Andrews and Boyle (2008) are magico-religious, scientific, and holistic. In reality, many people ascribe to a view that combines more than one of these belief systems, but it is helpful to examine them separately.

In the *magico-religious belief paradigm*, health and illness are determined by supernatural forces such as God, gods, magic, spirits, or fate. A miscarriage, for example, or the illness of a pregnant woman or of a child may be perceived as a punishment for actions. Children of preschool age and early school age usually have this view of illness; some adults also believe that higher or supernatural powers determine health and illness. It is wise to ask both children and their families what they think caused an illness or how they believe they can stay well. People who believe in this paradigm may gain comfort from prayer, healing rituals, and faith healing. Young children who, because of their developmental level, believe that they have caused their own illness can be expressly told that it was not something they did that caused the illness. This may help decrease their feelings of guilt.

The *scientific or biomedical health paradigm* assumes that physiology explains all illness and life itself (Andrews & Boyle, 2008). Biochemical reactions and the genomic code are used to explain all health states. Illness is always caused by viruses, bacteria, or damage to the body in this framework. This approach is often called "Western medicine." Families who hold this view expect a traditional Western medical intervention, such as medication, treatment, or surgery, to treat the specific health problem. Within this belief system, it is very difficult to understand certain health conditions. Families may struggle to "explain" an illness by wondering if the child was exposed to something harmful during fetal life or has been exposed to something in the environment. A reason for the condition is needed to understand it.

Most physicians, nurses, and other healthcare professionals adhere primarily to the biomedical or scientific theories to explain and treat illnesses. However, certain therapies such as therapeutic touch, biofeedback, and other nontraditional methods that are more common in a holistic health paradigm are gaining popularity within these professions. For the family with this belief system, health professionals sometimes need to emphasize that certain conditions have no known cause, and should suggest treatments other than traditional Western medicine if other approaches may be helpful.

Balance and harmony of the body and nature are important concepts in the *holistic health belief*. It is believed that illness results when the natural balance or harmony is disturbed. Infections and other illnesses gain entry into the body when it is not in balance. This health belief is most common in North American Indian and Asian cultures (Andrews & Boyle, 2008). Increasingly the ideas of holism are being integrated into Western health care and combined with other approaches. An example of integration of approaches is use of a medication or radiation for illness in combination with adequate rest and a diet that is designed to increase immune function.

An associated holistic health belief is the hot and cold theory of disease, which subscribes to the thought that illnesses and diseases are a result of disruption in the hot and cold balance of the body. Therefore, consuming foods of the opposite variety can cure or prevent specific hot and cold illnesses. Hot and cold therapies related to healing are practiced in some African American, Asian, Latino, Arab, Muslim, and Caribbean cultures (Andrews & Boyle, 2008); see Table 2–2.

HEALTHCARE PRACTITIONERS

The family seeking care for the child may choose one or a combination of magico-religious, holistic, or biomedical healthcare providers. The use of *folk healers* varies according to the culture. Though the healer's role and position in the community differ among cultures, healers do share commonalities. Healers speak the language of the cultural group, use common methods of communication for the culture, and live in the same community. They

Table 2–2 Hot and Cold Conditions and Foods

Hot Conditions	Cold Foods Used to Treat Hot Conditions	Cold Conditions	Hot Foods Used to Treat Cold Conditions
Diarrhea	Barley water	Cancer	Beef
Fever	Chicken	Earaches	Cheese
Constipation	Dairy products	Headaches	Eggs
Infection	Raisins	Musculoskeletal conditions	Grains
Kidney problems	Fish	Pneumonia	Liquor
Sore throats	Fresh fruits	Malaria	Onions
	Fresh vegetables		Spicy foods
	Goat meat		Chocolate

Data from Purnell, L. D., & Paulanka, B. J. (2005). *Guide to culturally competent health care.* Philadelphia: F. A. Davis; Giger, J. N., & Davidhizar, R. E (2008). *Transcultural nursing: Assessment & intervention* (5th ed.). St. Louis: Mosby Elsevier.

most often conduct healing in their homes or the homes of the individual or family. Cost is usually reasonable for the family, or some type of bartering may be common (Roy, Torrez, & Dale, 2004).

Mexican Americans and some Latino cultures may seek healing by a *curandero* (male healer) or *curandera* (female healer), who deals with all levels of illness, from minor colds to cancer (Spector, 2009). The curandero's holistic treatment may include use of herbs, laying on of hands, massaging the afflicted area, cleansing the body with herbs, preparing an amulet to be worn, burning a candle with a specific prayer printed on the candle jar, or calling the spirit of a saint to bless the individual. Essential to the curandero/a and the family is the faith the family has in his or her abilities. Families may combine curanderismo (Hispanic medical system) with a Western approach for some conditions. For example, a child with seizures may be given medications for the disorder obtained from Western care and may be fed a tea that the healer believes will treat the condition.

African Americans often combine Western and traditional beliefs about illness. Some believe in spirits as causes of illness and may use powders, oils, and ceremony to maintain health.

Native Americans may seek healing from a **shaman**, "a man or woman who enters an altered state of consciousness, at will, to contact and utilize another type of reality to acquire knowledge and power and to help other people" (Fontaine, 2005, p. 379). Because Native Americans generally believe in the balance of nature and a state of harmony, they seek advice to identify what they have done to disrupt their body harmony. The healer will then prescribe the required treatment for restoration of balance and harmony. Teas, other herbal products, sweats, smudges, meditation, and other approaches are common. Returning to one's family, home, and roots may produce a sense of balance.

IMPACT OF RELIGION AND SPIRITUALITY

The terms *religion* and *spirituality* mean different things to different people. Many people view religion, which is sometimes termed "faith-based belief," as an organized system that shares a common set of beliefs and practices about the significance, cause, and purpose of life and the universe. Religion is usually centered on the belief in or worshipping of a supernatural or supreme being (such as God or Allah). **Spirituality** refers to the individual's experience and own interpretation of his or her relationship with a supreme being. Children in general are more open than adults to their spirituality because they have not yet been exposed to cultural pressures. Spirituality helps children to establish their values and beliefs (Hufton, 2006). Prayer, one of the most common expressions of religious faith, is a frequently used therapy in which many children and families engage (NCCAM, 2005).

A family's religious beliefs, affiliation, and practices can deeply influence their experiences and attitudes toward health care, childbearing, and childrearing. Members of certain religious groups such as Christian Scientists may attempt to avoid all medical interventions, whereas others such as Jehovah's Witnesses may refuse specific interventions, such as blood transfusions. Roman Catholics may refuse contraception. In most cases, families gain comfort from acknowledgment of and respect for their religious beliefs and practices in the healthcare setting. However, the agnostic (one who has doubts about the existence of a transcendent being) or the atheist (one who believes that there is no higher power) may be offended if care providers assume that references to God or to a higher power will be comforting.

A religious or spiritual history is often completed when a woman is admitted to a clinic or labor setting or when a child is admitted to the hospital. The assessment can include questions about current spiritual beliefs and practices and preferences for religious rituals. Whenever possible the nurse should attempt to accommodate religious rituals and practices requested by the family.

Considering the diversity of religious beliefs, it is not unusual for nurses to encounter childbearing families whose beliefs conflict with their own. This is not problematic as long as the nurse avoids attempts to influence the family's decision making. For example, a nurse who does not believe in baptism should avoid revealing this to a Catholic seeking baptism for her stillborn infant. Nurses should also examine their religious beliefs related to genetic screening procedures, use of assisted reproductive technology to achieve pregnancy, abortion, use of technology to support life in a severely compromised newborn or a terminally ill child, and even less dramatic issues such as methods of contraception, circumcision, infant feeding, and disciplinary practices for children.

Although spirituality and faith-based belief are generally positive in supporting families to maintain and restore health, at times they can have potentially negative effects for children. Certain groups may blame individuals for their own illnesses, and children may develop guilt as a result. Abuse may result from parental religious beliefs about corporal punishment and discipline. If lifesaving treatments are denied by a religious group, courts may intervene to ensure care for the child.

Although adherence to a religious tradition is predominant in the United States, it should not be assumed that all individuals believe in or practice organized religion. The nurse should always ask the family if they follow a faith tradition and if they would like a leader from that faith to visit when in the hospital (Figure 2–4 ●). Adolescents may follow different faith traditions than their parents and should be asked the question individually.

Collaboration between the healthcare team and family is essential to providing care congruent with the child and family's

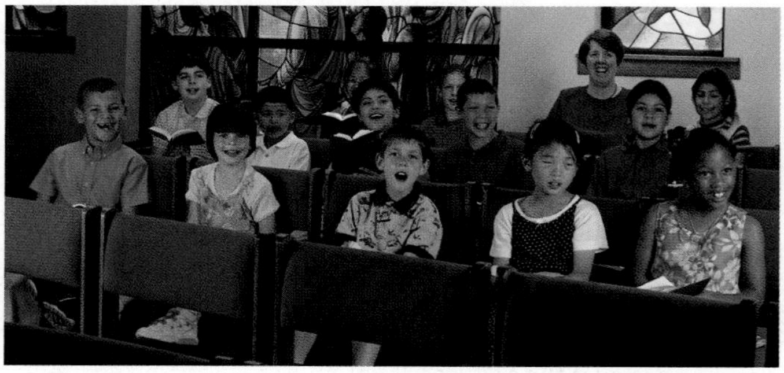

● **Figure 2–4** Today very few communities are limited to one culture. The children in this multicultural choir are representative of the changes in demographics of many Western countries. Even though they may differ in cultural background, a common thread is found in their religious preference.

expectations. While spirituality is important for many families, it is often overlooked as a healing strategy. Illness and injury may cause the family to turn to spiritual guidance as a method of understanding and coping. Trust in a higher being or purpose provides meaning for many children, supporting them as they deal with health problems (Elkins & Cavendish, 2004). The nurse must respect the family's view and avoid being judgmental toward their beliefs. Partnering with the child and family to incorporate their traditional practices and beliefs with prescribed therapies will help to ensure the delivery of safe and effective care for the child.

In many institutions, nurses can ask to be reassigned to a different client if their religious beliefs are in conflict because of health care being provided or refused by the client and family. However, if other personnel are not available, it is the nurse's responsibility to provide sensitive, appropriate, and nonjudgmental care to that client.

CHILDBEARING PRACTICES

Children are generally valued all over the world, not only for the joy they bring, but also because they ensure continuation of the family and cultural values. This valuing of children may manifest itself in different ways. Families in the United States and many Western countries commonly have only one or two children out of a desire to provide the children with the best home and education they can afford and to spend as much free time with them as possible. In contrast, in many cultures throughout the world, it is common to have as many children as possible.

In some cultures a woman who gives birth achieves a higher status, especially if the child is male (Safadi, 2005). This is especially true in the traditional Chinese culture and in some Middle Eastern cultures (Do, 2005). Similarly, in the western United States, people of the Mormon faith view motherhood as the most important aspect of a woman's life, comparable with the male role of priesthood (Faust, 2005). In Mexican American society and among many other Latino groups, having children is evidence of the male's virility and is a sign of manliness or *machismo,* a desired trait.

Culture may also influence attitudes and beliefs about contraception. For example, many Muslims from the Middle East may use birth control but do not believe in sterilization because it is a permanent method (Hammond, White, & Fetters, 2005). Other Muslims might not practice contraception because children are highly valued and it is believed that the traditional role of women is to bear children. In Chinese society, on the other hand, where state policy limits the number of children a couple can have, contraception is common.

Health values and beliefs are also important in understanding reactions and behavior. Certain behaviors can be expected if a culture views pregnancy as a sickness, whereas other behaviors can be expected if the culture views pregnancy as a natural occurrence. For example, because Native Americans, African Americans, and Mexican Americans generally view pregnancy as a natural and desirable condition, prenatal care may not be a priority. In Orthodox Judaism, for example, it is a man's responsibility to procreate, but it is a woman's right, not her obligation, to do so. This is because, according to Orthodox Jewish law, the health of the mother, both physically and mentally, is of primary concern, and she should never be obliged to do something that threatens her life (Semenic, Callister, & Feldman, 2004).

Individuals of many cultures take certain protective precautions based on their beliefs. For example, many Southeast Asian women fear that they will have a complicated labor and birth if they sit in a doorway or on a step. Thus they tend to avoid areas near doors in waiting rooms and examining rooms. In the Mexican American culture, the belief is common that *mal aire,* or bad air, may enter the body and cause harm. Preventive measures, such as keeping the windows closed or covering the head, are used. Some Latinos may place a raisin on the cord stump of a newborn to prevent drafts from entering their bodies.

A **taboo** is a behavior or thing that is to be avoided. Many cultures, including those found in the United States, have taboos centered on the unborn baby or newborn that are meant to ensure that the baby will survive. For example, it is common among Muslims to avoid naming the baby until after birth; similarly many Orthodox Jewish women wait to set up the nursery until after the baby is born.

In developing countries, mortality rates among infants and young children are extremely high; thus certain traditions focus on protecting the baby from evil spirits. For example, many Muslim parents will pin an amulet such as a blue stone or a verse from the Qu'ran to the newborn's clothing as protection. Following birth, it is common for a male family member to whisper prayers in the newborn baby's ear to declare faith and protect the baby (Cassar, 2006).

CHILDREARING PRACTICES

In some families children are expected to take on responsibilities early and may be expected to take on tasks such as management of their own chronic disease and nutritional intake. In other families, children are given long periods to grow up and are not expected to manage healthcare needs. Directing teaching to a child with diabetes in the latter family type may not be appropriate. Nurses often provide information and ask about developmental milestones for children; however, there may be variations in family goals and it is not unusual that families accomplish these tasks with children at younger or older ages. For example, it is commonly expected that children are weaned by 1 year of age and toilet trained at about 2 years of age, but this is not always the case. The nurse should ask about the norms in the family and whether the child is developing according to the parents' expectations. As long as the child is progressing in motor, language, and social tasks, some variation is expected due to cultural norms.

Views about alternative lifestyles such as sexual orientation and single parenting are also established by the family's values and beliefs. Understanding such values assists the nurse in providing sensitive care. Examples of childrearing practices common to particular cultures are listed in Table 2–3. Realize that the practices listed are common in these cultures, but not necessarily practiced by all members of that culture.

Table 2–3 Childrearing Practices of Selected Cultures

Culture	Childrearing Practices
African American	Grandmothers play an important role in the care of children Children are expected to demonstrate respectfulness, conformity to rules, obedience, and good behavior May use belly band or coin on umbilicus to prevent protrusion of umbilicus
Amish	Average of 7 children per family Childrearing is regarded as the highest priority for parents Grandparents often provide care to children Children are expected to continue with the Amish tradition Children are expected to follow the rules as prescribed by the church district
Appalachian	Large families are common Strict parenting practices Physical punishment is common Grandparents frequently provide care to children
Arab American	Father is typically the disciplinarian The child's character is considered a reflection of the family's influence Children are expected to respect their elders and to have good behavior Adolescents are expected to do well in their studies Discipline may include physical punishment and shaming Preference may be noted toward male children
Chinese American	Family may lavish resources on child Children typically depend on family for all needs and may not be expected to earn their own money as adolescents Male children are often more valued than female children Children may be taught to avoid displaying their emotions/feelings Children are expected to assist parents in the home (chores) High educational achievement is expected
Mexican American	Children are closely protected and are not encouraged to leave the home Extended family members frequently live close by Children are expected to demonstrate respect for parents and elder family members Discipline may include physical punishment Education is a priority
Navajo Indian	Children's name may not be revealed until their first laugh Infants may be kept in a cradleboard to protect them Grandmothers frequently are responsible for toilet training, disciplining, and weaning Children are allowed to make decisions about their care

Data from Purnell, L. D., & Paulanka, B. J. (2005). *Guide to culturally competent health care.* Philadelphia: F. A. Davis.

CULTURE AND NURSING CARE

Healthcare providers are often unaware of the cultural characteristics they themselves demonstrate. Without cultural awareness, caregivers tend to project their own cultural responses onto foreign-born clients; clients from different socioeconomic, religious, or educational groups; or clients from different regions of the country. This projection leads care providers to assume that the clients are demonstrating a specific behavior for the same reason that they themselves would. Moreover, healthcare providers often fail to realize that medicine has its own culture, which has been dominated historically by traditional middle-class values and beliefs.

Ethnocentrism is the conviction that the values and beliefs of one's own cultural group are the best or only acceptable ones. It is characterized by an inability to understand the beliefs and worldview of another culture. To a certain extent, everyone is guilty of ethnocentrism, at least some of the time. Thus, the nurse who values stoicism during labor may be uncomfortable with the more vocal response of some Latin American women. Another nurse may be disconcerted by a Southeast Asian woman who believes that pain is something to be endured rather than alleviated and who is intent on maintaining self-control in labor.

Healthcare providers sometimes believe that if members of other cultures do not share Western values and beliefs, they should adopt them. For example, a nurse who believes strongly in equality of the sexes may find it difficult to remain silent if a woman from a Middle Eastern culture defers to her husband in decision making. It is important to remember that pressure to

Developing Cultural Competence

CULTURE SHOCK

The experience that people have in attempting to understand or adapt to a culture that is fundamentally different from their own culture is known as culture shock. The person may experience feelings of discomfort, powerlessness, anxiety, and disorientation. Immigrants to the United States and Canada may experience culture shock when differences or conflicts arise between their own values, beliefs, and customs and the ways of their new surroundings. The nurse should assess childbearing women, children, and their families who have recently immigrated for indications of culture shock. Referring the family to counseling or support from representatives of the family's culture, such as a translator or community group, may be helpful.

defy cultural values and beliefs can be stressful and anxiety provoking for these women.

To address issues of cultural diversity in the provision of health care, emphasis is being placed on developing **cultural competence**—that is, ability to understand and effectively respond to the needs of individuals and families from different cultural backgrounds (Jirwe, Gerrish, & Emami, 2006; Spector, 2009). It involves identifying and integrating the family's beliefs about health and cultural values into their care (U.S. Department of Health and Human Services: Office of Minority Health, (2005).

CULTURALLY INFLUENCED RESPONSES

The nurse can begin developing cultural competence by becoming knowledgeable about the cultural differences and practices of various groups. Nurses who are knowledgeable of differences and who take them into account in planning and providing nursing care will be far more effective caregivers than those who do not.

Biologic Differences

Genetic and physical differences occur among cultural groups and can lead to disparity in needs and care. Differences include blood type, body build, skin color, drug metabolism, and susceptibility to certain diseases. Other disparities occur because of fundamental differences between genders, ages, and races. For example, male children are more likely to manifest pyloric stenosis and attention deficit disorder, whereas female children more often have congenital hip dysplasia and systemic lupus erythematosus. Age provides another biologic variation, as infants are more likely to manifest the cancer neuroblastoma, whereas adolescents have a higher incidence of Hodgkin's disease. Race is also connected with certain disease processes. Blacks are more likely to experience sickle cell anemia. Thalassemia, another type of anemia, is most common in Mediterranean people. Whites from certain geographic origins are more likely to manifest cystic fibrosis, celiac disease, and Crohn's disease. Hispanics have high rates of diabetes and lactose intolerance. Asians and Native Americans often do not metabolize alcohol readily and are more prone to either injury after alcohol ingestion or to alcohol abuse (Giger & Davidhizar, 2008).

Nurses need to understand other genetic characteristics in order to perform culturally competent nursing assessments and interventions. Differences in skin color and tone may make cyanosis, pallor, and jaundice difficult to recognize and describe. Mongolian spots are darkened skin on the lower back and buttocks of some babies with dark skin tones. Variations in texture of hair require different approaches to hygiene among various racial groups.

Communication Patterns

Communication is the method by which members of cultural groups share information and preserve their beliefs, values, norms, and practices. To ensure effective care, it is essential for families to be able to communicate with nurses and other healthcare providers. This becomes an issue when the family does not speak the language of the health professionals. In such cases it is best if the healthcare facility provides translators. Children are most likely to speak both the language of the parents and the healthcare providers and may appear to be likely interpreters. However, it is recommended that children never be used to interpret in healthcare situations due to the confidentiality needs of both parent and child. Additionally, if children are used as interpreters, it can create an imbalance in power that could adversely affect parental authority. Signs, posted literature, and brochures should also be available in the languages of the children and families served. Even when children speak the language of the healthcare providers, written material must be provided at a level that the family can read and understand.

Language can also affect health literacy skills as a large number of instructions are given in writing, including prescriptions and directions on medication bottles, signs hanging in health facilities, consent forms for procedures and surgery, insurance forms, directions for techniques or procedures, future appointment dates, and health promotion materials. Nurses need to verify what the client and family can read and whether alternative methods are needed. Nurses can verbally give the information and provide paper and pencil so that the family can take notes in their own language. Translation services should be available in all healthcare settings.

Variations in communication among cultures are reflected in their word meaning, voice inflection and quality, and verbal styles. Culture influences not only the manner in which feelings are expressed, but also which verbal and nonverbal expressions of

Nursing Practice

Speaking and reading may not occur in the same language. For example, an immigrant may read and speak fluently in his or her primary language and speak but not read the language of the new country. The immigrant's child may read and speak the language of the present country and speak but not read the native language of the family. Always ask about both reading and speaking preferences.

MyNursingKit Critical Thinking: Examine Your Cultural Influences communication are considered appropriate. An individual's willingness to discuss certain topics or to express or conceal certain thoughts and feelings is also influenced by the cultural norms. Some groups may be expected to remain quiet when experiencing pain, while other cultures may loudly and dramatically express pain.

Use of names varies among cultural groups. Assuming that each person wishes to be called by a first name can be disrespectful. Address family members respectfully, usually using terms such as Mr., Mrs., and Ms. If the person has a title such as doctor, judge, or senator, it should be used. The nurse should ask what the person prefers to be called and record this in the health record for future reference. In some cultures such as Korean, Cambodian, and Filipino, the first name used is actually the family name. Asking for the "family name" rather than the "last name" may clarify this practice.

Nonverbal communication. Nonverbal communication refers to body language such as posture, gestures, facial expressions, eye contact, and touch, as well as the use of silence. The nurse's use of nonverbal communication may hinder or help communication. Gestures and body language may be misunderstood or misinterpreted. Eye contact has different meanings among cultures. European Americans, for example, value eye contact with communication and interpret this as a sign of sincerity and interest. In other cultures, such as Asian and Native American, sustained eye contact may be considered rude or disrespectful.

Silence is considered a sign of respect in some cultures. Among those groups, offering an immediate response to a question may be viewed as being disrespectful since an instant reply could indicate that no thought was given to the matter. Nurses should watch for patterns in various cultures and alter their approach to be more congruent. For example, many nurses commonly nod and say "yes" or "oh, I see" when a health client is speaking. This may seem disruptive to some cultures. If the listener is silent and does not use such patterns of agreement, the nurse should alter his or her response to match more closely the acceptable method of communication for the family.

Touch. The appropriateness of touch varies with each culture. For example, an Asian may consider touching an unfamiliar person of the opposite gender to be inappropriate, whereas touch between men and women may be viewed as appropriate by another culture. Adults commonly feel that it is acceptable to touch children of all ages, but this may not be accurate. It is best to look for responses from the family to touch and progress accordingly.

Space. An individual's sense of personal space also differs by culture. Space refers to the physical distance and relationships between the individual and other persons and objects in the environment. Cultures may have specific spatial preferences, such as personal distance and social distance. Some cultures tend to prefer close contact with less space since they use touch as a form of communication. The nurse should be alert for how close a childbearing woman or a child comes to other individuals and try to maintain this space during interactions. Nursing procedures often cause the space barrier to be broken. Nurses need to touch clients to take vital signs, administer injections, change dressings, and the like. This does not mean that close touch is appropriate at all times. It is essential to tell all clients before touching them for procedures so they understand what is happening.

Time Orientation

Cultures have specific values and meanings regarding time orientation. Cultural groups may place emphasis on the events of the past, those events that occur in the present, or those events that will occur in the future. Children reflect the time orientation of their families and the cultures in which they live. Time is also influenced by development so that young children sometimes do not understand the use of clocks, the importance ascribed to being "on time," or other time orientations.

Cultures that are oriented predominantly to the past may want to begin healthcare encounters with lengthy descriptions of past healthcare treatments, family history of diseases, or individual past experiences with health. There may be little interest in learning methods of adapting to or maintaining a new plan of care.

For cultures that are oriented predominantly to the present, little consideration may be given to either the past or the future. For example, adolescents commonly focus on the present, and may not engage in preventive health practices for long-term health. Therefore, short-term goals often provide more incentive to adolescents.

Cultures that are oriented predominantly to the future, such as European American, may not focus on what is important at the present time. For example, the family focusing on the future may focus on the dreams they had for a child's education or sports performance and have trouble setting present goals for treatment of a disease such as juvenile arthritis. One commonly hears that it was a big adjustment to learn to "take one day at a time." Not living up to the family's expectation for their future success may be difficult for a child who has developed an illness that has a chronic course.

Time also refers to punctuality about schedules and appointments. In the United States and Canada, the predominant culture respects being on time and considers time valuable and not to be wasted. Other cultures may not emphasize a concern for time. This may be manifested by a family's inability to follow timed medication schedules or treatments, or to show up as scheduled for an appointment. In these cases it is not intended as a sign of disrespect.

Nutrition

Nutritional practices begin even before birth as many cultural groups have beliefs that determine foods that are healthy to eat or should be avoided during pregnancy. Nutritional habits and patterns vary among cultures and are related to both religious practices and health beliefs. Certain cultures and religions have restrictions on or prescriptions about specific foods and preparation methods. Ritualistic behaviors involving eating and drinking, for example on special occasions and holidays, are observed by most cultures. Many religions recommend fasts during specific holy seasons, such as Lent for Roman Catholics, Yom Kippur for Jews, and Ramadan for Muslims; however, in most cases, small children, pregnant women, the elderly, and sick individuals are not required to fast.

Additionally, some cultures value large size or may associate a healthy child with being "large." Other cultures value slimness and look down upon obese individuals. Both of these views influence family eating patterns and expectations for the child; the child's self-esteem can therefore be influenced. The U.S and Canadian cultures honor being slim in the media but reinforce eating and large size by the availability of fast food and positive image of large sports stars such as some football players, which can result in confusion about health and body image.

Nutrition may also be essential to the culture's practices for health promotion and care during illness. Health problems associated with specific cultures that may require dietary changes are also identified. Nutrition can be closely related to environmental situations, and families with few resources may not be able to obtain or eat cultural foods due to access or financial issues. Nutrition plays a powerful role in maintaining health, so resources for nutritious and desired foods may be needed.

NURSING MANAGEMENT

The focus of nursing care is assessment of cultural influences on the client's health. The nurse providing culturally competent care to the woman or child and family considers all facets of their culture. Identification of cultural influences as well as cultural barriers will enable the nurse to provide culturally competent nursing care in the management and support of culturally diverse clients and families.

NURSING ASSESSMENT

Mattson and Smith (2004) suggest that care providers conduct a cultural assessment to glean information about health practices based on the client's beliefs, values, and customs. This kind of assessment might include questions such as the following:

- Who in the family must be consulted before decisions are made about a person's care?
- Does the client, or do the parents of a child, see primarily in the present or do they have a futuristic time orientation?
- What type of health provider is most appropriate for (or preferred by) the woman, the child, or the family?
- Does the family have beliefs or traditions that may affect the plan of care?

Several cultural assessment tools are available to assist the nurse in gathering this information. These tools are becoming increasingly common at healthcare agencies as providers act in response to the expectation of culturally competent care. The nurse who respects cultural diversity is an asset to the childbearing and childrearing family as they adjust to their new role. Establishing a trusting relationship enables the nurse to assist the family in meeting educational needs.

The use of North American Nursing Diagnosis Association (NANDA) nursing diagnoses to describe situations specifically related to culture may in itself be culturally biased because the foci of these diagnoses are based on Western cultural beliefs. Diagnoses such as "impaired verbal communication" or "deficient knowledge" should not be used solely because a person does not speak English. Is someone who speaks a different language "impaired" in communication?

Specific nursing diagnoses are dependent upon the reason the family seeks contact with healthcare professionals, ranging from a pregnancy to a child's health promotion and health maintenance (e.g., immunizations) to the care of a chronic or terminally ill child. Examples include the following:

- *Ineffective Therapeutic Regimen Management* related to mistrust of healthcare personnel
- *Fear* related to separation from support system in stressful situation such as hospitalization
- *Spiritual Distress* related to discrepancy between spiritual beliefs and prescribed treatment
- *Interrupted Family Processes* related to a shift in family roles due to illness

The planning and implementation of nursing care for the culturally diverse family depends specifically on the findings of the previous assessments. Nurses need to partner with the family to establish a safe, effective, and desirable plan of care. Nurses can ensure access to an interpreter if needed and evaluate whether the match with a particular interpreter is appropriate for the child and family.

Recognizing the influence of culture on one's beliefs, values, and healthcare practices is essential for the nurse to deliver culturally competent care. Nurses demonstrate appropriate strategies to delivering culturally sensitive care when they develop techniques in assessing the influence of culture on the pregnant woman or the child and family and incorporate that information into an individualized plan of care.

Culturally competent nurses find effective ways to partner with the family to assist them in determining how they can incorporate prescribed therapies with their healthcare practices. Ensure that the woman herself or the child and family understand the problem or illness, treatment, and health promotion activities. Apply culturally sensitive techniques when dispelling any cultural myths.

Nurses can also collaborate with a multidisciplinary team, including social workers and language specialists, to assist the family in receiving assistance with barriers to care such as transportation, financial issues, remote access, and others.

COMPLEMENTARY AND ALTERNATIVE THERAPIES AND THE FAMILY

Through most of the 20th century in the United States, it was rare for European American childbearing families to consult anyone except their obstetrician for advice about their pregnancy, birth, and postpartum. Similarly, most childrearing families closely followed the advice of their pediatrician about all aspects of child care. Though such clients are still encountered

Evidence-Based Nursing

INVESTIGATING CULTURE AND HEALTHCARE BARRIERS

Clinical Question

What barriers to providing accessible health care exist among ethnically diverse families with children?

The Evidence

A study was conducted of 42 family members with Latino children and 42 family members of Euro-Americans with special healthcare needs. Both groups cited frustrations in care related to access to rehabilitation, and lack of integration of care within school systems. Latino families often cited need for more information and access to a support group, whereas Euro-American families cited a need for referral to day care and respite care resources (Gannotti, Kaplan, Handwerker, et al., 2004).

Shi and Stevens (2005) utilized data from the Household Component of the 1996 and 2000 Medical Expenditure Panel Survey cosponsored by the Agency for Healthcare Research and Quality and the National Center for Health Statistics to evaluate healthcare disparities among Asians, Hispanics, and Blacks. They found that compared to non-Hispanic whites, individuals in these minority groups were less likely to have a regular place for obtaining health care, and were less likely to have had a visit to the doctor or dentist in the past year. Some of the reasons cited for these differences included cost, availability of care, convenience, and cultural and language barriers.

A study of the child healthcare decision making and practices of 12 immigrant women from the Caribbean revealed concerns related to communication and trust with healthcare providers. The women shared feelings that they were not valued in the healthcare setting. Their use of herbs and folk practices was also frequently misunderstood or frowned upon, often resulting in a failure to disclose this information. The women also felt that they did not have the abilities to effectively navigate the healthcare system (Yearwood, 2007).

In another study of immigrants, Korean children were examined for completion of the hepatitis B vaccination series. Perception that hepatitis B was a serious disease was an incentive for completion of the series, although difficulty paying for the immunization was a major barrier to completion (Kim, 2004).

Best Practice

A theme in two of the previous studies was cost of care. Nurses need to refer families to sources for healthcare services and then follow up to be sure the families were able to access care. Referrals to community health centers and instructions for transportation to the health setting are important for many families.

A need for information is another theme among most groups. Explaining why an immunization is needed as well as providing information about the child's condition are important nursing roles. Referring the family to others from the same ethnic or racial group and assisting them in navigating complex systems such as school and social services may also be necessary.

Cultural differences and practices were also cited as a barrier to health care. It is essential that healthcare providers become familiar with other cultures and be accepting of practices that are safe for the child. By being open to practices of other cultures, healthcare providers will find families more willing to share openly about how they are treating their children. This may lead to an opportunity for education related to unsafe practices.

Critical Thinking

What is the process that immigrant families in your state or province must follow to secure health care for their children? How would you help to guide someone through this process? What cultural groups are common in your community? Do you speak their language? If not, what measures should you take to ensure that they understand the teaching offered in clinical settings? What type of support groups will be helpful for families when they have a child with special healthcare needs?

today, nurses are more likely to care for families who integrate other types of practitioners and therapies with traditional Western medicine.

Although the terms *complementary* and *alternative* are often used interchangeably, they have different meanings and applications. A **complementary therapy** may be defined as any procedure or product that is used as an adjunct to conventional medical treatment (National Center for Complementary and Alternative Medicine [NCCAM], 2007a). Although complementary therapies were absent from clinics and hospitals until the last few decades, therapies such as acupuncture, acupressure, and massage therapy are now often used with conventional medical care, and many health insurance plans cover at least a portion of the cost of such therapies.

In contrast, an **alternative therapy** is usually considered a substance or procedure that is used in place of conventional medicine (NCCAM, 2007a). It usually has not undergone rigorous scientific testing in this country, although it might have been thoroughly tested in other countries. Alternative therapies are not usually available in conventional clinics and hospitals, and their costs are not typically covered under most health insurance policies. An example of an alternative therapy is the use of herbal medicines instead of biomedicines for the treatment of a child's health condition. In other words, the child would not receive traditional Western medical care for the condition, such as surgery, radiation, prescribed medications, or other medical interventions. The dramatic increase in complementary and alternative therapies that began in the final decade of the 20th century was probably the result of a combination of several factors:

- Increased consumer awareness of the limitations of conventional Western medicine
- Increased international travel
- Increased media attention
- Advent of the Internet

In this new century, it seems clear that Western health care will see an ever-increasing integration between conventional medicine and complementary therapies. Some obvious examples of this new integration in perinatal settings include the acceptance of certain herbal teas for antepartum discomforts; the use of massage, Reiki, or therapeutic touch during the first stage of labor; music during childbirth; and the increased emphasis on skin-to-skin mother-to-baby bonding in the immediate postpartum period.

Further evidence of this increased integration is the establishment in 1992 of the Office of Alternative Medicine (OAM) at the National Institutes of Health. The OAM was mandated by Congress to promote research into complementary and alternative therapies and dissemination of information to consumers. In 1998 the OAM was incorporated into a new National Center for Complementary and Alternative Medicine (NCCAM) with an expanded mission and increased funding. Many studies of complementary and alternative therapies are currently under way at NCCAM.

BENEFITS AND RISKS

Complementary and alternative therapies undisputedly have many benefits for women and children. Many complementary and alternative therapies emphasize prevention and wellness, and place a higher value on holistic healing than on physical cure. Complementary and alternative medicine practices must be assessed for safety, including positive and negative benefits, cost, efficacy, and clinical usefulness. The use of herbs and natural products raises many issues, of which these are just a few: standards of products, misleading claims and safety related to megadoses of some products. Determine the family's use of complementary and/or alternative medicine such as the type of remedies and healthcare practices used. Also determine the side effects, risks, and other implications to the child receiving this type of therapy. Work with the family to ensure safe practices with the use of complementary and/or alternative modalities

TYPES OF COMPLEMENTARY AND ALTERNATIVE THERAPIES

Numerous forms of complementary and alternative therapies are available. Only a few of the most commonly used approaches are presented here.

Homeopathy

Homeopathy is a healing approach in which a person is treated with small doses of medicines that would cause illness when given to someone who is healthy. Traditional Western (or allopathic) medicine generally gives medicine or treatments that suppress symptoms. Analgesics for pain or antibiotics for infection are examples of such treatments. In homeopathy, the symptoms are viewed as the body's method of healing and small doses of medications are given to enhance the symptoms. For example, medications are chosen to promote fever and inflammation since they are thought to be healing forces (Fontaine, 2005; Spector, 2009).

Naturopathy

Naturopathy is a form of medicine that ascribes to the healing forces of nature. Naturopathic physicians focus on the restoration of health. They utilize opportunities to educate families about healthy lifestyles. A variety of interventions may be used, including herbs, nutrition, acupuncture, and stress management. Counseling is also a commonly used approach as it focuses on the holistic needs of the individual including mental, spiritual, and emotional factors (Fontaine, 2005).

Traditional Chinese Medicine

Traditional Chinese medicine (TCM) developed more than 3000 years ago in the Chinese culture and then gradually spread with modifications to other Asian countries. The underlying focus of TCM is prevention, although diagnosis and treatment of disease also play an important role.

TCM seeks to ensure the balance of energy, which is called *chi* or *qi* (pronounced "chee"). Chi is the invisible flow of energy in the body that maintains health and energy and enables the body to carry out its physiologic functions. Chi flows along certain pathways or meridians.

Another important concept in TCM is that of *yin* and *yang*, opposing internal and external forces that, together, represent the whole.

TCM includes the following therapeutic techniques:

- *Acupuncture* uses very fine (hairlike) stainless steel needles to stimulate specific acupuncture points, depending on the client's medical assessment and condition.
- *Acupressure* (Chinese massage) uses pressure from the fingers and thumbs to stimulate pressure points.
- *Herbal therapy* is an important part of TCM, but it is sometimes difficult to locate a skilled herbalist because there are relatively few in the United States and other English-speaking countries.
- *Qigong* (pronounced "chee-goong") is a self-discipline that involves the use of breathing, meditation, self-massage, and movement. Typically practiced daily, the movements are nontiring and are designed to stimulate the flow of chi.
- *Tai chi* (pronounced "ty chee") is a form of martial art. It originally focused on physical fitness and self-defense, but it is currently used to improve health as well (Fontaine, 2005).
- *Moxibustion* involves the application of heat from a small piece of burning herb called *moxa (Artemisia vulgaris)*. The moxa stick is typically burned at the lateral side of the little toe. In TCM moxibustion has many uses. For example, studies from China demonstrate good success when moxibustion is used to help turn a fetus who is breech to a vertex presentation. Controlled research on this use for moxibustion is underway (Grabowska, 2006).

Mind-Based Therapies

Biofeedback is a method used to help individuals learn to control their physiologic responses based on the concept that the mind controls the body. An individual is hooked up to a system of highly sensitive instruments that relay information about the body back to that person. Currently biofeedback has more than 150 applications for disease prevention and the restoration of health. The effectiveness of biofeedback has been proven in countless studies, and it is now considered a conventional therapy more than a complementary one.

Hypnosis, whether guided by a trained hypnotherapist or induced through self-hypnosis, is a state of great mental and physical relaxation during which a person is very open to suggestions. In this state the individual is able to modify body responses. Pregnant women who receive hypnosis before childbirth have reported shorter, less painful labors and births.

Visualization is a complementary therapy in which a person goes into a relaxed state and focuses on or "visualizes" soothing or positive scenes such as a beach or a mountain glade. Visualization helps reduce stress and encourage relaxation.

Guided imagery is a state of intense, focused concentration used to create compelling mental images. It is sometimes considered a form of hypnosis. Guided imagery is useful in imagining a desired effect such as weight loss or in mentally rehearsing a new procedure or activity.

Chiropractic

Chiropractic, the third largest independent health profession in the United States (behind medicine and dentistry), is based on concepts of manipulation to address health problems that are thought to be the result of abnormal nerve transmissions (subluxation) caused by misalignment of the spine. In the United States doctors of chiropractic perform more than 90% of all spinal manipulations (NCCAM, 2007b). Chiropractors also stress the importance of proper nutrition and regular exercise to good health. Chiropractic is widely available, and popular demand has earned it a higher level of insurance coverage than most other alternative therapies.

Massage Therapy

Massage has been used for centuries as a form of therapy. *Massage therapy* involves manipulation of the soft tissues of the body to reduce stress and tension, increase circulation, diminish pain, and promote a sense of well-being. Different techniques have been developed, including Swedish massage, shiatsu massage, Rolfing, and trigger point massage. Most forms use techniques such as pressing, kneading, gliding, circular motion, tapping, and vibrational strokes.

Certain massage therapists specialize in massage for women during pregnancy. Massage is often helpful as women adapt to the discomforts of their changing bodies. Certified nurse-midwives often use perineal massage prior to labor to stretch the muscles of the perineum around the vaginal opening and thereby prevent tearing of the tissues during childbirth. During labor, massage of the back and buttocks by the nurse, labor coach, or *doula* can help the woman relax and may help decrease her discomfort.

Infant massage is also growing in popularity in the United States, and many parents have learned to massage their infants and young children (Figure 2–5 ●). Massage also plays a role in therapy for children with a variety of conditions, including eczema.

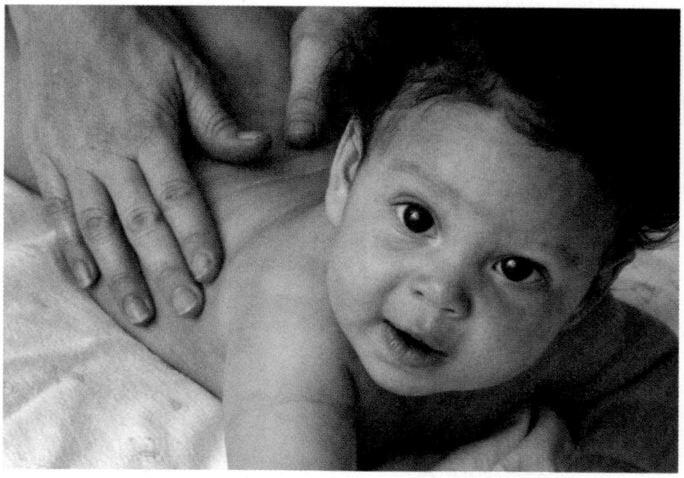

● **Figure 2–5** Infant massage.

Source: Peter Arnold, Inc./Laura Dwight.

Herbal Therapies

Herbal therapy or herbal medicine has been used since ancient times to treat illnesses and ailments. Well-known herbal remedies include, for example, ginger, rosemary, ginseng, ginkgo, chamomile, oil of evening primrose, *Echinacea,* garlic, lemon balm, and black cohosh.

Herbs are categorized as dietary supplements and are controlled by the Dietary Supplement Health Education Act. They do not require approval by the Food and Drug Administration (FDA) as prescripiton and over-the-counter medications do; however, the FDA does have the authority to pull a product off the market if it is proven to be dangerous (Cranwell-Bruce, 2008, Fontaine, 2005). Consequently most of what is known about herbs comes from Germany where they have been studied for some time (Fontaine, 2005). The use of herbs during pregnancy is an especially important consideration for nurses working with childbearing families. Pregnant and lactating women interested in using herbs are best advised to consult with their healthcare provider before taking any herbs, even as teas. Lists identifying common herbs that women are advised to avoid or use with caution during pregnancy and lactation are available.

Therapeutic Touch

Therapeutic touch is a complementary therapy meant to be used with conventional medical care. It was developed in the early 1970s by Dr. Delores Krieger, a nursing professor at New York University, and Dora Kunz, a clairvoyant healer. Therapeutic touch is grounded in the belief that people are a system of energy with a self-healing potential. The therapeutic touch practitioner, often a nurse, can unite his or her energy field with that of the client's, directing it in a specific way to promote well-being and healing. Proponents of ther-

Developing Cultural Competence

HERBALISM

The World Health Organization estimates that 80% of the earth's population depends on plants to treat common ailments. Herbalism is an essential part of traditional Indian, Asian, Native American, and naturopathic medicines. Many homeopathic remedies are also developed from herbs (Balch, 2006).

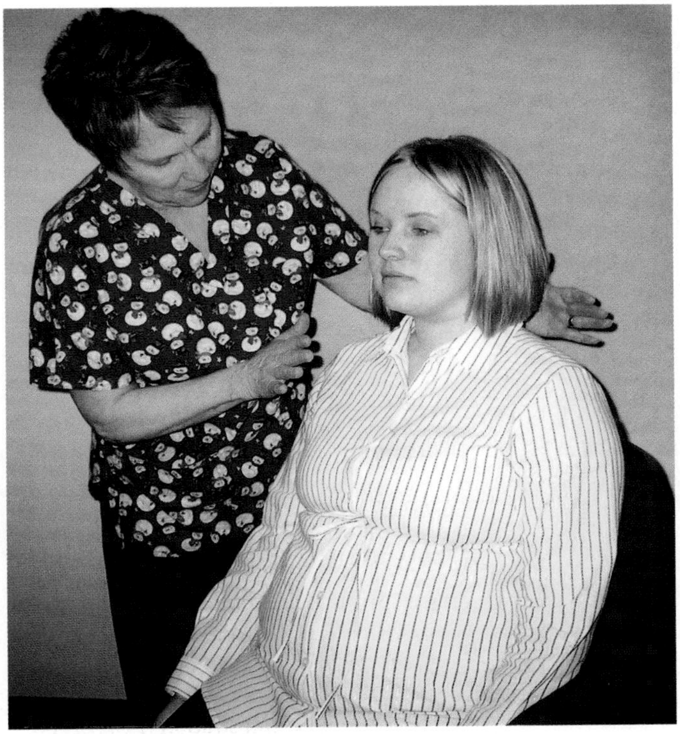

• **Figure 2–6** During pregnancy, therapeutic touch is often helpful in easing pain and reducing anxiety.

Used with permission from Nurse Healers—Professional Associates International, *the official organization for Therapeutic Touch*, http://www.therapeutic_touch.org

apeutic touch believe that a strong desire to help the recipient is essential, as is a conscious use of self to act as a link between the universal life energy and the other person (Fontaine, 2005). Impressive anecdotal evidence and many small studies suggest that therapeutic touch is effective in a variety of conditions. However, as yet, its effectiveness has not been scientifically proven in large, controlled studies (NCCAM, 2007b).

Like many other conventional and complementary therapies, therapeutic touch should be applied cautiously to pregnant women, newborns, and children by trained providers (Figure 2–6 ●).

Other Types of Complementary and Alternative Therapies

This discussion only touched on some of the most common forms of complementary and alternative therapies. Other examples include Ayurveda (the traditional medicine of India), meditation, craniosacral therapy, reflexology, hydrotherapy, Hatha yoga, regular physical exercise, aromatherapy, color and light therapy, music and sound therapies, magnetic therapy, and Reiki, to name a few. Readers interested in these therapies are referred to specialty texts.

NURSING CARE OF THE FAMILY USING COMPLEMENTARY THERAPIES

Some form of complementary and alternative medicine (CAM) is currently being used by 36% of adults in the United States. When prayer for health reasons and megavitamin therapy are added to the definition, that number increases to 62%. Women use CAM more often than men do, as do people with higher educational levels and people who have been hospitalized within the past year. By race, when megavitamin therapy and prayer are included in the definition, blacks are the greatest users of CAM. When those elements are excluded, Asians are the greatest users, followed by whites (NCCAM, 2007c).

The reality that families may use CAM and not reveal it raises some concern. Certain CAM modalities such as biofeedback, acupuncture, aromatherapy, and massage are not likely to cause adverse effects. However, the possibility exists that there might be interactions between herbal therapies and other medications prescribed by the care provider (Cranwell-Bruce, 2008; Fontaine, 2005)

Nurses need to become knowledgeable about CAM to be able to maximize its benefits and to protect pregnant women and children from any possible harm. The Society of Pediatric Nurses has affirmed that nurses must educate children and families about the benefits and risks of CAM (Asher, 2007). All healthcare providers must become knowledgeable about CAM therapies and the people who are providing these therapies in order to be able to balance risks and benefits to the child (Kemper & Cohen, 2004). The use of CAM in the care of children must be addressed because of the limited research with this age group and developmental variations that may influence efficacy and safety. While many CAM therapies may have been proven effective in adults, they may have little effect on children, or even be harmful.

Nurses who create a climate of respect and openness tend to be more effective in gathering information about a family's use of complementary or alternative therapies. The nurse should use a nonjudgmental approach in assessing pregnant women and families for the use of CAM. Ask specifically about the use of herbs and other supplements as the pregnant woman, parent, or child may not think to include them in their list of medications. The nurse should also identify the expected desired outcome of the use of herbal or dietary supplement (Cranwell-Bruce, 2008).

In working with childbearing and childrearing families, or indeed with any clients, nurses should use complementary modalities that are in the scope of their nursing practice and the nursing

Evidence in Action

A recent study examined the frequency of CAM use in general pediatric as compared to specialty pediatrics. Children with specific conditions such as epilepsy, cancer, and sickle cell disease were more likely to use CAM than those with acute illnesses or injury. This difference is perhaps related to recurring symptoms that are more likely to occur in children with chronic illnesses. Use of CAM in a child, however, was most directly related to whether or not CAM was used by the child's parents. Assessment of the child should include questions related to the use of CAM so that any concerns or questions related to their use can be addressed (Post-White, Fitzgerald, Hageness, et al., 2009).

practice act in their state and are not limited by the licensure of other providers (Radzyminski, 2007) Nurses should use CAM therapies that are supported by evidence-based research (Radzyminski). and considered somewhat mainstream. Nurses working with a pregnant woman might use acupressure wristbands for the treatment of nausea. Other therapies nurses often employ include progressive relaxation, exercise and movement, therapeutic touch, visualization and guided imagery, prayer, meditation, music therapy, massage, storytelling, aromatherapy, and journaling.

Modalities that are determined to be within the nurse's scope of practice should address a specific nursing diagnosis and these interventions should be documented appropriately. Thus, music therapy might be used for a child to help address the identified nursing diagnosis of "acute pain."

Nurses have a role in conducting and supporting research on CAM. Because of the variety of CAM therapies in use, research is needed in a host of areas. The results of research on CAM can be found in professional journals and at the National Institutes of Health (NIH) Web site. As the evidence supporting the use of certain interventions grows, nurses and other healthcare providers are incorporating the results as part of their evidence-based practice.

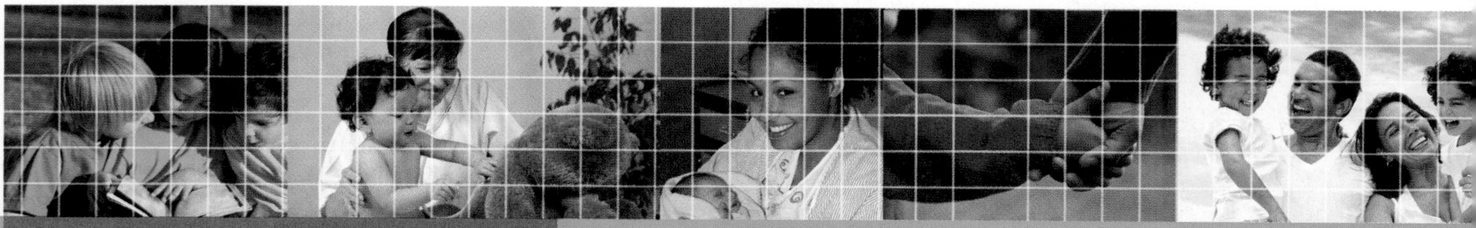

CRITICAL CONCEPT REVIEW

LEARNING OUTCOMES — CONCEPTS

2.1 Distinguish among several different types of families.

1. Nuclear families consist of a mother, father, and children.
2. Dual-career/dual-earner families make up the majority of contemporary families in the United States.
3. Childless families are a growing trend in American culture.
4. Extended family members can play an active role in family life, decision making, and family roles.
5. Single-parent families account for almost a third of all U.S. families, and stepparent and binuclear families are increasingly common.
6. Nonmarital heterosexual cohabitating family is often chosen for financial reasons or for companionship.
7. Gay and lesbian families have children who show no significant differences from children raised in more traditional families.

2.2 Identify the stages of a family life cycle.

1. Stage I: Beginning families.
2. Stage II: Childbearing families.
3. Stage III: Families with preschool children.
4. Stage IV: Families with school-age children.
5. Stage V: Families with teenagers.
6. Stage VI: Families launching young adults.
7. Stage VII: Middle-aged parents.
8. Stage VIII: Retirement and old age

2.3 Identify prevalent cultural norms related to childbearing and childrearing.

Childbearing and childrearing are influenced by the following cultural norms:

1. Status of the family unit:
   - Pregnancy may elevate the status of both the man and the woman depending upon the culture.
   - The role of extended family in the care of the child varies depending on the culture.
2. Contraception:
   - Culture may prohibit the use of contraception or may determine the type used.
3. View of pregnancy:
   - May be seen as an honor.
   - May be viewed as a sickness.
   - May determine the responsibilities of the mother or father.
4. Existence of taboos.
5. Discipline.

LEARNING OUTCOMES / CONCEPTS

LEARNING OUTCOMES	CONCEPTS
2.4 Summarize the importance of cultural competency in providing nursing care.	The nurse who provides culturally competent care: 1. Recognizes the importance of the childbearing family's value system. 2. Acknowledges that differences occur among people. 3. Seeks to respect and respond to ethnic diversity in a way that leads to mutually desirable outcomes.
2.5 Discuss the use of a cultural assessment tool as a means of providing culturally sensitive care.	A cultural assessment tool provides information of health practices based on: 1. Client beliefs. 2. Client values. 3. Client customs.
2.6 Identify key considerations in providing spiritually sensitive care.	To provide spiritually sensitive care, the nurse should: 1. Determine the current spiritual and religious beliefs and practices that will affect the mother and baby. 2. Accommodate these practices where possible. 3. Examine one's own spiritual or religious beliefs to be more aware and able to provide nonjudgmental care.
2.7 Distinguish between *complementary* and *alternative* therapies.	1. A complementary therapy is an adjunct to conventional medical treatment that has been through rigorous scientific testing, which shows that it has some reliability. 2. An alternative therapy is usually considered a substance or procedure that has not undergone rigorous scientific testing in this country, although it might have been thoroughly tested in other countries.
2.8 Identify the benefits and risks of complementary and alternative therapies.	1. CAM therapies have several benefits. Many of them emphasize prevention and wellness, place a higher value on holistic healing than on physical cure, are noninvasive, and have few side effects. In addition, many are more affordable and available than conventional therapies. 2. Risks of CAM therapies include lack of standardization, lack of regulation and research substantiating safety and effectiveness, inadequate training and certification of some healers, and financial and health risks of unproven methods.
2.9 Discuss complementary therapies appropriate for the nurse to use with childbearing and childrearing families.	Nurses may use the following CAM therapies: 1. Guided imagery. 2. Acupressure. 3. Prayer. 4. Music therapy. 5. Massage. 6. Storytelling. 7. Exercise and movement. 8. Meditation. 9. Aromatherapy. 10. Journaling. 11. Progressive relaxation

CRITICAL THINKING IN ACTION

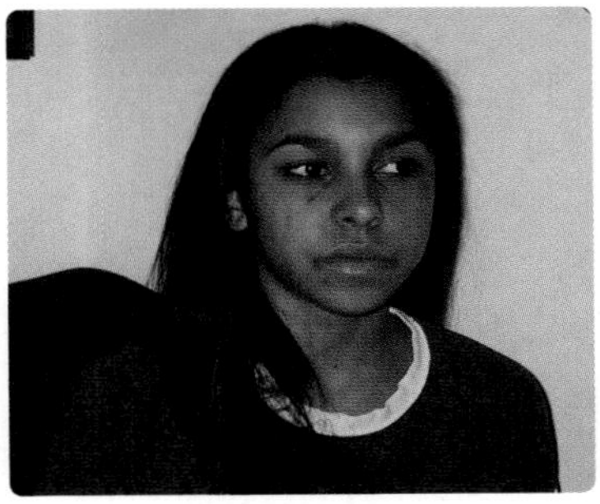

While working in an inner-city clinic for adolescents, you meet a new client, a 14-year-old Latina girl named Juanita. She is accompanied by her parents. None of them speak English. Through an interpreter, Juanita tells you that she recently moved here with her parents. They have brought her here today because she has a sore throat. The curandero they took her to see prescribed the herbal remedy *Echinacea,* but her throat is still sore. The rapid test you perform for strep throat is positive and the nurse practitioner prescribes an antibiotic.

1. According to the national standards for culturally and linguistically appropriate services in health care set by the government, what are examples of important standards of care you as the nurse can provide in the care of this adolescent?
2. How can you, as the nurse, take steps to achieve cultural competence?
3. How would you, as the nurse, be able to address some of the disparities that can exist when this client comes to the clinic?
4. What are some examples of common food preferences in the Latino-American culture?

See MyNursingKit for possible responses.

REFERENCES

American Psychological Association (2004). Sexual orientation, parents, and children: APA Policy Statement. Retrieved September 16, 2008, from www.apa.org/pi/lgbc/policy/parents.html

Andrews, M. M., & Boyle, J. S. (2008). *Transcultural concepts in nursing care* (5th ed.). Philadelphia: Lippincott Williams & Wilkins.

Asher, C. (2007). Position statement on complementary and alternative medicine in pediatrics. *Journal of Pediatric Nursing, 22*(2), 159–161.

Balch, P. A. (2006). *Prescription for Nutritional Healing* (4th ed.). New York: Avery.

Cassar, L. (2006). Cultural expectations of Muslims and Orthodox Jews in regard to pregnancy and the postpartum period: A study in comparison and contrast. *International Journal of Childbirth Education, 21*(2), 27–30.

Cranwell-Bruce, L. (2008). Herb-drug interactions. *MEDSURG Nursing, 17*(1), 52–54.

Denham, S. A. (2005). Family structure, function, and process. In S. M. H. Hanson, V. Gedaly-Duff, & J. R. Kaakinen, *Family health care nursing* (3rd ed., pp. 119–156), Philadelphia: F. A. Davis.

Do, H. (2005). Chinese culture *Ethnomed.* Retrieved November 29, 2005, from http://ethnomed.org

Duvall, E. M. (1977). *Marriage and family development* (5th ed.). New York: Harper & Row.

Duvall, E. M., & Miller, B. L. (1985). *Marriage and family development* (6th ed.). New York: Harper & Row.

Elkins, M., & Cavendish, R. (2004). Developing a plan for pediatric spiritual care. *Holistic Nursing Practice, 18,* 179–184.

Faust, J. E. (2005). Instruments in the hands of God. *Liahona Archives.* Retrieved January 4, 2008, from www.lds.org

Fontaine, K. L. (2005). *Healing practices: Alternative therapies for nursing practice* (2nd ed.). Upper Saddle River, NJ: Prentice-Hall Health.

Friedman, M. M., Bowden, V. R., & Jones, E. G. (2003). *Family nursing: Research, theory, and practice* (5th ed.). Upper Saddle River, NJ: Prentice Hall.

Gannotti, M. E., Kaplan, L. C., Handwerker, W. P., & Groce, N. E. (2004). Cultural influences on health care use: Differences in perceived unmet needs and expectations of providers by Latino and Euro-American parents of children with special health care needs. *Journal of Developmental and Behavioral Pediatrics, 25,* 156–165.

Gedaly-Duff, V., Heims, M. L., & Nielsen, A. E. (2005). Family child health nursing. In S. M. H. Hanson, V. Gedaly-Duff, & J. R. Kaakinen, *Family Health Care Nursing* (3rd ed., pp. 291–321). Philadelphia: F. A. Davis.

Giger, J. N., & Davidhizar, R. E (2008). *Transcultural nursing: Assessment & intervention* (5th ed.). St. Louis: Mosby Elsevier.

Grabowska, C. (2006). Turning the breech using moxibustion. *Midwives: The Official Journal of the Royal College of Midwives, 9*(12), 484–485.

Hammond, M. M., White, C. B., & Fetters, M. D. (2005). Opening cultural doors: Providing culturally sensitive health care to Arab American and American Muslim patients. *American Journal of Obstetrics & Gynecology, 193*(4), 1307–1311.

Hufton, E. (2006). Parting gifts: The spiritual needs of children. *Journal of Child Health Care,* 10 (3), 240–250.

Jirwe, M., Gerrish, K., & Emami, A. (2006). The theoretical framework of cultural competence. *The Journal of Multicultural Nursing & Health, 12*(3), 6–16.

Kemper, K. J., & Cohen, M. (2004). Ethics meet compementary and alternative medicine: New light on old principles. *Contemporary Pediatrics, 21*(3), 61–72.

Kim, Y. O. R. (2004). Access to hepatitis B vaccination among Korean American children in immigrant families. *Journal of Health Care for the Poor and Underserved, 15,* 170–174.

Mattson, S., & Smith, J. E. (2004). *Core curriculum for maternal-newborn nursing* (3rd ed.). Philadelphia: Saunders.

National Center for Complementary and Alternative Medicine. (2005). Prayer and Spirituality in Health: Ancient Practices, Modern Science. *CAM at the NIH: Focus on complementary and alternative medicine,* XII(1). Retrieved July 1, 2007, from http://nccam.nih.gov/news/newsletter/2005_winter/prayer.htm

National Center for Complementary and Alternative Medicine (NCCAM). (2007a). *What is CAM?* (NCCAM Publication No. D347). Retrieved July 1, 2007, from http://nccam.nih.gov

National Center for Complementary and Alternative Medicine. (2007b). *Backgrounder: Manipulative and body-based practices: An overview.* Retrieved January 4, 2008, from http://nccam.nih.gov

National Center for Complementary and Alternative Medicine. (2007c). *The use of CAM in the United States.* Retrieved January 4, 2008, from http://nccam.nih.gov

Pawelski, J. G., Perrin, E. D., Foy, J. M., Crawford, J., Del Monte, M., Kaufman, M., et al. (2006). The effects of marriage, civil union, and domestic partnership laws on the health and well-being of children. *Pediatrics, 118*(1), 349–364.

Post-White, J., Fitzgerald, M., Hageness, S., & Sencer, S. F. (2009). Complementary and alternative medicine use in children with cancer and general and specialty pediatrics. *Journal of Pediatric Oncology Nursing, 26*(1), 7–15.

Purnell, L. D., & Paulanka, B. J. (2005). *Guide to culturally competent health care.* Philadephia: F. A. Davis.

Radzyminski, S. (2007). Legal parameters of alternative-complementary modalities in nursing practice. *Nursing Clinics of North America, 42,* 189–212.

Roy, L. C., Torrez, C., & Dale, J. C. (2004). Ethnicity, traditional health beliefs, and health-seeking behavior: Guardians' attitudes regarding their children's medical treatment. *Journal of Pediatric Health Care, 18,* 22–30.

Safadi, R. (2005). Jordanian women: Perceptions and practices of first-time pregnancy. *International Journal of Nursing Practice, 11*(6), 269–276.

Semenic, S. E., Callister, L. C., & Feldman, P. (2004). Giving birth: The voices of Orthodox Jewish women living in Canada. *Journal of Obstetric, Gynecologic, and Neonatal Nursing, 33*(1), 80–87.

Shi, L., & Stevens, G. D. (2005). Disparities in access to care and satisfaction among U.S. children: The roles of race/ethnicity and poverty status. *Public Health Reports, 120*(4), 431–441.

Spector, R. E. (2009). *Cultural diversity in health and illness* (7th ed.). Upper Saddle River, NJ: Pearson Prentice Hall.

U.S. Census Bureau (2008). Definition: household and family. Retrieved September 20, 2008, from http://ask.census.gov

U.S. Department of Health and Human Services: Office of Minority Health. (2005). *What is cultural competency?* Retrieved September 20, 2008, from www.hhs.gov

Yearwood, E. L. (2007). Child health care decision making and experiences of Caribbean women. *Journal of Pediatric Health Care, 21*(2), 89–98.

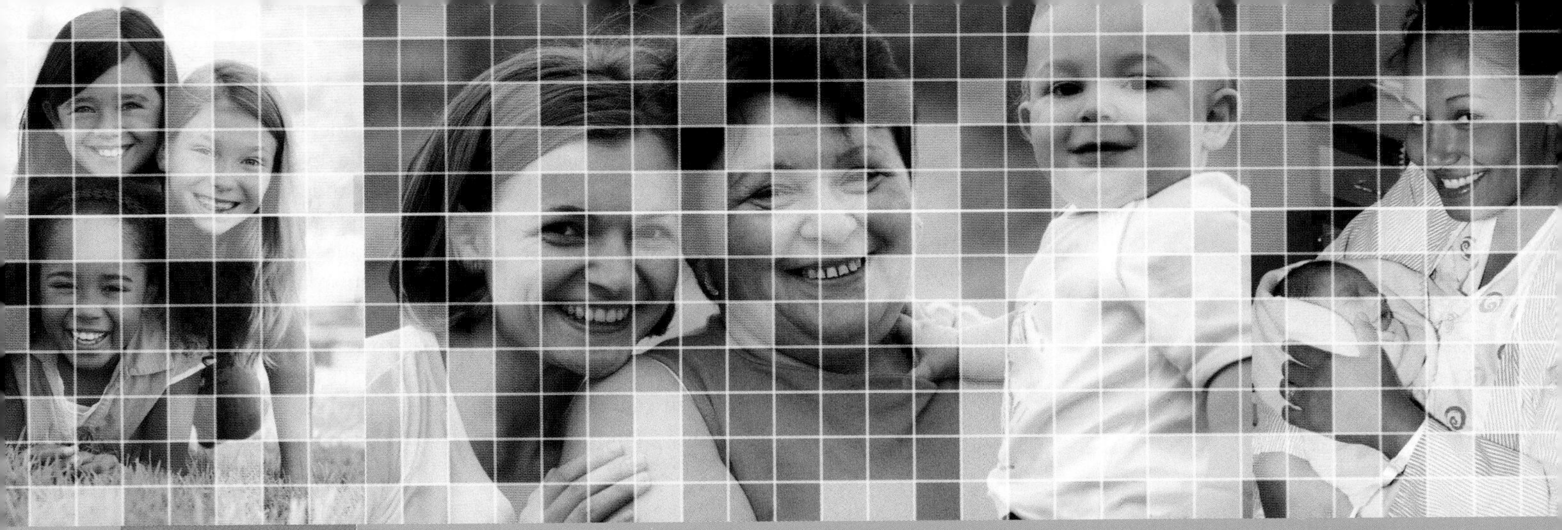

CHAPTER

3 Reproductive Anatomy and Physiology

I am amazed by how little many of our students know about anatomy, physiology, and reproduction. As nurses, we must use every opportunity we have to teach young people about their bodies and those of their partners. Information is the key to helping keep them safe and well! —University Health Clinic Nurse

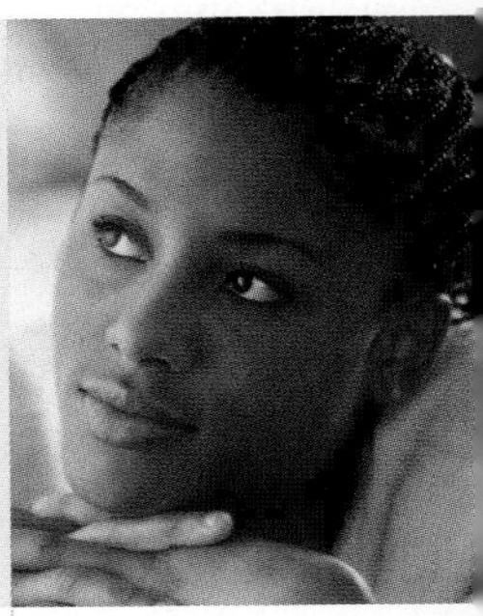

LEARNING OUTCOMES

3.1 Identify the structures and functions of the female reproductive system.

3.2 Identify the structures and functions of the male reproductive system.

3.3 Discuss the significance of specific female reproductive structures during childbirth.

3.4 Summarize the actions of the hormones that affect reproductive functioning.

3.5 Identify the two phases of the ovarian cycle and the changes that occur in each phase.

3.6 Describe the phases of the uterine (menstrual) cycle, their dominant hormones, and the changes that occur in each phase.

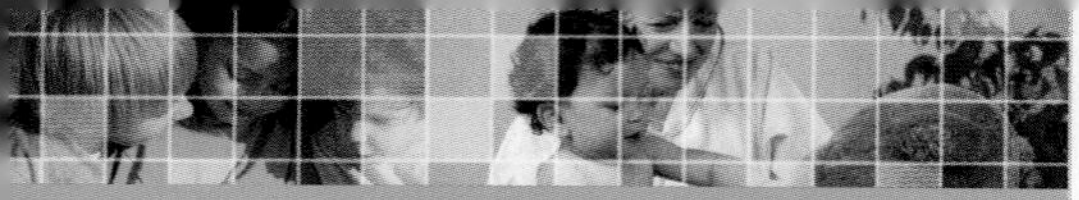

KEY TERMS

Ampulla, 47
Areola, 52
Breasts, 52
Broad ligament, 46
Cardinal ligaments, 46
Cervix, 46
Conjugate vera, 51
Cornua, 45
Corpus, 45
Corpus luteum, 54
Diagonal conjugate, 50
Endometrium, 46
Estrogens, 52
Fallopian tubes, 47
False pelvis, 49
Female reproductive cycle (FRC), 52
Fimbria, 47
Follicle-stimulating hormone (FSH), 40
Fundus, 45
Gonadotropin-releasing hormone (GnRH), 40
Graafian follicle, 55
Human chorionic gonadotropin (hCG), 55
Infundibulopelvic ligament, 46
Ischial spines, 48
Isthmus, 45
Luteinizing hormone (LH), 40
Myometrium, 45
Nidation, 45
Nipple, 52
Obstetric conjugate, 50
Ovarian ligaments, 46
Ovaries, 48
Ovulation, 54
Pelvic cavity, 49
Pelvic diaphragm, 49
Pelvic inlet, 50
Pelvic outlet, 51
Perimetrium, 45
Perineal body, 42
Progesterone, 54
Prostaglandins (PGs), 54
Pubis, 49
Puberty, 40
Round ligaments, 46
Sacral promontory, 49
Spermatogenesis, 58
Symphysis pubis, 49
Testosterone, 58
Transverse diameter, 51
True pelvis, 49
Uterosacral ligaments, 47
Uterus, 44
Vagina, 43
Vulva, 41

MyNursingKit Activity: Female Reproductive System

Understanding childbearing requires more than understanding sexual intercourse, or the process by which the female and male sex cells unite. The nurse must also become familiar with the structures and functions that make childbearing possible and the phenomena that initiate it. This chapter presents the anatomic and physiologic aspects of the female and male reproductive systems. Chapter 5∞ discusses the sexual and psychosocial aspects of human sexuality.

The female and male reproductive organs are *homologous;* that is, they are fundamentally similar in structure and function. The primary functions of both female and male reproductive systems are to produce sex cells and transport them to locations where their union can occur. The sex cells, called *gametes,* are produced by specialized organs called *gonads.* A series of ducts and glands within both male and female reproductive systems contributes to the production and transport of the gametes.

PUBERTY

The term **puberty** refers to the developmental period between childhood and attainment of adult sexual characteristics and functioning. Generally boys mature physically about two years later than girls. The age at onset and progress of puberty vary widely, physical changes overlap, and the sequence of events can vary from person to person. (For a detailed discussion of physical changes associated with puberty, see Chapter 35∞.) This diversity results from each individual's response to hormonal stimulation.

PHYSIOLOGY OF ONSET

Puberty is initiated by the maturation of the hypothalamic-pituitary-gonad complex (the *gonadostat*) and input from the central nervous system. The process, which begins during fetal life, is sequential and complex.

The central nervous system releases a neurotransmitter that stimulates the hypothalamus to synthesize and release **gonadotropin-releasing hormone (GnRH)**. GnRH is transmitted to the anterior pituitary, where it causes the synthesis and secretion of the gonadotropins **follicle-stimulating hormone (FSH)** and **luteinizing hormone (LH)** (Figure 3–1 ●).

Although the gonads do produce small amounts of *androgens* (male sex hormones) and *estrogens* (female sex hormones) before the onset of puberty, FSH and LH stimulate increased secretion of these hormones. Androgens and estrogens influence the development of secondary sex characteristics. FSH and LH stimulate the processes of spermatogenesis and maturation of ova.

Other hormones are involved in the onset of puberty. Although these hormones have a less direct effect, their action is essential. Abnormally high or low levels of adrenocorticotropic hormone (ACTH), thyroid hormone, or growth hormone (GH) can disrupt the onset of normal puberty (see Chapter 55∞ for a detailed discussion). The maturation process, beginning during fetal life development continues through puberty and the childbearing years. The external and internal female reproductive organs develop and mature in response to estrogen and progesterone.

FEMALE REPRODUCTIVE SYSTEM

The female reproductive system consists of the external and internal genitals and the accessory organs of the breasts. Because of its importance to childbearing, the bony pelvis is also discussed in this chapter.

EXTERNAL GENITALS

All the external reproductive organs except the glandular structures can be directly inspected. The appearance of the external genitalia varies greatly among women.

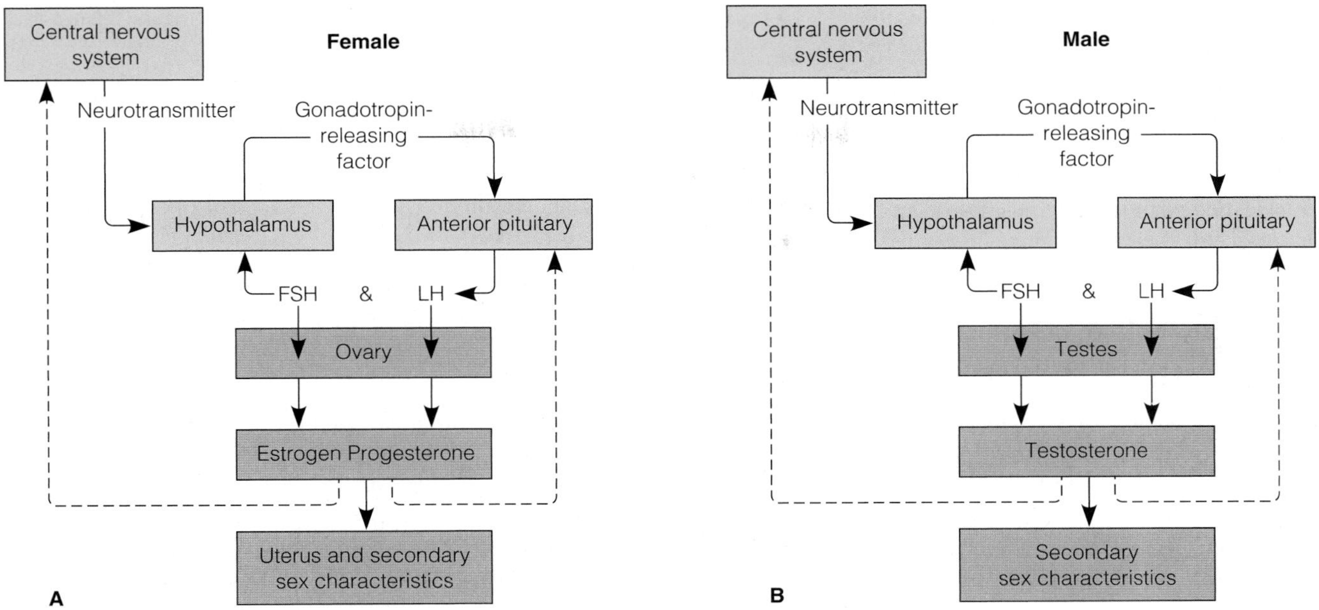

● **Figure 3–1** Physiologic changes leading to onset of puberty. ***A,*** In females, and ***B,*** in males. Solid lines illustrate stimulation of hormone production, and broken lines illustrate inhibition. Through a neurotransmitter the central nervous system stimulates the hypothalamus, which in turn produces a gonadotropin-releasing factor that causes the anterior pituitary to produce gonadotropins (follicle-stimulating hormone, FSH; or luteinizing hormone, LH). These hormones stimulate specific structures in the gonads to secrete steroid hormones (estrogen, progesterone, or testosterone). The rise in pituitary hormone production increases hypothalamus activity. Elevated steroid hormone levels stimulate the central nervous system and pituitary gland to inhibit hormone production.

Heredity, age, race, and the number of children a woman has borne influence the size, color, and shape of her external organs. The female external genitals, also referred to as the **vulva**, include the following structures (Figure 3–2 ●).

- Mons pubis
- Labia majora
- Labia minora
- Clitoris
- Urethral meatus and opening of the paraurethral (Skene's) glands
- Vaginal vestibule (vaginal orifice, vulvovaginal [Bartholin] glands, hymen, and fossa navicularis)
- Perineal body

Although they are not true parts of the female reproductive system, the urethral meatus and perineal body are considered here because of their proximity and relationship to the vulva. The vulva has a generous supply of blood and nerves. As a woman ages, estrogen secretions decrease, causing the vulvar organs to atrophy.

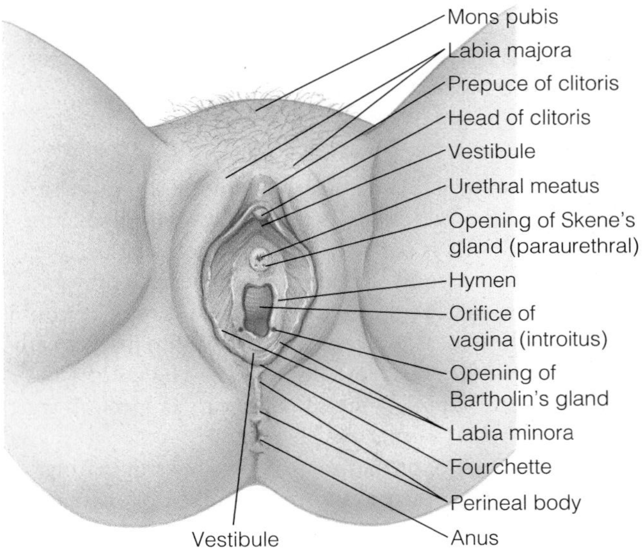

● **Figure 3–2** Female external genitals, longitudinal view.

Mons Pubis

The *mons pubis* is a softly rounded mound of subcutaneous fatty tissue beginning at the lowest portion of the anterior abdominal wall (see Figure 3–2). Also known as the *mons veneris,* this structure covers the front portion of the symphysis pubis. The mons pubis is covered with pubic hair, typically with the hairline forming a transverse line across the lower abdomen. The hair is short and varies from sparse and fine in Asian women to heavy, coarse, and curly in women of African descent. The mons pubis protects the symphysis pubis, especially during coitus.

Labia Majora

The *labia majora* are longitudinal, raised folds of pigmented skin, one on either side of the vulvar cleft. As the pair descend, they narrow and merge to form the posterior junction of the perineal skin. Their chief function is to protect the structures lying between them. The labia majora are covered by hair follicles and sebaceous glands, with underlying adipose and muscle tissue. The inner surface of the labia majora in women who have not had children is moist and looks like mucous membrane, whereas after many births it is more skinlike. With each pregnancy, the labia majora may become less prominent.

Because of the extensive venous network in the labia majora, varicosities may occur during pregnancy, and obstetric or sexual trauma may cause hematomas. The labia majora share an extensive lymphatic supply with the other structures of the vulva, which can facilitate the spread of cancer in the female reproductive organs. Because of the nerves supplying the labia majora (from the first lumbar and third sacral segment of the spinal cord), certain regional anesthesia blocks will affect them and cause numbness.

Labia Minora

The *labia minora* are soft folds of skin within the labia majora that converge near the anus, forming the *fourchette.* Each labium minus has the appearance of shiny mucous membrane, moist and devoid of hair follicles. The labia minora are rich in sebaceous glands, which lubricate and waterproof the vulvar skin and provide bactericidal secretions. Because the sebaceous glands do not open into hair follicles but open directly onto the surface of the skin, sebaceous cysts commonly occur in this area. Vulvovaginitis in this area is irritating because the labia minora have many tactile nerve endings. The labia minora increase in size at puberty and decrease after menopause because of changes in estrogen levels.

Clitoris

The *clitoris,* located between the labia minora, is about 5 to 6 mm long and 6 to 8 mm across. Its tissue is essentially erectile. The glans of the clitoris is partly covered by a fold of skin called the *prepuce,* or clitoral hood (an extension of the labia minora). This area resembles an opening to an orifice and may be confused with the urethral meatus. Accidental attempts to insert a catheter in this area produce extreme discomfort. The clitoris has rich blood and nerve supplies and is the primary erogenous organ of women. It secretes *smegma,* which along with other vulval secretions has a unique odor that may be sexually stimulating to the male. In some cultures, the clitoris is removed (see discussion in Chapter 5∞).

Urethral Meatus and Paraurethral Glands

The *urethral meatus* is located 1 to 2.5 cm beneath the clitoris in the midline of the vestibule; it often appears as a puckered, slitlike opening. At times the meatus is difficult to visualize because of the presence of blind dimples, small mucosal folds, or wide variations in location.

The paraurethral glands, or *Skene's glands,* open into the posterior wall of the urethra close to its opening (see Figure 3–2). Their secretions lubricate the vaginal opening, facilitating sexual intercourse.

Vaginal Vestibule

The vaginal vestibule is a boat-shaped depression enclosed by the labia majora and minora, which is visible when they are separated. The vestibule contains the vaginal opening, or *introitus,* which is the border between the external and internal genitals.

The *hymen* is a thin, elastic collar or semicollar of tissue that surrounds the vaginal opening. The appearance changes during the woman's lifetime. At birth, the hymen is essentially avascular. For thousands of years, some societies have perpetuated the belief that the hymen covers the vaginal opening and thus an intact hymen is a sign of virginity. However, modern studies of female genital anatomy have revealed that the hymen surrounds rather than entirely covers the vaginal opening, and can be torn not only through sexual intercourse but also through strenuous physical activity, masturbation, menstruation, or the use of tampons, thus dispelling old beliefs. For discussion of the nurse's role in discussing these topics see Chapter 5∞.

External to the hymen at the base of the vestibule are two small papular elevations containing the openings of the ducts of the *vulvovaginal (Bartholin's) glands.* They lie under the constrictor muscle of the vagina. These glands secrete a clear, thick, alkaline mucus that enhances the viability and motility of the sperm deposited in the vaginal vestibule. These gland ducts can harbor *Neisseria gonorrhea, Staphylococcus aureus,* and other bacteria, which can cause pus formation and abscesses in the Bartholin's glands.

The vestibular area is innervated predominantly by the perineal nerve from the sacral plexus. The area is not sensitive to touch generally; however, the hymen contains numerous free nerve endings as receptors to pain.

Perineal Body

The **perineal body** is a wedge-shaped mass of fibromuscular tissue found between the lower part of the vagina and the anus (Figure 3–2). The superficial area between the anus and the vagina is referred to as the *perineum.*

The muscles that meet at the perineal body are the external sphincter ani, both levator ani (the superficial and deep transverse perineal), and the bulbocavernosus. These muscles mingle with elastic fibers and connective tissue in an arrangement that allows a remarkable amount of stretching. During the last part of labor, the perineal body thins out until it is just a few centimeters thick. This tissue is often the site of lacerations or episiotomy during childbirth (see Chapter 23∞).

FEMALE INTERNAL REPRODUCTIVE ORGANS

The female internal reproductive organs—the vagina, uterus, fallopian tubes, and ovaries—are target organs for estrogenic hormones and they play a unique part in the reproductive cycle (Figure 3–3 ●). Certain internal reproductive organs can be palpated during vaginal examination and assessed with various instruments.

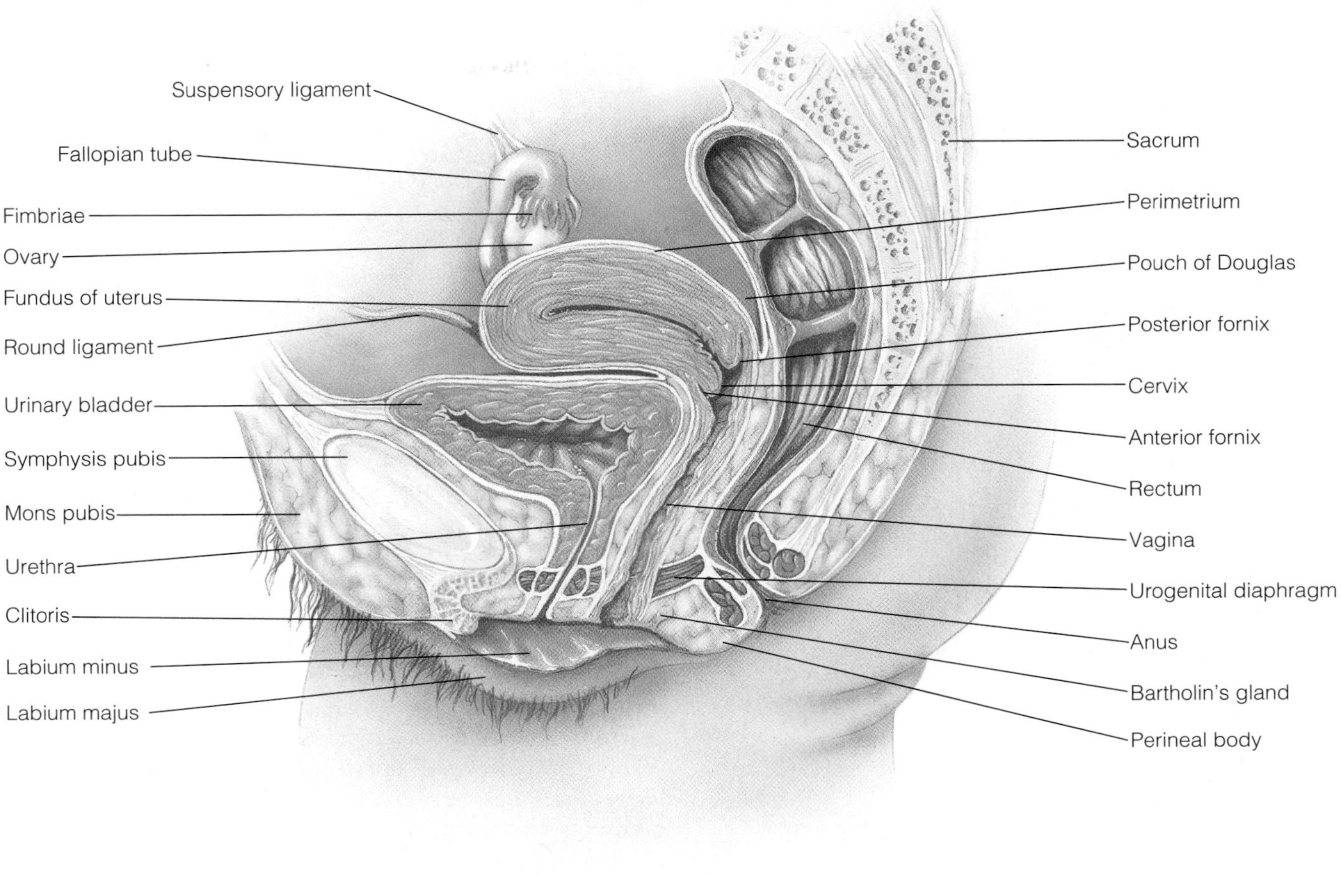

● **Figure 3–3** Female internal reproductive organs.

Vagina

The **vagina** is a muscular and membranous tube that connects the external genitals with the uterus. It extends from the vulva to the uterus in a position nearly parallel to the plane of the pelvic brim. The vagina is often called the *birth canal* because it forms the lower part of the pelvis through which the fetus must pass during birth.

Because the cervix of the uterus projects into the upper part of the anterior wall of the vagina, the anterior wall is approximately 2.5 cm shorter than the posterior wall. Measurements range from 6 to 8 cm for the anterior wall and from 7 to 10 cm for the posterior wall.

In the upper part of the vagina, which is called the *vaginal vault,* there is a recess or hollow around the cervix. This area is called the *vaginal fornix.* Since the walls of the vaginal vault are very thin, various structures can be palpated through the walls, including the uterus, a distended bladder, the ovaries, the appendix, the cecum, the colon, and the ureters. The upper fourth of the vagina is separated from the rectum by the pouch of Douglas (sometimes referred to as the cul-de-sac of Douglas). This deep pouch or recess is posterior to the cervix.

When a woman lies on her back after intercourse, the space in the fornix permits the pooling of semen. The collection of a large number of sperm near the cervix at or near the time of ovulation increases the chances of pregnancy.

The walls of the vagina are covered with ridges, or rugae, crisscrossing each other. These rugae allow the vaginal tissues to stretch enough for the fetus to pass through during childbirth as well as stretch for accommodation during coitus.

During a woman's reproductive life, an acidic vaginal environment is normal (pH 4–5). Secretion from the vaginal epithelium provides a moist environment. The acidic environment is maintained by a symbiotic relationship between lactic acid-producing bacilli (Döderlein bacillus or lactobacillus) and the vaginal epithelial cells. These cells contain glycogen, which is broken down by the bacilli into lactic acid. The amount of glycogen is regulated by the ovarian hormones. Any interruption of this process can destroy the normal self-cleaning action of the vagina. Such interruption may be caused by antibiotic therapy, douching, frequent intercourse, or use of vaginal sprays or deodorants. (For further discussion, see Chapter 5.) The acidic vaginal environment is normal only during the mature reproductive years and in the first days of life, when maternal hormones are operating in the infant. A relatively neutral pH of 7.5 is normal from infancy until puberty and after menopause.

Each third of the vagina is supplied by a distinct vascular pattern (Figure 3–4 ●). In addition to venous drainage going to the heart and lungs, anastomoses of the veins are present and make it possible for a pelvic embolism or carcinoma to bypass the heart and lungs and lodge in the brain, spine, or other remote part of the body.

Vaginal lymphatic fluids drain into the external and internal iliac nodes, the hypogastric nodes, and the inguinal glands. The posterior wall drains into nodes lying in the rectovaginal septum. Any vaginal infection follows these routes.

The pudendal nerve supplies what relatively little somatic innervation there is to the lower third of the vagina. Thus sensation during sexual excitement and coitus is reduced in this area, as is vaginal pain during the second stage of labor.

The vagina has three functions:

- To serve as the passage for sperm and for the fetus during birth
- To provide passage for the menstrual products from the uterine cavity to the outside of the body
- To protect against trauma from sexual intercourse and infection of the uterus, ovaries, and pelvis from pathogenic organisms

Uterus

As the core of reproduction and hence continuation of the human race, the uterus, or womb, has been endowed with a mystical aura. Numerous customs, taboos, mores, and values have evolved about women and their reproductive function. Although scientific knowledge has replaced much of this folklore, remnants of old ideas and superstitions persist. To provide effective care, nurses must be cognizant of their own attitudes and beliefs, as well as those of their clients.

The **uterus** is a hollow, muscular, thick-walled organ shaped like an upside-down pear (Figure 3–5 ●). It lies in the center of the pelvic cavity between the base of the bladder and the rectum and above the vagina. It is level with or slightly below the brim of the pelvis, with the external opening of the

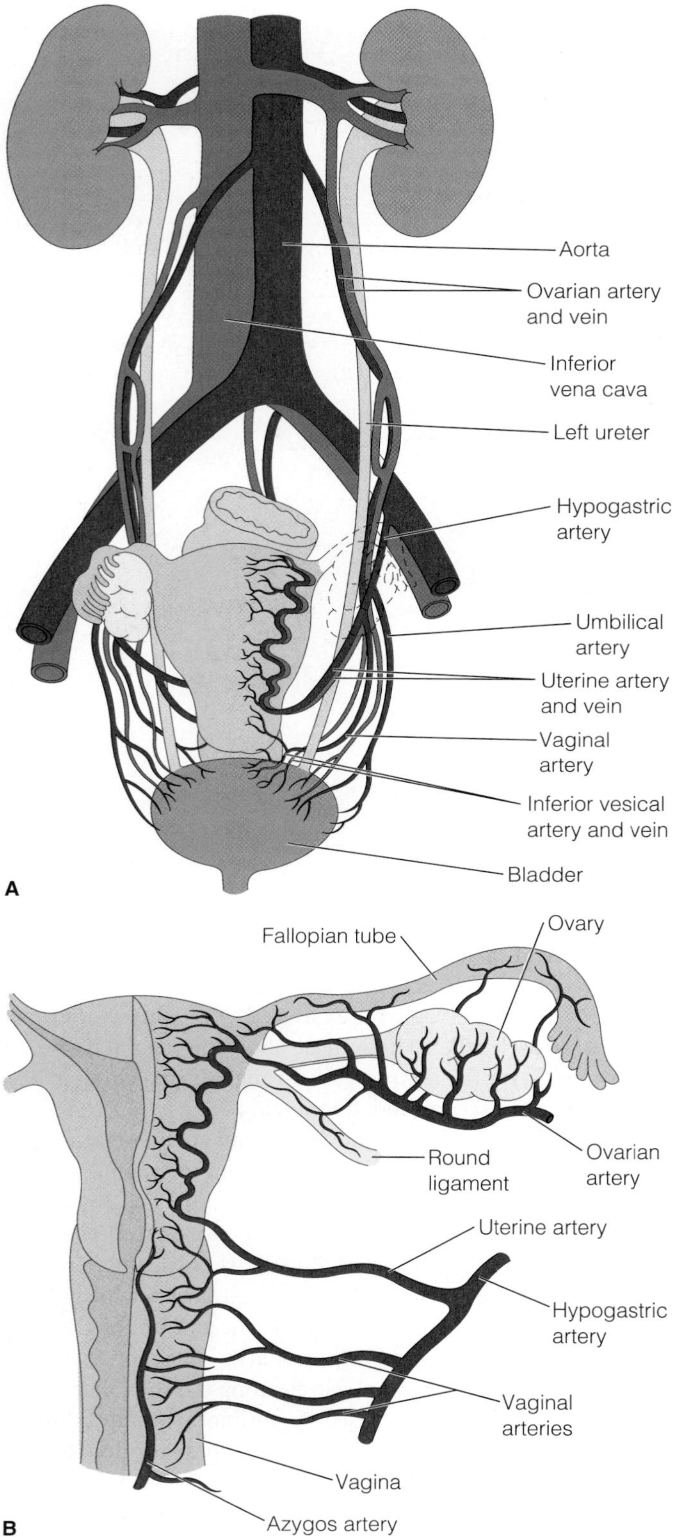

● **Figure 3–4** Blood supply to internal reproductive organs. ***A,*** Pelvic blood supply. ***B,*** Blood supply to vagina, ovaries, uterus, and fallopian tube.

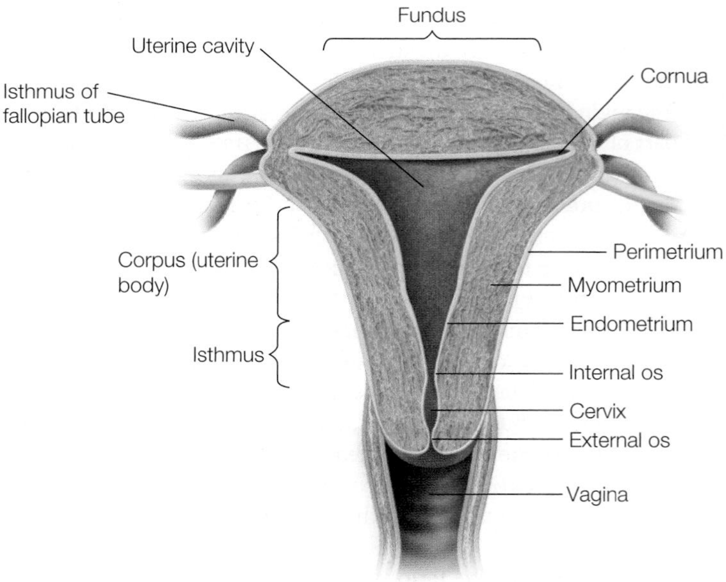

● **Figure 3–5** Structures of the uterus.

cervix (external os) about the level of the ischial spines. The uterus of the mature woman weighs about 40 to 70 g and is 6 to 8 cm long (Krantz, 2007).

The body of the uterus can move freely forward or backward. Only the cervix is anchored laterally. Thus the position of the uterus can vary, depending on a woman's posture and musculature, number of children borne, bladder and rectal fullness, and even normal respiratory patterns. Generally, the uterus bends forward, forming a sharp angle with the vagina. If there is a bend in the area of the isthmus of the uterus and from there the cervix points downward, the uterus is said to be anteverted or anteflexed. Four pairs of ligaments (i.e., the cardinal, uterosacral, round, and broad) support the uterus. Single anterior and posterior ligaments also support the uterus.

The uterus is divided into two major parts: the upper triangular portion called the **corpus**, or uterine body; and the lower cylindric portion called the cervix. The corpus comprises the upper two-thirds of the uterus and is composed mainly of a smooth muscle layer (myometrium). The lower third is the cervix, or neck. The rounded uppermost portion of the corpus that extends above the points of attachment of the fallopian tubes is called the **fundus**. The elongated portion of the uterus where the fallopian tubes enter is called the **cornua**.

The **isthmus** is that portion of the uterus between the internal cervical os and the endometrial cavity. The isthmus is about 6 mm above the uterine opening of the cervix (the internal os), and it is in this area that the uterine lining changes into the mucous membrane of the cervix; it joins the corpus to the cervix. The isthmus takes on importance in pregnancy because it becomes the lower uterine segment. At birth, this thin lower segment, situated behind the bladder, is the site for lower-segment cesarean births (see Chapter 23).

The blood and lymphatic supplies to the uterus are extensive. Innervation of the uterus is entirely by the autonomic nervous system. Even without an intact nerve supply, the uterus can contract adequately for birth; for example, hemiplegic women have adequate uterine contractions.

Pain of uterine contractions is carried to the central nervous system by the 11th and 12th thoracic nerve roots. Pain from the cervix and upper vagina passes through the ilioinguinal and pudendal nerves. The motor fibers to the uterus arise from the 7th and 8th thoracic vertebrae. Because the sensory and motor levels are separate, epidural anesthesia can be used during labor and birth.

The function of the uterus is to provide a safe environment for fetal development. The uterine lining is cyclically prepared by steroid hormones for implantation of the embryo, a process known as **nidation**. Once the embryo is implanted, the developing fetus is protected until it is expelled.

Both the body of the uterus and the cervix are changed permanently by pregnancy. The body never returns to its prepregnant size, and the external os changes from a circular opening of about 3 mm to a transverse slit with irregular edges.

Uterine corpus. The uterine corpus is made up of three layers. The outermost layer is the *serosal layer,* or **perimetrium**, which is composed of peritoneum. The middle layer is the *muscular uterine layer,* or **myometrium**. This muscular uterine layer is continuous with the muscle layers of the fallopian tubes and the vagina. This characteristic helps these organs present a unified reaction to various stimuli—ovulation, orgasm, or the deposit of sperm in the vagina. These muscle fibers also extend into the ovarian, round, and cardinal ligaments and minimally into the uterosacral ligaments, which helps explain the vague but disturbing pelvic "aches and pains" reported by many pregnant women.

The myometrium has three distinct layers of uterine (smooth) involuntary muscles (Figure 3–6 ●). The outer layer, found mainly over the fundus, is made up of longitudinal muscles that cause the descent of the fetus, which places pressure on the cervical fibers leading to cervical effacement and delivery of the fetus. The thick middle layer is made up of interlacing muscle fibers in figure-eight patterns, which assist the longitudinal fibers in expelling the fetus. These muscle fibers also surround large blood vessels, and their contraction produces a hemostatic action (a tourniquet-like action on blood vessels to stop bleeding) after birth. The inner muscle layer consists of circular fibers

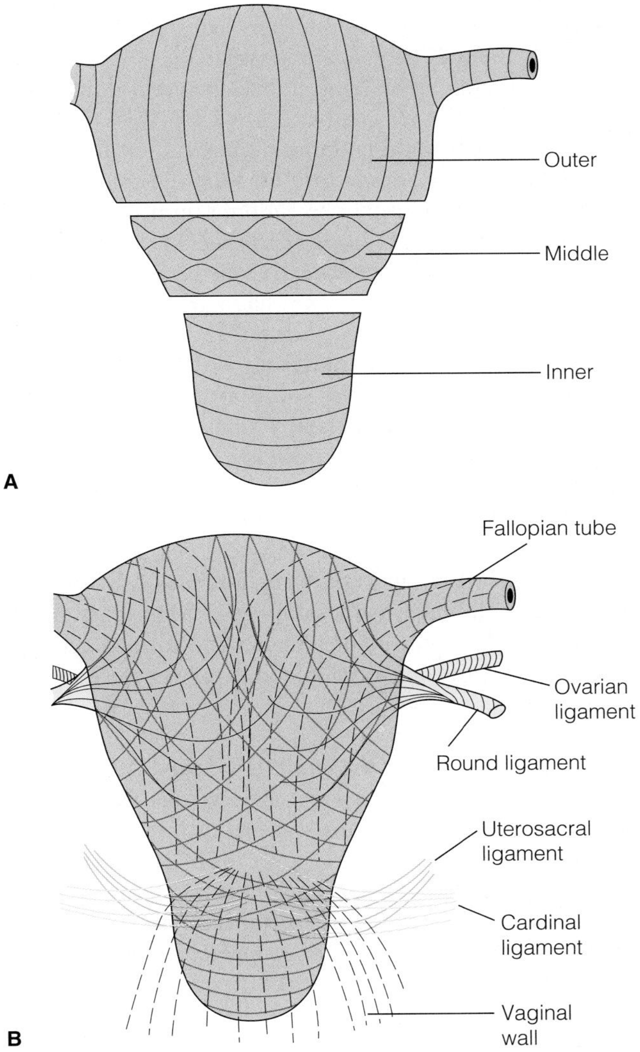

● **Figure 3–6** Uterine muscle layers. ***A,*** Muscle fiber placement. ***B,*** Interlacing of uterine muscle layers.

that form sphincters at the fallopian tube attachment sites and at the internal os. The internal os sphincter inhibits the expulsion of the uterine contents during pregnancy but relaxes in labor as cervical dilatation occurs. An incompetent cervical os can be caused by a torn, weak, or absent sphincter at the internal os. The sphincters at the fallopian tubes prevent menstrual blood from flowing backward into the fallopian tubes from the uterus.

Although each layer of muscle has been discussed as having a unique function, it must be remembered that the uterine musculature works as a whole. The uterine contractions of labor are responsible for the dilatation of the cervix and provide the major force for the passage of the fetus through the pelvis and vaginal canal at birth.

The *mucosal layer,* or **endometrium**, of the uterine corpus is the innermost layer. This single layer consists of columnar epithelium, glands, and stroma. From menarche to menopause, the endometrium undergoes monthly degeneration and renewal in the absence of pregnancy. As it responds to the governing hormonal cycle and prostaglandin influence, the endometrium varies in thickness from 0.5 to 5 mm.

The glands of the endometrium produce a thin, watery, alkaline secretion that keeps the uterine cavity moist. This endometrial milk not only helps sperm travel to the fallopian tubes but also nourishes the developing embryo before it implants in the endometrium (Chapter 4∞).

The blood supply to the endometrium is unique. In the myometrium, the radial arteries branch off from the arcuate arteries at right angles. Once inside the endometrium, they become the basal arteries supplying the zona basalis (a layer of the endometrium) and ultimately become the coiled arteries supplying the zona functionalis (also part of the endometrium). The basal arteries are not sensitive to cyclic hormonal control; hence, the zona basalis portion remains intact and is the site of new endometrial tissue generation. The coiled arteries are extremely sensitive to hormonal control. Their response is alternate relaxation and constriction during the ischemic, or terminal, phase of the menstrual cycle. These differing responses allow part of the endometrium to remain intact while other endometrial tissue is shed during menstruation.

When pregnancy occurs and the endometrium is not shed, the reticular stromal cells surrounding the endometrial glands become the decidual cells of pregnancy. The stromal cells are highly vascular, channeling a rich blood supply to the endometrial surface.

The cervix. The distal end of the uterus is the **cervix**. It meets the body of the uterus at the internal os and descends about 2.5 cm to connect with the vagina at the external os (see Figure 3–3). Thus it provides a protective entrance for the body of the uterus. The cervix is divided by its line of attachment into the vaginal and supravaginal areas. The vaginal cervix projects into the vagina at an angle of from 45 to 90 degrees. The *supravaginal* cervix is surrounded by the attachments that give the uterus its main support: the uterosacral ligaments, the transverse ligaments of the cervix (Mackenrodt's ligaments), and the pubocervical ligaments.

The vaginal cervix appears pink and ends at the external os. The cervical canal appears rosy red and is lined with columnar ciliated epithelium, which contains mucus-secreting glands. Most cervical cancer begins at this *squamocolumnar* junction. The specific location of the junction varies with age and number of pregnancies.

Elasticity is the chief characteristic of the cervix. Its ability to stretch results from both the high fibrous and collagenous content of the supportive tissues and the vast number of folds in the cervical lining.

The cervical mucus has three functions:

- To lubricate the vaginal canal
- To act as a bacteriostatic agent
- To provide an alkaline environment to shelter deposited sperm from the acidic vaginal secretions

At ovulation, cervical mucus is clearer, thinner, more profuse, and more alkaline than at other times.

Uterine Ligaments

The uterine ligaments support and stabilize the various reproductive organs. The ligaments shown in Figure 3–7 ● are described as follows:

1. The **broad ligament** keeps the uterus centrally placed and provides stability within the pelvic cavity. It is a double layer that is continuous with the abdominal peritoneum. The broad ligament covers the uterus anteriorly and posteriorly and extends outward from the uterus to enfold the fallopian tubes. The round and ovarian ligaments are at the upper border of the broad ligament. At its lower border, it forms the cardinal ligaments. Between the folds of the broad ligament are connective tissue, involuntary muscle, blood and lymph vessels, and nerves.
2. The **round ligaments** help the broad ligament keep the uterus in place. The round ligaments arise from the sides of the uterus near the fallopian tube insertions. They extend outward between the folds of the broad ligament, passing through the inguinal ring and canals and eventually fusing with the connective tissue of the labia majora. Made up of longitudinal muscle, the round ligaments enlarge during pregnancy. During labor the round ligaments steady the uterus, pulling downward and forward so that the presenting part of the fetus is moved into the cervix.
3. The **ovarian ligaments** anchor the lower pole of the ovary to the cornua of the uterus. They are surrounded by muscle fibers that allow the ligaments to contract. This contractile ability influences the position of the ovary to some extent, thus helping the fimbriae of the fallopian tubes to "catch" the ovum as it is released each month.
4. The **cardinal ligaments** are the chief uterine supports and suspend the uterus from the side walls of the true pelvis. These ligaments, also known as Mackenrodt's or transverse cervical ligaments, arise from the sides of the pelvic walls and attach to the cervix in the upper vagina. These ligaments prevent uterine prolapse and also support the upper vagina.
5. The **infundibulopelvic ligament** suspends and supports the ovaries. Arising from the outer third of the broad ligament,

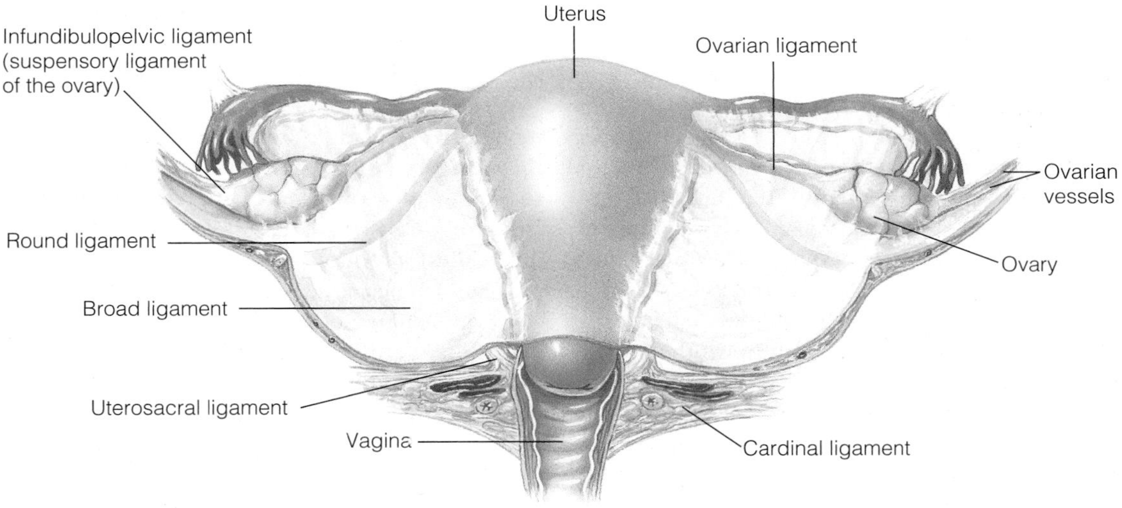

● **Figure 3–7** Uterine ligaments.

the infundibulopelvic ligament contains the ovarian vessels and nerves.

6. The **uterosacral ligaments** provide support for the uterus and cervix at the level of the ischial spines. Arising on each side of the pelvis from the posterior wall of the uterus, the uterosacral ligaments sweep back around the rectum and insert on the sides of the first and second sacral vertebrae. The uterosacral ligaments contain smooth muscle fibers, connective tissue, blood and lymph vessels, and nerves. They also contain sensory nerve fibers that contribute to dysmenorrhea (painful menstruation) (see Chapter 5∞).

Fallopian Tubes

The two **fallopian tubes**, also known as the *oviducts* or *uterine tubes*, arise from each side of the uterus and reach almost to the sides of the pelvis, where they turn toward the ovaries (Figure 3–8 ●). Each tube is approximately 8 to 13.5 cm long. A short section of each fallopian tube is inside the uterus; its opening into the uterus is only 1 mm in diameter. The fallopian tubes link the peritoneal cavity with the uterus and vagina. This linkage increases a woman's biologic vulnerability to disease processes in the pelvis.

Each fallopian tube may be divided into three parts: the *isthmus*, the *ampulla*, and the infundibulum or *fimbria*. The fallopian tube isthmus is straight and narrow, with a thick muscular wall and an opening (lumen) 2 to 3 mm in diameter. It is the site of tubal ligation, a surgical procedure to prevent pregnancy (see Chapter 5∞).

Next to the isthmus is the curved **ampulla**, which comprises the outer third of the tube. Fertilization of the secondary oocyte by a spermatozoon usually occurs here. The ampulla ends at the **fimbria**, which is a funnel-like enlargement with many fingerlike projections (fimbriae) reaching out to the ovary. The longest of

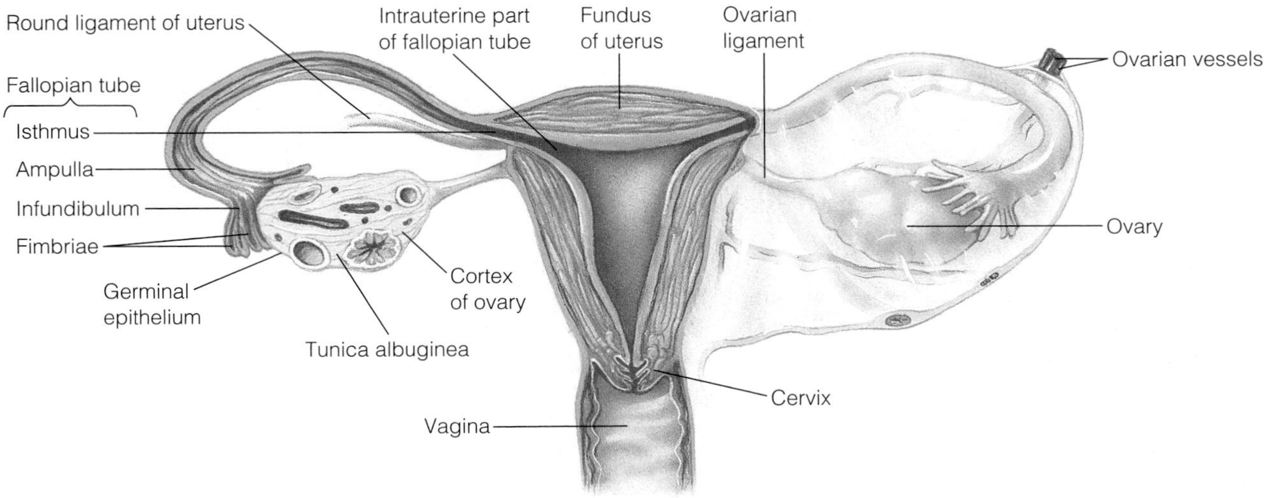

● **Figure 3–8** Fallopian tubes and ovaries.

these, the fimbria ovarica, is attached to the ovary to increase the chances of intercepting the ovum as it is released.

The wall of the fallopian tube consists of four layers: peritoneal (serous), subserous (adventitial), muscular, and mucous tissues. The peritoneum covers the tubes. The subserous layer contains the blood and nerve supply, and the muscular layer is responsible for the peristaltic movement of the tube. The mucosal layer, immediately next to the muscular layer, is composed of ciliated and nonciliated cells, with the number of ciliated cells more abundant at the fimbria. Nonciliated cells secrete a protein-rich, serous fluid that nourishes the ovum. The constantly moving tubal cilia propel the ovum toward the uterus. Because the ovum is a large cell, this ciliary action is needed to assist the tube's muscular layer peristalsis. Any malformation or malfunction of the tubes or cilia can result in infertility, ectopic pregnancy, or even sterility.

A well-functioning tubal transport system involves active fimbriae close to the ovary, peristalsis of the tube created by the muscular layer, ciliated currents beating toward the uterus, and the proximal contraction and distal relaxation of the tube caused by different types of prostaglandins.

A rich blood and lymphatic supply serves each fallopian tube. Thus the tubes have an unusual ability to recover from an inflammatory process (see Figure 3–4). The fallopian tubes have three functions:

- To provide transport for the ovum from the ovary to the uterus (transport time through the fallopian tubes varies from 3 to 4 days)
- To provide a site for fertilization
- To serve as a warm, moist, nourishing environment for the ovum or zygote (fertilized egg). (See Chapter 4 ∞ for further discussion.)

Ovaries

The **ovaries** are two almond-shaped structures just below the pelvic brim. One ovary is located on each side of the pelvic cavity. Their size varies among women and with the stage of the menstrual cycle. Each ovary weighs approximately 6 to 10 g and is 1.5 to 3 cm wide, 2 to 5 cm long, and 1 to 1.5 cm thick. The ovaries of girls are small, but they become larger after puberty and then decrease in size following menopause. They also change in appearance from a dull white, smooth-surfaced organ to a pitted gray organ as the woman ages. The pitting appearance on their surface is the result of scarring after ovulation. The ovaries are maintained in their position by the broad, ovarian, and infundibulopelvic ligaments. It is rare for both ovaries to be at the same level in the pelvic cavity.

There is no peritoneal covering for the ovaries. Although this lack of covering assists the mature ovum to erupt, it also allows easier spread of malignant cells from cancer of the ovaries. A single layer of cuboidal epithelial cells, called the germinal epithelium, covers the ovaries. The ovaries are composed of three layers: the tunica albuginea, the cortex, and the medulla. The *tunica albuginea* is dense and dull white and serves as a protective layer. The *cortex* is the main functional part because it contains ova, graafian follicles, corpora lutea, the degenerated corpora lutea (corpora albicantia), and degenerated follicles. The *medulla* is completely surrounded by the cortex and contains the nerves and the blood and lymphatic vessels.

The ovaries are the primary source of two important hormones: estrogen and progesterone. *Estrogens* are associated with those characteristics contributing to femaleness, including breast alveolar lobule growth and duct development. The ovaries secrete large amounts of estrogen, while the adrenal cortex (extraglandular sites) produces minute amounts of estrogen in nonpregnant women and the fat cells produce a secondary estrogen.

Progesterone is often called the *hormone of pregnancy* because it inhibits uterine contractions and relaxes smooth muscle to cause vasodilation allowing pregnancy to be maintained. The placenta is the primary source of progesterone during pregnancy. This hormone also inhibits the action of prolactin in alpha-lactalbumin synthesis, thereby preventing actual lactation during pregnancy (Lawrence & Lawrence, 2009).

The interplay between the ovarian hormones and other hormones such as follicle-stimulating hormone (FSH) and luteinizing hormone (LH) is responsible for the cyclic changes that allow pregnancy to occur. The hormonal and physical changes that occur during the female reproductive cycle are discussed in depth later in this chapter. Between the ages of 45 and 55, a woman's ovaries secrete decreasing amounts of estrogen. Eventually, ovulatory activity ceases and menopause occurs.

BONY PELVIS

The female bony pelvis has two unique functions:

- To support and protect the pelvic contents
- To form the relatively fixed axis of the birth passage

Because the pelvis is so important to childbearing, its structure must be understood clearly.

Bony Structure

The pelvis is made up of four bones: two innominate bones, the sacrum, and the coccyx. The pelvis resembles a bowl or basin; its sides are the innominate bones, and its back is the sacrum and coccyx. Lined with fibrocartilage and held tightly together by pelvic ligaments (Figure 3–9 ●), the four bones join at the symphysis pubis, the two sacroiliac joints, and the sacrococcygeal joints.

The *innominate bones,* also known as the hip bones, are made up of three separate bones: the ilium, ischium, and pubis. These bones fuse to form a circular cavity, the *acetabulum,* which articulates with the femur.

The *ilium* is the broad, upper prominence of the hip. The iliac crest is the margin of the ilium. The ischial spines, the foremost projections nearest the groin, are the site of attachment for ligaments and muscles.

The *ischium,* the strongest bone, is under the ilium and below the acetabulum. The L-shaped ischium ends in a marked protuberance, the ischial tuberosity, on which the weight of a seated body rests. The **ischial spines** arise near the junction of the ilium and ischium and jut into the pelvic cavity. The shortest diameter of the pelvic cavity is between the ischial spines. The ischial spines serve as reference points during labor to eval-

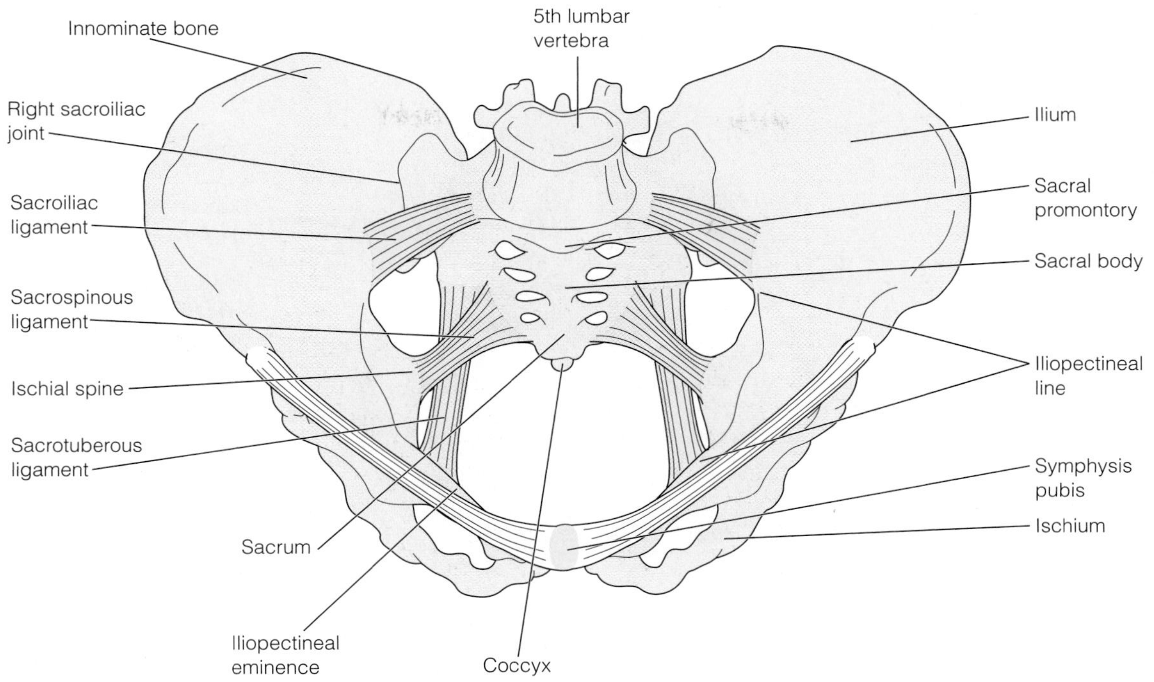

● **Figure 3–9** Pelvic bones with supporting pelvic ligaments.

uate the descent of the fetal head into the birth canal (see Chapter 17 and Figure 17–8∞).

The **pubis** forms the slightly bowed front portion of the innominate bone. Extending medially from the acetabulum to the midpoint of the bony pelvis, each pubis meets the other to form a joint called the **symphysis pubis**. The triangular space below this junction is known as the pubic arch. The fetal head passes under this arch during birth. The symphysis pubis is formed by heavy fibrocartilage and the superior and inferior pubic ligaments. The mobility of the inferior ligament increases during a first pregnancy and to a greater extent in subsequent pregnancies.

The sacroiliac joints also have a degree of mobility that increases near the end of pregnancy as the result of an upward, gliding movement. The pelvic outlet may be increased by 1.5 to 2 cm in the squatting and sitting positions. Relaxation of the pelvic joints is induced by relaxin, one of the hormones of pregnancy.

The *sacrum* is a wedge-shaped bone formed by the fusion of five vertebrae. The anterior upper portion of the sacrum has a projection into the pelvic cavity known as the **sacral promontory**. This projection is another obstetric guide in determining pelvic measurements. (For a discussion of pelvic measurements, see Chapter 10∞.)

The small triangular bone last on the vertebral column is the coccyx. It articulates with the sacrum at the sacrococcygeal joint. The coccyx usually moves backward during labor to provide more room for the fetus.

Pelvic Floor

The muscular floor of the bony pelvis is designed to overcome the force of gravity exerted on the pelvic organs. It acts as a buttress to the irregularly shaped pelvic outlet, thereby providing stability and support for surrounding structures.

Deep fascia, the levator ani, and coccygeal muscles form the part of the pelvic floor known as the **pelvic diaphragm**. The components of the pelvic diaphragm function as a whole, yet they are able to move over one another. This feature provides an exceptional capacity for relaxation during birth and return to prepregnancy condition following birth. Above the pelvic diaphragm is the pelvic cavity; below and behind it is the perineum.

The levator ani muscle makes up the major portion of the pelvic diaphragm and consists of four muscles: the iliococcygeus, pubococcygeus, puborectalis, and pubovaginalis. The iliococcygeal muscle, a thin muscular sheet underlying the sacrospinous ligament, helps the levator ani support the pelvic organs. Muscles of the pelvic floor are shown in Figure 3–10 ● and discussed in Table 3–1.

Pelvic Division

The **pelvic cavity** is divided into the false pelvis and the true pelvis (Figure 3–11A ●). The **false pelvis**, the portion above the pelvic brim, or linea terminalis, serves to support the weight of the enlarged pregnant uterus and direct the presenting fetal part into the true pelvis below.

The **true pelvis** is the portion that lies below the linea terminalis. The bony circumference of the true pelvis is made up of the sacrum, coccyx, and innominate bones and represents the bony limits of the birth canal. The relationship between the true pelvis and the fetal head is of paramount importance: The size and shape of the true pelvis must be adequate for normal fetal passage during labor and at birth. The true pelvis consists of three

MyNursingKit Animation: 3-D Female Pelvis

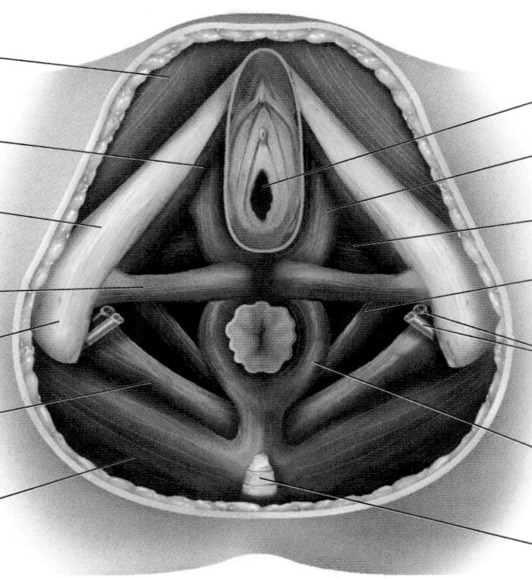

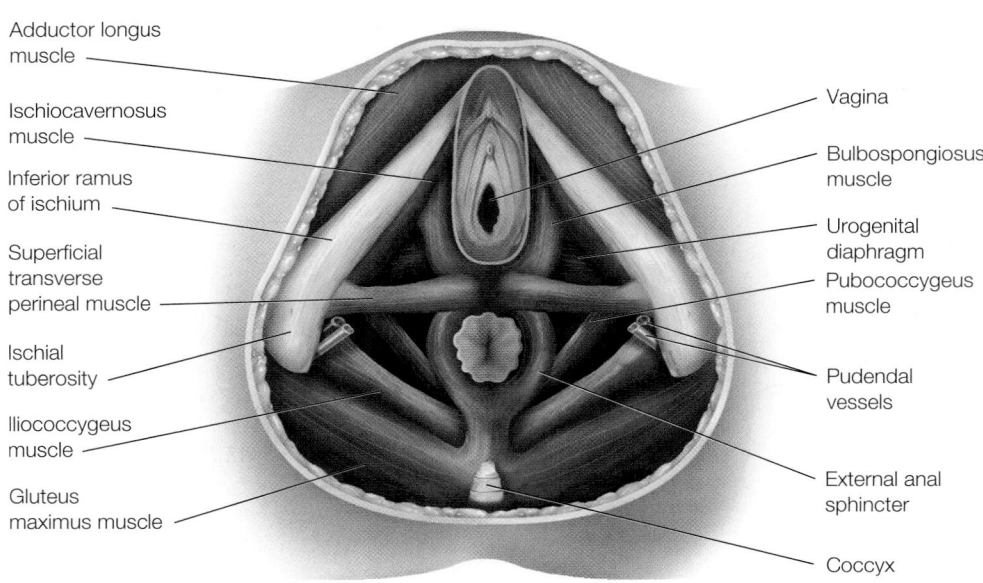

● **Figure 3–10** Muscles of the pelvic floor. (The puborectalis, pubovaginalis, and coccygeal muscles cannot be seen from this view.)

Table 3–1 Muscles of the Pelvic Floor

Muscle	Origin	Insertion	Innervation	Action
Levator ani	Pubis, lateral pelvic wall, and ischial spine	Blends with organs in pelvic cavity	Inferior rectal, second, and third sacral nerves, plus anterior rami of third and fourth sacral nerves	Supports pelvic viscera; helps form pelvic diaphragm
Iliococcygeus	Pelvic surface of ischial spine and pelvic fascia	Central point of perineum, coccygeal raphe, and coccyx		Assists in supporting abdominal and pelvic viscera
Pubococcygeus	Pubis and pelvic fascia	Coccyx		Forms part of levator ani and pelvic diaphragm
Puborectalis	Pubis	Blends with rectum; meets similar fibers from opposite side		Forms sling for rectum, just posterior to it; raises anus
Pubovaginalis	Pubis	Blends into vagina		Supports vagina
Coccygeus	Ischial spine and sacrospinous ligament	Lateral border of lower sacrum and upper coccyx	Third and fourth sacral nerves	Supports pelvic viscera; helps form pelvic diaphragm; flexes and abducts coccyx

parts: the inlet, the pelvic cavity, and the outlet (Figure 3–11B ●). Each part has distinct measurements that aid in evaluating the adequacy of the pelvis for childbirth. Measurement techniques are discussed in Chapter 10. The effects of inadequate or abnormal pelvic diameters on labor and birth are considered in Chapter 18.

The **pelvic inlet** is the upper border of the true pelvis and is typically rounded. Its size and shape are determined by assessing three anteroposterior diameters. The **diagonal conjugate** extends from the subpubic angle to the middle of the sacral promontory and is typically 12.5 cm. The diagonal conjugate can be measured manually during a pelvic examination. The **obstetric conjugate**

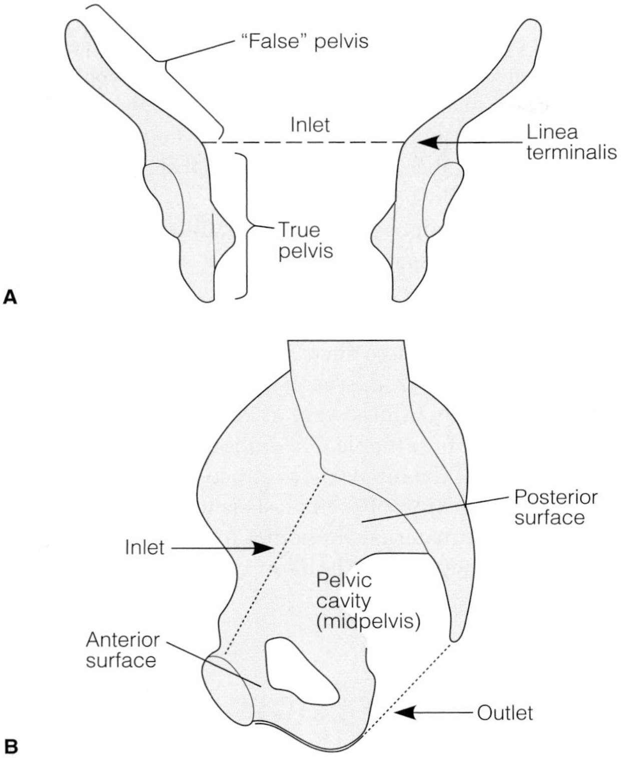

● **Figure 3–11** Female pelvis. ***A,*** False pelvis is a shallow cavity above the inlet; true pelvis is the deeper portion of the cavity below the inlet. ***B,*** True pelvis consists of inlet, cavity (midpelvis), and outlet.

extends from the middle of the sacral promontory to an area approximately 1 cm below the pubic crest. Its length is estimated by subtracting 1.5 cm from the length of the diagonal conjugate (Figure 3–12 ●). The fetus passes through the obstetric conjugate, and the size of this diameter determines whether the fetus can move down into the birth canal in order for engagement to occur. The true (anatomic) conjugate, or **conjugate vera**, extends from the middle of the sacral promontory to the middle of the pubic crest (superior surface of the symphysis). One additional measurement, the transverse diameter, helps determine the shape of the inlet. The **transverse diameter** is the largest diameter of the inlet and is measured by using the linea terminalis as the point of reference.

The *pelvic cavity* (canal) is a curved canal with a longer posterior than anterior wall. A change in the lumbar curve can increase or decrease the tilt of the pelvis and can influence the progress of labor because the fetus has to adjust itself to this curved path as well as to the different diameters of the true pelvis (see Figure 3–11B).

The **pelvic outlet** is at the lower border of the true pelvis. The size of the pelvic outlet can be determined by assessing the outlet *transverse diameter*. The anteroposterior diameter of the pelvic outlet increases during birth as the presenting part pushes the coccyx posteriorly at the mobile sacrococcygeal joint. Decreased mobility, a large head, and/or a forceful birth can cause the coccyx to break. As the infant's head emerges, the long diameter of the head (occipital frontal) parallels the long diameter of the outlet (anteroposterior).

The outlet transverse diameter *(bi-ischial or intertuberous)* extends from the inner surface of one ischial tuberosity to the other. It is the shortest diameter of the pelvic outlet and becomes even shorter if the woman has a narrowed pubic arch. The pubic arch is of great importance because the fetus must pass under it during birth. If it is narrow, the baby's head may be pushed backward

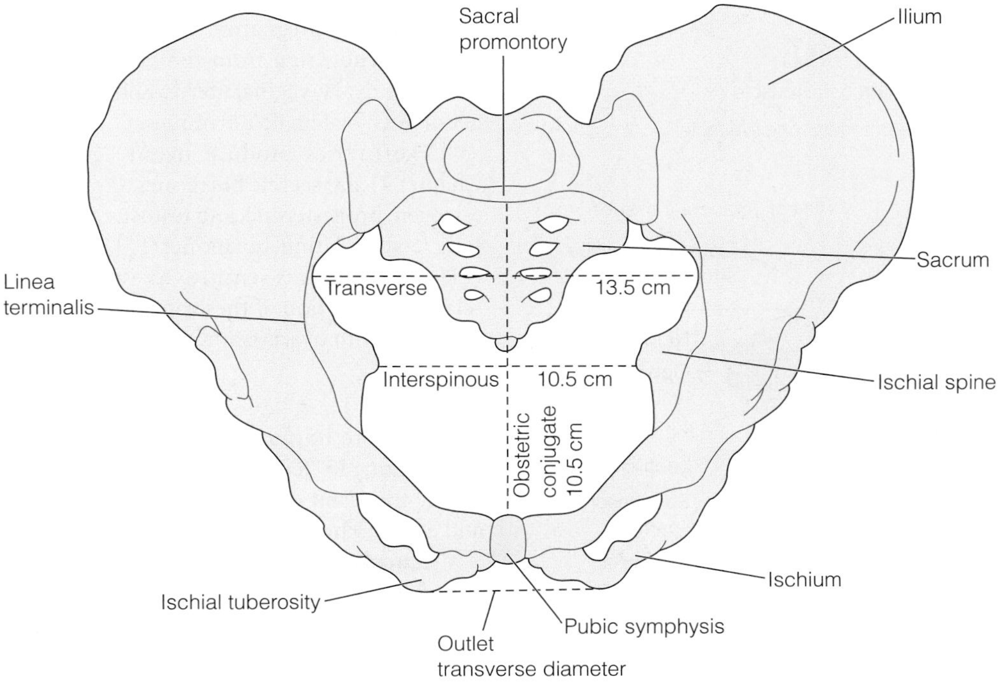

● **Figure 3–12** Pelvic planes: coronal section and diameters of the bony pelvis.

toward the coccyx, making extension of the head difficult. This situation, known as outlet dystocia, may require the use of forceps or a cesarean birth. The shoulders of a large baby may also become wedged under the pubic arch, making birth more difficult (see Chapter 23∞). The clinical assessment of each of these obstetrical diameters is discussed further in Chapter 10∞.

Pelvic Types

The Caldwell–Moloy classification of pelves is widely used to differentiate bony pelvic types (Caldwell & Moloy, 1933). The four basic types are *gynecoid, android, anthropoid*, and *platypelloid* (see Figure 17–1∞). However, variations in the female pelvis are so great that classic types are not usual. Each type has a characteristic shape, and each shape has implications for labor and birth which are discussed in detail in Chapter 22∞.

BREASTS

The **breasts**, or *mammary glands,* considered accessories of the reproductive system, are specialized sebaceous glands (Figure 3–13 ●). They are conical and symmetrically placed on the sides of the chest. The pectoral and anterior serratus muscles underlie each breast. Suspending the breasts are fibrous tissues, called *Cooper's ligaments,* which extend from the deep fascia in the chest outward to just under the skin covering the breast. Frequently, the left breast is larger than the right. In different racial groups breasts develop at slightly different levels in the pectoral region of the chest.

In the center of each mature breast is the **nipple**, a protrusion about 0.5 to 1.3 cm in diameter. The nipple is composed mainly of erectile tissue, which becomes more rigid and prominent during the menstrual cycle, sexual excitement, pregnancy, and lactation. The nipple is surrounded by the heavily pigmented **areola**, which is 2.5 to 10 cm in diameter. Both the nipple and the areola are roughened by small papillae called *tubercles of Montgomery.* As an infant suckles, these tubercles secrete a fatty substance that helps lubricate and protect the breasts.

The breasts are composed of glandular, fibrous, and adipose tissue. The glandular tissue is arranged in a series of 15 to 24 lobes separated by fibrous and adipose tissue. Each lobe is made up of several lobules composed of many alveoli clustered around tiny ducts. The lining of these ducts secretes the various components of milk. The ducts from several lobules merge to form the larger lactiferous ducts, which serve as reservoirs for milk and open on the surface of the nipple. The smooth muscle of the nipple causes erection of the nipple on contraction.

The biologic function of the breasts is to provide nourishment and protective maternal antibodies to infants through the lactation process. They can also be a source of pleasurable sexual sensation.

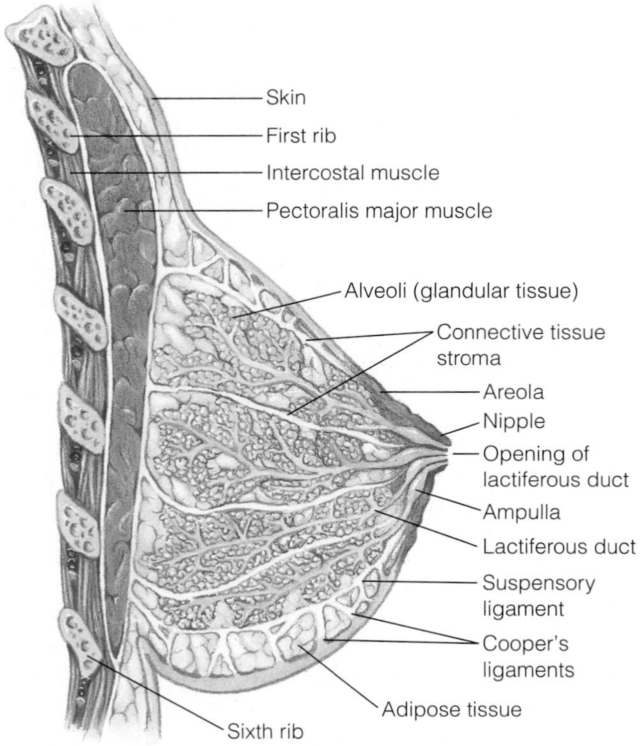

● **Figure 3–13** Anatomy of the breast: sagittal view of left breast.

THE FEMALE REPRODUCTIVE CYCLE

The **female reproductive cycle (FRC)** is composed of the ovarian cycle, during which ovulation occurs, and the uterine cycle, during which menstruation occurs. These two cycles take place simultaneously (Figure 3–14 ●).

EFFECTS OF FEMALE HORMONES

After menarche, a female undergoes a cyclic pattern of ovulation and menstruation for a period of 30 to 40 years. An orderly process under neurohormonal control, this cyclic pattern is disrupted only by pregnancy. Each month multiple oocytes mature, with one rupturing from the ovary, and entering the fallopian tube. The ovary, vagina, uterus, and fallopian tubes are major target organs for female hormones.

The ovaries produce mature gametes (see discussion in Chapter 4) and secrete hormones. Ovarian hormones include the estrogen, progesterone, and testosterone. The ovary is sensitive to follicle-stimulating hormone (FSH) and luteinizing hormone (LH). The uterus is sensitive to estrogen and progesterone. The relative proportion of these hormones to each other controls the events of both ovarian and menstrual cycles.

Estrogens

Estrogens are hormones that are associated with characteristics contributing to "femaleness." The major estrogenic effects are primarily the result of three classical estrogens: estrone, β-estradiol, and estriol. The major estrogen is β-estradiol.

Estrogens control the development of the female secondary sex characteristics: breast development, growth of body hair, widening of the hips, and deposits of tissue (fat) in the buttocks and mons pubis. Estrogens also assist in the maturation of the ovarian follicles and cause the endometrial mucosa to proliferate following menstruation. The amount of estrogens is greatest during the pro-

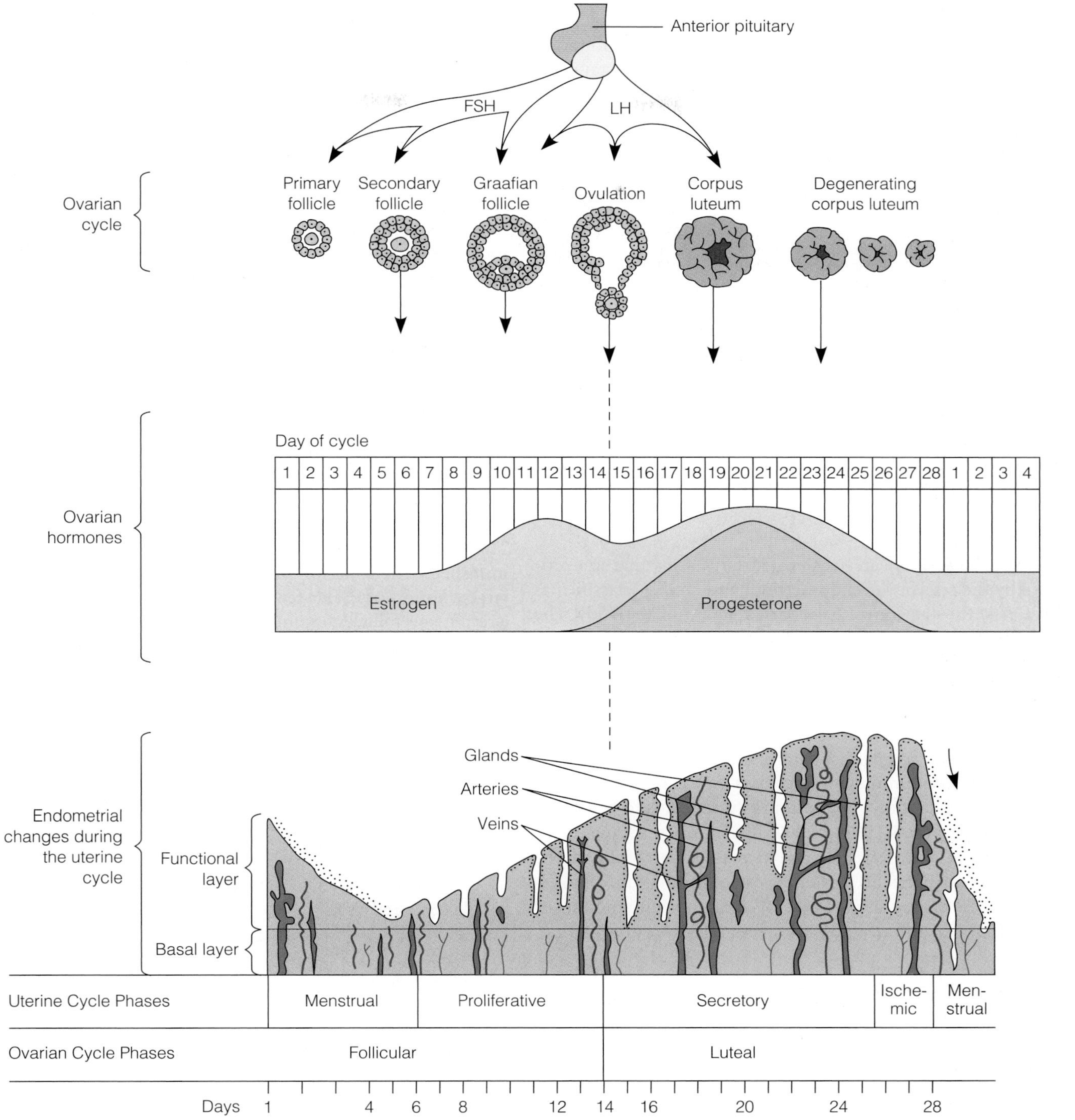

● **Figure 3–14** Female reproductive cycle: interrelationships of hormones with the four phases of the uterine cycle and the two phases of the ovarian cycle in an ideal 28-day cycle.

liferative (follicular or estrogenic) phase of the menstrual cycle. Estrogens also cause the uterus to increase in size and weight because of increased glycogen, amino acids, electrolytes, and water. Blood supply is expanded as well. Under the influence of estrogens, myometrial contractility increases in both the uterus and the fallopian tubes, and uterine sensitivity to oxytocin increases. Estrogens inhibit FSH production and stimulate LH production.

Estrogens have effects on many hormones and other carrier proteins, such as contributing to the increased amount of protein-bound iodine in pregnant women and women who use oral contraceptives containing estrogen. Estrogens may also increase libidinal feelings in humans. They decrease the excitability of the hypothalamus, which may cause an increase in sexual desire.

Progesterone

Progesterone is secreted by the corpus luteum and is found in greatest amounts during the secretory (luteal or progestational) phase of the menstrual cycle. It decreases uterine motility and contractility caused by estrogens, thereby preparing the uterus for implantation after the ovum is fertilized. The endometrial mucosa is in a ready state as a result of estrogenic influence. Progesterone causes the uterine endometrium to further increase its supply of glycogen, arterial blood, secretory glands, amino acids, and water.

This hormone is often called the *hormone of pregnancy* because its effects on the uterus allow pregnancy to be maintained. Under the influence of progesterone, the vaginal epithelium proliferates and the cervix secretes thick, viscous mucus. In the breast, progesterone stimulates development of lobules and alveoli and supports secretory function of the breast during lactation (Ganong, 2007).

The temperature rise of about 0.3°C to 0.6°C (0.5°F to 1.0°F) that accompanies ovulation and persists throughout the secretory phase of the menstrual cycle is due to progesterone.

Prostaglandins

Prostaglandins (PGs) are oxygenated fatty acids that are produced by the cells of the endometrium and are also classified as hormones. Prostaglandins have varied action in the body. The two primary types of prostaglandins are group E and F. Generally PGE relaxes smooth muscles and is a potent vasodilator; PGF is a potent vasoconstrictor and increases the contractility of muscles and arteries. Although the primary actions of PGE and PGF seem antagonistic, their basic regulatory functions in cells are achieved through an intricate pattern of reciprocal events.

Prostaglandin production increases during follicular maturation, is dependent on gonadotropins, and seems to be critical to follicular rupture (Ganong, 2007). Extrusion of the ovum, resulting from follicular swelling and increased contractility of the smooth muscle in the theca externa layer of the mature follicle, is thought to be caused in part by $PGF_{2\alpha}$. Significant amounts of PGs are found in and around the follicle at the time of ovulation.

NEUROHORMONAL BASIS OF THE FEMALE REPRODUCTIVE CYCLE

The female reproductive cycle is controlled by complex interactions between the nervous and endocrine systems and their target tissues. These interactions involve the hypothalamus, anterior pituitary, and ovaries.

The hypothalamus secretes *gonadotropin-releasing hormone (GnRH)* to the pituitary gland in response to signals received from the central nervous system. This releasing hormone is often called both luteinizing hormone-releasing hormone (LHRH) and follicle-stimulating hormone-releasing hormone (FSHRH) (Blackburn, 2007).

In response to GnRH, the anterior pituitary secretes the gonadotropic hormones *follicle-stimulating hormone (FSH)* and *luteinizing hormone (LH).* FSH is primarily responsible for the maturation of the ovarian follicle. As the follicle matures, it secretes increasing amounts of estrogen, which enhance the development of the follicle. (This estrogen is also responsible for the building or proliferation phase of the endometrium after it is shed during menstruation.)

MyNursingKit Activity: Ovulation

Final maturation of the follicle cannot come about without the action of LH. The anterior pituitary's production of LH increases six- to tenfold as the follicle matures. The peak production of LH can precede ovulation by as much as 12 hours. The LH is also responsible for the "luteinizing" of the theca and granulosa cells of the ruptured follicle. As a result, estrogen production is reduced and progesterone secretion continues. Thus estrogen levels fall a day before ovulation; tiny amounts of progesterone are in evidence. **Ovulation** takes place following the very rapid growth of the follicle, as the sustained high level of estrogen diminishes and progesterone secretion begins.

The ruptured follicle undergoes rapid change, complete luteinization is accomplished, and the mass of cells becomes the **corpus luteum**. The lutein cells secrete large amounts of progesterone with smaller amounts of estradiol. (Concurrently, the excessive amounts of progesterone are responsible for the secretory phase of the uterine cycle.) On day 7 or 8 following ovulation, the corpus luteum begins to involute, losing its secretory function. The production of both progesterone and estrogen is severely diminished. The anterior pituitary responds with increasingly large amounts of FSH; a few days later LH production begins. As a result, new follicles become responsive to another ovarian cycle and begin maturing.

Ovarian Cycle

The ovarian cycle has two phases: the *follicular phase* (days 1–14) and the *luteal phase* (days 15–28 in a 28-day cycle). Figure 3–15 ● depicts the changes that the follicle undergoes during the ovarian cycle. In women whose menstrual cycles vary, usually only the length of the follicular phase varies, because the luteal phase is of

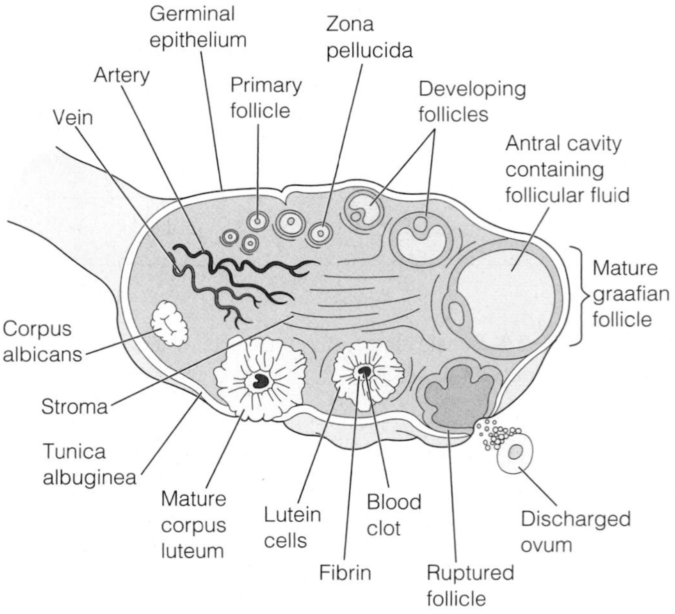

● **Figure 3–15** Various stages of development of the ovarian follicles.

fixed length. During the follicular phase, the immature follicle matures as a result of FSH. Within the follicle, the oocyte grows.

A mature **graafian follicle** appears on about the 14th day under dual control of FSH and LH. It is a large structure, measuring about 5 to 10 mm. The mature follicle produces increasing amounts of estrogen. In the mature graafian follicle, the cells surrounding the fluid-filled antral cavity are granulosa cells. The mass of granulosa cells surrounding the oocyte and follicular fluid is called the *cumulus oophorus.* In the fully mature graafian follicle, the zona pellucida, a thick elastic capsule, develops around the oocyte. Just before ovulation, the mature oocyte completes its first meiotic division (see Chapter 4 for a description of meiosis). As a result of this division, two cells are formed: a small cell, called a *polar body,* and a larger cell, called the *secondary oocyte.* The secondary oocyte matures into the ovum (see Figure 4–2).

As the graafian follicle matures and enlarges, it comes close to the surface of the ovary. The ovary surface forms a blisterlike protrusion 10 to 15 mm in diameter, and the follicle walls become thin. The secondary oocyte, polar body, and follicular fluid are pushed out. The ovum is discharged near the fimbria of the fallopian tube and is pulled into the tube to begin its journey toward the uterus.

In some women, ovulation is accompanied by midcycle pain known as *mittelschmerz.* This pain may be caused by a thick tunica albuginea or by a local peritoneal reaction to the expelling of the follicular contents. Vaginal discharge may increase during ovulation, and a small amount of blood (midcycle spotting) may be discharged as well.

The body temperature increases about 0.3°C to 0.6°C (0.5°F to 1.0°F) 24 to 48 hours after the time of ovulation. It remains elevated until the day before menstruation begins. There may be an accompanying sharp basal body temperature drop before the increase. These temperature changes are useful clinically to determine the approximate time ovulation occurs (Blackburn, 2007).

Generally the ovum takes several minutes to travel through the ruptured follicle to the fallopian tube opening. The contractions of the tube's smooth muscle and its ciliary action propel the ovum through the tube. The ovum remains in the ampulla, where, if it is fertilized, cleavage can begin. The ovum is thought to be fertile for only 6 to 24 hours. It reaches the uterus 72 to 96 hours after its release from the ovary.

The luteal phase begins when the ovum leaves its follicle. Under the influence of LH, the corpus luteum develops from the ruptured follicle. Within 2 or 3 days, the corpus luteum becomes yellowish and spherical and increases in vascularity. If the ovum is fertilized and implants in the endometrium, the fertilized egg begins to secrete **human chorionic gonadotropin (hCG)**, which is needed to maintain the corpus luteum. If fertilization does not occur, within about a week after ovulation the corpus luteum begins to degenerate, eventually becoming a connective tissue scar called the *corpus albicans.* With degeneration comes a decrease in estrogen and progesterone. This allows for an increase in LH and FSH, which trigger the hypothalamus.

UTERINE (MENSTRUAL) CYCLE

Menstruation is cyclic uterine bleeding in response to cyclic hormonal changes. Menstruation occurs when the ovum is not fertilized and begins about 14 days after ovulation in an ideal 28-day cycle. The menstrual discharge, also referred to as the *menses,* or *menstrual flow,* is composed of blood mixed with fluid, cervical and vaginal secretions, bacteria, mucus, leukocytes, and other cellular debris. The menstrual discharge is dark red and has a distinctive odor.

Menstrual parameters vary greatly among individuals. Generally, menstruation occurs every 29 days, but varies from 21 to 35 days. Some women normally have longer cycles, which can skew standard calculations of the estimated date of birth (EDB). Emotional and physical factors such as illness, excessive fatigue, stress or anxiety, and vigorous exercise programs can alter the cycle interval. Certain environmental factors such as temperature and altitude may also affect the cycle. The duration of menses is from 2 to 8 days, with the blood loss averaging 25 to 60 ml, and the loss of iron averaging 0.5 to 1 mg daily.

A review of the endometrium and its arterial blood supply provides further understanding of the menstrual process (Figure 3–16 ●). Blood flow from the spiral arterioles in the superficial endometrium is reduced, leading to a lack of blood and

MyNursingKit Care Plan Activity: Irregular Menses in a Client with Anxiety

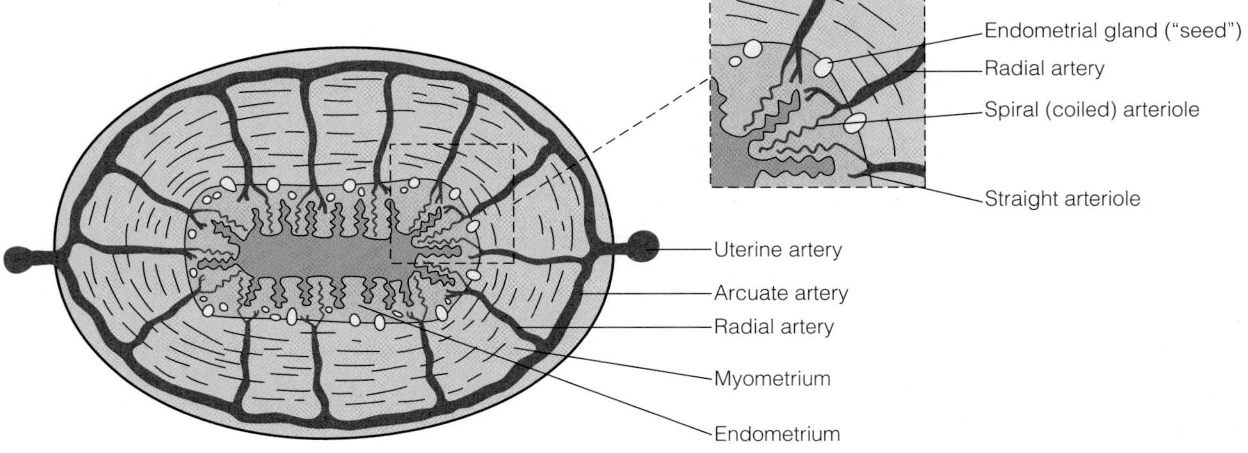

● **Figure 3–16** Blood supply to the endometrium (cross-sectional view of the uterus).

oxygen, which in turn produces tissue death (necrosis) and discharge of the superficial endometrium (menses). At the same time, the straight arterioles provide the basal endometrium with sufficient blood flow to maintain this layer of the endometrium and the endometrial glands (or seeds) that are responsible for the generation of the endometrium in the next female reproductive or menstrual cycle. Bleeding is controlled by vasospasm of the straight basal arterioles, resulting in coagulative necrosis at the vessel tips.

The uterine (menstrual) cycle has four phases: menstrual, proliferative, secretory, and ischemic (see Figure 3–14). Menstruation occurs during the *menstrual phase.* Some endometrial areas are shed, although others remain. Some of the remaining tips of the endometrial glands begin to regenerate. The endometrium is in a resting state following menstruation. Estrogen levels are low, and the endometrium is 1 to 2 mm deep. During this part of the cycle, the cervical mucosa is scanty, viscous, and opaque.

The *proliferative phase* begins when the endometrial glands enlarge, becoming twisted and longer in response to increasing amounts of estrogen. The blood vessels become prominent and dilated, and the endometrium increases in thickness six- to eightfold. This gradual process reaches its peak just before ovulation. The cervical mucosa becomes thin, clear, watery, and more alkaline, making the mucosa more favorable to spermatozoa. As ovulation nears, the cervical mucosa shows increased elasticity, called *spinnbarkeit.* At ovulation, the mucus will stretch more than 5 cm. The cervical mucosa pH increases from below 7.0 to 7.5 at the time of ovulation. On microscopic examination, the mucosa shows a characteristic ferning pattern (see Figure 7–3). This fern pattern is a useful aid in assessing ovulation time.

The *secretory phase* follows ovulation. The endometrium, under estrogenic influence, undergoes slight cellular growth. Progesterone, however, causes such marked swelling and growth that the epithelium is warped into folds. The amount of tissue glycogen increases. The glandular epithelial cells begin to fill with cellular debris, become twisted, and dilate. The glands secrete small quantities of endometrial fluid in preparation for a fertilized ovum. The vascularity of the entire uterus increases greatly, providing a nourishing bed for implantation. If implantation occurs, the endometrium, under the influence of progesterone, continues to develop and become even thicker (see Chapter 4 for a discussion of implantation).

If fertilization does not occur, the *ischemic phase* begins. The corpus luteum begins to degenerate, and as a result both estrogen and progesterone levels fall. Areas of necrosis appear under the epithelial lining. Extensive vascular changes also occur. Small blood vessels rupture, and the spiral arteries constrict and retract, causing a deficiency of blood in the endometrium, which becomes pale. This ischemic phase is characterized by the escape of blood into the stromal cells of the uterus. The menstrual flow begins, thus beginning the menstrual cycle again. After menstruation the basal layer remains, so that the tips of the glands can regenerate the new functional endometrial layer. For further discussion, see Table 3–2.

Table 3–2 Summary of Female Reproductive Cycle

Cycle	Phase	Days	Events
Ovarian Cycle	Follicular phase	Days 1–14	Primordial follicle matures under influence of FSH and LH up to the time of ovulation.
	Luteal phase	Days 15–28	Ovum leaves follicle; corpus luteum develops under LH influence and produces high levels of progesterone and low levels of estrogen.
Uterine (Menstrual) Cycle	Menstrual phase	Days 1–6	Estrogen levels are low. Cervical mucus is scant, viscous, and opaque. Endometrium is shed.
	Proliferative phase	Days 7–14	Endometrium and myometrium thickness increases. Estrogen peaks just before ovulation. Cervical mucus at ovulation: Is clear, thin, watery, alkaline Is more favorable to sperm; shows ferning pattern on microscopic exam Has spinnbarkeit greater than 5 cm Just before ovulation, body temperature may drop slightly, then at ovulation basal body temperature increases 0.3°C to 0.6°C (0.5°F to 1.0°F). Mittelschmerz and/or midcycle spotting may occur.
	Secretory phase	Days 15–26	Estrogen drops sharply, and progesterone dominates. Vascularity of entire uterus increases. Tissue glycogen increases, and the uterus is made ready for implantation.
	Ischemic phase	Days 27–28	Both estrogen and progesterone levels drop. Endometrium becomes pale, blood vessels rupture. Blood escapes into uterine stromal cells, gets ready to be shed.

MALE REPRODUCTIVE SYSTEM

The primary reproductive functions of the male genitals are to produce and transport sex cells (sperm) through and eventually out of the male genital tract and into the female genital tract. The external and internal genitals of the male reproductive system are shown in Figure 3–17 ●.

EXTERNAL GENITALS

The two external reproductive organs are the penis and scrotum.

Penis

The *penis* is an elongated, cylindrical structure consisting of a body, called the *shaft,* and a cone-shaped end, called the *glans.* The penis lies in front of the scrotum. The shaft of the penis is made up of three longitudinal columns of erectile tissue: the paired *corpora cavernosa* and the *corpus spongiosum.* These columns are covered by dense fibrous connective tissue and then enclosed by elastic tissue. The penis is covered by a thin outer layer of skin.

The corpus spongiosum contains the urethra and becomes the glans at the distal end of the penis. The urethra widens within the glans and ends in a slitlike opening, located in the tip of the glans, called the *urethral meatus.* A circular fold of skin arises just behind the glans and covers it. Known as the *prepuce,* or *foreskin,* it may be removed by the surgical procedure of circumcision (see Chapter 29∞). If the corpus spongiosum does not surround the urethra completely, the urethral meatus may occur on the ventral aspect of the penile shaft (hypospadias) or on the dorsal aspect (epispadias).

The penis is innervated by the pudendal nerve. Sexual stimulation causes the penis to elongate, thicken, and stiffen, a process called *erection.* The penis becomes erect when its blood vessels become engorged, a consequence of parasympathetic nerve stimulation. If sexual stimulation is intense enough, the forceful and sudden expulsion of semen occurs through the rhythmic contractions of the penile muscles. This phenomenon is called *ejaculation.*

The penis serves both the urinary and the reproductive systems. Urine is expelled through the urethral meatus. The reproductive function of the penis is to deposit sperm in the vagina so that fertilization of the ovum can occur.

Scrotum

The *scrotum* is a pouchlike structure that hangs in front of the anus and behind the penis. Composed of skin and the *dartos* muscle, the scrotum shows increased pigmentation and scattered hairs. The sebaceous glands open directly onto the scrotal surface; their secretion has a distinctive odor. Contraction of the dartos and cremasteric muscles shortens the scrotum and draws it closer to the body, thus wrinkling its outer surface. The degree of wrinkling is greatest in young men and at cold temperatures and is least in older men and at warm temperatures.

Inside the scrotum are two lateral compartments. Each compartment contains a testis with its related structures. Because the left spermatic cord grows longer, the left testis and its scrotal sac hang lower than the right. A ridge (raphe) on the external scrotal surface marks the position of the medial septum and continues anteriorly on the urethral surface of the penis, disappearing in the perineal area.

The function of the scrotum is to protect the testes and the sperm by maintaining a temperature lower than that of the body. Spermatogenesis cannot occur if the testes fail to descend and thus remain at body temperature. Because it is sensitive to touch, pressure, temperature, and pain, the scrotum defends against potential harm to the testes.

MALE INTERNAL REPRODUCTIVE ORGANS

The male internal reproductive organs include the gonads (testes or testicles), a system of ducts (epididymides, vas deferens, ejaculatory

MyNursingKit Animation: 3-D Male Pelvis

MyNursingKit Activity: Male Reproductive System

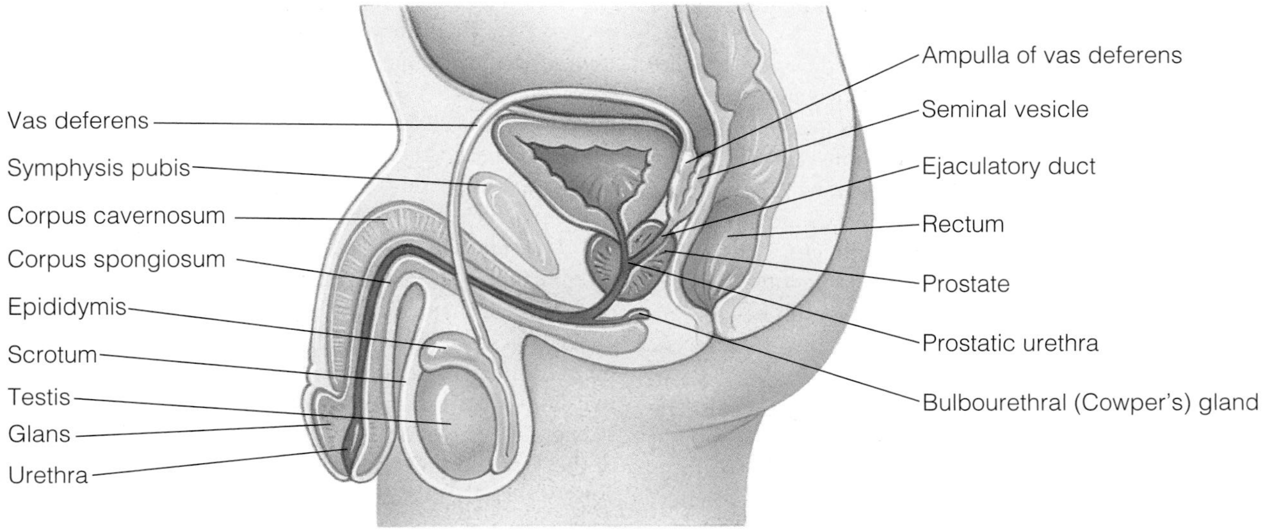

● **Figure 3–17** Male reproductive system, sagittal view.

Table 3–3 Summary of Male Reproductive Organ Functions

Organ	Structure	Function
Testes	Seminiferous tubules	Contain sperm cells in various stages of development and undergoing meiosis.
	Sertoli's cells	Nourish and protect spermatocytes (phase between spermatids and spermatozoa—see Chapter 4).
	Leydig's cells	Provide the main source of testosterone.
Ducts	Epididymides	Provide an area for maturation of sperm and a reservoir for mature spermatozoa.
	The vas deferens	Connects the epididymis with the prostate gland, then connects with ducts from the seminal vesicle to become an ejaculatory duct.
	Ejaculatory ducts	Provide a passageway for semen and seminal fluid into the urethra.
Accessory glands	Seminal vesicles	Secrete yellowish fluid rich in fructose, prostaglandins, and fibrinogen. This provides nutrition that increases motility and fertilizing ability of sperm. Prostaglandins also aid fertilization by making the cervical mucus more receptive to sperm.
	The prostate gland	Secretes thin, alkaline fluid containing calcium, citric acid, and other substances. Alkalinity counteracts acidity of ductus and seminal vesicle secretions.
	Bulbourethral (Cowper's) glands	Secrete alkaline, viscous fluid into semen, aiding in neutralization of acidic vaginal secretions.
	Urethral (Littré's) glands	Add secretions to those of the bulbourethral glands.

duct, and urethra), and accessory glands (seminal vesicles, prostate gland, bulbourethral glands, and urethral glands) (Table 3–3).

Testes

The *testes* are a pair of oval, compound glandular organs contained in the scrotum. In the sexually mature male, they are the site of spermatozoa (male gamete) production and the secretion of several male sex hormones.

Each testis is 4 to 6 cm long, 2 to 3 cm wide, and 3 to 4 cm thick and weighs about 10 to 15 g. Each is covered by an outer serous membrane and an inner capsule that is tough, white, and fibrous. The connective tissue sends projections inward to form septa, dividing the testis into 250 to 400 lobules. Each lobule contains one to three tightly packed, convoluted *seminiferous tubules* containing sperm cells in all stages of development.

The seminiferous tubules are surrounded by loose connective tissue that houses abundant blood and lymph vessels and *interstitial (Leydig's) cells.* The interstitial cells produce testosterone, the primary male sex hormone. The tubules also contain Sertoli's cells, which nourish and protect the spermatocytes. The seminiferous tubules come together to form 20 to 30 straight tubules, which in turn form an anastomotic network of thin-walled spaces, the *rete testis.* The rete testis forms 10 to 15 efferent ducts that empty into the duct of the epididymis.

Most of the cells lining the seminiferous tubules undergo **spermatogenesis**, a process of maturation in which spermatocytes become spermatozoa. (Chapter 4 further discusses the process of spermatogenesis.) Sperm production varies among and within the tubules, with cells in different areas of the same tubule undergoing different stages of spermatogenesis. The sperm are eventually released from the tubules into the epididymis, where they mature further.

Like the female reproductive cycle, the process of spermatogenesis and other functions of the testes are the result of complex neural and hormonal controls. The hypothalamus secretes releasing factors that stimulate the anterior pituitary to release the gonadotropins—FSH and LH. These hormones cause the testes to produce testosterone, which maintains spermatogenesis, increases sperm production by the seminiferous tubules, and stimulates production of seminal fluid.

Testosterone is the most prevalent and potent of the testicular hormones. It is also responsible for the development of secondary male characteristics and certain behavioral patterns. The effects of testosterone include structural and functional development of the male genital tract, emission and ejaculation of seminal fluid, distribution of body hair, promotion of growth and strength of long bones, increased muscle mass, and enlargement of the vocal cords. The action of testosterone on the central nervous system is thought to produce aggressiveness and sexual drive. The action of testosterone is constant, not cyclic like that of the female hormones. Its production is not limited to a certain number of years, but it is thought to decrease with age.

The testes have two primary functions:

- To serve as the site of spermatogenesis
- To produce testosterone

Epididymis

The *epididymis* (plural, *epididymides*) is a duct about 5.6 m long, although it is convoluted into a compact structure about 3.75 cm long. An epididymis lies behind each testis. It arises from the top of the testis, courses downward, and then passes upward, where it becomes the vas deferens.

The epididymis provides a reservoir for maturing spermatozoa. When discharged from the seminiferous tubules into the epididymis, the sperm are immotile and incapable of fertilizing an ovum. The spermatozoa usually remain in the epididymis for 2 to 10 days but can be stored in the body for up to 42 days. As the sperm move along the tortuous course of the epididymis they become both motile and fertile.

Vas Deferens and Ejaculatory Ducts

The *vas deferens,* also known as the *ductus deferens,* is about 40 cm long and connects the epididymis with the prostate. One vas deferens arises from the posterior border of each testis. It joins the spermatic cord and weaves over and between several pelvic structures until it meets the vas deferens from the opposite side. Each vas deferens terminus expands to form the *terminal ampulla.* It then unites with the seminal vesicle duct (a gland) to form the ejaculatory duct, which enters the prostate gland and ends in the prostatic urethra. The ejaculatory ducts serve as passageways for semen and fluid secreted by the seminal vesicles. The main function of the vas deferens is to rapidly squeeze the sperm from their storage sites (the epididymis and distal part of the vas deferens) into the urethra.

Men who choose to take total responsibility for birth control may elect to have a vasectomy. In this procedure, the scrotal portion of the vas deferens is surgically incised or cauterized. Although sperm continues to be produced for the next several years, they can no longer reach the outside of the body. Eventually, the sperm deteriorate and are reabsorbed.

Urethra

The *male urethra* is the passageway for both urine and semen. The urethra begins in the bladder and passes through the prostate gland, where it is called the *prostatic urethra.*

The urethra emerges from the prostate gland to become the *membranous urethra.* It terminates in the penis, where it is called the *penile urethra.* In the penile urethra, goblet secretory cells are present, and smooth muscle is replaced by erectile tissue.

Accessory Glands

The male accessory glands secrete a unique and essential component of the total seminal fluid in an ordered sequence.

The *seminal vesicles* are two glands composed of many lobes. Each vesicle is about 7.5 cm long. They are situated between the bladder and the rectum, immediately above the base of the prostate. The epithelium lining the seminal vesicles secretes an alkaline, viscous, clear fluid rich in high-energy fructose, prostaglandins, fibrinogen, and amino acids. During ejaculation, this fluid mixes with the sperm in the ejaculatory ducts. This fluid helps provide an environment favorable to sperm motility and metabolism.

The *prostate gland* encircles the upper part of the urethra and lies below the neck of the bladder. Made up of several lobes, it measures about 4 cm in diameter and weighs 20 to 30 g. The prostate is made up of both glandular and muscular tissue. It secretes a thin, milky, alkaline fluid containing high levels of zinc, calcium, citric acid, and acid phosphatase. This fluid protects the sperm from the acidic environment of the vagina and the male urethra, which would otherwise be spermicidal.

The *bulbourethral (Cowper's) glands* are a pair of small, round structures on either side of the membranous urethra. The glands secrete a clear, thick, alkaline fluid rich in mucoproteins that becomes part of the semen. This secretion also lubricates the penile urethra during sexual excitement and neutralizes the acid in the male urethra and the vagina, thereby enhancing sperm motility.

The *urethral (Littré's) glands* are tiny mucus-secreting glands found throughout the membranous lining of the penile urethra. Their secretions add to those of the bulbourethral glands.

Semen

The male ejaculate, *semen* or *seminal fluid,* is made up of spermatozoa and the secretions of all the accessory glands. The seminal fluid transports viable and motile sperm to the female reproductive tract. Effective transportation of sperm requires adequate nutrients, an adequate pH (about 7.5), a specific concentration of sperm to fluid, and an optimal osmolarity.

A spermatozoon is made up of a head and a tail (Figure 3–18 ●). The head's main components are the acrosome and nucleus. The

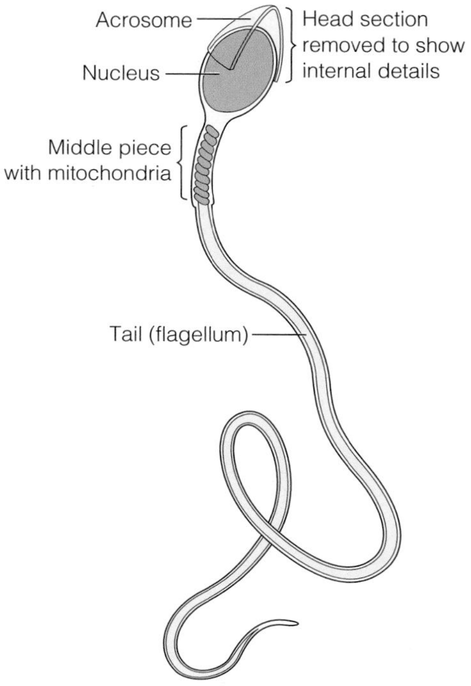

● **Figure 3–18** Schematic representation of a mature spermatozoon.

head carries the male's haploid number of chromosomes (23), and it is the part that enters the ovum at fertilization (see Chapter 4). The tail, or *flagellum,* is divided into the middle and end piece and is specialized for motility.

Sperm may be stored in the epididymis and distal vas deferens for up to 42 days, depending primarily on the frequency of ejaculations. The average volume of ejaculate following abstinence for several days is 2 to 5 ml but may vary from 1 to 10 ml. Repeated ejaculation results in decreased volume. Once ejaculated, sperm can live only 2 or 3 days in the female genital tract.

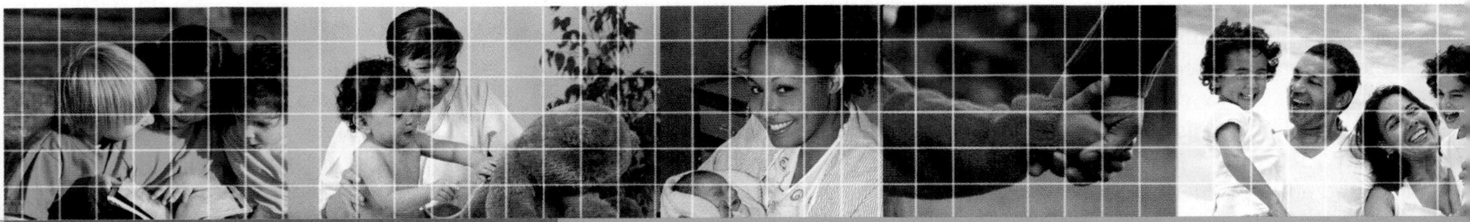

CRITICAL CONCEPT REVIEW

LEARNING OUTCOMES / CONCEPTS

3.1 Identify the structures and functions of the female reproductive system.

1. Ovaries:
   - Produce female gametes and female sex hormones.
2. Fallopian tubes:
   - Capture the ovum.
   - Allow transport of the ovum to the uterus.
3. Uterus:
   - Implantation site for the fertilized ovum.
4. Cervix:
   - Connection between the vagina and the uterus.
   - Protective portal for the body of the uterus.
5. Vagina:
   - Passageway from the external genitals to the uterus.
   - Provides for discharge of menstrual products out of the body.

3.2 Identify the structures and functions of the male reproductive system.

1. Penis:
   - Deposits sperm in the vagina so fertilization of the ovum can occur.
   - Reproductive organ of intercourse.
2. Scrotum:
   - Protects the testes and sperm by maintaining a temperature lower than the body.
3. Testes:
   - Serve as a site for spermatogenesis.
   - Produce testosterone.
   - Produce male gametes and male sex hormones.
4. Epididymis:
   - Provides a reservoir for maturing spermatozoa.
5. Vas deferens:
   - Rapidly squeeze the sperm from their storage sites into the urethra.
6. Ejaculatory duct:
   - Passageway for semen and fluid secreted by the seminal vesicles.
   - In conjunction with epididymis and vas deferens transport spermatozoa outside the body.
7. Urethra:
   - Passageway for both urine and semen.
8. Accessory glands:
   - Produce secretions necessary for sperm nutrition, survival, and transport.
9. Seminal fluid:
   - Provides environment favorable to sperm mobility and metabolism.
   - Transports viable and mobile sperm to the female reproductive tract.

LEARNING OUTCOMES	CONCEPTS
3.3 Discuss the significance of specific female reproductive structures during childbirth.	1. Ischial spines: ■ Serve as a reference point during labor to evaluate the descent of the fetal head. 2. Pubic arch (symphysis pubis): ■ Fetal head passes under this arch during birth. 3. False pelvis: ■ Serves to support the weight of the enlarged pregnant uterus and direct the presenting fetal part into the true pelvis. 4. True pelvis: ■ Shape and size must be adequate for normal fetal passage. ■ Fetus must change its position to move through the diameter of the true pelvis. 5. Pelvic cavity: ■ Can influence the length of labor.
3.4 Summarize the actions of the hormones that affect reproductive functioning.	1. Estrogen: ■ Controls development of female secondary sex characteristics. ■ Assists in the maturation of the ovarian follicles. ■ Causes endometrial mucosa to proliferate following menstruation. ■ Causes uterus to increase in size and weight. ■ Increases myometrial contractility in both the uterus and fallopian tubes. ■ Increases uterine sensitivity to oxytocin. ■ Inhibits FSH production. ■ Stimulates LH production. 2. Progesterone: ■ Decreases uterine motility and contractility. ■ Causes uterine endometrium to increase its supply of glycogen, arterial blood, secretory glands, amino acids, and water. ■ Vaginal epithelium proliferates. ■ Cervix secretes thick, viscous mucus. ■ Increases breast glandular tissue, both in size and in complexity. ■ Prepares breasts for lactation. 3. Prostaglandins: ■ Necessary for follicular rupture.
3.5 Identify the two phases of the ovarian cycle and the changes that occur in each phase.	1. Follicular phase: ■ Primordial follicle matures under the influence of FSH and LH until ovulation occurs. 2. Luteal phase: ■ Ovum leaves the follicle. ■ Corpus luteum develops under the influence of LH. ■ Corpus luteum produces high levels of progesterone and low levels of estrogen.
3.6 Describe the phases of the uterine (menstrual) cycle, their dominant hormones, and the changes that occur in each phase.	1. Menstrual phase: ■ Shedding of the endometrial lining. ■ Low estrogen levels. 2. Proliferative phase: ■ Enlargement of the endometrial glands under influence of estrogen. ■ Changes in cervical mucus; peak at ovulation. ■ Increasing estrogen levels. 3. Secretory phase: ■ Follows ovulation. ■ Influenced primarily by progesterone. ■ Increase in vascularity of the uterus to make ready for possible implantation. 4. Ischemic phase: ■ Decreasing levels of estrogen and progesterone. ■ Degeneration of the corpus luteum. ■ Constriction of the spiral arteries. ■ Escape of blood into the stromal cells of the endometrium.

CRITICAL THINKING IN ACTION

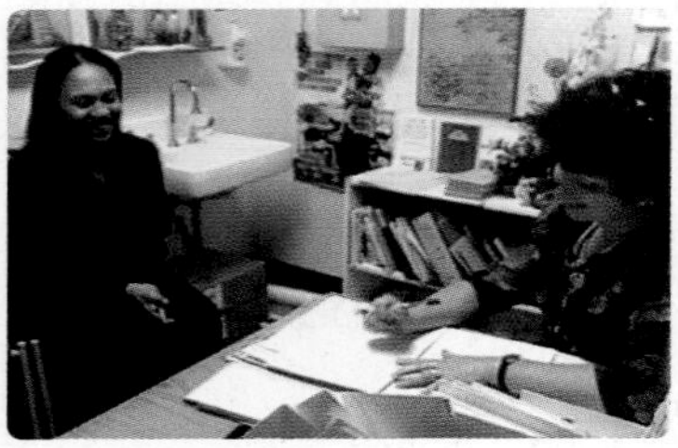

You are working in the OB/GYN clinic when Sally Smith, a 17-year-old teenager, comes in complaining of irregular menses. She believes her periods are really "messed up" and interfering with her active schedule. She wants them to be more regular and asks you for birth control. She tells you that she is a member of the swimming team and is a senior in high school. She says she is planning to start community college next year to obtain an associate degree in computer technology. You assess Sally's history as follows: menarche began at age 12; periods occur every 28 to 32 days. She usually experiences cramping in the first 2 days and the flow lasts 4 to 5 days. She uses an average of 4 to 5 tampons a day during her period. She has never been hospitalized, has no prior medical problems, and is up to date on her immunizations except for meningitis.

1. Based on your knowledge of menstruation, how would you describe Sally's menstrual cycle?
2. What is your primary goal in discussing Sally's menstrual cycle with her?
3. What information would you give Sally relating to her menstrual cycle?
4. What important request does Sally have?
5. Sally expresses problems dealing with the cramping she experiences with the first 2 days of her menses. What would you suggest to Sally to cope with the discomfort?

See MyNursingKit for possible responses.

REFERENCES

Blackburn, S. T. (2007). *Maternal, fetal, & neonatal physiology: A clinical perspective* (3rd ed.). St. Louis: Saunders.

Caldwell, W. E., & Moloy, H. C. (1933). Anatomical variations in the female pelvis and their effect on labor with a suggested classification [Historical article]. *American Journal of Obstetrics and Gynecology, 26,* 479–505.

Ganong, W. F. (2007). Physiology of reproduction in women. In A. H. Decherney, L. Nathan, T. M. Goodwin, & N. Laufer (Eds.), *Current diagnosis and treatment: Obstetrics & gynecology* (10th ed.). Boston: McGraw-Hill.

Krantz, K. E. (2007). Anatomy of the female reproductive system. In A. H. Decherney, L. Nathan, T. M. Goodwin, & N. Laufer (Eds.), *Current diagnosis and treatment: Obstetrics & gynecology* (10th ed.). Boston: McGraw-Hill.

Lawrence, R. M., & Lawrence, R. A. (2009). The breast and the physiology of lactation. In R. K. Creasy, R. Resnik, J. D. Iams, C J. Lockwood, & T. R. Moore (Eds.), *Creasy & Resnik's maternal-fetal medicine: Principles and practice* (6th ed.). St. Louis: Saunders.

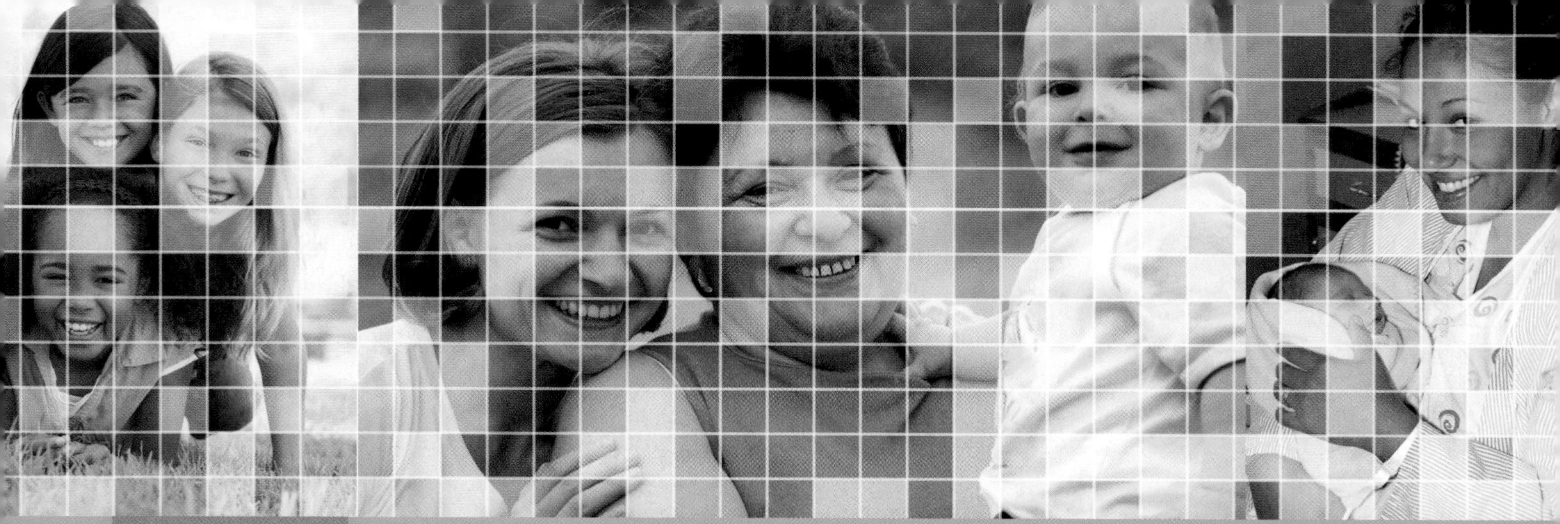

CHAPTER

4 Conception and Fetal Development

My friends tease me when I say this, but I know the moment my son was conceived. My husband and I had both been so busy at work, but finally we planned a getaway weekend. It was wonderful. We got back some of the magic as we took long walks and talked. Until that weekend, whenever we discussed having children it was always "maybe someday."

On the second night, we decided to skip the diaphragm for the first time. Our lovemaking seemed so special and magical—a true reflection of the emotional closeness we had recaptured. We are convinced that Michael is the result of that night together. —Michelle, 29

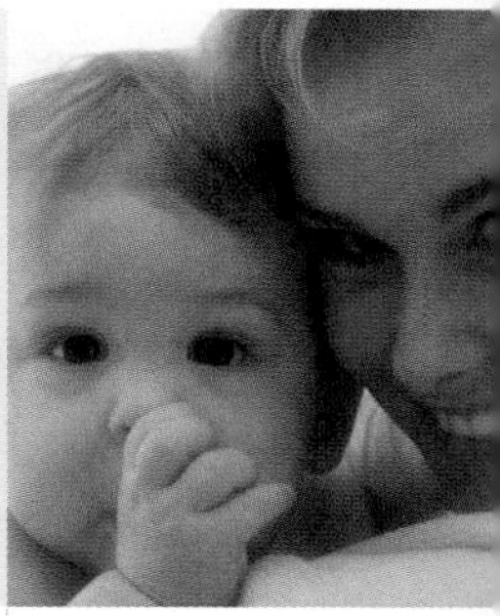

LEARNING OUTCOMES

4.1 Differentiate between meiotic cellular division and mitotic cellular division.

4.2 Compare the processes by which ova and sperm are produced.

4.3 Analyze the components of the process of fertilization as to how each may impact fertilization.

4.4 Analyze the processes that occur during the cellular multiplication and differentiation stages of intrauterine development and their effects on the structures that form.

4.5 Describe the development, structure, and functions of the placenta and umbilical cord during intrauterine life (embryonic and fetal development).

4.6 Compare the factors and processes by which fraternal (dizygotic) and identical (monozygotic) twins are formed.

4.7 Summarize the significant changes in growth and development of the fetus at 4, 6, 12, 16, 20, 24, 28, 36, and 40 weeks' gestation.

4.8 Identify the factors that influence congenital malformations of the various organ systems.

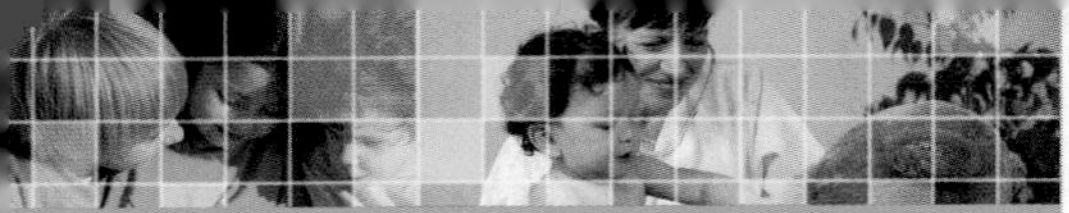

KEY TERMS

Acrosomal reaction, 66
Amnion, 70
Amniotic fluid, 70
Bag of waters (BOW), 70
Blastocyst, 68
Capacitation, 66
Chorion, 69
Cleavage, 68
Cotyledons, 73
Decidua basalis, 69
Decidua capsularis, 69
Decidua vera (parietalis), 69
Diploid number of chromosomes, 64
Ductus arteriosus, 77
Ductus venosus, 76
Ectoderm, 69
Embryo, 77
Embryonic membranes, 69
Endoderm, 69
Fertilization, 65
Fetus, 80
Foramen ovale, 76
Gametes, 65
Gametogenesis, 65
Haploid number of chromosomes, 64
Lanugo, 71
Meiosis, 64
Mesoderm, 69
Mitosis, 64
Morula, 68
Placenta, 72
Postconception age periods, 77
Teratogen, 82
Trophoblast, 69
Umbilical cord, 71
Vernix caseosa, 81
Wharton's jelly, 71
Zygote, 65

The human genome contains *genes,* which are units of genetic information. Genes are encoded in the DNA that makes up the chromosomes in the nucleus of each cell. These chromosomes, which determine the structure and function of organ systems and traits, are of the same biochemical substances. How then does each person become unique? The answer lies in the physiologic mechanisms of heredity, the processes of cellular division, and the environmental factors that influence our development from the moment we are conceived. This chapter explores the processes involved in conception and fetal development—the basis of human uniqueness.

CELLULAR DIVISION

Each human begins life as a single cell called a fertilized ovum, or zygote. This single cell reproduces itself, and in turn each resulting cell also reproduces itself in a continuing process. The new cells are similar to the cells from which they came. Cells are reproduced by either mitosis or meiosis, two different but related processes.

MITOSIS

During **mitosis**, the cell undergoes several changes, ending in cell division. As the last phase of cell division nears completion, a furrow develops in the cell cytoplasm, which divides it into two daughter cells, each with its own nucleus. Daughter cells have the same **diploid number of chromosomes** (46) and same genetic makeup as the cell from which they came. After a cell with 46 chromosomes goes through mitosis, the result is two identical cells, each with 46 chromosomes. Mitosis makes growth and development possible, and in mature individuals it is the process by which our body cells continue to divide and replace themselves.

MEIOSIS

Meiosis is a special type of cell division by which diploid cells in the testes and ovaries give rise to gametes (sperm and ova). Unlike cells produced during mitosis, the cells produced during meiosis contain only half the genetic material or number of chromsomes with the **haploid number of chromosomes**, which is 23.

Meiosis consists of two successive cell divisions. In the first division, the chromosomes replicate. Next, a pairing takes place between homologous chromosomes (Sadler, 2006). Instead of separating immediately, as in mitosis, the chromosomes become closely intertwined. At each point of contact, there is a physical exchange of genetic material between the chromatids (the arms of the chromosomes). New combinations are provided by the newly formed chromosomes; these combinations account for the wide variation of traits in people (e.g., hair or eye color). The chromosome pairs then separate, and the members of the pair move to opposite sides of the cell. (In contrast, during mitosis, the chromatids of each chromosome separate and move to opposite poles.) The cell divides, forming two daughter cells, each with 23 double-structured chromosomes—the same amount of deoxyribonucleic acid (DNA) as a normal somatic cell. In the second division, the chromatids of each chromosome separate and move to opposite poles of each of the daughter cells. Cell division occurs, resulting in the formation of four cells, each containing 23 single chromosomes (the haploid number of chromosomes). These daughter cells contain only half the DNA of a normal somatic cell (Sadler, 2006) (Table 4–1).

Mutations may occur during the second meiotic division, if two of the chromatids do not move apart rapidly enough when the cell divides. The still-paired chromatids are carried into one of the daughter cells and eventually form an extra chromosome. This condition, *autosomal nondisjunction* (chromosomal mutation), is harmful to the offspring that may result if fertilization occurs. Another type of chromosomal mutation can occur if chromosomes break during meiosis. If the broken segment is lost, the result is a shorter chromosome; this situation is known as *deletion.* If the broken segment becomes attached to another chromosome, a harmful mutation called a

Table 4–1 Comparison of Meiosis and Mitosis

Process	Purpose	Cell Division	Number of Daughter Cells
Meiosis	Produce reproductive cells (gametes). Reduction of chromosome number by half (from diploid [46] to haploid [23]), so that when fertilization occurs the normal diploid number is restored. Introduces genetic variability.	Two-stage reduction.	Four daughter cells, each containing one-half the number of chromosomes as the mother cell, or 23 chromosomes. Nonidentical to original cell.
Mitosis	Produce cells for growth and tissue repair. Cell division characteristic of all somatic cells.	One-stage cell division.	Two daughter cells identical to the mother cell, each with the diploid number (46 chromosomes).

translocation is the result. The implications of nondisjunction and the effects of translocation are described in Chapter 7∞.

GAMETOGENESIS

Meiosis occurs during **gametogenesis**, the process by which germ cells, or **gametes** *(ovum and sperm)*, are produced. These cells contain only half the genetic material of a typical body cell. The gametes must have a haploid number (23) of chromosomes so that when the female gamete (egg or ovum) and the male gamete (sperm or spermatozoon) unite to form the **zygote** (fertilized ovum), the normal human diploid number of chromosomes (46) is reestablished.

OOGENESIS

Oogenesis is the process that produces the female gamete, called an ovum (egg). As discussed in Chapter 3∞, the ovaries begin to develop early in the fetal life of the female. All the ova that the female will produce in her lifetime are present at birth. The ovary gives rise to oogonial cells, which develop into oocytes. Meiosis begins in all oocytes before the female fetus is born but stops before the first division is complete and remains in this arrested phase until puberty. During puberty, the mature primary oocyte proceeds (by oogenesis) through the first meiotic division in the graafian follicle of the ovary.

The first meiotic division produces two cells of unequal size with different amounts of cytoplasm but with the same number of chromosomes. These two cells are the *secondary oocyte* and a minute *polar body.* Both the secondary oocyte and the polar body contain 22 double-structured autosomal chromosomes and one double-structured sex chromosome (X).

At the time of ovulation, a second meiotic division begins immediately and proceeds as the oocyte moves down the fallopian tube. Division is again not equal, and the secondary oocyte moves into the metaphase stage of cell division, where its meiotic division is arrested until and unless the oocyte is fertilized.

When the secondary oocyte completes the second meiotic division after fertilization, the result is a mature ovum with the haploid number of chromosomes and virtually all the cytoplasm. In addition, the second polar body (also haploid) forms at this time. The first polar body has now also divided, producing two additional polar bodies. Thus, at the completion of meiosis, four haploid cells have been produced: the three polar bodies, which eventually disintegrate, and one ovum (Sadler, 2006) (Figure 4–1 ●).

MyNursingKit Animation: Spermatogenesis

MyNursingKit Animation: Oogenesis

SPERMATOGENESIS

During puberty, the germinal epithelium in the seminiferous tubules of the testes begins the process of spermatogenesis, which produces the male gamete (sperm). The diploid spermatogonium replicates before it enters the first meiotic division, during which it is called the *primary spermatocyte.* During this first meiotic division, the spermatogonium replicates and forms two cells called *secondary spermatocytes,* each of which contains 22 double-structured autosomal chromosomes and either a double-structured X sex chromosome or a double-structured Y sex chromosome. During the second meiotic division, they divide to form four spermatids, each with the haploid number of chromosomes. The spermatids undergo a series of changes during which they lose most of their cytoplasm and become sperm (spermatozoa) (Figure 4–1). The nucleus becomes compacted into the head of the sperm, which is covered by a cap called an *acrosome* that is, in turn, covered by a plasma membrane. A long tail is produced from one of the centrioles.

THE PROCESS OF FERTILIZATION

Fertilization is the process by which a sperm fuses with an ovum to form a new diploid cell, or zygote. The zygote begins life as a single cell with a complete set of genetic material, 23 chromosomes from the mother's ovum and 23 chromosomes from the father's sperm, for a total of 46 chromosomes. The following events lead to fertilization.

PREPARATION FOR FERTILIZATION

The mature ovum and spermatozoa have only a brief time to unite. Ova are considered fertile for about 12 to 24 hours after ovulation. Sperm can survive in the female reproductive tract for 48 to 72 hours, but are believed to be healthy and highly fertile for only about 24 hours.

The ovum's cell membrane is surrounded by two layers of tissue. The layer closest to the cell membrane is called the *zona pellucida.* It is a clear, noncellular layer whose thickness influences the

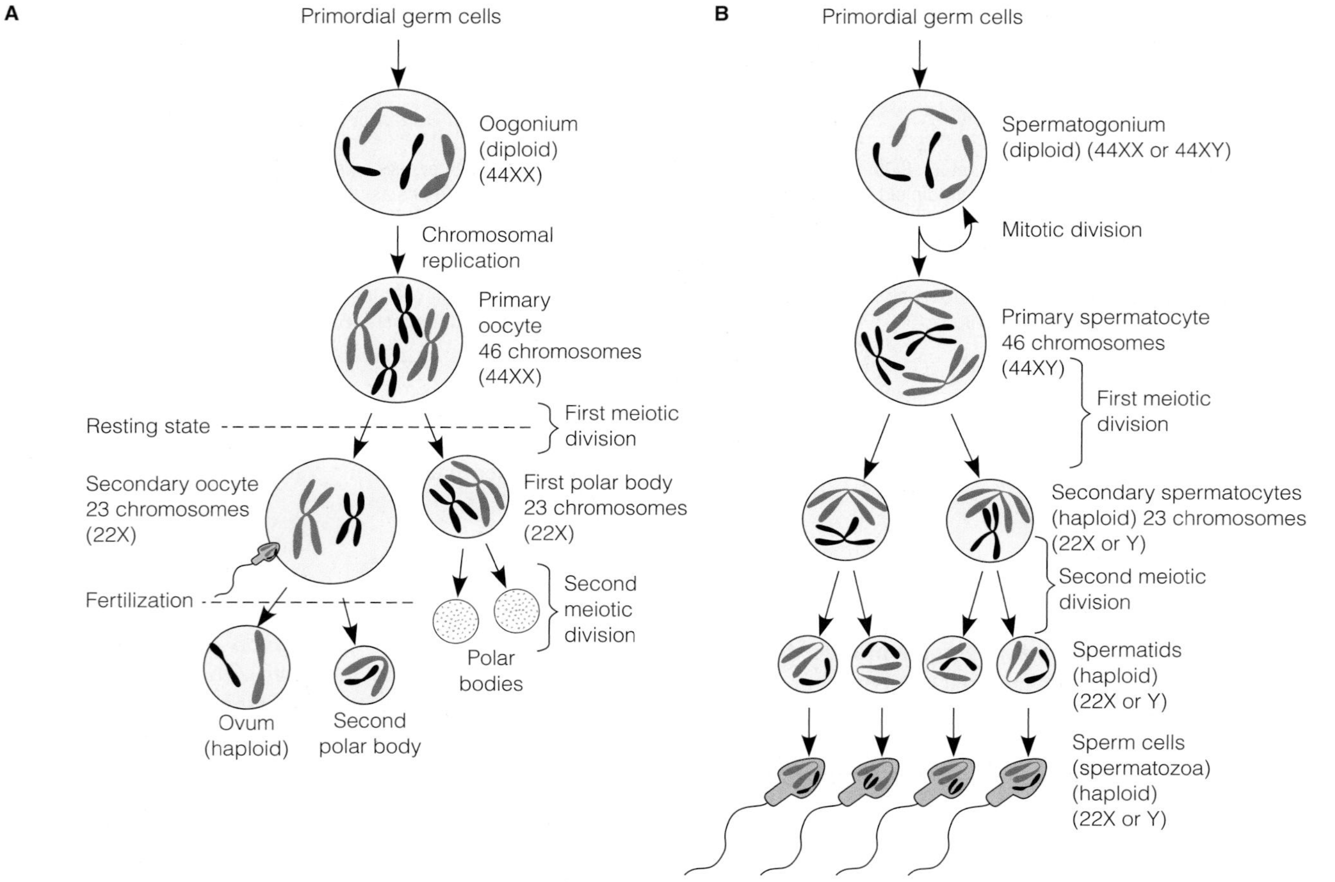

● **Figure 4–1** Result of gametogenesis. Gametogenesis involves meiosis within the ovary and testis. ***A,*** During meiosis each oogonium produces a single haploid ovum once some cytoplasm moves into the polar bodies. ***B,*** Each spermatogonium produces four haploid spermatozoa.

fertilization rate. Surrounding the zona pellucida is a ring of elongated cells, called the *corona radiata* because they radiate from the ovum like the gaseous corona around the sun. These cells are held together by hyaluronic acid. The ovum has no inherent power of movement. During ovulation, high estrogen levels increase peristalsis within the fallopian tubes, which helps move the ovum through the tube toward the uterus. The high estrogen levels also cause a thinning of the cervical mucus, facilitating movement of the sperm through the cervix, into the uterus, and up the fallopian tube.

The process of fertilization takes place in the ampulla (outer third) of the fallopian tube. In a single ejaculation, the male deposits approximately 200 to 300 million spermatozoa into the vagina, of which only hundreds of sperm actually reach the ampulla (Sadler, 2006). Fructose in the semen, secreted by the seminal vesicles, is the energy source for the sperm. The spermatozoa propel themselves up the female tract by the flagellar movement of their tails. Transit time from the cervix into the fallopian tube can be as short as 5 minutes but usually takes an average of 2 to 7 hours after ejaculation (Sadler, 2006). Prostaglandins in the semen may increase uterine smooth muscle contractions, which help transport the sperm. The fallopian tubes have a dual ciliary action that facilitates movement of the ovum toward the uterus and movement of the sperm from the uterus toward the ovary.

The sperm must undergo two processes before fertilization can occur: capacitation and the acrosomal reaction. **Capacitation** is the removal of the plasma membrane overlying the spermatozoa's acrosomal area and the loss of seminal plasma proteins. If the glycoprotein coat is not removed, the sperm will not be able to fertilize the ovum (Sadler, 2006). Capacitation occurs in the female reproductive tract (aided by uterine enzymes) and is thought to take about 7 hours. Sperm that undergo capacitation now take on three characteristics: (1) the ability to undergo the acrosomal reaction, (2) the ability to bind to the zona pellucida, and (3) the acquisition of hypermotility.

The **acrosomal reaction** follows capacitation, whereby the acrosomes of the sperms surrounding the ovum release their enzymes (hyaluronidase, a protease called acrosin, and trypsinlike substances) and thus break down the hyaluronic acid in the ovum's corona radiata (Sadler, 2006). Hundreds of acrosomes must rupture before enough hyaluronic acid is cleared for a single sperm to penetrate the ovum's zona pellucida successfully.

At the moment of penetration by a fertilizing sperm, the zona pellucida undergoes a reaction that prevents additional sperm from entering a single ovum (Figure 4–2 ●). This is known as the *block to polyspermy.* This cellular change is mediated by release of materials from the cortical granules, organelles found just below the ovum's surface, and is called the *cortical reaction.*

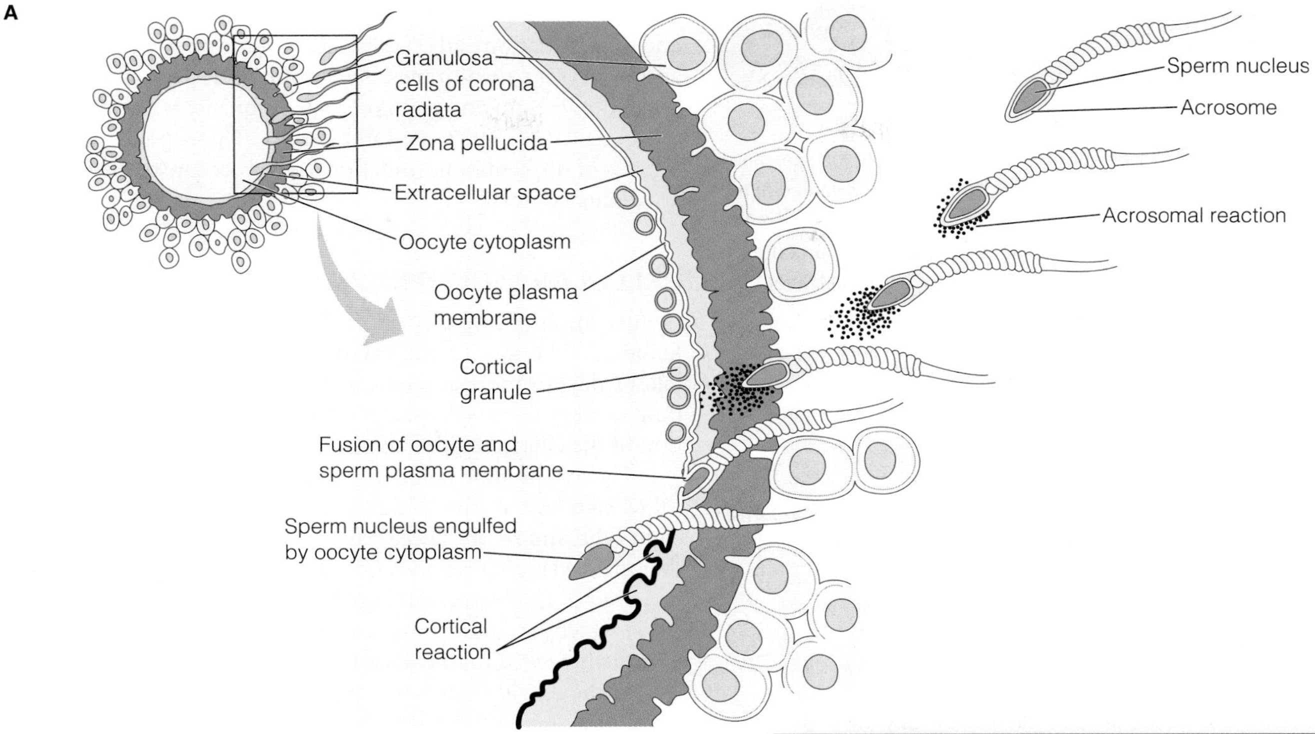

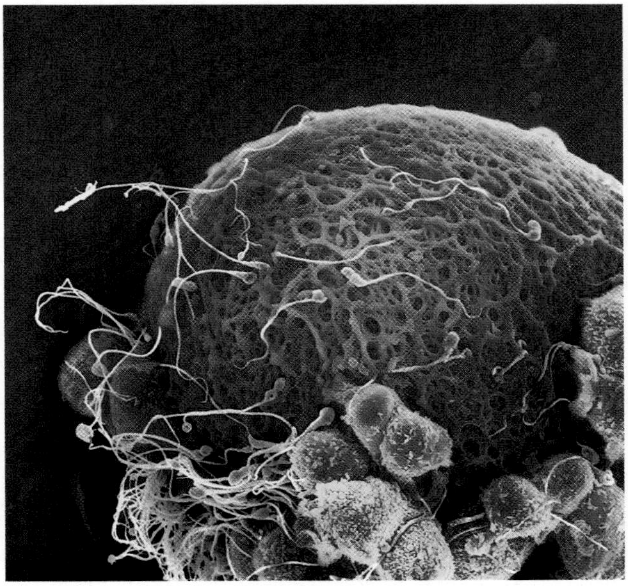

• **Figure 4–2** Sperm penetration of an ovum. ***A,*** The sequential steps of oocyte penetration by a sperm are depicted moving from top to bottom. ***B,*** Scanning electron micrograph of a human sperm surrounding a human ovum (750X). The smaller spherical cells are granulosa cells of the corona radiata.

Source: B, Scanning electron micrograph from Nilsson, L. (1990). *A child is born.* New York: Dell Publishing.

THE MOMENT OF FERTILIZATION

After the sperm enters the ovum, a chemical signal prompts the secondary oocyte to complete the second meiotic division, forming the nucleus of the ovum and ejecting the second polar body. Then the nuclei of the ovum and sperm swell and approach each other. The true moment of fertilization occurs as the nuclei unite. Their individual nuclear membranes disappear, and their chromosomes pair up to produce the diploid zygote. Because each nucleus contains a haploid number of chromosomes (23), this union restores the diploid number (46). The zygote contains a new combination of genetic material that results in an individual different from either parent and from anyone else.

The moment of fertilization is also when the sex of the zygote is determined. The two chromosomes (the sex chromosomes) of the 23rd pair—either XX or XY—determine the sex of an individual. The X chromosome is larger and bears more genes than the Y chromosome. Females have two X chromosomes, and males have an X and a Y chromosome. Whereas the mature ovum produced by oogenesis can have only one type of sex chromosome—an X—spermatogenesis produces two sperm with an X chromosome and two sperm with a Y chromosome. When each gamete contributes an X chromosome, the resulting zygote is female. When the ovum contributes an X and the sperm contributes a Y chromosome, the resulting zygote is male. Certain traits are termed *sex linked*

Developing Cultural Competence

IRAQI CHILDBIRTH CUSTOMS

"My sister, she did not have baby for very, very long time, you see. This is very sad where I am from [Iraq]. Her husband's family wanted him to leave her and we so feared he would. Then my sister became pregnant and it was very nice, we all so happy to see. Then I learned my sister birthed a baby girl and I cried and cried for a week. My mother cried too, so sad at this time no baby come and then finally to have a girl. I still feel sad for her."

(Excerpt from author's interview with an Iraqi woman on childbirth customs in Iraq)

because they are controlled by the genes on the X sex chromosome. Two examples of sex-linked traits are color blindness and hemophilia.

PREEMBRYONIC DEVELOPMENT

The first 14 days of development, starting the day the ovum is fertilized (conception), are called *the preembryonic stage,* or *the stage of the ovum.* Development after fertilization can be divided into two phases: cellular multiplication and cellular differentiation. These phases are characterized by rapid cellular multiplication, and differentiation and establishment of the primary germ layers and embryonic membranes. Synchronized development of both the endometrium and embryo is a prerequisite for implantation to succeed (Moore & Persaud, 2008). These phases and the process of implantation (nidation), which occurs between them, are discussed next.

CELLULAR MULTIPLICATION

Cellular multiplication begins as the zygote moves through the fallopian tube toward the cavity of the uterus. This transport takes 3 days or more and is accomplished mainly by a very weak fluid current in the fallopian tube resulting from the beating action of the ciliated epithelium that lines the tube.

The zygote now enters a period of rapid mitotic divisions called **cleavage**, during which it divides into two cells, four cells, eight cells, and so on. These cells, called *blastomeres,* are so small that the developing cell mass is only slightly larger than the original zygote. The blastomeres are held together by the zona pellucida, which is under the corona radiata. The blastomeres eventually form a solid ball of 12 to 16 cells called the **morula**.

As the morula enters the uterus, two things happen: The intracellular fluid in the morula increases, and a central cavity forms within the cell mass. Inside this cavity is an inner solid mass of cells called the **blastocyst**. The outer layer of cells that surrounds the cavity and replaces the zona pellucida is the

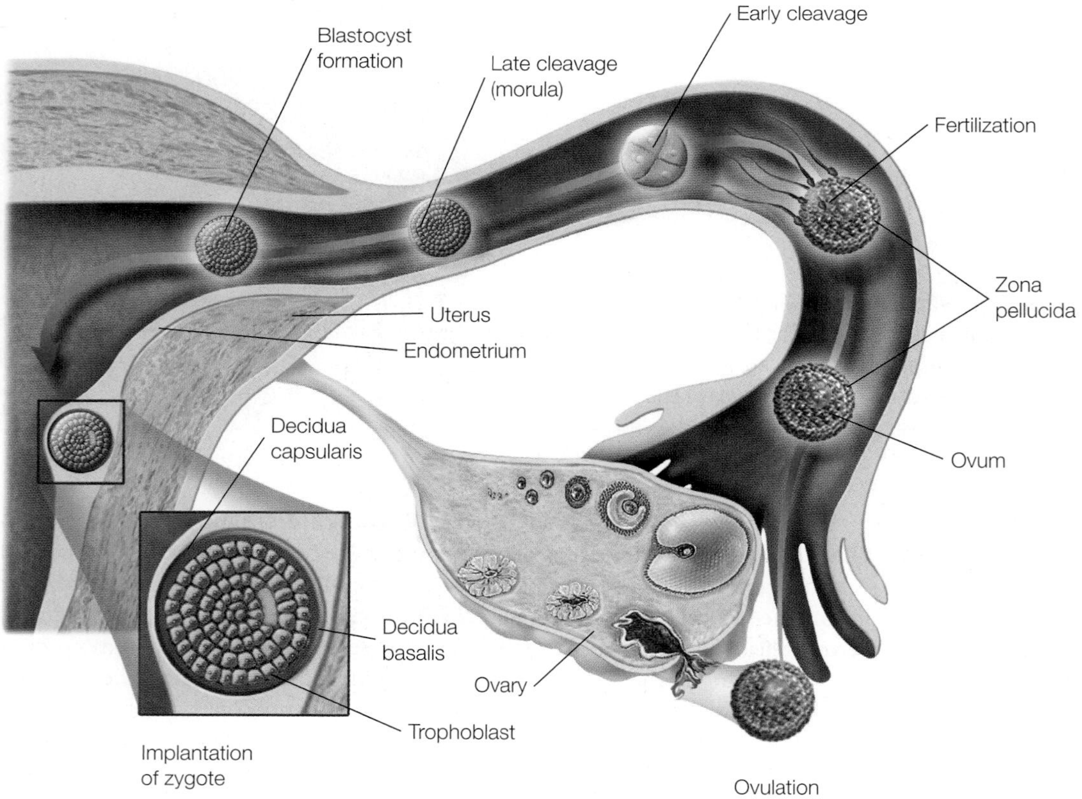

● **Figure 4–3** Changes in fertilized ovum from conception to implantation. During ovulation, the ovum leaves the ovary and enters the fallopian tube. Fertilization generally occurs in the outer third of the fallopian tube.

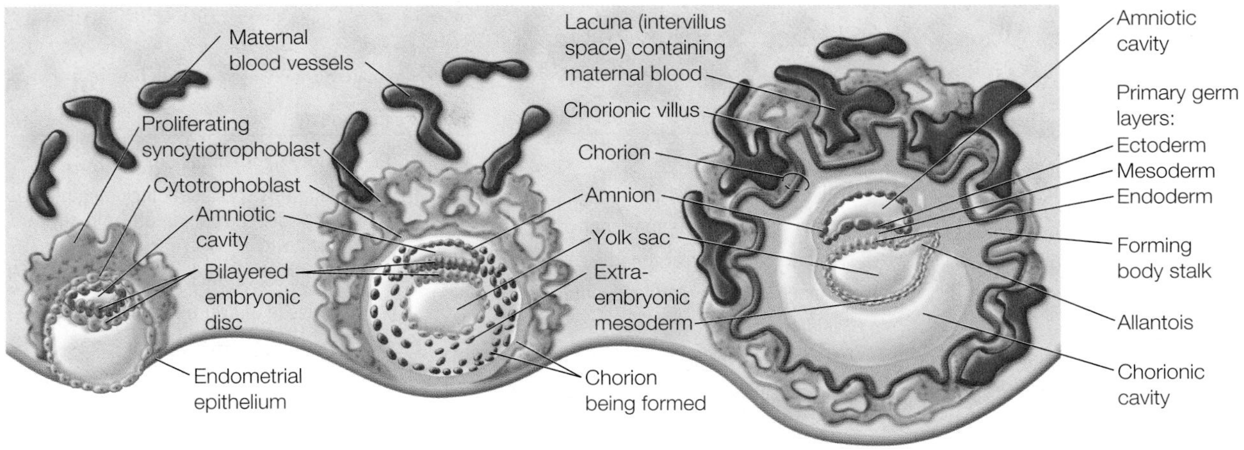

● **Figure 4–4** Formation of primary germ layers. ***A,*** Implantation of a 7½-day blastocyst in which the cells of the embryonic disc are separated from the amnion by a fluid-filled space. The erosion of the endometrium by the syncytiotrophoblast is ongoing. ***B,*** Implantation is completed by day 9, and extraembryonic mesoderm is beginning to form a discrete layer beneath the cytotrophoblast. ***C,*** By day 16 the embryo shows all three germ layers, a yolk sac, and an allantois (an outpouching of the yolk sac that forms the structural basis of the body stalk, or umbilical cord). The cytotrophoblast and associated mesoderm have become the chorion, and chorionic villi are developing.

trophoblast. Eventually, the trophoblast develops into one of the two embryonic membranes, the chorion. The blastocyst develops into a double layer of cells called the *embryonic disc,* from which the embryo and the amnion (embryonic membrane) will develop. Figure 4–3 ● shows the journey of the fertilized ovum to its destination in the uterus.

Early pregnancy factor (EPF), an immunosuppressant protein, is secreted by the trophoblastic cells. This factor appears in the maternal serum within 24 to 48 hours after fertilization and forms the basis of a pregnancy test during the first 10 days of development (Moore & Persaud, 2008).

IMPLANTATION (NIDATION)

While floating in the uterine cavity, the blastocyst is nourished by the uterine glands, which secrete a mixture of lipids, mucopolysaccharides, and glycogen. The trophoblast attaches itself to the surface of the endometrium for further nourishment. The most frequent site of attachment is the upper part of the posterior uterine wall. Between days 7 and 10 after fertilization, the zona pellucida disappears and the blastocyst implants itself by burrowing into the uterine lining and penetrating down toward the maternal capillaries until it is completely covered (Moore & Persaud, 2008). The lining of the uterus thickens below the implanted blastocyst, and the cells of the trophoblast grow down into the thickened lining, forming processes that will be called chorionic villi.

Under the influence of progesterone, the endometrium increases in thickness and vascularity in preparation for implantation and nutrition of the ovum. After implantation, the endometrium is called the decidua. The portion of the decidua that covers the blastocyst is called the **decidua capsularis**, the portion directly under the implanted blastocyst is the **decidua basalis**, and the portion that lines the rest of the uterine cavity is the **decidua vera (parietalis)**. The maternal part of the placenta develops from the decidua basalis, which contains large numbers of blood vessels (see magnified inset in Figure 4–3) (Benirschke, 2009a). The chorionic villi (discussed shortly) in contact with the decidua basalis will form the fetal portion of the placenta.

CELLULAR DIFFERENTIATION

Primary Germ Layers

About the 10th to 14th day after conception, the homogeneous mass of blastocyst cells differentiates into the primary germ layers (Figure 4–4 ●). These three layers, the **ectoderm**, **mesoderm**, and **endoderm**, are formed at the same time as the embryonic membranes. All tissues, organs, and organ systems will develop from these primary germ cell layers (see Table 4–2). For example, differentiation of the endoderm results in the formation of epithelium lining the respiratory and digestive tracts (Figure 4–5 ●).

MyNursingKit Animation: Cell Division

Embryonic Membranes

The **embryonic membranes** begin to form at the time of implantation (Figure 4–6 ●). These membranes protect and support the embryo as it grows and develops inside the uterus. The first and outermost membrane to form is the **chorion.** This thick membrane develops from the trophoblast, and has many fingerlike projections called *chorionic villi* on its surface. These chorionic villi can be used for early genetic testing of the embryo at 8 to 11 weeks' gestation by chorionic villi sampling (see Chapter 14 ∞). As the pregnancy progresses, the chorionic villi begin to degenerate, except for those just under the embryo, which grow and branch into depressions in the uterine wall, forming the fetal portion of the placenta. By the fourth month of pregnancy, the surface of the chorion is smooth except at the place of attachment to the uterine wall.

Table 4–2 Derivation of Body Structures from Primary Cell Layers

Ectoderm	Mesoderm	Endoderm
Epidermis	Dermis	Respiratory tract epithelium
Sweat glands	Wall of digestive tract	Epithelium (except nasal), including pharynx, tongue, tonsils, thyroid, parathyroid, thymus, tympanic cavity
Sebaceous glands	Kidneys and ureter (suprarenal cortex)	Lining of digestive tract
Nails	Reproductive organs (gonads, genital ducts)	Primary tissue of liver and pancreas
Hair follicles	Connective tissue (cartilage, bone, joint cavities)	Urethra and associated glands
Lens of eye	Skeleton	Urinary bladder (except trigone)
Sensory epithelium of internal and external ear, nasal cavity, sinuses, mouth, anal canal	Muscles (all types)	Vagina (parts)
Central and peripheral nervous systems	Cardiovascular system (heart, arteries, veins, blood, bone marrow)	
Nasal cavity	Pleura	
Oral glands and tooth enamel	Lymphatic tissue and cells	
Pituitary gland	Spleen	
Mammary glands		

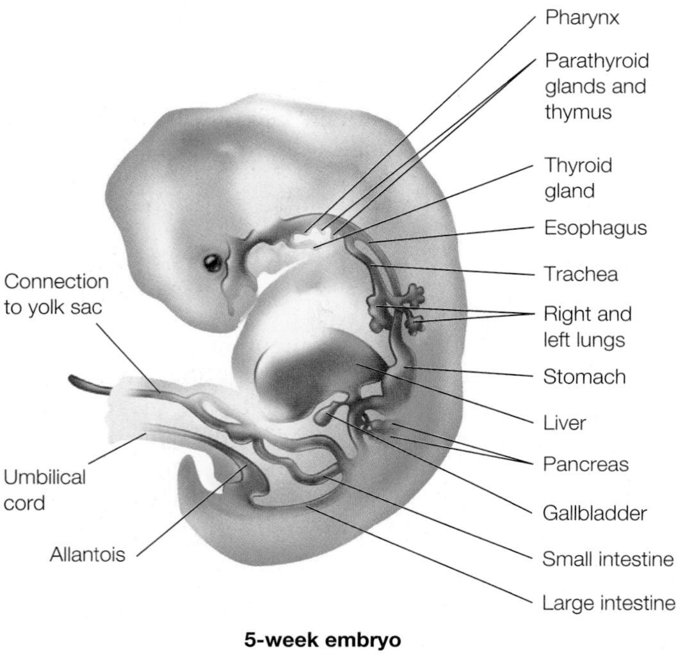

● **Figure 4–5** Differentiation of endoderm. Endoderm differentiates to form the epithelial lining of the digestive and respiratory tracts and associated glands.

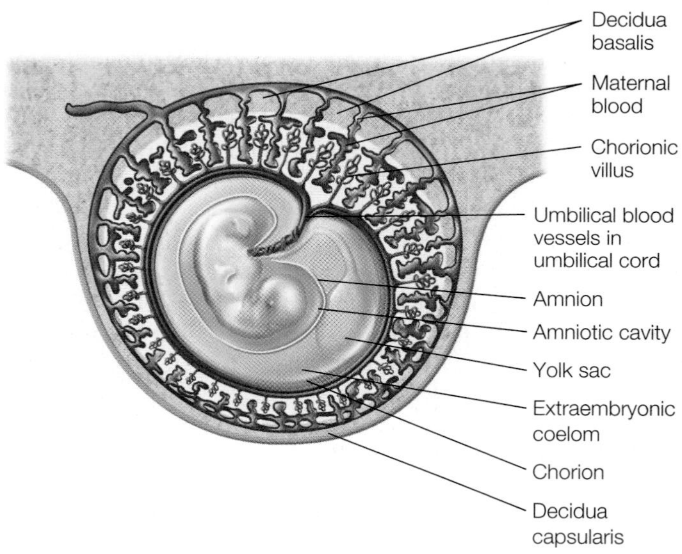

● **Figure 4–6** Early development of primary embryonic membranes. At 4½ weeks, the decidua capsularis (placental portion enclosing the embryo on the uterine surface) and decidua basalis (placental portion encompassing the elaborate chorionic villi and maternal endometrium) are well formed. The chorionic villi lie in blood-filled intervillous spaces within the endometrium. The amnion and yolk sac are well developed.

The second membrane to form, the amnion, originates from the ectoderm, a primary germ layer, during the early stages of embryonic development. The **amnion** is a thin protective membrane that contains amniotic fluid. The space between the membrane and the embryo is the *amniotic cavity.* This cavity surrounds the embryo and yolk sac, except where the developing embryo (germ-layer disc) attaches to the trophoblast via the umbilical cord. As the embryo grows, the amnion expands until it comes into contact with the chorion. These two slightly adherent membranes form the fluid-filled amniotic sac, also called the **bag of waters (BOW)**, which protects the floating embryo.

Amniotic Fluid

The *primary functions* of **amniotic fluid** are to:

- Act as a cushion to protect the embryo against mechanical injury

- Help control the embryo's temperature (relies on the mother to release heat)
- Permit symmetrical external growth and development of the embryo
- Prevent adherence of the embryo–fetus to the amnion (decreases chance of amniotic band syndrome) to allow freedom of movement so that the embryo–fetus can change position (flexion and extension), thus aiding in musculoskeletal development
- Allow the umbilical cord to be relatively free of compression
- Act as an extension of fetal extracellular space (hydropic infants have increased amniotic fluid)
- Act as a wedge during labor
- Provide fluid for analysis to determine fetal health and maturity

Amniotic fluid is slightly alkaline and contains albumin, uric acid, creatinine, lecithin, sphingomyelin, bilirubin, vernix, leukocytes, epithelial cells, enzymes, and fine hair called **lanugo**. The amount of amniotic fluid at 10 weeks is about 30 ml, and it increases to 350 ml at 20 weeks. After 20 weeks, the volume ranges from 700 to 1000 ml. The amniotic fluid volume is constantly changing as the fluid moves back and forth across the placental membrane. Water and solutes must pass between the amniotic fluid and fetus. As the pregnancy continues, the fetus contributes to the volume of amniotic fluid by excreting urine. The fetus also swallows up to 262 ml/kg/day. About 400 ml of lung fluid flows out of the fetal lungs each day (Gilbert, 2007). Abnormal variations in amniotic fluid volume are *oligohydramnios* (less than 400 ml of amniotic fluid) and *hydramnios* (more than 2000 ml or amniotic fluid index greater than 97.5 percentile for the corresponding gestational age). Hydramnios is also called *polyhydramnios*. See Chapter 22 for an in-depth discussion of alterations in amniotic fluid volume.

Yolk Sac

In humans, the yolk sac is small and functions early in embryonic life. It develops as a second cavity in the blastocyst on about day 8 or 9 after conception. It forms primitive red blood cells during the first 6 weeks of development, until the embryo's liver takes over the process. As the embryo develops, the yolk sac is incorporated into the umbilical cord, where it can be seen as a degenerated structure after birth.

Umbilical Cord

As the placenta is developing, the **umbilical cord** is also being formed from the amnion. The *body stalk,* which attaches the embryo to the yolk sac, contains blood vessels that extend into the chorionic villi. The body stalk fuses with the embryonic portion of the placenta to provide a circulatory pathway from the chorionic villi to the embryo. As the body stalk elongates to become the umbilical cord, the vessels in the cord decrease to one large vein and two smaller arteries. About 1% of umbilical cords have only two vessels, an artery and a vein; this condition may be associated with congenital malformations primarily of the renal, gastrointestinal, and cardiovascular systems. A specialized connective tissue known as **Wharton's jelly** surrounds the blood vessels in the umbilical cord. This tissue, plus the high blood volume pulsating through the vessels, prevents compression of the umbilical cord in utero. The umbilical cord has no sensory or motor innervation, so cutting the cord after birth is not painful. At term (38 to 42 weeks' gestation), the average cord is 2 cm (0.8 in.) across and about 55 cm (22 in.) long. The cord can attach itself to the placenta in various sites. Central insertion into the placenta is considered normal. (See Chapter 22 for a discussion of the various attachment sites.)

Umbilical cords appear twisted or spiraled, which is most likely caused by fetal movement. A true knot in the umbilical cord rarely occurs; if it does, the cord is longer than usual. More common are so-called false knots, caused by the folding of cord vessels. A *nuchal cord* is said to exist when the umbilical cord encircles the fetal neck.

TWINS

Twins normally occur in approximately 1 in 43 pregnancies, and triplets occur in 1 in 1341 pregnancies (Benirschke, 2009b). Among all groups, as parity (having given birth to a viable infant) increases, so does the chance for multiple births.

Twins may be either fraternal or identical (Figure 4–7 ●). If twins are fraternal (nonidentical), they are dizygotic, which means they arise from two separate ova fertilized by two separate spermatozoa. There are two placentas, two chorions, and two amnions; however, the placentas sometimes fuse and look as if they are one. Despite their birth relationship, fraternal twins are no more similar to each other than they would be to siblings born singly. They may be of the same or different sex.

Dizygotic twinning increases with maternal age up to about age 35 and then decreases abruptly. The chance of dizygotic twins increases with parity, in conceptions that occur in the first 3 months of marriage, and also with coital frequency. The chance of dizygotic twinning decreases during periods of malnutrition and during winter and spring for women living in the Northern Hemisphere. Studies indicate that dizygotic twins occur in certain families, perhaps because of genotype (genetic constitution) of the mother that results in elevated serum gonadotropin levels leading to double ovulation (Moore & Persaud, 2008). Fraternal (dizygotic) twins have been reported to occur more often among black than among white women and more often among white women than among women of Asian origin (Moore & Persaud, 2008).

Identical, or monozygotic, twins develop from a single fertilized ovum. They are of the same sex and have the same phenotype (appearance). Identical twins usually have a common placenta. Monozygosity is not affected by environment, race, physical characteristics, or fertility.

Monozygotic twins originate from division of the fertilized ovum at different stages of early development, after the zygote consists of thousands of cells. Complete separation of the cellular mass into two parts is necessary for twin formation. The number of amnions and chorions present depends on the timing of the division.

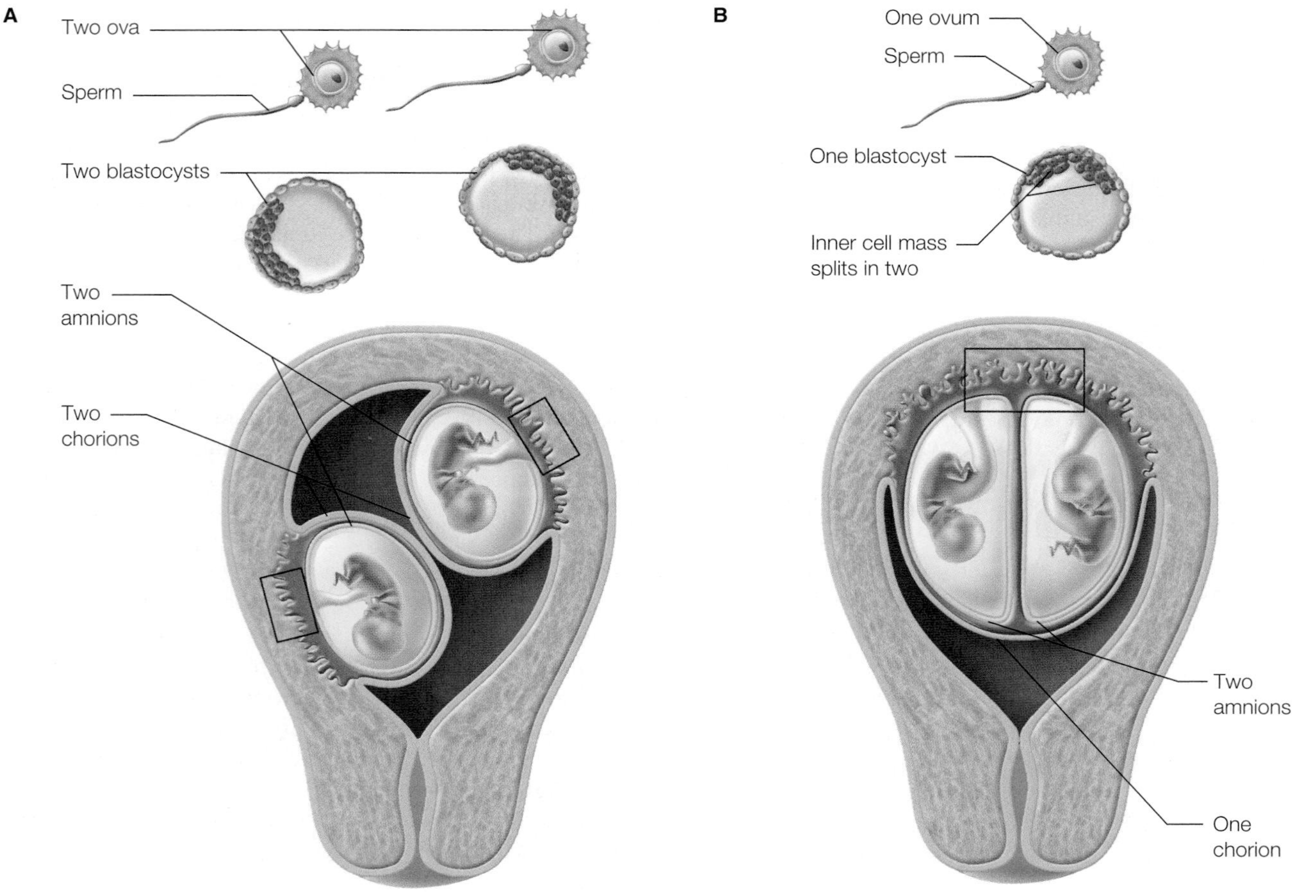

Figure 4–7 ***A,*** Formation of fraternal twins. (Note separate placentas.) ***B,*** Formation of identical twins.

1. If division occurs within 3 days of fertilization (before the inner cell mass and chorion are formed), two embryos, two amnions, and two chorions will develop. This dichorionic–diamniotic situation occurs about 20% to 30% of the time, and there may be two distinct placentas or a single fused placenta.
2. If division occurs about 5 days after fertilization (when the inner cell mass is formed and the chorion cells have differentiated but those of the amnion have not), two embryos develop with separate amnion sacs. These sacs will eventually be covered by a common chorion; thus there will be a monochorionic–diamniotic placenta (see Figure 4–7B).
3. If the amnion has already developed, approximately 7 to 13 days after fertilization, division results in two embryos with a common amnion sac and a common chorion (a monochorionic–monoamniotic placenta). This type rarely occurs.

Monozygotic twinning is considered a random event and occurs in approximately 3 to 4 per 1000 live births (Benirschke, 2009b). The survival rate of monozygotic twins is lower than that of dizygotic twins, and congenital anomalies are more prevalent. Both twins may have the same malformation.

DEVELOPMENT AND FUNCTIONS OF THE PLACENTA

The **placenta** is the means of metabolic and nutrient exchange between the embryonic and maternal circulations. Placental development and circulation do not begin until the third week of embryonic development. The placenta develops at the site where the embryo attaches to the uterine wall. Expansion of the placenta continues until about 20 weeks, when it covers approximately one-half of the internal surface of the uterus. After 20 weeks' gestation, the placenta becomes thicker but not wider. At 40 weeks' gestation, the placenta is about 15 to 20 cm (5.9 to 7.9 in.) in diameter and 2.5 to 3.0 cm (1.0 to 1.2 in.) in thickness. At that time, it weighs about 400 to 600 g (14 to 21 oz).

The placenta has two parts: the maternal and fetal portions. The maternal portion consists of the decidua basalis and its circulation. Its surface is red and fleshlike. The fetal portion consists of the chorionic villi and their circulation. The fetal surface of the placenta is covered by the amnion, which gives it a shiny, gray appearance (often called Shiny Schultz) (Figures 4–8 ● and 4–9 ●).

The placenta begins to form at implantation when the trophoblastic cells of the chorionic villi form spaces in the decidua basalis tissues. These spaces fill with maternal blood, and the chorionic villi grow into them. As the chorionic villi differenti-

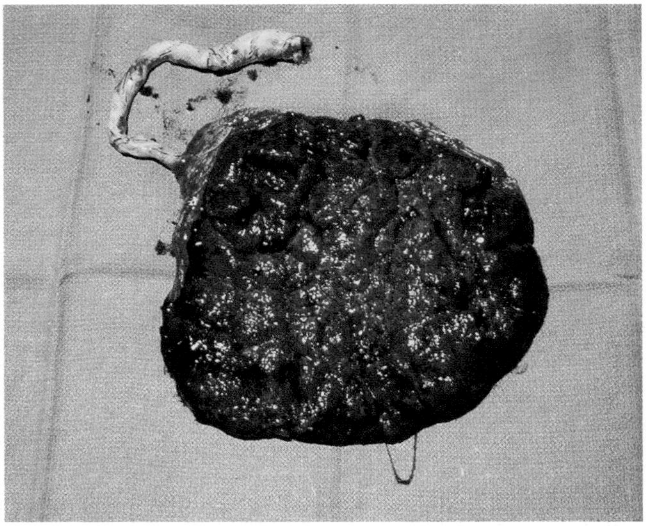

● **Figure 4–8** Maternal side of placenta.

Photo courtesy of Marcia London.

ate, two trophoblastic layers appear: an outer layer, called the *syncytium* (consisting of syncytiotrophoblasts), and an inner layer, known as the *cytotrophoblast* (see Figure 4–4). The cytotrophoblast thins out and disappears about the fifth month, leaving only a single layer of syncytium covering the chorionic villi. The syncytium is in direct contact with the maternal blood in the intervillous spaces. It is the functional layer of the placenta and secretes the placental hormones of pregnancy.

A third, inner layer of connective mesoderm develops in the chorionic villi, forming *anchoring villi.* These anchoring villi eventually form the *septa* (partitions) of the placenta. The septa divide the mature placenta into 15 to 20 segments called **cotyledons** (subdivisions of the placenta made up of anchoring villi and decidual tissue). In each cotyledon, the *branching villi* form a highly complex vascular system that allows compartmentalization of the uteroplacental circulation. The exchange of gases and nutrients takes place across these vascular systems.

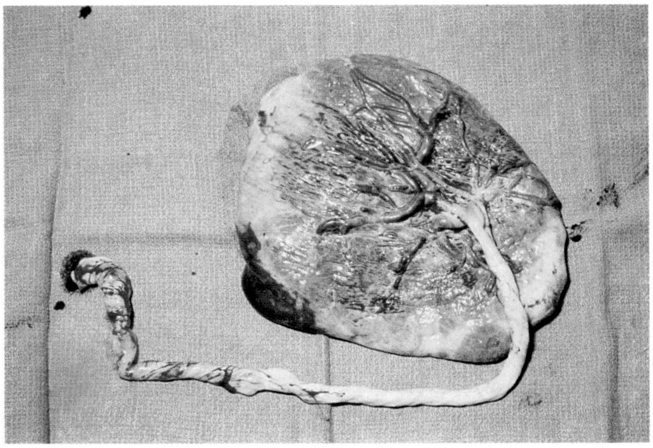

● **Figure 4–9** Fetal side of placenta.

Photo courtesy of Marcia London.

Exchange of substances across the placenta is minimal during the first 3 to 5 months of development because the villous membrane is initially too thick, which limits its permeability. As the villous membrane thins, placental permeability increases until about the last month of pregnancy, when permeability begins to decrease as the placenta ages. In the fully developed placenta, fetal blood in the villi and maternal blood in the intervillous spaces are separated by three to four thin layers of tissue.

PLACENTAL CIRCULATION

The completion of the maternal–placental–embryonic circulation occurs about 17 days after conception, when the embryonic heart begins functioning (Moore & Persaud, 2008). By the end of the fourth week, embryonic blood is circulating between the embryo and the chorionic villi. In the intervillous spaces, maternal blood supplies oxygen and nutrients to the embryonic capillaries in the villi. Waste products and carbonic dioxide diffuse into the maternal blood. By 14 weeks, the placenta is a discrete organ. It has grown in thickness as a result of growth in the length and size of the chorionic villi and accompanying expansion of the intervillous space.

In the fully developed placenta's umbilical cord, fetal blood flows through the two umbilical arteries to the capillaries of the villi, becomes oxygen enriched, and then flows back through the umbilical vein into the fetus (Figure 4–10 ●). Late in pregnancy, a soft blowing sound *(funic souffle)* can be heard over the area of the umbilical cord. The sound is synchronous with the fetal heartbeat and fetal blood flow through the umbilical arteries.

Maternal blood, rich in oxygen and nutrients, spurts from the spiral uterine arteries into the intervillous spaces. These spurts are produced by the maternal blood pressure. The spurt of blood is directed toward the chorionic plate, and as the blood loses pressure, it becomes lateral (spreads out). Fresh blood enters continuously and exerts pressure on the contents of the intervillous spaces, pushing blood toward the exits in the basal plate. The blood then drains through the uterine and other pelvic veins. A *uterine souffle,* timed precisely with the mother's pulse, is also heard just above the mother's symphysis pubis during the last months of pregnancy. This souffle is caused by the augmented blood flow entering the dilated uterine arteries.

Braxton Hicks contractions are intermittent painless uterine contractions that may occur every 10 to 20 minutes and occur more frequently near the end of pregnancy (see Chapter 17∞). These contractions are believed to facilitate placental circulation by enhancing the movement of blood from the center of the cotyledon through the intervillous space. Placental blood flow is enhanced when the woman is lying on her side because venous return from the lower extremities is not compromised (Blackburn, 2007).

PLACENTAL FUNCTIONS

Placental exchange functions occur only in those fetal vessels that are in intimate contact with the covering syncytial membrane. The syncytium villi have brush borders containing many microvilli, which greatly increase the exchange rate between maternal and fetal circulation (Sadler, 2006).

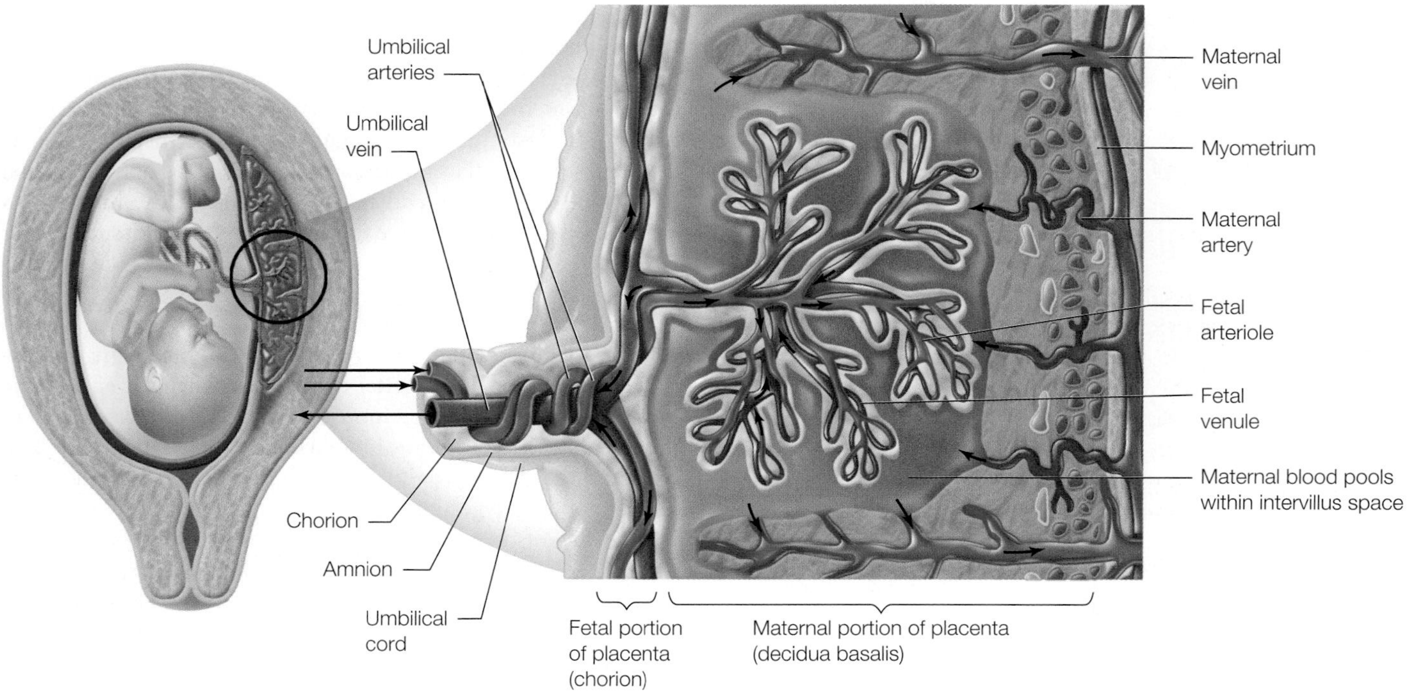

● **Figure 4–10** Vascular arrangement of the placenta. Arrows indicate the direction of blood flow. Maternal blood flows through the uterine arteries to the intervillous spaces of the placenta and returns through the uterine veins to maternal circulation. Fetal blood flows through the umbilical arteries into the villous capillaries of the placenta and returns through the umbilical vein to the fetal circulation.

The placental functions, many of which begin soon after implantation, include fetal respiration, nutrition, and excretion. To carry out these functions, the placenta is involved in metabolic and transfer activities. In addition, it has endocrine functions and special immunologic properties; see discussion later in this section.

Metabolic Activities

The placenta performs several essential metabolic activities:

- It continuously produces glycogen, cholesterol, and fatty acids for fetal use and hormone production.
- It produces numerous enzymes required for fetoplacental transfer, including:
  - sulfatase, which enhances excretion of fetal estrogen precursors,
  - insulinase, which increases the barrier to insulin
- It breaks down certain substances such as epinephrine and histamine (Blackburn, 2007).

In addition, the placenta also stores glycogen and iron.

Transport Function

The placental membranes actively control the transfer of a wide range of substances by a variety of transport mechanisms.

Simple diffusion moves substances from an area of higher concentration to an area of lower concentration. Substances that move across the placenta by simple diffusion include water, oxygen, carbon dioxide, electrolytes (sodium and chloride), anesthetic gases, and drugs. Insulin and steroid hormones originating from the adrenals, as well as thyroid hormones, also cross the placenta. However, this happens at a very slow rate. The rate of oxygen transfer across the placental membrane is greater than that allowed by simple diffusion, indicating that oxygen is also transferred by some type of facilitated diffusion transport. Unfortunately, many substances of abuse, such as cocaine and heroin, cross the placenta via simple diffusion.

Facilitated transport involves a carrier system to move molecules from an area of greater concentration to an area of lower concentration. Molecules such as glucose, galactose, and some oxygen are transported by this method. The glucose level in the fetal blood ordinarily is approximately 20% to 30% lower than the glucose level in the maternal blood, because the fetus is metabolizing glucose rapidly. This in turn causes rapid transport of additional glucose from the maternal blood into the fetal blood.

Active transport can work against a concentration gradient and allows molecules to move from areas of lower concentration to areas of higher concentration. Amino acids, calcium, iron, iodine, water-soluble vitamins, and glucose are transferred across the placenta in this way. The measured amino acid content of fetal blood is greater than that of maternal blood, and calcium and inorganic phosphate occur in greater concentration in fetal blood than in maternal blood (Blackburn, 2007).

Other modes of transfer also exist. *Pinocytosis* is important for transferring large molecules such as albumin and gamma globulin. Materials are engulfed by amoeba-like cells, forming plasma droplets. *Hydrostatic* and *osmotic pressures* allow the bulk flow of water and some solutes. Also fetal red blood cells can pass into the maternal circulation through breaks in the capillaries and placental membrane, particularly during labor and birth. Certain cells, such as maternal leukocytes, and microorganisms, such as viruses (e.g., the human immunodeficiency virus [HIV], which causes acquired immunodeficiency syndrome [AIDS]), rubella, cytomegalovirus, polio, and the bacterium *Treponema pallidum* (which causes syphilis), can also cross the placental membrane under their own power (Moore & Persaud, 2008). Some bacteria and protozoa infect the placenta by causing lesions and then entering the fetal blood system.

Reduction of the placental surface area, as with abruptio placentae (partial or complete premature separation of an abnormally implanted placenta), lessens the area that is functional for exchange. Placental diffusion distance also affects exchange. In conditions such as diabetes and placental infection, edema of the villi increases the diffusion distance, thus increasing the distance the substance has to be transferred.

Blood flow alteration changes the transfer rate of substances. Decreased blood flow in the intervillous space is seen in labor and with certain maternal diseases such as hypertension. Mild fetal hypoxia increases the umbilical blood flow, but severe hypoxia results in decreased blood flow.

As the maternal blood picks up fetal waste products and carbon dioxide, it drains back into the maternal circulation through the veins in the basal plate. Fetal blood is hypoxic by comparison; it therefore attracts oxygen from the mother's blood. Affinity for oxygen increases as the fetal blood gives up its carbon dioxide, which also decreases its acidity.

Endocrine Functions

The placenta produces hormones that are vital to the survival of the fetus. These include human chorionic gonadotropin (hCG); human placental lactogen (hPL); and two steroid hormones, estrogen and progesterone.

The hormone hCG is similar to luteinizing hormone (LH) and prevents the normal involution of the corpus luteum at the end of the menstrual cycle (see Chapter 3). If the corpus luteum stops functioning before the 11th week of pregnancy, spontaneous abortion occurs. The hCG also causes the corpus luteum to secrete increased amounts of estrogen and progesterone.

After the 11th week, the placenta produces enough progesterone and estrogen to maintain pregnancy. In the male fetus, hCG also exerts an interstitial cell-stimulating effect on the testes, resulting in the production of testosterone. This small secretion of testosterone during embryonic development is the factor that causes male sex organs to grow. Human chorionic gonadotropin may play a role in the trophoblast's immunologic capabilities (its ability to keep the mother's system from rejecting the placenta and embryo). This hormone is used as a basis for pregnancy tests (see Chapter 9).

Human chorionic gonadotropin is present in maternal blood serum 8 to 10 days after fertilization, just as soon as implantation has occurred, and is detectable in maternal urine at the time of missed menses. After reaching its maximum level at 50 to 70 days' gestation, hCG begins to decrease as placental hormone production increases.

Progesterone is an essential hormone for pregnancy. It increases the secretions of the fallopian tubes and uterus to provide appropriate nutritive matter for the developing morula and blastocyst. It also appears to aid in ovum transport through the fallopian tube. Progesterone causes decidual cells to develop in the uterine endometrium, and it must be present in high levels for implantation to occur. Progesterone also decreases the contractility of the uterus, thus preventing uterine contractions from causing spontaneous abortion.

Before stimulation by hCG, the corpus luteum's production of progesterone reaches a peak about 7 to 10 days after ovulation. Implantation occurs at about the same time as this peak. At 16 days after ovulation, progesterone reaches a level between 25 and 50 mg per day and continues to rise slowly in subsequent weeks. After 11 weeks, the placenta (specifically, the syncytiotrophoblast) takes over the production of progesterone and secretes it in tremendous quantities, reaching levels of more than 250 mg per day late in pregnancy.

By 7 weeks, the placenta produces more than 50% of the estrogens in the maternal circulation. *Estrogens* serve mainly a proliferative function, causing enlargement of the uterus, breasts, and breast glandular tissue. Estrogens also have a significant role in increasing vascularity and vasodilation, particularly in the villous capillaries toward the end of pregnancy. Placental estrogens increase markedly toward the end of pregnancy, to as much as 30 times the daily production in the middle of a normal monthly menstrual cycle. The primary estrogen secreted by the placenta is different from that secreted by the ovaries. The placenta secretes mainly *estriol,* whereas the ovaries secrete primarily estradiol. The placenta cannot synthesize estriol by itself. Essential precursors such as dehydroepiandrosterone sulfate (DHEA-S) is provided by the fetal adrenal glands, is processed by fetal liver, and is transported to the placenta for the final conversion to estrone, estradiol, and estriol (Blackburn, 2007; Knuppel, 2007).

The hormone human placental lactogen (hPL), also referred to as human chorionic somatomammotropin (hCS), is similar to human pituitary growth hormone in that hPL stimulates certain changes in the mother's metabolic processes. These changes ensure that more protein, glucose, and minerals are available for the fetus. Secretion of hPL can be detected by about 4 weeks after conception.

Immunologic Properties

The placenta and embryo are transplants of living tissue within the same species and are therefore considered *homografts.* Unlike other homografts, the placenta and embryo appear exempt from immunologic reaction by the host. Most recent data suggest that the placental hormones (progesterone and hCG) suppress cellular immunity during pregnancy (Knuppel, 2007). One theory suggests that chorionic villi syncytiotrophoblastic tissue is immunologically inert. The chorionic villi may lack major histocompatibility (MHC) antigens and thus do not evoke rejection responses. It does, however, protect against antibody formation. Extravillous trophoblast (EVT) cells, which invade the uterine deciduas, have

HLA-G, which is not readily recognized by sensitized T lymphocytes and natural killer cells (Moore & Persaud, 2008).

DEVELOPMENT OF THE FETAL CIRCULATORY SYSTEM

The circulatory system of the fetus has several unique features that, by maintaining the blood flow to the placenta, provide the fetus with oxygen and nutrients while removing carbon dioxide and other waste products.

Most of the blood supply bypasses the fetal lungs because they do not carry out respiratory gas exchange. The placenta assumes the function of the fetal lungs by supplying oxygen and allowing the fetus to excrete carbon dioxide into the maternal bloodstream. Figure 4–11 ● shows the fetal circulatory system. The blood from the placenta flows through the umbilical vein, which enters the abdominal wall of the fetus at the site that, after birth, is the umbilicus (belly button). As umbilical venous blood approaches the liver, a small portion of the blood enters the liver sinusoids, mixes with blood from the portal circulation, and then enters the inferior vena cava via hepatic veins. Most of the umbilical vein's blood flows through the **ductus venosus** directly into the fetal inferior vena cava, bypassing the liver. This blood then enters the right atrium, passes through the **foramen ovale** into the left atrium, and pours into the left ventricle, which pumps blood

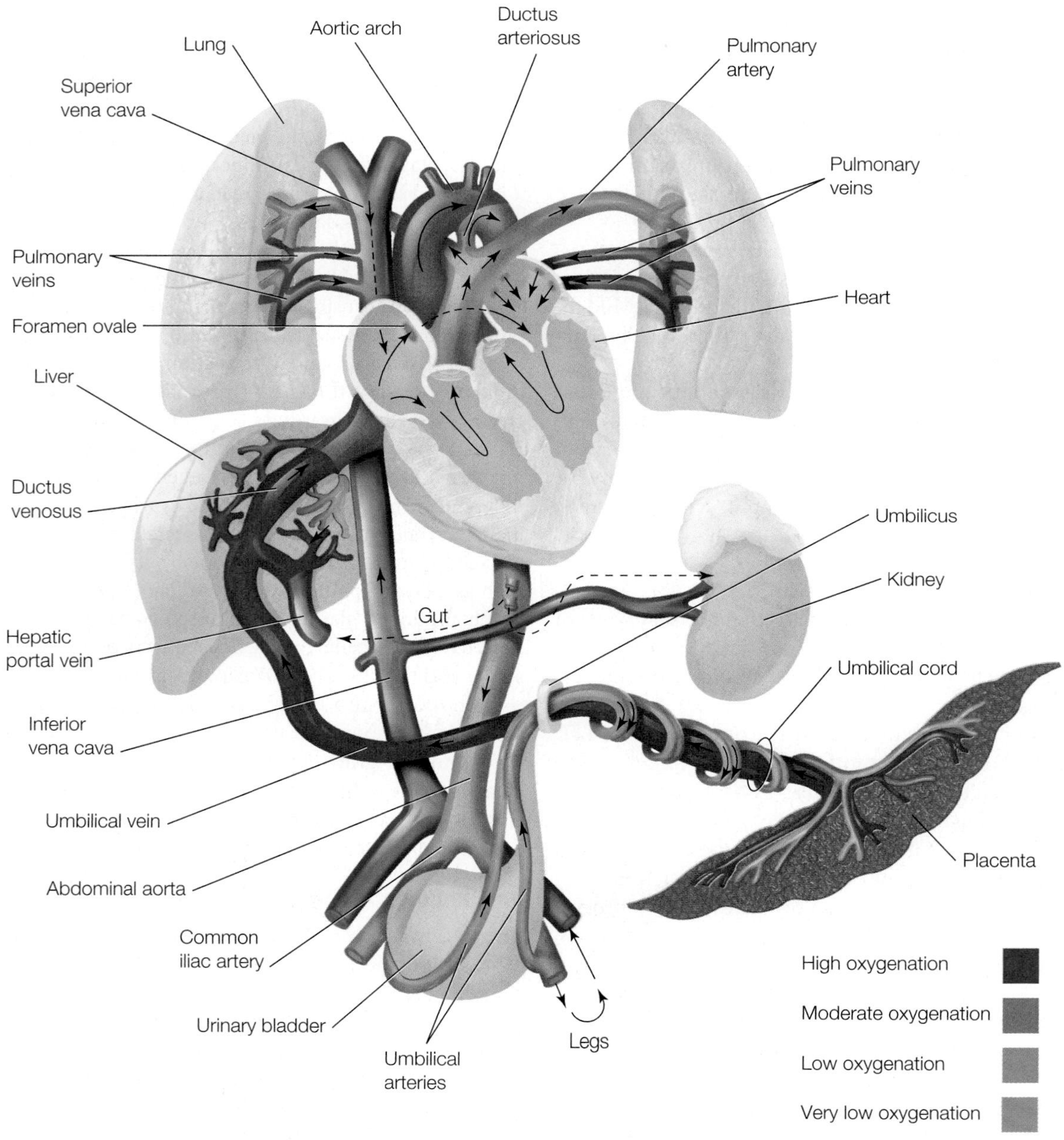

● **Figure 4–11** Fetal circulation. Blood leaves the placenta and enters the fetus through the umbilical vein. After circulating through the fetus, the blood returns to the placenta through the umbilical arteries. The ductus venosus, the foramen ovale, and the ductus arteriosus allow the blood to bypass the fetal liver and lungs.

into the aorta. Some blood returning from the head and upper extremities by way of the superior vena cava is emptied into the right atrium and passes through the tricuspid valve into the right ventricle. This blood is pumped into the pulmonary artery, and a small amount passes to the lungs for nourishment only. The larger portion of blood passes from the pulmonary artery through the **ductus arteriosus** into the descending aorta, bypassing the lungs. Finally, blood returns to the placenta through the two umbilical arteries, and the process is repeated.

The fetus obtains oxygen via diffusion from the maternal circulation because of the gradient difference of PO_2 of 50 mm Hg in maternal blood in the placenta to 30 mm Hg PO_2 in the fetus. At term the fetus receives oxygen from the mother's circulation at a rate of 20 to 30 ml per minute (Sadler, 2006). Fetal hemoglobin facilitates obtaining oxygen from the maternal circulation, because it carries as much as 20% to 30% more oxygen than adult hemoglobin. For further discussion, see Chapter 27 ∞.

Fetal circulation delivers the highest available oxygen concentration to the head, neck, brain, and heart (coronary circulation) and a lesser amount of oxygenated blood to the abdominal organs and the lower body. This circulatory pattern leads to cephalocaudal (head-to-tail) development in the fetus.

EMBRYONIC AND FETAL DEVELOPMENT

Pregnancy is calculated to last an *average* of 10 lunar months: 40 weeks, or 280 days. This period of 280 days is calculated from the onset of the last normal menstrual period to the time of birth. Estimated date of birth (EDB), sometimes referred to as the *estimated date of delivery (EDD)*, is usually calculated by this method. Most fetuses are born within 10 to 14 days of the calculated date of birth. The postconception age (fertilization age) of the fetus is calculated to be *about* 2 weeks less, or 266 days (38 weeks) or 9.5 calendar months. The latter measurement is more accurate because it measures time from the fertilization of the ovum, or conception.

The basic events of organ development in the embryo and fetus are outlined in Table 4–3. The time periods in the table are **postconception age periods**. During the period from fertilization to the end of the embryonic period (8 weeks), age is often expressed in days but can be given in weeks. During the fetal period (ninth week until birth) age is given in weeks (Moore & Persaud, 2008). The foldout poster in the middle of the book also summarizes fetal development.

In review, human development follows three stages. The preembryonic stage, as discussed earlier in the chapter, consists of the first 14 days of development after the ovum is fertilized; then the embryonic stage covers the period from day 15 until approximately the end of the eighth week postconception, and the fetal stage extends from the end of the eighth week until birth. (See the detailed discussion of the embryonic and fetal stages next.)

EMBRYONIC STAGE

The stage of the **embryo** starts on day 15 (the beginning of the third week after conception) and continues until approximately the eighth week, or until the embryo reaches a crown-to-rump (C–R) length of 3 cm (1.2 in.). This length is usually reached about 56 days after fertilization (the end of the eighth gestational week). During the embryonic stage, tissues differentiate into essential organs and the main external features develop. The embryo is the most vulnerable to *teratogens* during this period. These are discussed in more depth later in the chapter.

Three Weeks

In the third week, the embryonic disk becomes elongated and pear shaped, with a broad cephalic end and a narrow caudal end. The ectoderm has formed a long cylindrical tube for brain and spinal cord development. The gastrointestinal tract, created from the endoderm, appears as another tubelike structure communicating with the yolk sac. The most advanced organ is the heart. At 3 weeks, a single tubular heart forms just outside the body cavity of the embryo.

Four to Five Weeks

During days 21 to 32, *somites* (a series of mesodermal blocks) form on either side of the embryo's midline. The vertebrae that form the spinal column will develop from these somites. Before 28 days, arm and leg buds are not visible, but the tail bud is present. The pharyngeal arches—which will form the lower jaw, hyoid bone, and larynx—develop at this time. The pharyngeal pouches appear now; these pouches will form the eustachian tube and cavity of the middle ear, the tonsils, and the parathyroid and thymus glands. The primordia of the ear and eye are also present. By the end of 28 days, the tubular heart is beating at a regular rhythm and pushing its own primitive blood cells through the main blood vessels.

During the fifth week, the optic cups and lens vessels of the eye form and the nasal pits develop. Partitioning in the heart occurs with the dividing of the atrium. The embryo has a marked C-shaped body, accentuated by the rudimentary tail and the large head folded over a protuberant trunk (Figure 4–12 ●). By day 35,

(continued on page 80)

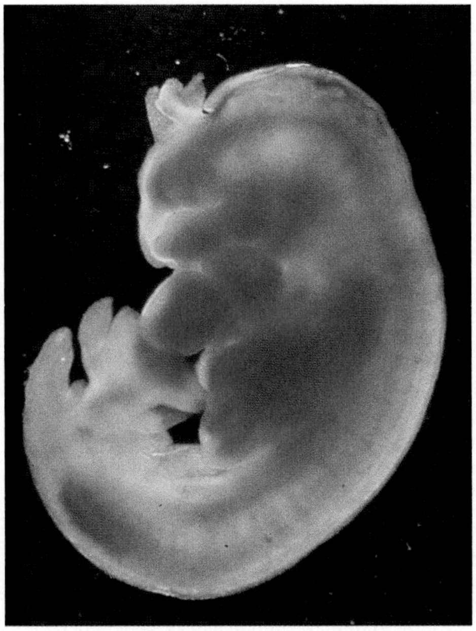

● **Figure 4–12** The embryo at 5 weeks. The embryo has a marked C-shaped body and a rudimentary tail.

Source: © Petit Format/Nestle/Science Source/Photo Researchers Inc.

Table 4–3 Timeline of Organ System Development in the Embryo and Fetus

Age: 2 to 3 Weeks

Length: 2 mm C–R (crown to rump)
Nervous system: Groove forms along middle back as cells thicken; neural tube forms from closure of neural groove.
Cardiovascular system: Beginning of blood circulation; tubular heart begins to form during third week.
Gastrointestinal system: Liver begins to function.
Genitourinary system: Formation of kidneys beginning.
Respiratory system: Nasal pits forming.
Endocrine system: Thyroid tissue appears.
Eyes: Optic cup and lens pit have formed; pigment in eyes.
Ears: Auditory pit is now enclosed structure.

Age: 4 Weeks

Length: 4 to 6 mm C–R
Weight: 0.4 g
Nervous system: Anterior portion of neural tube closes to form brain; closure of posterior end forms spinal cord.
Musculoskeletal system: Noticeable limb buds.
Cardiovascular system: Tubular heart beats at 28 days, and primitive red blood cells circulate through fetus and chorionic villi.
Gastrointestinal system: Mouth: formation of oral cavity; primitive jaws present; esophagotracheal septum begins division of esophagus and trachea. Digestive tract: stomach forms; esophagus and intestine become tubular; ducts of pancreas and liver forming.

Age: 5 Weeks

Length: 8 mm C–R
Weight: Only 0.5% of total body weight is fat (to 20 weeks).
Nervous system: Brain has differentiated and cranial nerves are present.
Musculoskeletal system: Developing muscles have innervation.
Cardiovascular system: Atrial division has occurred.

Age: 6 Weeks

Length: 12 mm C–R
Musculoskeletal system: Bone rudiments present; primitive skeletal shape forming; muscle mass begins to develop; ossification of skull and jaws begins.
Cardiovascular system: Chambers present in heart; groups of blood cells can be identified.
Gastrointestinal system: Oral and nasal cavities and upper lip formed; liver begins to form red blood cells.
Respiratory system: Trachea, bronchi, and lung buds present.
Ears: Formation of external, middle, and inner ear continues.
Sexual development: Embryonic sex glands appear.

Age: 7 Weeks

Length: 18 mm C–R
Cardiovascular system: Fetal heartbeats can be detected.
Gastrointestinal system: Mouth: tongue separates; palate folds. Digestive tract: stomach attains final form.
Genitourinary system: Separation of bladder and urethra from rectum.
Respiratory system: Diaphragm separates abdominal and thoracic cavities.
Eyes: Optic nerve formed; eyelids appear, thickening of lens.
Sexual development: Differentiation of sex glands into ovaries and testes begins.

Age: 8 Weeks

Length: 2.5 to 3 cm C–R
Weight: 2 g
Musculoskeletal system: Digits formed; further differentiation of cells in primitive skeleton; cartilaginous bones show first signs of ossification; development of muscles in trunk, limbs, and head; some movement of fetus now possible.
Cardiovascular system: Development of heart essentially complete; fetal circulation follows two circuits—four extraembryonic and two intraembryonic. Heartbeat can be heard with Doppler at 8 to 12 weeks.
Gastrointestinal system: Mouth: completion of lip fusion. Digestive tract: rotation in midgut; anal membrane has perforated.
Ears: External, middle, and inner ear assuming final forms.
Sexual development: Male and female external genitals appear similar until end of ninth week.

Age: 10 Weeks

Length: 5 to 6 cm C–R
Weight: 14 g
Nervous system: Neurons appear at caudal end of spinal cord; basic divisions of brain present.
Musculoskeletal system: Fingers and toes begin nail growth.
Gastrointestinal system: Mouth: separation of lips from jaw; fusion of palate folds. Digestive tract: developing intestines enclosed in abdomen.
Genitourinary system: Bladder sac formed.
Endocrine system: Islets of Langerhans differentiated.
Eyes: Eyelids fused closed; development of lacrimal duct.
Sexual development: Males: production of testosterone and physical characteristics between 8 and 12 weeks.

Age: 12 Weeks

Length: 8 cm C–R; 11.5 cm C–H
Weight: 45 g
Musculoskeletal system: Clear outlining of miniature bones (12 to 20 weeks); process of ossification is established throughout fetal body; appearance of involuntary muscles in viscera.
Gastrointestinal system: Mouth: completion of palate. Digestive tract: appearance of muscles in gut; bile secretion begins; liver is major producer of red blood cells.
Respiratory system: Lungs acquire definitive shape.
Skin: Pink and delicate.
Endocrine system: Hormonal secretion from thyroid; insulin present in pancreas.
Immunologic system: Appearance of lymphoid tissue in fetal thymus gland.

Table 4–3 Timeline of Organ System Development in the Embryo and Fetus—continued

Age: 16 Weeks

Length: 13.5 cm C-R; 15 cm C-H (crown to heel)
Weight: 200 g
Musculoskeletal system: Teeth beginning to form hard tissue that will become central incisors.
Gastrointestinal system: Mouth: differentiation of hard and soft palate. Digestive tract: development of gastric and intestinal glands; intestines begin to collect meconium.
Genitourinary system: Kidneys assume typical shape and organization.
Skin: Appearance of scalp hair; lanugo present on body; transparent skin with visible blood vessels; sweat glands developing.
Eyes, ears, and nose: Formed.
Sexual development: Sex determination possible.

Age: 18 Weeks

Musculoskeletal system: Teeth beginning to form hard tissue (enamel and dentine) that will become lateral incisors.
Cardiovascular system: Fetal heart tones audible with fetoscope at 16 to 20 weeks.

Age: 20 Weeks

Length: 19 cm C-R; 25 cm C-H
Weight: 435 g (6% of total body weight is fat).
Nervous system: Myelination of spinal cord begins.
Musculoskeletal system: Teeth beginning to form hard tissue that will become canine and first molar. Lower limbs are of final relative proportions.
Gastrointestinal system: Fetus actively sucks and swallows amniotic fluid; peristaltic movements begin.
Skin: Lanugo covers entire body; brown fat begins to form; vernix caseosa begins to form.
Immunologic system: Detectable levels of fetal antibodies (IgG type).
Blood formation: Iron is stored and bone marrow is increasingly important.

Age: 24 Weeks

Length: 23 cm C-R; 28 cm C-H
Weight: 780 g
Nervous system: Brain looks like mature brain.
Musculoskeletal system: Teeth are beginning to form hard tissue that will become the second molars.
Respiratory system: Respiratory movements may occur (24 to 40 weeks). Nostrils reopen. Alveoli appear in lungs and begin production of surfactant; gas exchange possible.
Skin: Reddish and wrinkled, vernix caseosa present.
Immunologic system: IgG levels reach maternal levels.

Age: 28 Weeks

Length: 27 cm C-R; 35 cm C-H
Weight: 1200 to 1250 g
Nervous system: Begins regulation of some body functions.
Skin: Adipose tissue accumulates rapidly; nails appear; eyebrows and eyelashes present.
Eyes: Eyelids open (26 to 29 weeks).
Sexual development: Males: testes descend into inguinal canal and upper scrotum.

Age: 32 Weeks

Length: 31 cm C-R; 38–43 cm C-H
Weight: 2000 g
Nervous system: More reflexes present.

Age: 36 Weeks

Length: 35 cm C-R; 42 to 48 cm C-H
Weight: 2500 to 2750 g
Musculoskeletal system: Distal femoral ossification centers present.
Skin: Pale; body rounded, lanugo disappearing, hair fuzzy or woolly; few sole creases; sebaceous glands active and helping to produce vernix caseosa (36 to 40 weeks).
Ears: Earlobes soft with little cartilage.
Sexual development: Males: scrotum small and few rugae present; descent of testes into upper scrotum to stay (36 to 40 weeks). Females: labia majora and minora equally prominent.

Age: 38 to 40 Weeks

Length: 40 cm C-R; 48 to 52 cm C-H
Weight: 3200+ g (16% of total body weight is fat).
Respiratory system: At 38 weeks, lecithin-sphingomyelin (L/S) ratio approaches 2:1 (indicates decreased risk of respiratory distress from inadequate surfactant production if born now).
Skin: Smooth and pink; vernix present in skin folds; moderate to profuse silky hair; lanugo on shoulders and upper back; nails extend over tips or digits; creases cover sole.
Ears: Earlobes firmer because of increased cartilage.
Sexual development: Males: rugous scrotum. Females: labia majora well developed and minora small or completely covered.

Note: Age refers to postfertilization or postconception age.
Source: Data from Sadler, T. W. (2006). *Langman's medical embryology* (10th ed). Baltimore: Lippincott Williams & Wilkins.

the arm and leg buds are well developed, with paddle-shaped hand and foot plates. The heart, circulatory system, and brain show the most advanced development. The brain has differentiated into five areas, and 10 pairs of cranial nerves are recognizable.

Six Weeks

At 6 weeks the head structures are more highly developed and the trunk is straighter than in earlier stages. The upper and lower jaws are recognizable, and the external nares are well formed. The trachea has developed, and its caudal end is bifurcated for beginning lung formation. The upper lip has formed, and the palate is developing. The ears are developing rapidly. The arms have begun to extend ventrally across the chest, and both arms and legs have digits, although they may still be webbed. There is a slight elbow bend in the arms, which are more advanced in development than the legs. Beginning at this stage, the prominent tail will recede. The heart now has most of its definitive characteristics, and fetal circulation begins to be established. The liver starts to produce blood cells.

Seven Weeks

At 7 weeks the head of the embryo is rounded and nearly erect (Figure 4–13 ●). The eyes have shifted and are closer together, and the eyelids are beginning to form. The palate is near completion, and the tongue is developing in the formed mouth. The gastrointestinal and genitourinary tracts undergo significant changes during the seventh week. Before this time the rectal and urogenital passages formed one tube that ended in a blind pouch; they now separate into two tubular structures. The intestines enter the extraembryonic coelom in the area of the umbilical cord (called umbilical herniation) (Moore & Persaud, 2008). The beginnings of all essential external and internal structures are present.

Eight Weeks

At 8 weeks the embryo is approximately 3 cm (1.2 in.) C–R length and clearly resembles a human being. Facial features continue to develop. The eyelids begin to fuse. Auricles of the external ears begin to assume their final shape, but they are still set low (Moore & Persaud, 2008). External genitals appear, but the embryo's sex is not clearly identifiable. The rectal passage opens with the perforation of the anal membrane. The circulatory system through the umbilical cord is well established. Long bones are beginning to form, and the large muscles are now capable of contracting.

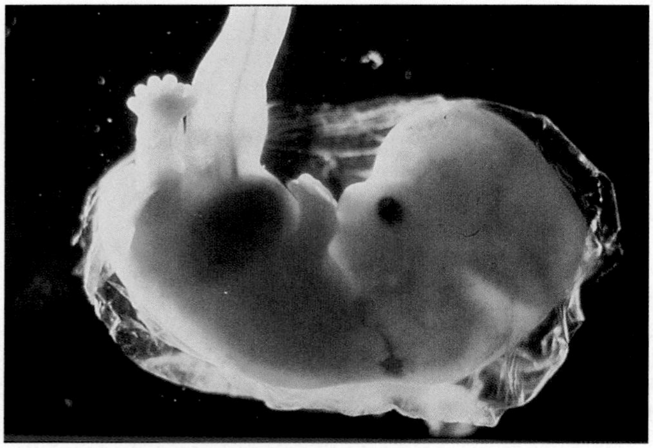

● **Figure 4–13** The embryo at 7 weeks. The head is rounded and nearly erect. The eyes have shifted forward and closer together, and the eyelids begin to form.

Source: © Petit Format/Nestle/Science Source/Photo Researchers Inc.

FETAL STAGE

By the end of the eighth week, the embryo is sufficiently developed to be called a **fetus**. Every organ system and external structure that will be found in the full-term newborn is present. The remainder of gestation is devoted to refining structures and perfecting function.

Nine to Twelve Weeks

By the end of the ninth week the fetus reaches a C–R length of 5 cm (2 in.) and weighs about 14 g (0.5 oz). The head is large and comprises almost half of the fetus's entire size (Figure 4–14 ●). At 12 weeks, the fetus reaches 8 cm (3.2 in.) C–R length and weighs about 45 g (1.6 oz). The face is well formed, with the nose protruding, the chin small and receding, and the ear acquiring a more adult shape. The eyelids close at about the 10th week and will not reopen until about the 26- to 29-week period. Some movement of the lips suggestive of the sucking reflex has been observed at 3 months. Tooth buds now appear for all 20 of the child's first teeth (baby teeth). The limbs are long and slender, with well-formed digits. The fetus can curl the fingers toward the palm and begins to make a tiny fist. The legs are still shorter and less developed than the arms. The urogenital tract completes its development, well-differentiated genitals appear, and the kidneys begin to produce urine. Red blood cells are produced primarily

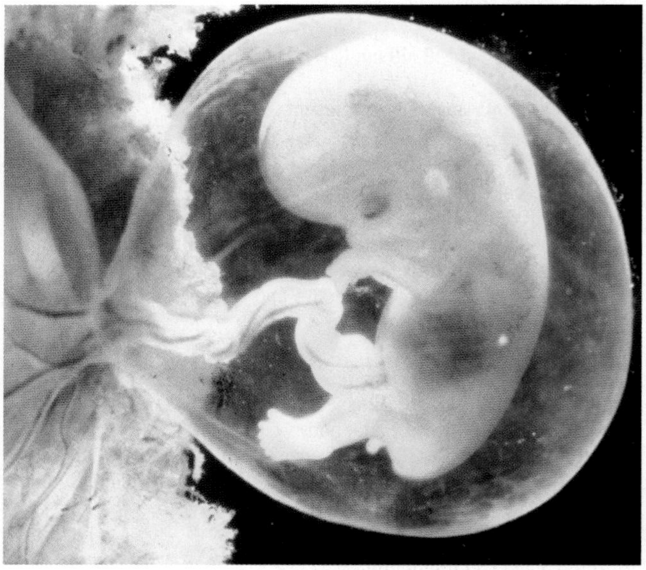

● **Figure 4–14** The fetus at 9 weeks. Every organ system and external structure is present.

Source: Nilsson, L. (1990). *A child is born.* New York: Dell Publishing.

by the liver. Spontaneous movements of the fetus now occur. Fetal heart rates can be ascertained by electronic devices between 8 and 12 weeks. The rate is 120 to 160 beats per minute.

Thirteen to Sixteen Weeks

This is a period of rapid growth. At 13 weeks, the fetus weighs 55 to 60 g (1.9 to 2.1 oz) and is about 9 cm (3.6 in.) in C–R length. Lanugo, or fine hair, begins to develop, especially on the head. The skin is so transparent that blood vessels are clearly visible beneath it. More muscle tissue and body skeleton have developed and hold the fetus more erect (Figure 4–15 ●). Active movements are present; the fetus stretches and exercises its arms and legs. It makes sucking motions, swallows amniotic fluid, and produces meconium in the intestinal tract. Bronchial tubes are branching out in the primitive lungs, and sweat glands are developing. The liver and pancreas now begin producing their appropriate secretions. By the beginning of week 16, skeletal ossification is clearly identifiable.

Twenty Weeks

The fetus doubles its C–R length and now measures 19 cm (8 in.) long. Fetal weight is between 435 and 465 g (15.2 and 16.3 oz). Lanugo covers the entire body and is especially prominent on the shoulders. Subcutaneous deposits of brown fat, which has a rich blood supply, make the skin less transparent. Nipples now appear over the mammary glands. The head is covered with fine, "woolly" hair, and the eyebrows and eyelashes are beginning to form. Nails are present on both fingers and toes. Muscles are well developed, and the fetus is active (Figure 4–16 ●). The mother feels fetal movement, known as *quickening*. The fetal heartbeat is audible through a fetoscope. Quickening and fetal heartbeat can help in validating the EDB.

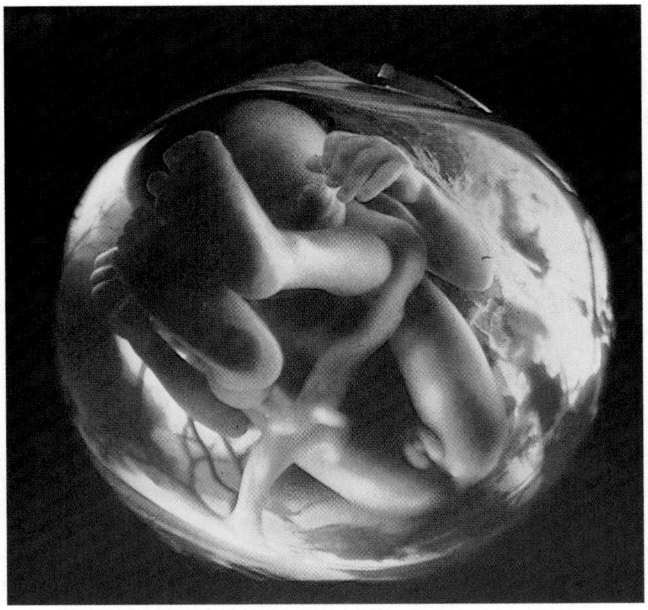

● **Figure 4–16** The fetus at 20 weeks. The fetus now weighs 435 to 465 g (15.2 to 16.3 oz) and measures about 19 cm (7.5 in.). Subcutaneous deposits of brown fat make the skin a little less transparent. "Woolly" hair covers the head, and nails have developed on the fingers and toes.

Source: Nilsson, L. (1990). *A child is born.* New York: Dell Publishing.

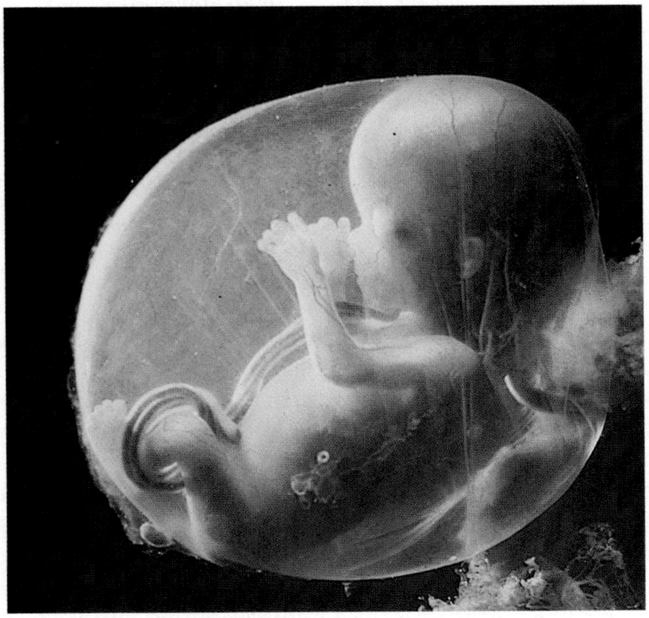

● **Figure 4–15** The fetus at 14 weeks. During this period of rapid growth the skin is so transparent that blood vessels are visible beneath it. More muscle tissue and body skeleton have developed, and they hold the fetus more erect.

Source: Nilsson, L. (1990). *A child is born.* New York: Dell Publishing.

Twenty-Four Weeks

The fetus at 24 weeks reaches a C–R of 23 cm (9.2 in.) or crown-to-heel (C–H) length of 28 cm (11.2 in.). It weighs about 780 g (1 lb, 10 oz). The hair on the head is growing long, and eyebrows and eyelashes have formed. The eye is structurally complete and will soon open. The fetus has a reflex hand grip (grasp reflex) and, by the end of 6 months, a startle reflex. Skin covering the body is reddish and wrinkled, with little subcutaneous fat. Skin on the hands and feet have thickened, with skin ridges on palms and soles forming distinct foot- and fingerprints. The skin over the entire body is covered with **vernix caseosa**, a protective cheeselike, fatty substance secreted by the sebaceous glands. The alveoli in the lungs are just beginning to form.

Twenty-Five to Twenty-Eight Weeks

At about 25 weeks the fetal skin is still red, wrinkled, and covered with vernix caseosa. The brain is developing rapidly, and the nervous system is complete enough to provide some degree of regulation of body functions. The eyelids, under neural control, open and close. The fetus has nails on both fingers and toes. In the male fetus, the testes begin to descend into the scrotal sac. Even though the lungs are still physiologically immature, they are sufficiently developed to provide gas exchange. A fetus born at this time will require immediate and prolonged intensive care to survive and then to decrease the risk of major handicap. The fetus at 28 weeks is about 27 cm (10.8 in.) C–R or 35 to 38 cm (14 to 15 in.) long C–H and weighs 1200 to 1250 g (2 lb, 10.5 oz to 2 lb, 12 oz).

Twenty-Nine to Thirty-Two Weeks

At 30 weeks the pupillary light reflex is present (Moore & Persaud, 2008). The fetus is gaining weight from an increase in body muscle and fat and weighs about 2000 g (4 lb, 6.5 oz), with a C–R of 31 cm (12.4 in.) or C–H length of about 38 to 43 cm (15 to 17 in.), by 32 weeks of age. The CNS has matured enough to direct rhythmic breathing movements and partially control body temperature; however, the lungs are not yet fully mature. Bones are fully developed but soft and flexible. The fetus begins storing iron, calcium, and phosphorus. In males the testicles may be located in the scrotal sac but are often still high in the inguinal canals.

Thirty-Five to Thirty-Six Weeks

The fetus begins to get plump, and less wrinkled skin covers the deposits of subcutaneous fat. Lanugo begins to disappear, and the nails reach the edge of the fingertips. By 35 weeks of age the fetus has a firm grasp and exhibits spontaneous orientation to light. By 36 weeks of age the weight is usually 2500 to 2750 g (5 lb, 12 oz to 6 lb, 11.5 oz), and the C–H length of the fetus is about 42 to 48 cm (17 to 19 in.) or C–R 35 cm (14 in.). An infant born at this time has a good chance of surviving but may require special care, especially if there is intrauterine growth restriction.

Thirty-Eight to Forty Weeks

The fetus is considered full term at 38 weeks and up to 40 weeks after conception. The C–H length varies from 48 to 52 cm (19 to 21 in.) or C–R of 40 cm (16 in.), with males usually longer than females. Males also usually weigh more than females. The weight at term is about 3000 to 3600 g (6 lb, 10 oz to 7 lb, 15 oz) and varies in different ethnic groups. The skin is pink and has a smooth, polished look. The only lanugo left is on the upper arms and shoulders. The hair on the head is no longer woolly but is coarse and about 1 in. long. Vernix caseosa is present, with heavier deposits remaining in the creases and folds of the skin. The body and extremities are plump, with good skin turgor, and the fingernails extend beyond the fingertips. The chest is prominent but still a little smaller than the head, and mammary glands protrude in both sexes. In males, the testes are in the scrotum or palpable in the inguinal canals.

As the fetus enlarges, amniotic fluid diminishes to about an average of 500 ml, and the fetal body mass fills the uterine cavity (Beall & Ross, 2009). The fetus assumes what is called its *position of comfort,* or lie. The head is generally pointed downward, following the shape of the uterus (and possibly because the head is heavier than the feet). The extremities, and often the head, are well flexed. After 5 months, patterns in feeding, sleeping, and activity become established, so at term the fetus has its own body rhythms and individual style of response. See Table 4–4 for important developmental milestones. For a detailed discussion of each body system's transition to and their functioning in the newborn see Chapter 27∞.

Table 4–4 Fetal Development: What Parents Want to Know

4 weeks:	The fetal heart begins to beat.
8 weeks:	All body organs are formed.
8 to 12 weeks:	Fetal heart rate can be heard by ultrasound Doppler device.
16 weeks:	Baby's sex can be seen. Although thin, the fetus looks like a baby.
20 weeks:	Heartbeat can be heard with fetoscope. Mother feels movement (quickening). Baby develops a regular schedule of sleeping, sucking, and kicking. Hands can grasp. Baby assumes a favorite position in utero. Vernix (lanolinlike covering) protects the body, and lanugo (fine hair) keeps oil on skin. Head hair, eyebrows, and eyelashes present.
24 weeks:	Weighs 780 g (1 lb, 10 oz). Activity is increasing. Fetal respiratory movements begin. Sucking movements.
28 weeks:	Eyes open and close. Baby can breathe at this time. Surfactant needed for breathing at birth is formed. Baby is two-thirds its final length.
32 weeks:	Baby has fingernails and toenails. Subcutaneous fat is being laid down. Baby appears less red and wrinkled.
38+ weeks:	Baby fills total uterus. Baby gets antibodies from mother.

FACTORS INFLUENCING EMBRYONIC AND FETAL DEVELOPMENT

Factors that may affect embryonic development include the quality of the sperm or ovum from which the zygote was formed, the genetic code established at fertilization, and the adequacy of the intrauterine environment. If the environment is unsuitable before cellular differentiation occurs, all the cells of the zygote are affected. The cells may die, which causes spontaneous abortion, or growth may be slowed, depending on the severity of the situation. When differentiation is complete and the fetal membranes have formed, an injurious agent has the greatest effect on those cells undergoing the most rapid growth. Thus the time of injury is critical in the development of anomalies.

Because organs are formed primarily during embryonic development, the growing organism is considered most vulnerable to hazardous agents during the first months of pregnancy. Any agent (e.g., drug, virus, or radiation) that can cause abnormal structures to develop in an embryo is called a **teratogen**. It is important to remember that the effects of teratogens depend on the

Evidence in Action

Cigarette smoking during pregnancy negatively impacts neurodevelopment of the fetus (Systematic review) (Shea & Steiner, 2008).

Thinking Critically

DRUGS IN PREGNANCY

Melodie Chong, in her third week of pregnancy, develops a fever of 104°F (40°C) but refuses to take any medication because she is afraid that drugs will harm her baby. Is she correct?

See MyNursingKit for possible responses.

(1) fetal genotype and maternal genome, (2) stage of development when exposure occurs, and (3) dose and duration of exposure of the agent (Chambers & Weiner, 2009). Chapter 9 discusses the effects of specific teratogenic agents on the developing fetus.

Adequacy of the maternal environment is also important during the periods of rapid embryonic and fetal development. Maternal nutrition can affect brain and neural tube development. The period of maximum brain growth and myelination begins with the fifth lunar month before birth and continues during the first 6 months after birth, when there is a twofold increase in myelination (Volpe, 2008). Amino acids, glucose, and fatty acids are considered to be the primary dietary factors in brain growth. A subtle type of damage that affects the associative capacity of the brain, possibly leading to learning disabilities, may be caused by nutritional deficiency at this stage. Vitamins and folic acid supplements taken before conception can reduce the incidence of neural tube defects (Volpe, 2008). The mother's nutrition may also predispose her offspring to developing adult coronary heart disease, hypertension, and diabetes if the baby was small or disproportionate at birth. Chapter 12 presents an in-depth discussion of maternal nutrition.

Another prenatal influence on the intrauterine environment is maternal hyperthermia associated with sauna or hot tub use. Studies of the effects of maternal hyperthermia during the first trimester have raised concern about possible CNS defects and failure of neural tube closure (Table 4–5). Maternal substance abuse also affects the intrauterine environment and is discussed in Chapters 15 and 31.

Table 4–5 Developmental Vulnerability Timetable

Weeks Since Conception	Potential Teratogen-Induced Malformation
3	Ectromelia (congenital absence of one or more limbs) Ectopia cordis (heart lies outside thoracic cavity)
4	Omphalocele (herniation of abdominal viscera into the umbilical cord) Tracheoesophageal fistula (abnormal connection between trachea and esophagus) (4 to 5 weeks) Hemivertebra (4 to 5* weeks)
5	Nuclear cataract Microphthalmia (abnormally small eyeballs) (5 to 6* weeks) Facial clefts Carpal or pedal ablation (5 to 6* weeks)
6	Gross septal or aortic abnormalities Cleft lip, agnathia (absence of the lower jaw)
7	Interventricular septal defects Pulmonary stenosis Cleft palate, micrognathia (smallness of the jaw) Epicanthus Brachycephalism (shortness of the head) (7 to 8* weeks) Mixed sexual characteristics
8	Persistent ostium primum (persistent opening in atrial septum) Digital stunting (shortening of fingers and toes)

Source: Modified from Danforth, D. N., & Scott, J. R. (1986). *Obstetrics and gynecology* (5th ed., p. 319). Philadelphia: Lippincott.
*May occur in several time periods after conception.

CRITICAL CONCEPT REVIEW

LEARNING OUTCOMES	CONCEPTS
4.1 Differentiate between meiotic cellular division and mitotic cellular division.	■ Mitosis produces cells that cause growth in the body. Results in daughter cells that are an exact copy of the parent cell. They contain a full diploid set (46) of chromosomes. ■ Meiosis produces cells called gametes that are necessary for reproduction of the species. Results in cells that contain only one half (haploid or 23) of the chromosomes of the parent cell.
4.2 Compare the processes by which ova and sperm are produced.	■ Ova are present in the female ovary at birth but are dormant until puberty. Meiosis initially produces via oogenesis two haploid cells (secondary oocyte and a minute polar body) that are released at ovulation. At the end of meiosis in the female, there are four haploid cells: the three polar bodies and one ovum. ■ Sperm are produced in the seminiferous tubules of the testes beginning at puberty. ■ Meiosis in the male creates four haploid sperm able to fertilize the ovum. Two sperm carry the Y chromosome and two sperm contain the X chromosome.
4.3 Analyze components of the process of fertilization as to how each may impact fertilization.	Preparation is the first component of fertilization: ■ Ovum released into fallopian tube—viable for 24 hr. ■ Sperm deposited into vagina—viable for 48 to 72 hr (highly fertile for 24 hr). ■ Sperm must undergo capacitation and acrosomal reaction. ■ Sperm penetration causes a chemical reaction that blocks more sperm penetration. Moment of fertilization is the second component of fertilization: ■ It occurs in the ampulla (outer third) of the fallopian tube. ■ Sperm enters ovum. The nuclei of the ovum and sperm swell, unite, and become a diploid zygote.
4.4 Analyze the processes that occur during the cellular multiplication and differentiation stages of intrauterine development and their effects on the structures that form.	Cellular multiplication: ■ Rapid mitotic division (cleavage). ■ Blastomeres grow to morula (solid ball of 12 to 16 cells). ■ Morula divides into a solid mass (blastocyst) surrounded by an outer layer of cells (trophoblast). ■ Implantation occurs in 7 to 10 days. Cellular differentiation: ■ At 10 to 14 days of age, blastocyst differentiates into three primary germ layers (ectoderm, mesoderm, and endoderm) from which all tissues, organs, and organ systems develop. ■ Embryonic membranes form at implantation and include the chorion and the amnion. ■ Amniotic fluid is created when the amnion and chorion grow and connect and form the amniotic sac and produce fluid. ■ Amniotic fluid cushions the fetus against mechanical injury, controls the embryo's temperature, allows symmetrical growth, permits freedom of movement, and prevents adherence to the amnion. ■ Yolk sac develops as part of the blastocyst and produces primitive red blood cells. It is soon incorporated into the umbilical cord. ■ After implantation, the endometrium is called the deciduas. Decidua capsularis is the portion that covers the blastocyst. Decidua basalis is the portion that is directly under the blastocyst.

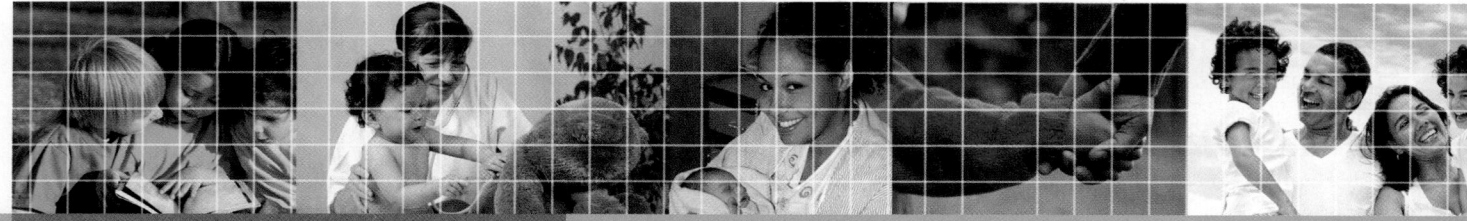

LEARNING OUTCOMES / CONCEPTS

LEARNING OUTCOMES	CONCEPTS
4.5 Describe the development, structure, and functions of the placenta and umbilical cord during intrauterine life (embryonic and fetal development).	Umbilical cord: ■ Develops from amnion. Contains two arteries and one vein and is surrounded by Wharton's jelly, which protects the vessels. ■ Function is to provide a circulatory pathway to the embryo. Placenta: ■ Develops at site of embryonic attachment to the uterus and is composed of two parts, the maternal side and the fetal side. The placenta is made up of 15 to 20 segments called cotyledons. ■ Serves as endocrine (production of hPL, hCG, estrogen, and progesterone), metabolic, and immunologic functions for the fetus. It acts as the fetus's respiratory organ, is an organ of excretion, and aids in the exchange of nutrients.
4.6 Compare the factors and processes by which fraternal (dizygotic) and identical (monozygotic) twins are formed.	Identical twins: ■ Develop from a single fertilized egg. Both fetuses are same sex with same characteristics. ■ Single placenta. Fraternal twins: ■ Develop from two separate ova fertilized by two separate sperm. ■ Two placentas.
4.7 Summarize the significant changes in growth and development of the fetus at 4, 6, 12, 16, 20, 24, 28, 36, and 40 weeks' gestation.	■ 4 weeks: 4 to 6 mm C-R, brain formed from anterior neural tube, limb buds seen, heart begins to beat. ■ 6 weeks: 12 mm C-R, primitive skeletal shape, chambers in heart, respiratory system begins, ear formation begins. ■ 12 weeks: 8 cm C-R, ossification of skeleton begins, liver produces red cells, palate complete in mouth, skin pink, thyroid hormone present, and insulin present in pancreas. ■ 16 weeks: 13.5 cm C-R, teeth begin to form, meconium begins to collect in intestines, kidneys assume shape, hair present on scalp. Sex can be determined. ■ 20 weeks: 19 cm C-R, myelination of spinal cord begins. Suck and swallow begins, lanugo covers body, vernix begins to form. ■ 24 weeks: 23 cm C-R, respiratory movement and surfactant production begins, brain appears mature. ■ 28 weeks: 27 cm C-R, nervous system begins regulation of some functions, adipose tissue accumulates rapidly. Nails, eyebrows, and eyelids are present. Eyes open and close. ■ 36 weeks: 35 cm C-R, earlobes soft with little cartilage, few sole creases. ■ 40 weeks: 40 cm C-R, adequate surfactant, vernix in skin folds and lanugo on shoulders, earlobes firm, and sex apparent.
4.8 Identify the factors that influence congenital malformations of the various organ systems.	■ Embryo is most vulnerable to teratogenesis during the first 8 weeks of cell differentiation and organ system development. ■ Effects of teratogens depend on the (1) maternal and fetal genotype, (2) stage of development when exposure occurs, and (3) dose and duration of exposure of the agent.

CRITICAL THINKING IN ACTION

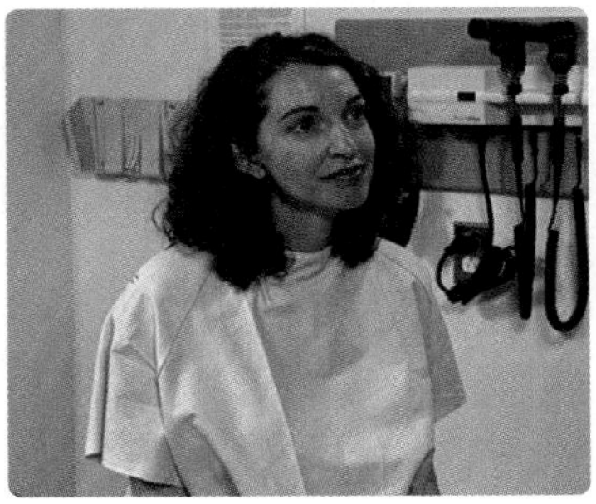

You are working at the local clinic when Frances, a 28-year-old G2 P1001 at 11 weeks' gestation, comes into the office. Frances tells you that early in the first trimester, her husband experienced a flulike syndrome and that he was later diagnosed with cytomegalovirus (CMV) pneumonia. She tells you that his physician found an enlarged supraclavicular lymph node and an ulcer on one tonsil. Laboratory testing revealed elevated liver enzymes. Further testing led to the discovery of positive cytomegalovirus (CMV) IgM levels. She has come today with symptoms including night sweats, persistent sore throat, joint pain, headache, vomiting, and fatigue. You obtain vital signs of temperature 99°F, pulse 90, respirations 14, BP 110/70. Her physical exam is normal; no lymphadenopathy are present. Her weight gain is 2 lb even with nausea and some vomiting. She is worried that her husband's illness could be related to her current symptoms.

1. How would you respond to Frances's concern?
2. Frances asks you if her baby is formed. How would you discuss the three stages of development?
3. Frances asks when her baby is most vulnerable for abnormal growth or structure. How would you answer?
4. Frances asks what stage her baby is in. What would you tell her?

See MyNursingKit for possible responses.

REFERENCES

Beall, M. H., & Ross, M. G. (2009). Amniotic fluid dynamics. In R. K. Creasy, R. Resnik, J. D. Iams, C. J. Lockwood, & T. R. Moore (Eds.). *Creasy & Resnik's maternal-fetal medicine: Principles and practice.* (6th ed., pp. 47–54). Philadelphia: Saunders Elsevier.

Benirschke, K. (2009a). Normal early development. In R. K. Creasy, R. Resnik, J. D. Iams, C. J. Lockwood, & T. R. Moore (Eds.). *Creasy & Resnik's maternal-fetal medicine: Principles and practice.* (6th ed., pp. 37–45). Philadelphia: Saunders Elsevier.

Benirschke, K. (2009b). Multiple gestation: The biology of twinning. In R. K. Creasy, R. Resnik, J. D. Iams, C. J. Lockwood, & T. R. Moore (Eds.). *Creasy & Resnik's maternal-fetal medicine: Principles and practice.* (6th ed., pp. 55–68). Philadelphia: Saunders Elsevier.

Blackburn, S. T. (2007). *Maternal, fetal, & neonatal physiology: A clinical perspective* (3rd ed.). St. Louis: Saunders.

Chambers, C., & Weiner, C. P. (2009). Teratogenesis and environmental exposure. In R. K. Creasy, R. Resnik, J. D. Iams, C. J. Lockwood, & T. R. Moore (Eds.). *Creasy & Resnik's maternal-fetal medicine: Principles and practice.* (6th ed., pp. 347–359). Philadelphia: Saunders Elsevier.

Gilbert, W. M. (2007). Amniotic fluid disorders. In S. G. Gabbe, J. R. Niebyl, & J. L. Simpson (Eds.). *Obstetrics: Normal and problem pregnancies* (5th ed., pp. 834–845). Philadelphia: Churchhill Livingstone Elsevier.

Knuppel, R. A. (2007). Maternal–placental–fetal unit: Fetal & early neonatal physiology. In A. H. Decherney, L. Nathan, T. M Goodwin, & N. Laufer (Eds.), *Current diagnosis and treatment: Obstetrics & gynecology* (10th ed.). Boston: McGraw-Hill.

Moore, K. L., & Persaud, T. V. N. (2008). *The developing human: Clinical oriented embryology* (8th ed.). Philadelphia: Saunders.

Sadler, T. W. (2006). *Langman's medical embryology* (10th ed.). Philadelphia: Lippincott Williams & Wilkins.

Shea, A. K., & Steiner, M. (2008). Cigarette smoking during pregnancy. *Nicotine & Tobacco Research, 10*(2), 267–278.

Volpe, J. J. (2008). *Neurology of the newborn* (5th ed.). Philadelphia: Saunders.

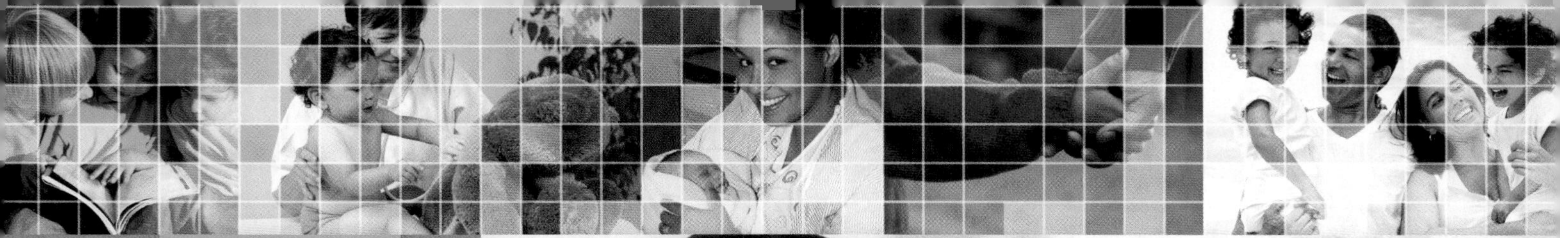

PART 2

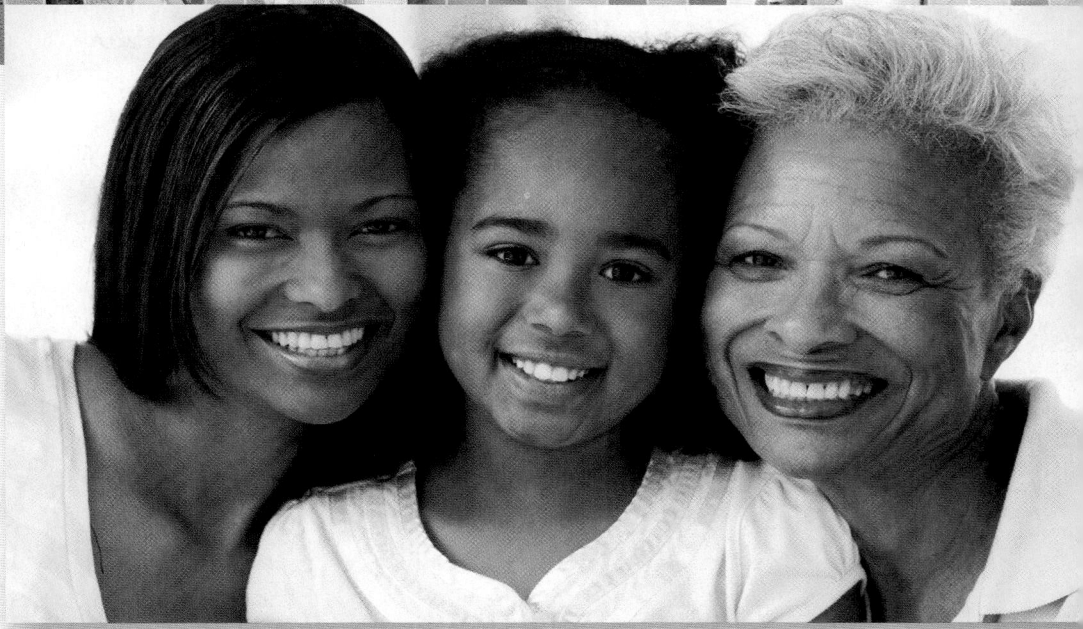

Women's Health

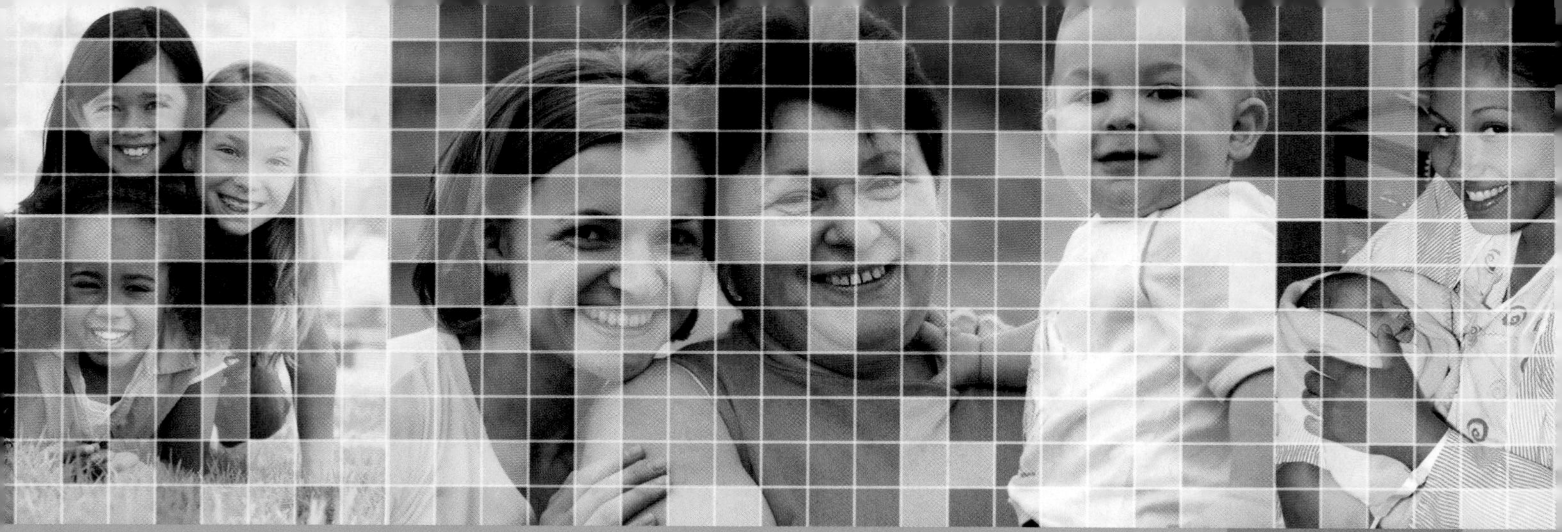

CHAPTER 5

Health Promotion for Women

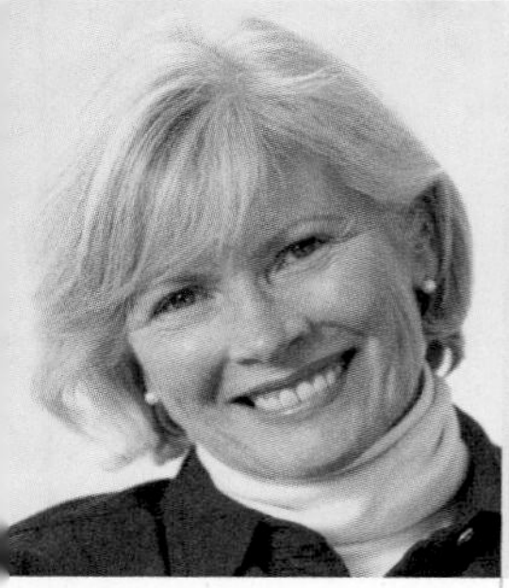

I am 61 now, an early baby boomer. I am astonished at the changes that have occurred in women's health care in my lifetime. I remember that my mom was shocked when our family doctor taught me to do a breast exam when I turned 18. What a farsighted man. Information on sexually transmitted infections was not as generally available. AIDS was beyond our imagination. Contraceptive options were more limited although the pill was gaining in popularity. Menopause seemed like the end of life—menopausal women were old. Today more and more of us women are becoming savvy healthcare consumers. We have more information, we have treatment options, we decide our own care. I think this is the most exciting change of all! —Alice

LEARNING OUTCOMES

5.1 Determine accurate information to be provided to girls and women so that they can implement effective self-care measures for dealing with menstruation.

5.2 Discriminate between the signs, symptoms, and nursing management of women with dysmenorrhea and premenstrual syndrome.

5.3 Compare the advantages, disadvantages, and effectiveness of the various methods of contraception available today.

5.4 Delineate basic gynecologic screening procedures indicated for well women.

5.5 Consider the physical and psychologic aspects and clinical treatment options of menopause when caring for menopausal women.

5.6 Delineate the nurse's role in screening and caring for women who have experienced domestic violence or rape.

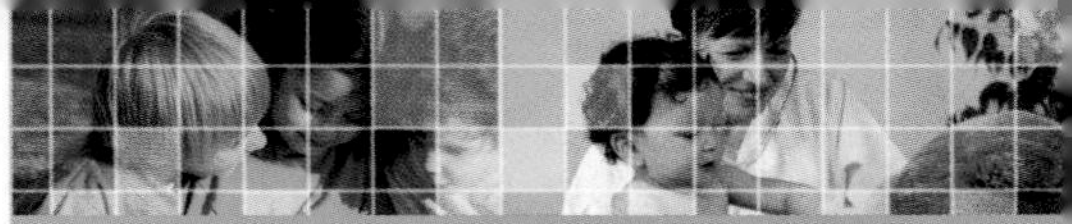

KEY TERMS

Amenorrhea, 91
Breast self-examination (BSE), 102
Cervical cap, 97
Coitus interruptus, 94
Combined oral contraceptives (COCs), 98
Condom, 94
Date rape, 111
Depo-Provera, 100
Diaphragm, 96
Domestic violence, 108
Dysmenorrhea, 91
Emergency contraception, 100
Fertility awareness-based methods, 93
Hormone replacement therapy (HRT), 106
Intimate partner violence, 108
Intrauterine device (IUD), 97
Mammogram, 103
Menopause, 103
Osteoporosis, 106
Perimenopause, 103
Premenstrual syndrome (PMS), 92
Rape, 110
Sexual assault, 110
Spermicide, 94
Sterilization, 100
Subdermal implant, 100
Tubal ligation, 100
Vasectomy, 100

A woman's healthcare needs change throughout her lifetime. As a young girl, she needs health teaching about menstruation, sexuality, and personal responsibility. As a teen she needs information about reproductive choices and safe sexual activity. During this time she should also be introduced to the importance of healthcare practices such as breast self-examination and regular Pap smears. The mature woman may need to be reminded of these self-care issues and prepared for the physical changes that accompany childbirth and aging. By educating women about their bodies, their healthcare choices, and their right to be knowledgeable consumers, nurses can help women assume responsibility for the health care they receive. This chapter provides information about selected aspects of women's health care with an emphasis on conditions typically addressed in a community-based setting.

NURSING CARE IN THE COMMUNITY

Women's health refers to a holistic view of women and their health-related needs within the context of their everyday lives. It is based on the awareness that a woman's physical, mental, and spiritual status are interdependent and affect her state of health or illness. The woman's view of her situation, her assessment of her needs, her values, and her beliefs are valid and important factors to be incorporated into any healthcare intervention.

Nurses can work with women to provide health teaching and information about self-care practices in schools, during routine examinations in a clinic or office, at senior centers, at meetings of volunteer organizations, through classes offered by local agencies or schools, or in the home. Nurses oriented to community-based care are especially effective in recognizing the autonomy of each individual and in dealing with clients holistically. This holistic approach is important in addressing not only physical problems but also major health issues such as violence against women, which may go undetected unless care providers are alert for signs of it.

THE NURSE'S ROLE IN ADDRESSING ISSUES OF SEXUALITY

Because sexuality and its reproductive implications are such intrinsic and emotion-laden parts of life, people have many concerns, problems, and questions about sex roles, behaviors, education, inhibitions, morality, and related areas such as family planning. The reproductive implications of sexual intercourse must also be considered. Some people desire pregnancy; others wish to avoid it. Health factors are another consideration. The increase in the incidence of sexually transmitted infections, especially HIV/AIDS and herpes, has caused many people to modify their sexual practices and activities. Women frequently ask questions or voice concerns about these issues to the nurse in a clinic or ambulatory setting. Thus, the nurse may need to assume the role of counselor or educator on sexual and reproductive matters.

Nurses who assume this role must recognize their own feelings, values, and attitudes about sexuality so they can be more sensitive when they encounter the values and beliefs of others. Nurses need to have accurate, up-to-date information about anatomy and physiology and about topics related to sexuality, sexual practices, and common gynecologic problems. In addition, when a woman is accompanied by her partner, it is important that the nurse be sensitive to the dynamics of the relationship and communication patterns between the two.

TAKING A SEXUAL HISTORY

Nurses are often responsible for taking a woman's initial history, including her gynecologic and sexual history. For the interview to be its most useful, the nurse must have effective communication skills and should conduct the interview in a quiet, private place free of distractions. It is important to phrase questions in a sensitive and nonjudgmental manner and to assure the woman of strict confidentiality.

Opening the discussion with a brief explanation of the purpose of such questions is often helpful. For example, the nurse might say, "As your nurse, I'm interested in all aspects of your well-being. Often women have concerns or questions about sexual matters, especially as their life situations change. I will be asking you some questions about your sexual history as part of your general health history." This explanation helps women understand the nature of this part of their history and encourages more open, honest answers.

It may be helpful to use direct eye contact as much as possible unless the nurse knows it is culturally unacceptable to the woman. The nurse should do little, if any, writing during the interview, especially if the woman seems ill at ease or is discussing very personal issues. Beginning with general questions such as, "What brings you here today?" before progressing to more sensitive topics will provide an opportunity for the woman to develop trust with the nurse. Open-ended questions are often useful in eliciting information. For example, "What, if anything, would you change about your sex life?" will elicit more information than "Are you happy with your sex life now?" The nurse needs to clarify terminology and proceed from easier topics to those that are more difficult to discuss.

Throughout the interview the nurse should be alert to body language and nonverbal cues. It is important that the nurse not assume that the client is heterosexual. Some women are open about lesbian relationships; others are more reserved until they develop a sense of trust in their caregivers.

After completing the sexual history, the nurse assesses the information obtained. If there is a problem that requires further medical tests and assessments, the nurse refers the woman to a nurse practitioner, certified nurse-midwife, physician, or counselor as necessary. In many instances the nurse alone will be able to develop a nursing diagnosis and then plan and implement therapy. The nurse must be realistic in making assessments and planning interventions. It requires insight and skill to recognize when a woman's problem requires interventions that are beyond a nurse's preparation and ability. In such situations it is essential that the nurse make appropriate referrals.

MENSTRUATION

Girls today begin to learn about puberty and menstruation at a young age. Unfortunately, the source of their "education" is sometimes their peers or the media; thus, the information is often incomplete, inaccurate, and sensationalized. Nurses who work with young girls and adolescents recognize this and are working hard to provide accurate health teaching and to correct misinformation about *menarche* (the onset of menses) and the menstrual cycle.

Cultural, religious, and personal attitudes about menstruation are part of the menstrual experience. Currently in the Western world, there are few customs associated with menstruation. Sexual intercourse during menses is a common practice and is not generally contraindicated. For most couples the decision is one of personal preference. (The physiology of menstruation is discussed in Chapter 3∞.)

COUNSELING THE PREMENSTRUAL GIRL ABOUT MENARCHE

Many young women find it embarrassing to discuss menstruation. However, the most critical factor in successful adaptation to menarche is the adolescent's level of preparedness. Information should be given to premenstrual girls over time rather than all at once. This allows them to absorb information and develop questions.

The following basic information is helpful for young clients:

- *Cycle length.* Cycle length is determined from the first day of one menses to the first day of the next menses. Initially a female's cycle length may be irregular. Once established, it is about 29 days, although may vary from 21 to 35 days. Cycle length frequently varies by a day or two from one cycle to the next, although greater normal variations may also occur.
- *Amount of flow.* The average flow is approximately 25 to 60 mL per period. Usually women characterize the amount of flow in terms of the number of pads or tampons used. Flow is often heavier at first and lighter toward the end of the period.
- *Length of menses.* Menses usually lasts from 2 to 8 days, although this may vary.

The nurse should make it clear that variations in age at menarche, length of cycle, and duration of menses are normal, because girls may worry if their experience varies from that of their peers. It also is helpful to acknowledge the negative aspects of menstruation (messiness, cramping, embarrassment) while stressing its positive role as a symbol of maturity and womanhood.

EDUCATIONAL TOPICS

Pads and Tampons

Since early times women have made pads and tampons from cloth or rags, which required washing but were reusable. Commercial tampons were introduced in the 1930s.

Today, adhesive-stripped, disposable minipads and maxipads and tampons are readily available. However, the deodorants and increased absorbency that manufacturers have added to both pads and tampons may prove harmful. The chemical used to deodorize can create irritation of the vulva and inner aspects of the vagina. Excessive or inappropriate use of tampons can produce dryness or even small sores or ulcers in the vagina.

Interest is also growing in the use of eco-friendly menstrual products, including reusable menstrual pads made of washable cotton, menstrual cups, and menstrual sponges. These products are becoming more readily available at major discount stores.

The use of superabsorbent tampons has been linked to the development of toxic shock syndrome (TSS) (see Chapter 6∞). Women can prevent problems by using tampons with the minimum absorbency necessary to control menstrual flow, changing them every 3 to 6 hours, and avoiding using them for vaginal discharge or light bleeding. Because *Staphylococcus aureus,* the causative organism of TSS, is frequently found on the hands, a woman should wash her hands before inserting a fresh tampon and should avoid touching the tip of the tampon when unwrapping it or before insertion.

In the absence of a heavy menstrual flow, tampons absorb moisture, leaving the vaginal walls dry and subject to injury. The absorbency of regular tampons varies. If the tampon is hard to pull out or shreds when removed, or if the vagina becomes dry, the tampon is probably too absorbent.

A woman may want to use tampons only during the day and switch to pads at night to avoid vaginal irritation. If a woman experiences vaginal irritation, itching, or soreness or notices an unusual odor while using tampons, she should stop using them and be evaluated for infection. The choice of sanitary protection—whether napkins or tampons—must meet the individual's needs and feel comfortable. Cultural factors may play a role in this decision and should be considered.

Vaginal Spray, Douching, and Cleansing

Vaginal sprays are unnecessary and can cause infections, itching (pruritus), burning, vaginal discharge, rashes, and other problems. If a woman chooses to use a spray, she needs to know that these sprays are for external use only, should be used infrequently, and should never be applied to irritated or itching skin.

Although douching is sometimes used to treat vaginal infections, douching as a hygiene practice is unnecessary because the vagina cleanses itself. Douching washes away the natural mucus and upsets the vaginal flora, which can make the vagina more susceptible to infection. Perfumed douches can cause allergic reactions, and too frequent use of an undiluted or strong douche solution can cause irritation or even tissue damage. Propelling water up the vagina may also erode the antibacterial cervical plug and force bacteria and germs from the vagina into the uterus. Women should avoid douching during menstruation because the cervix is dilated to permit the downward flow of menstrual fluids from the uterine lining. Douching is also contraindicated during pregnancy.

The mucous secretions that bathe the vagina are odor-free while they are in the vagina; odor develops only when they mingle with perspiration and are exposed to the air. Keeping one's skin clean and free of bacteria with plain soap and water is the most effective method of controlling odor. A soapy finger or soft washcloth should be used to wash gently between the vulvar folds. Although in the past some women felt that bathing was to be avoided during menses, bathing is as important during menses as at any other time. A long, leisurely soak in a warm tub promotes menstrual blood flow and relieves cramps by relaxing the muscles.

Developing Cultural Competence

USE OF TAMPONS

In certain religious or cultural groups unmarried women are expected to avoid the use of tampons. This is more common among those groups that highly value a girl's virginity, for fear of breaking the hymen. Thus it is wise to ask the girl (or her mother if the girl is uncertain) about the issue.

Keeping the vulva fresh throughout the day means keeping it dry and clean. A woman can ensure adequate ventilation by wearing cotton panties and clothes loose enough to permit the vaginal area to "breathe." After using the toilet, a woman should always wipe herself from front to back and, if necessary, follow up with a moistened paper towel or toilet paper. If an unusual odor persists despite these efforts, a visit to one's healthcare provider is indicated. Certain conditions such as vaginitis produce a foul-smelling discharge.

ASSOCIATED MENSTRUAL CONDITIONS

A variety of menstrual irregularities have been identified. An abnormally short duration of menstrual flow is termed *hypomenorrhea;* an abnormally long one is called *hypermenorrhea.* Excessive, profuse flow is called *menorrhagia,* and bleeding between periods is known as *metrorrhagia.* Infrequent and too frequent menses are termed *oligomenorrhea* and *polymenorrhea,* respectively. An *anovulatory cycle* is one in which ovulation does not occur. (*Note:* Anovulatory cycles often occur during the first year after menarche and during the perimenopause, the period around the time of menopause.) Generally, menstrual irregularities should be investigated to rule out disease.

Amenorrhea

Amenorrhea, the absence of menses, is classified as primary or secondary. Primary amenorrhea (menstruation has not been established by 16 years of age or within 4 years of breast development) necessitates a thorough assessment to determine its cause. Possible causes include congenital obstructions; Turner syndrome; congenital absence of the uterus, ovaries, or vagina; testicular feminization (external genitals appear female but uterus and ovaries are absent and testes are present); chronic anovulation related to polycystic ovarian syndrome, thyroid, or adrenal disorders; or absence or imbalance of hormones. Treatment depends on the causative factors. Some causes are not correctable.

Secondary amenorrhea is caused most frequently by pregnancy. Additional causes include lactation, hormonal imbalances, poor nutrition (anorexia nervosa, obesity, and fad dieting), ovarian lesions, strenuous exercise (associated with long-distance runners, dancers, and other athletes with low body fat ratios), debilitating systemic diseases, stress of high intensity or long duration, stressful life events, a change in season or climate, use of oral contraceptives, use of the phenothiazine and chlorpromazine group of tranquilizers, and syndromes such as Cushing and Sheehan.

The causative factors dictate treatment. The nurse can explain that once the underlying condition has been corrected—for example, when sufficient body weight is gained—menses will resume. Athletes and women who participate in strenuous exercise routines may be advised to increase their caloric intake or reduce their exercise levels for a month or two to see whether a normal cycle ensues. If it does not, medical referral is indicated.

Dysmenorrhea

Dysmenorrhea, or painful menstruation, occurs at, or a day before, the onset of menstruation and disappears by the end of menses. Dysmenorrhea is classified as primary or secondary.

Primary dysmenorrhea is defined as cramps without underlying disease. Prostaglandins F_2 and $F_{2\alpha}$, which are produced by the uterus in higher concentrations during menses, are the primary cause. They increase uterine contractility and decrease uterine artery blood flow, causing ischemia. The end result is the painful sensation of cramps. Dysmenorrhea typically disappears after a first pregnancy and does not occur if cycles are anovulatory. Treatment of primary dysmenorrhea includes combined oral contraceptives, which inhibit ovulation; nonsteroidal anti-inflammatory drugs (NSAIDs) (such as ibuprofen, aspirin, and naproxen), which act as prostaglandin inhibitors; and self-care measures such as regular exercise, rest, application of heat, and good nutrition. Some nutritionists suggest that vitamins B and E help relieve the discomforts associated with menstruation. Vitamin B_6 may help relieve the premenstrual bloating and irritability some women experience. Vitamin E, a mild prostaglandin inhibitor, may help decrease menstrual discomfort. Avoiding salt can decrease discomfort from fluid retention. Biofeedback has also been used with some success.

Secondary dysmenorrhea is associated with pathology of the reproductive tract and usually appears after menstruation has been established. Conditions that most frequently cause secondary dysmenorrhea include endometriosis; residual pelvic inflammatory disease; cervical stenosis, uterine fibroids, ovarian cysts, benign or malignant tumors of the pelvis or abdomen, and the presence of an intrauterine device. Because primary and secondary dysmenorrhea may coexist, accurate differential diagnosis is essential for appropriate treatment.

Premenstrual Syndrome

Premenstrual syndrome (PMS) refers to a symptom complex associated with the luteal phase of the menstrual cycle (2 weeks prior to the onset of menses). The symptoms must, by definition, occur between ovulation and the onset of menses. They repeat at the same stage of each menstrual cycle and include some or all of the following:

- *Psychologic:* irritability, lethargy, depression, low morale, anxiety, sleep disorders, crying spells, hostility
- *Neurologic:* classic migraine, vertigo, syncope
- *Respiratory:* rhinitis, hoarseness, and occasionally asthma
- *Gastrointestinal:* nausea, vomiting, constipation, abdominal bloating, craving for sweets
- *Urinary:* retention, oliguria
- *Dermatologic:* acne
- *Mammary:* swelling and tenderness

Most women experience only some of these symptoms. The symptoms usually are most pronounced 2 or 3 days before the onset of menstruation and subside as menstrual flow begins, with or without treatment. *Premenstrual dysphoric disorder* (PMDD) is a diagnosis that may be applied to a small subgroup of women with PMS whose symptoms are primarily mood related and severe.

The exact cause of PMS is unknown, although a variety of theories have been put forth to explain it. Currently researchers speculate that, in women who are susceptible, the fluctuating levels of estrogen and progesterone and the decreases in serotonin levels that occur premenstrually trigger symptoms (Reid, 2008).

> **Evidence in Action**
>
> Continuous versus intermittent dosing regimens of selective serotonin reuptake inhibitors (SSRIs) are effective in the treatment of premenstrual syndrome (PMS) and premenstrual dysphoric disorder (meta-analysis) (Shah, Jones, Aperi, et al., 2008).

Nursing management. Counseling for PMS may include advising the woman to restrict her intake of foods containing methylxanthines such as chocolate, cola, and coffee; restrict her intake of alcohol, nicotine, red meat, and foods containing salt and sugar; increase her intake of complex carbohydrates and protein; and increase the frequency of meals. For women whose primary symptoms are psychologic, supplementation with B-complex vitamins, especially B_6, may decrease anxiety and depression. Vitamin E supplements may help reduce breast tenderness. Supplementation with 1200 mg calcium daily may help relieve certain physical and psychologic symptoms. Magnesium supplements may help reduce fluid retention, breast tenderness, negative moods, food cravings, and pain.

A program of aerobic exercise such as fast walking, jogging, and aerobic dancing is generally beneficial. In addition to vitamin supplements, pharmacologic treatments for PMS include diuretics and prostaglandin inhibitors.

Women with PMDD may benefit from selective serotonin reuptake inhibitors (SSRI) such as fluoxetine hydrochloride (Prozac), sertraline hydrochloride (Zoloft), and paroxeline CR (Paxil CR) taken during the entire cycle or intermittently (half the cycle) (Endicott, 2007). The FDA has also approved the use of an oral contraceptive called YAZ for PMDD. YAZ may be a good choice for women who choose an oral contraceptive as their method of contraception and who experience side effects from SSRIs or dislike the idea of taking them (Rapkin, 2008).

Women with PMS may find it helpful to have an empathetic relationship with a healthcare professional to whom she feels free to voice concerns. Encourage the woman to keep a diary to help identify life events associated with PMS. Self-care groups and self-help literature both help women feel they have control over their bodies. Some women use complementary therapies such as homeopathic remedies or herbs. Women using such alternatives should seek advice from knowledgeable, experienced homeopaths or herbalists.

CONTRACEPTION

The decision to use a method of contraception may be made individually by a woman (or, in the case of vasectomy, by a man) or jointly by a couple. The decision may be motivated by a desire to avoid pregnancy, to gain control over the number of children conceived, or to determine the spacing of future children. In

Developing Cultural Competence

CONTRACEPTIVE USE

- Maternal morbidity and mortality remain a major health challenge in developing countries. In 2005 approximately 536,000 women died from pregnancy-related causes. Less than 1% of maternal deaths occur in developed countries (World Health Organization [WHO], 2007).
- Up to 100,000 maternal deaths per year could be avoided if contraception was available and used by women who did not desire children (WHO, 2005).
- In the developing world, 137 million women have an unmet need for contraception, and an additional 64 million have an unmet need for a modern contraceptive method. This is especially apparent in Sub-Saharan Africa where maternal mortality rates are very high (Sonfield, 2006).
- Most of the causes of maternal mortality are treatable or preventable with adequate health care, including contraceptive services. Thus, maternal healthcare services must improve if maternal mortality and morbidity are to be reduced.

choosing a specific method, consistency of use outweighs the absolute reliability of the given method.

Decisions about contraception should be made voluntarily, with full knowledge of available choices, advantages, disadvantages, effectiveness, side effects, contraindications, and long-term effects. Many outside factors influence this choice, including cultural practices, religious beliefs, attitudes and personal preferences, cost, effectiveness, misinformation, practicality of method, and self-esteem. Different methods of contraception may be appropriate at different times for individuals or couples.

FERTILITY AWARENESS METHODS

Fertility awareness-based methods, also known as *natural family planning,* are based on an understanding of the changes that occur throughout a woman's ovulatory cycle. All these methods require periods of abstinence and recording of certain events throughout the cycle, so cooperation of the partners is important.

Fertility awareness-based methods are free, safe, and acceptable to many whose religious beliefs prohibit other methods. They provide an increased awareness of the body, involve no artificial substances or devices, encourage a couple to communicate about sexual activity and family planning, and are useful in helping a couple plan a pregnancy.

However, these methods require extensive initial counseling to be used effectively. They may interfere with sexual spontaneity; they require extensive maintenance of records for several cycles before beginning to use them; they may be difficult or impossible for women with irregular cycles to use; and, although theoretically they should be very reliable, in practice they may not be as reliable in preventing pregnancy as other methods.

The *basal body temperature (BBT)* method to detect ovulation requires that a woman take her BBT every morning upon awakening (before any activity) and record the readings on a temperature graph. To do this she uses a BBT thermometer, which shows tenths of a degree rather than the two tenths shown on standard thermometers. She may also use tympanic thermometry (an "ear thermometer"). After 3 to 4 months of recording temperatures, a woman with regular cycles should be able to predict when ovulation will occur. The method is based on the fact that the temperature sometimes drops just before ovulation and almost always rises and remains elevated for several days after. The temperature rise occurs in response to the increased progesterone levels that occur in the second half of the cycle. Figure 7–2B∞ shows a sample BBT chart of an ovulating woman. To avoid conception, the couple abstains from intercourse on the day of the temperature rise and for 3 days after. Because the temperature rise does not occur until after ovulation, a woman who had intercourse just before the rise is at risk of pregnancy. To decrease this risk, some couples abstain from intercourse for several days before the *anticipated* time of ovulation and then for 3 days after.

The *calendar,* or *rhythm, method* is based on the assumptions that ovulation tends to occur 14 days (plus or minus 2 days) before the start of the next menstrual period, sperm are viable for up to 7 days, and the ovum is viable for up to 3 days. To use this method, the woman must record her menstrual cycles for 6 to 8 months to identify the shortest and longest cycles. The first day of menstruation is the first day of the cycle. The fertile phase is calculated from 18 days before the end of the shortest recorded cycle through 11 days from the end of the longest recorded cycle. For example, if a woman's cycle lasts from 24 to 28 days, the fertile phase would be calculated as day 6 through day 17. Once this information is obtained, the woman can identify the fertile and infertile phases of her cycle. For effective use of this method, she must abstain from intercourse during the fertile phase. The calendar method is the least reliable of the fertility awareness methods and has largely been replaced by other, more scientific approaches.

The *ovulation method,* sometimes called the *cervical mucus method* or the *Billings method,* involves the assessment of cervical mucus changes that occur during the menstrual cycle. The amount and character of cervical mucus change because of the influence of estrogen and progesterone. At the time of ovulation, the mucus (estrogen-dominant mucus) is clearer, more stretchable (a quality called *spinnbarkeit*), and more permeable to sperm. It also shows a characteristic fern pattern when placed on a glass slide and allowed to dry (see Figure 7–3∞). During the luteal phase, the cervical mucus is thick and sticky (progesterone-dominant mucus) and forms a network that traps sperm, making their passage more difficult.

To use the cervical mucus method, the woman abstains from intercourse for the first menstrual cycle. Each day she assesses her cervical mucus for amount, feeling of slipperiness or wetness, color, clearness, and spinnbarkeit, as she becomes familiar with varying characteristics.

The peak day of wetness and clear, stretchable mucus is assumed to be the time of ovulation. To use this method correctly, the woman should abstain from intercourse from the time she first notices that the mucus is becoming clear, more elastic, and slippery until 4 days after the last wet mucus (ovulation) day. Because this method evaluates the effects of hormonal changes, it can be used by women with irregular cycles.

The *symptothermal method* consists of various assessments made and recorded by the couple. These include information regarding cycle days, coitus, cervical mucus changes, and secondary signs such as increased libido, abdominal bloating, *mittelschmerz* (midcycle abdominal pain), and BBT. Through the various assessments, the couple learns to recognize signs that indicate ovulation. This combined approach tends to improve the effectiveness of fertility awareness as a method of birth control.

SITUATIONAL CONTRACEPTIVES

Abstinence can be considered a method of contraception, and, partly because of changing values and the increased risk of infection with intercourse, it is gaining increased acceptance.

Coitus interruptus, or *withdrawal,* is one of the oldest and least reliable methods of contraception. This method requires that the male withdraw from the female's vagina when he feels that ejaculation is impending. He then ejaculates away from the external genitalia of the woman. Failure tends to occur for two reasons: (1) this method demands great self-control on the part of the man, who must withdraw just as he feels the urge for deeper penetration with impending orgasm, and (2) some pre-ejaculatory fluid, which can contain sperm, may escape from the penis during the excitement phase prior to ejaculation. The fact that the quantity of sperm in this pre-ejaculatory fluid is increased after a recent ejaculation is especially significant for couples who engage in repeated episodes of intercourse within a short period of time. Couples who use this method should be aware of postcoital contraceptive options in case the man fails to withdraw in time.

Douching after intercourse is an ineffective method of contraception and is not recommended. It may actually facilitate conception by pushing sperm farther up the birth canal.

SPERMICIDES

The **spermicide** approved for use in the United States, nonoxynol-9 (N-9), is available as a cream, jelly, foam, vaginal film, and suppository. Spermicide is inserted into the vagina before intercourse. It destroys sperm by disrupting the cell membrane. Spermicides that effervesce in a moist environment offer more rapid protection, and coitus may take place immediately after they are inserted. Suppositories may require up to 30 minutes to dissolve and do not offer protection until they do so. The woman should be instructed to insert these spermicide preparations high in the vagina and maintain a supine position.

N-9 is minimally effective when used alone, but its effectiveness increases in conjunction with a diaphragm or condom. The major advantages of spermicides are their wide availability and low toxicity. Skin irritation and allergic reactions to spermicides are the primary disadvantages. N-9 does not offer protection against infection from the human immunodeficiency virus, which causes HIV/AIDS, or against any other sexually transmitted infection (STI). Moreover, N-9 may actually increase a woman's risk of HIV infection because it irritates vaginal tissue, making them more susceptible to invasion by organisms (FDA, 2007).

BARRIER METHODS OF CONTRACEPTION

Barrier methods of contraception prevent the transport of sperm to the ovum, immobilize sperm, or are lethal against sperm.

Male and Female Condoms

The male **condom** offers a viable means of contraception when used consistently and properly (Figure 5–1 ●). Acceptance has been increasing as a growing number of men are assuming responsibility for regulation of fertility. The condom is applied to the erect penis, rolled from the tip to the base of the shaft, before vulvar or vaginal contact. A small space must be left at the end of

A

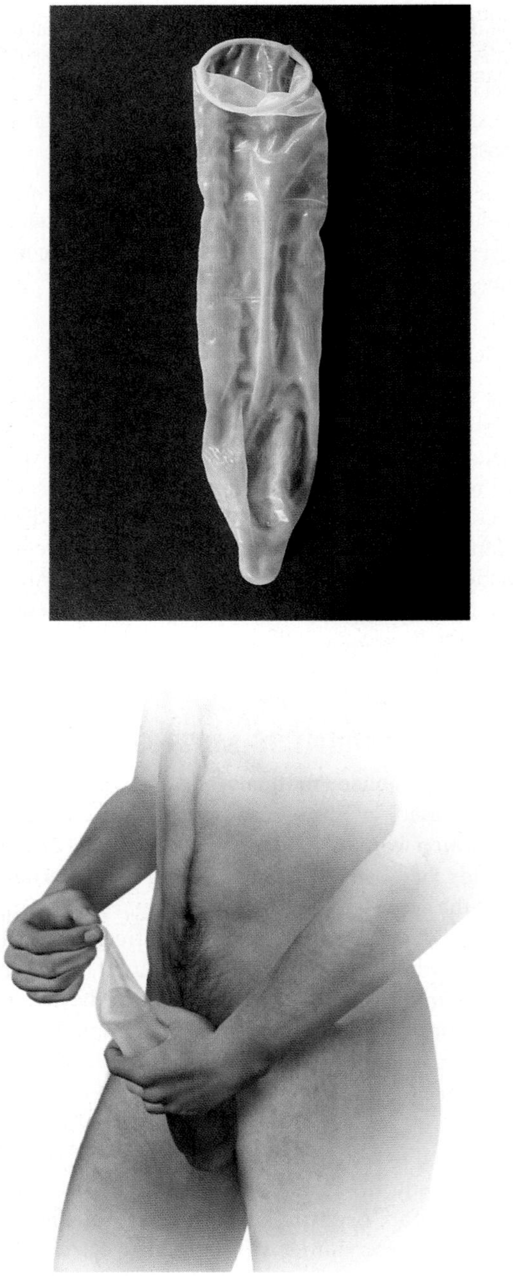

B

● **Figure 5–1** The male condom. ***A,*** Unrolled condom with reservoir tip. ***B,*** Correct use of a condom.

the condom to allow for collection of the ejaculate, so that the condom will not break at the time of ejaculation. If the condom or vagina is dry, a water-soluble lubricant such as K-Y jelly should be used to prevent irritation and possible condom breakage.

Couples should be careful when removing the condom after intercourse. For optimal effectiveness the man should withdraw his penis from the woman's vagina while it is still erect and hold the condom rim to prevent spillage. If after ejaculation the penis becomes flaccid while still in the vagina, the man should hold onto the edge of the condom while withdrawing to avoid spilling semen and to prevent the condom from slipping off.

The effectiveness of male condoms is determined by their use. The condom is small, disposable, and inexpensive; it has no side effects, requires no medical examination, and offers visual evidence of effectiveness. Most condoms are made of latex, although polyurethane and silicone rubber condoms are available for individuals allergic to latex. All condoms, except natural "skin" condoms, made from lamb's intestines, offer protection against both pregnancy and sexually transmitted infections (STIs). Breakage, displacement, perineal or vaginal irritation, and dulled sensation are possible disadvantages. Condoms deteriorate in hot conditions, making them susceptible to breaking. Thus, men should avoid placing them in their car glove box or in their wallets in a rear pant's pocket.

The male condom is becoming increasingly popular because of the protection it offers from infections. For women, an STI increases the risk of pelvic inflammatory disease (PID) and resultant infertility. Many women are beginning to insist that sexual partners use condoms, and many women carry condoms with them.

The *Reality female condom* (Figure 5–2 ●) is a thin polyurethane sheath with a flexible ring at each end. The inner ring, at the closed end of the condom, serves as the means of insertion and fits over the cervix like a diaphragm. The second ring

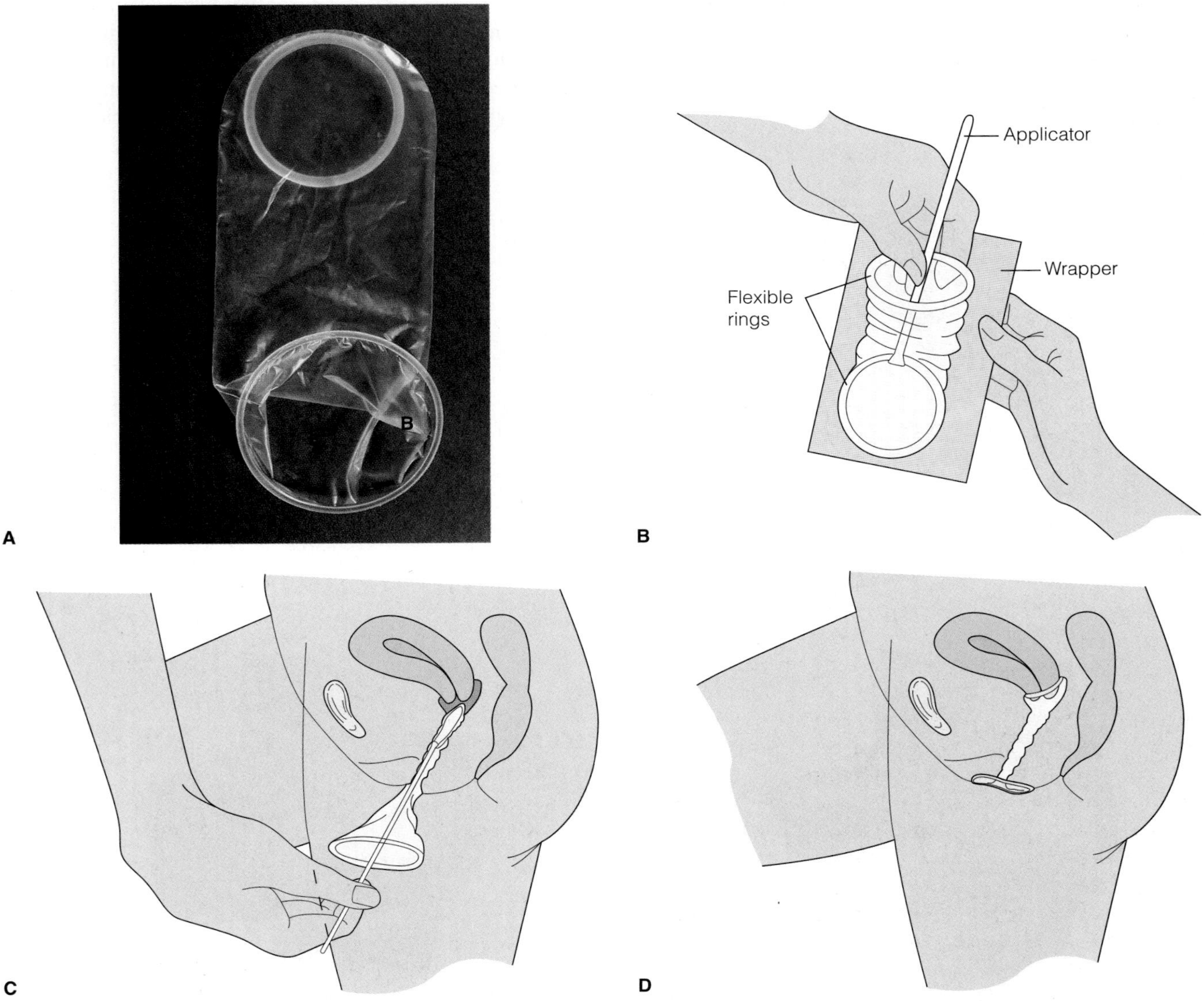

● **Figure 5–2** Application of the female condom. ***A,*** The condom. To insert: ***B,*** Remove condom and applicator from wrapper by pulling up on the ring. ***C,*** Insert condom slowly by gently pushing the applicator toward the small of the back. ***D,*** When properly inserted, the outer ring should rest on the folds of skin around the vaginal opening, and the inner ring (closed end) should fit loosely against the cervix.

remains outside the vagina and covers a portion of the woman's perineum. It also covers the base of the man's penis during intercourse. Available over the counter and designed for onetime use, the condom may be inserted up to 8 hours before intercourse. The inner sheath is prelubricated but does not contain spermicide and is not designed to be used with a male condom. Because it also covers a portion of the vulva, it probably provides better protection than other methods against some pathogens. High cost, noisiness during intercourse, and the cumbersome feel of the device make acceptability a problem for some couples.

In 2009 a second female condom, the FC2 Female Condom was approved by the Food and Drug Administration (FDA) (FDA, 2009). The new device is softer, less noisy during intercourse, and less expensive than the Reality female condom.

Diaphragm and Cervical Cap

The **diaphragm** (Figure 5–3 ●) is used with spermicidal cream or jelly and offers a good level of protection from conception. The woman must be fitted with a diaphragm and instructed in its use by trained personnel. The diaphragm should be rechecked for correct size after each childbirth and whenever a woman has gained or lost 10 to 15 lb or more.

The diaphragm must be inserted before intercourse, with approximately 1 teaspoon (or 1.5 inches from the tube) of spermicidal jelly placed around its rim and in the cup. This chemical barrier supplements the mechanical barrier of the diaphragm. The diaphragm is inserted through the vagina and covers the cervix. The last step in insertion is to push the edge of the diaphragm under the symphysis pubis, which may result in a "popping" sensation. When fitted properly and correctly in place, the diaphragm should not cause discomfort to the woman or her partner. Correct placement of the diaphragm can be checked by touching the cervix with a fingertip through the cup. The cervix feels like a small, firm, rounded structure and has a consistency similar to that of the tip of the nose. The center of the diaphragm should be over the cervix. If more than 6 hours elapse between insertion of the diaphragm and intercourse, additional spermicidal cream or jelly should be used. It is necessary to leave the diaphragm in place for at least 6 hours after coitus. The diaphragm should then be removed, cleaned with mild soap and water, and allowed to air dry before it is stored in its case. If intercourse is desired again within the 6 hours, another type of contraception must be used or additional spermicidal jelly placed in the vagina with an applicator, taking care not to disturb the placement of

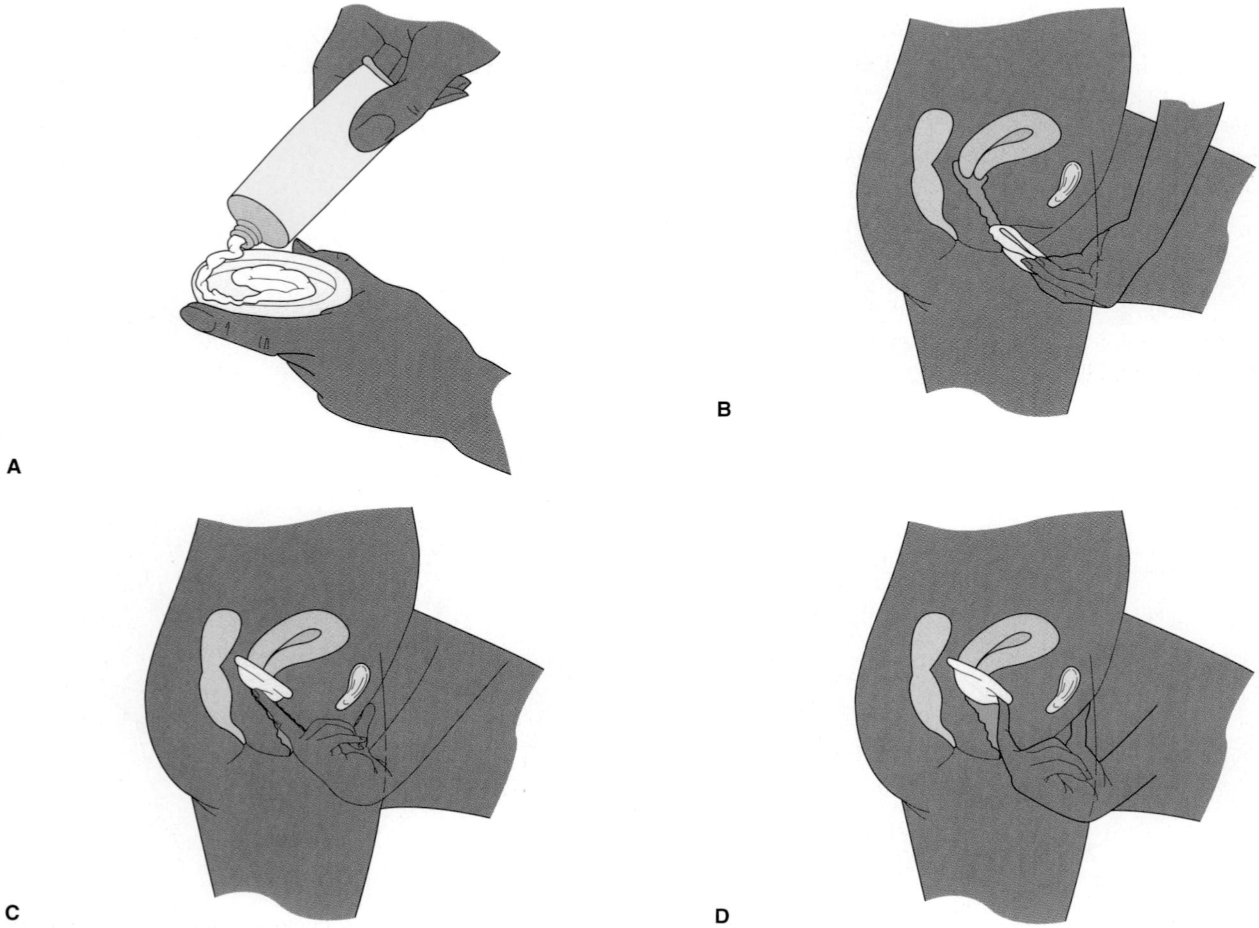

● **Figure 5–3** Inserting the diaphragm. ***A,*** Apply jelly to the rim and center of the diaphragm. ***B,*** Insert the diaphragm. ***C,*** Push the rim of the diaphragm under the symphysis pubis. ***D,*** Check placement of the diaphragm. Cervix should be felt through the diaphragm.

the diaphragm. Periodically the diaphragm should be held up to the light and inspected for tears or holes.

Some couples feel that the use of a diaphragm interferes with the spontaneity of intercourse. The nurse can suggest that the partner insert the diaphragm as part of foreplay. The woman can then easily verify the placement herself.

Diaphragms are an excellent contraceptive method for women who are lactating, who cannot or do not wish to use the pill (oral contraceptives), who are smokers over age 35, or who wish to avoid the increased risk of PID associated with intrauterine devices. A silicone diaphragm is available for women with latex allergies.

Women who object to manipulating their genitals to insert the diaphragm, check its placement, and remove it may find this method unsatisfactory. It is not recommended for women with a history of urinary tract infection, because pressure from the diaphragm on the urethra may interfere with complete bladder emptying and lead to recurrent urinary tract infections. Women with a history of toxic shock syndrome should not use diaphragms or any of the barrier methods because they are left in place for prolonged periods. For the same reason, the diaphragm should not be used during a menstrual period or if a woman has abnormal vaginal discharge.

The **cervical cap** (Figure 5–4 ●) is a cup-shaped device, used with spermicidal cream or jelly, that fits snugly over the cervix and is held in place by suction. Effectiveness rates and method of insertion are similar to those for the diaphragm. The cap may be left in place for up to 48 hours, and repeat acts of intercourse do not require additional spermicide. Advantages, disadvantages, and contraindications are similar to those associated with the diaphragm. The cervical cap may be more difficult to fit because of limited size options. It also tends to be more difficult for women to insert and remove. A newer form of cervical cap—the FemCap—is also available. It looks like a small sailor's cap and has a strap placed over the dome that allows easier removal.

Lea's shield is a reusable, silicone rubber barrier method that completely covers the cervix. It is similar to the cervical cap but contains a centrally located valve that permits the passage of cervical secretions and air. It can be used for up to 48 hours with a single application of spermicide. The device has been available over the counter in several European countries for over a decade because one size fits virtually all women. In the United States, a woman must see her practitioner to obtain one.

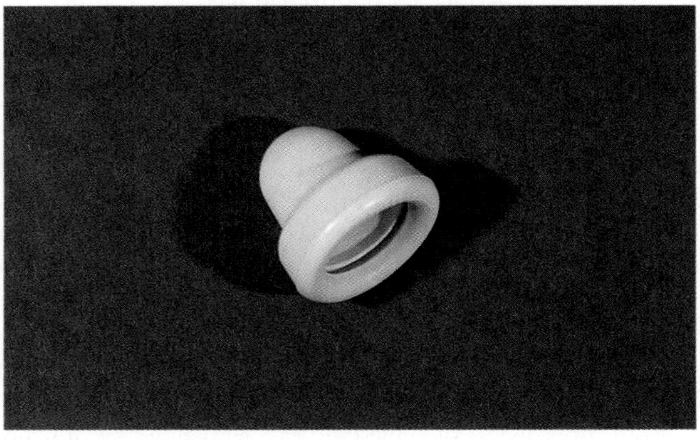

● **Figure 5–4** A cervical cap.

Vaginal Sponge

The *Today vaginal sponge,* available without a prescription, is a pillow-shaped, soft, absorbent synthetic sponge containing spermicide. It is made with a concave or cupped area on one side that fits over the cervix and has a loop for easy removal. The sponge is moistened thoroughly with water before insertion to activate the spermicide and then inserted into the vagina with the cupped side against the cervix (Figure 5–5 ●). It should be left in place for 6 hours following intercourse and may be worn for up to 24 hours, then removed and discarded.

Advantages include the following: professional fitting is not required, it may be used for multiple acts of coitus for up to 24 hours, one size fits all, and it acts as both a barrier and a spermicide. Disadvantages include problems associated with removing it and irritation or allergic reactions. Some women report a problem because the sponge absorbs vaginal secretions, contributing to vaginal dryness. For women without children the failure rate is comparable to that of the diaphragm and cervical cap. It is higher for women who have borne children, possibly because of changes in the shape of the cervix.

Intrauterine Devices

The **intrauterine device (IUD)** is a safe, effective method of reversible contraception that is designed to be inserted into the uterus by a qualified healthcare provider and left in place for an extended period, providing continuous contraceptive protection. Traditionally the IUD was believed to act by preventing the implantation of a fertilized ovum. Thus, the IUD was considered an abortifacient (abortion-causing) method. This belief is not accurate. IUDs truly are contraceptives; they trigger a spermicidal type reaction in the body, thereby preventing fertilization. The IUD is also known to have local inflammatory effects on the endometrium.

Advantages of the IUD include high rate of effectiveness, continuous contraceptive protection, no coitus-related activity,

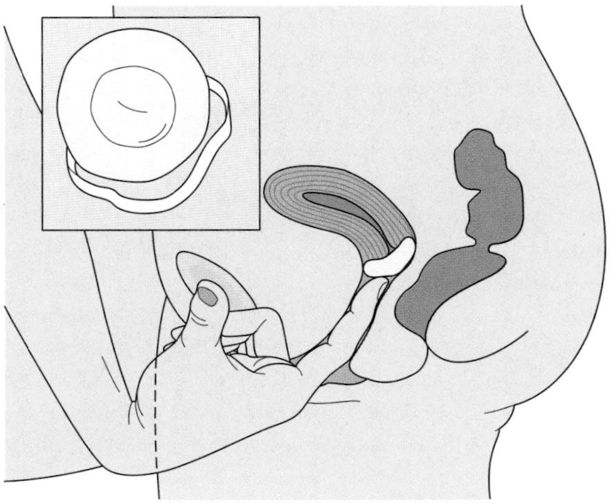

● **Figure 5–5** Application of the contraceptive sponge. The contraceptive sponge is moistened well with water and inserted into the vagina with the concave portion positioned over the cervix.

and relative inexpensiveness over time. Possible adverse reactions to the IUD include discomfort to the wearer, increased bleeding during menses, PID, perforation of the uterus, intermenstrual bleeding, dysmenorrhea, and expulsion of the device.

Two IUDs are currently available in the United States. The copper T380A (ParaGard) is a nonhormonal, highly effective IUD that can be left in place for up to 10 years. The levonorgestrel-releasing intrauterine system (LNG-IUS) (Mirena), which releases levonorgestrel gradually, is comparable in effectiveness to the copper T and may be left in place for up to 5 years (Figure 5–6 ●). The primary advantage of the LNG-IUS is that it produces diminished periods or even amenorrhea, which women welcome once they are advised that the absence of menses is safe and not an indication of pregnancy.

Formerly the IUD was recommended only for women who have at least one child and were in a stable, mutually monogamous relationship, because these women have the lowest risk of developing a pelvic infection. At the request of the company that manufactures the Copper T380A, the FDA removed a "patient or partner with multiple sexual partners" as a contraindication for its use. This change can apply as well to the LNG-IUS (Ogburn & Esprey, 2007). Research indicates that, contrary to common belief, the IUD is reliable and effective in women who have never been pregnant; it is effective against ectopic pregnancy because of its overall effectiveness in preventing any pregnancy. Moreover, the copper IUD is a good choice for women who cannot use hormonal forms of contraception (Jacobstein, 2007).

MyNursingKit | Animation: Oral Contraception

The IUD is inserted into the uterus with its string or tail protruding through the cervix into the vagina. It may be inserted at any time during a woman's cycle providing she is not pregnant or during the 4- to 6-week postpartum check. After insertion, the clinician instructs the woman to check for the presence of the string once a week for the first month and then after each menses. She is told that she may have some cramping or bleeding intermittently for 2 to 6 weeks and that her first few menses may be irregular. Follow-up examination is suggested 4 to 8 weeks after insertion.

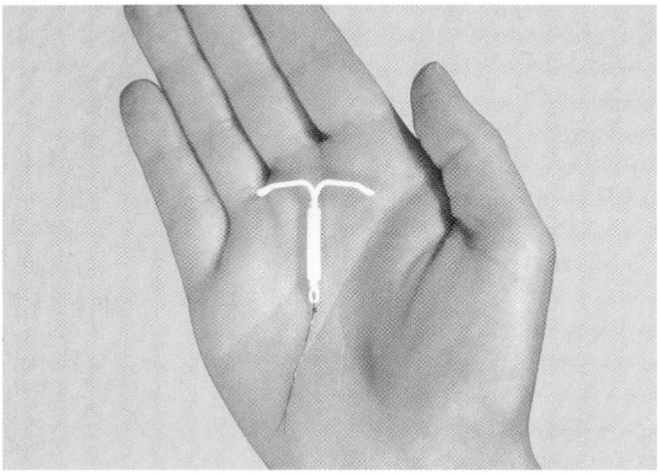

● **Figure 5–6** The Mirena Intrauterine System. This contraceptive device releases levonorgestrel gradually and may be left in place for up to 5 years.

Source: Used with permission from Berlex Laboratories, Inc.

Women with IUDs should contact their healthcare providers if they are exposed to an STI or if they develop the following warning signs: late period, abnormal spotting or bleeding, pain with intercourse, abdominal pain, abnormal discharge, signs of infection (fever, chills, and malaise), or missing string. If the woman becomes pregnant with an IUD in place, the device should be removed as soon as possible to prevent infection.

HORMONAL CONTRACEPTION

Hormonal contraceptives are available in a variety of forms. They may be progestin-only hormones, most often using a synthetic form of progesterone called progestin, or a combination of estrogen and a progestin.

Combined Estrogen-Progestin Approaches

Combined hormonal approaches work by inhibiting the release of an ovum, by creating an atrophic endometrium, and by maintaining thick cervical mucus that slows sperm transport and inhibits the process that allows sperm to penetrate the ovum.

Combined oral contraceptives. **Combined oral contraceptives (COCs)**, also called *birth control pills,* are typically a combination of the hormones estrogen and progesterone. COCs are safe, highly effective, and rapidly reversible. Many COCs are available. The pill is taken daily for 21 days, typically beginning on the Sunday after the first day of the menstrual cycle, although the woman can also start on day 1 of her menstrual cycle. In most cases menses occurs 1 to 4 days after the last pill is taken. Seven days after taking her last pill, the woman restarts the pill. Thus the woman always begins the pill on the same day. Some companies offer a 28-day pack with seven "blank" pills so that the woman never stops taking a pill. The pill should be taken at approximately the same time each day—usually upon arising or before retiring in the evening.

Research suggests that traditional 21/7 approaches may need to be modified. With today's low-dose COCs, the 7 hormone-free days may result in failure to completely suppress ovarian function, resulting in the development of an ovarian follicle and possible ovulation (Sulak, 2008). Consequently there is growing interest in extended oral contraceptives. Seasonale and Seasonique are the first FDA-approved extended cycle COCs. They both are 91-day regimens in which a woman takes an active pill daily for 84 consecutive days followed by 7 days of inactive tablets during which the woman has a period. Thus a woman has only four periods a year. Extended use reduces the side effects of COCs such as bloating, headache, breast tenderness, and cramping (Abboud, 2006). Another COC, Lybrel, has been approved by the FDA for continuous 365-day use with no scheduled hormone-free periods.

Although they are highly effective when taken correctly, COCs may produce a variety of side effects, which may be either progesterone or estrogen related (Table 5–1). The use of low-dose (35 mcg or less estrogen) preparations has reduced many of the side effects. The newer 20-mcg pills have even fewer side effects, but they may result in less contraceptive effectiveness.

Contraindications to the use of COCs include pregnancy, previous history of thrombophlebitis or thromboembolic disease, acute or chronic liver disease of cholestatic type with abnormal function, presence of estrogen-dependent carcinomas, undiagnosed uterine

Table 5–1 Side Effects Associated with Oral Contraceptives

Estrogen Effects	Progestin Effects
Alterations in lipid metabolism	Acne, oily skin
Breast tenderness, engorgement; increased breast size	Breast tenderness; increased breast size
Cerebrovascular accident	Decreased libido
Changes in carbohydrate metabolism	Decreased high-density lipoprotein (HDL) cholesterol levels
Chloasma (Melasma)	Depression
Fluid retention; cyclic weight gain	Fatigue
Headache	Hirsutism
Hepatic adenomas	Increased appetite; weight gain
Hypertension	Increased low-density lipoprotein (LDL) cholesterol levels
Leukorrhea, cervical erosion, ectopia	Oligomenorrhea, amenorrhea
Nausea	Pruritus
Nervousness, irritability	Sebaceous cysts
Telangiectasia	
Thromboembolic complications—thrombophlebitis, pulmonary embolism	

bleeding, heavy smoking, gallbladder disease, hypertension, diabetes, and hyperlipidemia. In addition, women with the following relative contraindications who use COCs need to be monitored frequently: migraine headaches, epilepsy, depression, oligomenorrhea, and amenorrhea. Women who choose this method of contraception should be fully advised of its potential side effects.

COCs also have some important noncontraceptive benefits. Many women experience relief of uncomfortable menstrual symptoms. Cramps are lessened, flow is decreased, and cycle regularity is increased. Mittelschmerz is eliminated, and the incidence of functional ovarian cysts is decreased. More important, there is a substantial reduction in the incidence of ectopic pregnancy, ovarian cancer, endometrial cancer, iron deficiency anemia, and benign breast disease. In addition, COCs are considered a good solution to the physiologic problems some women experience during the perimenopause. Because of the increased risk of myocardial infarction (heart attack), women over age 35 who smoke should not take COCs.

The woman using COCs should contact her healthcare provider if she becomes depressed, becomes jaundiced, develops a breast lump, or experiences any of the following warning signs: severe abdominal pain, severe chest pain or shortness of breath, severe headaches, dizziness, changes in vision (vision loss or blurring), speech problems, or severe leg pain.

Another oral contraceptive is the progesterone-only pill, also called the *minipill.* It is used primarily by nursing mothers and by women who have a contraindication to the estrogen component of the combination pills, such as history of thrombophlebitis, but are strongly motivated to use this form of contraception. The major problems with this preparation are amenorrhea or irregular spotting and bleeding patterns.

Other combined hormonal methods. Hormones can now be administered transdermally using a *contraceptive skin patch* called Ortho Evra. The patch is roughly the size of a silver dollar, but square. The woman applies it weekly for 3 weeks to one of four sites: her abdomen, buttocks, upper outer arm, or trunk (excluding the breasts). During the fourth week, no patch is worn and menses occurs. The patch is highly effective in women who weigh less than 198 lb. The patch is as safe and reliable as COCs and has a better rate of compliance. Questions of safety have arisen because skin absorption of transdermal estrogen is greater than oral absorption. However, research suggests that the incidence of stroke and MI is no greater in women using the patch than in women using 35 mcg COCs (Jick & Jick, 2007). Thus this method is currently considered a safe birth control option.

Evidence-Based Nursing

COC USE AND WEIGHT GAIN

Clinical Question

What is the effect of combination oral contraceptive use on weight gain?

The Evidence

Weight gain is often thought to be associated with combination hormonal contraceptives. When women are concerned about gaining weight, they may not use hormonal contraceptives effectively, or they may choose less effective methods to prevent pregnancy. However, a causal relationship between combination hormonal contraceptives and weight gain has not been empirically demonstrated. Five scientists conducted a systematic review of peer reviewed randomized trial for the Cochrane Collaborative, a rigorous peer reviewer focused on generating evidence for practice. Three randomized trials met the preset standards, representing the highest quality of evidence for practice. None of the three trials established a significant relationship between the use of combination hormonal contraceptives and substantive weight gain (Gallo, Lopea, Grimes, et al., 2008).

Best Practice

Combination oral contraceptives and/or patch delivery methods are not associated with weight gain. Women can be reassured that they may use appropriate combination hormonal contraceptives without gaining weight.

Critical Thinking

Is the lack of an association independent of the age of the woman? Is the demonstrated lack of association between hormonal contraceptives and weight gain a function of dosage?

See MyNursingKit for possible responses.

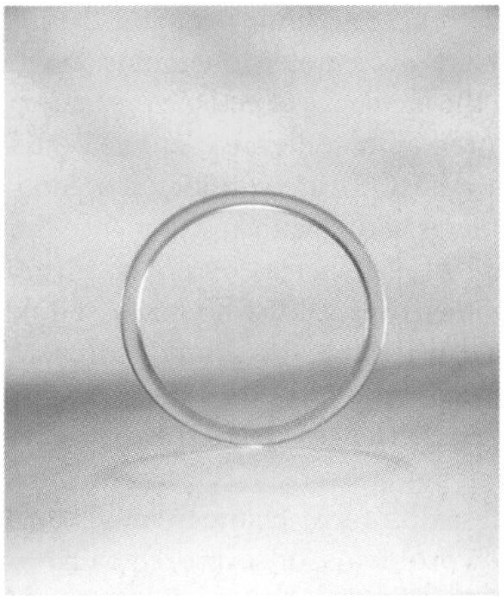

● **Figure 5–7** The NuvaRing vaginal contraceptive ring.
Source: Courtesy of Organon, Inc.

NuvaRing vaginal contraceptive ring (manufactured by Organon), another form of low-dose, sustained-release hormonal contraceptive, is a flexible soft ring that the woman inserts into her vagina (Figure 5–7 ●). The ring is left in place for 3 weeks and then removed for 1 week to allow for withdrawal bleeding. One size fits virtually all women. The ring is highly effective and has minimal side effects. The ring can be worn during intercourse and is comfortable for both the woman and her partner.

Lunelle, an injectable combination of medroxyprogesterone acetate (MPA) and estradiol cypionate (E_2C), is administered every 28 to 30 days (not to exceed 33 days) intramuscularly. Lunelle is a highly effective contraceptive that has a side-effect pattern similar to that of COCs. Lunelle is off the market in the United States and Canada but available in many other countries.

Long-Acting Hormonal Contraceptives

Norplant, a system consisting of six silastic capsules containing levonorgestrel, a progestin, which are implanted in a woman's arm, was the original **subdermal implant**. It is now off the market in the United States although some women still have the rods in place in their arm. Norplant II, which consists of a two-rod system that is effective for up to 5 years, has not been introduced in the United States, although it is marketed elsewhere as Jadelle.

Implanon, a single-capsule implant also inserted under the skin of the arm, is effective for up to 3 years. It is impregnated with etonogestrel, another progestin. Its release in the United States has been postponed, but remains anticipated.

Subdermal implants prevent ovulation in most women. They also stimulate the production of thick cervical mucus, which inhibits sperm penetration. Implants provide effective continuous contraception removed from the act of coitus. Possible side effects include spotting, irregular bleeding or amenorrhea, an increased incidence of ovarian cysts, weight gain, headaches, fluid retention, acne, mood changes, and depression.

Implants are mentioned in this chapter because some women may not have had their six Norplant rods removed or the nurse may care for women from foreign countries who use Jadelle or Implanon.

Depot-medroxyprogesterone acetate (DMPA) (**Depo-Provera**), another long-acting progestin that acts primarily by suppressing ovulation, provides effective birth control for 3 months when given as a single injection of 150 mg. Side effects include menstrual irregularities, headache, weight gain, breast tenderness, and depression. Prolonged use has been associated with significant, long-term loss of bone density, and many physicians have stopped prescribing it because of this. It should not be used for long-term birth control (longer than 2 years) without specific informed consent by the woman. Return of fertility may be delayed for an average of 9 months.

DepoProvera 104 mg SQ is an alternative to DepoProvera 150 mg. Because there is 30% less drug available compared with the 150 mg preparation, it may result in less bone density loss for long-term users. It is administered subcutaneously every 10 to 13 weeks.

EMERGENCY POSTCOITAL CONTRACEPTION

Emergency contraception is indicated when a woman is worried about pregnancy because of unprotected intercourse or possible contraceptive failure (e.g., broken condom, slipped diaphragm, or too long a time between DMPA injections). Plan B, a progestin-only approach (levonorgestrel), is the only emergency contraceptive currently available in the United States. In 2006 Plan B was approved by the FDA for over-the-counter sale to women 18 years and older. A prescription is still required for teens under age 18.

Though sometimes called the "morning-after pill," the phrase is misleading because the woman actually takes a dose as soon after intercourse as possible and a second dose 12 hours later. This regimen must be started within 72 hours after unprotected intercourse; the earlier the treatment is started, the greater the effectiveness. A woman can also use a regimen of COCs for emergency contraception if indicated.

OPERATIVE STERILIZATION

Operative **sterilization** refers to surgical procedures that permanently prevent pregnancy. Before sterilization is performed on either partner, the physician provides a thorough explanation of the procedure to both. Each needs to understand that sterilization is not a decision to be taken lightly or entered into when psychologic stresses, such as separation or divorce, exist. Even though both male and female procedures are theoretically reversible, the permanency of the procedure should be stressed and understood.

Male sterilization is achieved through a relatively minor procedure called a **vasectomy**. This procedure involves surgically severing the vas deferens in both sides of the scrotum. Following vasectomy it takes about 4 to 6 weeks and 6 to 36 ejaculations to clear the remaining sperm from the vas deferens. During that period the couple is advised to use another method of birth control and to bring in two or three semen samples for a sperm count. The man is rechecked at 6 and 12 months to ensure that fertility has not been restored by recanalization. Side effects of a vasectomy include pain, infection, hematoma, sperm granulomas, and spontaneous reanastomosis (reconnecting).

Female sterilization is most frequently accomplished by **tubal ligation**. The tubes are located through a small subumbilical incision or by minilaparotomy techniques and are clipped, ligated, electrocoagulated, banded, or plugged. Tubal ligation may be done at any time. However, the postpartum period is an ideal time to perform a tubal ligation because the tubes are somewhat enlarged and easily located.

Complications of female sterilization procedures include coagulation burns on the bowel, bowel perforation, pain, infection, hemorrhage, and adverse anesthesia effects. Reversal of a tubal ligation depends on the type of procedure performed.

The *Essure* method of permanent sterilization requires no surgical incision. Under hysteroscopy, stainless steel microinserts are inserted in the tubes stimulating the growth of local tissue, which then results in tubal blockage. Essure eliminates the need for transabdominal surgery but does take a few months to become effective so a backup method of contraception should be used until a hysterosalpingogram confirms that the tubes are occluded (Memmel & Gilliam, 2008).

MALE CONTRACEPTION

The vasectomy and the condom, discussed previously, are currently the only forms of male contraception available in the United States. Hormonal contraception for men has yet to be developed, although studies are under way.

Nursing management. In most cases the nurse who provides information and guidance about contraceptive methods works with the female partner, because most contraceptive methods are female oriented. Because men can purchase condoms without seeing a healthcare provider, counseling and interaction with a nurse are required only with vasectomy. As a nurse, you can play an important role in helping a woman choose a method of contraception acceptable to her and to her partner.

In addition to completing a history and assessing for any contraindications to specific methods, spend time with a woman learning about her lifestyle, personal attitudes about particular contraceptive methods, religious beliefs, personal biases, and plans for future childbearing, before helping the woman select a particular contraceptive method. Once the method is chosen, help the woman learn to use it effectively. Table 5–2 summarizes factors to consider in choosing an appropriate method of contraception.

Also review any possible side effects and warning signs related to the method chosen and counsel the woman about what action to take if she suspects she is pregnant. In many cases the nurse is involved in telephone counseling of women who call with questions and concerns about contraception. Thus, it is vital to be knowledgeable about this topic and have resources available to find answers to less common questions. "Teaching Highlights: Using a Method of Contraception" provides guidelines for helping women use a method of contraception effectively.

Table 5–2 Factors to Consider in Choosing a Method of Contraception

- Effectiveness of method in preventing pregnancy
- Safety of the method:
  - Are there inherent risks?
  - Does it offer protection against STIs or other conditions?
- Client's age and future childbearing plans
- Any contraindications in client's health history
- Religious or moral factors influencing choice
- Personal preferences, biases
- Lifestyle:
  - How frequently does client have intercourse?
  - Does she have multiple partners?
  - Does she have ready access to medical care in the event of complications?
  - Is cost a factor?
- Partner's support and willingness to cooperate
- Personal motivation to use method

CLINICAL INTERRUPTION OF PREGNANCY

Although abortion was legalized in the United States in 1973, controversy over moral and legal issues continues. Many people are opposed to abortion for religious, ethical, or personal reasons. Others feel that access to a safe, legal abortion is every woman's right. A number of physical and psychosocial factors influence a woman's decision to seek an abortion. Some situations may involve lack of knowledge about contraceptive options, contraceptive failure, rape, or incest.

Medical abortion provides an effective alternative to surgical abortion for many women with an unintended pregnancy. Mifepristone (Mifeprex), originally called RU-486, may be used to induce a medical abortion during the first 7 weeks of pregnancy (up to 49 days following conception). Mifepristone blocks the action of progesterone, thereby altering the endometrium. After the length of the woman's gestation is confirmed, she takes a dose of mifepristone (day 1). On day 3 she returns to her caregiver and takes a dose of the prostaglandin misoprostol, which induces contractions that expel the embryo/fetus. On day 14, the woman is seen a third time to confirm that the abortion was successful. Research suggests that a lower-dose regimen, which decreases both the cost and the side effects, is as effective as the original protocol and may be used up to 63 days' gestation (Holmquist & Gilliam, 2008).

Surgical abortion in the first trimester is technically easier and safer than abortion in the second trimester. It may be performed by dilation and curettage (D&C), minisuction, or vacuum curettage. Second-trimester abortion may be done using dilation and evacuation (D&E), hypertonic saline, systemic prostaglandins, and intrauterine prostaglandins.

Nursing management. Important aspects of nursing care for a woman who decides to have an abortion include providing information about the methods of abortion and associated risks; counseling regarding available alternatives to abortion and their implications; encouraging verbalization by the woman; providing counseling and emotional support before, during, and after the procedure; monitoring vital signs, intake, and output; providing for physical comfort and privacy throughout the procedure; and health teaching about self-care, the importance of the postabortion checkup, and contraception review.

Teaching Highlights

USING A METHOD OF CONTRACEPTION

- Discuss factors a woman should consider in choosing a method of contraception (see Table 5–2). Note that different methods may be appropriate at different times in a woman's life.
- Review the woman's reasons for choosing a particular method and confirm the absence of any contraindications to specific methods.
- Give a step-by-step description of the correct procedure for using the method chosen. Provide opportunities for questions.
- If a technique is to be learned, such as charting BBT or inserting a diaphragm, demonstrate and then have the woman do a return demonstration as appropriate. (*Note:* If certain aspects are beyond your level of expertise, such as fitting a cervical cap, review the content about its use and confirm that the woman understands what she is to do.)
- Provide information on what the woman should do if unusual circumstances arise (for example, she misses a pill or forgets a morning temperature). These can be presented in a written handout as well.
- Stress warning signs that may require immediate action by the woman and explain why these signs indicate a risk. (These should also be covered in the handout.)
- Arrange to talk with the woman again soon, either by phone or at a return visit, to see if she has any questions or has encountered any problems.

Thinking Critically

CHOOSING A METHOD OF CONTRACEPTION

Monique Hermann, age 37, was divorced 3 years ago. Her only son, now 19, is away at college. Recently, with some trepidation, Monique began dating, and she is now enjoying an active social life. She is being seen today for advice about contraception, which had not been an issue during her marriage because her husband had had a vasectomy. She reports that she is a little nervous about becoming sexually active because until this point her husband had been her only sexual partner. She is very attracted to two different men but does not prefer one over the other at this point. She states that she wants a reliable method that would permit her to have intercourse at any time without having to take action beforehand because she thinks that would be embarrassing for her. Similarly she is not interested in the patch, which is visible. She is not willing to consider a tubal ligation. She is a nonsmoker who drinks occasionally. She has no known contraindications to any available methods. Which methods of contraception might be appropriate for Monique?

See MyNursingKit for possible responses.

HEALTH PROMOTION FOR WOMEN

MyNursingKit Women's Health Web Links

Healthcare providers and consumers alike are becoming increasingly aware of the importance of activities that promote health and prevent illness, including lifestyle choices. In addition, the value of regular screenings to detect any health problems early cannot be overemphasized. Health screening recommendations vary by age. General screening and immunization guidelines for women can be found on the Companion Website.

This section focuses on some of the most commonly used screening procedures: breast self-examination and breast examination by a trained healthcare provider, mammography, Pap smear, and pelvic examination.

BREAST EXAMINATION

Like the uterus, the breast undergoes regular cyclic changes in response to hormonal stimulation. Each month, in rhythm with the cycle of ovulation, the breasts become engorged with fluid in anticipation of pregnancy, and the woman may experience sensations of tenderness, lumpiness, or pain. If conception does not occur, the accumulated fluid drains away via the lymphatic network. *Mastodynia* (premenstrual swelling and tenderness of the breasts) is common. It usually lasts for 3 to 4 days before the onset of menses, but the symptoms may persist throughout the month.

After menopause, adipose breast tissue atrophies and is replaced by connective tissue. Elasticity is lost, and the breasts may droop and become pendulous. The recurring breast engorgement associated with ovulation ceases. If estrogen replacement therapy is used to counteract other symptoms of menopause, breast engorgement may resume.

Monthly **breast self-examination (BSE)** is the best method for detecting breast masses early. A woman who knows the texture and feel of her own breasts is far more likely to detect changes that develop. Thus, it is important for a woman to develop the habit of doing routine BSE as early as possible, preferably as an adolescent. Women at high risk for breast cancer are especially encouraged to be attentive to the importance of early detection through routine BSE. Factors that predispose a woman to breast cancer include the following:

- Age. Incidence increases steadily with age. In fact, over 95% of new cases of breast cancer are diagnosed in women age 40 and over (American Cancer Society [ACS], 2006).
- Female gender.
- History of previous breast cancer.
- Family history of mother, sister, or daughter with breast cancer. The risk increases if two or more relatives develop breast cancer or if the relative developed breast cancer premenopausally or in both breasts.
- Long-term (more than 5 years) postmenopausal combined estrogen and progestin hormone replacement therapy (ACS, 2006).
- Being overweight or obese after menopause.
- Alcohol consumption. This risk increases with the amount of alcohol consumed (ACS, 2006).
- No history of pregnancy or first pregnancy after age 30.

- Never breastfeeding a child.
- Longer reproductive phase (early menarche [before age 12] and late menopause [after age 55]).
- History of high-dose radiation to the chest before age 30 (ACS, 2006).
- Physical inactivity.
- Ashkenazi Jewish descent.

The effectiveness of BSE is determined by the woman's ability to perform the procedure correctly. She should do a BSE on a regular monthly basis about 1 week after each menstrual period, when the breasts are typically not tender or swollen. After menopause she should perform BSE on the same day each month (as chosen by the woman). See "Teaching Highlights: Breast Self-Examination."

Clinical breast examination by a trained healthcare provider, such as a physician, nurse practitioner, or nurse-midwife, is an essential element of a routine gynecologic examination. Experience in differentiating among benign, suspicious, and worrisome breast changes lets the caregiver reassure the woman if the findings are normal or move forward with additional diagnostic procedures or referral if the findings are suspicious or worrisome.

MAMMOGRAPHY

A **mammogram** is a soft-tissue x-ray of the breast without the injection of a contrast medium. It can detect lesions in the breast before they can be felt. In 2009 a U. S. Preventive Services Task Force recommended against the use of routine mammograms for women ages 40 to 49. The Task Force recommended biennial screening mammograms for women ages 50 to 74. These recommendations sparked considerable controversy. Currently the American Cancer Society recommends that all women age 40 and over have an annual mammogram. The National Cancer Institute (2006) recommends mammograms every 1 to 2 years for women ages 40 to 49 and annually for all women age 50 and older.

PAP SMEAR AND PELVIC EXAMINATION

The Papanicolaou test (*Pap smear*) is a form of cervical cytology testing used to detect cellular abnormalities by examining a sample containing cells from the cervix and the endocervical canal.

Nursing Practice

Whenever you teach about pelvic examination and Pap smear, be sure the woman understands that she should not douche for at least 24 hours beforehand. Douching can interfere with the accuracy of the Pap smear. Occasionally a caregiver will specifically request that a woman use a douche before a Pap smear; douching should be done only in this circumstance.

For best test results, also advise women to avoid intercourse and the use of other female hygiene products and spermicidal agents immediately before a specimen is obtained. Specimens should not be obtained during menstruation or when visible cervicitis exists.

Traditionally the test has been done by preparing a Pap smear slide. A newer test, the liquid-based medium Pap smear, is now available. In this test, no slide is prepared. Instead the cervical cells, gathered in the same way as for the Pap smear, are transferred directly to a vial of preservative fluid, thereby preserving the entire specimen. The specimen is sent to a laboratory where a special processor prepares the slide. This test has become the method of choice for cervical cancer screening.

The pelvic examination lets the healthcare provider assess a woman's vagina, uterus, ovaries, and lower abdominal area. It is often performed after the Pap smear but may also be performed without a Pap for diagnostic purposes. Women sometimes perceive the pelvic examination as uncomfortable and embarrassing and may delay having yearly gynecologic examinations. This avoidance may pose a threat to life and health.

To make the pelvic examination less threatening and thus improve health-seeking behavior, caregivers can offer the woman a mirror to watch the procedure, point out anatomic parts to her, and position and drape her to allow eye-to-eye contact with the practitioner. Caregivers can encourage the woman to participate by asking questions and giving feedback.

Nurse practitioners, CNMs, and physicians all perform pelvic examinations. Nurses assist the practitioner and the woman during the examination. See "Skill 2–2: Assisting with a Pelvic Examination" in the Clinical Skills Manual.

MyNursingKit Video: Introduction to Mammography

MENOPAUSE

Menopause, defined as the absence of menses for a full year, is a time of transition for a woman, marking the end of her reproductive abilities. *Climacteric,* or *change of life* (often used synonymously with menopause), refers to the psychologic and physical alterations that occur around the time of menopause. Today the median age at menopause is 51.3 years, and the average life span of a woman in the United States is over 80 years. Thus the average woman will live one third of her life after menopause. A woman's psychologic adaptation to menopause and the climacteric is multifactorial. She is influenced by her own expectations and knowledge, physical well-being, family views, marital stability, and sociocultural expectations. As the number of women reaching menopause increases, the negative emotional connotations society once attached to menopause are diminishing, enabling menopausal women to cope more effectively and even encouraging them to view menopause as a time of personal growth.

Perimenopause is the term applied to the time before menopause, usually about 2 to 8 years, when ovarian function wanes and hormonal deficiencies begin to produce symptoms. Contraception remains a concern during perimenopause. Combined oral contraceptives (the pill, patches, and vaginal rings) are becoming increasingly popular among healthy nonsmokers because many women also benefit from the noncontraceptive effects, including regulation of menses, relief of symptoms of estrogen deficiency, and a decreased risk of endometrial and ovarian cancers. Other contraceptive options for perimenopausal women include sterilization, progestin-only methods, and barrier methods such as condoms, diaphragm, cervical cap, and spermicides.

Teaching Highlights

BREAST SELF-EXAMINATION

Begin by discussing the risk factors associated with breast cancer and the use of BSE in breast cancer detection. Then describe and demonstrate the correct procedure for BSE.

1. Timing—Instruct the woman to perform BSE on a monthly basis. Be specific based on whether she is premenopausal, pregnant, postmenopausal, or postmenopausal receiving hormone therapy.
2. Inspection—Instruct the woman to inspect her breasts by standing or sitting in front of a mirror. She should inspect them in three positions: both arms relaxed at her sides, both arms raised straight over her head, and both hands placed on her hips while she leans forward (Figure 5–8 ●). In these positions she should do the following:
   - Note size and symmetry of the breasts. Some size difference between breasts is normal. Breasts may vary but the variations should remain constant during rest or movement—note abnormal contours.
   - Note shape and direction of breasts. Breasts can be rounded or pendulous with some variation between breasts. Breasts should point slightly laterally.
   - Observe for color and venous patterns. Check for redness or inflammation. A blue hue with a marked venous pattern that is focal or unilateral may indicate an area of increased blood supply due to tumor. Symmetric venous patterns are normal.
   - Observe for thickening or edema. Skin edema is seen as thickened skin with enlarged pores ("orange peel"). It may indicate blocked lymph drainage due to tumor.
   - Note the surface of the skin. Skin dimpling, puckering, or retraction when the hands are pressed together in front of the chest or against the hips suggests malignancy. Striae (stretch marks) are normal.
   - Note nipple size, shape, and direction. Long-standing nipple inversion is normal, but an inverted nipple previously capable of erection is suspicious. Note any deviation, flattening, or broadening of the nipples.
   - Check for rashes, ulcerations, or discharge.

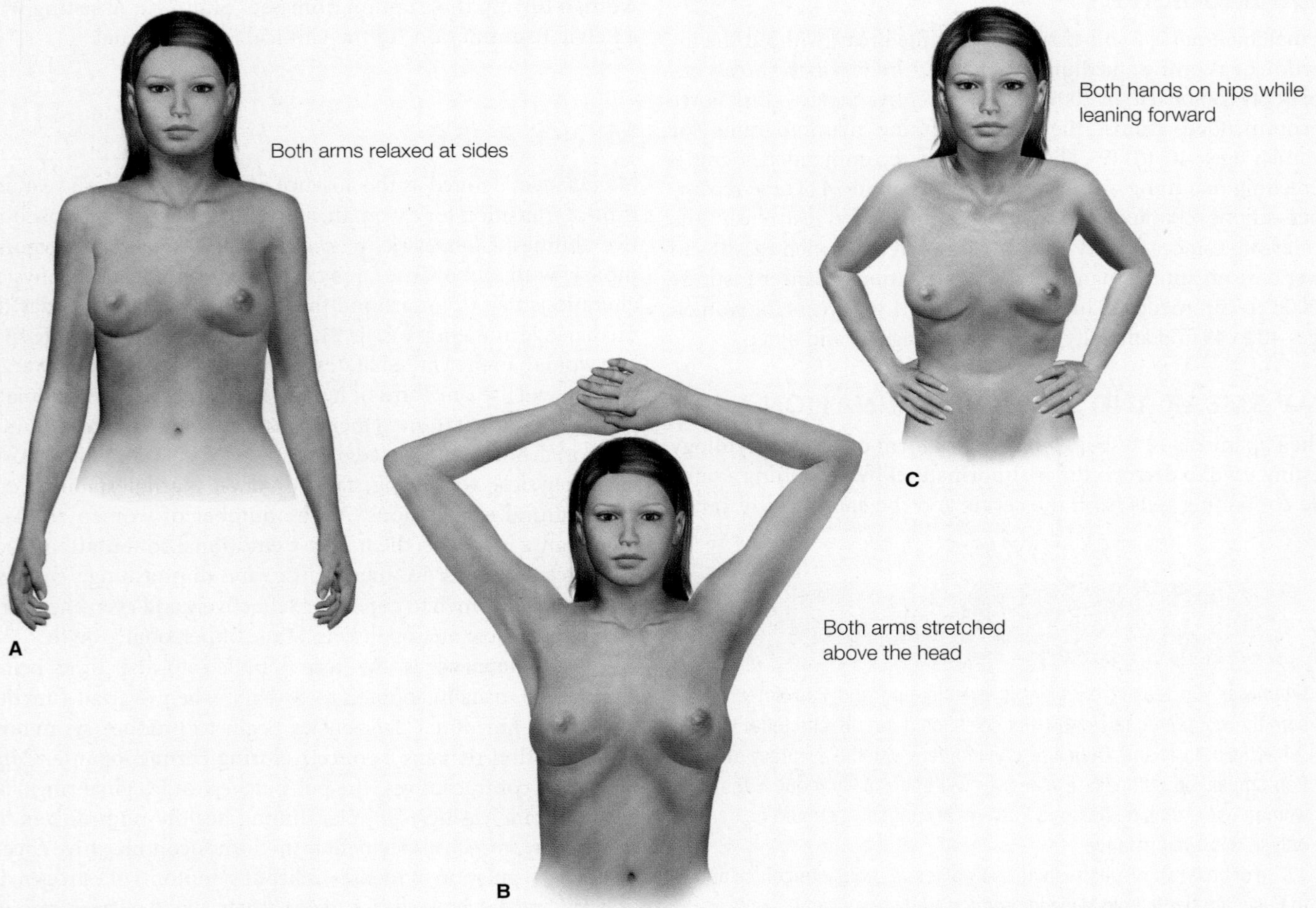

● **Figure 5–8** Positions for inspection of the breasts. ***A,*** Both arms relaxed at sides. ***B,*** Both arms stretched above the head. ***C,*** Both hands on hips while leaning forward.

Teaching Highlights—continued

3. Palpation—Instruct the woman to palpate (feel) her breasts as follows:
   - Lie down. Put one hand behind your head. With the other hand, fingers flattened, gently feel your breast. Press lightly (Figure 5–9A ●).
   - Figure 5–9B shows you how to check each breast. Begin as you see in B and follow the arrows, feeling gently for a lump or thickening. Remember to feel all parts of each breast, including the "tail" of tissue near the armpit. Repeat the process on the second breast.
   - Now repeat the same process on each breast sitting up, with your hand still behind your head (Figure 5–9C).
   - Squeeze the nipple between your thumb and forefinger. Look for any discharge—clear, bloody, or milky (Figure 5–9D).
4. Take the woman's hand and help her identify her "normal bumps" (e.g., mammary ridge, ribs, nodularity in the upper, outer quadrants).
5. Determine whether she has any questions about her findings during this examination. If she has questions, palpate the area and attempt to identify whether it is normal.
6. If a breast model is available, give the woman the opportunity to palpate it and identify the lumps.
7. Provide her with a monthly reminder, such as an American Cancer Society shower card.

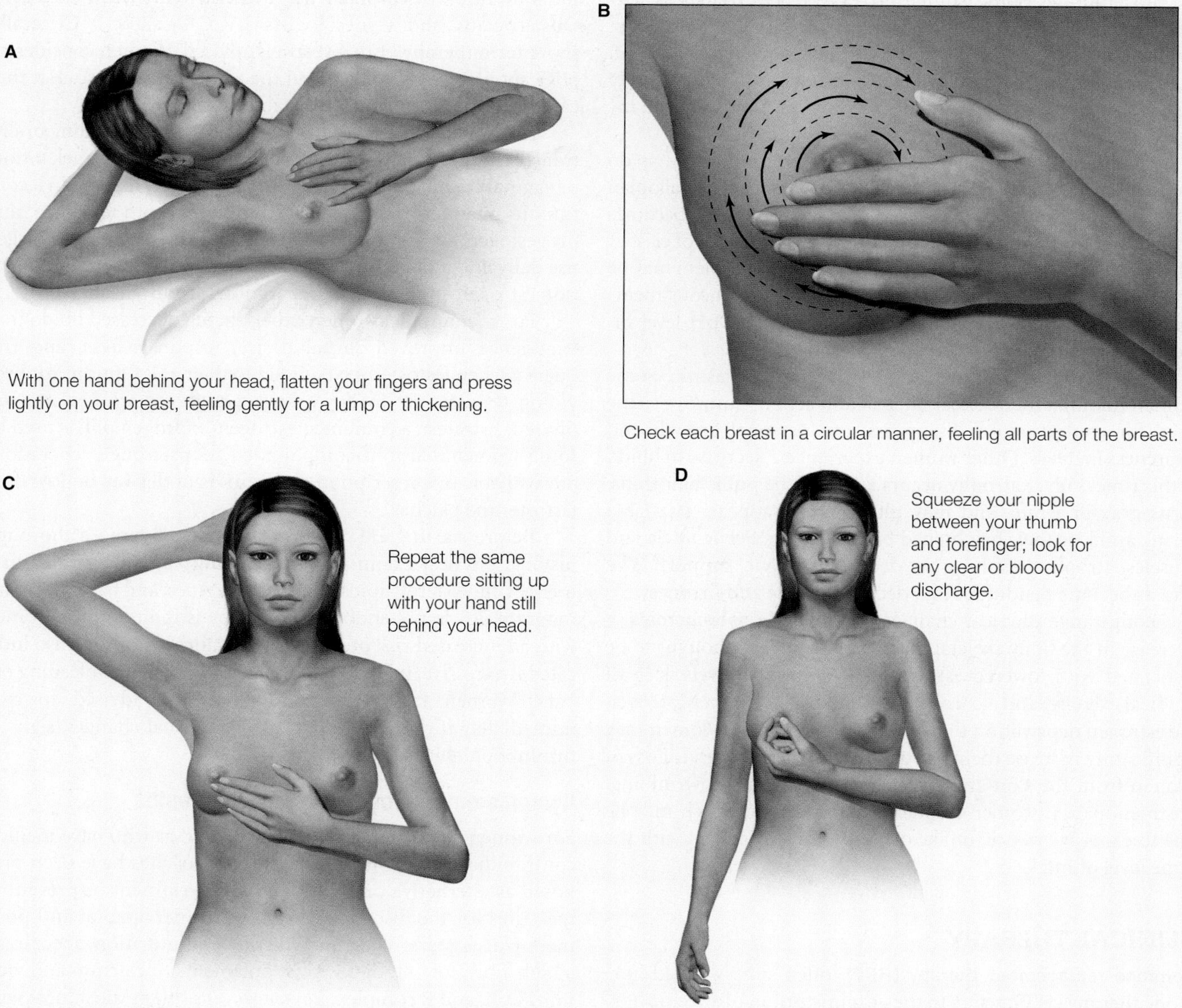
A
With one hand behind your head, flatten your fingers and press lightly on your breast, feeling gently for a lump or thickening.
B
Check each breast in a circular manner, feeling all parts of the breast.
C
Repeat the same procedure sitting up with your hand still behind your head.
D
Squeeze your nipple between your thumb and forefinger; look for any clear or bloody discharge.

● **Figure 5–9** Procedure for breast self-examination. ***A,*** With one hand behind your head, flatten your fingers and press lightly on your breast, feeling gently for a lump or thickening. ***B,*** Check each breast in a circular manner, feeling all parts of the breast. ***C,*** Repeat the same procedure sitting up with your hand still behind your head. ***D,*** Squeeze your nipple between your thumb and forefinger; look for any clear or bloody discharge.

The physical characteristics of menopause are linked to the shift from a cyclic to a noncyclic hormonal pattern. The age at onset may be influenced by nutritional, cultural, or genetic factors. The onset of menopause occurs when estrogen levels become so low that menstruation stops.

Generally, ovulation ceases 1 to 2 years before menopause, but individual variations exist. Atrophy of the ovaries occurs gradually. Follicle-stimulating hormone levels rise, and less estrogen is produced. Menopausal symptoms include atrophic changes in the vagina, vulva, and urethra and in the trigonal area of the bladder.

Many menopausal women experience a vasomotor disturbance commonly known as *hot flashes,* a feeling of heat arising from the chest and spreading to the neck and face. The hot flashes are often accompanied by sweating and sleep disturbances. These episodes may occur as often as 20 to 30 times a day and generally last 3 to 5 minutes. Some women also experience dizzy spells, palpitations, and weakness. Many women find their own most effective ways to deal with the hot flashes. Some report that using a fan or drinking a cool liquid helps relieve distress; others seek relief through hormone replacement therapy. In addition, many women use complementary therapies (see later discussion).

The uterine endometrium and myometrium atrophy, as do the cervical glands. The uterine cavity constricts. The fallopian tubes and ovaries atrophy extensively. The vaginal mucosa becomes smooth and thin, and the rugae disappear, leading to loss of elasticity. As a result, intercourse can be painful, but this problem may be overcome by using lubricating gel. Dryness of the mucous membrane can lead to burning and itching. The vaginal pH level increases as the number of Döderlein's bacilli decreases.

Postmenopausal women can still be multiorgasmic. Some women find that their sexual interest and activity improve as the need for contraception disappears and personal growth and awareness increase. Other women experience a decrease in libido at this time. Vulvar atrophy occurs late, and the pubic hair thins, turns gray or white, and may ultimately disappear. The labia shrink and lose their heightened pigmentation. Pelvic fascia and muscles atrophy, resulting in decreased pelvic support. The breasts become pendulous and decrease in size and firmness.

Long-range physical changes may include **osteoporosis**, a decrease in the bony skeletal mass. This change is thought to be associated with lowered estrogen and androgen levels, lack of physical exercise, and a chronic low intake of calcium. Moreover, the estrogen deprivation that occurs in menopausal women may significantly increase their risk of coronary heart disease. Loss of protein from the skin and supportive tissues causes wrinkling. Postmenopausal women frequently gain weight, which may be due to excessive caloric intake or to lower caloric need with the same level of intake.

CLINICAL THERAPY

Hormone replacement therapy (HRT), often simply called hormone therapy (HT), refers to the administration of specific hormones, usually estrogen with or without a progestin, to alleviate many menopausal symptoms, especially hot flashes, night sweats, and urogenital symptoms. HRT has also been recognized as very effective in preventing the development of osteoporosis. When estrogen is given alone, it can produce endometrial hyperplasia and increase the risk of endometrial cancer. Thus, in women who still have a uterus, estrogen is opposed by giving a progestin, often Provera, continuously or sequentially.

In 2002 the advisability of HRT was called into question because of the results of the Women's Health Initiative (WHI) study, which suggested that the risks of HRT outweigh the benefits, especially for long-term use, because of the slightly increased risk of breast cancer, thromboembolic disease, and stroke (Writing Group for the Women's Health Initiative Investigations, 2002). At present, the treatment of severe vasomotor symptoms (hot flashes and night sweats) is the primary indication for HT. It is also indicated for the treatment of moderate to severe symptoms of vulvar and vaginal atrophy (dyspareunia, vaginal dryness, and atrophic vaginitis). It is not currently recommended for the prevention of coronary heart disease (American College of Obstetricians and Gynecologists [ACOG], 2008). Generally, short-term therapy (1 to 4 years) is advised. Women considering HRT should clearly understand the associated risks so that they can make an informed decision about using it.

HT can be prescribed in a number of ways, including orally; transdermally (patch); intramuscularly; topically as a gel, lotion, or vaginal cream; and through a vaginal ring. It is given in a continuous manner, daily administration of both estrogen and progestogen, or as a cyclic or sequential therapy, with estrogen use daily and a progestogen added on a set sequence. Combination estrogen-progestogen preparations are also available.

Postmenopausal women experiencing decreased libido may experience improved sexual desire, responsiveness, and frequency when testosterone is added to their HT. Options for providing testosterone in doses low enough for women are still limited. Estratest, a combined estrogen-androgen pill, is used by some women. Custom-compounded testosterone preparations are available by prescription and work is underway on low dose testosterone patches.

Before starting HT, a woman should undergo a thorough history; physical examination, including Pap smear; measurement of cholesterol, lipids, and liver enzymes; and baseline mammogram. An initial endometrial biopsy is indicated for women with an increased risk of endometrial cancer; biopsy is also indicated if excessive, unexpected, or prolonged vaginal bleeding occurs. Women taking estrogen should be advised to stop immediately if they develop headaches, visual changes, signs of thrombophlebitis, or chest pain.

Complementary and Alternative Therapies

For women who do not wish to take HRT or who have medical contraindications to it, a variety of approaches have been proposed as alternative or complementary treatment or preventive measures for the discomforts of the perimenopausal and postmenopausal years. These include diet and nutrition, specifically a high-fiber, low-fat diet with supplements of calcium and vitamins D, E, and B complex. *Phytoestrogens* (plant substances with estrogen properties), found in a number of plant foods, especially soybean products, may be helpful. (See "Complementary Care: Use of Botanicals for Menopausal Symptoms" for a discussion of the use of botanicals.)

Evidence in Action

Soy isoflavone intake has been shown to increase the bone mineral density in the spine of menopausal women (meta-analysis) (Ma, Qin, Wang, & Katoh, 2008).

Weight-bearing exercises such as walking, jogging, tennis, and low-impact aerobics help increase bone mass and decrease the risk of osteoporosis. Exercise also improves cholesterol profiles and contributes to overall health. Stress management and relaxation techniques such as biofeedback, meditation, yoga, visualization, and massage may provide a sense of well-being. Some women also use homeopathic remedies and herbal treatments for symptom relief.

Prevention and Treatment of Osteoporosis

Osteoporosis is more common in women who are middle-aged or older. In fact, in the United States, 13% to 18% of women age 50 and older have osteoporosis (ACOG, 2004). Risk factors associated with osteoporosis include European American or Asian heritage; small-boned, thin build; low body weight (less than 127 lb); family history of osteoporosis; lack of regular weight-bearing exercise; never pregnant; early onset of menopause; consistently low intake of calcium; cigarette smoking; moderate to heavy alcohol intake; and the use of certain medications such as anticonvulsants, corticosteroids, or lithium.

Bone mineral density (BMD) testing is useful in identifying individuals who are at risk for osteoporosis. The National Osteoporosis Foundation (NOF) (2008) recommends BMD testing for the following:

- All postmenopausal women age 65 or older and men 70 years and older
- Postmenopausal women under age 65 and men ages 50 to 70 with one or more risk factors with a fracture
- Postmenopausal women and men who have had a fracture to determine the severity of the disease

A variety of conditions, including malabsorption syndrome, inflammatory bowel disease, AIDS, chronic obstructive pulmonary disease, certain cancers, eating disorders and inadequate diet, multiple sclerosis, and insulin-dependent diabetes mellitus may be associated with an increased risk of osteoporosis in adults. In addition, certain medications such as some anticonvulsants, lithium, long-term heparin use, glucocortico-steroids, and tamoxifen may also lead to osteoporosis.

Prevention of osteoporosis is a primary goal of care. Peri- and postmenopausal women are advised to have a daily calcium intake of 1200 mg (NAMS, 2006). Most women require supplements to achieve this level. Vitamin D supplements (800 to 1000 international units per day) may also be indicated for those at risk of deficiency (NOF, 2008). Women are also advised to participate regularly in exercise, to consume only modest quantities of alcohol and caffeine, and to stop smoking. Alcohol and smoking have a negative effect on the rate of bone resorption. Women's height should be measured at each visit, because a loss of height is often an early sign that vertebrae are being compressed because of reduced bone mass. The effectiveness of estrogen in preventing osteoporosis is well documented. However, because of the increased risks associated with long-term use of hormone replacement therapy, other pharmacologic agents are being used more frequently to prevent and treat osteoporosis. These include the following:

- *Bisphosphonates* are calcium regulators that act by inhibiting bone resorption and increasing bone mass. Alendronate (Fosamax) and risedronate (Actonel) are the two most commonly prescribed.

Complementary Care

USE OF BOTANICALS FOR MENOPAUSAL SYMPTOMS

The following botanicals were reviewed during a 2005 National Institutes of Health (NIH) State-of-the-Science conference on the management of menopausal symptoms. The panel found the following:

- *Black cohosh.* This substance has received the most attention of all the botanicals. It does not act as an estrogen, as was once believed. Studies of its effectiveness in relieving hot flashes have had mixed results but it has a good safety record over many years.
- *Red clover.* Five controlled studies found no conclusive or consistent evidence that hot flashes were reduced in women using red clover leaf extract. Few side effects have been reported and no serious health problems have been cited in the literature. Animal studies have raised a concern as to whether red clover might be harmful to estrogen-sensitive tissue such as the uterus and breasts.
- *Dong quai.* In the only randomized controlled study reported, dong quai was not found to be effective in reducing hot flashes. Because dong quai is known to interact with and increase the activity of warfarin (Coumadin), its use by women on warfarin can lead to bleeding problems.
- *Ginseng.* Although it has not been found to be effective in relieving hot flashes, ginseng may help with other menopausal symptoms such as sleep disturbances and mood swings.
- *Kava.* No evidence supports its effectiveness in relieving hot flashes, although it may decrease anxiety. The FDA has issued a warning about kava because it has been associated with liver disease.
- *Soy.* Results about the use of soy to relieve hot flashes (see discussion of phytoestrogens) are mixed. Its use as a dietary supplement for short periods of time is not associated with any serious side effects, although long-term use has been associated with a thickening of the uterine lining.

Source: National Center for Complementary and Alternative Medicine (NCCAM). (2006). Do CAM therapies help menopausal symptoms? Retrieved March 8, 2006, from http://nccam.nih.gov/health/menopauseandcam/

- *Selective estrogen receptor modulators (SERMs)* such as raloxifene (Evista) preserve the beneficial effects of estrogen, including its protection against osteoporosis, but do not stimulate uterine or breast tissue.
- *Calcitonin* is a calcium regulator that may inhibit bone loss. Generally administered as a nasal spray, although it is also available as an injection, its value is less clear than that of the other medications listed.
- *Parathyroid hormone*, taken daily as a subcutaneous injection, activates bone formation, which results in substantial increases in bone density.
- Ultra-low-dose estrogen patches (Menostar) can be used without a progestogen. These small doses can provide effective prevention of fracture without the increased side effects or risks of endometrial stimulation found in larger dose estrogen patches (Ettinger, 2004).

Women who are taking medication for osteoporosis should have BMD testing 2 years after beginning therapy and every 2 years thereafter (NOF, 2008).

Nursing management. Most menopausal women deal well with this developmental phase of life, although some women may need counseling to adjust successfully. Nurses and other health professionals can help menopausal women achieve high-level functioning at this time in life. Of major importance is the nurse's ability to understand and provide support for the woman's views and feelings. Use an empathetic approach in counseling, health teaching, and providing physical care.

Explore the question of the woman's comfort during sexual intercourse. In counseling, it may be appropriate to say, "After menopause many women notice that their vagina seems drier and intercourse can be uncomfortable. Have you noticed any changes?" This gives the woman information and may open discussion. Then go on to explain that dryness and shrinking of the vagina can be addressed by use of a water-soluble jelly. Use of estrogen, orally or in vaginal creams, may also be indicated. Increased frequency of intercourse will maintain some elasticity in the vagina. When assessing the menopausal woman, address the question of sexual activity openly but tactfully, because the woman may have been socialized to be reticent in discussing sex.

The crucial need of women in the menopausal period of life is for adequate information about the changes taking place in their bodies and their lives. Supplying that information provides both a challenge and an opportunity for nurses.

MyNursingKit Spousal Abuse Video

VIOLENCE AGAINST WOMEN

Violence against women is a major health concern in society today. Violence affects women of all ages, races, ethnic backgrounds, socioeconomic levels, educational levels, and walks of life. Two of the most common forms of violence are domestic violence and rape. Often people not only accept these forms of violence but also shift the blame for the violence to the women themselves by asking questions such as, "How did she make him so mad?" "Why does she stay?" "What was she doing out so late?" and "Why did she dress that way?"

Violence against women is also a major health concern. In addition to causing injuries, associated physical and mental health outcomes, and fatalities, violence costs the healthcare system millions of dollars annually. In response to this epidemic, healthcare providers are becoming more knowledgeable about actions they should take to identify women at risk, implement preventive measures, and provide effective care.

DOMESTIC VIOLENCE

Domestic violence is defined as a pattern of coercive behavior and methods used to exert power and control by one individual over another in an adult domestic or intimate relationship. It is also termed **intimate partner violence**. This section focuses on domestic violence experienced by women in heterosexual relationships, although gay and lesbian individuals do experience domestic violence in their relationships as well.

Although the incidence has decreased significantly in the last decade, domestic violence is still staggeringly common in the United States, where one in four women will experience domestice violence (National Coalition Against Domestic Violence [NCADV], 2007a). Worldwide, as many as one in three women will be the victim of violence or sexual coercion at some point in her life (NCADV, 2007c).

The woman may be married to her abuser, or she may be living with, dating, or divorced from him. Domestic violence takes many forms, including verbal attacks, insults, intimidation, threats, emotional abuse, social isolation, economic deprivation, intellectual derision, ridicule, stalking, and physical attacks and injury. Physical battering includes slapping, kicking, shoving, punching, forms of torture, attacks with objects or weapons, and sexual assault. Women who are physically abused can also suffer psychologic and emotional abuse.

Cycle of Violence

In an effort to explain the experience of battered women, Walker (1984) developed the theory of the *cycle of violence.* Battering takes place in a cyclic fashion through three phases:

1. In the *tension-building phase,* the batterer demonstrates power and control. This phase is characterized by anger, arguing, blaming the woman for external problems, and possibly minor battering incidents. The woman may blame herself and believe she can prevent the escalation of the batterer's anger by her own actions.
2. The *acute battering incident* is typically triggered by some external event or internal state of the batterer. It is an episode of acute violence distinguished by lack of control, lack of predictability, and major destructiveness. The cycle of violence can be interrupted before the acute battering incident if proper interventions take place.
3. The *tranquil, loving phase* is sometimes termed the honeymoon period. This phase may be characterized by

extremely kind and loving behavior on the part of the batterer as he tries to make up with the woman, or it may simply be manifested as an absence of tension and violence. Without intervention this phase will end and the cycle of violence will continue. Over time the violence increases in severity and frequency.

Characteristics of Battered Women

Battered women often hold traditional views of sex roles. Many were raised to be submissive, passive, and dependent and to seek approval from male figures. Some battered women were exposed to violence between their parents, whereas others first experienced it from their partners. Many battered women do not work outside the home. As part of the manipulation of batterers, they are isolated from family and friends and totally dependent on their partners for their financial and emotional needs.

Women with physically abusive partners nearly always experience psychologic abuse as well and have been told repeatedly by their batterers that the family's problems are all their fault. Many believe their batterers' insults and accusations. As these women become more isolated, they find it harder to judge who is right. Eventually they fully believe in their inadequacy, and their low self-esteem reinforces their belief that they deserve to be beaten. Battered women often feel a pervasive sense of guilt, fear, and depression. Their sense of hopelessness and helplessness reduces their problem-solving ability. Battered women may also experience a lack of support from family, friends, and their religious community.

Characteristics of Batterers

Batterers come from all backgrounds. They often have feelings of insecurity, socioeconomic inferiority, powerlessness, and helplessness that conflict with their assumptions of male supremacy. Emotionally immature and aggressive men have a tendency to express these overwhelming feelings of inadequacy through violence. Many batterers feel undeserving of their partners, yet they blame and punish the very women they value.

Battered women often describe their husbands or partners as lacking respect toward women in general, having come from homes where they witnessed abuse of their mothers or were themselves abused as children, and having a hidden rage that erupts occasionally. Batterers accept traditional macho values, yet when they are not angry or aggressive, they appear childlike, dependent, seductive, manipulative, and in need of nurturing. They may be well respected in the community. This dual personality of batterers reflects the conflict between their belief that they must live up to their macho image and their feelings of inadequacy in the role of husband or provider. Combined with low frustration tolerance and poor impulse control, their pervasive sense of powerlessness leads them to strike out at life's inequities by abusing women.

Nursing management. Nurses often come in contact with abused women but fail to recognize them, especially if their bruises are not visible. Women at high risk for battering often have a history of alcohol or drug abuse, child abuse, or abuse in the previous or present relationship. Other possible signs of abuse include expressions of helplessness and powerlessness; low self-esteem revealed by the woman's dress, appearance, and the way she relates to healthcare providers; signs of depression evidenced by fatigue, hopelessness, and somatic problems such as headache, insomnia, chest pain, back pain, or pelvic pain; and possible suicide attempts. In addition, the abused woman may have a history of missed or frequently changed appointments, perhaps because she had signs of abuse that kept her from coming in or because her partner prevented it.

Because female partner abuse is so prevalent, many caregivers now advocate *universal screening of all female clients at every health encounter.* Screening should be done privately, with only the caregiver and client present, in a safe and quiet place. Specific language leads to higher disclosure rates. Possible screening questions include the following:

1. During the past year, have you been slapped, kicked, hit, choked, or hurt physically by someone?
2. Has your partner or anyone else ever forced you to have sex?
3. Are you afraid of an ex-partner or anyone at home?

During the screening, assure the woman that her privacy will be respected (Figure 5–10 ●). It is essential to remain nonjudgmental. Create a warm, caring climate conducive to sharing, and demonstrate a willingness to talk about violence. A battered woman may interpret your willingness to discuss violence as permission for her to discuss it as well.

It is important to consider cultural and religious factors that may impact a woman's willingness to disclose abuse. See "Developing Cultural Competence: Supporting Immigrant Women Who Suffer Abuse."

When a woman seeks care for an injury, be alert to the following cues of abuse:

- Hesitation in providing detailed information about the injury and how it occurred

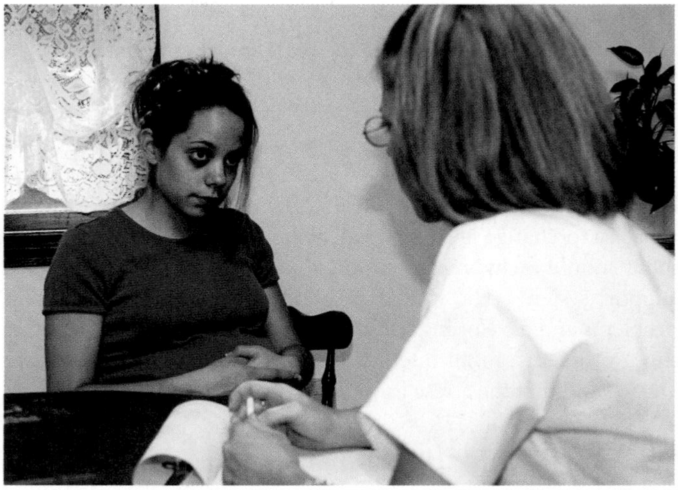

● **Figure 5–10** Domestic violence screening. Screening for domestic violence should be done privately.

Developing Cultural Competence

SUPPORTING IMMIGRANT WOMEN WHO SUFFER ABUSE

Nurses need to be aware that immigrant women who experience domestic violence may face barriers to seeking help including the following (NCADV, 2007b):

- *Language barriers* if English is not the primary language.
- *Fear of law enformcent or the legal system* if they have had negative experiences in their country of origin or if their abuser has given them misinformation.
- *Fear of deportation* if they are in the country illegally or if the abuser has led them to believe that it is possible if they complain or call the police.
- *Cultural or religious factors* if they were raised with strict guidelines about gender roles and the subservient position of women.

- Inappropriate affect for the situation
- Delayed reporting of symptoms
- Pattern of injury consistent with abuse, including multiple injury sites involving bruises, abrasions, and contusions to the head (eyes and back of the neck), throat, chest, abdomen, or genitals
- Inappropriate explanation for the injuries
- Lack of eye contact
- Signs of increased anxiety in the presence of the possible batterer, who frequently does much of the talking

When a battered woman comes in for treatment, she needs to feel safe physically and secure in talking about her injuries and problems. If a man is with her, ask or tell him to remain in the waiting room while the woman is examined. A battered woman also needs to regain a sense of predictability by knowing what to expect and how she can interact. Provide sufficient information about what to expect in terms the woman can understand.

In providing care, let the woman work through her story, problems, and situation at her own pace. Reassure the woman that she is believed and that her feelings are reasonable and normal. Anticipate the woman's ambivalence (due to her fear and possible love-hate relationship with her batterer), but also respect the woman's capacity to change and grow when she is ready. Thus any assessment should include information about a woman's strengths and support systems. The woman may need help identifying specific problems and developing realistic ideas for reducing or eliminating those problems. In all interactions, stress that no one should be abused and that the abuse is not the woman's fault.

Nursing Care in the Community

Inform any woman suspected of being in an abusive situation of the services available in the community. A battered woman may need the following:

- Medical treatment for injuries
- Temporary shelter to provide a safe environment for her and her children
- Counseling to raise her self-esteem and help her understand the dynamics of violence
- Legal assistance for protection, or prosecution of the batterer
- Financial assistance to obtain shelter, food, and clothing
- Job training or employment counseling
- An ongoing support group with counseling

If the woman returns to an abusive situation, encourage her to develop an exit plan for herself and her children, if any. As part of the plan, she should pack a change of clothing for herself and her children, including toiletries and an extra set of car and house keys. She should store these items away from the house with a friend or relative and ask a neighbor to call the police if violence begins. In planning she should be aware that her abuser may monitor mail, telephone, and Internet communication. If possible she should have money, identification papers (driver's license, social security card, and birth certificates for herself and her children), checkbook, savings account information, other financial information (such as mortgage papers, automobile papers, and pay stubs), court papers or orders, and information about the children to help her enroll them in school. She should also plan where she will go, regardless of the time of day. Ensure that the woman has a planned escape route and emergency telephone numbers she can call, including local police, a phone hotline, and a women's shelter if one is available in the community.

Working with battered women is challenging, and many healthcare providers feel frustrated and impotent when the women repeatedly return to their abusive situations. Nurses must realize that they cannot rescue battered women; battered women must decide on their own how to handle their situations. Effective nurses provide battered women with information that empowers them in decision making and supports their decisions, knowing that incremental assistance over the years may be the only alternative until the battered women are ready to explore other options.

SEXUAL ASSAULT AND RAPE

Broadly, **sexual assault** is involuntary sexual contact with another person. **Rape** is forced sexual intercourse as a result of physical force or psychologic coercion. Force sexual intercourse refers to vaginal, oral, or anal penetration by a body part or by an object.

Research indicates that one in six American women over age 12 has been the victim of an attempted or completed sexual assault or rape. However, the incidence of sexual assault is down by 69 percent since 1993 (Rape, Abuse, and Incest National Network [RAINN], 2008a).

No woman of any age or ethnicity is immune. Statistics indicate, however, that young, unmarried women, women who are unemployed or have a low family income, and students have the highest incidence of sexual assault or attempted assault. Like their victims, the assailants come from all ethnic backgrounds and walks of life. The majority are white (52%) with an average age of 31 years. Of those imprisoned for rape, 22 percent are married (RAINN, 2008b).

Why do men rape? Of the many theories put forth, none provides a completely satisfactory explanation. So few assailants are actually caught and convicted that a clear characteristic of the assailant has not been developed. However, rapists tend to be emotionally weak and insecure and may have difficulty maintaining interpersonal relationships. Many assailants also have trouble dealing with the stresses of daily life. Such men may become angry and overcome by feelings of powerlessness. They then commit a sexual assault as an expression of power or anger.

Acquaintance rape, which occurs when the assailant is someone with whom the victim has had previous nonviolent interaction, is the most common form of rape. In fact, in almost two-thirds of cases of rape or sexual assault, the assailant is known (RAINN, 2008b). One type of acquaintance rape, **date rape**, which occurs between a dating couple, is an increasing problem on high school and college campuses. In some cases an assailant uses alcohol or other drugs to sedate his intended victim. One drug, flunitrazepam (Rohypnol), has gained notoriety as a date rape drug because it frequently produces amnesia in its victims. In date rape situations, the male is usually determined to have sex and will do whatever he feels necessary if denied.

Responses to Sexual Assault

Sexual assault is a *situational crisis.* It is a traumatic event that the survivor cannot be prepared to handle because it is unforeseen. Following an assault the victim generally experiences a cluster of symptoms, described by Burgess and Holmstrom (1979) as the *rape trauma syndrome,* which last far beyond the rape itself. These phases are described in Table 5–3. Although the phases of response are listed individually, they often overlap, and individual responses and their duration may vary. A fourth phase—integration and recovery—has also been suggested (Holmes, 1998).

Research suggests that survivors of sexual assault may exhibit high levels of posttraumatic stress disorder, the same disorder that developed in many of the veterans of the Vietnam War. Posttraumatic stress disorder is marked by varying degrees of intensity. Assault victims with this disorder often require lengthy, intensive therapy to regain a sense of trust and feeling of personal control.

Care of the Sexual Assault Survivor

Survivors of sexual assault often enter the healthcare system by way of the emergency department. Thus, the emergency department nurse is often the first person to counsel them. Because the values, attitudes, and beliefs of the caregiver necessarily affect the competence and focus of the care, it is essential that nurses clearly understand their feelings about sexual assault and assault survivors and resolve any conflicts that may exist. In many communities a specially trained sexual assault nurse examiner (SANE) coordinates the care of survivors of sexual assault, gathers necessary forensic evidence, and is then available as an expert witness when assailants are tried for the crime.

The first priority in caring for a survivor of a sexual assault is to create a safe, secure environment. Admission information is gathered in a quiet, private room. The woman should be reassured that she is safe and not alone. The nurse assesses the survivor's appearance, demeanor, and ways of communicating for the purpose of planning care. Initially the woman is evaluated to determine the need for emergency care. Obtaining a careful, detailed history is essential. After the woman has received any necessary emergency care, a forensic chart and kit are completed.

The woman is given a thorough explanation of the procedures to be carried out and signs a consent form for the forensic examination and collection of materials. Sexual assault kits contain all the necessary supplies for collecting and labeling evidence. The woman's clothing is collected and bagged, swabs of stains and secretions are taken, hair samples and any fingernail scrapings are collected, blood samples are drawn, tissue swabs are obtained, and photographs are taken. Vaginal and rectal examinations are performed, along with a complete physical examination for trauma. If possible, photographs are taken of any injuries. The woman is offered prophylactic treatment for sexually transmitted infections. If the assailant's HIV status is not known, the woman may be offered postexposure prophylaxis with HIV antiviral medications. In such cases, consultation with an HIV specialist is advised. The woman is also questioned about

Table 5–3 Phases of Recovery Following Sexual Assault

Phase	Response
Acute phase (disorganization)	Fear, shock, disbelief, desire for revenge, anger, anxiety, guilt, denial, embarrassment, humiliation, helplessness, dependence, self-blame, wide variety of physical reactions, lost or distorted coping mechanisms
Outward adjustment phase (denial)	Survivor appears outwardly composed, denying and repressing feelings (e.g., she returns to work, buys a weapon); refuses to discuss the assault; denies need for counseling
Reorganization	Survivor makes many life adjustments, such as moving to a new residence or changing her phone number; uses emotional distancing; may engage in risky sexual behaviors; may experience sexual dysfunction, phobias, flashbacks, sleep disorders, nightmares, anxiety; has a strong urge to talk about or resolve feelings; may seek counseling or remain silent
Integration and recovery	Time of resolution; survivor begins to feel safe and be comfortable trusting others; places blame on assailant; may become an advocate for others

Nursing Practice

Strive to listen nonjudgmentally. Impartial listening can often make the difference in a victim's readiness to disclose the full details of the assault and can also assist her in the recovery process.

her menstrual cycle and contraceptive practices. If she could become pregnant as a result of the rape, she is offered postcoital contraceptive therapy.

Throughout the experience the nurse acts as the sexual assault survivor's advocate, providing support without usurping decision making. The nurse need not agree with all the survivor's decisions but should respect and defend her right to make them.

The family members and friends on whom the survivor calls also need nursing care. The reactions of the family will depend on the values to which they ascribe. Many families or mates blame the survivor for the assault and feel angry with her for not having been more careful. They may also incorrectly view the assault as a sexual act rather than an act of violence. They may feel personally wronged and see the survivor as devalued or unclean. Their reactions may compound the survivor's crisis. By spending some time with family members before their first interaction with the survivor, the nurse can perhaps reduce their anxiety and absorb some of their frustrations, sparing the woman further trauma.

Sexual assault counseling, provided by qualified nurses or other counselors, is a valuable tool in helping the survivor come to terms with her assault and its impact on her life. In counseling, the woman is encouraged to explore and identify her feelings and determine appropriate actions to resolve her problems and concerns. The counselor must avoid reinforcing the prevalent myth that the assault was somehow the woman's fault. The fault lies with the assailant. The counselor also plays an important role in emphasizing that the loss of control the woman experienced during the rape was temporary and that the woman can regain a feeling of control over life.

Prosecution of the Assailant

Legally, sexual assault is considered a crime against the state, and prosecution of the assailant is a community responsibility. The survivor, however, must begin the process by reporting the assault and pressing charges against her assailant. In the past, the police and the judicial system were notoriously insensitive in dealing with survivors. However, many communities now have classes designed to help officers work effectively with sexual assault survivors or have special teams to carry out this important task.

Many women who have sought to use the judicial process have had such a traumatic experience that they refer to it as a second assault. The woman may be asked repeatedly to describe the experience in intimate detail, and her reputation and testimony may be attacked by the defense attorney. In addition, publicity may intensify her feelings of humiliation, and, if her assailant is released on bail or found not guilty, she may fear retaliation.

The nurse acting as a counselor needs to be aware of the judicial sequence to anticipate rising tension and frustration in the survivor and her support system. The woman needs consistent, effective support at this crucial time.

CRITICAL CONCEPT REVIEW

LEARNING OUTCOMES	CONCEPTS
5.1 Determine accurate information to be provided to girls and women so that they can implement effective self-care measures for dealing with menstruation.	For effective self-care the woman may need information about: 1. Choice of sanitary protection: ■ Pads. ■ Tampons. 2. Use of vaginal sprays. 3. Douching practices. 4. Comfort measures: ■ Proper nutrition. ■ Exercise. ■ Use of heat and massage.

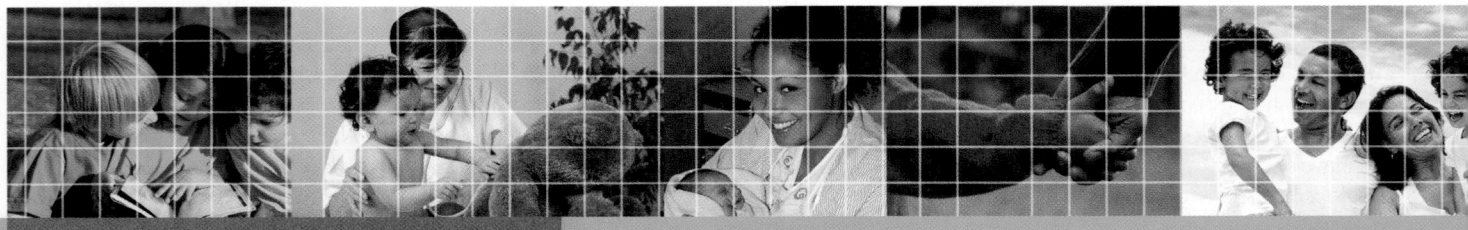

LEARNING OUTCOMES	CONCEPTS
5.2 Discriminate between the signs, symptoms, and nursing management of women with dysmenorrhea and premenstrual syndrome.	1. Dysmenorrhea: ■ Begins at onset of menstruation and disappears by the end of menstruation. ■ Treated with oral contraceptives, NSAIDs, or prostaglandin inhibitors. ■ Self-care measures include improved nutrition, exercise, heat application, and extra rest. 2. Premenstrual syndrome: ■ Symptoms are associated with the luteal phase (2 weeks prior to onset of menses). ■ Pronounced symptoms begin 2–3 days before onset of menstruation and subside as menstruation starts. ■ Symptoms disappear with or without treatment. ■ Treatment includes the use of progesterone agonists and prostaglandin inhibitors. ■ Self-care measures include use of vitamin B and E supplements, calcium, avoidance of sodium and caffeine, and increased aerobic exercise.
5.3 Compare the advantages, disadvantages, and effectiveness of the various methods of contraception available today.	1. Fertility awareness methods: ■ Advantages: Natural and noninvasive. ■ Disadvantages: Requires extensive initial counseling for effectiveness. Requires couple to practice abstinence during parts of each month. ■ Effectiveness: In practice, it may be less reliable than other methods. 2. Barrier contraceptives: ■ Advantages: Easy to use with no side effects. Condoms prevent spread of most venereal diseases. ■ Disadvantages: Some types must be fitted by a nurse practitioner or physician. Must be placed prior to intercourse. Must be used with spermicides. ■ Effectiveness: Excellent when used correctly. 3. Spermicides: ■ Advantages: Inexpensive and easy to obtain. ■ Disadvantages: Must be applied prior to intercourse. Considered "messy" by many people. ■ Effectiveness: Minimally effective when used alone. 4. Intrauterine devices: ■ Advantages: Effective for up to 5 years (Mirena) or 10 years (ParaGard) without removal. ■ Disadvantages: May cause cramping and bleeding for first 3–6 months. Woman must check for proper placement after each menses. Does not protect from STIs. May predispose woman to PID. ■ Effectiveness: Very effective while in place. 5. Hormonal contraceptives: ■ Advantages: Menstrual symptoms are lessened. Menstruation is very predictable. ■ Disadvantages: May increase chance of blood clots. Should not be used by anyone who smokes, has a heart condition, or has previous history of thromboembolic disease. Does not protect from STIs. ■ Effectiveness: Highly effective when used correctly. 6. Sterilization: ■ Advantages: Permanent form of birth control. No additional costs once procedure is completed. ■ Disadvantages: Considered nonreversible. Requires general anesthesia for the woman and local anesthesia for the man. Vasectomy does not produce immediate sterility; semen sample must be clear before other form of contraception is stopped. Does not protect against STIs. ■ Effectiveness: Considered completely effective.
5.4 Delineate basic gynecologic screening procedures indicated for well women.	1. Breast examination (yearly). 2. Mammography: Recommended every 1–2 years after age 40 and annually for women age 50 or older. 3. Pap smear and pelvic examination (yearly).

(continued)

LEARNING OUTCOMES / CONCEPTS

Learning Outcomes	Concepts
5.5 Consider the physical and psychologic aspects and clinical treatment options of menopause when caring for menopausal women.	1. Physical aspects of menopause: ■ Ovulation ceases 1–2 years prior to menopause. ■ Gradual atrophy of ovaries. ■ FSH levels rise. ■ Less estrogen is produced. ■ Atrophic changes of vagina, vulva, urethra, and bladder. ■ Vasomotor disturbances such as "hot flashes." ■ Atrophy of uterine endometrium and myometrium, and fallopian tubes. ■ Constriction of uterine cavity. ■ Vaginal tissue becomes smooth, thins, and loses elasticity. ■ Thinning of pubic hair. ■ Decreased pelvic support. ■ Decrease in breast firmness. ■ Possible development of osteoporosis. ■ Increased risk of coronary heart disease. 2. Psychologic aspects of menopause: ■ Possible helpless feelings at physical changes. ■ Fatigue from lack of sleep due to hot flashes. ■ Decreased libido. ■ Possible increase in enjoyment of sexual intercourse due to lack of worry about pregnancy.
5.6 Delineate the nurse's role in screening and caring for women who have experienced domestic violence or rape.	The nurse's role includes the following: 1. Create a safe, secure milieu. 2. Obtain a careful, detailed history. 3. Complete a forensic chart and kit. 4. Explain all procedures. 5. Act as the survivor's advocate.

CRITICAL THINKING IN ACTION

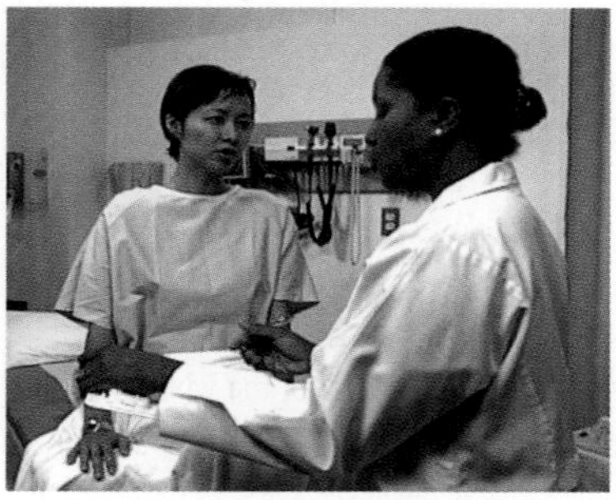

You are working at a local clinic when Joy Lang, age 20, presents for her first pelvic exam. You obtain the following GYN history: menarche age 12, menstrual cycle 28–30 days lasting 4–5 days, heavy one day, then lighter. She tells you that she needs to use superabsorbent tampons on the first day of her period and then she switches to a regular absorbency tampon for the remaining days. She confirms that she changes the tampon every 6 to 8 hours, never leaving it in overnight. She denies premenstrual syndrome, dysmenorrhea, or medical problems and says that she is not taking any medication on a regular schedule. She tells you that she recently got married, but would like to wait before getting pregnant. She'd like to discuss birth control methods. Joy tells you that doctors make her nervous and she admits to being anxious about her first pelvic exam.

1. What steps would you take to reduce Joy's anxiety relating to the pelvic exam?
2. What position is best to relax Joy's abdominal muscles for the pelvic exam?
3. What precaution should be taken when obtaining a Pap smear?
4. Explain the purpose of the Pap smear.
5. What factors do you include in a discussion of the type of birth control that Joy could practice?

See MyNursingKit for possible responses.

REFERENCES

Abboud, R. L. (2006). Delaying your period through oral contraceptives. Retrieved March 17, 2008, from www.mayoclinic.com/health/womens-health/WO00069/METHOD=print

American Cancer Society (ACS). (2006). *Breast cancer facts and figures 2005–2006*. Atlanta: American Cancer Society Inc.

American College of Obstetricians and Gynecologists (ACOG). (2004). *Osteoporosis.* (ACOG Practice Bulletin No. 50). Washington, DC: Author.

American College of Obstetricians and Gynecologists (ACOG). (2008). *Hormone therapy and heart disease.* (ACOG Committee Opinion No. 420). Washington, DC: Author.

Burgess, A. W., & Holmstrom, L. L. (1979). *Rape: Crisis and recovery.* Englewood Cliffs, NJ: Prentice-Hall.

Endicott, J. (2007). PMDD spotlight: Redefined expectations: Improving quality of life in women with PMDD. *Medscape Ob/Gyn & Women's Health.* Retrieved January 11, 2008, from www.medscape.com/viewarticle.567290_print

Food and Drug Administration (FDA). (2007). Over-the-counter vaginal contraceptive and spermicide drug products containing nonoxynol 9; required labeling. Final rule. *Federal Register, 72*(243), 71769–71785.

Food and Drug Administration (FDA). (2009). New device approval: FC2 Female Condom–P080002. Retrieved May 5, 2009, from www.fda.gov/cdrh/mda/docs/P080002.html

Gallo, M., Lopea, L., Grimes, D., Schula, K., & Helmerhorst, R. (2008). Combination contraceptives: Effects on weight. *Cochrane Database of Systematic Review.* Issue 4, Art. No. CD003987.

Holmes, M. M. (1998). The clinical management of rape in adolescents. *Contemporary OB/GYN, 43*(5), 62–78.

Holmquist, S., & Gilliam, M. (2008). Induced abortion. In R. S. Gibbs, B. Y. Karlan, A. F. Haney, & I. Nygaard (Eds.). *Danforth's Obstetrics and Gynecology* (10th ed.). Philadelphia: WoltersKluwer/Lippincott Williams & Wilkins.

Jacobstein, R. (2007). Long-acting and permanent sterilization: An international development, service delivery perspective. *Journal of Midwifery & Women's Health, 52*(4), 361–367.

Jick, S. S., & Jick, H. (2007). The contraceptive patch in relation to ischemic stroke and acute myocardial infarction. *Pharmacotherapy, 27*(2), 218–220.

Memmel, L., & Gilliam, M. (2008). Contraception. In R. S. Gibbs, B. Y. Karlan, A. F. Haney, & I. Nygaard (Eds.). *Danforth's Obstetrics and Gynecology* (10th ed.). Philadelphia: WoltersKluwer/Lippincott Williams & Wilkins.

National Cancer Institute. (2006). *Screening mammograms: Questions and answers.* Fact sheet retrieved July 6, 2006, from www.cancer.gov

National Coalition Against Domestic Violence (NCADV). (2007a). Domestic violence facts. Retrieved June 2, 2008, from www.ncadv.org

National Coalition Against Domestic Violence (NCADV). (2007b). Immigrant victims of domestic violence. Retrieved March 17, 2008, from www.ncadv.org

National Coalition Against Domestic Violence (NCADV). (2007c). International violence against women. Retrieved March 17, 2008, from www.ncadv.org

National Osteoporosis Foundation (NOF). (2008). *Clinician's Guide to prevention and treatment of osteoporosis.* Retrieved March 17, 2008, from www.nof.org

North American Menopause Society (NAMS). (2006). The role of calcium in peri- and postmenopausal women: 2006 position statement of The North American Menopause Society. *Menopause, 13*(6), 862–877.

North American Menopause Society (NAMS). (2007). Estrogen and progestogen use in peri- and postmenopausal women: March 2007 position statement of The North American Menopause Society. *Menopause, 14*(2), 168–182.

Ogburn, T., & Espey, E. (2007). Encouraging more patients to choose an IUD. *Contemporary OB/GYN, 52*(6), 72–77.

Rape, Abuse, & Incest National Network (RAINN). (2008a). Sexual assault statistics. Retrieved March 17, 2008, from www.rainn.org/print/81

Rape, Abuse, & Incest National Network (RAINN). (2008b). The offenders. Retrieved March 17, 2008, from www.rainn.org/print/289

Rapkin, A. J. (2008). YAZ® in the treatment of premenstrual dysphoric disorder. *Journal of Reproductive Medicine, 53,* 729–741.

Reid, R. L. (2008). Premenstrual syndrome. In R. S. Gibbs, B. Y. Karlan, A. F. Haney, & I. Nygaard (Eds.). *Danforth's Obstetrics and Gynecology* (10th ed.). Philadelphia: WoltersKluwer/Lippincott Williams & Wilkins.

Sonfield, A. (2006). Working to eliminate the world's unmet need for contraception. *Guttmacher Policy Review, 9*(1), 10–13.

Sulak, P. J. (2008). Continuous oral contraception: Changing times. *Best Practice & Research in Clinical Obstetrics and Gynaecology, 22*(2), 355–374.

U. S. Preventive Services Task Force. (2009). U. S. Preventive Services Task Force Recommendation Statement. Annals of *Internal Medicine, 151,* 716–726t.

Walker, L. (1984). *The battered woman syndrome.* New York: Springer.

World Health Organization (WHO). (2005). Facts and figures from the world health report, 2005. Retrieved January 6, 2006, from www.who.org

World Health Organization (WHO). (2007). Maternal mortality in 2005: Estimates developed by WHO, UNICEF, UNFPA, and the World Bank. Retrieved June 2, 2008, from www.who.org

Writing Group for the Women's Health Initiative Investigations. (2002). Risks and benefits of estrogen plus progestin in healthy postmenopausal women: Principal results from the Women's Health Initiative randomized controlled trial. *Journal of the American Medical Association, 288,* 321–333.

Zite, N., Gilliam, M., & Darney, P. (2004). Contraception choices for 2004. *Contemporary OB/GYN, 49*(2), 30–44.

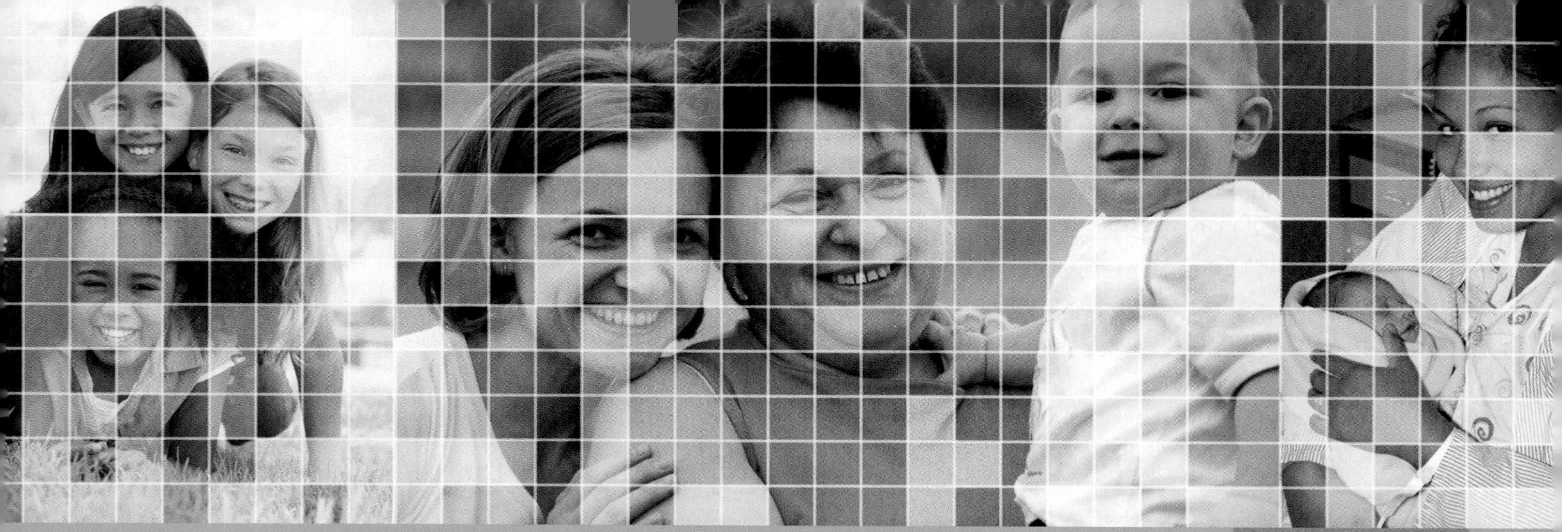

CHAPTER

Common Gynecologic Problems 6

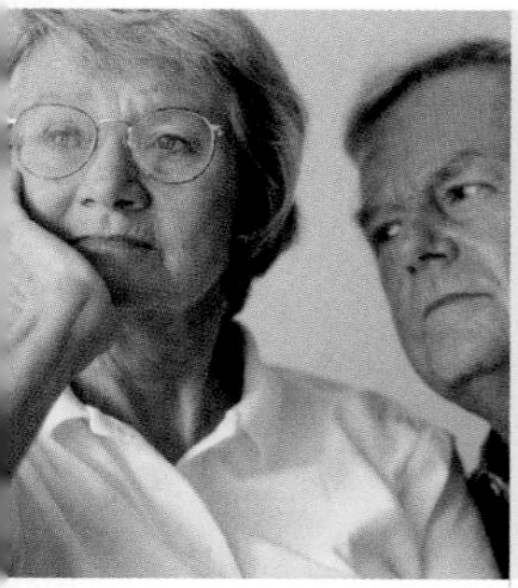

I was 58 when I learned that I had human papillomavirus infection. My first reaction was denial. I had been a virgin when I married and always thought I had the world's best marriage. When I confronted my husband of 30 years, I learned that he had been unfaithful to me with three different women over the course of our marriage. At first I was ready to walk away. But my husband begged for a second chance, we saw a counselor for almost 6 months, and eventually rebuilt our life together. Many women would call me a fool but I know that, for me, it was important to save something I had committed to—for better or for worse—and to practice the forgiveness so many preach but fail to follow. —Leonora

LEARNING OUTCOMES

6.1 Contrast the contributing factors, signs and symptoms, treatment options, and nursing care management of women with common benign breast disorders.

6.2 Consider the signs and symptoms, medical therapy, and implications for fertility in determining the nursing care management of a woman with endometriosis.

6.3 Identify the risk factors, treatment options, and nursing interventions for a woman with toxic shock syndrome.

6.4 Compare the causes, signs and symptoms, treatment options, and nursing care for women with vulvovaginal candidiasis versus bacterial vaginosis.

6.5 Compare the prevention, causes, treatment options, and nursing care of women for the common sexually transmitted infections.

6.6 Relate the implications of pelvic inflammatory disease (PID) for future fertility to its pathology, signs and symptoms, treatment, and nursing care.

6.7 Identify the cause and implications of an abnormal finding during a pelvic examination in the provision of nursing care.

6.8 Contrast the causes, signs and symptoms, treatment options, and nursing care for women with cystitis versus pyelonephritis.

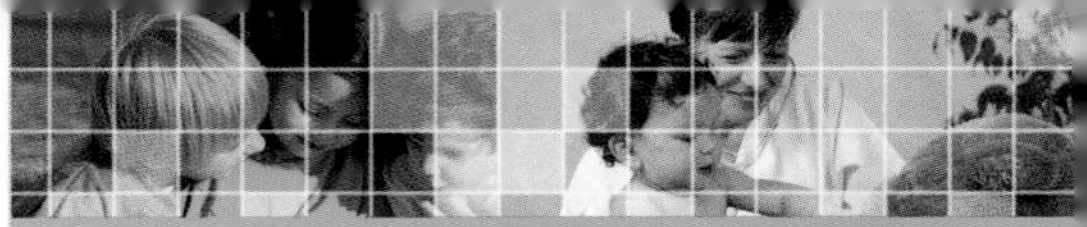

KEY TERMS

Chlamydial infection, 124

Colposcopy, 128

Condylomata acuminata, 125

Cystocele, 131

Dyspareunia, 119

Endometriosis, 118

Fibrocystic breast changes, 117

Hysterectomy, 132

Pelvic inflammatory disease (PID), 127

Polycystic ovarian syndrome (PCOS), 119

Rectocele, 132

Sexually transmitted infection (STI), 123

Toxic shock syndrome (TSS), 120

Urinary tract infection (UTI), 130

The contemporary woman is likely to encounter various major or minor gynecologic or urinary problems during her lifetime. Some may be minor and easily treated; others may be more serious. This chapter provides information about a variety of gynecologic conditions, with an emphasis on problems commonly addressed in community-based settings.

CARE OF THE WOMAN WITH A BENIGN DISORDER OF THE BREAST

This section deals with the most common breast disorders women encounter. For information on breast cancer, consult a medical-surgical nursing textbook.

FIBROCYSTIC BREAST CHANGES

Fibrocystic breast changes, the most common of the benign breast disorders, are most prevalent in women 30 to 50 years of age. *Fibrosis* is a thickening of the normal breast tissue. Cyst formation that may accompany fibrosis is considered a later change in the condition. The exact etiology of fibrocystic breast changes is unclear but they are probably caused by an imbalance in estrogen and progesterone that distorts the normal changes of the menstrual cycle. The symptoms often increase as the woman approaches menopause and generally decrease after menopause. However, if a postmenopausal woman is treated with hormone replacement therapy (HRT), the cyclic breast changes may resume. Only women whose fibrocystic breast changes are accompanied by certain cellular changes (usually found incidentally when a biopsy is done) have an increased risk of developing cancer.

The woman often reports pain, tenderness, and swelling that occur cyclically and are most pronounced just before menses. Physical examination may reveal only mild signs of irregularity, or the breasts may feel dense, with areas of irregularity and nodularity. Women often refer to this irregularity as "lumpiness." Some women may also have expressible nipple discharge. Although unilateral discharge and serosanguineous discharge are the most worrisome findings, all breast discharge should be investigated further.

If the woman has a large, fluid-filled cyst, she may experience a localized painful area as the capsule containing the accumulated fluid distends coincident with her cycle. However, if small cysts form, the woman may experience not a solitary tender lump but a diffuse tenderness. A cyst may often be differentiated from a malignancy because a cyst is more mobile (easily moved with palpation) and tender and is not associated with skin retraction (pulling) in the surrounding tissue.

Mammography, sonography, magnetic resonance imaging, palpation, and fine-needle aspiration are used to confirm fibrocystic breast changes. Often, fine-needle aspiration is the treatment as well, affording relief from the tenderness or pain. Treatment of palpable cysts is conservative; invasive procedures such as biopsy are used only if the diagnosis is questionable.

Women with mild symptoms may benefit from restricting sodium intake and taking a mild diuretic during the week before the onset of menses. This counteracts fluid retention, relieves pressure in the breast, and helps decrease the pain. In other cases a mild analgesic is necessary. In severe cases the hormone inhibitor danazol is often helpful because it suppresses FSH and LH, resulting in anovulation. However, it can cause undesirable side effects.

Some researchers suggest that methylxanthines (found in caffeine products, such as coffee, tea, colas, and chocolate, and in some medications) may contribute to the development of fibrocystic breast changes and that limiting intake of these substances will help decrease fibrocystic changes. Other research fails to demonstrate a clear association between methylxanthines and fibrocystic breast changes. Additional medical therapies that are helpful in varying degrees include combined oral contraceptives (COCs), progestins, bromocriptine, and the antiestrogen medication tamoxifen (although this is an "off-label" use for it). All of these therapies work on the principle of estrogen suppression and progesterone stimulation or augmentation. Oil of evening primrose may also be effective.

OTHER BENIGN BREAST DISORDERS

Fibroadenoma is a common benign tumor seen in women in their teens and early twenties. It has not been significantly associated with breast cancer. Fibroadenomas are freely movable, solid tumors that are well defined, sharply delineated, and rounded, with a rubbery texture. They are asymptomatic and nontender.

If there are any disquieting features to the appearance of a lump, fine-needle biopsy or excision of the mass may be indicated. Exercise caution when deciding on biopsy because excision of the mass in a young girl may interfere with normal breast development. Watchful observation and possible surgical excision are the only treatments for fibroadenomas. Surgery is often deferred, but when advisable because of severe symptoms or concerns about malignancy, it ends the treatment.

Intraductal papillomas, most often occurring during the menopausal years, are tumors growing in the terminal portion of a duct or, sometimes, throughout the duct system within a section of the breast. They are typically benign but have the potential to become malignant. Although relatively uncommon, they are the most frequent cause of nipple discharge in women who are not pregnant or lactating.

The majority of papillomas present as solitary nodules. These small, ball-like lesions may be detected on mammography but often are nonpalpable. A papilloma is often frightening to the woman, because her primary symptom is a discharge from the nipple that may be serosanguineous or brownish green due to old blood. The location of the papilloma within the duct system and its pattern of growth determine whether nipple discharge will be present.

If the woman reports a nipple discharge, the breast should be milked to obtain fluid. The fluid obtained is sent for a Pap smear. The diagnosis is confirmed if papilloma cells are present. The lesion must be excised and histologically examined because of the difficulty in differentiating between a benign papilloma and a papillary carcinoma. Treatment for benign intraductal papilloma is excision with follow-up care.

Duct ectasis (comedomastitis), an inflammation of the ducts behind the nipple, commonly occurs during or near the onset of menopause and is not associated with malignancy. The condition typically occurs in women who have borne and breastfed children. It is characterized by a thick, sticky nipple discharge and by burning pain, pruritus, and inflammation. Nipple retraction may also be noted, especially in postmenopausal women. Treatment is conservative, with drug therapy aimed at symptomatic relief. The major central ducts of the breast occasionally have to be excised.

NURSING MANAGEMENT

NURSING ASSESSMENT AND DIAGNOSIS

During the period of diagnosis of any breast disorder, the woman may be anxious about a possible change in body image or a diagnosis of cancer. Use therapeutic communication to assess the significance the woman places on her breasts; her current emotional status, coping mechanisms used during periods of stress, knowledge and beliefs about cancer; and other variables that may influence her coping and adjustment.

Nursing diagnoses that may apply to a woman with a benign disorder of the breast include the following:

- *Health-Seeking Behaviors: Information about Diagnostic Procedures for Breast Disorders* related to an expressed desire to understand procedures
- *Anxiety* related to threat to body image

PLANNING AND IMPLEMENTATION

During the prediagnosis period, clarify misconceptions and encourage the woman to express her anxiety. Once a diagnosis is made, ensure that the woman understands her condition, its association to breast malignancy, and the treatment options. Also point out that frequent professional breast examinations and regular mammograms help detect any abnormalities. Although recommendations about the importance of monthly breast self-examination (BSE) have modified in light of the fact that research failed to demonstrate that survival rates were improved in women who did regular BSE (Ruhl, 2007), most professionals agree that women should be familiar with their own breasts so that they are able to note changes should they occur.

EVALUATION

Expected outcomes of nursing care include the following:

- The woman is able to discuss her fears, concerns, and questions during the period of diagnosis.
- The diagnosis is made quickly and accurately, and treatment is initiated if indicated.

CARE OF THE WOMAN WITH ENDOMETRIOSIS

Endometriosis, a condition characterized by the presence of endometrial tissue outside the endometrial cavity, is present in 12% to 32% of women who undergo laparoscopy to determine the cause of pelvic pain (Schenken, 2008). Endometriosis has been found almost everywhere in the body, including the vagina, lungs, cervix, central nervous system, and gastrointestinal tract. The most common location, however, is the pelvis. This tissue responds to the hormonal changes of the menstrual cycle and bleeds in a cyclic fashion. The bleeding results in inflammation, scarring of the peritoneum, and formation of adhesions.

Endometriosis may occur at any age after puberty, but it is most common in women between ages 20 and 45. The exact cause of endometriosis is unknown. Leading theories include retrograde menstrual flow and inflammation of the endometrium, hereditary tendency, and a possible immunologic defect.

The most common symptom of endometriosis is pelvic pain, which is often dull or cramping. Usually the pain is related to menstruation and is thought to be dysmenorrhea by the affected woman. **Dyspareunia** (painful intercourse) and abnormal uterine bleeding are other common signs. The condition is often diagnosed when the woman seeks evaluation for infertility. Bimanual examination may reveal a fixed, tender, retroverted uterus and palpable nodules in the cul-de-sac. Diagnosis is confirmed by laparoscopy.

Treatment may be medical, surgical, or a combination of the two. During the laparoscopic examination, any visible implants of endometrial tissue are removed using excision, endocoagulation, electrocautery, or laser vaporization. Surgery is effective in relieving pain symptoms, at least for a time. In women with minimal disease and symptoms, treatment includes observation, analgesics, and nonsteroidal anti-inflammatory drugs (NSAIDs). If the woman does not currently desire pregnancy, she may be started on a combined oral contraceptive (COC), often in combination with an NSAID. The COC creates a pseudopregnancy state with decreased menstrual bleeding. If the COC does not relieve symptoms, therapy with medroxyprogesterone acetate (MPA), danazol, or a gonadotropin-releasing hormone (GnRH) agonist may be indicated.

MPA causes endometrial tissue to atrophy, thereby decreasing symptoms. It is administered intramuscularly every 3 months, and the effectiveness of treatment is evaluated every 3 to 6 months. Side effects include weight gain, bloating, acne, headaches, emotional lability, and irregular bleeding.

Danazol is a testosterone derivative that suppresses GnRH and has high-androgen and low-estrogen effects that inhibit the growth of the endometrium. It suppresses ovulation and causes amenorrhea. However, danazol has some significant side effects including hirsutism, vaginal bleeding, acne, oily skin, weight gain, reduced libido, voice changes and hoarseness, clitoral enlargement, and decreased breast size.

GnRH agonists such as nafarelin acetate (given as a metered nasal spray twice daily) and leuprolide acetate (Lupron) (given once a month as an intramuscular injection) are gaining popularity. Many women tolerate them better than danazol, and their results in treating endometriosis are comparable. GnRH agonists suppress the menstrual cycle through estrogen antagonism. This may result in the hypoestrogen side effects of hot flashes, vaginal dryness, decreased libido, pain in muscles and joints, and loss of bone density. These side effects can be reduced by adding an oral progestin or a combination of low-dose estrogen and progestin (Winkel, 2003). (*Note:* The estrogen dose should be comparable to that used for symptoms of menopause. COC estrogen levels are too high for add-back therapy.)

In more advanced cases, surgery may be done to remove endometrial implants and break up adhesions. If severe dyspareunia or dysmenorrhea are symptoms, the surgeon may perform a presacral neurectomy. In advanced cases in which childbearing is not an issue, treatment may be a hysterectomy (removal of the uterus) with bilateral salpingo-oophorectomy (removal of the fallopian tubes and ovaries).

NURSING MANAGEMENT

NURSING ASSESSMENT AND DIAGNOSIS

The nurse needs to know the symptoms of endometriosis and elicit an accurate history. If a woman is being treated for endometriosis, assess the woman's understanding of the condition, its implications, and the treatment alternatives.

Nursing diagnoses that may apply to a woman with endometriosis include the following:

- *Acute Pain* related to peritoneal irritation secondary to endometriosis
- *Compromised Family Coping* related to depression secondary to infertility

PLANNING AND IMPLEMENTATION

Be available to explain the condition, its symptoms, treatment alternatives, and prognosis. Help the woman evaluate treatment options and make appropriate choices. If the woman begins taking medication, review the dosage, schedule, possible side effects, and any warning signs. A woman with endometriosis is often advised not to delay pregnancy because of the increased risk of infertility. The woman may wish to discuss the implications of this decision on her life choices, relationship with her partner, and personal preferences. Be a nonjudgmental listener and help the woman consider her options.

EVALUATION

Expected outcomes of nursing care include the following:

- The woman is able to discuss her condition, its implications for fertility, and her treatment options.
- After considering the alternatives, the woman chooses appropriate treatment options.

CARE OF THE WOMAN WITH POLYCYSTIC OVARIAN SYNDROME

Polycystic ovarian syndrome (PCOS) is a complex endocrine disorder of ovarian dysfunction that is evidenced by amenorrhea or oligomenorrhea and clinical signs of androgen excess (typically hirsutism, acne) in the absence of other conditions that might have these same signs and symptoms (King, 2007).

The most common clinical signs and symptoms of PCOS include:

- *Menstrual dysfunction.* Irregular menses, ranging from total absence of periods (amenorrhea) to intermittent or infrequent periods (oligomenorrhea), to heavy periods (menorrhagia) are the hallmark of PCOS (Jackson, 2004/2005).

MyNursingKit Case Study: Toxic Shock Syndrome

- *Hyperandrogenism.* Women with PCOS consistently have elevated serum androgen levels, specifically testosterone and androsterone. These elevated androgen levels often lead to clinical manifestations such as acne, alopecia (male-patterned hair loss), hirsutism, deepening voice, increased muscle mass, and menstrual irregularities (King, 2007).
- *Obesity.* About half of women with PCOS are clinically obese. The obesity is generally of the android type, with an increased hip-to-waist ratio.
- *Hyperinsulinemia.* Women with PCOS are insulin resistant. This insulin resistance, characterized by the failure of insulin to enter the cells appropriately, places these women at increased risk for impaired glucose tolerance and type 2 diabetes mellitus (King, 2007).
- *Infertility.* Many women who have been diagnosed with PCOS struggle with some degree of infertility related to anovulation.
- The diagnosis of PCOS is one of exclusion of other conditions. The diagnostic process is four-fold: history, physical examination, laboratory studies, and endovaginal ultrasound to evaluate the uterus and ovaries.

CLINICAL THERAPY

The goals for treatment include decreasing the effects of hyperandrogenism (hirsutism, acne, etc.), restoring reproductive functioning for women desiring pregnancy, protecting the endometrium (increased risk for uterine cancer), and reducing long-term risks, specifically type 2 diabetes and cardiovascular disease.

If pregnancy is not an immediate goal, menstrual irregularities can be treated with a combined oral contraceptive or cyclic progesterone. Combined oral contraceptives help to regulate menstrual cycles; provide a balance between estrogen and progesterone, thereby protecting the endometrium and decreasing the risk of uterine cancer; and may improve acne by inhibiting ovarian androgen production. If pregnancy is an immediate goal, then another option is the use of medications that improve insulin sensitivity and use.

Antiandrogens such as spironolactone (Aldactone) may be used to decrease symptoms of androgen excess. Metformin (Glucophage) inhibits glucose production in the liver and improves glucose uptake by fat and muscle cells. It improves ovarian function, reduces the degree of hyperandrogenism, restores normal ovulation in women with PCOS, and is associated with an improved ability to lose weight. In addition, lifestyle changes are important. Modifications should include weight loss, regular exercise, balanced diet, and smoking cessation.

Long-term, PCOS may increase a woman's risk for developing type 2 diabetes, hypertension, cardiovascular disease, endometrial cancer, breast cancer, and ovarian cancer. Additionally, the woman with PCOS may struggle with significant emotional responses to this chronic disorder. She will likely face issues related to body image, infertility, problematic menses, and depression.

NURSING MANAGEMENT

The nurse plays a vital role in the identification, evaluation, management, and follow-up when caring for a woman with PCOS. The signs of PCOS, especially hirsutism, negatively impact women's feelings of femininity. Nurses can help women recognize these feelings and find ways to develop a more positive body image. The nurse also has an important role in providing accurate information, education, and counseling for a woman diagnosed with PCOS. Finally, because the woman with PCOS is at risk for developing long-term complications, the nurse can play a key role in follow-up and continuity of care throughout the life of a woman facing this challenging disorder.

CARE OF THE WOMAN WITH TOXIC SHOCK SYNDROME

Toxic shock syndrome (TSS) is primarily a disease of women at or near menses or during the postpartum period. The causative organism is a toxin released by a strain of *Staphylococcus aureus.* The use of superabsorbent tampons was once related to an increased incidence of TSS. That incidence has declined. Occluding the cervical os with a contraceptive device such as a diaphragm or cervical cap during menses may also increase the risk of TSS.

Early diagnosis and treatment are important in preventing death. The most common signs of TSS include fever (often greater than 38.9°C [102°F]); rash on the trunk initially followed by desquamation of the skin, especially the palms and soles, which usually occurs 1 to 2 weeks after the onset of symptoms; hypotension; and dizziness. Systemic symptoms often include vomiting, diarrhea, severe myalgia, and inflamed mucous membranes (oropharyngeal, conjunctival, or vaginal). Disorders of the central nervous system, including alterations in consciousness, disorientation, and coma, may also occur.

Women with TSS are generally hospitalized and given supportive therapy, including intravenous fluids to maintain blood pressure. Severe cases may require renal dialysis, administration of vasopressors, and intubation. Broad-spectrum antibiotic therapy (including antistaphylococcal agents) is initiated immediately until septicemia is excluded as a diagnosis; antibiotic therapy also reduces the risk of recurrence.

NURSING MANAGEMENT

Nurses play a major role in helping educate women about preventing the development of TSS. It is crucial that women understand the importance of avoiding prolonged use of tampons. Women who choose to continue using tampons may reduce their risk of TSS by alternating them with pads and avoiding overnight use of tampons. Women should avoid the use of tampons for 6 to 8 weeks after childbirth. Women who use diaphragms or cervical caps should not leave them in place for prolonged periods and should not use them during the postpartum period or when they are menstruating. Also, help make women aware of the signs and symptoms of TSS so that they will seek treatment promptly if symptoms occur.

CARE OF THE WOMAN WITH A VAGINAL INFECTION

Vaginitis is the most common reason women seek gynecologic care. Symptoms of vaginitis or vulvovaginitis may include increased vaginal discharge, vulvar irritation, pruritus, foul odor, and pain when urine touches irritated vulvar tissue. It may be caused directly by an infection or it may result from an alteration of normal flora, as in the case of bacterial vaginosis or *Candida albicans.*

BACTERIAL VAGINOSIS

Bacterial vaginosis (BV) is more prevalent among sexually active women, but it is not considered a sexually transmitted infection. BV is an alteration of normal vaginal bacterial flora that results in the loss of hydrogen peroxide-producing lactobacilli, which are normally the main vaginal flora. With the loss of this natural defense, bacteria such as *Gardnerella,* mycoplasmas, and anaerobes overgrow in large numbers, causing vaginitis. The cause of this overgrowth is not clear, although tissue trauma from douching, frequent sexual intercourse without condom use, and an upset in normal vaginal flora are predisposing factors.

The infected woman often notices an excessive amount of thin, watery, white or gray vaginal discharge with a foul odor described as "fishy." The characteristic "clue" cell is seen on a wet-mount preparation (Figure 6–1 ●). The addition of 10% potassium hydroxide (KOH) solution to the vaginal secretions, called a "whiff" test, releases a strong, fishy odor. The vaginal pH is usually greater than 4.5.

The nonpregnant, symptomatic woman is generally treated with metronidazole (Flagyl) orally or as a vaginal cream. (See "Drug Guide: Metronidazole.") If metronidazole is prescribed, the woman and her partner should be cautioned to avoid alcohol while taking it; the combination has an effect similar to that of alcohol and disulfiram (Antabuse)—abdominal pain, flushing, and tremors. Alternatively, clindamycin (Cleocin) vaginal cream may be used, although it is slightly less effective (Centers for Disease Control and Prevention [CDC], 2006).

Until recently, metronidazole was avoided during pregnancy because of its potential teratogenic effects. However, the CDC (2006) now reports that multiple studies failed to document a relationship between metronidazole use in pregnancy and teratogenesis in the newborn. Thus the recommended treatment for pregnant women with BV is either oral metronidazole or oral clindamycin. BV during pregnancy may be a factor in premature rupture of the membranes and preterm birth.

VULVOVAGINAL CANDIDIASIS

Vulvovaginal candidiasis (VVC), also called moniliasis or yeast infection, is one of the most common forms of vaginitis that women experience. Recurrences are frequent for some women. *Candida albicans* is the fungal species responsible for most vaginal yeast infections. Factors that contribute to VVC are the use of COCs, immunosuppressants, and antibiotics, which destroy normal bacteria that usually keep the yeast cells in check. Other factors are frequent douching, pregnancy, and diabetes mellitus.

The woman with VVC often complains of thick, curdy vaginal discharge, severe itching, dysuria, and dyspareunia. A male sexual partner may experience a rash or excoriation of the skin of the penis and possibly pruritus. The male may be symptomatic and the female asymptomatic.

On physical examination the woman's labia may be swollen and excoriated if pruritus has been severe. A speculum examination reveals thick, white, tenacious cheeselike patches adhering to the vaginal mucosa. Diagnosis is confirmed by microscopic examination of the vaginal discharge; hyphae and spores are usually seen on a wet-mount preparation (Figure 6–2 ●).

Treatment of VVC includes intravaginal butoconazole, miconazole, tioconazole, terconazole, clotrimazole, or nystatin suppositories, cream, or tablets. Single-dose and short-course

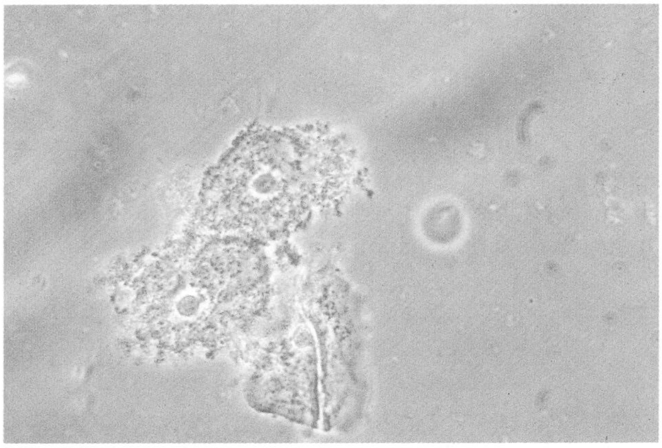

● **Figure 6–1** Clue cells characteristically seen in bacterial vaginosis. Unlike normal epithelial cells, which appear translucent and have a clear border, clue cells are desquamated epithelial cells with bacteria adhering to them. The presence of the bacteria makes the cell appear to be speckled with black dots. The borders are also obscured because of the bacteria.

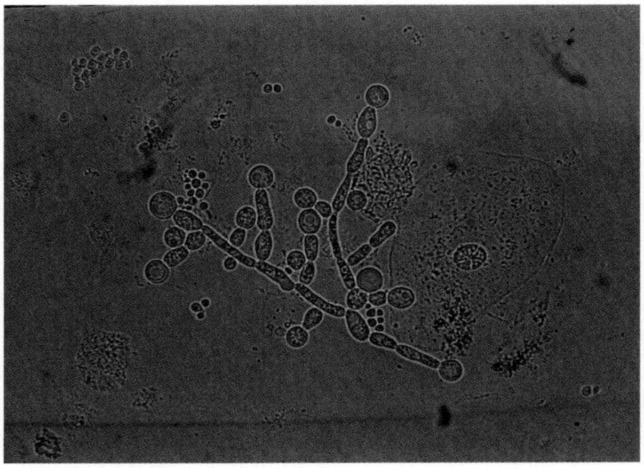

● **Figure 6–2** The hyphae and spores of *Candida albicans.* This is the fungus that is responsible for vulvovaginal candidiasis.

Source: Courtesy of Centers for Disease Control and Prevention.

Drug Guide

METRONIDAZOLE (FLAGYL)

Overview of Action

Metronidazole is an antiprotozoal and antibacterial agent. It possesses direct trichomonacidal and amebicidal activity against *T. vaginalis* and *E. histolytica.* Metronidazole is active in vitro against most obligate anaerobes but does not appear to possess any clinically relevant activity against facultative anaerobes or obligate aerobes. It is used in the treatment of various infections caused by organisms that are sensitive to this drug. It is used predominantly to treat the following infections in women: *T. vaginalis,* bacterial vaginosis, endometritis, endomyometritis, tubo-ovarian abscess, and postsurgical vaginal cuff infection.

Route, Dosage, Frequency

Trichomoniasis—1-day treatment: 2 g orally in a single dose; 7-day treatment: 500 mg orally twice a day for 7 consecutive days (CDC, 2006).

Amebiasis—Adults: 750 mg orally three times a day for 5–10 days; children: 35–50 mg/kg/24 hours orally divided into three doses for 10 days.

Bacterial vaginosis—500 mg orally twice a day for 7 consecutive days or one full applicator of metronidazole gel 0.75% intravaginally, once daily for 5 days (CDC, 2006).

Contraindications

Blood dyscrasias

Breastfeeding women (drug secreted in breast milk)

Impaired kidney or liver function

Active CNS disease

Side Effects

Convulsive seizures
Peripheral neuropathy
Nausea/vomiting
Weakness
Insomnia
Cystitis
Headache
Anorexia
Diarrhea
Epigastric distress
Abdominal cramping
Constipation
Metallic taste in mouth
Dizziness
Vertigo
Uncoordination
Ataxia
Confusion
Irritability
Dysuria
Reversible neutropenia and thrombocytopenia
Flattening of the T wave on ECG
Polyuria
Incontinence
Pelvic pressure
Proliferation of *Candida* in the vagina and mouth
Joint pains
Decreased libido
Dryness in the mouth, vulva, and vagina
Dyspareunia
Depression

Nursing Considerations

1. Inform woman about potential side effects.
2. Stress the importance of contraceptive compliance during course of treatment.
3. Obtain baseline renal and liver function tests as ordered.
4. Teach woman about the signs, symptoms, and treatment of vulvovaginal candidiasis.
5. Counsel the woman to avoid alcoholic beverages while taking the medication.
6. If the woman is taking oral contraceptives, a backup nonhormonal contraceptive method is recommended during treatment.
7. Take thorough history to rule out the woman's exposure to this medication within the last 6 weeks.
8. Teach woman to monitor the signs and symptoms of her infection.
9. Encourage cooperation with the entire course of treatment.

(3 days) approaches are effective for 80% to 90% of women with uncomplicated VVC. Oral fluconazole, 150 mg in a single dose, is also effective for uncomplicated VVC (CDC, 2006). If the vulva is also affected, the cream is applied topically. Some of the topical medications are available over the counter. They are indicated for women with a history of yeast infections who clearly recognize the symptoms.

Treatment of the male partner is generally not necessary unless candidal balanitis (inflammation of the glans penis) is present or if the man's partner has recurrent infection. Then treatment with a topical antifungal medication is indicated (CDC, 2006).

If a woman experiences recurrent VVC (four or more symptomatic episodes in one year), she should be tested for an elevated blood glucose level to determine whether a diabetic or prediabetic condition is present. Women at high risk for sexually transmitted infections should also be tested for HIV. Recurrent infection is then treated with an intensive regimen of oral and local agents for 7 to 14 days followed by maintenance antifungal therapy. Pregnant women with VVC are treated only with topical azole preparations applied for 7 days (CDC, 2006). Infection at the time of birth may cause *thrush* (a mouth infection) in the newborn.

NURSING MANAGEMENT

NURSING ASSESSMENT AND DIAGNOSIS

The nurse should suspect VVC if a woman complains of intense vulvar itching and a curdy, white discharge. Because pregnant women with diabetes mellitus are especially susceptible to this infection, be alert for symptoms in these women. In some areas, nurses are trained to do speculum examinations and wet-mount

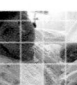

Nursing Practice

To distinguish among the common types of vaginitis and their treatments, it is useful to remember the following:

Vulvovaginal candidiasis (moniliasis)

Cause: *Candida albicans*

Appearance of discharge: Thick, curdy, like cottage cheese

Diagnostic test: Slide of vaginal discharge (treated with potassium hydroxide) shows characteristic hyphae and spores

Treatment: Clotrimazole vaginal cream or suppositories

Bacterial vaginosis (*Gardnerella vaginalis* vaginitis)

Cause: *Gardnerella vaginalis*

Appearance of discharge: Gray, milky

Diagnostic test: Slide of vaginal discharge shows characteristic "clue" cells

Treatment: Metronidazole

Trichomoniasis

- Cause: *Trichomonas vaginalis*
- Appearance of discharge: Greenish white and frothy
- Diagnostic test: Saline slide of vaginal discharge shows motile flagellated organisms
- Treatment: Metronidazole

preparations and can confirm the diagnosis themselves. In most cases, however, the nurse who suspects a vaginal infection reports it to the woman's healthcare provider.

Nursing diagnoses that might apply to the woman with VVC include the following:

- *Risk for Impaired Skin Integrity* related to scratching secondary to discomfort of the infection
- *Health-Seeking Behaviors: Information about Yeast Infection* related to an expressed desire to learn about ways of preventing VVC

PLANNING AND IMPLEMENTATION

If the woman is experiencing discomfort because of pruritus, recommend gentle bathing of the vulva with a weak sodium bicarbonate solution. If a topical treatment is being used, the woman will need to bathe the area before applying the medication.

Also discuss with the woman the factors that contribute to the development of VVC and suggest ways to prevent recurrences, such as wearing cotton underwear and avoiding vaginal powders or sprays that may irritate the vulva. Stress the importance of completing the course of medication even during menses. Some women report that the addition of yogurt to the diet or the use of activated culture of plain yogurt as a vaginal douche helps prevent recurrence by maintaining high levels of lactobacilli.

EVALUATION

Expected outcomes of nursing care include the following:

- The woman's symptoms are relieved, and the infection is cured.
- The woman is able to identify self-care measures to prevent further episodes of VVC.

CARE OF THE INDIVIDUAL WITH A SEXUALLY TRANSMITTED INFECTION

MyNursingKit Care Plan: Gynecologic Infection

The occurrence of **sexually transmitted infection (STI)**, or *sexually transmitted disease (STD)*, has increased over the past few decades. Centers for Disease Control and Prevention (CDC) analysis indicates that approximately 19 million new cases of STIs occur each year, with young people ages 15 to 24 years accounting for almost half the infections (CDC, 2009). In fact, vaginitis and STIs are the most common reasons for outpatient, community-based treatment of women.

Children and adolescents can also become infected with sexually transmitted organisms through sexual experimentation, sexual play, molestation, and sexual abuse. Of the 15 million new STI cases diagnosed each year, approximately 25% occur in adolescents. Results from the CDC National 2007 Youth Risk Behavior Survey revealed that 47.8% of high school students had engaged in sexual intercourse and 38.5% of sexually active adolescents had not used a condom at last sexual intercourse (CDC, 2008). Adolescents are considered an at-risk population because of their inexperience and lack of knowledge about STIs. They may disregard the importance of using barrier protection, may have multiple sexual partners, may have sex frequently, and often do not seek medical treatment until symptoms are well advanced.

Frequently diagnosed STIs include chlamydia, genital herpes (herpes simplex type 2), gonorrhea, genital warts (human papilloma virus), trichomoniasis, and syphilis. For more detailed information on the specific signs, symptoms, and treatment of males with STIs, consult a medical-surgical nursing textbook.

Developing Cultural Competence

RACIAL DISPARITY IN STIs

Racial disparities exist in all STIs, with the highest rates found among African Americans. Although African Americans comprise 12% of the population, they account for 70% of gonorrhea cases and almost half the cases of chlamydia and gonorrhea. Though less marked, disparities also exist among Hispanics. These disparities may result, in part, because people from minority populations are more likely to seek care in public health clinics, which report STIs more accurately than private providers do. However, socioeconomic barriers to high-quality health care and to STI prevention and treatment play a role. It is essential that these barriers be addressed if such disparities are to be eliminated (CDC, 2009).

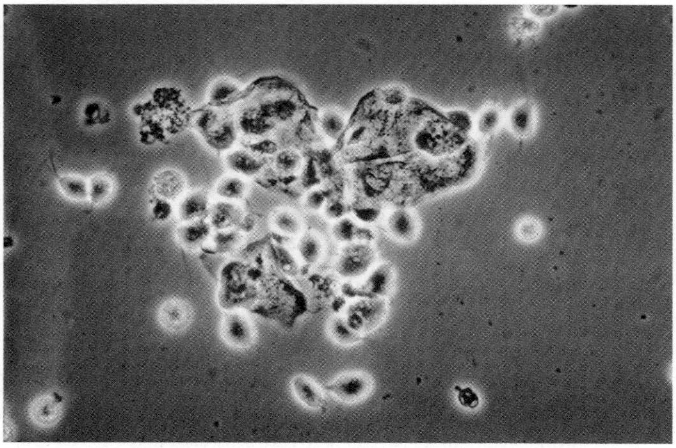

● **Figure 6–3** Microscopic appearance of *Trichomonas vaginalis*.
Source: Courtesy of Centers for Disease Control and Prevention.

TRICHOMONIASIS

Trichomoniasis is an infection caused by *Trichomonas vaginalis,* a microscopic motile protozoan that thrives in an alkaline environment. Almost all infections are acquired through sexual intimacy. Transmission by shared bath facilities, wet towels, or wet swimsuits, though possible, is unlikely.

In females, symptoms of trichomoniasis include a yellow-green, frothy, odorous discharge frequently accompanied by inflammation of the vagina and cervix, dysuria, and dyspareunia. Visualization of *T. vaginalis* under the microscope on a wet-mount preparation of vaginal discharge confirms the diagnosis (Figure 6–3 ●).

Treatment for trichomoniasis is metronidazole (Flagyl) administered in a single 2 g dose for both male and female sexual partners; a 7-day regimen is also available (CDC, 2006). Partners should avoid intercourse until both are cured.

Pregnant women with trichomoniasis may be at increased risk for premature rupture of the membranes, preterm birth, and low birth weight. Pregnant women who are symptomatic should be treated with a single 2-g dose of metronidazole (CDC, 2006).

CHLAMYDIAL INFECTION

Chlamydial infection, caused by *Chlamydia trachomatis,* is the most common reported STI in the United States (CDC, 2009). A strain of chlamydia is responsible for trachoma, the world's leading cause of preventable blindness.

In males, chlamydia is a major cause of nongonococcal urethritis (NGU). In females it can cause infections similar to those that occur with gonorrhea. It can infect the fallopian tubes, cervix, urethra, and Bartholin's glands. Pelvic inflammatory disease, infertility, and ectopic pregnancy are associated with chlamydia. The newborn of a woman with untreated chlamydia is at risk of developing ophthalmia neonatorum, which responds to erythromycin ophthalmic ointment prophylaxis at birth. The newborn may also develop chlamydia pneumonia.

MyNursingKit Video: Acyclovir

Both males and females may be asymptomatic. In females, symptoms of chlamydia include a thin or purulent discharge, burning and frequency of urination, and lower abdominal pain. Diagnosis is often made after treatment of a male partner for NGU or in a symptomatic woman with a negative gonorrhea culture. Of the laboratory tests available to diagnose chlamydia, nucleic acid amplification testing (NAAT) is the most sensitive. Other tests for diagnosis include culture, direct immunofluorescence, EIA, and nucleic acid hybridization tests (CDC, 2006). The recommended treatment is a single 1 g dose of azithromycin orally or doxycycline orally twice daily for 7 days. Sexual partners should be treated, and couples should abstain from intercourse for 7 days (CDC, 2006). Doxycycline is contraindicated in pregnancy. The CDC (2006) recommends that pregnant women be treated with azithromycin or amoxicillin.

GONORRHEA

Gonorrhea is an infection caused by the bacteria *Neisseria gonorrhoeae.* If a nonpregnant female contracts the disease, she is at risk of developing pelvic inflammatory disease. If a woman becomes infected after the third month of pregnancy, the mucous plug in the cervix will prevent the infection from ascending, and it will remain localized in the urethra, cervix, and Bartholin's glands until the membranes rupture. Then it can spread upward.

Often girls and women with gonorrhea are asymptomatic. Thus, it is routine to screen for this infection using a cervical culture during the initial prenatal examination. For women at high risk, the culture may be repeated during the last month of pregnancy. Cultures of the urethra, throat, and rectum may also be required for diagnosis, depending on the body orifices used for intercourse.

In females the most common symptoms of gonorrheal infection include a purulent, greenish yellow vaginal discharge, dysuria, and urinary frequency. Some women also develop inflammation and swelling of the vulva. The cervix may appear swollen and eroded and may secrete a foul-smelling discharge in which gonococci are present. Infections in the throat may cause a sore throat but are usually asymptomatic.

In males, urethritis, or inflammation of the urethra, is the cardinal symptom. This is marked by burning during urination and the presence of discharge from the urethra.

Treatment for nonpregnant females consists of antibiotic therapy with ceftriaxone or cefixime plus treatment for chlamydia if chlamydia has not been ruled out (CDC, 2007b). This combined approach is used because the two infections often occur together. Additional treatment may be required if the cultures remain positive 7 to 14 days after completion of treatment. All sexual partners must also be treated or the woman may become reinfected. Pregnant women should be treated with ceftriaxone intramuscularly or cefixime orally. This treatment is combined with azithromycin or amoxicillin to address the risk of coinfection with chlamydia (CDC, 2006).

Females should be informed of the need for reculture to verify cure and the need for abstinence or condom use until cure is confirmed. Both sexual partners should be treated if either has a positive test for gonorrhea.

HERPES GENITALIS

Herpes infections are caused by the herpes simplex virus (HSV). Two types of herpes infections can occur: HSV-1 (the cold sore), which can cause genital herpes through oral-genital contact, and HSV-2, which is usually associated with genital infections. The clinical symptoms and treatment of both types are the same. At least 50 million people in the United States have been diagnosed with genital HSV-2 infection—*herpes genitalis* (Hill-Brusselle, 2008).

The primary episode of herpes genitalis is characterized by the development of single or multiple blisterlike vesicles. In males these usually occur on the penis or anal area. In females the vesicles occur in the genital area and sometimes affect the vaginal walls, cervix, urethra, and anus. The vesicles may appear within a few hours to 20 days after exposure and rupture spontaneously to form painful, open, ulcerated lesions. Inflammation and pain secondary to the presence of herpes lesions can cause difficult urination and urinary retention. Inguinal lymph node enlargement may be present. Flulike symptoms and genital pruritus or tingling also may be noticed. Primary episodes usually last the longest and are the most severe. Lesions heal spontaneously in 2 to 4 weeks.

After the lesions heal, the virus enters a dormant phase, residing in the nerve ganglia of the affected area. Some individuals never have a recurrence, whereas others have regular recurrences. Recurrences are usually less severe than the initial episode and seem to be triggered by emotional stress, menstruation, ovulation, pregnancy, frequent or vigorous intercourse, poor health status or a generally run-down physical condition, tight clothing, or overheating. Although good diagnostic tests are available to detect HSV-2 infection, it is estimated that 80% to 90% of HSV infections are undiagnosed (Morrow, 2003). Diagnosis is most often made on the basis of the clinical appearance of the lesions, polymerase chain reaction (PCR) identification, and glycoprotein G-based Type-specific assays (Herpe Select™, Biokit HSV-2, and Sure Vue HSV-2) (CDC, 2006).

No known cure for herpes exists. The recommended treatment of the first clinical episode of genital herpes is oral acyclovir, valacyclovir, or famciclovir. These same medications, in somewhat different dosages, are also recommended for recurrent herpes infection and for daily suppression therapy for people who have frequent recurrences. Because there is more documented information on use of acyclovir during pregnancy, it may be administered orally to pregnant women with first-episode genital herpes or severe recurrent herpes. Its use in the third trimester may reduce the incidence of cesarean births by decreasing the incidence of recurrences at term (CDC, 2006).

Keeping the genital area clean and dry, wearing loose clothing, and wearing cotton underwear or none at all help promote healing. If herpes is present in the genital tract of a woman during childbirth, it can have a devastating effect on the newborn. See Chapter 16∞ for more information.

SYPHILIS

Syphilis is a chronic STI caused by the spirochete *Treponema pallidum.* Syphilis is divided into early and late stages. During the early stage (primary), a chancre appears at the site where the *T. pallidum* organism entered the body. Symptoms include slight fever, loss of weight, and malaise. The chancre persists for about 4 weeks and then disappears. In 6 weeks to 6 months, secondary symptoms appear. Skin eruptions called condylomata lata, which resemble wartlike plaques and are highly infectious, may appear on the vulva. Other secondary symptoms are acute arthritis, enlargement of the liver and spleen, nontender enlarged lymph nodes, iritis, and a chronic sore throat with hoarseness.

Syphilis may also be transmitted transplacentally. When infected in utero, the newborn exhibits secondary-stage symptoms of syphilis. Transplacentally transmitted syphilis may cause intrauterine growth restriction, preterm birth, and stillbirth. As a result of the disease's impact on the fetus in utero, serologic testing of every pregnant woman is recommended; some state laws require it. Testing is done at the initial prenatal screening and repeated in the third trimester. Blood studies in early pregnancy may be negative if the woman has only recently contracted the infection.

Diagnosis of syphilis is made by dark-field examination for spirochetes. Blood tests such as the Venereal Disease Research Laboratory (VDRL) test, the rapid plasma reagin (RPR) test, or the more specific fluorescent treponemal antibody absorption (FTA-ABS) test are commonly done.

For nonpregnant and pregnant women with syphilis of less than a year's duration, the CDC (2006) recommends 2.4 million units of benzathine penicillin G administered intramuscularly in a single dose. If syphilis is of long (more than a year) duration, 2.4 million units of benzathine penicillin G is given intramuscularly once a week for 3 weeks. For nonpregnant women allergic to penicillin, doxycycline or tetracycline can be given. The pregnant woman who is allergic to penicillin should be desensitized to penicillin and then treated with it (CDC, 2006). Maternal serologic testing may remain positive for 8 months, and the newborn may have a positive test for 3 months.

CONDYLOMATA ACUMINATA (VENEREAL WARTS)

The infection **condylomata acuminata**, also called *venereal warts,* is a common sexually transmitted condition caused by the human papillomavirus (HPV). Transmission can occur through vaginal, oral, or anal sex. The infection has received considerable attention because HPV is almost always the cause of cervical cancer (Schmidt, 2007).

Over 120 HPV subtypes have been identified. Of these about 30 can infect the genital tract (Scheinfeld & Lehman, 2006). HPV types 6 and 11 account for 90% of visible genital warts while HPV types 16 and 18 cause about 70% of cervical cancer (Schmidt, 2007).

Often an individual seeks medical care after noticing single or multiple soft, grayish pink, cauliflower-like lesions on the penis or in the genital area (Figure 6–4 ●). The moist, warm environment of the genital area is conducive to the growth of the warts, which may be present on the vulva, vagina, cervix, and anus. The incubation period following exposure is 3 weeks to 3 years.

Because condylomata sometimes resemble other lesions and malignant transformation is possible, all atypical, pigmented, and persistent warts should be biopsied and treatment should be instituted promptly. The CDC (2006) does not specify a treatment of choice for genital warts but recommends that treatment be determined based on client preference, available resources,

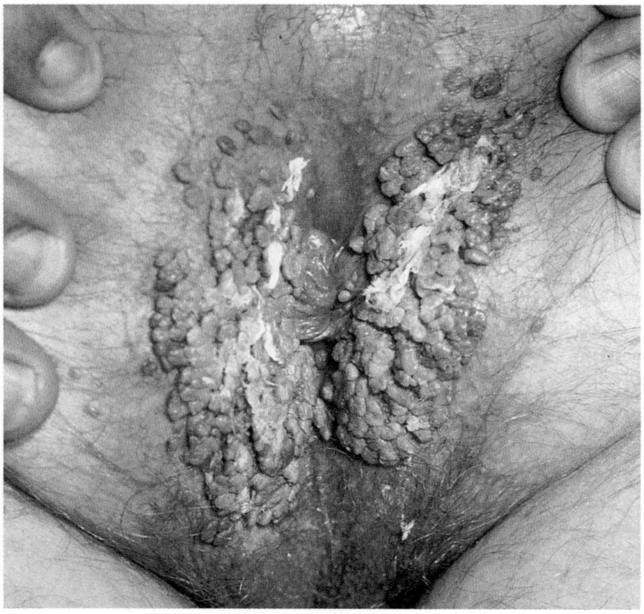

● **Figure 6–4** Condylomata acuminata on the vulva.
Source: Used with permission from Ken Greer/Visuals Unlimited.

and experience of the healthcare provider. Client-applied therapies include podofilox solution or gel or imiquimod cream. Provider-administered therapies include cryotherapy with liquid nitrogen or cryoprobe; trichloroacetic acid (TCA); bichloroacetic acid (BCA); intralesional interferon; surgical removal by tangential scissor excision, shave excision, or curettage; or laser surgery (CDC, 2006). Imiquimod, podophyllin, and podofilox are not used during pregnancy because they are thought to be teratogenic and in large doses have been associated with fetal death.

A vaccine, Gardasil, protects against four types of HPV. It is given in three doses and is recommended for females aged 9 to 26, preferably before they are sexually active. The vaccine does not treat existing infections. However, if a woman in this age group has already been diagnosed with one of the vaccine virus strains, she can still receive the vaccine because it offers protection against the other strains covered by the vaccine (CDC, 2007b).

Women who have received Gardasil should still receive regular Pap smears because the vaccine does not protect against all HPV types. Women with diagnosed HPV infections should have frequent Pap smears to monitor cervical cellular changes. Sex partners are probably infected but do not require treatment unless large lesions are present. The use of male or female condoms may reduce the risk of transmitting the virus to an uninfected partner.

ACQUIRED IMMUNODEFICIENCY SYNDROME

Acquired immunodeficiency syndrome (AIDS) is a serious, often fatal disorder caused by the human immunodeficiency virus (HIV). Medical-surgical texts more fully describe care of people with HIV/AIDS. However, because HIV/AIDS has profound implications for the pregnant woman's fetus, AIDS is discussed in more detail in Chapter 14.

NURSING MANAGEMENT

NURSING ASSESSMENT AND DIAGNOSIS

Nurses need to become adept at taking a thorough history and identifying people at risk for STIs. Risk factors include multiple sexual partners, a partner's involvement with other partners, high-risk sexual behaviors such as intercourse without barrier contraception or anal intercourse, partners with high-risk behaviors, treatment with antibiotics while taking oral contraceptives, and young age at onset of sexual activity. Be alert for signs and symptoms of STIs and be familiar with diagnostic procedures if an STI is suspected.

When children or adolescents have a possible STI, the nurse usually encounters them and their families in the emergency department, outpatient clinic, or nursing unit. Because adolescents are often afraid of the consequences of reporting symptoms, it is important to develop good assessment skills, particularly when asking questions about sexual activity, partners, and the possibility of abuse. When a child or adolescent is diagnosed with one STI, it is important to screen for others because these diseases may coexist. Adolescents who are symptomatic may postpone care because of their discomfort with examinations and cultures. Routine screening of sexually active adolescents is recommended because many have subclinical infections or are asymptomatic.

Although each STI has certain distinctive characteristics, the following complaints warrant further investigation: presence of a sore or lesion on the penis or vulva, increased vaginal discharge, malodorous vaginal discharge, urethral discharge (males), burning with urination, dyspareunia, bleeding after intercourse, and pelvic pain. In many instances a woman is asymptomatic but may report symptoms in her partner, especially painful urination or urethral discharge. It is often helpful to ask the woman whether her partner is experiencing any symptoms.

Nursing diagnoses that may apply when an STI is diagnosed include the following:

- *Interrupted Family Processes* related to the effects of a diagnosis of STI on the couple's relationship
- *Health-Seeking Behaviors: Information on Preventing STIs* related to an expressed desire to prevent infection

PLANNING AND IMPLEMENTATION

Provide the client who has an STI with information about the infection, methods of transmission, implications for pregnancy or future fertility, and the importance of thorough treatment, includ-

Nursing Practice

- When a child younger than 10 years of age is found to have gonorrhea or another STI, consider the possibility of sexual abuse.
- Whenever anorectal symptoms are found in a child, suspect molestation.

ing treatment of the partner if indicated. Partner notification is essential in order to provide treatment if the partner is infected, and to reduce the risk of reinfection. The person should also understand the need to abstain from sexual activity, if necessary, during treatment. Encourage sexually active adolescents to receive hepatitis B and HPV immunization if they haven't already done so.

Some STIs such as trichomoniasis or chlamydia may cause a woman concern but, once diagnosed, are rather easily treated. Other STIs may be simple to treat medically but may carry a stigma and be emotionally difficult to accept. Stress prevention with all clients and encourage them to require partners, especially new partners, to use condoms. See "Teaching Highlights: Preventing STIs and Their Consequences."

Teaching Highlights

PREVENTING STIs AND THEIR CONSEQUENCES

The risk of contracting an STI increases with the number of sexual partners. Because of the extended time between infection with HIV and evidence of infection, intercourse with an individual exposes a female or male to all the other sexual partners of that individual for the past 5 or more years. In light of this risk, it is important to take the following actions:

- Plan ahead and develop strategies to refuse sex (especially important for adolescents who may be less confident about saying "no" to casual sexual encounters). Abstinence is the best method of preventing STIs.
- Limit the number of sexual contacts and practice mutual monogamy with an uninfected partner.
- The condom is the best contraceptive method currently available (other than abstinence) for protection from STIs. Use one for every act of vaginal or anal intercourse. Other contraceptives such as the diaphragm, cervical cap, and spermicides also offer some protection against STIs.
- Plan strategies for negotiating condom use with a partner. Do not assume that a sexually experienced partner knows how to practice safe sex.
- Reduce high-risk behaviors. Use of recreational drugs and alcohol can increase sexual risk taking.
- Refrain from oral sex if your partner has active sores in the mouth, on the genitals, or around the anus.
- Refrain from sexual interaction when signs and symptoms of an STI are present.
- Seek care as soon as you notice symptoms and make sure your partner gets treatment if indicated. Absence of symptoms or disappearance of symptoms does not mean that treatment is unnecessary if you suspect an STI. Take all prescribed medications completely.
- The presence of a genital infection may lead to an abnormal Pap smear. Women with certain infections should have more frequent Pap smears according to a schedule recommended by their caregiver. Ask your healthcare provider if you need more frequent Paps.

Refer the child with signs of an STI for evaluation of sexual assault by a facility or healthcare provider specializing in collecting evidence and providing specialized care. Similarly refer any adolescent who has been sexually assaulted to a sexual assault nurse examiner or other healthcare provider who can collect evidence, coordinate medical treatment and coordinate mental health support.

As a nurse, you can be especially helpful in encouraging a client to explore feelings about the diagnosis. People may, for example, experience anger or feel betrayed by a partner, they may feel guilt or see their diagnosis as a form of punishment, or they may feel concern about the long-term implications for future childbearing or ongoing intimate relationships. Opportunities to discuss personal feelings in a nonjudgmental environment can be very helpful. Offer suggestions about support groups, if indicated, and assist the person in planning for future sexual activity.

An attitude of acceptance and matter-of-factness conveys the message that the individual is an acceptable person who happens to have an infection. See "Teaching Highlights" for key information about STIs.

EVALUATION

Expected outcomes of nursing care include the following:

- The infection is identified and cured, if possible; if not, supportive therapy is provided.
- The individual and partner can describe the infection, its method of transmission, its implications, and the therapy.
- The person copes successfully with the impact of the diagnosis on self-concept.

CARE OF THE WOMAN WITH PELVIC INFLAMMATORY DISEASE

Pelvic inflammatory disease (PID) is a clinical syndrome of inflammatory disorders of the upper female genital tract that includes any combination of endometritis, salpingitis (tubal infection), tubo-ovarian abscess, pelvic abscess, and pelvic peritonitis (CDC, 2006). In the United States an estimated 1 million cases of PID are diagnosed annually and more than 100,000 women become infertile as a result of it (CDC, 2004). The disease is more common in sexually active women younger than age 25. Other risk factors include multiple sexual partners, a history of PID, recent insertion of an intrauterine device, and regular douching (Mayo Clinic, 2009). Perhaps the greatest problem of PID is postinfection tubal damage, which is closely associated with infertility.

The organisms most frequently identified with PID are *Chlamydia trachomatis* and *Neisseria gonorrhoeae.* Symptoms of PID include bilateral sharp, cramping pain in the lower quadrants, fever, chills, purulent vaginal discharge, irregular bleeding, malaise, nausea, and vomiting. However, it is also possible to be asymptomatic and have normal laboratory values.

Diagnosis is based on examination, cultures for gonorrhea and chlamydia, a complete blood count with differential, and an RPR or VDRL to test for syphilis. The woman may have an elevated

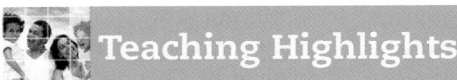

C-reactive protein and an elevated sedimentation rate. Physical examination usually reveals direct abdominal tenderness with palpation, adnexal tenderness, and cervical and uterine tenderness with movement (chandelier sign). A palpable mass is evaluated with ultrasound. Laparoscopy may confirm the diagnosis and enable the examiner to obtain cultures from the fimbriated ends of the fallopian tubes.

The decision to hospitalize is based on clinical judgment. Inpatient treatment includes intravenous fluids, pain medications, and intravenous antibiotics—often either cefoxitin or cefotetan, plus doxycycline or clindamycin plus gentamicin (CDC, 2002). Outpatient oral therapy usually includes ceftriaxone plus doxycycline with or without metronidazole (CDC, 2007a). Other antibiotic combinations may also be used. In addition, supportive therapy is often indicated for severe symptoms. The sexual partner should be treated. If the woman has an IUD, it is generally removed 24 to 48 hours after antibiotic therapy is started.

NURSING MANAGEMENT

NURSING ASSESSMENT AND DIAGNOSIS

Be alert to factors in a woman's history that put her at risk for PID. Question the woman who has an IUD about possible symptoms, such as aching pain in the lower abdomen, foul-smelling discharge, malaise, and the like. The woman who is acutely ill will have obvious symptoms, but a low-grade infection is more difficult to detect.

Nursing diagnoses that may apply to a woman with PID include the following:

- *Acute Pain* related to peritoneal irritation
- *Health-Seeking Behaviors: Information about the Possible Effects of PID on Fertility* related to a request for specific information

PLANNING AND IMPLEMENTATION

The nurse plays a vital role in helping to prevent or detect PID. Accordingly, spend time discussing risk factors related to this infection. The woman who uses an IUD for contraception and has multiple sexual partners needs to understand clearly the risk she faces. Discuss signs and symptoms of PID and stress the importance of early detection.

The woman who develops PID should be counseled on the importance of completing her antibiotic treatment and of returning for follow-up evaluation. She should also understand the possibility of decreased fertility following the infection.

EVALUATION

Expected outcomes of nursing care include the following:

- The woman describes her condition, her therapy, and the possible long-term implications of PID on her fertility.
- The woman completes her course of therapy and the PID is cured.

CARE OF THE WOMAN WITH AN ABNORMAL FINDING DURING PELVIC EXAMINATION

ABNORMAL PAP SMEAR RESULTS

As discussed in Chapter 5, a Papanicolaou (Pap) smear is a test done to screen for the presence of cellular anomalies of the cervix and endocervical canal. Although the Pap smear is useful in detecting a variety of abnormalities, it has had its greatest impact on the detection of cervical cancer. The *Bethesda system* (Table 6–1) has become the most widely used system in the United States for reporting Pap smear results. Early detection of abnormalities allows changes to be treated before cells reach the precancerous or cancerous stage. Notification of an abnormal Pap smear usually causes anxiety for a woman, so it is important that she be told in a caring way. The woman needs accurate, complete information about the meaning of the results and the next steps to be taken. She should also be given time to ask questions and express her concerns.

Diagnostic or therapeutic procedures used in cases of abnormalities include repetition of the Pap test using the liquid-based medium Pap smear, Pap tests at shorter intervals, colposcopy and endocervical biopsy, cryotherapy, laser conization, or loop electrosurgical excision procedure (LEEP). Management is based on the specific report.

Colposcopy has become a common second step in many cases of abnormal Pap smears. The examination, done in an office or clinic, permits more detailed visualization of the cervix in bright light, using a high-magnification microscope. The cervix can be visualized directly and again following application of acetic acid. The acetic acid causes abnormal epithelium to assume a characteristic white appearance. The colposcope can also be used to obtain a directed biopsy.

OVARIAN MASSES

Ovarian masses may be palpated during the pelvic examination. Between 70% and 80% of ovarian masses are benign. More than 50% are functional cysts (cysts that develop from ovarian follicles, from the corpus luteum, or from the theca luteum), occurring most commonly in women 20 to 40 years of age. Functional cysts are rare in women who take oral contraceptives. Ovarian cysts usually represent physiologic variations in the menstrual cycle. Dermoid cysts (cystic teratomas) and endometriomas, or "chocolate cysts," are common types of ovarian masses. No relationship exists between ovarian masses and ovarian cancer. However, ovarian cancer is the most fatal of all cancers in women because it is difficult to diagnose and often has spread throughout the pelvis before it is detected. Refer to medical-surgical nursing texts for an in-depth discussion of ovarian cancer.

Many women with a benign ovarian mass are asymptomatic; the mass may be noted on a routine pelvic examination. Others experience a sensation of fullness or cramping in the lower abdomen (often unilateral), dyspareunia, irregular bleeding, or delayed menstruation. Diagnosis is made on the basis of a

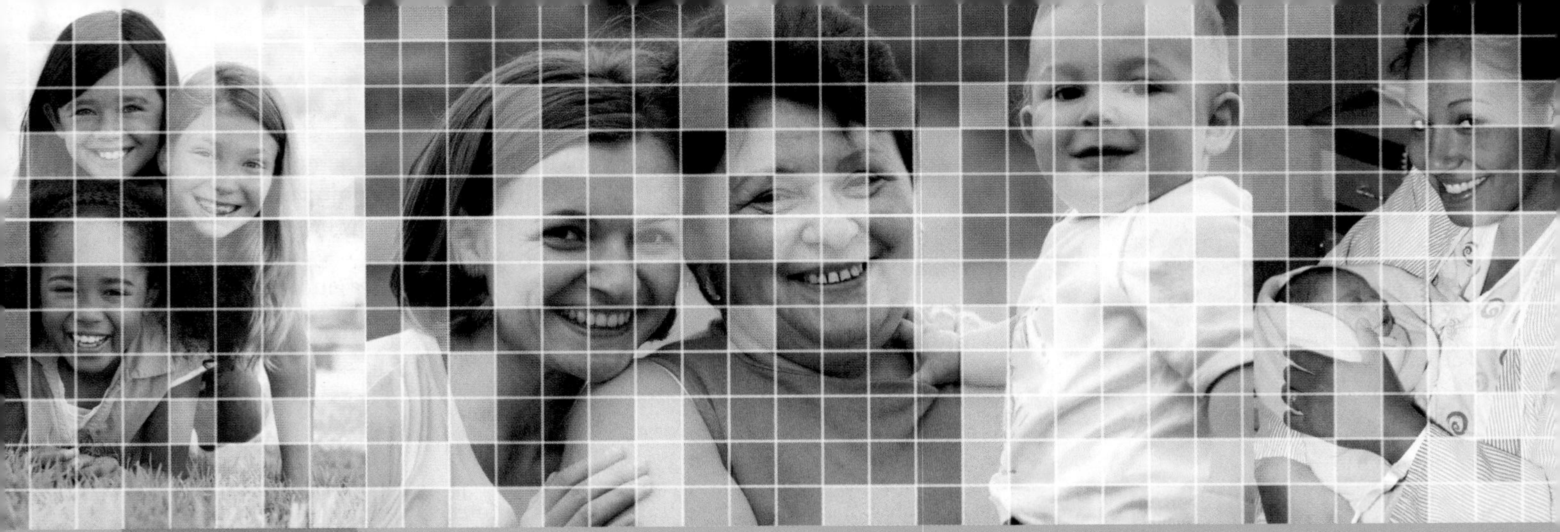

CHAPTER

7 Families with Special Reproductive Concerns

As we sat in the in vitro clinic waiting room, I felt great apprehension. For 4 years we had been unable to conceive. I'd been through two surgeries, dozens of blood tests, and hormone drugs that made me irrational and emotional. It was difficult at times—I blamed myself, felt out of control, and had surprisingly painful reactions to seeing mothers with babies. We were on the brink of the most expensive infertility treatment—the last resort for most infertile couples. Was this the right thing to do? —Samantha, 38

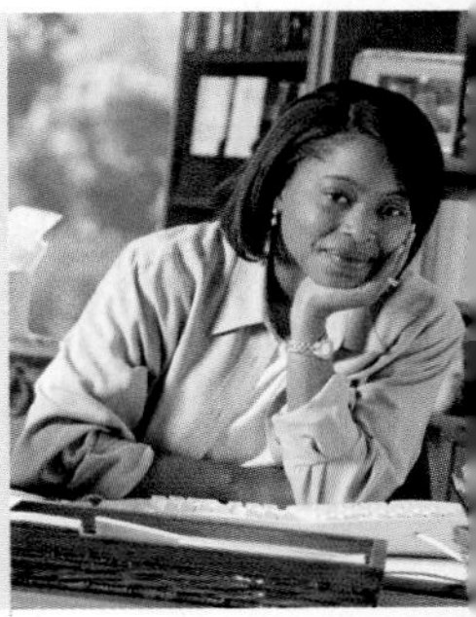

LEARNING OUTCOMES

7.1 Identify the essential components of fertility.

7.2 Describe the elements of the preliminary investigation of infertility and the nurse's role in supporting/teaching clients during this phase.

7.3 Summarize the indications for the tests and associated treatments, including assisted reproductive technologies, that are done in an infertility workup.

7.4 Relate the physiologic and psychologic effects of infertility on a couple to the nursing management of the couple.

7.5 Describe the nurse's role as counselor, educator, and advocate for couples during infertility evaluation and treatment.

7.6 Identify couples who may benefit from preconceptual chromosomal analysis and prenatal testing when providing care to couples with special reproductive concerns.

7.7 Identify the characteristics of autosomal dominant, autosomal recessive, and X-linked (sex-linked) recessive disorders.

7.8 Compare prenatal and postnatal diagnostic procedures used to determine the presence of genetic disorders.

7.9 Explore the emotional impact on a couple undergoing genetic testing or coping with the birth of a baby with a genetic disorder, and explain the nurse's role in supporting the family undergoing genetic counseling.

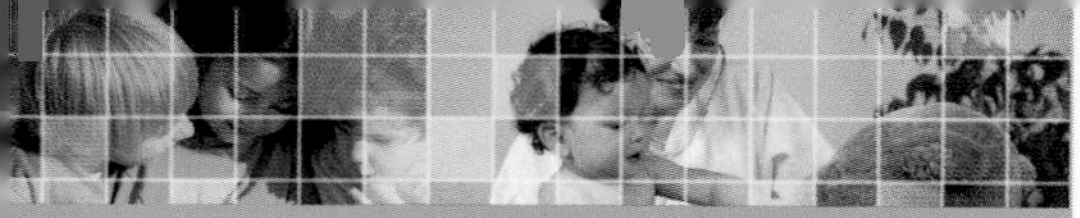

KEY TERMS

Autosomes, 154
Basal body temperature (BBT), 141
Chromosomes, 154
Endometrial biopsy, 144
Ferning capacity, 144
Gamete intrafallopian transfer (GIFT), 150
Genotype, 157
Hysterosalpingography (HSG), 145
Infertility, 138
In vitro fertilization (IVF), 149
Karyotype, 154
Laparoscopy, 145
Mendelian (single-gene) inheritance, 157
Monosomies, 156
Mosaicism, 156
Non-Mendelian (multifactorial) inheritance, 157
Pedigree, 158
Phenotype, 157
Postcoital test (PCI) or Huhner test, 145
Spinnbarkeit, 144
Subfertility, 138
Therapeutic insemination, 148
Transvaginal ultrasound, 144
Trisomies, 155
Tubal embryo transfer (TET), 150
Zygote intrafallopian transfer (ZIFT), 150

MyNursingKit Case Study: Infertility

Most couples who want children are able to conceive them with little difficulty. Pregnancy and childbirth usually take their normal course, and a healthy baby is born without problems. But some less fortunate couples are unable to fulfill their dream of having the desired baby because of infertility or genetic problems.

This chapter explores two particularly troubling reproductive problems facing some couples: the inability to conceive and the risk of bearing babies with genetic abnormalities.

INFERTILITY

Infertility, a lack of conception despite unprotected sexual intercourse for at least 12 months (Kumar, Ghadir, Eskandari, et al., 2007), has a profound emotional, psychologic, and economic impact on affected couples and society. The term *sterility* is applied when there is an absolute factor preventing reproduction. **Subfertility** is used to describe a couple who has difficulty conceiving because both partners have reduced fertility. The term *second infertility* is applied to couples who have been unable to conceive after one or more successful pregnancies or who cannot sustain a pregnancy.

Approximately 10–15% of couples in their reproductive years are infertile in the United States (Wright & Johnson, 2008). Public perception is that the incidence of infertility is increasing, but in fact there has been no significant change in the proportion of infertile couples in the United States. What has changed is the composition of the infertile population, which has increased in the age group 25 to 44 because of delayed childbearing and the entry of the baby boom cohort into this age range in Western society. The perception that infertility is on the rise may be related to the following factors:

- The deferring of marriage and then the desire to have a family shortly after marriage
- The increase in assisted reproductive techniques
- The increase in availability and use of infertility services
- The increase in insurance coverage of some ethnic groups for diagnosis of and treatment for infertility
- The increased number of childless women over age 35 seeking medical attention for infertility

ESSENTIAL COMPONENTS OF FERTILITY

Understanding the elements essential for normal fertility can help the nurse identify the many factors that may cause infertility. The components necessary for normal fertility are correlated with possible causes of deviation in Table 7–1. In addition, adequate reproductive hormones must be present. With timing and environment playing such a crucial role, it is an impressive natural phenomenon that the majority of couples in the United States are able to conceive. The remaining couples suffer infertility because of a male factor (40%), a female factor (40%), or either an unknown cause (unexplained infertility) or a problem with both partners (20%) (American Society of Reproductive Medicine, 2006b). Professional intervention can help approximately 65% of infertile couples achieve pregnancy.

Young couples with no history that is suggestive of reproductive disorders should be referred for infertility evaluation if they have been unable to conceive after at least 1 year of attempting to achieve pregnancy. An earlier workup is indicated in couples with positive history for fertility-lowering disease or advancing maternal age (Wright & Johnson, 2008). If the woman is over age 35, it may be appropriate to refer the couple after only 6 to 9 months of unprotected intercourse without conception. At age 25, when couples are the most fertile, in about 25% of cases, conception occurs within the first month of unprotected intercourse (Wright & Johnson, 2008).

Table 7–1 Possible Causes of Infertility

Necessary Norms	Deviations from Normal
	Female
Favorable cervical mucus	Cervicitis, cervical stenosis, use of coital lubricants, antisperm antibodies (immunologic response)
Clear passage between cervix and tubes	Myomas, adhesions, adenomyosis, polyps, endometritis, cervical stenosis, endometriosis, congenital anomalies (e.g., septate uterus, diethylstilbestrol [DES] exposure)
Patent tubes with normal motility	Pelvic inflammatory disease, peritubal adhesions, endometriosis, intrauterine device (IUD), salpingitis (e.g., chlamydia, recurrent sexually transmitted infections [STIs]), neoplasm, ectopic pregnancy, tubal ligation
Ovulation and release of ova	Primary ovarian failure, polycystic ovarian disease, hypothyroidism, pituitary tumor, lactation, periovarian adhesions, endometriosis, premature ovarian failure, hyperprolactinemia, Turner syndrome
No obstruction between ovary and tubes	Adhesions, endometriosis, pelvic inflammatory disease
Endometrial preparation	Anovulation, luteal phase defect, malformation, uterine infection, Asherman syndrome
	Male
Normal semen analysis	Abnormalities of sperm or semen, polyspermia, congenital defect in testicular development, mumps after adolescence, cryptorchidism, infections, gonadal exposure to X-rays, chemotherapy, smoking, alcohol abuse, malnutrition, chronic or acute metabolic disease, medications (e.g., morphine, aspirin [ASA], ibuprofen), cocaine, marijuana use, constrictive underclothing, heat
Unobstructed genital tract	Infections, tumors, congenital anomalies, vasectomy, strictures, trauma, varicocele
Normal genital tract secretions	Infections, autoimmunity to semen, tumors
Ejaculate deposited at the cervix	Premature ejaculation, impotence, hypospadias, retrograde ejaculation (e.g., diabetic), neurologic cord lesions, obesity (inhibiting adequate penetration)

INITIAL INVESTIGATION: PHYSICAL AND PSYCHOSOCIAL ISSUES

The easiest and least intrusive infertility testing approach is used first. Extensive testing for infertility is avoided until data confirm that the timing of intercourse and length of coital exposure have been adequate. The nurse provides information about the most fertile times to have intercourse during the menstrual cycle. Teaching the couple the signs and timing of ovulation, the most effective times for intercourse within the cycle, and other fertility awareness behaviors may solve the problem (see "Teaching Highlights: Suggestions for Improving Fertility"). Primary

Teaching Highlights

SUGGESTIONS FOR IMPROVING FERTILITY

Avoid douching and artificial lubricants (gels, oils, saliva) that can alter sperm motility. Prevent alteration of pH of vagina and introduction of spermicidal agents.

Promote retention of sperm. The male superior position with female remaining recumbent for at least 20 to 30 minutes after intercourse maximizes the number of sperm reaching the cervix.

Avoid leakage of sperm. Elevate the woman's hips with a pillow after intercourse for 20 to 30 minutes to allow liquefaction of seminal fluid and motility of the sperm toward the egg. Avoid getting up to urinate or shower for 1 hour after intercourse.

Maximize the potential for fertilization. Instruct the couple that it is optimal if sexual intercourse occurs every other day during the fertile period. Because each woman's menstrual cycle varies in length, the fertile period can extend from cycle day (CD) 7 through CD 17. Note CD 1 is considered the first day of actual menstrual flow.

Avoid emphasizing conception during sexual encounters to decrease anxiety and potential sexual dysfunction.

Maintain adequate nutrition and reduce stress. Stress-reduction techniques and good nutritional habits increase sperm production.

Explore other methods to increase fertility awareness, such as home assessment of cervical mucus and basal body temperature (BBT) recordings, and use of a home ovulation predictor kit (tests LH surge to time intercourse).

Consider incorporating culturally appropriate methods to enhance fertility.

assessment, including a comprehensive history (with a discussion of genetic conditions) and physical examination for any obvious causes of infertility, is done before a costly, time-consuming, and emotionally trying investigation is initiated.

During the first visit for the preliminary investigation, the nurse explains the basic infertility workup. The basic investigation depends on the couple's history and usually includes assessment of ovarian function, cervical mucus adequacy and receptivity to sperm, sperm adequacy, tubal patency, and the general condition of the pelvic organs. Because about 40% of infertility is related to a male factor, a semen analysis should be one of the first diagnostic tests done before moving on to more invasive diagnostic procedures involving the woman.

The mutual desire to have children is a cornerstone of many marriages. A fertility problem is a deeply personal, emotion-laden area in a couple's life. The self-esteem of one or both partners may be threatened if the inability to conceive is perceived as a lack of virility or femininity (Klock, 2004). It is never easy to discuss one's sexual activity, especially when potentially irreversible problems with fertility exist. The nurse can provide comfort to couples by offering a sympathetic ear, a nonjudgmental approach, and appropriate information and instructions throughout the diagnostic and therapeutic process. Because counseling includes discussion of very personal matters, nurses who are comfortable with their own sexuality are able to establish rapport and elicit relevant information from couples with fertility problems.

Table 7–2 Initial Infertility Physical Workup and Laboratory Evaluations

Screening	Female	Male
Physical Examination	Assessment of height, weight, blood pressure, temperature, and general health status Endocrine evaluation of thyroid for exophthalmos, lid lag, tremor, or palpable gland Optic fundi evaluation for presence of increased intracranial pressure, especially in oligomenorrheal or amenorrheal women (possible pituitary tumor) Reproductive features (including breast and external genital area) Physical ability to tolerate pregnancy	General health (assessment of height, weight, blood pressure) Endocrine evaluation (e.g., presence of gynecomastia) Visual fields evaluation for bitemporal hemianopia (blindness in one-half of the visual field) Abnormal hair patterns
Laboratory Examination	Complete blood count Sedimentation rate, if indicated Serology Urinalysis Rh factor and blood grouping Rubella IgG Follicle-stimulating hormone (FSH) level regardless of age and regularity of menstrual cycles If indicated depending on age and regularity of menstrual cycles: thyroid-stimulating hormone (TSH), prolactin levels (PRL), glucose tolerance test, hormonal assays including estradiol (E2), luteinizing hormone (LH), mid-luteal progesterone (MLP), dehydroepiandrosterone (DHEA), androstenedione, testosterone, 17 alpha-hydroxy progesterone (17-OHP).	Complete blood count Sedimentation rate, if indicated Serology Urinalysis Rh factor and blood grouping Semen analysis If indicated, testicular biopsy, buccal smear (to determine number of Barr bodies) Hormonal assays, FSH, LH, prolactin
Gender-specific Examinations	**Pelvic Examination** Papanicolaou (PAP) smear Culture for gonorrhea if indicated and possibly chlamydia or mycoplasma culture (opinions vary) Signs of vaginal infections (Chapter 6 ∞) Shape of escutcheon (e.g., does pubic hair distribution resemble that of a male?) Size of clitoris (enlargement caused by endocrine disorders) Evaluation of cervix: old lacerations, tears, erosion, polyps, condition and shape of os, signs of infections, cervical mucus (evaluate for estrogen effect of spinnbarkeit and cervical ferning) **Rectovaginal Examination** Presence of retroflexed or retroverted uterus Presence of rectouterine pouch masses Presence of possible endometriosis **Bimanual Examination** Size, shape, position, and motility of uterus Presence of congenital anomalies Evaluation for endometriosis Evaluation of adnexa: ovarian size, cysts, fixations, or tumors	**Urologic Examination** Presence or absence of phimosis (narrowing of the preputial orifice) Location of urethral meatus Size and consistency of each testis, vas deferens, and epididymis Presence of varicocele (enlargement of spermatic cord veins above testicles) **Rectal Examination** Size and consistency of prostate, with microscopic evaluation of prostate fluid for signs of infection Size and consistency of seminal vesicles

The first interview should involve both partners and include a comprehensive history and physical examination. Table 7–2 lists the items in a complete infertility physical workup and laboratory evaluation for both partners. Figure 7–1 ● outlines the couple's history and physical exam data, diagnostic tests usually performed, and healthcare interventions used in cases of infertility.

ASSESSMENT OF THE WOMAN'S FERTILITY

After a thorough history and physical examination, both partners may undergo tests to identify causes of infertility. A thorough female evaluation includes assessment of the hypothalamic–pituitary axis in terms of ovulatory function, as well as structure and function of the cervix, uterus, fallopian tubes, and ovaries. See Chapter 3∞ for an in-depth discussion of the fertility cycle.

Evaluation of Ovulatory Factors

MyNursingKit Activity: Ovulation

Ovulation problems account for approximately 15% of couples' infertility. For a review of female reproductive cycle characteristics, see Chapter 3∞.

Basal body temperature recording. One basic test of ovulatory function is the **basal body temperature (BBT)** recording, which aids in identifying follicular and luteal phase abnormalities. At the initial visit, the nurse instructs the woman in the technique of recording BBT on a special form. The woman is instructed to begin a new chart on the first day of every monthly cycle. The temperature can be taken with an oral or rectal thermometer that is calibrated by tenths of a degree, making slight temperature changes readily apparent. A special BBT thermometer may be used to measure temperatures only between 35.6°C and 37.8°C (96°F and 100°F). In addition to the traditional or digital thermometers, tympanic thermometry,

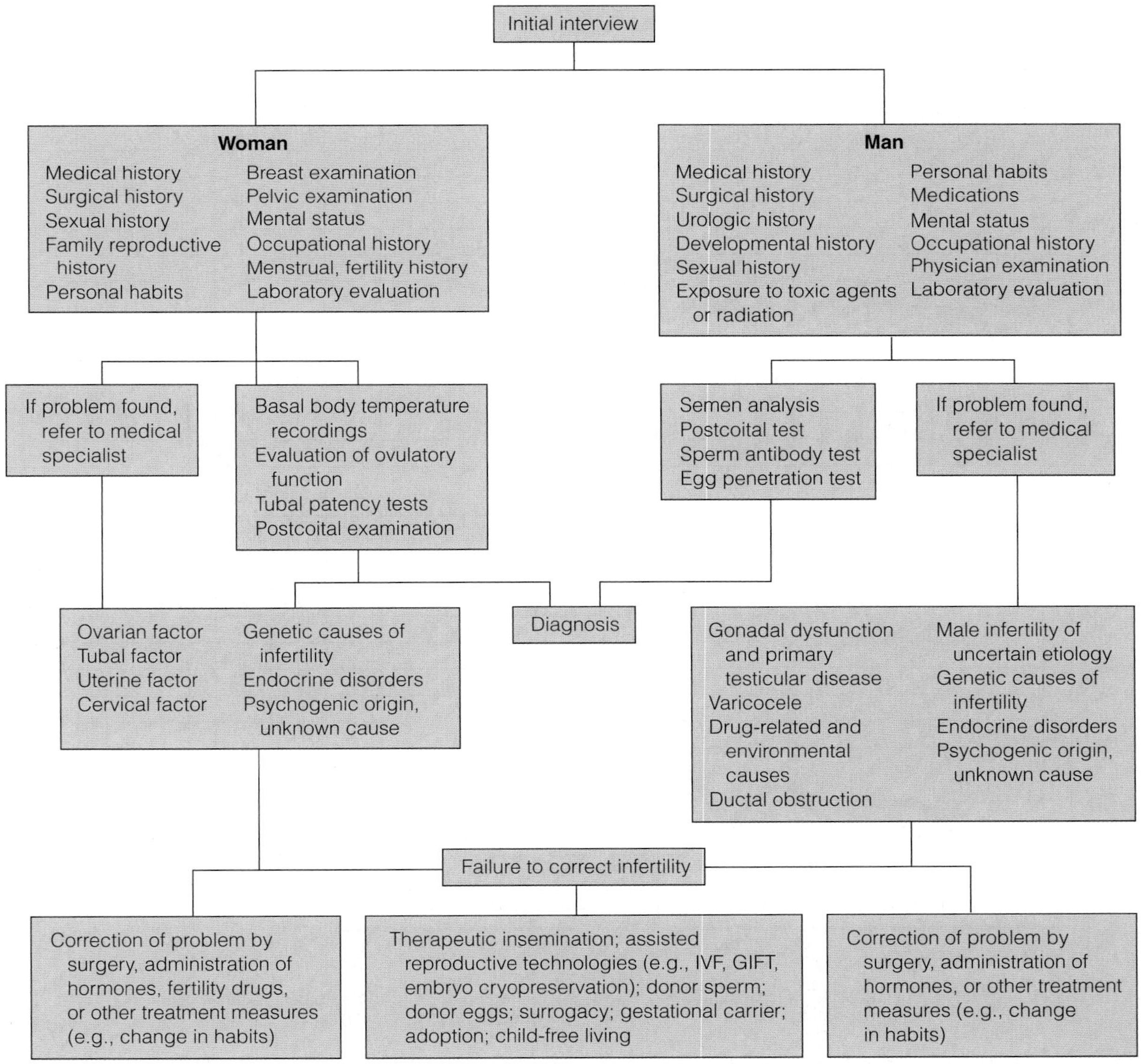

● **Figure 7–1** Flow chart for management of the infertile couple.

which provides a reading in only a few seconds, may also be a valid method.

The woman records daily variations on the temperature graph. The temperature graph shows a typical biphasic pattern during ovulatory cycles, whereas in anovulatory cycles it remains monophasic. The woman uses the readings on the temperature graph to detect ovulation and timing of intercourse (see Figure 7–2 ●).

Basal temperature for females in the preovulatory (follicular) phase is usually below 36.7°C (98°F). As ovulation approaches, production of estrogen increases and at its peak may cause a slight drop, then a rise, in the basal temperature. The slight drop in temperature before ovulation is often difficult to capture on the BBT chart. After ovulation, there is a surge of luteinizing hormone (LH), which stimulates production of progesterone. Because progesterone is thermogenic (produces heat), it causes a 0.3°C to 0.6°C (0.5°F to 1.0°F) sustained rise in basal temperature during the second half of the menstrual cycle (luteal phase). Immediately before or coincident with the onset of menses, the temperature again falls below 36.7°C (98°F). These changes in the basal temperature create the typical biphasic pattern. Figure 7–2B shows a biphasic ovulatory BBT chart. Temperature elevation does not predict the day of ovulation, but it does provide supportive evidence of ovulation about a day after it has occurred. Although there are other, more reliable methods to detect ovulatory function, BBT offers couples a low-tech, noninvasive, and inexpensive option. Based on serial BBT charts, the clinician might recommend sexual intercourse *every other day* beginning 3 to 4 days before and continuing for 2 to 3 days after the expected time of ovulation. See "Teaching Highlights: Methods of Determining Ovulation."

Hormonal assessments of ovulatory function. Hormonal assessments of ovulatory function fall into the following categories.

1. *Gonadotropin levels (FSH, LH).* Baseline hormonal assessment of FSH and LH provides valuable information about normal ovulatory function. Measured on cycle day (CD) 3, FSH is the single most valuable test of ovarian reserve (number of remaining oocytes or follicles in the

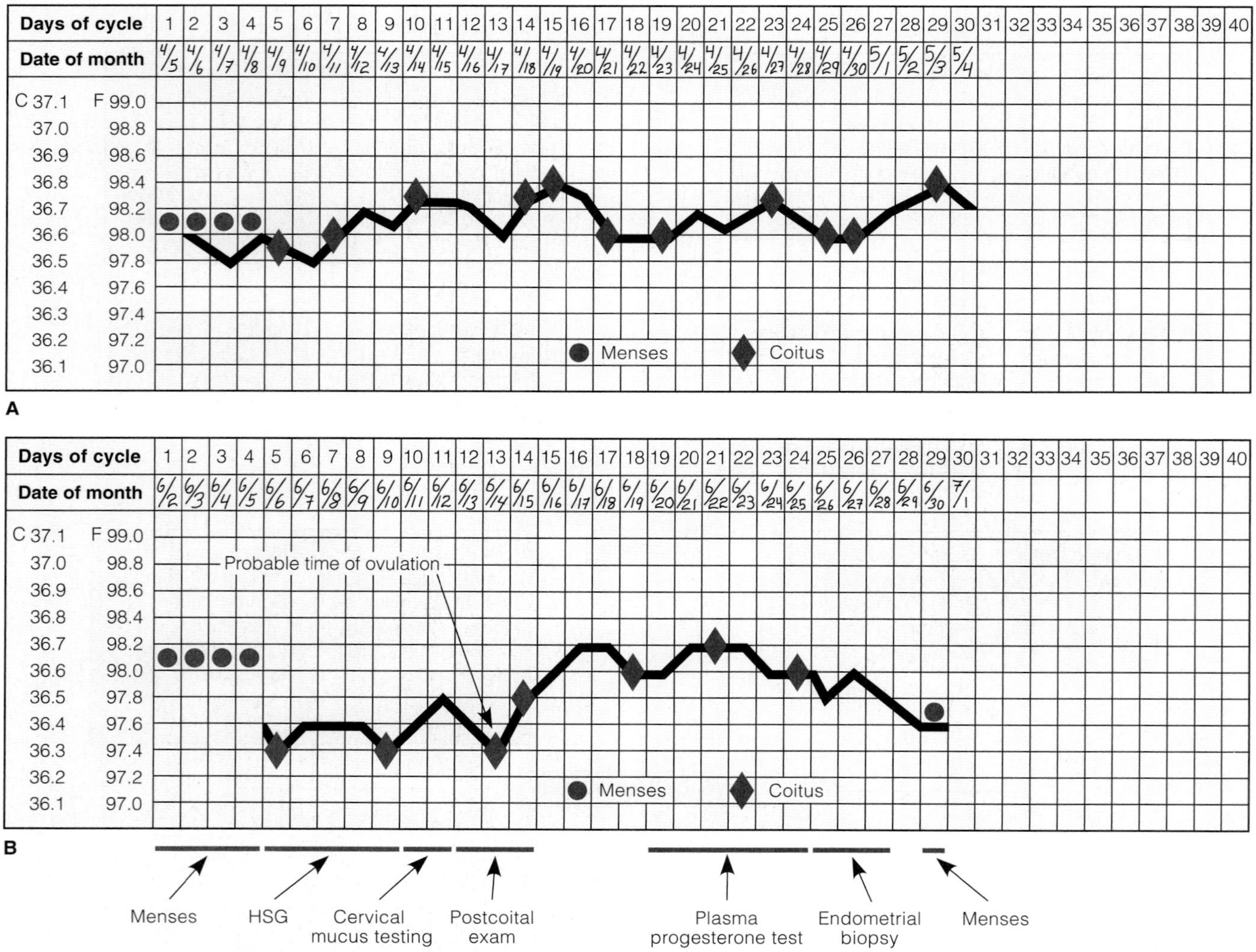

● **Figure 7–2** ***A,*** Monophasic, anovulatory basal body temperature (BBT) chart. ***B,*** Biphasic BBT chart illustrating probable time of ovulation, the different types of testing, and the time in the cycle that each would be performed.

Teaching Highlights

METHODS OF DETERMINING OVULATION

Basal Body Temperature (BBT) Method

The basal body temperature (BBT) method relies on assessing the woman's temperature pattern.

Describe the expected findings with an ovulatory (biphasic) cycle and stress the need to monitor BBT for 3 to 4 months to establish a pattern. BBT can be used to time intercourse if pregnancy is desired or as a method of natural family planning. Describe the timing of intercourse to achieve or avoid pregnancy.

Procedure for Measuring BBT

- Using a BBT thermometer, the woman chooses one site (oral, vaginal, or rectal), which she uses consistently.
- The woman takes her temperature every day before arising and before starting any activity, including smoking. Any activity can produce an increase in body temperature.

  Note: Read and follow manufacturers' instructions for each type of BBT thermometer in regard to the amount of time needed for an accurate reading.
- She then immediately records the result on a special BBT chart, and connects the temperature dots for each day to form a graph.
- She then shakes the thermometer down and cleans it in preparation for use the next day.

Explain that certain situations can disturb body temperature such as large alcohol intake, sleeplessness, fever, warm climate, jet lag, shift work, the use of an electric blanket, or use of a heated waterbed.

Cervical Mucus Method

Cervical mucus characteristics change throughout a woman's menstrual cycle, and the quality of the mucus can be used to predict ovulation elasticity (see Figure 7–3 ●).

Procedure for Assessing Cervical Mucus Changes

- Every day when she uses the bathroom the woman checks her vagina, either by dabbing the vaginal opening with toilet paper or by putting a finger in the opening.
- She notes the wetness (presence of mucus), collects some mucus, determines its color and consistency, and records her findings on a chart. For discussion of mucus characteristics, see page 144.
- She washes her hands before and after the procedure.

Stress that the presence and consistency of the mucus are altered by vaginal infection, vaginal medications, spermicides, lubricants, douching, sexual arousal, and semen.

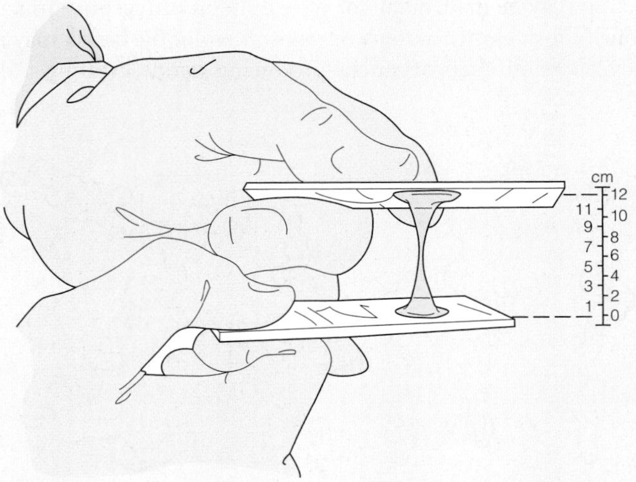

A

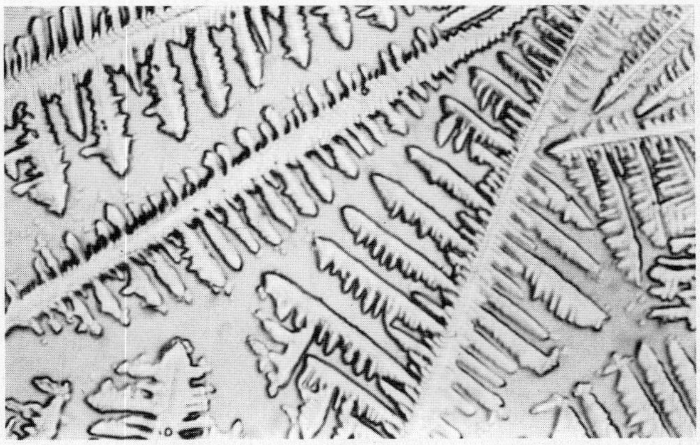

B

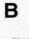

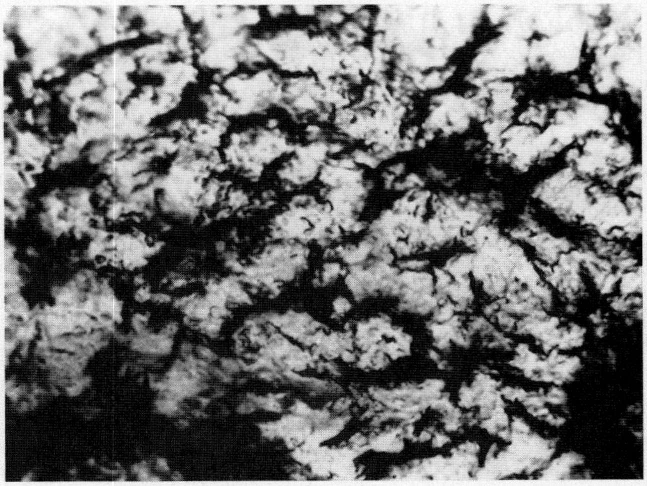

C

● **Figure 7–3** ***A,*** Spinnbarkeit (elasticity). ***B,*** Ferning pattern. ***C,*** Lack of ferning.

Source: B. Courtesy of Lavena Porter OB/GYN NP, *C.* Speroff, L., et al. (1994). *Clinical gynecologic endocrinology and infertility* (5th ed., p. 818). Baltimore: Williams & Wilkins.

ovary) and function. FSH should always be measured, particularly in women over age 30, to predict the potential for successful treatment with ovulation-induction treatment cycles (Wright & Johnson, 2008). LH levels may be measured early in the cycle to rule out androgen excess disorders, which disrupt normal follicular development and oocyte maturation. Daily sampling of LH at midcycle can detect the LH surge. The day of the LH surge is believed to be the day of maximum fertility. Ovulation occurs 24 to 36 hours after the onset of the LH surge and 10 to 12 hours after the peak of the LH surge. Urine LH ovulation prediction and serum LH assay kits are available for home use to better time postcoital testing, insemination, and intercourse (Kumar et al., 2007).

2. *Progesterone assays.* Progesterone levels furnish the best evidence of ovulation and corpus luteum function. Serum levels begin to rise with the LH surge and peak about 8 days later. A level of 3 ng/ml 3 days after the LH surge confirms ovulation (Wright & Johnson, 2008). On day 21 (7 days postovulation) a level of 10 ng/ml or higher indicates an adequate luteal phase.

Hormonal assessment may also be conducted for prolactin, thyroid-stimulating hormone, and androgen (testosterone, dehydroepiandrosterone [DHEAS], and androstenedione) levels.

Endometrial biopsy (EMB). **Endometrial biopsy** provides information about the effects of progesterone produced by the corpus luteum after ovulation and endometrial receptivity. EMB is reliable for determining the presence of ovulation. However, it is not effective for diagnosing luteal phase deficiency (Wright & Johnson, 2008).

The biopsy is performed not earlier than 10 to 12 days after ovulation (usually day 22 or 23 of a 28-day menstrual cycle), preferably 2 to 3 days before the expected onset of menses, and involves removing a sample of endometrium with a small pipette attached to suction (Kumar et al., 2007; Varney, Kriebs, & Gegor, 2004). The woman should be informed that some pelvic discomfort, cramping, and vaginal spotting are normal during and following the procedure. The woman should be pretreated with NSAIDs to help reduce the pain or cramping associated with the procedure (Speroff & Fritz, 2005). The onset of menses following biopsy should be disclosed for accurate interpretation of the biopsy report.

A dysfunction may exist if the endometrial lining does not show the expected amount of secretory tissue for that day of the woman's menstrual cycle. Historical evidence of a secretory endometrium detected by endometrial biopsy shows ovulation and corpus luteum formation.

Transvaginal ultrasound. **Transvaginal ultrasound** is the method of choice for follicular monitoring of women undergoing induction cycles, for timing ovulation for insemination and intercourse, for retrieving oocytes for in vitro fertilization (IVF), and for monitoring early pregnancy.

The use of a transvaginal color flow Doppler to investigate uterine blood flow may in the future help the endocrinologist evaluate the adequacy of the developing follicle, further assess oocyte maturity and endometrial development and patterns, and improve the diagnosis of luteal phase defects. For the procedure, the woman does not need to have a full bladder. In addition, if the woman finds it more comfortable to do so, she can insert the lubricated transvaginal probe herself (Storment, 2006).

Evaluation of Cervical Factors

The mucous cells of the endocervix consist predominantly of water. As ovulation approaches, the ovary increases its secretion of estrogen and produces changes in the cervical mucus. The amount of mucus increases tenfold, and the water content rises significantly. At ovulation, mucus elasticity (**spinnbarkeit**) increases to at least 5 cm in length and viscosity decreases. Excellent spinnbarkeit exists when the mucus can be stretched 8 to 10 cm or longer. Mucous elasticity is determined by using two glass slides (Figure 7–3A) or by grasping some mucus at the external os (see "Teaching Highlights: Methods of Determining Ovulation").

The **ferning capacity** (crystallization) (Figure 7–3B and 7–3C) of the cervical mucus also increases as ovulation approaches. Ferning is caused by decreased levels of salt and water interacting with the glycoproteins in the mucus during the ovulatory period and is thus an indirect indication of estrogen production. To test for ferning, mucus is obtained from the cervical os, spread on a glass slide, allowed to air dry, and examined under the microscope. Within 24 to 48 hours postovulation, rising levels of progesterone markedly decrease the quantity of cervical mucus and increase its viscosity and cellularity. The resulting absence of spinnbarkeit and ferning capacity decreases sperm survival.

To be receptive to sperm, cervical mucus must be thin, clear, watery, profuse, alkaline, and acellular. As shown in Figure 7–4 ●, the mazelike microscopic mucoid strands align in a parallel manner to allow for easy sperm passage. The mucus is termed *inhospitable* if these changes do not occur.

Cervical mucus inhospitable to sperm survival can have several causes, some of which are treatable. For example, estrogen secretion may be inadequate for development of receptive mucus. Cone biopsy, electrocautery, or cryosurgery of the cervix may remove large numbers of mucus-producing glands, creating a "dry

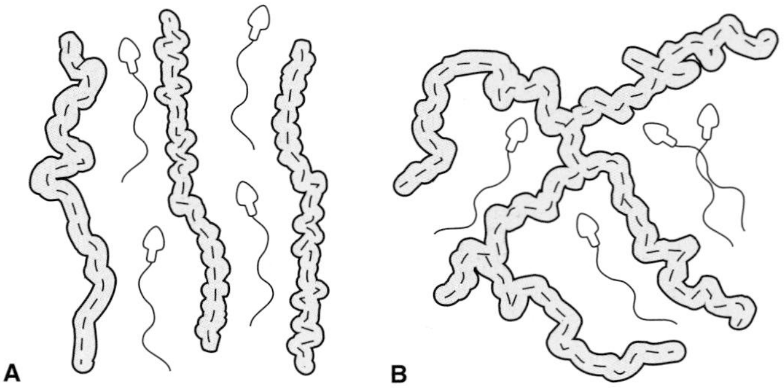

● **Figure 7–4** Sperm passage through cervical mucus. ***A,*** Appearance at the time of ovulation with channels favoring efficient sperm penetration and migration upward. ***B,*** Unfavorable mazelike configuration found at other times during the menstrual cycle.

Source: Corson, S. (1998). Conquering infertility, in *A guide for couples* (4th ed., p. 16). Vancouver, BC: EMIS-Canada.

cervix" that decreases sperm survival. Treatment with clomiphene citrate may have harmful effects on cervical mucus because of its antiestrogenic properties. Therapy with supplemental estrogen for approximately 6 days before expected ovulation encourages the formation of suitable spinnbarkeit. However, intrauterine insemination (IUI) is more often the most appropriate therapy to overcome these obstacles. When mucosal hostility to sperm is because of cervical infection, antimicrobial therapy may be effective.

The cervix can also be the site of secretory immunologic reactions in which antisperm antibodies are produced, causing agglutination or immobilization of sperm. The most widely used serum–sperm bioassay to detect specific classes of antibodies in serum and seminal fluid is immunobead testing (IBT) (Lu, Huang, & Lu, 2008; Kumar et al., 2007). The IBT is considered clinically significant when 50% of the sperm are coated with immunobeads. The treatment for antisperm antibodies may include IUI of the man's washed sperm to bypass the cervical factor.

The **postcoital test (PCT)**, also called the **Huhner test**, is performed 1 or 2 days before the expected date of ovulation as determined by previous BBT charts, the length of prior cycles, or a urinary LH kit. This examination evaluates the cervical mucus, the number of active sperm in the cervical mucus, and the length of sperm survival (in hours) after intercourse.

The couple can have intercourse 2 to 8 hours before the examination. If the results are abnormal, the test should be repeated at the optimal time of 2 to 3 hours after intercourse. A small plastic catheter attached to a 10 ml syringe is placed in the cervix. Mucus is aspirated from the endocervical canal, measured, and examined microscopically for signs of infection, spinnbarkeit, ferning, number and motility of active spermatozoa per high-power field (HPF), and number of sperm with poor or no motility. The focus of the postcoital exam on the timing of intercourse may promote sexual difficulties in some infertile couples. Its use is controversial and has limited use in infertility workups because its value in assessing cervical hostility to sperm has never been proven (Kumar et al., 2007). Tests that can potentially predict the fertilizing ability of sperm include the zona-free hamster egg penetration assay and the hemizona test.

Evaluation of Uterine Structures and Tubal Patency

Uterine abnormalities are a relatively uncommon cause of infertility but should be considered. A few tests offer the ability to evaluate the uterine cavity and tubal patency simultaneously. These tests are usually done after BBT evaluation, semen analysis, and other less invasive tests. Tubal patency and uterine structure are usually evaluated by hysterosalpingography or laparoscopy. Other invasive tests used to evaluate only the uterine cavity are hysteroscopy and sonohysterography. Hysteroscopy may be performed earlier in the evaluation if the woman's history suggests potential for adhesive disease or uterine abnormalities.

Hysterosalpingography. **Hysterosalpingography (HSG)**, or *hysterogram,* involves an instillation of a radiopaque substance into the uterine cavity. In addition, the oil-based dye and injection pressure used in HSG may have a therapeutic effect. This effect may be caused by the flushing of debris, breaking of adhesions, or induction of peristalsis by the instillation.

The HSG should be performed in the follicular phase of the cycle to avoid interrupting an early pregnancy. This timing also avoids the lush secretory changes in the endometrium that occur after ovulation, which may prevent the passage of the dye through the tubes and present a false picture of obstruction of the entry point of the fallopian tube into the uterus. HSG causes moderate discomfort. The pain is referred from the peritoneum (which is irritated by the subdiaphragmatic collection of gas) to the shoulder. The cramping may be decreased if the radiopaque dye is warmed to body temperature before instillation. Women can take an over-the-counter (OTC) prostaglandin synthesis inhibitor (such as ibuprofen) 30 minutes before the procedure to decrease the pain, cramping, and discomfort. HSG can also cause recurrence of pelvic inflammatory disease, so prophylactic antibiotics are recommended to prevent infection that could be triggered by the procedure (Wright & Johnson, 2008).

Hysteroscopy. *Hysteroscopy* is the definitive method for both diagnosis and treatment of intrauterine pathology (Speroff & Fritz, 2005). Hysteroscopy allows the physician to further evaluate any areas of suspicion within the uterine cavity or fallopian tubes revealed by the HSG. It can be done in conjunction with a laparoscopy or independently in the office and does not require general anesthesia. A fiberoptic instrument called a hysteroscope is placed into the uterus for further evaluation of polyps, fibroids, or structural variations (Goldstein, 2008).

Laparoscopy. **Laparoscopy** enables direct visualization of the pelvic organs and is not routinely advised after a normal HSG unless symptoms suggest the need for earlier evaluation (Wright & Johnson, 2008). Diagnostic laparoscopy is an outpatient procedure requiring the use of general anesthesia. Generally, a three-puncture approach is used, entry is made through the umbilical area, and supporting instruments are inserted in two suprapubic incisions. The peritoneal cavity is distended with carbon dioxide gas so that the pelvic organs can be directly visualized with a fiberoptic instrument. Tube patency can be assessed by instillation of dye into the uterine cavity through the cervix. The pelvis is evaluated for endometriosis, adhesions, organ fixations, pelvic inflammatory disease, tumors, and cysts. The intraperitoneal gas is usually manually expressed at the end of the procedure. In routine preanesthesia instructions, the woman is told that she may have some discomfort from organ displacement and shoulder and chest pain caused by gas in the abdomen. She should be informed that she can resume normal activities as tolerated after 24 hours. Using postoperative pain medication and assuming a supine position may help relieve discomfort caused by any remaining gas.

ASSESSMENT OF THE MAN'S FERTILITY

Male infertility can be caused by numerous factors and categorized as ductal obstruction or abnormalities of sperm production or sperm function (Speroff & Fritz, 2005). Sperm function abnormalities may result from problems with sperm binding or penetration of the egg, prostatitis, or varocele. Varocele accounts for approximately 40% of male infertility (Speroff & Fritz, 2005). If the man's history indicates the need, he may be referred to a urologist for testing. A semen analysis of sperm quality, quantity, and motility is the single most important initial diagnostic study of the man. It should be done early in the couple's evaluation, before invasive testing of the woman.

To obtain accurate results, the specimen is collected after 2 to 3 days of abstinence, usually by masturbation, to avoid contamination or loss of any ejaculate. If the man has difficulty producing sperm by masturbation, special medical-grade condoms are available to collect the sperm during intercourse. Regular latex and nonlatex condoms should not be used because they contain agents that impair the motility of sperm, which can result in sperm loss in the condom. Most lubricants also are spermicidal and should not be used unless approved by the andrology laboratory. If the specimen is obtained at home, it needs to be brought to the lab within 1 hour and kept at body temperature so as not to impair motility.

Both seasonal and incidental variability may be seen in count and motility in successive semen analyses from the same individual. Thus a repeat semen analysis may be required to assess the man's fertility potential adequately; a minimum of two separate analyses is recommended for confirmation. In cases in which a known testicular insult has occurred (infection, high fevers, or surgery), a repeat analysis may not be done for at least 2.5 months to allow for new sperm maturation.

Sperm analysis provides information about sperm motility and morphology and a determination of the absolute number of spermatozoa present (Table 7–3). Although low numbers and motility may indicate compromised fertility, other parameters, such as morphology, motion patterns, and progression, are important prognostic indicators. Values previously thought to indicate subfertility may in fact be compatible with normal fertility when morphology, motion patterns, and progression factors are considered (Kumar et al., 2007). The quality of sperm decreases with increasing paternal age and may result in chromosomal damage. For example, fathers older than 50 years have infants at increased risk for trisomies.

A variety of environmental factors can affect male fertility. Causes of increased scrotal heat, such as jockey shorts, hot tubs, or occupations requiring long hours of sitting, are thought to decrease fertility potential, but there are no clinical studies to substantiate this belief (Honig, 2005). Heavy use of marijuana, alcohol, or cocaine can depress sperm count and testosterone levels; cigarette smoking may depress sperm motility (Quallich, 2006). The use of anabolic steroids lowers the body's ability to make endogenous testosterone, causing low sperm counts, which may not be reversible (Honig, 2005). Neurologic ejaculatory dysfunction can be associated with the use of drugs such as alpha blockers; for example, phentolamine, methyldopa, guanethidine, and reserpine. Sperm quality may be affected by medicines such as calcium channel blockers, propranolol, cimetidine, nitrofurantoin, or allopurinol/colchicines (Honig, 2005). Heavy metals (lead) and pesticide exposure can also reduce sperm count (Denson, 2006). A low sperm count of at least 10 million/ml may benefit from IUI because an increased concentrated amount of sperm can be deposited directly into the uterine cavity. For a sperm count of less than 5% normal forms, IVF with intracytoplasmic sperm injection (ICSI) is recommended (Speroff & Fritz, 2005).

Table 7–3 Normal Semen Analysis

Factor	Value
Volume	Greater than 2 ml
pH	7.0 to 8.0
Total sperm count	Greater than 20 million/ml
Liquefaction	Complete in 1 hour
Motility	50% or greater forward progression
Normal forms	30% or greater
Round cells	Less than 5 million/ml
White cells	Less than 1 million/ml

Source: World Health Organization. (1993). *The WHO laboratory manual for the examination of human semen and sperm-cervical mucus interaction* (3rd ed.). Geneva: Author.

Spermatozoa have been shown to possess intrinsic antigens that can provoke male immunologic infertility. Immunologic infertility is especially apparent following vasectomy reversals or genital trauma, such as testicular torsion, in which autoimmunity to sperm (the man produces antibodies to his own sperm) develops. Research indicates that it is the actual presence of antibodies on the spermatozoal surface (not just the presence of antibodies in the serum) that affects sperm function and thus leads to subfertility. Antisperm antibodies can be screened for by an immunobead binding test (Kumar et al., 2007). Treatment for antisperm antibodies is directed toward preventing the formation of antibodies or arresting the underlying mechanism that compromises sperm function. Therapies such as immunosuppression with corticosteroids and IUI have not proved effective. The treatment of choice for clinically significant antisperm antibodies is intracytoplasmic sperm injection (ICSI) in conjunction with IVF.

METHODS OF INFERTILITY MANAGEMENT

Methods of managing infertility include pharmacologic agents, therapeutic insemination, in vitro fertilization, and other assisted reproductive techniques.

Pharmacological Agents

This section provides a brief overview of the drugs commonly used for ovarian stimulation in the follicular phase, control of midcycle release, and support of the luteal phase. The pharmacologic treatment chosen depends on the specific cause of infertility. Table 7–4 lists some of the drugs commonly used and indications for use.

Clomiphene citrate. If a woman has normal ovaries, a normal prolactin level, and an intact pituitary gland, *clomiphene citrate* (Clomid or Serophene) is often used. This medication induces ovulation in 70% of women by actions at both the hypothalamic

Table 7–4 Drugs Commonly Used to Treat Infertility

	INDICATIONS	
Drug	**Women**	**Men**
Clomiphene citrate (Clomid, Serophene)	PCOS Hyperandrogenemia Premature follicle rupture	Low levels of gonadotrophins Hypothalamic hypogonadism
Human menopausal gonadotropin (hMG), (Repronex, Bravelle)	Hypothalamic ovulatory dysfunction (after failure of clomiphene) Hypopituitarism PCOS (rarely) Luteinized unruptured follicle syndrome (after failure of hCG alone) Inadequate cervical mucus In vitro fertilization, GIFT, ZIFT Controlled super-ovulation	Hypothalamic pituitary failure due to Kallmann syndrome or delayed puberty Hypo-gonadotrophic hypogonadism (deficiency of FSH and LH)
Recombinant follicle-stimulating hormone (rFSH) (Follistim, Gonal-F)	PCOS Too long cycles In vitro fertilization, GIFT, ZIFT	
Human chorionic gonadotropin (hCG) (Pregnyl, Novarel, A.P.L)	Induces dominant follicle to release egg Luteinized unruptured follicle syndrome	
Bromocriptine (Parlodel)	Pituitary adenoma	Hyperprolactinemia (functional or pituitary adenoma)
Cabergoline (Dostinex)	Hyperpituitarism	
Gonadotropin releasing hormone (GnRh) (Factral, Lutre-pulse)	Hypothalamic ovulatory dysfunction—to ensure a pulsatile release of GnRH by a small pump	Hypothalamic pituitary failure due to Kallmann syndrome or delayed puberty (pulsed infusion)
GnRh analogs ■ Leuprolide acetate (Lupron) ■ Nafarelin acetate (Synarel) ■ Goserelin acetate (Zoladex)	Premature follicular rupture In vitro fertilization, GIFT, ZIFT Endometriosis	Hypogonadotrophic hypogonadism
GnRH antagonists ■ Ganirelix acetate (Antagon)	Same as GnRH analogs	
Progesterone (Crinone, Prometrium, progesterone in oil)	Luteal phase dysfunction Luteal phase support	

Source: Adapted from American Society for Reproductive Medicine Booklet. (2006). *Medications for inducing ovulation—A guide for patients.* http://www.org/patientbooklets/ovulation_drugs.pdf; Shane. J. (1993). Evaluation and treatment of infertility. *Clinical Symposia, 45(2)*; Wilson, B. A., Shannon, M. T., Shields, K. M., & Stang, C. L. (2009). *Prentice Hall nurse's drug guide 2009.* Upper Saddle River, NJ: Pearson Education.

and ovarian levels; 30% to 40% of these women will become pregnant. Approximately 10% of women develop multiple-gestation pregnancies, almost exclusively twins (Storment 2006). Clomiphene citrate works by stimulating the hypothalamus to secrete more gonadotropin-releasing hormone (GnRH). This increases the secretion of LH and FSH, which stimulates follicle growth and facilitates the release of ova (Speroff & Fritz, 2005).

For the first course the woman usually takes 50 mg/day orally for 5 days from cycle day (CD) 3 to day 7 or CD 5 to day 9. In nonresponders, the dose may be increased to 100 mg/day to a maximum of 250 mg/day, although doses in excess of 100 mg/day are not approved by the FDA (Wilson, Shannon, Shields et al., 2009). The woman may need to take estrogen simultaneously if a decrease in cervical mucus occurs.

The woman is informed that if ovulation occurs, it is expected 5 to 9 days after the last dose. The nurse determines if the couple has been advised to have sexual intercourse every other day for 1 week, beginning 5 days after the last day of medication. Upon a negative pregnancy test, another trial of clomiphene can be initiated. After the first treatment cycle, a pelvic ultrasound should be done to rule out ovarian enlargement, ovarian cysts, or hyperstimulation. Ovarian enlargement and abdominal discomfort (bloating) may result from follicular growth and formation of multiple corpora lutea. Persistence of ovarian cysts is a contraindication for further treatment regimens. Other side effects include hot flashes, abdominal distention, bloating, breast discomfort, nausea and vomiting, vision problems (such as visual spots), headache, and dryness or loss of hair (Wright & Johnson, 2008). Supplemental low-dose estrogen may be given to ensure appropriate quality and quantity of cervical mucus, or IUI may be employed to overcome this obstacle. Women can assess the presence of ovulation and possible response to clomiphene therapy by doing BBT and urinary LH tests. The woman should be knowledgeable about side effects and call her healthcare provider if they occur. When visual disturbances (flashes, blurring, or spots) occur, bright lighting should be avoided. This side effect disappears within a few days or weeks after discontinuation of therapy. The occurrence of hot flashes may be because of the antiestrogenic properties of clomiphene citrate. The woman can obtain some relief by increasing intake of fluids and using fans.

Gonadotropins. Therapy using *human menopausal gonadotropins (hMGs),* which include menotropins (Repronex and Menopur) and urofollitropin (Bravelle), is indicated as a first line of therapy for anovulatory infertile women with low to normal levels of gonadotropins (FSH and LH). It is a second line of therapy in women who fail to ovulate or conceive with clomiphene citrate therapy and in women undergoing controlled ovarian stimulation with assisted reproduction. Menotropin is a combination of FSH and LH, and urofollitropin is a further purified form and contains mainly FSH with trace amounts of LH. Immediately before injection, the powder is reconstituted with diluent and injected subcutaneously.

More recently, however, recombinant gonadotropins (rFSH and rLH) have been produced, giving rise to more consistent preparations. Recombinant FSH is homogenous and free of contaminants by proteins. Luveris, a recombinant form of LH, is used concomitantly with recombinant FSH in women with profound LH deficiency. It is thought that the use of recombinant gonadotropins will eventually become the preferred preparation and that the use of urinary preparations will be phased out.

Gonadotropin therapy requires close observation by means of serum estradiol levels and ultrasound. Monitoring of follicle development is necessary to minimize the risk of multiple fetuses and to avoid ovarian hyperstimulation syndrome. The daily dose of medication given is titrated based on serum estradiol and ultrasound findings. Then once follicle maturation has occurred, hCG may be administered by intramuscular or subcutaneous injection to induce final follicular maturation and stimulate ovulation. The couple is advised to have intercourse 24 to 36 hours after hCG administration and for the next 2 days. Women who elect to undergo ovarian stimulation with gonadotropins have usually passed through all other forms of management without conceiving. Strong emotional support and thorough education are needed because of the numerous office visits and injections. Often the male partner is instructed, with return demonstration, to administer the daily injections.

Bromocriptine. High prolactin levels may impair the glandular production of FSH and LH or block their action on the ovaries. When hyperprolactinemia accompanies anovulation, the infertility may be treated with bromocriptine (Parlodel). This medication acts directly on the prolactin-secreting cells in the anterior pituitary. It inhibits the pituitary's secretion of prolactin, thus preventing suppression of the pulsatile secretion of FSH and LH. This restores normal menstrual cycles and induces ovulation by allowing FSH and LH production. If treatment is successful, the tests of ovulatory function will indicate that ovulation is occurring with a normal luteal phase. Bromocriptine should be discontinued if pregnancy is suspected or at the anticipated time of ovulation because of its possible teratogenic effects. Other side effects include nausea, diarrhea, dizziness, headache, and fatigue, which can be attributed to the dopaminergic action of bromocriptine. To minimize side effects for women who are extremely sensitive, treatment may be initiated with a dose of 1.25 mg, slowly building tolerance toward the usual dose of 2.5 mg bid. An intravaginal preparation may also be used to decrease the occurrence of side effects (Wright & Johnson, 2008).

Aromatase inhibitors. Aromatase inhibitors (letrozole [Femara] and anastrozole [Arimidex]) are medications that reduce estrogen levels and have been successfully used for ovulation induction. They are currently FDA approved for postmenopausal breast cancer. Pregnancy rates have been reported to be comparable to clomiphene citrate (American Society of Reproductive Medicine, 2006c). Recent data have raised concern that letrozole may be associated with an increased risk of congenital abnormalities.

Other Pharmacologic Agents

Pharmacologic treatments for endometriosis-related infertility involve use of danazol (Danocrine), oral contraceptives or oral medroxyprogesterone acetate, and gonadotropin-releasing hormone (GnRH) agonists. The management and care of endometriosis is further discussed in Chapter 6 ∞. Treatment of luteal phase defects may include the use of progesterone to augment luteal phase progesterone levels. Ovulation-induction agents, such as clomiphene citrate or menotropins, may be used to augment proliferative phase FSH production in the developing follicle, as women with luteal phase defects have been found to have decreased FSH production in the proliferative phase. This is associated with a decline in luteal phase progesterone and estrogen production and is manifested by an out-of-phase endometrial biopsy. It is also common to use progesterone supplementation in conjunction with these ovulation-induction agents for luteal phase support, thereby increasing endometrial receptivity for embryonic implantation. Occasionally hCG therapy may be used in the luteal phase to stimulate corpus luteum production of progesterone.

Therapeutic Insemination

Therapeutic insemination has replaced the previously used term *artificial insemination* and involves the depositing of semen at the cervical os or in the uterus by mechanical means. *Therapeutic husband insemination (THI)* is the current term for use of the husband's semen, and *therapeutic donor insemination (TDI)* is the current term for use of donor semen.

THI is generally indicated for such seminal deficiencies as oligospermia (low sperm count), asthenospermia (decreased motility), and teratospermia (low percentage, abnormal morphology); for anatomic defects accompanied by inadequate deposi-

Complementary Care

COMMON TREATMENTS FOR INFERTILITY

Couples experiencing infertility may seek out alternative treatments. Some common treatments include acupuncture and herbs.

Acupuncture: Acupuncture is a therapy used in traditional Chinese medicine (TCM), and has become a popular complementary treatment. Acupuncture involves inserting sterile needles into specific points on the body to control the flow of chi, or life energy. Acupuncture treatment would focus on balancing the flow of chi in the kidneys and adrenal glands. Several clinical studies have shown acupuncture to be effective in treating infertility in both men and women (Cheong, Hung Yu Ng, & Ledger, 2008).

Herbal Treatments: Herbs frequently recommended to treat infertility include ginseng and astragalus. Herbalists cite the healing and hormone-balancing effects of these herbs. Ginseng has historically been used in TCM to enhance male virility and fertility. Several studies also cite ginseng, as well as astragalus, in enhancing in vitro sperm motility (Skidmore-Roth, 2006).

The nurse should be alert for signs that the couple is pursuing complementary therapies out of desperation. A sensitive, nonjudgmental approach will go a long way toward comforting a couple and assuring them that many complementary therapies used are helpful and not harmful.

tion of semen such as hypospadia (a congenital abnormal male urethral opening on the underside of the penis); and for ejaculatory dysfunction (such as retrograde ejaculation). THI is also indicated in cases of unexplained infertility and some cases of female factor infertility, such as scant or inhospitable mucus, persistent cervicitis, or cervical stenosis. In some cases, IUI would be indicated to bypass the cervical factor. Seminal fluid contains high levels of prostaglandins, which can cause nausea, severe cramps, abdominal pain, and diarrhea when absorbed by the uterine lining. Therefore, sperm preparation for IUI involves washing sperm from the seminal plasma. IUI, with or without ovulation-induction therapy, is an option for many couples before more aggressive treatments such as in vitro fertilization are employed.

TDI is considered in cases of azoospermia (absence of sperm), severe oligospermia or asthenospermia, inherited male sex-linked disorders, and autosomal dominant disorders. In the past several years, indications for donor insemination have expanded to include single women or lesbians who want to become pregnant. Some states have specified the parental rights of single women and donors, but most are silent on this issue.

TDI has become more complicated and expensive in the past decade because of the need for strict screening and processing procedures to prevent transmission of a genetic defect or sexually transmitted infection to the offspring or recipient. Guidelines have been established that include mandatory medical (genetic) and infectious disease screening of both donor and recipient, the need for informed consent from all parties, the need to limit the number of pregnancies per donor, and the need for accurate means of record keeping. Finally, because of the risk of transmitting infectious diseases, donated sperm must be frozen and quarantined for 6 months from the time of acquisition, and the donor must be retested before sperm can be released for use.

Numerous factors need to be evaluated before TDI is performed. Has every possible effort been made to diagnose and treat the cause of the male infertility? Do tests indicate normal fertility and sperm–ovum transport in the woman? Has the couple had an opportunity to discuss this option with an infertility counselor to explore the issues of secrecy, disclosure, and potential feelings of loss the couple (particularly the male partner) may feel about not having a genetic child? Are there any religious constraints? After making the decision, the couple should allow themselves time to further assess their concerns and explore their feelings individually and together to ensure that this option is acceptable to both.

In Vitro Fertilization

In vitro fertilization (IVF) is selectively used in cases when infertility has resulted from tubal factors, mucous abnormalities, male infertility, unexplained infertility, male and female immunologic infertility, and cervical factors. In IVF a woman's eggs are collected from her ovaries, fertilized in the laboratory, and placed into her uterus after normal embryo development has begun. If

Developing Cultural Competence

INFERTILITY TREATMENTS

The acceptance of infertility treatments varies widely around the world. Some belief systems do not allow various treatments, because using a treatment is considered interfering with God's design or because the treatment itself is seen as tainted or sinful. For example, fertility practices in Arab cultures are influenced by traditional Arab Bedouin values that support tribal dominance and beliefs that "God decides family sizes." In Arab cultures, procreation is the purpose of marriage.

If a couple is infertile, the approved methods for treating infertility are limited to use of therapeutic insemination using the husband's sperm and *in vitro* fertilization involving the fertilization of the wife's ovum by the husband's sperm because of lineage concerns (Purnell & Paulanka, 2008). Sterility in a woman can lead to rejection and divorce. Also with the use of ICSI, male-initiated divorce is becoming more common for aging wives of infertile husbands (Inhorn, 2002). Contemporary Islamic religious opinion forbids any kind of egg, embryo, or semen donation, as well as surrogacy (Inhorn, 2002).

In Jewish cultures, infertile couples are to try all possible means to have children, including egg and sperm donation. However, Orthodox Jewish opinion is virtually unanimous in prohibiting therapeutic insemination when the semen donor is a Jewish man other than the woman's husband, because it may constitute adultery (Purnell & Paulanka, 2008). If the infertility is because of a male factor, therapeutic insemination with sperm from a non-Jewish sperm donor is acceptable because "Jewishness" is conferred through the matriline. IVF and embryo transfer (ET) are also acceptable artificial insemination methods because they do not involve putting sperm into another's wife (Kahn, 2002).

the procedure is successful, the embryo continues to develop in the uterus, and pregnancy proceeds naturally.

The potential for a successful pregnancy with IVF is maximized when three to four embryos (rather than one) are placed into the uterus. For this reason, fertility drugs are used to induce ovulation before the process. Follicular development and oocyte maturity are monitored frequently with ultrasound and hormonal assays. Monitoring usually begins around cycle day 5, and medications are titrated according to individual response. When follicles appear mature, hCG is given to stimulate final egg maturation and control the induction of ovulation. Egg retrieval is performed approximately 35 hours later, before ovulation occurs.

In the majority of cases, egg retrieval is performed by a transvaginal approach under ultrasound guidance (Figure 7–5 ●). It is an outpatient procedure performed with intravenous sedation and a cervical block for anesthesia. Many follicles can be aspirated with only one puncture, and the procedure generally lasts no more than 30 minutes. Once the eggs are fertilized and progress to the embryo stage, the embryos are placed in the uterus. This occurs 1 to 2 days after conception. After the procedure, the woman is advised to engage in only minimal activity for 12 to 24 hours, and progesterone supplementation is prescribed. The progesterone supplementation is given to promote implantation and support the early pregnancy; therefore, she will not have a period even if she is not pregnant (the pregnancy is usually determined by transvaginal ultrasound).

Sperm used to fertilize the eggs in vitro can be obtained naturally or via microsurgical epididymal sperm aspiration (MESA) or testicular sperm aspiration (TESA). These are procedures that address severe male factor infertility. MESA and TESA involve the retrieval of sperm from the gonadal tissue of men who have azoospermia or an ejaculatory disorder (Figure 7–6 ●). Percutaneous epididymal sperm aspiration (PESA) and TESA are replacing MESA as the preferred techniques for retrieval of sperm because they are not surgical procedures. ICSI is a microscopic procedure to inject a single sperm into the outer layer of an ovum so that fertilization will occur (Devine, 2008).

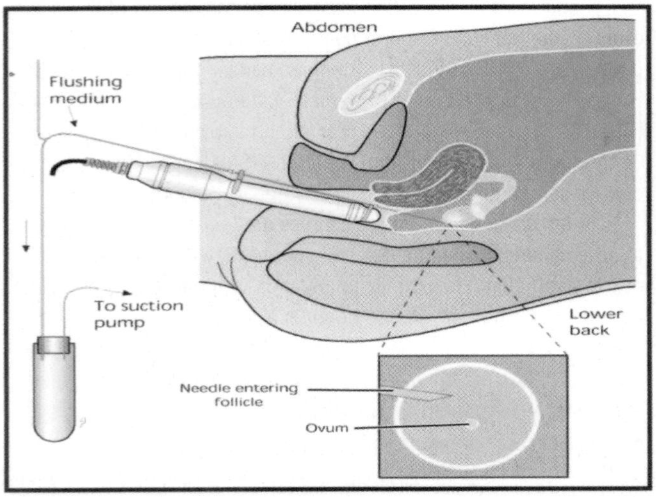

● **Figure 7–5** Transvaginal ultrasound-guided oocyte retrieval.

Source: Courtesy of Serone, Inc., Rockland, MA.

Evidence in Action

Acupuncture in conjunction with embryo transfer improves the rate of pregnancy and live birth in women undergoing in vitro fertilization (Systematic review and meta-analysis) (Manheimer, Zhang, Udoff, et al., 2008).

Success with IVF depends on many factors, but especially the woman's age and the specific indication. Women have a good chance of achieving pregnancy with an average of three cycles of IVF. Many couples find the emotional, physical, and financial costs of going beyond three cycles too great. Costs vary by treatment and by region of the country: one cycle of IVF-ET averages $12,400 (American Society of Reproductive Medicine, 2006a). Clinical birth rates reported by the Society of Assisted Reproductive Technology (SART) were 50% per egg donation for women regardless of age or indication in the United States (American Society of Reproductive Medicine, 2008). An increase in maternal and neonatal morbidity is associated with IVF because the rates of multiple fetuses remain an issue.

Other Assisted Reproductive Techniques

Other assisted reproductive techniques include procedures for transfer of gametes, zygotes, or embryos; cryo-preservation of embryos; IVF using donor oocytes; micromanipulation techniques; and use of a gestational carrier.

Gamete intrafallopian transfer. **Gamete intrafallopian transfer (GIFT)** involves three steps: (1) the retrieval of oocytes by laparoscopy; (2) immediate placement of the oocytes in a catheter with washed, motile sperm; and (3) placement of the gametes into the fimbriated end of the fallopian tube. Fertilization occurs in the fallopian tube as with normal conception (in vivo) rather than in the laboratory (in vitro). The fertilized egg then travels through the fallopian tube to the uterus for implantation as in normal reproduction. GIFT may be more acceptable than other procedures such as ZIFT to adherents of some religions (Roman Catholic Church), because fertilization does not occur outside the woman's body.

From the GIFT technology evolved procedures such as **zygote intrafallopian transfer (ZIFT)** and **tubal embryo transfer (TET)**. In these procedures eggs are retrieved and incubated with the man's sperm. However, the eggs are transferred back to the woman's body at a much earlier stage of cell division than in IVF and, as in GIFT, are placed in the fallopian tube or tubes and not the uterus. In TET the placement is done at the embryo stage. These procedures allow fertilization to be documented, which is not possible with GIFT, and the pregnancy rate is theoretically increased when the fertilized ovum is placed in the fallopian tube.

Preimplantation genetic diagnosis (PGD). Other recent advances in micromanipulation allow a single cell to be removed from the embryo for genetic study. Couples at risk for having a detectable single gene or chromosomal anomaly may wish to undergo such preimplantation genetic testing, called *blastomere analysis* or, more recently, *preimplantation genetic diagnosis (PGD)*. The single cell is

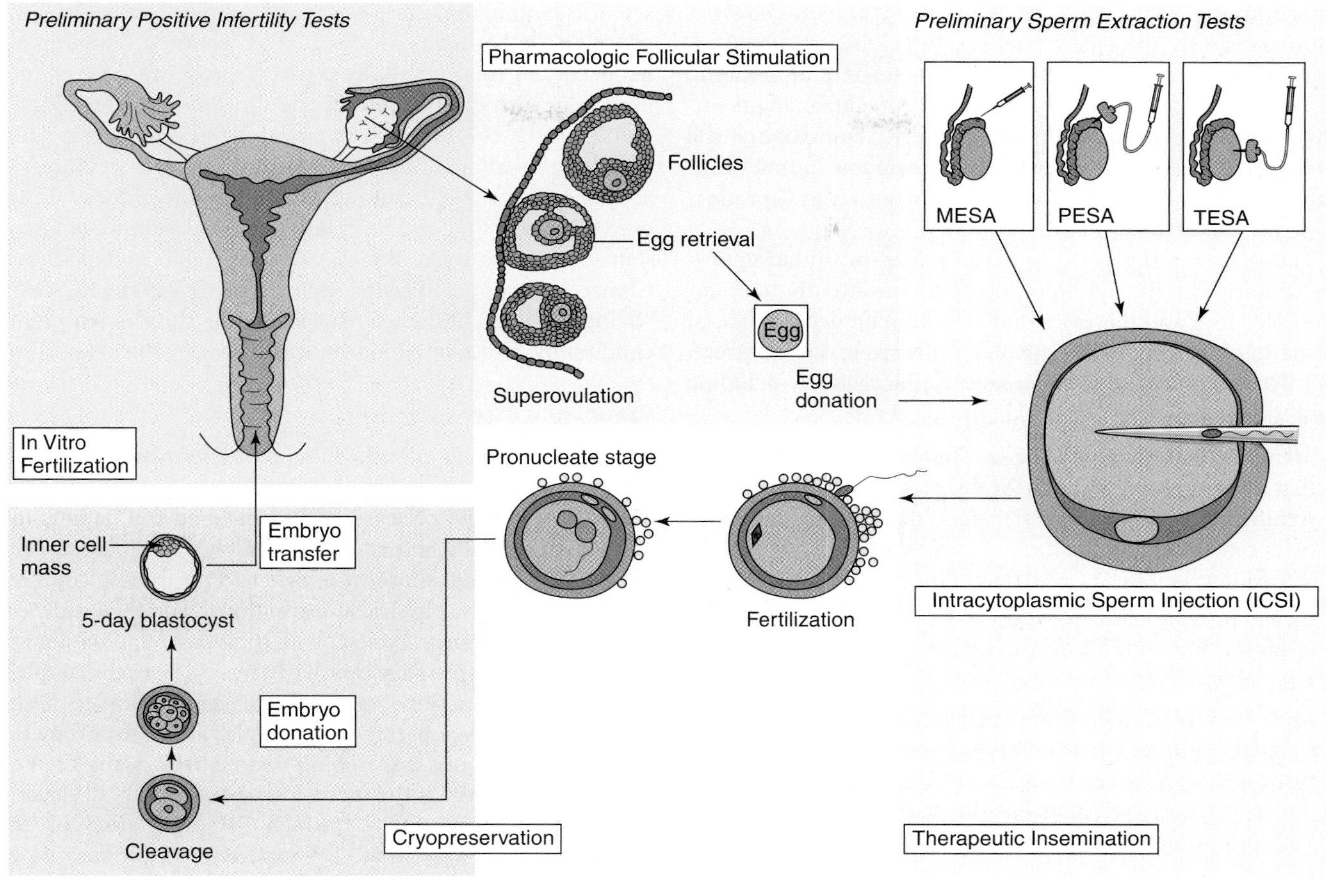

Figure 7–6 Assisted reproductive techniques.

Evidence-Based Nursing

ACUPUNCTURE AND ASSISTED CONCEPTION

Clinical Question

Is acupuncture effective in helping women conceive?

The Evidence

Families who have difficulty conceiving are often interested in any measures that may increase their chance of successful pregnancy and birth. Acupuncture has been studied as a potential adjunct to assisted reproductive treatment. Cheong, Hung, & Ledger (2008) appraised 13 randomized controlled trials of adjunct acupuncture during assisted reproductive treatments. A meta-analysis was conducted, which allows the authors to draw conclusions about the magnitude of effect that may be produced by the intervention. While these trials each had small samples, in aggregate they represent a strong level of evidence.

Best Practice

The data from this meta-analysis suggest that acupuncture may increase the live birth rate when combined with assisted reproductive treatment, but only when it is performed on the day of the embryo transfer. The live birth rate of those receiving acupuncture on the day of embryo transfer was 35% compared with 22% for those without acupuncture. However, the authors caution that it is difficult to control the placebo effect in studies of acupuncture, and so these numbers may be inflated. There is no benefit to performing acupuncture at the time of oocyte retrieval or in repeating the acupuncture 2 to 3 days after the transfer. No single acupuncture point or procedure was found to be the most effective. Acupuncture after conception and in early pregnancy should be avoided until evidence is generated that demonstrates no harm to mother or baby (Cheong, Hungy, & Ledger, 2008).

Critical Thinking

1. What is the best acupuncture procedure to assure optimal results?
2. What are potential complications of acupuncture in early pregnancy?

See MyNursingKit for possible responses.

obtained from a six- to eight-cell embryo by a process known as blastomere biopsy. The genetic content of the cell is examined using polymerase chain reaction (PCR) technique or fluorescence in situ (FISH). Results of genetic testing on the preimplantation embryos are available in 4 to 24 hours, so unaffected embryos may still be transferred during the required biologic window of time without the need for cryopreservation (American Society of Reproductive Medicine Practice Committee, 2008).

The diagnosis of genetic disorders before implantation provides couples with the option of foregoing the attempt to establish a pregnancy and thereby avoiding a difficult decision about terminating an affected pregnancy (Simpson & Holzgreve, 2007). This technology also raises several ethical issues, including the following:

- Identification of couples at risk. There is a need for criteria that identify couples at risk for diseases that constitute significant hardship and suffering so that "wrongful birth" cases can be avoided.
- Availability of and access to centers providing PGD. Should society provide access for those at risk for genetic transfer of disease but without the financial resources to pay for the services?
- Analysis of blastomeres for sex chromosome testing when a genetic disorder carried on the sex chromosomes is suspected. In X-linked diseases, the only way to prevent the disorder is to select against the blastomere with the Y chromosome.
- Identification of late-onset diseases. The Human Genome Project has aided in the identification of genetic markers for late-onset disease. Couples may wish to choose to implant blastomeres that do not carry these markers.
- Effect on the offspring as a result of removing cells from the embryo
- Selection for nonmedical reasons and potential concern of eugenics "designer babies"

A micromanipulation procedure called *assisted embryo hatching* has proved to be an effective adjunct therapy in IVF. In vitro fertilization using a *gestational carrier* (surrogacy) allows infertile women who are genetically sound but unable to carry a pregnancy to exercise the option of having their own biologic child. Other technologies involve oocyte donation and cryopreservation of the embryo.

Adoption

Infertile couples consider various alternatives for resolving their infertility, and adoption is one option that may be considered at several points during the treatment process. As couples begin to consider adoption, important aspects of this exploration are the gathering of information from magazines, books, informational websites, and organizations such as the National Adoption Information Clearinghouse; attending adoption support groups and conferences; and meeting with adoptive parents to discuss their experiences with adoption.

The adoption of a healthy American infant can be difficult and frustrating, often involving long waiting periods, continual setbacks, and high costs. Thus many couples seek international adoption or consider adopting older children, children with handicaps, or children of mixed parentage, because the adoption process in such cases is quicker and more children are available. Nurses in the community can assist couples considering adoption by providing information on community resources for adoption and support through the adoption process. Couples need support if they remain childless, either by choice or circumstance. Informational books, websites such as Childless by Choice, and support groups such as San Francisco RESOLVE's "living without children" are available for couples who remain childless by choice or circumstance at *www.resolve.org*.

Pregnancy After Infertility

The feeling of being infertile does not necessarily disappear with pregnancy. Although there may be initial ecstasy, couples may face a whole new arena of fear and anxiety, and the parents-to-be often do not know where they "fit in." They may feel a great sense of isolation because those who have had no trouble conceiving cannot relate to the physical and emotional pain they endured to achieve the pregnancy. Contact with their past support system of other infertile couples may vanish when peers learn the couple has resolved their infertility. Although the desperation to become pregnant may have superseded the couple's ability to acknowledge their concerns about undergoing various treatments or procedures, questions about the repeated cycle of fertility drugs or the achievement of pregnancy through IVF technology or cryopreservation may now arise. The expectant couple may be very concerned about the potential of these treatments to adversely affect the fetus (Wright & Johnson, 2008). Couples may need reassurance throughout the pregnancy to allay these anxieties. The nurse can assist couples who conceive after infertility by acknowledging their past experiences of infertility treatment; validating their fears and anxieties as they face childbirth classes, birth, and parenting issues; and providing support and education about what to anticipate physically and emotionally throughout the pregnancy. The nurse can also counsel couples that infertility because of nonstructural causes may correct itself following a successful pregnancy and birth; therefore, postchildbirth contraception counseling may be warranted. These interventions will go a long way toward normalizing the experience for the couple.

Nursing management. Infertility therapy taxes a couple's financial, physical, and emotional resources. Treatment can be costly, and insurance coverage is limited. Years of effort and numerous evaluations and examinations may take place before conception occurs, if it occurs at all. In a society that values children and considers them to be the natural result of marriage, infertile couples face a myriad of tensions and discrimination.

Clinic nurses need to be constantly aware of the emotional needs of the couple confronting infertility evaluation and treatment. Often an intact marriage will become stressed with intrusive infertility procedures and treatments. Constant attention to temperature charts and instructions about their sex life from a person outside the relationship naturally affects the spontaneity of a couple's interactions. Tests and treatments may heighten feelings of frustration or anger between partners. The need to share this intimate area of a relationship, especially when one or the other is identified as "the cause" of infertility, may precipitate feelings of guilt or shame. Infertility often becomes a central focus for role identity, especially for women (Devine, 2008).

The couple may experience feelings of loss of control, feelings of reduced competency and defectiveness, loss of status and ambiguity as a couple, a sense of social stigma, stress on the marital and sexual relationship, and a strained relationship with healthcare providers. The nurse's roles can be summarized as those of counselor, educator, and advocate.

Tasks of the infertile couple and appropriate nursing interventions are summarized in Table 7–5. Throughout the evaluation process nurses play a key role in lessening the stress these couples must endure by providing resources and accurate information about what is entailed in treatment and what physical, emotional, and financial demands they can anticipate throughout the process (Klock, 2004).

The nurse's ability to assess and respond to emotional and educational needs is essential to give infertile couples a sense of control and help them negotiate the treatment process. An assessment tool such as an infertility questionnaire (Table 7–6) may be helpful. Extensive and repeated explanations and written instruction may be necessary because the couple's anxiety often overwhelms their ability to retain all the information given. It is important to use a nursing framework that recognizes the multidimensional needs of the infertile individual or couple within physical, social, psychologic, spiritual, and environmental contexts.

Infertility may be perceived as a loss by one or both partners. Affected individuals have described this as a loss of their relationship with spouse, family, or friends; their health; their status or prestige; their self-esteem and self-confidence; their security; and

Table 7–5 Tasks of the Infertile Couple

Tasks	Nursing Interventions
Recognize how infertility affects their lives and express feelings (may be negative toward self or mate)	Supportive: Help to understand and facilitate free expression of feelings
Grieve the loss of potential offspring	Help to recognize feelings
Evaluate reasons for wanting a child	Help to understand motives
Decide about management	Identify alternatives; facilitate partner communication

Source: Sawatzky, M. (1981). Tasks of the infertile couple. *Journal of Obstetric, Gynecologic, and Neonatal Nursing, 10,* 132.

Table 7–6 Infertility Questionnaire

Self-Image

1. I feel bad about my body because of our inability to have a child.
2. Since our infertility, I feel I can do anything as well as I used to.
3. I feel as attractive as before our infertility.
4. I feel less masculine/feminine because of our inability to have a child.
5. Compared with others, I feel I am a worthwhile person.
6. Lately, I feel I am sexually attractive to my wife/husband.
7. I feel I will be incomplete as a man/woman if we cannot have a child.
8. Having an infertility problem makes me feel physically incompetent.

Guilt/Blame

1. I feel guilty about somehow causing our infertility.
2. I wonder if our infertility problem is because of something I did in the past.
3. My spouse makes me feel guilty about our problem.
4. There are times when I blame my spouse for our infertility.
5. I feel I am being punished because of our infertility.

Sexuality

1. Lately I feel I am able to respond to my spouse sexually.
2. I feel sex is a duty, not a pleasure.
3. Since our infertility problem, I enjoy sexual relations with my spouse.
4. We have sexual relations for the purpose of trying to conceive.
5. Sometimes I feel like a "sex machine," programmed to have sex during the fertile period.
6. Impaired fertility has helped our sexual relationship.
7. Our inability to have a child has increased my desire for sexual relations.
8. Our inability to have a child has decreased my desire for sexual relations.

Note: The questionnaire is scored on a Likert scale, with responses ranging from "strongly agree" to "strongly disagree." Each question is scored separately, and the mean score is determined for each section (Self-Image, Guilt/Blame, and Sexuality). The total mean score is then divided by 3. A final mean score of greater than 3 indicates distress.

Source: From Bernstein, J., Potts, N., & Mattox, J. H. (1985). Assessment of psychological dysfunction association with infertility. *Journal of Obstetric, Gynecologic, and Neonatal Nursing*, 14 (Suppl.), 64S, Table 1. Washington DC: Author. © 1985 by the Association of Women's Health, Obstetric and Neonatal Nurses. All rights reserved.

the potential child. Any one of these losses may lead to depression, but in many cases the crisis of infertility evokes feelings similar to those associated with all these losses (Klock, 2004). Each couple passes through several stages of feelings: surprise, denial, anger, isolation, guilt, grief, and resolution. The impact of these feelings on the couple and how fast they move into resolution, if ever, may depend on the cause and on the duration of treatment. Each partner may progress through the stages at different rates (Kumar et al., 2007). Nonjudgmental acceptance and a professional, caring attitude on the nurse's part can go far in dissipating the negative emotions the couple may experience while going through these stages. Recognition of these stages can assist the nurse in providing appropriate support and counseling or referral for additional therapy.

This is also a time when the nurse may assess the couple's relationship: Are both partners able and willing to communicate verbally and share feelings? Are the partners mutually supportive? The answers to such questions may help the nurse to identify areas of strength and weakness and to construct an appropriate plan of care.

Referral to mental health professionals is helpful when the emotional issues become too disruptive in the couple's relationship or life. The couple should be aware of infertility support and education organizations such as RESOLVE (National Infertility Association), which may help meet some of their needs and validate their feelings. Finally, individual or group counseling with other infertile couples can help the couple resolve feelings brought about by their own difficult situation.

GENETIC DISORDERS

Even when conception has been achieved, families can have special reproductive concerns. The desired and expected outcome of any pregnancy is the birth of a healthy, "perfect" baby. Parents experience grief, fear, and anger when they discover that their baby has been born with a defect or a genetic disease. Such an abnormality may be evident at birth or may not appear for some time. The baby may have inherited a disorder from one parent or both, creating guilt and strife within the family.

MyNursingKit Video: What Is a Gene?

Regardless of the type or scope of the problem, parents will have many questions: "What did I do?" "What caused it?" "How do I cope with it?" "Will it happen again?" The nurse must anticipate the couple's questions and concerns and guide, direct, and support the family. To do so, the nurse must have a basic knowledge of genetics and genetic counseling. Professional nurses can help expedite this process if they understand the principles involved and can direct the family to the appropriate resources.

CHROMOSOMES AND CHROMOSOMAL ANALYSIS

All hereditary material is carried on tightly coiled strands of DNA known as **chromosomes**. The chromosomes carry the *genes,* the smallest units of inheritance, as discussed in greater detail in Chapter 4. The Human Genome Project has made remarkable advances toward determining the exact DNA sequence of human genes and the precise genes that are associated with certain abnormalities such as fragile X syndrome and cystic fibrosis, as discussed in greater detail later in the chapter (Ward, 2008).

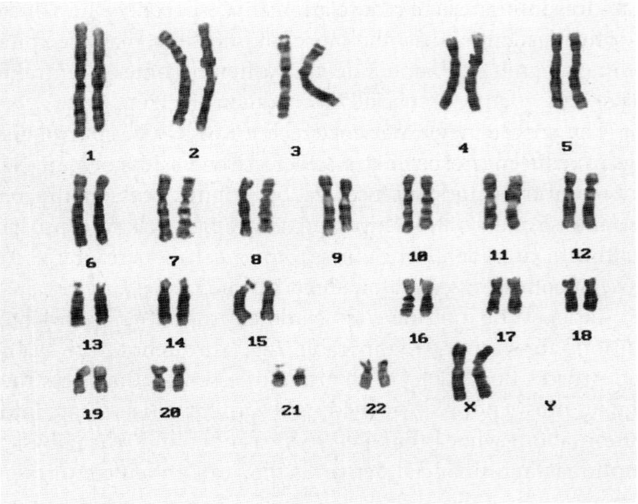

Figure 7–7 Normal female karyotype.

Source: Courtesy of David Peakman, Reproductive Genetics Center, Denver, CO.

All *somatic (body) cells* have 23 pairs of homologous chromosomes (a matched pair of chromosomes, one inherited from each parent) (see Chapter 4). Twenty-two of the pairs are **autosomes** (nonsex chromosomes), and one pair is made up of the sex chromosomes, X and Y. A normal female has a 46, XX chromosome constitution, the normal male, 46, XY (Figures 7–7 and 7–8 ●).

The **karyotype**, or pictorial analysis of these chromosomes, is usually obtained from specially treated and stained peripheral blood lymphocytes. Placental tissue taken from a site near the insertion of the cord and deep enough to include chorion can also be sent for karyotyping of the fetus.

Chromosome abnormalities can occur in either the autosomes or the sex chromosomes and can be divided into two categories: abnormalities of number and abnormalities of structure. Even small alterations in chromosomes can cause problems, especially those associated with delayed growth and development. Some of these abnormalities can be passed on to other offspring.

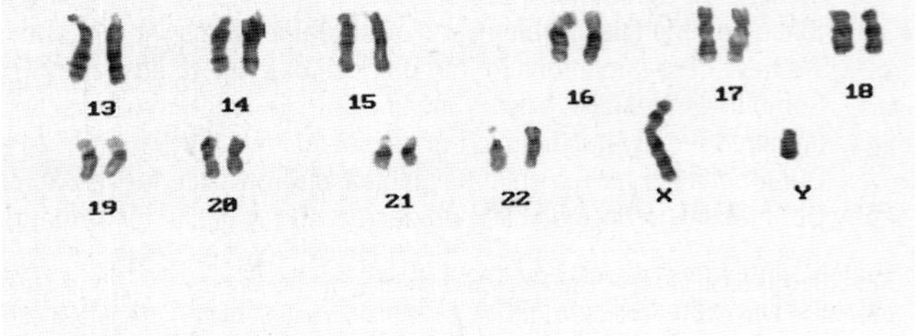

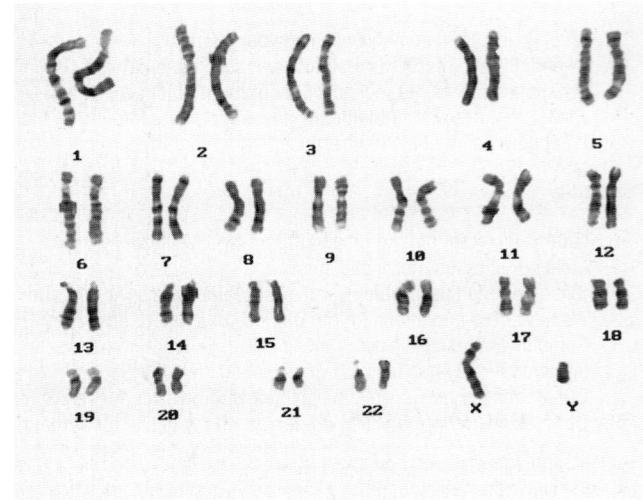

Figure 7–8 Normal male karyotype.

Source: Courtesy of David Peakman, Reproductive Genetics Center, Denver, CO.

Thus in some cases chromosomal analysis is appropriate even if clinical manifestations are mild.

Abnormalities of Chromosomal Number

Abnormalities of chromosomal number are most commonly seen as trisomies, monosomies, and mosaicism. In all three cases, the abnormality is most often caused by *nondisjunction,* a failure of paired chromosomes to separate during cell division. If nondisjunction occurs in either the sperm or the egg before fertilization, the resulting zygote (fertilized egg) will have an abnormal chromosome makeup in all of the cells (trisomy or monosomy). If nondisjunction occurs after fertilization, the developing zygote will have cells with two or more different chromosome makeups, evolving into two or more different cell lines (mosaicism).

Trisomies are the product of the union of a normal gamete (egg or sperm) with a gamete that contains an extra chromosome. The individual will have 47 chromosomes and be trisomic (has three copies of the same chromosome) for whichever chromosome is extra (Table 7–7). Down syndrome

Table 7–7 Chromosomal Syndromes

Altered chromosome: 21	Characteristics
Genetic defect: trisomy 21 (Down syndrome) (secondary nondisjunction or 14/21 unbalanced translocation) Incidence: average 1 in 700 live births, incidence variable with age of woman (Figures 7–9 and 7–10)	CNS: mental retardation; hypotonia at birth Head: flattened occiput; depressed nasal bridge; mongoloid slant of eyes; epicanthal folds; white specking of the iris (Brushfield spots); protrusion of the tongue; high, arched palate; low-set ears Hands: broad, short fingers; abnormalities of finger and foot; dermal ridge patterns (dermatoglyphics); transverse palmar crease (simian line) Other: congenital heart disease
Altered chromosome: 18	**Characteristics**
Genetic defect: trisomy 18 Incidence: 1 in 3,000 live births	CNS: mental retardation; severe hypotonia Head: prominent occiput; low-set ears; corneal opacities; ptosis (drooping eyelids) Hands: third and fourth fingers overlapped by second and fifth fingers; abnormal dermatoglyphics; syndactyly (webbing of fingers) Other: congenital heart defects; renal abnormalities; single umbilical artery; gastrointestinal tract abnormalities; rocker-bottom feet; cryptorchidism; various malformations of other organs
Altered chromosome: 13	**Characteristics**
Genetic defect: trisomy 13 Incidence: 1 in 5,000 live births	CNS: mental retardation; severe hypotonia; seizures Head: microcephaly; microphthalmia, and/or coloboma (keyhole-shaped pupil); malformed ears; aplasia of external auditory canal; micrognathia (abnormally small lower jaw); cleft lip and palate Hands: polydactyly (extra digits); abnormal posturing of fingers; abnormal dermatoglyphics Other: congenital heart defects; hemangiomas; gastrointestinal tract defects; various malformations of other organs
Altered chromosome: 5P	**Characteristics**
Genetic defect: deletion of short arm of chromosome 5 (cri du chat, or cat-cry syndrome) Incidence: 1 in 20,000 live births	CNS: severe mental retardation; a catlike cry in infancy Head: microcephaly; hypertelorism (widely spaced eyes); epicanthal folds; low-set ears Other: failure to thrive; various organ malformations
Altered chromosome: X (sex chromosome)	**Characteristics**
Genetic defect: only one X chromosome or partially missing second X chromosome in female (Turner syndrome) Incidence: 1 in 300 to 7,000 live female births (Figure 7–13 ●)	CNS: no intellectual impairment; some perceptual difficulties Head: low hairline; webbed neck Trunk: short stature; cubitus valgus (increased carrying angle of arm); excessive nevi (congenital discoloration of skin because of pigmentation); broad, shieldlike chest with widely spaced nipples; puffy feet; no toenails Other: fibrous streaks in ovaries; underdeveloped secondary sex characteristics; primary amenorrhea; usually infertile; renal anomalies; coarctation of the aorta
Altered chromosome: XXY (sex chromosome)	**Characteristics**
Genetic defect: extra X chromosome in male (Klinefelter syndrome) Incidence: 1 in 1,000 live male births	CNS: mild mental retardation Trunk: occasional gynecomastia (abnormally large male breasts); eunuchoid body proportions (lack of male muscular and sexual development) Other: small, soft testes; underdeveloped secondary sex characteristics; usually sterile

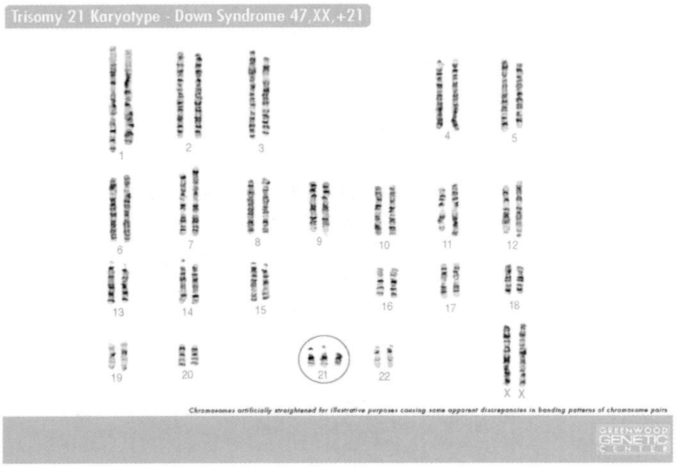

● **Figure 7–9** Karyotype of a female who has trisomy 21, Down syndrome. Note the extra 21 chromosome.

Source: Courtesy of Greenwood Genetics Center. (2002). *Genetic counseling aids*, 4th ed.

(formerly called mongolism) is the most common trisomy seen in children (see Figure 7–9 ●). The presence of the extra chromosome 21 produces distinctive clinical features (Figure 7–10 ●). Although children born with Down syndrome have a variety of physical ailments, advances in medical science have extended their life expectancy.

Two other common trisomies are trisomy 18 and trisomy 13 (refer to Table 7–7 and Figures 7–11 and 7–12 ●). The prognosis for both trisomies 13 and 18 is extremely poor. Most children (70%) die within the first 3 months of life secondary to complications related to respiratory and cardiac abnormalities. However, 10% survive the first year of life; therefore, the family needs to plan for the possibility of long-term care of a severely affected infant and for family support.

Monosomies occur when a normal gamete unites with a gamete that is missing a chromosome. In this case, the individual has only 45 chromosomes and is said to be monosomic. Monosomy of an entire autosomal chromosome is incompatible with life.

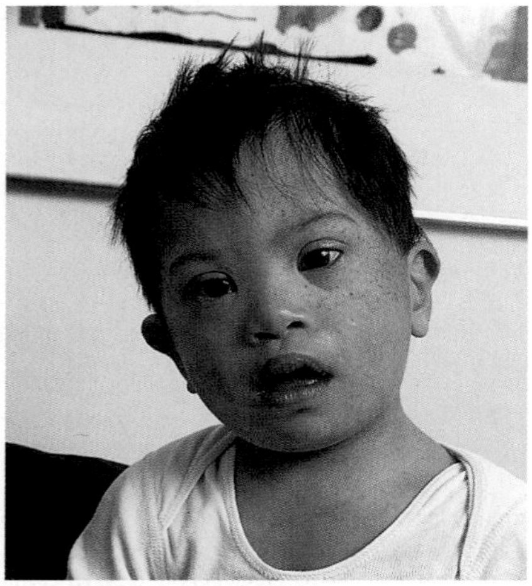

● **Figure 7–10** A boy with Down syndrome.

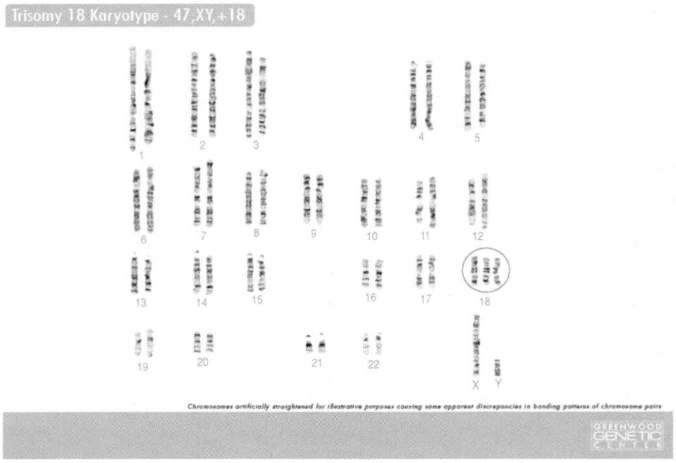

● **Figure 7–11** Karyotype of a male who has trisomy 18.

Source: Courtesy of Greenwood Center. (2002). *Genetic counseling aids*, 4th ed.

Mosaicism occurs after fertilization and results in an individual who has two different cell lines, each with a different chromosomal number. Mosaicism tends to be more common in the sex chromosomes than in the autosomes; when it occurs in the autosomes, it is most common in Down syndrome. An individual with many classic signs of Down syndrome but with normal or near-normal intelligence should be investigated for the possibility of mosaicism.

Abnormalities of Chromosome Structure

Abnormalities of chromosome structure involve only parts of the chromosome and occur in two forms: translocation and deletions or duplications. Some children born with Down syndrome have an abnormal rearrangement of chromosomal material known as a *translocation*. Clinically the two types of Down syndrome are indistinguishable; the only way to distinguish them is to do a chromosome analysis.

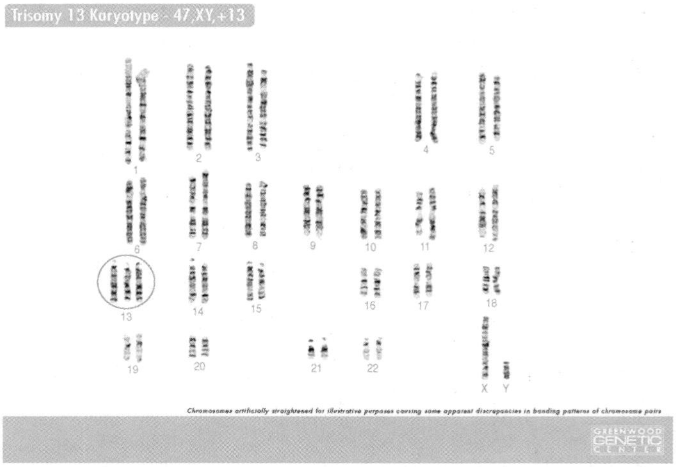

Trisomy 13 Karyotype - 47,XY,+13
Chromosomes artificially straightened for illustrative purposes causing some apparent discrepancies in banding patterns of chromosome pairs
GREENWOOD GENETIC CENTER

● **Figure 7–12** Karyotype of male with trisomy 13.

Source: Courtesy of Greenwood Center. (2002). *Genetic counseling aids*, 4th ed.

The translocation occurs when the carrier parent has 45 chromosomes, usually with one chromosome fused to another. For example, a common translocation is one in which a particle of chromosome 14 breaks and fuses to chromosome 21. The parent has one normal 14, one normal 21, and one 14/21 chromosome. Because all the chromosomal material is present and functioning normally, the parent is clinically normal. This individual is known as a *balanced translocation carrier.* When a person who is a balanced translocation carrier has a child with a partner who has a structurally normal chromosome constitution, the child can have a normal number of chromosomes, be a carrier, or have an extra chromosome 21. Such a child has an *unbalanced translocation* and has Down syndrome.

Structure abnormality is also caused by *duplications* or *deletions* of chromosomal material. Any portion of a chromosome may be lost or added, generally leading to some adverse effect. Depending on how much chromosomal material is involved, the clinical effects may be mild or severe. Many types of duplications and deletions have been described, such as the deletion of the short arm of chromosome 5 (*cri du chat,* or cat-cry syndrome) or the deletion of the long arm of chromosome 18 (Edwards syndrome). Table 7–7 lists other chromosomal syndromes.

Sex Chromosome Abnormalities

To better understand abnormalities of the sex chromosomes, the nurse should know that in a female, at an early embryonic stage, one of the two normal X chromosomes becomes inactive. The inactive X chromosome forms a dark staining area known as the *Barr body.* The normal female has one Barr body, because one of her two X chromosomes has been inactivated. The normal male has no Barr bodies because he has only one X chromosome.

The most common sex chromosome abnormalities are Turner syndrome in females (45, X with no Barr bodies present; see Figure 7–13●) and Klinefelter syndrome in males (47, XXY with one Barr body present). See Table 7–7 for clinical descriptions of these abnormalities.

The mosaic form of the X chromosome is associated with daughters of women who took the drug diethylstilbestrol (DES) during pregnancy. The fertility of women with the mosaic form of the XO chromosome may not be impaired; however, there is a higher percentage of uterine malformation and hormonal difficulty associated with it and therefore a high degree of miscarriage.

There is a concern that children born as a result of ICSI might be at increased risk for chromosomal and other major congenital anomalies, cancer, or infertility, because ICSI may override natural safeguards that serve to prevent fertilization. Therefore it is strongly recommended that karyotyping and Y chromosome deletion analysis be offered to all men with severe male factor infertility who are candidates for IVF and ICSI (Speroff & Fritz, 2005).

MODES OF INHERITANCE

Many inherited diseases are produced by an abnormality in a single gene or pair of genes. In such instances, the chromosomes are grossly normal. The defect is at the gene level. Some of these gene defects can be detected by technologies such as DNA and other

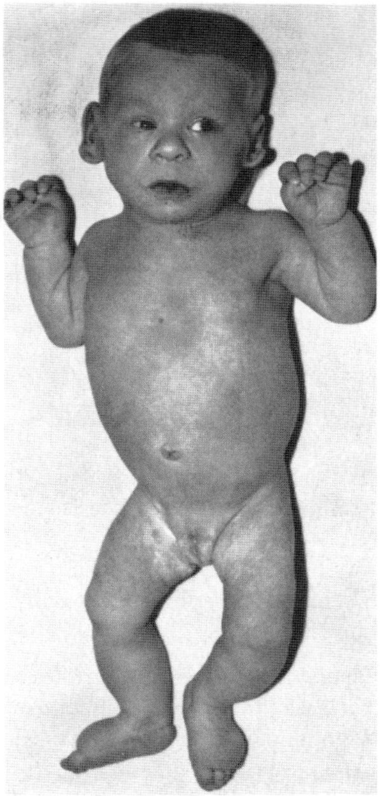

● **Figure 7–13** Infant with Turner syndrome at 1 month of age. Note prominent ears.

Source: Lemli, L., & Smith, D. W. (1963). The XO syndrome: A study of the differentiated phenotype in 25 patients. *Journal of Pediatrics, 63,* 577, with permission from Elsevier Science.

biochemical assays. The two major categories of inheritance are **Mendelian (single-gene) inheritance** and **non-Mendelian (multifactorial) inheritance**. Each single-gene trait is determined by a pair of genes working together. These genes are responsible for the observable expression of the traits (e.g., brown eyes, dark skin), referred to as the **phenotype**. The total genetic makeup of an individual is referred to as the **genotype** (pattern of the genes on the chromosomes).

One of the genes for a trait is inherited from the mother, the other from the father. An individual who has two identical genes at a given locus is considered to be *homozygous* for that trait. Individuals are considered to be *heterozygous* for a particular trait when they have two different alleles (alternate forms of the same gene) at a given locus on a pair of homologous chromosomes.

The best known modes of single-gene inheritance are autosomal dominant, autosomal recessive, and X-linked (sex-linked) recessive. There is also an X-linked dominant mode of inheritance, which is less common, and the new identified mode of inheritance, fragile X syndrome.

Autosomal Dominant Inheritance

A person is said to have an autosomal dominant inherited disorder if the disease trait is heterozygous—that is, the abnormal

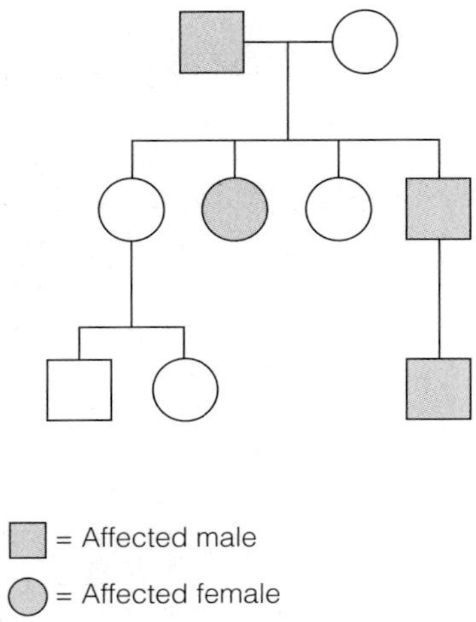

● **Figure 7–14** Autosomal dominant pedigree. One parent is affected. Statistically 50% of offspring will be affected regardless of sex.

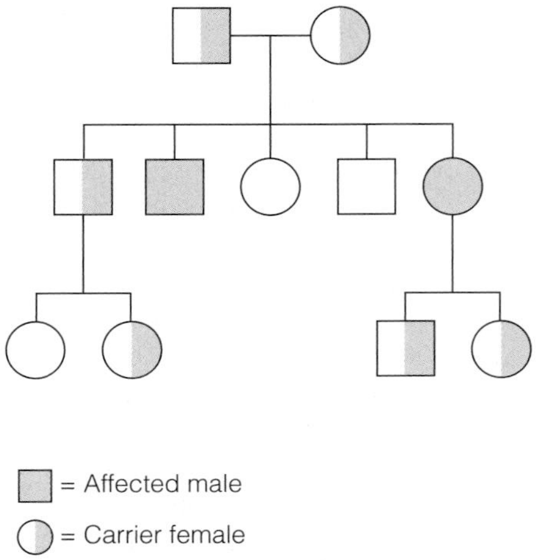

● **Figure 7–15** Autosomal recessive pedigree. Both parents are carriers. Statistically 25% of offspring are affected regardless of sex.

gene overshadows the normal gene of the pair to produce the trait. It is essential to remember that in autosomal dominant inheritance the following occurs:

- An affected individual generally has an affected parent. Thus the family **pedigree** (graphic representation of a family tree) usually shows multiple generations with the disorder.
- Affected individuals have a 50% chance of passing on the abnormal gene to each of their children (Figure 7–14 ●).
- Males and females are equally affected, and a father can pass the abnormal gene on to his son. This is an important principle when distinguishing autosomal dominant disorders from X-linked disorders.
- Autosomal dominant inherited disorders have varying degrees of presentation. This is an important factor when counseling families concerning autosomal dominant disorders. Although a parent may have a mild form of the disease, the child may have a more severe form.

Autosomal dominant conditions such as phocomelia (a developmental anomaly characterized by the absence of the upper portion of the limbs) can have minimal expression in a parent but severe effects in a child. Other common autosomal dominant inherited disorders are Huntington disease, polycystic kidney disease, neurofibromatosis (von Recklinghausen disease), and achondroplastic dwarfism.

Autosomal Recessive Inheritance

In an autosomal recessive inherited disorder, the individual must have two abnormal genes to be affected. The notion of a carrier state is appropriate here. A *carrier* is an individual who is heterozygous for the abnormal gene and clinically normal. It is not until two individuals mate and pass on the same abnormal gene that affected children may appear. It is essential to remember that in autosomal recessive inheritance the following occurs:

- An affected individual may have clinically normal parents, but both parents are carriers of the abnormal gene (Figure 7–15 ●).
- In the case where both parents are carriers, there is a 25% chance that the abnormal gene will be passed on to any of their offspring. Each pregnancy has a 25% chance of resulting in an affected child.
- If a child of two carrier parents is clinically normal, there is a 50% chance that the child is a carrier of the gene.
- Both males and females are equally affected.
- There is an increased history of consanguineous matings (mating of close relatives).

Some common autosomal recessive inherited disorders are cystic fibrosis, phenylketonuria (PKU), galactosemia, sickle cell anemia, Tay–Sachs disease, and most metabolic disorders.

X-Linked Recessive Inheritance

X-linked, or sex-linked, disorders are those for which the abnormal gene is carried on the X chromosome. Thus an X-linked disorder is manifested in a male who carries the abnormal gene on his X chromosome. His mother is considered to be a carrier when the normal gene on one X chromosome overshadows the abnormal gene on the other X chromosome. It is essential to remember that in X-linked recessive inheritance the following occurs:

- There is no male-to-male transmission. Affected males are related through the female line (see Figure 7–16 ●).
- There is a 50% chance that a carrier mother will pass the abnormal gene to each of her sons, who will thus be affected.
- There is a 50% chance that a carrier mother will pass the normal gene to each of her sons, who will thus be unaffected.
- There is a 50% chance that a carrier mother will pass the abnormal gene to each of her daughters, who become carriers.
- Fathers affected with an X-linked disorder cannot pass the disorder to their sons, but all their daughters become carriers of the disorder.

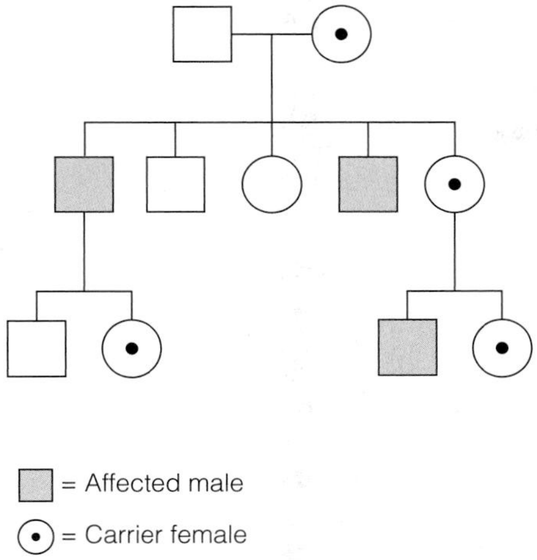

● **Figure 7–16** X-linked recessive pedigree. The mother is the carrier. Statistically 50% of male offspring are affected, and 50% of female offspring are carriers.

Common X-linked recessive disorders are hemophilia, Duchenne muscular dystrophy, and color blindness.

X-Linked Dominant Inheritance

X-linked dominant disorders are extremely rare, the most common being vitamin D–resistant rickets and fragile X syndrome. When X-linked dominance does occur, the pattern is similar to that of X-linked recessive inheritance except that heterozygous females are affected. It is essential to remember that in X-linked dominant inheritance there is no male-to-male transmission. Affected fathers will have affected daughters; however, because they pass only the Y chromosome to male offspring, any sons will not be affected.

Fragile X Syndrome

Fragile X syndrome is a common inherited form of mental retardation second only to Down syndrome among all causes of moderate mental retardation in males. Fragile X syndrome is a central nervous system disorder linked to a "fragile" site on the X chromosome. It is characterized by moderate mental retardation, large protuberant ears, and large testes after puberty. The carrier females do not have the abnormal features, but about one-third are mildly retarded.

Multifactorial Inheritance

Many common congenital malformations such as cleft palate, heart defects, spina bifida, dislocated hips, clubfoot, and pyloric stenosis are caused by an interaction of many genes and environmental factors. They are, therefore, multifactorial in origin. It is essential to remember that in multifactorial inheritance the following occurs:

- The malformations may vary from mild to severe. For example, spina bifida may range in severity from mild (spina bifida occulta) to more severe (myelomeningocele). It is believed that the more severe the defect, the greater the number of genes present for that defect.
- There is often a sex bias. For example, pyloric stenosis is more common in males, whereas cleft palate is more common in females. When a member of the less commonly affected sex shows the condition, a greater number of genes must usually be present to cause the defect.
- In the presence of environmental influences (such as seasonal changes, altitude, radiation exposure, chemicals in the environment, or exposure to toxic substances), fewer genes are needed to manifest the disease in the offspring.
- In contrast to single-gene disorders, there is an additive effect in multifactorial inheritance. The more family members who have the defect, the greater the risk that the next pregnancy will also be affected (Ward, 2008).

Although most congenital malformations are multifactorial, a careful family history should always be taken, because cleft lip and palate, certain congenital heart defects, and other malformations occasionally can be inherited as autosomal dominant or recessive traits. Other disorders thought to be within the multifactorial inheritance group are diabetes, hypertension, some heart diseases, and mental illness.

PRENATAL DIAGNOSTIC TESTS

Parent–child and family-planning counseling have become a major responsibility of professional nurses. To be effective counselors, nurses must have the most up-to-date information about prenatal diagnosis. Appropriate counseling should occur before prenatal screening is done. It is essential that couples be completely informed about the known and potential risks of each of the genetic diagnostic procedures. The prescreening counseling should include the conditions detectable by the screen, diagnostic test available if the screen is positive, risk to the mother and child of the test performed, accuracy of the test, and limitations of the test (Lashley, 2007). The nurse needs to recognize the emotional impact on the family of a decision to undergo or not to undergo a genetic diagnostic procedure.

The ability to diagnose certain genetic diseases has enormous implications for the practice of preventive health care. Several methods are available for prenatal diagnosis, although some are still experimental.

Genetic Ultrasound

Ultrasound may be used to assess the fetus for genetic or congenital problems. With ultrasound, one can visualize the fetal head for abnormalities in size, shape, and structure. (For a detailed discussion of ultrasound technology, see Chapter 14∞.) Craniospinal defects (anencephalus, microcephaly, hydrocephalus), thoracic malformations (diaphragmatic hernia), gastrointestinal malformations (omphalocele, gastroschisis), renal malformations (dysplasia or obstruction), and skeletal malformations (caudal regression, conjoined twins) are only some of the disorders that have been diagnosed in utero by ultrasound. Screening by ultrasound for congenital anomalies is best done at 18 to 20 weeks, when fetal structures have developed completely. With the addition of fetal nuchal translucency measurement at 10 to 13 weeks, there is high correlation with fetal chromosome abnormalities (Lashley, 2007). There is no information documenting harm to the fetus or long-term effects with exposure to ultrasound. However, there is no guarantee of complete safety; therefore, the practitioner and the parents must evaluate the risks against the benefits on an individual basis.

Genetic Amniocentesis

A major method of prenatal diagnosis is genetic amniocentesis (Figure 7–17 ●). The procedure is described in Chapter 14. The indications for genetic amniocentesis include the following:

1. *Maternal age 35 or older.* Women age 35 or older are at greater risk for having children with chromosomal abnormalities (see Chapter 9 for further discussion). Chromosomal abnormalities because of maternal age include trisomy 21, trisomy 13, trisomy 18, XXX, or XXY. The risk of having a live-born infant with a chromosome problem is 1 in 192 for a 35-year-old woman; the risk for trisomy 21 is 1 in 386. At age 44, the risks are 1 in 26 and 1 in 40, respectively (Ward, 2008).
2. *Previous child born with a chromosomal abnormality.* Young couples who have had a child with a trisomy 21, 18, or 13 have an approximately 1% to 2% risk of a future child having a chromosomal abnormality.
3. *Parent carrying a chromosomal abnormality (balanced translocation).* A woman who carries a balanced 14/21 translocation has a risk of approximately 10% to 15% that her children will be affected with the unbalanced translocation of Down syndrome; if the father is the carrier, there is a 2% to 5% risk.
4. *Mother carrying an X-linked disease.* In families in which the woman is a known or possible carrier of an X-linked disorder such as hemophilia A or B or Duchenne's muscular dystrophy, options may include genetic amniocentesis, chorionic villus sampling (CVS), or percutaneous umbilical blood sampling (PUBS). For a known female carrier, the risk of an affected male fetus is 50%. Now DNA testing may make it possible to identify affected males from nonaffected males in some disorders. In disorders in which female carriers can be distinguished from noncarriers, only the carrier females would be offered prenatal diagnosis.

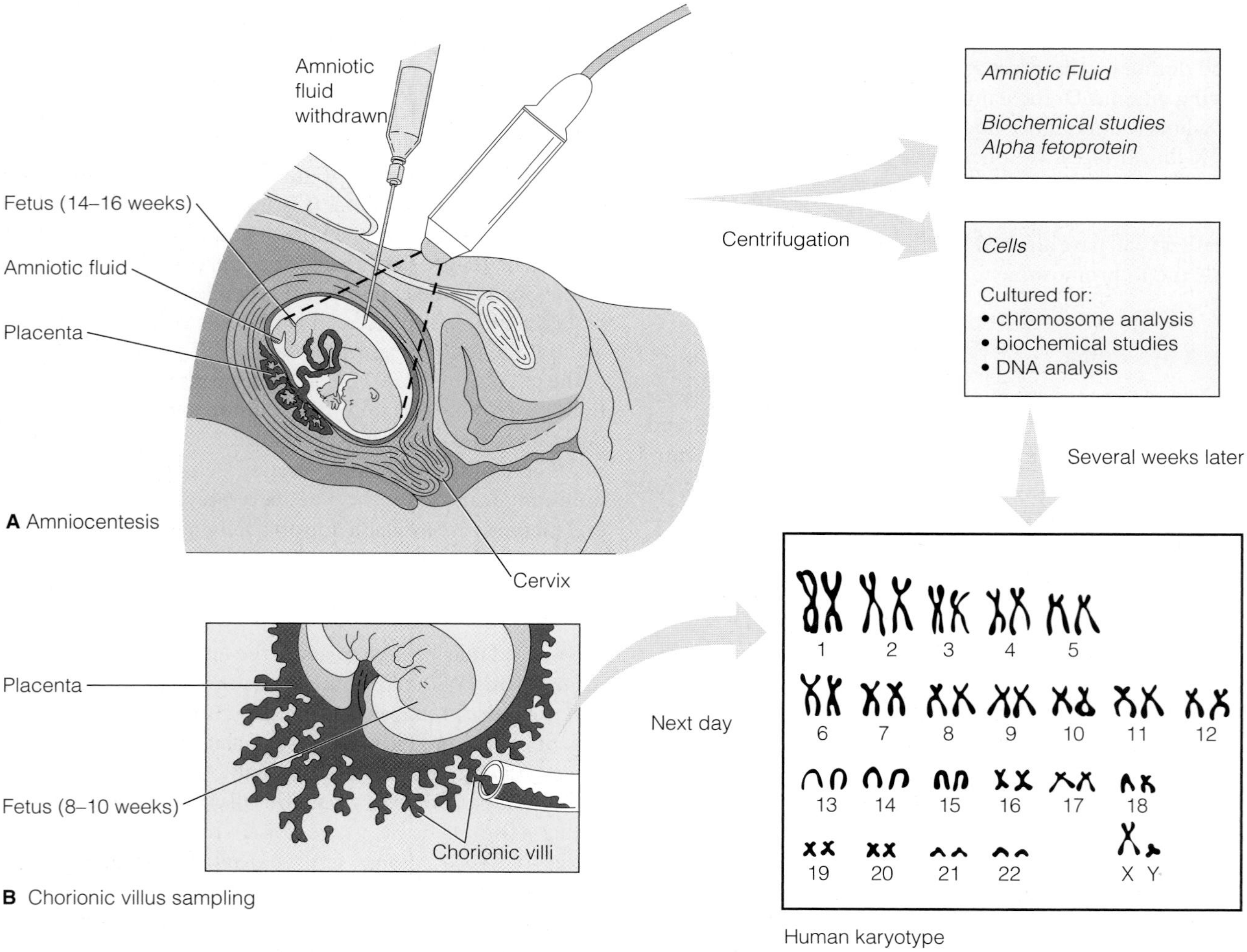

● **Figure 7–17** ***A,*** Genetic amniocentesis. This method used for prenatal diagnosis is done at 14 to 16 weeks' gestation. ***B,*** Chorionic villus sampling is done at 8 to 10 weeks, and the cells are karyotyped within 48 to 72 hours.

5. *Parents carrying an inborn error of metabolism that can be diagnosed in utero.* Inborn error of metabolism disorders detectable in utero include argininosuccinicaciduria, cystinosis, Fabry disease, galactosemia, Gaucher disease, homocystinuria, Hunter syndrome, Hurler syndrome, Krabbe disease, Lesch–Nyhan disease, maple syrup urine disease, metachromatic leukodystrophy, methylmalonic aciduria, Niemann–Pick disease, Pompe disease, Sanfilippo syndrome, and Tay–Sachs disease.
6. *Both parents carrying an autosomal recessive disease.* When both parents are carriers of an autosomal recessive disease, there is a 25% risk for *each pregnancy* that the fetus will be affected. Diagnosis is made by testing the cultured amniotic fluid cells (enzyme level, substrate level, product level, or DNA) or the fluid itself. Autosomal recessive diseases identified by amniocentesis are hemoglobinopathies such as sickle cell anemia, thalassemia, and cystic fibrosis (Dugoff, 2008).
7. *Family history of neural tube defects.* Genetic amniocentesis is available to couples who have had a child with neural tube defects or who have a family history of these conditions, which include anencephaly, spina bifida, and myelomeningocele. Neural tube defects are usually multifactorial traits.

Percutaneous Umbilical Blood Sampling and Chorionic Villus Sampling

Percutaneous umbilical blood sampling (PUBS) is a technique used for obtaining blood that allows for rapid chromosome diagnosis, genetic studies, or transfusion for Rh isoimmunization or hydrops fetalis. *Chorionic villus sampling (CVS)* is used in selected regional centers, and its diagnostic capability is similar to that of amniocentesis. Its advantage is that diagnostic information is available at 8 to 10 weeks' gestation and that products of conception are tested directly. Some potential risks include loss of pregnancy or limb-reduction defects especially if performed before 10 weeks gestation. For further discussion, see Chapter 14∞.

Alpha-Fetoprotein

The maternal circulation or amniotic fluid is tested for alpha-fetoprotein (AFP). The maternal serum AFP (MSAFP) level is elevated in cases of infants with open neural tube defects, anencephaly, omphalocele, or gastroschisis, and in multiple gestations (Lashley, 2007). Low MSAFP level has been associated with Down syndrome. MSAFP testing is done at 15 to 22 weeks' gestation (Lashley, 2007). In addition other screening labs may include maternal serum free beta human chorionic gonadotropin (hCG) and maternal serum-pregnancy-associated plasma protein (PAPP-A) to detect Down syndrome. Ultrasound and amniocentesis are offered to clients with low or high MSAFP levels. Inaccurate dating is the most common cause for abnormal AFP; therefore, ultrasound dating is very important. With high MSAFP levels, normal amniotic fluid AFP, and normal ultrasound, there is an increased risk for preterm labor, perinatal death, and intrauterine growth restriction.

Implications of Prenatal Diagnostic Testing

It is imperative that counseling precede any procedure for prenatal diagnosis. Many questions and points must be considered if the family is to reach a satisfactory decision. See "Developing Cultural Competence: Genetic Screening Recommendations for Various Ethnic and Age Groups."

With the advent of diagnostic techniques such as amniocentesis, at-risk couples who would not otherwise have a first child or additional children can decide to conceive. (See "Health Promotion: Couples Who May Benefit from Prenatal Diagnosis.") Following prenatal diagnosis, a couple can decide not to have a child with a genetic disease. For many couples, prenatal diagnosis is not a solution because they choose not to prevent the genetic disease by aborting the fetus. The decision about whether to use prenatal diagnosis can only be made by the family. Even when termination is not an option, prenatal diagnosis can give parents an opportunity to prepare for the birth of a child with special needs, contact the families of children with similar problems, or access support services before the birth.

HEALTH PROMOTION

COUPLES WHO MAY BENEFIT FROM PRENATAL DIAGNOSIS

- Women age 35 or over at time of birth
- Couples with a balanced translocation (chromosomal abnormality)
- Family history of known or suspected Mendelian genetic disorder (e.g., cystic fibrosis, hemophilia A and B, Duchenne muscular dystrophy)
- Couples with a previous child with chromosomal abnormality
- Couples in which either partner or a previous child is affected with, or in which both partners are carriers for, a diagnosable metabolic disorder
- Family history of birth defects and/or mental retardation (e.g., neural tube defects, congenital heart disease, cleft lip and/or palate)
- Ethnic groups at increased risk for specific disorders (see "Cultural Perspectives: Genetic Screening Recommendations for Various Ethnic and Age Groups" on page 162)
- Couples with history of two or more first trimester spontaneous abortions
- Women with an abnormal maternal serum alpha-fetoprotein (MSAFP or AFP) test
- Women with a teratogenic risk secondary to an exposure or maternal health condition (e.g., diabetes)

Developing Cultural Competence

GENETIC SCREENING RECOMMENDATIONS FOR VARIOUS ETHNIC AND AGE GROUPS

BACKGROUND OF POPULATION AT RISK	DISORDER	SCREENING TEST	DEFINITIVE TEST
Ashkenazic Jewish, French-Canadians, Cajuns	Tay-Sachs disease	Decreased serum hexosaminidase-A or DNA mutation analysis	CVS* or amniocentesis for hexosaminidase-A assay or DNA mutation analysis
African; Hispanic from Caribbean, Central America, or South America; Arabs; Egyptians; Asian Indians	Sickle cell anemia	Presence of sickle-cell hemoglobin; confirmatory hemoglobin electrophoresis	CVS or amniocentesis for DNA mutation analysis
Greek, Italian	Beta-thalassemia	Mean corpuscular volume less than 80%; confirmatory hemoglobin electrophoresis	CVS or amniocentesis for DNA mutation analysis
Southeast Asian (Vietnamese, Laotian, Cambodian), Filipino	Alpha-thalassemia	Mean corpuscular volume less than 80%; confirmatory hemoglobin electrophoresis	CVS or amniocentesis for DNA mutation analysis
Women over age 35 (all ethnic groups)	Chromosomal trisomies	Prenatal serum and/or ultrasound screening	CVS or amniocentesis for cytogenetic analysis
Women of any age (all ethnic groups; particularly suggested for women from British Isles, Ireland)	Neural tube defects and selected other anomalies	Maternal serum alpha-fetoprotein (MSAFP)	Amniocentesis for amniotic fluid, alpha-fetoprotein (AFP) and acetylcholinesterase assays
Ashkenazic Jewish	Gaucher disease	Decrease glucocerebrosidase	CVS
Caucasians (Northern Europeans, Celtic population), Ashkenazic Jewish	Cystic fibrosis	DNA mutation analysis of the (CFTR) gene	CVS or amniocentesis for DNA mutation analysis

*Chorionic villus sampling.
†Restriction fragment length polymorphism.

Every pregnancy has a 3% to 5% risk of resulting in an infant with a birth defect. When an abnormality is detected or suspected before birth, an attempt is made to determine the diagnosis by assessing the family health history (via the pedigree) and the pregnancy history and by evaluating the fetal anomaly or anomalies via ultrasound. Once experts on a specific disorder are consulted, healthcare professionals can then present the parents with options.

Treatment of prenatally diagnosed disorders may begin during the pregnancy, thus possibly preventing irreversible damage. For example, a mother carrying a fetus with galactosemia may follow a galactose-free diet. In light of the philosophy of preventive health care, information that can be obtained prenatally should be made available to all couples who are expecting a baby or who are contemplating pregnancy.

Postnatal Diagnosis

Questions concerning genetic disorders (cause, treatment, and prognosis) are most often first discussed in the newborn nursery or during the infant's first few months of life. When a child is born with anomalies, has a stormy newborn period, or does not progress as expected, a genetic evaluation may be warranted. An accurate diagnosis and an optimal treatment plan incorporate the following:

- Complete detailed history to determine whether the problem is prenatal (congenital), postnatal, or familial in origin
- Complete physical examination that includes a dermatoglyphics analysis (Figure 7–18 ●)
- Laboratory analysis, which includes chromosome analysis; enzyme assay for inborn errors of metabolism (see Chapter 31∞ for further discussion of these tests); DNA studies (both direct and by linkage); and antibody titers for infectious teratogens, such as toxoplasmosis, rubella, cytomegalovirus, and herpes virus (TORCH syndrome) (see Chapter 16∞).

To make an accurate diagnosis, the geneticist consults with other specialists and reviews the current literature. This lets the geneticist evaluate all the available information before arriving at a diagnosis and plan of action.

The Human Genome Project has significant implications for the identification and management of inherited disorders. Once genes are identified, it will be possible to detect their pres-

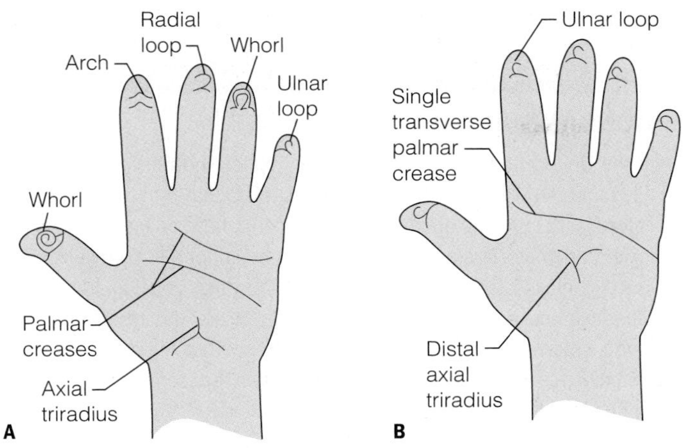

Figure 7–18 Dermatoglyphic patterns of the hands. ***A,*** Normal individual. ***B,*** Child with Down syndrome. Note the single transverse palmar crease, distally placed axial triradius, and increased number of ulnar loops.

ence in carriers and lead to better genetic counseling. New genetic material might be inserted into cells to provide important missing information (gene transfer) as may be possible in cystic fibrosis, or medications can be specifically designed to target the disease on a molecular level (Simpson & Holzgreve, 2007).

However, concerns have been voiced about ethical considerations with genetic research. What guidelines are needed to protect children and families so that genetic testing does not lead to discrimination in future employment or health insurance? Who should be tested for genetic diseases, and who should have access to the results? Because children cannot yet give informed consent for genetic testing (see Chapter 1 for discussion of informed consent), it is recommended that children and adolescents should have genetic testing only when medical treatment could help if the disease is identified, or when another family member might benefit from the knowledge for their own health and the child will not be harmed by testing (Simpson & Holzgreve, 2007). Whenever genetic testing is performed, counseling about the results must be available.

Perinatal and neonatal nurses must keep abreast of new genomic knowledge and prenatal/neonatal screening and testing that can be done to impact long-term health (Williams, Tripp-Reimer, Schutle, et al., 2004). Because of nursing's frontline position in healthcare systems and their emphasis on providing holistic, family-centered care, nurses are likely the first healthcare professionals individuals and families will turn to with questions about genetic risk and susceptibility, as well as to seek guidance regarding the complexities of genetic testing and interpretation. All health professionals at every level of education must have knowledge of genomics. In 2001 the National Coalition of Health Professional Education in Genetics (NCHPEG) published a list of core competencies for all health professionals in all disciplines (Jenkins, 2001). Currently a nursing group led by Dr. Jean Jenkins and colleagues are adapting these to reflect the nursing profession and care. Some nurses with a subspecialty in genomics enable them to act as a genetic counselor, informing families of their genetic risks, providing information, and giving support during the initial diagnosis and thorough follow-up.

GENETIC COUNSELING

MyNursingKit Human Genome Project

Genetic counseling is a communication process in which a genetic counselor, physician, or specially trained and certified nurse tries to provide a family with the most complete and accurate information about the occurrence or the risk of recurrence of a genetic disease in that family. Genetic counseling is thus an appropriate course of action for any family wondering, "Will it happen again?"

Referral

Genetic counseling referral is advised for any of the following categories:

- *Congenital abnormalities, including mental retardation.* Any couple who has a child or a relative with a congenital malformation may be at increased risk and should be so informed. If mental retardation of unidentified cause has occurred in a family, there may be an increased risk of recurrence. In some cases, the genetic counselor will identify the cause of a malformation as a teratogen (see Chapter 11). The family should be aware of teratogenic substances so they can avoid exposure during any subsequent pregnancy.
- *Familial disorders.* Families should be told that certain diseases may have a genetic component and that the risk of their occurrence in a particular family may be higher than that in the general population. Such disorders as diabetes, heart disease, cancer, and mental illness fall into this category.
- *Known inherited diseases.* Families may know that a disease is inherited but not know the mechanism or the specific risk for them. An important point to remember is that family members who are not at risk for passing on a disorder should be as well informed as family members who are at risk.
- *Metabolic disorders.* Any families at risk for having a child with a metabolic disorder or biochemical defect should be referred for genetic counseling. Because most inborn errors of metabolism are autosomal recessively inherited, a family may not be identified as being at risk until the birth of an affected child; for example, a child with cystic fibrosis or sickle cell anemia. Carriers of the sickle cell trait and cystic fibrosis can be identified before conception or a pregnancy has occurred, and the risk of having an affected child can be determined. Prenatal diagnosis of an affected fetus is available on an experimental basis only.
- *Chromosomal abnormalities.* As discussed previously, any couple who has had a child with a chromosomal abnormality may be at increased risk of having another child similarly affected. This group includes families in which there is concern about a possible translocation.

After a couple has been referred to the genetics clinic, they are sent a form requesting information on the health status of various family members. This information assists the genetic counselor in creating the family's pedigree.

Together, the pedigree and history facilitate identification of other family members who might also be at risk for the same

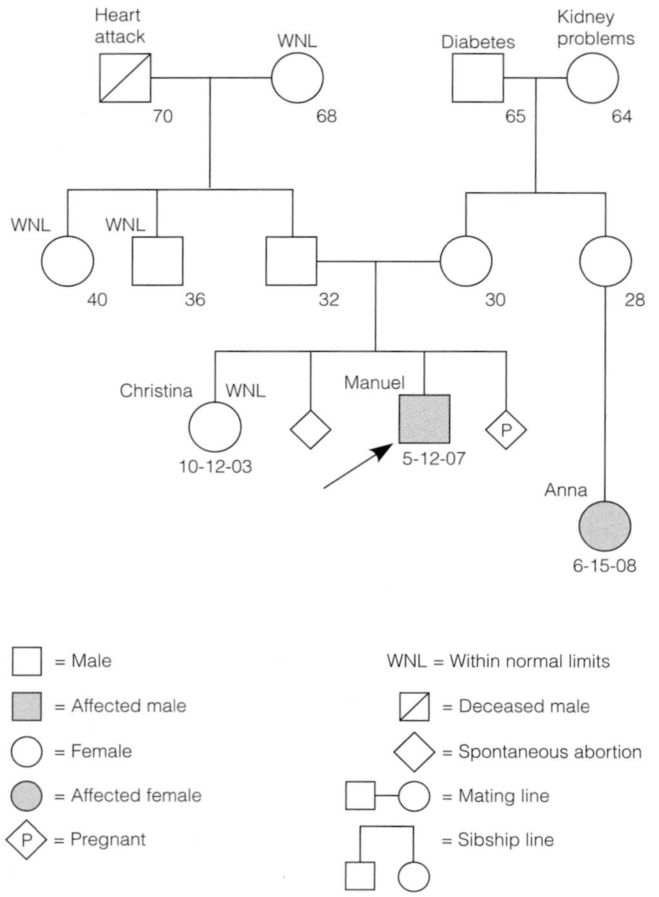

● **Figure 7–19** Screening pedigree. Arrow indicates the nearest family member affected with the disorder being investigated. Basic data have been recorded. Numbers refer to the ages of the family members.

Developing Cultural Competence

CONSANGUINEOUS MARRIAGES

In the United States, marriage between related individuals is generally taboo. In Western medicine, there is a concern that a child conceived by people who are related by blood may have an increased risk for birth defects. This has not, however, been supported by recent research unless the relationship is closer than first cousins. In many other cultures, marriage of first cousins and others who are related by blood is acceptable and even common. Egypt has a high rate of consanguineous (blood relationship) marriages. Reasons for consanguineous marriage include: "increase family links," "they knew each other and everything would be clear before marriage," "customs and traditions," and "less cost." The most common type of consanguineous marriage in Egypt is between first cousins.

disorder (Figure 7–19 ●). The family being counseled may wish to notify relatives at risk so that they, too, can begin genetic counseling. When done correctly, the family history and pedigree can be powerful tools for determining a family's risk.

Initial Session

During the initial session, the counselor gathers additional information about the pregnancy, the affected child's growth and development, and the family's understanding of the problem. The counselor also elicits information concerning ethnic background and family origin. Many genetic disorders are more common among certain ethnic groups or in particular geographic areas.

Generally the child undergoes a physical examination. Other family members may also be examined. If laboratory tests such as chromosomal analyses, metabolic studies, or viral titers are indicated, they are performed at this time. The genetic counselor may then give the parents some preliminary information based on the data at hand.

Follow-Up Counseling

When all the data have been carefully examined and analyzed, the couple returns for a follow-up visit. At this time, the genetic counselor gives the parents all the information available, including the medical facts, diagnosis, probable course of the disorder, and any available management; the inheritance pattern for this particular family and the risk of recurrence; and the options or alternatives for dealing with the risk of recurrence. The remainder of the counseling session is spent discussing the course of action that seems appropriate to the family in view of the risk and family goals. For couples who desire to become parents or who want a subsequent child, options include prenatal diagnosis, early detection and treatment, and, in some cases, adoption, therapeutic insemination, and delayed childbearing.

The couple may consider therapeutic donor insemination (TDI), discussed earlier in the chapter. This alternative is appropriate, for example, if the male partner has an autosomal dominant disease; TDI would decrease to zero the risk of having an affected child (if the sperm donor is not at risk) because the child would not inherit any genes from the affected parent. If the man has an X-linked disorder and does not wish to continue the gene in the family (all his daughters would be carriers), TDI is an alternative to terminating all pregnancies with a female fetus. If the man is a carrier for a balanced translocation and if termination of pregnancy is against family ethics, TDI is the most appropriate alternative. If both parents are carriers of an autosomal recessive disorder, TDI lowers the risk to a very low level or to zero if a carrier test is available. TDI also may be appropriate if the couple is at high risk for a multifactorial disorder.

Couples who are young and at risk may decide to delay childbearing. These couples may find in a few years that prenatal diagnosis is available or that a disease can be detected and treated early to prevent irreversible damage.

When the parents have completed the counseling sessions, the counselor sends them and their certified nurse-midwife or physician a letter detailing the contents of the sessions. The parents keep this document for reference.

Nursing management. In both prospective and retrospective genetic counseling, timely nursing intervention is a crucial factor. During annual exam and other clinical appointments, the nurse

Nursing Practice

Nursing responsibilities in Genetic Counseling include:

- Identify families at risk for genetic problems.
- Determine how the genetic problem is perceived and what information is desired before proceeding.
- Assist families in acquiring accurate information about the specific problem.
- Act as a liaison between the family and genetic counselor.
- Assist the family in understanding and dealing with information received.
- Provide information on support groups.
- Aid families in coping with this crisis.
- Provide information about known genetic factors.
- Assure continuity of nursing care to the family.

should interview all women of childbearing age to determine any family history or other risk factors for genetic disorders. If the woman is planning to conceive, genetic counseling should be encouraged before discontinuation of contraception.

The nurse has a key role in preventing recurrence. One cannot expect a couple who has just learned that their child has a birth defect or Down syndrome to take in any information concerning future risks. However, the couple should never be "put off" from genetic counseling for so long that they conceive another affected child because of lack of information. The perinatal nursing team frequently has the first contact with the family who has a newborn with a congenital abnormality. At the birth of an affected child, the nurse can inform the parents that genetic counseling is available.

After genetic counseling, the nurse with the appropriate knowledge of genetics is in an ideal position to help couples review what has been discussed during the counseling sessions and to answer any additional questions they might have. As families return to daily living, the nurse can provide helpful information on the day-to-day aspects of caring for a child, answer questions as they arise, support parents in their decisions, and refer families to other health and community agencies.

The family may return to the genetic counselor a number of times to ask questions and express concerns, especially if the couple is considering having more children, or if siblings want information about their affected brother or sister. It is most desirable for the nurse working with the family to attend many or all of these counseling sessions. Because the nurse has already established a rapport with the couple, she or he can act as a liaison between the family and the genetic counselor. Hearing directly what the genetic counselor says helps the nurse clarify the issues for the family, which in turn helps them formulate questions. Many genetic centers have found the public health nurse to be the ideal health professional to provide such follow-up care. Nurses must be careful not to assume a diagnosis, determine carrier status or recurrence risks, or provide genetic counseling without adequate information and training. Inadequate, inappropriate, or inaccurate information may be misleading or harmful. Healthcare professionals need to learn the appropriate referral systems and options for care in their region.

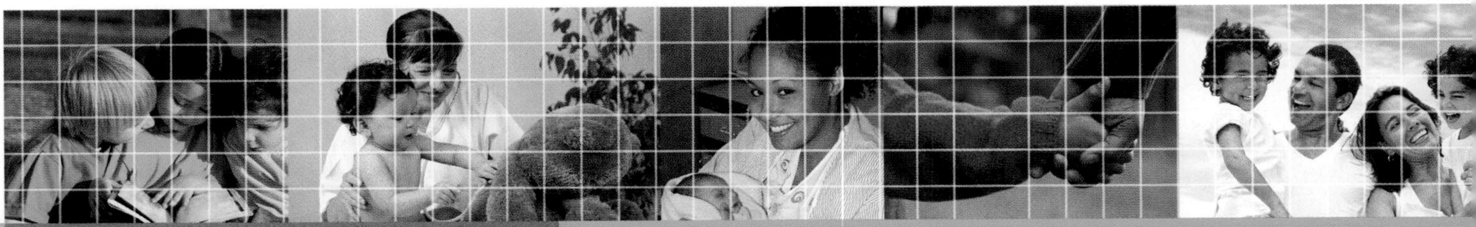

CRITICAL CONCEPT REVIEW

LEARNING OUTCOMES	CONCEPTS
7.1 Identify the essential components of fertility.	1. Female: ■ Cervical mucus must be favorable. ■ Fallopian tubes must be patent. ■ Ovaries must produce and release ova in a regular, cyclic fashion. ■ Endometrium must be prepared for implantation of the blastocyst. ■ Adequate reproductive hormones must be present. 2. Male: ■ Testes must produce adequate numbers of sperm. ■ Genital tract must be unobstructed. ■ Genital tract secretions must be normal. ■ Ejaculated sperm must reach cervix.

(continued)

LEARNING OUTCOMES	CONCEPTS
7.2 Describe the elements of the preliminary investigation of infertility and the nurse's role in supporting/teaching clients during this phase.	1. Information about most fertile times for intercourse. 2. Explanation of basic infertility workup. 3. Basic assessments: ■ Ovarian function. ■ Cervical mucus adequacy. ■ Receptivity to sperm. ■ Sperm adequacy. ■ Tubal patency. ■ General condition of pelvic organs. ■ Semen analysis. 4. Complete physical examination of both partners. 5. Laboratory examination: ■ CBC. ■ UA. ■ Hormonal assays. 6. Nurse's role: ■ Provide information about most fertile times to have intercourse. ■ Explain the basic infertility workup. Provide comfort to couples by using a nonjudgmental approach and information and instruction throughout the diagnostic and therapeutic process.
7.3 Summarize the indications for the tests and associated treatments, including assisted reproductive technologies that are done in an infertility workup.	1. If lack of ovarian function is suspected: ■ Basal body temperature recording. ■ Hormonal assessments. ■ Endometrial biopsy. ■ Transvaginal ultrasound. 2. If cervical problems are suspected: ■ Ferning capacity of cervical mucus. ■ Postcoital test. 3. If tubal or uterine problems are suspected: ■ Hysterosalpingography. ■ Hysteroscopy. ■ Laparoscopy. 4. If male's fertility is suspected: ■ Semen analysis. ■ Screening for antisperm antibodies. 5. Pharmacologic intervention is prescribed if ovarian or endometrial function is abnormal. 6. Therapeutic insemination is indicated for low or abnormal sperm counts or structural defects in the male reproductive tract. 7. In vitro fertilization (IVF) is used when infertility has resulted from tubal factors, mucus abnormalities, male infertility, female immunologic infertility, and cervical factors.
7.4 Relate the physiologic and psychologic effects of infertility on a couple to the nursing management of the couple.	1. Development of lack of spontaneity of sexual intercourse. 2. Feelings of loss of control. 3. Feelings of reduced competency. 4. Loss of status and ambiguity as a couple. 5. Sense of social stigma. 6. Stress on marital and sexual relationship. 7. Strained relationship with healthcare providers.
7.5 Describe the nurse's role as counselor, educator, and advocate for couples during infertility evaluation and treatment.	1. Support the couple and help them to understand and facilitate the free expressions of feelings. 2. Help the couple to recognize feelings. 3. Help the couple to understand motives. 4. Help the couple identify alternatives, and facilitate partner communication.

LEARNING OUTCOMES — CONCEPTS

Learning Outcomes	Concepts
7.6 Identify couples who may benefit from preconceptual chromosomal analysis and prenatal testing when providing care to couples with special reproductive concerns.	1. Women who are of advanced maternal age. 2. Family history of a chromosomal disorder, birth defects, or mental retardation. 3. Previous child with chromosomal disorder. 4. Ethnic group with history of chromosomal disorders. 5. Couples with a history of two or more first-trimester spontaneous abortions. 6. Women with an abnormal serum alpha-fetoprotein test.
7.7 Identify the characteristics of autosomal dominant, autosomal recessive, and X-linked (sex-linked) recessive disorders.	1. Autosomal dominant disorder: ■ An affected parent has a 50% chance of having an affected child with each pregnancy. 2. Autosomal recessive disorders: ■ Both parents must be carriers. ■ Each offspring has a 25% chance of having the disease and a 50% chance of being a carrier. 3. X-linked recessive disorders: ■ No male-to-male transmission. ■ Effects limited to males. ■ 50% chance a carrier mother will pass abnormal gene to her son. ■ 50% chance the daughter of a carrier mother will be a carrier. ■ 100% chance that daughter of an affected father will be a carrier.
7.8 Compare prenatal and postnatal diagnostic procedures used to determine the presence of genetic disorders.	1. Prenatal diagnostic tests: ■ Invasive procedure performed on mother, though it may affect the fetus. ■ Genetic ultrasound. ■ Serum alpha-fetoprotein tests. ■ Genetic amniocentesis. ■ Chorionic villus sampling. ■ Percutaneous umbilical blood sampling. 2. Postnatal diagnostic tests: ■ Physical examination and laboratory analysis is performed on the newborn.
7.9 Explore the emotional impact on a couple undergoing genetic testing or coping with the birth of a baby with a genetic disorder, and explain the nurse's role in supporting the family undergoing genetic counseling.	1. Emotional impact: ■ Concern for infant's survival and possible lifelong difficulties. ■ Fear of results of testing. ■ Blame for infant's disorder. 2. The nurse's role: ■ Help families to acquire adequate information and understand this information. ■ Act as a liaison between family and genetic counselor. ■ Provide information about support groups. ■ Provide continuity of care to the family.

CRITICAL THINKING IN ACTION

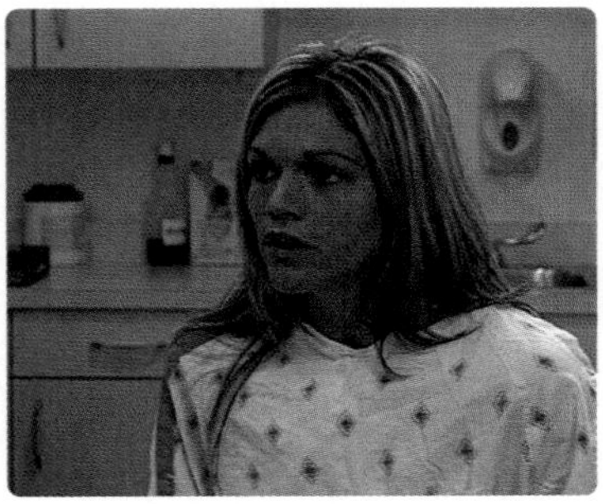

Marie Neives, age 19, presents while you are working at a Planned Parenthood Clinic. She is there for a GYN exam and tells you that she is sexually active with her boyfriend but doesn't want to become pregnant. Since she lives at home with her parents, she does not want to use "the pill" because her mother might find out. Marie tells you she has a family history of sickle cell anemia and is concerned that she will pass the disease on. Marie asks you for information concerning fertility awareness. You obtain a menstrual history as follows: menarche age 12, cycle every 28 days for 5 days, dysmenorrhea the first 2 days with moderate flow. She has had one sexual partner. She states her boyfriend doesn't like to use condoms and that she has been lucky so far in not getting pregnant. You assist the nurse practitioner with a physical and pelvic exam. The results show that Marie is essentially healthy. The nurse practitioner asks you to review with Marie the basal body temperature (BBT) method of fertility awareness.

1. Explore with Marie "natural family planning." How would you explain this to her?
2. Briefly explain why the basal body temperature (BBT) method can predict ovulation.
3. How would you describe to Marie the procedure for obtaining BBT?
4. After figuring out her menstruation cycle, to avoid conception when would you tell Marie to abstain from unprotected intercourse?

See MyNursingKit for possible responses.

REFERENCES

American Society of Reproductive Medicine (ASRM). (2006a). *Frequently asked questions about infertility*. Retrieved June 20, 2009, from www.asrm .org/patients/faqs.htm

American Society of Reproductive Medicine (ASRM). (2006b). *Frequently asked questions. The psychological component of infertility*. Retrieved June 20, 2009, from www.asrm.org/patients/ faqs.htm

American Society of Reproductive Medicine (ASRM). (2006c). *Medications for inducing ovulation: A guide for patients.* Retrieved June 20, 2009, from www.asrm.org/patientbooklets/ ovulation_drugs.pdf.

American Society of Reproductive Medicine (ASRM). (2008). *Assisted reproductive technologies: A guide for parents.* Retrieved June 20, 2009, from www.asrm.org/patientbooklets/ART

American Society of Reproductive Medicine Practice Committee (2008). Preimplantation genetic testing: A practice committee opinion. *Fertility and Sterility* 90(3), S136–43.

Cheong, Y. C., Hung, Yu Ng E., Ledger, W. L. (2008). Acupuncture and assisted conception. *Cochrane Database of Systematic Reviews*, Issue 4. Art. No. CD006920.

Denson, V. (2006). Diagnosis and management of infertility. *Journal for Nurse Practitioners, 2*(6), 380–386.

Devine, K. S. (2008). *Challenges and management of infertility, including assisted reproductive technologies.* White Plains, NY: March of Dimes Foundation.

Dugoff, L. (2008). Prenatal diagnosis. In R. S. Gibbs, B. Y. Karlan, A. F. Haney, & I. E. Nygaard (Eds.), *Danforth's obstetrics and gynecology* (10th ed., pp. 111–121). Philadelphia: Lippincott Williams & Wilkins.

Goldstein, S. R. (2008). Abnormal uterine bleeding. In R. S. Gibbs, B. Y. Karlan, A. F. Haney, & I. E. Nygaard (Eds.), *Danforth's obstetrics and gynecology* (10th ed., pp. 664–681). Philadelphia: Lippincott Williams & Wilkins.

Honig, S. (2005). Preventive medicine and male factor infertility: Facts & fiction. Retrieved December 17, 2005, from www.resolve.org/site/ PageServer?pagename=lrn_jfm_pm

Inhorn, M. C. (2002). "Local" confronts the "Global": Infertile bodies and the new reproductive technology in Egypt. In M. C. Inhorn & F. Van Balen (Eds.), *Infertility around the globe: New thinking on childness, gender, and reproductive technologies.* Berkeley and Los Angeles: University of California Press.

Jenkins, J. (2001). *Core competencies in genetics essential for all health care professionals.* Rockville, MD: National Coalition for Health Professional Education in Genetics (NCHPEG).

Kahn, S. M. (2002). Rabbis and reproduction: The uses of new reproductive technologies among ultraorthodox Jews in Israel. In M. C. Inhorn & F. Van Balen (Eds.), *Infertility around the globe: New thinking on childlessness, gender, and reproductive technologies.* Berkeley and Los Angeles: University of California Press.

Klock, S. C. (2004). Psychological issues related to infertility. In J. J. Sciarri (Ed.), *Gynecology and obstetrics* (Vol. 6, chap. 74, pp. 1–8). Philadelphia: Lippincott Williams & Wilkins.

Kumar, A., Ghadir, S., Eskandari, N., & DeCherney, A. H. (2007). Infertility. In A. H. DeCherney, L. Nathan, T. M. Goodwin, & N. Laufer (Eds.), *Current diagnosis and treatment: Obstetrics & gynecology* (10th ed.). Boston: McGraw-Hill.

Lashley, F. R. (2007). *Essentials of clinical genetics in nursing practice.* New York: Springer.

Lu, Jin-Chun, Huang, Yu-Feng, & Lu, Nian-Qing. (2008). Antisperm immunity and infertility. *Expert Review Clinical Immunology,* 4(1), 113–126

Manheimer, E., Zhang, G., Udoff, L., Haramati, A., Langenberg, P., Berman, B. M., et al. (2008). Effects of accupuncture on rates of pregnancy and live birth among women undergoing in vitro fertilisation: Systematic review and meta-analysis. *BMJ, 336,* 545–549.

Purnell, L. D., & Paulanka, B. J. (2008). *Transcultural health care: A culturally competent approach.* Philadelphia: F. A. Davis.

Quallich, S. (2006). Examining male infertility. *Urological Nurses 26*(4), 277–288.

Simpson, J. L., & Holzgreve, W. (2007). Genetic counseling and genetic screening. In S. G. Gabbe, J. R. Niebyl, & J. L. Simpson (Eds.), *Obstetrics: Normal and problem pregnancies* (5th ed., pp. 138–151). Philadelphia: Churchill Livingstone.

Skidmore-Roth, L. (2006). *Mosby's handbook of herbs & natural supplements.* St. Louis: Elsevier Mosby.

Speroff, L., & Fritz, M. (2005). *Clinical gynecologic endocrinology and infertility.* Philadelphia: Lippincott Williams & Wilkins.

Storment, J. M. (2006). Infertility and recurrent pregnancy loss. In M. G. Curtis, S. Overholt, & M. P. Hopkins, *Glass' office gynecology* (6th ed.). Philadelphia: Lippincott Williams & Wilkins.

Varney, H., Kriebs, J. M., & Gegor, C. L. (2004). *Varney's midwifery* (4th ed.). Boston: Jones and Bartlett.

Ward, K. (2008). Genetics in obstetrics and gynecology. In R. S. Gibbs, B. Y. Karlan, A. F. Haney, & I. E. Nygaard (Eds.), *Danforth's obstetrics and gynecology* (10th ed., pp. 88–110). Philadelphia: Lippincott Williams & Wilkins.

Williams, J. K., Tripp-Reimer, T., Schutle, D., & Barnette, J. J. (2004). Advancing genetic nursing knowledge. *Nursing Outlook, 52,* 73–79.

Wilson, B. A., Shannon, M. T., Shields, K. M., & Stang, C. L. (2009). *Prentice Hall nurse's drug guide—2009.* Upper Saddle River, NJ: Pearson Education.

Wright, K. P., Johnson, J. (2008). Infertility. In R. S. Gibbs, B. Y. Karlan, A. F. Haney, & I. E. Nygaard (Eds.), *Danforth's obstetrics and gynecology* (10th ed., pp. 705–715). Philadelphia: Lippincott Williams & Wilkins.

PEARSON

EXPLORE mynursingkit™

MyNursingKit is your one stop for online chapter review materials and resources. Prepare for success with additional NCLEX®-style practice questions, interactive assignments and activities, web links, animations and videos, and more!

Register your access code from the front of your book at **www.mynursingkit.com**

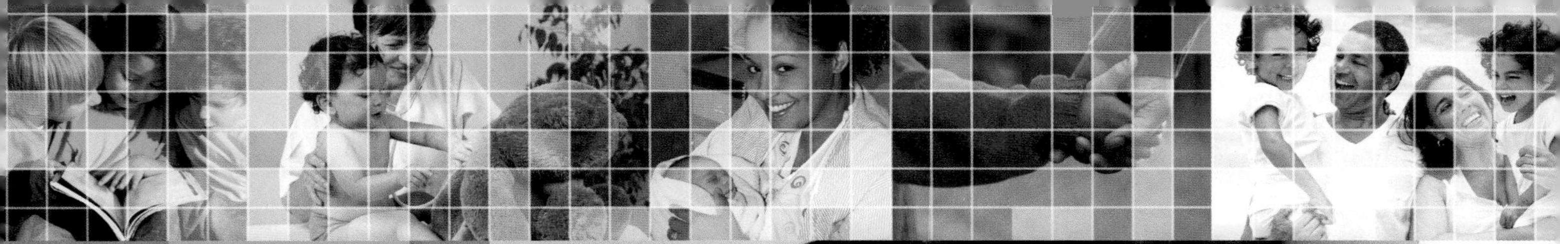

PART

3

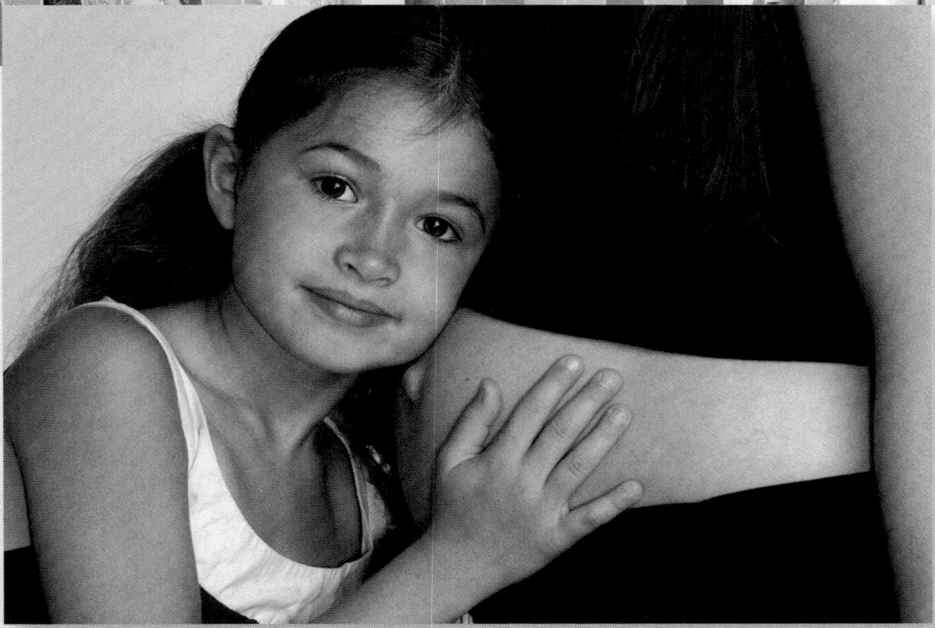

Pregnancy and Family

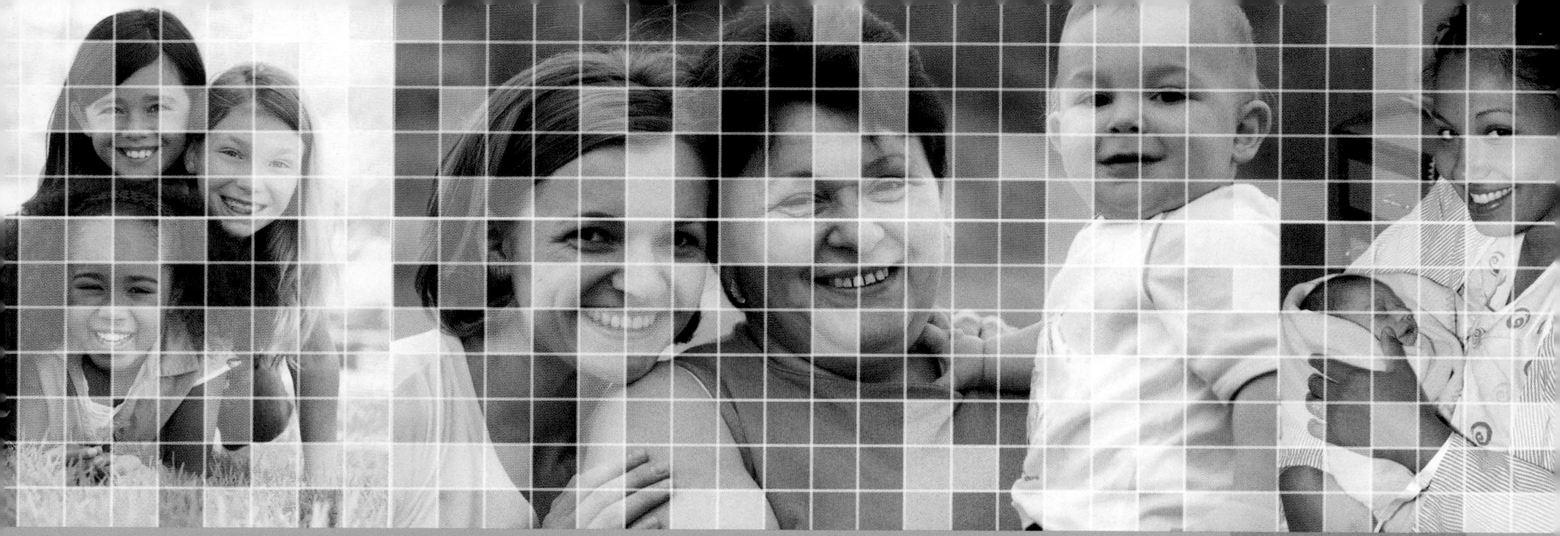

CHAPTER

Preparation for Parenthood 8

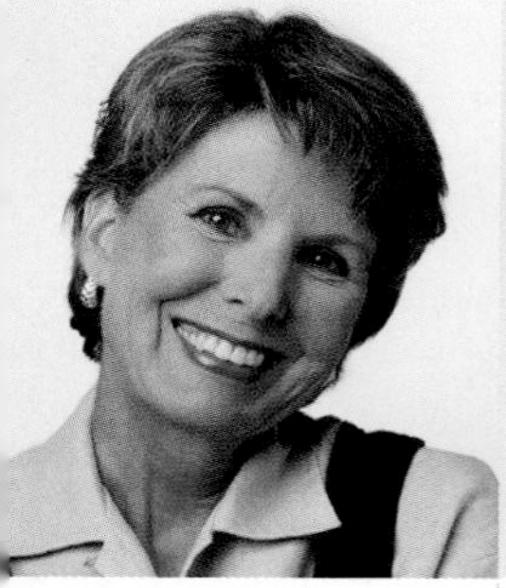

We took our childbirth education classes with seven other couples. Our instructor, who was a nurse, was great—warm and funny but very knowledgeable. After we all had given birth, she had everyone over to her house for a "reunion." We lined the babies up together on the sofa and took a picture. They leaned against each other, topsy-turvy. It was hilarious. My son is now 23 but I still love that picture of him. What memories it triggers of such a very special time!
—Trish, 47

LEARNING OUTCOMES

8.1 Determine the most appropriate nursing care for couples during preconception to help ensure their best possible health state.

8.2 Identify ways to assist expectant parents in making the best decisions possible about issues related to pregnancy, labor, and birth.

8.3 Summarize the goals and content of the various types of antepartal education programs when providing nursing care for expectant couples and their families.

8.4 Compare methods of childbirth preparation and the nursing interventions for each.

8.5 Explore ways in which the nurse conveys respect for client individuality in preparing for childbirth.

phy, and characteristics of practice of certified nurse-midwives, obstetricians, family practice physicians, and direct entry (lay) midwives. The nurse can encourage expectant parents to investigate the care provider's credentials, education and training, philosophy of childbirth, fee schedule or insurance plans accepted, availability to new clients, and on-call coverage issues. They can often get this information by telephoning the provider's office. The nurse can help the expectant parents develop a list of questions for their first visit to a care provider to help determine compatibility. These questions might include the following:

- Who is in practice with you, or who covers for you when you are unavailable?
- How do your partners' philosophies compare with yours?
- How do you feel about my partner, other support person, or other children coming to the prenatal visits?
- What are your feelings about ____ (fill in special desires for the birth event, such as different positions assumed during labor, episiotomy, induction of labor, other people present during the birth, breastfeeding immediately after the birth, no separation of infant and parents following birth, and so on)?
- If a cesarean birth is necessary, could my partner be present?
- Are you familiar with _____ (fill in complementary or alternative forms of health care that may be used if applicable)? How will this practice affect my plan of care?

Expectant parents also need to consider the qualities they want in a care provider for the newborn. They may want to visit several before the birth to select someone who will meet their needs and those of their child.

Pregnant women and couples will make many more choices. Some are explored in Table 8–1. A method that has helped many couples make these choices is a **birth preference plan**. By writing down preferences, prospective parents identify aspects of the childbearing experience that are most important to them (Figure 8–1 ●). Used as a tool for communication among the expectant parents, the healthcare provider, and the healthcare professionals at the birth setting, the written plan identifies options that are available as well as those that are not.

Birth Preference Plan

Choice

- Care provider:
  - Certified nurse-midwife
  - Obstetrician
  - Family physician
  - Direct entry midwife
- Birth setting:
  - Hospital:
    - Birthing room
    - Delivery room
  - Birth center
  - Home
- Support during labor and birth:
  - Partner present
  - Doula present
- During labor:
  - Ambulate as desired
  - Shower if desired
  - Wear own clothes
  - Use hot tub
  - Use own rocking chair
  - Have perineal prep
  - Have enema
- Membranes:
  - Rupture naturally
  - Amniotomy if needed
- Labor stimulation if needed
- Medication:
  - Identify type desired
- Fluids or ice as desired
- Music during labor and birth
- Massage
- Therapeutic touch
- Healing touch

Choice

- Position during birth:
  - On side
  - Hands and knees
  - Kneeling
  - Squatting
  - Birthing chair
  - Birthing bed
  - Other:
- Family present (siblings)
- Filming of birth (videotaping)
- Photography of birth
- Use of LeBoyer Method
- Episiotomy
- No sterile drapes
- Partner to cut umbilical cord
- Hold baby immediately after birth
- Breastfeed immediately after birth
- No separation after birth
- Save the placenta
- Collect cord blood for banking
- Newborn care:
  - Eye treatment for the baby
  - Vitamin K injection
  - Heptovac injection
  - Breastfeeding
  - Formula feeding
  - Pacifier use
  - Glucose water
  - Circumcision
- Postpartum care:
  - Short stay
  - 48-hour stay after vaginal birth
  - Home visits after discharge
  - Home doula
- Other:

● **Figure 8–1** Birth preference plan. The columns list the various choices that a couple may consider during their childbirth experience. Once the couple has considered each of the choices, they can circle the items they desire.

Although many birth experiences are very close to the desired experience, at times expectations cannot be met. This may be because of the unavailability of some choices in the community, limitations set by insurance providers, or unexpected problems during pregnancy or birth. It is important for the nurse to help expectant parents keep sight of what is realistic for their situation while also acting as an advocate for them.

BIRTH SETTING

The nurse can help expectant parents choose a birth setting by suggesting they tour facilities and talk with nurses there as well as with friends or acquaintances who are recent parents. However, the choice of healthcare provider may largely determine the birth setting. Questions that expectant parents might ask of new parents include the following:

- What kind of care and support did you receive during labor?
- If the setting has both labor and delivery rooms and birthing rooms, was a birthing room available when you wanted it?
- Were you encouraged to be mobile during labor or do what you wanted to do (walking, sitting in a rocking chair, sitting in a whirlpool bath, standing in a shower, and so on)? If not, were there reasonable circumstances that prevented you from doing so?
- Were you encouraged to be involved in your plan of care and kept well informed of progress or proposed changes?
- Was your labor partner or coach treated well?
- Were your birth preferences respected? Did you share them with the facility before the birth? If something did not work, why do you think there were problems?
- During labor, did the nurse offer or suggest a variety of comfort measures?
- How were medications handled during labor? Were you comfortable with this arrangement?

Table 8–1 Benefits and Risks of Some Consumer Decisions During Pregnancy, Labor, and Birth

Issue	Benefits	Risks
Breastfeeding	■ No additional expense ■ Contains maternal antibodies to decrease illnesses ■ Decreases incidence of infant otitis media, vomiting, diarrhea, hospitalizations during the first year of life, and allergies ■ Easier to digest than formula ■ Immediately after birth, promotes uterine contractions and decreases incidence of postpartum hemorrhage ■ Promotes maternal-infant bonding	■ Transmission of maternal infections such as HIV to newborn ■ Irregular ovulation and menses can cause false sense of security and nonuse of hormonal contraceptives ■ Increased nutritional requirement in mother ■ Limitation of birth control options in the postpartum period
Perineal prep	■ May decrease risk of infection ■ Facilitates episiotomy repair	■ Nicks can be portal for bacteria ■ Discomfort as hair grows back
Enema	■ May facilitate labor ■ Increases space for infant in pelvis ■ May increase strength of contractions ■ May prevent contamination of sterile field	■ Increases discomfort and anxiety

Ambulation during labor	■ Comfort for laboring woman
	■ May assist in labor progression by:
	  ■ Stimulating contractions
	  ■ Allowing gravity to help descent of fetus
	  ■ Giving sense of independence and control
		■ Cord prolapse with rupture of membranes unless engagement has occurred
		■ Birth of infant in undesirable locations (hallways, outdoors, waiting area)
		■ Inability to monitor fetal heart rate

Electronic fetal monitoring	■ Helps evaluate fetal well-being ■ Helps identify fetal stress ■ Useful in diagnostic testing ■ Helps evaluate labor progress	■ Supine postural hypotension ■ Intrauterine perforation (with internal uterine pressure device) ■ Infection (with internal monitoring) ■ Decreases personal interaction with mother because of attention paid to the machine ■ Mother is unable to ambulate or change her position freely
Whirlpool (jet hydrotherapy)	■ Increased relaxation ■ Decreased anxiety ■ Stimulation of labor ■ Provides pain relief ■ Slight decrease in blood pressure ■ Increased diuresis ■ Decreased incidence of vacuum and forceps births ■ Increased pain threshold ■ Higher satisfaction with birth ■ Decreased use of pain medication	■ May slow contractions if used before active labor is established ■ Possible risk of infection if membranes are ruptured ■ Slight increase in maternal temperature and pulse in tub ■ Hypothermia ■ Increases fetal heart rate by 10–20 beats per minute (Teschendorf & Evans, 2000)

Analgesia
Epidural anesthesia
	■ Maternal relaxation facilitates labor
	  ■ When effective, it eliminates the discomfort of labor and enables the woman to relax with loved ones
		■ All drugs reach the fetus in varying degrees and with varying effects
		  ■ Interferes with the woman's ability to push effectively
		  ■ May cause maternal hypotension

Episiotomy	■ Decreases irregular tearing of perineum ■ Easier to repair for practitioner	■ Increased pain after birth and for 1–3 months following birth ■ Dyspareunia ■ Infection ■ Increased frequency of third- and fourth-degree lacerations (Low, Seng, Murtland, et al., 2000)

- Were siblings welcomed in the birth setting? After the birth?
- Was the nursing staff helpful after the baby was born? Did you receive self-care and infant care information? Did you have a choice about what information was provided?

LABOR SUPPORT

Another important choice the expectant family faces is how active a support role the father or partner wants to take during labor and birth. Fathers often play a key role in the support of mothers during labor, birth, and the postpartum period. Although many partners are comfortable acting as the primary physical and emotional support for the laboring woman, some partners are not. In lieu of the partner, other options for labor support include asking a friend or family member to attend the birth and help with comfort needs, contacting a local childbirth advocate group for a volunteer referral, or hiring a specialized childbirth support person, known as a **doula**.

The doula attends to the needs of the childbearing family and acts as an advocate for them. Specially trained to assist with births and provide support to new parents and family members, the doula is an adjunct to the healthcare team. Doulas do not perform clinical tasks but they have a role in providing labor support, offering support and encouragement, building a good team relationship, helping the laboring woman cover gaps in her care, and encouraging good communication among the woman and her family and caregivers. In a managed care environment in which nursing staff are often stretched thinly, a doula can be an asset to the nurse by attending to the many comfort needs of the laboring mother and her family.

SIBLING PARTICIPATION IN THE BIRTH

Some expectant parents may wish to have their other children present at the birth. Children who will attend a birth can be prepared through books, audiovisual materials, use of models, discussion, and sibling classes. Nurses can assist parents with sibling preparation by helping them understand the stresses a child may experience. For example, the child may become frightened if the laboring mom is irritable and visibly showing discomfort, feel left out when there is a new child to love, or feel disappointed if a brother is born when a sister was expected.

During the birth it is important that a sibling have his or her own support person whose sole responsibility is tending to the child's needs. The support person needs to be familiar to the child; warm, sensitive, and flexible; knowledgeable about the birth process; and comfortable with sexuality and birth. This person must be prepared to interpret what is happening for the child and to intervene when necessary. For example, the support person needs to be prepared to remove the child from the birthing room at the child's request or if the situation warrants that action.

Siblings should be allowed to relate to the birth in whatever manner they choose, as long as it is not disruptive. They should understand that they can stay or leave the room as they choose. They should also feel free to ask questions and express feelings.

Siblings who are present at birth tend to have feelings of interest and the desire to nurture "our" baby, as opposed to jealousy and rivalry directed at "Mom's" baby. The mother does not disappear mysteriously into the hospital and return with a demanding outsider. Instead, the family attending the birth together finds a new opportunity for closeness and growth by sharing in the birth of a new member.

CLASSES FOR FAMILY MEMBERS DURING PREGNANCY

Prenatal education programs provide important opportunities to share information about pregnancy and childbirth and to enhance the parents' decision-making skills (Figure 8–2 ●). The content of each class is generally directed by the overall goals of the program. The nurse who knows the types of prenatal programs available in the community can direct expectant parents to programs that meet their special needs and learning goals.

From the expectant parents' point of view, class content is best presented in chronology with the pregnancy. Thus, prenatal classes are often divided into early and late classes (Table 8–2).

EARLY CLASSES: FIRST TRIMESTER

Early prenatal classes often include prepregnant women and couples as well as those in early pregnancy. The content that is typically covered is identified in Table 8–2. Early classes should also present information about breastfeeding and formula-feeding. Most women have made their infant feeding decision before the sixth month of pregnancy.

LATER CLASSES: SECOND AND THIRD TRIMESTERS

The later classes focus on preparation for the birth, postpartum self-care, infant care and feeding, and newborn safety issues. Since many expectant parents purchase a car seat before the birth of their child, later classes should also include information about the importance of car seats, how they work, and how to select an approved car seat.

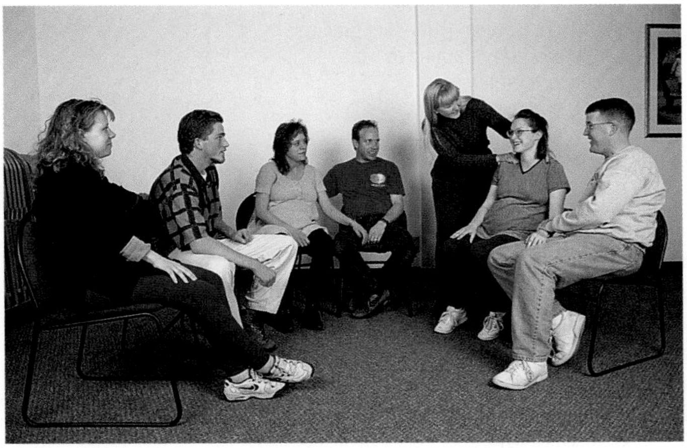

● **Figure 8–2** In a group setting with a nurse-instructor, expectant parents share information about pregnancy and childbirth.

Photographer: © Elena Dorfman.

Table 8–2 Possible Content of Classes for Childbirth Preparation

Early Classes (First Trimester)
Early gestational changes
Self-care during pregnancy
Fetal development, environmental dangers for the fetus
Sexuality in pregnancy
Birth settings and types of care providers
Nutrition, rest, and exercise suggestions
Relief measures for the common discomforts of pregnancy
Psychologic changes in pregnancy
Information for getting pregnancy off to a good start
Danger signs that warrant immediate medical attention
Feeding choices/benefits of breastfeeding
Later Classes (Second and Third Trimesters)
Preparation for birth process
Postpartum self-care
Birth choices (episiotomy, medications, fetal monitoring, perineal prep, enema, etc.)
Relaxation techniques
Breathing techniques
Alternative therapies in pregnancy and labor
Infant stimulation or infant massage
Newborn safety issues, such as car seats and sleeping positions
Sibling preparation and adjustment
Adolescent Preparation Classes
How to be a good parent
Newborn care
Health dangers for the baby
Weight gain issues and nutrition
How to recognize when baby is ill
Baby care: Physical and emotional
Sexuality
Peer relationships
Breastfeeding Programs
Advantages and disadvantages
Maternal nutrition
Techniques of breastfeeding
Methods of breast milk storage
Involvement of fathers in feeding process
Breastfeeding and returning to work
Cultural considerations

MyNursingKit | Case Study: Preparing for Pregnancy

Childbirth preparation classes are an ideal time to incorporate infant stimulation concepts. Tactile, vestibular, and auditory stimulation can be explained. As the uterine wall thins during the pregnancy, the mother and father are better able to feel the baby, and the fetus can sense the parents' stroking and patting through the abdominal wall. **Abdominal effleurage** (a light stroking movement made over the abdominal wall with the fingertips) can provide tactile stimulation to the fetus.

Vestibular stimulation through movement of the fetus is provided when the woman does the pelvic-tilt exercise. Rocking in a rocking chair is also a comfortable way to provide both relaxation for the expectant woman and vestibular stimulation for the fetus.

Nursing Practice

Advise parents of community resources available for inspecting the installation of car seats. Many police departments and fire stations have car-seat inspection clinics that are conducted within the community. Some fire stations have set times when parents can bring in their car seat and have it installed free of charge. Remind new parents that newborns should be in a rear-facing position until the age of 12 months.

Research indicates that auditory stimulation of the fetus and the newborn is important in promoting healthy auditory development (Graven & Browne, 2008). The fetus clearly responds to music and speech with heart rate accelerations and a motor response (Al-Qahtani, 2005). Thus it is helpful to have the pregnant woman speak to the fetus and expose the fetus to music in utero.

ADOLESCENT PARENTING CLASSES

Adolescents have special learning needs during pregnancy. Areas of concern for teens focus on how to be a good parent, how to care for a new baby, health dangers to the baby, and healthful foods to eat during pregnancy. Teens also need to learn how to recognize when the baby is sick, protect the baby from accidents, and make the baby feel happy and loved. Pregnant teens are often eager to hear more about the birth process (especially ways to cope with pain during the birth process), the personal health of the mother, the discomforts and life changes that accompany pregnancy, and sexuality.

BREASTFEEDING PROGRAMS

Programs offering information on breastfeeding are increasing. For many years a primary source of information has been **La Leche League**, a nonprofit organization that promotes breastfeeding. Certified lactation educators; clinical lactation consultants; and nurses at birthing centers, hospitals, and health clinics can also provide information. Online support groups can also be an important resource for new mothers. Expectant parents learn positioning and techniques of breastfeeding, advantages and disadvantages, and methods of breast pumping and milk storage. The father's support and encouragement of the mother is vital, so it is important to include him in the educational programs and decision making. Some fathers may feel ambivalent or resentful about breastfeeding and need opportunities in the prenatal period to discuss and share feelings and experiences.

SIBLING PREPARATION: ADJUSTMENT TO A NEWBORN

The birth of a new sibling is a significant event in a child's life. Attendance at sibling preparation classes can enhance positive adjustment (Figure 8–3 ●). The classes usually focus on reducing the child's anxiety, giving the child opportunities to express feelings and concerns, and encouraging realistic expectations of the

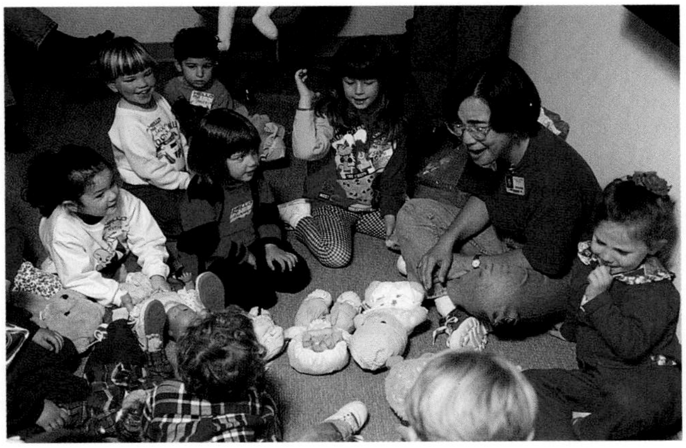

● **Figure 8–3** It is especially important that siblings be well prepared when they are going to be present for the birth. However, all siblings can benefit from information about birth and the new baby ahead of time.

newborn. Parents learn strategies to prepare the child for the birth and help the child cope with a new family member.

Sibling preparation can be addressed through a formal class or in a less formal way by providing a booklet for parents that addresses issues affecting both parents and children.

CLASSES FOR GRANDPARENTS

Grandparents are an important source of support and information for prospective and new parents. They are often included in the birthing process. Prenatal programs for grandparents can be a valuable source of information about current beliefs and practices in childbearing. The most useful content may include changes in birthing and parenting practices and helpful tips for being a supportive grandparent. Grandparents who will be integral members of the labor and birth team need information about that role.

EDUCATION OF THE FAMILY HAVING CESAREAN BIRTH

Cesarean birth is an alternative method of birth that now accounts for 31.8% of births in the United States (Hamilton, Martin, & Ventura, 2009). Consequently, although the need for a cesarean is not often known in advance, more and more childbirth preparation classes are integrating content on cesarean birth into the curriculum.

Class content should cover what the parents can expect to happen during a cesarean birth, what they might feel, and what choices are available. All pregnant women and couples should be encouraged to discuss with their certified nurse-midwife or physician the progression of events if a cesarean birth becomes necessary.

When expectant parents are anticipating a repeat cesarean birth, they have time to plan and prepare. Many birthing units provide preparation classes for repeat cesarean birth. Parents who have had previous negative experiences need an opportunity to describe what contributed to their feelings. They should be encouraged to identify what they would like to change and to list interventions that would make the experience more positive. Those who have had positive experiences require reassurance that their needs and desires will be met in a similar manner. All parents should be encouraged to air any fears or anxieties.

Often a woman facing a repeat cesarean is concerned about postoperative pain. She needs reassurance that subsequent cesarean births are often less painful than the first. In addition, planned cesarean births involve less fatigue than unplanned procedures because they are not preceded by a long, strenuous labor. Providing this information will help the woman cope more effectively with stressful stimuli, including pain.

PREPARATION FOR PARENTS DESIRING VAGINAL BIRTH AFTER CESAREAN

Vaginal birth after cesarean (VBAC) is discussed in detail in Chapter 23∞. Parents who have had a cesarean birth and are now anticipating a vaginal birth have unique needs. Because they may have unresolved questions and concerns about the last birth, it is helpful to begin the series of classes with an informational session. The nurse can supply information about the criteria necessary to attempt a trial of labor and identify decisions to be made regarding the birth experience. Some childbirth educators suggest that parents prepare two birth plans: one for vaginal birth and one for cesarean birth. Preparing birth plans seems to give parents some sense of control over the birth experience and tends to increase the positive aspects of the experience.

CHILDBIRTH PREPARATION METHODS

Childbirth preparation classes are usually taught by certified childbirth educators. Various types of childbirth preparation are available. Vital to each method is the educational component, which helps alleviate fear. The classes vary in coverage of subjects related to the maternity cycle, but all teach relaxation and coping techniques, as well as what to expect during labor and birth. Most classes also feature exercises to relax and condition muscles and breathing exercises for use in labor. The greatest differences among the methods lie in the theories of why they work and in the specific comfort techniques and breathing patterns they teach.

Developing Cultural Competence

CHILDBIRTH ATTENDANCE

Women from Latino cultures typically want their partner with them during labor. These women generally prefer both emotional and physical support, such as verbal reassurance, hand-holding, or assistance with ambulation. The woman may also want female relatives present during the labor and birth to provide additional support.

On the other hand, in most Middle Eastern countries, childbirth is exclusively attended by women. A woman in labor is commonly surrounded by female relatives and friends. It is customary for the husband to be excluded from the birthing area or delivery room.

Childbirth preparation offers several advantages. It helps a pregnant woman and her support person understand the choices and options available to them for a meaningful birth experience and provides tools for them to use during labor and birth. Another advantage is the satisfaction of the parents, for whom childbirth becomes a shared and profound emotional experience. In addition, each method has been shown to shorten labor. All nurses should know how these techniques differ, so that they can support each birth experience effectively.

PROGRAMS FOR PREPARATION

Some antepartal classes, specifically oriented to preparation for labor and birth, have a name associated with a theory of pain reduction in childbirth. The most common methods of this type are the Lamaze (psychoprophylactic), Kitzinger (sensory-memory), Bradley (partner-coached childbirth), and HypnoBirthing (deep relaxation). Table 8–3 identifies characteristics of each method.

Table 8–3 Summary of Selected Childbirth Preparation Methods

Method	Purpose or Philosophy	Goals	Techniques	Class Content
Bradley	To have the best, safest, and most rewarding birth experience possible.	■ Natural childbirth. ■ Active participation of the husband as coach. ■ Excellent nutrition. ■ Breastfeeding, beginning at birth.	■ Working in harmony with the body using controlled breathing and deep abdominopelvic breathing (American Academy of Husband-Coached Childbirth, 2008) ■ Promoting general body relaxation	■ Nutrition ■ Coach's role ■ Introduction to stages of labor ■ Birth planning ■ Variations and complications of labor ■ Postpartum preparation ■ Advanced first- and second-stage techniques ■ Preparation for the new family
Lamaze	Childbirth education empowers women to make informed choices in health care, to assume responsibility for their health, and to trust their inner wisdom.	■ Birth is normal, natural, and healthy. ■ The experience of birth profoundly affects women and their families. ■ Women's inner wisdom guides them through birth. ■ Women have the right to give birth free from routine medical interventions.	■ Disassociation relaxation ■ Controlled muscular relaxation ■ Breathing patterns	■ Nutrition ■ Gestational changes ■ Labor and birth techniques for easing pain ■ Breathing techniques ■ Positioning during labor
Kitzinger	■ Sheila Kitzinger campaigns for women to have the information they need to make choices about childbirth. ■ She is a strong believer in the benefits of home birth for women who are not at high risk.	■ Uses sensory memory to help the woman understand and work with her body in preparation for birth.	■ Uses chest breathing in conjunction with abdominal relaxation ■ Incorporates elements of the Stanislavsky method of acting in a way to teach relaxation	■ Antenatal care ■ Birth plans ■ Therapeutic touch during labor ■ Posttraumatic stress following childbirth ■ Breastfeeding
HypnoBirthing	Eliminate fear and experience birth in a stress-free, calm, and gentle environment that most resembles nature's own design.	■ With both mind and body relaxed, the muscles of the uterus work in complete neuromuscular harmony. ■ When in a relaxed state, the body releases endorphins, the body's natural anesthesia.	■ Relaxation techniques ■ Deep breathing ■ Slow breathing ■ Breathing the baby down ■ Maintaining comfort and eliminating pain	■ HypnoBirthing philosophy ■ Rapid, progressive relaxation/deepening techniques for transition ■ Visualizations for labor ■ Composing a birth plan ■ Early signs of labor ■ Birthing companion's integral role in labor ■ Pushing techniques ■ Postnatal bonding of parents with baby

Teaching Highlights

INTERNET RESOURCES

Explain to women who are using Internet childbirth education resources that some sites may not use health professionals or experts in the childbirth field and may be written by individuals who lack formal education and training. Advise women to look for resources that are supported by licensed professionals or well-known, credible organizations.

One of the most important components of childbirth education is instilling confidence in a woman's ability to give birth (Lothian, 2006). The Council of Childbirth Education Specialists encourages education that focuses on the interconnectedness of the body and spirit. After that connection is established and understood by pregnant women, coping strategies, stress reduction, and relaxation techniques can then be taught.

Another prominent organization that provides educational resources and certification for educators is the International Childbirth Education Association (ICEA). This organization does not advocate a particular method of childbirth preparation but rather promotes a philosophy of "freedom of choice based on knowledge of alternatives" (International Childbirth Education Association, 2006). Many expectant parents find this approach consistent with their own desires to experience birth as informed healthcare consumers. ICEA educators often teach a combination of techniques designed to meet individual needs.

BODY-CONDITIONING EXERCISES

Some body-conditioning exercises, such as the pelvic tilt, pelvic rock, and Kegel exercises, are taught in childbirth preparation classes. Other exercises strengthen the abdominal muscles for the expulsive phase of labor. (See Chapter 11 ∞ for a description of recommended exercises.)

RELAXATION EXERCISES

Relaxation during labor allows the woman to conserve energy and the uterine muscles to work more efficiently. Without practice it is difficult to relax the whole body in the midst of intense uterine contractions. Progressive relaxation exercises such as those taught to induce sleep can be helpful during labor. "Teaching Highlights: Touch Relaxation" provides information on one approach.

An additional exercise specific to Lamaze is disassociation relaxation. The woman is taught to become familiar with the sensation of contracting and relaxing the voluntary muscle groups throughout her body. She then learns to contract a specific muscle group and relax the rest of her body. The exercise conditions the woman to relax uninvolved muscles while the uterus contracts, creating an active relaxation pattern.

The relaxation techniques described are most effective if the woman practices them daily, both alone and with her support person. During a practice session, the partner begins by checking the woman's neck, shoulders, arms, and legs for relaxation. As tense areas are found, the helper encourages the woman to relax those body parts. By gentle touch and verbal cues, the woman learns to respond to her own perceptions of tense muscles and also to the suggestion from others. Relaxation may also be promoted by cutaneous stimulation. One type commonly used prior to the transitional phase of labor is abdominal effleurage, discussed previously (Figure 8–4 ●). This light abdominal stroking can relieve mild to moderate pain but not intense pain.

Teaching Highlights

TOUCH RELAXATION

Touch relaxation technique often combines patterned abdominal breathing with focused relaxation. It may be used to achieve relaxation of specific body parts or for general body relaxation.

Goals

The woman learns to release tension in the areas that her partner touches. The partner learns to watch his or her partner carefully and becomes attuned to tense, tightened muscles.

Technique

- The partner gently touches the woman's brow.
- The woman uses abdominal breathing. As she breathes in through her nose, her abdomen rises, and as she breathes out through her mouth, her abdomen falls. As each breath is released, she lets all tightness and tension flow out with the breath.
- The partner continues to lightly touch her brow until the woman feels relaxation. The partner may want to provide quiet encouragement such as, "You are doing fine, you are releasing the tension in your forehead." After at least five breaths, the partner may touch the woman's shoulders and repeat the pattern described earlier.
- The partner moves on to the arms, chest, abdomen, thighs, and calves. The last aspect is to breathe in, let the whole body relax and go limp, and slowly release the breath. It will be helpful at the end of each labor contraction to let the body go limp and release all tension.
- As the couple practices, it is important for the woman to relax each part of her body. When she is in labor, it will not be possible to go through the whole body; however, the woman can indicate what would be most helpful (e.g., touch her shoulder during each contraction). The partner can also be alert for signs of muscle tension and tightening. As the partner and woman practice touch relaxation, they may want to make the situation more realistic. They could decide that uterine contractions are occurring every 5 minutes and are lasting for 30 seconds. A clock will help the partner keep track of time. The partner can indicate that a contraction is beginning and suggest the woman begin her breathing. To help her focus, the partner may touch her shoulder or hand. In some instances, it is helpful for the partner to breathe along with the woman. Each couple can determine what works best for them.

MyNursingKit Video: Effleurage massage

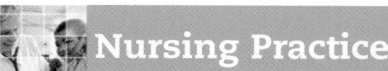

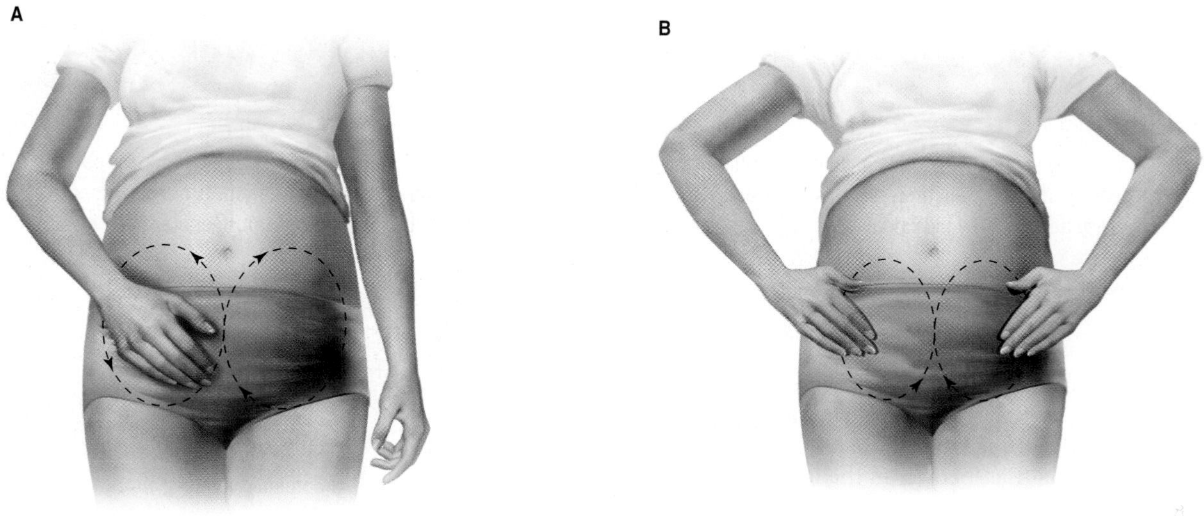

● **Figure 8–4** Effleurage is light stroking of the abdomen with the fingertips. ***A,*** Starting at the symphysis, the woman lightly moves her fingertips up and around in a circular pattern. ***B,*** An alternative approach involves using one hand in a figure-eight pattern. This light stroking can also be done by the support person.

BREATHING TECHNIQUES

Breathing techniques are a key element of most childbirth preparation programs. They help keep the mother and her unborn baby adequately oxygenated, and help the mother relax and focus her attention appropriately. Breathing techniques are best taught during the final trimester of pregnancy. The nurse then supports the mother's use of breathing techniques during labor. Breathing techniques are described in Chapter 19∞.

Nursing Practice

Identify the methods of childbirth preparation commonly used in your area and learn the basics of their approaches to relaxation and breathing. Then practice these methods so that you can support a laboring couple more effectively.

PREPARATION FOR CHILDBIRTH THAT SUPPORTS INDIVIDUALITY

Childbirth educators stress the value of individuality when providing information to expectant parents. The goal is to encourage women to incorporate their own natural responses into coping with the pain of labor and birth. Self-care activities that may be used include vocalization or "sounding" to relieve tension in pregnancy and labor, massage (light touch) to facilitate relaxation, use of warm water for showers or bathing during labor, visualization (imagery), relaxing music, subdued lighting, and the use of a birthing ball (see Chapter 19∞).

Nurses need to encourage expectant mothers and couples to make the birth a personal experience. A woman might choose to bring items from home that help create a more personal birthing space. These items might include warm socks, extra pillows, bath powder, lotion, or a favorite blanket. She may wish to bring photos of special people or places. Many expectant parents enjoy listening to tapes of favorite music or watching favorite home videos. Such personalization of the birth experience may give expectant parents feelings of increased serenity and empowerment.

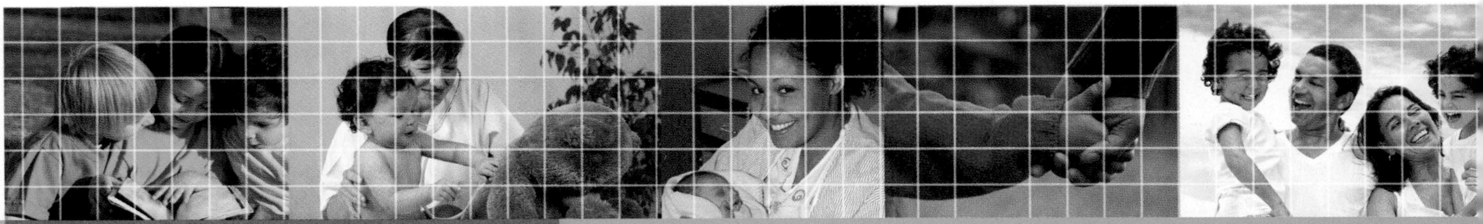

CRITICAL CONCEPT REVIEW

LEARNING OUTCOMES	CONCEPTS
8.1 Determine the most appropriate nursing care for couples during preconception to help ensure their best possible health state.	1. Information is a major nursing responsibility during the preconception period. Preconception counseling is designed to: ■ Teach the client about environmental and lifestyle hazards that could affect conception and pregnancy. ■ Identify any health problems that could impede a successful pregnancy. ■ Advise the client about contraception and fertility.
8.2 Identify ways to assist expectant parents in making the best decisions possible about issues related to pregnancy, labor, and birth.	1. Couples are faced with the need to make decisions about issues such as: ■ Choice of a healthcare provider. ■ Birth experience plan. ■ Choice of birth setting. ■ Choice of support person during labor. ■ Choice of who should be present during the birth, such as other family members and siblings.
8.3 Summarize the goals and content of the various types of antepartal education programs when providing nursing care for expectant couples and their families.	1. A broad range of classes are available, including: ■ Description of each stage of pregnancy. ■ Childbirth preparation. ■ Preparation for a cesarean birth. ■ Breastfeeding. ■ Sibling preparation. ■ Grandparent role preparation.
8.4 Compare methods of childbirth preparation and the nursing interventions for each.	1. There are many different methods to prepare clients for childbirth. They all emphasize measures that help to decrease anxiety and pain. The childbirth methods discussed in this chapter are: ■ Lamaze: uses breathing patterns, controlled muscular relaxation techniques (psychoprophylactic). ■ Bradley: partner-coached childbirth. ■ Kitzinger: sensory-memory techniques. ■ HypnoBirthing: deep relaxation techniques. 2. To support the approach the family has chosen.
8.5 Explore ways in which the nurse conveys respect for client individuality in preparing for childbirth.	1. Nurses convey respect during childbirth preparation by: ■ Emphasizing the uniqueness of each birth experience. ■ Providing the client with tools such as breathing and relaxation to choose the best childbirth methods.

CRITICAL THINKING IN ACTION

Terry Dole, a 38-year-old G1 P0000, at 6 weeks' gestation, presents to you at the OB clinic for her first prenatal visit with the certified nurse-midwife (CNM). One of the first decisions facing Terry is the selection of a healthcare provider. The midwife explains the various options available to Terry at the clinic related to the differences in educational preparation, skill level, practice characteristics, and general philosophy of CNMs and obstetricians. Terry tells you that she has been married for 6 years and works as a massage therapist. You obtain the following data: BP 110/70, temperature 97.0°F, pulse 76, respirations 12, weight 140 lb, height 5'7". The physical and pelvic exams are essentially normal. The CNM asks you to teach Terry about birth plans.

1. Discuss the advantages of a birth plan.
2. Discuss the disadvantages of a birth plan.
3. Explain the role of a doula.
4. What gender differences are there in moving toward parenthood?

See MyNursingKit for possible responses.

REFERENCES

Al-Qahtani, N. H. (2005). Foetal response to music and voice. *Australian and New Zealand Journal of Obstetrics and Gynaecology, 45*, 414–417.

American Academy of Husband-Coached Childbirth. (2008). The Bradley Method. Retrieved on February 11, 2008, from www.bradleybirth.com/Main.aspx

DiPietro, N. A. (2008). Preconception care: An overview. *U.S. Pharmacist, 33*(9), 340–342.

Graven, S. N., & Browne, J. V. (2008). Auditory development in the fetus and infant. *Newborn and Infant Nursing Reviews, 8*(4), 187–193.

Hamilton, B. E., Martin, J. A., & Ventura, S. J. (2009). Births: Preliminary data for 2007. *National Vital Statistics Resports, 57*(12), 1–17.

International Childbirth Education Association. (2006). ICEA philosophy statement. Retrieved on February 11, 2008, from http://www.icea.org

Lothian, J. A. (2006). Listening to mothers: Take two. *Journal of Perinatal Education, 15*(4), 41–43.

Low, L. K., Seng, J. S., Murtland, T. L., & Oakley, D. (2000). Clinician-specific episiotomy rates: Impact on perineal outcomes. *Journal of Nurse-Midwifery and Women's Health, 45*(2), 87–91.

O'Connor, M. J. (2008). Preconception care for reducing alcohol exposure in pregnancy. *The Female Patient, 33*(10), 14–20.

Teschendorf, M., & Evans, C. (2000). Hydrotherapy during labor: an example of a developing practice policy. *American Journal of Maternal-Child Nursing, 25*(4), 198–203.

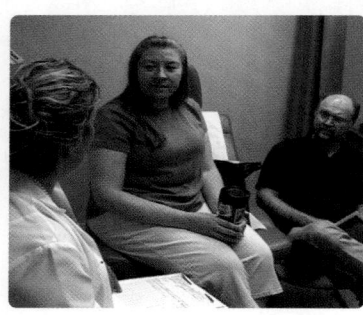

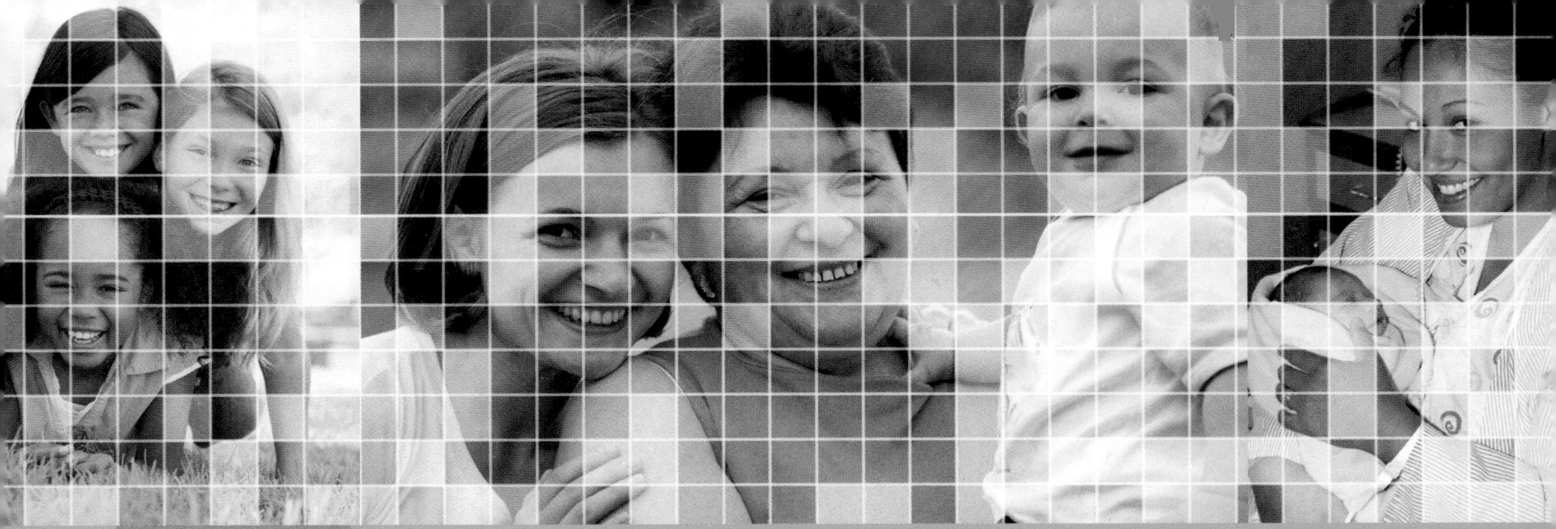

CHAPTER

9 Physical and Psychologic Changes of Pregnancy

Our son and his wife just told us they are pregnant. I am going to be a grandfather! I have tried to be a good father, to give my boy love, to teach him to respect others, to show him what it means to be a real man, someone a family can count on. Guess time will tell if the lessons took—I'm betting they have. —Martin, 52

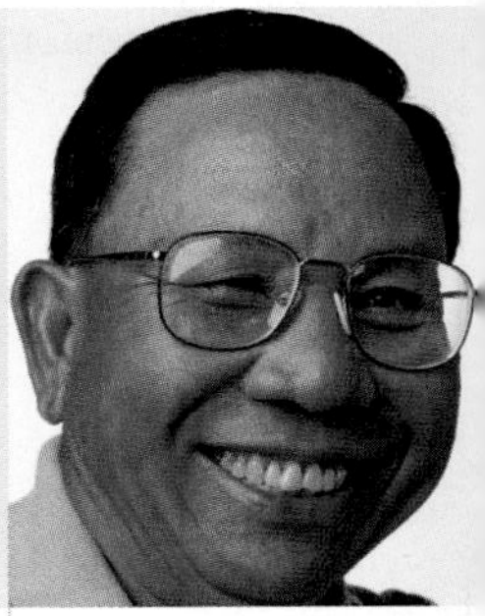

LEARNING OUTCOMES

9.1 Identify the anatomic and physiologic changes that occur during pregnancy.

9.2 Assess the subjective (presumptive), objective (probable), and diagnostic (positive) changes of pregnancy in clients.

9.3 Contrast the various types of pregnancy tests.

9.4 Address the emotional and psychologic changes that commonly occur in a woman, her partner, and her family during pregnancy when providing nursing care.

9.5 Recognize cultural factors that may influence a family's response to pregnancy in the provision of nursing care.

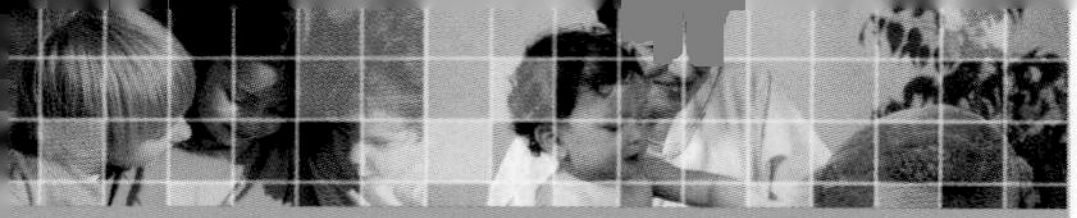

KEY TERMS

Ballottement, 190

Braxton Hicks contractions, 184

Chadwick's sign, 189

Chloasma (melasma gravidarum), 186

Couvade, 195

Diastasis recti, 187

Goodell's sign, 189

Hegar's sign, 189

Linea nigra, 186

McDonald's sign, 189

Morning sickness, 189

Mucous plug, 184

Physiologic anemia of pregnancy, 185

Quickening, 189

Striae (striae gravidarum), 186

Supine hypotensive syndrome (vena caval syndrome, aortocaval compression), 185

Pregnancy is divided into three trimesters, each approximately a 3-month period. Each trimester brings predictable changes for both the mother and the fetus. How does pregnancy affect the woman physically and psychologically? How does it affect her family, including siblings, partner, and grandparents? This chapter describes these physical and psychologic changes and the responses of the entire family to pregnancy. It also presents the various cultural factors that can affect a pregnant woman's well-being. Subsequent chapters build on this information in describing effective approaches to planning and providing care.

ANATOMY AND PHYSIOLOGY OF PREGNANCY

REPRODUCTIVE SYSTEM

Some of the most dramatic changes of pregnancy occur in the reproductive organs.

Uterus

Before pregnancy the uterus is a small, almost solid, pear-shaped organ measuring approximately 7.5 × 5 × 2.5 cm and weighing about 60 g (2 oz). At the end of pregnancy, it measures about 28 × 24 × 21 cm and weighs approximately 1100 g; its capacity has also increased from about 10 mL to 5000 mL (5 L) or more (Cunningham, Leveno, Bloom, et al., 2010). The change is primarily a result of the enlargement (hypertrophy) of the preexisting myometrial cells in response to the stimulating influence of estrogen and the distention caused by the growing fetus. Only a limited increase in cell number (hyperplasia) occurs. The fibrous tissue between the muscle bands increases markedly, which adds to the strength and elasticity of the muscle wall. The enlarging uterus, developing placenta, and growing fetus require additional blood flow to the uterus. By the end of pregnancy, one sixth of the total maternal blood volume is contained within the vascular system of the uterus.

Braxton Hicks contractions, which are irregular, generally painless contractions of the uterus, occur intermittently throughout pregnancy. They may be felt through the abdominal wall beginning about the fourth month of pregnancy. In later months these contractions become uncomfortable and may be confused with true labor contractions.

Cervix

Estrogen stimulates the glandular tissue of the cervix, which increases in cell number and becomes hyperactive. The endocervical glands secrete a thick, sticky mucus that accumulates and forms the **mucous plug**, which seals the endocervical canal and prevents the ascent of organisms into the uterus. This mucous plug is expelled when cervical dilatation begins. The hyperactivity of the glandular tissue also increases the normal physiologic mucorrhea, at times resulting in profuse discharge. Increased cervical vascularity also causes both the softening of the cervix (Goodell's sign) and its bluish discoloration (Chadwick's sign).

Ovaries

The ovaries stop producing ova during pregnancy, but the corpus luteum continues to produce hormones until about weeks 6 to 8. It secretes progesterone until about the seventh week of pregnancy, maintaining the endometrium until the placenta assumes the task. The corpus luteum then begins to disintegrate slowly.

Nursing Practice

Beginning early in pregnancy, have the woman feel her uterus periodically so that she becomes familiar with the size and the way it feels. As her pregnancy progresses, she then will be more likely to identify Braxton Hicks contractions and preterm labor, if it occurs.

Vagina

Estrogen causes a thickening of the vaginal mucosa, a loosening of the connective tissue, and an increase in vaginal secretions (leukorrhea). These secretions are thick, white, and acidic (pH 3.5 to 6.0). The acid pH helps prevent bacterial infection but favors the growth of yeast organisms. Thus, the pregnant woman is more susceptible to *Candida* infection than usual.

The supportive connective tissue of the vagina loosens throughout pregnancy. By the end of pregnancy, the vagina and perineal body are sufficiently relaxed to permit passage of the infant. Because blood flow to the vagina is increased, the vagina may show the same blue-purple color (Chadwick's sign) as the cervix.

Breasts

Estrogen and progesterone cause many changes in the mammary glands. The breasts enlarge and become more nodular as the glands increase in size and number in preparation for lactation. Superficial veins become more prominent, the nipples become more erectile, and the areolae darken. Montgomery's tubercles (sebaceous glands) enlarge, and striae (reddish stretch marks that slowly turn silver after childbirth) may develop.

Colostrum, an antibody-rich yellow secretion, may leak or be expressed from the breasts during the last trimester. Colostrum gradually converts to mature milk during the first few days after childbirth.

RESPIRATORY SYSTEM

Many respiratory changes occur to meet the increased oxygen requirements of a pregnant woman. The volume of air breathed each minute increases 30% to 40%. In addition, progesterone decreases airway resistance, permitting a 15% to 20% increase in oxygen consumption, as well as increases in carbon dioxide production and in the respiratory functional reserve.

As the uterus enlarges, it presses upward and elevates the diaphragm. The subcostal angle increases, so that the rib cage flares. The anteroposterior diameter increases, and the chest circumference expands by as much as 6 cm; as a result there is no significant loss of intrathoracic volume. Breathing changes from abdominal to thoracic as pregnancy progresses, and descent of the diaphragm on inspiration becomes less possible. Some hyperventilation and difficulty in breathing may occur.

Nasal stuffiness and epistaxis (nosebleeds) may also occur because of estrogen-induced edema, hypersecretion of mucus, and vascular congestion of the nasal mucosa.

CARDIOVASCULAR SYSTEM

Blood volume progressively increases beginning in the first trimester, increasing rapidly until about 30 to 34 weeks, and then plateauing until birth at about 40% to 50% above nonpregnant levels. This increase is a result of increases in both erythrocytes and plasma (Gordon, 2007).

During pregnancy, blood flow increases to organ systems with an increased workload. Thus, blood flow increases to the uterus, placenta, and breasts, whereas hepatic and cerebral flow remain unchanged. Cardiac output begins to increase early in pregnancy and peaks at 25 to 30 weeks' gestation at 30% to 50% above prepregnant levels. It generally remains elevated in the third trimester.

The pulse may increase by as many as 10 to 15 beats per minute at term. The blood pressure decreases slightly, reaching its lowest point during the second trimester. It gradually increases to near prepregnant levels by the end of the third trimester. This change is due to a decrease in systemic vascular resistance. The cause of the decrease in systemic vascular resistance is not well understood; however, progesterone-mediated smooth musculi relaxation may be a factor (Gordon, 2007).

The enlarging uterus puts pressure on pelvic and femoral vessels, interfering with returning blood flow and causing stasis of blood in the lower extremities. This condition may lead to dependent edema and varicosity of the veins in the legs, vulva, and rectum (hemorrhoids) in late pregnancy. This increased blood volume in the lower legs may also make the pregnant woman prone to postural hypotension.

When the pregnant woman lies supine, the enlarging uterus may press on the vena cava, thus reducing blood flow to the right atrium, lowering blood pressure, and causing dizziness, pallor, and clamminess. The enlarging uterus may also press on the aorta and its collateral circulation (Cunningham et al., 2010). This condition is called **supine hypotensive syndrome.** It may also be referred to as *vena caval syndrome* or *aortocaval compression* (Figure 9–1 ●). It can be corrected by having the woman lie on her side or by placing a pillow or wedge under her right hip.

The total erythrocyte (red blood cell) volume increases by about 30% in women who receive iron supplementation but only about 18% without iron supplementation. This increase in erythrocytes is necessary to transport the additional oxygen required during pregnancy. However, the increase in plasma volume during pregnancy averages about 50%. Because the plasma volume increase (50%) is greater than the erythrocyte increase (30%), the hematocrit, which measures the concentration of red blood cells in the plasma, decreases slightly (Gordon, 2007). This decrease is referred to as the **physiologic anemia of pregnancy** (pseudoanemia).

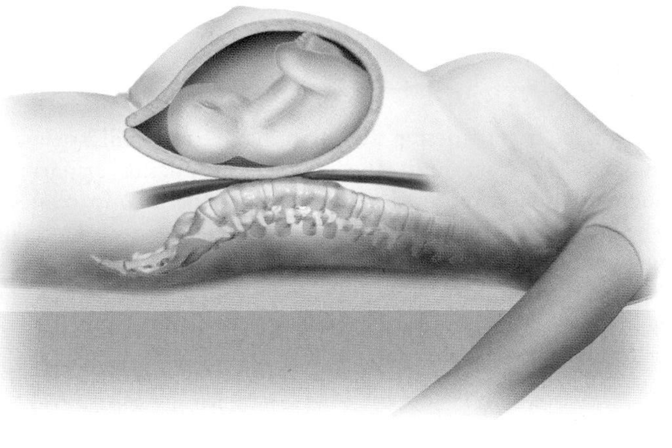

● **Figure 9–1** Supine hypotensive syndrome (vena caval syndrome). The gravid uterus compresses the vena cava when the woman is supine. This reduces the blood flow returning to the heart and may cause maternal hypotension.

Iron is necessary for hemoglobin formation, and hemoglobin is the oxygen-carrying component of erythrocytes. Thus, the increase in erythrocyte levels results in an increased need for iron by the pregnant woman. Even though the gastrointestinal absorption of iron is moderately increased during pregnancy, it is usually necessary to add supplemental iron to the diet to meet the expanded red blood cell and fetal needs.

Leukocyte production increases slightly to a range of 5600 to 12,200/mm^3. During labor and early postpartum, these levels may reach 20,000 to 30,000/mm^3 or higher (Gordon, 2007).

Both fibrin and plasma fibrinogen levels increase during pregnancy. Although the blood-clotting time of the pregnant woman does not differ significantly from that of the nonpregnant woman, clotting factors VII, VIII, IX, and X increase; thus, pregnancy is a somewhat hypercoagulable state. These changes, coupled with venous stasis in late pregnancy, increase the pregnant woman's risk of developing venous thrombosis.

GASTROINTESTINAL SYSTEM

Nausea and vomiting are common during the first trimester and may result from several factors, including elevated human chorionic gonadotropin (hCG) levels, relaxation of the smooth muscle of the stomach, and changed carbohydrate metabolism (Gordon, 2007). Gum tissue may soften and bleed easily. The secretion of saliva may increase and even become excessive (ptyalism).

Elevated progesterone levels cause smooth muscle relaxation, resulting in delayed gastric emptying and decreased peristalsis. As a result the pregnant woman may complain of bloating and constipation. These symptoms are aggravated as the enlarging uterus displaces the stomach upward and the intestines are moved laterally and posteriorly. The cardiac sphincter also relaxes, and heartburn (pyrosis) may occur because of reflux of acidic secretions into the lower esophagus. Hemorrhoids frequently develop in late pregnancy from constipation and from pressure on vessels below the level of the uterus.

The emptying time of the gallbladder is prolonged during pregnancy as a result of smooth muscle relaxation from progesterone. This, coupled with the elevated levels of cholesterol in the bile, can predispose the woman to gallstone formation.

URINARY TRACT

During the first trimester, the enlarging uterus is still a pelvic organ and presses against the bladder, producing urinary frequency. This symptom decreases during the second trimester, when the uterus becomes an abdominal organ and pressure against the bladder lessens. Frequency reappears during the third trimester, when the presenting part descends into the pelvis and again presses on the bladder, reducing bladder capacity, contributing to hyperemia, and irritating the bladder.

The ureters (especially the right ureter) elongate and dilate above the pelvic brim. The glomerular filtration rate rises by as much as 50% beginning in the second trimester and remains elevated until birth. To compensate for this increase, renal tubular reabsorption also increases. However, glycosuria is sometimes seen during pregnancy because of the kidneys' inability to reabsorb all the glucose filtered by the glomeruli. Glycosuria may be normal or may indicate gestational diabetes, so it always warrants further testing.

SKIN AND HAIR

Changes in skin pigmentation commonly occur during pregnancy. They are thought to be stimulated by increased estrogen, progesterone, and α-melanocytic-stimulating hormone levels. Pigmentation of the skin increases primarily in areas that are already hyperpigmented: the areolae, the nipples, the vulva, and the perianal area. The skin in the middle of the abdomen may develop a pigmented line, the **linea nigra**, which usually extends from the pubic area to the umbilicus or higher (Figure 9–2 ●). Facial **chloasma** (**melasma gravidarum**), also known as the "mask of pregnancy," a darkening of the skin over the forehead and around the eyes, may develop. Melasma is more prominent in dark-haired women and is aggravated by exposure to the sun. Fortunately, it fades or becomes less prominent soon after childbirth when the hormonal influence of pregnancy subsides. The sweat and sebaceous glands are often hyperactive during pregnancy. **Striae** (**striae gravidarum** when they result from pregnancy), or stretch marks, are reddish, wavy streaks that may appear on the abdomen, thighs, buttocks, and breasts. They result from reduced connective tissue strength because of elevated adrenal steroid levels.

Vascular spider nevi, small, bright-red elevations of the skin radiating from a central body, may develop on the chest, neck, face, arms, and legs. They may be caused by increased subcutaneous blood flow in response to elevated estrogen levels.

The proportion of hair in the growing phase increases during pregnancy compared with the number of hair follicles in the resting or dormant phase. After birth the number of hair follicles in the resting phase increases sharply, and the woman may notice increased hair shedding beginning 1 to 4 months postpartum.

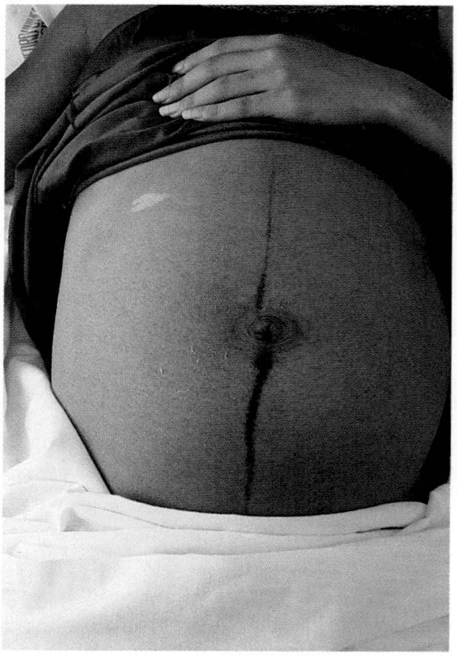

● **Figure 9–2** Linea nigra.

Practically all hair is replaced within 6 to 12 months, however (Cunningham et al., 2010).

MUSCULOSKELETAL SYSTEM

No demonstrable changes occur in the teeth of pregnant women. The dental caries that sometimes accompany pregnancy are probably caused by inadequate oral hygiene and dental care, especially if the woman has problems with bleeding gums or nausea and vomiting.

The joints of the pelvis relax somewhat because of hormonal influences. The result is often a waddling gait. As the pregnant woman's center of gravity gradually changes, the lumbar spinal curve becomes accentuated (lordosis), and her posture changes (Figure 9–3 ●). This posture change compensates for the increased weight of the uterus anteriorly and frequently results in low backache.

Pressure of the enlarging uterus on the abdominal muscles may cause the rectus abdominis muscle to separate, producing **diastasis recti**. If the separation is severe and muscle tone is not regained postpartally, subsequent pregnancies will not have adequate support and the woman's abdomen may appear pendulous.

CENTRAL NERVOUS SYSTEM

Pregnant women frequently describe decreased attention, concentration, and memory during and shortly after pregnancy, but few studies have explored this phenomenon. One study did find a decline in memory that could not be attributed to depression, anxiety, sleep deprivation, or other physical changes of pregnancy. This memory loss disappeared soon after childbirth (Cunningham et al, 2010).

METABOLISM

Most metabolic functions increase during pregnancy because of the increased demands of the growing fetus and its support system. For a detailed discussion of nutrient, vitamin, and mineral metabolism, see Chapter 12∞.

Weight Gain

The recommended weight gain for women of normal weight before pregnancy is 25 to 35 lb (11.4 to 15.9 kg), whereas women who are overweight should limit their gain to 15 lb (6.8 kg). Underweight women may gain up to 40 lb (18.1 kg) (Johnson, Gregory, & Niebyl, 2007). The average pattern of weight gain is 3.5 to 5 lb (1.6 to 2.3 kg) during the first trimester and 12 to 15 lb (5.5 to 6.8 kg) during each of the last two trimesters. Adequate nutrition and weight gain are important during pregnancy.

Water Metabolism

Increased water retention, a basic alteration of pregnancy, is caused by several interrelated factors. The increased level of steroid sex hormones affects sodium and fluid retention. The lowered serum protein also influences fluid balance, as do increased intracapillary pressure and permeability. The extra water is needed for the fetus, the placenta, amniotic fluid, and the mother's increased blood volume, interstitial fluids, and enlarged organs.

Nutrient Metabolism

The fetus makes its greatest protein and fat demands during the second half of pregnancy, doubling in weight during the last 6 to 8 weeks. Protein (contributing nitrogen) must be stored during pregnancy to maintain a constant level within the breast milk and to avoid depletion of maternal tissues. Carbohydrate needs also increase, especially during the second and third trimesters. Fats are more completely absorbed during pregnancy, and the level of free fatty acids increases in response to human placental lactogen (hPL). The levels of lipoproteins and cholesterol also increase. Because of these changes, increased levels of dietary fat or reduced carbohydrate production may lead to ketonuria in the pregnant woman.

MyNursingKit Case Study: Prenatal Education

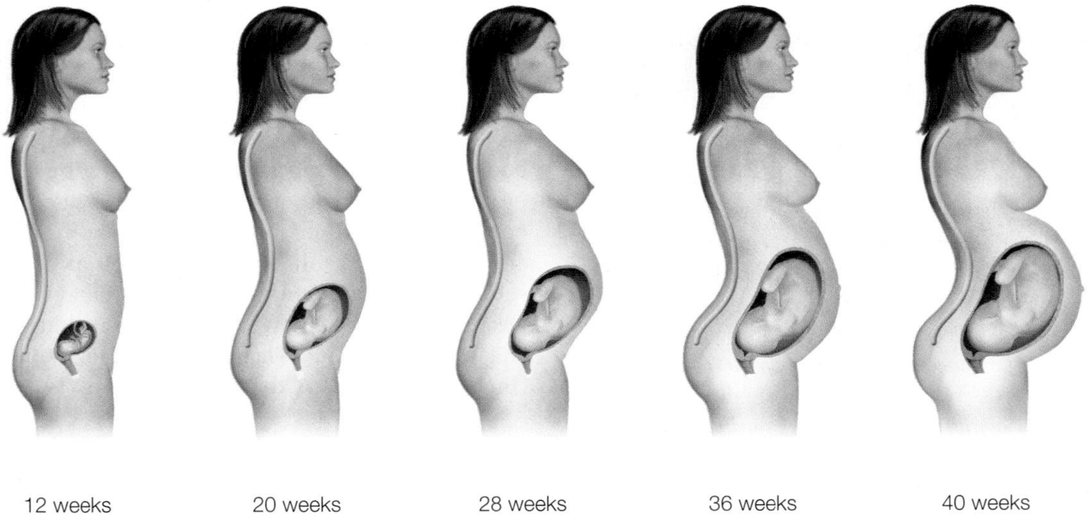

● **Figure 9–3** Postural changes during pregnancy. Note the increasing lordosis of the lumbosacral spine and the increasing curvature of the thoracic area.

ENDOCRINE SYSTEM

Thyroid

The thyroid gland often enlarges slightly during pregnancy because of increased vascularity and hyperplasia of glandular tissue. Estrogen increases its capacity to bind thyroxine, resulting in an increase in serum protein-bound iodine. The basal metabolic rate increases by as much as 20% to 25% during pregnancy. However, within a few weeks after birth, all thyroid function returns to normal limits.

Pituitary

Pregnancy is made possible by the hypothalamic stimulation of the anterior pituitary gland. The anterior pituitary produces follicle-stimulating hormone (FSH), which stimulates ovum growth, and luteinizing hormone (LH), which brings about ovulation. Stimulation of the pituitary also prolongs the ovary's corpus luteal phase. This maintains the endometrium in case conception occurs. Prolactin, another anterior pituitary hormone, is responsible for initial lactation.

The posterior pituitary secretes vasopressin (antidiuretic hormone) and oxytocin. Vasopressin causes vasoconstriction, which results in increased blood pressure; it also helps regulate water balance. Oxytocin promotes uterine contractility and stimulates ejection of milk from the breasts (the letdown reflex) in the postpartum period.

Adrenals

During pregnancy, circulating cortisol, which regulates carbohydrate and protein metabolism, increases in response to increased estrogen levels. Cortisol blood levels return to normal within 1 to 6 weeks postpartum. The adrenals secrete increased levels of aldosterone by the early part of the second trimester. This increase in aldosterone in a normal pregnancy may be the body's protective response to the increased sodium excretion associated with progesterone (Cunningham et al., 2010).

> **Complementary Care**
>
> **HERBS DURING PREGNANCY**
>
> Pharmaceutical companies have not included pregnant women in their studies of drug safety. As a result, very few over-the-counter or prescription drugs can claim to be safe for pregnant women and breastfeeding mothers. The same can be said for herbal medicines. Although many herbs have been researched extensively in Europe and Asia, there has been little clinical research done in the United States on the use of herbs in pregnancy. Nurses would do well to learn about many of the commonly used herbs so that they can provide pregnant women with accurate information. Pregnant or breastfeeding women must be cautious about everything they ingest—foods, liquids, medications, and herbs. If a problem warrants intervention, she and her primary healthcare provider should discuss the benefits and risks of all treatments, synthetic and natural.

Pancreas

The pregnant woman has increased insulin needs, and the pancreatic islets of Langerhans, which secrete insulin, are stressed to meet this increased demand. Any marginal pancreatic function quickly becomes apparent, and the woman may show signs of gestational diabetes.

Hormones in Pregnancy

Human chorionic gonadotropin. The trophoblast secretes hCG in early pregnancy. This hormone stimulates progesterone and estrogen production by the corpus luteum to maintain the pregnancy until the placenta is developed sufficiently to assume that function.

Human placental lactogen. Also called human chorionic somatomammotropin, hPL is produced by the syncytiotrophoblast. Human placental lactogen is an antagonist of insulin; it increases the amount of circulating free fatty acids for maternal metabolic needs and decreases maternal metabolism of glucose to favor fetal growth.

Estrogen. Secreted originally by the corpus luteum, estrogen is produced primarily by the placenta as early as the seventh week of pregnancy. Estrogen stimulates uterine development to provide a suitable environment for the fetus. It also helps develop the ductal system of the breasts in preparation for lactation.

Progesterone. Also produced initially by the corpus luteum and then by the placenta, progesterone plays the greatest role in maintaining pregnancy. It maintains the endometrium and inhibits spontaneous uterine contractility, thus preventing early spontaneous abortion. Progesterone also helps develop the acini and lobules of the breasts in preparation for lactation.

Relaxin. Relaxin is detectable in the serum of a pregnant woman by the time of the first missed menstrual period. Relaxin inhibits uterine activity, diminishes the strength of uterine contractions, aids in the softening of the cervix, and has the long-term effect of remodeling connective tissue, which is necessary for the uterus to accommodate pregnancy (Cunningham et al., 2010). Its primary source is the corpus luteum, but small amounts are believed to be produced by the placenta and uterine decidua.

Prostaglandins in Pregnancy

Prostaglandins are lipid substances that can arise from most body tissues but occur in high concentrations in the female reproductive tract and are present in the decidua during pregnancy. The exact functions of prostaglandins during pregnancy are still unknown, although it has been proposed that they are responsible for maintaining reduced placental vascular resistance. Decreased prostaglandin levels may contribute to hypertension and preeclampsia. Prostaglandins may also play a role in the complex biochemistry that initiates labor.

SIGNS OF PREGNANCY

Many of the changes women experience during pregnancy are used to diagnose the pregnancy itself. They may be grouped into three categories: the subjective, or presumptive, changes; the objective, or probable, changes; and the diagnostic, or positive, changes of pregnancy.

SUBJECTIVE (PRESUMPTIVE) CHANGES

The subjective changes of pregnancy are the symptoms the woman experiences and reports. Because they can be caused by other conditions, they cannot be considered proof of pregnancy (Table 9–1). Several subjective signs can be diagnostic clues when other signs and symptoms of pregnancy are also present.

Amenorrhea, or the absence of menses, is the earliest symptom of pregnancy. Missing more than one menstrual period, especially in a woman whose cycle is ordinarily regular, is an especially useful diagnostic clue.

Nausea and vomiting in pregnancy (NVP) occur frequently during the first trimester. It may be mild or may cause considerable distress. Because these symptoms often occur in the early part of the day, they are commonly referred to as **morning sickness**. In reality the symptoms may occur at any time and can range from a mere distaste for food to severe vomiting. Women who experience NVP often have a more favorable pregnancy outcome than those who do not.

Table 9–1 Differential Diagnosis of Pregnancy—Subjective Changes

Subjective Changes	Possible Alternative Causes
Amenorrhea	*Endocrine factors:* early menopause; lactation; thyroid, pituitary, adrenal, ovarian dysfunction *Metabolic factors:* malnutrition, anemia, climatic changes, diabetes mellitus, degenerative disorders, long-distance running *Psychologic factors:* emotional shock, fear of pregnancy or sexually transmitted infection, intense desire for pregnancy (pseudocyesis), stress Obliteration of endometrial cavity by infection or curettage Systemic disease (acute or chronic), such as tuberculosis or malignancy
Nausea and vomiting	Gastrointestinal disorders Acute infections such as encephalitis Emotional disorders such as pseudocyesis or anorexia nervosa
Urinary frequency	Urinary tract infection Cystocele Pelvic tumors Urethral diverticula Emotional tension
Breast tenderness	Premenstrual tension Chronic cystic mastitis Pseudocyesis Hyperestrogenism
Quickening	Increased peristalsis Flatus ("gas") Abdominal muscle contractions Shifting of abdominal contents

Nursing Practice

It is often helpful to give women who are pregnant for the first time a description of how quickening feels so that they can identify it more easily. Some women suggest that it is easiest to imagine the fluttering associated with quickening by letting the outer tips of the eyelashes brush a finger and then imagining that same sensation deep inside the abdomen.

Excessive fatigue may be noted within a few weeks after the first missed menstrual period and may persist throughout the first trimester.

Urinary frequency is experienced during the first trimester as the enlarging uterus presses on the bladder.

Changes in the breasts are frequently noted in early pregnancy. These changes include tenderness and tingling sensations, increased pigmentation of the areola and nipple, and changes in Montgomery's glands. The veins also become more visible and form a bluish pattern beneath the skin.

Quickening, or the mother's perception of fetal movement, occurs about 18 to 20 weeks after the last menstrual period in a woman pregnant for the first time but may occur as early as 16 weeks in a woman who has been pregnant before. Quickening is a fluttering sensation in the abdomen that gradually increases in intensity and frequency.

OBJECTIVE (PROBABLE) CHANGES

An examiner can perceive the objective changes that occur in pregnancy. Because these changes can have other causes, they do not confirm pregnancy (Table 9–2).

Changes in the pelvic organs—the only physical changes detectable during the first 3 months of pregnancy—are caused by increased vascular congestion. These changes are noted on pelvic examination. As noted earlier, there is a softening of the cervix called **Goodell's sign**. **Chadwick's sign** is a bluish, purple, or deep-red discoloration of the mucous membranes of the cervix, vagina, and vulva (some sources consider this a presumptive sign). **Hegar's sign** is a softening of the isthmus of the uterus, the area between the cervix and the body of the uterus (Figure 9–4 ●). **McDonald's sign** is an ease in flexing the body of the uterus against the cervix.

General enlargement and softening of the body of the uterus can be noted after the eighth week of pregnancy. The fundus of the uterus is palpable just above the symphysis pubis at about 10 to 12 weeks' gestation and at the level of the umbilicus at 20 to 22 weeks' gestation (Figure 9–5 ●).

Enlargement of the abdomen during the childbearing years is usually regarded as evidence of pregnancy, especially if it is continuous and accompanied by amenorrhea.

Braxton Hicks contractions can be palpated most commonly after the 28th week. As the woman approaches the end of pregnancy, these contractions may become uncomfortable. They are often called *false labor.*

Table 9–2 Differential Diagnosis of Pregnancy—Objective Changes

Objective Changes	Possible Alternative Causes
Changes in pelvic organs Goodell's sign Chadwick's sign Hegar's sign Uterine enlargement	Increased vascular congestion Estrogen-progestin oral contraceptives Vulvar, vaginal, cervical hyperemia Excessively soft walls of nonpregnant uterus Uterine tumors
Enlargement of abdomen	Obesity, ascites, pelvic tumors
Braxton Hicks contractions	Hematometra, pedunculated, submucous, and soft myomas
Uterine souffle	Large uterine myomas, large ovarian tumors, or any condition with greatly increased uterine blood flow
Pigmentation of skin Chloasma (melasma) Linea nigra Nipples/areolae	Estrogen-progestin oral contraceptives Melanocyte hormonal stimulation
Abdominal striae	Obesity, pelvic tumor
Ballottement	Uterine tumors/polyps, ascites
Pregnancy tests	Increased pituitary gonadotropins at menopause, choriocarcinoma, hydatidiform mole
Palpation for fetal outline	Uterine myomas

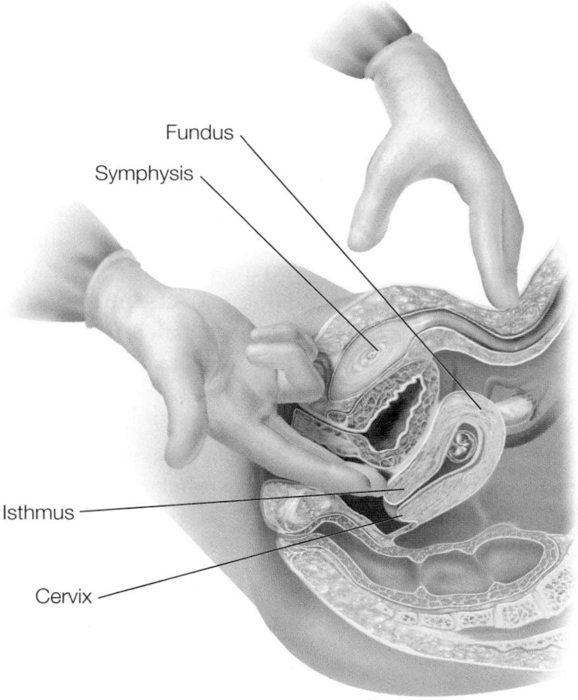

● **Figure 9–4** Hegar's sign. The presence of Hegar's sign, which is a softening of the isthmus of the uterus, can be determined by the examiner during a vaginal examination.

Uterine souffle may be heard when the examiner auscultates the abdomen over the uterus. It is a soft, blowing sound that occurs at the same rate as the maternal pulse and is caused by the increased uterine blood flow and blood pulsating through the placenta. It is sometimes confused with the funic souffle, a soft, blowing sound of blood pulsating through the umbilical cord. The funic souffle occurs at the same rate as the fetal heart rate.

Changes in pigmentation of the skin are common in pregnancy. The nipples and areolae may darken, and the linea nigra may develop. Facial melasma (chloasma) may become noticeable, and striae may appear.

The fetal outline may be identified by palpation in many pregnant women after 24 weeks' gestation. **Ballottement** is the passive fetal movement elicited when the examiner inserts two gloved fingers into the vagina and pushes against the cervix. This action pushes the fetal body up, and, as it falls back, the examiner feels a rebound.

Pregnancy tests detect the presence of hCG in the maternal blood or urine. These are not considered a positive sign of pregnancy because other conditions can cause elevated hCG levels.

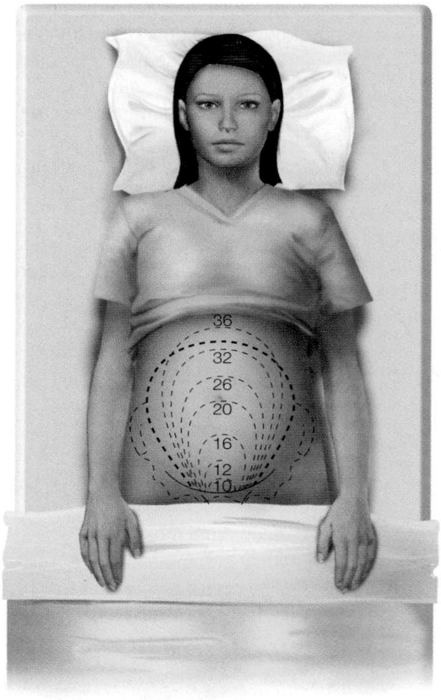

● **Figure 9–5** Approximate height of the fundus at various weeks of pregnancy.

Thinking Critically

EVALUATING FUNDAL HEIGHT

At 33 weeks' gestation, Elena Martinez, G2P1, who is 5 feet 4 inches tall and weighs 144 lb (prepregnancy weight of 120 lb), is examined by her certified nurse-midwife. At that time her fundal height is measured as 33 cm. Because of a vacation trip, she is not seen again by her midwife until 36 weeks' gestation. At that time her fundus measures 35 cm and she weighs 147 lb. Elena asks if there is something wrong with her baby's growth. What is your assessment?

See MyNursingKit for possible responses.

Clinical Pregnancy Tests

A variety of assay techniques are available to detect hCG during early pregnancy.

Hemagglutination-inhibition test (Pregnosticon R test), an immunoassay, is based on the fact that no clumping of cells occurs when the urine of a pregnant woman is added to the hCG-sensitized red blood cells of sheep.

Latex agglutination test (Gravindex and Pregnosticon slide tests), also an immunoassay, is based on the fact that latex particle agglutination is inhibited in the presence of urine containing hCG.

The two tests just described are done on the woman's first early morning urine because it is adequately concentrated. The tests become positive within 10 to 14 days after the first missed period.

Several pregnancy tests are done on maternal serum, including the following:

- *β-subunit radioimmunoassay (RIA)* uses an antiserum with specificity for the β-subunit of hCG in maternal blood. This very accurate pregnancy test has generally been replaced clinically by the technically simpler immunoradiometric assay.
- *Immunoradiometric assay (IRMA)* (Neocept, Pregnosis) uses a radioactive antibody to identify the presence of hCG in the serum. This test can detect very low concentrations of hCG and requires only about 30 minutes to perform.
- *Enzyme-linked immunosorbent assay (ELISA)* (Model Sensichrome, Quest Confidot) uses a substance that results in a color change after binding. The test is sensitive and quick. It can detect hCG levels as early as 7 to 9 days after ovulation and conception, which is 5 days before the first missed period.
- *Fluoroimmunoassay (FIA)* (Opus hCG, Stratus hCG) uses an antibody tagged with a fluorescent label to detect serum hCG. The test, which takes about 2 to 3 hours to perform, is extremely sensitive and is used primarily to identify and follow hCG concentrations.

Over-the-Counter Pregnancy Tests

Home pregnancy tests are available over the counter at a reasonable cost. These enzyme immunoassay tests, performed on urine, are quite sensitive and detect even low levels of hCG. Test instructions should be followed carefully. If the results are negative, the woman should repeat the test in 1 week if she has not started her period.

DIAGNOSTIC (POSITIVE) CHANGES

The positive signs of pregnancy are completely objective, cannot be confused with a pathologic state, and offer conclusive proof of pregnancy.

The *fetal heartbeat* can be detected with an electronic Doppler device as early as weeks 10 to 12 of pregnancy.

Fetal movement is actively palpable by a trained examiner after about the 20th week of pregnancy.

Visualization of the fetus by ultrasound examination confirms a pregnancy. The gestational sac can be observed by 4 to 5 weeks' gestation (2 to 3 weeks after conception). Fetal parts and fetal movement can be seen as early as 8 weeks' gestation. Transvaginal ultrasound has been used to detect a gestational sac as early as 10 days after implantation (Cunningham et al., 2005).

PSYCHOLOGIC RESPONSE OF THE EXPECTANT FAMILY TO PREGNANCY

Pregnancy is a turning point in a family's life, accompanied by stress and anxiety, whether the pregnancy is desired or not. For beginning families, pregnancy is the transition period from childlessness to parenthood. If the pregnancy results in the birth of a child, the couple enters a new, irreversible stage of their life together. The expectant couple may be unaware of the physical, emotional, and cognitive changes of pregnancy and may anticipate no problems from such a normal event. Thus, they may be confused and distressed by new feelings and behaviors that are essentially normal.

If the expectant woman is married or has a stable partner, she no longer is only a mate but must also assume the role of mother. Her partner will become a parent, too. Career goals and mobility may be affected, and the couple's relationship takes on a different meaning to them and their families and community. Routines and family dynamics are altered with each pregnancy, requiring readjustment and realignment. As pregnancy progresses, the couple must face the anxieties of labor and birth and must also deal with fears that the baby may be ill or disfigured. Classes in prepared childbirth can help the couple prepare.

If the pregnant woman has no stable partner, she must deal alone with the role changes, fears, and adjustments of pregnancy or seek support from family or friends. She also faces the reality of planning for the future as a single parent. Even if the pregnant woman plans to relinquish her infant, she must still deal with the adjustments of pregnancy. This adjustment can be especially difficult without a good support system.

In most pregnancies, finances are an important consideration. Traditional lore relegates to the father the role of primary breadwinner, and indeed finances are often a very real concern for fathers. In today's society, however, even pregnant women with stable partners recognize the financial impact of a child and may feel concern about financial issues. For the single mother, finances may be a major source of concern.

Decisions about financial matters need to be made at this time. Will the woman work during her pregnancy and return to work after her child is born? If so, who will provide child care? Couples may also need to decide about the division of domestic tasks. Any differences of opinion must be discussed openly and resolved so that the family can meet the needs of its members.

Pregnancy can be viewed as a developmental stage with its own distinct developmental tasks. For a couple it can be a time of support or conflict, depending on the amount of adjustment each is willing to make to maintain the family's equilibrium.

During a first pregnancy, the couple plans together for the child's arrival, collecting information on how to be parents. At the same time, each continues to participate in some separate activities with friends or family members. The availability of a social support network is an important factor in psychosocial well-being during pregnancy. The social network is often a major source of advice for the pregnant woman. However, both sound and unsound information may be conveyed.

During any pregnancy, the expectant parents both face significant changes and must deal with major psychosocial adjustments (Table 9–3). Other family members, especially other children of the woman or couple and the grandparents-to-be, must also adjust to the pregnancy.

For some, pregnancy is more than a developmental stage; it is a crisis. *Crisis* can be defined as a disturbance or conflict in which the individual cannot maintain a state of equilibrium. Pregnancy can be considered a maturational crisis, as it is a common event in the normal growth and development of the family. If the crisis is not resolved, it will result in maladaptive behaviors in one or more family members and possible disintegration of the family. Families that are able to resolve a maturational crisis will return successfully to normal functioning and can even strengthen the bonds in the family relationship.

THE MOTHER

Pregnancy alters body image and also necessitates a reordering of social relationships and changes in roles of family members. The way each woman meets the stresses of pregnancy is influenced by

Table 9–3 Parental Reactions to Pregnancy

First Trimester	Second Trimester	Third Trimester
Mother's Reactions	**Mother's Reactions**	**Mother's Reactions**
Informs father secretively or openly. Feels ambivalent toward pregnancy, anxious about labor and responsibility of child. Is aware of physical changes, daydreams of possible miscarriage. Develops special feelings for and renewed interest in her own mother, begins to form a personal identity as a mother.	Remains regressive and introspective, projects all preexisting problems with authority figures onto partner, may become angry as if lack of interest is sign of weakness in him. Continues to deal with feelings about motherhood and may start to look for furniture as a concrete action she can take. May have other extreme of anxiety and wait until ninth month to look for furniture and clothes for baby. Feels movement and is aware of fetus and incorporates it into herself. May dream that partner will be killed, telephones him often for reassurance. Experiences more distinct physical changes; sexual desires may increase or decrease.	Experiences more anxiety and tension, with physical awkwardness. Feels much discomfort and insomnia from physical condition. Prepares for birth, assembles layette, picks out names. Dreams often about misplacing baby or not being able to give birth, fears birth of deformed baby. Feels ecstasy and excitement, has spurt of energy during last month.
Father's Reactions	**Father's Reactions**	**Father's Reactions**
Differ according to age, parity, desire for child, economic stability. Acceptance of pregnant woman's attitude or complete rejection and lack of communication. Is aware of his own sexual feelings, may develop more or less sexual arousal. Accepts, rejects, or resents mother-in-law. May develop new hobby outside of family as sign of stress.	If he can cope, will give her extra attention she needs; if he cannot cope, will develop a new time-consuming interest outside of home. May develop a creative feeling and a "closeness to nature." May become involved in pregnancy and buy or make furniture. Feels for movement of baby, listens to heartbeat, or remains aloof, with no physical contact. May have fears and fantasies about himself being pregnant, may become uneasy with this feminine aspect in himself. May react negatively if partner is too demanding, may become jealous of physician and of physician's importance to partner and her pregnancy.	Adapts to alternative methods of sexual contact. Becomes concerned over financial responsibility. May show new sense of tenderness and concern, treats partner like doll. Daydreams about child as if older and not newborn, dreams of losing partner. Renewed sexual attraction to partner. Feels he is ultimately responsible for whatever happens.

her emotional makeup, her sociologic and cultural background, and her acceptance or rejection of the pregnancy. However, many women manifest similar psychologic and emotional responses during pregnancy, including ambivalence, acceptance, introversion, mood swings, and changes in body image.

A woman's attitude toward her pregnancy can be a significant factor in its outcome. Even if the pregnancy is planned, there is an element of surprise at first. Many women commonly experience feelings of ambivalence during early pregnancy. This ambivalence may be related to feelings that the timing is somehow wrong; worries about the need to modify existing relationships or career plans; fears about assuming a new role; unresolved emotional conflicts with the woman's own mother; and fears about pregnancy, labor, and birth. These feelings may be more pronounced if the pregnancy is unplanned or unwanted. Indirect expressions of ambivalence include complaints about considerable physical discomfort, prolonged or frequent depression, significant dissatisfaction with changing body shape, excessive mood swings, and difficulty accepting the life changes resulting from the pregnancy.

Many pregnancies are unintended, but not all unintended pregnancies are unwanted. For some women, an unintended pregnancy has more psychologic and social advantages than disadvantages. It provides purpose and direction to life and allows a woman to test the devotion and love of her partner and family. However, an unintended pregnancy can be a risk factor for depression. Women with an unintended pregnancy may perceive life events as being more stressful than women with an intended pregnancy—another contributor to depression. Depression, in turn, can negatively impact a woman's health choices and behaviors (Messer, Dole, Kaufman, et al., 2005).

Conflicts about adapting to pregnancy are no more pronounced for older pregnant women (age 35 and over) than for younger ones. Moreover, older pregnant women tend to be less concerned about the normal physical changes of pregnancy and are confident about handling issues that arise during pregnancy and parenting. This difference may result because mature pregnant women have more experience with problem solving. However, mature pregnant women may have fewer pregnant peers and thus may have fewer people with whom to share concerns and expectations.

Pregnancy produces marked changes in a woman's body within a relatively short period. Pregnant women experience changes in body image because of physical alterations and may feel a loss of control over their bodies during pregnancy and later during childbirth. These perceptions are related a certain extent to personality factors, social network responses, and attitudes toward pregnancy. Although changes in body image are normal, they can be stressful for the woman. Explanation and discussion of the changes may help both the woman and her partner deal with the stress associated with this aspect of pregnancy.

First Trimester

During the first trimester, feelings of disbelief and ambivalence are paramount. The woman's baby does not seem real, and she focuses on herself and her pregnancy. She may experience one or more of the early symptoms of pregnancy, such as breast tenderness or morning sickness, which are unsettling and at times unpleasant.

During this time, the expectant mother begins to exhibit some characteristic behavioral changes. She may become increasingly introspective and passive. She may be emotionally labile, with characteristic mood swings from joy to despair. She may fantasize about a miscarriage and feel guilt because of these fantasies. She may worry that these thoughts will harm the baby in some way.

Second Trimester

During the second trimester, quickening occurs. This perception of fetal movement helps the woman think of her baby as a separate person, and she generally becomes excited about the pregnancy even if earlier she was not. The woman becomes increasingly introspective as she evaluates her life, her plans, and her child's future. This introspection helps the woman prepare for her new mothering role. Emotional lability, which may be unsettling to her partner, persists. In some instances the partner may react by withdrawing. This withdrawal is especially distressing to the woman, because she needs increased love and affection. Once the couple understands that these behaviors are characteristic of pregnancy, they are easier to accept; however, they may be sources of stress to some extent throughout pregnancy.

As pregnancy becomes more noticeable, the woman's body image changes. She may feel great pride, embarrassment, or concern. Generally women feel best during the second trimester, which is a relatively tranquil time.

Third Trimester

In the third trimester, the woman feels pride about her pregnancy and anxiety about labor and birth. Physical discomforts increase, and the woman is eager for the pregnancy to end. She experiences increased fatigue, her body movements are awkward, and her interest in sexual activity may decrease. The woman tends to be concerned about the health and safety of her unborn child and may worry that she will not cope well during childbirth. Toward the end of this period, there is often a surge of energy as the woman prepares a "nest" for the infant. Many women report bursts of energy, during which they vigorously clean and organize their homes.

Psychologic Tasks of the Mother

Rubin (1984) identified four major tasks that the pregnant woman undertakes to maintain her intactness and that of her family and to incorporate her new child into the family system. These tasks form the foundation for a mutually gratifying relationship with her infant:

1. *Ensuring safe passage through pregnancy, labor, and birth.* The pregnant woman feels concern for both her unborn child and herself. She looks for competent maternity care to provide a sense of control. She may seek information from literature, observation of other pregnant women and new mothers, and discussion with others. She often engages in self-care activities related to diet, exercise, alcohol consumption, and so forth. In the third trimester, she becomes more aware of external threats in the environment—a toy on the stairs, the awkwardness of an escalator—that pose a threat to her well-being. Sleep becomes more difficult and she longs for birth even though it, too, is frightening.

2. *Seeking acceptance of this child by others.* The birth of a child alters a woman's primary support group (her family) and her secondary affiliative groups. The woman slowly and subtly alters her network to meet the needs of her pregnancy. In this adjustment the woman's partner is the most important figure. The partner's support and acceptance help form a maternal identity. If there are other children in the home, the mother also works to ensure their acceptance of the coming child. The woman without a partner looks to others such as a family member or friend for this support.
3. *Seeking commitment and acceptance of herself as mother to the infant (binding-in).* During the first trimester, the child remains a rather abstract concept. With quickening, however, the child begins to become a real person, and the mother begins to develop bonds of attachment. The mother experiences movement of the child within her in an intimate, exclusive way, and bonds of love form. The mother develops a fantasy image of her ideal child. This binding-in process, characterized by its strong emotional component, motivates the pregnant woman to become competent in her role and provides satisfaction for her in the role of mother.
4. *Learning to give of oneself on behalf of one's child.* Childbirth involves many acts of giving. The man "gives" a child to the woman; she in turn "gives" a child to him. Life is given to an infant; a sibling is given to older children of the family. The woman begins to develop a capacity for self-denial and learns to delay immediate personal gratification to meet the needs of another. Baby showers and gifts are acts of giving that increase the mother's self-esteem and help her recognize the separateness and needs of the coming baby.

Accomplishment of these tasks helps the pregnant woman develop her self-concept as mother. The expectant mother who was well nurtured by her own mother may view her as a role model and emulate her; the woman who views her mother as a "poor mother" may worry that she will make similar mistakes. A woman's self-concept as a mother expands with actual experience and continues to grow through subsequent childbearing and child rearing.

THE FATHER

For the expectant father, pregnancy is a psychologically stressful time because he, too, must make the transition from nonparent to parent or from parent of one or more to parent of two or more. Most men handle the transition to fatherhood well, and generally any anxieties they feel resolve over time. Fathers' feelings of anxieties often stem from inadequate preparation and can be addressed by recognizing paternal needs and including fathers more in antepartal education (Deave, Johnson, & Ingram, 2008).

Initially, expectant fathers may feel pride in their virility, which pregnancy confirms, but also have many of the same ambivalent feelings as expectant mothers. The extent of ambivalence depends on many factors, including the father's relationship with his partner, his previous experience with pregnancy, his age, his economic stability, and whether the pregnancy was planned.

In adjusting to his role, the expectant father must first deal with the reality of the pregnancy and then gain recognition as a parent from his partner, family, friends, coworkers, and society—and from his baby as well. The expectant mother can help her partner adjust if she has a definite sense of the experience as their pregnancy and their infant, and not her pregnancy and her infant.

The expectant father must establish a fatherhood role, just as the woman develops a motherhood role. Fathers who are most successful at this task generally like children, are excited about the prospect of fatherhood, are eager to nurture a child, and have confidence in their ability to be a parent. They also share the experiences of pregnancy and birth with their partners. (See Table 9–3.)

First Trimester

After the initial excitement attending the announcement of the pregnancy, an expectant father may begin to feel left out. He may be confused by his partner's mood changes. He might resent the attention she receives and her need to modify their relationship as she experiences fatigue and possibly a decreased interest in sex. He might also be concerned about what kind of father he will be. During this time, his child is a "potential" baby. Fathers often picture interacting with a child of 5 or 6 years, not a newborn. The pregnancy itself may seem unreal until the woman shows more physical signs.

Second Trimester

The father's role in the pregnancy is still vague, but his involvement may increase as he watches and feels fetal movement and listens to the fetal heartbeat during a prenatal visit. For many men, seeing their infant on ultrasound is an important experience in accepting the reality of pregnancy. Like expectant mothers, expectant fathers need to confront and resolve some of their conflicts about the parenting they received. A father needs to sort out which behaviors of his own father he wants to imitate and which he wants to avoid. Research indicates that a father's beliefs about the fathering role is a strong predictor of his competence in parenting (Schoppe-Sullivan, Brown, Cannon, et al., 2008).

The father-to-be's anxiety is lessened if both parents agree on the paternal role the man is to assume. For example, if both see his role as that of breadwinner, the man's stress is low. However, if the man views his role as that of breadwinner and the woman expects him to be actively involved in child care, his stress increases. An open, honest discussion about the expectations the parents have about their roles will help the father-to-be in his transition to fatherhood (Goodman, 2005).

As the woman's appearance begins to change, her partner may have several reactions. Her appearance may decrease his sexual interest, or it may have the opposite effect. Because of the variety of emotions both partners may feel, communication and acceptance remain important.

Third Trimester

If the couple's relationship has grown through effective communication of their concerns and feelings, the third trimester is often a rewarding time. They may attend childbirth classes and make concrete preparations for the arrival of the baby. If the father has developed a detached attitude about the pregnancy, however, it is unlikely he will become a willing participant, even though his role becomes more obvious.

Concerns and fears may recur. The father may worry about hurting the unborn baby during intercourse or become concerned about labor and birth. He may also wonder what kind of parents he and his partner will be.

Couvade

Couvade has traditionally referred to the observance of certain rituals and taboos by the male to signify the transition to fatherhood. This observance affirms his psychosocial and biophysical relationship to the woman and child. More recently the term has been used to describe the unintentional development of physical symptoms such as fatigue, increased appetite, difficulty sleeping, depression, headache, or backache by the partner of a pregnant woman. Men who demonstrate couvade syndrome tend to have a higher degree of paternal role preparation and be involved in more activities related to this preparation.

SIBLINGS

Bringing a new baby home often marks the beginning of sibling rivalry. The siblings view the baby as a threat to the security of their relationships with their parents. Parents who recognize this potential problem early in pregnancy and begin constructive actions can minimize the problem of sibling rivalry.

Preparation of the young child begins several weeks before the anticipated birth. Because they do not have a clear concept of time, young children should not be told too early about the pregnancy. From the toddler's point of view, several weeks is an extremely long time. The mother may let the child feel the baby moving in her uterus, explaining that the uterus is "a special place where babies grow." The child can help the parents put the baby clothes in drawers or prepare the baby's room.

Consistency is important in dealing with young children. They need reassurance that certain people, special things, and familiar places will continue to exist after the new baby arrives. The crib is often an important though transient object in a child's life. If it is to be given to the new baby, the parents should thoughtfully help the older child adjust to this change. Any move from crib to bed or from one room to another should precede the baby's birth by several weeks or more. If the new baby is to share a room with siblings, the parents must also discuss this situation with the older child or children.

Some parents advocate cosleeping (one or both parents sleeping with the baby or young child), and so the crib is less of an issue. Cosleeping, common in many non-Western cultures, is attracting more support in the United States. Opinion varies sharply about the advantages and risks of the practice, especially in light of an American Academy of Pediatrics policy statement (2005) recommending against cosleeping because of the increased risk of sudden infant death syndrome (SIDS). The AAP stresses that the infant can be brought to the bed to be comforted or for breastfeeding, but should be placed supine in a separate bed ("back to bed") to sleep. Parents who choose to cosleep must make decisions about the sleeping arrangements of other siblings following the birth of the baby.

If the child is ready, toilet training is most effective several months before or after the baby's arrival. It is not unusual for an older, toilet-trained child to regress to wetting or soiling because of the attention the newborn gets for such behavior. The older, weaned child may want to breast feed or drink from the bottle again after the baby arrives. If the new mother anticipates these behaviors, they will be less frustrating during her early postpartum days.

Pregnant women may find it helpful to bring their children on a prenatal visit to the certified nurse-midwife or physician to give them an opportunity to listen to the fetal heartbeat. Such a visit helps make the baby seem more real to the children.

If siblings are school-age children, pregnancy should be viewed as a family affair. Teaching should be suitable to the child's level of understanding and may be supplemented with appropriate books. Taking part in family discussions, attending sibling preparation classes, feeling fetal movement, and listening to the fetal heartbeat help the school-age child take part in the experience of pregnancy and not feel like an outsider.

Older children or adolescents may appear to have sophisticated knowledge but may have many misconceptions about pregnancy and birth. The parents should make opportunities to discuss their concerns and involve the children in preparations for the new baby.

MyNursingKit Care Plan: Prepare Siblings for New Baby

Even after birth, siblings need to feel that they are taking part. Having siblings visit their mother and the new baby at the hospital or birthing center will help. After the baby comes home, siblings can share in "showing off" the new baby.

Sibling preparation is essential, but other factors are equally important. These factors include how much parental attention the new arrival receives, how much attention the older child receives after the baby comes home, and how well the parents handle regressive or aggressive behavior.

GRANDPARENTS

The first relatives told about a pregnancy are usually the grandparents. The expectant grandparents often become increasingly supportive of the couple, even if conflicts previously existed. But it can be difficult for even sensitive grandparents to know how deeply to become involved in the childrearing process.

Because grandparenting can occur over a wide expanse of years, people's response to this role can vary considerably. Younger grandparents leading active lives may not demonstrate as much interest as the young couple would like. In other cases, expectant grandparents may give advice and gifts unsparingly. For grandparents, conflict may be related to the expectant couple's need to feel in control of their lives, or it may stem from events signaling changing roles in the grandparents' own lives (e.g., retirement, financial concerns, menopause, or death of a friend). Some parents of expectant couples may already be grandparents with a developed style of grandparenting. This influences their response to the pregnancy.

Because childbearing and childrearing practices have changed, family cohesiveness is promoted by effective communication and frank discussion between young couples and interested grandparents about the changes and the reasons for them. Classes for grandparents may provide information about changes in birth and parenting practices.

CULTURAL VALUES AND PREGNANCY

Cultures have a universal tendency to create ceremonial rituals or rites around important life events. The rituals and customs of a group are a reflection of the group's values. Thus, the identification of cultural values is useful in predicting reactions to pregnancy. An understanding of male and female roles, family lifestyles, religious values, or the meaning of children in a culture may explain reactions of joy or shame.

Generalization about cultural characteristics or values is difficult because not every individual in a culture may display these characteristics. Just as variations are seen between cultures, variations are also seen within cultures. For example, because of their exposure to the American culture, a third-generation Chinese-American family might have very different values and beliefs from those of a Chinese family that has recently immigrated to the United States. For this reason, the nurse needs to supplement a general knowledge of cultural values and practices with a complete assessment of the individual's values and practices. "Developing Cultural Competence: Providing Effective Prenatal Care to Families of Different Cultures" summarizes the key actions a nurse can take to become more culturally aware.

Cultural assessment is an important aspect of prenatal care. The nurse needs to identify the prospective parents' main beliefs, values, and behaviors about pregnancy and childbearing. This includes information about ethnic background, amount of affiliation with the ethnic group, patterns of decision making, religious preference, language, communication style, and common etiquette practices. The nurse can also explore the woman's (or family's) expectations of the healthcare system. Once this information is gathered, the nurse can then plan and provide care that is appropriate and responsive to family needs. See Chapter 2∞ for more detail on these topics.

Developing Cultural Competence

PROVIDING EFFECTIVE PRENATAL CARE TO FAMILIES OF DIFFERENT CULTURES

Nurses who are interacting with expectant families from a different culture or ethnic group can provide more effective, culturally sensitive nursing care by:

- Critically examining their own cultural beliefs.
- Identifying personal biases, attitudes, stereotypes, and prejudices.
- Making a conscious commitment to respect the values and beliefs of others.
- Using sensitive, current language when describing others' cultures.
- Learning the rituals, customs, and practices of the major cultural and ethnic groups with whom they have contact.
- Including cultural assessment and assessment of the family's expectations of the healthcare system as a routine part of prenatal nursing care.
- Incorporating the family's cultural and spiritual practices into prenatal care as much as possible.
- Fostering an attitude of respect for and cooperation with alternative healers and caregivers whenever possible.
- Providing for the services of an interpreter if language barriers exist.
- Learning the language (or at least several key phrases) of at least one of the cultural groups with whom they interact.
- Recognizing that ultimately it is the woman's right to make her own healthcare choices.
- Evaluating whether the woman's healthcare beliefs have any potential negative consequences for her health.

CRITICAL CONCEPT REVIEW

LEARNING OUTCOMES	CONCEPTS
9.1 Identify the anatomic and physiologic changes that occur during pregnancy.	1. Uterus: Increased amounts of estrogen and growing fetus cause enlargement in size and weight, strength, elasticity, and vascularity. 2. Cervix: Hyperplasia occurs (increase in cell number) due to increased estrogen level. Mucous plug forms to prevent organisms from entering uterus. 3. Vagina: Increased thickness of mucosa, increased vaginal secretions to prevent bacterial infections. Connective tissue relaxes. Caused by increased estrogen level. 4. Breasts: Estrogen and progesterone cause an increase in size and number of mammary glands; nipples more erectile, areolae darken, colostrum produced in last trimester. 5. Respiratory system: Increasing levels of progesterone cause increased volume of air, deceased airway resistance, increased anteroposterior diameter. Thoracic breathing occurs as uterus enlarges.

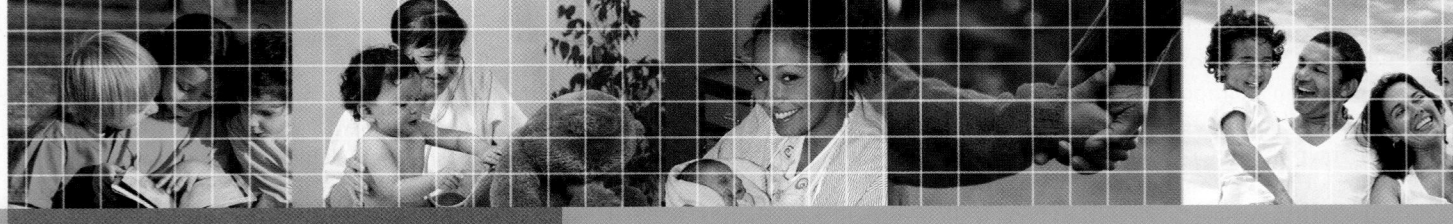

LEARNING OUTCOMES	CONCEPTS
	6. Cardiovascular system: Cardiac output increases, blood volume increases. Increased size of uterus interferes with blood return from lower extremities. Increased level of red cells to increase oxygen delivery to cells. Clotting factors increase. Caused by increased level of estrogen and progesterone. 7. Gastrointestinal system: Delayed gastric emptying and decreased peristalsis. Caused by increased progesterone levels. 8. Genitourinary system: Glomerular filtration rate and renal tubular reabsorption increase as a result of increased blood volume. 9. Skin and hair: Increased skin pigmentation caused by increased estrogen and progesterone. 10. Musculoskeletal: Relaxation of joints caused by increased estrogen and progesterone.
9.2 Assess the subjective (presumptive), objective (probable), and diagnostic (positive) changes of pregnancy in clients.	1. Subjective (presumptive) changes: ■ Amenorrhea ■ Nausea and vomiting ■ Fatigue ■ Urinary frequency ■ Breast changes ■ Quickening 2. Objective (probable) changes: ■ Goodell's and Chadwick's sign ■ Hegar's and McDonald's sign ■ Enlargement of the abdomen ■ Braxton Hicks contractions ■ Uterine souffle ■ Skin pigmentation changes ■ Pregnancy tests 3. Diagnostic (positive) changes: ■ Fetal heartbeat ■ Fetal movement ■ Visualization of the fetus
9.3 Contrast the various types of pregnancy tests.	1. Urine tests: Detect hCG during early pregnancy. 2. Serum tests: Also may detect hCG but may detect presence earlier than urine tests. 3. Home (OTC) tests: Urine tests designed to detect hCG.
9.4 Address the emotional and psychologic changes that commonly occur in a woman, her partner, and her family during pregnancy when providing nursing care.	1. Mother: ■ First trimester: Disbelief and ambivalence. ■ Second trimester: Quickening helps mother to view fetus as separate from herself. ■ Third trimester: Anxiety about labor and birth. Nesting (bursts of energy) occurs. ■ Rubin identified four tasks: Ensuring safe passage through pregnancy, labor, and birth Seeking acceptance of this child by others Seeking commitment and acceptance of herself as mother to infant Learning to give of oneself on behalf of one's child 2. Father/partner: ■ First trimester: May feel left out. Disbelief. ■ Second trimester: Begins to decide which behaviors of own father he wants to imitate or discard. ■ Third trimester: Anxiety about labor and birth. 3. Family: ■ Siblings' reaction depends upon age of siblings, but preparation is essential. ■ Grandparents are usually supportive and excited about the birth.
9.5 Recognize cultural factors that may influence a family's response to pregnancy in the provision of nursing care.	1. Cultural assessment should be done to determine the beliefs, wishes, and traditions of the family. Factors such as religious preference, language, and communication style will affect the family's plans for the pregnancy.

CRITICAL THINKING IN ACTION

Twenty-two-year-old Jean Simmons is an aerobics instructor, G0, P0000 in her first trimester of pregnancy. She presents to you at the local clinic complaining of frequent nausea, urinary frequency, and fatigue. You obtain her vital signs as: BP 108/60, temperature 97°F, pulse 68, respirations 12, weight 125 lb, height 64 inches. Her urine tests negative for ketones, albumin, leukocytes, and sugar. You note that Jean has lost 3 lb since her last visit. You assist the certified nurse-midwife with a physical exam, the findings of which are essentially normal. Jean says that while she knows it could become an issue, she would like to continue working as an aerobic instructor for as long as she possibly can during the pregnancy. You identify Jean's complaints as normal discomforts of pregnancy, and proceed with prenatal education.

1. What advice would you suggest to cope with the nausea of pregnancy?
2. What advice might you suggest to cope with urinary frequency?
3. What teaching would be important relating to exercise in pregnancy?
4. What symptoms related to exercise should Jean report to her physician?

See MyNursingKit for possible responses.

REFERENCES

American Academy of Pediatrics (AAP). (2005). Policy statement: The changing concept of sudden infant death syndrome: Diagnostic coding shifts, controversies regarding the sleeping environment, and new variables to consider in reducing risk. *Pediatrics, 116*(5), 1245–55.

Cunningham, F. G., Leveno, K. J., Bloom, S. L., Hauth, J. C., Rouse, D. J., & Spong, C. Y. (2010). *Williams obstetrics* (23rd ed.). New York: McGraw-Hill Medical.

Deave, T., Johnson, D., & Ingram, J. (2008). Transition to parenthood: the needs of parents in pregnancy and early parenthood. *Pregnancy and Childbirth, 8,* 30–35.

Goodman, J. H. (2005). Becoming an involved father of an infant. *Journal of Obstetric, Gynecologic, and Neonatal Nursing, 34*(2), 190–200.

Gordon, M. C. (2007). Maternal physiology. In S. G. Gabbe, J. R. Niebyl, & J. L. Simpson (Eds.), *Obstetrics: Normal and problem pregnancies* (5th ed.). Philadelphia: Churchill Livingstone.

Johnson, T. R. B., Gregory, K. D., & Niebyl, J. R. (2007). Preconception and prenatal care: Part of the continuum. In S. G. Gabbe, J. R. Niebyl, & J. L. Simpson (Eds.), *Obstetrics: Normal and problem pregnancies* (5th ed.). New York: Churchill-Livingstone.

Messer, L. C., Dole, N., Kaufman, J. S., & Savitz, D. A. (2005). Pregnancy intendedness, maternal psychosocial factors and preterm birth. *Maternal and Child Health Journal, 9*(4), 403–412.

Rubin, R. (1984). *Maternal identity and the maternal experience.* New York: Springer.

Schoppe-Sullivan, S. J., Brown, G. L., Cannon, E. A., Mangelsdorf, S. C., & Sokolowski, M. S. (2008). Maternal gatekeeping, coparenting quality, and fathering behavior in families with infants. *Journal of Family Psychology, 22*(3), 389–398.

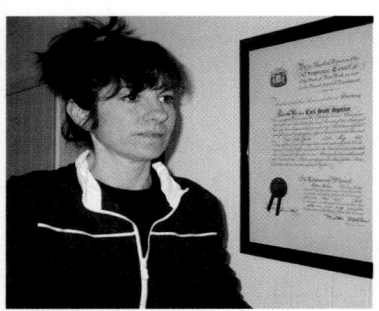

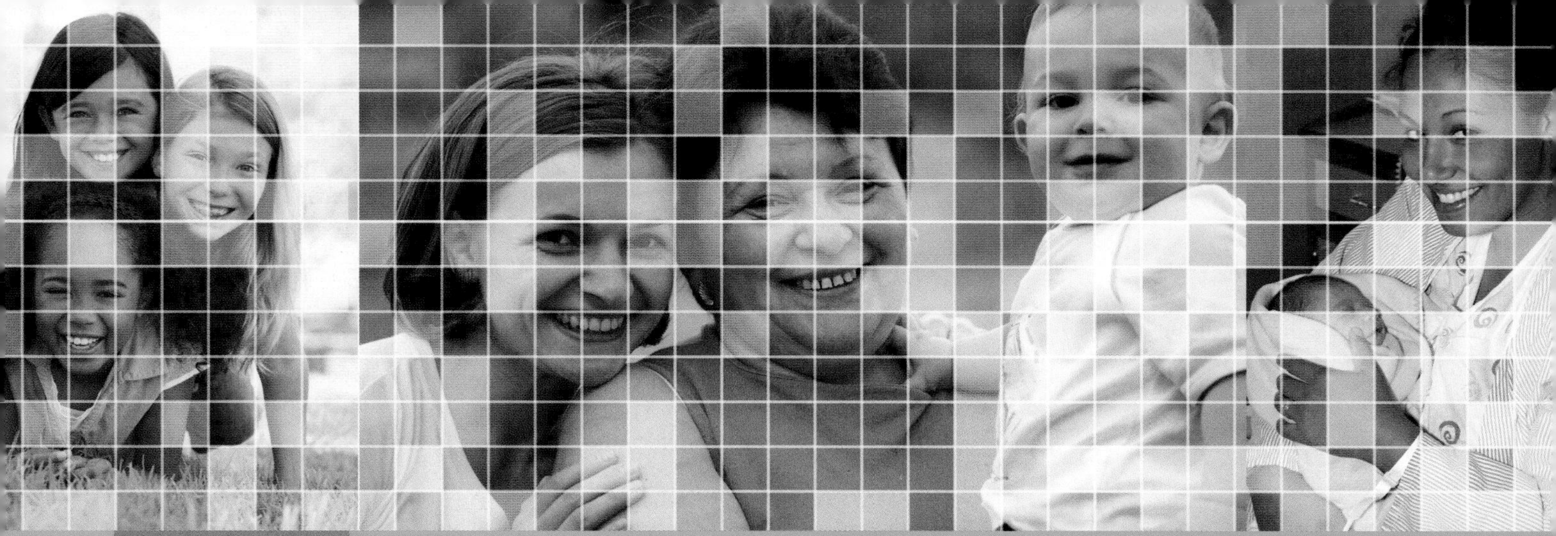

CHAPTER

10 Antepartal Nursing Assessment

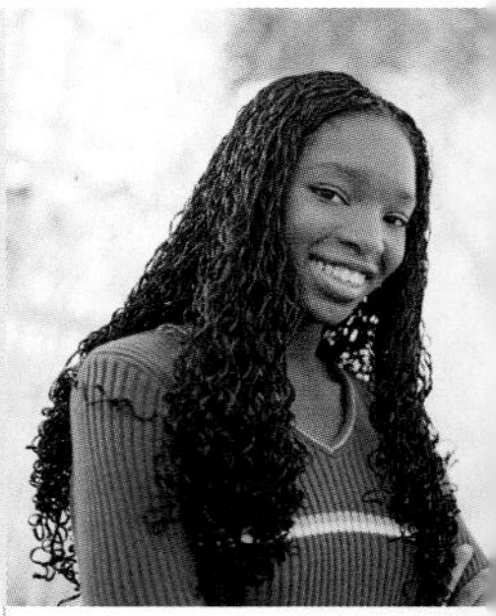

I'm 16—just got my license—so it was weird telling my friends that my mom is pregnant. I was embarrassed (and a little jealous) at first but now I kind of like the idea of having a baby sister. Mom had an amniocentesis because she is 37, so we know it's a girl. My mom has been great about including me and telling me what is going on. I've gone to a couple of her prenatal appointments so I got to hear the heartbeat and I saw the baby moving on ultrasound. I'm surprised by how interesting I am finding everything. Don't laugh, but I think I might like to be a nurse-midwife someday. —Krista, 16

LEARNING OUTCOMES

10.1 Use information provided on a prenatal history to identify risk factors for the mother and/or fetus.

10.2 Define common obstetric terminology found in the history of maternity clients.

10.3 Consider risk factors related to the father's health that are generally recorded on the prenatal record in assessing risk factors for the mother and/or fetus.

10.4 Evaluate those areas of the initial assessment that reflect the psychosocial and cultural factors related to a woman's pregnancy.

10.5 Predict the normal physiologic changes a nurse would expect to find when performing a physical assessment of a pregnant woman.

10.6 Calculate the estimated date of birth using the common methods.

10.7 Describe the essential measurements that can be determined by clinical pelvimetry.

10.8 Consider the results of the major screening tests used during the prenatal period in the assessment of the prenatal client.

10.9 Assess the prenatal client for any of the danger signs of pregnancy.

10.10 Relate the components of the subsequent prenatal history and assessment to the progress of pregnancy and the nursing care of the prenatal client.

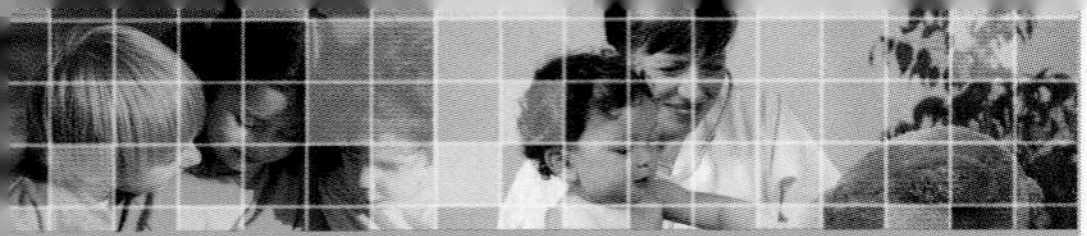

KEY TERMS

Abortion, 200
Antepartum, 200
Diagonal conjugate, 215
Estimated date of birth (EDB), 205
Gestation, 200
Gravida, 200
Intrapartum, 200
Multigravida, 200
Multipara, 200
Nägele's rule, 218
Nulligravida, 200
Nullipara, 200
Obstetric conjugate, 215
Para, 200
Postpartum, 200
Postterm labor, 200
Preterm or premature labor, 200
Primigravida, 200
Primipara, 200
Risk factors, 202
Stillbirth, 200
Term, 200

The RN may complete many areas of prenatal assessment. Advanced practice nurses such as certified nurse-midwives (CNMs) and nurse practitioners are able to perform complete antepartal assessments. This chapter focuses on the prenatal assessments completed initially and at subsequent visits to provide optimum care for the childbearing family.

INITIAL CLIENT HISTORY

The course of a pregnancy depends on a number of factors, including the woman's prepregnancy health, presence of disease states, emotional status, and past health care. A thorough history helps determine the status of a woman's prepregnancy health.

DEFINITION OF TERMS

The following terms are used in recording the history of maternity clients:

Gestation: the number of weeks of pregnancy since the first day of the last menstrual period

Abortion: birth that occurs before the end of 20 weeks' gestation or the birth of a fetus-newborn who weighs less than 500 g (Cunningham, Leveno, Bloom, et al., 2010). Abortion is abbreviated as ab.

Term: the normal duration of pregnancy (38 to 42 weeks' gestation)

Antepartum: time between conception and the onset of labor; usually used to describe the period during which a woman is pregnant; used interchangeably with *prenatal*

Intrapartum: time from the onset of true labor until the birth of the infant and placenta

Postpartum: time from the delivery of the placenta and membranes until the woman's body returns to a nonpregnant condition

Preterm or premature labor: labor that occurs after 20 weeks' but before completion of 37 weeks' gestation

Postterm labor: labor that occurs after 42 weeks' gestation

Gravida: any pregnancy, regardless of duration, including present pregnancy. Gravida is often abbreviated as G.

Nulligravida: a woman who has never been pregnant

Primigravida: a woman who is pregnant for the first time

Multigravida: a woman who is in her second or any subsequent pregnancy

Para: birth after 20 weeks' gestation regardless of whether the infant is born alive or dead. Para is often abbreviated as P.

Nullipara: a woman who has had no births at more than 20 weeks' gestation

Primipara: a woman who has had one birth at more than 20 weeks' gestation, regardless of whether the infant was born alive or dead

Multipara: a woman who has had two or more births at more than 20 weeks' gestation

Stillbirth: an infant born dead after 20 weeks' gestation

The terms *gravida* and *para* are used in relation to pregnancies, not to the number of fetuses. Thus twins, triplets, and so forth count as one pregnancy and one birth.

The following examples illustrate how these terms are applied in clinical situations:

1. Jean Sanchez has one child born at 38 weeks' gestation and is pregnant for the second time. At her initial prenatal visit, the nurse indicates her obstetric history as "gravida 2 para 1 ab 0." (She might also be identified as a G2P1Ab0). Jean Sanchez's present pregnancy terminates at 16 weeks' gestation. She is now "gravida 2 para 1 ab 1."
2. Tracy Hopkins is pregnant for the fourth time. At home she has a child who was born at term. Her second pregnancy ended at 10 weeks' gestation. She

then gave birth to twins at 35 weeks. One twin died soon after birth. At her antepartal assessment, the nurse records her obstetric history as "gravida 4 para 2 ab 1."

This approach is confusing, however, because it fails to identify the number of children that a woman might have. To provide comprehensive data, a more detailed approach is used in some settings. Using the detailed system, gravida keeps the same meaning, but the meaning of para changes because the detailed system counts each infant born rather than the number of pregnancies carried to viability (Varney, Kriebs, & Gegor, 2004). For example, triplets count as one pregnancy but three babies.

A useful acronym for remembering the system is TPAL:

T: number of term infants born—that is, the number of infants born after 37 weeks' gestation or more

P: number of preterm infants born—that is, the number of infants born after 20 weeks but before the completion of 37 weeks' gestation

A: number of pregnancies ending in either spontaneous or therapeutic abortion

L: number of currently living children

Using this approach the nurse would have initially described Jean Sanchez (see the first example) as "gravida 2 para 1001" or "G2P1001." Following Jean's spontaneous abortion, she would be "gravida 2 para 1011" or G2P1011." Tracy Hopkins would be described as "gravida 4 para 1212" or "G4P1212" (Figure 10–1 ●).

CLIENT PROFILE

The history is essentially a screening tool to identify factors that may place the mother or fetus at risk during the pregnancy. The following information is obtained for each pregnant woman at the first prenatal assessment:

1. Current pregnancy
   - First day of last normal menstrual period (LMP). Is she sure of the dates or uncertain? Do her cycles normally occur every 28 days, or do her cycles tend to be longer?
   - Presence of cramping, bleeding, or spotting since LMP
   - Woman's opinion about the time when conception occurred and when infant is due
   - Woman's attitude toward pregnancy (Is this pregnancy planned? Wanted?)
   - Results of pregnancy tests, if completed
   - Any discomforts since LMP such as nausea, vomiting, urinary frequency, fatigue, or breast tenderness
2. Past pregnancies
   - Number of pregnancies
   - Number of abortions, spontaneous or induced
   - Number of living children
   - History of previous pregnancies, length of pregnancy, length of labor and birth, type of birth (vaginal, forceps or vacuum-assisted birth, or cesarean), type of anesthesia used (if any), woman's perception of the experience, and complications (antepartal, intrapartal, and postpartal)
   - Neonatal status of previous children: Apgar scores, birth weights, general development, complications, and feeding patterns (breast milk or formula)
   - Loss of a child (miscarriage, elective or medically indicated abortion, stillbirth, neonatal death, relinquishment, or death after the neonatal period). What was the experience like for her? What coping skills helped? How did her partner, if involved, respond?
   - If Rh negative, was medication received after birth to prevent sensitization?
   - Prenatal education classes and resources (books)
3. Gynecologic history
   - Date of last Pap smear; any history of abnormal Pap smear; any follow-up therapy completed
   - Previous infections: vaginal, cervical, tubal, or sexually transmitted
   - Previous surgery
   - Age at menarche
   - Regularity, frequency, and duration of menstrual flow
   - History of dysmenorrhea
   - Sexual history
   - Contraceptive history (If birth control pills were used, did pregnancy occur immediately following cessation of pills? If not, how long after?)
   - Any issues related to infertility or fertility treatments
4. Current medical history
   - Weight
   - Blood type and Rh factor, if known
   - General health, including nutrition, normal dietary practices, and regular exercise program (type, frequency, and duration)
   - Any medications presently being taken (including prescription, nonprescription, homeopathic, or herbal medications) or taken since the onset of pregnancy

Nursing Practice

In general, it is best to avoid an initial discussion of a woman's gravida and para in front of her partner. It is possible that the woman had a previous pregnancy that she has not mentioned to her partner, and revealing the information could violate her right to privacy.

Name	Gravida	Term	Preterm	Abortions	Living Children
Jean Sanchez	2	1	0	1	1
Tracy Hopkins	4	1	2	1	2

● **Figure 10–1** TPAL. The TPAL approach provides detailed information about the woman's pregnancy history.

- Previous or present use of alcohol, tobacco, or caffeine (Ask specifically about the amounts of alcohol, cigarettes, and caffeine [specify coffee, tea, colas, or chocolate] consumed each day.)
- Illicit drug use or abuse (Ask about specific drugs such as cocaine, crack, methamphetamines, and marijuana.)
- Drug allergies and other allergies (Ask about latex allergies or sensitivities.)
- Potential teratogenic insults to this pregnancy such as viral infections, medications, x-ray examinations, surgery, or cats in the home (possible source of toxoplasmosis)
- Presence of disease conditions such as diabetes, hypertension, cardiovascular disease, renal problems, cancer, or thyroid disorder
- Record of immunizations (especially rubella)
- Presence of any abnormal symptoms

5. Past medical history
   - Childhood diseases
   - Past treatment for any disease condition (Any hospitalizations? History of hepatitis? Rheumatic fever? Pyelonephritis?)
   - Surgical procedures
   - Presence of bleeding disorders or tendencies (Has she received blood transfusions?)
6. Family medical history
   - Presence of diabetes, cardiovascular disease, cancer, hypertension, hematologic disorders, tuberculosis, or preeclampsia-eclampsia
   - Occurrence of multiple births
   - History of congenital diseases or deformities
   - Occurrence of cesarean births and cause, if known
7. Religious, spiritual, and cultural history
   - Does the woman wish to specify a religious preference on her chart? Does she have any spiritual beliefs or practices that might influence her health care or that of her child, such as prohibition against receiving blood products, dietary considerations, or circumcision rites?
   - What practices are important to maintain her spiritual well-being?
   - Might practices in her culture or that of her partner influence her care or that of her child?
8. Occupational history
   - Occupation
   - Physical demands (Does she stand all day, or are there opportunities to sit and elevate her legs? Any heavy lifting?)
   - Exposure to chemicals or other harmful substances
   - Opportunity for regular meals and breaks for nutritious snacks
   - Provision for maternity or family leave
9. Partner's history
   - Presence of genetic conditions or diseases
   - Age
   - Significant health problems
   - Previous or present alcohol intake, drug use, or tobacco use
   - Blood type and Rh factor
   - Occupation
   - Educational level; methods by which he learns best
   - Attitude toward the pregnancy
10. Personal information about the woman (Social history)
    - Age
    - Educational level; methods by which she learns best
    - Race or ethnic group (to identify need for prenatal genetic screening and racially or ethnically related risk factors)
    - Housing; stability of living conditions
    - Economic level
    - Acceptance of pregnancy, whether intended or unintended
    - Any history of emotional or physical deprivation or abuse of herself or children or any abuse in her current relationship (Ask specifically whether she has been hit, slapped, kicked, or hurt within the past year or since she has been pregnant. Is she afraid of her partner or anyone else? If yes, of whom is she afraid? [It is important to ask only when she is alone.])
    - History of emotional problems
    - Support systems available to her
    - Personal preferences about the birth (expectations of both the woman and her partner, presence of others, and so on). (For more information see Chapter 8∞.)
    - Plans for care of child following birth
    - Feeding preference for the baby (breast milk or formula?)

OBTAINING DATA

A questionnaire is used in many instances to obtain information. The woman should complete the questionnaire in a quiet place with a minimum of distractions. The nurse can get further information in an interview, which allows the pregnant woman to clarify her responses to questions and gives the nurse and client the opportunity to develop rapport.

The partner can be encouraged to attend the prenatal examinations. The partner is often able to contribute to the history and may use the opportunity to ask questions or express concerns.

HIGH-RISK SCREENING

Risk factors are any findings that suggest the pregnancy may have a negative outcome, for either the woman or her unborn child. Screening for risk factors is an important part of the prenatal assessment. Many risk factors can be identified during the initial assessment; others may be detected during subsequent prenatal visits. It is important to identify high-risk pregnancies early so that appropriate interventions can be started promptly. Not all risk factors threaten a pregnancy equally; thus, many agencies use a scoring sheet to determine the degree of risk. Information must be updated throughout pregnancy as necessary. Any pregnancy may begin as low risk and change to high risk because of complications.

Table 10–1 identifies the major risk factors currently recognized. The table also identifies maternal and fetal or newborn implications if the risk is present in the pregnancy.

Table 10–1	Prenatal High-Risk Factors	
Factor	**Maternal Implications**	**Fetal or Neonatal Implications**
	Social and Personal	
Low income level and/or low educational level	Poor antenatal care Poor nutrition ↑ risk preecalmpsia	Low birth weight Intrauterine growth restriction (IUGR)
Poor diet	Inadequate nutrition ↑ risk anemia ↑ risk of preeclampsia	Fetal malnutrition Prematurity
Living at high altitude	↑ hemoglobin	Prematurity IUGR ↑ hemoglobin (polycythemia)
Multiparity greater than 3	↑ risk antepartum or postpartum hemorrhage	Anemia Fetal death
Weight less than 45.5 kg (100 lb)	Poor nutrition Cephalopelvic disproportion Prolonged labor	IUGR Hypoxia associated with difficult labor and birth
Weight greater than 91 kg (200 lb)	↑ risk hypertension ↑ risk cephalopelvic disproportion ↑ risk diabetes	↓ fetal nutrition ↑ risk macrosomia
Age less than 16	Poor nutrition Poor antenatal care ↑ risk preeclampsia ↑ risk cephalopelvic disproportion	Low birth weight ↑ fetal demise
Age older than 35	↑ risk preeclampsia ↑ risk cesarean birth	↑ risk congenital anomalies ↑ chromosomal aberrations
Smoking one pack/day or more	↑ risk hypertension ↑ risk cancer	↓ placental perfusion → ↓ O_2 and nutrients available Low birth weight IUGR Preterm birth
Use of addicting drugs	↑ risk poor nutrition ↑ risk of infection with IV drugs ↑ risk HIV, hepatitis C	↑ risk congenital anomalies ↑ risk low birth weight Neonatal withdrawal Lower serum bilirubin
Excessive alcohol consumption	↑ risk poor nutrition Possible hepatic effects with long-term consumption	↑ risk fetal alcohol syndrome
	Preexisting Medical Disorders	
Diabetes mellitus	↑ risk preeclampsia, hypertension Episodes of hypoglycemia and hyperglycemia ↑ risk cesarean birth	Low birth weight Macrosomia Neonatal hypoglycemia ↑ risk congenital anomalies ↑ risk respiratory distress syndrome
Cardiac disease	Cardiac decompensation Further strain on mother's body ↑ maternal death rate	↑ risk fetal demise ↑ prenatal mortality
Anemia: hemoglobin less than 9 g/dL (white) Less than 29% hematocrit (white) Less than 8.2 g/dL hemoglobin (black) Less than 26% hematocrit (black)	Iron-deficiency anemia Low energy level Decreased oxygen-carrying capacity	Fetal death Prematurity Low birth weight
Hypertension	↑ vasospasm ↑ risk central nervous system irritability → convulsions ↑ risk cerebrovascular accident ↑ risk renal damage	↓ placental perfusion → low birth weight Preterm birth

(continued)

Table 10–1 Prenatal High-Risk Factors—continued

Factor	Maternal Implications	Fetal or Neonatal Implications
Thyroid disorder	↑ infertility	↑ spontaneous abortion
Hypothyroidism	↓ basal metabolic rate, goiter, myxedema	↑ risk congenital goiter
Hyperthyroidism	↑ risk postpartum hemorrhage ↑ risk preeclampsia Danger of thyroid storm	Mental retardation → cretinism ↑ incidence congenital anomalies ↑ incidence preterm birth ↑ tendency to thyrotoxicosis
Renal disease (moderate to severe)	↑ risk renal failure	↑ risk IUGR ↑ risk preterm birth
Diethylstilbestrol (DES) exposure	↑ infertility, spontaneous abortion ↑ cervical incompetence	↑ spontaneous abortion ↑ risk preterm birth
	Obstetric Considerations	
Previous Pregnancy		
Stillborn	↑ emotional or psychologic distress	↑ risk IUGR ↑ risk preterm birth
Habitual abortion	↑ emotional or psychologic distress ↑ possibility diagnostic workup	↑ risk abortion
Cesarean birth	↑ possibility repeat cesarean birth	↑ risk preterm birth ↑ risk respiratory distress
Rh or blood group sensitization	↑ financial expenditure for testing	Hydrops fetalis Icterus gravis Neonatal anemia Kernicterus Hypoglycemia
Large baby	↑ risk cesarean birth ↑ risk gestational diabetes	Birth injury Hypoglycemia
Current Pregnancy		
Rubella (first trimester)		Congenital heart disease Cataracts Nerve deafness Bone lesions Prolonged virus shedding
Rubella (second trimester)		Hepatitis Thrombocytopenia
Cytomegalovirus		IUGR Encephalopathy
Herpes virus type 2	Severe discomfort Concern about possibility of cesarean birth, fetal infection	Neonatal herpes virus type 2 2% hepatitis with jaundice Neurologic abnormalities
Syphilis	↑ incidence abortion	↑ fetal demise Congenital syphilis
Abruptio placenta and placenta previa	↑ risk hemorrhage Bed rest Extended hospitalization	Fetal or neonatal anemia Intrauterine hemorrhage ↑ fetal demise
Preeclampsia or eclampsia	See hypertension	↑ placental perfusion → low birth weight
Multiple gestation	↑ risk postpartum hemorrhage ↑ risk preterm labor	↑ risk preterm birth ↑ risk fetal demise
Elevated hematocrit Greater than 41% (white) Greater than 38% (black)	Increased viscosity of blood	Fetal death rate 5 times normal rate
Spontaneous premature rupture of membranes	↑ uterine infection	↑ risk preterm birth ↑ fetal demise

Evidence in Action

Periodontal disease and urinary tract infections are associated with an increase in the risk of preeclampsia (Systematic review and meta-analysis) (Conde-Agudelo, Villar, & Lindheimer, 2008).

INITIAL PRENATAL ASSESSMENT

The prenatal assessment focuses on the woman holistically by considering physical, cultural, and psychosocial factors that influence her health. The establishment of the nurse-client relationship is a chance to develop an atmosphere conducive to interviewing, support, and education. Because many women are excited and anxious at the first antepartal visit, the initial psychosocial-cultural assessment is general.

As part of the initial psychosocial-cultural assessment, discuss with the woman any religious or spiritual, cultural, or socioeconomic factors that influence the woman's expectations of the childbearing experience. It is especially helpful to be familiar with common practices of the members of various religious and cultural groups who reside in the community.

After obtaining the history, prepare the woman for the physical examination. The physical examination begins with assessment of vital signs; then the woman's body is examined. The pelvic examination is performed last.

Before the examination the woman should provide a clean urine specimen. When her bladder is empty, the woman is more comfortable during the pelvic examination and the examiner can palpate the pelvic organs more easily. After the woman empties her bladder, the nurse should ask her to disrobe and give her a gown and sheet or some other protective covering.

Increasing numbers of nurses, such as CNMs, nurse practitioners, and other nurses in advanced practice, are prepared to perform complete physical examinations. The nurse who is not an advanced practitioner assesses the woman's vital signs, explains the procedures to allay apprehension, positions her for examination, and assists the examiner as necessary.

Thoroughness and a systematic procedure are the most important considerations when performing the physical portion of an antepartal examination. See "Assessment Guide: Initial Prenatal Assessment." To promote completeness, the assessment guide is organized in three columns that address the areas to be assessed (and normal findings), the variations or alterations that may be observed, and nursing responses to the data. Certain organs and systems are assessed concurrently with others during the physical portion of the examination.

Nursing interventions based on assessment of the normal physical and psychosocial changes of pregnancy, evaluation of the cultural influences associated with pregnancy, and mutually defined client teaching and counseling needs are discussed further in Chapter 11∞.

Nursing Practice

In a clinic or office setting, gowns and goggles for the healthcare provider are usually not necessary because splashing of body fluids is unlikely. Gloves are worn for procedures that involve contact with body fluids such as drawing blood for lab work, handling urine specimens, and conducting pelvic examinations.

Thinking Critically

HOT TUB USE IN PREGNANCY

Karen Blade, a 23-year-old, G1P0, is 10 weeks' pregnant when she sees you for her first prenatal examination. She has been experiencing some mild nausea and fatigue but otherwise is feeling well. She asks you about continuing with her routine exercises (walking 3 miles a day and lifting light weights). She also asks about using the heated pool and a hot tub. What should you tell her?

See MyNursingKit for possible responses.

MyNursingKit Case Study: Initial Prenatal Assessment

DETERMINATION OF DUE DATE

Childbearing families generally want to know the "due date," or the date around which childbirth will occur. Historically the due date has been called the estimated date of confinement (EDC). However, the concept of confinement is rather negative, and many caregivers avoid it by referring to the due date as the estimated date of delivery (EDD). Childbirth educators often stress that babies are not "delivered" like a package; they are born. In keeping with a view that emphasizes the normality of the process, the authors of this text refer to the due date as the **estimated date of birth (EDB)**.

To calculate the EDB, it is helpful to know the date of the LMP. However, some women have episodes of irregular bleeding or fail to keep track of menstrual cycles. Thus, other techniques also help to determine how far along a woman is in her pregnancy—that is, at how many weeks' gestation she is. Techniques include evaluating uterine size, determining when quickening occurs, and auscultating fetal heart rate with a Doppler device or ultrasound.

Developing Cultural Competence

USING CULTURAL INFORMATION EFFECTIVELY

While it is important to avoid stereotyping, race and ethnicity may provide valuable starting information about cultural, behavioral, environmental, and medical factors that might affect a pregnant woman's health (American College of Obstetricians and Gynecologists [ACOG], 2005a). With this general knowledge as a framework, it is essential to ask the woman about specific practices in her culture to determine their meaning for her.

Assessment Guide

INITIAL PRENATAL ASSESSMENT

PHYSICAL ASSESSMENT/ NORMAL FINDINGS	ALTERATIONS AND POSSIBLE CAUSES*	NURSING RESPONSES TO DATA†
Vital Signs		
Blood pressure (BP): Less than or equal to 135/85 mm Hg	High BP (essential hypertension; renal disease; pregestational hypertension, apprehension or anxiety associated with pregnancy diagnosis, exam, or other crises; preeclampsia if initial assessment not done until after 20 weeks' gestation)	BP greater than 140/90 requires immediate consideration; establish woman's BP; refer to healthcare provider if necessary. Assess woman's knowledge about high BP; counsel on self-care and medical management
Pulse: 60–90 beats/min; rate may increase 10 beats/min during pregnancy	Increased pulse rate (excitement or anxiety, cardiac disorders)	Count for 1 full minute; note irregularities.
Respirations: 12–22 breaths/min (or pulse rate divided by four); pregnancy may induce a degree of hyperventilation; thoracic breathing predominant	Marked tachypnea or abnormal patterns	Assess for respiratory disease.
Temperature: 36.2°C–37.6°C (97°F–99.6°F)	Elevated temperature (infection)	Assess for infection process of disease state if temperature is elevated; refer to healthcare provider.
Weight		
Depends on body build	Weight less than 45 kg (100 lb) or greater than 91 kg (200 lb); rapid, sudden weight gain (preeclampsia)	Evaluate need for nutritional counseling; obtain information on eating habits, cooking practices, food regularly eaten, income limitations, need for food supplements, pica and other abnormal food habits. Note initial weight to establish baseline for weight gain throughout pregnancy.
Skin		
Color: Consistent with racial background; pink nail beds	Pallor (anemia); bronze, yellow (hepatic disease; other causes of jaundice) Bluish, reddish, mottled; dusky appearance or pallor of palms and nail beds in dark-skinned women (anemia)	The following tests should be performed: complete blood count (CBC), bilirubin level, urinalysis, and blood urea nitrogen (BUN). If abnormal, refer to healthcare provider.
Condition: Absence of edema (slight edema of lower extremities is normal during pregnancy)	Edema (preeclampsia); rashes, dermatitis (allergic response)	Counsel on relief measures for slight edema. Initiate preeclampsia assessment; refer to healthcare provider.
Lesions: Absence of lesions	Ulceration (varicose veins, decreased circulation)	Further assess circulatory status; refer to healthcare provider if lesion is severe.
Spider nevi common in pregnancy	Petechiae, multiple bruises, ecchymosis (hemorrhagic disorders; abuse) Change in size or color (carcinoma)	Evaluate for bleeding or clotting disorder. Provide opportunities to discuss abuse if suspected. Refer to healthcare provider.
Moles		
Pigmentation: Pigmentation changes of pregnancy include linea nigra, striae gravidarum, melasma		Assure woman that these are normal manifestations of pregnancy and explain the physiologic basis for the changes.
Café-au-lait spots	Six or more (Albright syndrome or neurofibromatosis)	Consult with healthcare provider.
Nose		
Character of mucosa: Redder than oral mucosa; in pregnancy nasal mucosa is edematous in response to increased estrogen, resulting in nasal stuffiness (rhinitis of pregnancy) and nosebleeds	Olfactory loss (first cranial nerve deficit)	Counsel woman about possible relief measures for nasal stuffiness and nosebleeds (epistaxis); refer to healthcare provider for olfactory loss.

Assessment Guide

INITIAL PRENATAL ASSESSMENT

PHYSICAL ASSESSMENT/ NORMAL FINDINGS	ALTERATIONS AND POSSIBLE CAUSES*	NURSING RESPONSES TO DATA†
Mouth		
May note hypertrophy of gingival tissue because of estrogen	Edema, inflammation (infection); pale in color (anemia)	Assess hematocrit for anemia; counsel regarding dental hygiene habits. Refer to healthcare provider or dentist if necessary. Routine dental care appropriate during pregnancy (no x-ray studies, no nitrous anesthesia).
Neck		
Nodes: Small, mobile, nontender nodes	Tender, hard, fixed, or prominent nodes (infection, carcinoma)	Examine for local infection; refer to healthcare provider.
Thyroid: Small, smooth, lateral lobes palpable on either side of trachea; slight hyperplasia by third month of pregnancy	Enlargement or nodule tenderness (hyperthyroidism)	Listen over thyroid for bruits, which may indicate hyperthyroidism. Question woman about dietary habits (iodine intake). Ascertain history of thyroid problems; refer to healthcare provider.
Chest and Lungs		
Chest: Symmetric, elliptic, smaller anteroposterior (AP) than transverse diameter	Increased AP diameter, funnel chest, pigeon chest (emphysema, asthma, chronic obstructive pulmonary disease [COPD])	Evaluate for emphysema, asthma, pulmonary disease (COPD).
Ribs: Slope downward from nipple line	More horizontal (COPD) angular bumps rachitic rosary (vitamin C deficiency)	Evaluate for COPD. Evaluate for fractures. Consult healthcare provider. Consult nutritionist.
Inspection and palpation: No retraction or bulging of intercostal spaces (ICS) during inspiration or expiration; symmetric expansion.	ICS retractions with inspirations, bulging with expiration; unequal expansion (respiratory disease)	Do thorough initial assessment. Refer to healthcare provider.
Tactile fremitus	Tachypnea, hyperpnea, Cheyne-Stokes respirations (respiratory disease)	Refer to healthcare provider.
Percussion: Bilateral symmetry in tone	Flatness of percussion, which may be affected by chest wall thickness	Evaluate for pleural effusions, consolidations, or tumor.
Low-pitched resonance of moderate intensity	High diaphragm (atelectasis or paralysis), pleural effusion	Refer to healthcare provider.
Auscultation: Upper lobes: bronchovesicular sounds above sternum and scapulas; equal expiratory and inspiratory phases	Abnormal if heard over any other area of chest	Refer to healthcare provider.
Remainder of chest: Vesicular breath sounds heard; inspiratory phase longer (3:1)	Rales, rhonchi, wheezes; pleural friction rub; absence of breath sounds; bronchophony, egophony, whispered pectoriloquy	Refer to healthcare provider.
Breasts		
Supple: Symmetric in size and contour; darker pigmentation of nipple and areola; may have supernumerary nipples, usually 5–6 cm below normal nipple line	"Pigskin" or orange-peel appearance, nipple retractions, swelling, hardness (carcinoma); redness, heat, tenderness, cracked or fissured nipple (infection)	Encourage monthly self-examination; instruct woman how to examine her own breasts.
Axillary nodes unpalpable or pellet sized	Tenderness, enlargement, hard node (carcinoma); may be visible bump (infection)	Refer to healthcare provider if evidence of inflammation.

(continued)

Assessment Guide

INITIAL PRENATAL ASSESSMENT

PHYSICAL ASSESSMENT/ NORMAL FINDINGS	ALTERATIONS AND POSSIBLE CAUSES*	NURSING RESPONSES TO DATA†
Pregnancy changes: 1. Size increase noted primarily in first 20 weeks. 2. Become nodular. 3. Tingling sensation may be felt during first and third trimester; woman may report feeling of heaviness. 4. Pigmentation of nipples and areolae darkens. 5. Superficial veins dilate and become more prominent. 6. Striae seen in multiparas. 7. Tubercles of Montgomery enlarge. 8. Colostrum may be present after 12th week. 9. Secondary areola appears at 20 weeks, characterized by series of washed-out spots surrounding primary areola. 10. Breasts less firm, old striae may be present in multiparas.		Discuss normalcy of changes and their meaning with the woman. Teach and/or institute appropriate relief measures. Encourage use of supportive, well-fitting brassiere.
Heart		
Normal rate, rhythm, and heart sounds ***Pregnancy changes:*** 1. Palpitations may occur due to sympathetic nervous system disturbance. 2. Short systolic murmurs that increase in held expiration are normal due to increased volume.	Enlargement, thrills, thrusts, gross irregularity or skipped beats, gallop rhythm or extra sounds (cardiac disease)	Complete an initial assessment. Explain normal pregnancy-induced changes. Refer to healthcare provider if indicated.
Abdomen		
Normal appearance, skin texture, and hair distribution; liver nonpalpable; abdomen nontender ***Pregnancy changes:*** 1. Purple striae may be present (or silver striae on a multipara) as well as linea nigra.	Muscle guarding (anxiety, acute tenderness); tenderness, mass (ectopic pregnancy, inflammation, carcinoma)	Assure woman of normalcy of diastasis. Provide initial information about appropriate prenatal and postpartum exercises. Evaluate woman's anxiety level. Refer to healthcare provider if indicated.
2. Diastasis of the rectus muscles late in pregnancy. 3. Size: Flat or rotund abdomen; progressive enlargement of uterus due to pregnancy. 10–12 weeks: Fundus slightly above symphysis pubis. 16 weeks: Fundus halfway between symphysis and umbilicus. 20–22 weeks: Fundus at umbilicus. 28 weeks: Fundus three finger breadths above umbilicus. 36 weeks: Fundus just below ensiform cartilage.	Size of uterus inconsistent with length of gestation (intrauterine growth restriction [IUGR], multiple pregnancy, fetal demise, hydatidiform mole)	Reassess menstrual history regarding pregnancy dating. Evaluate increase in size using McDonald's method. (See page 213.) Use ultrasound to establish diagnosis.
4. Fetal heart rate: 110–160 beats/min may be heard with Doppler at 10–12 weeks' gestation; may be heard with fetoscope at 17–20 weeks.	Failure to hear fetal heartbeat with Doppler (fetal demise, hydatidiform mole)	Refer to healthcare provider. Administer pregnancy tests. Use ultrasound to establish diagnosis.
5. Fetal movement palpable by a trained examiner after the 18th week.	Failure to feel fetal movements after 20 weeks' gestation (fetal demise, hydatidiform mole)	Refer to healthcare provider for evaluation of fetal status.
6. Ballottement: During fourth to fifth month fetus rises and then rebounds to original position when uterus is tapped sharply.	No ballottement (oligohydramnios)	Refer to healthcare provider for evaluation of fetal status.

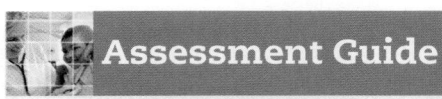

Assessment Guide

INITIAL PRENATAL ASSESSMENT

PHYSICAL ASSESSMENT/ NORMAL FINDINGS	ALTERATIONS AND POSSIBLE CAUSES*	NURSING RESPONSES TO DATA†
Extremities		
Skin warm, pulses palpable, full range of motion; may be some edema of hands and ankles in late pregnancy; varicose veins may become more pronounced; palmar erythema may be present	Unpalpable or diminished pulses (arterial insufficiency); marked edema (preeclampsia)	Evaluate for other symptoms of heart disease; initiate follow-up if woman mentions that her rings feel tight. Discuss prevention and self-treatment measures for varicose veins; refer to healthcare provider if indicated.
Spine		
Normal spinal curves: Concave cervical, convex thoracic, concave lumbar	Abnormal spinal curves; flatness, kyphosis, lordosis	Refer to healthcare provider for assessment of cephalopelvic disproportion (CPD).
In pregnancy, lumbar spinal curve may be accentuated	Backache	May have implications for administration of spinal anesthetics; see Chapter 20 for relief measures.
Shoulders and iliac crests should be even	Uneven shoulders and iliac crests (scoliosis)	Refer very young women to healthcare provider; discuss back-stretching exercise with older women.
Reflexes		
Normal and symmetric	Hyperactivity, clonus (preeclampsia)	Evaluate for other symptoms of preeclampsia.
Pelvic Area		
External female genitals: Normally formed with female hair distribution; in multiparas, labia majora loose and pigmented; urinary and vaginal orifices visible and appropriately located	Lesions, hematomas, varicosities, inflammation of Bartholin's glands; clitoral hypertrophy (masculinization)	Explain pelvic examination procedure. Encourage woman to minimize her discomfort by relaxing her hips. Provide privacy.
Vagina: Pink or dark pink, vaginal discharge odorless, nonirritating; in multiparas, vaginal folds smooth and flattened; may have episiotomy scar	Abnormal discharge associated with vaginal infections	Obtain vaginal smear. Provide understandable verbal and written instructions about treatment for woman and partner, if indicated.
Cervix: Pink color; os closed except in multiparas, in whom os admits fingertip	Eversion, reddish erosion, nabothian or retention cysts, cervical polyp; granular area that bleeds (carcinoma of cervix); lesions (herpes, human papilloma virus [HPV]); presence of string or plastic tip from cervix (intrauterine device [IUD] in uterus)	Provide woman with a hand mirror and identify genital structures for her; encourage her to view her cervix if she wishes. Refer to healthcare provider if indicated. Advise woman of potential serious risks of leaving an IUD in place during pregnancy; refer to healthcare provider for removal.
Pregnancy changes:		
1–4 weeks' gestation: Enlargement in anteroposterior diameter		
4–6 weeks' gestation: Softening of cervix (Goodell's sign); softening of isthmus of uterus (Hegar's sign); cervix takes on bluish coloring (Chadwick's sign)	Absence of Goodell's sign (inflammatory conditions, carcinoma)	Refer to healthcare provider.
8–12 weeks' gestation: Vagina and cervix appear bluish violet in color (Chadwick's sign)		
Uterus: Pear shaped, mobile; smooth surface	Fixed (pelvic inflammatory disease [PID]); nodular surface (fibromas)	Refer to healthcare provider.
Ovaries: Small, walnut shaped, nontender (ovaries and fallopian tubes are located in the adnexal areas)	Pain on movement of cervix (PID); enlarged or nodular ovaries (cyst, tumor, tubal pregnancy, corpus luteum of pregnancy)	Evaluate adnexal areas; refer to healthcare provider.

(continued)

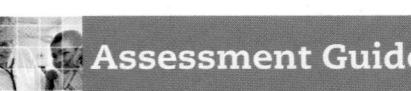

Assessment Guide

INITIAL PRENATAL ASSESSMENT

PHYSICAL ASSESSMENT/ NORMAL FINDINGS	ALTERATIONS AND POSSIBLE CAUSES*	NURSING RESPONSES TO DATA†
Pelvic Measurements		
Internal measurements:		
1. Diagonal conjugate at least 11.5 cm (Figure 10–5)	Measurement below normal	Vaginal birth may not be possible if deviations are present.
2. Obstetric conjugate estimated by subtracing 1.5–2 cm from diagonal conjugate	Disproportion of pubic arch	
3. Inclination of sacrum	Abnormal curvature of sacrum	
4. Motility of coccyx; external intertuberosity diameter greater than 8 cm	Fixed or malposition of coccyx	
Anus and Rectum		
No lumps, rashes, excoriation, tenderness; cervix may be felt through rectal wall	Hemorrhoids, rectal prolapse; nodular lesion (carcinoma)	Counsel about appropriate prevention and relief measures; refer to healthcare provider for further evaluation.
Laboratory Evaluation		
Hemoglobin: 12–16 g/dL; women residing in areas of high altitude may have higher levels of hemoglobin	Less than 11 g/dL in the first trimester, less than 10.5 g/dL in the second trimester, and less than 11 g/dL in the third trimester (anemia) (ACOG, 2008)	Note: Wear nonlatex gloves when drawing blood. Hemoglobin less than 12 g/dL requires nutritional counseling; less than 11 g/dL requires iron supplementation.
ABO and Rh typing: Normal distribution of blood types	Rh negative	If Rh negative, check for presence of anti-Rh antibodies. Check partner's blood type; if partner is Rh positive, discuss with woman the need for antibody titers during pregnancy, management during the intrapartal period, and possible need for Rh immune globulin. (See Chapter 16 ∞.)
Complete Blood Count (CBC)		
Hematocrit: 38%–47% physiologic anemia (pseudoanemia) may occur	Marked anemia or blood dyscrasias	Perform CBC and Schilling differential cell count.
Red blood cells (RBC): 4.2–5.4 million/microliter		
White blood cells (WBC): 5000–12,000/microliter	Presence of infection; may be elevated in pregnancy and with labor	Evaluate for other signs of infection.
Differential		
Neutrophils: 40%–60% Bands: up to 5% Eosinophils: 1%–3% Basophils: up to 1% Lymphocytes: 20%–40% Monocytes: 4%–8%		
First trimester aneuploidy screening: (testing to detect conditions related to abnormal chromosome number); If nuchal translucency (NT) testing is available, offer first-trimester screening for Down syndrome using nuchal translucency and serum markers (PAPP-A and free β-hCG). Normal range. ***Integrated screening:*** combines first-trimester aneuploidy screening results with second-trimester quad screen to detect aneuploidy and neural tube defects; may be used in areas in which NT testing is not available. (See discussion in "Subsequent Prenatal Assessment Guide.")	Increased nuchal translucency, elevated β-hCG, and reduced PAPP-A (Down syndrome, trisomy 18, trisomy 13, Turner syndrome)	If findings are positive, genetic counseling and diagnostic testing using chorionic villus sampling (CVS) or second-trimester amniocentesis is offered (ACOG, 2007).

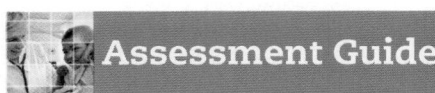

Assessment Guide

INITIAL PRENATAL ASSESSMENT

PHYSICAL ASSESSMENT/ NORMAL FINDINGS	ALTERATIONS AND POSSIBLE CAUSES*	NURSING RESPONSES TO DATA†
Syphilis tests: Serologic tests for syphilis (STS), complement fixation test, venereal disease research laboratory (VDRL) test—nonreactive	Positive reaction STS—tests may have 25%–45% incidence of biologic false-positive results; false results may occur in individuals who have acute viral or bacterial infections, hypersensitivity reactions, recent vaccinations, collagen disease, malaria, or tuberculosis	Positive results may be confirmed with the fluorescent treponemal antibody-absorption (FTA-ABS) test; all tests for syphilis give positive results in the secondary stage of the disease; antibiotic tests may cause negative test results.
Gonorrhea culture: Negative	Positive	Refer for treatment.
Urinalysis (u/a): Normal color, specific gravity; pH 4.6–8	Abnormal color (porphyria, hemoglobinuria, bilirubinemia): alkaline urine (metabolic alkalemia, *Proteus* infection, old specimen)	Repeat u/a; refer to healthcare provider.
Negative for protein, red blood cells, white blood cells, casts	Positive findings (contaminated specimen, kidney disease)	Repeat u/a; refer to healthcare provider.
Glucose: Negative (small degree of glycosuria may occur in pregnancy)	Glycosuria (low renal threshold for glucose, diabetes mellitus)	Assess blood glucose level; test urine for ketones.
Rubella titer: Hemagglutination-inhibition (HAI) test–1:10 or above indicates woman is immune	HAI titer less than 1:10	Immunization will be given on postpartum or within 6 weeks after childbirth. Instruct woman whose titers are less than 1:10 to avoid children who have rubella.
Hepatitis B screen: for hepatitis B surface antigen (HBsAg): negative	Positive	If negative, consider referral for hepatitis B vaccine. If positive, refer to physician. Infants born to women who test positive are given hepatitis B immune globulin soon after birth followed by first dose of hepatitis B vaccine.
HIV screen: Opt-out screening offered to all women; encouraged for those at risk; negative	Positive	Refer to healthcare provider.
Illicit drug screen: Offered to all women; negative	Positive	Refer to healthcare provider.
Sickle-cell screen for clients of African or Latino descent: Negative	Positive; test results would include a description of cells	Refer to healthcare provider.
Pap smear: Negative	Test results that show atypical cells	Refer to healthcare provider. Discuss with the woman the meaning of the findings and the importance of follow-up.

CULTURAL ASSESSMENT	VARIATIONS TO CONSIDER*	NURSING RESPONSES TO DATA†
Determine the woman's fluency in written and oral English.	Woman may be fluent in language other than English.	Work with a knowledgeable translator to provide information and answer questions.
Ask the woman how she prefers to be addressed.	Some women prefer informality; others prefer to use titles.	Address the woman according to her preference. Maintain formality in introducing oneself if that seems preferred.
Determine customs and practices regarding prenatal care:	Practices are influenced by individual preference, cultural expectations, or religious beliefs.	Honor a woman's practices and provide for specific preferences unless they are contraindicated because of safety.
■ Ask the woman if there are certain practices she expects to follow when she is pregnant.	Some women believe that they should perform certain acts related to sleep, activity, or clothing.	Have information printed in the language of different cultural groups that live in the area.
■ Ask the woman if there are any activities she cannot do while she is pregnant.	Some women have restrictions or taboos they follow related to work, activity, sexual, environmental, or emotional factors.	
■ Ask the woman whether there are certain foods she is expected to eat or avoid while she is pregnant. Determine whether she has lactose intolerance.	Foods are an important cultural factor. Some women may have certain foods they must eat or avoid; many women have lactose intolerance and have difficulty consuming sufficient calcium.	Respect the woman's food preferences, help her plan an adequate prenatal diet within the framework of her preferences, and refer to a dietitian if necessary.

(continued)

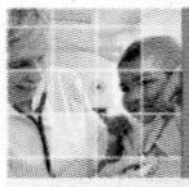

Assessment Guide

INITIAL PRENATAL ASSESSMENT

PHYSICAL ASSESSMENT/ NORMAL FINDINGS	ALTERATIONS AND POSSIBLE CAUSES*	NURSING RESPONSES TO DATA†
■ Ask the woman whether the gender of her caregiver is of concern.	Some women are comfortable only with a female caregiver.	Arrange for a female caregiver if it is the woman's preference.
■ Ask the woman about the degree of involvement in her pregnancy that she expects or wants from her support person, mother, and other significant people.	A woman may not want her partner involved in the pregnancy. For some the role falls to the woman's mother or a female relative or friend.	Respect the woman's preferences about her partner or husband's involvement; avoid imposing personal values or expectations.
■ Ask the woman about her sources of support and counseling during pregnancy.	Some women seek advice from a family member, *curandera,* tribal healer, and so forth.	Respect and honor the woman's sources of support.
Psychologic Status		
Excitement and/or apprehension, ambivalence	Marked anxiety (fear of pregnancy diagnosis, fear of medical facility)	Establish lines of communication. Active listening is useful. Establish trusting relationship. Encourage woman to take active part in her care.
	Apathy; display of anger with pregnancy diagnosis	Establish communication and begin counseling. Use active listening techniques.
Educational Needs		
May have questions about pregnancy or may need time to adjust to reality of pregnancy		Establish educational, supporting environment that can be expanded throughout pregnancy.
Support System		
Can identify at least two or three individuals with whom woman is emotionally intimate (partner, parent, sibling, friend)	Isolated (no telephone, unlisted number); cannot name a neighbor or friend whom she can call upon in an emergency; does not perceive parents as part of her support system	Institute support system through community groups. Help woman to develop trusting relationship with healthcare professionals.
Family Functioning		
Emotionally supportive Communications adequate Mutually satisfying Cohesiveness in times of trouble	Long-term problems or specific problems related to this pregnancy, potential stressors within the family, pessimistic attitudes, unilateral decision making, unrealistic expectations of this pregnancy or child	Help identify the problems and stressors, encourage communication, and discuss role changes and adaptations.
Economic Status		
Source of income is stable and sufficient to meet basic needs of daily lμiving and medical needs	Limited prenatal care; poor physical health; limited use of healthcare system; unstable economic status	Discuss available resources for health maintenance and the birth. Institute appropriate referral for meeting expanding family's needs—food stamps and so forth.
Stability of Living Conditions		
Adequate, stable housing for expanding family's needs	Crowded living conditions; questionable supportive environment for newborn	Refer to appropriate community agency. Work with family on self-help ways to improve situation.

*Possible causes of alterations are identified in parentheses.

†This column provides guidelines for further assessment and initial intervention.

NÄGELE'S RULE

The most common method of determining the EDB is **Nägele's rule**, which uses 280 days as the mean length of pregnancy. To use this method, begin with the first day of the LMP, subtract 3 months, and add 7 days. For example:

First day of LMP	November 21
Subtract 3 months	− 3 months
	August 21
Add 7 days	+ 7 days
EDB	August 28

It is simpler to change the months to numeric terms:

November 21 becomes	11–21
Subtract 3 months	− 3
	8–21
Add 7 days	+ 7
EDB	8–28

A gestation calculator or wheel lets the caregiver calculate the EDB even more quickly (Figure 10–2 ●).

Nägele's rule may be a fairly accurate determiner of the EDB if the woman has a history of menses every 28 days, remembers her LMP, and was not taking oral contraceptives before becoming pregnant.

However, Nägele's rule is not foolproof. A delay in ovulation affects the formula Nägele's rule uses to determine the EDB.

Ovulation usually occurs 14 days *before* the onset of the next menses, not 14 days after the previous menses. Consequently, if a woman's cycle is irregular, or more than 28 days long, the time of ovulation may be delayed. If a woman has been using oral contraceptives, ovulation may be delayed several weeks following her last menses. Then, too, a postpartum woman who is breastfeeding may resume ovulating but be amenorrheic for a time, making calculation based on LMP impossible.

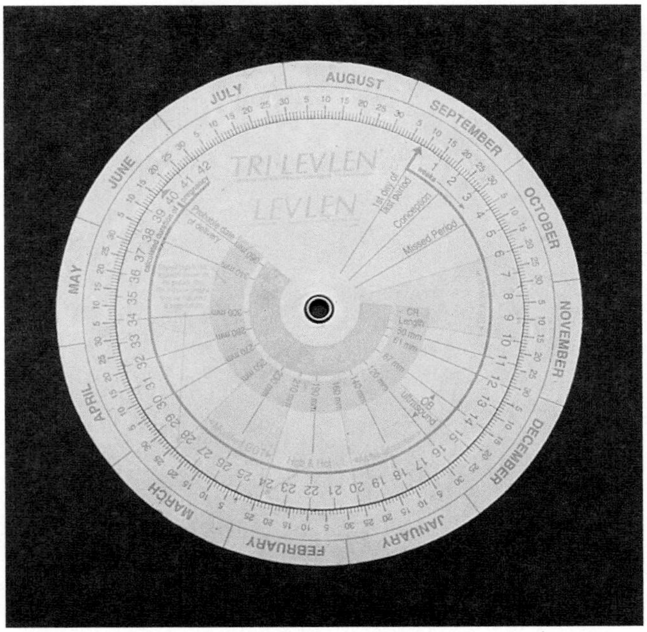

● **Figure 10–2** EDB wheel. The EDB wheel can be used to calculate the due date. To use it, place the "last menses began" arrow on the date of the woman's LMP. Then read the EDB at the arrow labeled 40. In this case the LMP is September 8, and the EDB is June 17.

UTERINE ASSESSMENT

Physical Examination

When a woman is examined in the first 10 to 12 weeks of her pregnancy and her uterine size is compatible with her menstrual history, uterine size may be the single most important clinical method for dating her pregnancy. In many cases, however, women do not seek maternity care until well into their second trimester, when it becomes much more difficult to evaluate specific uterine size. In obese women it is difficult to determine uterine size early in a pregnancy because the uterus is more difficult to palpate.

Fundal Height

Fundal height may be used as an indicator of uterine size, although this method is less accurate late in pregnancy. A centimeter tape measure is used to measure the distance abdominally from the top of the symphysis pubis to the top of the uterine fundus (McDonald's method) (Figure 10–3 ●). Fundal height in centimeters correlates well with weeks of gestation between 22 to 24 weeks and 34 weeks. Thus, at 26 weeks' gestation, fundal height is probably about 26 cm. If the woman is very tall or very short, fundal height will differ. To be most accurate, fundal height should be measured by the same examiner each time. The woman should have voided within one-half hour of the examination and should lie in the same position each time. In the third trimester, variations in fetal weight decrease the accuracy of fundal height measurements.

A lag in progression of measurements of fundal height from month to month and week to week may signal intrauterine growth restriction (IUGR). A sudden increase in fundal height may indicate twins or hydramnios (excessive amount of amniotic fluid).

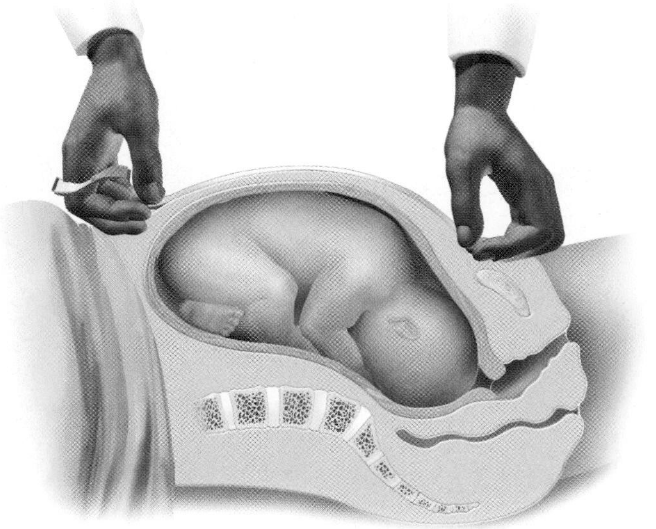

● **Figure 10–3** McDonald's method. A cross-sectional view of fetal position when McDonald's method is used to assess fundal height.

ASSESSMENT OF FETAL DEVELOPMENT

Quickening

Fetal movements felt by the mother, called quickening, may indicate that the fetus is nearing 20 weeks' gestation. However, quickening may be experienced between 16 and 22 weeks' gestation, so this method is not completely accurate.

Fetal Heartbeat

The ultrasonic Doppler device (Figure 10–4 ●) is the primary tool for assessing fetal heartbeat. It can detect fetal heartbeat, on average, at 8 to 12 weeks' gestation. If an ultrasonic Doppler is not available, a fetoscope may be used, although in current practice it is seldom necessary. The fetal heartbeat can be detected by fetoscope as early as week 16 and almost always by 19 or 20 weeks' gestation.

Ultrasound

In the first trimester, ultrasound scanning can detect a gestational sac as early as 5 to 6 weeks after the LMP, fetal heart activity by 6 to 7 weeks, and fetal breathing movement by 10 to 11 weeks of

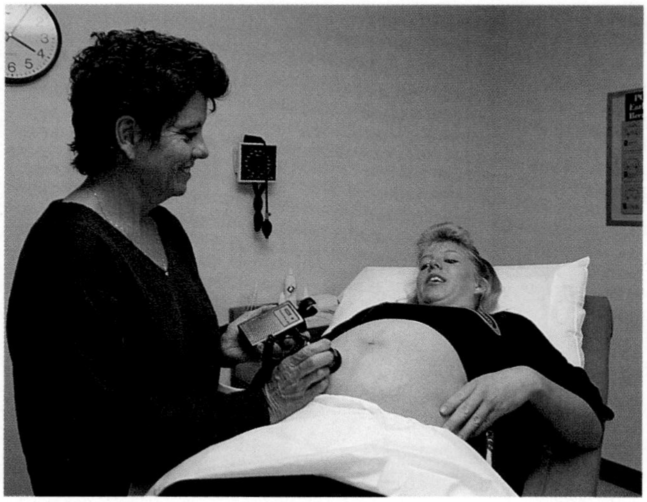

● **Figure 10–4** Ultrasonic Doppler device. This practitioner is using the device to listen to the fetal heartbeat.

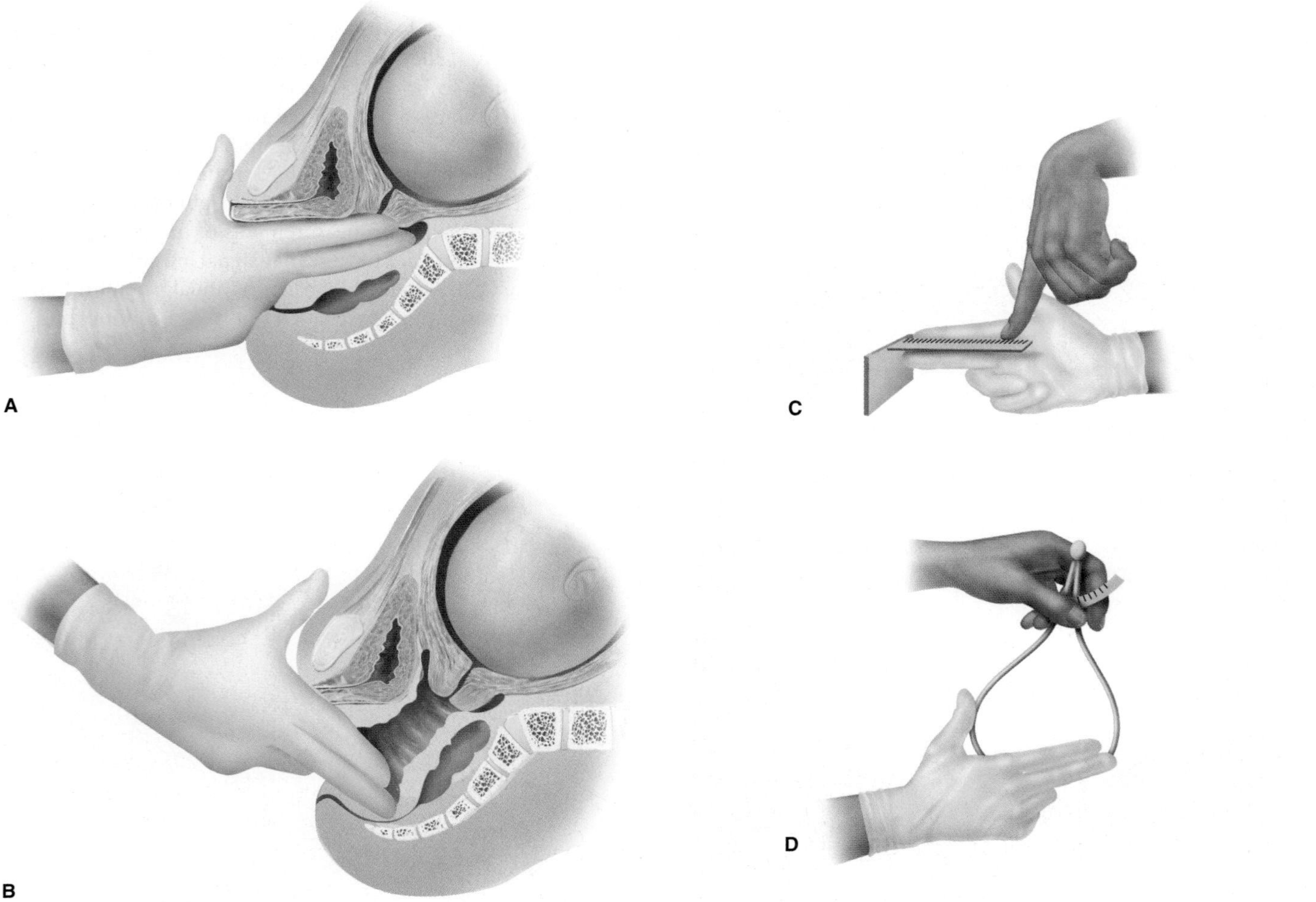

● **Figure 10–5** Manual measurement of inlet and outlet. ***A,*** Estimation of the diagonal conjugate, which extends from the lower border of the symphysis pubis to the sacral promontory. ***B,*** Estimation of the anteroposterior diameter of the outlet, which extends from the lower border of the symphysis pubis to the tip of the sacrum. ***C*** and ***D,*** Methods that may be used to check the manual estimation of anteroposterior measurements.

pregnancy. Crown-to-rump measurements can be made to assess fetal age until the fetal head can be visualized clearly. Biparietal diameter (BPD) can then be used. BPD measurements can be made by approximately 12 to 13 weeks and are most accurate between 20 and 30 weeks, when rapid growth in the biparietal diameter occurs. (See Chapter 14 for discussion of fetal ultrasound scanning.)

ASSESSMENT OF PELVIC ADEQUACY (CLINICAL PELVIMETRY)

The pelvis can be assessed vaginally to determine whether its size is adequate for a vaginal birth. This procedure, clinical pelvimetry, is performed by physicians or by advanced practice nurses such as CNMs or nurse practitioners. For a detailed description of clinical pelvimetry, refer to a nurse-midwifery text. This section provides basic information about the assessment of the inlet and outlet (see Figures 10–5 ● and 10–6 ●), which were described in Chapter 3.

1. Pelvic inlet (Figure 10–5)
   - **Diagonal conjugate** (the distance from the lower posterior border of the symphysis pubis to the sacral promontory) at least 11.5 cm
   - **Obstetric conjugate** (a measurement approximately 1.5 cm smaller than the diagonal conjugate) 10 cm or more
2. Pelvic outlet (Figures 10–5 and 10–6)
   - Anteroposterior diameter, 9.5 to 11.5 cm
   - Transverse diameter (bi-ischial or intertuberous diameter), 8 to 10 cm

The pelvic cavity (midpelvis) cannot be accurately measured by clinical examination. Examiners estimate its adequacy. However, that discussion is also beyond the scope of this text.

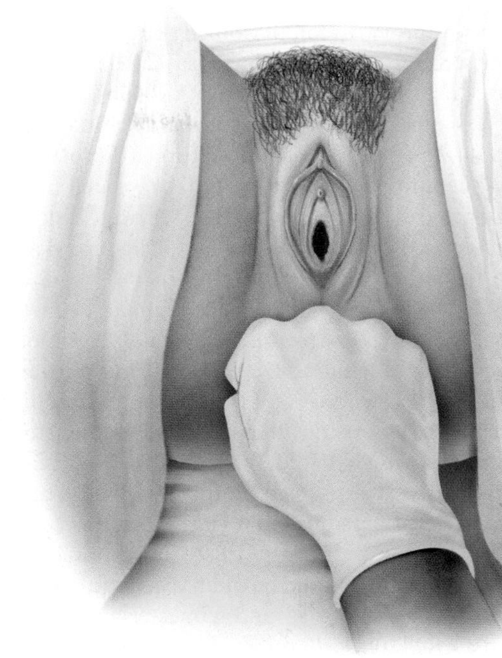

● **Figure 10–6** Use of a closed fist to measure the outlet. Most examiners know the distance between their first and last proximal knuckles. If they do not, they can use a measuring device.

SCREENING TESTS

Many screening tests are routinely performed either at the initial prenatal visit or at a specified time during pregnancy. These tests include a Pap smear, a complete blood count, hemoglobin, Rubella titer, ABO and Rh typing, and a hepatitis B screen as well as testing

Evidence-Based Nursing

MATERNAL OBESITY AND ULTRASOUND DETECTION

Clinical Question

Does maternal obesity interfere with the ultrasound detection of fetal problems?

The Evidence

Three physicians conducted a retrospective cohort study of more than 12,000 prenatal ultrasound examinations. Well-designed studies with large sample sizes provide some of the strongest evidence for practice. Obesity has been cited as the leading health problem confronting women, and its prevalence has increased dramatically in the last two decades. Obesity has the potential to affect prenatal diagnosis in several ways, and it has been suggested that excess body mass index may interfere with the accuracy of ultrasound detection of fetal abnormalities. In addition, obese women often present with gestational diabetes, which may interfere with the detection of fetal problems. In this study, detection of anomalous fetuses decreased with increasing body mass index and with gestational diabetes. In obese women, 1.0% of anomalies may go undiscovered by prenatal ultrasound; for the most obese women, 1 out of 4 anomalies may go undetected. In particular, visualization of the fetal heart was compromised by maternal obesity, and so cardiac anomalies such as ventricular septal defect, tetralogy of Fallot, and transposition of the great arteries were often undiscovered until after birth (Dashes, 2009).

Best Practice

The prevention of obesity is the best way to assure that prenatal ultrasound will be accurate in the detection of fetal problems. When obese women undergo ultrasound for the detection of fetal abnormalities, counseling may be needed to reflect the limitations on accurate diagnosis presented by excess body mass index.

Critical Thinking

Will additional imaging be of benefit in detecting abnormalities that may be missed by a single ultrasound examination?

for sexually transmitted infections such as syphilis and gonorrhea. A sickle cell screen is provided for all women of African or Latino descent. Prenatal screening for cystic fibrosis should be offered to all couples regardless of ethnicity or race (ACOG, 2005b).

The urine is screened for abnormal findings initially and at each prenatal visit. In addition, a urine culture at 12 to 16 weeks of pregnancy is recommended for all pregnant women to detect asymptomatic bacteriuria (U.S. Preventive Services Task Force, 2004). Other tests such as HIV screen and a drug screen are offered to all women.

ACOG (2007) recommends that all pregnant women, regardless of age, be offered screening for fetal chromosome anomolies *(aneuploidy)* including Down syndrome, trisomy 18, trisomy 13, and Turner syndrome. First trimester screening is available at many centers using ultrasound assessment of the thickness of the fetal nuchal fold (called *nuchal translucency* [NT]) combined with serum screening for free β-hCG and for pregnancy-associated plasma protein A (PAPP-A) Increased NT, elevated free β-hCG, and reduced PAPP-A suggest aneuploidy. Women with these findings should be offered genetic counseling and chorion villus sampling or second trimester amniocentesis for diagnosis (ACOG, 2007). If these tests are all negative no further testing is indicated. Instead, during the second trimester, the woman is simply offered a test for maternal serum alpha-fetoprotein to detect the risk of neural tube defects.

The *quadruple screen* (quad screen) is a safe, useful screening test performed on the mother's serum between weeks 15 and 20 of pregnancy. The test is used to detect levels of specific serum markers—alpha-fetoprotein (AFP), human chorionic gonadotropin (hCG), unconjugated estriol (UE), and inhibin-A (a placental hormone). Test results that reveal higher than normal AFP levels might indicate a fetal neural tube defect, a multiple gestation, or a pregnancy that is farther along than believed. Lower than normal AFP could indicate that the woman is at risk for Down syndrome or trisomy 18. Higher than normal levels of hCG and inhibin-A and lower than normal UE may also indicate that a woman is at increased risk of having a baby with Down syndrome. If the screening results are not in the normal range, follow-up testing using ultrasound and amniocentesis is often indicated (Cleveland Clinic, 2006).

NT evaluation requires a skilled ultrasonographer and specialized training. In areas where NT is not available, first trimester free ß-hCG screening and PAPP-A screening may be combined with second trimester quad screening in an integrated approach to detection of aneuploidy.

It is important for healthcare professionals to provide parents with factual information about the results of tests that detect chromosomal defects or fetal anomalies including the false-positive and detection rates and the implications of the findings (Nicolaides, 2005). Parents then need to decide on any course of action based on their own spiritual and cultural beliefs.

Between 24 and 28 weeks' gestation a 50 g 1-hour glucose screen is completed to detect gestational diabetes mellitus. Additional testing is indicated if abnormal results are obtained (See Chapter 15∞).

Group B streptococcus (GBS) can cause serious problems for a newborn. Consequently rectal and vaginal swabs of the mother are obtained at 35 to 27 weeks' gestation to screen for the infection.

SUBSEQUENT CLIENT HISTORY

At subsequent prenatal visits, continue to gather data about the course of the pregnancy to date and the woman's responses to it. Also ask about the adjustment of the support person and of other children, if any, in the family. As pregnancy progresses, inquire about the preparations the family has made for the new baby.

Ask specifically whether the woman has experienced any discomfort, especially the kinds of discomfort that are often seen at specific times during a pregnancy. Inquire about physical changes that relate directly to the pregnancy, such as fetal movement. Also ask about the danger signs in pregnancy (Table 10–2). (Note: Many of the danger signs indicate conditions that are potential complications. These conditions are discussed in the at-risk chapters, which are presented later in this text).

Other pertinent information includes any exposure to contagious illnesses, medical treatment and therapy prescribed for

Table 10–2 Danger Signs in Pregnancy

The woman should report the following danger signs in pregnancy immediately:

Danger Sign	Possible Cause
Sudden gush of fluid from vagina	Premature rupture of membranes
Vaginal bleeding	Abruptio placentae, placenta previa
	Lesions of cervix or vagina
	"Bloody show"
Abdominal pain	Premature labor, abruptio placentae
Temperature above 38.3°C (101°F) and chills	Infection
Dizziness, blurring of vision double vision, spots before eyes	Hypertension, preeclampsia
Persistent vomiting	Hyperemesis gravidarum
Severe headache	Hypertension, preeclampsia
Edema of hands, face, legs, and feet	Preeclampsia
Muscular irritability, convulsions	Preeclampsia, eclampsia
Epigastric pain	Preeclampsia, ischemia in major abdominal vessel
Oliguria	Renal impairment, decreased fluid intake
Dysuria	Urinary tract infection
Absence of fetal movement	Maternal medication, obesity, fetal death

nonpregnancy problems since the last visit, and any prescription, over-the-counter medications, or herbal supplements that were not prescribed as part of the woman's prenatal care.

Periodic prenatal examinations offer a chance to assess the childbearing woman's psychologic needs and emotional status. If the woman's partner attends the antepartal visits, they can also be a time to identify the partner's needs and concerns. The woman should have sufficient time to ask questions and air concerns. If a nurse provides the time and demonstrates genuine interest, the woman will be more at ease bringing up questions that she may believe are silly or has been afraid to verbalize.

Be sensitive to religious or spiritual, cultural, and socioeconomic factors that may influence a family's response to pregnancy, as well as to the woman's expectations of the healthcare system. One way to avoid stereotyping clients is simply to ask each woman about her expectations for the antepartal period. Although many women's responses may reflect what are thought to be traditional norms, other women will have decidedly different views or expectations that represent a blending of beliefs or cultures. During the antepartal period, it is also essential to begin assessing the readiness of the woman and her partner (if possible) to assume their responsibilities as parents successfully.

SUBSEQUENT PRENATAL ASSESSMENT

The "Assessment Guide: Subsequent Prenatal Assessment" provides a systematic approach to the regular physical examinations the pregnant woman should undergo for optimal antepartal care and also provides a model for evaluating both the pregnant woman and the expectant father, if he is involved in the pregnancy.

The recommended frequency of antepartal visits in an uncomplicated pregnancy is as follows:

Nursing Practice

When assessing blood pressure, have the pregnant woman sit up with her arm resting on a table so that her arm is at the level of her heart. Expect a decrease in blood pressure from baseline during the second trimester because of typical physiologic changes. If the decrease does not occur, evaluate further for signs of preeclampsia.

- Every 4 weeks for the first 28 weeks' gestation
- Every 2 weeks until 36 weeks' gestation
- After week 36, every week until childbirth

During the subsequent antepartal assessments, most women demonstrate ongoing psychologic adjustment to pregnancy. However, some women may exhibit signs of possible psychologic problems such as the following:

- Increasing anxiety
- Inability to establish communication
- Inappropriate responses or actions
- Denial of pregnancy
- Inability to cope with stress
- Intense preoccupation with the sex of the baby
- Failure to acknowledge quickening
- Failure to plan and prepare for the baby (e.g., living arrangements, clothing, and feeding methods)
- Indications of substance abuse

If the woman's behavior indicates possible psychologic problems, the nurse can provide ongoing support and counseling and also refer the woman to appropriate professionals.

Assessment Guide

SUBSEQUENT PRENATAL ASSESSMENT

PHYSICAL ASSESSMENT/ NORMAL FINDINGS	ALTERATIONS AND POSSIBLE CAUSES*	NURSING RESPONSES TO DATA†
Vital Signs		
Temperature: 36.2°C–37.6°C (97°F–99.6°F)	Elevated temperature (infection)	Evaluate for signs of infection. Refer to healthcare provider.
Pulse: 60–90/min Rate may increase 10 beats/min during pregnancy	Increased pulse rate (anxiety, cardiac disorders)	Note irregularities. Assess for anxiety and stress.
Respiration: 12–22/min	Marked tachypnea or abnormal patterns (respiratory disease)	Refer to healthcare provider.
Blood pressure: Less than or equal to 135/85 (falls in second trimester)	Greater than 140/90 or increase of 30 mm systolic and 15 mm diastolic (preeclampsia)	Assess for edema, proteinuria, and hyperreflexia. Refer to healthcare provider. Schedule appointments more frequently.

(continued)

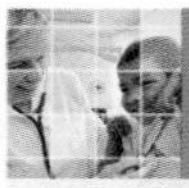

Assessment Guide

SUBSEQUENT PRENATAL ASSESSMENT

PHYSICAL ASSESSMENT/ NORMAL FINDINGS	ALTERATIONS AND POSSIBLE CAUSES*	NURSING RESPONSES TO DATA[†]
Weight Gain		
First trimester: 1.6–2.3 kg (3.5–5 lb)	Inadequate weight gain (poor nutrition, nausea, IUGR)	Discuss appropriate weight gain.
Second trimester: 5.5–6.8 kg (12–15 lb)	Excessive weight gain (excessive caloric intake, edema, preeclampsia)	Provide nutritional counseling. Assess for presence of edema or anemia.
Third trimester: 5.5–6.8 kg (12–15 lb)		
Edema		
Small amount of dependent edema, especially in last weeks of pregnancy	Edema in hands, face, legs, and feet (preeclampsia)	Identify any correlation between edema and activities, blood pressure, or proteinuria: Refer to healthcare provider if indicated.
Uterine Size		
See "Assessment Guide: Initial Prenatal Assessment" on page 209 for normal changes during pregnancy	Unusually rapid growth (multiple gestation, hydatidiform mole, hydramnios, miscalculation of EDB)	Evaluate fetal status. Determine height of fundus (page 213). Use diagnostic ultrasound.
Fetal Heartbeat		
120–160/min Funic souffle	Absence of fetal heartbeat after 20 weeks' gestation (maternal obesity, fetal demise)	Evaluate fetal status.
Laboratory Evaluation		
Hemoglobin: 12–16 g/dL Pseudoanemia of pregnancy	Greater than 11 g/dL (anemia)	Provide nutritional counseling. Hemoglobin is repeated at 7 months' gestation. Women of Mediterranean heritage need a close check on hemoglobin because of possibility of thalassemia.
Quad marker screen: Blood test performed at 15–20 weeks' gestation. Evaluates four factors—maternal serum alpha-fetoprotein (MSAFP), unconjugated estriol (UE), hCG, and inhibin-A: normal levels	Elevated MSAFP (neural tube defect, underestimated gestational age, multiple gestation). Lower than normal MSAFP (Down syndrome, trisomy 18). Higher than normal hCG and inhibin-A (Down syndrome). Lower than normal UE (Down syndrome).	Recommended for all pregnant women; especially indicated for women with any of the following risk factors: age 35 and over, family history of birth defects, previous child with a birth defect; insulin-dependent diabetes prior to pregnancy (Cleveland Clinic, 2006). If quad screen is abnormal, further testing such as ultrasound or amniocentesis may be indicated.
Indirect Coombs test done on Rh negative women: Negative (done at 28 weeks' gestation)	Rh antibodies present (maternal sensitization has occurred)	If Rh negative and unsensitized, Rh immune globulin given (see Chapter 16). If Rh antibodies present, Rh immune globulin not given; fetus monitored closely for isoimmune hemolytic disease.
50-g 1-hour glucose screen (done between 24 and 28 weeks' gestation)	Plasma glucose level greater than 140 mg/dL (gestational diabetes mellitus [GDM]) Note: Some facilities use level greater than 130 mg/d, which identifies 90% of women with GDM (American Diabetes Association, 2004)	Discuss implications of GDM. Refer for a diagnostic 100 g oral glucose tolerance test.
Urinalysis: See "Assessment Guide: Initial Prenatal Assessment" on page 211 for normal findings	See "Assessment Guide: Initial Prenatal Assessment" on page 211 for deviations	Repeat urinalysis at 7 months' gestation. Repeat dipstick test at each visit.

Assessment Guide

SUBSEQUENT PRENATAL ASSESSMENT

PHYSICAL ASSESSMENT/ NORMAL FINDINGS	ALTERATIONS AND POSSIBLE CAUSES*	NURSING RESPONSES TO DATA†
Protein: Negative	Proteinuria, albuminuria (contamination by vaginal discharge, urinary tract infection, preeclampsia)	Obtain dipstick urine sample. Refer to healthcare provider if deviations are present.
Glucose: Negative *Note:* Glycosuria may be present due to physiologic alterations in glomerular filtration rate and renal threshold	Persistent glycosuria (diabetes mellitus)	Refer to healthcare provider.
Screening for Group B streptococcus (GBS): Rectal and vaginal swabs obtained at 35–37 weeks' gestation for all pregnant women (Centers for Disease Control and Prevention [CDC], 2002).	Positive culture (maternal infection)	Explain maternal and fetal/neonatal risks (see Chapter 16). Refer to healthcare provider for therapy.

CULTURAL ASSESSMENT	VARIATIONS TO CONSIDER*	NURSING RESPONSES TO DATA†
Determine the mother's (and family's) attitudes about the sex of the unborn child.	Some women have no preference about the sex of the child; others do. In many cultures, boys are especially valued as firstborn children.	Provide opportunities to discuss preferences and expectations; avoid a judgmental attitude to the response.
Ask about the woman's expectations of childbirth. Will she want someone with her for the birth? Whom does she choose? What is the role of her partner?	Some women want their partner present for labor and birth; others prefer a female relative or friend. Some women expect to be separated from their partner once cervical dilation has occurred.	Provide information on birth options but accept the woman's decision about who will attend.
Ask about preparations for the baby. Determine what is customary for the woman.	Some women may have a fully prepared nursery; others may not have a separate room for the baby.	Explore reasons for not preparing for the baby. Support the mother's preferences and provide information about possible sources of assistance if the decision is related to a lack of resources.

Expectant Mother

Psychologic status	Increased stress and anxiety	Encourage woman to take an active part in her care.
First trimester: Incorporates idea of pregnancy; may feel ambivalent, especially if she must give up desired role; usually looks for signs of verification of pregnancy, such as increase in abdominal size or fetal movement ***Second trimester:*** Baby becomes more real to woman as abdominal size increases and she feels movement; she begins to turn inward, becoming more introspective ***Third trimester:*** Begins to think of baby as separate being; may feel restless and may feel that time of labor will never come; remains self-centered and concentrates on preparing place for baby	Inability to establish communication; inability to accept pregnancy; inappropriate response or actions; denial of pregnancy; inability to cope	Establish lines of communication. Establish a trusting relationship. Counsel as necessary. Refer to appropriate professional as needed.

(continued)

Assessment Guide

SUBSEQUENT PRENATAL ASSESSMENT

PHYSICAL ASSESSMENT/ NORMAL FINDINGS	ALTERATIONS AND POSSIBLE CAUSES*	NURSING RESPONSES TO DATA†
Educational needs: ***Self-care measures and knowledge about the following:*** Health promotion Breast care Hygiene Rest Exercise Nutrition Relief measures for common discomforts of pregnancy Danger signs in pregnancy (see Table 15–3)	Inadequate information	Provide information and counseling.
Sexual activity: Woman knows how pregnancy affects sexual activity	Lack of information about effects of pregnancy and/or alternative positions during sexual intercourse	Provide counseling.
Preparation for parenting: Appropriate preparation	Lack of preparation (denial, failure to adjust to baby, unwanted child)	Counsel. If lack of preparation is due to inadequacy of information, provide information.
Preparation for childbirth: Client aware of the following: 1. Prepared childbirth techniques 2. Normal processes and changes during childbirth		If couple chooses particular technique refer to classes (see Chapter 8 for description of childbirth preparation techniques). Encourage prenatal class attendance. Educate woman during visits based on current physical status. Provide reading list for more specific information.
3. Problems that may occur as a result of drug and alcohol use and of smoking	Continued abuse of drugs and alcohol; denial of possible effect on self and baby	Review danger signs that were presented on initial visit.
Woman has met other physician or nurse-midwife who may be attending her birth in the absence of primary caregiver	Introduction of new individual at birth may increase stress and anxiety for woman and partner	Introduce woman to all members of group practice.
Impending labor: Client knows signs of impending labor: 1. Uterine contractions that increase in frequency, duration, and intensity 2. Bloody show 3. Expulsion of mucous plug 4. Rupture of membranes	Lack of information	Provide appropriate teaching, stressing importance of seeking appropriate medical assistance.
Expectant Father		
Psychologic status ***First trimester:*** May express excitement over confirmation of pregnancy and of his virility; concerns move toward providing for financial needs; energetic, may identify with some discomforts of pregnancy and may even exhibit symptoms	Increasing stress and anxiety; inability to establish communication; inability to accept pregnancy diagnosis; withdrawal of support; abandonment of the mother	Encourage expectant father to come to prenatal visits. Establish line of communication. Establish trusting relationship.

Assessment Guide

SUBSEQUENT PRENATAL ASSESSMENT

PHYSICAL ASSESSMENT/ NORMAL FINDINGS	ALTERATIONS AND POSSIBLE CAUSES*	NURSING RESPONSES TO DATA†
Second trimester: May feel more confident and be less concerned with financial matters; may have concerns about wife's changing size and shape, her increasing introspection		Counsel. Let expectant father know that it is normal for him to experience these feelings.
Third trimester: May have feelings of rivalry with fetus, especially during sexual activity; may make changes in his physical appearance and exhibit more interest in himself; may become more energetic; fantasizes about child but usually imagines older child; fears mutilation and death of woman and child		Include expectant father in pregnancy activities as he desires. Provide education, information, and support. Increasing numbers of expectant fathers are demonstrating desire to be involved in many or all aspects of prenatal care, education, and preparation.

*Possible causes of alterations are identified in parentheses.

†This column provides guidelines for further assessment and initial intervention.

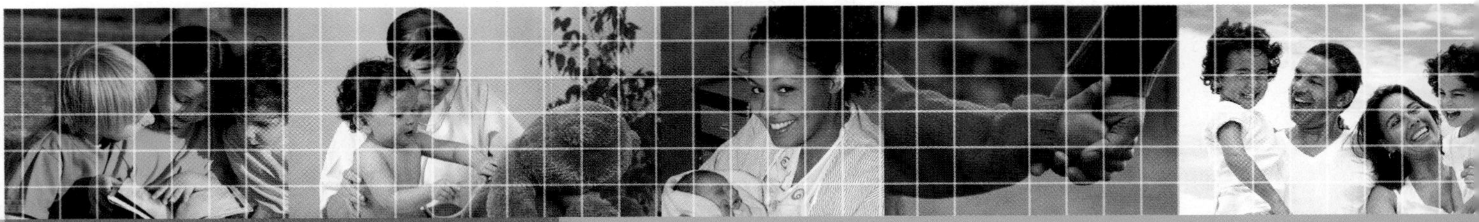

CRITICAL CONCEPT REVIEW

LEARNING OUTCOMES	CONCEPTS
10.1 Use information provided on a prenatal history to identify risk factors for the mother and/or fetus.	1. To identify all of the risk factors included in Table 10–1, all aspects of a women's history should be reviewed. A detailed prenatal history includes the following: ■ Details of current pregnancy (such as LMP). ■ History of past pregnancies. ■ Gynecologic history (such as last Pap and contraceptive use). ■ Current medical history (such as weight, prescription medications, chronic diseases). ■ Past medical history (past surgeries). ■ Family medical history (cancer or diabetes). ■ Religious, spiritual, and cultural history. ■ Occupational history (physical demands of present job). ■ Partner's history (genetic conditions, blood type). ■ Demographic information about woman (age, educational level, and ethnic background).
10.2 Define common obstetric terminology found in the history of maternity clients.	1. Terms about the number of pregnancies and births: gravida, parity, and TPAL. 2. Terms that denote the phase of pregnancy: ante-, intra-, and postpartum. 3. Terms that denote age and developmental status of fetus at birth: prematurity, postmaturity, and term (see page 200).
10.3 Consider risk factors related to the father's health that are generally recorded on the prenatal record in assessing risk factors for the mother and/or fetus.	1. Father's health details to be recorded: ■ History of chronic illness in father or immediate family member. ■ Blood type and Rh factor. ■ Present use of alcohol, tobacco, or recreational drugs. ■ Occupation. ■ Age.

(continued)

LEARNING OUTCOMES	CONCEPTS
10.4 Evaluate those areas of the initial assessment that reflect the psychosocial and cultural factors related to a woman's pregnancy.	1. Language preference. ■ Determine how woman should be addressed. ■ Determine food customs and preferences. ■ Determine significant people to woman, and degree of involvement of these persons. ■ Psychologic status. ■ Educational needs. ■ Support system. ■ Family functioning. ■ Economic status. ■ Stability of living conditions.
10.5 Predict the normal physiologic changes a nurse would expect to find when performing a physical assessment of a pregnant woman.	1. Vital signs: ■ Pulse may increase by 10 beats/min. ■ Respiration may be increased, and thoracic breathing predominant. ■ Temperature and blood pressure within normal limits. 2. Weight: ■ Varies, but should be proportional to the gestational age of the fetus. 3. Skin: ■ Linea nigra. ■ Striae gravidarum. ■ Melasma. ■ Spider nevi. 4. Nose: ■ Nasal stuffiness. 5. Mouth: ■ Gingival hypertrophy. 6. Neck: ■ Small, nontender nodes. ■ Slight hyperplasia of thyroid in third trimester. 7. Chest and lungs: ■ Transverse diameter greater than anteroposterior diameter. 8. Breasts: ■ Increasing size. ■ Pigmentation of nipples and areolae. ■ Tubercles of Montgomery enlarge. ■ Colostrum appears in third trimester. 9. Abdomen: ■ Progressive enlargement by Doppler. ■ Fetal heart rate heard by Doppler at approximately 12 weeks' gestation. 10. Extremities: ■ Possible edema late in pregnancy. 11. Spine: ■ Lumbar spinal curve may be accentuated. 12. Pelvic area: ■ Vagina without significant discharge. ■ Cervix closed. ■ Uterus shows progressive growth. 13. Laboratory tests: ■ Physiologic anemia may occur (hematocrit). ■ Small degree of glycosuria may occur.

LEARNING OUTCOMES / CONCEPTS

10.6 Calculate the estimated date of birth using the common methods.

1. Nägele's rule:
   - Date of LMP minus 3 months plus 7 days.
   - Accurate only if woman has 28-day cycles.
2. Physical examination:
   - Uterine size.
3. Fundal height:
   - Measurement should be made from the top of the symphysis pubis to the top of the uterine fundus.
4. Ultrasound:
   - BPD.

10.7 Describe the essential measurements that can be determined by clinical pelvimetry.

1. These measurements are estimates to determine probable adequacy of the pelvis to allow a vaginal birth:
   - Pelvic inlet:
     - Diagonal conjugate (should be at least 11.5 cm).
     - Obstetric conjugate (should be 10 cm or more).
   - Pelvic outlet:
     - Anteroposterior diameter (should be 9.5 to 11.5 cm).
     - Transverse diameter (should be 8 to 10 cm).

10.8 Consider the results of the major screening tests used during the prenatal period in the assessment of the prenatal client.

1. Screening tests are useful in identifying risk factors and potential complications.
   - Basic screening tests such as Pap smear, u/a, complete blood count, hemoglobin, Rubella titer, ABO and Rh typing, a hepatitis B screen, and tests for syphilis and gonorrhea.
   - Urine culture at 12–16 weeks
   - Other tests that may be indicated or are offered include drug screen, HIV testing, sickle cell screen, cystic fibrosis screen, screening for chromosomal anomolies, and neural tube defects.
   - 1-hr 50 g GTT at 24–28 weeks
   - Rectal and vaginal swabs for group B strep at 35 to 37 weeks

10.9 Assess the prenatal client for the danger signs of pregnancy.

1. The danger signs of pregnancy indicate that potential complications may be developing.
   - Ask client about the occurrence of any signs
   - Assess for danger signs at each visit

10.10 Relate the components of the subsequent prenatal history and assessment to the progress of pregnancy and the nursing care of the prenatal client.

1. At each visit the woman will be assessed for:
   - Vital signs.
   - Weight gain.
   - Edema.
   - Uterine size.
   - Fetal heartbeat.
   - Urinalysis.
   - Blood tests for alpha, fetoprotein, glucose.
   - Vaginal swab for group B streptococcus.
   - Expected psychologic stage of pregnancy.

CRITICAL THINKING IN ACTION

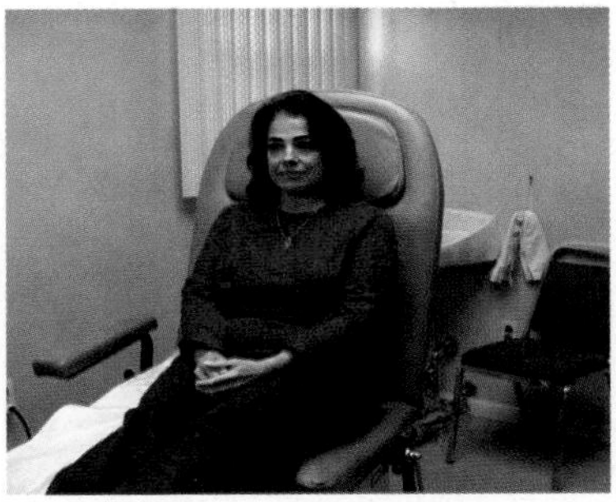

Wendy Stodard, age 40, G3, P0020 comes to the obstetrician's office where you are working for a prenatal visit. Wendy has experienced two spontaneous abortions followed by a D & C at 14 and 15 weeks' gestation during the previous year. She has a history of *Chlamydia trachomatis* infection 3 years ago, which was treated with azithromycin. She is at 10 weeks' gestation. Wendy tells you that she is afraid of losing this pregnancy as she did previously. She says that she has been experiencing some mild nausea, breast tenderness, and fatigue, which did not occur with her other pregnancies. You assist the obstetrician with an ultrasound. The gestational sac is clearly seen, fetal heartbeat is observed, and crown-to-rump measurements are consistent with gestational age of 10 weeks. The pelvic exam demonstrates a closed cervix, and positive Goodell's, Hegar's, and Chadwick's signs. You discuss with Wendy the signs of a healthy pregnancy.

1. What signs are reassuring with this pregnancy?
2. What symptoms should be reported to the obstetrician immediately?
3. What is the frequency of antepartal visits?

See MyNursingKit for possible responses.

REFERENCES

American College of Obstetricians and Gynecologists (ACOG). (2008). *Anemia in pregnancy* (ACOG Practice Bulletin No. 95). Washington, DC: Author.

American College of Obstetricians and Gynecologists. (2005a). *Racial and ethnic disparities in women's health* (ACOG Committee Opinion No. 317). Washington, DC: Author.

American College of Obstetricians and Gynecologists. (2005b). *Update on carrier screening for cystic fibrosis* (ACOG Committee Opinion No. 325). Washington, DC: Author.

American College of Obstetricians and Gynecologists. (2007). *Screening for fetal chromosomal abnormalities* (ACOG Practice Bulletin No. 77). Washington, DC: Author.

Cleveland Clinic. (2006). *Quad marker screen.* Retrieved December 31, 2007, from www.cchs.net/health/health-info/docs/0300/0386.asp?index=4698

Conde-Agudelo, A., Villar, J., & Lindheimer, M. (2008). Maternal infection and risk of preeclampsia: Systematic review and meta-analysis. *American Journal of Obstetrics & Gynecology, January,* 7–22.

Cunningham, F. G., Leveno, K. J., Bloom, S. L., Hauth, J. C., Rouse, D. J., & Spong, C. Y. (2010). *Williams obstetrics* (23rd ed.). New York: McGraw-Hill Medical.

Dashes, J., McIntire, D., & Twickler, D. 2009. Effect of maternal obesity on the ultrasound detection of anomalous fetuses. *Obstetrics and Gynecology.* 113: 1001–1007.

Nicolaides, K. H. (2005). First-trimester screening for chromosomal abnormalities. *Seminars in Perinatology, 29,* 190–194.

U.S. Preventive Services Task Force. (2004). Recommendation statement: Screening for asymptomatic bacteriuria. Retrieved December 31, 2007, from http://www.ahrq.gov

Varney, H., Kriebs, J. M., & Gegor, C. L. (2004). *Varney's midwifery* (4th ed.). Sudbury, MA: Jones and Bartlett.

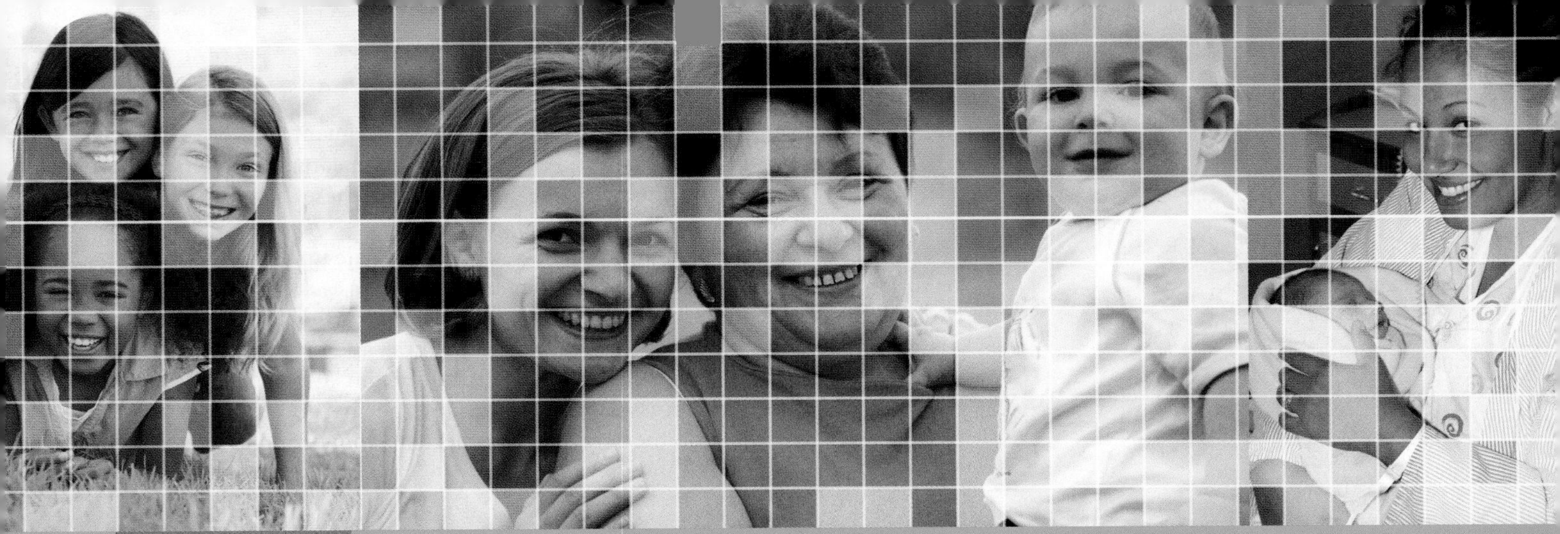

CHAPTER

11 The Expectant Family: Needs and Care

We have what I guess you would call a blended family. I have two college-age sons from my first marriage, and my wife has a 12-year-old boy. She is expecting our first child now. Because she is 38, she had an amniocentesis done and we know that this baby is a girl. How excited we all are! I don't think anything could have done more to unite us as a new family. Now if we can just agree on a name. —Ricardo, 46

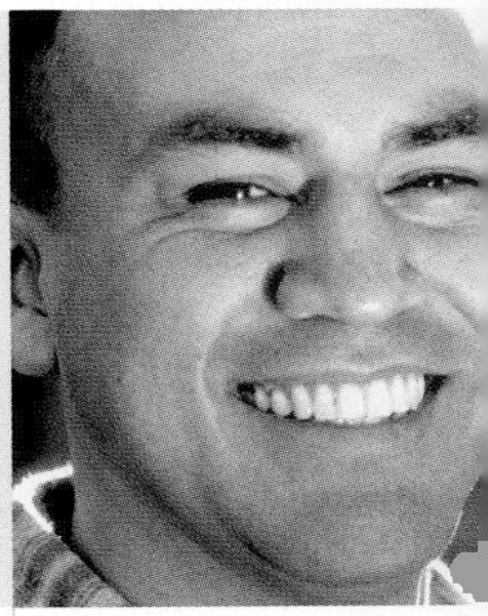

LEARNING OUTCOMES

11.1 Determine the most appropriate nursing care to help maintain the well-being of the expectant father and siblings during a family's pregnancy.

11.2 Recognize the causes of the common discomforts of pregnancy in each of the three trimesters.

11.3 Determine appropriate relief measures and interventions to alleviate the common discomforts of pregnancy.

11.4 Determine self-care measures that a pregnant woman can take to maintain and promote her well-being during pregnancy.

11.5 Address the concerns that an expectant couple might have about sexual activity.

11.6 Relate the medical risks and special concerns of the older expectant woman and her partner to the nursing management indicated in providing care for this population.

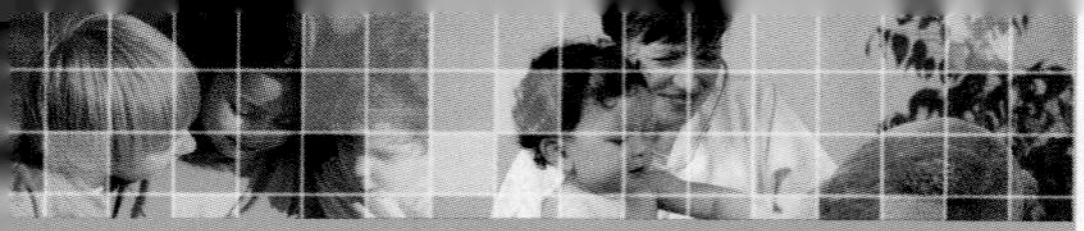

KEY TERMS

Fetal alcohol syndrome, 244
Fetal movement record, 236
Kegel exercises, 241
Leukorrhea, 231
Lightening, 235
Pelvic tilt, 240
Ptyalism, 233

From the moment a woman finds out she is pregnant, she faces a future marked by dramatic changes—changes in her appearance, in her relationships, and in her psychologic state. In coping with these changes, she and her loved ones need to make adjustments in their daily lives.

Nurses caring for pregnant women need an up-to-date understanding of pregnancy to be effective in implementing the nursing process as they plan and provide care. With this in mind, Chapter 9 provided a database for the nurse by presenting material related to the normal physical, social, cultural, and psychologic changes of pregnancy. Chapter 10 then used that database to begin discussing nursing care management by focusing on assessment. This chapter further addresses nursing care management as it relates to the needs of the expectant woman and her loved ones.

NURSING CARE DURING THE PRENATAL PERIOD

NURSING DIAGNOSIS DURING PREGNANCY

The nurse may see a pregnant woman only once every 3 to 4 weeks during the first several months of her pregnancy. Therefore, a written care plan or clinical path that incorporates the database, nursing diagnoses, and client goals is essential to ensure continuity of care.

The nurse can anticipate that, for many women with a low-risk pregnancy, certain nursing diagnoses will be made more frequently than others. The diagnoses will, of course, vary from woman to woman and according to the time in the pregnancy. After formulating an appropriate diagnosis, the nurse and woman establish related goals to guide the nursing plan and interventions.

PLANNING AND IMPLEMENTATION DURING PREGNANCY

Once nursing diagnoses have been identified, the next step is to establish priorities of nursing care. Sometimes priorities of care are based on the most immediate needs or concerns expressed by the woman. For example, during the first trimester, when she is experiencing nausea or is concerned about sexual intimacy with her partner, the woman is not likely to want to hear about labor and birth. At other times, priorities may develop from findings during a prenatal examination. For example, a woman who is showing signs of preeclampsia (a pregnancy complication discussed in Chapter 16 ∞) may feel physically well and find it hard to accept the nurse's emphasis on the need for frequent rest periods. It then becomes the responsibility of medical and nursing professionals to help the woman and her family to understand the significance of a problem and to plan interventions to deal with it.

Nursing Care in the Community

Prenatal care, especially for women with low-risk pregnancies, is community based, typically in a clinic or a private office. The nurse in a clinic or health maintenance organization may be the only source of continuity for the woman, who may see a different physician or certified nurse-midwife at each visit. The nurse can be extremely effective in working with the expectant family by answering questions; providing complete information about pregnancy, prenatal healthcare activities, and community resources; and supporting the healthcare activities of the woman and her family. Communities often have a wealth of services and educational opportunities available for pregnant women and their families, and the knowledgeable nurse can help expectant mothers to assess and access these services.

Throughout the prenatal period, the nurse shares information with the family, both verbally and through written materials. The nurse also provides anticipatory guidance to help the family plan for changes that will occur after childbirth. The nurse encourages the expectant couple to identify and discuss issues that could be sources of postpartum stress. Issues to be addressed beforehand may include the sharing of infant and household chores, help in the first few days after childbirth, options for babysitting to allow the mother (and couple) some free time, the mother's return to work after the baby's birth, and sibling rivalry. Couples resolve these issues in different ways, but postpartum adjustment tends to be easier for couples who address the issues than for couples who do not confront and resolve them.

Home care. Home care can be of benefit to any pregnant woman, but it is especially effective in removing barriers for women who have difficulty accessing health care. These barriers may include lack of locally available healthcare facilities, problems with transportation to the facility, or schedule conflicts with available appointment times because of employment hours or family responsibilities.

In-home nursing assessments vary according to the experience and preparation of the nurse and include current history, vital signs, weight, urine screen, physical activity, dietary intake, reflexes, tests of fetal well-being, and cervical examinations, if indicated. Once the assessments are completed, the nurse can determine the level of follow-up home care or telephone contact needed. See Chapter 25 for further discussion of home care of the childbearing family.

Currently, home care is most often used for women with prenatal complications that can be managed without hospitalization if effective nursing assessment and care are provided in the home.

CARE OF THE EXPECTANT FATHER AND SIBLINGS

The well-being of the pregnant woman is intertwined with the well-being of those to whom she is closest. Thus, the nurse also addresses the needs of the woman's family. Although the expectant father is often involved in the pregnancy, his presence cannot be assumed. If he is not part of the family structure, it is important to assess the woman's support system to determine which significant people in her life will play a major role during this childbearing experience.

Anticipatory guidance of the expectant father, if he is involved in the pregnancy, is a necessary part of any plan of care. He may need information about the anatomic, physiologic, and emotional changes that occur for the expectant mother and father during and after pregnancy; the couple's sexuality and sexual response; and the reactions that he is experiencing. He may wish to express his feelings about the sex of the child, his ability to parent, and other topics.

If it is culturally acceptable to the couple and personally acceptable to the expectant father, refer the couple to expectant parents' classes. These classes provide valuable information about pregnancy and childbirth, using a variety of teaching strategies such as discussion, films, demonstrations with educational models, and written handouts. Some classes even give the father the opportunity to get a "feel" for pregnancy by wearing a pregnancy simulator (Figure 11–1 ●). Such classes also offer the couple an opportunity to gain support from other couples.

The nurse assesses the father's intended degree of participation during labor and birth and his knowledge of what to expect. If the couple prefers that his participation be minimal or restricted, support their decision. With this type of consideration and collaboration, the father is less apt to develop feelings of alienation, helplessness, and guilt during the pregnancy. As the couple's relationship is strengthened and the father's self-esteem is raised, he is better able to provide physical and emotional support to his partner during labor and birth.

In the plan for prenatal care, the nurse also incorporates a discussion about the negative feelings older children may develop. Parents may be distressed to see an older child regress to "babyish" behavior or become aggressive toward the newborn. Parents who are unprepared for the older child's feelings of anger, jealousy, and rejection may respond inappropriately in their confusion and surprise. The nurse emphasizes that open communication between parents and children (or acting out feelings with a doll if the child is too young to verbalize) helps children master their feelings. Children may feel less neglected and more secure if they know that their parents are willing to help with their anger and aggressiveness.

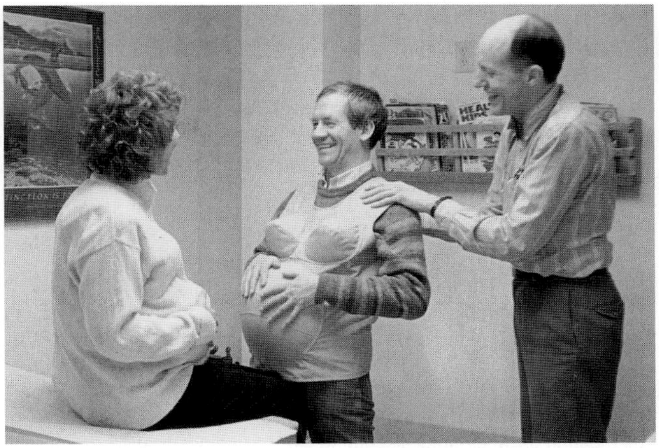

● **Figure 11–1** The Empathy Belly® is a pregnancy simulator that allows men and women to experience some of the symptoms of pregnancy. The "belly," which weighs 33 lb, produces symptoms such as shortness of breath, bladder pressure, shift in the center of gravity with resulting waddling gait, increased lordosis and backache, and fatigue. It also can simulate fetal kicking movements.

Used with permission from Birthways Childbirth Resource Center.

The nurse also addresses the couple's expectations of the grandparents and encourages the couple to explore ways of dealing with any conflicts that may arise over childrearing approaches. Couples resolve these issues in different ways. However, postpartum adjustment is easiest for couples who acknowledge potential problems and develop strategies to address them beforehand.

CULTURAL CONSIDERATIONS IN PREGNANCY

As discussed in Chapter 2, actions during pregnancy are often determined by cultural beliefs. Table 11–1 presents activities encouraged or forbidden by some specific cultures. The table is not meant to be all-inclusive, nor is it meant to imply that all members of a given culture hold these beliefs. Rather it offers a few examples of cultural activities that may be important to some women during the prenatal period.

In working with clients of other cultures, health professionals should be open to and respectful of other beliefs. Culturally competent nurses recognize that each childbearing family, shaped by culture and life experience, has expectations of both its members and the healthcare system during pregnancy and birth.

Language barriers often pose a challenge in providing effective prenatal nursing care. When possible, it is important to have an interpreter—family member, friend, or staff person—present at prenatal visits so that the nurse can provide basic information about

Table 11–1 Cultural Beliefs and Practices During Pregnancy

Here are a few examples of cultural beliefs and practices related to pregnancy. It is important not to make assumptions about a client's beliefs, because cultural norms vary greatly within a culture and from generation to generation. The nurse should observe the client carefully and take the time to ask questions. Clients will benefit greatly from the nurse's increased awareness of their cultural beliefs and practices.

Belief or Practice	Nursing Consideration
Home Remedies	
Pregnant women of Native American background may use herbal remedies. An example is the dandelion, which contains a milky juice in its stem believed to increase breast milk flow in mothers who choose to breastfeed (Spector, 2009). Clients of Chinese descent may drink ginseng tea for faintness after childbirth or as a sedative when mixed with bamboo leaves. Some people of African heritage may use self-medication for pregnancy discomforts—for example, laxatives to prevent or treat constipation (Spector, 2009).	Find out what medications and home remedies your client is using and counsel your client regarding overall effects. It is common for individuals to avoid telling healthcare workers about home remedies; the client may feel her use of home remedies will be judged unfavorably. Phrase your questions in a sensitive, accepting way.
Nutrition	
Some women of Italian background may believe that it is necessary to satisfy desires for certain foods in order to prevent congenital anomalies. Also, they may believe that they must eat food that they smell, or else the fetus will move "inside," which will result in a miscarriage. Pregnant women of African descent may continue the tradition of eating clay, dirt, or starch, which they believe will benefit the mother and fetus (Spector, 2009).	Discuss the woman's beliefs and practices in regard to nutrition during pregnancy. Obtain a diet history from her. Discuss the importance of a well-balanced diet during pregnancy, with consideration of the client's cultural beliefs and practices. In some cases, you might want to suggest remedies that may be more effective—for example, eating high-fiber foods to reduce constipation. If the home remedy is not harmful, there is no reason to ask a client to discontinue this practice.
Alternative Healthcare Providers	
Pregnant women of Mexican background may choose to seek out the care of a *partera* (midwife) for prenatal and intrapartal care. A *partera* speaks their language, shares a similar culture, and can help pregnant women give birth at home or in a birthing center instead of a hospital. Some people in Hispanic-American communities may use the *curandero,* the folk healer. The *curandero* frequently uses herbs, massage, and religious artifacts for treatment (Spector, 2009).	Discuss the variety of choices of healthcare providers available to the pregnant woman. Contrast the benefits and risks of different settings for prenatal care and birth. Provide reassurance that the goal of health care during pregnancy and birth is a healthy outcome for mother and baby, with respect for the specific cultural beliefs and practices of the client.
Exercise	
Pregnant women of Italian descent may fear changing their body position in certain ways because they believe doing so may cause the fetus to develop abnormally (Spector, 2009). Some people of European, African, and Mexican descent believe that reaching over the head during pregnancy can harm the baby.	Ask your client whether there are any activities she is afraid to do because of the pregnancy. Assure her that reaching over her head will not harm the baby and evaluate other activities related to their effect on the pregnancy.
Spirituality	
Navajo Indians are aware of the mind-soul connection and may try to follow certain practices to have a healthy pregnancy and birth. Practices could include focusing on peace and positive thoughts as well as certain types of prayers and ceremonies. A traditional healer may assist them (Purnell & Paulanka, 2005). Some people of European background may tend to pay more attention to spirituality in their life to alleviate fears and ensure a safe birth.	Encourage the use of support systems and spiritual aids that provide comfort for the mother.

pregnancy and prenatal care. The nurse should also give the woman opportunities to ask questions or express concerns. It is essential to have printed material available in the woman's language. (See "Nursing Care Plan: Language Barriers at First Prenatal Visit" on page 232.)

COMMON DISCOMFORTS OF PREGNANCY

The common discomforts of pregnancy result from physiologic and anatomic changes and are fairly specific to each of the three trimesters. Table 11–2 identifies the common discomforts of pregnancy, their possible causes, and self-care measures that often help relieve the discomfort.

FIRST TRIMESTER

Nausea and Vomiting

Nausea and vomiting of pregnancy (NVP) are early, common symptoms occurring in 60% to 80% of pregnant women (Krakow, 2008). These symptoms appear sometime after the first missed

Developing Cultural Competence

PREGNANT WOMEN OF AFRICAN AMERICAN HERITAGE

In caring for pregnant women of African American heritage, it is helpful to consider the following general points (Purnell & Paulanka, 2005):

- African American pregnant women may be guided by their extended family into common practices such as geophagia, the ingestion of dirt or clay, which is believed to reduce mineral deficiencies. This practice has implications for the focus of teaching a nurse offers.
- Many African American families are matriarchal. Women are respected and heeded in decision making and often stress good behavior and firm parenting with their children, especially to keep them safe in dangerous situations.
- Three-generation extended families are common, and the grandmother is often highly respected for her wisdom. She may play a critical role in the care of the children.
- Certain taboos may exist, such as the belief in the necessity to avoid taking pictures during pregnancy to prevent stillbirths. Some women of African American descent may also believe that the purchase of infant clothing or supplies can result in a stillbirth. Thus they may appear to be unprepared for the arrival of the baby.

Table 11–2 Self-Care Measures for Common Discomforts of Pregnancy

Discomfort	Influencing Factors	Self-Care Measures
	First Trimester	
Nausea and vomiting	Increased levels of human chorionic gonadotropin Changes in carbohydrate metabolism Emotional factors Fatigue	Avoid odors or causative factors. Eat dry crackers or toast before arising in morning. Have small but frequent meals. Avoid greasy or highly seasoned foods. Take dry meals with fluids between meals. Drink carbonated beverages.
Urinary frequency	Pressure of uterus on bladder in both first and third trimesters	Void when urge is felt. Increase fluid intake during the day. Decrease fluid intake only in the evening to decrease nocturia.
Fatigue	Specific causative factors unknown May be aggravated by nocturia due to urinary frequency	Plan time for a nap or rest period daily. Go to bed earlier. Seek family support and assistance with responsibilities so that more time is available to rest.
Breast tenderness	Increased levels of estrogen and progesterone	Wear well-fitting, supportive bra.
Increased vaginal discharge	Hyperplasia of vaginal mucosa and increased production of mucus by the endocervical glands due to the increase in estrogen levels	Promote cleanliness by daily bathing. Avoid douching, nylon underpants, and pantyhose; cotton underpants are more absorbent; powder can be used to maintain dryness if not allowed to cake.
Nasal stuffiness and nosebleed (epistaxis)	Elevated estrogen levels	May be unresponsive, but cool air vaporizer may help; avoid use of nasal sprays and decongestants.
Ptyalism (excessive, often bitter salivation)	Specific causative factors unknown	Use astringent mouthwashes, chew gum, or suck hard candy.
	Second and Third Trimesters	
Heartburn (pyrosis)	Increased production of progesterone, decreasing gastrointestinal motility and increasing relaxation of cardiac sphincter, displacement of stomach by enlarging uterus, thus regurgitation of acidic gastric contents into the esophagus	Eat small and more frequent meals. Use low-sodium antacids. Avoid overeating, fatty and fried foods, lying down after eating, and sodium bicarbonate.

(continued)

Table 11–2 Self-Care Measures for Common Discomforts of Pregnancy—continued

Discomfort	Influencing Factors	Self-Care Measures
Ankle edema	Prolonged standing or sitting Increased levels of sodium due to hormonal influences Circulatory congestion of lower extremities Increased capillary permeability Varicose veins	Practice frequent dorsiflexion of feet when prolonged sitting or standing is necessary. Elevate legs when sitting or resting. Avoid tight garters or restrictive bands around legs.
Varicose veins	Venous congestion in the lower veins that increases with pregnancy Hereditary factors (weakening of walls of veins, faulty valves) Increased age and weight gain	Elevate legs frequently. Wear supportive hose. Avoid crossing legs at the knees, standing for long periods, garters, and hosiery with constrictive bands.
Hemorrhoids	Constipation (see following discussion) Increased pressure from gravid uterus on hemorrhoidal veins	Avoid constipation. Apply ice packs, topical ointments, anesthetic agents, warm soaks, or sitz baths; gently reinsert into rectum as necessary.
Constipation	Increased levels of progesterone, which cause general bowel sluggishness Pressure of enlarging uterus on intestine Iron supplements Diet, lack of exercise, and decreased fluids	Increase fluid intake, fiber in the diet, and exercise. Develop regular bowel habits. Use stool softeners as recommended by physician.
Backache	Increased curvature of the lumbosacral vertebrae as the uterus enlarges Increased levels of hormones, which cause softening of cartilage in body joints Fatigue Poor body mechanics	Use proper body mechanics. Practice the pelvic-tilt exercise. Avoid uncomfortable working heights, high-heeled shoes, lifting heavy loads, and fatigue.
Leg cramps	Imbalance of calcium/phosphorus ratio Increased pressure of uterus on nerves Fatigue Poor circulation to lower extremities Pointing the toes	Practice dorsiflexion of feet to stretch affected muscle. Evaluate diet. Apply heat to affected muscles. Arise slowly from resting position.
Faintness	Postural hypotension Sudden change of position causing venous pooling in dependent veins Standing for long periods in warm area Anemia	Avoid prolonged standing in warm or stuffy environments. Evaluate hematocrit and hemoglobin.
Dyspnea	Decreased vital capacity from pressure of enlarging uterus on the diaphragm	Use proper posture when sitting and standing. Sleep propped up with pillows for relief if problem occurs at night.
Flatulence	Decreased gastrointestinal motility leading to delayed emptying time Pressure of growing uterus on large intestine Air swallowing	Avoid gas-forming foods. Chew food thoroughly. Get regular daily exercise. Maintain normal bowel habits.
Carpal tunnel syndrome	Compression of median nerve in carpal tunnel of wrist Aggravated by repetitive hand movements.	Avoid aggravating hand movements. Use splint as prescribed. Elevate affected arm.

Nursing Practice

At each prenatal visit, focus your teaching on changes or possible discomforts the woman might encounter during the coming month and the next trimester. If the pregnancy is progressing normally, spend a few minutes describing her baby at this stage of development.

menstrual period and usually cease by the fourth missed menstrual period. Some women develop an aversion to specific foods, many experience nausea when they get up in the morning, and others experience nausea throughout the day or in the evening.

The exact cause of NVP is unknown, but it is thought to be multifactorial. An elevated human chorionic gonadotropin (hCG) level is believed to be a major factor, but changes in carbohydrate metabolism, fatigue, and emotional factors may also play a role.

In addition to common self-care measures (see "Complementary Care: Ginger for Morning Sickness") and the use of acupressure wristbands (Figure 11–2 ●), some women find pyridoxine (vitamin B_6) or pyridoxine plus doxylamine (Unisom), an over-the-counter antihistamine, helpful in reducing symptoms. Antihistamine H_1 receptor blockers, benzamines, and phenothiazines are considered safe and effective for treating refractory cases. In severe cases, methylprednisolone, a steroid, may be used, but as a last resort, because it poses a potential risk to the fetus (ACOG, 2004).

The nurse should advise a woman to contact her healthcare provider if she vomits more than once a day or shows signs of dehydration such as dry mouth and concentrated urine. In such cases the physician or certified nurse-midwife might order an antiemetic. However, antiemetics should be avoided if possible during this time because of possible harmful effects on embryo development.

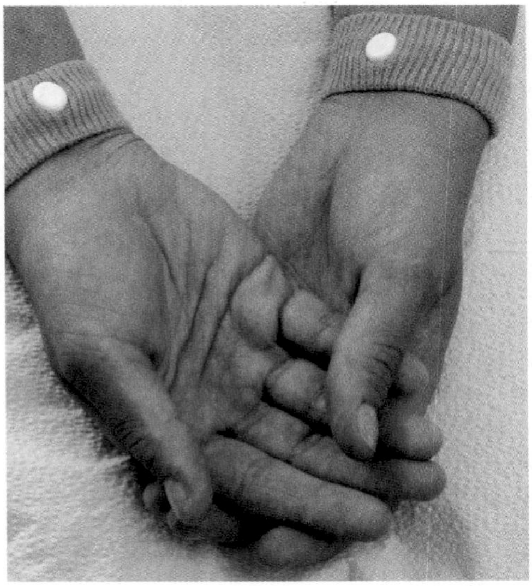

● **Figure 11–2** Morning sickness relief. Acupressure wristbands are sometimes used to help relieve nausea during early pregnancy.

Complementary Care

GINGER FOR MORNING SICKNESS

Ginger, long used in traditional Chinese medicine for a variety of maladies ranging from gastrointestinal problems to headaches, is becoming increasingly popular for the treatment of NVP, and its safety has been demonstrated in clinical trials (White, 2007). Ginger is available in a variety of forms, including the fresh root, capsules, tea, candy, cookies, crystals, inhaled powdered ginger, and sugared ginger (Lie, 2004). In the first trimester, the daily dosage should not exceed 2 g of dried ginger or 1 g of ginger syrup (Born & Barron, 2005).

Urinary Frequency

Urinary frequency, a common discomfort of pregnancy, occurs early in pregnancy and again during the third trimester because the enlarging uterus puts pressure on the bladder. Although frequency is considered normal during the first and third trimesters, advise the woman to tell her healthcare provider about signs of bladder infection such as pain, burning with voiding, or blood in the urine. Fluid intake should never be decreased to prevent frequency. The woman needs to maintain an adequate fluid intake—at least 2000 mL (eight to ten 8-oz glasses) per day. Also, encourage her to empty her bladder frequently (about every 2 hours while awake).

Fatigue

Marked fatigue is so common in early pregnancy that it is considered a presumptive sign of pregnancy. It is aggravated if the woman cannot sleep through the night because of urinary frequency. Typically it resolves after the end of the first trimester.

Breast Tenderness

Sensitivity of the breasts occurs early and continues throughout the pregnancy. Increased levels of estrogen and progesterone contribute to soreness and tingling of the breasts and increased sensitivity of the nipples.

Increased Vaginal Discharge

Increased whitish vaginal discharge, called **leukorrhea**, is common in pregnancy. It occurs as a result of hyperplasia of the vaginal mucosa and increased mucus production by the endocervical glands. The increased acidity of the secretions encourages the growth of *Candida albicans,* so the woman is more susceptible to monilial vaginitis.

Nasal Stuffiness and Epistaxis

Once pregnancy has progressed somewhat, elevated estrogen levels may produce edema of the nasal mucosa, which results in nasal stuffiness, nasal discharge, and obstruction. *Epistaxis* (nosebleeds) may also result. Cool air vaporizers and normal saline nasal sprays may help, but the problem is often unresponsive to treatment. Women experiencing these problems find it difficult to sleep and may resort to using medicated nasal sprays

Nursing Care Plan

LANGUAGE BARRIERS AT FIRST PRENATAL VISIT

INTERVENTION	RATIONALE	EXPECTED OUTCOME
1. Nursing Diagnosis: Ineffective Health Maintenance related to alteration in verbal and written communication skills		
NIC Intervention: Effective communication: Developing and providing prenatal instruction for a non-English-speaking client.		**NOC Outcome:** Effective communication occurs. The client will gain an understanding of basic prenatal information as evidenced by using hand gestures, by pointing to pictures on posters and translated phrases on handouts, and through an interpreter, if one is available.
Goal: Client will demonstrate understanding of health information received during prenatal visits.		
■ If no interpreter is available, refer to posters with pictures to explain routine care and procedures during the prenatal examination.	■ Posters put words into verbal images and are helpful in communicating information.	
■ Provide handouts and brochures about prenatal care in the woman's native language.	■ Translated handouts provide information that the client can refer to at home. This reinforces information discussed during the visit and helps the family understand what the woman will experience during the pregnancy and at each visit.	
■ Use teaching models to demonstrate procedures. Teaching models may include plastic pelvis, knitted uterus, fetal model, breast model, birth control devices, ultrasound equipment, and so forth.	■ Visual aids help to communicate information during the examination.	
■ Schedule an interpreter for subsequent prenatal visits.	■ If a family member cannot translate the health information to the client, an independent translator is essential to ensure that information is accurately provided. When an interpreter is used (especially a family member), the nurse should be sure that the interpreter is translating information received from the woman and not simply answering the questions for her.	
■ Refer the woman to prenatal classes taught in her own language, if available.	■ Prenatal classes taught in the woman's language enable her to receive health information that is easily understood, which will provide a better understanding of what she should expect during pregnancy, birth, and postpartum. Prenatal classes may also provide a social outlet for clients.	
■ Involve other members of the healthcare team in planning and providing care.	■ Cultures vary in language, nonverbal expression, dietary habits, use of time, spatial expectations, and so forth. Use of medication and blood products may also be influenced by cultural beliefs. Social workers who are familiar with the client's cultural beliefs, for example, may help the client adjust to different healthcare practices while providing suggestions to ensure prenatal care that is more in line with the woman's cultural beliefs. Dietitians may help the woman plan meals that are aligned with her cultural practices while meeting the nutritional needs of pregnancy.	

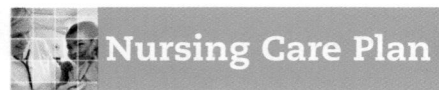

and decongestants. Such interventions may provide initial relief but can actually increase nasal stuffiness over time. Pregnant women should avoid using any medications, if possible.

Ptyalism

Ptyalism is a rare discomfort of pregnancy in which excessive, often bitter saliva is produced. The cause is unknown, and effective treatments are limited.

SECOND AND THIRD TRIMESTERS

The discomforts discussed in this section usually do not appear until the third trimester in primigravidas but may occur earlier with each succeeding pregnancy.

Heartburn (Pyrosis)

Heartburn is the regurgitation of acidic gastric contents into the esophagus. It creates a burning sensation in the esophagus and sometimes leaves a bad taste in the mouth. Heartburn during pregnancy appears to be primarily a result of the displacement of the stomach by the enlarging uterus. The increased production of progesterone in pregnancy, decreased gastrointestinal motility, and relaxation of the cardiac (esophageal) sphincter also contribute to heartburn.

Liquid forms of low-sodium antacids are often most effective in providing relief. However, many women prefer chewable over-the-counter antacid tablets. The nurse should advise women that antacids containing aluminum may cause constipation, and antacids containing magnesium can cause diarrhea. The nurse should also let women know that they should avoid sodium bicarbonate (baking soda) and Alka-Seltzer because they may lead to electrolyte imbalance.

If maternal heartburn is severe, not relieved by antacids, and accompanied by gastrointestinal reflux, an antisecretory agent (H_2 blocker) such as ranitidine (Zantac), cimetidine (Tagamet), or omeprazole (Losec) may be helpful. To date they have not been linked with an excessive risk of birth defects.

Ankle Edema

Most women experience ankle edema in the last part of pregnancy because of the increasing difficulty of venous return from the lower extremities. Prolonged standing or sitting and warm weather increase the edema. It is also associated with varicose veins. Ankle edema becomes a concern only when accompanied by hypertension or proteinuria or when the edema is not postural in origin.

Varicose Veins

Varicose veins are a result of weakening of the walls of veins or faulty functioning of the valves. Poor circulation in the lower extremities predisposes people to varicose veins in the legs and thighs, as does prolonged standing or sitting. The pregnant uterus puts pressure on the pelvic veins, preventing good venous return, so it may aggravate existing problems or contribute to obvious changes in the veins of the legs (Figure 11–3 ●).

Surgical correction of varicose veins is not generally recommended during pregnancy. The nurse should advise the woman that treatment may be needed after she gives birth because the problem will be aggravated by a succeeding pregnancy.

● **Figure 11–3** Relief from varicose veins. Swelling and discomfort from varicosities can be decreased by lying down with the legs and one hip elevated (to avoid compression of the vena cava).

Although less common, varicosities in the vulva and perineum may also develop. They produce aching and a sense of heaviness. Wearing one of the foam rubber commercial products that is placed across the perineum and held in place by a sanitary pad type belt can provide support for vulvar varicosities (Cunningham et al., 2010). It is important that the pelvic area be elevated to promote venous drainage into the trunk of the body. The woman may best relieve uterine pressure on the pelvic veins by resting on her side. Blocks may also be placed under the foot of her bed to elevate it slightly.

Flatulence

Flatulence results from decreased gastrointestinal motility, leading to delayed emptying, and from pressure on the large intestine by the growing uterus. Air swallowing may also contribute to the problem.

Hemorrhoids

Hemorrhoids are varicosities of the veins in the lower rectum and the anus. During pregnancy the gravid uterus presses on the veins and interferes with venous circulation. In addition, the straining that accompanies constipation is frequently a contributing cause of hemorrhoids.

Some women may not be bothered by hemorrhoids until the second stage of labor, when the hemorrhoids appear as they push. These hemorrhoids usually become asymptomatic a few days after childbirth. Symptoms of hemorrhoids include itching, swelling, pain, and bleeding. Women who have had hemorrhoids before pregnancy will probably experience difficulties with them during pregnancy.

Some women find relief by gently reinserting the hemorrhoid. The woman lies on her side, places some lubricant on her finger, and presses against the hemorrhoids, pushing them inside. She holds them in place for 1 to 2 minutes and then gently withdraws her finger. The anal sphincter should then hold them inside the

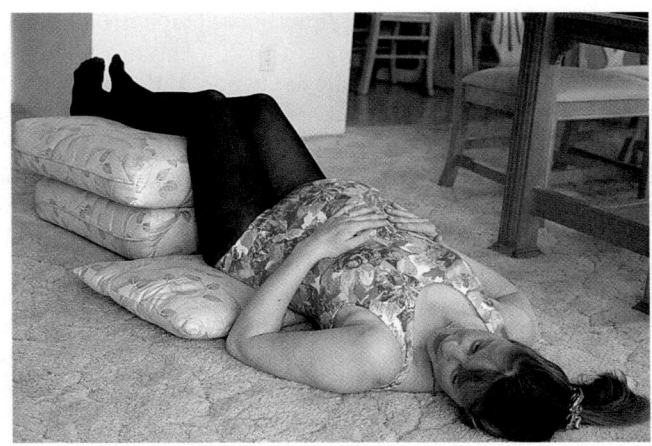

rectum. The woman will find it especially helpful if she can maintain a side-lying (Sims) position for a time, so this method is best done before bed or prior to a daily rest period.

The woman should contact her healthcare provider if the hemorrhoids become hardened and noticeably tender to touch. Rectal bleeding that is more than spotting following defecation should also be reported.

Constipation

Conditions that predispose the pregnant woman to constipation include general bowel sluggishness caused by increased progesterone and steroid metabolism; displacement of the intestines, which increases with growth of the fetus; and the oral iron supplements most pregnant women need. In severe or preexisting cases of constipation, the woman may need stool softeners, mild laxatives, or suppositories as recommended by her healthcare provider.

Backache

Over 50% of pregnant women experience backache (Johnson, Gregory, & Niebyl, 2007), due primarily to exaggeration of the lumbosacral curve that occurs as the uterus enlarges and becomes heavier. Maintaining good posture and using proper body mechanics throughout pregnancy can help prevent backache. Advise the pregnant woman to avoid bending over at the waist to pick up objects and to bend from the knees instead (Figure 11–4 ●). She should place her feet 12 to 18 inches apart to maintain body balance. If the woman uses work surfaces that require her to bend, advise her to adjust the height of the surfaces. (See "Complementary Care: Preventing and Treating Backache in Pregnancy for further information.)

Leg Cramps

Leg cramps are painful muscle spasms in the gastrocnemius muscles. They occur most often after the woman has gone to bed at night but may occur at other times. Extension of the foot can often cause leg cramps. The nurse should warn the pregnant woman not to extend the foot during childbirth preparation exercises or during rest periods. The exact cause of leg cramps is not known, but pressure of the enlarged uterus on pelvic nerves or blood vessels leading to the legs may be a contributing factor (Varney, Kriebs, & Gegor, 2004), especially during the third trimester.

Stretching provides immediate relief of the muscle spasm. With the woman lying on her back, another person presses the woman's knee down to straighten her leg while pushing her foot toward her leg. The woman may also stand and put her foot flat

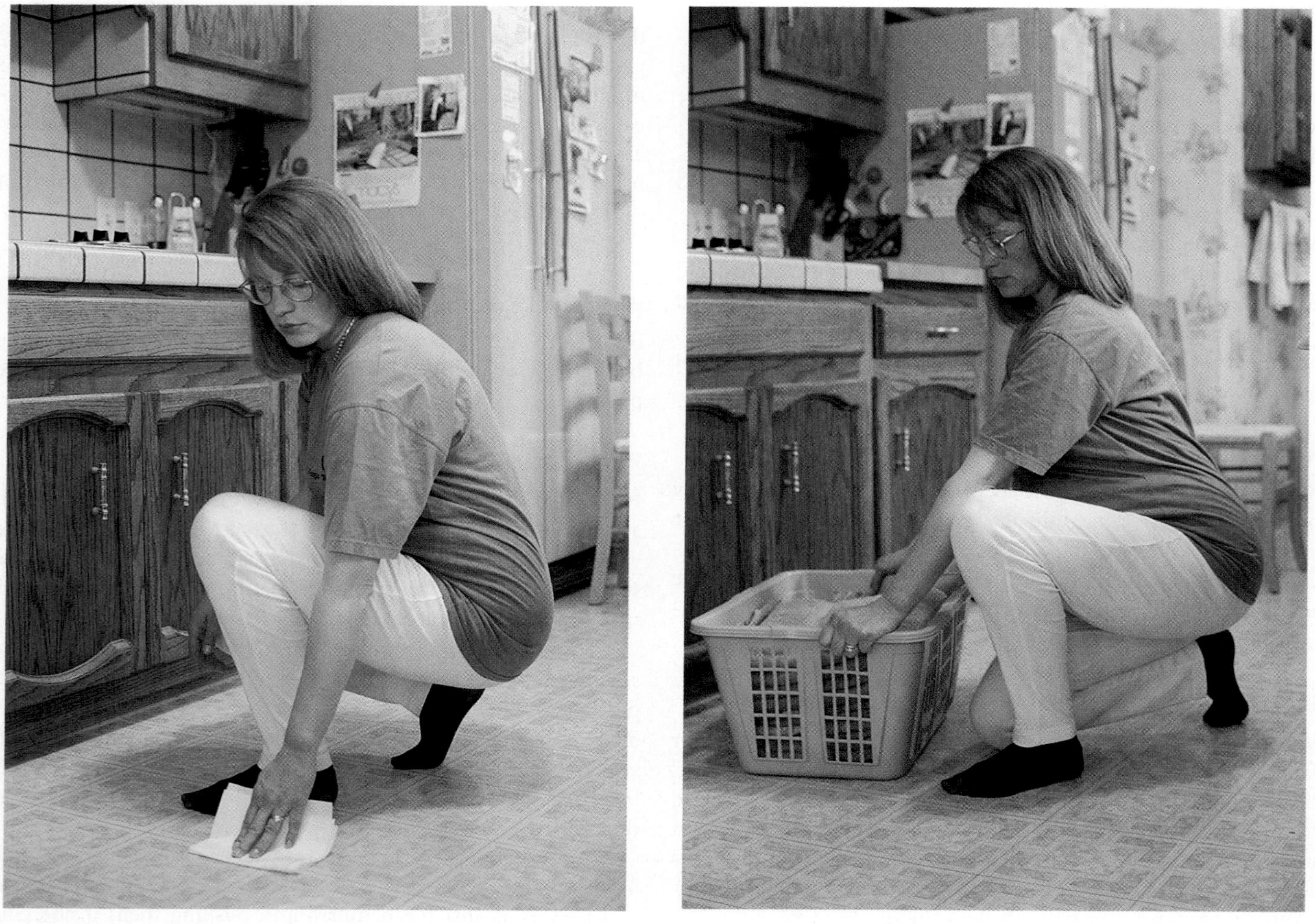

● **Figure 11–4** Body mechanics in pregnancy. When picking up objects from floor level or lifting objects, the pregnant woman must use proper body mechanics.

Complementary Care

PREVENTING AND TREATING BACK PAIN IN PREGNANCY

Exercises to strengthen the lower back, including pelvic tilt exercises, reduce pain intensity. Water aerobics reduce pain severity and also decrease the number of missed work days due to pain. Acupuncture reduces pain intensity and provides relief from evening pain, and so helps with sleep. Women who are considering acupuncture can be encouraged to pursue this option, as it has been shown to provide relief from pain, particularly in the evening. Supporting the back with standard bed pillows does not demonstrate any therapeutic effect. Helping mothers use these interventions may reduce their reliance on pharmacologic pain relievers (Granath, Hellgren, & Gunnarsson, 2006; Pennick & Young, 2007).

on the floor. Massage and warm packs can alleviate the discomfort of leg cramps (Figure 11–5 ●). A diet that includes daily portions of both calcium and phosphorus may help prevent leg cramps.

Faintness

Many pregnant women occasionally feel faint, especially in warm, crowded areas. Faintness is caused by a combination of changes in the blood volume and postural hypotension due to pooling of blood in the dependent veins. Sudden change of position or standing for prolonged periods can also cause this sensation, and the woman may faint.

If a woman begins to feel faint from prolonged standing or from being in a stuffy room, she should sit down and lower her head between her knees. If this procedure does not help, she should ask someone to help her to an area where she can lie down and get fresh air. The nurse should advise the woman that when getting up from a resting position, it is important to move slowly. Women whose jobs require standing in one place for long periods should march in place regularly to increase venous return from the legs.

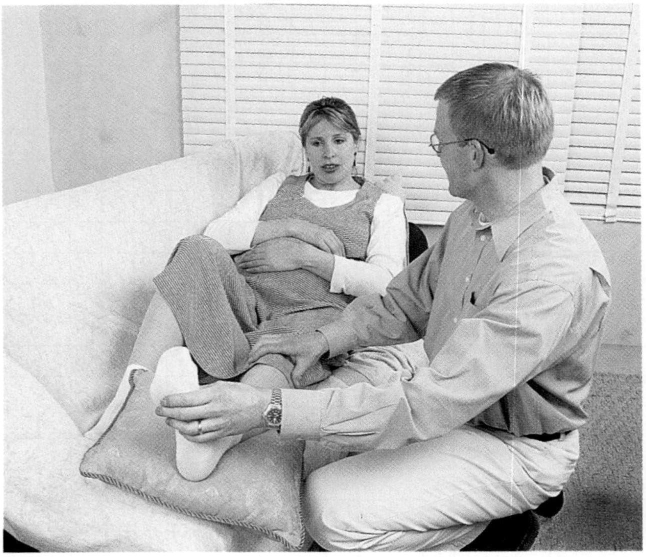

● **Figure 11–5** Leg cramp relief. The expectant father can help relieve the woman's painful leg cramps by flexing her foot and straightening her leg.

Shortness of Breath (Dyspnea)

Shortness of breath occurs as the uterus rises into the abdomen and causes pressure on the diaphragm. This problem worsens in the last trimester because the enlarged uterus presses directly on the diaphragm, decreasing vital capacity. The primigravida experiences considerable relief from shortness of breath in the last few weeks of pregnancy, when **lightening** occurs, and the fetus and uterus move down in the pelvis. Because the multigravida does not usually experience lightening until labor, she tends to feel short of breath throughout the latter part of her pregnancy.

Difficulty Sleeping

Many physical factors in late pregnancy may make sleeping difficult. The enlarged uterus may make it difficult to find a comfortable position for sleep, and an active fetus may aggravate the problem. Other discomforts of pregnancy such as urinary frequency, shortness of breath, and leg cramps may also make it hard to sleep.

Round Ligament Pain

As the uterus enlarges during pregnancy, the round ligaments stretch and hypertrophy as the uterus rises up in the abdomen, causing pain. The woman may feel concern when she first experiences round ligament pain, because it is often intense and causes a "grabbing" sensation in the lower abdomen and inguinal area. The nurse should warn the pregnant woman of this possible discomfort. Once it has been determined that the cause of the pain is not a medical complication such as appendicitis, the woman may find that applying a heating pad to the abdomen brings relief.

Carpal Tunnel Syndrome

Carpal tunnel syndrome, characterized by numbness and tingling of the hand near the thumb, occurs in about 25% to 50% of pregnant women (Johnson et al., 2007). It is caused by compression of the median nerve in the carpal tunnel of the wrist. The syndrome is aggravated by repetitive hand movements such as typing and may disappear following childbirth. Treatment usually involves splinting and avoiding aggravating movements, but surgery may be needed in severe cases if more conservative approaches are not effective.

PROMOTION OF SELF-CARE DURING PREGNANCY

FETAL ACTIVITY MONITORING

Many healthcare providers encourage pregnant women to monitor their unborn child's well-being by regularly assessing fetal activity beginning at 28 weeks' gestation. Vigorous activity generally provides reassurance of fetal well-being, but a marked decrease in activity or cessation of movement may indicate a problem that needs immediate evaluation. Fetal activity is affected by fetal sleep, sound, time of day, blood glucose levels, cigarette smoking, and some illicit drugs such as crack and cocaine. At times a healthy fetus may be minimally active or inactive. A variety of methods for tracking fetal activity have been developed. They focus on having the woman keep a **fetal movement record (FMR)** using a technique such as the Cardiff Count-to-Ten method. An FMR is noninvasive and lets the pregnant woman monitor and record movements easily and without expense. (See "Teaching Highlights: Assessing Fetal Activity".)

Teaching Highlights

ASSESSING FETAL ACTIVITY

- Explain that fetal movements are first felt around 18 weeks' gestation. From that time, the fetal movements get stronger and easier to detect. A slowing or stopping of fetal movement may be an indication that the fetus needs some attention and evaluation.
- Explain the procedure for the Cardiff Count-to-Ten method or for the daily fetal movement record. For both methods, advise the woman to:
  - Keep a daily record of fetal movement, beginning at about 27 weeks' gestation.
  - Try to begin counting at about the same time each day, about 1 hour after a meal if possible.
  - Lie quietly in a side-lying position.
- Using the Cardiff card, have the woman place an X for each fetal movement until she has recorded 10. Movement varies considerably, but most women feel fetal movement at least 10 times in 3 hours (see Figure 11–6 ●).

Sample Cardiff Count-to-Ten scoring card

Month: _________ Week of gestation at beginning of month: _________

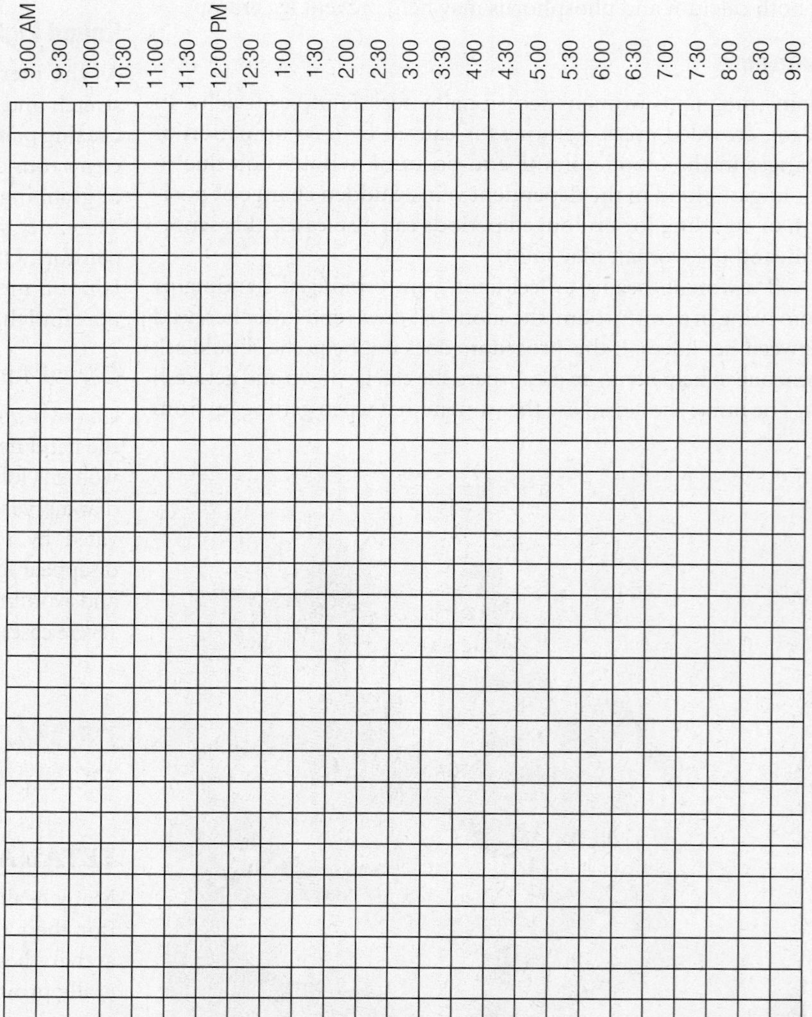

● **Figure 11–6** Fetal movement assessment method: the Cardiff Count-to-Ten scoring card (adaptation).

Teaching Highlights

ASSESSING FETAL ACTIVITY—continued

- Using the daily fetal movement record, have the woman count three times a day for 20 to 30 minutes each session. If there are fewer than 3 movements in a session, have the woman count for 1 hour or more.
- Explain when to contact the care provider:
  - If there are fewer than 10 movements in 3 hours
  - If overall the fetus's movements are slowing, and it takes much longer each day to note 10 movements
  - If there are no movements in the morning
  - If there are fewer than 3 movements in 8 hours
- Describe procedures and demonstrate how to assess fetal movement. Sit beside the woman and show her how to place her hand on the fundus to feel fetal movement.
- Provide a written teaching sheet for the woman's use at home.
- Demonstrate how to record fetal movements on the Cardiff Count-to-Ten scoring card or on the daily fetal movement record.
- Watch the woman fill out the record as examples are provided. Encourage her to complete the record each day and bring it with her to each prenatal visit. Assure her that the record will be discussed at each prenatal visit, and questions may be addressed at that time if desired.
- Provide the woman with a name and phone number in case she has further questions.
- Evaluate learning by having the woman explain the method and by asking the woman to fill the card in using a fictitious situation. At each prenatal visit, the expectant mother's record is reviewed. This provides another opportunity for evaluation of learning and for questions and clarification.

BREAST CARE

Whether the pregnant woman plans to formula-feed or breastfeed her infant, support of the breasts is important to promote comfort, retain breast shape, and prevent back strain, particularly if the breasts become large and pendulous. The sensitivity of the breasts in pregnancy is often relieved by good support.

A well-fitting, supportive brassiere has the following qualities:

- The straps are wide and do not stretch (elastic straps soon lose their tautness with the weight of the breasts and frequent washing).
- The cups hold all breast tissue comfortably.
- The brassiere has tucks or other devices that allow it to expand and accommodate the enlarging chest circumference.
- The brassiere supports the nipple line approximately midway between the elbow and shoulder but is not pulled up in the back by the weight of the breasts.

Cleanliness of the breasts is important, especially as the woman begins producing colostrum. Colostrum that crusts on the nipples can be removed with warm water. The nurse should advise the woman planning to breastfeed not to use soap on her nipples because of its drying effect.

Some women have flat or inverted nipples. True nipple inversion, which is rare, is usually diagnosed during the initial prenatal assessment. Breast shields designed to correct inverted nipples are effective for some women (Figure 11–7 ●) but others gain no benefit from them. For further discussion of inverted nipples, see Chapter 30 ∞.

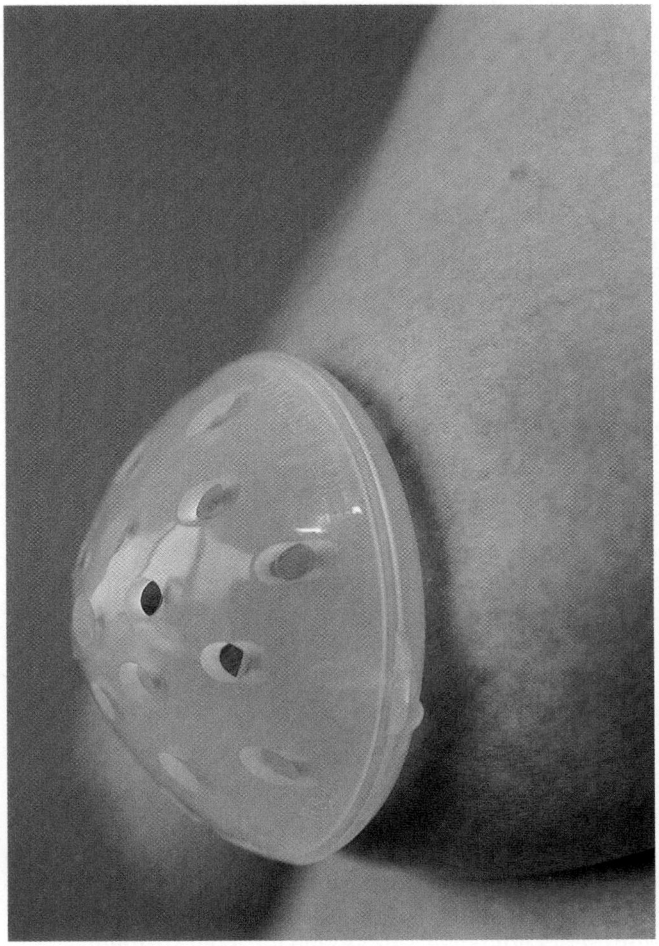

● **Figure 11–7** Help for inverted nipples. This breast shield is designed to increase the protractility of inverted nipples. Worn the last 3 to 4 months of pregnancy, it exerts gentle pulling pressure at the edge of the areola, gradually forcing the nipple through the center of the shield. It may be used after childbirth if still necessary.

CLOTHING

Traditionally maternity clothes have been constructed with fuller lines to allow for the increase in abdominal size that occurs during pregnancy. However, in recent years maternity clothing has changed and now also includes more clothes that are fitted with little attempt to hide the pregnant abdomen. Maternity clothing can be expensive and is worn for a relatively short time, so women can economize by sharing clothes with friends, sewing their own garments, or buying used maternity clothes.

High-heeled shoes tend to aggravate back discomfort by increasing the curvature of the lower back. Women who experience backache or have problems with balance do best to avoid them. Shoes should fit properly and feel comfortable.

BATHING

Hygiene is important because perspiration and mucoid vaginal discharge increase during pregnancy. Keep in mind, however, that cultural norms often influence bathing and cleansing practices. A pregnant woman may choose to cleanse only some portions of her body regularly or may elect to take showers or tub baths. Advise women to be careful in the tub because balance becomes a problem in late pregnancy. Rubber mats and hand grips are important safety devices. Vasodilation due to warm water may cause the woman to feel faint when she gets out of the tub, so she may need assistance, especially during the last trimester.

EMPLOYMENT

In general, women with low-risk pregnancies can continue working until the start of labor (American Academy of Pediatrics [AAP] & ACOG, 2008). Although pregnant women who are employed in jobs that require prolonged standing (more than 5 hours) do have a higher incidence of preterm births, this has no effect on fetal growth (Saade, 2007).

Overfatigue, excessive physical strain, fetotoxic hazards in the environment, and medical or obstetric complications are the major deterrents to certain types of employment during pregnancy. In the second half of pregnancy, women whose occupations involve balance should make adjustments as needed.

Fetotoxic hazards are always a concern to the expectant couple. The pregnant woman (or the woman contemplating pregnancy) who works in industry should contact her company physician or nurse about possible hazards in her work environment and should do her own reading and research on environmental hazards as well. Her partner can also find out how hazards in his workplace might affect his sperm.

TRAVEL

Pregnant women without complications can travel as usual. Pregnant women should avoid travel if they have a history of bleeding or preeclampsia or if multiple births are anticipated.

Travel by automobile can be tiring, aggravating many of the discomforts of pregnancy. The pregnant woman needs frequent opportunities to get out of the car and walk. (A good pattern is to stop every 2 hours and walk around for about 10 minutes.) She should wear both lap and shoulder belts. The lap belt should fit snugly and be positioned under the abdomen and across the upper thighs; the shoulder strap should rest comfortably between the woman's breasts. Seat belts play an important role in preventing fetal and maternal injury and death (Cesario, 2007). Fetal death in car accidents is sometimes caused by placental separation (abruptio placentae) as a result of uterine distortion. Shoulder belts decrease the risk of traumatic flexion of the woman's body, making placental separation less likely.

As pregnancy progresses, long-distance trips are best taken by plane or train. Before flying the woman should check with her airline to see if they have any travel restrictions. To avoid the development of phlebitis or blood clots, pregnant women should drink plenty of fluid to avoid dehydration and hemoconcentration. They should also walk about the plane at regular intervals and change position frequently (Saade, 2007). Currently flying is considered safe up to 36 weeks' gestation in the absence of any complications. Remind near-term women who travel to think about the availability of medical care at the destination.

ACTIVITY AND REST

Exercise during pregnancy helps maintain maternal fitness and muscle tone, leads to improved self-image, promotes regular bowel function, increases energy, improves sleep, relieves tension, helps control weight gain, and is associated with improved postpartum recovery. A woman with an uncomplicated pregnancy can and should continue normal participation in exercise. The woman can check with her certified nurse-midwife or physician about strenuous sports such as skiing and horseback riding. The skilled sportswoman should not usually be discouraged from participating in these activities if her pregnancy is uncomplicated. However, pregnancy is not the appropriate time to learn a new or strenuous sport.

Certain conditions contraindicate exercise. These conditions include rupture of the membranes, preeclampsia, incompetent cervix or cerclage placement, persistent vaginal bleeding, risk factors for preterm labor or a history of preterm labor in the prior or current pregnancy, placenta previa after 26 weeks' gestation, and chronic medical conditions that might be negatively affected by vigorous exercise such as significant heart disease (ACOG, 2002).

The following guidelines are helpful in counseling pregnant women about exercise. Even mild to moderate exercise is beneficial during pregnancy. Regular exercise—at least 30 minutes of moderate exercise daily or at least most days—is preferred (Penney, 2008). After the first trimester, women should avoid exercising in the supine position. In most pregnant women, the supine position is associated with decreased cardiac output. Because uterine blood flow is reduced during exercise as blood is shunted from the visceral organs to the muscles, the remaining cardiac output is further decreased. Similarly, women should also avoid standing motionless for prolonged periods (Penney, 2008).

Because decreased oxygen is available for aerobic exercise during pregnancy, women should modify the intensity of their exercise based on their symptoms, should stop when they become fatigued, and should avoid exercising to the point of exhaustion. Non-weight-bearing exercises such as swimming and cycling are recommended because they decrease the risk of injury and provide fitness with comfort.

As pregnancy progresses and the center of gravity changes, especially in the third trimester, women should avoid exercises in which the loss of balance could pose a risk to mother or fetus.

Similarly, women should avoid any type of exercise that might result in even mild abdominal trauma.

A normal pregnancy requires an additional 300 kcal per day. Women who exercise regularly during pregnancy should be careful to ensure that their diet is adequate. They should also avoid exercising in a fasting state (Lewis, Avery, Jennings, et al., 2008).

To avoid overheating, especially during the first trimester, pregnant women who exercise should wear clothing that is comfortable and loose, drink plenty of fluids, and avoid the prolonged overheating that can come from vigorous exercise in hot, humid weather. Hyperthermia may have teratogenic effects on the fetus (Berk, 2004). For the same reason, pregnant women are advised to avoid hot tubs and saunas.

Women should avoid reaching their maximum physical effort during pregnancy. If a pregnant, exercising woman is unable to maintain a conversation, then the exercise effort is too high (Saade, 2007).

The woman should wear a supportive bra and appropriate shoes when exercising. She should also warm up and stretch to help prepare the joints for activity and cool down with a period of mild activity to help restore circulation and avoid pooling of blood. A moderate, rhythmic exercise routine involving large muscle groups such as swimming, cycling, or brisk walking is best. Jogging or running is acceptable for women already conditioned to these activities as long as they avoid exercising at maximum effort and overheating.

When exercising, pregnant women should be alert for warning signs such as pain of any kind, decreased or absent fetal movement, difficulty walking, dizziness, headache, muscle weakness, dyspnea before exertion, uterine contractions, vaginal bleeding, or fluid loss from the vagina (ACOG, 2002). The woman should stop exercising if these symptoms occur, and modify her exercise program. If the symptoms persist, the woman should contact her caregiver.

Complementary Care

YOGA DURING PREGNANCY

The following advice is important for women who practice yoga during pregnancy (Fontaine, 2005):

- During pregnancy, some yoga poses or positions are contraindicated. In particular pregnant women should avoid those poses that put pressure on the uterus as well as any extreme stretching positions.
- Because of the changed center of gravity that occurs as pregnancy progresses, women need to be especially careful to maintain balance when doing stretching.
- Pregnant women should avoid stomach-lying for any poses. After 20 weeks' gestation, women should lie on their left side rather than their back for floor positions.
- Pregnant women should immediately stop any pose that is uncomfortable.
- Warning signs that indicate the need to contact the physician or certified nurse-midwife immediately include the following: dizziness, extreme shortness of breath, sudden swelling, vaginal bleeding.

Thinking Critically

COUNSELING ABOUT STRENUOUS PHYSICAL ACTIVITY

Constance Petrowski, a 24-year-old, G1P0, world-class marathon runner, is 11 weeks pregnant when she sees you, the nurse-midwife, for her first prenatal examination. Because of her low body fat, her menses have always been irregular, and it had not occurred to Constance that she might be pregnant. Constance tells you that she has just begun serious training for a marathon that is to take place when she is about 22 weeks pregnant. Constance says she has been told that it is fine to continue any physical activity at which one is proficient and says that she would like to compete in the marathon because she believes she has a chance to come in as one of the top three women runners. What should you tell Constance about competing in the marathon?

See MyNursingKit for possible responses.

During pregnancy, adequate rest is important for both physical and emotional health. Women need more sleep, particularly in the first and last trimesters, when they tire easily. Without enough rest, pregnant women have less resilience. Finding time to rest during the day may be difficult for women who work outside the home or who have small children. The nurse can help the expectant mother examine her daily schedule to develop a realistic plan for short periods of rest and relaxation.

Sleeping becomes more difficult during the last trimester because of the enlarged abdomen, increased frequency of urination, and greater activity of the fetus. Finding a comfortable position becomes difficult. Figure 11–8 ● shows a position most pregnant women find comfortable. Women can also prepare for sleep with progressive relaxation techniques similar to those taught in prepared childbirth classes.

EXERCISES TO PREPARE FOR CHILDBIRTH

Certain exercises help strengthen muscle tone in preparation for birth and promote more rapid restoration of muscle tone after

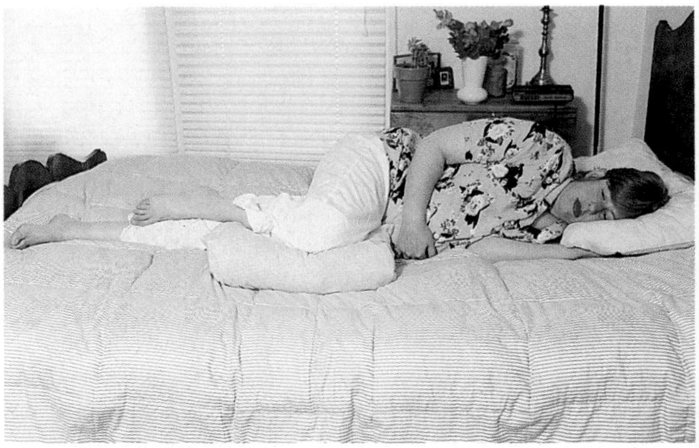

● **Figure 11–8** Position for relaxation and rest as pregnancy progresses.

birth. A few of the more common body-conditioning exercises for pregnancy are discussed here.

The **pelvic tilt**, or pelvic rocking, helps maintain pelvic flexibility and prevent or reduce back strain as it helps strengthen abdominal muscles. To do the pelvic tilt in early pregnancy, the pregnant woman lies on her back and puts her feet flat on the floor. This flexes the knees and helps prevent strain or discomfort. She decreases the curvature in her back by pressing her spine toward the floor. With her back pressed to the floor, the woman tightens her abdominal muscles as she tightens and tucks in her buttocks. In the second and third trimesters, the woman can also do the pelvic tilt on her hands and knees (Figure 11–9 ●), while sitting in a chair, or while standing with her back against a wall. The woman should maintain the body alignment that results when the pelvic tilt is done correctly as much as possible throughout the day.

Abdominal Exercises

A basic exercise to increase abdominal muscle tone is tightening abdominal muscles with each breath. It can be done in any position, but it is best learned while lying supine. With knees flexed and feet flat on the floor, the woman expands her abdomen and slowly takes a deep breath. Exhaling slowly, she gradually pulls in her abdominal muscles until they are fully contracted. She relaxes for a

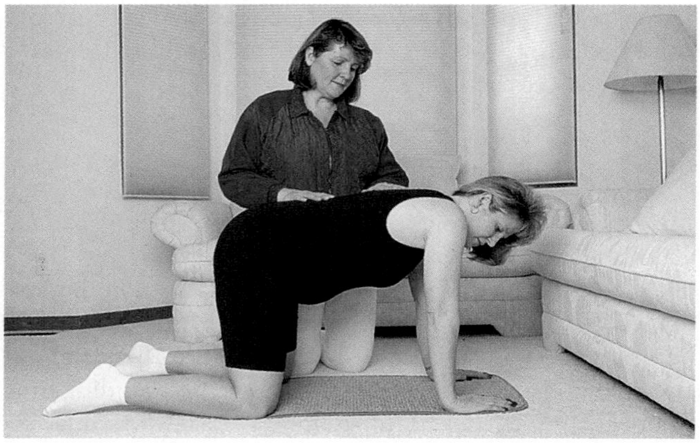

A

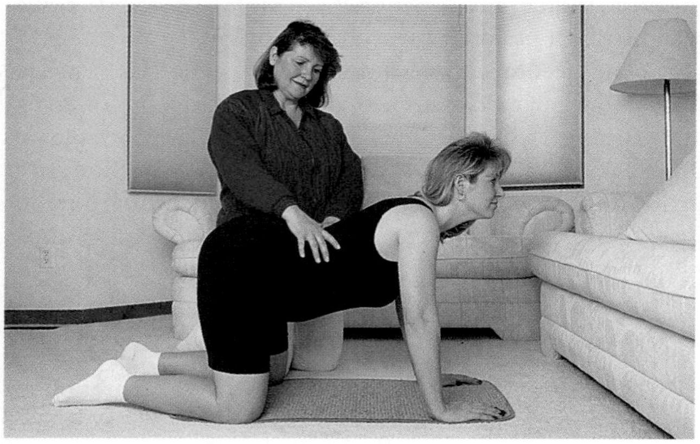

B

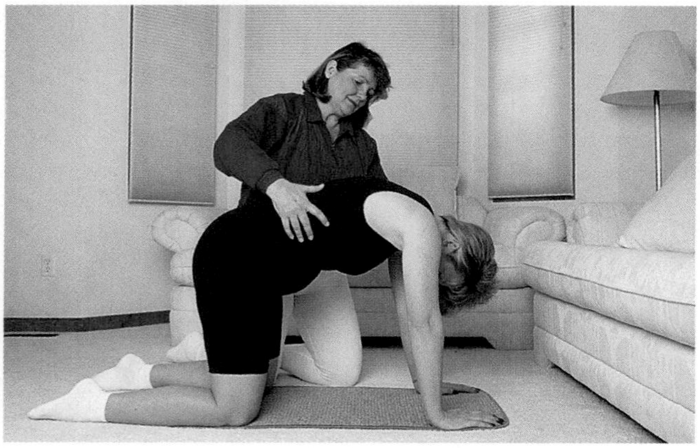

C

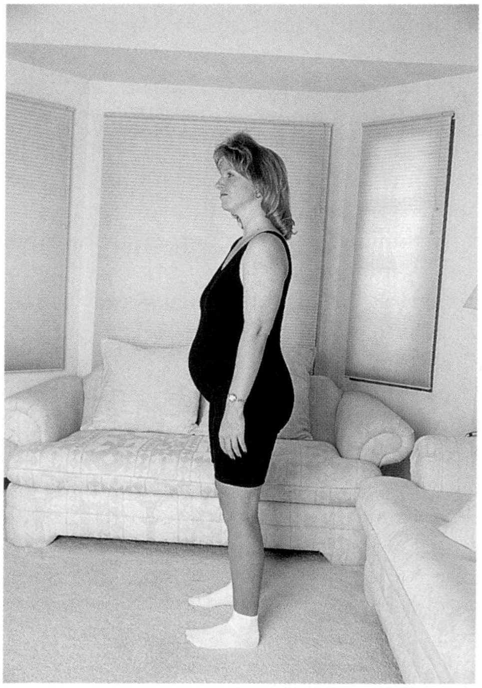

D

● **Figure 11–9** The pelvic tilt. ***A,*** Starting position when the pelvic tilt is done on hands and knees. The back is flat and parallel to the floor, the hands are below the head, and the knees are directly below the buttocks. ***B,*** A prenatal yoga instructor offers pointers for proper positioning for the first part of the tilt: head up, neck long and separated from the shoulders, buttocks up, and pelvis thrust back, allowing the back to drop and release on an inhaled breath. ***C,*** The instructor helps the woman assume the correct position for the next part of the tilt. It is done on a long exhalation, allowing the pregnant woman to arch her back, drop her head loosely, push away from her hands, and draw in the muscles of her abdomen to strengthen them. In this position the pelvis and buttocks are tucked under, and the buttock muscles are tightened. ***D,*** Proper posture. The knees are slightly bent but not locked, and the pelvis and buttocks are tucked under, thereby lengthening the spine and helping support the weighty abdomen. With her chin tucked in, this woman's neck, shoulders, hips, knees, and feet are all in a straight line perpendicular to the floor. Her feet are parallel. This is also the starting position for doing the pelvic tilt while standing.

Nursing Practice

Doing the pelvic tilt on hands and knees may aggravate back strain. Teach women with a history of minor back problems to do the pelvic rock only in the standing position.

few seconds and then repeats the exercise. The pregnant woman should avoid the supine position after the first trimester.

Partial sit-ups strengthen abdominal muscle tone and are done according to individual comfort levels. In early pregnancy, partial sit-ups may be done with the knees flexed and the feet flat on the floor to avoid strain on the lower back. The woman stretches her arms toward her knees as she slowly pulls her head and shoulders off the floor to a comfortable level (if she has poor abdominal muscle tone, she may not be able to pull up very far). She then slowly returns to the starting position, takes a deep breath, and repeats the exercise. To strengthen the oblique abdominal muscles, she repeats the process but stretches the left arm to the side of her right knee, returns to the floor, takes a deep breath, and then reaches with the right arm to the left knee. During the second and third trimesters these exercises can be done on a large exercise ball.

Women can do these exercises approximately five times in a sequence and repeat the sequence at other times during the day as desired. It is important to do the exercises slowly to prevent muscle strain and overtiring.

Perineal Exercises

Perineal muscle tightening, also called **Kegel exercises**, strengthens the pubococcygeus muscle and increases its elasticity (Figure 11–10 ●). The woman can feel the specific muscle group to be exercised by stopping urination midstream. Doing Kegel exercises while urinating is discouraged, however, because this practice has been associated with urinary stasis and urinary tract infection.

Childbirth educators sometimes use the following technique to teach Kegel exercises. They tell the woman to think of her perineal muscles as an elevator. When she relaxes, the elevator is on the first floor. To do the exercises, she contracts, bringing the elevator to the second, third, and fourth floors. She keeps the elevator on the fourth floor for a few seconds, and then gradually relaxes the area. If the exercise is properly done, the woman does not contract the muscles of the buttocks and thighs. Kegel exercises can be done at almost any time. Some women use ordinary events—for instance, stopping at a red light or talking on the telephone—as a cue to remember to do the exercise.

Inner Thigh Exercises

The nurse can advise the pregnant woman to assume a cross-legged sitting position whenever possible. This "tailor sit" stretches the muscles of the inner thighs in preparation for labor and birth.

SEXUAL ACTIVITY

Because of the physiologic, anatomic, and emotional changes of pregnancy, couples usually have many questions and concerns about sexual activity during pregnancy. Often these questions are about possible injury to the baby or the woman during intercourse and about changes in the desire each partner feels for the other.

In the past, couples were often warned to avoid sexual intercourse during the last 6 to 8 weeks of pregnancy to prevent complications such as infection or premature rupture of the membranes. However, these fears seem to be unfounded. In a healthy pregnancy, there is no medical reason to limit sexual activity. Intercourse is contraindicated for medical reasons such as threatened miscarriage or risk of preterm labor (Cunningham et al., 2010).

The expectant mother may experience changes in sexual desire and response. Often these changes are related to the various discomforts that occur throughout pregnancy. For instance, during the first trimester, fatigue or nausea and vomiting may decrease sexual desire. During the second trimester, many of these

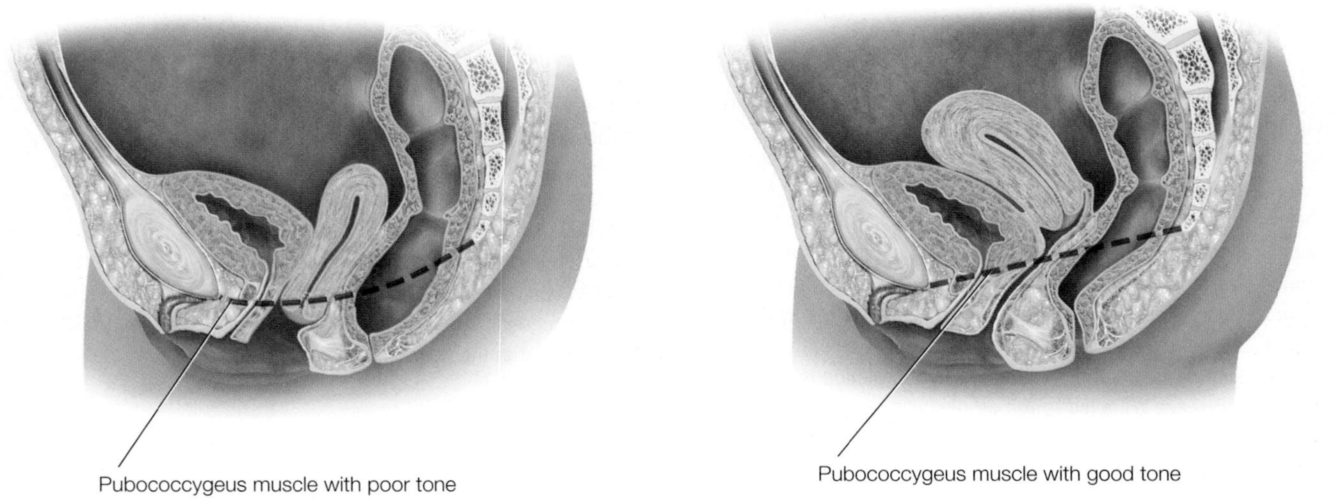

● **Figure 11–10** Kegel exercises. The woman learns to tighten the pubococcygeus muscle, which improves support to the pelvic organs.

discomforts are lessened and sexual satisfaction increases. During the third trimester, interest in sex may again decrease as the woman becomes more uncomfortable and tired. Shortness of breath, urinary frequency, leg cramps, and decreased mobility may also lessen sexual desire and activity. If they are not already doing so, the couple should consider coital positions other than male superior, such as side-by-side, female superior, and vaginal rear entry.

Sexual activity does not have to include intercourse. Many of the nurturing and sexual needs of the pregnant woman can be satisfied by cuddling, kissing, and being held. The warm, sensual feelings that accompany these activities can be an end in themselves. Her partner, however, may choose to masturbate more frequently than before.

Many factors in pregnancy also affect the sexual desires of men. The man's previous relationship with the partner, acceptance of the pregnancy, attitudes toward the partner's change of appearance, and concern about hurting the expectant mother or baby can all play a role. Some men find it difficult to view their partners as sexually appealing while they are adjusting to the concept of them as mothers. Other men find their partners' pregnancies arousing and experience feelings of increased happiness, intimacy, and closeness.

The expectant couple should be aware of their changing sexual desires, the normality of these changes, and the importance of communicating these changes to each other so that they can make nurturing adaptations. It is important that the couple feel free to express concerns about sexual activity. Use a relaxed manner when responding to questions and giving anticipatory guidance. (See "Teaching Highlights: Sexual Activity During Pregnancy".)

DENTAL CARE

Proper dental hygiene is important in pregnancy because ensuring a healthy oral environment is essential to overall health. In spite of such discomforts as nausea and vomiting, gum hypertrophy, and heartburn, it is important for pregnant women to maintain regular oral hygiene by brushing at least twice a day and flossing daily. It is important to encourage the woman to have a dental check-up early in pregnancy. She should inform her dentist that she is pregnant so that she is not exposed to teratogenic substances. (See "Evidence-Based Nursing" for a discussion of recommended dental care practices during pregnancy.)

IMMUNIZATIONS

Immunizations with attenuated live viruses, such as rubella vaccine, should not be given in pregnancy because of the teratogenic effect of the live viruses on the developing embryo. The most current recommendations on vaccines during pregnancy should be obtained from the Centers for Disease Control and Prevention website.

COMPLEMENTARY AND ALTERNATIVE THERAPIES

As discussed in Chapter 2, many women use complementary and alternative medicine (CAM) such as homeopathy, herbal medicine, acupressure and acupuncture, biofeedback, therapeutic touch, massage, and chiropractic as part of a holistic approach to their health care. Thus the nurse should inquire about the use of CAM as part of routine antepartal assessment. Nurses working with preg-

Evidence-Based Nursing

DENTAL CARE DURING PREGNANCY

Clinical Question

What is recommended dental care for women during pregnancy?

The Evidence

An advanced practice nurse and a dentist appraised multiple research studies for recommendations about appropriate oral care during pregnancy. Multiple studies with large samples were included in the review, which represents the strongest evidence for practice. Periodontitis has been linked to an increased risk of adverse birth outcomes, including preterm birth, low birth weight, and preeclampsia. Hormonal changes during pregnancy increase oral vascular permeability and decrease immunocompetence, and so increase susceptibility to oral infections. Furthermore, vomiting in early pregnancy changes the pH in the mouth, leaving it vulnerable to inflammation. The popular belief that pregnancy may weaken the teeth as a result of calcium depletion is unsupported; risk of oral disease is limited to soft tissues. Patterns of dental treatment are often altered during pregnancy, yet oral health can be safely maintained during pregnancy and the postpartum period (Russell & Mayberry, 2008).

Best Practice

Helping women appreciate the need for good dental health during pregnancy is important. Periodontal care is safe and effective throughout pregnancy. However, the best time for general dental procedures is during the second trimester, when the risk of pregnancy loss is lower. X-rays are safe as long as a lead apron with thyroid cuff is used. There is no evidence that the amount of mercury in dental amalgam (fillings) poses any risk to mother or fetus. Limitations on medications used for pain management are the same as those recommended during pregnancy in general. Local anesthetic is preferred, and should be carefully chosen, but a limited number can be used safely. Nitrous oxide should be avoided. Oral infections should be treated with antibiotics appropriate during pregnancy; tetracyclines and erythromycin in particular should be avoided, but the penicillins and cephalosporins are safe.

Critical Thinking

Are the benefits of postponing dental care to the second trimester outweighed by any risks associated with compromised oral health?

See MyNursingKit for possible responses.

Teaching Highlights

SEXUAL ACTIVITY DURING PREGNANCY

In starting a discussion about sexual activity during pregnancy, universal statements that give permission, such as "Many couples experience changes in sexual desire during pregnancy. What kind of changes have you experienced?" are often effective.

In your teaching, explain the following points to the woman and her partner:

- The pregnant woman may experience changes in desire during the course of pregnancy. During the first trimester, discomforts such as nausea, fatigue, and breast tenderness may make intercourse less desirable for many women. In the second trimester, as symptoms decrease, desire may increase. In the third trimester, discomfort and fatigue may lead to decreased desire in the woman.
- Men may notice changes in their level of desire, too. This may be related to feelings about their partner's changing appearance, their belief about the acceptability of sexual activity with a pregnant woman, or concern about hurting the woman or fetus. Some men find the changes of pregnancy erotic; others must adjust to the notion of their partners as mothers.
- The woman may notice that orgasms are much more intense during the last weeks of pregnancy and may be followed by cramping.
- Because of the pressure of the enlarging uterus on the vena cava, the woman should not lie flat on her back for intercourse after about the fourth month. If the couple prefer that position, a pillow should be placed under her right hip to displace the uterus. Alternative positions such as side-by-side, female superior, or vaginal rear entry may become necessary as her uterus enlarges.
- Sexual activities that both partners enjoy are generally acceptable. It is not advisable for couples who favor anal sex to go from anal penetration to vaginal penetration because of the risk of introducing *Escherichia coli* into the vagina.
- Alternative methods of expressing intimacy and affection such as cuddling, holding and stroking each other, and kissing may help maintain the couple's feelings of warmth and closeness. If the man feels desire for further sexual release, his partner may help him masturbate to ejaculation, or he may prefer to masturbate in private.
- Sexual intercourse is contraindicated once the membranes are ruptured or if bleeding is present. Women with a history of preterm labor may be advised to avoid intercourse because the oxytocin that is released with orgasm stimulates uterine contractions and may trigger preterm labor. Because oxytocin is also released with nipple stimulation, fondling the breasts may also be contraindicated in those cases.

Stress the importance of open communication so that the couple feel comfortable expressing their feelings, preferences, and concerns. Deal with any specific questions about the physical and psychologic changes that the couple may have.

nant women and childbearing families need to develop a general understanding of the more commonly used therapies to be able to answer basic questions and to provide resources as needed.

It is important for the pregnant woman to understand that herbs are considered dietary supplements and are not regulated as prescription or over-the-counter drugs are through the FDA. Herbal products have not been studied for potential harmful effect on the fetus during pregnancy and therefore should be avoided, particularly in the first trimester (Born & Barron, 2005). The website of the National Center for Complementary and Alternative Medicine is a reliable source of information about herbs, homeopathic remedies, and other alternative options.

TERATOGENIC SUBSTANCES

Substances that adversely affect the normal growth and development of the fetus are called teratogens (see Chapter 3 ∞). Many substances are known or suspected teratogens, including, for example, certain medications, psychotropic drugs, and alcohol. The harmful effects of others, such as some pesticides or exposure to x-rays in the first trimester of pregnancy, have also been documented. It is essential to provide pregnant women with information about recognized teratogens and environmental risks.

Medications

The use of medications during pregnancy, including prescriptions, over-the-counter drugs, and herbal remedies, is of great concern because maternal drug exposure is thought to account for at least 10% of all birth defects (Black & Hill, 2003). Many pregnant women need medication to treat infections, allergies, or other pathologic processes. In these situations the problem can be complex. Even when a woman is highly motivated to avoid taking any medications, she may have taken potentially teratogenic medications before her pregnancy was confirmed, especially if she has an irregular menstrual cycle.

The fetus is at highest risk for gross abnormalities during the first trimester of pregnancy, when fetal organs are first developing. The classic period of teratogenesis in a woman with a 28-day cycle extends from day 31 after the last menstrual period (17 days after fertilization) to day 71 (57 days after fertilization) (Niebyl & Simpson, 2007). Many factors influence teratogenic effects, including the type of teratogen and the dose, the stage of embryo development, and the genetic sensitivity of the mother and fetus. For example, the commonly prescribed acne medication isotretinoin (Accutane) is associated with a high incidence of spontaneous abortion and congenital malformations if taken early in pregnancy.

To provide information for healthcare providers and clients, the U.S. Food and Drug Administration has developed the following classification system for medications administered during pregnancy:

Category A: Controlled studies in women have demonstrated no associated fetal risk. Few drugs fall into this category.

Category B: Animal studies show no risk, but there are no controlled studies in women; or animal studies indicate a risk, but controlled human studies fail to demonstrate a risk. The penicillins fall into this category.

Category C: Either (1) no adequate animal or human studies are available or (2) animal studies show teratogenic effects, but no controlled studies in women are available. Many drugs fall into this category, which, because of the lack of information, is a problematic one for caregivers. Epinephrine, beta-blockers, and zidovudine (a drug used to decrease perinatal transmission of HIV) fall into this category.

Category D: Evidence of human fetal risk exists, but the benefits of the drug in certain situations are thought to outweigh the risks. Examples of drugs in this category include tetracycline, vincristine, lithium, and hydrochlorothiazide.

Category X: The demonstrated fetal risks clearly outweigh any possible benefit. Examples of drugs in this category include isotretinoin (Accutane), the acne medication, which can cause multiple central nervous system, facial, and cardiovascular anomalies.

Caregivers do not prescribe teratogenic medications to a pregnant woman. However, if a woman has taken a drug in category D or X, she should be informed of the risks associated with that drug and of her alternatives. A woman who has taken a drug in the safer categories can be reassured (Cunningham et al., 2010).

Although the first trimester is the critical period for teratogenesis, some medications are known to have a teratogenic effect when taken in the second and third trimesters. For example, tetracycline taken in late pregnancy is commonly associated with staining of teeth in children and has been shown to depress skeletal growth, especially in premature infants. Sulfonamides taken in the last few weeks of pregnancy are known to compete with bilirubin attachment of protein-binding sites, increasing the risk of jaundice in the newborn (Niebyl & Simpson, 2007).

Pregnant women need to avoid all medication—prescribed, homeopathic, or over-the-counter—if possible. If no alternative exists, it is wisest to select a well-known medication rather than a newer drug whose potential teratogenic effects may not be known. When possible, the oral form of a drug should be used, and it should be prescribed in the lowest possible therapeutic dose for the shortest time possible. Caution is the watchword for nurses caring for pregnant women who have been taking medications. It is essential that pregnant women check with their certified nurse-midwives or physicians about any herbs or medications they were taking when pregnancy began and about any nonprescription drugs they are thinking of using. The advantage of using a particular medication must outweigh the risks. Any medication with possible teratogenic effects is best avoided.

Tobacco

In the United States, smoking during pregnancy is one of the most significant, modifiable causes of poor pregnancy outcomes. It has a strong association with low birth weight infants. In addition, mothers who smoke have an increased risk of preterm birth, premature rupture of the membranes, fetal demise, placentae previa, and abruptio placentae (Hartmann, Wechter, Payne, et al., 2007). Pregnant women who smoke as well as participate in other unhealthy behaviors, such as alcohol use, further increase their risk for low birth weight infants (Okah, Cai, & Hoff, 2005). Research also links maternal smoking, both during pregnancy and afterward, with an increased risk of sudden infant death syndrome (SIDS). Maternal smoking exposes young children to other risks of secondhand smoke including middle ear infections, acute and chronic respiratory tract illnesses, and behavioral and learning disabilities (Albrecht, Maloni, Thomas, et al., 2004).

The specific mechanism of smoking's effect on the fetus is not known. However, the ingredients in cigarette smoke, such as carbon monoxide, nicotine, lead, and cotinine, are toxic to the fetus and decrease the availability of oxygen to maternal and fetal tissues (Cunningham et al., 2010).

In response to public health education campaigns in the United States, smoking during pregnancy has decreased significantly. In fact, approximately 46% of women who smoke quit during pregnancy. Unfortunately, 60% to 80% of women who quit smoking during their pregnancy resume smoking within a year after birth (ACOG, 2005). This finding suggests that although women are aware of the potential impact of smoking on the fetus, they may be less knowledgeable about the effects of passive smoke on the baby.

Quitting smoking early in pregnancy can help reverse the severe effects of smoking on the fetus. Recent research indicates that rates of spontaneous preterm birth and small-for-gestational-age infants are the same for women who quit smoking before 15 weeks' gestation as for non-smokers (McCowan, Dekker, Chan, et al., 2009). Any decrease in smoking during pregnancy most likely improves fetal outcome, and researchers continue to explore approaches designed to help women quit smoking. Pregnancy may be a difficult time for a woman to stop smoking, but the nurse should encourage her to reduce the number of cigarettes she smokes daily. The perceived need to protect her unborn child may increase her motivation.

Alcohol

Fetuses of women who drink heavily are at increased risk of developing **fetal alcohol syndrome** (see Chapter 28 ∞). This syndrome, which is characterized by growth restriction, facial anomalies, and central nervous system dysfunction of varying severity, is the major cause of mental retardation in the United States (Cunningham et al., 2010). Moreover, women who have more than three drinks per week have an increased risk for miscarriage, while those who have five or more drinks per week increase their risk for intrauterine death by two to three times that of nondrinkers (Wisner, Sit, Reynolds, et al., 2007).

The effects of moderate drinking during pregnancy are unclear. Research indicates an increased incidence of lowered birth weight and some neurologic effects, such as attention deficit disorder. Evidence suggests that the risk of teratogenic effects increases proportionately with increased average daily intake of alcohol. Although an occasional drink during pregnancy does not carry any known risk, no safe level of drinking during pregnancy has been identified; thus, healthcare providers recommend that pregnant women abstain from all alcohol during pregnancy. In most cases once a woman becomes aware of her pregnancy, she decreases her consumption of alcohol. However, the alcohol consumed after conception and before pregnancy is diagnosed remains a cause for concern.

Assessment of alcohol intake is a major part of every woman's medical history. The nurse should ask questions in a direct, nonjudgmental manner. All women need to be counseled about the role of alcohol in pregnancy. If heavy consumption is involved, the nurse should refer the pregnant woman immediately to an alcoholic treatment program. Counselors in these programs need to know about a woman's pregnancy before drug therapy is suggested, since certain drugs may be harmful to the developing fetus. For example, the drug disulfiram (Antabuse), often used in conjunction with alcohol treatment, is suspected to be a teratogenic agent.

Caffeine

Current research reveals no evidence that moderate caffeine intake has teratogenic effects in humans. However, high caffeine intake (greater than 3 cups per day) may be linked to an increased risk of miscarriage (Katz, 2008; Weng, Odouli, & Li, 2008). In addition, mothers who consume higher levels of caffeine may have a higher incidence of fetal growth restriction (CARE Study Group, 2008). (The average cup of brewed coffee has about 100 mg, a 12-oz can of cola has about 50 mg, and a cup of black tea has about 50 mg) (Niebyl & Simpson, 2007). Until more definitive data are available, nurses can advise women about common sources of caffeine, including coffee, tea, colas, and chocolate, and suggest that they limit their caffeine intake to less than the equivalent of 2 to 3 cups of coffee daily (Katz, 2008).

Marijuana

The prevalence of marijuana use raises many concerns about its effect on the fetus, but no teratogenic effects of marijuana use during pregnancy have yet been documented (Schempf, 2007). Research on marijuana use in pregnancy is difficult, however, because it is an illegal drug. Unreliability of reporting, lack of a representative population, inability to determine strength or composition of the marijuana used (including the presence of herbicides), and use of other drugs at the same time all complicate the research being done.

Cocaine

A woman who uses cocaine during pregnancy is at increased risk for acute myocardial infarction, cardiac arrhythmias, ruptured ascending aorta, seizures, cerebrovascular accidents, hyperthermia, bowel ischemia, and sudden death (Cunningham et al., 2010). Cocaine use during pregnancy has been related to abruptio placentae, premature rupture of the membranes, preterm birth, low birth weight, neonatal irritability, and neonatal depesssion (Schempf, 2007) as well as sudden infant death syndrome (SIDS) and developmental delays as a toddler (King, 2003). Several congenital anomalies have also been linked to maternal cocaine use, including genitourinary anomalies, congenital heart defects, limb reduction defects, and central nervous system anomalies (Cunningham et al., 2010).

As the number of women of childbearing age using cocaine increases, healthcare providers must be alert to early signs of cocaine use. It is often difficult for a nurse or physician to face the fact that a client is using cocaine, but ongoing alertness and an open, nonjudgmental approach are important in early detection. Urine screening for cocaine is valuable, but because cocaine is metabolized rapidly, the drug screen is negative within 24 to 48 hours after cocaine use. Thus, it is probable that many expectant mothers who use cocaine are not identified.

EVALUATION

Throughout the antepartal period, evaluation is an ongoing and essential part of effective nursing care. In evaluating the effectiveness of the interactions, try creative solutions that are logical and carefully thought out. Creative solutions are especially important in dealing with families from other cultures. If a practice is important to a woman and not harmful, the culturally competent nurse will not discourage it.

Be alert for situations that require referral for further evaluation. For example, a woman who has gained 4 lb in a single week does not require counseling about nutrition; she needs further assessment for preeclampsia. The nurse who has a sound knowledge of theory will recognize this need and act immediately.

Throughout the course of pregnancy, certain criteria determine the quality of care. In essence, nursing care has been effective if the following occur:

- The common discomforts of pregnancy are quickly identified and are relieved or lessened effectively.
- The woman is able to discuss the physiologic and psychologic changes of pregnancy.
- The woman uses self-care measures, if needed, during pregnancy.
- The woman avoids substances and situations that pose a risk to her or her child's well-being.
- The woman seeks regular prenatal care.

CARE OF EXPECTANT PARENTS OVER AGE 35

Today an increasing number of women are choosing to have their first baby after age 35. In the United States in 2005, more than 14.4% of all live births occurred to women age 35 and older (Martin, Hamilton, Sutton, et al., 2007). Many factors have contributed to this trend, including the following:

- The availability of effective birth control methods
- The expanded roles and career options available for women
- The increased number of women getting advanced education, pursuing careers, and delaying parenthood until they are established professionally
- The increased incidence of later marriage and second marriage
- The high cost of living, which causes some young couples to delay childbearing until they are more secure financially
- The increased number of women in this older reproductive age group due to the baby boom between 1946 and 1964
- The increased availability of specialized fertilization procedures, which may help women previously considered infertile

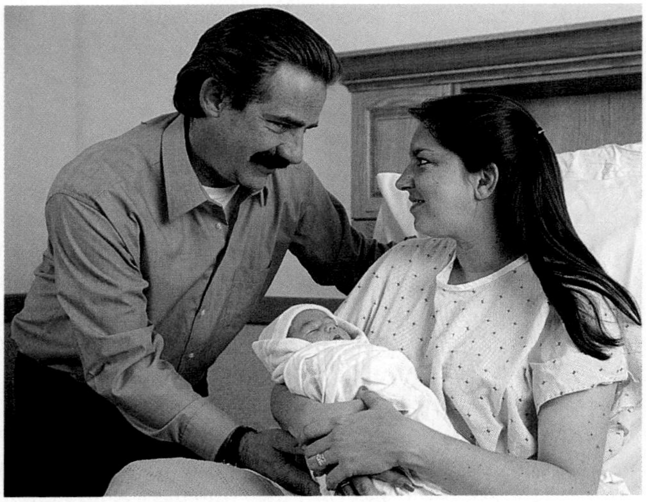

● **Figure 11–11** For many older couples, the decision to have a child may be very rewarding.

There are advantages to having a first baby after age 35. Single women or couples who delay childbearing until they are older tend to be well educated and financially secure. Usually their decision to have a baby was deliberately and thoughtfully made (Figure 11–11 ●). Because of their greater life experiences, they also are more aware of the realities of having a child and what it means to have a baby at their age. Many of the women have experienced fulfillment in their careers and feel secure enough to take on the added responsibility of a child. Some women are ready to make a change in their lives, wanting to stay home with a new baby. Those who plan to continue working typically can afford good child care.

MEDICAL RISKS

In the United States and Canada, the risk of fetal death has declined dramatically over the past 30 years for women of all ages. However, the risk of fetal death is significantly higher for women over age 35 and even higher for women age 40 and older. This is true regardless of a woman's parity, the time at which she begins prenatal care, and her level of education (Callaghan & Berg, 2003).

Women over age 35, especially those over age 40, are more likely to have chronic medical conditions that can complicate a pregnancy. Preexisting medical conditions such as hypertension or diabetes probably play a more significant role than age in maternal well-being and the outcome of pregnancy. The incidence of low birth weight infants, very preterm births, and perinatal deaths is higher among women age 35 and older (Delbaere, Verstraelen, Goetgeluk, et al., 2007). In addition, placenta previa, abruptio placentae, spontaneous abortion, macrosomia, and congenital malformations occur more frequently in pregnant women over 35 (Cunningham et al., 2010).

The cesarean birth rate is also increased in pregnant women over age 35. This may be related both to pregnancy complications and to increased concern by the woman and her physician about the pregnancy outcome (March of Dimes [MOD], 2006).

Recent research indicates that older maternal age (equal to or older than 35 years) and older paternal age (equal to or older than 40 years) are both independently associated with autism in the child. This association is even more significant in the firstborn children of two older parents (Durkin, Maenner, Newschaffer, et al., 2008).

The risk of conceiving a child with Down syndrome increases with age, especially over age 35. ACOG (2007) recommends that all pregnant women, regardless of age, be offered screening for Down syndrome. This screening typically includes a quadruple screen performed in the second trimester. However, more and more sites are now able to offer a first trimester assessment of the thickness of the fetal nuchal fold (*nuchal translucency* [NT]) combined with serum screening for free β-hCG and for pregnancy-associated plasma protein A (PAPP-A). See Chapter 10 ∞ for a discussion of screening tests.

Amniocentesis is routinely offered to all women over age 35 to permit the early detection of several chromosomal abnormalities, including Down syndrome. Genetic testing is not routinely offered to couples in whom there is only advanced paternal age, because there is not enough evidence to determine a paternal age at which to start genetic testing. However, advanced paternal age affects autosomal dominant inherited diseases, such as neurofibromatosis, achondroplasia, and Marfan syndrome.

SPECIAL CONCERNS OF EXPECTANT PARENTS OVER AGE 35

No matter what their age, most expectant parents have concerns about the well-being of the fetus and their ability to parent. Expectant parents over age 35 often have additional concerns about their age, especially the closer they are to age 40. Some couples are concerned about whether they will have enough energy to care for a new baby. Of greater concern is their ability to deal with the needs of the child as they age.

The financial concerns of the older couple are usually different from those of the younger couple. The older couple is generally more financially secure, but when their "baby" is ready for college, the older couple may be close to retirement and might not have the means to provide for their child. The older couple may also be forced to face their own mortality. Certainly the realization of one's mortality is not uncommon in midlife, but older expectant parents may confront the issue earlier as they consider what will happen as their child grows.

Older couples facing pregnancy in a late or second marriage or after therapy for infertility may find themselves somewhat isolated socially. They may feel different because they are often the only couple in their peer group expecting their first baby. In fact, many of their peers are likely to be parents of adolescents or young adults and may be grandparents as well.

Older couples who already have children may respond quite differently to learning that the woman is pregnant, depending on whether the pregnancy was planned or unexpected. Other factors influencing their response include their children's, family's, and friends' attitudes toward the pregnancy; the impact on their lifestyle; and the financial implications of having another child.

Sometimes couples who had previously been married to other mates will choose to have a child together. *Blended families* are formed when "her" children, "his" children, and "their" children come together as a new family group.

Healthcare professionals may treat older expectant parents differently than they would a younger couple. They may offer older women more medical procedures, such as amniocentesis and ultrasound, than younger women. They may also discourage an older woman from using a birthing room or birthing center even if she is healthy because her age is considered to put her at risk.

The woman who has delayed pregnancy may be concerned about the limited amount of time that she has to bear children. When pregnancy does not occur as quickly as she had hoped, the older woman may become increasingly anxious as time slips away on her "biological clock." When an older woman becomes pregnant but has a spontaneous abortion, her grief for the loss of her unborn child is exacerbated by anxiety about ability to conceive again in the time remaining to her.

NURSING MANAGEMENT

NURSING ASSESSMENT AND DIAGNOSIS

In working with a woman in her late 30s or 40s who is pregnant, make the same assessments as are indicated in caring for any woman who is pregnant. Assess physical status, the woman's understanding of pregnancy and its changes, the couple's attitudes about the pregnancy and their expectations of the impact a baby will have on their lives, their health teaching needs, the degree of support the woman has, and her knowledge of infant care.

The nursing diagnoses applicable to pregnant women in general apply to pregnant women over age 35. Examples of other nursing diagnoses that may apply include the following:

- *Decisional Conflict* related to unexpected pregnancy
- *Moderate Anxiety* related to uncertainty about fetal well-being

PLANNING AND IMPLEMENTATION

Once an older couple has made the decision to have a child, respect and support the couple in this decision. As with any client, discuss risks, identify concerns, and promote strengths. Do not make the woman's age an issue. It is helpful in promoting a sense of well-being to treat the pregnancy as normal unless the woman has specific health risks.

As the pregnancy continues, identify and discuss concerns the woman may have related to her age or to specific health problems. The older woman who has made a conscious decision to become pregnant often has carefully thought through potential problems and may actually have fewer concerns than a younger woman or one with an unplanned pregnancy.

Childbirth education classes are important in promoting adaptation to the event of childbirth for expectant parents of any age. However, older expectant parents often feel uncomfortable in classes in which most of the participants are much younger. Consequently, classes for expectant parents over age 35 are now available in many communities.

Women who are over age 35 and having their first baby tend to be better educated than other healthcare consumers. These clients frequently know the kind of care and services they want and may be assertive in their interactions with the healthcare system. You should not be intimidated by these individuals and should not assume that anticipatory guidance and support are not needed. Instead, support the couple's strengths and be sensitive to their individual needs.

In working with older expectant couples or an older single woman, the nurse should be sensitive to special needs. A particularly difficult issue these couples face is the possibility of bearing an unhealthy child or a child with a genetic disorder. As discussed previously, a quad screening test, also called multiple marker screen, is useful in assessing for Down syndrome. Because of the risk of Down syndrome in these families, amniocentesis is often suggested.

For couples who agree to amniocentesis, the first few months of pregnancy are a difficult time. Amniocentesis cannot be done until week 14 of pregnancy, and the chromosomal studies take roughly 2 weeks to complete. Their fear that the fetus is at risk may delay the successful completion of the psychologic tasks of early pregnancy.

You can support couples who decide to have amniocentesis by providing information and answering questions about the procedure and by providing comfort and emotional support during the amniocentesis. If the results indicate that the fetus has Down syndrome or another genetic abnormality, ensure that the couple has complete information about the condition, its range of possible manifestations, and its developmental implications.

EVALUATION

Expected outcomes of nursing care include the following:

- The woman and her partner are knowledgeable about the pregnancy and express confidence in their ability to make appropriate healthcare choices.
- The expectant parents (and their children) are able to cope with the pregnancy and its implications for the future.
- The woman receives effective health care throughout her pregnancy and during birth and the postpartum period.
- The woman and her partner develop skills in child care and parenting.

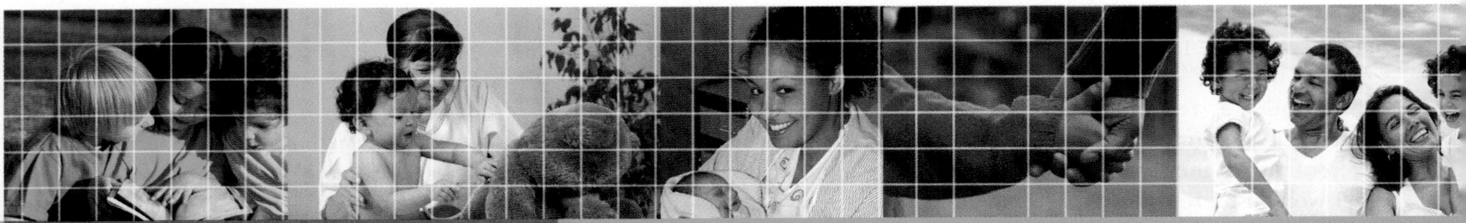

CRITICAL CONCEPT REVIEW

LEARNING OUTCOMES / CONCEPTS

11.1 Determine the most appropriate nursing care to help maintain the well-being of the expectant father and siblings during a family's pregnancy.

1. Father:
   - Provide information about expected changes (physical and emotional) during pregnancy.
   - Encourage the father to express feelings about pregnancy and other related topics such as feeding, ability to parent, and sexual activity.
   - Refer the couple to parenting classes for information about labor and birth. Also provide for support from other couples in the same situation.
   - Assess father's intended level of participation during labor and birth.
2. Siblings:
   - Discuss the possible negative feelings of siblings that may take place at the birth of a new child.
   - Teach parents to use open communication during the transition time.

11.2 Recognize the causes of common discomforts of pregnancy in each of the three trimesters.

1. In the first trimester:
   - Nausea and vomiting are caused by increased levels of hCG as well as changes in carbohydrate metabolism.
   - Urinary frequency is caused by pressure of the uterus on the bladder.
   - Fatigue may be caused by urinary frequency at night.
   - Breast tenderness is caused by increased estrogen and progesterone.
   - Increased vaginal discharge is caused by cervical hyperplasia and increased production of mucus by the endocervical gland.
   - Nasal stuffiness and epistaxis are caused by increased estrogen levels.
2. In the second and third trimesters:
   - Heartburn is caused by increased levels of progesterone as well as decreased gastric motility, increased relaxation of cardiac sphincter, and increased size of uterus, which displaces the stomach.
   - Ankle edema is caused by prolonged sitting or standing, slow venous return, increased capillary permeability, and increased level of sodium.
   - Varicose veins are caused by venous congestion and weight gain.
   - Hemorrhoids are caused by constipation and slow venous return of blood.
   - Constipation is caused by slow peristalsis due to increased level of progesterone. Constipation is also caused by decreased fluids, decreased exercise, increased level of iron, and pressure of the uterus on the intestines.
   - Backache is caused by increased lumbosacral vertebrae curve due to enlarging uterus.
   - Leg cramps are caused by an imbalance of calcium and phosphorus, fatigue, and poor lower extremity circulation.
   - Faintness is caused by a sudden change of position, which precipitates postural hypotension.
   - Dyspnea is caused by decreased vital capacity due to increasing size of uterus.
   - Flatulence is caused by decreased gastric motility and air swallowing.
   - Carpal tunnel syndrome is caused by compression of median nerve precipitated by edema.

11.3 Determine appropriate relief measures and interventions to alleviate the common discomforts of pregnancy.

1. In the first trimester:
   - For nausea and vomiting: avoid odors and eat dry crackers before arising in a.m. Drink fluids between meals and avoid greasy foods.
   - For urinary frequency: increase fluid intake during day and decrease in the evening.
   - For fatigue: plan rest periods and ask for help from family or support persons.
   - For breast tenderness: wear a well-supporting bra.
   - For increased vaginal discharge: bathe daily and wear cotton underwear.
   - For nasal stuffiness and epistaxis: use cool mist vaporizer.

LEARNING OUTCOMES | CONCEPTS

2. In the second and third trimester:
   - For heartburn: eat small, frequent meals, avoid overeating and lying down after eating.
   - For ankle edema: elevate legs while sitting or standing and dorsiflex feet frequently.
   - For varicose veins: elevate legs as much as possible and wear support hose.
   - For hemorrhoids: avoid constipation, use ice packs or sitz baths as necessary.
   - For constipation: increase fluid and fiber in diet. Develop regular bowel habits.
   - For backache: use good body mechanics and practice pelvic tilt exercises.
   - For leg cramps: apply heat to affected muscles and dorsiflex feet.
   - For faintness: change positions slowly, avoid standing for long periods of time.
   - For dyspnea: use good posture to sit and stand, and sleep in a semi-Fowler's position.
   - For flatulence: chew food completely and avoid gas-forming foods.
   - For carpal tunnel syndrome: avoid repetitive hand movement and elevate arm as needed.

11.4 Determine self-care measures that a pregnant woman can take to maintain and promote her well-being during pregnancy.

1. Fetal activity monitoring:
   - Cardiff Count-to-Ten Method: Lie quietly in the same position for 20–30 minutes each time. Should feel at least 10 fetal movements in 3 hours.
2. Breast care:
   - Wear a bra with good support and fit.
   - If breastfeeding, avoid soap on the nipples.
3. Clothing:
   - Should be loose and nonconstricting.
   - Wear low-heeled, comfortable, well-fitting shoes.
4. Bathing (be aware of cultural norms):
   - Be careful to avoid falls or feelings of faintness.
   - Shower may be easiest way to bathe in third trimester.
5. Employment:
   - Women with low-risk pregnancy can work until labor begins.
   - Workplace should be assessed for fetotoxic hazards.
6. Travel:
   - Avoid travel if woman has history of complications or has a multiple pregnancy.
   - With car travel, stop every 2 hours and walk. Position the seat belt under the abdomen.
7. Activity and rest:
   - Maintain regular exercise in uncomplicated pregnancy.
   - Avoid supine position.
   - Drink fluids and make sure to eat adequate amount of calories.
   - Avoid exercise during hot and humid weather.
   - Stop exercising with any suspicions of complications.
   - Plan for more sleep and regular rest periods.
   - Instruct in exercises to prepare for childbirth, including the pelvic tilt, partial sit-up, Kegel exercises, and the cross-legged sitting ("tailor sit") position.
8. Dental care:
   - Maintain regular dental checkups.
   - Dental work should be done in the second trimester.
   - Dental x-rays may be done if indicated as long as the woman is covered with a lead apron with a thyroid cuff.
9. Immunizations:
   - Avoid live virus vaccines.
10. Complementary and alternative therapies:
    - The nurse should develop understanding of most common ones.
    - The nurse should provide printed information about risks and benefits of homeopathic remedies and herbs.
11. Medications:
    - Avoid all OTC medications.
    - Take only medications approved by healthcare provider.
12. Substances to avoid during pregnancy:
    - All of the following should be avoided completely or decrease the amount of substance used: tobacco, alcohol, marijuana, and cocaine.
    - Caffeine has not been proven to impact pregnancy so women should be advised concerning common sources of caffeine and advised to moderate its use.

(continued)

LEARNING OUTCOMES / CONCEPTS

LEARNING OUTCOMES	CONCEPTS
11.5 Address the concerns that an expectant couple might have about sexual activity.	1. Traditional positions for intercourse may be uncomfortable; consider alternative positions. 2. Sexual desire may change during pregnancy. 3. Partners need to communicate feelings and needs. 4. Intercourse is contraindicated in: ■ Multiple pregnancy. ■ Threatened abortion. ■ Incompetent cervix. ■ Sexually transmitted infection. ■ Miscarriage following orgasm. ■ Rupture of membranes. ■ Preterm labor.
11.6 Relate the medical risks and special concerns of the older expectant woman and her partner to the nursing management indicated in providing care for this population.	1. Medical risks: ■ Fetal death risk is increased for all women older than 35. ■ Mother is more likely to have chronic medical conditions such as diabetes and hypertension that could pose a risk to the fetus. ■ Increased risk for cesarean birth. ■ Increased risk for autism when the mother and father are older, especially for first-born children. ■ Increased risk for Down syndrome and all autosomal dominant inherited disorders. 2. Special concerns: ■ Parents' ability to meet needs of child. ■ Not doing same things as peers, which could lead to social isolation. ■ Concern that "biological clock" continues to tick. ■ Fear of own mortality.

CRITICAL THINKING IN ACTION

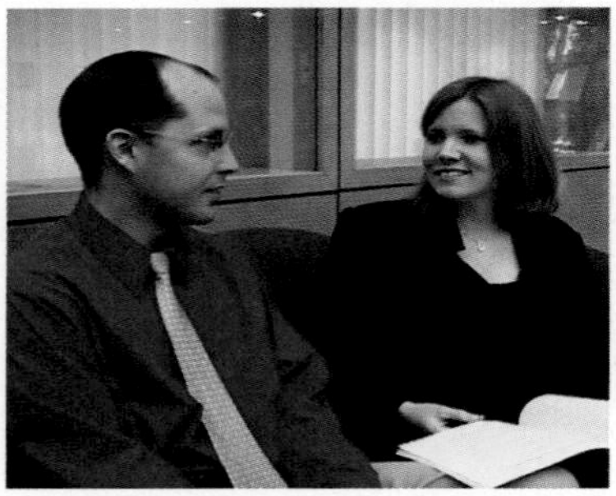

Thirty-seven-year-old Cathy Sommers, G1, P0000, presents to you, with her husband, at the OB physician's office at 32 weeks' gestation. Cathy tells you that she and her husband are practicing lawyers with their own firm. The couple delayed starting a family because it has been important to them to advance their careers and establish their firm. Cathy had an amniocentesis at 18 weeks' gestation because of her advanced maternal age, and the results ruled out chromosomal abnormalities. The couple knows that the baby is a boy, and are anticipating a vaginal birth. Cathy tells you that she is experiencing more fatigue, leg cramps, and shortness of breath when climbing stairs. The physical exam including a negative Homan's sign is within normal limits with the exception of slight ankle edema. Her weight is 150 lb, temperature 98.6°F, pulse 88, respirations 16, BP 126/70. You discuss pregnancy discomforts in the third trimester with Cathy and her husband.

1. What measures can you suggest to cope with fatigue?
2. Discuss measures to decrease leg cramps.
3. Discuss the physiologic changes underlying dyspnea.
4. Review Braxton Hicks contractions.

See MyNursingKit for possible responses.

REFERENCES

Albrecht, S. A., Maloni, J. A., Thomas, K. K., Jones, R., Halleran, J., & Osborne, J. (2004). Smoking cessation for pregnant women who smoke: Scientific basis for practice: AWHONN's SUCCESS Project. *Journal of Obstetric, Gynecologic, and Neonatal Nursing, 33*(3), 298–305.

American Academy of Pediatrics and the American College of Obstetricians and Gynecologists. (2008). *Guidelines for Perinatal Care* (6th ed.). Elk Grove Village, IL: Author.

American College of Obstetricians and Gynecologists (ACOG). (2005). *Smoking cessation during pregnancy* (Committee Opinion No. 316). Washington, DC: Author.

American College of Obstetricians and Gynecologists. (2002). *Exercise during pregnancy and the postpartum period* (ACOG Technical Bulletin No. 267). Washington, DC: Author.

American College of Obstetricians and Gynecologists. (2004). *Diagnosis and treatment of nausea and vomiting in pregnancy* (ACOG Practice Bulletin No. 52). Washington, DC: Author.

Baer, J. S., Sampson, P. D., Barr, H. M., Connor, P. D., & Streissguth, A. P. (2003). A 21-year longitudinal analysis of the effects of prenatal alcohol exposure on young adult drinking. *Archives of General Psychiatry, 60*(4), 377–385.

Berk, B. (2004). Recommended exercise during and after pregnancy: What the evidence says. *The International Journal of Childbirth Education, 19*(2), 18–22.

Black, R. A., & Hill, D. A. (2003). Over-the-counter medications in pregnancy. *American Family Physician, 67*(12), 2517–2524.

Born, D., & Barron, M. L. (2005). Herb use in pregnancy. *American Journal of Maternal Child Nursing, 30*(3), 201–206.

Callaghan, W. M., & Berg, C. J. (2003). Pregnancy-related mortality among women aged 35 years and older, United States, 1991–1997. *Obstetrics and Gynecology, 102*(5, Pt. 1), 1015–1021.

CARE Study Group (2008). Maternal caffeine intake during pregnancy and risk of fetal growth restriction: A large prospective observational study. *British Medical Journal, 337,* 2332–2333.

Cesario, S. K. (2007). Seat belt use in pregnancy. *Nursing for Women's Health, 11*(5), 474–481.

Cunningham, F. G., Leveno, K. J., Bloom, S. L., Hauth, J. C., Rouse, D. J., & Spong, C. Y. (2010). *Williams obstetrics* (23rd ed.). New York: McGraw-Hill.

Delbaere, I., Verstraelen, H., Goetgeluk, S., Martens, G., DeBacker, G., & Temmerman, M. (2007). Pregnancy outcome in primiparae of advanced maternal age. *European Journal of Obstetrics, Gynecology, and Reproductive Biology, 135*(1), 41–46.

Durkin, M. S., Maenner, M. J., Newschaffer, C. J., Lee, L. C., Cunniff, C. M., Daniels, J. L., et al. Advanced parental age and the risk of autism spectrum disorder. *American Journal of Epidemiology, 168*(11), 1268–1276.

Fontaine, K. L. (2005). *Healing practices: Alternative therapies for nursing* (2nd ed.). Upper Saddle River, NJ: Prentice Hall.

Granath, A., Hellgren, M., & Gunnarsson, R. 2006. Water aerobics reduces sick leave due to low back pain during pregnancy. *JOGNN: Journal of Obstetric, Gynecologic, & Neonatal Nursing,* 35(4): 465–471.

Hartmann, K. E., Wechter, M. E., Payne, P., Salisbury, K., Jackson, R. D., & Melvin, C. L. (2007). Best practice smoking cessation and resource needs of prenatal care providers. *Obstetrics & Gynecology, 110*(4), 765–770.

Johnson, T. R. B., Gregory, K. D., & Niebyl, J. R. (2007). Preconception and prenatal care: Part of the continuum. In S. G. Gabbe, J. R. Niebyl, & J. L. Simpson (Eds.), *Obstetrics: Normal and problem pregnancies* (5th ed.). New York: Churchill-Livingstone.

Katz, V. L. (2008). Prenatal care. In R. S. Gibbs, B. Y. Karlan, A. F. Haney, & I. E. Nygaard, (Eds.). *Danforth's Obstetrics and Gynecology* (10th ed.). Philadelphia: Wolters Kluwer/Lippincott Williams & Wilkins.

Krakow, D. (2008). Medical and surgical complications of pregnancy. In R. S. Gibbs, B. Y. Karlan, A. F. Haney, & I. E. Nygaard, (Eds.). *Danforth's Obstetrics and Gynecology* (10th ed.). Philadelphia: WoltersKluwer/Lippincott Williams & Wilkins.

Kuczkowski, K. M. (2003). Tobacco and ethanol use in pregnancy: Implications for obstetric and anesthetic management. *Female Patient, 28*(4), 16–22.

Lewis, B., Avery, M., Jennings, E., Sherwood, N., Martinson, B., & Crain, L. (2008). The effect of exercise during pregnancy on maternal outcomes: Practical implications for practice. *American Journal of Lifestyle Medicine, 2*(5), 441–455.

Lie, D. (2004). *Ginger helpful for nausea and vomiting of pregnancy. Medscape CME offering.* Retrieved January 13, 2004, from www.medscape .com/viewarticle/466746_print

March of Dimes (MOD). (2006). Pregnancy after 35. Retrieved January 16, 2006 from www.marchofdimes.com/printableArticles/ 14332_1155.asp

Martin, J. A., Hamilton, B. E., Sutton, P. D., Ventura, S. J., Menacker, F., Kirmeyer, S., & Munson, M. L. (2007). Births: Final data for 2005. *National Vital Statistics Reports, 56*(6), 1–108.

McCowan, L. M., Dekker, G. A., Chan, E., Stewart, A., Chappell, L. C., Hunter, M., et al. (2009). Spontaneous preterm birth and small for gestational age infants in women who stop smoking early in pregnancy: Prospective cohort study. *British Medical Journal, 338,* b1081.

Niebyl, J. R., & Simpson, J. L. (2007). Drugs and environmental agents in pregnancy and lactation: embryology, teratology, epidemiology. In S. G. Gabbe, J. R. Niebyl, & J. L. Simpson (Eds.), *Obstetrics: Normal and problem pregnancies* (5th ed.). New York: Churchill-Livingstone.

Okah, F. A., Cai, J., & Hoff, G. L. (2005). Term gestation low birth weight and health compromising behaviors during pregnancy. *Obstetrics and Gynecology, 105*(3), 543–550.

Penney, D. S. (2008). The effects of vigorous exercise during pregnancy. (2008). *Journal of Midwifery and Women's Health, 53*(2), 155–159.

Pennick, R., & Young, G. (2007). Interventions for preventing and treating pelvic and back pain in pregnancy. *Cochrane Database of Systematic Reviews,* 4.

Purnell, L. D., & Paulanka, B. J. (2005). *Guide to culturally competent health care.* Philadelphia: F. A. Davis.

Russell, S. L., & Mayberry, L. J. (2008). MCN *The American Journal of Maternal/Child Nursing 33*(1), 32–37.

Saade, G. R. (2007). Occupational Hazards. *Contemporary OB/Gyn, 52*(3), 59–68.

Schempf, A. H. (2007). Illict drug use and neonatal outcomes: A critical review. *Obstetrical & Gynecological Survey, 62*(11), 749–757.

Spector, R. E. (2009). *Cultural diversity in health and illness* (7th ed.). Upper Saddle River, NJ: Prentice Hall Health.

Varney, H., Kriebs, J. M., & Gegor, C. L. (2004). *Varney's midwifery* (4th ed.). Sudbury, MA: Jones & Bartlett.

Weng, X., Odouli, R., & Li, D-K. (2008). Maternal caffeine consumption during pregnancy and the risk of miscarriage: A prospective cohort study. *American Journal of Obstetrics & Gynecology, 198,* 279.e1–279.e8.

White, B. (2007). Ginger: An overview, *American Family Physician, 75,* 1689–1691.

Wisner, K. L., Sit, D. K. Y., Reynolds, S. K., Altemus, M., Bogen, D.L., Sunders, K. R., et al. (2007). Psychiatric disorders. In S. G. Gabbe, J. R. Niebyl, & J. L. Simpson (Eds.), *Obstetrics: Normal and problem pregnancies* (5th ed.). New York: Churchill-Livingstone.

EXPLORE PEARSON **mynursingkit**™

MyNursingKit is your one stop for online chapter review materials and resources. Prepare for success with additional NCLEX®-style practice questions, interactive assignments and activities, web links, animations and videos, and more!

Register your access code from the front of your book at
www.mynursingkit.com

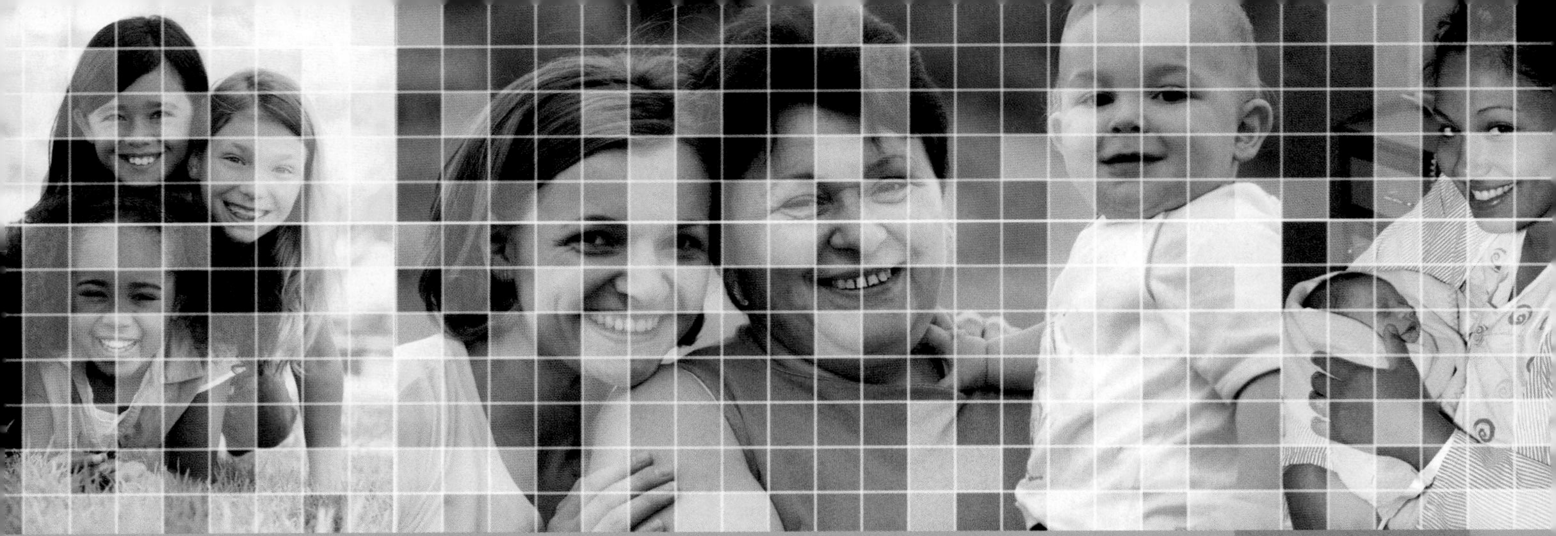

CHAPTER

Maternal Nutrition 12

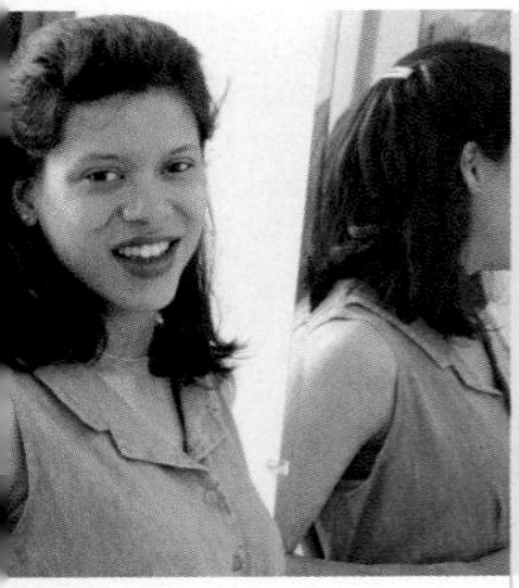

When I was young I thought nutrition was boring. Now that I am pregnant I find it endlessly fascinating. I realize how important good nutrition is for me, for my husband, and for the well-being of our child. My mother just laughs and reminds me about the times I resisted her efforts to help me develop better eating habits. Oh well, it is just another example of how smart our parents get as we get older! —Maria, 26

LEARNING OUTCOMES

12.1 Consider the recommended levels of weight gain during pregnancy when providing nursing care for pregnant women.

12.2 Recognize the significance of specific nutrients in the diet of the pregnant woman.

12.3 Compare nutritional needs during pregnancy, the postpartum period, and lactation with nonpregnant requirements.

12.4 Plan adequate prenatal vegetarian diets based on the nutritional requirements of pregnancy.

12.5 Consider ways in which various physical, psychosocial, and cultural factors can affect nutritional intake and status in the nursing care management of pregnant women.

12.6 Compare recommendations for weight gain and nutrient intakes in the pregnant adolescent with those for the mature pregnant adult.

12.7 Explore basic factors a nurse should consider when offering nutritional counseling to a pregnant adolescent.

12.8 Compare nutritional counseling issues for breastfeeding and formula-feeding mothers.

A woman's nutritional status before and during pregnancy can significantly influence her health and the health of her fetus. In most prenatal clinics and offices, nurses offer nutritional counseling directly or work closely with the nutritionist in providing nutritional assessment and teaching. This chapter focuses on the nutritional needs of the pregnant woman. Special sections consider the nutritional needs of the pregnant adolescent and the woman after giving birth.

Fetal growth occurs in three overlapping stages: (1) growth by increase in cell number, (2) growth by increase in cell number and cell size, and (3) growth by increase in cell size alone. Nutritional problems that interfere with cell division may have permanent consequences. If the nutritional deficit occurs when cells are mainly enlarging, the changes are usually reversible when normal nutrition resumes.

Growing fetal and maternal tissues require increased quantities of essential dietary components. These are listed in the **dietary reference intakes (DRIs)**, a broad array of dietary reference values developed jointly by the United States and Canada, as either the *recommended dietary allowance (RDA)* or *adequate intake (AI)*. An RDA is the daily dietary intake that is considered sufficient to meet the nutritional requirements of nearly all individuals in a specific life stage and gender group. An AI is a value cited for a nutrient when there is insufficient data to calculate an estimated average requirement. Women can get most of the recommended nutrients by eating a well-balanced diet each day. The basic food groups and recommended amounts during pregnancy and lactation are presented in Table 12–1.

MATERNAL WEIGHT GAIN

Maternal weight gain is an important factor in fetal growth and infant birth weight. Optimal weight gain depends on the woman's body mass index (BMI) (a measure of body fat based on height and weight) and her prepregnant nutritional state. An adequate weight gain indicates an adequate caloric intake. However, it does not ensure that the woman has a good diet nutritionally. The pregnant woman must maintain the nutritional quality of her diet as her weight gain progresses.

The Institute of Medicine (IOM, 2009) recommends that women should be within a normal BMI when they become pregnant and should limit their weight gain to the identified optimal ranges. The IOM's optimum ranges of weight gain based on a woman's BMI are as follows:

- Underweight woman: BMI less than 18.5, 28 to 40 lb (12.5 to 18 kg)
- Normal-weight woman: BMI between 18.5 and 24.9, 25 to 35 lb (11.5 to 16 kg)
- Overweight woman: BMI between 25 and 29.9, 15 to 25 lb (7 to 11.5 kg)
- Obese woman: BMI equal to or greater than 30, 11 to 20 lb (5 to 9.1 kg)

The average maternal weight gain is distributed as follows:

11 lb (5 kg)	Fetus, placenta, amniotic fluid
2 lb (0.9 kg)	Uterus
4 lb (1.8 kg)	Increased blood volume
3 lb (1.4 kg)	Breast tissue
5 to 10 lb (2.3 to 4.5 kg)	Maternal stores

The pattern of weight gain is important. For a normal-weight woman, the IOM recommendations are based on a first trimester weight gain of 1.1 to 4.4 lb (0.5 to 2 kg) followed by a gain of about 1 lb (0.45 kg) per week during the second and third trimesters. A normal-weight woman who is expecting twins should gain 37 to 54 lb (16.8 to 24.5 kg), women who are overweight should gain 31 to 50 lb (14 to 22.7 kg); women who are obese should gain 25 to 42 lb (7 to 19 kg) (IOM, 2009).

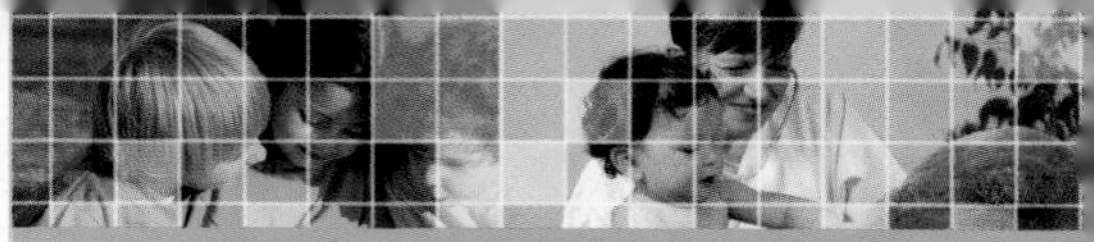

KEY TERMS

Calorie, 256

Dietary reference intakes (DRIs), 253

Folic acid, 256

Kilocalorie, 256

Lactase deficiency (lactose intolerance), 262

Lacto-ovovegetarians, 260

Lactovegetarians, 260

Pica, 263

Vegans, 260

Table 12–1 **Daily Food Plan for Pregnancy and Lactation**

Food Group	Nutrients Provided	Food Source	Recommended Daily Amount During Pregnancy	Recommended Daily Amount During Lactation
Dairy products	Protein; riboflavin; vitamins A, D, and others; calcium; phosphorus; zinc; magnesium	Milk—whole, 2%, skim, dry, buttermilk Cheeses—hard, semisoft, cottage Yogurt—plain, low-fat Soybean milk—canned, dry	Four (8 oz) cups (five for teenagers) used plain or with flavoring, in shakes, soups, puddings, custards, cocoa Calcium in 1 cup milk equivalent to 1 1/2 cups cottage cheese, 1 1/2 oz hard or semisoft cheese, 1 cup yogurt, 1 1/2 cups ice cream (high in fat and sugar)	Four (8 oz) cups (five for teenagers); equivalent amount of cheese, yogurt, etc.
Meat and meat alternatives	Protein; iron; thiamine, niacin, and other vitamins; and minerals	Beef, pork, veal, lamb, poultry, animal organ meats, fish, eggs; legumes; nuts, seeds, peanut butter, grains in proper vegetarian combination (vitamin B_{12} supplement needed)	Three servings (one serving = 2 oz), combination in amounts necessary for same nutrient equivalent (varies greatly)	Two servings
Grain products, whole grain or enriched	B vitamins; iron; whole grain also has zinc, magnesium, and other trace elements; provides fiber	Breads and bread products such as cornbread, muffins, waffles, hotcakes, biscuits, dumplings, cereals, pastas, rice	Six to 11 servings daily: one serving = one slice bread, 3/4 cup or 1 oz dry cereal, 1/2 cup rice or pasta	Same as for pregnancy
Fruits and fruit juices	Vitamins A and C; minerals; raw fruits for roughage	Citrus fruits and juices, melons, berries, all other fruits and juices	Two to four servings (one serving for vitamin C): one serving = one medium fruit, 1/2–1 cup fruit, 4 oz orange or grapefruit juice	Same as for pregnancy
Vegetables and vegetable juices	Vitamins A and C; minerals; provides roughage	Leafy green vegetables; deep yellow or orange vegetables such as carrots, sweet potatoes, squash, tomatoes; green vegetables such as peas, green beans, broccoli; other vegetables such as beets, cabbage, potatoes, corn, lima beans	Three to five servings (one serving of dark green or deep yellow vegetable for vitamin A): one serving = 1/2–1 cup vegetable, two tomatoes, one medium potato	Same as for pregnancy
Fats	Vitamins A and D; linoleic acid	Butter, cream cheese, fortified table spreads; cream, whipped cream, whipped toppings; avocado, mayonnaise, oil, nuts Butter, cream cheese, fortified table spreads; cream, whipped cream, whipped toppings; avocado, mayonnaise, oil, nuts	As desired in moderation (high in calories): one serving = 1 tbsp butter or enriched margarine	Same as for pregnancy
Sugar and sweets		Sugar, brown sugar, honey, molasses	Occasionally, if desired	Same as for pregnancy
Desserts		Nutritious desserts such as puddings, custards, fruit whips, and crisps; other rich, sweet desserts and pastries	Occasionally, if desired	Same as for pregnancy
Beverages	Fluid	Coffee, decaffeinated beverages, tea, bouillon, carbonated drinks	As desired, in moderation	Same as for pregnancy
Miscellaneous		Iodized salt, herbs, spices, condiments	As desired	Same as for pregnancy

Note: The pregnant woman should eat regularly: three meals a day, with nutritious snacks of fruit, cheese, milk, or other foods between meals if desired. (More frequent but smaller meals are also recommended.) Four to 6 (8 oz) glasses of water and a total of 8 to 10 (8 oz) cups total fluid intake should be consumed daily. Water is an essential nutrient.

Evidence in Action

Maternal obesity and high body mass increase the risk for a cesarean delivery (meta-analysis) (Chu, Kim, Schmid, Dietz, et al., 2007).

Nursing Practice

Weight varies with time of day, amount of clothing, inaccurate scale adjustment, or weighing error. Do not overemphasize a single weight, but pay attention to the overall pattern of weight gain.

Obesity is becoming a major health problem in many developed countries, and more women are entering pregnancy already overweight or obese. Obese pregnant women are at an increased risk for medical and pregnancy-related complications including:

- gestational diabetes
- preeclampsia
- induction of labor
- cesarean birth
- anesthesia complications
- venous thrombosis
- postpartum hemorrhage
- endometritis

They also have a higher incidence of fetal anomolies, macrosomia, birth injury, and stillbirth. They should be considered high risk and counseled accordingly (DiLillo, Hendrix, O'Neill, et al., 2008; Kominiarek, 2008).

Maternal obesity also has implications for children. The children of overweight and obese mothers are predisposed to developing obesity and its related health concerns. In fact, the child of an overweight mother is three times more likely to be overweight by the age of 7 than is a child of a normal-weight mother (Reece, 2008).

Because of the association between maternal weight gain and pregnancy outcome, most caregivers pay close attention to weight gain during pregnancy. Weight gain charts can be useful in monitoring the rate and pattern of weight gain over time.

Excessive weight gain during pregnancy also has long-term implications because weight gain during pregnancy is by far the most important predictor of the amount of weight that a woman will retain following childbirth (Walker, 2007). Counseling the pregnant woman to eat a variety of nutrients from each of the food groups places less emphasis on the amount of her weight gain and more on the quality of her intake. It may also be helpful to encourage her to begin a simple exercise program such as walking. The food group pyramid, MyPyramid, offers users a colorful plan that emphasizes variety, proportionality, moderation, and physical activity and is designed to help guide individuals to make healthier choices (Figure 12–1 ●).

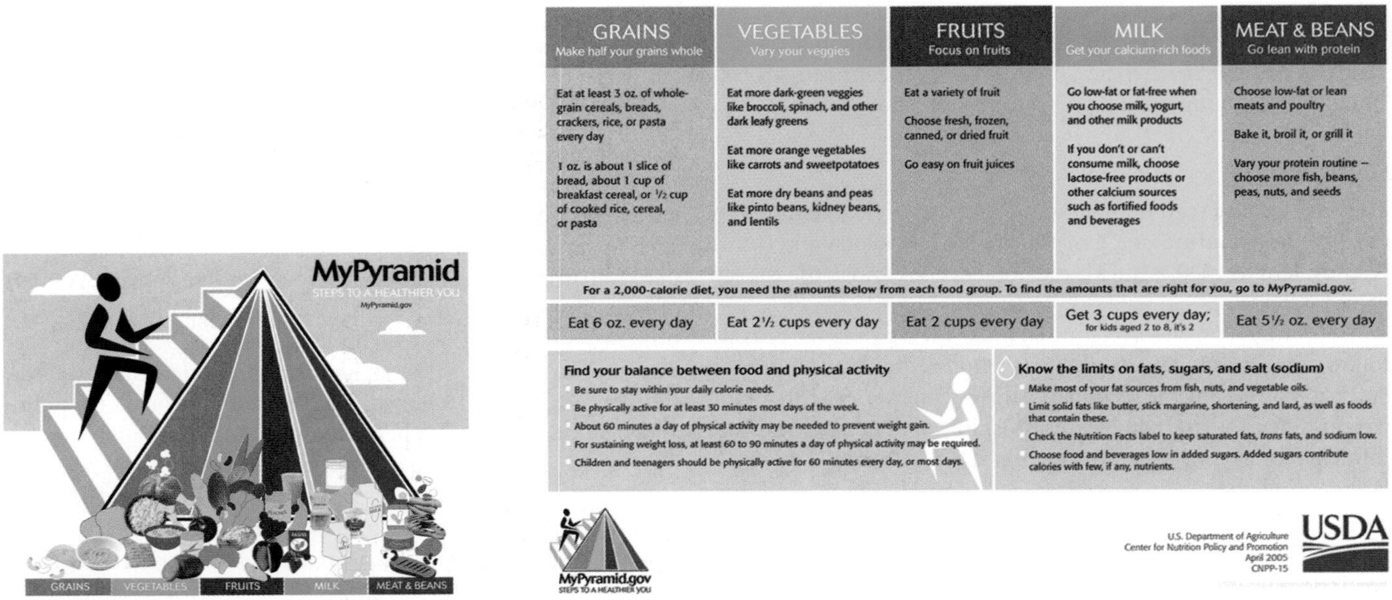

● **Figure 12–1** MyPyramid Food Guide. The "MyPyramid: Steps to a Healthier You" identifies the basic food groups and provides guidance about healthful eating. Grains, vegetables, fruits, and dairy products are emphasized, with slightly less emphasis on protein. The narrow yellow bar is designated for fats, sugar, and salt. People are encouraged to have most of their fat intake come from fish, nuts, and vegetable oils while limiting solid fats like butter, margarine, shortening, and lard. Emphasis is also placed on limiting added sugars, which contribute calories but few, if any, nutrients.

Source: Courtesy of the U.S. Department of Agriculture; U.S. Department of Health and Human Services.

Teaching Highlights

ADDING 300 KCAL DURING PREGNANCY

- The notion of "eating for two" may result in overeating.
- The additional 300 kcal/day recommended during pregnancy can be achieved by adding two milk servings and one serving of meat or alternative.
- The MyPyramid guide (see Figure 12–1) is helpful in planning healthy meals. It is designed to represent the food groups needed to make a balanced diet.
- A balanced diet includes the following:
  - Grains: Six to eleven servings (one serving = 1 slice bread, 1/2 hamburger roll, 1 oz dry cereal, 1 tortilla, 1/2 cup pasta, rice, grits)
  - Fruits: Two to four servings; one should be a good source of vitamin C (one serving = 1 medium-sized piece of fruit, 1/2 cup juice)
  - Vegetables: Three to five servings (one serving = 1 cup raw vegetable, 1 cup green leafy vegetable, 1/2 cup cooked vegetable)
  - Dairy: Two to three servings (one serving = 1 cup milk or yogurt, 1.5 oz hard cheese, 2 cups cottage cheese, 1 cup pudding made with milk)
  - Meats and alternatives: Two to three servings (one serving = 2 oz cooked lean meat, poultry, or fish; 2 eggs; 1/2 cup cottage cheese; 1 cup cooked legumes [kidney, lima, garbanzo, or soybeans, split peas]; 6 oz tofu; 2 oz nuts or seeds; 4 tbsp peanut butter)
- Not all foods that are nutritionally equivalent have the same number of calories; it is important to consider that when making food choices.
- Consider using low-fat milk, lean cuts of meat, or fish broiled or baked instead of fried.
- Foods can be combined. For example, 1 cup spaghetti with a 2-oz meatball would count as 1 serving meat, 3/4 cup spaghetti = 1 grain, and 1/4 cup tomato sauce = 1/2 serving vegetable.
- Use a calorie-counting guide to compare the calories in a variety of foods that are equivalent, such as 2 oz beef and 2 oz fish or 1 cup low-fat milk and 1 cup whole milk.

NUTRITIONAL REQUIREMENTS

The RDA for almost all nutrients increases during pregnancy, although the amount of increase varies with each nutrient. These increases reflect the additional requirements of both the mother and the developing fetus.

Folic acid and iron are the only nutritional supplements generally recommended during pregnancy. An adequate diet can usually meet the increased need for other vitamins and minerals. To avoid possible deficiencies, however, many healthcare professionals still recommend a daily vitamin supplement.

CALORIES

The term **calorie** (cal) designates the amount of heat required to raise the temperature of 1 g of water 1°C. The **kilocalorie** (kcal) is equivalent to 1000 cal and is the unit used to express the energy value of food.

The RDA for energy requirements during pregnancy is as follows: no increase during the first trimester but an increase of 300 kcal/day during the second and third trimesters. Prepregnant weight, height, maternal age, health status, and activity level all influence caloric needs, and weight should be monitored regularly during the pregnancy. See "Teaching Highlights: Adding 300 kcal During Pregnancy."

CARBOHYDRATES

Carbohydrates provide the body's main source of energy as well as the fiber necessary for proper bowel functioning. If the total caloric intake is not adequate, the body uses protein for energy. Protein then becomes unavailable for growth needs. In addition, protein breakdown leads to ketosis.

The carbohydrate and caloric needs of the pregnant woman increase, especially during the last two trimesters. Carbohydrate intake promotes weight gain and growth of the fetus, placenta, and other maternal tissues. Dairy products, fruits, vegetables, and whole-grain cereals and breads all contain carbohydrates and other important nutrients.

PROTEIN

Protein supplies the amino acids required for the growth and development of maternal tissues, such as the uterus and breasts, and to meet fetal needs. This is especially important during the last half of pregnancy, when fetal growth is greatest.

The protein requirement for a pregnant woman is 60 g/day, an increase of 14 g over nonpregnant levels. Animal products such as meat, fish, poultry, and eggs provide high-quality protein. Dairy products are also important protein sources. A quart of milk supplies 32 g of protein, more than half the average daily protein requirement. A woman can incorporate milk into her diet in a variety of dishes, including soups, puddings, custards, sauces, and yogurt. Beverages such as hot chocolate and milk-and-fruit drinks can also be included, but they are high in calories. Various kinds of hard and soft cheeses and cottage cheese are excellent protein sources, although cream cheese is considered a fat source only. Women who have allergies to milk, are lactose intolerant, or practice vegetarianism may find soy milk acceptable. It can be used in cooked dishes or as a beverage. Tofu, or soybean curd, can replace cottage cheese.

FAT AND FATTY ACIDS

Fats are valuable sources of energy for the body and aid in the absorption of fat-soluble vitamins. Fats are more completely absorbed during pregnancy, resulting in a marked increase in serum lipids, lipoproteins, and cholesterol, and decreased elimination of fat through the bowel. Fat deposits in the fetus increase from about 2% at midpregnancy to almost 12% at term. However, fat requirements are unchanged during pregnancy and should account for about 30% of daily caloric intake, of which less than 10% should be saturated fat.

The omega-3 fatty acids docosahexaenoic acid (DHA) and eicosapentaenoic acid (EPA) are important nutrients in pregnancy and during breastfeeding. They decrease the risk of preterm birth and also improve cognitive function, visual acuity, attention span, and sleep patterns in the infant. In the mother, an adequate intake (or supplementation) during pregnancy and the postpartal period may reduce the risk of postpartum depression (McGregor & French, 2008). The best sources of omega-3 fatty acids are flaxseeds and their oil, and fish oils. Consequently women need information about the importance of seafood in their diet and the need to consume seafood that is low in mercury. (See "Mercury in Fish" later in this chapter.) Eggs that have been enriched with omega-3 fatty acids can now be purchased in grocery stores.

MINERALS

Calcium and Phosphorus

Calcium and phosphorus are involved in the mineralization of fetal bones and teeth and acid-base buffering. The body absorbs and uses calcium more efficiently during pregnancy. Some calcium and phosphorus are required early in pregnancy, but most fetal bone calcification occurs during the last 2 to 3 months. Teeth begin to form at about 8 weeks' gestation and are formed by birth. The 6-year molars begin to calcify just before birth.

The identified AI for calcium for the pregnant or lactating woman, age 19 or older, is 1000 mg/day. It is 1300 mg/day for pregnant women younger than age 19. If calcium intake is low, fetal needs will be met at the mother's expense by demineralization of bone.

A diet that includes 4 cups of milk or an equivalent dairy alternative will provide sufficient calcium. Smaller amounts of calcium are supplied by legumes, nuts, dried fruits, and dark green leafy vegetables (such as kale, cabbage, collards, and turnip greens).

The RDA for phosphorus is 700 mg/day for the pregnant or lactating woman age 19 and older. It is 1250 mg/day for pregnant women younger than 19 years. Because phosphorus is so widely available in foods, the daily requirement is readily supplied through calcium- and protein-rich foods.

Iodine

Iodine is an essential part of the thyroid hormone thyroxine. The thyroid gland may become enlarged if iodine is not replaced by adequate dietary intake or an additional supplement. Moreover, cretinism may occur in the infant if the mother has a severe iodine deficiency. Pregnant women can meet the iodine allowance of 220 mcg/day by using iodized salt. When salt is restricted, the physician may prescribe an iodine supplement.

Sodium

Sodium is essential for proper metabolism and the regulation of fluid balance. Sodium intake in the form of salt is never entirely restricted during pregnancy, even when hypertension is present. The pregnant woman may season food to taste during cooking but should avoid using extra salt at the table. She can avoid excessive intake by eliminating salty foods such as potato chips, ham, sausages, and sodium-based seasonings.

Zinc

Zinc is needed for protein metabolism and the synthesis of DNA and RNA. It is essential for normal fetal growth and development as well as milk production during lactation. The RDA during pregnancy is 11 mg/day for women age 19 and older. This increases to 12 mg during lactation. Sources include meats, shellfish, poultry, whole grains, and legumes.

Magnesium

Magnesium is essential for cellular metabolism and structural growth. The RDA for pregnancy is 320 mg/day for women age 19 to 30. Good sources include milk, whole grains, dark green vegetables, nuts, and legumes.

Iron

Iron requirements increase during pregnancy because of the growth of the fetus and placenta and the increased maternal blood volume. Anemia in pregnancy is mainly caused by low iron stores, although it may also be caused by inadequate intake of other nutrients, such as vitamins B_6 and B_{12}, folic acid, ascorbic acid, copper, and zinc. Iron deficiency anemia is generally defined as a decrease in the oxygen-carrying capacity of the blood. Anemia leads to a significant reduction in hemoglobin in the volume of packed red cells per deciliter of blood (hematocrit) or in the number of erythrocytes. Iron deficiency anemia is associated with a higher incidence of preterm birth, low-birth-weight infants, and infant mortality (Gautam, Saha, Sekhri, et al., 2008).

Fetal demands for iron further contribute to symptoms of anemia in the pregnant woman. The fetal liver stores iron, especially during the third trimester. The infant needs this stored iron during the first 4 months of life to compensate for the normally inadequate levels of iron in breast milk and non-iron-fortified formulas.

To prevent anemia, the woman must balance iron requirements and intake. Adequate iron intake is a problem for nonpregnant women and a greater one for pregnant women. By carefully choosing foods high in iron, the woman can increase her daily iron intake considerably. Lean meats, dark green leafy vegetables, eggs, and whole-grain and enriched breads and cereals are the usual food sources of iron. Other iron sources include dried fruits, legumes, shellfish, and molasses.

Iron absorption is usually higher for animal products than for vegetable products. However, the woman can increase absorption of iron from nonmeat sources by combining them with meat or a food rich in vitamin C. The RDA for iron during pregnancy is 27 mg/day, but this intake is almost impossible to achieve through diet alone. Thus, in the second and third trimesters the pregnant woman should take a daily supplement of 30 mg elemental iron (Katz, 2008). Unfortunately, iron supplements often cause gastrointestinal discomfort, especially if taken on an empty stomach. Taking the iron supplement after a meal may help reduce this discomfort. Iron supplements may also cause constipation, so an adequate fluid intake is important in pregnancy.

VITAMINS

Vitamins are organic substances needed for life and growth. They are found in small amounts in specific foods and generally cannot be synthesized by the body in adequate amounts.

Vitamins are grouped according to solubility. Vitamins A, D, E, and K dissolve in fat; vitamin C and the B-complex vitamins dissolve in water. An adequate intake of all vitamins is essential during pregnancy; however, several are required in larger amounts to fulfill specific needs.

Fat-Soluble Vitamins

The fat-soluble vitamins, A, D, E, and K, are stored in the liver and thus are available if the dietary intake becomes inadequate. The major complication related to these vitamins is not deficiency but toxicity due to overdose. Unlike water-soluble vitamins, excess amounts of vitamins A, D, E, and K are not excreted in the urine. Symptoms of vitamin toxicity include nausea, gastrointestinal upset, dryness and cracking of the skin, and loss of hair.

Vitamin A is involved in the growth of epithelial cells, which line the entire gastrointestinal tract and make up the skin. It also plays a role in the metabolism of carbohydrates and fats. Without vitamin A the body cannot synthesize glycogen, and the body's ability to handle cholesterol is also affected. In addition, the protective layer of tissue surrounding nerve fibers does not form properly if vitamin A is lacking.

Probably the best known function of vitamin A is its effect on vision in dim light. A person's ability to see in the dark depends on the eye's supply of retinol, a form of vitamin A. Adequate vitamin A prevents night blindness. Vitamin A is associated with the formation and development of healthy eyes in the fetus. The RDA for vitamin A is 770 mcg/day for pregnant women age 19 and older.

Although routine supplementation with vitamin A is not recommended, supplementation with 5,000 international units is indicated for women whose dietary intake may be inadequate, such as strict vegetarians and recent emigrants from countries where deficiency of vitamin A is endemic. Rich sources of vitamin A include deep green, deep orange, and yellow vegetables; animal sources include egg yolk, cream, butter, and fortified margarine and milk.

Vitamin D is best known for its role in the absorption and use of calcium and phosphorus in skeletal development. To supply the needs of the developing fetus, the pregnant woman should have a vitamin D intake of 5 mcg/day. Main food sources of vitamin D include fortified milk, margarine, butter, and egg yolks. Drinking a quart of milk daily provides the vitamin D needed during pregnancy. Exposure to the ultraviolet rays of sunlight is also an important source of vitamin D. However, season, time of day, latitude, smog, cloud cover, and sunscreens affect ultraviolet ray exposure. (*Note:* It is still important to use sunscreens routinely.) For example, the average amount of sunlight in Boston and in points further north is insufficient to produce significant synthesis of vitamin D from November through February. Thus, it is vital for people with limited sun exposure to consume a diet that contains good sources of vitamin D (National Institutes of Health, 2007).

Excessive intake of vitamin D usually comes from high-potency vitamin preparations, not from the diet. Overdoses during pregnancy can cause hypercalcemia, or high blood calcium levels, due to withdrawal of calcium from the skeletal tissue. Symptoms of toxicity include excessive thirst, loss of appetite, vomiting, weight loss, irritability, and high blood calcium levels.

The major function of vitamin E, or tocopherol, is antioxidation. Antioxidants such as vitamin E protect the body's cells from the destructive effects of free radicals. Vitamin E takes on oxygen, thus preventing another substance from combining with the oxygen in a process called oxidation. For example, vitamin E helps spare vitamin A by preventing its oxidation in the intestinal tract and in the tissues. It decreases the oxidation of polyunsaturated fats, thus helping to retain the flexibility and health of the cell membrane. For this reason, vitamin E affects the health of all cells in the body.

Vitamin E is also involved in certain enzymatic and metabolic reactions. It is essential for the synthesis of nucleic acids required in the formation of red blood cells in the bone marrow. Vitamin E is useful in treating certain types of muscular pain and intermittent claudication, in surface healing of wounds and burns, and in protecting lung tissue from the damaging effects of smog. These functions may help explain the abundant claims and cures attributed to vitamin E, many of which have not been scientifically proved.

The recommended intake of vitamin E for pregnant women is unchanged at 15 mg/day. The vitamin E requirement varies with the polyunsaturated fat content of the diet. Vitamin E is widely distributed in foodstuffs, especially vegetable fats and oils, whole grains, greens, and eggs. Excessive intake of vitamin E has been associated with abnormal coagulation in the newborn.

Vitamin K, or menadione (as used synthetically in medicine), is essential for the synthesis of prothrombin, so its function is related to normal blood clotting. It is synthesized in the intestinal tract by the *Escherichia coli* bacteria normally found in the large intestine. However, the body's need for vitamin K is not totally met by synthesis. Green leafy vegetables are excellent sources. The RDA for vitamin K does not increase during pregnancy.

Intake of vitamin K is usually adequate in a well-balanced prenatal diet. Problems may arise if an illness is present that results in malabsorption of fats or if antibiotics are used for an extended period, which would inhibit vitamin K synthesis by destroying intestinal *E. coli.*

Water-Soluble Vitamins

Water-soluble vitamins are excreted in the urine. Since only small amounts are stored, adequate amounts must be consumed daily. During pregnancy the concentration of water-soluble vitamins in the maternal serum falls, whereas high concentrations are found in the fetus.

The RDA for vitamin C (ascorbic acid) increases in pregnancy from 75 to 85 mg. Vitamin C's major function is to aid in the formation and development of connective tissue and the vascular system. Ascorbic acid is essential to the formation of collagen, which binds cells together. If the collagen begins to disintegrate because of a lack of ascorbic acid, cell functioning is disturbed and cell structure breaks down, resulting in muscular weakness, capillary hemorrhage, and eventual death. These are symptoms of scurvy, the disease caused by vitamin C deficiency. Infants fed mainly cow's milk become deficient in vitamin C, and they are the main group that develops these symptoms. Surprisingly, newborns of women who have taken megadoses of vitamin C may have a rebound form of scurvy.

Maternal plasma levels of vitamin C progressively decrease during pregnancy, with values at term being about half those found at midpregnancy. It appears that ascorbic acid concentrates in the placenta; levels in the fetus are 50% or more above maternal levels.

A nutritious diet should meet the pregnant woman's needs for vitamin C without additional supplementation. Common food sources of vitamin C include citrus fruit, tomatoes, cantaloupe, strawberries, potatoes, broccoli, and other leafy greens. Ascorbic acid is readily destroyed by water and oxidation. Therefore, foods containing vitamin C must be stored and cooked properly.

The B vitamins include thiamine (B_1), riboflavin (B_2), niacin, folic acid, pantothenic acid, vitamin B_6, and vitamin B_{12}. These vitamins serve as vital coenzyme factors in many reactions such as cell respiration, glucose oxidation, and energy metabolism. The quantities needed increase as caloric intake increases to meet the metabolic and growth needs of the pregnant woman.

The thiamine requirement increases from the prepregnant level of 1.1 mg/day to 1.4 mg/day. Sources include pork, milk, potatoes, and enriched breads and cereals.

Riboflavin deficiency is manifested by cheilosis (fissures and cracks of the lips and corners of the mouth) and other skin lesions. During pregnancy, women may excrete less riboflavin and still require more because of increased energy and protein needs. An additional 0.3 mg/day, to 1.4 mg/day, is recommended for pregnant women age 19 and older. Sources include milk, eggs, enriched breads, and cereals.

Niacin intake should increase 4 mg/day during pregnancy to 18 mg/day. Sources of niacin include meat, fish, poultry, whole grains, enriched breads, cereals, and peanuts.

Folic acid, or folate, is required for normal growth, reproduction, and lactation and prevents the macrocytic, megaloblastic anemia of pregnancy. Megaloblastic anemia due to folate deficiency is rarely found in the United States, but it does occur.

Even more significantly, an inadequate intake of folic acid has been associated with neural tube defects (NTDs) (spina bifida, meningomyelocele) in the fetus or newborn. Although these defects are considered multifactorial (see Chapter 7), up to 70% of spina bifida and anencephaly could be prevented by adequate intake of folic acid (Spina Bifida Association, 2008). Consequently the U.S. Preventive Services Task Force (USPSTF) (2009) recommends that all women who are planning a pregnancy or who are capable of becoming pregnant consume 400 to 800 mcg of folic acid daily. This recommendation does not apply to women who are taking certain antiseizure medications or women who have had a previous pregnancy complicated by a neural tube defect because they may be advised by their caregiver to take a higher dose of folic acid (USPSTF, 2009). This recommendation is important because half of all U.S. pregnancies are unplanned and NTDs occur very early in pregnancy (3 to 4 weeks after conception), before most women realize they are pregnant (Centers for Disease Control and Prevention [CDC], 2009).

The best food sources of folates are fresh green leafy vegetables, liver, peanuts, and whole-grain breads and cereals. Folic acid can be made inactive by oxidation, ultraviolet light, and heating. It can easily be lost during improper storage and cooking. To prevent unnecessary loss, foods should be stored covered to protect them from light, cooked with only a small amount of water, and not overcooked.

No allowance has been set for pantothenic acid in pregnancy, but 5 mg/day is considered a safe, adequate intake. Sources include meats, egg yolk, legumes, and whole-grain cereals and breads.

Vitamin B_6 (pyridoxine) is associated with amino acid metabolism; thus, a higher-than-average protein intake requires increased pyridoxine intake. The RDA for vitamin B_6 during pregnancy is 1.9 mg/day, an increase of 0.6 mg over the allowance for nonpregnant women. Generally, the slightly increased need can be supplied by dietary sources, which include wheat germ, yeast, fish, liver, pork, potatoes, and lentils.

Vitamin B_{12}, or cobalamin, plays a role in the synthesis of DNA and red blood cells. It also is important in maintaining the myelin sheath of nerve cells. B_{12} is the cobalt-containing vitamin found only in animal sources. Women of reproductive age rarely have a B_{12} deficiency. Vegetarians (see later discussion on vegetarian diets) can develop a deficiency, however, so it is essential that their dietary intake be supplemented with this vitamin. The RDA during pregnancy is 2.6 mcg/day, an increase of 0.2 mcg. A deficiency may be due to a congenital inability to absorb vitamin B_{12}, resulting in pernicious anemia. Infertility is a complication of this type of anemia.

FLUID

Water is essential for life, and it is found in all body tissues. It is necessary for many biochemical reactions. It also serves as a lubricant, as a medium of transport for carrying substances in and out of the body, and as an aid in temperature control. A pregnant woman should consume at least 8 to 10 (8-oz) glasses of fluid each day, of which 4 to 6 glasses should be water. Because of their sodium content, diet sodas should be consumed in moderation. Caffeinated beverages have a diuretic effect, which is counterproductive to increasing fluid intake.

Nursing Practice

More women are consuming over-the-counter (OTC) vitamin, mineral, and food supplements today than in the past. Ask about the use of any OTC supplements to help avoid potentially harmful excess intakes.

Thinking Critically

WEIGHT GAIN IN PREGNANCY

Jaya Singh, a 28-year-old, G1P0, is 14 weeks pregnant. The rate and total amount of her weight gain during the first trimester have been consistent with recommendations. She has gained an average of 0.5 kg (1 lb) per week during both of the past 2 weeks. Her appetite is good, and she consumes three meals per day and snacks between meals on occasion.

Jaya has altered her diet because she is concerned about excessive weight gain. She told you that she has decreased her intake from the bread and dairy groups in order to limit her calorie intake. Because she has omitted most dairy products, she has increased her consumption of salads and broccoli to provide calcium sources.

A diet history revealed the following:

Grain	3-4 servings, mainly cereal and rice
Fruit	2-4 servings, fresh fruit
Vegetables	3-5 servings, salads, peas, corn, broccoli
Meat	4-5 servings, beef, pork, chicken
Dairy	occasionally cheese, ice cream, pudding
Fats, oils, sweets	occasionally salad dressings, margarine, desserts
Beverages	8-10 servings, soda, juices, water

After assessing her diet history, what is your evaluation of Jaya's diet? How would you counsel her?

See MyNursingKit for possible responses.

VEGETARIANISM

Vegetarianism is the dietary choice of many people for religious, health, or ethical reasons. There are several types of vegetarians. **Lacto-ovovegetarians** include milk, dairy products, and eggs in their diet. **Lactovegetarians** include dairy products but no eggs in their diets. **Vegans** are "pure" vegetarians who will not eat any food from animal sources.

The expectant mother who is vegetarian must eat the proper combination of foods to obtain adequate nutrients. If her diet allows, a woman can obtain ample and complete proteins from dairy products and eggs. An adequate, pure vegan diet contains protein from unrefined grains (brown rice, whole wheat), legumes (beans, split peas, lentils), nuts in large quantities, and a variety of cooked and fresh vegetables and fruits. Complete proteins can be obtained by eating different types of plant-based proteins such as beans and rice, peanut butter on whole-grain bread, and whole-grain cereal with soy milk, either in the same meal or over the day. Seeds may provide adequate protein in the vegetarian diet if the quantity is large enough. Obtaining sufficient calories to ensure adequate weight gain may be difficult because vegan diets tend to be high in fiber and therefore filling. Figure 12–2 ● depicts the vegetarian food pyramid.

Both lacto-ovovegetarians and vegans should eat four servings of vitamin B_{12}-fortified foods (meat substitutes, tofu, cereals, soy milk, and nutritional yeast) daily. A daily supplement of vitamin B_{12} is also recommended during pregnancy and while breastfeeding (Penney & Miller, 2008).

Because the best sources of iron and zinc are animal products, vegan diets may also be low in these minerals. In addition, a high fiber intake may reduce mineral (calcium, iron, and zinc) bioavailability. Nurses need to emphasize the use of foods containing these nutrients. A vegetarian food group guide appears in Table 12–2.

FACTORS INFLUENCING NUTRITION

It is important to consider the many factors that affect a client's nutrition. What are the age, lifestyle, and culture of the pregnant

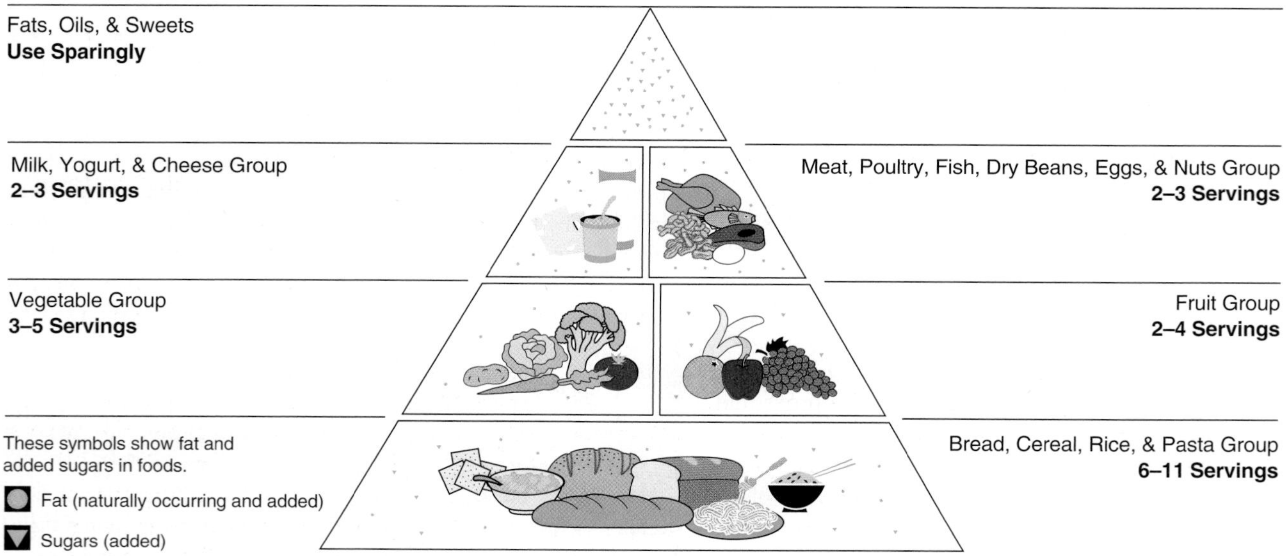

● **Figure 12–2** The vegetarian food pyramid.

Source: Adapted with permission from the Health Connection, 55 West Oak Ridge Drive, Hagerstown, MD 21740-7390.

Table 12–2 Vegetarian Food Groups

Food Group	Mixed Diet	Lacto-ovovegetarian	Lactovegetarian	Vegan
Grain	Bread, cereal, rice, pasta	Bread, cereal, rice, pasta	Bread, cereal, rice, pasta	Bread, cereal, rice, pasta
Fruit	Fruit, fruit juices	Fruit, fruit juices	Fruit, fruit juices	Fruit, fruit juices
Vegetable	Vegetables, vegetable juices	Vegetables, vegetable juices	Vegetables, vegetable juices	Vegetables, vegetable juices
Dairy and dairy alternatives	Milk, yogurt, cheese	Milk, yogurt, cheese	Milk, yogurt, cheese	Fortified soy milk, rice milk
Meat and meat alternatives	Meat, fish, poultry, eggs, legumes, tofu, nuts, nut butters	Eggs, legumes, tofu, nuts, nut butters	Legumes, tofu, nuts, nut butters	Legumes, tofu, nuts, nut butters

woman? What food beliefs and habits does she have? What a person eats is determined by availability, economics, and symbolism. These factors and others influence the expectant mother's acceptance of dietary recommendations.

COMMON DISCOMFORTS OF PREGNANCY

Gastrointestinal functioning can be altered at times during pregnancy, resulting in discomforts such as nausea, vomiting, heartburn, and constipation. Although these changes can be uncomfortable for the woman, they are seldom a major problem. These discomforts and dietary modifications that may provide relief are discussed in Chapter 11∞.

USE OF ARTIFICIAL SWEETENERS

Foods and beverages that contain artificial sweeteners are increasingly available. Sweeteners classified as Generally Recognized as Safe (GRAS) by the Food and Drug Administration are acceptable for use during pregnancy. As with other foods, moderation should be exercised when using artificial sweeteners, such as saccharin, which can cross the placenta and may remain in fetal tissues. Aspartame also appears to be safe if taken within FDA guidelines. Women affected by PKU should avoid aspartame, as phenylalanine intake needs to be monitored. Splenda, or sucralose, is the newest artificial sweetener to become available to the public. Tests have shown Splenda to have no effects on fetal or neonatal development, and support the safety of sucralose for use in pregnant or lactating women.

FOODBORNE ILLNESSES

Because of the risk of *Salmonella* contamination in raw eggs, pregnant women are advised to avoid eating or tasting foods that may contain raw or lightly cooked eggs. These foods include, for example, cake batter, cookie dough made with raw eggs, homemade eggnog, sauces made with raw eggs such as Caesar salad dressing, hollandaise sauce, and homemade ice cream (Food and Drug Administration [FDA], 2005).

Listeria monocytogenes is another bacterium that poses a threat to an expectant mother and her fetus. *Listeria* is especially challenging because the organism can be found in refrigerated, ready-to-eat foods such as unpasteurized milk and dairy products, meat, poultry, and seafood. To prevent listeria infection (listeriosis) pregnant women should be advised to do the following (FDA, 2005):

- Maintain refrigerator temperature at 40°F (4°C) or below and the freezer at 0°F (–18°C).
- Refrigerate or freeze prepared foods, leftovers, and perishables within 2 hours after eating or preparation.
- Do not eat hot dogs and luncheon meats unless they are reheated until they are steaming hot.
- Avoid soft cheeses such as feta, brie, Camembert, blue-veined cheeses, queso fresco or queso blanco (a soft cheese often used by Hispanic women in their cooking) unless the label clearly states that they are made with pasteurized milk.
- Do not eat refrigerated patés or meat spreads, foods that contain raw (unpasteurized) milk, or drink unpasteurized milk.
- Avoid eating refrigerated smoked seafood such as salmon, trout, cod, tuna, or mackerel unless it is in a cooked dish such as a casserole. Canned or shelf-stable patés, meat spreads, and smoked seafood are considered safe to eat.

Hepatitis E is a viral infection found most often in developing countries and spread through the feces of infected people or animals. It is transmitted most often through unclean drinking water but it can also be contracted by eating contaminated food. Hepatitis E is often more severe in pregnant women, especially during the third trimester, and may lead to maternal death (Bazaco, Albrecht, & Malek, 2008).

To prevent hepatitis E, pregnant women should wash their hands thoroughly after using the bathroom, changing diapers, or handling raw foods. When traveling to areas where the quality of the water is uncertain, they should avoid eating raw foods, unpeeled fruit, and uncooked fish. They should also avoid drinking tap water or using ice made with tap water. Rather they should use bottled or boiled water for drinking, tooth brushing, and formula preparation (Bazaco et al., 2008).

Evidence-Based Nursing

FISH CONSUMPTION DURING PREGNANCY

Clinical Question
Is the consumption of fish during pregnancy safe for the developing fetus?

The Evidence
Two researchers reviewed multiple research studies, longitudinal public health reports, and advice from regulatory agencies regarding the effects of maternal fish consumption on fetal health. Aggregation of research reports, and expert advice is the strongest level of evidence. Fetal exposure to mercury in utero causes widespread, sometimes devastating neurologic damage. The primary source of nonoccupational mercury exposure is the consumption of fish and seafood. The highest tissue concentrations of mercury are found in the longest-living, predatory fish. On the other hand, seafood is a primary source of the critical fatty acid docosahexaenoic acid (DHA) that is necessary for brain and eye development. Limiting all fish consumption, particularly in the third trimester when brain and eye development are rapid, may result in fetal harm. The evidence suggests that an average daily intake of at least 200 mg/day of DHA during pregnancy supports optimal brain and eye development, but this research demonstrated that few pregnant women consume this amount (Oken & Bellinger, 2008).

Best Practice
Pregnant women can be reassured that, on balance, there is no harm and some benefit from maternal fish consumption during pregnancy. The fatty acid provided by seafood is desirable during pregnancy to support optimal fetal development. In addition, fish consumption is desirable as an alternative to other protein sources that are higher in saturated fat. However, the mother should choose seafood low in mercury, avoiding the large, longer-living fish such as shark, swordfish, and tuna. It is recommended that women limit fish consumption to two, six-ounce servings per week, avoiding the fish that have the highest mercury content.

Critical Thinking
How can the nurse help the pregnant woman make good choices about seafood consumption during pregnancy?

See MyNursingKit for possible responses.

MERCURY IN FISH

Fish and shellfish are important parts of a healthy diet, but nearly all contain traces of mercury. Although this is not a concern for most people, some fish and shellfish contain higher levels of mercury than others, and mercury can pose a threat to the developing nervous system of an unborn baby or a young child. Mercury exposure can have a negative effect on cognitive functioning resulting in deficiencies in language, attention, motor function, memory, and visual-spatial abilities (Huffling, 2006). Because of this, the U.S. government issued the following guidelines for women who are pregnant or who may become pregnant, breastfeeding mothers, and young children (U.S. Department of Health and Human Services and U.S. Environmental Protection Agency, 2004):

- Do not eat swordfish, shark, tilefish, or king mackerel because these fish contain high levels of mercury.
- Eat up to 12 oz/week (two average meals) of a variety of shellfish and fish that are lower in mercury. (Commonly eaten fish that are lower in mercury include canned light tuna, shrimp, salmon, catfish, and pollack. Albacore [white] tuna has more mercury than canned light tuna, so only 6 oz/week of albacore tuna is recommended.)
- Check local advisories about the mercury content of fish caught locally by family and friends. If no information is available, limit fish caught in local areas to 6 oz/week and avoid consuming additional fish that week.
- Note, however, that fish oil supplements are available that have been lab tested for mercury. It is important to check labels for this lab certification when purchasing fish oil supplements.

LACTASE DEFICIENCY (LACTOSE INTOLERANCE)

Some individuals have difficulty digesting milk and milk products. This condition, known as **lactase deficiency (lactose intolerance)**, results from an inadequate amount of the enzyme lactase, which breaks down the milk sugar lactose into smaller digestible substances.

Lactase deficiency is found in most adults of African, Mexican, Native American, Ashkenazic Jewish, and Asian descent and, indeed, in many other adults worldwide. People of northern European heritage are usually not affected. Symptoms include abdominal distention, discomfort, nausea, vomiting, loose stools, and cramps.

In counseling pregnant women who might be intolerant of milk and milk products, be aware that even one glass of milk can produce symptoms. Milk in cooked form, such as custards, is sometimes tolerated, as are cultured or fermented dairy products such as buttermilk, some cheeses, kefir, and yogurt. Lactase deficiency need not be a problem for pregnant women because the enzyme is available over the counter in tablets or drops. Lactase-treated milk is also available commercially in some grocery stores.

CULTURAL, ETHNIC, AND RELIGIOUS INFLUENCES

Cultural, ethnic, and religious backgrounds determine people's experiences with food and influence food preferences and habits (Figure 12–3 ●). People of different nationalities are accustomed to eating different foods because of the kinds of foodstuffs available in their countries of origin. The way food is prepared varies,

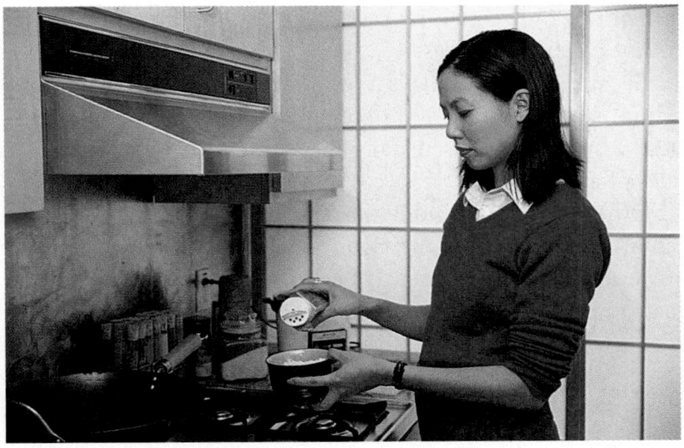

● **Figure 12–3** Culture and food preferences. Food preferences and habits are affected by cultural factors.

depending on the customs and traditions of the ethnic and cultural group. In addition, the laws of certain religions forbid the use of some foods and direct the preparation and serving of meals.

In each culture certain foods have symbolic meaning. Generally these symbolic foods are related to major life experiences such as birth, death, or developmental milestones. Although generalizations have been made about the food practices of ethnic and religious groups, there are many variations. The extent to which people continue to eat traditional ethnic foods and follow food-related ethnic customs is affected by their exposure to other cultures and the availability, quality, and cost of traditional foods.

When working with pregnant women from any ethnic background, it is important to understand the impact of the woman's cultural beliefs on her eating habits and to identify any beliefs she may have about food and pregnancy. Talking with the client can help determine the level of influence that traditional food customs exert. It is then possible to give dietary advice in a way that is meaningful to the woman and her family.

PSYCHOSOCIAL FACTORS

Various psychosocial factors may influence a woman's food choices. The sharing of food has long been a symbol of friendliness, warmth, and social acceptance in many cultures. Some foods and food practices are associated with status. Some foods are prepared "just for company"; others are served only on special occasions or holidays.

Socioeconomic level may be a determinant of nutritional status. Poverty-level families cannot afford the same foods that higher income families can. Thus, pregnant women with low incomes are frequently at risk for poor nutrition.

Knowledge about the basic components of a balanced diet is essential. Often educational level is related to economic status, but even people on very limited incomes can prepare well-balanced meals if they know enough about nutrition.

The expectant mother's attitudes and feelings about her pregnancy influence her nutritional status. For example, foods may be used as a substitute for the expression of emotions, such as anger or frustration, or as a way of expressing feelings of joy. The woman who is depressed or does not wish to be pregnant may manifest these feelings in loss of appetite or overindulgence in certain foods.

EATING DISORDERS

Two serious eating disorders, anorexia nervosa and bulimia nervosa, affect millions of men and women, although they develop most commonly in adolescent girls and young women. Both conditions are psychologic disorders that can have a major impact on physiologic well-being.

Anorexia nervosa is an eating disorder characterized by an extreme fear of weight gain and fat. People with this problem have distorted body images and perceive themselves as fat even when they are extremely underweight. Their dietary intake is very restrictive in both variety and quantity. They may also engage in excessive exercise to prevent weight gain.

Bulimia is characterized by bingeing (secretly consuming large amounts of food in a short time) and purging. Self-induced vomiting is the most common method of purging; laxatives or diuretics may also be used. Individuals with bulimia nervosa often maintain normal or near-normal weight for their height, so it is difficult to know whether bingeing and purging occur.

Individuals with anorexia nervosa do not often become pregnant because of the physiologic changes that affect their reproductive systems. Women with bulimia can become pregnant. Their self-induced vomiting may produce many of the same complications as hyperemesis gravidarum (see Chapter 16∞). In both anorexia nervosa and bulimia, a multidisciplinary approach to treatment, involving medical, nursing, psychiatric, and dietetic practitioners, is indicated. Pregnant women with eating disorders need to be closely monitored and supported throughout their pregnancies.

PICA

Pica is the persistent eating of substances, such as soil or clay (geophagia), powdered laundry starch or corn starch (amylophagia), soap, baking powder, ice (pagophagia), freezer frost, burned matches, or ashes that are not ordinarily considered edible or nutritionally valuable. In the United States, pica has been diagnosed among all socioeconomic and racial groups. However, pica is more common among economically disadvantaged women, women of African-American descent, women who live in rural areas, women who practiced pica before pregnancy, women from cultures where pica is commonly practiced, and women who have family members who also practice pica (Mills, 2007).

Women who practice pica may have nutrient deficiencies because they often consume a less varied diet than they might otherwise eat. Iron deficiency anemia is the most common concern in pica. Eating laundry starch or certain types of clay may contribute to iron deficiency because they interfere with iron absorption. The ingestion of large quantities of clay could fill the intestine and cause fecal impaction; eating starch may be associated with excessive weight gain.

Eating clay or soil is also a risk because of the possible presence of infectious microorganisms that can cause complications. For example, toxoplasmosis, a protozoan that can damage the fetal nervous system (see Chapter 16∞), is found in the soil as is the hookworm, a parasite that may contribute to maternal malnutrition (Mills, 2007).

Assessment for pica is an important part of a nutritional history. However, a woman may be embarrassed about her cravings or reluctant to discuss them for fear of criticism. Using a nonjudgmental approach, give the woman information that can help her decrease or eliminate this practice.

NUTRITIONAL CARE OF THE PREGNANT ADOLESCENT

Nutritional care of the pregnant adolescent is of particular concern to healthcare professionals. Many adolescents are nutritionally at risk because of a variety of complex emotional, social, and economic factors. Important nutrition-related factors to assess in pregnant adolescents include low prepregnant weight, low weight gain during pregnancy, young age at menarche, smoking, excessive prepregnant weight, anemia, unhealthy lifestyle (drugs or alcohol use), chronic disease, and history of an eating disorder.

The nutritional needs of adolescents are generally estimated by using the DRI for nonpregnant teenagers (ages 11 to 14 or 15 to 18) and adding nutrient amounts recommended for all women. If she is mature (more than 4 years since menarche), the pregnant adolescent's nutritional needs approach those reported for pregnant adults. However, adolescents who become pregnant less than 4 years after menarche are at risk due to their physiologic and anatomic immaturity. They are more likely than older adolescents to still be growing, which can affect the fetus's development. Thus, young adolescents (age 14 and younger) need to gain more weight than older adolescents (18 years and older) to produce babies of equal size.

In determining the optimal weight gain for the pregnant adolescent, add the recommended weight gain for an adult pregnancy to that expected during the postmenarcheal year in which the pregnancy occurs. If the teenager is underweight, additional weight gain is recommended to bring her to a normal weight for her height.

SPECIFIC NUTRIENT CONCERNS

Caloric needs of pregnant adolescents vary widely. Major factors in determining caloric needs include whether growth has been completed and the physical activity level of the individual. Figures as high as 50 kcal/kg have been suggested for young, growing teens who are very active physically. A satisfactory weight gain usually confirms an adequate caloric intake.

An inadequate iron intake is a major concern with the adolescent diet. Iron needs are high for the pregnant teen due to the requirement for iron by the enlarging maternal muscle mass and blood volume. Iron supplements are definitely indicated.

Calcium is another important nutrient for pregnant adolescents. Inadequate intake of calcium is often a problem in this age group. Adequate calcium intake is necessary to support normal growth and development of the fetus as well as growth and maintenance of calcium stores in the adolescent. An extra serving of dairy products is usually suggested for teenagers. Calcium supplementation is indicated for teens who dislike milk, unless they consume enough other dairy products or significant calcium sources.

Because folic acid plays a role in cell reproduction, it is also an important nutrient for pregnant teens. As previously indicated, a supplement is usually recommended for pregnant females of all ages.

Other nutrients and vitamins must be considered when evaluating the overall nutritional quality of the teenager's diet. Nutrients that have frequently been found to be deficient in this age group include zinc and vitamins A, D, and B_6. Eating a variety of foods—especially fresh and lightly processed foods—helps the teen get adequate amounts of trace minerals, fiber, and other vitamins.

DIETARY PATTERNS

Healthy adolescents often have irregular eating patterns. Many skip breakfast, and most tend to be frequent snackers. Teens rarely follow the traditional three-meals-a-day pattern. Their day-to-day intake often varies drastically, and they eat food combinations that may seem bizarre to adults. Despite these practices, adolescents usually achieve a better nutritional balance than most adults would expect.

In assessing the diet of the pregnant adolescent, it is important to consider the eating pattern over time, not simply a single day's intake. Once the pattern is identified, counseling can be directed toward correcting deficiencies.

COUNSELING ISSUES

Counseling about nutrition and healthy eating practices is an important element of care for pregnant teenagers. Nurses can effectively provide this counseling in a community setting. It may be individualized, involve other teens, or provide a combination of both approaches. If an adolescent's family member does most of the meal preparation, it may be useful to include that person in the discussion if the adolescent agrees. Involving the expectant father in counseling may also be helpful. Clinics and schools often offer classes and focused activities designed to address this topic.

The pregnant teenager's understanding of nutrition will influence not only her well-being but also that of her child. However, teens tend to live in the present, and counseling that stresses long-term changes may be less effective than more concrete approaches. In many cases, group classes are effective, especially those with other teens.

POSTPARTUM NUTRITION

Nutritional needs change following childbirth. Nutrient requirements vary depending on whether the mother decides to breastfeed. An assessment of postpartum nutritional status is necessary before nutritional guidance is given.

POSTPARTUM NUTRITIONAL STATUS

Postpartum nutritional status is determined by assessing the new mother's weight, hemoglobin and hematocrit levels, clinical signs, and dietary history. As mentioned previously, an ideal weight gain during pregnancy is 25 to 35 lb (11.5 to 16 kg). After birth there is a weight loss of approximately 10 to 12 lb. Additional weight loss is most rapid during the next few weeks as the body adjusts to the end of pregnancy. The mother's weight then begins to stabilize. This weight stabilization may take 6 months or longer. The mother's weight should be considered in terms of ideal weight, prepregnancy weight, and weight gain during pregnancy. Refer women who want information about weight reduction to a dietitian. Educational programs need to address a variety of issues such as the significance of the quality of food eaten rather than the quantity; the importance of regular physical activity in improving health, building lean muscle mass, and increasing metabolism; and the value of meal planning to ensure that healthy foods are readily available and to avoid pitfalls such as opting for fast foods, which are often high in fat (Smith, Hulsey, & Goodnight, 2008).

Hemoglobin and erythrocyte levels should return to normal within 2 to 6 weeks after childbirth. Iron supplements are generally continued for 2 to 3 months following childbirth to build stores depleted by pregnancy.

Constipation is a common problem following birth. To prevent it the woman should maintain a high fluid intake, which helps keep the stool soft. Dietary sources of fiber, such as whole grains, fruits, and vegetables, also help prevent constipation.

It is important to get specific information on dietary intake and eating habits directly from the woman. Visiting the mother during mealtimes provides an opportunity for unobtrusive nutritional assessment. Which foods has the woman selected? Is her diet nutritionally sound? A comment focusing on a positive aspect of her meal selection may initiate a discussion of nutrition.

Notify the dietitian about any woman whose cultural or religious beliefs require specific foods so that appropriate meals can be prepared for her. Also consider referring women with unusual eating habits or numerous questions about good nutrition to the dietitian. In addition, providing literature on nutrition ensures that the woman has a source of information at home.

NUTRITIONAL CARE OF FORMULA-FEEDING MOTHERS

After birth the formula-feeding mother's dietary requirements return to prepregnancy levels. If the mother has a good understanding of nutritional principles, it is sufficient to advise her to reduce her daily caloric intake by about 300 kcal and to return to prepregnancy levels for other nutrients.

If the mother has a limited understanding of nutrition, now is the time to teach her the basic principles and the importance of a well-balanced diet. Her eating habits and dietary practices will eventually be reflected in the diet of her child.

If the mother has gained excessive weight during pregnancy (or perhaps was overweight before pregnancy) and wishes to lose weight, a referral to the dietitian is appropriate. The dietitian can design weight reduction diets to meet nutritional needs and food preferences. Weight loss goals of 1 to 2 lb/week are usually suggested.

In addition to meeting her own nutritional needs, the new mother is usually interested in learning how to provide for her infant's nutritional needs. A discussion of infant feeding that includes topics such as selecting infant formulas, formula preparation, and vitamin and mineral supplementation are appropriate and generally well received.

Nursing Practice

Explain to breastfeeding mothers that liquids are especially important during lactation, because inadequate fluid intake may decrease milk volume. Encourage them to drink at least 8 to 10 (8-oz) glasses of fluid daily, including water, juice, milk, and soups.

NUTRITIONAL CARE OF BREASTFEEDING MOTHERS

A breastfeeding woman needs increased nutrients. Table 12–1 provides a sample daily food guide for lactating women. It is especially important for the breastfeeding mother to consume sufficient calories, because inadequate caloric intake can reduce milk volume. However, milk quality generally remains unaffected. The breastfeeding mother should increase her calories by about 200 kcal over her pregnancy requirement, or 500 kcal over her prepregnancy requirement. This results in a total of about 2500 to 2700 kcal/day for most women.

Because protein is an important ingredient in breast milk, an adequate intake while breastfeeding is essential. An intake of 65 g/day during the first 6 months of breastfeeding and 62 g/day during the second 6 months is recommended. As in pregnancy, it is important to consume adequate nonprotein calories to prevent the use of protein as an energy source.

Calcium is an important ingredient in milk production. Requirements during lactation remain the same as during pregnancy—an increase of 1000 mg/day. If the intake of calcium from food sources is not adequate, calcium supplements are recommended.

Iron is not a principal mineral component of milk; thus, the needs of lactating women are not substantially different from those of nonpregnant women. However, supplementation for 2 to 3 months after childbirth is advisable to replenish maternal stores depleted by pregnancy.

In addition to counseling breastfeeding mothers on how to meet their increased nutrient needs, the nurse should discuss a few issues related to infant feeding. For example, many mothers are concerned about how specific foods they eat will affect their babies during breastfeeding. Generally the breastfeeding mother need not avoid any foods except those to which she might be allergic. Occasionally, however, some breastfeeding mothers find that their babies are affected by certain foods. Onions, turnips, cabbage, chocolate, spices, and seasonings are commonly listed as offenders. The best advice to give the breastfeeding mother is to avoid those foods she suspects cause distress in her infant. For the most part, however, she should be able to eat any nourishing food she wants without fear that her baby will be affected. For further discussion of successful infant feeding, see Chapter 27.

NURSING MANAGEMENT

NURSING ASSESSMENT AND DIAGNOSIS

In order to plan an optimal diet with each woman, it is essential to assess nutritional status. The woman's chart and a client interview provide information about (1) the woman's height and weight, as well as her weight gain during pregnancy; (2) pertinent laboratory values, especially hemoglobin and hematocrit; (3) clinical signs that have possible nutritional implications, such as constipation, anorexia, or heartburn; and (4) dietary history to evaluate the woman's views on nutrition as well as her specific nutrient intake.

While gathering data, seek information about psychologic, cultural, and socioeconomic factors that may influence food intake. Also use the opportunity to discuss important aspects of nutrition within the context of the family's needs and lifestyle. A nutritional questionnaire is often useful in gathering and recording important facts. This information can be used to develop an intervention plan to fit the woman's individual needs. The sample questionnaire shown in Figure 12–4 ● has been filled in to demonstrate this process.

Once information is obtained, begin to analyze the information, formulate appropriate nursing diagnoses, and, with the woman, develop goals and desired outcomes. For a woman during the first trimester, for example, the diagnosis may be *Imbalanced Nutrition: Less than Body Requirements related to nausea and vomiting.* If a woman has excessive weight gain, the diagnosis might be *Imbalanced Nutrition: More Than Body Requirements related to excessive caloric intake.* Be specific in addressing issues such as inadequate intake of nutrients, including iron, calcium, or folic acid; problems with nutrition because of a limited food budget; problems related to physiologic alterations, including anorexia, heartburn, or nausea; and behavioral problems related to excessive dieting, binge eating, and so on. At other times the diagnosis *health-seeking behaviors* may seem most appropriate, especially if the woman asks for information about nutrition.

PLANNING AND IMPLEMENTATION

After determining the nursing diagnosis, plan an approach to address any nutritional deficiencies or improve the overall quality of the diet. To be truly effective, this plan must be made in cooperation with the woman. The following example demonstrates ways to plan with the woman based on the nursing diagnosis:

- Nursing Diagnosis: *Imbalanced Nutrition: Less than Body Requirements related to low intake of calcium*
- Goal: The woman will increase her daily intake of calcium to the minimum DRI level.
- Implementation:

  1. Plan with the woman how to add more milk or dairy products to the diet (specify amounts).
  2. Encourage the use of other calcium sources such as leafy greens and legumes.
  3. Plan for the addition of powdered milk in cooking and baking.
  4. If none of the preceding options are realistic or acceptable, consider the use of calcium supplements.

Most families can benefit from guidance about food purchasing and preparation. Advise women to plan food purchases thoughtfully by preparing general menus and a list before shopping. It is also helpful to monitor sales, compare brands, and be cautious when purchasing convenience foods, which tend to be expensive. Other techniques for keeping food costs down without jeopardizing quality include buying food in season, using bulk foods when appropriate, using whole-grain or enriched products, buying lower grade eggs (grading has no relation to the egg's nutritional value but indicates color of the shell, delicacy of flavor, and so forth), and avoiding foods from specialty shops and foods in elaborate packaging.

NURSING CARE IN THE COMMUNITY

Food is a significant portion of a family's budget, and meeting nutritional needs may be a challenge for families on limited incomes. Community-based services offered through clinics, local agencies, schools, and volunteer organizations address these needs. Increasingly nurses play an important role in managing such community-based services, especially services focusing on client education. Most communities offer special assistance to qualifying families to meet their nutritional needs. The Food Stamp Program provides stamps or coupons for participating households whose net monthly income is below a specified level. These stamps can be used to purchase food for the household each month.

The Special Supplemental Food Program for Women, Infants, and Children (WIC) is designed to assist pregnant or breastfeeding women with low incomes and their children younger than 5 years of age. The program provides food assistance, nutrition education, and referrals to healthcare providers. The food distributed, including dried beans and peas, peanut butter, eggs, cheese, milk, fortified adult and infant cereals, juice, and iron-fortified formula, is designed to provide good sources of iron, protein, and certain vitamins and minerals for people with an inadequate diet.

EVALUATION

Once a plan has been developed and implemented, work with the woman to identify ways of evaluating its effectiveness. This may involve keeping a food journal, writing out weekly menus, returning for weekly weigh-ins, and the like. If anemia is a special problem, periodic hematocrit assessments are also indicated. Refer women with serious nutritional deficiencies to a dietitian.

NUTRITIONAL QUESTIONNAIRE

Name Susan Longmont Date 2-18-10

Age 20

Ethnic group Caucasian

Religion Protestant

Gravida 1 Para 0 EDB 9-12-10

Age of youngest child? NA

Birth weights of previous children? NA

Usual nonpregnant weight 119 Present weight 125

Weight gain during last pregnancy? NA

Vitamin or herbal supplements? none

Current medications? aspirin for headache

Do you smoke? yes How much per day? 1-1$^1/_2$ packs

Have you ever had anorexia or bulimia? ______ Please describe the circumstances. ______

Eating patterns:

1. How many meals per day? 2 when 12:30 pm 6:30 pm
2. How many snacks per day? 3 when 10:30 am 4:00 pm 10:00 pm
3. What other foods are important to your usual diet? chocolate and candy bars
4. Amount per day 4 bars/week
5. Do you have any different food preferences now? no
6. Do you eat nonfoods such as:

		Amount
laundry starch	no	NA
ice	yes	10 cubes/day
other (name)	no	NA

7. What foods do you dislike or do not eat? spinach and dried beans
8. For added information complete a typical daily intake (24-hour recall is suggested).

Do you have special problems in food preparation such as:

1. Physical disability yes ______ no ✓ Explain ______
2. Cooking appliances yes ______ no ✓ Explain ______
3. Refrigeration of food yes ______ no ✓ Explain ______

Who does the meal planning? I do. shopping? We both do.

cooking? I do most of the time but my husband likes to help.

Are there transportation problems? We have only one car but we go in the evening.

Financial situation: My husband is working and going to school.

I am not working. Food Stamps yes WIC no

Do you have any previous nutritional problems? No. I have never paid much attention to food before, but now I have lots of questions.

Are there any problems with this pregnancy? Nausea Yes, in the morning.

Constipation No Other NA

Assessment by the nurse following the completion of the questionnaire.

Basic estimated nutrient and caloric value of typical daily intake.

Please circle one of the following:

Protein intake was	low	**adequate**	high
Caloric intake was	low	adequate	**high**
Calcium intake was	**low**	adequate	high
Iron intake was	**low**	adequate	high
Vitamin C intake was	low	**adequate**	high

● **Figure 12–4** Nutritional questionnaire. The form shown here is a sample nutritional questionnaire used in nursing management of a pregnant woman.

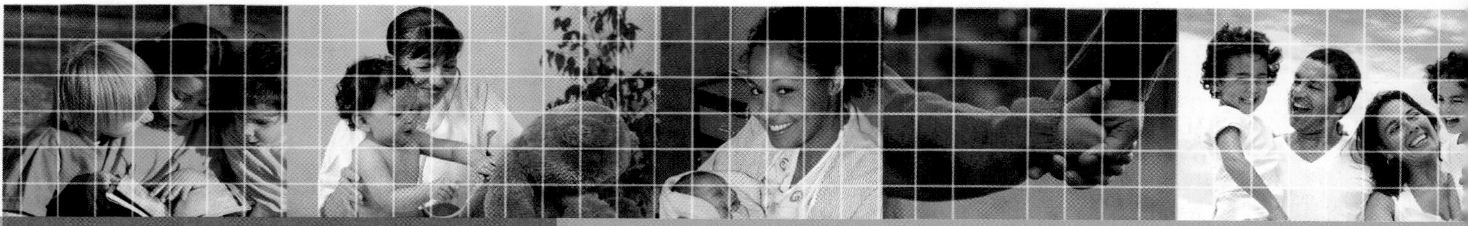

CRITICAL CONCEPT REVIEW

LEARNING OUTCOMES — CONCEPTS

12.1 Consider recommended levels of weight gain during pregnancy when providing nursing care for pregnant women.

1. Weight gain recommendations are dependent upon the woman's prepregnancy weight:
   - Underweight: 28–40 lb (12.5 to 18 kg)
   - Normal weight: 25–35 lb (11.5 to 16 kg)
   - Overweight: 15–25 lb (7 to 11.5 kg)
   - Obese: less than or equal to 15 lb (less than or equal to 7 kg)

12.2 Recognize the significance of specific nutrients in the diet of the pregnant woman.

1. Carbohydrates: The body's primary source of energy. Promotes weight gain and growth of the fetus and placenta.
2. Protein: Supplies needed amino acids for growth of tissue.
3. Fat: Source of maternal energy; also promotes fetal fat deposits.
4. Calcium and phosphorus: Promotes mineralization of fetal bones and teeth.
5. Iodine: Promotes fetal thyroid gland function.
6. Sodium: Regulates fluid balance and metabolism in the mother.
7. Zinc: Promotes growth of fetus and sufficient lactation.
8. Magnesium: Promotes cellular metabolism and bone mineralization.
9. Iron: Prevents maternal anemia and contributes to fetal and infant stores of iron.
10. Vitamins: Maintain good maternal health. Folic acid, taken prior to conception, may prevent neural tube defects in the fetus.

12.3 Compare nutritional needs during pregnancy, the postpartum period, and lactation with nonpregnant requirements.

1. During pregnancy and lactation, nutritional requirements increase significantly from nonpregnant requirements:
   - Calories in second and third trimester increase by 300 kcal/day, and during lactation, by another 200 kcal/day.
   - Protein increases by 14 mg to 60 g/day.
   - Calcium requirements for the pregnant or lactating woman increase to 1000–1300 mg/day depending upon the age of the woman.
   - Magnesium increases to 350 mg/day.
   - Iron increases to 27 mg/day. (It is very difficult to eat enough iron-rich foods in the regular diet, so iron supplements are commonly prescribed.)
   - Iodine increases to 220 mcg/day.
   - Zinc increases to 11 mg/day during pregnancy and 12 mg/day during lactation.
   - Vitamin A increases to 770 mcg/day.
   - Vitamin D increases to 5 mcg/day.
   - Vitamin C increases from 75 to 85 mg/day.
   - Thiamine increases from 1.1 mg to 1.4 mg/day.
   - Riboflavin increases from 1.1 mg to 1.4 mg/day.
   - Niacin increases from 14 to 18 mg/day.
   - Pantothenic acid increases to 5 mg/day.
   - Vitamin B_{12} increases from 2.4 to 2.6 mcg/day.
   - Fluid needs increase to 8–10 glasses of noncaffeinated beverages/day.
2. For nonbreastfeeding mothers, during the postpartum period, nutritional requirements return to prepregnancy levels.

12.4 Plan adequate prenatal vegetarian diets based on the nutritional requirements of pregnancy.

1. There are different types of vegetarian diets, which differ in the types of animal-based products that are eaten.
2. Vegans do not eat any animal-based products, but can obtain protein from beans, rice, peanut butter, soy products, and seeds. Most vegans need additional supplementation of vitamins B_{12} and D, and calcium.
3. Vegetarians' daily food requirements are:
   - 6–11 servings of whole grains, cereal, pasta, and rice.
   - 2–4 servings of fruit.
   - 3–5 servings of vegetables.
   - 2–3 servings of legumes, nuts, seeds, and meat alternatives.
   - 2–3 servings of milk products (unless vegan).

LEARNING OUTCOMES / CONCEPTS

LEARNING OUTCOMES	CONCEPTS
12.5 Consider ways in which various physical, psychosocial, and cultural factors can affect nutritional intake and status in the nursing care management of pregnant women.	1. Nausea, vomiting, constipation, and heartburn can limit a woman's intake of nutritional foods especially during the first trimester. 2. Lactose intolerance may cause diarrhea or bloating after intake of dairy products. 3. Cultural, ethnic, and religious influences may prohibit use of certain foods that are needed for adequate nutrition. 4. Socioeconomic level may limit amounts of nutritional foods available to the woman. 5. Lack of knowledge about proper nutrition may limit the woman's ability to prepare nutritional foods. 6. Clients with eating disorders may have nutritional and electrolyte imbalances due to starvation or vomiting. 7. Pica may result in iron deficiency anemia.
12.6 Compare recommendations for weight gain and nutrient intakes in the pregnant adolescent with those for the mature pregnant adult.	1. Weight gain: Add recommended weight gain of the adult pregnancy to the expected gain of the adolescent. 2. Nutrient needs: Adolescent needs more iron, calcium, and folic acid than the adult pregnant woman.
12.7 Explore basic factors a nurse should consider when offering nutritional counseling to a pregnant adolescent.	1. Basic factors to consider: ■ Number of years since adolescent reached menarche. ■ Whether growth has been completed. ■ Most adolescents have irregular eating patterns. ■ Adolescent may not be the one who regularly prepares meals, so the individual who prepares meals should be included in nutritional counseling. ■ Teens are present, not future, oriented, which impacts nutritional counseling.
12.8 Compare nutritional counseling issues for breastfeeding and formula-feeding mothers.	1. Formula-feeding mothers: ■ Eat a well-balanced diet. ■ Dietary requirements are the same as before pregnancy. ■ Weight loss of 1–2 lb/week is acceptable. 2. Breastfeeding mothers: ■ Calorie requirements increase by 200 kcal/day over needs during pregnancy. ■ Need 2500–2700 kcal/day. ■ Need 65 g/day of protein. ■ Need 1000 mg/day of calcium. ■ Should avoid foods that irritate the infant.

CRITICAL THINKING IN ACTION

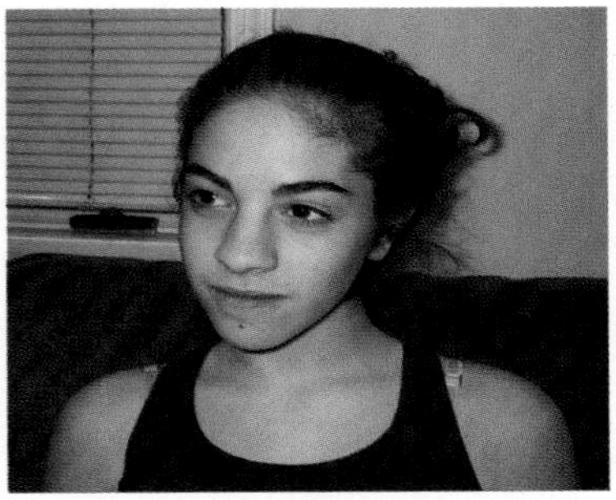

Sandra Hill is a 17-year-old at 19 weeks' gestation with her first pregnancy. She presents to you accompanied by her mother. Her mother tells you that Sandra is an active teenager who plays sports and has been taking dance lessons for 5 years. She maintains a B+ average in school. Sandra voices concern about potential weight gain during pregnancy. She tells you that this was not a planned pregnancy and she has ambivalent feelings about it. You become concerned as she tells you that she has reduced her caloric intake over the last few months to try to keep her weight down and camouflage her pregnancy. You do a nutritional assessment and find that she is deficient in calcium, iron, and protein. Sandra seems to have irregular eating patterns and she admits to skipping breakfast often. She asks why she has to gain so much weight when you explain the nutritional needs of her baby during the pregnancy.

1. Discuss weight distribution in pregnancy.
2. Discuss foods that will increase calcium, protein, and iron in her diet.
3. Explain why folate supplementation is important.
4. What criteria will measure adequate caloric intake during pregnancy?

See MyNursingKit for possible responses.

REFERENCES

Brazaco, M. C., Albrecht, S. A., & Malek, A. M. (2008). Preventing foodborne infection in pregnant women and infants. *Nursing for Women's Health, 12*(1), 46–54.

Centers for Disease Control and Prevention. (2009). *Women need 400 micrograms of folic acid every day.* Retrieved January 26, 2009, from www.cdc.gov/Features/FolicAcid/

Chu, S. Y., Kim, S. Y., Schmid, C. H., Dietz, P. M., Callaghan, W. M., Lau, J., et al. (2007). Maternal obesity and risk of cesarean delivery: A meta-analysis. *Obesity Reviews, 8*(5), 385–394.

DiLillo, M., Hendrix, N., O'Neill, M., & Berghella, V. (2008). Pregnancy in obese women: What you need to know. *Contemporary OB/GYN, 53*(11), 48–53.

Food and Drug Administration (FDA). (2005). *Food safety for mothers-to-be: Educator's resource guide.* College Park, MD: Center for Food Safety and Applied Nutrition.

Gautam, C. S., Saka, L., Sekhri, K., & Saha, P. (2008). Iron deficiency in pregnancy and the rationality of iron supplements prescribed during pregnancy. *Medscape Journal of Medicine.* 10(12): 283.

Huffling, K. (2006). The effects of environmental contaminants in food on women's health. *Journal of Midwifery and Women's Health, 51*(1), 19–25.

Institute of Medicine (IOM). (2009). *Weight gain during pregnancy: Reexamining the guidelines.* Washington, DC: National Academies Press.

Institute of Medicine, Subcommittee on Dietary Intake and Nutrient Supplements During Pregnancy, Committee on Nutrition Status During Pregnancy and Lactation, Food and Nutrition Board. (1990). *Nutrition during pregnancy: Weight gain and nutrient supplements.* Washington, DC: National Academy Press.

Katz, V. L. (2008). Prenatal care. In R. S. Gibbs, B. Y. Karlan, A. F. Haney, & I. E. Nygaard, (Eds.). *Danforth's Obstetrics and Gynecology* (10th ed.). Philadelphia: WoltersKluwer/Lippincott Williams & Wilkins.

Kominiarek, M. A. (2008). Obesity in pregnancy: Techniques for effective counseling. *The Female Patient, 33*(9), 17–26.

McGregor, J. A., & French, J. I. (2008). Optimizing perinatal and maternal nutrition: Omega-3 fatty acids and folic acid. *The Female Patient, June Supplement,* 19–23.

Mills, M. E. (2007). More than food: The implications of pica in pregnancy. *Nursing for Women's Health, 11*(3), 266–273.

National Institutes of Health. (2007). *Dietary Supplement Fact Sheet: Vitamin D.* Retrieved January 3, 2008, from www.ods.od.nih.gov/factsheets/vitamind.asp

Oken, E., & Bellinger, D. 2008. Fish consumption, methylmercury and child neurodevelopment. *Current Opinions in Pediatrics.* 20:178–183.

Penney, D. S., & Miller, K. G. (2008). Nutritional counseling for vegetarians during pregnancy. *Journal of Midwifery & Women's Health, 53,* 37–44.

Reece, E. A. (2008). Perspectives on obesity, pregnancy and bith outcomes in the United States: The scope of the problem. *American Journal of Obstetrics and Gynecology, 198*(1), 23–27.

Smith, S. A., Hulsey, T., & Goodnight, W. (2008). Effects of obesity on pregnancy. *JOGNN, 37*(2), 176–184.

Spina Bifida Association (2008). Folic acid. Retrieved January 26, 2009, from www.spinabifidaassociation.org

U.S. Department of Health and Human Services and U.S. Environmental Protection Agency. (2004). *What you need to know about mercury in fish and shellfish.* Retrieved April 24, 2004, from www.cfsan.fda.gov/~dms/admehg3.html

U.S. Preventive Services Task Force. (2009). Folic acid for the prevention of neural tube defects: U.S. Preventive Services Task Force Recommendation Statement. *Annals of Internal Medicine, 150*(9), 626–631.

Walker, L. O. (2007). Managing excessive weight gain during pregnancy and the postpartum period. *Journal of Obstetric, Gynecologic & Neonatal Nursing, 36*(5), 490–500.

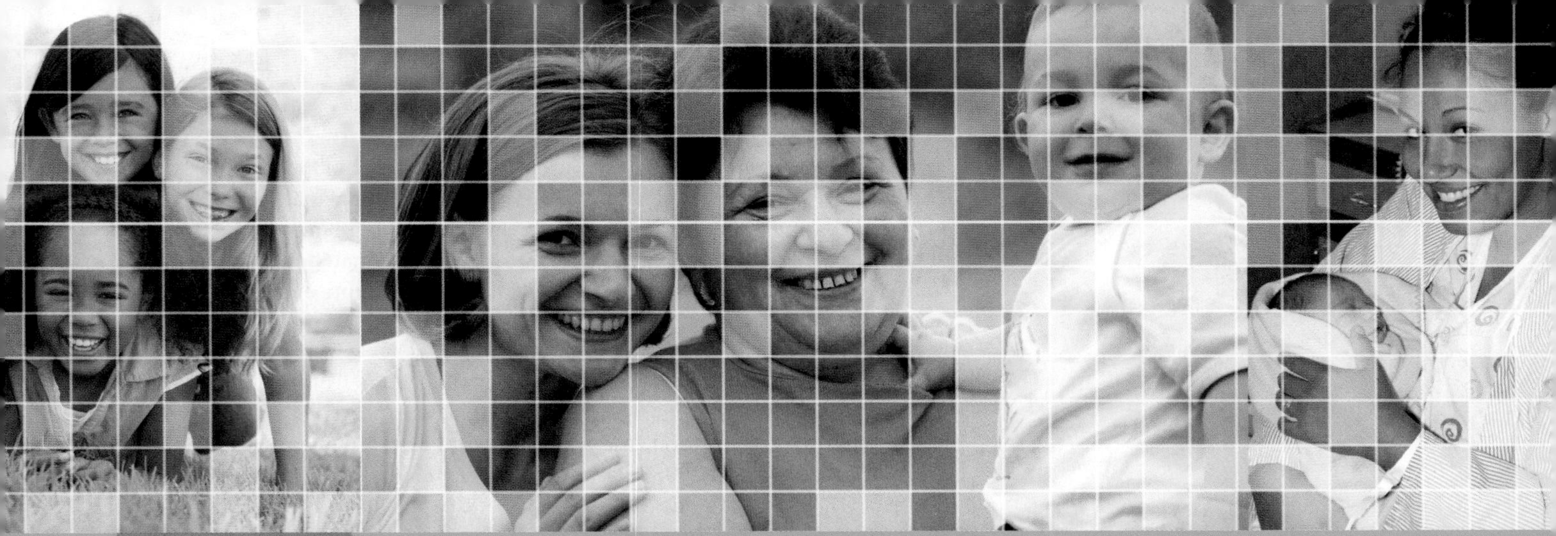

CHAPTER

13 Adolescent Pregnancy

I was a child when I had my daughter—just 16—and so afraid. I was one of the lucky ones though. My parents were wonderfully supportive and I went to a special teen clinic for my pregnancy. The nurses really taught me a lot about my body and about taking care of my baby. With help and encouragement from Mom and Dad, I got by. Last spring, at age 28 I graduated with a degree in nursing. I wanted a job with real security and opportunity, but more important, I want to give something back, to give others a little of the support I received. —*Joanna, 29*

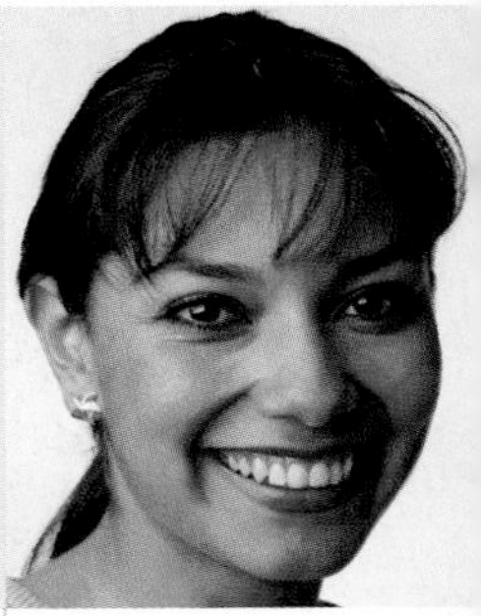

LEARNING OUTCOMES

13.1 Describe the scope of the problem and the impact of adolescent pregnancy.

13.2 Summarize factors contributing to adolescent pregnancy in the nursing care management of this population.

13.3 Assess the physical, psychologic, and sociologic risks a pregnant adolescent faces.

13.4 Delineate the characteristics of the fathers of children of adolescent mothers.

13.5 Discuss the range of reactions of the adolescent's family and social network to her pregnancy.

13.6 Formulate a plan of care to meet the needs of a pregnant adolescent.

13.7 Explore successful community approaches to prevention of adolescent pregnancy.

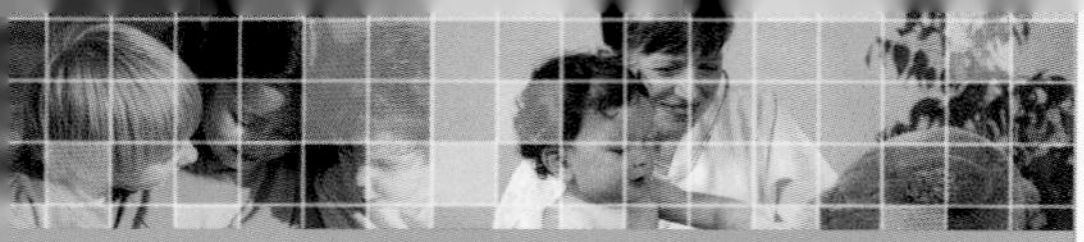

KEY TERMS

Early adolescence, 272
Late adolescence, 273
Middle adolescence, 273

Pregnancy can be challenging, and especially for the adolescent expectant mother. In the United States each year about 750,000 teenage girls (ages 15 to 19) become pregnant, and 8 out of 10 of these pregnancies are unplanned (National Campaign to Prevent Teen and Unplanned pregnancy [NCPTUP], 2006). Of these pregnancies, about one-third (34%) are terminated by therapeutic abortion (Alan Guttmacher Institute [AGI], 2006b). A portion of pregnancies end in miscarriage but more than half of teens who become pregnant give birth and keep their babies.

The U.S. birth rate (number of births per 1000 women) for adolescents ages 15 to 19 dropped by 34 percent from 1991 to 2005, which was an encouraging trend. From 2005 to 2007, however, the teen birth rate rose 5 percent to 42.5 births per 1000 teens from 40.5 in 2005 (Hamilton, Martin, & Ventura, 2009). This rate still is significantly lower than the 1991 rate of 61.8 per 1000 women (Hamilton et al., 2007) (Figure 13–1 ●). Much of this decline over the years is directly attributable to improved contraceptive use (Santelli, Lindberg, Finer, et al., 2007). Nevertheless, the United States continues to have one of the highest levels of adolescent childbearing among industrialized nations (NCPTUP, 2006). The incidence of sexual activity among teens in many other countries is as high as it is in the United States. These countries may have lower adolescent pregnancy rates because of family influences, a greater openness about sexuality, better access to contraceptives, and a more comprehensive approach to sex education.

This chapter explores the issue of adolescent pregnancy and the role of the nurse in meeting the special needs and concerns of pregnant adolescents and their families. It concludes with a discussion of efforts to prevent adolescent pregnancy.

OVERVIEW OF THE ADOLESCENT PERIOD

PHYSICAL CHANGES

Puberty—that period during which an individual becomes capable of reproduction—is a maturational process that can last from 1.5 to 6 years. The major physical changes of puberty include a growth spurt, weight change, and the appearance of secondary sexual characteristics. Menarche, or the time of the first menstrual period, usually occurs in the last half of this maturational process, with the average age between 12 and 13. The initial menstrual cycles are usually irregular and often anovulatory, although not always. Thus, contraception is important for all sexually active adolescents.

PSYCHOSOCIAL DEVELOPMENT

Many writers have described the developmental tasks of adolescence, based on a variety of classic theories. The following are major developmental tasks of this period (Steinberg, 2005):

- Developing a sense of identity
- Gaining autonomy and independence
- Developing intimacy in a relationship
- Developing comfort with one's own sexuality
- Developing a sense of achievement

Resolution of these tasks is a developmental process that occurs over time. Although average ages for the completion of tasks have been identified, these ages are somewhat arbitrary and are affected by many factors, including culture, religion, and socioeconomic status.

In **early adolescence** (age 14 and under) the teen still sees authority in his/her parents. However, he or she begins the process of gaining independence from the family by spending more time with friends. Conformity to peer group standards is important. The adolescent in this phase is very egocentric and is a concrete thinker,

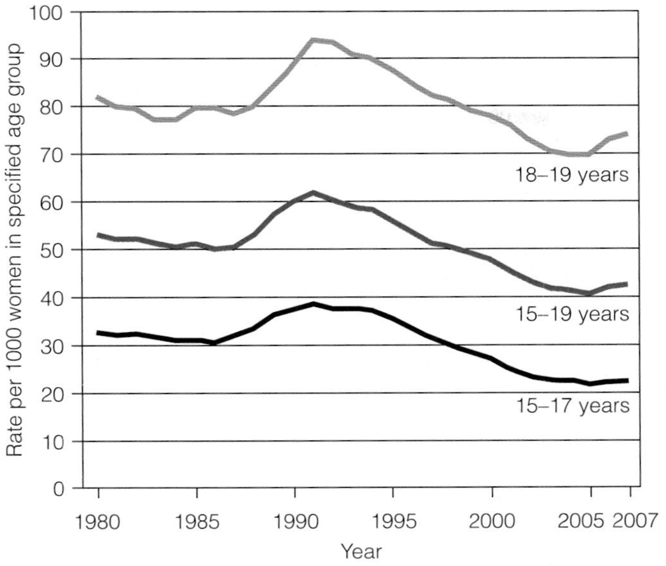

● **Figure 13–1** Birth rates for teenagers by age: United States, final 1980–2006 and preliminary 2007.

Source: Hamilton, B. E., Martin, J., & Ventura, S. J. (2007). Births: Preliminary data for 2007. *National Vital Statistics Reports, 57* (12), 1-23.

with only minimal ability to see him- or herself in the future or to foresee the consequences of his or her behavior. Teens perceive their locus of control as external; that is, their destinies are controlled by others such as parents and school authorities.

Middle adolescence (ages 15 to 17 years) is the time for challenging; experimenting with drugs, alcohol, and sex are common avenues for rebellion. Middle adolescents seek independence and turn increasingly to their peer groups. They begin to move from concrete thinking to formal operational thought but are not yet able to anticipate the long-term implications of all their actions. These years are often a time of great turmoil for the family as the adolescent struggles for independence and challenges the family's values and expectations.

In **late adolescence** (ages 18 to 19 years) teens are more at ease with their individuality and decision-making ability. They can think abstractly and anticipate consequences. Late adolescents are capable of formal operational thought. They learn to solve problems, to conceptualize, and to make decisions. These abilities help them see themselves as having control, which leads to the ability to understand and accept the consequences of their behavior.

FACTORS CONTRIBUTING TO ADOLESCENT PREGNANCY

SOCIOECONOMIC AND CULTURAL FACTORS

Poverty is a major risk factor for adolescent pregnancy. Adolescents who do not have access to middle-class opportunities tend to maintain their pregnancies, because they see pregnancy as their only option for adult status; 85% of births to unmarried teens occur to those from poor or low-income families (AGI, 2006a). Not surprisingly, research indicates that the more time high-school students spend without adult supervision, the greater their level of sexual activity.

In the United States, the adolescent birth rate is higher among African-American teens (63.7 per 1000) and Hispanic teens (83 per 1000) than among white teens (26.6 per 1000). However, until 2006 these pregnancy rates had been declining (Hamilton et al., 2007). To some degree, the higher teenage pregnancy rate in these groups reflects the impact of poverty, as a disproportionately higher number of African American and Hispanic youths live in poverty.

Low educational achievement is another major risk factor for adolescent pregnancy. Teenage girls who participate in after-school activities are less likely to be sexually experienced than girls who do not participate (Albert, Lippman, Franzetta, et al., 2005). Similarly, compared with other teens, teens with future goals (i.e., college or job) tend to use birth control more consistently; if they become pregnant, they are also more likely to have abortions.

The younger the teen when she first gets pregnant, the more likely she is to have another pregnancy in her teens. Moreover, the likelihood of repeat pregnancies increases when the teen is living with her sexual partner and has dropped out of school. Then, too, girls whose sister had a baby in her early teens and girls whose mother and sister both gave birth as teens are significantly more likely to have a teenage pregnancy themselves (East, Reyes, & Horn, 2007).

Internationally, adolescent women are more likely to welcome a pregnancy in a country in which Islam is the predominant religion, where large families are desired, where social change is slow in coming, and where most childbearing occurs within marriage. Early pregnancy is less desired in countries in which the reverse is true.

HIGH-RISK BEHAVIORS

Developmentally, adolescents, especially younger ones, are not yet able to foresee the consequences of their actions. As a result, they may have a sense of invulnerability that leads to the mistaken idea that harm will not befall them. This sense of invulnerability may also result in an overly optimistic view of the risks associated with their actions (King-Jones, 2008).

Among American adolescents there is great peer pressure to become sexually active during the teen years. Premarital sexual activity is commonplace, and teenage pregnancy is more socially acceptable today than it was in the past. In fact, nearly half (46%) of all teens ages 15 to 19 have had sex at least once (AGI, 2006a). Sexual innuendo permeates every aspect of the popular media, but issues of sexual responsibility are commonly ignored.

Developing Cultural Competence

IMPACT OF EDUCATION ON MARRIAGE AND CHILDBEARING

Throughout the world, the higher a woman's educational level, the more likely she is to delay marriage and childbirth.

High-risk sexual behaviors—for example, multiple partners and lack of contraceptive use—are of concern. Research indicates that young people 15 to 24 years of age comprise 25% of the sexually experienced population in the United States. However, they account for nearly half of the new cases of sexually transmitted infections (STIs) (AGI 2006b). This is particularly worrisome because many STIs, including human immunodeficiency virus (HIV), are asymptomatic. Thus, apparently healthy young people who are infected may not have a reason to seek health care.

Worldwide, people younger than 25 years of age account for the greatest proportion of STIs. Moreover, estimates suggest that 6000 young people are infected with HIV *daily* (Bearinger, Sieving, Ferguson, et al., 2007).

Statistics have demonstrated an increased use of condoms among the adolescent population, probably because of the tremendous educational efforts related to HIV. Nevertheless, adolescents remain inconsistent contraceptive users. Inconsistent contraceptive use is more common in girls who want to become pregnant, who have not established a pattern of consistent contraceptive use, who communicate less often with their partners about prevention issues, and who have an increased lifetime number of sexual partners (Davies, DiClemente, Wingood, et al., 2006).

Many teens lack accurate and adequate knowledge about contraceptive options. This is a common topic of sex education programs; however, debate continues about the appropriateness of such programs in schools. Proponents advocate early sex education to provide teens with the knowledge they need to avoid unwanted pregnancy and the risk of STIs. Opponents feel that sex education is the responsibility of parents and worry that sex education in the schools will promote sexual activity. However, a review of research on sex education reveals that it does not increase initiation of sexual activity at an earlier age. Other factors affecting the use of contraception include access or availability, cost of supplies, and concern about confidentiality.

PSYCHOSOCIAL FACTORS

Family dysfunction and poor self-esteem are also major risk factors for adolescent pregnancy. Some young teenagers deliberately plan to get pregnant. The adolescent girl may use pregnancy for various subconscious or conscious reasons: to punish her parents, to escape from an undesirable home situation, to gain attention, or to feel that she has someone to love and someone that loves her. Pregnancy may also be a young woman's form of acting out. In some circumstances, pregnancy could represent an important milestone that leads to positive lifestyle changes and healthier behaviors.

More teens who become pregnant have been physically, emotionally, or sexually abused, compared with teens who have not been pregnant. In fact, maltreatment of any kind is a high-risk contributor to early teen pregnancy (Francisco, Hicks, Powell, et al., 2008).

Teenage pregnancy can result from an incestuous relationship. In the very young adolescent, incest or sexual abuse should be suspected as a possible cause of pregnancy. Teenage pregnancy could also be caused by other nonvoluntary sexual experiences such as acquaintance rape.

Evidence-Based Nursing

IMPACT OF CHILDHOOD SEXUAL ABUSE ON PREGNANCY

Clinical Question

Is there an association between childhood sexual abuse and adolescent pregnancy?

The Evidence

Six clinician researchers reviewed 13 qualitative and quantitative research studies to develop an integrative review. Integrative review provides the strongest level of evidence, and is appropriate when the research question focuses on a sensitive subject that is difficult to measure, such as sexual abuse. Most of the studies identified a relationship between adolescent pregnancy and an experience of childhood sexual abuse. Three studies were unable to demonstrate a distinct link between childhood sexual abuse and pregnancy but did find strong relationships with risky sexual behaviors, including sexually transmitted diseases. Girls who were sexually abused by their mothers' boyfriends were more than twice as likely to become pregnant than those abused by family members. Other risk factors identified for both sexual abuse and adolescent pregnancy included family member substance abuse, parent-child conflict, and maternal disengagement (Francisco, Hicks, Powell, Styles, Tabor, & Hulton, 2008).

Best Practice

Nurses are in a special position to address sensitive topics with adolescents. Victimization should be treated as a condition, not an event that has an endpoint. Sexual assault assessment and treatment referral should be part of the healthcare encounter. Strategies for identifying adolescents at risk of pregnancy based on their sexual history is important for early intervention. When these at-risk youth are identified, an integrated interprofessional approach to pregnancy prevention is warranted. Shame is a key characteristic of childhood sexual abuse. Nurses should help victims attribute blame to the perpetrator rather than to themselves. Interventions that focus on helping adolescents form healthy peer relationships and maintain good school performance reduce the incidence of pregnancy in this population.

Critical Thinking

How can the nurse help adolescents reveal their experiences with sexual abuse in a sensitive and nonthreatening way? What interventions can help prevent adolescent pregnancy in those children with a history of sexual abuse?

See MyNursingKit for possible responses.

RISKS TO THE ADOLESCENT MOTHER

PHYSIOLOGIC RISKS

Adolescents older than 15 years who receive early, thorough prenatal care are at no greater risk during pregnancy than women older than age 20. Unfortunately, adolescents often begin prenatal care later in pregnancy than other age groups. Thus, risks for pregnant adolescents include preterm births, low-birth-weight infants, cephalopelvic disproportion, iron deficiency anemia, and preeclampsia and its sequelae. In the adolescent age group, prenatal care is the critical factor that most influences pregnancy outcome.

Teenagers aged 15 to 19 have a high incidence of STIs, including herpesvirus, syphilis, and gonorrhea. The incidence of chlamydial infection is also increased in this age group. The presence of such infections during a pregnancy greatly increases the risk to the fetus. Other problems seen in adolescents are cigarette smoking and drug use. By the time pregnancy is confirmed, the fetus may already have been harmed by these substances.

PSYCHOLOGIC RISKS

The major psychologic risk to the pregnant adolescent is the interruption of her developmental tasks. Adding the tasks of pregnancy to her own developmental tasks creates a huge amount of psychologic work, the completion of which will affect the adolescent's and her newborn's futures. Table 13–1 suggests typical behaviors of the adolescent when she becomes aware of her pregnancy. In reviewing these behaviors, the nurse should realize that other factors may influence individual response.

SOCIOLOGIC RISKS

Being forced into adult roles before completing adolescent developmental tasks causes a series of events that may result in prolonged dependence on parents, lack of stable relationships with the opposite sex, and lack of economic and social stability. Many teenage mothers drop out of school during their pregnancy and then are less likely to complete their schooling. Similarly, they are less likely to go to college, more likely to have big families, and more likely to be single. Lack of education in turn reduces the

Table 13–1 Initial Reaction to Awareness of Pregnancy

Age	Adolescent Behavior	Nursing Implications
Early adolescent (14 and younger)	Fears rejection by family and peers. Enters healthcare system with an adult, most likely mother (parents still seen as locus of control). Value system closely reflects that of parents, so teen turns to parents for decisions or approval of decisions. Pregnancy probably not a result of intimate relationship. Is self-conscious about normal adolescent changes in body. Self-consciousness and low self-esteem likely to increase with rapid breast enlargement and abdominal enlargement of pregnancy.	Be nonjudgmental in approach to care. Focus on needs and concerns of adolescent, but if parent accompanies daughter, include parent in plan of care. Encourage both to express concerns and feelings regarding pregnancy and options: abortion, maintaining pregnancy, adoption. Be realistic and concrete in discussing implications of each option. During physical exam of adolescent, respect increased sense of modesty. Explain in simple and concrete terms physical changes that are produced by pregnancy versus puberty. Explain each step of physical exam in simple and concrete terms.
Middle adolescent (15–17 years)	Fears rejection by peers and parents. Unsure of whom to confide in. May seek confirmation of pregnancy on own with increased awareness of options and services, such as over-the-counter pregnancy kits and Planned Parenthood. If in an ongoing, caring relationship with partner (peer), may choose him as confidant. Economic dependence on parents may determine if and when parents are told. Future educational plans and perception of parental support or lack of support are significant factors in decision regarding termination or maintenance of the pregnancy. Possible conflict between parental and own developing value system.	Be nonjudgmental in approach to care. Reassure the adolescent that confidentiality will be maintained. Help adolescent identify significant individuals in whom she can confide to help make a decision about the pregnancy. Be aware of state laws regarding requirement of parental notification if abortion intended. Also be aware of state laws regarding requirements for marriage: usually, minimum age for both parties is 18; 16- and 17-year-olds are, in most states, allowed to marry only with consent of parents. Encourage adolescent to be realistic about parental response to pregnancy.
Late adolescent (18–19 years)	Most likely to confirm pregnancy on own and at an earlier date due to increased acceptance and awareness of consequences of behavior. Likely to use pregnancy kit for confirmation. Relationship with father of baby, future educational plans, and personal value system are among significant determinants of decision about pregnancy.	Be nonjudgmental in approach to care. Reassure the adolescent that confidentiality will be maintained. Encourage adolescent to identify significant individuals in whom she can confide. Refer to counseling as appropriate. Encourage adolescent to be realistic about parental response to pregnancy.

quality of jobs available. Childbearing at an early age is a strong predictor that the children of teenage mothers will live in poverty (Kirby, 2007).

Adolescent mothers frequently fail to establish a stable family, especially if they have a second child while still in their teens. Their family structure tends to be single parent and matriarchal, often the same type in which the adolescents themselves were raised. Some pregnant adolescents choose to marry the father of the baby, who may also be a teenager. Unfortunately, most adolescent marriages end in divorce. This fact should not be surprising because pregnancy and marriage interrupt the adolescents' childhood and basic education. Lack of maturity in dealing with an intimate relationship also contributes to marital breakdown.

The increased incidence of maternal complications, preterm birth, and low-birth-weight babies among teen mothers also affects society because many of these mothers are on welfare. The need for increased financial support for good prenatal care and nutritional programs remains critical.

Table 13–2 identifies the early adolescent's response to the developmental tasks of pregnancy. Middle and older adolescents respond differently, reflecting their progression through developmental tasks. In addition to her maturational level, the amount of nurturing the pregnant adolescent receives is a critical factor in the way she handles pregnancy and motherhood.

RISKS FOR THE CHILD

Children of adolescent parents are at a disadvantage in many ways because teens are not developmentally or economically prepared to be parents. In general, children of teenage mothers are found to be at a developmental disadvantage compared with children whose mothers were older at the time of their birth. Many factors contribute to these differences, especially the adverse social and economic conditions many teenage mothers face. These factors result in high rates of family instability, disadvantaged neighborhoods, and high rates of behavior problems. In addition these children have an increased risk of academic problems, substance

Table 13–2 The Early Adolescent's Response to the Developmental Tasks of Pregnancy

Stage	Developmental Tasks of Pregnancy	Early Adolescent's Response to Pregnancy	Nursing Implications
First trimester	Pregnancy confirmation. Seeks early prenatal care as a confirmation tool. Begins to evaluate her diet and general health habits. Initial ambivalence common. Usually supportive partner.	May delay confirmation of pregnancy until late first trimester or later. Reasons for delay may include lack of awareness that she is pregnant, fear of confiding in anyone, and/or denial. Rapid enlargement and sensitivity of breasts are embarrassing and frightening to early adolescents—may be perceived as changes of puberty. If confiding in mother, may be experiencing family turmoil in response to pregnancy.	Explain physiologic changes of pregnancy versus those associated with puberty. Explain that ambivalence is normal with any pregnancy, but recognize it as a much greater concern with adolescent pregnancy. Emphasize need for good nutrition as important for her well-being as much as infant's (prevention of preeclampsia and anemia). Use simple explanations and lots of audiovisual aids. Have adolescent listen to fetal heart rate with Doppler.
Second trimester	Changes in physical appearance begin, and fetal movement is experienced, causing pregnancy to be experienced as a reality. Begins wearing maternity clothes to accommodate the physical changes. As a result of quickening, she perceives her fetus as a real baby and begins preparing for the maternal role and new relationships with her partner and members of her family.	Some teenagers may delay validation of pregnancy until now, with family turmoil occurring at this time. Abdominal enlargement and quickening may be perceived as loss of control over body image. May try to maintain prepregnant weight and wear restrictive clothing to control and conceal changing body. Becomes dependent on her own mother for support. Egocentric; unable to develop a maternal role at this time.	Continue to discuss importance of good nutrition and adequate weight gain as noted above. Discuss ways of wearing common teenage clothing (large sweatshirts, blouses) to promote comfort but preserve adolescent image to some degree. Discuss plans being made for baby, continued educational plans, and role of teen's parents.
Third trimester	At end of second trimester, begins to view fetus as separate from self. Buys baby clothes and supplies. Prepares a place for the baby. Realistic about what baby is like. Prepares to give birth to infant. Anxiety increases as labor and birth approach and has concerns about well-being of fetus.	May focus on "wanting it to be over." May have trouble individuating fetus. May have fantasies, dreams, or nightmares about childbirth. Natural fears of labor and birth greater than with older primigravida. Probably has not been in a hospital, and may associate this with negative experiences.	Assess whether adolescent is preparing for baby by buying supplies and preparing a place in the home. Childbirth education is important. Provide hospital tour. Assess for discomforts of pregnancy, such as heartburn and constipation. Adolescent may be uncomfortable mentioning these and other problems.

abuse, behavioral disorders, depression, and early sexual activity. Children born to adolescent mothers also have higher rates of abuse and neglect, and are more likely to become adolescent parents themselves (Klein & The Committee on Adolescence, 2005).

PARTNERS OF ADOLESCENT MOTHERS

Approximately two thirds of the fathers of infants of adolescent mothers are not teens but are 20 years of age or older. In particular, teens in poorer, recently immigrant populations have considerably older partners (Males, 2004).

Adolescent males are waiting longer than in the past to have sexual intercourse (average age at first intercourse is 17.5 years [AGI, 2008]). Nevertheless, adolescent males tend to become sexually active at an earlier age than females, and they have more sexual partners in their teenage years. Teen fatherhood varies significantly by race with rates among young black men (37 per 1000 males ages 15 to 19) more than double that among young white men (AGI, 2008).

When the father is an adolescent, he too has uncompleted developmental tasks for his age group and is no better prepared psychologically than his female counterpart to deal with the consequences of pregnancy. Consequently the adolescent who attempts to assume his responsibility as a father faces many of the same psychologic and sociologic risks as the adolescent mother. The mother and father are generally from similar socioeconomic backgrounds and have similar educational levels.

Although they may not be married, many adolescent couples have meaningful relationships. The male partners may be very involved in the pregnancy and may be present for the birth. In situations in which the adolescent father wants to assume some responsibility, healthcare providers should support him in his decision. If the adolescents perceive that they have a caring relationship, the adolescent father may want to be supportive and protective but not understand the physical and psychologic changes his partner is experiencing. The young man will need education about pregnancy, childbirth, child care, and parenting. It is also important to ensure that the pregnant adolescent has the opportunity to decide for herself whether she wants the father to participate in her health care.

The lack of responsibility shown by some unmarried fathers has caused a shift in cultural and community attitudes. Fathers are included on birth certificates far more frequently today than in the past. This inclusion helps ensure the fathers' rights and encourages them to meet their responsibilities to their children. In addition, legal paternity gives children access to military and social security benefits and to medical information about their fathers.

In some situations the pregnant adolescent may not want to identify or contact the father of the baby, and the male may not readily acknowledge paternity. Those situations include rape, exploitative sexual relations, incest, and casual sexual relations. If healthcare providers suspect any of the first three causes, further investigation into the situation is important for the well-being of the pregnant adolescent, and referral to other resources should be made as appropriate.

Even if the adolescent father has been included in the health care of the young woman throughout the pregnancy, it is not unusual for her to want her mother as her primary support person during labor and birth. Younger adolescents are especially likely to choose their mothers for this role. It is important to support the pregnant adolescent's wishes and to acknowledge and support the adolescent father's wishes as appropriate.

As a part of counseling, the nurse should assess the young man's stressors, his support systems, his plans for involvement in the pregnancy and childbearing, and his future plans. He should be referred to social services for counseling about his educational and vocational future. When the father is involved in the pregnancy, the young mother feels less deserted, more confident in her decision making, and better able to discuss her future.

Relationships among fathers, teenage mothers, and their infants appear prone to deterioration over time. Research suggests, however, that many young fathers genuinely want to be involved with their children and would have more contact and input if they could. Issues such as conflicts with the teen mother or maternal grandparents and a lack of financial resources may act as barriers for the young father (Bunting & McAuley, 2004).

REACTIONS OF FAMILY AND SOCIAL NETWORK TO ADOLESCENT PREGNANCY

The reactions of families and support groups to adolescent pregnancy vary widely. In families that foster children's educational and career goals, adolescent pregnancy is often a shock. Anger, shame, and sorrow are common reactions. The majority of pregnant adolescents from these families are likely to choose abortion, with the exception of teens whose cultural and religious beliefs prevent them from seeking abortions.

In populations in which adolescent pregnancy is more prevalent and more socially acceptable, family and friends may be more supportive of the adolescent parents. In many cases the teen's friends and mother are present at the birth. The expectant parents may also have friends who are already teen parents. Some male partners of these adolescent mothers see pregnancy and the birth of a baby as signs of adult status and increased sexual prowess—a source of pride.

The mother of the pregnant adolescent is usually among the first to be told about the pregnancy. She typically becomes involved with decision making, especially with the young adolescent, about issues such as maintaining the pregnancy, abortion, and dealing with the father-to-be and his family.

Once the pregnant adolescent decides how to proceed, it is often her mother who helps her access health care and accompanies her to her first prenatal visit. If the pregnancy is maintained, the mother may participate in prenatal care and classes and can be an excellent source of support for her daughter. She should be encouraged to participate if the mother-daughter relationship is positive. If the baby's father is involved in the pregnancy, he and the pregnant adolescent's mother may be able to work together to support the teenage mother. The nurse can update the pregnant adolescent's mother on childbearing practices to clarify any misconceptions she might have. During labor and birth, the mother may be a key figure for her daughter, offering reassurance and instilling confidence in the teen.

The younger the adolescent when she gives birth, the more she needs her mother's support. Children of adolescent parents experience more negative outcomes, including more aggressive behavior at a younger age, when the adolescent is in constant conflict with her mother and becomes less involved in parenting.

NURSING MANAGEMENT

NURSING ASSESSMENT AND DIAGNOSIS

Establish a knowledge base to plan interventions for the adolescent mother-to-be and family. Areas of assessment include history of family and personal physical health, developmental level and impact of pregnancy, and emotional and financial support. Also assess the family and social support network and the father's degree of involvement in the pregnancy.

As with all pregnant women, it is important to have information on the teen's general physical health. This may be the first time the adolescent has ever provided a health history. Consequently it may be helpful to ask specific questions and give examples if the young woman appears confused about a question. The teen's mother may be best able to answer questions about family history because the adolescent is often unaware of this information.

Assess the following areas: family and personal health history, medical history, menstrual history, obstetric and gynecologic history, and substance abuse history. It is also important to assess the maturational level of each person. The adolescent's development level and the impact of pregnancy are reflected in the degree of recognition of the realities and responsibilities involved in teenage pregnancy and parenting. Also assess the mother's self-concept (including body image), her relationship with the significant adults in her life, her attitude toward her pregnancy, and her coping methods in the situation, as well as the teen's knowledge of, attitude toward, and anticipated ability to care for the coming baby. Ask specifically about dating violence. Teens are not likely to reveal dating violence unless they are asked about it.

The socioeconomic status of the pregnant adolescent often places the baby at risk throughout life, beginning with conception. It is essential to assess family and social support systems, as well as the extent of financial support available.

The nursing diagnoses applicable to pregnant women in general apply to the pregnant adolescent. Other nursing diagnoses are influenced by the adolescent's age, support systems, socioeconomic situation, health, and maturity. Examples of nursing diagnoses specific to the pregnant adolescent may include the following:

- *Health-Seeking Behaviors:* Information about Child Care related to expressed desire to parent effectively
- *Imbalanced Nutrition:* Less than Body Requirements related to poor eating habits
- *Risk for Situational Low Self-Esteem* related to unanticipated pregnancy

PLANNING AND IMPLEMENTATION

Nursing Care in the Community

Nurses who work with adolescent girls can help them by providing the necessary information and guidance to enable each teen to make choices that are based on the development of a positive body image and a sense of herself as a sexual being with the ability to recognize the need for and to practice safe sex behaviors.

If pregnancy occurs, early, thorough prenatal care is the strongest and most critical determinant for reducing risk for the adolescent mother and her newborn. The nurse needs to understand the special needs of the adolescent mother to meet this challenge successfully.

Many new and innovative community-based programs have evolved to provide care for high-risk clients and their partners throughout the childbearing experience and beyond. Nurses in community-based agencies can help adolescents access the healthcare system as well as social services and other support services (e.g., food banks and the Special Supplemental Nutrition Program for Women, Infants, and Children [WIC]). These nurses are also involved extensively in counseling and client teaching.

Issue of Confidentiality

Most states have passed legislation that confirms the right of some minors to assume the rights of adults; they are then called *emancipated minors*. An adolescent may be considered emancipated if he or she is self-supporting and living away from home, married, pregnant, a parent, or in the military service. Even if a minor has not become formally "emancipated," all 50 states permit confidential testing and treatment for STIs but only half (25 states) explicitly permit minors (12 and older) to consent to contraception without a parent's knowledge or consent. Currently 32 states explicitly allow minors to consent to prenatal care; three states specify that "mature" minors can consent, whereas the remaining 15 states have no relevant law or policy. All states either explicitly allow minors to give consent for their children's medical care or have no explicit policy about it (AGI, 2009). If a pregnant minor is considered emancipated, she is entitled to confidentiality in her dealings with healthcare providers. Only with her agreement can other adults, including her parents, be included in communication.

Development of a Trusting Relationship with the Pregnant Adolescent

The first visit to the clinic or caregiver's office may make the young woman feel anxious and vulnerable. Making this first experience as positive as possible for the young woman will encourage the adolescent to return for follow-up care and to cooperate with her caregivers and will help her recognize the importance of healthcare for her and her baby. Developing a trusting relationship with the pregnant adolescent is essential. Honesty, respect, and a caring attitude promote self-esteem.

Nursing Practice

During the initial pelvic examination, with the consent of the examiner, offer the teen a handheld mirror. A mirror is helpful in enabling the young woman to see her cervix, thus educating her about her anatomy. It also gives her an active role in the exam if she so desires.

Depending on the adolescent's age, this may be her first pelvic examination, an anxiety-provoking experience for any woman. Provide explanations during the procedure. A gentle and thoughtful examination technique will help the young woman to relax.

Promotion of Self-Esteem and Problem-Solving Skills

Assist the adolescent in her decision-making and problem-solving skills so that she can proceed with her developmental tasks and begin to assume responsibility for her life and that of her newborn. Many adolescents are not aware of the legally available options to deal with an unplanned pregnancy. In an open, nonjudgmental way, without imposing personal values, educate the teen about her alternatives: terminating the pregnancy, maintaining the pregnancy and parenting the infant, or relinquishing the infant for adoption. The nurse can also provide information about community resources available to help with each alternative. Once the teen has decided on a course of action, healthcare providers should respect her decision and support her efforts to achieve her goals.

If the adolescent chooses to continue her pregnancy, describe what she can expect over the prenatal period and provide an explanation and rationale for each procedure as it occurs. This overview fosters the adolescent's understanding and gives her some control (Figure 13–2 ●).

Early adolescents tend to be egocentric and oriented to the present. They may not think it is important that their health and habits affect the fetus. Thus, it is often helpful to emphasize how these practices affect the teens themselves. Early adolescents also need help in problem solving and in visualizing the future so they can plan effectively.

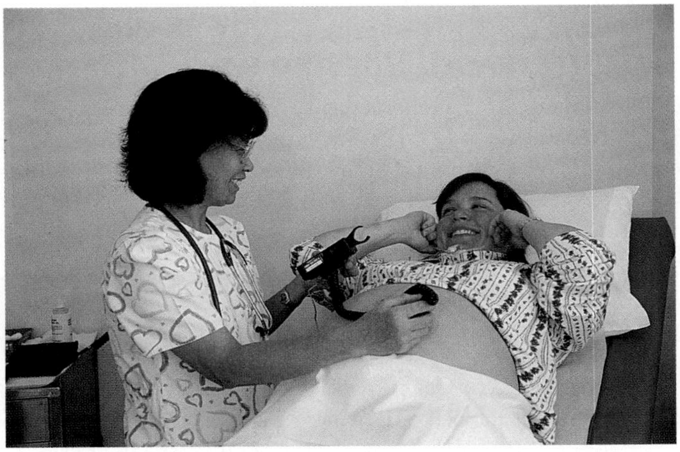

● **Figure 13–2** Promoting a sense of understanding and control. The nurse gives this young mother an opportunity to listen to her baby's heartbeat.

Middle adolescents are developing the ability to think abstractly and can recognize that actions may have long-term consequences. They may not yet have acquired assertive communication skills, however, and may be reluctant to ask questions. Therefore, ask teens directly if they have questions. Middle adolescents can absorb more detailed health teaching and apply it.

Late adolescents can usually think abstractly, plan for the future, and function in a manner comparable to older pregnant women. They can also handle complex information and apply it.

Promotion of Physical Well-Being

Baseline weight and blood pressure measurements are valuable in assessing weight gain and predisposition to preeclampsia. Encourage the adolescent to take part in her care by measuring and recording her own weight. Use this time as an opportunity for assisting the young woman in problem solving. Encourage her to ask herself the following questions: "Have I gained too much or too little weight?" "What influence does my diet have on my weight?" "How can I change my eating habits?"

Also introduce the subject of nutrition during measurement of baseline and subsequent hemoglobin and hematocrit values. Because the adolescent is at risk for anemia, she needs education about the importance of iron in her diet. Indeed, basic education about nutrition is a critical component of care for pregnant teens.

Preeclampsia is the most prevalent medical complication of pregnant adolescents. Blood pressure readings of 140/90 mm Hg are not acceptable as the determinant of preeclampsia in adolescents. Women ages 14 to 20 years without evidence of high blood pressure usually have diastolic readings between 50 and 66 mm Hg. Gradual increases from the prepregnant diastolic readings, along with excessive weight gain, must be evaluated as precursors to preeclampsia. Establishment of baseline readings is one reason early prenatal care is vital to management of the pregnant adolescent.

Adolescents have an increased incidence of STIs. The initial prenatal examination should include gonococcal and chlamydial cultures; wet-mount prep for *Candida, Trichomonas,* and *Gardnerella;* and tests for syphilis. Although today's teens are knowledgeable about HIV/AIDS, they know much less about other STIs, especially with regard to symptoms and risk reduction, so education is important. If the adolescent's history indicates that she is at increased risk for HIV, she should be given information about it and offered HIV screening.

Thinking Critically

A MOTHER CONSIDERING ADOPTION

Rachel Kalaras is an 18-year-old G1P0 who is 16 weeks pregnant when she arrives for her prenatal visit. When discussing her plans for the pregnancy, Rachel indicates that she is considering adoption. She has not discussed this plan with anyone but is seeking information about the process of relinquishment. What should you consider in discussing this issue with Rachel?

See MyNursingKit for possible responses.

Discuss substance abuse with the adolescent. It is important to review the risks associated with the use of tobacco, caffeine, drugs, and alcohol. The young woman should be aware of how these substances affect both her and her fetus's development.

Ongoing care should include the same assessments that an older pregnant woman receives. Pay special attention to evaluating fetal growth by determining when quickening occurs and by measuring fundal height, fetal heart rate, and fetal movement. If there is a question of size-date discrepancy by 2 cm either way when assessing fundal height, an ultrasound is warranted to establish fetal age so that instances of intrauterine growth restriction can be detected early.

Promotion of Family Adaptation

Assess the family situation during the first prenatal visit and find out the level of involvement the adolescent wants from each of her family members and the father of the child, as well as her perception of their present support. If the mother and daughter agree, the mother should be included in the client's care. Pregnancy may change a teen's relationship with her mother from one of antagonism to one of understanding and empathy. The opportunity to renew or establish a positive relationship with their mothers is welcomed by most teens. Help the teen's mother assess and meet her daughter's needs. Some adolescents become more dependent during pregnancy, and some become more independent. The mother can ease and encourage her daughter's self-growth by understanding how best to respond to and support the adolescent.

The adolescent's relationship with her father is also affected by her pregnancy. Provide information to the adolescent's father and encourage his involvement to whatever degree is acceptable to both daughter and father.

The father of the adolescent's infant should not be forgotten in promoting the family's adaptation to the pregnancy. He should be included in prenatal visits, classes, health teaching, and the birth itself to the extent that he wishes and that is acceptable to the teenage mother. He should also have the opportunity to express his feelings and concerns and to have his questions answered.

Facilitation of Prenatal Education

School systems attempt to meet prenatal education needs in many ways. The most effective method appears to be mainstreaming the pregnant adolescent in academic classes with her peers and adding classes appropriate to her needs during pregnancy and postpartum. Classes about growth and development beginning with the newborn and early infancy periods can help teenage parents to develop realistic expectations of their infants and may help decrease child abuse. Mainstreaming is an ideal way to help teens complete their education while learning the skills they need to cope. Vocational guidance in this setting is also beneficial as they plan for their futures.

Most childbirth educators believe that prenatal classes with other teens are best, even though they can be challenging to teach (Figure 13–3 ●). The pregnant teen may be accompanied by her mother, her boyfriend, or her girlfriends. Those who bring girlfriends may bring a different one each time, and giggling and side conversations may occur. Such activity reflects the short attention span of the teen and is fairly typical. Thus, to keep the attention of the participants, it is important to use a variety of teaching strategies including audiovisual aids, demonstrations, and games.

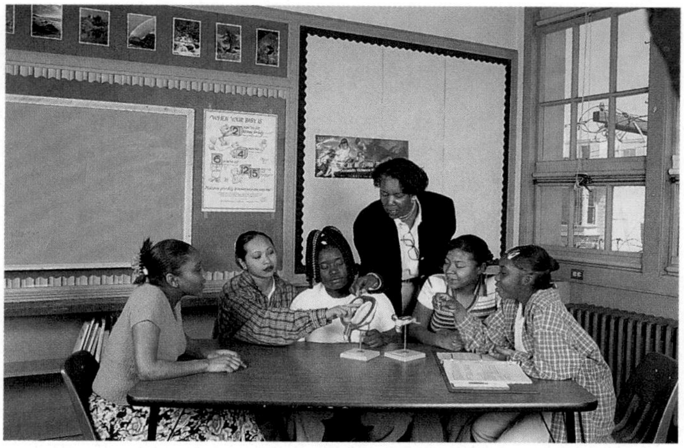

● **Figure 13–3** Prenatal classes for adolescents. Young adolescents may benefit from prenatal classes designed for them.

Goals for prenatal classes may include some or all of the following:

- Providing anticipatory guidance about pregnancy
- Preparing participants for labor and birth
- Helping participants identify the problems and conflicts of teenage pregnancy and parenting
- Promoting increased self-esteem
- Providing information about available community resources
- Helping participants develop adaptive coping skills

Although parenting topics are sometimes included in prenatal classes for adolescents, teens may not retain the information because they tend to be present oriented. Parenting skills are crucial, but adolescents generally are not ready to learn about these skills until birth makes the newborn—and thus parenting—a reality.

HOSPITAL-BASED NURSING CARE

As mentioned earlier, the adolescent's mother is often present during the teen's labor and birth. The father of the baby may also be involved. Close girlfriends may arrive soon after the teen is admitted. At admission, ask the teen who will be her primary support

Evidence in Action

To encourage breastfeeding in adolescent mothers, it is suggested that healthcare providers provide positive interpersonal relationships and in-person experiences (systematic review) (Hall Moran, Edwards, Dykes, et al., 2007).

Evidence in Action

The opinion of the American College of Obstetricians and Gynecologists (ACOG) is that the benefits and convenience of long-acting contraceptives are appropriate for sexually active adolescents (Opinion for Practice) (Tolaymat & Kaunitz, 2007).

person in labor and who she wants involved in the labor and birth. This information may also be included on her prenatal record.

The adolescent in labor has the same care needs as any pregnant woman. However, she may require more sustained care. Be readily available and answer questions simply and honestly, using lay terminology. Also help the adolescent's support people understand their roles in assisting the teen. If the father of the baby is involved, encourage him, at his own level of comfort, to play an active role in all phases of the birth process, perhaps by supporting the teen's relaxation techniques, feeding her ice chips, timing her contractions, and coaching her with her breathing. Recommend hand-holding, back rubs, and supportive touching.

During the postpartum period, most teens do not foresee that they will become sexually active in the near future and are often adamant that they will not become pregnant again for a long time. However, the statistics demonstrate a different reality. Consequently, predischarge teaching should include information about the resumption of ovulation and the importance of contraception.

Several safe and effective contraceptive options are available for adolescents. Condoms are by far the most common method of contraception among teens and, when used consistently and correctly, they offer the added advantage of protection against STIs. Increasingly, experts are recommending a dual approach to prevent pregnancy and STIs—a condom combined with a second method of contraception, typically a hormonal method such as a combined oral contraceptive (Hillard, 2005; WHO, 2004). The American College of Obstetricians and Gynecologists (ACOG) (2007) supports the use of intrauterine devices (IUDs) as a safe, first-line contraceptive choice for adolescents, stating that the IUD does not increase the adolescent's risk of PID or affect her fertility. The benefits and convenience of long-acting oral contraceptives also make them an appropriate choice for sexually active adolescents.

As part of discharge planning, ensure that the teen is aware of community resources available to assist her and her family. Postpartum classes, especially with peers, can be particularly beneficial. Such classes address a variety of topics, including postpartum adaptation, infant and child development, and parenting skills.

EVALUATION

Expected outcomes of nursing care include the following:

- A trusting relationship is established with the pregnant adolescent.
- The adolescent is able to use her problem-solving abilities to make appropriate choices.
- The adolescent follows the recommendations of the healthcare team and receives effective healthcare throughout her pregnancy, the birth, and the postpartum period.
- The adolescent, her partner (if he is involved), and their families are able to cope successfully with the effects of the pregnancy.
- The adolescent is able to discuss pregnancy, prenatal care, and childbirth.
- The adolescent develops skill in child care and parenting.

PREVENTION OF ADOLESCENT PREGNANCY

At the individual level, balanced and realistic sexual education, which includes information on both abstinence and contraception, can delay teens' onset of sexual activity, increase the use of contraception by sexually active teens, and reduce the number of their sexual partners. The American Academy of Pediatrics (2007) has issued a policy statement on contraception and adolescents that addresses the role of healthcare providers in working with adolescents. The statement stresses the importance of encouraging abstinence while also providing counseling on risk-reduction approaches, including the use of latex condoms for every act of sexual intercourse. It also emphasizes the need to ensure ready access to contraceptive services and appropriate follow-up.

At the national level, the National Campaign to Prevent Teen and Unplanned Pregnancy (NCPTUP), a private, nonprofit organization made up of a broad spectrum of religious, political, social, human services, health, and academic organizations, is working to reduce teenage pregnancy by one third between 2006 and 2015 (NCPTUP, 2006). The Association of Women's Health, Obstetric and Neonatal Nurses (AWHONN) is one of the many professional organizations that joined this group and made a commitment to focus on adolescent pregnancy prevention. Not surprisingly, the task forces have found that adolescent pregnancy is a multifaceted problem with no easy answers. The best approaches are local ones based on strong, community-wide involvement with a variety of programs directed at the multiple causes of the problem.

A major problem in local communities continues to be conflict among different groups about how to approach adolescent pregnancy prevention. Some groups believe that abstinence is the only answer, whereas others believe that abstinence programs do not work with the many teens who are already sexually active. The latter groups believe that sex education and easy availability of contraception are the answers. Many parents advocate an "abstinence-plus" approach that stresses abstinence as the best approach but includes information on condoms and contraception for those teens who do not abstain.

Recent research suggests that only 7% of people in the United States believe that sex education should not be provided in schools. Moreover, controversy about the type of sex education offered in schools seems to have decreased. Nearly three fourths (74%) of principals surveyed state that they have not had any recent discussions or debate (in school board, Parent-Teacher Association, or other public meetings) about what should be taught (National Public Radio [NPR], Kaiser Family Foundation, and John F. Kennedy School of Government, 2004).

Most Americans support providing education in junior and senior high schools with information about protection against unplanned pregnancy and STIs. Youth development programs that focus on meeting needs of adolescents by building on young person's capacities, assisting them to cultivate their own talent and to increase their feelings of self-worth, ease their transition into adulthood and can reduce sexual risk behaviors and unintended teen pregnancy (Advocates for Youth, 2005).

The National Campaign's task forces have identified characteristics shared by all successful programs, regardless of the type of offering or community. Effective adolescent pregnancy prevention programs are long term and intensive. They also involve adolescents in program planning, include good role models from the same cultural and racial backgrounds, and focus on the adolescent male.

Survey data from a representative sample of teens and adults provide some additional interesting insights (NCPTUP, 2006):

- Parents tend to underestimate their influence on their adolescents. Teens report that their parents, and not their friends, have the most influence on the teens' decisions about sex. However, a preponderance of teens also report that it would be easier to deal with issues related to sexuality and teen pregnancy if they could have more honest, open conversations with their parents.
- Teens' expressed attitudes about sexual activity reflect more cautious values and attitudes than generally believed. Teens report that their values, morals, religious beliefs, and concern for their future influence their decisions about sex more than concerns about becoming pregnant or developing a sexually transmitted infection.
- Almost all the adults and teens surveyed said that society should give teens a strong message that they should not have sex until they are at least out of high school.
- The majority of both groups advocate a message stressing abstinence while also providing information about contraception. They rejected the notion that such an approach sends a "mixed message."
- Teens want more information about sexuality, abstinence, and contraception.
- Teens tend to overestimate the percentage of their classmates and peers who have had sex.

In summary, although it is sometimes difficult for adults, it is important to address topics related to healthy relationships, abstinence, birth control, responsible sexual behavior, and the possible consequences of unsafe practices honestly and in a way that reflects adolescents' knowledge level, perspectives, and personal experience. Discussion about teenage pregnancy needs to reflect an awareness of teens' priorities related to the costs and rewards of having a baby. All such discussions need to be honest, frank, and open and based on a recognition of the developmental level of the teen (Herman, 2008).

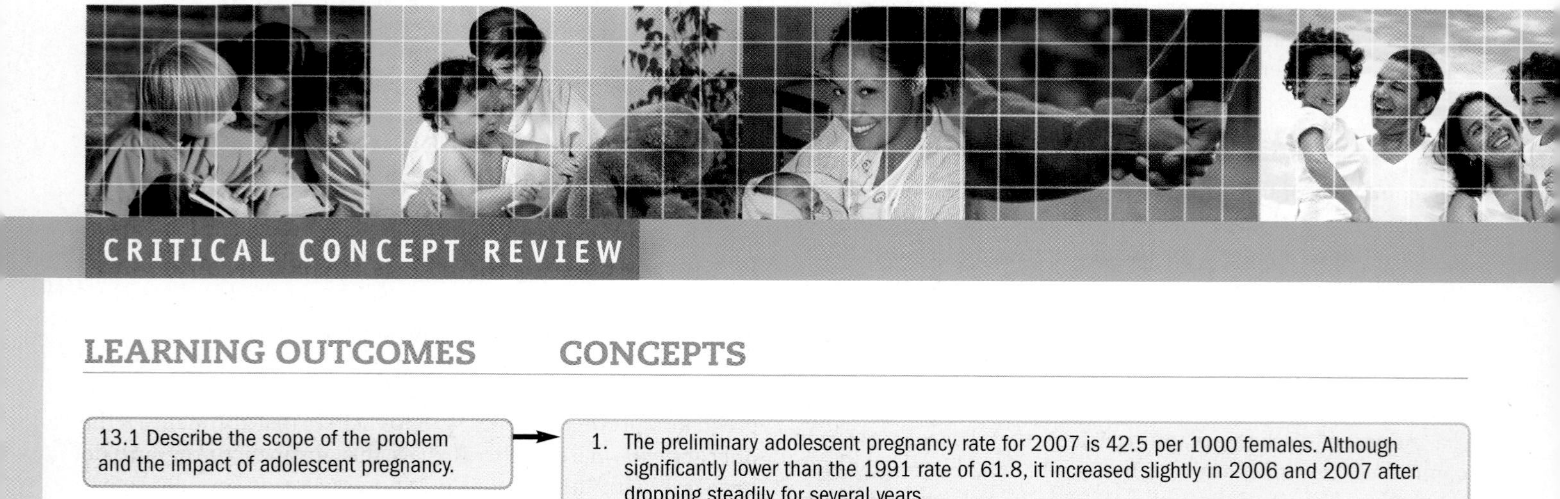

CRITICAL CONCEPT REVIEW

LEARNING OUTCOMES	CONCEPTS
13.1 Describe the scope of the problem and the impact of adolescent pregnancy.	1. The preliminary adolescent pregnancy rate for 2007 is 42.5 per 1000 females. Although significantly lower than the 1991 rate of 61.8, it increased slightly in 2006 and 2007 after dropping steadily for several years. 2. Despite the decline, the United States continues to have one of the highest levels of adolescent childbearing among industrialized nations.
13.2 Summarize factors contributing to adolescent pregnancy in the nursing care management of this population.	1. Many factors contribute to the high teenage pregnancy rate: ■ Earlier age at first experience with sexual intercourse. ■ Lack of knowledge about conception. ■ Lack of easy access to contraception. ■ Lessened stigma associated with adolescent pregnancy in some populations. ■ Poverty. ■ Early school failure. ■ Early childhood sexual abuse.

LEARNING OUTCOMES	CONCEPTS
13.3 Assess the physical, psychologic, and sociologic risks a pregnant adolescent faces.	1. Physical risks: ■ Preterm birth. ■ Low birth weight of infant. ■ Cephalopelvic disproportion of mother. ■ Iron deficiency anemia. ■ Preeclampsia. 2. Psychologic risks: ■ Interruption of the developmental tasks of adolescence. 3. Sociologic risks: ■ More likely to drop out of school. ■ Need for public assistance. ■ Low-paying employment. ■ Single parenthood. ■ Increased domestic violence.
13.4 Delineate the characteristics of the fathers of children of adolescent mothers.	1. Fathers of children of adolescent mothers: ■ 50% are greater than 20 years of age. ■ Generally from same socioeconomic and educational level as adolescent mother. ■ Often have experienced early school failure.
13.5 Discuss the range of reactions of the adolescent's family and social network to her pregnancy.	1. Families with high educational and career goals for their children experience: ■ Anger. ■ Shock. ■ Shame. ■ Sorrow. 2. Teen often chooses abortion unless cultural or religious beliefs prohibit this. 3. Teen receives more support from family and friends where adolescent pregnancy is more common and more socially acceptable. 4. Some adolescent fathers may view pregnancy as: ■ Sign of adult status. ■ Sign of increased sexual prowess. 5. The mother of the adolescent usually provides the most support.

13.6 Formulate a plan of care to meet the needs of a pregnant adolescent.	1. Nursing care of the pregnant adolescent includes:
	■ Obtaining consent for care.
	■ Developing a trusting relationship with the adolescent.
	■ Promoting self-esteem and problem-solving skills in the adolescent.
	■ Promoting the physical health of the adolescent, especially with information concerning:
	  ■ Regular prenatal visits.
	  ■ Signs of complications.
	  ■ Sexually transmitted diseases.
	  ■ Substance abuse.
	  ■ Promoting family adaptation.
	  ■ Facilitating prenatal education.

13.7 Explore successful community approaches to prevention of adolescent pregnancy.	1. Effective adolescent pregnancy prevention programs: ■ Are long term and intensive. ■ Involve adolescents in program planning. ■ Include good role models from the same cultural and racial backgrounds. ■ Include a focus on the adolescent male.

CRITICAL THINKING IN ACTION

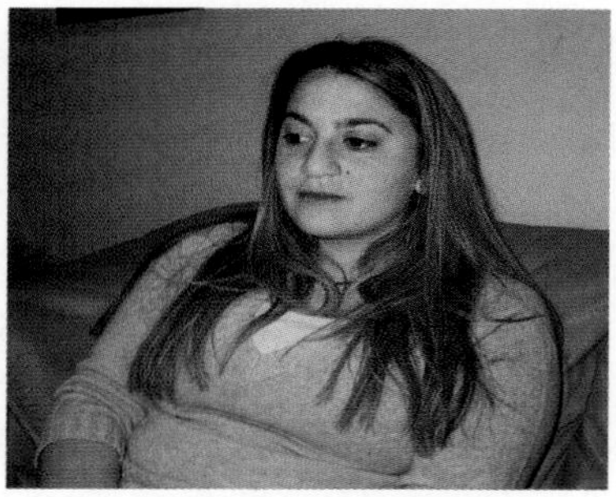

Sixteen-year-old Linda Perez and her mother present to you at the OB clinic for Linda's first prenatal visit. You determine that Linda is 20 weeks pregnant. Her weight is 135 lb, height 5'4", T 98°F, P 80, R 14, BP 100/64. You assess that Linda's mother has type 2 diabetes, and that her siblings are healthy. Linda admits to having one sexual partner and says she has never been hospitalized. Her immunizations are up to date and she's never used tobacco or recreational drugs. To date, the father of the baby is not involved. Mrs. Perez is clearly upset that Linda's pregnancy is so far advanced without her knowledge. Linda is quiet and speaks only when questioned directly. You do your best to try to establish a trusting relationship with Linda and her mother by providing an atmosphere where issues can be discussed.

1. What psychologic factors contribute to teenage pregnancy?
2. Explore reasons why teenagers delay prenatal care.
3. Linda's mother asks you what factors facilitate adolescent pregnancies.
4. You assess that Linda has some anxiety concerning the birth process. She states she is not interested in prenatal classes because she is single and does not want to have natural childbirth. Your best response would be:

See MyNursingKit for possible responses.

REFERENCES

Advocates for Youth. (2005). *Teenage Pregnancy, The case for prevention: An updated analysis of recent trends and federal expenditures associated with teenage pregnancy.* Retrieved October 7, 2005, from www.advocatesforyouth.org/publications/coststudy

Alan Guttmacher Institute. (2006a). *U.S. teenage pregnancy statistics: National and state trends and trends by race and ethnicity.* Retrieved January 11, 2008, from www.guttmacher.org

Alan Guttmacher Institute. (2006b). *Facts on American Teens' Sexual and Reproductive Health.* Retrieved January 11, 2008, from www.guttmacher.org

Alan Guttmacher Institute. (2008). *Facts on young men's sexual and reproductive health.* Retrieved May 22, 2009, from www.guttmacher.org

Alan Guttmacher Institute. (2009). State policies in brief: An overview of minors' consent law. Retrieved February 1, 2009 from www.guttmacher.org

Albert, B., Lippman, L., Franzetta, K., Ikramullah, E., Keith, E. D., Shwalb, R., et al. *Freeze frame: A snapshot of America's teens. (2005).* Retrieved February 1, 2009, from www.teenpregnancy.org

American Academy of Pediatrics. (2007). Policy Statement: Contraception and Adolescents. *Pediatrics, 120*(5), 1135–1148.

American College of Obstetricians and Gynecologists (ACOG). (2007). Intrauterine device and adolescents. Committee Opinion No. 392. Washington, DC: Author.

Bearinger, L. H., Sieving, R. E., Ferguson, J., & Sharma, V. (2007). Global perspectives on the sexual and reproductive health of adolescents: patterns, prevention, and potential. *The Lancet, 369,* 1220–1229.

Davies, S. L., DiClemente, R. J., Wingood, G. M., Person, S. D., Dix, E. S., Harrington, K., et al. (2006). Predictors of inconsistent contraceptive use among adolescent girls: Findings from a prospective study. *The Journal of Adolescent Health, 39*(1), 43–49.

East, P. L., Reyes, B. T., & Horn, E. J. (2007). Association between adolescent pregnancy and a family history of teenage births. *Perspectives on sexual and reproductive health, 39*(2), 108–115.

Francisco, M. A., Hicks, K., Powell, J., Styles, K., Tabor, J. L., & Hulton, L. J. (2008). The effect of childhood sexual abuse on adolescent pregnancy: An integrative research review. *Journal for specialists in pediatric nursing, 13*(4), 237–248.

Hall Moran, V., Edwards, J., Dykes, F., & Downe, S. (2007). A systematic review of the nature of support for breast-feeding adolescent mothers. *Midwifery, 23,* 157–171.

Hamilton, B. E., Martin, J., & Ventura, S. J. (2007). Births: Preliminary data for 2006. *National Vital Statistics Reports, 56*(7), 1–18.

Hamilton, B. E., Martin, J., & Ventura, S. J. (2009). Births: Preliminary data for 2007. *National Vital Statistics Reports, 57*(12), 1–23.

Herman, J. W. (2008). Adolescent perceptions of teen births. *JOGNN: Journal of Obstetric, Gynecologic, and Neonatal Nursing, 37*(1), 42–50.

King-Jones, T. C. (2008). Pregnant adolescents: Perils and pearls of communication. *Nursing for Women's Health, 12*(2), 114–119.

Kirby, D. (2007). Emerging answers: Research findings on programs to reduce teen pregnancy and sexually transmitted diseases. The National Campaign to Prevent Teen and Unplanned Pregnancy. Retrieved April 17, 2008, from http://www.thenationalcampaign.org/EA2007/EA2007–sum.pdf

Klein, J. D., & The Committee on Adolescence. (2005). Adolescent pregnancy: Current trends and issues. *Pediatrics, 116,* 281–286.

Males, M. (2004). Teens and older partners. Resource Center for Adolescent Pregnancy Prevention (ReCAPP). Retrieved January 15, 2008, from www.etr.org/recap/research/AuthoredPaPOlderPrtnrs0504.htm

National Campaign to Prevent Teen and Unplanned Pregnancy. (2006). *Teen sexual activity, contraceptive use, pregnancy, and childbearing: General facts and stats.* Retrieved January 11, 2008, from www.teenpregnancy.org

National Public Radio [NPR], Kaiser Family Foundation, and John F. Kennedy School of Government. (2004). *NPR/Kaiser/Kennedy School Poll: Sex education in America.* Retrieved April 18, 2004, from www.kff.org

Raneri, L. G., & Wiemann, M. (2007). Social ecological predictors of repeat adolescent pregnancy. *Perspectives on sexual and reproductive health, 39*(1), 39–47.

Santelli, J. S., Lindberg, L. D., Finer, L. B., & Singh, S. (2007). Explaining recent declines in adolescent pregnancy in the United States: The contribution of abstinence and improved contraceptive use. *American Journal of Public Health, 97*(1), 150–156.

Steinberg, L. (2005). *Adolescence* (6th ed.). New York: McGraw-Hill.

Tolaymat, L. L., & Kaunitz, A. M. (2007). Long-acting contraceptives in adolescents. *Current Opinion in Obstetrics and Gynecology, 19,* 453–460.

CHAPTER

14 Assessment of Fetal Well-Being

My first pregnancy was so tenuous that I didn't know from one moment to the next how it would end. I hoped for our baby's safety, but in the end the baby died. When I became pregnant the next time, I was very nervous. Being able to see the baby on ultrasound helped me so much. I knew then that our baby was alive and growing. —Sharon, 29

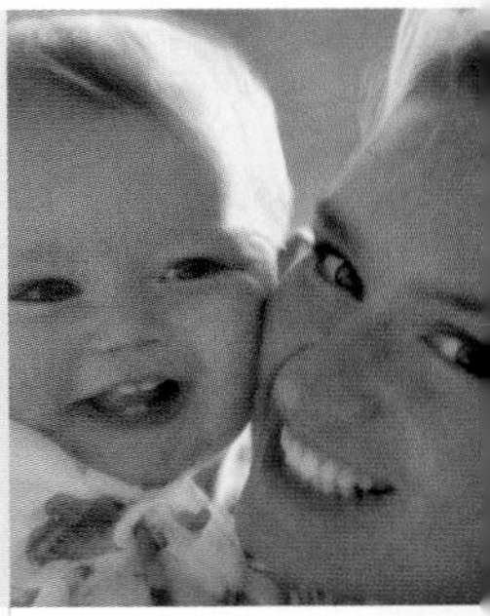

LEARNING OUTCOMES

14.1 Identify pertinent information to be discussed with the woman regarding her own assessment of fetal activity and methods of recording fetal activity.

14.2 Describe the methods, clinical applications, and results of ultrasound in the nursing care management of the pregnant woman.

14.3 Describe the use, procedure, information obtained, and nursing considerations for Doppler velocimetry, nonstress test, contraction stress test, and biophysical profile test.

14.4 Explain the use of amniocentesis as a diagnostic tool.

14.5 Describe the tests that can be done on amniotic fluid.

14.6 Compare the advantages and disadvantages of chorionic villus sampling (CVS).

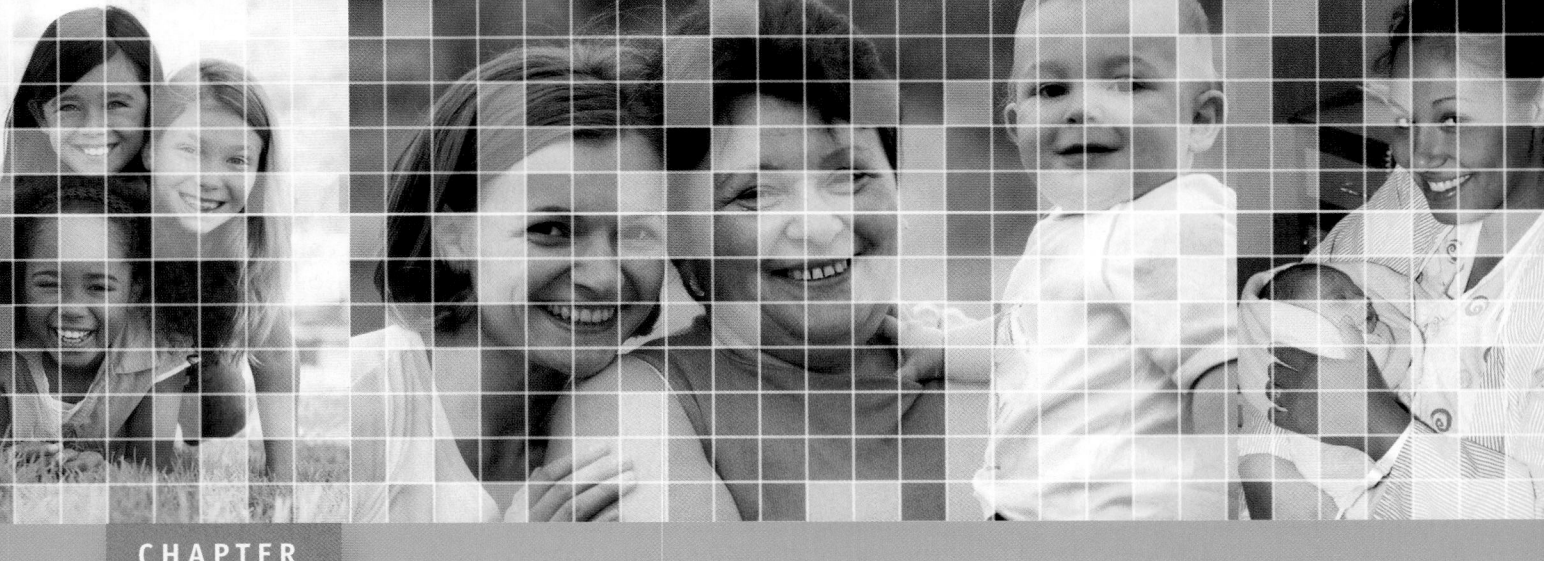

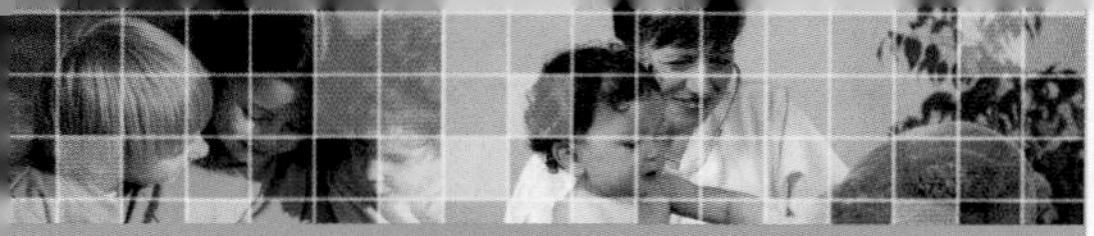

KEY TERMS

Amniocentesis, 296

Biophysical profile (BPP), 294

Chorionic villus sampling (CVS), 298

Contraction stress test (CST), 294

First-trimester combined screening, 290

Lamellar body count (LBC), 297

Lecithin/sphingomyelin (L/S) ratio, 297

Nonstress test (NST), 291

Nuchal translucency testing (NTT), 290

Phosphatidylglycerol (PG), 297

Quadruple screen, 296

Surfactant, 297

Ultrasound, 288

Umbilical velocimetry, 291

The past few decades have produced a notable increase in the number of techniques used to assess fetal well-being. From the relatively simple maternal assessment of fetal movement to more complex diagnostic tests guided by ultrasound, each technique is used to obtain accurate and helpful data about the developing fetus. For example, specialized diagnostic tests can provide information about the normal growth of the fetus, the presence of congenital anomalies, the location of the placenta, and fetal lung maturity (Table 14–1). At times just one test is done, and in other circumstances a combination of testing is needed.

Some of these assessment techniques pose risks to the fetus and possibly to the pregnant woman; the risk to both should be considered before deciding to perform the test. The healthcare provider must be certain that the advantages outweigh the potential risks and added expense. In addition, the diagnostic accuracy and applicability of these tests may vary.

Although some tests are for screening purposes, meaning that they indicate the fetus *may* be at risk for a certain disorder or abnormality, others are diagnostic, meaning that they can diagnose the abnormality. Certainly not all high-risk pregnancies require the same tests. Factors that indicate a pregnancy at risk include the following:

- Maternal age less than 16 or more than 35 years
- Chronic maternal hypertension, preeclampsia, diabetes mellitus, or heart disease
- Presence of Rh alloimmunization
- A maternal history of unexplained stillbirth
- Suspected intrauterine growth restriction (IUGR)
- Pregnancy prolonged past 42 weeks' gestation
- Multiple gestation
- Maternal history of preterm labor
- Previous cervical incompetence

See Chapter 9 for further discussion of prenatal at-risk factors and Chapters 15 and 16 for descriptions of various conditions that may threaten the successful completion of pregnancy.

Nursing care for the woman who is undergoing diagnostic testing focuses on outcomes to ensure that she understands the reasons for the test, the test results, and receives adequate support during the test (see Table 14–2). In addition, other objectives include completing the tests without complications and ensuring that the safety of the mother and her unborn child has been maintained.

MATERNAL ASSESSMENT OF FETAL ACTIVITY

Clinicians now generally agree that vigorous fetal activity provides reassurance of fetal well-being and that marked decrease in activity or cessation of movement may indicate possible fetal compromise (or even death) requiring immediate follow-up (Gabbe, Niebyl, & Simpson, 2007). Fetal activity is typically used to monitor fetal well-being beginning at approximately 28 gestational weeks. Fetal activity monitoring has been used for some time as a low technology, inexpensive means to evaluate fetal well-being. One study identified 19% of fetuses with intrauterine growth restriction on the basis of an initial report by the mother of decreased fetal movement (Sinha, Sharma, Nallaswamy, et al., 2007). A reduction of fetal movement has been associated with fetal hypoxia, fetal growth restriction, and fetal death (Heazell & Frøen, 2008). Another study showed that 5% to 15% of women report decreased fetal movement during their pregnancies (Heazell, Green, Wright, et al., 2008). Although more research is needed to determine if fetal activity assessment improves neonatal outcomes, the literature does suggest that maternal monitoring does result in a decrease in perinatal mortality (Heazell & Frøen, 2008; Mangesi & Hofmeyr,

Table 14–1 Summary of Screening and Diagnostic Tests

Goal	Test	Timing
To validate the pregnancy	Ultrasound: gestational sac volume	5 and 6 weeks after last menstrual period (LMP) by transvaginal ultrasound
To determine how advanced the pregnancy is	Ultrasound: crown–rump length Ultrasound: biparietal diameter, femur length, abdomen circumference	6 to 10 weeks' gestation 13 to 40 weeks' gestation
To identify normal growth of the fetus	Ultrasound: biparietal diameter Ultrasound: head/abdomen ratio Ultrasound: estimated fetal weight	Most useful from 20 to 30 weeks' gestation 13 to 40 weeks' gestation About 24 to 40 weeks' gestation
To detect congenital anomalies and problems	Nuchal translucency testing Ultrasound Chorionic villus sampling Amniocentesis Fetoscopy First trimester combination screening test or quadruple test	9 to 13 weeks' gestation 18 to 40 weeks' gestation 10 to 12 weeks' gestation 15 to 20 weeks' gestation 18 weeks' gestation Generally 15 to 20 weeks' gestation
To localize the placenta	Ultrasound	Usually in third trimester or before amniocentesis
To assess fetal status	Biophysical profile Maternal assessment of fetal activity Nonstress test Contraction stress test	Approximately 28 weeks to birth Approximately 28 weeks to birth Approximately 28 weeks to birth After 28 weeks
To diagnose cardiac problems	Fetal echocardiography	Second and third trimesters
To assess fetal lung maturity	Amniocentesis L/S ratio Phosphatidylglycerol Phosphatidylcholine Lamellar body counts	33 to 40 weeks 33 weeks to birth 33 weeks to birth 33 weeks to birth 33 weeks to birth
To obtain more information about breech presentation	Ultrasound	Just before labor is anticipated or during labor

Table 14–2 Suggested Nursing Approaches to Pretest Teaching

Assess if the woman knows the reason the screening or diagnostic test is being recommended.
Examples:
"What has your doctor or nurse-midwife told you about why this test is necessary?"
"Sometimes tests are done for many different reasons. Can you tell me why you are having this test?"
"What is your understanding about what the test will show?"

Provide an opportunity for questions.
Examples:
"What questions do you have about the test?"
"Is there anything that is not clear to you?"

Explain the test procedure, paying particular attention to any preparation the woman needs before the test.
Example:
"The test that has been ordered for you is designed to." (Add specific information about the particular test. Give the explanation using simple language.)

Validate the woman's understanding of the preparation.
Example:
"Tell me what you will have to do to get ready for this test."

Give permission for the woman to continue to ask questions if needed.
Example:
"I'll be with you during the test. If you have any questions at any time, please don't hesitate to ask."

Nursing Practice

Families undergoing fetal testing experience a wide range of emotions based on personal expectations, past experiences, fears, and cultural norms. Encouraging the family to verbalize concerns, ask questions, and express any apprehensions or fears can help put the family at ease.

2007). There is no precise definition of how many movements should occur within a specified time period. When explaining fetal activity monitoring, the mother is instructed to count fetal movements beginning the same time each day. If there are fewer than 10 movements in a 3-hour period or if the amount of movement is significantly less than normal, the woman should immediately notify her healthcare provider. The newest literature suggests that a maternal perception of decreased movement spanning a 24-hour period should cause concern and warrant antepartum fetal testing (Heazell et al., 2008).

Fetuses spend approximately 10% of their time making gross body movements. Fetal movements are directly related to the infant's sleep–wake cycles and vary from the maternal sleep–wake cycle (Blackburn, 2007). After 38 weeks, the fetus spends 75% of its time in a quiet sleep or active sleep state. In women with a multiple gestation, daily fetal movements are significantly higher. The expectant mother's perception of fetal movements and her commitment to completing a fetal movement record may vary. When a woman understands the purpose of the assessment, how to complete the form, whom to call with questions, and what to report—and has the opportunity for follow-up during each visit—she generally views completing the fetal movement record as an important activity. The nurse is available to answer questions and clarify areas of concern. (See earlier discussion and "Teaching Highlights: Assessing Fetal Activity," in Chapter 11 ∞.)

ULTRASOUND

Valuable information about the fetus may be obtained from **ultrasound** testing. Intermittent ultrasonic waves (high-frequency sound waves) are transmitted by an alternating current to a transducer, which is applied to the woman's abdomen. The ultrasonic waves deflect off tissues within the woman's abdomen, showing structures of varying densities (Figures 14–1 ● and 14–2 ●).

Diagnostic ultrasound has several advantages. It is noninvasive, and painless for both the woman and the fetus, and it has no known harmful effects to either. Serial studies (several ultrasound tests done over a span of time) may be done for assessment and comparison. Soft-tissue masses (such as tumors) can be differentiated, the fetus can be visualized, fetal growth can be followed (especially in the presence of multiple gestation), cervical length and impending cervical incompetence can be detected, and a number of other potential problems can be averted (Smith, Celik, To, et al., 2008; Verburg, Steegers, DeRidder, et al., 2008). In addition, the ultrasonographer or physician immediately obtains results.

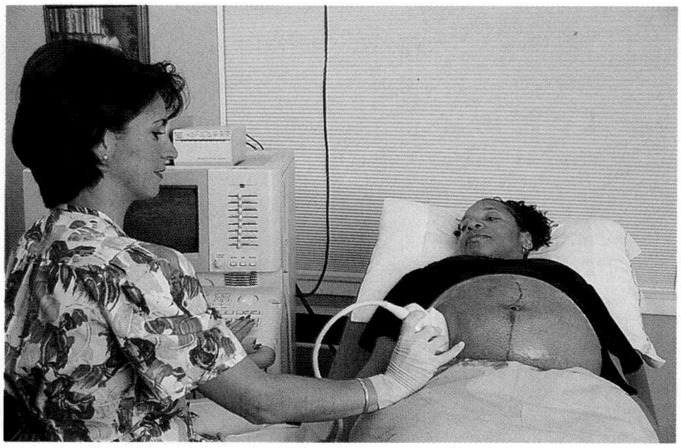

● **Figure 14–1** Ultrasound scanning permits visualization of the fetus in utero.

Future research in fetal well-being will be generated and enhanced by the use of the *four-dimensional ultrasound.* Four-dimensional ultrasound combines the components of three-dimensional ultrasound with a fourth dimension, time, because it monitors live action. The technology produces images of photolike quality, allowing healthcare providers to better visualize fetal structures, and providing better guidance during invasive intrauterine procedures such as amniocentesis and chorionic villus sampling (CVS) (discussed later in this chapter). Although ultrasound serves as a useful tool in monitoring the fetus throughout pregnancy, ultrasound has limitations and it cannot guarantee that a fetus does not have certain disorders or defects. Ultrasound is limited by fetal positioning, and technician or physician skill. Even though fetal problems can be diagnosed via the technology, there are times that abnormalities go unrecognized. A "normal" ultrasound is reassuring for the parents and healthcare team, but it is important that parents realize the ultrasound or sonogram is not 100% reliable.

PROCEDURES

The two most common methods of ultrasound scanning are transabdominal and transvaginal.

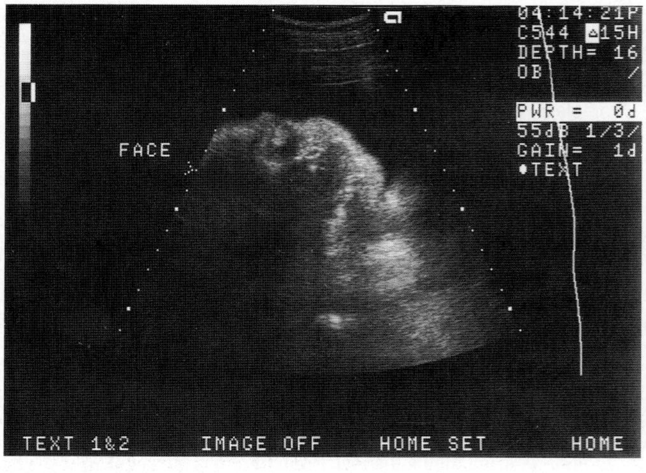

● **Figure 14–2** Ultrasound of fetal face.

Transabdominal Ultrasound

In the transabdominal approach, a transducer is moved across the woman's abdomen. The woman is often scanned with a full bladder. When the bladder is full, the examiner can assess other structures, especially the vagina and cervix, in relation to the bladder. The ability to see the lower portion of the uterus and cervix is particularly important when vaginal bleeding is noted and placenta previa is the suspected cause. The woman is advised to drink 1 to 1.5 quarts of water approximately 2 hours before the examination, and she is asked to refrain from emptying her bladder. If the bladder is not sufficiently filled, she is asked to drink three to four (8 oz) glasses of water and is rescanned 30 to 45 minutes later.

Mineral oil or a transmission gel is generously spread over the woman's abdomen, and the sonographer slowly moves a transducer over the abdomen to obtain a picture of the uterine contents. Ultrasound testing takes 20 to 30 minutes. The woman may feel discomfort caused by pressure applied over a full bladder. In addition, if the woman lies on her back during the test, shortness of breath can develop. This may be relieved by elevating her upper body during the test.

Transvaginal Ultrasound

The transvaginal approach uses a probe inserted into the vagina. Once inserted, the transvaginal probe is close to the structures being imaged and so produces a clearer, more defined image. The improved images obtained by transvaginal ultrasound have enabled sonographers to identify structures and fetal characteristics earlier in pregnancy. Internal visualization can also be used as a predictor for preterm birth in high-risk cases. Use of the ultrasound to detect shortened cervical length or funneling (a cone-shaped indentation in the cervical os) is helpful in predicting preterm labor, especially in women who have a history of preterm birth (ACOG, 2009).

After the procedure is fully explained to the woman, she is prepared in the same manner as for a pelvic examination: in the lithotomy position, with appropriate drapes to provide privacy and a female attendant in the room. It is important that her buttocks are at the end of the table so that, once inserted, the probe can be moved in various directions. A small, lightweight vaginal transducer is covered with a specially fitted sterile sheath, a condom, or one finger of a glove. Ultrasound coupling gel is then applied to both the inside and outside of the covering, making insertion into the vagina easier and providing a medium for enhancing the ultrasound image. The transvaginal procedure can be accomplished with an empty bladder, and most women do not feel discomfort during the exam. The probe is smaller than a speculum, so insertion is usually completed with ease. The woman may feel the movement of the probe during the exam as various structures are imaged. Some women may want to insert the probe themselves to enhance their comfort, whereas others would feel embarrassed even to be asked. The certified nurse-midwife, physician, or ultrasonographer offers the choice based on personal rapport with the woman.

CLINICAL APPLICATIONS

Ultrasound testing can be of benefit in the following ways:

- *Early identification of pregnancy.* Pregnancy may be detected as early as the fifth or sixth week after the last menstrual period (LMP) by assessing the gestational sac and the presence of a fetal heart rate after 6 gestational weeks.
- *Observation of fetal heartbeat and fetal breathing movements (FBMs).* FBMs have been observed as early as week 11 of gestation.
- *Identification of more than one embryo or fetus.*
- *Measurement of the biparietal diameter of the fetal head or the fetal femur length to assess growth patterns.* These measurements help determine the gestational age of the fetus and identify IUGR.
- *Clinical estimations of birth weight.* This assessment helps to identify macrosomia (infants greater than 4000 g at birth) and low-birth-weight infants (infants less than 2500 g at birth). Macrosomia has been identified as a predictor of birth-related trauma and is a risk factor for both maternal and fetal morbidity (ACOG, 2009).
- *Detection of fetal anomalies such as facial anomalies, anencephaly and hydrocephalus (ACOG, 2009).*
- *Examination of nuchal translucency in the first trimester to assess for Down syndrome and other fetal structural anomalies (ACOG, 2009).* Nuchal translucency describes an area in the back of the fetal neck that is measured via ultrasound during the first trimester of pregnancy. Fetuses with a nuchal translucency measurement of greater than 3 mm are at risk for certain birth defects, including trisomies 13, 18, and 21.
- *Examination of fetal cardiac structures (echocardiography).*
- *Length of fetal nasal bone.* The length of the fetal nasal bone during the nuchal translucency test is used to indicate a risk factor for Down syndrome. Fetuses with a nonvisualized or shortened nasal bone are more likely to have trisomy 21 than those with a normal length nasal bone (Cusick, Shevell, Duchan, et al., 2008).
- *Identification of amniotic fluid volume and amniotic fluid index (AFI).* Amniotic fluid volume (AFV) parameters measures the single largest pocket of amniotic fluid on ultrasonography, free of cord and fetal parts, and then measures either the greatest vertical dimension or the greatest vertical and horizontal dimensions. The vertical diameter of the largest amniotic fluid pocket in each of four quadrants is measured for AFI. The measurements are totaled to obtain the AFI in centimeters. Women with an AFI of more than 24 cm and amniotic fluid volume of equal to or greater than 8 cm are considered to have hydramnios, and women with less than 5 cm at term and the deepest vertical pocket of AFV of less than 2 cm are considered to have oligohydramnios (ACOG, 2009). After 39 weeks, the amniotic fluid volume begins to decline (Gabbe et al., 2007). Both hydramnios and oligohydramnios are associated with increased risk to the fetus, including nonreassuring fetal status, intrauterine growth restriction, meconium-stained amniotic fluid, and an increase in admissions to the neonatal intensive care unit.
- *Location of the placenta.* The placenta is located before amniocentesis to avoid puncturing the placenta.

Ultrasound is valuable in identifying and evaluating placenta previa.

- *Placental grading.* As the fetus matures, the placenta calcifies. These changes can be detected by ultrasound and graded according to the degree of calcification. Placenta grading can be used to identify internal placenta vasculature, which can be associated with preeclampsia and chronic hypertension. It can also identify disorders such as fetal growth abnormalities, triploidy, non-immune hydrops, and infections.
- *Detection of fetal death.* Inability to visualize the fetal heart beating and the separation of the bones in the fetal head are signs of fetal death.
- *Determination of fetal position and presentation.*
- *Accompanying procedures.* Amniocentesis, chorionic villus sampling, intrauterine procedures, and other procedures will be discussed shortly.

RISKS OF ULTRASOUND

Ultrasound has been used clinically for over 40 years; to date no clinical studies verify harmful effects to the mother, the fetus, or the newborn. Many pregnant clients themselves received diagnostic ultrasound in utero with no adverse effects.

Nursing Management

It is important for the nurse to ascertain whether the woman understands why the ultrasound is being suggested and that the ultrasound is an extremely valuable tool although it is not 100% reliable. The nurse provides an opportunity for the woman to ask questions and acts as an advocate if there are questions or concerns that need to be addressed before the ultrasound examination. The nurse discusses the options available to the woman and her partner for fetal evaluation. According to ACOG (2007), the option of fetal evaluation should be offered to all women, regardless of age. This includes both invasive testing, such as amniocentesis and chorionic villus sampling (CVS), and ultrasound screening. The nurse explains the preparation needed and ensures that adequate preparation is done. After the test is completed, the nurse can assist with clarifying or interpreting test results for the woman and her partner.

NUCHAL TRANSLUCENCY TESTING

Nuchal translucency testing (NTT), also known as nuchal testing (NT) or nuchal fold test, is performed at 11 1/7 to 13 6/7 gestational weeks to screen for trisomies 13, 18, and 21 (Wright, Kagan, Molina, et al., 2008). Although women over the age of 35 have a higher risk of chromosomal disorders, ACOG (2007) recommends that all women be offered first- and second-trimester screening. The test uses ultrasound to scan the translucent or clear area on the back of the fetal neck, measuring the diameter of the area. Fetuses with certain genetic disorders often have an excess accumulation of fluid that can be seen at the end of the first trimester. The results are computed using the nuchal measurement, exact gestational age, and maternal age. Fetuses that have a nuchal translucency measurement of greater than 3 mm are at risk for trisomies 13, 18, and 21 and should be offered an amniocentesis (to be discussed later). The NTT is a *screening test,* meaning it indicates that a fetus is at risk. Diagnostic testing, such as an amniocentesis, is a *diagnostic test,* which indicates that the fetus has the specific diagnosis.

The NTT test has several advantages over other testing options. It can be performed in the first trimester, early in a pregnancy, to determine if a fetus is *at risk* for chromosomal disorders. Unlike the chorionic villus sampling (CVS) or amniocentesis, it has no risk of spontaneous abortion because it is a noninvasive test. The NTT accurately detects 70% to 80% of fetuses with Down syndrome (DS) (Scott, 2007). When combined with serum testing, the accuracy level increases. Many women feel anxious during pregnancy. A normal result can provide reassurance to the woman that her baby is most likely without a chromosome disorder.

The disadvantage is that it can provide false positives and is not diagnostic. The combined test has a 5% false positive rate, meaning the test will indicate that the fetus is at risk for Down syndrome when in fact the fetus has normal chromosomes. Women who receive an abnormal test are then counseled to determine if they would like to have an amniocentesis for diagnostic purposes. The choice to proceed with testing is a very personal one. Some women will wish to obtain the test so they will be more prepared for the diagnosis; other women will want to discontinue the pregnancy. Some women may decide not to have additional testing.

Fetuses that have a nuchal translucency measurement above the 99th percentile are also at risk for congenital heart disease (Clur, Mathijssen, Pajkrt, et al., 2008). A fetal echocardiogram is ordered in these cases to determine if a cardiac anomaly is also present. Fetuses with a nuchal fold measurement equal to or greater than 6.5 mm had a 27.7% risk of having a congenital heart defect (Clur et al., 2008).

First-trimester combined screening is comprehensive screening testing that includes the NTT and serum screening for pregnancy-associated plasma protein-A (PAPP-A) and free beta human chorionic gonadotropin (β-hCG) to determine if a fetus is at risk for trisomies 13, 18, and 21. The combined test is more accurate than an NTT alone because it provides additional data. Using both the NTT and the serum testing, the accuracy rates for diagnosis improves to 91% for accurately assessing the risk of Down syndrome and 98% for assessing trisomy 18 (Clur et al., 2008).

Nursing Practice

When advising clients that a screening test, such as the NTT, is abnormal, make sure to explain that this does *not* mean their baby definitely has the disorder, but rather indicates that the baby *may* be at risk. It is imperative that parents understand an abnormal NTT, or any type of screening test, is only an indication that more testing is needed to make the actual diagnosis. Advise parents that some women with abnormal test results have normal fetuses and that because the test only screens and does not actually diagnose the fetus, a fetus that screens within the normal criteria could have an unrecognized anomaly.

DOPPLER BLOOD FLOW STUDIES (UMBILICAL VELOCIMETRY)

Umbilical velocimetry, a noninvasive ultrasound test, measures blood flow changes that occur in maternal and fetal circulation in order to assess placental function. An ultrasound beam, like that provided by the pocket Doppler (a handheld ultrasound device), is directed at the umbilical artery (in some cases a maternal vessel such as the arcuate can also be used). The signal is reflected off the red blood cells moving within the vessels and creates a "picture" (waveform) that looks like a series of waves (Figures 14–3 ● and 14–4 ●). The highest-velocity peak of the waves is the systolic measurement, and the lowest point is the diastolic velocity. To interpret the waveforms, the systolic (S) peak is divided by the end-diastolic (D) component. This calculation is called the S/D ratio. The normal S/D ratio is below 2.6 by 26 weeks' gestation and below 3 at term. A decrease in uteroplacental perfusion (because of narrowing of the vessels) causes an increase in placental bed resistance and a decrease in diastolic flow, resulting in an elevated S/D ratio (Kwon, 2006). Elevations of 3 and above are considered abnormal. Doppler blood flow studies are helpful in assessing and managing pregnancies with suspected uteroplacental insufficiency before asphyxia occurs (Kwon, 2006). Abnormal Doppler flow studies accompanied by a decrease in amniotic fluid have been associated with small-for-gestational-age fetuses, cesarean section for nonreassuring fetal status, 5 min Apgar score of less than 7 (7 to 10 is the normal range), respiratory distress syndrome, NICU admission, and perinatal death (Kwon, 2006).

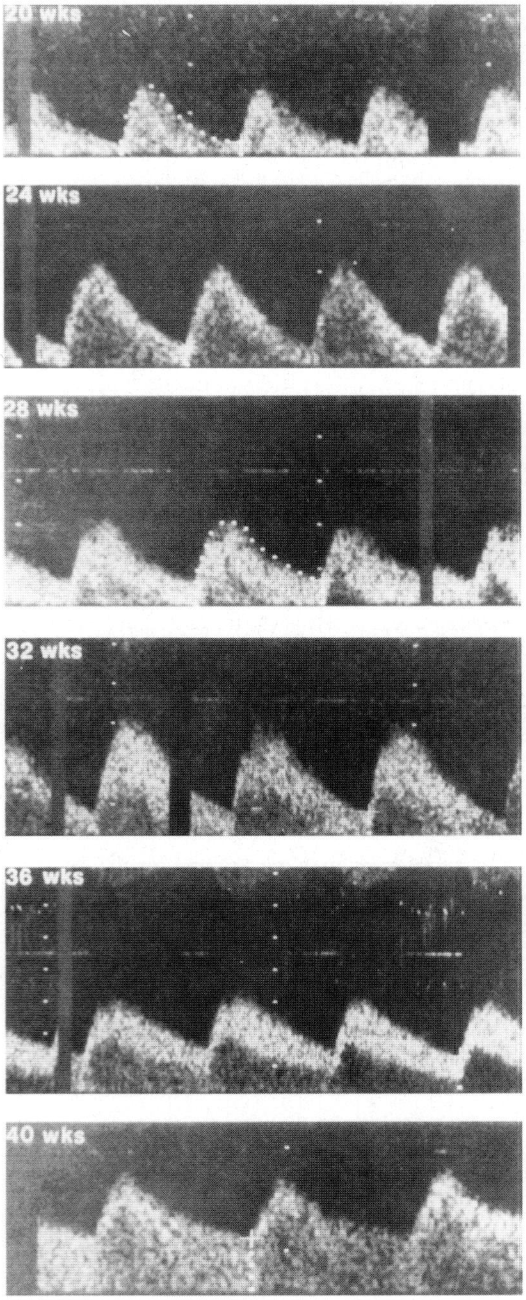

● **Figure 14–3** Serial studies of the umbilical artery velocity waveforms in a normal pregnancy from one client.

Source: AWHONN. (1990). Cundiff, J. L., Haybrich, K. L., & Hinzman, N. G. Umbilical artery Doppler flow studies during pregnancy. *Journal of Obstetric, Gynecologic, and Neonatal Nursing, 19*(6), 475–481 (Figure 3, p. 478). Washington, DC: Author.

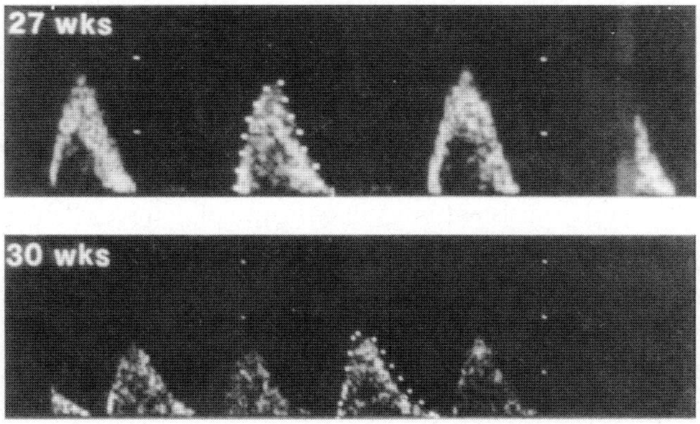

● **Figure 14–4** Two examples of abnormal umbilical artery velocity waveforms taken from a client with intrauterine growth restriction.

Source: AWHONN. (1990). Cundiff, J. L., Haybrich, K. L., & Hinzman, H. G. Umbilical artery Doppler flow studies during pregnancy. *Journal of Obstetric, Gynecologic, and Neonatal Nursing, 19*(6), 475–481 (Figure 4, p. 478). Washington, DC: Author.

Doppler blood flow studies are relatively easy to obtain. The woman lies supine with a wedge under the right hip (to promote uteroplacental perfusion). Warmed transducer gel is applied to the abdomen, and a pulsed-wave Doppler device is used to ascertain the blood flow. The Doppler flow study takes about 15 to 20 minutes. Doppler flow studies can be initiated at 16 to 18 weeks' gestation and are then scheduled at regular intervals for women at risk.

NONSTRESS TEST

The **nonstress test (NST)**, a widely used method of evaluating fetal status, may be used alone or as part of a more comprehensive diagnostic assessment called a biophysical profile (BPP). The nonstress test is based on the knowledge that when the fetus has adequate oxygenation and an intact central nervous system, there are accelerations of the fetal heart rate (FHR) with fetal movement (FM). An NST requires an electronic fetal monitor to observe and record these fetal heart rate accelerations (see discussion of acceleration in Chapter 18∞). A nonreactive NST is fairly consistent in identifying at-risk fetuses (Gabbe et al., 2007). The advantages of the NST are as follows:

- It is quick to perform, permits easy interpretation, and is inexpensive.
- It can be done in an office or clinic setting.
- There are no known side effects.

The disadvantages of the NST include the following:

- It is sometimes difficult to obtain a suitable tracing.
- The woman has to remain relatively still for at least 20 minutes.

PROCEDURE FOR NST

The test can be done with the woman in a reclining chair or in bed in a left-tilted semi-Fowler's or side-lying position. Research has shown that certain maternal positions can help produce more favorable results. Women in left-tilted semi-Fowler's, sitting positions, and left lateral positions have more fetal movement and are more likely to have a reactive tracing. Women should not be placed in a supine position because it is associated with less fetal movement, maternal back pain, and maternal shortness of breath (Alus, Okumus, Mete, et al., 2007). The nurse places the electronic fetal monitor under the woman's clothing. Privacy should be provided. The examiner places two elastic belts on the woman's abdomen. One belt (tocodynamometer) holds a device that detects uterine or fetal movement; the other belt holds the ultrasound transducer that detects the FHR. As the NST is done, each fetal movement is documented, so that associated or simultaneous FHR changes can be evaluated.

INTERPRETATION OF NST RESULTS

Women with a high-risk factor will probably begin having NSTs at 30 to 32 weeks' gestation and at frequent intervals for the remainder of the pregnancy. The results of the NST are interpreted as follows:

- *Reactive test.* A reactive NST shows at least two accelerations of FHR with fetal movements of 15 beats per minute, lasting 15 seconds or more, over 20 minutes (Figure 14–5 ●). This is the desired result. (See Table 14–3.)
- *Nonreactive test.* In a nonreactive test, the reactive criteria are not met. For example, the accelerations do not meet the requirements of 15 beats per minute or do not last 15 seconds (Figure 14–6 ●).
- *Unsatisfactory test.* An NST is unsatisfactory if the data cannot be interpreted or there was inadequate fetal activity.

Table 14–3 Nonstress Test

Diagnostic value: Demonstrates fetus's ability to respond to its environment by acceleration of FHR with movement.

Results:
- *Reactive test:* Accelerations (at least 2) of 15 bpm above the baseline, lasting 15 sec or more in a 20-min window, are present, indicating fetal well-being.
- *Nonreactive test:* Accelerations are not present or do not meet the above criteria indicating that the fetus is at risk or asleep.

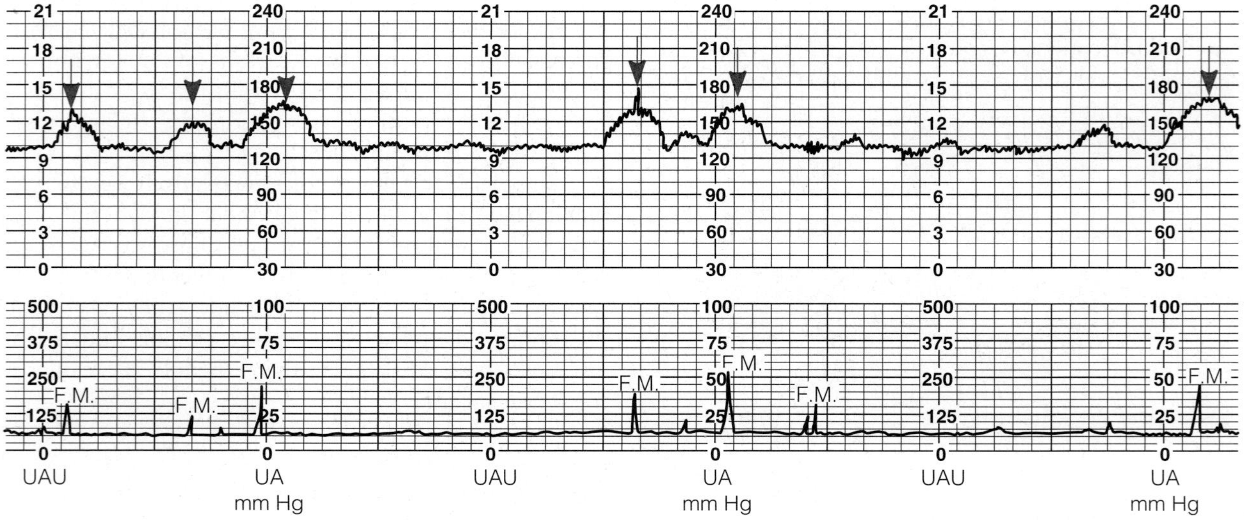

● **Figure 14–5** Example of a reactive nonstress test (NST). The test shows accelerations of 15 bpm lasting 15 seconds with each fetal movement (FM). Top of strip shows FHR; bottom of strip shows uterine activity tracing. Note that FHR increases (above the baseline) at least 15 beats and remains at that rate for at least 15 seconds before returning to the former baseline.

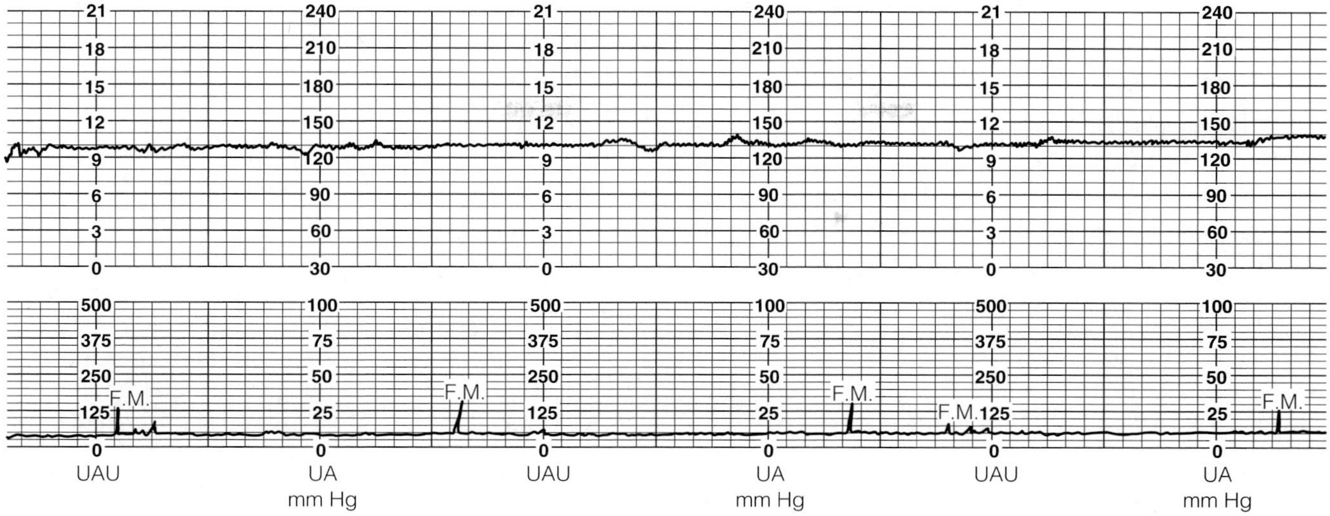

● **Figure 14–6** Example of a nonreactive NST. There are no accelerations of FHR with fetal movement (FM). Baseline FHR is 130 bpm. The tracing of uterine activity is on the bottom of the strip.

It is important that anyone who performs the NST understand the significance of any decelerations of the FHR during testing. If decelerations are noted, the certified nurse-midwife or physician should be notified for further evaluation of fetal status. (See Chapter 18 for further discussion of FHR decelerations.)

CLINICAL MANAGEMENT

The clinical management of potential nonreassuring fetal status may vary depending on the clinical judgment of the care provider. One commonly used protocol is as follows: If the NST is reactive in less than 30 minutes, the test is concluded and rescheduled as indicated by the high-risk condition that is present. If it is nonreactive, the test time is extended for 30 minutes until the results are reactive, and then the test is rescheduled as indicated. It is estimated that 80% to 90% of nonreactive NSTs happen because of fetal sleep states (Gabbe et al., 2007). If the FHR remains nonreactive for longer than 30 minutes, the test is typically repeated after the woman eats or the fetus is stimulated via vibroacoustic stimulation, a foot massage, or palpation. Such measures often wake a fetus so a reactive NST can be obtained. If a reactive test is not obtained within 30 minutes, additional testing (such as diagnostic ultrasound and BPP) or immediate birth is considered; if the NST is nonreactive and spontaneous decelerations of the FHR are present, diagnostic ultrasound and BPP are performed and birth is recommended (Figure 14–7 ●). Many testing guidelines vary in frequency, recommending a retest either once or twice a week, depending upon the at-risk condition that exists.

Nursing Practice

If a nonstress test fails to become reactive, a 3-minute foot massage has been shown to stimulate the fetus and increase fetal activity. It also helps the woman to relax during the test.

Nursing Management

The nurse evaluates the woman's understanding of the NST and the possible results. The reasons for the NST and the procedure are reviewed before beginning the test. The nurse administers the NST, interprets the results, and reports the findings to the certified nurse-midwife or physician and the expectant woman.

FETAL ACOUSTIC AND VIBROACOUSTIC STIMULATION TESTS

Acoustic (sound) and vibroacoustic (vibration and sound) stimulation of the fetus can be used as an adjunct to the NST. A handheld, battery-operated device is applied to the woman's abdomen over the area of the fetal head. This device generates a low-frequency vibration and a buzzing sound. These are intended to induce movement and associated accelerations of FHR in fetuses with a nonreactive NST and in fetuses with decreased variability of FHR during labor. (See discussion of variability in Chapter 18.) The sound stimulus persists for 2 to 5 seconds; if no accelerations occur, it is then repeated at 1-minute intervals up to three times. Whether the fetus responds more to the vibration or to the sound is not known. Two FHR accelerations of 15 beats per minute, lasting 15 seconds, in a 20-minute period indicate a reactive test (Gabbe et al., 2007). Advantages of the fetal acoustic stimulation test (FAST) and the vibroacoustic stimulation test (VST) are as follows:

- Both are noninvasive techniques and are easy to perform.
- Results are rapidly available.
- Time for the NST is shortened.

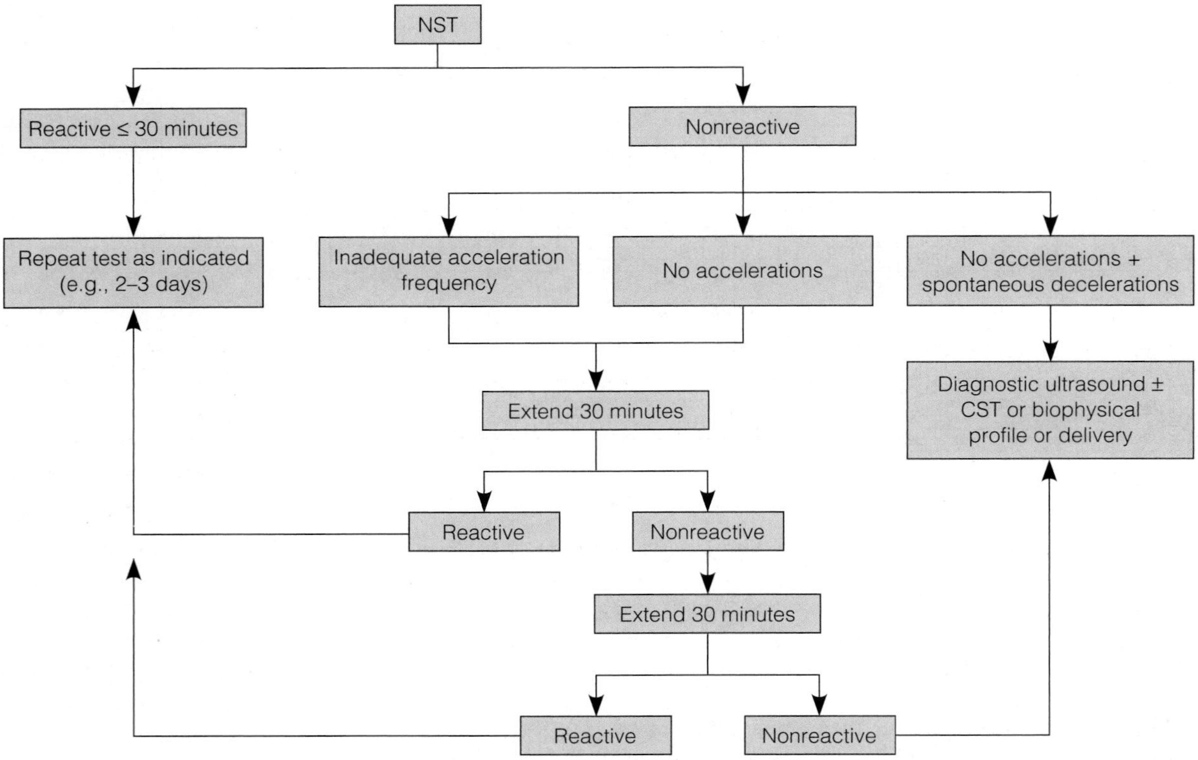

● **Figure 14–7** NST management scheme.

Source: Devoe, L. D. (1989). Nonstress and contraction stress testing. In R. Depp, D. A. Eschenbach, & J. J. Sciarri (Eds.), *Gynecology and obstetrics* (Vol. 3, p. 9, Figure 5). Philadelphia: Lippincott.

BIOPHYSICAL PROFILE

The **biophysical profile (BPP)** is a comprehensive assessment of five biophysical variables:

1. Fetal breathing movement
2. Fetal movements of body or limbs
3. Fetal tone (extension and flexion of extremities)
4. Amniotic fluid volume (visualized as pockets of fluid around the fetus)
5. Reactive FHR with activity (reactive NST)

The first four variables are assessed by ultrasound scanning; FHR reactivity is assessed with the NST. By combining these five assessments, the BPP helps to either identify the compromised fetus or confirm the healthy fetus and provides an assessment of placental functioning. Specific criteria for normal and abnormal assessments are presented in Table 14–4. A score of 2 is assigned to each normal finding, and 0 to each abnormal one, for a maximum score of 10. The absence of a specific activity is difficult to interpret, because it may indicate central nervous system (CNS) depression or simply the resting state of a healthy fetus. Scores of 8/10 (with normal amniotic fluid) and 10/10 are considered normal. Such scores have the least chance of being associated with a compromised fetus unless a decrease in the amount of amniotic fluid is noted, in which case the infant's birth may be indicated. The use of maximum vertical pocket depth, and not the four-quadrant AFI (amniotic fluid index), in traditional BPS is validated by current research (Harmon, 2009).

The BPP is indicated when there is risk of placental insufficiency or fetal compromise because of the following:

- Intrauterine growth restriction (IUGR)
- Maternal diabetes mellitus
- Maternal heart disease
- Maternal chronic hypertension
- Maternal preeclampsia or eclampsia
- Maternal sickle cell anemia
- Suspected fetal postmaturity (more than 42 weeks' gestation)
- History of previous stillbirths
- Rh sensitization
- Abnormal estriol excretion
- Hyperthyroidism
- Renal disease
- Nonreactive NST

CONTRACTION STRESS TEST

The **contraction stress test (CST)** is a means of evaluating the respiratory function (oxygen and carbon dioxide exchange) of the placenta. It enables the healthcare team to identify the fetus

Table 14–4 Criteria for Biophysical Profile Scoring

Component	Normal (score = 2)	Abnormal (score = 0)
Fetal breathing movements	≥ 1 episode of rhythmic breathing lasting ≥ 30 sec within 30 min	≤ 30 sec of breathing in 30 min
Gross body movements	≥ 3 discrete body or limb movements in 30 min (episodes of active continuous movement considered as single movement)	≤ 2 movements in 30 min
Fetal tone	≥ 1 episode of extension of a fetal extremity with return to flexion, or opening or closing of hand	No movements or extension/flexion
Amniotic fluid volume	Single vertical pocket > 2 cm AFI > 5 cm	Largest single vertical pocket ≤ 2 cm AFI < 5 cm
Nonstress test	≥ 2 accelerations of ≥ 15 beats/min for ≥ 15 sec in 20 min	0 or 1 acceleration in 20 min

at risk for intrauterine asphyxia by observing the response of the FHR to the stress of uterine contractions (spontaneous or induced). During contractions, intrauterine pressure increases. Blood flow to the intervillous space of the placenta is reduced momentarily, thereby decreasing oxygen transport to the fetus. A healthy fetus usually tolerates this reduction well and maintains a steady heart rate. If the placental reserve is insufficient, fetal hypoxia, depression of the myocardium, and a decrease in FHR occur.

In many areas, the CST has given way to the biophysical profile. It is still used in areas where the availability of other technology is reduced (such as during night shifts) or limited (such as at small community hospitals or birthing centers). It may also be used as an adjunct to other forms of fetal assessment.

The CST is contraindicated in third-trimester bleeding from placenta previa, marginal abruptio placentae or unexplained vaginal bleeding, previous cesarean with classical incision (vertical incision in the fundus of the uterus), premature rupture of the membranes, incompetent cervix, cerclage in place, anomalies of the maternal reproductive organs, history of preterm labor (if being done before term), or multiple gestation.

PROCEDURE

The critical component of the CST is the presence of uterine contractions. They may occur spontaneously (which is unusual before the onset of labor), or they may be induced (stimulated) with oxytocin (Pitocin) administered intravenously (also known as an oxytocin challenge test [OCT]). A natural method of obtaining oxytocin is through the use of breast stimulation (either via nipple self-stimulation or application of an electric breast pump); the posterior pituitary produces oxytocin in response to stimulation of the breasts or nipples.

An electronic fetal monitor is used to provide continuous data about the fetal heart rate and uterine contractions. After a 15-minute baseline recording of uterine activity and FHR, the tracing is evaluated for evidence of spontaneous contractions. If three spontaneous contractions of good quality and lasting 40 to 60 seconds occur in a 10-minute window, the results are evaluated, and the test is concluded. If no contractions occur or they are insufficient for interpretation, oxytocin is administered intravenously or breast self-stimulation or application of an electric breast pump is done to produce contractions of good quality. (See Chapter 23∞ for more information on nursing care management of oxytocin induction.) The CST should be conducted only in a setting where tocolytic medications are available if a hyperstimulation pattern occurs or if labor is stimulated from the test.

INTERPRETATION OF CST RESULTS

The CST is classified as follows:

- *Negative.* A negative CST shows three contractions of good quality lasting 40 or more seconds in 10 minutes without evidence of late decelerations. This is the desired result. It implies that the fetus can handle the hypoxic stress of uterine contractions.
- *Positive.* A positive CST shows repetitive persistent late decelerations with more than 50% of the contractions (Figure 14–8 ●). This is not a desired result. The hypoxic stress of the uterine contraction causes a slowing of the FHR. The pattern will not improve and will most likely get worse with additional contractions.
- *Equivocal or suspicious.* An equivocal or suspicious test has nonpersistent late decelerations or decelerations associated with hyperstimulation (contraction frequency of every 2 minutes or duration lasting longer than 90 seconds). When this test result occurs, more information is needed.

CLINICAL APPLICATION

A negative CST implies that the placenta is functioning normally, fetal oxygenation is adequate, and the fetus will probably be able to withstand the stress of labor. If labor does not occur in the ensuing week, further testing is done.

A positive CST with a nonreactive NST presents evidence that the fetus will not likely withstand the stress of labor. A positive CST may be able to identify compromised fetuses earlier

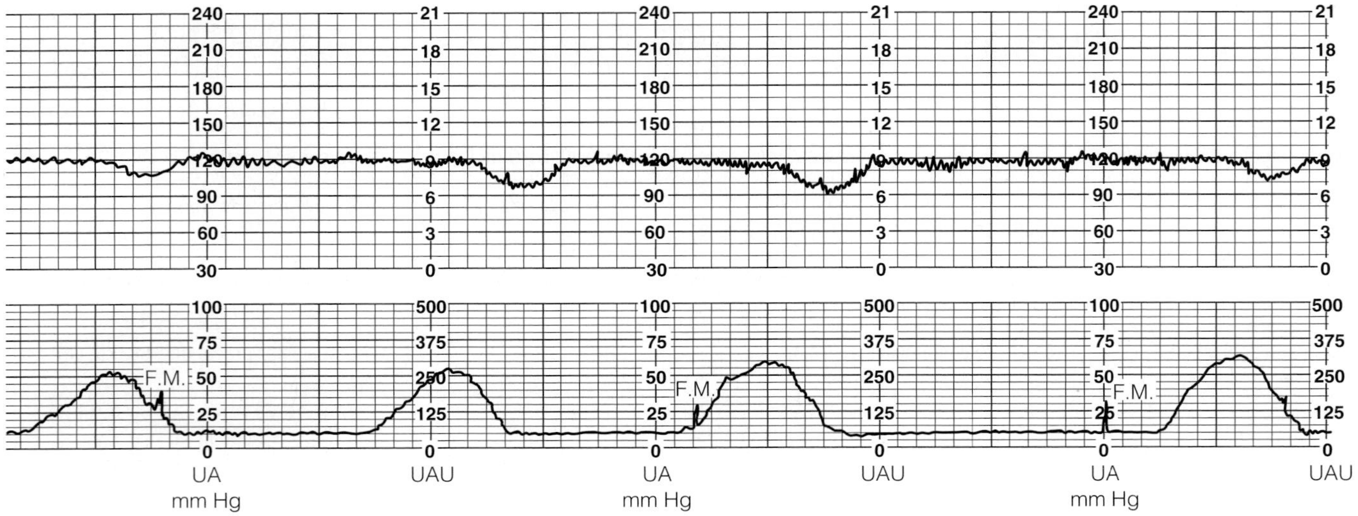

● **Figure 14–8** Example of a positive contraction stress test (CST). Repetitive late decelerations occur with each contraction. Note that there are no accelerations of FHR with three fetal movements (FM). The baseline FHR is 120 bpm. Uterine contractions (bottom half of strip) occurred four times in 12 minutes.

than a nonreactive NST because of the stimulated interruption of intervillous blood flow (Gabbe et al., 2007). Although a negative CST is reliable in predicting fetal status, a positive result needs to be verified, such as a biophysical profile (see Table 14–5).

Nursing Management

The nurse ascertains the woman's understanding of the CST, the reasons for the test, and the possible results before the test begins. Written consent is required in some settings. In this case, the certified nurse-midwife or physician is responsible for fully informing the woman about the test. The nurse administers the CST, interprets the results, and reports the findings to the certified nurse-midwife or physician and the expectant woman. In some settings, the presence of the CNM or physician is required because there is a risk of initiating labor or hypertonic uterine contractions. Throughout the procedure, the nurse performs critical assessments and provides continual reassurance to the woman and her support person.

Table 14–5 Contraction Stress Test

Diagnostic value: Demonstrates reaction of FHR to stress of uterine contraction.

Results:
- *Negative test:* Stress of uterine contraction shows three contractions of good quality lasting 40 or more seconds in 10 minutes without evidence of late decelerations.
- *Positive test:* Stress of uterine contraction shows repetitive persistent late deceleration with more than 50% of the uterine contractions.
- *Equivocal or suspicious:* Nonpersistent late decelerations or decelerations associated with hyperstimulation.

AMNIOTIC FLUID ANALYSIS

Amniocentesis is a procedure used to obtain amniotic fluid for genetic testing (early in pregnancy or between 15 to 16 weeks of pregnancy) for fetal abnormalities or to determine fetal lung maturity in the third trimester of pregnancy. During an amniocentesis, the physician scans the uterus using ultrasound to identify the fetal and placental positions and to identify adequate pockets of amniotic fluid. The skin is then cleaned with a Betadine solution. The use of a local anesthesia at the needle insertion site is optional. A 22-gauge needle is then inserted into the uterine cavity to withdraw amniotic fluid (Figure 14–9 ●). After 15 to 20 mL of fluid has been removed, the needle is withdrawn and the site is assessed for streaming (movement of fluid), which is an indication of bleeding. The fetal heart rate and maternal vital signs are then assessed. Rh immune globulin is given to all Rh-negative women. The analysis of amniotic fluid provides valuable information about fetal status. Amniocentesis is a fairly simple procedure, although complications do occur on rare occasions (fewer than 1% of cases). For nursing interventions during amniocentesis, see Clinical Skill 2–5 in the Clinical Skills Manual SKILLS.

DIAGNOSTIC USES OF AMNIOCENTESIS

A number of studies can be performed on amniotic fluid. These tests can provide information about fetal health, fetal lung maturity, and genetic disorders (see Chapter 7∞).

Evaluation of Fetal Health

Concentrations of certain substances in amniotic fluid provide information about the health status of the fetus. The **quadruple screen** is the most widely used test to screen for Down syndrome (trisomy 21), trisomy 18, and neural tube defects (NTDs). The serum test assesses for appropriate levels of alpha-fetoprotein

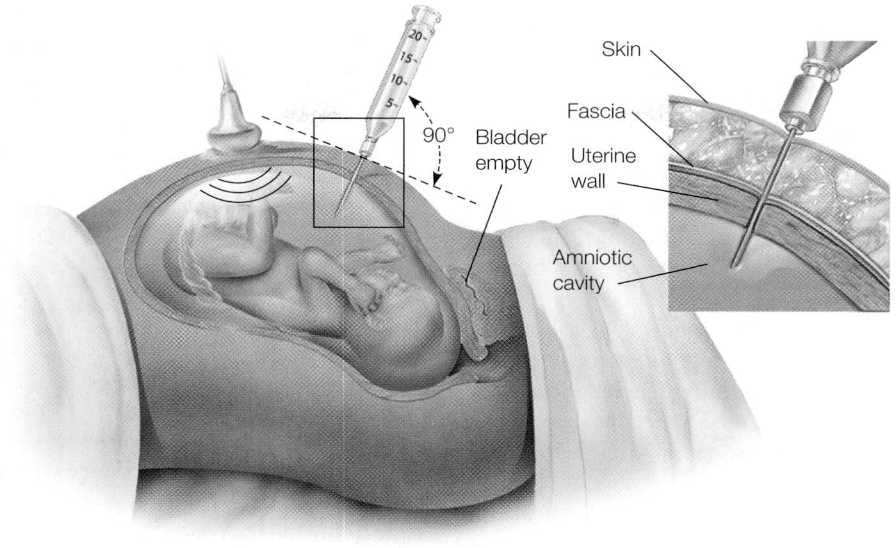

● **Figure 14–9** Amniocentesis. The woman is scanned by ultrasound to determine the placenta site and to locate a pocket of amniotic fluid. The needle is then inserted into the uterine cavity to withdraw amniotic fluid.

(AFP), human chorionic gonadotropin (hCG), and unconjugated estriol (UE3) and Diameric Inhibin-A. The quadruple screen offers the advantage of being noninvasive but is only a screening test (see Chapter 7∞). An amniocentesis is 99% accurate in diagnosing genetic abnormalities.

Evaluation of Fetal Maturity

Because gestational age, birth weight, and the rate of development of organ systems do not necessarily correspond, amniotic fluid may also be analyzed to determine the maturity of the fetal lungs. Fetal lung maturity determination in conjunction with gestational age is important when making clinical decisions regarding the timing of birth for women who may have complications, such as preeclampsia or diabetes.

Lecithin/Sphingomyelin (L/S) ratio. The alveoli of the lungs are lined with a substance called **surfactant**, which is composed of phospholipids. Surfactant lowers the surface tension of the alveoli when the newborn exhales. When a newborn with mature pulmonary function takes its first breath, a tremendously high pressure is needed to open the lungs. By lowering the alveolar surface tension, surfactant stabilizes the alveoli, and a certain amount of air always remains in the alveoli during expiration. Thus when the infant exhales, the lungs do not collapse. An infant born before synthesis of surfactant is complete is unable to maintain lung stability. Each breath requires the same effort as the first. This results in underinflation of the lungs and the development of respiratory distress syndrome (RDS).

Fetal lung maturity can be ascertained by determining the **lecithin/sphingomyelin (L/S) ratio**; lecithin and sphingomyelin are two components of surfactant. Early in pregnancy, the sphingomyelin concentration in amniotic fluid is greater than the concentration of lecithin, and so the L/S ratio is low (lecithin levels are low and sphingomyelin levels are high). At about 32 weeks' gestation, sphingomyelin levels begin to fall and the amount of lecithin begins to increase. By 35 weeks' gestation, an L/S ratio of 2:1 (also reported as 2.0) is usually achieved in the normal fetus. A 2:1 L/S ratio indicates that the risk of RDS is very low. Under certain conditions of stress (a physiologic problem in the mother, placenta, and/or fetus, such as hypertension or placental insufficiency), the fetal lungs mature more rapidly (Torrance, Voorbij, Wijnberger, et al., 2008).

Phosphatidylglycerol. **Phosphatidylglycerol (PG)** is another phospholipid in surfactant. Phosphatidylglycerol is not present in the fetal lung fluid early in gestation. It appears when fetal lung maturity has been attained, at about 35 weeks' gestation. Because the presence of PG is associated with fetal lung maturity, when it is present the risk of RDS is low. Phosphatidylglycerol determination is also useful in blood-contaminated specimens. Because PG is not present in blood or vaginal fluids, its presence is reliable in predicting fetal lung maturity. (See Table 14–6.)

Lamellar body count. **Lamellar body counts (LBC)** are present in amniotic fluid when phosphatidylglycerol (PG) is present (ACOG, 2008). When the LBC is 30,000–40,000 counts/UL,

Table 14–6 Fetal Lung Maturity Values

Diagnostic value: Provides information to help determine fetal lung maturity.

Results:
- L/S ratio of 2:1 and presence of PG correlate with 35 weeks' gestation.
- An L/S ratio lower than 2:1 and/or an absence of PG may indicate underinflation of lungs and an increased risk for development of RDS.
- An LBC of over 50,000 counts/UL is predictive of fetal lung maturity.

probable lung maturity is assumed. The laboratory analysis for LBC is considerably less costly than the previously discussed tests and can usually be performed at the acute care facility rather than a reference laboratory (ACOG, 2008).

CHORIONIC VILLUS SAMPLING

Chorionic villus sampling (CVS) involves obtaining a small sample of chorionic villi from the developing placenta. Chorionic villus sampling is performed in some medical centers for first-trimester diagnosis of genetic, metabolic, and deoxyribonucleic acid (DNA) studies. Chorionic villus sampling can be performed either transabdominally or transcervically. The fetal loss rate is the same regardless of the approach used although vaginal spotting is more common with the transcervical approach (Odibo, Dicke, Gray, et al., 2008).

The advantages of this procedure are early diagnosis and short waiting time for results. Whereas amniocentesis is not done until at least 16 weeks' gestation, CVS is typically performed between 10 and 12 weeks. Previous studies that evaluated the use of CVS at 9 weeks found a possible association between limb reduction birth defects and early CVS. Based on these findings, most practitioners do not recommend early CVS before 10 gestational weeks (Odibo et al., 2008). Risks of CVS include failure to obtain tissue, rupture of membranes, leakage of amniotic fluid, bleeding, intrauterine infection, maternal tissue contamination of the specimen, and Rh alloimmunization. Because CVS testing is performed so early in the pregnancy, it cannot detect neural tube defects. Women who desire testing for neural tube defects would need a quadruple screening at 15 to 20 weeks' gestation.

NURSING MANAGEMENT

The nurse assists the physician during the amniocentesis or CVS and supports the woman undergoing the procedure. Although the physician has explained the procedure in advance so that the woman can give informed consent, the woman is likely to be apprehensive both about the procedure itself and about the information it may reveal. She may become anxious during the procedure and need additional emotional support. The nurse can provide support by further clarifying the physician's instructions or explanations, by relieving the woman's physical discomfort when possible, and by responding verbally and physically to the woman's need for reassurance.

Nursing Practice

When explaining genetic testing options to expectant parents, inform the mother that even if a CVS shows no chromosomal abnormality, it cannot screen for neural tube defects. Women who have a normal CVS and an abnormal *quadruple screen test* would be offered amniocentesis. Women with risk factors for neural tube defects may want to consider amniocentesis instead of CVS because it screens for both types of disorders.

Following the procedure, the nurse reiterates explanations given by the physician and provides opportunities for questions. The nurse reviews the experience with the woman and presents self-care measures. Typically, the woman is monitored for a short time following the procedure. The nurse observes for contraction or uterine activity, amniotic fluid leakage, bleeding, or pain. The woman is advised of the warning signs of complications following the procedure.

Following an amniocentesis, approximately 1% to 2% of women develop complications such as amniotic fluid leakage from the puncture site or vaginal spotting. Approximately 1 in 1000 women develop infection. Needle puncture of the fetus rarely occurs during amniocentesis because of the use of ultrasound technology that allows for continuous visualization of the fetus (ACOG, 2007). Women should be reassured that although the complication rates are low, notification of her healthcare provider is necessary if any of these symptoms develop.

Because fetal loss occurs more commonly before 15 weeks, many practitioners theorize that the loss rates associated with CVS are higher than those associated with amniocentesis. Early amniocentesis before 15 weeks is associated with an increased risk of fetal loss when compared with performing the procedure after 15 weeks. Approximately 1 in 200 fetal losses occurs with CVS. When an amniocentesis is performed between 15 to 20 weeks, the risk of fetal loss is 1 in 300 to 1 in 500 (ACOG, 2007).

When an invasive procedure, such as an amniocentesis or a CVS, is performed, the nurse administers RhoGAM to the woman if she is Rh negative to prevent alloimmunization. Documentation should be charted and provided to the woman for future reference.

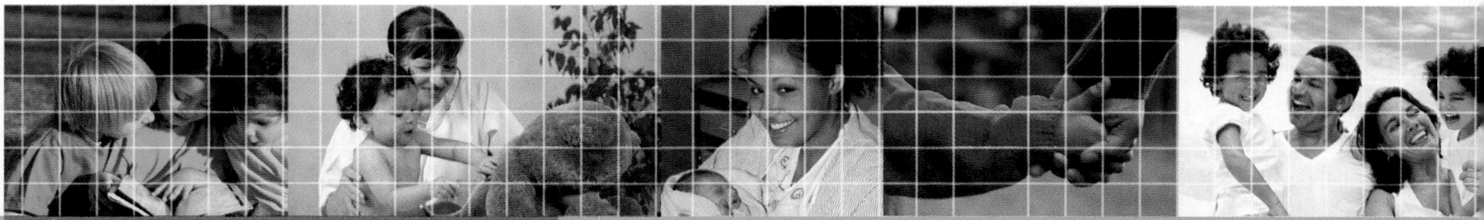

CRITICAL CONCEPT REVIEW

LEARNING OUTCOMES / CONCEPTS

14.1 Identify pertinent information to be discussed with the woman regarding her own assessment of fetal activity and methods of recording fetal activity.

1. Pertinent information to be discussed with the woman:
   - The purpose of the assessment.
   - How to complete the form.
   - Whom to call with questions.
   - What to report.
2. Provide the opportunity for follow-up during each visit.

14.2 Describe the methods, clinical applications, and results of ultrasound in the nursing care management of the pregnant woman.

1. Ultrasound offers a valuable means of assessing intrauterine fetal growth because the growth can be followed over a period of time.
2. It is noninvasive and painless.
3. It allows the certified nurse-midwife or physician to study the gestation serially.
4. It is nonradiating to both the woman and her fetus.It has no known harmful effects.

14.3 Describe the use, procedure, information obtained, and nursing considerations for Doppler velocimetry, nonstress test, contraction stress test, and biophysical profile tests.

1. Doppler blood flow studies are used to assess placental function and sufficiency.
   - It is noninvasive. The woman lies supine and the Doppler is placed on the abdomen.
2. A nonstress test is based on the knowledge that the FHR normally increases in response to fetal activity and to sound stimulation.
   - The woman is attached to an electronic fetal monitor for approximately 20 minutes. She is required to lie still during the test.
   - Desired result is a reactive test.
3. A contraction stress test evaluates respiratory function of the placenta.
   - The woman is attached to an electronic fetal monitor and contractions are stimulated. This evaluates the ability of the fetus to handle contractions. The procedure may precipitate labor prematurely.
   - Desired result is a negative test.
4. A biophysical profile includes five variables:
   - Fetal breathing movement.
   - Fetal body movement.
   - Fetal tone.
   - Amniotic fluid volume.
   - Fetal heart rate reactivity.

Biophysical profile is a combination of an ultrasound and a nonstress test to assess a fetus at risk for intrauterine compromise.

14.4 Explain the use of amniocentesis as a diagnostic tool.

1. Amniocentesis assesses amniotic fluid for the presence of genetic disorders, fetal health status, and evaluation of fetal maturity.

14.5 Describe the tests that can be done on amniotic fluid.

1. The quadruple screen measure substances contained in the amniotic fluid that provide information regarding the presence of fetal anomalies such as neural tube defects and Down syndrome.
2. The lecithin/sphingomyelin ratio, presence of phosphatidylglycerol, and level of lamellar body counts can be assessed to determine fetal lung maturity.

14.6 Compare the advantages and disadvantages of chorionic villus sampling (CVS).

1. Advantages:
   - Early detection of fetal disorders.
   - Decreased waiting time for results.
2. Disadvantages:
   - Increased risk of injury to fetus.
   - Inability to detect neural tube defects.
   - Potential for repeated invasive procedures.

CRITICAL THINKING IN ACTION

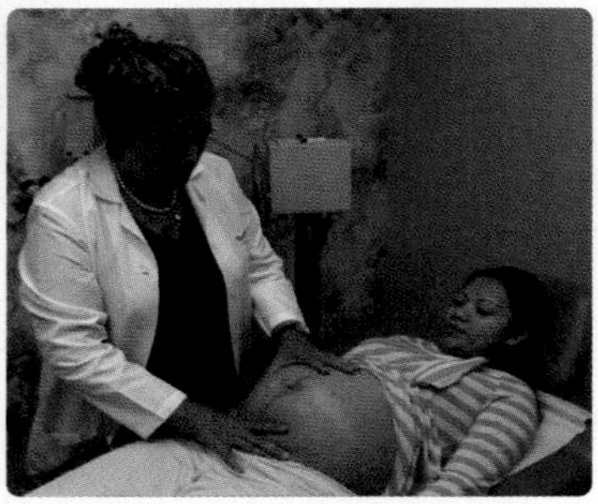

Patricia Adams is a 20-year-old, married, G2, P0010 at 36 weeks' gestation with gestational diabetes. She presents to you during her prenatal visit with a complaint of decreased fetal movement for the "last day or so." Her OB history includes a 13 lb weight gain, hematocrit of 29%, diastolic BP ranging 80–96 mm Hg, and 1+ proteinuria. A 19-week ultrasound demonstrated no fetal anatomic defects. A hemoglobin A_1c at 23 weeks was 5.8%. Patricia has had weekly NST since 28 weeks' gestation. You place Patricia on the fetal monitor for an NST. You obtain vital signs of T 97°F, P 88, R 14, BP 130/88. After 30 minutes you observe that the fetal heart rate baseline is 160–165, long-term variability is decreased, and repetitive variable decelerations are occurring. No contractions are noted. The fetus is very active. You notify the physician of the fetal heart rate baseline and unsatisfactory NST. The physician orders a biophysical profile (BPP) for fetal well-being. You describe and explain the biophysical profile test to Patricia.

1. How would you describe and explain the biophysical profile test?
2. To heighten Patricia's awareness of fetal movement, how would you instruct her to do a daily fetal movement record (FMR)?
3. Explain when Patricia should contact her care provider.
4. Discuss the significance of fetal movement.
5. Explore factors that decrease fetal movements.

See MyNursingKit for possible responses.

REFERENCES

Alus, M., Okumus, H., Mete, S., & Guclu, S. (2007, March). The effects of different maternal positions on non-stress test: An experimental study. *Journal Clinical Nursing. 16*(3), 562–568.

American College of Obstetricians & Gynecologists [ACOG]. (2007). First-trimester screening for fetal aneuploidy (ACOG Practice Bulletin No. 88). Washington, DC: Author.

American College of Obstetricians & Gynecologists [ACOG]. (2008). Fetal lung maturity (ACOG Practice Bulletin No. 97). *Obstetrics & Gynecology, 112*(3), 717–726.

American College of Obstetricians & Gynecologists [ACOG]. (2009). Ultrasonography in pregnancy. (ACOG Practice Bulletin No. 101). *Obstetrics & Gynecology, 113*(2) Part 1, 451–461.

Blackburn, S. T. (2007). *Maternal, fetal, & neonatal physiology: A clinical perspective* (3rd ed.). St. Louis: Saunders

Clur, S. A., Mathijssen, I. B., Pajkrt, E., Cook, A. L., Ottenkamp, J., & Bilardo, C. M. (2008). Structural heart defects associated with an increased nuchal translucency: 9 years experience in a referral centre. *Prenatal Diagnosis, 28*(4), 347–354.

Cusick, W., Shevell, T., Duchan, L. S., Lupinacci, C. A., Terranova, J., & Crombleholme, W. R. (2008). Likelihood ratios for fetal trisomy 21 based on nasal bone length in the second trimester: How best to define hypoplasia? *Ultrasound in Obstetrics & Gynecology, 30*(3), 271–274.

Gabbe, S. G., Niebyl, J. R., & Simpson, J. L. (2007). *Obstetrics: Normal and problem pregnancies pocket companion.* New York: Churchill Livingstone.

Harmon, C. R. (2009). Assessment of fetal health. In R. K. Creasy, R. Resnik, J. D. Iams, C. J. Lockwood, & T. R. Moore. *Creasy & Resnik's maternal-fetal medicine: Principles and practice* (6th ed., pp. 361–395). Philadelphia: Saunders.

Heazell, A. E., & Frøen, J. F. (2008). Methods of fetal movement counting and the detection of fetal compromise. *Journal of Obstetrics & Gynaecology, 28*(2), 147–154.

Heazell, A. E., Green, M., Wright, C., Flenady, V., & Frøen, J. F. (2008). Midwives' and obstetricians' knowledge and management of women presenting with decreased fetal movements. *Acta Obstetrics & Gynecology Scandavia, 87*(3), 331–339.

Kwon, J. Y. (2006). Abnormal Doppler velocimetry is related to adverse perinatal outcome for borderline amniotic fluid index during third trimester. *The Journal of Obstetrics and Gynaecology Research, 32*(6), 545–549.

Mangesi, L., & Hofmeyr, G. J. (2007). Fetal movement counting for assessment of fetal wellbeing. *Cochrane Database of Systematic Reviews* 2007, Issue 1. Art. No.: CD004909. DOI: 10.1002/14651858.CD004909.pub2.

Odibo, A. O., Dicke, J. M., Gray, D. L., Oberle, B., Stamilio, D. M., Macones, G. A., et al. (2008). Evaluating the rate and risk factors for fetal loss after chorionic villus sampling. *Obstetrics & Gynecology, 112*(4), 813–819.

Scott, A. (2007, June). Nuchal translucency in first trimester Down syndrome screening. *Issues in Emerging Health Technology, 100,* 1–6.

Sinha, D., Sharma, A., Nallaswamy, V., Jayagopal, N., & Bhatti, N. (2007). Obstetric outcome in women complaining of reduced fetal movements. *Journal of Obstetrics & Gynaecology, 27*(1), 41–43.

Smith, G. C., Celik, E., To, M., Khouri, O., & Nicolaides, K. H. (2008). Cervical length at mid-pregnancy and the risk for primary cesarean delivery. *New England Journal of Medicine, 358*(13), 1346–1353.

Torrence, H. L., Voorbij, H. A., Wijnberger, L. D., van Bel, F., & Visser, G. H. (2008). Lung maturation in small for gestational age fetuses from pregnancies complicated by placental insufficiency or maternal hypertension. *Early Human Development,* 84(7), 465–469.

Verburg, B. O., Steegers, E. A., De Ridder, M., Snijders, R. J., Smith, E., Hofman, A., et al. (2008). New charts for ultrasound dating of pregnancy and assessment of fetal growth: Longitudinal data from a population-based cohort study. *Ultrasound in Obstetrics & Gynecology, 31*(4), 388–396.

Wright, D., Kagan, K. O., Molina, F. S., Gazzoni, A., & Nicolaides, K. H. (2008). A mixture model of nuchal translucency thickness in screening for chromosomal defects. *Ultrasound in Obstetrics & Gynecology, 31*(4), 376–383.

PEARSON

EXPLORE mynursingkit™

MyNursingKit is your one stop for online chapter review materials and resources. Prepare for success with additional NCLEX®-style practice questions, interactive assignments and activities, web links, animations and videos, and more!

Register your access code from the front of your book at **www.mynursingkit.com**

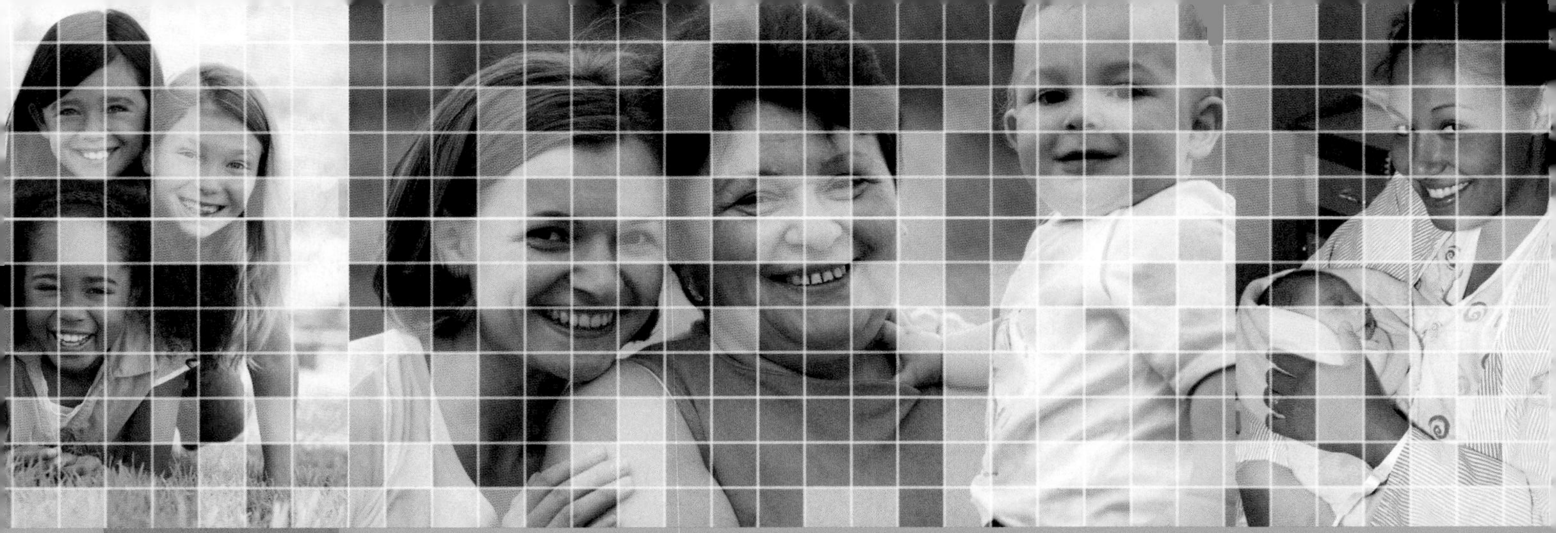

CHAPTER

15 Pregnancy at Risk: Pregestational Problems

When I learned I had gestational diabetes I felt panicky. My grandmother died of diabetes and it has always scared me. However, by taking each day as it came, cooperating with my doctors and nurses, and watching my diet, I did fine and gave birth to a beautiful 7 pound 10 ounce daughter. One good thing has come of the experience—I'm no longer so terrified of developing diabetes. I have become far more careful about taking care of myself, and I now think of diabetes as a chronic disease to be controlled. —*Ayisha, 34*

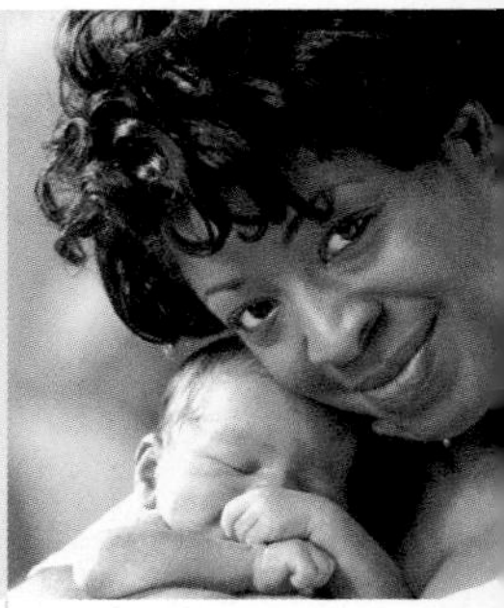

LEARNING OUTCOMES

15.1 Describe the effects of alcohol and illicit drugs in the nursing care management of the childbearing woman and her fetus/newborn.

15.2 Relate the pathology and clinical treatment of diabetes mellitus in pregnancy to the implications for nursing care.

15.3 Distinguish among the types of anemia associated with pregnancy regarding signs, treatment, and implications for pregnancy.

15.4 Describe acquired immunodeficiency syndrome (AIDS), including care of the pregnant woman who has tested positive for the human immunodeficiency virus (HIV), fetal/neonatal implications, and ramifications for the childbearing family.

15.5 Explain the effects of various heart disorders on pregnancy, including implications for nursing care management in the antepartum, intrapartum and postpartum periods.

15.6 Delineate the effects of selected pregestational medical conditions on pregnancy.

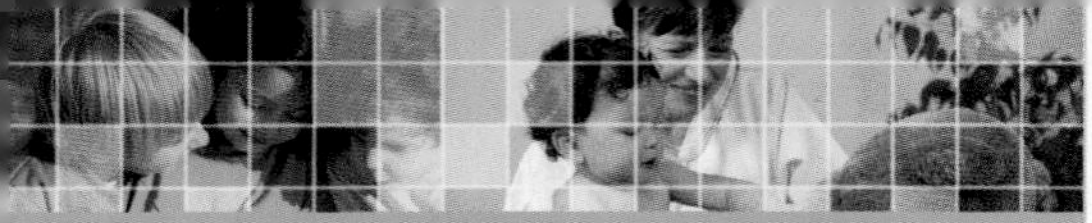

KEY TERMS

Acquired immunodeficiency syndrome (AIDS), 316

Gestational diabetes mellitus (GDM), 306

Human immunodeficiency virus (HIV), 316

Macrosomia, 308

For some women, pregnancy may become a life-threatening event because of potential or existing complications. These complications can be the result of factors such as age, parity, blood type, socioeconomic status, psychologic health, or preexisting chronic illnesses. This chapter focuses on women with pregestational medical disorders and their possible effects on the pregnancy.

CARE OF THE WOMAN WITH SUBSTANCE ABUSE PROBLEMS

Substance abuse occurs when a person experiences difficulties with work, family, social relations, and health as a result of alcohol or drug use. In general the rate of illicit drug use among pregnant women is significantly less than the rate among nonpregnant women. Approximately 5.2% of pregnant women ages 15 to 44 report having used an illicit drug in the past month as compared to 9.7% of nonpregnant women. However, illicit drug use varies significantly by age with higher rates among women ages 18 to 25 (7.2% for pregnant vs. 16% for nonpregnant women) than among women ages 26 to 44 (3% for pregnant vs. 6.5% for nonpregnant women). The findings were reversed among women ages 15 to 17. Those who were pregnant had a 22.6% rate of use while those who were not pregnant had a 13.3% rate (Substance Abuse and Mental Health Services Administration [SAMHSA], 2008).

Drugs that are commonly misused include tobacco, alcohol, cocaine, marijuana, amphetamines, barbiturates, hallucinogens, club drugs, heroin, and other narcotics. (Tobacco is discussed in Chapter 11 as a teratogenic substance.) Polydrug use involving multiple substances such as alcohol, tobacco, and illicit drugs is fairly common and contributes to the risks a pregnant woman faces. Table 15–1 identifies common addictive drugs and their effects on the fetus or newborn.

Drug use during pregnancy, particularly in the first trimester, may have a negative effect on the health of the woman and the growth and development of the fetus. Unfortunately, prenatal drug use may be the most frequently missed diagnosis in all of maternity care. Physicians and nurses may fail to ask women about drug and alcohol use because of their own lack of knowledge, discomfort, or biases. Often substance-abusing women wait until late in pregnancy to seek healthcare. Moreover, the substance-abusing woman who seeks early prenatal care may not voluntarily reveal her addiction, so healthcare providers should be alert for a history or physical signs that might indicate substance abuse.

Providing effective prenatal care to chemically dependent women is often challenging for clinicians. However, pregnancy is a time when most women are receptive to caring interventions.

SUBSTANCES COMMONLY ABUSED DURING PREGNANCY

Alcohol

Alcohol is a central nervous system (CNS) depressant and a potent teratogen. The incidence of alcohol abuse is highest among women ages 20 to 40 years, although alcoholism is also seen in teenagers. Among pregnant women aged 15 to 44, 11.6% used alcohol in a given month. This rate is significantly lower than the rate for nonpregnant women of that age (53.2%) (SAMHSA, 2008). This figure is of concern, however, because birth defects that are related to fetal alcohol exposure can occur in the first 3 to 8 weeks' gestation, often before the woman even knows she is pregnant. Alcohol use among pregnant women tends to decrease by trimester.

The effects of alcohol on the fetus may result in a group of signs known as *fetal alcohol spectrum disorders (FASD)*. The syndrome has characteristic physical and mental abnormalities that vary in severity. (See discussion in Chapter 28.) There is no final answer to how much alcohol a woman can safely drink during pregnancy. Consequently the expectant woman should avoid alcohol completely. Even low levels of alcohol cannot be recommended (Food and Drug Administration [FDA], 2005).

Table 15–1 Possible Effects of Selected Drugs of Abuse or Addiction on Fetus and Neonate

Maternal Drug	Effect on Fetus and Neonate
	Depressants
Alcohol	Mental retardation, microcephaly, midfacial hypoplasia, cardiac anomalies, intrauterine growth restriction (IUGR), potential teratogenic effects, fetal alcohol syndrome (FAS), fetal alcohol effects (FAE)
Narcotics	
Heroin	Withdrawal symptoms, convulsions, death, IUGR, respiratory alkalosis, hyperbilirubinemia
Methadone	Fetal distress, meconium aspiration; low birth weight; with abrupt termination of the drug, severe withdrawal symptoms, neonatal death
Barbiturates	Neonatal depression, increased anomalies; teratogenic effect (?); withdrawal symptoms, convulsions, hyperactivity, hyperreflexia, vasomotor instability
Phenobarbital	Bleeding (with excessive doses)
"T's and Blues" (combination of the following)	
Talwin (narcotic)	Safe for use in pregnancy; depresses respiration if taken close to time of birth
Amytal (barbiturate)	See barbiturates
Tranquilizers	
Phenothiazine derivatives	Withdrawal, extrapyramidal dysfunction, delayed respiratory onset, hyperbilirubinemia, hypotonia or hyperactivity, decreased platelet count
Diazepam (Valium)	Hypotonia, hypothermia, low Apgar score, respiratory depression, poor sucking reflex, possible cleft lip
Antianxiety drugs	
Lithium	Congenital anomalies, especially Ebstein anomaly; lethargy and cyanosis in the newborn
	Stimulants
Amphetamines	
Amphetamine sulfate (Benzedrine)	Generalized arthritis, learning disabilities, poor motor coordination, transposition of the great vessels, cleft palate
Dextroamphetamine sulfate (Dexedrine)	Congenital heart defects, hyperbilirubinemia
Cocaine	Cerebral infarctions, microcephaly, learning disabilities, poor state organization, decreased interactive behavior, central nervous system (CNS) anomalies, cardiac anomalies, IUGR, genitourinary anomalies, sudden infant death syndrome (SIDS)
Nicotine (half to one pack cigarettes/day)	Increased rate of spontaneous abortion, increased incidence of placental abruption, small for gestational age (SGA), cleft lip and palate, SIDS
	Psychotropics
PCP ("angel dust")	Flaccid appearance, poor head control, impaired neurologic development
LSD	Chromosomal breakage?
Marijuana	IUGR, SIDS

Chronic abuse of alcohol can undermine maternal health by causing malnutrition (especially folic acid and thiamine deficiencies), bone marrow suppression, increased incidence of infections, and liver disease. As a result of alcohol dependence, a woman may have withdrawal seizures in the intrapartal period as early as 12 to 48 hours after she stops drinking. Delirium tremens may occur in the postpartal period, and the newborn may suffer a withdrawal syndrome. Nurses in the maternal-newborn unit must be aware of the manifestations of alcohol abuse so they can prepare for the woman's special needs. Care includes sedation to decrease irritability and tremors, seizure precautions, intravenous (IV) fluid therapy for hydration, and preparation for an addicted newborn. Although high doses of sedatives and analgesics may be necessary for the woman, caution is advised because these medications can cause fetal depression.

Breastfeeding generally is not contraindicated, although alcohol is excreted in breast milk. Excessive alcohol consumption may intoxicate the infant and inhibit the maternal letdown reflex. Discharge planning for the alcohol-addicted mother and newborn needs to be correlated with the social service department of the hospital.

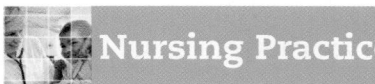

Nursing Practice

Keep in mind that at least 1 of 10 women in the United States, regardless of socioeconomic status or ethnic background, is currently abusing a substance. If you consider that possibility with every woman, you will ask the important questions about drug use and be alert for signs of substance abuse.

Cocaine and Crack

Cocaine acts at the nerve terminals to prevent the reuptake of dopamine and norepinephrine, which in turn results in vasoconstriction, tachycardia, and hypertension. Placental vasoconstriction decreases blood flow to the fetus. The onset of cocaine effects occurs rapidly, but the euphoria lasts only about 30 minutes. Euphoria and excitement are usually followed by irritability, depression, pessimism, fatigue, and a strong desire for more cocaine. This pattern often leads the user to take repeated doses to sustain the effect. Cocaine metabolites may be present in the urine of a pregnant woman for as long as 4 to 7 days after use.

Cocaine can be taken by IV injection or by snorting the powdered form. *Crack*, a form of freebase cocaine that is made up of baking soda, water, and cocaine mixed into a paste and microwaved to form a rock, can be smoked. Smoking crack leads to a quicker, more intense high because the drug is absorbed through the large surface area of the lungs.

The cocaine user is difficult to identify prenatally. Because cocaine is illegal, many women are reluctant to admit that they use it. The nurse may recognize subtle signs of cocaine use, including mood swings and appetite changes, and withdrawal symptoms such as depression, irritability, nausea, lack of motivation, and psychomotor changes.

Major adverse maternal effects of cocaine use include seizures and hallucinations, pulmonary edema, cerebral hemorrhage, respiratory failure, and heart problems. Women who use cocaine have an increased incidence of spontaneous abortion, abruptio placentae, preterm birth, and stillbirth (March of Dimes [MOD], 2006).

Fetal exposure to cocaine increases the risk of intrauterine growth restriction (IUGR), small head circumference, cerebral infarctions, altered brain development, shorter body length, malformations of the genitourinary tract, and lower Apgar scores. Newborns exposed to cocaine in utero may have neurobehavioral disturbances, marked irritability, an exaggerated startle reflex, labile emotions, and an increased risk of sudden infant death syndrome (SIDS). (See Chapter 28 for further discussion.) Most children who were exposed to cocaine in utero have normal intelligence. In some cases, cocaine-exposed children have subtle behavioral and learning problems; however, a good home environment seems to help reduce these effects (MOD, 2006).

Cocaine crosses into breast milk and may cause symptoms in the breastfeeding infant, including extreme irritability, vomiting, diarrhea, dilated pupils, and apnea. Thus, women who continue to use cocaine after childbirth should avoid breastfeeding.

Marijuana

Marijuana is the most widely used illicit drug among women, both pregnant and nonpregnant (SAMHSA, 2008). To date, there is no strong evidence that marijuana has teratogenic effects on the fetus although, following birth, some infants who were regularly exposed to marijuana in utero appear to have withdrawal symptoms including trembling and excessive crying (MOD, 2006). In reality the impact of heavy marijuana use on pregnancy is difficult to evaluate because of the variety of social factors that may influence the direct results of marijuana itself.

MDMA (Ecstasy)

Methylenedioxymethamphetamine (MDMA), better known as Ecstasy, is the most commonly used of a group of drugs referred to as *club drugs*, so called because they have become popular among adolescents and young adults who frequent dance clubs and "raves." Other club drugs include flunitrazepam (Rohypnol), gamma hydroxybutyrate (GHB), and ketamine hydrochloride. Phencyclidine (PCP) and LSD are sometimes classified as club drugs as well.

MDMA is the third most widely used illicit drug in the United States after marijuana and amphetamines. MDMA is taken by mouth, usually as a tablet. It produces euphoria and feelings of empathy for others. It has been widely perceived as a "safe" drug because of a relatively low incidence of adverse reactions. However, adverse responses are very unpredictable and the incidence is growing (Gamma, Jerome, Liechti, et al., 2005). Deaths have occurred among users.

Little is yet known about the effects of MDMA on pregnancy. Infants exposed to Ecstasy in utero may experience some of the same risks as infants exposed to other amphetamines during pregnancy, including the possibility of withdrawal-like symptoms such as drowsiness, jitteriness, and breathing problems (MOD, 2006).

Heroin

Heroin is an illicit CNS depressant narcotic that alters perception and produces euphoria. It is an addictive drug that is generally administered IV. Pregnancy in women who use heroin is considered high risk because of the increased incidence in these women of poor nutrition, iron deficiency anemia, and preeclampsia. Women addicted to heroin also have a higher incidence of sexually transmitted infections because many rely on prostitution to support their drug habit.

The fetus of a heroin-addicted woman is at increased risk for IUGR, meconium aspiration, and hypoxia. The newborn frequently shows signs of heroin addiction such as restlessness; shrill, high-pitched cry; irritability; fist sucking; vomiting; and seizures. Signs of withdrawal usually appear within 72 hours and may last for several days. The newborn may exhibit poor consolability for 3 months or more. These behaviors may interfere with successful maternal attachment and increase the risk for parenting problems or abuse in an already high-risk mother. (See discussion in Chapter 28.)

Methadone

Methadone is the most commonly used therapy for women dependent on opioids such as heroin. Methadone blocks withdrawal symptoms and reduces or eliminates the craving for narcotics. Dosage should be individualized at the lowest possible therapeutic level. Methadone crosses the placenta, but the effects on the newborn are inconsistent and do not seem to indicate as much of a dose-related effect on the newborn as previously believed (Jansson, DiPietro, & Elko, 2005). The therapeutic goal is to use methadone to help the mother recover from illicit drug abuse to optimize her health and that of her baby.

CLINICAL THERAPY

A team approach to the care of the pregnant woman with substance abuse problems ensures the management necessary to provide safe labor and birth for the woman and her child.

The management of drug addiction may include hospitalization if necessary to start detoxification. "Cold turkey" withdrawal is not advisable during pregnancy because of the possible risk to the fetus. Maintenance and support therapy are best individualized to the woman's history and condition. Urine screening is also done regularly throughout pregnancy if the woman has a known or suspected substance abuse problem and should include maternal informed consent. This testing helps to identify the type and amount of drug being abused.

NURSING MANAGEMENT

NURSING ASSESSMENT AND DIAGNOSIS

Because of the prevalence of substance abuse, it is important to screen all pregnant women for substance abuse during the health history. Several simple screening tools are available. In addition, be alert for clues in the history or appearance of the woman that suggest substance abuse. If abuse is suspected, ask direct questions, beginning with less threatening questions about use of tobacco, caffeine, and over-the-counter medications. Then progress to questions about alcohol intake and finally to questions focusing on past and current use of illegal drugs. A matter-of-fact, nonjudgmental approach is more likely to elicit honest responses.

When assessing a woman with a known substance abuse problem, focus on the woman's general health status, with specific attention to nutritional status, susceptibility to infections, and evaluation of all body systems. Also assess the woman's understanding of the impact of substance abuse on herself and on her pregnancy.

Nursing diagnoses that may apply to a woman at risk because of substance abuse include the following:

- *Imbalanced Nutrition: Less than Body Requirements* related to inadequate food intake secondary to substance abuse
- *Risk for Infection* related to use of inadequately cleaned syringes and needles secondary to IV drug use
- *Risk for Ineffective Health Maintenance* related to a lack of information about the impact of substance abuse on the fetus

PLANNING AND IMPLEMENTATION

Prevention of substance abuse during pregnancy is the ideal nursing goal and is best accomplished through education. Unfortunately, many women who abuse substances do not receive regular health care and may not seek care until they are far along in pregnancy.

Thus it is important to focus on ongoing assessment and client teaching. Consider providing information about the relationship between substance abuse and existing health problems and the implications for the woman's unborn child. Establishing a relationship of trust and support helps ensure the woman's cooperation. If possible, discuss strategies to help the woman quit (addiction treatment programs, 12-step programs, individual counseling) and suggest a referral for more in-depth assessment by a specialist.

Preparation for labor and birth should be part of prenatal planning. Nonnarcotic psychologic support and careful explanation of the labor process may help relieve the woman's fear, tension, and discomfort. If pain medication is necessary, it should not be withheld; the notion that it will contribute to further addiction is mistaken. Preferred methods of pain relief include the use of psychoprophylaxis and regional blocks, such as epidurals, or local anesthetics, such as pudendal block and local infiltration. Immediate intensive care should be available for the newborn, who is often depressed, small for gestational age (SGA), and premature. (For care of the addicted newborn, see Chapter 28∞.)

EVALUATION

Expected outcomes of nursing care include the following:

- The woman is able to describe the impact of her substance abuse on herself and her unborn child.
- The woman gives birth to a healthy infant.
- The woman accepts a referral to social services (or another appropriate community agency) for follow-up care after discharge.

CARE OF THE WOMAN WITH DIABETES MELLITUS

Diabetes mellitus (DM), an endocrine disorder of carbohydrate metabolism, results from inadequate production or use of insulin. Insulin, produced by the β-cells of the islets of Langerhans in the pancreas, lowers blood glucose levels by enabling glucose to move from the blood into muscle and adipose tissue cells. In the United States, over 8 million women have pregestational diabetes, and it occurs in 1% of pregnancies (American College of Obstetricians and Gynecologists [ACOG], 2005).

CARBOHYDRATE METABOLISM IN NORMAL PREGNANCY

In early pregnancy the rise in serum levels of estrogen, progesterone, and other hormones stimulates increased insulin production by the maternal pancreas and increased tissue response to insulin. Thus, an anabolic (building-up) state exists during the first half of pregnancy, with storage of glycogen in the liver and other tissues.

In the second half of pregnancy, placental secretion of human placental lactogen (hPL) and prolactin (from the decidua), as well as elevated cortisol and glycogen levels, cause increased resistance to insulin and decreased glucose tolerance. This decreased effectiveness of insulin results in a catabolic (destructive) state during fasting periods, such as during the night or after meal absorption. Because increasing amounts of circulating maternal glucose and amino acids are diverted to the fetus, maternal fat is metabolized much more readily during fasting periods than in a nonpregnant woman. As a result of this lipolysis (maternal metabolism of fat), ketones may be present in the urine.

The delicate system of checks and balances between glucose production and glucose use is stressed by the growing fetus, who derives energy from glucose taken solely from maternal stores. This stress is known as the *diabetogenic effect of pregnancy*. Thus, any preexisting disruption in carbohydrate metabolism is augmented by pregnancy, and any diabetic potential may precipitate gestational diabetes mellitus.

PATHOPHYSIOLOGY OF DIABETES MELLITUS

In DM the pancreas fails to produce insulin or does not produce enough insulin to allow necessary carbohydrate metabolism. Without adequate insulin, glucose does not enter the cells and they become energy depleted. Blood glucose levels remain high (hyperglycemia), and the cells break down their stores of fats and protein for energy. Protein breakdown results in a negative nitrogen balance; fat metabolism causes ketosis.

These pathologic developments cause the four cardinal signs and symptoms of DM: polyuria, polydipsia, polyphagia, and weight loss. Polyuria (frequent urination) results because water is not reabsorbed by the renal tubules due to the osmotic activity of glucose. Polydipsia (excessive thirst) is caused by dehydration from polyuria. Polyphagia (excessive hunger) is caused by tissue loss and a state of starvation, which results from the inability of the cells to use the blood glucose. Weight loss (seen with marked hyperglycemia) is due to the use of fat and muscle tissue for energy.

CLASSIFICATION

States of altered carbohydrate metabolism have been classified in several ways. Table 15–2 shows the classification of DM based on its cause. This classification contains four main categories: type 1 diabetes, type 2 diabetes, other specific types, and gestational diabetes mellitus. Type 1 diabetes develops because of β-cell destruction and generally results in an absolute insulin deficiency. Type 2 diabetes, which is the most common form, "may range from predominantly insulin resistance with relative insulin deficiency to a predominantly secretory defect with insulin resistance" (American Diabetes Association [ADA], 2007, p. S43).

Table 15–2 Etiologic Classification of Diabetes Mellitus

I	Type 1 diabetes* (β-cell destruction, usually leading to absolute insulin deficiency) A. Immune mediated B. Idiopathic
II	Type 2 diabetes* (may range from predominantly insulin resistance with relative insulin deficiency to a predominantly secretory defect with insulin resistance)
III	Other specific types†
IV	Gestational diabetes mellitus

Source: Adapted from the 1999 Report of the Expert Committee on the Diagnosis and Classification of Diabetes Mellitus. *Diabetes Care,* Suppl. 5.

*Patients with any form of diabetes may require insulin treatment at some stage of their disease. Such use of insulin does not classify the client.

†The more detailed classification, which can be found in medical-surgical texts and the original source, provides eight subcategories of type.

Table 15–3 shows White's classification of diabetes in pregnancy. This classification is useful for describing the extent of the disease.

Gestational diabetes mellitus (GDM) is defined as any degree of glucose intolerance that has its onset or is first diagnosed during pregnancy. It complicates about 4% of all pregnancies. Women who are markedly obese, have a prior history of GDM, have glycosuria, or have a strong family history of diabetes are at high risk (ADA, 2007). Diagnosis of GDM is very important because even mild diabetes causes increased risk for perinatal morbidity and mortality. Furthermore, many women with GDM progress over time to overt type 2 diabetes mellitus.

INFLUENCE OF PREGNANCY ON DIABETES

Pregnancy can affect diabetes significantly because the physiologic changes of pregnancy can drastically alter insulin requirements. Pregnancy may also alter the progress of vascular disease secondary to DM. Pregnancy can affect diabetes in the following ways:

- DM may be difficult to control because insulin requirements are changeable.
- During the first trimester, the need for insulin frequently decreases. Levels of hPL, an insulin antagonist, are low; fetal needs are minimal; and the woman may consume less food because of nausea and vomiting.
- Nausea and vomiting may cause dietary fluctuations and increase the risk of hypoglycemia, formerly called insulin shock.
- Insulin requirements begin to rise in the second trimester as glucose use and glucose storage by the woman and fetus increase. Insulin requirements may double or quadruple by the end of pregnancy as a result of placental maturation and hPL production.

MyNursingKit Case Study: Client with Gestational Diabetes

Table 15–3 White's Classification of Diabetes in Pregnancy

Class	Criterion
A	Chemical diabetes
B	Maturity onset (age over 20 years), duration under 10 years, no vascular lesions
C_1	Age 10 to 19 years at onset
C_2	10 to 19 years' duration
D_1	Under 10 years at onset
D_2	Over 20 years' duration
D_3	Benign retinopathy
D_4	Calcified vessels of legs
D_5	Hypertension
E	No longer sought
F	Nephropathy
G	Many failures
H	Cardiopathy
R	Proliferating retinopathy
T	Renal transplant (added by Tagatz and colleagues of the University of Minnesota)

Source: Used with permission from White, P. (1978). Classification of obstetric diabetes. *American Journal of Obstetrics and Gynecology, 130,* 228.

- Increased energy needs during labor may require increased insulin to balance IV glucose.
- Usually an abrupt decrease in insulin requirement occurs after passage of the placenta and the resulting loss of hPL in maternal circulation.
- A decreased renal threshold for glucose leads to a higher incidence of glycosuria.
- The risk of ketoacidosis, which may occur at lower serum glucose levels in the pregnant woman with DM than in the nonpregnant woman with diabetes, increases.
- The vascular disease that accompanies DM may progress during pregnancy.
- Hypertension may occur, contributing to vascular changes.
- Nephropathy may result from renal impairment, and retinopathy may develop.

INFLUENCE OF DIABETES ON PREGNANCY OUTCOME

The pregnancy of a woman who has diabetes carries a higher risk of complications, especially perinatal mortality and congenital anomalies. Tight metabolic control (fasting blood glucose less than 95 mg/dL and 2-hour postprandial glucose less than 120 mg/dL) reduces this risk (ACOG, 2005). New techniques for monitoring blood glucose level, delivering insulin, and monitoring the fetus have also helped reduce perinatal mortality.

Maternal Risks

The prognosis for the pregnant woman with gestational, type 1, or type 2 diabetes without significant vascular damage is positive. However, diabetic pregnancy still carries a higher risk of complications than normal pregnancy.

Hydramnios, or an increase in the volume of amniotic fluid, occurs in 10% to 20% of pregnant women with diabetes. It is thought to be a result of excessive fetal urination because of fetal hyperglycemia (Forsbach-Sanchez, Tamez-Perez, & Vazquez-Lara, 2005). Premature rupture of membranes and onset of labor may occasionally be a problem with hydramnios.

Preeclampsia-eclampsia occurs more often in diabetic pregnancies than in normal pregnancies, especially when vascular changes already exist.

Hyperglycemia can lead to *ketoacidosis* as a result of the increase in ketone bodies (which are acidic) released in the blood from the metabolism of fatty acids. Decreased gastric motility and the anti-insulin effects of hPL also predispose the woman to ketoacidosis. Ketoacidosis usually develops slowly but, if untreated, can lead to coma and death for mother and fetus.

Pregnancy can also worsen *retinopathy* in women with diabetes. However, good control of blood glucose levels lessens the impact. Hence, women with preexisting diabetes should be referred to an ophthalmologist for evaluation during pregnancy (ACOG, 2005).

The pregnant woman with diabetes is also at increased risk for monilial vaginitis and urinary tract infections because of increased glycosuria, which contributes to a favorable environment for bacterial growth.

Fetal-Neonatal Risks

Many of the problems of the newborn result directly from high maternal plasma glucose levels. In the presence of untreated maternal ketoacidosis, the risk of fetal death increases dramatically.

The incidence of *congenital anomalies* in diabetic pregnancies is 5% to 10% and is the major cause of death of infants born to women with diabetes. Research suggests that this increased incidence is related to multiple factors including high glucose levels in early pregnancy (Wyatt, Frias, Hoyme, et al., 2005). Most anomalies involve the heart, central nervous system, and skeletal system. One anomaly, *sacral agenesis,* appears almost exclusively in infants of diabetic mothers. In sacral agenesis, the sacrum and lumbar spine fail to develop and the lower extremities develop incompletely. Preconception counseling and strict diabetes control before conception help reduce the incidence of congenital anomalies.

Characteristically, infants of diabetic mothers on insulin therapy (or White's classes A, B, and C; see Table 15–3) are large for gestational age (LGA) as a result of the high maternal levels of blood glucose, from which the fetus derives its glucose. These elevated levels continually stimulate the fetal islets of Langerhans to produce insulin. This hyperinsulin state causes the fetus to use the available glucose, which leads to excessive growth (known as **macrosomia**) and fat deposits. If born vaginally, the macrosomic infant is at increased risk for shoulder dystocia and traumatic birth injuries; thus, cesarean birth may be indicated if birth weight is expected to exceed 4500 g (ACOG, 2005).

Once the umbilical cord is cut after birth, the generous maternal blood glucose supply stops. However, continued islet cell hyperactivity leads to high insulin levels and depleted blood glucose (hypoglycemia) in 2 to 4 hours. Macrosomia can be significantly reduced by strict maternal blood glucose control.

Infants of mothers with advanced diabetes (vascular involvement) may demonstrate IUGR, which occurs because vascular changes in the mother decrease the efficiency of placental perfusion and the fetus is not as well sustained.

Respiratory distress syndrome appears to result from high levels of fetal insulin, which inhibit some fetal enzymes necessary for surfactant production. *Polycythemia* (excessive number of red blood cells) in the newborn is mainly due to the diminished ability of glycosylated hemoglobin in the mother's blood to release oxygen. *Hyperbilirubinemia* is a direct result of the inability of immature liver enzymes to metabolize the increased bilirubin resulting from the polycythemia.

CLINICAL THERAPY

All pregnant women, regardless of risk factors, should have their risk for GDM assessed at the first prenatal visit. Women at low or normal risk should be screened for gestational diabetes at 24 to 28 weeks' gestation using a nonfasting 1-hour, 50-g oral glucose tolerance test (OGTT). Women with risk factors (such as marked obesity; history of diabetes in a first-degree relative; a prior macrosomic, malformed, or stillborn infant; hypertension; or glucosuria) should be screened earlier in pregnancy (Perkins, Dunn, & Jagasia, 2007).

To do the 1-hour OGTT, the woman drinks a 50-g oral glucose solution at any time during the day. One hour later a blood sample is obtained. If the plasma glucose level exceeds 130 to 140 mg/dL (depending on the lab used), a 3-hour OGTT is necessary (ADA, 2007).

To do this test, the woman eats a high-carbohydrate (at least 150 g carbohydrate daily) diet for 3 days before her scheduled test. She then drinks a 100-g oral glucose solution in the morning after an overnight fast. Plasma glucose levels are determined fasting and at 1, 2, and 3 hours. GDM is diagnosed if two or more of the following values are equaled or exceeded during an OGTT:

Fasting	95 mg/dL
1 hour	180 mg/dL
2 hours	155 mg/dL
3 hours	140 mg/dL

Laboratory Assessment of Long-Term Glucose Control

Measurement of glycosylated hemoglobin levels provides information about the long-term (previous 4 to 8 weeks) control of hyperglycemia. The test measures the percentage of glycohemoglobin in the blood. Glycohemoglobin, or HbA_{1c}, is the hemoglobin to which a glucose molecule is attached. Because glycosylation is a rather slow and essentially irreversible process, the test is not reliable for screening for gestational diabetes or for close daily control. HbA_{1c} values greater than 10% are associated with fetal anomaly rates of 20% to 25% (ACOG, 2005).

ANTEPARTAL MANAGEMENT OF DIABETES MELLITUS

To ensure an optimally healthy mother and newborn, good prenatal care using a team approach must be a top priority. The woman with gestational diabetes may find the diagnosis shocking and upsetting. She needs clear explanations and teaching to gain her cooperation in ensuring a good outcome. The nurse-educator plays a major role in this counseling. The woman with pregestational diabetes needs to understand what changes she can expect during pregnancy; she should receive such teaching in preconception counseling. In addition, preconception care focuses on stringent blood glucose control prior to conception and during the first trimester. Stringent glucose control during this period helps reduce the rate of infant malformations significantly (Slocum, 2007).

Dietary Regulation

The pregnant woman with diabetes needs to increase her caloric intake by about 300 kcal/day. During the first trimester, the normal-weight woman generally requires about 30 kcal/kg of ideal body weight. During the second and third trimesters, she needs about 35 kcal/kg of ideal body weight. Approximately 40% to 45% of the calories should come from complex carbohydrates, 12% to 20% from protein, and 35% to 40% from fats (Reece & Homko, 2008). The food is divided among three meals and three snacks. The bedtime snack is the most important and should include both protein and complex carbohydrates to prevent nighttime hypoglycemia. A nutritionist should work out meal plans with the woman based on the woman's lifestyle, culture, and food preferences. The woman needs to be familiar with the use of food exchanges so she can plan her own meals.

Glucose Monitoring

Glucose monitoring is essential to determine the need for insulin and to assess glucose control. Many physicians have the woman come in for weekly assessment of her fasting glucose levels and one or two postprandial levels. In addition, frequent self-monitoring of glucose levels is paramount in maintaining good glucose control. Self-monitoring is discussed on page 311.

Insulin Administration

Many women with gestational diabetes need insulin to maintain normal glucose levels. Those with pregestational diabetes typically have type 1 diabetes and are already on insulin. In either case, human insulin should be used because it is the least likely to cause an allergic reaction. Insulin is given either in multiple injections or by continuous subcutaneous infusion. Multiple injections are more common and generally produce excellent results. Many women receive a combination of intermediate and regular insulin.

Evidence-Based Nursing

DIETARY ADVICE FOR PREVENTING GESTATIONAL DIABETES MELLITUS

Clinical Question

What is effective dietary advice for preventing gestational diabetes?

The Evidence

Three researchers performed a systematic review of the research literature to develop a practice guideline for the Cochrane Collaborative. Cochrane reviews are held to a highly rigorous standard and represent the strongest level of evidence for practice. Three randomized trials were included in the review. One of the studies focused on a high-fiber diet and two of the studies assessed low glycemic index diets as compared to high glycemic index diets. Gestational diabetes increases the risk of significant problems for both mother and baby, and so prevention is a primary goal. Diet plays a significant part in the prevention and control of gestational diabetes. The high fiber diet was not effective in preventing gestational diabetes, but the low glycemic diets did appear to reduce the incidence of the disease (Tieu, et al., 2008).

Best Practice

Ideally, a pregnant woman's diet will provide adequate nutrition for fetal growth and maternal health. The aim of dietary advice is to prevent maternal hyperglycemia by relying on a diet with a low glycemic index. Low glycemic foods induce a gradual increase in blood glucose due to slow digestion and absorption. Foods that have a low glycemic index include whole grains, fruits, and vegetables. High glycemic diets should be avoided as these cause a rapid spike in blood glucose followed by a rapid decline. High glycemic foods include carbohydrates that are rapidly metabolized, including potatoes, white flour, and some breakfast cereals. Mothers should be encouraged to use a prenatal diet rich in whole grains, fruits, and vegetables and to minimize ingestion of highly processed, high-carbohydrate foods.

Critical Thinking

What educational methods and materials will help the nurse assist pregnant women in identifying the optimal diet during pregnancy?

See MyNursingKit for possible responses.

Recently, clinicians have moved away from the use of regular human insulin, replacing it with an insulin analog (either lispro or aspart), which mimics physiologic insulin action. These analogs are more effective than regular insulin in achieving desired glucose levels and in reducing the risk of fetal macrosomia (Perkins et al., 2007). The analogs are convenient because they can be given closer to a meal than regular insulin (5–10 minutes vs. 30–45 minutes). They are associated with a lower incidence of hypoglycemia, and they do not cross the placenta (Scollan-Koliopoulos, Guadagno, & Walker, 2006). Often a four-dose approach is used, with regular insulin or an analog taken before each meal and NPH or Lente insulin added at bedtime (ACOG, 2005). Other clinicians vary the NPH and regular insulin patterns slightly but still prefer a four-dose approach.

Oral hypoglycemics are not generally used during pregnancy because they cross the placenta and have not been well studied. However, glyburide, a sulfonylurea taken orally, is now being used as an alternative to insulin for women with GDM that is not controlled by diet and exercise alone. Glyburide enhances insulin secretion, but does not cross the placenta (Perkins et al., 2007).

Evaluation of Fetal Status

Information about the well-being, size, and maturation of the fetus is important for planning the course of pregnancy and the timing of birth. In pregnancies complicated by diabetes, the fetus is at increased risk of neural tube defects such as spina bifida, so maternal serum alpha-fetoprotein (MSAFP) screening is offered at 16 to 20 weeks' gestation.

Ultrasound is done at 18 weeks to determine gestational age and detect anomalies. It is then repeated at 28 weeks to monitor fetal growth for IUGR or macrosomia. Some agencies do *fetal biophysical profiles* (ultrasound evaluations of fetal well-being that assess fetal breathing movements, fetal activity, reactivity, muscle tone, and amniotic fluid volume) as part of an ongoing evaluation of fetal status.

Daily maternal evaluation of *fetal activity* is begun at about 28 weeks. Nonstress testing (NST) is usually begun weekly at 28 weeks and increased to twice weekly at 32 weeks' gestation. If the NST is nonreactive, a fetal biophysical profile or *contraction stress test* is performed. (For an explanation of these tests, see Chapter 14.) If the woman requires hospitalization for complications or to control blood glucose levels, NSTs may be done weekly.

INTRAPARTAL MANAGEMENT OF DIABETES MELLITUS

During the intrapartal period, medical therapy focuses on the following:

Timing of birth. Most pregnant women with diabetes, regardless of the type, are allowed to go to term, with spontaneous labor. Some clinicians opt to induce labor in a woman at term to avoid problems related to an aging placenta. Cesarean birth may be indicated if signs of fetal distress exist. Birth before term may be indicated for diabetic women with vascular changes and worsening hypertension or if evidence of IUGR exists (ACOG, 2005). To determine fetal lung maturity, amniotic fluid (obtained by amniocentesis) is evaluated for lecithin/sphingomyelin (L/S) ratio and the presence of phosphatidylglycerol (see Chapter 14). Preterm birth, often by cesarean, is considered if prenatal testing indicates that the fetus is deteriorating.

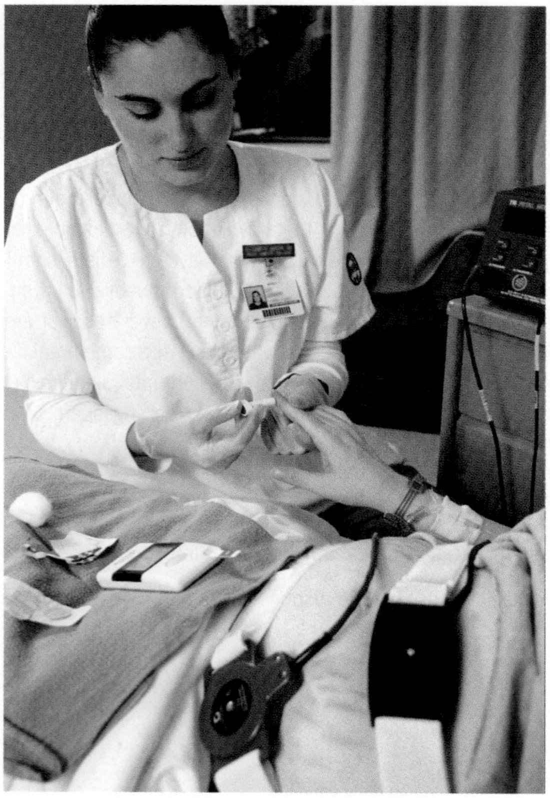

● **Figure 15–1** Maternal glucose levels. During labor the nurse closely monitors the blood glucose levels of the woman with diabetes mellitus.

Labor management. Frequently, maternal insulin requirements decrease dramatically during labor. Consequently maternal glucose levels are measured hourly to determine insulin need (Figure 15–1 ●). The primary goal in controlling maternal glucose levels intrapartally is to prevent neonatal hypoglycemia. Often two IV lines are used, one with a 5% dextrose solution and one with a saline solution. The saline solution is then available for piggybacking insulin or if a bolus is needed. Because insulin clings to plastic IV bags and tubing, the tubing should be flushed with insulin before the prescribed amount is added. During the second stage of labor and the immediate postpartal period, the woman may not need additional insulin. The IV insulin is discontinued at the end of the third stage of labor.

POSTPARTAL MANAGEMENT OF DIABETES MELLITUS

Generally maternal insulin requirements fall significantly during the postpartal period because, with placental separation, hormone levels fall and the anti-insulin effect ceases. For the first 24 hours postpartum, women with preexisting diabetes typically require very little insulin. They are usually managed with a sliding scale specifying dosage based on blood glucose levels. Afterward a more regular insulin dosage pattern can be reestablished. Women with mild diabetes not requiring insulin often have sufficient glucose control and do not require any therapy while they are hospitalized. Antihyperglycemics are contraindicated during breastfeeding. Consequently a breastfeeding woman with diabetes that is not controlled by diet alone may need insulin for a time (ACOG, 2005).

Women with GDM who did not require insulin during pregnancy generally do not need it during the postpartum period. Clinicians routinely discontinue insulin for women with GDM following childbirth and then monitor blood glucose levels (Menato, Bo, Signorite, et al., 2008). If elevated glucose levels develop, oral antihyperglycemic agents may be tried if the woman is not breastfeeding (ACOG, 2005). The woman should be reassessed 6 weeks postpartum to determine whether her glucose levels are normal. If the levels are normal, she should be reassessed at a minimum of 3-year intervals (ADA, 2006).

If the newborn requires a special care nursery, the nurse should provide the parents with ongoing information, support, and encouragement to visit and be involved in the newborn's care, since establishing parent-child relationships is a high priority during the postpartum.

The nurse should encourage breastfeeding as beneficial to both mother and baby. Maternal calorie needs increase during lactation to 500 to 800 kcal above prepregnant requirements, and insulin must be adjusted accordingly. Home blood glucose monitoring should continue for the woman with type 1 diabetes.

The woman and her partner should also receive information on family planning. Barrier methods of contraception (diaphragm, cervical cap, condom) used with a spermicide are safe, effective, economical, and the method of choice for insulin-dependent diabetic women. The use of combined oral contraceptives (COCs) by women with diabetes is somewhat controversial. Many physicians who prescribe low-dose COCs to women with diabetes restrict them to women who have no vascular disease and do not smoke. The progesterone-only pill may also be used as may Depo-Provera. Many couples who have completed their families choose elective sterilization.

NURSING MANAGEMENT

"Nursing Care Plan: The Woman with Diabetes Mellitus" on pages 312–314 addresses nursing management.

NURSING ASSESSMENT AND DIAGNOSIS

Whether diabetes has been diagnosed before pregnancy occurs or the diagnosis is made during pregnancy (GDM), careful assessment of the disease process and the woman's understanding of diabetes is important. Thorough physical examination—including assessment for vascular complications of the disease, any signs of infectious conditions, and urine and blood testing for glucose—is essential on the first prenatal visit. Follow-up visits are usually scheduled twice a month during the first two trimesters and once a week during the last trimester.

Assessment provides information about the woman's ability to cope with the combined stress of pregnancy and diabetes and to follow a recommended regimen of care. Determine the woman's knowledge about diabetes and self-care before developing a teaching plan.

Nursing diagnoses that may apply to the pregnant woman with diabetes include the following:

- *Risk for Imbalanced Nutrition: More than Body Requirements* related to imbalance between intake and available insulin
- *Risk for Injury* related to possible complications secondary to hypoglycemia or hyperglycemia
- *Interrupted Family Processes* related to the need for hospitalization secondary to DM

PLANNING AND IMPLEMENTATION

For the woman with preexisting diabetes, a nurse and a physician may provide prepregnancy counseling using a team approach. Ideally they see the couple before pregnancy so that the DM can be evaluated. The outlook for pregnancy is good if the diabetes is of recent onset without vascular complications, provided that glucose levels can be controlled.

For women with GDM, nursing care focuses heavily on client education about the condition, its implications, and its management.

NURSING CARE IN THE COMMUNITY

In many cases, women with GDM are stabilized in the hospital and necessary teaching for self-care is begun. Women with preexisting diabetes may also require hospitalization for stabilization of their diabetes. In either case the majority of ongoing teaching and supervision of pregnant women with diabetes is then carried out by nurses in clinics, community agencies, and the women's homes.

Effective Insulin Use

Ensure that the woman and her partner understand the purpose of insulin, the types of insulin to be used, and the correct procedure for administering it. Remember that regular (short-acting) insulin should be given about 30 minutes before a meal, but insulin lispro should be taken immediately before eating (ACOG, 2005). Instruct the woman's partner about insulin administration in case it becomes necessary for the partner to give it. For some highly motivated women whose glucose levels are not well controlled with multiple injections, a continuous infusion pump may improve glucose control.

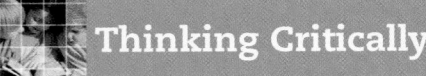

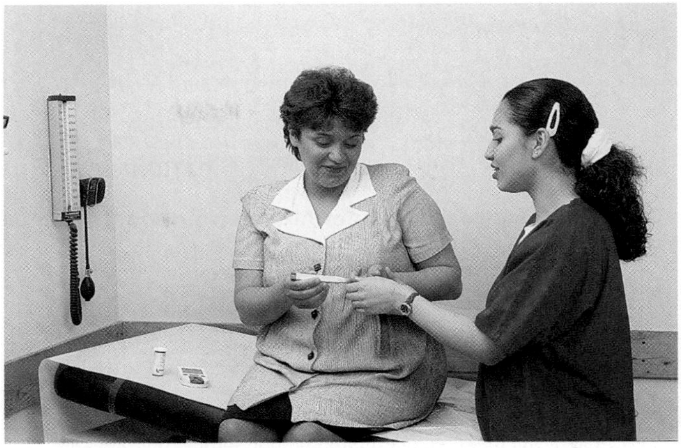

● **Figure 15–2** Home glucose monitoring. The nurse teaches the pregnant woman with gestational diabetes mellitus how to do home glucose monitoring.

Teach the woman how and when to monitor her blood glucose level, the desired range of blood glucose levels, and the importance of good control (Figure 15–2 ●). Most women use a glucose meter to monitor blood sugar level because the meter is more accurate. Teach the woman to follow the manufacturer's directions exactly; to wash her hands thoroughly before puncturing her finger; to touch the blood droplet, not her finger, to the test pad on the strip; and to store the test strips as directed and discard them after the expiration date. Clients with diabetes need to keep a record of each blood sugar reading. Specific record sheets are available for this purpose.

Planned Exercise Program

Regardless of the type of diabetes, unless otherwise medically contraindicated, exercise is important for the woman's overall well-being. If she is used to a regular exercise program, encourage her to continue. Advise the woman to exercise after meals when blood sugar levels are high, to wear diabetic identification, to carry a simple sugar such as hard candy (because of the possibility of exercise-induced hypoglycemia), to monitor her blood glucose levels regularly, and to avoid injecting insulin into an extremity that will soon be used during exercise.

Thinking Critically

GLUCOSE INTOLERANCE

Patti Chang, a 35-year-old G3P2, is a well-educated, active Chinese-American woman with no history of glucose intolerance. Her two children were born healthy at 36 weeks' gestation. She receives the usual 50-g glucose tolerance test at 26 weeks' gestation, and her plasma level is 160 mg/dL. She seems irritated and frustrated when her obstetrician tells her that it would be best to perform a 3-hour fasting glucose tolerance test. After the physician leaves the room, Patti asks you the following questions: "Will the glucose hurt my baby? What will the treatment be?" How will you answer the questions? Why does Patti seem so upset?

See MyNursingKit for possible responses.

Nursing Practice

It is essential to have a woman with GDM who is learning to test her blood glucose do a finger stick while you watch. For many women, actually sticking their finger can be a challenge to overcome. In addition this observation enables you to verify that correct technique is used.

Nursing Care Plan

THE WOMAN WITH DIABETES MELLITUS

INTERVENTION	RATIONALE	EXPECTED OUTCOME
1. Nursing Diagnosis: Risk for Altered Nutrition: Less than Body Requirements related to poor carbohydrate metabolism		
NIC Intervention: **Nutrition management:** Assistance with or provision of a balanced dietary intake of foods and fluids		**NOC Outcome:** **Nutritional status:** Extent to which nutrients are available to meet metabolic needs
Goal: Client will maintain adequate nutrition throughout pregnancy.		
■ Emphasize importance of regular prenatal visits for assessment of weight gain, blood sugar levels, fetal heart tones, urine ketones, and fundal height measurement.	■ Regular follow-up and assessment of weight, blood sugar levels, fetal heart tones, urine ketones, and fundal height will promote a healthy pregnancy and outcome, as well as allow for modifications in the treatment regimen if necessary.	■ The client will maintain adequate nutrition as evidenced by adequate weight gain, controlled blood sugar levels, verbalization of understanding of personal treatment regimen, and appropriate fetal growth and development during pregnancy.
■ Coordinate care with a dietitian to assist client in meal planning and educate client on the daily caloric needs of pregnancy.	■ A daily intake of high-quality foods promotes fetal growth and controls maternal glucose levels.	
■ Instruct client on signs and symptoms of hyperglycemia: polyphagia, nausea, hot flushes, polydipsia, polyuria, fruity breath, abdominal cramps, rapid deep breathing, headache, weakness, drowsiness, and general malaise. Instruct client on signs and symptoms of hypoglycemia: hunger, clammy skin, irritability, slurred speech, seizures, tachycardia, headache, pallor, sweating, disorientation, shakiness, blurred vision, and, if untreated, coma or convulsions.	■ Maintaining a euglycemic state throughout pregnancy aids in preventing diabetic complications and promotes a positive pregnancy outcome.	
■ Instruct client on management of hyperglycemia and hypoglycemia.		
■ Include family members in meal planning.	■ Gives the family member a sense of involvement and an understanding of the importance of adequate nutrition in pregnancy.	■ Client will recognize signs and intervene appropriately.
2. Nursing Diagnosis: Risk for Fetal Injury related to possible complications associated with altered tissue perfusion secondary to maternal diagnosis of diabetes mellitus		
NIC Intervention: **High-risk pregnancy care:** Identification and management of a high-risk pregnancy to promote healthy outcomes for mother and baby		**NOC Outcome:** **Risk control:** Actions to eliminate or reduce actual, personal, and modifiable health threats
Goal: Uncomplicated birth of a healthy newborn.		
■ Assess fetal heart tones for reassuring variability and accelerations.	■ Reassuring fetal heart rate variability and accelerations are interpreted as adequate placental oxygenation.	■ The fetus will not exhibit signs and symptoms of altered tissue perfusion as evidenced by positive fetal activity, reassuring fetal heart rate patterns, a biophysical profile score between 8 and 10, negative CST, L/S ratio indicating fetal lung maturity, and a reactive nonstress test.

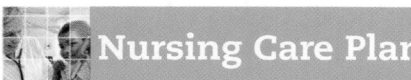

Nursing Care Plan—continued

THE WOMAN WITH DIABETES MELLITUS

INTERVENTION	RATIONALE	EXPECTED OUTCOME
■ Instruct mother on how to lie in a left recumbent position after eating and record how many fetal movements she feels in an hour.	■ More than five fetal kicks in an hour are indicative of fetal well-being.	
■ **Collaborative:** Perform oxytocin challenge test (OCT)/contraction stress test (CST) and nonstress tests as determined by physician.	■ Fetal surveillance testing assesses fetal well-being and adequate placental perfusion.	
■ Prepare client for frequent ultrasound assessments.	■ Ultrasonography is indicated at 18 and 28 weeks per physician order to confirm gestational age and fetal well-being. More frequent ultrasounds may be ordered depending on the woman's status.	
■ Prepare client for amniocentesis procedure.	■ A sample of amniotic fluid contains two phospholipids (lecithin/sphingomyelin) that can be used to detect fetal lung maturity and enables medical personnel to prepare for a potential preterm birth.	
■ Assist physician with biophysical profile assessment.	■ Helps assure fetal well-being and a positive fetal outcome.	

3. Nursing Diagnosis: Health-seeking Behaviors: Information about the effects of blood sugar on pregnancy related to an expressed desire to maintain stable blood glucose levels

NIC Intervention:

Health education: Developing and providing instruction and learning experiences to facilitate voluntary adaptation of behavior conducive to health in individuals, families, groups, or communities

NOC Outcome:

Health-seeking behavior: Actions to promote optimal wellness, recovery, and rehabilitation

Goal: The client and her family will verbalize the importance of maintaining blood sugar within prescribed ranges during pregnancy.

INTERVENTION	RATIONALE	EXPECTED OUTCOME
■ Assess the client and family's cognitive level and develop a teaching strategy that will facilitate learning at that level.	■ Behavior changes occur when teaching strategies are appropriate for the client and family's cognitive level.	■ The client and family members will verbalize understanding of the effects of blood sugar fluctuations on pregnancy as evidenced by asking questions and seeking health information when necessary. The client adheres to personal treatment regimen throughout pregnancy.
■ Teach blood glucose monitoring, insulin administration, and predicted insulin needs throughout pregnancy, and then have client and family members repeat the discussion.	■ Basic understanding of the relationship between blood sugar levels and how insulin needs change throughout pregnancy will foster compliance with prescribed regimen.	
■ Emphasize the importance of maintaining a healthy diet and exercise program during pregnancy. Encourage client and family to develop a sample diabetic diet and exercise regimen that is appropriate for pregnancy while present in the clinic or hospital and evaluate for appropriateness.	■ Involves the client and her family members in her care, and the evaluation method promotes positive reinforcement and a time for modifications of regimen if necessary.	
■ Emphasize the importance of prenatal care for the purpose of maternal and fetal surveillance.	■ Frequent prenatal visits allow for modifications in regimen and promote a healthy pregnancy outcome.	

(continued)

Nursing Care Plan—continued

THE WOMAN WITH DIABETES MELLITUS

INTERVENTION	RATIONALE	EXPECTED OUTCOME
4. Nursing Diagnosis: Risk for Infection related to increased levels of glucose in urine		
NIC Intervention: **Infection control:** Minimizing the acquisition and transmission of infectious agents		**NOC Outcome:** **Knowledge: Infection control:** Extent of understanding conveyed about prevention and control of infection
Goal: The client will have no urinary tract infections (UTIs) during pregnancy.		
■ Encourage client to use preventive measures to prevent UTIs: increasing intake of water and cranberry juice, wearing cotton underwear, wiping perineum from front to back, voiding frequently, and voiding before and immediately after sexual intercourse.	■ Using preventive measures decreases the likelihood of client acquiring a UTI.	■ Client will remain free of UTIs during pregnancy as evidenced by verbalizing and complying with appropriate preventive measures, increasing fluid intake, and negative urine samples during prenatal visits.
■ Instruct client on the signs and symptoms of UTIs: urinary frequency, dysuria, cloudy urine, hematuria, lower back pain, and foul-smelling urine.	■ Client will be aware of signs and symptoms of UTIs and report to physician for immediate intervention.	
Collaborative:		
■ Instruct client on how to obtain a clean-catch urine sample and send to lab for culture and sensitivity per physician's orders.	■ A clean-catch urine sample will contain bacteria if a UTI is present.	
■ Administer prescribed antibiotic therapy and teach client about medication, adverse effects, and appropriate dosage.	■ Antibiotic therapy is the appropriate treatment for a UTI. Compliance increases when a client fully understands medication regimen.	
■ Encourage client to drink 8–10 glasses of water each day.	■ Increased fluid intake assists in flushing bacteria out of the urinary tract system.	
5. Nursing Diagnosis: Anxiety related to unfamiliarity with diagnosis		
NIC Intervention: **Anxiety reduction:** Minimizing apprehension, dread, foreboding, or uneasiness related to an unidentified source of anticipated danger		**NOC Outcome:** **Anxiety control:** Ability to eliminate or reduce feelings of apprehension and tension from an unidentifiable source
Goal: The client expresses less anxiety.		
■ Assess client's level of anxiety (mild-1, moderate-2, or severe-3) and have client verbalize causes of anxiety.	■ Verbalization of anxiety provokers encourages expression of feelings and questions.	■ The client demonstrates appropriate coping strategies as evidenced by utilizing resources efficiently and verbalizing feelings of anxiety and the ways to deal with them.
■ Share information on diabetes care such as nutrition, exercise, and glucose control in a clear and concise manner.	■ Accurate information gives the client a sense of control and comfort.	
■ Instruct client on anxiety-reducing techniques such as imagery, breathing exercises, and massage used in pregnancy.	■ Gives client the tools necessary for decreasing anxiety.	
■ Refer client to a diabetes support group.	■ A support group allows clients with similar problems to express concerns and share information with each other.	

If the woman has not been following a regular exercise plan, encourage her to begin gradually. Due to alterations in metabolism with exercise, the woman's blood glucose should be well controlled before she begins an exercise program.

Teaching for Self-Care

Using the information gained during the nursing assessment of the pregnant woman with diabetes, provide appropriate teaching to the woman and her family so that she can meet her own healthcare needs as much as possible.

- *Glucose monitoring.* Home monitoring of blood glucose levels is the most accurate and convenient method to determine insulin dose and assess control. Women are taught self-monitoring techniques that they perform according to a specified schedule. Women with GDM typically measure their blood glucose 4 times a day (fasting and 1 to 2 hours after meals), while women with preexisting diabetes monitor their blood 5 to 7 times each day (Reece & Homko, 2008). They then regulate their insulin dosage based on blood glucose values and anticipated activity level. Women are encouraged to maintain blood glucose levels in normal ranges as follows: fasting (before eating or taking insulin), less than 95 mg/dL; 2 hours after each meal, less than 120 mg/dL (ADA, 2006).
- *Symptoms of hypoglycemia and ketoacidosis.* The pregnant woman with diabetes must recognize symptoms of changing glucose levels and take appropriate action by immediately checking her capillary blood glucose level. If it is less than 60 mg/dL, she is advised to take 20 g of carbohydrate, which she can obtain by drinking 1 cup of skim milk, 1/2 cup orange or apple juice, or 1/2 cup cola or by eating 4 to 6 pieces of hard candy or 1 tablespoon honey, corn syrup, or brown sugar. She should then wait 15 minutes and retest her glucose level. If it remains under 60 mg/dL she should ingest another 20 g of carbohydrate (Cleveland Clinic, 2006). Many people overtreat their symptoms by continuing to eat, but doing so can cause rebound hyperglycemia. The woman should carry a snack at all times and should have other fast sources of glucose (simple carbohydrates) at hand to treat an insulin reaction when milk or juice is not available. Family members also learn how to inject glucagon in case food does not work or is not feasible (e.g., in the presence of severe morning sickness).
- *Smoking.* Smoking has harmful effects on both the maternal vascular system and the developing fetus and is contraindicated for both pregnancy and diabetes.
- *Travel.* Insulin can be kept at room temperature while traveling. Insulin supplies should be kept with the traveler and not packed in the baggage. Special meals can be arranged by notifying most airlines a few days before departure. The woman should wear a diabetic identification bracelet or necklace and should check with her physician for any instructions or advice before traveling.
- *Support groups.* Many communities have diabetes support groups or education classes that are helpful to women with newly diagnosed diabetes.
- *Cesarean birth.* Chances for a cesarean birth increase if the pregnant woman is diabetic. The possibility should be anticipated; caregivers may suggest enrollment in cesarean birth preparation classes. The couple may prefer simply to discuss cesarean birth with the nurse and their obstetrician and read some books on the topic.

HOSPITAL-BASED NURSING CARE

Hospitalization may become necessary during the pregnancy to evaluate blood glucose levels and adjust insulin dosages. In such cases, monitor the woman's status and provide teaching so that she is knowledgeable about her condition and its management. See "Nursing Care Plan: The Woman with Diabetes Mellitus" starting on page 312.

During the intrapartum period, continue to monitor the woman's status, maintain her IV fluids, remain alert for signs of hypoglycemia, and provide the care indicated for any woman in labor. If a cesarean birth becomes necessary, provide appropriate care, as described in Chapter 22.

EVALUATION

Expected outcomes of nursing care include the following:

- The woman is able to discuss her condition and its possible impact on her pregnancy, labor and birth, and postpartum period.
- The woman participates in developing a healthcare regimen to meet her needs and follows it throughout her pregnancy.
- The woman avoids developing hypoglycemia or hyperglycemia.
- The woman gives birth to a healthy newborn.
- The woman is able to care for her newborn.

CARE OF THE WOMAN WITH ANEMIA

Anemia indicates inadequate levels of hemoglobin (Hb) in the blood. During pregnancy, anemia is defined as hemoglobin less than 11 g/dL in the first trimester, 10.5 g/dL in the second trimester, and 11g/dL in the third trimester (ACOG, 2008a). The common anemias of pregnancy are due either to insufficient hemoglobin production related to nutritional deficiency in iron or folic acid during pregnancy or to hemoglobin destruction in an inherited disorder such as sickle cell anemia. ACOG (2008a) recommends prenatal screening for anemia for all pregnant women. If a pregnant woman has iron deficiency anemia, she should receive iron supplements; if she has another type of anemia, she should be evaluated further. Table 15–4 describes these common anemias.

Table 15–4 Anemia and Pregnancy

Condition	Brief Description	Maternal Implications	Fetal/Neonatal Implications
Iron deficiency anemia	Condition caused by inadequate iron intake resulting in hemoglobin levels below 11 g/dL in the first trimester, 10.5 g/dL in the second, and 11 g/dL in the third (ACOG, 2008a). To prevent this, most women are advised to take supplemental iron during pregnancy.	A pregnant woman with this anemia tires easily, is more susceptible to infection, has increased chance of preeclampsia-eclampsia and postpartal hemorrhage, and cannot tolerate even minimal blood loss during birth. Healing of episiotomy or incision may be delayed.	Risk of low birth weight, preterm birth, nonreassuring fetal status, and perinatal mortality increases in women with severe iron deficiency anemia (maternal Hb less than 6 g/dL). Fetus may be hypoxic during labor due to impaired uteroplacental oxygenation. Consequently maternal blood transfusion may be indicated for fetal reasons (ACOG, 2008a).
Sickle cell anemia	Recessive autosomal disease in which normal adult hemoglobin, hemoglobin A, is abnormally formed. It occurs primarily in people of African descent. The disease is characterized by sickling of the RBCs in the presence of decreased oxygenation. Condition may be marked by crisis with profound anemia, jaundice, high temperature, infarction, and acute pain. Crisis is treated by rehydration with intravenous fluids, administration of oxygen, antibiotics, and analgesics. The fetus is monitored throughout.	Pregnancy may aggravate sickle cell anemia and bring on a vaso-occlusive crisis. Maternal mortality is rare but there is a significant risk of maternal infection, often urinary tract infection or pulmonary infection. Congestive heart failure or acute renal failure may also occur. Because the woman maintains her hemoglobin levels by intense erythropoiesis, additional folic acid supplements (1 mg/day) are necessary. Maternal infections are treated aggressively because dehydration and fever can trigger sickling and crisis. Oxygen supplementation is used throughout labor, and IV fluids are given to maintain hydration (Samuels, 2007). Fetal heart rate is monitored closely. Antiembolism stockings are indicated postpartally.	Abortion, fetal death, and prematurity may occur. IUGR is also a characteristic finding in newborns of women with sickle cell anemia.
Folic acid deficiency anemia	Folic acid deficiency is the most common cause of megaloblastic anemia. In the absence of folic acid, immature RBCs fail to divide, become enlarged (megaloblastic), and are fewer in number. Increased folic acid metabolism during pregnancy and lactation can result in deficiency. Because the condition is difficult to diagnose, the best approach is prevention. All women who could become pregnant should take a multivitamin containing 400 mcg daily (generally found in prenatal vitamins) before conception and through at least the first trimester of pregnancy. The condition is treated with 1 mg folate daily (see Chapter 12∞).	Folate deficiency is the second most common cause of anemia in pregnancy. Severe deficiency increases the risk that the mother may need a blood transfusion following birth due to anemia. She also has an increased risk of hemorrhage due to thrombocytopenia and is more susceptible to infection. Folic acid is readily available in foods such as fresh leafy green vegetables, red meat, fish, poultry, and legumes, but it is easily destroyed by overcooking or cooking with large quantities of water.	Maternal folic acid deficiency has been associated with an increased risk of neural tube defects (NTDs) such as spina bifida, meningomyelocele, and anencephaly in the newborn. Adequate folic acid intake can reduce the incidence of NTDs by 70% (Spina Bifida Association, 2008). Women who have already had one baby with a NTD are generally advised to take a larger dose of folic acid daily.

CARE OF THE WOMAN WITH HIV INFECTION

Human immunodeficiency virus (HIV) infection is one of today's major health concerns. It leads to a progressive disease that ultimately results in **acquired immunodeficiency syndrome (AIDS)**. In 2007, the estimated prevalence rate of adults and adolescents living with HIV infection (not AIDS) was 154.2 per 100,000, although this varies from 282 per 100,000 in New York City to 2.2 per 100,000 in American Samoa. In the 50 states and the District of Columbia, an estimated 455,636 people are currently living with AIDS (Centers for Disease Control and Prevention [CDC], 2009b). Men still make up the majority of cases (73%) (CDC, 2009b).

Among females 80% of the cases result from high-risk heterosexual contact, 19% from injection drug use, and 1% from other categories of transmission (CDC, 2008). Although about

Developing Cultural Competence

ETHNICITY AND AIDS INCIDENCE

The rate of HIV/AIDS-infected individuals varies significantly among races and ethnic groups. In 2007 it was 76.7 per 100,000 in the black/African American population, 34.6 per 100,000 in the native Hawaiian/other Pacific Islander population, 27.7 per 100,000 in the Hispanic/Latino population, 9.2 per 100,000 in the white population, and 7.7 per 100,000 in the Asian population (CDC, 2009).

24% of U.S. women are African American or Latino, these groups accounted for 82% of all female AIDS cases in 2005 (CDC, 2007).

PATHOPHYSIOLOGY OF HIV AND AIDS

HIV-1, which causes most cases of AIDS worldwide, typically enters the body through blood, blood products, or other body fluids such as semen, vaginal fluid, and breast milk. HIV affects specific T cells, thereby decreasing the body's immune responses. This makes the affected person susceptible to opportunistic infections such as *Pneumocystis carinii,* which causes a severe pneumonia, candidiasis, cytomegalovirus, tuberculosis, and toxoplasmosis.

Once infected with the virus, the individual develops antibodies that can be detected with the enzyme-linked immunosorbent assay (ELISA) and confirmed with the Western blot test. Antibodies can be detected in most individuals within 6 months after exposure, but in rare circumstances the latent period is longer. An asymptomatic period lasting from a few months to as long as 17 years (with a median length of 10 years) follows seroconversion. The majority of infected pregnant women fall into this category.

The diagnosis of AIDS is made when a person is HIV positive and has one of several specific opportunistic infections.

MATERNAL RISKS

AIDS-defining diseases that are more common in women than in men include wasting syndrome, esophageal candidiasis, and herpes simplex virus disease. Non-AIDS-defining gynecologic disorders, such as candidiasis or cervical pathology, are prevalent among women in all stages of HIV.

Many women who are HIV positive choose to avoid pregnancy because of the risk of infecting the fetus and the possibility of dying before the child is raised. Women who are asymptomatic and become pregnant should be advised that pregnancy is not believed to accelerate the progression of HIV/AIDS, that the use of antiretroviral (ARV) therapy during pregnancy significantly reduces the risk of transmitting the HIV-1 to the fetus, and that most medications used to treat HIV can be taken during the pregnancy.

Pregnant women who are HIV-positive should receive information about known risk factors for perinatal transmission and ways of reducing the risk. Risk factors include cigarette smoking, illicit drug use, genital tract infections, and unprotected sexual intercourse with multiple partners (Public Health Service Task Force, 2007).

FETAL-NEONATAL RISKS

HIV/AIDS may develop in infants whose mothers are seropositive, usually because of perinatal transmission. Perinatal transmission occurs transplacentally, at birth when the infant is exposed to maternal blood and vaginal secretions, and via breast milk. In the United States the rate of transmission has dropped dramatically and is now less than 2% because of the implementation of recommendations for universal prenatal HIV counseling and testing, the availability of antiretroviral prophylaxis, the use of scheduled cesarean birth, and the avoidance of breastfeeding (Public Health Service Task Force, 2007). Following birth, infants often have a positive antibody titer, which reflects the passive transfer of maternal antibodies and does not indicate HIV infection.

CLINICAL THERAPY

MyNursingKit Video: Zidovudine

CDC guidelines state that HIV screening, as early as possible in pregnancy, should be part of prenatal care for all women, with the understanding that a woman can "opt out" of screening should she so choose (Branson, Handsfield, Lampe, et al., 2006). If the results are positive, the Western blot test is used to confirm the diagnosis. Women who test positive should be counseled about the implications of the diagnosis for themselves and their fetus to ensure an informed reproductive choice.

Two rapid screening tests have been developed that are useful in assessing the HIV status of women who did not receive prenatal care prior to labor and for women in active labor who do not know their HIV status. These tests (OraQuick HIV-1 Antibody test and the SUDS HIV-1 test) require a small blood sample, can be read in 20 minutes, and are very sensitive and specific (Lachat, Scott, & Relf, 2006).

ACOG (2008c) recommends repeat HIV screening in the third trimester, using either conventional or rapid screening, for women known to be at high risk, namely women with a partner who is HIV-positive, a new partner during the current pregnancy, or multiple partners; women treated for another sexually transmitted infection in the past year; IV drug users; and sex trade workers. Third trimester screening is also recommended for women who live in areas with a high prevalence of HIV infection and those who declined testing earlier in pregnancy. In addition, rapid HIV screening is recommended for women in labor with an undocumented HIV status.

Antiretroviral prophylaxis or antiretroviral therapy should be recommended to all infected pregnant women regardless of CD4 count to reduce the rate of perinatal transmission. As more antiretroviral medications have been developed, a wide array of options exists. Highly active antiretroviral therapy (HAART) is a treatment approach that uses a minimum of three antiretroviral agents. It generally includes zidovudine (ZDV), a nucleoside reverse transcriptase inhibitor (NRTI), plus a second NRTI such as didanosine or lamivudine combined with a non-nucleoside reverse transcriptase inhibitor (NNRTI) such as nevirapine or a protease inhibitor such as indinavir, ritonavir, or saquinavir.

HIV antiretroviral drug resistance testing is recommended before beginning treatment in HIV-infected pregnant women who do not require treatment for their own health. When possible, treatment for these women is delayed until after the first trimester. HIV-infected women who are already receiving HAART when they become pregnant are advised to continue their current regimen if it is effective, but they should not receive drugs such as efavirenz (EFV), which have known teratogenic effects (Public Health Service Task Force, 2007).

Treatment recommendations have also been developed for the mother and infant for the intrapartum and postpartum periods. The decision about which regimen is most appropriate should be determined following discussion with the woman about the risks and benefits based on her individual HIV status.

HIV-infected women should be evaluated and treated for other sexually transmitted infections and for conditions occurring more commonly in women with HIV, such as tuberculosis, cytomegalovirus, toxoplasmosis, and cervical dysplasia. HIV-infected women with no history of hepatitis B should receive the hepatitis vaccine, which is not contraindicated prenatally, as well as the pneumococcal vaccine and an annual flu shot. In addition to routine prenatal laboratory tests, a platelet count and a complete blood count with differential should be obtained at the first prenatal visit and repeated each trimester to identify anemia, thrombocytopenia, and leukopenia, which are associated both with HIV infection and with antiviral therapy.

The woman with HIV also should be assessed regularly for serologic changes that indicate the disease is progressing. This is determined by the absolute CD4+ T-lymphocyte count, which provides the number of helper T4 cells. When CD4+ counts fall to 200/mm^3 or lower, opportunistic infections such as *Pneumocystis carinii* pneumonia are more likely to develop.

At each prenatal visit, asymptomatic, HIV-infected women are monitored for early signs of complications, such as weight loss in the second or third trimesters or fever. The clinician inspects the mouth for signs of infections such as thrush (candidiasis) or hairy leukoplakia; the lungs are auscultated for signs of pneumonia; and the lymph nodes, the liver, and the spleen are palpated for signs of enlargement. Each trimester the woman should have a visual examination and examination of the retina to detect such complications as toxoplasmosis retinitis.

A pregnancy complicated by HIV infection, even if asymptomatic, is considered high risk, and the fetus is monitored closely. Weekly nonstress testing is begun at 32 weeks' gestation, and serial ultrasounds are done to detect IUGR. Biophysical profiles are also indicated (see Chapter 14). Invasive procedures such as amniocentesis are avoided when possible to prevent the contamination of a noninfected fetus.

To reduce the risk of perinatal transmission, intrapartum intravenous ZDV is indicated for all pregnant women regardless of their prenatal therapy regimen. Scheduled cesarean birth at 38 weeks' gestation and before rupture of the membranes is recommended for women with elevated viral loads (Minkoff, 2008).

Women who are HIV positive are at increased risk for complications such as intrapartal or postpartal hemorrhage, postpartal infection, poor wound healing, and infections of the genitourinary tract. Thus they need careful monitoring and appropriate therapy as indicated.

Following childbirth, the HIV-positive woman should be referred to a physician knowledgeable about treating individuals with HIV infection. Because of the profound implications of HIV infection for the woman, her family, the fetus/newborn, and her healthcare providers, screening is recommended for all pregnant women, but especially those at increased risk, including the following: prostitutes; women with multiple sexual partners; women whose current or previous sex partners have been bisexual, have abused IV drugs, had hemophilia, or tested positive for HIV; women who are or have been IV drug users; and women from countries where heterosexual transmission is common. In addition, clinics located in areas with a large HIV-positive population may require routine HIV screening of all prenatal clients.

Complementary Care

EFFECTS OF A SPIRITUAL MANTRAM ON HIV OUTCOMES

Borman (2006) examined the effectiveness of the use of a psychosocial intervention—in this case a mantram repetition—on psychologic distress (anxiety, anger, depression and so forth), quality-of-life enjoyment and satisfaction, and spiritual well-being in HIV-infected adults. In this study a mantram is defined as a word or phrase that has spiritual associations for the individual. Subjects were asked to repeat the mantram silently throughout the day. A wrist counter was used to track the number of times the mantram was repeated each day. Over time, the mantram group showed significantly more improvement than the control group in reducing anger and in increased quality of life, peace, spiritual connectedness, and faith.

Clearly further study is warranted but the authors suggest that mantram practice may contribute to managing psychologic distress and enhancing spiritual well-being in people living with HIV/AIDS (Bormann, 2006).

NURSING MANAGEMENT

"Nursing Care Plan: The Woman with HIV Infection" on pages 319–320 addresses nursing management.

NURSING ASSESSMENT AND DIAGNOSIS

A woman who tests positive for HIV may be asymptomatic or may present with any of the following signs or symptoms: fatigue, anemia, malaise, progressive weight loss, lymphadenopathy, diarrhea, fever, neurologic dysfunction, cell-mediated immunodeficiency, or evidence of Kaposi's sarcoma (purplish, reddish brown lesions either externally or internally). If a woman

Nursing Care Plan

THE WOMAN WITH HIV INFECTION

INTERVENTION	RATIONALE	EXPECTED OUTCOME
1. Nursing Diagnosis: Risk for Infection related to inadequate defenses (leukopenia, suppressed inflammatory response) secondary to HIV-positive status		
NIC Intervention: **Infection control:** Minimizing the acquisition of infection		**NOC Outcome:** **Risk control:** Actions taken to eliminate or reduce risk of exposure to infection
Goal: Client will remain free of opportunistic infection during the course of pregnancy.		
■ Obtain a complete health history and physical examination during first prenatal visit.	■ A complete health history will help determine risk factors for the development of opportunistic infections, and a physical examination will assist in identifying any underlying problem symptoms or illnesses that may compromise the pregnancy or complicate the treatment of HIV.	■ Client will remain free of opportunistic infection as evidenced by CD4† lymphocyte count within normal limits; no complaints of chills, fever, or sore throat; normal weight gain throughout pregnancy.
■ Educate the woman as to the signs and symptoms of infection.	■ Early recognition of signs and symptoms of infection will allow for immediate treatment, which may decrease the severity of the infection. Signs and symptoms of infections include fever, weight loss, fatigue, persistent candidiasis, diarrhea, cough, and skin lesions (Kaposi's sarcoma and hairy leukoplakia in the mouth).	
■ Obtain nutritional history and monitor weight gain at each prenatal visit.	■ The HIV-infected woman needs to maintain optimal nutritional intake. A compromised nutritional status may affect maternal and fetal well-being. Depleted reserves of protein and iron may decrease the client's ability to fight infection, thereby making her more susceptible to opportunistic infections.	
Collaborative: Monitor the absolute CD4+ T lymphocyte count, erythrocyte sedimentation rate (ESR), complete blood count (CBC) with differential, and hemoglobin and hematocrit (H & H) at each prenatal visit.	■ Lab results provide information about the woman's immune system and the potential for disease progression. Opportunistic infections are more likely to occur when the CD4+ T lymphocyte count drops below a level of 200/mm^3. ESR can rise above 20 mm/hr with anemia and with acute and chronic inflammation. CBC with differential and platelet count helps identify anemia, thrombocytopenia, and leukopenia. H & H can also identify anemia.	
2. Nursing Diagnosis: Risk for Ineffective Health Maintenance related to lack of information about HIV/AIDS and its long-term implications for the woman, her unborn child, and her family		
NIC Intervention: **Health information:** Providing instruction and learning experiences to facilitate the woman's understanding of her condition and to enhance her self-care activities		**NOC Intervention:** **Health-promoting behavior:** Actions to promote optimal wellness and a healthy pregnancy and birth

(continued)

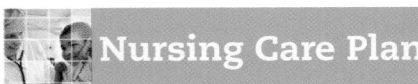

Nursing Care Plan—continued

THE WOMAN WITH HIV INFECTION

INTERVENTION	RATIONALE	EXPECTED OUTCOME
Goal: The client and her family will verbalize the importance of following her medication regimen and of regular prenatal care.		
■ Assess the client's and family's level of understanding of HIV infection, its methods of spread, and the long-term implications.	■ Knowledge of the woman's (and her family's) level of understanding about her HIV infection forms a starting point for further health teaching.	■ Woman will actively seek information about her condition, her treatment regimen, and her pregnancy and will cooperate with her caregivers.
■ Explain the risks of mother-to-child transmission of HIV infection.	■ In untreated women the risk of transmission is 21%. That risk has been reduced dramatically because of the availability of antiretroviral therapy, the use of cesarean birth when indicated, and formula-feeding rather than breastfeeding.	
■ Describe antiretroviral therapy. Include the regimen prescribed, its purposes, and the procedures for taking it.	■ ARV therapy approaches vary based on the health status of the individual woman and whether she is currently on ARV therapy. Generally it includes oral ZDV daily, IV ZDV during labor and until birth, and ZDV therapy for the infant for 6 weeks following birth.	
■ Discuss signs the woman should be alert for, including fever, fatigue, weight loss, persistent candidiasis, diarrhea, cough, skin lesions, and behavior changes.	■ These symptoms may indicate that the woman is developing symptomatic HIV infection.	

3. Nursing Diagnosis: Compromised Family Coping related to the implications of positive maternal HIV status on fetal/neonatal well-being and long-term family functioning

NIC Intervention:		NOC Outcome:
Emotional support: Provision of reassurance, acceptance, and encouragement during times of stress		**Family coping:** Family actions to manage stressors that tax family resources
Goal: Family is able to manage stressors related to the maternal diagnosis.		
■ Assess ability and readiness of family to learn about HIV and its long-term implications.	■ Readiness is a key element in the teaching-learning process.	■ Family members actively participate in the treatment plan, are involved in planning for labor and birth in light of a positive HIV status, and are able to express unresolved feelings about the diagnosis.
■ Provide woman and her family with accurate, reliable information about her diagnosis, its prognosis for her and for her baby, and the immediate and long-term implications for her care.	■ Fear and anxiety will lessen when the woman and her family understand her health status and the implications of the HIV diagnosis and can then plan for the future.	
■ Assess interactions between the woman and her family. Be alert for potentially destructive behaviors.	■ If the HIV diagnosis was not expected, the couple may have to deal with issues of blame, concerns about mortality, and worries about the status of the baby. If the HIV diagnosis was known, concerns may focus on fetal/neonatal well-being. In either case, negative responses can lead to destructive behaviors.	
■ Assist family in realistically identifying the needs of the woman and family unit.	■ Once needs are identified realistically, it is possible to plan interventions to meet the needs.	
Collaborative: Explore available community resources and family support systems.	■ Because HIV is a long-term condition, the family may require ongoing assistance.	

tests positive for HIV or is involved in a relationship that places her at high risk, assess the woman's knowledge level about the disease, its implications for her and her fetus, and self-care measures the woman can take.

Examples of nursing diagnoses that might apply for a pregnant woman who tests positive for HIV include the following:

- *Risk for Ineffective Health Maintenance* related to lack of information about HIV/AIDS and its long-term implications for the woman and her unborn child
- *Risk for Infection* related to altered immunity secondary to HIV infection
- *Compromised Family Coping* related to the implications of a positive HIV test in one of the family members

PLANNING AND IMPLEMENTATION

NURSING CARE IN THE COMMUNITY

Women need to understand that HIV/AIDS is a fatal disease. HIV infection can be avoided if women practice safe sex, including insisting that their partners wear a latex condom for each act of intercourse and avoiding sharing IV drug needles. Women at high risk for HIV/AIDS should be offered premarital and prepregnancy screening for HIV antibodies.

In monitoring the asymptomatic pregnant woman who is HIV positive, be alert for nonspecific symptoms such as fever, weight loss, fatigue, persistent candidiasis, diarrhea, cough, skin lesions, and behavior changes. These may be signs of developing symptomatic HIV infection. Laboratory findings such as increased viral load; decreased hemoglobin, hematocrit, and CD4+ lymphocytes; elevated erythrocyte sedimentation rate (ESR); and abnormal complete blood count, differential, and platelets may indicate complications such as infection or progression of the disease.

Education about optimal nutrition and maintenance of wellness is important; review the information frequently with the woman. Give her information about her ZDV prophylaxis and the importance of following the established regimen for herself during pregnancy and for her newborn after birth.

HOSPITAL-BASED NURSING CARE

Nurses who deal with childbearing families are exposed frequently to blood and body fluids and need to pay careful attention to the *standard precautions* addressed in introductory nursing courses as a preparation for clinical practice. Protocols have been established for postexposure treatment of a healthcare worker who experiences a needlestick or exposure to body fluids of a person with positive or unknown HIV status. The effectiveness of the therapy, usually a combined drug approach, depends on starting rapidly. Thus, such exposure should be reported immediately.

TEACHING FOR SELF-CARE

The psychologic implications of HIV/AIDS for the childbearing family are staggering. The woman is faced with the knowledge that she and her newborn, if infected, have a decreased life expectancy. If her infant is not infected, she must face the possibility that others will raise her child. She must also face the reality that she can only hope to lengthen her life by carefully following an expensive, exacting medical regimen. The couple must deal with the impact of the illness on the partner, who may or may not be infected, and on other children. The woman and her family may feel fearful, helpless, angry, and isolated.

It is important to preserve confidentiality and the woman's right to privacy. Help ensure that the woman receives complete, accurate information about her condition and ways she might cope. Teach about transmission prevention using language the woman and her partner understand. In addition, ensure that the woman is referred to a comprehensive program that includes social services, psychologic support, and appropriate health care.

> **Nursing Practice**
>
> Research indicates that prenatal care providers working in states with a low incidence of HIV/AIDS may not be as knowledgeable as they should be about follow-up when HIV testing is refused and about the disease itself as it relates to pregnancy and prenatal care (Olges, Murphy, Caldwell, et al., 2007). If you work with childbearing families it is crucial that you stay current on the diagnosis and treatment of pregnant women with HIV/AIDS, even if you live in an area where the incidence is low.

EVALUATION

Expected outcomes of nursing care include the following:

- The woman discusses the implications of her HIV infection (or diagnosis of AIDS), its implications for her unborn child and for herself, the method of transmission, and the treatment options.
- The woman uses information about social services (or other agency referral) for follow-up assistance and counseling.
- The woman begins to verbalize her feelings about her condition and its implications for her and her family.

CARE OF THE WOMAN WITH HEART DISEASE

Pregnancy results in increased cardiac output, heart rate, and blood volume. The normal heart is able to adapt to these changes without difficulty. The woman with heart disease, however, has decreased cardiac reserve, making it more difficult for her heart to handle the higher workload of pregnancy.

Cardiac disease complicates about 1% of pregnancies (Cunningham, Levon, Bloom, et al., 2010). It is the most common cause of maternal death overall (Burt & Durbridge, 2009). The pathology found in a pregnant woman with heart disease varies with the type of disorder. The more common conditions are discussed briefly here.

Congenital heart defects have become more common in pregnant women as improved surgical techniques enable females born with heart defects to live to childbearing age. Congenital heart defects most commonly seen in pregnant women include atrial septal defect, ventricular septal defect, patent ductus arteriosus, coarctation of the aorta, and tetralogy of Fallot.

For women with congenital heart disease, the impact of pregnancy depends on the specific defect. If the heart defect has been surgically repaired and no evidence of heart disease remains, the woman may undertake pregnancy with confidence. Because of the risk of subacute bacterial endocarditis, even in cases where the defect was corrected surgically, antibiotic prophylaxis is often recommended at the time of birth using IV or IM ampicillin, cefazolin, or ceftriaxone (Freeman & Foley, 2008). Women with congenital heart disease who experience cyanosis should be counseled to avoid pregnancy because the risk to mother and fetus is high.

Rheumatic fever, which may develop in untreated group A β-hemolytic streptococcal infections, is an inflammatory connective tissue disease that can involve the heart, joints, central nervous system, skin, and subcutaneous tissue. Once it occurs, rheumatic fever can recur; it is serious primarily because of the permanent damage it can do to the heart—rheumatic heart disease. Fortunately, rheumatic heart disease has declined rapidly in the past half century, primarily because of the availability of antibiotics for treatment.

Rheumatic heart disease results when recurrent inflammation from bouts of rheumatic fever causes scar tissue to form on the valves. The scarring results in stenosis (failure of the valve to open completely), regurgitation due to failure of the valve to close completely, or a combination of both, thereby increasing the workload of the heart. Although mitral valve stenosis is most common, the aortic and tricuspid valves may also be affected.

The increased blood volume of pregnancy, coupled with the pregnant woman's need for increased cardiac output, stresses the heart of a woman with mitral stenosis and increases her risk of developing congestive heart failure. Even the woman who has no symptoms at the onset of her pregnancy is at risk.

Mitral valve prolapse (MVP) is usually asymptomatic and commonly found in women of childbearing age. The condition is more common in women than in men and seems to run in families. In MVP the mitral valve leaflets tend to prolapse into the left atrium during ventricular systole because the chordae tendineae that support them are long, stretched, and thin. This produces a characteristic systolic click on auscultation. In more pronounced cases of MVP, mitral valve regurgitation occurs, producing a systolic murmur.

Women with MVP usually tolerate pregnancy well. Most women require assurance that they can continue with normal activities. A few women experience symptoms—primarily palpitations, chest pain, and dyspnea—which are often due to arrhythmias. They are usually treated with propranolol hydrochloride (Inderal). Limiting caffeine intake also helps decrease palpitations. Prophylactic antibiotics at the time of birth to prevent bacterial endocarditis are not usually necessary for women whose only sign of MVP is a systolic click. Antibiotics are recommended, however, for women with mitral valve regurgitation, valvular damage, or other risk factors (Cunningham et al., 2010).

Peripartum cardiomyopathy is a dysfunction of the left ventricle that occurs in the last month of pregnancy or the first 5 months postpartum in a woman with no previous history of heart disease. The cause is unknown, but the mortality rate is as high as 25% to 50% (Easterling & Stout, 2007). The symptoms are similar to those of congestive heart failure: dyspnea, orthopnea, fatigue, cough, chest pain, palpitations, and edema. The woman may have an enlarged heart, tachycardia, rales, and a third heart sound. Treatment includes digoxin, diuretics, vasodilators as necessary, anticoagulants, sodium restriction, and strict bed rest. The condition may resolve with bed rest as the heart gradually returns to normal size. Subsequent pregnancy is strongly discouraged because the disease tends to recur during pregnancy.

CLINICAL THERAPY

The primary goal of clinical therapy is early diagnosis and ongoing management of the woman with cardiac disease. Echocardiogram, chest x-ray, auscultation of heart sounds, and sometimes cardiac catheterization are essential for establishing the type and severity of the heart disease. The severity of the disease can also be determined by the individual's ability to perform ordinary physical activity. Table 15–5 outlines the classification of functional capacity that has been standardized by the Criteria Committee of the New York Heart Association (1994).

Women in classes I and II usually experience a normal pregnancy and have few complications, whereas those in classes III and IV are at risk for more severe complications. Because anemia increases the work of the heart, it should be diagnosed early and treated if present. Infections, even if minor, also increase cardiac workload and should be treated. As pregnancy progresses, the woman's activity should be limited to minimize cardiac workload. Similarly, weight gain and sodium intake may also be restricted.

Drug Therapy

The pregnant woman with heart disease may need drug therapy in addition to the iron and vitamin supplements ordinarily prescribed to maintain health during pregnancy. Antibiotics, usu-

Table 15–5 Severity of Heart Disease by Functional Capacity

Class	Functional Capacity
I	Asymptomatic. No limitation of physical activity.
II	Slight limitation of physical activity. Asymptomatic at rest; symptoms occur with ordinary physical activity.
III	Marked limitation of physical activity. Comfortable at rest but symptomatic during less-than-ordinary physical activity.
IV	Inability to carry on any physical activity without discomfort. Even at rest the person experiences symptoms of cardiac insufficiency or anginal pain; discomfort increases with any physical activity.

ally penicillin if not contraindicated by allergy, are used during pregnancy to prevent recurrent bouts of rheumatic fever and subsequent heart valve damage. Antibiotics are also recommended during labor and the early postpartum period to prevent bacterial endocarditis in women with either acquired or congenital disease. If the woman develops coagulation problems, the anticoagulant heparin may be used. Heparin is safest for the fetus because it does not cross the placenta. The thiazide diuretics and furosemide (Lasix) may be used to treat congestive heart failure if it develops. Digitalis glycosides and common antiarrhythmic drugs may be used to treat cardiac failure and arrhythmias. These agents cross the placenta but have no reported teratogenic effect.

LABOR AND BIRTH

Spontaneous natural labor with adequate pain relief is usually recommended for women in classes I and II. Special attention should be given to the prompt recognition and treatment of any signs of heart failure (Figure 15–3 ●). Those in classes III and IV may have labor induced and may need to be hospitalized before the onset of labor for cardiac stabilization. They also require invasive cardiac monitoring during labor.

Use of low forceps or vacuum assistance provides the safest method of birth, with lumbar epidural anesthesia to reduce the stress of pushing. Cesarean birth is used only if fetal or maternal indications exist, not on the basis of heart disease alone.

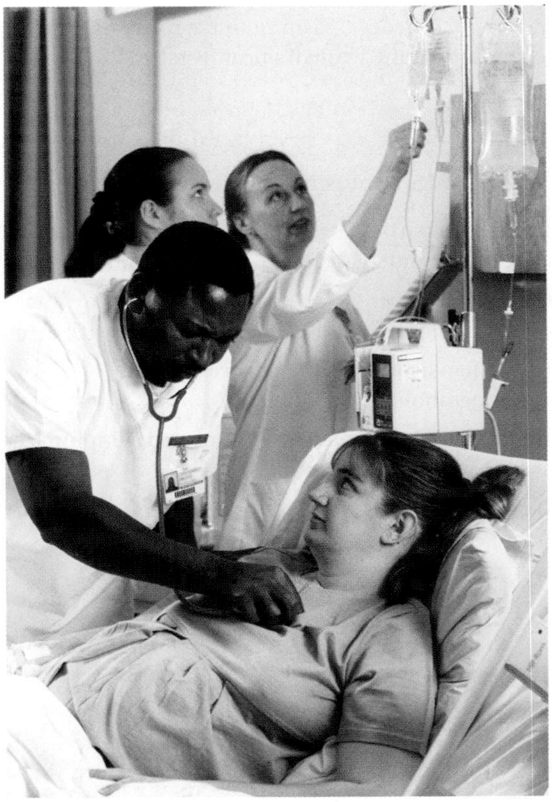

● **Figure 15–3** Monitoring for signs of heart failure. When a woman with heart disease begins labor, the nursing students and instructor monitor her closely for signs of congestive heart failure.

NURSING MANAGEMENT

NURSING ASSESSMENT AND DIAGNOSIS

Assess the stress of pregnancy on the heart's functioning during every antepartal visit. Note the category of functional capacity assigned to the woman; take the woman's pulse, respirations, and blood pressure; and compare the findings with the normal values expected during pregnancy. Then determine the woman's activity level, including rest, and any changes in the pulse and respirations since previous visits. Identify and evaluate other factors that would increase strain on the heart. These factors might include anemia, infection, anxiety, lack of a support system, and household and career demands.

The following signs and symptoms, if they are progressive, indicate congestive heart failure:

- Cough (frequent, with or without blood-stained sputum [hemoptysis])
- Dyspnea (progressive, on exertion)
- Edema (progressive, generalized, including extremities, face, eyelids)
- Heart murmurs (heard on auscultation)
- Palpitations
- Rales (auscultated in lung bases)
- Weight gain (related to fluid retention)

Progressiveness of the cycle is the critical factor because some of these same signs and symptoms are seen to a minor degree in a pregnancy without cardiac problems.

Nursing diagnoses that might apply to the pregnant woman with heart disease include the following:

- *Decreased Cardiac Output:* easy fatigability
- *Impaired Gas Exchange* related to pulmonary edema secondary to cardiac decompensation
- *Fear* related to the effects of the maternal cardiac condition on fetal well-being

PLANNING AND IMPLEMENTATION

Nursing care is directed toward maintaining a balance between cardiac reserve and cardiac workload.

ANTEPARTAL NURSING CARE

The priority of nursing action varies based on the severity of the disease process and the individual needs of the woman determined by the nursing assessment. Ensure that the woman and her family thoroughly understand her condition and its management and that they recognize signs of potential complications; this level of understanding will decrease their anxiety. Providing thorough explanations, using printed material, and giving frequent opportunities to ask questions and discuss concerns lets the woman better meet her own healthcare needs and seek assistance appropriately.

MyNursingKit Care Plan Activity: Antepartal Client at Risk

As part of health teaching, explain the purposes of the required dietary and activity changes. A diet high in iron, protein, and essential nutrients but low in sodium, with adequate calories to ensure normal weight gain, best meets the nutrition needs of the woman with cardiac disease. To help preserve her cardiac reserves, the woman may need to restrict her activities. In addition, 8 to 10 hours of sleep, with frequent daily rest periods, are essential. Because upper respiratory infections may tax the heart and lead to decompensation, the woman must avoid contact with sources of infection.

During the first half of pregnancy, the woman is seen approximately every 2 weeks to assess cardiac status. During the second half of pregnancy, the woman is seen weekly. These assessments are especially important between weeks 28 and 30, when the blood volume reaches its maximum. If symptoms of cardiac decompensation occur, prompt medical intervention is indicated to correct the cardiac problem.

INTRAPARTAL PERIOD

Labor and birth exert tremendous stress on the woman and her fetus. This stress could be fatal to the fetus of a woman with cardiac disease, because the fetus may be receiving a decreased oxygen and blood supply. Thus, the intrapartal care of a woman with cardiac disease is aimed at reducing physical exertion and the accompanying fatigue.

Evaluate maternal vital signs frequently to determine the woman's response to labor. A pulse rate greater than 100 beats per minute or respirations greater than 25 per minute may indicate the onset of cardiac decompensation and require further evaluation. Auscultate the woman's lungs frequently for evidence of rales and carefully observe for other signs that she is developing decompensation.

To ensure cardiac emptying and adequate oxygenation, encourage the laboring woman to assume either a semi-Fowler's or side-lying position, with her head and shoulders elevated. Oxygen by mask, diuretics to reduce fluid retention, sedatives and analgesics, prophylactic antibiotics, and digitalis may also be used as indicated by the woman's status. Remain with the woman to support her. It is essential to keep the woman and her family informed of labor progress and management plans, collaborating with them to fulfill their wishes for the birth experience as much as possible. Maintain an atmosphere of calm to lessen the anxiety of the woman and her family.

Continuous electronic fetal monitoring provides ongoing assessment of the fetal response to labor. To prevent overexertion and the accompanying fatigue, encourage the woman to sleep and relax between contractions and give her emotional support and encouragement. Epidural anesthesia is often used to decrease exertion. During pushing, encourage the woman to use shorter, more moderate open-glottis pushing, with complete relaxation between pushes. Forceps or vacuum extraction may be used if pushing is too difficult. Monitor vital signs closely during the second stage.

POSTPARTAL PERIOD

The postpartal period is a significant time for the woman with cardiac disease. As extravascular fluid returns to the bloodstream for excretion, cardiac output and blood volume increase. This physiologic adaptation places great strain on the heart and may lead to decompensation, especially in the first 48 hours after birth.

To detect any possible problems, the woman may remain in the hospital postpartally longer than the low-risk woman. Monitor her vital signs frequently, and assess for signs of decompensation. She stays in the semi-Fowler's or side-lying position, with her head and shoulders elevated, and begins a gradual, progressive activity program. Appropriate diet and stool softeners facilitate bowel movement without undue strain.

Give the woman opportunities to discuss her birth experience and help her deal with any feelings or concerns that distress her. Encourage maternal-infant attachment by providing frequent opportunities for the mother to interact with her child.

No evidence exists that breastfeeding stresses the heart. Thus, the only concern about breastfeeding for women with cardiovascular disease is related to medications the mother may be taking. These should be evaluated for the likelihood of passing into the milk or affecting lactation. Assist the breastfeeding mother to a comfortable side-lying position, with her head moderately elevated, or to a semi-Fowler's position. To conserve the mother's energy, position the newborn at the breast and be available to burp the baby and reposition him or her at the other breast.

In addition to providing the normal postpartal discharge teaching, ensure that the woman and her family understand the signs of possible problems from her heart disease or other postpartal complications. Work with the woman and her family to plan an activity schedule. Visiting nurse referrals may be necessary, depending on the woman's health status.

EVALUATION

Expected outcomes of nursing care include the following:

- The woman participates in developing an appropriate healthcare regimen and follows it throughout her pregnancy.
- The woman gives birth to a healthy infant.
- The woman avoids congestive heart failure, thromboembolism, and infection.
- The woman is able to identify signs and symptoms of possible postpartum complications.
- The woman is able to care effectively for her newborn infant.

OTHER MEDICAL CONDITIONS AND PREGNANCY

A woman with a preexisting medical condition needs to be aware of the possible impact of pregnancy on her condition, as well as the impact of her condition on the successful outcome of her pregnancy. Table 15–6 discusses some less common medical conditions in relation to pregnancy.

Table 15–6 Less Common Medical Conditions and Pregnancy

Condition	Brief Description	Maternal Implications	Fetal/Neonatal Implications
Asthma	Asthma, an obstructive lung condition, is the most common respiratory disease found in pregnancy, complicating 4% to 8% of all pregnancies (ACOG, 2008b). Typical symptoms include wheezing, dyspnea, and episodic coughing. A severe asthmatic attack often requires hospitalization. It is managed by long-term comprehensive drug therapy to prevent airway inflammation, combined with drug treatment to manage attacks or exacerbations and client education about triggers (such as cold air, dust, smoke, exercise, food additives), methods of prevention, and treatment options.	The goal of therapy is to maintain adequate oxygenation of the fetus by preventing maternal hypoxia. Thus it is safer to treat symptoms with asthma medications than to let the woman have untreated symptoms and exacerbations. The effects on pregnancy vary. Thus all pregnant women with asthma should be monitored by assessing their symptoms and measuring their peak expiratory flow rate and forced expiratory volume. The use of medication is individualized using the lowest amount possible to maintain normal lung function. During pregnancy, Budesonide is the preferred inhaled corticosteroid for regular control. Asthma medications should be continued during labor and birth. To decrease the risk of bronchospasm, the woman should be well hydrated and receive adequate analgesia (ACOG, 2008b).	Prematurity and low birth weight are more common in women with asthma (Dombrowski, 2006). Asthma has also been linked with higher rates of hyperemesis gravidarum, preeclampsia, uterine hemorrhage, and perinatal mortality. The goal of therapy is to prevent maternal exacerbations because even a mild exacerbation can cause severe hypoxia-related complications in the fetus. If an exacerbation occurs, inhaled albuterol is recommended as rescue therapy if needed. If symptoms and pulmonary function levels do not improve, hospitalization may be necessary (ACOG, 2008b).
Rheumatoid arthritis	Chronic inflammatory disease believed to be caused by a genetically influenced antigen-antibody reaction. Symptoms include fatigue, low-grade fever, pain and swelling of joints, morning stiffness, pain on movement. Treated with salicylates, physical therapy, and rest. Corticosteroids used cautiously if not responsive to above.	Usually there is remission of rheumatoid arthritis symptoms during pregnancy, often with a relapse postpartum. Anemia may be present due to blood loss from salicylate therapy. Mother needs extra rest, particularly to relieve weight-bearing joints, but needs to continue range-of-motion exercises. If in remission, may stop medication during pregnancy.	Possibility of prolonged gestation and longer labor with heavy salicylate use. Possible teratogenic effects of salicylates.
Epilepsy	Chronic disorder characterized by seizures; may be idiopathic or secondary to other conditions, such as head injury, metabolic and nutritional disorders such as phenylketonuria (PKU) or vitamin B_6 deficiency, encephalitis, neoplasms, or circulatory interferences. Treated with anticonvulsants.	Vast majority of pregnancies in women with seizure disorders are uneventful and have an excellent outcome. Women with more frequent seizures before pregnancy may have exacerbations during pregnancy, but this may be related to nausea and vomiting, lack of cooperation with drug regimen, or sleep deprivation (Samuels & Niebyl, 2007). During pregnancy the woman should continue to be treated with the medication that best controls her seizures. She should take a multivitamin with folate throughout pregnancy. Antiseizure medication is continued during labor (Krakow, 2008).	The risk of birth defects in infants of women with epilepsy is about 7% or more than double that of the general population (Krakow, 2008). These infants are also at increased risk for IUGR and stillbirth (Samuels & Niebyl, 2007). The goals of therapy are to maintain seizure control while minimizing fetal exposure to antiseizure medications. When possible the woman is maintained on single drug therapy at the lowest possible dose.

(continued)

Table 15–6 Less Common Medical Conditions and Pregnancy—continued

Condition	Brief Description	Maternal Implications	Fetal/Neonatal Implications
Hepatitis B	Hepatitis B, caused by the hepatitis B virus (HBV), is a major, growing health problem. Groups at risk include those from areas with a high incidence (primarily developing countries), illegal IV drug users, prostitutes, homosexuals, those with multiple sex partners, or occupational exposure to blood, although many infected people have no identifiable source of infection. HBV transmission is bloodborne, primarily sexually and perinatally transmitted. Because of the dramatic increase and the difficulty of vaccinating high-risk individuals before they become infected, the CDC now recommends (1) testing all pregnant women for the presence of hepatitis B surface antigen (HBsAg) preferably during the first trimester and prophylaxis of all infants born to women who are HBsAG-positive or whose status is unknown; (2) routine vaccination of all newborns; (3) universal vaccination of children and adolescents younger than 19 years of age who have not been vaccinated; (4) vaccination of unvaccinated adults at risk for hepatitis B including healthcare and public safety workers at risk for exposure to blood on the job (CDC, 2009b).	Hepatitis B does not usually affect the course of pregnancy. However, chronic HBV carriers have a great potential for infecting others when exposure to blood and body fluids occurs. In addition, chronic carriers may develop long-term sequelae, such as chronic liver disease and liver cancer. It is now recommended that all pregnant women be tested for the presence of HBsAg. A woman who is negative may be given the hepatitis B vaccine.	Perinatal transmission most often occurs at or near the time of childbirth. More important, the risk of becoming a chronic carrier of the HBV is inversely related to the age of the individual at the time of initial infection. Therefore, infants infected perinatally have the highest risk of becoming chronically infected if not treated. Recommendations now include routine vaccination of all newborns at birth. All newborns of HBsAg-positive women should also be given an injection of hepatitis B immunoglobulin (HBIG) at birth (CDC, 2009b).
Hyperthyroidism (thyrotoxicosis)	Enlarged, overactive thyroid gland; increased T_4:TBG ratio and increased basal metabolic rate (BMR). Symptoms include muscle wasting, tachycardia, excessive sweating, and exophthalmos. Treatment by antithyroid drug propylthiouracil (PTU) while monitoring free T_4 levels. Surgery used only if drug intolerance exists.	Mild hyperthyroidism is not dangerous. Increased incidence of preeclampsia and postpartum hemorrhage if not well controlled. Serious risk related to thyroid storm characterized by high fever, tachycardia, sweating, and congestive heart failure. Now occurs rarely. When diagnosed during pregnancy, may be transient or permanent.	Neonatal thyrotoxicosis is rare. Even low doses of antithyroid drug in mother may produce a mild fetal/neonatal hypothyroidism; higher dose may produce a goiter or mental deficiencies. Fetal loss not increased in euthyroid women. If untreated, rates of abortion, intrauterine death, and stillbirth increase. Breastfeeding contraindicated for women on antithyroid medication because it is excreted in the milk (may be tried by woman on low dose if neonatal T_4 levels are monitored).
Hypothyroidism	Characterized by inadequate thyroid secretions (decreased T_4:TBG ratio), elevated TSH, lowered BMR, and enlarged thyroid gland (goiter). Symptoms include lack of energy, excessive weight gain, cold intolerance, dry skin, and constipation. Treated by thyroxine replacement therapy.	Long-term replacement therapy usually continues at same dosage during pregnancy as before. Weekly nonstress test (NST) after 35 weeks' gestation.	If mother untreated, fetal loss 50%; high risk of congenital goiter or true cretinism. Therefore, newborns are screened for T_4 level. Mild TSH elevations present little risk because TSH does not cross the placenta.
Maternal phenylketonuria (PKU) (hyperphenylalaninemia)	Inherited recessive single gene anomaly causing a deficiency of the liver enzyme needed to convert the amino acid phenylalanine to tyrosine, resulting in high serum levels of phenylalanine. Brain damage and mental retardation occur if not treated early.	Low phenylalanine diet is mandatory before conception and during pregnancy. The woman should be counseled that her children will either inherit the disease or be carriers, depending on the zygosity of the father for the disease. Treatment at a PKU center is recommended.	Risk to fetus if maternal treatment not begun preconception. In untreated women, increased incidence of fetal mental retardation, microcephaly, congenital heart defects, and growth retardation. Fetal phenylalanine levels are approximately 50% higher than maternal levels.

Table 15–6 Less Common Medical Conditions and Pregnancy—continued

Condition	Brief Description	Maternal Implications	Fetal/Neonatal Implications
Multiple sclerosis	Neurologic disorder characterized by destruction of the myelin sheath of nerve fibers. The condition occurs primarily in young adults, more commonly in females, and is marked by periods of remission; progresses to marked physical disability in 10 to 20 years.	Generally associated with little symptom progression during pregnancy but flare-ups may occur postpartally (Krakow, 2008). Rest is important; help with child care should be planned. Uterine contraction strength is not diminished, but because sensation is frequently lessened, labor may be almost painless but the incidence of forceps or vacuum-assisted birth is higher because voluntary pushing is sometimes hindered (Samuels & Niebyl, 2007).	Increased evidence of a genetic predisposition. Therefore, reproductive counseling is recommended.
Systemic lupus erythematosus (SLE)	Chronic autoimmune collagen disease, characterized by exacerbations and remissions; symptoms range from characteristic rash to inflammation and pain in joints, fever, nephritis, depression, cranial nerve disorders, and peripheral neuropathies.	Women who conceive when the disease is in remission appear to have little risk for adverse outcomes but the risk of obstetric problems increases in women with active SLE. Thus women should be advised to delay pregnancy until they are in remission. With a planned pregnancy cytotoxic drugs are stopped before conception and long-term treatment with nonsteroidal antiinflammatory drugs is reduced or eliminated if possible. Maintenance therapy with low doses of glucocorticoids or hydroxychloroquine may continue. Prenatal visits are increased as is fetal testing (Holmgren & Branch, 2007).	Increased incidence of spontaneous abortion, stillbirth, prematurity, and IUGR. Infants born to women with SLE may have characteristic skin rash, which disappears as the infant metabolizes the maternal immunoglobulin. Infants are at increased risk for complete congenital heart block, a condition that can be diagnosed prenatally (Byron & Clancy, 2005). No known treatment exists although various therapies have been tried. The prognosis for the fetus varies but, because the heart damage is permanent, a pacemaker may be necessary if the infant is to survive (Branch, Silver, & Aagaard-Tillery, 2008).
Tuberculosis (TB)	Infection caused by *Mycobacterium tuberculosis;* inflammatory process causes destruction of lung tissue, increased sputum, and coughing. Associated primarily with poverty and malnutrition and may be found among refugees from countries where TB is prevalent. Treated with isoniazid and either ethambutol or rifampin or both.	The incidence of tuberculosis has begun to increase significantly since the late 1980s, and it is increasingly associated with HIV infection. If TB is inactive due to prior treatment, relapse rate is no greater than for nonpregnant women. When isoniazid is used during pregnancy, the woman should take supplemental pyridoxine (vitamin B_6). Extra rest and limited contact with others is required until disease becomes inactive.	If maternal TB is inactive, mother may breastfeed and care for her infant. If TB is active, newborn should not have direct contact with mother until she is noninfectious. Isoniazid crosses the placenta, but most studies show no teratogenic effects. Rifampin crosses the placenta. Possibility of harmful effects still being studied.

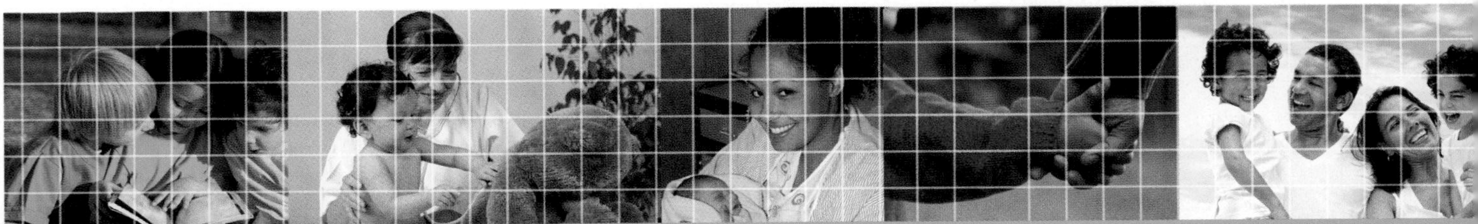

CRITICAL CONCEPT REVIEW

LEARNING OUTCOMES	CONCEPTS
15.1 Describe the effects of alcohol and illicit drugs on the nursing care management of the childbearing woman and her fetus/newborn.	1. Substance abuse (either drugs or alcohol) not only is detrimental to the mother's health but also may have profound, lasting effects on the fetus.

(continued)

LEARNING OUTCOMES / CONCEPTS

15.2 Relate the pathology and clinical treatment of diabetes mellitus in pregnancy to the implications for nursing care.

1. The key point in the care of the pregnant woman with diabetes is scrupulous maternal plasma glucose control. This is best achieved by home blood glucose monitoring, multiple daily insulin injections, and a careful diet.

15.3 Distinguish among the types of anemia associated with pregnancy regarding signs, treatment, and implications for pregnancy.

1. Anemia indicates inadequate levels of hemoglobin in the blood.
2. Signs include fatigue, paleness, and lack of energy.
3. Iron deficiency anemia is the most common form of anemia. Treatment is done through iron replacement by diet, iron supplement, or both.
4. Other forms of anemia include folic acid deficiency, sickle cell anemia, and thalassemia.
5. Implications for the infant include low birth weight, prematurity, and stillbirth.

15.4 Describe acquired immunodeficiency syndrome (AIDS), including care of the pregnant woman who has tested positive for the human immunodeficiency virus (HIV), fetal/neonatal implications, and ramifications for the childbearing family.

1. HIV infection, which is transmitted via blood and body fluids, may also be transmitted vertically from the mother to the fetus.
2. Vertical transmission of HIV infection has been reduced dramatically with the administration of ZDV to the mother prenatally and during labor, and to the newborn.
3. Nurses should employ blood and body fluid precautions in caring for all women to avoid potential spread of infection.

15.5 Explain the effects of various heart disorders on pregnancy, including their implications for nursing care management in the antepartum, intrapartum, and postpartum periods.

1. Cardiac disease during pregnancy requires careful assessment, limitation of activity, and reporting signs of impending cardiac decompensation by both client and nurse.

15.6 Delineate the effects of selected pregestational medical conditions on pregnancy.

1. All women with chronic medical conditions require increased vigilance of their condition during pregnancy.
2. Most chronic medical conditions will have some effect on the mother because pregnancy increases the stress on the mother's body.
3. Many chronic medical conditions in the mother increase risks to the newborn, such as premature birth, low birth weight, and growth retardation.

CRITICAL THINKING IN ACTION

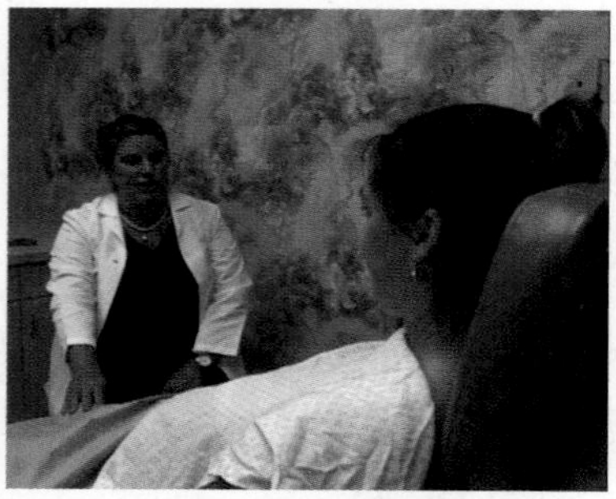

Jane Adams, a 23-year-old, G3 P2, at 37 weeks' gestation, presents to you in the birthing unit complaining of "vaginal pressure" but no contractions. You assess her and find that her history includes being HIV positive for 2 years, second-trimester cocaine and marijuana use, missed appointments, anemia (HCT 28%), and a positive syphilis serology. Jane tells you that she has other children and that they are being cared for by her mother, who has legal custody of them. You admit Jane and place her on the fetal monitor for evaluation of fetal well-being and contraction patterns. The monitor shows you that the fetal heart rate baseline is 120 to 130 with no decelerations; contractions are mild and irregular, lasting 20 to 30 seconds. You obtain vital signs of BP 130/88, temperature 97.0°F, P 88, R 14. A vaginal exam determines that Jane is 7 cm dilated at +1 station with intact membranes. She asks you if being HIV positive will affect her labor.

1. Discuss the prophylactic regimen for the prevention of HIV transmission to the fetus during labor.
2. Discuss the transmission of HIV to the fetus during pregnancy and birth.
3. Identify the emotional impact of HIV infection or other STIs on the woman.
4. On postpartum day 2 you inform Jane that her infant is HIV antibody positive. How would you clarify the results?

See MyNursingKit for possible responses.

REFERENCES

American College of Obstetricians and Gynecologists. (2005). *Pregestational diabetes mellitus* (ACOG Practice Bulletin No. 60). Washington, DC. Author.

American College of Obstetricians and Gynecologists (ACOG). (2008a). *Anemia in pregnancy* (ACOG Practice Bulletin No. 95). Washington, DC: Author.

American College of Obstetricians and Gynecologists (ACOG). (2008b). *Asthma in pregnancy* (ACOG Practice Bulletin No. 90). Washington, DC: Author.

American College of Obstetricians and Gynecologists (ACOG). (2008c). *Prenatal and perinatal human immunodeficiency virus testing: Expanded recommendations* (ACOG Committee Opinion No. 418). Washington, DC: Author.

American Diabetes Association (ADA). (2006). Position statement: Gestational diabetes mellitus. *Diabetes Care, 29*(Suppl. 1).

American Diabetes Association (ADA). (2007). Position statement: Diagnosis and classification of diabetes mellitus. *Diabetes Care, 30*(Suppl.), S42–S47.

Bormann, J. E. (2006). Effects of spiritual mantram repetition on HIV outcomes: a randomized controlled trial. *Journal of Behavioral Medicine, 29*(4), 359–376.

Branch, D. W., Silver, R. M., & Aagaard-Tillery, K. (2008). Immunologic disorders in pregnancy. In R. S. Gibbs, B. Y. Karlan, A. F. Haney, & I. E. Nygaard (Eds.), *Danforth's obstetrics and gynecology* (10th ed.). Philadelphia: WoltersKluwer/Lippincott Williams & Wilkins.

Branson, B. M., Handsfield, H. H., Lampe, M. A., Janssen, R. S., Taylor, A. W., Lyss, S. B., et al. (2006). Revised recommendations for HIV testing of adults, adolescents, and pregnant women in health-care settings. *Morbidity and Mortality Weekly Report, 55*(RR-14), 1–36.

Burt, C. C., & Durbridge, J. (2009). Management of cardiac disease in pregnancy. *Continuing Education in Anaesthesia, Critical Care & Pain.* Retrieved April 29, 2009, from www.medscape.com/viewarticle/590859_print

Byron, J. P., & Clancy, R. M. (2005). Neonatal lupus: Basic research and clinical perspectives. *Rheumatic diseases clinics of North America, 31*(2), 299–313.

Centers for Disease Control and Prevention (CDC). (2006, August 4). Sexually transmitted disease guidelines, 2006. *Morbidity and Mortality Weekly Report, 55*: No. RR-11, 1–93.

Centers for Disease Control and Prevention (CDC). (2007). *HIV/AIDS among women.* Retrieved May 18, 2008, from www.cdc.gov/hiv/topics/women/resources/factsheets/print/women.htm

Centers for Disease Control and Prevention (CDC). (2008). *HIV/AIDS in the United States.* CDC HIV/AIDS Facts. Retrieved May 18, 2008, from www.cdc.gov

Centers for Disease Control and Prevention (CDC). (2009a). *HIV/AIDS Surveillance Report, 2007.* Retrieved May 16, 2009, from www.cdc.gov/hiv/topics/surveillance/resources/reports/

Centers for Disease Control and Prevention (CDC). (2009b). *Viral Hepatitis: FAQs for the Public.* Retrieved May 18, 2009, from www.cdc.gov/hepatitis/B/bFAQ.htm

Cleveland Clinic. (2006). *Gestational diabetes. Hypoglycemia.* Retrieved July 7, 2007, from www.clevelandclinic.org/health/health-info/docs/2300/2354.asp?index=9012

Criteria Committee of the New York Heart Association. (1994). *Nomenclature and criteria for diagnosis of diseases of the heart and great vessels* (9th ed.). Dallas, TX: American Heart Association.

Cunningham, F. G., Leveno, K. L., Bloom, S. L., Hauth, J. C., Gilstrap, L. C., III, & Wenstrom, K. D. (2005). *Williams' obstetrics* (22nd ed.). New York: McGraw-Hill.

Dombrowski, M. P. (2006). Asthma and pregnancy. *Obstetrics and Gynecology, 108,* 667–681.

Easterling, T. R., & Stout, K. (2007). Heart disease. In S. G. Gabbe, J. R. Niebyl, & J. L. Simpson (Eds.). *Obstetrics: Normal and Problem Pregnancies* (5th ed.). Philadelphia: Churchill Livingstone.

Food and Drug Administration (FDA), (2005). Alcohol warning for pregnant women. *FDA Consumer, 39*(3), 4.

Forsbach-Sanchez, G., Tamez-Perez, H. E., & Vazquez-Lara, J. (2005, May–June) Diabetes and pregnancy. *Archives of Medical Research. 36*(3), 291–299.

Freeman, B. E., & Foley, M. R. (2008). Managing a pregnant patient with congenital heart disease. *Contemporary OB/GYN, 53*(10), 38–49.

Gamma, A., Jerome, L., Liechti, M. E., & Sumnall, H. R. (2005). Is ecstasy perceived to be safe? A critical survey. *Drug & Alcohol Dependence. 77*(2), 185–193.

Holmgren, C., & Branch, D. W. (2007). Collagen vascular diseases. In S. G. Gabbe, J. R. Niebyl, & J. L. Simpson (Eds.), *Obstetrics: Normal and problem pregnancies* (5th ed.). Philadelphia: Churchill Livingstone.

Jansson, L. M., Dipietro, J., & Elko, A. (2005). Fetal response to maternal methadone administration. *American Journal of Obstetrics & Gynecology. 193*(3 Pt 1), 611–617.

Krakow, D. (2008). Medical and surgical complications of pregnancy. In R. S. Gibbs, B. Y. Karlan, A. F. Haney, & I. E. Nygaard (Eds.), *Danforth's obstetrics and gynecology* (10th ed.). Philadelphia: WoltersKluwer/Lippincott Williams & Wilkins.

Lachat, M. F., Scott, C. A., & Relf, M. V. (2006). HIV and pregnancy: Considerations for nursing practice. *MCN, 31*(4), 233–240.

March of Dimes. (2006). Illicit drug use during pregnancy. *Fact sheet* retrieved June 27, 2007, from www.marchofdimes.com

Menato, G., Bo, S., Signorite, A., Gallo, M., Cotrino, I., Poala, C. B., et al. (2008). Current management of gestational diabetes. *Expert Review of Obstetrics and Gynecology, 3*(1), 73–91.

Minkoff, H. (2008). Human immunodeficiency virus. In R. S. Gibbs, B. Y. Karlan, A. F. Haney, & I. E. Nygaard (Eds.), *Danforth's obstetrics and gynecology* (10th ed.). Philadelphia: WoltersKluwer/Lippincott Williams & Wilkins.

Ogles, J. R., Murphy, B. S., Caldwell, G. G., & Thornton, A. C. (2007). Testing practices and knowledge of HIV among prenatal providers in a low seroprevalence state. *AIDS, Patient Care, and STDs, 21*(3), 187–194.

Perkins, J. M., Dunn, J. P., & Jagasia, S. (2007). Perspectives in gestational diabetes mellitus: A review of screening, diagnosis, and treatment. *Clinical Diabetes, 25*(2), 57–62.

Public Heatlh Service Task Force. (2007, November 2). Recommendations for use of antiretroviral drugs in pregnant HIV-infected women for maternal health and interventions to reduce perinatal HIV transmission in the United States. Retrieved May 19, 2008, from http://aidsinfo.nih.gov

Reece, E. A., & Homko, C. J. (2008). Diabetes mellitus and pregnancy. In R. S. Gibbs, B. Y. Karlan, A. F. Haney, & I. E. Nygaard (Eds.), *Danforth's obstetrics and gynecology* (10th ed.). Philadelphia: WoltersKluwer/Lippincott Williams & Wilkins.

Samuels, P. (2007). Hematologic complications of pregnancy. In S. G. Gabbe, J. R. Niebyl, & J. L. Simpson (Eds.), *Obstetrics: Normal and problem pregnancies* (5th ed.). Philadelphia: Churchill Livingstone.

Samuels, P., & Niebyl, J. R. (2007). Neurologic disorders. In S. G. Gabbe, J. R. Niebyl, & J. L. Simpson (Eds.), *Obstetrics: Normal and problem pregnancies* (5th ed.). Philadelphia: Churchill Livingstone.

Scollan-Koliopoulos, M., Guadagno, S., & Walker, E. A. (2006). Gestational diabetes management: Guidelines to a healthy pregnancy. *The Nurse Practitioner, 31*(6), 14–23.

Slocum, J. M. (2007). Preconception counseling and type 2 diabetes. *Diabetes Spectrum, 20,* 117–123.

Spina Bifida Association. (2008). Folic acid. Retrieved January 26, 2009, from www.spinabifidaassociation.org

Substance Abuse and Mental Health Services Administration (SAMHSA). (2008). *Results from the 2007 National Survey on Drug Use and Health: National Findings.* Rockville MD: Office of Applied Studies. Retrieved May 15, 2009, from http://oas.samhsa.gov

Tieu, J., Crowther, C., & Middleton, P. (2008). Dietary advice in pregnancy for preventing gestational diabetes mellitus. *Cochrane Database of Systematic Reviews.* Issues 2. Art. No.: CD006674.

Varney, H., Kriebs, J. M., & Gegor, C. L. (2004). *Varney's midwifery* (4th ed.). Sudbury, MA: Jones & Bartlett.

Wyatt, J. W., Frias, J. L., Hoyme, H. E., Jovanovic, L., Kaaja, R., Brown, F., et al. (2005). Congenital anomaly rate in offspring of mothers with diabetes treated with insulin lispro during pregnancy. *Diabetic Medicine, 22*(6), 803–807.

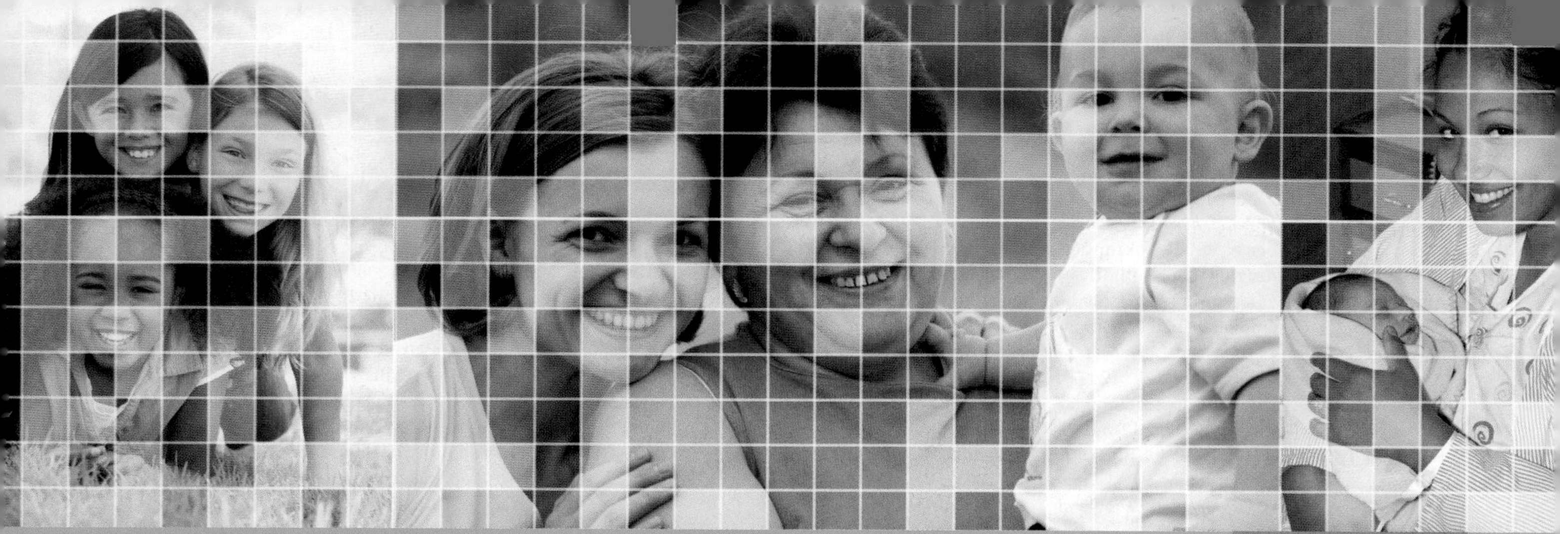

CHAPTER 16

Pregnancy at Risk: Gestational Problems

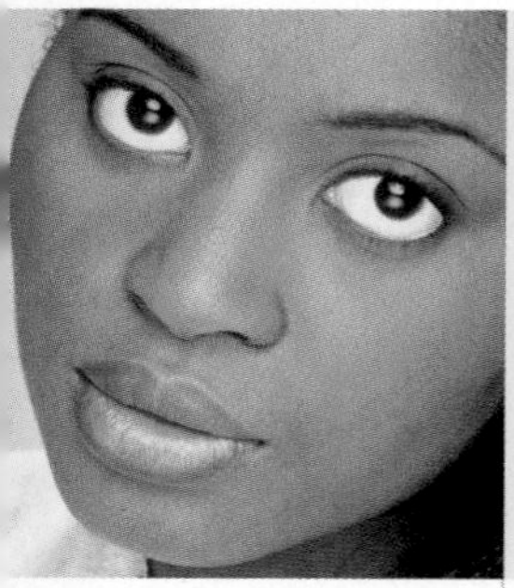

When we decided to have children we were so excited, so ready. I never expected that I would have two miscarriages. I can't tell you how hard that was to handle. Even today, with two healthy children, I remember the pain, the loss, the sense of failure, and I grieve for the children we will never know. —*Jasmine, 36*

LEARNING OUTCOMES

16.1 Summarize the etiology, medical therapy, and cultural perspectives to community-based and hospital-based nursing care management of women with a bleeding problem associated with pregnancy.

16.2 Describe the maternal and fetal-neonatal risks and medical therapy in the nursing care management of a woman with hyperemesis gravidarum.

16.3 Describe the maternal and fetal-neonatal risks, clinical manifestations, and diagnosis in determining the nursing care management of a pregnant woman with a hypertensive disorder.

16.4 Relate the cause, fetal-neonatal risks, prevention, and clinical therapy to the nursing care management of the woman at risk for Rh alloimmunization.

16.5 Explain the occurrence, cause, clinical treatment, and implications for the fetus or newborn in determining the nursing care management of a woman at risk for ABO incompatibility.

16.6 Examine the effects of surgical procedures in the nursing care management of the pregnant woman requiring surgery.

16.7 Relate the impact of trauma caused by an accident to the nursing care management of the pregnant woman or her fetus.

16.8 Delineate the needs and care of the pregnant woman who experiences abuse.

16.9 Explain the causes, fetal-neonatal risks, and clinical therapy in the nursing care management of the pregnant woman with a perinatal infection affecting the fetus.

In some pregnancies, problems arise that place the woman and her unborn child at risk. Regular prenatal care helps detect these complications quickly so that effective care can be provided. This chapter focuses on problems that develop during pregnancy, that is, problems with a *gestational onset.*

CARE OF THE WOMAN WITH A BLEEDING DISORDER

During the first and second trimesters, the major cause of bleeding is abortion. **Abortion** is the expulsion of the fetus prior to viability, which is considered to be 20 weeks' gestation or weight of less than 500 g. Definitions vary somewhat according to state reporting laws (Cunningham, Leveno, Bloom, et al., 2010). Abortions are either *spontaneous* (occurring naturally) or *induced* (occurring as a result of medical or surgical means). Because the term *abortion* may have a negative connotation, spontaneous abortion is often called **miscarriage**.

Other complications that can cause bleeding in the first half of pregnancy are ectopic pregnancy and gestational trophoblastic disease. In the second half of pregnancy, particularly in the third trimester, the two major causes of bleeding are placenta previa and abruptio placentae. (See Chapter 21 for more information ∞.) Regardless of the cause of bleeding, however, the nurse has certain general responsibilities in providing nursing care.

GENERAL PRINCIPLES OF NURSING INTERVENTION

Spotting is relatively common during pregnancy and usually occurs following sexual intercourse or exercise because of trauma to the highly vascular cervix. However, the woman is advised to report any spotting or bleeding that occurs during pregnancy so that it can be evaluated.

It is often the nurse's responsibility to make the initial assessment of bleeding. In general, the following nursing measures are indicated:

- Monitor blood pressure and pulse frequently.
- Observe the woman for behaviors indicative of shock, such as pallor, clammy skin, perspiration, dyspnea, or restlessness.
- Count and weigh pads to assess amount of bleeding over a given time period; save any tissue or clots expelled.
- If pregnancy is of 12 weeks' gestation or beyond, assess fetal heart tones with a Doppler.
- Prepare for intravenous (IV) therapy. There may be standing orders to begin IV therapy on clients who are bleeding.
- Prepare equipment for examination and have oxygen available.
- Collect and organize all data, including antepartal history, onset of bleeding episode, and laboratory studies (hemoglobin, hematocrit, Rh status, hormonal assays) for analysis.
- Notify other members of the healthcare team, including the physician or nurse-midwife and operating room staff if a surgical procedure is planned, and so forth.
- Obtain an order to type and crossmatch for blood if evidence of significant blood loss exists.
- Assess coping mechanisms of the woman in crisis. Give emotional support to enhance her coping abilities by continuous, sustained presence; by clear explanation of procedures; and by communicating her status to her family. Prepare the woman for possible fetal loss. Assess her expressions of anger, denial, silence, guilt, depression, or self-blame.
- Assess the family's response to the situation.

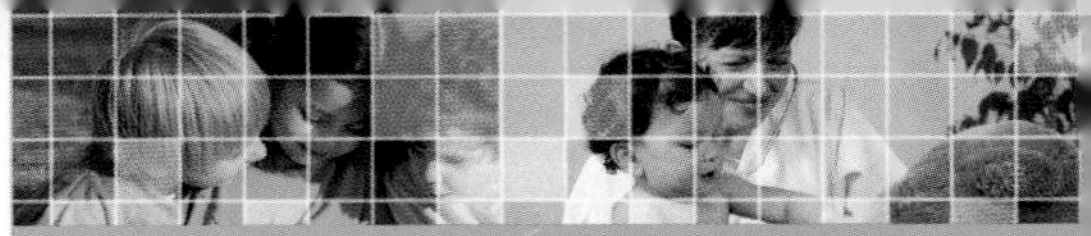

KEY TERMS

Abortion, 331
Eclampsia, 338
Ectopic pregnancy (EP), 334
Erythroblastosis fetalis, 349
Gestational trophoblastic disease (GTD), 335
HELLP syndrome, 339
Hydatidiform mole, 335
Hydrops fetalis, 349
Hyperemesis gravidarum, 337
Incompetent cervix, 337
Miscarriage, 331
Preeclampsia, 338
Rh immune globulin (RhoGAM), 349

SPONTANEOUS ABORTION (MISCARRIAGE)

The incidence of first-trimester spontaneous abortion is about 10% to 15% for clinically recognized pregnancies; however, maternal age influences this significantly. A 40-year-old woman has twice the risk of a 20-year old (Simpson & Jauniaux, 2007).

A majority of early miscarriages are related to chromosomal abnormalities. Other causes include teratogenic drugs, faulty implantation caused by abnormalities of the female reproductive tract, a weakened cervix, placental abnormalities, chronic maternal diseases, endocrine imbalances, and maternal infections. Women who use hot tubs or jacuzzis are twice as likely to have miscarriages as nonusers, probably because of the hyperthermia resulting from increased core body temperature (Li, Janevic, Odouli, et al., 2003).

Classification

Spontaneous abortions are subdivided into the following categories:

- *Threatened abortion* (Figure 16–1 ●). The embryo or fetus is jeopardized by unexplained bleeding, cramping, and backache. The cervix is closed. Bleeding may persist for days. It may be followed by partial or complete expulsion of the embryo or fetus, placenta, and membranes (sometimes called the "products of conception").
- *Imminent abortion* (Figure 16–1B). Bleeding and cramping increase. The internal cervical os dilates. Membranes may rupture. The term *inevitable abortion* also applies.
- *Complete abortion.* All the products of conception are expelled.
- *Incomplete abortion* (Figure 16–1C). Some of the products of conception are retained, most often the placenta. The internal cervical os is dilated slightly.
- *Missed abortion.* The fetus dies in utero but is not expelled. Uterine growth ceases, breast changes regress, and the woman may report a brownish vaginal discharge. The cervix is closed. If the fetus is retained beyond 6 weeks, the breakdown of fetal tissues results in the release of thromboplastin, and disseminated intravascular coagulation (DIC) may develop.
- *Recurrent (habitual) abortion.* Abortion occurs consecutively in three or more pregnancies.
- *Septic abortion.* Infection is present. It may occur with prolonged, unrecognized rupture of the membranes, pregnancy with an intrauterine device (IUD) in place, or attempts by unqualified individuals to end a pregnancy.

Clinical Therapy

Pelvic cramping and backache are reliable indicators of potential spontaneous abortion. These symptoms are usually absent in bleeding caused by polyps, ruptured cervical blood vessels, or cervical erosion.

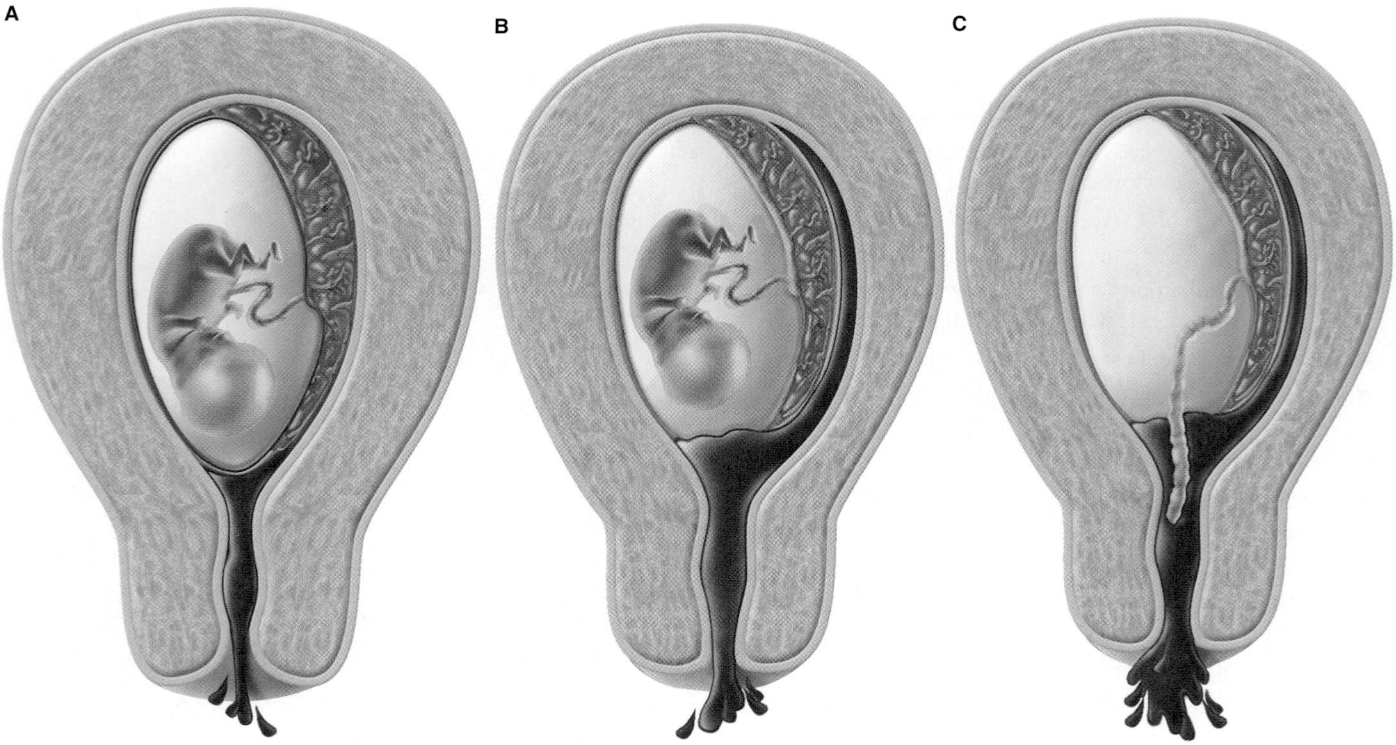

● **Figure 16–1** Types of spontaneous abortion. ***A,*** Threatened. The cervix is not dilated, and the placenta is still attached to the uterine wall, but some bleeding occurs. ***B,*** Imminent. The placenta has separated from the uterine wall, the cervix has dilated, and the amount of bleeding has increased. ***C,*** Incomplete. The embryo or fetus has passed out of the uterus, but the placenta remains.

Speculum examination is done to determine the presence of cervical polyps or cervical erosion. Ultrasound scanning may detect the presence of cardiac activity and a gestational sac, or may reveal a crown-rump length that is small for gestational age. Laboratory determination of hCG level can confirm a pregnancy, but because the hCG level falls slowly after fetal death, it cannot confirm a live embryo/fetus. Serial hCG levels may be indicated to confirm a diagnosis. Hemoglobin and hematocrit levels are obtained to assess blood loss. Blood is typed and cross-matched for possible replacement needs.

The therapy prescribed for the pregnant woman with bleeding is bed rest, abstinence from coitus, and emotional support. If bleeding persists and abortion is imminent or incomplete, the woman may be hospitalized, IV therapy or blood transfusions may be started to replace fluid, and dilation and curettage (D&C) or suction evacuation is performed to remove the remainder of the products of conception. If the woman is Rh negative and not sensitized, Rh immune globulin (RhoGAM) is given within 72 hours (see discussion on Rh alloimmunization beginning on page 348 in this chapter).

In missed abortions, the products of conception usually are expelled spontaneously. Diagnosis is based on history, pelvic examination, and a negative pregnancy test and may be confirmed by ultrasound if necessary. If this does not occur within 4 to 6 weeks after embryo or fetal death, hospitalization is necessary. If in the first trimester, D&C or suction evacuation is done. In the second trimester, labor is induced or dilation and evacuation (D&E) may be used.

Developing Cultural Competence

INDIVIDUAL RESPONSES TO FETAL LOSS

Remember that individual responses to fetal loss following miscarriage may vary greatly and may be influenced by ethnic or cultural norms.

- Miscarriage may be viewed in many ways. For example, it may be seen as a punishment from God, as the result of the evil eye or of a hex or curse by an enemy, or as a natural part of life.
- When grieving over a pregnancy loss, women from some cultures and ethnic groups may show their emotions freely, crying and wailing, whereas other women may hide their feelings behind a mask of stoicism.
- In some cultures the woman's partner is her primary source of support and comfort. In others, the woman turns to her mother or close female relatives for comfort.
- Avoid falling into the trap of stereotyping women according to culture. Individual responses are influenced by many factors, including the degree of assimilation into the dominant culture.

NURSING MANAGEMENT

NURSING ASSESSMENT AND DIAGNOSIS

Assess the woman's vital signs, amount and appearance of any bleeding, level of comfort, and general physical health. The woman's blood type and antibody status should be identified to determine the need for Rh immune globulin (see page 349). If the pregnancy is 10 to 12 weeks or more, determine fetal heart rates with a Doppler. It is also important to assess the responses of the woman and her family to this crisis, their coping mechanisms, and their ability to comfort each other.

Examples of nursing diagnoses that may apply include the following:

- *Acute Pain* related to abdominal cramping secondary to threatened abortion
- *Anticipatory Grieving* related to expected loss of unborn child

PLANNING AND IMPLEMENTATION

NURSING CARE IN THE COMMUNITY

If a woman in her first trimester of pregnancy begins cramping or spotting, she is often evaluated on an outpatient basis. Provide analgesics for pain relief if the woman's cramps are severe, and explain what is occurring throughout the process.

Feelings of shock or disbelief are normal. Couples who approached the pregnancy with joy and excitement now feel grief, sadness, and possibly anger. Because many women, even with planned pregnancies, feel some ambivalence initially, guilt is also a common emotion. These feelings may be even stronger for women who were negative about their pregnancies. The women may even believe that the miscarriage is a punishment for some wrongdoing.

Offer psychologic support to the woman and her family by encouraging them to talk about their feelings, allowing them the privacy to grieve, and listening sympathetically to their concerns about this pregnancy and future ones. To help decrease feelings of guilt or blame, inform the woman and her family about the causes of miscarriage. If the woman has older children, she may need guidance in how to help them understand and cope with what has occurred. Refer them to other healthcare professionals for additional help as necessary.

The grieving period following a miscarriage usually lasts 6 to 24 months. Many couples can be helped during this period by an organization or support group established for parents who have lost a fetus or newborn.

HOSPITAL-BASED NURSING CARE

A woman with an incomplete or missed abortion may need a D&C or other procedure, which is typically done on an outpatient basis. Barring any complications, the woman can return home a few hours after the procedure. Monitor the woman's condition closely and provide instruction for self-care. Administer Rh immune globulin if it is indicated. During discharge teaching, advise the woman to report heavy or bright red vaginal bleeding, to take the full course of antibiotics if they are prescribed, and to delay pregnancy for at least 2 months to allow sufficient time for healing.

EVALUATION

Expected outcomes of nursing care include the following:

- The woman is able to explain spontaneous abortion, the treatment measures employed in her care, and long-term implications for future pregnancies.
- The woman suffers no complications.
- The woman and her partner begin verbalizing their grief and acknowledge that the grieving process lasts several months.

ECTOPIC PREGNANCY

Ectopic pregnancy (EP) is the implantation of the fertilized ovum in a site other than the endometrial lining of the uterus. It has many causes, including tubal damage from pelvic inflammatory disease (PID), previous tubal surgery, congenital anomalies of the tube, endometriosis, previous EP, presence of an IUD, and in utero exposure to diethylstilbestrol (DES).

The exact incidence of EP in the United States is unknown although it seems to be increasing. This increase is related to better diagnostic measures, an increase in the associated risk factors, and the increased use of assisted reproductive technology, which carries a 5% risk of EP (Seeber & Barnhart, 2008). Although the incidence has increased, mortality rates have declined almost 90% as a result of better diagnostic techniques that allow detection before tubal rupture.

EP occurs when the fertilized ovum is prevented or slowed in its passage through the tube and thus implants before it reaches the uterus, usually in the ampulla of the fallopian tube. "Pathophysiology Illustrated: Ectopic Pregnancy" identifies other implantation sites.

Initially symptoms of pregnancy may be present, including amenorrhea, breast tenderness, and nausea. The hormone hCG is present in the blood and urine. As the pregnancy progresses, the chorionic villi grow into the tube wall or implantation site and establish a blood supply. When the embryo outgrows this space, the tube ruptures and there is bleeding into the abdominal cavity. This bleeding irritates the peritoneum, causing the characteristic symptoms of sharp, one-sided pain, syncope, and referred shoulder pain. The woman may also have lower abdominal pain. Vaginal bleeding occurs when the embryo dies and the decidua sloughs.

Physical examination usually reveals adnexal (area over each ovary and fallopian tube) tenderness. An adnexal mass is palpable about half the time. Bleeding tends to be slow and chronic, and the abdomen gradually becomes rigid and very tender. With bleeding into the abdominal cavity, pelvic examination is very painful, and a mass of blood may be palpated in the lower abdomen. Laboratory tests may reveal low hemoglobin and hematocrit levels and rising leukocyte levels.

Clinical Therapy

Diagnosis of EP begins with an assessment of menstrual history, including the date of the last menstrual period, followed by a pelvic examination to identify any pelvic masses and tenderness. A serum progesterone level is drawn. A viable intrauterine pregnancy can be diagnosed with 97.5% sensitivity if the progesterone level is 25 ng/mL or higher, whereas a serum progesterone

PATHOPHYSIOLOGY ILLUSTRATED

ECTOPIC PREGNANCY

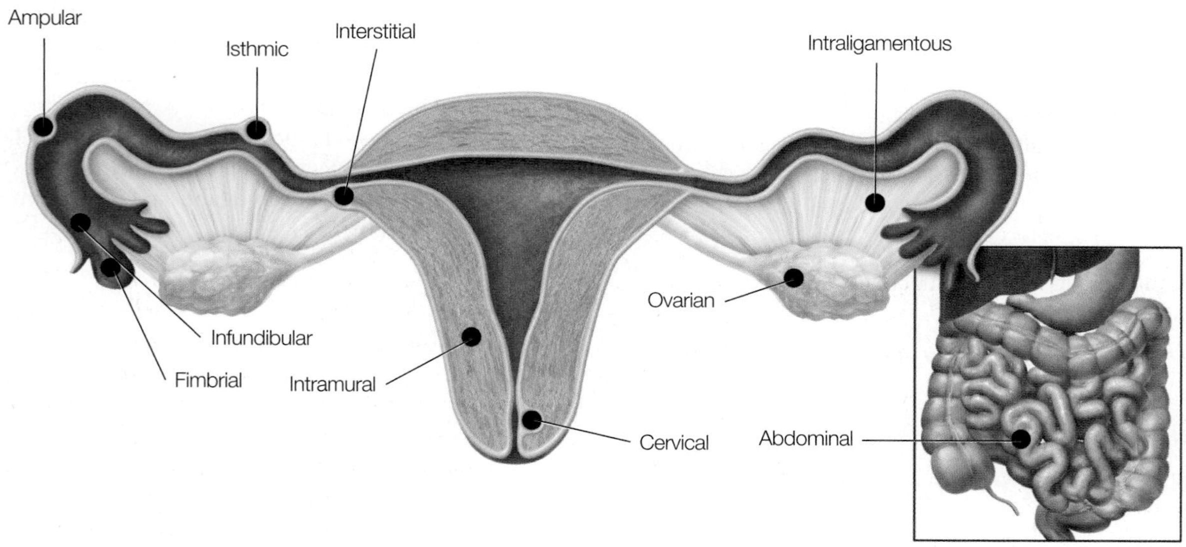

Various implantation sites in ectopic pregnancy. The most common site is within the fallopian tube, hence the name "tubal pregnancy."

lower than 5 ng/mL indicates a dead fetus or an ectopic pregnancy. Levels from 5 to 25 ng/mL are inconclusive (Cunningham, et al., 2010).

Serum β-hCG levels are drawn and reassessed in 48 hours if necessary. A woman with EP tends to have abnormally low hCG levels. In a normal pregnancy, hCG levels double every 48 to 72 hours. Nondoubling hCG levels occur in EP and in nonviable uterine pregnancies. If the β-hCG levels are above 1500 milli-international units/mm, transvaginal ultrasound is used to check for a uterine pregnancy or an adnexal mass. Confirming a uterine pregnancy nearly eliminates the diagnosis of EP.

Treatment may be medical or surgical. Methotrexate is used for the woman who desires future pregnancy, if her ectopic pregnancy is unruptured and of 4 cm size or less, and if her condition is stable. In addition, there must be no fetal heart motion and the woman must have no evidence of a blood disorder or kidney or liver disease. Methotrexate, a folic acid antagonist that interferes with DNA synthesis and cell multiplication, is given intramuscularly (IM). Although a single-dose approach requires fewer visits, a two-dose protocol has become increasingly popular because it has a lower failure rate. With the two-dose approach a second injection is given on day 4. A third dose can be given on day 7 if there has not been an appropriate drop in human chorionic gonadotropin (hCG) (Seeber & Barnhart, 2008). As an outpatient, the woman is monitored for increasing abdominal pain. β-hCG titers are monitored regularly. β-hCG titers typically increase for 1 to 4 days and then decrease (Lipscomb, Givens, Meyer, et al., 2005).

If surgery is indicated and the woman desires future pregnancies, treatment involves salpingostomy via a laparoscope. With this method an incision is made lengthwise in the fallopian tube and the products of conception are gently removed. The surgical incision is left open and allowed to close naturally. If the tube is ruptured or if future childbearing is not an issue, laparoscopic salpingectomy (removal of the tube) is performed, leaving the ovary in place unless it is damaged. With both medical and surgical therapies for EP, the Rh-negative nonsensitized woman is given Rh immune globulin to prevent sensitization.

NURSING MANAGEMENT

NURSING ASSESSMENT AND DIAGNOSIS

When the woman with a suspected ectopic pregnancy is admitted to the hospital, assess the appearance and amount of vaginal bleeding and monitor vital signs for developing shock. Assess the woman's emotional state and coping abilities, and determine the couple's informational needs. Determine the woman's level of pain, which can be significant. If surgery is necessary, complete the appropriate ongoing assessments postoperatively.

Nursing diagnoses that may apply for a woman with EP include the following:

- *Acute Pain* related to abdominal bleeding secondary to tubal rupture
- *Anticipatory Grieving* related to expected pregnancy loss
- *Health-Seeking Behaviors: Request for Information about Treatment of Ectopic Pregnancy and its Long-Term Implications* related to stated unfamiliarity with the condition

PLANNING AND IMPLEMENTATION

NURSING CARE IN THE COMMUNITY

Women with EP are often seen initially in a clinic or office setting. Be alert to the possibility of EP if a woman presents with complaints of abdominal pain and lack of menses for 1 to 2 months. A woman receiving medical treatment using methotrexate is followed as an outpatient. Advise the woman that some abdominal pain is common following the injection, but generally it is mild and lasts only 24 to 48 hours. More severe pain might indicate treatment failure and should be evaluated. The woman should also report heavy vaginal bleeding, dizziness, or tachycardia. Stress the need to return for follow-up β-hCG testing.

HOSPITAL-BASED NURSING CARE

Once a diagnosis of EP is made and surgery is scheduled, start an IV as ordered and begin preoperative teaching. Immediately report signs of developing shock. If the woman experiences severe abdominal pain, administer analgesics and evaluate their effectiveness.

Regardless of the treatment used, the woman and her family will need emotional support during this difficult time. Their feelings and responses to this crisis are generally similar to those that occur in cases of spontaneous abortion; similar nursing actions are required.

EVALUATION

Expected outcomes of nursing care include the following:

- The woman is able to explain ectopic pregnancy, treatment alternatives, and implications for future childbearing.
- The woman and her caregivers detect possible complications early and manage them successfully.
- The woman and her partner are able to begin verbalizing their loss.

GESTATIONAL TROPHOBLASTIC DISEASE

Gestational trophoblastic disease (GTD) is the pathologic proliferation of trophoblastic cells (the trophoblast is the outermost layer of embryonic cells). In the United States the incidence is approximately 1 per 1500 live births (Copeland & Landon, 2007). It includes hydatidiform mole, invasive mole (chorioadenoma destruens), and choriocarcinoma, a form of cancer.

Hydatidiform mole (molar pregnancy) is a disease in which (1) abnormal development of the placenta occurs, resulting in hydropic vesicles (a fluid-filled, grapelike cluster); and (2) the trophoblastic tissue proliferates. The disease results in the loss of the pregnancy and the possibility, though remote, of developing choriocarcinoma, a form of cancer, from the trophoblastic tissue.

Molar pregnancies are classified into two types, complete and partial, both of which meet the previously mentioned criteria. A *complete mole* develops from an ovum containing no maternal genetic material, an "empty egg," which is fertilized by a normal sperm. The embryo dies very early, no circulation is established, the hydropic vesicles are avascular, and no embryonic tissue is found. Choriocarcinoma seems to be associated exclusively with the complete mole.

The *partial mole* usually has a triploid karyotype (69 chromosomes). Most often a normal ovum with 23 chromosomes is fertilized by two sperm (dispermy) or by a sperm that has failed to undergo the first meiotic division and therefore contains 46 chromosomes. There may be a fetal sac or even a fetus with a heartbeat. The fetus has multiple anomalies and little chance for survival. Often partial moles are recognized only after miscarriage, and they may go unnoticed even then.

Invasive mole (chorioadenoma destruens) is similar to a complete mole, but it involves the uterine myometrium. Treatment is the same as for complete mole.

Clinical Therapy

Initially the clinical picture is similar to that of pregnancy. However, classic signs soon appear. Vaginal bleeding occurs almost universally. It is often brownish because of liquefaction of the uterine clot, but it may be bright red. Uterine enlargement greater than expected for gestational age is a classic sign of a complete mole, present in about 1/3 to 1/2 of cases (Li, 2008). In the remainder of cases, the uterus is appropriate or small for the gestational age. If hydropic vesicles are passed, they are diagnostic (Figure 16–2 ●). With a partial mole, the vesicles are often smaller and may not be noticed. Because serum hCG levels are higher with molar pregnancy than with normal pregnancy, the woman may experience hyperemesis gravidarum. Anemia occurs frequently as a result of blood loss and poor nutrition secondary to hyperemesis. Symptoms of preeclampsia prior to 24 weeks' gestation strongly suggest a molar pregnancy. No fetal heart tones are heard, and no fetal movement is palpated. Transvaginal ultrasound is used for diagnosis.

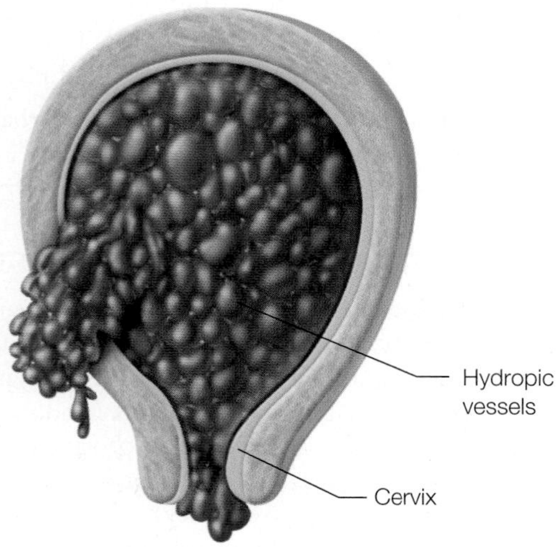

● **Figure 16–2** Hydatidiform mole. A common sign is vaginal bleeding, often brownish (the characteristic "prune juice" appearance) but sometimes bright red. In this figure, some of the hydropic vessels are being passed. This occurrence is diagnostic for hydatidiform mole.

Therapy begins with suction evacuation of the mole and curettage of the uterus to remove all fragments of the placenta. Early evacuation decreases the possibility of other complications. If the woman is older and has completed her childbearing, or if there is excessive bleeding, hysterectomy may be the treatment of choice to reduce the risk of choriocarcinoma.

Because of the risk of choriocarcinoma, the woman treated for hydatidiform mole should receive extensive follow-up therapy. Follow-up care includes a baseline chest x-ray to detect lung metastasis and a physical examination including a pelvic examination. Serum β-hCG levels are monitored every 1 to 2 weeks until negative results are obtained two consecutive times, then every 1 to 2 months for a year. Periodic pelvic exams are also indicated. The woman should avoid pregnancy during that time because the elevated hCG levels associated with pregnancy would cause confusion as to whether cancer had developed.

If hCG levels plateau for 3 to 6 consecutive weeks, or rise more than 50%, evaluation for metastatic disease should be undertaken and prompt chemotherapy initiated (Berman, Di Saia, & Tewari, 2004). Treatment at a center specializing in GTD is advised. Chemotherapy generally involves using methotrexate alone or with other chemotherapy agents. If, after a year of monitoring, the hCG serum titers are within normal limits, a couple may be assured that a normal pregnancy can be anticipated, with a low risk of recurring hydatidiform mole.

NURSING MANAGEMENT

NURSING ASSESSMENT AND DIAGNOSIS

Observe for symptoms of hydatidiform mole at each antepartal visit. The classic symptoms are found more frequently with the complete mole. Before evacuation the partial mole may be difficult to distinguish from a missed abortion. If a molar pregnancy is diagnosed, assess the woman's (or the couple's) understanding of the condition and its implications.

Nursing diagnoses that may apply include the following:

- *Fear* related to the possible development of choriocarcinoma
- *Anticipatory Grieving* related to the loss of the pregnancy secondary to GTD

PLANNING AND IMPLEMENTATION

NURSING CARE IN THE COMMUNITY

When a molar pregnancy is suspected, the woman needs emotional support. Answer questions about the condition and explain what ultrasound and other diagnostic procedures will entail. If a molar pregnancy is diagnosed, support the parents as they deal with their grief about the lost pregnancy. Healthcare counselors, a member of the clergy, or a professional counselor may also be of help.

HOSPITAL-BASED NURSING CARE

When the woman is hospitalized for removal of the mole, monitor vital signs and vaginal bleeding for signs of hemorrhage. Determine the presence of abdominal pain and evaluate the woman's emotional state and coping ability. Have typed and crossmatched blood available for surgery. Administer oxytocin as ordered to keep the uterus contracted and to prevent hemorrhage. If the woman is Rh negative and not sensitized, give Rh immune globulin to prevent antibody formation.

Stress the importance of follow-up visits. Advise the woman to delay another pregnancy until the follow-up program is completed.

EVALUATION

Expected outcomes of nursing care include the following:

- The woman has a smooth recovery following successful evacuation of the mole.
- The woman is able to explain GTD and its treatment, follow-up, and long-term implications for pregnancy.
- The woman and her partner are able to begin talking about their grief at the loss of their anticipated child.
- The woman can discuss the importance of follow-up care and indicates her willingness to cooperate with the regimen.

CARE OF THE WOMAN WITH AN INCOMPETENT CERVIX

Incompetent cervix refers to the premature dilatation of the cervix, usually in the fourth or fifth month of pregnancy. It is associated with repeated second-trimester abortions. Possible causes include cervical trauma, infection, congenital cervical or uterine anomalies, or increased uterine volume (as with a multiple gestation).

Diagnosis is based on a positive history of repeated, relatively painless and bloodless second-trimester abortions. Serial pelvic examinations early in the second trimester reveal progressive effacement and dilatation of the cervix and bulging of the membranes through the cervical os. If incompetent cervix is suspected, serial ultrasound provides information on dilatation of the internal cervical os before a dilated external os is detected.

Incompetent cervix is managed surgically with a Shirodkar procedure (cerclage)—or a modification of it by McDonald—which reinforces the weakened cervix by encircling it at the level of the internal os with suture material (Figure 16–3 ●). A purse-string suture is placed in the cervix in the first trimester or early in the second trimester. Once the suture is in place, a cesarean birth may be planned (to prevent repeating the procedure in subsequent pregnancies), or the suture may be cut at term and vaginal birth permitted. The effectiveness of cerclage for treating incompetent cervix has not been proven in controlled studies although there is some indication that cerclage plus bed rest is more effective than bed rest alone in decreasing fetal morbidity. Until research indicates otherwise, cerclage will remain the most common treatment for women who experience second trimester dilatation of at least 2 cm with no other emergency causes such as ruptured membranes, infection, or bleeding (Ludmir & Owen, 2007).

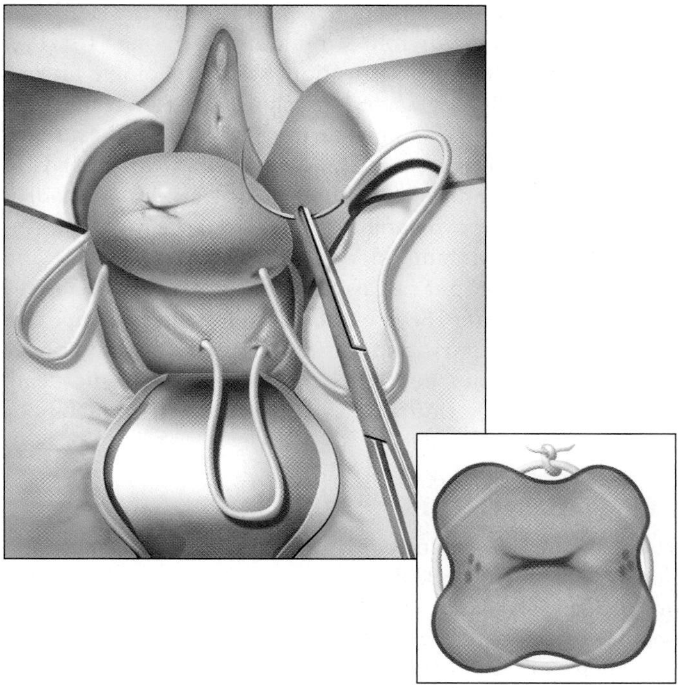

● **Figure 16–3** Management of incompetent cervix. A cerclage, or purse-string suture, is inserted in the cervix to prevent preterm cervical dilatation and pregnancy loss. After placement the string is tightened and secured anteriorly.

The woman must understand the importance of contacting her physician immediately if her membranes rupture or labor begins. The physician can remove the suture to prevent possible complications.

CARE OF THE WOMAN WITH HYPEREMESIS GRAVIDARUM

Hyperemesis gravidarum, which is excessive vomiting during pregnancy, occurs in one-half of 1% of pregnancies (Cappell, 2007). It may be mild at first, but true hyperemesis may progress to a point at which the woman not only vomits everything she swallows but also retches between meals.

Although the exact cause of hyperemesis is unclear, increased levels of hCG may play a role. Women with a history of migraine headaches, motion sickness, sickness related to oral contraceptives, and a family or personal history of hyperemesis are at increased risk. Other variables that may relate to hyperemesis include transient hyperthyroidism caused by the effect of hCG on the thyroid-stimulating hormone (TSH) receptor, *Helicobacter pylori* infection, and psychologic factors, although research suggests that psychologic findings may be a *response* to hyperemesis gravidarum rather than a cause. In severe cases, hyperemesis causes dehydration, which leads to fluid-electrolyte imbalance and alkalosis from loss of hydrochloric acid. Hypovolemia, hypotension, tachycardia, increased hematocrit and blood urea nitrogen (BUN), and decreased urine output can also occur. If untreated, metabolic acidosis may develop. Severe potassium loss may disrupt cardiac functioning. Starvation causes muscle wasting and severe protein and vitamin deficiencies. Fetal or embryonic death may result, and the woman may suffer irreversible metabolic changes or death.

CLINICAL THERAPY

The goals of treatment include control of vomiting and dehydration, restoration of electrolyte balance, and maintenance of adequate nutrition. If the woman does not respond to standard approaches to the control of nausea and vomiting in pregnancy (see Chapter 11 ∞), she may require IV fluids on an outpatient basis. If her symptoms do not improve, hospitalization may be indicated. Initially the woman is given nothing by mouth (NPO), and IV fluids are administered. Potassium chloride is often added to the IV to prevent hypokalemia. Thiamine and pyroxidine (vitamin B_6) may be replaced to correct deficiencies and prevent peripheral neuropathy. Antiemetics may also be administered. Typically the woman remains NPO for 48 hours. If her condition does not improve, total parenteral nutrition may be needed. She then begins controlled oral feedings.

NURSING MANAGEMENT

MyNursingKit Case Study: Client with Preeclampsia

NURSING ASSESSMENT AND DIAGNOSIS

When a woman is hospitalized for control of vomiting, assess the amount and character of any emesis, intake and output, fetal heart rate, signs of jaundice or bleeding, and her emotional state.

Nursing diagnoses that may apply include the following:

- *Imbalanced Nutrition: Less than Body Requirements* related to persistent vomiting secondary to hyperemesis
- *Fear* related to the effects of hyperemesis on fetal well-being

PLANNING AND IMPLEMENTATION

NURSING CARE IN THE COMMUNITY

Parenteral therapy provided at home in collaboration with a physician and a registered dietitian is sometimes used to enable the woman to remain in her home. This therapy also gives an opportunity to observe family interactions and evaluate the home environment. This assessment helps determine the pregnant woman's level of support, any significant stressors in her life, and her understanding of nutrition and self-care measures.

HOSPITAL-BASED NURSING CARE

Nursing care is supportive and directed at maintaining a relaxed, quiet environment away from food odors or offensive smells. Once oral feedings resume, food needs to be attractively served. Oral hygiene is important because the mouth is dry and may be irritated from vomitus. Monitor weight regularly. In some cases emotional factors have appeared to play a role, although that remains controversial. Nevertheless, psychotherapy may sometimes be recommended. With proper treatment, prognosis is favorable.

EVALUATION

Expected outcomes of nursing care include the following:

- The woman is able to explain hyperemesis gravidarum, its therapy, and its possible effects on her pregnancy.
- The woman's condition is corrected and complications are avoided.

CARE OF THE WOMAN WITH A HYPERTENSIVE DISORDER

A number of hypertensive disorders can occur during pregnancy. For clinical purposes, the following classification may be used (Sibai, 2007):

- Preeclampsia/eclampsia
- Chronic hypertension
- Chronic hypertension with superimposed preeclampsia or eclampsia
- Gestational (or transient) hypertension

PREECLAMPSIA AND ECLAMPSIA

Preeclampsia, the most common hypertensive disorder in pregnancy, occurs in 2% to 7% of pregnancies although the incidence is significantly higher (14%) in twin pregnancy (Habli & Sibai, 2008). Preeclampsia is defined as an increase in blood pressure after 20 weeks' gestation accompanied by proteinuria. Previously, edema was included in the definition but was removed because it is such a common finding in pregnancy. However, sudden onset of severe edema warrants close evaluation to rule out preeclampsia or other pathologic processes such as renal disease.

Preeclampsia, typically categorized as mild or severe, is a progressive disorder. In its most severe form, **eclampsia** (generalized seizures or coma), develops. Most often preeclampsia occurs in the last 10 weeks of gestation, during labor, or in the first 48 hours after childbirth. Although birth of the fetus and removal of the placenta is the only known cure for preeclampsia, it can be controlled with early diagnosis and careful management. Preeclampsia is seen more often in teenagers and in women over age 35, especially if they are primigravidas. Women with a history of preeclampsia are at increased risk, as are women with GTD, Rh incompatibility, diabetes, and a large placental mass (as in multiple gestation).

Pathophysiology of Preeclampsia

The cause of preeclampsia/eclampsia remains unknown, despite decades of research. Preeclampsia affects all the major systems of the body. The following pathophysiologic changes are associated with the disease:

- In normal pregnancy the lowered peripheral vascular resistance and the increased maternal resistance to the pressor effects of angiotensin II result in lowered blood pressure. In preeclampsia, blood pressure begins to rise after 20 weeks' gestation, probably in response to a gradual loss of resistance to angiotensin II. This response has been linked to the ratio between the prostaglandins prostacyclin and thromboxane. Prostacyclin is a potent vasodilator. It is decreased in preeclampsia, often several weeks before symptoms develop. This changes the ratio between the two prostaglandins, allowing the potent vasoconstriction and platelet-aggregating effects of thromboxane to dominate. These hormones are produced partially by the placenta, which helps explain the reversal of the condition when the placenta is removed and why the incidence is increased when there is a larger than normal placental mass.
- Nitric oxide, a potent vasodilator, plays a role in the pregnant woman's resistance to vasopressors. Decreased nitric oxide production in women with preeclampsia may contribute to the development of hypertension.
- The loss of normal vasodilation of uterine arterioles and the concurrent maternal vasospasm result in decreased placental perfusion (see "Pathophysiology Illustrated: Preeclampsia" on page 340). The effect on the fetus may be growth restriction, decrease in fetal movement, and chronic hypoxia or fetal distress.
- In preeclampsia, normal renal perfusion is decreased. With a reduction of the glomerular filtration rate, serum levels of creatinine, BUN, and uric acid begin to rise from normal pregnant levels, while urine output decreases. Sodium is retained in increased amounts, which results in increased extracellular volume, increased sensitivity to angiotensin II, and edema. Stretching of the capillary walls of the glomerular endothelial cells allows the large protein molecules, primarily albumin, to escape in the urine, decreasing serum albumin levels. The decreased serum albumin concentration causes decreased plasma colloid osmotic pressure. This lowered pressure results in a further movement of fluid to the extracellular spaces, which also contributes to the development of edema.
- The decreased intravascular volume causes increased viscosity of the blood and a corresponding rise in hematocrit.

HELLP syndrome (**h**emolysis, **e**levated **l**iver enzymes, and **l**ow **p**latelet count) is sometimes associated with severe preeclampsia. Women who experience this multiple-organ-failure syndrome have high morbidity and mortality rates, as do their offspring.

The hemolysis that occurs is termed *microangiopathic hemolytic anemia.* It is thought that red blood cells are fragmented during passage through small, damaged blood vessels. Elevated liver enzymes occur from blood flow that is obstructed by fibrin deposits. Hyperbilirubinemia and jaundice may also be seen. Liver distention causes epigastric pain. Thrombocytopenia (platelet count less than 100,000/mm^3) is a frequent finding in preeclampsia. It occurs when platelets aggregate at the sites of vascular damage associated with vasospasm. Symptoms may include nausea, vomiting, flulike symptoms, or epigastric pain. HELLP syndrome is sometimes complicated by disseminated intravascular coagulation (DIC).

The mother's condition should be assessed and stabilized, especially if her platelet counts are very low. Platelet transfusions are indicated for platelet counts below 20,000/mm^3. The fetus is also assessed, using a nonstress test and biophysical profile. Once HELLP syndrome is diagnosed and the woman's condition is stable, birth of the child is indicated.

Maternal Risks

Central nervous system changes associated with preeclampsia/eclampsia are hyperreflexia, headache, and seizures. Hyperreflexia may be a result of increased intracellular sodium and decreased intracellular potassium levels. Cerebral vasospasm causes headaches, and cerebral edema and vasoconstriction are responsible for seizures. There is also increased risk for thrombocytopenia, renal failure, abruptio placentae, DIC, ruptured liver, and pulmonary embolism.

Fetal-Neonatal Risks

Infants of women with preeclampsia tend to be small for gestational age (SGA). The cause is related specifically to maternal vasospasm and hypovolemia, which result in fetal hypoxia and malnutrition. In addition, the newborn may be premature because of the necessity for early birth. At birth, the newborn may be oversedated because of medications given to the mother. The newborn may also have hypermagnesemia resulting from treatment of the woman with large doses of magnesium sulfate.

Clinical Therapy

The goals of medical management include prompt diagnosis of the disease; prevention of cerebral hemorrhage, seizures, hematologic complications, and renal and hepatic diseases; and birth of an uncompromised newborn as close to term as possible. Reduction of elevated blood pressure is essential in accomplishing these goals.

Clinical Manifestations and Diagnosis

Mild Preeclampsia Women with mild preeclampsia may exhibit few, if any, symptoms. The blood pressure is elevated to 140/90 mm Hg or higher, 1+ proteinuria may occur, and liver

Evidence in Action

Even though the specific mechanisms are unknown, there is continued evidence that women with a history of preeclampsia/eclampsia have an increased risk of early cardiac, cerebrovascular and peripheral arterial disease and cardiovascular mortality (systematic review and meta-analyses) (McDonald, Malinowski, Zhou, et al., 2008).

PATHOPHYSIOLOGY ILLUSTRATED

PREECLAMPSIA

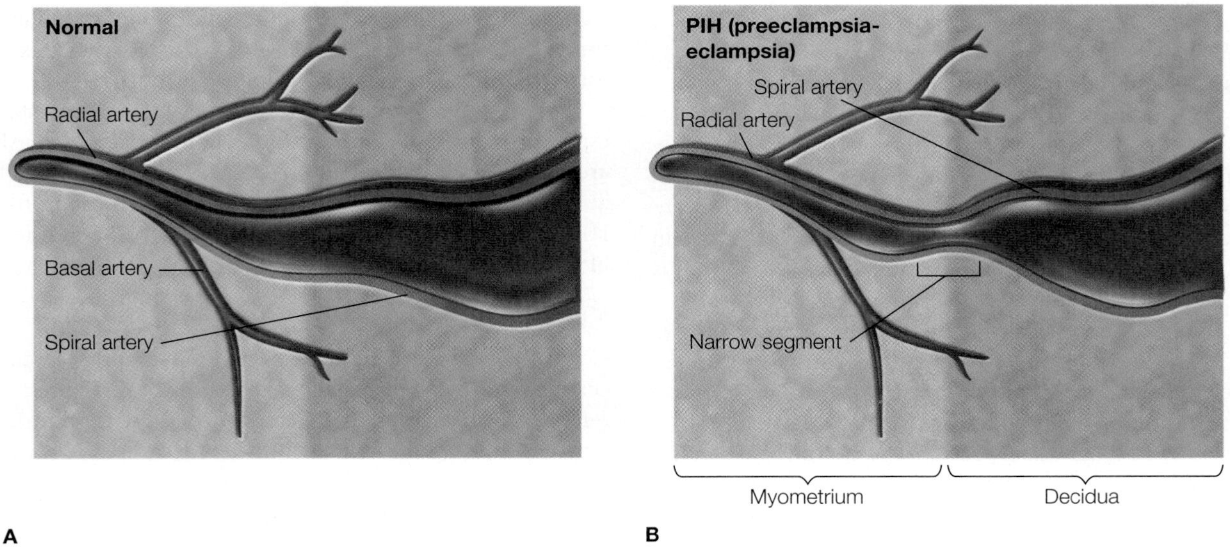

A, In a normal pregnancy, the passive quality of the spiral arteries permits increased blood flow to the placenta.
B, In preeclampsia, vasoconstriction of the myometrial segment of the spiral arteries occurs.

enzymes may be elevated minimally. Although no longer considered a diagnostic sign of preeclampsia, edema may be present.

Severe Preeclampsia Severe preeclampsia may develop suddenly. Blood pressure is 160/110 mm Hg or higher on two occasions at least 6 hours apart while the woman is on bed rest. Proteinuria of 5 g or higher is found in a 24-hour urine collection while a dipstick urine protein measurement is 3+ to 4+ on two random samples obtained at least 4 hours apart. Other characteristic symptoms include visual or cerebral disturbances (frontal headaches, blurred vision, scotomata [spots before the eyes]), cyanosis or pulmonary edema, epigastric or right upper quadrant pain, impaired liver function, thrombocytopenia or evidence of hemolysis or both, and intrauterine fetal growth restriction. Other signs or symptoms may include nausea, vomiting, irritability, hyperreflexia, and retinal edema (retinas appear wet and glistening), with narrowed segments on the retinal arterioles when examined with an ophthalmoscope. Epigastric pain is often the sign of impending convulsion and is thought to be caused by increased vascular engorgement of the liver.

Eclampsia Eclampsia, characterized by a grand mal convulsion, may occur before labor, during labor, or early in the postpartal period. Some women experience only one seizure; others have several.

Antepartal management. The clinical therapy for preeclampsia depends on the severity of the disease.

Home Care of Mild Preeclampsia For some women with mild preeclampsia, home care is an option. The woman monitors her blood pressure, weight, and urine protein daily. Weight gains of 1.4 kg (3 lb) in 24 hours or 1.8 kg (4 lb) in a 3-day period are generally a cause for concern. Remote nonstress tests (NSTs) are performed on a daily to biweekly basis. Nursing contact varies from daily to weekly, depending on physician request. It is extremely important to advise the woman to report to the doctor if she develops signs of worsening preeclampsia.

Hospital Care of Mild Preeclampsia The woman is placed on bed rest, primarily on her left side, to decrease pressure on the vena cava, thereby increasing venous return, circulatory volume, and placental and renal perfusion. She is weighed daily and evaluated for worsening edema, persistent headache, visual changes, or epigastric pain. Urine dipstick is done daily to assess for protein; blood pressure is checked at least 4 times per day. The woman's diet should be well balanced and moderate to high in protein (80 to 100 g/day, or 1.5 g/kg/day) to replace protein lost in the urine. Sodium intake should be moderate, not to exceed 6 g/day. Excessively salty foods should be avoided, but sodium restriction and diuretics are no longer used in treating preeclampsia.

To achieve a safe outcome for the fetus, tests to evaluate fetal status are done more frequently as preeclampsia progresses. The following tests are used:

- Fetal movement record
- Nonstress test
- Ultrasonography every 3 or 4 weeks for serial determination of growth
- Biophysical profile

Evidence-Based Nursing

ANTIOXIDANT THERAPY AND PREECLAMPSIA PREVENTION

Clinical Question

Is antioxidant therapy effective in preventing preeclampsia?

The Evidence

A possible contributing factor to the development of preeclampsia may be the presence of excessive amounts of free radicals, creating oxidative stress. It has been hypothesized that treating this stress with antioxidants (vitamins C and E, selenium, or lycopene) can neutralize the free radicals and prevent the effects of preeclampsia. Four health research specialists conducted a systematic review of the literature to determine if antioxidants were effective in preventing preeclampsia. They reviewed 10 trials involving 6533 mothers; the majority of the trials tested Vitamins C and E. Systematic reviews of multisite trials involving large samples provides the strongest level of evidence for practice.

Best Practice

Current evidence does not support the use of antioxidants to reduce the risk of preeclampsia or other complications of pregnancy. There was no significant difference in the rate of preeclampsia between groups of mothers receiving antioxidant therapy and mothers receiving a placebo. No differences were seen in the rate of preterm birth, small for gestational age infant, or neonatal death. Women who received antioxidants actually fared worse on some key measures. Women who received the antioxidants prenatally had more frequent complaints of abdominal pain and required more treatment for hypertension than did women who received a placebo, including a higher rate of antenatal hospital admission. There is limited evidence about the safety of giving antioxidants to women during pregnancy, although high doses of Vitamin E have demonstrated harmful effects in nonpregnant adults (Rumbold, Duley, Crowther, & Haslam, 2008).

Critical Thinking

Should nurses advise healthy mothers to avoid antioxidants during the prenatal period? What are the long-term effects of antioxidant therapy during the prenatal period?

See MyNursingKit for possible responses.

- Amniocentesis to determine fetal lung maturity
- Doppler velocimetry beginning at 30 to 32 weeks to screen for fetal compromise

Severe Preeclampsia In severe cases, birth may be the treatment of choice for both mother and fetus, even if the fetus is immature. Other medical therapies for severe preeclampsia include the following:

- *Bed rest.* Bed rest must be complete. Stimuli that may bring on a seizure should be reduced.
- *Diet.* A high-protein, moderate-sodium diet is given as long as the woman is alert and has no nausea or indication of impending seizure.
- *Anticonvulsants.* Magnesium sulfate is the treatment of choice for convulsions. Its depressant action on the central nervous system reduces the possibility of seizure (see "Drug Guide: Magnesium Sulfate" in Chapter 21).
- *Fluid and electrolyte replacement.* The goal of fluid intake is to achieve a balance between correcting hypovolemia and preventing circulatory overload. Fluid intake may be oral or supplemented with IV therapy. IV fluids may be started "to keep lines open" in case they are needed for drug therapy even when oral intake is adequate. Electrolytes are replaced as indicated by daily serum electrolyte levels.
- *Corticosteroids.* Betamethasone or dexamethasone is often administered to the woman whose fetus has an immature lung profile. Corticosteroids may also have a beneficial effect in women with HELLP syndrome.
- *Antihypertensives.* Antihypertensive medications are the most commonly used methods of treatment. Antihypertensive therapy is generally given for sustained systolic blood pressure of at least 160 to 180 mm Hg or diastolic blood pressures of 105 to 110 mm Hg or higher. Hydralazine (Apresoline) is the medication most commonly used. Methyldopa is often used for long-term control of mild to moderate hypertension in pregnancy because it is safe and effective. Research trials indicate that either intravenous labetalol or oral nifedipine is as effective as IV hydralazine and both have fewer side effects (Sibai, 2007). Labetalol should be avoided, however, in women with asthma or congestive heart failure (Habli & Sibai, 2008).

Eclampsia An eclamptic seizure requires immediate, effective treatment. A bolus of 4 to 6 g magnesium sulfate is given IV over 5 minutes to control convulsions. Antihypertensive agents are used to keep the diastolic blood pressure between 90 mm and 100 mm Hg, thus avoiding a potential reduction in uteroplacental blood flow or cerebral perfusion. A sedative such as diazepam or amobarbital is used only if the seizures are not controlled by magnesium sulfate. Phenytoin (Dilantin) may be used for seizure prevention. The lungs are auscultated for pulmonary edema. The woman is observed for circulatory and renal failure and signs of cerebral hemorrhage. Furosemide (Lasix) may be given for pulmonary edema; digitalis may be given for circulatory failure. Intake and output are monitored hourly.

The woman is assessed for signs of labor. She is also checked every 15 minutes for evidence of vaginal bleeding and abdominal rigidity, which might indicate abruptio placentae. While she is comatose, she is positioned on her side with the side rails up.

Because of the severity of her condition, the woman is often cared for in an intensive care unit. Invasive hemodynamic monitoring of either central venous pressure or pulmonary artery wedge pressure may be started using a Swan-Ganz catheter. Both of these procedures carry risk to the woman, and the decision to use them should be made judiciously. When the condition of the woman and the fetus are stabilized, induction of labor is considered, because birth is the only known cure for preeclampsia/eclampsia. The woman and her partner should be given a careful explanation about her status and that of her unborn child and the treatment they are receiving. Plans for further treatment and for birth must be discussed with them.

Intrapartal management. Labor may be induced by IV oxytocin when there is evidence of fetal maturity and cervical readiness. In very severe cases, cesarean birth may be necessary even if the fetus is immature.

Assessment for signs of worsening preeclampsia continues. The woman may receive IV oxytocin and magnesium sulfate simultaneously. Infusion pumps should be used, and bags and tubing must be carefully labeled.

Analgesics may be used to decrease discomfort, or the woman may have an epidural block administered by a skilled anesthesiologist who is knowledgeable about preeclampsia. However, spinal or epidural anesthesia is contraindicated in the presence of coagulopathy or a platelet count less than 50,000/mm (Sibai, 2007).

Birth in the Sims' or semisitting position should be considered. If the lithotomy position is used, a wedge should be placed under the right buttock to displace the uterus. The wedge should also be used if birth is by cesarean. Oxygen is administered to the woman during labor if the need is indicated by fetal response to the contractions.

A pediatrician or neonatal nurse practitioner must be available to care for the newborn at birth. This caregiver must be informed of all amounts and times of medication the woman has received during labor.

Postpartal management. The woman with preeclampsia usually improves rapidly after giving birth, although seizures can still occur during the first 48 hours postpartum. When the hypertension is severe, the woman may continue to receive antihypertensives or magnesium sulfate postpartally.

NURSING MANAGEMENT

See "Nursing Care Plan: The Woman with Preeclampsia" for information on nursing care.

NURSING ASSESSMENT AND DIAGNOSIS

Take and record the blood pressure during each antepartal visit. If the blood pressure rises, or if the normal decrease in blood pressure expected between 8 and 28 weeks of pregnancy does not occur, the woman should be followed closely. Also check the woman's urine for proteinuria at each visit.

If hospitalization becomes necessary, assess the following:

- *Blood pressure.* Assess every 1 to 4 hours, or more frequently if indicated by medication or other changes in the woman's status.
- *Temperature.* Take every 4 hours, or every 2 hours if elevated.
- *Pulse and respirations.* Determine pulse rate and respirations along with blood pressure.
- *Fetal heart rate.* Check the fetal heart rate with the blood pressure, or monitor continuously with the electronic fetal monitor if the situation indicates.
- *Urinary output.* Measure every voiding. The woman frequently has an indwelling catheter. In this case, urine output can be assessed hourly. Output should be 700 mL or greater in 24 hours, or at least 30 mL/hr.
- *Urine protein.* Evaluate urinary protein hourly if an indwelling catheter is in place or with each voiding. Readings of 3+ or 4+ indicate loss of 5 g or more of protein in 24 hours.
- *Urine specific gravity.* Check specific gravity of the urine hourly or with each voiding. Readings over 1.040 correlate with oliguria and proteinuria.
- *Weight.* Weigh the woman daily at the same time. She should be wearing the same robe or gown and slippers. Weighing may be omitted if the woman is to maintain strict bed rest.
- *Pulmonary edema.* Observe the woman for coughing. Auscultate the lungs for moist respirations.
- *Deep tendon reflexes.* Assess the woman for evidence of hyperreflexia in the brachial, wrist, patellar, or Achilles' tendons (Table 16–1). The patellar reflex is the easiest to assess. Clonus, an abnormal finding, is assessed by vigorously dorsiflexing the foot while the knee is held in a fixed position (Figure 16–4 ●). Normally, no clonus is present. Clonus is present if the foot "jerks" or taps the examiner's hand, at which time the examiner counts the number of taps or beats and records it as such. See Skill 2–3 in the Clinical Skills Manual SKILLS.
- *Placental separation.* Assess hourly for vaginal bleeding and uterine rigidity.
- *Headache.* Ask about the existence and location of any headache.
- *Visual disturbance.* Ask about any visual blurring or changes or scotomata. The results of the daily funduscopic examination should be recorded on the chart.

Table 16–1 Deep Tendon Reflex Rating Scale

Rating	Assessment
4+	Hyperactive; very brisk, jerky, or clonic response; abnormal
3+	Brisker than average; may not be abnormal
2+	Average response; normal
1+	Diminished response; low normal
0	No response; abnormal

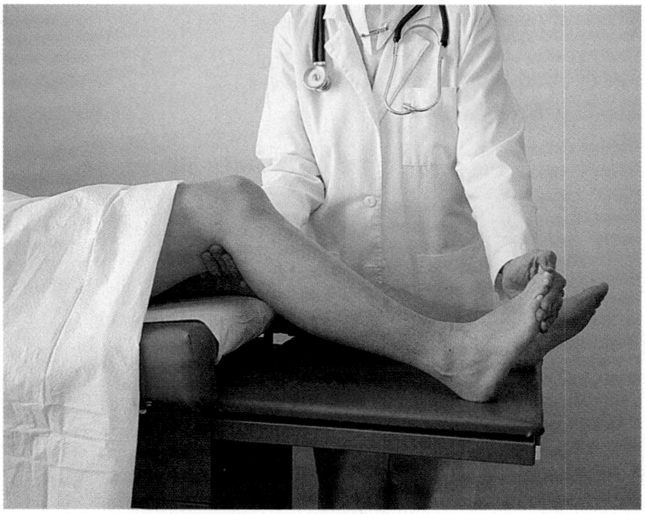

● **Figure 16–4** Assessing clonus. To elicit clonus, with the knee flexed and the leg supported, sharply dorsiflex the foot, hold it momentarily, and then release it. Normally the foot returns to its usual position of plantar flexion. Clonus is present if the foot "jerks" or taps against the examiner's hand. If so, the number of taps or beats of clonus is recorded.

- *Epigastric pain.* Ask about any epigastric pain. It is important to differentiate it from simple heartburn, which tends to be familiar and less intense.
- *Laboratory blood tests.* Daily tests of hematocrit to measure hemoconcentration; BUN, creatinine, and uric acid levels to assess kidney function; clotting studies for signs of thrombocytopenia or DIC; liver enzymes; and electrolyte levels are all indicated. Magnesium levels are monitored regularly in women receiving magnesium sulfate.
- *Level of consciousness.* Observe the woman for alertness, mood changes, and any signs of impending convulsion.
- *Emotional response and level of understanding.* Carefully assess the woman's emotional response so that support and teaching can be planned accordingly.

In addition, assess the effects of any medications administered. Become familiar with the more commonly used medications and their purpose, implications, and associated untoward or toxic effects.

Examples of nursing diagnoses that might apply include the following:

- *Deficient Fluid Volume* related to fluid shift from intravascular to extravascular space secondary to vasospasm
- *Risk for Injury* related to the possibility of seizure secondary to cerebral vasospasm or edema

PLANNING AND IMPLEMENTATION

NURSING CARE IN THE COMMUNITY

A woman with preeclampsia may fear losing her fetus, worry about her personal relationship with her other children and her personal and sexual relationship with her partner because of the limitations placed on her activities, be concerned about finances, and feel bored and a little resentful if she faces prolonged bed rest. If she has small children, she may have trouble providing for their care. Help couples identify and discuss these concerns. Offer information and explanations if certain aspects of therapy cause difficulty. Refer the woman and her family to community resources such as support groups or homemaker services as appropriate.

The woman needs to know which symptoms are significant and should be reported at once. Usually the woman with mild preeclampsia is seen once or twice weekly, but she may need to come in earlier than her next appointment if symptoms indicate that her condition is progressing.

HOSPITAL-BASED NURSING CARE

The development of severe preeclampsia is a cause for increased concern about the prognosis for the woman and her fetus. Explain medical therapy and its purpose and offer honest, hopeful information. Keep the couple informed of fetal status and discuss other concerns the couple may express. Provide as much information as possible and seek other sources of information or aid for the family as needed. Offer to contact a member of the clergy or hospital chaplain for additional support if the couple so chooses.

Maintain a quiet, low-stimulus environment for the woman. She should be in a private room in a quiet location where she can be watched closely. Limit visitors to close family members or main support persons. The woman should maintain the left lateral recumbent position most of the time, with side rails up for her protection.

Eliminate phone calls except for those that are planned because the phone ringing unexpectedly may be too jarring. To avoid a sense of isolation, however, some women find it preferable to limit calls to a certain time of day. Bright lights and sudden loud noises may precipitate seizures in the woman with severe preeclampsia.

Monitor the effectiveness of medications administered. Be alert for signs of untoward effects or developing toxic levels.

The occurrence of a convulsion is frightening to any family members who may be present, although the woman will not be

Nursing Practice

When caring for a woman with preeclampsia who is receiving IV magnesium sulfate, it is imperative to follow protocols for monitoring blood levels of magnesium. You are probably already aware of the common signs of increasing magnesium levels, such as diminished reflexes and decreased respiratory rate. However, you can also watch for some subtle clues that may suggest either the therapeutic or toxic range. When a woman's magnesium level is in the therapeutic range, she usually has some slurring of speech, awkwardness of movement, and decreased appetite. If the woman begins to have difficulty swallowing and begins to drool, she may be approaching the toxic range.

Nursing Care Plan

THE WOMAN WITH PREECLAMPSIA

INTERVENTION	RATIONALE	EXPECTED OUTCOME
1. Nursing Diagnosis: Deficient Fluid Volume related to fluid shift from intravascular to extravascular space secondary to vasospasm		
NIC Intervention: **Fluid management:** Promotion of fluid balance and prevention of complications related to fluid shifts		**NOC Outcome:** **Fluid balance:** Balance of fluid in the intracellular and extracellular compartments of the body
Goal: Client is restored to normal fluid volume levels.		
■ Encourage woman to lie in the left lateral recumbent position.	■ The left lateral recumbent position decreases pressure on the vena cava, thereby increasing venous return, circulatory volume, and placental and renal perfusion. Angiotensin II levels are decreased when there is improved renal blood flow, which helps to promote diuresis and lower blood pressure.	■ The signs and symptoms of preeclampsia will diminish as evidenced by decreased blood pressure, urine protein levels of zero, and a return of the deep tendon reflexes to normal.
■ Assess blood pressure every 1 to 4 hours as necessary.	■ Frequent monitoring will assess for progression of the disorder and allow for early intervention to ensure maternal and fetal health and well-being.	
■ Monitor urine for volume and proteinuria every shift or every hour per agency protocol.	■ Monitoring provides information to assess renal perfusion. Proteinuria is the last cardinal sign of preeclampsia to appear. As the disorder worsens, the capillary walls of the glomerular endothelial cells stretch, allowing protein molecules to pass into the urine. Normal urine does not contain protein. Reading of 3+ and 4+ indicate loss of 5 g or more protein in 24 hours. Urinary output decreases when there is a reduction of the glomerular filtration rate. Urinary output that falls below 30 mL per hour or less than 700 mL in a 24-hour period should be reported.	
■ Assess deep tendon reflexes and clonus.	■ Hyperreflexia may occur as preeclampsia worsens. Eliciting deep tendon reflexes provides information about CNS status and is also used to assess for magnesium sulfate toxicity. Reflexes are graded on a scale of 0 to 4+ using the Deep Tendon Reflex Rating Scale. A rating of 4+ is abnormal and indicates hyperreflexia. A rating of 0 or no response is also abnormal and is seen with high maternal serum magnesium levels. The presence of clonus is an abnormal finding that indicates a more pronounced hyperreflexia and is indicative of CNS irritability.	

Nursing Care Plan—continued

THE WOMAN WITH PREECLAMPSIA

INTERVENTION	RATIONALE	EXPECTED OUTCOME
■ Assess for edema.	■ Edema develops as fluid shifts from the intravascular to the extravascular spaces. Edema is assessed either by weight gain (more than 3.3 1b/month in the second trimester or more than 1.1 1b/week in the third trimester) or by assessing for pitting edema (assessed by using finger pressure to a swollen area, usually the lower extremities, and grading on a scale of 1+ to 4+).	
■ Administer magnesium sulfate per infusion pump as ordered.	■ As preeclampsia worsens, the risk of an eclamptic seizure increases. Magnesium sulfate is the treatment of choice for seizures because of its CNS depressant action. As a secondary effect, magnesium sulfate relaxes smooth muscles and may therefore decrease the blood pressure.	
■ Assess for magnesium sulfate toxicity.	■ Side effects of magnesium sulfate are dose related. Therapeutic levels are in the range of 4.8–9.6 mg/dL. As maternal serum magnesium levels increase, toxicity may occur. Signs of toxicity include decreased or absent DTRs, urine output below 30 mL/hr, respirations below 12, and confusion.	
■ Provide a balanced diet that includes 80–100 g/day or 1.5 g/kg/day of protein.	■ A diet rich in protein is necessary to replace protein that is excreted in the urine.	

2. Nursing Diagnosis: Risk for Injury to the Fetus related to uteroplacental insufficiency secondary to vasospasm

NIC Intervention:

High-risk pregnancy care: Identification and management of preeclampsia to promote healthy outcomes for mother and baby

NOC Outcome:

Risk control: Actions to manage signs and symptoms of preeclampsia and thereby reduce fetal risk

Goal: The fetus avoids complications related to uteroplacental insufficiency.

INTERVENTION	RATIONALE	EXPECTED OUTCOME
■ Instruct woman to count fetal movements 3 times a day for 20 to 30 minutes.	■ Fetal activity provides reassurance of fetal well-being. Decrease in fetal movement or cessation of movement may indicate fetal compromise.	■ The fetus will have an adequate supply of oxygen and nutrients as evidenced by absence of signs of fetal distress and fetal diagnostic test results within normal limits.
■ Encourage woman to rest in the left lateral recumbent position.	■ Lying in the left lateral recumbent position decreases pressure on the vena cava, which increases venous return, circulatory volume, and placental and renal perfusion. Blood flow to the fetus is increased, thereby reducing the risk of fetal hypoxia and malnutrition.	
Collaborative: Assist with serial ultrasounds.	■ Maternal vasospasm and hypovolemia result from preeclampsia, which may lead to SGA newborns. Ultrasound provides assessment of fetal growth by measuring the biparietal diameter of the fetal head or the fetal femur length.	

(continued)

THE WOMAN WITH PREECLAMPSIA

INTERVENTION	RATIONALE	EXPECTED OUTCOME
■ Perform nonstress test as ordered.	■ A nonstress test is performed to assess the fetal heart rate in response to fetal movement. Accelerations of fetal heart rate with fetal movement may indicate the fetus has adequate oxygenation and an intact central nervous system. (Refer to Chapter 14 for interpretation of NST results.)	
■ Describe for the woman the purposes of a biophysical profile (BPP).	■ Preeclampsia or eclampsia places the woman at risk for uteroplacental insufficiency resulting from the loss of normal vasodilation of uterine arterioles and maternal vasospasm. This results in decreased uteroplacental perfusion, which may lead to fetal hypoxia. A BPP is one assessment tool used to evaluate fetal well-being. Providing explanation of the diagnostic test helps relieve anxiety and ensures the woman understands what the test evaluates and what the results mean. (See discussion of BPP in Chapter 14.)	
■ Assist with amniocentesis to obtain lecithin/sphingomyelin (L/S) ratio.	■ Women with preeclampsia may give birth before term. Amniotic fluid may be analyzed to determine the maturity of the fetal lungs. An L/S ratio of 2:1 or greater indicates fetal lung maturity and is usually achieved by 35 weeks' gestation.	
■ Explain the purpose of Doppler flow studies.	■ Doppler flow studies (umbilical velocimetry) help to assess placental function and sufficiency. Uteroplacental insufficiency is a risk for a woman with preeclampsia. (See Chapter 14.)	

3. Nursing Diagnosis: Risk for Ineffective Health Maintenance related to deficient knowledge about new diagnosis (preeclampsia)

NIC Intervention:

Disease process teaching: Assisting the woman to understand information related to the diagnosis of preeclampsia

NOC Outcome:

Knowledge: Treatment regimen: Extent of understanding conveyed about treatment regimen for preeclampsia

Goal: The woman will describe the condition and treatment regimen.

INTERVENTION	RATIONALE	EXPECTED OUTCOME
■ Assess the woman and family's understanding of preeclampsia and its implications for pregnancy.	■ This assessment provides information about the woman's cognitive level and her understanding of her diagnosis. Behavior changes occur when teaching strategies are appropriate for the woman and family's cognitive level.	■ Woman will demonstrate understanding of preeclampsia and its implications as evidenced by verbalization of basic condition, signs and symptoms of progression, importance of sufficient rest in side-lying position, and need to follow prescribed diet.
■ Provide information about the disease process, impact on maternal well-being, risks of progression, implications for the fetus, and dangers of eclampsia.	■ Basic understanding of the condition and its implications is necessary for the woman to understand the treatment plan. A woman who shows signs of early preeclampsia often feels well and may have difficulty accepting the need to rest.	
■ Emphasize the importance of self-monitoring for signs that her condition is worsening and the importance of regular prenatal care for the purpose of maternal and fetal surveillance.	■ The woman should be able to identify signs of disease progression, including evidence of increasing edema, decreased urine output, signs of cerebral disturbance (frontal headache, blurred vision, scotomata), epigastric or right upper quadrant pain, nausea or vomiting, and increased irritability.	

able to recall it when she becomes conscious. Therefore, it is essential to offer explanations to the family members and the woman herself later.

A grand mal seizure has both a tonic phase, marked by pronounced muscular contraction and rigidity, and a clonic phase, marked by alternate contraction and relaxation of the muscles, which causes the woman to thrash about wildly. When the tonic phase of the contraction begins, turn the woman to her side (if she is not already in that position) to aid circulation to the placenta. Turn her head face down to allow saliva to drain from her mouth. Attempting to insert a padded tongue blade is no longer advocated in many facilities; in others, it is used if it can be inserted without force because it may prevent injury to the woman's mouth. The side rails should be padded or a pillow put between the woman and each side rail.

After 15 to 20 seconds, the clonic phase starts. When the thrashing subsides, intensive monitoring and therapy begin. An oral airway is inserted, the woman's nasopharynx is suctioned, and oxygen is administered by nasal catheter. Fetal heart tones are monitored continuously. Monitor maternal vital signs every 5 minutes until they are stable, then every 15 minutes.

Nursing Management During Labor and Birth

Keep the woman positioned on her left side as much as possible. Carefully monitor both the woman and the fetus throughout labor. Note the progress of labor and remain alert for signs of worsening preeclampsia or its complications.

During the second stage of labor, encourage the woman to push in the side-lying position if possible. If she is unable to do so comfortably or effectively, she can be helped to a semisitting position for pushing and can then resume the lateral position between contractions. Birth is in the side-lying position or in the lithotomy position with a wedge placed under the woman's right hip. Encourage a family member or other support person to stay with the woman as much as possible. Keep the woman and her support person informed of the progress and plan of care. Whenever possible, respect their wishes concerning the birth experience.

Nursing Management During the Postpartal Period

Because the woman with preeclampsia is hypovolemic, even normal blood loss can be serious. Assess the amount of vaginal bleeding and observe the woman for signs of shock. Monitor blood pressure and pulse every 4 hours for 48 hours. Check hematocrit daily. Assess the woman for any further signs of preeclampsia. Measure intake and output. Normal postpartum diuresis helps eliminate edema and is a favorable sign.

Postpartum depression can develop after such a difficult pregnancy. To help prevent it, provide opportunities for frequent maternal-infant contact and encourage family members to visit. The couple may have many questions, so be available for discussion. Give the couple family-planning information. Oral contraceptives may be used if the woman's blood pressure has returned to normal by the time they are prescribed (usually 4 to 6 weeks after birth).

EVALUATION

Expected outcomes of nursing care include the following:

- The woman is able to explain preeclampsia/eclampsia, its implications for her pregnancy, the treatment regimen, and possible complications.
- The woman suffers no eclamptic seizures.
- The woman and her caregivers detect early evidence of increasing severity of the preeclampsia or possible complications so that treatment measures can be instituted.
- The woman gives birth to a healthy newborn.

CHRONIC HYPERTENSION

Chronic hypertension exists when the blood pressure is 140/90 mm Hg or higher before pregnancy or before the 20th week of gestation, or when hypertension persists longer than 42 days following childbirth (Sibai, 2007). The cause of chronic hypertension has not been determined. In most women the disease is mild.

The goals of care are to prevent the development of preeclampsia and to ensure normal growth of the fetus. The woman is seen regularly for prenatal care (every 2 weeks until 28 weeks and then weekly until birth). The woman is taught the importance of daily rest periods in the left lateral recumbent position and also learns to monitor her blood pressure at home. Sodium is limited to about 2.4 g/day.

Antihypertensive medication is generally used only for women with blood pressure over 160/110. The drug of choice is methyldopa (Aldomet). Twenty-four-hour urines, serum creatinine, uric acid, hematocrit, and ultrasound examinations are repeated at least once in the second and third trimesters.

Nursing care is directed at providing information so that the woman can meet her healthcare needs. Provide information about her diet, the need for regular rest, her medications, the need for blood pressure control, and any procedures used to monitor the well-being of her fetus.

CHRONIC HYPERTENSION WITH SUPERIMPOSED PREECLAMPSIA

Preeclampsia develops in about 10% to 25% of women previously found to have chronic hypertension (Habli & Sibai, 2008). Close monitoring and careful management are indicated if the following signs develop: (1) elevations of systolic blood pressure 30 mm Hg above the baseline or diastolic blood pressure 15 to 20 mm Hg above the baseline, on two occasions at least 6 hours apart; (2) proteinuria; and (3) edema occurring in the upper half of the body. A woman with chronic hypertension who develops superimposed preeclampsia often progresses quickly to eclampsia, sometimes before 30 weeks of pregnancy.

GESTATIONAL HYPERTENSION

Gestational hypertension is characterized by hypertension occurring for the first time after midpregnancy without proteinuria. It is called transient hypertension if preeclampsia does not develop and if the blood pressure returns to normal within 12 weeks following childbirth.

DISSEMINATED INTRAVASCULAR COAGULATION

Disseminated intravascular coagulation (DIC) occurs more often in pregnancies complicated by preeclampsia, abruptio placentae, intrauterine fetal demise, amniotic fluid embolism, maternal liver disease, and septic abortion. Although DIC is not considered a component of severe preeclampsia, eclampsia, or HELLP syndrome, it can occur as a complication when any of these conditions exist. The incidence of DIC's occurrence when HELLP is the *only* risk factor is approximately 5% (Sibai, 2007).

DIC occurs when the normal clotting process is overactivated. In most instances, tissue factor entering the circulation is the primary trigger for DIC. When this occurs, there is an imbalance between the coagulation and the fibrinolytic systems. This mechanism leads to hemorrhage and shock. During these events, clots are being formed and fibrin is being deposited into the microcirculation, resulting in cell or tissue damage. This triggers further coagulation, which eventually depletes the plasma clotting factors. These fibrin clots can lead to intravascular obstruction and infarctions. In addition the fibrinolytic system is activated, which results in the formation of fibrin-fibrinogen degradation products or fibrin split products. The release of these products decreases platelet functioning and further inhibits coagulation.

DIC is diagnosed when thrombocytopenia, low fibrinogen levels, and elevated fibrin split products are found in the laboratory findings. Serial platelet and serum fibrin degradation product counts are performed to monitor the mother's hematologic status. Supportive measures and reversing the causative factors are the primary interventions used to manage DIC.

CARE OF THE WOMAN AT RISK FOR Rh ALLOIMMUNIZATION

The Rh blood group is present on the surface of erythrocytes of most of the population. When it is present, a person is said to be Rh positive. Those without the factor are Rh negative. If an Rh-negative individual is exposed to Rh-positive blood, an antigen-antibody response occurs, and the person forms anti-Rh agglutinin and is said to be sensitized. Subsequent exposure to Rh-positive blood can then cause a serious reaction that results in agglutination and hemolysis of red blood cells (RBCs). In the United States about 85% of white Americans, 92% to 95% of African Americans, and 1% to 2% of Asian and Native Americans are Rh positive (ACOG, 2006).

Rh alloimmunization (sensitization), also called *isoimmunization,* most often occurs when an Rh-negative woman carries an Rh-positive fetus, either to term or to termination by miscarriage or induced abortion. It can also occur if an Rh-negative nonpregnant woman receives an Rh-positive blood transfusion.

The RBCs from the fetus invade the maternal circulation, thereby stimulating the production of Rh antibodies. Because this transfer of RBCs usually occurs at birth, the first child is not affected. In a subsequent pregnancy, however, Rh antibodies cross the placenta and enter the fetal circulation, causing severe hemolysis. The destruction of fetal RBCs causes anemia in the fetus (Figure 16–5 ●).

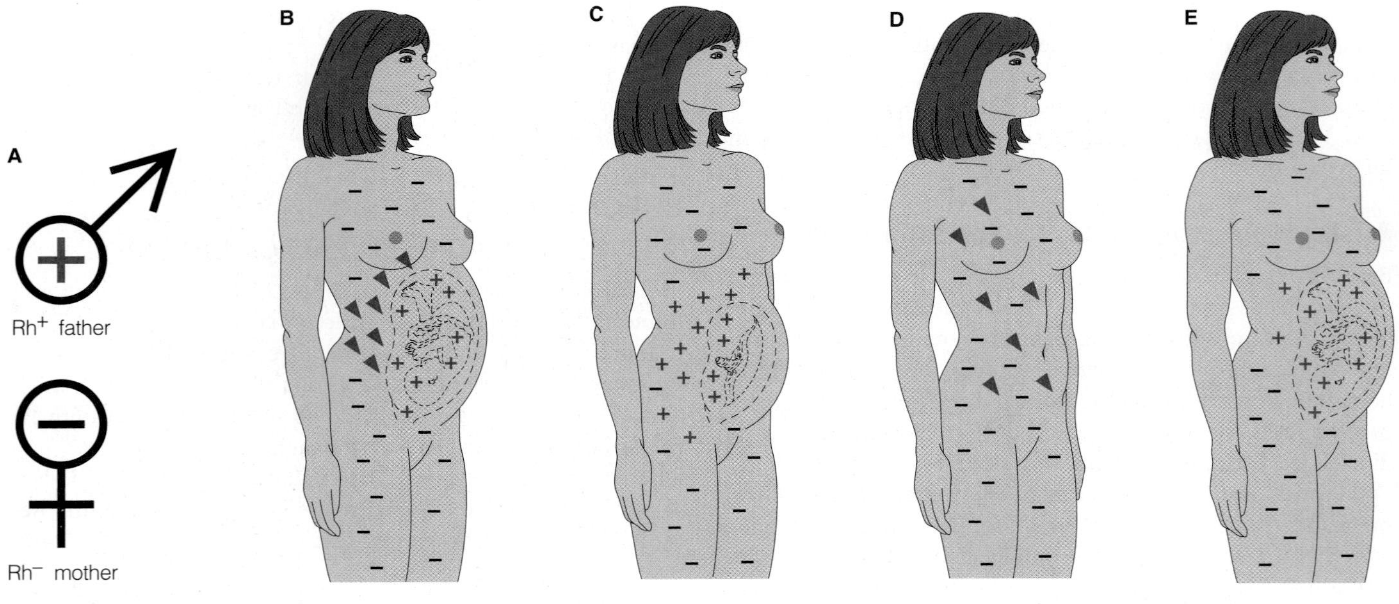

● **Figure 16–5** Rh alloimmunization sequence. ***A,*** Rh-positive father and Rh-negative mother. ***B,*** Pregnancy with Rh-positive fetus. Some Rh-positive blood enters the mother's bloodstream. ***C,*** As the placenta separates, the mother is further exposed to the Rh-positive blood. ***D,*** Anti-Rh-positive antibodies (triangles) are formed. ***E,*** In subsequent pregnancies with an Rh-positive fetus, Rh-positive red blood cells are attacked by the anti-Rh-positive maternal antibodies, causing hemolysis of the red blood cells in the fetus.

FETAL-NEONATAL RISKS

Although maternal sensitization can now be prevented by administration of **Rh immune globulin** (**RhoGAM**, or RhIgG), sensitization still occurs and infants still die of Rh hemolytic disease. If treatment is not initiated, the anemia resulting from this disorder can cause marked fetal edema, called **hydrops fetalis**. Congestive heart failure may result; marked jaundice (called *icterus gravis*), which can lead to neurologic damage (*kernicterus*), is also possible. This severe hemolytic syndrome is known as **erythroblastosis fetalis**.

SCREENING FOR Rh INCOMPATIBILITY AND SENSITIZATION

At the first prenatal visit, healthcare providers:

1. take a history of past pregnancies, previous sensitization, abortions, blood transfusions, or children who developed jaundice or anemia during the newborn period;
2. determine maternal blood type (ABO) and Rh factor and do a routine Rh antibody screen; and
3. identify other medical complications such as diabetes, infections, or hypertension.

When assessment identifies an Rh-negative woman who may be pregnant with an Rh-positive fetus, an antibody screen (indirect Coombs' test) is done to determine whether the woman is sensitized (has developed alloimmunization) to the Rh antigen. The indirect Coombs' test measures the number of antibodies in the maternal blood. If the pregnant woman is not sensitized, a second antibody screening test is done at 28 weeks' gestation. If the maternal antibody screen is positive, a maternal antibody titer is obtained. A woman with an elevated antibody titer should be considered sensitized and her pregnancy should be managed closely.

CLINICAL THERAPY

The goals of clinical management are the early identification and treatment of maternal conditions that predispose to hemolytic disease, evaluation of the Rh-sensitized woman, treatment for the affected newborn, and prevention of Rh sensitization if none is present.

Antepartal Management

Since transplacental hemorrhage is possible during pregnancy, an antibody screen is performed on an Rh-negative woman at 28 weeks' gestation. If she has no antibody titer, she is given an IM injection of 300 mcg Rh immune globulin (RhoGAM, HypRho-D). (*Note:* A new form of human Rh immune globulin—Rhophylac—is also available and can be administered either intravenously or intramuscularly.) The Rh immune globulin provides passive antibody protection against Rh antigens. This "tricks" the body, which does not then produce antibodies of its own (active immunity). As discussed later, Rh immune globulin is also given postpartally.

When the woman is Rh negative and not sensitized and the father is Rh positive or unknown, Rh immune globulin is also given after each abortion (whether spontaneous or induced), ectopic pregnancy, hydatidiform mole, chorionic villus sampling (CVS), amniocentesis, placenta previa with bleeding, blunt trauma to the abdomen, external cephalic version, suspected abruption, or stillbirth. When CVS is performed or if abortion or ectopic pregnancy occurs in the first trimester, a smaller (50 mcg) dose of Rh immune globulin (MICRhoGAM or Mini-Gamulin Rh) may be used; however, many clinical agencies no longer stock the lower dose preparation, which costs about the same as the standard dose. A full 300-mcg dose is used after the first trimester.

Two primary interventions can help the fetus whose blood cells are being destroyed by maternal antibodies: early birth and intrauterine transfusion. Both carry risks. Ideally, birth should be delayed until fetal maturity is confirmed at about 36 to 37 weeks.

Ultrasound is an invaluable tool in managing the pregnancy of a woman with alloimmunization. Ultrasound should be done at 14 to 16 weeks to determine gestational age. Then serial ultrasounds and amniotic fluid analysis can be used to follow fetal progress.

New technology, available in some clinical facilities, enables clinicians to use a Doppler to measure peak systolic middle cerebral artery (MCA) velocity in the fetus. The increased fetal cardiac output and decreased blood viscosity seen in fetal anemia result in increased MCA blood flow velocity. MCA Dopplers can be done starting as early as 18 weeks' gestation but are unreliable after 34 to 35 weeks. The test is valuable because it reduces the need for invasive diagnostic procedures such as amniocentesis (ACOG, 2006).

Ultrasound can also be used to detect ascites and subcutaneous edema, which are signs of severe fetal involvement. Other indicators of the fetal condition include an increase in fetal heart size and hydramnios.

As indicated previously, negative antibody titers and a negative indirect Coombs' test can identify the fetus not at risk. However, the titers cannot reliably point out the fetus in danger, since titer level does not correlate with the severity of the disease. Antibody titers are determined periodically throughout the pregnancy. If the maternal antibody titer is 1:16 or greater, a delta optical density (ΔOD) analysis of the amniotic fluid is performed. This ΔOD analysis measures the amount of pigment from the breakdown of RBCs and can determine the severity of the hemolytic process.

If ΔOD indicates severe anemia or if fetal hydrops is present, percutaneous umbilical blood sampling (PUBS) (see Chapter 14 ∞) is performed to determine fetal hematocrit. If the hematocrit is low (generally below 30%), the fetus is given an intrauterine blood transfusion. Severely sensitized fetuses may require birth at 32 to 34 weeks.

Postpartal Management

The Rh-negative mother who has no antibody titer (indirect Coombs' test negative, nonsensitized) and has given birth to an Rh-positive fetus (direct Coombs' test negative) is given an injection of Rh immune globulin within 72 hours of childbirth so that she does not have time to produce antibodies to fetal cells that entered her bloodstream when the placenta separated. Rh immune globulin provides her with temporary passive immunity, which prevents the development of permanent active immunity (antibody formation).

Table 16–2 Rh Alloimmunization

When trying to work through Rh problems, remember the following:

- A potential problem exists when an Rh-negative mother and an Rh-positive father conceive a child who is Rh positive.
- In this situation, the mother may become sensitized or produce antibodies to her fetus's Rh-positive blood.

The following tests are used to detect sensitization:

- Indirect Coombs' test—done on the mother's blood to measure the number of Rh-positive antibodies.
- Direct Coombs' test—done on the infant's blood to detect antibody-coated Rh-positive red blood cells.

Based on the results of these tests, the following may be done:

- If the mother's indirect Coombs' test is negative and the infant's direct Coombs' test is negative, the mother is given Rh immune globulin within 72 hours of birth.
- If the mother's indirect Coombs' test is positive and her Rh-positive infant has a positive direct Coombs' test, Rh immune globulin is not given; in this case the infant is carefully monitored for hemolytic disease.
- It is recommended that Rh immune globulin be given at 28 weeks antenatally to decrease possible transplacental bleeding concerns.

Rh immune globulin is also administered after each abortion (spontaneous or therapeutic), ectopic pregnancy, or amniocentesis.

Rh immune globulin is not given to the newborn or the father. It should not be given to a previously sensitized woman. However, sometimes after birth or an abortion the results of the blood test do not clearly show whether the mother is already sensitized to the Rh antigen. In such cases the Rh immune globulin is given; it will cause no harm (Table 16–2). (The treatment of the newborn is discussed in Chapter 29∞.)

NURSING MANAGEMENT

NURSING ASSESSMENT AND DIAGNOSIS

As part of the initial prenatal history, ask the mother if she knows her blood type and Rh factor. Many women are aware that they are Rh negative and that this status has implications for pregnancy. Ask the woman if she has ever received Rh immune globulin, if she has had any previous pregnancies and their outcomes, and if she knows her partner's Rh factor. If the partner is Rh negative, there is no risk to the fetus, who will also be Rh negative. If the woman does not know what Rh type she is, intervention begins after the initial laboratory data are obtained. Plan care based on the findings.

If the woman becomes sensitized during her pregnancy, nursing assessment focuses on the knowledge and coping skills of the woman and her family. After birth, review data about the Rh type of the fetus. If the newborn is Rh positive, the mother is Rh negative, and no sensitization has occurred, it is necessary to administer Rh immune globulin.

Nursing diagnoses that might apply include the following:

- *Health-Seeking Behaviors: Information about Rh Immune Globulin* related to an expressed need to understand the implications of being Rh negative and pregnant
- *Ineffective Coping* related to depression secondary to the development of indications of the need for fetal exchange transfusion

PLANNING AND IMPLEMENTATION

During the antepartal period, explain the mechanisms involved in alloimmunization (isoimmunization) and answer any questions the woman and her partner have. It is imperative that the woman understand the importance of receiving Rh immune globulin after every miscarriage, abortion, or ectopic pregnancy. In addition, explain the purpose of the Rh immune globulin administered at 28 weeks' gestation if the woman is not sensitized.

If the woman is sensitized to the Rh factor, it poses a threat to any Rh-positive fetus she carries. Provide emotional support to the family to help the members deal with their concern and any feelings of guilt about the infant's condition. If an intrauterine transfusion becomes necessary, provide support while also assuming responsibility as part of the healthcare team. During labor, when caring for an Rh-negative woman who has not been sensitized, ensure that the woman's blood is assessed for any antibodies and that it has also been crossmatched for Rh immune globulin. The postpartum nurse is usually responsible for administering the Rh immune globulin IM if the newborn is Rh positive. See Skill 2–4 in the Clinical Skills Manual **SKILLS**.

EVALUATION

Expected outcomes of nursing care include the following:

- The woman is able to explain the process of Rh sensitization and its implications for her unborn child and for subsequent pregnancies.
- If the woman has not been sensitized, she is able to discuss the importance of receiving Rh immune globulin when necessary and cooperates with the recommended dosage schedule.
- The woman gives birth to a healthy newborn.
- If complications develop for the fetus or newborn, they are detected quickly and therapy is instituted.

CARE OF THE WOMAN AT RISK FROM ABO INCOMPATIBILITY

In addition to the Rh antigen, human red blood cells may present one or more of the antigens of the ABO group, namely A or B. People with these antigens are then said to have type A, type B, or type AB blood. People whose blood cells present neither A nor B antigens have type O blood. In most cases ABO incompatibility is limited to type O mothers with a type A, B, or AB fetus. Group O infants, because they have no antigenic sites on the red blood cells, are never affected regardless of the mother's blood type. The incompatibility occurs as a result of the interaction of antibodies present in maternal serum and the antigen sites on the fetal red blood cells.

Anti-A and anti-B antibodies are naturally occurring; that is, women are naturally exposed to the A and B antigens through the foods they eat and through exposure to infection by gram-negative bacteria. As a result, some women have high serum anti-A and anti-B titers even before they become pregnant for the first time. Once they become pregnant, the maternal serum anti-A and anti-B antibodies cross the placenta and produce hemolysis of the fetal red blood cells. With ABO incompatibility, the first infant is often involved, and no relationship exists between the appearance of the disease and repeated sensitization from one pregnancy to the next.

Unlike Rh incompatibility, antepartal treatment is never warranted. As part of the initial assessment, however, note whether the potential for an ABO incompatibility exists (type O mother and type A or B father). This alerts healthcare providers so that, following birth, the newborn can be assessed carefully for the development of hyperbilirubinemia (see Chapter 29 ∞).

CARE OF THE WOMAN REQUIRING SURGERY DURING PREGNANCY

Although elective surgery should be delayed until the postpartum, essential surgery can generally be done during pregnancy. Surgery poses some risks, however. The incidence of miscarriage is increased for women who have surgery in the first trimester. Therefore, the early second trimester is the best time to operate because there is less risk of spontaneous abortion or early labor, and the uterus is not so large as to impinge on the abdominal field.

General preoperative and postoperative care is similar for pregnant and nonpregnant women; however special considerations must be kept in mind whenever the surgical client is pregnant. If a chest x-ray is done, the fetus should be shielded from radiation.

To prevent uterine compression of major blood vessels while the woman is supine, the caregiver must place a wedge under the woman's right hip to tilt the uterus during both surgery and recovery. The decreased intestinal motility and delayed gastric emptying that occur in pregnancy increase the risk of vomiting when anesthetics are given and during the postoperative period. Thus, a nasogastric tube is usually inserted before a pregnant woman has major surgery. An indwelling urinary catheter prevents bladder distention, decreases risk of injury to the bladder, and permits monitoring of output.

Pregnancy causes increased secretions of the respiratory tract and engorgement of the nasal mucous membrane, often making breathing through the nose difficult. Consequently, pregnant women often need an endotracheal tube to maintain an airway during surgery. Caregivers must guard against maternal hypoxia. During surgery, uterine circulation decreases, and fetal oxygenation may be reduced quickly. Fetal heart rate must be monitored electronically during and after surgery. Blood loss is also monitored throughout the procedure and following it.

Postoperatively, encourage the woman to turn, breathe deeply, and cough regularly and to use any ventilation therapy, such as incentive spirometry, to avoid developing pneumonia. The pregnant woman is at increased risk for thrombophlebitis, so apply antiembolism stockings, encourage leg exercises while the woman is in bed, and have her ambulate as soon as possible.

Discharge teaching is very important. The woman and her family should understand what to expect regarding activity level, discomfort, diet, medications, and any special considerations. In addition, they should know the warning signs they need to report to the physician immediately.

CARE OF THE WOMAN SUFFERING TRAUMA FROM AN ACCIDENT

MyNursingKit Animation: Premature Labor
MyNursingKit Care Plan: Client at Risk for Preterm Labor

Trauma complicates up to 8% of pregnancies and is the leading nonobstetric cause of maternal death (Lu & Curet, 2007). Trauma from motor vehicle accidents is the leading cause of fetal and maternal death. Falls and violence—including domestic violence—are the next most common causes of injury.

Late in pregnancy, when balance and coordination are affected, the woman may fall. Her protruding abdomen is vulnerable to a variety of minor injuries. The fetus is usually well protected by the amniotic fluid, which distributes the force of a blow equally in all directions, and by the muscle layers of the uterus and abdominal wall. In early pregnancy, while the uterus is still in the pelvis, it is shielded from blows by the surrounding pelvic organs, muscles, and bones.

Trauma that causes concern includes blunt trauma, penetrating abdominal injuries such as knife and gunshot wounds, and the complications of maternal shock, premature labor, and spontaneous abortion. Maternal mortality most often occurs from head trauma or hemorrhage. Uterine rupture is a rare but life-threatening complication of trauma. It may result from strong deceleration forces in an automobile accident, with or without seat belts. The most common serious complication of blunt trauma is placental abruption, which occurs in 20% to 50% of women with major injuries and causes a high rate of fetal mortality (Krakow, 2008). Premature labor, often following rupture of membranes during an accident, is another serious hazard to the fetus. Premature labor can begin even if the woman is not injured. To help prevent trauma from automobile accidents, all pregnant women should wear both lap seat belts and shoulder harnesses.

Penetrating trauma most often results from gunshot wounds and stab wounds. The mother generally fares better than the fetus if the penetrating trauma involves the abdomen, as the enlarged uterus is likely to protect the mother's bowel from injury. Unfortunately, the fetal injury rate is 59% to 89%, with fetal death occurring in 41% to 71% of cases (Krakow, 2008).

Treatment of major injuries during pregnancy focuses initially on lifesaving measures for the woman. Such measures include establishing an airway, controlling external bleeding, and administering IV fluid to alleviate shock. The woman must be kept on her left side to prevent further hypotension. Oxygen is administered. Fetal heart rate and fetal movement are monitored. Exploratory surgery may be necessary following abdominal trauma to determine the extent of injuries. If the fetus is near term and the uterus has been damaged, cesarean birth is indicated. If the fetus is still immature, the uterus can often be repaired, and the pregnancy can continue until term.

In cases of trauma in which the mother's life is not directly threatened, fetal monitoring for a minimum of 4 hours is suggested if there are no contractions, vaginal bleeding, uterine tenderness, or leaking amniotic fluid. Abruptio placentae may occur following a blow to the abdomen. Increased uterine irritability in the first few hours after trauma helps identify women who may be at risk for this potentially catastrophic complication.

When cardiopulmonary resuscitation (CPR) is performed on the pregnant woman late in gestation, perimortem cesarean birth is advocated if CPR is unsuccessful in the first 5 minutes. Chest compressions are less effective in the third trimester because of compression of the inferior vena cava by the gravid uterus. Cesarean birth alleviates this compression and improves resuscitation efforts in both the fetus and the mother. Research indicates that infants born by cesarean within 5 minutes of maternal death have no apparent neurologic damage. Overall fetal survival rates range from 50% to 70%. Mortality increases as the time from maternal arrest to infant birth increases (Lu & Curet, 2007).

CARE OF THE BATTERED PREGNANT WOMAN

Domestic violence, most often the intentional injury of a woman by her partner, often begins or increases during pregnancy. Up to 8% of women experience physical violence during pregnancy (National Coalition Against Domestic Violence [NCADV], 2007). Physical abuse may result in loss of pregnancy, preterm labor, low birth weight infants, and cesarean birth. Abused women often delay starting prenatal care and have higher rates of complications such as high blood pressure, vaginal bleeding, urinary tract infection, and sexually transmitted infections (NCADV, 2007).

The first step toward helping the battered woman is to identify her. Asking every woman about abuse at various times during pregnancy is crucial because a woman may not disclose abuse until she knows her caregivers better. Screening for abuse should be done at the first prenatal visit, at least once each trimester, and then again during the postpartum period.

Chronic psychosomatic symptoms can also be an indicator of abuse. The woman may have nonspecific or vague complaints. It is important to assess old scars around the head, chest, arms, abdomen, and genitalia. Any bruising or evidence of pain is also evaluated. Be especially alert for signs of bruising or injury to the woman's breasts, abdomen, or genitalia because these areas are common targets of violence during pregnancy. Other indicators include a decrease in eye contact; silence when the partner is in the room; and a history of nervousness, insomnia, drug overdose, or alcohol problems. Frequent visits to the emergency department and a history of accidents without understandable causes are possible indicators of abuse.

The goals of treatment are to identify the woman at risk, to increase her decision-making abilities to decrease the risk for further abuse, and to provide a safe environment for the woman and her unborn child. An environment that is private, accepting, and nonjudgmental is necessary so the woman can express her concerns. She needs to be aware of community resources available to her, such as emergency shelters; police, legal, and social services; and counseling. Ultimately it is the woman's decision to either seek assistance or return to old patterns.

Because abuse often begins during pregnancy, it may be a new, unexpected experience for the woman, one she believes is an isolated incident. She needs to know that battering may continue after childbirth and may extend to the child as well. This is an important time to provide information and establish a trusted link for the woman with a healthcare professional. (For further discussion see Chapter 5∞.)

CARE OF THE WOMAN WITH A PERINATAL INFECTION AFFECTING THE FETUS

Fetal infection may develop at any time during pregnancy. In general, perinatal infections are most likely to cause harm when the embryo is exposed during the first trimester when organ development is occurring. Infections that occur later in pregnancy create other concerns such as growth restriction, preterm birth, and neurologic changes. This section addresses several of the most commonly occurring viral and parasitic infections that may have an impact on the fetus if acquired during pregnancy.

TOXOPLASMOSIS

Toxoplasmosis is caused by the protozoan *Toxoplasma gondii.* It is barely noticeable in adults, but, when contracted in pregnancy, it can profoundly affect the fetus. The pregnant woman may contract the organism by eating raw or undercooked meat, by drinking unpasteurized goat's milk, or by contact with the feces of infected cats, either through the cat litter box or by gardening in areas frequented by cats.

Fetal-Neonatal Risks

The likelihood of fetal infection increases with each trimester of pregnancy, but the risk of serious impact on the fetus decreases. Thus, maternal infection contracted during the first trimester is associated with the lowest incidence of fetal infection (15%) but the highest risk of severe fetal disease or death (10%). The highest rate of fetal infection (60%) occurs when the mother contracts the infection in the third trimester, but most of these infants are born without clinical signs of infection (Davies & Gibbs, 2008). However, up to 85% of these infants will develop signs and symptoms if left untreated (Montoya & Rosso, 2005). The infection may vary from mild to severe. In mild cases, retinochoroiditis (inflammation of the retina and choroid of the eye) may be the only recognizable damage, and it and other manifestations may not appear until adolescence or young adulthood. Severe neonatal disorders associated with congenital infection include convulsions, coma, microcephaly, and hydrocephalus. The infant with a severe infection may die soon after birth. Survivors are often blind, deaf, and severely retarded. Treatment of the mother can reduce the incidence of fetal infection and decreases the late sequelae of the infection (Duff, 2007).

Clinical Therapy

Diagnosis can be made by serologic testing of antibody titers, specifically the IgG and IgM fluorescent antibody (IFA) tests. If a pregnant woman is positive for IgG antibodies and negative for IgM in the third trimester, it indicates that she had a toxoplasmosis infection in the past and the baby is not at risk. If she has a positive IgM, it indicates a more recent infection and it should be followed by confirmatory testing at a toxoplasma reference lab (Montoya & Rosso, 2005). Toxoplasmosis polymerase chain reaction (PCR) test of amniotic fluid is useful in diagnosing congenital toxoplasmosis. Ultrasound may be useful in detecting signs of fetal infection such as ascites, microcephaly, intracranial calcifications, and fetal growth restriction (Duff, 2007).

Women in whom maternal infection is established should receive spiramycin to decrease the frequency of vertical transmission, particularly in the first trimester. Spiramycin is not commercially available in the United States, but it can be obtained for treatment through the CDC. Spiramycin does not reliably cross the placenta. Thus if fetal infection is suspected, spiramycin should be replaced with pyrimethamine, folinic acid, and a sulfonamide after the 18th week of pregnancy (Duff, 2007).

NURSING MANAGEMENT

NURSING ASSESSMENT AND DIAGNOSIS

The incubation period for the disease is 10 days. The woman with acute toxoplasmosis may be asymptomatic, or she may develop myalgia, malaise, rash, splenomegaly, and enlarged posterior cervical lymph nodes. Symptoms usually disappear in a few days or weeks.

Nursing diagnoses that might apply include the following:

- *Risk for Ineffective Health Maintenance* related to lack of knowledge about ways in which a pregnant woman can contract toxoplasmosis
- *Anticipatory Grieving* related to potential effects on infant of maternal toxoplasmosis

PLANNING AND IMPLEMENTATION

During the antepartal period, discuss methods of preventing toxoplasmosis. The woman must understand the importance of avoiding poorly cooked or raw meat, especially pork, beef, lamb, and, in the Arctic region, caribou. Fruits and vegetables should be washed. She should avoid contact with the cat litter box and have someone else clean it frequently, since it takes approximately 48 hours for a cat's feces to become infectious. Stress the importance of wearing gloves when gardening and of avoiding garden areas frequented by cats.

EVALUATION

Expected outcomes of nursing care include the following:

- The woman is able to discuss toxoplasmosis, its methods of transmission, the implications for her fetus, and measures she can take to avoid contracting it.
- The woman implements health measures to avoid contracting toxoplasmosis.
- The woman gives birth to a healthy newborn.

RUBELLA

The effects of rubella (German measles) on the fetus and newborn are great, because rubella causes a chronic infection that begins in the first trimester of pregnancy and that may persist for months after birth. Fortunately, the success of the rubella vaccination program in the United States has led to a dramatic decrease in the incidence of rubella.

Fetal-Neonatal Risks

The period of greatest risk for the effects of rubella on the fetus is the first trimester. The most common clinical signs of congenital infection include congenital cataracts, sensorineural deafness, and congenital heart defects, particularly patent ductus arteriosus. Other abnormalities, such as mental retardation or cerebral palsy, may become evident in infancy. Diagnosis in the newborn can be made in the presence of these conditions and with an elevated rubella IgM antibody titer at birth. Infants born with congenital rubella syndrome are infectious and should be isolated.

The *expanded rubella syndrome* relates to effects that may develop for years after the infection. These include an increased incidence of type 1 diabetes mellitus, sudden hearing loss, glaucoma, and a slow, progressive form of encephalitis.

Clinical Therapy

The best therapy for rubella is prevention. Live attenuated vaccine is available and should be given to all children. Women of childbearing age should be tested for immunity and vaccinated if susceptible once it is established that they are not pregnant.

As part of the prenatal laboratory screen, the woman is evaluated for rubella using hemagglutination inhibition (HAI), a serology test. The presence of a 1:8 titer or greater is evidence of immunity. A titer less than 1:8 indicates susceptibility to rubella.

Because the vaccine is made with attenuated virus, pregnant women are not vaccinated. However, it is considered safe for newly vaccinated children to have contact with pregnant women. Women whose titers indicate that they are susceptible to rubella should be given the rubella vaccine postpartally.

If a woman becomes infected during the first trimester, therapeutic abortion is a legally available alternative.

NURSING MANAGEMENT

NURSING ASSESSMENT AND DIAGNOSIS

A woman who develops rubella during pregnancy may be asymptomatic or may show signs of a mild infection including a maculopapular rash, lymphadenopathy, muscular achiness, and joint pain. The presence of IgM antirubella antibody is diagnostic of a recent infection. These titers remain elevated for approximately 1 month after infection.

Nursing diagnoses that may apply to the woman who develops rubella early in her pregnancy include the following:

- *Ineffective Family Coping* resulting from an inability to accept the possibility of fetal anomalies secondary to maternal rubella exposure
- *Risk for Ineffective Health Maintenance* related to lack of knowledge about the importance of rubella immunization before becoming pregnant

PLANNING AND IMPLEMENTATION

Support is vital for the couple who are considering abortion because of a diagnosis of rubella. Such a decision may trigger a crisis for the couple. The parents need objective data to understand the possible effects on their unborn fetus and the long-term prognosis.

EVALUATION

Expected outcomes of nursing care include the following:

- The woman is able to describe the implications of rubella exposure during the first trimester of pregnancy.
- If exposure occurs in a woman who is not immune, she is able to identify her options and make a decision about continuing her pregnancy that is acceptable to her and her partner.
- The nonimmune woman receives the rubella vaccine during the early postpartal period.
- The woman gives birth to a healthy infant.

CYTOMEGALOVIRUS

Cytomegalovirus (CMV) belongs to the herpes virus group and causes both congenital and acquired infections that are referred to as cytomegalic inclusion disease (CID). This virus can be transmitted by asymptomatic women across the placenta to the fetus or by the cervical route during birth.

The virus can be found in virtually all body fluids. It can be passed between humans by any close contact, such as kissing, breastfeeding, and sexual intercourse. During pregnancy, infection occurs most often when the woman is exposed to infected children or through sexual contact (Davies & Gibbs, 2008). Asymptomatic CMV infection is particularly common in children and pregnant women. It is a chronic, persistent infection in that the individual may shed the virus continually over many years. The cervix can harbor the virus, and an ascending infection can develop after birth. Although the virus is usually innocuous in adults and children, it may be fatal to the fetus.

Accurate diagnosis in the pregnant woman is best documented by seroconversion. Routine screening of pregnant women is not recommended, however, because positive serology is so common. Identification of the virus in amniotic fluid by PCR or culture is the most specific way of diagnosing congenital infection (Bernstein, 2007). Ultrasound findings may include fetal hydrops, growth restriction, hydramnios, cardiomegaly, and fetal ascites.

CMV is the most frequent cause of viral infection in the human fetus, infecting 0.5% to 2% of all newborns. Of these, about 10% to 15% will have overt symptoms at birth and 20% to 30% of severely affected infants die; 90% of the survivors have significant neurologic complications (Hollier & Grissom, 2005). Subclinical infections in the newborn can produce mental retardation and hearing loss, sometimes not recognized for several months, or learning disabilities not seen until childhood. CMV may be the most common cause of mental retardation.

For the fetus, this infection can result in extensive intrauterine tissue damage that leads to fetal death; in survival with microcephaly, hydrocephaly, cerebral palsy, or mental retardation; or in survival with no damage at all. The infected newborn is often SGA.

At present, no treatment exists for maternal CMV or for the congenital disease in the newborn. Thus, prevention is important. The pregnant woman should be advised to avoid areas with high concentrations of young children such as day care centers, if possible, and to practice good handwashing techniques (Davies & Gibbs, 2008).

HERPES SIMPLEX VIRUS

Herpes simplex virus (HSV-1 or HSV-2) infection can cause painful lesions in the genital area. Lesions may also develop on the cervix. (This condition and its implications for nonpregnant women are discussed in Chapter 5∞.)

Fetal-Neonatal Risks

Primary infection poses the greatest risk to both the mother and her infant. Primary infection has been associated with spontaneous abortion, low birth weight, and preterm birth. Transmission to the fetus almost always occurs after the membranes rupture and the virus ascends or during birth through an infected birth canal. Transplacental infection is rare. Approximately 50% of all infants born vaginally to a mother experiencing a primary genital HSV infection develop some form of herpes infection. Exposure of the newborn to a *recurrent* infection drops the risk of transmission to between 1% and 5% (Hill & Roberts, 2005).

The infected infant is often asymptomatic at birth but develops symptoms of fever (or hypothermia), jaundice, seizures, and poor feeding after an incubation period of 2 to 12 days. Approximately half of infected infants develop the characteristic vesicular skin lesions. Infants who have neonatal herpes should be evaluated promptly and treated with acyclovir (Centers for Disease Control and Prevention [CDC], 2006).

Clinical Therapy

The vesicular lesions of herpes have a characteristic appearance, and they rupture easily. Definitive diagnosis is made by culturing active lesions.

Women with a primary HSV infection during pregnancy can be treated with oral acyclovir, valacyclovir, or famciclovir for 7 to 10 days (Bernstein, 2007). For a woman with either a primary or a secondary outbreak of genital herpes during labor, or symptoms that may indicate an impending outbreak, the preferred method of childbirth is cesarean birth. Although fetal transmission with recurrent outbreaks is low, a cesarean birth is warranted because of the serious nature of the disease in the newborn. The risk of neonatal transmission is low in women with a history of HSV in the current pregnancy or in the past. Thus cost-benefit analysis suggests that oral acyclovir prophylaxis and vaginal birth are appropriate for women with a history of HSV but who have no evidence of active genital disease at the time of childbirth (Davies & Gibbs, 2008).

NURSING MANAGEMENT

NURSING ASSESSMENT AND DIAGNOSIS

During the initial prenatal visit, it is important to learn whether the woman or her partner have had previous herpes infections. If so, ongoing assessment is indicated as pregnancy progresses.

Nursing diagnoses that may apply include the following:

- *Sexual Dysfunction* related to unwillingness to engage in sexual intercourse secondary to the presence of active herpes lesions
- *Ineffective Individual Coping* related to depression secondary to the risk to the fetus if herpes lesions are present at birth

PLANNING AND IMPLEMENTATION

Client education about this fast-spreading disease is crucial. Inform women of the association of HSV infection with spontaneous abortion, newborn mortality and morbidity, and the possibility of cesarean birth. A woman needs to inform all healthcare providers of her infection. She should also know of the possible association of genital herpes with cervical cancer and the importance of a yearly Pap smear.

The woman who acquired HSV infection as an adolescent may be devastated as a mature adult who wants to have a family. Counseling that allows her to express the negative feelings she may have about the infection may help. Literature may also help and is available from Planned Parenthood and public health agencies. The American Social Health Association has established the HELP program to provide information on genital herpes and has a quarterly journal, *The Helper*, for clients with HSV infection.

EVALUATION

Expected outcomes of nursing care include the following:

- The woman is able to describe her infection with regard to its method of spread, therapy and comfort measures, implications for her pregnancy, and long-term implications.
- The woman gives birth to a healthy infant.

GROUP B STREPTOCOCCAL INFECTION

Group B streptococcus (GBS) is a bacterial infection found in the lower gastrointestinal or urogenital tracts of 20% to 25% of pregnant women (Duff, 2007). Women may transmit GBS to their fetus in utero or during childbirth. GBS is one of the major causes of early-onset neonatal infection. Newborns become infected in one of two ways: by vertical transmission from the mother during birth or from horizontal transmission from colonized nursing personnel or colonized infants. GBS causes severe, invasive disease in infants. In newborns the majority of cases occur within the first week of life and are thus designated as early-onset disease. Late-onset disease occurs one week or more after birth.

Early-onset GBS is often characterized by signs of serious illness, including pneumonia and overwhelming septicemia. Late-onset GBS often manifests as meningitis or pneumonia. Long-term neurologic complications are common in both types of GBS.

Risk factors for GBS neonatal sepsis include preterm labor, maternal intrapartum fever, prolonged rupture of the membranes, previous birth of an infected infant, and GBS bacteriuria in the current pregnancy. Guidelines for the detection and preventive treatment of newborns at risk include the following (Duff, 2007):

- All pregnant women should be screened for both vaginal and rectal GBS colonization at 35 to 37 weeks' gestation. Treatment should be based on these results, even if cultures were done earlier in pregnancy.
- Positive GBS screening culture should be done during current pregnancy.
- Women with GBS in their urine in any concentration should receive antibiotic prophylaxis intrapartally because such women typically have heavy colonization with GBS and thus have an increased risk of giving birth to a newborn with early-onset disease. These women do not need vaginal and rectal cultures at 35 to 37 weeks because therapy is already indicated.
- Women who have already given birth to a newborn with invasive GBS disease should receive intrapartum antibiotic prophylaxis. Culture-based screening is not necessary for them.

- If the results of GBS screening are not known when labor begins, prophylaxis is indicated for women with any of the following risk factors: gestation less than 37 weeks, membranes ruptured 18 hours or longer, temperature equal to or greater than 38.0°C (100.4°F).

Intrapartum antibiotic therapy is recommended as follows: initial dose of penicillin G, 5 million units IV followed by 2.5 million units IV every 4 hours until childbirth. Alternatively, ampicillin 2 g initial dose IV followed by 1 g IV every 4 hours until childbirth may be used. Women at high risk for an anaphylactic reaction to penicillin because of marked allergy may be treated with clindamycin or erythromycin (Davies & Gibbs, 2008).

Thinking Critically

PREVENTING CYSTITIS

Your friend Jena Yoo, G1P0, is 6 months pregnant and mentions to you that she is developing symptoms of a bladder infection. She has had several bladder infections over the past few years and feels she has warded off others by increasing her fluid intake and drinking acidic juices. Jena tells you that she plans to use the same approach this time because she just had her prenatal appointment last week. She assures you that if symptoms persist, she will discuss it with her care provider at her next prenatal visit. What advice would you give her?

See MyNursingKit for possible responses.

OTHER INFECTIONS IN PREGNANCY

Table 16–3 summarizes other urinary tract, vaginal, and sexually transmitted infections that contribute to risk during pregnancy. (These are described in more detail in Chapter 6∞.) Spontaneous abortion is frequently the result of a severe maternal infection. Some evidence links infection and prematurity. If the pregnancy is carried to term in the presence of infection, the risk of maternal and fetal morbidity and mortality increases. Thus, it is essential to maternal and fetal health that infection be diagnosed and treated promptly.

Table 16–3 Infections That Put Pregnancy at Risk

Condition and Causative Organism	Signs and Symptoms	Treatment	Implications for Pregnancy
		Urinary Tract Infections (UTI)	
Asymptomatic bacteriuria (ASB): *Escherichia, Klebsiella, Proteus* most common	Bacteria present in urine on culture with no accompanying symptoms.	Oral sulfonamides early in pregnancy, ampicillin and nitrofurantoin (Furadantin) in late pregnancy. Antibody sensitivity results will guide the selection of an appropriate antibiotic.	Women with ASB in early pregnancy may go on to develop cystitis or acute pyelonephritis by third trimester if not treated. Oral sulfonamides taken in the last few weeks of pregnancy may lead to neonatal hyperbilirubinemia and kernicterus.
Cystitis (lower UTI): Causative organisms same as for ASB	Dysuria, urgency, frequency; low-grade fever and hematuria may occur. Urine culture (clean catch) shows ↑ leukocytes. Presence of 10^5 (100,000) or more colonies bacteria per mL urine.	Same.	If not treated, infection may ascend and lead to acute pyelonephritis.
Acute pyelonephritis: Causative organisms same as for ASB	Sudden onset. Chills, high fever, flank pain. Nausea, vomiting, malaise. May have decreased urine output, severe colicky pain, dehydration. Increased diastolic BP, positive fluorescent antibody (FA) test, low creatinine clearance. Marked bacteremia in urine culture, pyuria, WBC casts.	Hospitalization; IV antibiotic therapy. Other antibiotics safe during pregnancy include carbenicillin, methenamine, cephalosporins. Catheterization if output is ↓. Supportive therapy for comfort. Follow-up urine cultures are necessary.	Increased risk of premature birth and intrauterine growth restriction (IUGR). These antibiotics interfere with urinary estriol levels and can cause false interpretations of estriol levels during pregnancy.
		Vaginal Infections	
Vulvovaginal candidiasis (yeast infection): *Candida albicans*	Often thick, white, curdy discharge, severe itching, dysuria, dyspareunia. Diagnosis based on presence of hyphae and spores in a wet-mount preparation of vaginal secretions.	Intravaginal insertion of miconazole, butoconazole, or other topical azole preparation, clotrimazole suppositories at bedtime for 1 week. Cream may be prescribed for topical application to the vulva if necessary (CDC, 2006).	If the infection is present at birth and the fetus is born vaginally, the fetus may contract thrush.

Table 16–3 Infections That Put Pregnancy at Risk—continued

Condition and Causative Organism	Signs and Symptoms	Treatment	Implications for Pregnancy
Bacterial vaginosis: *Gardnerella vaginalis*	Thin, watery, yellow-gray discharge with foul odor often described as "fishy." Wet-mount preparation reveals "clue cells." Application of potassium hydroxide (KOH) to a specimen of vaginal secretions produces a pronounced fishy odor.	Metronidazole 250 mg PO TID × 7 days or metronidazole 500 mg PO BID × 7 days or clindamycin 300 mg PO BID × 7 days (CDC, 2006).	CDC (2006) reports that multiple studies have failed to demonstrate a teratogenic effect from metronidazole.
Trichomoniasis: *Trichomonas vaginalis*	Occasionally asymptomatic. May have frothy greenish gray vaginal discharge, pruritus, urinary symptoms. Strawberry patches may be visible on vaginal walls or cervix. Wet-mount preparation of vaginal secretions shows motile flagellated trichomonads.	Single 2-g dose of metronidazole orally (CDC, 2006).	Increased risk for PROM, preterm birth, and low birth weight.
	Sexually Transmitted Infections		
Chlamydial infection: *Chlamydia trachomatis*	Women are often asymptomatic. Symptoms may include thin or purulent discharge, urinary burning and frequency, or lower abdominal pain. Lab test available to detect monoclonal antibodies specific for *Chlamydia.*	Although nonpregnant women are treated with tetracycline, it may permanently discolor fetal teeth. Thus, pregnant women are treated with azithromycin or amoxicillin followed by repeat culture in 3 weeks (CDC, 2006).	Infant of woman with untreated chlamydial infection may develop newborn conjunctivitis, which can be treated with erythromycin eye ointment (but not silver nitrate). Infant may also develop chlamydial pneumonia. May be responsible for premature labor and fetal death.
Syphilis: *Treponema pallidum,* a spirochete	Primary stage: chancre, slight fever, malaise. Chancre lasts about 4 weeks, then disappears. Secondary stage: occurs 6 weeks to 6 months after infection. Skin eruptions (condyloma latal) also symptoms of acute arthritis, liver enlargement, iritis, chronic sore throat with hoarseness. Diagnosed by blood tests such as VDRL, RPR, FTA, ABS. Dark-field examination or spirochetes may also be done.	For syphilis less than 1 year in duration: 2.4 million units benzathine penicillin G IM. For syphilis of more than 1 year's duration or latent syphilis of unknown duration: 2.4 million units benzathine penicillin G once a week for 3 weeks. Sexual partners should also be screened and treated (CDC, 2006).	Syphilis can be passed transplacentally to the fetus. If untreated, one of the following can occur: second-trimester abortion, stillborn infant at term, congenitally infected infant, uninfected live infant.
Gonorrhea: *Neisseria gonorrhoeae*	Majority of women asymptomatic; disease often diagnosed during routine prenatal cervical culture. If symptoms are present they may include purulent vaginal discharge, dysuria, urinary frequency, inflammation, and swelling of the vulva. Cervix may appear eroded.	Pregnant women are treated with a cephalosporin (ceftriaxone, cefixime); if they cannot tolerate a cephalosporin, they should receive spectinomycin. They are also treated for chlamydia using azithromycin or amoxicillin (CDC, 2006). All sexual partners are also treated.	Infection at time of birth may cause ophthalmia neonatorum in the newborn.
Condyloma acuminata: caused by a papovavirus	Soft, grayish pink lesions on the vulva, vagina, cervix, or anus.	Podophyllin, podofilox, and imiquimod are contraindicated during pregnancy. Some caregivers recommend removing warts by surgical methods or laser because the warts can proliferate and become friable (bleed easily) during pregnancy (CDC, 2006).	Possible teratogenic effect of podophyllin. Large doses have been associated with fetal death.

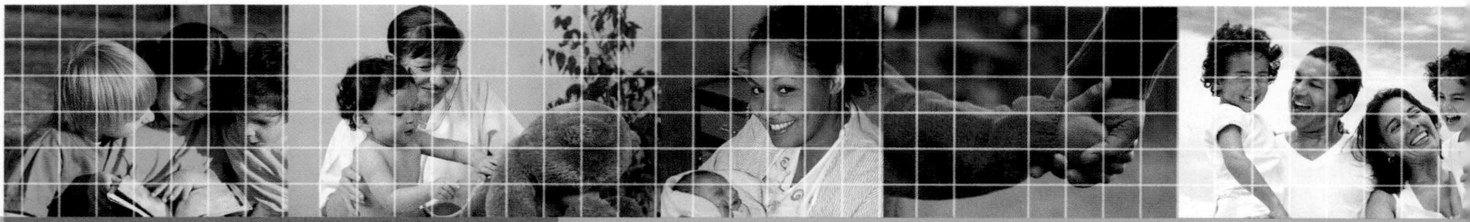

CRITICAL CONCEPT REVIEW

LEARNING OUTCOMES	CONCEPTS
16.1 Summarize the etiology, medical therapy, and cultural perspectives to community-based and hospital-based nursing care management of women with a bleeding problem associated with pregnancy.	1. Several health problems associated with bleeding arise from the pregnancy itself: ■ Spontaneous abortion. ■ Ectopic pregnancy. ■ Gestational trophoblastic disease. 2. The nurse needs to be alert to early signs of these situations: ■ Guard the woman against heavy bleeding and shock. ■ Facilitate the medical treatment. ■ Provide educational and emotional support.
16.2 Describe the maternal and fetal-neonatal risks and medical therapy in the nursing care management of a woman with hyperemesis gravidarum.	1. Treatment of hyperemesis gravidarum is aimed at: ■ Controlling the vomiting. ■ Correcting fluid and electrolyte imbalance. ■ Correcting dehydration. ■ Improving nutritional status. 2. Nursing care includes: ■ Maintain a relaxed, quiet environment. ■ Monitor weight. ■ Vigilant oral hygiene.
16.3 Describe the maternal and fetal-neonatal risks, clinical manifestations, and diagnosis in determining the nursing care management of a pregnant woman with a hypertensive disorder.	1. Hypertension may exist before pregnancy or, more often, may develop during pregnancy. 2. Preeclampsia can lead to growth retardation for the fetus. 3. Untreated preeclampsia may lead to seizures and death of the mother and infant. 4. It is important to educate the mother about the disease process. This may help motivate her to maintain the required rest periods in the left lateral recumbent position. 5. Antihypertensive and anticonvulsive drugs may be used.
16.4 Relate the cause, fetal-neonatal risks, prevention, and clinical therapy to the nursing care management of the woman at risk for Rh alloimmunization.	1. Rh incompatibility can occur when an Rh-negative woman and an Rh-positive partner conceive a child who is Rh positive. 2. Use of Rh immune globulin has greatly decreased the incidence of severe complications resulting from Rh incompatibility, because the drug "tricks" the body into thinking antibodies have been produced in response to the Rh antigens.
16.5 Explain the occurrence, cause, clinical treatment, and implications for the fetus or newborn in determining the nursing care management of a woman at risk for ABO incompatibility.	1. ABO incompatibility occurs when the mother has type O blood and the infant has A, B, or AB. 2. Unlike Rh incompatibility, no treatment exists to prevent the occurrence. 3. It creates hyperbilirubinemia in the infant, which is treated with phototherapy.
16.6 Examine the effects of surgical procedures in the nursing care management of the pregnant woman requiring surgery.	1. During surgery, a wedge is placed under the mother's hip to prevent compressing vessels while the mother is supine. 2. Pregnancy may hinder diagnosis because of the risk x-rays pose to the developing fetus. 3. Surgery increases the risk of miscarriage, preterm labor, and growth retardation in the fetus.
16.7 Relate the impact of trauma caused by an accident to the nursing care management of the pregnant woman or her fetus.	1. Trauma during pregnancy increases the risk of bleeding, a result of the increased blood volume of the mother. 2. The types of trauma that are of most concern are blunt trauma, penetrating injuries, and gunshot wounds. 3. Treatment centers on lifesaving measures to the mother. 4. Mother and fetus should be monitored after an accident even if no injury is apparent.

LEARNING OUTCOMES — CONCEPTS

16.8 Delineate the needs and care of the pregnant woman who experiences abuse.

1. The nurse needs to be alert for signs of abuse, including bruising or injury to the breasts, abdomen, or genitalia.
2. The woman should be given information about female partner abuse and about community resources available to assist her.

16.9 Explain the causes, fetal-neonatal risks, and clinical therapy in the nursing care management of the pregnant woman with a perinatal infection affecting the fetus.

1. Toxoplasmosis, rubella, cytomegalovirus, herpes, GBS, and other perinatal infections pose a grave threat to the fetus.
2. Prevention is the best therapy.
3. There is no known treatment for rubella or CMV, but antimicrobial drugs are available for toxoplasmosis, herpes, and GBS.

CRITICAL THINKING IN ACTION

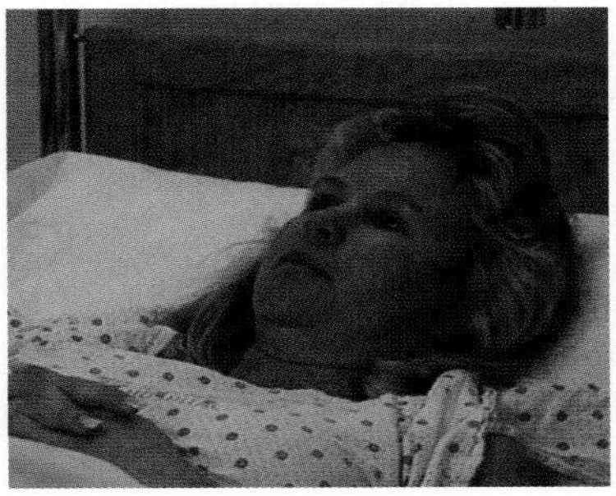

Carol Smith, a 40-year-old, single, G2, P0010, presents to you at 32 weeks' gestation while you are working in the birthing unit. Her chief complaint is severe headache, nausea, and trouble seeing. She describes "blackened areas" in her visual fields bilaterally. Her prenatal record reveals long-term substance abuse, depression, and hypertension currently treated with nifedipine 60 mg by mouth once in the morning. You note that she has had two prenatal visits with this pregnancy. You determine her blood pressure to be 170/110; deep tendon reflexes are 3+, clonus negative. She has general edema and 3+ proteinuria. You place Carol on the external fetal monitor to observe for fetal well-being and any contractions. You position her on her left side with her head elevated and use pillows for comfort. You observe that the fetal heart rate is 143–148 with decreased long-term variability. No fetal heart rate decelerations or accelerations are noted. The uterus is soft, and no contractions are palpated or noted on the fetal monitor.

Carol asks you why she should stay on her left side.

1. How would you explain the importance of the left side-lying position when on bed rest?
2. You administer nifedipine 10 mg sublingual and a loading dose of magnesium sulfate 4 gm IV piggyback to the main IV line of Ringer's lactate. What findings would indicate that Carol has therapeutic levels of magnesium?
3. What signs of magnesium toxicity should you monitor Carol for?
4. Carol asks if magnesium sulfate will affect her infant. How would you answer her?
5. Which signs of premature labor would you ask Carol to notify you of if she experiences?

See MyNursingKit for possible responses.

REFERENCES

American Academy of Pediatrics (AAP) & American College of Obstetricians and Gynecologists (ACOG). (2007). Obstetric and medical complications. In *Guidelines for perinatal care* (6th ed.). Elk Grove Village, IL: Author.

American College of Obstetricians and Gynecologists (ACOG). (1999a). *Domestic violence.* (ACOG Educational Bulletin No. 257). Washington, DC: Author.

American College of Obstetricians and Gynecologists (ACOG). (2004). *Diagnosis and treatment of gestational trophoblastic disease.* (ACOG Practice Bulletin No. 53). Washington, DC: Author.

American College of Obstetricians and Gynecologists (ACOG). (2004a). *Diagnosis and treatment of gestational trophoblastic disease.* (ACOG Practice Bulletin No. 53). Washington, DC: Author.

American College of Obstetricians and Gynecologists (ACOG). (2004b). *Nausea and vomiting of pregnancy.* (ACOG Practice Bulletin No. 52). Washington, DC: Author.

American College of Obstetricians and Gynecologists (ACOG). (2006). *Management of alloimmunization during pregnancy.* (ACOG Practice Bulletin No. 75). Washington, DC: Author.

Baxter, J. K., & Weinstein, L. (2004). HELLP syndrome: The state of the art. *Obstetrical & Gynecological Survey, 59*(12), 838–845.

Berkowitz, R. S., & Goldstein, D. P. (2005). Gestational trophoblastic diseases. In W. J. Hoskins, C. A. Perex, R. C. Young, , R. R. Barakat, M. Markman, & M. E. Randall (Eds.). *Principles and practice of gynecologic oncology.* Philadelphia: Lippincott Williams & Wilkins.

Berman, M. L., Di Saia, M. J., & Tewari, K. S. (2004). Pelvic malignancies, gestational trophoblastic neoplasia, and nonpelvic malignancies. In R. K. Creasy, R. Resnik, & J. Iams (Eds.). *Maternal fetal medicine* (5th ed.). Philadelphia: Saunders.

Bernstein, H. (2007). Maternal and perinatal infections—viral. In S. G. Gabbe, J. R. Niebyl, & J. L. Simpson (Eds.), *Obstetrics: Normal and problem pregnancies* (5th ed.). Philadelphia: Churchill Livingstone.

Bess, K. A., & Wood, T. L. (2006).Understanding gestational trophoblastic disease: How nurses can help those dealing with a diagnosis. *AWHONN Lifelines, 10*(4), 321–326.

Blackburn, S. T. (2007). *Maternal, fetal, and neonatal physiology: A clinical perspective* (3rd ed.). St. Louis: Saunders.

Briggs, G. G., Freeman, R. K., & Yaffee, S. J. (2005). Betamethasone. In G. G. Briggs, R. K. Freeman, & S. J. Yaffee (Eds.), *Drugs in pregnancy and lactation* (7th ed.). Philadelphia: Lippincott Williams & Wilkins.

Cappell, M. S. (2007). Hepatitis and gastrointestinal diseases. In S. G. Gabbe, J. R. Niebyl, and J. L. Simpson (Eds.). *Obstetrics: Normal and problem pregnancies* (5th ed.). Philadelphia: Churchill Livingstone.

Centers for Disease Control and Prevention (CDC). (2006). Sexually transmitted diseases treatment guidelines, 2006. *Morbidity and Mortality Weekly Report, 55*(RR-11), 1–93.

Copeland, L. J., & Landon, M. B. (2007). Malignant diseases and pregnancy. In S. G. Gabbe, J. R. Niebyl, and J. L. Simpson (Eds.). *Obstetrics: Normal and problem pregnancies* (5th ed.). Philadelphia: Churchill Livingstone.

Cunningham, F. G., Leveno, K. J., Bloom, S. L., Hauth, J. C., Rouse, D. J., & Spong, C. Y. (2010.) *Williams obstetrics* (23rd ed.). New York: McGraw-Hill Medical.

Davies, J. K., & Gibbs, R. S. (2008). Obstetric and perinatal infections. In R. S. Gibbs, B. Y. Karlan, A. F. Haney, & I. E. Nygaard (Eds.), *Danforth's obstetrics and gynecology* (10th ed.). Philadelphia: Wolters Kluwer/Lippincott Williams & Wilkins.

Dodds, L., Fell, D. B., Joseph, K. S., Allen, V. M., & Butler, B. (2006). Outcomes of pregnancy complicated by hyperemesis gravidarum. *Obstetrics and Gynecology, 107,* 285–292.

Duff, P. (2007). Maternal and perinatal infection—bacterial. In S. G. Gabbe, J. R. Niebyl, and J. L. Simpson (Eds.). *Obstetrics: Normal and problem pregnancies* (5th ed.). Philadelphia: Churchill Livingstone.

Easterwood, B. (2004). Silent lullabies: Helping parents cope with early pregnancy loss. *AWHONN Lifelines, 8*(4), 356–360.

Farag, K., Hassan, I., & Ledger, W. (2004). Prediction of preeclampsia: Can it be achieved? *Obstetrical & Gynecological Survey, 59*(6), 464–482.

Ghulmiyyah, L. M., & Sibai, B. M. (2006). Managing an eclamptic seizure and its aftermath. *Contemporary OB/GYN, 51*(3), 54–66.

Gibbs, R. S., Sweet, R. L., & Duff, W. P. (2004). Maternal and fetal infectious disorders. In R. K. Creasy, R. Resnik, & J. Iams (Eds.), *Maternal fetal medicine* (5th ed.). Philadelphia: Saunders.

Gonik, B., & Foley, M. R. (2004). Intensive care monitoring of the critically ill pregnant patient. In R. K. Creasy, R. Resnik, & J. Iams (Eds.), *Maternal fetal medicine* (5th ed.). Philadelphia: Saunders.

Habli, M., & Sibai, B. M. (2008). Hypertensive disorders of pregnancy. In R. S. Gibbs, B. Y. Karlan, A. F. Haney, & I. E. Nygaard (Eds.), *Danforth's obstetrics and gynecology* (10th ed.). Philadelphia: Wolters Kluwer/Lippincott Williams & Wilkins.

Harville, E. W., Wilcox, A. J., Bird, D. D., & Weinberg, C. R. (2004). Vaginal bleeding in very early pregnancy. *Obstetrical & Gynecological Survey, 59*(3), 172–173.

Hill, J., Roberts, S. (2005). Herpes simplex virus in pregnancy: New concepts in prevention and management. *Clinics in Perinatology, 32*(3), 657–670.

Hollier, L. M., & Grissom, H. (2005). Human herpes viruses in pregnancy: Cytomegalovirus, epstein-barr virus, and varicella zoster virus. *Clinics in Perinatology, 32*(3), 671–696.

Kady, D. E., Gilbert, W. M., Xing, G., & Smith, L. H. (2005). Maternal and neonatal outcomes of assaults during pregnancy. *Obstetrics & Gynecology, 105*(2), 357–363.

Katz, V., Balderston, K., & DeFreest, M. (2005). Perimortem cesarean delivery: Were our assumptions correct? *American Journal of Obstetrics & Gynecology, 192*(6), 1916–1921.

Krakow, D. (2008). Medical and surgical complications of pregnancy. In R. S. Gibbs, B. Y. Karlan, A. F. Haney, & I. E. Nygaard (Eds.), *Danforth's obstetrics and gynecology* (10th ed.). Philadelphia: Wolters Kluwer/Lippincott Williams & Wilkins.

Lagiou, P., Tamimi, R., Mucci, L. A., Trichopoulos, D., Adami, H-O., Shieh, C-C. (2003). Nausea and vomiting in pregnancy in relation to prolactin, estrogen, and progesterone: A prospective study. *Obstetrics & Gynecology, 101*(4), 639–644.

Landry, M. L. (2004). Viral infections. In G. N. Burrow, T. P. Duffy, & J. A. Copel (Eds.), *Medical complications during pregnancy* (6th ed.). Philadelphia: Elsevier Saunders.

Li, A. J. (2008). Gestational trophoblastic neoplasms. In R. S. Gibbs, B. Y. Karlan, A. F. Haney, & I. E. Nygaard (Eds.). *Danforth's obstetrics and gynecology* (10th ed.). Philadelphia: Wolters Kluwer/ Lippincott Williams & Wilkins.

Li, D., Janevic, T., Odouli, R., & Liyan, L. (2003). Hot tub use during pregnancy and the risk of miscarriage. *American Journal of Epidemiology, 158,* 931–937.

Lipscomb, G. H., Givens, V. M., Meyer, N. L., & Bran, D. (2005) Comparison of multidose and single-dose methotrexate protocols for the treatment of ectopic pregnancy. *American Journal of Obstetrics & Gynecology, 192*(6), 1844–1848.

Lu, E. J., & Curet, M. J. (2007). Surgical procedures in pregnancy. In S. G. Gabbe, J. R. Niebyl, & J. L. Simpson (Eds.), *Obstetrics: Normal and problem pregnancies* (5th ed.). Philadelphia: Churchill Livingstone.

Ludmir, J., & Owen, J. (2007). Cervical incompetence. In S. G. Gabbe, J. R. Niebyl, & J. L. Simpson (Eds.), *Obstetrics: Normal and problem pregnancies* (5th ed.). Philadelphia: Churchill Livingstone.

McDonald, S. D., Malinowski, A., Zhou, Q., Yusuf, S. & Devereaux, P. J. (2008) Cardiovascular sequelae of preeclampsia/eclampsia: A systematic review and meta-analyses. *American Heart Journal, 156*(5), 918–930.

Montoya, J. G., & Rosso, F. (2005). Diagnosis and management of toxoplasmosis. *Clinics in Perinatology, 32*(3), 705–726.

National Coalition Against Domestic Violence (NCADV). (2007). Reproductive health and pregnancy. Retrieved November 16, 2008, from www.ncadv.org

Okun, N., Gronau, K. A., & Hannah, M. E. (2005). Antibiotics for bacterial vaginosis or trichomonas vaginalis in pregnancy: A systematic review. *Obstetrics & Gynecology, 105*(4), 857–868.

Ramirez, M. M., & Mastrobattista, J. M. (2005). Diagnosis and management of human parvovirus B19 infection. *Clinics in Perinatology, 32*(3), 697–704.

Rumbold, A., Duley, L., Crowther, A., & Haslam, R. (2008). Antioxidants for preventing pre-eclampsia. *Cochrane Database of Systematic Reviews.* Issue 1. Art. No.: CD004227.

Schauberger, C. W., Mathiason, M. A., & Rooney, B. L. (2005). Ultrasound assessment of first-trimester bleeding. *Obstetrics & Gynecology, 105*(2), 333–338.

Scott, L. D., & Abu-Hamda, E. (2004). Gastrointestinal disease in pregnancy. In R. K. Creasy, R. Resnik, & J. Iams (Eds.), *Maternal fetal medicine* (5th ed.). Philadelphia: Saunders.

Seeber, B. E., & Barnhart, K. T. (2008). Ectopic pregnancy. In R. S. Gibbs, B. Y. Karlan, A. F. Haney, & I. E. Nygaard (Eds.). *Danforth's obstetrics and gynecology* (10th ed.). Philadelphia: Wolters Kluwer/Lippincott Williams & Wilkins.

Sibai, B. M. (2005). Diagnosis, prevention, and management of eclampsia. *Obstetrics and Gynecology, 105*(2), 402–410.

Sibai, B. M. (2007). Hypertension. In S. G. Gabbe, J. R. Niebyl, & J. L. Simpson (Eds.), *Obstetrics: Normal and problem pregnancies* (5th ed.). Philadelphia: Churchill Livingstone.

Simpson, J. L., & Jauniaux, R. M. (2007). Pregnancy loss. In S. G. Gabbe, J. R. Niebyl, and J. L. Simpson (Eds.). *Obstetrics: Normal and problem pregnancies* (5th ed.). Philadelphia: Churchill Livingstone.

Van Den Eeden, S. K., Shan, J., Bruce, C., & Glasser, M. (2005). Ectopic pregnancy rate and treatment utilization in a large managed care organization. *Obstetrics & Gynecology, 105*(5) pt. 1, 1052–1057.

Wiggens, D. A., & Elliott, M. (2005). Outcomes of pregnancies achieved by donor egg in vitro fertilization—A comparison with standard in vitro fertilization pregnancies. *American Journal of Obstetrics and Gynecology, 192*(6), 2002–2008.

Yudin, M. H. (2005). Bacterial vaginosis in pregnancy: Diagnosis, screening, and management. *Clinics in Perinatology, 32,* 617–627.

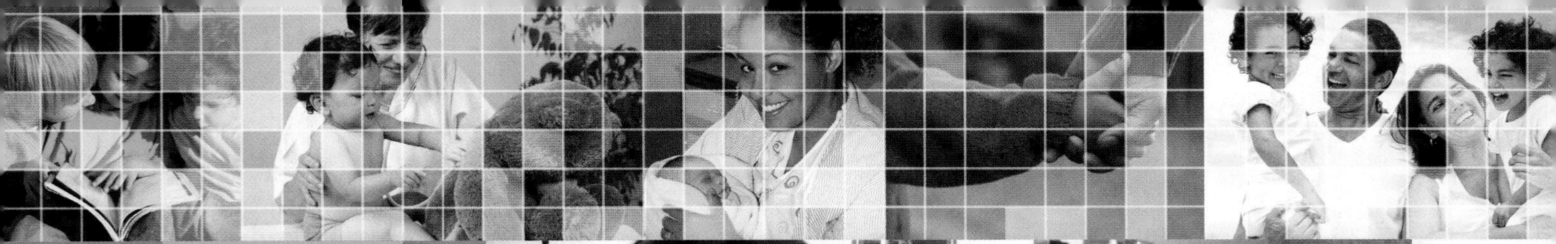

PART

4

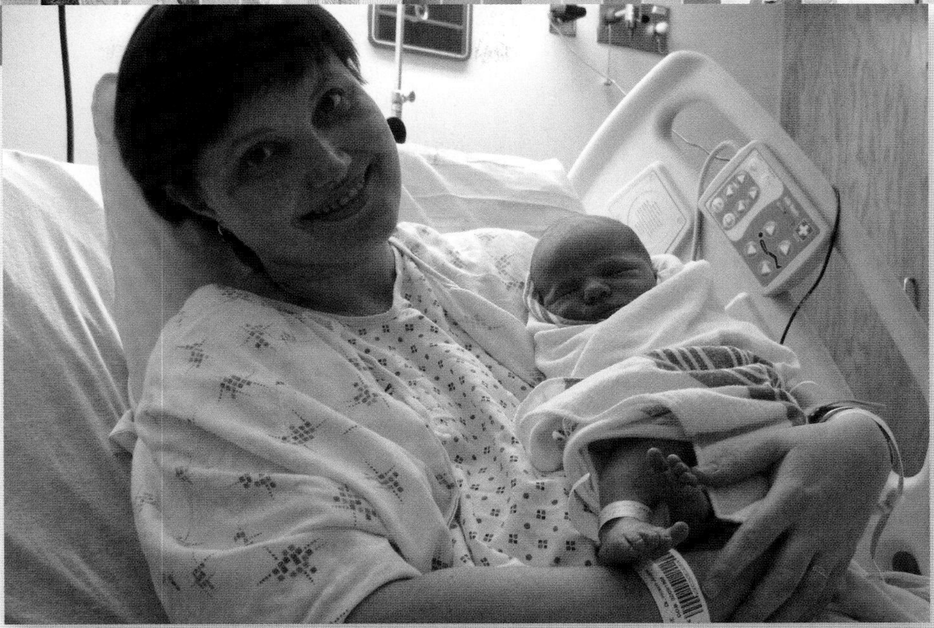

Birth and the Family

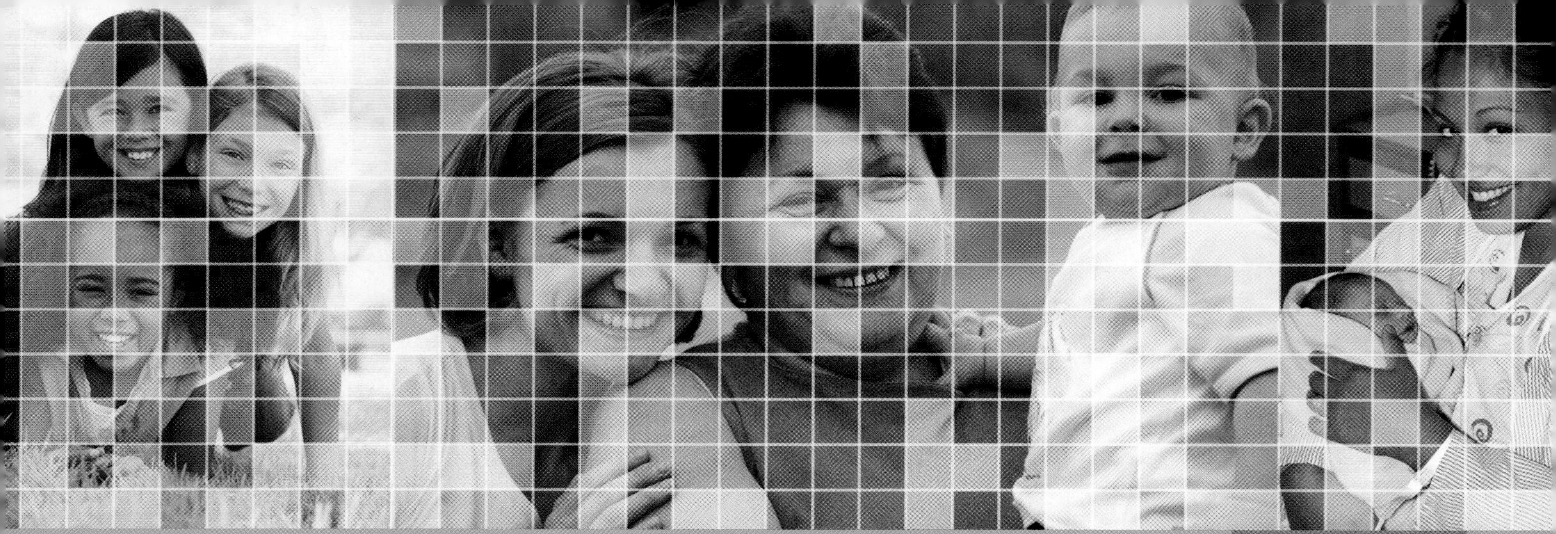

CHAPTER

Processes and Stages of Labor and Birth 17

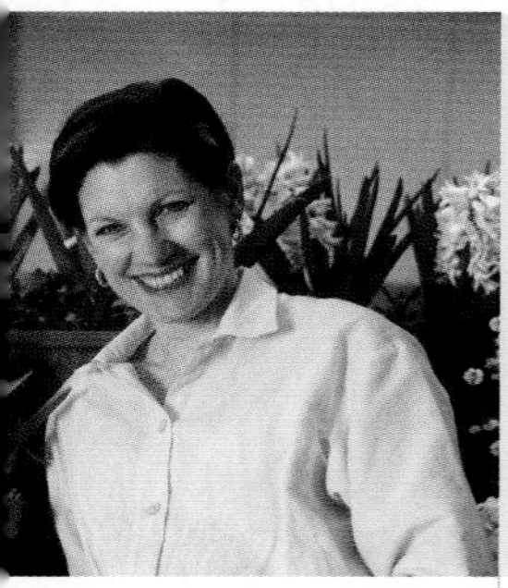

I think experts refer to us as a blended family. I have two sons, ages 12 and 9, from a previous marriage. They live part-time with us and part-time with their father. My husband has a 15-year-old daughter who lives with her mother. Here I am, 6 months pregnant with our first child together. It has been quite the time, getting used to the idea of a baby and trying to include our children in the pregnancy. They have all heard the heartbeat and felt the baby move. My sons are pretty blasé about it. I didn't know how Jack's daughter would respond but she has been great. Maybe this new baby will help us all grow closer together. I sure hope so. —*Letetia, 34*

LEARNING OUTCOMES

17.1 Describe the five critical factors that influence labor in the assessment of an expectant woman's and fetus's progress in labor and birth.

17.2 Examine an expectant woman's and fetus's response to labor based on the physiological processes that occur during labor.

17.3 Assess for the premonitory signs of labor when caring for the expectant woman.

17.4 Differentiate between false and true labor.

17.5 Describe the physiologic and psychologic changes occurring in an expectant woman during each stage of labor in the nursing care management of the expectant woman.

17.6 Explain the maternal systemic response to labor in the nursing care of an expectant woman.

17.7 Examine fetal responses to labor.

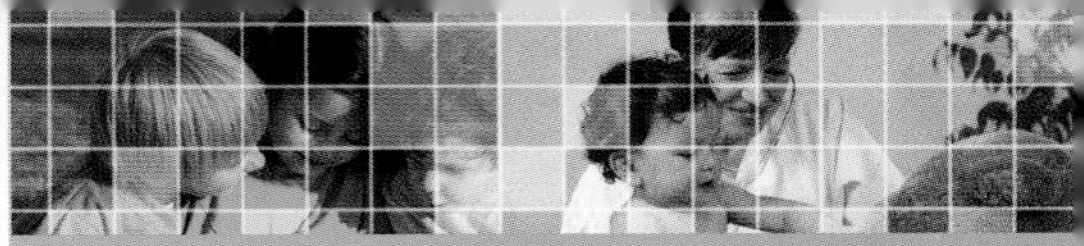

KEY TERMS

Artificial rupture of membranes (AROM), 374
Bloody show, 373
Breech presentation, 366
Cardinal movements, 376
Crowning, 375
Duration, 370
Effacement, 371
Engagement, 367
Fetal attitude, 366
Fetal lie, 366
Fetal position, 367
Fetal presentation, 366
Fontanelles, 364
Frequency, 370
Intensity, 370
Lightening, 373
Malpresentations, 366
Molding, 364
Presenting part, 366
Spontaneous rupture of membranes (SROM), 374
Station, 367
Sutures, 364

In the final weeks of pregnancy, both mother and baby begin to prepare for birth. The onset of labor begins a remarkable change in the relationship between the woman and her baby. In those hours and moments, the birth process may seem to carry all the power in the universe. The mother-to-be and her partner may feel stretched beyond their normal limits of concentration, purpose, endurance, and pain as they work to bring forth a precious new life.

This chapter focuses on the processes and stages of labor. Subsequent chapters describe intrapartum assessment and nursing care.

CRITICAL FACTORS IN LABOR

Five factors are of critical importance in the process of labor and birth: the passage, the fetus, the relationship between the passage and the fetus, the physiologic forces of labor, and the psychosocial considerations. Abnormalities that affect any component of these critical forces can alter the outcome of labor and jeopardize both the expectant woman and her baby. These factors are described in this section and summarized in Table 17–1. (Labor-related complications are discussed in Chapter 22.)

THE BIRTH PASSAGE

The true pelvis, which forms the bony canal through which the fetus must pass, is divided into three sections: the inlet, the pelvic cavity (midpelvis), and the outlet. (See Chapter 3 for discussion of the pelvis and Chapter 10 for assessment techniques.)

The Caldwell-Moloy classification of pelvises is widely used to differentiate bony pelvis types. The four classic types of pelvis are *gynecoid, android, anthropoid,* and *platypelloid* (Caldwell & Moloy, 1933) (Figure 17–1 ●). The gynecoid, or female, pelvis is most common. All diameters of the gynecoid are adequate for childbirth. Implications of each type of pelvis for childbirth are summarized in Table 17–2.

Table 17–1 Critical Factors in Labor

Critical Factors	Components
The birth passage	■ Size of the pelvis (diameters of the pelvic inlet, midpelvis or pelvic cavity, and outlet) ■ Type of pelvis (gynecoid, android, anthropoid, platypelloid, or a combination) ■ Ability of the cervix to dilate and efface and ability of the vaginal canal and the external opening of the vagina (the introitus) to distend
The fetus	■ Fetal head (size and presence of molding) ■ Fetal attitude (flexion or extension of the fetal body and extremities) ■ Fetal lie ■ Fetal presentation (the part of the fetal body entering the pelvis first in a single- or multiple-gestation pregnancy) ■ Placenta (implantation site)
The relationship between the passage and the fetus	■ Engagement of fetal presenting part ■ Station (location of fetal presenting part within the maternal pelvis) ■ Fetal position (relationship of the presenting part to one of the four quadrants of the maternal pelvis)
Physiologic forces of labor	■ Frequency, duration, and intensity of uterine contractions as the fetus moves through the birth passage ■ Effectiveness of the maternal pushing effort ■ Duration of labor
Psychosocial considerations	■ Physical preparation for childbirth ■ Sociocultural values and beliefs ■ Previous childbirth experience ■ Support from significant others ■ Emotional status

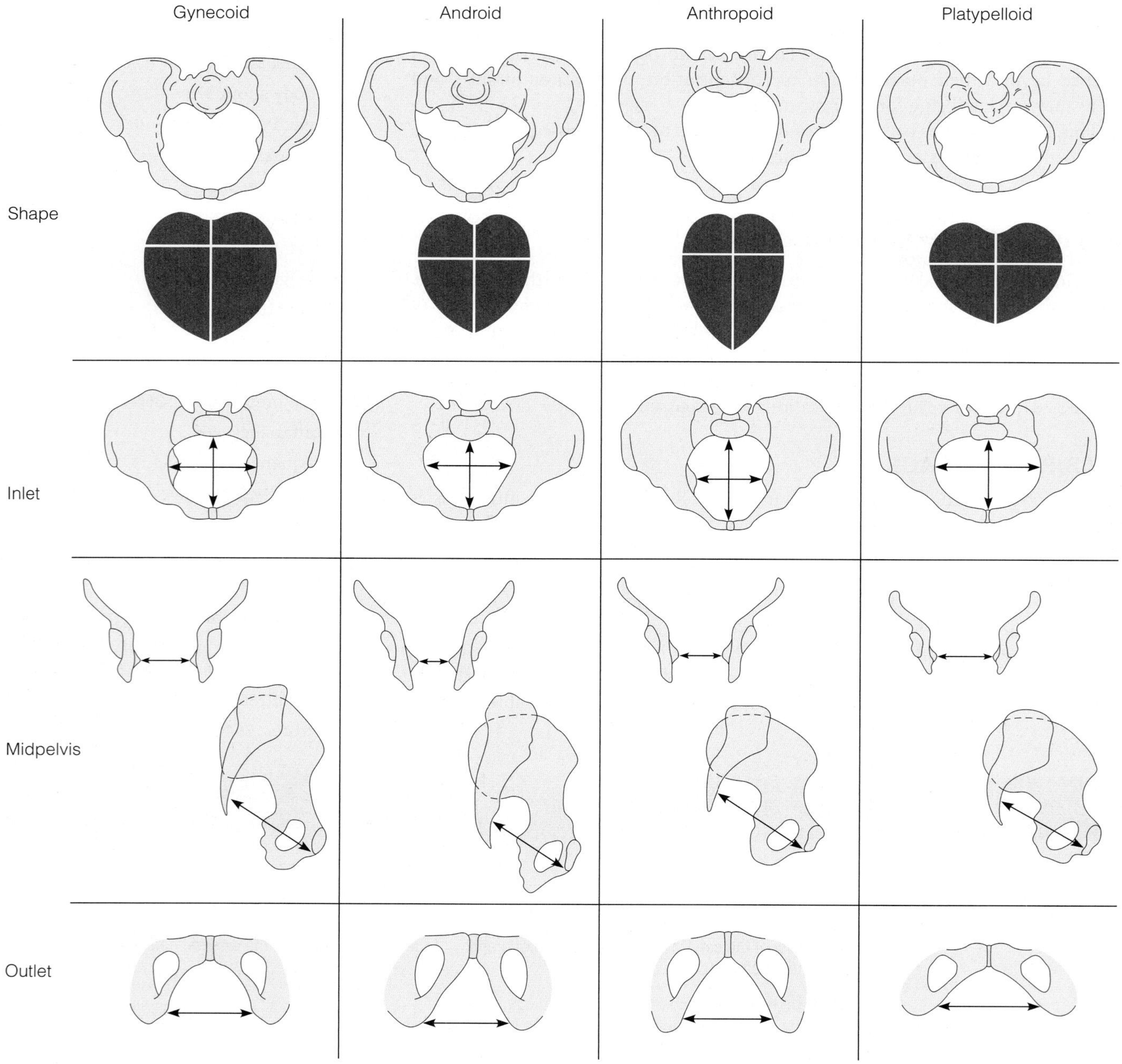

● **Figure 17–1** Comparison of Caldwell-Moloy pelvic types.

THE FETUS

Fetal Head

The fetal skull (cranium) has three major parts: the face, the base of the skull, and the vault of the cranium (roof). The bones of the face and cranial base are well fused and essentially fixed. The base of the cranium is composed of the two temporal bones, each with a sphenoid and ethmoid bone. The bones composing the vault are the two frontal bones, the two parietal bones, and the occipital bone (Figure 17–2 ●). These bones are not fused, so this portion of the head can adjust in shape as the presenting part passes through the narrow portions of the pelvis. The cranial bones overlap under pressure of the powers of labor and the demands of the unyielding pelvis. This overlapping is called **molding**. Once the head (the least compressible and largest part of the fetus) has been born, the birth of the rest of the body is rarely delayed.

The **sutures** of the fetal skull are membranous spaces between the cranial bones. The intersections of the cranial sutures are called **fontanelles**. These sutures allow for molding of the fetal head and help the clinician to identify the position of the fetal head during vaginal examination. The important sutures of the cranium are as follows (see Figure 17–2):

- *Frontal (mitotic) suture:* located between the two frontal bones; becomes the anterior continuation of the sagittal suture

Table 17–2 Implications of Pelvic Type for Labor and Birth

Pelvic Type	Pertinent Characteristics	Implications for Birth
Gynecoid	Inlet rounded with all inlet diameters adequate Midpelvis diameters adequate with parallel side walls Outlet adequate	Favorable for vaginal birth
Android	Inlet heart-shaped, with short posterior sagittal diameter Midpelvis diameters reduced Outlet capacity reduced	Not favorable for vaginal birth Descent into pelvis is slow Fetal head enters pelvis in transverse or posterior position, with arrest of labor frequent
Anthropoid	Inlet oval in shape, with long anteroposterior diameter Midpelvis diameters adequate Outlet adequate	Favorable for vaginal birth
Platypelloid	Inlet oval in shape, with long transverse diameters Midpelvis diameters reduced Outlet capacity inadequate	Not favorable for vaginal birth Fetal head engages in transverse position Difficult descent through midpelvis Frequent delay of progress at outlet of pelvis

Note: Description of pelvic shape is exaggerated for easier comprehension.

- *Sagittal suture:* located between the parietal bones; divides the skull into left and right halves; runs anteroposteriorly, connecting the two fontanelles
- *Coronal sutures:* located between the frontal and parietal bones; extend transversely left and right from the anterior fontanelle
- *Lambdoidal suture:* located between the two parietal bones and the occipital bone; extends transversely left and right from the posterior fontanelle

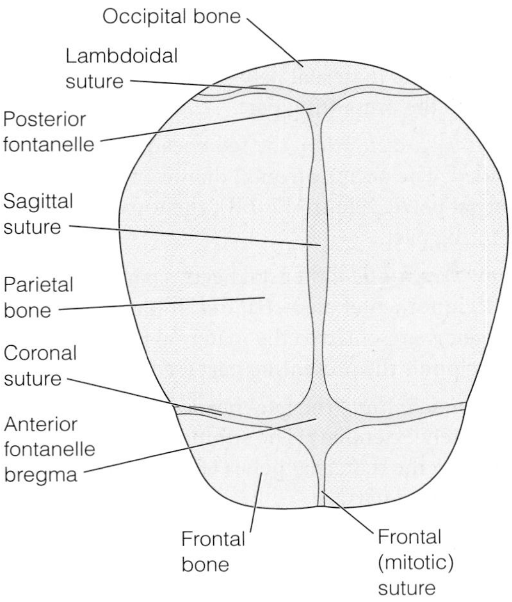

● **Figure 17–2** Superior view of the fetal skull.

The anterior and posterior fontanelles are clinically useful (along with the sutures) in identifying the position of the fetal head in the pelvis and in assessing the status of the newborn after birth. The anterior fontanelle is diamond shaped and measures about 2 cm by 3 cm. It permits growth of the brain by remaining unossified for as long as 18 months. The posterior fontanelle is much smaller and closes within 8 to 12 weeks after birth. It is shaped like a small triangle and marks the meeting point of the sagittal suture and the lambdoidal suture.

Following are several important landmarks of the fetal skull (Figure 17–3 ●):

- *Mentum:* fetal chin
- *Sinciput:* anterior area known as the brow

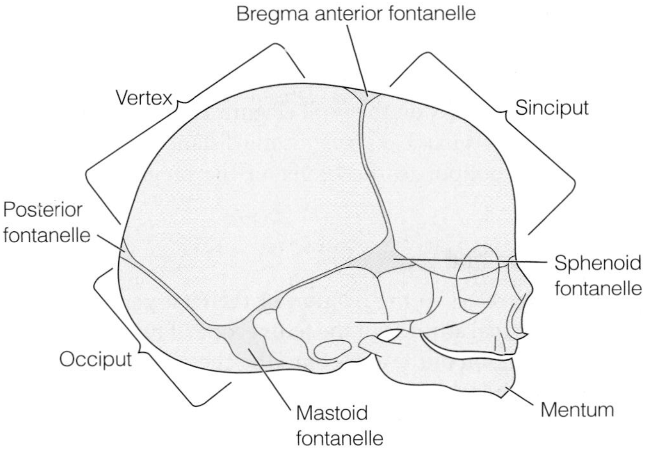

● **Figure 17–3** Lateral view of the fetal skull. This figure identifies the landmarks that have significance during birth.

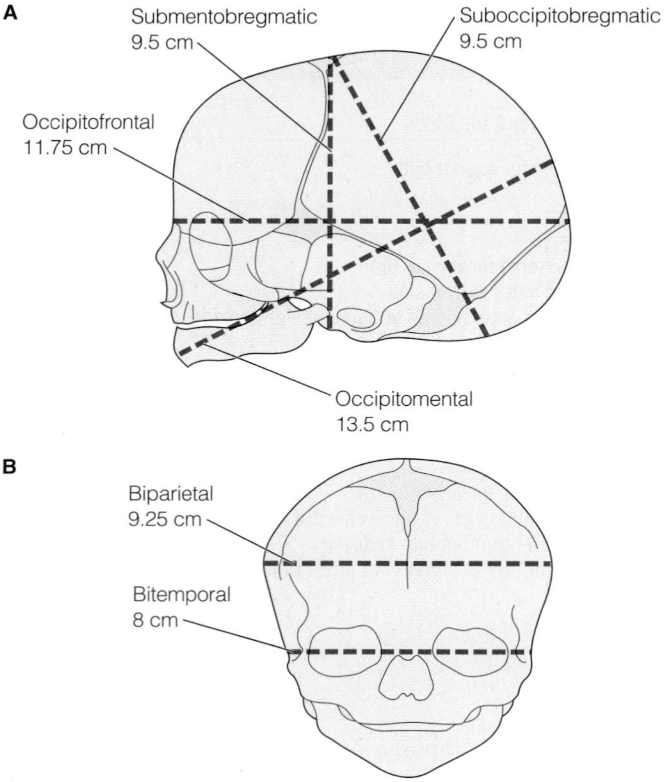

● **Figure 17–4** Fetal skull measurements. ***A,*** Typical anteroposterior diameters of the fetal skull. When the vertex of the fetus presents and the fetal head is flexed with the chin on the chest, the smallest anteroposterior diameter (suboccipitobregmatic) enters the birth canal. ***B,*** Transverse diameters of the fetal skull.

MyNursingKit Video: Fetal Lie

- *Bregma:* large diamond-shaped anterior fontanelle
- *Vertex:* area between the anterior and posterior fontanelles
- *Posterior fontanelle:* intersection between posterior cranial sutures
- *Occiput:* area of the fetal skull occupied by the occipital bone, beneath the posterior fontanelle

The diameters of the fetal skull vary considerably within normal limits. Some diameters shorten and others lengthen as the head is molded during labor. Fetal head diameters are measured between the various landmarks on the skull (Figure 17–4 ●). For example, the suboccipitobregmatic diameter is the distance from the undersurface of the occiput to the center of the bregma, or anterior fontanelle.

Fetal Attitude and Fetal Lie

Fetal attitude refers to the relation of the fetal parts to one another. The normal attitude of the fetus is one of moderate flexion of the head, flexion of the arms onto the chest, and flexion of the legs onto the abdomen (Figure 17–5 ●).

Fetal lie refers to the relationship of the cephalocaudal axis (spinal column) of the fetus to the cephalocaudal axis of the woman. The fetus may assume either a longitudinal or a transverse lie. A *longitudinal lie* occurs when the cephalocaudal axis of the fetus is parallel to the woman's spine. A *transverse lie* occurs when the cephalocaudal axis of the fetus is at a right angle to the woman's spine.

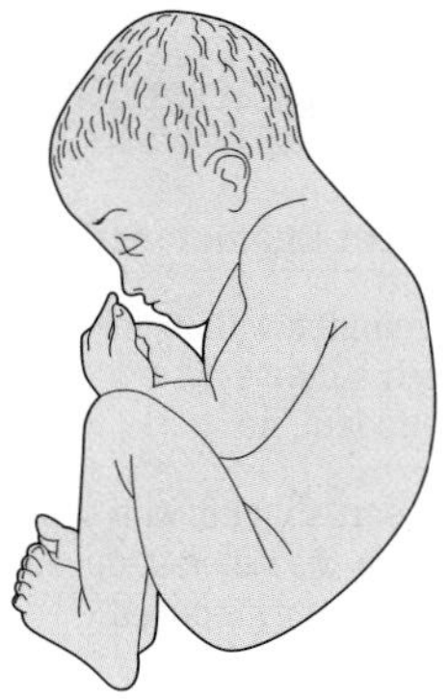

● **Figure 17–5** Fetal attitude. The attitude (or relationship of body parts) of this fetus is normal. The head is flexed forward, with the chin almost resting on the chest. The arms and legs are flexed.

Fetal Presentation

Fetal presentation is determined by fetal lie and by the body part of the fetus that enters the pelvic passage first. This portion of the fetus is referred to as the **presenting part**. Fetal presentation may be cephalic, breech, or shoulder. Cephalic presentation, in which the fetal head presents itself to the passage, occurs in approximately 97% of term births. When this presentation occurs, labor and birth are likely to proceed normally. Breech and shoulder presentations are associated with difficulties during labor, and labor does not proceed as expected; therefore, they are called **malpresentations** (see Chapter 22 ∞ for discussion).

The cephalic presentation can be further classified according to the degree of flexion or extension of the fetal head (attitude).

- In *vertex presentation,* the most common presentation, the fetal head is completely flexed onto the chest, and the smallest diameter of the fetal head (suboccipitobregmatic) presents to the maternal pelvis (Figure 17–6A ●). The occiput is the presenting part.
- In *military presentation,* the fetal head is neither flexed nor extended. The occipitofrontal diameter presents to the maternal pelvis (Figure 17–6B); the top of the head is the presenting part.
- In *brow presentation,* the fetal head is partially extended. The occipitomental diameter, the largest anteroposterior diameter, is presented to the maternal pelvis (Figure 17–6C); the sinciput is the presenting part (see Figure 17–3).
- In *face presentation,* the fetal head is hyperextended (completely extended). The submentobregmatic diameter presents to the maternal pelvis (Figure 17–6D); the face is the presenting part.

Breech presentation is a birth in which the buttocks and/or feet are the presenting part rather than the head. It occurs in 3% to 4% of term pregnancies. These presentations are classified according to the attitude of the fetus's hips and knees. In all varia-

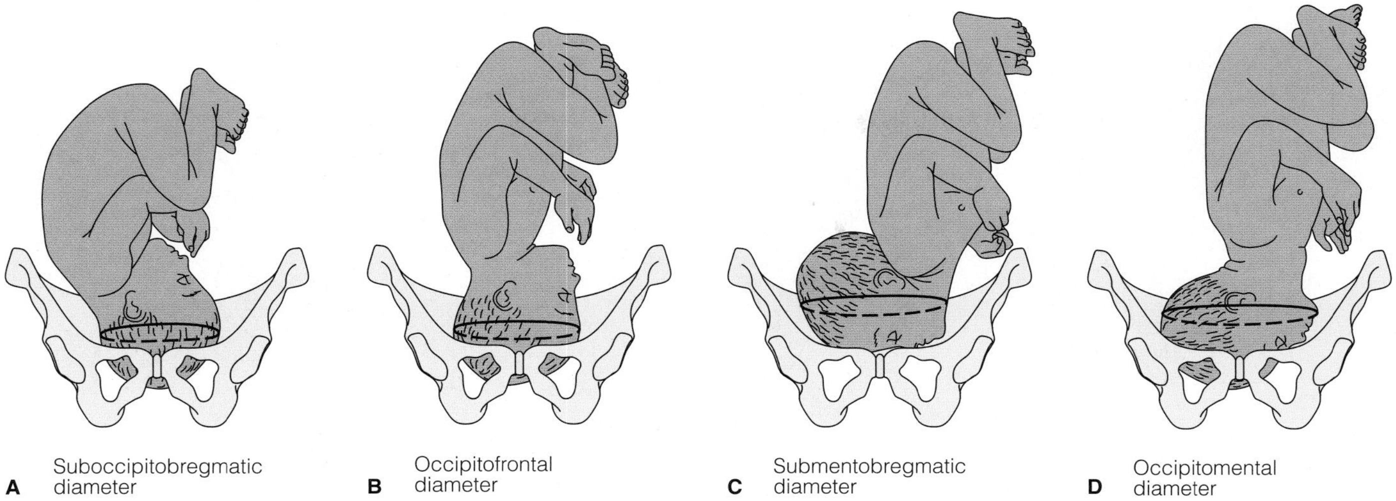

● **Figure 17–6** Cephalic presentation. ***A,*** Vertex presentation. Complete flexion of the head allows the suboccipitobregmatic diameter to present to the pelvis. ***B,*** Military (median vertex) presentation with no flexion or extension. The occipitofrontal diameter presents to the pelvis. ***C,*** Brow presentation. The fetal head is in partial (halfway) extension. The occipitomental diameter, which is the largest diameter of the fetal head, presents to the pelvis. ***D,*** Face presentation. The fetal head is in complete extension, and the submentobregmatic diameter presents to the pelvis.

tions of the breech presentation, the sacrum is the landmark to be noted.

In *complete breech,* the fetal knees and hips are both flexed; the thighs are on the abdomen, and the calves are on the posterior aspect of the thighs. The buttocks and feet of the fetus present to the maternal pelvis. (Refer to Figure 22–7∞.)

In *frank breech,* the fetal hips are flexed, and the knees are extended. The buttocks of the fetus present to the maternal pelvis.

In *footling breech,* the fetal hips and legs are extended, and the feet of the fetus present to the maternal pelvis. In a single footling, one foot presents; in a double footling, both feet present.

A shoulder presentation is also called a *transverse lie.* Most frequently the shoulder is the presenting part and the acromion process of the scapula is the landmark to be noted. However, the fetal arm, back, abdomen, or side may present in a transverse lie. (See Chapter 22∞.)

RELATIONSHIP BETWEEN THE MATERNAL PELVIS AND PRESENTING PART

Engagement

Engagement of the presenting part occurs when the largest diameter of the presenting part reaches or passes through the pelvic inlet (Figure 17–7 ●). Engagement can be determined by vaginal examination. In primigravidas, engagement occurs approximately 2 weeks before term. Multiparas, however, may experience engagement several weeks before the onset of labor or during the process of labor. Engagement confirms the adequacy of the pelvic inlet. Engagement does not, however, indicate whether the midpelvis and outlet are also adequate.

Station

Station refers to the relationship of the presenting part to an imaginary line drawn between the ischial spines of the maternal pelvis. In a normal pelvis, the ischial spines mark the narrowest diameter through which the fetus must pass. These spines are not sharp protrusions that harm the fetus but blunted prominences at the midpelvis. The ischial spines as a landmark have been designated as zero station (Figure 17–8 ●). If the presenting part is higher than the ischial spines, a negative number is assigned, noting centimeters above zero station. Positive numbers indicate that the presenting part has passed the ischial spines. Station –5 is at the pelvic inlet, and station +4 is at the outlet. If the presenting part can be seen at the woman's perineum, birth is imminent. During labor the presenting part should move progressively from the negative stations to the midpelvis at zero station and into the positive stations. If the presenting part fails to descend in the presence of strong contractions, there may be disproportion between the maternal pelvis and fetal presenting part.

MyNursingKit Animation: Vaginal Birth

Fetal Position

Fetal position refers to the relationship of a designated landmark on the presenting fetal part to the front, sides, or back of the maternal pelvis. The landmark chosen for vertex presentations is the occiput, and the landmark for face presentations is the mentum. In breech presentations the sacrum is the designated landmark, and the acromion process on the scapula is the landmark in shoulder presentations. If the landmark is directed toward the side of the pelvis, fetal position is designated as *transverse,* rather than anterior or posterior. Three notations are used to describe fetal position:

1. Right (R) or left (L) side of the maternal pelvis
2. The landmark of the fetal presenting part: occiput (O), mentum (M), sacrum (S), or acromion process (A)
3. Anterior (A), posterior (P), or transverse (T), depending on whether the landmark is in the front, back, or side of the pelvis

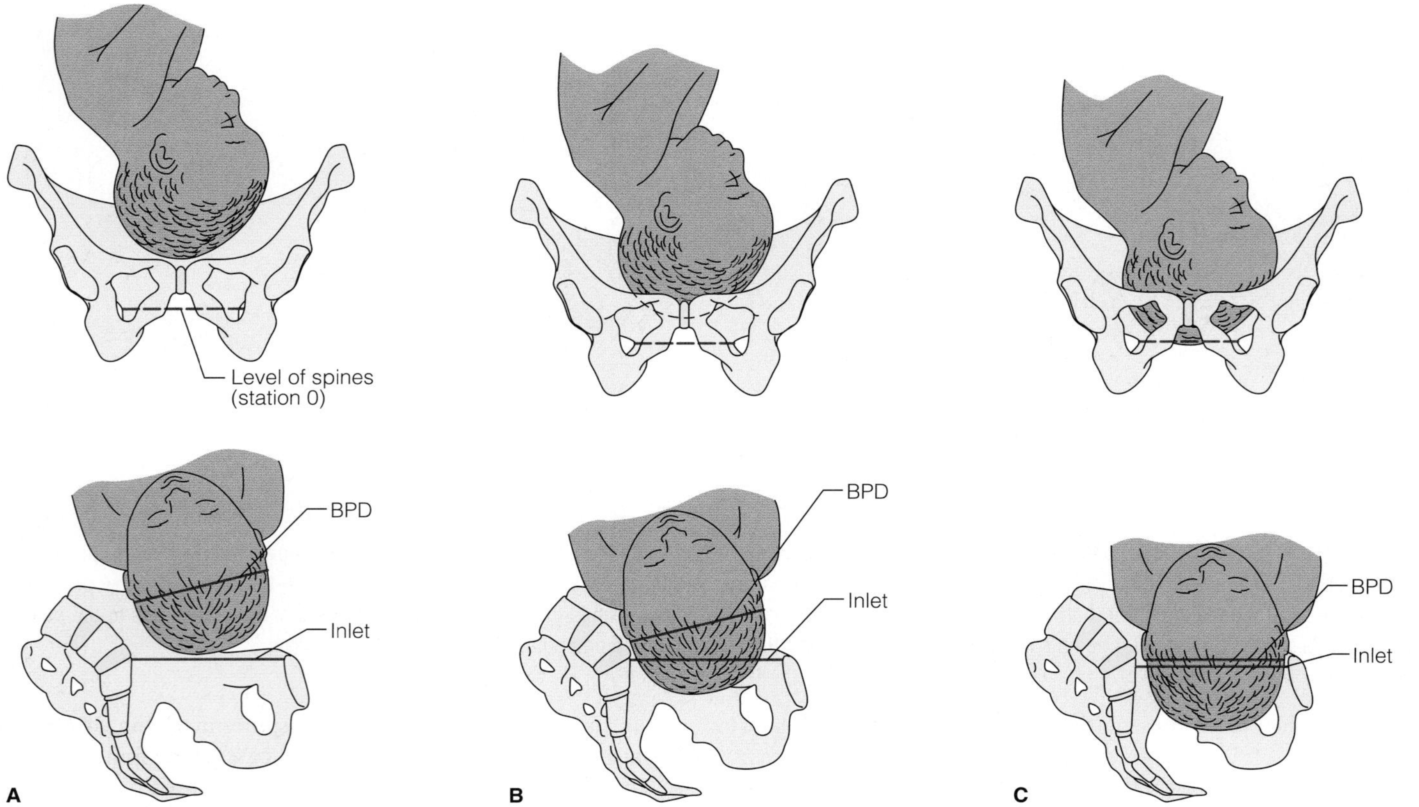

● **Figure 17–7** Process of engagement in cephalic presentation. ***A,*** Floating. The fetal head is directed down toward the pelvis but can still easily move away from the inlet. ***B,*** Dipping. The fetal head dips into the inlet but can be moved away by exerting pressure on the fetus. ***C,*** Engaged. The biparietal diameter (BPD) of the fetal head is in the inlet of the pelvis. In most instances the presenting part (occiput) is at the level of the ischial spines (zero station).

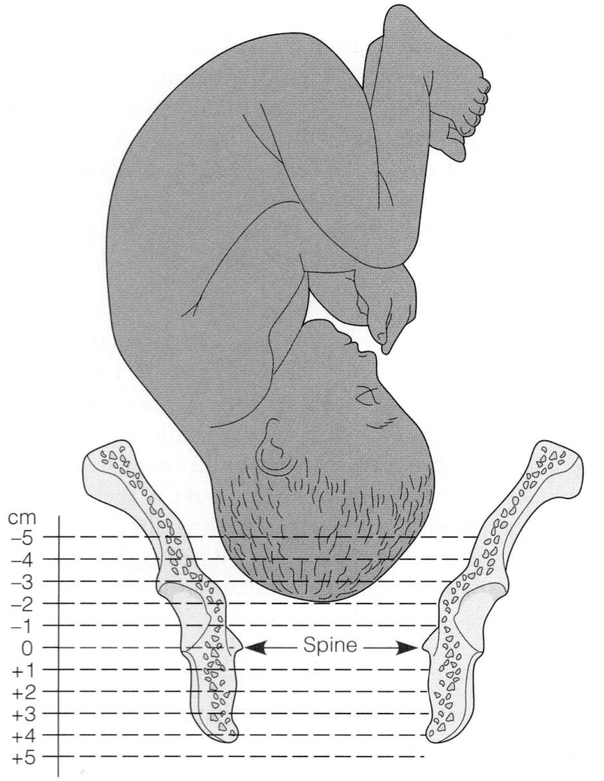

● **Figure 17–8** Measuring the station of the fetal head while it is descending. In this view the station is -2/-3.

These abbreviations help the health care team communicate the fetal position. Thus when the fetal occiput is directed toward the back and left of the birth passage, the abbreviation used is LOP (left occiput posterior). The term *dorsal* (D) is used when denoting the fetal position in a transverse lie; it refers to the fetal back. For example, RADA indicates that the acromion process of the scapula is directed toward the woman's right, and the fetus's back is anterior.

The most frequently occurring positions are illustrated in Figure 17–9 ●. The most common fetal position is occiput anterior. When this position occurs, labor and birth are likely to proceed normally. Positions other than occiput anterior are more frequently associated with problems during labor; therefore, they are called *malpositions.* (See Chapter 22 ∞.)

Assessment techniques to determine fetal position include inspection and palpation of the maternal abdomen and vaginal examination. They are discussed in Chapter 18 ∞.

PHYSIOLOGIC FORCES OF LABOR

Primary and secondary forces work together to achieve birth of the fetus, the fetal membranes, and the placenta. The *primary force* is uterine muscular contractions, which cause the complete effacement and dilatation of the cervix. The *secondary force* is the use of abdominal muscles to push during the second stage of labor. The pushing adds to the primary force after full dilatation.

In labor, uterine contractions are rhythmic but intermittent. Between contractions a period of relaxation occurs. This allows

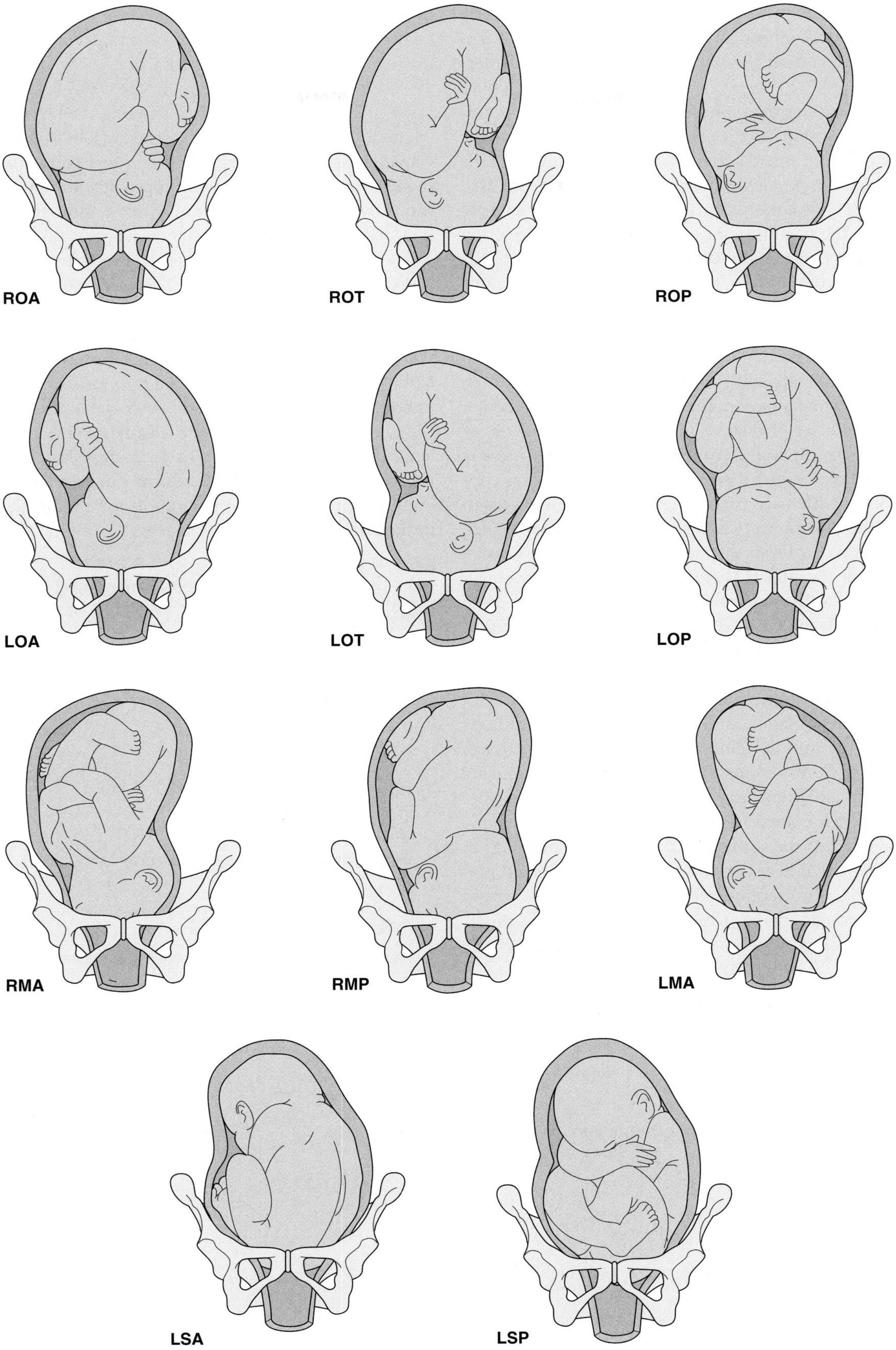

Figure 17–9 Categories of presentation.

uterine muscles to rest and provides relief for the laboring woman. It also restores uteroplacental circulation, which is important to fetal oxygenation and adequate circulation in the uterine blood vessels.

Each contraction has three phases: (1) *increment,* the building up of the contraction (the longest phase); (2) *acme,* or the peak of the contraction; and (3) *decrement,* or the letting up of the contraction. The terms *frequency, duration,* and *intensity* are used to describe uterine contractions during labor. **Frequency** refers to the time between the beginning of one contraction and the beginning of the next contraction. **Duration** is measured from the beginning of a contraction to the completion of that same contraction (Figure 17–10 ●). **Intensity** refers to the strength of the contraction during acme. In most instances, intensity is estimated by palpating the uterine fundus during a contraction, but it may be measured directly with an intrauterine catheter. When estimating intensity by palpation, the nurse determines whether it is mild, moderate, or strong by judging the amount of indentability of the uterine wall during the acme of a contraction. If the uterine wall can be indented easily, the contraction is considered mild. Strong intensity exists when the uterine wall cannot be indented. Moderate intensity falls somewhere between. When intensity is measured with an intrauterine catheter, the normal resting pressure in the uterus (between contractions) averages 10 to 12 mm Hg. During acme the intensity ranges from 25 to 40 mm Hg in early labor, 50 to 70 mm Hg in active labor, 70 to 90 mm Hg during transition, and 70 to 100 mm Hg while the woman is pushing in the second stage (Funai, Evans, & Lockwood, 2008). (See Chapter 18 ∞ for further discussion of assessment techniques.)

At the beginning of labor, contractions are usually mild. As labor progresses, the duration, intensity, and frequency of contractions increase. Contractions are involuntary; the laboring woman cannot control their duration, frequency, or intensity.

After the cervix is completely dilated, the maternal abdominal muscles contract as the woman pushes. This pushing action (called *bearing down*) aids in the expulsion of the fetus and placenta. If the cervix is not completely dilated, however, bearing down can cause cervical edema (which retards dilatation), possible tearing and bruising of the cervix, and maternal exhaustion.

PSYCHOSOCIAL CONSIDERATIONS

The final critical factor influencing labor outcome is the parents' psychosocial readiness. Similar psychosocial factors affect the mother and the father if he is involved. Both are making a transition to a new role, and both have expectations of themselves during the labor and birth experience.

Although many expectant mothers and fathers attend childbirth preparation classes, they still tend to be concerned about what labor will be like, whether they will be able to perform the way they expect, whether the discomfort and pain will be more than the mother expects or can cope with, and whether the father can provide helpful support. A woman approaching her first labor faces a totally new experience, whereas the woman who has given birth before knows that each labor is unique and different. Most women wonder if they will live up to their expectations for themselves; whether they will be injured through laceration, episiotomy, or cesarean incision; and whether loved ones will be supportive. They must also deal with concerns about loss of control of body functions, emotional responses to an unfamiliar situation, and reactions to the pain associated with labor.

Various factors influence a woman's reaction to the challenge of labor (Table 17–3). Her accomplishment of the tasks of pregnancy, usual coping mechanisms in response to stressful life events, support system, preparation for childbirth, and cultural influences are all significant factors.

Table 17–3 Factors Associated with a Positive Birth Experience

Motivation for the pregnancy
Attendance at childbirth education classes
A sense of competence or mastery
Self-confidence and self-esteem
Positive relationship with mate
Perception of maintaining control during labor
Support from mate or other person during labor
Not being left alone in labor
Trust in the medical and nursing staff
Having personal control of breathing patterns, comfort measures
Choosing a physician or certified nurse-midwife who has a similar philosophy of care
Receiving clear information regarding procedures

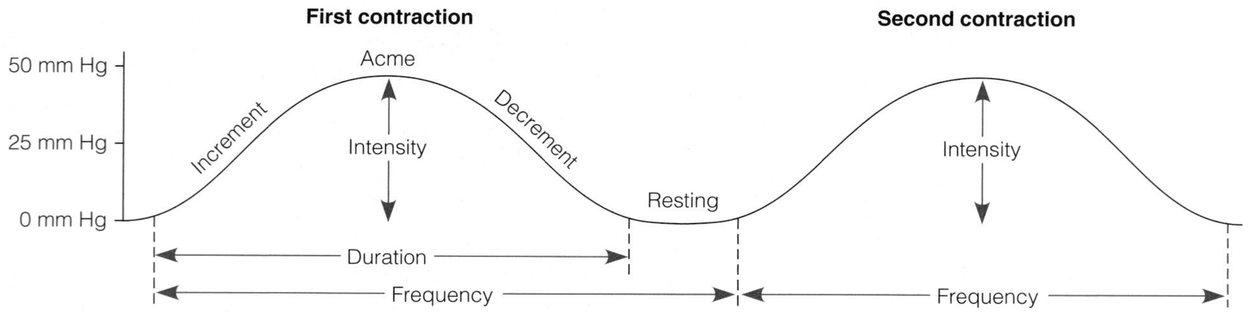

● **Figure 17–10** Characteristics of uterine contractions.

Pregnant women mentally prepare for labor through meaningful actions and imaginary rehearsal. The actions frequently consist of "nesting behavior" (housecleaning, decorating the nursery) and a "psyching up" for the labor, which varies depending on the woman's self-confidence, self-esteem, and previous experiences with stress. Specific actions to prepare for labor may focus on becoming better informed and prepared. Just as a woman tries on the maternal role during pregnancy, fantasizing about labor seems to help her understand and become better prepared for it. Fantasies about the excitement of the baby's birth and the sharing of the experience are positive forms of preparation. Many pregnant women have dreams about their infant, labor, birth, and parenting. These dreams may result from sleep deprivation, rapid eye movement sleep deprivation, and altered hormone levels (Nielson & Paquette, 2007).

Some women fear the pain of contractions and associate it with a loss of control over their bodies and emotions. Other women see pain as a rite of passage to motherhood and a necessary means to an end. It is helpful for women to realize that the discomfort and stresses of labor are natural. Assurances that labor is progressing normally and that the woman is "doing a good job" can go a long way toward reducing anxiety and thereby reducing pain. Women are likely to feel empowered and better able to cope with labor if they recognize that maintaining control is not important or perhaps even possible. A wide variety of coping techniques to assist both the laboring woman and her partner are discussed in Chapter 19 ∞ and Chapter 20 ∞.

The laboring woman's support system may also influence the course of labor and birth. Although some women prefer not to have a support person or family member with them, most women choose to have a significant person or persons (partner, family member, close friend) with them for support and encouragement. A labor partner's presence at the bedside provides a means to enhance communication and to demonstrate feelings of love. Communication needs may include talking and the use of affectionate and understanding words from the partner. Showing love may take the form of holding hands, hugging, or touching or gentle reassurance for the woman.

How the woman views the birth experience in hindsight may have implications for mothering behaviors. It appears that any activities by the expectant mother or by healthcare providers that enhance the birth experience are beneficial to the mother-baby connection. The father's experience of childbirth and his opportunities for bonding may have important implications for fathering as well.

Complementary Care

MUSIC DURING CHILDBIRTH

The therapeutic use of music to help with pain management is becoming increasingly popular. Research suggests that soft music can help decrease both the sensation of labor pain and a woman's response to it. With this in mind, the woman should choose her music selections in advance so that she is prepared when labor begins. She can also be advised to bring her own MP3, MP4, or CD player, so she does not have to rely on the availability of equipment in the birthing area (Zwelling, Johnson, & Allen, 2006).

THE PHYSIOLOGY OF LABOR

POSSIBLE CAUSES OF LABOR ONSET

The process of labor usually begins between the 38th and the 42nd week of gestation, when the fetus is mature and ready for birth. The exact cause of labor onset is not clearly understood. However, some important aspects have been identified: progesterone relaxes smooth muscle tissue, estrogen stimulates uterine muscle contractions, and connective tissue loosens to permit the softening, thinning, and eventual opening of the cervix (Blackburn, 2007). Currently, researchers are focusing on the role of fetal membranes (chorion and amnion), the decidua, and the effect of progesterone withdrawal, of prostaglandin, and of corticotropin-releasing hormone in relation to labor onset (Blackburn, 2007).

Progesterone Withdrawal Hypothesis

Progesterone, produced by the placenta, relaxes uterine smooth muscle by interfering with the conduction of impulses from one cell to the next. During pregnancy, progesterone exerts a quieting effect and the uterus generally does not have coordinated contractions. Toward the end of gestation, biochemical changes decrease the availability of progesterone to myometrial cells and may be associated with an antiprogestin that inhibits the relaxant effect but allows other progesterone actions such as lactogenesis. With the decreased availability of progesterone, estrogen is better able to stimulate contractions (Blackburn, 2007). Interestingly, progesterone administration is now used as a mechanism to prevent preterm labor and birth (Szekeres-Bartho, Wilczynski, Basta, et al., 2008).

Prostaglandin Hypothesis

Although the exact relationship between prostaglandin and the onset of labor is not yet known, the effect is clinically demonstrated by the successful induction of labor after vaginal application of prostaglandin E. Preterm labor may be stopped by using an inhibitor of prostaglandin synthesis. Oxytocin may also play a role in the process in two ways: first by direct stimulation of uterine contractions and second, indirectly, by stimulating prostaglandin production by the amnion and decidua (Kilpatrick & Garrison, 2007).

Corticotropin-Releasing Hormone

Corticotropin-releasing hormone (CRH) has a possible role in labor onset. It increases throughout pregnancy, with a sharp increase at term. Plasma CRH is also increased before preterm labor, and CRH levels are elevated in multiple gestation. CRH is known to stimulate the synthesis of prostaglandin F and prostaglandin E by amnion cells (Vogel, Thorsen, Currey, et al., 2005).

MYOMETRIAL ACTIVITY

In true labor the muscles of the upper uterine segment shorten and exert a longitudinal pull on the cervix with each contraction, causing effacement. **Effacement** is the drawing up of the internal os and the cervical canal into the side walls of the uterus. The

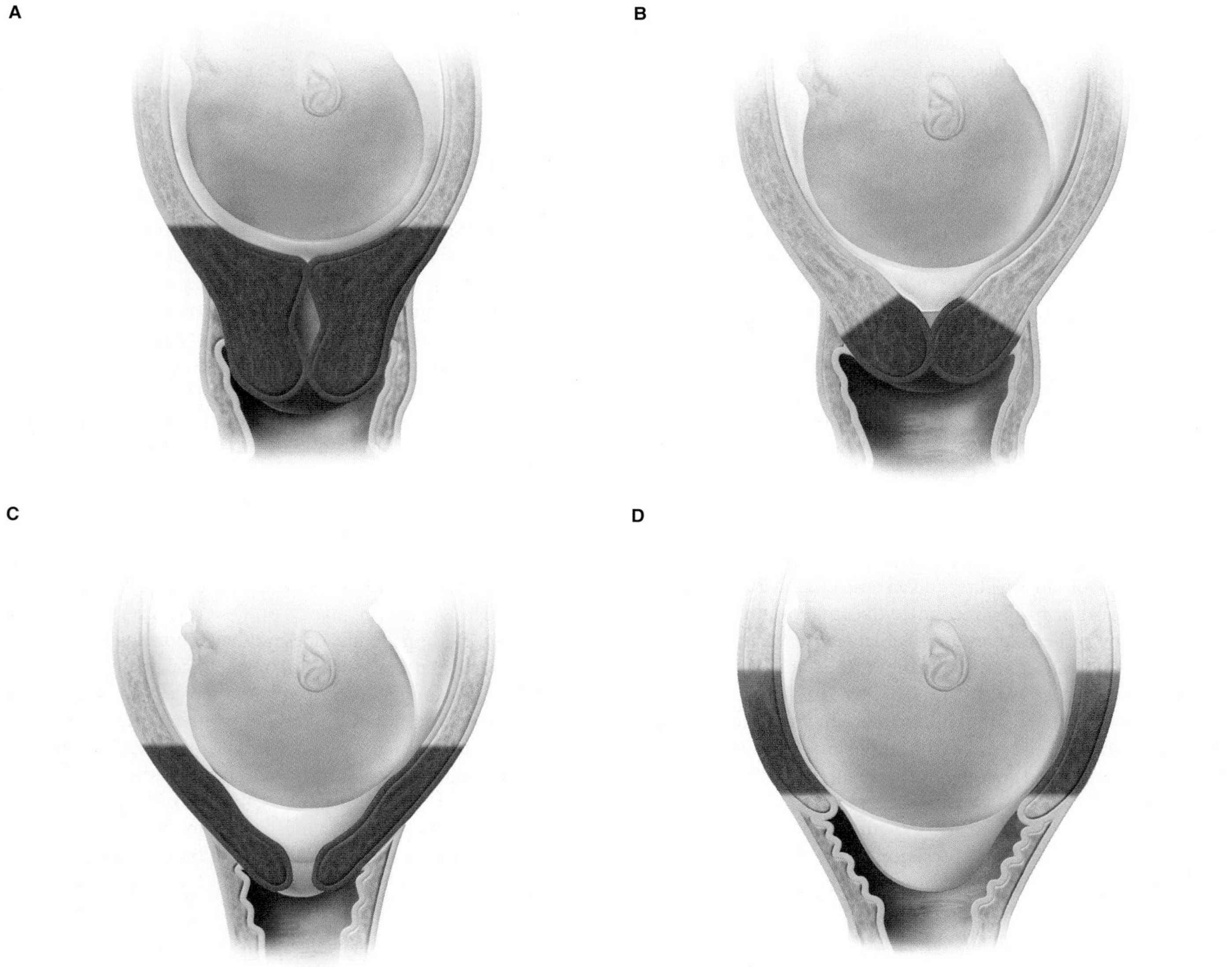

● **Figure 17–11** Effacement of the cervix in the primigravida. ***A,*** Beginning of labor. There is no cervical effacement or dilatation. The fetal head is cushioned by amniotic fluid. ***B,*** Beginning cervical effacement. As the cervix begins to efface, more amniotic fluid collects below the fetal head. ***C,*** Cervix about one half effaced and slightly dilated. The increasing amount of amniotic fluid exerts hydrostatic pressure. ***D,*** Complete effacement and dilatation.

cervix changes progressively from a long, thick structure to one that is tissue-paper thin (Figure 17–11 ●). In primigravidas, effacement usually occurs before dilatation.

The uterus elongates with each contraction, decreasing the horizontal diameter. This elongation causes a straightening of the fetal body, pressing the upper portion against the fundus and thrusting the presenting part down toward the lower uterine segment and the cervix. The pressure exerted by the fetus is called the *fetal axis pressure.* As the uterus elongates, the longitudinal muscle fibers are pulled upward over the presenting part. This action and the hydrostatic pressure of the fetal membranes cause cervical dilatation. The cervical os and cervical canal widen from less than 1 cm to approximately 10 cm, allowing birth of the fetus. When the cervix is completely dilated and retracted up into the lower uterine segment, it can no longer be palpated. At the same time, the round ligament pulls the fundus forward, aligning the fetus with the bony pelvis.

MUSCULATURE CHANGES IN THE PELVIC FLOOR

The levator ani muscle and fascia of the pelvic floor draw the rectum and vagina upward and forward with each contraction, along the curve of the pelvic floor. As the fetal head descends to the pelvic floor, the pressure of the presenting part causes the perineal structure, which was once 5 cm in thickness, to thin, to less than 1 cm. The anus everts, exposing the interior rectal wall as the fetal head descends forward (Blackburn, 2007).

PREMONITORY SIGNS OF LABOR

Most primigravidas and many multiparas experience the following signs and symptoms of impending labor.

Nursing Practice

Encourage expectant mothers who experience a sudden burst of energy to eat small, frequent, nutritious meals during this period, and to rest. Encourage the pregnant woman to have her significant other or a friend do chores and activities that she feels are essential to complete before the baby arrives.

Lightening

Lightening describes the effects that occur when the fetus begins to settle into the pelvic inlet (engagement). With fetal descent the uterus moves downward, and the fundus no longer presses on the diaphragm, which allows breathing to become easier. However, with increased downward pressure of the presenting part, the woman may notice the following:

- Leg cramps or pains due to pressure on the nerves that pass through the obturator foramen in the pelvis
- Increased pelvic pressure
- Increased venous stasis, leading to edema in the lower extremities
- Increased vaginal secretions resulting from congestion of the vaginal mucous membranes

Braxton Hicks Contractions

Before the onset of labor, *Braxton Hicks contractions* (the irregular, intermittent contractions that have been occurring throughout the pregnancy) may become uncomfortable. The pain seems to be focused in the abdomen and groin but may feel like the "drawing" sensations experienced by some women with dysmenorrhea. When these contractions are strong enough for the woman to believe she is in labor, she is said to be in *false labor.* False labor is uncomfortable and may be exhausting. Since the contractions can be fairly regular, the woman has no way of knowing if they are true labor.

Cervical Changes

Considerable change occurs in the cervix during the prenatal and intrapartal period. At the beginning of pregnancy, the cervix is rigid and firm, and it must soften so it can stretch and dilate to allow the fetus passage. This softening of the cervix is called *ripening.*

As term approaches, collagen fibers in the cervix are broken down by certain enzymes. As the fibers change, their ability to bind together decreases, while the water content of the cervix increases. All these changes result in a weakening and softening of the cervix.

Bloody Show

During pregnancy, cervical secretions accumulate in the cervical canal to form a barrier called a *mucous plug.* With softening and effacement of the cervix, the mucous plug is often expelled, resulting in a small amount of blood loss from the exposed cervical capillaries. The resulting pink-tinged secretions are called **bloody show.** Bloody show is considered a sign that labor will begin within 24 to 48 hours. Vaginal examination that includes manipulation of the cervix may also result in a blood-tinged discharge, which may be confused with bloody show.

Rupture of Membranes

Approximately 8% of women at term (38 through 41 weeks' gestation) experience rupture of the amniotic membranes (ROM) before the onset of labor. After the membranes rupture, 50% of these women gave birth within 5 hours and 95% gave birth within 28 hours (ACOG, 2007). Women who are 34 weeks' gestation or more and who present with ruptured membranes without contractions are often started on an oxytocin infusion to decrease the incidence of chorioamnionitis. Women with preterm gestations of less than 34 weeks are managed conservatively provided both the mother and the fetus are stable (ACOG, 2007).

When the membranes rupture, the amniotic fluid may be expelled in large amounts. If engagement has not occurred, there is danger of the umbilical cord washing out with the fluid (prolapsed cord). In addition, the open pathway into the uterus increases the risk of infection. Because of these risks, when the membranes rupture, the woman is advised to call her certified nurse-midwife or physician and proceed to the hospital or birthing center. In some instances the fluid is expelled in small amounts and may be confused with episodes of urinary incontinence associated with urinary urgency, coughing, or sneezing. The discharge should be checked to determine its source and the appropriate action. (See Chapter 18 ∞ for assessment techniques.)

Sudden Burst of Energy

Some women report a sudden burst of energy approximately 24 to 48 hours before labor. The cause of the energy spurt is unknown. In prenatal teaching it is important to warn prospective mothers not to overexert themselves during this energy burst to avoid being overtired when labor begins.

Other Signs

Additional premonitory signs include the following:

- Weight loss of 1 to 3 lb resulting from fluid loss and electrolyte shifts produced by changes in estrogen and progesterone levels
- Diarrhea, indigestion, or nausea and vomiting just before onset of labor

The causes of these signs are unknown.

DIFFERENCES BETWEEN TRUE AND FALSE LABOR

The contractions of true labor produce progressive dilatation and effacement of the cervix. They occur regularly and increase in frequency, duration, and intensity. The discomfort of true labor contractions usually starts in the back and radiates around to the abdomen. The pain is not relieved by ambulation (in fact, walking may intensify the pain).

MyNursingKit Animation: Rupturing Membranes

Table 17–4 Comparison of True and False Labor

True Labor	False Labor
Contractions occur at regular intervals.	Contractions are irregular.
Interval between contractions gradually shortens.	Usually no change.
Contractions increase in duration and intensity.	Usually no change.
Discomfort begins in back and radiates around to abdomen.	Discomfort is usually in abdomen.
Intensity usually increases with walking.	Walking has no effect on or lessens contractions.
Cervical dilatation and effacement are progressive.	No change.

MyNursingKit Case Study: Client in First Stage of Labor

The contractions of false labor do not produce progressive cervical effacement and dilatation. Classically, they are irregular and do not increase in frequency, duration, and intensity. The contractions may be perceived as a hardening or "balling up" without discomfort, or discomfort may occur mainly in the lower abdomen and groin. The discomfort may be relieved by ambulation, changes of position, drinking a large amount of water, or a warm shower or tub bath (Edwards & Byrom, 2007). Many times the only way to differentiate accurately between true and false labor is to assess dilatation. The woman must feel free to come in for accurate assessment of labor and should be counseled not to feel foolish if the labor is false. She can be reassured that false labor is common and that it often cannot be distinguished from true labor except by vaginal examination (Table 17–4).

STAGES OF LABOR AND BIRTH

The labor process is divided into phases and stages of labor. These represent theoretic separations in the process. A laboring woman does not usually experience distinct differences from one stage to the next.

The *first stage* begins with the onset of true labor and ends when the cervix is completely dilated to 10 cm. The *second stage* begins with complete dilatation and ends with the birth of the baby. The *third stage* begins with the birth of the baby and ends with the expulsion of the placenta. Some clinicians identify a *fourth stage.* During this stage, which lasts 1 to 4 hours after expulsion of the placenta, the uterus contracts to control bleeding at the placental site (Edwards & Byrom, 2007).

MyNursingKit Video: First Stage of Labor and Transition

FIRST STAGE

The first stage of labor is divided into the *latent, active,* and *transition* phases. Each phase of labor is characterized by physical and psychologic changes.

Latent Phase

The *latent phase* starts with the beginning of regular contractions, which are usually mild. The woman feels able to cope with the discomfort. She may be relieved that labor has finally started. Although she may be anxious, she is able to recognize and express those feelings of anxiety. The woman is often talkative and smiling and is eager to talk about herself and answer questions. Excitement is high, and her partner or other support person is often as elated as she is.

Uterine contractions become established during the latent phase and increase in frequency, duration, and intensity. They may start as mild contractions lasting 30 seconds with a frequency of 10 to 30 minutes and progress to moderate ones lasting 30 to 40 seconds with a frequency of 5 to 7 minutes. As the cervix begins to dilate, it also effaces, although little or no fetal descent is evident. For a woman in her first labor (nullipara), the latent (or early) phase of the first stage of labor averages 8.6 hours but should not exceed 20 hours. The latent phase in multiparas averages 5.3 hours but should not exceed 14 hours.

At the beginning of labor, the amniotic membranes bulge through the cervix in the shape of a cone. **Spontaneous rupture of membranes (SROM)** generally occurs at the height of an intense contraction with a gush of fluid out of the vagina. In many instances the membranes are ruptured by the certified nurse-midwife or physician, using an instrument called an *amniohook.* This procedure is called *amniotomy,* or **artificial rupture of membranes (AROM)**.

Active Phase

When a woman enters the early *active phase,* her anxiety tends to increase as she senses the intensification of contractions and pain. She begins to fear a loss of control and may use a variety of coping mechanisms. Some women show decreased ability to cope and a sense of helplessness. Women who have support people and family available may feel greater satisfaction and less anxiety than those without support. During this phase the cervix dilates from about 4 cm to 7 cm. Fetal descent is progressive. Cervical dilatation averages 1.2 cm/hr in nulliparas and 1.5 cm/hr in multiparas.

Transition Phase

The *transition phase* is the last part of the first stage of labor. When the woman enters transition, she may show significant anxiety. She becomes acutely aware of the increasing force and intensity of the contractions. She may become restless, frequently changing posi-

Evidence in Action

Twelve contractions an hour is considered a meaningful signal that spontaneous birth is beginning or is imminent (prospective observational cohort study) (Pates, McIntire, & Leveno, 2006).

tion. By the time the woman enters the transition phase, she is inner directed and often tired. She may fear being left alone at the same time the support person may be feeling the need for a break. The nurse should reassure the woman that she will not be left alone. It is important to be available as relief support at this time and to keep the woman informed about where her labor support people are, if they leave the room.

During the active and transition phases, contractions become more frequent and longer in duration, and they increase in intensity. During transition, contractions have a frequency of about every 1 1/2 to 2 minutes, a duration of 60 to 90 seconds, and strong intensity. Cervical dilatation slows as it progresses from 8 to 10 cm, and the rate of fetal descent dramatically increases. The average rate of descent is 1.6 cm/hr and at least 1 cm/hr in nulliparas; the average rate is 5.4 cm/hr and at least 2.1 cm/hr in multiparas. The transition phase does not usually last longer than 3 hours for nulliparas or longer than 1 hour for multiparas (Edwards & Byrom, 2007).

As dilatation approaches 10 cm, the woman may feel increased rectal pressure and an uncontrollable desire to bear down, the amount of bloody show may increase, and the membranes may rupture (if it has not already occurred). The woman may also fear that she will be "torn open" or "split apart" by the force of the contractions. With the peak of a contraction, she may experience a sensation of pressure so great that it seems to her that her abdomen will burst open with the force. The nurse should inform the woman that what she is feeling is normal. The woman may doubt her ability to cope with labor and may become apprehensive, irritable, and withdrawn. She may be terrified of being left alone, though she does not want anyone to talk to or touch her. However, with the next contraction she may ask for verbal and physical support. Other characteristics of this phase may include the following:

- Increasing bloody show
- Hyperventilation, as the woman increases her breathing rate
- Generalized discomfort, including low backache, shaking and cramping in legs, and increased sensitivity to touch
- Increased need for partner's or nurse's presence and support
- Restlessness
- Increased apprehension and irritability
- Difficulty understanding directions
- A sense of bewilderment, frustration, and anger at the contractions

Developing Cultural Competence

PRESENCE OF THE FATHER

The presence of the father during labor and at birth, although common in countries such as the United States, Canada, and Australia, is not a universal norm. Rather it is strongly influenced by cultural practices. The father is not present at the birth in many countries, including Algeria, Brazil, China, Ethiopia, and Korea. Similarly, Orthodox Jews do not allow men to attend the labor and birth (Spector, 2009).

- Requests for medication
- Hiccuping, belching, nausea, or vomiting
- Beads of perspiration on the upper lip or brow
- Increasing rectal pressure and an urge to bear down

The woman in this phase is anxious to "get it over with." She may be amnesic and sleep between her frequent contractions. Her support persons may start to feel helpless and may turn to the nurse for increased help as their efforts to alleviate her discomfort seem less effective.

SECOND STAGE

MyNursingKit Video: Second Stage of Labor

The second stage of labor begins with complete cervical dilatation and ends with birth of the infant. The second stage is usually completed within 3 hours after the cervix becomes fully dilated for primigravidas; the stage averages 15 minutes for multiparas. Contractions continue with a frequency of about every 1 1/2 to 2 minutes, duration of 60 to 90 seconds, and strong intensity. Descent of the fetal presenting part continues until it reaches the perineal floor.

As the fetal head descends, the woman usually has the urge to push because of pressure of the fetal head on the sacral and obturator nerves. As she pushes, contraction of the maternal abdominal muscles exerts intra-abdominal pressure. As the fetal head continues its descent, the perineum begins to bulge, flatten, and move anteriorly. The amount of bloody show may increase. The labia begin to part with each contraction. Between contractions the fetal head appears to recede. With succeeding contractions and maternal pushing effort, the fetal head descends farther. **Crowning** occurs when the fetal head is encircled by the external opening of the vagina (introitus), and it means birth is imminent.

The woman may feel some relief that the acute pain she felt during the transition phase is over (Table 17–5). She may also be relieved that the birth is near and she can push. Some women feel a sense of purpose that they can be actively involved. Others, particularly those without childbirth preparation, may become frightened and fight each contraction. Such behavior may be disconcerting to the woman's support persons. The woman may feel she has lost her ability to cope and become embarrassed, or she may demonstrate extreme irritability toward the staff or her supporters as she attempts to regain control over forces against which she feels helpless. Most women feel acute, increasingly severe pain and a burning sensation as the perineum distends.

Table 17–5 Characteristics of Labor

	First Stage			Second Stage
	Latent Phase	Active Phase	Transition Phase	
Nullipara	8.6 hr	4.6 hr	3.6 hr	Up to 3 hr
Multipara	5.3 hr	2.4 hr	Variable	Less than 1 hr; averages 15 min
Cervical dilatation	0–3 cm	4–7 cm	8–10 cm	
Contractions				
Frequency	Every 10–30 min, progressing to every 5 to 7 min	Every 2–3 min	Every 1 1/2–2 min	Every 1 1/2–2 min
Duration	30–40 sec	40–60 sec	60–90 sec	60–90 sec
Intensity	Begin as mild and progress to moderate; 25–40 mm Hg by intrauterine pressure catheter (IUPC)	Begin as moderate and progress to strong; 50–70 mm Hg by IUPC	Strong by palpation; 70–90 mm Hg by IUPC	Strong by palpation; 70–100 mm Hg by IUPC

MyNursingKit Care Plan Activity: Labor Progress

Spontaneous Birth (Vertex Presentation)

As the fetal head distends the vulva with each contraction, the perineum becomes extremely thin and the anus stretches and protrudes. With time the head extends under the symphysis pubis and is born. When the anterior shoulder meets the underside of the symphysis pubis, a gentle push by the mother aids in the birth of the shoulders. The body then follows (Figure 17–12 ●). (Birth of a fetus in other than a vertex presentation is discussed in Chapter 22∞.)

Cardinal Movements of Labor

For the fetus to pass through the birth canal, the fetal head and body must adjust to the passage by certain positional changes. These changes, called **cardinal movements** or mechanisms of labor, are described in the order in which they occur (Figure 17–13 ●).

Descent. Descent occurs because of four forces: (1) pressure of the amniotic fluid, (2) direct pressure of the uterine fundus on the breech, (3) contraction of the abdominal muscles, and (4) extension and straightening of the fetal body. The head enters the inlet in the occiput transverse or oblique position because the pelvic inlet is widest from side to side. The sagittal suture is an equal distance from the maternal symphysis pubis and sacral promontory.

MyNursingKit Video: Third Stage of Labor

Flexion. Flexion occurs as the fetal head descends and meets resistance from the soft tissues of the pelvis, the muscles of the pelvic floor, and the cervix. As a result of the resistance, the fetal chin flexes downward onto the chest.

Internal rotation. The fetal head must rotate to fit the diameter of the pelvic cavity, which is widest in the anteroposterior diameter. As the occiput of the fetal head meets resistance from the levator ani muscles and their fascia, the occiput rotates—usually from left to right—and the sagittal suture aligns in the anteroposterior pelvic diameter.

Extension. The resistance of the pelvic floor, and the mechanical movement of the vulva opening anteriorly and forward, assist with extension of the fetal head as it passes under the symphysis pubis. With this positional change, the occiput, then brow and face, emerge from the vagina.

Restitution. The shoulders of the fetus enter the pelvic inlet obliquely and remain oblique when the head rotates to the anteroposterior diameter through internal rotation. Because of this rotation, the neck becomes twisted. Once the head is born and is free of pelvic resistance, the neck untwists, turning the head to one side (restitution), and aligns with the position of the back in the birth canal.

External rotation. As the shoulders rotate to the anteroposterior position in the pelvis, the head turns farther to one side (external rotation).

Expulsion. After the external rotation, and through the pushing efforts of the laboring woman, the anterior shoulder meets the undersurface of the symphysis pubis and slips under it. As lateral flexion of the shoulder and head occurs, the anterior shoulder is born before the posterior shoulder. The body follows quickly.

THIRD STAGE

Placental Separation

After the infant is born, the uterus contracts firmly, decreasing its capacity and the surface area of placental attachment. The placenta begins to separate because of this decreased surface area. As separation occurs, bleeding results in the formation of a hematoma between the placental tissue and the remaining decidua. This hematoma speeds the separation process. The membranes are the last to separate. They are peeled off the uterine wall as the placenta descends into the vagina. Signs of placental separation usually ap-

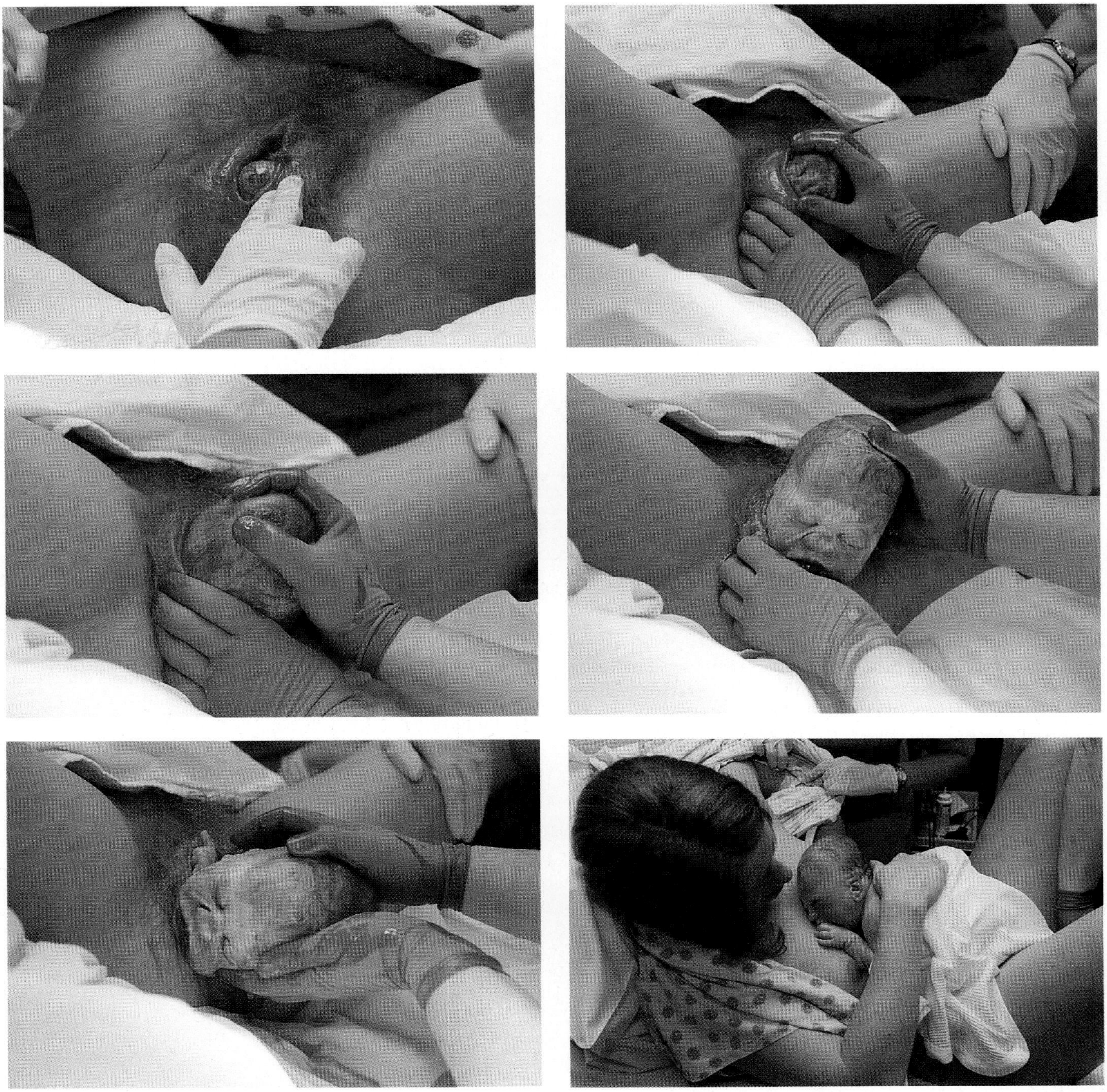

● **Figure 17–12** The birth sequence.

© Stella Johnson (www.stellajohnson.com)

pear about 5 minutes after the birth of the newborn. These signs are (1) a globular-shaped uterus, (2) a rise of the fundus in the abdomen, (3) a sudden gush or trickle of blood, and (4) further protrusion of the umbilical cord out of the vagina.

Placental Delivery

When the signs of placental separation appear, the woman may bear down to aid in placental expulsion. If this fails and the certified nurse-midwife or physician has ascertained that the fundus is firm, gentle traction may be applied to the cord while pressure is exerted on the fundus. The weight of the placenta as it is guided into the placental collection pan aids in the removal of the membranes from the uterine wall. A placenta is considered to be retained if 30 minutes have elapsed from completion of the second stage of labor.

If the placenta separates from the inside to the outer margins, it is expelled with the fetal (shiny) side presenting (Figure 17–14 ●).

MyNursingKit Animation: Placenta Delivery

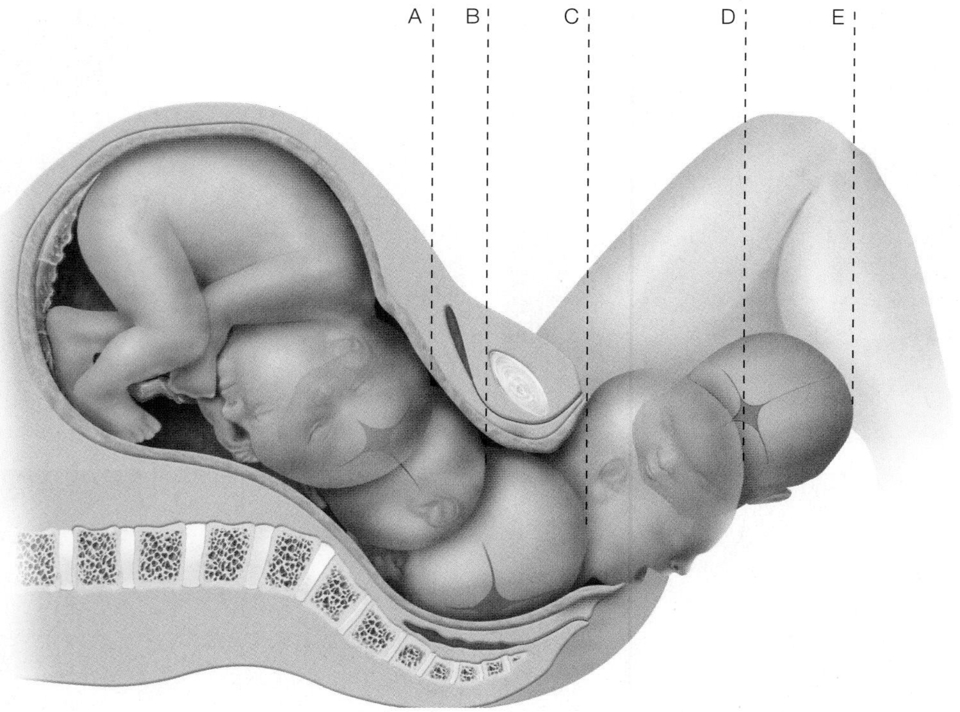

● **Figure 17–13** Mechanisms of labor. ***A*** and ***B,*** Descent. ***C,*** Internal rotation. ***D,*** Extension. ***E,*** External rotation.

This is known as the Schultze mechanism of placental delivery or, more commonly, "shiny Schultze." If the placenta separates from the outer margins inward, it rolls up and presents sideways with the maternal surface expelled first. This is known as the Duncan mechanism and is commonly called "dirty Duncan" because the placental surface is rough. (Interventions for the third stage are discussed in Chapter 19∞.)

FOURTH STAGE

The fourth stage of labor is the time, from 1 to 4 hours after birth, during which physiologic readjustment of the mother's body begins. With the birth, hemodynamic changes occur. Blood loss ranges from 250 to 500 mL. With this blood loss and removal of the weight of the pregnant uterus from the surrounding vessels, blood is redistributed into venous beds. This results in a moderate drop in both systolic and

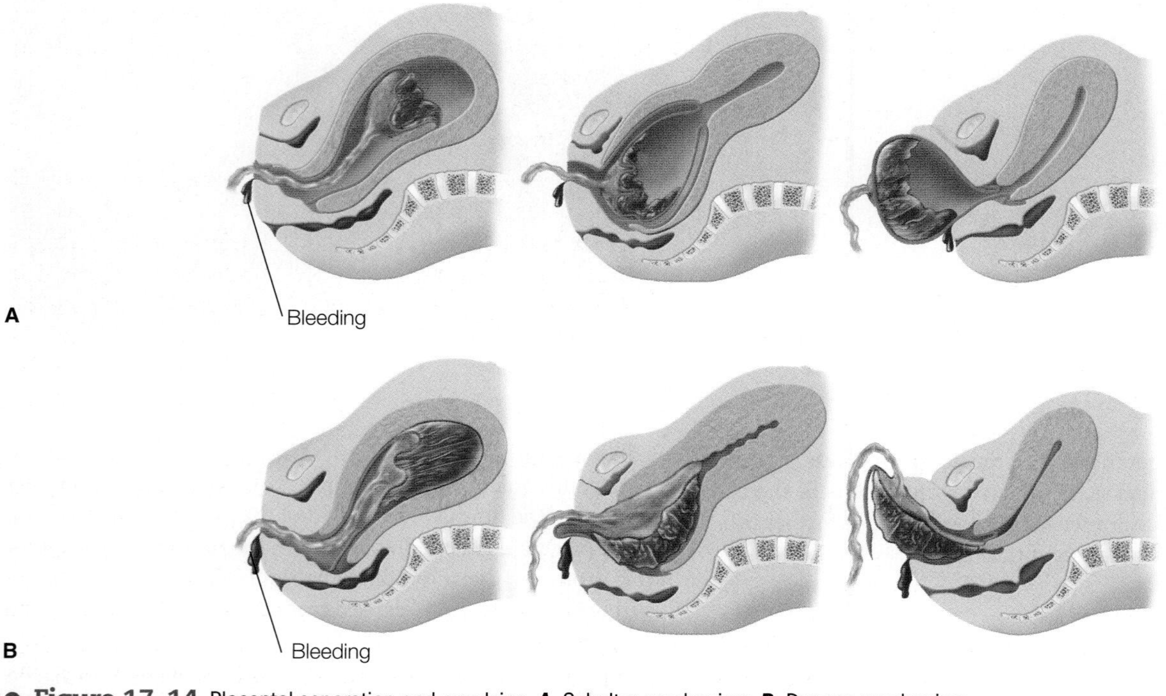

● **Figure 17–14** Placental separation and expulsion. ***A,*** Schultze mechanism. ***B,*** Duncan mechanism.

diastolic blood pressure, increased pulse pressure, and moderate tachycardia (Cunningham, Leveno, Gilstrap, et al., 2010).

The uterus remains contracted in the midline of the abdomen. The fundus is usually midway between the symphysis pubis and umbilicus. Its contracted state constricts the vessels at the site of placental implantation. Immediately after expulsion of the placenta, the cervix is widely spread and thick.

Nausea and vomiting usually cease. The woman may be thirsty and hungry. She may experience a shaking chill, which is thought to be associated with the ending of the physical exertion of labor. The bladder is often hypotonic due to trauma during the second stage or the administration of anesthetics that decrease sensations. Hypotonic bladder can lead to urinary retention.

MATERNAL SYSTEMIC RESPONSE TO LABOR

The process of labor and birth affects almost all maternal physiologic systems.

CARDIOVASCULAR SYSTEM

Uterine contractions and the pain, anxiety, and apprehension a laboring woman experiences stress her cardiovascular system. With each contraction, 300 to 500 mL of blood volume is forced back into the maternal circulation, which results in an increase in cardiac output of as much as 10% to 15% over the typical third trimester levels (Blackburn, 2007). Cardiac output increases more as the laboring woman experiences pain with uterine contractions and her anxiety and apprehension increase.

Maternal position also affects cardiac output. In the supine position, cardiac output lowers, heart rate increases, and stroke volume decreases. When the woman turns to a lateral (side-lying) position, cardiac output increases (Blackburn, 2007).

Blood Pressure

As a result of increased cardiac output, blood pressure rises during uterine contractions. In the first stage, systolic pressure increases by 35 mm Hg and diastolic pressure increases by about 25 mm Hg. There may be further increases in the second stage during pushing (Blackburn, 2007).

RESPIRATORY SYSTEM

Oxygen demand and consumption increase when labor begins because of the presence of uterine contractions. As anxiety and pain from contractions increase, hyperventilation frequently occurs. With hyperventilation there is a fall in $PaCO_2$, and respiratory alkalosis results (Tomimatsu, Peña, & Longo, 2007).

By the end of the first stage, most women have developed a mild metabolic acidosis compensated by respiratory alkalosis. As they push in the second stage of labor, their $PaCO_2$ levels may rise along with blood lactate levels (due to muscular activity), and mild respiratory acidosis occurs. By the time the baby is born (end of second stage), the woman has metabolic acidosis uncompensated for by respiratory alkalosis. The changes in acid-base status that occur in labor are quickly reversed in the fourth stage because of changes in women's respiratory rates. Acid-base levels return to pregnancy levels by 24 hours after birth, and to nonpregnant values a few weeks after birth (Blackburn, 2007).

RENAL SYSTEM

During labor there is an increase in maternal renin, plasma renin activity, and angiotensinogen. This elevation is thought to be important in the control of uteroplacental blood flow during birth and the early postpartal period. Structurally the base of the bladder is pushed forward and upward when engagement occurs. The pressure from the presenting part may impair blood and lymph drainage from the base of the bladder, leading to edema (Cunningham et al., 2010).

GASTROINTESTINAL SYSTEM

During labor, gastric motility and absorption of solid food are reduced. Gastric emptying time is prolonged, and gastric volume (amount of contents that remain in the stomach) remains increased, regardless of the time the last meal was taken. Some narcotics also delay gastric emptying time and add to the risk of aspiration if general anesthesia is used.

IMMUNE SYSTEM AND OTHER BLOOD VALUES

The white blood cell (WBC) count increases to 25,000 to 30,000/mm^3 during labor and the early postpartum. The change in WBC count is mostly due to increased neutrophils resulting from a physiologic response to stress. The increased WBC count makes it difficult to identify an infection. Maternal blood glucose levels decrease because the body uses glucose as an energy source during contractions. Decreased blood glucose levels lead to a decrease in insulin requirements.

PAIN

Pain during labor comes from a complexity of physical causes. Each woman will experience and cope with pain differently. Multiple factors affect a woman's reaction to labor pain.

Causes of Pain During Labor

The pain associated with the first stage of labor is unique in that it accompanies a normal physiologic process. Even though perception of the pain of childbirth varies among women, there is a physiologic basis for discomfort during labor. Pain during the first stage of labor arises from (1) dilatation of the cervix, which is the primary source of pain; (2) stretching of the lower uterine segment; (3) pressure on adjacent structures; and (4) hypoxia of the uterine muscle cells during contraction (Blackburn, 2007). The areas of pain include the lower abdominal wall and the areas over the lower lumbar region and the upper sacrum.

During the second stage of labor, discomfort is due to (1) hypoxia of the contracting uterine muscle cells, (2) distention of the vagina and perineum, and (3) pressure on adjacent structures. The area of pain increases as shown in Figures 17–15 ● and 17–16 ●.

Pain during the third stage results from uterine contractions and cervical dilatation as the placenta is expelled. This stage of labor is short, and after it anesthesia is needed primarily for episiotomy repair.

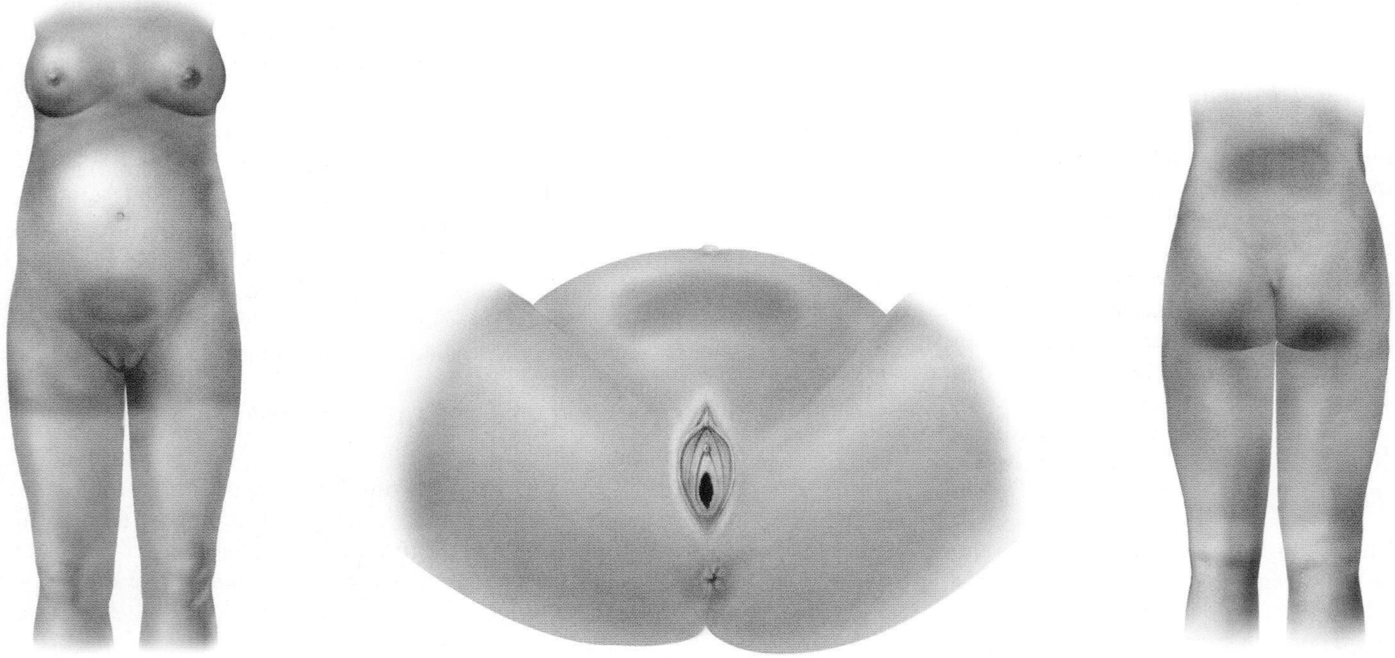

● **Figure 17–15** Distribution of labor pain during the later phase of the first stage and early phase of the second stage. The darkest colored areas indicate the location of the most intense pain, moderate color indicates moderate pain, and lighter color indicates mild pain. The uterine contractions, which at this stage are very strong, produce intense pain.

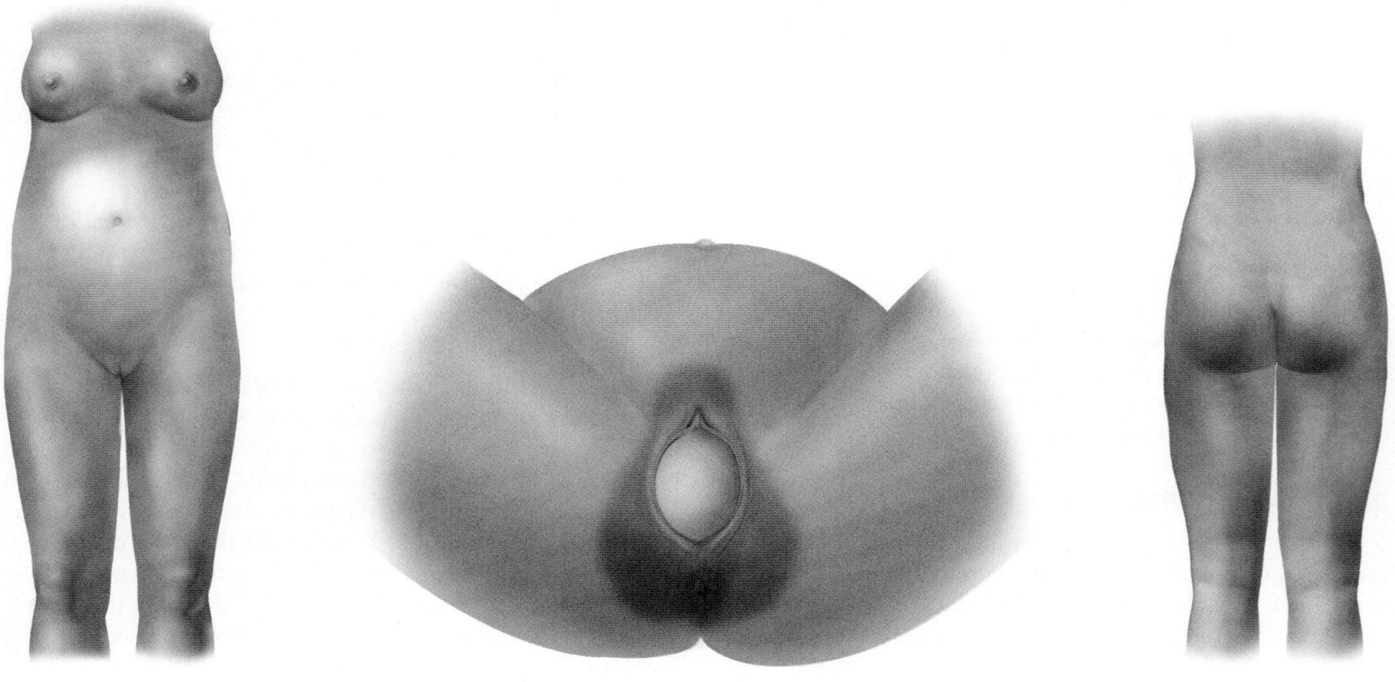

● **Figure 17–16** Distribution of labor pain during the later phase of the second stage and actual birth. The perineal component is the primary cause of discomfort. Uterine contractions contribute much less to the level of pain.

Factors Affecting Response to Pain

Many factors affect the individual's perception of and response to pain. For example, childbirth preparation classes may reduce the need for analgesia during labor. People tend to respond to painful stimuli in the way that is acceptable in their culture. In some cultures it is natural to communicate pain, no matter how mild, whereas members of other cultures stoically accept pain. Fatigue and sleep deprivation may also influence response to pain. The tired woman has less energy and ability to use such strategies as distraction or imagination to deal with pain. As a result she may lose her ability to cope with labor and choose analgesics or other medications to relieve the discomfort.

The woman's previous experience with pain and her anxiety level also affect her ability to manage current and future pain. Those who have had experience with pain seem more sensitive to painful stimuli than those who have not. Unfamiliar surroundings and events can increase anxiety, as does separation from family and loved ones. Anticipation of discomfort and questions about whether she can cope with the contractions may also increase anxiety.

Both attention and distraction influence the perception of pain. When pain sensation is the focus of attention, the perceived intensity is greater. A sensory stimulus such as a back rub can be a distraction that focuses the woman's attention on the stimulus rather than on the pain.

FETAL RESPONSE TO LABOR

When the fetus is healthy, the mechanical and hemodynamic changes of normal labor have no adverse effects. Certain physiologic responses do occur, however.

- *Heart rate changes.* Early fetal heart rate decelerations can occur with intracranial pressures of 40 to 55 mm Hg, as the head pushes against the cervix. This early deceleration is believed to be due to hypoxic depression of the central nervous system, which is under vagal control. The absence of head compression decelerations in some fetuses during labor is explained by a threshold reached more gradually in the presence of intact membranes and lack of maternal resistance. These early decelerations are harmless in a normal fetus.
- *Acid-base status in labor.* Blood flow is decreased to the fetus at the peak of each contraction, which leads to a slow decrease in pH. During the second stage of labor, as uterine contractions become longer and stronger and the woman holds her breath to push, the fetal pH decreases more rapidly. The base deficit increases, and fetal oxygen saturation drops about 10% (Blackburn, 2007).
- *Hemodynamic changes.* The adequate exchange of nutrients and gases in the fetal capillaries and intervillous spaces depends in part on the fetal blood pressure. Fetal blood pressure protects the normal fetus during the anoxic periods caused by the contracting uterus during labor. The fetal and placental reserve is usually enough to see the fetus through these anoxic periods unharmed (Blackburn, 2007).
- *Fetal sensation.* Beginning at about 37 or 38 weeks' gestation, the fetus is able to experience sensations of light, sound, and touch. The full-term fetus is able to hear music and the maternal voice. Even in utero the fetus is sensitive to light and will move away from a bright light source. The term baby is aware of pressure sensations during labor such as the touch of the care provider during a vaginal examination or pressure on the head as a contraction occurs. Although the fetus may not be able to process this input, the fetus is experiencing labor as the woman labors.

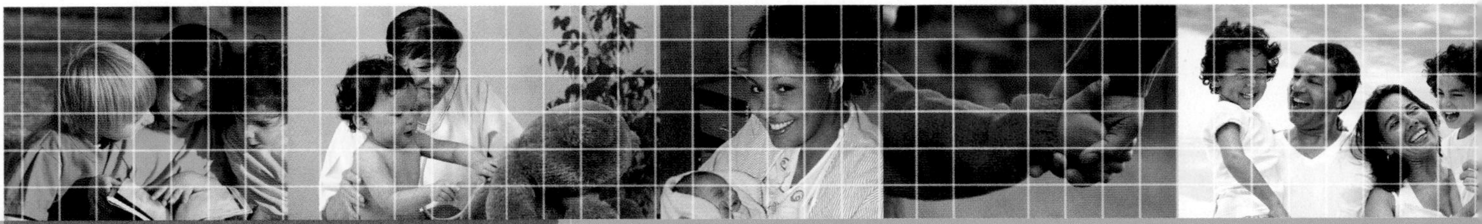

CRITICAL CONCEPT REVIEW

LEARNING OUTCOMES	CONCEPTS
17.1 Describe the five critical factors that influence labor in the assessment of an expectant woman's and fetus's progress in labor and birth.	1. Birth passage: ■ The ability of the pelvis and cervix to accommodate the passage of the fetus. 2. Fetus: ■ The ability of the fetus to complete the birth process. 3. Relationship between the passage and the fetus: ■ The position of the fetus in relation to the pelvis. 4. Physiologic forces of labor: ■ Characteristics of contractions and the effectiveness of expulsion methods. 5. Psychosocial considerations: ■ Understanding and preparing for the childbirth experience. ■ Amount of support from others. ■ Present emotional status. ■ Beliefs and values.

(continued)

LEARNING OUTCOMES	CONCEPTS
17.2 Examine an expectant woman's and fetus's responses to labor based on the physiologic processes that occur during labor.	1. Progesterone causes relaxation of smooth muscle tissue. 2. Estrogen causes stimulation of uterine muscle contractions. 3. Connective tissue loosens and permits the softening, thinning, and opening of the cervix. 4. Muscles of the upper uterine segment shorten and cause the cervix to thin and flatten. 5. Fetal body is straightened as the uterus elongates with each contraction. 6. Pressure of the fetal head causes cervical dilatation. 7. Rectum and vagina are drawn upward and forward with each contraction. 8. During the second stage, the anus everts.
17.3 Assess for the premonitory signs of labor when caring for the expectant woman.	1. Lightening: ■ Fetus descends into the pelvic inlet. 2. Braxton Hicks contractions: ■ Irregular, intermittent contractions that occur during pregnancy. ■ Cause more discomfort closer to onset of labor. 3. Cervical changes: ■ Cervix begins to soften and weaken (ripening). 4. Bloody show: ■ Loss of the cervical mucous plug. ■ Causes blood-tinged discharge. 5. Rupture of membranes: ■ If membranes rupture prior to the onset of labor, there is a good chance labor will begin within 24 hours. 6. Sudden burst of energy: ■ Known as nesting. ■ Usually occurs 24–48 hours before the start of labor. 7. Other signs: ■ Loss of 1–3 pounds. ■ Diarrhea, indigestion, nausea, and vomiting may occur prior to the onset of labor.
17.4 Differentiate between false and true labor.	1. True labor is characterized by: ■ Contractions that occur at regular intervals and increase in duration and intensity. ■ Discomfort that begins in the back and radiates to the front of the abdomen. ■ Walking intensifies contractions. ■ Resting or relaxing in warm water does not decrease the intensity of contractions. ■ Contractions that produce cervical dilatation. 2. False labor is characterized by: ■ Irregular contractions that do not increase in duration or intensity. ■ Contractions that may be lessened by walking, rest, or warm water. ■ Discomfort that is felt primarily in the abdomen. ■ Contractions that produce no effect on cervix.
17.5 Describe the physiologic and psychologic changes occurring in an expectant woman during each of the stages of labor in the nursing care management of the expectant woman.	1a. Latent phase *physiologic* changes: ■ Regular, mild contractions begin and increase in intensity and frequency. ■ Cervical effacement and dilatation begins. 1b. Latent phase *psychologic* changes: ■ Relief that labor has begun. ■ High excitement with some anxiety. 2a. Active phase *physiologic* changes: ■ Contractions increase in intensity, frequency, and duration. ■ Cervical dilatation increases from 4 to 7 cm. ■ Fetus begins to descend into the pelvis. 2b. Active phase *psychologic* changes: ■ Fear of loss of control. ■ Anxiety increases. ■ Possible decrease in coping skills. 3a. Transition phase *physiologic* changes: ■ Contractions continue to increase in intensity, duration, and frequency. ■ Cervix dilates from 8 to 10 cm. ■ Fetus descends rapidly into the birth passage. ■ Woman may experience rectal pressure. ■ Woman may experience nausea, vomiting, or both.

LEARNING OUTCOMES	CONCEPTS

3b. Transition phase *psychologic* changes:
- Increased feelings of anxiety.
- Irritability.
- Eager to complete birth experience.
- Need to have support person or nurse at bedside.

4a. Second stage *physiologic* changes:
- Begins with complete cervical dilatation and ends with the birth of the infant.
- Woman pushes due to pressure of fetal head on sacral and obturator nerves.
- Woman uses intra-abdominal pressure.
- Perineum begins to bulge, flatten, and move anteriorly as fetus descends.

4b. Second stage *psychologic* changes:
- May feel a sense of purpose.
- May feel out of control, frightened, and irritable.

5a. Third stage *physiologic* changes:
- Placental separation: uterus contracts and the placenta begins to separate.
- Placental expulsion: woman bears down and expels the placenta. Physician may put slight traction on the cord to assist the expulsion of the placenta.

5b. Third stage *psychologic* changes:
- Woman may feel relief at the completion of the birth.
- Woman is usually focused on welfare of the infant and may not recognize that placental expulsion is occurring.

6a. Fourth stage *physiologic* changes:
- Woman experiences increased pulse and decreased blood pressure due to redistribution of blood from uterus and blood loss.
- Uterus remains contracted and is located between umbilicus and symphysis pubis.
- Woman may experience a shaking chill.
- Urine may be retained due to decreased bladder tone and possible trauma to the bladder.

6b. Fourth stage *psychologic* changes:
- May experience euphoria and be energized at birth of child.
- May be thirsty and hungry.

17.6 Explain the maternal systemic responses to labor in the nursing care of the expectant woman.

1. Cardiovascular changes:
   - Increase in cardiac output.
2. Blood pressure:
   - Rises with each contraction.
   - May rise further with pushing.
3. Respiratory system:
   - Increase in oxygen demand and consumption.
   - Mild respiratory acidosis usually occurs by time of birth.
4. Renal system:
   - Increase in renin, plasma renin activity, and angiotensinogen.
   - Edema may occur at base of bladder due to pressure of fetal head.
5. Gastrointestinal system:
   - Gastric motility decreased.
   - Gastric emptying is prolonged.
   - Gastric volume remains increased.
6. Immune system and other blood values:
   - WBC count increases.
   - Blood glucose decreases.
7. Pain:
   - In the first stage: Arises from dilatation of cervix, stretching of lower uterine segment, pressure, and hypoxia of uterine muscle cells during contractions.
   - In the second stage: Arises from hypoxia of contracting uterine muscle cells, distention of the vagina and perineum, and pressure.
   - In the third stage: Arises from contractions and dilatation of cervix as placenta is expelled.

17.7 Examine fetal responses to labor.

1. Labor may cause no adverse effects in the healthy fetus.
2. FHR may decrease as the head pushes against the cervix.
3. Blood flow decreases to the fetus at the peak of each contraction, leading to a decrease in pH.
4. Further decrease of pH occurs during pushing due to the woman holding her breath.

CRITICAL THINKING IN ACTION

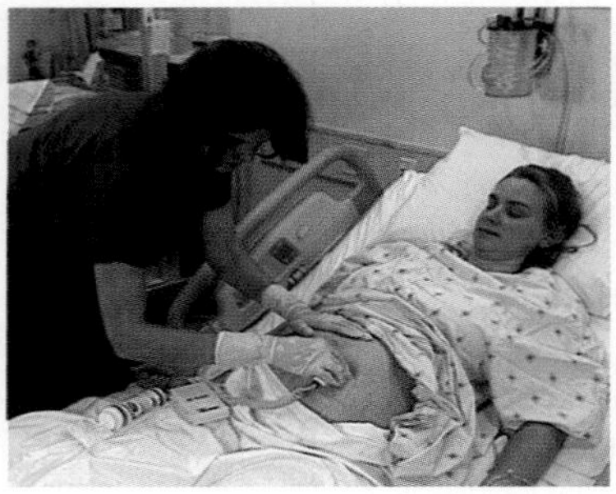

Ann Nelson, a 28-year-old, G2, P0010 at 41 weeks' gestation, is admitted to the birthing unit where you are working. She is here for cervical ripening and induction of labor due to postdate pregnancy and decreased amniotic fluid volume. A review of her prenatal chart reveals a pertinent history of infertility (Clomid-induced pregnancy) and asthma (treated with inhalers on a PRN basis). The Doppler picks up a fetal heart rate of 120 bpm. You place Ann on the electronic fetal monitor and obtain the following data: BP 126/76, T 98°F, P 82, R 16; vaginal exam reveals a 20% effaced cervix, 1 cm dilatation in the posterior position, and vertex at –2 station. The fetal monitor shows a fetal heart rate baseline of 120 to 128 with occasional variable decelerations, accelerations to 140 with fetal activity. No contractions are noted on the monitor or palpated. Ann asks you what to expect with "cervical ripening" using prostaglandin gel.

1. Discuss the action of prostaglandin gel.
2. Ann asks you why cervical ripening and induction of labor are recommended for her and her baby. How would you best respond to her?
3. Ann asks how she will know if she is getting contractions. How would you answer her?
4. Discuss the difference between mild, moderate, and strong contractions.
5. Describe the latent phase of labor.

See MyNursingKit for possible responses.

REFERENCES

American College of Obstetricians & Gynecologists. [ACOG]. (2007). *Premature rupture of membranes* (ACOG Practice Bulletin No. 80). Washington, DC: ACOG.

Blackburn, S. T. (2007). *Maternal, fetal, and neonatal physiology: A clinical perspective* (3rd ed.). Philadelphia: Saunders.

Caldwell, W. E., & Moloy, H. C. (1933). Anatomical variation in the female pelvis and their effect on labor with a suggested classification. *American Journal of Obstetrics and Gynecology, 26*, 479–487.

Cunningham, F. G., Leveno, K. J., Bloom, S. L., Hauth, J. C., Rouse, D. J., & Spong, C. Y. (2010). *Williams obstetrics* (23rd ed.). New York: McGraw-Hill.

Edwards, G., & Byrom, S. (2007). *Essential midwifery practice: Public health*. Hoboken, NJ: Wiley-Blackwell.

Funai, E. F., Evans, M., & Lockwood, C. J. (2008). *High risk obstetrics: The requisites in obstetrics & gynecology*. Mosby: St. Louis.

Kilpatrick, S., Garrison, E. (2007). Normal labor and delivery. In S. G. Gabbe, J. R. Niebyl, & J. L. Simpson (Eds.). *Obstetrics: Normal and problem pregnancies* (5th ed.). Philadelphia: Churchill Livingstone.

Nielson, T., & Paquette, T. (2007). Dream-associated behaviors affecting pregnant and postpartum women. *Sleep, 30*(9), 1162–1169.

Pates, J. A., McIntire, D. D., & Leveno, K. J. (2007). Uterine contractions preceding labor. *Obstetrics & Gynecology, 110*(3), 566–569.

Spector, R. E. (2009). *Cultural diversity in health and illness* (7th ed). Upper Saddle River, NJ: Pearson/Prentice Hall.

Szekeres-Bartho, J., Wilczynski, J. R., Basta, P., & Kalinka. J. (2008). Role of progesterone and progestin therapy in threatened abortion and preterm labour. *Front Bioscience, 1*(13), 1981–1990.

Tomimatsu, T., Peña, J. P., & Longo, L. D. (2007). Fetal cerebral oxygenation: The role of maternal hyperoxia with supplemental CO_2 in sheep. *American Journal of Obstetrics & Gynecology, 196*(4), 359. e1–5.

Vogel, I., Thorsen, P., Curry, A., Sandager, P., & Uldbjerg, N. (2005). Biomarkers for the prediction of preterm delivery. *Acta obstetrician et Gynecologica Scandinavica, 84*(6), 516–525.

Zwelling, E., Johnson, K., & Allen, J. (2006). How to implement complementary therapies for laboring women. *MCN The American Journal of Maternal-Child Nursing, 31*(6), 364–370.

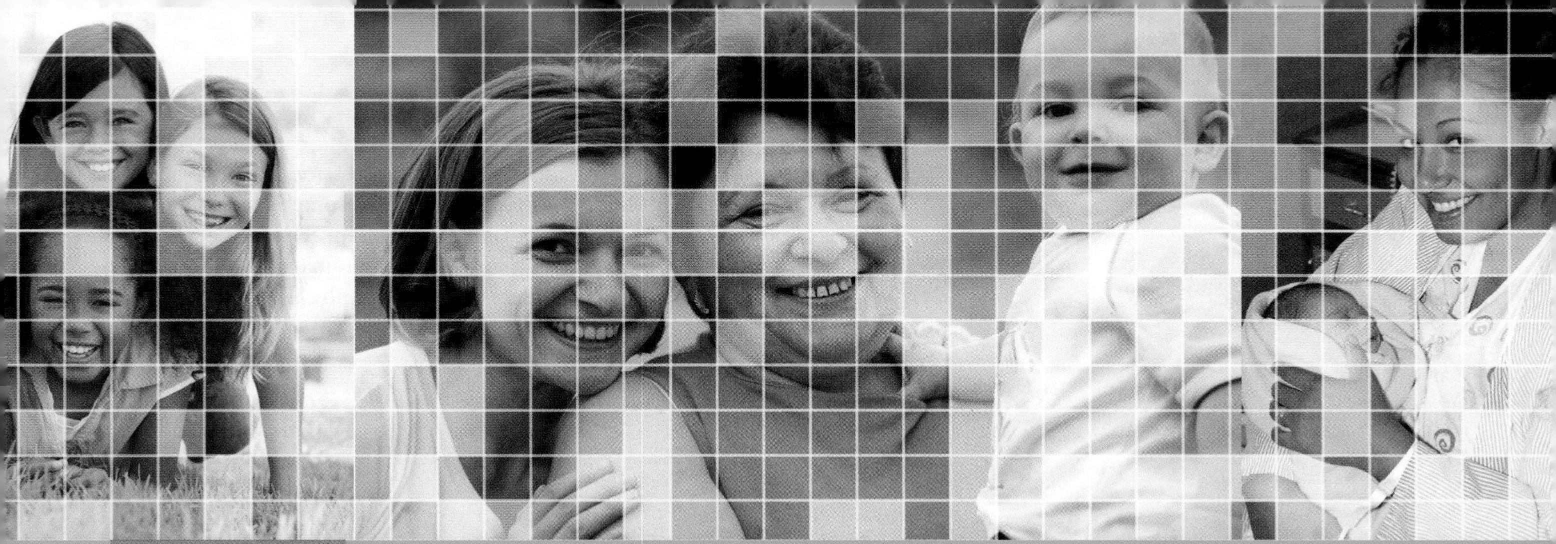

CHAPTER

18 Intrapartal Nursing Assessment

It was strange. After months of waiting for my baby's birth, labor took me by surprise. I wasn't quite ready to move from being pregnant to being a mother. Not that I had any choice!
—Malika, 23

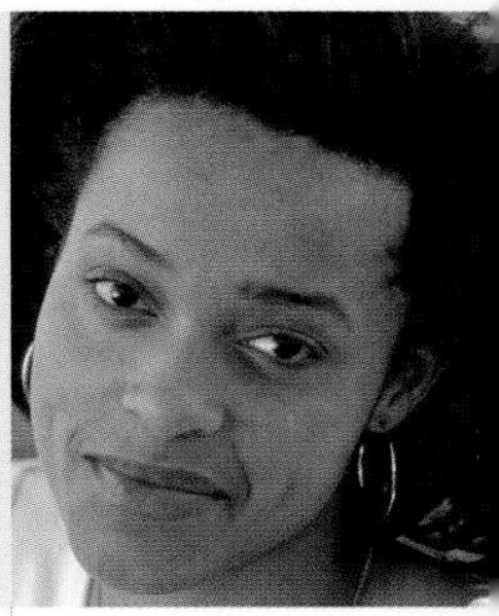

LEARNING OUTCOMES

18.1 Describe a maternal assessment of the laboring woman that includes the client history, high-risk screening, and physical and psychosociocultural factors.

18.2 Evaluate the progress of labor by assessing the laboring woman's contractions, cervical dilatation, and effacement.

18.3 Describe the steps and frequency for performing auscultation of fetal heart rate.

18.4 Delineate the procedure for performing Leopold's maneuvers and the information that can be obtained.

18.5 Distinguish between baseline and periodic changes in fetal heart rate monitoring, and the appearance and significance of each.

18.6 Evaluate fetal heart rate tracings using a systematic approach.

18.7 Compare nonreassuring fetal heart rate patterns to appropriate nursing responses.

18.8 Explain the family's responses to electronic fetal monitoring in nursing care management.

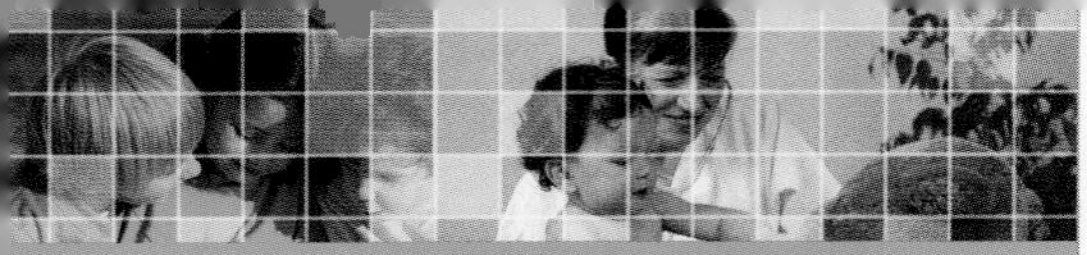

KEY TERMS

Accelerations, 403
Baseline rate, 400
Baseline variability, 401
Decelerations, 403
Early deceleration, 403
Electronic fetal monitoring (EFM), 398
Fetal blood sampling, 406
Fetal bradycardia, 400
Fetal tachycardia, 400
Intrauterine pressure catheter, 395
Late deceleration, 403
Leopold's maneuvers, 397
Variable decelerations, 403

The physiologic events during labor call for many adaptations by the mother and the fetus. Thus, frequent and accurate assessments are crucial. The woman's partner or chosen support person is also an integral part of the childbirth experience. Moreover, the traditional assessment techniques of observation, palpation, and auscultation are augmented by the judicious use of technology such as ultrasound and electronic monitoring. However, the technology only provides data; it is the nurse who monitors the mother and her baby.

MATERNAL ASSESSMENT

HISTORY

Obtain a brief oral history when the woman is admitted to the birthing area. Each agency has its own admission forms, but they usually include the following information:

- Woman's name and age
- Last menstrual period (LMP) and estimated date of birth (EDB)
- Attending physician or certified nurse-midwife (CNM)
- Personal data: blood type; Rh factor; results of serology testing; prepregnant and present weight; allergies to medications, foods, or other substances; prescribed and over-the-counter medications taken during pregnancy; and history of drug and alcohol use and smoking during the pregnancy
- History of previous illness, such as tuberculosis, heart disease, diabetes, and other serious conditions that could influence the pregnancy
- Problems in the prenatal period, such as elevated blood pressure, bleeding problems, recurrent urinary tract infections, other infections
- Pregnancy data: gravida, para, abortions, and perinatal deaths
- The method chosen for infant feeding
- Type of prenatal education classes (childbirth education classes)
- Woman's preferences about labor and birth, such as no episiotomy, no analgesics or anesthetics, or the presence of the father or others at the birth
- Pediatrician or family practice physician
- Additional data: history of special tests such as nonstress test (NST), biophysical profile (BPP), or ultrasound; history of any preterm labor; onset of labor; amniotic fluid membrane status; and brief description of previous labor and birth
- Onset of labor
- Status of amniotic membranes (Are they intact or ruptured? If ruptured, time of rupture, color of fluid, and odor.)

The psychosocial history is a critical component of assessment. An estimated one-third of all pregnant women are exposed to some type of psychotropic medication during their pregnancies. In addition, up to 70% report depressive symptoms while pregnant (American College of Obstetricians and Gynecologists [ACOG], 2008). It is also not uncommon for adults to be diagnosed with eating disorders, autism, learning disabilities, and attention deficit or attention deficit hyperactivity disorder. All of these diagnoses can play a role in how the woman copes with labor and birth and should be assessed by the admitting nurse.

Because of the prevalence of domestic violence in our society (see Chapter 5), the nurse needs to consider the possibility that the woman may have experienced abuse at some point in her life. Many victims of domestic violence, sexual assault, or childhood abuse may have anxiety about the labor process before it begins, or the anxiety may arise during labor. Therefore, it is essential to be alert for information that may indicate abuse or a history of victimization of violence. Antepartal assessment for domestic violence is discussed in Chapter 10.

Nursing Practice

Many nurses have difficulty asking questions about domestic violence, sexual abuse, and drug or alcohol use during pregnancy. However, this information is necessary to provide effective care. To create a relationship of trust with the woman, the following tips may be helpful:

- Explore your own beliefs and values.
- Use open-ended questions.
- Be receptive to the answers.
- Be accepting of others' life experiences.

Thinking Critically

IDENTIFYING DOMESTIC VIOLENCE

You are the birthing center nurse and you have reason to suspect that Lynn Ling, who has just been admitted in labor, may be in an abusive relationship. How could you set up an interview so that the partner would leave the room (and take any accompanying children) without feeling that you are possibly increasing the risk to the woman? What communication techniques would you use to encourage Lynn to reveal if her partner is abusive?

See MyNursingKit for possible responses.

INTRAPARTAL HIGH-RISK SCREENING

Screening for intrapartal high-risk factors is an integral part of assessment. As the history is obtained, note the presence of any factors that may be associated with a high-risk condition. For example, the woman who reports a physical symptom such as intermittent bleeding needs further assessment to rule out abruptio placentae or placenta previa before the admission process continues. It is also important to recognize the implications of a high-risk condition for the laboring woman and her fetus. For example, if there is an abnormal fetal presentation, labor may be prolonged, prolapse of the umbilical cord is more likely, and the possibility of a cesarean birth is increased.

Although physical conditions are major factors that increase risk in the intrapartal period, sociocultural variables such as poverty, nutrition, the amount of prenatal care, cultural beliefs about pregnancy, and communication patterns may also precipitate a high-risk situation. In addition, women who suffer from posttraumatic stress disorder may be at increased risk for some pregnancy complications (Griebenow, 2006). Other risk factors include smoking, drug use, and consumption of alcohol during pregnancy.

Begin gathering data about sociocultural factors as the woman enters the birthing area. Observe the communication pattern between the woman and her support person or people and their responses to admission questions and initial teaching. If the woman and those supporting her do not speak English and translators are not available among the birthing unit staff, the course of labor and the ability of caregivers to interact and provide support and education are affected. The couple must receive information in their primary language to make informed decisions. Communication may also be affected by cultural practices such as beliefs about when to speak, who should ask questions, or whether it is acceptable to let others know about discomfort. In some countries such as Algeria, Brazil, China, and Korea, and among orthodox Jews, the father is not expected to be in the birthing area. Culturally sensitive nurses realize that this should not be interpreted as a lack of interest in the mother, the infant, or the birth itself (Spector, 2009).

Table 18–1 provides a partial list of intrapartal risk factors to keep in mind during the intrapartal assessment.

INTRAPARTAL PHYSICAL AND PSYCHOSOCIOCULTURAL ASSESSMENT

A physical examination is part of the admission procedure and part of the ongoing care of the woman. Although the intrapartal physical assessment is not as complete and thorough as the initial prenatal physical examination (see Chapter 10∞), it does involve assessment of some body systems and of the actual labor process. See "Assessment Guide: Intrapartal—First Stage of Labor" for a framework to use when examining the laboring woman.

Table 18–1 Intrapartal High-Risk Factors

Factor	Maternal Implications	Fetal-Neonatal Implications
Abnormal presentation	↑ Incidence of cesarean birth ↑ Incidence of prolonged labor	↑ Incidence of placenta previa Prematurity ↑ Risk of congenital abnormality Neonatal physical trauma ↑ Risk of intrauterine growth restriction (IUGR)
Multiple gestation	↑ Uterine distention → ↑ risk of postpartum hemorrhage ↑ Risk of cesarean birth ↑ Risk of preterm labor	Low birth weight Prematurity ↑ Risk of congenital anomalies Feto-fetal transfusion
Hydramnios	↑ Discomfort ↑ Dyspnea ↑ Risk of preterm labor Edema of lower extremities	↑ Risk of esophageal or other high-alimentary-tract atresias ↑ Risk of CNS anomalies (myelocele)

(continued)

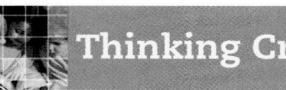

Table 18–1 Intrapartal High-Risk Factors—continued

Factor	Maternal Implications	Fetal-Neonatal Implications
Oligohydramnios	Maternal fear of "dry birth"	↑ Incidence of congenital anomalies ↑ Incidence of renal lesions ↑ Risk of IUGR ↑ Risk of fetal acidosis ↑ Risk of cord compression Postmaturity
Meconium staining of amniotic fluid	Psychologic stress due to fear for baby	↑ Risk of fetal asphyxia ↑ Risk of meconium aspiration ↑ Risk of pneumonia due to aspiration of meconium
Premature rupture of membranes	↑ Risk of infection (chorioamnionitis) ↑ Risk of preterm labor ↑ Anxiety Fear for the baby Prolonged hospitalization ↑ Incidence of tocolytic therapy	↑ Perinatal morbidity Prematurity ↑ Birth weight ↑ Risk of respiratory distress syndrome Prolonged hospitalization
Induction of labor	↑ Risk of hypercontractility of uterus ↑ Risk of uterine rupture Length of labor if cervix not ready ↑ Anxiety	Prematurity if gestational age not assessed correctly Hypoxia if hyperstimulation occurs
Abruptio placentae/placenta previa	Hemorrhage Uterine atony ↑ Incidence of cesarean birth	Fetal hypoxia/acidosis Fetal exsanguination ↑ Perinatal mortality
Failure to progress in labor	Maternal exhaustion ↑ Incidence of augmentation of labor ↑ Incidence of cesarean birth	Fetal hypoxia/acidosis Intracranial birth injury
Precipitous labor (less than 3 hours)	Perineal, vaginal, cervical lacerations ↑ Risk of postpartum hemorrhage	Tentorial tears
Prolapse of umbilical cord	↑ Fear for baby Cesarean birth	Acute fetal hypoxia/acidosis
Fetal heart aberrations	↑ Fear for baby ↑ Risk of cesarean birth, forceps, vacuum Continuous electronic monitoring and intervention in labor	Tachycardia, chronic asphyxic insult, bradycardia, acute asphyxic insult Chronic hypoxia Congenital heart block
Uterine rupture	Hemorrhage Cesarean birth for hysterectomy ↑ Risk of death	Fetal anoxia Fetal hemorrhage Neonatal morbidity and mortality
Postdates (greater than 42 weeks)	↑ Anxiety ↑ Incidence of induction of labor ↑ Incidence of cesarean birth ↑ Use of technology to monitor fetus ↑ Risk of shoulder dystocia	Postmaturity syndrome ↑ Risk of fetal-neonatal mortality and morbidity ↑ Risk of antepartum fetal death ↑ Incidence or risk of large baby
Diabetes	↑ Risk of hydramnios ↑ Risk of hypoglycemia or hyperglycemia ↑ Risk of preeclampsia-eclampsia	↑ Risk of malpresentation ↑ Risk of macrosomia ↑ Risk of IUGR ↑ Risk of respiratory distress syndrome ↑ Risk of congenital anomalies
Preeclampsia-eclampsia	↑ Risk of seizures ↑ Risk of stroke ↑ Risk of HELLP	↑ Risk of small-for-gestational-age baby ↑ Risk of preterm birth ↑ Risk of mortality
AIDS/sexually-transmitted infection (STI)	↑ Risk of additional infections	↑ Risk of transplacental transmission

Assessment Guide

INTRAPARTAL—FIRST STAGE OF LABOR

PHYSICAL ASSESSMENT/ NORMAL FINDINGS	ALTERATIONS AND POSSIBLE CAUSES*	NURSING RESPONSES TO DATA†
Vital Signs		
Blood pressure (BP): less than or equal to 135 systolic and 85 diastolic in adult 18 years of age or older or no more than 15–20 mm Hg rise in systolic pressure over baseline BP during early pregnancy	High BP (essential hypertension, preeclampsia, renal disease, apprehension or anxiety), Low BP (supine hypotension)	Evaluate history of preexisting disorders and check for presence of other signs of preeclampsia. Do not assess during contractions; implement measures to decrease anxiety and reassess. Turn woman on her side and recheck BP. Provide quiet environment. Have O_2 available.
Pulse: 60–90 beats per minute (bpm)	Increased pulse rate (excitement or anxiety, cardiac disorders, early shock)	Evaluate cause, reassess to see if rate continues; report to physician.
Respirations: 16–24/minute (or pulse rate divided by 4)	Marked tachypnea (respiratory disease), hyperventilation in transition phase Hyperventilation (anxiety)	Assess between contractions; if marked tachypnea continues, assess for signs of respiratory disease.
Pulse oximeter (if used) 95% or greater	Less than 90% (hypoxia, hypotension, hemorrhage)	Encourage slow breaths if woman is hyperventilating. Apply O_2; notify physician
Temperature: 36.2–37.6°C (98–99.6°F)	Elevated temperature (infection, dehydration, prolonged rupture of membranes, epidural regional block)	Assess for other signs of infection or dehydration.
Weight		
25–35 lb greater than prepregnant weight	Weight gain greater than 35 lb (fluid retention, obesity, large infant, diabetes mellitus, preeclampsia), weight gain less than 15 lb (SGA, substance abuse, psychosocial problems).	Assess for signs of edema. Evaluate pattern from prenatal record.
Lungs		
Normal breath sounds, clear and equal	Rales, rhonchi, friction rub (infection), pulmonary edema, asthma	Reassess; refer to physician.
Fundus		
At 40 weeks' gestation fundus is located just below xiphoid process	Uterine size not compatible with estimated date of birth (small for gestational age [SGA], large for gestational age [LGA], hydramnios, multiple pregnancy, placental/fetal anomalies, malpresentation)	Reevaluate history regarding pregnancy dating. Refer to physician for additional assessment.
Edema		
Slight amount of dependent edema	Pitting edema of face, hands, legs, abdomen, sacral area (preeclampsia)	Check deep tendon reflexes for hyperactivity; check for clonus; refer to physician.
Hydration		
Normal skin turgor, elastic	Poor skin turgor (dehydration)	Assess skin turgor; refer to physician for deviations.
Perineum		
Tissues smooth, pink color (see "Assessment Guide: Initial Prenatal Assessment," Chapter 10)	Varicose veins of vulva, herpes lesions, genital warts	Exercise care while doing a perineal prep; note on client record need for follow-up in postpartal period; reassess after birth; refer to physician/CNM.

(continued)

Assessment Guide—continued

INTRAPARTAL—FIRST STAGE OF LABOR

PHYSICAL ASSESSMENT/ NORMAL FINDINGS	ALTERATIONS AND POSSIBLE CAUSES*	NURSING RESPONSES TO DATA†
Clear mucus; may be blood tinged with earthy or human odor	Profuse, purulent, foul-smelling drainage	Suspected gonorrhea or chorioamnionitis; report to physician/CNM; initiate care to newborn's eyes; notify neonatal nursing staff and pediatrician.
Presence of small amount of bloody show that gradually increases with further cervical dilatation	Hemorrhage	Assess BP and pulse, pallor, diaphoresis; report any marked changes. (*Note:* Gaping of vagina or anus and bulging of perineum are signs that suggest the onset of the second stage of labor.) Follow universal precautions.
Labor Status		
Uterine contractions: regular pattern	Failure to establish a regular pattern, prolonged latent phase; hypertonicity; hypotonicity; dehydration	Evaluate whether woman is in true labor; ambulate if in early labor. Evaluate client status and contractile pattern. Obtain a 20-minute EFM strip. Notify physician or CNM. Provide hydration.
Cervical dilation: progressive cervical dilatation from size of fingertip to 10 cm (see Skill 3–1 in the Clinical Skills Manual that accompanies this text SKILLS)	Rigidity of cervix (frequent cervical infections, scar tissue, failure of presenting part to descend)	Evaluate contractions, fetal engagement, position, and cervical dilatation. Inform woman of progress.
Cervical effacement: progressive thinning of cervix (see Skill 3–1 SKILLS)	Failure to efface (rigidity of cervix, failure of presenting part to engage); cervical edema (pushing effort by woman before cervix is fully dilated and effaced, trapped cervix)	Evaluate contractions, fetal engagement, and position. Notify physician or CNM if cervix is becoming edematous; work with woman to prevent pushing until cervix is completely dilated. Keep vaginal exams to a minimum.
Fetal descent: progressive descent of fetal presenting part from station -5 to +4 (see Skill 3–1 SKILLS)	Failure of descent (abnormal fetal position or presentation, macrosomic fetus, inadequate pelvic measurement)	Evaluate fetal position, presentation, and size. Evaluate maternal pelvic measurements.
Membranes: may rupture before or during labor	Rupture of membranes more than 12–24 hours before onset of labor	Assess for ruptured membranes using Nitrazine test tape before doing vaginal exam. Follow universal precautions. Instruct woman with ruptured membranes to remain on bed rest if presenting part is not engaged and firmly down against the cervix. Keep vaginal exams to a minimum to prevent infection. When membranes rupture in the birth setting, **immediately assess FHR** to detect changes associated with prolapse of umbilical cord (FHR slows).
Findings on Nitrazine test tape: Membranes probably intact Yellow pH 5.0 Olive pH 5.5 Olive green pH 6.0 Membranes probably ruptured Blue-green pH 6.5 Blue-gray pH 7.0 Deep blue pH 7.5	False-positive results may be obtained if large amount of bloody show is present, previous vaginal examination has been done using lubricant, or tape is touched by nurse's fingers.	Assess fluid for consistency, amount, odor, assess FHR frequently. Assess fluid at regular intervals for presence of meconium staining. Follow universal precautions while assessing amniotic fluid. Reassure woman that amniotic fluid is continually produced (to allay fear of "dry birth"). Teach woman that she may feel amniotic fluid trickle or gush with contractions. Change chux pads often.

Assessment Guide—continued

INTRAPARTAL—FIRST STAGE OF LABOR

PHYSICAL ASSESSMENT/ NORMAL FINDINGS	ALTERATIONS AND POSSIBLE CAUSES*	NURSING RESPONSES TO DATA†
Amniotic fluid clear, with earthy or human odor, no foul-smelling odor	Greenish amniotic fluid (fetal stress) Bloody fluid (abruptio placentae)	Assess FHR; do vaginal exam to evaluate for prolapsed cord; apply fetal monitor for continuous data; report to physician/CNM.
	Strong or foul odor (amnionitis)	Take woman's temperature and report to physician/CNM.
Fetal Status		
FHR: 110–160 bpm	Less than 110 or greater than 160 bpm (nonreassuring fetal status); abnormal patterns on fetal monitor: decreased variability, late decelerations, variable decelerations, absence of accelerations with fetal movement	Initiate interventions based on particular FHR pattern.
Presentation: Cephalic, 97% Breech, 3%	Face, brow, breech, or shoulder presentation	Report to physician/CNM; after presentation is confirmed as face, brow, breech, or shoulder, woman may be prepared for cesarean birth.
Position: left occiput anterior (LOA) most common	Persistent occipital posterior (OP) position; transverse arrest	Carefully monitor maternal and fetal status. Reposition mother to sidelying or hands and knees to promote rotation of fetal head.
Activity: fetal movement	Hyperactivity (may precede fetal hypoxia) Complete lack of movement (fetal distress or fetal demise)	Carefully evaluate FHR; apply fetal monitor. Carefully evaluate FHR; apply fetal monitor. Report to physician or CNM.
Laboratory Evaluation		
Hematologic tests: *Hemoglobin:* 12–16 g/dL	Less than 11 g/dL (anemia, hemorrhage)	Evaluate woman for problems due to decreased oxygen-carrying capacity caused by lowered hemoglobin.
Complete blood count (CBC): *Hematocrit:* 38%–47% *Red blood cell count (RBC):* 4.2–5.4 million/mm^3 *White blood cell count (WBC):* 4,500–11,000/mm^3, although leukocytosis to 20,000/mm^3 is not unusual *Platelets:* 150,000–400,000/mm^3	Presence of infection or blood dyscrasias, loss of blood (hemorrhage, disseminated intravascular coagulation [DIC])	Evaluate for other signs of infection or for petechiae, bruising, or unusual bleeding.
Serologic testing: Serologic test for syphilis (STS) or Venereal Disease Research Laboratory (VDRL) test: nonreactive	Positive reaction (see "Assessment Guide: Initial Prenatal Assessment," Chapter 10 ∞)	For reactive test, notify newborn nursery and pediatrician.
Rh factor	Rh-positive fetus in Rh-negative woman	Assess prenatal record for titer levels during pregnancy. Obtain cord blood for direct Coombs' at birth.
Urinalysis Glucose: negative	Glycosuria (low renal threshold for glucose, diabetes mellitus)	Assess blood glucose level; test urine for ketones; ketonuria and glycosuria require further assessment of blood sugar levels.‡
Ketones: negative	Ketonuria (starvation ketosis)	

(continued)

Assessment Guide—continued

INTRAPARTAL—FIRST STAGE OF LABOR

PHYSICAL ASSESSMENT/ NORMAL FINDINGS	ALTERATIONS AND POSSIBLE CAUSES*	NURSING RESPONSES TO DATA†
Proteins: negative	Proteinuria (urine specimen contaminated with vaginal secretions, fever, kidney disease); proteinuria of 2+ or greater found in uncontaminated urine may be a sign of ensuing preeclampsia	Instruct woman in collection technique; incidence of contamination from vaginal discharge is common. Report any increase in proteinuria to physician/CNM.
Red blood cells: negative	Blood in urine (calculi, cystitis, glomerulonephritis, neoplasm)	Assess collection technique (may be bloody show).
White blood cells: negative	Presence of white blood cells (infection in genitourinary tract)	Assess for signs of urinary tract infection.
Casts: none	Presence of casts (nephrotic syndrome)	

CULTURAL ASSESSMENT§	VARIATIONS TO CONSIDER	NURSING RESPONSES TO DATA†
Cultural influences determine customs and practices regarding intrapartal care	Individual preferences may vary.	
Ask the following questions:		
Who would you like to remain with you during your labor and birth?	She may prefer only her partner/significant other to remain or may also want family and/or friends.	Provide support for her wishes by encouraging desired people to stay. Provide information to others (with the woman's permission) who are not in the room.
What would you like to wear during labor?	She may be more comfortable in her own clothes.	Offer supportive materials such as chux pad if needed to protect her own clothing. Avoid subtle signals to the woman that she should not have chosen to remain in her own clothes. Have other clothing available if the woman desires. If her clothing becomes contaminated, it will be simple to place it in a plastic bag. The nurse can soak soiled clothing in cool water. The nurse needs to remember to wear disposable gloves and a plastic apron if splashing is anticipated.
What activity would you like during labor?	She may want to ambulate most of the time, stand in the shower, sit in the Jacuzzi, sit in a chair or on a stool, remain on the bed, and so forth.	Support the woman's wishes; provide encouragement and complete assessments in a manner so her activity and positional wishes are disturbed as little as possible.
What position would you like for the birth?	She may feel more comfortable in lithotomy with stirrups and her upper body elevated, or side-lying or sitting in birthing bed, or standing, or squatting, or on hands and knees.	Collect any supplies and equipment needed to support her in her chosen birthing position. Provide information to the coach regarding any changes that may be needed based on the chosen position.
Is there anything special you would like?	She may want the room darkened or to have curtains and windows open, music playing, a Leboyer birth, certain scents, her coach to cut the umbilical cord, to save a portion of the umbilical cord, to save the placenta, to videotape the birth, and so forth.	Support requests and communicate requests to any other nursing or medical personnel (so requests can continue to be supported and not questioned). If another nurse or physician does not honor the request, act as advocate for the woman by continuing to support her unless her desire is truly unsafe.
Ask the woman if she would like fluids and ask what temperature she prefers.	She may prefer clear fluids other than water (tea, clear juice). She may prefer iced, room-temperature, or warmed fluids.	Provide fluids as desired.

Assessment Guide—continued

INTRAPARTAL—FIRST STAGE OF LABOR

PHYSICAL ASSESSMENT/ NORMAL FINDINGS	ALTERATIONS AND POSSIBLE CAUSES*	NURSING RESPONSES TO DATA†
Observe the woman's response when privacy is difficult to maintain and her body is exposed.	Some women do not seem to mind being exposed during an exam or procedure; others feel acute discomfort.	Maintain privacy and respect the woman's sense of privacy. If the woman is unable to provide specific information, the nurse may draw from general information regarding cultural variation: a Southeast Asian woman may not want any family member in the room during exams or procedures. Her partner may not be involved with coaching activities during labor or birth. Muslim women may need to remain covered during the labor and birth and avoid exposure of any body part. The husband may need to be in the room but remain behind a curtain or screen so he does not view his wife at this time.
If the woman is to breastfeed, ask if she would like to feed her baby immediately after birth.	She may want to feed her baby right away or may want to wait a little while.	
Preparation for Childbirth		
Woman has some information regarding process of normal labor and birth.	Some women do not have any information regarding childbirth.	Add to present information base.
Woman has breathing and/or relaxation techniques to use during labor.	Some women do not have any method of relaxation or breathing to use, and some do not desire them.	Support breathing and relaxation techniques that client is using; provide information if needed.
Response to Labor		
Latent phase: relaxed, excited, anxious for labor to be well established *Active phase:* becomes more intense, begins to tire *Transitional phase:* feels tired, may feel unable to cope, needs frequent coaching to maintain breathing patterns	May feel unable to cope with contractions because of fear, anxiety, or lack of information May remain quiet and without any sign of discomfort or anxiety, may insist that she is unable to continue with the birthing process	Provide support and encouragement; establish trusting relationship. Provide support and coaching if needed.
Coping mechanisms: ability to cope with labor through utilization of support system, breathing, relaxation techniques	May feel marked anxiety and apprehension, may not have coping mechanisms that can be brought into this experience, or may be unable to use them at this time. Survivors of sexual abuse may demonstrate fear of IVs or needles, may recoil when touched, may insist on a female caregiver, may be very sensitive to body fluids and cleanliness, and may be unable to labor lying down.	Support coping mechanisms if they are working for the woman; provide information and support if she exhibits anxiety or needs alternative to present coping methods. Encourage participation of coach or significant other if a supportive relationship seems apparent. Establish rapport and a trusting relationship. Provide information that is true and offer your presence.
Anxiety		
Some anxiety and apprehension is within normal limits	May show anxiety through rapid breathing, nervous tremors, frowning, grimacing, clenching of teeth, thrashing movements, crying, increased pulse and blood pressure.	Provide support, encouragement, and information. Teach relaxation techniques; support controlled breathing efforts. May need to provide a paper bag to breathe into if woman says her lips are tingling. Note FHR.

(continued)

Assessment Guide—continued

INTRAPARTAL—FIRST STAGE OF LABOR

PHYSICAL ASSESSMENT/ NORMAL FINDINGS	ALTERATIONS AND POSSIBLE CAUSES*	NURSING RESPONSES TO DATA†
Sounds During Labor		
	Some women are very quiet; others moan or make a variety of noises.	Provide a supportive environment. Encourage woman to do what is right for her.
Support System		
Physical intimacy between mother and father (or mother and support person); caretaking activities such as soothing conversation, touching	Some women would prefer no contact; others may show clinging behaviors.	Encourage caretaking activities that appear to comfort the woman; encourage support to the woman; if support is limited, the nurse may take a more active role.
Support person stays in close proximity	Limited interaction may come from a desire for quiet.	Encourage support person to stay close (if this seems appropriate).
Relationship between mother and father (or support person): involved interaction	The support person may seem to be detached and maintain little support, attention, or conversation.	Support interactions; if interaction is limited, the nurse may provide more information and support. Ensure that coach or significant other has short breaks, especially prior to transition.

*Possible causes of alterations are placed in parentheses.
†This column provides guidelines for further assessment and initial nursing intervention.
‡Glycosuria should not be discounted. The presence of glycosuria necessitates follow-up.
§These are only a few suggestions. We do not mean to imply that this is a comprehensive cultural assessment; rather, it is a tool to encourage cultural sensitivity.

The physical assessment portion includes assessments performed immediately on admission as well as ongoing assessments. When labor is progressing very quickly, there may not be time for a complete nursing assessment. In that case the critical physical assessments include maternal vital signs, labor status, fetal status, and laboratory findings.

The cultural assessment portion provides a starting point for this increasingly important aspect of assessment. Individualized nursing care can best be planned and implemented when the values and beliefs of the laboring woman are known and honored. It is sometimes challenging to achieve a balance between cultural awareness and the risk of stereotyping because cultural responses are influenced by so many factors. Nurses are most effective when they combine an awareness of the major cultural values and beliefs of a specific group with the recognition that individual differences have an impact.

The final section of the assessment guide addresses psychosocial factors. The laboring woman's psychosocial status is an important part of the total assessment. The woman has previous ideas, knowledge, and fears about childbearing. By assessing her psychosocial status, the nurse can meet the woman's needs for information and support.

While performing the intrapartal assessment, it is crucial to follow the Centers for Disease Control and Prevention (CDC) guidelines to prevent exposure to body substances. Provide information about the precautions in a factual manner.

Developing Cultural Competence

USE OF PROTECTIVE AMULETS

Placing a protective amulet on the baby or in the crib is common practice among people from many countries including, for example, Greece, Iran, Iraq, Israel, Italy, Malaysia, and Russia (Spector, 2009).

MyNursingKit Case Study: Maternal Assessment during Labor

METHODS OF EVALUATING LABOR PROGRESS

The nurse assesses the woman's contractions and cervical dilatation and effacement to evaluate labor progress.

Contraction Assessment

Uterine contractions may be assessed by palpation or continuous electronic monitoring.

Palpation. Assess contractions for frequency, duration, and intensity by placing one hand on the uterine fundus. Keep the hand relatively still because excessive movement may stimulate contractions or cause discomfort. Determine the frequency of the contractions by noting the time from the beginning of one contraction to the beginning of the next. If contractions begin at 7:00, 7:04, and 7:08, for example, their frequency is every 4 minutes. To determine contraction duration, note the time when tensing of the fundus is first felt (beginning of contraction) and again as relaxation occurs (end of contraction). During the acme of the contraction, intensity can be

Table 18–2 Contraction and Labor Progress Characteristics

Contraction Characteristics	
Latent phase:	Every 10–30 min × 30 sec; mild, progressing to Every 5–7 min × 30–40 sec; moderate
Active phase:	Every 2–5 min × 40–60 sec; moderate to strong
Transition phase:	Every 1 1/2–2 min × 60–90 sec; strong
Labor Progress Characteristics	
Primipara:	At least 1.2 cm/hr dilatation At least 1 cm/hr descent Less than 2 hr in second stage
Multipara:	At least 1.5 cm/hr dilatation At least 2.1 cm/hr descent Less than 1 hr in second stage

evaluated by estimating the indentability of the fundus. Assess at least three successive contractions to gain enough data to determine the contraction pattern. See Table 18–2 for a review of contraction characteristics in different phases of labor.

This is also a good time to assess the laboring woman's perception of pain. How does she describe the pain? What is her affect? Is this contraction more uncomfortable than the last one? Note and chart the woman's affect and response to the contractions.

Electronic monitoring of contraction. Electronic monitoring of uterine contractions provides continuous data. In many birth settings, electronic monitoring is routine for high-risk clients and women having oxytocin-induced labor. Other facilities monitor all laboring women.

Electronic monitoring may be done externally with a device placed against the maternal abdomen, or internally with an **intrauterine pressure catheter**. When monitoring by external means, the portion of the monitoring equipment called a tocodynamometer, or "toco," is positioned against the fundus of the uterus and held in place with an elastic belt (Figure 18–1 ●). The toco contains a flexible disk that responds to pressure. When the uterus contracts, the fundus tightens and the change in pressure against the toco is amplified and transmitted to the electronic fetal monitor. The monitor displays the uterine contraction as a pattern on graph paper.

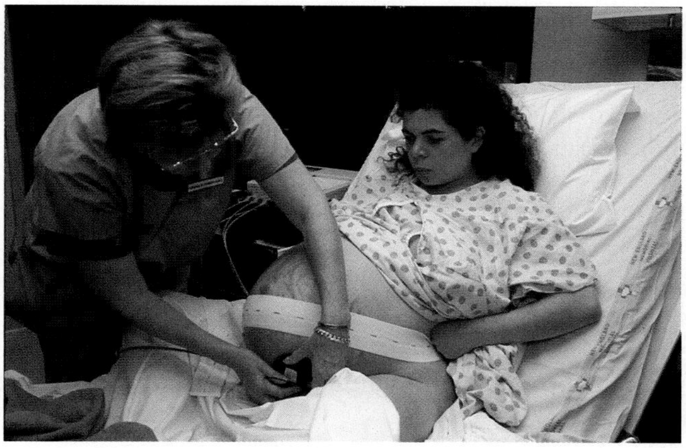

● **Figure 18–1** Woman in labor with external monitor applied. The tocodynamometer placed on the uterine fundus is recording uterine contractions. The lower belt holds the ultrasonic device that monitors the fetal heart rate. The belts can be adjusted for comfort.

External monitoring provides a continuous recording of the frequency and duration of uterine contractions and is noninvasive. However, it does not accurately record the intensity of the uterine contraction, and it is difficult to obtain an accurate fetal heart rate (FHR) in some women, such as those who are very obese, those who have hydramnios (an abnormally large amount of amniotic fluid), or those whose fetus is very active. In addition, the belt may bother the woman if it requires frequent readjustment when she changes position.

Internal intrauterine monitoring provides the same data and also provides accurate measurement of uterine contraction intensity (the strength of the contraction and the actual pressure within the uterus). After membranes have ruptured, the certified nurse-midwife or physician inserts the intrauterine pressure catheter into the uterine cavity and connects it by a cable to the electronic fetal monitor. A small micropressure device located in the tip of the catheter measures the pressure within the uterus in the resting state and during each contraction. Internal electronic monitoring is

Nursing Practice

Many experienced nurses note that when palpating a woman's uterus, mild contractions feel similar in consistency to the tip of the nose, moderate contractions feel more like the chin, and with strong contractions, there is little indentability, much like the forehead. When palpating during a contraction, compare the consistency to your nose, chin, and forehead to determine the intensity.

Complementary Care

AROMATHERAPY IN CHILDBIRTH

Aromatherapy is the use of aromas for physical, mental, and emotional healing. The primary sources of healing aromas are essential oils distilled from herbs and flowers. During labor, essential oils such as jasmine or lavender may be used as an environmental fragrance or added to a hydrotherapy bath. They may also be diluted with a carrier oil or lotion for massage. Therapeutic grade oils may help promote relaxation, improve a woman's ability to cope, and decrease the perception of pain (Zwelling, Johnson, & Allen, 2006).

used when it is imperative to have accurate intrauterine pressure readings to evaluate the stress on the uterus.

In addition, it is important to evaluate the woman's labor status by palpating the intensity and resting tone of the uterine fundus during contractions.

Cervical Assessment

Cervical dilatation and effacement are evaluated directly by vaginal examination (see Skill 3–1 in the Clinical Skills Manual **SKILLS**). The vaginal examination can also provide information about membrane status, characteristics of amniotic fluid, fetal position, and station. See Figures 18–2 ●, 18–3 ●, and 18–4 ●.

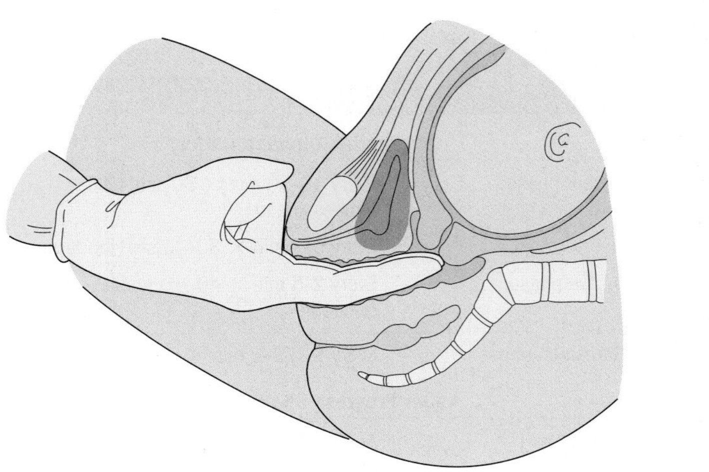

● **Figure 18–2** Gauging cervical dilatation. To gauge cervical dilatation, the nurse places the index and middle fingers against the cervix and determines the size of the opening. Before labor begins, the cervix is long (approximately 2.5 cm), the sides feel thick, and the cervical canal is closed, so an examining finger cannot be inserted. During labor the cervix begins to dilate, and the size of the opening progresses from 1 cm to 10 cm in diameter.

FETAL ASSESSMENT

FETAL POSITION AND PRESENTATION

Fetal position and presentation are determined by inspecting the woman's abdomen, palpating it, performing a vaginal examination, and auscultating FHR. Ultrasound may also be used.

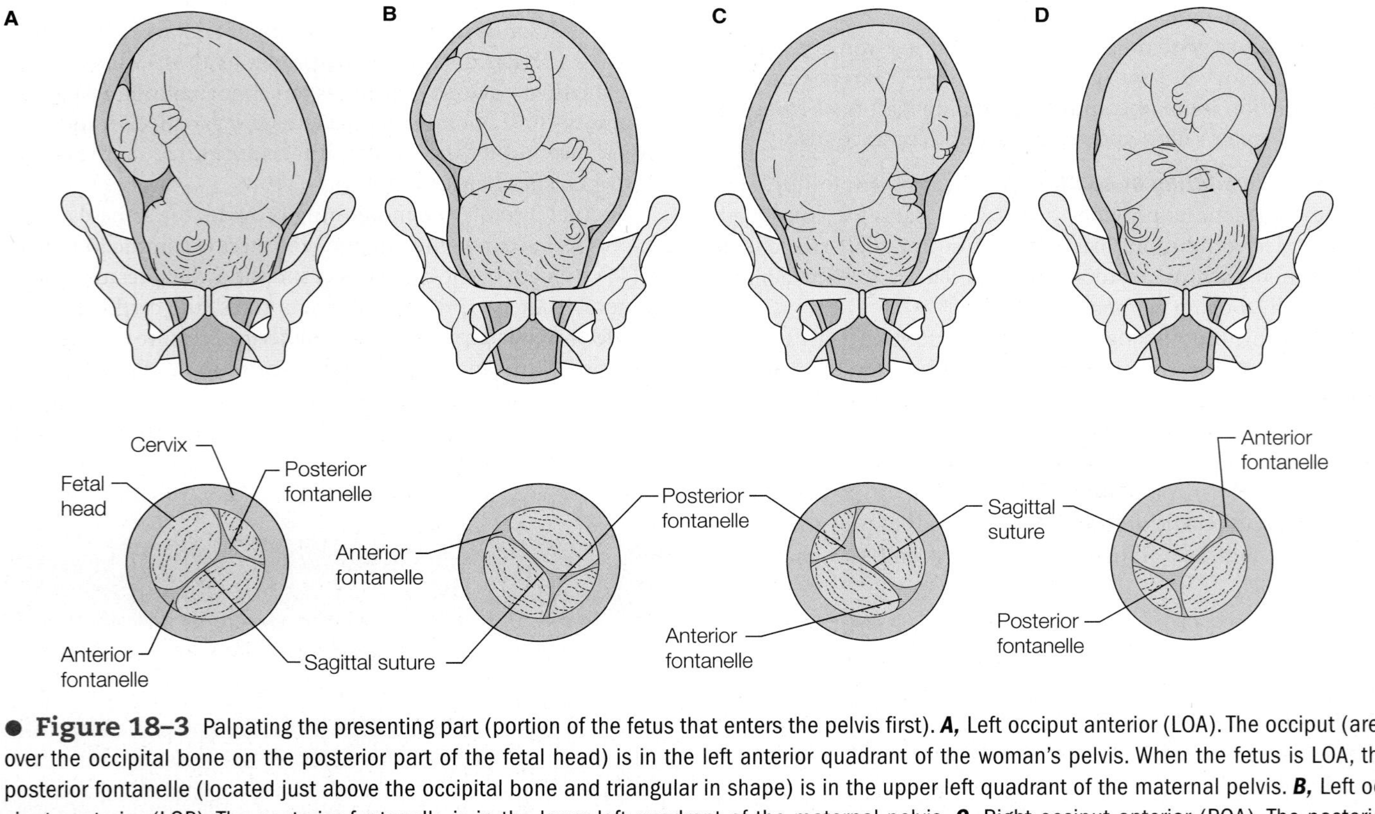

● **Figure 18–3** Palpating the presenting part (portion of the fetus that enters the pelvis first). ***A,*** Left occiput anterior (LOA). The occiput (area over the occipital bone on the posterior part of the fetal head) is in the left anterior quadrant of the woman's pelvis. When the fetus is LOA, the posterior fontanelle (located just above the occipital bone and triangular in shape) is in the upper left quadrant of the maternal pelvis. ***B,*** Left occiput posterior (LOP). The posterior fontanelle is in the lower left quadrant of the maternal pelvis. ***C,*** Right occiput anterior (ROA). The posterior fontanelle is in the upper right quadrant of the maternal pelvis. ***D,*** Right occiput posterior (ROP). The posterior fontanelle is in the lower right quadrant of the maternal pelvis.

Note: The anterior fontanelle is diamond shaped. Because of the roundness of the fetal head, only a portion of the anterior fontanelle can be seen in each of the views, so it appears to be triangular in shape.

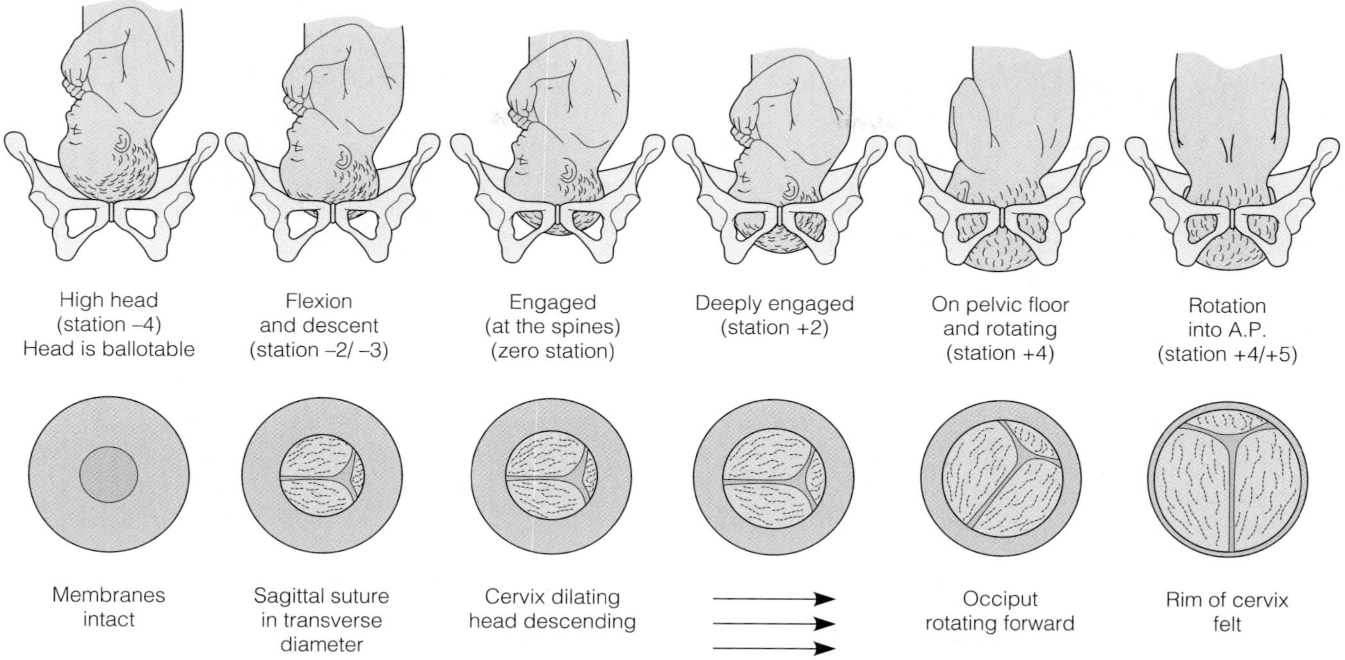

● **Figure 18–4** Assessing fetal position and station. *Top:* The fetal head progressing through the pelvis. *Bottom:* The changes the nurse will detect on palpation of the occiput through the cervix while doing a vaginal examination.

Source: Used with permission from Myles, M. F. (1975). Textbook for midwives *(p. 246), by permission of the publisher: Churchill-Livingstone.*

Inspection

Observe the woman's abdomen for size and shape. Assess the lie of the fetus by noting whether the uterus projects up and down (longitudinal lie) or left to right (transverse lie).

Palpation: Leopold's Maneuvers

Leopold's maneuvers are a systematic way to evaluate the maternal abdomen. Frequent practice increases the examiner's skill in determining fetal position by palpation. Leopold's maneuvers may be difficult to perform on an obese woman or on a woman who has excessive amniotic fluid (hydramnios). Before performing Leopold's maneuvers, have the woman empty her bladder and lie on her back with her feet on the bed and her knees bent. (See Figure 18–5 ● for technique. Also see Clinical Skills Manual that accompanies this text **SKILLS**.)

Vaginal Examination and Ultrasound

During a vaginal examination, the examiner can palpate the presenting part if the cervix is dilated. The examination also provides information about the position of the fetus and the degree of flexion of its head (in cephalic presentations). Visualization by ultrasound is used when the fetal position cannot be determined by abdominal palpation.

AUSCULTATION OF FETAL HEART RATE

The handheld Doppler ultrasound or the fetoscope is used to auscultate the FHR between, during, and immediately after uterine contractions. Instead of listening haphazardly over the woman's abdomen for the FHR, it is useful to perform Leopold's maneuvers first. Leopold's maneuvers not only indicate the probable location of the FHR but also help determine the presence of multiple fetuses, fetal lie, and fetal presentation. The FHR is heard most clearly at the fetal back (Figure 18–6 ●). Thus, in a cephalic presentation, the FHR is best heard in the lower quadrant of the maternal abdomen. In a breech presentation, it is heard at or above the level of the maternal umbilicus. In a transverse lie, FHR may be heard best just above or just below the umbilicus. As the presenting part descends and rotates through the pelvic structure during labor, the location of the FHR tends to descend and move toward the midline.

After the FHR is located, it is usually counted for 30 seconds and multiplied by 2 to obtain the number of beats per minute (bpm). Check the woman's pulse against the fetal sounds. If the rates are the same, readjust the Doppler or fetoscope. Occasionally listen for a full minute, through and just after a contraction, to detect any abnormal heart rate, especially if the FHR is over 160 bpm (tachycardia), under 110 bpm (bradycardia), or irregular. If the FHR is irregular or has changed markedly from the last assessment, listen for a full minute through and immediately after a contraction. In these situations, continuous electronic fetal monitoring is warranted (American College of Obstetricians & Gynecologists, 2009) (see Skill 3–4 **SKILLS** in the Clinical Skills Manual that accompanies this text and Table 18–3 for guidelines on how often to auscultate the FHR).

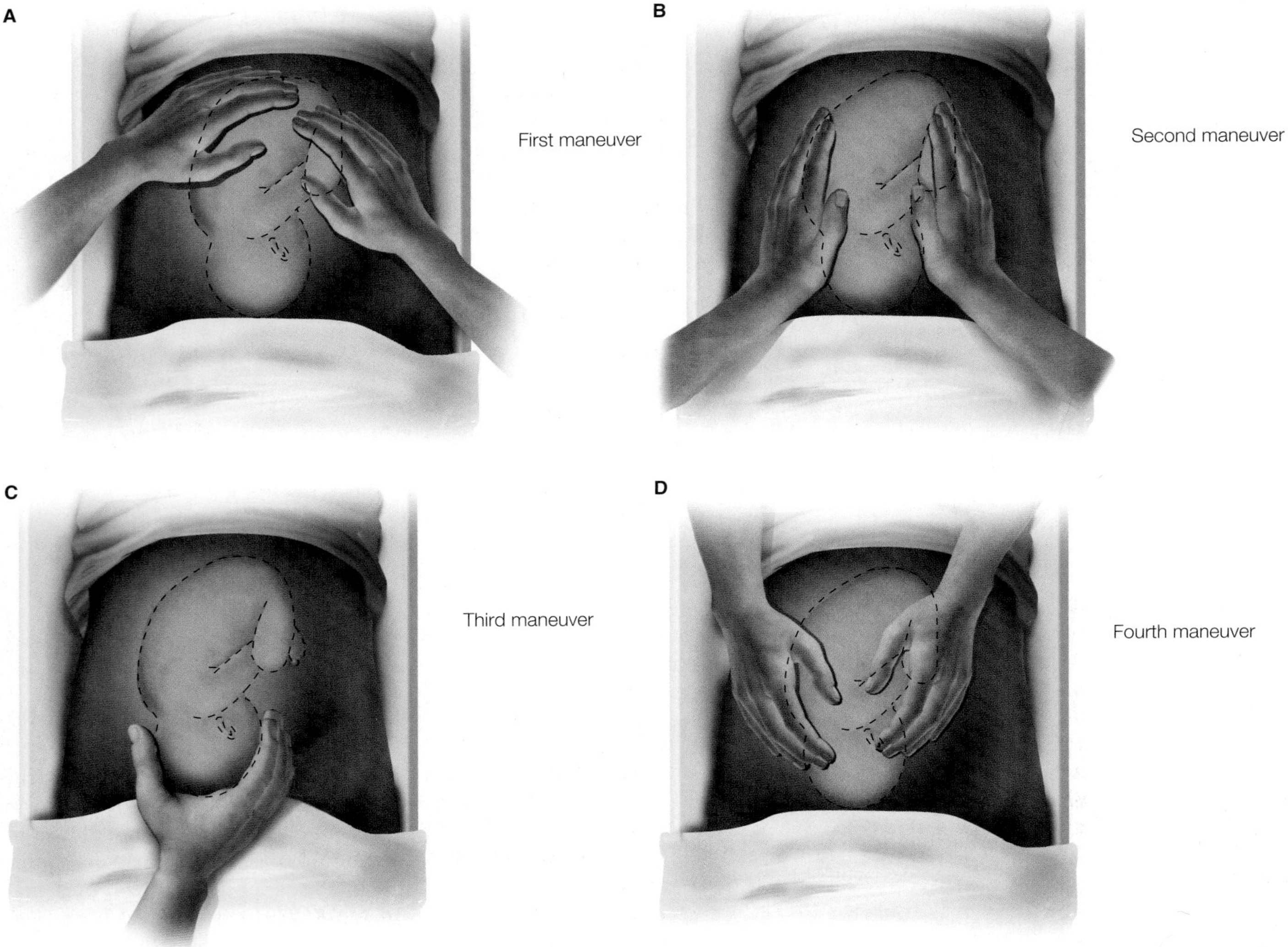

● **Figure 18–5** Leopold's maneuvers for determining fetal position and presentation. ***A,*** First maneuver: Facing the woman, palpate the upper abdomen with both hands. Note the shape, consistency, and mobility of the palpated part. The fetal head is firm and round and moves independently of the trunk. The buttock feels softer, and it moves with the trunk. ***B,*** Second maneuver: Moving the hands on the pelvis, palpate the abdomen with gentle but deep pressure. The fetal back, on one side of the abdomen, feels smooth, and the fetal extremities on the other side feel knobby. ***C,*** Third maneuver: Place one hand just above the symphysis. Note whether the part palpated feels like the fetal head or the breech and whether it is engaged. ***D,*** Fourth maneuver: Facing the woman's feet, place both hands on the lower abdomen and move hands gently down the sides of the uterus toward the pubis. Note the cephalic prominence or brow.

Intermittent auscultation has been found to be as effective as the electronic method for fetal surveillance. A growing number of healthcare professionals, doctors and nurses alike, are beginning to question the widespread use of a technology that has not proven its overall worth.

ELECTRONIC MONITORING OF FETAL HEART RATE

Electronic fetal monitoring (EFM) produces a continuous tracing of the FHR, which allows visual assessment of many characteristics of the FHR (see Skill 3–6 **SKILLS** in the Clinical Skills Manual that accompanies this text).

Indications for Electronic Monitoring

If one or more of the following factors are present, the FHR and contractions are monitored by electronic fetal monitoring:

- Previous history of a stillborn (fetus dies in the uterus) at 38 or more weeks' gestation
- Presence of a complication of pregnancy (e.g., preeclampsia-eclampsia, placenta previa, abruptio placentae, multiple gestation, prolonged or premature rupture of membranes)
- Induction of labor (labor that is begun as a result of some type of intervention such as an intravenous infusion of oxytocin [Pitocin])

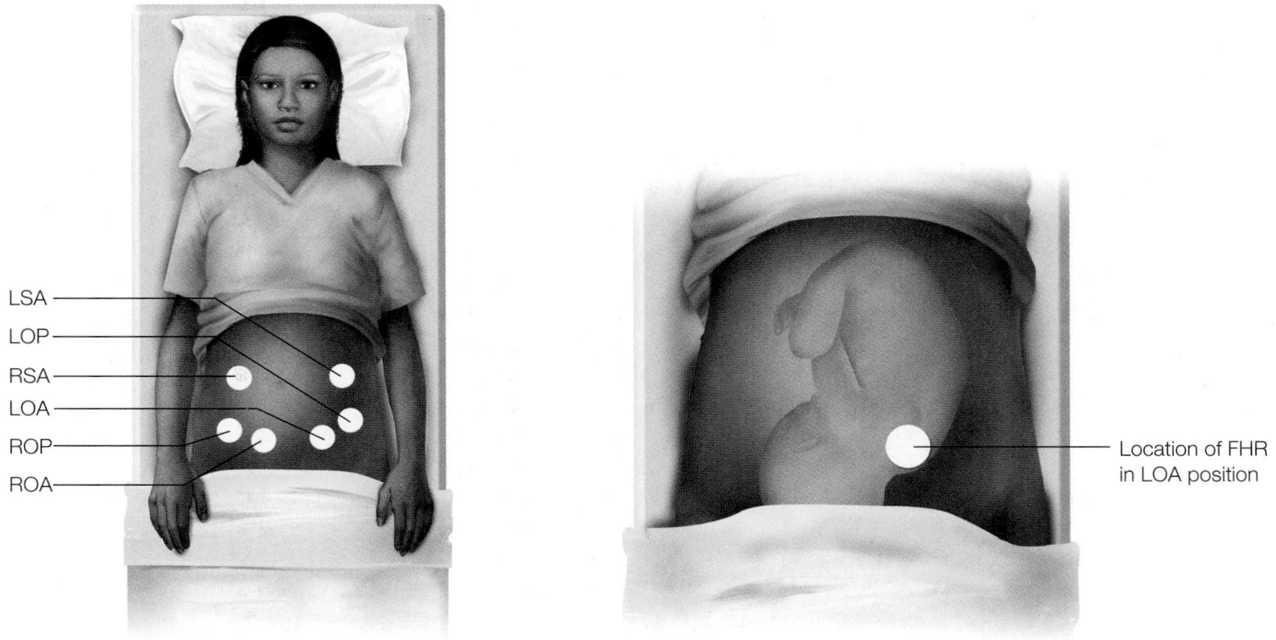

● **Figure 18–6** Location of FHR in relation to the more commonly seen fetal positions.

Table 18–3 Frequency of Auscultation: Assessment and Documentation

Low-Risk Women	High-Risk Women
First stage of labor: q30 min Second stage of labor: q15 min	First stage of labor: q15 min Second stage of labor: q5 min

Labor Events

Assess FHR before:
- Initiation of labor-enhancing procedures (e.g., artificial rupture of membranes)
- Periods of ambulation
- Administration of medications
- Administration or initiation of analgesia or anesthesia

Assess FHR following:
- Rupture of membranes
- Recognition of abnormal uterine activity patterns, such as increased basal tone or tachysystole
- Evaluation of oxytocin (maintenance, increase, or decrease of dosage)
- Administration of medications (at time of peak action)
- Expulsion of enema
- Urinary catheterization
- Vaginal examination
- Periods of ambulation
- Evaluation of analgesia and/or anesthesia (maintenance, increase, or decrease of dosage)

Note: Adopted from American College of Obstetricians & Gynecologists. (2005). *Intrapartum fetal heart rate monitoring.* ACOG Practice Bulletin, No. 70. Washington, DC.

- Preterm labor (gestation less than 37 completed weeks)
- Decreased fetal movement
- Nonreassuring fetal status
- Meconium staining of amniotic fluid (meconium has been released into the amniotic fluid by the fetus, which may indicate a problem)
- Trial of labor following a previous cesarean birth (American Academy of Pediatrics & American College of Obstetricians and Gynecologists [AAP & ACOG], (2007).

Methods of Electronic Monitoring of FHR

External monitoring of the fetus is usually accomplished by ultrasound. A transducer, which emits continuous sound waves, is placed on the maternal abdomen. When the transducer is placed correctly, the sound waves bounce off the fetal heart and are picked up by the electronic monitor. The actual moment-by-moment FHR is displayed graphically on a screen (Figure 18–7 ●). In some instances the monitor may track the maternal heart rate instead of the fetal heart rate. Avoid this error by comparing the maternal pulse to the FHR.

Recent advances in technology have led to the development of new ambulatory methods of external monitoring. Using a telemetry system, a small, battery-operated transducer transmits signals to a receiver connected to the monitor. This system, held in place with a shoulder strap, allows the woman to ambulate, helping her to feel more comfortable and less confined during labor. In contrast the system depicted in Figure 18–7 requires the woman to remain close to the electrical power source for the monitor.

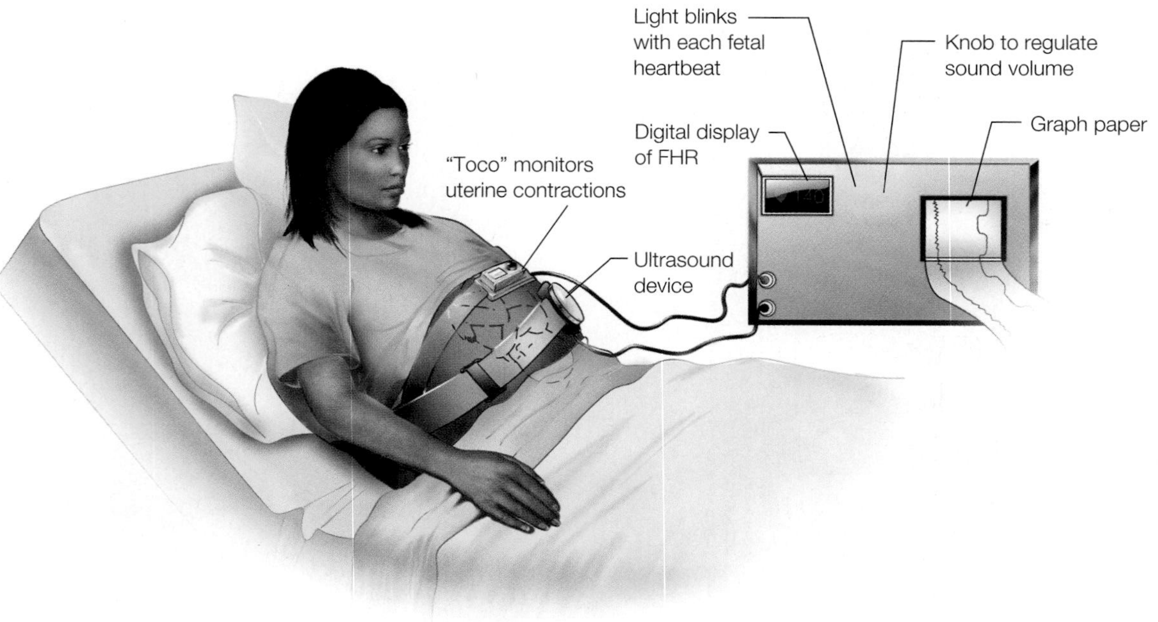

● **Figure 18–7** Electronic fetal monitoring by external technique. The tocodynamometer ("toco") is placed over the uterine fundus. The toco provides information that can be used to monitor uterine contractions. The ultrasound device is placed over the area of the fetal back. This device transmits information about the FHR. Information from both the toco and the ultrasound device is transmitted to the electronic fetal monitor. The FHR is displayed in a digital display (as a blinking light), on the special monitor paper, and audibly (by adjusting a button on the monitor). The uterine contractions are displayed on the special monitor paper as well.

Internal monitoring requires an internal spiral electrode. To place the spiral electrode on the fetal occiput, the amniotic membranes must be ruptured, the cervix must be dilated at least 2 cm, the presenting part must be down against the cervix, and the presenting part must be known (that is, the examiner must be able to detect the actual part of the fetus that is down against the cervix). If all these factors are present, the labor and birth nurse, the physician, or the certified nurse-midwife inserts a sterile internal spiral electrode into the vagina and places it against the fetal presenting part. The spiral electrode is rotated clockwise until it is attached to the presenting part. Wires that extend from the spiral electrode are attached to a leg plate (which is placed on the woman's thigh) and then attached to the electronic fetal monitor. This method of monitoring the FHR provides more accurate continuous data than external monitoring, because the signal is clearer and movement of the fetus or the woman does not interrupt it (Figure 18–8 ●). The FHR tracing at the top of Figure 18–9 ● was obtained by internal monitoring with a spiral electrode; the uterine contraction tracing at the bottom of the figure was obtained by external monitoring with a toco.

Baseline Fetal Heart Rate

The **baseline rate** refers to the average FHR rounded to increments of 5 bpm observed during a 10-minute period of monitoring. Normal FHR (baseline rate) ranges from 110 to 160 bpm. This excludes periodic or episodic changes, periods of marked variability, greater than 25 bpm. The duration should be at least 2 minutes (Macones, Hankins, Spong, et al., 2008). There are two abnormal variations of the baseline rate—those above 160 bpm (tachycardia) and those below 110 bpm (bradycardia). Another change affecting the baseline is called *variability,* a change in FHR over a few seconds to a few minutes.

Fetal tachycardia is a sustained rate of 161 bpm or above. *Marked tachycardia* is 180 bpm or above. Causes of tachycardia include the following (Cunningham, Leveno, Bloom, et al., 2010):

- Early fetal hypoxia, which leads to stimulation of the sympathetic system as the fetus compensates for reduced blood flow
- Maternal fever, which accelerates the metabolism of the fetus
- Maternal dehydration
- Beta-sympathomimetic drugs such as ritodrine, terbutaline, atropine, and isoxsuprine, which have a cardiac stimulant effect
- Amnionitis (fetal tachycardia may be the first sign of developing intrauterine infection)
- Maternal hyperthyroidism (thyroid-stimulating hormones may cross the placenta and stimulate FHR)
- Fetal anemia (the heart rate is increased to improve tissue perfusion)

Tachycardia is considered an ominous sign if it is accompanied by late decelerations, severe variable decelerations, or decreased variability. If tachycardia is associated with maternal fever, treatment may include antipyretics and/or antibiotics.

Fetal bradycardia is a rate less than 110 bpm during a 10-minute period or longer. Causes of fetal bradycardia include the following (Cunningham et al., 2010):

- Late (profound) fetal hypoxia (depression of myocardial activity)

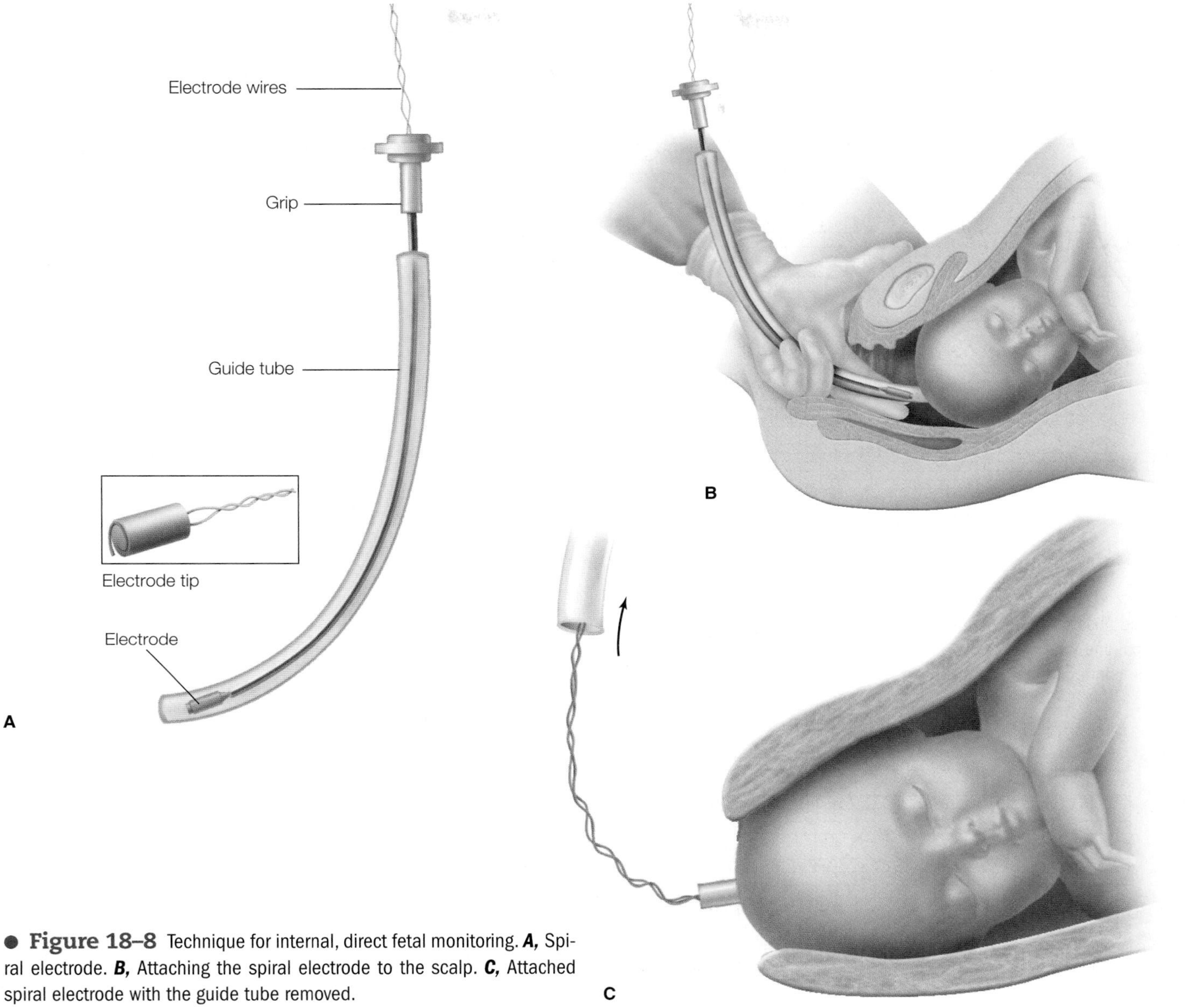

● **Figure 18–8** Technique for internal, direct fetal monitoring. ***A,*** Spiral electrode. ***B,*** Attaching the spiral electrode to the scalp. ***C,*** Attached spiral electrode with the guide tube removed.

- Maternal hypotension, which results in decreased blood flow to the fetus
- Prolonged umbilical cord compression; fetal baroreceptors are activated by cord compression and this produces vagal stimulation, which results in decreased FHR
- Fetal arrhythmia, which is associated with complete heart block in the fetus
- Uterine hyperstimulation
- Abruptio placentae
- Uterine rupture
- Vagal stimulation in the second stage (since this does not involve hypoxia, the fetus can recover)
- Congenital heart block
- Maternal hypothermia

Bradycardia may be a benign or an ominous sign. If average long-term variability exists, the bradycardia is considered benign. When bradycardia is accompanied by decreased long-term variability and late decelerations, it is considered a sign of nonreassuring fetal status (Cunningham et al., 2010).

Baseline Variability

Baseline variability is a measure of the interplay (the push-pull effect) between the sympathetic and parasympathetic nervous systems over a 10-minute period. It reflects baseline fluctuations that are irregular in frequency and amplitude.

Fetal heart rate variability is defined as follows (Macones et al., 2008) (see Figure 18–10 ●):

- *Absent:* amplitude undetectable
- *Minimal:* amplitude detectable but 5 bpm or less

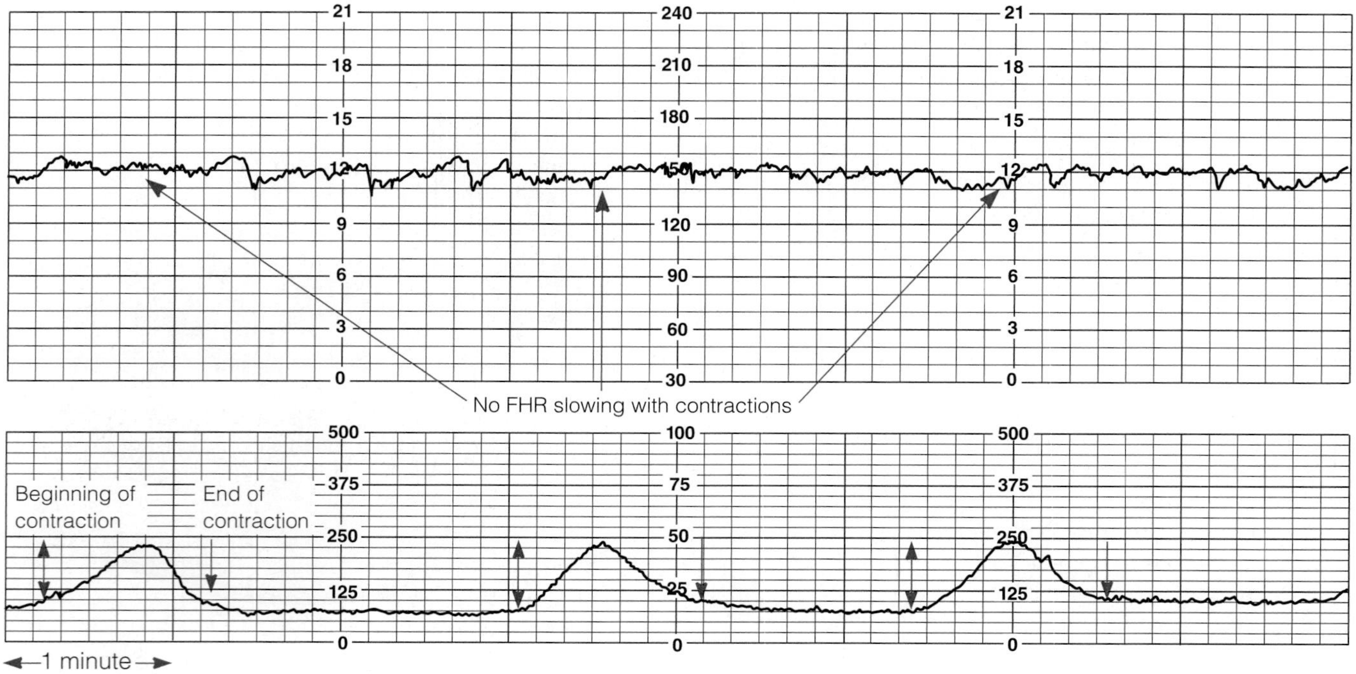

● **Figure 18–9** Normal FHR pattern obtained by internal monitoring. Note normal FHR, 140 to 158 bpm, presence of long- and short-term variability, and absence of deceleration with adequate contractions. The bottom portion depicts uterine contractions obtained by external monitoring. Each dark vertical line marks 1 minute, and each small rectangle represents 10 seconds. The contraction frequency is about every 2½ minutes, and the duration of the contractions is 50 to 60 seconds. Arrows on the bottom of tracing indicate beginnings of uterine contractions.

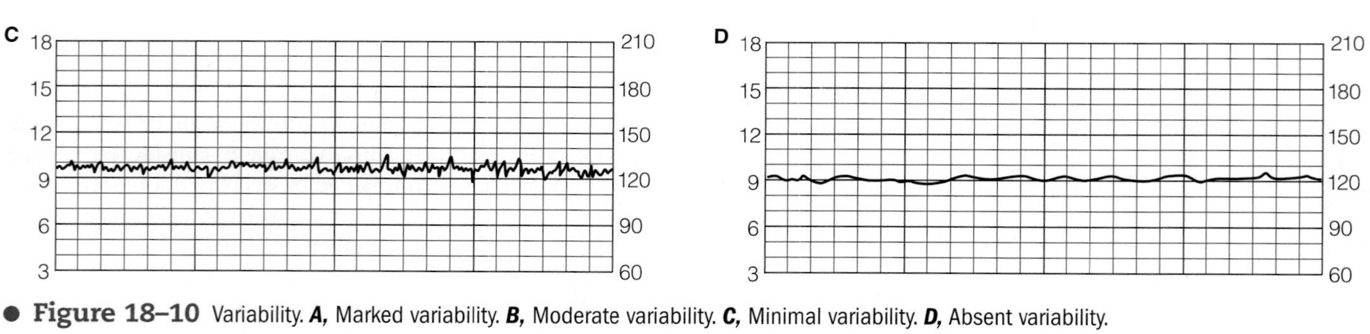

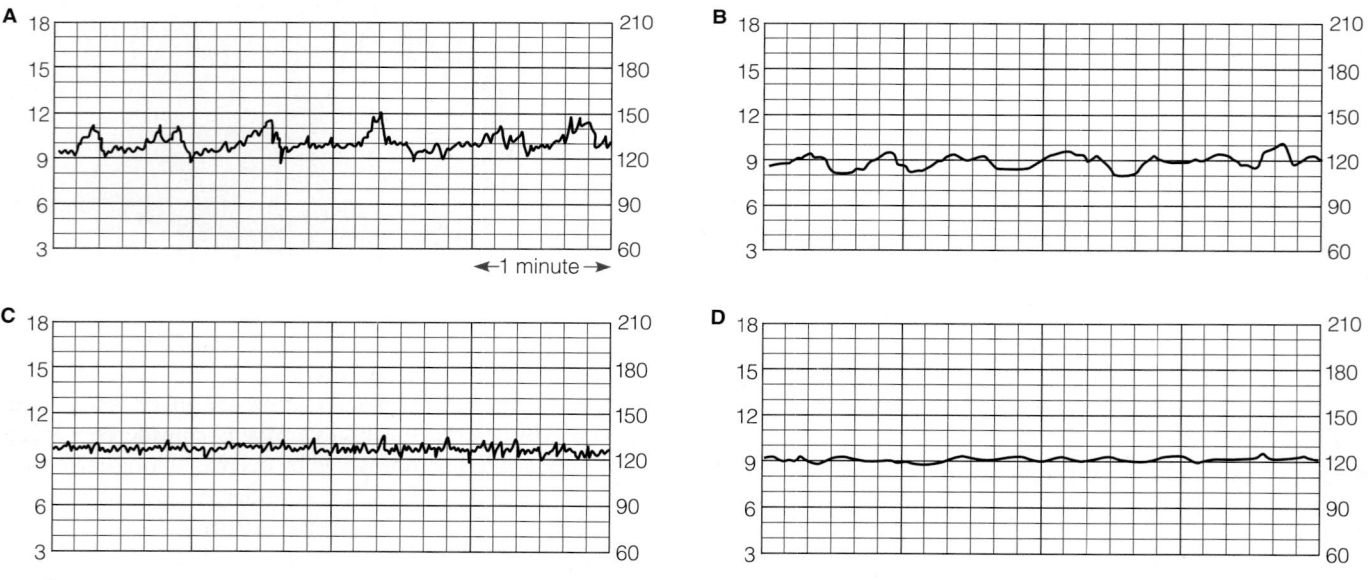

● **Figure 18–10** Variability. ***A,*** Marked variability. ***B,*** Moderate variability. ***C,*** Minimal variability. ***D,*** Absent variability.

- *Moderate:* amplitude 6 to 25 bpm
- *Marked:* amplitude greater than 25 bpm

Reduced variability is the best single predictor for determining fetal compromise (Cunningham et al., 2010). Fetal acidosis and subsequent hypoxia are highest in fetuses that have absent or minimial variability (Siira, Ojala, Ekholm, et al., 2007).

Causes of decreased variability include the following (Cunningham et al., 2010):

- Hypoxia and acidosis (decreased blood flow to the fetus)
- Administration of drugs such as meperidine hydrochloride (Demerol), diazepam (Valium), or hydroxyzine (Vistaril), which depress the fetal central nervous system

- Fetal sleep cycle (during fetal sleep, variability is decreased; fetal sleep cycles usually last for 20 to 40 minutes each hour)
- Fetus of less than 32 weeks' gestation (fetal neurologic control of heart rate is immature)
- Fetal anomalies affecting the heart, central nervous system, or autonomic nervous system
- Fetal dysrhythmias or fetal anomalies affecting the heart, central nervous system, or autonomic nervous system
- Previous neurologic insult
- Tachycardia

Causes of marked variability include the following (Cunningham et al., 2005):

- Early mild hypoxia (variability increases as a result of compensatory mechanism)
- Fetal stimulation or activity (stimulation of autonomic nervous system because of abdominal palpation, maternal vaginal examination, application of spiral electrode on fetal head, or acoustic stimulation)
- Fetal breathing movements
- Advancing gestational age (greater than 30 weeks' gestation)

Absent variability that does not appear to be associated with a fetal sleep cycle or the administration of drugs is a warning sign of nonreassuring fetal status. It is especially ominous if absent or minimal variability is accompanied by late decelerations, explained shortly.

External electronic fetal monitoring is not an adequate method to assess variability. If decreased variability is noted on monitoring, application of a spiral electrode should be considered to obtain more accurate information.

Accelerations

Accelerations are transient increases in the FHR normally caused by fetal movement. When the fetus moves, the heart rate increases, just as the heart rates of adults increase during exercise. Often, accelerations accompany uterine contractions, usually due to fetal movement in response to the pressure of the contractions. Accelerations of this type are thought to be a sign of fetal well-being and adequate oxygen reserve. The accelerations with fetal movement form the basis for nonstress tests (see Chapter 16∞.)

Decelerations

Decelerations are periodic decreases in FHR from the normal baseline. They are categorized as early, late, and variable according to the time of their occurrence in the contraction cycle and their waveform (Figure 18–11 ●). When the fetal head is compressed, cerebral blood flow is decreased, which leads to central vagal stimulation and results in early deceleration. The onset of **early deceleration** occurs before the onset of the uterine contraction. This type of deceleration is of uniform shape, is usually considered benign, and does not require intervention.

Late deceleration is caused by uteroplacental insufficiency resulting from decreased blood flow and oxygen transfer to the fetus through the intervillous spaces during uterine contractions. The most common causes of late decelerations are maternal hypotension resulting from the administration of epidural anesthesia and uterine hyperstimulation associated with oxytocin infusion (Caracostea, Stamatian, Lerintiu, et al., 2007). The onset of the deceleration occurs after the onset of a uterine contraction and is of a uniform shape that tends to reflect associated uterine contractions. The late deceleration pattern is considered a nonreassuring sign but does not necessarily require immediate childbirth. However, if they continue and birth is not imminent, a cesarean birth may be indicated.

Variable decelerations occur if the umbilical cord becomes compressed, thus reducing blood flow between the placenta and fetus. The resulting increase in peripheral resistance in the fetal circulation causes fetal hypertension. The fetal hypertension stimulates the baroreceptors in the aortic arch and carotid sinuses, which slow the FHR. The onset of variable decelerations varies in timing with the onset of the contraction, and the decelerations are variable in shape. This pattern requires further assessment. Nursing interventions for late and variable decelerations in FHR are presented in Table 18–4.

A *sinusoidal pattern* appears similar to a waveform. The characteristics of this pattern include absence of variability and the presence of a smooth, wavelike undulating shape. This pattern is associated with Rh alloimmunization, fetal anemia, severe fetal hypoxia, or a chronic fetal bleed. It may also occur with the administration of medications such as meperidine (Demerol) or butorphanol tartrate (Stadol). When it appears in association with medication, the pattern is usually temporary and is commonly referred to as *pseudosinusoidal* (Cunningham et al., 2005).

Decelerations are also classified based on the rate in which the FHR leaves the baseline FHR. *Episodic decelerations* occur independently of the uterine contractions and are frequently the result of external stimulations, such as vaginal exams. *Intermittent decelerations* refer to decelerations that occur with less than 50% of contractions and are considered recurrent if they occur with 50% or more of the contractions (Macones et al., 2008). Accelerations that leave the baseline for more than 2 minutes but less than 10 minutes are known as *prolonged decelerations.*

Psychologic Reactions to Electronic Monitoring

Responses to electronic fetal monitoring can be varied and complex. Many women have little knowledge of monitoring unless they have attended a prenatal class that dealt with this subject.

MyNursingKit Care Plan Activity: Client with Decelerations

Nursing Practice

The presence of repetitive early decelerations may be a sign of advanced dilatation or the beginning of the second stage of labor. If the monitoring strip shows recurring early decelerations, ask the laboring woman if she is experiencing any pressure. Pressure that occurs only with the contractions typically indicates advanced dilatation. Intense pressure that does not change or ease up when the contractions cease may indicate the beginning of the second stage. A vaginal examination may be performed to establish the dilatation.

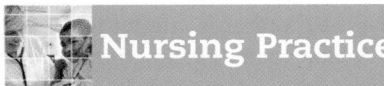

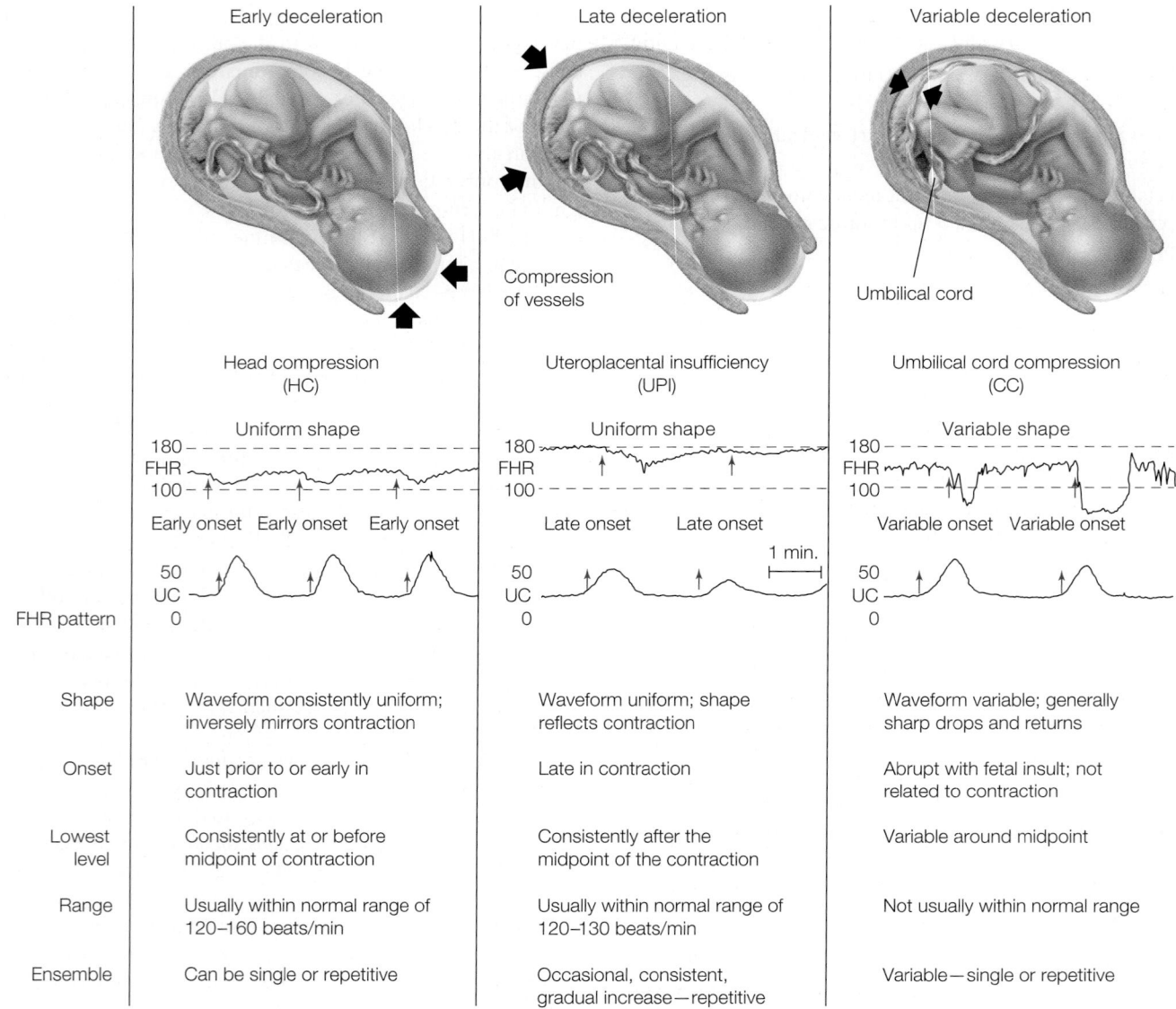

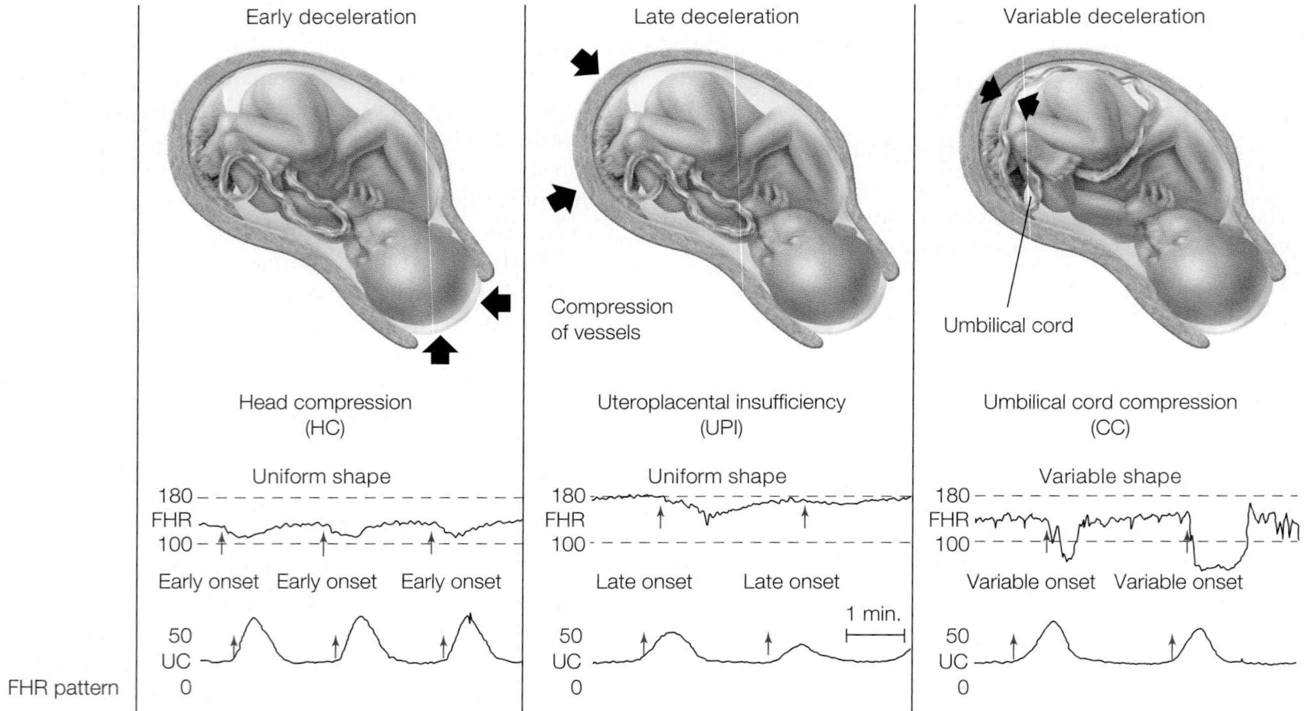

	Early deceleration	Late deceleration	Variable deceleration
Shape	Waveform consistently uniform; inversely mirrors contraction	Waveform uniform; shape reflects contraction	Waveform variable; generally sharp drops and returns
Onset	Just prior to or early in contraction	Late in contraction	Abrupt with fetal insult; not related to contraction
Lowest level	Consistently at or before midpoint of contraction	Consistently after the midpoint of the contraction	Variable around midpoint
Range	Usually within normal range of 120–160 beats/min	Usually within normal range of 120–130 beats/min	Not usually within normal range
Ensemble	Can be single or repetitive	Occasional, consistent, gradual increase—repetitive	Variable—single or repetitive

• **Figure 18–11** Types and characteristics of early, late, and variable decelerations.

Source: Used with permission from Hon, E. (1976). An introduction to fetal heart rate monitoring *(2nd ed., p. 29). Los Angeles: University of Southern California School of Medicine.*

Some women react to electronic monitoring positively, viewing it as a reassurance that "the baby is OK." They may also feel that the monitor helps identify problems that develop in labor. Other women may have ambivalent or even negative feelings about the monitor. They may think that the monitor is interfering with a natural process, and they do not want the intrusion. Some women may find that the equipment, wires, and sounds increase their anxiety. The discomfort of lying in one position and fear of injury to the baby are other objections.

NURSING MANAGEMENT

A key strength of technology is its ability to explain and possibly predict health patterns or problems. However, this advantage has the potential to dehumanize the nurse-client relationship. It is crucial that nurses balance technology with holistic nursing practice. Therefore, it is important to recognize that every encounter with the childbearing family offers an opportunity to provide education and empowerment to the laboring woman and her partner. Helping to provide information when needed, answering questions, and encouraging the woman to make decisions establishes a trusting nurse-client relationship.

Before using the electronic fetal monitor, explain the reason for its use and the information that it can provide. After applying the monitor, record basic information on the monitor strip. These data should include the date, client's name, physician or certified nurse-midwife's name, hospital identification number, age, gravida, para, estimated date of birth, membrane status, and maternal vital signs. As the monitor strip runs and care is provided, occurrences during labor should be recorded not only in the medical record but also on the monitor strip. This information helps the healthcare team assess current status and evaluate the tracing.

Table 18–4 Guidelines for Management of Variable, Late, and Prolonged Deceleration Patterns

Pattern	Nursing Interventions
Variable decelerations Isolated or occasional Moderate	Report findings to physician or CNM and document in chart. Provide explanation to woman and partner. Change maternal position to one in which FHR pattern is most improved. Discontinue oxytocin if it is being administered and other interventions are unsuccessful. Perform vaginal examination to assess for prolapsed cord or change in labor progress. Monitor FHR continuously to assess current status and for further changes in FHR pattern.
Variable decelerations Severe and uncorrectable	Administer oxygen at 7 to 10 L/min. Report findings to physician or CNM and document in chart. Provide explanation to woman and partner. Prepare for probable cesarean birth. Follow interventions listed above. Prepare for vaginal birth unless baseline variability is decreasing or FHR is progressively rising—then cesarean, forceps, or vacuum birth is indicated. Assist physician with fetal scalp sampling if ordered. Prepare for cesarean birth if scalp pH shows acidosis or downward trend.
Late decelerations	Administer oxygen by face mask at 7 to 10 L/min. Report findings to physician or CNM and document in chart. Provide explanation to woman and partner. Monitor for further FHR changes. Maintain maternal position on left side. Maintain good hydration with IV fluids (normal saline or lactated Ringer's). Discontinue oxytocin if it is being administered and late decelerations persist despite other interventions. Monitor maternal blood pressure and pulse for signs of hypotension; possibly increase flow rate of IV fluids to treat hypotension. Follow physician's orders for treatment for hypotension if present. Assess labor progress (dilatation and station). Assist physician with fetal blood sampling: If pH stays above 7.25, physician will continue monitoring and resample; if pH shows downward trend (between 7.25 and 7.2) or is below 7.2, prepare for birth by most expeditious means.
Late decelerations with tachycardia or decreasing variability	Report findings to physician or CNM and document in chart. Maintain maternal position on left side. Administer oxygen by face mask at 7 to 10 L/min. Discontinue oxytocin if it is being administered. Assess maternal blood pressure and pulse. Increase IV fluids (normal saline or lactated Ringer's). Assess labor progress (dilatation and station). Prepare for immediate cesarean birth. Explain plan of treatment to woman and partner. Assist physician with fetal blood sampling (if ordered).
Prolonged decelerations	Perform vaginal examination to rule out prolapsed cord or to determine progress in labor status. Change maternal position as needed to try to alleviate decelerations. Discontinue oxytocin if it is being administered. Notify physician or CNM of findings and initial interventions and document in chart. Provide explanation to woman and partner. Increase IV fluids (normal saline or lactated Ringer's). Administer tocolytic if hypertonus noted and ordered by physician or CNM. Anticipate normal FHR recovery following deceleration if FHR previously normal. Anticipate intervention if FHR previously abnormal or deceleration lasts more than 3 minutes.

Note the following information on the tracing (AAP & ACOG, 2007):

- Vaginal examination (dilatation, effacement, station, position)
- Amniotomy or spontaneous rupture of membranes, color and amount of amniotic fluid, presence of any odor
- Maternal vital signs
- Maternal position in bed and changes of position
- Application of spiral electrode or intrauterine pressure catheter
- Medications given
- Oxygen administration
- Maternal behaviors (emesis, coughing, hiccups)
- Fetal scalp stimulation or fetal scalp blood sampling
- Vomiting
- Pushing
- Administration of anesthesia blocks

If the monitor does not automatically add the time on the strip at specific intervals, include the time when recording any information on the strip. If more than one nurse is adding information to the monitor strip, it is essential to initial each note. The tracing is considered a legal part of the woman's medical record and is submissible as evidence in court.

The fetal monitoring strip should be reviewed regularly—at least every 30 minutes in the first stage and every 15 minutes during the second stage (ACOG, 2009).

The laboring woman needs to feel that what is happening to her is the central focus. Acknowledge this need by always speaking to and looking at the woman when entering the room, before looking at the monitor.

Evaluation of FHR Tracings

It is important to use a systematic approach in evaluating FHR tracings. Evaluation of the electronic monitor tracing begins by looking at the uterine contraction pattern:

- Determine the uterine resting tone.
- Assess the contractions: What is the frequency? What is the duration? What is the intensity?

The next step is to evaluate the FHR tracing:

- Determine the baseline: Is the baseline within the normal range? Is there evidence of tachycardia? Of bradycardia?
- Determine FHR variability: Is variability absent? minimal? moderate? marked?
- Determine if a sinusoidal pattern is present.
- Determine if there are periodic changes: Are accelerations present? Do they meet the criteria for a reactive NST? Are decelerations present? Are they uniform in shape? If so, determine if they are early or late decelerations. Are they nonuniform in shape? If so, determine whether they are variable decelerations.

After evaluating the FHR tracing for the factors just listed, classify the tracing as reassuring (normal) or nonreassuring (worrisome). Reassuring patterns contain normal parameters and do not require additional treatment or intervention.

Characteristics of reassuring FHR patterns include the following:

- Baseline rate is 110 to 160 bpm.
- Variability is present.
- Variability is at least two cycles per minute. Periodic patterns consist of accelerations with fetal movement, and early decelerations may be present.

Nonreassuring patterns may indicate that the fetus is becoming stressed and intervention is needed. Characteristics of nonreassuring patterns include the following:

- Severe variable decelerations (FHR drops below 70 bpm for longer than 30 to 45 seconds and is accompanied by rising baseline or decreasing variability or slow return to baseline)
- Late decelerations of any magnitude
- Absence of variability
- Prolonged deceleration (a deceleration that lasts 60 to 90 seconds or more)
- Severe (marked) bradycardia (FHR baseline of 70 bpm or less)

Nonreassuring patterns may require continuous monitoring and more involved treatment and intervention (see Table 18–4).

Guidelines for the interpretation of fetal heart rate monitoring results have been developed that classify findings into three categories: I, II, and III. Category I is considered normal while category III is considered abnormal and predictive of compromised fetal status (ACOG, 2009; Macones, Hankins, Spong, et al., 2008). See Evidence-Based Nursing: Catergories of Fetal Heart Rate Monitoring Findings for detailed information about each category.

Provision of Emotional Support

It is vital to provide information to the laboring woman about the FHR pattern and the interventions, if necessary, that will help her fetus. Most women are aware that something is happening. Sharing information with them provides reassurance that a potential or actual problem is identified and that they are active participants in the interventions. Occasionally a problem arises that requires immediate intervention. In that case it may be helpful to say something like, "It is important for you to turn on your left side right now because the baby is having a little difficulty. I'll explain what is happening in just a few moments." This type of response lets the woman know that although an action needs to be accomplished rapidly, information will soon be provided. In the haste to act quickly, nurses and other caregivers must not forget that it is the woman's body and her baby.

SCALP STIMULATION TEST

When there is a question about fetal status, a scalp stimulation test can be used before the more invasive **fetal blood sampling**. In this test the examiner applies pressure to the fetal scalp while doing a vaginal examination. The fetus who is not in any stress or distress responds with an acceleration of the FHR (Spong, 2008).

Fetal vibroacoustic stimulation using a handheld artificial larnynx applied to the maternal abdomen may also be used to assess fetal status. As with scalp stimulation, fetal heart rate accelerations in response are a sign of fetal well-being (Spong, 2008).

CORD BLOOD ANALYSIS AT BIRTH

In cases where significant abnormal FHR patterns have been noted, meconium-stained amniotic fluid is present, or the infant is depressed at birth, umbilical cord blood may be analyzed immediately following the birth to determine if acidosis is present. AAP and ACOG (2007) recommend performing cord blood analysis in cases in which the Apgar score is below 7 at 5 minutes of age. (Normal Apgar score is 7 to 10.)

The cord is clamped before the infant takes the first breath. A small amount of blood is aspirated with a syringe from one of the umbilical arteries. If the cord blood will not be analyzed immediately, a heparinized syringe should be used. Normal fetal blood pH should be above 7.25 (AAP & ACOG, 2002). Lower levels indicate acidosis and hypoxia. Many practitioners obtain cord blood analysis to minimize medicolegal exposure.

Evidence-Based Nursing

CATEGORIES OF FHR MONITORING PATTERNS

Clinical Question

How should fetal heart rate patterns relate to nursing interventions?

The Evidence

The National Institute of Child Health and Human Development, the American College of Obstetricians, and the Society for Maternal-Fetal Medicine partnered to sponsor a workshop to develop recommendations for intrapartum electronic fetal heart rate monitoring. The participants included numerous obstetric experts that reviewed the research literature relative to fetal monitoring. The resulting guidelines are a combination of multiple research studies and clinical expertise that represents the strongest level of evidence (Macones et al., 2008).

Best Practice

A baseline fetal heart rate (FHR) of 110 to 160 beats per minute with moderate variability, no decelerations, and any accelerations is normal. These are considered Category I and no interventions are indicated. Bradycardia or tachycardia in the baseline FHR with minimal or absent variability, or, conversely, marked variability, are considered Category II. This category includes the absence of induced accelerations after fetal stimulation, and recurrent or prolonged (more than 2 minutes but less than 10 minutes) decelerations. Category II FHR tracings are indeterminate. This category has not been shown to predict abnormal fetal acid-base status, yet there is inadequate evidence to consider Category II normal. These mothers should be assessed frequently, taking into account the associated maternal condition and clinical circumstances. Category III FHR tracings include *either* absent baseline FHR variability and late or variable decelerations, absent baseline variability and bradycardia, or a sinusoidal pattern. Category III FHR tracings are abnormal and predictive of compromised fetal acid-base status. Category III tracings require prompt evaluation of the maternal and fetal conditions. Interventions may include provision of maternal oxygen, change in maternal position, discontinuation of labor stimulants, and/or treatment of maternal hypothension.

Critical Thinking

How long can Category II FHR tracings continue before they are considered truly abnormal?

See MyNursingKit for possible responses.

CRITICAL CONCEPT REVIEW

LEARNING OUTCOMES / CONCEPTS

18.1 Describe a maternal assessment of the laboring woman that includes the client history, high-risk screening, and physical and psychosociocultural factors.

1. High-risk screening is completed to determine if there are any factors present that may be associated with a high-risk condition.
2. Maternal physical factors include:
   - Vital signs.
   - Labor status.
   - Fetal status.
   - Laboratory findings.
3. Cultural assessment:
   - Individual beliefs and preferences.
4. Psychosocial factors:
   - Childbearing fears.
   - Childbearing knowledge and fantasies.
   - Previous history of psychological disorders.

18.2 Evaluate the progress of labor by assessing the laboring woman's contractions, cervical dilatation, and effacement.

Progress of labor is evaluated by:

1. Assessment of strength and frequency of contractions:
   - Hand palpation.
   - Electronic monitoring.
   - External and internal pressure catheters.
2. Cervical assessment:
   - Determination of cervical dilatation – from 1 cm to 10 cm
   - Determination of effacement – measured in percentage. Full effacement is 100%.

(continued)

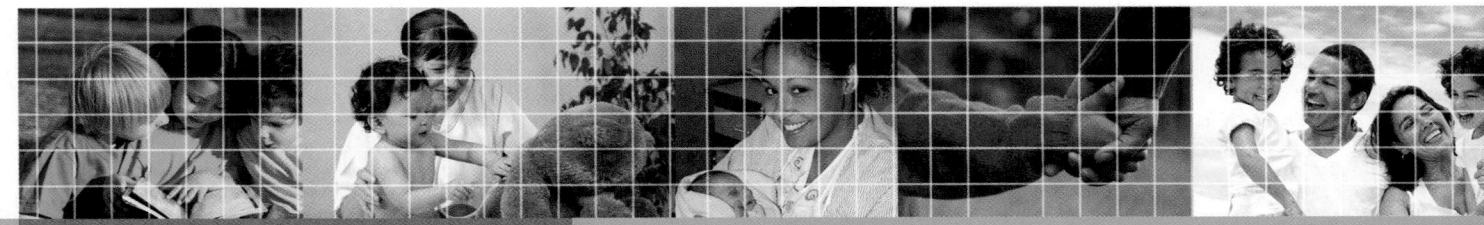

LEARNING OUTCOMES	CONCEPTS
18.3 Describe the steps and frequency for performing auscultation of fetal heart rate.	1. Location of fetal heart rate: ■ Heard best at the fetal back. 2. Assessment may be intermittent: ■ Handheld Doppler ultrasound auscultates the FHR between, during, and after a contraction. ■ Fetoscope may be used. 3. Most assessment is continuous: ■ External. ■ Internal scalp electrode.
18.4 Delineate the procedure for performing Leopold's maneuvers and the information that can be obtained.	1. Leopold's maneuvers evaluate the position, presentation, and lie of the fetus by palpation of the woman's abdomen: ■ Woman empties her bladder and lies on her back with her knees flexed. ■ The practitioner palpates the abdomen gently but deeply using the palms of the hands. ■ One hand is held steady while the other explores one side of the abdomen, then the action of the hands is switched.
18.5 Distinguish between baseline and periodic changes in fetal heart rate monitoring, and the appearance and significance of each.	1. Baseline fetal heart rate: ■ Average FHR observed during a 10-minute period of monitoring. ■ Should be between 110 and 160 bpm. ■ Baseline changes of the FHR include tachycardia, bradycardia, and variability. Periodic changes: 1. Accelerations: ■ Usually caused by fetal movement. ■ Reassuring sign of fetal well-being when it occurs during a contraction. 2. Decelerations: ■ Early deceleration occurs before a contraction and usually requires no intervention. ■ Later deceleration occurs during and after a contraction and indicates insufficient blood flow to the fetus. It is a nonreassuring sign. ■ Variable decelerations occur due to umbilical cord compression and require further assessment. ■ Sinusoidal pattern appears when there are no periods of normal fetal heart rate. It is associated with Rh problems, fetal anemia, severe fetal hypoxia, or a chronic fetal bleed.
18.6 Evaluate fetal heart rate tracings using a systematic approach.	1. Evaluate the uterine contraction pattern. 2. Determine the baseline FHR. 3. Determine FHR variability. 4. Determine if a sinusoidal pattern is present. 5. Determine if there are periodic changes.
18.7 Compare nonreassuring fetal heart rate patterns to appropriate nursing responses.	1. Severe variable decelerations. 2. Late decelerations of any magnitude. 3. Absence of variability. 4. Prolonged deceleration. Nursing responses include: 1. Notify the physician or CNM. 2. Administer maternal oxygen. 3. Turn mother to the left side. 4. Discontinue oxytocin if being administered. 5. Monitor FHR continuously. 6. Provide explanation to the mother and partner.
18.8 Explain the family's responses to electronic fetal monitoring in nursing care management.	1. Explain the use of EFM. 2. Look at mother prior to looking at monitor. 3. Record pertinent data on monitor strip.

CRITICAL THINKING IN ACTION

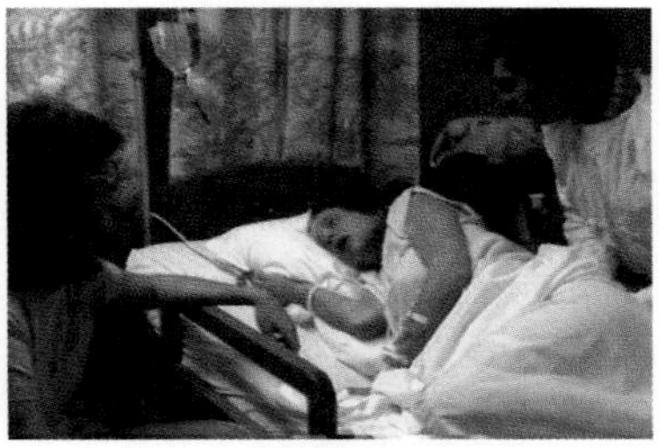

Cindy Bell, a 20-year-old gravida 2, para 1 at 40 weeks' gestation, presents to you in the birthing unit with contractions every 5 to 7 minutes. She is accompanied by her husband. Spontaneous rupture of membranes occurred 2 hours prior to admission. Cindy tells you that the fluid was colorless and clear. You orient Cindy and her family to the birthing room and perform a physical assessment, documenting the following data: vital signs are normal. A vaginal exam demonstrates the cervix is 75% effaced, 4 cm dilated with a vertex at -1 station in the LOP position. You place Cindy on an external fetal monitor. The fetal heart rate baseline is 140–147 with accelerations to 156; no decelerations are noted. Contractions are 5–6 minutes apart, moderate intensity and lasting 40–50 seconds. Cindy states she would like to stay out of bed as long as possible because lying down seems to make the contractions more painful, especially in her back.

1. Discuss the benefits of ambulation in labor.
2. Cindy would like her daughter to be present for the baby's birth. What would you discuss with her about the impact of having a young sibling present during labor and birth?
3. What fetal heart rate assessment will best ensure fetal well-being during the period Cindy is ambulating?
4. When a nonreassuring fetal heart pattern is detected, what remedial nursing intervention is carried out?
5. What are indications for continuous fetal monitoring in labor?

See MyNursingKit for possible responses.

REFERENCES

American Academy of Pediatrics & American College of Obstetricians and Gynecologists. (2007). *Guidelines for perinatal care* (6th ed.).Washington, DC: Author.

American College of Obstetricians and Gynecologists [ACOG]. (2008). *Use of psychiatric medications during pregnancy and lactation.* ACOG Practice Bulletin No. 92. Washington, DC: Author.

American College of Obstetricians and Gynecologists [ACOG]. (2009). *Intrapartum fetal heart rate monitoring: Nomenclature, interpretation, and general management principles.* ACOG Practice Bulletin No. 106. Washington, DC: Author.

Bloom, S. L., Spong, C. Y., Thom, E., Varner, M. W., Rouse, D. J., Weininger, S., et al. (2006). Fetal pulse oximetry and cesarean delivery. *New England Journal of Medicine, 355,* 2195–2202.

Caracostea, G., Stamatian, F., Lerintiu, M., & Herghea, D. (2007). The influence of maternal epidural anesthesia upon intrapartum fetal oxygenation. *Journal of Maternal Fetal Neonatal Medicine, 20*(2), 161–165.

Cunningham, F. G., Leveno, K. J., Bloom, S. L., Hauth, J. C., Rouse, D. J., & Spong, C. Y. (2010). *Williams obstetrics* (23rd ed.). New York: McGraw-Hill Medical.

Griebenow, J. J. (2006). Healing the trauma: Entering motherhood with posttraumatic stress disorder (PTSD). *Midwifery Today International Midwife, 80,* 28–31, 68.

Macones, G. A., Hankins, G. D. V., Spong, C. Y., Hauth, J., & Moore, T. (2008). The 2008 National Institute of Child Health and Human Development Workshop Report on Electronic Fetal Monitoring: Update on definitions, interpretation, and research guidelines. *JOGNN: The Journal of Obstetric, Gynecologic, and Neonatal Nursing, 37*(5), 510–515.

Macones, G., Hankins, G., Spong, C., Hauth, J., & Moore, T. (2008). The 2008 National Institute of Child Health and Human Development Workshop Report on Electronic Fetal Monitoring. *Obstetrics and Gynecology, 112*(34), 661–666.

Siira, S., Ojala, T., Ekholm, E., Vahlberg, T., Blad, S., & Rosen, K. G. (2007). Change in heart rate variability in relation to a significant ST-event associates with newborn metabolic acidosis. *British Journal of Obstetrics & Gynecology, 114*(7), 819–823. Epub 2007 May 16.

Spector, R. E. (2009). *Cultural diversity in health and illness* (7th ed.). Upper Saddle River, NJ: Prentice Hall Health.

Spong, C. Y. (2008). Assessment of fetal well-being. In R. S. Gibbs, B. Y. Karlan, A. F. Haney, & I. E. Nygaard (Eds.), *Danforth's obstetrics and gynecology* (10th ed.). Philadelphia: Wolters Kluwer/Lippincott Williams & Wilkins.

Zwelling, E., Johnson, K., & Allen, J. (2006). How to implement complementary therapies for laboring women. *MCN The American Journal of Maternal-Child Nursing, 31*(6), 364–370.

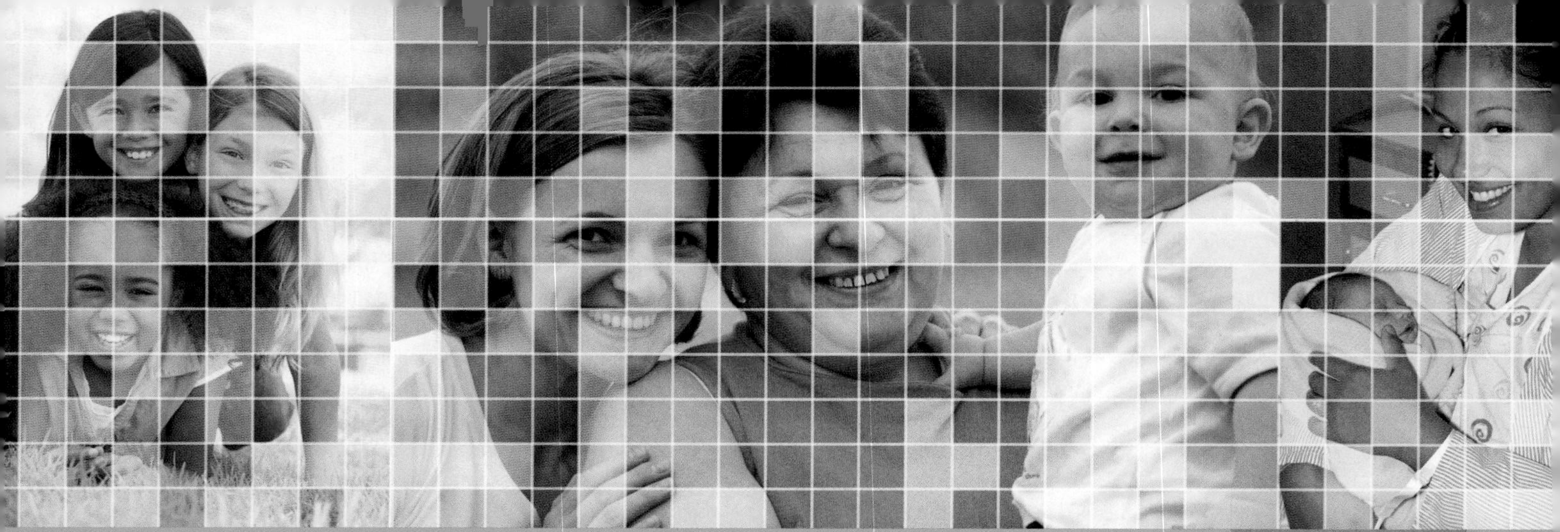

CHAPTER 19

The Family in Childbirth: Needs and Care

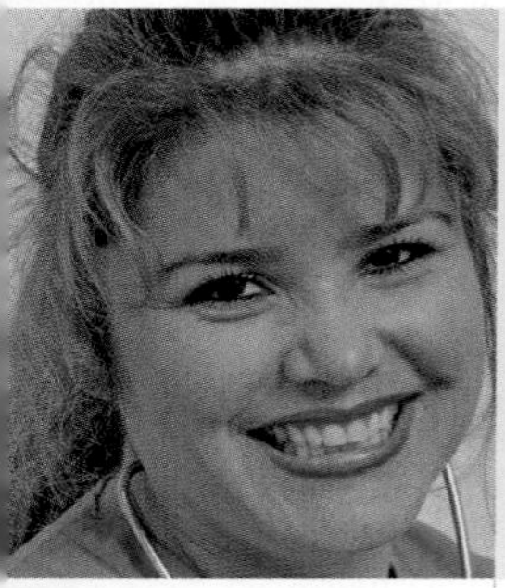

For as long as I can remember, I have been fascinated with birth. Currently, I am a labor and delivery nurse at our town's only hospital. I'm still fascinated with birth but a little nervous, too. You see, I was just admitted in early labor with my first child. Before I got here I worried that I would be a "bad" patient or that I would lose my cool. How silly I was. All that matters is that my baby is healthy and that I am able to take care of him effectively. (Yes. We know it is a boy!) —Amanda, 31

LEARNING OUTCOMES

19.1 Identify admission data that should be noted when a woman is admitted to the birthing area.

19.2 Describe the nursing care of a woman and her partner/family upon admission to the birthing area.

19.3 Use assessment data to determine the nursing interventions to meet the psychologic, social, physiologic, and spiritual needs of the woman during each stage of labor.

19.4 Compare methods of promoting comfort during the first and second stages of labor.

19.5 Explain the immediate needs and physical assessment of the newborn following birth in the provision of nursing care.

19.6 Examine the unique needs of the adolescent during birth in the provision of nursing care.

19.7 Describe the role and responsibilities of the nurse in the management of a precipitous birth.

It is time for a child to be born. The parents are about to undergo one of the most meaningful and stressful events of their lives. The adequacy of their preparation for childbirth, including the coping mechanisms, communication, and support systems that they have established, will be put to the test. Like Amanda, the child-bearing woman may feel that her psychologic and physical limits are about to be challenged. These events may be even more challenging for the single woman, especially if she lacks a strong support system.

Family-centered care is a model of care based on the philosophy that physical, sociocultural, spiritual, and economic needs of the family are combined and considered collectively when planning care for the childbearing family (Chai-Chen, 2007). To reflect the consumer demand for family-centered care, most birthing centers now have **birthing rooms**, single rooms where the woman and her partner or other family members will stay for the labor, birth, recovery, and possibly the postpartum period. These rooms may be called *labor, delivery, recovery, and postpartum (LDRP) rooms* or *single-room maternity care (SRMC).*

The birthing room atmosphere is more relaxed than a traditional labor room, and families seem to feel more comfortable in it. Not having to be transferred from one area to another for birth helps the laboring woman create her own space to labor in and enhances the family's involvement. Birthing rooms usually have beds that can be adapted for birth by removing a small section near the foot. The room's decor is designed to produce a homelike atmosphere in which families can feel both safe and at ease.

The previous two chapters provided information about physiologic and psychologic changes during labor and birth and needed nursing assessments. This chapter focuses on nursing care during labor and birth. See "Clinical Pathway: For Intrapartal Stages" on page 412.

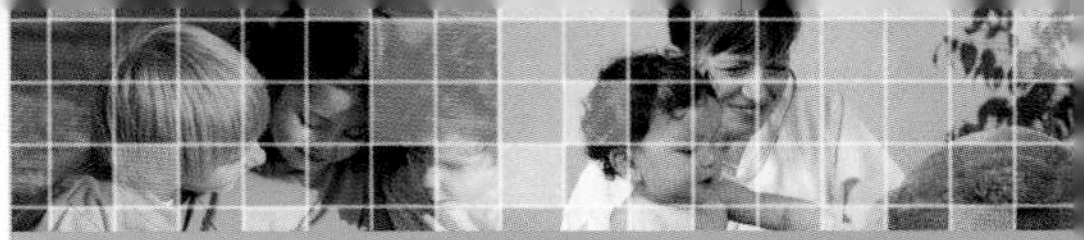

KEY TERMS

Apgar score, 430

Birthing room, 411

Doula, 425

Family-centered care, 411

Precipitous birth, 436

NURSING DIAGNOSIS DURING LABOR AND BIRTH

When devising a plan of care for the intrapartal period, the nurse can develop a general plan that encompasses the total process, from the beginning of labor through the fourth stage, or a more specific plan that identifies nursing diagnoses for each stage of labor and birth.

Examples of appropriate nursing diagnoses may include the following:

- *Fear* related to uncertainty about the outcome of the birth process
- *Acute Pain* related to uterine contractions, cervical dilatation, and fetal descent
- *Health-seeking Behaviors: Information About the Fetal Monitor* related to an expressed desire to understand equipment used
- *Readiness for Enhanced Family Processes* related to opportunity to incorporate newborn into the family

NURSING CARE DURING ADMISSION

During prenatal visits, instruct the woman to come to the birthing unit if any of the following occurs:

- Rupture of membranes (ROM)
- Regular, frequent uterine contractions (nulliparas, 5 minutes apart for 1 hour; multiparas, 6 to 8 minutes apart for 1 hour)
- Vaginal bleeding
- Decreased fetal movement

The woman in labor and her partner or support person(s) tend to be concerned about arriving at the birth center in time for the birth. Sometimes the labor is advanced and birth is imminent, but usually the woman is in early labor at admission. If time permits and the family is not familiar with what will occur during labor, provide necessary information. (See "Teaching Highlights: What to Expect During Labor" on page 415.)

Clinical Pathway

FOR INTRAPARTUM STAGES

CATEGORY	FIRST STAGE	SECOND AND THIRD STAGES	FOURTH STAGE BIRTH TO 1 HOUR PAST BIRTH
Referral	Review prenatal record Advise physician/CNM of admission	Labor record for first stage	Report to recovery room nurse **EXPECTED OUTCOMES** Appropriate resources identified and used
Assessments	*Admission Assessments:* Ask about problems since last prenatal visit; labor status (contraction frequency and duration), membrane status (intact or ruptured); coping level; support; woman's desires during labor and birth; ability to verbalize needs; laboratory testing (blood and UA) Intrapartum assessments: cervical assessment: from 1 to 10 cm dilatation; nullipara (1.2 cm/h), multipara (1.5 cm/h) Cervical effacement: from 0% to 100% Fetal descent: progressive descent from -4 to +4 Membrane assessment: intact or ruptured; when ruptured, Nitrazine positive, fluid clear, no foul odor Comfort level: woman states she is able to cope with contractions Behavioral characteristics: facial expressions, tone of voice, and verbal expressions are consistent with comfort level and ability to cope *Latent Phase:* ■ BP, P, R q1h if in normal range (BP less than or equal to 135/85 or not more than 30 mm Hg systolic or 15 mm Hg diastolic over baseline; pulse 60–90; respirations 16–24/min, quiet, easy) ■ Temp q4h unless greater than 37.6°C (99.6°F) or membranes ruptured then q2h ■ Uterine contractions q30 min (contractions q5–10 min, 15–40 sec, mild intensity) ■ FHR q60 min (for low-risk women) and q30min (for high-risk women) if reassuring (reassuring FHR has: baseline 110-variability present, accelerations with fetal movement, no late decelerations); if nonreassuring, position on side, start O_2, assess for hypotension, monitor continuously, notify physician/CNM	*Second-Stage Assessments:* ■ BP, P, R q5–15 min ■ Uterine contractions palpated continuously ■ FHR q15 min (for low-risk women) and q5 min (for high-risk women) if reassuring; if nonreassuring, monitor continuously Fetal descent: descent continues to birth Comfort level: woman states she is able to cope with contractions and pushing Behavioral characteristics: response to pushing, facial expressions, verbalization *Third-Stage Assessments:* ■ BP, P, R q 5min ■ Uterine contractions, palpate occasionally until placenta is expelled, fundus maintains tone, and contraction pattern continues to expulsion of placenta Newborn assessments: ■ Assess Apgar score of newborn ■ Respirations: 30–60, irregular ■ Apical pulse: 110–160 and somewhat irregular ■ Temperature: Skin temp above 36.5°C (97.8°F) ■ Umbilical cord: two arteries, one vein (if one artery, assess for anomalies and urine output) ■ Gestational age: 38–42 weeks	*Immediate Postbirth Assessments of Mother q15 min for 1h:* ■ BP: less than 135/85; should return to prelabor level ■ Pulse: slightly lower than in labor; range is 60–90 ■ Respirations: 16–24/min; easy; quiet ■ Temperature: 36.2–37.6°C (97–99.6°F) ■ Fundus firm, in midline, at the umbilicus ■ Lochia rubra; moderate amount; less than 2 pad/hr; no free flow or passage of clots with massage ■ Perineum: sutures intact; no bulging or marked swelling; minimal bruising may be present; no c/o severe pain or rectal pain ■ Bladder nondistended; spontaneous void of more than 100 mL clear, straw-colored urine; bladder nondistended following voiding ■ If hemorrhoids present, no tenseness or marked engorgement; less than 2 cm diameter Comfort level: pain less than 3 on scale of 1 to 10 Energy level: awake and able to hold newborn Newborn assessments if newborn remains with parents: ■ Respirations: 30–60; irregular ■ Apical pulse: 110–160 and somewhat irregular ■ Temperature: skin temperature above 36.5°C (97.8°F); skin feels warm to touch ■ Skin color noncyanotic ■ Mucus: small amount, clear, easily suctioned with bulb syringe without skin color change ■ Behavioral: newborn opens eyes widely if room is slightly darkened ■ Movements rhythmic; no hand tremors present

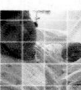

Clinical Pathway—continued

FOR INTRAPARTUM STAGES

CATEGORY	FIRST STAGE	SECOND AND THIRD STAGES	FOURTH STAGE BIRTH TO 1 HOUR PAST BIRTH
	Active Phase: ■ BP, P, R q1h if WNL ■ Temp as above ■ Uterine contractions q15–30 min: contractions q2–5 min, 40–60 sec, moderate to strong ■ FHR q30 min (for low-risk women) and q15 min (for high-risk women) if reassuring; if nonreassuring institute interventions and continuous electronic monitoring *Transition:* ■ BP, P, R, q30 min ■ Uterine contractions q15 min: contractions q1/2–2 min, 60–90 sec, strong ■ FHR q15 min if nonreassuring, see above		**EXPECTED OUTCOMES** Findings indicate normal progression with absence of complications
Teaching/ psychosocial	Establish rapport Orient to environment, expected assessments, and procedures Answer questions and provide information Orient to EFM if used Teach relaxation, visualization, and breathing pattern if needed Explain comfort measures available Assume advocacy role for woman/family during labor and birth	Orient to expected assessments and procedures Answer questions and provide information Explain comfort measures available Continue advocacy role	Explain immediate assessments and care after this first hour Teach self-massage of fundus and expected findings Instruct to call for assistance if mother desires to get OB Begin newborn teaching; bulb syringe, positioning; maintaining warmth Assist parents in exploring their newborn Assist with first breastfeeding experience **EXPECTED OUTCOMES** Client and partner verbalize/demonstrate understanding of teaching
Nursing care management and report	Straight cath prn if bladder distended If regional block administered monitor BP, FHR, sensation per protocol Provide continuing status reports to physician/CNM Perform sterile vaginal examination as indicated	Straight cath prn if bladder distended Continue monitoring VS, FHR, and sensation if regional block has been given	Straight cath if bladder distended and woman unable to void Monitor return of motor ability and sensation if regional block has been given Weigh perineal pads if lochia flow greater than 1 saturated pad in 15 min, presence of boggy uterus and clots; ↓ BP, ↑ P **EXPECTED OUTCOMES** ■ Maternal/fetal well-being maintained and supported ■ Mother and newborn experience safe labor and birth ■ Family participates in process as desired
Activity	Encourage ambulation unless contraindicated Maintain bed rest immediately after administration of IV pain medication, or following regional block Woman rests comfortably between contractions	Position comfortably for birth Woman rests comfortably between pushing efforts and while awaiting expulsion of placenta	Position of comfort **EXPECTED OUTCOMES** ■ Activity maintained as desired unless contraindicated ■ Comfort enhanced by positioning/movement

(continued)

Clinical Pathway—continued

FOR INTRAPARTUM STAGES

CATEGORY	FIRST STAGE	SECOND AND THIRD STAGES	FOURTH STAGE BIRTH TO 1 HOUR PAST BIRTH
Comfort	Institute comfort measures: ambulation, frequent position change, effleurage, focal point, patterned-paced breathing, visualization, therapeutic touch, back rub, moist cloths to face, holding hand, words of encouragement, changing underpad, shower, whirlpool, staying with the woman/family, warmed blanket at back, sacral pressure Offer pain medication or administer if requested Assist with administration of regional block	Institute comfort measures: ■ Second stage: cool cloth to forehead, encouragement, coaching, help support legs while pushing, position of comfort for pushing and birth ■ Third stage: cool cloth to forehead, assist parents to see newborn, position mother to hold newborn, provide encouragement	Institute comfort measures: ■ Perineal discomfort: gently cleanse and apply ice pack; position to decrease pressure on perineum ■ Uterine discomfort: palpate fundus gently ■ Hemorrhoids: ice pack ■ General fatigue: position of comfort, encourage rest ■ Administer pain medication PRN **EXPECTED OUTCOMES** ■ Optimal comfort level maintained ■ Active reduction of pain/discomfort achieved
Nutrition	Ice chips and clear fluids Evaluate for signs of dehydration	Ice chips and clear fluids	Regular diet if assessments are WNL Encourage fluids **EXPECTED OUTCOMES** Nutritional needs met
Elimination	Voids at least q2h; urine clear, straw-colored, negative for protein Bladder nondistended May have bowel movement Monitor I & O with IVs	May void spontaneously with pushing May pass stool with pushing	Voids spontaneously **EXPECTED OUTCOMES** Urinary bladder and bowel function unimpaired
Medications	Administer pain medication per woman's request	Local infiltration of anesthetic agent for birth by physician/CNM Pitocin 10–20 units IM, IVP per IV tubing, or added to IV fluids	Continue Pitocin infusion Administer pain medication PRN **EXPECTED OUTCOMES** Comfort enhanced by pain-relieving techniques, administration of analgesia agent, or an analgesic or anesthetic block
Discharge planning	Evaluate knowledge of labor and birth process Evaluate support system and need for referral after birth		Provide information if mother to be moved from LDR room Provide opportunity for parents to ask questions regarding newborn Evaluate knowledge of normal postpartum, newborn care **EXPECTED OUTCOMES** Mother and newborn transferred to low-risk postpartum and newborn care
Family involvement	Identify available support person(s) Recognize possible impact of culture on responses Observe interaction between woman and partner Create moment alone with woman to identify possible abuse Assess current parenting skills	Provide opportunities for woman and support person(s) to watch newborn assessments Perform newborn assessment on mother's abdomen/chest if possible	Provide opportunity for parents to be with baby Encourage skin-to-skin contact Darken room to encourage eye-to-eye contact Provide quiet time for new family Parenting: demonstrates early culturally expected parenting behaviors **EXPECTED OUTCOMES** Incorporation of newborn into family Family verbalizes comfort with newborn care
Date			

CNM, certified nurse-midwife; BP, blood pressure; FHR, fetal heart rate; STV, short-term variability; LTV, long-term variability; WNL, within normal limits; VS, vital signs; EFM, electronic fetal monitoring; IV, intravenous; I & O, intake & output; IM, intramuscularly; IVP, intravenous push; LDR, labor, delivery, and recovery; OB, out of bed; UA, urinary analysis; PRN, as needed; c/o, complains of.

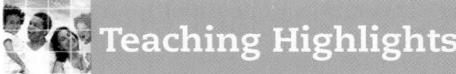

Teaching Highlights

WHAT TO EXPECT DURING LABOR

Describe aspects of the admission process:

- Abbreviated history
- Physical assessment (maternal vital signs, fetal heart rate, contraction status, status of membranes)
- Assessment of uterine contractions (frequency, duration, intensity)
- Orientation to surroundings
- Introductions to other staff
- Determination of the woman's and support person's expectations of the nurse

Present aspects of ongoing physical care, such as when to expect assessment of maternal vital signs, fetal heart rate, and contractions.

If an electronic fetal monitor is used, describe how it works and the information it provides. Orient the woman to sights and sounds of the monitor.

Explain what "normal" data look like and what characteristics are being watched for.

Be sure to note that assessments will increase as the labor progresses, especially during the transition phase, to help keep the mother and baby safe by noting any changes from the normal course.

Explain the vaginal examination and the information it can provide.

Review comfort techniques that may be used in labor and ascertain what the woman thinks will promote comfort.

Review breathing techniques the woman has learned so that you can support her technique.

Review comfort and support measures such as positioning, back rub, effleurage, touch, distraction techniques, and ambulation.

If the woman is in early labor, offer her a tour of the birthing area.

Have printed materials available for reference, especially for the partner or support person.

If time permits, a brief video describing procedures may be helpful.

The way the maternity nurse greets the woman and her partner influences the course of the woman's hospital stay. The sudden environmental change and the sometimes impersonal and technical aspects of admission can produce significant stress. If women and their families are greeted in a brusque, harried manner, they are less likely to look to the nurse for support. A calm, pleasant manner indicates to the woman that she is important. It helps to instill a sense of confidence in the staff's ability to provide quality care during this critical time.

Following the initial greeting, escort the woman to the birthing room and provide a quick yet thorough orientation to the facility, including the location of the restrooms, public phones, and nurse-call or emergency-call system. These simple steps can go a long way toward helping the woman and her partner feel more at ease. Explain the monitoring equipment or other unfamiliar technology and make every effort to make the environment less frightening for the laboring woman and her support person(s).

Some women prefer that their partner remain with them during the admission process, and others prefer to have the partner wait outside. While helping the woman undress and get into a hospital gown, begin to develop rapport and establish a nursing database. The experienced labor and birth nurse can obtain essential information about the woman and her pregnancy within a few minutes after admission, initiate any immediate interventions needed, and establish individualized priorities.

The woman may be facing a number of unfamiliar procedures that seem routine for healthcare providers. Remember that all women have the right to determine what happens to their bodies. The woman's informed consent should be obtained prior to any procedure that involves touching her.

If indicated, assist the woman into bed. A side-lying or semi-Fowler's position rather than a supine position is most comfortable and avoids supine hypotensive syndrome (vena caval syndrome). After obtaining the essential information from the woman and her records, begin the intrapartal assessment. (See Chapter 18.) Once the assessment is complete, it is possible to make effective nursing decisions about care, such as the following:

- Should ambulation, bed rest, or a combination of both be encouraged?
- Is more frequent or continuous electronic fetal monitoring needed?
- What does the woman want during her labor and birth?
- Is a support person available?
- What special needs do this woman and her partner have?

Auscultate the fetal heart rate (FHR). (See Chapter 18.) Determine the woman's blood pressure, pulse, respirations, and oral temperature and assess contraction frequency, duration, and intensity (possibly while gathering other data). Before the vaginal examination, inform the woman about the procedure and its purpose; afterward, report the findings. If signs of advanced labor exist (frequent contractions, an urge to bear down, and so on), a vaginal examination must be done immediately. If there are signs of excessive bleeding or if the woman reports episodes of painless bleeding in the last trimester, suspect placenta previa. *Do not do a vaginal examination, and notify the physician or certified nurse-midwife (CNM) immediately.*

Results of FHR assessment, uterine contraction evaluation, and the vaginal examination help determine whether the rest of the admission process can proceed at a leisurely pace or whether additional interventions are required. For example, an FHR of less than 110 beats per minute on auscultation indicates that a fetal monitor should be applied immediately to obtain additional data. The woman's vital signs can be assessed once the monitor is in place.

After obtaining admission data, collect a clean voided midstream urine specimen. The woman with intact membranes may collect her specimen in the bathroom. If the membranes are ruptured and the presenting part is not engaged, the woman generally remains in bed to avoid prolapse of the umbilical cord. Views vary about the wisdom of ambulation once the membranes are ruptured. The decision is generally based on history and physical findings (for example, history of precipitous labors, indications for continuous fetal monitoring, presence of meconium), clinician orders, the woman's desires, agency policy, and safety concerns.

Use a dipstick to test the woman's urine for the presence of protein, ketones, and glucose before sending the sample to the laboratory. This procedure is especially important if edema or elevated blood pressure is noted on admission. Proteinuria of 1+ or more may be a sign of impending preeclampsia. Glycosuria (sugar in the urine) is found frequently in pregnant women because of the increased glomerular filtration rate in the proximal tubules and the inability of these tubules to increase reabsorption of glucose. However, it may also be associated with gestational diabetes, so do not discount it. While the woman is collecting the urine specimen, gather the equipment needed for any procedures ordered by the CNM or physician.

Laboratory tests are done during early admission. Hemoglobin and hematocrit values help determine the oxygen-carrying capacity of the circulatory system and the woman's ability to withstand blood loss at birth. Elevation of the hematocrit may reveal hemoconcentration of blood, which occurs with edema or dehydration. A low hemoglobin, in the absence of other evidence of bleeding, suggests anemia. Blood may be typed and cross-matched if the woman is in a high-risk category. Platelets are also evaluated because low platelets can lead to bleeding problems. Additional serologic testing may be performed as indicated. HIV testing should be offered to all women who have not been previously screened (Perinatal HIV Guidelines Working Group, 2006).

MyNursingKit Care Plan Activity: Presence of Extended Family

Depending on how rapidly labor is progressing, notify the CNM or physician before or after completing the admission procedures. The report should include the following information: parity, cervical dilatation and effacement, station, presenting part, status of the membranes, contraction pattern, FHR, vital signs that are not in the normal range, any significant prenatal history, the woman's birth preferences, and her reaction to labor.

Enter a nursing admission note into the computer or the charting system. The admission note should include the reason for admission, the date and time of the woman's arrival and notification of the CNM or physician, the condition of the woman and her baby, and labor and membrane status.

NURSING CARE DURING THE FIRST STAGE OF LABOR

After completing the nursing assessment and diagnosis steps, create a plan of care to achieve identified nursing goals. For instance, if the woman and her support person did not have the opportunity to attend childbirth preparation classes, the nursing goal would be to provide desired information. To accomplish this goal, the nurse would assess the current level of the couple's understanding and then plan to provide brief explanations as labor progresses.

INTEGRATION OF FAMILY EXPECTATIONS

Families come into the birth setting with basic expectations that they will not be harmed and that the labor and birth will be safe for the mother and baby. In addition, women look for the following from their nurses:

- Emotional support, which includes sustained presence of the nurse, praise, encouragement, reassurance, and companionship
- Comfort measures such as the use of touch, provision of ice chips and fluids, massage, assistance with care, and a bath or shower
- Information and advice, which includes offering information about procedures, interventions as they occur, and reports of labor progress
- Advocacy to help the woman and her partner achieve their goals, hopes, and dreams for their labor and birth experience
- Support of the partner, including encouragement, praise for his or her efforts, an opportunity for rest breaks, and role modeling

INTEGRATION OF CULTURAL BELIEFS

Knowledge of values, customs, and practices of different cultures is as important during labor as it is in the prenatal period. Without this knowledge a nurse is less likely to understand a family's behavior and may attempt to impose personal values and beliefs on them. As cultural sensitivity increases, so does the likelihood of providing high-quality care.

The following sections briefly present a few possible cultural responses to labor. General examples about any culture or belief system should be viewed as background information only. An individual example of a birthing practice will never be pertinent to all women in a given group. Within every culture, each person develops his or her own beliefs, values, and behaviors. Culture is also discussed in Chapter 2.

Modesty

Modesty is an important consideration for women regardless of culture. However, some women may be more uncomfortable than others with the degree of exposure needed for certain procedures during labor and the birth process. Some women may be particularly uncomfortable when men are present and feel more comfortable with women; others may be uncomfortable with exposure of personal body parts regardless of the gender of the caregivers. The nurse should be alert to the woman's responses to examinations and procedures and provide the draping and privacy the woman needs. It is more prudent to assume that embarrassment will occur with exposure and take measures to provide privacy than to assume that it will not matter to the woman if she is exposed during procedures.

Pain Expression

The manner in which a woman chooses to deal with the discomfort of labor varies widely. Some women seem to turn inward and remain very quiet during the whole process. They speak only to ask others to leave the room or cease conversation. Others may be very vocal, with behaviors such as counting out loud, moaning quietly, crying, or use of loud vocalization. They may also turn from side to side or change positions frequently.

In many Asian cultures, it is important for individuals to act in a way that will not bring shame on the family. Therefore, the Korean woman may not express pain outwardly for fear of shaming herself or her family. Silence is valued in Chinese society, so a woman of that heritage is usually quiet and stoic to avoid dishonoring herself or her family. Mexican women often chant the phrase "Aye yie yie" while in labor, which is actually a form of "folk lamaze." Repeating the phrase in succession several times necessitates taking long, slow, deep breaths. Thus, it is a cultural method for alleviating pain (St. Elizabeth's Medical Center, 2007). European Americans demonstrate a wide variety of behaviors in response to pain, from silence to shouting. It is important to support a woman's individual expression, whatever it may be (as long as harm is not done to another), in order to enhance the birthing experience for mother, baby, and family.

Cultural Beliefs: Some Examples

It is essential to avoid stereotyping in providing care. The four examples that follow give insight into the variety of responses nurses may encounter.

Squatting during labor is common for Hmong women from Laos. They may also prefer to be active and move about. The husband is frequently present and involved in providing comfort. The woman may ask that the amniotic membranes not be ruptured until just before birth. It is thought that the escape of fluid at this time makes the birth easier. During labor the woman usually prefers only "hot" foods and warm water to drink (Spector, 2009) (see Chapter 2). As soon as the baby is born, the family may request that a soft-boiled egg be given to the mother to restore her energy.

Vietnamese women usually maintain self-control and may even smile throughout labor. They may prefer to walk about and to give birth in a squatting position. In labor the woman may prefer cold beverages because pregnancy is viewed as a "hot" condition. However, during the postpartum, which is viewed as a "cold" condition, she may prefer warm liquids (Ethnomed, 2007). The newborn is protected from praise to prevent jealousy (Spector, 2009).

Latina women have identified expectations of their partners during labor and birth such as wanting their partners to stay with them and to reassure them that everything will be all right. As they labor, the women want their partners to show their love and to speak using affectionate words.

Muslim women may have their husband, a female friend or relative, or a male relative with them during childbirth. If a specialist such as an anesthesiologist or neonatologist is needed, it is best to speak to the husband first and obtain his permission. Family support is important but does not preclude the importance of the nurse's presence. The woman may want to retain her head covering (*khimar*) and may prefer to wear two long-sleeved gowns to enhance modesty. It is important for a female nurse, physician, or CNM to perform examinations whenever possible. After the birth Muslim fathers may call praise to Allah (*adhan*) in the newborn's right ear and clean the newborn.

Maternity nurses can provide culturally sensitive care by first becoming acquainted with the beliefs and practices of the various subcultures in their communities. In the birthing situation, the truly effective nurse supports the family's cultural practices as long as it is safe to do so.

PROVISION OF CARE IN THE FIRST STAGE OF LABOR

Latent Phase

As discussed in Chapter 18, it is important to assess the physical well-being of the woman and her fetus. Monitor maternal temperature every 4 hours unless the temperature is over 37.5°C (99.6°F); in such cases take it every hour. Monitor blood pressure, pulse, and respirations every hour. If the woman's blood pressure is over 135/85 mm Hg or her pulse is more than 100, notify the CNM or physician and reevaluate the blood pressure and pulse more frequently.

Palpate uterine contractions for frequency, intensity, and duration every 30 minutes. Auscultate the FHR every 60 minutes for low-risk women and every 30 minutes for high-risk women as long as it remains between 110 and 160 beats per minute and is reassuring (American College of Obstetricians & Gynecologists [ACOG], 2005). Auscultate the FHR throughout one contraction and for about 15 seconds after the contraction to ensure that there are no decelerations. If the FHR baseline is not in the 110 to 160 range or if decelerations are heard, continuous electronic monitoring is recommended (Table 19–1).

Offer the woman fluids in the form of clear liquids or ice chips frequently, unless complications exist that may result in a cesarean birth. Some certified childbirth educators advise the woman to bring lollipops to help combat the dryness that occurs with some of the labor breathing patterns. Avoiding both liquids and solids during labor, which was once a standard of practice, is

Developing Cultural Competence

NATIVE AMERICAN WOMEN AND LABOR

Native American women typically view labor pain as natural, and may use meditation, self-control, or indigenous plants or herbs, such as black cohosh, throughout their labor as well as to aid them during birth (Spector, 2009).

Thinking Critically

GENDER-SPECIFIC CARE PREFERENCE

Fatima Al Ahala is a 22-year-old, G1 who presents in labor. Fatima and her husband Samir are from Pakistan. The couple has stated that they can accept care only from female providers. The couple is being attended by a female nurse-midwife, and the backup physician is also a female. When her labor intensifies, Fatima requests an epidural. The only anesthesiologist available is a male physician. What actions can you take to help this family meet their cultural preferences?

See MyNursingKit for possible responses.

Table 19–1 Nursing Assessments in the First Stage

Phase	Mother	Fetus
Latent	Blood pressure, respirations each hour if in normal range Temperature every 4 hours unless over 37.5°C (99.6°F) or membranes ruptured, then every hour Uterine contractions every 30 minutes	Fetal heart rate (FHR) every 60 minutes for low-risk women and every 30 minutes for high-risk women if normal characteristics present (average variability, baseline in the 110–160 beats per minute range, without late or variable decelerations). Note fetal activity. If electronic fetal monitor in place, assess for reactive nonstress test (NST).
Active	Blood pressure, pulse, respirations every hour if in normal range Uterine contractions every 15 to 30 minutes	FHR every 30 minutes for low-risk women and every 15 minutes for high-risk women if normal characteristics are present.
Transition	Blood pressure, pulse, respirations every 30 minutes Uterine contractions at least every 15 minutes	FHR every 30 minutes for low-risk women and every 15 minutes for high-risk women if normal characteristics are present.

no longer so as evidence-based practice research and new guidelines indicate that clear fluids can be consumed throughout labor and up to 2 hours before an elective cesarean birth. Current guidelines suggest avoiding solids for 6 to 8 hours before an elective cesarean birth (American Society of Anesthesiologists [ASA], 2006). Eating during labor has not been associated with an increase in aspiration but some institutions continue to limit oral intake in labor (Gennaro, Mayberry, & Kafulafula, 2007). Previously, it was believed that drinking fluids should be avoided because it can lead to vomiting caused by the decreased gastric emptying time. Although vomiting is common during the first stage of labor, many women have more energy and tolerate labor better with oral intake and have higher satisfaction with their labor and birth experience (ASA, 2006).

Active Phase

During the active phase, contractions have a frequency of 2 to 5 minutes, a duration of 40 to 60 seconds, and a moderate to strong intensity. Palpate contractions every 15 to 30 minutes. As the contractions become more frequent and intense, vaginal exams assess cervical dilatation and effacement and fetal station and position. During the active phase, the cervix dilates from 4 to 7 cm, and vaginal discharge and bloody show increase. Monitor maternal blood pressure, pulse, and respirations every hour for low-risk women (unless elevated, as previously noted) and every 30 minutes for high-risk women. Auscultate the FHR every 30 minutes for low-risk women and every 15 minutes for high-risk women (ACOG, 2005).

A woman who has been ambulatory up to this point may wish to sit in a chair or on a bed. If the woman wants to lie on the bed, encourage her to assume a side-lying position, help her into a comfortable position, and place pillows to support her body. To increase comfort, offer a back rub or effleurage or place a cool cloth on the woman's forehead or across her neck. Because vaginal discharge increases, change the chux pad frequently. Washing the perineum with warm soapy water removes secretions and increases comfort. During such procedures it is essential to wear disposable gloves to avoid exposure to vaginal discharge.

If the amniotic membranes have not ruptured previously, they may do so during this phase. When the membranes rupture, note the color, odor, and consistency of the amniotic fluid and the time of rupture, and immediately note the FHR on the monitor if one is being used. If the woman is not on a monitor, auscultate FHR. The fluid should be clear, with no odor. Fetal stress leads to intestinal and anal sphincter relaxation, and meconium may be released into the amniotic fluid, which turns the fluid greenish brown. Whenever meconium-stained fluid is present, apply an electronic monitor to assess the FHR continuously. Note the time of rupture because medical practice suggests that birth should occur within 24 hours of the rupture of membranes.

Prolapse of the umbilical cord is a possible risk when membranes rupture and the fetus is not engaged, because the amniotic fluid coming through the cervix might wash the umbilical cord out through the cervix. With each contraction the cord would then become trapped between the presenting part and the maternal pelvis. The FHR is auscultated because a drop in the rate might indicate an undetected prolapsed cord. Immediate intervention is necessary to remove pressure on a prolapsed umbilical cord (see Chapter 21∞). (See Table 19–2 for additional deviations from normal.)

Transition

During transition the contraction frequency is every 1 1/2 to 2 minutes, duration is 60 to 90 seconds, and intensity is strong. Cervical dilatation increases from 8 to 10 cm, effacement is complete (100%), and there is usually a heavy amount of bloody show. Palpate contractions at least every 15 minutes. Sterile vaginal examinations may be done more frequently because this stage of labor usually is accompanied by rapid change. Take the maternal blood pressure, pulse, and respirations at least every 30 minutes, and auscultate FHR every 15 minutes.

Comfort measures are important in this phase of labor, but continual assessment is required to intervene appropriately. The woman may rapidly change from wanting a back rub and other hands-on care to wanting to be left completely alone. The support person and the nurse need to follow her cues and change

Table 19–2 Deviations from Normal Labor Process Requiring Immediate Intervention

Problem	Immediate Action
Woman admitted with vaginal bleeding or history of painless vaginal bleeding	Do not perform vaginal examination. Assess fetal heart rate (FHR). Evaluate amount of blood loss. Evaluate labor pattern. Notify physician or certified nurse-midwife (CNM) immediately.
Presence of greenish or brownish amniotic fluid	Continuously monitor FHR. Evaluate dilatation of cervix and determine if umbilical cord is prolapsed. Evaluate presentation (vertex or breech). Maintain woman on complete bed rest on left side. Notify physician or CNM immediately.
Absence of FHR and fetal movement	Notify physician or CNM. Provide truthful information and emotional support to laboring couple. Remain with the couple.
Prolapse of umbilical cord	Relieve pressure on cord manually. Continuously monitor FHR; watch for changes in FHR pattern. Notify physician or CNM. Assist woman into knee-chest position or place in Trendelenburg position. Administer oxygen.
Woman admitted in advanced labor; birth imminent	Prepare for immediate birth. Obtain critical information: Estimated date of birth (EDB) History of bleeding problems History of medical or obstetric problems Past or present use or abuse of prescription, over-the-counter (OTC), or illicit drugs Problems with this pregnancy FHR and maternal vital signs Whether membranes are ruptured and how long since rupture Blood type and Rh Direct another person to contact physician or CNM. Do not leave woman alone. Provide support to couple. Put on gloves.

interventions as needed. Because the woman is breathing more rapidly, increase her comfort by offering small spoonfuls of ice chips to moisten her mouth or offer an emollient for her dry lips. Encourage the woman to rest between contractions. If analgesics have been administered, a quiet environment enhances the quality of rest between contractions. Awaken the woman just before a contraction begins so that she can begin patterned breathing.

Some women have difficulty coping during this time and need help with their breathing. Either the support person or the nurse can breathe along with the woman during each contraction to help her maintain her pattern. It is helpful to encourage the woman and to assure her that she is doing a good job. The woman will begin to feel increased rectal pressure as the fetal presenting part moves down the birth canal. To help prevent cervical edema, encourage the woman to refrain from pushing until the cervix is completely dilated.

The end of transition and the beginning of the second stage may be indicated by a change in the woman's voice or the sounds she is making. As the fetus moves down and she feels increased pressure and a bearing-down sensation, her voice tends to deepen. A moan during a contraction takes on a more guttural quality.

PROMOTION OF COMFORT IN THE FIRST STAGE

The first step in planning care is to talk with the woman and her partner or support person to identify their goals. Usually the woman or couple is concerned with discomfort, so it is helpful to identify factors that may contribute to it. These factors include uncomfortable positions, diaphoresis, continual leaking of amniotic fluid, a full bladder, a dry mouth, anxiety, and fear. Nursing interventions can minimize the effects of these factors. These interventions are described later in this section.

As the intensity of the contraction increases with the progress of labor, the woman becomes less aware of the environment and may have difficulty hearing and understanding verbal instructions. The pattern of coping with labor contractions varies from the use of highly structured breathing techniques to turning inward. Low moaning that begins deep in the throat, rocking or swaying, facial grimacing, and using loud vocalizations are all effective means of dealing with the power of labor and birth. Some women feel that making sounds helps them cope and do the work of labor, whereas others make loud sounds only as they lose their perception of control.

The most frequent physiologic manifestations of pain are increased pulse and respiratory rates, dilated pupils, increased blood pressure, and muscle tension. In labor these reactions are transitory because the pain is intermittent. Increased muscle tension is most significant because it may impede the progress of labor. Women in labor often tighten skeletal muscles voluntarily during a contraction and remain motionless. This method of dealing with the contractions may actually increase the level of discomfort because of muscular tension, but the women may believe it is the only acceptable way to cope with the pain.

A woman generally wants touching, massage, effleurage (see Chapter 8 ∞), and other forms of physical contact during the first part of labor, but when she moves into the transition phase, she may pull away. Women may provide verbal and nonverbal signs such as crying, moaning, and beseeching the coach or nurse to hold their hand or rub their back. Some women are uncomfortable with being touched at all, regardless of the phase of labor. It is important to confirm the woman's preferences and to meet each family on its own terms, always keeping in mind that this is their experience.

Nonpharmacologic Pain Relief

The nurse can introduce the following nonpharmacologic pain relief techniques in labor to encourage maternal comfort and facilitate coping: massage, effleurage, hydrotherapy, position changes, hypnosis, aromatherapy, sitting in a rocking chair/glider/birthing ball, walking, leaning against the bed or her partner, use of a TENs unit, visualization, relaxation techniques, the use of prayer or meditation, and breathing techniques. See "Complementary Care: Acupressure During Labor."

Many nurses readily respond to the woman's needs. As the nurse and woman or couple work together to increase comfort during contractions, a ritual of supportive measures begins to develop. The nurse watches for cues and nonverbal behaviors and asks for feedback from the woman. As labor progresses, the

Complementary Care

ACUPRESSURE DURING LABOR

Acupressure is an ancient Chinese medical treatment that involves using the fingers to press key pressure points on the surface of the skin. This pressure ultimately stimulates the immune system to promote healing by triggering the release of endorphins, reducing stress through muscle relaxation, and promoting circulation. The specific acupressure point used in laboring women is the San Yin-Jiao (SP-6) acupressure point. The SP-6 acupressure point is located on the medial side of the leg, in the calf region, approximately 3 cm (1.2 in.) superior to the prominence of the inner malleus. The use of acupressure in labor has been associated with shorter labors and lower subjective and objective pain scores. Women who receive acupressure typically use less pain medication than those who do not receive acupressure (Smith, Collins, Cyna, et al., 2006).

Evidence-Based Nursing

MATERNAL POSITIONS DURING THE FIRST STAGE OF LABOR

Clinical Question

What maternal positions during the first stage of labor are associated with optimal outcomes for mother and baby?

The Evidence

Five researchers conducted a systematic review of 21 studies representing 3706 women. The resulting guideline was reviewed and published by the Cochrane Collaboration, which provides a rigorous appraisal process. The recommendations from a Cochrane review represent the strongest level of evidence. Women in the developed world often labor in the reclining position in bed during the first stage of labor. This position is more convenient for the staff to assess the mother and conduct procedures, but has not been linked to better outcomes for the mother or baby. Physiologically, the supine position puts the weight of the pregnant uterus on abdominal blood vessels. Contractions may be weaker when lying down. These researchers found that the first stage of labor may be up to an hour shorter for women who walk around versus those who maintain the supine position in bed. The length of the second stage of labor and the number of spontaneous (versus assisted) births were the same regardless of first stage position. Opioid usage was no different based on position in the first stage, but women who walked had less epidural analgesia (Lawrence, Lewis, Hofmeyr, et al., 2009).

Best Practice

Women should be encouraged to walk or remain upright during the first stage of labor to speed the progress of cervical dilation. When lying in bed, the mothers should choose the position most comfortable to them, but should be encouraged to avoid the supine position. When in bed, the lateral position will reduce pressure on the abdominal blood vessels and enhance contractions.

Critical Thinking

What is the effect of maternal position on satisfaction? Is maternal position during the first stage of labor associated with better neonatal outcomes?

See MyNursingKit for possible responses.

nurse and couple use their experience and growing rapport to change comfort measures as needed. Nursing measures used to decrease pain include the following:

- Ensuring general comfort
- Providing information to decrease anxiety
- Using specific supportive relaxation techniques
- Encouraging controlled breathing
- Administering pharmacologic agents as ordered by the physician or CNM

General Comfort

General comfort measures are of great importance during labor. By relieving minor discomforts, the nurse helps the woman optimize her ability to cope with pain. Encourage the woman to ambulate as long as there are no contraindications, such as vaginal bleeding or rupture of membranes before the fetus is engaged in the pelvis. Ambulation can increase comfort and aid in fetal descent (Figure 19–1 ●).

Even if the woman prefers not to walk around, upright positions such as sitting in a rocker or leaning against a wall or bed can enhance comfort. If she stays in bed, encourage the woman

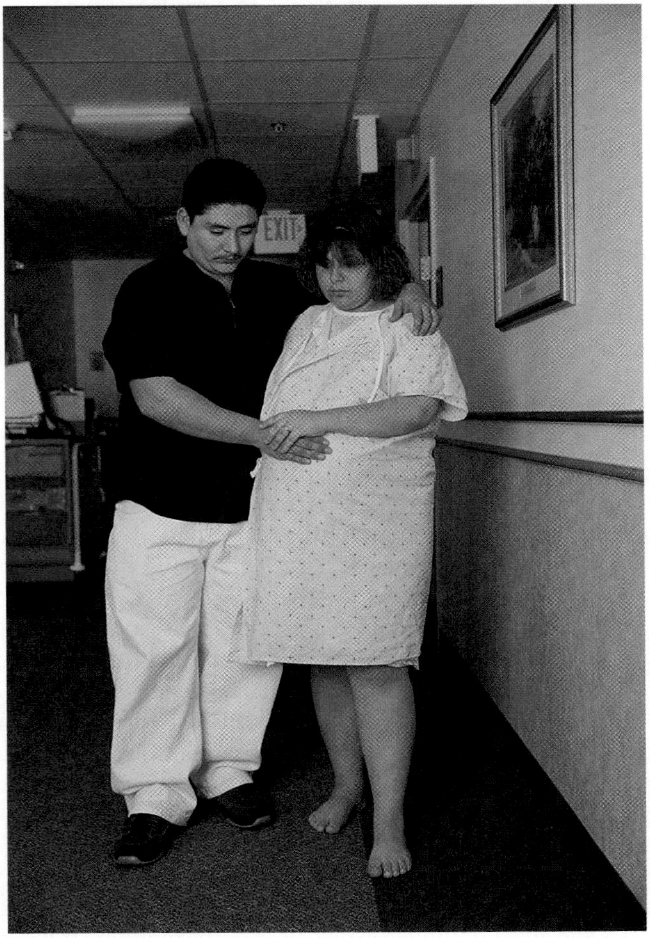

● **Figure 19–1** Increasing comfort and aiding in fetal descent. This woman and her partner are walking in the hospital during labor.

Evidence in Action

A review of the research supports the use of the hands-and-knees posture to relieve persistent back pain during labor (Cochrane Review) (Hunter, Hofmeyr, & Kulierm, 2007).

to assume positions that she finds comfortable (Figure 19–2 ●). A side-lying position is generally the most advantageous for the laboring woman, although frequent position changes seem to achieve more efficient contractions. It is important to support all body parts, with the joints kept slightly flexed. For instance, when the woman is in a side-lying position, pillows may be placed against her chest and under the uppermost arm. Place a pillow or folded bath blanket between her knees to support the uppermost leg and relieve tension or muscle strain. A pillow placed at the woman's midback also helps provide support. If the woman is more comfortable on her back, elevate the head of the bed to relieve the pressure of the uterus on the vena cava.

Pillows may be placed under each arm and under the knees to provide further support. Because a pregnant woman is at increased risk for thrombophlebitis, excessive pressure behind the knee and calf should be avoided. Assess pressure points frequently.

Back rubs and frequent changes of position contribute to comfort and relaxation. Wearing socks or slippers may alleviate cold feet, just as adjusting the room's thermostat can offset excessive warmth. Attention to such details allows the woman to focus on the more important issues of giving birth.

Diaphoresis and the constant leaking of amniotic fluid can dampen the woman's gown and bed linen. Fresh, smooth, dry bed linen promotes comfort. To avoid having to change the bottom sheet following rupture of the membranes, replace chux pads at frequent intervals (following body substance isolation precautions). Keep the woman's perineal area as clean and dry as possible to promote comfort and to prevent infection.

A full bladder adds to the discomfort during a contraction and may prolong labor by interfering with the descent of the fetus. The bladder should be kept as empty as possible. Even if the woman is voiding, urine may be retained because of the pressure of the fetal presenting part. To detect a full bladder, palpate directly over the symphysis pubis. Some regional analgesia procedures contribute to

Nursing Practice

Support persons and family members need to be encouraged to maintain their own comfort. Because they are paying attention to the laboring woman, they may forget their own needs. It may be necessary to encourage them to take breaks, to eat and drink, and to rest. However, they may be reluctant to leave the woman unattended while they meet their own personal needs. Offer to stay with the woman during their absence. This provides reassurance that the woman will be well cared for in their absence.

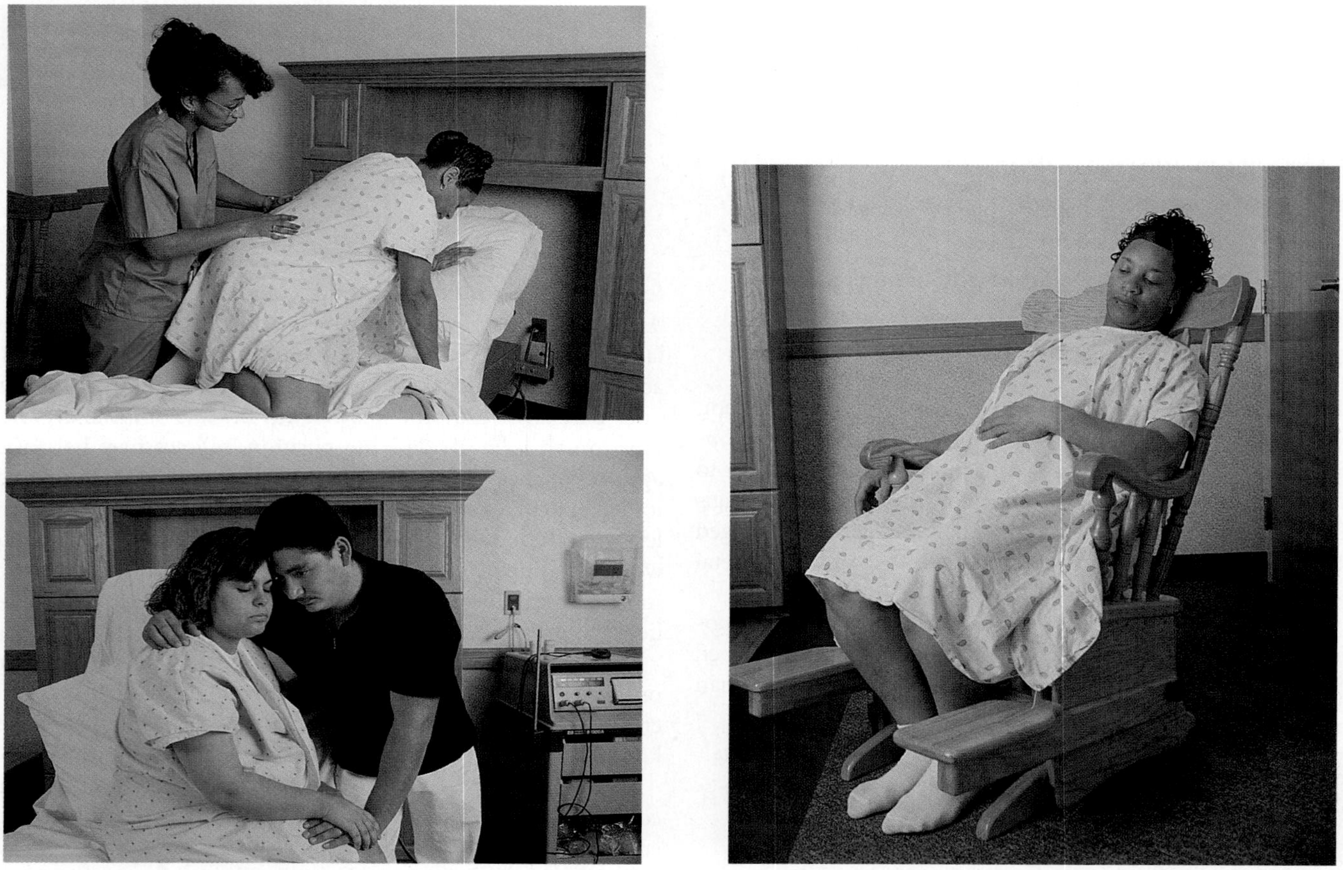

● **Figure 19–2** General comfort. The laboring woman is encouraged to choose a comfortable position. The nurse modifies assessments and intervention as necessary.

the inability to void, and catheterization may be necessary. Encourage the woman to empty her bladder every 1 to 2 hours.

Handling Anxiety

A woman's anxiety as she begins labor is related to a combination of factors inherent to the process. A moderate amount of anxiety about the pain enhances the woman's ability to deal with it. In contrast, an excessive degree of anxiety decreases her ability to cope. Women who have increased anxiety about safety and their ability to cope are much more likely to describe their pain as unbearable.

To decrease anxiety not related to pain, give information (which eases fear of the unknown), establish rapport with the couple (which helps them preserve their personal integrity), and express confidence in the couple's ability to work with the labor process. Remaining with the woman as much as possible conveys a caring attitude and dispels fears of abandonment. Praise for breathing, relaxation, and pushing efforts not only encourages repetition of the behavior but also decreases anxiety about the ability to cope with labor.

Client Teaching

Providing truthful information about the nature of the discomfort that will occur during labor is important. Stressing the intermittent nature and maximum duration of the contractions can be most helpful. The woman can cope with pain better when she knows that a period of relief will follow.

Descriptions of sensations are best accompanied by information on specific comfort measures. Some women experience the urge to push during transition, when the cervix is not fully dilated and effaced. Panting can control this sensation (it is difficult to pant and bear down at the same time). If time permits, explain the purpose of panting and have the woman practice before the technique is needed.

Thorough orientation and explanation of surroundings, procedures, and equipment being used also decrease anxiety, thereby reducing pain. Explain beeps, clicks, and other strange noises and give a simplified explanation of the monitor strip, emphasizing that the use of the fetal monitor provides a way to assess the well-being of the fetus during labor. It helps to show the

Teaching Highlights

ANXIETY ABOUT VAGINAL EXAMINATION

If a woman is experiencing severe fear or anxiety about a vaginal examination, advise her to slowly count to 10 during the examination while continually wiggling her toes. This source of distraction may lessen her fear and anxiety. It also enables the woman to have a sense of control.

woman and her partner or support person how the monitor can identify the beginnings of contractions. At the onset of each contraction, encourage the woman to begin her breathing technique to lessen her perception of pain.

Labor and childbirth may be a critical time for the woman with a history of childhood sexual abuse or rape. All women entering the healthcare arena need to be evaluated for a history of sexual abuse or rape. However, a woman may or may not be able to address this issue with the nurse, because sharing such personal information with a stranger is difficult. It is especially important to be alert for nonverbal cues, such as unexplained anxiety, unrelenting pain, or fear during vaginal examinations, and to be prepared to offer additional teaching and relaxation support to help offset the woman's anxiety.

Supportive Relaxation Techniques

Tense muscles increase resistance to the descent of the fetus and contribute to maternal fatigue. This fatigue increases pain perception and decreases the woman's ability to cope with the pain. Comfort measures, massage, water therapy using immersion in a Jacuzzi or spa, techniques for decreasing anxiety, and client teaching can contribute to relaxation. Adequate sleep and rest are also important. Encourage the laboring woman to use the periods between contractions for rest and relaxation. A prolonged prodromal phase of labor may have kept her awake. Moreover, a woman beginning labor is naturally excited, making it difficult for her to sleep even if her contractions are mild and infrequent.

Distraction helps increase relaxation and ability to cope with discomfort. During early labor, conversation or activities such as light reading or playing cards or other games serve as distractions. It may be helpful to have the woman concentrate on a pleasant experience she has had in the past. Other techniques include the use of a specific visual or mental focal point, breathing techniques, counting or humming, or visualization.

Touch is another type of distraction (Figure 19–3 ●). Although some women regard touching as an invasion of privacy or threat to their independence, many want to touch and be touched during a painful experience. Nurses can make themselves available to the woman who desires touch by placing a hand on the side of the bed within the woman's reach. The person who needs touch will reach out for contact. (See "Complementary Care: Intuitive Touch.")

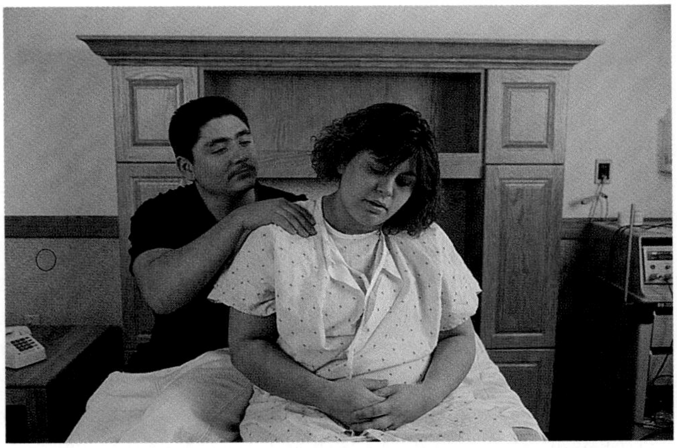

● **Figure 19–3** Touch as a distraction technique. The woman's partner provides support and encouragement during labor.

Complementary Care

INTUITIVE TOUCH

Intuitive touch is the nurse's intentional use of physical contact with the woman with the intent of helping to slow down and regulate the breathing pattern. (*Note:* Therapeutic touch, a complementary therapy that focuses on energy fields, is a different process. See discussion in Chapter 2 ∞.) Evidence suggests that touch induces the relaxation response, which is mediated through the neuroendocrine and sympathetic nervous systems.

A variety of techniques can be used. These include hand-holding; stroking or patting of a woman's arm, face, or legs; placing one hand on her shoulder; putting an arm around her shoulders; and hugging. To implement intuitive touch, use long, slow, up-and-down strokes on the woman's limbs. You do not need special training to use this intervention; all that is needed is the intention to help regulate the breathing pattern and the willingness to use a little time to achieve this goal.

Mild to moderate abdominal discomfort during contractions may be relieved or lessened by effleurage. Firm pressure on the lower back or sacral area may relieve back pain associated with labor. To apply firm pressure, place a hand or a rolled, warmed towel or blanket in the small of the woman's back. In addition to the measures just described, enhance the woman's relaxation by providing encouragement and support for her controlled breathing techniques.

Breathing Techniques

Breathing techniques may help the laboring woman. Used correctly they increase the woman's pain threshold, permit relaxation, enhance the woman's ability to cope with the uterine contractions, and allow the uterus to function more efficiently.

Many women learn patterned-paced breathing during childbirth preparation classes. This type of controlled breathing often has three levels. The woman tends to begin with the first level and then proceed to the next when she feels the need. Regardless of the level of breathing used, a cleansing breath begins and ends each pattern. A cleansing breath involves only the chest. It consists of inhaling through the nose and exhaling through pursed lips (Table 19–3).

The first pattern may also be called slow, deep breathing or slow-paced breathing. During the breathing movements, only the chest moves. The woman inhales slowly through her nose. She moves her chest up and out during the inhalation. She exhales through pursed lips. The breathing rate is 6 to 9 breaths a minute.

The second pattern is called shallow or modified-paced breathing. The woman begins with a cleansing breath and at the end of the cleansing breath pushes out a short breath. She then inhales and exhales through the mouth at a rate of about 4 breaths every 5 seconds. This pattern can be altered into a more rapid rate that does not exceed 2 to 2 1/2 breaths every second.

Table 19–3 Nursing Support of Patterned-Paced Breathing

Determine which breathing method the woman (couple) has learned. Provide encouragement as needed in maintaining breathing pattern. Provide support to the labor coach and assist as needed.

Lamaze Breathing Pattern Levels

First level (slow paced)
Pattern begins and ends with a cleansing breath (in through the nose and out through pursed lips as if cooling a spoonful of hot food). While inhaling through the nose and exhaling through pursed lips, slow breaths are taken, moving only the chest. The rate should be approximately 6-9 / minute or 2 breaths / 15 seconds. The coach or nurse may assist by reminding the woman to take a cleansing breath, and then the breaths could be counted out if needed to maintain pacing. The woman inhales as someone counts "one one thousand, two one thousand, three one thousand, four one thousand." Exhalation begins and continues through the same count.

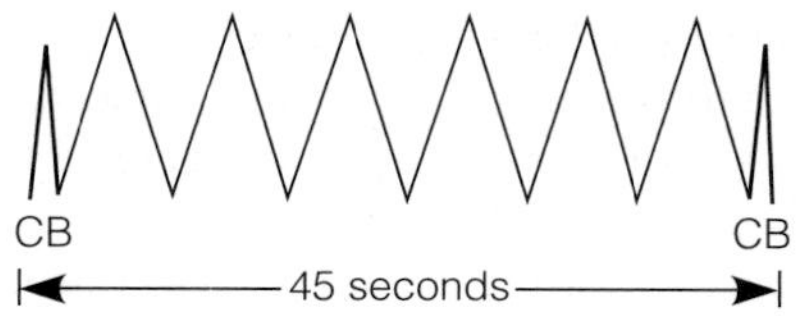

Second level (modified paced)
Pattern begins and ends with a cleansing breath. Breaths are then taken in and out silently through the mouth at approximately 4 breaths / 5 seconds. The jaw and entire body need to be relaxed. The rate can be accelerated to 2-2 1/2 breaths/second. The rhythm for the breaths can be counted out as "one and two and one and two and . . ." with the woman exhaling on the numbers and inhaling on "and."

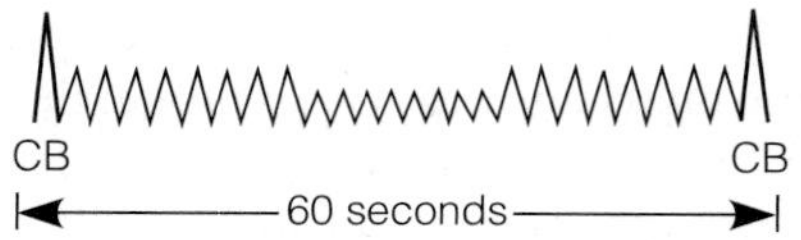

Third level (pattern paced)
Pattern begins and ends with a cleansing breath. All breaths are rhythmic, in and out through the mouth. Exhalations are accompanied by a "hee" or "hoo" sound in a varying pattern, 2:1, which begins as 3:1 (hee hee hee hoo) and can change to 2:1 (hee hee hoo) or 1:1 (hee hoo) as the intensity of the contraction changes. The rate should not be more rapid than 2-2 1/2 breaths/second. The rhythm of the breaths would match a "one and two and . . ." count.

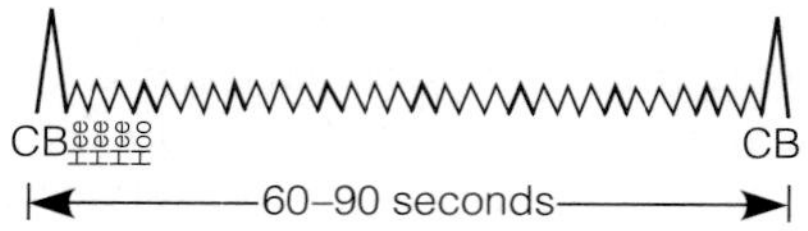

Abdominal Breathing Pattern Cues

The abdomen moves outward during inhalation and downward during exhalation. The rate remains slow, with approximately 6-9 breaths/minute.

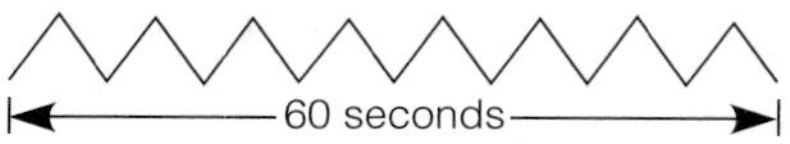

Quick Method

When the woman has not learned a particular method and is in the active phase of labor, the nurse may teach her a combination of two patterns. Abdominal breathing may be used until labor is more advanced. Then a more rapid pattern consisting of two short blows from the mouth followed by a longer blow can be used. (This pattern is called "pant-pant-blow" even though all exhalations are a blowing motion.)

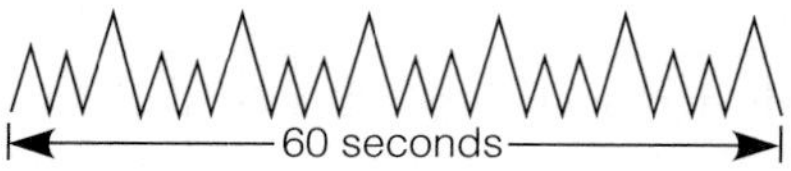

First level for use during uterine contractions. (The level begins and ends with a cleansing breath [CB].)
Second level
Third level (Darkened spike represents "hoo.")
Breathing sequence for abdominal breathing.
Pant-pant-blow breathing pattern

The third pattern is called pant-blow or patterned-paced breathing. It is similar to modified-paced breathing except the breathing is punctuated every few breaths by a forceful exhalation through pursed lips. A pattern of 4 breaths may be used to begin. All breaths are kept equal and rhythmic. As the contraction becomes more intense, the woman may adjust the pattern as needed to 3:1, 2:1, and finally 1:1.

If the woman has not learned a controlled breathing technique, teaching her may be difficult when she is admitted in active labor. In this instance, teach abdominal and pant-pant-blow breathing (see Table 19–3). In abdominal breathing the woman moves the abdominal wall upward as she inhales and downward as she exhales. This method tends to lift the abdominal wall off the contracting uterus and thus may provide some pain relief. The breathing is deep and rhythmic. As transition approaches, the woman may feel the need to breathe more rapidly. To avoid breathing too rapidly, the woman can use the pant-pant-blow breathing pattern.

Hyperventilation is the result of an imbalance of oxygen and carbon dioxide (i.e., too much carbon dioxide is exhaled, and too much oxygen remains in the body). Hyperventilation may occur when a woman breathes very rapidly over a prolonged period. The signs and symptoms of hyperventilation are tingling or numbness in the tip of the nose, lips, fingers, or toes; dizziness; spots before the eyes; or spasms of the hands or feet (carpal-pedal spasms). If hyperventilation occurs, encourage the woman to slow her breathing rate and take shallow breaths. With instruction and encouragement, many women are able to change their breathing to correct the problem. It may also help to count out loud for the woman so she can pace her breathing during contractions. If the signs and symptoms continue or become more severe (they progress from numbness to spasms), the woman can breathe into a paper surgical mask or a paper bag until symptoms go away. Breathing into a mask or bag causes rebreathing of carbon dioxide. During this time remain with the woman to reassure her.

In some instances, analgesics or regional anesthetic blocks may be used to increase comfort and relaxation during labor. (See Chapter 18.) Table 19–4 summarizes labor progress, possible responses of the laboring woman, and support measures.

Role of the Doula

Throughout the first stage of labor, assess and support the interactions between the woman and her support person or partner. In the absence of a partner, or when the partner wants a less active role in the support of the laboring woman, it is becoming more common for women to employ a paid care provider, often called a **doula**, who has experience in caring for laboring women. The doula typically has received special training and may even be certified. The role of the doula is to enhance the comfort and decrease the anxiety of the laboring woman. A doula can be a valuable advocate to the laboring woman and her family, as well as an asset to the labor nurse. For example, the doula might support the woman by helping identify the beginning of each contraction and encouraging her as she breathes through it.

NURSING CARE DURING THE SECOND STAGE OF LABOR

The second stage is reached when the cervix is fully dilated (10 cm). The contractions continue as in the transition phase. Maternal pulse is assessed at the onset of the second stage. Blood pressure is assessed every 30 minutes, but may be done more frequently if fetal decelerations or bradycardia occur. The FHR is assessed every 15 minutes in low-risk women and every 5 minutes in women with high-risk complications (ACOG, 2005). Once the second stage is reached, the nurse remains with the woman continually and does not generally leave the room.

As the woman pushes during the second stage, she may make a variety of sounds. A low-pitched, grunting sound ("uhhh") usually indicates that the woman is working with the pushing. The nurse who feels comfortable with maternal sounds and stays sensitive to changes in the sounds may be able to detect if the woman is losing her ability to cope. For instance, if the woman feels afraid of the sensations produced by her pushing effort, her sound may change to a high-pitched cry or whimper. During the second stage, the woman may interpret rectal pressure as a need to move her bowels. The instinctive response is to resist and to tighten muscles rather than bear down (push). A sensation of splitting apart also occurs in the latter part of the second stage, and the woman may fear the urge to push. The woman who expects these sensations and understands that bearing down contributes to progress at this stage is more likely to do so effectively.

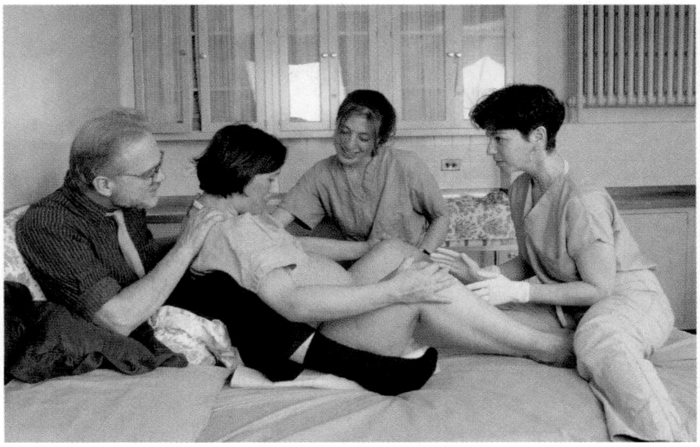

● **Figure 19–4** Care during the second stage of labor. The nurse provides encouragement and support during pushing efforts.

When the urge to bear down becomes uncontrollable and pushing begins, the nurse can help by encouraging the woman and by assisting with positioning (Figure 19–4 ●). Most women spontaneously push very effectively in response to messages from their body. However, in some settings sustained, forceful pushing is still advocated. In that case, when the contraction begins, the woman is told to take a cleansing breath or two, then to take a third large breath and hold it while pushing down with her abdominal muscles (called the Valsalva maneuver). A more natural approach that lets the mother wait to bear down until she feels an urge to push may shorten the pushing phase, reducing the incidence of physiologic stress in the mother and acidosis in the newborn.

A nullipara is usually prepared for birth when perineal bulging is noted. A multipara usually progresses far more quickly, so she may be prepared for the birth when the cervix is dilated 7 to 8 cm. As the birth approaches, the woman's partner or support person also prepares for the birth.

Monitor the woman's blood pressure and the FHR between contractions, and palpate the contractions at least every 5 minutes until the birth. Continue to assist the woman in her pushing efforts, keep both the woman and the coach informed of procedures and progress, and support them both throughout the birth.

PROMOTION OF COMFORT IN THE SECOND STAGE

Most of the comfort measures used during the first stage remain appropriate at this time. Applying cool cloths to the face and forehead may help cool the woman involved in the intense physical

Nursing Practice

Birth is imminent if the woman shows the following changes:

- Bulging of the perineum
- Uncontrollable urge to bear down
- Increased bloody show

Table 19–4 Normal Progress. Psychologic Characteristics, and Nursing Support During the First and Second Stages of Labor

Phase	Cervical Dilatation	Uterine Contractions	Woman's Response	Support Measures
Stage 1 **Latent phase**	1–4 cm	Every 10–20 minutes, 15–20 seconds' duration Mild intensity *progressing to* Every 5–7 minutes, 30–40 seconds' duration Moderate intensity	Usually happy, talkative, and eager to be in labor Exhibits need for independence by taking care of own bodily needs and seeking information	Establish rapport on admission and continue to build during care. Assess information base and learning needs. Be available to consult regarding breathing technique if needed; teach breathing technique if needed and in early labor. Orient family to room, equipment, monitors, and procedures. Encourage woman and partner to participate in care as desired. Provide needed information. Assist woman into position of comfort; encourage frequent change of position; encourage ambulation during early labor. Offer fluids or ice chips. Keep couple informed of progress. Encourage woman to void every 1 to 2 hours. Assess need for an interest in using visualization to enhance relaxation, and teach if appropriate.
Active phase	4–7 cm	Every 2–3 minutes, 40–60 seconds' duration Moderate to strong intensity	May experience feelings of helplessness Exhibits increased fatigue and may begin to feel restless and anxious as contractions become stronger Expresses fear of abandonment Becomes more dependent because she is less able to meet her needs	Encourage woman to maintain breathing patterns. Provide quiet environment to reduce external stimuli. Provide reassurance, encouragement, support; keep couple informed of progress. Promote comfort by giving back rubs, sacral pressure, cool cloth on forehead, assistance with position changes, support with pillows, effleurage. Provide ice chips, ointment for dry mouth and lips. Encourage to void every 1 to 2 hours. Offer shower, whirlpool, or warm bath if available.
Transition phase	8–10 cm	Every 2 minutes, 60–75 seconds' duration Strong intensity	Tires and may exhibit increased restlessness and irritability May feel she cannot keep up with labor process and is out of control Physical discomforts Fear of being left alone May fear tearing open or splitting apart with contractions	Encourage woman to rest between contractions. If she sleeps between contractions, wake her at beginning of contraction so she can begin breathing pattern (increases feeling of control). Provide support, encouragement, and praise for efforts. Keep couple informed of progress; encourage continued participation of support persons. Promote comfort as listed earlier but recognize that many women do not want to be touched when in transition. Provide privacy. Provide ice chips, ointment for lips. Encourage to void every 1 to 2 hours.
Stage 2	Complete	Every 2 minutes	May feel out of control, helpless, panicky	Assist woman in pushing efforts. Encourage woman to assume position of comfort. Provide encouragement and praise her efforts. Keep couple informed of progress. Provide ice chips. Maintain privacy as woman desires.

exertion of pushing. The woman may feel hot and want to remove some covers. Care still needs to be taken to provide privacy even though covers are removed. Encourage the woman to rest and relax all muscles during the periods between contractions. With the support person(s), help the woman into a pushing position with each contraction. Sips of fluids or ice chips may relieve dry mouth. Continually provide encouragement and positive reinforcement.

ASSISTING DURING BIRTH

In addition to assisting the woman and her partner, the nurse also assists the physician or CNM in preparing for the birth. The physician or CNM dons a sterile gown and gloves and may place sterile drapes over the woman's abdomen and legs. An episiotomy may be done just before the actual birth if needed. (See the discussion of episiotomy in Chapter 23∞.)

Shortly before the birth, the birthing room or delivery room is prepared with the equipment and materials that may be needed. Family members do not need to change into other clothing if the birth occurs in a birthing room; they don a disposable scrub suit or scrubs provided by the facility if the birth is to occur in a delivery room or surgery suite. Thorough handwashing is required of the nurses and CNM or physician. Nurses who will be in direct contact with the mother at the time of birth need to wear protective clothing such as an apron or gown with a splash apron, disposable gloves, and eye covering. The CNM or physician also needs to wear a plastic apron or a gown with a splash apron, eye covering, and sterile gloves.

If the laboring woman is to give birth in a location other than the birthing room (such as in the case of a cesarean birth), she is moved onto her bed or a cart shortly before birth. To ensure the woman's safety, the side rails should be raised into a locked position. It is important that the woman move from one bed to another between contractions. During the contraction the woman feels increased discomfort and may be involved in pushing efforts. Take care to preserve her privacy during the transfer. The labor bed or transfer cart must be carefully braced against the delivery table to ensure the woman's safety during the transfer.

Even though there are differences in the delivery room setting, the family can still be together during the birth. Encourage family members to participate, because the delivery room environment may seem intimidating. The family member may hesitate to continue providing support because of fear of interfering or being in the way.

Maternal Birthing Positions

Until modern times the upright posture for birth was considered normal in most societies. Women chose to squat, kneel, stand, or sit for birth. The recumbent position (lithotomy) became more usual in the Western world because of the convenience it offers in applying technology. The lithotomy position has thus become the conventional manner in which North American women give birth in hospitals. In seeking alternative positions, consumers and professionals alike are refocusing on the comfort of the laboring woman rather than on the convenience of the CNM or physician (Figure 19–5 ● and Table 19–5).

The woman is typically positioned for birth on a bed with leg supports, in a squatting position, or perhaps on her hands and knees. If a birthing bed is used, the back is elevated 30 to 60 degrees to help the woman bear down. Stirrups, if needed and used,

MyNursingKit Case Study: Labor and Birth

A

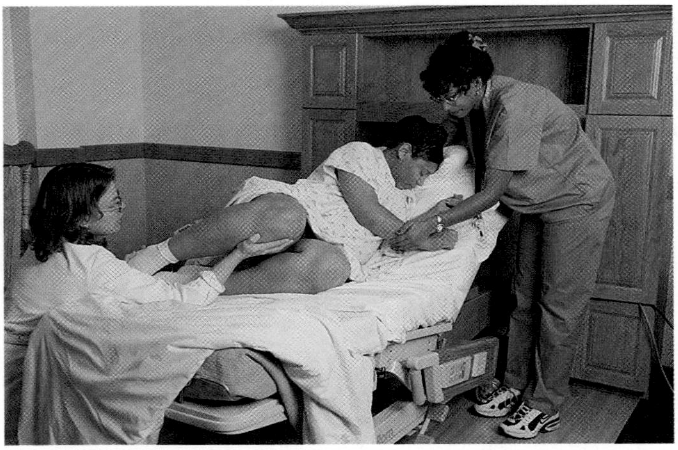

C

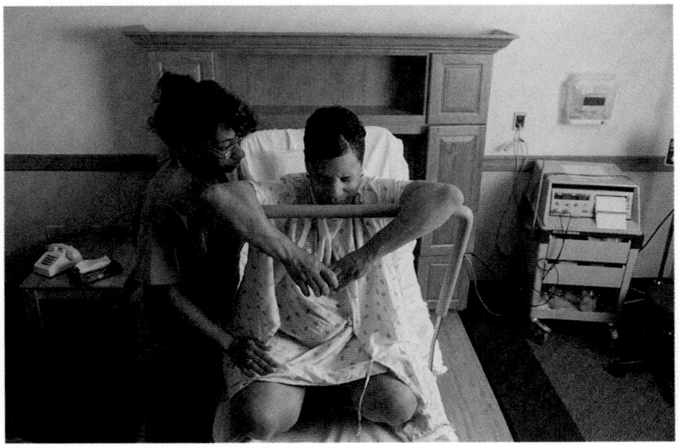

B

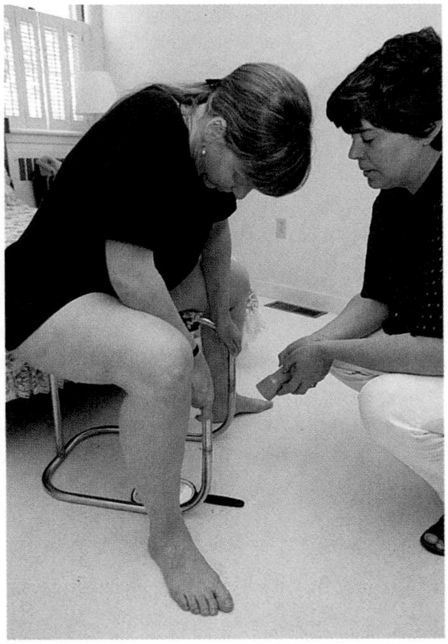

● **Figure 19–5** Birthing positions. ***A,*** Side-lying (also known as left lateral Sims') position. ***B,*** Using a birthing stool. ***C,*** Using a birthing bar.

Table 19–5 Comparison of Birthing Positions

Position	Advantages	Disadvantages	Nursing Actions
Sitting on birthing stool	Gravity aids descent and expulsion of infant. Does not compromise venous return from lower extremities. Woman can view birth process.	It is difficult to provide support for the woman's back.	Encourage woman to sit in a position that increases her comfort.
Semi-Fowler's	Does not compromise venous return from lower extremities. Woman can view birth process.	If legs are positioned wide apart, relaxation of perineal tissues is decreased.	Assess that upper torso is evenly supported. Increase support of body by changing position of bed or using pillows as props.
Left lateral Sims'	Does not compromise venous return from lower extremities. Increases perineal relaxation and decreases need for episiotomy. Appears to prevent rapid descent.	It is difficult for the woman to see the birth.	Adjust position so that the upper leg lies on the bed (scissor fashion) or is supported by the partner or on pillows.
Squatting	Size of pelvic outlet is increased. Gravity aids descent and expulsion of newborn. Second stage may be shortened.	It may be difficult to maintain balance while squatting.	Help woman maintain balance. Use a birthing bar if available.
Sitting in birthing bed	Gravity aids descent and expulsion of the fetus. Does not compromise venous return from lower extremities. Woman can view the birth process. Leg position may be changed at will.		Ensure that legs and feet have adequate support.
Hands and knees	Increases perineal relaxation and decreases need for episiotomy. Increases placental and umbilical blood flow and decreases fetal distress. Improves fetal rotation. Better able to assess the perineum. Better access to fetal nose and mouth for suctioning at birth. Facilitates birth of infant with shoulder dystocia.	Woman cannot view birth. There is decreased contact with birth attendant. Caregivers cannot use instruments. There may be increased maternal fatigue.	Adjust birthing bed by dropping the foot down. Supply extra pillows for increased support.

are padded to avoid pressure. In helping the woman place her legs in the stirrups, lift both legs simultaneously to avoid strain on abdominal, back, and perineal muscles. Adjust the stirrups to fit the woman's legs. The feet are supported in the stirrup holders. The height and angle of the stirrups are adjusted so there is no pressure on the backs of the knees or the calves, which might cause discomfort and postpartal vascular problems. When stirrups are not used for the birth, the woman's legs may be placed in stirrups after the birth to enhance visibility if a perineal repair is needed.

Cleansing the Perineum

After the woman has been positioned for the birth, her vulvar and perineal areas are cleansed to increase her comfort and to remove any bloody discharge. Depending on agency protocol or on physician or CNM orders, perineal cleansing methods range from use of soapy water to aseptic technique. Once the cleansing is completed, the woman returns to the desired birthing position.

Continued Labor Support

Both the woman's partner and the nurse who has been with the woman during the labor continue to provide support during contractions. The woman is encouraged to push with each contraction and, as the fetal head emerges, is asked to take shallow breaths or to pant to prevent pushing. While supporting the head, the physician or certified nurse-midwife assesses whether the umbilical cord is around the fetal neck and removes it if it is, then suctions the mouth and nose with a bulb syringe. The mouth is suctioned first to prevent reflex inhalation of mucus when the nostrils are touched with the bulb syringe tip. The woman is encouraged to push again as the rest of the newborn's body is born. Figure 19–6 ● depicts a birth.

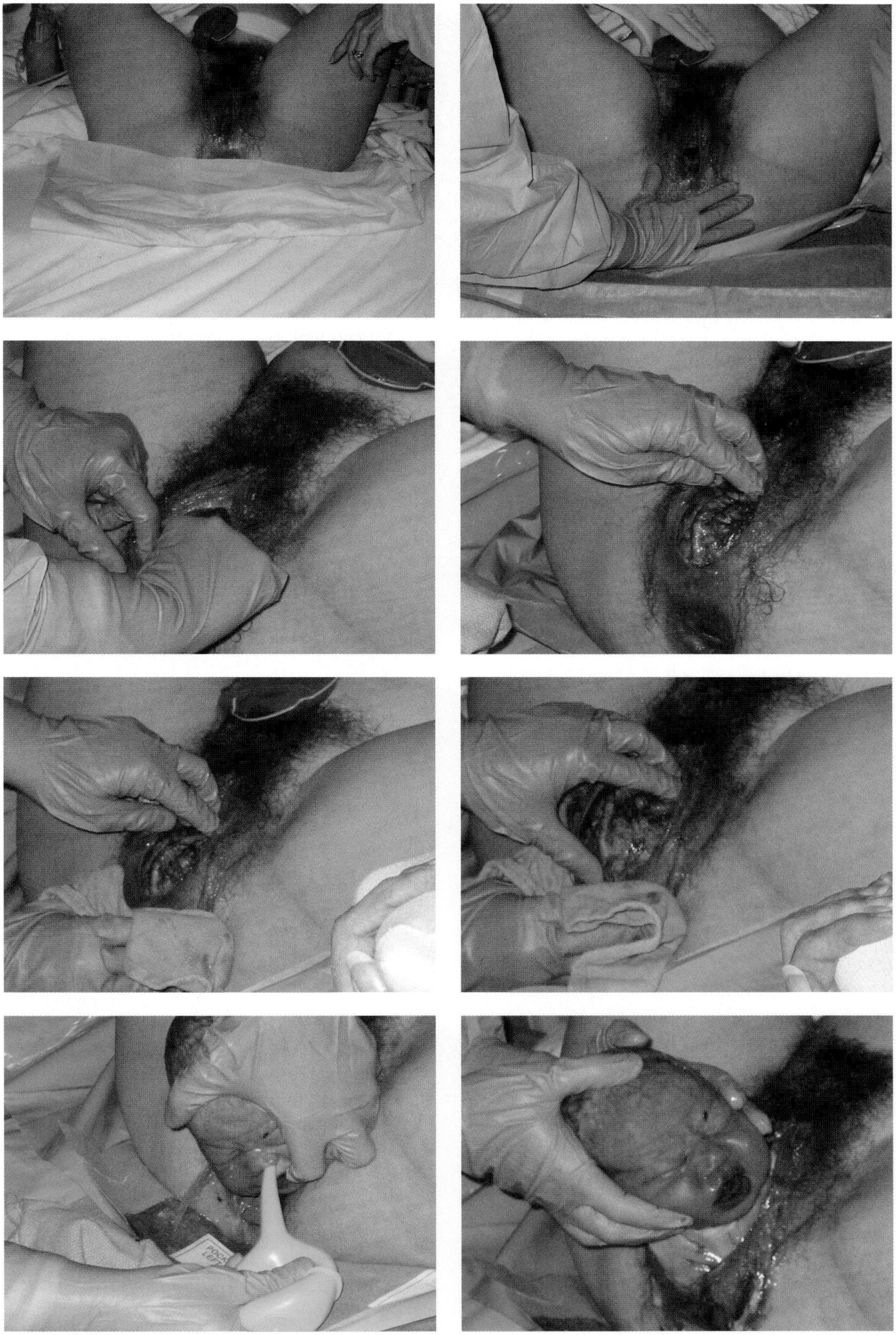

Figure 19–6 A birthing sequence.

MyNursingKit Video: Newborn Assessment

NURSING CARE DURING THE THIRD AND FOURTH STAGES OF LABOR

INITIAL CARE OF THE NEWBORN

The CNM or physician places the newborn on the mother's abdomen, which promotes attachment, or in the radiant-heated unit. The newborn is maintained in a modified Trendelenburg position. In this position, gravity aids drainage of mucus from the nasopharynx and trachea. Dry the newborn immediately and help keep the infant warm by placing warmed blankets over the newborn or by placing him or her in skin-to-skin contact with the mother. If the newborn is in a radiant-heated unit, he or she is dried, placed on a dry blanket, and left uncovered. Because radiant heat warms the outer surface of objects, a newborn wrapped in blankets will receive no benefit from the unit.

Suction the newborn's nose and mouth with a bulb syringe as needed. Most immediate care of the newborn can be done while the newborn is in the parent's arms or in the radiant-heated unit.

Apgar Scoring System

The Apgar scoring system (Table 19–6) evaluates the physical condition of the newborn at birth. The newborn is rated 1 minute after birth and again at 5 minutes and receives a total score (**Apgar score**) ranging from 0 to 10 based on the following assessments:

1. *Heart rate* is auscultated or palpated at the junction of the umbilical cord and skin. This is the most important assessment. A heart rate above 100 is scored as 2, a heart rate below 100 receives a 1, and a score of 0 is assigned if there is no heartbeat. A newborn heart rate of less than 100 beats per minute indicates the need for immediate resuscitation.
2. *Respiratory effort* is the second most important Apgar assessment. A vigorous cry indicates adequate respirations and is scored as 2, whereas a slow, irregular respiratory effort receives a 1. Complete absence of respirations is termed apnea (scored 0).
3. *Muscle tone* is determined by evaluating the degree of flexion and resistance to straightening of the extremities. A normal newborn's elbows and hips are flexed, with the knees positioned up toward the abdomen (scored as 2). Some flexion of the extremities is scored as 1, while a flaccid infant receives a 0.
4. *Reflex irritability* is evaluated by stroking the baby's back along the spine or by flicking the soles of the feet. A cry merits a full score of 2. A grimace is 1 point, and no response is 0.
5. *Skin color* is inspected for cyanosis and pallor. Generally, newborns have blue extremities, with a pink body, which merits a score of 1. This condition is termed *acrocyanosis* and is present in many normal newborns at 1 minute after birth. A totally pink newborn scores a 2, and a totally cyanotic, pale infant scores 0. Newborns with darker skin are not pink in color. Their skin color is assessed for pallor and acrocyanosis.

Table 19–6 The Apgar Scoring System

	Score		
Sign	**0**	**1**	**2**
Heart rate	Absent	Slow—below 100	Above 100
Respiratory effort	Absent	Slow—irregular	Good crying
Muscle tone	Flaccid	Some flexion of extremities	Active motion
Reflex irritability	None	Grimace	Vigorous cry
Color	Pale blue	Body pink, blue extremities	Completely pink

Data from Apgar, V. (1968, August). The newborn (Apgar) scoring system, reflections and advice. *Pediatric Clinics of North America, 13,* 645.

A score of 7 to 10 indicates a newborn in good condition who requires only nasopharyngeal suctioning and perhaps some oxygen near the face (called "blow-by" oxygen). If the Apgar score is below 7, resuscitative measures may be needed. (See the discussion in Chapter 28.) Apgar scores of less than 3 at 5 minutes postbirth may correlate with neonatal mortality (ACOG, 2006).

Care of Umbilical Cord

Delayed cord clamping is associated with positive outcomes for the infant and is now the preferred approach (Levy & Blickstein, 2006). If the physician or CNM has not placed some type of cord clamp on the newborn's umbilical cord, the nurse does so. Before applying the cord clamp, examine the cut end of the cord for the presence of two arteries and one vein. The umbilical vein is the largest vessel, and the arteries are seen as smaller vessels. Record the number of vessels on the birth and newborn records. The cord is clamped approximately 1/2 to 1 inch from the abdomen to allow room between the abdomen and clamp as the cord dries. Abdominal skin must not be clamped, because this will cause necrosis of the tissue. The most common type of cord clamp is the plastic Hollister cord clamp (Figure 19–7 ●). The Hollister clamp is removed in the nursery about 24 hours after the cord has dried.

Cord Blood Collection for Banking

A growing number of parents are arranging for cord blood banking with individual cord blood registries (see discussion in Chapter 1). These registries provide the parents with a special container for the cord blood, which they bring with them to the birth. The parents should have received directions from the registry about the storage and care of the container prior to the birth. Immediately after the newborn's umbilical cord is clamped and cut and the placenta is expelled, the CNM or physician withdraws blood from the remaining umbilical cord and the placenta and places it in the special container. The cord blood remains with the mother until it is picked up by the cord blood registry.

Physical Assessment of the Newborn

The nurse performs an abbreviated systematic physical assessment in the birthing area to detect any abnormalities (Table 19–7). First, note the size of the newborn and the contour and size of the head

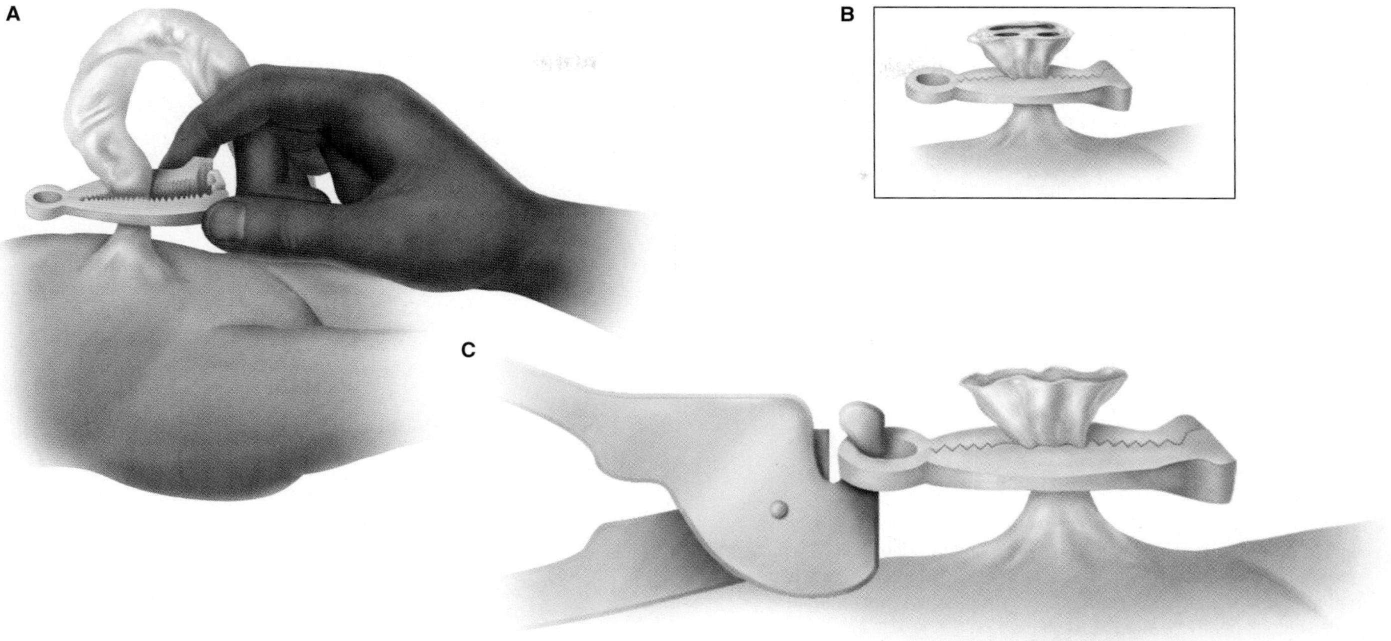

● **Figure 19–7** Hollister cord clamp. ***A,*** Clamp is positioned 1/2 to 1 inch from the abdomen and then secured. ***B,*** Cut cord. The one vein and two arteries can be seen. ***C,*** Plastic device for removing clamp after cord has dried. After the cord is cut, the nurse grasps the Hollister clamp on either side of the cut area and gently separates it.

in relationship to the rest of the body. The newborn's posture and movements indicate tone and neurologic functioning.

Inspect the skin for discoloration, presence of vernix caseosa and lanugo, and signs of trauma and desquamation (peeling of skin). Vernix caseosa is a white, cheesy substance found normally on newborns. It is absorbed within 24 hours after birth. Vernix is abundant on preterm infants and absent on postterm newborns. Fine hair (lanugo) is often seen on preterm newborns' shoulders, foreheads, backs, and cheeks. Desquamation is seen in postterm newborns.

Observe the nares (nostrils) for flaring and, as the newborn cries, inspect the palate for cleft palate. Look for mucus in the nose and mouth, and remove it with a bulb syringe as needed. Inspect the chest for respiratory rate and the presence of retractions. If retractions are present, assess the newborn for grunting or stridor. A normal respiratory rate is 30 to 60 per minute. Auscultate the lungs bilaterally for breath sounds. Absence of breath sounds on one side could mean pneumothorax. Rales may be heard immediately after birth because a small amount of fluid may remain in the lungs; this fluid will be absorbed. Rhonchi indicate aspiration of oral secretions. If there is excessive mucus or respiratory distress, suction the newborn with a mucus trap. (See Figure 19–8 ● as well as Skill 4–2 **SKILLS** in the Clinical Skills Manual that accompanies this text.) Note and record elimination of urine or meconium on the newborn record.

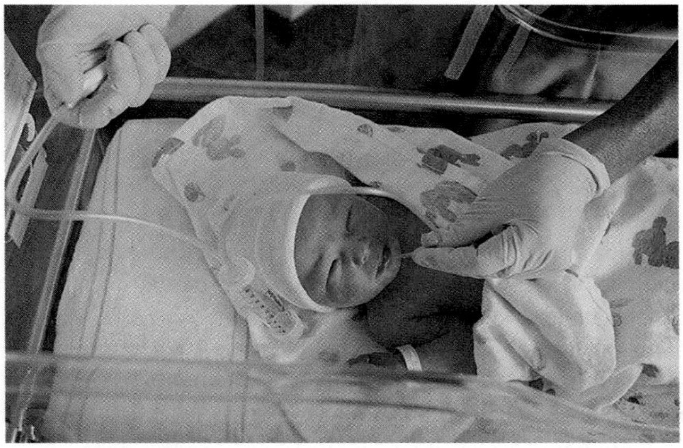

● **Figure 19–8** Clearing secretions. To clear secretions from the newborn's nose or oropharynx, a DeLee mucus trap (shown here) or other suction device is used. One end of the suction tubing is connected to low suction, and the other end of the tubing is inserted 3 to 5 inches into the newborn's nose or mouth. Suction is applied as the tubing is pulled out. The process is repeated for as long as fluid is aspirated.

Newborn Identification

Place two ID bands on the newborn—one on the wrist and one on the ankle. The bands must fit snugly so they will not be lost. To ensure correct identification, while still in the birthing or delivery room, give the mother and her partner each a band that matches that of the baby. The bands allow access to the infant care areas and must not be removed until the infant is discharged.

Some facilities now use an umbilical cord clamp that includes an infant security alarm. The cord clamp and alarm are left in place until the mother and baby are discharged home. The alarm sounds if the infant is removed from the hospital unit or if the cord clamp or alarm is cut or disengaged (Figure 19–9 ●).

Table 19–7 Initial Newborn Evaluation

Assess	Normal Findings
Respirations	Rate 36–60, irregular No retractions, no grunting
Apical pulse	Rate 120–160 and somewhat irregular
Temperature	Skin temp above 36.5°C (97.8°F)
Skin color	Body pink with bluish extremities
Umbilical cord	Two arteries and one vein
Gestational age	Should be 38–42 weeks to remain with parents for extended time
Sole creases	Sole creases that involve the heel

In general, expect scant amount of vernix on upper back, axilla, groin; lanugo only on upper back; ears with incurving of upper 2/3 of pinnae and thin cartilage that springs back from folding; male genitals—testes palpated in upper or lower scrotum; female genitals—labia majora larger, clitoris nearly covered

In the following situations, newborns should generally be stabilized rather than remaining with parents in the birth area for an extended period of time:

- Apgar less than 8 at 1 minute and less than 9 at 5 minutes or baby requires resuscitation measures (other than whiffs of oxygen)
- Respirations below 30 or above 60, with retractions and/or grunting
- Apical pulse below 120 or above 160 with marked irregularities
- Skin temperature below 36.5°C (97.8°F)
- Skin color pale blue or circumoral pallor
- Baby less than 38 weeks or more than 42 weeks' gestation
- Baby very small or very large for gestational age
- Congenital anomalies involving open areas in the skin (meningomyelocele)

MyNursingKit Video: Fourth Stage of Labor

MyNursingKit Animation: Placental Delivery

Additional hospital security measures are now commonplace in maternity settings. This includes mandating that all staff wear appropriate identification at all times. The nurse advises the parents to place the infant on the side of the bed away from the window, and to have the baby returned to the nursery whenever the mother naps or showers and no other family member is present.

Although hospital infant abductions are rare, they are catastrophic to the family, hospital, and community. Many abductors pose as medical personnel to gain access to the infant. Women should be advised to ask all hospital personnel for proper identification. If the mother or family feels unsure of the individual, they should immediately call on the call bell to alert the nurse and ask for other verification. If a woman is reluctant to allow a student nurse to transport her infant, the staff nurse should be asked to assist the student.

DELIVERY OF THE PLACENTA

After birth the certified nurse-midwife or physician prepares for the delivery of the placenta. The following signs suggest placental separation:

1. The uterus rises upward in the abdomen.
2. As the placenta moves downward, the umbilical cord lengthens.

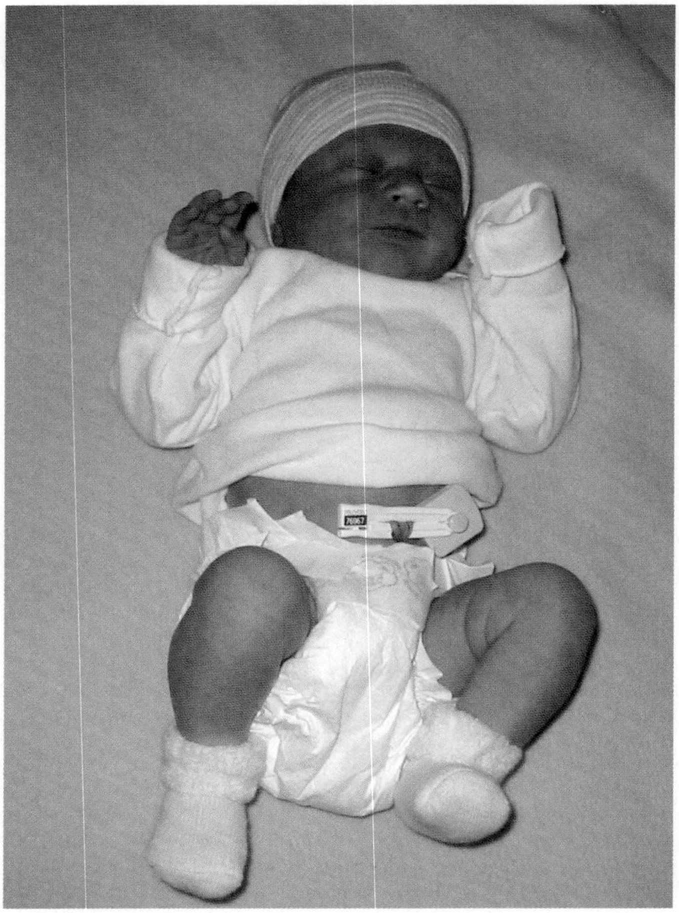

● **Figure 19–9** Umbilical alarm in place on a newborn infant.

3. A sudden trickle or spurt of blood appears.
4. The shape of the uterus changes from a disk to a globe.

While waiting for these signs, palpate the uterus to check for ballooning caused by uterine relaxation and subsequent bleeding into the uterine cavity. After the placenta has separated, the woman may be asked to bear down to aid delivery of the placenta.

Oxytocics are frequently given at the time of the delivery of the placenta, so the uterus will contract and bleeding will be minimized. Oxytocin (Pitocin), 10 to 20 units, may be added to an intravenous (IV) infusion, or 10 units may be given intramuscularly. Some physicians order methylergonovine maleate (Methergine), 0.2 mg administered intramuscularly, or carboprost tromethamine (Hemabate), 250 mcg/mL administered intramuscularly. (See "Drug Guide: Carboprost Tromethamine (Hemabate)" on page 434). In addition to administering the ordered medications, it is essential to assess and record maternal blood pressure before and after administration of oxytocics. For further information, refer to "Drug Guide: Oxytocin" (in Chapter 23) and "Drug Guide: Methylergonovine Maleate" (in Chapter 31). After expulsion of the placenta, the CNM or physician inspects the placental membranes to make sure they are intact and that all cotyledons are present. If there is a defect or a part missing from the placenta, a manual uterine examination is done. On the birth record, note the time of delivery of the placenta.

Evidence in Action

Infant to mother skin-to-skin contact immediately following birth supports breastfeeding and bonding (meta-analysis) (Moore, Anderson, & Bergman, 2007).

After the placenta is expelled, the physician or CNM inspects the vagina and cervix for lacerations and makes any necessary repairs. The episiotomy may be repaired if it has not been done previously (see Chapter 23).

ENHANCING ATTACHMENT

The first few hours and even minutes after birth are an important period for the attachment of mother and infant. If this period of contact can occur during the first hour after birth, the newborn will be in the quiet state and able to interact with parents by looking at them. Newborns also turn their heads in response to a spoken voice. (For further discussion of newborn states, see Chapter 24.)

The first parent-newborn contact may be brief (a few minutes), to be followed by a more extended contact after uncomfortable procedures (expulsion of the placenta and suturing of the episiotomy) are completed. When the newborn is returned to the mother, help her begin breastfeeding if she so desires. The baby may seek out the mother's breast, and early contact between the two can greatly affect breastfeeding success. Even if the newborn does not actively nurse, he or she can lick, taste, and smell the mother's skin. This activity by the newborn stimulates the maternal release of prolactin, which promotes the onset of lactation.

Darkening the birthing room by turning out most of the lights causes newborns to open their eyes and gaze around. This in turn enhances eye-to-eye contact with the parents. (*Note:* If the physician or CNM needs a light source, the spotlight can be left on.) Treatment of the newborn's eyes may also be delayed. Many parents who establish eye contact with the newborn are content to quietly gaze at their infant. Others may show more active involvement by touching or inspecting the newborn. Some mothers talk to their babies in a high-pitched voice, which seems to be soothing to newborns. Some couples verbally express amazement and pride when they see they have produced a beautiful, healthy baby. Their verbalization enhances feelings of accomplishment and ecstasy.

Both parents need to be encouraged to do whatever they feel most comfortable doing. Some parents prefer only limited contact with the newborn immediately after birth and instead want private time together in a quiet environment. In spite of the current zeal for providing immediate attachment opportunities, nursing personnel need to be aware of parents' wishes. The desire to delay interaction with the newborn does not necessarily imply a decreased ability of the parents to bond with their newborn. (For further discussion of parent-newborn attachment, see Chapter 26.)

PROVISION OF CARE IN THE FOURTH STAGE

The period of 1 to 4 hours immediately following the expulsion of the placenta, during which the mother's condition stabilizes, is often referred to as the fourth stage of labor and birth. This is actually the initial recovery period.

After childbirth it is critical that the uterine fundus stay well contracted to clamp off uterine blood vessels at the placental site and thereby prevent hemorrhaging. Consequently, palpate the uterine fundus at frequent intervals for the first 4 hours to ensure that it remains firmly contracted. Normally the fundus is located in the midline and at or below the umbilicus. Palpate the fundus (Figure 19–10 ●) but do not massage it unless it is soft (boggy). When a uterus becomes boggy, pooling of blood occurs within it, causing clots. Anything left in the uterus prevents it from contracting effectively. Thus, if the uterus becomes boggy or appears to rise in the abdomen, massage the fundus until firm; then with one hand supporting the uterus at the symphysis pubis, use the other hand to exert steady pressure on the fundus to express retained clots. The uterus is very tender at this time so all palpation and massage must be done as gently as possible.

In some women the uterus becomes so relaxed that it cannot be found when palpation is attempted. In this case, place one hand in the midline of the abdomen at about the level of the umbilicus and begin to make kneading motions. This motion generally stimulates the uterus to contract, and it then feels like a firm, hard object.

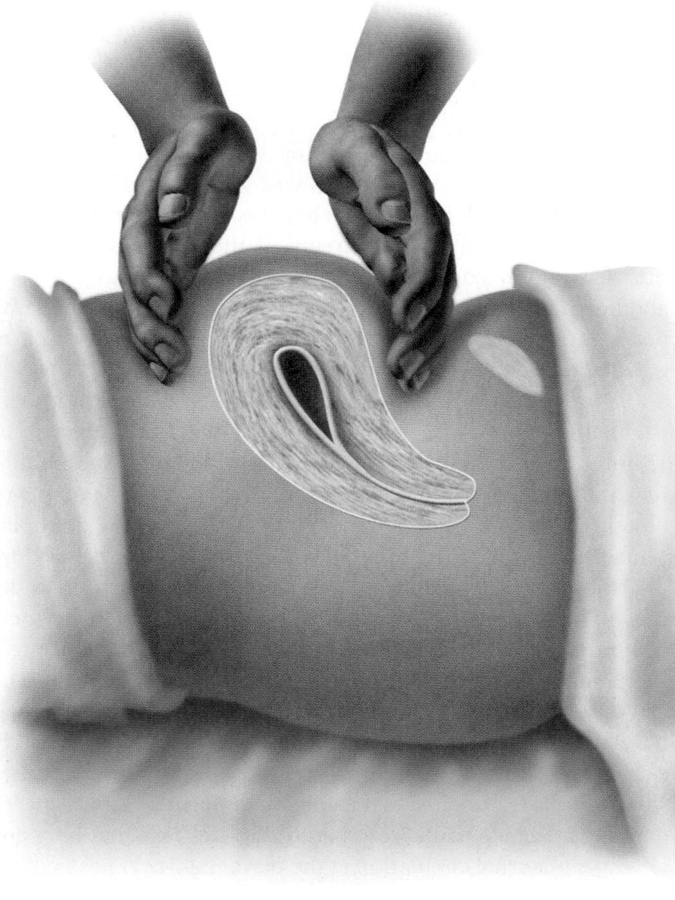

● **Figure 19–10** Suggested method of palpating the fundus of the uterus during the fourth stage. The left hand is placed just above the symphysis pubis, and gentle downward pressure is exerted. The right hand is cupped around the uterine fundus.

Drug Guide

CARBOPROST TROMETHAMINE (HEMABATE)

Pregnancy Risk Category: D

Overview of Action

Carboprost tromethamine (Hemabate) is used to reduce blood loss secondary to uterine atony. It stimulates myometrial contractions to control postpartum hemorrhaging that is unresponsive to usual techniques. Carboprost tromethamine can also be used to induce labor in women desiring an elective termination of a pregnancy. The drug is also used to induce labor in cases of intrauterine fetal death and hydatidiform mole (Wilson, Shannon, & Shields, 2009).

Route, Dosage, Frequency

In cases of immediate postpartum hemorrhage, the usual intramuscular dose is 250 mcg (1 mL), which can be repeated every 1 1/2 to 3 1/2 hours if uterine atony persists. The dosage can be increased to 500 mcg (2 mL) if uterine contractility is inadequate after several doses of 250 mcg. The total dosage should not exceed 12 mg. The maximum duration of use is 48 hours (Wilson et al., 2009).

Contraindications

The drug is contraindicated in women with active cardiac, pulmonary, or renal disease. It should not be administered during pregnancy or in women with acute pelvic inflammatory disease. It should be used with caution in women with asthma, adrenal disease, hypotension, hypertension, diabetes mellitus, epilepsy, fibroids, cervical stenosis, or previous uterine surgery (Wilson et al., 2009).

Side Effects

The most common side effects are nausea and diarrhea. Fever, chills, and flushing can occur. Headache, muscle, joint, abdominal, or eye pain can also occur (Wilson et al., 2009).

Nursing Considerations

1. The injection should be given in a large muscle. Aspiration should be performed to avoid injection into a blood vessel, which can result in bronchospasm, tetanic contractions, and shock.
2. After administration, monitor uterine status and bleeding carefully.
3. Report excess bleeding to the physician/CNM.
4. Check vital signs routinely, observing for an increase in temperature, elevated pulse, and decreased blood pressure.
5. Breastfeeding should be delayed for 24 hours after administration (Wilson et al., 2009).

Wash the woman's perineum with gauze squares and warmed solution and dry the area well with a towel before placing the maternity pad. If stirrups have been used, remove both of the woman's legs from the stirrups at the same time to avoid muscle strain. Encourage the woman to move her legs gently up and down in a bicycle motion. The woman remains in the same bed or is transferred to a recovery room bed. Help her don a clean gown and offer her something to drink.

During the recovery period, it is essential to monitor maternal vital signs closely. Check the maternal blood pressure at 5- to 15-minute intervals to detect any changes. Blood pressure should return to the prelabor level as a result of an increased volume of blood returning to the maternal circulation from the uteroplacental shunt. Pulse rate should be slightly lower than it was during labor. Baroreceptors cause a vagal response, which slows the pulse. A rise in blood pressure may be a response to oxytocic drugs or may be caused by preeclampsia. A lowered blood pressure and a rising pulse rate may reflect blood loss (Table 19–8).

Also monitor the woman's temperature. Frequently, women have tremors in the immediate postpartum period, possibly caused by a difference in internal and external body temperatures (higher temperature inside the body than outside). Another theory is that the woman is reacting to the fetal cells that have entered the maternal circulation at the placental site. A heated bath blanket placed next to the woman is helpful and can be replaced as often as the mother desires.

Inspect the bloody vaginal discharge for amount and chart it as minimal, moderate, or heavy and with or without clots. This discharge, lochia rubra, should be bright red. A soaked perineal pad contains approximately 100 mL of blood. If the perineal pad becomes soaked in a 15-minute period or if blood pools under the buttocks, continuous observation is necessary (see Skill 5–1 SKILLS in the Clinical Skills Manual that accompanies this text). When the fundus is firm, a continuous trickle of blood may sig-

Table 19–8 Maternal Adaptations Following Birth

Characteristic	Normal Finding
Blood pressure	Returns to prelabor level
Pulse	Slightly lower than in labor
Uterine fundus	In the midline at the umbilicus or one to two finger-breadths below the umbilicus
Lochia	Red (rubra), small to moderate amount (from spotting on pads to 1/4–1/2 of pad covered in 15 minutes) Does not exceed saturation of one pad in first hour
Bladder	Nonpalpable
Perineum	Smooth, pink, without bruising or edema
Emotional state	Wide variation, including excited, exhilarated, smiling, crying, fatigued, verbal, quiet, pensive, and sleepy

nal laceration of the vagina or cervix or an unligated vessel in the episiotomy.

If the fundus rises and displaces to the right, it is important to consider two factors:

1. As the uterus rises, the uterine contractions become less effective and increased bleeding may occur.
2. The most common cause of uterine displacement is bladder distention.

Palpate the bladder to determine whether it is distended. The bladder fills rapidly with the extra fluid volume returned from the uteroplacental circulation (and with any fluid received intravenously during labor and birth). The postpartal woman may not realize that her bladder is full because trauma to the bladder and urethra during childbirth and the use of regional anesthesia decrease bladder tone and the urge to void.

Use a variety of measures to help the mother to void. Place a warm towel across the lower abdomen or pour warm water over the perineum to relax the urinary sphincter and facilitate voiding. If the woman is unable to void, catheterization is necessary.

The perineum is inspected for edema and hematoma formation. An ice pack often reduces the swelling and alleviates the discomfort of an episiotomy.

The couple may be tired, hungry, and thirsty. Some agencies serve the couple a meal. The tired mother will probably drift off into a welcome sleep. The partner can also be encouraged to rest, since the supporting role is physically and mentally tiring. If the mother is not in a birthing room, she is usually transferred from the birthing unit to the postpartal or mother-baby area after 2 hours or more, depending on agency policy and whether the following criteria are met:

- Stable vital signs
- No bleeding
- Undistended bladder
- Firm fundus
- Sensations fully recovered from any anesthetic agent received during birth

SUPPORT OF THE ADOLESCENT DURING BIRTH

As with all women, each adolescent in labor is different. Assess what each teen brings to the experience by considering the following:

- Has the young woman received prenatal care?
- What are her attitudes and feelings about the pregnancy?
- Who will attend the birth and what is the person's relationship to her?
- What preparation has she had for the experience?
- What are her expectations and fears regarding labor and birth?
- How has her culture influenced her?
- What are her usual coping mechanisms?
- Does she plan to keep the newborn?

Adolescent women are at highest risk for pregnancy and labor complications and must be assessed carefully. Fetal well-being is established by fetal monitoring. Be especially alert for any physiologic complications of labor. The young woman's prenatal record is carefully reviewed for risks, and she is screened for preeclampsia, cephalopelvic disproportion, anemia, drugs ingested during pregnancy, sexually transmitted infections, and size-date discrepancies.

The support role of the nurse depends on the young woman's support system during labor. The adolescent may not be accompanied by someone who will stay with her during childbirth, or she may have her mother, the father of the baby, or a close friend as her labor partner. Regardless of whether the teen has a support person, it is important to establish a trusting relationship with her. In this way it is possible to help the teen understand what is happening to her. The adolescent given positive reinforcement for "work well done" will leave the experience with increased self-esteem, despite the emotional problems that may accompany her situation. If a support person accompanies the adolescent, that person also needs encouragement and support. Explain changes in the young woman's behavior and describe ways the support person can be of help.

The adolescent who has taken childbirth education classes is generally better prepared for labor than the adolescent who has not. However, the younger the adolescent, the less she may be able to participate actively in the process, even if she has taken prenatal classes. See Figure 19–11 ●.

The very young adolescent (age 14 and under) has fewer coping mechanisms and less experience to draw on than her older counterparts. Because her cognitive development is incomplete, the younger adolescent may have fewer problem-solving capabilities. She may be more threatened by the experience, and she may be more vulnerable to stress and discomfort.

The very young adolescent needs someone to rely on at all times during labor. She may be more childlike and dependent than older teens. Instructions and explanations should be simple and concrete. During the transition phase, the young teenager may become withdrawn and unable to express her need to be nurtured. Touch, soothing encouragement, and

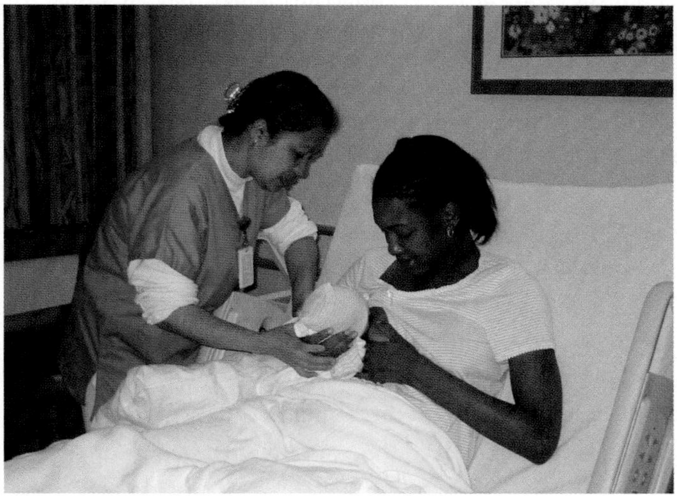

● **Figure 19–11** Breastfeeding assistance. An adolescent mother receives breastfeeding assistance in the immediate postpartum period.

measures to provide comfort help her maintain control and meet her needs for dependence. During the second stage of labor, the young adolescent may feel as if she is losing control and may reach out to those around her. It is important to remain calm and give clear, simple directions to help the teen cope with feelings of helplessness.

The middle adolescent (age 15 to 17 years) often attempts to remain calm and unflinching during labor. Nevertheless, a caring attitude still helps the young woman. Many older adolescents believe that they "know it all," but they may be no more prepared for childbirth than their younger counterparts. Positive reinforcement and a nonjudgmental manner will help them save face. If the adolescent has not taken childbirth preparation classes, she may require preparation and explanations. The older teenager's (age 18 to 19) response to the stresses of labor, however, is similar to that of the adult woman.

Even if the adolescent is planning to relinquish her newborn, she should be given the option of seeing and holding the infant. She may be reluctant to do this at first, but the mother's grieving process is facilitated if she sees the infant. However, seeing or holding the newborn should be the young woman's choice. (See Chapter 22∞ for further discussion of the relinquishing mother and the adolescent parent.)

NURSING CARE DURING PRECIPITOUS BIRTH

Occasionally labor progresses so rapidly that the maternity nurse is faced with the task of managing the actual birth of the baby. This is called a **precipitous birth**. The attending nurse has the primary responsibility for providing a physically and psychologically safe experience for the woman and her baby. A woman whose certified nurse-midwife or physician is not present may feel disappointed, frightened, abandoned, angry, and cheated. She may fear what is going to happen and feel that everything is out of her control. In working with the woman, the nurse provides support by keeping her informed about the labor progress and assuring her that the nurse will stay with her.

If birth is imminent, the nurse must not leave the mother alone. The nurse can direct auxiliary personnel to contact the CNM or physician and retrieve the emergency birth pack ("precip pack"), which should be readily accessible to birthing rooms. A typical pack contains the following items:

- A small drape that can be placed under the woman's buttocks to provide a sterile field
- A bulb syringe to clear mucus from the newborn's mouth
- Two sterile clamps (Kelly or Rochester) to clamp the umbilical cord before applying a cord clamp
- Sterile scissors to cut the umbilical cord
- A sterile umbilical cord clamp, either Hesseltine or Hollister
- A baby blanket to wrap the newborn in after birth
- A package of sterile gloves

At all times during the birth, the nurse remains calm, provides suggestions such as when to maintain a controlled breathing pattern and when to push, supports the woman's efforts, and provides reassurance.

The nurse assists in the precipitous birth as follows: The woman is encouraged to assume a comfortable position. If time permits, the nurse scrubs his or her hands with soap and water and puts on sterile gloves. Sterile drapes are placed under the woman's buttocks. The nurse may place an index finger inside the lower portion of the vagina and the thumb on the outer portion of the perineum and gently massage the area to help stretch perineal tissues and prevent perineal lacerations. This procedure is called "ironing the perineum."

When the infant's head crowns, the nurse instructs the woman to pant, which decreases her urge to push. The nurse checks whether the amniotic sac is intact. If it is, the nurse tears the sac so the newborn will not breathe in amniotic fluid with the first breath.

With one hand the nurse applies gentle pressure against the fetal head to prevent it from popping out rapidly. The nurse does not hold the head back forcibly. Rapid birth of the head may result in tears in the woman's perineal tissues. The rapid change in pressure within the fetal head may cause subdural or dural tears. The nurse supports the perineum with the other hand and allows the head to be born between contractions.

As the woman continues to pant, the nurse inserts one or two fingers along the back of the fetal head to check for the umbilical cord. If there is a nuchal cord (umbilical cord around the neck), the nurse bends his or her fingers like a fish hook, grasps the cord, and pulls it over the baby's head. It is important to check that the cord is not wrapped around the neck more than one time. If the cord is tightly looped and cannot be slipped over the baby's head, two clamps are placed on the cord, the cord is cut between the clamps, and the cord is unwound.

Immediately after birth of the head, the nurse suctions the baby's mouth, throat, and nasal passages. The nurse then places one hand on each side of the head and exerts gentle downward traction until the anterior shoulder passes under the symphysis pubis. Then gentle upward traction aids the birth of the posterior shoulder. The nurse then instructs the woman to push gently so that the rest of the body can be born quickly. The newborn must be supported as he or she emerges.

The newborn is held at the level of the uterus to facilitate blood flow through the umbilical cord. The combination of amniotic fluid and vernix makes the newborn very slippery, so the nurse must be careful to avoid dropping the baby. The nose and mouth of the newborn are suctioned again, using a bulb syringe. The nurse then dries the newborn to prevent heat loss. As soon as the nurse determines that the newborn's respirations are adequate, the infant can be placed on the mother's abdomen. The newborn's head should be slightly lower than the body to aid drainage of fluid and mucus. The weight of the newborn on the mother's abdomen stimulates uterine contractions, which aid in placental separation. The umbilical cord should not be pulled. The nurse is alert for signs of placental separation (slight gush of dark blood from the vagina, lengthening of the cord, or a change in uterine shape from discoid to globular). When these signs are present, the nurse tells the mother to push so that the placenta can be delivered. The nurse inspects the placenta to determine whether it is intact.

The nurse checks the firmness of the uterus. The fundus may be gently massaged to stimulate contractions and decrease bleeding. Putting the newborn to breast also stimulates uterine contractions through release of oxytocin from the pituitary gland.

The umbilical cord may now be cut. The nurse places two sterile Kelly clamps approximately 1 to 3 inches from the newborn's abdomen. The cord is cut between the Kelly clamps with sterile scissors. The nurse places a sterile umbilical cord clamp adjacent to the clamp on the newborn's cord, between the clamp and the newborn's abdomen. The clamp must not be placed snugly against the abdomen, because the cord will dry and shrink.

The nurse cleanses the area under the mother's buttocks and inspects her perineum for lacerations. Bleeding from lacerations may be controlled by pressing a clean perineal pad against the perineum and instructing the woman to keep her thighs together.

If the CNM or physician's arrival is delayed or if the newborn is having respiratory distress, the newborn should be transported immediately to the nursery. The newborn must be properly identified before he or she leaves the birth area. The nurse notes and places on a birth record the following information:

- Position of fetus at birth
- Presence of cord around neck or shoulder (nuchal cord)
- Time of birth
- Apgar scores at 1 and 5 minutes after birth
- Gender of newborn
- Time of expulsion of placenta
- Method of placental expulsion
- Appearance and intactness of placenta
- Mother's condition
- Any medications given to mother or newborn (per agency protocol)

EVALUATION

As a result of comprehensive nursing care during the intrapartal period, the following outcomes may be anticipated:

- The mother's physical and psychologic well-being has been maintained and supported.
- The baby's physical and psychologic well-being has been protected and supported.
- The couple have had input into the birth process and have participated as much as they desired.
- The mother and her baby have had a safe birth.

CRITICAL CONCEPT REVIEW

LEARNING OUTCOMES	CONCEPTS
19.1 Identify admission data that should be noted when a woman is admitted to the birthing area.	1. Information obtained during admission is used to develop a clinical pathway for the four stages of labor: ■ Prenatal information. ■ Current assessments. ■ Expected teaching. ■ Nursing care expected for each stage. ■ Expected activity level. ■ Proposed comfort measures. ■ Elimination and nutritional needs. ■ Level of family involvement.
19.2 Describe the nursing care of a woman and her partner/family upon admission to the birthing area.	1. The nursing care at admission focuses on providing an orientation to the unit and obtaining an overall physical assessment of the mother that focuses on the well-being of the mother and fetus: ■ Assess the maternal vital signs and FHR. ■ Perform a vaginal exam to determine stage of cervical dilatation and state of membranes. ■ Determine frequency and intensity of contractions. ■ Review systems such as respiratory and neurological. ■ Assess any recent symptoms experienced by the woman. ■ Assess the woman's understanding of the labor process and identification of the woman's support system.

(continued)

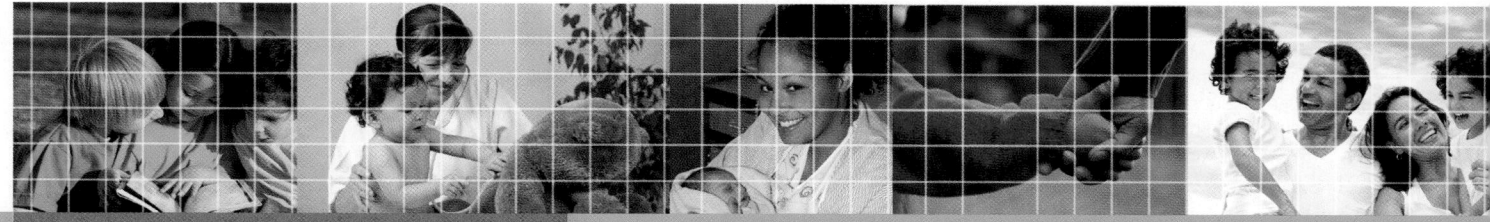

LEARNING OUTCOMES / CONCEPTS

LEARNING OUTCOMES	CONCEPTS
19.3 Use assessment data to determine the nursing interventions to meet the psychologic, social, physiologic, and spiritual needs of the woman and her partner/family during each stage of labor.	1. First stage of labor: ■ Establish rapport with the woman and support person. ■ Discuss expectations of labor and birth. ■ Provide for privacy. ■ Discuss individual expression of pain and discomfort. 2. Second stage of labor: ■ Provide as much privacy as possible. ■ Encourage the woman and support person to decide who should be present at the birth. ■ Provide praise and encouragement of progress. 3. Third and fourth stages of labor: ■ Encourage the woman and support person to hold and look at infant as much as possible. ■ Teach the woman the care to be performed after the baby is born. ■ Provide the woman with food and fluids as allowed.
19.4 Compare methods of promoting comfort during the first and second stages of labor.	1. Comfort measures common to the first and second stages of labor include: ■ Assist the woman to reduce anxiety. ■ Teach the woman about what to expect during the labor experience. ■ Promote relaxation techniques. ■ Instruct in appropriate controlled breathing pattern. ■ Give instruction to the woman's support person. 2. Comfort measures specific to the first stage of labor: ■ Administer pharmacologic agents as ordered by the physician or certified nurse-midwife. ■ Assist with the placement of an epidural for pain control. 3. Comfort measures specific to the second stage of labor: ■ Help the woman find an effective pushing pattern. ■ Support the woman's attempt to rest between pushes.
19.5 Explain the immediate needs and physical assessment of the newborn following birth in the provision of nursing care.	1. Immediate care of the newborn includes: ■ Maintain respiration. ■ Promote warmth. ■ Prevent infection. ■ Provide accurate identification.
19.6 Examine the unique needs of the adolescent during birth in the provision of nursing care.	1. The adolescent is unique in that she has developmental needs as well as physical needs that must be addressed.
19.7 Describe the role and responsibilities of the nurse in the management of a precipitous birth.	1. A precipitous birth is one that occurs rapidly without a physician or certified nurse-midwife in attendance. 2. The nurse attends to the woman, guides the infant's passage through the birth canal, clamps the umbilical cord, and immediately transports the infant to the nursery for care. 3. The nurse focuses care on the woman and the expulsion of the placenta and contraction of the uterus.

CRITICAL THINKING IN ACTION

Anita Grey, a 22-year-old primigravida at 40 weeks' gestation, is admitted by you to the birthing center in labor. Anita was sent from her physician's office after being evaluated at her prenatal visit. While in the office, she was assessed to be 4 cm dilated, 100% effaced, vertex at 0 station with bulging membranes. She tells you that her husband is on his way to the birthing center and that she is anxious for him to arrive. A review of her prenatal record shows no complications affecting this pregnancy. Anita's vital signs are within normal limits. You assess the fetal heart rate and contraction pattern with the fetal monitor and observe a fetal heart rate of 140 to 150 bpm with accelerations to 160s. Contractions are every 3 to 4 minutes $\times$ 30 seconds of moderate intensity by palpation. Anita seems to be tolerating the contractions well, but still seems anxious about her husband's arrival.

1. What steps can you take to reduce the stress and anxiety of the laboring woman and her family?

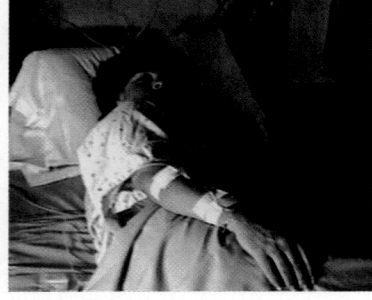

2. When you notify the physician/midwife, what pertinent information should the report contain?
3. What support measures can you give in the active phase of labor?
4. What measures can be used to decrease discomfort/pain as labor progresses?
5. What observations reflect the physiologic manifestations of pain?

See MyNursingKit for possible responses.

REFERENCES

American College of Obstetricians & Gynecologists (ACOG). (2005). *Intrapartum fetal heart rate monitoring.* (ACOG Practice Bulletin No. 70). Washington, DC: Author.

American College of Obstetricians & Gynecologists (ACOG). (2006a). *Apgar score* (Committee Opinion No. 333). Washington, DC: Author.

American Society of Anesthesiologists (ASA). (2006). *Practice guidelines for obstetric anesthesia.* Park Ridge, IL: Author.

Chai-Chen, A. (2007). Family-centered care. *Journal for Specialists in Pediatric Nursing, 12*(2), 119–122.

Ethnomed. (2007). Peripartum and infant care issues and practices among refugee groups. Retrieved April 15, 2007, at http://ethnomed.org/ethnomed/clin_topics/peri.html

Gennaro, S., Mayberry, L. J., & Kafulafula, U. (2007). The evidence supporting nursing management of labor. *JOGNN, 36*(6), 598–604.

Hunter, S., Hofmeyr, G. J., & Kulier, R. (2007). Hands and knees posture in late pregnancy of labour for fetal malposition (lateral or posterior). [Cochrane Review]. In *Cochrane Database of Systematic Reviews.* 2007. Retrieved May 19, 2008, from The Cochrane Library, Wiley Interscience.

Lawrence, A., Lewis, L., Hofmeyr, G., Dowswell, T., & Styles, C. (2009). Maternal positions and mobility during first stage labor. *Cochrane Database of Systematic Reviews. Issue 2. Art. No.: CD003034.*

Levy, T., & Blickstein, I. (2006). Timing of cord clamping revisited. *Journal of Perinatal Medicine, 34*(4), 293–297.

Moore, E. R., Anderson, G. C., Bergman, N. (2007). Early skin-to-skin contact for mothers and their healthy newborn infants. [Cochrane Review]. In *Cochrane Database of Systematic Reviews.* 2007. Retrieved April 10, 2008, from The Cochrane Library, Wiley Interscience.

Perinatal HIV Guidelines Working Group. (2006). Public Health Service Task Force recommendations for use of antiretroviral drugs in pregnant HIV-1 infected women for maternal health and interventions to reduce perinatal HIV-1 transmission in the United States. October 12, 2006, 1–65. Retrieved April 17, 2007, at http://aidsinfo.nih.gov/ContentFiles/PerinatalGL.pdf

Smith, C. A., Collins, C. T., Cyna, A. M., & Crowther, C. A. (2006). Complementary and alternative therapies for pain management in labour. *Cochrane Database Systematic Review, 18*(4), CD003521.

Spector, R. E. (2009). *Cultural diversity in health and illness* (7th ed.). Upper Saddle River, NJ: Prentice Hall Health.

St. Elizabeth's Medical Center. (2007). Cultural diversity: Latinos. Retrieved April 17, 2007, from http://www.stemc.org/about_stemc/cultural_diversity/latinos.php?id=294

Wilson, B. A., Shannon, M. T., & Shields, K. M. (2009). *Nurse's drug guide 2009.* Upper Saddle River, NJ: Pearson Education.

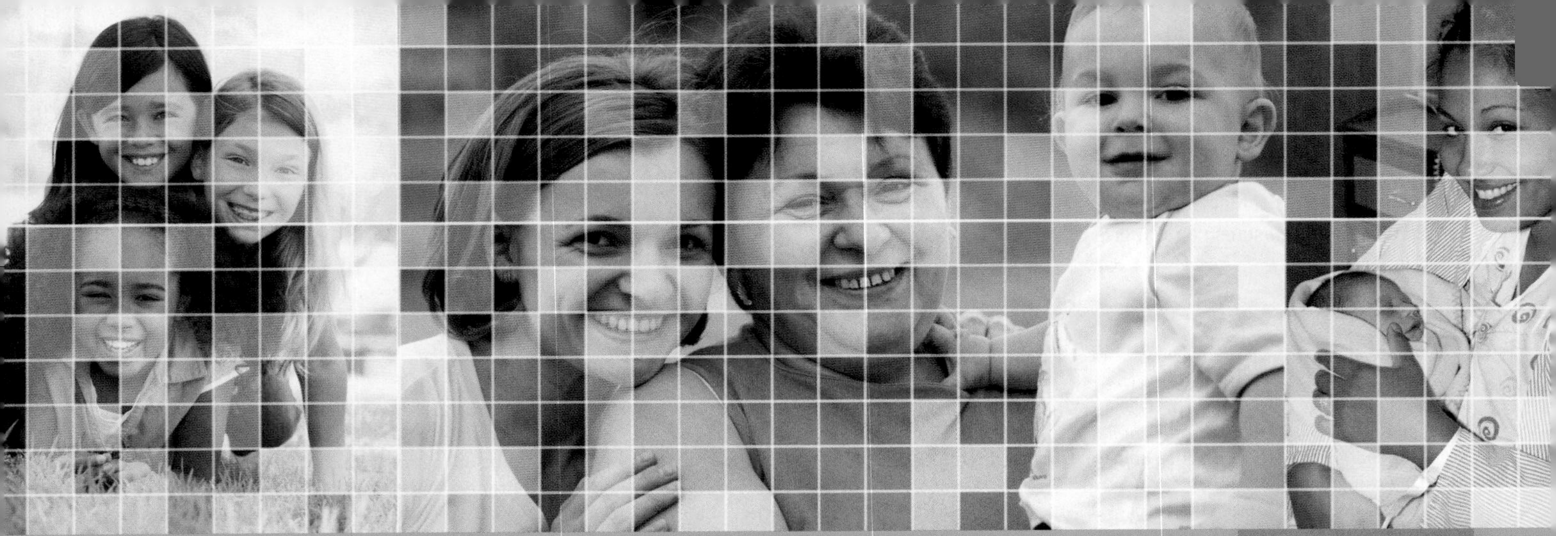

CHAPTER 20

Pharmacologic Pain Management

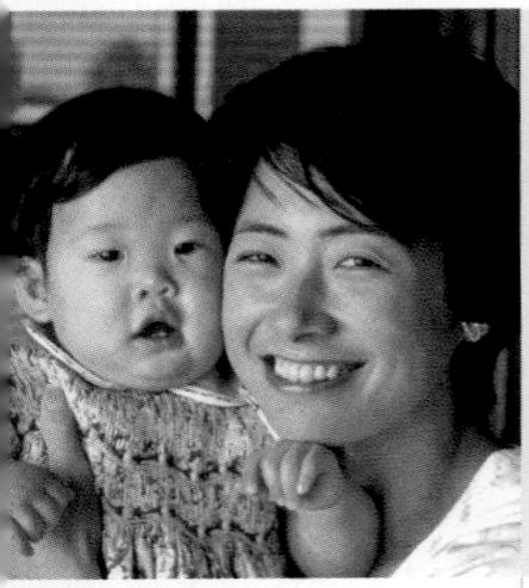

We had attended our classes and practiced through the last few weeks, but I was not ready for the amount of discomfort that I felt during my labor. I've always been able to handle pain much better, but this pain was very different. I had hoped to go through all of labor and birth without medications, but we had talked about it and I knew that if I felt I needed something, it would be all right. My nurse was also helpful and supportive of my decision. She helped me feel that I was making a good decision and that I wasn't failing somehow. —Kyung-aie, 36

LEARNING OUTCOMES

20.1 Describe the use, administration, dose, onset of action, and adverse effects of systemic drugs to promote pain relief during the nursing care management of the woman in labor and her fetus.

20.2 Compare the major types of regional analgesia and anesthesia, including area affected, advantages, disadvantages, techniques, and nursing care management of the laboring woman and her fetus.

20.3 Explain the possible complications of regional anesthesia in nursing care management of the laboring woman and her fetus.

20.4 Describe the nursing care management for the laboring woman and her fetus related to general anesthesia.

20.5 Describe the major complications of general anesthesia during labor in nursing care management of the woman in labor and her fetus.

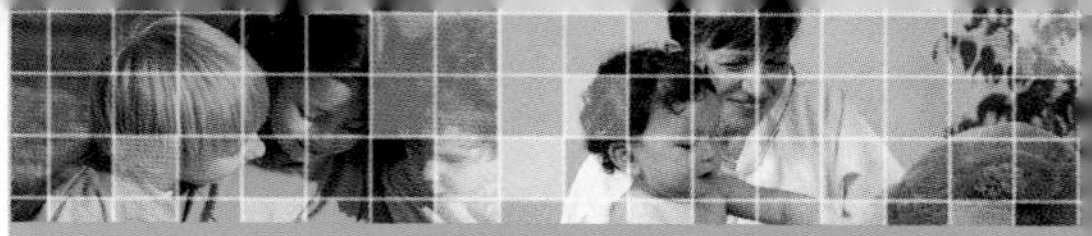

KEY TERMS

Childbearing women experience varying levels of pain and other demanding sensations during labor and birth. As discussed in Chapter 19, nursing interventions directed toward pain relief begins with psychologic measures such as providing information, support, and encouragement. Measures to promote physical comfort include back rubs, showers, whirlpools (Jacuzzi), and the application of cool cloths. Some laboring women need no further interventions.

For other women, the progression of labor brings increasing pain that interferes with their ability to cope. These women may elect to use pharmacologic agents such as systemic medications, regional nerve blocks (epidural, spinal, or combined epidural-spinal), and local anesthetic blocks (pudendal and perineal) to decrease discomfort, increase relaxation, and reestablish their ability to participate more effectively in the labor and birth experience. The methods are not all mutually exclusive, and any of them may be used in combination with nonpharmacologic comfort measures. The use of general anesthesia has very limited use in modern obstetrics. It is occassionally used during emergency cesarean births although this trend continues to decrease because of the associated adverse maternal and fetal effects.

Although systemic analgesics and regional anesthetic blocks may affect the fetus, so do the laboring woman's pain and stress. During labor, maternal respirations and oxygen consumption increase, and this decreases the amount of oxygen available to the fetus. In addition, the pain and stress can lead to metabolic acidosis and the release of catecholamines, which causes maternal blood vessels to constrict, lessening oxygen and nutrient supply to the fetus (Hawkins, Goetzl, & Chestnut, 2007).

There is a good deal of peer pressure on expectant parents to have the "ideal" birth experience. They may plan a natural childbirth, in which case the need for analgesia may make them feel inadequate and guilty. The nurse has a special role in helping a woman and her partner accept alterations in their original plan and recognize the unique qualities of their birth experience. Reassurance that accepting analgesia for discomfort is not a failure can help maintain the woman's self-esteem. The emphasis should be on achieving a healthy, satisfying outcome for the family. Evidence has shown that women who have continuous one-to-one support during labor were more likely to have a spontaneous vaginal birth, less likely to require analgesia, and less likely to report dissatisfaction with their childbirth experience (O'Sullivan, 2009). Also, ACOG has concluded that a woman's request is sufficient justification for pain relief during labor (ACOG, 2006).

SYSTEMIC MEDICATIONS

It should be noted that this discussion of obstetric analgesia and anesthesia applies only to a healthy woman and fetus. Pain relief during labor and birth for women with high-risk conditions, such as preterm labor, preeclampsia, blood disorders, or diabetes mellitus, requires skilled decision making, close observation, and awareness of all the potential threats to both the woman and her baby. The goal of pharmacologic analgesia during labor is to provide maximum pain relief at minimum risk for the mother and fetus. To reach this goal, clinicians must consider a number of factors, including the following:

- All systemic medications used for pain relief during labor cross the placental barrier by simple diffusion, but some medications cross more readily than others.
- Medication action in the body depends on the rate at which the substance is metabolized by liver enzymes and excreted by the kidneys.
- High medication doses may remain in the fetus for long periods because fetal liver enzymes and kidney excretion are inadequate for metabolizing analgesic agents.

Thinking Critically

ANESTHESIA DURING LABOR

Luisa Silva, a 33-year-old G1P0, is 32 weeks pregnant. She is trying to decide whether she should accept any analgesia during her labor. She has finished childbirth education classes and wants an unmedicated labor and birth. She says, "I want to do this on my own, but I'm afraid it may be too much. Will it be OK if I need to take something?" What will you tell her?

See MyNursingKit for possible responses.

Teaching Highlights

WHAT WOMEN NEED TO KNOW ABOUT PAIN-RELIEF MEDICATIONS

Before receiving medications, the woman should understand the following:

- Type of medication administered
- Route of administration
- Expected effects of medication
- Implications for fetus or newborn
- Safety measures needed (e.g., remain in bed with side rails up)

Developing Cultural Competence

CULTURAL INFLUENCE ON RESPONSES TO PAIN

A woman's cultural background may influence her responses to pain. Following are generalizations of how some cultures perceive pain and pain responses:

- Mexican American women may moan rhythmically and massage their thighs and abdomen when in pain.
- Haitian women may prefer massage, movement, and position changes to increase comfort.
- Filipino women may lie quietly because they believe that noise and activity increase labor pain.
- Black, Puerto Rican, and Middle Eastern women are often verbally expressive of pain.
- Native American women may be viewed as stoic, using meditation, self-control, and traditional herbs.
- Thai women's silent but restless behavior can reflect high levels of pain.
- Japanese, Chinese, Vietnamese, Laotian, and other women of Asian descent may feel that crying out during labor is shameful.
- Samoan women may believe no verbal response is allowed.

NURSING MANAGEMENT

Analgesic medications provide pain relief for the laboring woman but also affect the fetus and the labor process. Pain medication given too early may prolong labor and depress the fetus; if given too late it is of minimal use to the woman and may lead to respiratory depression in the newborn. The nurse assesses the mother and fetus and also evaluates the contraction pattern before administering prescribed systemic medications.

Maternal assessment parameters include:

- The woman is willing to receive medication after being advised about the risks and benefits of the medication.
- Maternal vital signs are stable.
- Contraindications (such as specific medication allergy, respiratory compromise, or current medication dependence) are not present.

Fetal assessment parameters include:

- The fetal heart rate (FHR) baseline is between 110 and 160 beats per minute, and no late decelerations or nonreassuring FHR patterns are present.
- Variability is present.
- The fetus exhibits normal movement, and accelerations are present with fetal movement.
- The fetus is term.

Assessment of labor includes:

- Documentation of the contraction pattern.
- The cervical status including cervical position, consistency, effacement, dilatation, and station.

Before administering the medication, the nurse once again ascertains whether the woman has a history of any medication reactions or allergies and provides information about the medication. (See "Teaching Highlights: What Women Need to Know About Pain-Relief Medications.") Maternal vital signs, FHR, contraction pattern, and pain level should be assessed and documented before administering any pain medication. After giving the medication, the nurse records the medication name, dose, route, and site, as well as the woman's blood pressure (BP) and pulse, on the FHR monitor strip and on the woman's medical record. If the woman is alone, side rails should be raised to provide safety. The nurse assesses the FHR for possible adverse effects of the medication. After the medication has been administered, the nurse should document the woman's pain level, the effectiveness of the medication, and any adverse effects if they occurred.

When an analgesic medication is administered by intramuscular or subcutaneous route, it takes a few minutes for the effect to be felt. The nurse can continue with other supportive measures to enhance comfort, such as ensuring a quiet environment, providing a back rub or cool cloth, assisting with relaxation and visualization exercises, or providing therapeutic touch until the woman feels the effect of the medication. Often, continued reassurance and verbal praise have a calming effect. When the medication begins to take effect, the woman may sleep between contractions. This short period of rest helps her relax and can restore her energy. When the physician/CNM orders an intravenous route, the effect of the medication will be felt within a few minutes, so if any change of position is necessary or if the woman needs to void, the nurse may suggest that the woman complete these activities before receiving the medication. Some women may be so uncomfortable that they do not want anything except the medication. In this case, administering the medication first would be more helpful for the woman.

OPIOID ANALGESICS

Opioid analgesic agents that are injected into the circulation have their primary action at sites in the brain, activating the neurons that descend to the spinal cord. The opioid analgesics used in early labor are given in either intermittent doses or, less commonly, by patient-controlled administration. These medications work by providing some analgesic effect and by inducing sedation (Hawkins, 2008). See Table 20–1 for a list of analgesics used in labor.

Butorphanol Tartrate (Stadol) and Nalbuphine Hydrochloride (Nubain)

Butorphanol tartrate (Stadol) is a synthetic agonist-antagonist opioid analgesic agent. The medication has been proven effective in reducing pain intensity in laboring women. A study that compared butorphanol (Stadol) with meperidine (Demerol) found that both medications relieved pain intensity, although the magnitude of pain following the administration of butorphanol (Stadol) was less (Nelson & Eisenach, 2005). Respiratory depression of both the mother and fetus or newborn can occur but can be reversed with naloxone (Narcan).

The most common side effect associated with butorphanol (Stadol) is drowsiness. Dizziness, fainting, and hypotension can also occur (Wilson, Shannon, & Shields, 2010). If these symptoms do occur, the woman should remain in bed with the side rails up to prevent injury. Urinary retention following administration of butorphanol is not common but does occur. Therefore, the nurse should be alert for bladder distention when a woman has received butorphanol for analgesia during labor, has IV fluids infusing, and receives regional anesthesia for the birth. Butorphanol needs to be protected from light and stored at room temperature (Wilson et al., 2010).

Like butorphanol, nalbuphine hydrochloride (Nubain) is a synthetic agonist-antagonist opioid analgesic and may precipitate medication withdrawal if the woman is physically dependent on opioids. It also crosses the placenta to the fetus and can cause a nonreassuring fetal heart rate and neonatal respiratory depression. In the birth setting, Nubain may be given directly into the tubing of a running IV infusion and 10 mg should be administered over 3 to 5 minutes (Wilson et al., 2010). Both Nalbuphine and Butorphanol can have a ceiling effect where the pain reduction qualities do not increase, but the side effects increase. Nalbuphine is often the medication of choice because it is associated with less nausea and vomiting, and a lower incidence of respiratory depression. Nalbuphine is also associated with increased maternal sedation, which allows the mother an opportunity to rest between contractions. See "Drug Guide: Nalbuphine Hydrochloride (Nubain)."

Table 20–1 Drug Guide: Analgesics Used in Labor

Drug/Class	Dosage, Route, Frequency	Common Side Effects	Life-Threatening Reactions	Contraindications
Stadol (butorphanol tartrate): CNS agent, analgesic, narcotic agonest/antagonist	IM 1–2 mg every 4 hours IV 0.5–2 mg every 4 hrs; rapid onset; peak: 30–60 min; duration 3–4 hrs Intranasal: 1 mg (1 puff) may repeat in 90 seconds (max dose every 3–4 hours)	Sedation, dizziness, fainting, hypotension, hypertension	Respiratory depression	Narcotic dependency, Breastfeeding, women with chronic hypertension or preeclampsia
Nubain (nalbuphine hydrochloride): CNS aµgent analgesic, narcotic agonist	10–20 mg every 3–6 hours prn SC/IM/IV	Sedation; sweaty, clammy skin; nausea and vomiting	Respiratory depression	Hypersensitivity to the drug
Demerol (meperidine hydrochloride): CNS agent, analgesic, narcotic agonist	IV 2.5–15 mg every 4 hours IM/SC 5–20 mg every 4 hours	Pruritus, dizziness, sedation, nausea, constipation	Respiratory depression, convulsions, cardiovascular collapse, cardiac arrest, respiratory depression in newborn, bronchoconstriction	Hypersensitivity to the drug, convulsive disorders, breastfeeding, undiagnosed acute abdomen
Fentanyl (Sublimaze): Short-acting opiate agonist, analgesic	50–100 mcg every 2 hrs IV/IM IV give over 1–2 min.; immediate onset; peak 30–60 min., duration limited to 30–60 min. IM onset 7–15 min.	Bradycardia, hypotension, nausea, vomiting, and respiratory depression	Muscle rigidity, especially in the respiratory muscles.	Women with opioid dependency

Drug Guide

NALBUPHINE HYDROCHLORIDE (NUBAIN)

Overview of Action

Nubain is a synthetic opioid analgesic with agonist and weak antagonist properties. Analgesic properties are equal to those produced by morphine. Nubain's potency is three to four times greater than pentazocine. The incidence of respiratory depression that occurs is equivalent to morphine.

Dosage, Route

Nubain is indicated for moderate to severe pain. Adults: 10 to 20 mg every 3 to 6 hours PRN subcutaneous/IM/IV. Commonly given IV, onset in 2–3 min, peaks in 15-20 min, duration 3–6 hrs. IM or subcutaneous, onset in less than 15 min, peaks 30–60 min, duration 3–6 hrs (Wilson et al., 2010).

Maternal Contraindications

Hypersensitivity or allergy to nalbuphine hydrochloride, respiratory depression, acute asthma attack, bradycardia, inflammatory bowel disease, and substance abuse.

Maternal Side Effects

Sedation, clammy sweaty skin, abdominal pain with cramps, nausea and vomiting, dizziness, vertigo, fainting, nervousness, restlessness, depression; false sense of well-being, hallucinations, headache, nightmares, allergic dermatitis, allergic reactions, anorexia, blurred vision, diplopia, bradycardia, tachycardia, asthma, dyspnea, flushing, general weakness, hypertension, hypotension, impaired cognition, malaise, pruritus, urinary urgency.

Nursing Considerations

- Assess client's allergy, sensitivity, or dependence to opioids on admission.
- Inform woman of potential side effects.
- Monitor and evaluate analgesic effect. Ask client about comfort level and notify analgesia provider of inadequate pain relief.
- Observe for symptoms of hypersensitivity: pruritus, urticaria, and/or burning sensation.
- May produce an allergic response in clients with sulfite sensitivity.
- If allergic reaction (urticaria, edema, or respiratory difficulties) occurs, administer naloxone or diphenhydramine per physician order.
- Assess respiratory rate before administration. Notify healthcare provider if respirations are less than 12 per minute.
- Monitor urinary output and assess bladder for distention. Assist client to void.
- Maintain bed rest or assist client with ambulation after administration.
- Counsel client that use with alcohol or other central nervous system depressants may increase medication effects.
- Prolonged use with abrupt discontinuation can result in symptoms consistent with opioid withdrawal in both the mother and infant.

Fentanyl (Sublimaze)

Fentanyl is a short-acting opiate that has been used during labor to relieve pain and induce sedation. Fentanyl is 50 to 100 times more potent than morphine. Fentanyl has less neonatal neurobehavioral depression than Demerol because it does not cross the placenta. However, neonatal depression can still occur, although at much lower rates when compared with Demerol. Fentanyl results in less sedation, nausea, vomiting, and pruritis compared with Demerol. See Table 20–1.

ANALGESIC POTENTIATORS

The use of **analgesic potentiators**, also known as *ataractics*, can decrease anxiety and increase the effectiveness of analgesics when given simultaneously. These medications, which are classified as tranquilizers, have no specific properties that decrease pain; however, they do work well to potentiate the effects of opioid analgesics without increasing unwanted side effects. This enhancement enables the woman to receive a smaller dose of the opioid being administered. These medications can also be used to manage unpleasant side effects, such as nausea or vomiting, associated with the administration of opioid analgesics.

Commonly used analgesic potentiators include promethazine (Phenergan), hydroxyzine (Vistaril), propiomazine (Largon), and promazine (Sparine). The main side effect is sedation, which may be helpful in promoting rest in women who have had a prolonged labor or who have had little sleep; however, the effect may be undesirable to other women.

OPIATE ANTAGONIST: NALOXONE (NARCAN)

Because naloxone is an antagonist with little or no agonistic effect, it exhibits little pharmacologic activity in the absence of opioids. Naloxone can be used to reverse the mild respiratory depression that follows administration of small doses of opiates such as fentanyl and meperidine, as well as butorphanol tartrate and nalbuphine hydrochloride. Naloxone is the medication of choice when the depressant is unknown because it will cause no further depression (Wilson et al., 2010). An initial dose of 0.4 to 2 mg may be administered intravenously to the laboring woman. If the woman is nonresponsive, the medication can be readministered every 2 to 3 minutes. The nurse should be prepared to provide basic airway management, including chin lift, jaw thrust maneuver, and initiation of respirations through a bag valve mask device when the woman is not immediately responsive and respiratory depression is occurring. It is typically administered to mothers who have received opioids within 4 hours of the birth (Wilson et al., 2010). When naloxone is given, other resuscitative measures may be indicated, and trained personnel should be readily available. The duration of the medication's effect is shorter than that of

Complementary Care

ACUPRESSURE FOR LABOR PAIN

Acupressure can lessen pain during the first stage of labor (Chung, Hung, Kuo, et al., 2003). The acupressure point for labor and birth is found in the webbing between the thumb and index finger. This point should never be stimulated during pregnancy since it stimulates uterine contractions. The mother places her right thumb on the back of her left hand and her right index finger on the front of the left hand at the acupressure point. She can rub the point to stimulate labor and squeeze the point to decrease labor pain. Another acupressure point is found between the inner ankle bone and the Achilles' tendon. Squeezing for 1 minute on each ankle reduces labor pain. See MyNursingKit at http://www.prenhall.com/london for more information on acupressure, including an interview with a labor and delivery nurse on her use of acupressure to relieve labor pain.

the analgesic medication for which it is acting as an antagonist, so the nurse must be alert to the return of respiratory depression and the need for repeated doses. Naloxone should not be given in women with known or suspected opiate dependency because it may precipitate severe withdrawal (Wilson et al., 2010). Naloxone may be given to the newborn if needed after birth. The newborn dose is 0.1 mg/kg and may need to be repeated. (See "Drug Guide: Naloxone Hydrochloride (Narcan)," in Chapter 29 ∞).

REGIONAL ANESTHESIA AND ANALGESIA

Regional anesthesia is the temporary loss of sensation produced by injecting an anesthetic agent (called a *local*) into direct contact with nervous tissue. Loss of sensation happens because the local agents stabilize the cell membrane, which prevents initiation and transmission of nerve impulses. The regional anesthetic blocks most commonly used in childbirth include the epidural, spinal, and combined epidural-spinal blocks. Epidural blocks may be used for analgesia during labor and vaginal birth and for anesthesia during cesarean birth.

An epidural relieves pain associated with the first stage of labor by blocking the sensory nerves supplying the uterus. Pain associated with the second stage of labor and with birth can be alleviated with epidural, combined epidural-spinal, and pudendal blocks (see Figure 20–1 ●).

Until recently, the same anesthetic agents used for regional epidurals were also used to produce **regional analgesia** (pain relief to a body region) during labor. This practice was problematic because the anesthetic agents used alter the transmission of impulses to the bladder, making voiding difficult. The agents also interfere with blood pressure stability and leg movement. The descent of the fetus is slowed and an increased risk of perineal lacerations occurs more commonly in women with epidural anesthesia (Fitzgerald, Weber, Howden et al., 2007; Sheiner, Walfisch, Hollak, et al., 2006). To address these difficulties, regional analgesia is now obtained by injecting an opioid such as fentanyl along with only a small amount of anesthetic agent. New medication combinations relieve the woman's pain while minimizing the side effects just mentioned (Hawkins et al., 2007).

MyNursingKit Complementary Care: Acupressure Information

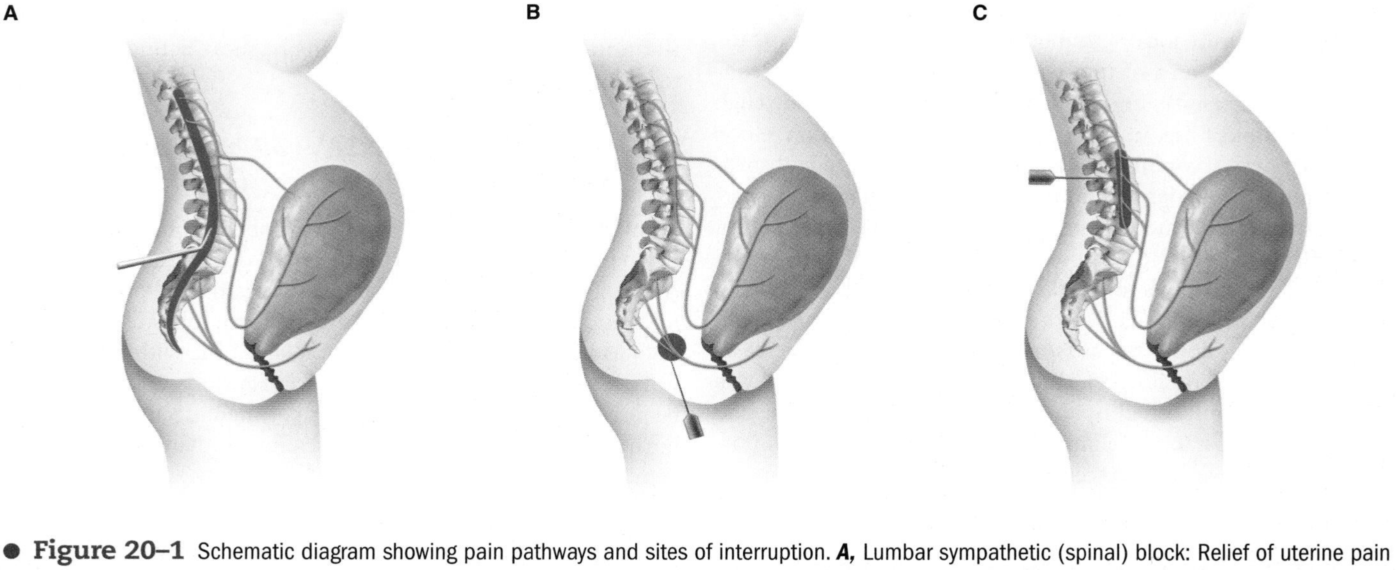

● **Figure 20–1** Schematic diagram showing pain pathways and sites of interruption. ***A,*** Lumbar sympathetic (spinal) block: Relief of uterine pain only. ***B,*** Pudendal block: Relief of perineal pain. ***C,*** Lumbar epidural block: Dark area demonstrates peridural (epidural) space and nerves affected, and the gray tube represents a continuous plastic catheter.

Source: Bonica, J. J. (1972). *Principles and practice of obstetric analgesia and anesthesia* (pp. 492, 512, 521, 614). Philadelphia: F. A. Davis.

The intrathecal injection of opioids results in another type of regional analgesia. In this case, the opioid is injected into the subarachnoid space. It is important for the anesthesia provider to provide a test dose before giving the entire dose to determine that the catheter is correctly placed. Fentanyl citrate and preservative-free morphine are the most commonly used medications. This typically results in more effective pain relief over the subsequent 24 hours after birth, although the incidence of nausea may be increased in some women (Vasudevan, Snowman, Sundar, et al., 2007).

Nursing care during administration of regional analgesia is directed toward helping the woman void before administration, assisting her with positioning during and after the procedure, monitoring and assessing vital signs and respiratory status, monitoring analgesic effect, and determining fetal well-being. Reassurance and thorough explanations help decrease anxiety and fear. Additional measures may be needed to address pruritus, nausea and vomiting, and urinary retention.

As with other procedures, the woman needs to know how the block is given, the expected effect on her and the fetus, advantages and disadvantages, and possible complications. Many women discuss possible anesthetic blocks with their care provider at some point in the pregnancy. If they have not, it is important to give them an opportunity to ask questions and obtain information before receiving the block while in labor.

ANESTHETIC AGENTS FOR REGIONAL BLOCKS

MyNursingKit Case Study: Relief Therapies during Birth

Local anesthetic agents block the conduction of nerve impulses from the periphery to the central nervous system by preventing the propagation of an action potential from the source of pain (Hawkins, 2008). The types of nerve fibers are differentially sensitive to the various anesthetic agents. In general, the smaller the fiber, the more sensitive it is to local agents. For example, it is possible to block the small C and A delta fibers, which transmit pain and temperature, without blocking the larger A alpha, A beta, and A gamma fibers, which continue to maintain a sense of pressure, muscle tone, position sense, and motor function.

Absorption of local anesthetics depends primarily on the vascularity of the area of injection. The agents themselves contribute to increased blood flow by causing vasodilation. High concentrations of medications cause greater vasodilation. Good maternal physical condition or a high metabolic rate aids absorption. Malnutrition, dehydration, electrolyte imbalance, and cardiovascular and pulmonary problems increase the potential for toxic effects. The pH of tissues affects the rate of absorption, which has implications for fetal complications such as acidosis. The addition of vasoconstrictors such as epinephrine delays absorption and prolongs the anesthetic effect because it decreases uteroplacental blood flow. The breakdown of local anesthetics in the body is accomplished by the liver and plasma esterase, and the resulting substance is eliminated by the kidneys. It is important to use the weakest concentration and the smallest amount necessary to produce the desired results.

MyNursingKit Video: Epidural Placement

TYPES OF LOCAL ANESTHETIC AGENTS

Two types of local anesthetic agents are currently available: esters and amides. The ester type includes procaine hydrochloride (Novocain), chloroprocaine hydrochloride (Nesacaine), and tetracaine hydrochloride (Pontocaine). Esters are rapidly metabolized; therefore, toxic maternal levels are not as likely to be reached, and placental transfer to the fetus is prevented. Ester-linked agents have a higher incidence of allergic reactions when compared with amides. However, they do not appear to have a higher incidence of fetal effects (Hawkins, 2008).

Amide types include lidocaine hydrochloride (Xylocaine), mepivacaine hydrochloride (Carbocaine), and bupivacaine hydrochloride (Marcaine). Amide types are more powerful and longer-acting agents. They readily cross the placenta, can be measured in the fetal circulation, and affect the fetus for a prolonged period. Lidocaine (Xylocaine) has been associated with major neurological and minor neurological toxicity; therefore, the dose of lidocaine should not exceed 75 mg.

Ropivacaine (Naropin) is a new generation amide that is now being used in labor. The pain relief effects are similar to other amides. However, the blockade effect is slightly lower than other amides, thus increasing the rates of vaginal births and decreasing instrument-assisted births. Levobupivacaine (Chirocaine) has less toxicity than ropivacaine and is safer in longer surgical procedures because it has decreased toxicity.

ADVERSE MATERNAL REACTIONS TO ANESTHETIC AGENTS

Reactions to local anesthetic agents range from mild symptoms to cardiovascular collapse. Mild reactions include palpitations, tinnitus, apprehension, confusion, and a metallic taste in the mouth. Moderate reactions include more severe degrees of mild symptoms plus nausea and vomiting, hypotension, and muscle twitching, which may progress to convulsions. Severe reactions are sudden loss of consciousness, coma, severe hypotension, bradycardia, respiratory depression, and cardiac arrest. Anesthetic agents should not be used unless an intravenous line is in place.

The preferred treatment for a mild toxic reaction is administration of oxygen and IV injection of a short-acting barbiturate to diminish anxiety.

NEONATAL NEUROBEHAVIORAL EFFECTS OF ANESTHESIA AND ANALGESIA

Many studies have focused on the neurobehavioral effects on the newborn of pharmacologic agents used during labor and birth. Although analgesic and anesthetic agents may alter the behavioral and adaptive function of the newborn, physiologic factors such as hunger, degree of hydration, and time within the sleep-wake cycle may also exert an influence (Hawkins, 2008). It should be noted that more neurological impairment occurs in the newborn resulting from normal birth process than from epidural complications.

EPIDURAL BLOCK

A lumbar **epidural block** involves injection of an anesthetic agent into the epidural space to provide pain relief throughout labor. The epidural space, a potential space between the dura mater and the ligamentum flavum, is accessed through the lumbar area (Figure 20–2 ●). The epidural is most frequently used as a continuous block to provide analgesia and anesthesia from active labor through episiotomy repair (Figure 20–3 ●).

Epidurals have become a relatively common method of analgesia and anesthesia during labor and birth in the United States. It is estimated that 68% of all women in the United States receive an epidural during their labor. Non-Hispanic white women had the highest rates of epidural use (70.2%), followed by non-Hispanic black women (65.6%). Hispanic women used epidural anesthesia the least (57.8%). Epidural use did not differ among age groups (Martin & Menacker, 2007). An epidural can be given as soon as active labor is established.

Advantages

The epidural block relieves discomfort during labor and birth, and the woman is fully awake and a part of the birth process. Epidural anesthesia results in less adverse fetal effects when compared with intravenous analgesia or general anesthesia. It can also allow the woman to rest and regain strength before the woman needs to push during the second stage. The continuous epidural allows different blocking for each stage of labor, so that the fetus is able to descend and rotate in the maternal pelvis; many times the woman's urge to bear down is preserved. Epidurals that combine anesthesia and an opioid agent are often effective in providing postoperative pain relief for longer periods of time.

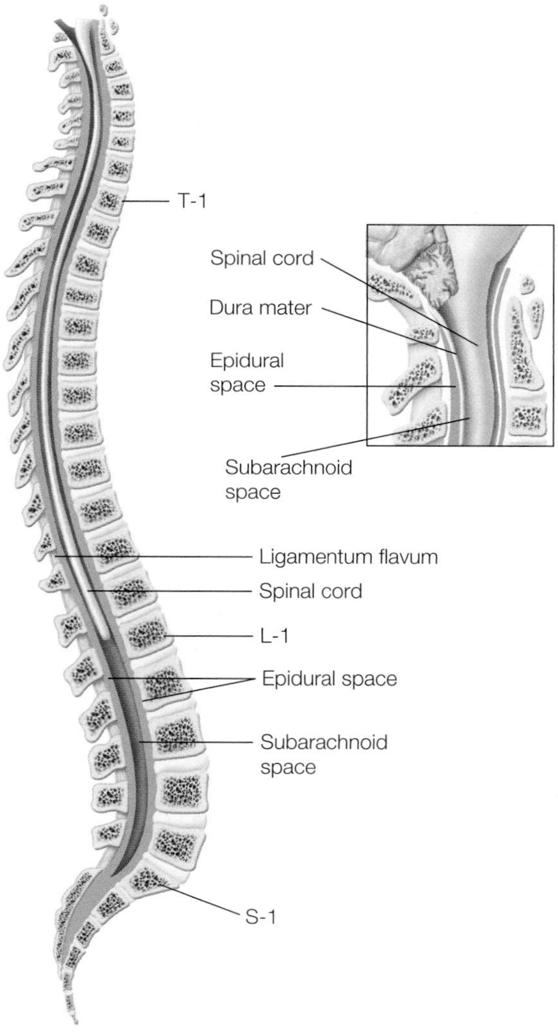

● **Figure 20–2** Epidural space. The epidural space lies between the dura mater and the ligamentum flavum, extending from the base of the skull to the end of the sacral canal.

Opioids are used with epidural blocks for labor. Some of the agents used include morphine, fentanyl, butorphanol, and meperidine (Hawkins, 2008). When only opioids are used epidurally, rather than in combination with another type of agent, the amount of pain relief is not as effective, especially toward the end of labor; therefore, a combination of opioids and a low dose of local are given (Hawkins, 2008).

Disadvantages

The most common complication of an epidural block is maternal hypotension, which is generally prevented by administering intravenous fluid before epidural placement, left uterine displacement, and maternal positioning on her side. In some instances, labor progress and fetal descent may be slowed, and pushing efforts in the second stage may be less effective because of a decrease in sensation. There does not appear to be an increase in forceps or vacuum use or in cesarean section births related to epidural anesthesia (Hawkins, 2008). Delay in return of bladder sensation may result in urinary retention and the need for catheterization during labor and in the fourth stage (Musselwhite, Faris, Moore, et al., 2007). Low back pain can also occur after an epidural and is usually more common in women who underwent vaginal deliveries. Typically, epidurals do not cause chronic low back pain, although the woman can have soreness at the insertion site for a few days.

Contraindications

The absolute contraindications for epidural block are client refusal, infection at the site of the needle puncture, maternal problems with blood coagulation (coagulopathies), raised intracranial pressure, specific medication allergy to the agent being used, and hypovolemic shock (Hawkins, 2008).

Nursing management. Assessment of the woman's knowledge level about an epidural block is essential. Before providing information, the nurse determines the woman's current knowledge and evaluates factors related to learning, such as primary language spoken, ability to hear and interpret information, and the presence of anxiety. Although the nurse is an integral person in providing information, the anesthesia provider is the essential person to provide information and to obtain written informed consent.

In preparation for the epidural, the nurse encourages the woman to empty her bladder, because the block may interfere with her ability to void. The nurse assesses the woman's pain level, maternal blood pressure, pulse, respirations, and FHR to determine that normal parameters are present and to establish a baseline. Continuous electronic fetal monitoring to assess fetal status and frequent monitoring of maternal blood pressure and pulse

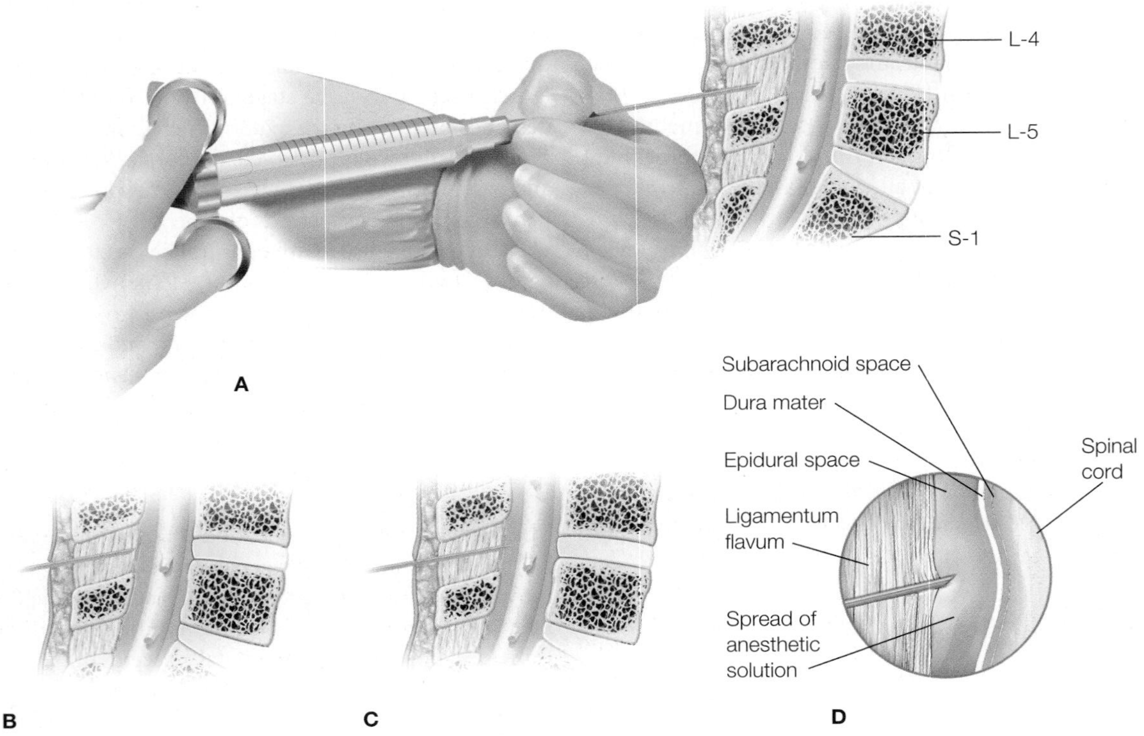

● **Figure 20–3** Technique for lumbar epidural block. ***A,*** Proper position for insertion. ***B,*** Needle in the ligamentum flavum. ***C,*** Tip of needle in epidural space. ***D,*** Force of injection pushing dura away from tip of needle.

Source: Bonica, J. J. (1972). *Principles and practice of obstetric analgesia and anesthesia* (p. 631). Philadelphia: F. A. Davis.

Evidence-Based Nursing

PATIENT-CONTROLLED EPIDURAL ANALGESIA

Clinical Question

What is the most effective use of patient-controlled epidural analgesia during labor?

The Evidence

Two authors conducted a systematic review of the literature to determine the most effective use of patient-controlled epidural analgesia during labor (Halpern & Carvalho, 2009). This represents the strongest level of evidence for practice. Patient-controlled epidural analgesia (PCEA) has demonstrated benefits when compared with continuous epidural infusion, including a lower overall dose of anesthetic and a reduction in the need for clinician intervention. There were no significant differences in fetal or maternal outcomes when PCEA was used versus continuous infusion. Various regimens can produce effective labor analgesia; bolus doses from 4 mL to 12 mL were shown to provide sufficient analgesia and maternal satisfaction. Lockout periods of up to 25 minutes were found to be adequate for pain control, although the longer time periods between doses required larger bolus doses to achieve adequate pain control. Dilute anesthetic solutions with opioids resulted in smaller requirements for anesthesia and less motor block, without compromising analgesia.

Best Practice

PCEA is a reliable and effective method of maintaining epidural analgesia during labor. A wide variety of drugs, dosages, combinations, and settings have been used successfully; there does not appear to be a singular ideal dose or lockout interval setting for PCEA during labor. More dilute solutions are recommended, as they result in less motor block and still provide good pain control.

Critical Thinking

What is the optimal method for customizing PCEA to each mother? Can PCEA be used to maximize the mother's sense of control during labor?

See MyNursingKit for possible responses.

for hypotension are essential. An intravenous infusion is usually begun with an 18-gauge plastic indwelling catheter. A large-gauge catheter is used so that IV fluids can be administered quickly if hypotension occurs. A bolus of 500 to 1000 mL of IV fluid is given before beginning the epidural block to decrease the incidence of hypotension. See "Evidence-Based Nursing" above.

Either of two positions can be used to achieve epidural placement: side-lying or sitting. If the side-lying position is used, the nurse assists the woman to move to the edge of the bed, where the mattress is firmer and provides more support. The woman's head is supported with a small pillow so it remains in alignment with the spine. A pillow may also be placed in front of her chest

Nursing Practice

Advise the woman to identify when uterine contractions are occurring. Reassure her that the anesthesiologist will administer the injection between contractions when she is comfortable. Provide encouragement and reposition the woman as needed after a contraction occurs, since it is common for the woman to slouch during intense uterine contractions.

to provide support for her upper arm. Her back needs to remain straight, with the shoulders square. Her legs are bent and her knees kept together so that the upper hip does not roll forward and cause the spine to twist.

The block may also be given with the woman in a sitting position, with her back flexed and her feet supported on a stool. The woman should be advised to push her back toward the anesthesia provider. The nurse typically stands directly in front of the woman with hands placed on the woman's shoulders. The woman is encouraged to arch her back and push back toward the analgesia provider. After positioning, the nurse continues to provide support and tries to ensure that the woman does not move during the procedure. After the needle and catheter are placed, the woman is assisted into a reclining position.

Maternal vital signs are assessed frequently per protocol until the block wears off. The blood pressure can be monitored by a mechanical blood pressure device or directly by the nurse. The vital signs are recorded on the fetal monitor strip and/or on the client record. The nurse encourages the woman to maintain a side-lying position to maximize uteroplacental blood flow and changes her position (from side to side) frequently to increase circulation, promote comfort, and avoid a one-sided block. The nurse assesses the woman's ability to lift her legs and her level of sensation every 30 minutes to monitor the effects of the nerve block.

The nurse assesses the woman's bladder for distention at frequent intervals because the epidural block decreases the urge to urinate. During the second stage of labor, the woman with an epidural block may need assistance with pushing. The nurse may need to tell the woman when contractions begin and give extra assistance by holding her legs during pushing efforts. The woman's legs need to be protected from pressure applied to them while sensation is diminished. If the woman has little or no control of her legs, stirrups may be needed to avoid injury.

The most common side effect of epidural regional block is hypotension. The risk can be minimized by a preload fluid bolus of crystalloid solution (Segal, 2009). If hypotension occurs, the nurse increases the IV flow rate (to increase intravascular volume and raise the blood pressure), ensures or verifies left uterine displacement (to increase circulation), and administers oxygen (to improve oxygenation). If blood pressure is not restored in 1 to 2 minutes, ephedrine 5 to 10 mg IV, is administered (Segal, 2009). After ephedrine is administered, the blood pressure is continually monitored and the maternal and fetal responses are recorded.

The epidural may cause elevation of maternal temperature (pyrexia). Pyrexia may be confused with maternal infection and frequently results in additional testing of the newborn to rule out infection (Segal, 2009).

Headache (which may occur with spinal blocks) is not a side effect of epidural anesthesia because the dura mater of the spinal canal has not been penetrated and there is no leakage of spinal fluid. Motor control of the legs is weak but not totally absent after birth. Return of complete sensation and the ability to control the legs are essential before ambulation is attempted. Recovery may take several hours, depending on the anesthetic agent and the dose given.

To assess sensation the nurse can touch various parts of the woman's legs and abdomen bilaterally to determine if the touch can be felt. The nurse can evaluate motor control by asking the woman to raise her knees, to lift her feet (one at a time) off the bed, or to dorsiflex her foot. Even though assessments may indicate that sensation and motor control have returned, the nurse needs to be ready to support the woman's weight as she stands and quickly return her to bed if motor control is inadequate. In addition, blood pressure assessments help the nurse determine the safety of ambulation. The nurse assesses blood pressure while the woman is lying down, then sitting in the bed. As long as blood pressure values remain stable (no evidence of orthostatic hypotension), a standing blood pressure is assessed. It is advisable to have additional assistance when the woman stands for the first time, to maintain safety.

CONTINUOUS EPIDURAL INFUSION

MyNursingKit Care Plan Activity: Client with an Epidural

Epidural anesthesia may be given with a continuous infusion pump. Some of the benefits include good to excellent analgesia, infrequent nausea, minimal sedation, decreased anxiety, earlier mobilization, retained cough reflex, decreased risk of deep vein thrombosis, decreased myocardial oxygen demand, and ease of administration. A continuous infusion reduces the use of bolus dosages, which may provide intermittent pain control.

Obviously, ease of administration does not imply lack of need for close observation. Malfunctioning equipment with subsequent overdose is always a possibility. Fortunately, infusion pumps designed specifically for use in epidural anesthesia have safety factors incorporated. Continuous epidural infusions should be administered with the same precautions used for intermittent injections.

Some of the potential problems of epidural infusions include breakthrough pain, sedation, nausea and vomiting, pruritus, and hypotension. Breakthrough pain may occur at any time during the epidural infusion but usually occurs when the infusion rate of the agent is below the recommended therapeutic rate. It may also occur when the infusion pump rate is altered or the integrity of the epidural line is broken. When breakthrough pain occurs, the nurse checks the integrity of the epidural infusion line and notifies the analgesia provider. There may be standing orders for treatment of breakthrough pain, but it is best to inform the analgesia provider of any problems that occur. Often, breakthrough pain can be corrected with a bolus dose of medication. In rare circumstances, the epidural itself may need to be replaced.

Some women may experience *hot spots,* or areas of incomplete anesthesia coverage. Nursing interventions include position changes. If the hot spot becomes too uncomfortable, an anesthesia provider can administer additional medication. In some cases, the epidural will need to be replaced.

General sedation and resulting respiratory depression may occur from the systemic effect of the epidural agents as they are absorbed into the circulation. The respiratory rate, along with the quality of respirations, should be assessed no less frequently than every 15 to 30 minutes. The nurse should notify the anesthetist of any significant decreases in respiratory rate or respiratory pattern change. If respiratory rate decreases below 14 respirations per minute, naloxone may be given to counteract the effect of the anesthetic agent; typically respirations then return to a normal rate.

Nausea and vomiting can occur at any time during or after epidural infusion. The nurse should give an antiemetic if one is ordered and notify the analgesia provider. The nausea and vomiting can make the woman very uncomfortable, and the infusion rate of the epidural may need to be decreased or terminated to alleviate this discomfort. Nausea and vomiting can sometimes occur as a result of transition rather than as a direct side effect of the epidural infusion.

Pruritus (itching and rash) may occur at any time during the epidural infusion. It usually appears first on the face, neck, or torso and is usually the result of the agent in the epidural infusion. Treatment generally involves administration of diphenhydramine hydrochloride (Benadryl). If no standing order exists, the nurse notifies the anesthetist and identifies the problem. The epidural infusion may need to be decreased or terminated.

Hypotension may occur from hypovolemia or from the effect of the epidural. Treatment involves administering oxygen by mask, administering a bolus of crystalloid fluid, and notifying the anesthetist. Usually standing orders for treatment of hypotension are graded in terms of the degree of hypotension. The epidural infusion may have to be terminated and the woman placed in the Trendelenburg position.

EPIDURAL OPIOID ANALGESIA AFTER BIRTH

To provide analgesia for approximately 24 hours after the birth, the analgesia provider may inject an opioid, such as morphine sulfate (Duramorph) or fentanyl (Sublimaze), into the epidural space immediately after the birth. The analgesic effect begins approximately 30 to 60 minutes after the injection. The side effects include pruritus, nausea and vomiting, and urinary retention (Wilson et al., 2010). The onset seems to occur early, and it resolves within 14 to 16 hours after the birth. (See "Drug Guide: Postpartum Epidural Morphine" in Chapter 31∞.)

SPINAL BLOCK

In a **spinal block**, a local anesthetic agent is injected directly into the spinal fluid in the spinal canal to provide anesthesia for cesarean birth and occasionally for vaginal birth. This technique involves passing through the epidural space and dura mater and injecting the medication directly into the cerebral spinal fluid. The technique of administration varies depending on whether the spinal block is being given for a cesarean or vaginal birth (Figure 20–4 ●).

Advantages

The advantages of spinal block are immediate onset of anesthesia, relative ease of administration, a need for smaller medication volume, and maternal compartmentalization of the medication.

Disadvantages

The primary disadvantage of spinal block is blockade of sympathetic nerve fibers, resulting in a high incidence of hypotension; maternal hypotension may lead to alterations in the fetal heart rate and fetal hypoxia. In addition, uterine tone is maintained, which makes intrauterine manipulation difficult.

Contraindications

Contraindications for spinal block include severe hypovolemia, regardless of the cause; central nervous system disease; infection over the puncture site; allergy to local anesthetic agents; coagulation problems; and client refusal (Hawkins, 2008).

Nursing management. If an intravenous infusion is not already in place, it is started with a 16- to 18-gauge plastic catheter. A bolus of 500 to 1000 mL is infused rapidly. The nurse assesses maternal vital signs, pain level, and the FHR to establish a baseline and then positions the woman in a sitting (or a side-lying) posi-

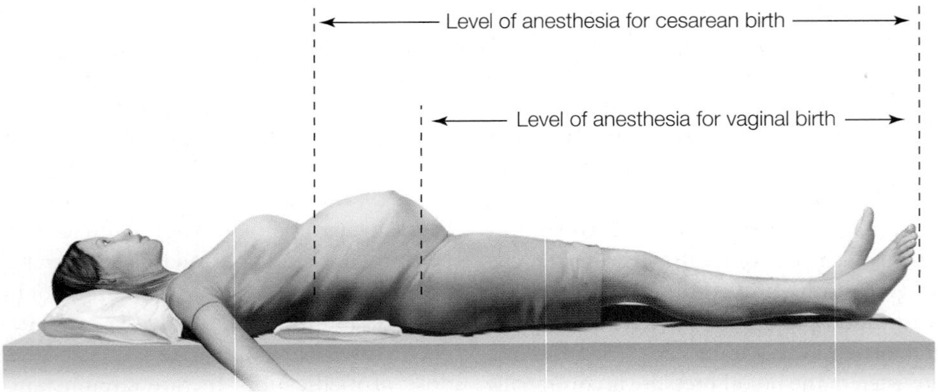

● **Figure 20–4** Levels of spinal anesthesia for vaginal and cesarean births.

Source: Reprinted with permission of Ross Laboratories, Columbus, OH. From Clinical Education Aid No. 17.

tion. The woman sits on the side of the bed or operating room table and places her feet on a stool. The woman places her arms between her knees or up around the nurse's shoulders, places her head to her chest, and arches her back to widen the intervertebral spaces. The nurse supports the woman in this position and palpates the uterus to identify the beginning of uterine contractions (if labor is present). The analgesia provider injects the anesthetic agent between contractions. If the anesthetic agent is injected during a contraction, the level of anesthesia obtained is higher and may compromise respirations.

The woman remains in a sitting position for 30 seconds and then returns to a lying position, with a rolled towel or blanket under her right hip to displace the uterus from the vena cava. The nurse monitors maternal blood pressure and pulse frequently per protocol or physician's order. The blood pressure is also reassessed when the woman is moved after birth, because movement may lower blood pressure.

If the spinal block is being used during vaginal birth, the nurse monitors uterine contractions and instructs the woman to bear down during a contraction. The block may reduce the woman's ability to push, although the new combinations of medications tend to decrease this side effect. Sometimes, the birth may be assisted with forceps or vacuum extractor (see Chapter 23 ∞).

After birth, the temporary motor paralysis of the woman's legs continues. The nurse needs to exercise caution when moving the woman from the birthing bed (or operating room table) to protect her from injury. The woman remains in bed for 6 to 12 hours following the block; she may not regain sensation and control of her bladder for 8 to 12 hours and may need to be catheterized. An indwelling bladder catheter is usually inserted before surgery for women undergoing cesarean birth.

The epidural or spinal catheter is removed by either an analgesia provider or the nurse. The tape used to secure the block is removed. The catheter is then grasped between the fingers and slowly removed with gentle traction. The catheter should be inspected to ensure the tip did not break off. A band-aid or gauze and tape is placed over the site. It is not unusual for a small amount of bleeding to occur initially upon removal. Continuous bleeding warrants a call to the anesthesia provider. The nurse documents removal of the catheter and any adverse effects.

COMBINED SPINAL-EPIDURAL BLOCK

Spinal anesthesia may be combined with an epidural block. The combined spinal-epidural (CSE) block can be used for labor analgesia and for cesarean birth. The anesthetic and analgesic agents used differ according to the purpose of the CSE block. A CSE is accomplished by inserting an epidural needle into the epidural space. A narrow-gauge atraumatic (24- to 27-gauge pencil point) needle is inserted through the epidural needle, through the dura, and into the cerebral spinal fluid. A small amount of local anesthetic agent, opioid, or both is injected, and the atraumatic needle is withdrawn. An epidural catheter is then threaded through the epidural needle and into the epidural space. The epidural needle is removed, and the epidural catheter is secured.

An advantage of CSE block is that the spinal (intrathecal) anesthetic and/or analgesic agent has a faster onset than medications that are injected into the epidural space. Most medications are used in low dose, so spinal analgesia may be given in early labor to assist in alleviating labor pain. The epidural is activated when active labor begins. Another advantage of a CSE block is that laboring women can ambulate after the CSE is placed.

Nursing Practice

Advise women with a CSE in place always to have assistance during ambulation to prevent falls.

PUDENDAL BLOCK

A **pudendal block**, administered by a transvaginal method, intercepts signals to the pudendal nerve (Figure 20–5 ●). The pudendal block provides perineal anesthesia for the latter part of the first stage of labor, the second stage, birth, and episiotomy repair. The pudendal block relieves the pain of perineal distention and typically relieves pain in the lower vagina, vulva, and perineum but not the discomfort of uterine contractions (Hawkins, 2008).

Advantages of the pudendal block are ease of administration and absence of maternal hypotension. It also may be used to decrease the discomfort of low forceps or vacuum-assisted birth. Because a pudendal block does not alter maternal vital signs or

A

B

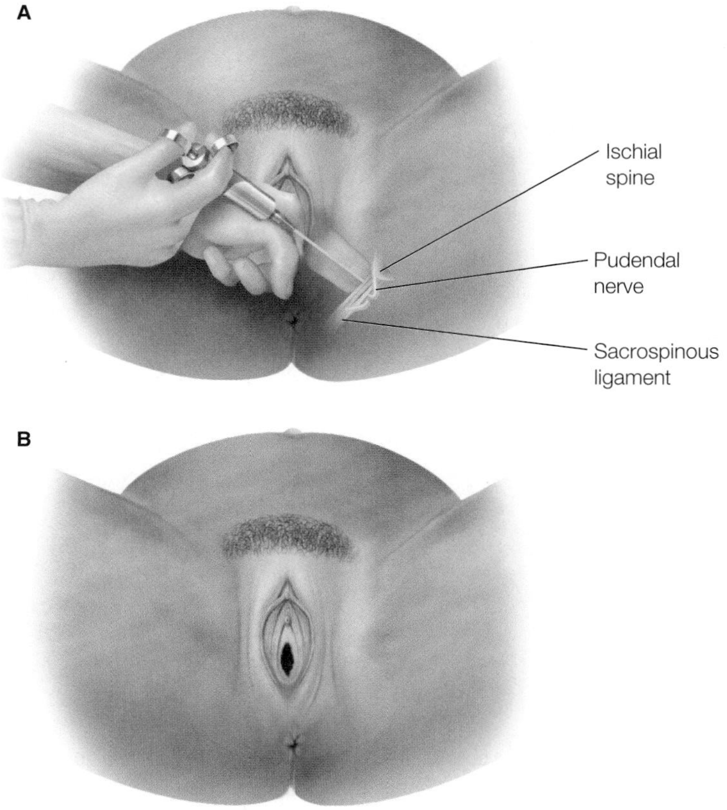

● **Figure 20–5** Pudendal block. ***A,*** Pudendal block by the transvaginal approach. ***B,*** Area of perineum affected by pudendal block.

FHR, additional assessments are not necessary. The nurse explains the procedure and answers any questions.

The disadvantages of the pudendal block include possible broad ligament hematoma, perforation of the rectum, and trauma to the sciatic nerve. A moderate dose of anesthetic agent has minimal ill effects on the course of labor, but the urge to push may decrease.

LOCAL INFILTRATION ANESTHESIA

Local infiltration anesthesia is accomplished by injecting an anesthetic agent into the intracutaneous, subcutaneous, and intramuscular areas of the perineum (Figure 20–6 ●). It is generally used at the time of birth, both in preparation for an episiotomy if one is needed and for the episiotomy repair. Women who have followed some type of prepared childbirth method and want minimal analgesia and anesthesia usually do not object to local anesthesia for the episiotomy or laceration repair. The administration procedure is technically uncomplicated and is practically free from complications.

A disadvantage of local infiltration is that large amounts of local anesthetic must be used to infuse the tissues. Although any local anesthetic may be used, chloroprocaine hydrochloride (Nesacaine), lidocaine hydrochloride (Xylocaine), tetracaine hydrochloride (Pontocaine), and mepivacaine hydrochloride (Carbocaine) are the agents of choice because of their capacity for diffusion. Because local anesthetic agents have no effect on maternal vital signs or FHR, additional assessments are unnecessary.

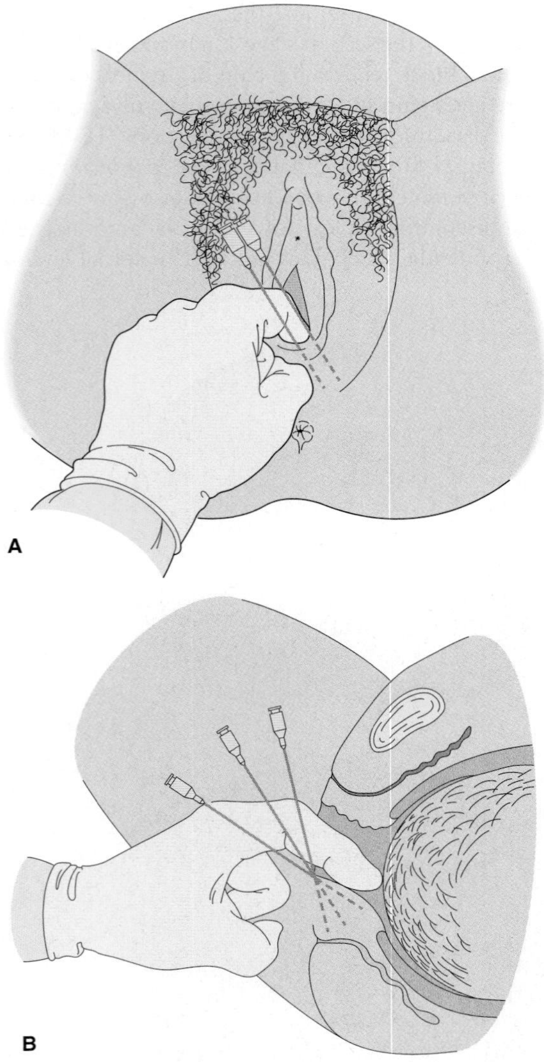

● **Figure 20–6** Local infiltration anesthesia. ***A,*** Technique of local infiltration for episiotomy and repair. ***B,*** Technique of local infiltration showing fan pattern for the fascial planes.

Source: Bonica, J. J. (1972). *Principles and practice of obstetric analgesia and anesthesia* (p. 505). Philadelphia: F. A. Davis.

GENERAL ANESTHESIA

Occasionally, **general anesthesia** (induced unconsciousness) may be needed for cesarean birth. The method used to achieve general anesthesia is usually a combination of intravenous injection and inhalation of anesthetic agents. Maternal complications include: difficulty in maternal intubation resulting in increased incidence of vomiting and aspiration (Munnur & Suresh, 2009), increased blood loss because of uterine relaxation (Gaiser, 2009); and may experience difficulty remembering events in the early postpartum period.

Common fetal complication is fetal depression.The depression in the fetus is directly proportional to the depth and duration of the anesthesia. Infants born to mothers who have received general anesthesia have lower 1 minute Apgar scores than those who are given regional anesthesia for an emergency cesarean birth (Gori, Pasqualucci, Corradetti, et al., 2007). General anesthesia is not advocated when the fetus is considered to be at high risk, particularly in preterm birth.

Nursing management. Because pregnancy results in decreased gastric motility, and the onset of labor halts the process almost entirely, food eaten hours earlier may remain undigested in the stomach. The nurse must find out when the laboring woman last ate and record this information on the client's chart and on her anesthesia record. Even when food and fluids have been withheld, the gastric juice produced during fasting is highly acidic and can cause chemical pneumonitis if aspirated. Prophylactic antacid therapy to reduce the acidic content of the stomach before general anesthesia is common

Nursing Practice

Some women may wake from general anesthesia with an awareness of events that occurred during a cesarean birth. A small number of women experience unpleasant thoughts or nightmares as a result. If a woman expresses anxiety or states she has unpleasant memories of the birth, the nurse should encourage her to discuss her feelings and the experiences she remembers. The analgesia provider and physician should be notified so they can establish a therapeutic dialogue with the woman. Some women may have to be referred for counseling to prevent or treat posttraumatic stress disorder.

practice. A nonparticulate antacid (such as bicitra); H2-receptor antagonists (such as Cimetidine [Tagamet] or Famotidine); or the use of prokinetic medications (such as metoclopramide), may also help empty gastric contents.

Before induction of anesthesia, the nurse places a wedge under the woman's right hip to displace the uterus and prevent vena caval compression in the supine position. The woman should also be preoxygenated with 3 to 5 minutes of 100% oxygen. Intravenous fluids are started so that access to the intravascular system is immediately available. During the preparation, the woman should be counseled on what to expect and should be told that the baby will have limited exposure to the anesthesia agents.

During the process of rapid induction of anesthesia, the nurse applies cricoid pressure to occlude the esophagus and prevent possible aspiration; the esophagus is occluded by applying 1 to 2 kg before the loss of consciousness and increasing that to 2 to 4 kg after the induction of anesthesia. The amount of pressure applied is critical because too much pressure can result in difficulty in performing a successful intubation. Too little pressure can result in aspiration. Cricoid pressure is maintained until the anesthesia provider has placed the endotracheal tube and indicates that the pressure can be released. Figure 20–7 ● shows the appropriate technique.

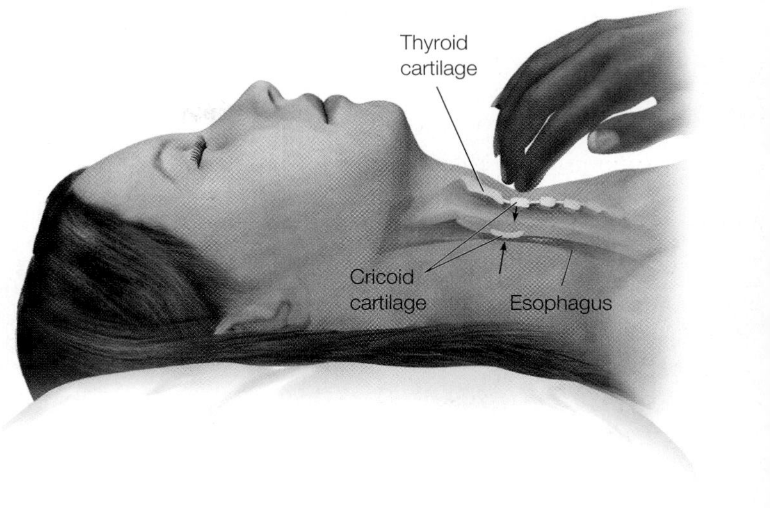

● **Figure 20–7** Cricoid pressure technique. Proper position for fingers in applying cricoid pressure until a cuffed endotracheal tube is placed by the analgesia provider or certified nurse-anesthetist. The cricoid cartilage is depressed 2 to 3 cm posteriorly so that the esophagus is occluded.

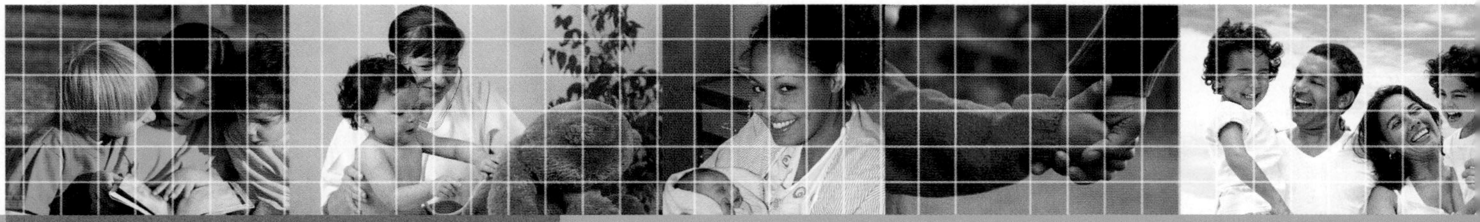

CRITICAL CONCEPT REVIEW

LEARNING OUTCOMES	CONCEPTS
20.1 Describe the use, administration, dose, onset of action, and adverse effects of systemic drugs to promote pain relief during the nursing care management of the woman in labor and her fetus.	1. The goal is to provide maximum pain relief with minimum risk to the mother and fetus. 2. After complete assessment, an analgesia agent is generally administered when cervical change has occurred. 3. Drugs may cause fetal respiratory depression at birth if given too late in labor. 4. Maternal and fetal vital signs must be stable before systemic drugs may be administered. 5. Naloxone (Narcan) should be available at birth to treat respiratory depression in the newborn.
20.2 Compare the major types of regional analgesia and anesthesia, including area affected, advantages, disadvantages, techniques, and nursing care management of the laboring woman and her fetus.	1. Epidural: ■ Injection of anesthetic agent into the epidural space. ■ Produces little or no feeling to the area from the uterus downward. ■ Pushing during second stage of labor may be impaired due to lack of sensation. ■ Hypotension is the most common side effect. ■ May preload with crystalloid solution bolus. ■ Woman may need urinary catheterization due to the loss of bladder sensation. ■ Assess sensation, motor control, and orthostatic blood pressure. 2. Continuous epidural analgesia: ■ Provides good analgesia. ■ Produces less nausea and provides a greater ability to cough. ■ May produce breakthrough pain, sedation, and respiratory depression. ■ Itching and hypotension are side effects.

(continued)

LEARNING OUTCOMES	CONCEPTS
	3. Spinal block: ■ A local anesthetic agent is injected directly into spinal canal. The level of anesthesia is dependent upon level of administration. May be administered higher for cesarean birth or lower for vaginal birth. ■ The onset of anesthesia is immediate. ■ Side effects include maternal hypotension, which can lead to fetal hypoxia. ■ Requires frequent blood pressure monitoring with changes in position. ■ Indwelling urinary catheter is usually needed due to decreased bladder sensation and tone. ■ Woman's legs must be protected from injury for 8 to 12 hours after birth of baby due to decreased movement and sensation. 4. Pudendal block: ■ Local anesthesia is injected directly into the pudendal nerve, which produces anesthesia to the lower vagina, vulva, and perineum. ■ Produces pain relief only at the end of labor. ■ Has no effect on fetus or the progress of labor. ■ May cause hematoma, perforation of the rectum, or trauma to the sciatic nerve. 5. Local infiltration anesthesia: ■ Local anesthesia is injected into the perineum prior to an episiotomy. ■ Provides pain relief only for the episiotomy incision. ■ There is no effect on maternal or fetal vital signs. ■ Requires large amounts of local anesthetic agents.
20.3 Explain the possible complications of regional anesthesia in nursing care management of the laboring woman and her fetus.	Regional anesthesia administered per spinal or epidural route has similar possible complications: 1. Maternal hypotension. 2. Bladder distention. 3. Inability to push during second stage of labor. 4. Severe headache with spinal anesthesia. 5. Elevated temperature with epidural anesthesia. 6. Possible neurologic damage.
20.4 Describe the nursing care management for the laboring woman and her fetus related to general anesthesia.	The nurse should: 1. Assess when the mother ate or drank last. 2. Administer prescribed premedications such as an antacid. 3. Place a wedge under the mother's right hip to displace the uterus and prevent vena cava compression. 4. Provide oxygen prior to the start of the surgery. 5. Ensure that IV access is established. 6. Assist the anesthesiologist by applying cricoid pressure during the placement of the endotracheal tube.
20.5 Describe the major complications of general anesthesia during labor in nursing care management of the woman in labor and her fetus.	Major complications of general anesthesia are: 1. Fetal depression. 2. Uterine relaxation. 3. Vomiting. 4. Aspiration.

CRITICAL THINKING IN ACTION

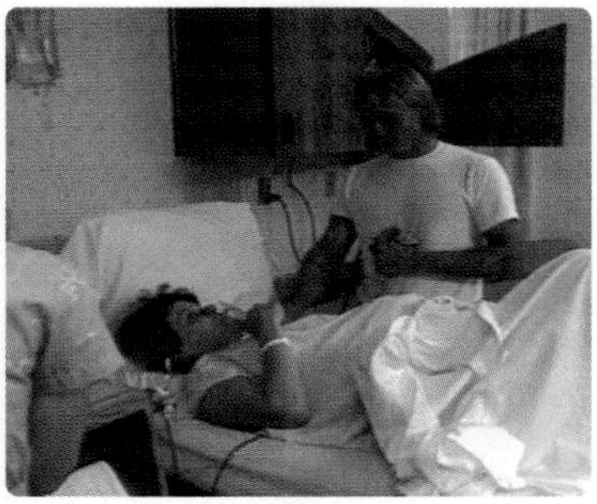

Sandra, a 26-year-old G1 P0000, is in active labor when she presents to you at the birthing center. She has been in labor for 5 hours and is clearly tired and seems to be having difficulty coping with the pain. Her contractions are occurring every 2 to 4 minutes lasting 50 to 60 seconds, and are moderate to strong in intensity. You assess the fetal heart rate of 120 to 130 with early decelerations; moderate long-term variability is present. Sandra's vital signs are stable and her laboratory results are within normal limits. She is requesting an epidural analgesia for pain control. A vaginal exam demonstrates the cervix is 100% effaced, 6 cm dilated with the vertex at 0 station in the LOT position. You notify the physician of Sandra's wish for pain relief and labor progress. You review the client's record for written consent for regional analgesia and assist the anesthesiologist with the procedure.

1. Discuss the advantages of regional analgesia.
2. Describe the nursing responsibility during the administration of regional analgesia.
3. Discuss the side effects of regional analgesia.
4. What are the absolute contraindications for an epidural block?
5. How do you assist Sandra with the second stage of labor when she cannot feel her contractions?

See MyNursingKit for possible responses.

REFERENCES

American College of Obstetricians and Gynecologists [ACOG]. (2006). ACOG committee opinion. No. 339: Analgesia and cesarean delivery rates. *Obstetrics & Gynecology, 107*(6), 1487–1488.

Chung, U. L., Hung, L. C., Kuo, S. C., & Huang, C. L. (2003). Effects of L14 and BL 67 acupressure on labor pain and uterine contractions in the first stage of labor. *Journal of Nursing Research, 11*(4), 251–260.

Fitzgerald, M. P., Weber, A. M., Howden, N., Cundiff, G. W., Brown, M. B., and Pelvic Floor Disorders Network. (2007). Risk factors for anal sphincter tear during vaginal delivery. *Obstetrics & Gynecology, 109*(1), 29–34.

Gaiser, R. (2009). Anesthesia for cesarean delivery. In B. A. Bucklin, D. R. Gambling, & D. Wlody (Eds.). *A practical approach to obstetric antesthesia* (pp. 185–207). Philadelphia: Lippincott Williams & Wilkins.

Gori, F., Pasqualucci, A., Corradetti, F., Milli, M., & Peduto, V. A. (2007). Maternal and neonatal outcome after cesarean section: The impact of anesthesia. *Journal of Maternal Fetal Neonatal Medicine, 20*(1), 53–57.

Halpern, S., & Carvalho, B. (2009). Patient controlled epidural analgesia for labor. *Anesthesia and Analgesia, 108*(3), 921–928.

Hawkins, J. L. (2008). Obstetric analgesia and anesthesia. In R. S. Gibbs, B. Y. Karlan, A. F. Haney, & I. E. Nygaard (Eds.). *Dansforth's obstetrics and gynecology* (10th ed., pp. 43–60). Philadelphia: Lippincott Williams & Wilkins.

Hawkins, J. L., Goetzl, L., & Chestnut, D. H. (2007). Obstetric anesthesia. In S. G. Gabbe, J. R. Niebyl, & J. L. Simpson (Eds.). *Obstetrics: Normal and problem pregnancies* (5th ed., pp. 396–427). Philadelphia: Churchill Livingstone.

Martin, J. A., & Menacker, F. (2007). Expanded health data from the new birth certificate, 2004. *National Vital Statistics Report, 55*(12), 1–23.

Munnur, U., & Suresh, M. S. (2009). Difficult airway management in the pregnant patient. In B. A. Bucklin, D. R. Gambling, & D. Wlody (Eds.). *A practical approach to obstetric antesthesia* (pp. 209–222). Philadelphia: Lippincott Williams & Wilkins.

Musselwhite, K. L., Faris, P., Moore, K., Berci, D., & King, K. M. (2007). Use of epidural anesthesia and the risk of acute postpartum urinary retention. *American Journal of Obstetrics & Gynecology, 196*(5), 472.e 1–5.

Nelson, K. E., & Eisenach, J. C. (2005). Intravenous butorphanol, meperidine, and their combination relieve pain and distress in women in labor. *Anesthesiology, 102*(5), 1008–1013.

O'Sullivan, G. (2009). Non-neuraxial analgesic techniques. In B. A. Bucklin, D. R. Gambling, & D. Wlody (Eds.). *A practical approach to obstetric antesthesia* (pp. 131–142). Philadelphia: Lippincott Williams & Wilkins.

Segal, S. (2009). Choice of neuraxial analgesia and local anesthetics. In B. A. Bucklin, D. R. Gambling, & D. Wlody (Eds.). *A practical approach to obstetric antesthesia* (pp. 143–168). Philadelphia: Lippincott Williams & Wilkins.

Sheiner, E., Walfisch, A., Hallak, M., Harlev, S., Mazor, M., & Shoham-Vardi, I. (2006). Length of the second stage of labor as a predictor of perineal outcome after vaginal delivery. *Journal of Reproductive Medicine, 51*(2), 115–119.

Vasudevan, A., Snowman, C. E., Sundar, S., Sarge, T. W., & Hess, P. E. (2007). Intrathecal morphine reduces breakthrough pain during labour epidural analgesia. *British Journal of Anaesthia, 98*(2), 241–245. Epub 2007, Jan 8.

Wilson, B. A., Shannon, M. T., & Shields, K. L., (Eds.). (2010). *Nurse's drug guide: 2010.* Upper Saddle River, NJ: Prentice Hall.

PEARSON

EXPLORE mynursingkit™

MyNursingKit is your one stop for online chapter review materials and resources. Prepare for success with additional NCLEX®-style practice questions, interactive assignments and activities, web links, animations and videos, and more!

Register your access code from the front of your book at **www.mynursingkit.com**

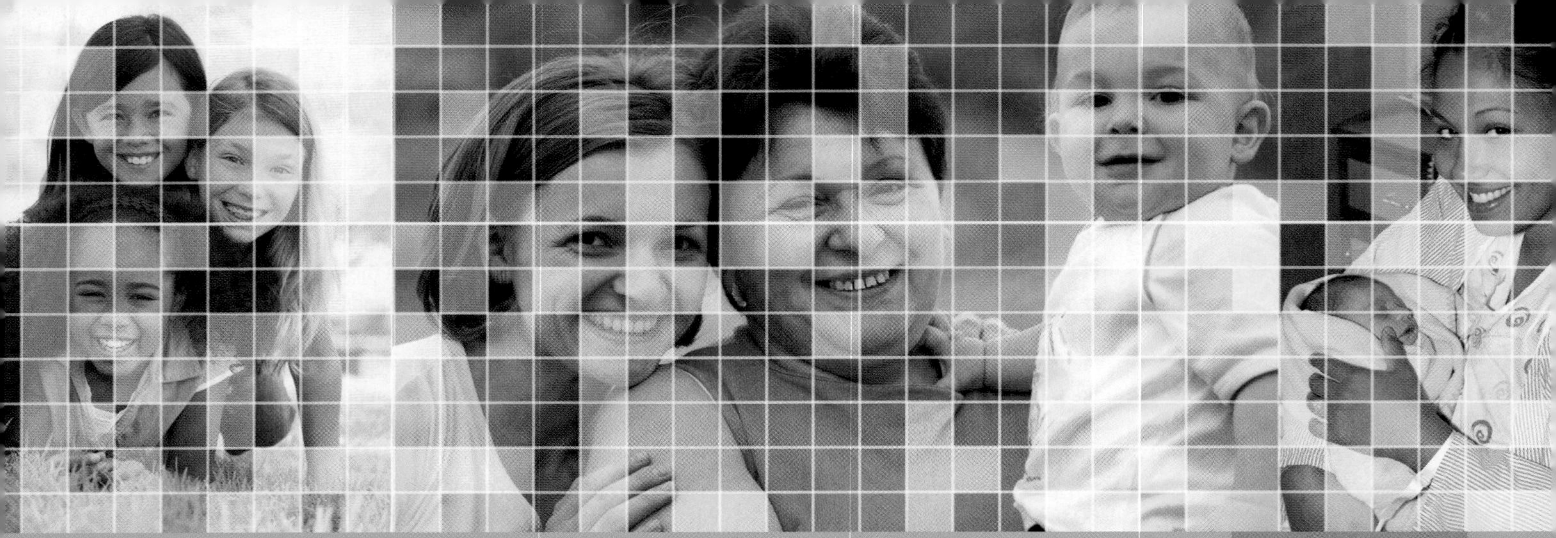

CHAPTER 21

Childbirth at Risk: Prelabor Complications

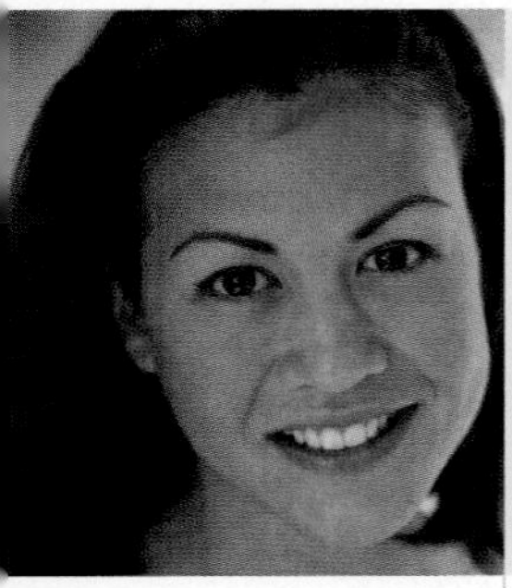

When I learned that we were going to have twins I was stunned. How would we ever manage? Our daughters were born 2 weeks early but both weighed over 5 pounds and did well. The early days were far from easy, especially breastfeeding. I was always tired and it seemed that at least one of the girls was always awake. But they shared a room and after a while they got on the same schedule. That made things easier. They are 2 years old now and such amazing little people. Marcel and I feel that we are blessed with double joy! —Monique, 31

LEARNING OUTCOMES

21.1 Explain the possible causes, risk factors, and clinical therapy for premature rupture of the membranes or preterm labor in determining the nursing care management of the woman and her fetus-newborn.

21.2 Compare placenta previa and abruptio placenta, including implications for the mother and fetus, as well as nursing care.

21.3 Explain the maternal and fetal-neonatal implications and the clinical therapy in determining the nursing care management of the woman with multiple gestation.

21.4 Compare the identification, maternal and fetal-neonatal implications, clinical therapy, and nursing care management of the woman with hydramnios and oligohydramnios.

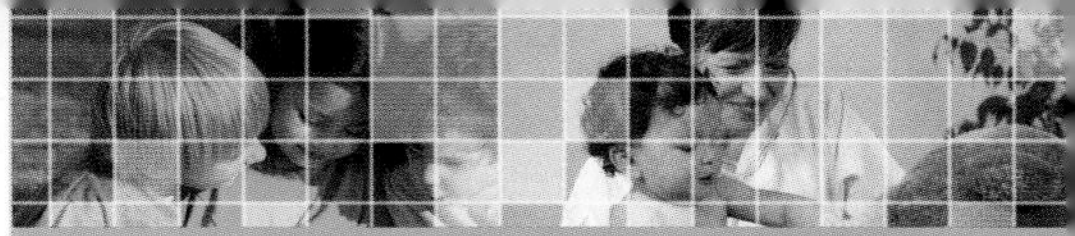

KEY TERMS

Abruptio placentae, 466

Hydramnios, 473

Oligohydramnios, 473

Placenta previa, 464

Premature rupture of membranes (PROM), 457

Preterm labor (PTL), 459

Tocolysis, 461

After the first trimester, the majority of pregnancies progress smoothly to term. In some cases, however, complications can occur before the onset of labor that significantly impact the outcome of pregnancy. This chapter presents content related to the most common of these conditions. It also serves as a prelude to the complications discussed in Chapter 22.

CARE OF THE WOMAN WITH PREMATURE RUPTURE OF MEMBRANES

Premature rupture of membranes (PROM) is spontaneous rupture of the membranes before the onset of labor. PROM affects approximately 5% to 10% of all pregnancies. *Preterm PROM (PPROM),* which affects approximately 3% of all pregnancies, is the rupture of membranes occurring before 37 weeks' gestation (Mercer, 2007). Although the exact cause is unknown, PPROM is associated with infection, previous history of PPROM, hydramnios, multiple pregnancy, urinary tract infection (UTI), amniocentesis, placenta previa, abruptio placentae, trauma, incompetent cervix, history of laser conization or LEEP procedure, bleeding during pregnancy, and maternal genital tract anomalies.

Maternal risk is related to infection, specifically *chorioamnionitis* (intra-amniotic infection resulting from bacterial invasion before birth) and *endometritis* (postpartal infection of the endometrium). In addition, abruptio placentae occurs more frequently in women with PROM. Other rare complications include retained placenta and hemorrhage, maternal sepsis, and maternal death.

Fetal-newborn implications include risk of respiratory distress syndrome (with PPROM), fetal sepsis caused by ascending pathogens, malpresentation, prolapse of the umbilical cord, nonreassuring fetal heart rate tracings, compression of the umbilical cord related to oligohydramnios, premature birth, and increased perinatal morbidity and mortality. PROM that occurs at term is associated with favorable outcomes. Gestations from 32 to 36 weeks generally have favorable outcomes although there may be some complications caused by prematurity. In general, infants born before 32 weeks have some complications, including respiratory distress syndrome (RDS), necrotizing enterocolitis, intraventricular hemorrhage, and sepsis. The earlier the gestational age, the greater the likelihood of infant complications (Mercer, 2007).

CLINICAL THERAPY

A sterile speculum examination is done to detect the presence of amniotic fluid in the vagina. If fluid is not obviously pooling, information can be gained by using nitrazine paper, which turns deep blue when amniotic fluid is present. Because certain bacterial pathogens can also result in a positive nitrazine test, a microscopic examination (ferning test) should be used as a confirmation of rupture. It is considered a definitive test. Digital examination increases the risk of infection and is not recommended until a management plan has been determined.

Fetal well-being is assessed through a fetal heart rate tracing or biophysical profile. In addition, the gestational age of the fetus is calculated to develop a management plan. The gestational age of the fetus and the presence or absence of infection determine the direction of treatment for PROM. If maternal signs and symptoms of infection are evident, antibiotic therapy (usually by intravenous infusion) is begun immediately, and the fetus is born vaginally or by cesarean regardless of the gestational age. Prophylactic antibiotics are often administered for the first 48 hours while awaiting culture results. Upon admission to the nursery, the newborn is assessed for sepsis and placed on antibiotics. (Chapter 29 provides further information about the newborn with sepsis.)

Management of PROM in the absence of infection and gestation of less than 37 weeks is usually conservative. The woman is hospitalized on bed rest. On admission, complete blood cell count (CBC), C-reactive protein, and urinalysis are obtained, as are cultures, including chlamydia, gonorrhea, and group B streptococcus. An ultrasound is done to determine gestational age, amniotic fluid level, and fetal well-being. Continuous electronic fetal monitoring may be ordered at the beginning of treatment but usually is discontinued after a few hours, unless the fetus is estimated to be very low birth weight (VLBW) or if the tracing is of concern. Regular nonstress tests (NSTs) or biophysical profiles are used to monitor fetal well-being. (These tests are discussed in Chapter 14.) Maternal blood pressure, pulse, temperature, and fetal heart rate (FHR) are assessed every 4 hours. Regular laboratory evaluations are done to detect maternal infection. Vaginal exams are avoided to decrease the chance of infection. As the gestation approaches 34 weeks, fetal lung maturity studies are indicated (see Chapter 14).

Maternal corticosteroid administration promotes fetal lung maturity and helps to prevent respiratory distress syndrome and other complications. Currently a single course of corticosteroids is recommended (see "Drug Guide: Betamethasone"). Repeat courses of corticosteroids should not be routinely used because they have not been shown to improve neonatal outcomes and are associated with an increased incidence of chorioamnionitis (Gibbs, 2008). Research has not yet determined whether a repeat dose at 30 to 32 weeks may help stimulate alveoli that were not formed when the initial dose was given (Mercer, 2007).

NURSING MANAGEMENT

NURSING ASSESSMENT AND DIAGNOSIS

Determining the duration of the rupture of the membranes is a significant component of the intrapartal assessment. Ask the woman when her membranes ruptured and when labor began, because the risk of infection is related to the time involved. De-

Drug Guide

BETAMETHASONE (CELESTONE SOLUSPAN)

Overview of Maternal-Fetal Action

Studies have provided ample evidence that glucocorticoids such as betamethasone are capable of inducing pulmonary maturation and decreasing the incidence of respiratory distress syndrome in preterm infants. The mechanism by which corticosteroids accelerate fetal lung maturity is unclear, but it is related to the stimulation of enzyme activity by the drug. The enzyme is required for biosynthesis of surfactant by the type II pneumocytes. Surfactant is of major importance to the proper functioning of the lung in that it decreases the surface tension of the alveoli. Glucocorticoids also increase the rate of glycogen depletion, which leads to thinning of the interalveolar septa and increases the size of the alveoli. The thinning of the epithelium brings the capillaries into closer proximity with the air spaces and improves oxygen exchange.

Route, Dosage, Frequency

Prenatal maternal intramuscular injections of 12 mg of betamethasone are given once a day for 2 days. Dexamethasone has also been given in doses of 6 mg every 12 hours for four doses (Iams & Romero, 2007). To obtain maximum results, birth should be delayed for at least 24 hours after completing the first round of treatment. The effect of corticosteroids may be transient. Repeat courses of corticosteroids should not be used routinely (Gibbs, 2008).

Contraindications

Inability to delay birth

Adequate L/S ratio

Presence of a condition that necessitates immediate birth (e.g., maternal bleeding)

Presence of maternal infection, diabetes mellitus (relative contraindication)

Gestational age greater than 34 completed weeks

Maternal Side Effects

Increased risk for infection has not been supported in large studies. There may, however, be some increase in the incidence of infection in women with premature rupture of the membranes. Maternal hyperglycemia may occur during corticosteroid administration. Insulin-dependent diabetics may require insulin infusions for several days to prevent ketoacidosis. Corticosteroids possibly may increase the risk of pulmonary edema, especially when used concurrently with tocolytics (Briggs, Freeman, & Yaffee, 2005).

Effects on Fetus/Newborn

Lowered cortisol levels at birth, but rebound occurs by 2 hours of age.

Hypoglycemia

Increased risk of neonatal sepsis

Animal studies have shown serious fetal side effects such as reduced head circumference and decreased placental weight. Human studies have not shown these effects, however (Briggs et al., 2005).

Nursing Considerations

- Assess for presence of contraindications.
- Provide education regarding possible side effects.
- Administer betamethasone deep into gluteal muscle, avoiding injection into deltoid (high incidence of local atrophy). (Dexamethasone may be administered IM or IV.)
- Periodically evaluate BP, pulse, weight, and edema.
- Assess lab data for electrolytes and blood glucose.
- Although concomitant use of betamethasone and tocolytic agents has been implicated in increased risk of pulmonary edema, the betamethasone has little mineral corticoid activity; therefore, it probably doesn't add significantly to the salt and water retention effects of beta-adrenergic agonists. Other causes of noncardiogenic pulmonary edema should also be investigated if pulmonary edema develops during administration of betamethasone to a woman in preterm labor.

termine gestational age to prepare for the possibility of a preterm birth. Observe the mother for signs and symptoms of infection, especially by reviewing her white blood cell (WBC) count, temperature, pulse rate, and the character of her amniotic fluid. If the mother has a fever, check hydration status. When a preterm or cesarean birth is anticipated, evaluate the childbirth preparation and coping abilities of the woman and her partner.

Nursing diagnoses that may apply to a woman with PROM include the following:

- *Risk for Infection* related to premature rupture of membranes
- *Impaired Gas Exchange* in the fetus related to compression of the umbilical cord secondary to prolapse of the cord
- *Risk for Ineffective Individual Coping* related to unknown outcome of the pregnancy

PLANNING AND IMPLEMENTATION

Nursing actions should focus on the woman, her partner, and the fetus. Monitor for and report signs of infection to the certified nurse-midwife or physician. Evaluate uterine activity and fetal response to the labor, but vaginal exams are not done unless absolutely necessary because this increases the risk of infection. Encourage the woman to rest on her left side to promote optimal uteroplacental perfusion. Use comfort measures to help promote rest and relaxation. Also ensure that hydration is maintained, particularly if the woman's temperature is elevated.

Education is another important aspect of nursing care. The woman and her partner, if he is involved, need to understand the implications of PROM and all treatment methods. It is important to address side effects and alternative treatments. The couple needs to know that although the membranes are ruptured, amniotic fluid continues to be produced.

Providing psychologic support for the couple is critical. Help reduce anxiety by listening empathetically, relaying accurate information, and providing explanations of procedures. Preparing the couple for a cesarean birth, a preterm newborn, and the possibility of fetal or newborn demise may be necessary. Consultation with the neonatologist or pediatric provider can give the woman and her partner an opportunity to ask questions if a preterm birth is anticipated.

Teaching Highlights

EXPLAINING AMNIOTIC MEMBRANES

To help a laboring woman and her family understand how the amniotic membranes provide protection, use a color chart that shows a side view of the fetus in the uterus with the membranes intact. Ask the couple to visualize what would happen if the membranes rupture. They will be able to see that pathogens have direct access to the uterus, increasing the risk of infection. They will also see that, when the membranes rupture and the fluid escapes, the cord could "wash out" with the fluid and become trapped between the pelvis and fetal head, causing cord compression.

EVALUATION

Expected outcomes of nursing care include the following:

- The woman's risk of infection and of cord prolapse decrease.
- The couple is able to discuss the implications of PROM and all treatments and alternative treatments.
- The couple verbalizes understanding that they did not cause the event.
- The pregnancy is maintained without trauma to the mother or fetus.

CARE OF THE WOMAN AT RISK BECAUSE OF PRETERM LABOR

Labor that occurs between 20 and 36 completed weeks of pregnancy is called **preterm labor (PTL)**. Prematurity continues to be the number one perinatal and neonatal problem in the United States, with 12.7% of all live births occurring prematurely. In fact, the incidence of premature birth has risen by more than 20% since 1990 (March of Dimes, 2007). Often PTL is related to multiple risk factors; only rarely is there a single cause. Table 21–1 presents a list of risk factors for spontaneous preterm labor.

Maternal implications of PTL include psychologic stress related to the baby's condition and physiologic stress related to medical treatment for preterm labor.

Fetal-neonatal implications include increased morbidity and mortality, especially caused by respiratory distress syndrome (RDS), increased risk of trauma during birth, and maturational deficiencies (fat storage, heat regulation, immaturity of organ systems).

CLINICAL THERAPY

Women who are at risk for PTL are taught to recognize its symptoms and, if any symptoms are present, to notify their certified nurse-midwife or physician immediately. Prompt diagnosis is necessary to stop preterm labor before it progresses to the point where intervention is ineffective.

Prompt diagnosis of PTL is often difficult because many of the symptoms are common in normal pregnancy. The strongest predictors of preterm birth include the following: cervicovaginal fibronectin, abnormal cervical length on ultrasound, history of previous preterm birth, and the presence of infection (Iams & Romero, 2007).

Fetal fibronectin (fFN) is a protein normally found in the fetal membranes and decidua. It is in the cervicovaginal fluid in early pregnancy but is not usually present in significant quantities between 22 and 37 weeks' gestation (Ness, Visintine, Ricci, et al., 2007). A positive fFN test (fFN found in the cervicovaginal fluid) during this time puts the woman at increased risk for preterm birth. Conversely, a negative fFN in a woman with preterm contractions is associated with a very low risk of birth within 7 to 14 days (Ness et al., 2007). The test is over 99% accurate for predicting no preterm birth within 7 days. The procedure

Table 21–1 Risk Factors for Spontaneous Preterm Labor

Multiple gestation	Cervical shortening / 1 cm
DES exposure	Uterine irritability
Known cervical incompetence	Age (less than 17 or over 35)
Hydramnios	Low socioeconomic status
Uterine anomaly	Cigarettes—more than 10/day
Cervix dilated / 1 cm at 32 weeks	Substance abuse
Second-trimester abortion	Low maternal weight
Fetal abnormality	Poor weight gain
Febrile illness	More than two first-trimester abortions
Bleeding after 12 weeks	Non-white race
History of pyelonephritis or other maternal infection	Cervical cerclage in situ
Diabetes	In vitro fertilization (singleton or multiple gestation)
Previous preterm birth	STI (trichomoniasis, chlamydia)
Previous preterm labor with term birth	Anemia
Abdominal surgery during second or third trimester	Abdominal trauma
History of cone biopsy	Foreign body (IUD)
Uteroplacental ischemia	Bacterial vaginosis, *E. coli* (ascending intrauterine infection)
Stress	Periodontal disease
Inadequate or no prenatal care	Domestic violence
Lack of social support	Long work hours with prolonged standing
Hypertension (preeclampsia, gestational hypertension, chronic hypertension)	Clotting disorders
Obesity	Interval of less than 6 to 9 months between pregnancies

for collecting a sample is similar to that of the Pap smear; results can be available within 1 hour.

The length of the cervix can be measured fairly reliably after 16 weeks' gestation using an ultrasound probe inserted into the vagina. A cervix that is shorter than expected may help a physician to identify a woman at increased risk for PTL. In such cases, research indicates that vaginal progesterone gel can be used prophylactically to increase gestational age (Ross, 2009). Some clinicians consider that a shorter-than-anticipated cervix reveals the need for a cerclage to prevent preterm birth because of incompetent cervix (Iams & Romero, 2007). However, opinion varies as to the value of cerclage as compared with expectant management (Carey & Gibbs, 2008).

Diagnosis of preterm labor is confirmed if the pregnancy is between 20 and 37 weeks, there are documented uterine contractions (four in 20 minutes or eight in 1 hour), and documented cervical change or cervical dilatation of greater than 1 cm (0.4 in.) or cervical effacement of 80% or more.

Labor is not interrupted if one or more of the following conditions are present: severe preeclampsia or eclampsia, chorioamnionitis, hemorrhage, maternal cardiac disease, poorly controlled diabetes mellitus or thyrotoxicosis, severe abruptio placentae, fetal anomalies incompatible with life, fetal death, nonreassuring fetal status, or fetal maturity.

Evidence in Action

Progesterone therapy should be offered to women with a history of spontaneous preterm labor for the prevention of preterm birth (Systematic review of latest research) (Da Fonseca, Bittar, Damião, et al., 2009).

The goal of clinical therapy is to prevent preterm labor from advancing to the point that it no longer responds to medical treatment. The initial management is directed toward maintaining good uterine blood flow, detecting uterine contractions, and ensuring that the fetus is stable. The mother is asked to lie on her side to increase placental profusion, an IV infusion is started to promote maternal hydration, and maternal laboratory studies including CBC, C-reactive protein, vaginal cultures, fetal fi-

Evidence-Based Nursing

PRENATAL SCREENING AND TREATMENT OF LOWER GENITAL TRACT INFECTIONS

Clinical Question

Can antenatal genital tract infection screening and treatment programs reduce preterm birth and its associated morbidities?

The Evidence

A lower genital tract infection can cross into the amniotic fluid prenatally and cause rupture of the membranes. This may happen before 37 weeks of gestation and so cause a preterm birth. Two reviewers appraised research studies that focused on antenatal lower genital tract infection screening and treatment. While only one study met the preset quality criteria, it had a large sample size (n = 4155) and was of high methodological quality; as such it represents strong evidence for practice.

More than 2000 women were screened in early pregnancy for bacterial vaginosis, trichomonas vaginalis, and candidiasis. When the presence of these infectious agents was detected, the mothers were treated. The rate of preterm birth (before 37 weeks' gestation) of these women was compared with women who did not receive routine screening and treatment for these conditions. The women in the screening/ intervention group had significantly lower rates of preterm birth. The intervention group also had significantly lower rates of low birth weight (less than 2500 g) and very low birth weight (less than 1500 g) babies. No adverse effects from the treatment were reported for either mother or baby (Sangkomkamhang, Lumbiganon, Prasertcharoensook, and Laopaiboon, 2008).

Best Practice

A simple infection screening and treatment program during routine antenatal care may reduce the rate of preterm births, low birth weight, and very low birth weight neonates. The reduction in risk was from 5% in the group that did not receive screening and treatment to 3% in the group that did.

Critical Thinking

Are there other antenatal genital tract infections that could generate similar results if treated early in pregnancy?

See MyNursingKit for possible responses.

bronectin (fFN), and urine culture are completed. An ultrasound may be obtained to determine cervical shortening or funneling, as well as assess fetal well-being.

Tocolysis is the use of medications in an attempt to stop labor. Drugs currently used as tocolytics include the β-adrenergic agonists (also called β-mimetics), cyclooxygenase (prostaglandin synthetase) inhibitors, and calcium channel blockers such as nifedipine (Procardia). The β-mimetics terbutaline sulfate (Brethine) and magnesium sulfate are the most widely used tocolytics.

Although tocolytic drugs suppress uterine contractions and allow pregnancy to continue, they may cause maternal side effects; the most serious is maternal pulmonary edema. Reducing the dose and duration of therapy sometimes reduces the side effects.

The selection of magnesium sulfate, calcium channel blockers, or β-mimetics also depends on the experience of the healthcare providers. For magnesium sulfate, the recommended loading dose is 4 g IV in 100 mL of IV fluid using an infusion pump over 30 minutes, followed by a maintenance dose of 1 to 4 g/hr titrated to response and side effects (Iams & Romero, 2007). The therapy is continued for 12 hours after uterine contractions have stopped.

Side effects with the loading dose may include flushing, a feeling of warmth, headache, nystagmus, nausea, and dizziness. Other side effects include lethargy, sluggishness, and pulmonary edema (see "Drug Guide: Magnesium Sulfate"). Fetal side effects may include hypotonia and lethargy that persists for 1 or 2 days following birth. Respiratory depression in the newborn can also occur (Iams & Romero, 2007).

One calcium channel blocker, nifedipine (Procardia), is becoming increasingly popular in treating preterm labor because it is easily administered orally or sublingually and has few serious maternal side effects. It decreases smooth muscle contractions by blocking the slow calcium channels at the cell surface. The most common side effects are related to arterial vasodilation and include hypotension, tachycardia, facial flushing, and headache. Nifedipine may be coadministered with the β-mimetics. However, it should *not* be used with magnesium because both drugs block calcium and simultaneous administration has been implicated in serious maternal side effects related to low calcium levels.

Prostaglandin synthesis inhibitors (PSIs) such as indomethacin (Indocin) have been used for tocolysis in selected instances. Although this medication has been highly effective in delaying birth, potential fetal side effects, such as constriction of the ductus arteriosus, necrotizing enterocolitis (NEC), and intraventricular hemorrhage (IVH), have made it an uncommon treatment modality (Gill, 2004).

The American College of Obstetricians and Gynecologists (ACOG) (2003a) recommends that corticosteroids (typically betamethasone or dexamethasone) be administered antenatally to women at risk for preterm birth because of their beneficial effect on preventing neonatal respiratory distress syndrome (RDS), intraventricular hemorrhage (IVH), necrotizing enterocolitis (NEC), and neonatal mortality (ACOG, 2003a). Women who are candidates for tocolysis are candidates for antenatal corticosteroids, regardless of fetal gender, race, or availability of surfactant therapy for the newborn, especially between 24 and 34 weeks' gestation (see

Evidence in Action

Prostaglandin inhibitors as tocolytics are more effective before 32 weeks' gestation, and calcium-channel blockers are best after 32 weeks' gestation (Meta-analysis) (Haas, Imperiale, Kirkpatrick, et al., 2009).

Drug Guide

MAGNESIUM SULFATE

Pregnancy Risk Category: B

Overview of Obstetric Action

Magnesium sulfate acts as a CNS depressant by decreasing the quantity of acetylcholine released by motor nerve impulses and thereby blocking neuromuscular transmission. This action reduces the possibility of convulsion, which is why magnesium sulfate is used in the treatment of preeclampsia. Because magnesium sulfate secondarily relaxes smooth muscle, it may decrease the blood pressure, although it is not considered an antihypertensive. Magnesium sulfate may also decrease the frequency and intensity of uterine contractions; as a result it is also used as a tocolytic in the treatment of preterm labor.

Route, Dosage, Frequency

Magnesium sulfate is generally given intravenously to control dosage more accurately and prevent overdosage. The intravenous route allows for immediate onset of action. It must be given by infusion pump for accurate dosage.

For Treatment of Preterm Labor

Loading dose: 4 to 8 g magnesium sulfate in a 10% to 20% solution administered over a 20- to 60-minute period.

Maintenance dose: 2 to 4 g/hr via infusion pump (Carey & Gibbs, 2008).

For Treatment of Preeclampsia

Loading dose: 4 to 6 g magnesium sulfate administered over a 20- to 30-minute period.

Maintenance dose: 2 to 3 g/hr via infusion pump (Habli & Sibai, 2008).

Note: Magnesium sulfate is excreted via the kidneys. Because women in preterm labor typically have normal renal function, they generally require higher levels of magnesium to achieve a therapeutic range than women who have preeclampsia and may have compromised renal function. Maintenance dose may need to be adjusted based on serum magnesium levels.

Maternal Contraindications

Diagnosed maternal myasthenia gravis is the only absolute contraindication to the administration of magnesium sulfate. A history of myocardial damage or heart block is a relative contraindication to use of the drug because of the effects on nerve transmission and muscle contractility. Extreme care is necessary in administration to women with impaired renal function because the drug is eliminated by the kidneys, and toxic magnesium levels may develop quickly.

Maternal Side Effects

Most maternal side effects are dose related. Lethargy and weakness related to neuromuscular blockade are common. Sweating, a feeling of warmth, flushing, and nasal congestion may be related to peripheral vasodilation. Other common side effects include nausea and vomiting, constipation, visual blurring, headache, and slurred speech. Signs of developing toxicity include depression or absence of reflexes, oliguria, confusion, respiratory depression, circulatory collapse, and respiratory paralysis. Rapid administration of large doses may cause cardiac arrest. If any of these occur, the drip should be stopped immediately.

Effects on Fetus/Newborn

The drug readily crosses the placenta. Some authorities suggest that transient decrease in FHR variability may occur; others report that no change occurred. In general, magnesium sulfate therapy does not pose a risk to the fetus. Occasionally, the newborn may demonstrate neurologic depression or respiratory depression, loss of reflexes, and muscle weakness. Ill effects in the newborn may actually be related to fetal growth retardation, prematurity, or perinatal asphyxia.

Nursing Considerations

- Monitor the blood pressure every 10 to 15 minutes during administration.
- Monitor maternal serum magnesium levels as ordered (usually every 6 to 8 hours). Therapeutic levels are in the range of 4 to 8 mg/dL. Reflexes often disappear at serum magnesium levels of 9 to 13 mg/dL; respiratory depression occurs at levels of 14 mg/dL; cardiac arrest occurs at levels above 30 mg/L (Rideout, 2005).
- Monitor respirations closely. If the rate is less than 12/minute, magnesium toxicity may be developing, and further assessments are indicated. Many protocols require stopping the medication if the respiratory rate falls below 12/minute.
- Assess knee jerk (patellar tendon reflex) for evidence of diminished or absent reflexes. Loss of reflexes is often the first sign of developing toxicity. Also note marked lethargy or decreased level of consciousness and hypotension.
- Determine urinary output. Output less than 30 mL/hr may result in the accumulation of toxic levels of magnesium.
- If the respirations or urinary output fall below specified levels or if the reflexes are diminished or absent, no further magnesium should be administered until these factors return to normal.
- The antagonist of magnesium sulfate is calcium. Consequently, an ampule of calcium gluconate should be available at the bedside. The usual dose is 1 g given IV over a period of about 3 minutes.
- Monitor fetal heart tones continuously with IV administration.
- Continue magnesium sulfate infusion for approximately 24 hours after birth as prophylaxis against postpartum seizures if given for preeclampsia.
- If the mother has received magnesium sulfate close to birth, the newborn should be closely observed for signs of magnesium toxicity for 24 to 48 hours.
- The antidote for magnesium sulfate is calcium gluconate. Calcium gluconate should always be on hand in case the magnesium levels get too high.

Note: Protocols for magnesium sulfate administration may vary somewhat according to agency policy. Consequently, individuals are referred to their own agency protocols for specific guidelines.

Teaching Highlights

PRETERM LABOR

- Describe the dangers of preterm labor, especially the risk of prematurity in the infant, and all the potential problems.
- Explain that many of the early symptoms of labor, such as backache and increased bloody show, may be subtle initially.
- Summarize self-care measures (see Table 21–2) the woman can take to prevent preterm labor.
- Teach the woman how to palpate for uterine contractions. Demonstrate and ask for a return demonstration.

"Drug Guide: Betamethasone" on page 458). Betamethasone is primarily used and should be administered in two intramuscular doses. When dexamethasone is used, four doses are given.

NURSING MANAGEMENT

NURSING ASSESSMENT AND DIAGNOSIS

During the antepartal period, identify the woman at risk for preterm labor by noting the presence of risk factors. During the intrapartal period, assess the progress of labor and the physiologic impact of labor on the mother and fetus.

Nursing diagnoses that may apply to the woman with preterm labor include the following:

- *Fear* related to risk of early labor and birth
- *Ineffective Individual Coping* related to need for constant attention to pregnancy
- *Acute Pain* related to uterine contractions

PLANNING AND IMPLEMENTATION

NURSING CARE IN THE COMMUNITY

Once the woman at risk for preterm labor has been identified, she needs to be taught about the importance of recognizing the onset of labor (see "Teaching Highlights: Preterm Labor").

Periodic home visits by a home care nurse are also a common part of care. During these visits it is important to complete physical assessments similar to those done in the hospital and assess the woman's emotional state. Provide information about support groups and other community resources for women at risk for preterm birth.

Teaching the woman to be aware of the signs and symptoms of preterm labor is a primary objective. She should be alert for the following:

- Uterine contractions that occur every 10 minutes or less, with or without pain
- Mild menstrual-like cramps felt low in the abdomen
- Constant or intermittent feelings of pelvic pressure that feel like the baby pressing down
- Rupture of membranes
- Constant or intermittent low, dull backache
- A change in the vaginal discharge (an increase in amount, a change to more clear and watery, or a pinkish tinge)
- Abdominal cramping with or without diarrhea

Teach the woman to evaluate contraction activity once or twice a day. She does so by lying down tilted to one side with a pillow behind her back for support. The woman places her fingertips on the fundus of the uterus, which is above the umbilicus (navel). She checks for contractions (hardening or tightening in the uterus) for about 1 hour. It is important for the pregnant woman to know that uterine contractions occur occasionally throughout the pregnancy. If they occur every 10 minutes for 1 hour, however, the cervix could begin to dilate, and labor could ensue.

Ensure that the woman knows when to report signs and symptoms. If contractions occur every 10 minutes (or more frequently) for 1 hour, if any of the other signs and symptoms are present for 1 hour, or if clear fluid begins leaking from the vagina, the woman should telephone her physician or certified nurse-midwife, clinic, or hospital birthing unit and make arrangements to be checked for ongoing labor. Caregivers need to be aware that the woman's call must be taken seriously. When a woman is at risk for preterm labor, she may have many episodes of contractions and other signs or symptoms. If she is treated positively, she will feel freer to report problems as they arise.

Preventive self-care measures are also important. The nurse has a vital role in communicating the self-care measures described in Table 21–2.

HOSPITAL-BASED NURSING CARE

Supportive nursing care is important to the woman in preterm labor during hospitalization. This care consists of promoting bed rest, monitoring vital signs (especially blood pressure and respirations), measuring intake and output, and continuous monitoring of FHR and uterine contractions. Placing the woman on her left side facilitates maternal-fetal circulation. Keep vaginal examinations to a minimum. If medications are being used, administer them and monitor the mother and fetus for any adverse effects.

Whether preterm labor is arrested or proceeds, the woman and her partner, if involved, experience intense psychologic stress. Decreasing the anxiety associated with the risk of a preterm newborn by providing emotional support is a primary aim of the nurse. It is important to recognize the stress of prolonged bed rest and of lack of sexual contact and to help the couple find satisfactory ways of dealing with those stresses. With empathetic communication, it is possible to assist the woman and her partner to express their feelings, which commonly include guilt and anxiety, thereby helping them identify and implement coping mechanisms. Keep them informed about the labor progress, the treatment regimen, and the status of the fetus. In the event of imminent vaginal or cesarean birth, the woman or

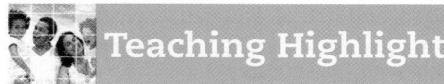

Table 21–2 Self-Care Measures to Prevent Preterm Labor

- Rest two or three times a day lying on your left side.
- Drink 2 to 3 quarts of water or fluid each day. Avoid caffeine drinks. Filling a quart container and drinking from it will eliminate the need to keep track of numerous glasses of fluid.
- Empty your bladder at least every 2 hours during waking hours.
- Avoid lifting heavy objects. If small children are in the home, work out alternatives for picking them up, such as sitting on a chair and having them climb on your lap.
- Avoid prenatal breast preparation such as nipple rolling or rubbing nipples with a towel. This is not meant to discourage breastfeeding but to avoid the potential increase in uterine irritability.
- Pace necessary activities to avoid overexertion.
- Curtail or eliminate sexual activity that involves nipple stimulation or leads to orgasm.
- Find pleasurable ways to help compensate for limitations of activities and boost the spirits.
- Try to focus on 1 day or 1 week at a time rather than on longer periods of time.
- If on bed rest, get dressed each day and rest on a couch rather than becoming isolated in the bedroom.

Source: Prepared in consultation with Susan Bennett, RN, ACCE, Coordinator of the Prematurity Prevention Program.

couple should be offered brief but ongoing explanations to prepare them for the actual birth process and the events following the birth. Arrange for consultations with the neonatologist or pediatrician to assist the woman and her partner in anticipating potential neonatal complications and risks for the newborn.

EVALUATION

Expected outcomes of nursing care include the following:

- The woman is able to discuss the cause, identification, and treatment of preterm labor.
- The woman states that she feels comfortable in her ability to cope with her situation and has resources available to her.
- The woman can describe appropriate self-care measures and can identify characteristics that need to be reported to her caregiver.
- The woman successfully gives birth to a healthy infant.

CARE OF THE WOMAN AT RISK BECAUSE OF BLEEDING DURING PREGNANCY

Bleeding during pregnancy always requires assessment. The most common causes of bleeding during the first and second trimesters, namely spontaneous abortion, ectopic pregnancy, gestational trophoblastic disease, and incompetent cervix, are addressed in Chapter 16∞. The two most clinically significant causes of bleeding in the second half of pregnancy, placenta previa and abruptio placentae, are discussed here. Other placental problems are addressed in Chapter 22∞.

PLACENTA PREVIA

In **placenta previa**, the placenta is implanted in the lower uterine segment rather than the upper portion of the uterus. This implantation may be on a portion of the lower segment or over the internal cervical os. As the lower uterine segment contracts and dilates in the later weeks of pregnancy, the placental villi are torn from the uterine wall, exposing the uterine sinuses at the placental site. Bleeding begins, but because its amount depends on the number of sinuses exposed, initially it may be either scanty or profuse (Figure 21–1 ●). Placenta previa is categorized as being *complete* (the internal os is completely covered), *partial* (the internal os is partially covered), *marginal* (the edge of the placenta is covered), or *low-lying* (the placenta is implanted in the lower

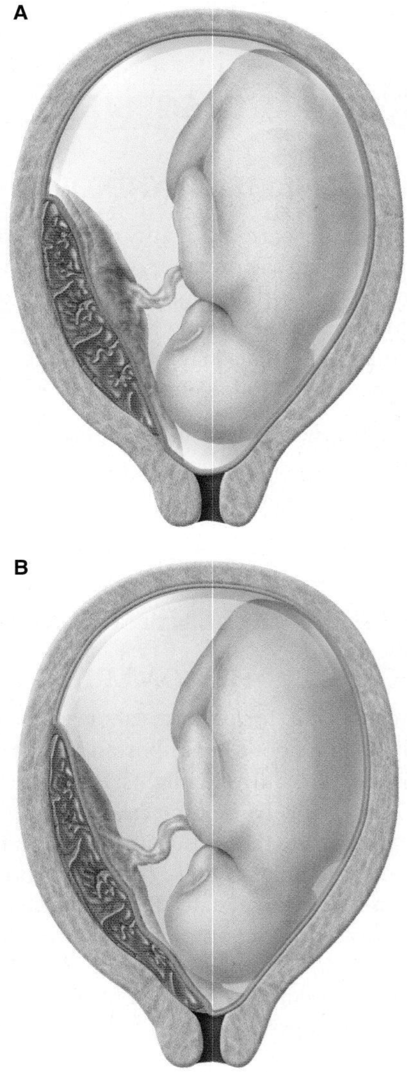

● **Figure 21–1** Classification of placenta previa. ***A***, Marginal placental implantation. ***B***, Placenta previa.

uterine segment in close proximity to but not covering the os) (Cunningham, Leveno, Bloom, et al., 2010).

The cause of placenta previa is unknown. Statistically it occurs in about 4 per 1000 births (Francois & Foley, 2007). Women who are black or minorities and women who have undergone a prior cesarean birth are at higher risk of placenta previa. Other risk factors include high gravidity, high parity, advanced maternal age, previous miscarriage, previous induced abortion, cigarette smoking, and male fetus (Kay, 2010).

Fetal-Neonatal Implications

The prognosis for the fetus depends on the extent of placenta previa. In cases of a marginal previa or a low-lying placenta, the woman may be allowed to labor. Changes in the FHR and meconium staining of the amniotic fluid may be apparent. In a profuse bleeding episode, the fetus is compromised and suffers some hypoxia. FHR monitoring is imperative when the woman is admitted, particularly if a vaginal birth is anticipated, because the presenting part of the fetus may obstruct the flow of blood from the placenta or umbilical cord. If nonreassuring fetal status occurs, cesarean birth is indicated. Women who are diagnosed with a complete or partial previa will undergo a cesarean birth because the risk of intrapartum hemorrhage is high. After birth, blood sampling should be done to determine whether the intrauterine bleeding episodes of the woman have caused anemia in the newborn.

Clinical Therapy

The goal of medical care is to identify the cause of bleeding and to provide treatment that will ensure birth of a mature newborn. Indirect diagnosis is made by localizing the placenta through tests that require no vaginal examination, such as a transabdominal ultrasound scan. Until placenta previa is ruled out, vaginal examinations should never be performed on a woman with bleeding because the examiner's fingers could perforate the placenta if cervical dilatation has occurred. Once placenta previa is ruled out, a vaginal examination can be performed with a speculum to determine the cause of bleeding (such as cervical lesions).

The differential diagnosis of placental or cervical bleeding takes careful consideration. Partial separation of the placenta may also present with painless bleeding, and true placenta previa may not demonstrate overt bleeding until labor begins, thus confusing the diagnosis.

Care of the woman with painless late-gestational bleeding depends on (1) the week of gestation during which the first bleeding episode occurs and (2) the amount of bleeding (see Figure 21–2 ●). If the pregnancy is less than 37 weeks' gestation, expectant management is used to delay birth until about 37 weeks' gestation to allow the fetus time to mature. Expectant management involves the following:

1. Providing bed rest with bathroom privileges as long as the woman is not bleeding
2. Performing no vaginal exams
3. Monitoring blood loss, pain, and uterine contractility
4. Evaluating FHR with an external fetal monitor
5. Monitoring maternal vital signs
6. Performing a complete laboratory evaluation: hemoglobin, hematocrit, Rh factor, and urinalysis
7. Providing intravenous fluid (lactated Ringer's solution)
8. Having two units of cross-matched blood available for transfusion

If frequent, recurrent, or profuse bleeding persists, or if fetal well-being appears threatened, a cesarean birth may be needed.

NURSING MANAGEMENT

NURSING ASSESSMENT AND DIAGNOSIS

Assessment of the woman with placenta previa must be ongoing to prevent or treat complications that are potentially lethal to the mother and fetus. Painless, bright-red vaginal bleeding is the most accurate diagnostic sign of placenta previa. If this sign develops during the last 3 months of pregnancy, placenta previa should always be considered until ruled out by ultrasound examination. The first bleeding episode is generally scanty. If no vaginal examinations are performed, it often subsides spontaneously. However, each subsequent hemorrhage is more profuse.

The uterus remains soft; if labor begins, it relaxes fully between contractions. The FHR usually remains stable unless profuse hemorrhage and maternal shock occur. As a result of the placement of the placenta, the fetal presenting part is often unengaged, and transverse lie is common.

It is important to assess blood loss, pain, and uterine contractility both subjectively and objectively. Maternal vital signs and the results of blood and urine tests provide additional data about the woman's condition. Evaluate the FHR with continuous external fetal monitoring. Observe and verify the family's ability to cope with the anxiety associated with an unknown outcome.

Nursing diagnoses that may apply include the following:

- *Fluid Volume Deficit* related to hypovolemia secondary to excessive blood loss
- *Risk for Impaired Gas Exchange* of the fetus related to decreased blood volume and maternal hypotension
- *Anxiety* related to concern for own personal status and the baby's safety

PLANNING AND IMPLEMENTATION

Monitor the woman and her fetus to determine the status of the bleeding and the responses of the mother and baby. Vital signs, intake and output, and other pertinent assessments must be made frequently. Use the electronic monitor tracing to evaluate

> **Nursing Practice**
>
> The amount of bleeding from the vagina is not a reliable guide to the degree of placental separation.

fetal status. A whole-blood setup should be ready for intravenous infusion and a patent intravenous line established before caregivers undertake any invasive procedures. Monitor maternal vital signs every 15 minutes in the absence of hemorrhage and every 5 minutes with active hemorrhage. The external tocodynamometer should be connected to the maternal abdomen to continuously monitor uterine activity.

Provision of emotional support for the family is an important nursing care goal. During active bleeding, the assessments and management are directed toward physical support. However, emotional aspects need to be addressed simultaneously. Explain the assessments and treatment measures needed. Provide time for questions, and act as an advocate in obtaining information for the family. Emotional support can also be offered by staying with the family and using touch.

Promotion of neonatal physiologic adaptation is another important nursing responsibility. Check the newborn's hemoglobin, cell volume, and erythrocyte count immediately and then monitor them closely. The newborn may require oxygen, administration of blood, and admission into a special-care nursery.

EVALUATION

Anticipated outcomes of nursing care include the following:

- The cause of hemorrhage is recognized promptly and corrective measures are taken.
- The woman's vital signs remain in the normal range.
- Any other complications are recognized and treated early.
- The family understands what has happened and the implications and associated problems of placenta previa.
- The woman and her baby have a safe labor and birth.

MyNursingKit Case Study: Client with Hemorrhage

ABRUPTIO PLACENTAE

Abruptio placentae is the premature separation of a normally implanted placenta from the uterine wall. Premature separation, the leading cause of perinatal mortality, is considered a catastrophic event because of the severity of the resulting hemorrhage. The incidence of abruptio placentae is 0.5% to 1.0% of all pregnancies but it accounts for 10% to 15% of all perinatal deaths (Kay, 2008).

The cause of abruptio placentae is largely unknown. Risk factors associated with placental abruption include increased maternal age, increased parity, cigarette smoking, cocaine abuse, trauma, maternal hypertension, rapid uterine decompression associated with hydramnios and multiple gestation, PPROM, uterine malformations or fibroids, placental anomalies, previous abruption, and inherited thrombophilia (Francois & Foley, 2007).

Abruptio placentae is subdivided into three types (Figure 21–2):

- *Marginal.* In this case the placenta separates at its edges, the blood passes between the fetal membranes and the uterine wall, and the blood escapes vaginally (also called marginal sinus rupture).

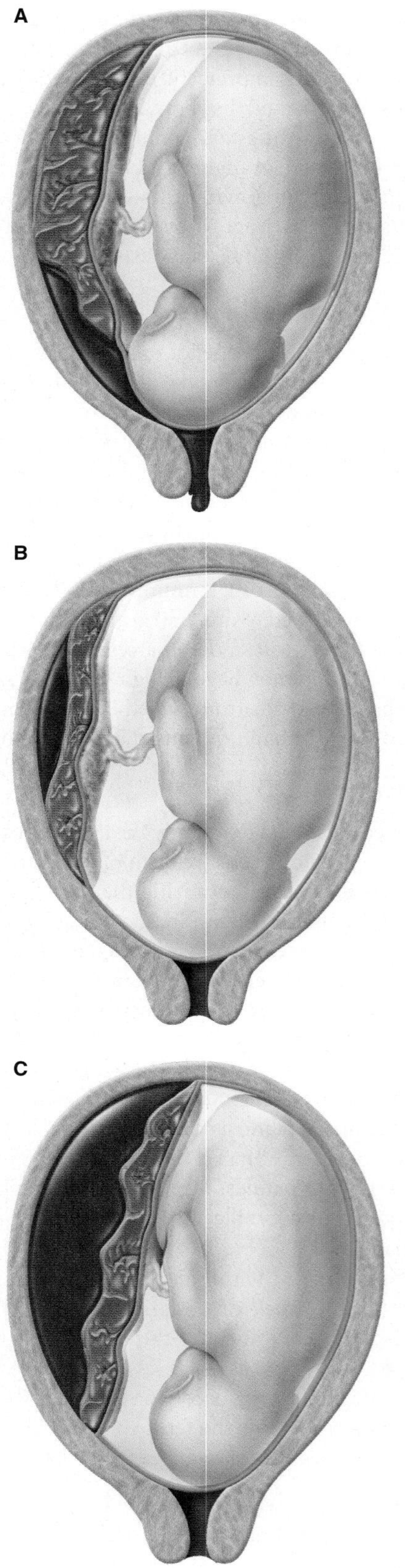

● **Figure 21–2** Abruptio placentae. ***A***, Marginal abruption with external hemorrhage. ***B***, Central abruption with concealed hemorrhage. ***C***, Complete separation.

- *Central.* In this situation, the placenta separates centrally, and the blood is trapped between the placenta and the uterine wall. Entrapment of the blood results in concealed bleeding.
- *Complete.* Massive vaginal bleeding is seen in the presence of total separation.

Abruptio placentae may also be graded according to the severity of clinical and laboratory findings as follows (Francois & Foley, 2007):

Grade 1. Mild separation with slight vaginal bleeding. Fetal heart rate (FHR) pattern and maternal blood pressure unaffected. Accounts for 40% of abruptions.

Grade 2. Partial abruption with moderate bleeding. Significant uterine irritability is present. Maternal pulse may be elevated although blood pressure is stable. Signs of fetal compromise evident in FHR. Accounts for 45% of abruptions.

Grade 3. Large or complete separation with moderate to severe bleeding. Maternal shock and painful uterine contractions present. Fetal death common. Accounts for about 15% of abruptions.

The signs and symptoms of placental abruption are listed in Table 21–3. In severe cases of central abruptio placentae, the blood invades the myometrial tissues between the muscle fibers. This occurrence accounts for the uterine irritability that is a significant sign of abruptio placentae. If hemorrhage continues, eventually the uterus turns entirely blue because the muscle fibers are filled with blood. After birth the uterus contracts poorly. This condition is known as a *Couvelaire uterus* and frequently necessitates hysterectomy.

Maternal Implications

As a result of the damage to the uterine wall and the retroplacental clotting with central abruption, large amounts of thromboplastin are released into the maternal blood supply. This thromboplastin in turn triggers the development of disseminated intravascular coagulation (DIC) and resultant hypofibrinogenemia. Fibrinogen levels, which are ordinarily elevated in pregnancy, may drop in minutes to the point at which blood will no longer coagulate.

Maternal mortality is now uncommon, although maternal morbidity still occurs (Cunningham et al., 2010). Postpartal problems depend in large part on the severity of the intrapartal bleeding, coagulation defects (DIC), hypofibrinogenemia, and time between separation and birth. Moderate to severe hemorrhage results in hemorrhagic shock, which may prove fatal to the mother if it is not rapidly reversed. In the postpartal period, women with this disorder are at risk for hemorrhage and renal failure caused by shock, vascular spasm, intravascular clotting, or a combination of these factors.

Fetal-Neonatal Implications

Perinatal mortality associated with abruptio placentae is about 25% (Cunningham et al., 2010). In severe cases, in which most of the placenta has separated, the infant mortality rate is near 100%. In less severe separation, fetal outcome depends on the level of maturity and the length of time to birth. The most serious complications in the newborn arise from preterm labor, anemia, and hypoxia. If fetal hypoxia progresses unchecked, irreversible brain damage or fetal demise may result. Thorough assessment and prompt action on the part of the healthcare team can improve both fetal and maternal outcomes.

Table 21–3 Differential Signs and Symptoms of Placenta Previa and Abruptio Placentae

	Placenta Previa	Abruptio Placentae
Onset	Quiet and sneaky	Sudden and stormy
Bleeding	External	External or concealed
Color of blood	Bright red	Dark venous
Anemia	= to blood loss	Greater than apparent blood loss
Shock	= to blood loss	Greater than apparent blood loss
Toxemia	Absent	May be present
Pain	Only labor	Severe and steady
Uterine tenderness	Absent	Present
Uterine tone	Soft and relaxed	Firm to stony hard
Uterine contour	Normal	May enlarge and change shape
Fetal heart tones	Usually present	Present or absent
Engagement	Absent	May be present
Presentation	May be abnormal	*No relationship*

Source: Oxorn, H. (1986). *Human labor and birth* (5th ed., p. 507). Norwalk, CT: Appleton & Lange.

Clinical Therapy

Because of the risk of DIC, evaluating the results of coagulation tests is imperative. In DIC, fibrinogen levels and platelet counts usually decrease; prothrombin times and partial thromboplastin times are normal to prolonged. If the values are not markedly abnormal, serial testing may be helpful in establishing an abnormal trend indicative of coagulopathy. Another test determines levels of fibrin-degradation products; these values rise with DIC.

After establishing the diagnosis, immediate priorities are maintaining the cardiovascular status of the mother and developing a plan for the birth of the fetus. The birth method selected depends on the condition of the woman and fetus and the speed in which the birth will occur; in many circumstances, cesarean birth will be the safest option.

If the separation is mild and the pregnancy is late preterm, labor may be induced and the fetus born vaginally with as little trauma as possible. If rupture of membranes and oxytocin infusion by pump do not initiate labor, a cesarean birth is required. A long delay would raise the risk of increased hemorrhage, with resulting hypofibrinogenemia. Supportive actions to decrease the risk of DIC include typing and crossmatching for blood transfusions (at least three units), evaluating the clotting mechanism, and providing intravenous fluids.

In cases of moderate to severe placental separation, a cesarean birth is done after treatment of hypofibrinogenemia by intravenous infusion of cryoprecipitate or fresh frozen plasma. Vaginal birth is impossible with a Couvelaire uterus, because the uterus would not contract properly in labor, and a hysterectomy is often needed.

The hypovolemia that accompanies severe abruptio placentae is life threatening and must be combated with whole blood. If the fetus is alive but experiencing stress, emergency cesarean birth is the method of choice. With a stillborn fetus, vaginal birth is preferable if bleeding has stabilized, unless maternal shock from hemorrhage is uncontrollable. Intravenous fluids are administered. Central venous pressure (CVP) monitoring may be needed to evaluate intravenous fluid replacement. An absolute level is not as important as the response to fluid replacement. CVP is evaluated hourly, and the results are communicated to the physician. Elevations of CVP may indicate fluid overload and pulmonary edema. Laboratory testing is ordered to provide ongoing data regarding hemoglobin, hematocrit, and coagulation status. The hematocrit is maintained at 30% through the administration of packed red blood cells or whole blood (Cunningham et al., 2010). Measures are taken to stimulate labor to effect a vaginal birth, if possible. An amniotomy may be performed, and oxytocin is given. Progressive dilatation and effacement usually occur.

Nursing management. Electronic monitoring of the uterine contractions and resting tone between contractions provides information about the labor pattern and effectiveness of the oxytocin induction. Because uterine resting tone is frequently increased with abruptio placentae, it must be evaluated frequently for further increase. Abdominal girth measurements may be ordered hourly and are obtained by placing a tape measure around the maternal abdomen at the level of the umbilicus. Another method of evaluating uterine size, which increases as more bleeding occurs at the site of abruption, involves placing a mark at the top of the uterine fundus; the distance from the symphysis pubis to the mark may then be measured hourly. Overdistention of the uterus can lead to a ruptured uterus, another life-threatening complication. See the "Nursing Care Plan: Hemorrhage in the Third Trimester."

CARE OF THE WOMAN WITH MULTIPLE GESTATION

In part because of advances in infertility treatments, the incidence of twins in the United States has increased by 65% since 1980 (ACOG, 2004). In 2004, the rate of twins was 32.2 per 1000 births. Multifetal births account for only 3% of all births in the United States (ACOG, 2004). The incidence of spontaneous twins varies but is highest among African Americans, women of greater age and parity, women with a family history of fraternal twins, and women who are tall and overweight. The incidence is low in the Asian and Hispanic populations (Martin, Hamilton, Sutton, et al., 2006). The physiology of multiple gestation is discussed in Chapter 4.

Twins that occur from two separate ova are called dizygotic (two zygotes), or fraternal, twins. The fetuses may be the same sex or different sexes and are no more closely related genetically than any other siblngs. In contrast, 33% of twins are monozygotic, or identical, twins; they develop from one fertilized ovum. They are genetically identical and always the same sex (Blackburn, 2007).

During the prenatal period, visualization of two gestational sacs at 5 to 6 weeks, fundal height greater than expected for the length of gestation, and auscultation of heart rates that differ by at least 10 beats per minute are the most likely clues to multiple-gestation pregnancies. In addition, the alpha-fetoprotein level on the quadruple screen is usually elevated and many women experience severe nausea and vomiting (caused by elevated levels of the human chorionic gonadotropin [hCG] hormone) (Blackburn, 2007).

MATERNAL IMPLICATIONS

During her pregnancy, the woman may experience physical discomfort such as shortness of breath, dyspnea on exertion, backaches and musculoskeletal disorders, and pedal edema. Other associated problems include urinary tract infections, threatened abortion, anemia, gestational hypertension, preeclampsia, preterm labor and birth, premature rupture of membranes, thromboembolism, and placenta previa, placenta abruption, and other types of placenta disorders (Blackburn, 2007; Cleary-Goldman, Chitkara, & Berkowitz, 2007). Complications during labor include abnormal fetal presentations, uterine dysfunction, prolapsed cord, and hemorrhage at birth or shortly after (Blackburn, 2007; Cleary-Goldman et al., 2007).

FETAL-NEONATAL IMPLICATIONS

The perinatal mortality rate is approximately three times greater for twins than for a single fetus, although the mortality rate for triplets and higher-order multiple births is four times higher (MacDorman, Hoyert, Martin, et al., 2007). The perinatal mortality rate for monoamniotic siblings has been estimated to be as

Nursing Care Plan

HEMORRHAGE IN THE THIRD TRIMESTER

INTERVENTION	RATIONALE	EXPECTED OUTCOME
1. Nursing Diagnosis: High Risk for Fluid Volume Deficit related to excessive vascular loss during pregnancy		
NIC Intervention: **Fluid management:** Promotion of fluid balance and prevention of complications resulting from abnormal or undesired fluid levels		**NOC Outcome:** **Fluid balance:** Balance of water in the intracellular and extracellular compartments of the body
Goal: Woman will not experience significant fluid volume deficit during the third trimester of pregnancy.		
■ Monitor vital signs (i.e., temperature—normal range is 96.8–100.4° F, pulse—normal is 60–90, respirations—normal is 12–22, blood pressure—normal range is 110/70 to 135/85, central venous pressure—normal range is 5–10 mm H_2O). Compare present blood pressure with woman's baseline blood pressure. Note pulse pressure.	■ Any deviations in a woman's baseline vital signs could indicate intravascular fluctuations.	■ The woman will show signs of adequate fluid volume during pregnancy as evidenced by vital signs within normal limits, capillary refill in less than 3 seconds, adequate sensorium, and urine output greater than 30 mL/hr.
■ Weigh pads and chux. If the woman has bathroom privileges, instruct her on initiating pad counts. Teach woman how to weigh pads and chux, with each gram = to approximately 1 mL of blood loss.	■ The combination of weighing and counting pads and chux assists medical personnel in determining the woman's blood loss.	
■ Report amount of blood loss within a specific period of time (e.g., 50 mL of bright-red blood on pad in 20 minutes).		
■ Monitor urinary output hourly and measure urine specific gravity (normal: 1.010–1.025).	■ A decrease in urinary output (less than 30 ml/hr) and an increase in specific gravity suggest dehydration and a need for an increase in fluid intake.	
■ Palpate bilateral peripheral pulses (normal: equal and strong) and note capillary refill (normal: less than 3 seconds). Also, assess skin color and temperature (normal: pink, warm, dry, and intact).	■ Helps determine signs of circulatory loss or hypovolemic shock that include weak pulses, capillary refill greater than 3 seconds, skin color that is cyanotic or pallor, and skin temperature that is cool and clammy.	
■ Assess mental status at frequent intervals.	■ Excessive blood loss can lead to changes in mentation.	
■ Assess woman for signs and symptoms of disseminated intravascular coagulation.	■ Provides vital information on maternal status.	
■ Instruct the woman on importance of strict bed rest and avoidance of any sexual activity that involves nipple stimulation or that might lead to orgasm.	■ Bleeding may cease with limited activity. Pressure on the abdomen and orgasms can stimulate uterine activity, thereby causing bleeding. Nipple stimulation may result in uterine contractions, as can orgasm.	
■ Monitor fetal status and uterine activity by continuous fetal monitoring.	■ May determine origin of bleeding and fetal well-being.	

(continued)

Nursing Care Plan—continued

HEMORRHAGE IN THE THIRD TRIMESTER

INTERVENTION	RATIONALE	EXPECTED OUTCOME
Collaborative:		
Collect and review blood work: complete blood count (CBC), type and cross-match, Rh titer, fibrinogen levels, platelet count, activated partial thromboplastin time (APTT), prothrombin time (PT), and hCG levels.	■ Determines blood loss and need for intervention if blood work is abnormal.	
■ Administer appropriate isotonic IV solutions and blood products (e.g., plasma expanders, whole blood, serum albumin, or packed red blood cells) as ordered by physician.	■ Reverses shock symptoms by increasing blood volume.	
■ Insert Foley catheter.	■ Close monitoring of urinary output will aid in determining adequate renal perfusion.	
2. Nursing Diagnosis: Risk for Ineffective Tissue Perfusion (uteroplacental) related to hypovolemia secondary to excessive maternal blood loss		
NIC Intervention: **Electronic fetal monitoring:** Electronic evaluation of fetal heart rate response to movement, external stimuli, or uterine contractions during antepartum testing		**NOC Outcome:** **Circulation status:** Extent to which blood flows unobstructed, unidirectionally, and at an appropriate pressure through large vessels of the systemic and pulmonary circuits
Goal: The fetus will have no evidence of hypoxia during pregnancy.		
■ Assess maternal vital signs.	■ Closely monitoring maternal physiologic status and circulatory status will assist in determining if an episode of bleeding has occurred and allow for interventions to protect maternal and fetal well-being.	
■ Monitor fetal heart tones continuously, assessing for variability, accelerations, and decelerations, and record.	■ Continuous electronic fetal monitoring will aid in detecting signs of fetal hypoxia and allow time for appropriate intervention.	■ Fetus will demonstrate adequate tissue perfusion as evidenced by fetal heart tones that remain within 110–160 bpm, long-term variability and short-term variability present, positive periodic changes (no variable or late decelerations), and fetal scalp blood pH greater than 7.25.
■ Encourage woman to adhere to a strict lateral-lying bed rest regimen.	■ Promotes good placental/fetal oxygen exchange because pressure on the inferior vena cava is relieved.	
■ Assess fundal height.	■ Determines an approximate gestational age.	
■ Assess labor progression by determining cervical dilatation and effacement if contractions are present.	■ This provides information on maternal labor status.	
Collaborative:		
■ Perform scalp stimulation to assess fetal accelerations.	■ FHR acceleration is considered 15 beats above the baseline lasting for 15 seconds and is indicative of fetal well-being.	
■ Assess amniotic fluid for meconium.	■ Impaired gas exchange relaxes fetal intestinal motility, causing expulsion of meconium into amniotic fluid.	
■ Assist physician during ultrasonography and amniocentesis for lecithin/sphingomyelin [LS] ratio sample.	■ Determines viability and alerts appropriate medical personnel of fetal age if birth is imminent.	

Nursing Care Plan—continued

HEMORRHAGE IN THE THIRD TRIMESTER

INTERVENTION	RATIONALE	EXPECTED OUTCOME
3. Nursing Diagnosis: Fear/Anxiety related to personal and fetal well-being secondary to third-trimester hemorrhage		
NIC Intervention: **Anxiety reduction:** Minimizing apprehension, dread, foreboding, or uneasiness related to an unidentified source of anticipated danger		**NOC Outcome:** **Fear control:** Ability to eliminate or reduce disabling feelings of alarm aroused by an identifiable source
Goal: The woman will verbalize a decrease in fear and anxiety.		
■ Maintain frequent contact with the woman and family members.	■ Establishes trust with the woman and her family members, so the patient will not feel alone or abandoned.	■ The woman will actively seek information about diagnosis and prognosis.
■ Provide woman with accurate, reliable information concerning diagnosis and prognosis.	■ Fear and anxiety will lessen when the woman is informed of health status and is allowed to make decisions based on present situation.	■ The woman and her family members develop appropriate coping strategies that decrease fear and anxiety.
■ Allow woman and family members to verbalize origin of fears.	■ Recognizing the origin of fear gives the woman and her family the appropriate tool to begin the process of developing coping strategies for dealing with the fears.	
■ Explain all procedures in an easy-to-understand, nonthreatening manner, and allow woman and family members to ask questions.	■ Accurate information prepares the woman and family members for the impending procedures, thereby reducing fear of the unknown.	

high as 10% to 32% (Cleary-Goldman et al., 2007). Fetal problems include decreased intrauterine growth rate for each fetus, increased incidence of fetal anomalies, increased risk of prematurity and its associated problems, abnormal presentations, increase in cord accidents, and an increase in cerebral palsy (Blackburn, 2007; Cleary-Goldman et al., 2007). Twins are more likely to have long-term disabilities when compared with children who were singleton births. Primiparous women who are pregnant with twins have higher rates of complications and prematurity than multiparous women (Erez, Mayer, Shoham-Vardi, et al., 2007). Multifetal pregnancies that are conceived spontaneously have better outcomes than those achieved with assisted reproductive technology (Kor-anantakul, Suwanrath, Suntharasaj, et al., 2007).

CLINICAL THERAPY

Once the presence of twins has been detected, preventing and treating problems that infringe on the development and birth of normal fetuses is the most significant clinical goal. Prenatal visits are more frequent for women with twins than for those with one fetus. Women with multiple-gestation pregnancies need to understand the nutritional implications of multiple fetuses, the assessment of fetal activity, the signs of preterm labor, and the danger signs of pregnancy.

If the initial ultrasound scan performed at 18 to 20 weeks' gestation is normal and no risk factors are identified, serial ultrasounds performed every 3 to 4 weeks are used to assess the growth of each fetus. If the pregnancy has identified risks, including monochorionic diamniotic placentation, ultrasounds are performed every 2 to 3 weeks to detect possible twin-to-twin transfusion syndrome (Cleary-Goldman et al., 2007).

A systematic review of studies of hospitalization and bed rest for multiple pregnancy showed insufficient evidence to support routine bed rest (ACOG, 2004). More recent strategies include work leave, lifestyle modifications, and avoidance of sexual activity, although well-designed controlled studies supporting the use of these interventions is lacking in the current literature.

Third trimester testing usually begins at 32 to 34 weeks' gestation and may include NST or BPP. A reactive NST is associated with good fetal outcome if birth occurs within 1 week of the testing. The NST is done every 3 to 7 days until birth or until results become nonreactive. The BPP is also accurate in assessing fetal status with twin pregnancies. A biophysical profile of 8 or better for each fetus is considered reassuring, and weekly or biweekly BPPs and NSTs continue until birth.

Intrapartal management requires careful attention to maternal and fetal status. The mother should have an IV with a large-bore needle in place. Anesthesia and cross-matched blood should be readily available. The twins are monitored by continuous dual electronic fetal monitoring.

The decision about method of birth, which depends on a variety of factors, may not be made until labor occurs. The presence of maternal complications such as placenta previa, abruptio placentae, or severe preeclampsia usually indicates the need for cesarean birth. Fetal factors such as severe intrauterine growth restriction (IUGR), preterm birth, fetal anomalies, nonreassuring fetal status, and unfavorable fetal position or presentation also require cesarean birth.

Any combination of presentations and positions can occur with multiple births. Figure 21–3 ● shows some possible presentations of twins. When the presenting fetus is in a nonvertex position, cesarean birth is indicated.

Nursing Management

Community-based nursing care. During pregnancy the woman may need counseling about diet and daily activities. The nurse can help her plan meals to meet her increased needs. Nutritional requirements vary somewhat based on the mother's prepregnancy weight and the estimated weight of the twins. A daily intake of 3500 kcal (minimum) and 175 g protein is recommended for a woman with normal-weight twins although an intake of 4000 kcal and 200 g of protein is recommended if the twins are underweight. A prenatal vitamin and 1 mg of folic acid should also be taken daily. A total weight gain of 40 to 45 lb, with a 24-lb gain by 24 weeks, is recommended for women with multiple-gestation pregnancy (Newman & Rittenberg, 2008).

Counseling about daily activities may include encouraging the woman to plan frequent rest periods during the day. The rest period is most effective if the woman rests in a side-lying position (which increases uteroplacental blood flow) and elevates her lower legs and feet to reduce edema. Back discomfort may be relieved by pelvic rocking, maintaining good posture, consistent use of a pregnancy belt to support the abdomen and lower back, and using good body mechanics when lifting objects and moving about.

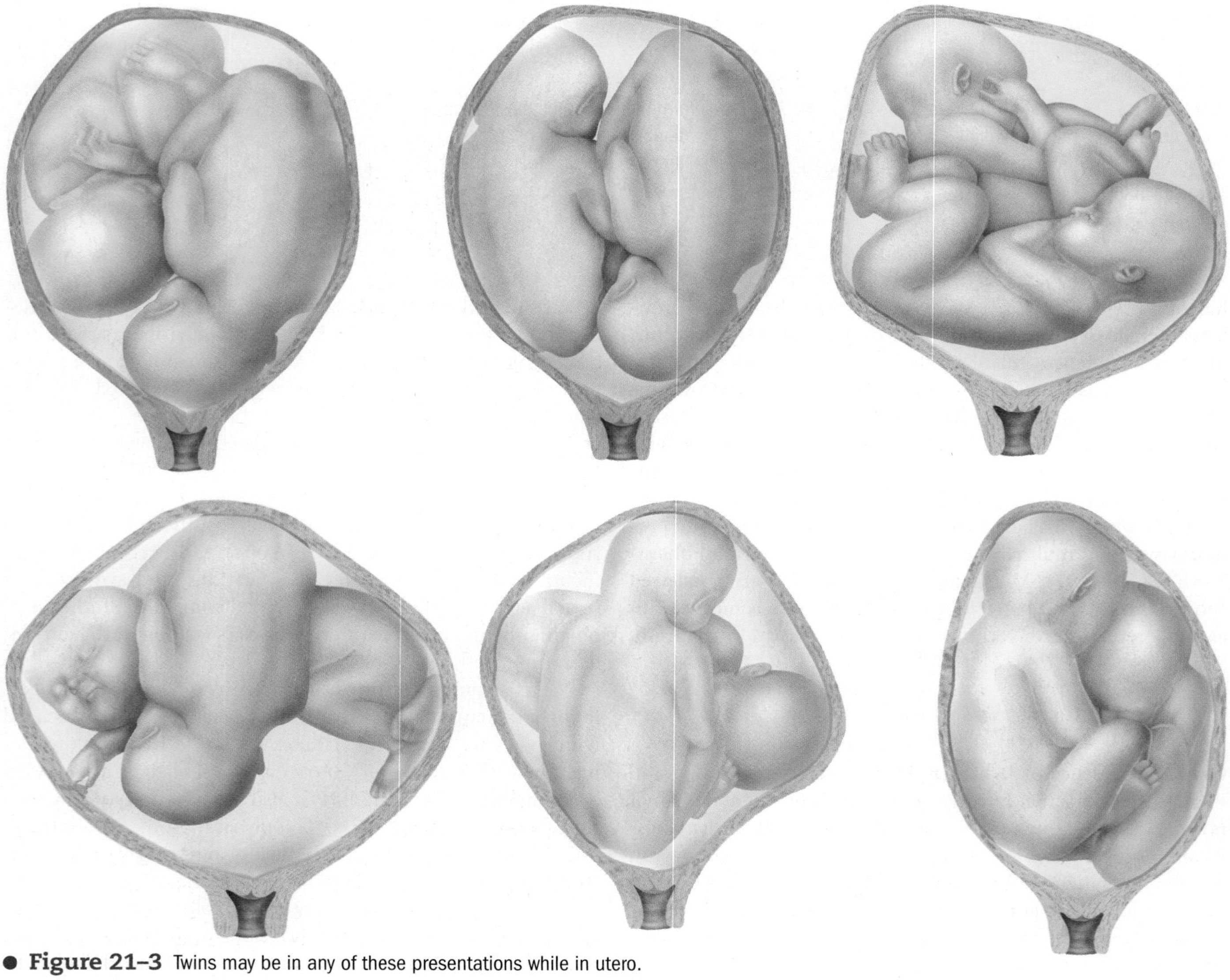

● **Figure 21–3** Twins may be in any of these presentations while in utero.

Hospital-based nursing care. During labor, the FHRs of the siblings are monitored continuously by an electronic fetal monitor (EFM). Electronic monitoring equipment now makes it possible to monitor the fetuses simultaneously. They are monitored throughout labor and vaginal birth or up to the time of abdominal incision if a cesarean is done. Most multiple gestations are now delivered via cesarean birth.

After birth, prepare to receive two or more newborns instead of one. This means duplicating everything, including resuscitation equipment, radiant warmers, and newborn identification papers and bracelets. Additional staff members should be available for newborn resuscitation, monitoring, and newborn care. Special precautions should be taken to ensure correct identification of the newborns. The first born is usually tagged Baby A; the second, Baby B; and so on.

CARE OF THE WOMAN WITH ABNORMAL AMNIOTIC FLUID VOLUME

Amniotic fluid serves many important functions during pregnancy. However, some pregnancies are complicated by either an excessive amount of amniotic fluid or a reduced amount of fluid.

HYDRAMNIOS

Hydramnios (also called *polyhydramnios*), a situation in which there is more than 2000 mL of amniotic fluid, occurs in about 1% of all pregnancies (Cunningham et al., 2010). The exact cause of hydramnios is unknown; however, it often occurs in cases of major congenital anomalies.

During the second half of a normal pregnancy, the fetus begins to swallow and inspire amniotic fluid and to urinate, which contributes to the amount of amniotic fluid present. In cases of hydramnios, no pathology has been found in the amniotic epithelium. However, hydramnios is associated with fetal malformations that affect the fetal swallowing mechanism and neurologic disorders in which the fetal meninges are exposed in the amniotic cavity. This condition is also found in cases of anencephaly, in which the fetus is thought to urinate excessively because of overstimulation of the cerebrospinal centers. When monozygotic twins manifest hydramnios, it is because the twin with the increased blood volume urinates excessively. Because the weight of the placenta has been found to be increased in some cases of hydramnios, increased functioning of the placental tissue may be a factor.

There are two types of hydramnios: chronic and acute. In the chronic type, the fluid volume gradually increases and is a problem of the third trimester. Most cases are of this variety. In acute cases, the volume increases rapidly over a period of a few days. The acute type is usually diagnosed between 20 and 24 weeks' gestation.

Maternal Implications

When the amount of amniotic fluid is over 3000 mL, the woman experiences shortness of breath and edema in the lower extremities from compression of the vena cava. Milder forms of hydramnios occur more frequently and are associated with minimal symptoms. Hydramnios is associated with maternal disorders such as diabetes and Rh sensitization and with multiple-gestation pregnancies. It can also occur as a result of infections such as syphilis, toxoplasmosis, cytomegalovirus, herpes, and rubella.

If the amniotic fluid is removed rapidly before birth, abruptio placentae can result from too sudden a change in the size of the uterus. Because of overdistention of uterine muscles, uterine dysfunction can occur in the intrapartal period, and the incidence of postpartal hemorrhage increases.

Fetal-Neonatal Implications

Fetal malformations and preterm birth are common with hydramnios; thus the perinatal mortality rate is fairly high. Prolapsed cord can occur when the membranes rupture, creating a further complication for the fetus. The incidence of malpresentations also increases. In addition, the incidence of preterm labor and cesarean birth is significantly increased in pregnancies complicated by hydramnios.

Clinical Therapy

Hydramnios is managed with supportive treatment unless the intensity of the woman's distress and symptoms dictates otherwise. If the accumulation of amniotic fluid is severe enough to cause maternal dyspnea and pain, hospitalization and removal of the excessive fluid are required. Fluid can be removed vaginally or by amniocentesis. The dangers of performing the technique vaginally are prolapsed cord and the inability to remove the fluid slowly. If amniocentesis is performed, it should be done with the aid of sonography to prevent inadvertent damage to the fetus and placenta. In addition, the fluid should be removed slowly to prevent abruption.

Nursing management. Hydramnios should be suspected when the fundal height increases out of proportion to the gestational age. As the amount of fluid increases, it may be difficult to palpate the fetus and auscultate the FHR. In more severe cases, the maternal abdomen appears extremely tense and tight on inspection. On sonography, large spaces can be identified between the fetus and the uterine wall.

When amniocentesis is performed, it is vital to maintain sterile technique to prevent infection. Offer support to the woman and her partner by explaining the procedure to them.

If the fetus has been diagnosed with a congenital defect in utero or is born with a defect, the family needs psychologic support. Often the nurse collaborates with social services to offer the family this additional help.

OLIGOHYDRAMNIOS

Oligohydramnios is defined as a less-than-normal amount of amniotic fluid (approximately 500 mL is considered normal). This condition affects 1% to 3% of all pregnancies (Gilbert, 2007). Oligohydramnios is diagnosed when the largest vertical pocket of amniotic fluid visible on ultrasound examination is 5 cm (2 in.) or less (Cunningham et al., 2010).

The exact cause of this condition is unknown. It is found in cases of postmaturity; maternal hypertensive disorders, with IUGR secondary to placental insufficiency; and in fetal conditions associated with major renal malformations, including renal aplasia with dysplastic kidneys and obstructive lesions of the lower urinary tract. If oligohydramnios occurs in the first part of pregnancy, there is a danger of fetal adhesions (one part of the fetus may adhere to another part).

Maternal Implications

When oligohydramnios exists, labor can be dysfunctional, and progress is slow. The woman should be monitored for hypertensive disorders.

Fetal-Neonatal Implications

During the gestational period, fetal skin and skeletal abnormalities may occur because fetal movement is impaired as a result of reduced amniotic fluid volume. Because there is less fluid available for the fetus to use during fetal breathing movements, pulmonary hypoplasia may develop. During the labor and birth, oligohydramnios reduces the cushioning effect for the umbilical cord, and cord compression is more likely to occur. Decreased amniotic fluid also contributes to fetal head compression.

Clinical Therapy

During the antepartum period oligohydramnios may be suspected when the uterus does not increase in size according to the dates, the fetus is easily palpated and outlined by the examiner, and the fetus is not ballottable. The fetus can be assessed by biophysical profiles, nonstress tests, and serial ultrasounds. As soon as the fetus is term, induction is typically scheduled because the fetus is at an increased risk for intrauterine fetal demise. During labor, the fetus is monitored by continuous EFM to detect cord compression, which is indicated by variable decelerations. Some clinicians advocate the use of an *amnioinfusion* (a transcervical instillation of 250 mL of warmed sterile saline, followed by a continuous infusion rate of 100 to 200 mL/hr) after membranes have ruptured to decrease the frequency and severity of variable decelerations in the FHR during labor. The fluid is administered in a blood warmer to maintain a constant temperature. It is imperative to monitor for expulsion of the fluid to prevent overdistention of the uterus. The infusion of saline provides more fluid for the umbilical cord to float in and thereby lessens or prevents cord compression. Amnioinfusions are also used in cases of thick meconium to decrease the consistency and decrease the incidence of meconium below the infant's vocal cords (Gilbert, 2007).

Nursing management. Continuous electronic fetal monitoring is an important part of the assessment during the labor and birth. Evaluate the EFM tracing for the presence of variable decelerations or other nonreassuring signs (such as increasing or decreasing baseline, decreased variability, presence of late decelerations). If variable decelerations are noted, the woman's position can be changed (to relieve pressure on the umbilical cord), and the physician/CNM is notified. If the tracing is not reassuring, a cesarean birth is performed. After the birth, the newborn is evaluated for signs of congenital anomalies, pulmonary hypoplasia, and postmaturity.

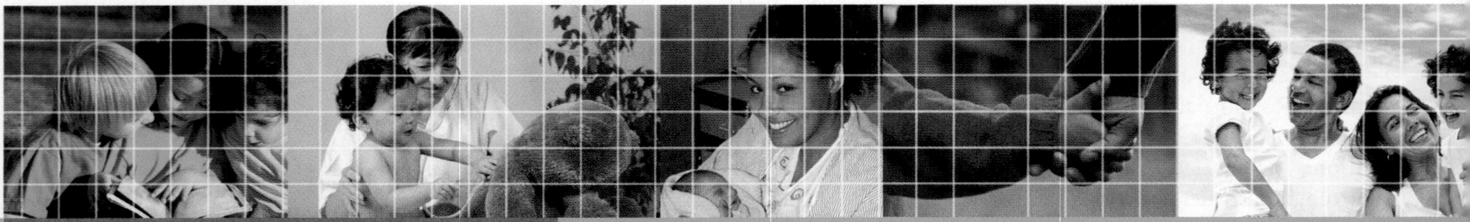

CRITICAL CONCEPT REVIEW

LEARNING OUTCOMES	CONCEPTS
21.1 Explain the possible causes, risk factors, and clinical therapy for premature rupture of the membranes or preterm labor in determining the nursing care management of the woman and her fetus-newborn.	1. PROM: ■ Although the exact cause is unknown, PPROM is associated with infection, multiple pregnancy, bleeding during pregnancy, trauma, and a variety of other factors. ■ PROM nursing care focuses on prevention of infection such as limiting vaginal exams and changing the bed pads frequently. ■ The fetus is monitored carefully. 2. Preterm labor: ■ Nursing care during preterm labor focuses on administration of tocolytics and monitoring for progression of labor.

LEARNING OUTCOMES / CONCEPTS

21.2 Compare placenta previa and abruptio placentae, including implications for the mother and fetus, as well as nursing care.

1. Abruptio placentae:
   - Condition in which the placenta prematurely separates from the uterine wall.
   - May result in severe hemorrhage.
   - May cause death to mother, fetus, or both.
   - May lead to clotting disorders in the mother.
   - Nursing care involves frequent assessment of uterine tone and measurement of abdominal girth.
2. Placenta previa:
   - Condition in which the placenta implants in the lower segment of the uterus. It may partially or completely cover the cervical os.
   - Bleeding occurs as the cervix begins to dilate. Bleeding may be mild to severe, depending upon how much of the placenta covers the cervical os.
   - Fetus may develop hypoxia, anemia, or both from bleeding episode.
   - Nursing care involves assessing blood loss, pain, and uterine contractions.
   - The nurse should NEVER perform a vaginal examination if placenta previa is suspected.

21.3 Explain the maternal and fetal-neonatal implications and the clinical therapy in determining the nursing care management of the woman with multiple gestation.

1. Care of the woman with more than one fetus includes:
   - Frequent assessment of the fetal heart tones of each fetus.
   - Education of the mother about signs and symptoms of preterm labor.
   - Encouraging the mother to rest frequently.
   - Prior to birth, preparation of equipment needed to care for each individual newborn.

21.4 Compare the identification, maternal and fetal-neonatal implications, clinical therapy, and nursing care management of the woman with hydramnios and oligohydramnios.

1. Hydramnios:
   - In this condition, the woman has greater than 2000 mL of amniotic fluid.
   - Associated with fetal swallowing and neurologic disorders.
   - Also associated with maternal gestational diabetes, Rh disorders, and multiple-gestation pregnancies.
   - Woman may experience shortness of breath and lower extremity edema.
   - Amniocentesis may be performed to remove some of the excess fluid.
   - The nurse monitors the mother for complications of the amniocentesis and supports the family if fetal disorders are the cause of the excess fluid.
2. Oligohydramnios:
   - In this condition the amount of amniotic fluid is reduced and concentrated.
   - Often found with some renal fetal disorders, fetal postmaturity, and placental insufficiency.
   - May cause fetal respiratory and skeletal abnormalities.
   - May cause prolonged labor.
   - Amnioinfusion may be used during labor to help to cushion the fetus and umbilical cord.
   - The nurse must continuously monitor the labor pattern for any sign of fetal distress.

CRITICAL THINKING IN ACTION

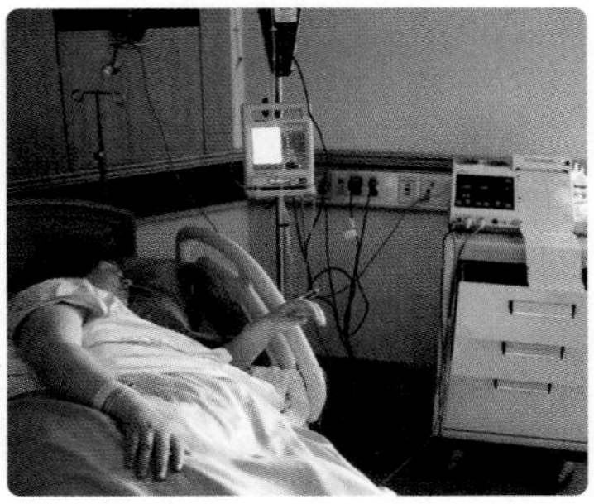

Monique Waleski, a 34-year old G1 P0000, at 32-weeks' gestation, contacts her physician's office because she has been experiencing labor contractions that have gradually increased in frequency. She reports that she has been having about 8 contractions an hour for the past two hours. She is instructed to meet her doctor at the birthing unit for further evaluation.

At the birthing unit a vaginal examination reveals that Monique's cervix is dilated 3 cm and 80% effaced. Contractions continue to occur every 7 to 8 minutes. Her fFN test is positive. She is diagnosed with preterm labor.

You position her on her left side and start an IV infusion.

Her physician tells Monique that she wants to begin tocolysis using magnesium sulfate and then prescribes two doses of betamethasone. You explain to Monique and her partner that you will be giving her the magnesium sulfate by infusion pump and the betamethasone by IM injection once a day today and tomorrow. She asks you about the two medications including their specific purposes.

1. Explain the concept of tocolysis and the purpose of magnesium sulfate.
2. Describe the concept of a loading dose and maintenance dose.
3. How will you know if Monique is developing toxic levels of magnesium?
4. Describe the role of corticosteroids used during preterm labor.

See MyNursingKit for possible responses.

REFERENCES

American College of Obstetricians and Gynecologists (ACOG). (2003a). *Management of preterm labor.* ACOG Practice Bulletin No. 43. Washington, DC: Author.

American College of Obstetricians & Gynecologists (ACOG). (2004). *Multiple gestation: Complicated twin, triplet, and higher-order multifetal pregnancy.* ACOG Practice Bulletin No. 56. Washington, DC: Author.

Blackburn, S. T. (2007). *Maternal, fetal, and neonatal physiology: A clinical perspective* (3rd ed.). Philadelphia: Saunders.

Briggs, G. G., Freeman, R. K., & Yaffee, S. J. (2005). *Drugs in pregnancy and lactation* (7th ed.). Philadelphia: Lippincott Williams & Wilkins.

Carey, J. C., & Gibbs, R. S. (2008). Preterm labor and postterm delivery. In R. S. Gibbs, B. Y. Karlan, A. F. Haney, & I. E. Nygaard (Eds.), *Danforth's obstetrics and gynecology* (10th ed.). Philadelphia: Wolters Kluwer/Lippincott Williams & Wilkins.

Cleary-Goldman, J., Chitkara, U., & Berkowitz, R. L. (2007). Multiple gestations. In S. G. Gabbe, J. R. Niebyl, & J. L. Simpson (Eds.), *Obstetrics: Normal and problem pregnancies* (5th ed.). Philadelphia: Churchill Livingstone.

Cunningham, F. G., Leveno, K. J., Bloom, S. L., Hauth, J. C., Rouse, D. J., & Spong, C. Y. (2010). *Williams obstetrics* (23rd ed.). New York: McGraw-Hill Medical.

Da Fonseca, E. B., Bittar, R. E., Damião, R., & Zugaib, M. (2009). Prematruity prevention: The role of progesterone. *Current Opinions in Obstetrics and Gynecology, 21,* 142–147.

Erez, O., Mayer, A., Shoham-Vardi, I., Dukler, D., & Mazor, M. (2007). Primiparity, assisted reproduction, and preterm birth in twin pregnancies: A population based study. *Archives of Gynecology & Obstetrics* (2007 Oct 31) [Epub ahead of print].

Francois, K. E., & Foley, M. R. (2007). Antepartum and postpartum hemorrhage. In S. G. Gabbe, J. R. Niebyl, & J. L. Simpson (Eds.), *Obstetrics: Normal and problem pregnancies* (5th ed.). Philadelphia: Churchill Livingstone.

Gibbs, R. S. (2008). Premature rupture of the membranes. In R. S. Gibbs, B. Y. Karlan, A. F. Haney, & I. E. Nygaard (Eds.), *Danforth's obstetrics and gynecology* (10th ed.). Philadelphia: Wolters Kluwer/Lippincott Williams & Wilkins.

Gilbert, W. M. (2007). Amniotic fluid disorders. In S. G. Gabbe, J. R. Niebyl, & J. L. Simpson (Eds.), *Obstetrics: Normal and problem pregnancies* (5th ed.). Philadelphia: Churchill Livingstone.

Gill, G. (2004). Etiology and prevention of preterm labor. Retrieved November 4, 2007, from www.acog.org/acog_sections/download/EtiologyandPreventionofPretermLabor.pdf - 2004-05-17

Haas, D. M., Imperiale, T. F., Kirkpatrick, P. R., Klein, R. W., Zollinger, T. W., & Golichowski (2009). Tocolytic therapy: A meta-analysis and decision analysis. *Obstetrics & Gynecology, 113*(3), 585–594.

Habli, M., & Sibai, B. (2008). Hypertensive disorders of pregnancy. In R. S. Gibbs, B. Y. Karlan, A. F. Haney, & I. E. Nygaard (Eds.), *Danforth's obstetrics and gynecology* (10th ed.). Philadelphia: Wolters Kluwer/Lippincott Williams & Wilkins.

Iams, J. D., & Romero, R. (2007). Preterm birth. In S. G. Gabbe, J. R. Niebyl, & J. L. Simpson (Eds.), *Obstetrics: Normal and problem pregnancies* (5th ed.). Philadelphia: Churchill Livingstone.

Kay, H. H. (2008). Placenta previa and abruption. In R. S. Gibbs, B. Y. Karlan, A. F. Haney, & I. E. Nygaard (Eds.), *Danforth's obstetrics and gynecology* (10th ed.). Philadelphia: Wolters Kluwer/Lippincott Williams & Wilkins.

Kor-anantakul, O., Suwanrath, C., Suntharasaj, T., Getpook, C., & Leetanaporn, R. (2007). Outcomes of multifetal pregnancies. *Journal of Obstetric & Gynaecology Research, 33*(1), 49–55.

MacDorman, M. F., Hoyert, D. L., Martin, J. A., Munson, M. L., & Hamilton, B. E. (2007). Fetal and perinatal mortality, United States, 2003. *National Vital Statistics Reports, 55*(6), 1–18.

March of Dimes (MOD). (2007). March of Dimes Peristats: More babies born prematurely, new report shows. Retrieved August 20, 2008, from www.marchofdimes.com

Martin, J. A., Hamilton, B. E., Sutton, P. D., Ventura, S. J., Menacker, F., & Kirmeyer, S. (2006). Births: Final data for 2004. *National Vital Statistics Reports, 55*(1), 1–102.

Mercer, B. M. (2007). Premature rupture of the membranes. In S. G. Gabbe, J. R. Niebyl, & J. L. Simpson (Eds.), *Obstetrics: Normal and problem pregnancies* (5th ed.). Philadelphia: Churchill Livingstone.

Ness, A., Visintine, J., Ricci, E., & Berghella, V. (2007). Does knowledge of cervical length and fetal fibronectin affect management of women with threatened preterm labor? A randomized trial. *American Journal of Obstetricians & Gynecologists, 197*(4), 426–427.

Newman, R. B. (2005). Uterine contraction assessment. *Obstetrics & Gynecology Clinics in North America, 32*(3), 341–367.

Newman, R. B., & Rittenberg, C. (2008). Multiple gestation. In R. S. Gibbs, B. Y. Karlan, A. F. Haney, & I. E. Nygaard (Eds.), *Danforth's obstetrics and gynecology* (10th ed.). Philadelphia: Wolters Kluwer/Lippincott Williams & Wilkins.

Rideout, S. L. (2005). Tocolytics for pre-term labor: What nurses need to know. *AWHONN Lifelines, 9*(1), 56–61.

Ross, M. G. (2009). Preventing preterm birth: Progesterone and cervical length assessments. *The Female Patient, 34*(3), 38–40.

PEARSON

EXPLORE mynursingkit™

MyNursingKit is your one stop for online chapter review materials and resources. Prepare for success with additional NCLEX®-style practice questions, interactive assignments and activities, web links, animations and videos, and more!

Register your access code from the front of your book at
www.mynursingkit.com

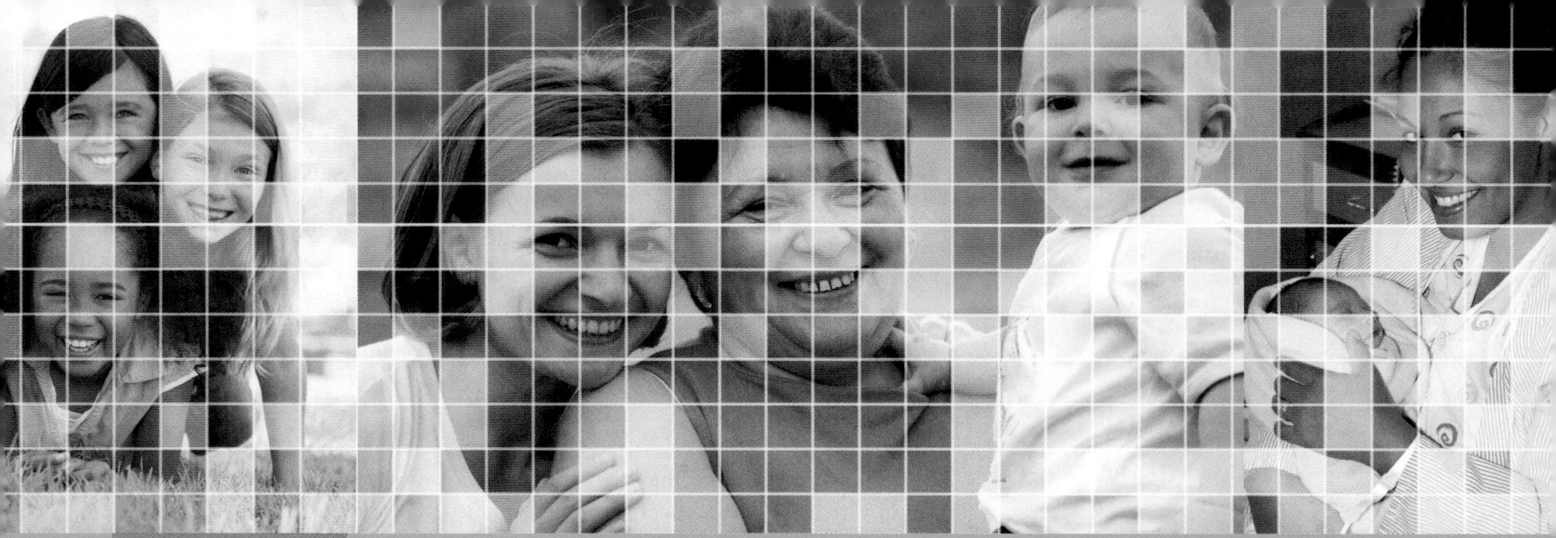

CHAPTER

22 Childbirth at Risk: Labor-Related Complications

We arrived at the birthing unit with such wonderful plans for the birth of our first baby. I was able to do my breathing with the assistance of my husband and the nurse. Then suddenly my baby's heart rate dropped. It lasted for about 20 seconds but it felt like a lifetime. The nurse helped me to my side, and just stayed with us while we waited and watched the fetal monitor. There were no further problems, but I will never forget that moment. —Yolanda, 26

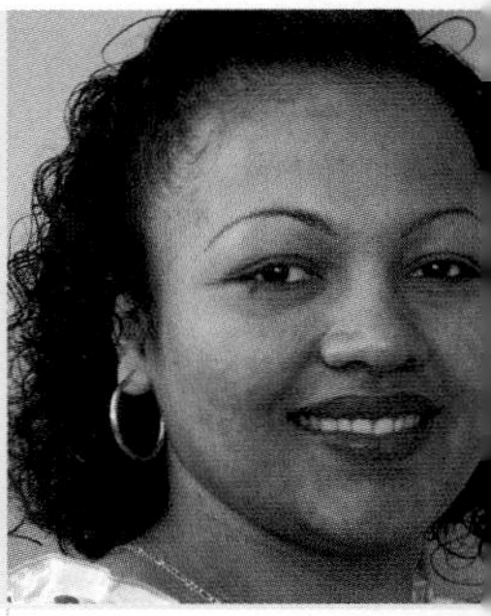

LEARNING OUTCOMES

22.1 Compare hypertonic and hypotonic labor patterns, including the risks, clinical therapy, and nursing care management.

22.2 Describe the risks and clinical therapy in determining the nursing care management of postterm pregnancy on the childbearing family.

22.3 Relate the various types of fetal malposition and malpresentation to the nursing management for each.

22.4 Explain the identification, risks, and clinical therapy in determining the nursing care management of the woman and fetus at risk for fetal macrosomia.

22.5 Relate the maternal implications, clinical therapy, prenatal history, and conditions that may be associated with nonreassuring fetal status to the nursing care of the mother and fetus.

22.6 Describe the nursing care for the mother and fetus with a prolapsed umbilical cord.

22.7 Summarize the identification, maternal and fetal-neonatal implications, clinical therapy, and nursing care management of women with amniotic fluid embolism.

22.8 Explain the types, maternal and fetal-neonatal implications, and clinical therapy in determining the nursing care management of the woman with cephalopelvic disproportion.

22.9 Identify common complications of the third and fourth stages of labor.

22.10 Explain the etiology, diagnosis, and phases of grief in determining the nursing care management of the family experiencing perinatal loss.

22.11 Explain the psychologic factors that may contribute to complications during labor and birth in determining the nursing care management.

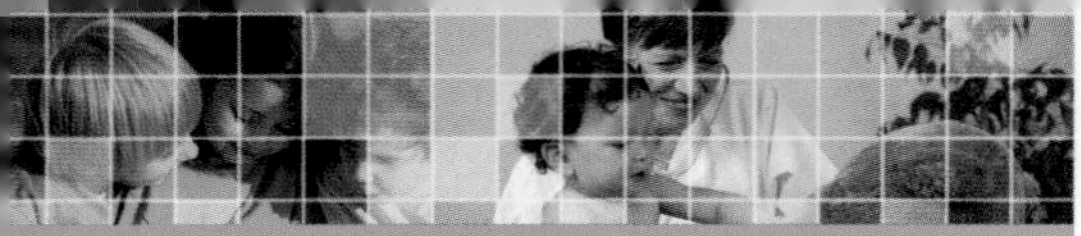

KEY TERMS

Amniotic fluid embolism, 493
Cephalopelvic disproportion (CPD), 493
Dystocia, 478
Intrauterine resuscitation, 491
Macrosomia, 490
Perinatal loss, 495
Persistent occiput posterior (POP) position, 483
Precipitous labor, 481
Prolapsed umbilical cord, 491
Prolonged (postterm) pregnancy, 482
Retained placenta, 494

Successful completion of a pregnancy requires the harmonious functioning of the five critical factors discussed in the "Critical Factors in Labor" section in Chapter 17: the birth passage, the fetus, the relationship between the passage and the fetus, the forces of labor, and psychosocial considerations. Disruptions in any of these components may cause dystocia (abnormal or difficult labor). The most common of these disruptions are discussed in this chapter.

CARE OF THE WOMAN WITH DYSTOCIA RELATED TO DYSFUNCTIONAL UTERINE CONTRACTIONS

Dystocia, or difficult labor, may be caused by a wide variety of problems, the most common of which is dysfunctional (or uncoordinated) uterine contractions. These uncoordinated contractions result in a prolonged labor. Contractions that result in a more normal progression of labor tend to be moderate to strong when palpated and occur regularly (two to four contractions in 10 minutes in early labor and four to five per 10 minutes in later phases). Dysfunctional contractions are typically irregular in strength, timing, or both. These irregular uterine contractions often arrest cervical dilatation.

HYPERTONIC LABOR PATTERNS

A normal contraction pattern is shown in Figure 22–1A ●. In hypertonic labor patterns, ineffectual uterine contractions of poor quality occur in the latent phase of labor, and the resting tone of the myometrium increases. Contractions usually become more frequent, but their intensity may decrease (Figure 22–1B). The con-

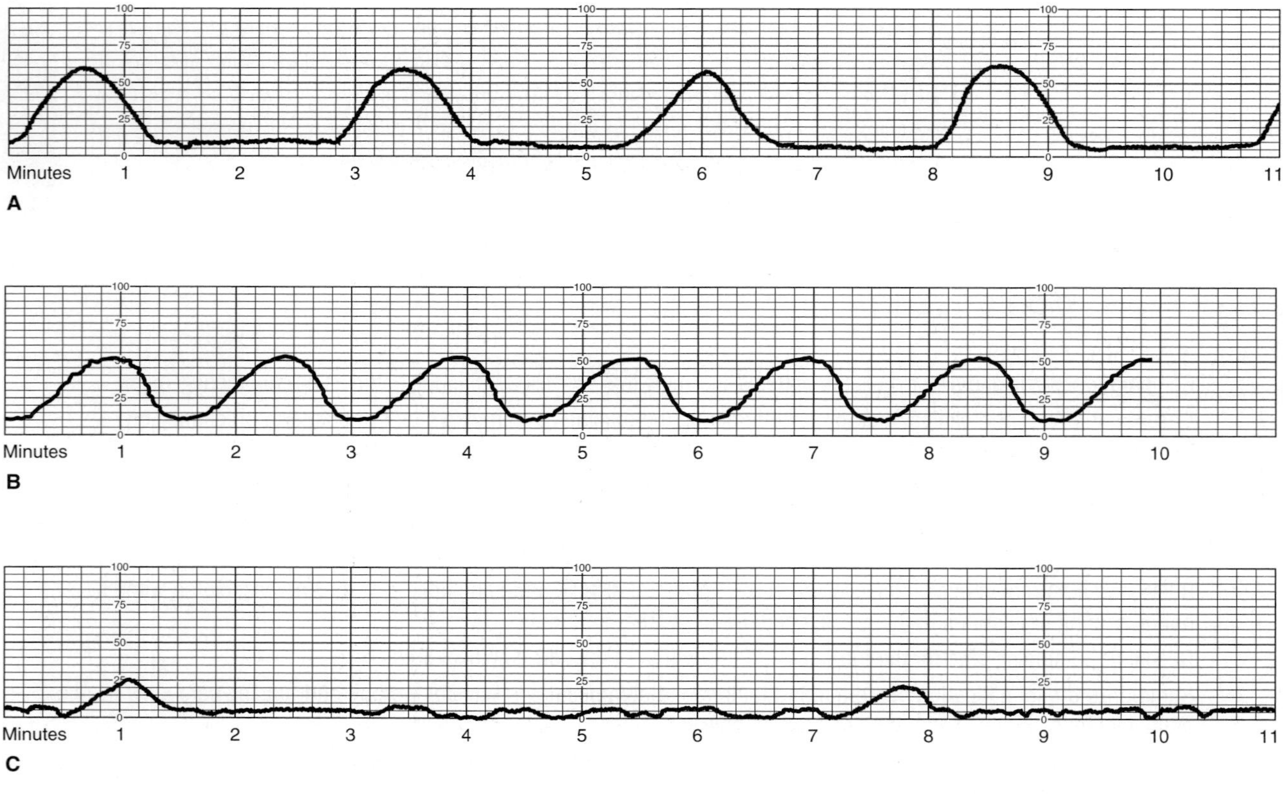

● **Figure 22–1** Comparison of labor patterns. ***A,*** Normal uterine contraction pattern. In this example, contraction frequency is every 3 minutes; duration is 60 seconds. The baseline resting tone is below 10 mm Hg. ***B,*** Hypertonic uterine contraction pattern. Note that the contraction frequency is every 1 1/2 minutes, duration is 90 seconds. The baseline resting tone is 10 mm Hg. ***C,*** Hypotonic uterine contraction pattern. In this example, the contraction frequency is every 7 minutes (with some uterine activity between contractions), duration is 50 seconds, and intensity increases approximately 25 mm Hg during contractions.

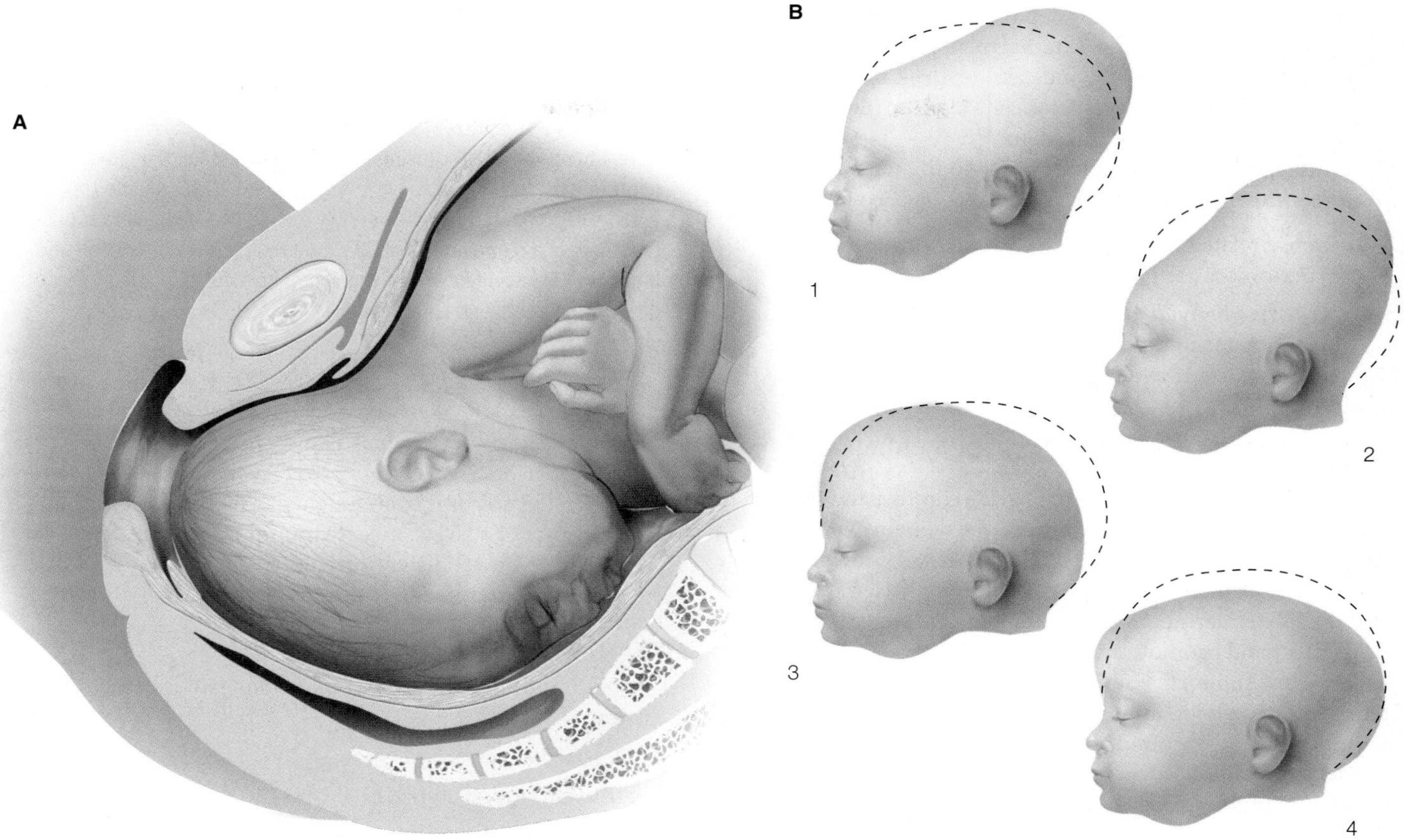

● **Figure 22–2** Effects of labor on the fetal head. ***A,*** Caput succedaneum formation. The presenting portion of the scalp area is encircled by the cervix during labor, causing swelling of the soft tissue. ***B,*** Molding of the fetal head in cephalic presentations: (1) occiput anterior, (2) occiput posterior, (3) brow, (4) face.

tractions are painful but ineffective in dilating and effacing the cervix, and a prolonged latent phase may result.

Risks of Hypertonic Labor

Maternal risks of hypertonic labor include the following:

- Increased discomfort due to uterine muscle cell anoxia
- Fatigue as the pattern continues and no labor progress results
- Stress on coping abilities
- Dehydration and increased incidence of infection if labor is prolonged

Fetal-neonatal risks include the following:

- Nonreassuring fetal status because contractions and increased resting tone interfere with the uteroplacental exchange of gases and nutrients
- Prolonged pressure on the fetal head, which may result in cephalohematoma, caput succedaneum, or excessive molding (Figure 22–2 ●)

Clinical Therapy

Management of hypertonic labor may include bed rest and sedation to promote relaxation and reduce pain. Often pharmacologic intervention to promote sedation will stop these contractions. If the hypertonic pattern continues and develops into a prolonged latent phase, oxytocin (Pitocin) infusion or amniotomy may be considered (see "Care of the Woman During Labor Induction" in Chapter 23∞). These methods are instituted only after cephalopelvic disproportion (CPD) and fetal malpresentation have been ruled out. If the maternal pelvic diameters are less than average, or if the fetus is particularly large or is in a malpresentation or malposition, CPD is said to be present. In such cases, labor is not stimulated because vaginal birth is not possible. Instead a cesarean birth will be performed.

> **Nursing Practice**
>
> To determine whether the fetal heart rate (FHR) is reassuring, look for the following: baseline FHR of 110 to 160 bpm, presence of variability, and spontaneous accelerations.

NURSING MANAGEMENT

NURSING ASSESSMENT AND DIAGNOSIS

As part of the labor assessment, evaluate the relationship between the intensity of the pain being experienced and the degree to which the cervix is dilating and effacing. Also note whether anxiety is negatively affecting labor progress. Evidence of increasing frustration and discouragement on the part of the mother and her partner may indicate the need to provide some additional information or assurance. Monitor the fetus closely for signs of nonreassuring fetal status.

Nursing diagnoses that may apply to the woman in hypertonic labor include the following:

- *Fatigue* related to inability to relax and rest secondary to a hypertonic labor pattern
- *Ineffective Individual Coping* related to ineffectiveness of breathing techniques to relieve discomfort
- *Anxiety* related to slow labor progress

PLANNING AND IMPLEMENTATION

A key nursing responsibility is to provide comfort and support to the laboring woman and her partner. The woman experiencing a hypertonic labor pattern will probably be very uncomfortable because of the increased force of contractions. Her anxiety level and that of her partner may be high. Work to reduce the woman's discomfort and promote a more effective labor pattern.

Suggest supportive measures such as a change of position: left lateral side-lying, high Fowler's, or on her knees in the bed with her arms up around the top of the bed while it is in high Fowler's, rocking in a rocking chair, sitting up, and walking. It may be helpful to offer soothing measures such as a quiet environment, use of music the woman finds calming, back rubs, therapeutic touch, and visualization, as well as comfort measures such as mouth care, change of linens, effleurage, and relaxation exercises. The use of tub baths or a warm shower can help promote comfort and uterine relaxation. If sedation is ordered, ensure that the environment is conducive to relaxation. The labor partner may also need assistance in helping the woman cope. A calm, understanding approach offers the woman and her partner further support. Providing information about the cause of the hypertonic labor pattern and assuring the woman that she is not overreacting to the situation are important nursing actions.

Client education is key for the woman experiencing hypertonic labor. She needs information about the dysfunctional labor pattern and the possible implications for her and her baby. Information will help relieve anxiety and thereby increase relaxation and comfort. Explain treatment options and offer opportunities to ask questions.

EVALUATION

Expected outcomes of nursing care include the following:

- The woman has increased comfort and decreased anxiety.
- The woman and her partner are able to cope with the labor.
- The woman experiences a more effective labor pattern.

HYPOTONIC LABOR PATTERNS

A hypotonic labor pattern usually develops in the active phase of labor, after labor has been well established. Hypotonic labor is characterized by fewer than two to three contractions in a 10-minute period (see Figure 22–1C). Hypotonic labor may occur when the uterus is overstretched from a twin gestation, or in the presence of a large fetus, hydramnios, or grand multiparity. Bladder or bowel distention and CPD may also be associated with this pattern.

Thinking Critically

FETAL HEART RATE TRACING

A fetal heart rate (FHR) tracing demonstrates the following: baseline heart rate of 140 with variability of 6 to 10 beats per minute (bpm). When you compare the FHR with the uterine contractions, you note that there is a slowing of the FHR at the time of the contraction and that the FHR tracing looks like the contraction curve, but it is upside down. Based on this tracing, what would you do?

See MyNursingKit for possible responses.

Risks of Hypotonic Labor

Maternal implications of hypotonic labor patterns include the following risks:

- Maternal exhaustion
- Stress on coping abilities
- Postpartum hemorrhage from insufficient uterine contractions following birth
- Intrauterine infection if labor is prolonged

Fetal-neonatal implications include the following:

- Nonreassuring fetal status due to prolonged labor pattern
- Fetal sepsis from pathogens that ascend from the birth canal

Clinical Therapy

The goals of clinical therapy are to improve the quality of the uterine contractions and to ensure a safe outcome for the woman and her baby. Uterine contractions can be stimulated in several ways, including the use of Pitocin, amniotomy, or stimulation of the nipples, which causes the release of oxytocin. Before initiating treatment for hypotonic labor, the physician or certified nurse-midwife (CNM) validates the adequacy of pelvic measurements and completes tests to establish gestational age if fetal maturity is in question. After CPD, fetal malpresentation, and fetal immaturity have been ruled out, Pitocin may be given intravenously (IV) via an infusion pump to improve the quality of uterine contractions. Intravenous fluid is useful to maintain adequate hydration and prevent maternal exhaustion. Amniotomy may be used to stimulate the labor process. The application of an electric breast pump or manual stimulation of the nipples may help strengthen uterine contractions, and is an excellent starting point for women who want an unmedicated birth.

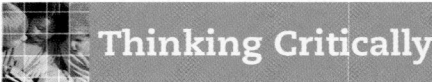

Some physicians support the use of *active management of labor (AMOL)*, a process whereby labor is managed from the beginning with amniotomy, timed cervical examinations are performed, and augmentation of labor with IV administration of Pitocin is begun if a specified level of progress is not met. Supporters of AMOL contend that it is a preventive treatment that reduces the chance for protracted labor and decreases the cesarean birth rate. Opponents argue that the use of AMOL increases the incidence of infection (because of frequent vaginal examinations), necessitates the use of additional interventions, and increases the incidence of instrument-assisted births (Albers, 2007).

An improvement in the quality of uterine contractions is demonstrated by noticeable progress in the labor. If the labor pattern does not become effective or if other complications develop, further interventions, including cesarean birth, may be necessary.

NURSING MANAGEMENT

NURSING ASSESSMENT AND DIAGNOSIS

Assessment of contractions (for frequency, intensity, and duration), maternal vital signs, and FHR provides data to evaluate maternal-fetal status. Also be alert for signs and symptoms of infection and dehydration. Because of the stress associated with a prolonged labor, observe the woman and her partner's success in implementing coping mechanisms.

Nursing diagnoses that may apply to the woman in hypotonic labor include the following:

- *Acute Pain* related to uterine contractions secondary to dysfunctional labor
- *Ineffective Individual Coping* related to unanticipated discomfort and slow progress in labor
- *Fatigue* related to prolonged labor and discomfort

PLANNING AND IMPLEMENTATION

Nursing measures to promote maternal-fetal physical well-being include frequent monitoring of contractions, maternal vital signs, and FHR. If amniotic membranes are ruptured, assess for the presence of meconium, which makes close observation of fetal status more critical because it often indicates that the fetus is experiencing some form of stress. An intake and output record provides a way of determining maternal hydration or dehydration. Encourage the woman to void every 2 hours, and check her bladder for distention. Because labor may be prolonged, continue to monitor the woman for signs of infection (elevated temperature, chills, foul-smelling amniotic fluid, and fetal tachycardia). Vaginal examinations should be kept to a minimum to decrease the risk of introducing an infection.

Women experiencing a hypotonic labor pattern require emotional support. Help the couple cope with the frustration of a lengthy labor process. Combine a warm, caring approach with techniques to reduce anxiety and discomfort.

The teaching plan needs to include information about the dysfunctional labor process and implications for the mother and baby. Disadvantages of and alternatives to treatment also need to be discussed and understood.

EVALUATION

Expected outcomes of nursing care include the following:

- The woman maintains comfort during labor.
- The woman understands the type of labor pattern that is occurring and the treatment plan.

CARE OF THE WOMAN EXPERIENCING PRECIPITOUS LABOR

Precipitous labor is labor that lasts less than 3 hours and results in rapid birth. Contributing factors in precipitous labor are multiparity, large pelvis, previous precipitous labor, a small fetus in a favorable position, and recent maternal cocaine use. One or more of these factors, plus strong contractions, result in a rapid descent of the infant through the birth canal.

Precipitous labor and precipitous birth are not the same. A precipitous birth is an unexpected, sudden, and often unattended birth. (See Chapter 19∞.)

RISKS OF PRECIPITOUS LABOR

Maternal risks of precipitous labor include the following:

- Loss of coping abilities
- Lacerations of the cervix, vagina, and perineum due to rapid descent and birth of the fetus
- Postpartum hemorrhage due to undetected lacerations or inadequate uterine contractions after birth

Fetal-neonatal implications include the following:

- Nonreassuring fetal status or hypoxia from decreased uteroplacental circulation due to intense uterine contractions
- Cerebral trauma from rapid descent through the birth canal
- Brachial plexus injuries from rapid descent and uncontrolled birth

CLINICAL THERAPY

Any woman with a history of precipitous labor requires close monitoring in the last few weeks of pregnancy. If the cervix softens and begins to dilate, the woman may be scheduled for immediate induction of labor.

NURSING MANAGEMENT

NURSING ASSESSMENT AND DIAGNOSIS

During the intrapartum nursing assessment, identify a woman at increased risk of precipitous labor (e.g., a previous history of precipitous or short labor places the woman at risk as does recent cocaine use). During labor the presence of one or both of the following factors may indicate potential problems:

- Accelerated cervical dilatation (more than 2 cm/hr in multigravidas and more than 1.2 cm/hr in primigravidas) and fetal descent
- Intense uterine contractions with little uterine relaxation between contractions

Nursing diagnoses that may apply to the woman with precipitous labor include the following:

- *Risk for Injury* related to rapid labor and birth
- *Acute Pain* related to rapid labor process

PLANNING AND IMPLEMENTATION

If the woman has a history of precipitous labor, monitor her closely and keep an emergency birth pack at hand. Stay in constant attendance if possible and promote comfort and rest by assisting the woman to a comfortable position, providing a quiet environment, and administering sedatives as needed. Give information and support before and after the birth.

To avoid possible precipitous labor and hyperstimulation of the uterus during Pitocin administration, be alert to the dangers of Pitocin overdosage (see "Drug Guide: Oxytocin" in Chapter 23∞). If the woman receiving Pitocin develops an accelerated labor pattern, the Pitocin is discontinued immediately, and the woman is turned on her left side to improve uterine perfusion. Oxygen may be administered to increase the available oxygen in the maternal circulating blood, which in turn increases the amount available for exchange at the placental site. The fetus is monitored for signs of hypoxia and other indications of nonreassuring fetal status such as late decelerations, loss of variability, or change in the FHR baseline rate.

EVALUATION

Expected outcomes of nursing care include the following:

- The woman and her baby are closely monitored during labor, and a safe birth occurs.
- The woman maintains optimal comfort.

CARE OF THE WOMAN WITH PROLONGED (POSTTERM) PREGNANCY

A **prolonged (postterm) pregnancy** is one that extends more than 294 days or 42 weeks past the first day of the last menstrual period (LMP). It is distinct from a *postdate* pregnancy, which means that the pregnancy has gone beyond the estimated date of birth (EDB) at 40 weeks. Approximately 4% to 19% of pregnancies reach or exceed 42 completed weeks but only 2% to 7% reach 43 completed weeks (Divon, 2007). The cause of true postterm pregnancy is unknown, but it seems to occur more frequently in primigravidas, women with a history of prolonged pregnancy, and in the presence of fetal anencephaly or placental sulfatase deficiency (Divon, 2007).

RISKS OF PROLONGED PREGNANCY

Maternal risks associated with prolonged pregnancy include the following (Blackburn, 2007):

- Probable labor induction
- Increased risk for large-for-gestational-age (LGA) infant and resultant perineal trauma
- Increased incidence of forceps-assisted, vacuum-assisted, or cesarean birth
- Increased psychologic stress as the due date passes and concern for the baby increases
- Increased risk of infection

Fetal risks include the following (Blackburn, 2007):

- Decreased perfusion from the placenta
- Oligohydramnios (decreased amount of amniotic fluid), which increases the risk of cord compression
- Meconium aspiration (aspiration of meconium-stained amniotic fluid by the fetus at the time of birth), which is more likely if oligohydramnios and thick meconium are present
- Low 5-minute Apgar score

Some fetuses continue to grow beyond the 42nd week of pregnancy and can be excessively large at birth (macrosomia). In other cases the intrauterine environment becomes unfavorable for growth, uteroplacental insufficiency occurs, and at birth the infant has lost muscle mass and subcutaneous fat. This is known as *dysmaturity syndrome*. The macrosomic fetus is at risk for birth trauma, whereas the small-for-gestational-age (SGA) fetus is at risk for nonreassuring fetal status during labor because there is often associated oligohydramnios (Blackburn, 2007).

CLINICAL THERAPY

In managing prolonged pregnancy, some caregivers prefer induction at 41 weeks; others advocate expectant management by doing a nonstress test (NST) and biophysical profile (BPP) (especially the amniotic fluid volume portion of the BPP – the amniotic fluid index) two to three times a week to evaluate fetal well-being (Carey & Gibbs, 2008). If the fetal assessment tests indicate a problem, interventions are begun to accomplish the birth.

NURSING MANAGEMENT

NURSING ASSESSMENT AND DIAGNOSIS

When the woman is admitted into the birthing area, ongoing assessments of fetal well-being begin as soon as the postterm condition has been verified. Identify reassuring FHR characteristics and evaluate for the presence of nonreassuring patterns, such as non-

Evidence-Based Nursing

INTERVENTIONS FOR POSTTERM PREGNANCY

Clinical Question
When is intervention warranted in a postterm pregnancy?

The Evidence
Three authors conducted systematic reviews of research literature regarding postterm pregnancy complications and recommendations for intervention. This represents the strongest level of evidence. The continuation of pregnancy beyond 41 weeks poses an increased risk of adverse outcomes for both baby and mother. Postterm stillbirths account for more perinatal deaths than prematurity. A range of neonatal morbidities is associated with postterm pregnancy, including fetal distress, birth injury, and meconium aspiration syndrome. Complications for mothers include prolonged labor, cephalopelvic disproportion, perineal lacerations, and hemorrhage. The rates of postterm pregnancy complications are dropping, but this is likely a result of better methods for dating pregnancy and not better interventions.

Best Practice
Establishing an accurate gestational age should occur as early as possible during pregnancy. Routine use of ultrasound for dating significantly reduces the incidence of postterm pregnancy. Tests of fetal health are recommended after 42 weeks' gestation, but no specific method of testing fetal health has been found to be superior to other methods. Birth, either via induction or cesarean, is indicated when the risks associated with continuing the pregnancy are greater than those presented from the birth method. Favorable outcomes have been reported when birth is accomplished at 41 weeks of dated gestation (Caughey, A., Engovskikh, V., & Norwitz, E. 2008).

Critical Thinking
What is the best way to counsel a mother whose pregnancy has passed 40 weeks but who is hesitant to undergo induction or cesarean? How can the nurse support the mother's autonomy while encouraging a decision that will maximize the health of both baby and mother?

See MyNursingKit for possible responses.

periodic variable decelerations (which may indicate cord compression or oligohydramnios), so that corrective actions can be taken. When the amniotic membranes rupture, assess the fluid for meconium. In addition, assess the woman's knowledge about the condition, implications for her baby, risks, and possible interventions.

Nursing diagnoses that may apply to the woman with postterm pregnancy include the following:

- *Fear* related to the unknown outcome for the baby
- *Ineffective Individual Coping* related to anxiety about the status of the baby

PLANNING AND IMPLEMENTATION

NURSING CARE IN THE COMMUNITY

If the woman has not been assessing fetal movement every day, teach her how to do so. It is vital to stress the importance of identifying inadequate fetal movement and immediately contacting her healthcare provider. (See "Fetal Activity Monitoring" in Chapter 11 for further discussion of techniques to detect fetal movement.)

Client education about the postterm pregnancy is another important nursing responsibility. Address the implications and associated risks for the baby, as well as possible treatment plans. The woman and her partner need opportunities to ask questions and clarify information.

HOSPITAL-BASED NURSING CARE

Promoting fetal well-being requires careful assessment of the response of the fetus during labor. If oligohydramnios exists, obtain a continuous FHR tracing and evaluate it frequently. Variable decelerations are often associated with oligohydramnios because the decreased amount of fluid may allow compression of the umbilical cord. If the fetus is macrosomic, carefully assess labor progress (contraction characteristics, progressive cervical dilatation, and fetal descent).

Emotional support is a key nursing intervention for women with pregnancies that extend past the due date. Women experiencing postterm pregnancy frequently feel increased stress and anxiety and have difficulty coping. Encouragement, support, and recognition of the woman's anxiety are helpful strategies.

EVALUATION

Expected outcomes of nursing care include the following:

- The woman has knowledge about the postterm pregnancy.
- The woman and her partner feel supported and able to cope with the postterm pregnancy.
- Fetal status is maintained, any abnormalities are quickly identified, and supportive measures are initiated.

CARE OF THE WOMAN AND FETUS AT RISK BECAUSE OF FETAL MALPOSITION

Persistent occiput posterior (POP) position is the most common fetal malposition and occurs when the fetus does not rotate but is born in the OP position. This position may be normal in women with small pelvises. It may also be related to poor contractions, abnormal flexion of the head, inadequate maternal pushing efforts usually related to epidural anesthesia, or a large fetus. Labor may be prolonged; however, most POP fetuses are born without the aid of forceps.

RISKS OF FETAL MALPOSITION

Maternal risks related to the persistent POP position include the following:

- Risk of third- or fourth-degree perineal lacerations during birth
- Risk of extension of a midline episiotomy

Fetal implications do not include an increased mortality risk unless labor is prolonged or additional interventions such as forceps-assisted, vacuum-assisted, or cesarean birth are required.

CLINICAL THERAPY

Clinical treatment focuses on close monitoring of maternal and fetal status and labor progress to determine whether vaginal or cesarean birth is the safer method. A cesarean birth is chosen if maternal or fetal problems make a vaginal birth unwise or if CPD is present. The majority of POP fetuses are born vaginally, either spontaneously or with the assistance of forceps. The forceps can be used to assist in the birth of the fetus while it is still in the occiput posterior position or to rotate the occiput to an anterior position (called Scanzoni's maneuver). (See Chapter 23∞ for further discussion of forceps.)

NURSING MANAGEMENT

NURSING ASSESSMENT AND DIAGNOSIS

Signs and symptoms of a POP position include complaints of intense back pain by the laboring woman, a dysfunctional labor pattern, hypotonic labor (the fetal head does not put adequate pressure on the cervix), arrest of dilatation, or arrest of fetal descent. The back pain is caused by the fetal occiput compressing the sacral nerves. Further assessment may reveal a depression in the maternal abdomen above the symphysis. FHR is typically heard far laterally on the abdomen. On vaginal examination the physician or CNM finds the wide, diamond-shaped anterior fontanelle in the anterior portion of the pelvis. This fontanelle may be difficult to feel because of molding of the fetal head.

Nursing diagnoses that may apply to women with POP position fetuses include the following:

- *Acute Pain* related to back discomfort secondary to the OP position
- *Ineffective Individual Coping* related to unanticipated discomfort and slow progress in labor

PLANNING AND IMPLEMENTATION

Changing maternal posture has been used for many years to enhance rotation of OP or occiput transverse (OT) to OA. A number of position changes may be tried. For instance, the woman may be asked to lie on one side and then asked to move to the other side as the fetus begins to rotate. This side-lying position may promote rotation; it also enables the support person to apply counterpressure on the sacral area to decrease discomfort. A knee-chest position provides a downward slant to the vaginal canal, directing the fetal head downward on descent. A hands-and-knees position is often effective in rotating the fetus. In addition to maintaining a hands-and-knees position on the bed, the woman may try pelvic rocking, and the support person may firmly stroke the abdomen. The stroking begins over the fetal back and swings around to the other side of the abdomen. After the fetus has rotated, the woman lies in a Sims' position on the side opposite the fetal back.

EVALUATION

Expected outcomes of nursing care include the following:

- The woman's discomfort is decreased.
- The coping abilities of the woman and her partner are strengthened.

CARE OF THE WOMAN AND FETUS AT RISK BECAUSE OF FETAL MALPRESENTATION

In a normal presentation, the occiput is the presenting part (Figure 22–3A ●). *Fetal malpresentations* include brow, face, breech, shoulder (transverse lie), and compound presentation.

BROW PRESENTATION

In a *brow presentation*, the forehead of the fetus becomes the presenting part. In the *military presentation*, the fetal head is between flexion and extension (Figure 22–3B), whereas in the *occipitomental presentation*, the fetal head enters the birth canal with the widest diameter of the head (approximately 13.5 cm) foremost (Figure 22–3C).

The brow presentation occurs more often in multiparas than in nulliparas and is thought to be due to lax abdominal and pelvic musculature. Many brow presentations spontaneously convert to face or occipital presentations. Brow presentations are the least common types of abnormal presentations.

Risks of Brow Presentation

Maternal implications of brow presentation include increased risk of the following:

- Longer labor due to ineffective contractions and slow or arrested fetal descent
- Cesarean birth if brow presentation persists

Fetal-neonatal risks include increased mortality because of cerebral and neck compression and damage to the trachea and larynx. In addition, facial edema, bruising, and exaggerated molding of the newborn's head may be observed.

Clinical Therapy

If a brow presentation fails to convert to occipital or face presentation, cesarean birth is indicated in most cases (Lanni & Seeds,

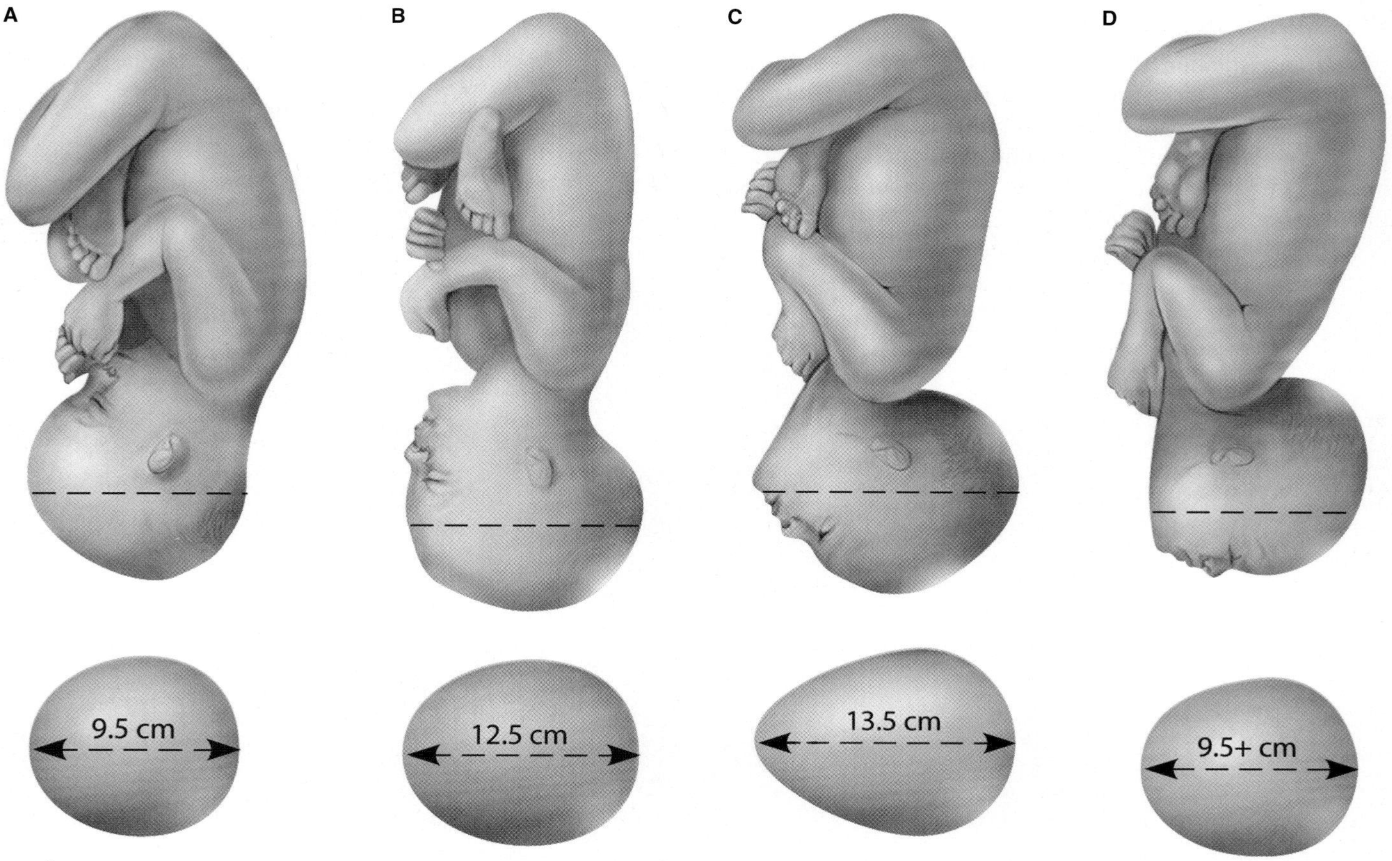

● **Figure 22–3** Types of cephalic presentations. ***A,*** The occiput is the presenting part because the head is flexed and the fetal chin is against the chest. The largest anteroposterior (AP) diameter that presents and passes through the pelvis is approximately 9.5 cm. ***B,*** Military presentation. The head is neither flexed nor extended. The presenting AP diameter is approximately 12.5 cm. ***C,*** Brow presentation. The largest diameter of the fetal head (approximately 13.5 cm) presents in this situation. ***D,*** Face presentation. The AP diameter is 9.5 cm.

Source: Used with permission from Danforth, D. N., & Scott, J. R. (Eds.). (1990). Obstetrics and gynecology *(5th ed., p. 170, fig. 8–9). New York: Lippincott.*

2007). If a vaginal birth is attempted, the woman is closely monitored for CPD, facial edema, and nonreassuring fetal status. Attempts to convert brow presentations manually or through the use of forceps or vacuum are contraindicated, as is the use of oxytocin. The use of oxytocin can result in dystocia. Scalp electrodes should not be placed when the fetus is in a brow presentation (Family Practice Notebook, 2007)

NURSING MANAGEMENT

NURSING ASSESSMENT AND DIAGNOSIS

A brow presentation can be detected on vaginal examination by palpation of the diamond-shaped anterior fontanelle on one side and orbital ridges and root of the nose on the other side.

Nursing diagnoses that may apply to a woman with a brow presentation include the following:

- *Health-Seeking Behaviors* related to lack of information about the possible maternal-fetal effects of brow presentation
- *Risk for Injury* to the fetus related to pressure on fetal structures secondary to brow presentation

PLANNING AND IMPLEMENTATION

Closely observe the woman for labor problems and the fetus for signs of hypoxia as evidenced by late decelerations and bradycardia. Provide emotional support to the family. Explain the fetal position to the woman and her support person or interpret what the physician or CNM has told them. Stay close at hand to reassure the couple, inform them of any changes, and assist them with labor-coping techniques. In face and brow presentations, the newborn's face may be edematous. The couple may need help in beginning the attachment process because of the newborn's facial appearance. After the infant is inspected for any abnormalities, the pediatrician and nurse can assure the couple that the facial edema is only temporary and will subside in 3 or 4 days and that the molding will be much less visible in a few days (even though completion of the process takes several weeks).

EVALUATION

Expected outcomes of nursing care include the following:

- The woman and her partner understand the implications and associated problems of brow presentation.
- The mother and her baby have a safe labor and birth.

FACE PRESENTATION

In a face presentation, the face of the fetus is the presenting part (Figure 22–3D and Figure 22–4 ●). The fetal head is hyperextended even more than in the brow presentation. Face presentation occurs most frequently in multiparas, in preterm birth, and in the presence of anencephaly. The incidence of face presentation is about 1 in 600 births.

Risks of Face Presentation

Maternal risks related to face presentation include the following:

- Increased risk of CPD and prolonged labor
- Increased risk of infection (with prolonged labor)
- Cesarean birth if fetal chin is posterior (mentum posterior)

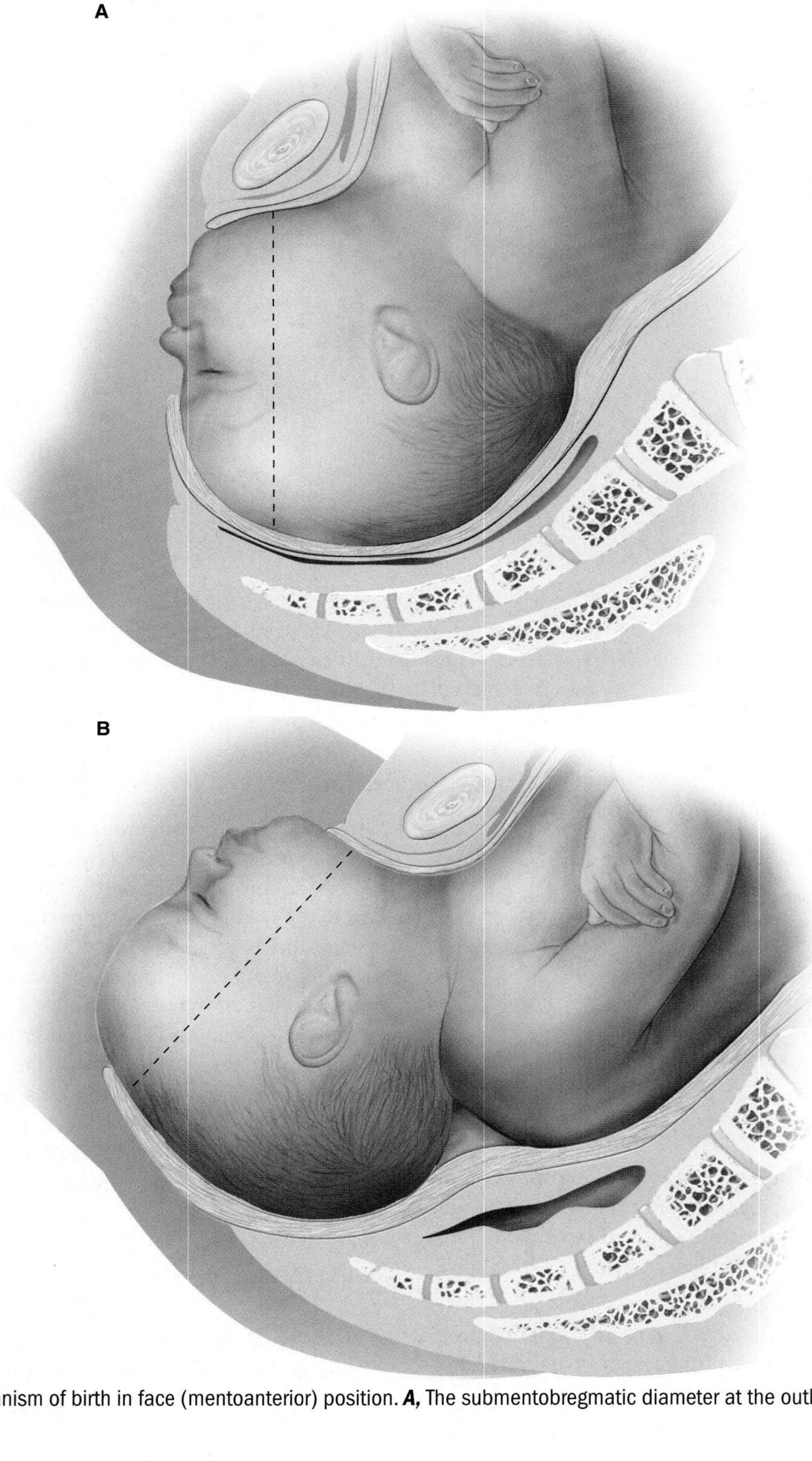

● **Figure 22–4** Mechanism of birth in face (mentoanterior) position. ***A,*** The submentobregmatic diameter at the outlet. ***B,*** The fetal head is born by the movement of flexion.

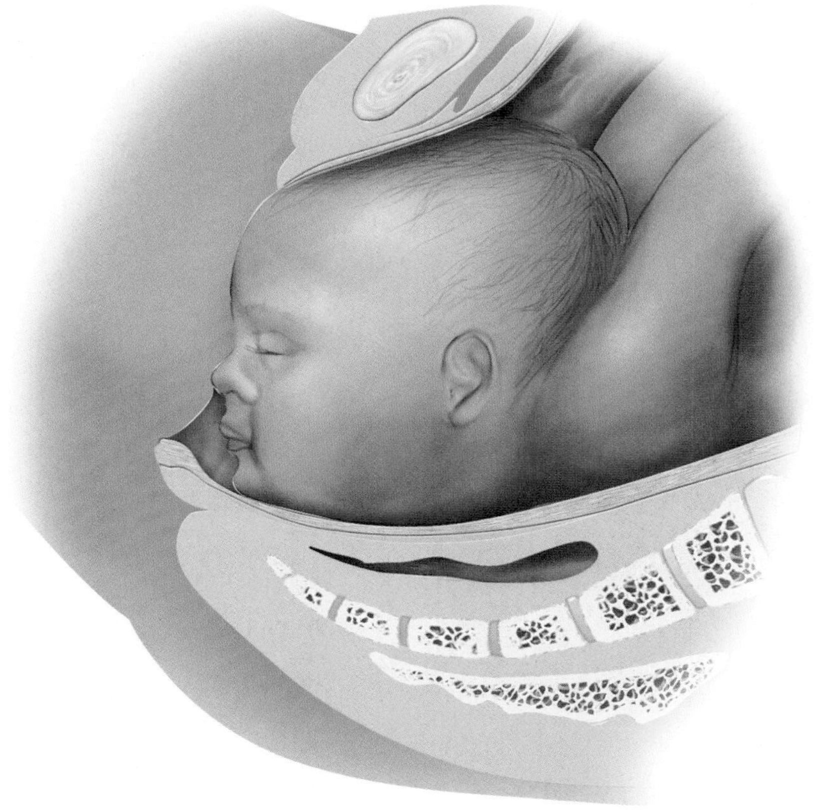

● **Figure 22–5** Face presentation. Mechanism of birth in mentoposterior position. Fetal head is unable to extend farther. The face becomes impacted.

Fetal-neonatal risks include the following:

- Cephalohematoma
- Edema of the face and throat if the fetal chin is anterior (mentum anterior)
- Pronounced molding of the head
- Nonreassuring fetal status

Clinical Therapy

A vaginal birth may be anticipated if no CPD is present, the chin (mentum) is anterior, the labor pattern is effective, and the fetal status is reassuring. Many mentum posterior presentations spontaneously convert to anterior in the late stages of labor. If the mentum remains posterior, a vaginal birth is not possible and a cesarean birth is necessary (Figure 22–5 ●).

NURSING MANAGEMENT

NURSING ASSESSMENT AND DIAGNOSIS

When performing Leopold's maneuvers, the back of the fetus is difficult to outline with a face presentation, and a deep furrow can be palpated between the hard occiput and the fetal back (Figure 22–6 ●). Fetal heart tones are audible on the side where the fetal feet are palpated. It may be difficult to determine by vaginal examination whether a breech or face is presenting, especially if facial edema is already present. During the vaginal examination, palpation of the saddle of the nose and the gums should be attempted. When assessing engagement, remember that the face has to be deep within the pelvis before the biparietal diameters have entered the inlet.

Nursing diagnoses that may apply to the woman with a fetus in face presentation include the following:

- *Fear* related to unknown outcome of the labor and a possible instrument-assisted or cesarean birth
- *Risk for Injury to the Newborn's Face* related to edema secondary to the birth process

PLANNING AND IMPLEMENTATION

Nursing interventions are the same as those indicated for the brow presentation.

EVALUATION

Expected outcomes of nursing care include the following:

- The woman and her partner understand the implications and associated problems of face presentation.
- The mother and her baby have a safe labor and birth.

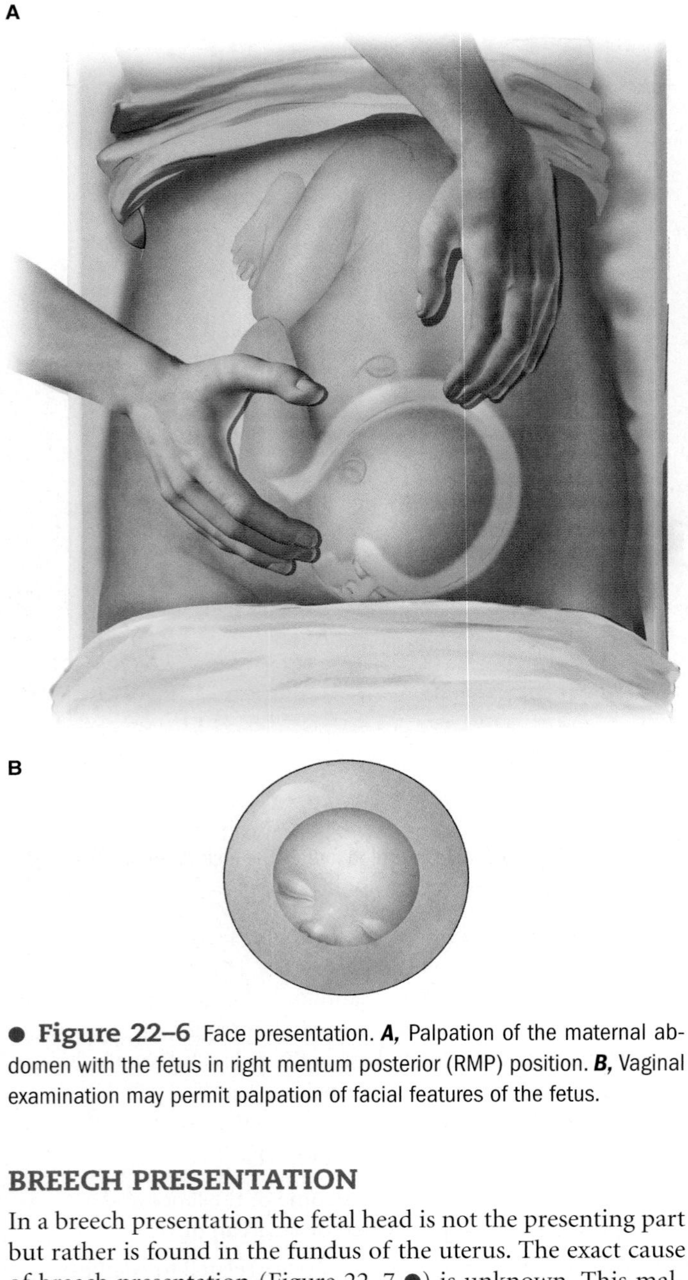

● **Figure 22–6** Face presentation. ***A,*** Palpation of the maternal abdomen with the fetus in right mentum posterior (RMP) position. ***B,*** Vaginal examination may permit palpation of facial features of the fetus.

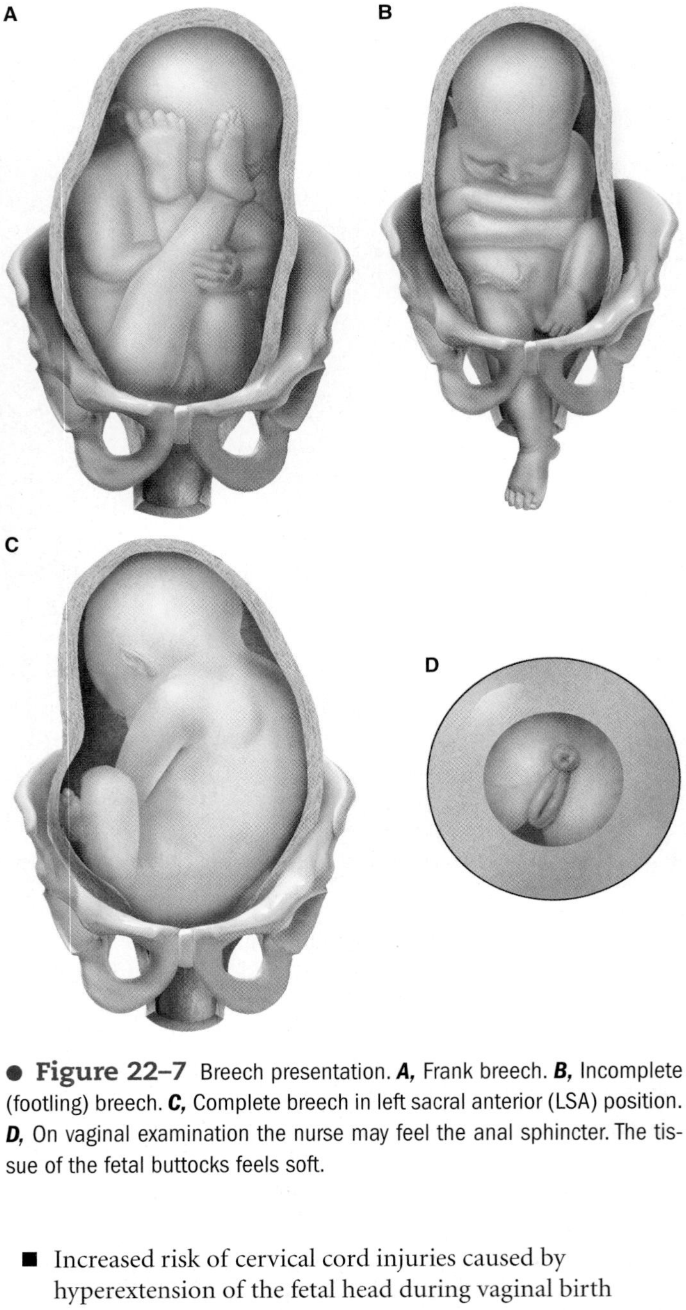

● **Figure 22–7** Breech presentation. ***A,*** Frank breech. ***B,*** Incomplete (footling) breech. ***C,*** Complete breech in left sacral anterior (LSA) position. ***D,*** On vaginal examination the nurse may feel the anal sphincter. The tissue of the fetal buttocks feels soft.

BREECH PRESENTATION

In a breech presentation the fetal head is not the presenting part but rather is found in the fundus of the uterus. The exact cause of breech presentation (Figure 22–7 ●) is unknown. This malpresentation occurs in about 3% to 4% of labors and is frequently associated with preterm birth, placenta previa, hydramnios, multiple gestation, uterine anomalies (such as bicornuate uterus), and fetal anomalies (especially anencephaly and hydrocephaly) (Lanni & Seeds, 2007).

Risks of Breech Presentation

The maternal implication of breech presentation is a likelihood of cesarean birth. Fetal-neonatal implications include the following (Lanni & Seeds, 2007):

- Higher perinatal morbidity and mortality rates
- Increased risk of prolapsed cord, especially in incomplete breeches, because space is available between the cervix and presenting part
- Increased risk of cervical cord injuries caused by hyperextension of the fetal head during vaginal birth
- Increased risk of asphyxia and nonreasssuring fetal status
- Increased risk of birth trauma (especially of the head) during either vaginal or cesarean breech birth

Clinical Therapy

Current clinical therapy is directed toward converting the breech presentation to a cephalic presentation prior to the beginning of labor. Some physicians attempt an external cephalic version (ECV) at 36 to 38 weeks' gestation as long as the woman is not in labor. (See Chapter 23∞ for discussion of external version.) ACOG recommends a planned cesarean birth for the fetus in a breech presentation because of the significant increase in complications associated with breech vaginal births (ACOG, 2006).

NURSING MANAGEMENT

NURSING ASSESSMENT AND DIAGNOSIS

Frequently it is the nurse who first recognizes a breech presentation. On palpation the firm fetal head is felt in the uterine fundus and the wider sacrum in the lower part of the abdomen. If the sacrum has not descended, ballottement causes the entire fetal body to move. Furthermore, FHR is usually auscultated above the umbilicus. Passage of meconium into the amniotic fluid due to compression of the fetus's intestinal tract is common.

If membranes are ruptured, be particularly alert for a prolapsed umbilical cord, especially in footling breeches, because there is space between the cervix and presenting part through which the cord can slip. If the infant is small and the membranes rupture, the danger is even greater. The risk of a prolapsed umbilical cord is one reason any woman with ruptured membranes should not ambulate until a full assessment, including vaginal examination, has been performed.

Nursing diagnoses that may apply to a woman with a breech presentation include the following:

- *Impaired Gas Exchange in the Fetus* related to interruption in umbilical blood flow secondary to compression of the cord
- *Health-Seeking Behaviors* related to lack of information about the implications and associated complications of breech presentation for the mother and fetus

PLANNING AND IMPLEMENTATION

During labor, promote maternal-fetal physical well-being by frequently assessing fetal and maternal status. Since the fetus is at increased risk for prolapse of the cord, agency protocols may call for continuous fetal monitoring. If the head is not completely engaged, continuous monitoring is warranted and the woman should maintain complete bed rest. Provide teaching and information about the breech presentation and the nursing care needed.

Most physicians perform cesarean births because of the increased fetal risks associated with breech vaginal birth. Vaginal birth is more common in multiparous women with a proven pelvis (prior birth of a normal or large size fetus without difficulty). The nurse assists with the vaginal birth by including Piper forceps (used to guide the after-coming fetal head) in the birth table setup. The nurse may assist the physician if forceps are needed for the birth.

Vaginal breech births commonly occur in the operating room with a "double setup" in place. If difficulties arise with the birth, the room is already prepared for a cesarean so the procedure can be performed quickly. If the family and physician or CNM decide on a cesarean birth, provide assistance as with any cesarean birth.

EVALUATION

Expected outcomes of nursing care include the following:

- The woman and her partner understand the implications and associated problems of breech presentation.
- Major complications are recognized early and corrective measures are instituted.
- The mother and baby have a safe labor and birth.

TRANSVERSE LIE (SHOULDER PRESENTATION) OF A SINGLE FETUS

A transverse lie occurs in approximately 1 in 300 term births (Lanni & Seeds, 2007). Maternal conditions associated with a transverse lie are grand multiparity with relaxed uterine muscles, preterm fetus, abnormal uterus, excessive amniotic fluid, placenta previa, and contracted pelvis (Figure 22–8 ●).

Clinical Therapy

The management of shoulder presentation depends on the gestational age. If discovered before term, the management is expectant (watchful), because some fetuses may change presentation without intervention. When a shoulder presentation is still evident at 37 completed weeks of gestation, an external cephalic version (ECV) attempt (followed, if successful, by induction of labor) is recommended, because the associated risk of prolapsed cord is significant. Intrapartum ECV is often successful in early labor and can reduce the need for cesarean birth. If it is unsuccessful, cesarean birth is indicated.

Nursing Management

The nurse can identify a transverse lie by inspection and palpation of the abdomen, by auscultation of FHR, and by vaginal

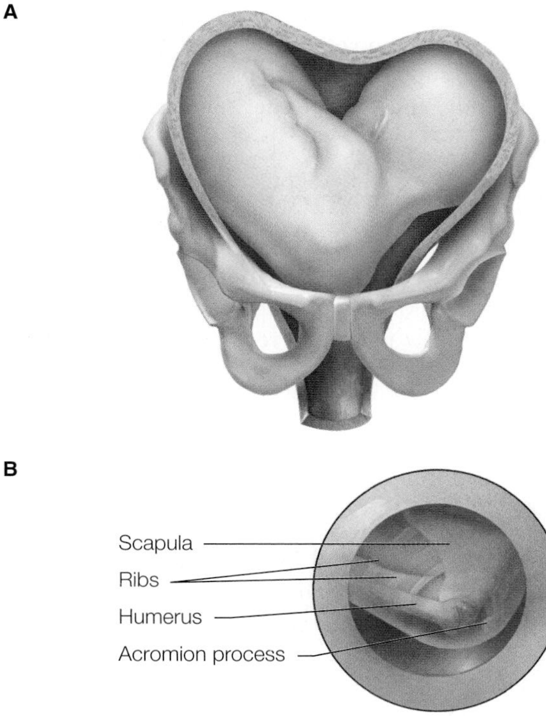

● **Figure 22–8** Transverse lie. ***A,*** Shoulder presentation. ***B,*** On vaginal examination the nurse may feel the acromion process as the fetal presenting part.

Complementary Care

MOXIBUSTION TO PROMOTE VERSION IN BREECH PRESENTATIONS

Traditional Chinese medicine uses the herb mugwort in the form of moxa to promote version in a breech presentation. Moxa is a system of treatment, often combined with acupuncture, in which an herb is dried, rolled into cones (like incense cones), and placed on certain meridian points of the body. The moxa is then lit and allowed to burn close to the skin, hence the *bustion* component of the name. The heat and pungency of mugwort stimulates the point, and it is believed that the energy moves through the body and increases fetal activity.

The meridian point that is used in moxibustion to promote version in breech presentation is acupoint BL 67, located beside the outer corner of the fifth toenail. Treatment may take from 7 days to 2 weeks. There is limited evidence suggesting that moxibustion is an effective modality in managing breech presentations (Coyle, Smith, & Peat, 2005).

examination. On inspection the woman's abdomen appears widest from side to side as a result of the long axis of the infant's body lying parallel to the ground and across the mother's uterus.

On palpation no fetal part is felt in the fundal portion of the uterus or above the symphysis. The head may be palpated on one side and the breech on the other. Fetal heart rate is usually auscultated just below the midline of the umbilicus. If a presenting part is palpated on vaginal examination, it is the ridged thorax or possibly an arm compressed against the chest.

Assist in the interpretation of the fetal presentation and provide information and support to the couple. Assess maternal and fetal status frequently, and prepare the woman for a cesarean birth (see Chapter 23).

COMPOUND PRESENTATION

A compound presentation is one in which there are two presenting parts, such as the occiput and fetal hand or the complete breech and fetal hand. Most compound presentations resolve themselves spontaneously, but others require additional manipulation at birth.

CARE OF THE WOMAN AND FETUS AT RISK FOR MACROSOMIA

Fetal **macrosomia** is defined as a birth weight of more than 4500 g (Cunningham, Leveno, Bloom, et al., 2010) (Note: some sources say 4000 g). The condition is more common with prepregnancy maternal obesity, excessive maternal weight gain, maternal diabetes, prior history of macrosomia, a male fetus, grand multiparity, prolonged gestation, and in women of Hispanic ethnic background (Luo & Copel, 2009). Macrosomia is also more common in fetuses who have erythroblastosis fetalis (Mahony, Foley, McAuliffe et al., 2007).

RISKS OF MACROSOMIA

Maternal implications of macrosomia include increased risk of the following:

- CPD
- Dysfunctional labor and prolonged labor
- Soft-tissue laceration during vaginal birth
- Postpartum hemorrhage

Fetal-neonatal implications include increased risk of the following:

- Meconium aspiration
- Asphyxia
- Shoulder dystocia, in which, after birth of the head, the anterior shoulder fails to deliver either spontaneously or with gentle traction (unresolved shoulder dystocia can lead to fetal death)
- Upper brachial plexus injury and fractured clavicles
- Hypoglycemia, polycythemia, and hyperbilirubinemia

CLINICAL THERAPY

The occurrence of maternal and fetal problems associated with excessively large infants may be lessened somewhat by identifying macrosomia before the onset of labor. If a large fetus is suspected, the maternal pelvis should be evaluated carefully. Fetal size can be estimated by palpating the crown-to-rump length of the fetus in utero and by ultrasound or x-ray pelvimetry. Studies indicate that palpation and ultrasound are equally effective assessments of fetal weight. When the uterus appears excessively large, hydramnios, an oversized fetus, or multiple gestation must be considered as the possible cause.

When fetal weight is estimated to be 4500 g or more, a cesarean birth is usually planned. The best method of birth for an estimated fetal weight of 4000 to 4500 g is debatable. The discussion centers primarily on the incidence of shoulder dystocia during vaginal birth and the difficulty in accurately estimating the fetal weight. Unexpected shoulder dystocia during vaginal birth can be a grave problem. As an emergency measure, the physician or CNM may ask the nurse to assist the woman into the McRoberts maneuver (sharp flexion of the thighs toward the hips and abdomen) or to apply gentle suprapubic pressure in an attempt to aid in the birth of the fetal shoulders. Fundal pressure should never be used because it can further wedge the anterior shoulder under the symphysis pubis.

Nursing Management

Assist in identifying women who are at risk for carrying a large fetus and those who exhibit signs of macrosomia. Because these women are prime candidates for dystocia and its complications, frequently assess the FHR for indications of nonreassuring fetal status and evaluate the rates of cervical dilatation and fetal descent.

Apply the fetal monitor for continuous fetal evaluation. Early decelerations (caused by fetal head compression) could mean size disproportion at the bony inlet. Report any sign of labor dysfunction or nonreassuring fetal status to the physician or CNM immediately. Lack of fetal descent is another indicator that should alert the nurse to the possibility that the infant is too large for a vaginal birth.

The nurse provides support for the laboring woman and her partner and information about the implications of macrosomia and possible associated problems. During the birth, continue to provide support and encouragement to the woman or the couple.

Inspect macrosomic newborns after birth for cephalohematoma, Erb's palsy, and fractured clavicles, and inform the nursery staff of any problems so that the newborn can be closely monitored for cerebral, neurologic, and motor problems.

In a woman with a macrosomic fetus, the uterus has been stretched farther than it would have been with an average-sized fetus. The overstretching may lead to contractile problems during labor or after birth. After birth the overstretched uterus may not contract well (uterine atony) and will feel boggy (soft). In this case, uterine hemorrhage is likely. The fundus of the uterus is massaged to stimulate contraction; IV or IM Pitocin may be needed. Monitor maternal vital signs closely for deviations suggestive of shock.

CARE OF THE WOMAN AND FETUS IN THE PRESENCE OF NONREASSURING FETAL STATUS

When the oxygen supply is insufficient to meet the physiologic needs of the fetus, a nonreassuring fetal status may result. This status may be transient or chronic, and may be prompted by a variety of factors. The most common are cord compression and uteroplacental insufficiency, possibly caused by preexisting maternal or fetal disease or placental abnormalities. If the resulting hypoxia persists and metabolic acidosis occurs, the situation could cause permanent damage to or be life threatening for the fetus.

MATERNAL IMPLICATIONS

Indications of nonreassuring fetal status greatly increase the psychologic stress of a laboring woman and her family members. Professional staff members may become so involved in assessing fetal status and initiating corrective measures that they fail to provide the woman and her partner with explanations and emotional support. It is imperative to offer both. In many instances, if birth is not imminent, the woman must undergo cesarean birth. This method of birth may be a source of fear and frustration, too, if the couple prepared for a shared vaginal birth experience.

CLINICAL THERAPY

The most common initial signs of nonreassuring fetal status are variations from the normal heart rate pattern and decreased fetal movement. Meconium-stained amniotic fluid and the presence of ominous FHR patterns such as persistent late decelerations (regardless of the depth of deceleration), persistent and severe variable decelerations (especially if the return to baseline is prolonged), and prolonged decelerations are signs of nonreassuring fetal status. When these patterns are detected, **intrauterine resuscitation** (corrective measures used to optimize the oxygen exchange within the maternal-fetal circulation) should be started without delay.

Treatment of maternal hypotension involves having the woman turn to a left lateral position (right lateral may also be tried), beginning an IV infusion or increasing the flow rate if an infusion is already in place, or, if cord prolapse is suspected, having the woman assume a knee-chest position. Position changes that result in an increase in the fetal heart rate should be maintained. Perform a vaginal examination to attempt to detect a prolapsed cord. Decrease uterine activity by discontinuing IV Pitocin administration or administering a tocolytic agent (such as terbutaline) to decrease contraction frequency and intensity. Administer oxygen to the woman via facial mask.

Caregivers can obtain additional information about the condition of the fetus by fetal scalp blood sampling, fetal scalp stimulation, or fetal acoustic stimulation (see "Fetal Acoustic Stimulation Test" and "Vibroacoustic Stimulation Test" in Chapter 14∞). The management of nonreassuring fetal status is illustrated in Figure 22–9 ●.

Nursing Management

Review the woman's prenatal history and notes the presence of any conditions (such as preeclampsia, diabetes, renal disease, or IUGR) that may be associated with decreased uteroplacental-fetal blood flow. When the membranes rupture, assess the FHR immediately and note the characteristics of the amniotic fluid. As labor progresses, be especially alert to suspicious changes in the FHR. At all times, encourage and support maternal positioning that maximizes utero-placental-fetal blood flow.

MyNursingKit Care Plan Activity: Prevention of Cord Prolapse

CARE OF THE WOMAN AND FETUS WITH A PROLAPSED UMBILICAL CORD

A **prolapsed umbilical cord** results when the umbilical cord precedes the fetal presenting part. When this occurs, pressure is placed on the umbilical cord as it is trapped between the presenting part and the maternal pelvis. Consequently the vessels carrying blood to and from the fetus are compressed (Figure 22–10 ●). Prolapse of the cord may occur with rupture of the membranes if the presenting part is not well engaged in the pelvis.

RISKS OF PROLAPSED UMBILICAL CORD

Although a prolapsed cord does not directly precipitate physical alterations in the woman, her immediate concern for the baby creates enormous stress. The woman may need to deal with some unusual interventions, a cesarean birth, and, in some circumstances, the death of her baby.

For the fetus, compression of the cord results in decreased blood flow and leads to nonreassuring fetal status. If labor is under way, the cord is compressed further with each contraction. If the pressure on the cord is not relieved, the fetus will die.

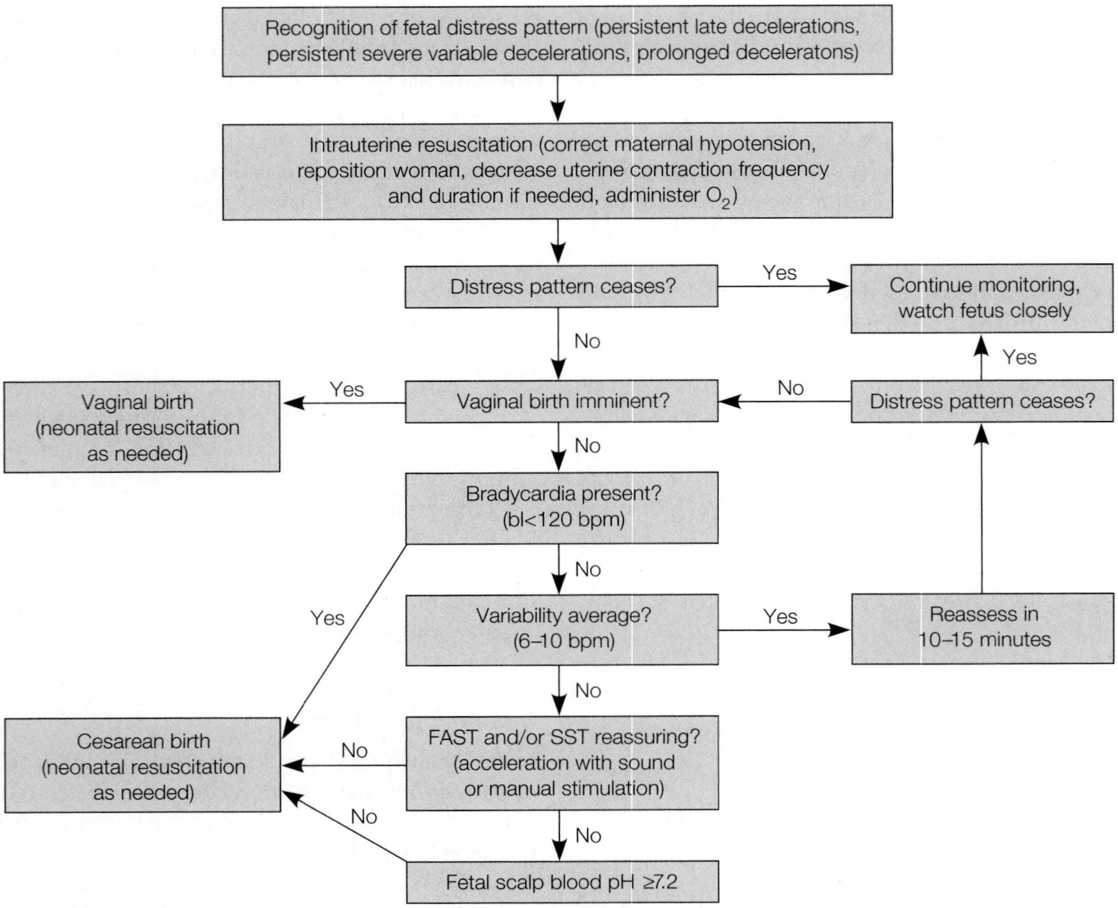
Recognition of fetal distress pattern (persistent late decelerations, persistent severe variable decelerations, prolonged deceleratons)
Intrauterine resuscitation (correct maternal hypotension, reposition woman, decrease uterine contraction frequency and duration if needed, administer O_2)
Distress pattern ceases?
Yes
Continue monitoring, watch fetus closely
No
Yes
Vaginal birth (neonatal resuscitation as needed)
Yes
Vaginal birth imminent?
No
Distress pattern ceases?
No
Bradycardia present? (bl<120 bpm)
No
Yes
Variability average? (6–10 bpm)
Yes
Reassess in 10–15 minutes
No
Cesarean birth (neonatal resuscitation as needed)
No
FAST and/or SST reassuring? (acceleration with sound or manual stimulation)
No
No
Fetal scalp blood pH ≥7.2

● **Figure 22–9** Intrapartum management of nonreassuring fetal status. Note: bl = baseline; FAST = fetal acoustic stimulation test; SST = scalp stimulation test.

Source: Used with permission from Zuspan, F. P., & Quilligan, E. J. Handbook of obstetrics, gynecology, and primary care. Copyright 1998, Mosby. Reprinted with permission from Elsevier Science.

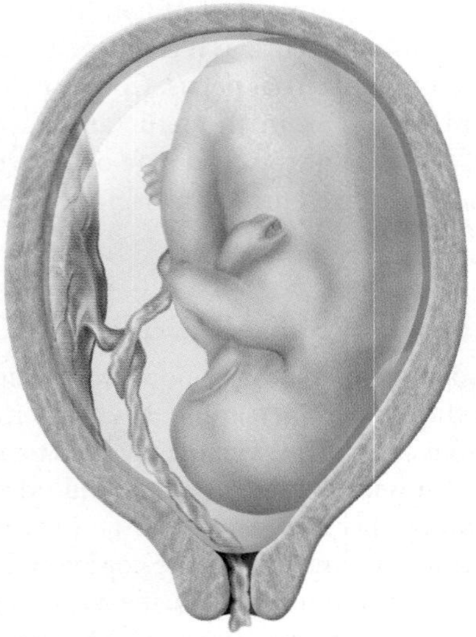

● **Figure 22–10** Prolapse of the umbilical cord.

CLINICAL THERAPY

Preventing prolapse of the cord is the preferred medical approach. A laboring woman with a confirmed rupture of membranes will be kept horizontal, usually in bed, until the fetal head is well engaged and the risk of a prolapse is significantly decreased. If a prolapse occurs, relieving the compression on the cord is critical to fetal outcome. The medical and nursing team must work together to facilitate birth.

Bed rest is indicated for all laboring women with a history of ruptured membranes, until engagement with no cord prolapse has been documented. Furthermore, with spontaneous rupture of membranes or amniotomy, the FHR should be auscultated for at least a full minute and at the beginning and end of contractions for several contractions. If fetal bradycardia is detected on auscultation, perform a vaginal examination to rule out cord prolapse. In the presence of cord prolapse, electronic monitor tracings show severe, moderate, or prolonged variable decelerations with baseline bradycardia.

If a loop of cord is discovered, the examiner's gloved fingers must remain in the vagina to provide firm pressure on the fetal head (to relieve compression) until the physician or CNM arrives. This is a lifesaving measure. Give the mother oxygen via

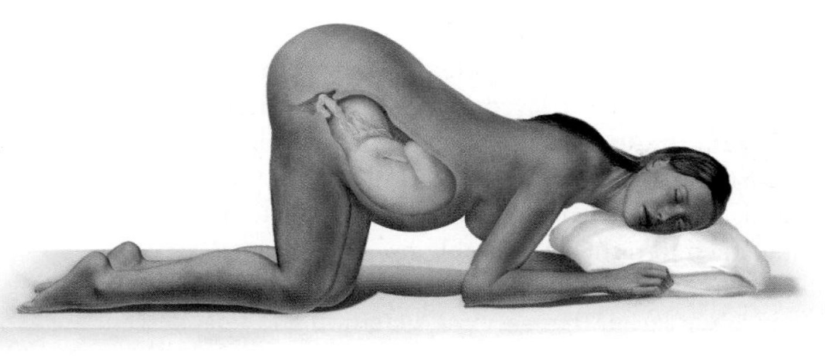

● **Figure 22–11** Knee-chest position is used to relieve cord compression during cord prolapse emergency.

face mask, and monitor the FHR to determine whether the cord compression is adequately relieved.

The force of gravity can be employed to relieve umbilical cord compression. The nurse can instruct the woman to assume the knee-chest position or can adjust the bed to the Trendelenburg position, and transport the woman to the delivery or operating room in this position (Figure 22–11 ●). The cord may be occultly prolapsed with an actual loop extending into the vagina or lying alongside the presenting part. It may be pulsating strongly or so weakly that it is difficult to determine upon palpation of the cord whether the fetus is alive.

NURSING MANAGEMENT

Because there are few outward signs of cord prolapse, each pregnant woman is advised to call her physician or CNM when the membranes rupture and to go to the office, clinic, or birthing facility. Perform a sterile vaginal examination to determine if there is danger of cord prolapse. If the presenting part is well engaged, the risk of cord prolapse is minimal, and the woman may ambulate as desired. If the presenting part is not well engaged, bed rest is recommended to prevent cord prolapse.

Because cord prolapse can be associated with fetal death, some physicians and CNMs insist that bed rest be maintained after rupture of membranes regardless of fetal engagement. This can lead to conflict if the laboring woman and her partner do not hold the same opinions. Ease this situation by helping the physician or CNM and the couple communicate.

During labor any alteration of the FHR or the presence of meconium in the amniotic fluid indicates the need to assess for cord prolapse. Vaginal birth is possible with prolapsed cord if the cervix is completely dilated and pelvic measurements are adequate. If these conditions are not present, cesarean birth is the method of choice.

CARE OF THE WOMAN AND FETUS AT RISK DUE TO AN AMNIOTIC FLUID EMBOLISM

In the presence of a small tear in the amnion or chorion high in the uterus, a small amount of amniotic fluid may leak into the chorionic plate and enter the maternal system as an **amniotic fluid embolism**. The fluid can also enter at areas of placental separation or cervical tears. Under pressure from the contracting uterus, the fluid is driven into the maternal circulation and then the maternal lungs. The more debris in the amniotic fluid (such as meconium), the greater the maternal problems. This condition, although rare, can be catastrophic. Risk factors associated with it include a tumultuous labor, placental abruption, trauma, induction of labor, eclampsia, operative vaginal birth, cesarean birth, and multiple gestation among other things (Gilstrap & Yeomans, 2008).

MATERNAL IMPLICATIONS

The woman with an amniotic fluid embolism experiences sudden onset of respiratory distress, circulatory collapse, acute hemorrhage, and cor pulmonale (failure of the right ventricle) as the embolism blocks the vessels of the lungs. She exhibits dyspnea and cyanosis leading to hemorrhagic shock and coma and may develop seizures. Birth must be facilitated immediately to obtain a live fetus.

CLINICAL THERAPY

Any woman exhibiting chest pain, dyspnea, cyanosis, frothy sputum, tachycardia, hypotension, and massive hemorrhage requires the cooperation of every member of the health team if her life is to be saved. Medical interventions are supportive. Recovery is contingent on return of the mother's cardiovascular and respiratory stability. If necessary, a cesarean birth is performed.

NURSING MANAGEMENT

In the absence of the physician or CNM, the nurse administers oxygen under positive pressure until medical help arrives. An intravenous line is quickly established. If respiratory and cardiac arrest occurs, initiate cardiopulmonary resuscitation (CPR) immediately.

Ready the equipment necessary for blood transfusion and for the insertion of the CVP line. As the blood volume is replaced, using fresh whole blood to provide clotting factors, the CVP must be monitored frequently. In the presence of cor pulmonale, fluid overload could easily occur.

CARE OF THE WOMAN WITH CEPHALOPELVIC DISPROPORTION

The birth passage includes the maternal bony pelvis, beginning at the pelvic inlet and ending at the pelvic outlet, and the maternal soft tissues within these anatomic areas. A contracture (narrowed diameter) in any of the described areas can result in **cephalopelvic disproportion (CPD)** if the fetus is larger than the pelvic diameters. Abnormal fetal presentations and positions occur in CPD as the fetus moves to accommodate its passage through the maternal pelvis.

The gynecoid and anthropoid pelvic types are usually adequate for vertex birth, but the android and platypelloid types are predisposed to CPD. Certain combinations of types also can result in pelvic diameters inadequate for vertex birth. (See Chapter 17∞ or a description of pelvic types and their implications for childbirth.)

TYPES OF CONTRACTURES

The pelvic inlet is contracted if the shortest anterior-posterior diameter is less than 10 cm or the greatest transverse diameter is less than 12 cm. The anterior-posterior diameter may be approximated by measuring the diagonal conjugate, which in the contracted inlet is less than 11.5 cm. Clinical and x-ray pelvimetry are used to determine the smallest anterior-posterior diameter through which the fetal head must pass.

The treatment goal is to allow the natural forces of labor to push the biparietal diameter of the fetal head beyond the potential interspinous obstruction. Although forceps may be used, they cause difficulty because pulling on the head destroys flexion, and the space is further diminished. A bulging perineum and crowning indicate that the obstruction has been passed.

An interischial tuberous diameter of less than 8 cm constitutes an outlet contracture. Outlet and midpelvic contractures frequently occur simultaneously. Whether vaginal birth can occur depends on the woman's interischial tuberous diameters and the fetal posteriosagittal diameter.

RISKS OF CEPHALOPELVIC DISPROPORTION

When CPD is present, the mother experiences prolonged labor. Membrane rupture can result from the force of the unequally distributed contractions being exerted on the fetal membranes. In obstructed labor, in which the fetus cannot descend, uterine rupture can occur. With delayed descent, necrosis of maternal soft tissues can result from pressure exerted by the fetal head. Eventually necrosis can cause fistulas from the vagina to other nearby structures. Difficult, forceps-assisted births can also result in damage to maternal soft tissue.

If the membranes rupture and the fetal head has not entered the inlet, there is a danger of cord prolapse. Excessive molding of the fetal head can result. Traumatic, forceps-assisted birth can damage the fetal skull and central nervous system.

CLINICAL THERAPY

Fetopelvic relationships can be assessed by comparing pelvic measurements obtained by a manual examination before labor and by computed tomography (CT). An estimated weight of the fetus is obtained by ultrasound measurements.

When the pelvic diameters are borderline or questionable, a *trial of labor* (TOL) may be advised. In this process the woman continues to labor, and careful, frequent assessments of cervical dilatation and fetal descent are made. As long as there is continued progress, the TOL continues. If progress ceases, the decision for a cesarean birth is made.

NURSING MANAGEMENT

The adequacy of the maternal pelvis for a vaginal birth should be assessed both during and before labor. During the intrapartum assessment, the size of the fetus and its presentation, position, and lie must also be considered. (See Chapter 18∞ for intrapartum assessment techniques.)

The nurse should suspect CPD when labor is prolonged, cervical dilatation and effacement are slow, and engagement of the presenting part is delayed. The couple may need support in coping with the stresses of this complicated labor. Keep the couple informed of what is happening and explain the procedures being used. This knowledge reassures the couple that measures are being taken to resolve the problem.

Nursing actions during the TOL are similar to care during any labor except that cervical dilatation and fetal descent are assessed more frequently. Both contractions and the fetus should be monitored continuously. Report any signs of nonreassuring fetal status to the physician or CNM immediately.

The mother may be positioned in a variety of ways to increase the pelvic diameters. Sitting or squatting increases the outlet diameters and may be effective when there is failure of, or slow, fetal descent. Changing from one side to the other or maintaining a hands-and-knees position may assist the fetus in the occiput posterior position to change to an occiput anterior position. The mother may instinctively want to assume one of these positions. If not, the nurse can encourage a change of position.

CARE OF THE WOMAN WITH A COMPLICATION OF THE THIRD OR FOURTH STAGE OF LABOR

Common complications of the third and fourth stages of labor include retained placenta, lacerations, and placenta accreta.

RETAINED PLACENTA

Retention of the placenta beyond 30 minutes after birth is termed **retained placenta**. It occurs in 1 in 100 to 1 in 200 vaginal births (Francois & Foley, 2007). Bleeding as a result of a retained placenta can be excessive. If placenta expulsion does not occur, the physician or CNM attempts to remove the placenta manually. In women who do not have an epidural in place, intravenous sedation may be required because of the discomfort caused by the procedure. Failure to retrieve the placenta via manual removal usually necessitates surgical removal by curettage. If the woman does not have an epidural in place, the procedure can be performed under general anesthesia. Retained placenta may be a symptom of an accreta, increta, or percreta (to be discussed shortly).

LACERATIONS

Lacerations of the cervix or vagina may be indicated when bright-red vaginal bleeding persists in the presence of a well-contracted uterus. The incidence of lacerations is higher when the childbearing woman is young or a nullipara, has an epidural, has forceps-assisted birth and an episiotomy, and has not done perineal massage or preparation during pregnancy. Vaginal and perineal lacerations are often categorized in terms of degree, as follows:

- First-degree laceration is limited to the fourchette, perineal skin, and vaginal mucous membrane.

- Second-degree laceration involves the perineal skin, vaginal mucous membrane, underlying fascia, and muscles of the perineal body; it may extend upward on one or both sides of the vagina.
- Third-degree laceration extends through the perineal skin, vaginal mucous membranes, and perineal body and involves the anal sphincter; it may extend up the anterior wall of the rectum.
- Fourth-degree laceration is the same as third-degree but extends through the rectal mucosa to the lumen of the rectum; it may be called a third-degree laceration with a rectal wall extension.

PLACENTA ACCRETA

The chorionic villi attach directly to the myometrium of the uterus in *placenta accreta.* Two other types of placental adherence are *placenta increta,* in which the myometrium is invaded, and *placenta percreta,* in which the myometrium is penetrated. The adherence itself may be total, partial, or focal, depending on the amount of placental involvement. The incidence of placenta accreta is 1 in 533 births (Francois & Foley, 2007). It is the most common type, accounting for almost three-fourths of adherent placentas.

The primary complication with placenta accreta is maternal hemorrhage and failure of the placenta to separate following birth of the infant. An abdominal hysterectomy may be necessary, depending on the amount and depth of involvement.

CARE OF THE WOMAN AND FETUS WITH PLACENTAL PROBLEMS

The most common types of placental problems—placenta previa and abruptio placentae—are discussed in Chapter 21 ∞. Other problems of the placenta are presented in Table 22–1.

CARE OF THE FAMILY EXPERIENCING PERINATAL LOSS

Perinatal loss is death of a fetus or infant from the time of conception through the end of the newborn period 28 days after birth. Spontaneous abortion (miscarriage) in the antepartum period is discussed in Chapter 16 ∞; this section discusses intrauterine fetal death (IUFD) after 20 weeks' gestation, often referred to as *stillbirth* or *fetal demise.*

Table 22–1 Placental and Umbilical Cord Variations

Placental Variation	Maternal Implications	Fetal-Neonatal Implications	
		Succenturiate Placenta	
One or more accessory lobes of fetal villi will develop on the placenta.	Postpartum hemorrhage from retained lobe	None, as long as all parts of the placenta remain attached until after birth of the fetus	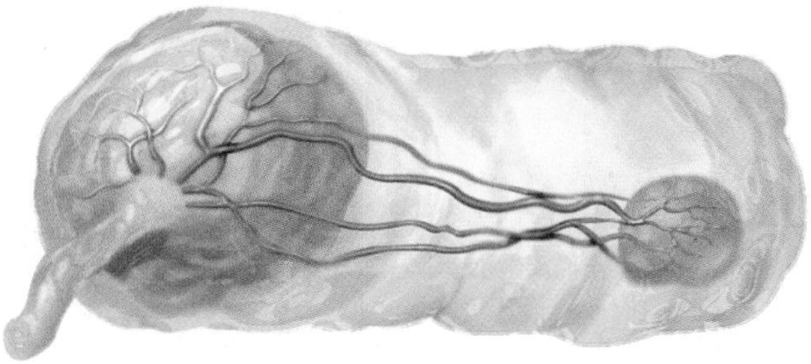
		Circumvallate Placenta	
A double fold of chorion and amnion form a ring around the umbilical cord, on the fetal side of the placenta.	Increased incidence of late abortion, antepartum hemorrhage, and preterm labor	Intrauterine growth restriction, prematurity, fetal death	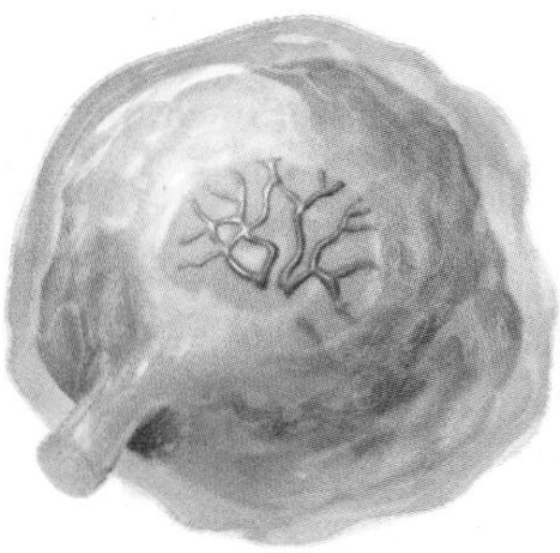

(continued)

Table 22–1 Placental and Umbilical Cord Variations—continued

Placental Variation	Maternal Implications	Fetal-Neonatal Implications	
Battledore Placenta			
The umbilical cord is inserted at or near the placental margin.	Increased incidence of preterm labor and bleeding	Prematurity, nonreassuring fetal status	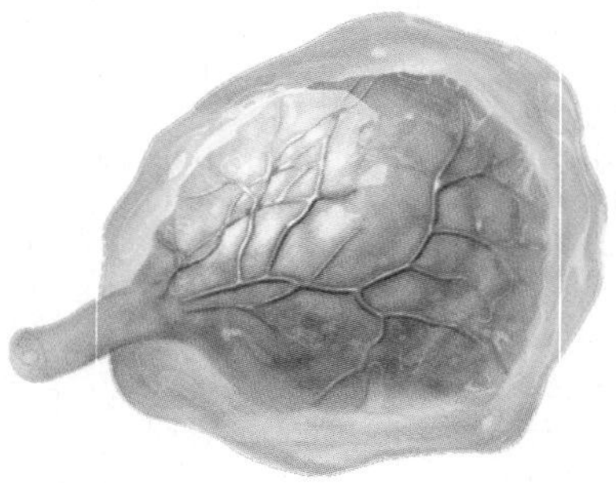
Velamentous Insertion of the Umbilical Cord			
The vessels of the umbilical cord divide some distance from the placenta in the placental membranes.	Hemorrhage if one of the vessels is torn	Nonreassuring fetal status, hemorrhage	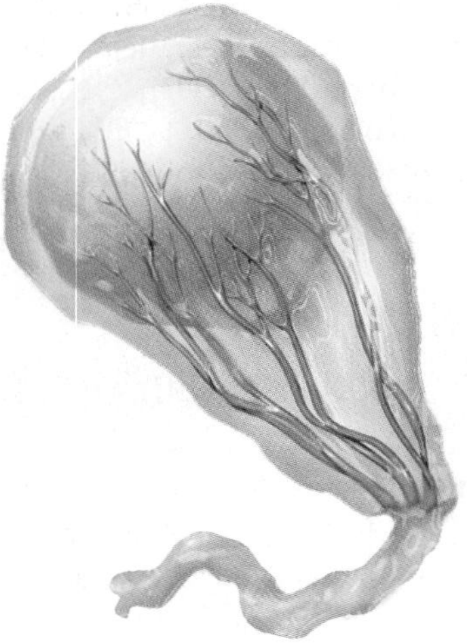

COMMON CAUSES OF PERINATAL LOSS

Antepartal fetal deaths, although infrequent, account for about half of all perinatal mortality in the United States. About 70% to 90% of all stillbirths occur before the onset of labor, with more than half occurring between 20 and 28 weeks' gestation (Druzin, Smith, Jr., Gabbe, et al., 2007). The cause may be unknown, or it may be related to fetal factors such as chromosomal disorders, birth defects, exposure to teratogens, infections, or complications of multiple gestation or fetal growth restriction; maternal factors such as chronic hypertension, preeclampsia or eclampsia, diabetes, advanced maternal age, Rh disease, uterine rupture, or ascending maternal infection; or placental factors such as placenta previa, abruptio placentae, or a cord accident. In 25% of fetal deaths, the cause remains unknown even after autopsy (Lindsay, 2006).

Perinatal loss in industrialized countries has declined in recent years as early diagnosis of congenital anomalies and advances in genetic testing techniques have increased the use of elective termination. Fetal death occurs more frequently in monochorionic twins and in pregnancies conceived by assisted reproductive technologies (Shevell, Malone, Vidaver, et al., 2005). Certain genetic testing procedures such as amniocentesis and chorionic villus sampling (CVS) can actually cause fetal loss.

In developing countries, infection plays a significant role in fetal deaths. Ascending bacterial organisms include *Escherichia coli,* group B streptococci, and *Ureaplasma urealyticum.* These infections can occur either before or after the membranes have ruptured, resulting in fetal demise. Viral causes of fetal demise include parvovirus and coxsackievirus. *Toxoplasma gondii, Listeria monocytogenes,* and the organisms that cause leptospirosis, Q fever, and Lyme disease have also been identified as causative factors for stillbirth. Untreated syphilis is associated with a high stillborn rate as are malaria infections when contracted for the first time by the mother during pregnancy (Gibbs & Roberts, 2007). These infections carry a much higher morbidity and mortality rate in developing countries.

Paternal causes of fetal death are also being examined. One recent study determined that paternal exposure to pesticides resulted in a high rate of fetal anomalies and fetal deaths when compared with pregnancies fathered by men who were not exposed to pesticides occupationally (Ronda, Regidor, Garcia et al., 2005).

Certain maternal conditions can also be associated with higher rates of fetal death. Past maternal exposure to certain bacterial and viral antigens can produce an autoimmune response that can result in fetal death (Silver, 2007). Women with acquired and immune thrombophilia have higher rates of miscarriage and fetal demise than those without hematologic alterations (Michels & Tiu, 2007).

MATERNAL PHYSIOLOGIC IMPLICATIONS

Prolonged retention of the dead fetus may lead to the development of disseminated intravascular coagulation (DIC), also called consumption coagulopathy, in the mother. After the release of thromboplastin from the degenerating fetal tissues into the maternal bloodstream, the extrinsic clotting system is activated, triggering the formation of multiple tiny blood clots. Fibrinogen and factors V and VII are subsequently depleted, and the woman begins to display symptoms of DIC. Fibrinogen levels begin a linear descent 3 to 4 weeks after the death of the fetus and continue to decrease in the absence of appropriate medical intervention.

Besides DIC, other adverse outcomes can occur if the onset of labor and subsequent birth are delayed. Women with prolonged retention of a dead fetus are more prone to infection. A resulting infection can cause endometritis or sepsis. The longer the pregnancy continues, the higher the incidence of maternal infection.

Although immediate induction is routinely performed, there may be situations in which induction is delayed, such as maternal refusal or the presence of a multiple gestation. In these cases, fibrinogen levels are monitored weekly or biweekly to recognize and prevent progressive coagulopathy from occurring (Lindsey, 2006).

CLINICAL THERAPY

When fetal death has occurred, abdominal x-ray examination may reveal Spalding's sign, an overriding of the fetal cranial bones. In addition, maternal estriol levels fall. Diagnosis of IUFD is confirmed by absence of heart action on ultrasound. Without medical intervention, most women have spontaneous labor within 2 weeks of fetal death. The once common practice of waiting for the onset of labor has largely been abandoned in recent years since the risks of complications increase with delaying the birth. Prompt birth also increases the ability to identify the cause of death.

In modern practice, most women with a diagnosed fetal demise are given the option of waiting a few days or scheduling an induction procedure immediately. Most women will elect for an induction within a day or two of the final diagnosis. The mode of induction is dependent upon the gestational age of the fetus, the readiness of the cervix, and previous mode of birth. In women who have had a previous cesarean birth, a repeat cesarean may be performed since the use of Pitocin or prostaglandin agents can increase the risk of a uterine rupture.

Women with an unfavorable cervix may be given vaginal prostaglandin agents, misoprostol, or laminaria tents. *Laminaria tents*, made from dried seaweed, work by drawing water out of the cervical tissue, allowing the cervix to soften and dilate. They are commonly used to dilate the cervix in preterm gestations when induction is warranted.

Women less than 28 weeks' gestation are typically given prostaglandin E_2 (PGE_2) vaginal suppositories every 4 to 6 hours or oral or vaginal misoprostol every 4 to 6 hours until spontaneous labor occurs (Lindsey, 2006). Because PGE_2 suppositories can cause severe vomiting and diarrhea, women are commonly pretreated with antiemetic and antidiarrheal preparations to prevent or lessen these unpleasant side effects (Lindsey, 2006).

POSTBIRTH EVALUATION

Identifying the causative factor of fetal loss assists many families in progressing through the grieving process. Information obtained from a postmortem examination or postmortem studies can provide vital information related to the cause of the fetal death, the possibility for reoccurrence, and closure for the couple. The types of studies and tests performed depend on the parents' past history, medical history, and preferences for the depth of testing desired. Chromosome studies should be considered if the couple has a history of other second- or third-trimester losses or if either parent has a suspected balanced translocation or mosaic chromosomal pattern (Lindsey, 2006).

If an intra-amniotic infection is the suspected cause, cultures of both the placenta and the fetus should be obtained. If specific infections are being considered, both IgM and IgG antibodies should be drawn to determine if an acute infectious process has occurred.

All stillborn infants should have a careful visual inspection at the time of birth for obvious defects or abnormalities. The placenta and membranes should also be closely examined, and the placenta should be sent to pathology for further testing. The umbilical cord should be inspected for true knots, a velamentous insertion, lack of Wharton's jelly, or a short cord to determine if a cord accident was the cause. If a specific cause is suspected, blood tests and x-rays can be performed. An autopsy is the best mechanism to determine the cause of death; however, in the event that the parents decline an autopsy, magnetic resonance imaging (MRI) can also provide detailed information (Lindsey, 2006).

Most practitioners perform a CBC and antibody screen upon admission. Because diabetes is a causative factor, a random

Table 22–2 Tests to Determine Cause of Fetal Loss

Fetal Testing	Maternal Testing
Fetal blood tests and x-rays	Diabetes testing
Autopsy or MRI	CBC with platelet count
Placental studies	Kleihauer-Betke test
Chromosomal studies (if indicated)	Abnormal antibody testing (lupus anticoagulant, anticardiolipin antibodies)
	TSH levels
	Infectious disease testing (rubella, syphilis, malaria, toxoplasmosis, cytomegalovirus)
	Hereditary thrombophilia testing
	Toxicology testing

or postpartum glucose level can be obtained to rule out this cause. Additional maternal factors that can also be evaluated are listed in Table 22–2.

PHASES OF GRIEF

Grief is an individual's total response to a loss, including physical symptoms, thoughts, feelings, functional limitations, and spiritual reactions. It may be manifested by certain behaviors and rituals of *mourning,* such as weeping or visiting a gravesite, which help the person experience, accept, and adjust to the loss. The period of adjustment to loss is known as *bereavement.* (Note: grief as it relates to the birth of an at-risk newborn is discussed in Chapter 32∞.)

The behaviors that couples exhibit while mourning may be associated with the five stages of grieving described by Kubler-Ross (1969). Often the first stage is *denial* of the death of the fetus. Even when the initial healthcare provider suspects fetal demise, the couple is hoping that a second opinion may be different. Some couples may not be convinced of the death until they see and hold the stillborn infant after birth. The second stage is *anger,* resulting from feelings of loss, loneliness, and perhaps guilt. The anger may be projected at significant others and healthcare team members, or it may be absent when the death is sudden and unexpected. The mother may attempt to identify a specific event that caused the death and may blame herself. *Bargaining,* the third stage, may or may not be present, depending on the couple's preparation for the death of the fetus. If the death is unanticipated, the couple may not have time for bargaining. When the death is expected, such as in the case of a known lethal congenital anomaly, bargaining is more commonly seen. It is marked by the couple making mental trade-offs in exchange for the fetus being healthy. In the fourth stage, *depression* is evidenced by preoccupation, weeping, and withdrawal. Changing hormonal levels in the first 24 to 48 hours after birth may compound the depression and associated grief.

Nursing Practice

No matter who you are or how much nursing experience you have, when an expectant family is in pain because of their loss, it can be difficult to know the right thing to say. A good start is to say "I'm so sorry, I don't know what to say."

The final stage, *acceptance,* occurs when resolution occurs. This stage is highly individualized and may take months to years to complete.

NURSING MANAGEMENT

NURSING ASSESSMENT AND DIAGNOSIS

Cessation of fetal movement reported by the mother to the nurse is frequently the first indication of fetal death. It is followed by a gradual decrease in the signs and symptoms of pregnancy. Fetal heart tones are absent, and fetal movement is no longer palpable. Once fetal demise is established, assess the family members' ability to adapt to their loss. Open communication between the mother, her partner, and the healthcare team members contributes to a realistic understanding of the medical condition and its associated treatments. Discuss prior experiences the family has had with loss and what they feel were their perceived coping abilities at that time. Identifying the family's social supports and resources is also important.

Perinatal loss may also occur in the intrapartum period as a result of an intrapartum complication, such as an unresolved shoulder dystocia, prolapsed umbilical cord, abruptio placentae, or other complication. In such emergency situations, healthcare team members often focus on the physical needs of the mother and an attempt to save the fetus's life. Commonly, the family is not informed that a perinatal death has occurred until the infant is born. Thus, the parents are faced with the sudden and completely unanticipated death of their infant. The most common reaction is protest or disbelief.

Although the physician or CNM informs the family of the death, the nurse continues one-on-one care with the family, providing both physical and emotional support throughout this crucial period. Assist the family in the grief process and explore their immediate wishes for viewing and holding their deceased child.

Nursing diagnoses that may apply include the following:

- *Anticipatory Grieving* related to imminent loss of a child
- *Compromised Family Coping* related to the death of a child/unresolved feelings regarding perinatal loss
- *Hopelessness* related to sudden, unexpected fetal loss
- *Risk for Spiritual Distress* related to intense suffering secondary to unexpected fetal loss

PLANNING AND IMPLEMENTATION

Most facilities have an established protocol to follow in the event of perinatal death. It typically provides a holistic focus for family-centered nursing care. It is important that the entire healthcare team is notified so multidisciplinary care can be initiated. When fetal death has been confirmed before admission, the entire staff on the unit is informed so they can avoid making inappropriate remarks. Many facilities have a symbol, such as a card with a leaf or a cluster of flowers, that is placed on the mother's door so all staff members are aware of the loss.

PREPARING THE FAMILY FOR THE BIRTH

Upon arrival to the facility, the couple with a known or suspected fetal demise should immediately be placed in a private room. When possible the woman should be in a room that is farthest away from other laboring women. Take care not to leave the couple in the waiting room with other expectant parents or visitors waiting for news from other women in labor.

The couple should be allowed to remain together as much as they wish. Provide privacy as needed and maintain a supportive environment. Give the couple complete information about what to expect and what will happen. Encourage and answer questions. Stay with the couple so they do not feel alone and isolated; however, continuously assess cues from the couple that they want to be alone. Some couples may want outside support, such as family members or friends, to be present during the labor. Facilitate the couple's wishes.

When possible the same nurse should provide care for the couple so a therapeutic relationship can be established. As the relationship develops, provide solace by listening to the couple without offering explanations. Also provide ongoing opportunities for the couple to ask questions. It is not uncommon for the family to ask the same questions repeatedly as part of the initial grief process. Provide clear explanations and straightforward answers.

Consider cultural factors in providing care. Although not everyone from a given culture responds to loss in the same way, responses to fetal death are often influenced by culture and personal beliefs. Similarly, responses to loss may be influenced by spiritual beliefs. In considering religious practices, it is prudent simply to ask the family how they can best be helped to meet their religious needs. Some families may desire to see a spiritual advisor. If so, offer to contact the hospital chaplain or another cleric for them. It is important to let the family process their own beliefs and feelings about the meaning, purpose, and significance of the life and death of their infant.

If a grief counselor is available, arrange an initial interaction with the couple if they are willing. A social worker is commonly involved. Coordinate members of the multidisciplinary team so a comprehensive plan of care can be initiated.

Explain details of the plan of care and allow the family to ask questions and make decisions for their labor and birth preferences. Review the availability of anesthesia and analgesia. The woman typically can have pain medication whenever she desires. Facilitate the participation of the woman and her partner in the labor and birth process.

Developing Cultural Competence

GRIEF RESPONSES AND INTERACTIONS

- Cultures that are stoic in nature can be difficult to assist. Stoicism may stem from family or cultural background, shock, or denial. It is important to ascertain the underlying reason so that appropriate interventions, where warranted, can occur.
- In male-dominant cultures, mothers experiencing perinatal loss may tend to focus on their "failure" as a woman to successfully reproduce. Reassure these women (while respecting cultural beliefs) that nothing they did or did not do affected the outcome. A reiteration of known medical causes may be helpful.
- In cultures in which the extended family is the couple's main source of support, it is important to allow as much interaction with family members as possible. In cultures where privacy is valued above all, help the family limit visitors if that is their preference.
- Avoidance is not therapeutic. If you are not certain what the family needs, simply ask them how you can help to accommodate their wishes. Families appreciate an honest and caring attitude.

Remember that, in contrast to a typical birth experience, the birth of a stillborn infant marks both the beginning and the end. It is imperative that the couple and family have all wishes and preferences respected. However, the family may have difficulty making decisions in this period. Assist the couple to explore their feelings and help them to make decisions about who is present and what rituals will occur during and following the birth. Examples of birth preferences include the following:

- Use of music, dimmed lighting, or other environmental preferences
- Laboring or birthing in a specific position
- Having the infant placed on the mother's chest immediately after birth
- Allowing the father to cut the umbilical cord
- Presence of other family members or friends at the birth

Sometimes couples worry that others may view their preferences as "strange" or "wrong." Reassure the family that it is their experience and that there are no right or wrong feelings or wishes.

The couple may have waves of overwhelming grief, disbelief, or sadness. Encourage the couple to experience the grief that they feel. It is not uncommon for one partner to attempt to put on a "brave front," feeling that by showing grief he or she will make the other partner feel worse. It is also not uncommon for partners to have intense feelings that they are unable to share. Encourage partners to express their emotions freely to the extent they are able. Help them understand that they may each experience different feelings.

SUPPORTING THE FAMILY IN VIEWING THE STILLBORN INFANT

Advocates of seeing the stillborn infant believe that viewing assists in dispelling denial and enables the couple to progress to the next step in the grieving process. If they choose to see their stillborn infant, prepare the couple for what they will see by saying "she is going to feel cold," "he is going to be blue," or other appropriate statements. If the parents have shared with you the name they had chosen for their baby, use that name in discussing the baby, for example, "Jessie's face is bruised." Another common practice is to wrap the infant in a blanket or apply a hat to cover birth defects. This allows the parents an opportunity to view the infant before seeing the birth defect. Most parents will eventually remove the covering to inspect the infant; however, applying a covering allows them time to adjust to the appearance at their own pace.

Some families will hold their infant for a short time before returning him or her to the nurse, whereas others will wish to spend a great deal of time with their infant. Allow the infant to remain with the family for as long as the family desires. Some parents may elect to bathe or dress their stillborn baby; support them in their choice. Some couples may want other family members, friends, or their other children to see the infant. Act as an advocate to ensure that the family's wishes are respected.

PROVIDING DISCHARGE CARE

Most facilities prepare a remembrance box or package for the family to take home. This typically consists of a photograph taken of the infant or the family, a card with the baby's footprints, a crib card, identification band, a lock of hair, and possibly a blanket or clothing worn by the infant. In the event that the couple declines the package, it is common for the hospital to retain these items for a specific period in case they change their minds.

After the birth, give the option of an early discharge (as early as 6 to 8 hours after the birth) to the couple. Facility protocol will dictate where mothers are transferred after a perinatal loss. Some hospitals have the women remain on the birthing unit; others give the mother the option of choosing a postpartum room or one on a medical unit. If the mother is transferred to a postpartum room, select a room for her that is far away from other rooms and the newborn nursery. It is imperative that all staff members, as well as student nurses, are notified of the mother's status.

Include information on the grief process in discharge information. Prepare the couple to return home by stressing that others may not know what to say, and that even loved ones may make inappropriate comments because they do not know how to respond to grief and loss. This can prepare the couple for the reactions of others. If there are siblings, each will usually progress through age-appropriate grieving. Provide the parents with information about normal mourning reactions, both psychologic and physiologic.

When caring for a family suffering from a perinatal loss, it is important to remember that the nurse experiences many of the same grief reactions as the parents of a stillborn infant. It is important to have colleagues and family members available for counseling and support.

FACILITATING THE FAMILY'S GRIEF WORK

The parents of a stillborn infant suffer a devastating experience that precipitates an intense emotional trauma. During pregnancy the couple has already begun the attachment process, which now must be ended through the grieving process. Facilitating the family's grief work is thus a critical nursing intervention—one that requires skill, sensitivity, and compassion.

Following discharge, some families may need closure of the intrapartum event in order to continue the grief work. A consultation can be scheduled with the practitioner who cared for them during the pregnancy and birth. Families may also wish to read the results of tests performed during the intrapartum period and the autopsy report. Provide a copy of the medical record to the couple and encourage them to ask questions, express their feelings, and ask for clarification.

Families are routinely referred for counseling services after a perinatal loss has occurred. A counselor who specializes in perinatal issues can provide expertise and assist the couple in their grieving. Partners should be allowed to verbalize fears and concerns about future pregnancies. When appropriate, also provide referrals to genetic counselors, religious support persons, and social service agencies.

Besides referral information, the woman should receive scheduled, follow-up phone calls to assess the family's functioning and their progress with grief work. Use these follow-up phone calls to provide pertinent information and identify additional resources for the family.

As the grief process ensues, encourage families to implement cultural, religious, or social customs that will assist them in grieving and mourning. Advise the family that certain upcoming milestones, such as holidays, future birthdays, baby showers, Mother's Day, Father's Day, and other social events may trigger their grief. The family can better cope with these events if they are adequately prepared.

REFERRING THE FAMILY TO COMMUNITY SERVICES

Although most facilities have an established protocol for families experiencing perinatal loss, more comprehensive intervention programs are being established in communities to assist these families. Community support groups that focus on perinatal loss can provide an important support network and resources. Specialized groups, such as those focused on early pregnancy loss, stillbirth, and perinatal loss associated with specific congenital anomalies, allow families the opportunity to interact with peers who have lost infants under similar circumstances. Provide the group name, contact person (if possible), and phone number. Various books written by mothers who have lost children are available in bookstores and are valuable resources for grieving parents.

Internet technology has allowed large numbers of individuals to share resources and information, and participate in online support groups. Internet resources can be effective for all families and may be the only resources available for families in rural, underserved areas.

Specialized community outreach programs are another resource that can provide assistance to grieving families; some provide early counseling to parents whose fetus has a known lethal congenital anomaly. In perinatal hospice programs, parents are given the opportunity to explore options, such as elective termination or waiting for the onset of spontaneous labor or a medically indicated induced labor. For families wishing to continue their pregnancies, the program typically assigns a multidisciplinary team who provides compassionate care, ongoing counseling, referral to support groups, and spiritual guidance (Ramer-Chrastek & Thygesen, 2005).

CARE OF THE COUPLE WHO HAS EXPERIENCED LOSS IN A PREVIOUS PREGNANCY

Couples who have had previous perinatal loss typically enter a subsequent pregnancy with conflicting feelings and may experience ambivalence, fear, and anxiety. Many times, their past experience is relived when another pregnancy occurs. Some couples conceive soon after a loss while others wait years. Some couples enter a subsequent pregnancy with grief work largely completed while others are still experiencing unresolved grief.

The nurse caring for a couple who has had a previous loss needs to be kind, compassionate, and patient. Couples need specific information and clear explanations of all prenatal information. Make referrals to genetic counselors when appropriate. Some couples may wish to have a consultation with a perinatologist. If unresolved grief issues are present or the family experiences extreme anxiety, counseling may be beneficial.

Interventions to decrease anxiety can help the couple tremendously. At the first visit, an early ultrasound can be performed to verify the presence of the fetal heart. In early pregnancy, women may be fearful when first-trimester pregnancy symptoms begin to resolve. It may be helpful for these women to come in for weekly visits for a period of time simply to hear the fetal heartbeat. This intervention may continue to be helpful until the woman begins to feel fetal movement. Throughout the pregnancy, the office or clinic nurse can play a key role by providing reassurance and answer questions that the woman may have.

Women with a previous loss typically receive additional antepartum testing throughout the pregnancy. Ultrasounds can be used to provide reassurance and assess fetal growth and development, placental functioning, and cord variations. Nonstress testing and biophysical profiles can be performed weekly after 32 weeks to ensure fetal well-being. Fetal kick counts should be initiated at 28 weeks and continue until the birth occurs. Women with a previous loss should give birth at their expected date of birth or when the pregnancy is at term and should not go over their due date, since placental functioning can decline in post-date pregnancies.

EVALUATION

Expected outcomes of nursing care for the family experiencing perinatal loss include the following:

- Family members express their feelings about the death of their baby.
- Family members participate in the decision making regarding preferences for the labor, birth, and the immediate postpartum period.
- Family members participate in the decision of whether to see their baby and other decisions about the baby.
- The family has resources available for continued support.
- Family members know the community resources available and have names and phone numbers to use if they choose.
- The family is moving into and through the grieving process.

CARE OF THE WOMAN WITH A PSYCHOLOGIC DISORDER

The onset of labor is a time of mixed emotions. Joy, excitement, happiness, fear of the unknown, and anxiety related to pain may all occur. These reactions are expected and pose no health risk in women with adequate coping mechanisms. In contrast, laboring women with psychologic disorders face additional emotional challenges and require additional nursing support in the intrapartum period.

The prevalence of psychologic disorders among adults in the United States is 26.2%, or roughly 1 in 4 adults (National Institute of Mental Health, 2008). Psychologic disorders are characterized by alterations in thinking, mood, or behavior. Although many such disorders can affect labor and birth, only the most common are discussed here. Postpartum psychologic disorders are discussed in Chapter 26∞.

The psychologic disorders that most commonly affect pregnant women are depression, bipolar disorder, anxiety, phobias, obsessive-compulsive disorder, posttraumatic stress disorder, and schizophrenia. These disorders may manifest themselves in different ways during the birth process; however, all require the nurse to provide compassionate and consistent nursing care.

RISKS OF PSYCHOLOGIC DISORDERS

Depression can reduce the woman's ability to concentrate or process information being provided by healthcare team members. The labor process may feel overwhelming to her, and she may feel hopelessness about the outcome of her labor. Women with bipolar disorder experience the symptoms of depression during the depressive phase, but if labor occurs during a manic phase, the woman may be hyperexcitable. Anxiety disorders may cause the laboring woman to experience physical symptoms such as chest pain, shortness of breath, faintness, fear, or even terror. In general, laboring women with psychologic disorders tend to exhibit behaviors characteristic of their disorder, but these behaviors may be somewhat exaggerated.

CLINICAL THERAPY

The goal of clinical therapy is to provide strategies that will help decrease the anxiety of the woman and her partner, keep her oriented to reality, and promote optimal functioning while in labor.

The woman should be oriented to her new environment. All questions and concerns should be addressed promptly. When needed, pharmacologic measures such as sedatives, analgesics, or antianxiety medications may be ordered.

NURSING MANAGEMENT

The nurse uses therapeutic communication and sharing of information to allay anxiety for both the woman and her support person. Consistent care enables the woman to adjust to a new environment and begin to establish a relationship with her nurse.

NURSING ASSESSMENT AND DIAGNOSIS

Unless birth is imminent or severe complications exist, begin the assessment by reviewing the woman's background. Factors such as age, marital and socioeconomic status, culture, methods of coping, support system, and understanding of the labor process contribute to the woman's psychologic response to labor. Ask the woman if she has ever been diagnosed with a psychologic disorder. If the woman has, also ask her if she is currently receiving any treatment, including medications or psychotherapy.

Assess the woman for objective cues indicating a psychologic disorder. Monotone replies or flat affect may indicate depression. Women with schizophrenia may lack orientation to person, time, and place. Objective cues indicating acute anxiety or signs of panic attack include tachycardia and hyperventilation.

As labor progresses, remain alert to the woman's verbal and nonverbal behavior responses to the pain and anxiety of labor. The woman who is too quiet and compliant, is disoriented, is agitated and seems uncooperative, or is experiencing acute anxiety symptoms may require further appraisal for psychologic disorders. These rare circumstances require one-on-one nursing care. A consultation with a psychiatrist is often warranted.

Nursing diagnoses that may apply to the woman with a psychologic disorder include the following:

- *Anxiety* related to stress of the labor process, unfamiliar environment, and unknown care providers.
- *Fear* related to unknown outcome of labor and invasive medical procedures.
- *Ineffective Individual Coping* related to increased anxiety and stress.

PLANNING AND IMPLEMENTATION

The primary nursing interventions center on providing support to the laboring woman and her partner or family. Families that have had the opportunity to attend prenatal classes may benefit from encouragement as they employ some of the coping techniques they have learned (see Chapter 8). If the woman begins to lose her ability to cope or her orientation to reality, assist her in regaining control and orientation by explaining where she is, why she is there, and what is currently happening. Provide reassurance, decrease stimuli, and acknowledge her fears, concerns, and symptoms.

The nurse's ability to help the woman and her partner cope with the stress of labor is directly related to the rapport they have established. By employing a calm, caring, confident, nonjudgmental approach, you may be able not only to acknowledge the anxiety or other emotions the woman is feeling but also to identify the source of the distress. Once the causative factors are known, implement appropriate interventions such as offering information, comfort measures, touch, or therapeutic communication. Some women with severe psychologic disorders may have excessive symptoms during their labor and birth. Although providing emotional support is imperative, focus your care of these women on maintaining a safe environment and ensuring maternal and fetal well-being. Pharmacologic interventions may be necessary for excessive symptoms.

EVALUATION

Expected outcomes of nursing care include the following:

- The woman experiences a decrease in physiologic and psychologic stress and an increase in physical and psychologic comfort.
- The woman remains oriented to person, time, and place.
- The woman uses effective coping mechanisms to manage her stress and anxiety in labor.
- The woman is able to verbalize feelings about her labor.
- The woman's and her family's fear is decreased.

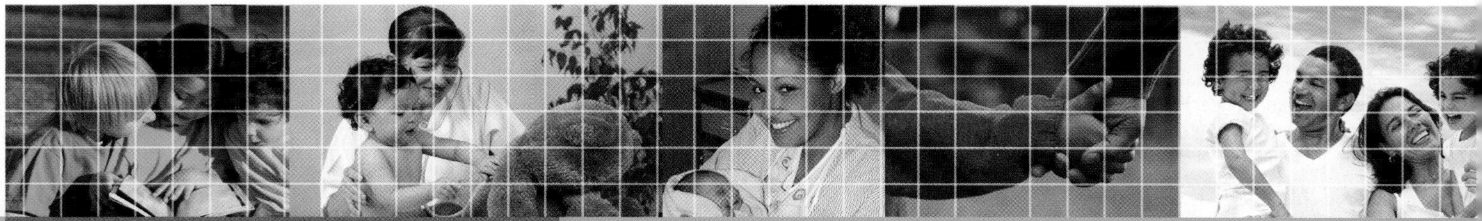

CRITICAL CONCEPT REVIEW

LEARNING OUTCOMES	CONCEPTS
22.1 Compare hypertonic and hypotonic labor patterns, including the risks, clinical therapy, and nursing care management.	1. Hypertonic labor patterns: ■ Characterized by increased frequency but decreased effectiveness of contraction in effacing and dilating the cervix. Usually leads to a prolonged latent phase. ■ May cause mother to become fatigued and have difficulty coping with stress of labor. ■ Pattern may cause prolonged pressure on the fetal head. ■ Clinical therapy may involve sedation, pain medication, and bed rest. Pitocin may be given only if CPD and fetal malpresentation are ruled out. ■ Nursing management includes decreasing environmental stimuli, decreasing anxiety, and promoting comfort. 2. Hypotonic labor patterns: ■ Characterized by fewer than 2–3 contractions in a 10-minute period during the active phase of labor. ■ Mother may experience fatigue and coping difficulties. ■ Mother is at risk for intrauterine infection and postpartal hemorrhage. ■ Fetus is at risk for sepsis. ■ Clinical therapy includes assessment of adequacy of pelvic measurement and fetal maturity; the use of Pitocin or nipple stimulation once CPD and fetal malpresentation are ruled out. ■ Nursing management includes close monitoring for signs and symptoms of infection and dehydration, and keeping vaginal exams to a minimum.
22.2 Describe the risks and clinical therapy in determining the nursing care management of postterm pregnancy on the childbearing family.	1. Postterm pregnancy may result in an increased possibility of: ■ Probable labor induction. ■ Forceps or vacuum-assisted or cesarean birth. ■ Decreased perfusion to the placenta. ■ Decreased amount of amniotic fluid and possible cord compression. ■ Increased possibility of meconium aspiration. ■ Increased risk for macrosomia or a loss of fat and muscle mass resulting in small-for-gestational age (SGA).
22.3 Relate the various types of fetal malposition and malpresentation to the nursing management for each.	1. Occiput posterior position: ■ Baby is face up instead of face down as it enters the vagina. ■ May prolong labor. ■ Baby is usually able to be born vaginally but may need forceps assistance to turn baby. 2. Brow presentation: ■ Forehead of the fetus becomes the presenting part. ■ May cause labor to be prolonged. ■ Cesarean birth necessary if brow presentation persists. 3. Face presentation: ■ Face of the fetus is the presenting part. ■ Vaginal birth may be possible, but cesarean birth remains a significant possibility. 4. Breech presentation: ■ Fetal buttocks or foot/feet are the presenting part. ■ 90% of breech presentations result in cesarean birth. 5. Transverse lie: ■ Fetal shoulder is the presenting part. ■ Fetus must be born by cesarean.

(continued)

LEARNING OUTCOMES / CONCEPTS

22.4 Explain the identification, risks, and clinical therapy in determining the nursing care management of the woman and fetus at risk for fetal macrosomia.

1. Identification of fetal macrosomia is conducted through:
   - Palpation of fetus in utero.
   - Ultrasound of fetus.
   - X-ray pelvimetry.
2. Management of fetal macrosomia involves the following:
   - Cesarean birth performed if fetus is greater than 4500 g.
   - Continuous fetal monitoring if labor is allowed to progress.
   - Notification of physician for early decelerations, labor dysfunction, or nonreassuring fetal status.
3. Care of newborn with macrosomia requires:
   - Assessment of newborn for cephalohematoma, Erb's palsy, and fractured clavicles.
4. Care of the mother after birth of newborn with macrosomia requires:
   - Fundal massage to prevent maternal hemorrhage from overstretched uterus.
   - Close monitoring of vital signs.

22.5 Relate the maternal implications, clinical therapy, prenatal history, and conditions that may be associated with nonreassuring fetal status to the nursing care of the mother and fetus.

1. Nursing actions (intrauterine resuscitation) include:
   - Turn the woman to left lateral position to treat hypotension.
   - Begin or increase IV flow rate.
   - Perform vaginal exam to check for cord prolapse.
   - Have woman assume knee-chest position if cord prolapse is suspected.
   - Discontinue Pitocin or administer a tocolytic agent to decrease contraction frequency and intensity.
   - Administer oxygen.
   - Notify physician.
   - Obtain additional information about fetus by fetal scalp blood sampling or fetal acoustical stimulation.

22.6 Describe the nursing care for the mother and fetus with a proplapsed umbilical cord.

1. Umbilical cord precedes fetal presenting part, placing pressure on cord and diminishing blood flow to the fetus.
2. Bed rest is recommended if engagement has not occurred and membranes have ruptured.
3. Assess for nonreassuring fetal status.

22.7 Summarize the identification, maternal and fetal-neonatal implicateons, clinical therapy, and nursing care management of a woman with amniotic fluid embolism.

1. Amniotic fluid embolism:
   - Caused by a small tear in the chorion or amnion high in the uterus, which may allow amniotic fluid to enter the maternal circulatory system.
   - Usually occurs during or after birth.
   - The woman experiences sudden symptoms of respiratory distress leading to severe hemorrhage.
   - This disorder is life threatening, so medical management and nursing care is aimed at delivering lifesaving treatments such as CPR and transfusion until the woman is stabilized.

22.8 Explain the types, maternal and fetal-neonatal implications, and clinical therapy in determining the nursing care management of a woman with cephalopelvic disproportion.

1. Labor is usually prolonged in the presence of CPD.
2. Vaginal birth may be possible depending upon the type of CPD.
3. Woman may increase pelvic diameter during labor by squatting, sitting, rolling from side to side, or maintaining a knee-chest position.
4. CPD may make cesarean birth the only available method of birth.

22.9 Identify common complications of the third and fourth stages of labor.

1. The most common complications are:
   - Retained placenta:
     - If not expelled, the placenta must be manually removed from the uterus.
   - Lacerations:
     - Suspected when there is bright-red bleeding in the presence of a contracted uterus.
     - Usually repaired immediately after birth of child.
   - Placenta accreta:
     - In this condition, the chorionic villi attach directly to the myometrium of the uterus.
     - May result in maternal hemorrhage and failure of the placenta to separate from the uterus.
     - May result in the need for hysterectomy at time of birth.

LEARNING OUTCOMES / CONCEPTS

22.10 Explain the etiology, diagnosis, and phases of grief in determining the nursing care management of the family experiencing perinatal loss.

1. Perinatal loss results from three factors:
   - Fetal factors: The fetus has or develops a disorder that is incompatible with life.
   - Maternal factors: The mother has a disorder such as diabetes or preeclampsia that creates a hostile environment for the fetus.
   - Placental or other factors: Certain conditions such as abruptio placentae or cord accident cut off blood supply to the fetus, leading to death.
2. Diagnosis may be made when the mother notices lack of movement in the fetus or at a regularly scheduled physician's visit when a fetal heart tone cannot be found.
3. Nursing care involves supporting the family through the grief work:
   - Assist the family through the labor and birth.
   - Provide for the woman's physical needs after the birth.
   - Encourage family members to express and share their thoughts and feelings about the loss.
   - Give the family an opportunity to view, hold, and name the infant.
   - Prepare items for the family to keep to remember the infant.
   - Provide opportunities for religious or spiritual counseling and cultural practices.
   - Visit or phone the family after discharge to assist in closure.
   - Make referrals to appropriate perinatal loss counseling services if indicated.

22.11 Explain the psychologic factors that may contribute to complications during labor and birth in determining the nursing care management.

1. Psychologic disorders such as depression and acute anxiety may have a profound effect on labor, particularly when complications occur that might jeopardize the mother or fetus.

CRITICAL THINKING IN ACTION

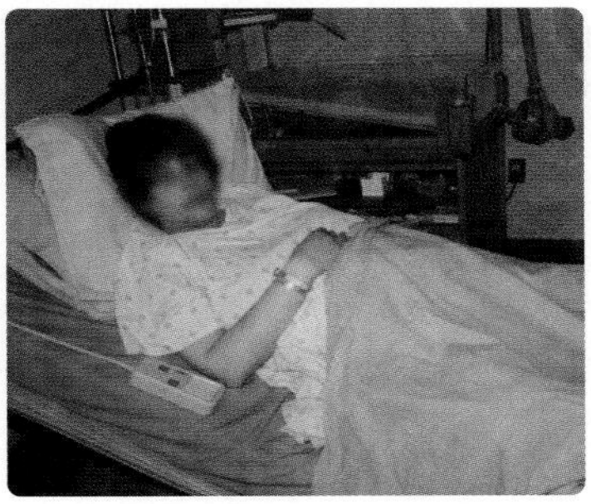

June Dice, a 25-year-old G3, P1011, is admitted to you in labor and delivery at 38 weeks with a moderate amount of dark red vaginal bleeding. June's prenatal history is significant for late prenatal care (20 weeks' gestation by ultrasound) and cocaine abuse. An ultrasound is done upon admission that demonstrates a marginal placenta abruption. You place June on the fetal monitor and observe a fetal heart rate baseline of 146 to 155 with accelerations to 166 with fetal movement. There are occasional mild variable decelerations with a quick return to baseline. Contraction pattern is interpreted as an irritable uterus. An intravenous infusion with Ringer's lactate is started with a #18 intracath. June's vital signs are within normal limits. Her hematocrit is 29%. You assist the physician with a vaginal exam to rupture membranes and insert a fetal scalp electrode and intrauterine pressure catheter. A small amount of light yellow-green amniotic fluid is observed. The exam shows June is 4 cm dilated, 50% effaced, vertex at –1 station. You follow protocol and start an oxytocin induction/augmentation. June is asking why oxytocin is needed.

1. Explain the goal of labor induction/augmentation in response to June's question.
2. Explain potential risk factors associated with oxytocin induction of labor.
3. You observe a nonreassuring fetal heart rate of 144 to 150 with decreased variability, and persistent late decelerations with each contraction. What interventions would you immediately take?
4. What supportive actions are taken to decrease the risk of hypofibrinogenemia?
5. What complications might be present in the newborn at birth?

See MyNursingKit for possible responses.

REFERENCES

Albers, L. L. (2007). The evidence for physiologic management of the active phase of the first stage of labor. *Journal of Midwifery & Womens Health, 52*(3), 207–215.

American College of Obstetricians & Gynecologists (ACOG). (2006). *Mode of term singleton breech delivery*. ACOG Committee Opinion No. 340. Washington, DC: Author.

Battista, L. R., & Wing, D. H. (2007). Abnormal labor and induction of labor. In S. G. Gabbe, J. R. Niebyl, & J. L. Simpson (Eds.), *Obstetrics: Normal and problem pregnancies* (5th ed.). Philadelphia: Churchill Livingstone.

Blackburn, S. T. (2007). *Maternal, fetal, and neonatal physiology: A clinical perspective* (3rd ed.). Philadelphia: Saunders.

Carey, J. C., & Gibbs, R. S. (2008). Preterm labor and post-term delivery. In R. S. Gibbs, B. Y. Karlan, A. F. Haney, & I. Nygaard (Eds.). *Danforth's Obstetrics and Gynecology* (10th ed.). Philadelphia: WoltersKluwer/Lippincott Williams & Wilkins.

Coyle, M. E., Smith, C. A., & Peat, B. (2005). Cephalic version by moxibustion for breech presentation. *Cochrane Database of Systematic Reviews,* Issue 2. Art. No.: CD003928. DOI: 10.1002/14651858.CD003928.pub2.

Cunningham, F. G., Leveno, K..J., Bloom, S. L., Hauth, J. C., Rouse, D. J., & Spong, C. Y. (2010). *Williams' obstetrics* (23rd ed.). New York: McGraw-Hill Medical.

Divon, M. Y. (2007). Prolonged pregnancy. In S. G. Gabbe, J. R. Niebyl, & J. L. Simpson (Eds.), *Obstetrics: Normal and problem pregnancies* (5th ed.). Philadelphia: Churchill Livingstone.

Druzin, M. L., Smith, J. F., Gabbe, S. G., & Reed, K. L. (2007) Antepartum fetal evaluation. In S. G. Gabbe, J. R. Niebyl, & J. L. Simpson (Eds.), *Obstetrics: Normal and problem pregnancies* (5th ed.). Philadelphia: Churchill Livingstone.

Family Practice Notebook. (2007). Brow presentation. Retrieved November 9, 2007, from http://www.fpnotebook.com/OB102.htm

Francois, K. E., & Foley, M. R. (2007). Antepartum and postpartum hemorrhage. In S. G. Gabbe, J. R. Niebyl, & J. L. Simpson (Eds.), *Obstetrics: Normal and problem pregnancies* (5th ed.). Philadelphia: Churchill Livingstone.

Gibbs, R. S., & Roberts, D. J. (2007). Case records of the Massachusetts General Hospital. Case 27-2007. A 30-year-old pregnant woman with intrauterine fetal death. *New England Journal of Medicine, 357*(9), 918–925.

Gilstrap, L. C., & Yeomans, E. R. (2008). Complications of delivery. In R. S. Gibbs, B. Y. Karlan, A. F. Haney, & I. Nygaard (Eds.). *Danforth's Obstetrics and Gynecology* (10th ed.). Philadelphia: WoltersKluwer/Lippincott Williams & Wilkins.

Kubler-Ross, E. (1969). *On death and dying.* New York: MacMillian.

Lanni, S. M., & Seeds, J. W. (2007). Malpresentations. In S. G. Gabbe, J. R. Niebyl, & J. L. Simpson (Eds.), *Obstetrics: Normal and problem pregnancies* (5th ed.). Philadelphia: Churchill Livingstone.

Le Ray, C., Serres, P., Schmitz, T., Cabrol, D., & Goffinet, F. (2007). Manual rotation in occiput posterior or transverse positions: Risk factors and consequences on the cesarean delivery rate. *Obstetrics & Gynecology, 110*(4), 873–879.

Lindsey, J. L. (2006). Evaluation of fetal death. *E-medicine.* Retrieved November 27, 2007, from http://www.emedicine.com/med/topic3235.htm

Luo, G., & Copel, J. A. (2009). Using U/S to assess macrosomia: Are we there yet? *Conmtemporary OB/GYN, 54*(1), 26–34.

Mahony, R., Foley, M., McAuliffe, F., & O'Herlihy, C. (2007). Maternal weight characteristics influence recurrence of fetal macrosomia in women with normal glucose tolerance. *The Australian & New Zealand Journal of Obstetrics & Gynaecology, 47*(5), 399–401; PMID: 17877598.

Michels, T. C., & Tiu, A. Y. (2007). Second trimester pregnancy loss. *American Family Physician, 1*;76(9), 1341–1346.

National Institute of Mental Health (NIMH). (2008). Statistics. Retrieved August 20, 2008, from www.nimh.gov/health/statistics/index.shtml

Ramer-Chrastek, J., & Thygesen, N. V. (2005). A perinatal hospice for an unborn child with a life-limiting condition. *International Journal of Palliative Nursing, 11*(6), 274–276.

Ronda, E., Regidor, E., García, A. M., & Domínguez, V. (2005). Association between congenital anomalies and paternal exposure to agricultural pesticides depending on mother's employment status. *Journal of Occupational Environmental Medicine, 47*(8), 826–828.

Shevell, T., Malone, F. D., Vidaver, J., Porter, T. F., Luthy, D. A., Comstock, C. H., et al. (2005). Assisted reproductive technology and pregnancy outcome. *Obstetrics & Gynecology, 106*(5 Pt 1), 1039–1045.

Silver, R. M. (2007). Fetal death. *Obstetrics & Gynecology, 109*(1), 153–167.

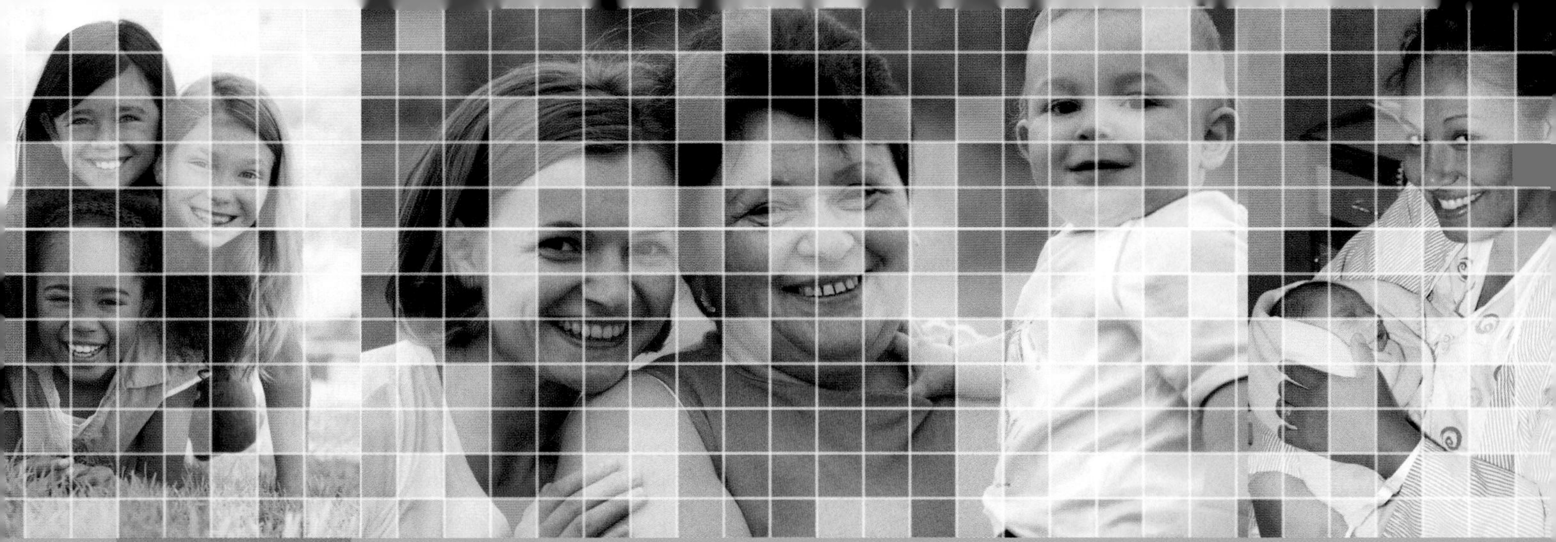

CHAPTER

23 Birth-Related Procedures

With our first baby, all of a sudden I had to have a cesarean. Everything happened so fast but our son was OK, and that's all that mattered. With our second baby, I wanted to try a vaginal birth. Even though I wanted to, I was afraid. I don't know what I would have done without my nurse. She stayed with me the whole time and kept giving me support. She explained what was happening and gave encouragement. I felt safe. I had a beautiful baby girl after 8 hours of labor. —Marianne, 22

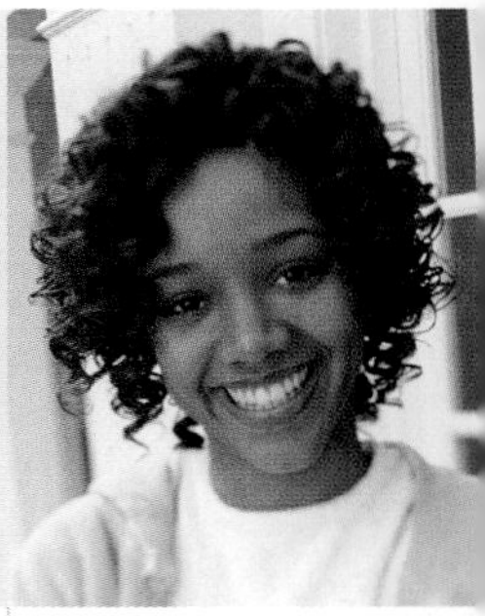

LEARNING OUTCOMES

23.1 Explain the methods, purpose, and contraindications of external and podalic versions that determine nursing care management.

23.2 Describe the use of amniotomy and the nursing care management of woman and fetus.

23.3 Compare the methods for inducing labor, explaining their advantages and disadvantages in determining the nursing management for women during labor induction.

23.4 Describe the measures to prevent episiotomy, and the types of episiotomy and associated nursing care management.

23.5 Explain the indications, maternal, and neonatal risks that impact nursing care management during forceps-assisted birth.

23.6 Describe the use of and risk of vacuum extraction use to assist birth.

23.7 Explain the indications for cesarean birth, impact on the family unit, preparation and teaching needs, and associated nursing care.

23.8 Examine the risks, guidelines, and nursing care of the woman undergoing vaginal birth following cesarean birth.

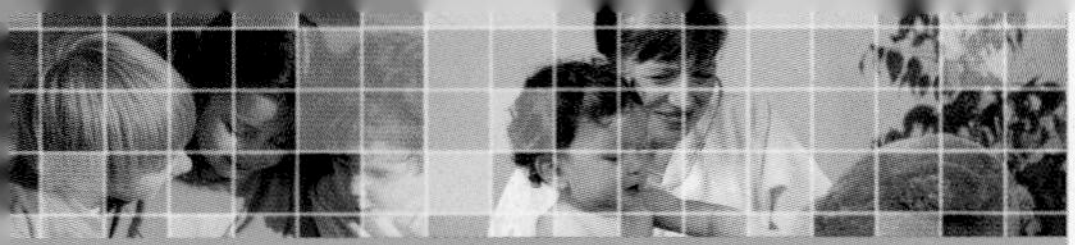

KEY TERMS

Amniotomy, 509
Cervical ripening, 510
Cesarean birth, 522
Episiotomy, 518
External cephalic version (ECV), 508
Forceps-assisted birth, 519
Funic presentation, 512
Labor induction, 512
Podalic version, 508
Vacuum-assisted birth, 521
Vaginal birth after cesarean (VBAC), 527

Most births occur without the need for operative obstetric intervention. In some instances, however, procedures are necessary to maintain the safety of the woman and the fetus. The most common of these procedures are amniotomy, induction of labor, episiotomy, cesarean birth, and vaginal birth following a previous cesarean birth.

Generally, women are aware of the possible need for an obstetric procedure during their labor and birth. However, some women expect to have a "natural" experience and feel disappointed, angry, or even guilty when an unanticipated procedure is needed. This conflict between expectation and the need for intervention presents a challenge to maternity nurses. The nurse provides information regarding any procedure to help the woman and her partner understand what is proposed, the anticipated benefits and possible risks, and any alternatives.

CARE OF THE WOMAN DURING VERSION

Version, or turning the fetus, is a procedure used to change the fetal presentation by abdominal or intrauterine manipulation. The most common type of version is **external cephalic version (ECV)**, in which the fetus is changed from a breech to a cephalic presentation by external manipulation of the maternal abdomen (Figure 23–1 ●). A less common type of version, called **podalic version**, is used only with the second fetus during a vaginal twin birth and only if the twin does not descend readily or if the heart rate is nonreassuring. The use of podalic versions are declining as more women with a second twin in a non-vertex presentation are counseled to undergo a cesarean birth (Bjelic-Radisic, Pristauz, Haas, et al., 2007). The success rates of ECV in singleton pregnancies ranges from 51% to 65% (Zeck, Walcher, & Lang, 2008).

CRITERIA FOR EXTERNAL VERSION

If breech or shoulder presentation (transverse lie) is detected in the later weeks of pregnancy, an external version may be attempted. Before the external version is begun, an ultrasound is used to locate the placenta and to confirm fetal presentation.

The following criteria should be met before performing external version:

- The pregnancy is 36 or more weeks' gestation. A version may result in complications that require immediate birth by cesarean (Thorp, 2009).
- A nonstress test (NST), obtained immediately before performing the version, is reactive. A reactive NST indicates fetal well-being.
- The fetal breech is not engaged. Once the presenting part is engaged it is difficult, if not impossible, to do a version.

CONTRAINDICATIONS FOR EXTERNAL VERSION

Contraindications include the following:

- Maternal problems, such as uterine anomalies, uncontrolled preeclampsia, or third-trimester bleeding
- Complications of pregnancy, such as rupture of membranes, oligohydramnios, hydramnios, or placenta previa or vasa previa
- Previous cesarean birth or other significant uterine surgery
- Multiple gestations
- Nonreassuring fetal heart rate (FHR) or other evidence of uteroplacental insufficiency
- Fetal abnormalities, such as intrauterine growth restriction (IUGR) or nuchal cord

Before the external version begins, an intravenous line may be established to administer medications in case of difficulty. The woman may receive terbutaline subcutaneously to relax the uterus. Some physicians may also order regional anesthesia for the

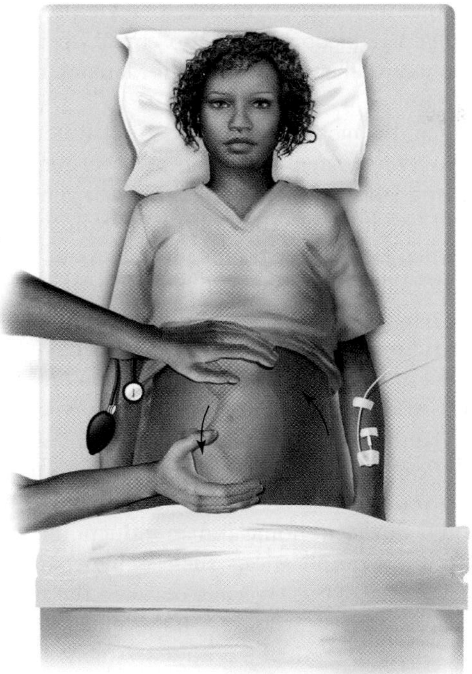

● **Figure 23–1** External (or cephalic) version of the fetus. A new technique involves applying pressure to the fetal head and buttocks so that the fetus completes a "backward flip" or "forward roll."

procedure. Both tocolytics and regional anesthesia have been associated with higher success rates and lower cesarean births (Thorp, 2009). Ultrasound is frequently used to provide information about the fetal position. The version is discontinued in the presence of severe maternal pain or significant fetal bradycardia or decelerations.

Nursing Management

On admission the nurse begins a thorough assessment by verifying that there are no contraindications to the version procedure. Maternal vital signs and a reactive NST are obtained. This initial assessment period provides an ideal time for educating the woman and her partner and for addressing their concerns. They can be encouraged to express their understanding and expectations of the procedure. At the same time, the nurse can discuss the possibility of failure of the ECV and slight risk of cesarean birth if the FHR becomes nonreassuring. Explaining what will occur in either of these circumstances will better prepare the woman and her partner if intervention becomes necessary. Although the physician is ultimately responsible for obtaining informed consent, it is also the nurse's role to ensure that the woman understands the procedure and has the opportunity to ask questions and voice her concerns or fears.

Evidence in Action

External cephalic version is considered a safe procedure but should be performed only when there is the ability to provide a cesarean delivery if necessary (Meta-analysis) (Grootscholten, Kok, Oei, et al., 2008).

Nursing Practice

Because the ECV procedure can be uncomfortable, encourage the woman to take slow, deep breaths. Using distraction and speaking in a calm, reassuring voice can help decrease fear and anxiety.

The nurse places an intravenous line before beginning the procedure to maintain intravenous (IV) access in case of a complication. Throughout the procedure, the nurse continues to monitor maternal blood pressure, pulse, and comfort level frequently (because the mother may experience pain during the procedure). Fetal well-being is ascertained before, intermittently during, and for (at least) 30 minutes following the procedure, using electronic fetal monitoring (EFM), ultrasound, or both. The nurse also assesses maternal-fetal response to the tocolytic. Aftercare instructions, which may include maternal monitoring for contractions and fetal movement (fetal kick counts), are provided as well.

CARE OF THE WOMAN DURING AMNIOTOMY

Amniotomy is the artificial rupture of the amniotic membranes (AROM). It is probably the most common invasive procedure in obstetrics. Because the amniotomy requires that an instrument, called an amnihook, be inserted through the cervix, at least 2 cm (0.8 in.) of cervical dilatation is required.

Amniotomy has been used as a means to shorten labor. A recent study that examined amniotomy and the length of labor did show a reduction in the first stage of labor as well as differences in maternal satisfaction or low Apgar scores (Smyth, Alldred, & Markham, 2007). Amniotomy can also be used at any time during the first stage to augment labor (accelerate the progress). Amniotomy is more effective in multiparous women. This is because the cervix is more pliable. Amniotomy manipulates both hormones and mechanical factors to stimulate labor. Upon rupturing the membranes, natural prostaglandins are released that stimulate uterine contractions. The escape of amniotic fluid allows the presenting part to descend and place direct pressure on the cervix, thus resulting in an acceleration of dilatation.

Amniotomy may also be done during labor to apply an internal fetal heart monitoring electrode to the scalp, to insert an intrauterine pressure catheter, or to obtain a fetal scalp blood sample for acid-base determination and fetal pH monitoring. In addition, amniotomy allows assessment of the color and composition of amniotic fluid. Amniotomy performed when the presenting part is not well applied to the cervix increases the risk of umbilical cord prolapse (see Chapter 22∞).

AROM PROCEDURE

While performing a vaginal examination, the physician or certified nurse-midwife (CNM) introduces an amnihook into the vagina and makes a small tear in the amniotic membrane, which allows amniotic fluid to escape.

Nursing Practice

Before the AROM procedure, place several layers of disposable pads under the woman's buttocks and a folded towel between her legs. The towel readily absorbs the fluid released during the procedure and prevents soiling of the bed linens. After the procedure, remove the towel as well as all layers of absorbent pads that have been soiled. To increase the woman's comfort, place several clean absorbent pads under her buttocks because amniotic fluid will continue to leak from the vagina.

Nursing Management

The nurse explains the AROM procedure to the woman and then assesses fetal presentation, position, and station, because amniotomy is usually delayed until engagement has occurred. The woman is asked to assume a semi-reclining position and is draped to provide privacy. The FHR is assessed just before and immediately after the amniotomy, and the two FHR assessments are compared. If there are marked changes, the nurse should check for prolapse of the cord (see Chapter 22 ∞). The amniotic fluid is inspected for amount, color, odor, and the presence of meconium or blood. While wearing disposable gloves, the nurse cleanses and dries the perineal area and changes the underpads as needed. Because there is now an open pathway for organisms to ascend into the uterus, the number of vaginal exams must be kept to a minimum to reduce the chance of introducing an infection. In addition, the woman's temperature is monitored a minimum of every 2 hours. The nurse needs to provide information regarding the expected effects of the amniotomy. It is important for the woman to know that amniotic fluid is constantly produced, because some women may worry that they will experience a "dry birth."

CARE OF THE WOMAN DURING CERVICAL RIPENING

Cervical ripening is softening and effacing of the cervix. It may be used for the pregnant woman who is at term or late preterm when there is a medical or obstetric indication for induction of labor. Pharmacologic methods of cervical ripening include prostaglandin agents and Cytotec.

PROSTAGLANDIN AGENTS

The most commonly used ripening agent is Prepidil gel, which contains 0.5 mg dinoprostone, a prostaglandin E_2 (PGE_2) agent. It is placed either intracervically or intravaginally. Prostaglandin agents placed intravaginally are superior to intracervical placement (Boulvain, Kelly, & Irion, 2008). A similar agent called Cervidil is packaged as a 2 cm (0.8 in.) square vaginal insert that resembles a thin piece of cardboard. It releases 10 mg of dinoprostone at a rate of 0.3 mg/hour over 12 hours. In a study by Facchinetti and colleagues (2007), women who received the Cervidil vaginal insert had more vaginal births within 24 hours of administration and shorter hospitalizations than those who received the prostaglandin gel. There is often a reduction of time to childbirth in multiparous women who receive the gel preparation (Marconi, Bozzetti, Morabito, et al., 2008).

Prostaglandin agents have been demonstrated to cause cervical ripening, to shorten labor, and to lower requirements for Pitocin during labor induction (Facchinetti, Venturini, Fazzio, et al., 2007; Marconi et al., 2008). Prostaglandin agents are typically used when labor induction is indicated, but not emergent, such as maternal gestational diabetes, postdates, or large-for-gestational-age fetuses who warrant birth occurring in the near future. For example, a woman who is over 41 weeks of gestation but has a very unfavorable cervix may be given prostaglandin gel to ripen her cervix before a Pitocin induction is scheduled.

Prostaglandin gel is administered in a hospital setting where women can be monitored for approximately 2 hours (depending on agency protocol) after the administration of the medication. The woman is then sent home and an induction is scheduled in the near future. Complications such as hyperstimulation and nonreassuring fetal status typically occur in the first hour after administration and peak at 4 hours. If the fetal heart rate remains unchanged during the initial 2 hour assessment and uterine activity has not become regular, the woman may be discharged once appropriate follow-up instructions and warning signs are provided. See "Drug Guide: Dinoprostone (Prepidil) Vaginal Gel" on page 511 for additional information.

Women receiving the Cervidil vaginal insert are observed in the hospital setting and have continuous fetal monitoring while the insert is in place. The woman should remain incumbent for 2 hours after administration. The insert should be removed immediately if uterine hyperstimulation or nonreassuring fetal status occurs. A beta-adrenergic agent should also be administered if hyperstimulation occurs (Forrest Pharmaceuticals, 2007).

MISOPROSTOL (CYTOTEC)

Misoprostol (Cytotec) is a synthetic PGE_1 analogue that some healthcare agencies use to ripen the cervix and induce labor. It is available as a tablet and can be administered using several routes including the following: oral, vaginal, rectal, sublingually, or buccally. Although the last two routes are effective, they are rarely used. The rectal route is primarily used when attempting to control postpartum hemorrhaging (Tang, Gemzell-Danielsson, & Ho, 2007). Practitioners may opt to administer the medication using different routes. One study

Nursing Practice

Advise the woman that prostaglandin agents commonly cause uterine stimulation after insertion. Review the signs of labor that warrant further assessment after discharge home. Teach the woman the difference between common reactions to the prostaglandin agents (such as cramping, uterine irritability, and gel leakage) and the true signs of labor (strong regular contractions, rupture of membranes) before she leaves the hospital.

Drug Guide

DINOPROSTONE (PREPIDIL) VAGINAL GEL

Pregnancy Risk Category: C

Overview of Maternal-Fetal Action

Dinoprostone is a naturally occurring form of prostaglandin E_2. Dinoprostone can be used at term to ripen the cervix and can stimulate the smooth muscle of the uterus to enhance uterine contractions. Prepidil can be administered endocervically (Pfizer Pharmaceuticals, Inc., 2008).

Route, Dosage, Frequency

The gel contains 0.5 mg of dinoprostone. The gel is placed in the posterior fornix of the vagina, and the client is kept supine for 2 hours, after which time she may ambulate. Continuous electronic monitoring is typically used for 2 hours after administration. Women who show no signs of labor and have a reassuring fetal monitoring strip may be discharged after 2 hours of administration.

Contraindications

- Client with known sensitivity to prostaglandins
- Presence of nonreassuring fetal status
- Unexplained bleeding during pregnancy
- Strong suspicion of cephalopelvic disproportion
- Client already receiving Pitocin
- Client who is not anticipated to be able to give birth vaginally
- Previous cesarean birth, uterine scar, or uterine rupture.

Dinoprostone vaginal gel should be used with CAUTION in clients with ruptured membranes, a fetus in breech presentation, presence of glaucoma, or history of asthma (Pfizer Pharmaceuticals, Inc., 2008).

Maternal Side Effects

Uterine hyperstimulation with or without nonreassuring fetal status has occurred in a very small number (6.6%) of clients. Other reported maternal side effects include gastrointestinal disturbance (fewer than 1% of clients have experienced fever, nausea, vomiting, diarrhea, or abdominal pain) (Wilson, Shannon, & Shields, 2010).

Effects on Fetus/Newborn

Nonreassuring fetal heart rate patterns

Nursing Considerations

- Assess for presence of contraindications.
- Monitor maternal vital signs, cervical dilatation, and effacement carefully.
- Monitor fetal status for presence of reassuring fetal heart rate pattern (baseline 110 to 160 bpm, presence of variability, presence of accelerations with fetal movement, absence of late or variable decelerations).
- Prepare to administer terbutaline if uterine hyperstimulation, sustained uterine contractions, nonreassuring fetal status, or any other adverse reactions occur.

showed that oral administration reduced hyperstimulation and had a lower cesarean birth rate when compared with vaginal administration (Cheng, Ming, & Lee, 2008). However, previous studies stated the opposite, that the vaginal route had higher rates of vaginal births (Cunningham, Leveno, Bloom, et al., 2010). Other studies report that the low dosages used in current practice are all associated with a lower incidence of hyperstimulation (Weeks, Alfirevic, Faúndes, et al., 2007). Although conflicting research findings can be confusing, it is important to note that Cytotec is delivered via various routes and yields successful results.

Since the 1990s, cytotic has been contraindicated for inducing labor in women who have had a previous cesarean birth or have a scar on their uterus (Cheng et al., 2008). Although quite rare, Cytotec has also been associated with uterine rupture in women who have no previous scar on their uterus (Matsuo, Scanlon, Atlas, et al., 2008). Other risk factors for uterine rupture include a high-dose regimen (100 mcg or higher), advanced gestational age, and five or more previous pregnancies (ACOG, 2003; FDA, 2008). After a careful review of the literature and current studies, ACOG (2003) issued the following recommended guidelines for Cytotec administration:

- Use only during the third trimester for cervical ripening or labor induction.
- One-fourth tablet or 25 mcg should be the initial dosage.
- Recurrent administration should not exceed dosing intervals of more than 3 to 6 hours.
- Pitocin should not be administered less than 4 hours after the last Cytotec dose.
- Continuous fetal and uterine monitoring should be performed in a hospital setting.

Absolute contraindications for the use of Cytotec include the following:

- Presence of uterine contractions three times in 10 minutes
- Significant maternal asthma (Shiraishi, Asano, Niimi, et al., 2008)
- History of previous cesarean birth or other uterine scar
- Bleeding during the pregnancy
- Presence of placenta previa
- Fetal tachycardia, nonreassuring fetal heart rate tracing, meconium passage (FDA, 2008)

Nursing Management

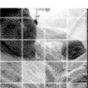

Physicians, certified nurse-midwives (CNMs), and birthing room nurses who have had special education and training may administer agents for cervical ripening. Provide the woman and her support person(s) information about the procedure, and answer any questions they may have. Assess baseline maternal vital signs, and apply an electronic fetal monitor (EFM). The EFM tracing should indicate minimal or absent uterine activity, a reassuring FHR pattern, and a reactive NST. If uterine contractions are not occurring regularly, the ripening agent is inserted into the vagina. Prepidil can be administered every 6 hours. If prescribed, Cytotec is administered every 3 to 6 hours until adequate cervical change occurs (Cheng et al., 2008). The nurse instructs the woman to lie supine with a right hip wedge for a specified time (usually at least 1 hour). The woman can then assume any comfortable position. As discussed previously, the nurse monitors the woman for uterine hyperstimulation and FHR abnormalities (changes in baseline rate, variability, presence of decelerations) for at least 2 hours following insertion. During administration of PGE_2, if nausea and vomiting are present or if contractions occur more frequently than every 2 minutes (and/or last greater than 75 seconds), remove the gel.

CARE OF THE WOMAN DURING LABOR INDUCTION

MyNursingKit Case Study: Client Undergoing Labor Induction

ACOG defines **labor induction** as the stimulation of uterine contractions before the spontaneous onset of labor, with or without ruptured fetal membranes, for the purpose of accomplishing birth. Induction may be indicated in the presence of the following (Thorp, 2009):

- Diabetes mellitus
- Preeclampsia/eclampsia
- Premature rupture of membranes (PROM) with established fetal maturity
- Chorioamnionitis
- Postterm gestation, especially in association with oligohydramnios
- Intrauterine fetal demise (IUFD)
- Intrauterine fetal growth restriction (IUGR)
- Alloimmunization
- Nonreassuring antepartum testing

Relative indications include chronic hypertension, systemic lupus erythematosus, gestational diabetes, hypercoagulation disorders, cholestasis of pregnancy, polyhydramnios, fetal anomalies requiring specialized neonatal care, logistical factors (risk of rapid birth, distance from hospital, psychologic factors, advanced cervical dilatation), and previous stillbirth (Thorp, 2009).

All contraindications to spontaneous labor and vaginal birth are contraindications to the induction of labor. Maternal contraindications include but are not limited to the following (Thorp, 2009):

- Client refusal
- Placenta previa or vasa previa
- Floating fetal presenting part
- Prior uterine incision that would preclude a trial of labor
- Active genital herpes infection
- Umbilical cord prolapse
- Acute severe fetal distress
- Absolute cephalopelvic disproportion

Relative contraindications include cervical carcinoma; malpresentation, such as breech; and funic presentation. A **funic presentation** is when the umbilical cord is interposed between the cervix and the presenting part. It can be located by clinical evaluation or by ultrasound (Thorp, 2009).

LABOR READINESS

Before attempting an induction, assess fetal maturity and cervical readiness to ensure that both the woman and fetus are ready for the onset of labor.

Fetal Maturity

The gestational age of the fetus is best evaluated by accurate maternal menstrual dating and early ultrasounds. Amniotic fluid studies also provide valuable information in assessing fetal lung maturity (see Chapter 14∞).

Cervical Readiness

The findings on vaginal examination help determine whether cervical changes favorable for induction have occurred. Bishop (1964) developed a prelabor scoring system that is helpful in predicting the potential success of induction (Table 23–1). Components evaluated are cervical dilatation, effacement, consistency, and position, as well as the station of the fetal presenting part. A score of 0, 1, 2, or 3 is given to each assessed characteristic. The higher the total score for all the criteria, the more likely it is that labor will occur. The lower the total score, the higher the failure rate. A favorable cervix is the most important criterion for a successful induction (Cheng et al., 2008). The presence of a cervix that is anterior, soft, 50% effaced, and dilated at least 2 cm (0.8 in.), with the fetal head at −1 to +1 station or lower (Bishop score of 8 or 9), is favorable for successful induction (Mbele, Makin, & Pattinson, 2007). If the cervix is unfavorable, a method of cervical ripening may be tried.

METHODS OF INDUCING LABOR

When the cervix is favorable, the most frequently used methods of induction are amniotomy (discussed previously), stripping the amniotic membranes, intravenous Pitocin infusion, and complementary methods.

Stripping the Membranes

A nonpharmacologic method of induction frequently used by physicians/CNMs is *stripping* (or *sweeping*) *the amniotic membranes.* The practitioner inserts a gloved finger into the internal os and rotates it 360 degrees twice, separating the amniotic membranes that are lying against the lower uterine segment. This is thought to release prostaglandins that stimulate uterine contractions. The procedure is usually uncomfortable and can result in cramping, uterine contractions, and vaginal bleeding.

Table 23–1 Prelabor Status Evaluation Scoring System

	ASSIGNED VALUE			
Factor	**0**	**1**	**2**	**3**
Cervical dilatation	Closed	1 to 2 cm	3 to 4 cm	5 cm or more
Cervical effacement	0% to 30%	40% to 50%	60% to 70%	80% or more
Fetal station	−3	−2	−1, 0	+1, or lower
Cervical consistency	Firm	Moderate	Soft	
Cervical position	Posterior	Midposition	Anterior	

Source: Bishop, E. H. (1964). Pelvic scoring for elective inductions. *Obstetrics & Gynecology, 24,* 266.

Pitocin Infusion

Administration of Pitocin is an effective method of initiating uterine contractions to induce labor and may also be used to enhance ineffective contractions (*labor augmentation*). A primary line of 1000 mL of electrolyte solution (e.g., lactated Ringer's solution) is started intravenously. Ten units of Pitocin are added to a secondary line of intravenous (IV) fluid so the resulting mixture will contain 10 milliunits/mL of Pitocin (1 milliunit/min, or 6 mL/h), and the prescribed dose can be calculated easily. After the primary infusion is started, the Pitocin solution is piggybacked into the primary tubing port closest to the catheter insertion. The infusion is then administered using an infusion pump to control the flow rate precisely. The rate of infusion is based on physician/CNM protocol and careful assessment of the contraction pattern. The goal for induction is to achieve stable contractions every 2 to 3 minutes that last 40 to 60 seconds. The uterus should relax to full baseline resting tone between each contraction. Progress is determined by changes in the effacement and dilatation of the cervix and station of the presenting part.

Pitocin induction is not without some associated risks, including hyperstimulation of the uterus, resulting in uterine contractions that are too frequent or too intense, with an increased resting tone. Hypertonic contractions may lead to decreased placental perfusion and nonreassuring fetal status. Other risks include uterine rupture, water intoxication, fetal hypoxia, and in rare circumstances fetal death (Wilson et al., 2010).

Complementary Methods

Although not frequently presented in medical (allopathic) or nursing texts, a variety of more natural, noninvasive methods of inducing labor can be effective. These methods include sexual intercourse; self or partner nipple or breast stimulation; the use of herbs, castor oil, or enemas; acupuncture; and mechanical dilatation of the cervix with balloon catheters (Tenore, 2003). Many CNMs and their clients desire a less medical approach to birth and want to use natural methods when possible. The cautions and contraindications for these natural methods are the same as those for medical induction of labor. And it's important to understand that some of them may not have undergone as rigorous scientific research as pharmacologic agents.

Sexual intercourse is a logical method of inducing cervical ripening and uterine contractions; female orgasm stimulates contractions, and male ejaculate is a rich source of prostaglandins. Penetration during intercourse can also stimulate the lower uterine segment and cause uterine contractions. In addition, breast and nipple stimulation, which are often part of lovemaking, cause the production of endogenous oxytocin, which in turn stimulates the uterus to contract (Tenore, 2003).

Herbal preparations and other homeopathic solutions have not been scientifically studied to the same extent as other natural methods. The caregiver needs a thorough personal knowledge or ongoing consultation with a homeopathic physician to safely recommend the use of these approaches during late pregnancy (Tenore, 2003).

Although castor oil has been used for many years it has not been frequently studied as a method of labor induction. The mechanism by which castor oil stimulates uterine contractions is not understood. Some practitioners consider it to be an old-fashioned, nonuseful substance, whereas others have noted that it is especially effective for primigravidas.

MyNursingKit Care Plan Activity: Client with Pitocin for Labor Augmentation

Complementary Care

EVENING PRIMROSE OIL

Evening primrose oil is a natural substance that is extracted from the plant's seeds. It has been widely used for centuries by midwives as a means of softening the cervix, vagina, and perineum to facilitate the onset of labor. Evening primrose oil contains a fatty acid called gamma linolenic acid, which is converted into a prostaglandin compound. Prostaglandins play a key role in ripening the cervix so labor can begin. Women can be advised to begin evening primrose oil supplementation during the 36th week of pregnancy. The recommended dose is 2500 mg per day taken either orally or vaginally until birth. Side effects are rare but can include headaches, nausea, or skin rashes. Women who experience side effects should be counseled to discontinue the supplement unless advised otherwise by their physician (Midwifery Today E-News, 2007).

Thinking Critically

DETERMINING INFUSION RATE

You are a birthing center nurse caring for Wendy Johnson, G2P1, during a Pitocin infusion to induce her labor. Wendy has been receiving the medication via infusion pump for 4 hours and currently is receiving 6 milliunits/min (36 mL/hr). You have just completed your assessments and found the following: BP 120/80, pulse 80, respirations 16; contractions every 3 minutes lasting 60 seconds and of strong intensity; the FHR baseline is 144 to 150 with average variability; and cervical dilatation is 6 cm (2.4 in.). Will you continue the same infusion rate, increase the rate, or decrease the rate?

See MyNursing Kit for possible responses.

Nursing management. Aspects to address during client teaching about induction of labor include the purpose, the procedure itself, nursing care that will be provided, assessments, comfort measures, and a review of breathing techniques that may be used during labor. Regardless of the induction method used, close observation and accurate, ongoing assessments are mandatory to provide safe, optimal care for both woman and fetus. A qualified clinician should be readily accessible to manage any complications that may occur.

As contractions are established, perform vaginal examinations to evaluate cervical dilatation, effacement, and station. The frequency of vaginal examinations primarily depends on the woman's parity, comfort level, and strength of her contractions. If evaluating the need for analgesia, perform a vaginal examination to avoid giving the medication too early and increasing the risk of prolonging labor. This examination also helps identify advanced dilatation and imminent birth.

Pitocin induction protocols recommend obtaining baseline data (maternal temperature, pulse, respirations, blood pressure), a 20- to 30-minute EFM recording demonstrating a reassuring FHR, a reactive NST, and the contraction status before starting an induction. Use a fetal monitor to provide continuous data.

Before each increase of the Pitocin infusion rate the nurse assesses the following:

- Maternal blood pressure, pulse, respirations, temperature, and pain level
- Contraction status including frequency, duration, intensity, and resting tone
- FHR baseline, variability, and reactivity, noting the presence of accelerations, any decelerations, or bradycardia

For additional information about nursing interventions during use of Pitocin, see "Drug Guide: Oxytocin (Pitocin)" and the "Clinical Pathway for Induction of Labor."

Drug Guide

OXYTOCIN (PITOCIN)

Overview of Obstetric Action

Oxytocin (Pitocin) exerts a selective stimulatory effect on the smooth muscle of the uterus and blood vessels. Oxytocin affects the myometrial cells of the uterus by increasing the excitability of the muscle cell, increasing the strength of the muscle contraction, and supporting propagation of the contraction (movement of the contraction from one myometrial cell to the next). Its effect on the uterine contraction depends on the dosage used and on the excitability of the myometrial cells. During the first half of gestation, there is little excitability of the myometrium, and the uterus is fairly resistant to the effects of oxytocin. However, from midgestation on, the uterus responds increasingly to exogenous intravenous oxytocin. Cautious use of diluted oxytocin administered intravenously at term results in a slow rise of uterine activity.

The circulatory half-life of oxytocin is 3 to 5 minutes. It takes approximately 40 minutes for a particular dose of oxytocin to reach a steady-state plasma concentration (Wilson et al., 2010).

The effects of oxytocin on the cardiovascular system can be pronounced. Blood pressure initially may decrease but after prolonged administration increase by 30% above the baseline. Cardiac output and stroke volume increase. With doses of 20 milliunits/min or above, oxytocin exerts an antidiuretic effect decreasing free water exchange in the kidney and markedly decreasing urine output.

Oxytocin is used to induce labor at term and to augment uterine contractions in the first and second stages of labor. Oxytocin may also be used immediately after birth to stimulate uterine contraction and thereby control uterine atony.

Route, Dosage, Frequency

For induction of labor: Add 10 units of Pitocin (1 mL) to 1000 mL of intravenous solution. (The resulting concentration is 10 mU oxytocin per 1 mL of intravenous fluid.) Using an infusion pump, administer IV, starting at 0.5–1 milliunit/min and increase by 1–2 milliunits/min every 40–60 minutes. Alternatively, start at 1–2 milliunits/min and increase by 1 milliunit/min every 15 minutes until a good contraction pattern (every 2–3 minutes and lasting 40–60 seconds) is achieved.

Maternal Contraindications

- Severe preeclampsia-eclampsia
- Predisposition to uterine rupture (in nullipara over 35 years of age, multigravida 4 or more, overdistention of the uterus, previous major surgery of the cervix or uterus)
- Cephalopelvic disproportion
- Malpresentation or malposition of the fetus, cord prolapse

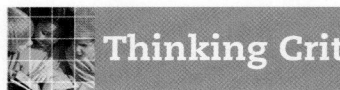

Drug Guide—continued

- More than 1 previous cesarean birth
- Preterm infant
- Rigid, unripe cervix; total placenta previa
- Presence of nonreassuring fetal status

Maternal Side Effects

Hyperstimulation of the uterus results in hypercontractility, which in turn may cause the following:

- Abruptio placentae
- Impaired uterine blood flow, leading to fetal hypoxia
- Rapid labor, leading to cervical lacerations
- Rapid labor and birth, leading to lacerations of cervix, vagina, or perineum, uterine atony; fetal trauma
- Uterine rupture
- Water intoxication (nausea, vomiting, hypotension, tachycardia, cardiac arrhythmia) if oxytocin is given in electrolyte-free solution or at a rate exceeding 20 milliunits/min; hypotension with rapid IV bolus administration postpartum

Effect on Fetus-Newborn

- Fetal effects are primarily associated with the presence of hypercontractility of the maternal uterus. Hypercontractility decreases the oxygen supply to the fetus, which is reflected by irregularities or decrease in fetal heart rate (FHR), and hypoxia
- Hyperbilirubinemia (Wilson et al., 2010)
- Trauma from rapid birth
- Hypoxia as an effect of maternal hypotension

Nursing Considerations

- Explain induction or augmentation procedure to client.
- Apply fetal monitor, and obtain 15- to 20-minute tracing and nonstress test (NST) to assess FHR before starting IV oxytocin.
- For induction or augmentation of labor, start with primary IV, and piggyback secondary IV with oxytocin and infusion pump.
- Ensure continuous monitoring of the fetus and uterine contractions.
- The maximum rate is 40 milliunits/min (Blackburn, 2007). Not all protocols recommend a maximum dose. When indicated, the maximum dose is generally between 16 and 40 milliunits/min. Decrease oxytocin by similar increments once labor has progressed to 5–6 cm dilatation. Protocols may vary from one agency to another.

0.5 milliunit/min = 3 mL/hr	8 milliunit/min = 48 mL/hr
1.0 milliunit/min = 6 mL/hr	10 milliunit/min = 60 mL/hr
1.5 milliunit/min = 9 mL/hr	12 milliunit/min = 72 mL/hr
2 milliunit/min = 12 mL/hr	15 milliunit/min = 90 mL/hr
4 milliunit/min = 24 mL/hr	18 milliunit/min = 108 mL/hr
6 milliunit/min = 36 mL/hr	20 milliunit/min = 120 mL/hr

- Assess FHR, maternal blood pressure, pulse, frequency and duration of uterine contractions, presence of decelerations, and uterine resting tone before each increase in the oxytocin infusion rate.
- Record all assessments and IV rate on monitor strip and on client's chart.
- Record oxytocin infusion rate in milliunits/min and mL/hr (e.g., 0.5 milliunits/min [3 mL/hr]).
- Record on monitor strip all client activities (such as change of position, vomiting), procedures done (amniotomy, sterile vaginal examination), and administration of analgesic agents to allow for interpretation and evaluation of tracing.
- Assess cervical dilatation as needed.
- Apply nursing comfort measures.
- Discontinue IV oxytocin infusion and infuse primary solution when (1) nonreassuring fetal status is noted (bradycardia, late or variable decelerations); (2) uterine contractions are more frequent than every 2 minutes; (3) duration of contractions exceeds more than 60 seconds; or (4) insufficient relaxation of the uterus between contractions or a steady increase in resting tone are noted (Blackburn, 2007). In addition to discontinuing IV oxytocin infusion, turn client to side, and if nonreassuring fetal status is present, administer oxygen by tight face mask at 7–10 L/min; notify physician.
- Maintain intake and output record.

For Augmentation of Labor

Prepare and administer IV Pitocin as for labor induction. Increase rate until labor contractions are of good quality, duration, and frequency. The flow rate is gradually increased at no less than every 30 minutes to a maximum of 10 milliunits/min (Blackburn, 2007). In some settings or in a situation when limited fluids may be administered, a more concentrated solution may be used. When 10 units Pitocin are added to 500 mL IV solution, the resulting concentration is 1 milliunit/min = 3 mL/hr. If 10 units Pitocin are added to 250 mL IV solution, the concentration is 1 milliunit/min = 1.5 mL/hr.

For Administration After Expulsion of Placenta

- One dose of 10 units of Pitocin (1 mL) is given intramuscularly or added to IV fluids for continuous infusion.
- Assess maternal blood pressure, pulse, and uterine resting tone before each increase in oxytocin infusion rate.
- Record all assessments and IV rate on client's chart. Record oxytocin infusion rate in milliunits/min and mL/hr (e.g., 0.5 milliunits/min [3 mL/hr]).
- Record all client activities and procedures.
- Apply nursing comfort measures.
- If bleeding is well controlled, often oxytocin is discontinued after the initial postpartum infusion.

Clinical Pathway

CLINICAL PATHWAY FOR INDUCTION OF LABOR

CATEGORY	IMMEDIATE CARE	OUTCOMES
Referral	Review prenatal record Advise certified nurse-midwife (CNM) or physician of admission Anesthesia	**EXPECTED OUTCOMES** Appropriate resources identified and utilized
Assessments	Previous pregnancies, present pregnancy, and childbirth preparation Estimated gestational age of the fetus Assess woman's feelings regarding induction as well as knowledge base regarding the induction process Assess knowledge of breathing techniques; if woman does not have a method to use, teach breathing techniques before starting oxytocin infusion	**EXPECTED OUTCOMES** Potential/actual complications identified
Teaching/ psychosocial	Provide emotional support through teaching and answering all questions	**EXPECTED OUTCOMES** Woman verbalizes or demonstrates understanding of information given
Nursing care management and reports	Examination of pregnant uterus (Leopold's maneuvers to determine fetal size and position) Vaginal examination to evaluate cervical readiness: ■ Ripe cervix feels soft to the examining finger, is located in a medial to anterior position, is more than 50% effaced, and is 2–3 cm dilated ■ Unripe cervix feels firm to the examining finger, is long and thick, is perhaps in a posterior position, and is dilated little or not at all Presence of contractions Membranes intact or ruptured Maternal vital signs and a 20-minute baseline fetal monitoring strip prior to induction to determine fetal well-being Diagnostic studies: ■ Fetal maturity tests (lecithin/sphingomyelin [L/S] ratio, creatinine concentrations, ultrasonography), NST, CST, BPP ■ Maternal blood studies (complete blood count [CBC], hemoglobin, hematocrit, blood type, Rh factor) ■ Urinalysis Monitor for nausea, vomiting, hypotension, tachycardia, cardiac arrhythmias, headache, mental confusion, decreased urinary output Monitor FHR by continuous electronic fetal monitoring; do not start oxytocin infusion or advance rate (if induction has already begun) if FHR is not in range of 110–160 bpm, if decelerations are present, or if variability decreases Evaluate and document maternal BP and pulse before beginning induction and then before each increase in infusion rate; do not advance infusion rate in presence of maternal hypertension or hypotension or radical changes in pulse rate If the woman becomes hypotensive: ■ Keep her on her side; may change to other side ■ Discontinue oxytocin infusion ■ Increase rate of primary IV line ■ Monitor FHR ■ Notify physician ■ Assess for cause of hypotension Evaluate and document contraction frequency, duration, and intensity prior to each increase in oxytocin infusion rate Discontinue oxytocin infusion if: ■ Contractions are more frequent than every 2 minutes ■ Contraction duration exceeds 90 seconds ■ Uterus does not relax between contractions	**EXPECTED OUTCOMES** Progression of labor and birth without difficulty Potential/actual complications minimized

Clinical Pathway—continued

CLINICAL PATHWAY FOR INDUCTION OF LABOR

CATEGORY	IMMEDIATE CARE	OUTCOMES
Nursing care management and reports—continued	Increase oxytocin IV infusion rate every 20 minutes until adequate contractions are achieved. Do not exceed an infusion rate of 20–40 mL/min. (*Note:* Protocols directing how often oxytocin is increased may vary from 15 to 60 minutes. See institutional protocols.) Check infusion pump to ensure oxytocin is infusing. Check whether pump is on, chamber refills and empties, level of fluid in IV bottle becomes lower. If problem is found, correct and restart infusion at beginning dose. Check main IV site frequently. Check piggyback connection to primary tubing to ensure solution is not leaking. Evaluate cervical dilatation by vaginal examination as indicated. Monitor FHR continuously (normal range is 110–160 bpm). In episodes of bradycardia (<110 bpm) lasting for more than 30 seconds, administer oxygen by face mask at 7–10 L/min. Stop oxytocin infusion. Position woman on left side if quick recovery of FHR does not occur. Carefully evaluate fetal tachycardia (>160 bpm). Sustained tachycardia may necessitate discontinuation of oxytocin infusion. Assess for presence of meconium staining. Notify physician.	
Activity	Ambulate until 5–10 cm. dilated, then bed Position woman in left lateral or semi-Fowler's position Encourage her to avoid supine position	**EXPECTED OUTCOMES** Activity individualized for woman
Comfort	Provide support to woman as she uses breathing techniques Encourage use of effleurage, back rub, and other supportive measures Assess need for analgesia or anesthesia	**EXPECTED OUTCOMES** Optimal comfort level maintained
Nutrition	IV or lactated Ringer's solution Ice chips, clear fluids	**EXPECTED OUTCOMES** Nutritional and hydration needs met
Elimination	Encourage voiding every 2 hours; monitor and record intake and output	**EXPECTED OUTCOMES** Intake and output WNL
Medications	Start primary IV as ordered Administer oxytocin in electrolyte solution (piggyback oxytocin onto primary IV at closest site to IV needle insertion) Pain medications prn	**EXPECTED OUTCOMES** Induction or augmentation of labor occurs within expected parameters
Discharge planning/ home care	Photo packet Birth certificate worksheet Sibling visitation Car seat	**EXPECTED OUTCOMES** Individualized discharge teaching completed
Family involvement	Family visitation policy per institutional protocol Encourage significant other to stay close and assist the woman with breathing techniques	**EXPECTED OUTCOMES** Family or support person involvement maximized
Date		

BP, blood pressure; bpm, beats per minute; BPP, biophysical profile; CBC, complete blood count; CST, contraction stress test; FHR, fetal heart rate; I&O, intake and output; IV, intravenous; NST, nonstress test; prn, as needed; WNL, within normal limits

CARE OF THE WOMAN DURING AN EPISIOTOMY

An **episiotomy** is a surgical incision of the perineal body to enlarge the outlet. It is the second-most-common procedure in maternal-child care and has long been thought to minimize the risk of lacerations of the perineum and the overstretching of perineal tissues. However, episiotomy may actually increase the risk of fourth-degree perineal lacerations (Dudding, Vaizey, &, Kamm, 2008). Though very common, the routine use of episiotomy has been seriously questioned for several years. Research suggests that (1) rather than protecting the perineum from lacerations, the presence of an episiotomy makes it more likely that the woman will have anal sphincter tears and (2) perineal lacerations heal more quickly than deep perineal tears (Wheeler & Richter, 2007). In clinical practice, research has shown that the incidence of major perineal trauma (extension to or through the anal sphincter) is more likely to happen if a midline episiotomy is done (Roberts, Ely, & Ward, 2007). Women with previous episiotomies that resulted in a third- or fourth-degree extension were more likely to have a repeat occurrence when episiotomy was used initially compared with those women who had a spontaneous laceration without the use of episiotomy (Edwards, Grotegut, Harmanli et al., 2006). Additional complications associated with episiotomy are blood loss, infection, pain, and perineal discomfort that may continue for days or weeks past birth, including painful intercourse (Ejegård, Ryding, & Sjögren, 2008).

FACTORS THAT PREDISPOSE WOMEN TO EPISIOTOMY

Overall factors that place a woman at increased risk for episiotomy are primigravid status, large or macrosomic fetus, occiput-posterior position, use of forceps or vacuum extractor, and shoulder dystocia. Other factors that may be mitigated by nurses and physicians/CNMs include the following:

- Use of lithotomy and other recumbent positions (causes excessive and uneven stretching of the perineum)
- Encouraging or requiring sustained breath holding during second-stage pushing (causes excessive and rapid perineal stretching, can adversely affect blood flow in mother and fetus, and requires woman to be responsive to caregiver directions rather than to her own urges to push spontaneously)
- Arbitrary time limit placed by the physician/CNM on the length of the second stage

PREVENTIVE MEASURES

These general tips help reduce the incidence of routine episiotomies:

- Perineal massage during pregnancy for nulliparous women
- Natural pushing during labor, and avoiding the lithotomy position or pulling back on legs (which tightens the perineum)

Nursing Practice

Some practitioners routinely perform episiotomy as a standard of care. Therefore, nurses should provide information about episiotomy and encourage women to talk to their practitioner about the incidence of its use within the practice. Encourage women who are opposed to an episiotomy to discuss their objection to the procedure with their healthcare provider at a prenatal visit before the onset of labor.

- Side-lying position for pushing, which helps slow birth and diminish tears
- Warm or hot compresses on the perineum and firm counterpressure
- Encouraging a gradual expulsion of the infant at the time of birth by encouraging the mother to "push, take a breath, push, take a breath" thereby easing the infant out slowly
- Avoiding immediate pushing after epidural placement

EPISIOTOMY PROCEDURE

The two types of episiotomy in current practice are midline and mediolateral (Figure 23–2 ●). Just before birth, when approximately 3 to 4 cm (1.2 to 1.6 in.) of the fetal head is visible during a contraction, the episiotomy is performed using sharp scissors with rounded points (Kilpatrick & Garrison, 2007). The midline incision begins at the bottom center of the perineal body and extends straight down the midline to the fibers of the rectal sphincter. The mediolateral incision begins in the midline of the posterior fourchette and extends at a 45-degree angle downward to the right or left.

The episiotomy is usually performed with regional or local anesthesia but may be done without anesthesia in emergency situations. It is generally proposed that as crowning occurs, the distention of the tissues causes numbing. Repair of the episiotomy (episiorrhaphy) and any lacerations is completed either during the period between birth of the newborn and expulsion of the placenta or after expulsion of the placenta. Adequate anesthesia must be given for the repair.

Nursing Management

The woman needs to be supported during the episiotomy and the repair because she may feel some pressure or pulling or tugging sensations. If anesthesia is inadequate, she may feel pain. Placing a hand on the woman's shoulder and talking with her can provide comfort and distraction from the repair process. If the woman is having more discomfort than she can handle, the nurse needs to act as an advocate in communicating the woman's needs to the physician/CNM. At all times the woman needs to be the one who decides whether the amount of discomfort she is experiencing is tolerable. She should never be

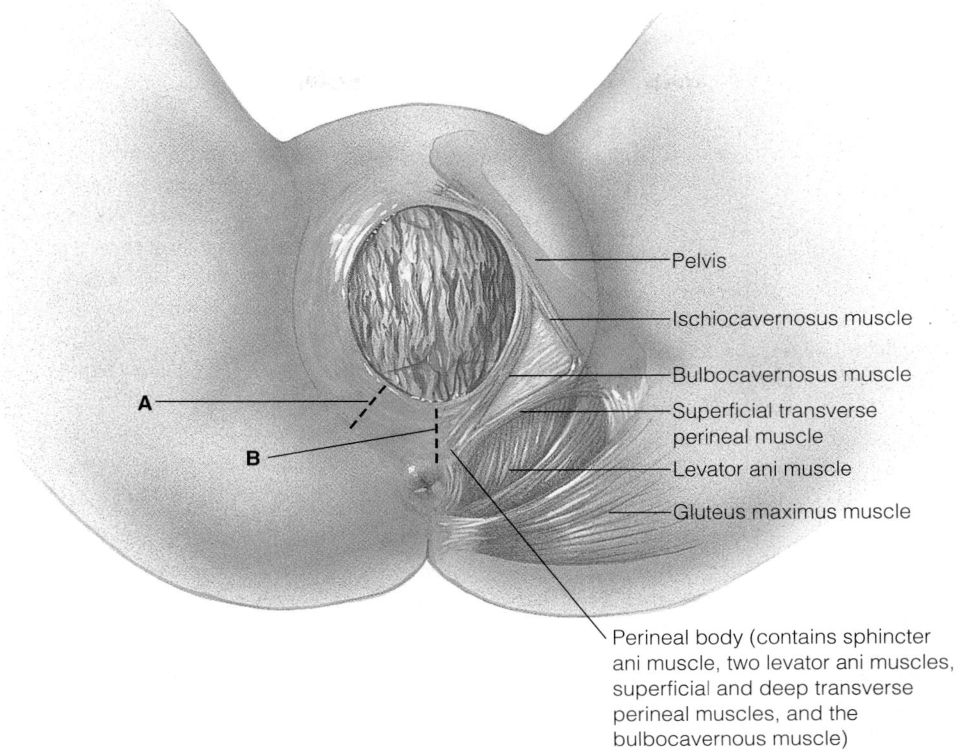

● **Figure 23–2** Common types of episiotomies. The two most common types of episiotomies are midline and mediolateral. ***A,*** Right mediolateral. ***B,*** Midline.

told, "This doesn't hurt." She is the person experiencing the discomfort, and her evaluation needs to be respected.

The type of episiotomy is recorded on the birth record. This information should also be included in a report to subsequent caregivers so that adequate assessments can be made and relief measures can be instituted.

Comfort measures may begin immediately after birth with the application of an ice pack to the perineum. For optimal effect the ice pack should be applied for 20 to 30 minutes and removed for at least 20 minutes before being reapplied. The nurse assesses the perineal tissues frequently to prevent injury from the ice pack. The episiotomy site should be inspected every 15 minutes during the first hour after the birth for redness, swelling, tenderness, bruising, and hematomas. As part of postpartal care the mother will need instruction in perineal hygiene, self-care, and comfort measures (see further discussion on nursing care after episiotomy in Chapters 30 and 31∞).

It is important for nurses to recognize that perineal pain continues for a period of time, and it may be significant. This pain should not be discounted: Women who experience prolonged perineal pain tend to have problems with breastfeeding and depression and are reluctant to reestablish sexual activity.

Nursing advocacy is needed to promote selective rather than routine episiotomy. It is imperative that each nurse stay current regarding new information and research in order to maintain current practice standards.

CARE OF THE WOMAN DURING FORCEPS-ASSISTED BIRTH

Forceps are surgical instruments designed to assist in the birth of a fetus by providing either traction or the means to rotate the fetal head to an occiput-anterior position. In medical literature and practice, **forceps-assisted birth** is also known as *instrumental delivery* or *operative vaginal delivery.* Three categories of forceps application exist:

1. Outlet forceps are applied when the fetal skull has reached the perineum, the fetal scalp is visible, and the sagittal suture is not more than 45 degrees from the midline.
2. Low forceps are applied when the leading edge (presenting part) of the fetal skull is at a station of +2 or more.
3. Midforceps are applied when the fetal head is engaged.

INDICATIONS FOR FORCEPS-ASSISTED BIRTH

Forceps may be indicated in the presence of any condition that threatens the mother or fetus and that can be relieved by birth. Conditions that put the woman at risk include heart disease, pulmonary edema, infection, and exhaustion. Fetal conditions include premature placental separation and nonreassuring fetal status. Forceps may be used to shorten the second stage of labor and assist the woman's pushing effort. They may also be used

Evidence-Based Nursing

EPISIOTOMY FOR VAGINAL BIRTH

Clinical Question

How does the restrictive use of episiotomy during birth compare to routine episiotomy?

The Evidence

The most common injuries during birth are due to tears around the vagina that occur as the baby's head passes through. These tears may range from minor discomforts to major injuries extending to the anus. Traditionally, routine episiotomy has been used to substitute a surgical enlargement for a traumatic tear; it has become the most commonly performed birth procedure. Carroli and Mignini (2009) reviewed eight studies comparing routine episiotomy to restrictive (medically indicated) episiotomy for the Cochrane Database, a source of rigorous evidence-based reviews. More than 5000 women were represented by these studies; 75% of the women in the "routine" group had an episiotomy performed, compared to 28% of the "restrictive" group. Multiple studies with large samples represent the strongest level of evidence.

Best Practice

There is clear evidence to recommend a restrictive episiotomy policy based on medical necessity when compared with the routine use of this procedure. Performing an episiotomy only when medically indicated results in less severe perineal trauma, less posterior perineal trauma, less suturing, and fewer healing complications at seven days post-birth. There was no difference in the occurrence of pain, urinary incontinence, painful sex, or severe vagina/perineal trauma after birth when episiotomy was restricted to medical necessity versus routinely applied. Women did experience more anterior perineal trauma with restrictive application, although this type of trauma is usually less serious than posterior trauma. A restrictive episiotomy policy was also more cost-effective than routine episiotomy.

Critical Thinking

What is the effect of restrictive episiotomy with other birth procedures such as forceps or vacuum, or in special cases such as breech position? See MyNursing Kit for possible responses.

when regional anesthesia has affected the woman's motor innervation and she cannot push effectively.

Before forceps are used, the following conditions must be met (Nielsen, Galan, Kilpatrick et al., 2007):

- The cervix must be completely dilated and the exact position and station of the fetal head known.
- Membranes must be ruptured to allow a firm grasp on the fetal head, which must be engaged and in vertex or face presentation.
- The type of pelvis should be known, because certain pelvic types do not permit rotation.
- The maternal bladder should be empty and adequate anesthesia given.
- No degree of cephalopelvic disproportion can be present.
- The operator must have the knowledge to perform the procedure.
- Maternal anesthesia is available.
- Adequate staff is available with the ability to perform a cesarean birth if indicated.
- Maternal consent has been obtained.

NEONATAL AND MATERNAL RISKS

Some newborns may develop a small area of ecchymosis and/or edema along the sides of the face as a result of forceps application. Facial lacerations and brachial plexus can also occur (Doumouchtsis & Arulkumaran, 2008). Caput succedaneum or cephalohematoma (with subsequent hyperbilirubinemia) may occur, as may transient facial paralysis. Although rare, cerebral hemorrhages, fractures, brain damage, and fetal death have also been reported (Doumouchtsis & Arulkumaran, 2008).

Maternal risks include possible lacerations of the birth canal; extensions of a midline episiotomy into the anus; increased bleeding, bruising, and perineal edema; and anal incontinence (Pretlove, Thompson, Toozs-Hobson, et al., 2008).

Nursing Management

By using ongoing assessment, the nurse may note the variables that are associated with an increased rate of instrument-assisted or operative birth. Nursing care measures can then be directed toward variables that may reduce the incidence of these factors. For example, labor dystocia may be corrected by changing maternal position, ambulation, use of breast/nipple stimulation or an electric breast pump, and frequent bladder emptying. FHR abnormalities may be improved by position changes, increased fluid intake, and/or adequate oxygen exchange.

If a forceps-assisted birth is required, the nurse explains the procedure briefly to the woman. With adequate regional anesthesia the woman should feel only pressure during the procedure. The nurse ensures that adequate anesthesia is provided by alerting the physician if the woman experiences discomfort or pain. The nurse encourages the woman to use breathing techniques that help prevent her from pushing during application of the forceps (Figure 23–3 ●). The nurse monitors contractions and advises the physician when one is present. With each contraction the physician provides traction on the forceps as the woman pushes. The nurse reinforces to the woman that she needs to push while traction is being applied, explaining that the combined efforts help with expulsion of the fetus. It is not uncommon to observe mild fetal bradycardia as traction is being applied to the forceps. This bradycardia results from head compression and is transient.

Immediately following birth, the newborn is assessed for facial edema, bruising, caput succedaneum, cephalohe-

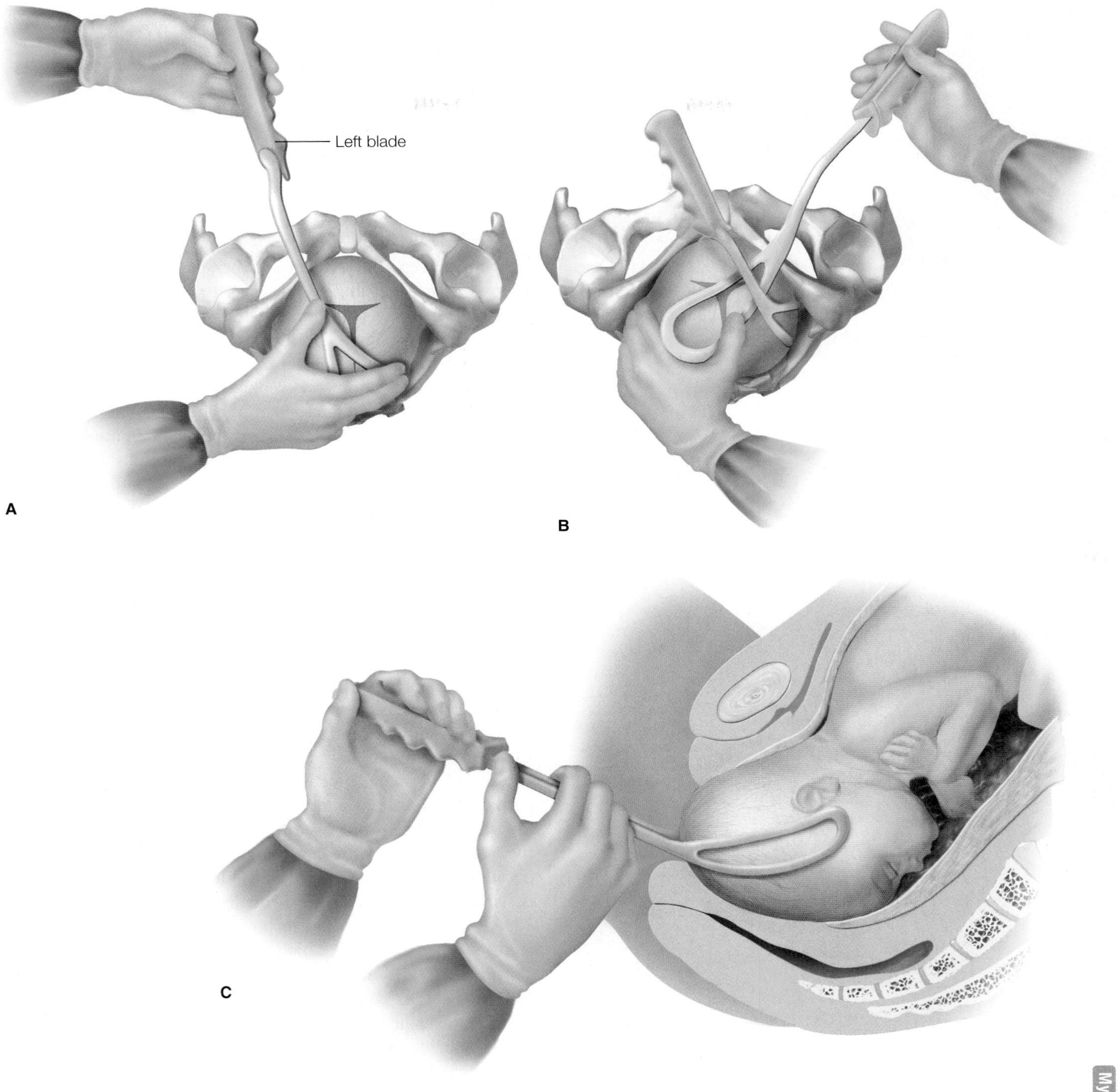

● **Figure 23–3** Application of forceps in occiput-anterior (OA) position. ***A,*** The left blade is inserted along the left side wall of the pelvis over the parietal bone. ***B,*** The right blade is inserted along the right side wall of the pelvis over the parietal bone. ***C,*** With correct placement of the blades, the handles lock easily. During uterine contractions, traction is applied to the forceps in a downward and outward direction to follow the birth canal.

MyNursingKit Video: Vacuum Extraction

matoma, and any signs of cerebral edema. In the fourth stage the nurse assesses the woman for perineal swelling, bruising, hematoma, excessive bleeding, and hemorrhage. In the postpartum period it is important to assess for signs of infection if lacerations occurred during the procedure. The nurse provides an opportunity for questions and reiterates explanations provided.

CARE OF THE WOMAN DURING VACUUM-ASSISTED BIRTH

Vacuum-assisted birth is an obstetric procedure used to facilitate the birth of a fetus by applying suction to the fetal head. The vacuum extractor is composed of a soft suction cup attached to a suction bottle (pump) by tubing. The suction cup, which comes

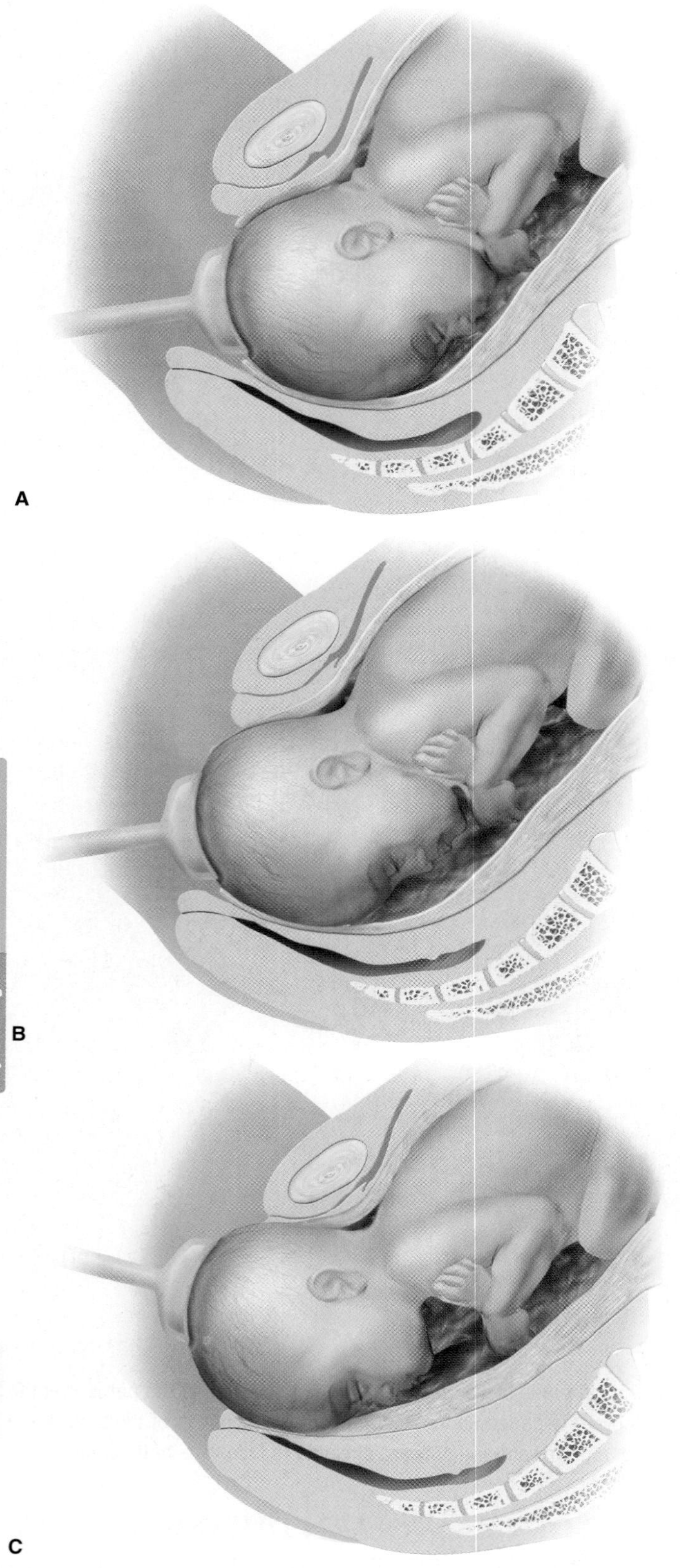

● **Figure 23–4** Vacuum extractor traction. ***A,*** The cup is placed on the fetal occiput, creating suction. Traction is applied in a downward and outward direction. ***B,*** Traction continues in a downward direction as the fetal head begins to emerge from the vagina. ***C,*** Traction is maintained to lift the fetal head out of the vagina.

MyNursingKit Video: Cesarean Birth

in various sizes, is placed against the fetal occiput, and the pump is used to create negative pressure (suction) inside the cup. Traction is applied in coordination with uterine contractions, descent occurs, and the fetal head is born (Figure 23–4 ●). General recommendations include that there should be progressive descent with the first two pulls and that the procedure should be limited to prevent cephalohematomas, brain injury, and fetal death (Doumouchtsis & Arulkumaran, 2008).

Nursing Management

The nurse keeps the woman and her partner informed about what is happening during the procedure. If adequate regional anesthesia has been administered, the woman feels only pressure during the procedure. The nurse assesses FHR by continuous EFM. Assessment of the newborn should include inspection and continued observation for cephalohematomas, intracerebral hemorrhage, and retinal hemorrhages (Doumouchtsis & Arulkumaran, 2008). Because infants born via vacuum are at increased risk for jaundice, the nurse should carefully assess the infant's skin color. Finally, the nurse should reassure the parents that the caput (chignon) on the baby's head will disappear within 2 to 3 days.

CARE OF THE FAMILY DURING CESAREAN BIRTH

Cesarean birth, the birth of the infant through an abdominal and uterine incision, is one of the oldest surgical procedures known. Until the twentieth century cesarean procedures were primarily used in an attempt to save the fetus of a dying woman. As the maternal and perinatal morbidity and mortality rates associated with cesarean birth steadily decreased throughout the 20th century, the proportion of cesarean births increased. Beginning in the early 1970s the cesarean birth rate rose steadily for almost two decades. In 1989, however, in an effort to control healthcare costs, the number of cesarean births began to decline. But in 2006, the number of cesarean births performed in the United States reached an all-time high of 31.1% (Hamilton, Martin, & Ventura, 2007). Canada's cesarean section rate is also at an all-time high at 23.7% (Chaillet & Dumont, 2007).

Cesarean birth rates differ dramatically around the globe. The worldwide rate is estimated to be 12% (Thomas, 2006). Cesarean birth is the least common in the Sub-Sahara African countries with rates averaging 0.3%. In these areas, however, many women do not have access to cesarean births, which leads to the world's highest maternal and infant morbidity (Ronsmans, Holtz, & Stanton, 2006). The cesarean birth rate in East Asia, the Caribbean, and Latin America averages 26%. Brazil (36%) and Chile (40%) have the highest cesarean birth rates in the world (Tang, Wang, Hsu, et al., 2006). Other countries with cesarean rates over 30% include China, Iran, South Korea, Taiwan, and the Dominican Republic (Tang et al., 2006; Thomas, 2006). Worldwide, women living in urban areas were three times more likely to have a cesarean than women living in rural areas (Thomas, 2006). Countries with low cesarean birth rates include Austria

(14.5%), the Netherlands (13.6%), and Norway (15.7%) (Häger, Øian, Nilsen, et al., 2006; Kwee, Elferink-Stinkens, Reuwer et al., 2007). Overall, the incidence of cesarean birth has continued to increase around the world.

The increasing rate in the United States is linked to a rise in repeat cesarean births fueled by concerns regarding the risk of uterine rupture with a vaginal birth after a previous cesarean birth. There is also an increase in requests from women for cesarean births so that they can avoid the pain of labor and vaginal birth. The trend increased further when some medical literature stated that vaginal births could result in pelvic floor damage during the birth process (Samarasekera, Bekhit, Wright, et al., 2008). There is also an emerging trend to "schedule" birth into busy routines to meet specific needs of the parents, such as coordinating work projects, arranging for babysitting of older children, or arranging for relatives who live in other geographic locations to travel to be present for the birth itself.

Over the last few years, there has been a rise in the number of nulliparous women requesting cesarean births (Wiklund, Edman, Ryding, et al., 2008). This trend has led to further increases in the cesarean birth rate. Although cesarean birth on request is associated with a reduction in maternal hemorrhage risk, it is also associated with increases in neonatal respiratory problems, longer hospitalizations, and an increase in complications in subsequent pregnancies, including placenta implantation problems and uterine rupture (ACOG, 2007). Therefore, cesarean birth without medical indications should not be recommended for women desiring several children, for women less than 39 gestational weeks, or when pregnancy dating is unknown or may be inaccurate. It should also not be motivated by the lack of anesthesia availability in an institution (National Institutes of Health, 2006). In some developing countries, such as Nigeria, cesarean by request is viewed as a guarantee that a woman will deliver a live infant (Chigbu & Iloabachie, 2007).

Many other factors have contributed to the rise in the cesarean birth rate and need to be considered in any discussion about decreasing the rate. These factors include an increased use of epidural anesthesia, maternal age over 35, failed inductions, decline in vaginal breech deliveries, decreases in operative vaginal deliveries, increased repeat cesarean rates, reduced vaginal birth after cesarean birth rates, increased physician scheduling of cesarean births for personal convenience, policy statements from professional organizations encouraging cesarean birth, political pressure from malpractice insurance carriers who attempt to dictate practice standards, and fear of litigation (ACOG, 2007; Landon, 2007).

INDICATIONS

Commonly accepted indications for cesarean birth include complete placenta previa, cephalopelvic disproportion, placental abruption, active genital herpes, umbilical cord prolapse, failure to progress in labor, nonreassuring fetal status, previous classical incision on the uterus (either previous cesarean birth or myomectomy), more than one previous cesarean birth, benign and malignant tumors that obstruct the birth canal, and cervical cerclage. Certain maternal medical conditions are contraindications to a vaginal birth and warrant a cesarean birth. These include cardiac disorders; severe maternal respiratory disease; central nervous system disorders that increase intracranial pressure; mechanical vaginal obstruction, such as an ovarian mass or lower uterine segment fibroids; and severe mental illness that results in an altered state of consciousness (Landon, 2007). Other indications that are now commonly associated with cesarean birth, although in some circumstances they may be able to be delivered vaginally, include breech presentation, previous cesarean birth, major congenital anomalies, and severe Rh alloimmunization.

MATERNAL MORTALITY AND MORBIDITY

Cesarean births have a higher maternal mortality rate than vaginal births. Women giving birth via cesarean are 3.6 times more likely to die in the postpartum period compared with women who give birth vaginally (Deneux-Tharaux, Carmona, Bouvier-Colle, et al., 2006). Whereas approximately 2.1 per 100,000 women die during a vaginal birth, mortality is 5.9 per 100,000 for women who undergo an elective cesarean birth. Women who undergo an emergency cesarean birth face a significantly higher incidence of death, 18.2 per 100,000 (Hannah, 2004). Perinatal morbidity is often associated with infection, hypertensive disorders, reaction to anesthesia, blood clots, and bleeding problems (Moodley, 2008).

Countries vary widely regarding the percentage of women who die from birth-related complications. The worldwide maternal morbidity rate is 402 per 100,000 births, with the most occurring in the Sub-Saharan Africa countries and in Asia (Hill, Thomas, AbouZahr, et al., 2007). In the United States, 12.1 women per 100,000 giving birth to a live infant die in childbirth (Hoyert, 2007). In Albania, 6.9 women per 100,000 live births die annually as a result of childbirth, which is significantly lower than the reported 22.9 deaths in 2000 (World Health Organization, 2007).

In addition to the complications associated with cesarean birth, there are also risks that increase maternal mortality and morbidity in subsequent pregnancies. Women who have previously given birth via cesarean have a 1% risk of uterine rupture in subsequent pregnancies (Shipp, Zelop, & Lieberman, 2008). Women who have had a previous cesarean birth have an increased risk of bleeding problems in future pregnancies. The risk of placenta previa in subsequent pregnancies is 15 per 1000, while the risk of abruptio placentae is 13 per 1000 (Odibo, Cahill, Stamilio, et al., 2007). There is also an increase in fetal demise and in neonatal respiratory distress and the need for oxygen administration in fetuses whose mothers have previously given birth via cesarean (Gray, Quigley, Hockley, et al., 2007).

Evidence in Action

One dose of cefazolin before the surgical incision or after cord clamp (extended regimen of antibiotic) is associated with a reduced incidence of postcesarean maternal infections (Systematic review) (Tita, Rouse, Blackwell, et al., 2009).

SKIN INCISIONS

The skin incision for a cesarean birth is either transverse (Pfannenstiel) or vertical and is not indicative of the type of incision made into the uterus. The transverse incision is made across the lowest and narrowest part of the abdomen. Because the incision is made just below the pubic hairline, it is almost invisible after healing. The limitation of this type of skin incision is that it does not allow for extension of the incision if needed. This incision is used when time permits (e.g., with failure to progress and stable fetal and maternal status), because it usually requires more time to make and repair.

The vertical incision is made between the navel and the symphysis pubis. This type of incision is quicker and is therefore preferred in cases of nonreassuring fetal status when rapid birth is indicated, with preterm or macrosomic infants, or when the woman is significantly obese (Landon, 2007). Time factors, client preference, previous vertical skin incision, or physician preference determines the type of skin incision.

UTERINE INCISIONS

The type of uterine incision depends on the need for the cesarean. The choice of incision affects the woman's opportunity for a subsequent vaginal birth and her risks of a ruptured uterine scar with a subsequent pregnancy.

The two major locations of uterine incisions are in the lower uterine segment and in the upper segment of the uterine corpus. The most common lower uterine segment incision is a transverse incision (Figure 23–5 ●). The lower uterine segment incision is preferred for the following reasons (Cunningham et al., 2010):

1. The lower segment is the thinnest portion of the uterus and involves less blood loss.
2. It requires only moderate dissection of the bladder from underlying myometrium.
3. It is easier to repair, although repair takes longer.

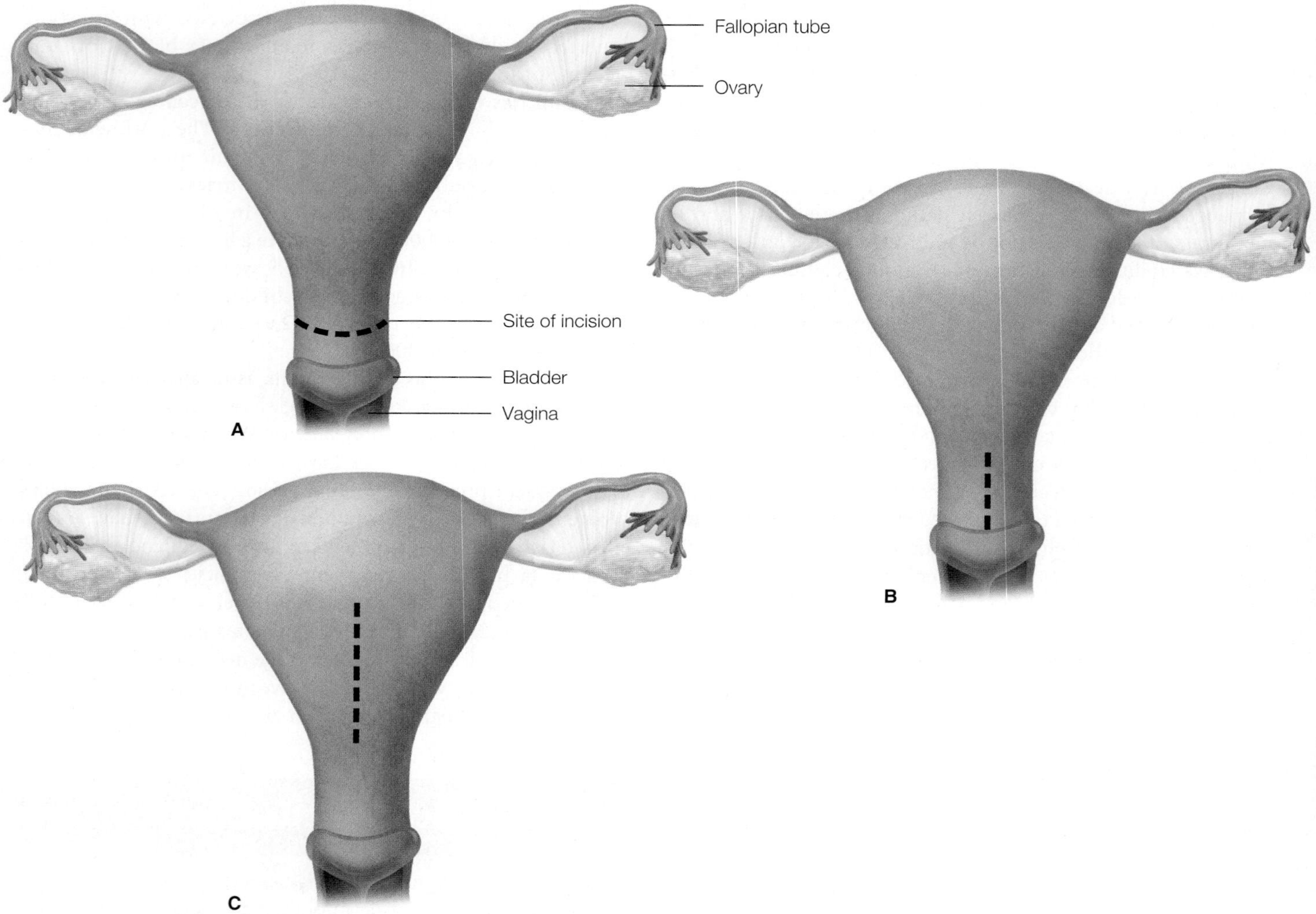

● **Figure 23–5** Uterine incisions for a cesarean birth. ***A,*** This transverse incision in the lower uterine segment is called a Kerr incision. ***B,*** The Sellheim incision is a vertical incision in the lower uterine segment. ***C,*** This view illustrates the classic uterine incision that is done in the body (corpus) of the uterus. The classic incision was commonly done in the past and is associated with increased risk of uterine rupture in subsequent pregnancies and labor.

Developing Cultural Competence

TRANSLATING OPERATIVE REPORTS

Women from other countries who have had a previous cesarean birth typically have a vertical skin incision; however, the skin incision does not provide data on the type of uterine incision that was performed. Obtain an operative report if possible. Operative reports in other languages need to be translated by personnel familiar with medical terminology. If an operative report cannot be obtained, which is common, provide the woman with a thorough explanation regarding the need for a repeat cesarean.

4. The site is less likely to rupture during subsequent pregnancies.
5. There is a decreased chance of adherence of bowel or omentum to the incision line.

Disadvantages are as follows:

1. It takes longer to make a transverse incision.
2. It is limited in size because of the presence of major vessels on either side of the uterus.
3. It has a greater tendency to extend laterally into the uterine vessels.
4. The incision may stretch and become a thin window, but it usually does not create problems clinically until subsequent labor ensues.

The lower uterine segment vertical incision is preferred for multiple gestation, abnormal presentation, placenta previa, nonreassuring fetal status, and preterm and macrosomic fetuses. A disadvantage of this incision is that once a vertical incision is performed, future births need to be via cesarean.

One other incision, the classic incision, was the method of choice for many years but is used infrequently now. The classic vertical incision was made into the upper uterine segment. More blood loss resulted and it was more difficult to repair. Most important, it carried an increased risk of uterine rupture with subsequent pregnancy, labor, and birth because the upper uterine segment is the most contractile portion of the uterus.

ANALGESIA AND ANESTHESIA

There is no perfect anesthesia for cesarean birth. Each has its advantages, disadvantages, possible risks, and side effects. Goals for analgesia and anesthesia administration include safety, comfort, and emotional satisfaction for the client (see Chapter 20).

NURSING MANAGEMENT

PREPARATION FOR CESAREAN BIRTH

Because one of every four births is a cesarean, preparation for this possibility should be an integral part of all prenatal education. Pregnant women and their partners should be encouraged to discuss the possibility of a cesarean birth with their physician/CNM and at the same time discuss their specific needs and desires under those circumstances. Their preferences may include the following:

- Participating in the choice of anesthetic
- Father or significant other being present during the procedures and/or birth
- Father or significant other being present in the recovery or postpartum room
- Video recording and/or taking pictures of the birth
- Delayed instillation of eye drops to promote eye contact between parent and infant in the first hours after birth
- Physical contact or holding the infant while in the operating and/or recovery room (by the father if the mother cannot hold the newborn)
- Breastfeeding in the recovery area within the first hour of birth

Information that couples need about cesarean birth includes the following:

- What preparatory procedures to expect
- Description or viewing of the birthing room
- Types of anesthesia for birth and analgesia available postpartum
- Sensations that may be experienced
- Roles of significant others
- Interaction with newborn
- Immediate recovery phase
- Postpartum phase

Preparing the woman and her family for birth involves more than the procedures of establishing an intravenous line, instilling a urinary indwelling catheter, and performing an abdominal prep. As discussed previously, good communication skills are essential for preparing the woman and her support person. Use therapeutic touch and direct eye contact (if culturally acceptable and possible) to assist the woman in maintaining a sense of control and to lessen anxiety.

If the cesarean birth is scheduled and not an emergency, the nurse has ample time for preoperative teaching. The context in which this information is relayed should be birth oriented rather than surgery oriented. This provides an opportunity for the woman to express her concerns, ask questions, and develop a relationship with the nurse.

In preparation for surgery, the woman is given nothing by mouth. To reduce the likelihood of serious pulmonary damage if gastric contents are aspirated, antacids may be administered within 30 minutes of surgery. If epidural anesthesia is used, the nurse may assist with the procedure, monitor the woman's blood pressure and response, and continue EFM. The nurse performs an abdominal and perineal prep, inserts an indwelling catheter to prevent bladder distention, and starts an intravenous line with a large-bore needle to permit blood administration if it becomes

Nursing Practice

Women undergoing elective cesarean birth can be taught many aspects of postoperative teaching before their birth experience. Important components of client education that can be emphasized before birth include dealing with postoperative discomfort, splinting the incision to decrease pain, frequent deep breathing and coughing, and the importance of early ambulation. Women who receive this information before the birth are more apt to remember it when it is reviewed in the early postpartum period.

necessary. The nurse also orders preoperative medication, notifies the pediatrician, and prepares to receive the new baby. The nurse ensures that the infant warmer is working and that resuscitation equipment is available.

The nurse assists in positioning the woman on the operating table. Fetal heart rate is assessed before surgery and during preparation because fetal hypoxia can result from the supine position. The operating room table is adjusted so it slants slightly to one side or a hip wedge (folded blanket or towels) is placed under the right hip to tip the uterus slightly and reduce compression of blood vessels. The uterus should be displaced 15 degrees from the midline. This helps relieve the pressure of the heavy uterus on the vena cava and lessens the incidence of vena cava compression and maternal supine hypotension. The suction should be in working order and the urine collection bag should be positioned under the operating table to obtain proper drainage. Auscultation or EFM of the fetal heart rate is continued until immediately before the procedure. A last-minute check is done to ensure that the fetal scalp electrode has been removed if the fetus was internally monitored.

The nurse continues to provide reassurance and describe the various procedures being performed along with a rationale to ease anxiety and give the woman a sense of control.

PREPARATION FOR REPEAT CESAREAN BIRTH

When a couple is anticipating a repeat cesarean birth, they have a general understanding of what will occur, which can help them make informed choices about their birth experience. Couples who have had previous negative experiences need an opportunity to describe what they felt. Encourage them to identify what they would like to do differently and to list options that would make the experience more positive. Those who have already had positive experiences need reassurance that their needs and desires will be met in a similar manner and should be allowed to discuss any fears or anxieties. For women who previously labored and then had an unexpected cesarean birth, the experience may be perceived as negative. Positive aspects that can be emphasized include participation in selecting the birth date, lack of fatigue related to labor, ability to prepare and make arrangements for other children, and ability for other family members or friends to be present at the hospital during or immediately after birth if desired by the couple.

PREPARATION FOR EMERGENCY CESAREAN BIRTH

When the need for a cesarean birth emerges suddenly, the period preceding surgery must be used to its greatest advantage. It is imperative that caregivers use their most effective communication skills in supporting the couple. The nurse describes what the couple may anticipate during the next few hours. Asking the couple "What questions or concerns do you have about the decision?" gives them an opportunity for clarification. The nurse can prepare the woman in stages, giving her information and the rationale for interventions before beginning any procedure. It is essential to tell the woman (1) what is going to happen, (2) why it is being done, and (3) what sensations she may experience. This allows the woman to be informed and to consent to the procedure, which gives her a sense of control and reduces her feelings of helplessness.

SUPPORTING THE FATHER OR PARTNER

Every effort should be made to include the father or partner in the birth experience. When attending the cesarean birth, the partner wears protective coverings similar to those worn by others in the operating suite. A stool can be placed beside the woman's head so that the partner can sit nearby to provide physical touch, visual contact, and verbal reassurance.

To promote the participation of the father who chooses not to be in the operating suite, the nurse can do the following:

1. Allow the father to be nearby, where he can hear the newborn's first cry.
2. Encourage the father to carry or accompany the infant to the nursery for the initial assessment.
3. Involve the father in postpartum care in the recovery room.

In some emergency circumstances, a support person may not be permitted in the operating room. Some facilities have policies that prohibit a support person from being in the operating room if the woman requires general anesthesia or if an emergency birth is being performed. In these situations, the support person should receive a thorough explanation of what is happening and why, be advised when the staff will return to provide information, know the expected length of time for the procedure, and be reassured that the mother is receiving the care she and the baby need. Because this exclusion is stressful for family members, staff should try to provide information as soon as possible after providing emergency care to the mother.

IMMEDIATE POSTNATAL RECOVERY PERIOD

After birth the nurse assesses the Apgar score and completes the same initial assessment and identification procedures used for vaginal births. Infant identification bands must be placed on the infant and the mother (as well as the father or support person, if present) before removing the infant from the operating room. Every effort should be made to assist the parents in bonding with their infant. If the mother is awake, one of her arms can be freed to enable her to touch and stroke the infant. The newborn may be placed on the mother's chest or held in an *en face* position. If physical contact is not possible, the nurse can provide a running

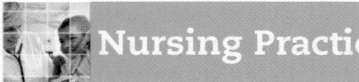

Nursing Practice

Promote bonding by allowing the mother to hold or nurse the infant during this time period. If the infant has been moved to a separate area, such as the nursery, encourage maternal participation by allowing the support person to visit the infant and report back to the mother. The support person can take digital pictures or bring back the blanket that was used to wrap up the baby immediately after the birth. Frequent updates from the nurse such as "Your baby's doing just fine" provide reassurance to the mother if separation is needed.

narrative so the mother knows what is happening with her baby. The nurse assists the anesthesiologist or nurse anesthetist with raising the mother's head so she can see her infant immediately after birth. The parents can be encouraged to talk to the baby, and the father can hold the baby until she or he is taken to the nursery.

The nurse caring for the postpartum woman assesses the mother's vital signs every 5 minutes until they are stable, then every 15 minutes for an hour, then every 30 minutes until she is discharged to the postpartum unit. The nurse should remain with the woman until she is stable.

The nurse evaluates the dressing and perineal pad every 15 minutes for at least an hour. The fundus should be gently palpated to determine whether it is remaining firm; it may be palpated by placing a hand to support the incision. Intravenous Pitocin is usually administered to promote the contractility of the uterine musculature. If the woman has been under general anesthesia, she should be positioned on her side to facilitate drainage of secretions, turned, and assisted with coughing and deep breathing every 2 hours for at least 24 hours. If she has received a spinal or epidural anesthetic, the level of anesthesia is checked every 15 minutes until full sensation has returned. It is important for the nurse to monitor intake and output and to observe the urine for a bloody tinge, which could mean surgical trauma to the bladder. The physician prescribes medication to relieve the mother's pain and nausea, and it is administered as needed.

CARE OF THE WOMAN UNDERGOING VAGINAL BIRTH AFTER CESAREAN (VBAC)

In the late 1990s there was an increasing trend to have a trial of labor and attempt **vaginal birth after cesarean (VBAC)** in cases of nonrecurring indications for a cesarean (such as umbilical cord prolapse, breech, placenta previa, or nonreassuring fetal status). This trend was influenced by consumer demand and studies that supported VBAC as a viable alternative to repeat cesarean. It resulted in a reduction in the cesarean section rate to 20.7% in 1996.

Recent media reports identifying risks of VBAC (discussed shortly) have reintroduced the debate regarding its safety. At the same time, trends in counseling women to have an elective repeat cesarean birth are driving cesarean births to an all-time high in the United States.

The ACOG (2004) guidelines update states that the following aspects need to be considered for VBAC:

- A woman with one previous cesarean birth and a low transverse uterine incision may be counseled and encouraged to attempt VBAC.
- A clinically adequate pelvis is a requirement for VBAC.
- A woman with two previous cesareans who has also had a previous vaginal birth may attempt VBAC.
- It must be possible to perform a cesarean within 30 minutes.
- A physician, adequate staff, anesthesia, and facilities must be readily available throughout active labor to perform a cesarean birth if needed.
- A classic or T uterine incision is a contraindication to VBAC.

The most common risks associated with failed VBAC births are hemorrhage, uterine scar separation or uterine rupture, hysterectomy, surgical injuries, infant death, and neurologic complications (see Chapter 21). It should be noted that these complications occur as a result of a uterine rupture. The incidence of uterine rupture is 0.9% of all trials of labors when the mother has had a previous cesarean birth (Shipp, Zelop, & Lieberman, 2008). Women who go into spontaneous labor have a much lower incidence of uterine rupture (1 per 100) compared with women who undergo Pitocin induction (1.4 per 100) (Grossetti, Vardon, Creveuil, et al., 2007). Prostaglandin agents should not be used in women attempting a VBAC because of the increased risk of uterine rupture. The incidence of uterine rupture in women who receive a prostaglandin agent is as high as 2.2 per 100 (Grossetti et al., 2007). Conservative policies, such as awaiting spontaneous labor, avoiding prostaglandin agents, and avoiding elective inductions, can assist in reducing the incidence of uterine rupture. The incidence of uterine rupture in women before labor is 3 per 1000 (Grossetti et al., 2007).

Women who have a successful VBAC have lower incidences of infection, less blood loss, fewer blood transfusions, and shorter hospital stays. Healthcare costs are considerably lower for women who have a VBAC than for those who have a repeat cesarean birth (Odibo & Macones, 2003). After a woman had one successful VBAC, the risks of neonatal and maternal complications was low in subsequent attempts. An increasing number of VBACs are associated with greater VBAC success (Mercer, Gilbert, Landon, et al., 2008).

Research shows a close correlation between maternal weight and success for VBACs (Juhasz,, Gyamfi, Gyamfi, et al., 2005). Obese women with a body mass index greater than 29 were 50% less likely to have a successful VBAC (Juhasz et al., 2005).

NURSING MANAGEMENT

The nursing care of a woman undergoing VBAC varies according to institutional protocols. Generally, a saline lock is inserted for IV access if needed or an intravenous infusion of fluids is started, continuous EFM is used, and clear fluids may be taken. A woman at higher risk may require additional precautionary measures, such as internal monitoring after the membranes have ruptured.

Take care to ensure that the woman and her partner feel safe but not unduly restricted by the VBAC status.

Supportive and comfort measures are very important. The woman may be excited about this opportunity to experience labor and vaginal birth, or she may be hesitant and frightened about the possibility of complications. The presence of the nurse is important in providing information and encouragement for the laboring woman and her partner.

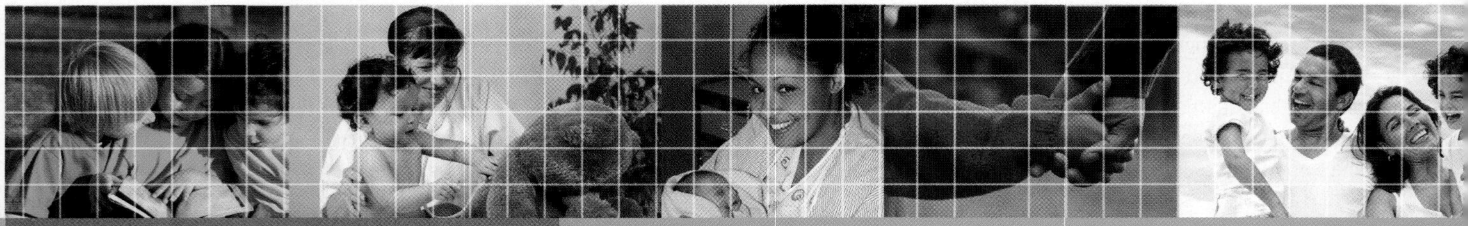

CRITICAL CONCEPT REVIEW

LEARNING OUTCOMES	CONCEPTS
23.1 Explain the methods, purpose, and contraindications of external and podalic version that impact nursing care management.	1. An external version (cephalic version) may be done after 36 weeks' gestation to change a breech presentation to a cephalic presentation. ■ Physician applies external manipulation to the maternal abdomen. ■ Fetal part must not be engaged. ■ NST performed to establish fetal well-being. ■ Tocolytic given during procedure to relax uterus. 2. Podalic version is used to turn a second twin during a vaginal birth. ■ Used only if second fetus does not descend readily and heartbeat is not reassuring. ■ Physician reaches into uterus and grabs feet of fetus and pulls them down through cervix. ■ A tocolytic is given to relax uterus.
23.2 Describe the use of amniotomy in the nursing care management of woman and fetus.	1. There are several reasons an amniotomy (artificial rupture of the amniotic membranes) is used: ■ To induce labor. ■ To accelerate labor. ■ To apply an internal fetal monitor or insert an intrauterine pressure catheter. 2. Risks include prolapse cord and infection.
23.3 Compare the methods for inducing labor, explaining their advantages and disadvantages in determining the nursing management for women during labor induction.	1. Cervical ripening: ■ May hasten the beginning of labor or shorten the course of labor. ■ May cause hyperstimulation of the uterus. 2. Stripping the membranes: ■ May not induce labor; if labor is initiated, it typically begins within 48 hours. ■ May cause bleeding. 3. Pitocin infusion: ■ Usually effective at producing contractions. ■ May cause hyperstimulation of uterus.
23.4 Describe the measures to prevent episiotomy, the types of episiotomy performed, and the associated nursing interventions.	1. Preventive measures ■ Perineal massage during pregnancy ■ Natural pushing during labor ■ Side-lying position for pushing; avoid lithotomy position or pulling back on legs ■ Avoid immediate pushing after epidural placement ■ Encourage a gradual expulsion of the infant by doing controlled breathing pattern 2. There are two types of episiotomy used: ■ Midline. ■ Mediolateral. 3. During the episiotomy the nurse supports the woman, explaining the procedure. 4. After the birth: ■ Place an ice pack to the perineum. ■ Inspect the perineum frequently. ■ Instruct the woman in perineal hygiene, self-care, and comfort measures.

LEARNING OUTCOMES	CONCEPTS
23.5 Explain the indications, maternal and neonatal risks that impact nursing care management during forceps-assisted birth.	Indications: 1. To shorten the second stage of labor. ■ Used in the presence of nonreassuring fetal status and premature placental separation. 2. To assist woman's pushing effort. ■ Used in the presence of maternal exhaustion, or when regional anesthesia impairs woman's ability to push effectively. Maternal and neonatal risks: 1. Newborn bruising, facial edema, facial lacerations, cephalohematoma, and transient facial paralysis. 2. Woman may experience vaginal lacerations, increased bleeding, bruising, and perineal edema.
23.6 Describe the use and risk of vacuum extraction use to assist birth.	1. Vacuum extractor assists birth by applying suction to the fetal head. ■ May cause cephalhematoma. ■ Increases risk for jaundice.
23.7 Explain the indications for cesarean birth, impact on the family unit, preparation and teaching needs, and associated nursing care.	1. Most common indications for cesarean birth are: ■ Nonreassuring fetal status. ■ Lack of labor progression. ■ Maternal infection. ■ Pelvic size disproportion. ■ Placenta previa. ■ Previous cesarean birth. 2. Couples should be encouraged to participate in as many choices as possible concerning the surgical birth. 3. Preparation for cesarean birth requires: ■ Establishing IV lines. ■ Placing an indwelling catheter. ■ Performing an abdominal prep. 4. Teaching needs include: ■ What to expect before, during, and after birth. ■ Role of significant others. ■ Interaction with newborn. 5. Associated nursing care: ■ Routine postpartal care including fundal checks. ■ Care of incision. ■ Monitoring intake and output. ■ Assessment of respiratory system and returning bowel sounds. ■ Assessment of maternal pain level and provision of pain relief.
23.8 Examine the risks and nursing care of the woman undergoing vaginal birth following cesarean birth.	1. Most common risks are: ■ Hemorrhage. ■ Uterine rupture. ■ Infant death. 2. Nursing care: ■ Continuous EFM. ■ Internal monitoring. ■ IV fluid. 3. Prostaglandin agents induction should be avoided if possible.

CRITICAL THINKING IN ACTION

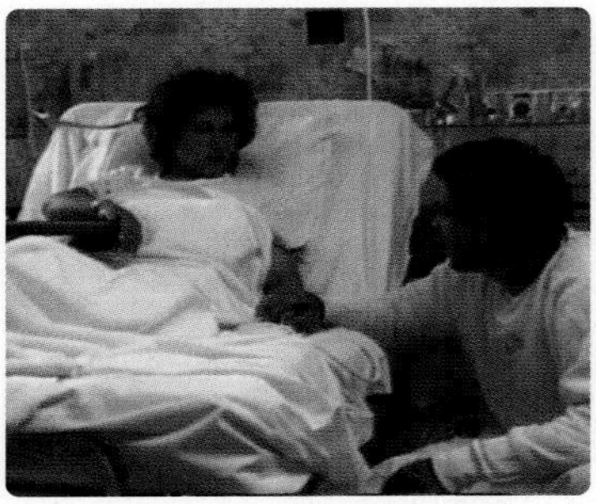

Betsy Jones, a 28-year-old G1 P0 is at 39 weeks' gestation, and her husband present to you in the labor suite for an external cephalic version procedure by her obstetrician. You introduce yourself and review her prenatal record for any significant risk factors or contraindications to the version procedure. Her prenatal chart is significant in that the fetus has been in a persistent frank breech position. You encourage Betsy and her husband to express their understanding and expectations of the procedure. You discuss certain criteria to be met prior to the procedure and obtain vital signs as follows: T 98.8°F, P 88, R 14, BP 110/80, urine screening negative for sugar, albumin, and ketones. You place Betsy on the external electronic fetal monitor, which demonstrates a fetal heart rate baseline of 140 to 152 with moderate long-term variability. There are no contractions observed by the monitor or Betsy. After explaining how to record fetal movement on the monitor, you proceed with an NST.

1. Explain the contraindications to the version procedure.
2. Discuss the criteria that should be met prior to performing external version.
3. How would you explain to Betsy and her husband what to expect during the version procedure?
4. What support would you give Betsy during the procedure?
5. Explain postversion discharge teaching.

See MyNursing Kit for possible responses.

REFERENCES

American College of Obstetricians and Gynecologists (ACOG). (2003). *New U.S. Food and Drug Administration labeling on Cytotec (misoprostol) use and pregnancy* (ACOG Committee Opinion No. 283). Washington, DC: Author.

American College of Obstetricians and Gynecologists (ACOG). (2004). *Vaginal birth after previous cesarean delivery* (Practice Bulletin No. 54). Washington, DC: Author. Reaffirmed June 2009.

American College of Obstetricians and Gynecologists (ACOG). (2007). *Cesarean delivery upon maternal request* (ACOG Committee Opinion No. 394). Washington, DC: Author.

Bishop, E. H. (1964). Pelvic scoring for elective inductions. *Obstetrics and Gynecology, 24,* 266.

Bjelic-Radisic, V., Pristauz, G., Haas, J., Giuliani, A., Tamussino, K., Bader, A., et al. (2007). Neonatal outcome of second twins depending on presentation and mode of delivery. *Twin Research & Human Genetics, 10*(3), 521–527.

Blackburn, S. (2007). *Maternal-fetal-neonatal physiology: A clinical perspective* (3rd ed.). Philadelphia: Saunders.

Boulvain, M., Kelly, A., & Irion, O. (2008). Intracervical prostaglandins for induction of labour. *Cochrane Database Systematic Review, 23*(1), CD006971.

Carroli, G., & Mignini, L.(2009). Episiotomy for vaginal birth. *Cochrane Database of Systematic Reviews*, Issue 1. Art. No.: CD000081.

Chaillet, N., & Dumont, A. (2007). Evidence-based strategies for reducing cesarean section rates: A meta-analysis. *Birth, 34*(1), 53–64.

Cheng, S. Y., Ming, H., & Lee, J. C. (2008). Titrated oral compared with vaginal misoprostol for labor induction: A randomized controlled trial. *Obstetrics & Gynecology, 111*(1), 119–125.

Chigbu, C. O., & Iloabachie, G. C. (2007). The burden of caesarean section refusal in a developing country setting. *British Journal Obstetrics & Gynecology, 114*(10), 1261–1265.

Cunningham, F. G., Leveno, K. J., Bloom, S. L., Hauth, J. C., Gilstrap, L. C., & Wenstrom, K. D. (2010). *Williams obstetrics* (23rd ed.). Norwalk, CT: Appleton & Lange.

Deneux-Tharaux, C., Carmona, E., Bouvier-Colle, M. H., & Bréart, G. (2006). Postpartum maternal mortality and cesarean delivery. *Obstetrics & Gynecology, 108*(3), 541–548.

Doumouchtsis, S. K., & Arulkumaran, S. (2008). Head trauma after instrumental births. *Clinics in Perinatology, 35*(1), 69–83.

Dudding, T., Vaizey, C. & Kamm, M. (2008). Obstetrics anal sphincter injury: Incidence, risk factors, and management. *Annuals Surgery 247*(2), 224–237.

Edwards, H., Grotegut, C., Harmanli, O. H., Rapkin, D., & Dandolu, V. (2006). Is severe perineal damage increased in women with prior anal sphincter injury? *Journal of Maternal, Fetal & Neonatal Medicine, 19*(11), 723–727.

Ejegård, H., Ryding, E. L., & Sjögren, B. (2008). Sexuality after delivery with episiotomy: A long-term follow-up. *Gynecologic and Obstetric Investigation 66*(1), 1–7.

Facchinetti, F., Venturini, P., Fazzio, M., & Volpe, A. (2007). Elective cervical ripening in women beyond the 290th day of pregnancy: A randomized trial comparing 2 dinoprostone preparations. *Journal of Reproductive Medicine, 52*(10), 945–949.

Food & Drug Administration (FDA). (2008). Cytotec. Retrieved February 18, 2008, from http://www.fda.gov/cder/foi/label/2002/19268slr037.pdf

Forrest Pharmaceuticals, Inc. (2007). *Cervidil dinoprostone 10 mg vaginal insert.* St. Louis: Forrest Pharmaceutical Laboratories.

Grootscholten, K., Kok, M., Oei, S. G., Mol, B. W., & van der Post, J. A. (2008) External cephalic version—related risks: A meta-analysis. *Obstetrics & Gynecology, 112*(5), 1143–1151.

Grossetti, E., Vardon, D., Creveuil, C., Herlicoviez, M., & Dreyfus, M. (2007). Rupture of the scarred uterus. *Acta Obstet Gynecol Scand, 86*(5), 572–578.

Gray, R., Quigley, M. A., Hockley, C., Kurinczuk, J. J., Goldacre, M., & Brocklehurst, P. (2007). Caesarean delivery and risk of stillbirth in subsequent pregnancy: A retrospective cohort study in an English population. *British Journal of Obstetrics & Gynecology, 114*(3), 264–270.

Häger, R., Øian, P., Nilsen, S. T., Holm, H. A., & Berg, A. B. (2006). The breakthrough series on Cesarean section. *Tidsskr Nor Laegeforen, 126*(2), 173–175.

Hamilton, B. E., Martin, J. A., & Ventura, S. J. (2007). Births: Preliminary data for 2006. *National Vital Statistics Reports, 56*(7), 1–50.

Hannah, M. E. (2004). Planned elective cesarean: A reasonable choice for some women. *Canadian Medical Association Journal, 170*(5), 813–814.

Hill, K., Thomas, K., AbouZahr, C., Walker, N., Say, L., Inoue, M., et al. (2007). Estimates of maternal mortality worldwide between 1990 and 2005: An assessment of available data. *Lancet, 13; 370*(9595), 1311–1319.

Hoyert, D. L. (2007). Maternal mortality and related concepts. National Center for Health Statistics. *Vital Health Statistics, 3*(33), 1–15.

Juhasz, G., Gyamfi, C., Gyamfi, P., & Stone, C. L. (2005). Effect of body mass index and excessive weight gain on success of vaginal birth after cesarean. *Obstetrics & Gynecology, 106*(4), 741–746.

Kilpatrick, S., & Garrison, E. (2007). Normal labor and delivery. In S. G. Gabbe, J. R. Niebyl, & J. L. Simpson (Eds.), *Obstetrics: Normal and problem pregnancies* (5th ed., pp. 303–321). Philadelphia: Churchill Livingston/Elsevier.

Kwee, A., Elferink-Stinkens, P. M., Reuwer, P. J., & Bruinse, H. W. (2007). Trends in obstetric interventions in the Dutch obstetrical care system in the period 1993–2002. *European Journal of Obstetrics, Gynecology & Reproductive Biology, 132*(1), 70–75.

Landon, M. B. (2007). Cesarean delivery. In S. G. Gabbe, J. R. Niebyl, & J. L. Simpson (Eds.), *Obstetrics: Normal and problem pregnancies* (5th ed., pp. 486–520). Philadelphia: Churchill Livingston/Elsevier.

Marconi, A. M., Bozzetti, P., Morabito, A., & Pardi, G. (2008). Comparing two dinoprostone agents for cervical ripening and induction of labor: A randomized trial. *European Journal Obstetric Gynecology Reproductive Biology, 138*(20), 135–140.

Matsuo, K., Scanlon, J. T., Atlas, R. O., & Kopelman, J. N. (2008). Staircase sign: A newly described uterine contraction pattern seen in rupture of unscarred gravid uterus. *Journal of Obstetrics & Gynaecology, 34*(1), 100–104.

Mbele, A. M., Makin, J. D., & Pattinson, R. C. (2007). Can the outcome of induction of labour with oral misoprostol be predicted? *South Africa Medical Journal, 97*(4), 289–292.

Mercer, B. M., Gilbert, S., Landon, M. B., Spong, C. Y., Leveno, K. J., Rouse, D. J., et al. (2008). Labor outcomes with increasing number of prior vaginal births after cesarean delivery. *Obstetrics & Gynecology, 111*(2), 285–291.

Midwifery Today E-News. (2007). *Herbs. Midwifery Today Forums, 9*, 3. Retrieved June 19, 2007, from http://www.midwiferytoday.com/enews

Moodley, J. (2008). Maternal deaths due to hypertensive disorders in pregnancy. *Best Practices in Research & Clinical Obstetrics & Gynaecology* (2008 Feb 15); E-pub ahead of print.

National Institutes of Health. (2006). NIH State-of-the-Science Conference Statement on cesarean delivery on maternal request. *NIH Consensus State Science Statements, 23*(1), 1–29.

Nielson, P. E., Galan, H. L., Kilpatrick, S., & Garrison, E. (2007). Operative vaginal delivery. In S. G. Gabbe, J. R. Niebyl, & J. L. Simpson (Eds.), *Obstetrics: Normal and problem pregnancies* (5th ed., pp. 344–363). Philadelphia: Churchill Livingston/Elsevier.

Odibo, A. O., Cahill, A. G., Stamilio, D. M., Stevens, E. J., Peipert, J. F., & Macones, G. A. (2007). Predicting placental abruption and previa in women with a previous cesarean delivery. *American Journal of Perinatology, 24*(5), 299–305.

Odibo, A. O., & Macones, G. A. (2003). Current concepts regarding vaginal birth after cesarean delivery. *Current Opinion in Obstetrics and Gynecology, 15*(6), 479–482.

Pfizer Pharmaceuticals, Inc. (2008). Dinoprostone (Prepidil) Vaginal Gel insert. New York: Pfizer Pharmaceutical Laboratories.

Pretlove, S. J., Thompson, P. J., Toozs-Hobson, P. M., Radley, S., & Khan, K. S. (2008). Does the mode of delivery predispose women to anal incontinence in the first year postpartum? A comparative systematic review. *British Journal of Obstetrics & Gynecology, 115*(4), 421–434.

Roberts, L. L., Ely, J. W., & Ward, M. M. (2007). Factors contributing to maternal birth-related trauma. *American Journal of Medical Quality, 22*(5), 334–343.

Ronsmans, C., Holtz, S., & Stanton, C. (2006). Socioeconomic differentials in caesarean rates in developing countries: A retrospective analysis. *The Lancet, 368*(9546), 1472–1473.

Samarasekera, D. N., Bekhit, M. T., Wright, Y., Lowndes, R. H., Stanley, K. P., Preston, J. P., Preston, P., & Speakman, C. T. (2008). Long-term anal continence and quality of life following postpartum anal sphincter injury. *Colorectal Disease, 10*(8), 793–799.

Shipp, T. D., Zelop, C., & Lieberman, E. (2008). Assessment of the rate of uterine rupture at the first prenatal visit: A preliminary evaluation. *Journal of Maternal Fetal & Neonatal Medicine, 21*(2), 129–133.

Shiraishi, Y., Asano, K., Niimi, K., Fukunaga, K., Wakaki, M., Kagyo, J., et al. (2008). Cyclooxygenase-2/prostaglandin D2/CRTH2 pathway mediates double-stranded RNA-induced enhancement of allergic airway inflammation. *Journal of Immunology, 180*(1), 541–549.

Smyth, R. M. D., Alldred, S. K., & Markham, C. (2007). Amniotomy for shortening spontaneous labor. *Cochrane Database of Systematic Reviews 2007*, Issue 4, Art. No.: CD006167. DOI: 10.1002/14651858.CD006167.pub2

Tang, C. H., Wang, H. I., Hsu, C. S., Su, H. W., Chen, M. J., & Lin, H. C. (2006). Risk-adjusted cesarean section rates for the assessment of physician performance in Taiwan: A population-based study. *Bio-Medical Central Public Health, 6*, 246.

Tang, O. S., Gemzell-Danielsson, K., & Ho, P. C. (2007). Misoprostol: Pharmacokinetic profiles, effects on the uterus and side-effects. *International Journal of Gynaecology & Obstetrics, 99,* Suppl 2: S160-7. E-pub 2007 Oct 26.

Tenore, J. L. (2003). Methods for cervical ripening and induction of labor. *American Family Physician*, 67, 2123–2128.

Thomas, J. (2006). Rates of cesarean delivery in developing countries suggest unequal access. *International Family Planning Perspectives, 32*(2). Retrieved June 19, 2009, from http://www.guttmacher.org/pubs/journals/3210506.html

Thorpe, J. M. (2009). Clinical aspects of normal and abnormal labor. In R. K. Creasy, R. Resnik, & J. D. Iams (Eds.), *Obstetrics: Normal and problem pregnancies* (6th ed., pp. 691–724). Philadelphia: Saunders.

Tita, A. T., Rouse, D. J., Blackwell, S., Saade, G. R., Spong, C. Y., & Andrews, W. W. (2009). Emerging concepts in antibiotic prophylaxis for cesarean delivery. *Obstetrics & Gynecology, 113*(3), 675–682.

Weeks, A., Alfirevic, Z., Faúndes, A., Hofmeyr, G. J., Safar, P., & Wing, D. (2007). Misoprostol for induction of labor with a live fetus. *International Journal of Gynaecology & Obstetrics, 99* Suppl 2: S194-7. E-pub 2007 Oct 25.

Wheeler, T. L., & Richter, H. E. (2007). Delivery method, anal sphincter tears and fecal incontinence: New information on a persistent problem. *Current Opinions in Obstetrics & Gynecology, 19*(5), 474–479.

Wilkund, I., Ryding, E. G., & Andolf, E. (2008). Expectation and experience of childbirth in primiparae with caesarean section. *British Journal of Obstetrics and Gynaecology 115*(3), 324–331.

Wilson, B. A., Shannon, M. T., & Shields, K. M. (Eds.). (2009). *Nursing drug guide: 2009.* Upper Saddle River, NJ: Prentice Hall.

World Health Organization [WHO]. (2007). *Making pregnancy safer towards the European strategy for making pregnancy safer: Improving maternal and perinatal health.* Country profile: Albania. Copenhagen, Denmark: WHO.

Zeck W., Walcher, W., & Lang, U. (2008). External cephalic version in singleton pregnancies at term: A retrospective analysis. *Gynecology & Obstetric Investigation, 66*(1), 18–21.

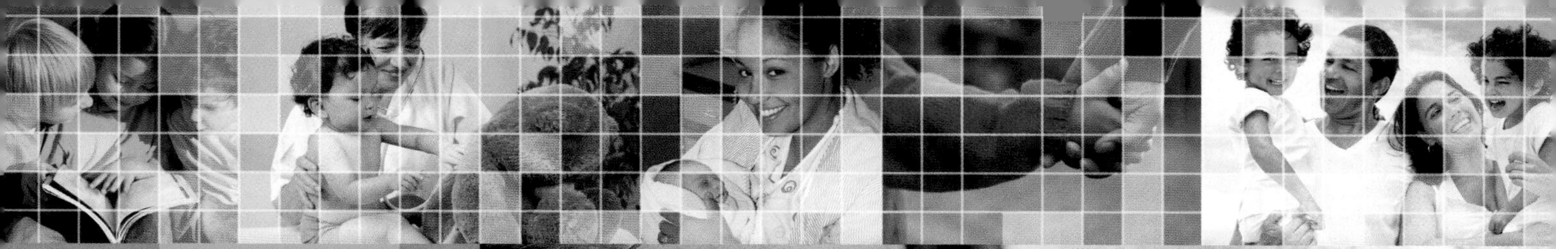

PART

5

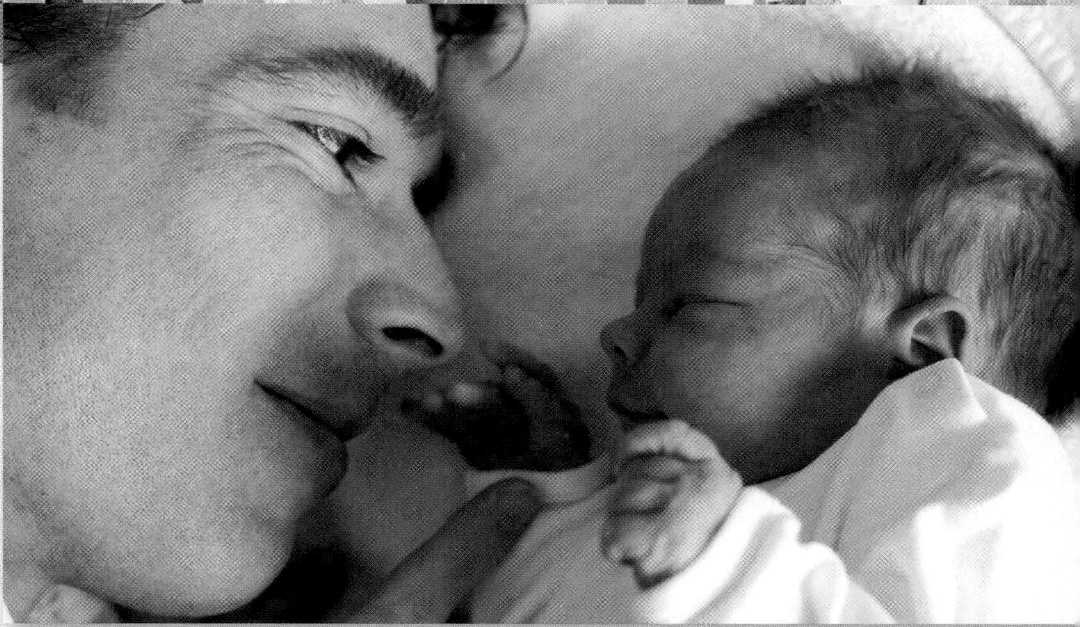

The Postpartal Family and the Newborn

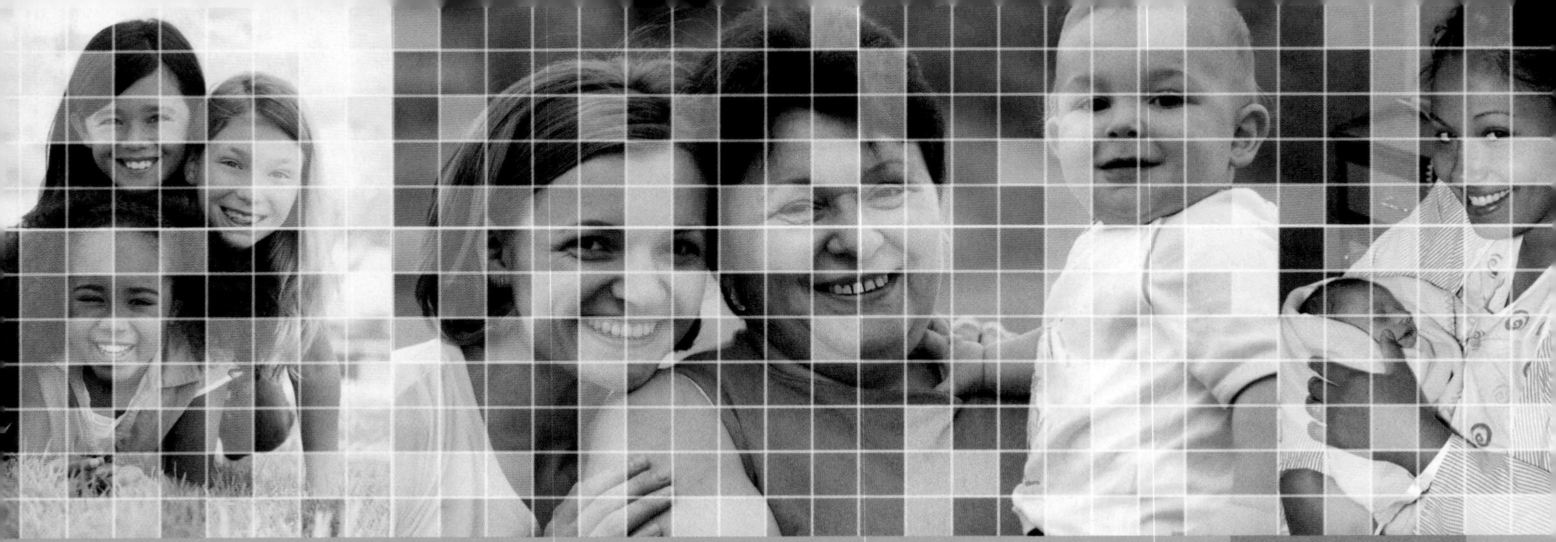

CHAPTER 24

The Physiologic Responses of the Newborn to Birth

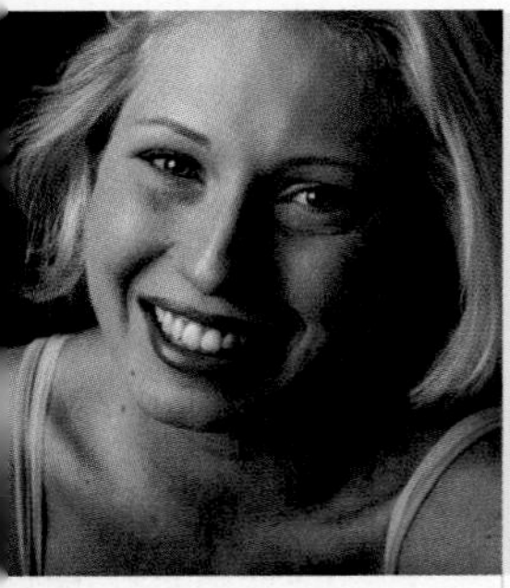

I remember clearly when they held him up for us to see and my husband and I cried and laughed and it was so amazing. He was 9 1/2 pounds and was so beautiful. Even though my labor was long, his Apgars were high, and he didn't even cry—not until we dressed him, anyway. —*Crystal, 26*

LEARNING OUTCOMES

24.1 Explain the respiratory and cardiovascular changes that occur during the newborn's transition to extrauterine life and during stabilization in determining the nursing care of the newborn.

24.2 Compare the factors that modify the newborn's blood values to the corresponding results.

24.3 Relate the process of thermogenesis in the newborn and the major mechanisms of heat loss to the challenge of maintaining newborn thermal stability.

24.4 Explain the steps involved in conjugation and excretion of bilirubin in the newborn.

24.5 Identify the reasons a newborn may develop jaundice and nursing interventions to decrease the probability of jaundice.

24.6 Delineate the functional abilities of the newborn's gastrointestinal tract and liver.

24.7 Relate the development of the newborn's kidneys to the newborn's ability to maintain fluid and electrolyte balance.

24.8 Describe the immunologic response available to the newborn.

24.9 Explain the physiologic and behavioral characteristics of newborn neurologic function, patterns of behavior during the periods of reactivity, and possible nursing interventions.

24.10 Describe the normal sensory-perceptual abilities and behavioral states seen in the newborn period and the associated nursing care.

The newborn period is the time from birth through the 28th day of life. During this period, the newborn adjusts from intrauterine to extrauterine life. The nurse needs to be knowledgeable about a newborn's normal physiologic and behavioral adaptations and to be able to recognize alterations from normal.

The first few hours of life, in which the newborn stabilizes respiratory and circulatory functions, are called **neonatal transition**. All other newborn body systems change their level of functioning and become established over a longer period of time during the neonatal period.

RESPIRATORY ADAPTATIONS

To begin life as a separate being, the baby must immediately establish respiratory gas exchange in conjunction with marked circulatory changes. These radical and rapid changes are crucial to the maintenance of extrauterine life.

INTRAUTERINE FACTORS SUPPORTING RESPIRATORY FUNCTION

Even before the significant respiratory events occur at birth, certain intrauterine factors also enhance the newborn's ability to breathe. Adequate fetal lung development allows the newborn to expand his or her lungs and exchange oxygen and carbon dioxide gases. Even before birth the fetus practices breathing movements, which allow him or her to breathe immediately after birth.

Fetal Lung Development

The respiratory system is in an ongoing state of development during fetal life, and lung development continues into early childhood. During the first 20 weeks' gestation, development is limited to the differentiation of pulmonary, vascular, and lymphatic structures. At 20 to 24 weeks, alveolar ducts begin to appear, followed by primitive alveoli at 24 to 28 weeks. During this time, the alveolar epithelial cells begin to differentiate into type I cells (structures necessary for gas exchange) and type II cells (structures that provide for the synthesis and storage of surfactant). **Surfactant** is composed of surface-active phospholipids (lecithin and sphingomyelin), which are critical for alveolar stability.

At 28 to 32 weeks' gestation, the number of type II cells increases further, and surfactant is produced by a choline pathway within them. Surfactant production by this pathway peaks at about 35 weeks' gestation and remains high until term, paralleling late fetal lung development. At this time, the lungs are structurally developed enough to permit maintenance of lung expansion and adequate exchange of gases.

Clinically, the peak production of lecithin—one component of surfactant—corresponds closely to the marked decrease in the incidence of respiratory distress syndrome for babies born after 35 weeks' gestation. Production of sphingomyelin (the other component of surfactant) remains constant during gestation. The newborn who is born before the lecithin/sphingomyelin (L/S) ratio is 2:1 will have varying degrees of respiratory distress. (See discussion of L/S ratio and respiratory distress syndrome in Chapter 29.)

Fetal Breathing Movements

The newborn's ability to breathe air immediately after his or her birth appears to result from weeks of intrauterine practice. In this respect, breathing can be seen as a continuation of an intrauterine process; the lungs convert from a fluid-filled organ to a gas-filled organ capable of gas exchange.

Fetal breathing movements (FBMs) occur as early as 11 weeks' gestation (see "Biophysical Profile" in Chapter 14 for discussion). These breathing movements are essential for developing the chest wall muscles and the diaphragm and, to a lesser extent, for regulating lung fluid volume and resultant lung growth.

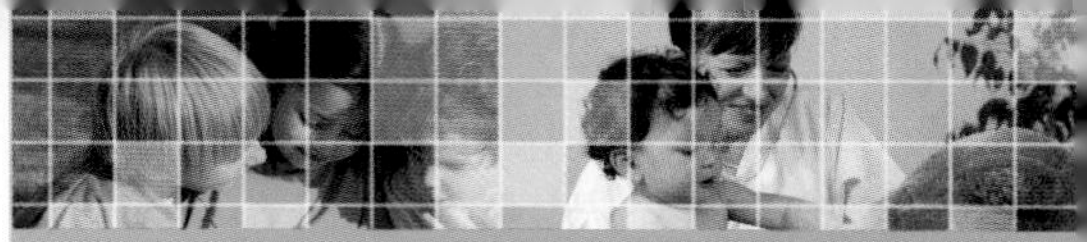

KEY TERMS

INITIATION OF BREATHING

To maintain life, the lungs must function immediately after birth. Two radical changes must take place for the lungs to function:

1. Pulmonary ventilation must be established through lung expansion following birth.
2. A marked increase in the pulmonary circulation must occur.

The first breath of life—the gasp in response to mechanical and reabsorptive, chemical, thermal, and sensory changes associated with birth—initiates the serial opening of the alveoli. So begins the transition from a fluid-filled environment to an air-breathing, independent, extrauterine life (Knuppel, 2007). Figure 24–1 ● summarizes the initiation of respiration.

Mechanical and Reabsorptive Processes

During the latter half of gestation, the fetal lungs continuously produce fluid. This fluid expands the lungs almost completely, filling the air spaces. Some of the lung fluid moves up into the trachea and into the amniotic fluid and is then swallowed by the fetus.

In preparation for birth, lung fluid production normally decreases and fetal breathing movement decreases 24 to 36 hours before the onset of true labor (Knuppel, 2007). However, approximately 80 to 100 mL of lung fluid remains in the respiratory passages of a normal full-term fetus at the time of birth. This lung fluid must be removed from the lungs to permit adequate movement of air (Polin, Fox, & Abman, 2004).

As the fetus experiences labor there is a fetal gasp and active exhalation that initiates the removal of fluid from the lungs (Rosenberg, 2007). During birth the fetal chest is compressed, increasing intrathoracic pressure, and squeezing a small amount of the fluid out of the lungs. After the birth of the newborn's trunk, the chest wall recoils. This chest recoil creates a negative intrathoracic pressure, which is thought to produce a small, passive inspiration of air that replaces the fluid in the large airways that is squeezed out. The significance of the "thoracic squeeze" is controversial and it is now thought that the process of labor is primarily responsible for the initial expulsion of lung fluid (Rosenberg, 2007).

After this first inspiration, the newborn exhales, with crying, against a partially closed glottis, creating positive intrathoracic pressure. The high positive intrathoracic pressure distributes the inspired air throughout the alveoli and begins to establish *functional residual capacity* (FRC), the air left in the lungs at the end of a normal expiration. The higher intrathoracic pressure also increases absorption of fluid via the capillaries and lymphatic system. The negative intrathoracic pressure created when the diaphragm moves down with inspiration causes lung fluid to flow from the alveoli across the alveolar membranes into the pulmonary interstitial tissue.

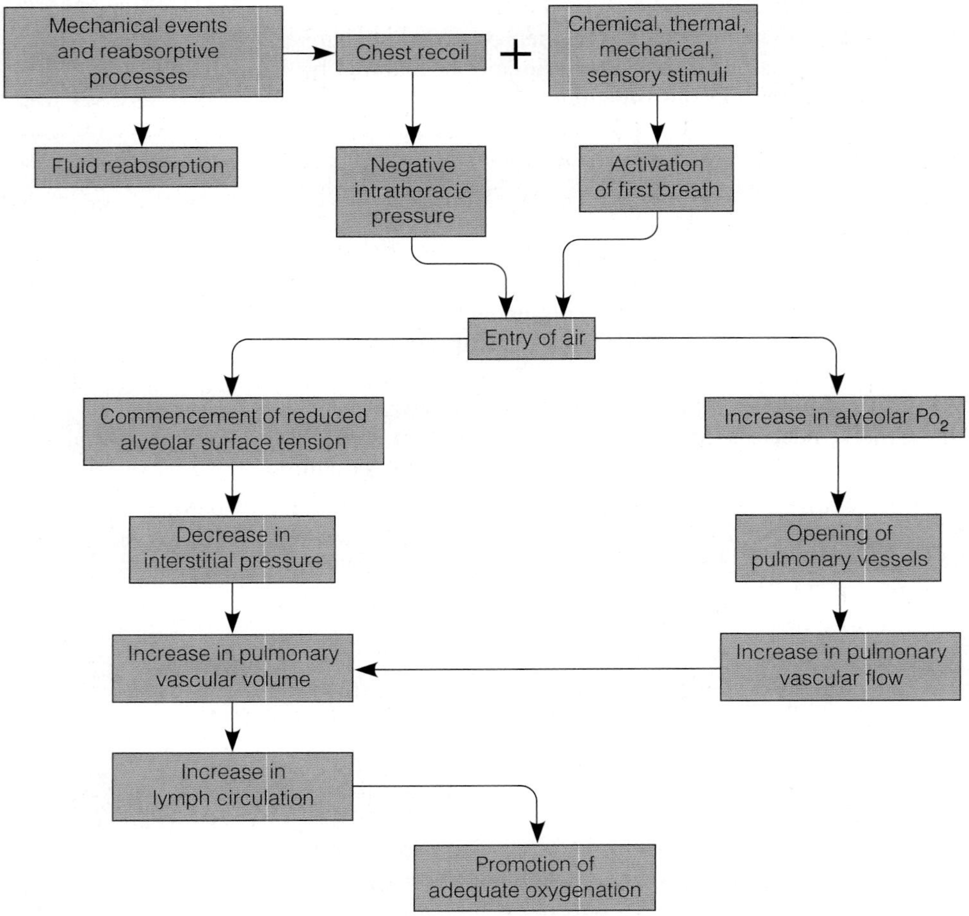

● **Figure 24–1** Initiation of respiration in the newborn.

At birth the alveolar epithelium is temporarily more permeable. This, combined with decreased cellular resistance at the onset of breathing, may facilitate passive liquid absorption. With each succeeding breath, the lungs continue to expand, stretching the alveolar walls and increasing the alveolar volume. Protein molecules are too large to pass through capillary walls. The presence of more protein molecules in the pulmonary capillaries than in the interstitial tissue creates oncotic pressure. This pressure draws the interstitial fluid into the capillaries and lymphatic tissue to balance the concentration of protein. Lung expansion helps the remaining lung fluid move into the interstitial tissue. As pulmonary vascular resistance decreases, pulmonary blood flow increases, and more interstitial fluid is absorbed into the bloodstream. In the healthy term newborn, lung fluid moves rapidly into the interstitial tissue but may take several hours to move into the lymph and blood vessels. Most of the lung fluid is reabsorbed within 2 hours after birth, and it is completely absorbed within 12 to 24 hours after birth (Rosenberg, 2007).

Although the initial chest recoil assists in clearing the airways of accumulated fluid and permits further inspiration, most clinicians believe mucus and fluid should be suctioned from the newborn's mouth, nose, and throat. They use a bulb or mucous trap attached to suction as soon as the newborn's head and shoulders are born and again as the newborn adapts to extrauterine life and stabilizes (see Clinical Skills Manual, "Performing Nasal Pharyngeal Suctioning" SKILLS).

Newborns may have problems clearing the fluid from their lungs and beginning respiration for a variety of reasons:

- The lymphatic system may be underdeveloped, thus decreasing the rate at which the fluid is absorbed from the lungs.
- Complications that occur before or during labor and birth can interfere with adequate lung expansion and cause failure to decrease pulmonary vascular resistance, resulting in decreased pulmonary blood flow. These complications include inadequate compression of the chest wall in very small newborns (small for gestational age [SGA] or very low birth weight [VLBW]) because of immature muscular development; the absence of chest wall compression in a newborn born by cesarean birth, although this compression can be externally applied by skilled physicians as they deliver the newborn from the uterus; respiratory depression because of maternal analgesia or anesthesia agents; or aspiration of amniotic fluid, meconium, or blood.

Chemical Stimuli

An important chemical stimulator that contributes to the onset of breathing is transitory asphyxia of the fetus and newborn. The first breath is an inspiratory gasp, the result of CNS reaction to sudden pressure, temperature change, and other external stimuli (Knuppel, 2007). This first breath is triggered by the slight elevation in PCO_2 and decrease in pH and PO_2, which are the natural result of a normal vaginal labor and birth. These changes, which are present in all newborns to some degree, stimulate the aortic and carotid chemoreceptors, initiating impulses that trigger the medulla's respiratory center. Although this brief period of asphyxia is a significant stimulator, prolonged asphyxia is abnormal and depresses respiration. Another chemical factor may result from clamping the umbilical cord that may cause a drop in levels of a prostaglandin that inhibits respirations (Bloom, 2006). As a result newborns can vigorously cry and be active before the cord is clamped or the placenta separates.

Thermal Stimuli

A significant decrease in environmental temperature after birth, 37°C to 21°C–23.9°C (98.6°F to 70°F–75°F), results in sudden chilling of the moist newborn (Cheffer, 2004). The cold stimulates skin nerve endings, and the newborn responds with rhythmic respirations. Normal temperature changes that occur at birth are apparently within acceptable physiologic limits. Excessive cooling may result in profound depression and evidence of cold stress (see Chapter 29 for discussion of cold stress).

Sensory Stimuli

During intrauterine life, the fetus is in a dark, sound-dampened, fluid-filled environment and is nearly weightless. After birth the newborn experiences light, sounds, and the effects of gravity for the first time. As the fetus moves from a familiar, comfortable, quiet environment to one of sensory abundance, a number of physical and sensory influences help respiration begin. They include the numerous tactile, auditory, and visual stimuli of birth. Joint movement also results in enhanced proprioreceptor stimulation to the respiratory center to sustain respirations.

FACTORS OPPOSING THE FIRST BREATH

Three major factors may oppose the initiation of respiratory activity: (1) the contracting force between alveoli—called *alveolar surface tension;* (2) viscosity of lung fluid within the respiratory tract, which is influenced by surfactant levels; and (3) the ease with which the lung is able to fill with air—called *lung compliance.*

Alveolar surface tension is the contracting force between the moist surfaces of the alveoli. This tension, which is necessary for healthy respiratory function, would nevertheless cause the small airways and alveoli to collapse between each inspiration were it not for the presence of surfactant. By reducing the attracting force between alveoli, surfactant prevents the alveoli from completely collapsing with each expiration and thus promotes lung expansion. Similarly, surfactant promotes lung compliance, the ability of the lung to fill with air easily. When surfactant decreases, compliance also decreases, and the pressure needed to expand the alveoli with air increases.

Nursing Practice

Gentle physical contact by thoroughly drying the newborn and placing the baby in skin-to-skin contact with the mother's chest and abdomen is emphasized when using external stimulation means for the first breaths. These methods provide ample stimulation in a comforting way and also decrease heat loss.

Resistive forces of the fluid-filled lung, combined with the small radii of the airways, necessitate pressures of 30 to 40 cm (11.8 to 15.7 in.) of water to open the lung initially (Thureen, Deacon, Hernandez, et al., 2005). The first breath usually establishes FRC that is 30% to 40% of the fully expanded lung volume. This FRC allows alveolar sacs to remain partially expanded on expiration, decreasing the need for continuous high pressures for each of the following breaths. Subsequent breaths require only 6 to 8 cm H_2O pressure to open alveoli during inspiration. Therefore, the first breath of life is usually the most difficult.

CARDIOPULMONARY PHYSIOLOGY

The onset of respiration stimulates changes in the cardiovascular system necessary for successful transition to extrauterine life, hence the term **cardiopulmonary adaptation**. As air enters the lungs, Po_2 rises in the alveoli, which stimulates the relaxation of the pulmonary arteries and triggers a decrease in pulmonary vascular resistance. As pulmonary vascular resistance decreases, the vascular flow in the lung increases rapidly and achieves 100% normal flow at 24 hours of life. This delivery of greater blood volume to the lungs contributes to the conversion from fetal circulation to newborn circulation.

After pulmonary circulation is established, blood is distributed throughout the lungs, although the alveoli may or may not be fully open. For adequate oxygenation to occur, the heart must deliver sufficient blood to functional, open alveoli. Shunting of blood is common in the early newborn period. Bidirectional blood flow, or right-to-left shunting through the ductus arteriosus, may divert a significant amount of blood away from the lungs, depending on the pressure changes of respiration, crying, and the cardiac cycle. This shunting in the newborn period is also responsible for the unstable transitional period in cardiopulmonary function.

OXYGEN TRANSPORT

The transportation of oxygen to the peripheral tissues depends on the type of hemoglobin in the red blood cells. In the fetus and newborn, a variety of hemoglobins exist, the most significant being fetal hemoglobin (HbF) and adult hemoglobin (HbA). Approximately 70% to 90% of the hemoglobin in the fetus and newborn is of the fetal variety. The greatest difference between HbF and HbA relates to the transport of oxygen.

Because HbF has a greater affinity for oxygen than does HbA, the oxygen saturation in the newborn's blood is greater than in the adult's, but the amount of oxygen available to the tissues is less. This situation is beneficial prenatally, because the fetus must maintain adequate oxygen uptake in the presence of very low oxygen tension (umbilical venous Po_2 cannot exceed the uterine venous Po_2). Because of this high concentration of oxygen in the blood, hypoxia in the newborn is particularly difficult to recognize. Clinical manifestations of cyanosis do not appear until low blood levels of oxygen are present. In addition, alkalosis (increased pH) and hypothermia can result in less oxygen being available to the body tissues, whereas acidosis, hypercarbia, and hyperthermia can result in less oxygen being bound to hemoglobin and more oxygen being released to the body tissues.

MAINTAINING RESPIRATORY FUNCTION

The lung's ability to maintain oxygenation and ventilation (the exchange of oxygen and carbon dioxide) is influenced by such factors as lung compliance and airway resistance. Lung compliance is influenced by the elastic recoil of the lung tissue and anatomic differences in the newborn. The newborn has a relatively large heart and mediastinal structures that reduce available lung space. Also, the newborn chest is equipped with weak intercostal muscles and a rigid rib cage with horizontal ribs and a high diaphragm, which restricts the space available for lung expansion. The large abdomen further encroaches on the high diaphragm to decrease lung space. Another factor that limits ventilation is airway resistance, which depends on the radii, length, and number of airways. Airway resistance is increased in the newborn when compared with adults.

CHARACTERISTICS OF NEWBORN RESPIRATION

The normal newborn respiratory rate is 30 to 60 breaths per minute. Initial respirations may be largely diaphragmatic, shallow, and irregular in depth and rhythm. The abdomen's movements are synchronous with the chest movements. When the breathing pattern is characterized by pauses lasting 5 to 15 seconds, **periodic breathing** is occurring. Periodic breathing is rarely associated with differences in skin color or heart rate changes, and it has no prognostic significance. Tactile or other sensory stimulation increases the inspired oxygen and converts periodic breathing patterns to normal breathing patterns during neonatal transition. With deep sleep, the pattern is reasonably regular. Periodic breathing occurs with rapid-eye-movement (REM) sleep, and grossly irregular breathing is evident with motor activity, sucking, and crying. Cessation of breathing lasting more than 20 seconds is defined as *apnea* and is abnormal in term newborns. Apnea may or may not be associated with changes in skin color or heart rate (drop below 100 beats per minute). Apnea always needs to be further evaluated.

Newborns tend to be obligatory nose breathers because the nasal route is the primary route of air entry. This is because of the high position of the epiglottis and the position of the soft palate (Blackburn, 2007). Although many term newborns can breathe orally, with nasal occlusion, nasal obstructions can cause respiratory distress. Therefore, it is important to keep the nose and throat clear. Immediately after birth, and for about the next 2 hours, respiratory rates of 60 to 70 breaths per minute are normal. Some cyanosis and acrocyanosis are normal for several hours; thereafter the infant's color improves steadily. If respirations drop below 30 or exceed 60 per minute when the infant is at rest, or if retractions, cyanosis, or nasal flaring and expiratory grunting occur, the clinician should be notified. Any increased use of the intercostal muscles (retractions) may indicate respiratory distress. (See Chapter 29 and Table 29–1 ∞ for signs of respiratory distress.)

CARDIOVASCULAR ADAPTATIONS

As described earlier, the onset of respiration triggers increased blood flow to the lungs after birth. This greater blood volume contributes to the conversion from fetal circulation to neonatal circulation.

FETAL-NEWBORN TRANSITIONAL PHYSIOLOGY

During fetal life, blood with the higher oxygen content is diverted to the heart and brain. Blood in the descending aorta is less oxygenated and supplies the kidney and intestinal tract before it is returned to the placenta. Limited amounts of blood, pumped from the right ventricle toward the lungs, enter the pulmonary vessels. In the fetus, increased pulmonary resistance forces most of this blood through the ductus arteriosus into the descending aorta (Table 24–1). See the fetal heart animation in My Nursing Kit.

Marked changes occur in the cardiovascular system at birth. Expansion of the lungs with the first breath decreases pulmonary vascular resistance and increases pulmonary blood flow. Pressure in the left atrium increases as blood returns from the pulmonary veins. Pressure in the right atrium drops, and systematic vascular resistance increases as umbilical venous blood flow is halted when the cord is clamped. These physiologic mechanisms mark the transition from fetal to neonatal circulation and show the interplay of cardiovascular and respiratory systems (Figure 24–2 ●).

Five major areas of change occur in cardiopulmonary adaptation (Figure 24–3 ●):

1. *Increased aortic pressure and decreased venous pressure.* Clamping of the umbilical cord eliminates the placental vascular bed and reduces the intravascular space. Consequently, aortic (systemic) blood pressure increases. At the same time, blood return via the inferior vena cava

Table 24–1 Fetal and Neonatal Circulation

System	Fetal	Neonatal
Pulmonary blood vessels	Constricted, with very little blood flow; lungs not expanded	Vasodilation and increased blood flow; lungs expanded; increased oxygen stimulates vasodilation.
Systemic blood vessels	Dilated, with low resistance; blood mostly in placenta	Arterial pressure rises because of loss of placenta; increased systemic blood volume and resistance.
Ductus arteriosus	Large, with no tone; blood flow from pulmonary artery to aorta	Reversal of blood flow; now from aorta to pulmonary artery because of increased left atrial pressure. Ductus is sensitive to increased oxygen and body chemicals and begins to constrict.
Foramen ovale	Patent, with increased blood flow from right atrium to left atrium	Increased pressure in left atrium attempts to reverse blood flow and shuts one-way valve.

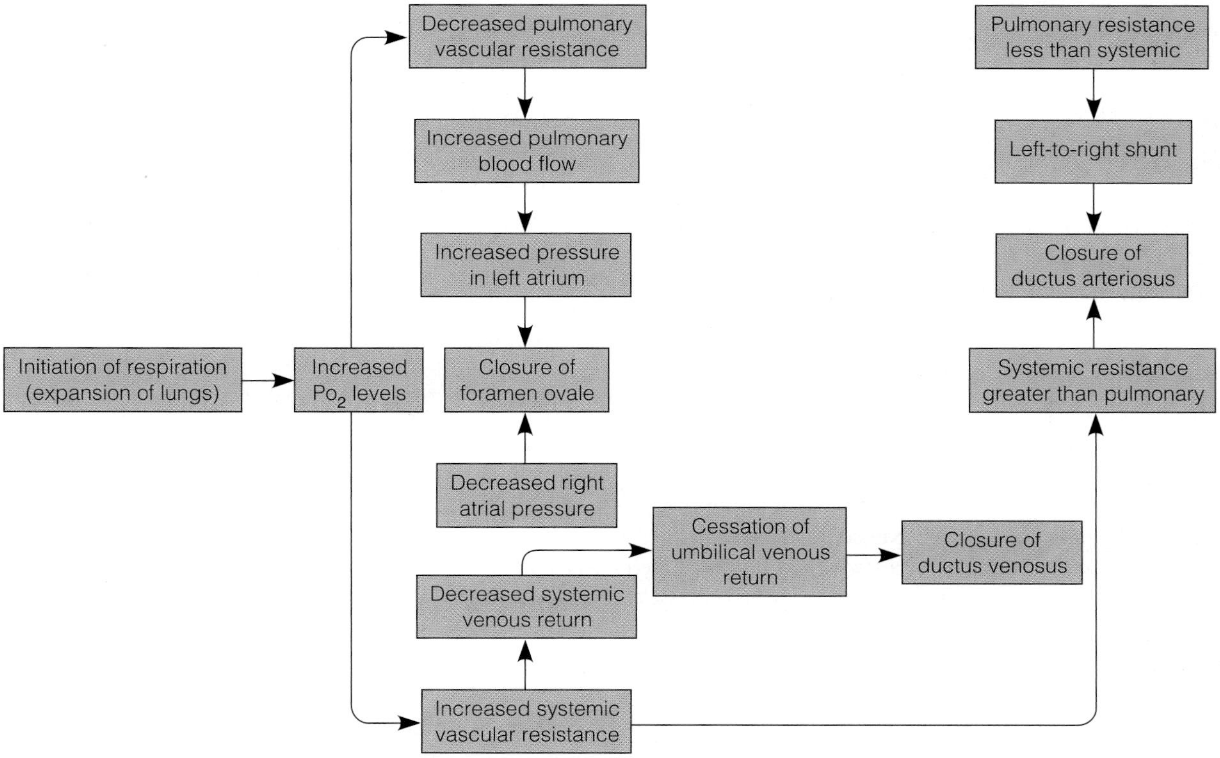

● **Figure 24–2** Transitional circulation: Conversion from fetal to neonatal circulation.

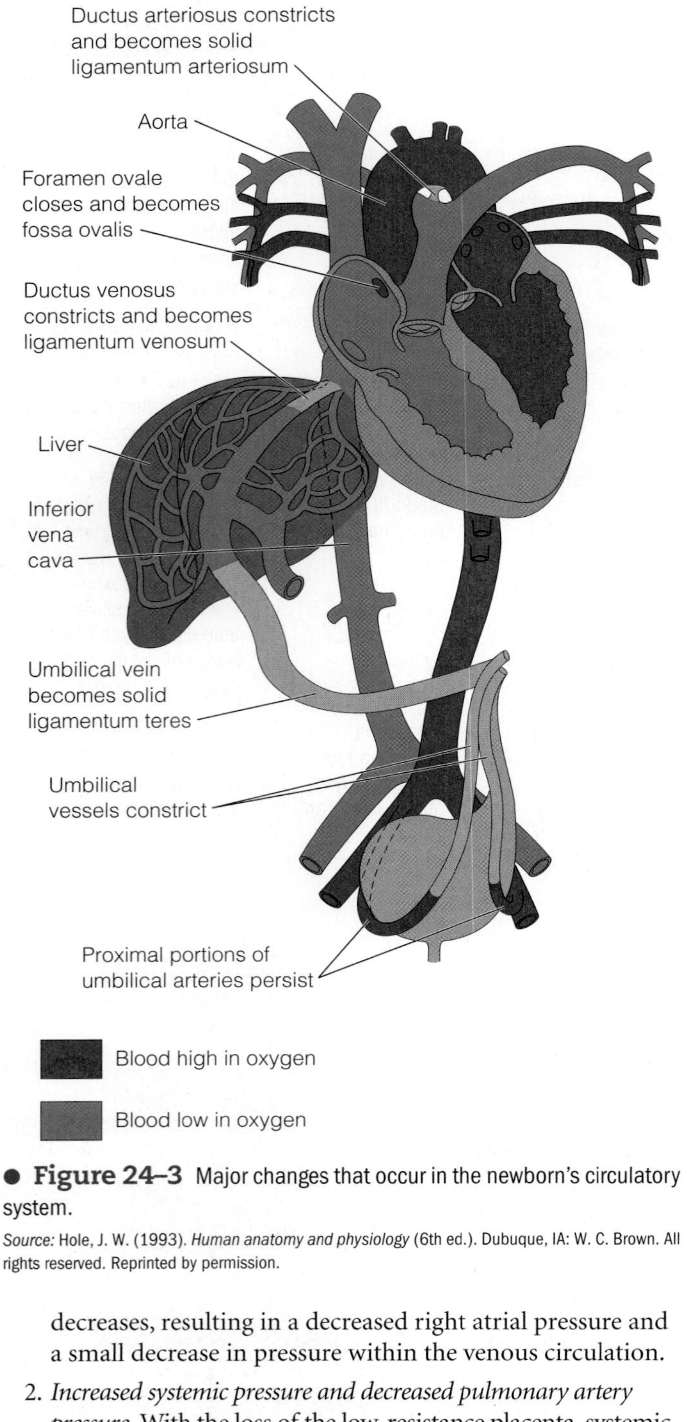

• **Figure 24–3** Major changes that occur in the newborn's circulatory system.

Source: Hole, J. W. (1993). *Human anatomy and physiology* (6th ed.). Dubuque, IA: W. C. Brown.

decreases, resulting in a decreased right atrial pressure and a small decrease in pressure within the venous circulation.

2. *Increased systemic pressure and decreased pulmonary artery pressure.* With the loss of the low-resistance placenta, systemic resistance pressure increases, resulting in greater systemic pressure. At the same time, lung expansion increases pulmonary blood flow, and the increased blood Po_2 associated with initiation of respirations dilates pulmonary blood vessels. The combination of vasodilation and increased pulmonary blood flow decreases pulmonary artery resistance. As the pulmonary vascular beds open, the systemic vascular pressure increases, enhancing perfusion of the other body systems.
3. *Closure of the foramen ovale.* Closure of the foramen ovale is a function of changing atrial pressures. In utero, pressure is greater in the right atrium, and the foramen ovale is open after birth. Decreased pulmonary resistance and increased pulmonary blood flow increase the pulmonary venous return into the left atrium, thereby increasing left atrial pressure slightly. The decreased pulmonary vascular resistance and the decreased umbilical venous return to the right atrium also decrease right atrial pressure. The pressure gradients across the atria are now reversed, with the left atrial pressure now greater, and the foramen ovale is functionally closed 1 to 2 hours after birth. However, a slight right-to-left shunting may occur in the early newborn period. Any increase in pulmonary resistance or right atrial pressure, such as occurs with crying, acidosis, or cold stress, may cause the foramen ovale to reopen, resulting in a temporary right-to-left shunt. Anatomical closure occurs within 30 months (Blackburn, 2007).
4. *Closure of the ductus arteriosus.* Initial elevation of the systemic vascular pressure above the pulmonary vascular pressure increases pulmonary blood flow by reversing the flow through the ductus arteriosus. Blood now flows from the aorta into the pulmonary artery. Furthermore, although the presence of oxygen causes the pulmonary arterioles to dilate, an increase in blood Po_2 triggers the opposite response in the ductus arteriosus—it constricts.

   In utero, the placenta provides prostaglandin E_2 (PGE_2), which causes ductus vasodilation. With the loss of the placenta and increased pulmonary blood flow, PGE_2 levels drop, leaving the active constriction by Po_2 unopposed. If the lungs fail to expand or if Po_2 levels drop, the ductus remains patent. Functional closure starts by 10 to 15 hours after birth, and fibrosis of the ductus occurs within 4 weeks after birth (Blackburn, 2007).
5. *Closure of the ductus venosus.* Although the mechanism initiating closure of the ductus venosus is not known, it appears to be related to mechanical pressure changes after severing of the cord, redistribution of blood, and cardiac output. Closure of the bypass forces perfusion of the liver. Fibrosis of the ductus venosus occurs within 2 months. Figure 24–3 depicts the changes in blood flow and oxygenation as the fetal cardiopulmonary circulation adapts to extrauterine life.

CHARACTERISTICS OF CARDIAC FUNCTION

Evaluation of the newborn's heart rate, blood pressure, heart murmurs, and cardiac workload provides data for evaluating cardiac function.

Heart Rate

Shortly after the first cry and the start of changes in cardiopulmonary circulation, the newborn heart rate can accelerate to 180 beats per minute. The average resting heart rate in the first week of life is 120 to 160 beats per minute in a healthy, full-term newborn but may vary significantly during deep sleep or active awake states. In the full-term newborn, the heart rate may drop to 80 to 100 beats per minute during deep sleep (Creehan, 2008).

Apical pulse rates should be obtained by auscultation for a full minute, preferably when the newborn is asleep. The heart rate should be evaluated for abnormal rhythms or beats. Peripheral pulses of all extremities should also be evaluated to detect any inequalities or unusual characteristics (Creehan, 2008). Peripheral pedal pulses may be difficult to palpate in the newborn. They can be assessed when blood pressure is measured if blood pressure readings are taken on all four extremities.

Blood Pressure

The blood pressure tends to be highest immediately after birth and then descends to its lowest level at about 3 hours of age. By days 4 to 6, the blood pressure rises and plateaus at a level approximately the same as the initial level. Blood pressure is sensitive to the changes in blood volume that occur in the transition to newborn circulation (Figure 24–4 ●). Peripheral perfusion pressure is a particularly sensitive indicator of the newborn's ability to compensate for alterations in blood volume before changes in blood pressure. Capillary refill should be less than 2 to 3 seconds when the skin is blanched.

Blood pressure values during the first 12 hours of life vary with the birth weight and gestational age. The average mean blood pressure is 50 to 55 mm Hg in the full-term, resting newborn over 3 kg during the first 12 hours of life (Thureen et al., 2005). In the preterm newborn, the average blood pressure varies according to weight. Crying may cause an elevation of 20 mm Hg in both the systolic and diastolic blood pressure; thus accuracy is more likely in the quiet newborn. Four point extremity blood pressure assessment is warranted in the presence of any cardiovascular symptoms (tachycardia, persistent murmur, abnormal pulses, poor perfusion, or abnormal precordial activity) (Creehan, 2008). Blood pressure in the lower extremities is usually higher than that in the upper extremities.

Heart Murmurs

Murmurs are produced by turbulent blood flow. Murmurs may be heard when blood flows across an abnormal valve or across a stenosed valve, when there is an atrial or ventricular septal defect, or when there is increased flow across a normal valve.

In newborns, 90% of all murmurs are transient *and not associated with anomalies*. They usually involve incomplete closure of the ductus arteriosus or foramen ovale. Soft murmurs may be heard as the pulmonary branch arteries increase their blood flow from 7% to 50% of the combined ventricular output during transition, causing a physiologic peripheral pulmonary stenosis. Clicks may normally be heard at the lower left sternal border as the great vessels dilate to accommodate systolic blood flow in the first few hours of life. Because of the current practice of early discharge, murmurs associated with ventricular septal defect and patent ductus arteriosus are not often picked up until the first well-baby checkup at 4 to 6 weeks of age. Murmurs are sometimes absent even in seriously malformed hearts.

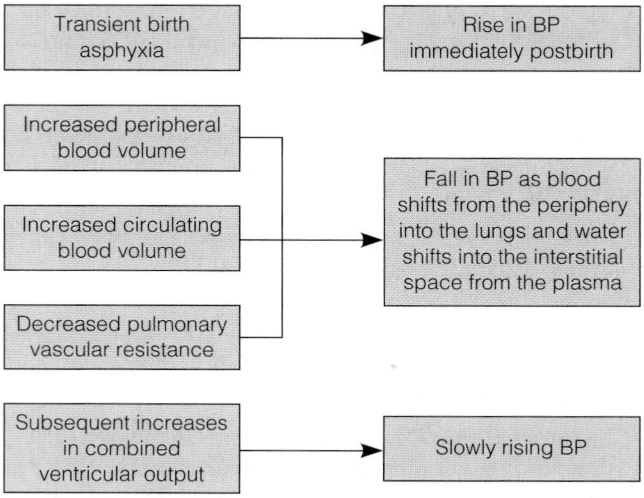

● **Figure 24–4** Response of blood pressure (BP) to neonatal changes in blood volume.

Cardiac Workload

Before birth, the right ventricle does approximately two-thirds of the cardiac work, resulting in increased size and thickness of the right ventricle at birth. In the first 2 hours after birth, when the ductus arteriosus remains mostly patent, about one-third of the left ventricular output is returned to the pulmonary circulation. As a result, the left ventricle has a significantly greater increase in volume load than the right ventricle after birth and it needs to progressively increase in size and thickness. This may explain why right-sided heart defects are better tolerated than left-sided ones and why left-sided heart defects rapidly become symptomatic after birth.

HEMATOPOIETIC SYSTEM

In the first days of life, hematocrit may rise 1 to 2 g/dL above fetal levels as a result of placental transfusion, low oral fluid intake, and diminished extracellular fluid volume. By 1 week postnatally, peripheral hemoglobin is comparable to fetal blood counts. The hemoglobin level declines progressively over the first 2 months of life (Polin, Fox, & Abman, 2004). This initial decline in hemoglobin creates a phenomenon known as **physiologic anemia of infancy**. A factor that influences the degree of physiologic anemia is the nutritional status of the newborn. Supplies of vitamin E, folic acid, and iron may be inadequate given the amount of growth in the later part of the first year of life. Hemoglobin values fall, mainly from a decrease in red cell mass rather than from the dilutional effect of increasing plasma volume. The fact that red cell survival is lower in newborns than in adults, and that red cell production is less, also contributes to this anemia. Neonatal RBCs have a life span of 80 to 100 days, approximately two-thirds the life span of adult RBCs. The normal RBC count in a term newborn is in the range of 5.1 to 5.3 million per milliliter during the first 24 to 48 hours of life (Bagwell, 2007).

Leukocytosis is a normal finding, because the stress of birth stimulates increased production of neutrophils during the first few days of life. Neutrophils then decrease to 35% of the total leukocyte count by 2 weeks of age. Lymphocytes play a role in antibody formation and eventually become the predominant type of leukocyte and the total white blood cell count falls.

Developing Cultural Competence

ABORIGINAL CULTURE

In aboriginal cultures, cords and placentas were sometimes left to dry attached to the newborn.

Blood volume is approximately 85 mL/kg of body weight for a term infant (Bagwell, 2007). For example, a 3.6 kg (8 lb) newborn has a blood volume of 306 mL. Blood volume varies based on the amount of placental transfusion received during the delivery of the placenta, as well as other factors, including the following:

1. *Delayed cord clamping and the normal shift of plasma to the extravascular spaces.* Newborn hemoglobin and hematocrit values are higher when a placental transfusion occurs after birth. Placental vessels contain about 75 to 125 mL of blood at term, most of which can be transfused into the newborn by holding the newborn below the level of the placenta and delaying clamping of the cord. Blood volume increases by 61% with delayed cord clamping (Bagwell, 2007). The increase is reflected by a rise in hemoglobin level and an increase in the hematocrit. For greatest accuracy, the initial hemoglobin and hematocrit levels should be measured in the cord blood, although this is not a routine practice. In term newborns a delay in clamping the umbilical cord appears to offer protection from anemia without harmful effects (Mercer, Erickson-Owens, Graves, et al., 2007). In preterm or SGA newborns delay in cord clamping may have risks. It can speed and worsen symptoms of hyperbilirubinemia and cause hypervolemia.
2. *Gestational age.* There appears to be a positive association between gestational age, RBC numbers, and hemoglobin concentration.
3. *Prenatal and/or perinatal hemorrhage.* Significant prenatal or perinatal bleeding decreases the hematocrit level and causes hypovolemia.
4. *The site of the blood sample.* Hemoglobin and hematocrit levels are significantly higher in capillary blood than in venous blood. Sluggish peripheral blood flow creates RBC stasis, thereby increasing RBC concentration in the capillaries. Consequently, blood samples taken from venous blood sites are more accurate than those from capillary sites.

The concentration of serum electrolytes in the blood indicates the fluid and electrolyte status of the newborn. See Table 24–2 for normal term newborn electrolyte and blood values.

Table 24–2 Normal Term Newborn Cord Blood Values

Laboratory Data	Normal Range
Hemoglobin	14 to 20 g/dL
Hematocrit	43% to 63%
WBC	10,000 to 30,000/mm^3
Neutrophils	40% to 80%
Platelets	150,000 to 350,000/mm^3
RBC	5,100,000 to 5,300,000/mL
Reticulocytes	3% to 7%
Blood volume	82.3 mL/kg (third day after early cord clamping) 92.6 mL/kg (third day after delayed cord clamping)
Sodium	129 to 144 mEq/L
Potassium	3.4 to 9.9 mEq/L
Chloride	103 to 111 mEq/L
Calcium	8.2 to 11.1 mg/dL
Glucose	45 to 96 mg/dL

Source: Fanaroff, A. A., & Martin, R. J. (Eds.). (2006). *Neonatal-perinatal medicine* (7th ed., pp. 1801, 1810). St. Louis: Mosby.

TEMPERATURE REGULATION

Temperature regulation is the maintenance of thermal balance by the loss of heat to the environment at a rate equal to the production of heat. Newborns are *homeothermic;* they attempt to stabilize their internal (core) body temperatures within a narrow range in spite of significant temperature variations in their environment.

Thermoregulation in the newborn is closely related to the rate of metabolism and oxygen consumption. Within a specific environmental temperature range, called the **neutral thermal environment (NTE)** zone, the rates of oxygen consumption and metabolism are minimal, and internal body temperature is maintained because of thermal balance (Thureen et al., 2005) (See Neutral Thermal Environmental Temperature table on My Nursing Kit). For an unclothed, full-term newborn, the NTE is an ambient environmental temperature range of 32°C to 34°C (89.6°F to 93.2°F) within 50% relative humidity. The limits for an adult are 26°C to 28°C (78.8°F to 82.4°F) (Polin, Fox, & Abman, 2004). Thus, the normal newborn requires higher environmental temperatures to maintain a thermoneutral environment.

Several newborn characteristics affect the establishment of thermal stability:

- The newborn has less subcutaneous fat than an adult and a thin epidermis.
- Blood vessels in the newborn are closer to the skin than those of an adult. Therefore, the circulating blood is influenced by changes in environmental temperature and in turn influences the hypothalamic temperature-regulating center.

- The flexed posture of the term newborn decreases the surface area exposed to the environment, thereby reducing heat loss.

Size and age may also affect the establishment of a NTE. For example, the preterm or small-for-gestational-age (SGA) newborn has less adipose tissue and is hypoflexed, and therefore requires higher environmental temperatures to achieve a neutral thermal environment. Larger, well-insulated newborns may be able to cope with lower environmental temperatures. If the environmental temperature falls below the lower limits of the NTE, the newborn responds with increased oxygen consumption and metabolism, which results in greater heat production. Prolonged exposure to the cold may result in depleted glycogen stores and acidosis. Oxygen consumption also increases if the environmental temperature is above the NTE.

HEAT LOSS

A newborn is at a distinct disadvantage in maintaining a normal temperature. With a large body surface in relation to mass and a limited amount of insulating subcutaneous fat, the full-term newborn loses about four times the heat of an adult. The newborn's poor thermal stability is primarily because of excessive heat loss rather than impaired heat production. Because of the risk of hypothermia and possible cold stress, minimizing heat loss in the newborn after birth is essential (See "Provision of Initial Newborn Care" in Chapters 19 and 26∞ for nursing measures).

Two major routes of heat loss are from the internal core of the body to the body surface and from the external surface to the environment. Usually the core temperature is higher than the skin temperature, resulting in continuous transfer or conduction of heat to the surface. The greater the difference in temperature between core and skin, the more rapidly heat transfers. The transfer is accomplished through an increase in oxygen consumption, depletion of glycogen stores, and metabolization of brown fat.

Heat loss from the body surface to the environment takes place in four ways—by convection, radiation, evaporation, and conduction (Figure 24–5 ●).

- **Convection** is the loss of heat from the warm body surface to the cooler air currents. Air-conditioned rooms, air currents with a temperature below the infant's skin temperature, oxygen by mask, and removal from an incubator for procedures increase convective heat loss in the newborn.
- **Radiation** losses occur when heat transfers from the heated body surface to cooler surfaces and objects not in direct contact with the body. The walls of a room or of an incubator are potential causes of heat loss by radiation, even if the ambient temperature of the incubator is within the thermal neutral range for that infant. Placing cold objects (such as ice for blood gases) onto the incubator or near the infant in the radiant warmer will increase radiant losses.
- **Evaporation** is the loss of heat incurred when water is converted to a vapor. The newborn is particularly prone to lose heat by evaporation immediately after birth (when the

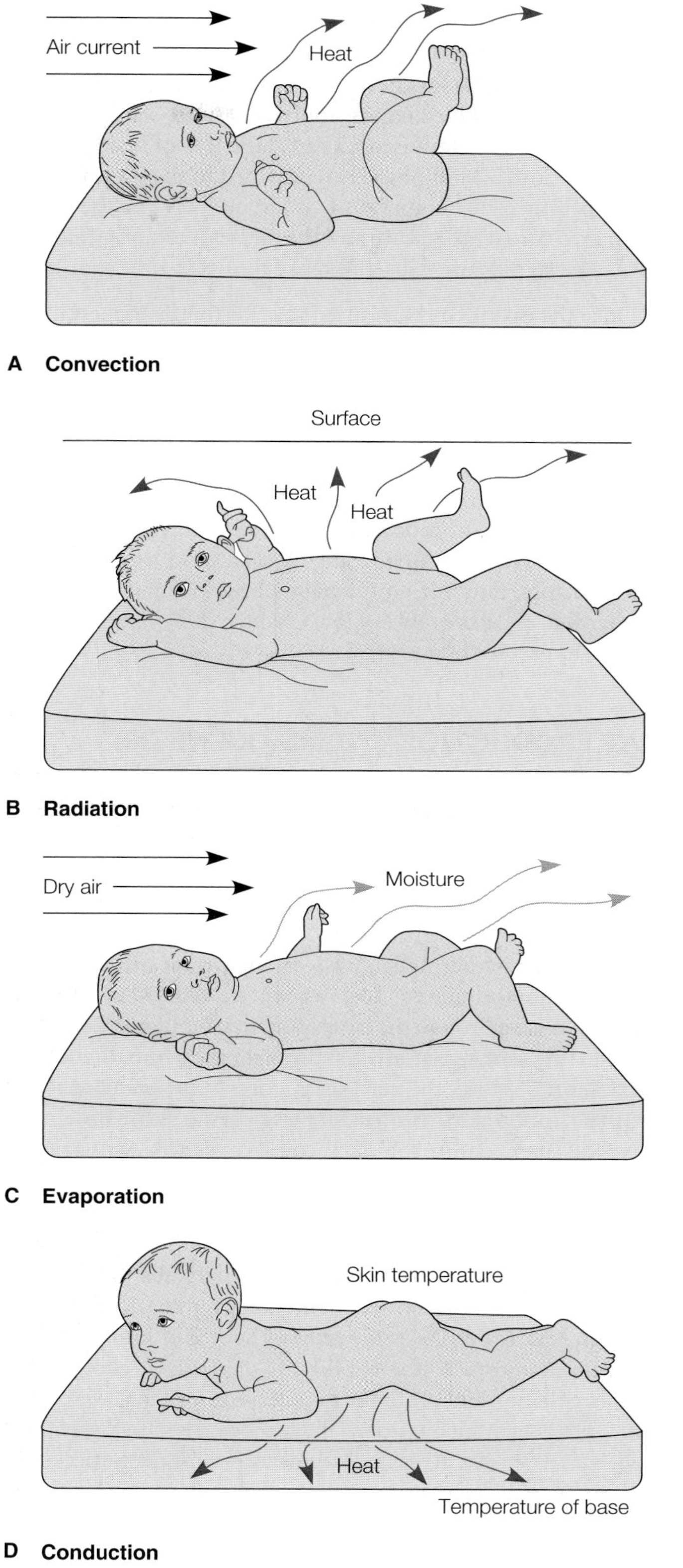

● **Figure 24–5** Methods of heat loss. ***A,*** Convection. ***B,*** Radiation. ***C,*** Evaporation. ***D,*** Conduction.

baby is wet with amniotic fluid), and during baths; thus, drying the newborn is critical.

- **Conduction** is the loss of heat to a cooler surface by direct skin contact. Chilled hands, cool scales, cold examination tables, and cold stethoscopes can cause loss of heat by conduction. Even if objects are warmed to the incubator temperature, the temperature difference between the infant's core temperature and the ambient temperature may be significant. This difference results in heat transfer.

Once the infant has been dried after birth, the highest losses of heat generally result from radiation and convection, because of the newborn's large body surface compared with weight, and from thermal conduction, because of the marked difference between core temperature and skin temperature. The newborn can respond to the cooler environmental temperature with adequate peripheral vasoconstriction, but this mechanism is not entirely effective because of the minimal amount of fat insulation present, the large body surface, and ongoing thermal conduction. Because of these factors, minimizing the baby's heat loss and preventing hypothermia are imperative. (See Chapter 29 for nursing measures to prevent hypothermia.)

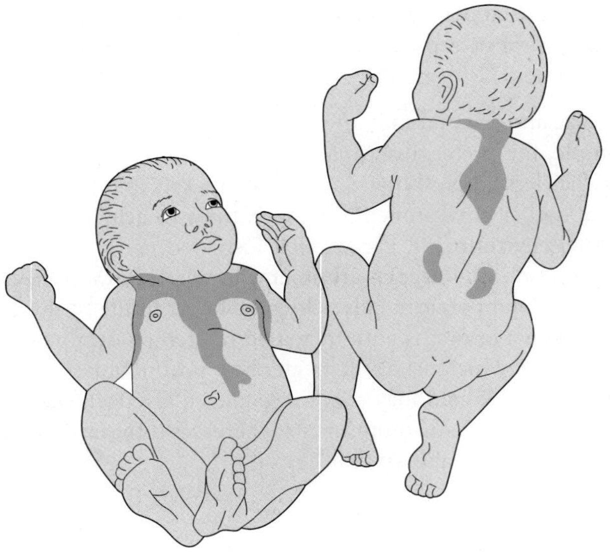

● **Figure 24–6** The distribution of brown adipose tissue (brown fat) in the newborn.

Source: Adapted from Davis, V. (1980, November-December). Structure and function of brown adipose tissue in the neonate. *Journal of Obstetric, Gynecologic, and Neonatal Nursing, 9,* 364.

HEAT PRODUCTION (THERMOGENESIS)

When exposed to a cool environment, the newborn requires additional heat. The newborn has several physiologic mechanisms that increase heat production, or *thermogenesis.* These mechanisms include increased basal metabolic rate, muscular activity, and chemical thermogenesis (also called *nonshivering thermogenesis [NST]*) (Rosenberg, 2007).

Nonshivering thermogenesis is an important mechanism of heat production unique to the newborn. It occurs when skin receptors perceive a drop in the environmental temperature and, in response, transmit sensations to stimulate the sympathetic nervous system. NST uses the newborn's stores of **brown adipose tissue (BAT)** (also called brown fat) to provide heat. Brown fat receives its name from the dark color caused by its enriched blood supply, dense cellular content, and abundant nerve endings. These characteristics of brown fat cells promote rapid metabolism, heat generation, and heat transfer to the peripheral circulation. The large numbers of brown fat cells increase the speed with which triglycerides are metabolized to produce heat.

Thus, NST from BAT is the primary source of heat in the hypothermic newborn. It first appears in the fetus at about 26 to 30 weeks' gestation and continues to increase until 2 to 5 weeks after the birth of a term infant, unless the fat is depleted by cold stress. Brown fat is deposited in the midscapular area, around the neck, and in the axillas, with deeper placement around the trachea, esophagus, abdominal aorta, kidneys, and adrenal glands (Figure 24–6 ●). BAT constitutes 2% to 6% of the newborn's total body weight.

Shivering, a form of muscular activity common in the cold adult, is rarely seen in the newborn, although it has been observed at ambient temperatures of 15°C (59°F) or less (Polin et al., 2004). If the newborn shivers, it means the newborn's metabolic rate has already doubled. The extra muscular activity does little to produce needed heat.

Thermographic studies of newborns exposed to cold show an increase in the skin heat produced over the newborn's brown fat deposits between 1 and 14 days of age (Polin et al., 2004). However, if the brown fat supply has been depleted, the metabolic response to cold is limited or lacking. An increase in basal metabolism as a result of hypothermia results in an increase in oxygen consumption. A decrease in the environmental temperature of 2°C, from 33°C to 31°C, is a drop sufficient to double the oxygen consumption of a term newborn. Keeping the normal newborn warm promotes normal oxygen requirements, whereas chilling can cause the newborn to show signs of respiratory distress.

When exposed to cold, the normal term newborn is usually able to cope with the increase in oxygen requirements, but the preterm newborn may be unable to increase ventilation to the necessary level of oxygen consumption. (See Chapter 29 for a discussion of cold stress.) Because oxidation of fatty acids depends on the availability of oxygen, glucose, and adenosine triphosphate (ATP), the newborn's ability to generate heat can be altered by pathologic events such as hypoxia, acidosis, and hypoglycemia or by medication that blocks the release of norepinephrine. Meperidine (Demerol) given to a laboring woman or as a newborn analgesic could slow or prevent metabolism of newborn brown fat and

Developing Cultural Competence

NEWBORN BATHS IN JORDAN

In Jordan, the birth of a male infant is a much celebrated event. The newborn is bathed daily during the first week of life. During the final bath, salt is added to the water to help the newborn's skin adjust to the external environment and protect it from changes in the weather.

can lead to a greater fall in the newborn's body temperature during the neonatal period. The potential effect of meperidine on brown fat can be lessened if the mother and the newborn are well hydrated and in a neutral thermal environment. Newborn hypothermia prolongs as well as potentiates the effects of many analgesic and anesthetic drugs in the newborn.

RESPONSE TO HEAT

Sweating is the term newborn's usual initial response to hyperthermia. The newborn sweat glands have limited function until after the fourth week of extrauterine life; heat is lost through peripheral vasodilation and evaporation of insensible water loss. The term infant will be flaccid and assume a position of extension to facilitate heat loss (Blackburn, 2007). Oxygen consumption and metabolic rate also increase in response to hyperthermia. Severe hyperthermia can lead to death or to gross brain damage if the baby survives.

HEPATIC ADAPTATIONS

In the newborn, the liver is frequently palpable 2 to 3 cm below the right costal margin. It is relatively large and occupies about 40% of the abdominal cavity. The newborn liver plays a significant role in iron storage, carbohydrate metabolism, conjugation of bilirubin, and coagulation.

IRON STORAGE AND RBC PRODUCTION

As RBCs are destroyed after birth, the iron is stored in the liver until needed for new RBC production. Newborn iron stores are determined by total body hemoglobin content and length of gestation. The term newborn has about 270 mg of iron at birth, and about 140 to 170 mg of this amount is in the hemoglobin. If the mother's iron intake has been adequate, enough iron will be stored to last until the infant is about 5 months of age.

CARBOHYDRATE METABOLISM

At term, the newborn's cord blood glucose level is 15 mg/dL lower than maternal blood glucose level (Rosenberg, 2007). Newborn carbohydrate reserves are relatively low. One-third of this reserve is in the form of liver glycogen. Newborn glycogen stores are twice those of the adult. The newborn enters an energy crunch at the time of birth, with the removal of the maternal glucose supply and the increased energy expenditure associated with the birth process and extrauterine life. Fuel sources are consumed at a faster rate because of the work of breathing, loss of heat when exposed to cold, activity, and activation of muscle tone. Glucose is the main source of energy in the first 4 to 6 hours after birth. During the first 2 hours of life, the serum blood glucose level declines, then rises, and finally reaches a steady state by 3 hours after birth (Rosenberg, 2007).

The nurse may assess the glucose level on admission if risk factors are present or per agency protocol. As stores of liver and muscle glycogen and blood glucose decrease, the newborn compensates by changing from a predominantly carbohydrate metabolism to fat metabolism. Energy can be derived from fat and protein, as well as from carbohydrates. The amount and availability of each of these "fuel substrates" depend on the ability of immature metabolic pathways (which lack specific enzymes or hormones) to function in the first few days of life.

CONJUGATION OF BILIRUBIN

Conjugation of bilirubin is the conversion of yellow lipid-soluble pigment into water-soluble pigment. Unconjugated (indirect) bilirubin is a breakdown product derived from hemoglobin released primarily from destroyed RBCs. Unconjugated bilirubin is not in excretable form and is a potential toxin. **Total serum bilirubin** is the sum of conjugated (direct) and unconjugated (indirect) bilirubin.

Fetal unconjugated bilirubin crosses the placenta to be excreted, so the fetus does not need to conjugate bilirubin. Total bilirubin at birth is usually less than 3 mg/dL unless an abnormal hemolytic process has been present in utero. After birth the newborn's liver must begin to conjugate bilirubin. This produces a normal rise in serum bilirubin levels in the first few days of life.

The bilirubin formed after RBCs are destroyed is transported in the blood bound to albumin. The bilirubin is transferred into the hepatocytes and bound to intracellular proteins. These proteins determine the amount of bilirubin held in a liver cell for processing and consequently determine the amount of bilirubin uptake into the liver. The activity of uridine-diphosphoglucuronosyl transferase (UDPGT) enzyme results in the attachment of unconjugated bilirubin to glucuronic acid (product of liver glycogen), producing conjugated (direct) bilirubin. Direct bilirubin is excreted into the tiny bile ducts, then into the common duct and duodenum. The conjugated bilirubin then progresses down the intestines, where bacteria transform it into urobilinogen (urine bilirubin) and stercobilinogen. Stercobilinogen is not reabsorbed but is excreted as a yellow-brown pigment in the stools.

Even after the bilirubin has been conjugated and bound, it can be changed back to unconjugated bilirubin via the enterohepatic circulation. In the intestines β-glucuronidase enzyme acts to split off (deconjugate) the bilirubin from glucuronic acid if it has not first been acted on by gut bacteria to produce urobilinogen; the free bilirubin is reabsorbed through the intestinal wall and brought back to the liver via portal vein circulation. This recycling of the bilirubin and decreased ability to clear bilirubin from the system are prevalent in babies with very high β-D-glucuronidase activity levels, those who are exclusively breastfed, and those with delayed bacterial colonization of the gut (such as with the use of antibiotics). This further increases the newborn's susceptibility to jaundice (Figure 24–7 ●).

The newborn liver has relatively less glucuronyl transferase activity in the first few weeks of life than an adult liver. This reduction in hepatic activity, along with a relatively large bilirubin load, decreases the liver's ability to conjugate bilirubin and increases susceptibility to jaundice.

PHYSIOLOGIC JAUNDICE

Physiologic jaundice is caused by accelerated destruction of fetal RBCs, impaired conjugation of bilirubin, and increased bilirubin reabsorption from the intestinal tract. This condition does not

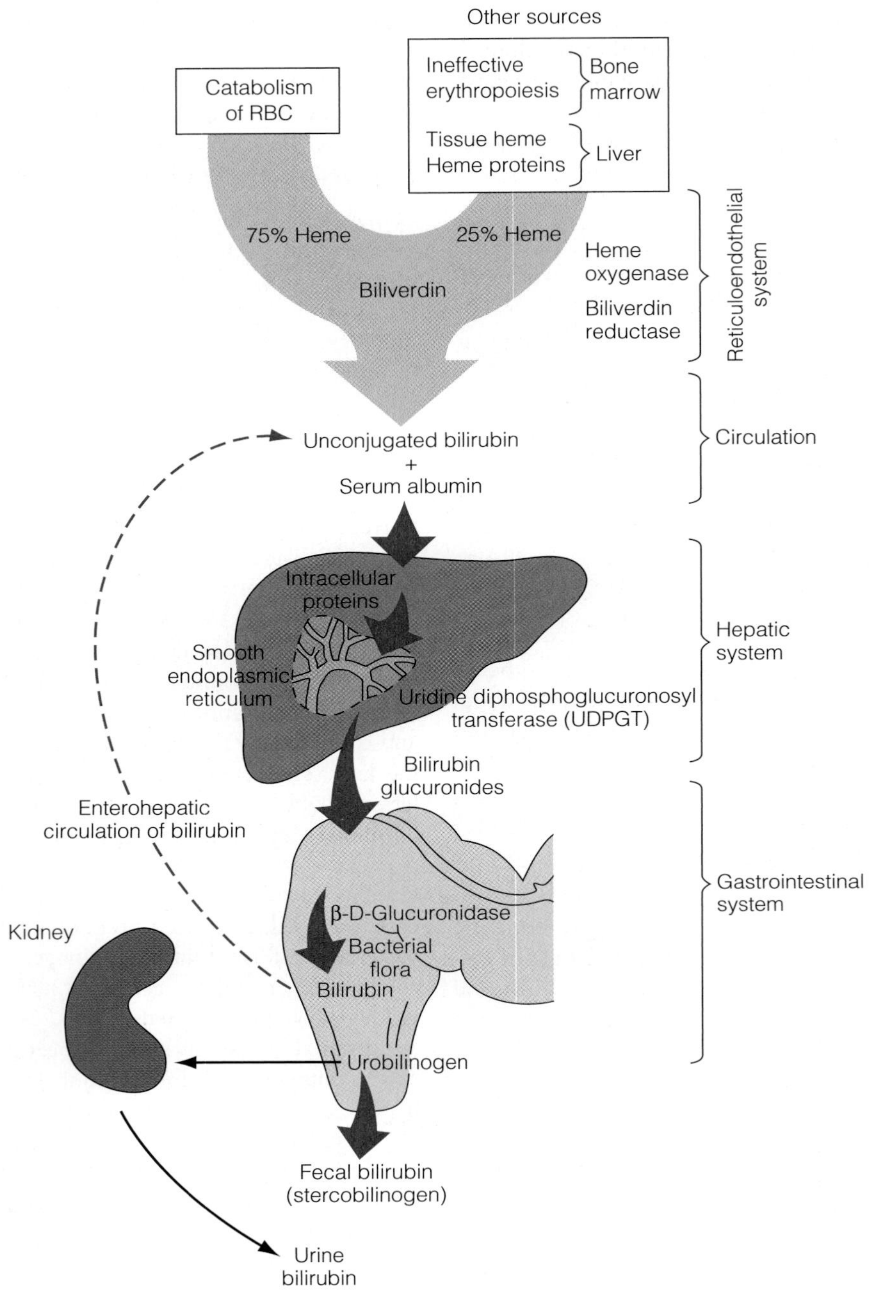

• **Figure 24–7** Conjugation of bilirubin in newborns.

Source: Adapted from Avery, G. B., Fletcher, M. A., & MacDonald, M. G. (1999). *Neonatology: Pathophysiology and management of the newborn* (5th ed., p. 767, Fig. 38-5). Philadelphia: Lippincott Williams & Wilkins.

have a pathologic basis but is a normal biologic response of the newborn.

Maisels (2005) describes six factors—several of which can also be related to pathologic events—that may interact to create physiologic jaundice.

1. *Increased amounts of bilirubin delivered to the liver.* The increased blood volume because of delayed cord clamping combined with faster RBC destruction in the newborn leads to an increased bilirubin level in the blood. A proportionately larger amount of nonerythrocyte bilirubin forms in the newborn. Therefore, newborns have two to three times greater production or breakdown of bilirubin than do adults. The use of forceps or vacuum extraction, which sometimes causes facial bruising or cephalohematoma (entrapped hemorrhage), can increase the amount of bilirubin to be handled by the liver.
2. *Defective hepatic uptake of bilirubin from the plasma.* If the newborn does not ingest adequate calories, the formation of hepatic binding proteins diminishes, resulting in higher bilirubin levels.

3. *Defective conjugation of the bilirubin.* Decreased uridine-diphosphoglucuronosyl activity as in hypothyroidism or inadequate caloric intake causes the intracellular binding proteins to remain saturated and results in greater unconjugated bilirubin levels in the blood. The fatty acids in breast milk are thought to compete with bilirubin for albumin-binding sites and therefore impede bilirubin processing.
4. *Defect in bilirubin excretion.* A congenital infection may cause impaired excretion of conjugated bilirubin. Delay in introduction of bacterial flora and decreased intestinal motility can also delay excretion and increase enterohepatic circulation of bilirubin.
5. *Inadequate hepatic circulation.* Decreased oxygen supplies to the liver associated with neonatal hypoxia or congenital heart disease lead to a rise in the bilirubin level.
6. *Increased reabsorption of bilirubin from the intestine.* Reduced bowel motility, intestinal obstruction, or delayed passage of meconium increases the circulation of bilirubin in the enterohepatic pathway, thereby resulting in higher bilirubin values.

About 50% of full-term and 80% of preterm newborns exhibit physiologic jaundice on about the second or third day after birth. The characteristic yellow color results from increased levels of unconjugated (indirect) bilirubin, which are a normal product of RBC breakdown and reflect the body's temporary inability to eliminate bilirubin. Serum levels of bilirubin are about 4 to 6 mg/dL before the yellow coloration of the skin and sclera appear. *The signs of physiologic jaundice appear after the first 24 hours postnatally.* This time frame differentiates physiologic jaundice from pathologic jaundice (see Chapter 29), which is clinically seen at birth or within the first 24 hours of postnatal life. Major risk factors for developing severe hyperbilirubinemia in late preterm and term infants are total serum (TSB) or transcutaneous (TcB) level in the high-risk zone on the bilirubin nomogram (Figure 24–8 ●).

There is no consistent definition of neonatal hyperbilirubinemia; what is considered to be in that range varies with population characteristics and postbirth age (Blackburn, 2007). Peak bilirubin levels are reached between days 3 and 5 in the full-term infant and between days 5 and 7 in the preterm infant. These values are established for European and American Caucasian newborns. Chinese, Japanese, Korean, and Native American newborns have considerably higher bilirubin

Evidence in Action

Universal screening for hyperbilirubinemia versus visual inspection alone is necessary to identify elevated bilirubin levels in newborns (AWHONN, Clinical Position Statement, 2005).

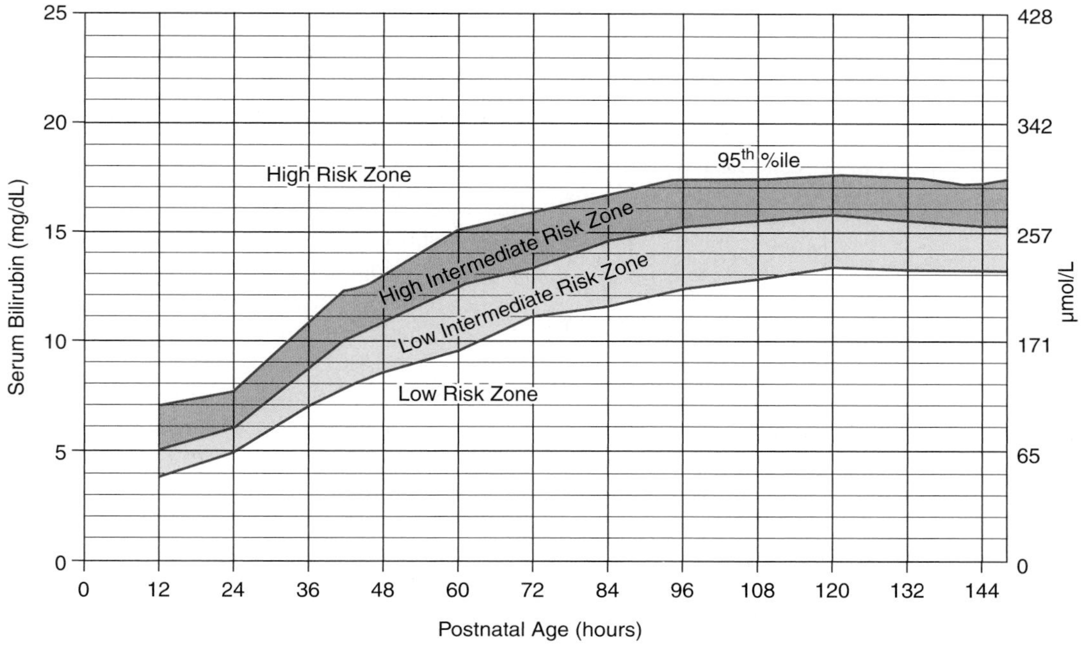

● **Figure 24–8** Postnatal hour-specific bilirubin nomogram. Note: Nomogram for designation of risk in 2840 well newborns at 36 or more weeks' gestational age with birth weight of 2000 g or more or 35 or more weeks' gestational age and birth weight of 2500 g or more based on the hour-specific serum bilirubin values. The serum level was obtained before discharge, and the zone in which the value fell predicted the likelihood of a subsequent bilirubin level exceeding the 95th percentile (high-risk zone) as shown in Appendix 3, Table 4. Used with permission from Bhutani et al. See Appendix 1 for additional information about this nomogram, which should not be used to represent the natural history of neonatal hyperbilirubinemia.

Source: American Academy of Pediatrics Subcommittee on Hyperbilirubinemia. (2004). Management of hyperbilirubinemia in the newborn infant 35 or more weeks of gestation. *Pediatrics, 114*(1), 297–316 (Fig. 2. p. 301).

levels that are not as apparent and that persist for longer periods with no apparent ill effects (Maisels, 2005).

The nursery or postpartum environment, including lighting, may hinder the early detection of the degree and type of jaundice. Pink walls and artificial lights mask the beginning of jaundice in newborns but daylight can help to recognize jaundice early as it eliminates distortions from artificial light.

If jaundice is suspected, the nurse can assess the newborn's coloring by pressing the skin, on the forehead or nose, with a finger. As blanching occurs, the nurse can observe the icterus (yellow coloring).

Several newborn care procedures will decrease the probability of high bilirubin levels.

- Maintain the newborn's skin temperature at 36.5°C (97.8°F) or above; cold stress results in acidosis. Acidosis decreases available serum albumin-binding sites, weakens albumin-binding powers, and causes elevated unconjugated bilirubin levels.
- Monitor stool for amount and characteristics. Bilirubin is eliminated in the feces; inadequate stooling may result in reabsorption and recycling of bilirubin. Early breastfeeding should be encouraged because the laxative effect of colostrum increases excretion of meconium and transitional stool.
- Encourage early feedings to promote intestinal elimination and bacterial colonization and provide caloric intake necessary for hepatic binding proteins to form.

If jaundice becomes apparent, nursing care is directed toward keeping the newborn well hydrated and promoting intestinal elimination. (For specific nursing management and therapies, see "Nursing Care Plan: Newborn with Hyperbilirubinemia" in Chapter 29.)

Physiologic jaundice may upset parents; provide emotional support and thorough explanation of the condition. If the baby is placed under phototherapy (see Chapter 29), a few additional days of hospitalization may be required, which may also upset parents. Encourage them to meet the emotional needs of their newborn by continuing to feed, hold, and caress the infant. If the mother is discharged, encourage the parents to return for feedings and to telephone or visit when possible. In many instances, the mother, especially if she is breastfeeding, may elect to remain hospitalized with her newborn; the nurse should support this decision. If insurance limitations make this unrealistic, it may be possible to find an empty room for the discharged mother and her family to use while visiting the newborn. As an alternative to continued hospitalization, the newborn may be treated with home phototherapy. (See "Phototherapy" in Chapter 29 for more information.)

BREASTFEEDING JAUNDICE AND BREAST MILK JAUNDICE

Breastfeeding is implicated in prolonged jaundice in some newborns. *Breastfeeding jaundice* occurs in the first days of life in breastfed newborns. It appears to be associated with poor feeding practices and not with any abnormality in milk composition (Shrago, 2006). Prevention of early breastfeeding jaundice includes encouraging frequent (every 2 to 3 hours) breastfeeding, avoiding supplementation, and accessing maternal lactation counseling.

In *breast milk jaundice,* the bilirubin level begins to rise after the first week of life, when physiologic jaundice is waning after the mother's milk has come in. The level peaks at 5 to 10 mg/dL at 2 to 3 weeks of age and declines over the first several months of life (Maisels, 2005).

In contrast to breastfeeding jaundice, breast milk jaundice is related to milk composition. Some women's breast milk contains several times the normal concentration of certain free fatty acids. These free fatty acids may compete with bilirubin for binding sites on albumin and inhibit the conjugation of bilirubin or increase lipase activity, which disrupts the RBC membrane. Increased lipase activity enhances absorption of bile across the gastrointestinal tract membrane, thereby increasing the enterohepatic circulation of bilirubin. In the past it was thought that the breast milk of women whose newborns have breast milk jaundice contained an enzyme that inhibited glucuronyl transferase, but this hypothesis has not been proven (Thureen et al., 2005).

Newborns with breastfeeding jaundice appear well, and at present development of kernicterus (toxic levels of bilirubin in the brain) has not been documented. Temporary cessation of breastfeeding may be advised if bilirubin reaches presumed toxic levels of approximately 20 mg/dL or if the interruption is necessary to establish the cause of the hyperbilirubinemia. Most physicians believe that breastfeeding may be resumed once other causes of jaundice have been ruled out and as long as serum bilirubin levels remain below 20 mg/dL. In cases of breast milk jaundice, within 24 to 36 hours after breastfeeding is discontinued, the newborn's serum bilirubin lev-

Developing Cultural Competence

INTERPRETING ILLNESS THROUGH CULTURAL BELIEFS

Cultural beliefs lead mothers to interpret illness within their cultural framework, especially when left without clear and understood explanations (Hannon, Willis, & Scrimshaw, 2001). For example, some Latina women believe that showing strong maternal emotions during pregnancy and during breastfeeding can be detrimental. They blame jaundice in their newborn on "bili" associated with anger. Such maternal reactions can be lessened by careful explanations to the mothers about the diagnosis, prognosis, duration, and management options for jaundice, and possibility for recurrence.

Nursing Practice

Encourage and support mothers who desire to breastfeed their infants. Assist and instruct them on how to pump and express milk during the interrupted breastfeeding period. Reassure them that nothing is wrong with their milk or mothering abilities.

Table 24–3 Factors in Physiologic, Breast Milk, and Breastfeeding Jaundice

Physiologic Jaundice
Physiologic jaundice occurs after the first 24 hours of life. During the first week of life, bilirubin should not exceed 13 mg/dL. Some pediatricians allow levels up to 15 mg/dL. Bilirubin levels peak at 3 to 5 days in term infants.
Breast Milk Jaundice
Bilirubin levels begin to rise after the first week of life when mature breast milk comes in. Peak of 5 to 10 mg/dL is reached at 2 to 3 weeks of age. It may be necessary to interrupt breastfeeding for a short period when bilirubin reaches 20 mg/dL.
Breastfeeding Jaundice
Bilirubin levels rise after the first 24 hours of age. Peaks on third or fourth day of life and declines through first month to normal levels. Incidence can be decreased by increasing the number of breastfeeding episodes to 8 to 12 in 24 hours.

els begin to fall dramatically. With resumption of breastfeeding, the bilirubin concentration may have a slight rise of 2 to 3 mg/dL, with a subsequent decline (Table 24–3).

COAGULATION

The liver plays an important part in blood coagulation during fetal life and continues this function following birth. Coagulation factors II, VII, IX, and X (synthesized in the liver) are activated under the influence of vitamin K and therefore are considered vitamin K dependent. The absence of normal flora needed to synthesize vitamin K in the newborn gut results in low levels of vitamin K and creates a transient blood coagulation alteration between the second and fifth day of life. From a low point at about 2 to 3 days after birth, these coagulation factors rise slowly, but they do not approach adult levels until 9 months of age or later (Luchtman-Jones, Schwartz, & Wilson, 2006). Other coagulation factors with low umbilical cord blood levels are XI, XII, and XIII. Fibrinogen and factors V and VII are near adult.

Although newborn bleeding problems are rare, an injection of vitamin K (AquaMEPHYTON) is given prophylactically on the day of birth to combat potential clinical bleeding problems. (Chapter 26∞ discusses administration of vitamin K to newborns and Chapter 29∞ discusses hemorrhagic disease of the newborn in greater depth.)

Platelet counts at birth are in the same range as for older children, but newborns may manifest mild transient difficulty in platelet aggregation functioning. This platelet problem is accentuated by phototherapy. Prenatal maternal therapy with phenytoin sodium (Dilantin) or phenobarbital also causes abnormal clotting studies and newborn bleeding in the first 24 hours after birth. Infants born to mothers receiving warfarin (Coumadin) compounds may bleed, because these agents cross the placenta and accentuate existing vitamin K-dependent factor deficiencies. Transient neonatal thrombocytopenia may occur in infants born to mothers with severe hypertension or HELLP syndrome (hemolysis, elevated liver enzymes, and low platelet count) and in infants born to mothers who have idiopathic isoimmune thrombocytopenic purpura.

GASTROINTESTINAL ADAPTATIONS

By 36 to 38 weeks' gestation, the gastrointestinal system is adequately mature, with enzymatic activity and the ability to transport nutrients.

DIGESTION AND ABSORPTION

The full-term newborn has sufficient intestinal and pancreatic enzymes to digest most simple carbohydrates, proteins, and fats. The carbohydrates requiring digestion in the newborn are usually disaccharides (lactose, maltose, sucrose), which are split into monosaccharides (galactose, fructose, and glucose) by the enzymes of the intestinal mucosa. Lactose is the primary carbohydrate in the breastfeeding newborn and is generally easily digested and well absorbed. The only enzyme lacking is pancreatic amylase, which remains relatively deficient during the first few months of life. Newborns have trouble digesting starches (changing more complex carbohydrates into maltose) so they should not eat until after the first few months of life.

Although proteins require more digestion than carbohydrates, they are well digested and absorbed from the newborn intestine. The newborn digests and absorbs fats less efficiently because of the minimal activity of the pancreatic enzyme lipase. The newborn excretes about 10% to 20% of the dietary fat intake, compared with 10% for the adult. The newborn absorbs the fat in breast milk more completely than the fat in cows' milk, because breast milk consists of more medium-chain triglycerides and contains lipase. (See Chapter 27∞ for further discussion of newborn nutrition.)

By birth, the newborn has experienced swallowing, gastric emptying, and intestinal propulsion. In utero, fetal swallowing is accompanied by gastric emptying and peristalsis of the fetal intestinal tract. By the end of gestation, peristalsis becomes much more active in preparation for extrauterine life. Fetal peristalsis is also stimulated by anoxia, causing the expulsion of meconium into the amniotic fluid in more mature fetuses.

Air enters the stomach immediately after birth. The small intestine is filled with air within 2 to 12 hours and the large bowel within 24 hours. The salivary glands are immature at birth, and the newborn produces little saliva until about 3 months of age. The newborn's stomach can hold 50 to 60 mL. It empties intermittently, starting within a few minutes of the beginning of a feeding and ending 2 to 4 hours after feeding. Bowel sounds are present within the first 30 to 60 minutes of birth and the newborn can successfully feed during this time. The newborn's gastric pH becomes less acidic about a week after birth and remains less acidic than that of adults for the next 2 to 3 months.

The cardiac sphincter is immature, as is neural control of the stomach, so some regurgitation may be noted in the newborn period. Regurgitation of the first few feedings during the first day or two of life can usually be lessened by avoiding overfeeding and by burping the newborn well during and after the feeding.

When no other signs and symptoms are evident, vomiting is limited and ceases within the first few days of life. Continuous vomiting or regurgitation should be observed closely. If the newborn has swallowed bloody or purulent amniotic fluid, lavage of the stomach may be indicated in the term newborn to relieve the problem. Bilious vomiting is abnormal and must be evaluated thoroughly because it might represent a condition that warrants prompt surgical intervention.

Adequate digestion and absorption are essential for newborn growth and development. If optimal nutritional support is available, postnatal growth should parallel intrauterine growth; that is, after 30 weeks' gestation, the fetus gains 30 g per day and adds 1.2 cm (0.5 in.) to body length daily. To gain weight at the intrauterine rate, the term newborn requires 120 cal/kg/day. After birth, caloric intake is often insufficient for weight gain until the newborn is 5 to 10 days old. During this time, there may be a weight loss of 5% to 10% in term newborns. A shift of intracellular water to extracellular space and insensible water loss accounts for the 5% to 10% weight loss; thus failure to lose weight when caloric intake is inadequate may indicate fluid retention.

ELIMINATION

Term newborns usually pass meconium within 8 to 24 hours of life and almost always within 48 hours. **Meconium** is formed in utero from the amniotic fluid and its constituents, intestinal secretions, and shed mucosal cells. It is recognized by its thick, tarry black, or dark green appearance. Transitional (thin brown to green) stools consisting of part meconium and part fecal material are passed for the next day or two, and then the stools become entirely fecal. Generally the stools of a breastfed newborn are pale yellow (but may be pasty green); they are more liquid and more frequent than those of formula-fed newborns, whose stools are paler (Figure 24–9 ●). Frequency of bowel movement varies but ranges from one every 2 to 3 days to as many as 10 daily. Totally breastfed infants often progress to stools that occur every 5 to 7 days. Mothers should be counseled that the newborn is not constipated as long as the bowel movement remains soft (Table 24–4).

Table 24–4 Physiologic Adaptations to Extrauterine Life

Periodic breathing may be present.
Desired skin temperature 36°C to 36.5°C (96.8°F to 97.7°F) stabilizes 4 to 6 hours after birth.
Desired blood glucose level reaches 60 to 70 mg/dL by third postnatal day.
Stools (progress from): Meconium (thick, tarry, black) Transitional stools (thin, brown to green) Breastfed infants (yellow-gold, soft, or mushy) Formula-fed infants (pale yellow, formed, and pasty)

URINARY TRACT ADAPTATIONS

KIDNEY DEVELOPMENT AND FUNCTION

Certain physiologic features of the newborn's kidneys influence the newborn's ability to handle body fluids and excrete urine.

1. The term newborn's kidneys have a full complement of functioning nephrons by 34 to 36 weeks' gestation.
2. The glomerular filtration rate of the newborn's kidney is low compared with the adult rate. Because of this physiologic decrease in kidney glomerular filtration, the newborn's kidney is unable to dispose of water rapidly when necessary.
3. The juxtamedullary portion of the nephron has limited capacity to reabsorb HCO_3^+ and H^+ and concentrate urine (reabsorb water back into the blood). The limitation of tubular reabsorption can lead to inappropriate loss of substances present in the glomerular filtrate, such as amino acids, bicarbonate, glucose, and sodium.

Full-term newborns are less able than adults to concentrate urine because the tubules are short and narrow. Also the reduced

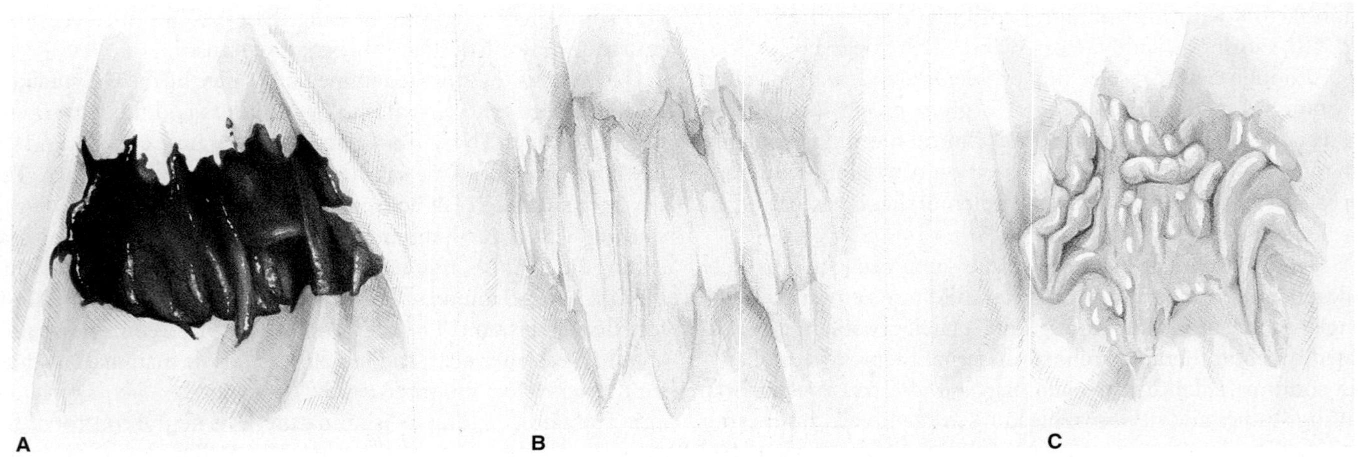

● **Figure 24–9** Newborn stool samples. ***A,*** Meconium stool. ***B,*** Breast milk stool. ***C,*** Cow's milk stool.

ability to concentrate urine is caused by the limited tubular reabsorption of water and limited excretion of solutes (principally sodium, potassium, chloride, bicarbonate, urea, and phosphate) in the growing newborn. The ability to concentrate urine fully is attained by 3 months of age. Feeding practices may affect the osmolarity of the urine but have limited effect on concentration of the urine.

Because the newborn has difficulty concentrating urine, the effect of excessive insensible water loss or restricted fluid intake is unpredictable. The newborn kidney is also limited in its dilutional capabilities. The concentrating and dilutional abilities of the kidneys are an important consideration in monitoring fluid therapy to prevent dehydration or overhydration.

CHARACTERISTICS OF NEWBORN URINARY FUNCTION

Many newborns void immediately after birth, and the voiding frequently goes unnoticed. Among normal newborns, 93% void by 24 hours after birth and 99% void by 48 hours after birth (Knuppel, 2007). A newborn who has not voided by 48 hours should be assessed for adequacy of fluid intake, bladder distention, restlessness, and symptoms of pain. The appropriate clinical personnel should be notified if indicated.

The initial bladder volume is 6 to 44 mL of urine. Unless edema is present, normal urinary output is often limited, and the voidings are scanty until fluid intake increases. (The fluid of edema is eliminated by the kidneys, so infants with edema have a much higher urinary output.) The first 2 days postnatally, the newborn voids two to six times daily, with a urine output of 15 mL/kg/day. The newborn subsequently voids 5 to 25 times every 24 hours, with a volume of 25 mL/kg/day.

Following the first voiding, the newborn's urine frequently appears cloudy (because of mucus content) and has a high specific gravity, which decreases as fluid intake increases. Occasionally pink stains ("brick dust spots") appear on the diaper. These are caused by urates and are innocuous. Blood may occasionally be observed on the diapers of female newborns. This *pseudomenstruation* is related to the withdrawal of maternal hormones. Males may have bloody spotting from a circumcision if performed. In the absence of apparent causes for bleeding, the clinician should be notified. During early infancy, normal urine is straw colored and almost odorless, although odor occurs when certain drugs are given, metabolic disorders exist, or infection is present. Table 24–5 contains urinalysis values for the normal newborn.

Table 24–5	Newborn Urinalysis Values
Protein less than 5 to 10 mg/dL	
WBC less than 2 to 3/hpf	
RBC 0	
Casts 0	
Bacteria 0	
Color pale yellow	

IMMUNOLOGIC ADAPTATIONS

The newborn's immune system is not fully activated until sometime after birth. Limitations in the newborn's inflammatory response result in failure to recognize, localize, and destroy invasive bacteria. Thus the signs and symptoms of infection are often subtle and nonspecific in the newborn. The newborn also has a poor hypothalamic response to pyrogens; therefore fever is not a reliable indicator of infection. In the neonatal period, hypothermia is a more reliable sign of infection.

Of the three major types of immunoglobulins that are primarily involved in immunity—IgG, IgA, and IgM—only IgG crosses the placenta. The pregnant woman forms antibodies in response to illness or immunization. This process is called **active acquired immunity**. When IgG antibodies are transferred to the fetus in utero, **passive acquired immunity** results, because the fetus does not produce the antibodies itself. IgG antibodies are very active against bacterial toxins.

Because the maternal IgG is transferred primarily during the third trimester, preterm newborns (especially those born before 34 weeks' gestation) may be more susceptible to infection. In general, newborns have immunity to tetanus, diphtheria, smallpox, measles, mumps, poliomyelitis, and a variety of other bacterial and viral diseases. The period of resistance varies: Immunity against common viral infections such as measles may last 4 to 8 months, whereas immunity to certain bacteria may disappear within 4 to 8 weeks.

The normal newborn can produce a protective immune response to vaccines, such as hepatitis B immunoglobulin vaccine, given as early as a few hours after birth. It is customary to begin most routine immunizations at 2 months of age so that the infant can develop active acquired immunity. For discussion of newborn immunization see Chapter 26∞.

IgM antibodies are produced in response to blood group antigens, gram-negative enteric organisms, and some viruses in the expectant mother. Because IgM does not normally cross the placenta, most or all of it is produced by the fetus beginning at 10 to 15 weeks' gestation. Elevated levels of IgM at birth may indicate placental leaks or, more commonly, antigenic stimulation in utero. Consequently elevations suggest that the newborn was exposed to an intrauterine infection such as syphilis or TORCH syndrome (toxoplasmosis, rubella, cytomegalovirus, herpesvirus hominis type 2 infection). (For further discussion, see Chapter 16∞.) The lack of available maternal IgM in the newborn also accounts for the susceptibility to gram-negative enteric organisms such as *Escherichia coli*.

The functions of IgA immunoglobulins are not fully understood. IgA appears to provide protection mainly on secreting surfaces such as the respiratory tract, gastrointestinal tract, and eyes. Serum IgA does not cross the placenta and is not normally produced by the fetus in utero. Unlike the other immunoglobulins, IgA is not affected by gastric action. Colostrum, the forerunner of breast milk, is very high in the secretory form of IgA. Consequently it may be of significance in providing some passive immunity to the infant of a breastfeeding mother. Newborns begin to produce secretory IgA in their intestinal mucosa about 4 weeks after birth.

NEUROLOGIC AND SENSORY-PERCEPTUAL FUNCTIONING

The newborn's brain is about one-quarter the size of an adult's, and myelination of nerve fibers is incomplete. Unlike the cardiovascular and respiratory systems, which undergo tremendous changes at birth, the nervous system is minimally influenced by the actual birth process.

Because many biochemical and histologic changes have yet to occur in the newborn's brain, the postnatal period is considered a time of risk with regard to the development of the brain and nervous system. For neurologic development—including development of intellect—to proceed, the brain and other nervous system structures must mature in an orderly, unhampered fashion. (For discussion of cranial nerves, see Chapter 25∞.)

INTRAUTERINE ENVIRONMENT INFLUENCE ON NEWBORN BEHAVIOR

Newborns respond to and interact with the environment in a predictable pattern of behavior that is somewhat shaped by their intrauterine experience. This intrauterine experience is affected by intrinsic factors such as maternal nutrition and external factors such as the mother's physical environment. Depending on the newborn's intrauterine experience and individual temperament, neonatal behavioral responses to different stresses vary. Some newborns react quietly to stimulation, others become overreactive and tense, and some may exhibit a combination of the two.

Factors such as exposure to intense auditory stimuli in utero can eventually be manifested in the behavior of the newborn. For example, the fetal heart rate (FHR) initially increases when the pregnant woman is exposed to auditory stimuli, but repetition of the stimuli leads to decreased FHR. Thus the newborn who was exposed to intense noise during fetal life is significantly less reactive to loud sounds postnatally.

CHARACTERISTICS OF NEWBORN NEUROLOGIC FUNCTION

Normal newborns are usually in a position of partially flexed extremities with the legs near the abdomen. When awake, the newborn may exhibit purposeless, uncoordinated bilateral movements of the extremities. The organization and quality of the newborn's motor activity are influenced by a number of factors, including the following (Brazelton, 1984):

- Sleep-alert states
- Presence of environmental stimuli, such as heat, light, cold, and noise
- Conditions causing a chemical imbalance, such as hypoglycemia
- Hydration status
- State of health
- Recovery from the stress of labor and birth

Eye movements are observable during the first few days of life. An alert newborn is able to fixate on faces and geometric objects or patterns such as black-and-white stripes. A bright light shining in the newborn's eyes elicits the blinking reflex.

The cry of the newborn should be lusty and vigorous. High-pitched cries, weak cries, and no cries are causes for concern.

The newborn's body growth progresses in a cephalocaudal (head-to-toe), proximal-distal fashion. The newborn is somewhat hypertonic; that is, there is resistance to extending the elbow and knee joints. Muscle tone should be symmetrical. Diminished muscle tone and flaccidity may indicate neurologic dysfunction.

Specific symmetrical deep tendon reflexes can be elicited in the newborn. The knee-jerk reflex is brisk; a normal ankle clonus may involve three to four beats. Plantar flexion is present. Other reflexes, including the Moro, grasping, Babinski, rooting, and sucking reflexes, are characteristic of neurologic integrity. (For discussion of reflexes see Chapter 25∞.)

PERIODS OF REACTIVITY

The newborn usually shows a predictable pattern of behavior during the first several hours after birth, characterized by two **periods of reactivity** separated by a sleep phase.

First Period of Reactivity

The first period of reactivity lasts approximately 30 minutes after birth. During this period the newborn is awake and active and may appear hungry and have a strong sucking reflex. This is a natural opportunity to initiate breastfeeding if the mother has chosen it. Bursts of random, diffuse movements alternating with relative immobility may occur. Respirations are rapid, as high as 80 breaths per minute, and there may be retraction of the chest, transient flaring of the nares, and grunting. The heart rate is rapid, and the rhythm may be irregular. Bowel sounds are usually absent.

Period of Inactivity to Sleep Phase

After approximately half an hour the newborn's activity gradually diminishes, and the heart rate and respirations decrease as the newborn enters the sleep phase. The sleep phase may last from a few minutes to 2 to 4 hours. During this period, the newborn will be difficult to awaken and will show no interest in sucking. Bowel sounds become audible, and cardiac and respiratory rates return to baseline values.

Second Period of Reactivity

During the second period of reactivity, the newborn is again awake and alert. This period lasts 4 to 6 hours in the normal newborn. Physiologic responses are variable during this stage. The heart and respiratory rates increase; however, the nurse must be alert for apneic periods, which may cause a drop in the heart rate. The newborn is stimulated to continue breathing during such times. The newborn may develop rapid color changes and become mildly cyanotic or mottled during these fluctuations. Production of respiratory and gastric mucus increases, and the newborn responds by gagging, choking, and regurgitating.

Continued close observation and intervention may be required to maintain a clear airway during this period of reactivity. The gastrointestinal tract becomes more active. The newborn often passes the first meconium stool and may also have an initial voiding. The newborn will indicate readiness for feeding by such behaviors as sucking, rooting, and swallowing. If feeding was not initiated in the first period of reactivity, it is done at this time. (See Chapter 27∞ for further discussion of this first feeding.)

BEHAVIORAL STATES OF THE NEWBORN

The behavior of the newborn can be divided into two categories, the sleep state and the alert state (Brazelton, 1999). These postnatal behavioral states are similar to those that have been identified during pregnancy. Subcategories are identified under each major category.

Sleep States

The sleep states are as follows:

1. **Deep** or *quiet* **sleep**. Deep sleep is characterized by closed eyes with no eye movements; regular, even breathing; and jerky motions or startles at regular intervals. Behavioral responses to external stimuli are likely to be delayed. Startles are rapidly suppressed, and changes in state are not likely to occur. Heart rate may range from 100 to 120 beats per minute.
2. **Light sleep** (active rapid eye movement [REM]). The baby has irregular respirations; eyes closed, with REM; irregular sucking motions; minimal activity; and irregular but smooth movement of the extremities. Environmental and internal stimuli may initiate a startle reaction and a change of state.

Newborn sleep cycles have been recognized and defined according to duration. The length of the sleep cycle depends on the age of the newborn. At term, REM active sleep and quiet sleep occur in intervals of 50 to 60 minutes (Gardner & Goldson, 2006). About 45% to 50% of the newborn's total sleep is active sleep, 35% to 45% is quiet sleep, and 10% is transitional between these two periods. Growth hormone secretion depends on regular sleep patterns. Any disturbance of the sleep-wake cycle can result in irregular spikes of growth hormone. REM sleep stimulates the highest peaks of growth hormone and the growth of the neural system. Over time, the newborn's sleep-wake patterns become diurnal; that is, the newborn sleeps at night and stays awake during the day. (See "Newborn Behavioral Assessment" in Chapter 25∞ for a short discussion of Brazelton's assessment of newborn states.)

Alert States

In the first 30 to 60 minutes after birth, many newborns display a quiet alert state, characteristic of the first period of reactivity (Figure 24–10 ●). Nurses should use these alert states to encourage bonding and breastfeeding. These periods of alertness tend to be short the first 2 days after birth to allow the baby to recover from the birth process. Subsequent alert states are of choice or of necessity (Brazelton, 1999). Increasing choice of wakefulness by the newborn indicates a maturing capacity to achieve and maintain consciousness. Heat, cold, and hunger are but a few of the stimuli that can cause wakefulness by necessity. Once the disturbing stimuli are removed, the newborn tends to fall back asleep.

The following are subcategories of the alert state (Brazelton, 1999).

1. **Drowsy** or *semidozing*. The behaviors common to the drowsy state are open or closed eyes; fluttering eyelids; semidozing appearance; and slow, regular movements of the extremities. Mild startles may be noted from time to time. Although the reaction to a sensory stimulus is delayed, a change of state often results.

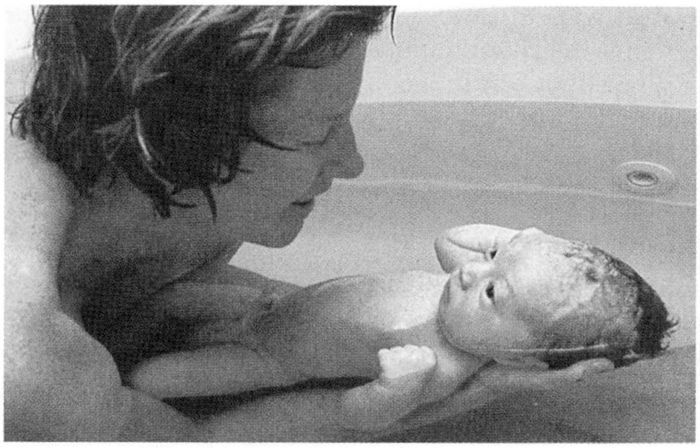

● **Figure 24–10** Mother and newborn gaze at each other. This quiet, alert state is the optimum state for interaction between baby and parents.

2. **Quiet alert** or *wide awake*. In the wide-awake state, the newborn is alert and follows and fixates on attractive objects, faces, or auditory stimuli. Motor activity is minimal, and the response to external stimuli is delayed.
3. **Active alert**. In the active alert awake state the newborn's eyes are open and motor activity is quite intense, with thrusting movements of the extremities. Environmental stimuli increase startles or motor activity, but individual reactions are difficult to distinguish because of the generally high activity level.
4. *Crying*. Intense crying is accompanied by jerky motor movements. Crying serves several purposes for the newborn. It may be a distraction from disturbing stimuli such as hunger and pain. Fussiness often allows the newborn to discharge energy and reorganize behavior. Most important, crying elicits an appropriate response of help from the parents.

BEHAVIORAL AND SENSORY CAPACITIES OF THE NEWBORN

Performance of complex behavioral patterns reflects the newborn's neurologic maturation and integration. The newborn has several behavioral capacities that assist in adaptation to extrauterine life. Newborns who can bring a hand to their mouth may be demonstrating motor coordination as well as a self-quieting technique, thus increasing the complexity of the behavioral response. For example, **self-quieting ability** is the ability of newborns to use their own resources to quiet and comfort themselves. Their repertoire includes hand-to-mouth movements, sucking on a fist or tongue, and attending to external stimuli. Neurologically impaired newborns are unable to use self-quieting activities and require more frequent comforting from caregivers when stimulated. For example, drug-positive newborns often exhibit abnormal sleep and feeding patterns and irritability.

Habituation is the newborn's ability to process and respond to complex stimulation. For example, when a bright light is flashed into the newborn's eyes, the initial response is blinking, constriction of the pupil, and perhaps a slight startle reaction.

However, with repeated stimulation, the newborn's response repertoire gradually diminishes and disappears. The capacity to ignore repetitious disturbing stimuli is a newborn defense mechanism readily apparent in the noisy, well-lit nursery.

Sensory abilities include visual, auditory, olfactory, taste, and tactile capacities.

Visual Capacity

Orientation is the newborn's ability to be alert to, to follow, and to fixate on appealing and attractive complex visual stimuli. The newborn prefers the human face and eyes and bright shiny objects. As the face or object comes into the line of vision, the newborn responds with bright, wide eyes, still limbs, and fixed staring. This intense visual involvement may last several minutes, during which time the newborn is able to follow the stimulus from side to side. Figure 24–11 ● illustrates this response. The newborn uses this sensory capacity to become familiar with family, friends, and surroundings.

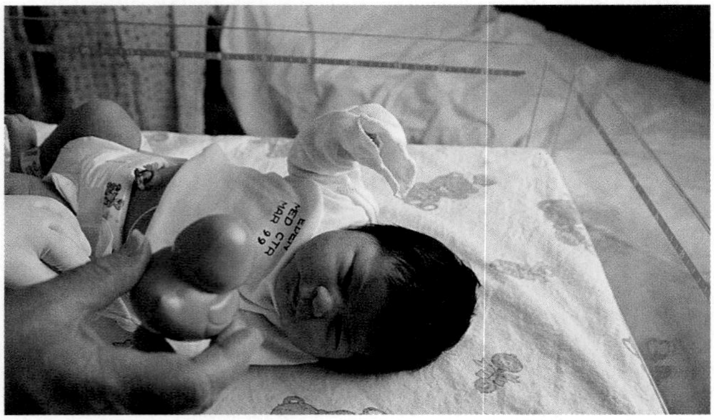

● **Figure 24–11** Head turning to follow movement.

Auditory Capacity

The newborn responds to auditory stimulation with a definite, organized behavior repertoire. The stimulus used to assess auditory response should be selected to match the state of the newborn. A rattle is appropriate for light sleep, a voice for an awake state, and a clap for deep sleep. As the newborn hears the sound, the cardiac rate rises, and a minimal startle reflex may be seen. If the sound is appealing, the newborn will become alert and search for the site of the auditory stimulus. Lack of auditory development is associated with an increased risk of SIDS.

Olfactory Capacity

Newborns can select their mother by smell and are apparently able to select people by smell (Klaus, Kennell, & De Pompei, 2006). Newborns are able to distinguish their mothers' breast pads from those of other mothers at just 1 week postnatally.

Taste and Sucking

The newborn responds differently to varying tastes. Sugar, for example, increases sucking. Newborns fed with a rubber nipple versus the breast also show sucking pattern variations. While breastfeeding, the newborn sucks in bursts, with frequent regular pauses. The bottle-fed newborn tends to suck at a regular rate, with infrequent pauses.

When awake and hungry, the newborn displays rapid searching motions in response to the rooting reflex. Once feeding begins, the newborn establishes a sucking pattern according to the method of feeding. Finger sucking is seen in utero as well as after birth. The newborn frequently uses nonnutritive sucking as a self-quieting activity, which assists in the development of

Evidence-Based Nursing

NEWBORN NURSERY NOISE LEVELS

Clinical Question

What is an acceptable noise level in the newborn nursery?

The Evidence

Neonates respond to sound in a variety of ways, including changes in heart and respiratory rates, oxygenation, and intracranial pressure. These changes are not dependent upon chronic exposure; neonatal reactions have been documented in response to periodic bursts of sound as well as to continuous ambient noise. The newborn residing in a nursery may experience many fluctuations in sound on a daily basis, at a time when rapid brain growth is occurring. The deleterious effects may be even greater for preterm neonates, whose auditory systems have not had the benefit of uterine dampening of sound during the critical final weeks of gestation. Criteria for acceptable noise levels were developed by a group of experts in audiology, acoustical engineering, nursing, and neonatology. The recommendations were based on multiple research studies focused on the effects of the sound environment on auditory health. This combination of literature aggregation and expert panel review provides the strongest level of evidence for practice.

Best Practice

The sound level in a newborn nursery should exceed 55 decibels only 10% of the time, or 6 minutes in an hour. Sounds greater than 55 decibels interfere with the ability to hear normal speech at a distance of 12 feet. Sounds less than 55 decibels enable caregivers at nearby bedspaces to speak at normal conversation levels and be clearly understood 12 feet away more than 90% of the time. Louder sounds, even if only periodic, should be avoided whenever possible.

Critical Thinking

Should these sound levels vary by time of day to support sleep-wake cycles? How can we protect newborns from periodic sounds greater than 55 decibels, which are likely inevitable in a busy newborn nursery?

See MyNursingKit for possible responses.

self-regulation. For bottle-fed infants, there is no reason to discourage nonnutritive sucking with a pacifier. Pacifiers should be offered to breastfed infants only after breastfeeding is well established. If the pacifier is offered too soon, a phenomenon called "nipple confusion" may occur in which the breastfed infant has difficulty learning to suck from the breast and will nurse less (see "Supplementary Bottle Feeding" in Chapter 27).

Tactile Capacity

The newborn is very sensitive to being touched, cuddled, and held. Often a mother's first response to an upset or crying newborn is touching or holding. Swaddling, placing a hand on the abdomen, or holding the arms to prevent a startle reflex are other methods of soothing the newborn. The quieted newborn is then able to attend to and interact with the environment.

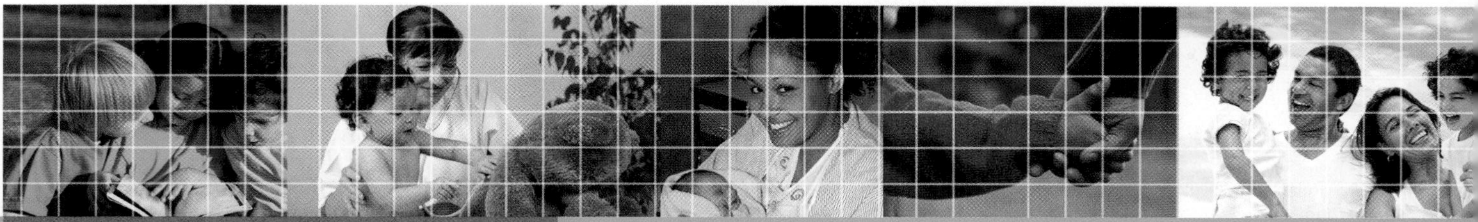

CRITICAL CONCEPT REVIEW

LEARNING OUTCOMES	CONCEPTS
24.1 Explain the respiratory and cardiovascular changes that occur during the newborn's transition to extrauterine life and during stabilization in determining the nursing care of the newborn.	1. Newborn respiration is initiated primarily by chemical, mechanical, and reabsorptive processes associated with thermal and sensory stimulation. 2. Onset of respirations stimulates cardiovascular changes: ■ Air enters the lungs, oxygen content rises in alveoli and stimulates relaxation of pulmonary arteries ■ This leads to a decrease in pulmonary vascular resistance, which allows complete vascular flow to lungs ■ With increased oxygenated pulmonary blood flow and loss of the placenta, systemic flood flow increases and the foramen ovale and ductus arteriosus begin to close.
24.2 Compare the factors that modify the newborn's blood values to the corresponding results.	1. Newborn blood values are affected by: ■ Site of the blood sample: venous versus capillary ■ Gestational age ■ Prenatal and/or perinatal hemorrhage ■ Timing of the clamping of the umbilical cord
24.3 Relate the process of thermogenesis in the newborn and the major mechanisms of heat loss to the challenge of maintaining newborn thermal stability.	1. Thermogenesis is achieved by: ■ Increased basal metabolic rate ■ Muscular activity ■ Nonshivering thermogenesis ■ Metabolizing of brown adipose fat 2. Heat loss is created by: ■ Evaporation (infant is wet from amniotic fluid and/or bath) ■ Convection ■ Radiation ■ Conduction
24.4 Explain the steps involved in the conjugation and excretion of bilirubin in the newborn.	1. Unconjugated bilirubin is a by-product of the destruction of red blood cells. 2. Bilirubin is bound to albumin. It is transferred into liver cells and bound to intracellular proteins. These proteins determine the amount of bilirubin uptake into the liver. 3. UDGPT causes unconjugated bilirubin to attach to glucuronic acid, producing conjugated bilirubin. This is excreted into bile ducts, then into common duct, and into duodenum. 4. In the intestines, bacteria transforms the conjugated bilirubin into urobilinogen (urine bilirubin) and stercobilinogen, and is excreted as a pigment in the stools.

(continued)

LEARNING OUTCOMES	CONCEPTS
24.5 Identify the reasons a newborn may develop jaundice and nursing interventions to decrease the probability of jaundice.	1. Newborn may develop jaundice because of: ■ Accelerated destruction of fetal RBCs ■ Impaired conjugation of bilirubin ■ Increased bilirubin reabsorption from the intestinal tract 2. Early nursing interventions to decrease jaundice are: ■ Maintain newborn's skin temperature ■ Monitor stool for amount and characteristics for excretion of meconium ■ Encourage early feedings to promote intestinal elimination
24.6 Delineate the functional abilities of the newborn's gastrointestinal tract and liver.	1. At birth the newborn is able to digest most simple carbohydrates, proteins, and fats. They have trouble digesting starches. 2. The newborn usually passes meconium within 24–48 hours after birth and begins to have normal bowel movements. 3. The newborn liver is slightly less active than the adult liver, which is indicative in the liver's decreased ability to conjugate all of the bilirubin produced by the destruction of fetal RBCs. 4. The liver plays a crucial role in iron storage, carbohydrate metabolism, and coagulation.
24.7 Relate the development of the newborn's kidneys to the newborn's ability to maintain fluid and electrolyte balance.	1. The following characteristics of a newborn's kidneys cause difficulty in maintaining fluid and electrolyte balance: ■ Decreased rate of glomerular flow and limited excretion of solutes ■ Limited tubular reabsorptions ■ Limited ability to concentrate urine 2. Most newborns void within 48 hours of birth.
24.8 Describe the immunologic responses available to the newborn.	1. The newborn is unable to recognize, localize, and destroy invasive bacteria. 2. The newborn has passive acquired immunity from the mother, lasting from 4 weeks to 8 months. 3. The newborn begins to produce own immunity at about 4 weeks of age.

24.9 Explain the physiologic and behavioral responses of newborns during the periods of reactivity and identify possible interventions.	1. Periods of reactivity:
	■ First period of reactivity (lasts 30 minutes after birth):
	  ■ The newborn is awake and active, appears hungry, and has a strong suck.
	  ■ The nurse should help mother to initiate breastfeeding.
	  ■ Vital signs are elevated at this time.
	■ Period of inactivity to sleep (30 minutes to 4 hours after birth):
	  ■ The newborn is difficult to awaken.
	  ■ Vital signs return to normal.
	■ Second period of reactivity (lasts 4–6 hours after period of inactivity):
	  ■ The newborn is awake and alert.
	  ■ Vital signs are variable and the nurse must observe the newborn closely during this time for periods of apnea, gagging, and regurgitation.
	  ■ The newborn often passes meconium stool.
	  ■ The newborn shows a readiness to feed.
	2. Behavioral states:
	■ Sleep state:
	  ■ Deep or quiet sleep: closed eyes with no eye movement
	  ■ Light sleep (active rapid eye movements)
	■ Alert state:
	  ■ Subcategories include: drowsy or semidozing, quiet alert, active alert, and crying.
	  ■ The mother and nurse should use this time to facilitate feedings.

24.10 Describe the normal sensory-perceptual abilities and behavioral states seen in the newborn period and the associated nursing care.	1. The normal sensory-perceptual abilities of the newborn are:
	■ Visual:
	  ■ The newborn is able to be alert to, follow, and fixate on complex visual stimuli for short periods of time.
	■ Auditory:
	  ■ The newborn is able to be alert to and search for an appealing auditory stimulus.
	■ Olfactory:
	  ■ The newborn is able to select people by smell.
	■ Taste and sucking:
	  ■ The newborn is able to respond selectively to different tastes.
	■ Tactile:
	  ■ The newborn is very sensitive to being touched, cuddled, and held.
	  ■ The newborn is able to attend to and interact with the environment.
	2. Some of the behavioral capabilities of the newborn that assist in adaptation to extrauterine life include self-quieting ability and habituation.

CRITICAL THINKING IN ACTION

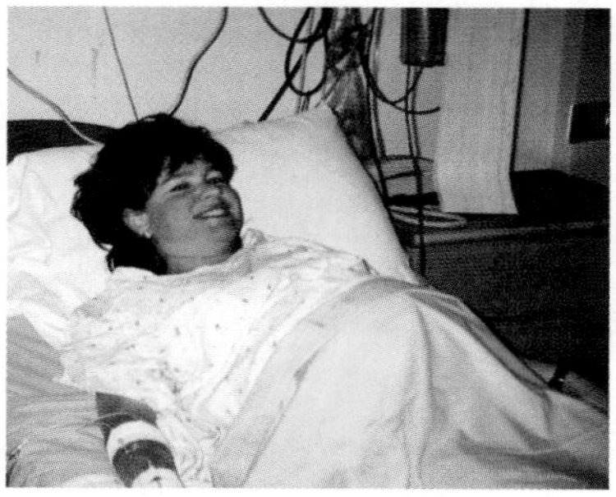

Sandra Dee, a 21-year-old, G1, P0000, at 36 weeks' gestation, has been in labor for the last 12 hours and is fully dilated with caput visible on the perineum. The fetal heart rate is 148 to 152 with early deceleration down to 142 with contraction and pushing. Her contractions are 4 to 5 minutes apart of good quality. Sandra's mother and sister are present for the birth. Her prenatal record shows no significant pregnancy problems or complications, and her vital signs have been stable within normal limits. Sandra has received two doses of Stadol for a total of 2 mg IV for pain relief during her labor. The last dose was given 2 hours ago. You assist with the vaginal birth of a live baby without an episiotomy. You observe the sex and time as the midwife places the infant girl on the mother's abdomen, suctions out the baby's mouth and nose, and proceeds to clamp the cord. You dry and stimulate the infant to breathe, remove the wet blanket and replace it with a dry one, and place the infant skin to skin on the mother's chest. You assess the need for infant resuscitation. The baby has a lusty cry spontaneously less than 30 seconds after birth. You palpate the cord, obtaining a heart rate of 120, and observe that the baby's chest and face are pink, and the legs and arms are flexed with open fist.

1. Explain the changes that must occur in the infant's cardiopulmonary system at birth.
2. What criteria do you look for when you assess the newborn for adequate cardiopulmonary adaptation at birth?
3. What steps do you take to maintain a neutral thermal environment at birth?
4. Sandra plans to breastfeed. When would you initiate the first feeding?
5. Discuss nursing actions that can decrease the probability of high bilirubin levels in the newborn.

See MyNursingKit for possible responses.

REFERENCES

Bagwell, G. A. (2007). Hematologic system. In C. Kenner & J. W. Lott, *Comprehensive neonatal care: An interdisciplinary approach* (4th ed., pp. 221–253). St. Louis: Saunders.

Blackburn, S. T. (2007). *Maternal, fetal, & neonatal physiology: A clinical perspective* (3rd ed.). St. Louis: Saunders.

Bloom, R. (2006). Delivery room resuscitation of the newborn: Part I Overview and initial management. In A. A. Fanaroff, R. J. Martin, & M. C. Walsh (Eds.), *Fanaroff and Martin's neonatal-perinatal medicine* (8th ed., pp. 483–491). St. Louis: Mosby.

Brazelton, T. B. (1984). *Neonatal behavioral assessment scale* (2nd ed.). London: Heineman.

Brazelton, T. B. (1999). Behavioral competence. In G. B. Avery, M. A. Fletcher, & M. G. MacDonald (Eds.), *Neonatology: Pathophysiology and management of the newborn* (5th ed., pp. 321–332). Philadelphia: Lippincott.

Cheffer, N. D. (2004). Adaptation to extrauterine life and immediate nursing care. In S. Mattson & J. E. Smith (Eds.), *Core curriculum for maternal-newborn nursing* (3rd ed., pp. 421–436). St. Louis: Saunders.

Creehan, P. A. (2008). Newborn physical assessment. In K. R. Simpson & P. A. Creehan, *Perinatal nursing* (3rd ed., pp. 546–574). Philadelphia: Lippincott Williams & Wilkins.

Gardner, S. L., & Goldson, E. (2006). The neonate and the environment: Impact on development. In G. B. Merenstein & S. L. Gardner (Eds.), *Handbook of neonatal intensive care* (6th ed., pp. 273–349). St. Louis: Mosby.

Hannon, P. R., Willis, S. K., & Scrimshaw, S. C. (2001). Persistence of maternal concerns surrounding neonatal jaundice: An exploratory study. *Archives of Pediatrics & Adolescent Medicine*, 155, 1357–1363.

Klaus, M. H., Kennell, J. H., & De Pompei, P. M. (2006). Care of the mother, father, and infant. In A. A. Fanaroff, R. J. Martin, & M. C. Walsh (Eds.), *Fanaroff and Martin's neonatal-perinatal medicine* (8th ed., pp. 645–659). St. Louis: Mosby.

Knuppel, R. A. (2007). Maternal-placental-fetal unit: Fetal & early neonatal physiology. In A. H. DeCherney, L. Nathan, T. M. Goodwin, & N. Laufer (Eds.), *Current obstetric & gynecologic diagnosis & treatment* (10th ed., pp. 159–186). New York: Lang Medical Books/McGraw-Hill.

Luchtman-Jones, L., Schwartz, A., & Wilson, D. (2006). Hematologic problems in the fetus and neonate. In R. Martin, A. Fanaroff, & M. Walsh (Eds.), *Fanaroff and Martin's neonatal-perinatal medicine* (8th ed., pp. 1287–1343). St. Louis: Mosby.

Maisels, M. J. (2005). Jaundice. In M. G. MacDonald, M. D. Mullett, & M. Seshia (Eds.), *Avery's neonatology: Pathophysiology & management of the newborn* (6th ed., pp. 768–846). Philadelphia: Lippincott Williams & Wilkins.

Mercer, J. S., Erickson-Owens, D. A., Graves, B., & Haley, M. (2007). Evidence-based practices for the fetal to newborn transition. *Journal of Midwifery and Women's Health, 52*(3), 262–272.

Philbin, M., Robertson, A., & Hall, J. (2008). Recommended permissible noise criteria for occupied, newly constructed, or renovated hospital nurseries. *Advances in Neonatal Care.* 8(5S): S11-S15.

Polin, R. A., Fox, W. W., & Abman, S. H. (2004). *Fetal and neonatal physiology* (3rd ed.). Philadelphia: Saunders.

Rosenberg, A. A. (2007). The neonate. In S. G. Gabbe, J. R. Niebyl, & J. L. Simpson (Eds.), *Obstetrics: Normal and problem pregnancies* (5th ed., pp. 523–565). Philadelphia: Churchill Livingstone/Elsevier.

Shrago, L. C., Reisnider, E., & Insel, E. (2006). The neonatal bowel output study: Indicators of adequate breast milk intake neonates. *Pediatric Nursing, 32*(3), 195–201.

Thureen, P. J., Deacon, J., Hernandez, J., & Hall, D. M. (2005). *Assessment and care of the well newborn* (2nd ed.). Philadelphia: Saunders.

EXPLORE PEARSON **mynursingkit™**

MyNursingKit is your one stop for online chapter review materials and resources. Prepare for success with additional NCLEX®-style practice questions, interactive assignments and activities, web links, animations and videos, and more!

Register your access code from the front of your book at **www.mynursingkit.com**

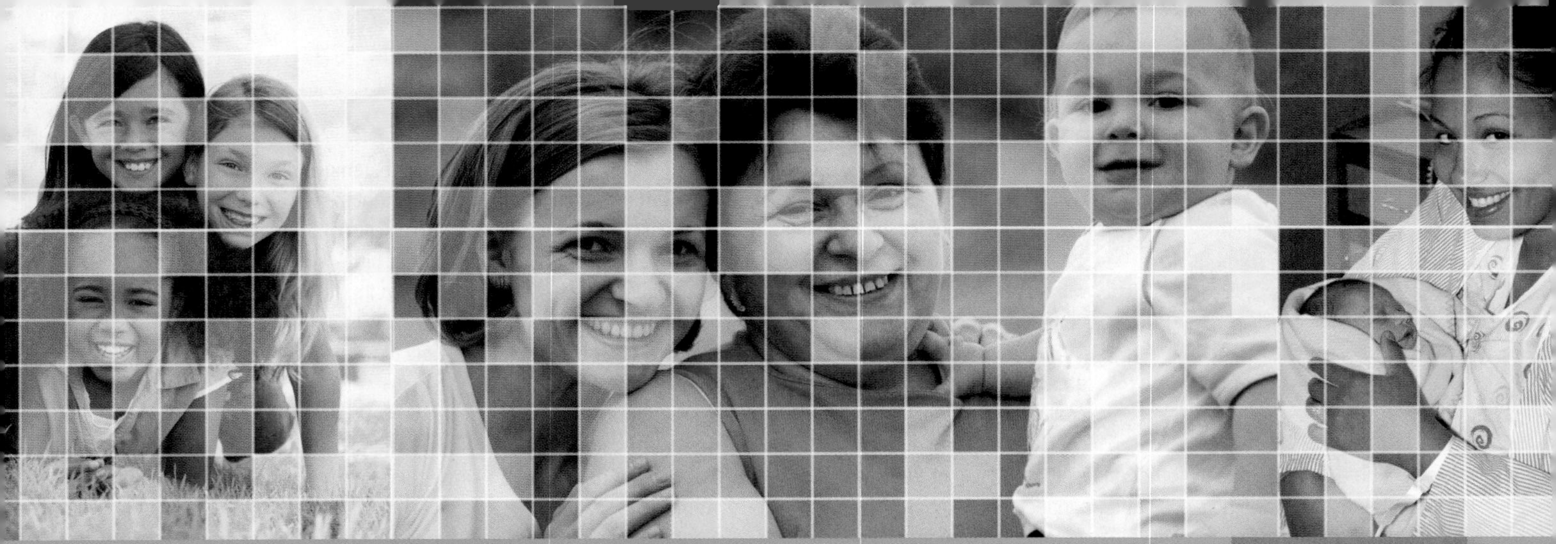

CHAPTER 25

Nursing Assessment of the Newborn

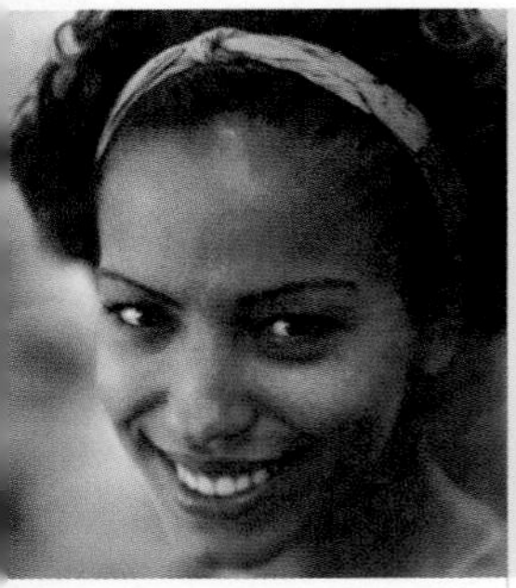

Like most parents, when I held my son for the first time, I checked that all his fingers and toes were present. Then he looked at me with wide, bright, serious eyes and began my introduction to his unique personality. —*Leah, 23*

LEARNING OUTCOMES

25.1 Describe the physical and neuromuscular maturity characteristics assessed to determine the gestational age of the newborn.

25.2 Identify the components of a systematic physical assessment of the newborn.

25.3 Describe the normal physical characteristics and normal variations of the newborn and compare abnormal findings to possible causes and nursing responses.

25.4 Describe the components of a neurologic assessment, and the neurologic and neuromuscular characteristics of the newborn and the reflexes that may be present at birth.

25.5 Describe the components of the newborn behavioral assessment and the normal behavioral characteristics and normal variations of the newborn.

25.6 Correlate findings in a newborn behavioral assessment to nursing responses and to teach and involve parents in the care of their newborn.

Newborns communicate their needs primarily by behavior. Because nurses are the most consistent professional observers of the newborn, they can translate this behavior into information about a newborn's condition and respond with appropriate nursing interventions. This chapter focuses on the assessment of the newborn and the interpretation of these findings.

Newborn assessment is a continuous process designed to evaluate development and adjustments to extrauterine life. In the birth setting, the Apgar scoring procedure (see Chapter 19 for discussion) and careful observation form the basis of assessment and are correlated with information such as the following:

- Maternal prenatal care and medical history
- Birthing history
- Maternal analgesia and anesthesia
- Complications of labor or birth
- Treatment instituted immediately after birth, in conjunction with determination of clinical gestational age
- Consideration of the classification of newborns by weight and gestational age and by neonatal mortality risk
- Physical examination of the newborn

The nurse incorporates data from these sources with the assessment findings during the first 1 to 4 hours after birth to formulate a plan for nursing intervention.

The various newborn assessments and the data obtained from them are valuable only to the degree to which they are shared with the parents. The parents must be included in the assessment process from the moment of their child's birth. The *Apgar score* and its meaning should be explained immediately to the family (see Chapter 19). As soon as possible, the parents should take part in the physical and behavioral assessments as well.

The nurse encourages the parents to identify the unique behavioral characteristics of their newborn and to learn nurturing activities. Attachment is promoted when parents have an opportunity to explore their newborn in private and identify individual physical and behavioral characteristics. The nurse's supportive responses to parents' questions and observations are essential throughout the assessment process. The newborn physical examination is the beginning of newborn health surveillance and health education for the newborn's family that continues into the community setting.

TIMING OF NEWBORN ASSESSMENTS

During the first 24 hours of life, the newborn makes the critical transition from intrauterine to extrauterine life. The risk of mortality and morbidity is statistically high during this period. Assessment of the newborn is essential to ensure that the transition proceeds successfully.

There are three major time frames for assessments of newborns while they are in the birth facility.

1. The first assessment is done in the birthing area immediately after birth to determine the need for resuscitation or other interventions. The stable newborn can stay with the family after birth to initiate early attachment. The newborn with complications is usually taken to the nursery for further evaluation and intervention.
2. A second assessment is done as part of routine admission procedures. During this assessment, the nurse carries out a brief physical examination to estimate gestational age and evaluate the newborn's adaptation to extrauterine life. No later than 2 hours after birth, the admitting nurse should evaluate the newborn's status and any problems that place the newborn at risk (American Academy of Pediatrics [AAP] & American College of Obstetricians and Gynecologists [ACOG], 2007).
3. Before discharge, a certified nurse-midwife, physician, or nurse practitioner will carry out a behavioral state organizational assessment and a complete physical

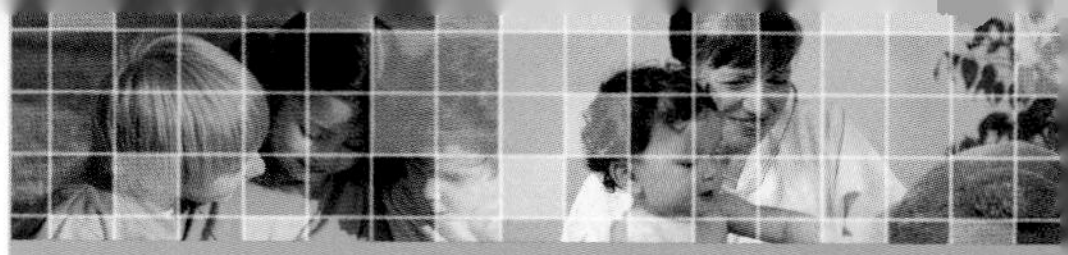

KEY TERMS

Acrocyanosis, 571
Barlow's maneuver, 583
Brazelton Neonatal Behavioral Assessment Scale, 586
Caput succedaneum, 575
Cephalohematoma, 574
Chemical conjunctivitis, 576
Dubowitz tool, 560
Epstein's pearls, 577
Erb-Duchenne paralysis (Erb's palsy), 582
Erythema toxicum, 572
Forceps marks, 573
Gestational age assessment tools, 560
Grasping reflex, 585
Harlequin sign, 572
Jaundice, 572
Lanugo, 562
Milia, 572
Molding, 574
Mongolian spots, 573
Moro reflex, 585
Mottling, 571
New Ballard Score (NBS), 560
Nevus flammeus (port-wine stain), 573
Nevus vasculosus (strawberry mark), 573
Ortolani's maneuver, 582
Pseudomenstruation, 581
Rooting reflex, 585
Skin turgor, 572
Subconjunctival hemorrhage, 576
Sucking reflex, 585
Telangiectatic nevi (stork bites), 573
Thrush, 577
Tonic neck reflex, 584
Trunk incurvation (Galant reflex), 585
Vernix caseosa, 573

Table 25–1 Timing and Types of Newborn Assessments

Assess immediately after birth:
- Need for resuscitation
- If newborn is stable and can be placed with parents to initiate early attachment and bonding.

Assessments within 1 to 4 hours after birth:
- Progress of newborn's adaptation to extrauterine life
- Determination of gestational age
- Ongoing assessment for high-risk problems

Assessment procedures within first 24 hours or before discharge:
- Complete physical examination (Depending on agency protocol, the nurse may complete some components independently, with the certified nurse-midwife, physician, or nurse practitioner completing the exam before discharge.)
- Nutritional status and ability to formula-feed or breastfeed satisfactorily
- Behavioral state organization abilities

examination to detect any emerging or potential problems. A general assessment is also done at this time (Table 25–1).

This chapter presents the procedures for estimating gestational age and performing the complete physical examination and behavioral assessment. Chapter 19 discusses the immediate postbirth assessment.

ESTIMATION OF GESTATIONAL AGE

The nurse must establish the newborn's gestational age in the first 4 hours after birth so that careful attention can be given to age-related problems. Traditionally, a newborn's gestational age was determined from the date of the pregnant woman's last menstrual period. However, this method was accurate only 75% to 85% of the time. Because of the problems that develop with the preterm newborn or the newborn whose weight is inappropriate for gestational age, a more accurate system was developed to postnatally evaluate the newborn. Once learned, the procedure can be done in a few minutes. *It is essential that the nurse wear gloves when assessing the newborn in these early hours after birth and before the first bath until amniotic fluid, as well as vaginal and bloody secretions on the skin, are removed.*

Clinical **gestational age assessment tools** have two components: (1) external physical characteristics and (2) neurologic or neuromuscular development. Physical characteristics generally include plantar (sole) creases, amount of breast tissue, amount of lanugo, cartilaginous development of the ear, and testicular descent and scrotal rugae or labial development. These objective clinical criteria are not influenced by labor and birth and do not change significantly within the first 12 hours after birth.

Neurologic examination facilitates assessment of functional or physiologic maturation in addition to physical development. However, the newborn's nervous system is unstable during the first 24 hours of life; neurologic evaluation findings based on reflexes or assessments dependent on the higher brain centers may not be reliable. If the neurologic findings drastically deviate from the gestational age derived by evaluation of external characteristics, a second assessment is done in 24 hours.

The neurologic assessment components (excluding reflexes) can aid in assessing the gestational age of newborns of less than 34 weeks' gestation. Between 26 and 34 weeks, neurologic changes are significant, whereas significant physical changes are less evident. One significant neuromuscular change is that muscle tone progresses from extensor tone to flexor tone in the extremities as the neurological system matures in a *caudocephalad* (tail-to-head) progression.

Ballard, Khoury, Wedig, et al. (1991) developed the *estimation of gestational age by maturity rating*, a simplified version of the well-researched **Dubowitz tool**. The Ballard tool omits some of the neuromuscular tone assessments, such as head lag, ventral suspension (which is difficult to assess in very ill newborns or those on respirators), and leg recoil. In the Ballard tool, each physical and neuromuscular finding is given a value, and the total score is matched to a gestational age (Figure 25–1 ●). The maximum score on the Ballard tool is 50, which corresponds to a gestational age of 44 weeks.

For example, on completion of a gestational assessment of a 1-hour-old newborn, the nurse gives a score of 3 to all the physical characteristics, for a total of 18, and gives a score of 3 to all neuromuscular assessments, for a total of 18. The physical characteristics score of 18 is added to the neurologic score of 18 for a total score of 36, which correlates with 38+ weeks' gestation. Because all newborns vary slightly in the development of physical characteristics and maturation of neurologic function, scores usually vary instead of all being 3, as in this example.

Postnatal gestational age assessment tools can overestimate preterm gestational age and underestimate postterm gestational age. The tools have been shown to lose accuracy when newborns of less than 28 weeks' or more than 43 weeks' gestation are assessed. Ballard et al. (1991) in the **New Ballard Score (NBS)** added criteria for more accurate assessment of the gestational age of newborns between 20 and 28 weeks' gestation and less than 1500 g. They suggest that the assessments should be made within 12 hours of birth to optimize accuracy, especially in infants of less than 26 weeks' gestational age. Also the Ballard assessment may be overstimulating to infants of less than 27 weeks' gestation. Some maternal conditions, such as preeclampsia, diabetes, and maternal analgesia and anesthesia, may affect certain gestational assessment components and warrant further evaluation (see Chapters 14, 15, and 20). Maternal diabetes, although it appears to accelerate fetal physical growth, seems to retard maturation. Maternal hypertension states, which retard fetal physical growth, seem to speed maturation.

Newborns of women with preeclampsia have a poor correlation with the criteria involving active muscle tone and edema. Maternal analgesia and anesthesia may cause respiratory depression in the baby. Babies with respiratory distress syndrome (RDS) tend to be flaccid and edematous and to assume a "froglike" posture (see Chapter 28). These characteristics affect the scoring of the neuromuscular components of the assessment tool used. The NBS gestational age assessment tool will be used throughout the chapter to demonstrate the assessment of the physical and neuromuscular criteria associated with gestational age.

NEWBORN MATURITY RATING & CLASSIFICATION

ESTIMATION OF GESTATIONAL AGE BY MATURITY RATING

Symbols: X - 1st Exam O - 2nd Exam

NEUROMUSCULAR MATURITY

	−1	0	1	2	3	4	5
Posture							
Square Window (wrist)	>90°	90°	60°	45°	30°	0°	
Arm Recoil		180°	140°–180°	110°–140°	90°–110°	<90°	
Popliteal Angle	180°	160°	140°	120°	100°	90°	<90°
Scarf Sign							
Heel to Ear							

Gestation by Dates ________________ wks

Birth Date ____________ Hour ____________ am pm

APGAR ____________ 1 min ____________ 5 min

MATURITY RATING

score	weeks
−10	20
−5	22
0	24
5	26
10	28
15	30
20	32
25	34
30	36
35	38
40	40
45	42
50	44

PHYSICAL MATURITY

	−1	0	1	2	3	4	5
Skin	sticky friable transparent	gelatinous red, translucent	smooth pink, visible veins	superficial peeling &/or rash, few veins	cracking pale areas rare veins	parchment deep cracking no vessels	leathery cracked wrinkled
Lanugo	none	sparse	abundant	thinning	bald areas	mostly bald	
Plantar Surface	heel-toe 40–50mm:–1 <40mm:–2	>50mm no crease	faint red marks	anterior transverse crease only	creases ant. 2/3	creases over entire sole	
Breast	imperceptible	barely perceptible	flat areola no bud	stippled areola 1–2mm bud	raised areola 3–4mm bud	full areola 5–10mm bud	
Eye/Ear	lids fused loosely:–1 tightly:–2	lids open pinna flat stays folded	sl. curved pinna; soft; slow recoil	well curved pinna; soft but ready recoil	formed & firm instant recoil	thick cartilage ear stiff	
Genitals male	scrotum flat, smooth	scrotum empty faint rugae	testes in upper canal rare rugae	testes descending few rugae	testes down good rugae	testes pendulous deep rugae	
Genitals female	clitoris prominent labia flat	prominent clitoris small labia minora	prominent clitoris enlarging minora	majora & minora equally prominent	majora large minora small	majora cover clitoris & minora	

SCORING SECTION

	1st Exam = X	2nd Exam = 0
Estimating Gest Age by Maturity Rating	______Weeks	______Weeks
Time of Exam	Date ________ Hour______ am pm	Date ________ Hour______ am pm
Age at Exam	______ Hours	______ Hours
Signature of Examiner	____________ M.D.	____________ M.D.

● **Figure 25–1** Newborn maturity rating and classification. If a 1-hour-old newborn is given a score of 3 for each of the physical characteristics and neuromuscular assessments, the newborn's total score would be 36. A total score of 36 correlates with 38 or more weeks' gestation.

Source: Ballard, J. L., Khoury, J. C., Wedig, K., Wang, L., Eilers-Walsmann, B. L., & Lipp, R. (1991). New Ballard score, expanded to include extremely premature infants. *Journal of Pediatrics, 119*(3), 417.

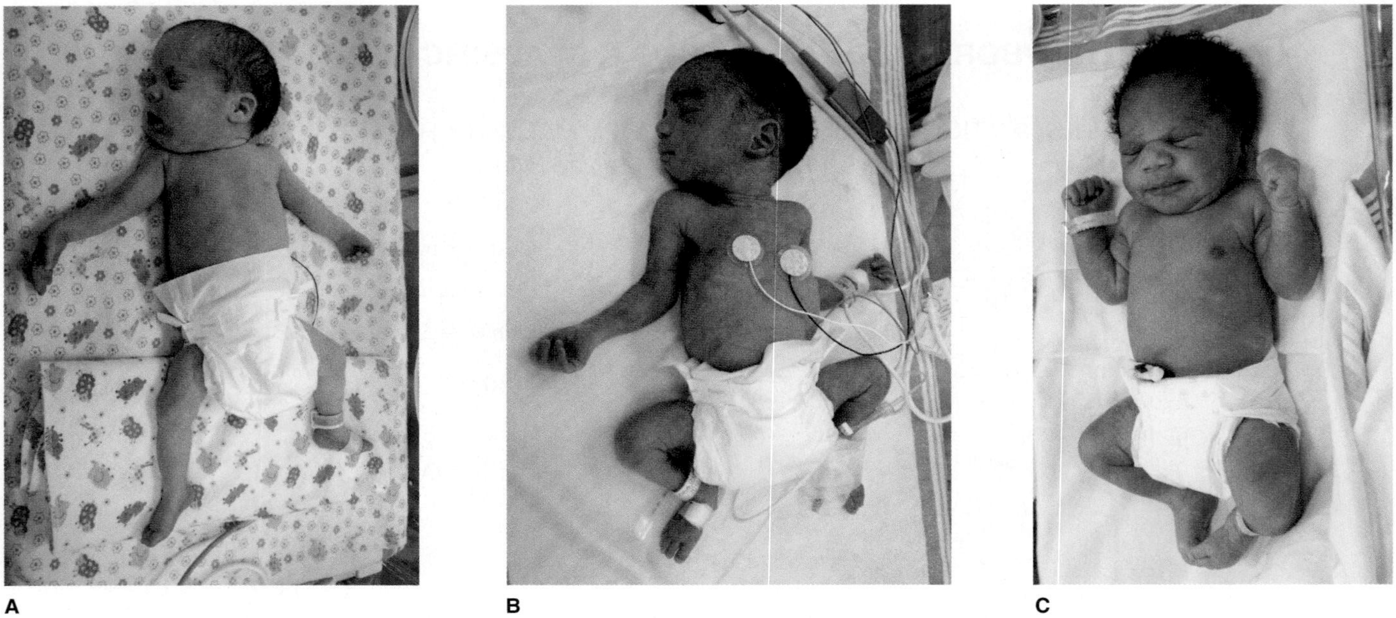

● **Figure 25–2** Resting posture. ***A,*** Newborn exhibits beginning of flexion of the thigh (score 1 or 2). The gestational age is approximately 31 weeks. Note the extension of the upper extremities. ***B,*** Newborn exhibits stronger flexion of the arms, hips, and thighs (score 3). The gestational age is approximately 35 weeks. ***C,*** The full-term newborn exhibits hypertonic flexion of all extremities (score 4).

MyNursingKit Case Study: Newborn Maturity Assessment

ASSESSMENT OF PHYSICAL MATURITY CHARACTERISTICS

The nurse first evaluates observable characteristics without disturbing the baby. Selected physical characteristics common to the Dubowitz and Ballard gestational assessment tools are presented here in the order in which they might be most effectively evaluated:

1. *Resting posture,* although a neuromuscular component, should be assessed as the baby lies undisturbed on a flat surface (Figure 25–2 ●).
2. *Skin* in the preterm newborn appears thin and transparent, with veins prominent over the abdomen early in gestation. As the newborn approaches term, the skin appears opaque because of increased subcutaneous tissue. Disappearance of the protective vernix caseosa promotes skin desquamation; this is commonly seen in postmature infants (infants of more than 42 weeks' gestational age) and those showing signs of placental insufficiency; see Chapter 28∞).
3. *Lanugo,* a fine hair covering, decreases as gestational age increases. The amount of **lanugo** is greatest at 28 to

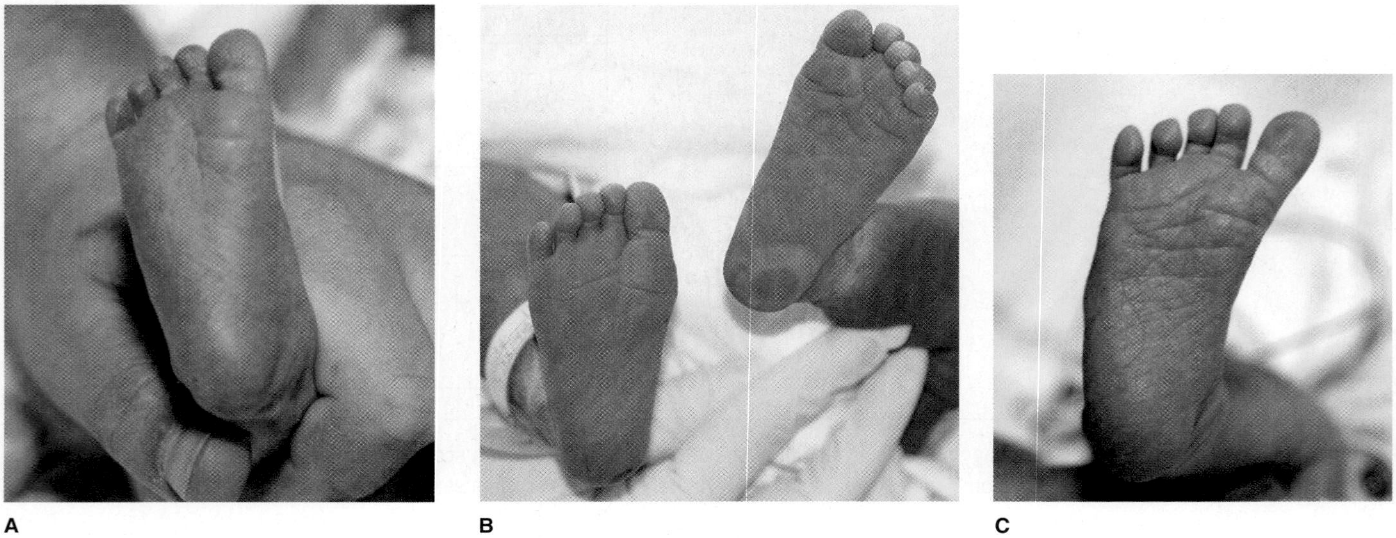

● **Figure 25–3** Sole creases. ***A,*** Newborn has a few sole creases on the anterior portion of the foot. Note the slick heel (score 2). The gestational age is approximately 35 weeks. ***B,*** Newborn has a deeper network of sole creases on the anterior two-thirds of the sole. Note the slick heel (score 3). The gestational age is approximately 37 weeks. ***C,*** The term newborn has deep sole creases down to and including the heel as the skin loses fluid and dries after birth (score 4). Sole (plantar) creases can be seen even in preterm newborns.

30 weeks and then disappears, first from the face and then from the trunk and extremities.

4. *Plantar (sole) creases* are reliable indicators of gestational age in the first 12 hours of life. Later the skin of the foot begins drying, and superficial creases appear. Development of plantar creases begins at the top (anterior) portion of the sole and, as gestation progresses, proceeds to the heel (Figure 25–3 ●). Peeling may also occur. Plantar creases vary with race. In newborns of African descent, plantar creases may be less developed at term.
5. The nurse inspects the *areola* and gently palpates the *breast bud tissue* by applying the forefinger and middle finger to the breast area and measuring the tissue between them in centimeters or millimeters (Figure 25–4 ●). At term gestation, the tissue measures between 0.5 and 1 cm (5 and 10 mm). During the assessment, the nipple should not be grasped firmly because skin and subcutaneous tissue will prevent accurate estimation of size. The nurse must do this procedure gently to avoid causing trauma to the breast tissue.

   As gestation progresses, the breast tissue mass and areola enlarge. However, a large breast tissue mass can occur as a result of specific conditions other than advanced gestational age or the effects of maternal hormones on the baby. In the large-for-gestational-age infant, a diabetic mother's accelerated development of breast tissue is a reflection of subcutaneous fat deposits. Small-for-gestational-age (SGA) term or postterm newborns may have used subcutaneous fat (which would have been deposited as breast tissue) to survive in utero; as a result, their lack of breast tissue may indicate a gestational age of 34 to 35 weeks, even though other factors indicate a term or postterm newborn.
6. *Ear form and cartilage distribution* develop with gestational age. The cartilage gives the ear its shape and substance (Figure 25–5 ●). In a newborn of less than 34 weeks' gestation, the ear is relatively shapeless and flat; it has little cartilage, so the ear folds over on itself and remains folded. By approximately 36 weeks' gestation, some cartilage and incurving of the upper pinna are present, and the pinna springs back slowly when folded. (The nurse tests this response by holding the top and bottom of the pinna together with the forefinger and thumb and then releasing them or by folding the pinna of the ear forward against the side of the head, releasing it, and observing the response.) By term, the newborn's pinna is firm, stands away from the head, and springs back quickly from the folding.
7. *Male genitals* are evaluated for size of the scrotal sac, presence of rugae (wrinkles and ridges in the scrotum), and descent of the testes (Figure 25–6 ●). Before 36 weeks, the scrotum has few rugae, and the testes are palpable in the inguinal canal. By 36 to 38 weeks, the testes are in the upper scrotum, and rugae have developed over the anterior portion of the scrotum. By term, the testes are generally in the lower scrotum, which is pendulous and covered with rugae.
8. The appearance of the *female genitals* depends in part on subcutaneous fat deposition and therefore relates to fetal nutritional status (Figure 25–7 ●). The clitoris varies in size, and occasionally is so swollen that it is difficult to identify the sex of the newborn. This swelling may be caused by adrenogenital syndrome, which causes the adrenals to secrete excessive amounts of androgen and other hormones. At 30 to 32 weeks' gestation, the clitoris is prominent, and the labia majora are small and widely separated. As gestational age

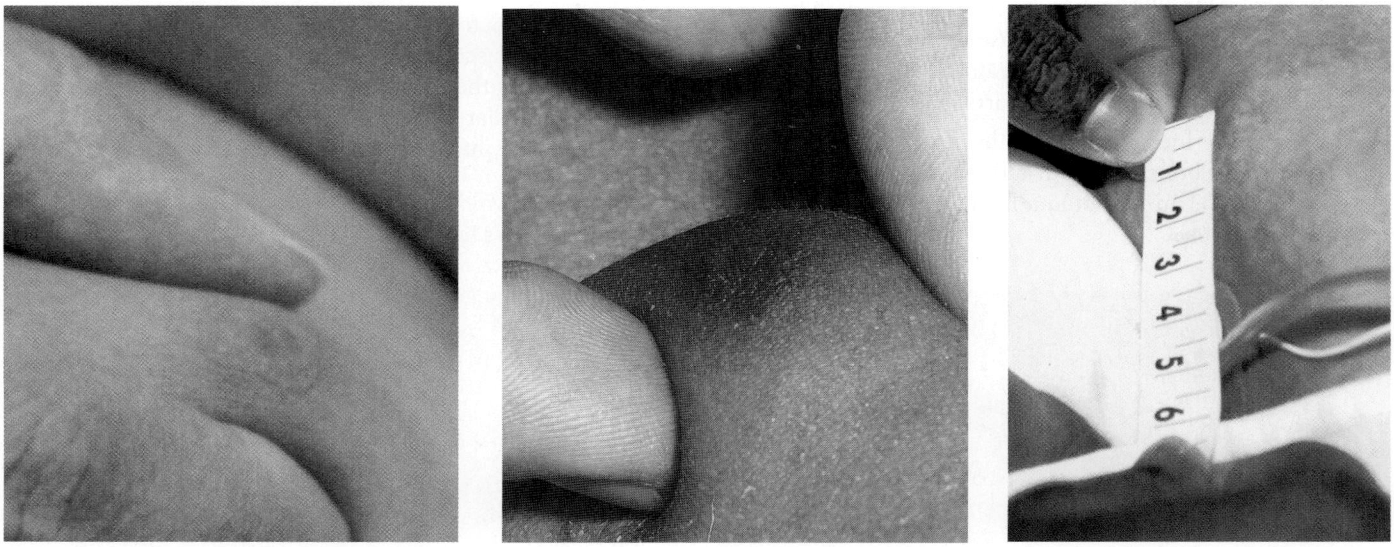

A B C

● **Figure 25–4** Breast tissue. ***A,*** Newborn has stippled areola, a visible raised area of 0.75 cm (0.3 in.) diameter (score 3). The gestational age is 38 weeks. ***B,*** Newborn has 10 mm breast tissue area (score 4). The gestational age is 40 to 44 weeks. ***C,*** Gently compress the tissue between the middle and index fingers and measure the tissue in centimeters or millimeters. Absence of or decreased breast tissue often indicates premature or small-for-gestational-age newborn.

Source: B is from Dubowitz, L., & Dubowitz, V. (1977). *The gestational age of the newborn.* Menlo Park, CA: Addison-Wesley. Reprinted by permission of V. Dubowitz, MD, Hammersmith Hospital, London, England.

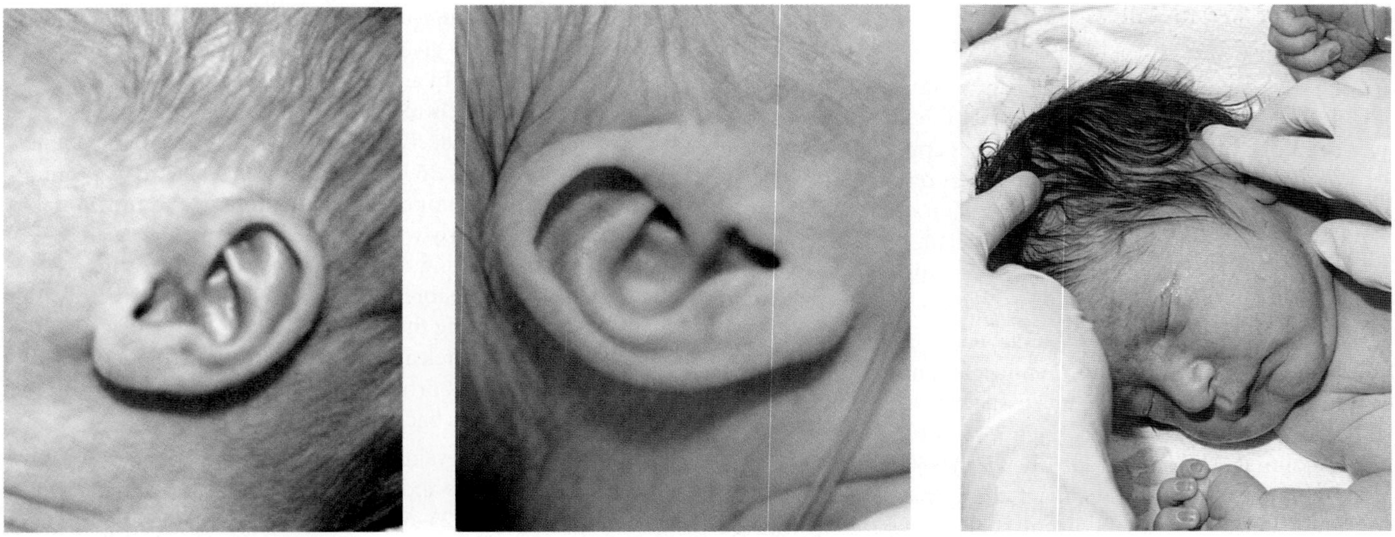

A B C

● **Figure 25–5** Ear form and cartilage. ***A,*** The ear of the infant at approximately 36 weeks' gestation shows incurving of the upper two-thirds of the pinna (score 2). ***B,*** Infant at term shows well-defined incurving of the entire pinna (score 3). ***C,*** If the auricle stays in the position in which it is pressed or returns slowly to its original position, it usually means the gestational age is less than 38 weeks.

increases, the labia majora increase in size. At 36 to 40 weeks, they nearly cover the clitoris. At 40 weeks and beyond, the labia majora cover the labia minora and clitoris.

Other physical characteristics assessed by some gestational age scoring tools include the following:

1. *Vernix* covers the preterm newborn. The postterm newborn has no vernix. After noting vernix distribution, the birthing area nurse (wearing gloves) dries the newborn to prevent evaporative heat loss, thus disturbing the vernix and potentially altering this gestational age criterion.
2. *Hair* of the preterm newborn has the consistency of matted wool or fur and lies in bunches rather than in the silky, single strands of the term newborn's hair.
3. *Skull firmness* increases as the fetus matures. In a term newborn the bones are hard, and the sutures are not easily displaced. The nurse should not attempt to displace the sutures forcibly.
4. *Nails* appear and cover the nail bed at about 20 weeks' gestation. Nails extending beyond the fingertips may indicate a postterm newborn.

ASSESSMENT OF NEUROMUSCULAR MATURITY CHARACTERISTICS

The central nervous system of the fetus matures at a fairly constant rate. Tests have been designed to evaluate neurologic status as manifested by development of neuromuscular tone. As noted earlier, neuromuscular tone in the fetus develops in a caudocephalic direction, from the lower to the upper extremities.

The neuromuscular evaluation requires more manipulation and disturbances than the physical evaluation of the newborn. The neuromuscular evaluation (see Figure 25–1) is best performed when the infant has stabilized.

1. The *square window sign* is elicited by gently flexing the newborn's hand toward the ventral forearm until

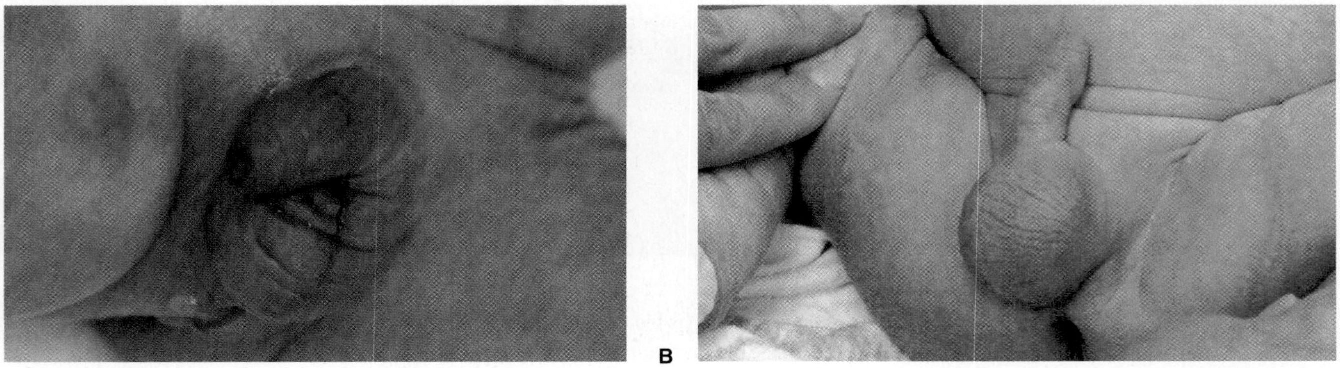

A B

● **Figure 25–6** Male genitals. ***A,*** Preterm newborn's testes are not within the scrotum. The scrotal surface has few rugae (score 2). ***B,*** Term newborn's testes are generally fully descended. The entire surface of the scrotum is covered by rugae (score 3).

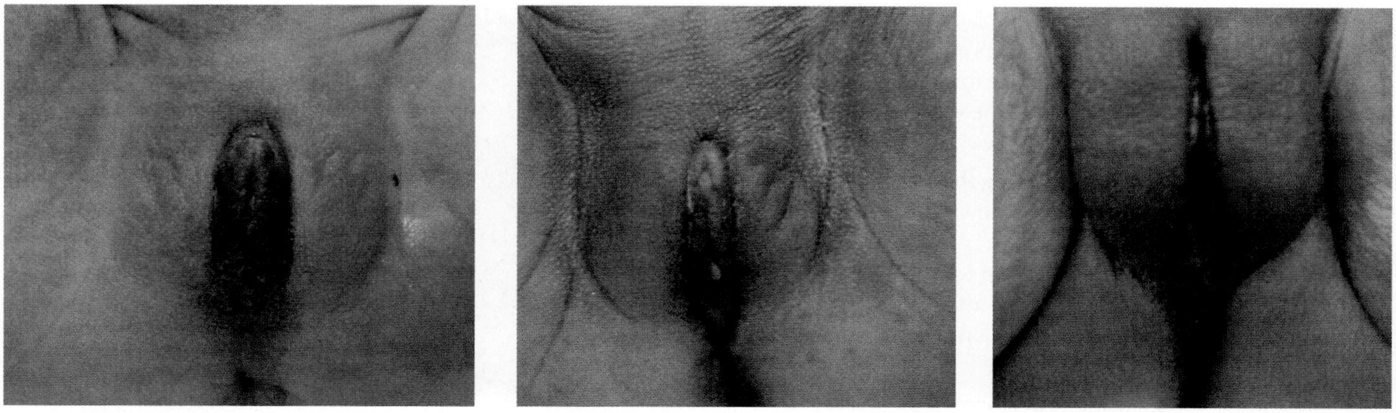

A B C

● **Figure 25–7** Female genitals. ***A,*** Newborn has a prominent clitoris. The labia majora are widely separated, and the labia minora, viewed laterally, would protrude beyond the labia majora (score 1). The gestational age is 30 to 36 weeks. ***B,*** The clitoris is still visible. The labia minora and labia majora are equally prominent (score 2). The gestational age is 36 to 40 weeks. ***C,*** The term newborn has developed large labia majora that cover both clitoris and labia minora (score 3).

resistance is felt. The angle formed at the wrist is measured (Figure 25–8 ●).

2. *Recoil* is a test of flexion development. Because flexion first develops in the lower extremities, recoil is first tested in the legs. Place the newborn on its back on a flat surface. With a hand on the newborn's knees, the nurse places the baby's legs in flexion, then extends them parallel to each other and flat on the surface. The response to this maneuver is recoil of the newborn's legs. According to gestational age, they may not move or they may return slowly or quickly to the flexed position. Preterm infants have less muscle tone than term infants, so preterm infants have less recoil.

   Test arm recoil by flexion at the elbow and extension of the arms at the newborn's side. While the baby is in the supine position, the nurse completely flexes both elbows, holds them in this position for 5 seconds, extends the arms at the baby's side, and releases them. On release, the elbows of a full-term newborn form an angle of less than 90 degrees and rapidly recoil back to a flexed position. The elbows of a preterm newborn have slower recoil time and form an angle greater than 90 degrees. Arm recoil is also slower in healthy but fatigued newborns after birth; therefore arm recoil is best elicited after the first hour of birth, when the baby has had time to recover from the stress of the birth. The deep sleep state also decreases the arm recoil response. Assessment of arm recoil should be bilateral to rule out brachial palsy.

3. The *popliteal angle* (degree of knee flexion) is determined with the newborn flat on its back. The thigh is flexed on the

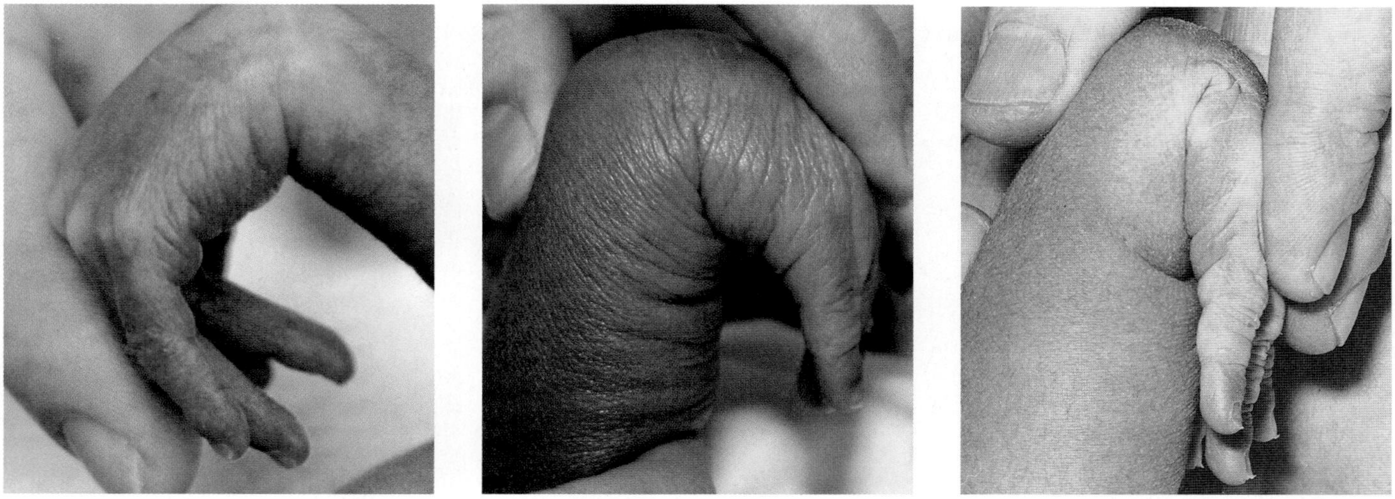

A B C

● **Figure 25–8** Square window sign. ***A,*** This angle is 90 degrees and suggests an immature newborn of 28 to 32 weeks' gestation (Score 0). ***B,*** A 30- to 40-degree angle is commonly found from 38 to 40 weeks' gestation (score 2 to 3). ***C,*** A 0-degree angle can occur from 40 to 42 weeks' gestation (score 4).

Source: C is from Dubowitz, L, & Dubowitz, V. (1977). *The gestational age of the newborn.* Menlo Park, CA: Addison-Wesley. Reprinted by permission of V. Dubowitz, MD, Hammersmith Hospital, London, England.

abdomen and chest, and the nurse places the index finger of the other hand behind the newborn's ankle to extend the lower leg until resistance is met. The angle formed is then measured. Results vary from no resistance in the very immature newborn to an 80-degree angle in the term newborn.

4. The *scarf sign* is elicited by placing the newborn supine and drawing an arm across the chest toward the newborn's opposite shoulder until resistance is met. The location of the elbow is then noted in relation to the midline of the chest (Figure 25–9 ●). A preterm infant's elbow will cross the midline of the chest, whereas a full-term infant's elbow will not cross midline.
5. The *heel-to-ear extension* is performed by placing the newborn in a supine position and then gently drawing the foot toward the ear on the same side until resistance is felt. The nurse should allow the knee to bend during the test. It is important to hold the buttocks down to keep from rolling the baby. Both the proximity of foot to ear and the degree of knee extension are assessed. A preterm, immature newborn's leg will remain straight and the foot will go to the ear or beyond (Figure 25–10 ●). With advancing gestational age, the newborn demonstrates increasing resistance to this maneuver. Maneuvers involving the lower extremities of newborns who had frank breech presentation should be delayed to allow for resolution of leg positioning.
6. *Ankle dorsiflexion* is determined by flexing the ankle on the shin. The nurse uses a thumb to push on the sole of the newborn's foot while the fingers support the back of the leg. Then the angle formed by the foot and the interior leg is measured (Figure 25–11 ●). Intrauterine position and congenital deformities can influence this sign.
7. *Head lag* (neck flexor) is measured by pulling the newborn to a sitting position and noting the degree of head lag. Total lag is common in newborns up to 34 weeks' gestation, whereas postterm newborns (42+ weeks) hold their heads in front of their body lines. Full-term newborns can support their heads momentarily.

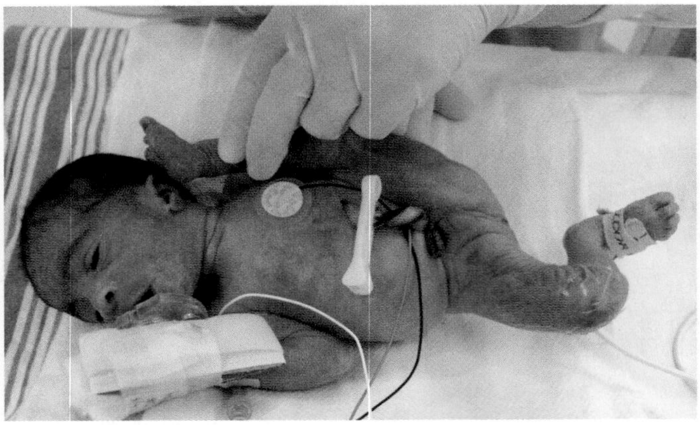

● **Figure 25–10** Heel to ear. No resistance. Leg fully extended (score 0).

8. *Ventral suspension* (horizontal position) is evaluated by holding the newborn prone on the nurse's hand. The position of the head and back and the degree of flexion in the arms and legs are noted. Some flexion of arms and legs indicates 36 to 38 weeks' gestation; fully flexed extremities, with head and back even, are characteristic of a term newborn.
9. *Major reflexes* such as *sucking, rooting, grasping, Moro, tonic neck,* and others are evaluated during the newborn exam. These reflexes are discussed later in the chapter.

A supplementary method for estimating gestational age (done by the physician or nurse practitioner) is to view the vascular network of the cornea with an ophthalmoscope. The nurse may need to delay administration of prophylactic eye ointment in preterm infants until after this vascular eye exam is done. The amount of vascularity present over the surface of the lens assists in identifying infants of 27 through 34 weeks' gestational age.

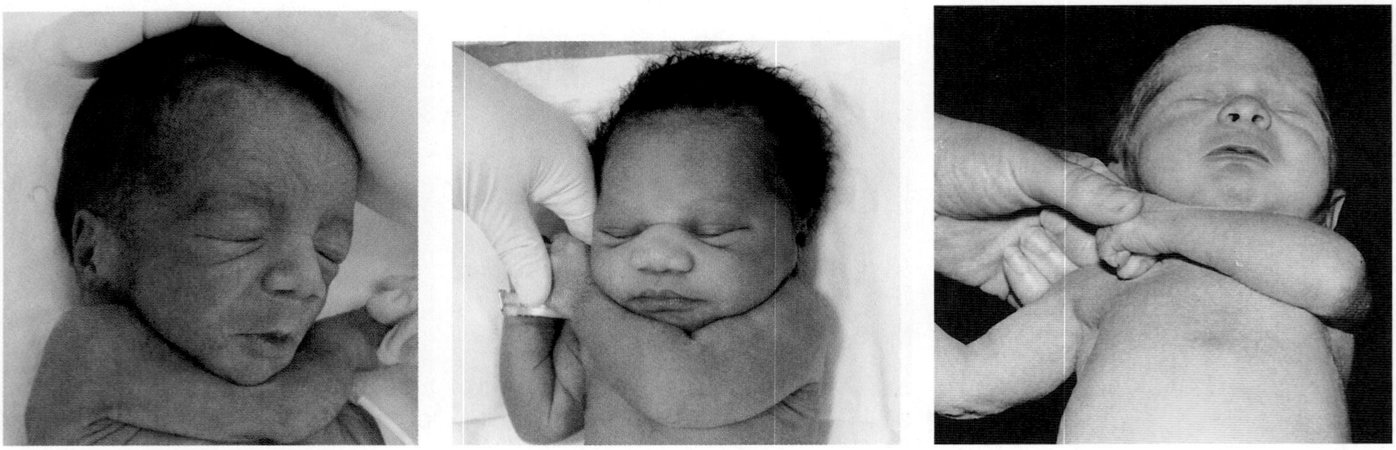

A B C

● **Figure 25–9** Scarf sign. ***A,*** No resistance is noted until after 30 weeks' gestation. The elbow moves readily past the midline (score 1). ***B,*** The elbow is at midline at 36 to 40 weeks' gestation (score 2). ***C,*** Beyond 40 weeks' gestation the elbow will not reach the midline (score 4).

Source: C is from Dubowitz, L, & Dubowitz, V. (1977). *The gestational age of the newborn.* Menlo Park, CA: Addison-Wesley. Reprinted by permission of V. Dubowitz, MD, Hammersmith Hospital, London, England.

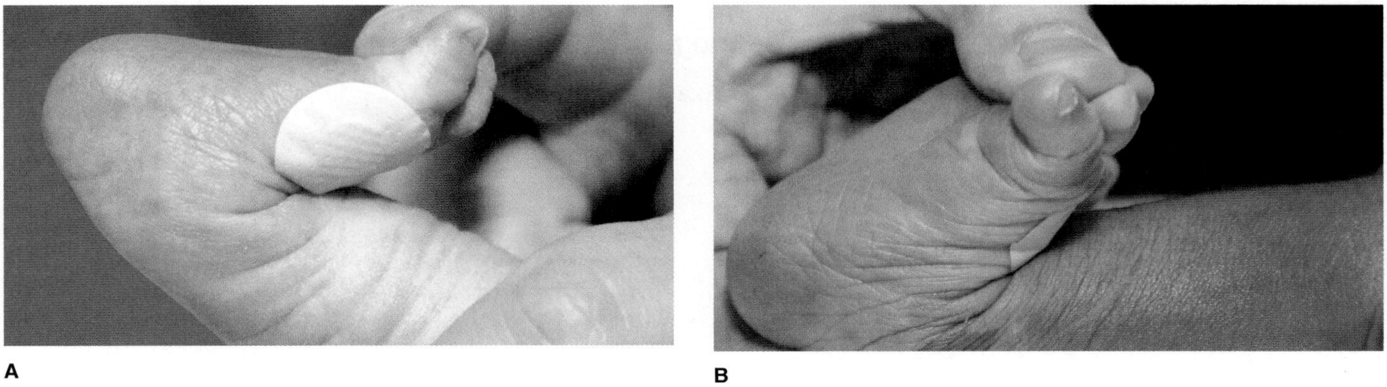

● **Figure 25–11** Ankle dorsiflexion. ***A,*** A 45-degree angle indicates 32 to 36 weeks' gestation. A 20-degree angle indicates 36 to 40 weeks' gestation (score 2 to 3). ***B,*** A 15- to 0-degree angle is common at 40 weeks' or more gestational age (score 4).

When the gestational age determination and birth weight are considered together, the newborn can be identified as one whose growth is *below the 10th percentile, or small for gestational age (SGA); appropriate for gestational age (AGA); or above the 90th percentile, which is large for gestational age (LGA)* (Figure 25–12 ●). This determination enables the nurse to anticipate possible physiologic problems. This information is used in conjunction with a complete physical examination, to establish a

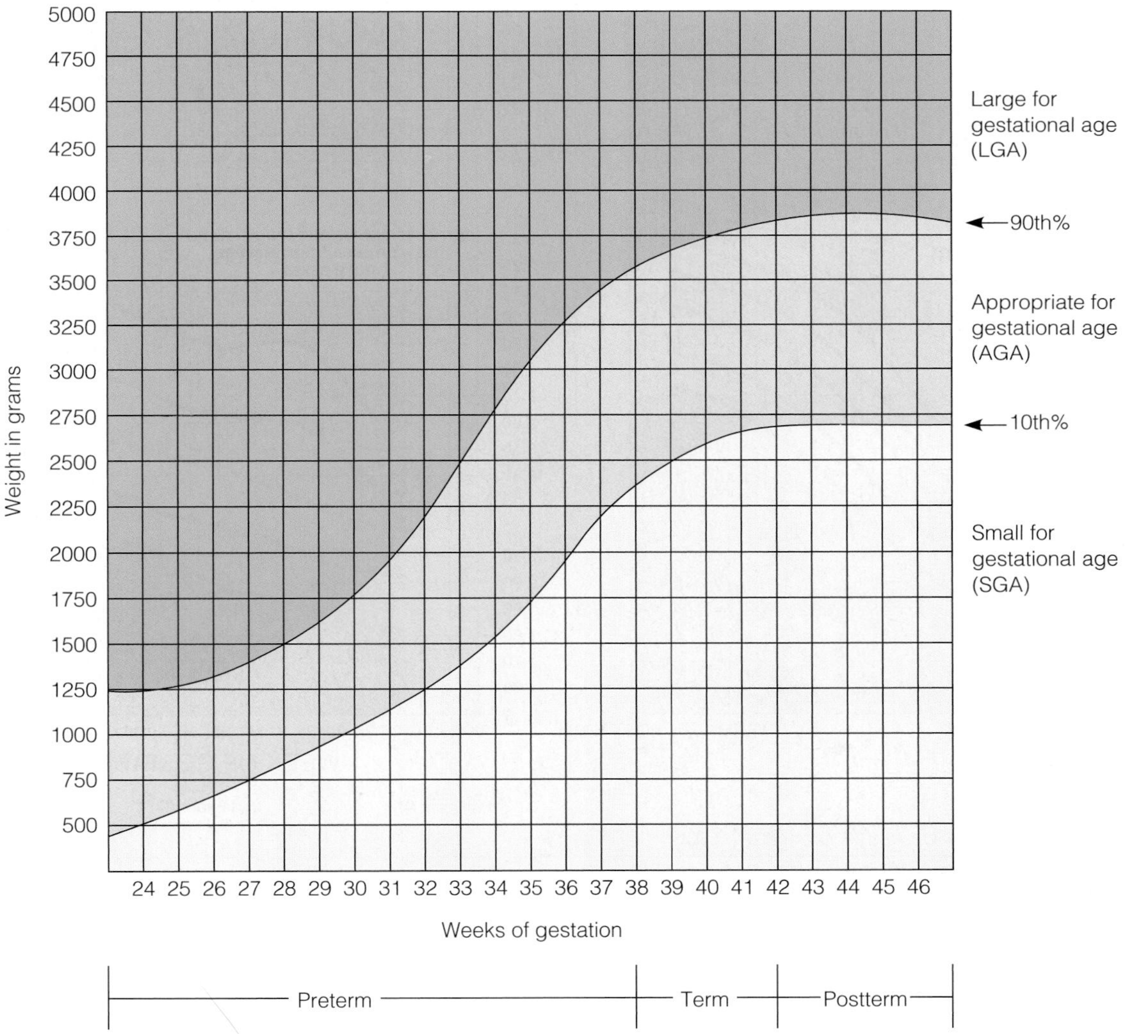

● **Figure 25–12** Classification of newborns by birth weight and gestational age. The nurse places the newborn's birth weight and gestational age on the graph and classifies the newborn as large for gestational age (LGA), appropriate for gestational age (AGA), or small for gestational age (SGA).

Source: Battaglia, F. C., & Lubchenco, L. O. (1967). A practical classification of newborn infants by weight and gestational age. *Journal of Pediatrics, 71,* 161.

CLASSIFICATION OF NEWBORNS— BASED ON MATURITY AND INTRAUTERINE GROWTH

Symbols: X-1st Exam O-2nd Exam

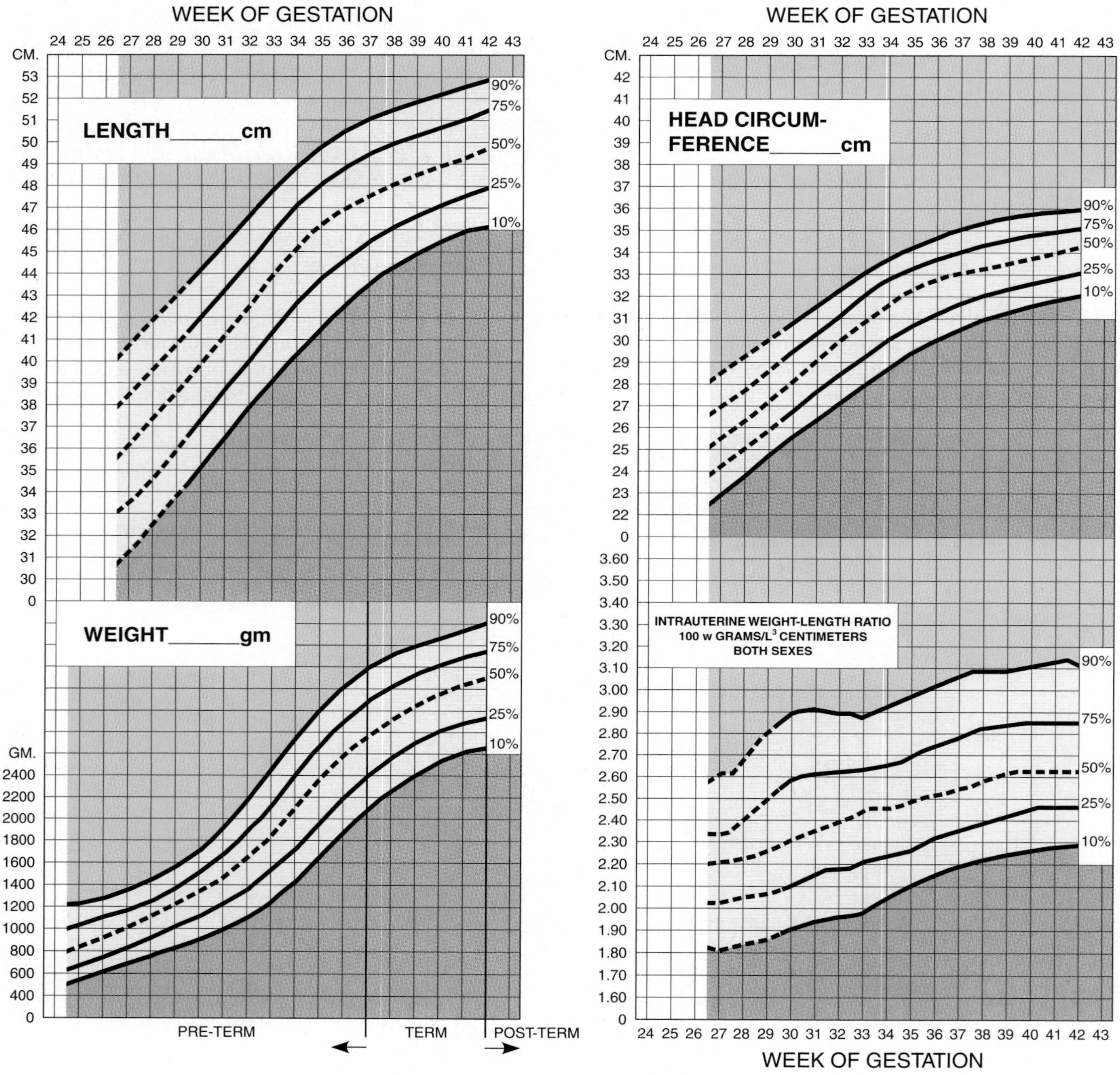

	1st Exam (X)	2nd Exam (O)
LARGE FOR GESTATIONAL AGE **(LGA)**		
APPROPRIATE FOR GESTATIONAL AGE **(AGA)**		
SMALL FOR GESTATIONAL AGE **(SGA)**		
Age at Exam	hrs	hrs
Signature of Examiner	M.D.	M.D.

• **Figure 25–13** Classification of newborns based on maturity and intrauterine growth.

Sources: Adapted from Lubchenco, L. O., Hansman, C., & Boyd, E. (1966). Intrauterine growth in length and head circumference as estimated from live births at gestational ages from 26 to 42 weeks. *Pediatrics, 37,* 403–408; Battaglia, F. C., & Lubchenco, L. O. (1967). A practical classification of newborn infants by weight and gestational age. *Journal of Pediatrics, 71,* 159.

Nursing Practice

Measuring weight and height often aggravates newborns and may alter their vital signs. For better accuracy, take the newborn's vital signs before weighing and measuring the infant.

plan of care appropriate for the individual newborn. For example, an SGA or LGA newborn often requires frequent glucose monitoring and early feedings started soon after birth as they are at risk for hypoglycemia. (See Chapter 28 for more complete discussion of these categories and the potential problems associated with them.)

The nurse also plots the gestational age against the newborn's length, head circumference, and weight on the appropriate growth chart to determine if these measurements fall within the average range—the 10th to 90th percentile for the corresponding gestational age (Figure 25–13 ●). These correlations further document the level of maturity and appropriate category for the newborn. The comparison of the infant's weight-length ratio further facilitates identification of SGA infants as having symmetrical or asymmetrical growth restriction.

PHYSICAL ASSESSMENT

After the initial determination of gestational age and related potential problems, the nurse carries out a more extensive physical assessment in a warm, well-lit area that is free of drafts. Completing the physical assessment in the presence of the parents provides an opportunity to acquaint them with their unique newborn. The examination is performed in a systematic, head-to-toe manner, and all findings are recorded. When assessing the physical and neurologic status of the newborn, the nurse should first consider general appearance and then proceed to specific areas.

The "Assessment Guide: Newborn Physical Assessment" on pages 588–599 outlines how to systematically assess the newborn. Normal findings, alterations, and related causes are presented and correlated with suggested nursing responses. The findings are typical for a full-term newborn.

GENERAL APPEARANCE

The newborn's head is disproportionately large for its body. The neck looks short because the chin rests on the chest. Newborns have a prominent abdomen, sloping shoulders, narrow hips, and rounded chests. The center of the baby's body is the umbilicus rather than the symphysis pubis as in the adult. The body appears long and the extremities short.

Newborns tend to stay in a flexed position similar to the one maintained in utero and will offer resistance when the extremities are straightened. This flexed position contributes to the short appearance of the extremities. The hands are tightly clenched. After a breech birth, the feet are usually dorsiflexed, and it may take several weeks for the infant to assume the typical newborn posture.

WEIGHT AND MEASUREMENTS

The normal full-term Caucasian newborn has an average birth weight of 3405 g (7 lb, 8 oz). Newborns of African, Asian, or Mexican American descent are usually somewhat smaller at term whereas Native American infants are often heavier at term (Mandleco, 2004; Wu & Daniel, 2001). Other factors that influence weight are age, size and genetic makeup of parents, health of mother (smoking and malnutrition decrease birth weight), and the interval between pregnancies (short intervals, such as every year, result in lower birth weight). After the first week, and for the first 6 months, the newborn's weight increases about 198 g (7 oz) weekly.

Approximately 70% to 75% of the newborn's body weight is water. During the initial newborn period (the first 3 or 4 days), term newborns have a physiologic weight loss of about 5% to 10% because of fluid shifts. This weight loss may reach 15% for preterm newborns. Large babies also tend to lose more weight because of greater fluid loss in proportion to birth weight. If weight loss is greater than 10%, clinical reappraisal is indicated. Factors contributing to weight loss include insufficient fluid intake resulting from delayed breastfeeding or a slow adjustment to the formula, increased volume of meconium excreted, and urination. Weight loss may be marked in the presence of temperature elevation (because of associated dehydration) or consistent chilling (because of nonshivering thermogenesis).

The length of the normal newborn is difficult to measure because the legs are flexed and tensed. To measure length, the nurse should place newborns flat on their backs with their legs extended as much as possible (Figure 25–14 ●). The average length is 50 cm (20 in.), and the range is 46 to 56 cm (18 to 22 in.). The newborn will grow approximately 2.5 cm (1 in.) a month for the next 6 months. This is the period of most rapid growth.

At birth the newborn's head is one-third the size of an adult's head. The circumference (biparietal diameter) of the newborn's head is 32 to 37 cm (12.5 to 14.5 in.). For accurate measurement, the nurse places the tape over the most prominent part of the occiput and brings it just above the eyebrows

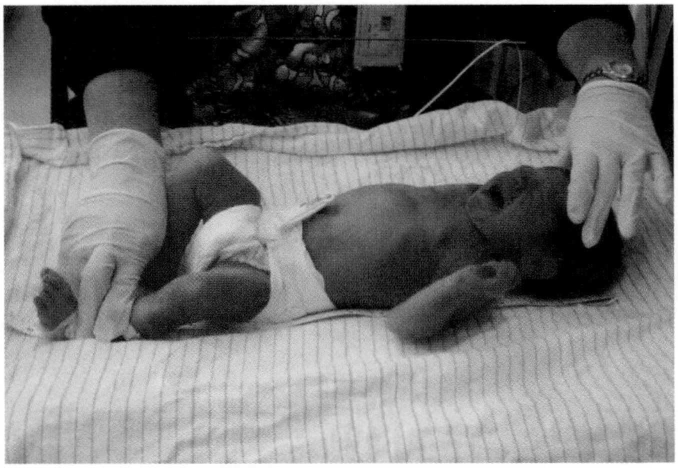

● **Figure 25–14** Measuring the length of the newborn.

Source: Courtesy of Vanessa Howell, RNC, MSN

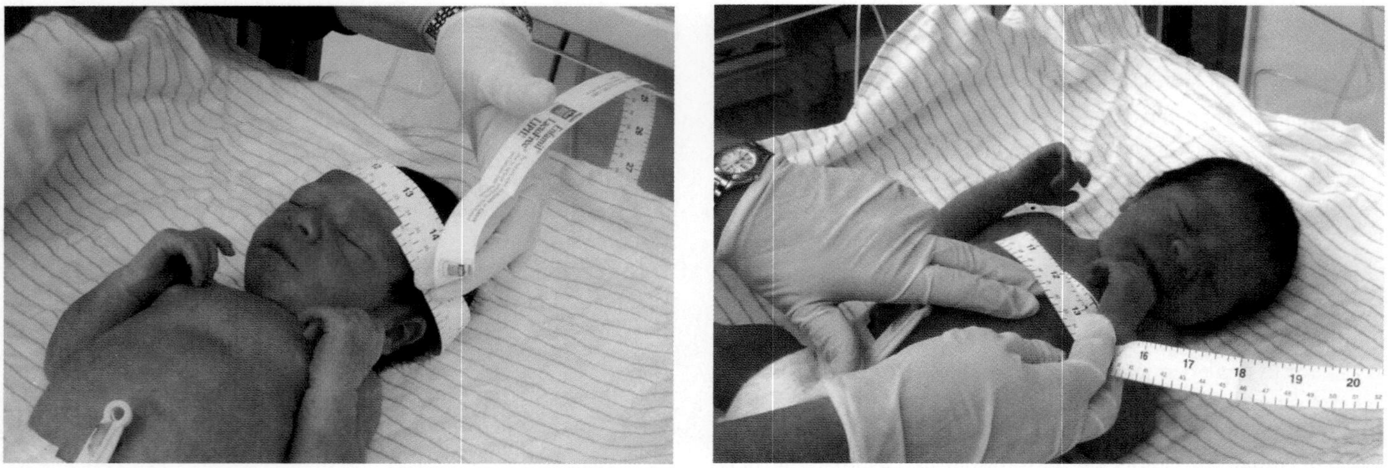

A B

● **Figure 25–15** Head and chest measurements. ***A,*** Measuring the head circumference of the newborn. ***B,*** Measuring the chest circumference of the newborn.

Source: Courtesy of Vanessa Howell, RNC, MSN.

(Figure 25–15A ●). The circumference of the newborn's head is approximately 2 cm (0.8 in.) greater than the circumference of the newborn's chest at birth, and will remain in this proportion for the next few months. (Factors that alter this measurement are discussed in the section titled "Head" later in this chapter.) It is best to take another head circumference on the second day if the newborn experienced significant head molding or developed a caput from the birth process.

The average circumference of the chest is 32 cm (12.5 in.) and ranges from 30 to 35 cm (12 to 14 in.). Chest measurements are taken with the tape measure placed at the lower edge of the scapulas and brought around anteriorly, directly over the nipple line (Figure 25–15B). The abdominal circumference, or girth, may also be measured at this time, by placing the tape around the newborn's abdomen at the level of the umbilicus, with the bottom edge of the tape at the top edge of the umbilicus (Table 25–2).

TEMPERATURE

Initial assessment of the newborn's temperature is critical. In utero, the temperature of the fetus is about the same as, or slightly higher than, the expectant mother's. When babies enter the outside world, their temperature can suddenly drop as a result of exposure to cold drafts and the skin's heat loss mechanisms.

If no heat conservation measures are started, the normal term newborn's deep body temperature falls 0.1°C (0.2°F) per minute; skin temperature drops 0.3°C (0.5°F) per minute. Skin temperature markedly decreases within 10 minutes after exposure to room air. The temperature should stabilize within 8 to 12 hours. Temperature is monitored at least every 30 minutes until the newborn's status has remained stable for 2 hours. Thereafter, the nurse should assess temperature at least once every 8 hours, or according to institutional policy (AAP & ACOG, 2007). In infants who have been exposed to group B hemolytic streptococcus, more frequent temperature monitoring

Table 25–2 Newborn Measurements

Measurement	Average	Range	Growth
Weight (Weight is influenced by racial origin and maternal age and size. Physiologic weight loss 5% to 10% for term newborns, up to 15% for preterm newborns.)	3405 g (7 lb, 8 oz)	2500–4000 g (5 lb, 8 oz–8 lb, 13 oz)	198 g (7 oz) per week for first 6 mo
Length	50 cm (20 in.)	46–56 cm (18–22 in.)	2.5 cm (1 in.) per month for first 6 mo
Head circumference (Approximately 2 cm larger than chest circumference)	33–35 cm (13–14 in.)	32–37 cm (12.5–14.5 in.)	
Chest circumference	32 cm (12.5 in.)	30–35 cm (12–14 in.)	

may be required (see Chapter 24∞ for a discussion of the physiology of temperature regulation).

Temperature is usually assessed in the birthing unit by the axillary skin method, a continuous skin probe, or may be via the rectal route. Axillary temperature reflects body (core) temperature and the body's compensatory response to the thermal environment. Axillary temperatures are the preferred method and are considered to be a close estimation of the rectal temperature. In preterm and term newborns, there is less than 0.1°C (0.2°F) difference between temperatures between the two sites. With the axillary method, the thermometer must remain in place at least 3 minutes unless an electronic thermometer is used (Figure 25–16 ●). Axillary temperature ranges from 36.4°C to 37.2°C (97.5°F to 99°F). The nurse should keep in mind that axillary temperatures can be misleading because the friction caused by apposition of the inner arm skin and upper chest wall and the nearness of brown fat to the probe may elevate the temperature.

Skin temperature is measured most accurately by means of continuous skin probe, especially for small newborns or newborns maintained in incubators or under radiant warmers. Normal skin temperature is 36°C to 36.5°C (96.8°F to 97.7°F). Continuous assessment of skin temperature allows time for initiation of interventions before a more serious fall in core temperature occurs (Figure 25–17 ●).

Rectal temperature is assumed to be the closest approximation to core temperature, but the accuracy of this method depends on the depth to which the thermometer is inserted. Normal rectal temperature is 36.6°C to 37.2°C (97.8°F to 99°F). The rectal route is *not* recommended as a routine method because it may irritate the rectal mucosa and increase chances of perforation (Blackburn, 2007).

Temperature instability, a deviation of more than 1°C (2°F) from one reading to the next, or a subnormal temperature may indicate an infection. In contrast to an elevated temperature in older children, an increased temperature in a newborn may indicate a reaction to too many coverings, too hot a room, or dehydration. Dehydration, which tends to increase body temperature, occurs in newborns whose feedings have been delayed for any reason. Newborns may respond to overheating (a temperature greater than 37.5°C [99.5°F]) by increased restlessness and eventually by perspiration after 35 to 40 minutes of exposure (Blackburn, 2007). The perspiration appears initially on the head and face and then on the chest.

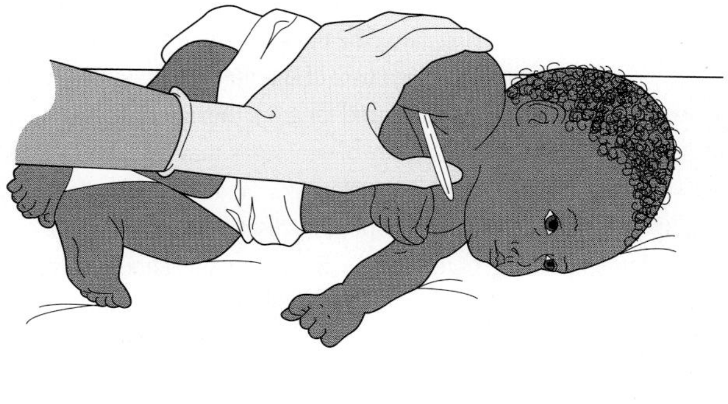

● **Figure 25–16** Axillary temperature measurement. The thermometer should remain in place for 3 minutes. The nurse presses the newborn's arm tightly but gently against the thermometer and the newborn's side, as illustrated.

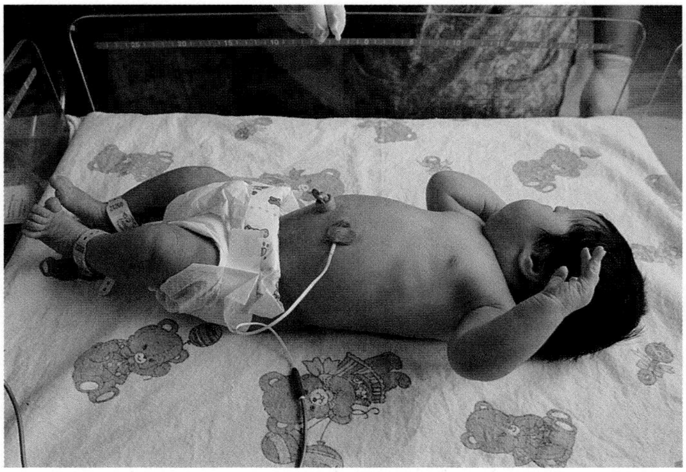

● **Figure 25–17** Temperature monitoring for the newborn. A skin thermal sensor is placed on the newborn's abdomen, upper thigh, or arm and secured with porous tape or a foil-covered foam pad.

SKIN CHARACTERISTICS

Although the newborn's skin color varies with genetic background, all healthy newborns have a pink tinge to their skin. The ruddy hue results from increased red blood cell concentrations in the blood vessels and limited subcutaneous fat deposits.

Skin pigmentation is slight in the newborn period, so color changes may be seen even in darker skinned babies. Caucasian newborns have a pinkish red skin tone a few hours after birth, and African-American newborns have a reddish-brown skin color. Hispanic and Asian newborns have an olive or yellow skin tone (Creehan, 2008). Skin pigmentation deepens over time; therefore, variations in skin color indicating illness are more difficult to evaluate in African-American and Asian newborns (Creehan, 2008). A newborn who is cyanotic at rest and pink only with crying may have *choanal atresia* (congenital blockage of the passageway between the nose and pharynx). If crying increases the cyanosis, heart or lung problems should be suspected. Very pale newborns may be anemic or have hypovolemia (low BP) and should be evaluated for these problems.

Acrocyanosis (bluish discoloration of the hands and feet) may be present in the first 2 to 6 hours after birth (Figure 25–18 ●). This condition is caused by poor peripheral circulation, which results in vasomotor instability and capillary stasis, especially when the baby is exposed to cold. If the central circulation is adequate, the blood supply should return quickly (2 to 3 seconds) to the extremity after the skin is blanched with a finger. The nurse assesses the face and mucous membranes for pinkness that reflects adequate oxygenation.

Mottling (lacy pattern of dilated blood vessels under the skin) occurs as a result of general circulation fluctuations. It may last several hours to several weeks or may come and go periodically. Mottling may be related to chilling or prolonged apnea, sepsis, or hypothyroidism.

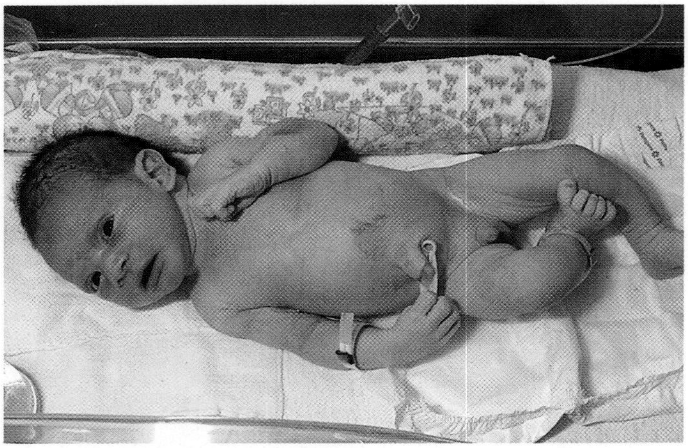

● **Figure 25–18** Acrocyanosis.

Harlequin sign (clown) color change is occasionally noted: A deep red color develops over one side of the newborn's body while the other side remains pale, so that the skin resembles a clown's suit. This color change results from a vasomotor disturbance in which blood vessels on one side dilate while the vessels on the other side constrict. It usually lasts from 1 to 20 minutes. Affected newborns may have single or multiple episodes, but they are transient and clinically insignificant. The nurse should document each occurrence.

Jaundice (yellowish discoloration of skin and mucous membrane) is first detectable on the face (where skin overlies cartilage) and the mucous membranes of the mouth and has a head-to-toe progression (Creehan, 2008). Jaundice advances from head to toe and regresses in the opposite direction. It is evaluated by blanching the tip of the nose, the forehead, the sternum, or the gum line. This procedure must be carried out in appropriate lighting. If jaundice is present, the area will appear yellowish immediately after blanching. Another area to assess for jaundice is the sclera. Evaluation and determination of the cause of jaundice must be initiated immediately to prevent possibly serious sequelae. The jaundice may be related to immature liver function, hematomas, bruises from forceps, blood incompatibility, oxytocin (Pitocin) augmentation or induction, or a severe hemolysis process. Any jaundice noted before a newborn is 24 hours of age should be reported to the physician or neonatal nurse practitioner. Breastfeeding is a possible cause of late onset jaundice. (For discussion of various types of jaundice see Chapter 24∞ and for detailed discussion of causes and treatment for jaundice, see Chapter 29∞.)

Erythema toxicum is an eruption of lesions in the area surrounding a hair follicle that are firm, vary in size from 1 to 3 mm, and consist of a white or pale yellow papule or pustule with an erythematous base. It is often called "newborn rash" or "flea bite" dermatitis. The rash may appear suddenly, usually over the trunk and diaper area, and is frequently widespread (Figure 25–19 ●). The lesions do not appear on the palms of the hands or the soles of the feet. The peak incidence is at 24 to 48 hours of life. The condition rarely presents at birth or after 5 days of life. The cause is unknown, and no treatment is necessary. Some clinicians believe it may be caused by irritation from clothing. The lesions disappear in a few hours or days. If a maculopapular rash appears, a smear of the aspirated papule will show numerous eosinophils on staining; no bacteria will be cultured.

Milia, which are exposed sebaceous glands, appear as raised white spots on the face, especially across the nose (Figure 25–20 ●). No treatment is necessary, because they will clear spontaneously within the first month. Infants of African heritage have a similar condition called transient neonatal pustular melanosis (Thureen, Deacon, Hernandez, et al., 2005).

Skin turgor is assessed to determine hydration status, the need to initiate early feedings, and the presence of any infectious processes. The usual place to assess skin turgor is over the ab-

Evidence-Based Nursing

HYPOXIA IN THE NEWBORN

Clinical Question

How should the nurse assess the newborn for signs of hypoxia?

The Evidence

Rohan & Golombek (2009), a neonatal nurse practitioner and a neonatologist, reviewed existing research and developed a guideline for assessing the newborn for signs of hypoxia. Seventeen research studies were used as support for the guideline, making this the strongest level of evidence for practice. During the transitional stage from intrauterine to extrauterine life, neonates require close monitoring so that the nurse can recognize signs of hypoxia and intervene appropriately. Hypoxia means inadequate oxygenation is occurring at the cellular level and is most commonly characterized by cyanosis. The blue discoloration typical of cyanosis may be exhibited on the skin, tongue, or mucous membranes. Lack of cyanosis does not always mean the baby is healthy, though, because newborns can tolerate a large decrease in oxygenation without evidence of cyanosis.

Best Practice

Assessment of the neonate should begin with as many noninvasive and nonintrusive measures as possible, so that the baby's respiratory status can be evaluated in his or her noncrying state. The nurse should distinguish between acrocyanosis (normal peripheral cyanosis of the hands and feet) and central cyanosis (of mucous membranes and tongue). The latter is a much more serious sign. A decrease in the stability of vital signs may be the first sign of hypoxia when cyanosis is absent. Either tachycardia or bradycardia may indicate problems with oxygenation. Respiratory distress may be evidenced by tachypnea, grunting, flaring, or retractions. Breath sounds should be auscultated over all lung fields. O_2 saturation levels should be measured at both preductal (right hand) and postductal (left arm and lower extremities) sites.

Critical Thinking

What conditions in the maternal or birth history might indicate to the nurse that the neonate is at risk of hypoxia?

See MyNursingKit for possible responses.

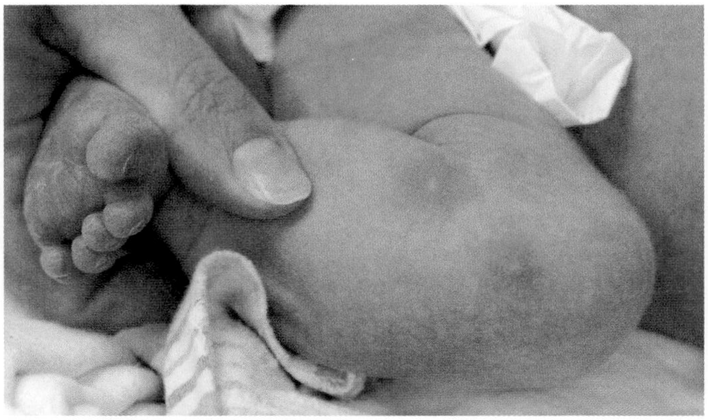

● **Figure 25–19** Erythema toxicum on leg.

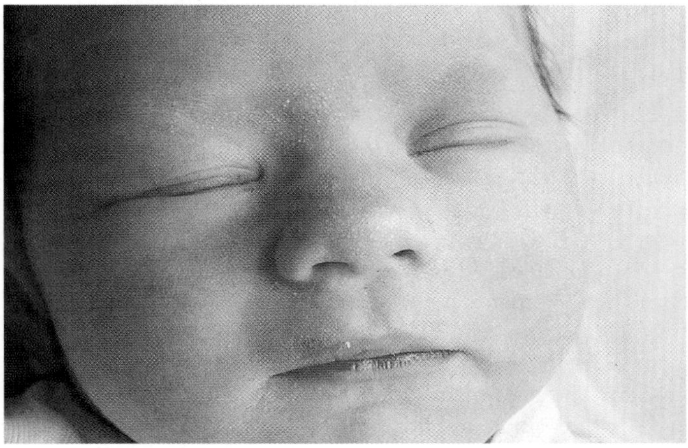

● **Figure 25–20** Facial milia.

domen, forearm, or thigh. Skin should be elastic and should return rapidly to its original shape.

Vernix caseosa, a whitish, cheeselike substance, covers the fetus while in utero and lubricates the skin of the newborn. The skin of the term or postterm newborn has less vernix and is frequently dry; peeling is common, especially on the hands and feet.

Forceps marks may be present after a difficult forceps birth. The newborn may have reddened areas over the cheeks and jaws. It is important to reassure the parents that these marks will disappear, usually within 1 or 2 days. Transient facial paralysis resulting from the forceps pressure is a rare complication. Vacuum extractor suction marks on the vertex of the scalp are often seen when vacuum extractors are used to assist with the birth. These marks are benign and do not indicate underlying brain lesions.

BIRTHMARKS

Telangiectatic nevi (stork bites) appear as pale pink or red spots and are frequently found on the eyelids, nose, lower occipital bone, and nape of the neck (Figure 25–21 ●). These lesions are common in newborns with light complexions and are more noticeable during periods of crying. These areas have no clinical significance and usually fade by the second birthday.

Mongolian spots are macular areas of bluish black or gray-blue pigmentation on the dorsal area and the buttocks (Fig-

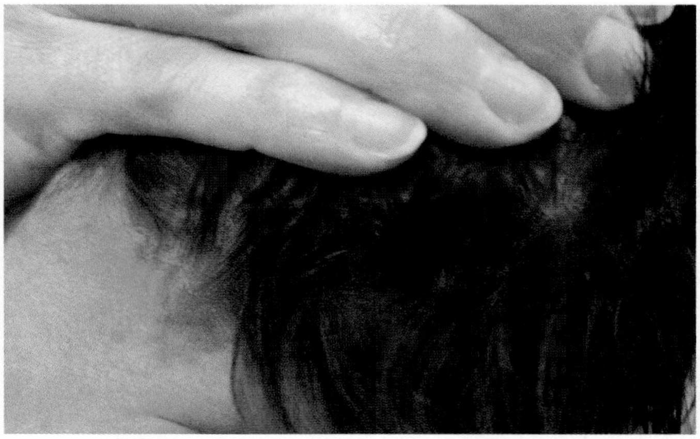

● **Figure 25–21** Stork bites on nape of neck.

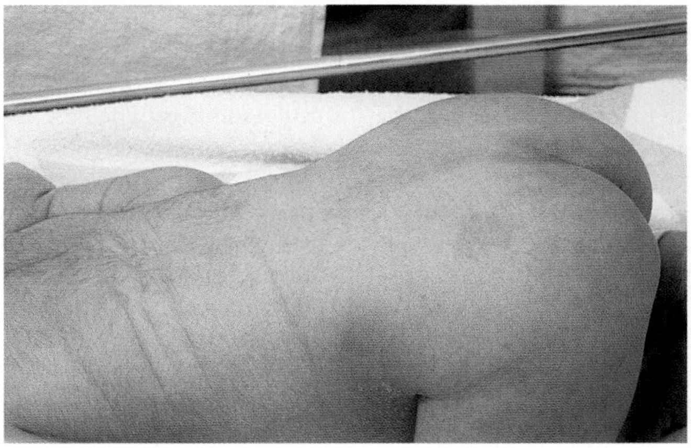

● **Figure 25–22** Mongolian spots.

ure 25–22 ●). They are common in newborns of Asian, Hispanic, and African descent and other dark-skin races. They gradually fade during the first or second year of life. They may be mistaken for bruises and should be documented in the newborn's chart.

Nevus flammeus (port-wine stain) is a capillary angioma directly below the epidermis. It is a nonelevated, sharply demarcated, red-to-purple area of dense capillaries (Figure 25–23 ●). In infants of African descent, it may appear as a purple-black stain. The size and shape vary, but it commonly appears on the face. It does not grow in size, does not fade with time, and does not blanch as a rule. The birthmark may be concealed by using an opaque cosmetic cream. If convulsions and other neurologic problems accompany the nevus flammeus, the clinical picture is suggestive of *Sturge-Weber syndrome,* with involvement of the fifth cranial nerve (the ophthalmic branch of the trigeminal nerve).

Nevus vasculosus (strawberry mark) is a capillary hemangioma. It consists of newly formed and enlarged capillaries in the dermal and subdermal layers. It is a raised, clearly delineated, dark red, rough-surfaced birthmark commonly found in the head region. Such marks usually grow (often rapidly) starting during the second or third week of life and may not reach their fullest size for 1 to 3 months (Thureen, et al., 2005). They begin to shrink and start to resolve spontaneously several weeks to months after they

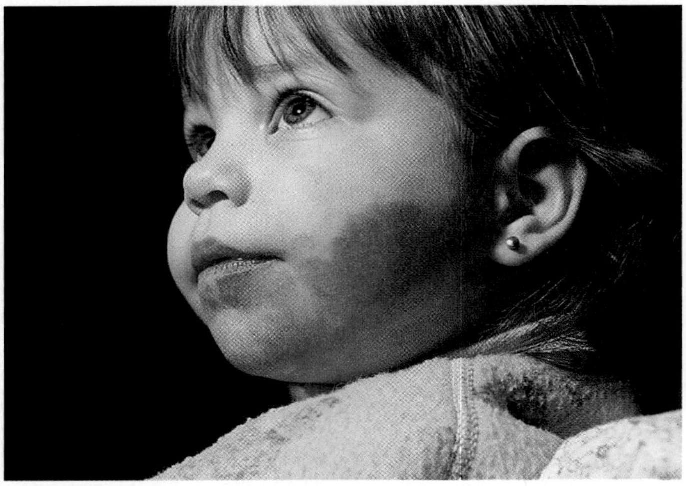

● **Figure 25–23** Port-wine stain.

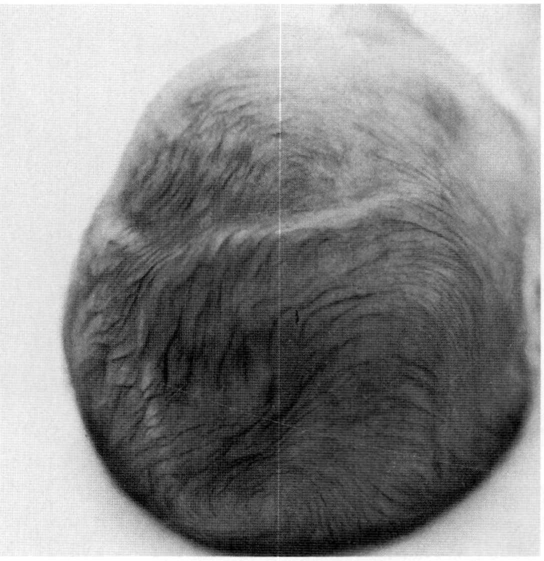

● **Figure 25–24** Molding. Overlapped cranial bones produce a visible ridge in a small, premature newborn. Easily visible overlapping does not occur often in term infants.

Source: Korones, S. B. (1986). *High-risk newborn infants* (4th ed.). St. Louis: Mosby.

reach peak growth. A pale purple or gray spot on the surface of the hemangioma signals the start of resolution. The best cosmetic effect is achieved when the lesions are allowed to resolve spontaneously.

Birthmarks are frequently a cause of concern for parents. The mother may be especially anxious, fearing that she is to blame ("Is my baby 'marked' because of something I did?"). Guilt feelings are common in the presence of misconceptions about the cause. Birthmarks should be identified and explained to the parents. By providing appropriate information about the cause and course of birthmarks, the nurse frequently relieves the fears and anxieties of the family. The nurse should note any bruises, abrasions, or birthmarks seen on admission to the nursery.

HEAD

General Appearance

The newborn's head is large (approximately one-fourth of the body size), with soft, pliable cranial skull bones. For most term infants, the occipital-frontal circumference (OFC) is 32 to 37 cm (12.6 to 14.6 in.). The head may appear asymmetrical in the newborn of a vertex birth. This asymmetry, called **molding**, is caused by the overriding of the cranial bones during labor and birth (Figure 25–24 ●). The degree of molding varies with the amount and length of pressure exerted on the head. Within a few days after birth, the overriding usually diminishes and the suture lines become palpable. Because head measurements are affected by molding, a second measurement is indicated a few days after birth. The heads of breech-born newborns and those born by elective cesarean are characteristically round and well-shaped because no pressure was exerted on them during birth. Any extreme differences in head size may indicate microcephaly (abnormally small head) or hydrocephalus (an abnormal buildup of fluid in the brain). Variations in the shape, size, or appearance of the head measurements may be caused by *craniosynostosis* (premature closure of the cranial sutures), which will need to be corrected through surgery to allow brain growth, and *plagiocephaly* (asymmetry caused by pressure on the fetal head during gestation) (Thureen, et al., 2005).

Two *fontanelles* ("soft spots") may be palpated on the newborn's head. Fontanelles, which are openings at the juncture of the cranial bones, can be measured with the fingers. Accurate measurement necessitates that the examiner's finger be measured in centimeters. The assessment should be carried out with the newborn in a sitting position and not crying. The *diamond-shaped anterior fontanelle* is approximately 3 to 4 cm long by 2 to 3 cm wide. It is located at the juncture of the frontal and parietal bones. The *posterior fontanelle,* smaller and triangular, is formed by the parietal bones and the occipital bone and is 0.5 by 1 cm. Because of molding, the fontanelles are smaller immediately after birth than several days later. The anterior fontanelle closes within 18 months, whereas the posterior fontanelle closes within 8 to 12 weeks.

The fontanelles are a useful indicator of the newborn's condition. The anterior fontanelle may swell when the newborn cries or passes a stool or may pulsate with the heartbeat, which is normal. A bulging fontanelle usually signifies increased intracranial pressure, and a depressed fontanelle indicates dehydration (Creehan, 2008).

The sutures between the cranial bones should be palpated for the amount of overlapping. In newborns whose growth has been restricted the sutures may be wider than normal, and the fontanelles may also be larger because of impaired growth of the cranial bones. In addition to inspecting the newborn's head for degree of molding and size, the nurse should evaluate it for soft tissue edema and bruising.

Cephalohematoma

Cephalohematoma is a collection of blood resulting from ruptured blood vessels between the surface of a cranial bone (usually parietal) and the periosteal membrane (Figure 25–25 ●). The scalp in these areas feels loose and slightly edematous. These areas emerge as defined hematomas between the first and second day. Although external pressure may cause the mass to fluctuate, it does not increase in size when the newborn cries. Cephalohematomas may be unilateral or bilateral and do not cross suture lines. They are relatively common in vertex births and may disappear within 2 weeks to 3 months. They may be associated with physiologic jaundice, because extra red blood cells are being destroyed within the cephalohematoma. A large cephalohematoma can lead to anemia and hypotension.

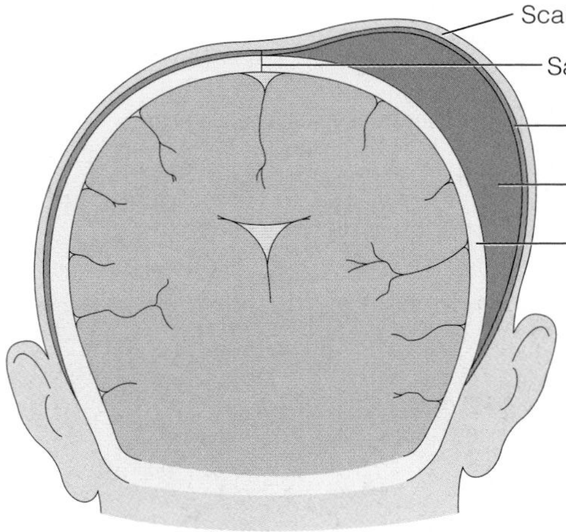

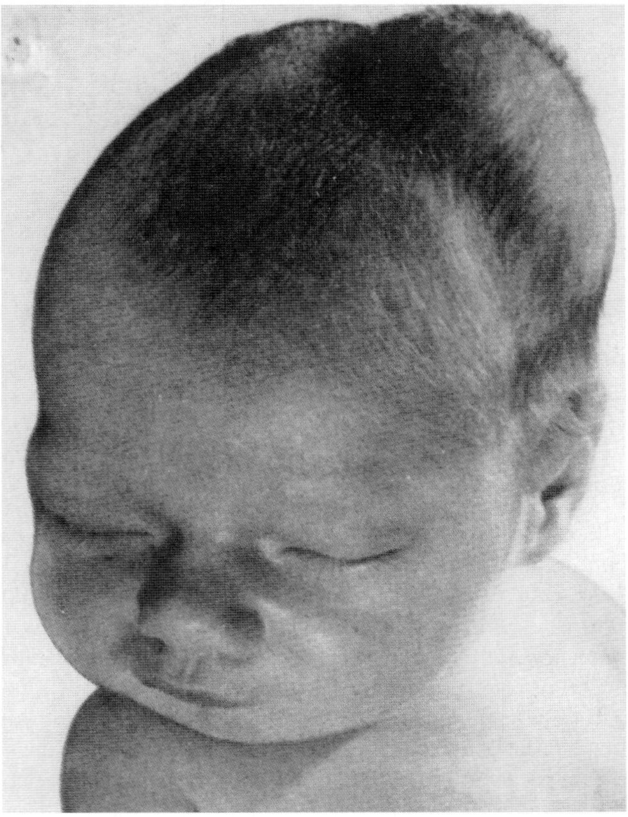

● **Figure 25–25** Cephalohematoma. Cephalohematoma is a collection of blood between the surface of a cranial bone and the periosteal membrane. This is a cephalohematoma over the left parietal bone.

Source: Potter, E. L., & Craig, J. M. (1975). *Pathology of the fetus and infant* (3rd ed.). Chicago: Year Book Medical Publishers. Reproduced with permission.

Caput Succedaneum

Caput succedaneum is a localized, easily identifiable, soft area of the scalp, generally resulting from a long and difficult labor or vacuum extraction. The sustained pressure of the presenting part against the cervix results in compression of local blood vessels, and venous return is slowed. Slowed venous return in turn causes an increase in tissue fluids, an edematous swelling, and occasional bleeding under the periosteum. The caput may vary from a small area to a severely elongated head. The fluid in the caput is reabsorbed within 12 hours to a few days after birth. Caputs resulting from vacuum extractors are sharply outlined, circular areas up to 2 cm (0.8 in.) thick. They disappear more slowly than naturally occurring edema. It is possible to distinguish between a cephalohematoma and a caput because the caput overrides suture lines (Figure 25–26 ●), whereas the cephalohematoma, because of its location, never crosses a suture line. Also, caput succedaneum is present at birth, whereas cephalohematoma generally is not. See Table 25–3.

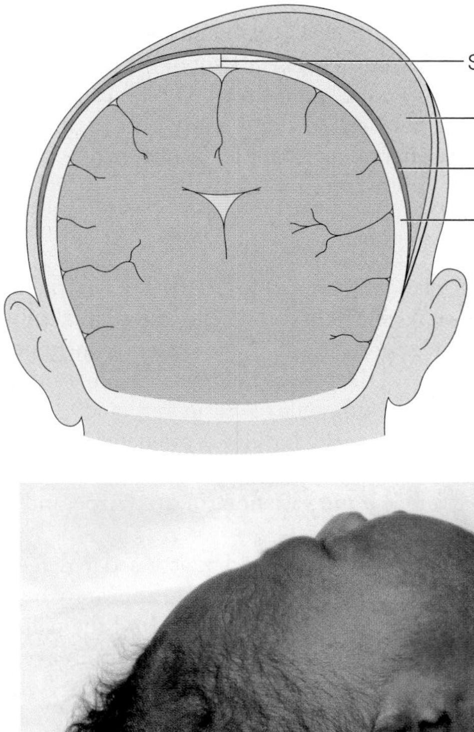

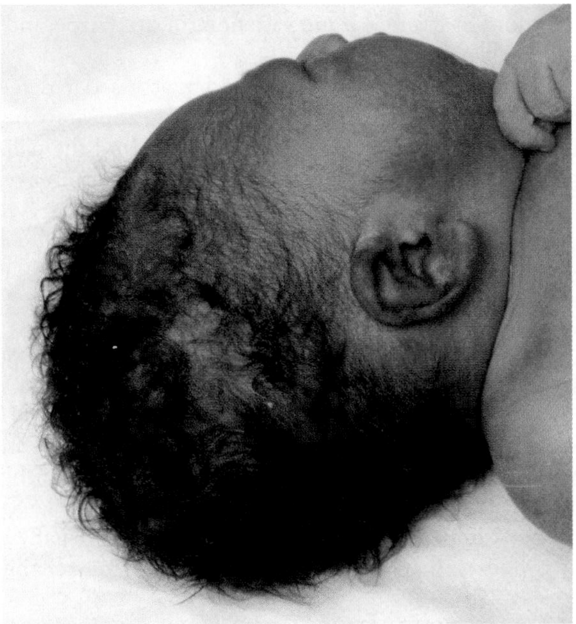

● **Figure 25–26** Caput succedaneum. Caput succedaneum is a collection of fluid (serum) under the scalp.

Table 25–3 Comparison of Cephalohematoma and Caput Succedaneum

Cephalohematoma	Caput Succedaneum
Collection of blood between cranial (usually parietal) bone and periosteal membrane	Collection of fluid, edematous swelling of the scalp
Caused by subperiosteal hemorrhage	Causes by pressure of the fetal head against the cervix during labor, which decreases blood flow to the area and results in edema
Does not cross suture lines	Crosses suture lines
Appears on first and second day, increases in size for 2–3 days	Present at birth or shortly thereafter, does not increase in size
Disappears after 2 to 3 weeks or may take months	Reabsorbed within 12 hours or a few days after birth

HAIR

The term newborn's hair is smooth with texture variations depending on ethnic background (Creehan, 2008). Scalp hair is usually high over the eyebrows. Assessment of the newborn's hair characteristics such as color, quantity, texture, hairlines, direction of growth, and hair whorls can identify genetic, metabolic, and neurologic disorders. For example, coarse, brittle, and dry hair may indicate hypothyroidism.

FACE

The newborn's face is well designed to help the newborn suckle. Sucking (fat) pads are located in the cheeks, and a labial tubercle (sucking callus) is frequently found in the center of the upper lip. The chin is recessed, and the nose is flattened. The lips are sensitive to touch, and the sucking reflex is easily initiated.

Symmetry of the eyes, nose, and ears is evaluated. See the "Assessment Guide: Newborn Physical Assessment" on pages 588–599 for deviations in symmetry and variations in size, shape, and spacing of facial features.

Facial movement symmetry should be assessed to determine the presence of facial palsy. Facial paralysis appears when the newborn cries; the affected side is immobile, and the palpebral (eyelid) fissure widens (Figure 25–27 ●). Paralysis may result from forceps-assisted birth or pressure on the facial nerve from the maternal pelvis during birth. Facial paralysis usually disappears within a few days to 3 weeks, although in some cases it may be permanent.

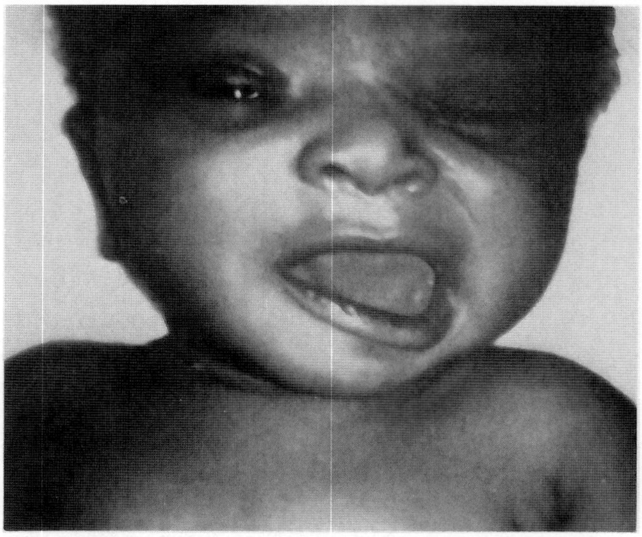

● **Figure 25–27** Facial paralysis. Paralysis of the right side of the face from injury to right facial nerve.

Source: Courtesy of Dr. Ralph Platow. From Potter, E. L., & Craig, J. M. (1975). *Pathology of the fetus and infant* (3rd ed.). Chicago: Year Book Medical Publishers. Reproduced with permission.

EYES

The eyes of the newborn of northern European descent are a blue-gray or slate blue-gray color. Dark-skin newborns tend to have dark eyes at birth. Scleral color tends to be bluish white because of its relative thinness. A blue sclera is associated with osteogenesis imperfecta. The infant's eye color is usually established at approximately 3 months, although it may change any time up to 1 year.

The eyes should be checked for size, equality of pupil size, reaction of pupils to light, blink reflex to light, and edema and inflammation of the eyelids. The eyelids are usually edematous during the first few days of life because of the pressure associated with birth.

Erythromycin is frequently used prophylactically instead of silver nitrate and usually does not cause chemical irritation of the eye (see Chapter 26 ∞). The instillation of silver nitrate drops in the newborn's eyes may cause edema, and **chemical conjunctivitis** may appear a few hours after instillation, but it disappears in 1 to 2 days. Tetracycline is still used in some institutions (AAP & ACOG, 2007). If infectious conjunctivitis exists, the newborn has the same purulent (greenish yellow) discharge exudate as in chemical conjunctivitis, but it is caused by gonococcus, *Chlamydia,* staphylococci, or a variety of gram-negative bacteria. It requires treatment with ophthalmic antibiotics. Onset is usually after the second day. Edema of the orbits or eyelids may persist for several days, until the newborn's kidneys can eliminate the fluid.

Small **subconjunctival hemorrhages** appear in about 10% of newborns and are commonly found on the sclera. These hemor-

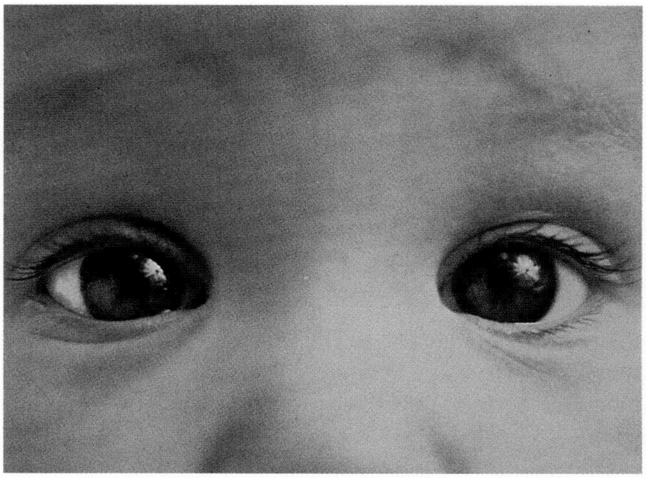

● **Figure 25–28** Transient strabismus. Transient strabismus may be present in the newborn because of poor neuromuscular control.

Source: Photo courtesy of Mead Johnson Laboratories, Evansville, IN.

rhages are caused by the changes in vascular tension or ocular pressure during birth. They will remain for a few weeks and are of no pathologic significance. Parents need reassurance that the newborn is not bleeding from within the eye and that vision will not be impaired.

The newborn may demonstrate transient strabismus caused by poor neuromuscular control of eye muscles (Figure 25–28 ●). It gradually regresses in 3 to 4 months. The "doll's eye" phenomenon is also present for about 10 days after birth. As the newborn's head position is changed to the left and then to the right, the eyes move to the opposite direction. "Doll's eye" results from underdeveloped integration of head-eye coordination.

The nurse should observe the newborn's pupils for opacities or whiteness and for the absence of a normal red retinal reflex. Red retinal reflex is a red-orange flash of color observed when an ophthalmoscope light reflects off the retina. In a newborn with dark skin color, the retina may appear paler or more grayish. The color of the red reflex can also be abnormal with retinoblastoma. Absence of red reflex occurs with cataracts. Congenital cataracts should be suspected in newborns of mothers with a history of rubella, cytomegalic inclusion disease, or syphilis. Brushfield spots (black or white spots on the periphery of the iris) can be associated with Down syndrome (Creehan, 2008).

The cry of the newborn is commonly tearless because the lacrimal structures are immature at birth and are not usually fully functional until the second month of life. However, some babies produce tears during the newborn period.

Poor oculomotor coordination and absence of accommodation limit visual abilities, but newborns have peripheral vision, can fixate on objects near (20.3 to 25.4 cm [8 to 10 in.]) and in front of their face for short periods, can accommodate to large objects (7.6 cm [3 in.] tall by 7.6 cm [3 in.] wide), and can seek out high-contrast geometric shapes. Newborns can perceive faces, shapes, and colors and begin to show visual preferences early. Newborns generally blink in response to bright lights, to a tap on the bridge of the nose (glabellar reflex), or to a light touch on the eyelids. Pupillary light reflex is also present. Examination of the eye is best accomplished by rocking the newborn from an upright position to the horizontal a few times or by other methods, such as diminishing overhead lights, which elicit an opened-eye response.

NOSE

The newborn's nose is small and narrow. Infants are characteristically nose breathers for the first few months of life and generally remove obstructions by sneezing. Nasal patency is ensured if the newborn breathes easily with the mouth closed. If respiratory difficulty occurs, the nurse checks for choanal atresia (congenital blockage of the passageway between nose and pharynx). Historically, choanal atresia can be checked by attempting to gently pass a soft #5 French catheter into both nostrils. Because of possible trauma from the catheter, a cold, flat metal object may instead be held under the nose to observe for fogging (Thureen et al., 2005).

The newborn has the ability to smell after the nasal passages are cleared of amniotic fluid and mucus. Newborns demonstrate this ability by the search for milk. Newborns turn their heads toward a milk source, whether bottle or breast. Newborns react to strong odors, such as alcohol, by turning their heads away or blinking.

MOUTH

The lips of the newborn should be pink, and a touch on the lips should produce sucking motions. Saliva is normally scant. The taste buds develop before birth, and the newborn can easily discriminate between sweet and bitter flavors.

The easiest way to examine the mouth completely is to stimulate infants to cry such as by gently depressing their tongue, thereby causing them to open the mouth fully. It is extremely important to examine the entire mouth to check for a cleft palate, which can be present even in the absence of a cleft lip. The examiner moves a gloved index finger along the hard and soft palate to feel for any openings (Figure 25–29 ●). Glove powder should always be removed before examining the newborn's mouth.

Occasionally, an examination of the gums will reveal *precocious teeth* over the area where the lower central incisor will erupt. If they appear loose, they should be removed to prevent aspiration. Gray-white lesions (inclusion cysts) on the gums may be confused with teeth. On the hard palate and gum margins, **Epstein's pearls**, small glistening white specks (keratin-containing cysts) that feel hard to the touch, are often present. They usually disappear in a few weeks and are of no significance. **Thrush** may appear as white patches that look like milk curds adhering to the mucous membranes and bleeding may occur when patches are removed. Thrush is caused by *Candida albicans,* often acquired from an infected vaginal tract during birth, antibiotic use, or poor handwashing when the mother handles her newborn. Thrush is treated with a preparation of nystatin (Mycostatin).

A newborn who is tongue-tied has a ridge of frenulum tissue attached to the underside of the tongue at varying lengths from its base, causing a heart shape at the tip of the tongue. "Clipping the tongue," or cutting the ridge of tissue, is not currently

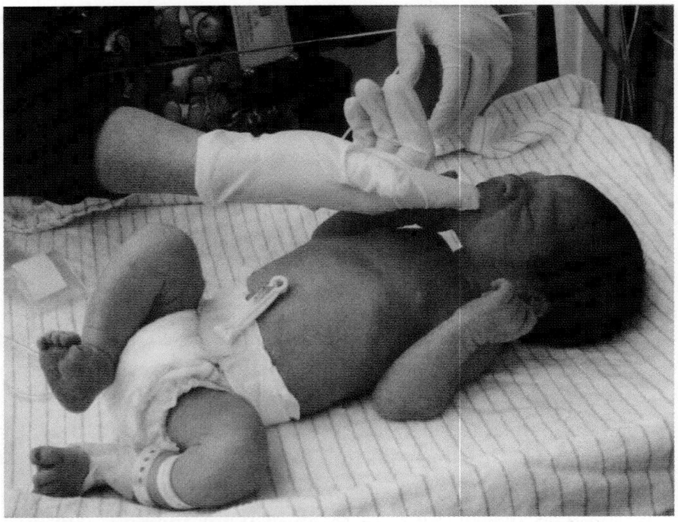

● **Figure 25–29** Examining the mouth. The nurse inserts a gloved index finger into the newborn's mouth and feels for any openings along the hard and soft palates.

Note: Gloves or a finger cot are always worn to examine the palate.

Source: Courtesy of Vanessa Howell, RNC, MSN.

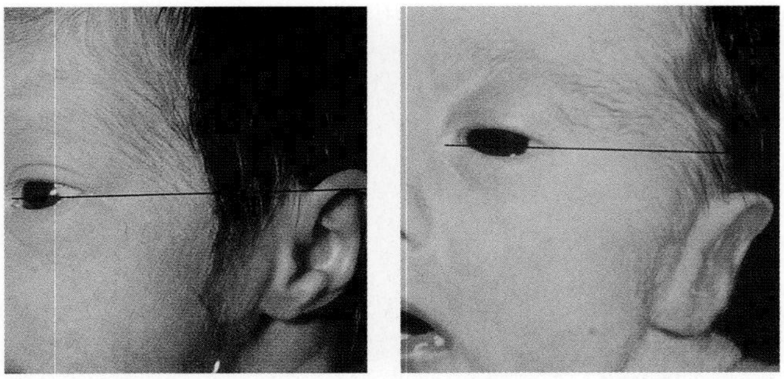

● **Figure 25–30** External ear position. The position of the external ear may be assessed by drawing a line across the inner and outer canthus of the eye to the insertion of the ear. ***A,*** Normal position. ***B,*** True low-set position.

Source: Photo courtesy of Mead Johnson Laboratories, Evansville, IN.

recommended. This ridge does not usually affect speech or eating, but cutting creates an entry for infection (Kliegman, Behrman, Jenson, et al., 2007).

Transient nerve paralysis resulting from birth trauma may be manifested by asymmetrical mouth movements when the newborn cries or by difficulty with sucking and feeding.

EARS

The ears of the newborn are soft and pliable and should recoil readily when folded and released. In the normal newborn, the top of the ear (pinna) should be parallel to the outer and inner canthus of the eye. The ears should be inspected for shape, size, firmness of cartilage, and position. *Low-set ears* are characteristic of many syndromes and may indicate chromosomal abnormalities (especially trisomies 13 and 18), mental retardation, and internal organ abnormalities, especially bilateral renal agenesis as a result of embryologic developmental deviations (Figure 25–30 ●). *Preauricular skin tags* may be present just in front of the ear. Visualization of the tympanic membrane is not usually done soon after birth because blood and vernix block the ear canal.

Following the first cry, the newborn's hearing becomes acute as mucus from the middle ears is absorbed, the eustachian tubes become aerated, and the tympanic membranes become visible. The newborn's hearing initially can be evaluated by noting the baby's response to loud or moderately loud noises that are not accompanied by vibrations. The sleeping newborn should stir or awaken in response to nearby sounds. (This is not a very accurate test, but it may alert the examiner to a possible problem.) The newborn can discriminate the individual characteristics of the human voice and is especially sensitive to sound levels within the normal conversational range. The newborn in a noisy nursery may habituate to the sounds and not stir unless the sound is sudden or much louder than usual.

The AAP has endorsed universal newborn hearing screening (UNHS) before discharge from the birthing unit as the standard of care (Creehan, 2008). If the birth occurs in the home or an alternative birthing center, referral for screening should be made within 1 month of birth.

NECK

A short neck, creased with skin folds, is characteristic of the normal newborn. Because muscle tone is not well developed, the neck cannot support the full weight of the head, which rotates freely. The head lags considerably when the newborn is pulled from a supine to a sitting position, but the prone newborn is able to raise the head slightly. The neck is palpated for masses and the presence of lymph nodes and is inspected for webbing. Adequacy of range of motion and neck muscle function is determined by fully extending the head in all directions. Injury to the sternocleidomastoid muscle (congenital torticollis) must be considered in the presence of neck rigidity.

The nurse evaluates the clavicles for evidence of fractures, which occasionally occur during difficult births or in newborns with broad shoulders. The normal clavicle is straight. If fractured, a lump and a grating sensation (crepitus) during movements may be palpated along the course of the side of the break. The nurse also elicits the Moro reflex (page 585) to evaluate bilateral equal movement of the arms. If the clavicle is fractured, the response will be demonstrated only on the unaffected side.

CHEST

The thorax is cylindric and symmetric at birth, and the ribs are flexible. The general appearance of the chest should be assessed. A protrusion at the lower end of the sternum, called the xiphoid cartilage, is frequently seen. It is under the skin and will become less apparent after several weeks as adipose tissue accumulates.

Engorged breasts occur frequently in both male and female newborns. This condition, which occurs by the third day, is a result of maternal hormonal influences and may last up to 2 weeks (Figure 25–31 ●). A whitish secretion from the nipples may also

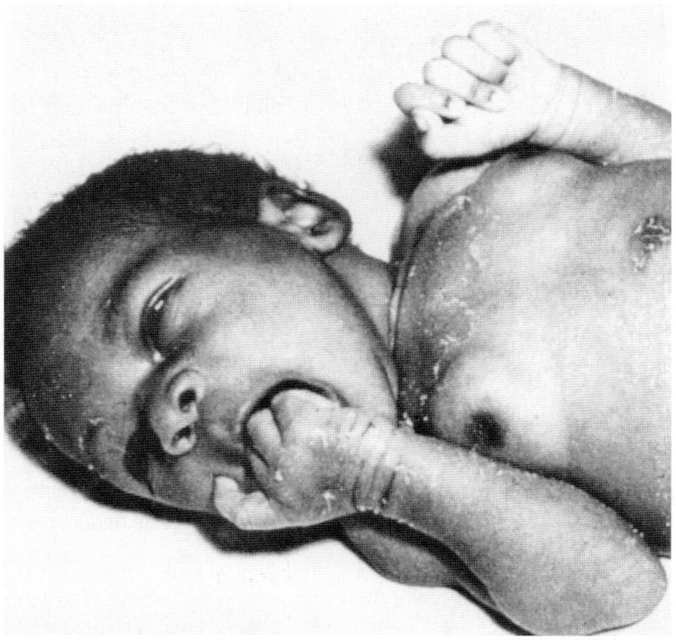

Figure 25–31 Breast hypertrophy.

Source: Korones, S. B. (1986). *High-risk newborn infants* (4th ed.). St. Louis: Mosby.

be noted. The newborn's breast should not be massaged or squeezed, because this may cause a breast abscess. Supernumerary nipples are occasionally noted below and medial to the true nipples. These harmless pink or brown (in dark-skin newborns) spots vary in size and do not contain glandular tissue. Accessory nipples can be differentiated from a pigmented nevi (mole) by placing the fingertips alongside the accessory nipple and pulling the adjacent tissue laterally. The accessory nipple will appear dimpled. At puberty the accessory nipple may darken.

CRY

The newborn's cry should be strong, lusty, and of medium pitch. A high-pitched, shrill cry is abnormal and may indicate neurologic disorders or hypoglycemia. Periods of crying usually vary in length after consoling measures are used. Babies' cries are an important method of communication and alert caregivers to changes in their condition and needs (see Chapter 31 ∞).

RESPIRATION

Normal breathing for a term newborn is 30 to 60 respirations per minute and is predominantly diaphragmatic, with associated rising and falling of the abdomen during inspiration and expiration. The nurse should note any signs of respiratory distress, nasal flaring, intercostal or xiphoid retraction, expiratory grunt or sigh, seesaw respirations, or tachypnea (greater than 60 breaths per minute). Hyperextension (chest appears high) or hypoextension (chest appears low) of the anteroposterior diameter of the chest should also be noted. Both the anterior and posterior chest are auscultated. Some breath sounds are heard best when the newborn is crying, but localizing and identifying breath sounds is difficult in the newborn. Upper airway noises and bowel sounds can be heard over the chest wall, making auscultation difficult. Because sounds may be transmitted from the unaffected lung to the affected lung, the absence of breath sounds may not be diagnosed. Air entry may be noisy in the first couple of hours until lung fluid resolves, especially after cesarean births. Brief periods of apnea (episodic breathing) occur, but no color or heart rate changes occur in healthy, term newborns. Sepsis should be suspected in full-term newborns experiencing apneic episodes.

Nursing Practice

Vital sign assessments are most accurate if the newborn is at rest, so measure pulse and respirations first if the baby is quiet. To soothe a crying baby, try placing your moistened gloved finger in the baby's mouth, and then complete your assessment while the baby suckles.

HEART

Heart rates can be as rapid as 180 beats per minute in newborns and fluctuate a great deal, especially if the baby moves or is startled. The normal range is 120 to 160 beats per minute. The heart is examined for rate and rhythm, position of the apical impulse, and heart sound intensity. Dysrhythmias should be evaluated by the physician.

The pulse rate is variable and is influenced by physical activity, crying, state of wakefulness, and body temperature. Auscultation is performed over the entire heart region (precordium), below the left axilla, and below the scapula. Apical pulse rates are obtained by auscultation for a full minute, preferably when the newborn is asleep.

The placement of the heart in the chest should be determined when the newborn is in a quiet state. The heart is relatively large at birth and is located high in the chest, with its apex somewhere between the fourth and fifth intercostal space.

A shift of heart tones in the mediastinal area to either side may indicate pneumothorax, dextrocardia (heart placement on the right side of the chest), or a diaphragmatic hernia. The experienced nurse can detect these and many other problems early with a stethoscope. Auscultate heart sounds using both the bell and diaphragm of the stethoscope. Normally, the heart beat has a "toc tic" sound. A slur or slushing sound (usually after the first sound) may indicate a *murmur.* Although 90% of all murmurs are transient and are considered normal, they should be monitored closely by a physician. Many murmurs are secondary to closing of patent ductus arteriosus or patent foramen ovale, which should close 1 to 2 days after birth.

In newborns, a low-pitched, musical murmur just to the right of the apex of the heart is fairly common. Occasionally, significant murmurs are heard, such as the murmur of a patent ductus arteriosus, aortic or pulmonary stenosis, or small ventricular septal defect. (See Chapters 28 and 49 ∞ for a discussion of congenital heart defects.)

Peripheral pulses (brachial, femoral, pedal) are also evaluated to detect any lags or unusual characteristics. Brachial

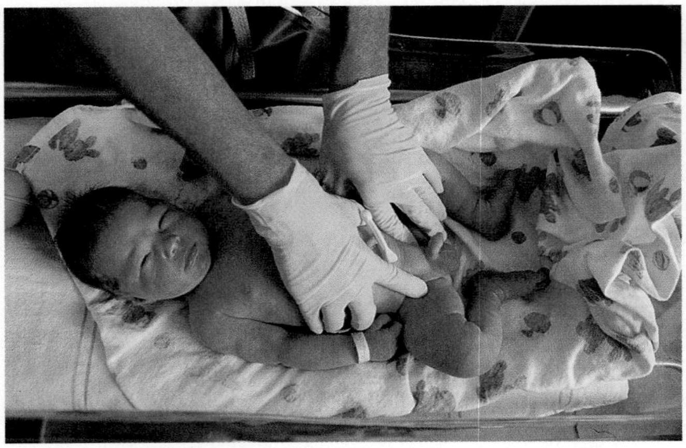

A

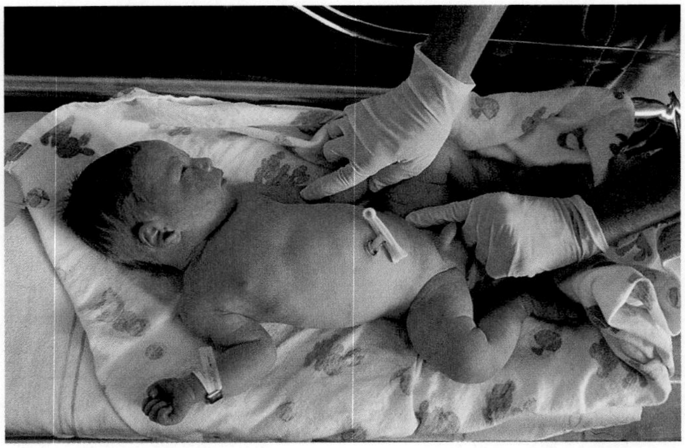

B

● **Figure 25–32** Palpating femoral pulses. ***A,*** Bilaterally palpate the femoral arteries for rate and intensity of the pulses. Press fingertip gently at the groin as shown. ***B,*** Compare the femoral pulses to the brachial pulses by palpating the pulses simultaneously for comparison of rate and intensity.

pulses are palpated bilaterally for equality and compared with the femoral pulses. Femoral pulses are palpated by applying gentle pressure with the middle finger over the femoral canal (Figure 25–32 ●). Decreased or absent femoral pulses may indicate coarctation of the aorta or hypovolemia and require additional evaluation. A wide difference in blood pressure between the upper and lower extremities also indicates coarctation of aorta.

The measurement of blood pressure is best accomplished by using a noninvasive blood pressure device (Figure 25–33 ●). If a blood pressure cuff is used, the newborn's extremities must be immobilized during the assessment, and the cuff should cover two-thirds of the upper arm or upper leg. Movement, crying, and inappropriate cuff size can give inaccurate measurements of the blood pressure.

Blood pressure may not be measured routinely on healthy newborns, but it is essential for newborns who are having distress, are premature, or are suspected of having a cardiac anomaly (Thureen et al., 2005). Infants who have birth asphyxia and are on ventilators have significantly lower systolic and diastolic blood pressures than healthy infants. If a cardiac anomaly is suspected, blood pressure is measured in all four extremities (Table 25–4). At birth, systolic values usually range from 70 to 50 mm Hg and diastolic values from 45 to 30 mm Hg. By the tenth day of life, blood pressure rises to 90/50 mm Hg.

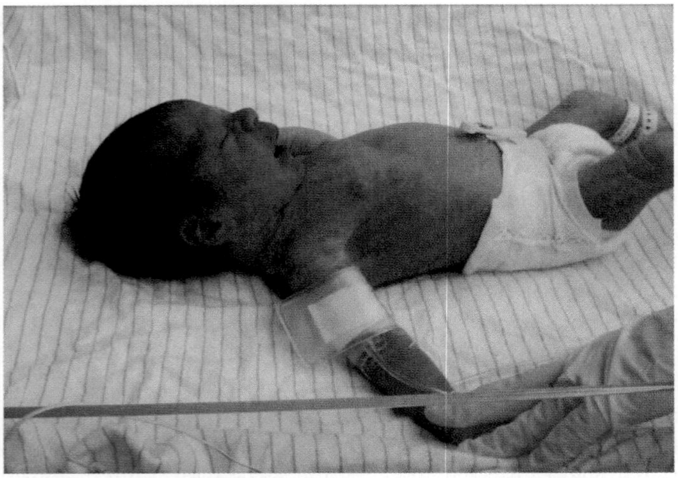

● **Figure 25–33** Blood pressure measurement using a Doppler device. The cuff can be applied to the upper arm or thigh.

Source: Courtesy of Vanessa Howell, RNC, MSN.

Nursing Practice

If possible, obtain blood pressure measurement during quiet sleep or sleep state. Place the cuff on the infant's arm or leg and give the infant time to quiet. Obtain an average of two to three measurements when making clinical decisions. Follow mean blood pressure to monitor changes, as it is less likely to be erroneous. Noninvasive blood pressure may overestimate blood pressure in very low birth weight infants.

ABDOMEN

The nurse can learn a great deal about the newborn's abdomen without disturbing the infant. The abdomen should be cylindrical, protrude slightly, and move with respiration. A certain amount of laxness of the abdominal muscles is normal. A scaphoid (hollow-shaped) appearance suggests the absence of abdominal contents, often seen in diaphragmatic hernias. No cyanosis should be present, and few if any blood vessels should be apparent to the eye. There should be no gross distention or bulging. The more distended the abdomen, the tighter the skin becomes, with engorged vessels appearing. Distention is the first sign of many gastrointestinal abnormalities.

Before palpation of the abdomen, the nurse should auscultate for the presence or absence of bowel sounds in all four quadrants. Bowel sounds may be present by 1 hour after birth. Palpation can cause a transient decrease in bowel sounds intensity.

Table 25–4 Newborn Vital Signs

Pulse
120–160 bpm During sleep as low as 80–100 bpm; if crying, up to 180 bpm Apical pulse counted for 1 full minute
Respirations
30–60 respirations/minute Predominantly diaphragmatic but synchronous with abdominal movements Respirations are counted for 1 full minute
Blood Pressure
70–50/45–30 mm Hg at birth 90/50 mm Hg at day 10
Temperature
Normal range: 36.5°C to 37.5°C (97.7°F to 99.4°F) Axillary: 36.4°C to 37.2°C (97.5°F to 99°F) Skin: 36°C to 36.5°C (96.8°F to 97.7°F) Rectal: 36.6°C to 37.2°C (97.8°F to 99°F)

Abdominal palpation should be done systematically. The nurse palpates each of the four abdominal quadrants and moves in a clockwise direction until all four quadrants have been palpated for softness, tenderness, and the presence of masses. The nurse should place one hand under the back for support during palpation.

UMBILICAL CORD

Initially the umbilical cord is white and gelatinous in appearance, with the two umbilical arteries and one umbilical vein readily apparent. Because a single umbilical artery is frequently associated with congenital anomalies, the nurse should count the vessels during the newborn assessment. The cord begins drying within 1 or 2 hours of birth and is shriveled and blackened by the second or third day. Within 7 to 10 days it sloughs off, although a granulating area may remain for a few days longer. (Care of the umbilical cord is discussed in Chapter 26.)

Cord bleeding is abnormal and may result because the cord was inadvertently pulled or the cord clamp was loosened. Foul-smelling drainage is also abnormal and is generally caused by infection, which requires immediate treatment to prevent septicemia. If the newborn has a patent urachus (abnormal connection between the umbilicus and bladder), moistness or draining urine may be apparent at the base of the cord. Another umbilical cord anomaly that can occur is umbilical cord hernia and associated patent omphalomesenteric duct (Figure 25–34 ●). Umbilical hernias are more common in infants of African American descent than in Caucasian infants (Thureen et al., 2005).

Serous or serosanguineous drainage that continues after the cord falls off may indicate a granuloma. It appears as a small red button deep in the umbilicus. Treatment involves cauterization by a healthcare provider with a topical silver nitrate stick (Thureen et al., 2005).

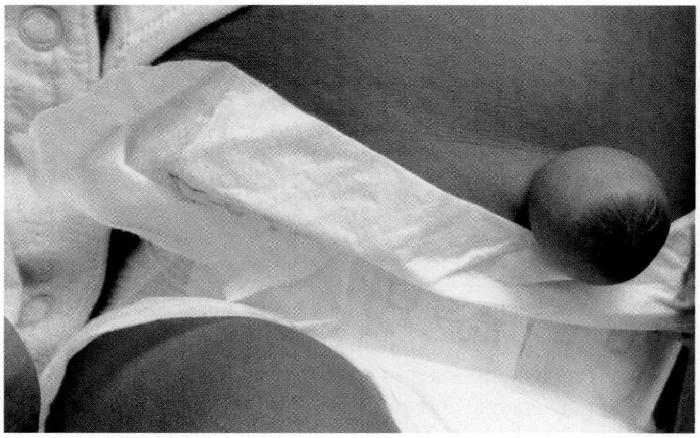

● **Figure 25–34** Umbilical hernia.

Developing Cultural Competence

RITUALS INVOLVING THE UMBILICAL CORD

In the Woodland Indian tribe, upon birth, the umbilical cord is tied and a small piece is saved. This section of the umbilical cord is sewn into a deerskin diamond-shaped pocket. The pocket is hung over the infant's crib to provide protection for the infant.

GENITALS

Female Infants

Examine the labia majora, labia minora, and clitoris and note the size of each as appropriate for gestational age. A vaginal tag or hymenal tag is often evident and will usually disappear in a few weeks. During the first week of life, the female newborn may have a vaginal discharge composed of thick, whitish mucus. This discharge, which can become tinged with blood, is called **pseudomenstruation** and is caused by the withdrawal of maternal hormones. *Smegma,* a white, cheeselike substance, is often present between the labia. Do not remove it because it may traumatize tender tissue.

Male Infants

The nurse inspects the penis to determine whether the urinary orifice is correctly positioned. *Hypospadias* occurs when the urinary meatus is located on the ventral surface of the penis or *epispadias* (meatus is on the dorsal surface of the glans). Hypospadias occurs most commonly among people of Western European descent. *Phimosis* is a condition in which the opening of the foreskin (prepuce) is small and the foreskin cannot be pulled back over the glans at all. This condition may interfere with urination, so the adequacy of the urinary stream should be evaluated.

The scrotum is inspected for size and symmetry. Scrotal color variations are especially prominent in African American, Indian, and Hispanic newborns (Creehan, 2008). The scrotum should be

Nursing Practice

Always examine more closely any infant who is reluctant to move an extremity. Fractures are often asymptomatic in the newborn. Paralytic injuries are characterized by immobility of an extremity.

palpated to verify the presence of both testes and to rule out *cryptorchidism* (failure of testes to descend). The testes are palpated separately between the thumb and forefinger, with the thumb and forefinger of the other hand placed together over the inguinal canal. Scrotal edema and discoloration are common in breech births. *Hydrocele* (a collection of fluid surrounding the testes in the scrotum) is common in newborns and should be identified. It usually resolves without intervention. The presence of a discolored or dusky scrotum and solid testis should raise the suspicion of testicular torsion which should be reported immediately.

ANUS

The anal area is inspected to verify that it is patent and has no fissure. Imperforate anus and rectal atresia may be ruled out by observation. Digital examination, if necessary, is done by a physician or nurse practitioner. The nurse also notes the passage of the first meconium stool. Atresia of the gastrointestinal tract or meconium ileus with resultant obstruction must be considered if the newborn does not pass meconium in the first 24 hours of life.

EXTREMITIES

Extremities are examined for gross deformities, extra digits or webbing, clubfoot, and range of motion. Normal newborn extremities appear short, are generally flexible, and move symmetrically.

Arms and Hands

Nails extend beyond the fingertips in term newborns. The nurse should count fingers and toes. *Polydactyly* is the presence of extra digits on either the hands or the feet. *Syndactyly* refers to fusion (webbing) of fingers or toes. The hands are inspected for normal palmar creases. A single palmar crease, called *simian line* (see Chapter 7, Figure 7–18B), is frequently present in children with Down syndrome.

Brachial palsy, paralysis of portions of the arm, results from trauma to the brachial plexus during a difficult birth. It occurs commonly when strong traction is exerted on the head of the newborn in an attempt to deliver a shoulder lodged behind the symphysis pubis in the presence of shoulder dystocia. Brachial palsy may also occur during a breech birth if an arm becomes trapped over the head and traction is exerted.

The portion of the arm affected is determined by the nerves damaged. **Erb-Duchenne paralysis (Erb's palsy)** involves damage to the upper arm (fifth and sixth cervical nerves) and is the most common type. Injury to the eighth cervical and first thoracic nerve roots and the *lower portion* of the plexus produces the relatively rare lower arm injury. The *whole-arm type* results from damage to the entire plexus.

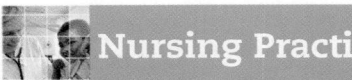

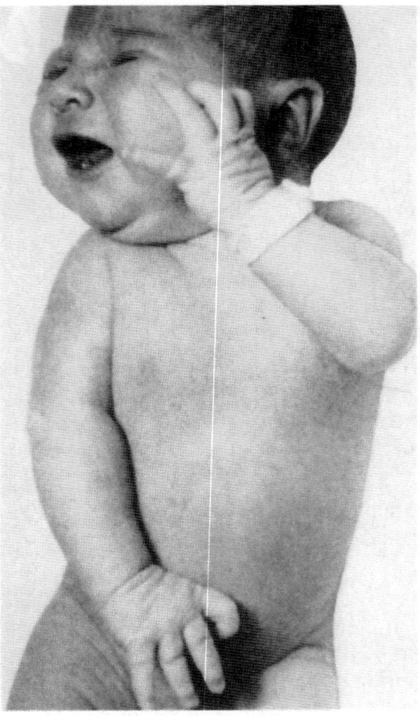

● **Figure 25–35** Right Erb's palsy. This palsy resulting from injury to the fifth and sixth cervical roots of the brachial plexus.

Source: Potter, E. L., & Craig, J. M. (1975). *Pathology of the fetus and infant* (3rd ed.). Chicago: Year Book Medical Publishers. Reproduced with permission.

With Erb-Duchenne paralysis the newborn's arm lies limply at the side. The elbow is held in extension, with the forearm pronated. The newborn is unable to elevate the arm, and the Moro reflex cannot be elicited on the affected side (Figure 25–35 ●). Lower arm injury causes paralysis of the hand and wrist; complete paralysis of the limb occurs with the whole-arm type.

Carefully instruct the parents in the correct method of performing passive range of motion exercises (to prevent muscle contractures and restore function) and arrange supervised practice sessions for the parents and referral to physical therapy follow-up within 2 weeks of discharge. In more severe cases, splinting of the arm is indicated until the edema decreases. The arm is held in a position of abduction and external rotation with the elbow flexed 90 degrees, often called the "Statue of Liberty" position and a "Statue of Liberty" splint is commonly used. Prognosis is related to the degree of nerve damage resulting from trauma and hemorrhage within the nerve sheath. Complete recovery occurs within a few months with minimal trauma. Moderate trauma may result in partial paralysis. Recovery is unlikely with severe trauma, and muscle wasting may develop.

Legs and Feet

The legs of the newborn should be of equal length, with symmetrical skin folds. However, they may assume a "fetal posture" secondary to position in utero, and it may take several days for the legs to relax into a normal position. To evaluate for hip dislocation or hip instability, the Ortolani and Barlow maneuvers are performed. The nurse (or more commonly, the physician or nurse practitioner) performs the **Ortolani's maneuver** to rule out the possibility of developmental dysplastic hip, also called congenital hip dysplasia (hip dislocatability). With the newborn relaxed and quiet on a firm surface, with hips and knees flexed at a 90-degree angle, the experienced nurse grasps the infant's thigh with the middle finger over the greater trochanter and lifts the thigh to bring the femoral head from its posterior position toward the acetabulum. With gentle abduction of the thigh, the femoral head is returned to the acetabulum. Simultaneously, the examiner feels a sense of reduction or a "clunk" as the femoral head returns. This reduction is palpable and may be heard. With **Barlow's maneuver**, the healthcare provider grasps and adducts the infant's thigh and applies gentle downward pressure. Dislocation is felt as the femoral head slips out of the acetabulum. The femoral head is then returned to the acetabulum using the Ortolani maneuver, confirming the diagnosis of an unstable or dislocatable hip (Figure 25–36 ●).

Examine the feet for evidence of a talipes deformity (clubfoot). Intrauterine position frequently causes the feet to appear to turn inward (Figure 25–37 ●); this is termed a "*positional*" *clubfoot*. If the feet can easily be returned to the midline by manipulation, no treatment is indicated and the nurse teaches range of motion exercises to the family. Further evaluation is indicated when the foot will not turn to a midline position or align readily. This is considered the most severe type of "true clubfoot," or talipes equinovarus.

BACK

With the newborn prone, examine the back. The spine should appear straight and flat, because the lumbar and sacral curves do not develop until the newborn begins to sit. The base of the spine is examined for a dermal sinus. A nevus pilosus ("hairy nerve")

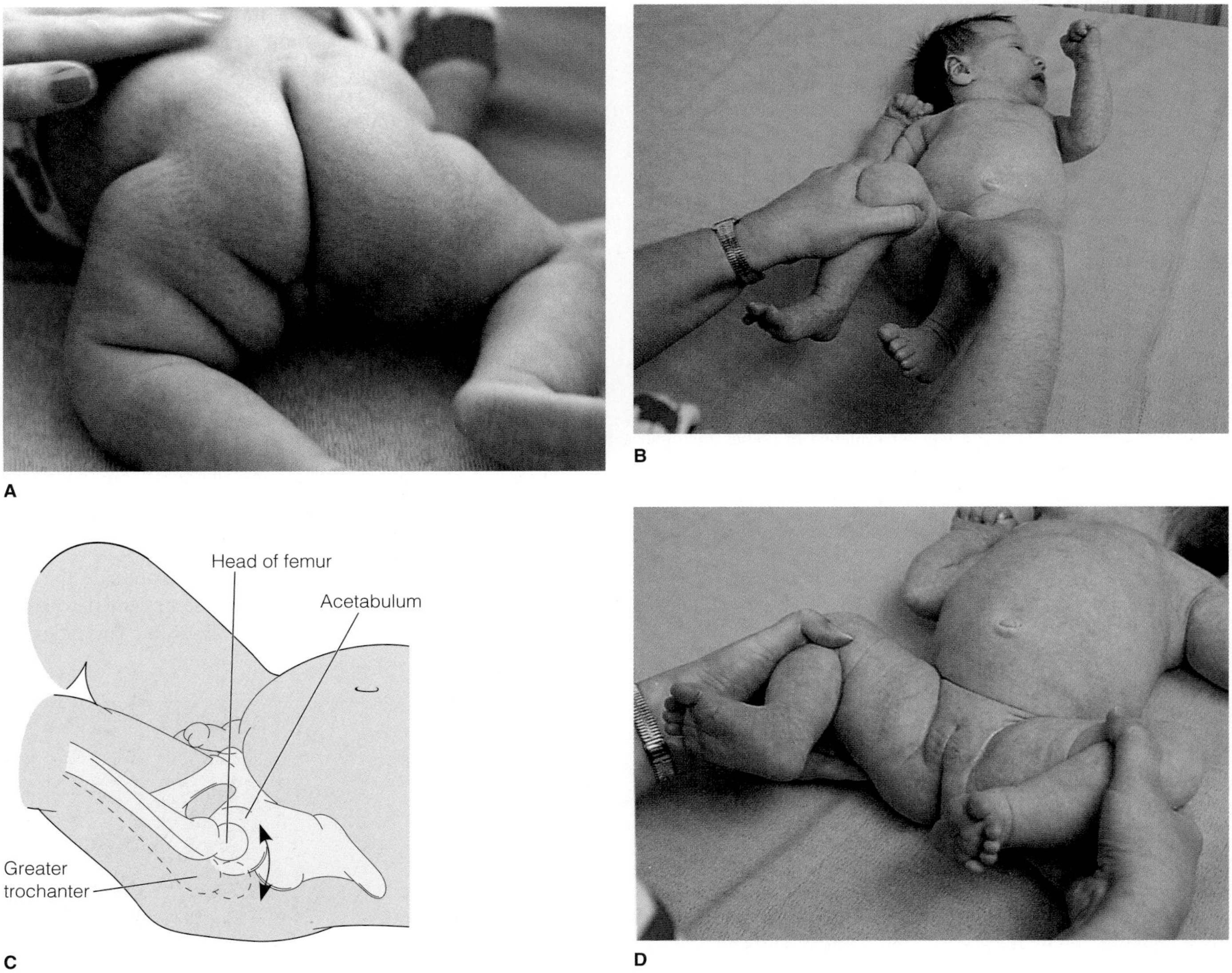

● **Figure 25–36** Barlow and Ortolani maneuvers. ***A,*** The asymmetry of gluteal and thigh fat folds seen in infant with left developmental dysplasia of the hip. ***B,*** Barlow's (dislocation) maneuver. Baby's thigh is grasped and adducted (placed together) with gentle downward pressure. ***C,*** Dislocation is palpable as femoral head slips out of acetabulum. ***D,*** The Ortolani maneuver puts downward pressure on the hip and then inward rotation. If the hip is dislocated, this maneuver will force the femoral head back into the acetabular rim with a noticeable "clunk."

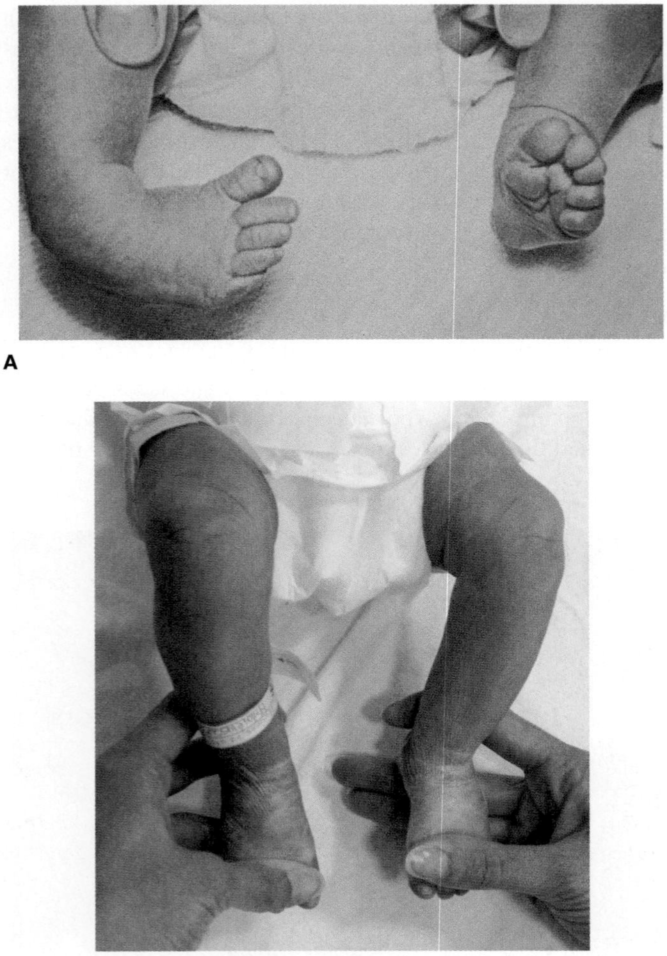

A

B

● **Figure 25–37** Examining feet for evidence of talipes deformity. ***A,*** Unilateral talipes equinovarus (clubfoot). ***B,*** To determine the presence of clubfoot, the nurse moves the foot to the midline. Resistance indicates true clubfoot.

Source: ***A.*** Used with permission from Mead Johnson Nutritionals, Evansville, IN.

is occasionally found at the base of the spine in newborns. It is significant because it is frequently associated with spina bifida.

ASSESSMENT OF NEUROLOGIC STATUS

MyNursingKit Newborn Reflex Videos

The neurologic examination should begin with a period of observation, noting the general physical characteristics and behaviors of the newborn. Important behaviors to assess are the *state of alertness, resting posture, cry,* and *quality of muscle tone and motor activity.*

The usual position of the newborn is with partially flexed extremities, with the legs abducted to the abdomen. When awake, the newborn may exhibit purposeless, uncoordinated bilateral movements of the extremities. If these movements are absent, minimal, or obviously asymmetrical, neurologic dysfunction should be suspected. Eye movements are observable during the first few days of life. An alert newborn is able to fixate on faces and brightly colored objects. Shining a bright light in the newborn's eyes elicits the blinking response.

Evaluate muscle tone by moving various parts of the body while the head of the newborn is in a neutral position. The newborn is somewhat hypertonic; that is, there should be resistance to extending the elbow and knee joints. Muscle tone should be symmetrical. Diminished muscle tone and flaccidity require further evaluation.

Tremors or jitteriness (tremor-like movements) in the full-term newborn must be evaluated to differentiate the tremors from convulsions. Tremors may also be related to hypoglycemia, hypocalcemia, or substance withdrawal. Environmental stimuli may initiate tremors. Jitteriness may be distinguished from tonic-clonic seizure activity because it usually can be stopped by the infant's sucking on the extremity or by the nurse holding or flexing the involved extremity. A fine jumping of the muscle is likely to be a central nervous system disorder and requires further evaluation. Newborn seizures may consist of no more than chewing or swallowing movements, deviations of the eyes, rigidity, or flaccidity because of CNS immaturity. In contrast to tremors, seizures are not usually initiated by stimuli, and cannot be stopped by holding.

Specific deep tendon reflexes can be elicited in the newborn but have limited value unless they are obviously asymmetric. The knee jerk is typically brisk; a normal ankle clonus may involve three or four beats. Plantar flexion is present.

The immature CNS of the newborn is characterized by a variety of reflexes. Because the newborn's movements are uncoordinated, methods of communication are limited, and control of bodily functions is restricted, the reflexes serve a variety of purposes. Some are protective (blink, gag, sneeze), some aid in feeding (rooting, sucking) and may not be very active if the infant has eaten recently, and some stimulate human interaction (grasping). See the "Assessment Guide: Newborn Physical Assessment" on pages 588–599 in this chapter for a summary of stimulus for, alternations for, and possible causes of common newborn reflexes.

The most common reflexes found in the normal newborn are the following:

- The **tonic neck reflex** (fencer position) is elicited when the newborn is supine and the head is turned to one side. In response, the extremities on the same side straighten, whereas on the opposite side they flex (Figure 25–38 ●). This reflex

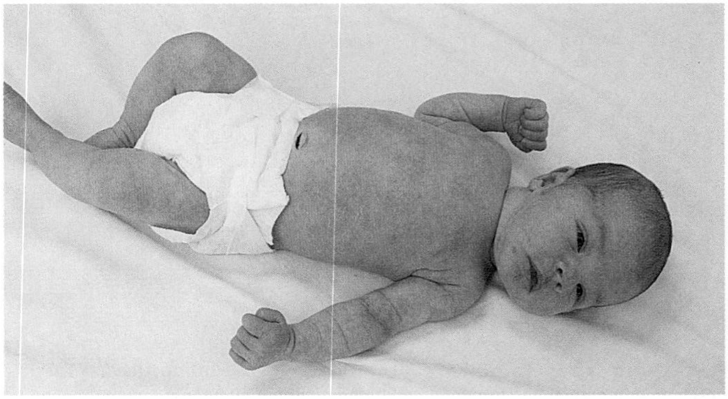

● **Figure 25–38** Tonic neck reflex.

Source: © Stella Johnson (www.stellajohnson.com).

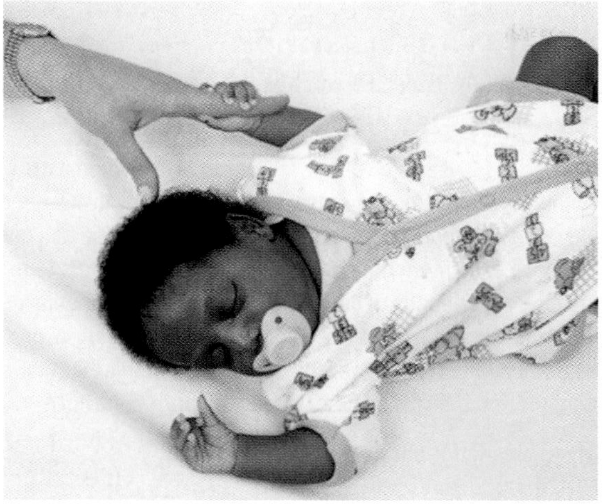

● **Figure 25–39** Palmar grasp.

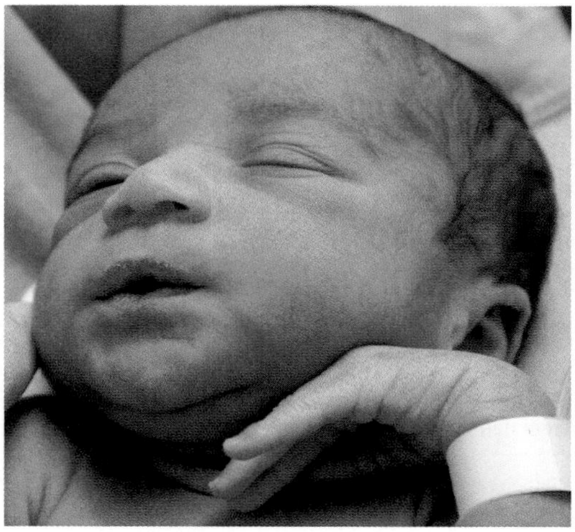

● **Figure 25–41** Rooting reflex.

may not be seen during the early newborn period, but once it appears it persists until about the third month.

- The palmar **grasping reflex** is elicited by stimulating the newborn's palm with a finger or object; the newborn grasps and holds the object or finger firmly enough to be lifted momentarily from the crib (Figure 25–39 ●).
- The **Moro reflex** is elicited when the newborn is startled by a loud noise or lifted slightly above the crib and then suddenly lowered. In response, the newborn straightens arms and hands outward while the knees flex. Slowly the arms return to the chest, as in an embrace. The fingers spread, forming a C, and the newborn may cry (Figure 25–40 ●). This reflex may persist until about 6 months of age.
- The **rooting reflex** is elicited when the side of the newborn's mouth or cheek is touched. In response, the newborn turns toward that side and opens the lips to suck (if not fed recently) (Figure 25–41 ●).
- The **sucking reflex** is elicited when an object is placed in the newborn's mouth or anything touches the lips. Newborns suck even while sleeping; this is called nonnutritive sucking, and it can have a quieting effect on the baby.
- **Trunk incurvation (Galant reflex)** is seen when the newborn is prone. Stroking the spine causes the pelvis to turn to the stimulated side.

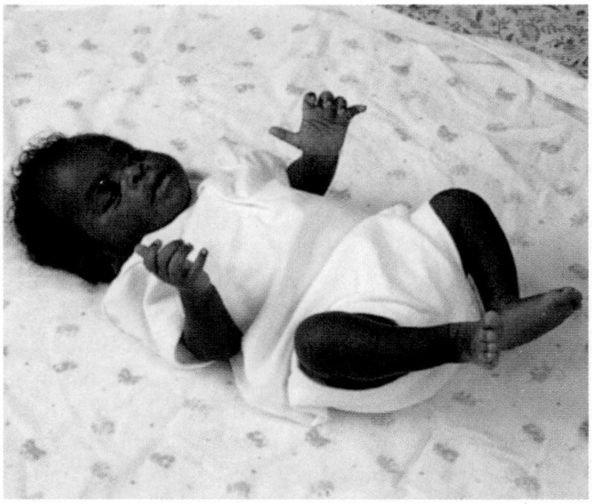

● **Figure 25–40** Moro reflex.

In addition to these reflexes, newborns can *blink, yawn, cough, sneeze,* and *draw back from pain* (protective reflexes). They can even move a little on their own. When placed on their stomachs, they push up and try to crawl (prone crawl). When held upright with one foot touching a flat surface, the newborn puts one foot in front of the other and "walks" (*stepping reflex*) (Figure 25–42 ●). This reflex is more pronounced at birth and is lost in 4 to 8 weeks.

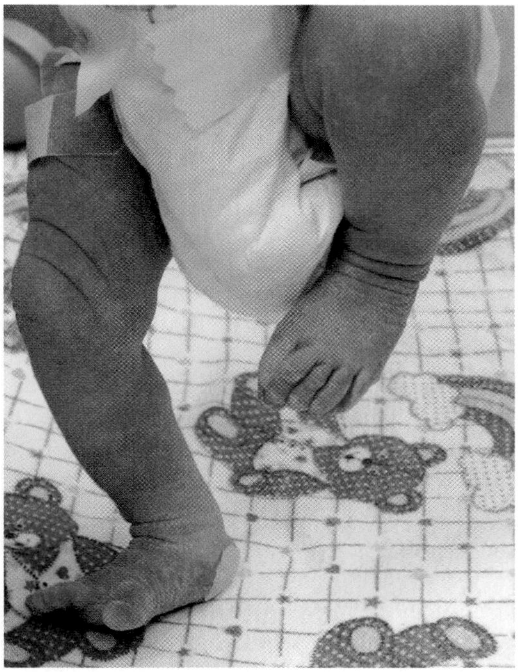

● **Figure 25–42** Stepping reflex. The stepping reflex disappears after about 4 to 8 weeks of age.

Table 25–5 Potential Birth Injuries

Classification	Examples*
Soft-tissue injuries	Lacerations, abrasions, bruising, fat necrosis
Skull injuries	Cephalohematoma,* fractures
Scalp laceration	Fetal scalp electrode
Scalp abscess	Fetal scalp electrode
Intracranial hemorrhage	Subdural, subarachnoid
Eye injuries	Subconjunctival* and retinal hemorrhages
Fractures	Clavicle,* facial bones, humerus, femur
Dislocations	Hips
Torticollis	Sternocleidomastoid muscle
Nerve injuries	Facial nerve,* brachial plexus,* phrenic nerve, recurrent laryngeal nerve (vocal cord paralysis), Horner syndrome
Spinal cord injuries	Spina bifida
Visceral rupture	Liver, spleen

*Most common birth injuries seen in newborns.

MyNursingKit Care Plan Activity: Assessment of the Newborn

The nurse uses the following steps to assess CNS integration:

1. Insert a gloved finger into the newborn's mouth to elicit a sucking reflex.
2. As soon as the newborn is sucking vigorously, assess hearing and vision responses by noting changes in sucking in the presence of a light, a rattle, and a voice.
3. The newborn should respond to such stimuli with a brief cessation of sucking, followed by continuous sucking with repetitious stimulation.

This CNS integration exam demonstrates auditory and visual integrity as well as the capability of complex behavioral interactions.

As healthcare providers carry out the newborn physical and neurologic assessment, they are always on the alert to recognize possible alterations and possible injuries related to the birth process that require further investigation and intervention. (See Table 25–5 for potential birth injuries.)

NEWBORN PHYSICAL ASSESSMENT GUIDE

Following is a guide for systematically assessing the newborn (pages 588–599). Normal findings, alterations, and related causes are presented and correlated with suggested nursing responses. The findings are typical for a full-term newborn.

Thinking Critically

NEWBORN BEHAVIOR

Maria Reyes, a 19-year-old G2 (now P2) mother, delivered a 40-week-old female newborn 24 hours ago. The newborn exam was normal. Mrs. Reyes asks about the newborn's exam. She says she has noticed that the baby cries more than her first child did and seems to require holding for longer periods of time after feeding before "quieting down." She is concerned that there is something she is doing wrong and wants to know when her newborn will start to act like her first baby. What should you discuss with her about newborn behavior?

See MyNursingKit for possible responses.

NEWBORN BEHAVIORAL ASSESSMENT

Two conflicting forces influence parents' perceptions of their newborn. One is their preconception, based on hopes and fears, of what their newborn will be like. The other is their initial reaction to the baby's temperament, behaviors, and physical appearance. Nurses can assist parents in identifying their baby's specific behaviors.

The **Brazelton Neonatal Behavioral Assessment Scale** provides valuable guidelines for assessing the newborn's state changes, temperament, and individual behavior patterns. It provides a way for the nurse, in conjunction with the parents (primary caregivers), to identify and understand the individual newborn's states and capabilities. Families learn which responses, interventions, or activities best meet the special needs of their newborn, and this understanding fosters positive attachment experiences.

The assessment tool identifies the newborn's repertoire of behavioral responses to the environment and also documents the newborn's neurologic adequacy and capabilities. The examination usually takes 20 to 30 minutes and involves about 30 tests. Some items are scored according to the newborn's response to specific stimuli. Others, such as consolability and alertness, are scored as a result of continuous behavioral observations throughout the assessment. (For a complete discussion of all test items and maneuvers, see Brazelton & Nugent, 1995.)

Because the first few days after birth are a period of behavioral disorganization, the complete assessment should be done on the third day after birth. The nurse should make every effort to elicit the best response. This may be accomplished by repeating tests at different times or by testing during situations that facilitate the best possible response, such as when the parents are holding, cuddling, rocking, and/or singing to their baby.

Assessment of the newborn should be carried out initially in a quiet, dimly lighted room, if possible. The nurse first determines the newborn's state of consciousness, because scoring and introduction of the test items are correlated with the sleep or waking state. The newborn's state depends on physiologic variables, such as the amount of time from the last feeding, positioning, environmental temperature, and health status; presence of such external stimuli as noises and bright lights; and the wake-sleep cycle of the infant. An important characteristic of the newborn period is the pattern of states, as well as the transitions from one state to another. The pattern of states is a predictor of the newborn's receptivity and ability to respond to stimuli in a cognitive manner. Babies learn best in a quiet, alert state and in an environment that is supportive and protective and that provides appropriate stimuli.

Observe the newborn's sleep-wake patterns (as discussed in Chapter 24), including the rapidity with which the newborn moves from one state to another, the ability to be consoled, and the ability to diminish the impact of disturbing stimuli. The following questions may provide the nurse with a framework for assessment:

- Does the newborn's response style and ability to adapt to stimuli indicate a need for parental interventions that will alert the newborn to the environment so that he or she can grow socially and cognitively?
- Are parental interventions necessary to lessen the outside stimuli, as in the case of the baby who responds to sensory input with intensity?
- Can the baby control the amount of sensory input that he or she must deal with?

The behaviors, and the sleep-wake states in which they are assessed, are categorized as follows:

- *Habituation.* The nurse assesses the newborn's ability to diminish or shut down innate responses to specific repeated stimuli, such as a rattle, bell, light, or pinprick to heel.
- *Orientation to inanimate and animate visual and auditory assessment stimuli.* The nurse observes how often and where the newborn attends to auditory and visual stimuli. Orientation to the environment is determined by an ability to respond to clues given by others and by a natural ability to fix on and follow a visual object horizontally and vertically. This capacity and parental appreciation of it are important for positive communication between infant and parents; the parents' visual (*en face*) and auditory (soft, continuous voice) presence stimulates their newborn to orient to them. Inability or lack of response may indicate visual or auditory problems. It is important for parents to know that their newborn can turn to voices soon after birth or by 3 days of age and can become alert at different times with a varying degree of intensity in response to sounds.
- *Motor activity.* Several components are evaluated. Motor tone of the newborn is assessed in the most characteristic state of responsiveness. This summary assessment includes overall use of tone as the newborn responds to being handled—whether during spontaneous activity, prone placement, or horizontal holding—and overall assessment of body tone as the newborn reacts to all stimuli.

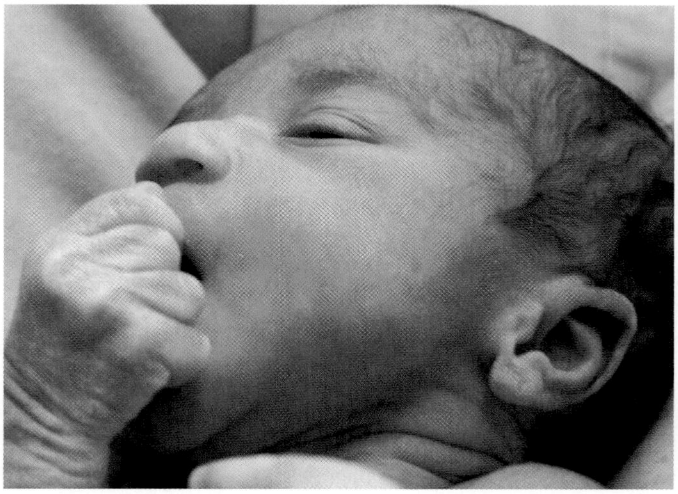

● **Figure 25–43** Self-soothing. The newborn can bring hand to mouth as a self-soothing activity.

- *Variations.* Frequency of alert states, state changes, color changes (throughout all states as examination progresses), activity, and peaks of excitement are assessed.
- *Self-quieting activity.* This assessment is based on how often, how quickly, and how effectively newborns can use their resources to quiet and console themselves when upset or distressed. Considered in this assessment are such self-consolatory activities as putting hand to mouth, sucking on a fist or the tongue, and attuning to an object or sound (Figure 25–43 ●). The newborn's need for outside consolation must also be considered (e.g., seeing a face; being rocked, held, or dressed; using a pacifier; being swaddled).
- *Cuddliness or social behaviors.* This area encompasses the newborn's need for, and response to, being held. Also considered is how often the newborn smiles. These behaviors influence the couple's self-esteem and feelings of acceptance or rejection. Cuddling also appears to be an indicator of personality. Cuddlers appear to enjoy, accept, and seek physical contact; are easier to placate; sleep more; and form earlier and more intense attachments. Noncuddlers are active, restless, have accelerated motor development, and are intolerant of physical restraint. Smiling, even as a grimace reflex, greatly influences parent-newborn feedback. Parents identify this response as positive.

Assessment Guide

NEWBORN PHYSICAL ASSESSMENT

PHYSICAL ASSESSMENT/ NORMAL FINDINGS	ALTERATIONS AND POSSIBLE CAUSES*	NURSING RESPONSES TO DATA†
Vital Signs		
Blood pressure (BP): At birth: 70–50/45–30 mm Hg Day 10: 90/50 mm Hg (may be unable to measure diastolic pressure with standard sphygmomanometer)	Low BP (hypovolemia, shock)	Monitor BP in all cases of distress, prematurity, or suspected anomaly. Low BP: Refer to physician immediately so measures to improve circulation are begun.
Pulse: 120 to 160 bpm (if asleep, as low as 100 bpm; if crying, up to 180 bpm)	Weak pulse (decreased cardiac output) Bradycardia (severe asphyxia) Tachycardia (over 160 bpm at rest) (infection, CNS problems, arrhythmia, stress, hypovolemia)	Assess skin perfusion by blanching (capillary refill test-normal 2–3 sec.). Correlate finding with BP assessments; refer to physician. Carry out neurologic and thermoregulation assessments. Check blood pressure and Hct.
Respirations: 30 to 60 breaths/minute Synchronization of chest and abdominal movements Diaphragmatic and abdominal breathing	Tachypnea (pneumonia, respiratory distress syndrome [RDS]) Rapid, shallow breathing (hypermagnesemia caused by large doses given to mothers with preeclampsia) Respirations below 30 breaths/minute (maternal anesthesia or analgesia)	Identify sleep-wake state; correlate with respiratory pattern. Evaluate for all signs of respiratory distress; report findings to physician.
Transient tachypnea	Expiratory grunting, subcostal and substernal retractions; flaring of nares (respiratory distress); apnea (cold stress, respiratory disorder)	Evaluate for cold stress. Report findings to physician/neonatal nurse practitioner.
Crying: Strong and lusty Moderate tone and pitch Cries vary in length from 3 to 7 minutes after consoling measures are used	High pitched, shrill (neurologic disorder, hypoglycemia) Weak or absent (CNS disorder, laryngeal problem)	Discuss newborn's use of cry for communication. Assess and record abnormal cries. Reduce environmental noises.
Temperature: Axilla 36.4°C to 37.2°C (97.5°F to 99°F)	Elevated temperature (room too warm, too much clothing or covers, dehydration, sepsis, brain damage) Subnormal temperature (brainstem involvement, cold, sepsis)	Notify physician of elevation or drop. Counsel parents on possible causes of elevated or low temperatures, appropriate home-care measures, when to call physician.
Heavier newborns tend to have higher body temperatures	Swings of more than 2°F from one reading to next or subnormal temperature (infection)	Teach parents how to take rectal and/or axillary temperature; assess parents' information regarding use of thermometer; provide teaching as needed.
Weight: 2500 to 4000 g (5 lb, 8 oz to 8 lb, 13 oz)	Less than 2748 g (less than 6 lb) = SGA or preterm infant Greater than 4050 g (greater than 9 lb) = LGA or infants of diabetic mothers	Plot weight and gestational age on growth chart to identify high-risk infants. Ascertain body build of parents. Counsel parents regarding appropriate caloric intake.
Within first 3 to 4 days, normal weight loss of 5% to 10% Large babies tend to lose more because of greater fluid loss in proportion to birth weight except infants of diabetic mother	Loss greater than 15% (low fluid intake, loss of meconium and urine, feeding difficulties, diabetes insipidus)	Notify physician of net losses or gains. Calculate fluid intake and losses from all sources (insensible water loss, radiant warmers, and phototherapy lights).

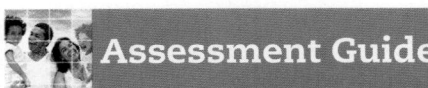

Assessment Guide—continued

NEWBORN PHYSICAL ASSESSMENT

PHYSICAL ASSESSMENT/ NORMAL FINDINGS	ALTERATIONS AND POSSIBLE CAUSES*	NURSING RESPONSES TO DATA†
Length: 46–56 cm (18–22 in.) Grows 10 cm (3 in.) during first 3 months	Less than 45 cm (congenital dwarf) Short/long bones proximally (achondroplasia) Short/long bones distally (Ellis-van Creveld syndrome)	Assess for other signs of dwarfism. Determine other signs of skeletal system adequacy. Plot progress at subsequent well-baby visits.
Posture		
Body usually flexed, hands may be tightly clenched, neck appears short as chin rests on chest	Only extension noted, inability to move from midline (trauma, hypoxia, immaturity)	Record spontaneity of motor activity and symmetry of movements.
In breech births feet are usually dorsiflexed	Constant motion (maternal caffeine intake or drug withdrawal)	If parents express concern about newborn's movement patterns, reassure and evaluate further if appropriate.
Skin		
Color: Color consistent with genetic background Newborns of European descent: pink-tinged or ruddy color over face, trunk, extremities Newborns of African or Native American descent: pale pink with yellow or red tinge Newborns of Asian descent: pink or rosy red to yellow tinge	Pallor of face, conjunctiva (anemia, hypothermia, anoxia) Beefy red (hypoglycemia, immature vasomotor reflexes, polycythemia)	Discuss with parents common skin color variations to allay fears. Document extent and time of occurrence of color change.
Common variations: acrocyanosis, circumoral cyanosis, Mongolian spots, or harlequin color change	Meconium staining (nonreassuring fetal status) Jaundice (hemolytic reaction from blood incompatibility within first 24 hours, sepsis)	Obtain Hgb and hematocrit values, obtain bilirubin levels. Assess for respiratory difficulty. Differentiate between physiologic and pathologic jaundice.
Mottled when undressed	Cyanosis (choanal atresia, CNS damage or trauma, respiratory or cardiac problem, cold stress)	Assess degree of (central or peripheral) cyanosis and possible causes; refer to physician.
Minor bruising: over buttocks in breech presentation and over eyes and forehead in facial presentations		Discuss with parents cause and course of minor bruising related to labor and birth.
Texture: Smooth, soft, flexible, may have dry, peeling hands and feet	Generalized cracked or peeling skin (SGA or postterm; blood incompatibility; metabolic, kidney dysfunction) Seborrheic-dermatitis (cradle cap) Absence of vernix (postmature) Yellow vernix (bilirubin staining)	Report to physician. Instruct parents to shampoo the scalp and anterior fontanelle areas daily with soap; rinse well; avoid use of oil.
Turgor: Elastic, returns to normal shape after pinching	Maintains tent shape (dehydration)	Assess for other signs and symptoms of dehydration.
Pigmentation: Clear; milia across bridge of nose, forehead, or chin will disappear within a few weeks Café-au-lait spots (one or two) Mongolian spots common over dorsal area and buttocks in dark-skin infants	Six or more (neurologic disorder such as von Recklinghausen's disease, cutaneous neurofibromatosis)	Advise parents not to pinch or prick these pimplelike areas. If there are six or more café-au-lait spots, refer for genetic and neurologic consult. Assure parents of normalcy of this pigmentation; it will fade in first year or two.

(continued)

Assessment Guide—continued

NEWBORN PHYSICAL ASSESSMENT

PHYSICAL ASSESSMENT/ NORMAL FINDINGS	ALTERATIONS AND POSSIBLE CAUSES*	NURSING RESPONSES TO DATA†
Skin—continued		
Erythema toxicum	Impetigo (group β-hemolytic streptococcus or *Staphylococcus aureus* infection)	If impetigo occurs, instruct parents about handwashing and linen precautions during home care.
Telangiectatic nevi	Hemangiomas: Nevus flammeus (port-wine stain) Nevus vascularis (strawberry hemangioma) Cavernous hemangiomas	Collaborate with physician. Counsel parents about birthmark's progression to allay misconceptions. Record size and shape of hemangiomas. Refer for follow-up at well-baby clinic.
Rashes	Rashes (infection)	Assess location and type of rash (macular, papular, vesicular). Obtain history of onset, prenatal history, and related signs and symptoms.
Petechiae of head or neck (breech presentation, cord around neck)	Generalized petechiae (clotting abnormalities)	Determine cause; advise parents if further health care is needed.
Head		
General appearance, size, movement Round, symmetric, and moves easily from left to right and up and down; soft and pliable	Asymmetric, flattened occiput on either side of the head (plagiocephaly) Head held at angle (torticollis)	Instruct parents to change infant's positions frequently when awake. When awake, needs to spend "tummy time." Infants should be placed supine for sleep per "back to sleep" guidelines.
	Unable to move head side to side (neurologic trauma)	Determine adequacy of all neurologic signs.
Circumference 32–37 cm (12.5–14.5 in.); 2 cm greater than chest circumference Head one-fourth of body size	Extreme differences in size may be microencephaly (Cornelia de Lange syndrome, cytomegalic inclusion disease [CID], rubella, toxoplasmosis, chromosome abnormalities), hydrocephalus (meningomyelocele, achondroplasia), anencephaly (neural tube defect) Head is 3 cm or more larger than chest circumference (preterm, hydrocephalus)	Measure circumference from occiput to frontal area using metal or paper tape. Measure chest circumference using metal or paper tape and compare to head circumference. Record measurements on growth chart. Reevaluate at well-baby visits.
Common variations: Molding Breech and cesarean newborns' heads are round and well shaped	Cephalohematoma (trauma during birth, may persist up to 3 months) Caput succedaneum (long labor and birth; disappears in 1 week)	Evaluate neurologic response. Observe for hyperbilirubinemia. Check Hct. Reassure parents regarding common manifestations caused by birth process and when they should disappear.
Fontanelles: Palpation of juncture of cranial bones Anterior fontanelle: 3–4 cm long by 2–3 cm wide, diamond shaped	Overlapping of anterior fontanelle (malnourished or preterm newborn) Premature closure of sutures (craniosynostosis)	Discuss normal closure times with parents and care of "soft spots" to allay misconceptions. Refer to physician.
Posterior fontanelle: 1–2 cm at birth, triangle shaped	Late closure (hydrocephalus)	Observe for signs and symptoms of hydrocephalus.
Slight pulsation	Moderate to severe pulsation (vascular problems)	Refer to physician.
Moderate bulging noted with crying, stooling, or pulsations with heartbeat	Bulging (increased intracranial pressure, meningitis) Sunken (dehydration)	Evaluate hydration status. Evaluate neurologic status. Report to physician.

Assessment Guide—continued

NEWBORN PHYSICAL ASSESSMENT

PHYSICAL ASSESSMENT/ NORMAL FINDINGS	ALTERATIONS AND POSSIBLE CAUSES*	NURSING RESPONSES TO DATA†
Hair		
Texture: Smooth with fine texture variations (Note: Variations depend on ethnic background.)	Coarse, brittle, dry hair (hypothyroidism) White forelock (Waardenburg syndrome)	Instruct parents regarding routine care of hair and scalp.
Distribution: Scalp hair high over eyebrows (Spanish, Mexican hairline begins mid-forehead and extends down back of neck.)	Low forehead and posterior hairlines may indicate chromosomal disorders	Assess for other signs of chromosomal aberrations. Refer to physician.
Face		
Symmetric movement of all facial features, normal hairline, eyebrows and eyelashes present		Assess and record symmetry of all parts, shape, regularity of features, sameness or differences in features.
Spacing of features: Eyes at same level, nostrils equal size, cheeks full, and sucking pads present	Eyes wide apart—ocular hypertelorism (Apert syndrome, Cri du chat, Turner syndrome)	Observe for other signs and symptoms indicative of disease states or chromosomal aberrations.
Lips equal on both sides of midline	Abnormal face (Down syndrome, cretinism, gargoylism)	
Chin recedes when compared with other bones of face	Abnormally small jaw—micrognathia (Pierre Robin syndrome, Treacher Collins syndrome)	Maintain airway; do not position supine. Initiate surgical consultation and referral.
Movement: Makes facial grimaces	Inability to suck, grimace, and close eyelids (cranial nerve injury)	Initiate neurologic assessment and consultation.
Symmetric when resting and crying	Asymmetry (paralysis of facial cranial nerve)	Assess and record symmetry of all parts, shape, regularity of features, and sameness or differences in features.
Eyes		
General placement and appearance: Bright and clear; even placement; slight nystagmus (involuntary cyclical eye movements)	Gross nystagmus (damage to third, fourth, and sixth cranial nerves)	
Concomitant strabismus	Constant and fixed strabismus	Reassure parents that strabismus is considered normal up to 6 months.
Move in all directions		
Blue or slate blue-gray	Lack of pigmentation (albinism) Brushfield spots may indicate Down syndrome (a light or white speckling of the outer two-thirds of the iris)	Discuss with parents any necessary eye precautions. Assess for other signs of Down syndrome.
Brown color at birth in dark-skin infants		Discuss with parents that permanent eye color is usually established by 3 months of age.
Eyelids: Position: above pupils but within iris, no drooping	Elevation of (hydrocephalus) or retraction of upper lid (hyperthyroidism) "Sunset sign" lid elevation and downward gaze (hydrocephalus), ptosis (congenital or paralysis of oculomotor muscle)	Assess for signs of hydrocephalus and hyperthyroidism. Evaluate interference with vision in subsequent well-baby visits.
Eyes on parallel plane	Upward slant in non-Asians (Down syndrome)	Assess for other signs of Down syndrome
Epicanthal folds in Asians and 20% of newborns of northern European descent	Epicanthal folds (Down syndrome, Cri du chat syndrome)	

(continued)

NEWBORN PHYSICAL ASSESSMENT

PHYSICAL ASSESSMENT/ NORMAL FINDINGS	ALTERATIONS AND POSSIBLE CAUSES*	NURSING RESPONSES TO DATA†
Eyes—continued		
Movement: Blink reflex in response to light stimulus Eyes open wide in dimly lighted room	Blink absent (CNS injury)	Evaluate neurologic status. Refer to physician.
Inspection: Edematous for first few days of life, resulting from birth; no lumps or redness	Purulent drainage (infection); infectious conjunctivitis (gonococcus, chlamydia, staphylococcus, or gram-negative organisms) Marginal blepharitis (lid edges red, crusted, scaly)	Initiate good handwashing. Refer to physician. Evaluate infant for seborrheic dermatitis; scales can be removed easily.
Cornea: Clear Corneal reflex present	Ulceration (herpes infection); large cornea or corneas of unequal size (congenital glaucoma) Clouding, opacity of lens (cataract)	Refer to ophthalmologist. Assess for other manifestations of congenital herpes; institute nursing care measures.
Sclera: May appear bluish in newborn, then white; slightly brownish color frequent in newborns of African descent	True blue sclera (osteogenesis imperfecta)	Refer to physician.
Pupils: Pupils equal in size, round, and react to light by accommodation	Anisocoria—unequal pupils (CNS damage) Dilation or constriction (intracranial) damage, retinoblastoma, glaucoma; Pupils nonreactive to light or accommodation (brain injury)	Refer for neurologic examination.
Slight nystagmus in newborn who has not learned to focus Pupil light reflex demonstrated at birth or by 3 weeks of age	Nystagmus (labyrinthine disturbance, CNS disorder)	
Conjunctiva: Chemical conjunctivitis Subconjunctival hemorrhage	Pale color (anemia)	Obtain hematocrit and hemoglobin. Reassure parents that chemical conjunctivitis will subside in 1 to 2 days and subconjunctival hemorrhage disappears in a few weeks.
Palpebral conjunctiva (red but not hyperemic)	Inflammation or edema (infection, blocked tear duct)	
Vision: 20/200 Tracks moving object to midline Fixed focus on objects at a distance of about 10 to 20 in.; may be difficult to evaluate in newborn Prefers faces, geometric designs, and black and white to colors	Cataracts (congenital infection)	Record any questions about visual acuity, and initiate follow-up evaluation at first well-baby checkup.
Lashes and lacrimal glands: Presence of lashes (lashes may be absent in preterm newborns)	No lashes on inner two-thirds of lid (Treacher Collins syndrome); bushy lashes (Hurler syndrome); long lashes (Cornelia de Lange syndrome)	
Cry commonly tearless	Excessive tearing (plugged lacrimal duct, natal narcotic withdrawal), glaucoma	Demonstrate to parents how to milk blocked tear duct. Refer to ophthalmologist if tearing is excessive before third month of life.
Nose		
Appearance of external nasal aspects: May appear flattened as a result of birth process	Continued flat or broad bridge of nose (Down syndrome)	Arrange consultation with specialist.
Small and narrow in midline, even placement in relationship to eyes and mouth	Low bridge of nose, beaklike nose (Apert syndrome, Treacher Collins syndrome) Upturned (Cornelia de Lange syndrome)	Initiate evaluation of chromosomal abnormalities.

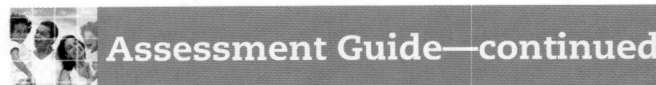

Assessment Guide—continued

NEWBORN PHYSICAL ASSESSMENT

PHYSICAL ASSESSMENT/ NORMAL FINDINGS	ALTERATIONS AND POSSIBLE CAUSES*	NURSING RESPONSES TO DATA†
Patent nares bilaterally (nose breathers)	Blockage of nares (mucus and/or secretions), choanal atresia	Inspect for obstruction of nares.
Sneezing common to clear nasal passages	Flaring nares (respiratory distress)	Maintain oral airway until surgical correction is made.
Responds to odors, may smell breast milk	No response to stimulating odors	Inspect for obstruction of nares.
Mouth		
Function of facial, hypoglossal, glossopharyngeal, and vagus nerves: Symmetry of movement and strength	Mouth draws to one side (transient seventh cranial nerve paralysis caused by pressure in utero or trauma during birth, congenital paralysis) Fishlike shape (Treacher Collins syndrome)	Initiate neurologic consultation. Administer artificial tears if eye on affected side of face is unable to close.
Presence of gag, swallowing, coordinated with sucking reflexes Adequate salivation	Suppressed or absent reflexes	Evaluate other neurologic functions of these nerves.
Palate (soft and hard): Hard palate dome-shaped Uvula midline with symmetrical movement of soft palate	High-steepled palate (Treacher Collins syndrome), bifid uvula (congenital anomaly)	Assess for other congenital anomalies.
Palate intact, sucks well when stimulated	Clefts in either hard or soft palate (polygenic disorder)	Initiate a surgical consultation referral.
Epithelial (Epstein's) pearls appear on mucosa		Assure parents that these are normal and will disappear at 2 or 3 months of age.
Esophagus patent, some drooling common in newborn	Excessive drooling or bubbling (esophageal atresia)	Test for patency of esophagus.
Tongue: Free moving in all directions, midline	Tongue-tied Lack of movement or asymmetric movement (neurologic damage) Fasciculations (fine tremors) Spinal muscular atrophy	Further assess neurologic functions. Test reflex elevation of tongue when depressed with tongue blade.
Pink color, smooth to rough texture, noncoated	Deviations from midline (cranial nerve damage) White cheesy coating (thrush) Tongue has deep ridges	Check for signs of weakness or deviation. Differentiate between thrush and milk curds by wiping patches: if white patches don't come off easily, it is thrush. Reassure parents that tongue pattern may change from day to day.
Tongue proportional to mouth	Large tongue with short frenulum (cretinism, Down syndrome, other syndromes)	Evaluate in well-baby clinic to assess development delays. Initiate referrals.
Ears		
External ear: Without lesions, cysts, or nodules	Nodules, cysts, or sinus tracts in front of ear. Adherent earlobes Low set ears (genetic anomaly or syndrome) Preauricular skin tags	Evaluate characteristics of lesions. Counsel parents to clean external ear with washcloth only; discourage use of cotton-tip applicators. Refer to physician for ligation.
Hearing: Eustachian tubes are cleared with first cry		
Absence of all risk factors for hearing loss	Presence of one or more risk factors	Assess history of risk factors for hearing loss.
Attends to sounds; sudden or loud noise elicits Moro reflex	No response to sound stimuli (deafness)	Test for Moro reflex.

(continued)

Assessment Guide—continued

NEWBORN PHYSICAL ASSESSMENT

PHYSICAL ASSESSMENT/ NORMAL FINDINGS	ALTERATIONS AND POSSIBLE CAUSES*	NURSING RESPONSES TO DATA†
Neck		
Appearance: Short, straight, creased with skin folds	Abnormally short neck (Turner syndrome) Arching or inability to flex neck (meningitis, congenital anomaly)	Report findings to physician.
Posterior neck lacks loose extra folds of skin	Webbing of neck (Turner syndrome, Down syndrome, trisomy 18)	Assess for other signs of the syndromes.
Clavicles: Straight and intact	Knot or lump on clavicle (fracture during difficult birth)	Obtain detailed labor and birth history; apply figure-8 bandage. Consider oral analgesics.
Moro reflex elicitable	Unilateral Moro reflex response on unaffected side (fracture of clavicle, brachial palsy, Erb-Duchenne paralysis)	Collaborate with physician.
Symmetric shoulders	Hypoplasia	
Chest		
Appearance and size: Circumference: 32.5 cm (12.8 in.), 1–2 cm (0.4–0.8 in.) less than head		Measure at level of nipples after exhalation.
Wider than it is long Normal shape without depressed or prominent sternum Lower end of sternum (xiphoid cartilage) may be protruding; is less apparent after several weeks Sternum 8 cm (3.1 in.) long	Funnel chest (congenital or associated with Marfan syndrome) Continued protrusion of xiphoid cartilage (Marfan syndrome, "pigeon chest") Barrel chest	Determine adequacy of other respiratory and circulatory signs. Assess for other signs and symptoms of various syndromes.
Expansion and retraction: Bilateral expansion	Unequal chest expansion (pneumonia, pneumothorax, respiratory distress)	Assess respiratory effort regularity, flaring of nares, difficulty on both inspiration and expiration.
No intercostal, subcostal, or supracostal retractions	Retractions (respiratory distress) See-saw respirations (respiratory distress)	
Auscultation: Breath sounds are louder in infants	Decreased breath sounds (decreased respiratory activity, atelectasis, pneumothorax)	Obtain transillumination. Record finding and consult physician. Perform assessment and report to physician any positive findings.
Chest and axillae clear on crying	Increased breath sounds (resolving pneumonia or in cesarean births)	
Bronchial breath sounds (heard where trachea and bronchi closest to chest wall, above sternum and between scapulae): Bronchial sounds bilaterally Air entry clear Rales may indicate normal newborn atelectasis Cough reflex absent at birth, appears in 2 or more days	Adventitious or abnormal sounds (respiratory disease or distress)	Evaluate color for pallor or cyanosis. Report to physician.
Breasts: Flat with symmetric nipples Breast tissue diameter 5 cm (2 in.) or more at term Distance between nipples 8 cm (3.1 in.) Breast engorgement occurs on third day of life; liquid discharge may be expressed in term newborns	Lack of breast tissue (preterm or SGA) Discharge Enlargement Breast abscesses Supernumerary nipples Dark-colored nipples	Evaluate for infection. Reassure parents of normality of breast engorgement. No intervention is necessary.

Assessment Guide—continued

NEWBORN PHYSICAL ASSESSMENT

PHYSICAL ASSESSMENT/ NORMAL FINDINGS	ALTERATIONS AND POSSIBLE CAUSES*	NURSING RESPONSES TO DATA[†]
Heart		
Auscultation: Location: lies horizontally, with left border extending to left of midclavicle Regular rhythm and rate Determination of point of maximal impulse (PMI)	Arrhythmia (anoxia), tachycardia, bradycardia Malpositioning (enlargement, abnormal placement, pneumothorax, dextrocardia, diaphragmatic hernia)	Refer all arrhythmia and gallop rhythms. Initiate cardiac evaluation.
Functional murmurs No thrills	Location of murmurs (possible congenital cardiac anomaly)	Evaluate murmur: location, timing, and duration; observe for accompanying cardiac pathology symptoms; ascertain family history.
Horizontal groove at diaphragm shows flaring of rib cage to mild degree	Marked rib flaring (vitamin D deficiency) Inadequacy of respiratory movement	Initiate cardiopulmonary evaluation; assess pulses and blood pressures in all four extremities for equality and quality.
Abdomen		
Appearance: Cylindrical with some protrusion, appears large in relation to pelvis, some laxness of abdominal muscles No cyanosis, few vessels seen Diastasis recti—common in infants of African descent	Distention, shiny abdomen with engorged vessels (gastrointestinal abnormalities, infection, congenital megacolon) Scaphoid abdominal appearance (diaphragmatic hernia) Increased or decreased peristalsis (duodenal stenosis, small bowel obstruction) Localized flank bulging (enlarged kidneys, ascites, or absent abdominal muscles)	Examine abdomen thoroughly for mass or organomegaly. Measure abdominal girth. Report deviations of abdominal size. Assess other signs and symptoms of obstruction. Refer to physician.
Umbilicus: No protrusion of umbilicus (protrusion of umbilicus common in infants of African descent)	Umbilical hernia Patent urachus (congenital malformation)	Measure umbilical hernia by palpating the opening and record; it should close by 1 year of age; if not, refer to physician.
Bluish white color	Omphalocele (covered defect) Gastroschisis (uncovered defect)	Cover omphalocele and gastroschisis with sterile, moist dressing or plastic sterile bag.
Cutis navel (umbilical cord projects), granulation tissue present in navel	Redness or exudate around cord (infection) Yellow discoloration (hemolytic disease, meconium staining)	Instruct parents on cord care and hygiene.
Two arteries and one vein apparent Begins drying 1 to 2 hours after birth No bleeding	Single umbilical artery (congenital anomalies) Discharge or oozing of blood from the cord	Refer anomalies to physician.
Auscultation and percussion all four gradients	Bowel sounds in chest (diaphragmatic hernia)	Collaborate with physician.
Soft bowel sounds heard shortly after birth every 10 to 30 seconds	Absence of bowel sounds Hyperperistalsis (intestinal obstruction)	Assess for other signs of dehydration and/or infection.
Femoral pulses: Palpable, equal bilateral	Absent or diminished femoral pulses (coarctation of aorta)	Monitor blood pressure in upper and lower extremities.
Inguinal area: No bulges along inguinal area No inguinal lymph nodes felt	Inguinal hernia	Initiate referral. Continue follow-up in well-baby clinic.
Bladder: Percusses 1-4 cm (0.4-1.6 in.) above symphysis Emptied about 3 hours after birth; if not, at time of birth Urine—inoffensive, mild odor	Failure to void within 24 to 48 hours after birth Exposure of bladder mucosa (exstrophy of bladder) Foul odor (infection)	Check whether baby voided at birth. Obtain urine specimen if infection is suspected. Consult with clinician.

(continued)

Assessment Guide—continued

NEWBORN PHYSICAL ASSESSMENT

PHYSICAL ASSESSMENT/ NORMAL FINDINGS	ALTERATIONS AND POSSIBLE CAUSES*	NURSING RESPONSES TO DATA†
Genitals		
Gender clearly delineated	Ambiguous genitals	Refer for genetic consultation.
Male		
Penis: Slender in appearance, about 2.5 cm (1 in.) long, 1 cm (0.4 in.) wide at birth Normal urinary orifice, urethral meatus at tip of penis	Micropenis (congenital anomaly) Meatal atresia Hypospadias, epispadias	Observe and record first voiding. Collaborate with physician in presence of abnormality. Delay circumcision.
Noninflamed urethral opening	Urethritis (infection)	Palpate for enlarged inguinal lymph nodes and record painful urination.
Foreskin adheres to glans	Ulceration of meatal opening (infection, inflammation)	Evaluate whether ulcer is because of diaper rash; counsel regarding care.
Uncircumcised foreskin tight for 2 to 3 months Circumcised Erectile tissue present	Phimosis—if still tight after 3 months	Instruct parents on how to care for uncircumcised penis. Teach parents how to care for circumcision.
Scrotum: Skin loose and hanging or tight and small; extensive rugae and normal size Normal skin color Scrotal discoloration common in breech	Large scrotum containing fluid (hydrocele) Minimal rugae, small scrotum Red, shiny scrotal skin (orchitis)	Shine a light through scrotum (transilluminate) to verify diagnosis. Assess for prematurity.
Testes: Descended by birth; not consistently found in scrotum	Undescended testes (cryptorchidism)	If testes cannot be felt in scrotum, gently palpate femoral, inguinal, perineal, and abdominal areas for presence.
Testes size 1.5–2 cm (0.6–0.8 in.) at birth	Enlarged testes (tumor) Small testes (Klinefelter syndrome or adrenal hyperplasia)	Refer and collaborate with physician for further diagnostic studies.
Female		
Mons: Normal skin color, area pigmented in dark-skin infants Labia majora cover labia minora in term and postterm newborns; symmetric size appropriate for gestational age	Hematoma, lesions (trauma) Labia minora prominent	Evaluate for recent trauma. Assess for prematurity.
Clitoris: Normally large in newborn Edema and bruising in breech birth	Hypertrophy (hermaphroditism)	Refer for genetic workup.
Vagina: Urinary meatus and vaginal orifice visible (0.5 cm [0.2 in.] circumference)	Inflammation; erythema and discharge (urethritis)	Collect urine specimen for laboratory examination.
Vaginal tag or hymenal tag disappears in a few weeks	Congenital absence of vagina	Refer to physician.
Discharge; smegma under labia	Foul-smelling discharge (infection)	Collect data and further evaluate reason for discharge.
Bloody or mucoid discharge	Excessive vaginal bleeding (blood coagulation defect)	
Buttocks and Anus		
Buttocks symmetric	Pilonidal dimple	Examine for possible sinus. Instruct parents about cleansing this area.
Anus patent and passage of meconium within 24 to 48 hours after birth	Imperforate anus, rectal atresia (congenital gastrointestinal defect)	Evaluate extent of problems. Initiate surgical consultation. Perform digital examination to ascertain patency if patency uncertain.
No fissures, tears, or skin tags	Fissures	

Assessment Guide—continued

NEWBORN PHYSICAL ASSESSMENT

PHYSICAL ASSESSMENT/ NORMAL FINDINGS	ALTERATIONS AND POSSIBLE CAUSES*	NURSING RESPONSES TO DATA†
Extremities and Trunk		
Short and generally flexed, extremities move symmetrically through range of motion but lack full extension	Unilateral or absence of movement (spinal cord involvement) Fetal position continued or limp (anoxia)	Review birth record to assess possible cause.
All joints move spontaneously; good muscle tone, of flexor type, birth to 2 months	Spasticity when infant begins using extensors (cerebral palsy)	Collaborate with physician.
Arms: Equal in length Bilateral movement Flexed when quiet	Brachial palsy (difficult birth) Erb-Duchenne paralysis Muscle weakness, fractured clavicle Absence of limb or change of size (phocomelia, amelia)	Report to clinician.
Hands: Normal number of fingers	Polydactyly (Ellis-van Creveld syndrome) Syndactyly—one limb (developmental anomaly) Syndactyly—both limbs (genetic component)	Report to clinician.
Normal palmar crease Normal size hands	Simian line on palm (Down syndrome) Short fingers and broad hand (Hurler syndrome)	Refer for genetic workup.
Nails present and extend beyond fingertips in term newborn	Cyanosis and clubbing (cardiac anomalies) Nails long or yellow stained (postterm)	Evaluate for history of distress in utero. Carry out cardiac and respiratory assessments. Check pulse oximetry.
Spine: C-shaped spine Flat and straight when prone Slight lumbar lordosis Easily flexed and intact when palpated At least half of back devoid of lanugo	Spina bifida occulta (nevus pilosus) Dermal sinus Myleomeningocele	Evaluate extent of neurologic damage; initiate care of spinal opening. Elicit reflex to assess degree of involvement.
Full-term infant in ventral suspension should hold head at 45-degree angle, back straight	Head lag, limp, floppy trunk (neurologic problems)	
Hips: No sign of instability	Sensation of abnormal movement, jerk, or snap of hip dislocation	Physician or nurse practitioner examines all newborn infants for dislocated hip before discharge from birthing center.
Hips abduct to more than 60 degrees	Limited abduction (developmental dysplasia of hip)	If this is suspected, refer to orthopedist for further evaluation. Reassess at well-baby visits.
Inguinal and buttock skin creases: Symmetric inguinal and buttock creases	Asymmetry (dislocated hips)	Refer to orthopedist for evaluation. Counsel parents regarding symptoms of concern, and discuss therapy.
Legs: Legs equal in length Legs shorter than arms at birth	Shortened leg (dislocated hips) Lack of leg movement (fractures, spinal defects)	Refer to orthopedist for evaluation. Counsel parents regarding symptoms of concern, and discuss therapy.
Feet: Foot is in straight line Positional clubfoot—based on position in utero	Talipes equinovarus (true clubfoot)	Discuss differences between positional and true clubfoot with parents. Teach parents passive manipulation of foot.
Fat pads and creases on soles of feet	Incomplete sole creases in first 24 hours of life (premature)	Refer to orthopedist if not corrected by 3 months of age.
Talipes planus (flat feet) normal under 3 years of age		Reassure parents that flat feet are normal in infants.
Neuromuscular		
Motor function: Symmetric movement and strength in all extremities	Limp, flaccid, or hypertonic (CNS disorders, infection, dehydration, fracture)	Appraise newborn's posture and motor functions by observing activities and motor characteristics.

(continued)

Assessment Guide—continued

NEWBORN PHYSICAL ASSESSMENT

PHYSICAL ASSESSMENT/ NORMAL FINDINGS	ALTERATIONS AND POSSIBLE CAUSES*	NURSING RESPONSES TO DATA†
Neuromuscular—continued		
May be jerky or have brief twitchings	Tremors (hypoglycemia, hypocalcemia, infection, neurologic damage)	Evaluate for electrolyte imbalance, hypoglycemia, and neurologic functioning.
Head lag not over 45 degrees	Delayed or abnormal development (preterm, neurologic involvement)	
Neck control adequate to maintain head erect briefly	Asymmetry of tone or strength (neurologic damage)	Refer for genetic evaluation.
Reflexes		
Blink: Stimulated by flash of light; response is closure of eyelids	Lack of blink response (damage to cranial nerve, CNS injury)	Assess neurologic status.
Pupillary reflex: Stimulated by flash of light; response is constriction of pupil	Lack of reflex (damage to cranial nerve, CNS injury)	
Moro: Response to sudden movement or loud noise should be one of symmetric extension and abduction of arms with fingers extended; then return to normal relaxed flexion. Infant lying on back: slightly raised head suddenly released; infant held horizontally, lowered quickly about 6 in., and stopped abruptly. Fingers form a C. Present at birth; disappears by 6 months of age	Asymmetry of body response (fractured clavicle, injury to brachial plexus) Consistent absence (brain damage)	Discuss normality of this reflex in response to loud noises and/or sudden movements. Absence of reflex requires neurologic evaluation.
Rooting and sucking: Turns in direction of stimulus to cheek or mouth; opens mouth and begins to suck rhythmically when finger or nipple is inserted into mouth; difficult to elicit after feeding; disappears by 4 to 7 months of age Sucking is adequate for nutritional intake and meeting oral stimulation needs	Poor sucking or easily fatigable (preterm, breastfed infants of drug-addicted mothers, possible cardiac problem) Absence of response (preterm, neurologic involvement, depressed newborns)	Evaluate strength and coordination of sucking. Observe newborn during feeding, and counsel parents about mutuality of feeding experience and newborn's responses.
Palmar grasp: Fingers grasp adult finger when palm is stimulated and held momentarily; lessens at 3 to 4 months of age	Asymmetry of response (neurologic problems)	Evaluate other reflexes and general neurologic functioning.
Plantar grasp :Toes curl downward when sole of foot is stimulated; lessens by 8 months	Absent (defects of lower spinal column)	Assess for other lower extremity neurologic problems.
Stepping: When held upright and one foot touching a flat surface, will step alternately; disappears at 4 to 8 weeks of age	Asymmetry of stepping (neurologic abnormality)	Evaluate muscle tone and function on each side of body. Refer to specialist.
Babinski: Fanning and extension of all toes when one side of sole is stroked from heel upward across ball of foot; disappears at about 12 months	Absence of response (low spinal cord defects)	Refer for further neurologic evaluation.
Tonic neck: Fencer position—when head is turned to one side, extremities on same side extend and on opposite side flex; this reflex may not be evident during early neonatal period; disappears at 3 to 4 months of age Response often more dominant in leg than in arm	Absent after 1 month of age or persistent asymmetry (cerebral lesion)	Assess neurologic functioning.

Assessment Guide—continued

NEWBORN PHYSICAL ASSESSMENT

PHYSICAL ASSESSMENT/ NORMAL FINDINGS	ALTERATIONS AND POSSIBLE CAUSES*	NURSING RESPONSES TO DATA†
Prone crawl: While on abdomen, newborn pushes up and tries to crawl	Absence or variance of response (preterm, weak, or depressed newborns)	Evaluate motor functioning. Refer to specialist.
Trunk incurvation (Galant): In prone position, stroking of spine causes pelvis to turn to stimulated side	Failure to rotate to stimulated side (neurologic damage)	

*Possible causes of alterations are identified in parentheses.
†This column provides guidelines for further assessment and initial nursing interventions.

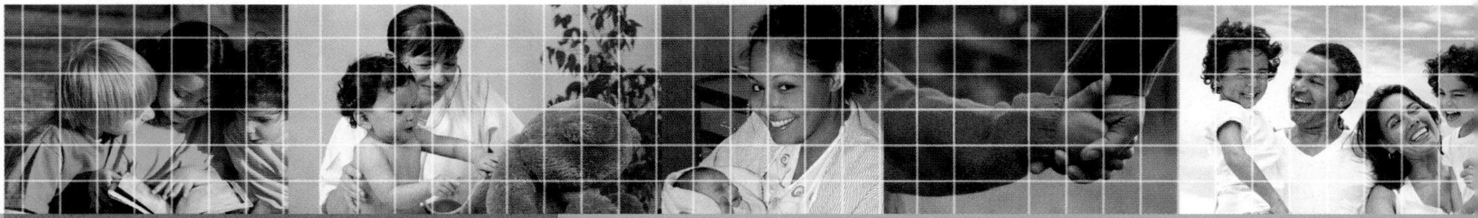

CRITICAL CONCEPT REVIEW

LEARNING OUTCOMES — CONCEPTS

25.1 Describe the physical and neuromuscular maturity characteristics assessed to determine the gestational age of the newborn.

1. The common physical characteristics included in the gestational age assessment are:
   - Skin
   - Lanugo
   - Plantar (sole) creases
   - Breast tissue and size
   - Ear form and cartilage
   - Genitalia
2. The neuromuscular components of gestational age scoring tools are:
   - Posture
   - Square window sign
   - Popliteal angle
   - Arm recoil
   - Heel-to-toe extension
   - Scarf sign
3. By assessing the physical and neuromuscular components specified in a gestational age tool, the nurse determines the gestational age of the newborn and identifies the newborn as SGA, AGA, or LGA and prioritizes individual needs.

25.2 Identify the components of a systematic physical assessment of the newborn.

1. Basis for complete newborn assessment include:
   - Perinatal history
   - Determination of gestational age
   - Physical assessment
   - Behavioral assessment
2. Components of a complete newborn physical assessment include:
   - Vital signs
   - Weight length, and head circumference
   - Skin appearance and presence of birthmarks
   - Examination of the head for size, appearance, symmetry, presence, and status of fontanels
   - Hair appearance
   - Appearance, condition, and symmetry of face, eyes, and ears
   - Appearance and condition of nose and mouth
   - Appearance of chest and auscultation of lungs and heart
   - Appearance of abdomen and presence of bowel sounds
   - Inspection of umbilical stump for 2 arteries and 1 vein
   - Appearance of appropriate genitalia
   - Condition and patency of anus
   - Position and condition of extremities, trunk, and spine

(continued)

LEARNING OUTCOMES | CONCEPTS

25.3 Describe the normal physical characteristics and normal variations of the newborn and compare abnormal findings to possible causes and nursing responses.

1. Normal ranges for newborn vital signs include:
   - heart rate, 120 to 160 beats per minute
   - respirations, 30 to 60 respirations per minute
   - axillary temperature, 36.4°C to 37.2°C (97.5°F to 99°F); skin temperature, 36°C to 36.5°C (96.8°F to 97.7°F); rectal temperature, 36.6°C to 37.2°C (97.8°F to 99°F)
   - blood pressure at birth, 70–50/45–30 mm Hg.
2. Normal newborn measurements include:
   - weight range, 2500 to 4000 g (5 lb, 8 oz to 8 lb, 13 oz), with weight dependent on maternal size and age
   - length range, 46 to 56 cm (18 to 22 in.)
   - head circumference range, 32 to 37 cm (12.5 to 14.5 in.)—approximately 2 cm larger than the chest circumference.
3. The newborn infant should have a head that appears large for its body.
4. The normal newborn has a prominent abdomen, sloping shoulders, narrow hips, and rounded chest. The body appears long and the extremities short.
5. Newborns tend to stay in a flexed position and will resist straightening of the extremities. Hands remain clenched.
6. The nurse should be knowledgeable about variations that are indicative of normal newborn responses as well as those that indicate a need for further investigation.
7. See newborn physical assessment guide for possible causes of abnormal findings and possible nursing responses.
8. An important role of the nurse during the physical assessments of the newborn is to teach parents about their newborn and involve them in their baby's care.

25.4 Describe the components of a neurologic assessment, and the neurologic and neuromuscular characteristics of the newborn and the reflexes that may be present at birth.

1. Neurologic assessment characteristics are:
   - State of alertness
   - Resting position
   - Muscle tone
   - Cry
   - Motor activity
2. Neuromuscular assessment characteristics are:
   - Symmetric movements and strength of all extremities
   - Head lag less than 45 degrees
   - Ability to hold head erect briefly
3. Normal reflexes
   - Blink
   - Pupillary reflex
   - Moro
   - Rooting and sucking
   - Palmar grasp
   - Plantar grasp
   - Stepping
   - Babinski
   - Tonic neck
   - Prone crawl
   - Trunk incurvation

25.5 Describe the components of the newborn behavioral assessment and the normal behavioral characteristics and normal variations of the newborn.

1. Components of Brazelton Neonatal Behavioral Assessment include:
   - Newborn state changes
   - Temperament
   - Individual behavioral patterns
2. The categories of the newborn behavioral characteristics are:
   - Habitation
   - Orientation to inanimate and animate visual and auditory assessment stimuli
   - Motor activity
   - Variations. Frequency of alert states, state changes, color changes, activity, and peaks of activity
   - Self-quieting activity
   - Cuddliness or social behavior

LEARNING OUTCOMES | CONCEPTS

25.6 Correlate findings in a newborn behavioral assessment to possible nursing responses and to teach and involve parents in the care of their newborn.

1. Behaviorally, the infant will sleep the majority of the time and wake for feeding. The infant should be easily consoled when upset.
2. An important role of the nurse during the behavioral assessments of the newborn is to teach parents about their newborn and involve them in their baby's care. This involvement facilitates the parents' identification of their newborn's uniqueness, allays their concerns, and fosters positive attachment experiences.

CRITICAL THINKING IN ACTION

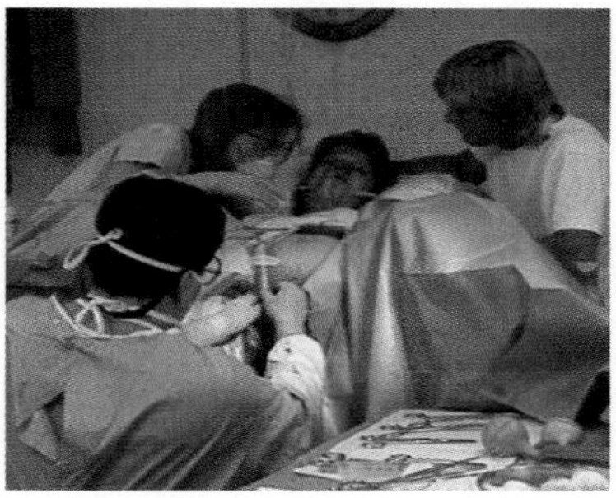

Susan Pine, a 21-year-old G2, now P1011, delivers a 39 2/7-weeks gestation female newborn. The vaginal birth is assisted with a vacuum extractor. The prenatal record is significant for an increase of maternal blood pressure to 140/90 on the day of birth. Susan is treated with magnesium sulfate during her labor and has an epidural analgesia for the pain of labor. The baby's Apgar is 8 and 9 at 1 and 5 minutes, and she has been admitted to the newborn nursery. The newborn's admission exam is normal except for a 2-cm round caput succedaneum. Now, 8 hours later, the baby's condition is stable and she needs to be bottle-fed. You take her to her mother's room where you observe that Susan does not reach out to take her from you. She seems unsure when handling her baby. Susan asks you about the swelling on her baby's head and wonders if it will ever go away.

1. How would you explain the cause of Susan's baby's caput succedaneum?
2. Compare the difference between a cephalohematoma and caput succedaneum.
3. Explore with Susan her baby's reflexes and state of alertness.
4. Susan asks you how she will know what her baby needs. How would you respond?

See MyNursingKit for possible responses.

REFERENCES

American Academy of Pediatrics (AAP), Committee on Fetus and Newborn, & American College of Obstetricians and Gynecologists (ACOG), Committee on Obstetrics. (2007). *Guidelines for perinatal care* (6th ed.). Evanston, IL: Author.

Ballard, J. L., Khoury, J. C., Wedig, K., Wang, L., Eilers-Walsmann, B. L., & Lipp, R. (1991). New Ballard score, expanded to include extremely premature infants. *Journal of Pediatrics, 119*(3), 417–423.

Blackburn, S. T. (2007). *Maternal, fetal, neonatal physiology: A clinical perspective* (3rd ed.). St. Louis: Saunders.

Brazelton, T. B., & Nugent, J. K. (1995). *The neonatal behavioral assessment scale* (3rd ed.). London: MacKeith.

Creehan, P. A. (2008). Newborn physical assessment. In K. R. Simpson & P. A. Creehan, *Perinatal nursing* (3rd ed., pp. 546–574). Philadelphia: Lippincott Williams & Wilkins.

Kliegman, R. M., Behrman, R. E., Jenson, H. B., Stanton, B. F. (Eds.). (2007). Nelson textbook of pediatrics. (18th ed.). Philadelphia: Saunders.

Mandleco, B. L. (2004). *Growth and development handbook: Newborn through adolescence.* Clifton Park, NY: Thomson/Delmar Learning.

Rohan, A., & Golombek, S. (2009). Hypoxia in the newborn: cardiopulmonary physiology and assessment. *Maternal Child Nursing,* 34(2), 106–112.

Thureen, P. J., Deacon, J., Hernandez, J. A., & Hall, D. M. (2005). *Assessment and care of the well newborn* (2nd ed.). St. Louis: Elsevier.

Wu, T.-Y., & Daniel, L. (2001). Growth of immigrant Chinese infants in the first year of life. *American Journal of Maternal Child Nursing, 26*(4), 202–207.

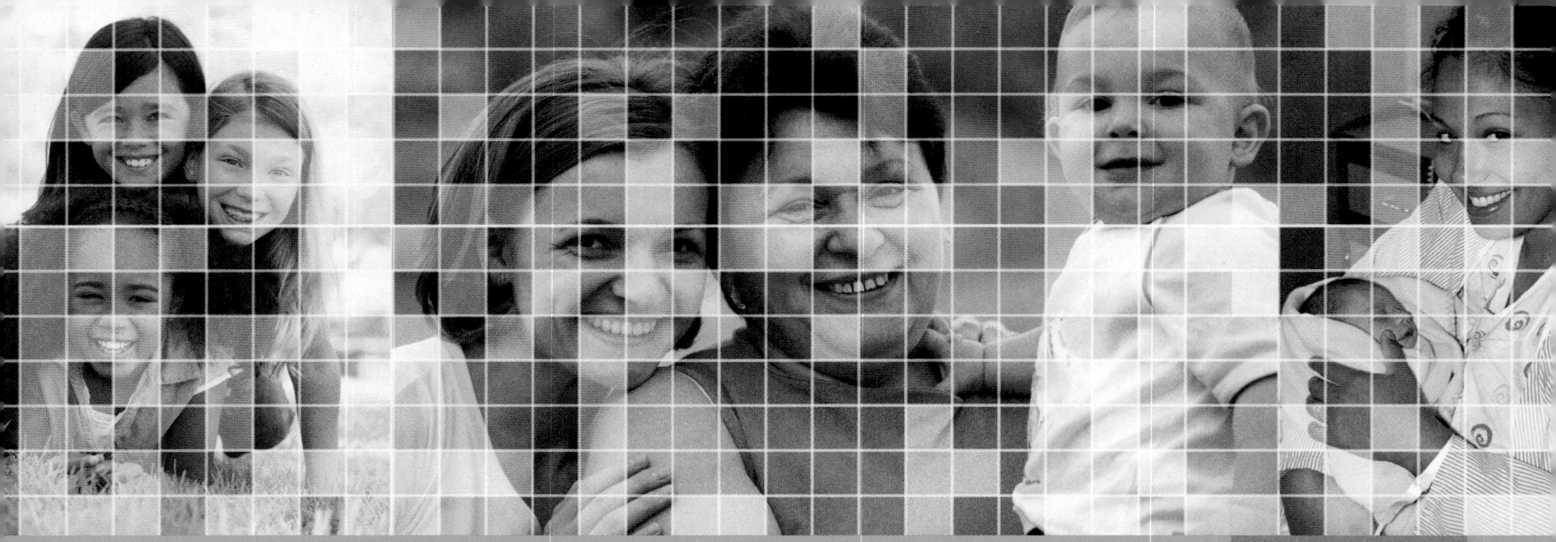

CHAPTER

The Normal Newborn: Needs and Care 26

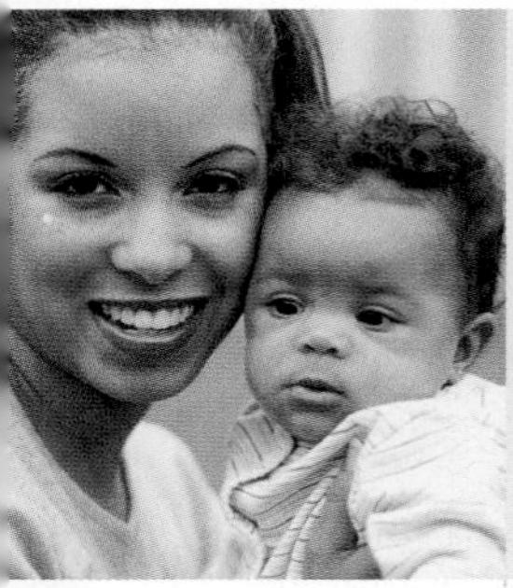

When our daughter was laid in my arms right after birth she was so delicate. I had not dared to hope that we would be blessed with a girl because there were so few girls in my husband's family. Our 2-year-old niece was the first girl in 107 years, so I had pretty much decided that another boy would be just fine. But here she was, right here in my arms. —Catherine, 32

LEARNING OUTCOMES

26.1 Summarize essential information to be obtained about a newborn's birth experience and immediate postnatal period.

26.2 Explain how the physiologic and behavioral responses of the newborn during the first 4 hours after birth (admission and transitional period) determine the nursing care of the newborn.

26.3 Describe the major nursing considerations and activities to be carried out after the transitional period until discharge based on the physiologic and behavioral responses of the newborn.

26.4 Describe common concerns of families and related content to be included in parent teaching on daily newborn and infant care and discharge planning.

26.5 Discuss opportunities to individualize parent teaching and enhance each parent's abilities and confidence while providing infant care in the birthing unit.

At the moment of birth, numerous physiologic adaptations begin to take place in the newborn's body. Because of these dramatic changes, newborns require close observation to determine how smoothly they are making the transition to extrauterine life. Newborns also require specific care that enhances their chances of making the transition successfully.

The two broad goals of nursing care during this period are: (1) to promote the physical well-being of the newborn, and (2) to support the establishment of a well-functioning family unit. To meet the first goal, the nurse provides comprehensive care to the newborn in the mother-baby unit. To meet the second goal, the nurse teaches family members how to care for their new baby and supports their efforts so that they feel confident and competent. Thus, the nurse must be knowledgeable about necessary family adjustments as well as the healthcare needs of the newborn. It is important that the family return home confident, knowing that they have the support, information, and skills to care for their newborn. Equally important is the need for each member of the family to begin a unique relationship with the newborn. The cultural and social expectations of individual families and communities affect the way in which normal newborn care is implemented.

The previous two chapters presented an informational database of the physiologic and behavioral changes occurring in the newborn and the pertinent nursing assessments that are needed. This chapter discusses the nursing care management while the newborn is in the birthing unit.

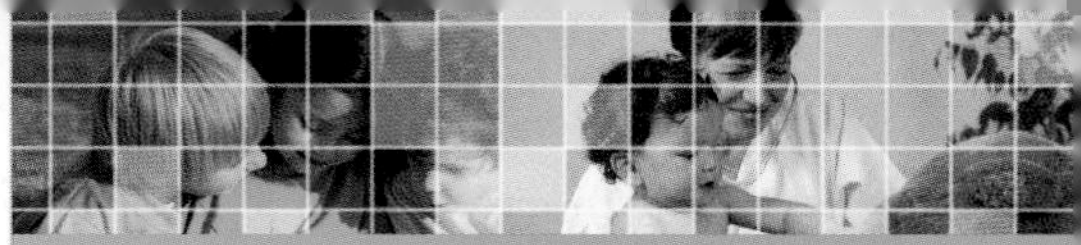

KEY TERMS

Circumcision, 614

Newborn screening tests, 621

Parent-newborn attachment, 611

NURSING CARE DURING ADMISSION AND THE FIRST FOUR HOURS OF LIFE

Immediately after birth, the baby is formally admitted to the healthcare facility.

NURSING ASSESSMENT AND DIAGNOSIS

Before the birth of an infant, the nurse reviews the mother's prenatal record for information concerning possible risk factors for the infant. These include infectious diseases screening results, drug or alcohol use by the mother, gestational diabetes, and any other data determined to be of use in anticipating the needs of the newborn. Review the birth record for prolonged rupture of membranes, instrument or vacuum childbirth, use of narcotic analgesia, presence of meconium, and any other data that may impact the infant's ability to successfully transition to the extrauterine environment.

During the first 4 hours after birth, the nurse carries out a preliminary physical examination, including an assessment of the newborn's physiologic adaptations. In many birthing units, the nurse performs and documents the initial head-to-toe physical assessment during the first hour of transition. The nurse is responsible for notifying the physician or nurse practitioner of anything abnormal. A complete physical examination is also performed later by the physician or nurse practitioner, within 24 hours after birth and within 24 hours before discharge. This can be accomplished with one physical examination (American Academy of Pediatrics [AAP] & American College of Obstetricians and Gynecologists [ACOG], 2007) (see Chapter 25∞).

Nursing diagnoses are based on an analysis of the assessment findings. Physiologic alterations of the newborn form the basis of many nursing diagnoses, as does the family members' incorporation of them in caring for their newborn. Nursing diagnoses that may apply to newborns include the following:

- *Ineffective Airway Clearance* related to presence of mucus and retained lung fluid
- *Risk for Imbalanced Body Temperature* related to evaporative, radiant, conductive, and convective heat losses
- *Acute Pain* related to heel sticks for glucose or hematocrit tests or vitamin K injection

MyNursingKit Video: Newborn Care

Table 26–1 Signs of Newborn Transition

Normal findings for the newborn during the first few days of life include the following: Pulse: 120 to 160 beats/minute During sleep as low as 100 beats/minute If crying, up to 180 beats/minute Apical pulse is counted for 1 full minute because rate may fluctuate
Respirations: 30 to 60 respirations/minute Predominantly diaphragmatic but synchronous with abdominal movements Brief periods of apnea (less than 15 seconds) with no color or heart rate changes
Temperature: Axillary: 36.4°C to 37.2°C (97.5°F to 99°F) Skin: 36°C to 36.5°C (96.8°F to 97.7°F)
Blood pressure: 90–60/50–40 mm Hg at birth; 100/50 mm Hg at day 10 Blood glucose: greater than or equal to 40 mg% Hematocrit: less than 65% to 70% central venous sample

As discussed in Chapter 24∞, the newborn's physiologic adaptation to extrauterine life occurs rapidly and all body systems are affected (Table 26–1). Therefore, many of these nursing diagnoses and associated interventions must be identified and implemented in a short period.

MyNursingKit Care Plan Activity: Initial Newborn Care

NURSING PLAN AND IMPLEMENTATION

The nurse initiates newborn admission procedures and evaluates the newborn's need to remain under observation. This evaluation may take place in a special transition area or at the mother's bedside. It includes the following:

- Maternal and birth history
- Airway clearance
- Vital signs
- Body temperature
- Neurologic status
- Ability to feed
- Evidence of complications

If the evaluation is normal, the newborn is successfully transitioning to extrauterine life and may need less frequent observations. In some settings, it may be an appropriate time for moving the mother and newborn to another care unit.

Initiating Admission Procedures

After birth, the newborn is formally admitted to the healthcare facility. The admission procedures include a review of prenatal and birth information for possible risk factors, a gestational age assessment, and an assessment to ensure that the newborn's adaptation to extrauterine life is proceeding normally. This evaluation of the newborn's status and risk factors must be done no later than 2 hours after birth (AAP & ACOG, 2007).

If the initial assessment indicates that the newborn is not at risk physiologically, the nurse performs many of the routine admission procedures in the presence of the parents in the birthing area. Some care measures indicated by the assessment findings may be performed by the nurse or by the family members under the guidance of the nurse in an effort to educate and support the family. Other interventions may be delayed until the newborn has been transferred to an observational nursery.

The nurse responsible for the newborn first checks and confirms the newborn's identification with the mother's identification and then obtains and records all significant information. The essential data to be recorded on the newborn's chart are as follows:

1. *Condition of the newborn.* Include the newborn's Apgar scores at 1 and 5 minutes, resuscitative measures required in the birthing area, physical examination, vital signs, voidings, and passing of meconium. Complications to be noted are excessive mucus, delayed spontaneous respirations or responsiveness, abnormal number of cord vessels, and obvious physical abnormalities.
2. *Labor and birth record.* A copy of the labor and birth record should be placed in the newborn's chart or be accessible on the computer. The record contains the significant data about the birth, for example, duration, course, and status of mother and fetus throughout labor and birth and any analgesia or anesthesia administered to the mother. The nurse notes any variation or difficulties, such as prolonged rupture of membranes, abnormal fetal position, presence or absence of meconium-stained amniotic fluid, signs of nonreassuring fetal heart rate during labor, nuchal cord (cord around the newborn's neck at birth), precipitous birth, use of forceps or vacuum extraction assisted device, maternal analgesics and anesthesia received within 1 hour before birth, and administration of antibiotics during labor.
3. *Antepartal history.* Any maternal problems that may have compromised the fetus in utero are of immediate concern in newborn assessment and can include the following: preeclampsia, spotting, illness, recent infections (evidence of chorioamnionitis), blood type, rubella status, serology results, hepatitis B screen results, colonization with group B streptococci or intrapartum maternal antibiotic therapy; maternal medications (including tocolytics and corticosteroids), a history of maternal substance abuse. The chart should also include information about maternal age, estimated date of birth (EDB), previous pregnancies, and presence of any congenital anomalies. A human immunodeficiency virus (HIV) test result, if obtained, is also relevant (AAP & ACOG, 2007).
4. *Parent-newborn interaction information.* The nurse notes parents' interactions with their newborn and their desires regarding care, such as rooming-in, circumcision, and the type of feeding. Information about other children in the home, available support systems, interactional patterns within each family unit, situations that compromise lactation (breast surgery, previous lactation failure), and any high risk circumstances (adolescent mother, domestic

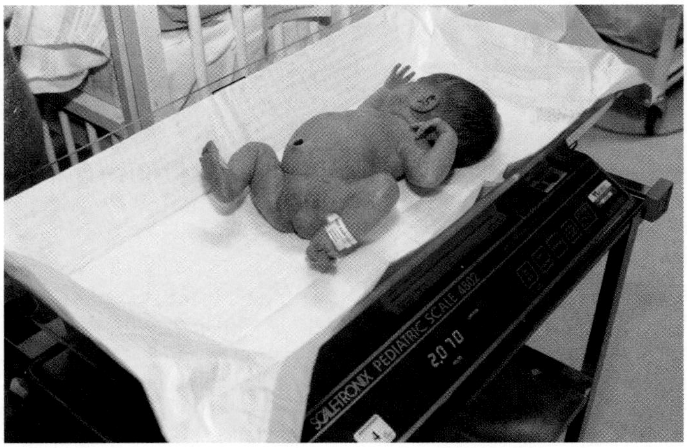

● **Figure 26–1** Weighing of newborn: The scale is cleaned and balanced before each weighing, with the protective pad in place.

violence, history of child abuse) help in providing comprehensive care (AAP & ACOG, 2007).

As part of the admission procedure, the nurse weighs the newborn in both grams and pounds. In the United States, parents understand weight best when it is stated in pounds and ounces (Figure 26–1 ●). The nurse cleans and covers the scales each time a newborn is weighed to prevent cross infection and heat loss from conduction.

The nurse then measures the newborn, recording the measurements in both centimeters and inches. The three routine measurements are length, head circumference, and chest circumference. In some facilities, abdominal girth may also be measured. Rapidly assesses the baby's color, muscle tone, alertness, and general state. Remember that the first period of reactivity may have concluded, and the baby may be in the sleep-inactive phase, which makes the infant hard to arouse. Do basic assessments for estimating gestational age and complete the physical assessment (see Chapter 25∞).

In addition to obtaining vital signs, perform a hematocrit and blood glucose evaluation on at-risk newborns or as clinically indicated (such as for small-for-gestational-age [SGA] or large-for-gestational-age [LGA] infants, or if the newborn is jittery). These procedures may be done on admission or within the first 2 hours after birth (AAP & ACOG, 2007.) (See the Clinical Skills Manual: Performing a Heel Stick on a Newborn SKILLS and Chapter 29, see "Clinical Pathway: Newborn Care" feature starting on page 606.)

Maintaining a Clear Airway and Stable Vital Signs

Free flow oxygen should be readily available. The nurse positions the newborn on his or her back (or side, if infant has copious secretions). If necessary, the nurse should use a bulb syringe or DeLee wall suction (see Chapter 19, Figure 19–8∞ and in the Clinical Skills Manual SKILLS) to remove mucus from the stomach to help prevent possible aspiration. When possible, this procedure should be delayed for 10 to 15 minutes after birth, reducing the potential for severe vasovagal reflex apnea.

In the absence of any newborn distress, continue with the admission by taking the newborn's vital signs. The initial temperature is taken by the axillary method. A wider range of normal exists for axillary temperature, specifically 36.4°C to 37.2°C (97.5°F to 99°F).

Once the initial temperature is taken, the nurse monitors the core temperature either by obtaining axillary temperatures at intervals or by placing a skin sensor on the newborn for continuous reading. The usual skin sensor placement site is the newborn's abdomen, but placement on the upper thigh or arm can give a reading closely correlated with the mean body temperature. The vital signs for a healthy term newborn should be monitored at least every 30 minutes until the newborn's condition has remained stable for 2 hours (AAP & ACOG, 2007). The newborn's respirations may be irregular yet still be normal. Brief periods of apnea, lasting only 5 to 10 seconds with no color or heart rate changes, are considered normal. The normal pulse range is 120 to 160 beats per minute (bpm), and the normal respiratory range is 30 to 60 respirations per minute.

Thinking Critically

EARLY RESPIRATORY EFFORTS

You overhear Mr. Johannson speaking to his mother on the phone. He is telling her about the "cute little noises" his 30-minute-old baby makes. The infant is in the room with the mother. What is your best course of action?

See MyNursingKit for possible responses.

Maintaining a Neutral Thermal Environment

A neutral thermal environment is essential to minimize the newborn's need for increased oxygen consumption and use of calories to maintain body heat in the optimal range of 36.4°C to 37.2°C (97.5°F to 99°F). If the newborn becomes hypothermic, the body's response can lead to metabolic acidosis, hypoxia, and shock.

A neutral thermal environment is best achieved by performing the newborn assessment and interventions with the newborn unclothed and under a radiant warmer. The radiant warmer's thermostat is controlled by the thermal skin sensor taped to the newborn's abdomen, upper thigh, or arm (Figure 26–2 ●). The sensor indicates

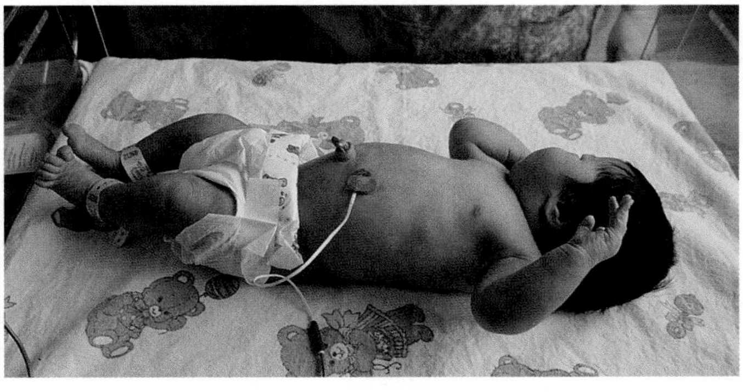

● **Figure 26–2** Temperature monitoring for the newborn. A skin thermal sensor is placed on the newborn's abdomen, upper thigh, or arm and secured with porous tape or a foil-covered foam pad.

Source: Photographer, Elena Dorfman.

Clinical Pathway

NEWBORN CARE

CATEGORY	FIRST 4 HOURS	4 TO 8 HOURS PAST BIRTH	8 TO 24 HOURS PAST BIRTH
Referral	Review labor/birth record Review transitional nursing record Check ID bands and security alarms if present Consult prn: orthopedics, genetics, infectious disease	Check ID bands and security alarms Transfer to mother-baby care at 4 to 6 hours of age if stable As parents desire, obtain circumcision permit after their discussion with physician Lactation consult prn	Check ID bands and security alarm q shift **EXPECTED OUTCOMES** Mother/baby ID bands correlate at time of discharge, security alarms in place at all times; consults completed prn
Assessments	Continue assessments begun first hour after birth Vital sign: TPR, BP prn, q1h × 4 (skin temp 36°C to 36.5°C [96.8°F to 97.7°F], resp may be irregular but within 30 to 60 per min) **NEWBORN ASSESSMENTS** ■ Respiratory status with resp. distress scale × 1 then prn. If resp. distress, assess q5–15 min ■ Cord: bluish white color, clamp in place and free from skin ■ Color: skin, mucous membranes, extremities, trunk pink with slight acrocyanosis of hands and feet ■ Wt (5 lb, 8 oz to 8 lb, 13 oz) 2,500 to 4,000 g, length (18 to 22 in.) 46 to 56 cm, HC (12.5 to 14.5 in.) 32 to 37 cm, CC (32.5 cm, 1 to 2 cm less than head) ■ Extremity movement—may be jerky or brief twitches ■ Gestational age classification—term AGA ■ Anomalies (cong. anomalies can interfere with normal extrauterine adaptation)	Assess newborn's progress through periods of reactivity Vital signs: TPR q8h and prn, or per agency protocol, BP prn **NEWBORN ASSESSMENTS** ■ Skin color q4h prn (circulatory system stabilizing, acrocyanosis decreased) ■ Eyes for drainage, redness, hemorrhage ■ Auscultate lungs q4h (noisy, wet breath sounds clear and equal) ■ Increased mucus production (normal in second period of reactivity) ■ Check apical pulse q4h ■ Check umbilical cord base for redness, drainage, foul odor, drying, clamp in place ■ Extremity movements q4h ■ Check for expected reflexes (suck, rooting, Moro, grasp, blink, yawn, sneeze, tonic neck, Babinski) ■ Note common normal variations ■ Assess suck and swallow during feeding ■ Note behavioral characteristics ■ Check temp before and after admission bath	VS q8h; normal ranges: T, 36.4°C to 37.2°C (97.5°F to 99°F) P, 120 to 160; R, 30 to 60; BP, 90–60/50–40 mm Hg **CONTINUE NEWBORN ASSESSMENTS** ■ Skin color q4h ■ Signs of drying or infection in cord area ■ Check that clamp is in place until removed before discharge ■ Check circ. for bleeding after procedure, then q30min × 2, then q4h and prn Observe for jaundice. Obtain total serum bili (TsB) if infant visibly jaundiced before 24 hours of age. Obtain transcutaneous bili on all infants not previously tested before discharge. **EXPECTED OUTCOMES** Vital signs medically acceptable, color pink, assessments WNL, circ. site without s/s infection, cord site without s/s of infection and clamp removed; newborn behavior WNL
Teaching/ psychosocial	Admission activities performed at mother's bedside if possible, orient to nursery prn, handwashing, assess teaching needs Teach parents use of bulb syringe, signs of choking, positioning, and when to call for assistance Teach reasons for use of radiant warmer, infant hat, and warmed blankets when out of warmer Discuss/teach infant security, identification	Reinforce teaching about choking, bulb syringe use, positioning, temperature maintenance with clothing and blankets Teach infant positioning to facilitate breathing and digestion Teach new parents holding and feeding skills Teach parents soothing and calming techniques Teach parents about introducing newborn to sibling	Final discharge teaching: diapering, normal void and stool patterns, bathing, nail and cord care, circumcision/uncircumcised penis/genital care and normal characteristics, rashes, jaundice, sleep-wake cycles, soothing activities, taking temperatures, thermometer reading Explain s/s of illness and when to call healthcare provider Infant safety: car seats, immunizations, metabolic screening **EXPECTED OUTCOMES** Mother/family verbalize comprehension of teaching; demonstrate care capabilities

Clinical Pathway—continued

NEWBORN CARE

CATEGORY	FIRST 4 HOURS	4 TO 8 HOURS PAST BIRTH	8 TO 24 HOURS PAST BIRTH
Nursing care management and reports	Place under radiant warmer Place hat on newborn (decreases convection heat loss) Suction nares/mouth with bulb syringe prn Keep bulb syringe with infant Attach security sensor Obtain lab tests: blood glucose; as needed Obtain blood type, Rh, Coombs on cord blood, HSV culture if parental hx Notify physician's office of infant's birth and any change in status Maintain Standard Precautions	Wean from radiant warmer (T 37°C [98°F] axillary) Chemstrips prn; BP prn Oxygen saturation prn Bathe infant if temp > 36.5°C (97.7°F) Position on side Suction nares prn (esp. during second period of reactivity) Obtain peripheral Hct per protocol Cord care per protocol Fold diaper below cord (for plastic diapers, turn plastic layer away from skin)	Check for hearing test results Weigh before discharge Cord assessment q shift DC cord clamp before discharge Perform newborn metabolic screening blood tests before discharge Circumcision if indicated; circumcision care: change diaper prn, noting ability to void; follow policy for circumcision damp or Plastibell care **EXPECTED OUTCOMES** Newborn maintains temp, lab test WNL, cord dry without s/s infection and clamp removed, screening tests accomplished, circ. site without s/s of infection or bleeding
Activity and comfort	Place under radiant warmer or wrap in prewarmed blankets until stable or maintain skin-to-skin contact with mother Soothe baby as needed with voice, touch, cuddling, nesting in radiant warmer	Leave in warmer until stable, then swaddle Position on back after each feeding	Place in open crib Swaddle to allow movement of extremities in blanket, including hands to face **EXPECTED OUTCOMES** Infant maintains temp WNL in open crib, infant attempts self-calming behaviors
Nutrition	Assist newborn to breastfeed as soon as mother/baby condition allows Supplement breast only when medically indicated or per agency policy Initiate formula-feeding within first hour Gavage feed if necessary to prevent hypoglycemia	Breastfeed on demand, at least q3–4h Teach positions, observe/assist with feeding, breast/nipple care, establishing milk supply, breaking suction, feeding cues, latching-on techniques, nutritive suck, burping Formula-feed on demand, at least q3–4h Determine readiness to feed and feeding tolerance	Continue breastfeeding or formula-feeding pattern Assess feeding tolerance q4h Discuss normal feeding requirements, signs of hunger and satiation, handling feeding problems, and when to seek help **EXPECTED OUTCOMES** Mother verbalizes knowledge of feeding information; breastfeeds on demand without supplement; bottle—tolerates formula-feeding, nipples without problems
Elimination	Note first void and stool if not noted at birth	Note all voids, amount and color of stools q4h	Evaluate all voids and stool color q8h **EXPECTED OUTCOMES** Voids qs; stools qs without difficulty; stool character WNL diaper area without s/s of skin breakdown or rashes
Medication	Prophylactic ophthalmic ointment both eyes after baby makes eye contact with parents within 1 hr after birth Administer AquaMEPHYTON IM, dosage according to infant weight per MD/NP order.	Hepatitis B injection as ordered by physician after consent signed by parents	Hepatitis B vaccine within 2 hrs of birth or before discharge **EXPECTED OUTCOMES** Baby has received ophthalmic ointment and vitamin K injection; baby has received first Hep B vaccine if ordered and parental permission received

(continued)

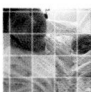

Clinical Pathway—continued

NEWBORN CARE

CATEGORY	FIRST 4 HOURS	4 TO 8 HOURS PAST BIRTH	8 TO 24 HOURS PAST BIRTH
Discharge planning/ home care	Hepatitis B consent signed Hearing screen consent signed Plan discharge call with parent or guardian in 24 hr to 2 days Assess parents' discharge plans, needs, and support systems	Review/reinforce teaching with mother and significant other Review home preparedness Present birth certificate instructions	Initial newborn screening tests (hearing, blood tests, metabolic screen [i.e., PKU]) before discharge Bath and feeding classes, videos, or written information given Give written copy of discharge instructions Newborn photographs Set up appointment for follow-up PKU test Have car seat available before discharge All discharge referrals made, follow-up appt scheduled **EXPECTED OUTCOMES** Infant discharged home with family; mother verbalizes follow-up appt time/date
Family involvement	Facilitate early investigation of baby's physical characteristics (maintain temp during unwrapping), hold infant *en face* Dim lights to help infant keep eyes open	Assess parents' knowledge of newborn behaviors, such as alertness, suck and rooting, attention to human voice, response to calming techniques Facilitate parent interaction with infant by performing care in presence of parents and encouraging parents to participate in care	Assess mother-baby bonding/interaction Incorporate father and siblings in care Enhance parent-infant interaction by sharing characteristics and behavioral assessment Support positive parenting behaviors Identify community referral needs and refer to community agencies **EXPECTED OUTCOME** Demonstrates caring and family incorporation of infant
Date			

AGA, average for gestational age; Appt, appointment; CC, chest circumference; cong., congenital; esp., especially; HC, head circumference; Hct, hematocrit; Hx, history; ID, identification; PKU, phenylketonuria; qs, quantity sufficient; s/s, signs and symptoms; temp, temperature; TPR, temperature, pulse, respirations; VS, vital signs; WNL, within normal limits.

when the newborn's temperature exceeds or falls below the acceptable temperature range. The nurse should be aware that leaning over the newborn may block the radiant heat waves from reaching the newborn. It is common practice in some institutions to cover the newborn's head with a cap made of insulated fabrics, wool, or polyolefin; lined with Gamgee; or insulated with a plastic liner to prevent further evaporative heat loss, in addition to placing the newborn under a radiant warmer (Blackburn, 2007).

When the newborn's temperature is normal and vital signs are stable (about 2 to 4 hours after birth), the newborn may be bathed. However, this admission bath may be postponed for some hours if the newborn's condition dictates or the parents wish to give the first bath. In light of early discharge practices (12 to 48 hours), healthy term infants can be safely bathed immediately after the admission assessment is completed. The newborn is bathed while still under the radiant warmer; bathing may be done in the parents' room and by the parents (Medves & O'Brien, 2004). Bathing the newborn offers an excellent opportunity for teaching and welcoming parents' involvement in the care of their newborn.

> **Nursing Practice**
>
> A cap can be fashioned from a piece of stockinette to help reduce heat loss from the head.

The nurse rechecks the newborn's temperature after the bath and, if it is stable, dresses the newborn in a shirt, diaper, and cap; wraps the baby; and places the newborn in an open crib at room temperature. If the newborn's axillary temperature is below 36.5°C

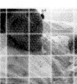

Table 26–2	Maintenance of Stable Newborn Temperature
Take action to help the newborn maintain a stable temperature:	
■ Keep the newborn's clothing and bedding dry.	
■ Double-wrap the newborn and put a stocking cap on him or her.	
■ Use the radiant warmer during procedures.	
■ Reduce the newborn's exposure to drafts.	
■ Warm objects that will be in contact with the newborn (e.g., stethoscope).	
■ Encourage the mother to snuggle with the newborn under blankets or to breastfeed the newborn with hat and light cover on.	

(97.7°F), the nurse returns the newborn to the radiant warmer. The rewarming process should be gradual to prevent hyperthermia. Once the newborn is rewarmed, the nurse implements measures to prevent further neonatal heat loss, such as keeping the newborn dry, swaddled in one or two blankets with hat on, and away from cool surfaces or instruments. The nurse also protects the newborn from drafts, open windows or doors, and air conditioners. Blankets and clothing are stored in a warm place. (See Chapter 25∞ and Table 26–2.) Newborns are often "double-wrapped" in two or more blankets for temperature maintenance.

Preventing Vitamin K Deficiency Bleeding

A prophylactic injection of vitamin K_1 (AquaMEPHYTON) is recommended to prevent hemorrhage, which can occur because of low prothrombin levels in the first few days of life (see "Drug Guide: Vitamin K_1 Phytonadione [AquaMEPHYTON]" on page 610). The potential for hemorrhage is considered to result from the absence of gut bacterial flora, which influences the production of vitamin K_1 in the newborn (see Chapter 29∞ for further discussion). Newborns should receive a single parenteral dose of 0.5 to 1 mg of natural vitamin K_1 oxide (phytonadione) within 1 hour of birth or this dose may be delayed until after the first breastfeeding in the childbirth/birthing area (AAP & ACOG, 2007; Wilson, Shannon, & Shields, 2010). Current recommendations underscore the need for treatment in infants who are exclusively breastfed (Blackburn, 2007).

The vitamin K_1 injection is given intramuscularly in the middle third of the vastus lateralis muscle, located in the lateral aspect of the thigh (Figure 26–3 ●). Before injecting, the nurse must thoroughly clean the newborn's skin site for the injection with a small alcohol swab. The nurse uses a 25-gauge, 5/8-in. needle for the injection. An alternate site is the rectus femoris muscle in the anterior aspect of the thigh. However, this site is near the sciatic nerve and femoral artery; therefore, injections here should be done with caution (Figure 26–4 ●).

Preventing Eye Infection

The nurse is also responsible for giving the legally required prophylactic eye treatment for *Neisseria gonorrhoeae,* which may have infected the newborn of an infected mother during the birth process. A variety of topical agents appear to be equally effective. Ophthalmic ointments that are used include 0.5% erythromycin (Ilotycin Ophthalmic) (see "Drug Guide: Erythromycin Ophthalmic Ointment [Ilotycin Ophthalmic]" on page 611), 1% tetracycline, or per agency protocol (AAP & ACOG, 2007). All are also effective against chlamydia, which has a higher incidence rate than gonorrhea.

Successful eye prophylaxis requires that the medication be instilled into the lower conjunctival sac of each eye (Figure 26–5 ●).

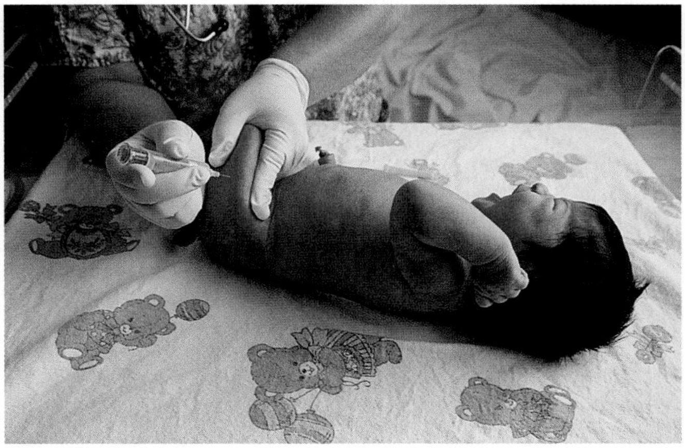

● **Figure 26–3** Procedure for vitamin K injection. Cleanse area thoroughly with alcohol swab and allow skin to dry. Bunch the tissue of the upper outer thigh (vastus lateralis muscle) and quickly insert a 25-gauge, 5/8-in. needle at a 90-degree angle to the thigh. Aspirate, then slowly inject the solution to distribute the medication evenly and minimize the baby's discomfort. Remove the needle and gently massage the site with an alcohol swab.

Source: Photographer, Elena Dorfman.

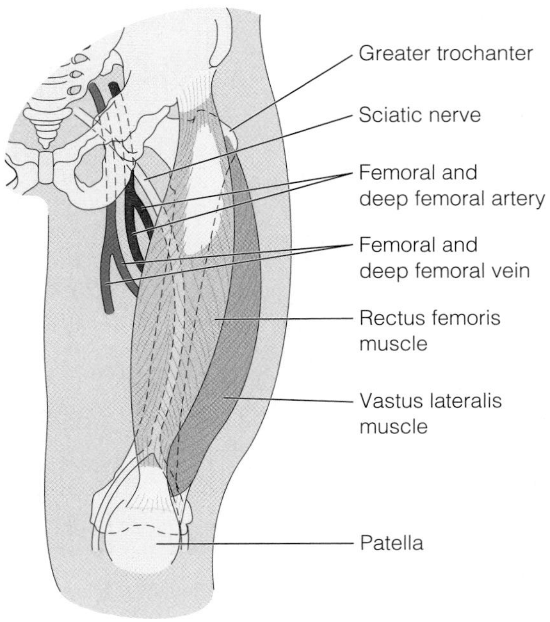

● **Figure 26–4** Injection sites. The middle third of the vastus lateralis muscle is the preferred site for intramuscular injection in the newborn. The middle third of the rectus femoris is an alternate site, but its proximity to major vessels and the sciatic nerve requires caution in using this site for injection.

Drug Guide

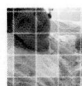

VITAMIN K_1 PHYTONADIONE (AQUAMEPHYTON)

Pregnancy Risk Category: C

Overview of Neonatal Action

Phytonadione is used in prophylaxis and treatment of vitamin K deficiency bleeding (VKDB), formerly known as hemorrhagic disease of the newborn. It promotes liver formation of the clotting factors II, VII, IX, and X. At birth, the newborn does not have the bacteria in the colon that are necessary for synthesizing fat-soluble vitamin K_1. Therefore, the newborn may have decreased levels of prothrombin during the first 5 to 8 days of life, reflected by a prolongation of prothrombin time.

Route, Dosage, Frequency

Intramuscular injection is given in the vastus lateralis thigh muscle. A one-time-only prophylactic dose of 0.5 to 1 mg is given intramuscularly within 1 hour of birth or may be delayed until after the first breastfeeding in the delivery/birthing area (AAP & ACOG, 2007; Wilson, Shannon, & Shields, 2010).

If the mother received anticoagulants during pregnancy, an additional dose may be ordered by the physician and is given 6 to 8 hours after the first injection. IM concentration: 1 mg/0.5 mL (neonatal strength); can use 10 mg/mL concentration to minimize volume injected.

Neonatal Side Effects

Pain and edema may occur at the injection site. Allergic reactions, such as rash and urticaria, may also occur.

Nursing Considerations

- Protect drug from light
- Give vitamin K_1 before circumcision procedure
- Observe for signs of local inflammation
- Observe for bleeding (usually occurs on second or third day). Bleeding may be seen as generalized ecchymoses or bleeding from umbilical cord, circumcision site, nose, or gastrointestinal tract. Results of serial prothrombin time (PT) and international normalized ratio (INR) should be assessed.
- Observe for jaundice and kernicterus, especially in preterm infants.

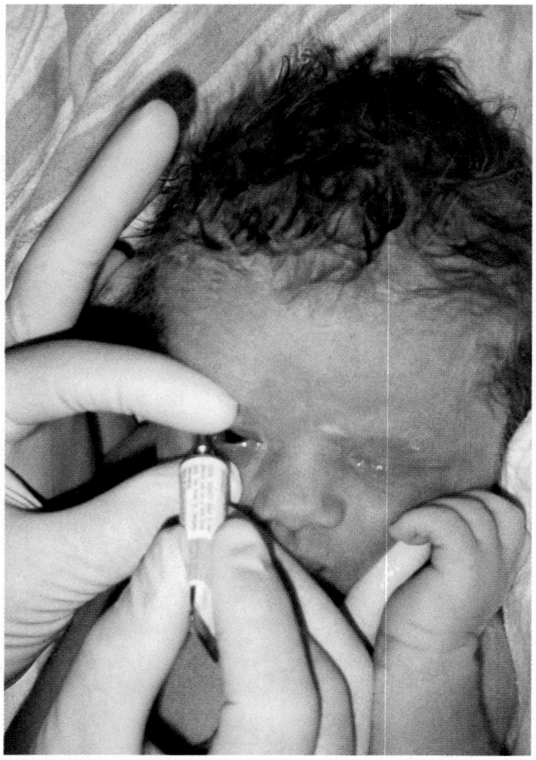

● **Figure 26–5** Ophthalmic ointment. Retract the lower eyelid outward to instill a 1/4-in. (1 cm) long strand of ointment from a single-dose tube along the lower conjunctival surface. *Make sure that the tip of the tube does not touch the eye.*

The nurse massages the eyelid gently to distribute the ointment. Instillation may be delayed up to 1 hour after birth to allow eye contact during parent-newborn bonding.

Eye prophylaxis medications can cause chemical conjunctivitis, which gives the newborn some discomfort and may interfere with the ability to focus on the parents' faces. The resulting edema, inflammation, and discharge may cause concern if the parents have not been informed that the side effects will clear in 24 to 48 hours and that this prophylactic eye treatment is necessary for the newborn's well-being.

Early Assessment of Neonatal Distress

During the first 24 hours of life, be constantly alert for signs of distress. If the newborn is with the parents during this period, the nurse must take extra care to teach them how to maintain their newborn's temperature, recognize the hallmarks of newborn distress, and respond immediately to signs of respiratory problems. The parents learn to observe the newborn for changes in color or activity, grunting or "sighing" sounds with breathing, rapid breathing with chest retractions, or facial grimacing. Their interventions include nasal and oral suctioning with a bulb syringe, positioning, and vigorous fingertip stroking of the newborn's spine to stimulate respiratory activity if necessary. The nurse must be available immediately if the newborn develops distress (Table 26–3).

A common cause of neonatal distress is early onset group B streptococcal (GBS) disease. Infected mothers transmit GBS infection to their infants during labor and birth; thus it is recommended that at-risk mothers receive intrapartum antimicrobial prophylaxis (IAP) for GBS disease. All infants of mothers identified as at risk should be assessed and observed for signs and symptoms of sepsis (see Chapter 16∞ for discussion of maternal care).

Drug Guide

ERYTHROMYCIN OPHTHALMIC OINTMENT (ILOTYCIN OPHTHALMIC)

Pregnancy Risk Category: B

Overview of Neonatal Action

Erythromycin (Ilotycin Ophthalmic) is used as prophylactic treatment of ophthalmia neonatorum, which is caused by the bacteria *Neisseria gonorrhoeae.* Preventive treatment of gonorrhea in the newborn is required by law. Erythromycin is also effective against ophthalmic chlamydial infections. It is either bacteriostatic or bactericidal, depending on the organisms involved and the concentration of drug.

Route, Dosage, Frequency

Ophthalmic ointment (0.5%) is instilled as a narrow ribbon or strand, 1 cm long, along the lower conjunctival surface of each eye, starting at the inner canthus. It is instilled only once in each eye (AAP & ACOG, 2007). The ointment may be administered in the birthing area or, alternatively, later in the nursery so that eye contact between infant and parent is facilitated and the bonding process immediately after birth is not interrupted. After administration, gently close the eye and manipulate to ensure the spread of ointment (Wilson, Shannon, & Shields, 2010).

Neonatal Side Effects

Sensitivity reaction; may interfere with ability to focus and may cause edema and inflammation. Side effects usually disappear in 24 to 48 hours.

Nursing Considerations

- Wash hands immediately before instillation to prevent introduction of bacteria.
- Do not irrigate the eyes after instillation. Use new tube or single-use container for ophthalmic ointment administration shortly after birth. May wipe away excess after 1 minute with sterile cotton (AAP & ACOG, 2007).
- Observe for hypersensitivity.
- Teach parents about need for eye prophylaxis. Educate them regarding side effects and signs that need to be reported to the healthcare provider.

Table 26–3 Signs of Newborn Distress

Increased respiratory rate (more than 60/minute) or difficult respirations
Sternal retractions
Nasal flaring
Grunting
Excessive mucus
Facial grimacing
Cyanosis (central: skin, lips, tongue)
Abdominal distention or mass
Vomiting of bile-stained material
Absence of meconium elimination within 24 hours of birth
Absence of urine elimination within 24 hours of birth
Jaundice of the skin within 24 hours of birth or because of a hemolytic process
Temperature instability (hypothermia or hyperthermia)
Jitteriness or glucose less than 40 mg%

Source: Adapted from Tappero, E. P., & Honeyfield, M. E. (1996). *Physical assessment of the newborn* (2nd ed.). Petaluma, CA: NICU Inc.

Initiating First Feeding

The timing of the first feeding varies depending on whether the newborn is to be breastfed or formula-fed and whether there were any complications during pregnancy or birth, such as maternal diabetes or intrauterine growth restriction (IUGR). Mothers who choose to breastfeed their newborns should be encouraged to put their baby to the breast during the first period of reactivity. This practice should be encouraged because successful, long-term breastfeeding during infancy appears to be related to beginning breastfeedings in the first few hours of life. Sleep-wake states affect feeding behavior and need to be considered when evaluating the newborn's sucking ability (Karl, 2004).

Formula-fed newborns usually begin the first feedings by 5 hours of age, during the second period of reactivity when they awaken and appear hungry. Signs indicating newborn readiness for the first feeding are licking of the lips, placing a hand in or near the mouth, active bowel sounds, absence of abdominal distention, and a lusty cry that quiets with rooting and sucking behaviors when a stimulus is placed near the lips. Observing the earlier, more subtle cues that the newborn is ready to nurse provides an opportunity for the nurse to teach the parents to recognize these cues and respond before the newborn is frustrated and crying.

Facilitating Parent-Newborn Attachment

To facilitate **parent-newborn attachment,** eye-to-eye contact between the parents and their newborn is extremely important during the early hours after birth when the newborn is in the first period of reactivity. The newborn is alert during this time, the eyes are wide open, and the baby often makes direct eye contact with human faces within optimal range for visual acuity (7 to 8 in.). It is theorized that this eye contact is an important foundation in establishing attachment in human relationships (Klaus & Klaus, 1985). Consequently, administration of the prophylactic eye medication is often delayed, but no more than 1 hour, to provide an opportunity for a period of eye contact between parents and their newborn, thus facilitating the attachment process (AAP & ACOG, 2007). Parents who cannot be with their newborns in this first period because of maternal or infant distress may need reassurance that the bonding process can proceed normally as soon as both mother and baby are stable.

Another situation that can facilitate attachment is the interactive bath. While bathing their newborn for the first time, parents attend closely to their baby's behavior. In this way, the newborn becomes an active participant and parents are drawn into an interaction with their newborn. The nurse can interpret the infant's behavior, model ways to respond to the behavior, and support parental strategies for doing so (Karl, 2004).

EVALUATION

When evaluating the nursing care provided during the period immediately after birth, the nurse may anticipate the following outcomes:

- The newborn's adaptation to extrauterine life is successful as demonstrated by all vitals within acceptable parameters.
- The newborn's physiologic and psychologic integrity is supported.
- Positive interactions between parent and infant will be supported.

NURSING CARE OF THE NEWBORN FOLLOWING TRANSITION

MyNursingKit Care Plan Activity: Infant Care During Transition

Once a healthy newborn has demonstrated successful adaptation to extrauterine life, he or she needs appropriate observations for the first 6 to 12 hours after birth and the remainder of the stay in the birthing facility.

NURSING DIAGNOSIS

Examples of nursing diagnoses that may apply during daily care of the newborn include the following:

- *Risk for Ineffective Breathing Pattern* related to periodic breathing
- *Imbalanced Nutrition: Less than Body Requirements* related to limited nutritional and fluid intake and increased caloric expenditure
- *Impaired Urinary Elimination* related to meatal edema secondary to circumcision
- *Risk for Infection* related to umbilical cord healing, circumcision site, immature immune system, or potential birth trauma (forceps or vacuum extraction birth)
- *Health-Seeking Behaviors* related to lack of information about basic newborn care, male circumcision, and breastfeeding and/or formula-feeding
- *Interrupted Family Processes* related to integration of newborn into family or demands of newborn care and feeding

NURSING PLAN AND IMPLEMENTATION

Maintaining Cardiopulmonary Function

Assess vital signs every 6 to 8 hours or more, depending on the newborn's status. The newborn should be placed on the back (supine) for sleeping. A bulb syringe is kept within easy reach should the newborn need oral-nasal suctioning. If the newborn has respiratory difficulty, the nurse clears the airway. Vigorous fingertip stroking of the baby's spine will frequently stimulate respiratory activity. A cardiorespiratory monitor can be used on newborns that are not being observed at all times and are at risk for decreased respiratory or cardiac function. Indicators of risk are pallor, cyanosis, ruddy color, apnea, and other signs of instability. Changes in skin color may indicate the need for closer assessment of temperature, cardiopulmonary status, hematocrit, glucose, and bilirubin levels.

> **Thinking Critically**
>
> **NEWBORN BREATHING DIFFICULTIES**
>
> Aisha Khan gave birth to a healthy girl 2 hours ago; she calls you to her room. She sounds frightened and says her baby cannot breathe. You find Aisha cradling her newborn in her arms. The baby is mildly cyanotic, is waving her arms, and has mucus coming from her nose and mouth. What would you do?
>
> *See* MyNursingKit for possible responses.

Maintaining a Neutral Thermal Environment

Make every effort to maintain the newborn's temperature within the normal range. The nurse must make certain the newborn is dried completely after the bath, dressed, and exposed to the air as little as possible. A head covering should be used for the small newborn that has less subcutaneous fat to act as insulation in maintaining body heat. Ambient temperature of the room where the newborn is kept should be monitored to prevent excessive cooling. Parents may be advised to dress the newborn in one more layer of clothing than is necessary for an adult to maintain thermal comfort. The use of layering allows for flexibility as the infant is moved from one area to another.

A newborn whose temperature falls below optimal level uses calories to maintain body heat rather than for growth. Chilling also decreases the affinity of serum albumin for bilirubin, thereby increasing the likelihood of newborn jaundice. In addition, it increases oxygen use and may cause respiratory distress.

An overheated newborn will increase activity and respiratory rate in an attempt to cool the body. Both measures deplete caloric reserves, and the increased respiratory rate leads to increased insensible fluid loss (Blackburn, 2007).

Promoting Adequate Hydration and Nutritional Status

Newborn nutrition is addressed in depth in Chapter 27∞. Record caloric and fluid intake and enhance adequate hydration by maintaining a neutral thermal environment and offering early and frequent feedings. Early feedings promote gastric emptying and increase peristalsis, thereby decreasing the potential for hyperbilirubinemia by decreasing the amount of time fecal material is in contact with enzyme β-glucuronidase in the small intestine. This enzyme frees the bilirubin from the feces, allowing it to be reabsorbed into the vascular system. The nurse records voiding and stooling patterns. The first voiding should occur within 24 hours and the first passage of stool within 48 hours. When they do not occur, the nurse continues the normal observation routine while assessing for abdominal distention, bowel sounds, hydration, fluid intake, and temperature stability.

The newborn is weighed at the same time each day for accurate comparisons and must be kept warm during the weighing. A weight loss of up to 10% for term newborns is considered within normal limits during the first week of life. This weight loss is the result of limited intake, loss of excess extracellular fluid, and passage of meconium. Parents should be told about the expected weight loss, the reason for it, and the expectations for regaining the birth weight. Birth weight is usually regained by 2 weeks if feedings are adequate.

Excessive handling can cause an increase in the newborn's metabolic rate and caloric use and cause fatigue. The nurse should be alert to the newborn's subtle cues of fatigue, including a decrease in muscle tension and activity in the extremities and neck, as well as loss of eye contact, which may be manifested by fluttering or closure of the eyelids. The nurse quickly ceases stimulation when signs of fatigue appear. The nurse should demonstrate to parents the need to be aware of newborn cues and to wait for periods of alertness for contact and stimulation. Assess the woman's comfort and latching-on techniques if breastfeeding, or the bottle-feeding techniques.

Promoting Skin Integrity

Newborn skin care, including bathing, is important for the health and appearance of the individual newborn and for infection control within the nursery. Ongoing skin care involves cleansing the buttock and perianal areas with fresh water and cotton or a mild soap and water with diaper changes. If commercial baby wipes are used, those without alcohol should be selected. Perfumed and latex-free wipes are also available.

The umbilical cord is assessed for signs of bleeding or infection. Removal of the cord clamp within 24 to 48 hours of birth reduces the chance of tension injury to the area. Keeping the umbilical stump clean and dry can reduce the chance for infection (Figure 26–6 ●).

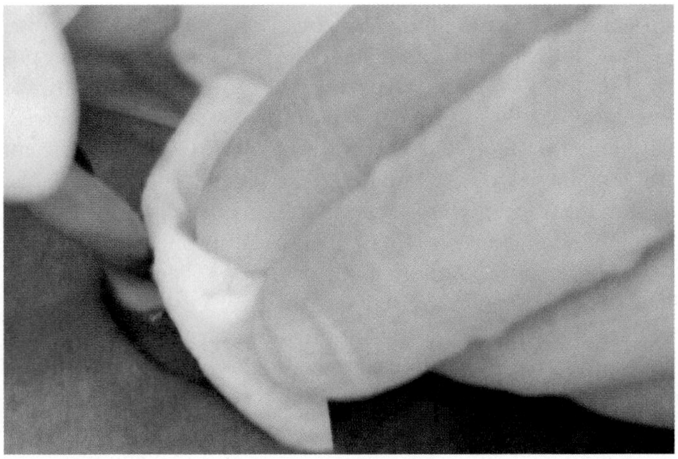

● **Figure 26–6** Routine umbilical cord care. The umbilical cord base is carefully cleansed.

Many types of routine cord care are practiced, including the use of triple dye, an antimicrobial agent such as bacitracin, or application of 70% alcohol to the cord stump. These practices are largely based on tradition rather than current research findings. The skin absorption and toxicity of triple-dye agents in newborns have not been carefully studied. No single method of umbilical cord care (topical antimicrobials [triple-dye, iodophor ointment, or hexachlorophene powder] or alcohol) has been proven to be superior in preventing colonization and disease (AAP & ACOG, 2007). The use of sterile water or air drying results in umbilical cords separating more quickly than those treated with alcohol (Askin, 2008).

Folding the diaper down to avoid covering the cord stump can prevent contamination of the area and promote drying. The nurse is responsible for cord care per agency policy. It is also the nurse's responsibility to instruct parents in caring for the cord and observing for signs and symptoms of infection after discharge, such as foul smell, redness and greenish yellow drainage, localized heat and tenderness, or bright red bleeding or if the area remains unhealed 2 to 3 days after the cord stump has sloughed off.

Promoting Safety

Safety of the newborn is paramount. It is essential that the nurse and other caregivers verify the identity of the newborn by comparing the numbers and names on the identification bracelets of mother and newborn before giving a newborn to a parent (AAP & ACOG, 2007; Askin, 2008). An additional form of identification band has a built-in sensor unit that sounds an alarm if the newborn is transported beyond set birthing-unit boundaries. Individual birthing units should practice safety measures to prevent infant abduction and provide information to parents regarding their role in this area and in general newborn safety measures (Vincent, 2009). Parental measures to prevent abduction and provide for safety include the following:

Security

- Check that identification bands are in place as they care for their newborn and, if missing, they should ask that they be replaced immediately.
- Allow only people with proper birthing unit picture identification to bring and/or remove the baby from the room. If parents do not know the staff person, they should call the nurse for assistance.
- Report the presence of any suspicious people on the birthing unit.

Safety

- Never leave their newborn alone in their room. If they walk in the halls or take a shower, parents should have a family member watch the newborn or return the newborn to the nursery.
- If a parent feels weak, faint, or unsteady on his or her feet, he or she should not lift the newborn. Instead, the parent should call for assistance.
- Always keep an eye and hand on the newborn when he or she is out of the crib.

- Protect from infection even though they do possess some immunity. Parents should ask visitors to leave if they have any of the following: cold, diarrhea, discharge from sores, or contagious disease.

Preventing Complications

Newborns are at continued risk for the complications of hemorrhage, late-onset cardiac symptoms, and infection. Pallor may be an early sign of hemorrhage and must be reported to the physician. The newborn is placed on a cardiorespiratory monitor to permit continuous assessment. Several newborn conditions put newborns at risk for hemorrhage. Cyanosis that is not relieved by oxygen administration requires emergency intervention, may indicate a congenital cardiac condition or shock, and requires ongoing assessment.

Infection in the nursery is best prevented by requiring that all personnel who have direct contact with newborns scrub for 2 to 3 minutes from the fingertips up to and including the elbows at the beginning of each shift. The hands must also be washed with soap and rubbed vigorously for 15 seconds before and after contact with every newborn and after touching any soiled surface such as the floor or one's hair or face. Parents are instructed to practice good handwashing and/or use of an antiseptic hand cleaner before touching the newborn. They are also instructed that anyone holding the baby should practice good handwashing, even after the family returns home. In some clinical settings family members are asked to wear gowns (preferably disposable) over their street clothes during their contact with infants. These are good opportunities for the nurse to reinforce the efficacy of handwashing in preventing the spread of infection.

Jaundice occurs in most newborn infants. Most jaundice is benign, but because of the potential toxicity of bilirubin, newborn infants must be monitored to identify those who might develop severe hyperbilirubinemia and, in rare cases, acute bilirubin encephalopathy or kernicterus (see Chapter 29∞ for more detailed discussion) (AAP & ACOG, 2007). Current recommendations include obtaining a total serum bilirubin level in any infant that is visibly jaundiced in the first 24 hours of life, and obtaining either a serum or transcutaneous bilirubin level before discharge. Nomograms for evaluating risk factors based on bilirubin levels and age of infant are available (see Chapter 24∞ for discussion).

Circumcision

Circumcision is a surgical procedure in which the prepuce, an epithelial layer covering the penis, is separated from the glans penis and excised. This procedure permits exposure of the glans for easier cleaning.

Circumcision was originally a religious rite practiced by Jews and Muslims. Families make the decision about circumcision for their newborn male child. The practice gained widespread cultural acceptance in the United States but is much less common in Europe. Many parents choose circumcision because they want their male child to have a physical appearance similar to that of his father or the majority of other children or they may feel that it is expected by society. Another commonly cited reason for circumcising newborn males is to prevent the need for anesthesia, hospitalization, pain, and trauma if the procedure is needed later in life (AAP & ACOG, 2007). To ensure informed consent, parents should be advised during the prenatal period about possible long-term medical effects of circumcision and noncircumcision.

Current recommendations for circumcision. The 2005 AAP policy statement reaffirmed that it does not recommend *routine* circumcision but acknowledges that medical indications for circumcision still exist (AAP & ACOG, 2007). The policy recommends that analgesia (dorsal penile nerve block [DPNB], or subcutaneous ring block) be used during circumcision to decrease procedural pain. The DPNB and subcutaneous ring block are the most effective options (AAP & CPS, 2006). If a circumcision is to be performed, it should be done using the least painful method. Recent studies show that using oral sucrose for painful procedures can be effective in reducing pain for newborns and it should be used with other nonpharmacologic measures to enhance its effectiveness (AAP & CPS, 2006).

Circumcision *should not be performed* if the newborn is premature or compromised, has a known bleeding problem, or is born with a genitourinary defect such as hypospadias or epispadias, which may necessitate the use of the foreskin in future surgical repairs.

Nurse's role. A well-informed nurse can allay parents' anxiety by sharing information and allowing them to express their concerns. In order for parents to make a truly informed decision, they must be knowledgeable about the potential risks and outcomes of circumcision. Hemorrhage, infection, difficulty in voiding, separation of the edges of the circumcision, discomfort, and restlessness are early potential problems. Later there is a risk that the glans and urethral meatus may become irritated and inflamed from contact with the ammonia from urine. Ulcerations and progressive stenosis may develop. Adhesions, entrapment of the penis, and damage to the urethra are all potential complications that could require surgical correction (AAP & ACOG, 2007).

The parents of an uncircumcised male infant require information from the nurse about good hygienic practices. They are told that the foreskin and glans are two similar layers of cells that separate from each other. The separation process begins prenatally and is normally completed between 3 to 5 years of age. In the process of separation, sterile sloughed cells build up between the layers. This buildup looks similar to the smegma secreted after puberty, and it is harmless. Occasionally during the daily bath, the parent can gently test for retraction. If retraction has occurred, daily gentle washing of the glans with soap and water is sufficient to maintain adequate cleanliness. The parents should teach the child to incorporate this practice into his daily self-care activities. Most uncircumcised males have no difficulty doing so.

If circumcision is desired, the procedure is performed when the newborn is well stabilized and has received his initial physical examination by a healthcare provider. The parents may also choose to have the circumcision done after discharge. However, they need to be advised that if the baby is older than 1 month, the current practice is to hospitalize him for the procedure.

Before a circumcision, the nurse ensures that the physician has explained the procedure, determined whether the parents have any further questions about the procedure, and verified that the circumcision permit is signed. As with any surgical procedure, the infant's identification band should be checked to verify his identity before the procedure begins. The nurse gathers the equipment and prepares the newborn by removing the diaper and placing him on a padded circumcision board or some other type of restraint, but restraining only the legs. These restraint measures along with the application of warm blankets to the upper body increase infant comfort during the procedure (Thureen, Deacon, Hernandez, et al., 2005). In Jewish circumcision ceremonies, the infant is held by the father or godfather and given wine before the procedure.

A variety of devices (Gumco clamp, Plastibel, Mogen clamp) are used for circumcision (Figures 26–7 ● and 26–8 ●), and all produce minimal bleeding. Therefore, make special note of infants with a family history of bleeding disorders or with mothers who took anticoagulants, including aspirin, prenatally. During the procedure, assess the newborn's response. One important consideration is pain experienced by the newborn. A DPNB or ring block using 1% lidocaine without epinephrine or similar anesthetic significantly minimizes the pain and shifts in behavioral patterns such as crying, irritability, and erratic sleep cycles associated with circumcision. Other studies are investigating the use of topical anesthetic applied 60 to 90 minutes before prepuce removal, acetaminophen, and cryoanalgesia. Studies indicate that a combination of methods is most effective in reducing pain during circumcision (AAP & CPS, 2006).

During the procedure, provide comfort measures such as swaddling, lightly stroking the newborn's head, providing a pacifier for nonnutritive sucking, and talking to him. Following the circumcision, the infant should be held and comforted by a family member or the nurse. Be alert to any behavioral cues that these measures are overstimulating the newborn instead of comforting him. Such cues include turning away of the head, increased generalized body movement, skin color changes, hyperalertness, and hiccoughing.

Ideally, the circumcision should be assessed every 30 minutes for at least 2 hours following the procedure. It is important to observe for the first voiding after a circumcision to evaluate for urinary obstruction related to penile injury and/or edema. Petroleum ointment and gauze may be applied to the site immediately following the procedure to help prevent bleeding and can be used to protect the healing tissue afterward.

Teach family members how to assess for unusual bleeding, how to respond if it is present, and how to care for the newly circumcised penis. Parents of newborns circumcised with a method other than Plastibell should receive the following information:

- Clean with warm water with each diaper change.
- Apply petroleum ointment for the next few diaper changes to help prevent further bleeding (Figure 26–9 ●).

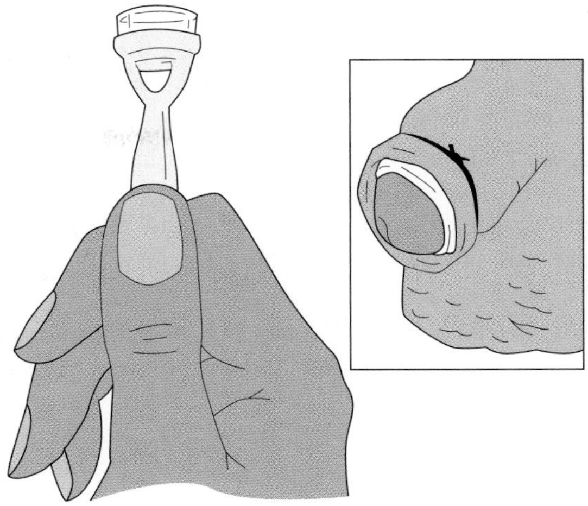

● **Figure 26–8** Circumcision using the Plastibell. The bell is fitted over the glans. A suture is tied around the bell's rim and the excess prepuce is cut away. The plastic rim remains in place for 3 to 4 days until healing occurs. The bell may be allowed to fall off; it is removed if still in place after 8 days.

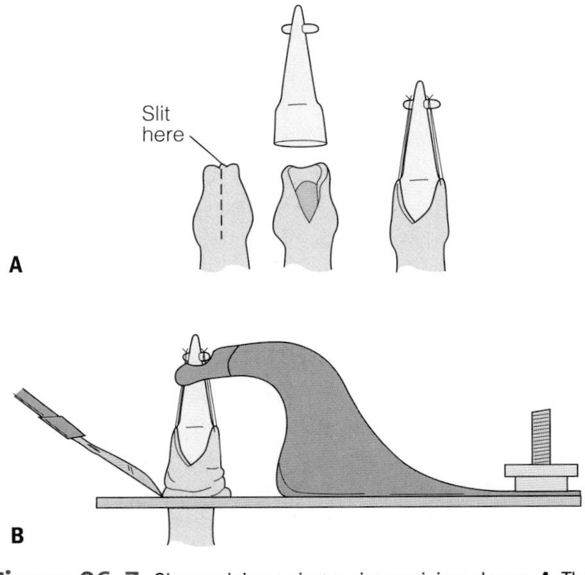

● **Figure 26–7** Circumcision using a circumcision clamp. ***A,*** The prepuce is drawn over the cone and ***B,*** the clamp is applied. Pressure is maintained for 3 to 4 minutes, and then excess prepuce is cut away.

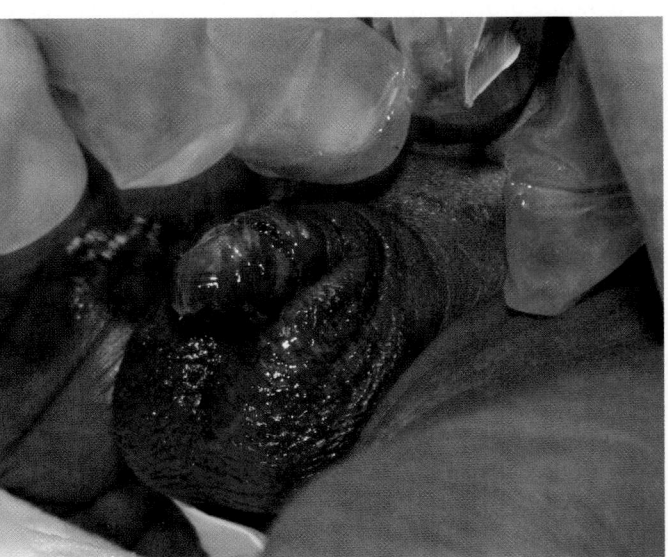

● **Figure 26–9** Following circumcision, petroleum ointment may be applied to the site for the next few diaper changes.

- If bleeding does occur, apply light pressure with a sterile gauze pad to stop the bleeding within a short time. If this is not effective, contact the physician immediately, or take the newborn to the caregiver's office.
- The glans normally has granulation tissue (a yellowish film) on it during healing. Continued application of a petroleum ointment (or ointment suggested by the healthcare provider) can help protect the granulation tissue that forms as the glans heals.
- Report to the care provider any signs or symptoms of infection, such as increasing swelling, pus drainage, and cessation of urination.
- When diapering, ensure that the diaper is not too loose to cause rubbing with movement, or too tight to cause pain.
- If the infant's care provider recommends oral analgesics, follow instructions for proper measuring and administration.

If the Plastibell is used, parents should receive information about normal appearance and how to observe for infection. The parents are informed that the Plastibell should fall off within 8 days. If it remains on after 8 days, they should consult with the newborn's physician. Though no ointments or creams should be used while the bell remains, application of petroleum ointment may protect granulation tissue afterward.

Enhancing Parent-Newborn Attachment

The nurse encourages parent-newborn attachment by involving all family members with the new member of the family. (For specific interventions see Chapters 19 and 31∞ and "Teaching Highlights: What Parents Need to Know About Enhancing Attachment.") Infant massage is a common childcare practice in many parts of the world, especially Africa and Asia, and has recently gained attention in the United States. Parents can be taught to use infant massage as a method to facilitate the bonding process and to reduce the stress and pain associated with teething, constipation, inoculations, and colic. Infant massage not only induces relaxation for the infant but also provides a calming and "feel-good" interaction for the parents that foster the development of warm, positive relationships. See Developing Cultural Competence: Infant Naming in Kenya.

The nurse can discuss waking activities such as talking with the newborn while making eye contact, holding the newborn in an upright position (sitting or standing), gently bending the newborn back and forth while grasping under the knees and supporting the head and back with the other hand, or gently rubbing the newborn's hands and feet. Quieting activities may include swaddling or bundling the baby to increase a sense of security; using slow, calming movements; and talking softly, singing, or humming to the newborn (Figure 26–10 ●).

Caring for newborns in the birthing setting means that the nurse will have contact with clients from a wide variety of racial, religious, and cultural backgrounds. Though it may not be possible to be conversant with all cultures, the nurse can demonstrate cultural competence with both colleagues and patients. The nurse must be sensitive to the cultural beliefs and values of the family and be aware of cultural variations in newborn care such as naming the newborn, giving compliments about the newborn, and using good luck charms (see "Developing Cultural Competence: Examples of Cultural Beliefs and Practices Regarding Baby Care" on page 618).

Teaching Highlights

WHAT PARENTS NEED TO KNOW ABOUT ENHANCING ATTACHMENT

- Information on the periods of reactivity, expected newborn responses, and normal newborn physical characteristics (see Chapter 25∞).
- The gradual developmental nature of the bonding process and the reciprocal interactive nature of the process.
- The infant's capabilities for interaction such as nonverbal communication abilities. Nonverbal communications include movement, gaze, touch, facial expressions, and vocalizations—including crying. Eye contact is considered one of the cardinal factors in developing infant-parent attachment and will be integrated with touching and vocal behaviors.
- Touching, including stroking, patting, massaging, and kissing, will progress to interactive touch between parent and infant; parents need to assimilate these and other comforting behaviors (sound, swaddling, rocking) into daily routines with their baby.
- The infant's behaviors will change as the infant matures, and it is important for parents to be consistent in response to their infant's cues and needs.
- Information about pamphlets, videos, and support groups in the community should be available.

Developing Cultural Competence

INFANT NAMING IN KENYA

In Kenya, the naming of a child is an important event. Names are commonly selected to mirror important or current events. For example, an infant who is born while traveling may be given a name that means "wanderer" or "traveler." Other names may be chosen after a relative who is among the "living-dead" (deceased). It is believed that this results in a partial reincarnation of that relative, especially if the child has characteristics in common with that individual. It is also believed there is a connection between newborns and the spirit world. In some parts of the country, the name is chosen when the child is crying. Different names of the living-dead are called, and if the child quits crying when a particular name is called, that is the given name. In some areas, the name is given on the third day and is marked by a celebration with feasting and rejoicing. On the fourth day, the father of the child commonly hangs an iron necklace on the child's neck. It is at this time that the infant is considered a full human being and the connection with the spirit world is lost.

A Letter From Your Baby

Dear Parents:

I come to you a small, immature being with my own style and personality. I am yours for only a short time; enjoy me.

1. Please take time to find out who I am, how I differ from you, and how much I can bring you joy.
2. Please feed me when I am hungry. I never knew hunger in the womb, and clocks and time mean little to me.
3. Please hold, cuddle, kiss, touch, stroke, and croon to me. I was always held closely in the womb and was never alone before.
4. Please don't be disappointed when I am not the perfect baby that you expected, nor disappointed with yourselves that you are not the perfect parents.
5. Please don't expect too much from me as your newborn baby, or too much from yourself as a parent. Give us both six weeks as a birthday present—six weeks for me to grow, develop, mature, and become more stable and predictable, and six weeks for you to rest and relax and allow your body to get back to normal.
6. Please forgive me if I cry a lot. Bear with me and in a short time, as I mature, I will spend less and less time crying and more time socializing.
7. Please watch me carefully and I can tell you the things that soothe, console, and please me. I am not a tyrant who was sent to make your life miserable, but the only way I can tell you that I am not happy is with my cry.
8. Please remember that I am resilient and can withstand the many natural mistakes you will make with me. As long as you make them with love, you cannot ruin me.
9. Please take care of yourself and eat a balanced diet, rest, and exercise so that when we are together, you have the health and strength to take care of me.
10. Please take care of your relationship with others. Relationships that are good for you support both you and me.

Although I may have turned your life upside down, please realize that things will be back to normal before long.

Thank you,

Your Loving Child

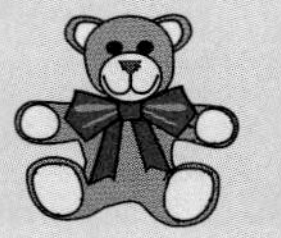

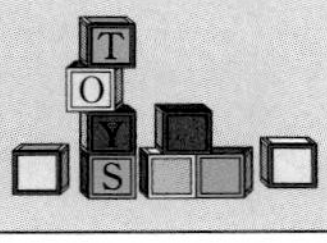

● **Figure 26–10** A letter from your baby.

EVALUATION

When evaluating the nursing care provided during the newborn period, the nurse may anticipate the following outcomes:

- The baby's physiologic and psychologic integrity is supported by maintaining stable vital signs and interactions based on normal newborn behaviors.
- The newborn feeding pattern will be satisfactorily established.
- The parents express understanding of the bonding process and display attachment behaviors.

NURSING MANAGEMENT IN PREPARATION FOR DISCHARGE

Although the adjustment to parenting is a normal process, going home presents a critical transition for the family. The parents become the primary caregivers for the newborn and must provide a nurturing environment in which the emotional and physical needs of the newborn can be met. Nursing interventions focus on promoting health and preventing possible problems.

NURSING ASSESSMENT AND DIAGNOSIS

When preparing for discharge, assess whether parents have realistic expectations of the newborn's behavior and the depth of their knowledge in caring for their newborn.

Nursing diagnoses that may apply to the newborn's family include the following:

- *Readiness for Enhanced Parenting* related to appropriate behavioral expectations for the newborn.
- *Readiness for Enhanced Family Processes* related to integration of newborn into family unit or demands of newborn care and feeding.

PLANNING AND IMPLEMENTATION

Parent Teaching

To meet the parent's need for information, the nurse who is responsible for the care of the mother and newborn should assume the primary responsibility for parent education. Nearly every contact with the parents presents an opportunity for sharing information that can facilitate their sense of competence in newborn care. The nurse also needs to recognize and respect the many good ways of providing safe care. Unless their care methods are harmful to the newborn, the parents' methods of giving care should be reinforced rather than contradicted.

The information that follows is provided to increase the nurse's knowledge of newborn care and can also be used to meet parents' needs for information. Parents may be familiar with handling and caring for infants, or this may be their first time to interact with a newborn. If they are new parents, the sensitive nurse gently teaches them by example and provides instructions geared to their needs and previous knowledge about the various aspects of newborn care.

Developing Cultural Competence

EXAMPLES OF CULTURAL BELIEFS AND PRACTICES REGARDING BABY CARE*

Umbilical Cord

People of Latin American, Filipino, Haitian cultural background may use an abdominal binder or bellyband to protect against dirt, injury, and umbilical hernia. They may also apply oils to the stump of the cord or tape metal to the umbilicus to ward off evil spirits (D'Avanza & Geissler, 2008).

People of northern European ancestry may expect a sterile cutting of the cord at birth. They may allow the stump to air-dry and discard the cord once it falls off.

Some Latin American parents cauterize the stump with a candle flame, hot coal, or burning stick (WHO, 1999).

In Ecuador, the cord stump is left long in girls to prevent a small uterus and problems with childbirth (WHO, 1999).

Parent-Infant Contact

People of Asian ancestry may pick up the newborn as soon as it cries, or they may carry the newborn at all times.

Several native North American nations people, notably the Navajos, may use cradle boards, so the infant can be with family even during work and feel secure (Andrews, 2008).

The Muslim father traditionally calls praise to Allah in the newborn's right ear and cleans the infant after birth (Hedayat, 2001).

Feeding

Some women of Asian heritage may breastfeed their newborns for the first 1 to 2 years of life. Many Cambodian refugees practice breastfeeding on demand without restriction, or, if formula-feeding, provide a "comfort bottle" in between feedings (Lipson & Dibble, 2008).

People of Iranian heritage may breastfeed females longer than males. Many Muslim women will not breastfeed in public.

Some people of African ancestry may wean their newborns after they begin to walk.

Some Asians, Haitian, Hispanics, Eastern Europeans, and Native Americans may delay breastfeeding because they believe colostrum is "bad" (D'Avanzo & Geissler, 2008).

Haitian mothers may believe that "strong emotions" spoil breast milk (Lipson & Dibble, 2008).

Circumcision

People of Muslim and Jewish ancestry practice circumcision as a religious ritual (Ott, Al-Khadhuri, & Al-Junaibi, 2003; Lipson & Dibble, 2008).

Many natives of Africa and Australia practice circumcision as a puberty rite.

Native Americans and people of Asian and Latin American cultures rarely perform circumcision (Lipson & Dibble, 2008).

As of 2006, global estimates are that about 30% of males are circumcised (WHO, 2008).

Health and Illness

Some people from Latin American cultural backgrounds may believe that touching the face or head of an infant when admiring it will ward off the "evil eye." They may also neglect to cut the baby's nails to avoid nearsightedness and instead put mittens on the newborn's hands to prevent scratching. They also may believe that fat newborns are healthy.

Some people of Asian heritage may not allow anyone to touch the newborn's head without asking permission.

Some Orthodox Jews believe that saying the newborn's name before the formal naming ceremony will harm the baby.

Some Asians and Haitians delay naming their infants until after confinement month (D'Avanzo & Geissler, 2008).

Some people of Vietnamese ancestry believe that cutting a baby's hair or nails will cause illness.

**Note: The information is meant only to provide examples of the behaviors that may be found within certain cultures. Not all members of a culture practice the behaviors described.*

The nurse observes how parents interact with their newborn during feeding and caregiving activities. Even during a short stay (48 hours or less), there are opportunities for the nurse to provide information and observe whether the parents are comfortable with changing the diapers of, wrapping, handling, and feeding their newborn (Figure 26–11 ●). Do both parents get involved in the newborn's care? Is the mother depending on someone else to help her at home? Does the mother give reasons (e.g., "I'm too tired," "My stitches hurt," or "I'll learn later") for not wanting to be involved in her baby's care? As the family provides care, the nurse can enhance parental confidence by giving them positive feedback. If the parents encounter problems, the nurse can express confidence in their abilities to master the new skill or information, suggest alternatives, and serve as a role model. All these factors need to be considered when evaluating the educational needs of the parents. Providing mother-baby care and home care instruction on the night shift assists with education needs for early discharge parents.

Several methods may be used to teach families about newborn care. Daily newborn care videos and classes are nonthreatening ways to convey general information. Individual instruction is helpful to answer specific questions or to clarify an item that may have been confusing in class. Currently many birthing centers have 24-hour educational video channels or videos to be viewed in the mother's room on a variety of postpartum and newborn care issues. One-to-one teaching while the nurse is in the

Nursing Practice

For clients who are hearing impaired, videotapes with information in both spoken and signed formats are most helpful. Birthing centers should have handouts available for families who do not speak English and either birthing center interpreters (not family members) or language interpreter phones.

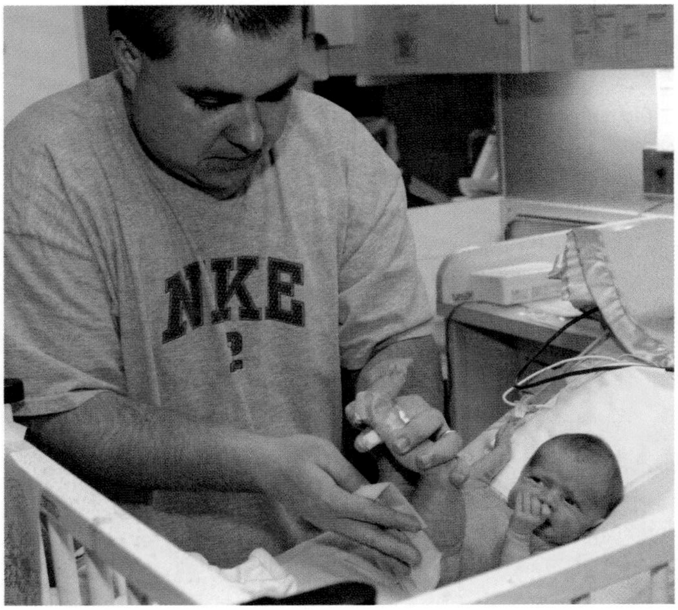

● **Figure 26–11** Parental confidence. A father demonstrates competence and confidence in diapering his newborn daughter.

mother's room is the most effective educational method. Both first-time and experienced postpartum parents rate individual teaching as the most effective method of instruction. Individual instruction is helpful both to answer specific questions and to clarify something that the parents may have found confusing in the educational video. With shorter stays, most teaching unfortunately tends to focus on infant feeding and immediate physical care needs of the mothers, with limited anticipatory guidance provided in other areas.

General Instructions for Newborn Care

One of the first concerns of anyone who has not had the experience of picking up a baby is how to do it correctly. The newborn is easily picked up by sliding one hand under the neck and shoulders and the other hand under the buttocks or between the newborn's legs and then gently lifting upward. This technique provides security and support for the head (which the newborn is unable to support until 3 or 4 months of age) (see Chapter 31 ∞ for more detail).

The nurse can be an excellent role model for families in the area of safety. Safety topics include the proper positioning of the newborn on the back to sleep and correct use of the bulb syringe. The baby should never be left alone anywhere but in the crib. The mother is reminded that while she and her newborn are together in the birthing unit, she should never leave her baby alone for security reasons and because newborns spit up frequently the first day or two after birth. Other newborn safety measures are discussed in detail in Chapter 31 ∞.

Demonstrating a bath (see Chapter 31 ∞), cord care, and temperature assessment is the best way for the nurse to provide information on these topics to parents.

The nurse demonstrates and reviews the taking of axillary or tympanic temperatures and discourages the use of mercury thermometers. It is important that families understand the differences and know how to select a thermometer. The newborn's temperature needs to be taken only when signs of illness are present. Parents are advised to call their physician or pediatric nurse practitioner immediately if they observe any signs of illness.

(See "Teaching Highlights: What Parents Need to Know about Newborn Care" on page 620, which includes a broad range of information important to share with new parents. These topics are discussed in detail here.)

Nasal and Oral Suctioning

Most newborns are obligatory nose breathers for the first months of life. They generally maintain air passage patency by coughing or sneezing. During the first few days of life, however, the newborn has increased mucus, and gentle suctioning with a bulb syringe may be indicated. The nurse can demonstrate the use of the bulb syringe in the mouth and nose and have the parents do a return demonstration. The parents should repeat this demonstration of suctioning and cleansing the bulb before discharge so they feel confident in performing the procedure. Care should be taken to apply only gentle suction to prevent nasal bleeding.

To suction the newborn, the bulb syringe is compressed before the tip is placed in the nostril. The nurse or parent must take care not to occlude the passageway. The bulb is permitted to reexpand slowly by releasing the compression on the bulb (Figure 26–12 ●). The bulb syringe is removed from the nostril, and drainage is then compressed out of the bulb and onto a tissue. The bulb syringe may also be used in the mouth if the newborn is spitting up and unable to handle the excess secretions. The bulb is compressed, the tip of the bulb syringe is placed about 1 inch to one side of the newborn's mouth, and compression is released. This draws up the excess secretions. The procedure is repeated on the other side of the mouth. The roof of the mouth and the back of the throat are avoided because suction in these areas might stimulate the gag reflex. The bulb syringe should be washed in warm, soapy water and rinsed in warm water daily and as needed after use. Rinsing with a half-strength white vinegar

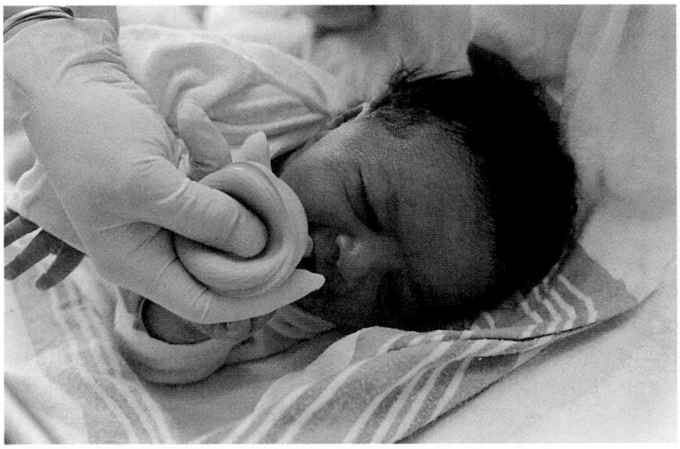

● **Figure 26–12** Nasal and oral suctioning. The bulb is compressed, the tip is placed in either the mouth or the nose, and the bulb is released.
Source: © Stella Johnson (www.stellajohnson.com).

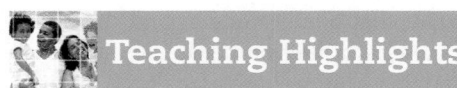

Teaching Highlights

WHAT TO TELL PARENTS ABOUT INFANT CARE

Immediate Safety Measures for the Newborn

Watch for excessive mucus: use bulb syringe to remove mucus.

Have baby sleep on his or her back in crib or in someone's arms.

Voiding and Stool Characteristics and Patterns

Urine is straw to amber color without foul smell. Small amounts of uric acid crystals are normal in first days of life (may be mistaken by parents as blood in diaper because of reddish "brick dust" appearance).

At least 6 to 10 wet diapers a day after the first few days of life.

Normal progression of stool changes: (1) meconium (thick, tarry, dark green); (2) transitional stools (thin, brown to green); (3a) breastfed infant: yellow gold, soft or mushy stools; (3b) formula-fed infant: pale yellow, formed and pasty stools.

Only one to two stools a day for formula-fed baby.

Six to 10 small, loose yellow stools per day or only one stool every few days after breastfeeding is well established (after about 1 month).

Cord Care

Wash hands with clean water before and after care. Keep the cord dry and exposed to air or loosely covered with clean clothes. (If cultural custom demands binding of the abdomen, a sanitary method such as the use of a clean piece of gauze can be recommended.)

Clean cord and skin around base with a cotton swab or cotton ball. Clean two to three times a day or with each diaper change. Touching the cord, applying unclean substances to it, and applying bandages should be avoided. Do not give tub baths until cord falls off in 7 to 14 days.

Fold diapers below umbilical cord to air-dry the cord (contact with wet or soiled diapers slows the drying process and increases the possibility of infection).

Check cord each day for any odor, oozing of greenish yellow material, or reddened areas around the cord. Expect tenderness around the cord and darkening and shriveling of cord. Report to healthcare provider any signs of infection.

Normal changes in cord: Cord should look dark and dry up before falling off. A small drop of blood may present when cord falls off.

Never pull the cord or attempt to loosen it.

Care Required for Circumcision and Uncircumcised Infants

Circumcision Care

Squeeze water over circumcision site once a day.

Rinse area off with warm water and pat dry.

Apply a small amount of petroleum jelly (unless a Plastibell is in place) with each diaper change.

Fasten diaper over penis snugly enough so that it does not move and rub the tender glans.

Because the glans is sensitive, avoid placing baby on his stomach for the first day after the procedure.

Check for any foul-smelling drainage or bleeding at least once a day.

Let Plastibell fall off by itself (about 8 days after circumcision).

Plastibell should not be pulled off.

Light, sticky, yellow drainage (part of healing process) may form over head of penis.

Uncircumcised Care

Clean uncircumcised penis with water during diaper changes and with bath.

Do not force foreskin back over the penis; foreskin will retract normally over time (may take 3 to 5 years).

Techniques for Waking and Quieting Newborns

Techniques for Waking Baby

Loosen clothing, change diaper.

Hand-express milk onto baby's lips.

Talk with baby while making eye contact.

Hold baby in upright position (sitting or standing).

Have baby do sit-ups (gently and rhythmically bend baby back and forth while grasping the baby under his or her knees and supporting baby's head and back with your other hand).

Play patty-cake with baby.

Stimulate rooting reflex (brush one cheek with hand or nipple).

Increase skin contact (gently rub hands and feet).

Techniques for Quieting Baby

Check for soiled diaper.

Hold swaddled baby upright against mid-chest, supporting bottom and back of head. Baby can hear heartbeat, feel warmth, and hear your softly spoken words or calming sounds.

Use slow, calming movements with baby.

Softly talk, sing, or hum to baby.

Signs of Illness

See Table 26–4 "When Parents Should Call Their Healthcare Provider" on page 624.

solution followed by clear water may help to extend the useful life of the bulb syringe by inhibiting bacterial growth. A bulb syringe should always be kept near the newborn. New parents and nurses who are inexperienced with babies may fear that the baby will choke and are relieved to know how to take action if such an event occurs. They should be advised to turn the newborn's head to the side or hold the newborn with his or her head down as soon as there is any indication of gagging or vomiting and to use the bulb syringe as needed.

Some infants may have transient edema of the nasal mucosa following suctioning of the airway after birth. The nurse can demonstrate the use of normal saline to loosen secretions, and instruct parents in the gentle and moderate use of the bulb syringe to avoid further irritation of the mucous membranes. If parents will be using humidifiers at home, they should be instructed to follow the manufacturer's cleaning instructions carefully so that molds, spores, and bacteria from a dirty humidifier do not enter the baby's environment.

Thinking Critically

NEWBORN VAGINAL DRAINAGE

You are caring for Sarah Feldstein, who had her first child, a daughter, about 4 hours ago. She appears visibly upset when changing her infant's diaper and says she thinks something is wrong because her daughter has tissue protruding from her vagina and some bleeding in her diaper. What would you do?

See MyNursingKit for possible responses.

Swaddling the Newborn

Swaddling (wrapping) helps the newborn maintain body temperature, provides a feeling of closeness and security, and may be effective in quieting a crying baby by having the newborn's hands near their mouth to allow for sucking (Roach, 2004). A blanket is placed on the crib (or secure surface) in the shape of a diamond. The top corner of the blanket is folded down slightly, and the newborn's body is placed with the head at the upper edge of the blanket. The right corner of the blanket is wrapped around the newborn and tucked under the left side (not too tightly—the newborn needs a little room to move and to allow for hands to get to the mouth). The bottom corner is then pulled up to the chest, and the left corner wrapped around the baby's right side (Figure 26–13 ●). The nurse can show this wrapping technique to a new mother so she will feel more skilled in handling her baby.

Nursing Practice

Remember that left-handed people tend to hold the baby over their right shoulder, and right-handed people do the opposite. This keeps the dominant hand free. However, most health personnel wear their nametags on the left side. To avoid scratching the baby's face, wear your nametag on the same side as your dominant hand.

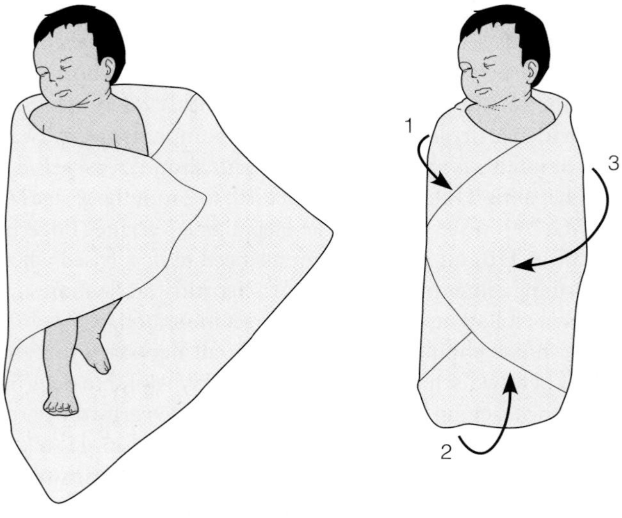

● **Figure 26–13** Steps in wrapping a baby.

Evidence in Action

Newborns should be placed in the supine position during sleep to reduce the risk of SIDS (Organization Guidelines) (American Academy of Pediatrics: Task force on Sudden Infant Death Syndrome, 2005).

Sleep and Activity

The National Institute of Child Health and Human Development and the American Academy of Pediatrics recommend that healthy term infants be placed on their back to sleep. Parents are taught the importance of following "Back to Sleep Guidelines" to reduce the incidence of sudden infant death syndrome (SIDS) (American Academy of Pediatrics [AAP] Task Force on Sudden Infant Death Syndrome, 2005). Though infants may need to be placed on their sides initially because of copious or thick secretions, placing them on their backs in the newborn period serves to educate parents regarding infant positioning. Studies indicate that parents position their babies in the same positions they observe in the hospital setting, so nurses must demonstrate this behavior to reduce the risk of SIDS. If exceptions are warranted, these should be explained to families so they do not misinterpret what they observe. The placement of babies in a prone position during wakeful play sessions "tummy time" should be encouraged as well (AAP & ACOG, 2007).

Perhaps nothing is more individual to each baby than the sleep-activity cycle. It is important for the nurse to recognize the individual variations of each newborn and to assist parents as they develop sensitivity to their infant's communication signals and rhythms of activity and sleep. See Chapter 25 ∞ for a more detailed discussion of sleep-wake activity.

Car Safety Considerations

Half of the children killed or injured in automobile accidents could have been protected by the use of federally approved car seats. Newborns must go home from the birthing unit in a car seat adapted to fit them (Figure 26–14 ●). Babies should never be placed in the front seat of a car equipped with a passenger-side airbag. The car seat should be positioned to face the rear of the car until the baby is 1 year old or weighs 9.09 kg (20 lb) (AAP, 2008). Nurses need to ensure that all parents are knowledgeable about the benefits of child safety seat use and proper installation. Nurses can encourage parents to have their infant safety seats checked by local groups trained specifically for that purpose. The Seat Check Initiative provides locations and information about child safety seats. For more detail, see "Injury Prevention Strategies" Chapter 36 ∞.

Newborn Screening and Immunization Programs

Before the newborn and mother are discharged from the birthing unit, the nurse informs the parents about the **newborn screening tests** and tells them when to return to the birthing center or clinic if further tests are needed.

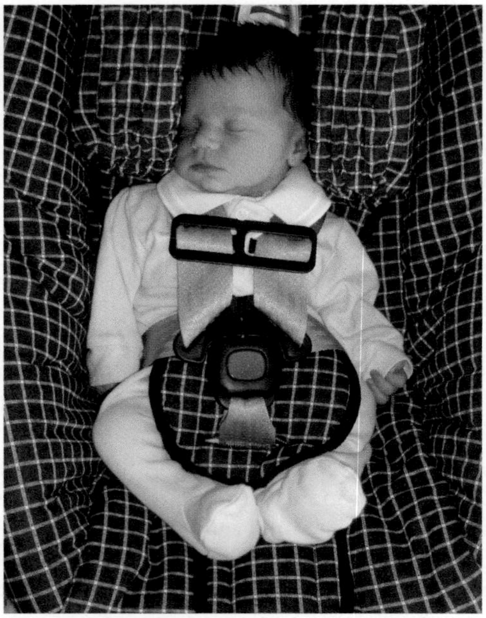

● **Figure 26–14** Newborn car seat. An infant car restraint such as this one should be used from birth to about 12 months of age.

Several disorders that can be identified from a few drops of blood obtained by a heel stick are cystic fibrosis, galactosemia, congenital adrenal hyperplasia, congenital hypothyroidism, maple syrup urine disease, phenylketonuria (PKU), sickle cell trait, biotinidase deficiency, and hemoglobinopathies. The Expanded Newborn Screening Program allows parents to have their babies screened for more than 20 disorders. Although controversy exists over the need for such comprehensive testing, it is recommended that states test for a core panel of 29 treatable congenital conditions and an additional 25 conditions that may be detected by screening (AAP, Newborn Screening Authoring Committee, 2008).

Phenylketonuria and congenital hypothyroidism are the only tests that are performed in all 50 states and the District of Columbia (ACOG Committee on Genetics, 2003). Early newborn discharge puts infants at risk for delayed or even missed diagnosis of PKU and congenital hypothyroidism because of decreased sensitivity of screening before 24 hours of age. The likelihood of detecting PKU increases as the infant grows older; the infant must be at least 24 hours old for a valid test. A second test is required in most states, usually between 1 week and 1 month of age, to minimize the chance of a positive child going undetected. PKU and other inborn errors of metabolism are discussed further in Chapter 55.

Evidence in Action

Routine screening of newborns for metabolic and other disorders that are initially asymptomatic has been elevated from a Level II (good evidence category) to a Level I (best evidence) based on latest evidence. (Institute for Clinical Systems Improvement Guidelines; Maternal Child Health Bureau Recommendations), (Institute for Clinical Systems Improvement, 2008).

Nursing Practice

As many as 50% of parents whose infants failed the initial hearing test do not arrange for a rescreening. Many parents do not understand the importance of rescreening or how early diagnosis of hearing loss can impact early speech and development. Explain the importance of rescreening to the parents and encourage them to verbalize their questions. Few infants who are rescreened have actual hearing loss, but early detection can greatly improve the development of infants with hearing loss or those who are hard of hearing.

Hearing loss is found in 1 to 3 per 1000 infants in the normal newborn population (Thureen et al., 2005). Hearing screenings before discharge are now conducted in all 50 states. The recommended initial newborn hearing screening should be accomplished before discharge from the birthing unit with appropriate follow-up if the newborn fails to pass the initial screen in all hospitals providing obstetric services (AAP & ACOG, 2007; Creehan, 2008).

According to the National Center for Hearing Assessment & Management (2007), 95.7% of all infants obtained hearing screening in the United States. Sometimes infants fail to pass these tests for reasons other than hearing loss. Amniotic fluid in the ear canals is a frequent cause of suboptimal test results. In these cases, infants are retested in a week or two. The current goal is to screen all infants by 1 month of age, confirm hearing loss with audiologic examination by 3 months of age, and treat with comprehensive early intervention services before 6 months of age (AAP & ACOG, 2007).

Parents need to be advised whether their birthing center provides newborn hepatitis vaccination so that an adequate follow-up program can be set in motion (AAP & ACOG, 2007). For more detailed discussion of newborn screening and immunization needs see Chapters 26 and 45. Immunization programs against the hepatitis B virus during the newborn period and infancy are in place in many states, at least 20 countries, and high-incidence areas such as American Samoa. Universal vaccination of infants is recommended. Infants should receive the first dose of hepatitis B (Hep B) vaccine at birth to 2 months of age (AAP & ACOG, 2007). See Drug Guide: Hepatitis B Vaccine (Engerix-B, Recombivax HB) on page 624. Parents need to be advised whether their birthing center provides newborn hepatitis vaccination so that an adequate follow-up program can be set in motion.

The nurse should teach the family all necessary caregiving methods before discharge. A checklist may be helpful to determine whether the teaching has been completed and to verify the parents' knowledge on leaving the birthing unit (Figure 26–15 ●). The nurse needs to review all areas for understanding or answer outstanding questions with the mother and father, without rushing,

FOR NURSES ONLY

NURSERY TEACHING CHECKLIST

Please read the *Mother/Baby* information booklet given to you after birth. After reading it, please go through the following list and check whether you understand each topic or need to know more.

		I know this already	Doesn't apply to me	I need to know more	Taught/ reviewed/ demonstrated (For nurses only)
Baby Care	What to do if baby is choking or gagging				
	Safety				
	How to do skin care/cord care				
	How to take care of the circumcision or genital area				
	How to know if my baby is sick and what to do				
	What is jaundice and how to detect it				
	Use of thermometer				
	Use of bulb syringe				
	How and when to burp baby				
	Newborn behavior: crying/comforting				
	How to position baby after feeding				
	What does demand scheduling mean?				
Breastfeeding	I attended breastfeeding class/watched breastfeeding video	YES ☐	NO ☐		
	How to position baby for feeding				
	How to get baby to latch on to my nipple properly				
	When and how long to breastfeed				
	Removal of baby from my nipple				
	What is the supply and demand concept?				
	What is the let-down reflex?				
	When does breast milk come in?				
	Supplementing				
	Proper diet for breastfeeding mothers				
	Prevention and comfort measures for sore nipples				
	Prevention and comfort measures for engorgement				
	When and how to use a breast pump				
	How to express milk by hand				
	How to go back to work and continue to breastfeed				
Bottle-Feeding	How to feed my baby a bottle				
	Reasons for NOT propping bottles				
	How to clean nipple/bottle				
	How to prepare formula				
	What formula should my baby drink				
Safety	**Use of infant car seat**				
	Back to Sleep				
	Shaken Baby Syndrome				

Other information: ______________________

I have received and understand the instructions given on the above topics.

______________________ ______________

MOTHER'S SIGNATURE DATE

Videos viewed/ Literature given: ______________________

Language Spoken by Mother:

☐ English ☐ Spanish ☐ Other ______________

Interpreter Used? ☐ Yes ☐ No ☐ Family Interprets

Nurse's Signature(s): ______________________

● **Figure 26–15** Nursery teaching checklist. An infant teaching checklist is completed by the time of discharge.

Source: Adapted from Presbyterian/St. Luke's Medical Center, Denver, CO.

Drug Guide

HEPATITIS B VACCINE (ENGERIX-B, RECOMBIVAX HB)

Pregnancy Risk Category: C

Overview of Neonatal Action

Recombinant hepatitis B vaccine is used as a prophylactic treatment against all subtypes of hepatitis B virus. It provides passive immunization for newborns of HBsAg-negative and HBsAg-positive mothers. Hepatitis B can be transmitted across the placenta, but most newborns are infected during birth.

The vaccine is produced from baker's yeast and plasmid containing the HBsAg gene.

Hepatitis B (thimerosal free) vaccine contains more than 95% HBsAg protein and is an inactivated (noninfective) product. Universal immunization is recommended.

Infants of HBsAg-positive mothers should concurrently receive 0.5 mL of hepatitis B immunoglobulin (HBIG) prophylaxis at separate injection sites (AAP & ACOG, 2007; Wilson, Shannon, & Shields, 2009).

Route, Dosage, Frequency

The first dose of 0.5 mL (10 mcg) is given intramuscularly into the anterolateral thigh within 12 hours of birth for infants born to HBsAg-positive mothers. The second dose of vaccine is given at least 1 month after the first dose and followed by a final dose at least 4 months after the first dose and at least 3 months after the second dose, but not before 6 months of age.

Infants born to HBsAg-negative mothers receive their first dose of vaccine at birth, the second dose at 1 to 2 months, and the third dose at 6 to 18 months (AAP & ACOG, 2007).

Infants whose mother's HBsAg status is unknown should receive the same doses of vaccine as infants born to HBsAg-positive mothers.

Neonatal Side Effects

The only common side effect is soreness at the injection site. Occasionally, there is erythema, swelling, warmth, and induration at the injection site, irritability, or a low-grade fever (37.7°C [99.8°F]).

Nursing Considerations

Delay administration during active infection, as the vaccine will not prevent infection during its incubation period.

- The vaccine should be used as supplied. Do not dilute. Shake well.
- Do not inject intravenously or interdermally.
- Monitor for adverse reactions. Monitor temperature closely.
- Have epinephrine available to treat possible allergic reactions.
- Responsiveness to the vaccine is age dependent. Preterm infants weighing less than 1000 g have lower seroconversion rates. Consider delaying the first dose until the infant is term postconceptual age (PCA) or use a four-dose schedule.

and take time to resolve all queries. Any concerns of the parents or nurse are noted.

Community-Based Nursing Care

The nurse discusses with parents ways to meet their newborn's needs, ensure safety, and appreciate the newborn's unique characteristics and behaviors. By assisting parents in establishing links with their community-based healthcare provider, the nurse can get the new family off to a good start. Parents also need to know the signs of illness, how to reach the pediatrician or after-hours clinic, and the importance of follow-up after discharge (Table 26–4). Parents should also check with their clinician for advice about over-the-counter medications to be kept in the medicine cabinet.

The family should have the care provider's phone number, address, and any specific instructions. Having the birthing unit or nursery phone number is also reassuring to a newborn's family. They are encouraged to call with questions.

Some institutions have initiated postpartum and/or newborn follow-up home visits especially for infants discharged before 48 hours after birth. The follow-up infant examination should be within 48 hours of discharge (AAP & ACOG, 2007) when the family is unable to visit their primary care physician within that time period. The home visit focuses on normal newborn care, assessment for hyperbilirubinemia (jaundice), ex-

Table 26–4 When Parents Should Call Their Healthcare Provider

Temperature above 38°C (100.4°F) axillary or below 36.6°C (97.8°F) axillary
Continual rise in temperature
More than one episode of forceful vomiting or frequent vomiting over a 6-hour period
Refusal of two feedings in a row
Lethargy (listlessness), difficulty in awakening baby
Cyanosis (bluish discoloration of skin) with or without a feeding
Absence of breathing longer than 20 seconds
Inconsolable infant (quieting techniques are not effective) or continuous high-pitched cry
Discharge or bleeding from umbilical cord, circumcision, or any opening (except vaginal mucus or pseudomenstruation)
Two consecutive green, watery stools or black stools or increased frequency of stools
No wet diapers for 18 to 24 hours or fewer than six to eight wet diapers per day after 4 days of age
Development of eye drainage

treme weight loss, feeding problems, and knowledge related to newborn care and feeding within the family unit.

Routine well-baby visits should be scheduled with the clinic, pediatric nurse practitioner, or physician. Regardless of the type of follow-up services available in the community, the nurse contributes to the newborn's health by stressing the importance of routine care and by helping families who have no follow-up plans to connect to local resources for care. (For detailed discussion of home care, see Chapter 31∞.)

EVALUATION

When evaluating the nursing care provided in preparation for discharge, the nurse may anticipate the following outcomes:

- The parents demonstrate safe techniques in caring for their newborn.
- Parents verbalize developmentally appropriate behavioral expectations of their newborn and knowledge of community-based newborn follow-up care.

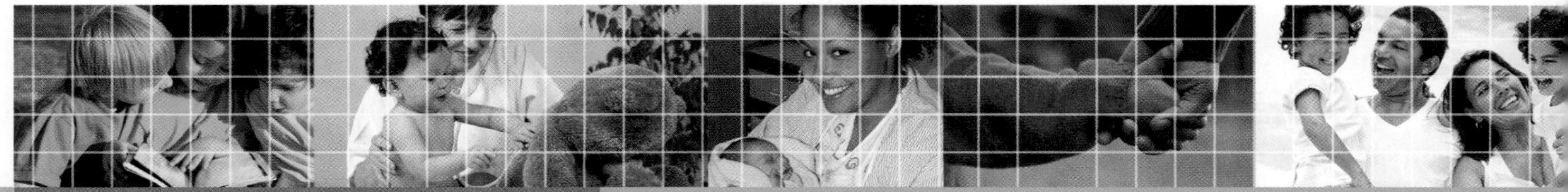

CRITICAL CONCEPT REVIEW

LEARNING OUTCOMES	CONCEPTS
26.1 Summarize essential information to be obtained about a newborn's birth experience and immediate postnatal period.	Information is gathered from these sources: 1. Condition of the newborn: ■ Apgar scores. ■ Any resuscitation effort. ■ Vital signs. ■ Voiding. ■ Passage of meconium. 2. Labor and birth record: ■ Length and course of labor. ■ Type of delivery. ■ Conditions at delivery. ■ Medications given during labor. 3. Antepartal record: ■ Infections during pregnancy. ■ EDB. ■ Previous pregnancies. ■ Any congenital anomalies. ■ HIV test result. 4. Parent-newborn interaction information: ■ Type of infant feeding desired. ■ Desire for circumcision if infant is male. ■ Support system available. ■ Whether rooming-in is desired.

(continued)

LEARNING OUTCOMES	CONCEPTS
26.2 Explain how the physiologic and behavioral responses of the newborn during the first 4 hours after birth (admission and transitional period) determine the nursing care of the newborn.	1. Maintaining a clear airway and stable vital signs: ■ The infant's cardiovascular and respiratory systems are changing rapidly. ■ The infant is dried and stimulated to breathe. ■ Free flow oxygen is available if needed, to assist the infant's transition. ■ Apgar score and vital signs are used to assess the infant's transition. 2. Maintaining a neutral thermal environment: ■ The infant is stressed by the change from the warm, moist environment of the uterus to the dry, drafty environment of the birthing room and nursery. ■ A neutral thermal environment is needed to prevent the need for increased oxygen and calories. ■ The newborn is dried and placed under a radiant warmer. ■ A cap is placed on the infant's head to prevent heat loss. ■ Temperature is checked frequently and the infant is kept from drafts and open windows. 3. Preventing hemorrhagic disease in the newborn: ■ Newborn lacks intestinal bacterial flora, which is necessary for the production of Vitamin K. ■ Prothrombin levels are low during the first few days of life. ■ Vitamin K injection is given IM quickly after birth. 4. Preventing eye infection: ■ Infant may come in contact with infected material during birth. ■ Eye prophylaxis is given to all newborns to prevent serious eye infection. 5. Assessment of neonatal distress: ■ The nurse assesses and teaches parents signs and symptoms of respiratory distress such as tachypnea, grunting, retractions, or change in color. ■ Parents are taught to use the bulb syringe and proper positioning to prevent respiratory problems. 6. Expected periods of reactivity: ■ The infant is usually alert for the first hour after birth. ■ The nurse should encourage eye-to-eye contact between the infant and parents. ■ The nurse should initiate first feedings if the infant is stable. 7. Nursing interventions during the first 4 hours after birth include: ■ Monitor vital signs: every hour, four times daily. ■ Assess and monitor skin color, including acrocyanosis. ■ Assess condition of cord (note number and type of vessels). ■ Assess weight, length, and head circumference. ■ Determine gestational age classification. ■ Assess for the presence of any anomalies. ■ Identify infant and initiate security system. ■ Check for expected reflexes. ■ Assess ability to suck and swallow. ■ Bathe infant when temperature is stable. ■ Assist mother to feed as soon as infant is stable. ■ Administer necessary medications.
26.3 Describe the major nursing considerations and activities to be carried out after the transitional period until discharge based on the physiologic and behavioral responses of the newborn.	1. Subsequent daily care includes: ■ Monitor vital signs every 6 to 8 hours. ■ Assess weight. ■ Assess overall color. ■ Assess and care for umbilical cord and circumcision, if performed. ■ Assess intake and output. ■ Assess infant's ability to void and stool. ■ Assess nutritional status. ■ Determine if infant is feeding adequately. ■ Swaddle infant to provide for warmth. ■ Initiate necessary immunizations. ■ Initiate newborn screening tests such as hearing test, if applicable. ■ Assess parent attachment. ■ Provide teaching to parents concerning newborn care.

LEARNING OUTCOMES	CONCEPTS
26.4 Describe common concerns of families and related content to be included in parent teaching on daily newborn and infant care and discharge planning.	Parent concerns and teaching about newborn and infant care include: 1. Immediate health status of the newborn. 2. Measures to ensure infant safety: ■ How to properly use bulb syringe. ■ Place baby on back to sleep. ■ How to safely position infant in crib. 3. Voiding and stool characteristics and patterns: ■ Normal color of urine and appropriate number of voidings. ■ Color, type, and number of expected stools. 4. How to provide general infant care. Cord care: ■ How to keep cord clean and dry. ■ How to keep diapers from irritating cord. ■ Normal changes of cord. ■ Possible cord complications. Male genitalia care: ■ Care of circumcision site. ■ Signs and symptoms of complications from circumcision. ■ Care and cleaning of uncircumcised infant. How to awaken infant: ■ Dress, undress, or bathe hands and feet of infant. ■ Change diaper. ■ Talk to infant, place in upright position. ■ Increase skin contact. How to quiet infant: ■ Move infant slowly and calmly. ■ Burp infant or change soiled diaper. ■ Swaddle infant. ■ Talk to or coo to infant. Prior to discharge, review with parents about: 1. How to properly feed infant. Breastfeeding, if applicable: ■ Position of baby. ■ Supply and demand. ■ Latching on and breaking suction. ■ Supplementing. ■ Care of sore nipples and engorgement. ■ How to express milk by hand and the use of a breast pump. Bottle-feeding, if applicable: ■ Position for feeding and burping the baby. ■ How to prepare formula and how to clean bottles and nipples. ■ Determination of proper formula. 2. General baby care: ■ Safety measures. ■ Skin and cord care. ■ How to detect jaundice. ■ Normal newborn behavior. ■ How to know if infant is sick, take a temperature, and phone number of and when to call infant's healthcare provider. ■ The proper use of car seats. ■ Remaining newborn screenings. ■ Schedule for newborn immunizations. ■ Appointment for infant's next visit with healthcare provider.
26.5 Discuss opportunities to individualize parent teaching and enhance each parent's abilities and confidence while providing infant care in the birthing unit.	Individualized parent teaching is best accomplished by: 1. Observation and demonstration of common infant activities such as: ■ Feeding. ■ Bathing. ■ Diaper changing. ■ Cord care. ■ Circumcision care. 2. Videotapes of selected infant care activities. 3. Written handouts of selected infant care activities. 4. Return demonstration of parents completing selected infant care activities.

CRITICAL THINKING IN ACTION

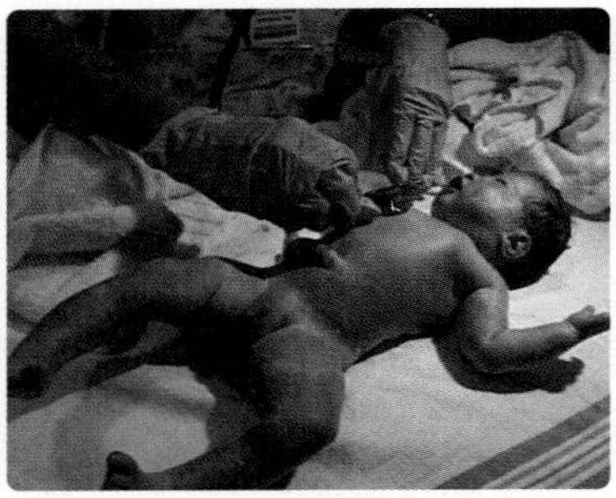

Alice Fine, age 32, G1, now P1001, spontaneously delivers a 7.25 pound baby girl over a median episiotomy. The baby's Apgars are 7 and 9 at 1 and 5 minutes. The baby is suctioned, stimulated, and given free flow oxygen at birth. As the nurse on duty, you admit baby Fine to the newborn nursery, place her under a radiant heater, and perform a newborn assessment. You obtain the vital signs of temperature 97°F, heart rate 128, respiration 55. A physical exam demonstrates no abnormalities, and you note that there were no significant problems with the pregnancy, the mother's blood type is A+, and she plans to bottle-feed. You monitor the baby until her vital signs are stable and then take her to the mother's room for her first bottle-feeding at 60 minutes old.

1. How would you review measures to promote the safety of the newborn from abduction?
2. How would you explain the technique to suction the newborn with a bulb syringe?
3. Describe the care of the newborn's cord.
4. How would you review bottle-feeding with the mother?

See MyNursingKit for possible responses.

REFERENCES

American Academy of Pediatrics (AAP). (2008). Car safety seats: A guide for families 2008. Retrieved April 20, 2008, from www.aap.org/family/carseatguide

American Academy of Pediatrics (AAP) & Canadian Paediatric Society (CPS). (2006). Prevention and management of pain in the neonate: An update. *Pediatrics, 118*(5), 2231–2241.

American Academy of Pediatrics (AAP), Committee on Fetus and Newborn & American College of Obstetricians and Gynecologists (ACOG) Committee on Obstetrics. (2007). *Guidelines for perinatal care* (6th ed.). Evanston, IL: Author.

American Academy of Pediatrics (AAP), Newborn Screening Authoring Committee. (2008). Newborn screening expands: Recommendations for pediatricians and medical homes—implications for the system. *Pediatrics, 121*(1), 192–217.

American Academy of Pediatrics (AAP). Task Force on Sudden Infant Death Syndrome. (2005). The changing concept of sudden infant death syndrome: Diagnostic coding shifts, controversies regarding the sleeping environment, and new variables to consider in reducing risk. *Pediatrics, 116*(5), 1245–1255.

American College of Obstetricians and Gynecologists (ACOG), Committee on Genetics. (2003). Newborn screening (ACOG Committee Opinion No. 287). *Obstetrics & Gynecology, 102,* 887–889.

Andrews, M. M. (2008). Transcultural perspectives in the nursing care of children and adolescents. In M. M. Andrews & J. S. Boyle (Eds.), *Transcultural concepts in nursing care* (5th ed., pp. 116–145). Philadelphia: Lippincott.

Askin, D. (2008). Newborn adaptations to extrauterine life. In K. R. Simpson & P. A. Creehan, *Perinatal nursing* (3rd ed., pp. 527–545). Philadelphia: Lippincott Williams & Wilkins.

Blackburn, S. T. (2007). *Maternal, fetal, & neonatal physiology: A clinical perspective* (3rd ed.). St. Louis: Saunders.

Creehan, P. A. (2008). Newborn physical assessment. In K. R. Simpson & P. A. Creehan, *Perinatal nursing* (3rd ed., pp. 546–574). Philadelphia: Lippincott Williams & Wilkins.

D'Avanzo, C. E., & Geissler, E. M. (2008). *Pocket guide to cultural assessment* (4th ed.). St. Louis: Mosby.

Hedayat, K. M. (2001). Issues in Islamic biomedical ethics: A primer for the pediatrician. *Pediatrics, 108*(4), 965–971.

Institute for Clinical Systems Improvement (2008). Preventive services for children and adolescents, *Institute for Clinical Systems Improvement,* 2008 October. Retrieved March 31, 2009, from www.guidelines.gov/summary/summary.aspx?doc_id=13314&nbr=006758&string=%22preventive+services+for+children%22+and+adolescents

Karl, D. J. (2004). Using principles of newborn behavioral state organization to facilitate breastfeeding. *MCN American Journal of Maternal Child Nursing, 29*(5), 292–298.

Klaus, M., & Klaus, P. (1985). *The amazing newborn.* Menlo Park, CA: Addison-Wesley.

Lipson, J. G., & Dibble, S. L. (2008). *Culture & Clinical Care* (7th ed.). San Francisco, CA: The Regents, University of California.

Medves, J. M., & O'Brien, B. (2004). The effect of bather and location of first bath on maintaining thermal stability in newborns. *Journal of Obstetric, Gynecologic, and Neonatal Nursing, 33*(2), 175–182.

Ott, B., Al-Khadhuri, J., & Al-Junaibi, S. (2003). Preventing ethical dilemmas: Understanding Islamic health care practices. *Pediatrics, 29*(3), 227–230.

Roach, J. A. (2004). Newborn stimulation: Preventing over-stimulation is key for optimal growth & well-being. *AWHONN Lifelines, 7*(6), 531–535.

Thureen, P. J., Deacon, J., Hernandez, J. A., & Hall, D. M. (2005). *Assessment and care of the well newborn* (2nd ed.). St. Louis: Elsevier Saunders.

Vincent, J. L. (2009). Infant hospital abduction: Security measures to aid in prevention. *American Journal of Maternal/Child Nursing, 34*(3), 179–183.

Wilson, B. A., Shannon, M. T., & Shields, K. M. (2010). *Prentice Hall nurse's drug guide 2010.* Upper Saddle River, NJ: Pearson Education, Inc.

World Health Organization. (1999). Care of the umbilical cord: A review of the evidence [On-line]. Retrieved June 21, 2008, from www.who.int/rht/documents/MSM98-4

World Health Organization. (2008). Male circumcision information package. [On-line]. Retrieved June 20, 2008, from www.who.int/hiv/pub/malecircumcision/infopack/en/index.html

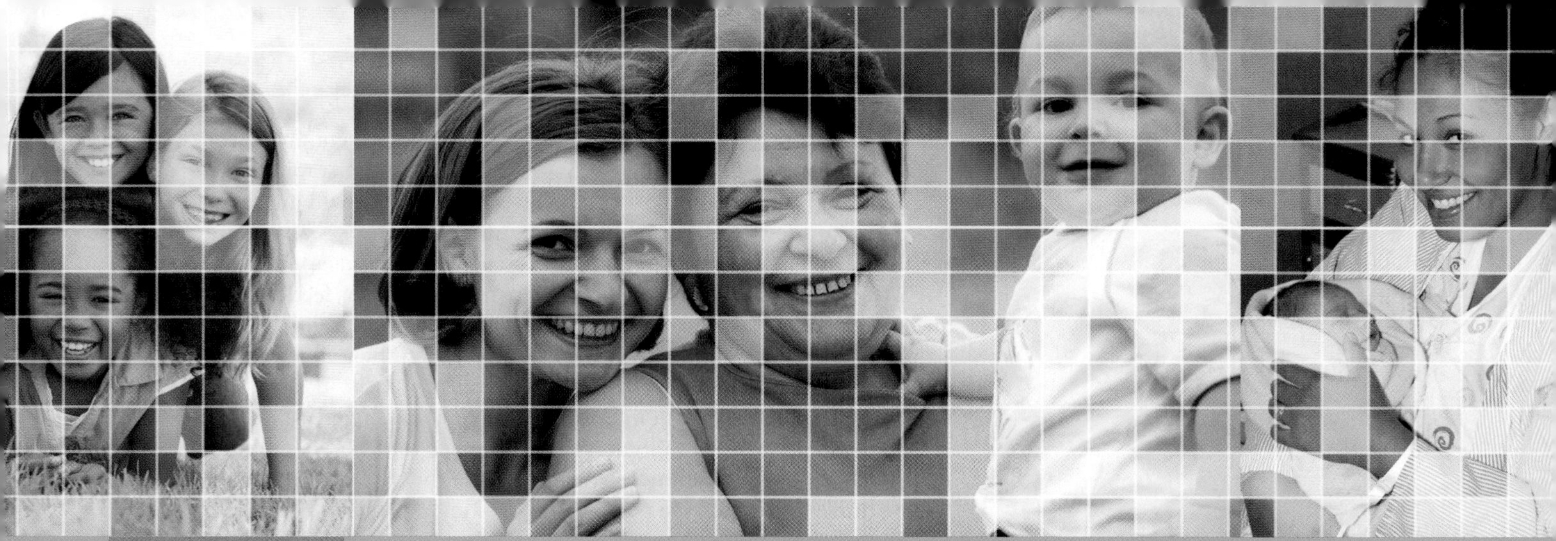

CHAPTER

27 Newborn Nutrition

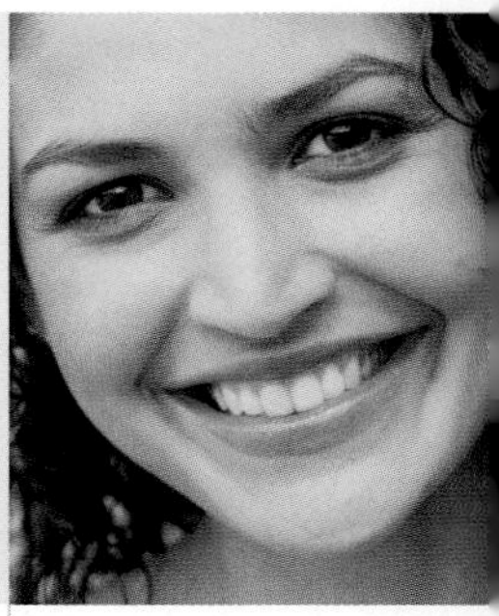

I had been told that most babies ate every 3 to 4 hours and slept the rest of the time. But not my son! He wanted to nurse every 2 hours, and sometimes more often than that. I wanted to meet his needs but felt consumed by them. It was hard to adjust to the fact that I could not get done what I usually accomplished. Once I accepted this fact, I felt free to enjoy the time I was spending with my son. —*Ryan's mother, 30*

LEARNING OUTCOMES

27.1 Compare the nutritional value and composition of breast milk and formula preparations in relation to the nutritional needs of the newborn.

27.2 Explain the advantages and disadvantages of breastfeeding and formula-feeding in determining the nursing care of both mother/family and newborn.

27.3 Develop guidelines for helping both breast- and formula-feeding mothers to feed their newborns successfully in hospital and community-based settings.

27.4 Explain the influence of cultural values on infant care, especially feeding practices, in nursing care of the newborn, mother, and family.

27.5 Explain the nutritional needs and normal growth patterns of infants and educate parents on these topics.

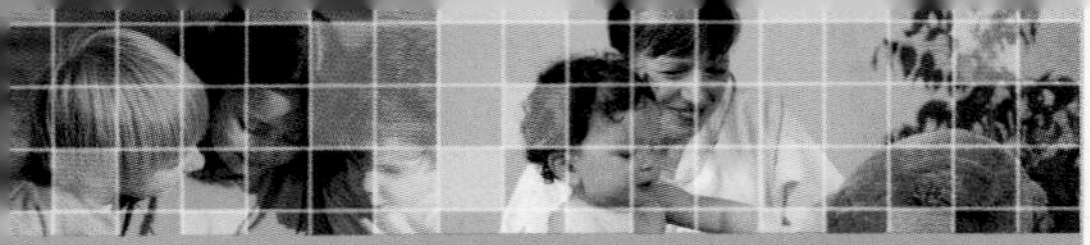

KEY TERMS

Colostrum, 636
Foremilk, 635
Hindmilk, 635
La Leche League International, 655
Let-down reflex, 635
Mature milk, 636
Oxytocin, 635
Prolactin, 635
Transitional milk, 636

Early nutrition has a significant impact on the present and future health and well-being of the infant because this is a period of rapid growth and brain development. Good nutrition fosters physical growth and helps maintain a healthy immune system. In addition, infant feeding itself is an important component of newborn socialization that promotes cognitive and emotional development.

Whether choosing to breastfeed or use infant formula, feeding their newborn is an exciting and satisfying, but often worrisome, task for parents. Meeting this essential need of their new child helps parents strengthen their attachment to their baby and fosters their self-images as nurturers and providers. It is important that the nurse is well informed about infant nutrition and feeding methods because the parents look to the nurse for this guidance. They need to learn the skills to feed their infant successfully. Through each interaction with the parents, there is an opportunity for the nurse to support the parents and promote the family's sense of confidence.

In this chapter an emphasis is placed on feeding the full-term healthy infant of normal birth weight during the neonatal period. We will look at the nutritional needs of the newborn in the context of both breast milk and formula composition, discuss feeding methods, explore community-based nursing care, and finally look at a nutritional assessment of the newborn.

NUTRITIONAL NEEDS AND MILK COMPOSITION

The newborn's diet must supply all the nutrients required by the body in the proper quantities to meet the newborn's rapid rate of physical and neurologic growth and development. A newborn's diet should provide adequate hydration and sufficient calories and must include protein, carbohydrates, fat, vitamins, and minerals. Exclusive breast milk and/or iron-fortified 20-calorie/ounce formula are sufficient as sole sources of nutrition to meet the dietary needs of the newborn from birth up to 6 months of age. Complementary solid foods are introduced in the second half of the first year, and the infant continues to receive breast milk and/or formula until at least 12 months of age (American Academy of Pediatrics Section on Breastfeeding, 2005).

DIETARY REFERENCE INTAKES

Before discussing the nutritional needs of the infant, the nurse should note that the new title *dietary reference intake (DRI)* is an updated generic term that replaces the well-known nutritional reference term *recommended dietary allowances (RDAs).* RDA previously served as a benchmark for nutritional adequacy in the United States, but it reflected primarily disease prevention from nutrient deficiency. The term *DRI* encompasses four aspects of nutrient-based reference values: (1) estimated average requirement (EAR), (2) recommended dietary allowance (RDA), (3) adequate intake (AI), and (4) tolerable upper intake level (UL). The DRIs represent a framework that links nutrition and health across the lifespan (Gregory, 2005).

GROWTH

It is normal for both breastfed and formula-fed infants to lose weight in the first 3 to 4 days of life. Formula-feeding infants generally lose up to 3.5% of their birth weight; breastfeeding infants should not exceed a weight loss greater than 7% of their birth weight (Association of Women's Health, Obstetric and Neonatal Nurses (AWHONN, 2007). Infants lose weight with the passage of meconium and because their fluid intake is normally low in the first few days while transitioning to enteral feedings. This loss is normal and does not result in dehydration, as infants draw on their extracellular water reserves. Infants should begin gaining weight by day of life 5 or sooner and should be at or above birth weight by 10 to 14 days of age. North American breastfed infants gain an average of 35 gm (approximately 1 oz) per day at 1 month whereas formula-fed infants gain an average of 34.4 gm per day at 1 month (Riodan & Wambach, 2010). In general infants gains about 10 g/kg/day or 5 to 7 oz/week (Riordan & Wambach, 2010).

Nursing Practice

Newborn caloric and fluid needs are:

- Caloric intake: 45.5 to 52.5 kcal/lb/day or 100 to 115 kcal/kg/day
- Fluid requirements: 64 to 73 mL/lb/day or 140 to 160 mL/kg/day
- First 6 months weight gain: Formula-fed—1 oz/day;
- Breastfed—0.5 oz/day

Breastfed and formula-fed babies have different growth rates. This is understandable because the compositions of breast milk and formula are different. See comparing breast milk and formula compositions table on MyNursingKit. Most health care providers (as well as formula companies) consider breastfeeding as the "gold standard" from which to compare nutritional outcomes (AAP, 2005; Lawrence & Lawrence, 2005).

Formula-fed infants tend to regain their birth weight earlier than breastfed infants because the formula-fed infant has a greater fluid intake early on. The breastfeeding infant's fluid intake depends on the mother's milk supply and breastfeeding efficiency. It is noteworthy that breastfeeding infants born to multiparous mothers often do not lose as much weight as infants born to primiparous mothers, because the multiparous mother's milk typically "comes in" quicker (Lawrence & Lawrence, 2005). If a healthy full-term infant with normal birth weight has a weight loss exceeding 7%, then a feeding evaluation is indicated. If an infant has a weight loss of 10% or greater then an evaluation, intervention, and follow-up is indicated to make certain that the infant receives sufficient fluid and calories. In this case, a follow-up weight check is recommended to ascertain if the feeding problem is resolved.

Growth rates for breastfed and formula-fed infants are also somewhat different once feedings are established. Exclusively breastfed infants have the same or slightly higher weight gain than their formula-fed and mixed-fed peers in the first 3 to 4 months. Thereafter, formula-fed and mixed-fed infants have a greater weight gain pattern compared with breastfed infants. This characteristic weight gain pattern results in a leaner body build in the breastfed group by the latter half of the first year of life (Riordan & Wambach, 2010). Measurements of length and head circumference are the same for both groups. An infant typically grows 2.5 cm (1 in.) per month in the first 6 months, and then 1.3 cm (0.5 in.) for the next 6 months. Length is a greater indicator of growth than is weight. Infants generally double their birth weight by 5 months, triple their birth weight by 1 year of age, and quadruple their birth weight by 2 years (Riordan & Wambach, 2010). Growth charts for tracking an infant's weight, length, and head circumference can be downloaded from the Centers for Disease Control website (see MyNursingKit).

FLUID

Fluid requirements during the neonatal period are high (140 to 160 mL/kg/day) because of the newborn's decreased ability to concentrate urine and increased overall metabolic rate. Although the infant's total body water content is high (75% to 80%) compared with an adult (60%), the infant has an increased surface area-to-mass ratio and decreased renal absorptive capacity that makes the infant more susceptible to dehydration from insufficient fluid intake or increased fluid loss caused by diarrhea, vomiting, or another source of fluid loss. Parents and caretakers should be aware of the signs of dehydration. Dry or chapped lips, dry oral cavity, decreased urine output, concentrated urine, general weakness, lethargy, poor skin turgor, sunken eyes, and sunken fontanelle are some of the signs of dehydration. The infant's fluid intake will need to be increased above the baseline fluid needs when the infant has a fever or is in a warm environment for an extended period of time. For infants under 6 months of age, increased fluid requirements should be met with additional breast milk or formula, rather than water. Feeding supplemental water is not recommended routinely for infants under 6 months of age who are still on an exclusively milk diet (breast milk or formula), because the increased water can cause hyponatremia and may result in seizures if water consumption is excessive.

ENERGY (CALORIES)

The basal metabolic rate (BMR) refers to the energy needed for thermoregulation, cardiorespiratory function, cellular activity, and growth. The healthy full-term infant's BMR is about twice that of an adult, based on body weight (Rolfes, Pinna, & Whitney, 2006). A newborn requires 100 to 115 kcal/kg/day at 1 month and 85 to 95 kcal/kg/day from 6 to 12 months of age. When infants do not receive sufficient calories, they risk losing weight, may experience tissue breakdown, and are at risk for delayed growth and development (Gregory, 2005).

FATS

Infants receive approximately 50% of their calories from fat. Fats also help the body absorb the fat-soluble vitamins A, D, E, and K. Fats are a precursor of prostaglandins and other hormones. Essential fatty acids and their derivitives, long-chain polyunsaturated fatty acids (LCPUFAs), namely docosahexaenoic acid (DHA) for brain development and arachidonic acid (ARA) for visual acuity (Cloherty, Eichenwald, & Stark, 2008; Riordan & Wambach, 2010).

Milk Composition

Fat content is the most variable component in breast milk, ranging from 30 to 50 grams/liter. Approximately 98% of the human milk fat is in the form of triglycerides, and a very small but clinically significant amount is from cholesterol. Some researchers believe that the cholesterol in breast milk may play a role in myelination and neurologic development. Cholesterol levels in breast milk may also stimulate the production of enzymes that lead to more efficient metabolism of cholesterol, thereby reducing its harmful long-term effects on the cardiovascular system.

Fatty acids are another key component to brain development. Prenatally, fatty acids transfer across the placenta. Postnatally, they are obtained from the diet. Omega-3 and omega-6 fatty acids are two classes of essential fatty acids found in breast milk, although the level can vary with maternal diet. Fish is a rich source of these kinds of fatty acids. Docosahexaenoic acid (DHA) and arachidonic acid (ARA) are long-chain polyunsaturated fatty acids (LCPUFAs) derived from linoleic acid and α-linolenic acid. They are major components of the cell membranes of the retina, brain, and other neural tissues. Along with oleic acid, these LCPUFAs are needed for myelination of the spinal cord and other nerves, and they have an impact on visual acuity and cognitive and behavioral functions.

It is influenced by maternal parity, duration of pregnancy, the stage of lactation, diurnally regulation, and changes in fat content even during a single feeding. Multiparous mothers produce milk with a lower content of fatty acids. For example, the milk of a mother who delivers a preterm infant has a greater concentration of DHA and ARA than does the milk of a mother who gives birth to a full-term infant. Babies born prematurely miss receiving the continuous placental transfer of DHA and ARA while developing during the third trimester. By receiving breast milk, these preterm infants receive the increased concentrations of DHA and ARA intended for the premature infant (Lawrence & Lawrence, 2005).

Phospholipids and cholesterol levels are higher in colostrum compared with mature milk, although overall fat content is higher in mature breast milk compared with colostrum. Fat content is generally higher in the evening and lower in the early morning. Within a single feeding session an infant initially receives the low-fat foremilk before receiving the higher calorie, high-fat hindmilk. Finally, the fat content of breast milk is also affected by maternal diet and maternal fat stores. Mothers on low-fat diets have increased production of medium chain fatty acids (C6–C10), and mothers with high levels of body fat produce breast milk with a higher fat content (Lawrence & Lawrence, 2005).

The fats in the milk-based formulas are modified to parallel the fat profile of breast milk by removing the butterfat from cow's milk and adding vegetable oils. The different blends of fats used by major formula brands all provide a fatty acid profile in the end that is similar to breast milk in terms of amount of saturated, monounsaturated, and polyunsaturated fats present. Since 2002 some infant formulas have been supplemented with DHA and ARA. However, breast milk also contains 167 other fatty acids of uncertain function, and these are absent from formula (Cloherty et al., 2008).

CARBOHYDRATES

Carbohydrates (sugars) serve as the other main source of energy for the infant, providing about 40% of the calories in the infant's diet. By weight, both breast milk and formula contain more carbohydrate than fat.

Lactose is the primary carbohydrate in mammalian milk and plays a crucial role in the nourishment of our offspring. Human milk has a very high lactose content compared with the milk of other mammal species. After lactose is hydrolyzed into galactose and glucose, the galactose is used in the formation of cerebral galactolipids and contributes to brain and central nervous system development. Glucose is used by many tissues, but especially by the brain, which consumes 20% of the body's energy requirements and derives this almost exclusively from glucose. In addition to providing a cellular energy source, lactose enhances the absorption of calcium, magnesium, and zinc (Lawrence & Lawrence, 2005).

Breast milk also contains trace amounts of other carbohydrates such as glucosamines and nitrogen-containing oligosaccharides. Glucosamines are one of the building blocks for connective tissues and help strengthen and hold together ligaments and tendons. Oligosaccharides promote the growth of *Lactobacillus bifidus,* which promotes an intestinal acidic environment creating a hostile environment for bacteria to thrive (Riordan & Wambach, 2010).

In comparing carbohydrates among the milk-based formulas, both Enfamil® and Similac® provide all of their carbohydrate calories from lactose. Carnation Good Start® uses a blend of 70% lactose and 30% maltodextrin (a table sugar–like carbohydrate) (Sears, 2009).

PROTEIN

Proteins are the building blocks for muscle and organ structure. They are key to just about every metabolic process in the body including energy metabolism, cell-signaling, growth, and immune function. The protein requirement for an infant is about 0.8 to 0.9 grams per deciliter (Riordan & Wambach, 2010).

Milk proteins are often grouped into whey proteins and casein. Casein is the major phosphoprotein found in milk. Cow's milk contains a high amount of casein (a low ratio of whey to casein—approximately 20:80) compared with human milk (60:40 whey: casein). Because of its tendency to form curds, milk with high amounts of casein is less easily digested. Cow's-milk–based formulas are usually modified to get closer to the whey:casein ratio of human milk. For example, the whey:casein ratio in Enfamil® is 60:40. Although Similac® has a ratio of 48:52, the company claims this produces an amino acid profile in the blood that is closer to that found in the breastfeeding infant. Carnation Good Start® contains hydrolyzed whey protein, which the company states decreases the incidence of constipation, but which makes comparison difficult (Sears, 2009). It should also be noted that the whey and casein components in breast milk are not static and change over time to meet the needs of the growing infant. In early lactation, the whey:casein ratio is 90:10. As lactation progresses, the whey:casein ratio in mature breast milk is 60:40. Finally, during late lactation, the whey: casein ratio is 50:50 (Riordan & Wambach, 2010).

Whey protein in breast milk is composed of five major components: (1) alpha-lactalbumin, (2) serum albumin, (3) lactoferrin, (4) immunoglobulins, and (5) lysozyme. The latter three components are involved in immunologic activities. Breast milk contains many other kinds of proteins as well. These include enzymes, growth modulator, and hormones (Blackburn, 2007). The major whey components in cow's-milk–based formula are beta-lactoglobulin and alpha-lactalbumin. The former can trigger allergic reactions in some infants (Vonlanthen, 1998).

VITAMINS, MINERALS, AND TRACE ELEMENTS

Vitamins can be grouped into fat-soluble and water-soluble vitamins. The fat-soluble vitamins A, D, E, and K are found in both cow's-milk–based formula and breast milk. Vitamin K is also synthesized in the infant's intestinal tract by bacteria that are colonized there. Excessive amounts of fat-soluble vitamins may result in toxicity, and there is general agreement that no routine fat-soluble vitamin supplementation is needed with the exception of vitamin D. To prevent rickets the AAP recommends that deeply pigmented breastfed infants or those with inadequate exposure to sunlight receive 200 international units of oral vitamin D drops daily during the first 2 months of life (AAP & ACOG, 2007). The infants should continue to take the vitamin supplement until feeding at least 500 mL per day (about 16.6 oz/day) of vitamin D-fortified formula or milk. Most healthy, full-term formula-feeding infants of average birth weight will receive sufficient vitamin D intake before they are 2 months old, and therefore may not require vitamin D supplementation.

Milk composition. Breast milk is naturally low in vitamin D (25 international units/L or less), and may be a cause of concern particularly among breastfed infants who have limited sunlight exposure. Factors that place an infant at high risk for vitamin D deficiency include having increased skin pigmentation, living in a geographic location where there is little sunlight, having their skin consistently covered with clothing or sunscreen, not spending much time outdoors, living in an area that consistently has heavy pollution that blocks sunlight, and having a mother who is vitamin D deficient. (See Chapter 34∞ for discussion of vitamin and mineral deficiencies.)

The vitamin B complex and vitamin C are water-soluble vitamins that pass readily from serum to breast milk. However, mothers who follow a strict vegetarian diet or macrobiotic diet may have insufficient vitamin B_{12} in their milk. In that case the exclusively breastfed infant should receive vitamin B_{12} supplementation. Formula is fortified with adequate amounts of the water-soluble vitamins to meet the DRI.

Minerals

Minerals have diverse regulatory functions throughout the body. For example, calcium is important in the clotting mechanisms; phosphorus is a component in ATP, DNA, RNA, and phospholipids; calcium and phosphorus are necessary for bone formation; sodium is involved in fluid balance; calcium, sodium, and potassium are needed for nerve and muscle function; chlorine is involved in acid-base balance; cobalt works with vitamin B_{12} to form blood cells; copper and iron aid in extracting energy from the citric acid cycle and are also involved in blood production; iodine is needed for thyroid hormone synthesis; and magnesium, manganese, and zinc are needed to help with many enzymatic processes.

Milk composition. Both breast milk and infant formulas contain several major and trace minerals to satisfy the needs of the growing infant. Breast milk provides newborns with minerals in more appropriate doses than do formulas (Blackburn, 2007). The mineral content of breast milk does not appear to be influenced by maternal diet. The vitamins and minerals among the three formulas being compared are essentially the same, although all generally contain higher levels of minerals than breast milk to compensate for their lower bioavailability.

The amount of iron transferred to the fetus during the third trimester of pregnancy is influenced by maternal iron status (Riordan & Wambach, 2010). Iron is an important mineral required by the body to make hemoglobin and is needed for neurologic function. Neurotransmitters require adequate iron levels to function properly and therefore infants with chronic anemia are at risk for cognitive and developmental delays. Infants deficient in iron may look pale, appear sleepy or tire easily while feeding, and be tachycardic or tachypneic at rest. The infant's iron status is affected by the amount of iron accumulated in utero, the infant's diet after birth, and the general health of the infant.

The American Academy of Pediatrics does not advocate the use of low-iron fortified formulas because of the increased risk for anemia associated with their use (AAP & ACOG, 2007). Low-iron formula is fortified with only 2 mg of iron per liter compared with "iron-fortified" formula, which is fortified with 12 mg of iron per liter. It should be noted that the iron concentration in breast milk is 0.5 to 1.0 mg per liter, which is considerably lower than in iron-fortified formulas.

However, the iron in breast milk is much more completely absorbed—the infant receiving breast milk absorbs 50% to 80% of the iron in breast milk compared with less than 12% of the iron in formula. Healthy term infants with normal birth weights receiving breast milk or an iron-fortified infant formula during the first 5 to 6 months of life are unlikely to develop iron-deficiency anemia because these infants have sufficient iron stores to sustain them until they start solid feedings in the second half of the first year of life (Riordan & Wambach, 2010). (See Chapter 34∞.)

Some parents have a misconception that infants fed iron-fortified formula are likely to have constipation. Nurses have a responsibility to educate parents and help them understand that the iron added to formula is in an ionic form and does not cause constipation (Katz, Levin, Cotton, et al., 2007). The casein in formula (which is different from the casein in breast milk) creates large, rubbery curds that are slow to metabolize and have been associated with constipation in formula-fed infants. In addition, there is evidence that palm olein oil (an additive to some formulas) also may contribute to constipation. Palm olein oil is added to some formulas to provide palmitic acid in an attempt to match the natural palmitic acid profile in breast milk. However, the chemical arrangements are different. Palmitic acid derived from olein oil is poorly absorbed. The unabsorbed palmitic acid in formula reacts with calcium to create insoluble soaps during digestion (Ross Products Division, 2007).

Trace Elements

Other additives to formulas not yet mentioned include nucleotides (building blocks for DNA and RNA that appear to enhance the immune system, among other things), carnitine (derived from the amino acid lysine and functioning in part to transport fatty acids to the mitochondria for oxidation), and taurine (a conditionally essential non-protein sulfur amino acid with a number of functions including a role in growth, and in CNS and auditory function development). There are many other breast milk components not yet duplicated in formula and not all components in breast milk have been identified. In general, though, formula companies are always striving to improve their products to develop the best "humanized" milk possible. There is no question that formulas today are far superior to formulas from the past.

SPECIALTY FORMULAS

If an infant has medical problems related to inability to metabolize components of breast milk or standard cow's-milk formula, or if the parents are vegans, the family should consult with the baby's healthcare provider to discuss the issue of supplements or switching their infant to another infant formula. Switching to cow's-milk–based formula will not always help as the infant may react to the cow's-milk proteins in the formula. Often these infants will have cross-reaction to other types of proteins and will not tolerate soy-based formulas either. These babies may need to be on an expensive specialty formula such as a "predigested" hydrolysate formula if the mother quits breastfeeding.

Soy Formulas

Soy protein–based formulas (e.g., Enfamil Prosobee LIPIL®, Isomil®, Isomil Advance®, Isomil DF®, and Good Start Supreme Soy®) use a soy protein harvested from soybeans and supplemented with methionine (an essential amino acid), carnitine, and taurine. Soy protein–based formulas do not contain any bovine protein or lactose. Because soy protein–based formulas do not contain lactose, the formula is usually sweetened with corn syrup or sucrose. The latter may cause dental decay after teeth have erupted. Phytates present in soy formulas decrease the absorption of iron, calcium, and zinc, so greater concentrations of minerals and vitamins are added to soy formulas.

Soy protein-based formula is not intended as a first-choice formula except for infants with primary lactase deficiency or galactosemia and for term infants of formula-feeding vegan parents. According to the AAP, there is no proof that soy protein–based formula will prevent or lessen the symptoms of colic or prevent atropic disease, and infants who have a sensitivity to cow's-milk protein may have a sensitivity to soy protein as well. Therefore, the AAP does not recommend routinely switching an infant from cow's-milk–based formula to soy-based formula (Greer, Sicherer, Burks, & Committee on Nutrition and Section on Allergy and Immunology, 2008).

Other Specialized Formulas

Infants with an allergic response to standard formulas may require a hypoallergenic "hydrolysate" formula. Hydrolyzed formulas (e.g. Nutramigen®, Alimentum®, and Pregestimil®) are sometimes referred to as "predigested" formulas because the dietary proteins have been broken down in a process that mimics digestion (hydrolysis). The simple protein compounds are usually too small to be recognized by the infant's immune system as an antigen, thereby decreasing the infant's allergic response. These formulas are also used in infants who have difficulties with normal digestion or absorption.

The other group of hypoallergenic formulas is the elemental amino acid-based formulas, such as Neocate® and Elecare®. The proteins in these formulas have been completely broken down to their amino acid constituents. These formulas are the most hypoallergenic formulas available and virtually eliminate the possibility of allergic reaction. They are intended for severely allergenic infants with multiple dietary protein intolerances or infants with severe absorption disorders. (See Chapter 34∞ for discussion of lactose intolerance.)

Other specialized formulas are intended for infants with particular medical conditions and should be fed to infants only under a physician's supervision. There are specific specialized formulas intended for infants born prematurely to promote rapid growth. There are other specialized formulas for infants with heart disease, kidney disease, malabsorption syndromes, metabolic diseases, and allergies. These formulas vary in caloric content, nutrient composition and ingredients, digestibility, taste/odor, and cost.

CHOICE OF FEEDING: BREAST VERSUS FORMULA

Feeding their newborn is an exciting, satisfying, but often worrisome task for parents. Meeting this essential need of their new child helps parents strengthen their attachment to their child and fosters their self-images as nurturers and providers, yet carries great responsibility. Whether a woman chooses to breastfeed or formula feed, she can be reassured that she can adequately meet her infant's needs. As questions about feeding arise, the nurse works with the woman to help her develop skill in her chosen method. In every interaction, it is the nurse's responsibility to support the parents and promote the family's sense of confidence.

The mother usually decides to breastfeed or formula feed by the sixth month of pregnancy and often even before conception. However, she may not make her final decision until admission to the birth center. The decision is often influenced by relatives, especially the baby's father and maternal grandmother (Chezen, Friesen, & Boettcher, 2003), by friends, and by social customs rather than being based on knowledge about the nutritional and psychologic needs of the mother and her newborn.

The goals of *Healthy People 2010* continue to be 75% of infants breastfeeding in the early postpartal period and 50% taking in at least some human milk until age 6 months (Riordan & Wambach, 2010). A recent survey of breastfeeding in the United States showed a slow rise to 77% of hospital-born infants received some breastmilk but the continuation of breastfeeding until 6 months of age still falls short of the desired goal (McDowell, Wang, & Kennedy-Stephenson, 2008). It is the health care provider's responsibility to provide the parents with accurate information about the distinct advantages of breastfeeding to the mother and infant. In these times of short stays, the Baby-Friendly Hospital Initiative program promotes breastfeeding by designating hospitals as centers for breastfeeding education.

Once the parents have made an informed choice of feeding method, the nurse's primary responsibilities are to support the family's decision and to help the family achieve a positive result. No woman should be made to feel either inadequate or superior because of her choice in feeding. There are advantages and disadvantages to breastfeeding and bottle-feeding, but positive bonds in parent-child relationships can be developed with either method.

BREASTFEEDING

THE BREASTFEEDING PROCESS

Breast Milk Production

Breast anatomy. The female breast is divided into 15 to 20 lobes, separated from one another by fat and connective tissue, and interspersed with blood vessels, lymphatic vessels, and nerves. These lobes are subdivided into connected lobules composed of small units called alveoli where milk is synthesized by the alveolar secretory epithelium. The lobules have a system of lactiferous ducts that branches into mammary ducts that open onto the nipple surface (Riordan & Wambach, 2010). Mothers are often surprised to see milk coming out multiple nipple pores when they express their milk. See Figure 27–1 ● to view the anatomy of the breast.

Physiologic and endocrine control of lactogenesis. During pregnancy, increased levels of estrogen stimulate breast duct proliferation and development, and elevated progesterone levels promote the development of lobules and alveoli in preparation for lactation. Prolactin levels rise from approximately 10 ng/mL prepregnancy to 200 ng/mL at term. However, lactation is suppressed during pregnancy by elevated progesterone levels secreted by the placenta. Once the placenta is expelled at birth, progesterone levels fall and the inhibition is removed, triggering milk production. This occurs whether the mother has breast stimulation or not. However, if by the third or fourth day breast stimulation is not occurring, prolactin levels begin to drop.

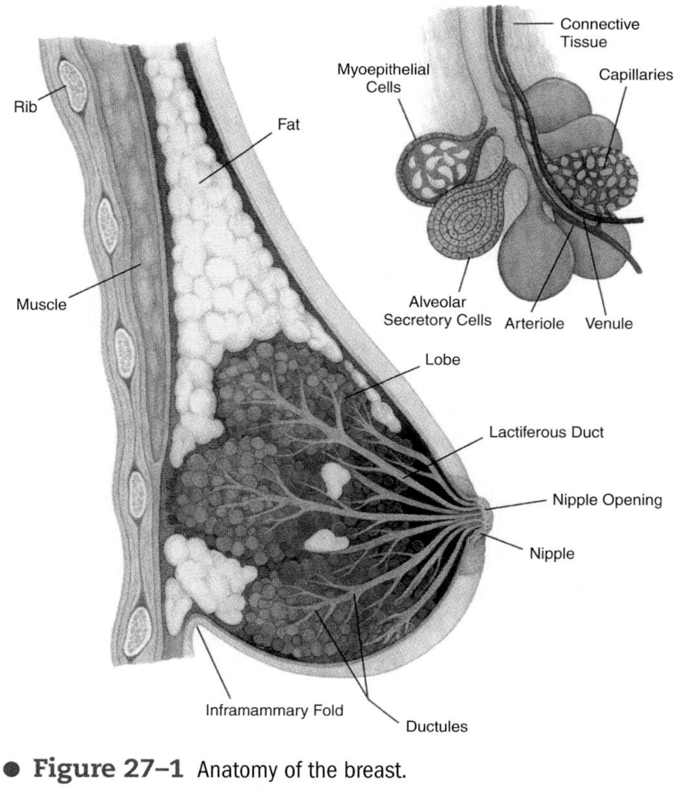

● **Figure 27–1** Anatomy of the breast.

Source: From Riordan, J. (2005). *Breastfeeding and human lactation* (3rd ed.). Boston: Jones & Bartlett. Copyright 2005 Jones and Bartlett Publishers, Sudbury, MA, www.jbpub.com. Reprinted with permission.

Initially, lactation is under endocrine control. The hormone **prolactin** is released from the anterior pituitary in response to breast stimulation from suckling or the use of a breast pump. Prolactin levels double each time the infant suckles at the breast, regardless of the age of the infant or duration of lactation. Prolactin stimulates the milk secreting cells in the alveoli to produce milk, then rapidly drops back to baseline. If more than approximately 3 hours occurs between stimulation, prolactin levels begin to drop below baseline. To reverse the overall decline in prolactin level, the mother can be encouraged to stimulate her breasts more frequently (e.g., every 1.5 to 2 hours). Mothers should be strongly encouraged to stimulate their breasts frequently if their infants are not effective feeders or if they are separated from their infants. Prolactin receptors are established during the first 2 weeks postpartum in response to frequency of breast stimulation (Human Milk Banking Association of North America, 2005). Inadequate development of prolactin receptors during this time is likely to negatively impact the mother's long-term milk volume. By 2 weeks postpartum, prolactin levels will be back to prepregnancy levels and milk production will cease if stimulation of the breasts by breastfeeding or pumping does not occur (Lawrence & Lawrence, 2005).

The milk that flows from the breast at the start of a feeding or pumping session is called **foremilk**. The foremilk is watery milk high in protein and low in fat (1% to 2%). This milk has trickled down from the alveoli between feedings to fill the lactiferous ducts. It is low-fat milk because the fat globules made in the alveoli stick to each other and to the walls of the alveoli and do not trickle down. If a mother does not stimulate her breasts by breastfeeding or pumping, her prolactin levels return to prepregancy levels by 14 days postpartum (Lawrence & Lawrence, 2005).

In addition to prolactin release, stretching of the nipple and compression of the areola signal the hypothalamus to trigger the posterior pituitary gland to release oxytocin. **Oxytocin** acts on the myoepithelial cells surrounding the alveoli in the breast tissue to contract, ejecting milk, including the fat globules present, into the ducts. This process is called the *"milk-ejection reflex,"* better known in lay terms as the **"let-down" reflex** *(response).* The average initial let-down response occurs about 2 minutes after an infant begins to suckle, and there will be 4 to 10 let-down responses during a feeding session. The milk that flows during "let-down" is called hindmilk. **Hindmilk** is rich in fat (can exceed 10%) and therefore high in calories. In a sample of expressed breast milk, the average total fat concentration is about 4% and the total caloric content is about 20 calories/ounce.

By 6 months of breastfeeding, prolactin levels are only 5 to 10 ng/mL, yet milk production continues. A whey protein called feedback inhibitor of lactation (FIL) has been identified as influencing milk production through a negative feedback loop. FIL is present in breast milk and functions to decrease milk production. The more milk that remains in the breast for a longer period of time, the more milk production is decreased. On the other hand, the more often the breasts are emptied, the lower the level of FIL and the faster milk is produced. This mechanism of regulating milk at the local level is called autocrine control. This process is key to understanding how a mother maintains or loses her milk supply (Riordan & Wambach, 2010).

MyNursingKit Video Activity: Nursing in Action: Breastfeeding

There are a number of factors that can delay or impair lactogenesis. Maternal factors include cesarean birth, postpartum hemorrhage, type 1 diabetes, untreated hypothyroidism, obesity, polycystic ovary syndrome, retained placenta fragments, vitamin B_6 deficiency, history of previous breast surgery, insufficient glandular breast tissue, and significant stress (Riordan & Wambach, 2010). Other factors that can interfere with breastfeeding include smoking and use of alcohol, as well as some prescription and over-the-counter medications (e.g., antihistamines, combined birth control pills).

Stages of human milk. During the establishment of lactation there are three stages of human milk: colostrum, transitional milk, and mature milk.

Colostrum is the initial milk that begins to be secreted during midpregnancy and is immediately available to the baby at birth. It provides the infant with all the nutrition required until the mother's milk becomes more abundant in a few days. Colostrum is a thick, creamy yellowish fluid with concentrated amounts of protein, fat-soluble vitamins, and minerals, and it has lower amounts of fat and lactose compared with mature milk. It also contains antioxidents and high levels of lactoferrin and secretory IgA. It promotes the establishment of *Lactobacillus bifidus* flora in the digestive tract, which helps to protect the infant from disease and illness. Colostrum also has a laxative effect on the infant, which helps the baby pass meconium stools, which in turn helps decrease hyperbilirubinemia.

Between day 2 and day 5, maternal milk production normally becomes noticeably more abundant. The milk "coming in" is called transitional milk. **Transitional milk** has qualities intermediate to colostrum and mature milk. It is still light yellow in color but is more copious than colostrum and contains more fat, lactose, water-soluble vitamins, and calories. By day 5, most mothers are producing about 500 mL/day.

Mature milk is white or slightly blue-tinged in color. It is present by 2 weeks postpartum and continues thereafter until lactation ceases. Mature milk contains about 13% solids (carbohydrates, proteins, and fats) and 87% water. Although mature human milk appears similar to skim cow's milk and may cause mothers to question whether their milk is "rich enough," mothers should be reassured that this is the normal appearance of mature human milk and that it provides the infant with all the necessary nutrients. Although gradual changes in composition do occur continuously over periods of weeks to accommodate the needs of the growing newborn, in general the composition of mature milk is fairly consistent with the exception of the fat content as noted previously. Milk production continues to increase slowly over the first month. By 6 months postpartum a mother produces about 800 mL/day (Blackburn, 2007).

ADVANTAGES OF BREAST MILK

In their breastfeeding policy statement, the American Academy of Pediatrics recommends exclusive breastfeeding as the preferred feeding for all infants, with a few exceptions, for the first 6 months and continued breastfeeding during the introduction of solids until the infant is 12 months old or older, as desired. There is overwhelming scientific evidence that shows that breastfeeding provides newborns and infants with specific nutritional, immunologic, and psychosocial advantages over formula-feeding (AAP & ACOG, 2007).

Nutritional Advantages

Human milk provides optimum nutrition for the human infant because it is species specific. The macronutrients such as protein, fat, and carbohydrates (lactose) are synthesized by the mother in the alveoli of the breasts by specialized secretory cells. Micronutrient elements such as vitamins and minerals derive from the circulating maternal plasma. There are more than 200 distinct components in breast milk, with more remaining to be identified (Lawrence & Lawrence, 2005). (See earlier discussion of milk composition in this chapter.)

Additional health advantages for breastfed infants include reduced risk of developing type 1 or type 2 diabetes melitus, lymphoma, leukemia, Hodgkin's disease, obesity, hypercholesterolemia, and asthma. The mother who breastfeeds has health advantages such as burns additional calories making milk (quicker return to prepregnancy weight), has a decreased risk of developing breast cancer and ovarian cancer, and may have a decreased risk of developing postmenopausal osteoporosis (AWHONN, 2007) .

Immunologic Advantages

The immunologic advantages of breast milk include varying degrees of protection from respiratory tract and gastrointestinal tract infections, necrotizing enterocolitis, urinary tract infections, otitis media, bacterial meningitis, bacteremia, and allergies (AWHONN, 2007). Transplacental passage of maternal immunoglobulin gradually diminishes over the first 6 months of life until the infant can begin to produce his or her own immunoglobulins.

Secretory IgA, an immunoglobulin present in colostrum and breast milk, has antiviral, antibacterial, and antigenic-inhibiting properties, specifically across mucosal surfaces such as the intestinal tract. Secretory IgA plays a role in decreasing the permeability of the small intestine to help prevent large protein molecules from triggering an allergic response. Other constituents of colostrum and breast milk that act to inhibit the growth of bacteria or viruses are *Lactobacillus bifidus,* lysozymes, lactoperoxidase, lactoferrin, transferrin, and various immunoglobulins.

Some mothers wonder if there are special considerations for breastfed infants regarding immunizations, in particular the oral poliovirus vaccination because it is a live virus vaccine. The Centers for Disease Control states that there is no indication for withholding breastfeeding (Lawrence and Lawrence, 2005). (See Chapter 45∞ for discussion of immunizations.)

Psychosocial Benefits of Breastfeeding

The psychosocial advantages of breastfeeding are primarily those associated with maternal-infant attachment. For some mothers the attachment process begins when the decision to become pregnant is made. The hormonal changes associated with pregnancy strengthen that bond. Events that occur during pregnancy, such as hearing the fetal heart beat, feeling the fetus move within her, and watching her abdomen grow bigger, further promote the bonding. At delivery there may be intense bonding. For other mothers

Evidence in Action

Infant to mother skin-to-skin care immediately following birth supports breastfeeding and bonding (Moore, Anderson, & Bergman, 2007; Ramano & Lothian, 2008).

bonding develops over the next few days (Lawrence & Lawrence, 2005). Some hospital practices inadvertently interfere with the attachment process. Rooming-in and breastfeeding have been shown to increase maternal-infant attachment.

When a mother chooses to breastfeed, she often has more frequent direct skin-to-skin contact with her infant than if she were bottle feeding. (Bottle-feeding parents should be encouraged to have frequent skin-to-skin contact too.) Infants with skin-to-skin contact have greater physiologic stability, cry less, sleep longer, and tend to breastfeed better. The newborn's sense of touch is highly developed at birth and is a primary means of communication. The tactile stimulation associated with breastfeeding can communicate warmth, closeness, and comfort. The increased closeness provides both newborn and mother with the opportunity to learn each other's behavioral cues and needs. Mothers may feel more affectionate toward their newborns, have improved let-down response while pumping, and breastfeed more frequently and for longer periods of time (Klaus, 1998; Mohrbacher & Stock, 2003).

The mother who breastfeeds has a different hormonal state compared with the mother who does not breastfeed. Prolactin increases feelings of relaxation and euphoria. Oxytocin levels also increase with breastfeeding. Oxytocin produces feelings of relaxation and sleepiness, heightens responsiveness and receptivity toward the infant, and increases the frequency of nurturing behaviors (Lawrence & Lawrence, 2005).

Another psychological advantage to the breastfeeding mother is satisfaction derived from the knowledge that she is providing her infant with the optimal nutritional start in life. For many mothers breastfeeding takes effort, understanding, and an emotional commitment to endure the demands of this lifestyle choice. The mother's sense of accomplishment in being able to satisfy her baby's needs for nourishment and comfort can be a tremendous source of personal satisfaction.

There are significant cost savings for the family that chooses breastfeeding; healthcare cost savings for families resulting from the decreased incidence of illness in the infant and potential societal benefits to breastfeeding include decreased spending on public assistance programs (e.g., WIC), and environmental benefits in terms of use of natural resources and solid waste disposal (see Table 27–1 for comparison of breastfeeding and formula feeding) (AWHONN, 2007).

POTENTIAL DISADVANTAGES AND CONTRAINDICATIONS TO BREASTFEEDING

Disadvantages

The following is a list of sometimes cited potential disadvantages to breastfeeding:

1. *Pain with breastfeeding.* Breastfeeding is a natural process but requires a certain knowledge base that formerly was passed on from generation to generation. Nipple tenderness is the most common source of discomfort and is usually related to improper positioning and/or not obtaining a proper attachment of the infant on the breast. Pain can also be related to engorgement or infection. Breastfeeding with proper technique should not hurt and these mothers should be encouraged to seek assistance from a knowledgeable person skilled in lactation.
2. *Leaking milk.* Some women will leak milk when their breasts are full and it is nearly time to breastfeed again or whenever they experience "let-down," which can be triggered by hearing, seeing, or even thinking of their babies. If this causes concern to the mother, the nurse can instruct the mother on how to apply gentle pressure directly over her nipple for a minute or so to stop the leaking momentarily. The use of nursing pads (with instructions to change wet pads frequently), wearing printed tops that camouflage small leaks, and reassurance that the problem lessens with time may help alleviate this problem.
3. *Embarrassment.* Some mothers feel uncomfortable about breastfeeding because they are modest, or they may feel embarrassed because our society views breasts as sexual objects. In addition, an unfriendly social environment may make it difficult to breastfeed in public. This is not an easy issue to overcome. Some mothers will feel some reassurance after learning how to breastfeed discreetly while in public.
4. *Stress.* Finding time and feeling tied down to the demands of breastfeeding can be stressful, especially for the mother attending school or working outside of the home. This is a common reason mothers cite for weaning their infant prematurely. Mothers can be offered the option to decrease the frequency of pumping rather than quitting altogether. Of course this will decrease the mother's milk supply, but babies who receive some breast milk are still healthier than babies who do not receive any breast milk at all. Nurses can encourage mothers to breastfeed or pump as long as possible.
5. *Unequal feeding responsibilities/fathers left out.* Some parents want feedings to be a shared responsibilty. The parents should be informed that it is advisable for the father to wait to bottle-feed the baby with expressed breast milk until after breastfeeding is established. In the meantime, encourage the father to be supportive of the breastfeedng mother, to have a lot of skin-to-skin contact with his infant, and to share the responsibilities of all other aspects of infant care (bathing, dressing, diapering, burping, rocking, etc.).
6. *Diet restriction.* Some mothers think that they have to give up eating certain foods when they breastfeed. This is, for the most part, a myth. Generally, mothers can still eat all the foods they are accustomed to eating. There are rare instances in which some infants are intolerant to something in the mother's milk. The most common problem comes from dairy products. Again, this is not a

Table 27–1 Comparison of Breastfeeding and Formula Feeding

Breastfeeding	Formula (Iron-Enriched) Feeding
INFANT NUTRITION	
An ideal balance of nutrients, efficiently absorbed. High bioavailability of iron leaves lower iron for bacterial growth, cell injury. Higher levels of essential fatty acids, lactose, cystine, and cholesterol, necessary for brain and nerve growth. Composition varies according to gestational age and stage of lactation, meeting changing nutritional needs. Long-term decreased incidence of diabetes, cancer, obesity, asthma. Contains unsaturated fats. Infants determine the volume of milk consumed. Frequency of feeding is determined by infant cues. May feed more frequently as milk digests faster.	Derived from bovine milk and/or plant sources. Lower bioavailability of nutrients requires higher concentrations in milk. Additives may cause intolerance. Still missing numerous ingredients. Formulas do not contain cholesterol. Soy and hydrolysate formulas do not contain lactose. DHA & ARA now added. Nutritional value not varied. Nutritional adequacy depends on proper preparation/dilution. Contains saturated fats. Parents or healthcare provider determine the volume consumed. Overfeeding may occur if caregiver is determined that baby empty bottle. Frequency of feeding is determined by infant's cues. May feed less frequently as milk digestion slower.
IMMUNOLOGIC PROPERTIES	
Contains immunoglobulins, enzymes, and leukocytes that protect against pathogens. Nutrients promote growth of *Lactobacillus,* protective bacteria. Lower rates of urinary tract infections, otitis media, and other infectious diseases. Anti-infective properties present in the milk permit longer storage duration. Breast milk is hypoallergenic, with minimal risk of protein allergy/intolerance.	No anti-infective properties. Formula is linked to an increased incidence of gastrointestinal and respiratory tract infections. Potential for bacterial contamination exists during preparation and storage. Cow's milk protein allergy relatively common.
MATERNAL HEALTH	
Faster return to prepregnancy weight. Breastfeeding associated with lower risk of breast, ovarian cancer. Concerns over breastfeeding and medications.	Provides infant nutrition when breast milk not available because of maternal illness, medication/drug use, or lactation failure (breast surgery, endocrine disease)
PSYCHOSOCIAL ASPECTS	
Skin-to-skin contact enhances bonding. Hormones of lactation promote maternal feelings and sense of well-being. Some mothers may feel ashamed or embarrassed because of the value system of modern society. Leaking of breastmilk. Breastfeeding after returning to work may be difficult.	Both parents can participate in positive parent-infant interaction during feeding. Father can assume feeding responsibilities.
COST	
Healthy diet for mother. Savings for infant medical costs: approximately $400 average in first year of life. Ancillary costs: nursing pads, nursing bras. A breast pump may be needed. Refrigeration is necessary for storing expressed milk.	Formula cost per year: $1200 for standard formula, $2500/year for hypoallergenic formulas. Ancillary costs: bottles or bottle liners, nipples, cleaning costs. Refrigeration is needed if preparing more than one bottle at a time.
CONVENIENCE	
Milk is always the perfect temperature. No preparation time is needed. The mother must be available to feed or will need to provide expressed milk to be given in her absence. If she misses a feeding, the mother must express milk to maintain lactation. The mother may experience breast tenderness and engorgment in the early days of lactation. Limited birth control options and vaginal dryness.	Formula must be purchased commercially. Preparation is time consuming. Less convenient for traveling or for night feedings. Mother need not be present—anyone can feed the infant

common problem, but when it comes up, it is advisable to refer the mother to a lactation consultant for its management.

7. *Limited hormonal birth control options.* Some mothers think that they cannot use a hormonal method of birth control while breastfeeding. Mothers should be informed that using birth control pills containing progesterone and estrogen can cause a decrease in milk volume and may affect the quality of breast milk. It is preferred that the mother who wants to use a hormonal birth control method consider using the progestin-only mini pill (i.e., Nicronor®, Nor-QD®, Aygestin®, or Norlutate®); receive Depo-Provera®, a progestin-only injection administered every 90 days; or have a progestin-only implant. Although progestin-only hormonal birth control is compatible with lactation, it should not be started at the time of discharge. It is recommended that the mother wait 6 weeks before taking the hormonal medication to ensure a good milk supply (AAP & ACOG, 2007). Mothers can be reassured that barrier methods of birth control and natural family planning do not interfere with lactation at all and are good options to consider as well.
8. *Vaginal dryness associated with breastfeeding.* Some mothers experience vaginal dryness related to a low level of estrogen while lactating. Mothers can be given reassurance that this is only a temporary side effect while breastfeeding. A water-based lubricant such as K-Y® jelly or Astroglide® can be used during intercourse until the mother weans and estrogen levels increase again.
9. *Medications and breastfeeding.* Some mothers are concerned about the safety of breastfeeding while they are taking medications. For additional information on medications and their compatibility with breastfeeding, see the list of resources on MyNursingKit.

Medications

It has long been recognized that medications taken by the breastfeeding mother may penetrate breast milk to some degree. But having a better understanding of the kinetics of drug entry into breast milk, as well as factors influencing its bioavailability to the nursing infant is important, because use of medication has been identified as a barrier to breastfeeding and a major reason women cite for discontinuing it (Hale, 2008).

It should be noted that (1) most drugs pass into breast milk, (2) almost all medications appear in only small amounts in human milk (usually less than 1% of the maternal dosage), and (3) very few drugs are contraindicated for breastfeeding women (AAP Committee on Drugs, 2001; Briggs, Freeman, & Yaffe, 2008; Hale, 2008). The properties of a drug influence its passage into breast milk, as does the amount of the drug taken, the frequency and route of administration, and the timing of the dose in relationship to infant feeding. The drug's effects are influenced by the infant's age, the feeding frequency, the volume of milk taken, and the degree of absorption through the gastrointestinal tract.

Five adjustments should be made when administering drugs to a nursing mother to decrease the effects on the infant (Blackburn, 2007).

1. Avoid long-acting forms of drugs. The infant may have difficulty metabolizing and excreting them, and accumulation may be a problem.
2. Consider absorption rates and peak blood levels in scheduling the administration of the drugs. Less of the drug crosses into the milk if the infant is fed before the mother is given the oral medication.
3. Use preparations that can be given at longer intervals (once versus three to four times per day).
4. When alternatives are available, select the drug that shows the least tendency to pass into breast milk.
5. Use single-symptom drugs versus multisymptom drugs (e.g., a decongestant for allergy rather than a multisymptom drug, especially because liquid forms may contain alcohol).

The mother should be advised to inform her healthcare provider that she is breastfeeding when a drug is prescribed for her. In counseling the breastfeeding mother, the healthcare provider should weigh the benefits of the medication against the possible risk to the infant and its possible effects on the breastfeeding process (see Table 27–1.) Mothers can be reassured that most prescription and over-the-counter medications are safe for the breastfeeding infant.

Potential Contraindications

There are some instances when breastfeeding is or may be contraindicated:

- If mother is HIV-positive or has AIDS, she is counseled against breastfeeding except in countries where the risk of neonatal death from diarrhea and other disease (excluding AIDS) is high (AWHONN, 2007).
- If mother has active, untreated tuberculosis, has varicella, or mother is HTLV1–positive (human T-cell leukemia virus type 1).
- When mother has active herpes on her breast—the infant may still feed on the unaffected side only until the lesion has healed.
- If mother has other illness, on a case-by-case basis.
- When mother uses illicit drugs (e.g., cocaine, heroin) or is an alcoholic.
- Maternal smoking can result in breast milk concentrations of nicotine of 1.5 to 3 times the maternal plasma concentration. Although there is no documented infant health risk related to breastfeeding and smoking, smoking cessation is urged for maternal health reasons (Riordan & Wambach, 2010).
- Specific medications (e.g., radioactive isotopes, antimetabolites, chemotherapy drugs, and a few others) may cause concerns. A mother with a diagnosis of breast cancer should not breastfeed so that she can begin treatment immediately.
- If infant has galactosemia.

MyNursingKit Actions and Effects of Selected Drugs During Breastfeeding

In addition, there is concern about whether women with breast implants should breastfeed or are able to breastfeed. Some research on breast augmentation using the periareolar approach suggests increased incidence of lactation insufficiency (inadequate expressed milk volume and/or infant growth). Factors that may influence the ability of a mother with breast augmentation to breastfeed include the surgical approach used, alterations in nipple sensation, amount of breast tissue present, and lack of or little breast changes during pregnancy with little or no postpartum engorgement (Hill, Wihelm, Aldag, et al., 2004).

Another concern is related to the possible toxicity of the silicone in some breast implants. The silicone concentrations in formula and cow's milk is higher than that found in the milk of mothers with implants; therefore silicone breast implants are not a contraindication to breastfeeding (Riordan & Wambach, 2010).

Potential Problems in Breastfeeding

Because mothers are discharged from the birthing unit before breastfeeding is well established, they are frequently alone when they encounter changes in the breastfeeding process. Many women stop nursing if the situations they encounter seem to pose problems. Nurses can offer anticipatory guidance regarding common breastfeeding phenomena and provide resources for the woman's use after discharge. (See Chapter 31 for a detailed discussion of self-care measures the nurse can suggest to a woman with a breastfeeding problem after discharge from the birthing unit.)

MyNursingKit Case Study: Breastfeeding Client

TIMING OF NEWBORN FEEDINGS

The timing of newborn feedings is ideally determined by physiologic and behavioral cues rather than a set schedule.

Initial Feeding

The nurse should assess for active bowel sounds, absence of abdominal distention, and a lusty cry that quiets and is replaced with rooting and sucking behaviors when a stimulus is placed near the lips. These signs indicate that the newborn is hungry and physically ready to tolerate the initial feeding.

If there are no complications at the birth and the mother is not overly sedated, the infant may be placed on the mother's chest after birth. Throughout the first 2 hours after birth, but especially during the first hour of life, the infant is usually alert and ready to breastfeed. Because colostrum is not irritating if aspirated (which may occur because of the newborn's initial uncoordinated sucking and swallowing abilities) and is readily absorbed by the respiratory system, breastfeeding can usually begin immediately after birth. The mother benefits psychologically from early breastfeeding through enhancement of maternal-infant bonding and physiologically by the release of oxytocin, which helps contract the uterus, expelling the placenta and decreasing the risk of postpartum hemorrhage. Early feedings benefit the newborn because they enhance maternal-infant attachment; stimulate peristalsis, helping to eliminate the by-products of bilirubin conjugation (which decreases the risk of jaundice); help prevent hypoglycemia; promote the passage of meconium; provide the immunologic protection of colostrum; and begin to stimulate further maternal milk production, helping prevent later feeding difficulties.

Complementary Care

HERBS FOR BREASTFEEDING

Herbs (galactagogues) thought to increase milk supply include alfalfa, dandelion, fennel seeds, horsetail, red raspberry, fenugreek, goat's rue, milk thistle, basil, blessed thistle, marshmallow, caraway, and anise to name a few (Academy of Breastfeeding Medicine [ABM], 2004). The mother may drink caraway tea to reduce colic in the breastfeeding infant. Caraway tea also may be given directly to infants to treat colic (Skidmore-Roth, 2006). Most of the herbal galactogogues are taken as a tea, although capsules are also available. Fenugreek is probably the most commonly used herbal galactagogue because it seems to have the fewest adverse side effects. Women who drink it as a tea generally drink 2 to 3 cups per day. The tea is made by adding ¼ teaspoon of fenugreek seeds steeped in 8 ounces of water for 10 minutes. Women who take the capsules generally take one to four capsules (580 to 610 mg capsules) three to four times per day (ABM, 2004). Mothers usually notice an increase in their milk production in 2 to 3 days. Goat's rue, fennel seed, or milk thistle (not blessed thistle) tea is made with 1 teaspoon of dried leaves steeped in 8 ounces of water for 10 minutes; women usually have 2 to 3 cups of tea per day (Wagner, Graham, & Hope, 2006).

There are anti-galactogogue herbs (e.g., sage, parsley, and peppermint) that may or may not be used in combination with cabbage leaves and ice to decrease severe engorgement, to diminish an oversupply, and to "dry up" when weaning an infant from the breast. The following anti-galactagogue herbs may decrease milk supply, so they should be avoided until a woman is no longer breastfeeding: black walnut, sage, parsley, and yarrow (Skidmore-Roth, 2006). Black cohosh, blessed thistle, cascara sagrada, horseradish, garlic, cinnamon bark, kava kava, and senna are also contraindicated during lactation.

If the mother plans to formula-feed, she and her newborn can still enjoy skin-to-skin contact initially. Formula feedings are not typically initiated in the birthing room. Formula-feeding newborns are offered formula as soon as they show an interest/feeding cues or per hospital policy.

Assessment of the newborn's physiologic status is a primary and ongoing concern to the nurse throughout the first feeding. Extreme fatigue coupled with rapid respiration, circumoral cyanosis, and diaphoresis of the head and face may indicate cardiovascular complications and should be assessed further.

The first feeding also provides an opportunity for the nurse to assess the effectiveness of the newborn's suck, swallow, and gag reflexes. The nurse should also remain alert to the possibility of medical problems during this time, including respiratory disorders, congenital cardiovascular problems, or more rare disorders such as tracheoesophageal fistula and esophageal atresia (see Chapter 28). Findings associated with esophageal anomalies include maternal polyhydramnios and increased oral mucus in the infant. In cases of esophageal atresia, the feeding is taken well initially, but as the esophageal pouch fills, the feeding is quickly regurgitated unchanged by stomach contents. If a fistula is present, the infant gags, chokes, regurgitates mucus, and may become cyanotic as fluid passes through the fistula into the lungs.

It is not unusual for the newborn to regurgitate some mucus and water following a feeding, even if it was taken without difficulty, because of initial uncoordinated suck and swallow abilities. It is important to observe the newborn closely and position the baby on the side after the feeding to aid drainage and facilitate gastric emptying. Once the infant is tolerating feeding, the child's normal position after feeding is on his or her back.

Establishing a Feeding Pattern

An "on-demand" feeding program facilitates each baby's own rhythm and helps a new mother establish lactation. The newborn rapidly digests breast milk and may want to nurse 8 to 10 times in a 24-hour period. After the initial period of alertness and eagerness to suckle, the infant progresses to light sleep, then deep sleep, followed by increased wakefulness and interest in breastfeeding. As wakefulness and interest in nursing increase, the infant will often cluster 5 to 10 feeding episodes over 2 to 3 hours, followed by a 4- to 5-hour deep sleep. After this cluster of minifeeds and deep sleep, the infant will feed frequently but at more regular intervals. Often newborn arousal from sleep is the first sign of hunger. Early feeding cues include rooting, smacking, or attempting to suck on anything near his mouth (especially his hand). Crying is considered a late feeding cue. Although people often accept crying as normal and healthy behavior for newborns, it may actually delay the transition to extrauterine life. Crying involves a Valsalva maneuver that increases pulmonary vascular pressure, which may cause unoxygenated blood to be shunted into systemic circulation through the foramen ovale and ductus arteriosus. If no one has responded to the newborn by this time, then the infant may begin to fuss and eventually work up to a full cry. A newborn that is left to cry and not given the opportunity to feed at this point may subsequently become very disorganized and have a difficult time latching on to the breast or coordinating his suck correctly.

Certain hospital practices/policies may contribute to delays in feeding by prolonging the feeding intervals and even decreasing the number of feedings in a 24-hour period. Couplet care or rooming-in practices promote cue-based feedings. Therefore, it may be advantageous for the baby to be in the room with the mother; she will respond to the baby's needs more quickly than the nursery staff may be able to, resulting in less infant crying.

Couplet care permits the mother to learn about and respond to her infant's early feeding cues. Early cues that indicate a newborn is interested in feeding include hand-to-mouth or hand-passing-mouth motion, whimpering, sucking, and rooting (Mulford, 1992).

Satiety behaviors are the same for formula-fed babies as for breastfed babies. These behaviors include longer pauses toward the end of the feeding and noticeable total body relaxation (the baby lies limp with hands down at his side and unclenched). The infant may also release his mother's nipple or the bottle nipple, and may fall asleep. If a baby is satiated and content following feedings, is meeting daily output expectations, and is gaining weight as expected, then feedings are going well.

When couplet care is not available, a supportive nursing staff and flexible nursery policies allow the mother to feed her infant on cue, that is, nurses bring babies to the mothers when the babies are awake and showing signs of hunger. Nurseries that use feeding schedules rather than on-cue feedings cause frustration for the new mother. It is very frustrating to attempt to feed a newborn who is sound asleep because he or she is either not hungry or exhausted from crying.

Feeding intervals are counted from the start of one feeding to the start of the next feeding. Breastfeeding babies typically feed every 1.5 to 3 hours (8 to 12 times in a 24-hour period), but often in an irregular pattern known as "cluster feeding," in which the infant feeds as frequently as every hour for a few feedings followed by a longer sleep period. The normal newborn sleeps a total of 16 to 18 hours per day, but generally with no more than one sleep stretch of up to 5 hours in length. It is more important to focus on the number of feedings in 24 hours than the exact feeding interval time. Formula-fed infants generally eat every 3 to 4 hours and typically 6 to 8 times per day. It is important that families are taught about the normal feeding/sleeping pattern of a newborn, as many parents are distressed by their infant's early erratic feeding pattern. Parents need to be informed that their infant will have a more predictable sleep and feeding pattern when she is 2 to 4 months of age.

Maternal medications received during labor may affect newborn feeding behavior by delaying these early cluster feedings. Delays in normal feeding patterns depend on the specific drug and its half-life. Newborns whose mothers received epidural analgesia have been noted to be irritable and demonstrate reduced motor organization, poor self-quieting skills, and decreased visual skills and alertness. Because breastfeeding infants generally have only one long sleep stretch in a 24-hour period, parents can help their infant to take the long sleep stretch at night if they attempt to awaken their infant during the day when the infant is in a light state of sleep and has already slept longer than 3 hours. Parents can attempt to encourage cluster feedings during the day, and, after a while, the infant may sleep a 5-hour sleep stretch at night. In the meantime, the mother can be encouraged to take "cat naps" during the day while her infant is sleeping. At night the mother can keep stimulation down (lights low, noise low, and diaper change only when necessary).

Breastfeeding and formula-feeding infants have the same fluid requirements, but because they have different diets, their rates of digestion are different. Digestion of formula produces large, rubbery curds that take about 4 hours to digest compared with the softer, smaller curds produced by breast milk. For this reason formula-fed newborns generally sleep longer at a stretch and awaken to feed every 3 to 4 hours. It is not uncommon that formula-fed newborns may take one or two 5-hour sleep stretches in a 24-hour period. As a result they will often take a larger volume at each feed. Babies may begin skipping the night feeding about 8 to 12 weeks after birth. The need for a night feeding is individual and depends on the infant's size and development.

Both breastfed and formula-fed infants experience growth spurts at certain times and require increased feeding. The breastfeeding mother may meet these increased demands by nursing more frequently to increase her milk supply. It takes about 72 hours for the milk supply to increase adequately to meet the new demand. A slight increase in feedings meets the formula-fed infant's needs.

Some mothers may find fixed feeding schedules attractive. These mothers should be informed that although strict feeding schedules may work for some babies, they often do not work for all babies because they do not take into account differences among breastfeeding women and differences among infants. There are documented cases of infants diagnosed with failure to thrive, poor weight gain, dehydration, breast milk supply failure, and involuntary early weaning associated with this feeding method (Aney, 1998). The American Academy of Pediatrics released a Media Alert reaffirming its position that "the best feeding schedules are ones babies design themselves. Scheduled feedings designed by parents may put babies at risk for poor weight gain and dehydration" (AAP, 1998).

Nourishing her newborn is a major concern of the new mother. Her feelings of success or failure may influence her self-concept as she assumes her maternal role. With proper instruction, support, and encouragement from professionals, breastfeeding becomes a source of pleasure and satisfaction to both the parents and infant.

CULTURAL CONSIDERATIONS IN INFANT FEEDING

All groups of people are influenced by their cultural background. Every culture shares a set of values, beliefs, behaviors, and a language unique for that group. These are learned characteristics shared among their members. A person's culture influences every aspect of his or her life. By learning about other cultures, the nurse will gain an understanding of the "context," or unstated assumptions that influence behavior, thus avoiding misunderstanding and improving the nurse's ability to communicate with the person. Of course, it is also true that not all individuals within a particular cultural group subscribe to each of the values, beliefs, and behaviors characteristic of that group. People need to be seen as individuals within the context of their culture (Callister, 2008).

Within the United States, many people agree that breastfeeding is the optimum infant feeding method. However, breast exposure is often viewed in a sexual context, leading to disapproval of the mother who attempts to breastfeed in public. Although this norm may be changing, it is important for the nurse to recognize that not only do "others" often hold these views, but the mother herself may feel this way. It is therefore important to determine the attitudes of the mother—based on her feelings, it may be very important or not important at all to spend time discussing methods of breastfeeding discreetly.

In Black women, higher rates of initiation of breastfeeding were associated with increased age, education, and income (McCarter-Spaulding & Gore, 2009). Social support for breastfeeding primarily came from other women, especially maternal grandmothers, but the social support was very limited and early formula and cereal supplementation is common. In many ethnic groups self efficacy has been shown to predict breastfeeding duration and pattern (exclusive breastfeeding or breastfeeding in combination with formula feeding (McCarter-Spaulding & Gore, 2009).

With regard to the feeding of colostrum, although many recognize that it has properties uniquely suited to the newborn, there are people who consider colostrum "unclean" and do not offer it to their newborns. This belief is found among some groups of Hispanics, Navajo Indians, Filipinos, and Vietnamese (Galanti, 2004; D'Avanzo & Geissler, 2008). In a situation like this, in which a cultural custom is harmful or denies the infant benefits, it is the nurse's responsibility to try to educate the family about the value of colostrum. A possible approach to this situation is as follows. First, reinforce the parents' desire to protect their baby from infection. Next, validate the assumption that since colostrum looks similar to pus from a wound, it makes sense that one might think it is also unclean. Next, point out that the reason pus looks the way it does is because of the white cells that the body sends to fight infection. Last, explain that as in the case of a wound, colostrum *is* one of the body's ways of helping fight infection—only in this case it is sending the white cells to the baby even before there is an infection. This last point again reinforces the initial validation of the parents' concern for infection but now uses that concern as motivation to feed the colostrum, rather than avoid it.

In these cultures and in some countries (Guinea, Pakistan, Bagladesh), breastfeeding begins only after milk flow is established (Riordan & Wambach, 2010). In many Asian cultures, the newborn is given boiled water until the mother's milk flows. The newborn is fed on demand, and cries are responded to immediately. If the crying continues, evil spirits may be blamed and a priest's blessing may be sought. Although many of the Hmong women of Laos combine breastfeeding with some formula feeding, they usually find expressing their milk or pumping their breasts unacceptable. Thus other methods of providing relief should be suggested if breast engorgement develops. Most Muslim mothers breastfeed because the Qur'an (Koran) encourages it until the child is 2 years old (Ott, Al-Khadhuri, & Al-Junaibi, 2003). Japanese women are returning to breastfeeding as the method of feeding for the baby's first year.

Language is one of the most culturally sensitive behaviors and the source of much confusion. African Americans may refer to their infant as "greedy," which may be interpreted by the nurse as a concern that the infant is taking too much. However, rather than an expression of concern, this term is often used as an expression of approval of the infant's vigorous feeding. African American culture tends to emphasize plentiful feeding, and solid foods are introduced early—possibly even added to the infant's formula. If the nurse misinterprets the expression, he or she may think that the mother is limiting the baby's feeding and may attempt to convince the mother that she should be encouraging higher intake, which could lead to overfeeding. African American mothers view frequent feeding as an expression of hardiness and a positive behavioral characteristic for their children for the future. For traditional Mexicans, a fat baby is considered healthy and infants are fed on demand.

These are but a few of the multitude of cultural influences related to feeding (see "Developing Cultural Competence: Breastfeeding in Other Cultures" on page 643). When faced with an infant care practice different from the ones to which they are accustomed, nurses need to evaluate the effect of the practice. Different practices are not necessarily inferior. The nurse should intervene only if the practice is actually harmful to the mother or baby.

Developing Cultural Competence

BREASTFEEDING IN OTHER CULTURES

Some people of Asian heritage may breastfeed their babies for the first 1 to 2 years of life. Many Cambodian refugees practice breastfeeding on demand without restriction, or, if formula-feeding, provide a "comfort bottle" in between feedings (Lipson & Dibble, 2008).

People of Iranian heritage may breastfeed female babies longer than male babies. Many Muslim women will not breastfeed in public (Hedayat, 2001; Ott, Al-Khadhuri, & Al-Junaibi, 2003).

Some people of African ancestry may wean their babies after they begin to walk.

Some Asians, Hispanics, Eastern Europeans, and Native Americans may delay breastfeeding because they believe colostrum is "bad" (D'Avanzo & Geissler, 2008; Riordan & Wambach, 2010).

Haitian mothers may believe that "strong emotions" spoil breast milk; and that thick breastmilk causes skin rashes and thin milk results in diarrhea (Callister, 2008; Lipson & Dibble, 2008).

In Malaysia, the ingestion of breast milk represents a great deal more than simple nutrition for newborn infants. It is believed that the mother's milk enters the baby's blood. This is thought to cultivate a long life. Breast milk is thought to bind the mother and baby together, creating a sense of respect and closeness. Although milk develops the infant's spirit and body, it also develops faith and character. It is thought that the consumption of breast milk formulates a maternal-infant bond that lasts throughout life. This bond cannot be broken by any means. Breastfeeding mothers drink "jamu" (a drink consisting of egg yolk, palm sugar, tamarind, and herbs) to ensure an adequate milk supply.

BREASTFEEDING TECHNIQUE

Breastfeeding Positions and Latching On

Breastfeeding is not instinctive, it is learned. It is a natural process, but it takes "know-how." Ideally, each breastfeeding mother should have a breastfeeding evaluation to determine any knowledge deficits, acknowledge any concerns, provide instructions, and assist with breastfeeding.

Positioning. There are many breastfeeding positions, but only the four classic breastfeeding positions will be discussed here: (1) modified cradle position, (2) cradle position, (3) football (or clutch) hold position, and (4) side-lying position (Figures 27–2 through 27–5 ●). In addition, there are minor variations of hand placement and body position even among the four classic positions. After a mother has fed using one position, encourage her to try a different position when she offers her second breast.

Nursing Practice

The cradle position is challenging, especially when attempted during early lactation by inexperienced mothers, because the mother is attempting to support her baby's head near the crook of her arm. This makes it difficult to control the head position and may allow the baby's head to bend forward (chin toward chest) making attachment difficult. It is better to have the infant's head lag slightly backward (chin tilted slightly upward) so that the infant leans into the breast chin first. Some mothers find it easier to start in the modifed cradle position and then switch into the cradle position.

Modified cradle position

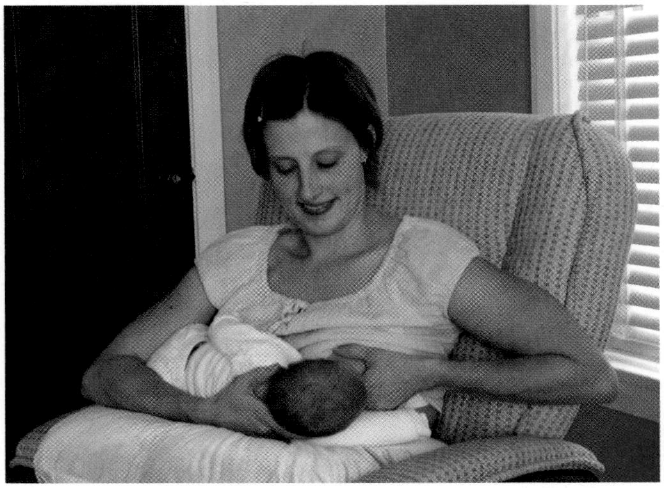

- Have the mother sit comfortably in upright position using good body alignment. Use pillows for support (may use Boppy, body pillow, or standard bed pillows). Lap pillow should help bring the baby up to breast level so the mother does not lean over baby.
- Place the baby on the mother's lap and turn the baby's entire body toward the mother (the baby is in side-lying position). Position the baby's body so that the baby's nose lines up to the nipple. Maintain the baby's body in a horizontal alignment.
- To feed at left breast, the mother supports the baby's head with her right hand at nape of the baby's neck (allow head to slightly lag back); the mother's right thumb by the baby's left ear, and right forefinger near the baby's right ear.
- With the mother's free left hand, she can offer her left breast.

● **Figure 27–2** Modified cradle position.

Source: Courtesy of Brigette Hall, MSN, IBCLC.

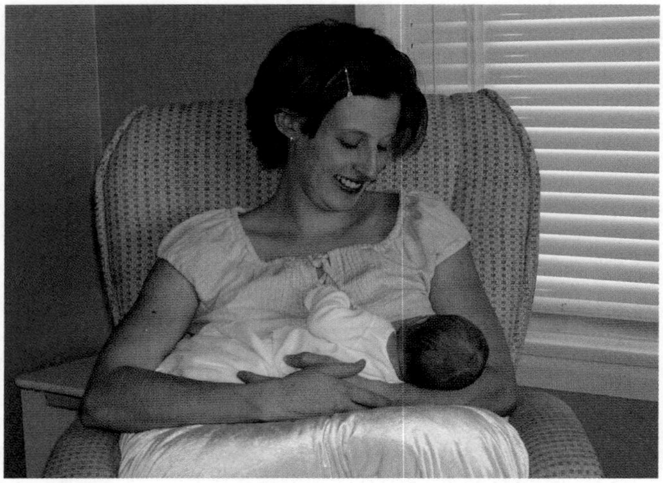

● **Figure 27–3** Cradle position.

Source: Courtesy of Brigette Hall, MSN, IBCLC.

- Have the mother sit comfortably in upright position using good body alignment. Use pillows for support (may use Boppy, body pillow, or standard bed pillows). Lap pillow should help bring the baby up to breast level so the mother does not lean over the baby.
- Place the baby on the mother's lap and turn the baby's entire body toward the mother (the baby is in side-lying position). Position the baby's body so that the baby's nose lines up to the nipple. Maintain the baby's body in a horizontal alignment.
- If feeding from the left breast, have the mother cradle the baby's head near the crook of her left arm while supporting her baby's body with her left forearm.
- With the mother's free right hand, she can offer her left breast.

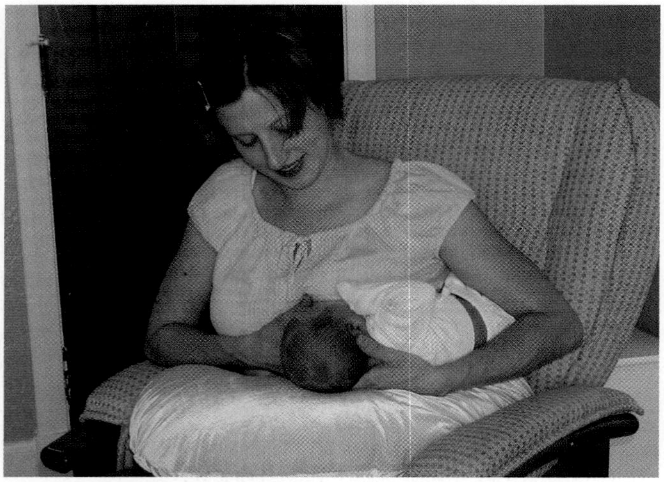

● **Figure 27–4** Football hold position.

Source: Courtesy of Brigette Hall, MSN, IBCLC.

- Have the mother sit comfortably and use pillows to raise the baby's body to breast level. If using a Boppy and the Boppy is in "normal" position on the mother's lap, turn it counterclockwise slightly (if feeding at left breast) to provide extended support for the baby's body resting along the mother's left side and near the back of the mother's chair.
- If feeding at left breast, place the baby on the left side of the mother's body, heading the baby into position feet first. The baby's bottom should rest on the pillow near the mother's left elbow.
- Turn the baby slightly on her side so that she faces the breast.
- The mother's left arm clutches the baby's body close to the mother's body. The baby's body should feel securely tucked in under the mother's left arm.
- Have the mother support the baby's head with her left hand. With the mother's free right hand, she can offer her breast. (Good position for the mother with c-section.)

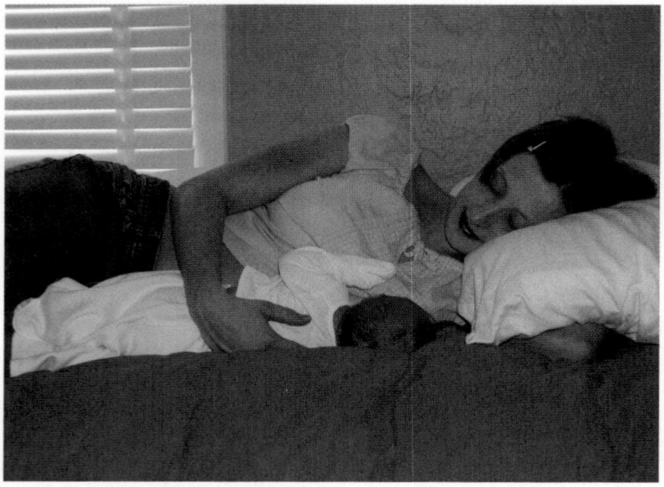

● **Figure 27–5** Side-lying position.

Source: Courtesy of Brigette Hall, MSN, IBCLC.

- Have the mother rest comfortably lying on her side (left side for this demonstration). Use pillows to support the mother's head and back, and provide support for the mother's hips by placing a pillow between her bent knees.
- Place the baby in side-lying position next to the mother's body. The baby's body should face the mother's body. The baby's nose should line up to the mother's nipple. Place a roll behind the baby's back, if desired.
- With the mother's free right hand, she can offer her left breast. After the baby is securely attached, mom can rest her right hand anywhere that is comfortable for her.

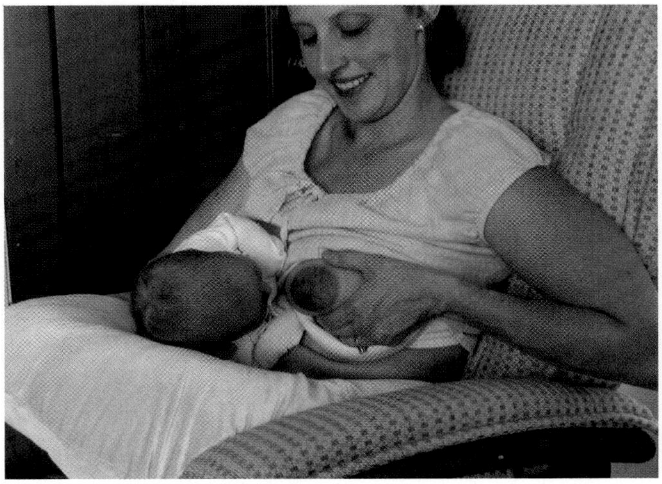

To be ready to draw the baby's mouth onto the mother's breast, as soon as the baby opens her mouth widely enough, the mother needs to have her hand supporting her breast in the ready position. She can use various hand holds, but she needs to keep her fingers well behind the areola. One such hand position is called the "C-hold." In this hold, the thumb is placed on top of the breast near 12:00 position and the other four fingers are placed on the underside of the breast near the 6:00 position (depends on mother's hand size and length of fingers). The key point is to keep the fingers at least 1 1/2 inches back from the base of the nipple as the fingers support the breast. Mothers are not often aware of where they place their fingers especially on the underside of the breast. If the fingers are too far forward (too close to the nipple), then the infant cannot grasp a large amount of areola in her mouth and this results in a "shallow" latch. A shallow latch is associated with nipple pain and ineffective drainage of the breast.

An alternate hand hold not shown is a "U-hold" hand position. The thumb and forefinger are near the 3 and 9 position on the breast again with fingers at least 1 1/2 inches back from the base of the nipple; the body of the hand rests on the lower portion of the breast. Using this hand hold, the mother's arm position is down at her side rather than sticking outward as it is when supporting the breast using the C-hold position.

● **Figure 27–6** C-hold hand position.

Source: Courtesy of Brigette Hall, MSN, IBCLC.

Alternating positions facilitates drainage of the breasts and changes the pressure points on the breast. This will provide some relief to the mother with sore nipples.

Latching on. It is important to have the mother and baby positioned properly in order to achieve an optimal attachment. If, for example, the infant is lying flat on his back (supine position) to feed in the modified cradle position, cradle position, or side-lying position, the infant can obtain only a shallow latch (not attached far back onto the areola). The infant's shoulder becomes an obstacle putting distance between the infant's mouth and his mother's breast. Anything that contributes to a shallow latch is going to cause sore nipples and other complications. Nipple trauma, although relatively common, is not normal. (See Chapter 31 ∞ for a discussion of breastfeeding with inverted or flat nipples.)

The infant needs to attach his lips onto the breast or, rather more accurately, far back onto the areola, not on the nipple. If the infant attaches just to the nipple, the mother will have sore nipples and pain may inhibit the let-down reflex. To obtain a deep latch, the mother needs to be taught how to elicit the infant's rooting reflex, stimulating the infant to open his mouth as widely as possible (like a big yawn). Once the infant does this, the mother should quickly but gently draw her baby in toward her. During the first few days of life, the newborn typically only opens his mouth widely for a second or so, and then he begins to close his mouth again. If the mother misses her chance to get her baby latched on, she needs to simply start over again.

Figures 27–6 through 27–11 ● demonstrate various positions and techniques used in latching on.

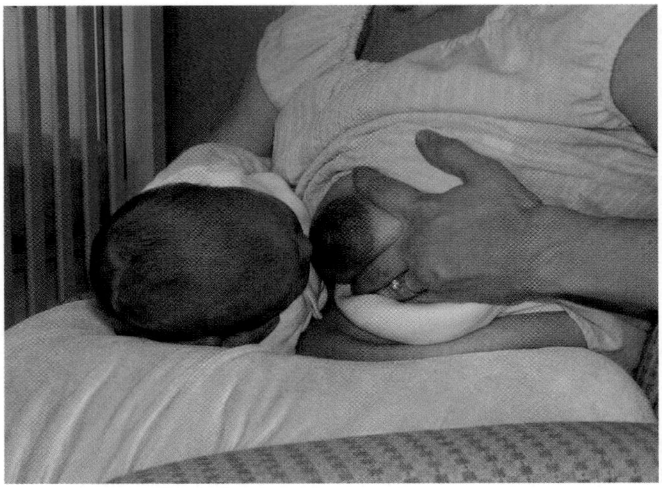

The scissor hold is often discouraged because mothers (especially mothers with small hands) have a difficult time keeping their fingers off the areola or at least 1 1/2 inches back from the base of the areola. Here, the mother is able to support her breast well without letting her fingers encroach onto the areola.

The mother should be instructed to gently support the breast and not press too deeply, which can obstruct the flow of milk through the ducts.

● **Figure 27–7** Scissor hold hand position.

Source: Courtesy of Brigette Hall, MSN, IBCLC.

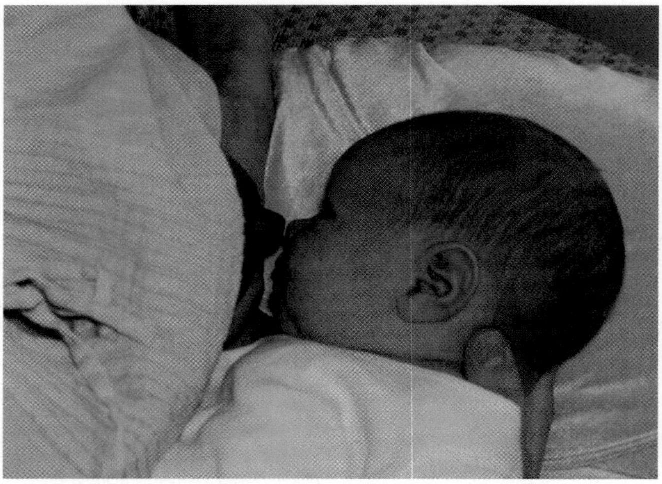

● **Figure 27–8** Nose to nipple.
Source: Courtesy of Brigette Hall, MSN, IBCLC.

Before eliciting the rooting reflex, it is important to have the baby in good alignment. When the infant opens his mouth to latch on, the goal is to achieve a deep, asymmetric latch attachment. The goal is *not* to center the nipple in the baby's mouth. The rationale for this is to optimize oral-motor function. The jaw is a hinge joint. The upper jaw is immobile; the lower jaw compresses the breast. The breast is efficiently drained if more areola is drawn into the baby's mouth from the inferior aspect of the breast and a smaller amount drawn in from the superior aspect of the areola. Aligning the infant to the mother with baby's nose facing mother's nipple permits the jaw to be in a lower position. The next step is to let the infant drop his head back (head in "sniff position"), so that the infant leads into the breast with the chin.

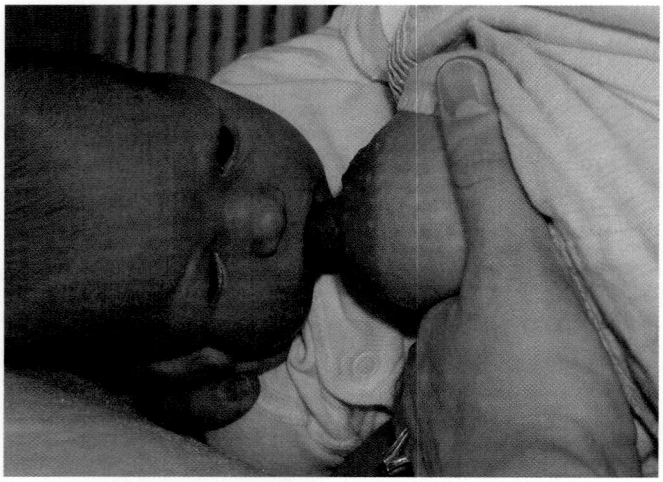

● **Figure 27–9** Initial attempt to elicit the rooting reflex.
Source: Courtesy of Brigette Hall, MSN, IBCLC.

To trigger the rooting reflex, teach the mother to use her nipple to stroke downward in a vertical motion across the middle of baby's lower lip. Initially, the infant may respond by licking or smacking. This is a normal response to the stimulus. Encourage the mother to keep stimulating the infant's lower lip until the infant finally opens his mouth widely. If the infant is not responding at all, then the infant is probably too sleepy and may need help waking up. After trying wake up techniques, the infant may be ready to try breastfeeding again.

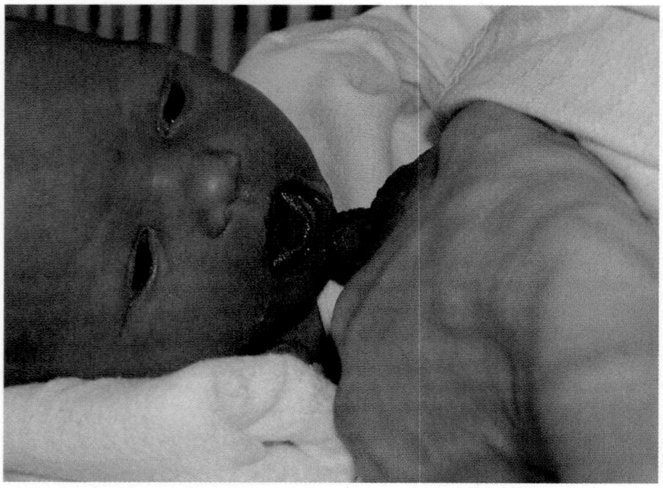

● **Figure 27–10** Continued attempt to elicit rooting reflex.
Source: Courtesy of Brigette Hall, MSN, IBCLC.

Teach the mother to be patient and wait for the infant's mouth to gape open as widely as possible. Here the infant needs to open the mouth even wider before the mother draws her baby toward the breast. The mother should be encouraged to continue stroking the infant's lip until the infant opens the mouth wider.

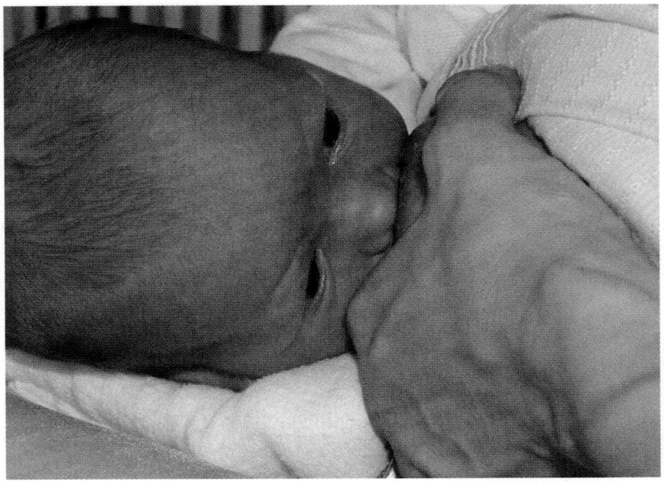

● **Figure 27–11** Baby is latched-on.

Source: Courtesy of Brigette Hall, MSN, IBCLC.

Once the baby has latched onto the breast, the mother should check that the baby is latched-on properly. The infant's chin should be embedded into the mother's breast. The infant's nose should be very close but not actually touching the breast. The nose should be centered. If the mother feels a little pinch on her areola, she can slowly release the hand supporting her breast so she can have a free hand to attempt to move her baby's jaw gently downward. To do this maneuver, the mother needs to place the thumb or forefinger of her free hand (the hand that just released the breast) on the baby's lower jaw (there is a horizontal groove to use as leverage—the groove on the baby's chin is parallel with the baby's lips). With gentle downward pressure the mother should feel relief of any persistent tenderness. This procedure opens the jaw wider and it also helps to roll out the infant's lower lip that may have been inadvertently drawn into the baby's mouth. As the baby begins to suckle, there should be no dimpling of the infant's cheeks and no smacking or clicking noises.

Nursing Practice

As you assist new mothers with breastfeeding, it is important to create a relaxed environment and approach to breastfeeding. Encourage the mother to get into a comfortable position, well supported with pillows. Remind her to bring the baby to her breast rather than leaning forward to the baby.

Nursing Practice

With a sleepy baby, unwrap the baby, encourage lots of skin-to-skin contact between the mother and baby, and have the mother rest with her baby near her breast so that the baby can feel and smell the breast. Encourage the mother to watch for feeding cues, such as hand-to-mouth activity, fluttering eyelids, vocalization (but not necessarily crying), and mouthing activities.

Breastfeeding Assessment

During the birthing unit stay, the nurse must carefully monitor the progress of the breastfeeding pair. A systematic assessment of several breastfeeding episodes provides the opportunity to teach the new mother about lactation and the breastfeeding process, provide anticipatory guidance, and evaluate the need for follow-up care after discharge. Criteria for evaluating a breastfeeding session include maternal and infant cues, latch-on, position, letdown, nipple condition, infant response, and maternal response. The literature provides various tools to guide the assessment and documentation of the breastfeeding efforts. The LATCH Scoring System is one example (Figure 27–12 ●).

Breastfeeding Efficiency

Parents are often concerned because they have no visual assurance of the amount of breast milk consumed. The mother should be taught to observe the infant for effective breastfeeding. The infant should have a rhythmic suckling pattern (the slight pause between jaw compressions on the breast permits the mouth to fill with milk before swallowing). To note if the jaw compressions are strong enough, the mother should observe or feel if there is movement at the bilateral temporomandibular joints located in front of the infant's ears.

The infant should maintain a rhythmic feeding pattern with only brief pauses (lasting only seconds, not minutes) between spurts of active feeding, with the feeding session typically lasting for 10 to 20 minutes on the first breast. The infant may feed only a few minutes on the second breast or not at all; so the mother should alternate the first breast at the next feeding. The mother should visually observe for swallowing and later, as her milk is abundant, she will hear the infant's swallows. Discourage the mother from watching the clock to determine when the infant needs to switch breast sides but rather encourage her to watch the newborn's feeding pattern to note when active feeding ceases. When the infant is satiated, she will either pull away from the breast or fall asleep. The infant will be extremely relaxed at the end of the feeding and will sleep until the next feeding is due (at least an hour). As the infant matures, the feeding intervals will lengthen.

Another indicator of breastfeeding efficiency is softening of the mother's breasts, although this is not a reliable indicator in the first few days postpartum while breast milk volume is low. Within a week, however, this is a good indicator of milk transfer.

	0	1	2
L Latch	Too sleepy or reluctant No latch achieved	Repeated attempts Hold nipple in mouth Stimulate to suck	Grasps breast Tongue down Lips flanged Rhythmic sucking
A Audible swallowing	None	A few with stimulation	Spontaneous and intermittent > 24 hours old Spontaneous and frequent < 24 hours old
T Type of nipple	Inverted	Flat	Everted (after stimulation)
C Comfort (breast/ nipple)	Engorged Cracked, bleeding, large blisters or bruises Severe discomfort	Filling Reddened/small blisters or bruises Mild/moderate discomfort	Soft Nontender
H Hold (positioning)	Full assist (staff holds infant at breast)	Minimal assist (e.g., elevate head of bed, place pillows for support) Teach one side; mother does other Staff holds and then mother takes over	No assist from staff Mother able to position and hold infant

● **Figure 27–12** LATCH Scoring System. A breastfeeding charting and documentation tool, LATCH was created to provide a systematic method for breastfeeding assessment and charting. It can be used to assist the new mother in establishing breastfeeding and define areas of needed intervention.

Source: Used with permission from AWHONN. (1994). Jensen, D., Wallace, S., & Kelsay, P. A breastfeeding charting system and documentation tool. *Journal of Obstetric, Gynecologic, and Neonatal Nursing*, *23*(1), 27–32. (Table 1 Latch Scoring Table, p. 29.) Washington, DC: Author. © 1994 by the Association of Women's Health, Obstetric and Neonatal Nurses. All rights reserved.

Nursing Practice

Babies are probably getting enough milk if:

- They are nursing at least eight times in 24 hours.
- In a quiet room, their mothers can hear them swallow while nursing.
- Their mothers' breasts appear to soften after breastfeeding.
- The number of wet diapers increases daily until the fourth or fifth day after birth, and there are at least six to eight wet diapers every 24 hours after day 5.
- Their stools are beginning to lighten in color by the third day after birth, or have changed to yellow no later than day 5.
- Offering a supplemental bottle is not a reliable indicator because most babies will take a few ounces even if they are getting enough breast milk.

The infant who feeds well will have a characteristic output. See Figure 27–13 ● for breastfeeding intake and output expectations. The infant should also have the characteristic weight loss followed by weight gain pattern discussed earlier in this chapter.

Finally, the most reliable measurement of effective breastfeeding is measuring the breast milk that actually transfers. This is done by obtaining pre- and post-breastfeeding weight checks of the infant using an accurate infant scale. The difference in pre-feed and post-feed weights is the amount of milk transferred to the infant and may be useful with assessing weight gain in late preterm infants.

Bottle-Feeding Breast Milk

There are a number of different reasons for bottle-feeding breast milk. The nurse should evaluate the indications in order to recommend the best technique for the mother and her particular need.

Hand expression. Some mothers prefer to hand express their milk rather than use a breast pump, and many find that in the immediate postpartum period hand expression of milk may be a more effective method of removing drops of colostrum than using an electric breast pump. Nurses should teach all mothers the skill of hand expressing breast milk, as it is possible the mother will find herself in a situation without a breast pump but needing to relieve herself from engorgement.

To help the mother hand express breast milk, have her follow steps 1 to 4 of the pumping instructions provided on MyNursingKit. The mother should then use the Marmet Technique of hand expression described next. It is important that the mother take care to place her hands exactly as directed. The steps are as follows:

1. The mother will position her thumb at the 12:00 position on the top edge of the areola (about 1 to 1½ inches back from the tip of her nipple) and her forefinger and middle finger pads at the 6:00 position on the bottom edge of the

(continued on page 650)

Breastfeeding Intake and Output Expectations

- Baby should breastfeed 8 to 12 times/day and appear satisfied after feeding.
- Colostrum is all that the newborn needs in the first few days of life in most cases.
- It is normal for the infant to lose up to 7% (or between 5% and 10%) of birth weight in the first few days of life.
- Baby should gain 10 grams/kg/day after the milk is abundant (about day 4 of life).
- Baby should be back to birth weight by 2 weeks of age.
- Baby's stool should change in color, consistency, and frequency during the first few days of life. The color of stools changes from tarry black to dark greenish-black, to greenish-brown, to brownish-yellow, to light greenish-yellow, to bright yellow or yellowish-orange. The consistency of stools changes from tarry-sticky to thinner consistencies to curdy or seedy and "explosive." Volume of stool increases as volume of intake increases.

Day 1 and Day 2

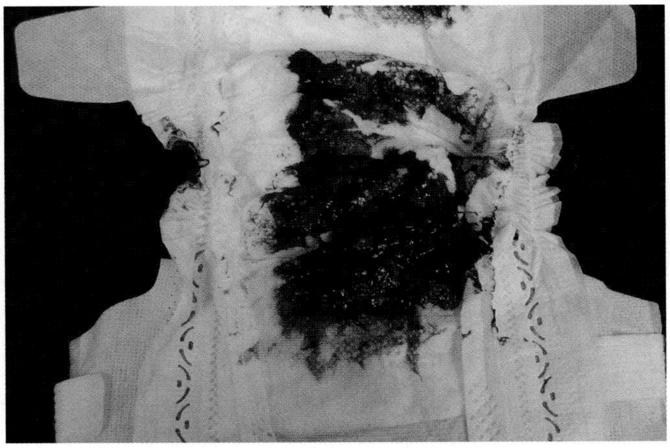

Minimum Output:

On day 1, the infant should produce at least one wet diaper and one meconium stool by 24 hours of age.

On day two, the infant should produce at least two wet diapers and 2 meconium stools. The stools may be thinning but remain dark (tarry black to greenish-brown).

Day 3 and Day 4

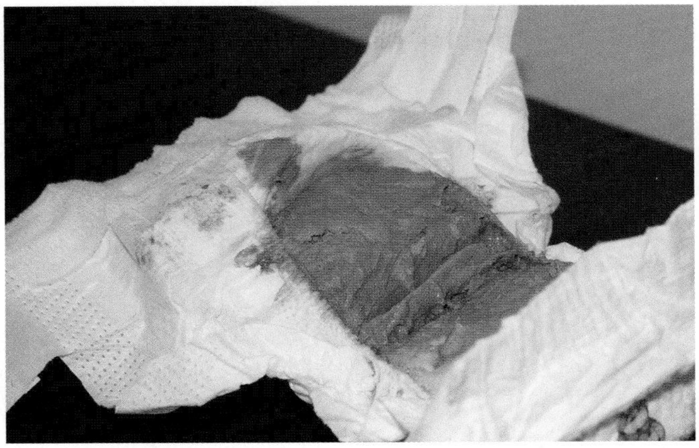

On day 3, the infant should produce at least three wet diapers and three transitional stools.

On day 4, the infant should produce at least four wet diapers and three to four transitional stools. The transitional stools are greenish-brown to greenish-yellow. Some infants will have transitioned to bright yellow milk stools by now.

Day 5

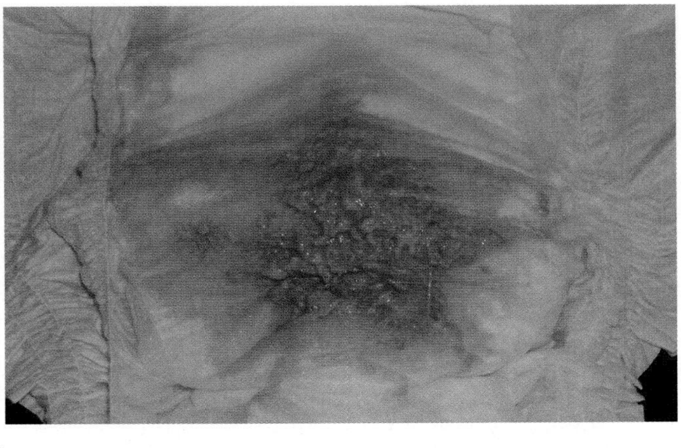

On day 5, the infant should produce at least five wet diapers and three to four yellow milk stools.

Hereafter, breastfeeding babies will always produce at least six well-saturated wet diapers per day. They typically produce at least three to four stools per day (not uncommon to have up to 10 stools per day) for the first month of life. After a month of age, breastfeeding infants may drastically reduce the number of stools per day, even skipping several days.

Because stools are an indicator of caloric intake, low stool output (especially in the first couple of weeks of life) warrants a weight check and evaluation.

● **Figure 27–13** Breastfeeding intake and output (stool characterics) expectations.

Source: Courtesy of Brigette Hall MSN, IBCLC.

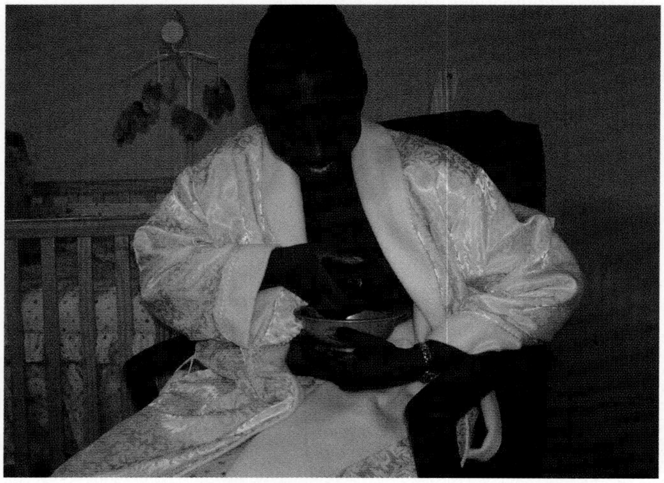

● **Figure 27–14** Hand expression.

Source: Courtesy of Brigette Hall, MSN, IBCLC.

areola (about 1 to 1½ inches from the tip of her nipple). If positioned correctly, a line between the thumb and fingers will cross the nipple (see Figure 27–14 ●).

2. Next the mother will stretch her areola back toward her chest wall without lifting her fingers off her breast.
3. Now she should roll her thumb and fingers simultaneously forward. This action compresses the ducts beneath the areola and stimulates the breast to empty both manually and by triggering the let-down reflex.
4. The mother should repeat the sequence multiple times to completely drain her breasts. She should try to maintain a steady rhythm, cycling 45 to 60 times/minute. It is also more effective if the mother repositions her fingers to other positions on the same breast (3:00 and 9:00, 1:00 and 7:00, etc.) when the milk flow slows.

The mother should take care not to traumatize her breasts or nipples. Hand expression should not be painful. Most mothers will need assistance in learning this technique initially. Reassure the mother that this skill is learned; with practice, she can become an expert at hand expression.

Breast pump. Although hand expression can be efficient, many mothers will choose to use a mechanical breast pump to express their milk. Not all breast pumps are of the same quality, even within the same category (see Table 27–2 and Figures 27–15 and 27–16 ●). Pumps generally cycle from low to high suction at a frequency similar to that of a breastfeeding infant (about 45 to 60 cycles per minute). However, differences in the quality of the pump motor or the presence or absence of controls over suction pressure mean that some pumps will generate inadequate pressure or cycle too slowly to be effective, whereas others may exert too high a suction that can cause injury. Flange size, proper fit, and comfort are other variables to consider. The nurse should refer the mother to a lactation consultant or other person knowledgeable regarding different breast pumps.

Storing expressed breast milk. There are different guidelines for storage of expressed breast milk (EBM) depending on whether the infant is a healthy full-term infant or a premature or sick infant in the hospital. The guidelines in Table 27–3 are intended as a resource for the mother of a healthy, full-term infant.

Table 27–2 Types of Breast Pumps and Indications for Use

Indication	Manual Breast Pump (Figure 27–15)	Small Battery/ Electric Breast Pump	Individual Double Electric Breast Pump	Hospital-Grade Multiuser Double Electric Breast Pump (Figure 27–16)
A missed feeding	•	•		
An evening out	•	•		
Working part-time	•	•		
Convenience—occasional use	•	•		
Working full-time			•	•
Premature/hospitalized infant				•
Low milk supply				•
Sore nipples/engorgement			•	•
Latch-on problems/infection			•	•
Drawing out flattish nipples	•	•	•	•

Modified from the *Medela Breastfeeding Information Guide Tips and Products* (2002). Table: Which Breastpump Is Best for You? Pg. 3. Medela, Inc.

• Good • Better • Best

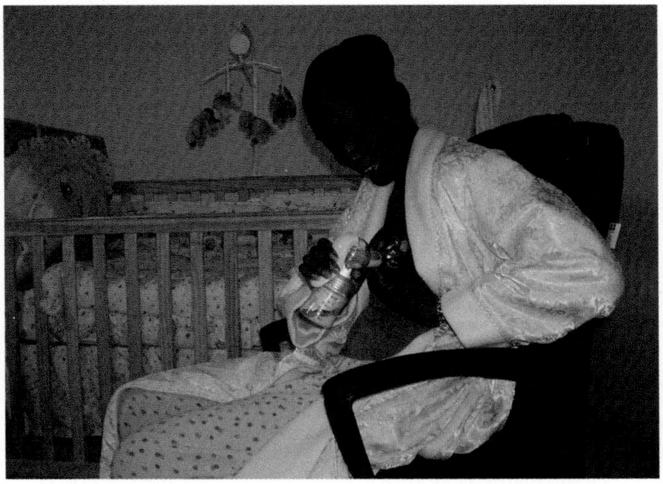

● **Figure 27–15** Manual breast pump.
Source: Courtesy of Brigette Hall, MSN, IBCLC.

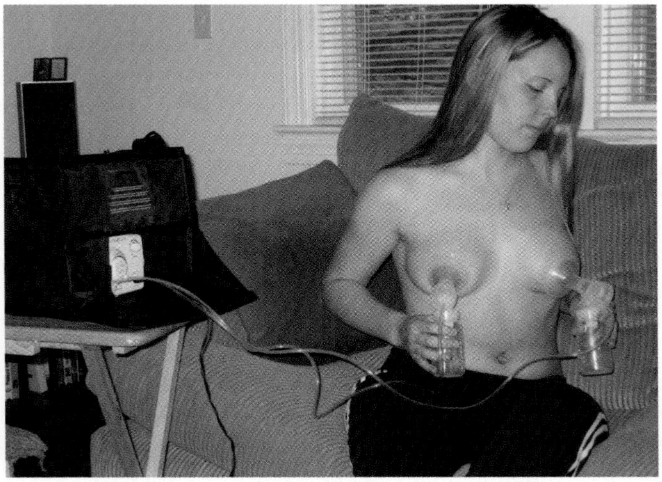

● **Figure 27–16** New mom using double electric breast pump at home.

Supplementary Formula Feeding

Supplementary formula feedings for the breastfeeding infant after birth are not recommended. Routine supplementation has been strongly implicated in early breastfeeding termination (AWHONN, 2007). Routine supplements are not only unnecessary, they can also contribute to maternal and infant health problems, including delayed early maternal milk production, maternal engorgement after her milk production has increased, infant milk-protein intolerance, and difficulties with learning to breastfeed.

"Nipple confusion" or "nipple preference" can occur in some babies causing them to develop an incorrect sucking technique, or to simply refuse to breastfeed again. This potential problem occurs because the techniques for breastfeeding and formula feeding are different. In breastfeeding, the infant has to open his mouth very wide in order to latch on. To transfer milk she has to extend her tongue forward, cupping the nipple and drawing it from back to front in a milking motion. With bottle-feeding, the infant keeps the tongue retracted and uses the tip of the tongue to block the flow of milk, which otherwise drips rapidly. Some babies can switch back and forth between breast and bottle without obvious difficulty, but for other infants, it is a problem. To reduce this possibility, lactation experts recommend introducing the

Table 27–3 Storage Guidelines for Breast Milk and Formula

Milk	Environment	Time Until Discard
Breast milk or Formula, opened/reconstituted	Being fed	Finish feed within 1 hour
Breast milk or Formula, opened/reconstituted	Environment/79 degrees	1 hour
Breast milk or Formula, opened/reconstituted	Room temperature	4 hours
Breast milk or Formula, opened/reconstituted	Cooler pack/59 degrees	24 hours
Thawed breast milk	Refrigerator	24 hours
Formula, opened/reconstituted	Refrigerator	24 to 48 hours (see label)
Fresh breast milk	Refrigerator	8 days
Formula powder, opened can	Room temperature	1 month
Fresh breast milk	Freezer	3 months
Formula/powder in sealed container	Avoid excessive heat	Printed expiration date
Thawed breast milk	Freezer	Do not refreeze
Formula	Freezer	Do not freeze

Sources: Adapted from Human Milk Banking Association of North America (HMBANA). (2005). *Best practice for expressing, storing and handling human milk in hospitals, homes and child care settings.* Raleigh, NC: Author; Mead-Johnson Nutritionals. (2007). *Pediatric products handbook.* New York: Bristol-Myers Squibb Company and Ross Products Division. (2007). *Pediatric nutritionals product guide.* Columbus, OH: Abbott Laboratories. http://www.ROSS.com

bottle only after the infant is able to latch on and breastfeeding is well established, usually after 1 month of age (AWHONN, 2007).

At times there are valid medical indications for supplementation of the breastfeeding infant. These include delayed lactogenesis; unavailability of the mother because of severe illness or separation; primary lactation failure; hypoglycemia; significant dehydration; weight loss of 8% to 10% with exclusive breastfeeding; delayed passage of stool (presence of meconium on day 5); hyperbilirubinemia related to poor intake, prematurity, or low birth weight; and refusal of or ineffective breastfeeding.

For those times when supplementation is indicated, the first choice is to use the mother's own milk (fresh, previously expressed, or frozen/thawed). If maternal breast milk is not available, pasteurized donor milk is the next choice, and then formula. The method of supplementation chosen is based on the particular situation and parental preference (see Chapter 34∞). Breastfed babies transition best going from breast to bottle and back to breast again when using a bottle nipple that has a relatively wide base (to help maintain a wide open latch) and a medium to long nipple length.

FORMULA FEEDING

With more attention placed on promoting and assisting breastfeeding mothers, the teaching needs of the mother who is formula-feeding may inadvertently get overlooked. Nurses may assume that families can simply follow the formula preparation instructions on the side of the formula containers. However, research shows that these parents also need teaching, counseling, and support. In a systematic review of five studies from developed countries looking at how parents prepare formula, all the studies revealed "errors in reconstitution with a tendency to over-concentrate feeds, although under-concentrating also occurred" (Renfrew, Ansell, & Macleod, 2003). Parents need to learn about the feeding pattern for a formula-feeding infant, the intake and output expectations, the recommended type of formula for their infant, how to prepare and store formula, what equipment they will need, feeding technique, and safety precautions. (See Table 27–1.)

FORMULA-FEEDING TECHNIQUE

Commercial formulas are available in three forms: powder, concentrate, and ready-to-feed. There are situations in which one formula may be better to use than another, but in general, convenience and cost usually influence the parents' decision.

- *Powdered formula* is the least expensive type of formula. This formula can be made up one bottle at a time, or multiple bottles can be prepared, but they must be used within 24 to 48 hours. Standard powdered formula is made by adding one level scoop of powdered formula to 60 mL of water (the powder is added to the water). Powdered formulas are not sterile. Powdered formula is made from pasteurized liquid that is then freeze-spray dried into a powder; contamination with microorganisms can occur in the final stages of production. Preparation of any infant formula, but especially powdered formulas, requires careful handling to avoid contamination with microorganisms.
- *Formula concentrate* is more expensive than powder but is not as expensive as ready-to-feed formula. Formula concentrate is commercially sterile. This formula must be diluted with an equal part of water. By adding boiled water that has been cooled, sterility can be maintained.
- *Ready-to-feed* formula is the easiest to use because it does not require any mixing; however, this convenience comes at a cost—it is the most expensive formula. It is indicated for use when adequate water is not available, when the infant is immunocompromised and requires commercially sterile (pasteurized) formula, when an inexperienced babysitter will be feeding the infant, and for convenience.

Whatever the type of formula chosen, the nurse should underscore the importance of proper preparation and prompt refrigeration. Parents will need to be briefed on safety precautions during formula preparation. A primary concern is proper mixing to reconstitute formula. Parents need clear instructions to avoid unintentional harm to their infant. Parents should be instructed to follow the directions on the formula can label precisely as written. They should know that adding too much water during preparation dilutes the nutrients and caloric density. This contributes to undernourishment, insufficient weight gain, and possibly water intoxication, which can cause hyponatremia and seizures. Not adding enough water concentrates nutrients and calories and can tax an infant's immature kidneys and digestive system as well as cause dehydration (Morin, 2005). See Table 27–3 for storage guidelines for formula.

Some recommended sanitary precautions and additional safety precautions are listed here:

- Check the expiration date on the formula container.
- Ensure good handwashing before preparing formula; never dip into the can without clean hands.
- Clean bottles, nipples, rings, disks, and bottle caps.
  a. Washing in a dishwasher when available (small items and heat-sensitive items on top rack secured in a basket), or
  b. Boiling briefly (1 to 2 minutes) in a pot of water, or
  c. Cleaning using a microwave sterilization kit, or
  d. Cleaning using very warm soapy water and a nipple and bottle brush.
- Wash the top of the formula container before piercing the lid.
- Shake the liquid formulas well before pouring off the desired amount.
- Shake prepared milk that has been sitting in the refrigerator before feeding.
- Allow tap water to run for 1 minute before obtaining water to use for mixing—this helps clear any lead standing in the pipes. Also, always use cold tap water, as warm water tends to contain higher levels of lead as well. Water should be warmed (or cooled after boiling) before being added to the formula.

- Use only the scoop supplied in the can of formula when formula preparation instructions call for a "scoop" of powdered formula.
  a. A scoop should not be "packed" and should be leveled off (e.g., with the back of a knife).
- Do not add anything else to the bottle, except under direction of the baby's healthcare provider.
- Milk in a bottle should be warmed by placing the bottle in a bowl of warm tap water. Do not fill the bowl with water higher than the rim of the bottle. (Babies can take cold formula but most young infants will prefer it warm.)
- Do not freeze formula.
- Allow freshly prepared (unused) formula to sit out at room temperature for no longer than 2 hours; use an insulated pack to transport formula. Milk left over in the bottle after a feeding should be discarded.
- In warm weather, transport reconstituted or formula concentrate from an open can in an insulated pack with frozen gel packs.
- Travel with water and formula separated—carry premeasured water bottles and bottles with premeasured amounts of powdered formula, or carry premeasured commercially prepared formula packets, or have the can of formula available.
- Inspect and replace bottle nipples as soon as they show wear—worn nipples can break apart and can become a choking hazard.
- Holding the infant during feeding (even when the infant can hold the bottle for himself) promotes bonding and prevents supine feedings.
- Do not allow the infant to formula-feed in a supine position because this increases the risk of otitis media and dental caries in the older infant.
- Never prop a bottle—this is a choking hazard.
- Allow infants to take what they want AND to stop when they want. Overfeeding can lead to obesity.

Parents also need guidance about what kind of water to use to reconstitute formula (see Table 27–4 to review types of water sources) and should discuss with their infant's healthcare provider whether to boil the water before use. If boiling is used, parents need to be instructed to heat the water until it reaches a rolling boil, continue to let the water boil for 1 to 2 minutes, and, most importantly, to allow the water to cool before using it to reconstitute the formula. Parents should also be instructed not to let the water boil down to a low level in the pan because this can cause minerals in the water to become concentrated.

Use of distilled bottle water and filtered tap water raises concerns with regard to fluoride. The American Academy of Pediatrics recommends that no fluoride supplements be given to an infant before 6 months of age, but does recommend supplementary fluoride for infants and children ages 6 months to 3 years of age if the water source contains less than 0.3 ppm (AAP & ACOG, 2007). Parents should be encouraged to read the labels on bottled water to see if fluoride has been added and to determine if the water source is suitable for their infant depending on his or her age (Table 27–4).

Parents often have questions about the kind of bottles and nipples to purchase. Plastic, glass, or disposable bottle bags may all be used based on preference. Mothers who bottle-feed expressed breast milk may want to avoid the use of bottle liners/bottle bags, especially if they have a fragile infant. Research shows that up to 60% of secretory immunoglobulin A (SIgA) found in breast milk binds to the polyethylene material used in these and is therefore lost to the infant (Lawrence & Lawrence, 2005). There are no human antibodies in formula so this is not a concern for bottle-feeding formula.

Table 27–4 Water Sources

Type	Description
Distilled water	Minerals and most other impurities have been removed. It will not contain any flouride. An acceptable water source for reconstituting formula.
Filtered tap water	Some minerals and impurities removed during filtration, including fluoride. This is an acceptable water source for reconstituting formula.
Natural mineral water	Comes from protected ground water and by law cannot be treated. Naturally contains high levels of minerals and sodium and so is not suitable for infants or for reconstituting formula.
Spring water	Comes from a single nonpolluted groundwater source, but unlike natural mineral water, it can be further treated. Because there is no regulation requiring the mineral content to be printed on the bottle label, it is best to avoid this water source for reconstituting formula.
Tap water	Water from the municipal water supply, and regulated by drinking water regulations. It is treated and considered safe for use in reconstituting formula.
Well water	Needs to be tested before use. Higher risk of nitrate poisoning. Untested water is not recommended for use in reconstituting formula.

There are many different bottle nipples on the market. Parents will want to consider a slow-flow nipple for all newborns and for older breastfeeding babies learning to formula-feed—over time the infant will graduate to medium-flow and high-flow nipples. Another variable to consider is nipple construction. Nipples are generally made from either rubber or silicone. Families with a sensitivity to latex are advised to use silicone nipples. Silicone nipples also have less of an odor, which may be an issue for some infants who are breastfed.

Many newly designed bottles are marketed to lessen air intake while an infant feeds. There is not a particular bottle design that is best for all babies. Different families find different bottles and nipple assembly products better than others. A key point to emphasize to the families is feeding technique. Parents should try to avoid situations in which an infant is crying for a prolonged time. Crying results in increased ingestion of air even before the infant has started feeding. Infants who are very hungry also gulp more air. For these situations, instruct the parents to burp their infant frequently to prevent the infant from having a large emesis (see Figure 27–17 ●). The parent may even want to attempt to pat the baby's back briefly before starting the feeding to calm the infant and possibly burp as well. Another tip to avoid excessive ingestion of air is to have the parent hold his or her infant cradled in the arms while formula-feeding and have the parent tilt the baby's bottle at a 45-degree angle (at least) in order for fluid to cover the nipple. This prevents the infant from sucking in air and swallowing it. See Figure 27–18 ● to view this technique.

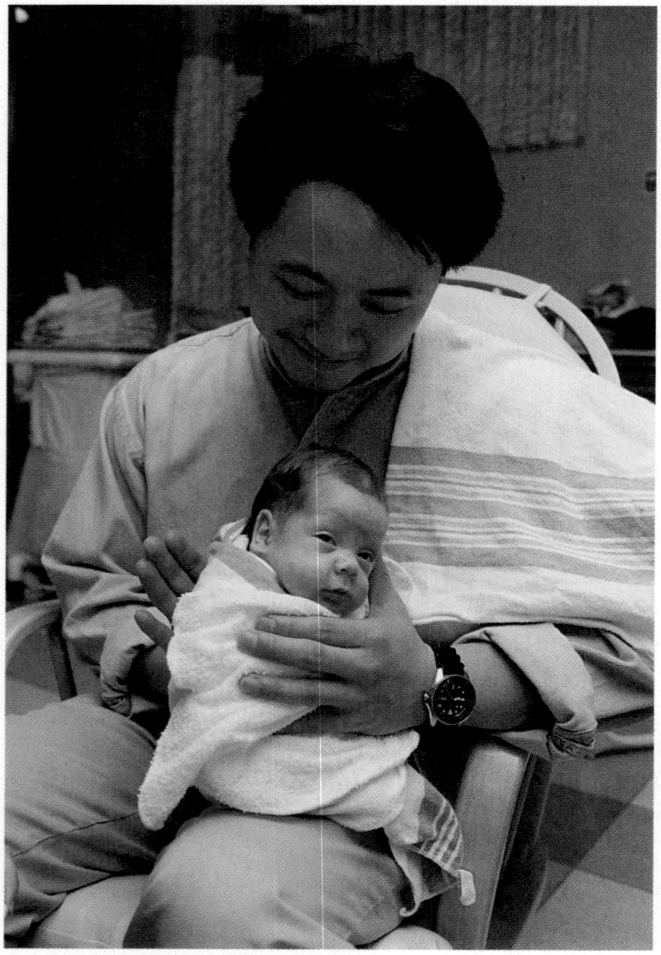

● **Figure 27–17** Burping time.

Source: Stella Johnson (www.stellajohnson.com)

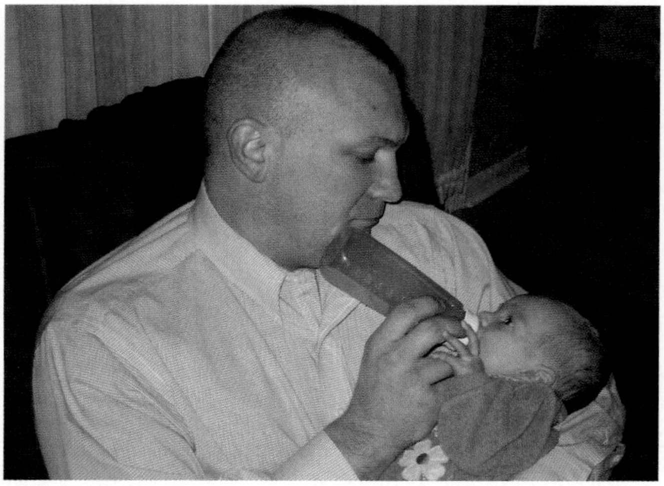

● **Figure 27–18** Dad feeding his baby a bottle.

To know if an infant is formula-feeding well, the nurse needs to observe a formula-feeding session. Parents should be informed that if the infant is sucking effectively, the parents should observe bubbles rising in the fluid (except if they are using plastic-lined bottles, which contract as they empty). If the parent unintentionally placed the bottle nipple under the infant's tongue, preventing him from sucking, the infant may make sucking efforts but will not receive any fluid and no bubbles will be visualized. Infants who persistently leak milk from the side of the mouth may be getting fluid too quickly. The nurse could suggest using a slower flowing nipple. If symptoms persist, the infant should have an oral evaluation. The infant could have a short lingual frenulum (tongue-tie) and not be able to properly cup his tongue under the nipple and channel fluid to the back of his throat, or she may have an oral-motor dysfunction and need speech therapy or occupational therapy evaluation. Evidence suggests that pacifier use may have a protective effect against SIDS. At 1 month of age, parents should consider offering a pacifier at nap and bedtime (Janke, 2008). To decrease risk of infection, pacifiers should be cleaned often and replaced regularly.

Nursing Practice

Parents should be instructed not to put honey or corn syrup on their infant's pacifier to encourage an infant to accept it. Honey and possibly corn syrup may be contaminated with *Clostridium botulinum*, a bacteria that causes infantile botulism. This is not a risk for the older child. Botulism is rare, but when it occurs it causes serious illness.

COMMUNITY-BASED NURSING CARE

PROMOTION OF SUCCESSFUL INFANT BREASTFEEDING

To promote a supportive hospital environment for breastfeeding, the Baby-Friendly Hospital Initiative recognizes hospitals and birthing centers that offer optimal lactation services and comply with the 10 steps outlined in Table 27–5 (WHO/UNICEF, 1994). Baby-Friendly status is not easy to achieve. One obstacle to achieving Baby-Friendly status, among many, is having to agree not to accept free or low-cost formula. Currently there are approximately 82 hospitals in the United States with Baby-Friendly designation as of July 2009 according to an update on the Baby-Friendly Hospital Initiative USA website (BFHI USA, 2009).

Childbirth and the beginning of motherhood are critical times in a woman's life, so physical, psychologic, and social supports are of paramount importance. The nurse needs to explore the family's social support base. The father or other partner is the most important support person for her, although the baby can also provide some support in the form of positive feedback.

Many families will have adequate income, a good knowledge base, and good coping skills to handle problems. Some families will have support from a large extended family group, friends, church, or other organization. However, that is not the case for everyone; as evidenced by the frequent discontinuing of breastfeeding in the early postpartum weeks, there is a need for assistance and follow-up in this area. Mothers, mothers-in-law, sisters, and other females who could mentor and care for the new mother may live at a distance or work full-time. When inadequate support is identified, it may be beneficial to request a referral for the family to have an outpatient case manager involved to make sure the mother knows how to access the community resources (mother-to-mother support groups), provide consistent, timely information and support, and to attend to the new mother's special needs.

Breastfeeding mothers who work outside the home and are supported in their decision tend to breastfeed their infants for longer periods than mothers who work but do not receive support. A baby-friendly workplace needs to be seen as another item in a benefit package offered by a company. Families and nurses who believe in breastfeeding need to be part of the solution to breastfeeding and workplace issues by educating employers in their communities (Riordan & Wambach, 2010).

With a national nursing shortage and the trend toward earlier discharge from the birthing center, there is limited time for inpatient education. Teaching moments, when they occur, may not be optimal because of the distraction of visitors and the mother's being sleep deprived, uncomfortable, or feeling the effects of an analgesic. It is important that parents receive verbal and written instructions and community resource information to which they can later refer. (See also Chapter 31 for a complete discussion of self-care measures the nurse can suggest to a woman with a breastfeeding problem after discharge from the birthing center.)

When breastfeeding mothers leave the birthing center, the center staff need to provide a list of lactation resources available in the community. If no resource handout is available, the mother should be given the phone number to **La Leche League International** or the International Lactation Consultant Association (see MediaLink), which can provide assistance with finding the closest lactation support. Many hospitals around the country have a lactation program and may provide lactation services for a fee to anyone seeking services. Some cities have outpatient lactation centers that provide comprehensive lactation services including consultation services, breastfeeding classes, and an infant scale for assessing baby's weight, as well as telephone-based lactation advice. The Women Infant Children (WIC) Supplemental Nutrition Program may have a lactation consultant on staff or may have a contract with a lactation consultant in private practice in the community. Some military facilities provide lactation services to their service members and dependents. The local library is also an excellent resource, and there are many books available commercially. Finally, the Internet can be a tremendous resource, although the quality of information cannot always be ensured. It is very helpful to have a handout listing some good sites that have been reviewed for accuracy.

Table 27–5 Baby-Friendly Requirements

Baby-Friendly 10 Steps to Successful Breastfeeding
■ Have a written breastfeeding policy that is routinely communicated to all healthcare staff.
■ Train all healthcare staff in skills necessary to implement this policy.
■ Inform all pregnant women about the benefits and management of breastfeeding.
■ Help mothers initiate breastfeeding within one hour of birth.
■ Show mothers how to breastfeed and maintain lactation, even if they should be separated from their infants.
■ Give newborn infants no food or drink other than breast milk, unless medically indicated.
■ Practice rooming in—that is, allow mothers and infants to remain together 24 hours a day.
■ Encourage breastfeeding on demand.
■ Give no artificial teats or pacifiers (also called dummies or soothers) to breastfeeding infants.
■ Foster the establishment of breastfeeding support groups and refer mothers to them on discharge from the hospital or clinic.

Source: World Health Organization/United Nations Children's Emergency Fund (WHO/UNICEF). (1994). *U.S. committee for UNICEF interim program in the United States to promote the Baby-Friendly ten steps to successful breastfeeding.* Washington, DC: Government Printing Office.

WIC

Both breastfeeding and formula-feeding mothers who may be eligible for WIC should be encouraged to enroll themselves and their infants in the WIC nutrition program. WIC provides a specific number of cans of powdered formula to eligible mothers free of charge. The number of cans the mother receives is based on the current government contract with one of the two major formula companies (Mead-Johnson, the maker of Enfamil®; or Ross, the maker of Similac®) and whether a mother is partially breastfeeding or entirely formula-feeding. The breastfeeding mother can also receive additional food vouchers for herself. The amount of formula the mother receives *does not* increase as the infant grows and will need to purchase additional formula. Mothers with an extremely low income who lack family support may need the numbers for emergency food assistance programs in the area. Low-income mothers also need to be reminded to enroll their infant in the Food Stamp Program so they can receive additional food vouchers each month.

NUTRITIONAL ASSESSMENT

A nutritional assessment is an integral part of a thorough health appraisal and is commonly performed by the infant's primary care provider, a nurse, or a lactation consultant.

The nutritional assessment includes the infant nutritional history obtained from the parents, growth chart percentiles, and physical exam.

Parents will be asked to present a feeding diary for the provider to review, or the parents will need to recall the infant's feeding pattern over the last 24 to 48 hours. The healthcare professional is interested in the infant's behavior pattern, especially during and immediately after feeding. If the infant is breastfeeding, a relevant maternal history is needed to determine if the mother is having breastfeeding difficulties and to help determine the root cause of the problem. If the infant is formula-feeding, the healthcare professional will first want to investigate the family's formula-feeding practices (including formula preparation technique). While gathering this data, the healthcare professional should be sensitive to the family's cultural practices. However, if a cultural practice has harmful effects, then the provider needs to tactfully educate the family to that fact.

The provider should plot the infant's measurements for length, head circumference, and weight on a growth chart denoting the infant's individual percentile measurement compared with the general population. Because there are variations among infants at the same age, it is important to monitor the infant's individual growth pattern over time. A drop of 20 percent or more on the growth curve is cause for concern and increase assessment of feeding history and assessment parameters. (See "Nutritional Assessment" in Chapter 34 for more in-depth discussion of infant nutrition.)

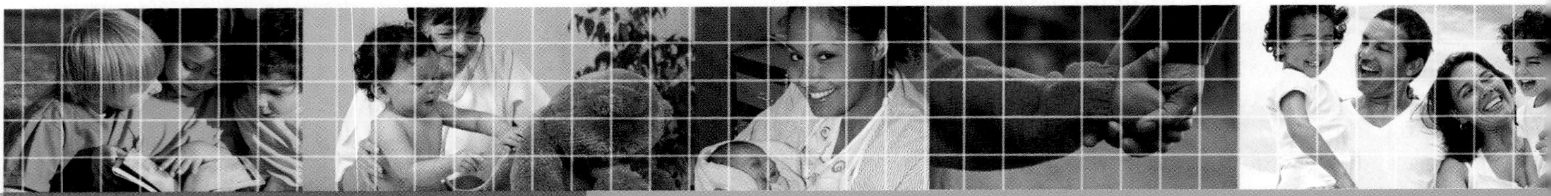

CRITICAL CONCEPT REVIEW

LEARNING OUTCOMES	CONCEPTS
27.1 Compare the nutritional value and composition of breast milk and formula preparations in relation to the nutritional needs of the newborn.	1. Composition of breast milk: ■ 10% solids consisting of carbohydrates, proteins, and fats ■ 90% is water 2. Breast milk has immunologic and nutritional (biodegradable) properties that make it the optimal food for first year of life. 3. Most common cow's-milk protein–based formulas attempt to duplicate the same concentration of carbohydrates, proteins, and fats as 20 kcal/oz breast milk.
27.2 Explain the advantages and disadvantages of breastfeeding and formula feeding in determining nursing care of both mother/family and newborn.	1. Advantages of breastfeeding: ■ Provides immunologic protection. ■ Infant digests and absorbs components of breast milk easier. ■ Provides most vitamins to infant if mother's diet is adequate. ■ Strengthens the mother-infant attachment. ■ No additional cost. ■ Breast milk requires no preparation. 2. Disadvantages of breastfeeding: ■ Many medications pass through to breast milk. ■ Father is unable to participate equally in actual feeding of infant. ■ Mother may have difficulty being separated from infant. 3. Advantages of bottle feeding: ■ Provides good nutrition to infant. ■ Father can participate in infant feeding activities. 4. Disadvantages of bottle feeding: ■ May need to try different formulas before finding one that is well-tolerated by the infant. ■ Formula must be purchased and prepared. ■ Proper preparation is necessary for nutritional adequacy.

LEARNING OUTCOMES / CONCEPTS

Learning Outcomes	Concepts
27.3 Develop guidelines for helping both breast- and formula-feeding mothers to feed their newborns successfully in hospital and community-based settings.	1. The breastfeeding mother needs to know: ■ How breast milk is produced. ■ How to correctly position and facilitate "latching on" by the infant for feeding. ■ The procedure for feeding the infant. ■ How to express, pump, and store breast milk. ■ How and when to supplement with formula. ■ How to care for the breasts. ■ Medications that pass through breast milk. ■ Support groups for breastfeeding. 2. The bottle-feeding mother needs to know: ■ Types of formula available and how to prepare each type. ■ The procedure for feeding the infant. ■ How to correctly position the infant for bottle-feeding. ■ How to safely store the formula. ■ How to safely care for bottles and nipples.
27.4 Describe the influence of cultural values on infant care, especially feeding practices in the nursing care of the newborn, mother, and family.	Nurses must: 1. Describe how cultural values influence infant feeding practice. 2. Be sensitive to ethnic backgrounds of minority populations. 3. Understand that the dominant culture in any society defines normal maternal infant feeding interactions.
27.5 Explain the nutritional needs and normal growth patterns of infants and educate parents on these topics.	Parents need to know: 1. Amount of formula to feed infant at each feeding and how often to feed infant. 2. Number of times per day the breastfed infant should be put to the breast. 3. The expected weight gain of both formula and breastfed infants.

CRITICAL THINKING IN ACTION

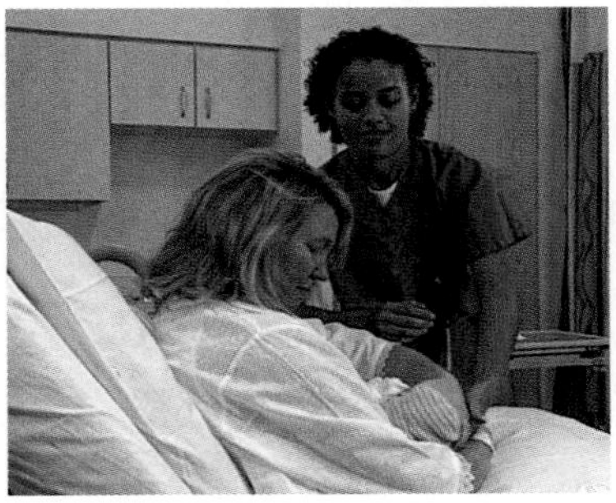

Patty Kline, age 28, G1, now P1, delivers a 7.3 pound baby girl by spontaneous vaginal birth over a median episiotomy. The newborn's Apgar scores are 8 and 9 at 1 and 5 minutes. The infant is suctioned in the nose and mouth and given free-flow oxygen on the mother's abdomen. Patty received an epidural during her labor and birth. Patty initiated breastfeeding within the first hour after the birth, but at that time the newborn did not latch on. The infant was held to the mother's breast, rooted, and licked the nipple. You are the nurse caring for the infant at 2 hours of age. The admission assessment is significant for asymmetric head with a 3-cm caput succedaneum. The infant's temperature is stable. You bring the infant to the mother's room to assist her with breastfeeding.

1. Describe clues that indicate the infant is ready to breastfeed with the mother.
2. How would you explain how to position the infant at the breast?
3. Explain what to observe for the infant's proper latch-on.
4. Explain the basics of milk production.
5. Explore helpful measures the mother can attempt in support of breastfeeding.

See MyNursingKit for possible responses.

REFERENCES

Academy of Breastfeeding Medicine (ABM). (2004). Protocol #9: Use of galactogogues initiating or augmenting maternal milk supply. *ABM News and Views, 10*(3), 20–22. Retrieved July 20, 2009, from http://www.bfmed.org/

American Academy of Pediatrics (AAP), Committee on Drugs. (2001). Transfer of drugs and other chemicals into human milk. *Pediatrics, 108*(3), 776–789. Retrieved July 20, 2009, from http://www.aap.org/healthtopics/breastfeeding.cfm

American Academy of Pediatrics (AAP), Committee on Fetus and Newborn & American College of Obstetricians and Gynecologists (ACOG), Committee on Obstetrics. (2007). *Guidelines for perinatal care* (6th ed.). Evanston, IL: Author.

American Academy of Pediatrics (AAP), Media Alert. (1998, April 20). *AAP addresses scheduled feedings vs. demand feedings.* Retrieved July 20, 2009, from http://www.ezzo.info/Aney/aaspmediaalert.pdf

American Academy of Pediatrics (AAP), Section on Breastfeeding. (2005). Policy statement: Breastfeeding and the use of human milk. *Pediatrics, 115*(2), 496–506. Retrieved July 20, 2009, from http://www.aappolicy.aappublications.org

Aney, M. (1998). Commentary: 'Babywise' advice linked to dehydration, failure to thrive. *AAP News, 14*(4), 21. Retrieved July 20, 2009, from http://aapnews.aappublications.org/contentvol14/issue4/#COMMENTARY

Association of Women's Health, Obstetric and Neonatal Nurses (AWHONN). (2007) *Breastfeeding support: Prenatal care through the first year. Evidence-based clinical practice guideline* (2nd ed., pp. 1–89). Washington, DC: AWHONN.

Baby-Friendly Hospital Initiative USA (BFHI USA). (2009). *Implementing the UNICEF/WHO baby-friendly hospital initiative in the U.S.* Retrieved July 20, 2009, from http://www.babyfriendlyusa.org/eng/03.html

Blackburn, S. T. (2007). *Maternal, fetal, & neonatal physiology: A clinical perspective* (3rd ed.). St. Louis: Saunders.

Briggs, G. G., Freeman, R. K., & Yaffe, S. J. (2008). *Drugs in pregnancy and lactation: A reference guide to fetal and neonatal risk* (8th ed.). Baltimore: Lippincott Williams & Wilkins.

Callister, L. C. (2008). Integrating cultural beliefs and practices when caring for childbearing women and families. In K. R. Simpson & P. A. Creehan, *Perinatal nursing* (3rd ed., pp. 29–57). Philadelphia: Lippincott Williams & Wilkins.

Chezem, J., Friesen, C., & Boettcher, J. (2003). Breastfeeding knowledge, breastfeeding confidence, and infant feeding plans: Effects on actual feeding practices. *Journal of Obstetric, Gynecologic, & Neonatal Nursing, 32*(1), 40–47.

Cloherty, J. P., Eichenwald, E. C., & Stark, A. R. (2008). *Manual of neonatal care* (6th ed.). Philadelphia: Lippincott Williams & Wilkins.

D'Avanzo, C. E., & Geissler, E. M. (2008). *Pocket guide to cultural assessment* (4th ed.). St. Louis: Mosby.

Galanti, G. A. (2004). *Caring for patients from different cultures* (3rd ed.). Philadelphia: University of Pennsylvania Press.

Greer, F. R., Sicherer, S. H., Burks, W., & Committee on Nutrition and Section on Allergy and Immunology. (2008). Effects of early nutritional interventions on the development of atropic disease in infants and children: The role of maternal dietary restriction, breastfeeding, timing of introduction of complementary foods, and hydrolyzed formulas. *Pediatrics, 121*(1), 183–191.

Gregory, K. (2005). Update on nutrition for preterm and full-term infants. *Journal of Obstetric, Gynecologic, & Neonatal Nursing, 34*(1), 98–108.

Hale, T. W. (2008). *Medications and mothers' milk.* (13th ed.). Amarillo, TX: Pharmasoft.

Hedayat, K. M. (2001). Issues in Islamic biomedical ethics: A primer for the pediatrician. *Pediatrics, 108*(4), 965–991.

Hill, P. D., Wilhelm, P. A., Aldag, J. C., & Chatterton, R. T. (2004). Breast augmentation & lactation outcome: A case report. *American Journal of Maternal Child Nursing, 29*(4), 238–242.

Human Milk Banking Association of North America (HMBANA). (2005). *Best practice for expressing, storing and handling human milk in hospitals, homes and child care settings.* Raleigh, NC: Author.

Janke, J. (2008). Newborn nutrition. In K. R. Simpson & P. A, Creehan, *Perinatal nursing.* (3rd ed., pp. 582–611). Philadelphia: Lippincott Williams & Wilkins.

Katz, N., Levin, M. B., Cotton, J. M., Patrick-Miller, T. J., Tesoro, L. J., & Rose, H. M. (2007). *The pediatric group brochure on formula feeding: Formula feeding information.* Retrieved July 20, 2009, from http://www.pedgroup.com/frmlabrc.htm

Klaus, M. (1998). Mother and infant: Early emotional ties. *Pediatrics, 102*(5), 1244–1246.

Lawrence, R. A., & Lawrence, R. M. (2005). *Breastfeeding: A guide for the medical profession* (6th ed.). Philadelphia: Mosby.

Lipson, J. G., & Dibble, S. L. (2008). *Culture & Clinical Care* (7th ed.). San Franciso: The Regents, University of California.

McCarter-Spaulding, D., & Gore, R. (2009). Brestfeeding self-efficacy in women of African descent. *JOGNN, 38(2),* 230–243.

McDowell, M. M., Wang, C. Y., Kennedy-Stephenson, J. (2008). Breastfeeding in the United States: findings from the National Heaalth and Nutrition Examination Surveys 1999–2006. *NCHS Data Brief,* No. 5, April 2008.

Mead-Johnson Nutritionals. (2007). *Pediatric products handbook.* New York: Bristol-Myers Squibb Company.

Mohrbacker, N., & Stock, J. (2003). *La Leche League International: The breastfeeding answer book* (3rd ed.). Schaumburg, IL: La Leche League International.

Moore, E. R., Anderson, G. C., & Bergman, N. (2007). Early skin-to-skin contact for mothers and their healthy newborn infants. [Cochrane Review]. In *Cochrane Database of Systemic Reviews*, 2007. Retrieved July 20, 2009, from The Cochrane Library, Wiley Interscience.

Morin, K. (2005). Information parents need about preparing formula. *The American Journal of Maternal/Child Nursing, 30*(5), 334.

Mulford, C. (1992). The mother-baby assessment (MBA): An "Apgar score" for breastfeeding. *Journal of Human Lactation, 8*(2), 79–82.

Ott, B. B., Al-Khadhuri, J., & Al-Junaibi, S. (2003). Preventing ethical dilemmas: Understanding Islamic health care practices. *Pediatric Nursing, 29*(3), 227–230.

Renfrew, M. J., Ansell, P. L., & Macleod, K. L. (2003). Formula feed preparation: Helping reduce risks; a systematic review. *Archives of Diseases of Children, 88*, 855–858.

Riordan, J., & Wambach, K. (2010). *Breastfeeding and human lactation* (4th ed.). Boston: Jones & Bartlett.

Rolfes, S. R., Pinna, K., & Whitney, E. (2006). *Understanding normal and clinical nutrition* (7th ed.). Belmont, CA: Thomson Wadsworth, a part of The Thomson Corporation. experience. *MCN. American Journal of Maternal Child Nursing, 29*(4), 222–228.

Romano, A. M., & Lothian, J. A. (2008). Promoting, protecting, and supporting normal birth: A look at the evidence. *Journal of Obstetric, Gynecologic & Neonatal Nursing, 37*(1), 94–105.

Ross Products Division. (2007). *Pediatric nutritionals product guide.* Columbus, OH: Abbott Laboratories.

Sears, W. (2009). *A word about bottle-feeding.* Retrieved July 20, 2009, from http://www.askdrsears.com/html/0/T000100.asp#T031010

Skidmore-Roth, L. (2006). *Mosby's handbook of herbs and natural supplements.* St. Louis: Mosby.

Vonlanthen, M. (1998). Lactose intolerance, diarrhea, and allergy. *Breastfeeding Abstracts, 18*(2), 11–12.

Wagner, C. L., Graham, E. M., & Hope, W. W. (2006). Counseling the breastfeeding mother. *e-Medicine.com., Inc.* Retrieved July 20, 2009, from http://www.emedicine.com/ped/topic2774.htm

World Health Organization/United Nations Children's Emergency Fund (WHO/UNICEF). (1994). *U.S. committee for UNICEF interim program in the United States to promote the Baby Friendly ten steps to successful breastfeeding.* Washington, DC: Government Printing Office.

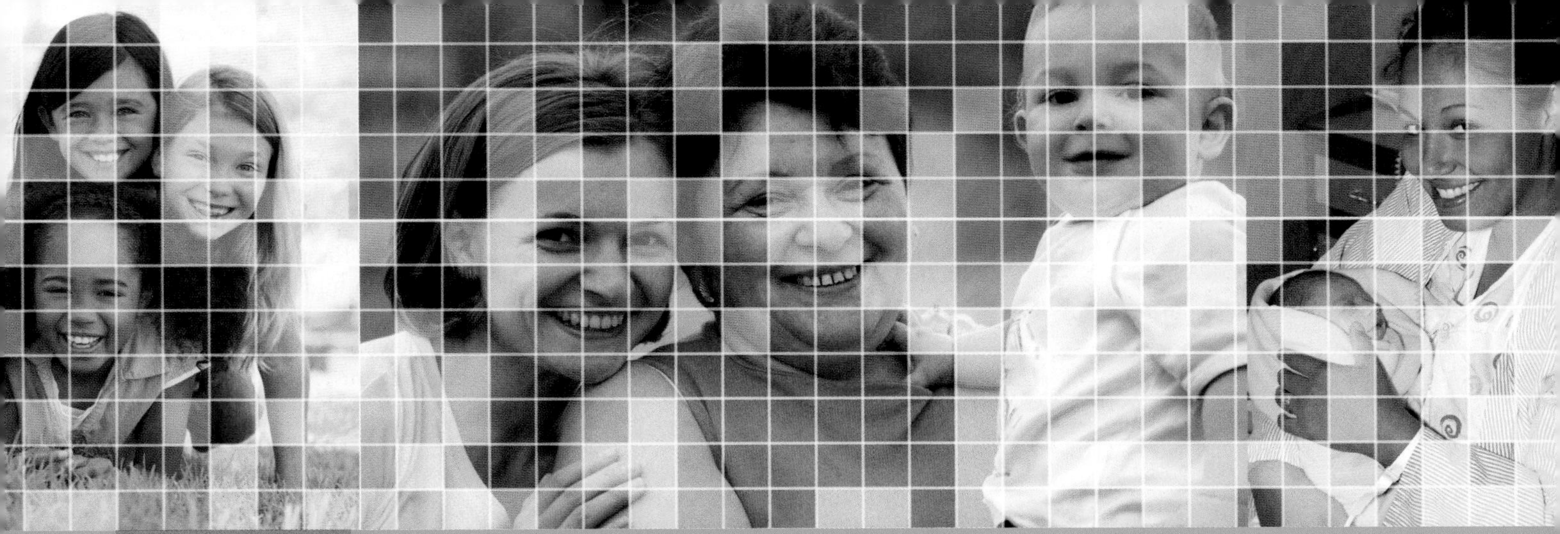

CHAPTER

28 The Newborn at Risk: Conditions Present at Birth

There is an initial flurry of activity when my baby is taken into the NICU. Now my entire universe, everything that I am, constricts down to focus on our little one. She hardly dents this world, a withery face that shows a kind of infinitely pained acceptance, breath and heartbeat almost nothing, and a pose that moves to rest, resisting nothing. I look at my small daughter with eyes naked with amazement and unsure joy. —*Jontelle, 42*

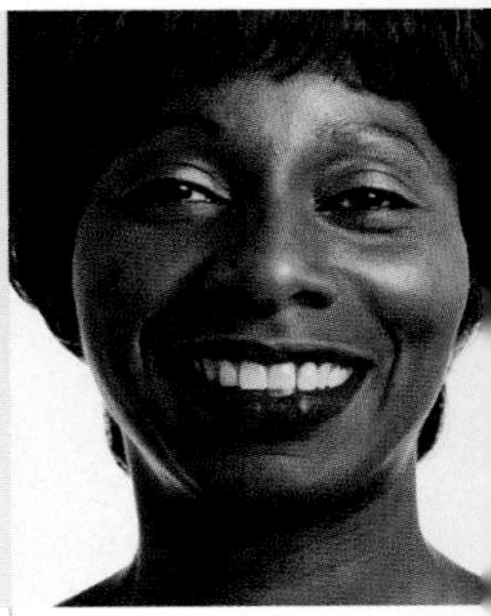

LEARNING OUTCOMES

28.1 Explain the factors present at birth that indicate an at-risk newborn.

28.2 Compare the underlying etiologies of the physiologic complications of small-for-gestational-age (SGA) newborns and preterm appropriate-for-gestational-age (Pr AGA) newborns and the nursing care management for each.

28.3 Describe the impact of maternal diabetes mellitus on the newborn.

28.4 Compare the characteristics and potential complications that influence nursing care management of the postterm newborn and the newborn with postmaturity syndrome.

28.5 Discuss the physiologic characteristics of the preterm newborn that predispose each body system to various complications and that are used in developing a plan of care that includes nutritional management.

28.6 Summarize the nursing assessments of and initial interventions for a newborn with selected congenital anomalies.

28.7 Explain the special care needed by an alcohol- or drug-exposed newborn.

28.8 Correlate the effects of maternal HIV/AIDS on the infant in the neonatal period and the issues for caregivers of infants at risk for HIV/AIDS in determining hospital-based and community-based nursing care management.

28.9 Identify the physical examination findings during the early newborn period that would make the nurse suspect a congenital cardiac defect or congestive heart failure.

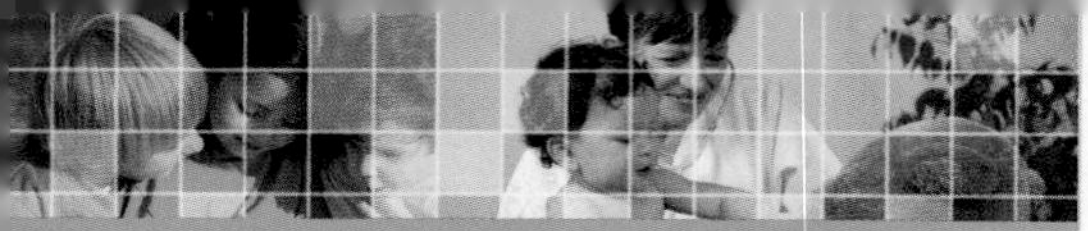

KEY TERMS

Fetal alcohol spectrum disorder (FASD), 686

Fetal alcohol syndrome (FAS), 686

Infant of a diabetic mother (IDM), 670

Infant of a substance-abusing mother (ISAM), 686

Intrauterine drug-exposed infants, 692

Intrauterine growth restriction, (IUGR), 663

Large for gestational age (LGA), 665

Neonatal mortality risk, 662

Postmaturity, 672

Postterm newborn, 672

Preterm infant, 673

Small for gestational age (SGA), 663

The field of neonatology has expanded greatly. Many levels of nursery care have evolved in response to increasing knowledge about at-risk newborns: special care, intensive care, and convalescent or transitional care. Along with the newborn's parents, the nurse is an important caregiver in all these settings. As a member of the multidisciplinary healthcare team, the nurse is a technically competent professional who contributes the high-touch human care necessary in the high-tech perinatal environment.

In addition to the availability of a high level of newborn care, various other factors influence the outcome of at-risk infants, including the following:

- Birth weight
- Gestational age
- Type and length of newborn illness
- Environmental factors
- Maternal factors
- Maternal-infant separation

IDENTIFICATION OF AT-RISK NEWBORNS

An at-risk newborn is one susceptible to illness (morbidity) or even death (mortality) because of dysmaturity, immaturity, physical disorders, or complications during or after birth. In most cases, the infant is the product of a pregnancy involving one or more predictable risk factors, including the following:

- Low socioeconomic level of the mother
- Limited access to health care or no prenatal care
- Exposure to environmental dangers, such as toxic chemicals and illicit drugs
- Preexisting maternal conditions such as heart disease, diabetes, hypertension, hyperthyroidism, and renal disease
- Maternal factors such as age and parity
- Medical conditions related to pregnancy and their associated complications
- Pregnancy complications such as abruptio placentae, oligohydramnios, preterm labor, premature rupture of membranes, preeclampsia

Various risk factors and their specific effects on the pregnancy outcome are listed in Table 10–1 ∞. Because these factors and the perinatal risks associated with them are known, the birth of at-risk newborns can often be anticipated. The pregnancy can be closely monitored, treatment can be started as necessary, and arrangements can be made for birth to occur at a facility with appropriate resources to care for both mother and baby.

Whether or not prenatal assessment indicates that the fetus is at risk, the course of labor and birth, and the infant's ability to withstand the stress of labor cannot be predicted. Thus, the nurse's use of electronic fetal heart monitoring or fetal heart auscultation by Doppler plays a significant role in detecting stress or distress in the fetus. Immediately after birth the Apgar score is a helpful tool for identifying the at-risk newborn, but it is not the only indicator of possible long-term outcome.

The newborn classification and neonatal mortality risk chart is another useful tool for identifying newborns at risk. Before this classification tool was developed, birth weight of less than 2500 g was the sole criterion for determining immaturity. Clinicians then recognized that a newborn could weigh more than 2500 g and still be immature. Conversely, an infant weighing less than 2500 g might be functionally at term or beyond. Thus birth weight and gestational age together are now the criteria used to assess neonatal maturity, morbidity, and mortality risk.

According to the newborn classification and neonatal mortality risk chart, gestation (posmenstrual age) is divided as follows:

- *Preterm:* less than 37 (completed) weeks
- *Term:* 37 to 41 6/7 (completed) weeks
- *Postterm:* greater than 42 weeks

Late preterm is an emerging classification that refers to subgroups of infants between 34 and 37 weeks' gestation; however, it is not yet used consistently for a single age range (Cloherty, Eichenwald, & Stark, 2008).

As shown in Figure 28–1 ●, large-for-gestational-age (LGA) newborns are those who plot above the 90th percentile curve on intrauterine growth curves. Appropriate-for-gestational-age (AGA) newborns are those that plot between the 10th percentile and 90th percentile growth curves. Small-for-gestational-age (SGA) newborns are those that plot below the 10th percentile growth curve. A newborn is assigned to a category depending on birth weight, length, occipital-frontal head circumference, and gestational age. For example, a newborn classified as Pr SGA is preterm and small for gestational age. The full-term newborn whose weight is appropriate for gestational age is classified FAGA. It is important to note that intrauterine growth charts are influenced by altitude and the ethnicity of the newborn population used to create the chart. Also, the assigned newborn classification may vary according to the intrauterine growth curve chart used; therefore, the chart used should correlate with the characteristics of the client population.

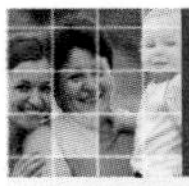

Evidence in Action

According to the American Academy of Pediatrics, Apgar scores that are low at 1 and 5 minutes are not definite indications of an acute intrapartum hypoxic event (policy statement) (Martin & Hankins, 2006).

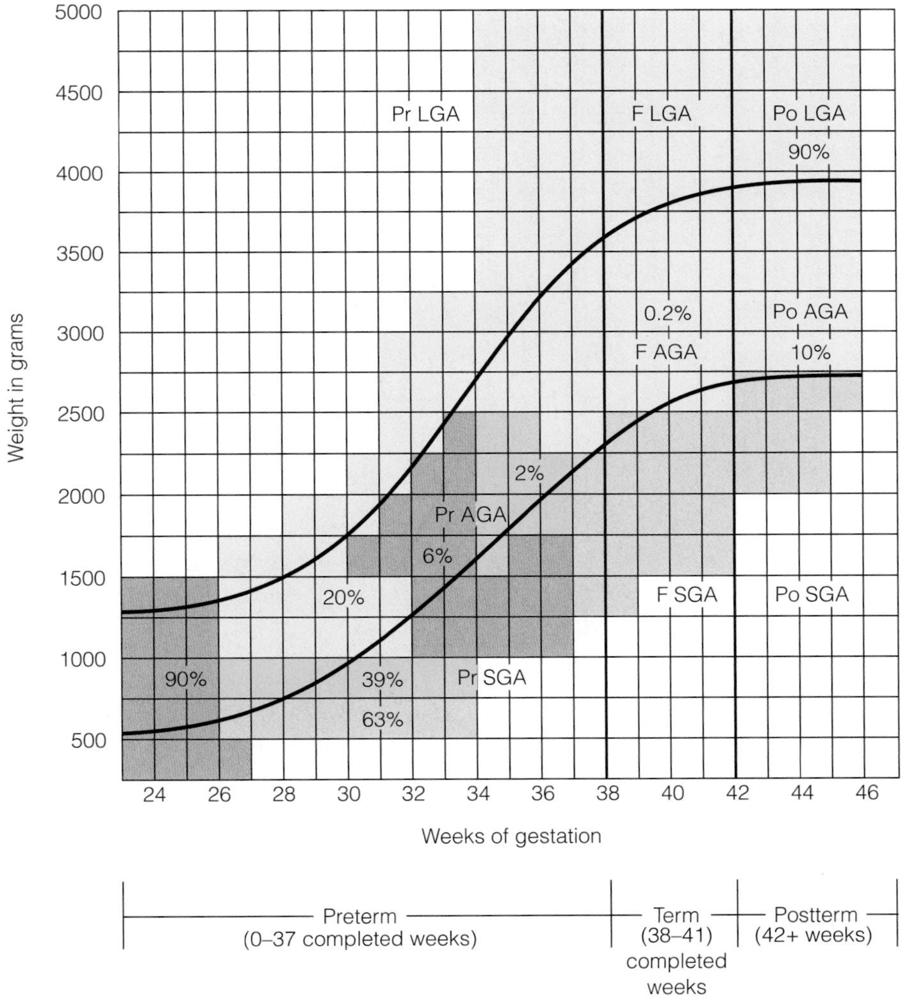

● **Figure 28–1** Newborn classification and neonatal mortality risk chart. Infants are classified according to weight as small for gestational age (SGA), appropriate for gestational age (AGA), or large for gestational age (LGA) and by weeks of newborn as preterm (Pr), term (F), or postterm (Po). Corresponding neonatal mortality risks are indicated by the percentage in the various colored regions.

Source: Koops, B. L., Morgan, L. P., & Battaglia, F. C. (1982). Neonatal mortality risk in relationship to birth weight and gestational age. *Journal of Pediatrics, 101*(6), 969.

Neonatal mortality risk is the infant's chance of death within the newborn period—that is, within the first 28 days of life. As indicated in Figure 28–1, the neonatal mortality risk decreases as both gestational age and birth weight increase. Infants who are preterm and small for gestational age have the highest neonatal mortality risk. The previously high mortality rates for LGA newborns have decreased at most perinatal centers because of both improved management of diabetes in pregnancy and increased recognition of potential complications of LGA newborns.

Neonatal morbidity can be anticipated based on birth weight and gestational age. In Figure 28–2 ●, the infant's birth weight is located on the vertical axis, and the gestational age in weeks is found along the horizontal axis. The area where the two meet on the graph identifies common problems. This tool assists in determining the needs of particular infants for special observation and care. For example, an infant of 2000 g at 40 weeks' gestation should be carefully assessed for evidence of neonatal distress, hypoglycemia, congenital anomalies, congenital infection, and polycythemia.

Identifying the nursing care needs of the at-risk newborn depends on minute-to-minute observations of the changes in the newborn's physiologic status. The organization of nursing care must be directed toward the following:

- Decreasing physiologically stressful situations
- Constantly observing for subtle signs of change in clinical condition
- Interpreting laboratory data and coordinating interventions
- Conserving the infant's energy for healing and growth
- Providing for developmental stimulation and maintenance of sleep cycles

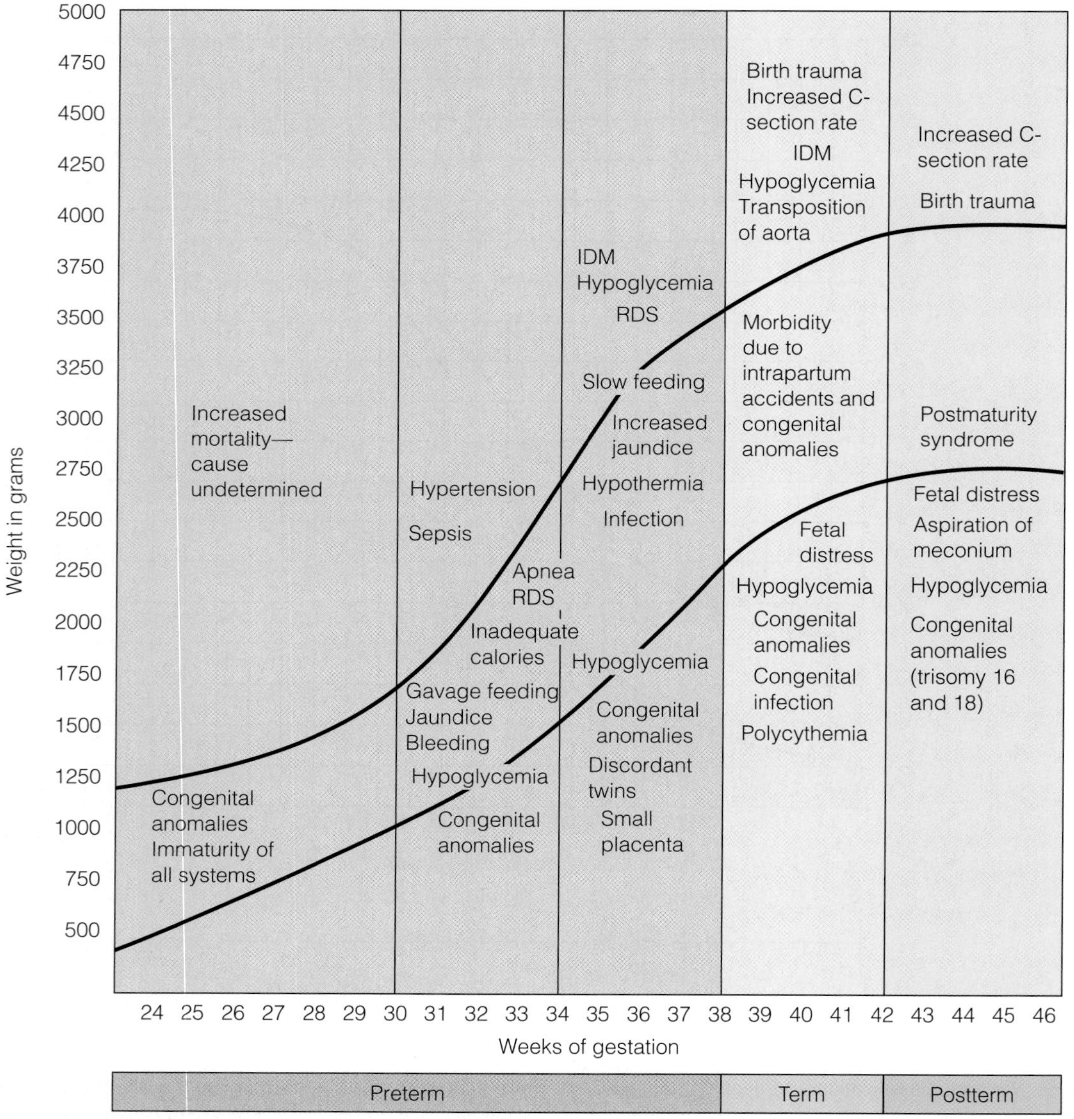

● **Figure 28–2** Neonatal morbidity by birth weight and gestational age.

Source: Lubchenco, L. O. (1976). *The high-risk infant* (p. 122). Philadelphia: Saunders.

- Assisting the family in developing attachment behaviors
- Involving the family in planning and providing care

CARE OF THE SMALL-FOR-GESTATIONAL-AGE/INTRAUTERINE GROWTH RESTRICTION NEWBORN

Currently infants are considered **small for gestational age (SGA)** when they are less than the 10th percentile for birth weight; very small for gestational age is when they are two standard deviations below the population norm or less than the third percentile (Baschat, Galan, Ross, et al., 2007) (Figure 28–3 ●). When possible, the birth weight charts used to assign the SGA classification to a newborn should be based on the local population into which the newborn is born (Baschat et al., 2007). A SGA newborn may be preterm, term, or postterm. An undergrown newborn may also be said to have **intrauterine growth restriction (IUGR)**, which describes pregnancy circumstances of advanced gestation and limited fetal growth. This classification of abnormal growth is also enhanced by looking at growth potential by adjusting birth-weight reference limits for first trimester maternal height, birth order, and fetal neonatal sex. The terms *SGA* and *IUGR* are not necessarily interchangeable.

SGA infants are commonly seen with mothers who smoke or have high blood pressure, causing these infants to have an increased incidence of perinatal asphyxia and perinatal mortality when compared with AGA infants (Baschat et al., 2007). The incidence of polycythemia and hypoglycemia is also higher in this group of infants.

FACTORS CONTRIBUTING TO IUGR

IUGR may be caused by maternal, placental, or fetal factors and may not be apparent antenatally. Intrauterine growth is linear in the normal pregnancy from approximately 28 to 38 weeks' gestation. After 38 weeks, growth is variable, depending on the growth potential of the fetus and placental function (Baschat et al., 2007). The most common causes of growth restriction are as follows:

- *Maternal factors.* Primiparity, grand multiparity, multiple-gestation pregnancy (twins and higher-order multiples), lack of prenatal care, age extremes (< 16 years or > 40 years), and low socioeconomic status (which can result in inadequate health care, inadequate education, and inadequate living conditions) affect IUGR (Baschat et al., 2007). Before the third trimester, the nutritional supply to the fetus far exceeds its needs. Only in the third trimester are maternal malnutrition and drug abuse limiting factors in fetal growth.
- *Maternal disease.* Maternal heart disease, substance abuse (drugs, tobacco, alcohol), sickle cell anemia, phenylketonuria (PKU), lupus erythematosus, and asymptomatic pyelonephritis are associated with SGA. Complications associated with preeclampsia, chronic hypertensive vascular disease, and advanced diabetes mellitus can diminish blood flow to the uterus, thereby decreasing oxygen delivery to the fetus.
- *Environmental factors.* High altitude, exposure to x-rays, excessive exercise, work-related exposure to toxins, hyperthermia, and maternal use of drugs that have teratogenic effects, such as nicotine, alcohol, antimetabolites, anticonvulsants, narcotics, and cocaine, affect fetal growth (Baschat et al., 2007).
- *Placental factors.* Placental conditions such as small placenta, infarcted areas, abnormal cord insertions, placenta previa, and thrombosis may affect circulation to the fetus, which becomes more deficient with increasing gestational age.
- *Fetal factors.* Congenital infections such as TORCH infections (*t*oxoplasmosis, *o*ther, *r*ubella, *c*ytomegalovirus, *h*erpes simplex virus), syphilis congenital malformations, discordant twins (see Chapter 4), sex of the fetus (females tend to be smaller), chromosomal syndromes (trisomies 13, 18, 21), two-vessel umbilical cord, and inborn errors of metabolism can predispose a fetus to fetal growth disturbances.

Identifying fetuses with IUGR is the first step in detecting common disorders associated with affected newborns. The perinatal history of maternal conditions, early dating of pregnancy by first-trimester ultrasound measurements, antepartal testing (nonstress test, contraction stress test, biophysical profile, see Chapter 14), Doppler velocimetry of placenta, gestational age assessment, and the physical and neurologic assessment of the newborn are also important (Cloherty et al., 2008).

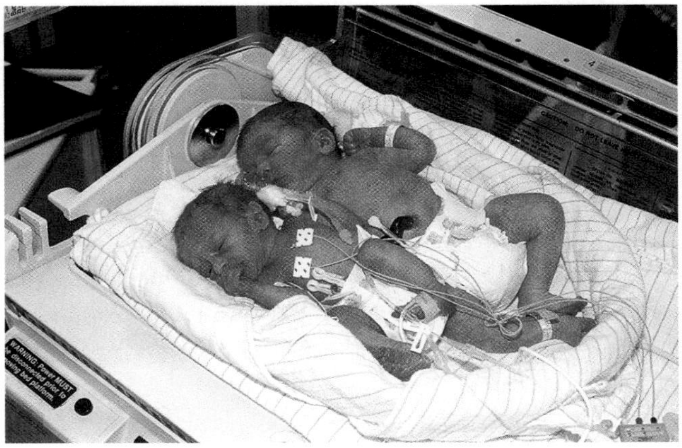

● **Figure 28–3** Thirty-five-week gestational age twins. Twin B (on left) is SGA and weighs 1260 g and twin A (on right) is AGA and weighs 2605 g.

Source: Courtesy of Carol Harrigan, RNC, MSN, NNP.

Nursing Practice

In assessing a growth-restricted infant resulting from unexplained maternal etiology (e.g., hypertension, placental insufficiency), an in utero viral infection may be the cause.

PATTERNS OF IUGR

Intrauterine growth occurs by an increase in both cell number and cell size. If insult occurs early during the critical period of organ development in the fetus, fewer new cells are formed, organs are small, and organ weight is subnormal. In contrast, growth failure that begins later in pregnancy does not affect the total number of cells, only their size. The organs are normal, but their size is diminished. There are two clinical pictures of IUGR newborns:

- *Symmetric (proportional) IUGR* is caused by long-term maternal conditions (such as chronic hypertension, severe malnutrition, chronic intrauterine viral infection, substance abuse [drugs, alcohol, tobacco], anemia) or fetal genetic abnormalities (Baschat et al., 2007). Symmetric IUGR can be noted by ultrasound in the first half of the second trimester. In symmetric IUGR there is chronic, prolonged restriction of growth in the size of organs, weight, length, and, especially, head circumference.
- *Asymmetric (disproportional) IUGR* is associated with an acute compromise of uteroplacental blood flow. Some associated causes are placental infarcts, preeclampsia, and poor weight gain in pregnancy. The growth restriction is usually not evident before the third trimester because, although weight is decreased, length and head circumference (used as a growth indicator) remain appropriate for that gestational age. After 36 weeks' gestation, the abdominal circumference of a normal fetus becomes larger than the head circumference. In asymmetric IUGR, the head circumference remains larger than the abdominal circumference. Thus measuring only the biparietal diameter on ultrasound will not reveal asymmetric IUGR. An early indicator of asymmetric SGA is a decrease in the growth rate of the abdominal circumference, reflecting subnormal liver growth, a reduction in glycogen stores, and a scarcity of subcutaneous fat (Baschat et al., 2007). Birth weight is below the 10th percentile, whereas head circumference and/or length may be between the 10th and 90th percentiles. Asymmetric SGA newborns are particularly at risk for asphyxia, pulmonary hemorrhage, hypocalcemia, and hypoglycemia in the newborn period.

Despite growth restriction, physiologic maturity develops according to gestational age. The SGA newborn's chances for survival are better than those of the preterm AGA newborn because of organ maturity, although this newborn still faces many potential difficulties.

COMMON COMPLICATIONS OF THE SGA NEWBORN

The complications occurring most frequently in the SGA newborn include the following:

- *Asphyxia.* The SGA newborn suffers chronic hypoxia in utero, which leaves little reserve to withstand the demands of normal labor and birth. Thus, intrauterine asphyxia, and its potential systemic problems, can occur. Cesarean birth may be necessary.
- *Aspiration syndrome.* In utero hypoxia can cause the fetus to gasp during birth, resulting in aspiration of amniotic fluid into the lower airways. It can also lead to relaxation of the anal sphincter and passage of meconium. This may result in aspiration of the meconium in utero or with the first breaths after birth.
- *Hypothermia.* Diminished subcutaneous fat (used for survival in utero), depletion of brown fat in utero, and a large surface area decrease the SGA newborn's ability to conserve heat. The flexed position assumed by the term SGA newborn diminishes the effect of surface area.
- *Hypoglycemia.* An increase in metabolic rate in response to heat loss and poor hepatic glycogen stores causes hypoglycemia. In addition, the newborn is compromised by inadequate supplies of enzymes to activate gluconeogenesis (conversion of nonglucogen sources such as fatty acids and proteins to glucose).
- *Polycythemia.* The number of red blood cells is increased in the SGA newborn. This finding is considered a physiologic response to in utero chronic hypoxic stress. Polycythemia may contribute to hypoglycemia.

Newborns who have significant IUGR tend to have a poor prognosis, especially when born before 37 weeks' gestation. Factors contributing to poor outcome include the following:

- *Congenital malformations.* Congenital malformations occur in 5% of SGA infants (Cloherty et al., 2008). The more severe the IUGR, the greater the chance for malformation as a result of impaired mitotic activity and cellular hypoplasia.
- *Intrauterine infections.* When fetuses are exposed to intrauterine infections such as rubella and cytomegalovirus, they are profoundly affected by direct invasion of the brain and other vital organs by the offending virus, resulting in IUGR.
- *Continued growth difficulties.* SGA newborns tend to be shorter than newborns of the same gestational age. Asymmetric IUGR infants can be expected to catch up in weight and approach their inherited growth potential when given an optimal environment. Symmetric IUGR infants reportedly have varied growth potential but tend not to catch up to their peers (Baschat et al., 2007).
- *Cognitive difficulties.* Often SGA newborns can exhibit subsequent learning disabilities. The disabilities are characterized by hyperactivity, short attention span, and poor fine motor coordination (writing and drawing). Some hearing loss and speech deficits also occur (Kahn, Hobbins, & Galan, 2008).

CLINICAL THERAPY

The goal of medical therapy for SGA infants is early recognition and implementation of the medical management of potential problems.

NURSING MANAGEMENT

NURSING ASSESSMENT AND DIAGNOSIS

The nurse is responsible for assessing gestational age and identifying signs of potential complications associated with SGA infants. All body parts of the symmetric IUGR infant are in proportion, but they are below normal size for the baby's gestational age. Therefore the head does not appear overly large or the length excessive in relation to the other body parts. These newborns are generally vigorous.

The asymmetric IUGR infant appears long, thin, and emaciated, with loss of subcutaneous fat tissue and muscle mass. The baby may have loose skin folds; dry, desquamating skin; and a thin and often meconium-stained cord. The head appears relatively large (although it approaches normal size) because the chest size and abdominal girth are decreased. The baby may have a vigorous cry and appear alert and wide-eyed.

Nursing diagnoses that may apply to the SGA newborn include the following:

- *Impaired Gas Exchange* related to aspiration of meconium
- *Hypothermia* related to decreased subcutaneous fat
- *Risk for Injury to Tissues* related to decreased glycogen stores and impaired gluconeogenesis
- *Altered Nutrition: Less than Body Requirements* related to SGA newborn's increased metabolic rate
- *Risk for Altered Parenting* related to prolonged separation of newborn from parents secondary to illness

PLANNING AND IMPLEMENTATION

HOSPITAL-BASED NURSING CARE

Hypoglycemia, the most common metabolic complication of IUGR, produces such sequelae as CNS abnormalities and mental retardation (intellectual disability). Conditions such as asphyxia, hyperviscosity, and cold stress may also affect the baby's outcome. Meticulous attention to physiologic parameters is essential for immediate nursing management and reduction of long-term disorders. (See "Nursing Care Plan for a Small-for-Gestational-Age Newborn" on pages 666–669).

COMMUNITY-BASED NURSING CARE

The long-term needs of the SGA newborn include careful follow-up evaluation of patterns of growth and possible disabilities that may later interfere with learning or motor functioning. Long-term follow-up care is essential for infants with congenital malformations, congenital infections, and obvious sequelae from physiologic problems. Parents of the IUGR newborn need support, because a positive atmosphere can enhance the baby's growth potential and the child's ultimate outcome.

EVALUATION

Expected outcomes of nursing care include the following:

- The SGA newborn is free from respiratory compromise.
- The SGA newborn maintains a stable temperature.
- The SGA infant is free from hypoglycemic episodes and maintains glucose homeostasis.
- The SGA newborn gains weight and takes breast or formula feedings without developing physiologic distress or fatigue.
- The parents verbalize their concerns about their baby's health problems and understand the rationale behind management of their newborn.

CARE OF THE LARGE-FOR-GESTATIONAL-AGE (LGA) NEWBORN

A newborn whose birth weight is at or above the 90th percentile on the intrauterine growth curve (at any week of gestation) is considered **large for gestational age (LGA)**. Some AGA newborns have been incorrectly categorized as LGA because of miscalculation of the date of conception caused by postconceptual bleeding. Careful gestational age assessment is essential to identify the potential needs and problems of these infants.

The most well-known condition associated with excessive fetal growth is maternal diabetes (White's classes A to C; see Chapter 15, Table 15–3∞); however, only a small fraction of large newborns are born to diabetic mothers. The cause of the majority of cases of LGA newborns is unclear, but certain factors or situations have been found to correlate with their birth (Cloherty et al., 2008):

- Genetic predisposition is correlated proportionately to the mother's prepregnancy weight and to weight gain during pregnancy. Large parents tend to have large infants.
- Multiparous women have two to three times the number of LGA infants as primigravidas.
- Male infants are typically larger than female infants.
- Infants with erythroblastosis fetalis, Beckwith-Wiedemann syndrome (a genetic condition associated with omphalocele and neonatal hypoglycemia and hyperinsulinemia), or transposition of the great vessels are usually large.

The increase in the LGA infant's body size is characteristically proportional, although head circumference and body length are in the upper limits of intrauterine growth. The exception to this rule is the infant of the diabetic mother, whose body weight increases while length and head circumference may remain in the normal range. Macrosomic infants have poor motor skills and have difficulty in regulating behavioral states. LGA infants tend to be more difficult to arouse to a quiet alert state. They may also have feeding difficulties.

(continued on page 669)

Nursing Care Plan

THE SMALL-FOR-GESTATIONAL-AGE NEWBORN

INTERVENTION	RATIONALE	EXPECTED OUTCOME
1. Nursing Diagnosis: Risk for Impaired Gas Exchange related to meconium aspiration		
NIC Intervention: **Respiratory monitoring:** Collection and analysis of patient data to ensure airway patency and adequate gas exchange		**NOC Outcome:** **Respiratory status:** Gas exchange: Alveolar exchange of CO_2 or O_2 to maintain arterial blood gas concentrations
Goal: The newborn's respirations will be stable and maintained within normal limits.		
■ Obtain maternal prenatal, labor, and birth records.	■ Provides information of fetal stress that may have occurred during the prenatal or intrapartum period. In addition, the birth record will provide information concerning infant's respiratory status at birth; for example, the Apgar score.	■ The infant will maintain adequate respiratory gas exchange as evidenced by respirations of 30–60/min with no periods of apnea or evidence of worsening distress.
■ Maintain airway patency through judicious suctioning.	■ Respiratory distress in SGA newborns is due to in utero hypoxia and aspiration of meconium.	
■ Observe for worsening signs of respiratory distress such as generalized cyanosis; worsening retractions, grunting, and nasal flaring, as evidenced by Silverman respiratory index; sustained tachypnea; apnea episodes; inequality of breath sounds; presence of rales and rhonchi.		
■ Monitor and maintain adequate body temperature (36°C+/−0.2°C [97.7°F+/−0.5°F]) to avoid increased oxygen consumption.	■ Temperature elevation may cause metabolic rate and oxygen needs to increase when associated with meconium aspiration.	
■ Administer oxygen per order for relief of respiratory distress signs (see "Care of the Newborn with Respiratory Distress" in Chapter 29 ∞ for nursing care and treatment of meconium aspiration, infant resuscitation).	■ Provides healthcare personnel with cardiac and pulmonary status.	
■ Implement treatment plan for respiratory distress.		
■ Monitor glucose levels.	■ Respiratory distress increases consumption of glucose.	
■ **Collaborative:** Obtain arterial blood gases per physician's orders.		
■ Monitor infant's cardiac status and pulmonary status; pulse oximetry and arterial blood gases (ABGs).	■ Oxygen demands increase with meconium aspiration. Obtaining ABGs will provide medical personnel baseline information of infant's respiratory status, and effective medical interventions can be initiated.	
2. Nursing Diagnosis: Risk for Ineffective Thermoregulation and Cold Stress secondary to decreased subcutaneous fat		
NIC Intervention: **Temperature regulation:** Attaining and/or maintaining body temperature within a normal range		**NOC Outcome:** **Thermoregulation:** Newborn: Balance among heat production, heat gain, and heat loss during the neonatal period
Goal: The infant's temperature will be stable and maintained within normal limits.		

Nursing Care Plan—continued

THE SMALL-FOR-GESTATIONAL-AGE NEWBORN

INTERVENTION	RATIONALE	EXPECTED OUTCOME
■ Provide neutral thermal zone (NTZ) range for infant based on postnatal weight.	■ Neutral thermal environment charts used for preterm infant are not reliable for weight of SGA infant.	■ The infant will not exhibit signs and symptoms of hypothermia as evidenced by temperature maintenance of 97.7°F–99.1°F and no signs and symptoms of respiratory distress.
■ Use a skin probe to maintain infant's skin temperature at 36°C–36.5°C.	■ A neutral thermal environment requires minimal oxygen consumption to maintain a normal core temp.	
■ Obtain axillary temps and compare to registered skin probe temp. If discrepancy exists evaluate potential cause.	■ Discrepancies between axillary and skin probe monitor temp may be due to mechanical causes or the burning of brown fat.	
■ Adjust and monitor incubator or radiant warmer to maintain skin temp.		
■ Minimize heat losses and prevent cold stress by: ■ Warming and humidifying oxygen without blowing over face in order to avoid increasing oxygen consumption. ■ Keeping skin dry. ■ Keeping isolettes, radiant warmers, and cribs away from windows and cold external walls and out of drafts. ■ Avoiding placing infant on cold surfaces such as metal treatment tables, cold x-ray plates. ■ Padding cold surfaces with diapers and using radiant warmers during procedures. ■ Warming blood for exchange transfusions.	■ Physical principles of heat loss effects include: ■ Evaporation—lungs and skin when cooling occurs as a result of water evaporation. ■ Convection—air currents. ■ Conduction—skin contact with cooler object. ■ Radiation—loss of warmth to cooler surrounding objects.	
■ Observe for signs and symptoms of cold stress: decreased temperature, lethargy, pallor (for further discussion see Chapter 29 ∞).	■ Hypothermia is a potential problem for SGA infant because: ■ SGA infant has decreased stores of brown fat available for thermogenesis, because SGA infant has used these stores in utero for survival. ■ SGA infant has poor insulation due to use of subcutaneous tissues in utero for survival.	

3. Nursing Diagnosis: Risk for Injury to Tissues related to decreased glycogen stores and impaired gluconeogenesis

NIC Intervention:

High-risk infant care: Identification and management of a high-risk infant to promote healthy outcomes for the baby

NOC Outcome:

Risk control: Actions to eliminate or reduce actual, personal, and modifiable health threats

Goal: Newborn will have a normal blood glucose level.

INTERVENTION	RATIONALE	EXPECTED OUTCOME
■ Monitor chemstrip per SGA protocol and report values <45 mg/dL.	■ Combined with depletion of glycogen stores, impaired gluconeogenesis predisposes SGA infants to profound hypoglycemia within first 2 days of life.	■ The fetus will not exhibit signs and symptoms of hypoglycemia as evidenced by a euglycemic state and blood glucose greater than 20 mg/dL.

(continued)

Nursing Care Plan—continued

THE SMALL-FOR-GESTATIONAL-AGE NEWBORN

INTERVENTION	RATIONALE	EXPECTED OUTCOME
■ Observe, record, and report signs of hypoglycemia: cyanosis, lethargy, jitteriness, seizure activity, and apnea.	■ Hypoglycemia in SGA infant is indicated by whole blood sugar less than 20 mg/dL.	
■ Initiate feeding schedule for SGA newborns per agency protocol.	■ Frequent monitoring of Dextrostix assists in identifying decreasing glucose levels.	
■ Provide glucose intake either through early enteral feeding (before 4 hr) or by IV per physician's order. See further discussion of hypoglycemia in Chapter 29 ∞.	■ Provision of glucose through early feedings (begin before 4 hr of age) assists in maintaining glucose levels.	

4. Nursing Diagnosis: Altered Nutrition: Less than Body Requirements related to increased metabolic needs in the infant

NIC Intervention:

Newborn monitoring: Measurement and interpretation of physiologic status of the newborn for the first 24 hours

NOC Outcome:

Nutritional status: Food and fluid intake: Amount of food and fluid taken into the body over a 24-hr period

Goal: Infant will gain weight and tolerate nipple-feedings without tiring.

INTERVENTION	RATIONALE	EXPECTED OUTCOME
■ Assess suck, swallow, gag, and cough reflexes.	■ Prevents feeding problems and assists in determining the best method of feeding for infant.	■ The infant will maintain steady weight gain as evidenced by < 2%/day weight loss, tolerates oral feedings, and urine output is 1–3 mL/kg/hr.
■ Initiate test water feeding at 1 hour of age, then proceed to 5% glucose/water. Move early to formula-feeding q2–3 hr.	■ Sterile water is desirable for first feedings because it causes fewer pulmonary complications in the presence of gastrointestinal tract abnormalities or aspiration of feeding. ■ SGA newborns require more calories/kg for growth than AGA newborns because of increased metabolic activity and oxygen consumption secondary to increased percentage of body weight made up by visceral organs.	
■ Supplement oral feedings with intravenous intake per orders. ■ Use concentrated formulas that supply more calories in less volume, such as Similac 24.	■ Small, frequent feedings of high-caloric formula are used because of limited gastric capacity and decreased gastric emptying.	
■ Promote growth by providing caloric intake of 120–150 cal/kg/day in small amounts.	■ Growth is evaluated by increase in weight, length, and body measurements. ■ Decrease in exhaustion is an important consideration in feeding SGA infant.	
■ Observe, record, and report signs of respiratory distress or fatigue occurring during feedings.	■ Adequate nutritional intake promotes growth and prevents such complications as metabolic catabolism and hypoglycemia.	
■ Supplement gavage or nipple-feedings with intravenous therapy per physician order until oral intake is sufficient to support growth.	■ Gavage feedings require less energy expenditure on the part of the newborn.	
■ Establish a nipple-feeding program that is begun slowly and progresses slowly, such as nipple-feed once per day, nipple-feed once per shift, and then nipple-feed every other feeding.		

Nursing Care Plan—continued

THE SMALL-FOR-GESTATIONAL-AGE NEWBORN

INTERVENTION	RATIONALE	EXPECTED OUTCOME
■ Monitor daily weight with anticipation of small amount of weight loss when nipple-feedings start.	■ Nipple-feeding, an active rather than passive intake of nutrition, requires energy expenditure and burning of calories by infant.	

5. Nursing Diagnosis: Risk for Altered Parenting related to lack of knowledge of infant care and prolonged separation of infant and parents secondary to illness

NIC Intervention:

Teaching: Infant care: Instruction on nurturing and physical care needed during the first year of life

NOC Outcome:

Parenting: Provision of an environment that promotes optimum growth and development of dependent children.

Goal: Parents will bond with infant and have realistic expectations about infant. Parents are comfortable taking infant home. They are able to demonstrate normal infant care and assessments of possible complications, and know when to return for follow-up.

INTERVENTION	RATIONALE	EXPECTED OUTCOME
■ Support emotionally the psychologic well-being of family, including positive parent-infant bonding and sensory stimulation of infant. ■ Include parents in determining infant's plan of care and encourage their participation. Encourage parents to visit frequently. Provide opportunities for parents to touch, hold, talk to, and care for infant. Determine the type and amount of appropriate sensory stimulation and implement sensory stimulation program.	■ Parent-infant bonding begins in first few hours or days following birth. SGA infants may experience prolonged periods of separation from their parents, which necessitates intervention to ensure parent-infant bonding.	■ The parent will demonstrate ability to perform basic infant care tasks as evidenced by exhibiting appropriate attachment behaviors (e.g., talking and holding infant), feeding infant, and bathing infant.
■ Prepare for discharge by instructing parents in such areas as feeding techniques, formula preparation, and breastfeeding; bathing, diapering, and hygiene; temperature monitoring; administration of vitamins, care of complications, and preventing exposure to infections; normal elimination patterns, normal reflexes and activity, and how to promote normal growth and development without being overprotective; returning for continued medical care; and availability of community resources if indicated.	■ Parents should receive the same postpartum teaching as any parent taking a new infant home. ■ Parents need to understand the changes to expect in color of the infant's stool and number of bowel movements plus odor from formula- or breastfeeding in order to avoid unnecessary concern. SGA infants usually do not require referral to community agencies such as visiting nurse associations unless there is a specific problem requiring assistance.	

COMMON COMPLICATIONS OF THE LGA NEWBORN

Complications of the LGA newborn can include the following:

- *Birth trauma caused by cephalopelvic disproportion (CPD).* Often LGA newborns have a biparietal diameter greater than 10 cm (4 in.) or are associated with a maternal fundal height measurement greater than 42 cm (16 in.) without the presence of polyhydramnios. Because of their excessive size, there are more breech presentations and shoulder dystocia. These complications may result in asphyxia, fractured clavicles, brachial palsy, facial paralysis, phrenic nerve palsy, depressed skull fractures, cephalohematoma, and intracranial hemorrhage caused by birth trauma.
- *Increased incidence of cesarean births and oxytocin-induced births* because of fetal size. Mothers and infants have all the risk factors associated with cesarean births.
- *Hypoglycemia, polycythemia, and hyperviscosity.* These disorders are most often seen in infants of diabetic mothers, infants with erythroblastosis fetalis, or infants with Beckwith-Wiedemann syndrome.

Nursing Management

The perinatal history, in conjunction with ultrasonic measurement of fetal skull (biparietal diameter) and gestational age testing, is important in identifying an at-risk LGA newborn. Nursing care is directed toward early identification and immediate treatment of the common disorders. Essential components of the nursing assessment are monitoring vital signs, screening for hypoglycemia and polycythemia, and observing for signs and symptoms related to birth trauma. The nurse should address parental concerns about the visual signs of birth trauma and the potential for continuation of the overweight pattern. The nurse helps parents learn to arouse and console their newborn and facilitate attachment behaviors. Mothers of LGA infants with facial or head bruising may be reluctant to interact with their newborns because they fear hurting their infants. The nursing care involved in the complications associated with LGA newborns is similar to the care needed by the infant of a diabetic mother and is discussed in the next section.

CARE OF THE INFANT OF A DIABETIC MOTHER

MyNursingKit Care Plan Activity: Infant of a Diabetic Mother

The **infant of a diabetic mother (IDM)** is considered at risk and requires close observation during the first few hours to the first few days of life. Mothers with severe diabetes or diabetes of long duration associated with vascular complications may give birth to SGA infants. The typical IDM, when the diabetes is poorly controlled or gestational, is LGA. The infant is macrosomic, ruddy in color, and has excessive adipose (fat) tissue (Figure 28–4 ●). The umbilical cord is thick and the placenta is large. There is a higher incidence of macrosomic infants born to certain ethnic groups (Native Americans, Mexican Americans, African Americans, Pacific Islanders).

IDMs have decreased total body water, particularly in the extracellular spaces, and are therefore not edematous. Their excessive weight is because of increased weight of the visceral organs, cardiomegaly (hypertrophy), and increased body fat. The only organ not affected is the brain.

The excessive fetal growth of the IDM is caused by exposure to high levels of maternal glucose, which readily crosses the placenta. The fetus responds to these high glucose levels with increased insulin production and hyperplasia of the pancreatic beta cells. The main action of the insulin is to facilitate the entry of glucose into muscle and fat cells. Once in the cells, glucose is converted to glycogen and stored. Insulin also inhibits the breakdown of fat to free fatty acids, thereby maintaining lipid synthesis; increases the uptake of amino acids; and promotes protein synthesis. Insulin is an important regulator of fetal metabolism and has a "growth hormone" effect that results in increased linear growth. Infants of diabetic mothers may be obese as children (Landon, Catalano, & Gabbe, 2008).

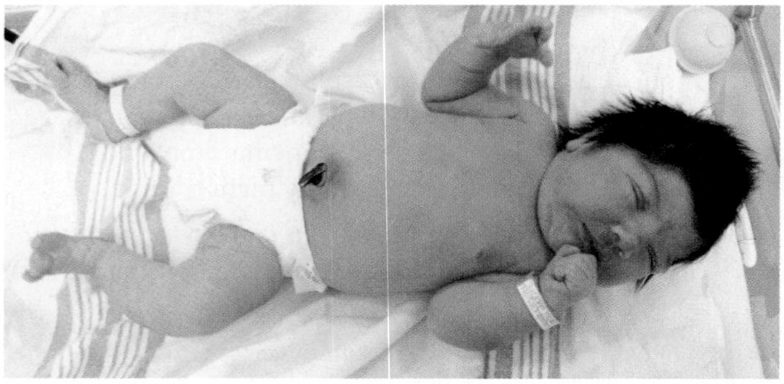

● **Figure 28–4** Macrosomic infant of a Class B insulin-dependent diabetic mother born at 38 weeks' gestation weighing 3402 grams.

Source: Courtesy of Carol Harrigan, RNC, MSN, NNP.

COMMON COMPLICATIONS OF THE IDM

Although IDMs are usually large, they have immature physiologic functions and exhibit many of the problems of the preterm (premature) infant. The complications most often seen in an IDM are as follows:

- *Hypoglycemia.* Hypoglycemia is defined as a blood sugar less than 40 mg/dL. Even though the high maternal blood supply is lost, the IDM continues to produce high levels of insulin, which deplete the infant's blood glucose within hours after birth. IDMs also have less ability to release glucagon and catecholamines, which normally stimulate glucagon breakdown and glucose release. The incidence of hypoglycemia in IDMs varies according to the degree of success in controlling the maternal diabetes, the maternal blood sugar level at the time of birth, the length of labor, the class of maternal diabetes, and early versus late feedings of the newborn. Signs and symptoms of hypoglycemia include tremors, cyanosis, apnea, temperature instability, poor feeding, and hypotonia. Seizures may occur in severe cases.
- *Hypocalcemia.* Tremors are the obvious clinical sign of hypocalcemia. They may be caused by the IDM's increased incidence of prematurity and by the stresses of difficult pregnancy, labor, and birth. Diabetic women tend to have decreased serum magnesium levels at term secondary to increased urinary calcium excretion, which causes secondary hypoparathyroidism in their infants. Other factors may include vitamin D antagonism, which results from elevated cortisol levels, hypophosphatemia from tissue catabolism, and decreased serum magnesium levels.
- *Hyperbilirubinemia.* This condition may be seen at 48 to 72 hours after birth. It may be caused by slightly decreased extracellular fluid volume, which increases the hematocrit level. This elevation facilitates an increase in red blood cell breakdown thereby increasing bilirubin levels. The presence

Nursing Practice

When beginning fluids on an IDM, it is sometimes best to start at a higher concentration of dextrose to avoid hypoglycemia episodes.

of hepatic immaturity may impair bilirubin conjugation. Enclosed hemorrhages resulting from complicated vaginal birth may also cause hyperbilirubinemia.

- *Birth trauma.* Because most IDMs are macrosomic, trauma may occur during labor and birth from shoulder dystocia.
- *Polycythemia.* Fetal hyperglycemia and hyperinsulinism result in increased oxygen consumption, which can lead to fetal hypoxia (Landon et al., 2008). Hemoglobin A_{1c} binds to oxygen, decreasing the oxygen available to the fetal tissues. This tissue hypoxia stimulates increased erythropoietin production, which increases both the hematocrit level and the potential for hyperbilirubinemia. See Chapter 15 for discussion of hemoglobin A_{1c}.
- *Respiratory distress syndrome (RDS).* This complication occurs especially in newborns of diabetic mothers in White's classes A to C who are not well controlled (Cloherty et al., 2008). Insulin antagonizes the cortisol-induced stimulation of lecithin synthesis that is necessary for lung maturation. Therefore, IDMs may have less mature lungs than expected for their gestational age. There is also a decrease in the phospholipid phosphatidylglycerol (PG), which stabilizes surfactant. The insufficiency of PG increases the incidence of RDS. Therefore, it is important to test for the presence of PG in the amniotic fluid before birth.

  RDS does not appear to be a problem for infants born of diabetic mothers in White's classes D to F; instead, the stresses of poor uterine blood supply may lead to increased production of steroids, which accelerates lung maturation. IDMs may also have a delay in closure of the ductus arteriosus and decreases in postnatal pulmonary artery pressure (Cloherty et al., 2008).
- *Congenital birth defects.* These may include congenital heart defects (transposition of the great vessels, ventricular septal defect, patent ductus arteriosus), small left colon syndrome, renal anomalies, neural tube defects, and sacral agenesis (caudal regression) (Cloherty et al., 2008). Early close control of maternal glucose levels before and during pregnancy decreases the risk of birth defects. See Chapter 15.

CLINICAL THERAPY

Prenatal management is directed toward controlling maternal glucose levels, which minimizes the common complications of IDMs. Because the onset of hypoglycemia occurs between 1 and 3 hours after birth in IDMs (with a spontaneous rise to normal levels by 4 to 6 hours), blood glucose determinations should be done on cord blood or by heel stick hourly during the first 4 hours after birth and then at 4-hour intervals until the risk period (about 48 hours) has passed or per agency protocol.

IDMs whose serum glucose level falls below 40 mg/dL should have early feedings with formula or breast milk (colostrum). If normal glucose levels cannot be maintained with oral feedings an intravenous (IV) infusion of glucose will be necessary. An infusion of $D_{10}W$ usually maintains normoglycemia in the IDM. If higher glucose concentrations are needed to maintain normal serum glucose levels, a central line will be placed to minimize tissue extravasation. Newborns with refractory hypoglycemia may benefit from the administration of intravenous corticosteroids. Once the blood glucose level has been stable for 24 hours, the infusion rate can be decreased as oral feedings are increased. The newborn's blood glucose levels must be carefully monitored. Repeat dextrose as bolus infusion is contraindicated because it may lead to severe rebound hypoglycemia following an initial brief increase in glucose level.

NURSING MANAGEMENT

NURSING ASSESSMENT AND DIAGNOSIS

The nurse should not be lulled into thinking that a big baby is a mature baby. In almost every case, because of the infant's large size, the IDM will appear older than gestational age scoring indicates. The nurse must consider both the gestational age and whether the baby is AGA or LGA in planning and providing safe care. In caring for the IDM, the nurse assesses for signs of respiratory distress, hyperbilirubinemia, birth trauma, and congenital anomalies.

Nursing diagnoses that may apply to IDMs include the following:

- *Altered Nutrition: Less than Body Requirements* related to increased glucose metabolism secondary to hyperinsulinemia
- *Impaired Gas Exchange* related to respiratory distress secondary to impaired production of surfactant
- *Increased Incidence of Congenital Anomalies* related to poor maternal metabolic control
- *Ineffective Family Coping: Compromise* related to the illness of the baby

PLANNING AND IMPLEMENTATION

Nursing care of the IDM is directed toward early detection and ongoing monitoring of hypoglycemia (by performing glucose tests) and polycythemia (by obtaining central hematocrits), RDS, and hyperbilirubinemia. (These conditions are presented in Chapter 29.) The nurse also assesses for signs of birth trauma and congenital anomalies.

Parent teaching is directed toward preventing macrosomia and the resulting fetal-neonatal problems by instituting early and ongoing diabetic control. Parents are advised that with early identification and care, most IDMs' neonatal problems have no significant sequelae.

EVALUATION

Expected outcomes of nursing care include the following:

- The IDM's respiratory distress and metabolic problems are minimized.

- The parents understand the effects of maternal diabetes on the baby's health and preventive steps they can initiate to decrease its impact on subsequent pregnancies.
- The parents verbalize their concerns about their baby's health problems and understand the rationale behind management of their newborn.

CARE OF THE POSTTERM NEWBORN

The **postterm newborn** is any newborn born after 42 completed weeks of gestation. Postterm or prolonged pregnancy occurs in less than 12% of all pregnancies (Cloherty et al., 2008). The cause of postterm pregnancy is not completely understood, but several factors are known to be associated with it. (See Chapter 21∞ for discussion of maternal factors.) Many pregnancies classified as prolonged are thought to be a result of inaccurate estimates of date of birth (EDB). Postterm pregnancy is more common in Australian, Greek, and Italian ethnic groups.

Most babies born as a result of prolonged pregnancy are of normal size and health; some continue growing and are over 4000 g at birth, which supports the contention that the postterm fetus can remain well nourished. Potential intrapartal problems for these healthy but large fetuses are cephalopelvic disproportion (CPD) and shoulder dystocia. See Chapter 22∞ for discussion of the necessary assessments and interventions for CPD and shoulder dystocia.

COMMON COMPLICATIONS OF THE NEWBORN WITH POSTMATURITY SYNDROME

The term **postmaturity** applies only to the infant who is born after 42 completed weeks of gestation and also demonstrates characteristics of *postmaturity syndrome.* Only about 5% of postterm newborns show signs of postmaturity syndrome.

The truly postmature newborn is at high risk for morbidity and has a mortality rate two to three times greater than that of term infants. Although today the percentages are extremely low, the majority of postmature fetal deaths occur during labor, because the fetus uses up necessary body reserves.

Decreased placental function, which impairs nutrition transport and oxygenation, leaves the fetus prone to hypoglycemia and asphyxia when the stresses of labor begin. The following are common disorders of the postmature newborn:

- Hypoglycemia, from nutritional deprivation and depleted glycogen stores
- Meconium aspiration in response to in utero hypoxia (The presence of oligohydramnios increases the danger of aspirating thick meconium. Severe meconium aspiration syndrome increases the baby's chance of developing persistent pulmonary hypertension, pneumothorax, and pneumonia. See detailed discussion of meconium aspiration in Chapter 29∞.)
- Polycythemia caused by increased production of red blood cells (RBCs) in response to hypoxia
- Congenital anomalies of unknown cause
- Seizure activity because of hypoxic insult
- Cold stress because of loss or poor development of subcutaneous fat

The long-term effects of postmaturity syndrome are unclear. At present, studies do not agree on the effect of postmaturity syndrome on weight gain and IQ scores (Divon, 2007).

Prolonged pregnancy itself is not solely responsible for the postmaturity syndrome. The characteristics of postmature newborns are primarily caused by a combination of advanced gestational age, placental aging and subsequent insufficiency, and continued exposure to amniotic fluid.

CLINICAL THERAPY

The aim of antenatal management is to differentiate the fetus who has postmaturity syndrome from the fetus who at birth is large, well nourished, alert, and tolerating the prolonged (postterm) pregnancy. Antenatal tests that are done to evaluate fetal status and determine obstetric management and their use in postterm pregnancy are discussed in more depth in Chapters 15 and 21∞. If the amniotic fluid is meconium stained, an amnioinfusion may be done during labor. This procedure dilutes the meconium by directly infusing either normal saline or Ringer's lactate into the uterus, decreasing the risk of meconium aspiration syndrome. (For detailed discussion of clinical management and care of the newborn at risk for meconium aspiration, see Chapter 29∞.)

Hypoglycemia is monitored by serial glucose determinations per agency protocols. The baby may be placed on glucose infusions or given early feedings if respiratory distress is not present, but these measures must be instituted with caution because of the frequency of asphyxia in the first 24 hours. Postmature newborns are often voracious eaters.

For the SGA infant who is postmature, peripheral and central hematocrits are tested to determine the presence of polycythemia. Fluid resuscitation can be initiated. In extreme cases a partial exchange transfusion may be necessary to prevent polycythemia and adverse sequelae such as hyperviscosity. Oxygen is provided for respiratory distress. In addition, temperature instability and excessive loss of heat can result from decreased liver glycogen stores. (See Chapter 29∞ for thermoregulation techniques.)

NURSING MANAGEMENT

NURSING ASSESSMENT AND DIAGNOSIS

The newborn with postmaturity syndrome appears alert. This wide-eyed, alert appearance is not necessarily a positive sign because it may indicate chronic intrauterine hypoxia. The infant typically has dry, cracking, parchmentlike skin without vernix or lanugo (Figure 28–5 ●). Fingernails are long, and scalp hair is profuse. The infant's body appears long and thin. The wasting involves depletion of previously stored subcutaneous tissue, causing the skin to be loose. Fat layers are almost nonexistent.

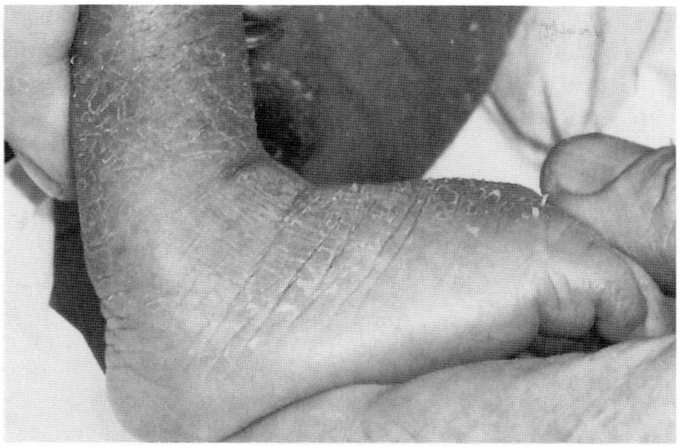

● **Figure 28–5** Postterm infant demonstrates deep cracking and peeling of skin.

Source: Dubowitz, L., & Dubowitz, V. (1977). *The gestational age of the newborn.* Redwood City, CA: Addison-Wesley. Reprinted by permission of V. Dubowitz, MD, Hammersmith Hospital, London, England.

Postmature newborns frequently have meconium staining, which colors the nails, skin, and umbilical cord. The varying shades (yellow to green) of meconium staining can give some clue as to whether the expulsion of meconium in utero was a recent or chronic problem. Green coloring indicates a more recent event.

Nursing diagnoses that may apply to the postmature newborn include the following:

- *Hypothermia* related to decreased liver glycogen and brown fat stores
- *Altered Nutrition: Less than Body Requirements* related to increased use of glucose secondary to in utero stress and decreased placenta perfusion
- *Impaired Gas Exchange in the Lungs and at the Cellular Level* related to airway obstruction from meconium aspiration

PLANNING AND IMPLEMENTATION

Nursing interventions are primarily supportive measures. The nurse needs to do the following:

- Monitor cardiopulmonary status because the stresses of labor are poorly tolerated and can result in hypoxemia in utero and possible asphyxia at birth.
- Provide warmth to counterbalance the infant's poor response to cold stress and decreased liver glycogen and brown fat stores.
- Frequently monitor blood glucose and initiate early feeding (at 1 or 2 hours of age) or intravenous glucose per physician order.
- Obtain a central line hematocrit to determine accurately the presence of polycythemia.

The nurse encourages parents to express their feelings and fears about the newborn's condition and potential long-term problems. The nurse gives careful explanations of procedures, includes the parents in the development of care plans for their baby, and encourages follow-up care as needed.

EVALUATION

Expected outcomes of nursing care include the following:

- The postterm newborn establishes effective respiratory function.
- The postmature baby is free of metabolic alterations (hypoglycemia) and maintains a stable temperature.

CARE OF THE PRETERM (PREMATURE) NEWBORN

A **preterm infant** is any infant born at 36 6/7 or less weeks' gestation (Figure 28–6 ●). With the help of modern technology, infants are surviving at younger gestational ages, but not without significant morbidity. The incidence of all preterm births in the United States is approximately 12%. In addition, 18% of African American newborns are preterm (Vargo & Trottter, 2007). The rise in multiple birth rates has markedly influenced overall rates of low-birth-weight (LBW) infants. Prematurity and low birth weight are common in single women and adolescents. (See Chapter 16 for a discussion of preterm labor.)

The major problem of the preterm newborn is the variable immaturity of all systems. The degree of immaturity depends on the length of gestation. The preterm newborn must traverse the same complex, interconnected pathways from intrauterine to extrauterine life as the term newborn. Immaturity means the premature newborn is ill equipped to make this transition smoothly.

ALTERATION IN RESPIRATORY AND CARDIAC PHYSIOLOGY

The preterm newborn is at risk for respiratory problems because the lungs are not fully mature and not fully ready to take over the

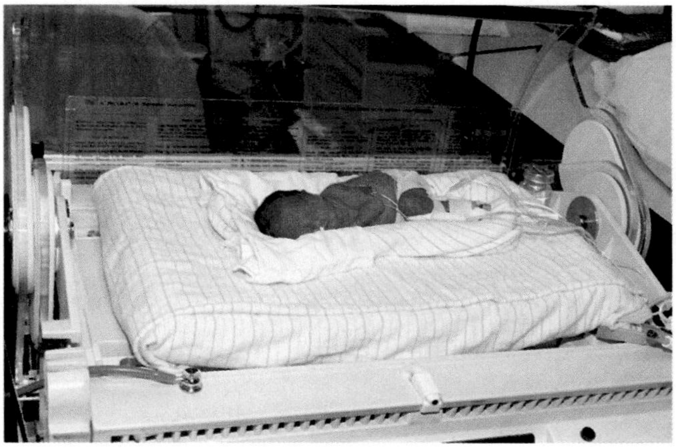

● **Figure 28–6** A 6-day-old, 28-week gestational age, 960 g preterm infant.

Source: Courtesy of Carol Harrigan, RNC, MSN, NNP.

process of oxygen and carbon dioxide exchange without assistance until 37 to 38 weeks' gestation. Critical factors in the development of respiratory distress include the following:

1. The preterm infant is unable to produce adequate amounts of surfactant. (See Chapter 24 for discussion of respiratory adaptation and development.) Inadequate surfactant lessens compliance (ability of the lung to fill with air easily), thereby increasing the inspiratory pressure needed to expand the lungs with air. The collapsed (or atelectatic) alveoli will not facilitate an exchange of oxygen and carbon dioxide. As a result, the infant becomes hypoxic, pulmonary blood flow is inefficient, and the preterm newborn's available energy is depleted.
2. The muscular coat of pulmonary blood vessels is incompletely developed. Because of this, the pulmonary arterioles do not constrict as well in response to decreased oxygen levels. This lowered pulmonary vascular resistance leads to left-to-right shunting of blood through the ductus arteriosus, which increases the blood flow back into the lungs.
3. Normally the ductus arteriosus responds to increasing oxygen levels and prostaglandin E levels by vasoconstriction; in the preterm infant, who is more susceptible to hypoxia, the ductus may remain open. A patent ductus increases the blood volume to the lungs, causing pulmonary congestion, increased respiratory effort, carbon dioxide retention, and bounding femoral pulses.

The common complications of the cardiopulmonary system in preterm infants are discussed later in this chapter and in Chapter 29.

ALTERATION IN THERMOREGULATION

Heat loss is a major problem in preterm newborns that the nurse can do much to prevent. Two factors limiting heat production, however, are the availability of glycogen in the liver and the amount of brown fat available for heat production. Both of these limiting factors appear in the third trimester. In the cold-stressed baby, norepinephrine is released which in turn stimulates the metabolism of brown fat for heat production. As a complicating factor, the hypoxic newborn cannot increase oxygen consumption in response to cold stress because of the already limited reserves and thereby becomes progressively colder. Because the muscle mass is small in preterm infants, and muscular activity is diminished (they are unable to shiver), heat production is further limited.

Five physiologic and anatomic factors increase heat loss in the preterm infant:

1. The preterm baby has a higher ratio of body surface to body weight. This means that the baby's ability to produce heat (based on body weight) is much less than the potential for losing heat (based on surface area). The loss of heat in a preterm infant weighing 1500 g is five times greater per unit of body weight than in an adult.
2. The preterm baby has very little subcutaneous fat, which is the human body's insulation. Without adequate insulation, heat is easily conducted from the core of the body (warmer temperature) to the surface of the body (cooler temperature). Heat is lost from the body as the blood vessels, which lie close to the skin surface in the preterm infant, transport blood from the body core to the subcutaneous tissues.
3. The preterm baby has thinner, more permeable skin than the term infant. This increased permeability contributes to a greater insensible water loss as well as to heat loss.
4. The posture of the preterm baby influences heat loss. Flexion of the extremities decreases the amount of surface area exposed to the environment. Extension increases the surface area exposed to the environment and thus increases heat loss. The gestational age of the infant influences the amount of flexion, from completely hypotonic and extended at 28 weeks to strong flexion displayed by 36 weeks.
5. The preterm baby has a decreased ability to vasoconstrict superficial blood vessels and conserve heat in the body core.

In summary, gestational age is directly proportional to the ability to maintain thermoregulation; thus the more preterm the newborn, the less able the infant is to maintain heat balance. Preventing heat loss by providing a neutral thermal environment is one of the most important considerations in nursing management of the preterm infant (see "Maintenance of Neutral Thermal Environment" later in the chapter). Cold stress, with its accompanying severe complications, can be prevented (see Chapter 29).

ALTERATION IN GASTROINTESTINAL PHYSIOLOGY

The basic structure of the gastrointestinal (GI) tract is formed early in gestation. Maturation of the digestive and absorptive process is more variable, however, and occurs later in gestation. As a result of GI immaturity, the preterm newborn has the following ingestion, digestive, and absorption problems:

- A marked danger of aspiration and its associated complications because of the infant's poorly developed gag reflex, incompetent esophageal cardiac sphincter, and poor sucking and swallowing reflexes.
- Difficulty in meeting high caloric and fluid needs for growth because of small stomach capacity.
- Limited ability to convert certain essential amino acids to nonessential amino acids. Certain amino acids, such as histidine, taurine, and cysteine, are essential to the preterm infant but not to the term infant.
- Inability to handle the increased osmolarity of formula protein because of kidney immaturity. The preterm infant requires a higher concentration of whey protein than of casein.
- Difficulty absorbing saturated fats because of decreased bile salts and pancreatic lipase. Severe illness of the newborn may also prevent intake of adequate nutrients.

Evidence in Action

Studies support the use of probiotics (in forms that can be administered in small amounts) for the prevention of necrotizing enterocolitis in preterm infants (AlFaleh & Bassler, 2008; Zupancic, 2009).

- Difficulty with lactose digestion initially because processes may not be fully functional during the first few days of a preterm infant's life. The preterm newborn can digest and absorb most simple sugars.
- Deficiency of calcium and phosphorus may exist because two-thirds of these minerals are deposited in the last trimester. Rickets and significant bone demineralization caused by deficiency of calcium and phosphorus, which are deposited primarily in the last trimester, are also problems.
- Increased basal metabolic rate and increased oxygen requirements caused by fatigue associated with sucking.
- Feeding intolerance and necrotizing enterocolitis (NEC) as a result of diminished blood flow and tissue perfusion to the intestinal tract because of prolonged hypoxia and hypoxemia at birth.

ALTERATION IN RENAL PHYSIOLOGY

The kidneys of the preterm infant are immature compared with those of the full-term infant, which poses clinical problems in the management of fluid and electrolyte balance. Specific characteristics of the preterm infant include the following:

- The glomerular filtration rate (GFR) is lower because of decreased renal blood flow. The GFR is directly related to lower gestational age, so the more preterm the newborn, the lower the GFR. The GFR is also decreased in the presence of diseases or conditions that decrease the renal blood flow and perfusion, such as severe respiratory distress, hypotension, and asphyxia. Anuria and oliguria may also be observed.
- The preterm infant's kidneys are limited in their ability to concentrate urine or to excrete excess amounts of fluid. This means that if excess fluid is administered, the infant is at risk for fluid retention and overhydration. If too little is administered, the infant will become dehydrated because of the inability to retain adequate fluid.
- The preterm kidneys begin excreting glucose (glycosuria) at a lower serum glucose level than those of the term infant. Therefore, glycosuria with hyperglycemia can lead to osmotic diuresis and polyuria.
- The kidney's buffering capacity of the kidney is reduced, predisposing the infant to metabolic acidosis. Bicarbonate is excreted at a lower serum level, and acid is excreted more slowly. Therefore, after periods of hypoxia or insult, the preterm infant's kidneys require a longer time to excrete the lactic acid that accumulates. Sodium bicarbonate is frequently required to treat the metabolic acidosis.
- The immaturity of the renal system affects the preterm infant's ability to excrete drugs. Because excretion time is longer, many drugs are given over longer intervals (e.g., every 24 hours instead of every 12 hours). Urine output must be carefully monitored when the infant is receiving nephrotoxic drugs such as gentamicin and vancomycin. In the event that urine output is poor, drugs can become toxic in the infant much more quickly than in the adult.

ALTERATION IN IMMUNOLOGIC PHYSIOLOGY

The preterm infant is at a much greater risk for infection than the term infant. This increased susceptibility may be the result of an infection acquired in utero that may have precipitated preterm labor and birth. However, all preterm infants have immature specific and nonspecific immunity.

In utero the fetus receives passive immunity against a variety of infections from maternal IgG immunoglobulins, which cross the placenta (see Chapter 29 ∞). Because most of this immunity is acquired in the last trimester of pregnancy, the preterm infant has few antibodies at birth.

The other immunoglobulin significant for the preterm infant is secretory IgA, which does not cross the placenta but is found in breast milk in significant concentrations. Breast milk's secretory IgA provides immunity to the mucosal surfaces of the GI tract, protecting the newborn from enteric infections such as those caused by *Escherichia coli* and *Shigella*.

ALTERATION IN NEUROLOGIC PHYSIOLOGY

Because the period of most rapid brain growth and development occurs during the third trimester of pregnancy, the closer to term an infant is born, the better the neurologic prognosis. A common interruption of neurologic development in the preterm infant is caused by intraventricular hemorrhage (IVH) and intracranial hemorrhage (ICH). Hydrocephalus may develop as a consequence of an IVH caused by the obstruction at the cerebral aqueduct (Volpe, 2008).

ALTERATION IN REACTIVITY PERIODS AND BEHAVIORAL STATES

The newborn infant's response to extrauterine life is characterized by two periods of reactivity (see Chapter 24 ∞). The preterm infant's periods of reactivity are delayed. In the very ill infant, these periods of reactivity may not be observed at all because the infant may be hypotonic and unreactive for several days after birth. As the preterm newborn grows and the condition stabilizes, identifying behavioral states and traits unique to each infant becomes

Nursing Practice

The sudden onset of apnea and bradycardia, coupled with metabolic acidosis in an otherwise healthy, growing premature infant, may be suggestive of bacterial sepsis, especially if there is a central line present.

Teaching Highlights

OPTIMAL TIMING FOR TEACHING

After observing an infant's pattern of behavior and responses, especially the sleep-wake states, the nurse uses the time when the infant is alert and best able to attend to help parents learn about and provide newborn care and form a positive attachment with their child.

increasingly possible. In general, stable preterm infants do not demonstrate the same behavioral states as term infants. Preterm infants tend to be more disorganized in their sleep-wake cycles and are unable to attend as well to the human face and objects in the environment. Neurologically, their responses (sucking, muscle tone, states of arousal) are weaker than full-term infants' responses.

MANAGEMENT OF NUTRITION AND FLUID REQUIREMENTS

Early feedings are extremely valuable in maintaining normal metabolism and lowering the possibility of such complications as hypoglycemia, hyperbilirubinemia, and azotemia. However, the preterm infant is at risk for complications that may develop because of immaturity of the digestive system.

Nutritional Requirements

Oral (enteral) caloric intake necessary for growth in a healthy preterm newborn is 95 to 130 kcal/kg/day (Blackburn, 2007). In addition to these relatively high caloric needs, the preterm newborn requires more protein than the full-term infant. To meet these needs, many institutions use breast milk or special preterm formulas.

Whether breast milk or formula is used, feeding regimens are established based on the infant's weight and estimated stomach capacity (Table 28–1). Initial formula feedings are gradually increased as the infant tolerates them. It may be necessary to supplement oral feedings with parenteral fluids to maintain adequate hydration and caloric intake until the baby is on full oral feedings. Preterm infants who cannot tolerate any oral (enteral) feedings are given nutrition by total parenteral nutrition (TPN).

In addition to a higher calorie and protein formula, preterm infants should receive supplemental multivitamins, including vitamin A, D, and E, iron, and trace minerals. A diet high in polyunsaturated fats (which preterm infants tolerate best) increases the requirement for vitamin E. Preterm infants fed iron-fortified formulas have higher red cell hemolysis and lower vitamin E concentrations and thus require additional vitamin E. Preterm formulas also need to contain medium-chain triglycerides (MCT) and additional amino acids such as cysteine, as well as calcium, phosphorus, and vitamin D supplements to increase mineralization of bones. Nutritional intake is considered adequate when there is consistent weight gain of 20 to 30 g/day. Initially, no weight gain may be noted for several days, but total weight loss should not exceed 15% of the total birth weight or more than 1% to 2% per day. Some institutions add the criteria of head circumference growth and increase in body length of 1 cm (0.4 in.) per week, once the newborn is stable.

Methods of Feeding

The preterm infant is fed by various methods depending on the infant's gestational age, health and physical condition, and neurologic status. The three most common oral feeding methods are bottle, breast, and gavage.

Bottle-feeding. Preterm infants who have a coordinated as well as rhythmic suck-swallow-breathing pattern are usually between 35 and 36 weeks' postconceptual age and may be fed by bottle.

Table 28–1 Suggested Feeding Guidelines for the Preterm Infant

Weight	< 1000 Grams	1000 to 1500 Grams	1501 to 1800 Grams Sick†	1501 to 1800 Grams Healthy†	> 1800 grams sick†
Feeding interval	Every 3 hours	Every 3 hours	Every 3 hours	Every 3 hours	Every 3 hours
Beginning interval	10 to 20 mL/kg/d	10 to 20 mL/kg/d	10 to 20 mL/kg/d	20 to 40 mL/kg/d	20 to 40 mL/kg/d
Feeding increments (mL/kg/d)	10 to 20 mL/kg/d	15 to 20 mL/kg/d	20 to 30 mL/kg/d	30 to 50 mL/kg/d	30 to 75 mL/kg/d
Time required to attain full feedings	16 to 13 days	10 to 7 days	7 to 5 days	5 to 3 days	5 to 2 days
Advancement of feedings	■ Start infants on either full-strength human milk or 24 kcal/oz premature infant formula. ■ A full feeding is 120 kcal/kg/day of either a 24 kcal/oz formula or human milk. ■ Advance feedings to the next level only when the infant demonstrates the ability to tolerate enternal feedings. ■ If the caregiver observed clinical signs of feeding intolerances or illness, do not advance feedings.				
Other feeding instructions	■ Add fortifier to human milk when feeding advances to 100 to 120 mL/kg. ■ For an infant fed human milk at full feeds, add iron supplements at 2 to 4 mg/kg/day.				

†A *sick* infant is one who has had symptoms of any medical or surgical condition other than uncomplicated prematurity. A *healthy* term or preterm infant has had no symptomatic medical or surgical conditions.

Source: Adapted from *Neonatal nutrition survival guide for the practitioner* by Lisa R. Vanatta, MS, RD, CSP, Clinical Nutrition Services, Phoenix Children's Hospital.

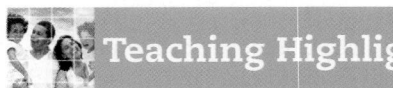

Oral readiness to feed is best described by the following behaviors: remaining engaged in the feeding, organizing oral-motor functioning, coordinating the suck-swallow-breath skill, and maintaining physiologic stability (Thomas, 2007). Those premature infants who root when their cheek is stroked and actively search for the nipple are neurodevelopmentally ready to initiate oral feeding. To avoid excessive expenditure of energy, a soft, yellow, single-hole nipple is usually used (milk flow is less rapid). The infant is fed in a semisitting position and burped gently after each ½ to 1 oz. The feeding should take no longer than 15 to 20 minutes (nippling requires more energy than other methods). Premature infants who are progressing from gavage feedings to bottle-feeding should start with one session of bottle-feeding a day and slowly increase the number of times a day a bottle is given until the baby tolerates all feedings from a bottle.

Sucking may be affected by age, asphyxia, sepsis, intraventricular hemorrhage, or other neurologic insult. Before initiating nipple feeding, the nurse observes for signs of stress, such as tachypnea (more than 60 respirations per minute), respiratory distress, or hypothermia, which may increase the risk of aspiration. During the feeding the nurse observes the infant for signs of feeding difficulty (tachypnea, cyanosis, bradycardia, lethargy, uncoordinated suck and swallow). Difficulty in bottle feeding is often associated with a milk bolus that is too large for the infant's oral cavity that can lead to aspiration. Demand feeding protocols, based on the infant's hunger cues, should be considered for a growing premature infant only when there is sufficient caloric intake to promote consistent weight gain (Kenner & Lott, 2007).

Breastfeeding. Mothers who wish to breastfeed their preterm infants are given the opportunity to put the infant to the breast as soon as the infant has demonstrated a coordinated suck and swallow reflex, is showing consistent weight gain, and can control body temperature outside of the incubator, regardless of weight. Preterm infants tolerate breastfeeding with higher transcutaneous oxygen pressures and better maintenance of body temperature than during bottle-feeding. Besides breast milk's many benefits for the infant, it allows the mother to contribute actively to the infant's well-being (Figure 28–7 ●). It is important for the nurse to be aware of the advantages of breastfeeding, as well as the possible disadvantages of breast milk as the sole source of food for the preterm infant (see Chapter 27∞).

By initiating skin-to-skin holding of premature infants in the early intensive care phase, mothers can significantly increase milk volume, thereby overcoming lactation problems (Turnage-Carrier, 2010). Many mothers of preterm infants seem to find the football hold position the most convenient breastfeeding for preterm infants. Feeding may take up to 45 minutes, and babies should be burped as they alternate breasts. The length of feeding time is monitored so that the preterm infant does not burn too many calories.

The nurse should coordinate a flexible feeding schedule so babies can nurse during alert times and be allowed to set their own pace. Feedings should be on demand, but a maximum number of hours between feedings should be set. The mother begins with one feeding at the breast and then gradually increases the number of times during the day that the baby breastfeeds. Even if the infant cannot be put to the breast, mothers can pump their breasts, and the breast milk can be given via gavage. Use of the double-pumping system produces higher levels of prolactin than sequential pumping of the breasts. When breastfeeding is not possible because the infant is too small or too weak to suck at the breast, an option for the mother may be to express her breast milk into a cup. The milk touches the infant's lips and is lapped by the protruding motions of the tongue.

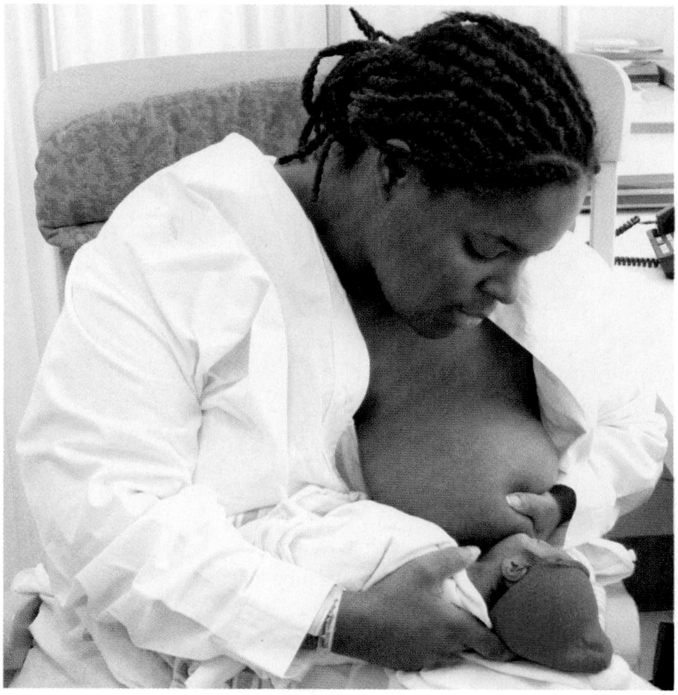

● **Figure 28–7** Breastfeeding. This mother is breastfeeding her premature infant.

Gavage feeding. The gavage feeding method is used with preterm infants (less than 34 weeks' gestation) who lack or have a poorly coordinated suck and swallow reflex or are ill and ventilator dependent. Gavage feeding may be used as an adjunct to nipple feeding if the infant tires easily or as an alternative if an infant is losing weight because of the energy expenditure required for nippling (see Clinical Skills Manual: Performing Gavage Feeding SKILLS). Gavage feedings are administered by either the nasogastric or orogastric route and by intermittent bolus or continuous drip method (Figures 28–8 and 28–9 ●). Currently, there are no conclusive studies supporting one method (bolus versus

Nursing Practice

For an otherwise healthy, growing, premature infant who is receiving total enteral intake and has started to experience apnea and bradycardia, one differential diagnosis to think about is reflux rather than sepsis, although sepsis may need to be ruled out.

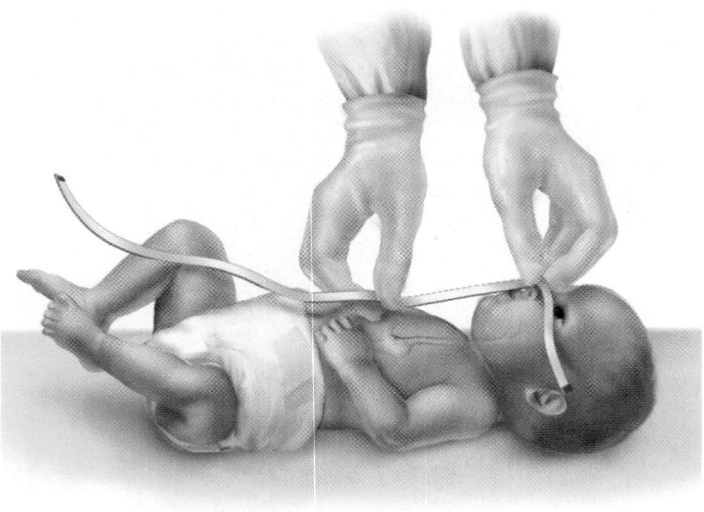

● **Figure 28–8** Measuring gavage tube length.

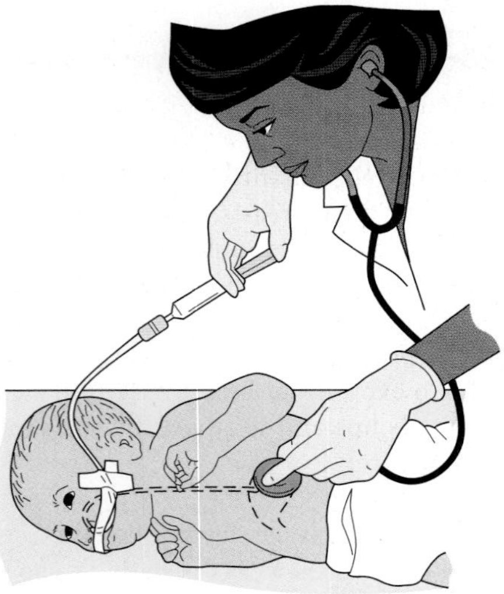

● **Figure 28–9** Auscultation for placement of gavage tube.

continuous) over the other. In common practice, bolus feedings are usually initiated, but if intolerance occurs, then the feedings are changed to continuous (Kenner & Lott, 2007).

Early initiation of minimal enteral nutrition (MEN) via gavage is now advocated as a supplement to parenteral nutrition. MEN refers to small-volume feedings of formula or human milk (usually less than 24 mL/kg/day) which are designed to "prime" the intestinal tract, thereby stimulating many of its hormonal and enzymatic functions (AAP & ACOG, 2007; Kenner & Lott, 2007). Benefits of early feeding (as early as 24 to 72 hours of life) include the following: no increased incidence in NEC; fewer days on TPN, thereby decreasing the incidence of cholestatic jaundice; increased weight gain; increased muscle maturation of the gut function which can lead to improved feeding tolerance; lower risk of osteopenia; and a possible decrease in the total number of hospital days in the NICU (Kenner & Lott, 2007). TPN (total parenteral nutrition) provides complete nutrition and is used in situations that do not allow feeding the infant through the GI tract.

> **Nursing Practice**
>
> Orogastric gavage catheter placement is preferable to nasogastric because most infants are obligatory nose breathers. If nasogastric is used, a #5 French catheter should be used to minimize airway obstruction.

Fluid Requirements

The calculation of fluid requirements must take into account the infant's weight and postnatal age. Recommendations for fluid therapy in the preterm infant are approximately 80 to 100 mL/kg/day for day 1, 100 to 120 mL/kg/day for day 2, and 120 to 150 mL/kg/day by day 3 of life. These amounts may be increased up to 200 mL/kg/day if the infant is very small, receiving phototherapy, or under a radiant warmer because of the increased insensible water losses. Fluid losses can be minimized through the use of heat shields and added humidification in the incubator. Daily weights, and sometimes twice-a-day weights, are the best indicator of fluid status in the preterm infant. The expected weight loss during the first 3 to 5 days of life in a preterm infant is 15% to 20% of birth weight.

COMMON COMPLICATIONS OF PRETERM NEWBORNS AND THEIR CLINICAL MANAGEMENT

The goals of medical and nursing care are to meet the preterm infant's growth and development needs and to anticipate and manage the complications associated with prematurity. The most common complications associated with prematurity are as follows:

1. *Apnea of prematurity.* Apnea of prematurity refers to cessation of breathing for 20 seconds or longer or for less than 20 seconds when associated with cyanosis, pallor, and bradycardia. Apnea is a common problem in the preterm infant presenting between day 2 and day 7 of life. The etiology of apnea is multifactorial but is thought to be primarily a result of neuronal immaturity, a factor that contributes to the preterm infant's irregular breathing patterns (central apnea). Obstructive apnea can occur when there is cessation of airflow associated with blockage

> **Nursing Practice**
>
> A growing premature infant showing clinical signs of worsening respiratory status (e.g., increased oxygen needs, increased ventilatory settings), acidosis, and hypotension may be exhibiting signs and symptoms of a PDA.

of the upper airway (small airway diameter, increased pharyngeal secretions, altered body alignment and positioning). Gastroesophageal reflux (GER) is defined as a movement of gastric contents into the lower esophagus caused by poor esophageal sphincter tone, causing laryngospasm, which leads to bradycardia and apnea. Apnea of prematurity is then a diagnosis of exclusion.

2. *Patent ductus arteriosus (PDA).* The ductus arteriosus fails to close because of decreased pulmonary arteriole musculature and hypoxemia. Symptomatic PDA is often seen around the time when premature infants are recovering from RDS. Patent ductus arteriosus often prolongs the course of illness in a preterm newborn and leads to chronic pulmonary dysfunction. Premature infants who are being treated for complications such as respiratory distress syndrome or patent ductus arteriosus may be on diuretics that can influence their fluid requirements.
3. *Respiratory distress syndrome (RDS).* Respiratory distress results from inadequate surfactant production (see Chapter 29).
4. *Intraventricular hemorrhage (IVH).* Intraventricular hemorrhage is the most common type of intracranial hemorrhage in small preterm infants, especially those weighing less than 1500 g or of less than 34 weeks' gestation. Up to 34 weeks' gestation the preterm's brain ventricles are lined by the germinal matrix, which is highly susceptible to hypoxic events such as respiratory distress, birth trauma, and birth asphyxia. The germinal matrix is highly vascular, and these blood vessels rupture in the presence of hypoxia.
5. *Anemia of prematurity.* The preterm infant is at risk for anemia because of the rapid rate of growth required, shorter red blood cell life, excessive blood sampling, decreased iron stores, and deficiency of vitamin E. The hemoglobin usually reaches its lowest level by 3 to 12 weeks and remains low for 3 to 6 months.

Other common problems of preterm infants such as NEC are briefly discussed earlier in the physiologic sections. (For an in-depth discussion of RDS, hyperbilirubinemia, hypoglycemia, and sepsis, see Chapter 29.)

LONG-TERM NEEDS AND OUTCOME

The care of preterm infants and their families does not stop on discharge from the nursery. Follow-up care is extremely important because many developmental problems are not noted until an infant is older and begins to demonstrate motor delays or sensory disability.

Nursing Practice

An extremely premature, low-birth-weight infant who presents with a sudden drop in hemoglobin along with the onset of severe metabolic acidosis, a "waxy" color, and hypotension may have experienced an intracranial hemorrhage.

Within the first year of life, low-birth-weight preterm infants face higher mortality rates than term infants. Causes of death include sudden infant death syndrome (SIDS)—which occurs about five times more frequently in the preterm infant—respiratory infections, and neurologic defects. Morbidity is also much higher among preterm infants, with those weighing less than 1500 g at highest risk for long-term complications.

The most common long-term needs observed in preterm infants include the following:

- *Retinopathy of prematurity (ROP).* Premature newborns are particularly susceptible to characteristic retinal changes, known as ROP, which can result in visual impairment. Increased survival of very-low-birth-weight (VLBW) infants may be the most important factor in the increased incidence of ROP.
- *Bronchopulmonary dysplasia (BPD).* Long-term lung disease is a result of damage to the alveolar epithelium secondary to positive pressure respirator therapy and high oxygen concentration. These infants have long-term dependence on oxygen therapy and an increased incidence of respiratory infection during their first few years of life.
- *Neurologic problems.* The most common neurologic defects include cerebral palsy, hydrocephalus, seizure disorders, lower IQ, and learning disabilities. However, the socioeconomic climate and family support systems are extremely important influences on the child's ultimate school performance in the absence of major neurologic defects.
- *Auditory problems.* Preterm infants have a 1% to 4% incidence of moderate to profound hearing loss and should have a formal audiologic exam before discharge and at 3 to 6 months (corrected age). Any infant with repeated abnormal results should be referred to speech-and-language specialists.
- *Speech problems.* The most frequently observed speech defects involve delayed development of receptive and expressive ability that may persist into the school-age years.

When evaluating the infant's abilities and disabilities, parents must understand that developmental progress must be evaluated based on chronological age from the expected date of birth, not from the actual date of birth (corrected age). In addition, the parents need the consistent support of healthcare professionals in the long-term management of their infants. Many new and ongoing concerns arise as the high-risk infant grows and develops; the goal is to promote the highest quality of life possible.

NURSING MANAGEMENT

NURSING ASSESSMENT AND DIAGNOSIS

The nurse needs to assess the physical characteristics and gestational age of the preterm newborn accurately to anticipate the special needs and problems of the baby. Physical characteristics vary greatly depending on gestational age, but the following characteristics are frequently present:

- *Color* is usually pink or ruddy but may show acrocyanosis. (Cyanosis, jaundice, and pallor are abnormal and should be noted.)
- *Skin* is reddened and translucent, blood vessels are readily apparent, there is little subcutaneous fat.
- *Lanugo* is plentiful and widely distributed.
- *Head size* appears large in relation to the body.
- *Skull bones* are pliable; fontanelle is smooth and flat.
- *Ears* have minimal cartilage and are pliable, folded over.
- *Nails* are soft, short.
- *Genitals* are small; testes may not be descended and scrotum nonrugated; clitoris and labia minora are prominent.
- *Resting position* is flaccid, froglike.
- *Cry* is weak, feeble.
- *Reflexes* (sucking, swallowing, gag) are poor.
- *Activity* consists of jerky, generalized movements. (Seizure activity is abnormal.)

Determining gestational age in preterm newborns requires knowledge and experience in administering gestational assessment tools. The tool used should be specific, reliable, and valid. (For a discussion of gestational age assessment tools, see Chapter 25∞.)

Nursing diagnoses that may apply to the preterm newborn include the following:

- *Impaired Gas Exchange* related to immature pulmonary vasculature and inadequate surfactant production
- *Ineffective Breathing Pattern* related to immature central nervous system
- *Altered Nutrition: Less than Body Requirements* related to weak suck and swallow reflexes and decreased ability to absorb nutrients
- *Ineffective Thermoregulation* related to hypothermia secondary to decreased glycogen and brown fat stores
- *Fluid Volume Deficit* related to high insensible water losses and inability of kidneys to concentrate urine
- *Ineffective Family Coping* related to anger or guilt at having given birth to a premature baby

PLANNING AND IMPLEMENTATION

MAINTENANCE OF RESPIRATORY FUNCTION

Preterm newborns have an increased danger of respiratory obstruction because their bronchi and trachea are so narrow that mucus can obstruct the airway. The nurse must maintain patency through judicious suctioning, but only on an as-needed basis.

Positioning can also affect respiratory function. If the baby is in the supine position, the nurse should slightly elevate the infant's head to maintain the airway, being careful to avoid hyperextension of the neck because the trachea will collapse. Also, because the newborn has weak neck muscles and cannot control head movement, the nurse should ensure that this head position is maintained by placing a small roll under the shoulders. Because the prone position splints the chest wall and decreases the amount of respiratory effort used to move the chest wall, it facilitates chest expansion and improves air entry and oxygenation. Weak or absent cough or gag reflexes increase the chance of aspiration in the premature newborn. The nurse should ensure that the infant's position facilitates drainage of mucus or regurgitated formula.

Monitors heart and respiratory rates with cardiorespiratory monitors and observes the newborn to identify alterations in cardiopulmonary status. Signs of respiratory distress include the following:

- Cyanosis (serious sign when generalized)
- Tachypnea (sustained respiratory rate greater than 60/minute after first 4 hours of life)
- Retractions
- Expiratory grunting
- Nasal flaring
- Apneic episodes
- Presence of rales or rhonchi on auscultation
- Diminished air entry

If respiratory distress occurs, the nurse administers oxygen per physician or nurse practitioner order to relieve hypoxemia. If hypoxemia is not treated immediately, it may result in patent ductus arteriosus or metabolic acidosis. If oxygen is administered to the newborn, the nurse monitors the oxygen concentration with devices such as the transcutaneous oxygen monitor ($tcPO_2$) or the pulse oximeter. Periodic arterial blood gas sampling to monitor oxygen concentration in the baby's blood is essential because hyperoxemia may lead to ROP.

The nurse also needs to consider respiratory function before initiation of feedings as well as during feeding. To prevent aspiration as well as increased energy expenditure and oxygen consumption, the nurse must ensure that the infant's gag and suck reflexes are intact before starting oral feedings.

MAINTENANCE OF NEUTRAL THERMAL ENVIRONMENT

Providing a neutral thermal environment minimizes the oxygen consumption required to maintain a normal core temperature; it also prevents cold stress and facilitates growth by decreasing the calories needed to maintain body temperature. The preterm infant's immature central nervous system, as well as small brown fat stores, provides poor temperature control. A small infant (less than 1200 g) can lose 80 kcal/kg/day through radiation of body heat. Implement all the usual thermoregulation measures discussed in Chapter 26∞.

In addition, to minimize heat loss and temperature instability effects:

1. Allow skin-to-skin contact between mother and newborn to maintain warmth and faster security (see kangaroo care, described later).

2. Warm and humidify oxygen to minimize evaporative heat loss and decrease oxygen consumption.
3. Place the baby in a double-walled incubator or use a Plexiglas heat shield over small preterm infants in single-walled incubators to avoid radiative heat losses. Some institutions use radiant warmers and plastic wrap over the baby and pipe in humidity (swamping). Use warmed ambient humidity. Humidity can decrease insensible and transdermal water loss especially in VLBW infants (Blackburn, 2007). Do not use Plexiglas shields on radiant warmer beds because they block the infrared heat.
4. Avoid placing the baby on cold surfaces such as metal treatment tables and cold x-ray plates (conductive heat loss). Pad cold surfaces with diapers and use radiant warmers during procedures, place the preterm infant on prewarmed mattresses, and warm hands before handling the baby to prevent heat transfer via conduction.
5. Keep the skin dry (evaporative heat loss) and place a cap on the baby's head. The head makes up 25% of the total body size.
6. Keep radiant warmers, incubators, and cribs away from windows and cold external walls (radiative heat loss) and out of drafts (conductive heat loss).
7. Open incubator portholes and doors only when necessary, and use plastic sleeves on portholes to decrease convective heat loss.
8. Use a skin probe to monitor the baby's skin temperature. Correlate ambient temperatures with the skin probe in the incubator using the servocontrol rather than the manual mode. The temperature should be 36°C to 37°C (96.8°F to 98.6°F). Temperature fluctuations indicate hypothermia or hyperthermia. Be careful not to place skin temperature probes over bony prominences, areas of brown fat, poorly vasoreactive areas such as extremities, or excoriated areas.
9. Warm formula or stored breast milk before feeding.
10. Use reflector patch over the skin temperature probe when using a radiant warmer bed so that the probe does not sense the higher infrared temperature as the baby's skin temperature and therefore decrease the heater output.

Once preterm infants are medically stable, they can be clothed with a double-thickness cap, cotton shirt, and diaper and, if possible, swaddled in a blanket. The nurse should be familiar with the individual institution's protocol for weaning preterm infants to a crib.

Evidence in Action

Preventing hypothermia in preterm infants can be achieved with the use of plastic wraps, heated mattresses, and skin-to-skin contact and should be considered in the care of these infants (Cochrane Review) (McCall, Alderdice, Halliday, et al., 2008).

MAINTENANCE OF FLUID AND ELECTROLYTE STATUS

Keep the newborn hydrated by providing adequate intake based on weight, gestational age, chronologic age, and volume of sensible and insensible water losses. Adequate fluid intake should compensate for increased insensible losses and the amount needed for renal excretion of metabolic products. Insensible water losses can be minimized by providing high ambient humidity, humidifying oxygen, using heat shields, covering the skin with plastic wrap, and placing the infant in a double-walled incubator.

Evaluate the hydration status of the baby by assessing and recording signs of dehydration such as:

- Sunken fontanelle
- Loss of weight
- Poor skin turgor (skin returns to position slowly when squeezed gently)
- Dry oral mucous membranes
- Decreased urine output
- Increased specific gravity (greater than 1.013)

The nurse must also identify signs of overhydration by observing the newborn for edema or excessive weight gain and by comparing urine output with fluid intake.

The nurse weighs the preterm infant at least once daily at the same time each day. *Weight change is one of the most sensitive indicators of fluid balance.* Weighing diapers is also important for accurate input and output measurement (1 mL = 1 g). A comparison of intake and output measurements over an 8- or 24-hour period provides important information about renal function and fluid balance. Assessment of patterns and whether they show a net gain or loss over several days is also essential to fluid management. In addition, the nurse monitors blood serum levels and pH to evaluate for electrolyte imbalances.

Accurate hourly intake calculations are needed when administering intravenous fluids. Because the preterm infant is unable to excrete excess fluid, it is essential that the nurse maintain the correct amount of IV fluid to prevent overload. Accuracy can be ensured by using neonatal or pediatric infusion pumps. To prevent electrolyte imbalance and dehydration, take care to give the correct intravenous (IV) solutions, as well as the correct volumes and concentrations of formulas. Urine-specific gravity and pH are obtained periodically. Hydration is considered adequate when the urine output is 1 to 3 mL/kg/hr.

PROVISION OF ADEQUATE NUTRITION AND PREVENTION OF FATIGUE DURING FEEDING

The feeding method depends on the preterm newborn's feeding abilities and health status. Both nipple and gavage methods are initially supplemented with intravenous therapy until oral intake is sufficient to support growth (110 to 130 kcal/kg/day). Early, small-volume enteral feedings called *minimal enteral nutrition via gavage* have proved to be of benefit to the very-low-birth-weight infant (see "Methods of Feeding" earlier in the chapter). Formula or breast milk (with or without fortifiers to increase caloric

Nursing Practice

Residual feeding may indicate early NEC and should be called to the attention of the clinician.

content) is incorporated into the feedings slowly. This is done to avoid overtaxing the digestive capacity of the preterm newborn. Carefully watch for other signs of feeding intolerance including guaiac-positive stools (occult blood in stools, lactose in the stools (reducing substance in the stools), vomiting, and diarrhea.

Before each feeding, the nurse measures abdominal girth and auscultates the abdomen to determine the presence and quality of bowel sounds. Such assessments permit early detection of abdominal distention, visible bowel loops, and decreased peristaltic activity, which may indicate necrotizing enterocolitis (NEC) or paralytic ileus. The nurse also checks for residual formula in the stomach before feeding when the newborn is fed by gavage. This procedure also can be performed when the nipple-fed newborn presents with abdominal distention. The presence of increasing residual formula is an indication of intolerance to the type or amount of feeding or the increase in amount of feeding.

Preterm newborns who are ill or who fatigue easily with nipple feedings are usually fed by gavage. The infant is essentially passive with these methods, thus conserving energy and calories. As the baby matures, gavage feedings are replaced with nipple (breast or formula) feedings to assist in strengthening the sucking reflex and in meeting oral and emotional needs. Signs that indicate readiness for oral feedings are a strong gag reflex, presence of nonnutritive sucking, and rooting behavior. Both low-birth-weight and preterm infants nipple-feed more effectively in a quiet state. The nurse establishes a gradual nipple-feeding program, such as one nipple feeding per day, then one nipple feeding per shift, and then a nipple feeding every other feeding. Daily weights are monitored because often there is a small weight loss when nipple feedings are started. After feedings, the nurse places the baby on the right side (with support to maintain this position) or on the abdomen. These positions facilitate gastric emptying and decrease the chance of aspiration if regurgitation occurs. Gastroesophageal reflux is not uncommon in preterm newborns. Long-term gavage feeding may create nipple aversion that will require developmental occupational therapy interventions.

The nurse involves the parents in feeding their preterm baby (Figure 28–10 ●). This is essential to the development of attachment between parents and infant. In addition, it increases parental knowledge about the care of their infant and helps them cope with the situation.

PREVENTION OF INFECTION

The nurse is responsible for minimizing the preterm newborn's exposure to pathogenic organisms. The preterm newborn is susceptible to infection because of an immature immune system and thin and permeable skin. Invasive procedures, techniques such as umbilical catheterization and mechanical ventilation, and prolonged hospitalization place the infant at greater risk for infection.

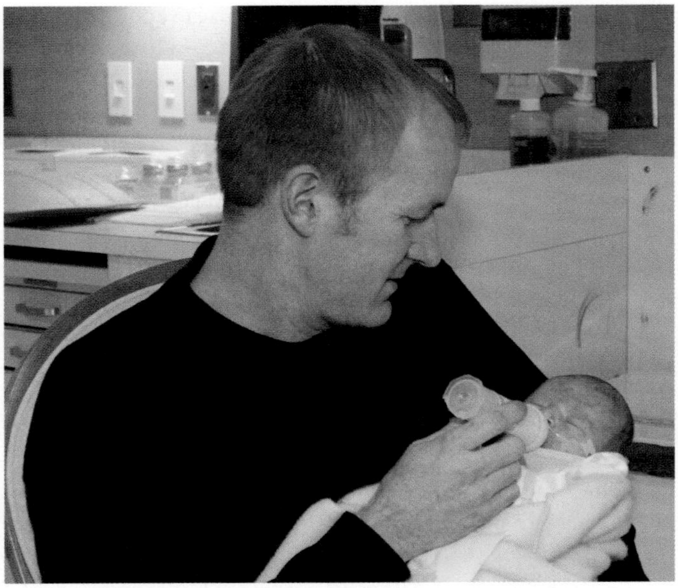

● **Figure 28–10** Father participating in feeding experience with his premature infant.

Strict handwashing and use of separate equipment for each infant help minimize the preterm newborn's exposure to infectious agents. Most nurseries have adopted the Centers for Disease Control and Prevention (CDC) standard precautions of isolating every baby and the Joint Commission on Accreditation of Healthcare Organization (JCAHO) requirement that staff members have short-trimmed nails and no artificial nails. Staff members are required to complete a 2- to 3-minute scrub using iodine-containing antibacterial solutions, which inhibit growth of gram-positive cocci and gram-negative rod organisms. Other specific nursing interventions include limiting visitors, requiring visitors to wash their hands, maintaining strict aseptic practices when changing IV tubing and solutions (IV solutions and tubing should be changed every 24 hours or per agency protocols), administering parenteral fluids, and assisting with sterile procedures. Incubators and radiant warmers should be changed weekly. The nurse prevents pressure-area breakdown by changing the baby's position regularly, doing range of motion exercises, and using water-bed pillows or an air mattress. To avoid skin tears, a protective transparent covering can be applied over vulnerable joints; however, this method is used sparingly (Blackburn, 2007). Chemical skin preps and tape may cause skin trauma and should be avoided as much as possible.

If infection (sepsis) occurs in the preterm newborn, the nurse may be the first to identify its subtle clinical signs, such as lethargy and increased episodes of apnea and bradycardia. The nurse informs the clinician of the findings immediately and implements the treatment plan per clinician orders in the presence of infection. (For specific nursing care required for the newborn with an infection, see Chapter 29∞.)

PROMOTION OF PARENT-INFANT ATTACHMENT

Preterm newborns can be separated from their parents for prolonged periods after illness or complications that are detected in the first few hours or days following birth. The resultant interruption in parent-newborn bonding necessitates intervention to ensure successful attachment.

Nurses need to take measures to promote positive parental feelings toward the preterm newborn. They can give photographs of the baby to parents to take home. These can also be given to the mother if she is in a different hospital or too ill to come to the nursery and visit. The infant's first name is placed on the incubator as soon as it is known to help the parents feel that their infant is a unique and special person. Parents are given a weekly card with the baby's footprint, weight, and length. The parents are also given the telephone number of the nursery or intensive care unit and the names of staff members so that parents have access to information about their baby at any time of the day or night. Visits from siblings and grandparents are encouraged to foster attachment.

Early involvement in the care of and decisions about their baby provides the parents with realistic expectations for their baby. The individual personality characteristics of the infant and the parents influence the bonding and contribute to the interactive process for the family. By observing each infant's patterns of behavior and responses, especially sleep-wake states, the nurse can teach parents optimal times for interacting with their infants. Parents need education to develop caregiving skills and to understand the premature infant's behavioral characteristics. Their daily participation (if possible) is encouraged, as are early and frequent visits. The nurse should provide opportunities for parents to touch, hold, talk to, and care for the baby. Skin-to-skin holding *(kangaroo care)* helps parents feel close to their small infant (Figure 28–11 ●). Kangaroo care has been shown to improve sleep periods and parents' perception of their caregiving ability (Turnage-Carrier, 2010). (See "Complementary Care: Complementary and Alternative Medicine (CAM) in the NICU" on page 685.)

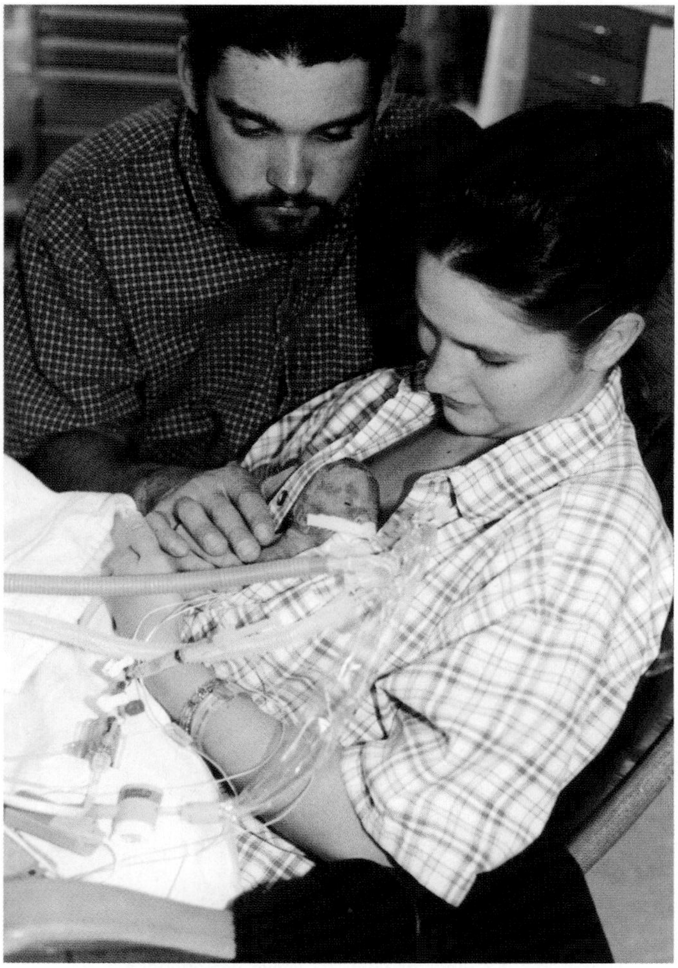

● **Figure 28–11** Kangaroo (skin-to-skin) care facilitates closeness and attachment between parents and their premature infant.

Source: Courtesy of Carol Harrigan, RNC, MSN, NNP.

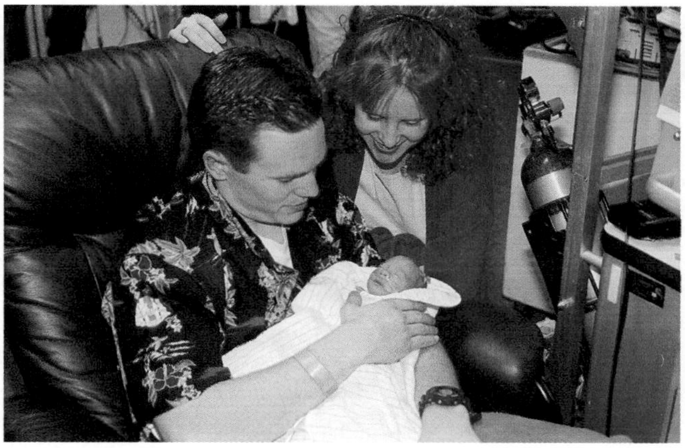

● **Figure 28–12** Family bonding occurs when parents have opportunities to spend time with their infant.

Source: Courtesy of Carol Harrigan, RNC, MSN, NNP.

The parents and nurse can plan nursing care around the times when the infant is alert and best able to attend. The more knowledge parents have about the meaning of their infant's responses, behaviors, and cues for interaction, the better prepared they will be able to meet their newborn's needs and form a positive attachment with their child. Parental involvement in difficult care decisions is essential and discussed in greater detail in Chapter 29∞.

Some parents may progress easily to touching and cuddling their infant; however, others will not. Parents need to know that their feelings are normal and that the progression of acquaintanceship is slow. Rooming-in can provide another opportunity for the stable preterm infant and family to get acquainted; it offers both privacy and readily available help (Figure 28–12 ●).

PROMOTION OF DEVELOPMENTALLY SUPPORTIVE CARE

Prolonged separation and the NICU environment necessitate individualized baby sensory stimulation programs. The nurse plays a key role in determining the appropriate type and amount of visual, tactile, and auditory stimulation.

Some preterm infants are not developmentally able to deal with more than one sensory input at a time. The Assessment of Preterm Infant Behavior (APIB) scale identifies individual preterm newborn behaviors according to five areas of development (Als, Lester, Tronick, et al., 1982). The preterm baby's behavioral reactions to stimulation are observed, and developmental interventions are then based on reducing detrimental environmental stimuli to

Evidence-Based Nursing

KANGAROO CARE

Clinical Question

Does kangaroo care—the skin-to-skin contact between mother and newborn—provide benefits for premature infants?

The Evidence

Ludington, Morgan, & Abouelfettoh (2008), nurse researchers, developed a clinical guideline based on extensive research focused on the physiologic, psychosocial, and behavioral effects of kangaroo care (KC.) This type of systematic review of the literature based on multiple studies is the strongest level of evidence for practice. The effects of KC appear universally beneficial for premature babies as well as their normal counterparts. Heart rate and respiratory rate are stable when premature babies are held in kangaroo care. Painful procedures such as heel sticks resulted in less cardiorespiratory instability when in KC than in the isolette. Oxygen saturation improved when in KC, and episodes of apnea decreased. There was no documented increase in nosocomial infections in the premature babies. Behaviorally, crying was reduced and positive sleep patterns enhanced with KC. Skin-to-skin contact improved breastfeeding success, enhanced neurobehavioral development, and enhanced parental bonding. Overall, when criteria for appropriateness are applied, kangaroo care is safe for premature babies.

Best Practice

Stable premature infants are eligible for kangaroo care, and its benefits are well supported. Stable means no deterioration of condition within the 24 hours preceding the Kangaroo Care. All neonatal lines and tubes must be well secured. Supplemental oxygen or CPAP are not contraindications for KC, and babies on ventilators can be eligible once they are past the first 24 hours and are stable. Some lines—such as arterial lines, thoracostomy tubes, and intracardiac lines—render the infant ineligible until removed. Parents should be educated about KC and its benefits, and their readiness assessed. Initially, KC should be given for at least an hour to allow the infant to complete a sleep cycle. After that, KC can be delivered at any time; continuous KC is acceptable.

Critical Thinking

How can the nurse help parents reduce their anxiety regarding transferring their premature infant from the isolette to their skin? What will be the elements of the patient education plan?

See MyNursingKit for possible responses.

the lowest possible level and providing appropriate opportunities for development (Blackburn, 2007).

Providing developmentally supportive, as well as family-centered, care has been proven to improve the outcomes of the critically ill newborn (Bowie, Hall, Faulkner, et al., 2003). With this in mind, specially designed NICUs with the single-room care concept are being developed to minimize lighting and noise as well as to provide privacy for the parents of the convalescing newborn.

The NICU environment contains many detrimental stimuli that the nurse can help reduce. Noise levels can be lowered by replacing alarms with lights or silencing alarms quickly and keeping conversations away from the baby's bedside. Dimmer switches should be used to shield the baby's eyes from bright lights, and blankets may be placed over the top portion of the incubator. Dimming the lights may encourage infants to open their eyes and be more responsive to their parents. Nursing care should be planned to decrease the number of times the baby is disturbed. Signs (e.g., "Quiet Please") can be placed near the bedside to allow the baby some periods of uninterrupted sleep (Blackburn, 2007). Some other suggested developmentally supportive interventions include the following:

- Facilitate handling by using containment measures when turning or moving the infant or doing procedures such as suctioning. Use the hands to hold the infant's arms and legs flexed close to the midline of the body. This helps stabilize the infant's motor and physiologic subsystems during stressful activities.
- Touch the infant gently and avoid sudden postural changes.
- Promote self-consoling and soothing activities, such as placing blanket rolls or approved manufactured devices next to the infant's sides and against the feet to provide "nesting." Swaddle the infant to maintain extremities in a flexed position while ensuring that the hands can reach the face. This permits the infant to do hand-to-mouth activities, which can be consoling (Figure 28–13 ●).
- Simulate the kinesthetic advantages of the intrauterine environment by using sheepskin and approved water beds. Water bed and pillow use has been reported to improve sleep and decrease motor activity as well as lead to more mature motor behavior, fewer state changes, and a decreased heart rate.

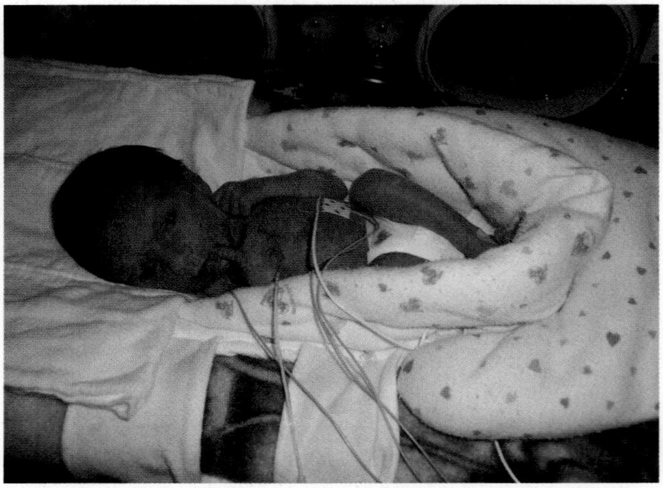

● **Figure 28–13** An 8-day-old, 30 weeks' gestational age, 860-gram IUGR infant is "nested." Hand-to-mouth behavior facilitates self-consoling and soothing activities.

Source: Courtesy of Carol Harrigan, RNC, MSN, NNP.

Complementary Care

COMPLEMENTARY AND ALTERNATIVE MEDICINE (CAM) IN THE NICU

As NICUs are becoming more and more "developmentally" friendly, complementary and alternative medicine (CAM) has become an adjunct to that nurturing environment. This holistic approach in caring for the low-birth-weight infant attempts not only to mimic the intrauterine environment, but also to foster parent-infant bonding by simultaneously caring for the body, spirit, and mind.

Aromatherapy is the use of scent to alter mood or behavior to produce a calming and sedating effect. There is an enhanced bonding process between mothers and newborns associated with the natural body odor emitted from the mother (Turnage-Carrier, 2010). Aromatherapy is utilized in the NICU by placing an article of clothing belonging to the mother next to the infant to produce a soothing and consoling effect on the infant in her absence. Researchers are also investigating other aromatherapies, including peppermint as a respiratory stimulant, chamomile as a method to regulate sleep–wake cycles, Brazilian guava for its analgesic effects, and lavender sitz baths for management of diaper rash.

Skin-to-skin (kangaroo) care is becoming more prevalent in NICUs across the United States. Skin-to-skin care is defined as the practice of holding infants skin-to-skin next to their parents. The infant is usually naked, except for a diaper, and placed on his/her parent's bare chest. They are then both covered with a blanket. Benefits of skin-to-skin care as a developmental intervention include the following: improved oxygenation as evidenced by an increase in transcutaneous oxygen levels, enhanced temperature regulation, a decline in the episodes of apnea and bradycardia, increased periods of quiet sleep, stabilization of vital signs, positive interaction between parent and infant that enhances attachment and bonding, increased growth parameters, and early discharge (Kledzik, 2005). Limitations to skin-to-skin care may be because of staff uneasiness when moving the infant while attached to multiple IV lines, monitor leads, and a ventilator. The limited confines of the nursery may be another limiting factor.

Infant massage and gentle human touch (GHT) have been practiced for many centuries. The types of stimulation include massage with stroking, gentle touch without stroking, and therapeutic touch or "hands on" containment. Practitioners report such physiologic benefits as stimulating blood and lymphatic flow, promoting weight gain in premature infants, and regulating sleep patterns (Turnage-Carrier, 2010). Many emotional and behavioral benefits are also cited by practitioners. Classes are available to teach parents how to perform massage on their infants. Massage demonstrates compassion while increasing the parent's empathy and understanding of the baby. It helps parents learn to interpret their baby's behavioral cues such as facial expression, various crying patterns, and other body language. At the same time it helps infants learn about their various body parts and boundaries and feel how they integrate into the whole. Therapeutic touch reduces motor activity and energy expenditure by the infant and also promotes comfort.

- Provide opportunities for nonnutritive sucking with a pacifier. This improves transcutaneous oxygen saturation; decreases body movements; improves sleep, especially after feedings; and increases weight gain.
- Provide objects for the infant to grasp (e.g., a piece of blanket, oxygen tubing, a finger) during caregiving. Grasping may comfort the baby.

Teaching the parents to read behavioral cues will help them move at their infant's own pace when providing stimulation. Parents are ideally equipped to meet the baby's need for stimulation. Stroking, rocking, cuddling, quiet singing, and talking to the baby can all be integral parts of the baby's care. Visual stimulation in the form of *en face* interaction with caregivers and mobiles is also important.

PREPARATION FOR HOME CARE

Parents are often anxious when their premature infant is transferred out of the NICU or is discharged home. Parents of preterm babies should receive the same postpartal teaching as any parent taking a new infant home. In preparing for discharge, the nurse encourages the parents to spend time caring directly for their baby. This familiarizes them with their baby's behavior patterns and helps them establish realistic expectations about the infant. Some hospitals have a special room near the nursery where parents can spend the night with their baby before discharge.

Discharge instruction includes breastfeeding and formula-feeding techniques, formula preparation, and vitamin administration. If the mother wishes to breastfeed, the nurse teaches her to pump her breasts to keep the milk flowing and provide milk even before discharge. Give information on bathing, diapering, hygiene, and normal elimination patterns and prepare the parents to expect changes in the color of the baby's stool, number of bowel movements, and timing of elimination if the infant is switched from formula to breast milk. This information can prevent unnecessary concern by the parents. The nurse also discusses normal growth and development patterns, reflexes, and activity for preterm infants. In these discussions, the nurse should emphasize ways to promote bonding behaviors and deal with newborn crying. Care of the preterm infant with complications, feeding problems, preventing infections, recognizing signs of a sick baby and the need for continued medical follow-up, and if the parents seem unable to cope with an at-risk baby are other key issues.

Parents of preterm infants can benefit from meeting with others in a similar situation to share common experiences and concerns. Nurses should refer parents to support groups sponsored by the hospital or by others in the community and make connections for parents with early education intervention centers.

Preterm and low-birth-weight infants are at greater risk of increased morbidity from vaccine-preventable diseases (AAP & ACOG, 2007). Preterm infants who weigh less than 2000 g that are medically stable and thriving do show consistently high rates of seroconversion following the first dose of hepatitis B vaccine even when the first dose is given as early as 1 month after birth (AAP & ACOG, 2007). The medically stable preterm infant and LBW infant should receive full doses of diphtheria, tetanus, acellular pertussis, *Haemophilus influenzae* type b, poliovirus, and pneumococcal conjugate vaccines at a chronologic age consistent with the schedule recommended for full-term infants (AAP & ACOG, 2007). The influenza vaccine should be administered at 6 months of age before the beginning of and during the influenza season. Palivizumab for respiratory syncytial (RSV) should be administered during the local RSV season and before hospital discharge to preterm newborns born at less than 35 weeks of gestation as well as those with BPD or congenital heart disease (AAP & ACOG, 2007). Immunoprophylaxis should be continued on a monthly basis until the local RSV season ends.

EVALUATION

Expected outcomes of nursing care include the following:

- The preterm newborn is free of respiratory distress and establishes effective respiratory function.
- The preterm newborn gains weight and shows no signs of fatigue or aspiration during feedings.
- The preterm newborn demonstrates a serial head circumference growth rate of 1 cm (0.4 in.) per week.
- The parents are able to verbalize their anger and guilt feelings about the birth of a preterm baby and show attachment behavior such as frequent visits and growing confidence in their participatory care activities.

CARE OF THE NEWBORN WITH CONGENITAL ANOMALIES

The birth of a baby with a congenital defect places both newborn and family at risk. Many congenital anomalies can be life threatening if not corrected within hours after birth; others are very visible and cause the families emotional distress. When one congenital anomaly is found, healthcare providers should look for others, particularly in body systems that develop at the same time during gestation. Table 28–2 identifies common anomalies and their early management and nursing care in the newborn period.

CARE OF THE INFANT OF A SUBSTANCE-ABUSING MOTHER

An **infant of a substance-abusing mother (ISAM)** may also be alcohol or drug dependent. After birth, when an infant's connection with the maternal blood supply is severed, the newborn may suffer withdrawal. In addition, the drugs ingested by the mother may be teratogenic, resulting in congenital anomalies or in developmental problems.

ALCOHOL DEPENDENCE

The **fetal alcohol syndrome (FAS),** a leading cause of mental retardation that is potentially preventable, includes a group of physical, behavioral, and cognitive abnormalities frequently found in infants exposed to alcohol in utero (Pitts, 2010). It is estimated that complete FAS occurs in 0.5 to 2 per 1000 live births annually in the United States (Pitts, 2010). FAS rates are higher among Native Americans, Alaska natives, African Americans, and women of low socioeconomic status. Children exposed to binge drinking are 1.7 times more likely to have mental retardation and 2.5 times more likely to demonstrate delinquent behavior than unexposed children (Wisner, Sit, Reynolds, et al., 2007).

A new set of guidelines for diagnosis and referral of infants and children with FAS have been developed (Pitts, 2010). The term *fetal alcohol effects* (FAE) was used to describe children who had some, but not all, of the characteristics of FAS; however, it was vague. Recently the term **fetal alcohol spectrum disorder (FASD)** has been used to include all categories of prenatal alcohol exposure, including FAS. FASD, however, is an umbrella term and not meant to be used as a clinical diagnosis. The new diagnostic categories for FAS take into consideration the various clinical manifestations of FAS, the social and family environment, and, if available, the maternal alcohol history. Five diagnostic categories are used to describe effects of alcohol exposure:

1. FAS with a confirmed history of maternal alcohol intake.
2. FAS with phenotypic features but no confirmed history of maternal alcohol intake.
3. Partial FAS with confirmed history of maternal alcohol intake, some facial abnormalities, and one of the following: CNS abnormalities, growth restriction, or behavioral or cognitive disabilities.
4. *Alcohol-related birth defects (ARBD)* are usually determined only by a positive maternal drinking history. They present with one or more birth defects including malformations and dysplasias of the heart, bone, kidney, vision, or hearing systems and do not exhibit the classic facial dysmorphology of the FAS infant (Pitts, 2010).
5. *Alcohol related neurodevelopmental disorder (ARND).* These children have CNS neurodevelopmental abnormalities and complex behavior and cognitive abnormalities (Pitts, 2010). ARBD and ARND can both occur together.

Although it is known that ethanol freely crosses the placenta to the fetus, it is still not known whether the alcohol alone or the breakdown products of alcohol cause the damage. (Chapter 15 ∞ discusses alcohol abuse in pregnancy.) The effects of other substances often combined with alcohol, such as nicotine, diazepam (Valium), marijuana, and caffeine, as well as poor diet, enhance the likelihood of FAS.

Long-Term Complications for the Infant with FAS

The long-term prognosis for the FAS newborn is less than favorable. Because of the failure-to-thrive appearance, many FAS infants are often evaluated for deficiencies in organic and inorganic amino acids. These infants have a delay in oral feeding development but have a normal progression of oral motor function. Many FAS infants nurse poorly and have persistent vomiting until 6 to 7 months of age. They have difficulty adjusting to solid foods and show little spontaneous interest in food.

CNS dysfunctions are the most common and serious problem associated with FAS. Hypertonicity and increased placidity are seen in these infants. They also have a decreased ability to block out repetitive stimuli. Children exhibiting FAS can have either severe mental retardation or normal intelligence. The degree of mental retardation is directly proportional to the severity of the dysmorphic findings, meaning the more abnormal the facial features, the lower the IQ scores will be (Jones, 2003). Often there is little improvement in intelligence (as measured by IQ) despite positive environmental and educational factors (Moran, 2004). These children show impulsivity, cognitive impairment, and speech and language abnormalities indicative of CNS involvement (Moran, 2004). As they progress through the adolescent years, they change from a very thin and underweight child to one who is overweight and often obese. Short stature and microcephaly persist.

Table 28–2 Congenital Anomalies: Identification and Care in the Newborn Period

Congenital Anomaly	Nursing Assessments	Nursing Goals and Interventions
Congenital Hydrocephalus (Enlarged head)	Enlarged or full fontanelles Split or widened sutures "Setting sun" eyes Head circumference greater than 90% on growth chart	Assess presence of hydrocephalus: Measure and plot occipital-frontal baseline measurements; then measure head circumference once a day. Check fontanelle for bulging and sutures for widening. Assist with head ultrasound and transillumination. Maintain skin integrity: Change position frequently. Clean skin creases after feeding or vomiting. Use sheepskin pillow under head. Postoperatively, position head off operative site. Watch for signs of infection.
Choanal Atresia (Occlusion of posterior nares)	Cyanosis and retractions at rest Noisy respirations Difficulty breathing during feeding Obstruction by thick mucus	Assess patency of nares: Listen for breath sounds while holding baby's mouth closed and alternately compressing each nostril. Assist with passing feeding tube to confirm diagnosis. Maintain respiratory function: Assist with taping airway in mouth to prevent respiratory distress. Position with head elevated to improve air exchange.
Cleft Lip (Unilateral or bilateral visible defect)	May involve external nares, nasal cartilage, nasal septum, and alveolar process Flattening or depression of midfacial contour 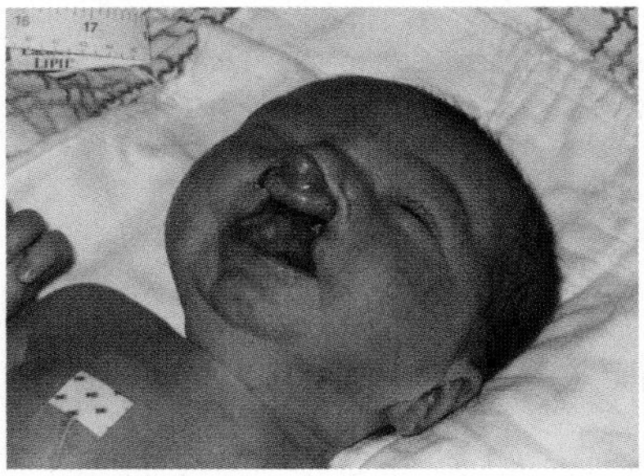	Provide nutrition: Feed with special nipple. Burp frequently (increased tendency to swallow air and reflex vomiting). Clean cleft with sterile water (to prevent crusting on cleft before repair). Support parental coping: Assist parents with grief over loss of idealized baby. Encourage verbalization of their feelings about visible defect. Provide role model in interacting with infant: Parents internalize others' responses to their newborn. (At left) Bilateral cleft lip with cleft abnormality involving both hard and soft palates. *Source:* Courtesy of Carol Harrigan, RNC, MSN, NNP.
Cleft Palate (Fissure connecting oral and nasal cavity)	May involve uvula and soft palate May extend forward to nostril involving hard palate and maxillary alveolar ridge Difficulty in sucking Expulsion of formula through nose	Prevent aspiration/infection: Place prone or in side-lying position to facilitate drainage. Suction nasopharyngeal cavity (to prevent aspiration or airway obstruction). During newborn period feed in upright position with head and chest tilted slightly backward (to aid swallowing and discourage aspiration). Provide nutrition: Feed with special nipple that fills cleft and allows sucking. Also decreases chance of aspiration through nasal cavity. Clean mouth with water after feedings. Burp after each ounce (tend to swallow large amounts of air). Thicken formula to provide extra calories. Plot weight gain patterns to assess adequacy of diet. Provide parental support: Refer parents to community agencies and support groups. Encourage verbalization of frustrations because feeding process is long and frustrating. Praise all parental efforts. Encourage parents to seek prompt treatment for upper respiratory infection (URI) and teach them ways to decrease URI.

(continued)

Table 28–2 Congenital Anomalies: Identification and Care in the Newborn Period—continued

Congenital Anomaly	Nursing Assessments	Nursing Goals and Interventions
Tracheoesophageal Fistula (type 3) (Connection between trachea and esophagus)	History of maternal polyhydramnios Excessive oral secretions Constant drooling Abdominal distention beginning soon after birth Periodic choking and cyanotic episodes Immediate regurgitation of feeding Clinical symptoms of aspiration pneumonia (tachypnea, retractions, rhonchi, decreased breath sounds, cyanotic spells) Inability to pass nasogastric tube	Maintain respiratory status and prevent aspiration. Withhold feeding until esophageal patency is determined. Quickly assess patency before putting to breast in birth area. Place on low intermittent suction to control saliva and mucus (to prevent aspiration pneumonia). Place in warmed, humidified incubator (liquefies secretions, facilitating removal). Elevate head of bed 20–40 degrees (to prevent reflux of gastric juices). Keep quiet (crying causes air to pass through fistula and to distend intestines, causing respiratory embarrassment). Maintain fluid and electrolyte balance. Give fluids to replace esophageal drainage and maintain hydration. Provide parent education: Explain staged repair—provision of gastrostomy and ligation of fistula, then repair of atresia. Keep parents informed; clarify and reinforce physician's explanations regarding malformation, surgical repair, pre- and postoperative care, and prognosis (knowledge is ego strengthening). Involve parents in care of infant and in planning for future; facilitate touch and eye contact (to dispel feelings of inadequacy, increase self-esteem and self-worth, and promote incorporation of infant into family).
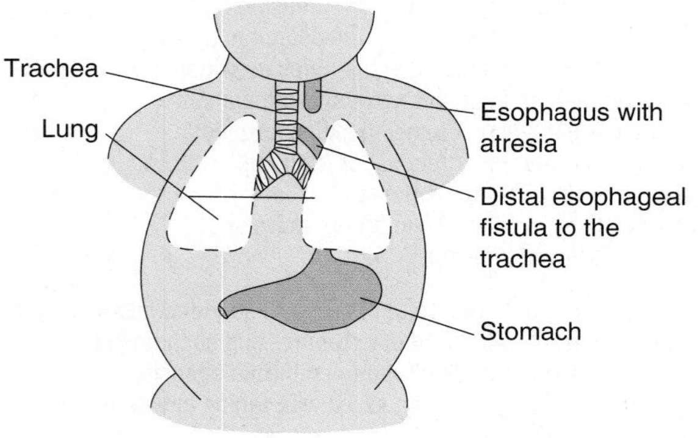		(At left) The most frequently seen type of congenital tracheoesophageal fistula and esophageal atresia. *Source:* Courtesy Nancy Houck, RNC, BSN, NNP.
Diaphragmatic Hernia (Portion of intestines in the thoracic cavity through abnormal opening in diaphragm)	Difficulty initiating respirations Gasping respirations with nasal flaring and chest retraction Barrel chest and scaphoid abdomen Asymmetric chest expansion Breath sounds may be absent, usually on left side Heart sounds displaced to right Spasmodic attacks of cyanosis and difficulty in feeding Bowel sounds may be heard in thoracic cavity.	Nurse should never ventilate with bag and mask O_2 because the stomach will inflate, further compressing the lungs. Maintain respiratory status: Immediately administer oxygen. Initiate gastric decompression. Place in high semi-Fowler's position (to use gravity to keep abdominal organs' pressure off diaphragm). Turn to affected side to allow unaffected lung expansion. Carry out interventions to alleviate respiratory and metabolic acidosis. Assess for increased secretions around suction tube (denotes possible obstruction). Aspirate and irrigate tube with air or sterile water.
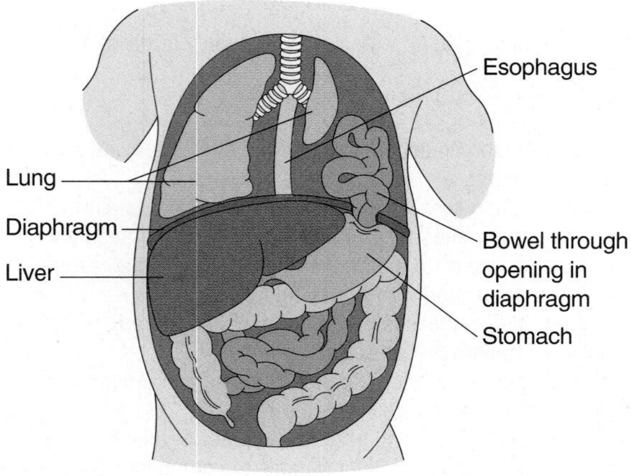		(At left) Diaphragmatic hernia. Note compression of the lung by the intestine on the affected side. *Source:* Courtesy Nancy Houck, RNC, BSN, NNP.

Table 28–2 Congenital Anomalies: Identification and Care in the Newborn Period—continued

Congenital Anomaly	Nursing Assessments	Nursing Goals and Interventions
Omphalocele (Herniation of abdominal contents into base of umbilical cord) 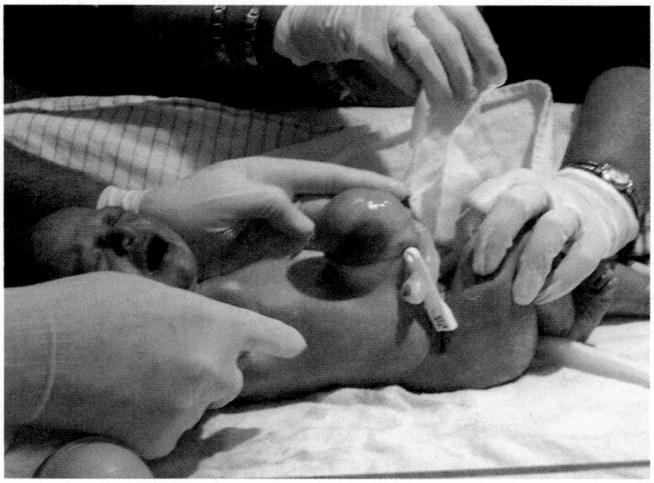	May have an enclosed transparent sac covering	Maintain hydration and temperature. Provide D5LR and albumin for hypovolemia. Place infant in sterile bag up to and covering defect. Initiate gastric decompression by insertion of nasogastric tube attached to low suction (to prevent distention of lower bowel and impairment of blood flow). Prevent infection and trauma to defect. Position to prevent trauma to defect. Administer broad-spectrum antibiotics. (At left) Newborn with omphalocele. *Source:* Courtesy of Carol Harrigan, RNC, MSN, NNP.
Gastroschisis (Full-thickness defect in abdominal wall allowing viscera outside the body to the right of an intact umbilical cord.) 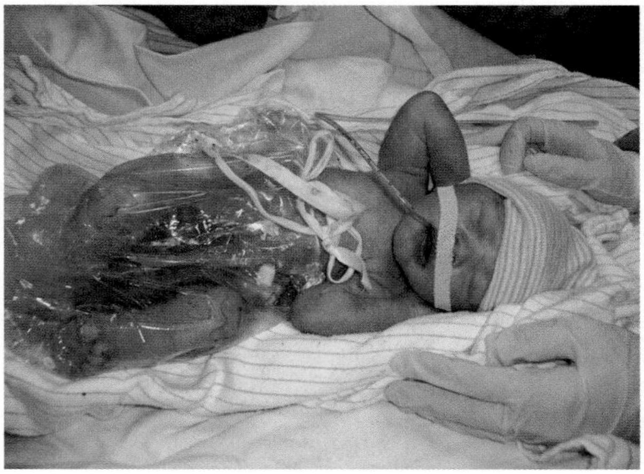	No sac covering. Intestines exposed to the caustic amniotic fluid. Associated with intestinal atresia, malrotation	Maintain hydration and temperature. Prevent trauma and infection to defect. Provide D5LR normal saline, and/or albumin for hypovolemia. Place infant in sterile bag up to axilla. Initiate gastric decompression by insertion of nasogastric tube attached to low suction. Administer broad-spectrum antibiotics. (At left) Term newborn with gastroschisis. Note the externalized loops of bowel visible through the bag. *Source:* Courtesy of Carol Harrigan, RNC, MSN, NNP.

(continued)

Table 28–2 Congenital Anomalies: Identification and Care in the Newborn Period—continued

Congenital Anomaly	Nursing Assessments	Nursing Goals and Interventions
Prune Belly Syndrome (Congenital absence of one or more layers of abdominal muscles)	Oligohydramnios leading to pulmonary hypoplasia common Deficiency of the abdominal wall musculature causing the abdomen to be shapeless Skin hangs loosely and is wrinkled in appearance Associated with urinary abnormalities (urethral obstruction) In males, cryptorchidism is common; rarely occurs in females 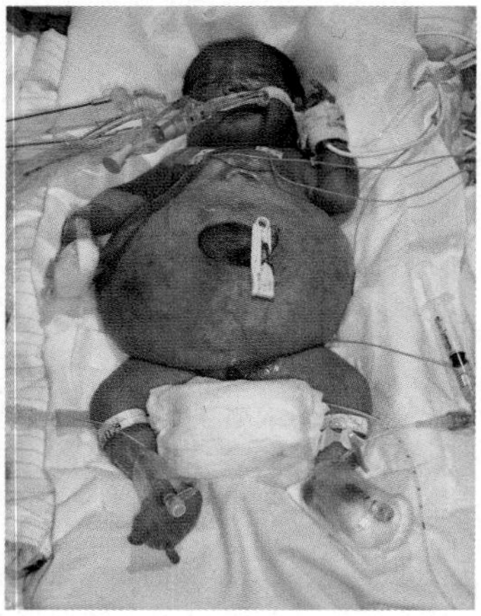	Maintain respiratory status: May need to be immediately intubated and ventilated. Prevent trauma and infection. Administer broad-spectrum antibiotics. Place a urinary catheter and monitor urinary output. Carry out interventions to alleviate respiratory and metabolic acidosis. Keep parents updated and informed about prognosis. (At left) Prune belly syndrome. *Source:* Courtesy of Carol Harrigan, RNC, MSN, NNP.
Myelomeningocele (Saclike cyst containing meninges, spinal cord, and nerve roots in thoracic and/or lumbar area)	Myelomeningocele directly connects to subarachnoid space so hydrocephalus often associated No response or varying response to sensation below level of sac May have constant dribbling of urine Incontinence or retention of stool Anal wink may or may not be present 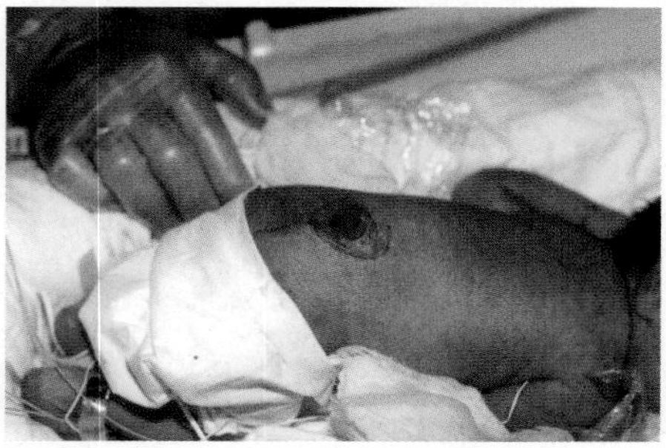	Prevent trauma and infection. Position on abdomen or on side and restrain (to prevent pressure and trauma to sac). Meticulously clean buttocks and genitals after each voiding and defecation (to prevent contamination of sac and decrease possibility of infection). May put protective covering over sac (to prevent rupture and drying). Observe sac for oozing of fluid. Credé bladder (apply downward pressure on bladder with thumbs, moving urine toward the urethra) as ordered to prevent urinary stasis. Assess amount of sensation and movement below defect. Observe for complications. Obtain occipital-frontal circumference baseline measurements; then measure head circumference once a day (to detect hydrocephalus). Check fontanelle for fullness and bulging. (At left) Newborn with lumbar myelomeningocele. *Source:* Courtesy of Carole Harrigan, RNC, MSN, NNP.
Imperforate Anus, Congenital Dislocated Hip, and Clubfoot	See Chapters 53 and 58∞.	Identify defect and initiate appropriate referral early.

NURSING MANAGEMENT

NURSING ASSESSMENT AND DIAGNOSIS

Newborns with FAS show the following characteristics:

- *Abnormal structural development and CNS dysfunction.* This includes mental retardation, microcephaly, and hyperactivity.
- *Growth deficiencies.* The growth of infants with FAS is often restricted in regard to weight, length, and head circumference. These infants continue to show a persistent postnatal growth deficiency, with head circumference and linear growth most affected.
- *Distinctive facial abnormalities.* These include short palpebral fissures; epicanthal folds; broad nasal bridge; flattened midfacies; short, upturned, or beaklike nose; micrognathia (abnormally small lower jaw); hypoplastic maxilla; thin upper lip or vermilion border; and smooth philtrum (groove on upper lip) (Kenner & Lott, 2007).
- *Associated anomalies.* Abnormalities affecting the heart (primarily septal and valvular defects), eyes (optic nerve hypoplasia), ears (conductive and sensorineural hearing loss), kidneys, and skeleton (especially involving joints, such as congenital dislocated hips) systems are often noted.

An alcohol-exposed newborn in the first week of life may show symptoms that include sleeplessness, excessive arousal states, inconsolable crying, abnormal reflexes, hyperactivity with little ability to maintain alertness and attentiveness to environment, jitteriness, abdominal distention, and exaggerated mouthing behaviors such as hyperactive rooting and increased nonnutritive sucking. Seizures may be common. These symptoms commonly persist throughout the first month of life but may continue longer. Alcohol dependence in the infant is physiologic, not psychologic. Signs and symptoms of withdrawal often appear within 6 to 12 hours and at least within the first 3 days of life. Seizures after the neonatal period are rare.

Nursing diagnoses that may apply to the FAS include the following:

- *Altered Nutrition: Less than Body Requirements* related to decreased food intake and hyperirritability
- *Alteration in Neurodevelopmental Status* related to central nervous system involvement secondary to maternal alcohol use
- *Ineffective Coping* related to dysfunctional family dynamics and substance-dependent mother

PLANNING AND IMPLEMENTATION

HOSPITAL-BASED NURSING CARE

Nursing care of the FAS newborn is aimed at avoiding heat loss, providing adequate nutrition, and reducing environmental stimuli. The FAS baby is most comfortable in a quiet, dimly lit environment. Because of their feeding problems, these infants require extra time and patience during feedings. It is important to provide consistency in the staff working with the baby and parents and to keep personnel and visitors to a minimum at any one time.

The nurse should inform the alcohol-dependent mother that breastfeeding is not contraindicated but that excessive alcohol consumption may intoxicate the newborn and inhibit the letdown reflex. The nurse should monitor the newborn's vital signs closely and observe for evidence of seizure activity and respiratory distress.

COMMUNITY-BASED NURSING CARE

Infants affected by maternal alcohol abuse are also at risk psychologically. Restlessness, sleeplessness, agitation, resistance to cuddling or holding, and frequent crying can be frustrating to parents because their efforts to relieve the distress are unrewarded. Feeding difficulties can also result in frustrations for the caregiver and digestive upsets for the infant. Frustration may cause the parents to punish the baby or result in the unconscious desire to stay away from the infant. Either outcome may create an unstable family environment and result in failure to thrive.

The nurse should focus on providing support for the parents and reinforcing positive parenting activity. Before discharge, parents should be given opportunities to provide baby care so that they can feel confident in their interpretations of their baby's cues and ability to meet the baby's needs. Referring the family to social services and visiting nurse or public health nurse associations is essential for the well-being of the infant. Follow-up care and teaching can strengthen the parents' skill and coping abilities and help them create a stable, healthy environment for their family. The infant with FAS should be involved in intervention programs that monitor the child's developmental progress, health, and home environment.

EVALUATION

Expected outcomes of nursing care include the following:

- The FAS newborn is able to tolerate feedings and gain weight.
- The FAS infant's hyperirritability or seizures are controlled, and the baby has suffered no physical injuries.
- The parents are able to identify the special needs of their newborn and accept outside assistance as needed.

DRUG DEPENDENCE

Drugs abused by pregnant women can include the following substances, used singularly or in combination: tobacco, cocaine, phencyclidine (PCP), methamphetamines, inhalants, marijuana, heroin, and methadone. Patterns of abuse of alcohol, marijuana, and heroin in childbearing women have changed very little in the past few years. The incidence of cocaine (especially "crack") use has stabilized, OxyContin use has risen dramatically (see "Substances Commonly Abused During Pregnancy" in Chapter 15∞ for more discussion of maternal substance abuse).

Marijuana, alcohol, and nicotine are sometimes used in conjunction with cocaine.

Intrauterine drug-exposed infants are predisposed to a number of problems. Because almost all narcotic drugs cross the placenta and enter the fetal circulatory system, the fetus can develop problems in utero or soon after birth. The effects of polydrug use on the newborn must always be taken into consideration.

The greatest risks to the fetus of the drug-abusing mother are as follows:

- *Intrauterine asphyxia.* Asphyxia is often a direct result of fetal withdrawal secondary to maternal withdrawal. Fetal withdrawal is accompanied by hyperactivity, with increased oxygen consumption. Insufficiency of oxygen can lead to fetal asphyxia. Moreover, women addicted to narcotics tend to have a higher incidence of preeclampsia, abruptio placentae, and placenta previa, resulting in placental insufficiency and fetal asphyxia.
- *Intrauterine infection.* Sexually transmitted infection, HIV infection, and hepatitis are often connected with the pregnant addict's lifestyle. Such infections can involve the fetus.
- *Alterations in birth weight.* These alterations may depend on the type of drug the mother uses. Women using predominantly heroin have infants of lower birth weight who are SGA. Women maintained on methadone have higher-birth-weight infants, some of whom are LGA.
- *Low Apgar scores.* Low scores may be related to the intrauterine asphyxia or the medication the woman received during labor. The use of a narcotic antagonist (nalorphine or naloxone) to reverse respiratory depression is contraindicated because it may precipitate acute withdrawal in the infant.

COMMON COMPLICATIONS OF THE DRUG-EXPOSED NEWBORN

The newborn of a woman who abused drugs during her pregnancy is predisposed to the following problems:

- *Respiratory distress.* The heroin-addicted newborn frequently suffers respiratory stress, mainly meconium-aspiration pneumonia and transient tachypnea. Meconium aspiration is usually secondary to increased oxygen consumption and activity experienced by the fetus during intrauterine withdrawal. Transient tachypnea may develop secondary to the inhibitory effects of narcotics on the reflex responsible for clearing the lungs. Respiratory distress syndrome, however, occurs less often in heroin-addicted newborns, even in those who are premature, because they have tissue-oxygen-unloading capabilities comparable to those of a 6-week-old term infant.
- *Jaundice.* Newborns of methadone-addicted women may develop jaundice because of prematurity. By contrast, infants of mothers addicted to heroin or cocaine have a lower incidence of hyperbilirubinemia because these substances contribute to early maturity of the liver.
- *Congenital anomalies and growth restriction.* Infants of cocaine-addicted mothers exhibit congenital malformations involving bony skull defects, such as microencephaly, and symmetric intrauterine growth restriction, cardiac defects, and genitourinary defects. Infants exposed to methamphetamines during gestation may show a higher incidence of cleft lip and palate, cardiac anomalies, microcephaly, and LBW (Kenner & Lott, 2007). Congenital anomalies, however, are rare.
- *Behavioral abnormalities.* Babies exposed to cocaine have poor state organization. They exhibit decreased interactive behaviors when tested with the Brazelton Neonatal Behavioral Assessment Scale. These infants also have difficulty moving through the various sleep and wake states and have problems attending to and actively engaging in auditory and visual stimuli.
- *Withdrawal.* The most significant postnatal problem of the drug-exposed newborn is opiate withdrawal (usually from heroin or methadone). The onset of the withdrawal manifestations often occurs after discharge, especially with short birthing-unit stays. See "Clinical Manifestations: Newborn Withdrawal" for withdrawal symptoms.

Long-Term Effects

During the first 2 years of life, many cocaine-exposed infants demonstrate susceptibility to behavior lability and the inability to express strong feelings such as pleasure, anger, or distress, or even a strong reaction to being separated from their parents. Cocaine-exposed infants are at higher risk for motor development problems, delays in expressive language skills, and feeding difficulties because of swallowing problems (Kenner & Lott, 2007). Behavioral state control is poorly developed in drug-exposed infants, who tend to rapidly progress from sleep to the awake state of crying without a smooth transition from one state to the next. As a result, these infants have poor social interaction skills; cannot habituate to external stimuli; and become easily overstimulated, having difficulty sleeping.

These infants also have a higher incidence of gastrointestinal and respiratory illnesses. These illnesses can be related not to drug exposure but to the mother's lack of education regarding proper infant care, feeding, and hygiene. After birth the infant born to a drug-dependent mother may also be subject to neglect or abuse, or both.

Clinical Therapy

For optimal fetal and neonatal outcome, the heroin-addicted woman should receive complete prenatal care as early as possible to reduce maternal morbidity and mortality rates and to promote fetal stability and growth (Kenner & Lott, 2007). For those women dependent on narcotics, the woman should not be withdrawn completely while pregnant because it induces fetal withdrawal with poor newborn outcomes. Unfortunately, however, pregnant women may be denied access to programs for substance abusers (Lester & Twomey, 2008).

Newborn treatment may include management of complications; serologic tests for syphilis, HIV, and hepatitis B; urine drug

Clinical Manifestations

NEWBORN WITHDRAWAL

CENTRAL NERVOUS SYSTEM SIGNS
- Hyperactivity
- Hyperirritability (persistent shrill cry)
- Increased muscle tone
- Exaggerated reflexes
- Tremors and myoclonic jerks
- Sneezing, hiccups, yawning
- Short, unquiet sleep
- Fever (accompanies the increased neuromuscular activities)

RESPIRATORY SIGNS
- Tachypnea (greater than 60 breaths per minute when quiet)
- Excessive secretions

GASTROINTESTINAL SIGNS
- Disorganized, vigorous suck
- Vomiting
- Drooling
- Sensitive gag reflex
- Hyperphagia
- Diarrhea
- Poor feeding (less than 15 mL on first day of life; takes longer than 30 minutes per feeding)

VASOMOTOR SIGNS
- Stuffy nose, yawning, sneezing
- Flushing
- Sweating
- Sudden, circumoral pallor

CUTANEOUS SIGNS
- Excoriated buttocks, knees, elbows
- Facial scratches
- Pressure-point abrasions

screen and meconium analysis; and social service referral. Screening of meconium provides a more comprehensive and accurate indication of exposure over a longer gestational period than does screening of neonatal urine (AAP & ACOG, 2007). Drugs used to control withdrawal symptoms vary and may be regionally based. They include oral morphine sulfate solution, paregoric, tincture of opium, oral methadone, phenobarbital, and diazepam (Pitts, 2010). Nutritional support is important in light of the increase in energy expenditure that withdrawal may entail.

NURSING MANAGEMENT

NURSING ASSESSMENT AND DIAGNOSIS

Early identification of the newborn needing clinical or pharmacologic interventions decreases the incidence of neonatal mortality and morbidity. The identification of substance-exposed newborns is determined primarily by clinical indicators in the prenatal period including maternal presentation, history of substance use or abuse, medical history, or toxicology results. During the newborn period, nursing assessment focuses on the following:

- Discovering the mother's last drug intake and dosage level. Women may be reluctant to disclose this information; therefore, a nonjudgmental interview technique is essential (AAP & ACOG, 2007).
- Assessing for congenital malformations and the complications related to intrauterine withdrawal such as SGA, asphyxia, meconium aspiration, and prematurity.
- Identifying the signs and symptoms of newborn withdrawal or neonatal abstinence syndrome (see Table 28–3).

Although many of the signs and symptoms of drug withdrawal are similar to those seen with hypoglycemia and hypocalcemia, glucose and calcium values are reported to be within normal limits.

Neonatal abstinence syndrome includes both physiologic and behavioral responses. A number of useful systematic scoring systems are available for assessing severity (AAP & ACOG, 2007). Assess the severity of withdrawal with a scoring system such as the Finnegan scale that is based on observations and measurement of the responses to neonatal abstinence. It evaluates the infant on potentially life-threatening signs such as vomiting, diarrhea, weight loss, irritability, tremors, and tachypnea (Table 28–3).

Nursing diagnoses that may apply to drug-dependent newborns include the following:

- *High Risk for Infant CNS Injury* related to perinatal substance abuse
- *Risk for Ineffective Airway Clearance* related to suppression of respiratory system
- *Altered Nutrition: Less than Body Requirements* related to vomiting and diarrhea, uncoordinated suck and swallow reflex, and hypertonia secondary to withdrawal
- *Impaired Skin Integrity* related to constant activity, diarrhea
- *Sleep Pattern Disturbance* related to CNS excitation secondary to drug withdrawal
- *Altered Parenting* related to hyperirritable behavior of the infant and lack of knowledge of infant care

PLANNING AND IMPLEMENTATION

HOSPITAL-BASED NURSING CARE

Care of the drug-dependent newborn is based on reducing withdrawal symptoms and promoting adequate respiration, temperature, and nutrition. See "Nursing Care Plan: Newborn of a

Table 28–3 Neonatal Abstinence Score Sheet

Neonatal Abstinence Scoring System

System	Signs and Symptoms	Score	AM	PM	Comments
Central Nervous System Disturbances	Excessive high-pitched (or other) cry Continuous high-pitched (or other) cry	2 3			Daily weight:
	Sleeps < 1 hour after feeding Sleeps < 2 hours after feeding Sleeps < 3 hours after feeding	3 2 1			
	Hyperactive Moro reflex Markedly hyperactive Moro reflex	2 3			
	Mild tremors disturbed Moderate-severe tremors disturbed	1 2			
	Mild tremors undisturbed Moderate-severe tremors undisturbed	3 4			
	Increased muscle tone	2			
	Excoriation (specific area)	1			
	Myoclonic jerks	3			
	Generalized convulsions	5			
Metabolic/Vasomotor/ Respiratory Disturbances	Sweating	1			
	Fever < 101 (99° to 100.8°F/ 37.2°C to 38.2°C) Fever > 101 (38.4°C [101.1°F] and higher)	1 2			
	Frequent yawning (> 3 to 4 times/interval)	1			
	Mottling	1			
	Nasal stuffiness	1			
	Sneezing (> 3 to 4 times/interval)	1			
	Nasal flaring	2			
	Respiratory rate > 60/min Respiratory rate > 60/min with retractions	1 2			
Gastrointestinal Disturbances	Excessive sucking	1			
	Poor feeding	2			
	Regurgitation Projectile vomiting	2 3			
	Loose stools Watery stools	2 3			
	Total Score				
	Initials of Scorer				

Source: Finnegan, L. P. (1990). Neonatal abstinence syndrome. In N. Nelson (Ed.), *Current therapy in neonatal-perinatal medicine* (2nd ed.). Ontario: BC Decker.

Substance-Abusing Mother" on pages 696–697 for specific nursing measures. Some general nursery care measures include the following (Crocetti, Amin, & Jansson, 2007; Pitts, 2010):

- Performing neonatal abstinence scoring per hospital protocol
- Monitoring temperature for hypothermia
- Carefully monitoring pulse and respirations every 15 minutes until stable; stimulation if apnea occurs
- Providing small, frequent feedings, especially in the presence of vomiting, regurgitation, and diarrhea
- Proper positioning on the right side-lying or semi-Fowler's to avoid possible aspiration of vomitus or secretions

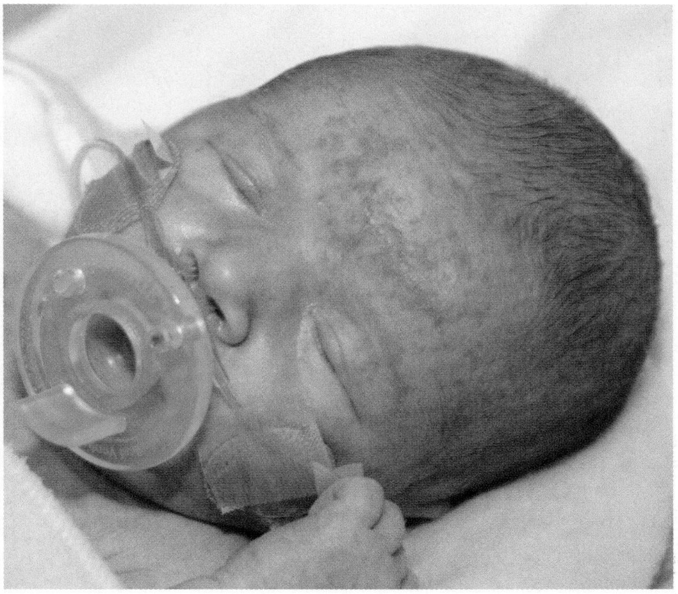

● **Figure 28–14** Nonnutritive sucking on a pacifier has a calming effect on the newborn.

- Administering medications as ordered, such as oral morphine, tincture of opium, and paregoric
- Monitoring frequency of diarrhea and vomiting, and weighing infant every 8 hours during withdrawal
- Swaddling with hands near mouth to minimize injury and help achieve a more organized behavioral state. (Offer a pacifier for nonnutritive, excessive sucking. Gentle, vertical rocking can be successful in calming an infant who is out of control.) (See Figure 28–14 ●.)
- Protecting face and extremities from excoriation by using mittens, and soft sheets or sheepskin. Applying protective skin emollient to the groin area with each diaper change
- Placing the newborn in a quiet, dimly lit area of the nursery

COMMUNITY-BASED NURSING CARE

Parents need assistance to prepare for what they can expect for the first few months at home. At the time of discharge, the mother should be instructed to anticipate mild jitteriness and irritability in the newborn, which may persist from 6 days to 8 weeks, depending on the initial severity of the withdrawal (Blackburn, 2007). Infants with neonatal abstinence syndrome are at significantly higher risk for SIDS when the mother used heroin or cocaine. The infant should sleep supine and home apnea monitoring should be implemented. The nurse should help the mother learn feeding techniques, comforting measures, how to recognize newborn cues, and appropriate parenting responses. Parents are to be counseled regarding available resources, such as support groups, as well as signs and symptoms that indicate the need for further care. Ongoing evaluation is necessary because of the potential for long-term problems. Follow-up on missed appointments can bring parents back into the healthcare system, thereby improving parent and infant outcomes and promoting a positive, interactive environment after birth (AAP & ACOG, 2007).

EVALUATION

Expected outcomes of nursing care include the following:

- The newborn tolerates feedings, gains weight, and has a decreased incidence of diarrhea.
- The parents learn innovative ways to comfort their newborn.
- The parents are able to cope with their frustrations and begin to use outside resources as needed.

INFANTS OF MOTHERS WHO ARE TOBACCO DEPENDENT

Despite increased knowledge about the dangers to the fetus and newborn of smoking mothers, 15% to 20% of these women continue to smoke during pregnancy (Pitts, 2010). The common consequence of tobacco use is addiction to nicotine. Most smokers report true enjoyment, associated with a sense of relaxation during stress, especially with the first cigarette of the day (CDC, 2005).

Risks of Tobacco to the Fetus and Newborn

Preconceptual cigarette smoking has been found to increase infertility. Fortunately, the reduction in fertility is reversible if the woman stops smoking. Smoking during pregnancy has been associated with spontaneous abortion, placenta previa, and abruptio placentae. See "Tobacco" in Chapter 11 ∞ for discussion of maternal care. The most studied compound found in cigarette smoking that can adversely affect the intrauterine environment is carbon monoxide. Carbon monoxide binds hemoglobin to form carboxyhemoglobin which reduces the oxygen-carrying capacity of the blood. It also increases the binding of hemoglobin to oxygen, which impairs the release of oxygen to the tissues. Therefore the fetus can experience intrauterine hypoxia and ischemia. Mothers who smoke during pregnancy are more likely to have IUGR infants and preterm infants (Pitts, 2010). These infants typically weigh 150 to 250 g or less than infants of nonsmokers (Cloherty et al., 2008). The nicotine in cigarettes acts as a neuroteratogen that interferes with fetal development, specifically the developing nervous system. The greatest risks to the fetus and newborn of the mother who smokes include the following (Barron, 2008):

- *Intrauterine growth restriction and/or prematurity* secondary to cigarette metabolites crossing the placenta causing vasoconstriction and decreased placental blood flow
- *Intrauterine distress* presenting as meconium staining and low Apgar scores
- *Neonatal neurobehavioral abnormalities* such as impaired habituation, orientation, consolability, orientation to sound
- *Hypertonia or hypotonia, increase in tremors, increased Moro reflex*
- *Signs of nicotine toxicity* (tachycardia, irritability, poor feeding)
- *Sudden infant death syndrome*

Nursing Care Plan

THE NEWBORN OF A SUBSTANCE-ABUSING MOTHER

INTERVENTION	RATIONALE	EXPECTED OUTCOME
1. Nursing Diagnosis: High Risk for Infant CNS Injury related to perinatal substance abuse		
NIC Intervention: **Newborn monitoring:** Measurement and interpretation of physiologic status of the newborn the first 24 hours after birth		**NOC Outcome:** **Neurologic status:** Extent to which the peripheral and central nervous systems receive, process, and respond to internal and external stimuli
Goal: The newborn will be free of signs and symptoms of CNS injury.		
■ Obtain prenatal records and question patient about history of drug addiction. Include duration, type of drug or drugs used, and time and amount of last dose taken prior to birth.	■ Noting the mother's last drug ingestion will provide the medical staff with an approximate time frame to expect the infant to exhibit withdrawal symptoms.	■ Infant will have no signs and symptoms of CNS injury as evidenced by reduced hyperactivity and irritability, normal sleep-wake pattern, no jitteriness, and no seizure activity.
■ Assess newborn for signs and symptoms of withdrawal (e.g., high-pitched shrill cry, sneezing, vomiting, diarrhea, hypertonicity, restlessness, and wakefulness).	■ The average symptoms of withdrawal occur 72 hours after birth; however, symptoms may appear as early as 6–24 hours after birth.	
■ Provide a quiet and calm environment. Swaddle infant tightly and place in a side-lying or prone position.	■ Providing a quiet environment decreases stimuli, therefore reducing CNS symptoms.	
■ Carefully plan tests and treatments to avoid excessive stimuli.	■ Planning care promotes rest and reduces external stimuli.	
■ Use soothing techniques such as rocking, cuddling, soft music, and soft tones when speaking.	■ These activities promote comfort, security, and infant bonding.	
■ Administer appropriate medications as ordered by physician. Monitor efficacy and side effects of these medications, which may include paregoric and phenobarbital.	■ These medications aid patient in alleviating symptoms related to withdrawal.	

INTERVENTION	RATIONALE	EXPECTED OUTCOME
2. Nursing Diagnosis: Risk for Ineffective Airway Clearance related to suppression of respiratory system		
NIC Intervention: **Respiratory monitoring:** Collection and analysis of patient data to ensure airway patency and adequate gas exchange		**NOC Outcome:** **Respiratory status:** Gas exchange: Alveolar exchange of CO_2 or O_2 to maintain arterial blood gas concentrations
Goal: Infant will be free of signs and symptoms of respiratory distress after birth.		
■ Obtain maternal prenatal, labor, and birth records.	■ Provides information of fetal stress that may have occurred during the prenatal or intrapartum period. In addition the birth record will provide information concerning infant's respiratory status at birth; for example, the Apgar score.	■ The infant will maintain adequate respiratory gas exchange as evidenced by: respirations are 30–60 breaths/min and arterial blood gases are within normal range.
■ Assess infant's respiratory rate and effort, skin color, heart rate, presence or absence of cough reflex, and symptoms of respiratory distress.	■ Maternal narcotic consumption may depress the cough reflex and respiratory center of the infant after birth. Symptoms such as cyanosis, tachycardia, grunting, retractions, and nasal flaring may indicate hypoxia.	
■ Position infant in a side-lying or semi-Fowler's position.	■ Prevents aspiration.	
■ Monitor infant for temperature elevation.	■ Temperature elevation may cause metabolic rate and oxygen needs to increase when associated with CNS stimulation.	

Nursing Care Plan—continued

THE NEWBORN OF A SUBSTANCE-ABUSING MOTHER

INTERVENTION	RATIONALE	EXPECTED OUTCOME
Collaboration: Obtain arterial blood gases (ABGs) as ordered by physician.	■ Oxygen demands increase with drug withdrawal. Obtaining ABGs will provide medical personnel baseline information of infant's respiratory status, and effective medical interventions can be initiated.	
■ Monitor infant's cardiac status and pulmonary status using ECG and pulse oximetry	■ Provides medical personnel with cardiac and pulmonary status.	

3. Nursing Diagnosis: Altered Nutrition: Less than Body Requirements related to vomiting and diarrhea, uncoordinated suck and swallow reflex, and hypertonia secondary to withdrawal

NIC Intervention:		NOC Outcome:
Nutrition therapy: Administration of food and fluids to support metabolic processes of a patient who is malnourished or at high risk for becoming malnourished		**Nutritional status:** Extent to which nutrients are available to meet metabolic needs

Goal: The infant will gain or maintain weight.

■ Review gestational age assessment. ■ Assess infant's sucking and swallowing reflexes. ■ Monitor regurgitation, vomiting, and diarrhea. ■ Use bulb syringe before feedings if having problems with nasal stuffiness and congestion. ■ Initiate appropriate feedings per physician's orders (i.e., oral, gavage, or IV feedings). ■ Provide small frequent feedings of a high-calorie formula. ■ Position infant on right side after feedings. ■ Monitor infant's weight and document on graph.	■ Oral feeding may be difficult due to CNS hyperactivity and GI hypermobility. ■ GI hypermobility, irritation, and CNS stimulation can increase nutritional needs. ■ Allows infant to breathe easier by ridding the nasal passages of excessive mucus. ■ Facilitates nutritional intake because SGA infants require 110–120 kcal/kg/day for adequate nutrition. ■ Prevents regurgitation and promotes gastric emptying. ■ Identifies abnormalities in weight gain or loss and allows for early intervention when necessary.	■ The infant will tolerate feedings, maintain weight, or gain weight as evidenced by no regurgitation or aspiration of feedings, and adequate weight gain according to weight graph.

4. Nursing Diagnosis: Risk for Altered Parenting related to lack of knowledge of infant care

NIC Intervention:		NOC Outcome:
Teaching: Infant care: Instruction on nurturing and physical care needed during the first year of life		**Parenting:** Provision of an environment that promotes optimum growth and development of dependent children

Goal: The parent will demonstrate ability to independently provide infant care.

■ Assess mother's desire to learn infant care tasks. Evaluate her present physical and emotional stability. ■ Instruct mother on coping strategies (e.g., exercise, listening to music, and discussing concerns openly) to manage stressful situations. ■ Assess mother's insight into her own chemical dependency. ■ Instruct mother on signs and symptoms of withdrawal and treatment interventions. ■ Encourage mother and family members to perform basic infant care tasks.	■ Will provide knowledge of mother's ability to care for infant. ■ Will give mother the tools to handle stress, thereby decreasing the chances of exhibiting abusive behavior. ■ Assistance in enrollment into a chemical dependency program may be necessary before mother can independently care for infant. ■ Assists the mother in understanding infant's behaviors and gives her the tools to intervene without feeling anxious. ■ Facilitates attachment and increases parenting competence.	■ The parent will demonstrate ability to perform basic infant care tasks as evidenced by exhibiting appropriate attachment behaviors (e.g., talking and holding infant), feeding infant, and bathing infant.

Clinical Therapy

Inquiry into tobacco and smoke exposure should be a routine part of the prenatal history. Preconception and prenatal counseling about the effects of cigarette smoking on pregnancy and the fetus should occur. An estimated 5% reduction in perinatal mortality would occur if smoking during pregnancy were eliminated (AAP & ACOG, 2007).

Cotinine, a metabolite of nicotine, has been found in fetal body fluids. There is also a positive correlation between the number of cigarettes smoked per day and the concentration of cotinine in maternal urine. Other factors that influence fetal and maternal serum cotinine concentrations are nicotine content of the cigarette and the time elapsed between the last cigarette smoked and the sampling. These findings indicate that cotinine may be used as a marker of maternal-fetal tobacco exposure during pregnancy (Kenner & Lott, 2007).

Nursing management. Mothers should be counseled that eliminating or reducing smoking even late in pregnancy can improve fetal growth. The use of nicotine patches (instead of smoking) reduces the absorption of nicotine and thereby may increase the birth weight of the fetus. See "Tobacco" in Chapter 11∞ for further discussion of prenatal smoking cessation and other intervention programs. Newborns of mothers who are tobacco dependent may be screened with the NICU Network Neurobehavioral Scale (NNNS) to assess their neurologic, behavioral, and stress/abstinence neurobehavioral function (Kenner & Lott, 2007).

The potential for long-term respiratory problems such as asthma, as well as cognitive and receptive language delays that may persist into school age, should be evaluated.

CARE OF THE NEWBORN EXPOSED TO HIV/AIDS

An increasing number of newborns are being born infected with HIV or are at risk for acquiring it in the newborn period or early infancy. More than 90% of transmissions during the perinatal and neonatal periods can occur across the placenta or through breast milk or contaminated blood (Cloherty et al., 2008). The risk of vertical transmission can be decreased in mothers taking antiretroviral drug regimens during gestation to a rate of less than 2% (American Academy of Pediatrics [AAP] and American College of Obstetricians and Gynecologists [ACOG], 2007). (For discussion of maternal and fetal HIV/AIDS, see Chapter 15∞).

NURSING MANAGEMENT

Many newborns exposed to HIV/AIDS are premature or SGA, or both, and show evidence of failure to thrive during neonatal and infant periods. They can show signs and symptoms of disease within days of birth.

Nursing care of the newborn exposed to HIV/AIDS includes all the care normally given to any newborn in a nursery. In addition, the nurse must include care for a newborn suspected of having a blood-borne infection, as with hepatitis B. Standard precautions should be used when caring for the newborn immediately after birth and when obtaining blood samples via vein puncture or heel stick. (The blood of all newborns must be considered potentially infectious because the status of the infant's blood is often not known until after the infant is discharged. Most institutions recommend that their caregivers wear gloves during all diaper changes, especially in the presence of diarrhea, because blood may be in the stool and should be considered part of standard precautions [AAP & ACOG, 2007]. There is a window of time before seroconversion occurs when the baby is still considered infectious. See Table 28–4 for some general issues for all caregivers of newborns at risk for HIV/AIDS.) In addition, the nurse provides for comfort; keeps the newborn well nourished and protected from opportunistic infections; good skin care to prevent skin rashes; and facilitates growth, development, and attachment. For the infant with HIV/AIDS see "Acquired Immune Deficiency Syndrome" in Chapter 50∞.

CARE OF THE NEWBORN WITH A CONGENITAL HEART DEFECT

Congenital heart defects occur in 3% to 8% of live births (depending on the severity of structural defects). Because accurate diagnosis and surgical treatment are now available, many deaths can be prevented (Cloherty et al., 2008). Corrective cardiac surgery is being done at earlier ages; for example, more than half the children undergoing surgery are less than 1 year of age, and one-fourth are less than 1 month old. It is crucial for the nurse to have comprehensive knowledge of congenital heart disease to detect deviations from normal and initiate interventions.

OVERVIEW OF CONGENITAL HEART DEFECTS

In the majority of cases of congenital heart malformations, the cause is multifactorial with no specific trigger. Other factors that might influence development of congenital heart malformation can be classified as environmental or genetic. Infections of the pregnant woman, such as rubella, cytomegalovirus, coxsackie B, and influenza, have been implicated. Steroids, alcohol, lithium, and some anticonvulsants have been shown to cause malformations of the heart. Seasonal spraying of pesticides has also been linked to an increase in congenital heart defects. Clinicians are also beginning to see cardiac defects in infants of mothers with PKU who do not follow their diets. Infants with Down syndrome, Turner syndrome, and Holt-Oram syndrome, as well as trisomy 13 and trisomy 18, frequently have heart lesions. Increased incidence and risk of recurrence of specific defects occur in families.

The most common cardiac defects seen in the first 6 days of life are left ventricular outflow obstructions (mitral stenosis, aortic stenosis or atresia), hypoplastic left heart, coarctation of the aorta, patent ductus arteriosus (PDA, the most common defect in premature infants), transposition of the great vessels, tetralogy of Fallot, and large ventricular septal defect or atrial septal defects. Many cardiac defects may not manifest themselves until after discharge from the birthing unit.

Thinking Critically

CASE STUDY: A NEWBORN WITH HIV

Mrs. Jean Corrigan, a 23-year-old GIPI positive for HIV, has just given birth to a 7 lb, 1 oz baby girl. As she watches you assessing her daughter in the birthing room, she asks why you are wearing gloves and whether her daughter will have to be in isolation. What will your response be?

See MyNursingKit for possible responses.

NURSING MANAGEMENT

The primary goal of the neonatal nurse is to identify cardiac defects early and initiate referral to the physician. The three most common manifestations of cardiac defect are cyanosis, detectable heart murmur, and congestive heart failure signs (tachycardia, tachypnea, diaphoresis, hepatomegaly, cardiomegaly). See Chapter 49∞ for detailed discussion of the clinical manifestations and medical–surgical management of these specific cardiac defects.

Initial repair of heart defects in the newborn period is becoming more commonplace. The NICU staff is now involved in both the preoperative and postoperative care of newborns. The benefits for the cardiac infant of being cared for by NICU staff include the staff's knowledge of neonatal anatomy and physiology, experience in supporting the family, and an awareness of the newborn's developmental needs.

After the baby is stabilized, decisions are made about ongoing care. The parents need careful and complete explanations and the opportunity to take part in decision making. They also require ongoing emotional support. Families with a baby born with any congenital anomaly also need genetic counseling about future conception. Parents need opportunities to verbalize their concerns about their baby's health maintenance and their understanding of the rationale for follow-up care.

Nursing Practice

When cyanosis occurs in an otherwise healthy 12- to 24-hour-old newborn displaying no respiratory distress and is not resolved with oxygen, think about cardiac issues, especially a ductal-dependent lesion.

Table 28–4 Issues for Caregivers of Infants at Risk for HIV/AIDS

Resuscitation	For suctioning use a bulb syringe, mucus extractor, or meconium aspirator with wall suction on low setting. Use masks, goggles, and gloves.
Admission care	To remove blood from baby's skin, give warm water–mild soap bath using gloves as soon as possible after admission.
Handwashing	Thorough handwashing is indicated before and after caring for infant. Hands must be washed immediately if contaminated with blood or body fluids. Wash hands after removal of gloves.
Gloves	Gloves are indicated with touching blood or other high-risk fluids. Gloves should also be worn when handling newborns before and during their initial baths, cord care, eye prophylactics, and vitamin K administration.
Mask, goggle, and gown	Not routinely needed unless coming in contact with placenta or the blood and amniotic fluid on the skin of the newborn.
Needles and syringes	Used needles should not be recapped or bent; they should be disposed of in a puncture-resistant plastic container belonging specifically to that baby. After the newborn is discharged the container is discarded.
Specimens	Blood and other specimens should be double-bagged and/or sealed in an impervious container and labeled according to agency protocol.
Equipment and linen	Articles contaminated with blood or body fluids should be discarded or bagged according to isolation or institution protocol.
Body fluid spills	Blood and body fluids should be cleaned promptly with a solution of 5.25% sodium hypochlorite (household bleach) diluted 1:10 with water. Apply for at least 30 seconds then wipe after the minimum contact time.
Education and support	Provide education and psychologic support for family and staff. Caregivers who avoid contact with a baby at risk or who overdress in unnecessary isolation garb subtly exacerbate an already difficult family situation. Information resources include the National AIDS Hotline (1-800-342-2437) and HIV/AIDS Treatment Enforcement Service Website http://www.hevatis.org
Exempted personnel	Immunologically compromised staff (pregnant women may be included in this group) and possibly infectious staff members should not care for these infants.

Source: Adapted from American Academy of Pediatrics, Committee on Pediatric AIDS and Committee on Infectious Diseases. (1999). Issues related to human immunodeficiency transmission in schools, child care, medical settings, the home, and community. *Pediatrics, 104*(2), 318–324; Mendez, H., & Jule, J. E. (1990). Care of the infant born exposed to AIDS. *Obstetric and Gynecologic Clinics of North America, 17*(3), 637; Krist, A. H., & Crawford-Faucher, A. (2002). Management of newborns exposed to maternal HIV infection. *American Family Physician, 65*(10), 2049–2056.

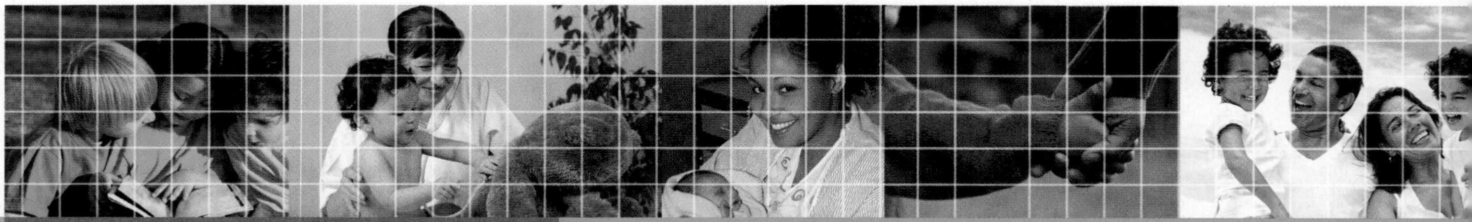

CRITICAL CONCEPT REVIEW

LEARNING OUTCOMES / CONCEPTS

28.1 Explain the factors present at birth that indicate an at-risk newborn.

Factors present at birth that may place an infant at risk include:

1. Maternal low socioeconomic level:
   - Decreased access to healthcare.
2. Exposure to environmental dangers:
   - Toxic chemicals.
   - Illicit drugs.
3. Preexisting maternal conditions:
   - Heart disease.
   - Diabetes.
   - Hypertension.
   - Renal disease.
4. Maternal age and parity.
5. Pregnancy complications:
   - Abruptio placenta.
   - Placenta previa.
   - Preeclampsia.

28.2 Compare the underlying etiologies of the physiologic complications of small-for-gestational-age (SGA) newborns and preterm appropriate-for-gestational-age (Pr AGA) newborns and the nursing care management for each.

Many of the same factors contribute to the common complications of the SGA newborn and the Pr AGA newborn:

1. Maternal factors:
   - Grand multiparity.
   - Multiple gestation pregnancy.
   - Low socioeconomic status.
   - Poor maternal nutrition.
2. Maternal disease:
   - Heart disease.
   - Hypertension.
   - Preeclampsia.
3. Environmental factors:
   - Maternal use of drugs.
   - Exposure to toxins.
   - High altitude.
4. Placental factors:
   - Small placenta.
   - Placenta previa.
   - Abnormal cord insertions.
5. Fetal factors:
   - Congenital infections.
   - Chromosomal syndromes.

28.3 Describe the impact of maternal diabetes mellitus on the newborn.

The most common complications of maternal diabetes mellitus are:

1. Hypoglycemia.
2. Hypocalcemia.
3. Hyperbilirubinemia.
4. Birth trauma.
5. Polycythemia.
6. Respiratory distress syndrome.
7. Congenital birth defects:
   - Cardiac anomalies.
   - Gastrointestinal anomalies.
   - Sacral agenesis.

LEARNING OUTCOMES	CONCEPTS
28.4 Compare the characteristics and potential complications that influence nursing care management of the postterm newborn and the newborn with postmaturity syndrome.	1. Postmaturity: ■ Applies to any newborn born after 42 weeks' gestation. ■ Most are of normal size and health. ■ Large fetus may have difficult time passing through birth passage. 2. Postmaturity syndrome, in which the fetus is exposed to poor placental function, which impairs nutrition and oxygenation and has the following characteristics: ■ Hypoglycemia. ■ Meconium aspiration. ■ Polycythemia. ■ Congenital anomalies. ■ Seizure activity. ■ Cold stress.
28.5 Discuss the physiologic characteristics of the preterm newborn that predispose each body system to various complications and that are used in developing a plan of care that includes nutritional management.	1. Respiratory difficulties: ■ Lack of surfactant causes the alveoli to collapse and infant becomes hypoxic. ■ Incomplete development of the muscular coat of the pulmonary blood vessels, which leads to left to right shunting of blood through the ductus arteriosus back into lungs. 2. Cardiac difficulties: ■ Ductus arteriosus remains open due to low oxygen levels and low prostaglandin E levels. ■ Patent ductus remains open, causing more blood to flow to lungs, increased respiratory effort, carbon dioxide retention, and bounding femoral pulses. 3. Temperature control difficulties: ■ Less able to produce heat because of the higher ratio of body surface to body weight. ■ Lack of brown fat. ■ Thin skin, which causes greater insensible water loss. ■ Lack of flexion increases heat loss. 4. Gastrointestinal difficulties: ■ Poor suck effort. ■ High caloric needs and limited ability to take in nutrition. ■ Increased basal metabolic rate and oxygen needs related to increased effort at sucking. ■ Increased chance of aspiration. ■ Decreased ability to convert amino acids. ■ Decreased ability to handle increased osmolarity of formula protein. ■ Difficulty absorbing saturated fats. ■ Difficulty digesting lactose. ■ Diminished blood flow to the intestines resulting in necrotizing enterocolitis. 5. Renal difficulties: ■ Decreased glomerular filtration rate due to decreased renal blood flow. ■ Inability to concentrate urine. ■ Decreased ability of kidney to buffer. ■ Delayed drug excretion time. ■ Spilling of glucose at a lower serum glucose rate. 6. Reactivity and behavioral state difficulties: ■ Delayed or lack of periods of reactivity due to poor condition of newborn. ■ More disorganized in sleep-wake cycle.
28.6 Summarize the nursing assessments of and initial interventions for a newborn with selected congenital anomalies.	Nursing assessments and initial interventions focus on: 1. Respiratory: ■ Ability of infant to breathe. ■ Maintain respiratory function. 2. Nutritional: ■ Is infant able to suck and swallow? ■ Does feeding cause respiratory distress? ■ Provide calories by breast, nipple, gastrointestinal tube, or IV. 3. Neurologic: ■ Is infant able to move all extremities? ■ Is there a visible defect present on the spine? ■ Is head circumference normal size and does it maintain normal size? ■ Keep infant in prone position if necessary. ■ Keep defect covered with sterile saline soaks until surgery. ■ Keep HOB elevated if head circumference is larger than normal.

LEARNING OUTCOMES / CONCEPTS

4. Parental involvement:
   - Assess parents' knowledge of infant's anomaly.
   - Keep parents informed about infant's condition.
   - Teach parents appropriate home care of infant.

28.7 Explain the special care needed by an alcohol- or drug-exposed newborn.

Special care of the infant who was exposed to drugs or alcohol focuses on:
1. Assessment of the mother's last drug intake and dosage.
2. Assessment for congenital anomalies and complications.
3. Assessment for signs and symptoms of withdrawal.

28.8 Correlate the effects of maternal HIV/AIDS on the infant in the neonatal period and the issues for caregivers of infants at risk for HIV/AIDS in determining hospital-based and community-based nursing care management.

Infant of the mother who has HIV/AIDS receives the same care as all newborn infants. The nurse also includes the following aspects of care:
1. Uses standard precautions when drawing blood samples.
2. Uses disposable gloves when changing diapers.
3. Protects infant from opportunistic diseases.
4. Keeps newborn well-nourished to prevent failure to thrive.

28.9 Identify the physical examination findings during the early newborn period that would make the nurse suspect a congenital cardiac defect or congestive heart failure.

The three most common manifestations of cardiac defects are:
1. Cyanosis.
2. Detectable heart murmur.
3. Signs of congestive heart failure:
   - Tachycardia.
   - Tachypnea.
   - Diaphoresis.
   - Hepatomegaly.
   - Cardiomegaly.

CRITICAL THINKING IN ACTION

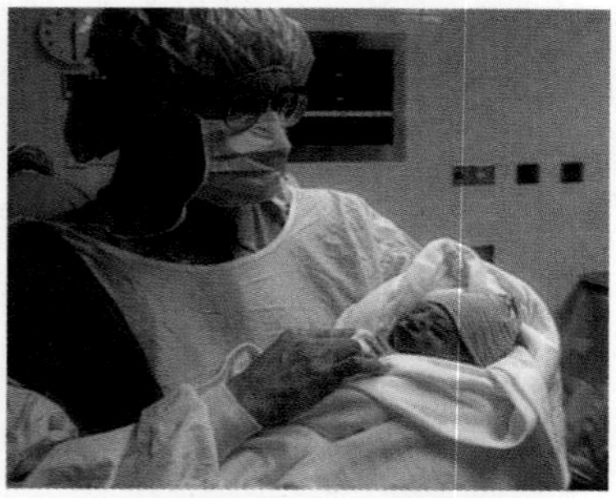

As the nurse on duty, you are caring for baby Erin, a 38-week IDM female born by repeat cesarean birth to a 32-year-old G3 now P3 mother. Erin's Apgar scores are 7 and 9 at 1 and 5 minutes. At 2 hours of age, the baby has an elevated respiratory rate of 100 to 110, heart rate of 165 with Grade II/VI intermittent machinery murmur, and mild cyanosis. She is now receiving 30% oxygen and has a respiratory rate of 70 to 80. The baby's clinical course, chest x-ray, and lab results are all consistent with transient tachypnea of the newborn and patent ductus arteriosus. The mother calls you to ask about how her baby is doing. She tells you that her last child was born at 30 weeks and had to be hospitalized for 6 weeks. She says, "I really tried to do it right this time," and asks you if this baby will have the same respiratory problem.

1. What should you tell the mother?
2. What can you do to facilitate mother–infant attachment?
3. Discuss the emotional response of parents to the birth of an ill or at-risk infant. (See Chapter 29 for additional information.)
4. Discuss the four psychologic tasks essential for coping with the stress of an at-risk newborn and providing a basis for the maternal-infant relationship. (See Chapter 29.)
5. Baby Erin is being discharged tomorrow. Review the elements of discharge and home care instructions.

See MyNursingKit for possible responses.

REFERENCES

AlFaleh, K. M., & Bassler, D. (2008). Probiotics for prevention of necrotizing enterocolitis in preterm infants. *Cochrane Database of Systematic Reviews*, Issue 1.

Als, H., Lester, B. M., Tronick, E., & Brazelton, T. B. (1982). Assessment of preterm infant behavior (APIB). In B. M. Fitzgerald Lester, & M. W. Yogman (Eds.), *Theory and research in behavioral pediatrics* (Vol. 1). New York: Plenum.

American Academy of Pediatrics (AAP) Committee on Fetus and Newborn & American College of Obstetricians and Gynecologists (ACOG) Committee on Obstetrics. (2007). *Guidelines for perinatal care* (6th ed.). Elk Grove Village, IL: Author.

Barron, M. L. (2008). Antenatal care. In K. R. Simpson & P. A. Creehan, *AWHONN perinatal nursing* (3rd ed., pp. 88–124). Philadelphia: Lippincott Williams & Wilkins.

Baschat, A. A., Galan, H. L., Ross, M. G., & Gabbe, S. G. (2007). Intrauterine growth restriction. In S. G. Gabbe, J. R. Niebyl, & J. L. Simpson (Eds.), *Obstetrics: Normal and problem pregnancies* (5th ed., pp. 771–814). Philadelphia: Churchill Livingstone/Elsevier.

Blackburn, S. (2007). *Maternal-fetal-neonatal physiology: A clinical perspective* (3rd ed.). Philadelphia: Saunders.

Bowie, B., Hall, R., Faulkner, J., & Anderson, B. (2003). Single-room infant care: Future trends in special care nursery planning and design. *Neonatal Network, 22*(3), 27–34.

Centers for Disease Control and Prevention (CDC), National Center for Chronic Disease Prevention and Health Promotion. (2005). Pattern of tobacco use among women and girls: Fact sheet. Retrieved January 31, 2005, from www.cdc.gov/tobacco/sgr_forwomen/factsheet

Cloherty, J. R., Eichenwald, E. C., & Stark, A. R. (2008). *Manual of neonatal care.* Philadelphia: Lippincott Williams & Wilkins.

Crocetti, M. T., Amin, D. D., & Jansson, L. M. (2007). Variability in the evaluation and management of opiate-exposed newborns in Maryland. *Clinical Pediatrics, 46*(7), 632–635.

Divon, M. Y. (2007). Prolonged pregnancy. In S. G. Gabbe, J. R. Niebyl, & J. L. Simpson (Eds.), *Obstetrics: Normal and problem pregnancies* (5th ed., pp. 846–860). Philadelphia: Churchill Livingstone/Elsevier.

Jones, M. (2003). Fetal alcohol syndrome. *Neonatal Network, 22*(3), 63–69.

Kahn, B. F., Hobbins, J. C., & Galan, H. L. (2008). Intrauterine growth restriction. In R. S. Gibbs, B. Y. Karlan, A. F. Haney, & I. Nygaard, *Danforth's obstetrics and gynecology* (10th ed., pp. 198–219). Philadelphia: Lippincott Williams & Wilkins.

Kenner, C., & Lott, J. W. (2007). *Comprehensive neonatal care: An interdisciplinary approach* (4th ed.). St. Louis: Saunders/Elsevier.

Kledzik, T. (2005). Holding the very low birth weight infant: Skin-to-skin techniques. *Neonatal Network, 24*(1), 7–14.

Landon, M. B., Catalano, P. M., & Gabbe, S. G. (2008). Diabetes mellitus complicating pregnancy. In R. S. Gibbs, B. Y. Karlan, A. F. Haney, & I. Nygaard, *Danforth's obstetrics and gynecology* (10th ed., pp. 976–1010). Philadelphia: Lippincott Williams & Wilkins.

Lester, B. M., & Twomey, J. E. (2008). Treatment of substance abuse during pregnancy. *Women's Health, 4*(1), 67–77.

Ludington, S., Morgan, K., & Abouelfettoh, A. (2008). A clinical guideline for implementation of Kangaroo Care with premature infants of 30 or more weeks postmenstrual age. *Advances in Neonatal Care,* 8(3S): S3–S23.

Martin, G. L., & Hankins, G. D. (2006). The Apgar score. *Advances in Neonatal Care, 6*(4), 220–223.

McCall, E. M., Alderdice, F., Halliday, H. L., Jenkins, J. G., & Vohra, S. (2008). Interventions to prevent hypothermia at birth in preterm and/or low birthweight infants. *Cochrane Database of Systematic Reviews,* Issue 1.

Moran, B. A. (2004). Substance abuse in pregnancy. In S. Mattson & J. E. Smith (Eds.), *Core curriculum for maternal-newborn nursing* (3rd ed., pp. 750–770). St. Louis: Elsevier Saunders.

Pitts, K. (2010). Perinatal substance abuse. In M. T. Verklan & M. Walden (Eds.), *Core curriculum for neonatal intensive care nursing* (4th ed., pp. 41–71). St. Louis: Saunders/Elsevier.

Thomas, J. A. (2007). Guidelines for bottle feeding your premature baby. *Advances in Neonatal Care, 7*(6), 311–318.

Turnage-Carrier, C. S. (2010). Development support. In M. T. Verklan & M. Walden (Eds.), *Core curriculum for neonatal intensive care nursing* (4th ed., pp. 208–232). St. Louis: Saunders/Elsevier.

Vargo, L. E., & Trotter, C. W. (2007). *The premature infant: Nursing assessment and management* (2nd ed.). White Plains, NY: March of Dimes Foundation.

Volpe, J. J. (2008). *Neurology of the newborn* (5th ed.). Philadelphia: Saunders.

Wisner, K. L., Sit, D., Reynolds, S. K., Altemus, M., Bogen, D. L., Sunder, K. R., Misra, D., et al. (2007). Psychiatric disorders. In S. G. Gabbe, J. R. Niebyl, & J. L. Simpson (Eds.), *Obstetrics: Normal and problem pregnancies* (5th ed., pp. 1249–1288). Philadelphia: Churchill Livingstone/Elsevier.

Zupancic, J. (2009). Probiotic use in neonates. *Nursing for Women's Health, 13*(1), 59–64.

EXPLORE PEARSON **mynursingkit**™

MyNursingKit is your one stop for online chapter review materials and resources. Prepare for success with additional NCLEX®-style practice questions, interactive assignments and activities, web links, animations and videos, and more!

Register your access code from the front of your book at **www.mynursingkit.com**

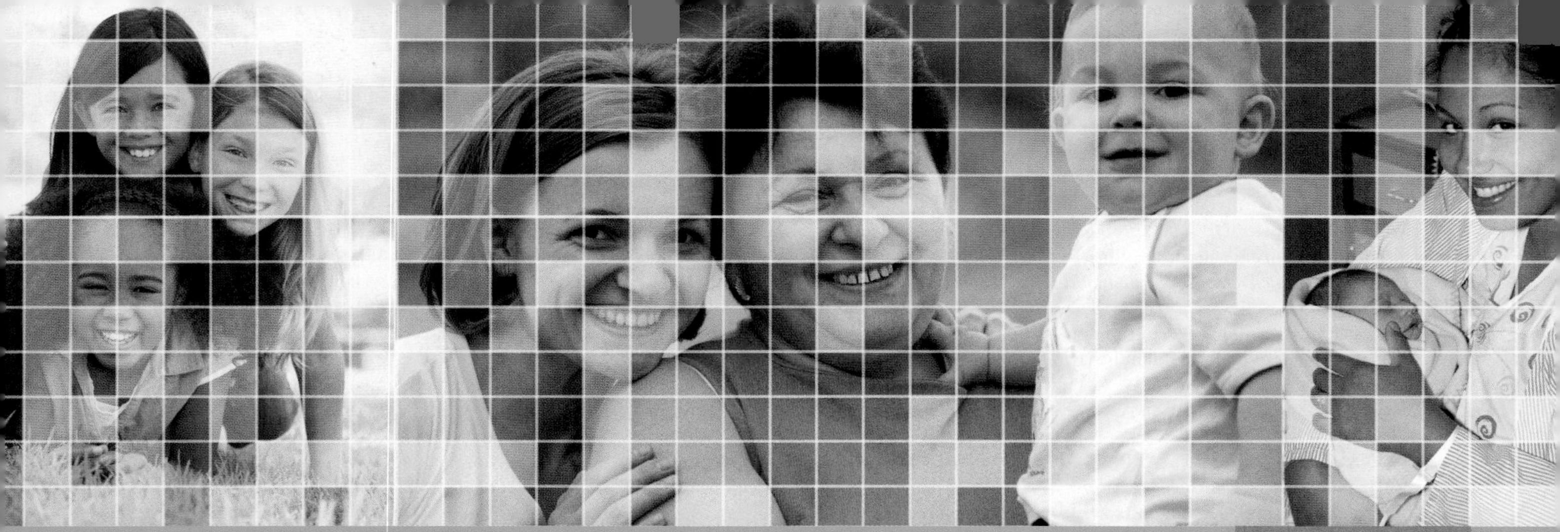

CHAPTER 29

The Newborn at Risk: Birth-Related Stressors

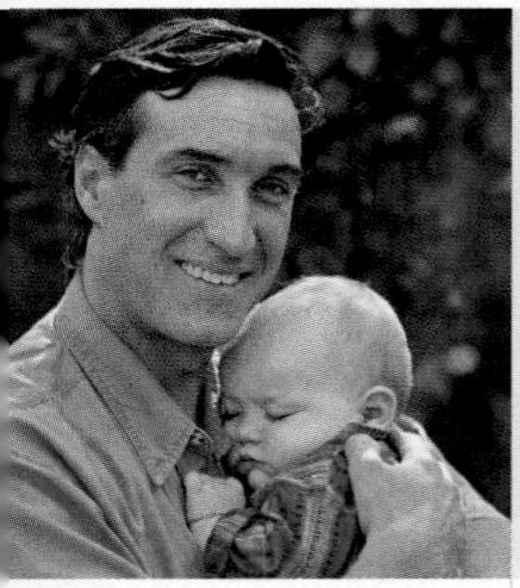

We watched him breathe every precious breath. He was covered with wires and tubes. The rhythmic tides of his sleeping and feeding spaciously measured his days and nights. We kept watch. He was special to us and we would say over and over, "Daddy and Mommy are here and we love you." —Alan and Claudia, parents of a baby with RDS

LEARNING OUTCOMES

29.1 Discuss how to identify infants in need of resuscitation and the appropriate method of resuscitation based on the labor record and observable physiologic indicators.

29.2 Based on clinical manifestations, differentiate among the various types of respiratory distress (respiratory distress syndrome, transient tachypnea of the newborn, and meconium aspiration syndrome) in the newborn and their related nursing care.

29.3 Discuss selected metabolic abnormalities (including cold stress and hypoglycemia), their effects on the newborn, and the nursing implications.

29.4 Explain the causes, pathophysiology, risks for developing, possible sequelae, clinical therapy, and the difference between physiologic and pathologic jaundice in determining the hospital and community-based nursing care management of the infant with jaundice.

29.5 Explain how Rh incompatibility or ABO incompatibility can lead to the development of hyperbilirubinemia.

29.6 Identify nursing responsibilities and rationale in caring for the newborn receiving phototherapy.

29.7 Explain the causes and nursing care of infants with anemia or polycythemia.

29.8 Describe the nursing assessments that would lead the nurse to suspect newborn sepsis and the nursing care of the newborn with an infection.

29.9 Relate the consequences of maternally transmitted infections, such as maternal syphilis, gonorrhea, herpesviridae family (HSV or CMV), and chlamydia, to the nursing care of infants in the neonatal period.

29.10 Describe the interventions to facilitate parental attachment and meet the special initial and long-term needs of parents of at-risk infants.

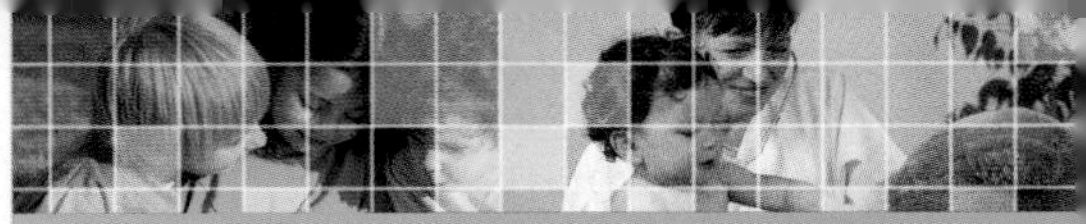

Marked homeostatic changes occur during the infant's transition from fetal to neonatal life. Because the most rapid anatomic and physiologic changes occur in the cardiopulmonary system, most major problems of the newborn are usually related to this system. These problems include asphyxia, respiratory distress syndrome (RDS), cold stress, jaundice, hemolytic disease, and anemia. Ideally, most problems are anticipated and identified prenatally. Some treatment may be initiated in the prenatal period, whereas other intervention measures are begun at or immediately after birth.

KEY TERMS

Acute bilirubin encephalopathy, 726

Cold stress, 722

Erythroblastosis fetalis, 726

Hemolytic disease of the newborn, 726

Hydrops fetalis, 727

Hyperbilirubinemia, 726

Hypoglycemia, 723

Jaundice, 726

Kernicterus, 726

Meconium aspiration syndrome (MAS), 720

Phototherapy, 728

Physiologic anemia of infancy, 735

Polycythemia, 735

Respiratory distress syndrome (RDS), 710

Sepsis neonatorum, 736

CARE OF THE NEWBORN AT RISK FROM ASPHYXIA

Neonatal asphyxia occurs in 1% to 1.5% of live births, and the incidence increases as the gestational age decreases (Cloherty, Eichenwald, & Stark, 2008). Neonatal asphyxia results in circulatory, respiratory, and biochemical changes. Circulatory patterns that accompany asphyxia indicate an inability of the newborn to make the transition to extrauterine circulation—in effect, a return to fetal circulatory patterns. Failure of lung expansion and establishment of respiration rapidly produces serious biochemical changes, including hypoxemia (decreased oxygen in the blood), metabolic acidosis (increased acidity of blood reflected by low pH), and hypercarbia (excess levels of carbon dioxide in the blood).

These biochemical changes produce the following results:

- pulmonary vasoconstriction and high pulmonary vascular resistance in relation to lower systemic vascular resistance (following birth the pulmonary vascular resistance should be markedly lower than the systemic vascular resistance);
- hypoperfusion of the lungs;
- a large right-to-left shunt through the ductus arteriosus, bypassing the lungs and impeding oxygenation of the blood.

As right atrial pressure exceeds left atrial pressure, the foramen ovale reopens, allowing blood to flow from right to left. (See Chapter 24 for a review of normal newborn cardiopulmonary adaptation.)

However, the most serious biochemical abnormality is a change from aerobic to anaerobic metabolism in the presence of hypoxia. This change results in the buildup of lactate, which combines with hydrogen to form lactic acid, and the development of metabolic acidosis. Lactic acidosis can develop after prolonged tissue hypoxia (oxygen starvation) as active cells rely on anaerobic metabolism.

Simultaneous respiratory acidosis may also occur because of a rapid increase in carbon dioxide (P_{CO_2}) during asphyxia. In response to hypoxia and anaerobic metabolism, the amounts of free fatty acids (FFAs) and glycerol in the blood increase. Glycogen stores are also mobilized to provide a continuous glucose source for the brain. Hepatic and cardiac stores of glycogen may be used up rapidly during an asphyxial incident.

The newborn is supplied with several protective mechanisms against hypoxic insults. These include:

- a relatively immature brain
- a resting metabolic rate lower than that of adults
- an ability to mobilize substances within the body for anaerobic metabolism and to use energy more efficiently
- an intact circulatory system able to redistribute lactate and hydrogen ions in tissues still being perfused

Severe prolonged hypoxia overcomes these protective mechanisms, resulting in brain damage or death of the newborn. The newborn suffering apnea requires immediate resuscitative efforts. The need for resuscitation can be anticipated if specific risk factors are present during the pregnancy or labor and birth period.

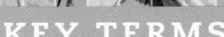

RISK FACTORS PREDISPOSING TO ASPHYXIA

The need for resuscitation may be anticipated if the mother demonstrates the antepartal and intrapartal risk factors described in Tables 10–1 and 18–1. Fetal-neonatal risk factors for resuscitation are as follows (Cloherty et al., 2008; Pappas & Walker, 2010):

- Nonreassuring fetal heart rate (FHR) pattern/sustained bradycardia
- Difficult birth, prolonged labor
- Fetal scalp/capillary blood sample—acidosis pH less than 7.2
- Significant intrapartum bleeding
- Maternal infection/sepsis with cardiovascular collapse
- Male infant
- Prematurity
- Small for gestational age or macrosomia
- Multiple births
- Structural lung abnormality/oligohydramnios (congenital diaphragmatic hernia, lung hypoplasia)
- Congenital heart disease
- Narcotic use in labor

At times no risk factors may be apparent prenatally. Particular attention must be paid to all at-risk pregnancies during the intrapartal period. Certain aspects of labor and birth challenge the oxygen supply to the fetus, and often the at-risk fetus has less tolerance for the stress of labor (indicated by decelerations or lack of variability of the FHR) and birth.

CLINICAL THERAPY

The initial goal of clinical management is to identify the fetus at risk for asphyxia, so that resuscitative efforts can begin at birth.

Fetal biophysical assessment (see Chapter 14), combined with monitoring of fetal pH, FHRs, and fetal oximeter if available during the intrapartal period, may help identify the presence of nonreassuring fetal status. If nonreassuring fetal status is present, appropriate measures can be taken to deliver the fetus immediately, before major damage occurs, and to treat the asphyxiated newborn.

The fetal biophysical profile enhances the ability to predict an abnormal perinatal outcome. In addition to the fetal biophysical profile, fetal scalp blood sampling may indicate asphyxic insult and the degree of fetal acidosis, when considered in relation to the stage of labor, uterine contractions, and the presence of nonreassuring FHR patterns. The stress of labor causes an intermittent decrease in exchange of gases in the placental intervillous space, which causes the fall in pH and fetal acidosis. The acidosis is primarily metabolic.

During labor, a fetal pH of 7.25 or higher is considered normal (nonacidemia). A pH value of 7.20 or less is considered an ominous sign of intrauterine asphyxia (acidemia), whereas a pH of less than 7 is considered pathologic acidemia (Cloherty et al., 2008). However, low fetal pH without associated hypoxia can be caused by maternal acidosis secondary to prolonged labor, dehydration, and maternal lactate production.

Assessment of the newborn's need for resuscitation begins at the time of birth. The nurse should note the time of the first gasp, first cry, and onset of sustained respirations in the order of occurrence. The Apgar score (see Chapter 19) may be helpful in describing the status of the newborn at birth and his or her subsequent adaptation to the extrauterine environment but should not be used to determine whether certain steps need to be taken during resuscitation. If indicated, resuscitation should be started before the 1-minute Apgar score is obtained. The AAP Committee on Fetus and Newborn has recommended the use of an assisted Apgar scoring system that documents the assistance the infant is receiving at the time his or her score is assigned (AAP & ACOG, 2007).

As many as 10% of all newborns require some assistance at birth (Cloherty et al., 2008). The AAP and ACOG (2007, pg. 207) recommend identification of newborns who *do not* require resuscitation by carrying out a rapid assessment of these four characteristics:

1. Is the baby full term?
2. Is the amniotic fluid clear of meconium and evidence of infection?
3. Is the baby breathing or crying?
4. Does the baby have good muscle tone?

If the answer to these questions is "yes" then the baby does not need resuscitation and should not be separated from the mother. If the answer to *any* of the previous questions is "no," the infant should receive resuscitative assistance (Pappas & Walker, 2010). The infant should receive one or more of the following categories of action:

- initial steps in stabilization (warmth, positioning, clearing the airway as necessary, drying, stimulating, and repositioning);
- oxygen administration;
- positive pressure ventilation;
- chest compressions, and
- administration of epinephrine, volume expansion, or both (AAP & ACOG, 2007).

In the birthing room exposure to blood or other body fluids is inevitable. Standard precautions must be practiced by wearing caps, goggles or glasses, gloves, and impervious gowns until the cord is cut and the newborn is dried and wrapped (Cloherty et al., 2008).

RESUSCITATION MANAGEMENT

Suctioning (clearing airway) is always performed before resuscitation measures are started so that mucus, blood, or meconium is not aspirated into the lungs. Caregivers should keep the infant in a head-down position to avoid aspiration of oropharyngeal secretions and should suction the oropharynx and nasopharynx immediately. Clearing the nasal and oral passages of obstructive fluid, using a bulb syringe or suction catheter attached to low continuous suction, establishes a patent airway. Vigorous suctioning of the posterior pharynx should be avoided because it can produce significant reflex bradycardia and damage the oral mucosa (Pappas & Walker, 2010). Although clear mucus routinely is suctioned from the mouth in most birthing units, there is no evidence to support the value of this practice (AAP & ACOG, 2007).

Breathing is established by employing the simplest form of resuscitative measures initially, with progression to more complicated methods as required. For example:

1. Position and clear the airway only as necessary. Simple stimulation is provided by rubbing the newborn's back with a blanket or towel, while simultaneously drying the baby.
2. If respirations have not been initiated or are inadequate (gasping or occasional respirations), the lungs must be inflated with positive pressure. The proper size mask is positioned securely on the face (over nose and mouth, avoiding the eyes), with *the infant's head in a "sniffing" or neutral position* (Figure 29–1 ●). Hyperextension of the infant's neck obstructs the trachea and must be avoided. An airtight connection is made between the baby's face and the mask (thus allowing the bag to inflate). The lungs are inflated rhythmically by squeezing the bag. Oxygen can be delivered at 100% with an anesthesia bag or modified self-inflating bag with reservoir and adequate liter flow of at least 8 L/min. The self-inflating (Ambu or Hope) bag delivers only 40% oxygen unless it has been adapted with an attached oxygen reservoir (Cloherty et al., 2008). It may not be possible to maintain adequate inspiratory pressure with self-inflating bags. In a crisis situation, it is crucial that 100% oxygen be delivered with adequate pressure.

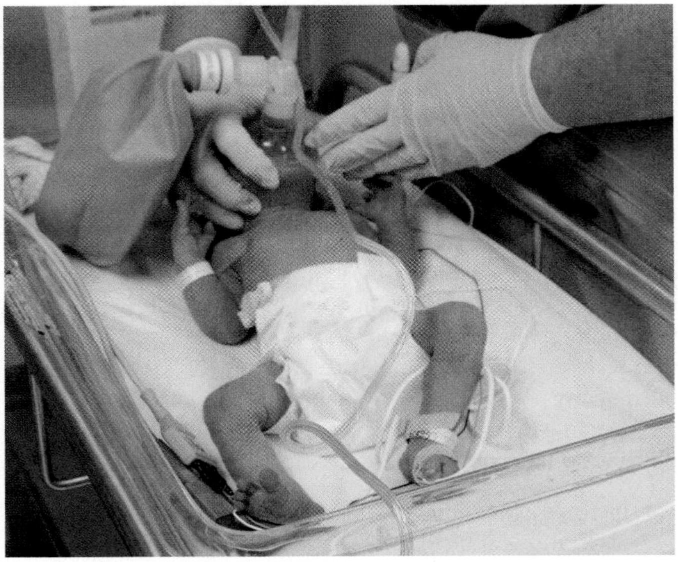

● **Figure 29–1** Demonstration of resuscitation of a newborn with bag and mask. Note that the mask covers the nose and mouth, and the head is in a neutral "sniff" position. The resuscitating bag is placed to the side of the baby so that chest movement can be seen.

3. Chest movement is observed for proper ventilation. Air entry and heart rate are checked by auscultation. Heart rate may be quickly checked by palpating the base of the umbilical cord stump and counting the pulsations for 6 seconds and then multiplying by 10. Manual resuscitation is coordinated with any voluntary efforts. During positive pressure ventilation, the nurse should squeeze the resuscitation bag just enough to improve heart rate, color, and muscle tone. The rate of ventilation should be between 40 and 60 breaths per minute. Pressure should be adequate to move the chest wall. The pressure gauge (manometer) must be in place to avoid overdistention of the newborn's lungs and other problems such as pneumothorax or abdominal distention. Increasing the pressure to 30 cm H_2O or greater is occasionally necessary if there is no improvement in these parameters (heart rate, color, muscle tone) (American Academy of Pediatrics [AAP] & American Heart Association [AHA], 2006). If ventilation is adequate, the chest moves with each inspiration, bilateral breath sounds are audible, and the lips and mucous membranes become pink. Distention of the stomach is controlled by inserting a nasogastric tube for decompression.
4. Endotracheal intubation may be needed. However, most newborns, except for very-low-birth-weight (VLBW) (< 1500 g) infants, can be resuscitated by bag and mask ventilation.

Once breathing has been established, the heart rate should increase to more than 100 beats per minute. If the heart rate is absent or the heart rate remains less than 60 beats per minute after 30 seconds of effective positive pressure ventilation with 100% oxygen, external cardiac massage (chest compression) is begun. Chest compressions are started immediately if there is no detectable heartbeat. The following procedure is used for performing chest compressions:

1. The infant is positioned properly on a firm surface.
2. The resuscitator stands at the foot or head of the infant and places both thumbs over the lower third of the sternum (just below an imaginary line drawn between the nipples), with the fingers wrapped around and supporting the back (Figure 29–2A ●). Alternatively, the resuscitator can use two fingers instead of thumbs (Figure 29–2B). The two-thumb method is preferred because it may provide better coronary perfusion pressure; however, it decreases thoracic expansion during ventilation and makes access to the umbilical cord for medication administration more difficult (Cloherty et al., 2008).
3. The sternum is depressed to sufficient depth to generate a palpable pulse or approximately one-third of the anterior-posterior diameter of the chest at a rate of 90 compressions per minute (AAP & AHA, 2006; Cloherty et al., 2008). Nurses use a 3:1 ratio of heartbeat to assisted ventilation.

Drugs that should be available in the birthing area include those needed in the treatment of shock, cardiac arrest, and narcosis. Oxygen, because of its effective use in ventilation, is the

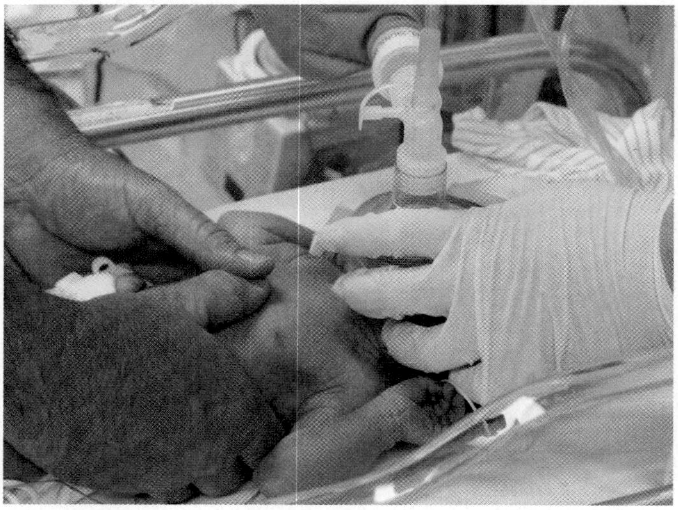

A

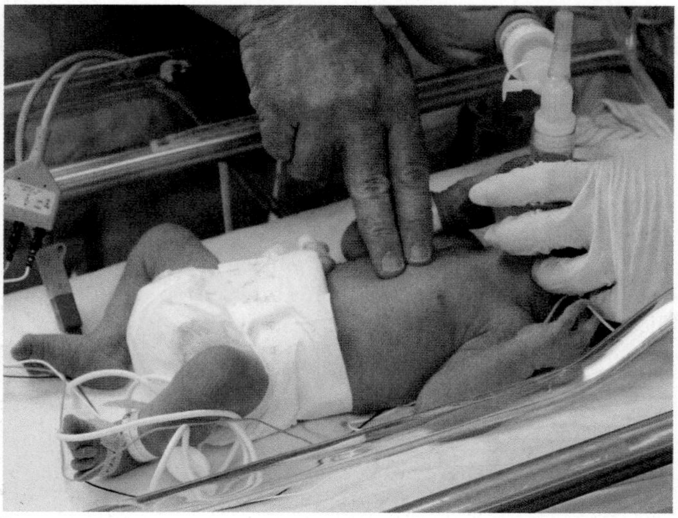

B

● **Figure 29–2** External cardiac massage. The lower third of the sternum is compressed with two fingertips or thumbs at a rate of 90 beats per minute. ***A,*** In the thumb method, the fingers support the infant's back and both thumbs compress the sternum. ***B,*** In the two-fingers method, the tips of two fingers of one hand compress the sternum, and the other hand or a firm surface supports the infant's back.

drug most often used. After 30 seconds of ventilation and cardiac compression, the nurse will reassess the newborn's cardiopulmonary status by palpating the umbilical cord for a pulse. If the newborn has not responded with spontaneous respirations and a heart rate above 60 beats per minute, resuscitative medications are necessary (Cloherty et al., 2008). The most accessible route for administering medications is the umbilical vein (give intravenously [IV]). When the heart rate remains below 60 beats per minute despite 30 seconds of assisted ventilation followed by another 30 seconds of coordinated chest compression, then epinephrine, a cardiac stimulant, is indicated (AAP & AHA, 2006). If bradycardia is present, an intravenous dose of epinephrine (0.1 to 0.3 mL/kg [up to 1.0 mL] of a 1:10,000 solution) is given through the umbilical vein catheter as rapidly as possible. Endotracheal administration may be considered while IV access is being established. When epinephrine is administered by endotracheal tube, consider a higher dose (0.3 to 1 mL/kg). The endotracheal route is associated with unreliable absorption and may not be effective at the lower dose (AAP & AHA, 2006). *Sodium bicarbonate is rarely given in the birthing room.* Sodium bicarbonate is given only to correct metabolic acidosis that results from lactic acid buildup caused by insufficient tissue oxygenation and after effective ventilation is established. Dextrose (2 mL/kg) is given to prevent progression of hypoglycemia. A 10% dextrose in water intravenous solution is usually sufficient to prevent or treat hypoglycemia in the birthing area. Naloxone hydrochloride (0.1 mg/kg), a narcotic antagonist, is used to reverse known iatrogenic narcotic depression (AAP & AHA, 2006). (See "Drug Guide: Naloxone Hydrochloride [Narcan]" on page 709.)

If shock develops (low blood pressure, pallor, or poor peripheral perfusion), the baby may be given a volume expander such as normal saline or lactated Ringer's in a dose of 10 mL/kg via umbilical vein route. If there is a known fetal hemorrhage or fetal anemia, whole blood (O Rh-negative cross-matched against the mother's blood) and packed red blood cells (RBCs) given over a 5- to 10-minute period can also be used for volume expansion and treatment of hypovolemic shock. In some instances of prolonged resuscitation associated with shock and poor response to resuscitation, dopamine (5 mcg/kg/min) may be necessary.

NURSING MANAGEMENT

NURSING ASSESSMENT AND DIAGNOSIS

Communication between the obstetric office or clinic and the birthing area nurse facilitates the identification of newborns who may need resuscitation. When the woman arrives in the birthing area, the nurse should have the antepartal record, note any contributory perinatal history factors, and assess present fetal status. As labor progresses, continue ongoing monitoring of fetal heartbeat and its response to contractions, assisting with fetal scalp blood sampling, and observing for the presence of meconium in the amniotic fluid to assess for fetal asphyxia. Alert the resuscitation team and the practitioner responsible for care of the newborn of any potential high-risk laboring women.

Nursing diagnoses that may apply to the newborn with asphyxia and the newborn's parents include:

- *Ineffective Breathing Pattern* related to lack of spontaneous respirations at birth secondary to in utero asphyxia
- *Decreased Cardiac Output* related to impaired oxygenation
- *Ineffective Family Coping: Compromised* related to baby's lack of spontaneous respirations at birth and fear of losing their newborn

Drug Guide

NALOXONE HYDROCHLORIDE (NARCAN)

Overview of Neonatal Action

Naloxone hydrochloride (Narcan) is used to reverse respiratory depression caused by acute narcotic toxicity when the mother received a narcotic within 4 hours of birth. It displaces morphine-like drugs from receptor sites on the neurons; therefore the narcotics can no longer exert their depressive effects. It is essentially a pure opioid antagonist. Naloxone reverses narcotic-induced respiratory depression, analgesia, sedation, hypotension, and pupillary constriction.

Route, Dosage, Frequency

Intravenous dose is 0.1 mg/kg (0.25 mL/kg of 0.4 mg/mL concentration) at birth, including for premature infants. This drug is usually given through the umbilical vein or endotracheal tube (ET), although naloxone can be given intramuscularly (delays onset of action) if adequate perfusion exists. For IV push, infuse over at least 1 minute; for ET administration, dilute in 1 to 2 millimeters of normal saline (NS).

Reversal of drug depression occurs within 1 to 2 minutes after IV administration and within 15 minutes of IM administration. The duration of action is variable (minutes to hours) and depends on the amount of the drug present and the rate of excretion. Duration of narcotic often exceeds that of the naloxone. The dose may be repeated in 3 to 5 minutes. If there is no improvement after two or three doses, discontinue naloxone administration. If the initial reversal occurs, repeat the dose as needed (Young & Mangum, 2009).

Neonatal Contraindications

Naloxone should not be administered to infants of mothers who chronically use narcotics or those on methadone maintenance, because it may precipitate acute withdrawal syndrome (increased heart rate and blood pressure, vomiting, seizures, tremors).

Respiratory depression may result from nonmorphine drugs, such as sedatives, hypnotics, anesthetics, or other nonnarcotic central nervous system (CNS) depressants.

Neonatal Side Effects

Excessive doses may result in irritability, increased crying, and possible prolongation of partial thromboplastin time (PTT).
Tachycardia may occur.

Nursing Considerations

- Monitor respirations—rate and depth—closely for improved respiratory effort.
- Assess for return of respiratory depression when naloxone effects wear off and effects of longer-acting narcotics.
- Assess for continued respiratory depression after positive-pressure ventilation has restored normal heart rate and color.
- Have resuscitative equipment, O_2, and ventilatory equipment available.
- Note that naloxone is incompatible with alkaline solutions such as sodium bicarbonate.
- Store at room temperature and protect from light.
- Compatible with heparin.

PLANNING AND IMPLEMENTATION

HOSPITAL-BASED NURSING CARE

Following identification of possible high-risk situations, the next step in effective resuscitation is assembling the necessary equipment and ensuring proper functioning.

Check and maintain equipment to ensure its reliability before an emergency arises, and the equipment must be restocked immediately after use and rechecked before every birth. Inspect all equipment—bag and mask, oxygen and flowmeter, laryngoscope, and suction machine—for damaged or nonfunctioning parts before a birth or when setting up an admission bed. A systematic check of the emergency cart and equipment is a routine responsibility of each shift. Resuscitative equipment in the birthing room must be sterilized after each use. It is desirable to assemble equipment for pH and blood gas determination as well.

During resuscitation, it is essential to keep the newborn warm. The newborn should be dried quickly with warmed towels or blankets and a hat placed on the newborn's head to prevent evaporative heat loss, then placed under a prewarmed radiant warmer with servocontrol set at 36.5°C (97.7°F). This device provides an overhead radiant heat source. (A thermostatic mechanism that is secured to the infant's abdomen, over a solid organ like the liver, triggers the radiant warmer to turn on or off to maintain a constant temperature.) An open bed is necessary for easy access to the newborn.

Training and knowledge about resuscitation are vital to personnel in the birth setting for both normal and at-risk births. Resuscitation is at least a two-person effort and the nurse should call for additional support as needed. One member must have the skill to perform airway management and ventilation. Resuscitative efforts are recorded on the newborn's chart so that all members of the healthcare team have access to the information.

PARENT TEACHING

The new newborn resuscitation guidelines favor family members being present during resuscitation in the birthing room and in the neonatal intensive care unit (NICU), but nurses should be aware that the procedure is particularly distressing for parents. If the need for resuscitation is anticipated, the parents should be assured that a team will be present at the birth to care specifically for their newborn. Nurses should advise parents that a support person will be available for them as well if resuscitation is necessary. As soon as the infant's condition has stabilized, a member of the interdisciplinary team needs to discuss the newborn's condition with the parents. The parents may have many fears about the reasons for resuscitation and the condition of their baby following resuscitation.

EVALUATION

Expected outcomes of nursing care include the following:

- The newborn requiring resuscitation is promptly identified, and intervention is started early.
- The newborn's metabolic and physiologic processes are stabilized, and recovery is proceeding without complications.
- The parents can verbalize the reason for resuscitation and what was done to resuscitate their newborn.
- The parents can verbalize their fears about the resuscitation process and potential implications for their baby's future.

> **Teaching Highlights**
>
> **UNDERSTANDING RESPIRATORY DISTRESS**
>
> You can help parents understand their baby's respiratory distress by having them think of the air sacs (alveoli) of the lungs as tiny balloons filled with water and no air. When the tiny balloon (alveoli) is emptied (as in expiration), water droplets can remain inside the balloon and the sides of the balloons stick together (increasing the surface tension between the sides of the balloon). This increased surface tension makes the next reinflation very difficult and requires an increased amount of energy.

MyNursingKit Weblink Application: Infant Respiratory Distress Syndrome

CARE OF THE NEWBORN WITH RESPIRATORY DISTRESS

Respiratory distress syndrome is an inappropriate respiratory adaptation to extrauterine life. The nurse caring for a baby with respiratory distress needs to understand the normal pulmonary and circulatory physiology (Chapter 24), the pathophysiology of the disease process, clinical manifestations, and supportive and corrective therapies. Only with this knowledge can the nurse make appropriate observations about responses to therapy and development of complications. Unlike the verbalizing adult client, the newborn communicates needs only by behavior or physiologic parameters that must be interpreted by the NICU nurse. The neonatal nurse interprets this behavior as clues about the individual baby's condition. This section discusses respiratory distress syndrome, transient tachypnea of the newborn, and meconium aspiration syndrome.

RESPIRATORY DISTRESS SYNDROME

Respiratory distress syndrome (RDS) also referred to as *hyaline membrane disease (HMD),* is the result of a primary absence, deficiency, or alteration in the production of pulmonary surfactant. It is a complex disease that affects approximately 24,000 infants a year in the United States, most of whom are preterm (Nash & Smith, 2008). The syndrome occurs more frequently in premature Caucasian infants than in infants of African or Hispanic descent and almost twice as often in males as in females.

All the factors precipitating the pathologic changes of RDS have not been determined, but the main factors associated with its development include:

1. *Prematurity.* All preterm newborns—whether AGA, SGA, or LGA—and especially infants of diabetic mothers (IDM) are at risk for RDS. The incidence of RDS increases with the degree of prematurity, and most deaths occur in newborns weighing less than 1500 g. The maternal and fetal factors resulting in preterm labor and birth, complications of pregnancy, cesarean birth (and its indications), and familial tendency are all associated with RDS.
2. *Surfactant deficiency disease.* Normal pulmonary adaptation requires adequate surfactant, a lipoprotein that coats the inner surfaces of the alveoli. Surfactant provides alveolar stability by decreasing the alveoli's surface tension and tendency to collapse. Surfactant is produced by type II alveolar cells starting at about 24 weeks' gestation. In the normal or mature newborn lung, it is continuously synthesized, oxidized during breathing, and replenished. Adequate surfactant levels lead to better lung compliance and permit breathing with less work. RDS is caused by alterations in surfactant quantity, composition, function, or production.

Development of RDS indicates a failure to synthesize surfactant, which is required to maintain alveolar stability (see Factors Opposing the First Breath in Chapter 24). Upon expiration this instability increases atelectasis, which causes hypoxia and acidosis because of the lack of gas exchange. These conditions further inhibit surfactant production and cause pulmonary vasoconstriction. The resulting lung instability causes the biochemical problems of hypoxemia (decreased Po_2), hypercarbia (increased Pco_2), and acidemia (decreased pH), primarily metabolic, which further increase pulmonary vasoconstriction and hypoperfusion; alveolar endothelial and epithelial damage; and subsequent protein-rich interstitial and alveolar edema (Nash & Smith, 2008). The cycle of events of RDS leading to eventual respiratory failure is diagrammed in "Pathophysiology Illustrated: Respiratory Distress Syndrome (RDS)."

Because of these pathophysiologic conditions, the newborn must expend increasing amounts of energy to reopen the collapsed alveoli with every breath, so that each breath becomes more difficult than the last. The progressive expiratory atelectasis upsets the physiologic homeostasis of the pulmonary and cardiovascular systems and prevents adequate gas exchange (Cole, Nogee, & Hamvas, 2006). Breathing becomes progressively harder as lung compliance decreases, which makes it more difficult to inflate the lungs and breathe.

PATHOPHYSIOLOGY ILLUSTRATED

RESPIRATORY DISTRESS SYNDROME (RDS)

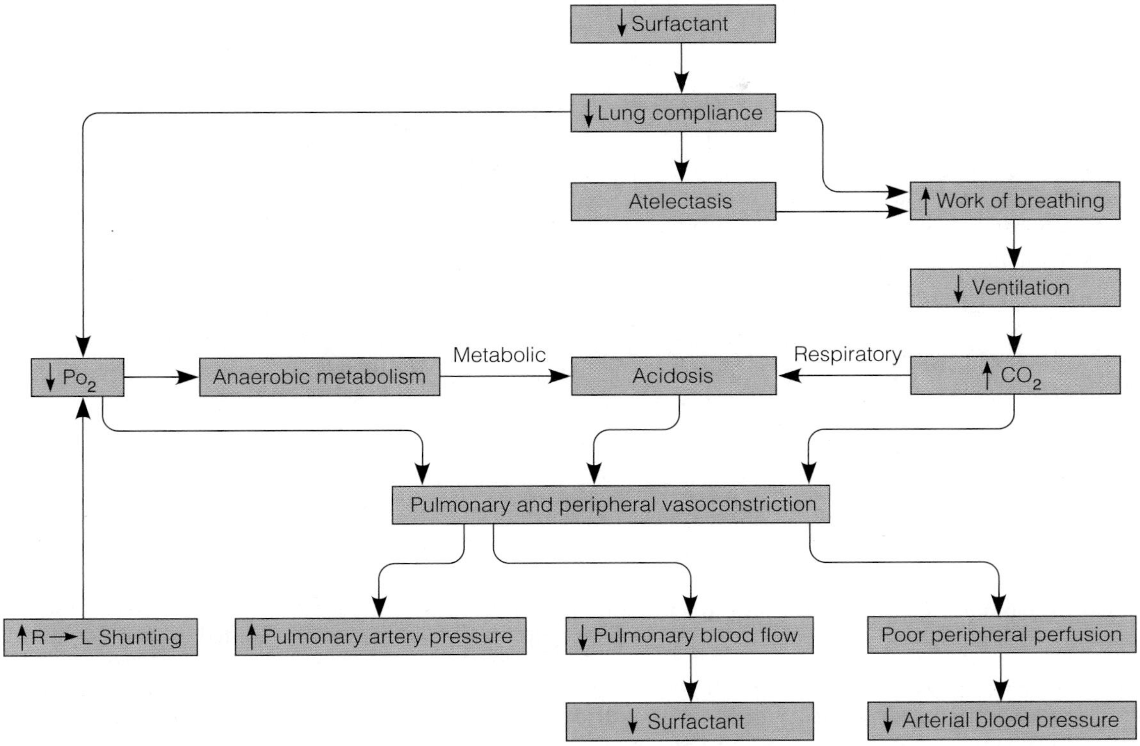

Cycle of events of RDS leading to eventual respiratory failure.

Modified from Gluck, L., & Kulovich, M. V. (1973). Fetal lung development. *Pediatric Clinics of North America, 20,* 375.

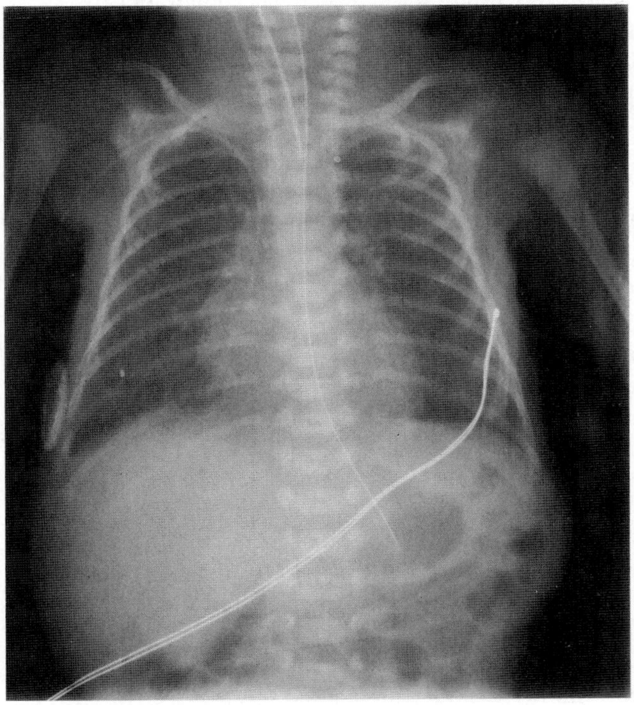

RDS chest x-ray. Chest radiograph of respiratory distress syndrome characterized by a reticulogranular pattern with areas of microatelectasis of uniform opacity and air bronchograms.

Courtesy of Carol Harrigan, RNC, MSN, NNP.

The physiologic alterations of RDS produce the following complications:

1. *Hypoxia.* As a result of hypoxia, the pulmonary vasculature constricts, pulmonary vascular resistance increases, and pulmonary blood flow is reduced. Increased pulmonary vascular resistance may precipitate a return to fetal circulation as the ductus opens and blood flow is shunted around the lungs in a right-to-left blood flow. This shunting increases the hypoxia and further decreases pulmonary perfusion. Hypoxia also causes impairment or absence of metabolic response to cold; reversion to anaerobic metabolism, resulting in lactate accumulation (acidosis); and impaired cardiac output, which decreases perfusion to vital organs.
2. *Respiratory acidosis.* Increased P_{CO_2} and decreased pH are results of alveolar hypoventilation. A persistent rise in P_{CO_2} is a poor prognostic sign of pulmonary function and adequacy because the increased P_{CO_2} and decreased pH are results of alveolar hypoventilation.
3. *Metabolic acidosis.* Because of the lack of oxygen at the cellular level, the newborn begins an anaerobic pathway of metabolism, with an increase in lactate levels and a resulting base deficit (loss of bicarbonate). As the lactate levels increase, the pH decreases in an attempt to maintain acid-base homeostasis.

The classic radiologic picture of RDS is diffuse bilateral reticulogranular (ground glass appearance) density, with portions of the air-filled tracheobronchial tree (air bronchogram) outlined by the opaque ("white-out") lungs with widespread atelectasis, potentially obliterating the heart borders (Cloherty et al., 2008; Thureen, Deacon, Hernandez et al., 2005). (See "Pathophysiology Illustrated Respiratory Distress Syndrome (RDS).") The progression of x-ray findings parallels the pattern of resolution, which usually occurs in 7 to 10 days, and the time of surfactant reappearance, unless surfactant replacement therapy has been used (Blackburn, 2007). Echocardiography is a valuable tool in diagnosing vascular shunts that move blood either away from or toward the lungs.

Clinical Therapy

The primary goal of prenatal management is to prevent preterm birth through early assessment of fetal lung maturity, aggressive treatment of preterm labor, and administration of glucocorticoids to enhance fetal lung development (see Chapter 16∞). Antenatal steroids reduce the incidence and severity of RDS and improve survivability of the 24 to 34 weeks' gestation and extremely low birth weight newborn (less than 1250 grams) (Cloherty et al., 2008).

Postnatal surfactant replacement therapy is available for infants to decrease the severity of RDS in low birth weight newborns. This is one of the best studied therapies in newborns. Surfactant replacement therapy is delivered through an endotracheal tube and may be given in either the birthing room or the nursery as indicated by the severity of RDS. Repeat doses are often required. The most frequent reported response to treatment is rapidly improved oxygenation and decreased need for ventilatory support (AAP & ACOG, 2007).

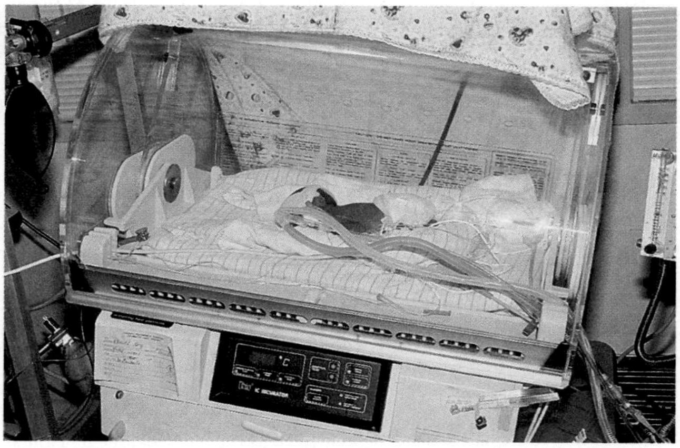

● **Figure 29–3** Mechanical ventilatory assistance. One-day-old, 29 weeks' gestational age, 1450 g baby on respirator and in isolette.
Source: Courtesy of Carol Harrigan, RNC, MSN, NNP.

Supportive medical management consists of ventilation therapy, transcutaneous oxygen and carbon dioxide monitoring, blood gas monitoring, correction of acid-base imbalance, environmental temperature regulation, adequate nutrition, and protection from infection. Ventilation therapy is directed toward preventing hypoventilation and hypoxia. Mild cases of RDS may require only increased humidified oxygen concentrations. Use of continuous positive airway pressure (CPAP) may be required in moderately afflicted infants. Babies with severe RDS require mechanical ventilatory assistance from a respirator (Figure 29–3 ●).

High-frequency ventilation (HFV) can be tried when conventional ventilator therapy has not been successful, and it sometimes can be the primary mode of ventilation to minimize lung injury in very small and/or sick infants (Cloherty et al., 2008). In some institutions, morphine or fentanyl is used for its analgesic and sedative effects. Sedation may be indicated for infants who have air leak respiratory problems. Using pancuronium (Pavulon) for muscle relaxation in infants with RDS is controversial.

NURSING MANAGEMENT

The nurse should look for characteristics of RDS such as increasing cyanosis, tachypnea (greater than 60 respirations per minute),

Nursing Practice

In babies with RDS who are on ventilators, increased diuresis or urination (determined by weighing diapers) may be an early clue that the baby's condition is improving. As fluid moves out of the lungs into the bloodstream, alveoli open and kidney perfusion increases; this results in increased voiding. At this point, the nurse must monitor chest expansion closely. If chest expansion is increasing, pulmonary compliance is improving and ventilator settings may have to be decreased, sometimes quite soon after surfactant dosing. Too high a ventilator setting may "blow the lung," resulting in pneumothorax.

Evidence-Based Nursing

NURSING CARE OF THE NEWBORN WITH NCPAP

Clinical Question

What are guidelines for care of the newborn with nasal continuous positive airway pressure (CPAP)?

The Evidence

McCoskey (2008), a clinical expert, was asked by the National Association of Neonatal Nurses to review research and develop guidelines for nursing care of neonates who are receiving CPAP treatment. More than 30 research studies were systematically reviewed to develop comprehensive clinical care guidelines. Nasal CPAP benefits neonates with inadequately developed lungs by increasing lung volume and preventing atelectasis. This is achieved by supplying continuous pressure at the alveolar level, thus increasing functional oxygenation capacity. Use of nasal CPAP has proved beneficial in many studies, primarily by improving oxygenation and decreasing the work of breathing. Complications may also occur, particularly if clinical management is inappropriate. Primary adverse effects include skin breakdown, nasal/nares/septum damage, and the potential for delayed surfactant therapy.

Best Practice

Clinical assessment of the neonate on CPAP falls under three categories: observation signs of respiratory distress; auscultation of breath sounds; and assessment of the skin and mucus membranes of the nasal area. Inspection of the nasal area includes skin breakdown, symmetry of the nares, and position of the septum. Nasal prongs will tend to cause nasal wall and septal breakdown, whereas nasal CPAP masks tend to cause breadown low on the septum at the base of the nares. Obtain an appropriate fitting hat and mask and place the nasal circuit so that it does not increase pressure points. Position the neonate prone and with the neonate's hand tucked under the chin to help keep the mouth closed. Nasal prongs should fill the entire nare without causing blanching of the external nare; a small space should be present between nares and prong base. All tubes and straps should be secure but without creating undue pressure on any sites.

Critical Thinking

What are the long-term outcomes for neonates who have been treated with CPAP with appropriate clinical management?

See MyNursingKit for possible responses.

grunting respirations, nasal flaring, significant retractions, and apnea. Table 29–1 reviews clinical findings associated with respiratory distress in general. The Silverman-Andersen index (Figure 29–4 ●) may be helpful in evaluating the signs of respiratory distress used in the birthing area.

Based on clinical parameters, the neonatal nurse implements therapeutic approaches to maintain physiologic homeostasis and provides supportive care to the newborn with RDS. (See "Nursing Care Plan: Care of Newborn with Respiratory Distress Syndrome," on pages 717–719.)

Nursing interventions and criteria for instituting mechanical ventilation depend on institutional protocol. Noninvasive oxygen monitoring provides real-time trend information that is particularly useful in infants showing frequent swings in PaO_2 and oxygen saturation. These methods (pulse oximetry, transcutaneous oxygen monitor) can also reduce the frequency of

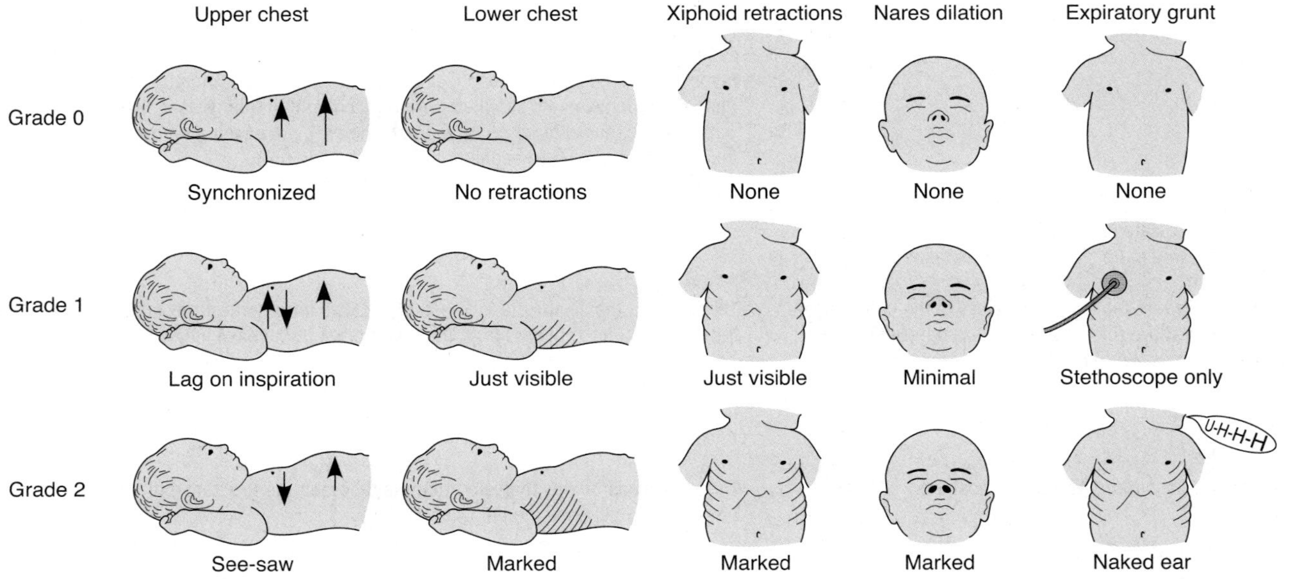

● **Figure 29–4** Evaluation of respiratory status using the Silverman-Andersen index. The baby's respiratory status is assessed. A grade of 0, 1, or 2 is determined for each area, and a total score is charted in the baby's record or on a copy of this tool and placed in the chart.

Source: Used with permission: Clinical Education Series No. 2: Columbus, OH: Ross Products Division, Abbott Laboratories.

Table 29–1 Clinical Assessments Associated with Respiratory Distress

Clinical Picture	Significance
SKIN COLOR	
Pallor or mottling	These represent poor peripheral circulation caused by systemic hypotension and vasoconstriction and pooling of independent areas (usually in conjunction with severe hypoxia).
Cyanosis (bluish tint)	Depending on hemoglobin concentration, peripheral circulation, intensity and quality of viewing light, and acuity of observer's color vision, this is frankly visible in advanced hypoxia. Central cyanosis is most easily detected by examination of mucous membranes and tongue.
Jaundice (yellow discoloration of skin and mucous membranes caused by presence of unconjugated [indirect] bilirubin)	Metabolic alterations (acidosis, hypercarbia, asphyxia) of respiratory distress predispose a newborn to dissociation of bilirubin from albumin-binding sites and deposition in the skin and central nervous system.
Edema (presents as slick, shiny taut skin)	This is characteristic of preterm infants because their total protein concentration is low, with a decrease in colloidal osmotic pressure and transudation of fluid. Edema of hands and feet is frequently seen within first 24 hours and resolved by fifth day in infants with severe RDS.
RESPIRATORY SYSTEM	
Tachypnea (normal respiratory rate [RR] 30 to 60/minute, sustained, elevated respiratory rate 60+/minute)	Increased respiratory rate is the easiest detectable sign of respiratory distress after birth. Because of the premature infant's very compliant chest wall, it is more energy efficient to increase the respiratory rate than the depth of respirations. This compensatory mechanism attempts to increase respiratory dead space to maintain alveolar ventilation and gas exchange in the face of an increase in mechanical resistance. As a decompensatory mechanism it increases workload and energy output by increasing respiratory rate, which causes increased metabolic demand for oxygen and thus increases alveolar ventilation on an already overstressed system. During shallow, rapid respirations, there is an increase in dead space ventilation, thus decreasing alveolar ventilation.
Apnea (episode of nonbreathing for more than 20 seconds; periodic breathing, a common "normal" occurrence in preterm infants, is defined as apnea of 5 to 10 seconds alternating with 10 to 15 seconds of ventilation)	This poor prognostic sign indicates cardiorespiratory disease, CNS disease, metabolic alterations, intracranial hemorrhage, sepsis, or immaturity. Physiologic alterations include decreased oxygen saturation, respiratory acidosis, and bradycardia.
CHEST	
	Inspection of the thoracic cage includes shape, size, and symmetry of movement. Respiratory movements should be symmetrical and diaphragmatic; asymmetry reflects pathology (pneumothorax, diaphragmatic hernia). Increased anteroposterior diameter indicates air trapping (meconium aspiration syndrome).
Labored respirations (Silverman-Andersen index in Figure 29–6 indicates severity of retractions, grunting, and nasal flaring, which are signs of labored respirations)	Indicates marked increase in the work of breathing.
Retractions (inward pulling of soft parts of the chest cage—suprasternal (above the sterum), substernal (below xiphoid process), intercostals (between the ribs)—at inspiration)	These reflect the significant increase in negative intrathoracic pressure necessary to inflate stiff, noncompliant lungs. Infants attempt to increase lung compliance by using accessory muscles. Lung expansion markedly decreases. Seesaw respirations are seen when the chest flattens with inspiration and the abdomen bulges. Retractions increase the work of breathing and O_2 need. As a result, assisted ventilation may be necessary because of exhaustion.
Nasal flaring (inspiratory dilation of nostrils)	This compensatory mechanism attempts to lessen the resistance of the narrow nasal passage and increase the inflow of air.
Expiratory grunt (Valsalva maneuver in which the infant exhales against a partially closed glottis, thus producing an audible moan)	This increases intrapulmonary pressure, which decreases or prevents atelectasis, thus improving oxygenation and alveolar ventilation. It allows more time for the passage of oxygen into the circulatory system. Intubation should not be attempted unless the infant's condition is rapidly deteriorating, because it prevents this maneuver and allows the alveoli to collapse.

Table 29–1 Clinical Assessments Associated with Respiratory Distress—continued

Clinical Picture	Significance
Rhythmic body movement with labored respirations (chin tug, head bobbing, retractions of anal area)	This is a result of using abdominal and other respiratory accessory muscles during prolonged forced respirations.
Auscultation of chest reveals decreased air exchange, with harsh breath sounds or fine inspiratory rales; rhonchi may be present	Decrease in breath sounds and distant quality may indicate interstitial or intrapleural air or fluid.
CARDIOVASCULAR SYSTEM	
Continuous systolic murmur may be audible	Patent ductus arteriosus is a common occurrence with hypoxia, pulmonary vasoconstriction, right-to-left shunting, and congestive heart failure.
Heart rate usually within normal limits (fixed heart rate may occur with a rate of 110 to 120/minute)	A fixed heart rate indicates a decrease in vagal control.
Point of maximal impulse usually located at fourth to fifth intercostal space, left sternal border	Displacement may reflect dextrocardia, pneumothorax, or diaphragmatic hernia.
HYPOTHERMIA	
	This is inadequate functioning of metabolic processes that require oxygen to produce necessary body heat.
MUSCLE TONE	
Flaccid, hypotonic, unresponsive to stimuli Hypertonia and/or seizure activity	These may indicate deterioration in the newborn's condition and possible CNS damage caused by hypoxia, acidemia, or hemorrhage.

blood gas sampling. Methods of noninvasive oxygen monitoring and nursing interventions are included in Table 29–2. (The nursing care of infants on ventilators or with umbilical artery catheters is not discussed here. These infants have severe respiratory distress and are cared for in neonatal intensive care units by nurses with advanced knowledge and training.) Ventilatory assistance with high-frequency ventilators shows positive results. The parents of a baby with respiratory distress should be provided with a very supportive environment (Figure 29–5 ●).

TRANSIENT TACHYPNEA OF THE NEWBORN

Some newborns, primarily LGA and late preterm infants, may develop progressive respiratory distress that clinically can resemble RDS. They may have had intrauterine or intrapartal asphyxia caused by maternal oversedation, maternal bleeding, prolapsed cord, breech birth, or maternal diabetes. The newborn then fails to clear the airway of lung fluid, mucus, and other debris or an excess of fluid in the lungs caused by aspiration of amniotic or tracheal fluid. Transient tachypnea of the newborn (TTN), which occurs in 11 per 1000 live births (Nash & Smith, 2008), is also more prevalent in cesarean-birth newborns who have not had the thoracic squeeze that occurs during vaginal birth and removes some of the lung fluid (Blackburn, 2007).

Usually the newborn experiences little or no difficulty at the onset of breathing. However, shortly after birth, expiratory grunting, flaring of the nares, and mild cyanosis may be noted in the newborn breathing room air. Air will become trapped and an increase

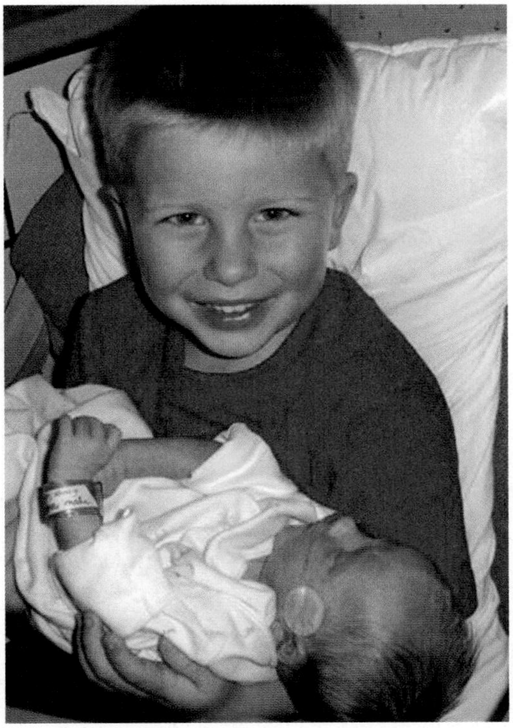

● **Figure 29–5** This baby born at 36 weeks' gestational age had severe RDS. He has ongoing oxygen needs provided by a nasal cannula but still can be held by his proud big brother.

Source: Courtesy of Lisa Smith-Pedersen, RNC, MSN, NNP.

(continued on page 720)

Table 29–2 Oxygen Monitors

Type	Function and Rationale	Nursing Interventions
PULSE OXIMETRY—SPo_2		
Estimates beat-to-beat arterial oxygen saturation.	Calibration is automatic.	Understand and use oxyhemoglobin dissociation curve.
Microprocessor measures saturation by the absorption of red and infrared light as it passes through tissue.	Less dependent on perfusion than $TcPo_2$ and $TcPco_2$, however, functions poorly if peripheral perfusion is decreased due to low cardiac output.	Monitor trends over time and correlate with arterial blood gases. Check disposable sensor at least q8h.
Changes in absorption related to blood pulsation through vessel determine saturation and pulse rate.	Much more rapid response time than $TcPo_2$—offers real-time readings. Can be located on extremity, digit, or palm of hand, leaving chest free; not affected by skin characteristics. Requires understanding of oxyhemoglobin dissociation curve. Pulse oximeter reading of 85% to 95% reflects clinically safe range of saturation. Extreme sensitivity to movement; decreases if average of 7th or 14th beat is selected rather than beat to beat. Poor correlation with extreme hyperoxia.	Use disposable cuffs (reusable cuffs allow too much ambient light to enter, and readings may be inaccurate).
TRANSCUTANEOUS OXYGEN MONITOR—$TcPo_2$		
Measures oxygen diffusion across the skin. Clark electrode is heated to 43°C (preterm) or 44°C (term) to warm the skin beneath the electrode and promote diffusion of oxygen across the skin surface. Po_2 is measured when oxygen diffuses across the capillary membrane, skin, and electrode membrane.	When transcutaneous monitors are properly calibrated and electrodes are appropriately positioned, they will provide reliable, continuous, noninvasive measurements of Po_2, Pco_2, and oxygen saturation. Readings vary when skin perfusion is decreased. Reliable as trend monitor. Frequent calibration necessary to overcome mechanical drift. Following membrane change, machine must "warm up" 1 hour prior to initial calibration; otherwise, after turning it on, it must equilibrate for 30 minutes prior to calibration. When placed on infant, values will be low until skin is heated; approximately 15 minutes required to stabilize.	Use $TcPo_2$ to monitor trends of oxygenation with routine nursing care procedures. Clean electrode surface to remove electrolyte deposits; change solution and membrane once a week. Allow machine to stabilize before drawing arterial gases; note reading when gases are drawn and use values to correlate. Ensure airtight seal between skin surface and electrode; place electrodes on clean, dry skin on upper chest, abdomen, or inner aspect of thigh; avoid bony prominences.
	Second-degree burns are rare but can occur if electrodes remain in place too long. Decreased correlations noted with older infants (related to skin thickness), with infants with low cardiac output (decreased skin perfusion), and with hyperoxic infants.	Change skin site and recalibrate at least every 4 hours; inspect skin for burns; if burns occur, use lowest temperature setting and change position of electrode more frequently.
	The adhesive that attaches the electrode may abrade the fragile skin of the preterm infant. May be used for both preductal and postductal monitoring of oxygenation for observations of shunting.	Adhesive disks may be cut to a smaller size, or skin prep may be used under the adhesive circle only; allow membrane to touch skin surface at center.

Nursing Care Plan

THE NEWBORN WITH RESPIRATORY DISTRESS SYNDROME

INTERVENTION	RATIONALE	EXPECTED OUTCOME
1. Nursing Diagnosis: Risk for Ineffective Breathing Pattern related to immature lung development		
NIC Intervention: **Respiratory monitoring:** Collection and analysis of patient data to ensure airway patency and adequate gas exchange		**NOC Outcome:** **Respiratory status:** Ventilation: Movement of air in and out of the lungs
Goal: The infant will maintain an effective breathing pattern.		
■ Review maternal birth records noting medications given to mother prior to birth and the infant's condition at birth such as Apgar scores and resuscitative measures.	■ Several drugs suppress respiratory function in the newborn.	■ The infant will maintain an effective breathing pattern as evidenced by: respirations are 30–60 breaths/min, arterial blood gases are within a normal range, infant is free of signs of retractions or nasal flaring, and blood pH is 7.35–7.45.
■ Initiate cardiac and respiratory monitoring and calibrate these monitors every 8 hours.	■ Close monitoring detects periodic apneic spells and allows for medical intervention if necessary.	
■ Monitor infant's respiratory rate and rhythm, pulse, blood pressure, and activity.	■ Increases in respiratory rate and pulse, alteration in rhythm, and blood pressure may indicate respiratory distress.	
■ Assess skin color; note signs of cyanosis, duskiness, and pallor.	■ Any changes in the normal skin color may indicate a physiologic change occurring.	
■ Clear infant's airway by suctioning prn with bulb syringe.	■ Opens airway by clearing mucus and allows maximum respiratory effort.	
■ Administer warmed, humidified oxygen by oxygen hood and monitor the oxygen concentrations every 30 minutes.	■ Prevents mucosal dryness and maintains an even level of oxygen administration.	
■ Do not allow oxyhood to touch infant's face; maintain a stable oxygen concentration by increasing and decreasing oxygen by 5%–10% increments.	■ Allowing oxyhood to touch infant's face may cause apnea by stimulating the facial nerve.	
Collaborative: Obtain arterial blood gases (ABGs) per physician orders. 1. Maintain constant O_2 concentration for 15–30 minutes before sample is obtained. 2. Avoid stimulating infant 15 minutes prior to obtaining sample. 3. Avoid suctioning infant prior to obtaining sample. 4. Obtain sample in heparinized tuberculin syringe and maintain the temperature of the sample. 5. Assess the patency of the IV line to prevent clot formation, then replace blood used to clear line. 6. Flush line with 2 mL heparinized solution before restarting flow of IV fluids. 7. Monitor transcutaneous pulse oximeter continuously or hourly and record. Rotate sensor site every 3–4 hours.	■ Obtaining arterial blood gases is essential in managing an infant receiving oxygen. Suctioning may cause a discrepancy in ABG readings and should be avoided.	
■ Assess infant's need for mechanical ventilation: apnea present, hypoxia ($PaO_2 < 50$ mm Hg), hypercapnia ($PaCO_2 > 60$ mm Hg), respiratory acidosis ($pH < 7.2$).	■ Mechanical ventilation improves oxygenation and ventilation, resulting in rise in PaO_2 and decrease in $PaCO_2$.	
■ Administer mechanical ventilation per hospital protocol.	■ CPAP or PEEP can be administered by nasal prongs or by nasopharyngeal or oral intubation.	

(continued)

Nursing Care Plan—continued

THE NEWBORN WITH RESPIRATORY DISTRESS SYNDROME

INTERVENTION	RATIONALE	EXPECTED OUTCOME
2. Nursing Diagnosis: Ineffective Thermoregulation related to increased respiratory effort		
NIC Intervention:		**NOC Outcome:**
Temperature regulation: Attaining or maintaining body temperature within a normal range		**Thermoregulation: Newborn:** Balance among heat production, heat gain, and heat loss during the neonatal period
Goal: The infant will exhibit no signs of hypothermia.		
■ Review maternal prenatal and intrapartum records. Note any medications mother received during these times.	■ Medications such as Demerol and magnesium sulfate used by the mother during the prenatal or intrapartum periods significantly interfere with the infant's ability to retain heat.	■ The infant will not exhibit signs and symptoms of hypothermia as evidenced by temperature maintenance of 97.7–99.1°F and no signs and symptoms of respiratory distress.
■ Assess infant's temperature frequently.	■ Hypothermia leads to pulmonary vasoconstriction because of the increase in oxygen consumption.	
■ Observe for signs of increased oxygen consumption and metabolic acidosis.	■ Cold stress leads to increased oxygen needs; thereby, brown fat is used to maintain body temperature. Hypoxia and acidosis further depresses surfactant production.	
■ Warm all inspired gases and record temperature of delivered gases.	■ Cold air/oxygen blown in face of newborn is stimulus for consumption of oxygen and glucose and increased metabolic rate.	
■ Use radiant warmers or isolettes with servocontrols, incubators, and open cribs with appropriate clothing.	■ Maintains neutral thermal environment.	
■ Note signs and symptoms of respiratory distress, including tachypnea, apnea, cyanosis, acrocyanosis, bradycardia, lethargy, weak cry, and hypotonia.	■ These signs can predispose the infant to metabolic acidosis.	
3. Nursing Diagnosis: Altered Nutrition: Less than Body Requirements related to increased metabolic needs in the infant		
NIC Intervention:		**NOC Outcome:**
Newborn monitoring: Measurement and interpretation of physiologic status of the newborn the first 24 hours		**Nutritional status: Food and fluid intake:** Amount of food and fluid taken into the body over a 24-hour period
Goal: Infant will gain weight in a normal curve.		
■ Assess suck, swallow, gag, and cough reflexes.	■ Prevents feeding problems and assists in determining the best method of feeding for infant.	■ The infant will maintain steady weight gain as evidenced by < 2%/day weight loss, tolerates oral feedings, and urine output is 1–3 mL/kg/hour.
■ Assess respiratory status of infant. If problems are noted, notify physician.	■ In the presence of respiratory distress, avoid oral fluids and initiate parenteral nutrition per physician's orders.	
■ Monitor IV rates per infusion pump (starting at 60 mL/kg/day) or as ordered by physician.	■ Allows for close monitoring of fluid intake.	
■ Record hourly intake and output (I&O) and daily weights.	■ IV fluids are administered to replace sensible and insensible water loss, as well as evaporative water loss secondary to infant respiratory distress. Monitoring I&O will prevent circulatory system overload that can lead to pulmonary edema and cardiac problems.	

Nursing Care Plan—continued

THE NEWBORN WITH RESPIRATORY DISTRESS SYNDROME

INTERVENTION	RATIONALE	EXPECTED OUTCOME
■ Provide total parenteral nutrition (TPN) when indicated.	■ TPN is used as nutritional alternative if bowel sounds are not present and/or infant remains in acute distress.	
■ Advance, based on tolerance, from intravenous to gastrointestinal (GI) feedings. Gavage or nipple-feedings are used, and IV is used as supplement (discontinued when oral intake is sufficient).	■ If IV is discontinued before oral intake is established, baby will not receive adequate calories. ■ Formula or breast milk stimulate GI hormones necessary for a functional absorptive GI tract. ■ Avoid complications associated with nutrition by IV route only.	
■ Provide adequate caloric intake: consider amount of intake, type of formula, route of administration, and need for supplementation of intake by other routes.	■ Calories are essential to prevent catabolism of body proteins, and metabolic acidosis due to starvation or inadequate caloric intake.	
■ Assess infusion site for signs and symptoms of infection, including erythema, edema, and drainage with a foul odor.	■ Appropriate intervention can be initiated when signs and symptoms of infection are detected early. Treatment may avoid infection and sepsis in the infant.	

4. Nursing Diagnosis: Risk for Fluid Volume Deficit related to increased insensible water losses

NIC Intervention:

Fluid monitoring: Collection and analysis of patient data to regulate fluid balance

NOC Outcome:

Fluid balance: Balance of water in the intracellular and extracellular compartments of the body

Goal: The infant will not exhibit signs of dehydration and will display appropriate weight gain.

INTERVENTION	RATIONALE	EXPECTED OUTCOME
■ Observe for weight fluctuations by obtaining daily weights.	■ Fluctuations in weight may indicate water imbalance or inadequate caloric intake.	■ The infant will be free of signs and symptoms of dehydration as evidenced by intake equaling output, urine specific gravity in normal range, and a weight gain of at least 20–30 grams/day.
■ Document cumulative balances of intake (IV fluid administration and feedings) and output (urine collection bags, weighing or counting diapers) hourly.	■ Balanced fluid intake and output suggest homeostasis.	
■ Obtain urinalysis, monitor closely specific gravity and nitrites.	■ Specific gravity $>$ 1.013 and nitrites present in the urine are indicative of not enough fluid intake.	
■ Monitor vital signs, including blood pressure, pulse, temperature, and mean arterial pressure (MAP).	■ A MAP of less than 20 mm Hg may indicate hypotension.	
■ Assess client for signs of dehydration (i.e., poor skin turgor, pale mucous membranes, and sunken anterior fontanelle).	■ Detecting signs and symptoms of dehydration early in the infant is important because early intervention is vital to prevent further damage.	
■ Assess IV site for signs of infection (erythema and edema) and infiltration.	■ If signs and symptoms of infection are noted, intervention is necessary and IV site should be changed.	
Collaborative: Obtain labs for Hct, serum calcium, serum magnesium, serum potassium, blood urea nitrogen (BUN), creatinine, and uric acid levels.	■ Determines necessity for TPN administration. ■ Replaces low nutrient stores and treats anemia if present.	
■ Administer fluids, blood products, and electrolytes as ordered by physician.		

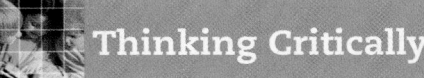

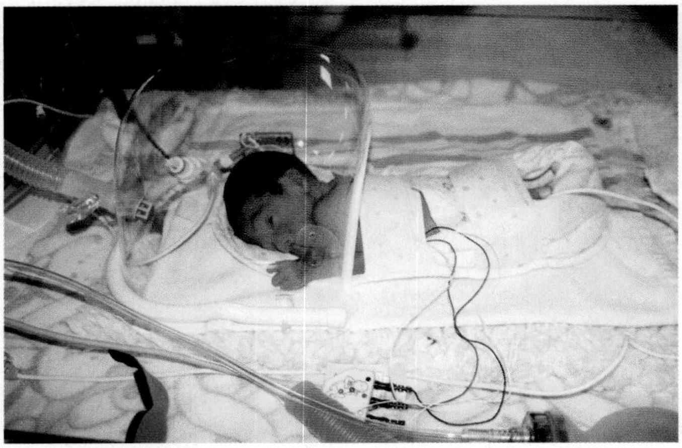

● **Figure 29–6** Premature infant under oxygen hood. Infant is nested and has a nonnutritive sucking pacifier.

Source: Courtesy of Lisa Smith-Pedersen, RNC, MSN, NNP.

in the anterior/posterior diameter of the chest will be observed (Blackburn, 2007). Tachypnea is usually present by 6 hours of age, with respiratory rates consistently greater than 60 breaths per minute. Mild respiratory and metabolic acidosis may be present at 2 to 6 hours. These clinical signs usually persist for 12 to 24 hours. In mild TTN, the signs can improve within 24 hours but may continue for 48 to 72 hours when more severe (Cloherty et al., 2008).

Clinical Therapy

Initial x-ray findings may be identical to those showing RDS within the first 3 hours. However, radiographs of infants with transient tachypnea usually reveal a generalized overexpansion of the lungs (hyperaeration of alveoli), which is identified principally by flattened contours of the diaphragm. Dense streaks (increased vascularity) radiate from the hilar region and represent engorgement of the lymphatic vessels, which clear alveolar fluid on initiation of air breathing. Within 48 to 72 hours, the chest x-ray examination is normal (Cloherty et al., 2008).

Ambient oxygen concentrations of less than 40%, usually under an oxyhood, may be required to correct the hypoxemia (Cloherty et al., 2008) (Figure 29–6 ●). Fluid and electrolyte requirements should be met with IV during the acute phase of the disease. Oral feedings are contraindicated because of rapid respiratory rates and the subsequent risk of aspiration.

When hypoxemia is severe and tachypnea continues, persistent pulmonary hypertension must be considered and treatment measures initiated. If pneumonia is suspected initially, antibiotics may be administered prophylactically.

Nursing management. For nursing actions, see the "Nursing Care Plan: The Newborn with Respiratory Distress Syndrome" on pages 717–719.

CARE OF THE NEWBORN WITH MECONIUM ASPIRATION SYNDROME

Because the body's physiologic response to asphyxia is increased intestinal peristalsis, relaxation of the anal sphincter and presence of meconium in the amniotic fluid indicates that the fetus may be suffering from asphyxia. However, if the fetus is in a breech position, the presence of meconium in the amniotic fluid *does not necessarily* indicate asphyxia.

Approximately 8% to 15% of all live-born, late preterm or term infants are born through meconium-stained amniotic fluid (MSAF). Of the newborns born through MSAF, an average of 5% develop **meconium aspiration syndrome (MAS)** (Cloherty et al., 2008). This fluid may be aspirated into the tracheobronchial tree in utero or during the first few breaths taken by the newborn. This syndrome primarily affects term, SGA, and postterm newborns and those who have experienced a long labor.

Presence of meconium in the lungs produces:

- Mechanical obstruction of airways: ball-valve action (air is allowed in but not exhaled), so that alveoli overdistend.
- Chemical pneumonitis; with oxygen and carbon dioxide trapping and hyperinflation, air leaks such as pneumothorax are common, occurring in 15% to 33% of babies with MAS; secondary bacterial pneumonia can occur.
- Vasoconstriction of pulmonary vessels; allowing development of persistent hypertension (PPHN).
- Inactivation of natural surfactant (Cloherty et al., 2008).

Clinical Manifestations of MAS

Clinical manifestations of MAS include (1) fetal hypoxia in utero a few days or a few minutes before birth, indicated by a sudden increase in fetal activity followed by diminished activity, slowing of FHR or weak and irregular heartbeat, loss of beat-to-beat variability, and meconium staining of amniotic fluid or particulate meconium; and (2) presence of signs of distress at birth, such as pallor, cyanosis, apnea, slow heartbeat, and low Apgar scores (below 6) at 1 and 5 minutes. Newborns with intrauterine asphyxia, meconium-stained newborns, or newborns who have aspirated

---

Thinking Critically

TRANSIENT TACHYPNEA OF THE NEWBORN

You are caring for baby girl Linn, who is a 39-week, AGA female born by repeat cesarean birth to a 34-year-old G3, now P3 mother. Baby Linn's Apgar scores were 7 at 1 minute and 9 at 5 minutes. At 2 hours of age, you note an elevated respiratory rate of 70 to 80 and mild cyanosis. The infant is now receiving 30% oxygen and has a respiratory rate of 100 to 120. The baby's clinical course, chest x-ray examination, and lab work are all consistent with transient tachypnea of the newborn. Her mother calls you to ask about her baby. She tells you that her last child was born at 30 weeks' gestation, had respiratory distress syndrome requiring ventilator support, and was hospitalized for 6 weeks. She asks you, "Is this the same respiratory distress?" What will you tell her?

See MyNursingKit for possible responses.

Evidence in Action

It is no longer recommended that suctioning of the oropharynx and nasopharynx be done before the delivery of the shoulders in the incidence of a meconium-stained amniotic fluid (Organization Guidelines) (American Academy of Pediatrics (AAP), Committee on Fetus and Newborn, & American College of Obstetricians and Gynecolgists (ACOG), Committee on Obstetrics, 2007).

particulate meconium often have respiratory depression at birth and require resuscitation to establish adequate respiratory effort.

After the initial assessment and stabilization, the severity of the ongoing clinical symptoms correlates with the extent of aspiration. Many infants require mechanical ventilation at birth because of immediate signs of distress (generalized cyanosis, tachypnea, and severe retractions). An overdistended, barrel-shaped chest with increased anteroposterior diameter is common. Auscultation reveals diminished air movement, with prominent rales and rhonchi. Abdominal palpation may reveal a displaced liver caused by diaphragmatic depression resulting from the overexpansion of the lungs. Yellowish/pale green staining of the skin, nails, and umbilical cord is usually present, especially if the incident occurred some time before birth.

The MAS chest x-ray film reveals asymmetric, coarse, patchy densities and possible hyperinflation (9 to 11 rib expansion), which may predispose the newborn to air leak syndrome such as pneumothorax or pneumomediastinum (Cloherty, 2008). Evidence of pulmonary air leak is frequently present. These infants have serious biochemical alterations, which include (1) extreme metabolic acidosis resulting from the cardiopulmonary shunting and hypoperfusion; (2) extreme respiratory acidosis caused by shunting and alveolar hypoventilation; and (3) extreme hypoxia, even in 100% O_2 concentration and with ventilatory assistance. Extreme hypoxia is also caused by the cardiopulmonary shunting and resultant failure to oxygenate and can lead to PPHN.

Clinical Therapy

The combined efforts of the maternity and pediatric team are needed to prevent MAS. Previously, the most effective form of preventive management was intrapartum suctioning after the head of the newborn was delivered but the shoulders and chest were still in the birth canal. Current evidence does not support this practice, as routine intrapartum oropharyngeal and nasopharyngeal suctioning does not prevent or alter the course of MAS (AAP & ACOG, 2007; Wiedemann, Saugstad, Barnes-Powell, et al., 2008).

If the infant is vigorous even if there is meconium-stained amniotic fluid, no subsequent special resuscitation such as tracheal suctioning is indicated. Injury to the vocal cords is also more likely to occur during attempts to intubate a vigorous newborn.

If the infant has absent or depressed respirations, heart rate less than 100 beats per minute, or poor muscle tone, direct tracheal suctioning by specially trained personnel such as a neonatal nurse practitioner, an experienced NICU nurse trained in those skills, a respiratory therapist, or a nurse anesthetist is recommended. The glottis is visualized and the trachea suctioned to remove meconium or other aspirated material from beneath the glottis with use of a DeLee attached to low-pressure wall suction to decrease the possibility of human immunodeficiency virus (HIV) transmission. When using mechanical suction, the suction pressure should be set so that negative pressure does not exceed 100 mm Hg. (This is also done with a cesarean birth.)

Further resuscitative efforts are undertaken as indicated, following the same principles of clinical therapy used for asphyxia (discussed earlier in this chapter). Resuscitated newborns should be transferred immediately to the nursery for closer observation. The infant should be maintained in a neutral thermal environment and tactile stimulation should be minimized. An umbilical arterial line may be used for direct monitoring of arterial blood pressures, as well as blood sampling for pH and blood gases. An umbilical venous catheter may be placed for infusion of IV fluids, blood, or medications.

Treatment usually involves delivery of high levels of oxygen and high-pressure ventilation. Low positive end-expiratory pressures (PEEPs) are preferred to avoid air leaks such as pneumothorax. Unfortunately, high pressures may be needed to cause sufficient expiratory expansion of obstructed terminal airways or to stabilize airways that are weakened by inflammation so that the most distal atelectatic alveoli are ventilated.

Naturally occurring surfactant may be inactivated by the presence of meconium and the subsequent inflammatory response that occurs. Surfactant replacement therapy is most effective when used prophylactically. It improves oxygenation and decreases the incidence of air leaks (Cloherty et al., 2008). Systemic blood pressure and pulmonary blood flow must be maintained. Dopamine or dobutamine and/or volume expanders may be used to maintain systemic blood pressure.

Newborns with respiratory failure who are not responding to conventional ventilator therapy may require treatment with high-frequency ventilation and/or nitric oxide therapy or extracorporeal membrane oxygenation (ECMO) if the baby weighs more than 2 kg (Cloherty et al., 2008). Inhaled nitric oxide has proven successful for newborns with meconium aspiration, pneumonia, and PPHN who are not responding to traditional treatment modalities, and it avoids the need for ECMO.

Treatment includes chest physiotherapy (chest percussion, vibration, and drainage) to remove debris. Prophylactic intravenous antibiotics are frequently given. Continuous infusion of bicarbonate to correct metabolic acidosis may be necessary for several days for severely ill newborns. Mortality in term or postterm infants is very high because the cycle of hypoxemia and acidemia is difficult to break.

NURSING MANAGEMENT

NURSING ASSESSMENT AND DIAGNOSIS

During the intrapartal period, the nurse should observe for signs of fetal hypoxia and meconium staining of amniotic fluid. At birth, the nurse assesses the newborn for signs of distress. During the ongoing assessment of the newborn, the nurse carefully observes for complications such as pulmonary air leaks; anoxic cerebral injury manifested by seizure and/or convulsions; myocardial injury evidenced by congestive heart failure or cardiomegaly; disseminated intravascular coagulation (DIC) resulting from hypoxic hepatic damage with depression of liver-dependent clotting factors; anoxic renal damage demonstrated by hematuria, oliguria, or anuria; fluid overload; sepsis secondary to bacterial pneumonia; and any signs of intestinal necrosis from ischemia, including GI obstruction or hemorrhage.

Nursing diagnoses that may apply to the newborn with MAS and the infants' parents include the following:

- *Ineffective Gas Exchange* related to aspiration of meconium and amniotic fluid during birth
- *Altered Nutrition: Less than Body Requirements* related to respiratory distress and increased energy requirements
- *Ineffective Family Coping: Compromised* related to life-threatening illness in term newborn

PLANNING AND IMPLEMENTATION

HOSPITAL-BASED NURSING CARE

Initial interventions are aimed at early identification of meconium aspiration. When significant aspiration occurs, therapy is supportive with the primary goals of maintaining appropriate gas exchange and minimizing complications. Nursing interventions after resuscitation should include maintaining adequate oxygenation and ventilation, regulating temperature, performing glucose testing by glucometer to check for hypoglycemia, observing IV fluid administration, calculating necessary fluids (which may be restricted in the first 48 to 72 hours because of cerebral edema), providing caloric requirements with TPN, and monitoring IV antibiotic therapy.

EVALUATION

Expected outcomes of nursing care include the following:

- The newborn at risk for MAS is promptly identified and early intervention is initiated.
- The newborn is free of respiratory distress and metabolic alterations.
- The parents verbalize their concerns about their baby's health problem and survival and understand the rationale behind the management of their newborn.

CARE OF THE NEWBORN WITH COLD STRESS

Cold stress is excessive heat loss resulting in the use of compensatory mechanisms (such as increased respirations and nonshivering thermogenesis/use of brown fat stores) to maintain core body temperature. Heat loss that results in cold stress occurs in the newborn through the mechanisms of evaporation, convection, conduction, and radiation. (See Chapter 24 for types of thermoregulation.) Heat loss at birth that leads to cold stress can play a significant role in the severity of RDS and the ultimate outcome for the infant. Both preterm and SGA newborns are at risk for cold stress because they have decreased adipose tissue, brown fat stores, and glycogen available for metabolism.

As discussed in Chapter 24, the newborn infant's major source of heat production in nonshivering thermogenesis (NST) is brown fat metabolism. The ability of an infant to respond to cold stress by NST is impaired in the presence of several conditions:

- Hypoxemia (Po_2 less than 50 torr)
- Intracranial hemorrhage or any CNS abnormality
- Hypoglycemia (blood glucose level less than 40 mg/dL)

When these conditions occur, the infant's temperature should be monitored more closely and the neutral thermal environment conscientiously maintained. The nurse must recognize these conditions and treat them as soon as possible. The metabolic consequences of cold stress can be devastating and potentially fatal to an infant. Oxygen requirements rise; even before noting a change in temperature, glucose use increases, acids are released into the bloodstream, and surfactant production decreases (Blackburn, 2007). The effects are graphically depicted in Figure 29–7 ●.

NURSING MANAGEMENT

The amount of heat an infant loses depends to a large extent on the actions of the nurse or caregiver. During the transfer of an NICU newborn from one bed to another, a transient (although not significant) decrease in temperature may be noted for up to 1 hour. Prevention of heat loss is especially critical in the very low birth weight (VLBW) infant. Placing the VLBW newborn in a polyethylene wrapping immediately following birth can decrease the postnatal fall in temperature that normally occurs. Using head coverings made of insulated fabrics, wool, polyolefin, or those lined with Gamgee can significantly decrease heat loss after childbirth (Blackburn, 2007). Convective, radiant, and evaporative heat loss can all be reduced (Blackburn, 2007). Swaddling and nesting maintain flexion, which reduces exposed surface area and thus convective and radiant losses.

Observe all newborns for signs of cold stress, including increased movement and respirations, decreased skin temperature and peripheral perfusion, development of hypoglycemia, and possibly development of metabolic acidosis.

Vasoconstriction is the initial response to cold stress; because it initially decreases skin temperature, the nurse should monitor and assess skin temperature instead of rectal temperature. A decrease in rectal temperature means that the infant has long-standing cold stress. By monitoring skin temperature, a possible decrease will become apparent before the infant's core temperature is affected.

If skin temperature is decreased, determine whether hypoglycemia is present. **Hypoglycemia** is a result of the metabolic effects of cold stress and is suggested by glucometer values below 40 mg/dL, tremors, irritability or lethargy, apnea, or seizure activity.

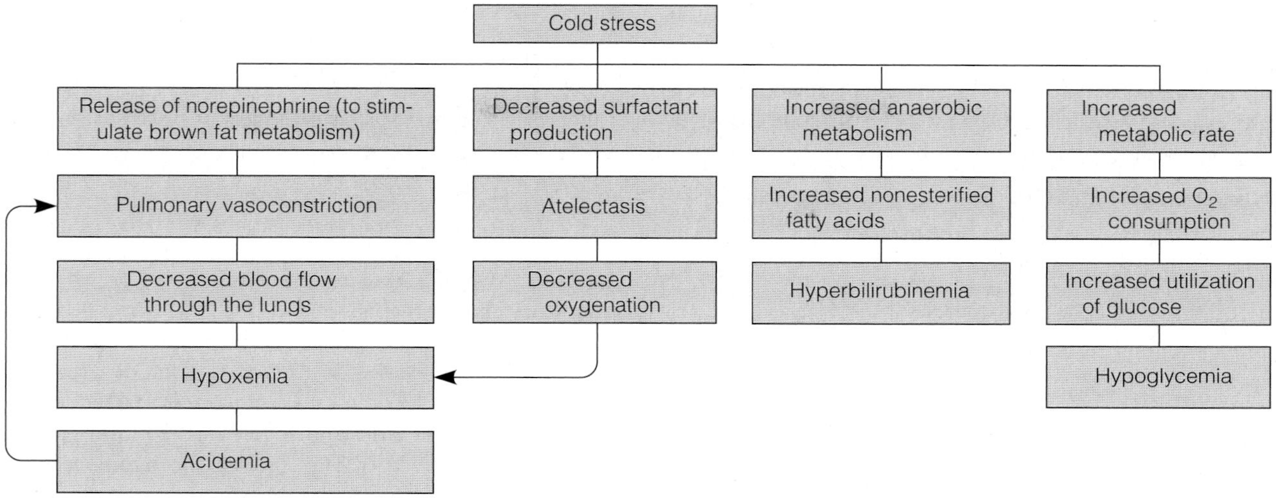

● **Figure 29–7** Cold stress chain of events. The hypothermic, or cold-stressed, newborn attempts to compensate by conserving heat and increasing heat production. These physiologic compensatory mechanisms initiate a series of metabolic events that result in hypoxemia and altered surfactant production, metabolic acidosis, hypoglycemia, and hyperbilirubinemia.

If the newborn becomes hypothermic, initiate the following nursing interventions (Blackburn, 2007; Cloherty et al., 2008):

- Maintain a neutral thermal environment (NTE); adjust based on the gestational age and postnatal age.
- Warm the newborn slowly because rapid temperature elevation may cause hypotension and apnea.
- Increase the air temperature in hourly increments of 1°C (33.8°F) until the infant's temperature is stable.
- Monitor skin temperature every 15 to 30 minutes to determine if the newborn's temperature is increasing.
- Remove plastic wrap, caps, and heat shields while rewarming the infant so that neither cool air nor warm air is trapped.
- Warm IV fluids before infusion.
- Initiate efforts to block heat loss by evaporation, radiation, convection, and conduction and maintain the newborn in NTE such as a heated incubator for transport and radiant heater for procedures.

Assess for the presence of anaerobic metabolism and initiate interventions for the resulting metabolic acidosis. Burning brown fat increases oxygen consumption, lactic acid levels, and metabolic acidosis. Hypoglycemia may be reversed by adequate glucose intake, as described in the following section.

CARE OF THE NEWBORN WITH HYPOGLYCEMIA

An operational threshold for intervention in newborn **hypoglycemia** is a plasma glucose concentration of less than 40 mg/dL at any time in any newborn. It requires follow-up glucose measurement to document normal values (Cloherty et al., 2008). Within the first hours of life, normal asymptomatic newborns may have a transient glucose level in the 30s (mg/dL) that will increase either spontaneously or with feedings. Plasma glucose values less than 20 to 25 mg/dL should be treated with parenteral glucose $D_{10}W$, regardless of the age or gestation to raise plasma glucose to greater than 45 mg/dL. *There is no absolute threshold that can be applied to all babies. Glucose concentrations must be looked at in conjunction with clinical manifestations.*

Hypoglycemia is the most common metabolic disorder occurring in IDMs, SGA infants, the smaller of twins, infants born to mothers with preeclampsia, male infants, and preterm AGA infants. The pathophysiology of hypoglycemia differs for each classification.

AGA preterm infants have not been in utero a sufficient time to store glycogen and fat. As a result, they have decreased ability to carry out gluconeogenesis. This situation is further aggravated by increased use of glucose by the tissues (especially the brain and heart) during stress and illness (chilling, asphyxia, sepsis, RDS).

Infants of White's classes A–C or type 1 diabetic mothers have increased stores of glycogen and fat (see Chapter 31). Circulating insulin and insulin responsiveness are also higher when compared with other newborns. Because the high glucose loads present in utero stop at birth, the newborn experiences rapid and profound hypoglycemia (Blackburn, 2007). Infants with recurrent episodes of hypoglycemia resulting from congenital hyperinsulinism showed that 50% have long-term neurological deficits (Nash & Smith, 2008).

The SGA infant has used up glycogen and fat stores because of intrauterine malnutrition and has a blunted hepatic enzymatic response with which to produce and use glucose. Any newborn stressed at birth from asphyxia or cold also quickly uses up available glucose stores and becomes hypoglycemic. Epidural anesthesia may alter maternal-fetal glucose homeostasis, resulting in hypoglycemia.

CLINICAL THERAPY

The goal of management includes early identification of hypoglycemia through observation and screening of newborns at risk (Cloherty et al., 2008; Mileic, 2008; Nash & Smith, 2008). The newborn may be asymptomatic, or any of the following may occur:

- Lethargy, apathy, and limpness
- Poor feeding, poor sucking, vomiting
- Pallor, cyanosis
- Hypothermia in LBW infants
- Apnea, irregular respirations, respiratory distress
- Hypotonia, possible loss of swallowing reflex
- Tremors, jerkiness, jitteriness, seizure activity
- High-pitched or weak cry
- Exaggerated Moro reflex

Aggressive treatment is recommended after a single low blood glucose value if the infant shows any of these symptoms. In at-risk infants, routine screening should be done frequently during the first 4 hours of life and then at 4-hour intervals until the risk period has passed.

Hypoglycemia may also be defined as a *glucose oxidase reagent strip with reflectance meter* below 40 mg/dL, but only when corroborated with laboratory plasma glucose testing (see Clinical Skills Manual: "Performing a Heel Stick on a Newborn"). **SKILLS** Common bedside methods use whole blood, an enzymatic reagent strip, and a reflectance meter or color chart. Bedside glucose oxidase strip tests may be used for screening for hypoglycemia, but laboratory determinations *must confirm* the results before a diagnosis of hypoglycemia can be made. Glucose reagent strips should not be used by themselves to screen for and diagnose hypoglycemia, because their results depend on the baby's hematocrit (they react to the glucose in the plasma, not the red blood cells) and there is a wide variance (5 to 15 mg/dL) when compared with laboratory plasma determinations.

Blood glucose sampling techniques can significantly affect the accuracy of the blood glucose value. It is important to note that whole blood glucose concentrations are 10% to 15% lower than plasma glucose concentrations (Cloherty et al., 2008). The higher the hematocrit, the greater the difference between whole blood and plasma values. Also, venous blood glucose concentrations are approximately 15% to 19% lower than arterial blood glucose concentrations because the tissues extract some glucose before the blood enters the venous system. Newer point of care techniques, such as using a glucose oxidase analyzer or an optical bedside glucose analyzer, are more reliable for bedside screening but must also be validated with laboratory chemical analysis.

Evidence in Action

There is not significant evidence to support the use of heel warmers preceding a capillary heelstick of an infant and no evidence of an increased yield of blood with the use of heel warmers (National Association of Neonatal Nurses' Guidelines) (Folk, 2007).

Nursing Practice

Blood samples for the laboratory should be placed on ice and analyzed within 30 minutes of drawing to prevent the RBCs from continuing to metabolize glucose and giving a falsely low reading.

Adequate caloric intake is important. Early formula-feeding or breastfeeding is one of the major preventive approaches. If early feeding or IV glucose is started to meet the recommended fluid and caloric needs, the blood glucose concentration is likely to remain above the hypoglycemic level. During the first hours after birth, asymptomatic newborns may also be given oral glucose contained in formula or breast milk (glucose water should not be used because it causes a rapid increase in glucose followed by an abrupt decrease), and then another plasma glucose measurement is obtained within 30 to 60 minutes after feeding.

IV infusions of a dextrose solution D_5W to $D_{10}W$ (5% to 10%) begun immediately after birth should prevent hypoglycemia. Plasma glucose levels are obtained when the parenteral infusion is started. However, in the very small AGA infant, infusions of 10% dextrose solution may cause hyperglycemia to develop, requiring an alteration in the glucose concentration. An IV glucose solution should be calculated based on the infant's body weight and fluid requirements and correlated with blood glucose tests to determine adequacy of the infusion treatment.

A rapid infusion of greater than 25% dextrose or the use of glucose water in place of formula is contraindicated because it may lead to profound rebound hypoglycemia following an initial brief increase. In more severe cases of hypoglycemia, corticosteroids may be administered (Cloherty et al., 2008).

NURSING MANAGEMENT

NURSING ASSESSMENT AND DIAGNOSIS

The objectives of nursing assessment are to identify newborns at risk and to screen symptomatic infants. For newborns diagnosed with hypoglycemia, assessment is ongoing and includes careful monitoring of glucose values. Glucose strips, urine dipstick, and urine volume tests (monitor only if above 1 to 3 mL/kg/hr) may be evaluated frequently for osmotic diuresis and glycosuria.

Nursing diagnoses that may apply to the newborn with hypoglycemia include the following:

- *Altered Nutrition: Less than Body Requirements* related to increased glucose use secondary to physiologic stress
- *Ineffective Breathing Pattern* related to tachypnea and apnea
- *Acute Pain* related to frequent heel sticks secondary to glucose monitoring

Complementary Care

PAIN RELIEF IN THE NICU

The newborn relies on the nurse's observational, assessment, and interventional skills for anticipation and prevention of pain if possible and then prompt, safe, and effective pain relief. It is vital that the nurse assist infants to cope with and recover from necessary painful clinical procedures (Saniski, 2005). A variety of nonpharmacologic pain-prevention and relief techniques have been shown to be effective in reducing pain from minor procedures in newborns.

Pain can be managed effectively by limiting or avoiding noxious stimuli and by providing analgesia. Any unnecessary stimuli (i.e., noise, visual, tactile, and vestibular) of the newborn should be avoided, if possible (AAP & ACOG, 2007). Developmental care, which includes limiting environmental stimuli, lateral positioning, the use of supportive bedding, and attention to behavioral cues, assists the newborn to cope with painful procedures (AAP & CPS, 2006).

Containment with swaddling or facilitated tucking (holding the arms and legs in a flexed position) is effective in reducing excessive immature motor responses. Swaddling also may provide comfort through other senses, such as thermal, tactile, and proprioceptive senses. Breastfeeding and skin-to-skin contact with the mother during the painful procedure may help to relieve pain. Nonnutritive sucking (NNS) refers to the provision of a pacifier into the infant's mouth to promote sucking without the provision of breast milk or formula for nutrition. NNS is thought to produce analgesia through stimulation of orotactile and mechanoreceptors when the pacifier is placed into the infant's mouth. Allowing nonnutritive sucking with a pacifier aids in the reduction of procedural pain and stress. Unfortunately a rebound in distress occurs when the NNS pacifier is removed from the infant's mouth (Walden, 2007).

A wide range of oral sucrose doses has been used for procedural pain relief (heel sticks, venipuncture, IM injections), but no optimal dose has been established (AAP & CPS, 2006). The sweetness of the sucrose, a disaccharide, elevates the pain threshold through endogenous opioid release in the CNS and produces a calming effect (AAP & CPS, 2006). A range of 0.05 to 0.5 mL of 24% sucrose is administered on the anterior part of the tongue via a syringe or nipple approximately 2 minutes before the procedure (Walden, 2007). Some authors have suggested that multiple doses, such as giving a dose 2 minutes before and 1 to 2 minutes after a procedure, is more effective. It is important to be careful with repeated doses of sucrose, as the concern for hyperglycemia may arise. Also, repeated use of sucrose analgesia in preterm infants may affect their neurologic development and behavioral outcomes. Until further research is done, repeated doses of sucrose are not recommended (AAP & CPS, 2006). Because oral sucrose reduces but does not eliminate pain, it should be used with other nonpharmacologic measures to enhance effectiveness.

PLANNING AND IMPLEMENTATION

Infants in at-risk groups should be monitored within 30 to 60 minutes after birth and before feedings or whenever there are abnormal clinical manifestations (Nash & Smith, 2008). The IDM should be monitored within 30 minutes of birth. Once an at-risk infant's blood sugar level is stable, glucose testing every 2 to 4 hours (or per agency protocol), or before feedings, adequately monitors glucose levels. See Figures 29–8 ● and 29–9 ● and Clinical Skills Manual: "Performing a Heel Stick on a Newborn" **SKILLS**.

The method of feeding greatly influences glucose and energy requirements; thus careful calculating glucose requirements, and attention to glucose monitoring is required during the transition from IV to oral feedings. Titration of IV glucose may be required until the infant is able to take adequate amounts of formula or breast milk to maintain a normal blood sugar level. Decrease the concentration of parenteral glucose gradually to 5% (D_5W), then reduce the rate of infusion (mg/kg/min) and slowly discontinue

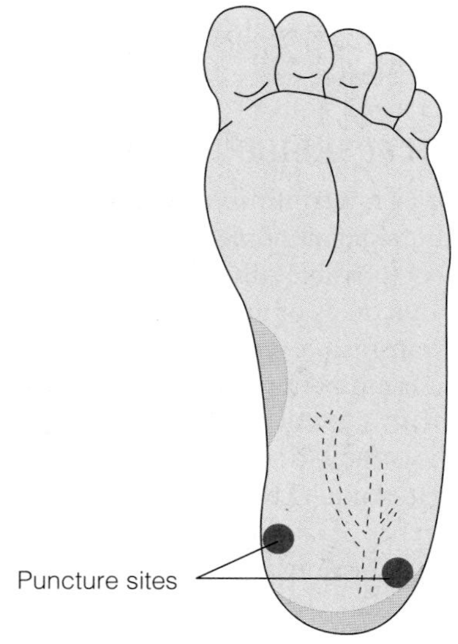

● **Figure 29–8** Potential puncture sites for heel sticks. Avoid gray-shaded areas to prevent injury to arteries and nerves in the foot.

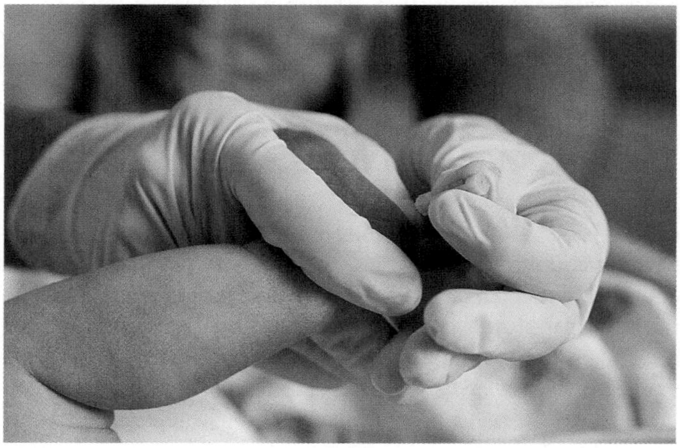

● **Figure 29–9** Heel stick.

it over 4 to 6 hours. Enteral feedings are increased to maintain an adequate glucose and caloric intake and maintain normal blood glucose levels.

The therapeutic nursing measure of nonnutritive sucking during gavage feedings has been reported to increase the baby's daily weight gain and lead to earlier formula feeding or breastfeeding and discharge. Nonnutritive sucking may also lower activity levels, which allows newborns to conserve their energy stores. Hypothermia and activity can increase energy requirements; crying alone can double the baby's metabolic rate.

EVALUATION

Expected outcomes of nursing care include the following:

- The newborn at risk for hypoglycemia is identified, and prompt intervention is started.
- The newborn's glucose level is stabilized, and recovery is proceeding without sequelae.

CARE OF THE NEWBORN WITH JAUNDICE

The most common abnormal physical finding in newborns is jaundice *(icterus neonatorum)*. Some degree of jaundice, resulting from elevated unconjugated bilirubinemia, occurs in approximately 60–70% of term infants and 80% of preterm infants (Glomella, 2009; Bradshaw, 2010). **Jaundice** is a yellowish coloration of the skin and sclera of the eyes that develops from deposit of the yellow pigment bilirubin in lipid/fat containing tissues as described in Chapter 24. Fetal unconjugated (indirect) bilirubin is normally cleared by the placenta in utero, so total bilirubin at birth is usually less than 3 mg/dL unless an abnormal hemolytic process has been present. Postnatally, the infant must conjugate bilirubin (convert a lipid-soluble pigment into a water-soluble pigment) in the liver.

The rate and amount of conjugation of bilirubin depend on the rate of hemolysis, the bilirubin load, the maturity of the liver, and the presence of albumin-binding sites. (See Chapter 24 for discussion of conjugation of bilirubin.) The liver of a normal, healthy term infant is usually mature enough and producing enough glucuronyl transferase that the total serum bilirubin does not reach a pathologic level.

PHYSIOLOGIC JAUNDICE

Physiologic or *neonatal jaundice* is a normal process that occurs during transition from intrauterine to extrauterine life and appears after 24 hours of life. It is caused by the newborn's shortened red blood cell lifespan (90 days as compared with 120 days in the adult), slower uptake by the liver, lack of intestinal bacteria, and/or poorly established hydration from initial breastfeeding (Glomella, 2009).

Lab tests reveal a predominance of unconjugated bilirubin. The average level of unconjugated bilirubin in cord blood is approximately 2 mg/dL at birth. This level rises to an average level of 5 to 6 mg/dL between the third and fifth days of life. The jaundice is usually not visible after 14 days. The pattern of physiologic jaundice differs between breastfed and formula-fed newborns (for further discussion of physiologic jaundice, see Chapter 24). Physiologic jaundice remains a common problem for the term newborn and may require treatment with phototherapy.

PATHOPHYSIOLOGY OF HYPERBILIRUBINEMIA

Serum albumin-binding sites are usually sufficient to conjugate enough bilirubin to meet the normal demands of the newborn. However, certain conditions tend to decrease the sites available. Fetal or neonatal asphyxia and neonatal drugs such as indomethacin decrease the binding affinity of bilirubin to albumin, because acidosis impairs the capacity of albumin to hold bilirubin. Hypothermia and hypoglycemia release free fatty acids that dislocate bilirubin from albumin. Maternal medications such as sulfa drugs and salicylates compete with bilirubin for these sites. Finally, premature infants have less albumin available for binding with bilirubin. Neurotoxicity is possible because unconjugated bilirubin has a high affinity for extravascular tissue, such as fatty tissue (subcutaneous tissue) and cerebral tissue.

Bilirubin not bound to albumin can cross the blood-brain barrier, damage cells of the CNS, and produce kernicterus or **acute bilirubin encephalopathy** (ABE). **Kernicterus** (meaning "yellow nucleus") refers to the deposition of indirect or unconjugated bilirubin in the basal ganglia of the brain and to the permanent neurologic sequelae of untreated **hyperbilirubinemia** (elevation of bilirubin level) (Cloherty et al., 2008).

The classic acute bilirubin encephalopathy of kernicterus most commonly found with Rh and ABO blood group incompatibility is less common today because of aggressive treatment with phototherapy and exchange transfusions. But cases of kernicterus are reappearing as a result of early discharge and the increased incidence of dehydration (as a result of discharge before the mother's milk is established). Current therapy can reduce the incidence of kernicterus encephalopathy but cannot distinguish all infants who are at risk.

CAUSES OF HYPERBILIRUBINEMIA

A primary cause of hyperbilirubinemia is **hemolytic disease of the newborn**. All pregnant women who are Rh negative or who have blood type O (possible ABO blood incompatibility) should be asked about outcomes of any previous pregnancies and history of blood transfusion. Prenatal amniocentesis with spectrophotographic examination may be indicated in some cases. Cord blood from newborns is evaluated for bilirubin level, which normally does not exceed 5 mg/dL. Newborns of Rh-negative and O blood type mothers are carefully assessed for appearance of jaundice and levels of serum bilirubin.

Alloimmune hemolytic disease, also known as **erythroblastosis fetalis**, occurs when an Rh-negative mother is pregnant with an Rh-positive fetus and maternal antibodies cross the placenta. Maternal antibodies enter the fetal circulation, then attach to and destroy the fetal RBCs. The fetal system responds by increasing RBC production. Jaundice, anemia, and compensatory erythropoiesis result. A marked increase in immature RBCs (erythroblasts) also occurs, hence the designation erythroblastosis fetalis. Because of the widespread use of Rh immune globulin (RhoGAM), the incidence of erythroblastosis fetalis has dropped dramatically.

Hydrops fetalis, the most severe form of erythroblastosis fetalis, occurs when maternal antibodies attach to the Rh site on the fetal RBCs, making them susceptible to destruction; severe anemia and multiorgan system failure result. Cardiomegaly with severe cardiac decompensation and hepatosplenomegaly occurs. Severe generalized massive edema (anasarca) and generalized fluid effusion into the pleural cavity (hydrothorax), pericardial sac, and peritoneal cavity (ascites) develops. Jaundice is not present until the newborn period because the bilirubin pigments are excreted through the placenta into the maternal circulation. The hydropic hemolytic disease process is also characterized by hyperplasia of the pancreatic islets, which predisposes the infant to neonatal hypoglycemia similar to that of IDMs. These infants have increased bleeding tendencies because of associated thrombocytopenia and hypoxic damage to the capillaries. Hydrops is a frequent cause of intrauterine death among infants with Rh disease.

ABO incompatibility (the mother is blood type O and the baby is blood type A or B) may result in jaundice, although it rarely results in hemolytic disease severe enough to be clinically diagnosed and treated. Hepatosplenomegaly may be found occasionally in newborns with ABO incompatibility, but hydrops fetalis and stillbirth are rare.

During pregnancy, maternal conditions that predispose the fetus to neonatal hyperbilirubinemia include hereditary spherocytosis, diabetes, intrauterine infections, and gram-negative bacilli infections that stimulate production of maternal alloimmune antibodies, drug ingestion (such as sulfas, salicylates, novobiocin, diazepam), and oxytocin administration. Early prenatal identification of the fetus at risk for Rh or ABO incompatibility allows prompt treatment.

In addition to Rh or ABO incompatibility, other newborn conditions can predispose to hyperbilirubinemia: polycythemia (central hematocrit 65% or more), pyloric stenosis, obstruction or atresia of the biliary duct or of the lower bowel, low-grade urinary tract infection, sepsis, hypothyroidism, enclosed hemorrhage (cephalohematoma, large bruises), asphyxia neonatorum, hypothermia, acidemia, and hypoglycemia. Neonatal hepatitis, atresia of the bile ducts, and GI atresia all can alter bilirubin metabolism and excretion (Glomella, 2009). See risk factors for development of severe hyperbilirubinemia in their approximate order of importance table on MyNursingKit.

The prognosis for a newborn with hyperbilirubinemia depends on the extent of the hemolytic process and the underlying cause. Severe hemolytic disease results in fetal and early neonatal death from the effects of severe anemia—cardiac decompensation, edema, ascites, and hydrothorax. Hyperbilirubinemia that is not aggressively treated may lead to kernicterus. The resultant neurologic damage is responsible for death, cerebral palsy, possible mental retardation, or hearing loss or, to a lesser degree, perceptual impairment, delayed speech development, hyperactivity, muscle incoordination, or learning difficulties.

CLINICAL THERAPY

The best treatment for hemolytic disease is prevention by early recognition of prenatal risk factors such as Rh and ABO incompatibility (see Chapter 16 for discussion of in utero management of this condition); and then neonatal conditions.

Laboratory and Diagnostic Assessments

Neonatal hyperbilirubinemia can be considered pathologic and requires further investigation if any of the following criteria are met (Bhutani, Johnson, & Keren, 2004; Glomella, 2009):

1. Clinically evident jaundice appearing before 24 hours of life or if jaundice seems excessive for the newborn's age in hours
2. Serum bilirubin concentration rising by more than 0.2 mg/dL per hour
3. Total serum bilirubin concentration exceeding the 95th percentile on the nomogram
4. Conjugated bilirubin concentrations greater than 2 mg/dL or more than 10–20% of the total serum bilirubin concentration
5. Clinical jaundice persisting for more than 2 weeks in a term newborn

Initial diagnostic procedures are aimed at differentiating jaundice resulting from increased bilirubin production, impaired conjugation or excretion, increased intestinal reabsorption, or a combination of these factors.

Transcutaneous bilirubin (TcB) measurements are a noninvasive method of assessing bilirubin levels and may be used for predischarge risk assessment. A TcB can be performed quickly and painlessly, and repeated measures are easily obtained. TcB can quantify the amount of bilirubin pigment in the infant's skin. Nurses need to measure bilirubin levels to confirm the presence, absence, or suspicion of jaundice. However, it is important to remember that total serum bilirubin levels remain the standard of care for confirmation or diagnosis of hyperbilirubinemia (Glomella, 2009).

Because of the shorter lifespan of red blood cells in the newborn, a significant bilirubin load is produced. When bilirubin breaks down, carbon monoxide (CO) is released. This production of carbon monoxide is being investigated as a marker in the study of bilirubin production. Measuring end-tidal CO (ETCO) has been shown to provide results similar to those of laboratory bilirubin; however, devices to measure CO are not widely available (Glomella 2009).

Essential laboratory evaluations are Coombs' test, serum bilirubin levels (direct and total), hemoglobin, reticulocyte

Nursing Practice

Because of exposure to sunlight, sternal area TcB measurements may be more accurate than those taken on the forehead. The sternum, in a dressed infant, is less likely to be affected by the influence of ambient light (such as sunlight) on the skin.

percentage, white cell count, and positive smear for cellular morphology.

The Coombs' test is performed to determine whether jaundice is because of Rh or ABO incompatibility. The indirect Coombs' test measures the amount of Rh-positive antibodies in the mother's blood. Rh-positive red blood cells are added to the maternal blood sample. If the mother's serum contains antibodies, the Rh-positive red blood cells will agglutinate (clump) when rabbit immune antiglobulin is added, which is a positive test result.

The direct Coombs' test reveals the presence of antibody-coated (sensitized) Rh-positive red blood cells in the newborn. Rabbit immune antiglobulin is added to the specimen of neonatal blood cells. If the neonatal red blood cells agglutinate, they have been coated with maternal antibodies, a positive result.

If the hemolytic process is caused by Rh sensitization, laboratory findings reveal the following: (1) an Rh-positive newborn with a positive Coombs' test; (2) increased erythropoiesis with many immature circulating red blood cells (nucleated blastocysts); (3) anemia, in most cases; (4) elevated levels (5 mg/dL or more) of bilirubin in cord blood; and (5) a reduction in albumin-binding capacity. Maternal data may include an elevated anti-Rh titer and spectrophotometric evidence of a fetal hemolytic process.

If the hemolytic process is caused by ABO incompatibility, laboratory findings reveal an increase in reticulocytes. The resulting anemia is usually not significant during the newborn period and is rare later on. The direct Coombs' test may be negative or mildly positive, whereas the indirect Coombs' test may be strongly positive. Infants with a positive direct Coombs' test have increased incidence of jaundice, with bilirubin levels in excess of 10 mg/dL. Increased numbers of spherocytes (spherical, plump, mature erythrocytes) are seen on a peripheral blood smear. Increased numbers of spherocytes are not seen on blood smears from Rh disease infants.

Therapeutic Management

Whatever the cause of hyperbilirubinemia, management of these infants is directed toward alleviating anemia, removing maternal antibodies and sensitized erythrocytes, increasing serum albumin levels, reducing serum bilirubin levels, and minimizing the consequences of hyperbilirubinemia. Early discharge of newborns from birthing centers has significantly influenced the diagnosis and management of neonatal jaundice, increasing the emphasis on outpatient and home care management.

If hemolytic disease is present, it may be treated with phototherapy, exchange transfusion, and drug therapy. When determining the appropriate management of hyperbilirubinemia caused by hemolytic disease, the three relevant variables are the newborn's (1) serum bilirubin level, (2) birth weight, and (3) age in hours. If a newborn has hemolysis with an unconjugated bilirubin level of 14 mg/dL, weighs less than 2500 g (birth weight), and is 24 hours old or less, an exchange transfusion may be the best management. However, if that same newborn is over 24 hours of age, which is past the time during which an increase in bilirubin would occur because of pathologic causes, phototherapy may be the treatment of choice to prevent the possible complication of kernicterus.

Phototherapy

Phototherapy is the exposure of the newborn to high-intensity light. It may be used alone or in conjunction with exchange transfusion to reduce serum bilirubin levels. Exposure of the newborn to high-intensity light (a bank of fluorescent light bulbs or bulbs in the blue-light spectrum) decreases serum bilirubin levels in the skin by facilitating biliary excretion of unconjugated bilirubin. Phototherapy decreases serum bilirubin levels by changing bilirubin from the nonwater-soluble (lipophilic) form to water-soluble by-products that can then be excreted via urine and bile. Photoisomerization occurs when the natural form of bilirubin is exposed to light at a certain wavelength and the bilirubin is converted to a less toxic form. The new isomer, photobilirubin, is created rapidly but is quite unstable. The photobilirubin is bound to albumin, transported to the liver, and incorporated into bile. If it is not quickly eliminated from the bowel, then it can convert back to its original form and return to the bloodstream. In addition, the photodegradation products formed when light oxidizes bilirubin can be excreted in the urine.

Phototherapy is an intervention that is used to prevent hyperbilirubinemia in order to halt bilirubin levels from climbing dangerously high. The decision to start phototherapy is based on two factors: gestational age and age in hours. Phototherapy is the most effective in the first 24 to 48 hours of usage; frequently the light can be discontinued during or immediately after this time frame. Phototherapy does not alter the underlying cause of jaundice, and hemolysis may continue to produce anemia. Many authors have recommended initiating phototherapy "prophylactically" in the first 24 hours of life in high-risk, VLBW, or severely bruised infants. Figure 29–10 ● shows guidelines for the use of phototherapy.

Phototherapy can be provided by halogen spotlights (although these are not widely used because of the risk of thermal burns), conventional banks of fluorescent tube phototherapy lights, a fiberoptic blanket attached to a halogen light source around the trunk of the newborn, by a fiberoptic mattress placed under the baby, or by a combination of these delivery methods. Banks of fluorescent bilirubin lights utilize light in the blue spectrum. This is the most effective source available but can mask cyanosis and causes dizziness and nausea in the staff.

With the fiberoptic blanket, the light stays on at all times, and the newborn is accessible for care, feeding, and diaper changes; greater surface area is exposed and there are no thermoregulation issues. The eyes are not covered. The babies do not get overheated, and fluid and weight loss are not complications of this system. Furthermore, it makes the infant accessible to the parents and is less alarming to parents than standard phototherapy. Many institutions and pediatricians use fiberoptic blankets for home care. A combination of a fiberoptic light source in the mattress under or around the baby and a standard light source above has also been recommended. This is termed *intensive phototherapy*. Intensive phototherapy should show a drop in total serum bilirubin (TSB) within 4 to 8 hours. Levels should continue to decline when phototherapy covers a wider surface area. If a drop in bilirubin levels is not reached, then an

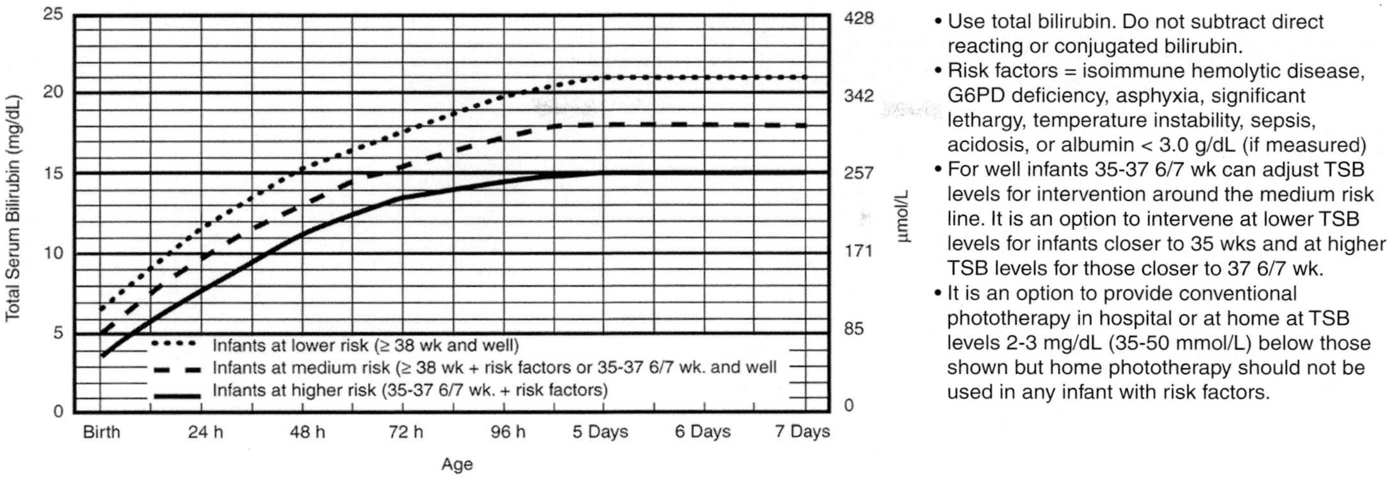
25
20
15
10
5
0
Total Serum Bilirubin (mg/dL)
428
342
257
171
85
0
μmol/L
Infants at lower risk (≥ 38 wk and well)
Infants at medium risk (≥ 38 wk + risk factors or 35-37 6/7 wk. and well
Infants at higher risk (35-37 6/7 wk. + risk factors)
Birth
24 h
48 h
72 h
96 h
5 Days
6 Days
7 Days
Age
• Use total bilirubin. Do not subtract direct reacting or conjugated bilirubin.
• Risk factors = isoimmune hemolytic disease, G6PD deficiency, asphyxia, significant lethargy, temperature instability, sepsis, acidosis, or albumin < 3.0 g/dL (if measured)
• For well infants 35-37 6/7 wk can adjust TSB levels for intervention around the medium risk line. It is an option to intervene at lower TSB levels for infants closer to 35 wks and at higher TSB levels for those closer to 37 6/7 wk.
• It is an option to provide conventional phototherapy in hospital or at home at TSB levels 2-3 mg/dL (35-50 mmol/L) below those shown but home phototherapy should not be used in any infant with risk factors.

• **Figure 29–10** Guidelines for phototherapy in hospitalized infants of 35 or more weeks' gestation.

Note: These guidelines are based on limited evidence and the levels shown are approximations. The guidelines refer to the use of intensive phototherapy, which should be used when the TSB (total serum bilirubin) exceeds the line indicated for each category. Infants are designated as "higher risk" because of the potential negative effects of the conditions listed on albumin binding of bilirubin, the blood-brain barrier, and the susceptibility of the brain cells to damage by bilirubin.

From American Academy of Pediatrics Subcommittee on Hyperbilirubinemia. (2004). Management of hyperbilirubinemia in the newborn infant 35 or more weeks of gestation. *Pediatrics, 114*(1), 297–316, Fig. 3, p. 304.

exchange transfusion should be considered. The nurse uses a photometer to measure and maintain desired irradiance levels. The nurse keeps track of the number of hours each lamp is used so that each can be replaced before its effectiveness is lost (Bradshaw, 2010).

Exchange Transfusion

Exchange transfusion is the withdrawal and replacement of the newborn's blood with donor blood. It is used to treat anemia with red blood cells that are susceptible to maternal antibodies, remove sensitized red blood cells that would soon be lysed, remove serum bilirubin, and provide bilirubin-free albumin and increase the binding sites for bilirubin. Concerns about exchange transfusion are related to the use of blood products and associated potential for HIV infection and hepatitis. If the TSB is at or approaching the exchange level, send blood for immediate type and crossmatch. Blood for exchange transfusion is modified whole blood (red cells and plasma) crossmatched against the mother and compatible with the infant.

NURSING MANAGEMENT

NURSING ASSESSMENT AND DIAGNOSIS

Assessment is aimed at identifying prenatal and perinatal factors that predispose the newborn to the development of jaundice and at recognizing the jaundice as soon as it is apparent. Clinically, ABO incompatibility presents as jaundice and occasionally as hepatosplenomegaly. Fetal hydrops or erythroblastosis is rare (see Chapter 16∞). Hemolytic disease of the newborn is suspected if the placenta is enlarged; if the newborn is edematous, with pleural and pericardial effusion plus ascites; if pallor or jaundice is noted during the first 24 to 36 hours; if hemolytic anemia is diagnosed; or if the spleen and liver are enlarged. The nurse carefully notes changes in behavior and observes for evidence of bleeding. If laboratory tests indicate elevated bilirubin levels, the nurse checks the newborn for jaundice about every 2 hours and records observations.

To check for jaundice in lighter skinned babies, the nurse blanches the skin over a bony prominence (forehead, nose, sternum) by pressing firmly with the thumb. After pressure is released, if jaundice is present, the area appears yellow before normal color returns. The nurse checks oral mucosa and the posterior portion of the hard palate and conjunctival sacs for yellow pigmentation in darker skinned babies. Jaundice progresses in a cephalocaudal direction from the face to the trunk and then to the lower extremities. The overall progression of jaundice should be noted. Assessment in daylight gives the best results, because pink walls and surroundings may mask yellowish tints and yellow light makes differentiation of jaundice difficult. The time at onset of jaundice is recorded and reported. If jaundice appears, careful observation of the increase in depth of color and of the newborn's behavior is mandatory. In addition to visual inspection, reflectance photometers that measure transcutaneous bilirubin (TcB) should be used to screen and monitor neonatal jaundice. Some hospitals have developed a mandatory screening policy for all newborns before discharge using the TcB monitor. If the level comes back elevated then a follow-up TSB will be performed. Another portable screening tool is the analysis for end-tidal carbon monoxide (ETCO). This analysis allows for rapid identification of newborns with significant hemolytic disease who may be at risk for the sequelae of unconjugated hyperbilirubinemia.

The nurse assesses the newborn's behavior for neurologic signs associated with hyperbilirubinemia, which are rare but may include hypotonia, diminished reflexes, lethargy, or seizures.

Developing Cultural Competence

ETHNIC VARIATIONS AND JAUNDICE

East Asian infants (Japanese, Chinese, and Filipino ethnic groups) have a higher occurrence of hyperbilirubinemia than Caucasian infants. In addition, infants with Asian fathers and Caucasian mothers have a higher incidence of jaundice than if both parents are Caucasian. Other ethnic groups at risk for increased bilirubinemia are Navajo, Eskimo, and Sioux Native American newborns; Greek newborns; Sephardic-Jewish (Asian ancestry) newborns; and some Hispanic newborns.

MyNursingKit Nursing in Action: Infant Receiving Phototherapy

Nursing diagnoses that may apply to care of a newborn with jaundice include the following:

- *Risk for Fluid Volume Deficit* related to increased insensible water loss and frequent loose stools
- *Potential for Injury* related to use of phototherapy
- *Sensory-Perceptual Alterations* related to neurologic damage secondary to kernicterus
- *Risk for Altered Parenting* related to deficient knowledge of infant care and prolonged separation of infant and parents secondary to illness

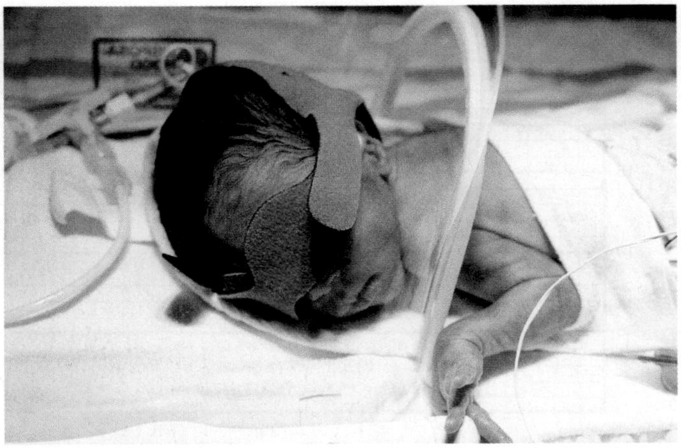

● **Figure 29–11** Infant receiving phototherapy. The phototherapy light is positioned over the incubator. Bilateral eye patches are always used during photo light therapy to protect the baby's eyes.

Courtesy of Lisa Smith-Pedersen, RNC, MSN, NNP.

Nursing Practice

If the area of jaundice around the eyes begins to disappear, it is probable that the eye patches are allowing light to enter and better eye protection is needed.

PLANNING AND IMPLEMENTATION

HOSPITAL-BASED NURSING CARE

Hospital-based care is described in the "Nursing Care Plan: For a Newborn with Hyperbilirubinemia," on pages 732–735. If banks of phototherapy lights are used, the nurse exposes the entire skin surface of the newborn to the light. Minimal covering may be applied over the genitals and buttocks to expose maximum skin surface while still protecting the bedding from soiling. Phototherapy success is measured every 12 hours or with daily serum bilirubin levels (more frequently if there is hemolysis or a higher level before initiation of phototherapy). The nurse must turn lights off while blood is drawn to ensure accurate serum bilirubin levels. Because it is not known if phototherapy injures the delicate eye structures, particularly the retina, the nurse applies eye patches over the newborn's closed eyes during exposure to banks of phototherapy lights (Figure 29–11 ● and Clinical Skills Manual: "Infant Receiving Phototherapy" SKILLS). Conventional phototherapy is discontinued and the eye patches are removed at least once per shift to assess the eyes for conjunctivitis. Patches are also removed to allow eye contact during feeding (social stimulation) or when parents are visiting (to promote parental attachment).

Some parents may feel guilty about their baby's condition and think they have caused the problem. Under stress, parents may not be able to understand the physician's first explanations. The nurse must expect that the parents will need explanations repeated and clarified and that they may need help in voicing their questions and fears. Eye and tactile contact with the newborn is encouraged. The nurse can coach parents when they visit with the baby. After the mother's discharge, parents are kept informed of their infant's condition and are encouraged to return to the hospital or telephone at any time so that they can be fully involved in the care of their infant. Parents are advised that after discontinuation of phototherapy, a rebound of 1 to 2 mg/dL can be expected and a follow-up bilirubin test may be done (Cloherty et al., 2008; Bradshaw, 2010).

While the mother is still hospitalized, phototherapy can also be carried out in the parents' room if the only problem is hyperbilirubinemia. The parents must be willing to keep the baby in the room for 24 hours a day, be able to take emergency action (e.g., for choking) if necessary, and complete instruction checklists. Some institutions require that parents sign a consent form. The nurse instructs the parents but also continues to monitor the infant's temperature, activity, intake and output, and positioning of eye patches (if conventional light banks are used) at regular intervals. See "Teaching Highlights: Instructional Checklist for In-Room Phototherapy."

COMMUNITY-BASED NURSING CARE

Some studies have shown that the early discharge of newborns and their mothers comes with an increase in hospital readmission and elevated risk of pathologic hyperbilirubinemia. Home phototherapy use is recommended only if the bilirubin level is plotted on the nomogram and found to be in the "optional phototherapy" range. Any newborn with a level in the higher range

Teaching Highlights

INSTRUCTIONAL CHECKLIST FOR IN-ROOM PHOTOTHERAPY

Explain and demonstrate the placement of eye patches and explain that they must be in place when the infant is under the lights.

Explain the clothing to be worn (diaper under lights, dress and wrap when away from the lights).

Explain the importance of taking the infant's temperature regularly.

Explain the importance of adequate fluid intake.

Explain the charting flow sheet (intake, output, eyes covered).

Explain how to position the lights at a proper distance.

Explain the need to keep the infant under phototherapy except during feeding and diaper change.

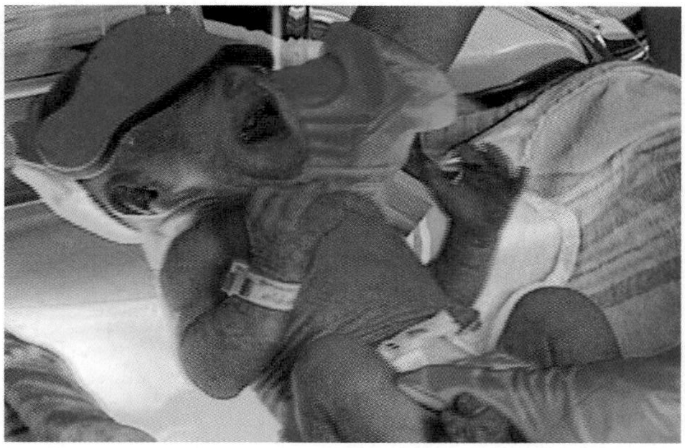

● **Figure 29–12** Newborn on fiberoptic "bili" mattress and under phototherapy lights. A combination of fiberoptic light source mattress and standard phototherapy light source above may also be used.

Note: The color is distorted because of the reflection of the bililight mattress.

should be hospitalized for continual phototherapy and serum bilirubin levels closely monitored on a regular schedule (Bhutani et al., 2004).

Jaundice and its treatment (phototherapy, exchange transfusion) can be disturbing to parents and may generate feelings of guilt and fear. The parent's perception of and/or misconceptions about jaundice can affect parent-infant interactions. The nurse should explain the causes of jaundice and emphasize that it is usually a transient problem and one to which all infants must adapt after birth. Reassurance and support are vital especially for the breastfeeding mother, who may question her ability to adequately nourish her newborn.

It is essential that the impact of cultural beliefs be considered. Some Latina women believe that showing strong maternal emotions during pregnancy and breastfeeding can be detrimental. Some Latina women may blame "bilis" associated with maternal anger for the jaundice. Cultural beliefs lead mothers to interpret illness within their cultural framework, especially when left without clear and understood explanations.

If the baby is to receive phototherapy at home, the nurse teaches the parents to record the infant's temperature, weight, fluid intake and output, stools, and feedings and to use the phototherapy equipment. In addition, if banks of phototherapy lights are being used, parents must agree that the baby will be exposed to the lights for long periods of time; that they will hold the baby for only short periods for feeding, comforting, and cleansing of the perineal area; and that the room temperature will be regulated to minimize heat loss. Fiberoptic phototherapy blankets eliminate the need for eye patches, decrease heat loss because the baby is clothed, and provide more opportunities for interaction between the baby and parents. The best method of home phototherapy depends on the cause of the hyperbilirubinemia and the rate of progression of the jaundice. A combination of phototherapy lights and fiberoptic mattress may be used (Figure 29–12 ●). Ongoing monitoring of bilirubin levels is essential with home phototherapy and can be carried out in the home, in the follow-up clinic, or in the clinician's office.

EVALUATION

Expected outcomes of nursing care include the following:

- The newborn at risk for development of hyperbilirubinemia is identified, and action is taken to minimize the potential impact of hyperbilirubinemia.
- The baby does not have any corneal irritation or drainage, skin breakdown, or major fluctuations in temperature.
- Parents understand the rationale for, goal of, and expected outcome of therapy.
- Parents verbalize concerns about their baby's condition and identify how they can facilitate their baby's improvement.

CARE OF THE NEWBORN WITH ANEMIA

Neonatal anemia is often difficult to recognize by clinical evaluation alone. The hemoglobin concentration in a term newborn is 14 to 20 g/dL, slightly higher than that in premature newborns. Infants with hemoglobin values of less than 14 g/dL (term) and less than 12 g/dL (preterm) are usually considered anemic. The most common causes of neonatal anemia are blood loss, hemolysis/erythrocyte destruction, and impaired red blood cell production (Aher, Malwatkar & Kadam, 2008).

Blood loss (hypovolemia) occurs in utero from placental bleeding (placenta previa or abruptio placentae). Intrapartal blood loss may be fetomaternal, fetofetal, or the result of umbilical cord bleeding. Birth trauma to abdominal organs (adrenal hemorrhage) or the cranium (subgaleal bleed) may produce significant blood loss, and cerebral bleeding may occur because of hypoxia.

Excessive hemolysis of red blood cells is usually a result of blood group incompatibilities but may be caused by infections. The most common cause of impaired red blood cell production is a genetically transmitted deficiency in glucose-6-phosphate dehydrogenase (G-6-PD). Anemia and jaundice are the presenting signs.

Nursing Care Plan

THE NEWBORN WITH HYPERBILIRUBINEMIA

INTERVENTION	RATIONALE	EXPECTED OUTCOME
1. Nursing Diagnosis: Impaired Tissue Integrity related to predisposing factors associated with hyperbilirubinemia		
NIC Intervention: **High–risk newborn care:** Identification and management of a high-risk newborn to promote healthy outcomes for baby		**NOC Outcome:** **Risk control:** Actions to eliminate or reduce actual, personal, and modifiable health threats
Goal: Babies at risk for jaundice and early signs of jaundice will be identified.		
■ Evaluate baby's history for predisposing factors for hyperbilirubinemia.	■ Early identification of risk factors enables the nurse to monitor babies for early signs of hyperbilirubinemia. Acidosis, hypoxia, and hypothermia increase the risk of hyperbilirubinemia at lower bilirubin levels.	■ Baby's jaundice is identified early.
■ Observe color of amniotic fluid at time of rupture of membranes.	■ Amber-colored amniotic fluid indicates hyperbilirubinemia.	
■ Assess baby for developing jaundice in daylight if possible.	■ Early detection is affected by nursery environment. Artificial lights (with pink tint) may mask beginning of jaundice.	
1. Observe sclera.	1. Most visible sign of hyperbilirubinemia is jaundice noted in skin, sclera, or oral mucosa. Onset is first seen on face and then progresses down trunk.	
2. Observe skin color and assess by blanching.	2. Blanching the skin leaves a yellow color to the skin immediately after pressure is released.	
3. Check oral mucosa, posterior portion of hard palate, and conjunctival sacs for yellow pigmentation in dark-skinned newborns.	3. Underlying pigment of dark-skinned people may normally appear yellow.	
4. Report jaundice occurring within 24 hours of birth.		
2. Nursing Diagnosis: Risk for Fluid Volume Deficit related to phototherapy		
NIC Intervention: **Fluid monitoring:** Collection and analysis of patient data to regulate fluid balance		**NOC Outcome:** **Fluid balance:** Balance of water in the intracellular and extracellular compartments of the body
Goal: The infant will not exhibit signs of dehydration and will display appropriate weight gain.		
■ Offer feedings every 2 to 3 hr. Breastfeed on demand with no supplementation unless excessive weight loss or increasing TSB with adequate feeding.	■ Adequate hydration increases peristalsis and excretion of bilirubin.	■ Baby will have good skin turgor, clear amber urine output of 1–3 mL/kg/hr, six to eight wet diapers/day, and will maintain weight.
■ Provide 25% extra fluid intake.	■ Replace fluid losses due to watery stools, if under phototherapy.	
■ Assess for dehydration: 1. Poor skin turgor 2. Depressed fontanelles 3. Sunken eyes 4. Decreased urine output 5. Weight loss 6. Changes in electrolytes	■ Phototherapy treatment may cause liquid stools and increased insensible water loss, which increases risk of dehydration.	

Nursing Care Plan—continued

THE NEWBORN WITH HYPERBILIRUBINEMIA

INTERVENTION	RATIONALE	EXPECTED OUTCOME
■ Monitor intake and output (I & O). ■ Weigh daily. ■ Report signs of dehydration. ■ Administer IV fluids: 1. Monitor flow rates. 2. Assess insertion sites for signs of infection.	■ Prevents fluid overload. IV fluids may be used if baby is dehydrated or in presence of other complications. IV may be started if exchange transfusion is to be done. ■ Prevents fluid overload. IV fluids may be used if baby is dehydrated or in presence of other complications. IV may be started if exchange transfusion is to be done.	

3. Nursing Diagnosis: Potential for Injury related to use of banks of phototherapy lights

NIC Intervention:

Newborn monitoring: Measurement and interpretation of physiologic status of the newborn the first 24 hr after birth

NOC Outcome:

Risk Control: Actions to eliminate or reduce actual, personal, and modifiable health threats

Goal: Baby will not have any corneal irritation or drainage, skin breakdown, or major fluctuations in temperature.

INTERVENTION	RATIONALE	EXPECTED OUTCOME
■ Cover baby's eyes with eye patches while under banks of phototherapy lights. Cover testes/penis in male infants.	■ Protects retina from damage due to high-intensity light and testes from damage from heat.	■ Baby's eyes are protected, skin is intact, and baby maintains a stable temperature.
■ Make certain that eyelids are closed prior to applying eye patches.	■ Prevents corneal abrasions.	
■ Remove baby from under phototherapy and remove eye patches during feedings.	■ Provides visual stimulation and facilitates attachment behaviors.	
■ Inspect eyes each shift for conjunctivitis, drainage, and corneal abrasions due to irritation from eye patches.	■ Prevents or facilitates prompt treatment of purulent conjunctivitis.	
■ Administer thorough perianal cleansing with each stool or change of perianal protective covering.	■ Frequent stooling increases risk of skin breakdown. Prevents infection.	
■ Provide minimal coverage—only of diaper area.	■ Provides maximal exposure. Shielded areas become more jaundiced, so maximum exposure is essential.	
■ Avoid the use of oily applications on the skin.	■ Prevents superficial burns to skin.	
■ Reposition baby q 2 hours.	■ Provides equal exposure of all skin areas and prevents pressure areas.	
■ Observe for bronzing of skin.	■ Bronzing is related to use of phototherapy with increased direct bilirubin levels or liver damage; may last for 2 to 4 months.	
■ Place Plexiglas shield between baby and light. Monitor baby's skin and core temperature frequently until temperature is stable.	■ Hypothermia and hyperthermia are common complications of phototherapy. Hypothermia results from exposure to lights, subsequent radiation, and convection losses.	
■ Check axillary temperature with readings on servo-controlled unit on incubator. Regulate incubator temperature as needed.	■ Hyperthermia may result from the increased environmental heat. Additional heat from phototherapy lights frequently causes a rise in the baby's and incubator's temperatures. Fluctuations in temperature may occur in response to radiation and convection.	

(continued)

Nursing Care Plan—continued

THE NEWBORN WITH HYPERBILIRUBINEMIA

INTERVENTION	RATIONALE	EXPECTED OUTCOME
4. Nursing Diagnosis: Risk for Impaired Parenting related to deficient knowledge of infant care and prolonged separation of infant and parents secondary to illness		
NIC Intervention: **Teaching:** Infant care: Instruction on nurturing and physical care needed during the first year of life		**NOC Outcome:** **Parenting:** Provision of an environment that promotes optimum growth and development of dependent children
Goal: Parents will bond with infant and have realistic expectations about their infant. Parents are comfortable taking their infant home. They are able to demonstrate normal infant care and assessments of possible complications, and they know when to return for follow-up.		
■ Encourage parents to provide tactile stimulation during feeding and diaper changes.	■ Newborn has normal needs for tactile stimulation.	■ The parents will demonstrate ability to perform basic infant care tasks as evidenced by exhibiting appropriate attachment behaviors (e.g., talking to and holding infant), feeding infant, and caring for infant under home bili therapy.
■ Encourage cuddling and eye contact during feedings.	■ Provides opportunity for parents to bond with their newborn.	
■ Offer suggestions to comfort restless infant: 1. Nesting when beneath bili lights 2. Talking softly and singing quietly to infant 3. Taped music or tape recording of evening activities from home 4. Rhythmic patting of buttocks 5. Firm, nonstroking touch, assisting with control of extremities 6. Pacifier for nonnutritive sucking	■ Provides comfort and decreases sensory deprivation. Presence of equipment may discourage parents from interacting with newborn.	
■ Encourage family/friend support of mother/parents (e.g., meals, rest, child care for siblings, allow expressions of concerns/feelings).	■ Decreases strain on mother/parents by assisting with other responsibilities and allows for additional time with newborn for bonding, care, etc.	
■ Evaluate additional psychosocial needs.	■ Parents may not understand what is happening or why.	
■ Discuss rationale for treatment and possible side effects of phototherapy with family (stool changes, increased fluid loss, possible temp instability, slight lethargy, rash, altered sleep-wake patterns). Instruct family on infant's care while undergoing phototherapy: 1. Safety precautions—bili mask, incubator door closed and latched, covering genitalia per policy if under banks of phototherapy lights. 2. Skin care, cord care, circumcision care as appropriate. 3. Lab draws, rationale for intake and output.	■ Physician preference of treatment modalities may vary. Parents may not understand why their newborn is not receiving a treatment that another with the same condition is receiving.	■ Parents verbalize understanding of rationale and possible side effects from phototherapy; parents/family demonstrate safety precautions when caring for infant; parents getting meals and rest; parents verbalize support given.
■ Encourage parent/significant other/sibling involvement in infant care as possible.		
■ Evaluate family's understanding of information.		
■ Give explanation of equipment being used and changes in bilirubin levels. Allow parents an opportunity to ask questions; reinforce or clarify information as needed.		

Nursing Care Plan—continued

THE NEWBORN WITH HYPERBILIRUBINEMIA

INTERVENTION	RATIONALE	EXPECTED OUTCOME
■ As necessary, review role of pumping breasts and offering formula for limited time. ■ Assist mother to pump her breasts to maintain milk supply.	■ The etiology of breast milk jaundice remains uncertain. The serum bilirubin levels begin to fall within 48 hr after discontinuation of breastfeeding. Opinion of physicians varies regarding the need for discontinuing breastfeeding. ■ If breastfeeding is temporarily discontinued, assess mother's knowledge of pumping her breasts and provide information and support as needed.	

A condition known as **physiologic anemia of infancy** exists as a result of the normal gradual drop in hemoglobin for the first 6 to 12 weeks of life or corresponds with the decline in fetal hemoglobin. Theoretically, the bone marrow stops production of RBCs in response to higher oxygen levels that result from breathing changes after birth. When the amount of hemoglobin decreases, reaching levels of 9 to 11 g/dL at about 8 to 12 weeks of age (the average is 70 days) in term infants, the bone marrow begins production of RBCs again, and the anemia disappears (Diehl-Jones & Askin, 2010).

Anemia in preterm newborns is seen earlier than in term newborns, and increased production of red blood cells does not start until hemoglobin is 7 to 9 g/dL. The preterm baby's hemoglobin reaches a low sooner (by 4 to 8 weeks after birth) than does a term newborn's (6 to 12 weeks) because a preterm infant's red blood cell survival time is shorter than that of a term newborn (Cloherty et al., 2008). This difference is a result of several factors: the preterm infant's rapid growth rate, decreased iron stores, and an inadequate production of erythropoietin (EPO).

CLINICAL THERAPY

Hematologic problems can be anticipated based on the pregnancy history and clinical manifestations. The age at which anemia is first noted is also of diagnostic value. Clinically, light-skinned anemic infants are very pale in the absence of other symptoms of shock and usually have abnormally low red blood cell counts. In acute blood loss, symptoms of shock such as pallor, low arterial blood pressure, and a decreasing hematocrit value may be present.

The initial laboratory workup should include hemoglobin and hematocrit measurements, reticulocyte count, ferritin concentrations, examination of peripheral blood smear, bilirubin determinations, direct Coombs' test of infant's blood, and examination of maternal blood smear for fetal erythrocytes (Kleihauer-Betke test). Clinical management depends on the severity of the anemia and on whether blood loss is acute or chronic. The baby should be placed on constant cardiac and respiratory monitoring. Mild or slow chronic anemia may be treated adequately with iron supplements alone or with iron-fortified formulas. Frequent determinations of hemoglobin, hematocrit, and bilirubin levels (in hemolytic disease) are essential. In severe cases of anemia, transfusions with O-negative or typed and cross-matched irradiated packed red cells are the treatment of choice. The nurse should try to prevent iron deficiency by limiting phlebotomy losses and starting iron therapy at 2 weeks of postnatal age (Aher et al., 2008; Diehl-Jones & Askin, 2010). Management of anemia of prematurity includes treating the causative factor (e.g., antibiotics/antivirals used for infection, steroid therapy for disorders of erythrocyte production) and supplemental iron. Blood transfusions (dedicated units of blood) are kept to a minimum. Evidence supports use of recombinant human erythropoietin (rEPO) in only selected cases. For example, infants in whom it is desirable to maintain a relatively high hematocrit such as infants with bronchopulmonary dysplasia (Cloherty et al., 2008).

Nursing Management

The nurse assesses the newborn for symptoms of anemia (pallor). If the blood loss is acute, the baby may exhibit signs of shock (a capillary filling time greater than 3 seconds, decreased pulses, tachycardia, low blood pressure). Continued observation is necessary to identify physiologic anemia as the preterm newborn grows. Signs of compromise include poor weight gain, tachycardia, tachypnea, and apneic episodes. The nurse promptly reports any symptoms indicating shock. The amount of blood drawn for all laboratory tests is recorded in tenths of a milliliter, so that total blood removed can be assessed and replaced by transfusion when necessary. For long-term management, see "Normocyctic Anemia" in Chapter 51∞.

CARE OF THE NEWBORN WITH POLYCYTHEMIA

Polycythemia, a condition in which blood volume and hematocrit values are increased, is more common in intrauterine growth restricted (IUGR), full-term, or late preterm infants; placental transfusion caused by delayed cord clamping or cord stripping; infants receiving maternal-fetal and twin-to-twin transfusions; infants exposed to intrauterine hypoxia; and babies of mothers who smoke, or who take propranolol during pregnancy. Other conditions that present with polycythemia are chromosomal anomalies such as trisomies 21, 18, and 13; endocrine disorders such as hypoglycemia and hypocalcemia; and births at altitudes over 5000 feet. The incidence ranges from 1.5% to 4%, and the condition is uncommon in newborns less than 34 weeks' gestation (Rosenberg, 2007). An infant is considered polycythemic when the central venous hematocrit value is greater than 65% (Cloherty et al., 2008). A potential complication of polycythemia is hyperviscosity, which results in impaired perfusion of the capillary vessels (Rosenberg, 2007).

CLINICAL THERAPY

The goal of therapy is to reduce the peripheral venous hematocrit value to a range of 55% to 60% in symptomatic infants. To decrease the red blood cell mass, the symptomatic infant receives a partial exchange transfusion in which blood is removed from the infant and replaced millimeter for millimeter with fresh frozen plasma or 5% albumin, or crystalloids such as isotonic saline. The preference is to use crystalloids because of their decreased promotion of infection, incidence of necrotizing enterocolitis (NEC), and hypoallergenic properties. Supportive treatment of presenting symptoms is required until resolution, which usually occurs spontaneously following the partial exchange transfusion.

Nursing Management

Assess, record, and report symptoms of polycythemia. The nurse also does an initial screening of the newborn's hematocrit value on admission to the nursery. The peak of a term newborn's hematocrit will occur at 2 hours of age and begin to drop slowly by 12 to 18 hours. A capillary hematocrit may be done (see Clinical Skills Manual: "Performing a Heel Stick on a Newborn" SKILLS); however, peripheral free-flowing venous hematocrit samples are usually obtained from the antecubital fossa for confirmation.

Many infants are asymptomatic, but as symptoms develop, they are related to the increased blood volume, hyperviscosity (thickness) of the blood, and decreased deformability of red blood cells, all of which result in poor perfusion of tissues. The infants have a characteristic plethoric (ruddy) appearance. The most common symptoms observed include the following:

- *Cardiopulmonary.* Tachycardia and congestive heart failure caused by the increased blood volume
- *Respiratory.* Respiratory distress with grunting, tachypnea, and cyanosis; increased oxygen need; or respiratory hemorrhage caused by pulmonary venous congestion, edema, and hypoxemia
- *Hematologic.* Hyperbilirubinemia caused by increased numbers of RBCs breaking down; thrombocytopenia; or elevated reticulocytes and nucleated RBCs
- *Gastrointestinal.* Feeding intolerance, poor feeding, vomiting, or NEC
- *Renal.* Renal vein thrombosis with decreased urine output, hematuria, or proteinuria caused by thromboembolism; or renal tubular damage
- *Central nervous system.* Jitteriness, irritability, decreased activity and tone, lethargy, stroke (rare), or seizures caused by decreased perfusion of the brain and increased vascular resistance secondary to sluggish blood flow, which can result in neurologic or developmental problems

Observe closely for the signs of distress or change in vital signs during the partial exchange. The nurse assesses carefully for potential complications resulting from partial exchange transfusion, such as transfusion overload (which may result in congestive heart failure), irregular cardiac rhythm, bacterial infection, hypovolemia, and anemia. Parents need specific explanations about polycythemia and its treatment.

CARE OF THE NEWBORN WITH INFECTION

Newborns up to 1 month of age are particularly susceptible to an infection, referred to as **sepsis neonatorum**, caused by organisms that do not cause significant disease in older children. Once any infection occurs in the newborn, it can spread rapidly through the bloodstream, regardless of its primary site. The incidence of primary neonatal sepsis is 1 to 5 per 1000 live births (0.1% to 0.5) (Nash & Smith, 2008). The risk of mortality is 5% to 15% in this population. Nosocomial infection frequency is less in normal newborn infants and increases in infants in the neonatal intensive care unit (NICU).

Prematurity and low birth weight are associated with nosocomial infection rates up to 15 times higher than average. The general debilitation and underlying illnesses often associated with prematurity necessitate invasive procedures such as umbilical catheterization, intubation, resuscitation, ventilator support, monitoring, parenteral alimentation (especially lipid emulsions), and prior broad-spectrum antibiotic therapy.

However, even full-term infants are susceptible, because their immunologic systems are immature. Their immune systems lack the complex factors involved in effective phagocytosis and the ability to localize infection or to respond with a well-defined, recognizable inflammatory response. In addition, all newborns lack IgM immunoglobin, which is necessary to protect against bacteria, because it does not cross the placenta (refer to Chapter 24∞ for immunologic adaptations in the newborn period).

Most nosocomial infections in the NICU present as bacteremia/sepsis, urinary tract infections, meningitis, or pneumonia. Maternal antepartal infections such as rubella, toxoplasmosis, cytomegalic inclusion disease, and herpes may cause congenital infections and resulting disorders in the newborn. Intrapartal maternal infections, such as amnionitis and those resulting from premature rupture of membranes (PROM) and precipitous birth, are sources of neonatal infection (see Chapter 16∞ for more detailed information). Passage through the birth canal and contact with the vaginal flora (β-hemolytic streptococci, herpes, *Listeria,* gonococci) expose the infant to infection (Table 29–3). With infection anywhere in the fetus or newborn,

Table 29–3 Maternally Transmitted Newborn Infections

Infection	Nursing Assessment	Planning and Implementation
GROUP B STREPTOCOCCUS		
1% to 2% colonized with 1 in 10 developing disease. Early onset—usually within hours of birth or within first week. Late onset—1 week to 3 months (Nash & Smith, 2008).	Severe respiratory distress (grunting and cyanosis). May become apneic or demonstrate symptoms of shock. Meconium-stained amniotic fluid seen at birth.	Early assessment of clinical signs necessary. Assist with x-ray examination—shows aspiration pneumonia or respiratory distress syndrome. Immediately obtain blood, gastric aspirate, external ear canal, and nasopharynx cultures. Administer antibiotics, usually aqueous penicillin or ampicillin combined with gentamicin, as soon as cultures are obtained. Early assessment and intervention are essential to survival.
CONGENITAL SYPHILIS		
Spirochetes (*Treponemia pallidum*) cross placenta after 16th to 18th week of gestation. The more recent the maternal infection the more likelihood of transmission. Most are asymptomatic at birth but develop symptoms within first 3 months of life.	Check perinatal history for positive maternal serology. Assess infant using screening nontreponemal titer (RPR or VDRL) tests; then use treponemal (FTA-ABS or TP-PA) tests on infant serum to confirm diagnosis (AAP & ACOG, 2007). Rhinitis (sniffles). Fissures on mouth corners and excoriated upper lip. Red rash around mouth and anus. Copper-colored rash over face, palms, and soles. Irritability; generalized edema, particularly over joints; bone lesions; painful extremities, hepatosplenomegaly, jaundice, congenital cataracts, SGA, and failure to thrive.	Initiate standard precautions until infants have been on antibiotics for at least 24 hours. Administer penicillin. Initiate referral to evaluate for blindness, deafness, learning or behavioral problems. Provide emotional support for parents because of their feelings about mode of transmission and potential long-term sequelae.
GONORRHEA		
Approximately 30% to 35% of newborns born vaginally to infected mothers acquire the infection.	Assess for Ophthalmia neonatorum (conjunctivitis). Purulent discharge and corneal ulcerations. Neonatal sepsis with temperature instability, poor feeding response, and/or hypotonia, jaundice.	Administer prophylaxis ophthalmic antibiotic ointment (see "Drug Guide: Erythromycin [Ilotycin] Ophthalmic Ointment" in Chapter 29) or tetracycline. If positive maternal test, single dose systemic antibiotic therapy (AAP & ACOG, 2007). Initiate follow-up referral to evaluate any loss of vision.
HERPES TYPE 2		
Usually transmitted during vaginal birth; a few cases of in utero transmission have been reported.	Check perinatal history for active herpes genital lesions. Small cluster vesicular skin lesions over all the body about 6 to 9 days of life. Disseminated form—Pneumonia, DIC, hepatitis with jaundice, hepatosplenomegaly, and neurologic abnormalities. Without skin lesions, assess for fever or subnormal temperature, respiratory congestion, tachypnea, and tachycardia.	Carry out careful handwashing and contact precautions (gown and glove isolation with linen precautions) (AAP & ACOG, 2007). Obtain throat, conjunctiva, urine, stool, and lesion cultures to identify herpesvirus type 2 antibiotics in serum IgM fraction. Cultures positive in 24 to 48 hours after birth. Administer intravenous acyclovir (Zovirax). Make a follow-up referral to evaluate potential sequelae of microcephaly, spasticity, seizures, deafness, or blindness. Encourage parental rooming-in and touching of their newborn. Show parents appropriate handwashing procedures and precautions to be used at home if mother's lesions are active.
CYTOMEGALOVIRUS (CMV)		
Most common cause of congenital infection in the United States—approximately 1% of all newborn infants (AAP & ACOG, 2007). Transmission occurs in utero, during labor, or may happen postnatally through breast milk.	Congenital CMV disease, including intrauterine growth restriction, jaundice, hepatosplenomegaly, petechiae or purpura (blueberry muffin spots), thrombocytopenia, and pneumonia. CNS manifestations are very common and include lethargy and poor feeding, hypertonia or hypotonia, microcephaly, intracranial calcifications, chorioretinitis, and sensorineural deafness.	Diagnosis of congenital CMV infection is established by isolating virus from urine, saliva, or tissue obtained during the first 3 weeks of life. All infants in whom the diagnosis is suspected should have a viral culture performed; a CT scan of the brain is particularly important to document the extent of CNS involvement; eye exam and hearing test; close long-term follow-up evaluating for developmental effects.

(continued)

Table 29–3 Maternally Transmitted Newborn Infections—continued

Infection	Nursing Assessment	Planning and Implementation
ORAL CANDIDAL INFECTION (THRUSH)		
Acquired during passage through birth canal.	Assess newborn's buccal mucosa, tongue, gums, and inside the cheeks for white plaques (seen 5 to 7 days of age). Check diaper area for bright red, well-demarcated eruptions. Assess for thrush periodically when newborn is on long-term antibiotic therapy.	Differentiate white plaque areas from milk curds by using cotton tip applicator (if it is thrush, removal of white areas causes raw, bleeding areas). Maintain cleanliness of hands, linen, clothing, diapers, and feeding apparatus. Instruct breastfeeding mothers on treating their nipples with nystatin. Administer nystatin swabbed on oral lesions 1 hour after feeding or nystatin instilled in baby's oral cavity and on mucosa. Swab skin lesions with topical nystatin. Discuss with parents that gentian violet stains mouth and clothing. Avoid placing gentian violet on normal mucosa; it causes irritation.
CHLAMYDIA TRACHOMATIS		
Acquired during passage through birth canal.	Assess for perinatal history of preterm birth. Symptomatic newborns present with conjunctivitis and pneumonia. Chlamydial conjunctivitis presents with inflammation, yellow discharge, and eyelid swelling 5 to 14 days after birth. Chronic follicular conjunctivitis (corneal neovascularization and conjunctival scarring).	Instillation of prophylactic ophthalmic erythromycin is controversial (AAP & ACOG, 2007). Treat chlamydial conjunctivitis or pneumonia with oral erythromycin for 14 days. Monitor for hypertrophic pyloric stenosis. Initiate follow-up referral for eye complications and late development of pneumonia at 4 to 11 weeks postnatally.

the adjacent tissues or organs are easily penetrated, and the blood-brain barrier is ineffective. Septicemia is more common in males, except for infections caused by group B β-hemolytic streptococcus.

Gram-negative organisms (especially *Escherichia coli, Enterobacter, Proteus,* and *Klebsiella*) and the gram-positive organism β-hemolytic streptococcus are the most common causative agents. *Pseudomonas* is a common fomite contaminant of ventilator support and oxygen therapy equipment. Gram-positive bacteria, especially coagulase-negative staphylococci, are common pathogens in nosocomial bacteremias, pneumonias, and urinary tract infections. Other gram-positive bacteria frequently isolated are enterococci and *Staphylococcus aureus* (Vargo & Trotter, 2007).

Protection of the newborn from infections starts prenatally and continues throughout pregnancy and birth. Prenatal prevention should include maternal screening for sexually transmitted infections and monitoring of rubella titers in women who test negative. Intrapartally, sterile technique is essential. Smears from genital lesions are taken, and placenta and amniotic fluid cultures are obtained if amnionitis is suspected. If genital herpes is present toward term, cesarean birth may be indicated. All newborns' eyes should be treated with an antibiotic ophthalmic ointment to prevent damage from gonococcal (occurring 3 days following birth) infection. Prophylactic antibiotic therapy, for asymptomatic women who test positive for group B streptococcus (GBS) during the intrapartum period, helps prevent early-onset sepsis (Nash & Smith, 2008).

CLINICAL THERAPY

Cultures should be taken as soon after birth as possible for infants with a history of possible exposure to infection in utero (e.g., PROM more than 24 hours before birth or questionable maternal history of infection, maternal fever/chorioammionitis, or high-risk behavior (such as multiple sexual partners or illicit drug use). Cultures are obtained before antibiotic therapy is begun.

1. Anaerobic and aerobic blood cultures are taken from a peripheral site rather than an umbilical vessel, because catheters have yielded false-positive results caused by contamination. The skin is prepared by cleaning with a unit antiseptic solution and allowed to dry; the specimen is obtained with a sterile needle and syringe to lessen the likelihood of contamination.
2. Spinal fluid culture is done following a spinal tap/lumbar puncture if there are concerns about CNS symptoms/pathology.
3. The specimen for urine culture is best obtained by a suprapubic bladder aspiration or sterile catheterization.
4. Skin cultures are taken of any lesions or drainage from lesions or reddened areas.
5. Tracheal aspirate cultures, if intubated, may be obtained.

Other laboratory investigations include a complete blood count, C-reactive protein (CRP), chest x-ray examination, serology, and Gram stains of cerebrospinal fluid, urine, skin exudate, and umbilicus. White blood cell (WBC) count with differential may indicate the presence or absence of sepsis. A level of 30,000 to 40,000 mm^3 WBCs may be normal in the first 24 hours of life, whereas low WBC (less than 5000 to 7500/mm) may indicate sepsis. A low neutrophil count and a high band (immature white blood cells) count indicate that an infection is present. Stomach aspirate should be sent for culture and smear if a gonococcal infection or amnionitis is suspected. The C-reactive protein, an acute-phase reactant protein synthesized in response to inflammation, may or may not be elevated. Other inflammatory responses may cause an elevation in the CRP, so it should not be used as the only indicator of infection (Hawk, 2008; Nash & Smith, 2008; Lott, 2010). The CRP may be helpful in watching for improvement once antibiotic therapy is initiated.

Serum IgM levels are elevated (normal level less than 20 mg/dL) in response to transplacental infections (Blackburn, 2007). If available, counterimmunoelectrophoresis tests for specific bacterial antigens are performed. In the future repetitive sequence-based polymerase chain reactions (rep-PCR) will be used to identify specific infectious organisms within hours instead of days (Cloherty et al., 2008; Lott, 2010). Evidence of congenital infections may be seen on skull x-ray films for cerebral calcifications (cytomegalovirus, toxoplasmosis), on bone x-ray films (syphilis, cytomegalovirus), and in serum-specific IgM levels (rubella). Cytomegalovirus infection is best diagnosed by urine culture.

Because neonatal infection causes high mortality, therapy is instituted before results of the septic workup are obtained. A combination of two broad-spectrum antibiotics, such as ampicillin and gentamicin, is given in large doses until a culture with sensitivities is obtained.

After the pathogen and its sensitivities are determined, appropriate specific antibiotic therapy is begun. Combinations of penicillin or ampicillin and kanamycin have been used in the past, but new kanamycin-resistant enterobacteria and penicillin-resistant staphylococcus necessitate increasing use of gentamicin. Rotating aminoglycosides has been suggested to prevent development of resistance. Use of cephalosporins and, in particular, cefotaxime has emerged as an alternative to aminoglycoside therapy in the treatment of neonatal infections. Duration of therapy varies from 7 to 14 days (Table 29–4). If cultures are negative and symptoms subside, antibiotics may be discontinued after 2 days/48 hours of negative blood cultures. Supportive physiologic care may be required to maintain respiratory, hemodynamic, nutritional, and metabolic homeostasis.

NURSING MANAGEMENT

NURSING ASSESSMENT AND DIAGNOSIS

Symptoms of infection are most often noticed by the nurse during daily care of the newborn. The infant may deteriorate rapidly in the first 12 to 24 hours after birth if β-hemolytic streptococcal infection is present, with signs and symptoms mimicking RDS. In other cases, the onset of sepsis may be gradual, with more subtle signs and symptoms (Nash & Smith, 2008). The most common signs observed include the following:

1. Subtle behavioral changes; the infant "is not doing well" and is often lethargic or irritable (especially after the first 24 hours) and hypotonic; color changes may include pallor, duskiness, cyanosis, or a "shocky" appearance; skin is cool and clammy
2. Temperature instability, manifested by either hypothermia (recognized by a decrease in skin temperature) or, rarely in newborns, hyperthermia (elevation of skin temperature) necessitating a corresponding increase or decrease in incubator temperature to maintain a neutral thermal environment
3. Feeding intolerance, as evidenced by a decrease in total intake, abdominal distention, vomiting, poor sucking, lack of interest in feeding, and diarrhea
4. Jaundice, petechial hemorrhages, hepatosplenomegaly
5. Tachycardia initially, followed by spells of apnea or bradycardia

Other signs and symptoms may suggest CNS disease such as jitteriness, tremors, seizure activity. A differential diagnosis is necessary because of the similarity of symptoms to other more specific conditions.

Nursing diagnoses that may apply to the infant with sepsis neonatorum and the family include the following:

- *Risk for Infection* related to newborn's immature immunologic system
- *Deficient Fluid Volume* related to feeding intolerance
- *Ineffective Family Coping: Compromised* related to present illness resulting in prolonged hospital stay for the newborn

PLANNING AND IMPLEMENTATION

In the nursery, environmental control and prevention of acquired infection are the responsibilities of the neonatal nurse. An infected newborn can be isolated effectively in an isolette and receive close observation. The nurse must promote strict handwashing technique for all who enter the nursery, including nursing colleagues; physicians; laboratory, x-ray, and respiratory therapists; and parents. Visits by unnecessary personnel should be discouraged. Be prepared to assist in the aseptic collection of specimens for laboratory investigations. Scrupulous care of equipment—changing and cleaning of incubators at least every 7 days, removing and sterilizing wet equipment every 24 hours, preventing cross use of linen and equipment, cleaning sinkside equipment such as soap containers periodically, and taking special care with the open radiant warmers (access without prior handwashing is much more likely than with the closed incubator)—will prevent contamination.

PROVISION OF ANTIBIOTIC THERAPY

Administer antibiotics as ordered by the nurse practitioner or physician. It is the nurse's responsibility to be knowledgeable about the following:

- The proper dose to be administered, based on the weight of the newborn and desired peak and trough levels

Table 29–4 Neonatal Sepsis Antibiotic Therapy

Drug	Dose (mg/kg) Total Daily Dose	Schedule for Divided Doses	Route	Comments
Acyclovir (Zovirax)	20 mg/kg	Every 8 hours	IV	Length of treatment is 14 days for skin/eye/mouth (SEM) or 21 days for CNS and disseminated disease: *Herpes.*
Ampicillin	50 to 100 mg/kg	Every 12 hours* Every 8 hours†	IM or IV	Effective against gram-positive microorganisms, *Haemophilus influenzae,* and most *Escherichia coli* strains. Higher doses indicated for meningitis. Used with aminoglycoside for synergy.
Cefotaxime	50 mg/kg 100 to 150 mg/kg/day	Every 12 hours* Every 8 hours†	IM or IV	Active against most major pathogens in infants; effective against aminoglycoside-resistant organisms; achieves CSF bactericidal activity; lack of ototoxicity and nephrotoxicity; wide therapeutic index (levels not required); resistant organisms can develop rapidly if used extensively; ineffective against *Pseudomonas, Listeria.*
Gentamicin	2.5 to 3 mg/kg 5 to 7.5 mg/kg/day 4 to 5 mg/kg/dose (first week of life)	Every 12 to 24 hours*‡ Every 8 to 24 hours† Every 24 to 48 hours	IM or IV	Effective against gram-negative rods and staphylococci; may be used instead of kanamycin against penicillin-resistant staphylococci and *E. coli* strains and *Pseudomonas aeruginosa.* May cause ototoxicity and nephrotoxicity. Need to follow serum levels. Must never be given as IV push. Must be given over at least 30 to 60 minutes. In presence of oliguria or anuria, dose must be decreased or discontinued. In infants less than 1000 g or 29 weeks, lower dosage 2.5 to 3 mg/kg/day. Monitor serum levels before administration of second dose. Peak 5 to 12 mcg/mL. Trough 0.5 to 1 mcg/mL.
Nafcillin	25 to 50 mg/kg dependent on age	Every 8 to 12 hours* Every 6 to 8 hours†	IM or IV	Effective against penicillinase-resistant staphylococci aureus. Avoid IM if possible. Monitor CBC, UA, LFTs. Caution in presence of jaundice.
Penicillin G (aqueous crystalline)	25,000 to 50,000 units/kg 50,000 to 125,000 units/kg/day Up to 400,000 units/kg/day for group β strep. Meningitis	Every 12 hours* Every 8 hours†	IM or IV	Initial sepsis therapy effective against most gram-positive microorganisms except resistant staphylococci; can cause heart block in infants.
Vancomycin	10 to 20 mg/kg 30 mg/kg/day	Every 12 to 24 hours*‡ Every 8 hours†	IV	Effective for methicillin-resistant strains (*Staphylococcus epidermis*); must be administered by slow intravenous infusion to avoid prolonged cutaneous eruption. For smaller infants, $<$ 1200 g, $<$ 29 weeks, smaller dosages and longer intervals between doses. Nephrotoxic, especially in combination with aminoglycosides. Slow IV infusion over at least 60 minutes. Peak 25 to 40 mcg/mL. Trough 5 to 10 mcg/mL.

*Up to 7 days of age. †Greater than 7 days of age. ‡ Dependent on GA.

- The appropriate route of administration, because some antibiotics cannot be given intravenously
- Admixture incompatibilities, because some antibiotics are precipitated by intravenous solutions or by other antibiotics
- Side effects and toxicity

For term infants being treated for infections, neonatal home infusion of antibiotics should be considered as a viable alternative to continued hospitalization. The infusion of antibiotics at home by skilled RNs facilitates parent-infant bonding while meeting the infant's ongoing healthcare needs.

PROVISION OF SUPPORTIVE CARE

In addition to antibiotic therapy, physiologic supportive care is essential in caring for a septic infant. The nurse should carry out the following:

- Observe for resolution of symptoms or development of other symptoms of sepsis.
- Maintain neutral thermal environment with accurate regulation of humidity and oxygen administration.
- Provide respiratory support: administer oxygen and observe and monitor respiratory effort.
- Provide cardiovascular support: observe and monitor pulse and blood pressure; observe for hyperbilirubinemia, anemia, and hemorrhagic symptoms.
- Provide adequate calories, because oral feedings may be discontinued because of increased mucus, abdominal distention, vomiting, and aspiration.
- Provide fluids and electrolytes to maintain homeostasis; monitor weight changes, urine output, and urine specific gravity.
- Observe for the development of hypoglycemia, hyperglycemia, acidosis, hyponatremia, and hypocalcemia.

Restricting parental visits has not been shown to have any effect on the rate of infection and may be harmful for the newborn's psychologic development. With instruction and guidance from the nurse, both parents should be allowed to handle the baby and participate in daily care. Support of the parents is crucial. They need to be informed of the newborn's prognosis as treatment continues and to be involved in care as much as possible. They also need to understand how infection is transmitted.

EVALUATION

Expected outcomes of nursing care include the following:

- The risks for development of sepsis are identified early, and immediate action is taken to minimize the development of the illness.
- Appropriate use of aseptic technique protects the newborn from further exposure to illness.
- The baby's symptoms are relieved, and the infection is treated.
- The parents verbalize concerns about their baby's illness and understand the rationale behind the management of their newborn.

CARE OF THE FAMILY WITH BIRTH OF AN AT-RISK NEWBORN

The birth of a preterm or ill infant or an infant with a congenital anomaly is a serious crisis for a family. Throughout the pregnancy, both parents, together and separately, have felt excitement, experienced thoughts of acceptance, and pictured what their baby would look like. Both parents have wished for a perfect baby and feared an unhealthy one. Each parent and family member must accept and adjust when the fantasized fears become reality.

PARENTAL RESPONSES

Family members have acute grief reactions to the loss of the idealized baby they have envisioned. In a preterm birth, the mother is denied the last few weeks of pregnancy that seem to prepare her psychologically for the stress of birth and the attachment process. Attachment at this time is fragile, and interruption of the process by separation can affect the future mother-child relationship. Parents express grief as shock and disbelief, denial of reality, anger toward self and others, guilt, blame, and concern for the future. Self-esteem and feelings of self-worth are jeopardized.

Feelings of guilt and failure often plague mothers of preterm newborns. Guilt fantasies may lead her to wonder what she might have done to cause the early labor. She might ask herself questions such as: "Why did labor start?" "What did I do (or not do)?" "Was it because I had sexual intercourse with my husband (a week, 3 days, a day) ago?" "Was it because I carried three loads of wash up from the basement?" "Am I being punished for something done in the past—even in childhood?"

The period of waiting between suspicion and confirmation of abnormality or dysfunction is a very anxious one for parents because it is difficult, if not impossible, to begin attachment to the infant if the newborn's future is questionable. During the waiting period, parents need support and acknowledgment that this is an anxious time. They must be kept informed about tests and efforts to gather additional data, as well as efforts to improve their baby's outcome. It is helpful to tell both parents about the problem at the same time, with the baby present. An honest discussion of the problem and anticipatory management at the earliest possible time by health professionals help the parents (1) maintain trust in the physician and nurse, (2) appreciate the reality of the situation by dispelling fantasy and misconception, (3) begin the grieving process, and (4) mobilize internal and external support.

Nurses need to be aware that anger is a universal response by parents to a preterm birth. It is best that the parents direct it outward because holding it in check requires great energy which is then diverted away from grieving and physical recovery from pregnancy and giving birth. Anger may be directed at the physician and/or nurse, at the food, at nursing care, or at hospital regulations and routines. Parents rarely show anger with the baby; such responses can precipitate guilt feelings.

Although reactions and steps of attachment are altered by the birth of at-risk infants, a healthy parent-child relationship can occur. Kaplan and Mason (1974) have identified four psychologic tasks as essential for coping with the stress of an at-risk newborn and for providing a basis for the maternal-infant relationship:

1. Anticipatory grief as a psychologic preparation for possible loss of the child while still hoping for his or her survival
2. Acknowledgment of maternal failure to produce a term or perfect newborn expressed as anticipatory grief and depression and lasting until the chances of survival seem secure
3. Resumption of the process of relating to the infant may be impaired by continuous threat of death or abnormality, and the mother may be slow in her response of hope for the infant's survival

4. Understanding of the special needs and growth patterns of the at-risk newborn, which are temporary and yield to normal patterns

Solnit and Stark (1961) postulate that grief and mourning over the loss of the loved object—the idealized child—mark parental reactions to a child with abnormalities. *Grief work*, the emotional reaction to a significant loss, must occur before adequate attachment to the actual child is possible. Parental detachment precedes parental attachment. The parents must first grieve the loss of the wished-for perfect child, and then must adopt the imperfect child as the new love object.

Parental responses to a child with health problems may be viewed as a five-stage process (Klaus & Kennell, 1982):

1. *Shock* is felt at the reality of the birth of this child. This stage may be characterized by forgetfulness, amnesia about the situation, and a feeling of desperation.
2. There is *disbelief (denial)* of the reality of the situation, characterized by a refusal to believe the child is defective. This stage is exemplified by assertions that "It didn't really happen!" or "There has been a mistake; it's someone else's baby."
3. *Depression* over the reality of the situation and a corresponding grief reaction follows acceptance of the situation. This stage is characterized by much crying and sadness. Anger may also emerge at this stage. A projection of blame on others or on self and feelings of "not me" are characteristic of this stage.
4. *Equilibrium and acceptance* are characteristic of a decrease in the emotional reactions of the parents. This stage is variable and may be prolonged by a continuing threat to the infant's survival. Some parents experience chronic sorrow in relation to their child.
5. *Reorganization* of the family is necessary to deal with the child's problems. Mutual support of the parents facilitates this process, but the crisis of the situation may precipitate alienation between the mother and father.

Postpartal depression in new mothers and stressful events can exaggerate the problem (see Chapter 32∞). Fathers also may suffer from depression both before and after the birth of their child, adding to the discord in the family unit and compounding the perceived stress experienced by the mother.

DEVELOPMENTAL CONSEQUENCES

The baby who is born prematurely, is ill, or has a malformation or disorder is at risk for emotional, intellectual, and cognitive development delays. The risk is directly proportional to the seriousness of the problem and the length of treatment. Necessary physical separation of family and infant and the tremendous emotional and financial burdens may adversely affect the parent-child relationship. The recent trend to involve the parents with their newborn early, repeatedly, and over protracted periods of time has done much to facilitate positive parent-child relationships.

Parents must have a clear picture of the reality of the handicap and the types of developmental hurdles ahead. Unexpected behaviors and responses from the baby because of his or her defect or disorder can be upsetting and frightening. The demands of care for the child and disputes regarding management of behavior stress family relationships. The entire multidisciplinary team may need to pool their resources and expertise to help parents of children born with problems or disorders so that both parents and children can thrive.

A variety of behavioral patterns may occur. For example, one or more members of the family may make a scapegoat of the child. Another may become the youngster's champion to the exclusion of others. One or the other spouse may feel pushed aside or denied attention, and thus may withdraw or leave the family unit. Parents or siblings may feel that their own needs (schooling, material goods, freedom of movement) are being set aside while all assets (financial and other) go to support the one child's needs. There may also be an increase in child abuse.

NURSING MANAGEMENT

NURSING ASSESSMENT AND DIAGNOSIS

A concurrent illness of the mother or other family members or other concurrent stress (lack of hospitalization insurance, loss of job, age of parents) may alter the family response to the baby. Feelings of apprehension, guilt, failure, and grief expressed verbally or nonverbally are important aspects of the nursing history. These observations enable all professionals to be aware of the parental state, coping behaviors, and readiness for attachment, bonding, and caretaking. Appropriate nursing observations during interviewing and relating to the family include the following:

1. *Level of understanding.* Observations concerning the family's ability to assimilate the information given and to ask appropriate questions; the need for constant repetition of information
2. *Behavioral responses.* Appropriateness of behavior in relation to information given; lack of response; flat affect
3. *Difficulties with communication.* Deafness (reads lips only); blindness; dysphagia; understanding only a non-English language
4. *Paternal and maternal education level.* Parents unable to read or write; parents with eighth-grade-level education or lower; parents with a graduate-level degree or healthcare background

Documentation of such information, gathered through continuing contact and development of a therapeutic nurse-family relationship, lets all professionals understand and use the nursing history to provide continuous individual care.

A record of visits, caretaking procedures, affect (in relating to the newborn), and telephone calls indicate the level or lack of parental attachment. Serial observations, rather than just isolated observations that cause concern, must be obtained. Grant (1978)

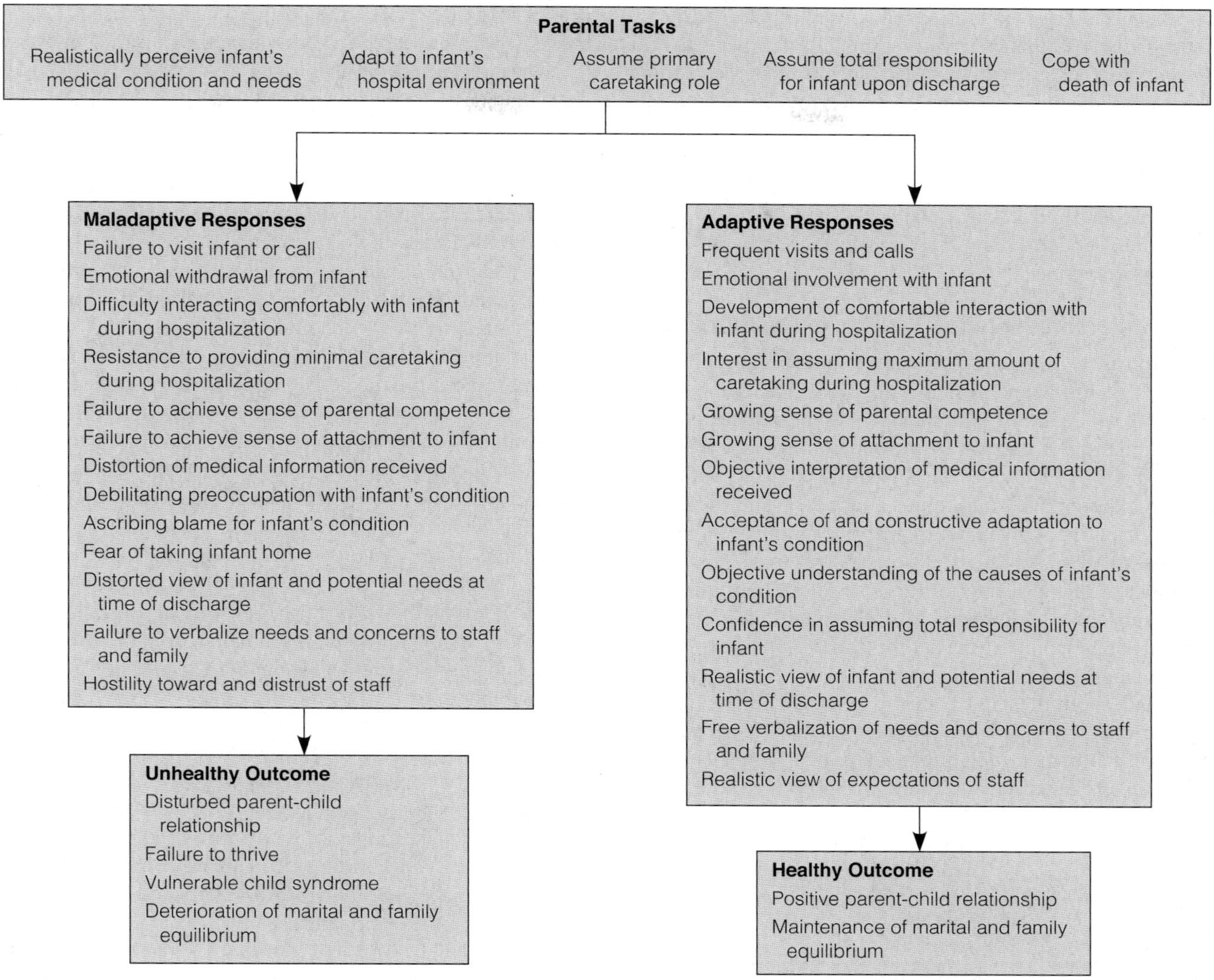

Parental Tasks
Realistically perceive infant's medical condition and needs
Adapt to infant's hospital environment
Assume primary caretaking role
Assume total responsibility for infant upon discharge
Cope with death of infant
Maladaptive Responses
Failure to visit infant or call
Emotional withdrawal from infant
Difficulty interacting comfortably with infant during hospitalization
Resistance to providing minimal caretaking during hospitalization
Failure to achieve sense of parental competence
Failure to achieve sense of attachment to infant
Distortion of medical information received
Debilitating preoccupation with infant's condition
Ascribing blame for infant's condition
Fear of taking infant home
Distorted view of infant and potential needs at time of discharge
Failure to verbalize needs and concerns to staff and family
Hostility toward and distrust of staff
Adaptive Responses
Frequent visits and calls
Emotional involvement with infant
Development of comfortable interaction with infant during hospitalization
Interest in assuming maximum amount of caretaking during hospitalization
Growing sense of parental competence
Growing sense of attachment to infant
Objective interpretation of medical information received
Acceptance of and constructive adaptation to infant's condition
Objective understanding of the causes of infant's condition
Confidence in assuming total responsibility for infant
Realistic view of infant and potential needs at time of discharge
Free verbalization of needs and concerns to staff and family
Realistic view of expectations of staff
Unhealthy Outcome
Disturbed parent-child relationship
Failure to thrive
Vulnerable child syndrome
Deterioration of marital and family equilibrium
Healthy Outcome
Positive parent-child relationship
Maintenance of marital and family equilibrium

● **Figure 29–13** Parental response patterns during crisis period. Maladaptive and adaptive parental responses during crisis period, showing unhealthy and healthy outcomes.

Source: Grant, P. (1978). Psychological needs of families of high-risk infants. *Family and Community Health, 11*, 93, Fig. 1. Philadelphia: Lippincott Williams & Wilkins.

has developed a conceptual framework depicting adaptive and maladaptive responses to parenting of an infant with an actual or potential problem (Figure 29–13 ●).

If a pattern of distancing behaviors evolves, the nurse should institute appropriate interventions. Follow-up studies have found that a statistically significant number of preterm, sick, and congenitally defective infants suffer from failure to thrive, battering, or other parenting disorders (Grant, 1978). Early detection and intervention will prevent these aberrations in parenting behaviors from leading to irreparable damage or death.

Nursing diagnoses that may apply to the family of a newborn at risk include the following:

- *Dysfunctional Grieving* related to loss of idealized newborn
- *Fear* related to emotional involvement with an at-risk newborn
- *Altered Parenting* related to impaired bonding secondary to feelings of inadequacy about caretaking activities

PLANNING AND IMPLEMENTATION

HOSPITAL-BASED NURSING CARE

In their sensitive and vulnerable state, parents are acutely perceptive of others' responses and reactions (particularly nonverbal) to the child. Parents can be expected to identify with the responses of others. Therefore, it is imperative that medical and nursing staff be fully aware of and come to terms with their own feelings so they are comfortable and at ease with the baby and grieving family.

Nurses may feel uncomfortable, may not know what to say to parents, or may fear confronting their own feelings as well as those of the parents. Each nurse must work out personal reactions with instructors, peers, clergy, parents, or significant others. It is helpful to have a stockpile of therapeutic questions and statements to initiate meaningful dialogue with parents. Opening statements might include the following: "You must be wondering what could have caused this," "Are you thinking that you (or someone else) may have done something?" "How can I help?" and "Are you wondering how you are going to manage?" Avoid statements such as: "I understand how you feel," "It could have been worse," "It's God's will," "You have other children," and "You are still young and can have more." This child is important now.

Support of Parents for Initial Viewing of the Newborn

Before parents see their child, the nurse must prepare them for the visit. It is important to maintain a positive, realistic attitude regarding the infant. An overly negative, fatalistic attitude further alienates the parents from their infant and retards attachment behaviors. Instead of beginning to bond with their child, the parents will anticipate their loss and begin the process of grieving. Once started, the grieving process is difficult to reverse.

Before preparing parents for the first view of their infant, the nurse should observe the baby. All infants exhibit strengths as well as deficiencies; prepare the parents to see both the deviations and the normal aspects of their infant. The nurse may say, "Your baby is small, about the length of my two hands. She weighs 2 lb, 3 oz, but is very active and cries when we disturb her. She is having some difficulty breathing but is breathing without assistance and is in only 35% oxygen and room air is 21%."

Many NICUs have booklets for parents to read before entering the units. Through explanations and pictures, the parents are better prepared to deal with the feelings they may experience when they see their infant for the first time (Figure 29–14 ●). Describe the equipment being used for the at-risk newborn and its purpose before the parents enter the intensive care unit.

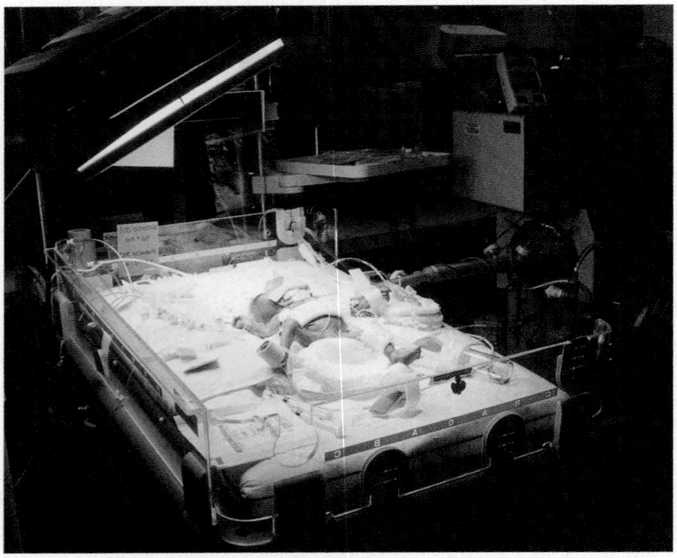

● **Figure 29–14** Preparing parents for first visit to at-risk newborn. This 25 weeks' gestational age infant with respiratory distress syndrome may be frightening for her parents to see for the first time because of the technology that is attached to her.

Source: Courtesy of Lisa Smith-Pedersen, RNC, MSN, NNP.

Upon entering the unit, parents may be overwhelmed by the sounds of monitors, alarms, and respirators, as well as by the unfamiliar language and "foreign" atmosphere. The primary nurse and physician caring for the newborn need to be with the parents when they first visit their baby. Parental reactions vary, but initially there is usually an element of shock. Providing chairs and time to regain composure assists the parents. Slow, complete, and simple explanations—first about the infant and then about the equipment—allay fear and anxiety.

Concern about the infant's physical appearance is common yet may remain unvoiced. Parents may express such concerns as: "He looks so small and red—like a drowned rat," "Why do her genitals look so abnormal?" and "Will that awful-looking mouth [cleft lip and palate] ever be normal?" The nurse needs to anticipate and address such questions. Use of pictures, such as of an infant after cleft lip repair, may be reassuring to doubting parents. Knowledge of the development of a "normal" preterm infant allows the nurse to make reassuring statements such as, "The baby's skin may look very red and transparent with lots of visible veins, but it is normal for her maturity. As she grows, subcutaneous fat will be laid down, and these superficial veins will begin to disappear."

The nursing staff set the tone of the NICU. Nurses foster the development of a safe, trusting environment by viewing the parents as essential caregivers, not as visitors or nuisances in the unit. It is important to provide parents privacy when needed and easy access to staff and facilities. An uncrowded and welcoming atmosphere lets parents know, "You are welcome here." However, even in crowded physical surroundings, the nurses can convey an attitude of openness and trust.

A trusting relationship is essential for collaborative efforts in caring for the infant. Nurses need to therapeutically use their own responses to relate to the parents on a one-to-one basis. Each individual has different needs, different ways of adapting to crisis, and different means of support. Nurses can use techniques that are real and spontaneous to them and avoid words or actions that are foreign to them. Nurses must also gauge their interventions so that they match the parents' pace and needs.

Nurses show concern and support by planning time to spend with the parents, by being psychologically as well as physically present, by encouraging open discussion and grieving, by repetitious explanations (as necessary), by providing privacy as needed, and by encouraging contact with the newborn. Identifying and clarifying feelings and fears decrease distortions in perception, thinking, and feeling. Nurses invest the baby with value in the eyes of the parents when they provide meticulous care to the newborn, talk and coo (especially in the face-to-face position) while holding or providing care to the newborn, refer to the child by gender or name, and relate the newborn's activities ("He took a whole ounce of formula," "She took hold of the blanket and just wouldn't let go"). Nurses should note the "normal" characteristics and capabilities of each newborn as well as the newborn's needs. The nurse should also learn the baby's name and refer to him or her by name.

Facilitation of Attachment If Neonatal Transport Occurs

Transport to a regional referral center some distance from the parents may be necessary. It is essential that the mother see and touch her infant before the infant is transported. Bring the mother to the nursery or take the infant in a warmed transport incubator to the mother's bedside to allow her to see the infant before transportation to the center. When the infant reaches the referral center, a staff member should call the parents with information about the infant's condition during transport, safe arrival at the center, and present condition.

Support of parents, with explanations from the professional staff, is crucial. Occasionally the mother may be unable to see the infant before transport (e.g., if she is still under general anesthesia or experiencing complications such as shock, hemorrhage, or seizures). In these cases, the infant should be photographed before transport. The picture should be given to the mother, along with an explanation of the infant's condition, present problems, and a detailed description of the infant's characteristics, to facilitate the attachment process until the mother can visit. An additional photograph is also helpful for the father to share with siblings or extended family. With the increased attention on improved fetal outcome, prenatal maternal transports, rather than neonatal transports, are occurring more frequently. This practice gives the mother of an at-risk infant the opportunity to visit and care for her infant during the early postpartal period.

Promotion of Touching and Parental Caretaking

Parents visiting a preterm, SGA or sick infant may need several visits to become comfortable and confident in their ability to touch the infant without injuring her or him. Barriers such as incubators, incisions, monitor electrodes, and tubes may delay the mother's development of comfort in touching the newborn.

Klaus and Kennell (1982) have demonstrated a significant difference in the amount of eye contact and touching behaviors of mothers of normal newborns and mothers of preterm infants. Whereas mothers of normal newborns progress within minutes to palm contact of the infant's trunk, mothers of preterm infants are slower to progress from fingertip to palm contact and from the extremities to the trunk. The progression to palm contact with the infant's trunk may take several visits to the nursery.

Use support, reassurance, and encouragement to help the mother develop positive feelings about her ability and importance to her infant. Touching facilitates "getting to know" the infant and thus establishes a bond with the infant. Touching and seeing the infant help the mother realize the "normals" and potential of her baby (Figure 29–15 ●).

The nurse can also encourage parents to meet their newborn's need for stimulation. Stroking, rocking, cuddling, singing, and talking should be an integral part of the parents' caretaking responsibilities. Bonding can be facilitated by encouraging parents to visit and become involved in their baby's care (Figure 29–16 ●). When visiting is impossible, the parents should feel free to phone when they wish to receive information about their baby. A nurse's warm, receptive attitude provides support. Nurses can also facilitate parenting by personalizing a baby to the parents, by referring to the infant by name, or relating personal behavioral characteristics. Remarks such as "Jenny loves her pacifier" help make the infant seem individual and unique.

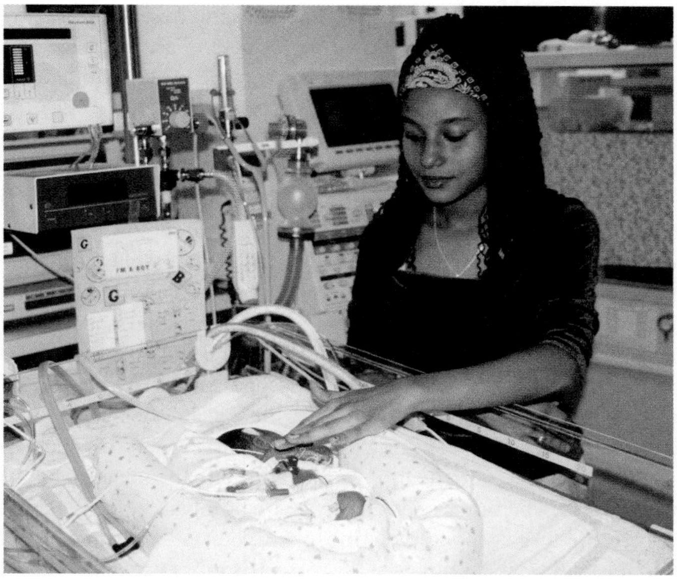

● **Figure 29–15** Beginnings of attachment. Mother of this 26 weeks' gestational age 600 g baby begins attachment through fingertip touch.

Source: Courtesy of Lisa Smith-Pedersen, RNC, MSN, NNP.

The variety of equipment needed for life support is hardly conducive to anxiety-free caretaking by the parents. However, even the sickest infant may be cared for, if only in a small way, by the parents. Demonstration and explanation, followed by support of the parents in initial caretaking behaviors, positively reinforce parents' sense of success. Changing their infant's diaper, providing skin or oral care, or helping the nurse turn the infant may at first provoke anxiety, but the parents will become more comfortable and confident in caretaking and feel satisfied by the baby's reactions and their ability "to do something." Complimenting the parents' competence in caretaking also increases their self-esteem,

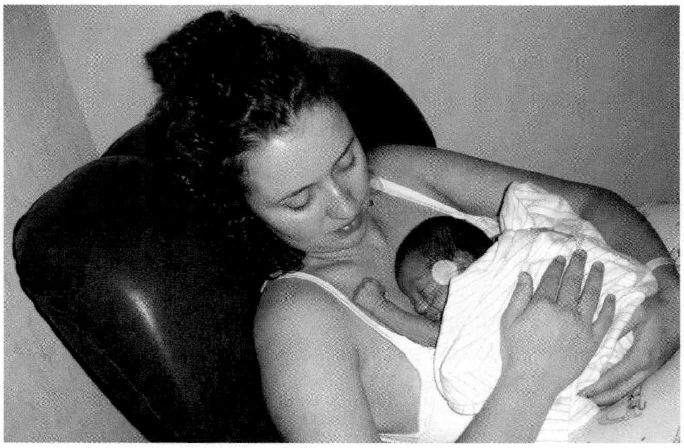

● **Figure 29–16** Facilitating bonding. This mother of a 31 weeks' gestational age infant with respiratory distress syndrome is spending time with her newborn and meeting the baby's need for cuddling.

Source: Courtesy of Lisa Smith-Pedersen, RNC, MSN, NNP.

which has received recent "blows" of guilt and failure. *Never give the parents a task that they might not be able to accomplish.* Cues that the parents are ready to become involved with the child's care include their reference to the baby by name and their questioning as to amount of feeding taken, sleeping patterns, appearance today, and the like (Loo, Espinosa, Tyler, et al., 2003).

Often parents of high-risk infants have ambivalent feelings toward the nurse. These feelings may take the form of criticism of the care of the infant, manipulation of staff, or personal guilt. The nurse should accept this behavior, but continue to remind the parents that it is okay and natural to feel disappointment, a sense of failure, helplessness, or anger about the birth. The overprotectiveness and overoptimism are defense mechanisms. To deny the negative feelings only entrenches them further, delays their resolution, and delays realistic planning. Instead of fostering (by silence) nurses need to intervene appropriately to enhance parent-infant attachment. The nurse needs to deal with ambivalent feelings that contribute to a competitive atmosphere. For example, the nurse should avoid making unfavorable comparisons between the baby's responses to parental and nursing caretaking. It is an essential and easy task for the nurse to make statements that will help improve the parents' self-esteem. The nurse can point out that, in addition to physiologic use, breast milk is important because of the emotional investment of the mother. Pumping, storing, labeling, and delivering quantities of breast milk is a time-consuming "labor of love" for mothers. Positive remarks about breast milk reinforce the maternal behavior of caretaking and providing for her infant: "Breast milk is something that only you can give your baby," "You really have brought a lot of milk today," "Look how rich this breast milk is," or "Even small amounts of milk are important, and look how rich it is." If the infant begins to gain weight while being fed breast milk, it is important that the nurse point this correlation out to the mother. Parents should also be advised that initial weight loss with beginning nipple feedings is common because of the increased energy expended when the infant begins active rather than passive nutritional intake.

During a quiet time it may help for the nurse to encourage the parents to talk about their hopes and fears and to facilitate their involvement in parent groups. Encourage parents to provide care for their infant even if the baby is very sick and likely to die. Detachment is easier after attachment, because the parents are comforted by the knowledge that they did all they could for their child while he or she was alive.

Facilitation of Family Adjustment

During crisis, it is difficult to maintain interpersonal relationships. Yet in a newborn intensive care area, the parents are expected to relate to many different care providers. It is important that parents have as few professionals as possible relaying information to them. A primary nurse should coordinate care and provide continuity for parents. Care providers are individuals and thus will use different terms, inflections, and attitudes. These subtle differences are monumental to parents and may confuse, confound, and produce anxiety. Parents are also often anxious when their baby is transferred from the NICU to a step-down unit or the "regular nursery" or transport back to the home hospital provokes parental anxiety because they must now deal with new healthcare professionals. They may feel that their infant is not being cared for as proficiently because the nurses are not at the infant's bedside as often as they were in the NICU. The nurse not only functions as a liaison between the parents and the various professionals interacting with the infant and parents but also offers clarification, explanation, interpretation of information, and support to the parents.

The nurse encourages parents to deal with the crisis with help from their support system. The support system attempts to meet the emotional needs and to provide support for the family members in crisis and stress situations. Biologic kinship is not the only valid criterion for a support system; an emotional kinship is the most important factor. In our mobile society of isolated nuclear families, the support system may be a next-door neighbor, a best friend, or perhaps a schoolmate. The nurse needs to search out the significant others in the lives of the parents and help them understand the problems so that they can be a constant parental support.

The impact of the crisis on the family is individual and varied. To institute appropriate interventions, the nurse must view the birth of any infant (normal newborn, preterm infant, infant with congenital anomaly) as defined by the family. The nurse obtains information about the family's ability to adapt to the situation through interaction with the family. It is important for the nurse to encourage open intrafamily communication. The nurse should discourage the family from keeping secrets from one another, especially between spouses, because secrets undermine the trust of relationships. Well-meaning rationales such as "I want to protect her," "I don't want him to worry about it," and so on can be destructive to open communication and to the basic element of a relationship—trust.

Open communication is especially important when the mother is hospitalized apart from the infant. The first person to visit the infant relays information regarding the infant's care and condition to the mother and family. In this situation, the mother has had minimal contact, if any, with her infant. Because of her anxiety and isolation, she may mistrust all those who provide information (the father, nurse, physician, or extended family) until she sees the infant for herself. This can put tremendous stress on the relationship between spouses. The parents (and family) should be given information together. This practice helps overcome misunderstandings and misinterpretations and promotes cooperative "working through" of problems.

The nurse should encourage the entire family—siblings as well as other relatives—to visit and obtain information about the baby. Methods of intervention in helping the family cope with the situation include providing support, confronting the crisis, and understanding the reality. Support, explanations, and the helping role must extend to the kin network, as well as to the nuclear family, to aid the extended family in communication and support ties with the nuclear family.

The needs of siblings should not be overlooked. Siblings have been looking forward to the new baby, and they, too, suffer a degree of loss. Young children may react with hostility and older ones with shame at the birth of an infant with an anomaly. Both reactions may make siblings feel guilty. Parents, who may be preoccupied with working through their own feelings, often cannot give the other children the attention and support they need.

Sometimes another child becomes the focus of family tension. Anxiety thus directed can take the form of finding fault or of overconcern. This is a form of denial; the parents cannot face the real worry—the infant at risk. After assessing the situation, the observant nurse can ensure that another family member or friend steps in to support the siblings of the affected baby.

The nurse must respect and seek to meet the desires and needs of the individuals involved and understand that differences can exist side by side. The nurse can often elicit the parents' feelings about the experience by asking "How are you doing?" The emphasis is on "you," and the interest must be sincere.

Parents from minority cultures must deal with language barriers and cultural differences that can make feelings of isolation and uncertainty more acute. Healthcare providers have the professional responsibility to be aware of cultural needs of all clients and to ensure their needs are met. Feelings of isolation and uncertainty influence not only the parent's emotional responses to the ill newborn, but also the utilization of services and their interaction with health professionals. Hospital cultural interpreter programs can assist families with interactions with staff, as well as provide translation during family meetings, multidisciplinary family conferences, and parent support groups (Lipson & Dibble, 2008).

Families with children in the NICU may become friends and support one another. To encourage the development of these friendships and to provide support, many units have established parent groups. The core of the groups consists of parents whose infants were once in the intensive care unit. Most groups make contact with families within a day or two of the infant's admission to the unit, through either phone calls or visits to the hospital. Early one-on-one parent contacts are more effective than discussion groups in helping families work through their feelings. This personalized method gives the grieving parents an opportunity to express personal feelings about the pregnancy, labor, and birth and their "different from expected" infant with others who have experienced the same feelings and with whom they can identify.

COMMUNITY-BASED NURSING CARE

Predischarge planning begins once the infant's condition becomes stable and it seems likely the newborn will survive. Discharge preparation and care conferences should involve a multidisciplinary team approach (Hummel & Cronin, 2004). NICU nursing staff is the fulcrum for aiding in the transition of high-risk infants from the intensive care unit to the home. Effective open communication with the families during the entire discharge-planning phase of care empowers the families to assume the role of primary caregiver for their children.

Adequate predischarge teaching helps parents transform any feelings of inadequacy they may have into feelings of self-assurance and attachment. From the beginning the parents should be taught about their infant's special needs and growth patterns. This teaching and involvement are best facilitated by a nurse who is familiar with the infant and his or her family over a period of time and who has developed a comfortable and supportive relationship with them.

Cobedding of twins is often used in the NICU to provide comfort, decrease stress to the twins, and provide a form of developmentally supportive care. Cobedding is also a strategy to maximize the synchronization of sleep-wake cycles (Bowers, Curran, Freda, et al., 2008). Parents of multiples may desire cobedding at home to allow for clustering of care and to facilitate the parents' ability to spend time with both of their children (Figure 29–17 ●). If twins or other multiples experienced cobedding in the NICU, the nurse needs to discuss the advantages and disadvantages of continuing the practice at home. Currently, there is no evidence to establish cobedding of multiples outside the NICU as a safe or unsafe sleep practice (Gromada & Bowers, 2005). The high incidence of prematurity and LBW in multiple birth infants and the corresponding risks for SIDS should be considered. As with all families at discharge, parents of multiples should be taught SIDS risk-reduction practices. SIDS reduction practices include supine positioning, babies sleeping in parents' room, firm bedding surface, no loose coverings/items and no barriers between infants (Bowers et al., 2008).

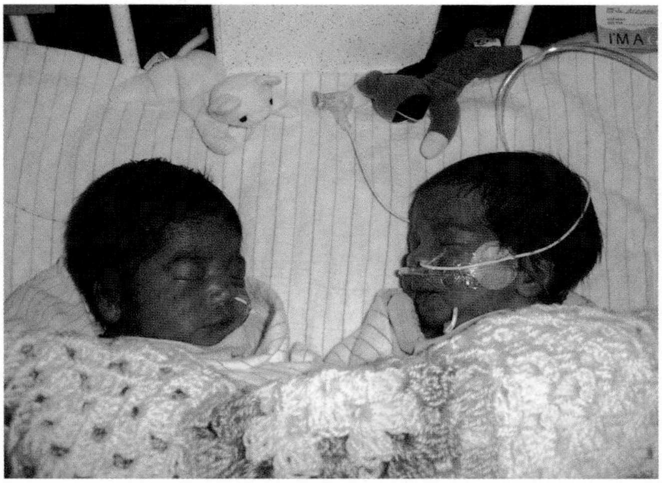

● **Figure 29–17** Cobedding. Cobedding of twins facilitates delivery of care and parent interaction with healthcare members. These twins were born at 33 weeks' gestation and required oxygen and gavage feeding while in the NICU.

Source: Courtesy of Lisa Smith-Pedersen, RNC, MSN, NNP.

The nurse's responsibility is to provide home care instructions in an optimal environment for parental learning. Learning should take place over time, to avoid bombarding the parents with instructions in the day or hour before discharge. Parents often enjoy performing minimal caretaking tasks, with gradual expansion of their role. Many NICUs provide facilities for parents to room in with their infants for a few days before discharge. This allows parents a degree of independence in the care of their infant with the security of nursing help nearby. This practice is particularly helpful for anxious parents, parents who have not had the opportunity to spend extended time with their infant, or parents who will be giving complex physical care at home, such as gastrostomy feeding and care (Collins, Makrides, & McPhee, 2008).

The families are able to interact with staff while gradually transitioning to sole caretakers of their medically complex high-risk infant. When discharging a medically fragile infant to home, schedule a predischarge home visit by a public health nurse or home health agency. This discharge visit evaluates the home for any possible issues that may complicate the parents' ability to care for their at-risk infant, especially if there are multiple monitoring equipment needs.

The basic elements of discharge and home care instruction are as follows:

1. Teach the parents routine well-baby care, such as bathing, taking a temperature, preparing formula, and breastfeeding.
2. Help parents learn to do special procedures as needed by the newborn, such as gavage or gastrostomy feedings, tracheostomy or enterostomy care, medication administration, CPR, and operation of the apnea monitor. Before discharge, the parents should be as comfortable as possible with these tasks and should demonstrate independence. Written tools and instructions are useful for parents to refer to once they are home with the infant, but they should not replace actual participation in the infant's care.
3. Make sure that all applicable screening (metabolic, vision, hearing) tests, immunizations, and respiratory syncytial virus (RSV) prophylaxis are done before discharge and that all records are given to the primary care provider and parents.
4. Refer parents to community health and support organizations. The Visiting Nurse Association, public health nurses, or social services can assist the parents in the stressful transition from hospital to home by providing the necessary home teaching and support. Some NICUs have their own parent support groups to help bridge the gap between hospital and home care. Parents can also find support from a variety of community organizations, such as mothers-of-twins groups, March of Dimes Birth Defects Foundation, handicapped children services, and teen mother and child programs. Each community has numerous agencies capable of assisting the family in adapting emotionally, physically, and financially to the chronically ill infant. The nurse should be familiar with community resources and help the parents identify which agencies may benefit them.
5. Help parents recognize the growth and development needs of their infant. A development program begun in the hospital can be continued at home, or parents may be referred to an infant development program in the community.
6. Arrange medical follow-up care before discharge. The infant will need to be followed up by a family pediatrician, a well-baby clinic, or a specialty clinic. The first appointment should be made before the infant is discharged from the hospital.
7. Evaluate the need for special equipment for infant care (such as a respirator, oxygen, apnea monitor, feeding pump) in the home. Any equipment or supplies should be placed in the home before the infant's discharge.
8. Arrange for neonatal hospice support for parents of the medically fragile infant as needed.

Further evaluation after the infant has gone home is useful in determining whether the crisis has been resolved satisfactorily.

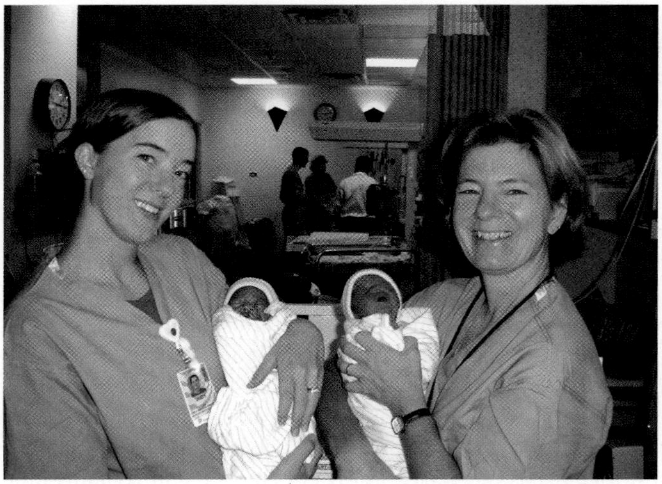

● **Figure 29–18** Discharge day. These 33 weeks' gestational age twins are being held by staff in the NICU on the happy day of discharge. This is what is so rewarding about working in the NICU: healthy babies going home to their families.

Source: Courtesy of Lisa Smith-Pedersen, RNC, MSN, NNP.

The parents are usually given the intensive care nursery's telephone number to call for support and advice. The staff can follow up with each family with visits or telephone calls at intervals for several weeks to assess and evaluate the infant's (and parents') progress (Fig. 29–18 ●).

EVALUATION

Expected outcomes of nursing care include the following:

- The parents are able to verbalize their feelings of grief and loss.
- The parents verbalize their concerns about their baby's health problems, care needs, and potential outcome.
- The parents are able to participate in their infant's care and show attachment behaviors.

CONSIDERATIONS FOR THE NURSE WHO WORKS WITH AT-RISK NEWBORNS

The birth of a baby with a problem is a traumatic event with the potential for either both disruption and growth of the involved family. The NICU staff nurses may never see the long-term results of the specialized sensitive care they give to parents and their newborns. Their only immediate evidence of effective care may be the beginning resolution of parental grief; or discharge of a recovered, thriving infant to the care of happy parents; and the beginning of reintergration of family life.

Nurses cannot provide support unless they themselves are supported. Working in an emotional environment of "lots of living and lots of dying" takes its toll on staff. NICUs are among the most stressful areas in health care for patients, families, and nurses. Nurses bear most of the stress and largely determine the atmosphere of the NICU. The nurse's ability to cope with stress is the key to creating an emotionally healthy environment and a positive working atmosphere. The emotional needs and feelings of the staff must be recognized and dealt with so that staff can support the parents. An environment of openness to feelings and support in dealing with their human needs and emotions is essential for staff.

As caregivers, nurses may be unaware of their need to grieve for their own losses in the NICU. Nurses must also go through the grief work that parents experience. Techniques such as group meetings, individual support, and primary care nursing may assist in maintaining staff mental health. Reunions in some nurseries are beneficial for the families and healthcare professionals so they are able to see the children after discharge.

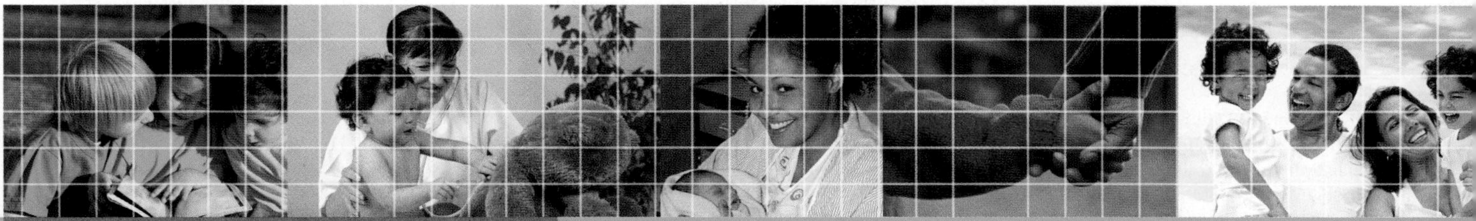

CRITICAL CONCEPT REVIEW

LEARNING OUTCOMES — CONCEPTS

29.1 Discuss how to identify infants in need of resuscitation and the appropriate method of resuscitation based on the labor record and observable physiologic indicators.

1. Infants at risk for resuscitation include:
   - Nonreassuring fetal heart pattern, meconium-stained amniotic fluid and/or acidosis detected by fetal scalp sample.
   - Cardiac disease diagnosed prenatally.
   - Other congenital abnormality diagnosed prenatally.
   - Premature birth.
   - Infant of multiple pregnancy.
   - Prolonged or difficult delivery.
2. Infants needing resuscitation:
   - Weak cry at birth.
   - Poor respiratory effort at birth.
   - Retractions at birth.
3. Resuscitation methods:
   - Stimulation by rubbing the newborn's back. (Done initially to all infants.)
   - Use of positive pressure to inflate the lungs. (Used if respirations are inadequate or have not been initiated.)
   - Endotracheal intubation. (Used immediately for severely premature infants, infants with known congenital anomalies, and infants who do not respond to stimulation or bag and mask.)
   - Medications: Naloxone (Narcan) may be used to reverse effects of narcotics given to mother prior to birth.

29.2 Based on clinical manifestations, differentiate among the various types of respiratory distress (respiratory distress syndrome, transient tachypnea of the newborn, and meconium aspiration syndrome) in the newborn and their related nursing care.

1. Respiratory distress syndrome:
   - Lack of sufficient surfactant causes labored respirations and increased work at breathing.
   - Seen most frequently in premature newborns.
   - Nursing care involves administration of surfactant, close assessment, and supportive care if mechanical ventilation is needed.
2. Transient tachypnea of the newborn (TTNB):
   - Usually results from excess fluid in the lungs.
   - Infant breathes normally at birth, but develops symptoms of respiratory distress by 4-6 hours of age.
   - Nursing care involves initiating oxygen therapy and restricting oral feedings until respiratory status improves.
3. Meconium aspiration syndrome:
   - Signs and symptoms of respiratory distress beginning at birth.
   - May depend upon the amount of meconium that is aspirated and the activity level of the newborn.
   - Initial nursing care involves:
     - If infant is vigorous even in presence of meconium—no subsequent special resuscitation
     - If infant has absent or depressed respirations, HR less than 100 beats per minute, or poor muscle tone—direct tracheal suctioning by specially trained personnel
   - After initial suctioning and/or resuscitation efforts, nursing care involves ongoing assessment for signs and symptoms of respiratory distress and supportive care of the infant requiring mechanical ventilation or ECMO.

LEARNING OUTCOMES	CONCEPTS
29.3 Discuss selected metabolic abnormalities (including cold stress and hypoglycemia), their effects on the newborn, and the nursing implications.	1. Cold stress sets up the chain of physiologic events of hypoglycemia, pulmonary vasconstriction, hyperbilirubinemia, respiratory distress, and metabolic acidosis. 2. Nursing interventions include: ■ Keep infant warmed during any transport. ■ Observe for any signs of hypoglycemia. ■ Have infant go to breast or feed early in neonatal period. ■ Assess blood glucose frequently.
29.4 Explain the causes, pathophysiology, risks for developing, possible sequelae, clinical therapy, and the difference between physiologic and pathologic jaundice in determining the hospital and community-based nursing care management of the infant with jaundice.	1. Physiologic jaundice: ■ Occurs in 50% of all newborns. ■ Appears after 24 hours of age. ■ Not visible after 10 days of age. ■ May require phototherapy. 2. Pathologic jaundice: ■ Usually caused by ABO or Rh incompatibility. ■ Jaundice may be present within 24 hours of birth. ■ Treatment begins with phototherapy, but may progress to exchange transfusions. 3. Untreated hyperbilirubinemia (due to either type of jaundice) may result in neurotoxicity.
29.5 Explain how Rh incompatibility or ABO incompatibility can lead to the development of hyperbilirubinemia.	1. Rh incompatibility: ■ Maternal antibodies enter the fetal circulation, then attach to and destroy fetal red blood cells. ■ Fetal system produces more RBCs. ■ Hyperbilirubinemia, anemia, and jaundice result. 2. ABO incompatibility: ■ Mother is type O and infant is type A or B. ■ Less severe than Rh incompatibility.
29.6 Identify nursing responsibilities and rationale in caring for the newborn receiving phototherapy.	Nursing responsibilities for the newborn receiving phototherapy include: 1. Expose maximum amount of skin surface for optimal therapeutic results. 2. Apply eye patches while banks of phototherapy lights are in progress. 3. Assess eyes for signs/symptoms of conjunctivitis per agency protocol. 4. Frequently monitor temperature. 5. Offer infant water and formula frequently to assist in excretion of bilirubin. 6. Keep parents informed of need for phototherapy and encourage parents to hold and care for infant while undergoing phototherapy.
29.7 Explain the causes and nursing care of infants with anemia or polycythemia.	1. Anemia in newborns results from prenatal blood loss, birth trauma, infection, or blood group incompatibility: ■ Nursing assessments for signs and symptoms of anemia. ■ Record all amounts of blood taken during laboratory testing. 2. Polycythemia may result from delayed cord clamping, twin-to-twin transfusion, or chronic intrauterine hypoxia: ■ Nursing assessments for signs and symptoms of polycythemia.
29.8 Describe the nursing assessments that would lead the nurse to suspect newborn sepsis and the nursing care of the newborn with an infection.	The most common signs of newborn sepsis include: 1. Lethargy or irritability. 2. Pallor or duskiness. 3. Hypothermia. 4. Feeding intolerance. 5. Hyperbilirubinemia. 6. Tachycardia, bradycardia, or apneic spells. The nursing care includes: ■ Obtain cultures before antibiotic therapy starts ■ Carry out laboratory sepsis workup ■ Administer antibiotics as prescribed ■ Provide supportive care to include: NTE, respiratory and cardiovascular support, nutrition, monitor fluid and electrolyte homeostasis, and observe for complications.

LEARNING OUTCOMES / CONCEPTS

29.9 Relate the consequences of maternally transmitted infections, such as maternal syphilis, gonorrhea, herpesviridae family (HSV or CMV), and chlamydia, to the nursing care of infants in the neonatal period.

1. All infants receive eye prophylaxis with opthalmic antibiotic due to possibility of transmission of gonorrhea or chlamydia during the birth process.
2. Maternal syphilis requires that the infant be isolated from other newborns and receive antibiotics at birth.
3. Maternal herpes virus infection requires administration of IV antiviral medications in the immediate newborn period as well as multiple cultures (skin, spinal fluid) for presence of herpesvirus.

29.10 Describe the interventions to facilitate parental attachment and meet the special initial and long-term needs of parents of at-risk infants.

1. Assess the parent's level of understanding of the infant's problem. Initially, the parents need to understand the infant's problem, including expected treatments.
2. Prepare and facilitate the parents' viewing of the infant.
3. Promote touching and facilitate parental participation in care of the infant.
4. Ensure parents understand routine well-baby care, normal growth and development of infants and have referral for normal infant screening procedures.
5. Have medical follow-up arranged.
6. Facilitate parental adjustment to the infant's special needs.
7. Parents have referral for any special equipment required at home and understand how to perform any special procedures needed to care for the infant.

CRITICAL THINKING IN ACTION

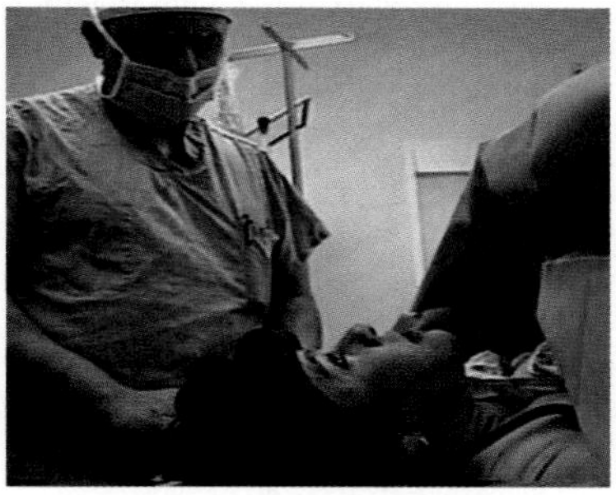

Rebecca Prince, age 21, G2 now P2, gives birth to a 5 pound baby at 38 weeks' gestation by primary cesarean birth for fetal distress. The infant's Apgars are 7 and 9 at 1 and 5 minutes. The infant is suctioned and given free-flow oxygen at birth, then is admitted to the newborn nursery for transitional care and does well. You are the nurse caring for baby Prince at 36 hours old. You review the newborn's record and note that the baby's blood type is A+ and his mother is O+. Rebecca wants to breastfeed. You are performing a shift assessment on baby Prince when you observe that the infant has a unilateral cephalhematoma and is lethargic. You blanch the skin over the sternum and observe a yellow discoloration of the skin. Lab tests reveal a serum bilirubin level of 12 mg/dl, hematocrit 55%, a mildly positive direct Coombs' test, and a positive indirect Coombs' test. Baby Prince is diagnosed with hyperbilirubinemia secondary to ABO incompatibility and cephalhematoma. You provide phototherapy by fiberoptic blanket around the trunk of the infant and take the baby to his mother's room.

1. How would you explain the purpose of phototherapy with the mother?
2. Describe the care the mother can give to the newborn.
3. Discuss the advantage of the fiberoptic blanket phototherapy for the newborn.
4. Newborns up to 1 month of age are susceptible to organisms that do not cause significant disease in older children. Explore the circumstances that cause susceptibility to infection.
5. Describe how to distinguish between oral thrush and milk curds.

See MyNursingKit for possible responses.

REFERENCES

Aher, S., Malwatkar, K., & Kadam, S. (2008). Neonatal anemia. *Seminars in Fetal & Neonatal Medicine 13*, 239–247.

American Academy of Pediatrics [AAP] & American Heart Association [AHA]. (2006). *Neonatal resuscitation: Instructor manual* (5th ed.). Evanston, IL: Author.

American Academy of Pediatrics (AAP) & Canadian Paediatric Society. (2006). Prevention and management of pain in the neonate: An update. *Pediatrics, 118*(5), 2231–2241.

American Academy of Pediatrics (AAP), Committee on Fetus and Newborn, & American College of Obstetricians and Gynecolgists (ACOG), Committee on Obstetrics. (2007). *Guidelines for perinatal care* (6th ed.). Evanston, IL: Author.

Bhutani, V. K., Johnson, L. H., & Keren, R. (2004). Diagnosis and management of hyperbilirubinemia in the term neonate: For a safer first week. *Pediatric Clinics of North America, 51*(4), 843–861.

Blackburn, S. T. (2007). *Maternal, fetal, & neonatal physiology: A clinical perspective* (3rd ed.). St. Louis: Saunders.

Bowers, N. A., Curran, C. A., Freda, M. C., Poole, J. H., Slocum, J., & Sosa, M. E. (2008). High-risk pregancy. In K. R. Simpson & P. A. Creehan, *AWHONN perinatal nursing* (3rd ed., pp. 125–299). Philadelphia: Lippincott Williams & Wilkins.

Bradshaw, W. T. (2010). Gastrointestinal disorders. In M. T. Verklan & M. Walden, *Core curriculum for neonatal intensive care nursing* (4th ed., pp. 589–637). St. Louis: Saunders/Elsevier.

Cloherty, J. P., Eichenwald, E. C., & Stark, A. R. (2008). *Manual of neonatal care* (6th ed.). Philadelphia: Lippincott Williams & Wilkins.

Cole, F. S., Nogee, L. M., & Hamvas, A. (2006). Defects in surfactant synthesis: Clinical implications. *Pediatrics Clinics of North America, 53*(5), 911–927.

Collins, C. T., Makrides, M. E., & McPhee, A. J. (2008). Early discharge with home support of gavage feeding for stable preterm infants who have not established full oral feeds. *Cochrane database of systematic reviews.* 2, ID #CD003743.

Diehl-Jones, W. & Askin, D. F. (2010). Hematologic disorders. In M. T. Verklan & M. Walden, *Core curriculum for neonatal intensive care nursing* (4th ed., pp. 666–693). St. Louis: Saunders/Elsevier.

Folk, L. A. (2007). Guide to capillary heelstick blood sampling in infants. *Advances in Neonatal Care, 7*(4), 171–178.

Glomella, T. L. (2009). *Neonatology: Management, procedures, on-call problems, diseases, and drugs* (6th ed.). New York, NY: McGraw Hill.

Grant, P. (1978). Psychological needs of families of high-risk infants. *Family and Community Health, 11*(3), 93–97.

Gromada, K. K., & Bowers, N. A. (2005). Care of the multiple-birth family: *Postpartum through infancy* (Nursing Module). New York: March of Dimes Birth Defects Foundation.

Hawk, M. (2008). C-Reactive protein in neonatal sepsis. *Neonatal Network, 27*(2), 117–123.

Hummel, P., & Cronin, J. (2004). Home care of the high-risk infant. *Advances in Neonatal Care, 4*(6), 354–364.

Kaplan, D. M., & Mason, E. A. (1974). Maternal reactions to premature birth viewed as an acute emotional disorder. In H. J. Parad (Ed.), *Crisis intervention* (Ch. 9, pp. 118–128). New York: Family Services Association of America.

Klaus, M. H., & Kennell, J. H. (1982). *Maternal-infant bonding* (2nd ed.). St. Louis: Mosby.

Lipson, J. G., & Dibble, S. L. (2008). *Culture & clinical care.* (7th ed.). San Francisco: The Regents, University of California.

Loo, K. K., Espinosa, M., Tyler, R., & Howard, J. (2003). Using knowledge to cope with stress in the NICU: How parents integrate learning to read the physiologic and behavioral cues of the infant. *Neonatal Network, 22*(1), 31–37.

Lott, J. W. (2010). Immunology and infectious disease. In M. T. Verklan & M. Walden, *Core curriculum for neonatal intensive care nursing* (4th ed., pp. 694–723). St. Louis: Saunders/Elsevier.

McCoskey, L. (2008). Nursing care guidelines for prevention of nasal breakdown in neonates receiving nasal CPAP. *Advances in Neonatal Care, 8*(2), 116 –124.

Mileic, T. L. (2008). Neonatal glucose homeostasis. *Neonatal Network, 27*(3), 203–207.

Nash, P., & Smith, J. R. (2008). Common neonatal complications. In K. R. Simpson & P. A. Creehan, *AWHONN perinatal nursing* (3rd ed., pp. 612–646). Philadelphia: Lippincott Williams & Wilkins.

Pappas, B. E., & Walker, B. (2010). Neonatal delivery room resuscitation. In M. T. Verklan & M. Walden, *Core curriculum for neonatal intensive care nursing* (4th ed., pp. 91–109). St. Louis: Saunders/Elsevier.

Rosenberg, A. A. (2007). The neonate. In S. G. Gabbe, J. R. Niebyl, & J. L. Simpson (Eds.), *Obstetrics: Normal and problem pregnancies* (5th ed., pp. 523–565). Philadelphia, PA: Churchill Livingstone/Elsevier.

Saniski, D. (2005). Neonatal pain relief protocols in their infancy. *Nurse Week News.* Retrieved November 3, 2005, from www.nurseweek.com/news/features/05-02/Clinical_Babypain

Solnit, A., & Stark, M. (1961). Mourning and the birth of a defective child. *Psychoanalytic Study of the Child, 16,* 505.

Thureen, P. J., Deacon, J., Hernandez, J. A., & Hall, D. M. (2005). *Assessment and care of the well newborn* (2nd ed.). St. Louis: Elsevier Saunders.

Vargo, L. E., & Trotter, C. W. (2007). *The premature infant: Nursing assessment and management.* (2nd ed.). White Plains, NY: March of Dimes.

Walden, M. (2007). Pain in the newborn and infant. In C. Kenner & J. W. Lott. *Comprehensive neonatal care: An interdisciplinary approach* (4th ed., pp. 350–371). St. Louis: Elsevier Saunders.

Wiedemann, J. R., Saugstad, A. M., Barnes-Powell, L., & Duran, K. (2008). Meconium aspiration syndrome. *Neonatal Network, 27*(2), 81–87.

Young, T. E., & Mangum, O. B. (2009). *Neofax®: A manual of drugs used in neonatal care* (22nd ed.). Raleigh, NC: Acorn.

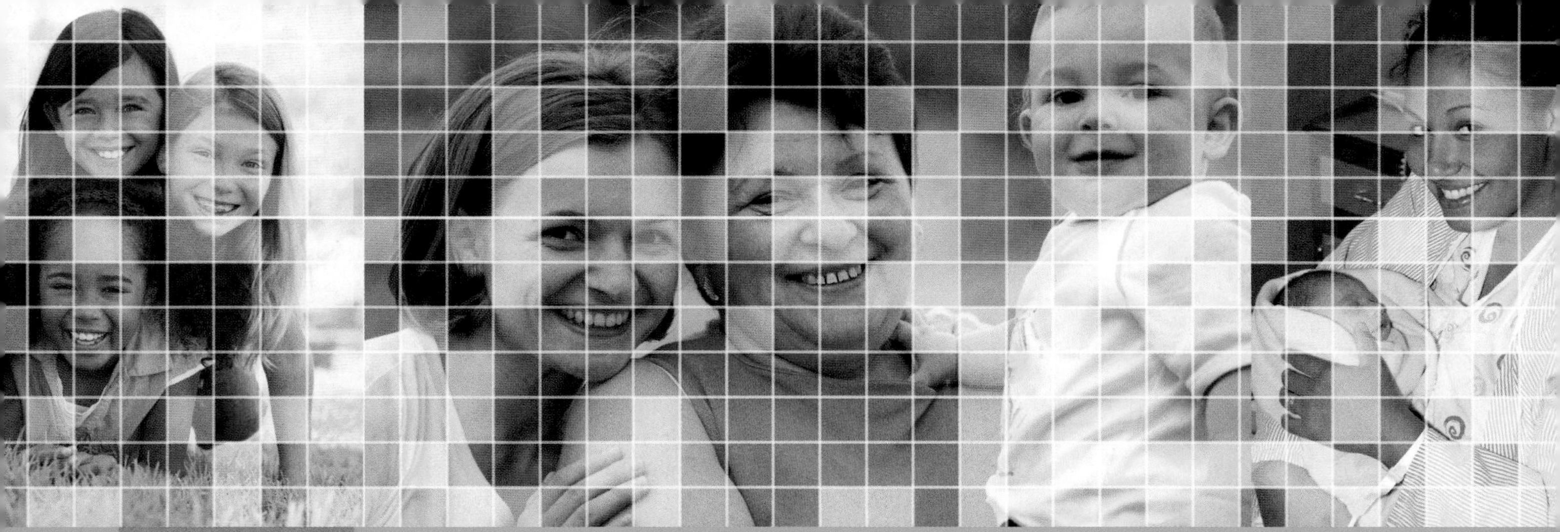

CHAPTER

30 Postpartal Adaptation and Nursing Assessment

I acutely felt the fatigue and sense of loss of the relationship with my baby that I had during pregnancy. But then the wonderful part happened with the reuniting with my new daughter. Holding her, having her latch on to my breast to get nourishment, and her looking into my eyes to say "hello Mom." —Susan, 34

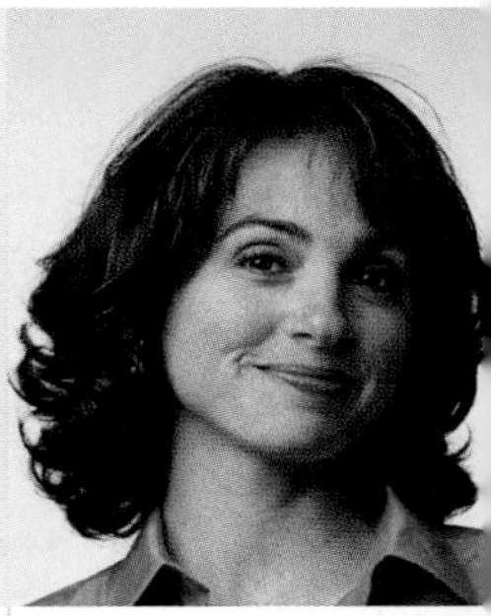

LEARNING OUTCOMES

30.1 Describe the basic physiologic changes that occur in the postpartal period as a woman's body returns to its prepregnant state.

30.2 Describe the psychologic adjustments that normally occur during the postpartal period.

30.3 Explain the components and methods of a systematic postpartal assessment.

30.4 Describe the normal characteristics and common concerns of the mother considered in a postpartal assessment.

30.5 Examine the physical and developmental tasks that the mother must accomplish during the postpartal period.

30.6 Explain the factors that influence the development of parent-infant attachment in the nursing assessment of early attachment.

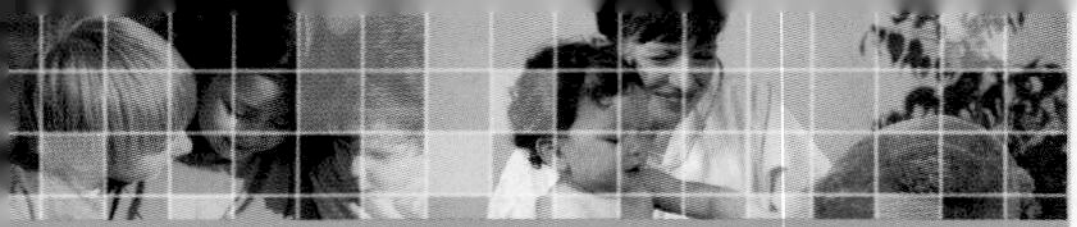

KEY TERMS

Afterpains, 760
Becoming a mother (BAM), 761
Boggy uterus (uterine atony), 755
Diastasis recti abdominis, 757
En face, 762
Engrossment, 763
Fundus, 754
Involution, 754
Lochia, 756
Lochia alba, 756
Lochia rubra, 756
Lochia serosa, 756
Postpartum blues, 761
Puerperium, 754
Reciprocity, 763
Subinvolution, 756

During the **puerperium**, or postpartal period, the woman readjusts, physically and psychologically, from pregnancy and birth. The period begins immediately after birth and continues for approximately 6 weeks, or until the body has returned to a near prepregnant state.

This chapter describes the physiologic and psychologic changes that occur postpartally and the basic aspects of a thorough postpartal assessment.

POSTPARTAL PHYSICAL ADAPTATIONS

Comprehensive nursing assessment is based on a sound understanding of the normal anatomic and physiologic processes of the puerperium. These processes involve the reproductive organs and other major body systems.

REPRODUCTIVE SYSTEM

Involution of the Uterus

The term **involution** is used to describe the rapid reduction in size and the return of the uterus to a nonpregnant state. Following separation of the placenta, the decidua of the uterus is irregular, jagged, and varied in thickness. The spongy layer of the decidua is cast off as lochia, and the basal layer of the decidua remains in the uterus to become differentiated into two layers. This occurs within the first 48 to 72 hours after birth. The outermost layer becomes necrotic and is sloughed off in the lochia. The layer closest to the myometrium contains the fundi of the uterine endometrial glands, and these glands lay the foundation for the new endometrium. Except at the placental site, this process is completed in approximately 3 weeks. Healing at the placenta site occurs gradually over 6 weeks, at which point the site is completely healed (Blackburn, 2007). Bleeding from the larger uterine vessels of the placenta site is controlled by compression of the retracted uterine muscle fibers. The clotted blood is gradually absorbed by the body. Some of these vessels are eventually obliterated and replaced by new vessels with smaller lumens.

The placenta site heals by a process of exfoliation and growth of endometrial tissue. This occurs with upward endometrial growth in the decidua basalis under the placental site, with simultaneous growth of endometrial tissue from the margins of the site. The infarcted superficial tissue then becomes necrotic and is sloughed off (Blackburn, 2007). *Exfoliation* is a very important aspect of involution; if healing of the placenta site leaves a fibrous scar, the area available for future implantation is limited, as is the number of possible pregnancies.

With the dramatic decrease in the levels of circulating estrogen and progesterone following placental separation, the uterine cells atrophy, and the hyperplasia of pregnancy begins to reverse. Proteolytic enzymes are released, and macrophages migrate to the uterus to promote autolysis (self-digestion). Protein material in the uterine wall is broken down and absorbed. Factors that enhance involution include an uncomplicated labor and birth, complete expulsion of the placenta or membranes, breastfeeding, manual removal of the placenta during a cesarean birth, and early ambulation. Factors that slow uterine involution and rationale for each factor are listed in Table 30–1.

Changes in Fundal Position

The **fundus** (top portion of the uterus) is situated in the midline midway between the symphysis pubis and the umbilicus (Figure 30–1 ●). Immediately following the birth of the placenta, the uterus contracts to the size of a large grapefruit. The walls of the contracted uterus are in close proximity, and the uterine blood vessels are firmly compressed by the myometrium. Within 6 to 12 hours after birth, the fundus of the uterus rises to the level of the umbilicus because of blood and clots that remain within the uterus and changes in support of the uterus by the ligaments. A fundus that is above the umbilicus and boggy (feels soft and spongy rather than firm and well contracted)

Table 30–1 Factors That Retard Uterine Involution

Factor	Rationale
Prolonged labor	Muscles relax because of prolonged time of contraction during labor.
Anesthesia	Muscles relax.
Difficult birth	The uterus is manipulated excessively.
Grand multiparity	Repeated distention of uterus during pregnancy and labor leads to muscle stretching, diminished tone, and muscle relaxation.
Full bladder	As the uterus is pushed up and usually to the right, pressure on it interferes with effective uterine contraction.
Incomplete expulsion of placenta or membranes	The presence of even small amounts of tissue interferes with the ability of the uterus to remain firmly contracted.
Infection	Inflammation interferes with the uterine muscle's ability to contract effectively.
Overdistention of uterus	Overstretching of uterine muscles with conditions such as multiple gestation, hydramnios, or a very large baby may set the stage for slower uterine involution.

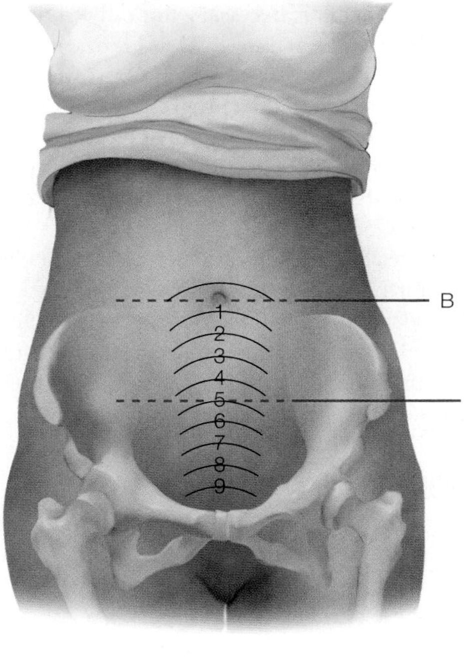

● **Figure 30–1** Involution of the uterus. ***A,*** Immediately after delivery of the placenta, the top of the fundus is in the midline and approximately halfway between the symphysis pubis and the umbilicus. About 6 to 12 hours after birth, the fundus is at the level of the umbilicus. ***B,*** The height of the fundus then decreases about one finger breadth (approximately 1 cm) each day.

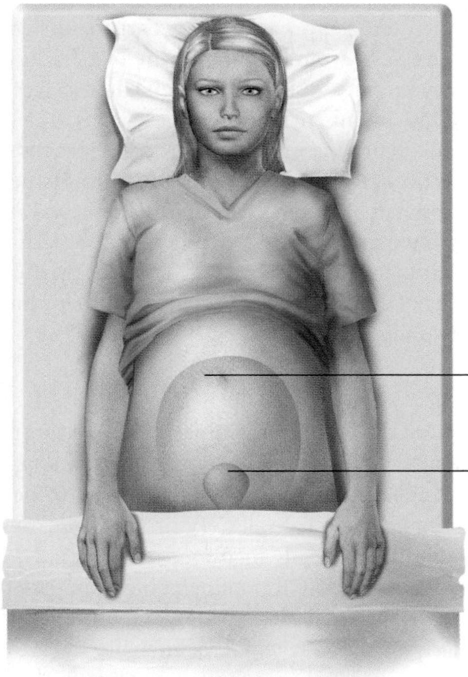

● **Figure 30–2** Displacement and deviation of the uterus. The uterus becomes displaced and deviated to the right when the bladder is full.

is associated with excessive uterine bleeding. As blood collects and forms clots within the uterus, the fundus rises; firm contractions of the uterus are interrupted, causing a **boggy uterus (uterine atony)**. When the fundus is higher than expected on palpation and is not in the midline (usually deviated to the right), distention of the bladder should be suspected; the bladder should be emptied immediately and the uterus remeasured (Figure 30–2 ●). If the woman is unable to void, in-and-out catheterization of the bladder may be required. In the immediate postpartum period many women may not be aware of a full bladder. Because the uterine ligaments are still stretched, a full bladder can move the uterus. By the end of the puerperium these ligaments have regained their nonpregnant length and tension.

Thinking Critically

VARIATION IN FUNDUS STATUS

You have completed your assessment of Patty Clark, a 24-year-old, G2P2 woman who is 24 hours past childbirth. The fundus is just above the umbilicus and slightly to the right. Lochia rubra is present, and a pad is soaked every 2 hours. What would you do?

See MyNursingKit for possible responses.

After birth the top of the fundus remains at the level of the umbilicus for about half a day. On the first postpartum day, the top of the fundus is located about 1 cm below the umbilicus. The top of the fundus descends approximately one finger breadth (width of index, second, or third finger), or 1 cm, per day until it descends into the pelvis on about the 10th day. If the mother is breastfeeding, the release of endogenous oxytocin from the posterior pituitary in response to suckling hastens involution of the uterus. Barring complications, such as infection or retained placental fragments, the uterus approaches its prepregnant size and location by 5 to 6 weeks. In women who had an oversized uterus during the pregnancy (because of hydramnios, birth of a large-for-gestational-age [LGA] infant, or multiple gestation), the time frame for an immediate uterine involution process is lengthened. If intrauterine infection is present, in addition to foul-smelling lochia or vaginal discharge, the uterine fundus descends much more slowly. When infection is suspected, other clinical signs such as fever and tachycardia in addition to delay in involution must be assessed. Any slowing of descent is called **subinvolution** (for further discussion of subinvolution, see Chapter 32).

Lochia

The uterus rids itself of the debris remaining after birth through a discharge called **lochia**, which is classified according to its appearance and contents. **Lochia rubra** is dark red. It occurs for the first 2 to 3 days and contains epithelial cells, erythrocytes, leukocytes, shreds of decidua, and occasionally fetal meconium, lanugo, and vernix. Clotting is often the result of pooling of blood in the upper portion of the vagina. A few small clots (no larger than a nickel) are common, particularly in the first few days after birth. However, lochia should not contain large (plum-size) clots; if it does the cause should be investigated without delay. **Lochia serosa** is a pinkish color. It follows from about day 3 until day 10. Lochia serosa is composed of serous exudate (hence the name), shreds of degenerating decidua, erythrocytes, leukocytes, cervical mucus, and numerous microorganisms (Blackburn, 2007).

The red blood cell (RBC) component decreases gradually, and a creamy or yellowish discharge persists for an additional week or two. This final discharge, termed **lochia alba** from the Latin word for *white*, is composed primarily of leukocytes, decidual cells, epithelial cells, fat, cervical mucus, cholesterol crystals, and bacteria. Recent studies examining lochia patterns have found that the lochia rubra phase lasts longer than generally assumed and that it varies according to breastfeeding practice and parity (Blackburn, 2007). Variation in the duration of lochia discharge is not uncommon; however, the trend should be toward a lighter amount of flow and a lighter color of discharge. When the lochia flow stops, the cervix is considered closed, and chances of infection ascending from the vagina to the uterus decrease.

Like menstrual discharge, lochia flow has a musty, stale odor that is not offensive. Microorganisms are always present in the vaginal lochia, and by the second day following birth the uterus is contaminated with the vaginal bacteria. It is thought that an infection does not develop because the organisms involved are relatively nonvirulent. Any foul smell to the lochia or used peripad suggests infection and the need for prompt additional assessment, such as white blood cell (WBC) count and differential and assessment for uterine tenderness and fever.

The total average volume of lochia is about 225 mL, and the daily volume gradually decreases (Blackburn, 2007). Discharge is greater in the morning because of pooling in the vagina and uterus while the mother lies sleeping. The amount of lochia may also be increased by exertion or breastfeeding. Multiparous women usually have more lochia than first-time mothers. Women who undergo a cesarean birth typically have less lochia than women who give birth vaginally (Blackburn, 2007).

Evaluation of lochia is necessary not only to determine the presence of hemorrhage but also to assess uterine involution. The type, amount, and consistency of lochia determines the stage of healing of the placenta site, and a progressive change from bright red at birth to dark red to pink to white or clear discharge should be observed. Persistent discharge of lochia rubra or a return to lochia rubra indicates subinvolution or late postpartal hemorrhage (see Chapter 32).

The nurse should exercise caution in evaluating bleeding immediately after birth. The continuous seepage of blood is more consistent with cervical or vaginal lacerations and may be effectively diagnosed when the bleeding is evaluated in conjunction with the consistency of the uterus. Lacerations should be suspected if the uterus is firm and of expected size and if no clots can be expressed.

Cervical Changes

Following birth the cervix is flabby, formless, and may appear bruised. The lateral aspects of the external os are frequently lacerated during the birth process (Cunningham, Leveno, Bloom, et al., 2010). The external os is markedly irregular and closes slowly. It admits two fingers for a few days following birth, but by the end of the first week it admits only a fingertip.

The shape of the external os is permanently changed by the first childbearing. The characteristic dimplelike os of the nullipara changes to the transverse slit (fish-mouth) os of the multipara (Blackburn, 2007). After significant cervical laceration or several lacerations, the cervix may appear lopsided. Because of the slight change in the size of the cervix, a diaphragm or cervical cap will need to be refitted if the woman is using one of these methods of contraception.

Vaginal Changes

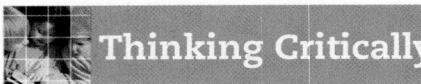

Following birth the vagina appears edematous and may be bruised. Small superficial lacerations may be evident, and the rugae are obliterated. The apparent bruising is caused by pelvic congestion and trauma and will quickly disappear. The hymen, torn and jagged, heals irregularly, leaving small tags called *carunculae myrtiformes.*

The size of the vagina decreases and rugae return within 3 to 4 weeks (Blackburn, 2007). This facilitates the gradual return to smaller, although not nulliparous, dimensions. By 6 weeks the nonbreastfeeding woman's vagina usually appears normal. The lactating woman is in a hypoestrogenic state because of ovarian suppression, and her vaginal mucosa may be pale and without rugae; the effects of the lowered estrogen level may lead to dyspareunia (painful intercourse), which may be reduced by the addition of a water-soluble personal lubricant. Tone and contractility of the vaginal orifice may be improved by perineal tightening exercises such as Kegel exercises (see Chapter 11∞), which may begin soon after birth. The labia majora and labia minora are more flaccid in the woman who has borne a child than in the nullipara.

Perineal Changes

During the early postpartal period the soft tissue in and around the perineum may appear edematous, with some bruising. If an episiotomy or a laceration is present, the edges should be drawn together. Occasionally, ecchymosis occurs, and this may delay healing. Initial healing of the episiotomy or laceration occurs in 2 to 3 weeks after the birth, although complete healing may take up to 4 to 6 months (Blackburn, 2007). Perineal discomfort may be present during this time.

Recurrence of Ovulation and Menstruation

The return of ovulation and menstruation varies for each postpartal woman. In nonbreastfeeding mothers, menstruation generally returns between 4 and 6 weeks after birth. The first postpartum menstrual cycles may be anovulatory, although up to 25% of these cycles are preceded by ovulation (Blackburn, 2007). The return of ovulation is directly associated with a rise in the serum progesterone level. In nonlactating mothers the average time to first ovulation can be as early as 27 days with a mean time of 70 to 75 days (Lipscomb & Novy, 2007).

The return of ovulation and menstruation in breastfeeding mothers is usually prolonged and is associated with the length of time the woman breastfeeds and whether formula supplements are used. If a mother breastfeeds for less than 1 month, the return of menstruation and ovulation is similar to that of the nonbreastfeeding mother. In women who exclusively breastfeed, menstruation is usually delayed for at least 3 months. Suckling by the infant typically results in alterations in the gonadotropin releasing hormone (GnRH) production, which is thought to be the cause of amenorrhea (Blackburn, 2007). Although exclusive breastfeeding helps to reduce the risk of pregnancy for the first 6 months after birth, it should be relied upon only temporarily and if it meets the observed criteria for lactational amenorrhea method (LAM). Furthermore, because ovulation precedes menstruation and women often supplement breastfeeding with bottles and pacifiers, breastfeeding is not considered a reliable means of contraception.

ABDOMEN

The uterine ligaments (notably the round and broad ligaments) are stretched and require the length of the puerperium to recover. Although the stretched abdominal wall appears loose and flabby, it responds to exercise within 2 to 3 months. However, the abdomen may fail to regain good tone and will remain flabby in the grand multipara, in the woman whose abdomen is overdistended, or in the woman with poor muscle tone before pregnancy. **Diastasis recti abdominis**, a separation of the abdominal muscle, may occur with pregnancy, especially in women with poor abdominal muscle tone (Figure 30–3 ●). If diastasis occurs, part of the abdominal wall has no muscular support but is formed only by skin, subcutaneous fat, fascia, and peritoneum. This may be especially pronounced in women who have undergone a cesarean section, as the rectus abdominis muscles are manually separated to access the uterine muscle. Improvement depends on the physical condition of the mother, the total number of pregnancies, pregnancy spacing, and the type and amount of physical exercise. This may result in a pendulous abdomen and increased maternal backache. Fortunately, diastasis responds well to exercise, and abdominal muscle tone can improve significantly.

The striae (stretch marks), which occurred as a result of stretching and rupture of the elastic fibers of the skin, take on different colors based on the mother's skin color. The striae of Caucasian mothers are red to purple at the time of birth and gradually fade to silver or white. The striae of mothers with darker skin, in contrast, are darker than the surrounding skin and remain darker. These marks gradually fade after a time but remain visible.

LACTATION

During pregnancy, breast development in preparation for lactation results from the influence of both estrogen and progesterone. After birth, the interplay of maternal hormones leads to milk production. (For further details, see the section on breastfeeding in Chapter 27∞.)

GASTROINTESTINAL SYSTEM

Hunger following birth is common, and the mother may enjoy eating a light meal. Frequently, she is quite thirsty and will drink large amounts of fluid. Drinking fluids helps replace fluids lost during labor, in the urine, and through perspiration.

The bowels tend to be sluggish following birth because of the lingering effects of progesterone, decreased abdominal muscle tone, and bowel evacuation associated with the labor and birth process. Women who have had an episiotomy, lacerations, or hemorrhoids may tend to delay elimination for fear of increasing their pain or because they believe their stitches will be torn if they bear down. In refusing or delaying the bowel movement, the woman may cause increased constipation and more pain when bowel elimination finally occurs.

The woman with a cesarean birth may receive clear liquids shortly after surgery; once bowel sounds are present, her diet is quickly advanced to solid food. In addition, the woman may experience some initial discomfort from flatulence, which is relieved

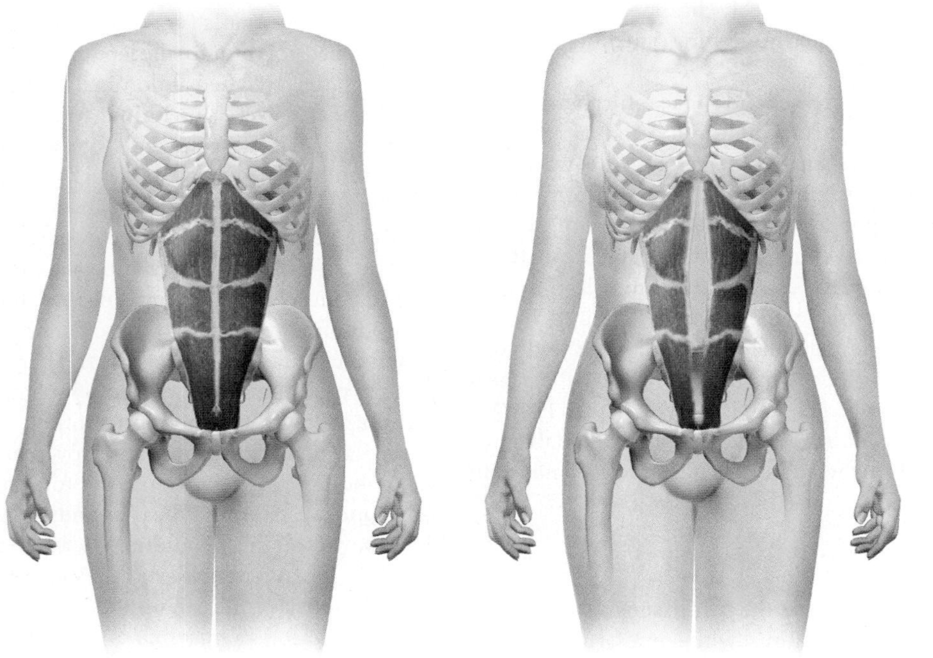

● **Figure 30–3** Diastasis recti abdominis. This condition, which involves a separation of the abdominal musculature, commonly occurs after pregnancy.

by early ambulation and use of antiflatulent medications. Chamomile tea and peppermint tea may also be helpful in reducing discomfort from flatulence. It may take a few days for the bowel to regain its tone, especially if general anesthesia was used. The woman who has had a cesarean or a difficult birth may benefit from stool softeners.

URINARY TRACT

The postpartal woman has an increased bladder capacity, swelling and bruising of the tissue around the urethra, decreased sensitivity to fluid pressure, and a decreased sensation of bladder filling. Consequently, she is at risk for overdistention, incomplete bladder emptying, and a buildup of residual urine. Women who have had an anesthetic block have inhibited neural functioning of the bladder and are more susceptible to bladder distention, difficulty voiding, and bladder infections. In addition, immediate postpartal use of oxytocin to facilitate uterine contractions following expulsion of the placenta has an antidiuretic effect. Following cessation of the oxytocin the woman will experience rapid bladder filling (Cunningham et al., 2010).

Urinary output increases during the early postpartal period (first 12 to 24 hours) because of *puerperal diuresis.* The kidneys must eliminate an estimated 2000 to 3000 mL of extracellular fluid with the normal pregnancy, which causes rapid filling of the bladder. Thus adequate bladder elimination is an immediate concern. Women with preeclampsia, chronic hypertension, and diabetes experience greater fluid retention than other women, and postpartal diuresis is increased accordingly.

If urine stasis exists, chances for urinary tract infection increase because of bacteriuria and the presence of dilated ureters and renal pelves, which persist for about 6 weeks after birth. A full bladder may also increase the tendency of the uterus to relax by displacing the uterus and interfering with its contractility, leading to hemorrhage. In the absence of infection, the dilated ureters and renal pelves return to prepregnant size by the end of the sixth week.

VITAL SIGNS

During the postpartal period, with the exception of the first 24 hours, the woman should be afebrile. Epidural anesthesia for labor, which can interfere with heat dissipation, has a direct effect on maternal temperature but rarely results in overt fever (Alexander, 2005). A maternal temperature of up to 38°C (100.4°F) may occur after childbirth as a result of the exertion and dehydration of labor. An increase in temperature to between 37.8°C and 39°C (100°F to 102.2°F) may also occur during the first 24 hours after the mother's milk comes in (Cunningham et al., 2010). However, in women not meeting these criteria, infection must be considered in the presence of an increased temperature (see discussion in Chapter 32).

Immediately following childbirth, many women experience a transient rise in both systolic and diastolic blood pressure, which spontaneously returns to the prepregnancy baseline over the next few days (James, 2008). A decrease may indicate physiologic readjustment to decreased intrapelvic pressure, or it may be related to uterine hemorrhage. Orthostatic hypotension, as indicated by

Nursing Practice

During the first few hours after birth, the woman may have some orthostatic hypotension; it will cause her to have a lower blood pressure reading in a sitting position. For the most accurate reading, be sure to measure the woman in the same position each time, preferably lying on her back with her arm at her side.

feelings of faintness or dizziness immediately after standing up, can develop in the first 48 hours as a result of abdominal engorgement that may occur after birth. A low or decreasing blood pressure may reflect hypovolemia secondary to hemorrhage, but it is a late sign. Blood pressure elevations may result from excessive use of oxytocin or vasopressor medications. Because preeclampsia can persist into or occur first in the postpartum period, routine evaluation of blood pressure is needed. If a woman complains of headache, hypertension must be ruled out before analgesics are administered.

Puerperal bradycardia with rates of 50 to 70 beats per minute (bpm) commonly occurs during the first 6 to 10 days of the postpartal period. It may be related to decreased cardiac effort, the decreased blood volume following placental separation and contraction of the uterus, and increased stroke volume. A pulse rate greater than 100 bpm may be indicative of hypovolemia, infection, fear, or pain and requires further assessment.

BLOOD VALUES

Blood values should return to the prepregnant state by the end of the postpartal period. Pregnancy-associated activation of coagulation factors may continue for variable amounts of time after birth. This condition, in conjunction with trauma, immobility, or sepsis, predisposes the woman to the development of thromboembolism. The incidence of thromboembolism is reduced by early mobilization.

Nonpathologic leukocytosis often occurs during labor and in the immediate postpartum period, with white blood cell counts of 25,000 to 30,000/mm^3 (James, 2008). WBC values typically return to normal levels by the end of the first postpartum week. Leukocytosis combined with the normal increase in erythrocyte sedimentation rate may obscure the diagnosis of acute infection at this time (James, 2008).

Hemoglobin and hematocrit levels may be difficult to interpret in the first 2 days after birth because of the changing blood volume. This loss in blood in the first 24 hours accounts for half of the RBC volume gained during the course of the pregnancy. Blood loss averages 400 mL with a vaginal birth and nearly 1000 mL with a cesarean birth (Lipscomb & Novy, 2007). Lochia constitutes less than 25% of this blood loss (Varney, et al., 2004). As extracellular fluid is excreted, hemoconcentration occurs, with a concomitant rise in hematocrit. A drop in values indicates an abnormal blood loss. The following is a convenient rule to remember: A two to three percentage point drop in hematocrit equals a blood loss of 500 mL (James, 2008). After 3 to 4 days, mobilization of interstitial fluid leads to a slight increase in plasma volume. This hemodilution leads to a decrease in hemoglobin, hematocrit, and plasma protein by the end of the first postpartum week. Decreases in plasma volume reach nonpregnant levels by 4 to 6 weeks postpartum (Blackburn, 2007).

Platelet levels typically fall as a result of placental separation. They then begin to increase by the third to fourth postpartum day, gradually returning to normal by the sixth postpartum week. Fibrinolytic activity typically returns to normal during the hours following birth. The hemostatic system as a whole reaches its normal prepregnant status by 3 to 4 weeks postpartum; however, the diameter of deep veins can take up to 6 weeks to return to prepregnant levels (Blackburn, 2007). This is why there is a prolonged risk of thromboembolism in the first 6 weeks following birth.

CARDIOVASCULAR CHANGES

The cardiovascular system undergoes dramatic changes during the birth that can result in cardiovascular instability because of an increase in the cardiac output. The cardiac output typically stabilizes and returns to pregnancy levels within an hour following birth. Maternal hypervolemia acts to protect the mother from excessive blood loss. Cardiac output declines by 30% in the first 2 weeks and reaches normal levels by 6 to 12 weeks (Blackburn, 2007). For a more detailed description of cardiovascular changes that occur immediately following birth, consult a perinatal physiology text. Diuresis in the first 2 to 5 days assists to decrease the extracellular fluid and results in a weight loss of 3 kg (James, 2008). Failure to diuresis in the immediate postpartum period can lead to pulmonary edema and subsequent cardiac problems. This is seen more commonly in women with a history of preeclampsia or preexisting cardiac problems (Cunningham et al., 2010; James, 2008).

NEUROLOGIC AND IMMUNOLOGIC CHANGES

Neurologic problems and disorders can predispose women to higher rates of morbidity and mortality during pregnancy and in the postpartum period. Headaches are the most common neurologic symptoms encountered by postpartum women. Headaches may result from fluid shifts in the first week after birth, leakage of cerebrospinal fluid into the extradural space during spinal anesthesia, gestational hypertension, or stress (James, 2008). Migraine headaches, although less frequent during pregnancy, tend to resume in the postpartum period. Women with epilepsy are at a 1% to 2% risk of having a seizure in the immediate postpartum period (Tatum, Liporace, Benbadis, et al., 2004). It is nine times more likely that a woman will have a seizure during labor or in the first 24 hours after birth than it is during the pregnancy (Shehata & Okosun, 2004). Women with epilepsy also have more feeding difficulties, irritability, and lethargy. Women with MS or Guillain-Barré syndrome are more likely to have symptoms in the postpartum period than during pregnancy (Cunningham et al., 2010). Myasthenia gravis is an autoimmune disease that affects the neuromuscular junctions. The exacerbation of symptoms during pregnancy is variable; however, the first month of pregnancy and the first month of the postpartal period is the most critical (Cunningham et al., 2010).

WEIGHT LOSS

An initial weight loss of about 10 to 12 lb occurs as a result of the birth of the infant, placenta, and amniotic fluid. Diuresis accounts for the loss of an additional 5 lb during the early puerperium. By the sixth to eighth week after birth, many women have returned to approximately prepregnant weight if they gained the average 25 to 30 lb. For others, a return to prepregnant weight may take longer. Women often express concern about the slow pace of their postpartum weight loss. Multiparas tend to be more positive than primiparas, probably because the multipara's previous experience has prepared her for the fact that the body does not immediately return to a prepregnant state.

POSTPARTAL CHILL

Frequently the mother experiences intense tremors that resemble shivering from a chill immediately after birth. Several theories have been offered to explain this shivering: It is the result of sudden release of pressure on the pelvic nerves after birth, a response to a fetus-to-mother transfusion that occurred during placental separation, a reaction to maternal adrenaline production during labor and birth, or a reaction to epidural anesthesia. If not followed by fever, this chill is of no clinical concern, but it is uncomfortable for the woman. The nurse can increase the woman's comfort by covering her with a warmed blanket and reassuring her that the shivering is a common, self-limiting situation. If she allows herself to go with the shaking, the shivering will last only a short time. Some women may also find a warm beverage helpful. Later in the puerperium, chill and fever indicate infection and require further evaluation.

POSTPARTAL DIAPHORESIS

The elimination of excess fluid and waste products via the skin during the puerperium produces increased perspiration. Diaphoretic (sweating) episodes frequently occur at night, and the woman may awaken drenched with perspiration. This perspiration is not significant clinically, but the mother should be protected from chilling.

AFTERPAINS

Afterpains are more common in multiparas than in primiparas and are caused by intermittent uterine contractions. Although the uterus of the primipara usually remains consistently contracted, the lost tone of the multiparous uterus results in alternate contraction and relaxation. This phenomenon also occurs if the uterus has been markedly distended, as with a multiple-gestation pregnancy or hydramnios, or if clots or placental fragments were retained. These afterpains may cause the mother severe discomfort for 2 to 3 days after birth. The administration of oxytocic agents (intravenous infusion with Pitocin or oral administration of Methergine) stimulates uterine contraction and increases the discomfort of the afterpains. Because endogenous oxytocin is released when the infant suckles, breastfeeding also increases the frequency and severity of the afterpains. A warm water bottle placed against the low abdomen may reduce the discomfort of afterpains. In addition, the breastfeeding mother may find it helpful to take a mild analgesic agent approximately 1 hour before feeding her infant. The nurse can assure the nursing mother that the prescribed analgesics are not harmful to the newborn and help improve the quality of the breastfeeding experience. An analgesic is also helpful at bedtime if the afterpains interfere with the mother's rest.

POSTPARTAL PSYCHOLOGIC ADAPTATIONS

The postpartal period is a time of readjustment and adaptation for the entire childbearing family, but especially for the mother. The woman experiences a variety of responses as she adjusts to a new family member, postpartal discomforts, changes in her body image, and the reality that she is no longer pregnant.

TAKING-IN AND TAKING-HOLD

Initially after birth during the *"taking-in"* period, the woman tends to be passive and somewhat dependent. She follows suggestions, hesitates to make decisions, and is still rather preoccupied with her needs (Rubin, 1961). She may have a great need to talk about her perceptions of her labor and birth. This helps her work through the process, sort out the reality from her fantasized experience, and clarify anything that she did not understand. Food and sleep are major needs.

After the taking-in period, Rubin (1961) observed that new mothers were ready to resume control of their bodies, mothering, and life in general. Rubin labeled this the *taking-hold* period. If she is breastfeeding, she may worry about her technique or the quality of her milk. If her baby spits up after a feeding, she may view it as a personal failure. She may also feel demoralized by the fact that the nurse or an older family member handles her baby proficiently while she feels unsure and tentative. She requires assurance that she is doing well as a mother. Today's mothers seem to be more independent and adjust more rapidly, exhibiting behaviors of "taking-in" and "taking-hold" in shorter time periods.

BECOMING A MOTHER (BAM)

Maternal role attainment is the process by which a woman learns mothering behaviors and becomes comfortable with her identity as a mother. As the mother grows to know her child and forms a relationship, the mother's maternal identity gradually and systematically evolves and she "binds in" to the infant (Rubin, 1984). Formation of a maternal identity occurs with each child a woman bears.

Maternal role attainment often occurs in four stages (Mercer, 1995):

1. The *anticipatory stage* occurs during pregnancy. The woman looks to role models, especially her own mother, for examples of how to mother.
2. The *formal stage* begins when the child is born. The woman is still influenced by the guidance of others and tries to act as she believes others expect her to act.
3. The *informal stage* begins when the mother begins to make her own choices about mothering. The woman begins to

develop her own style of mothering and finds ways of functioning that work well for her.

4. The *personal stage* is the final stage of maternal role attainment. When the woman reaches this stage, she is comfortable with the notion of herself as "mother."

In most cases, maternal role attainment occurs within 3 to 10 months after birth. Social support, the woman's age and personality traits, the marital relationship, the presence of underlying anxiety or depression, the woman's previous childcare skills, the temperament of her infant, and the family's socioeconomic status all influence the woman's success in attaining the maternal role. The postpartum woman faces a number of challenges as she adjusts to her new role (Mercer, 1995):

- For many women, finding time for themselves is one of the greatest challenges. It is often difficult for the new mother to find time to read a book, talk to her partner, or even eat a meal without interruption.
- Women also report feelings of incompetence because they have not mastered all aspects of the mothering role. Often they are unsure of what to do in a given situation.
- The next greatest challenge involves fatigue resulting from sleep deprivation. The demands of nighttime care are tremendously draining, especially if the woman has other children.
- Another challenge faced by the new mother involves the feeling of responsibility that having a child brings. Women experience a sense of lost freedom, an awareness that they will never again be quite as carefree as they were before becoming mothers.
- For women with older children, finding time for them is a challenge. Many women feel guilty because the new baby takes up so much of their time. Sibling rivalry or ill feelings about the baby from other children can put additional stress on the mother.
- Mothers sometimes cite the infant's behavior as a challenge, especially when the child is about 8 months old. Stranger anxiety develops, the infant begins crawling and getting into things, teething may cause fussiness, and the baby's tendency to put everything in his or her mouth requires constant vigilance by the parent.

In 2004, Mercer proposed replacing the term *maternal role attainment* (MRA) with the term **becoming a mother (BAM)**. She stated that BAM "more accurately encompasses the dynamic transformation and evolution of a woman's persona than does MRA, and the term MRA should be discontinued" (p. 226) (Mercer, 2004). BAM more accurately reflects the transition process of becoming a mother that changes throughout the maternal-child relationship. Postpartal nurses need to be aware of the long-term adjustments and stresses that the childbearing family faces as its members adjust to new and different roles. They can help by providing anticipatory guidance about the realities of being a parent, and by giving the postpartal family parenting literature for reference at home. Nursing interventions that foster the process of becoming a mother include the following categories: instructions for infant care giving, building awareness of and responsiveness to infant interactive capabilities, promoting maternal-infant attachment, maternal/social role preparation, and interactive therapeutic nurse-client relationships (Mercer & Walker, 2006). Interactive therapeutic nurse-client relationships and maternal/social role preparation have a greater impact on the progress of becoming a mother than formal teaching. Instructions without nurse input were ineffective. Ongoing parenting groups give parents an opportunity to discuss problems and become comfortable in new roles.

POSTPARTUM BLUES

The **postpartum blues** consist of a transient period of depression that occurs during the first few days of the puerperium in 70% of all postpartal women (Varney et al., 2004). It may be manifested by mood swings, anger, weepiness, anorexia, difficulty sleeping, and a feeling of letdown. This mood change frequently occurs while the woman is still hospitalized, but it may occur at home as well. Changing hormone levels are certainly a factor; psychologic adjustments, an unsupportive environment, and insecurity also have been identified as potential causes. In addition, fatigue, discomfort, and overstimulation may play a role. The postpartum blues usually resolve naturally within 10 to 14 days, but if they persist or symptoms worsen, the woman may need evaluation for postpartum depression (see Chapter 32∞). Ideally a depression assessment should be completed each trimester to update a pregnant woman's risk status (Beck, 2002). If not done previously, the nurse assesses the woman for predisposing factors during labor and the postpartum stay. Several depression scales are available for assessing postpartum depression. The routine use of a screening tool such as the Edinburgh Postnatal Depression Scale or Postpartum Depression Predictors Inventory-Revised in a matter-of-fact approach significantly increases the diagnosis (Beck, 2008).

IMPORTANCE OF SOCIAL SUPPORT

The psychologic outcomes of the postpartal period are far more positive when the parents have access to a support network. Women and their partners may find that family relationships become increasingly important. The attention that their infant receives from family members is a source of satisfaction to the new parents. In many cases, the ties to the woman's family become especially good. Fathers may report that their relationships with their in-laws become far more positive and supportive. However, the increased family interaction can be a source of stress, especially for the new mother, who tends to have more contact with the families.

The new parents may also have increasing contact with other parents of small children although contact with coworkers declines.

Of great concern are women and their partners who have no family or friends with whom to form a social network. Isolation at a time when the woman feels an increased need for support can result in tremendous stress and is often a contributing factor in situations of postpartum depression, child neglect, or abuse.

MyNursingKit Case Study: Mother–Infant Bonding

Developing Cultural Competence

MIDDLE EAST INITIAL POSTPARTUM EXPERIENCE

In many countries in the Middle East that follow a patriarchal system, the new mother and her infant stay with the husband's family following the birth of the infant. Frequent visits from the woman's family are discouraged and may even be viewed as burdensome by the husband's family. Typically, only women visit the new mother during the postpartum period. For the birth of the first baby, the wife's parents are expected to purchase all of the baby's supplies and clothing.

New mother support groups are helpful for women who lack a social support system.

Postpartum doulas are professionals trained to help the new mother after the birth of the baby. As a "mother helper," postpartum doula services are tailored to help the new mother feel as rested as possible and well-nourished, and to place her household in good order so that she can focus her energy on her new baby.

DEVELOPMENT OF FAMILY ATTACHMENT

A mother's first interaction with her infant is influenced by many factors, including her involvement with her family of origin, her relationships, the stability of her home environment, the communication patterns she developed, and the degree of nurturing she received as a child. These factors have shaped the person she has become. The following personal characteristics are also important.

- *Level of trust.* What level of trust has this mother developed in response to her life experiences? What is her philosophy of childrearing? Will she be able to treat her infant as a unique individual with changing needs that should be met as much as possible?
- *Level of self-esteem.* How much does she value herself as a woman and as a mother? Does she feel generally able to cope with the adjustments of life?
- *Capacity for enjoying herself.* Is the mother able to find pleasure in everyday activities and human relationships?
- *Adequacy of knowledge about childbearing and childrearing.* What beliefs about the course of pregnancy, the capabilities of newborns, previous experiences with infants/children, and the nature of her emotions may influence her behavior at first contact with her infant and later?
- *Prevailing mood or usual feeling tone.* Is the woman predominantly content, angry, depressed, or anxious? Is she sensitive to her own feelings and those of others? Will she be able to accept her own needs and to obtain support in meeting them?
- *Reactions to the present pregnancy.* Was the pregnancy planned? Did it go smoothly? Were there ongoing life events that enhanced her pregnancy or depleted her reserves of energy? How have other life roles changed because of her pregnancy and motherhood?

By the time of birth each mother has developed an emotional orientation of some kind to the baby based on these factors.

INITIAL MATERNAL ATTACHMENT BEHAVIOR

After labor and birth, a new mother will demonstrate a fairly regular pattern of maternal behaviors as she continues to familiarize herself with her newborn. In a progression of touching activities, the mother proceeds from fingertip exploration of the newborn's extremities toward palmar contact with larger body areas and finally to enfolding the infant with the whole hand and arm. The time taken to accomplish these steps varies from minutes to days. The mother increases the proportion of time spent in the ***en face*** position (Figure 30–4 ●). She arranges herself or the newborn so that she has direct face-to-face and eye-to-eye contact. There is an intense interest in having the infant's eyes open. When the infant's eyes are open, the mother characteristically greets the newborn and talks in high-pitched tones to him or her.

In most instances the mother relies heavily on her senses of sight, touch, and hearing in getting to know what her baby is really like. She tends also to respond verbally to any sounds emitted by the newborn, such as cries, coughs, sneezes, and grunts. The sense of smell may be involved as well.

While interacting with her newborn, the mother may be experiencing shock, disbelief, or denial. She may state, "I can't believe she's finally here" or "I feel like he is a stranger." On the other hand, feelings of connectedness between the newborn and the rest of the family can be expressed in positive or negative terms: "She's got your cute nose, Daddy" or "Oh, no! He looks just like Matthew, and he was an impossible baby." A mother's facial expressions or the frequency and content of her questions may demonstrate concerns about the infant's general condition or normality, especially if her pregnancy was complicated or if a previous baby was not healthy.

During the first few days after her child's birth, the new mother applies herself to the task of getting to know her baby.

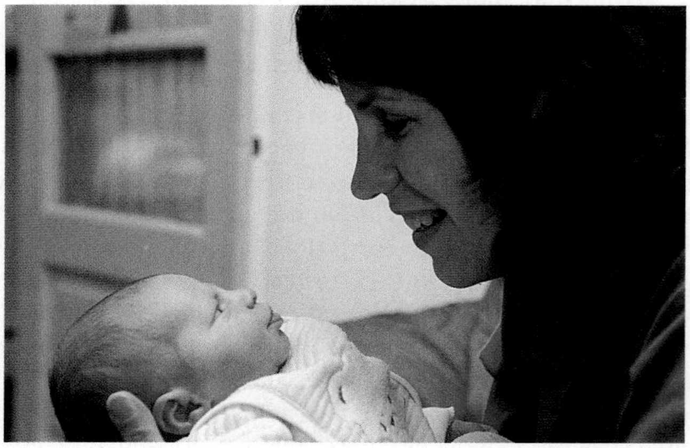

● **Figure 30–4** *En face* position. The mother has direct face-to-face and eye-to-eye contact in the *en face* position.

Source: © Stella Johnson (www.stellajohnson.com).

Nursing Practice

Newborns are sometimes taken from their parents immediately after birth and placed in a special care or intensive care nursery. This separation can interfere with the normal attachment process. If this occurs, parents should be brought to the nursery as soon as possible to interact with their infants, and should be allowed to hold and care for their infant as much as possible. If the infant is in an incubator and cannot be held, encourage the parents to stroke the infant's hand, foot, or cheek. Provide reassurance that this will not hurt the infant and is in fact beneficial.

This is termed the *acquaintance phase.* If the infant gives clear behavioral cues about needs, the infant's responses to mothering will be predictable, which will make the mother feel effective and competent. Other behaviors that make an infant more attractive to caretakers are smiling, grasping a finger, nursing eagerly, and being easy to console.

During this time the newborn is also becoming acquainted. Within a few days after birth, infants show signs of recognizing recurrent situations and responding to changes in routine. To the extent that their mother is their world, it can be said that they are actively acquainting themselves with her.

During the *phase of mutual regulation,* mother and infant seek to determine the degree of control each partner in their relationship will exert. In this phase of adjustment, a balance is sought between the needs of the mother and the needs of the infant. The most important consideration is that each should obtain a good measure of enjoyment from the interaction. During this phase, negative maternal feelings are likely to surface or intensify. Because "everyone knows that mothers love their babies," these negative feelings often go unexpressed and are allowed to build up. If they are expressed, the response of friends, relatives, or healthcare personnel is often to deny the feelings to the mother: "You don't mean that." Some negative feelings are normal in the first few days after birth, and the nurse should be supportive when the mother vocalizes these feelings.

When mutual regulation arrives at the point where both mother and infant primarily enjoy each other's company, reciprocity has been achieved. **Reciprocity** is an interactional cycle that occurs simultaneously between mother and infant. It involves mutual cuing behaviors, expectancy, rhythmicity, and synchrony. The mother develops a new relationship with an individual who has a unique character and evokes a response entirely different from the fantasy response of pregnancy. When reciprocity is synchronous, the interaction between mother and infant is mutually gratifying and is sought and initiated by both partners.

Father-Infant Interactions

In Western cultures, commitment to family-centered maternity care has fostered interest in understanding the feelings and experiences of the new father. Evidence suggests that the father has a strong attraction to his newborn and that the feelings he experiences are similar to the mother's feelings of attachment

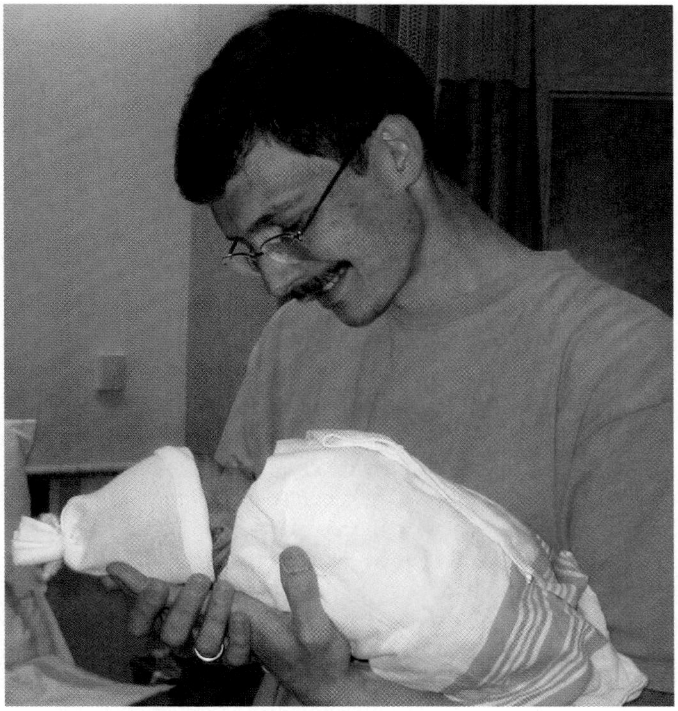

● **Figure 30–5** Engrossment. The father experiences strong feelings of attraction during engrossment.

(Figure 30–5 ●). The characteristic sense of absorption, preoccupation, and interest in the infant demonstrated by fathers during early contact is termed **engrossment**. Differences in involvement still exist among fathers in Western culture and may be influenced by factors other than culture (e.g., previous experience with paternal role or exposure to male/father role models).

Siblings and Others

Infants are capable of maintaining a number of strong attachments without loss of quality. These attachments may include siblings, grandparents, aunts, and uncles. The social setting and personality of the individual seem to be significant factors in the development of multiple attachments. Birth centers are especially geared toward the inclusion of the family in the birth process. In the hospital setting, the advent of open visiting hours and rooming-in permits siblings and others to participate in the attachment process.

Developing Cultural Competence

MUSLIM PATERNAL ATTACHMENT

In some cultures, there may be little involvement of the father in newborn care. In the Muslim culture, for example, emphasis on childrearing and infant care activities is on the mother and extended female family members. Nurses need to be aware of cultural differences when evaluating a father's interaction with his newborn.

CULTURAL INFLUENCES IN THE POSTPARTAL PERIOD

Whereas Western culture places primary emphasis on the events of birth, many other cultures place greater emphasis on the postpartum period. For women not of the dominant American culture, the new mother's culture and personal values influence her beliefs about her postpartal care. Her expectations about food, fluids, rest, hygiene, medications and relief measures, support, and counsel—as well as other aspects of her life—will be influenced by the beliefs and values of her family and cultural group. Sometimes, a new mother's wishes will differ from the expectations of the certified nurse-midwife (CNM), physician, or nurse. (See Chapter 2 for an in-depth discussion.)

All nurses belong to their particular ethnoculture and also share in the culture of health care. Thus their nursing care may include practices that support the general beliefs of these groups, such as offering food and fluids in the recovery period after birth, expecting the woman to ambulate as soon as possible, and assuming the woman will want to shower and perhaps wash her hair soon after giving birth. It is important for nurses to recognize that they are approaching their client's care from their own perspective and that, to individualize care for each mother, they need to assess the woman's preferences, her level of acculturation and assimilation to Western culture, her linguistic abilities, and her educational level (Lauderdale, 2008). In addition, the nurse should have the mother exercise her choices when possible, and support those choices, with the help of cultural awareness and a sound knowledge base.

Although describing particular practices of differing cultural groups always involves some generalization, it is helpful for nurses to understand some of the possible differences in beliefs and practices. The woman of European heritage may expect to eat a full meal and have large amounts of iced fluids after the birth, in the belief that the food restores energy and the fluids help replace fluid lost during the labor. She may want to ambulate shortly after the birth, shower, wash her hair, and put on a fresh gown. She may expect a short stay in the hospital and may or may not be interested in educational classes. Women of the Islamic faith may have specific modesty requirements; the woman must be completely covered, with only her feet and hands exposed, and no man, other than the husband or a family member, may be alone with her (Al-Oballi Kridli, 2002; Lauderdale, 2008).

MyNursingKit Video: Postpartum Assessment

Some cultures emphasize certain postpartal routines or rituals for mother and baby that are designed to restore the hot-cold balance of the body. Some women of Hispanic, African, and Asian cultures may avoid cold after birth. This prohibition includes cold air, wind, and all water (even if heated). On the other hand, some women of traditional Mexican descent may avoid eating "hot" foods such as pork just after the birth of a baby (considered a "hot" experience). It is important to note that each individual or cultural group may define hot and cold conditions and foods differently. The nurse should ask each woman what she can eat and what foods she thinks would be helpful for healing. The nurse may encourage family members to bring preferred foods and drinks for the mother. For more detailed discussion of the hot-cold balance concept see "Cultural Influences Affecting the Family" in Chapter 2.

In many cultures, the extended family plays an essential role during the puerperium. The grandmother is often the primary helper to the mother and newborn. She brings wisdom and experience, allowing the new mother time to rest and giving her ready access to someone who can help with problems and concerns as they arise. It is important to ensure access of all family members to the mother and newborn. Visiting hours may be waived to allow family members or authority figures access to the mother and newborn. These practices show respect and foster a blending of old and new behaviors to meet the goals of all concerned (Purnell & Paulanka, 2008). African American mothers model their mothering skills after their older female relatives. In addition, these same older female relatives usually provide child care as needed (Purnell & Paulanka, 2008). People of Jewish faith observe a Sabbath from sundown Friday to sundown Saturday. During this time, Orthodox Jews do not perform any manual labor; for the postpartal woman, this includes turning on or off the lights, pressing the call bell, or raising/lowering the head of the bed (Zauderer, 2009). If the mother is to be discharged on Saturday, she will not be able to leave the birthing unit until the Sabbath is over (Zauderer, 2009). Jewish clients may also request a kosher diet. Some traditional Jewish couples avoid physical contact while the woman is experiencing any vaginal discharge; unfortunately, the man following this custom may be viewed as unsupportive by the staff during the postpartal period (D'Avanzo & Geissler, 2008).

POSTPARTAL NURSING ASSESSMENT

Comprehensive care is based on a thorough assessment that identifies individual needs or potential problems. See the accompanying "Assessment Guide: Postpartal—First 24 Hours After Birth."

RISK FACTORS

Ongoing assessment and client education during the puerperium is designed to meet the needs of the childbearing family and to detect and treat possible complications. Table 30–2 identifies factors that may place the new mother at risk during the postpartal period. The nurse uses this knowledge during the assessment and is particularly alert for possible complications associated with identified risk factors.

PHYSICAL ASSESSMENT

The nurse should remember the following principles in preparing for and completing the assessment of the postpartal woman.

- Select a time that will provide the most accurate data. Palpating the fundus when the woman has a full bladder, for example, may give false information about the progress of involution. Ask the woman to void before assessment.
- Explain the purpose of regular assessment.
  - Ensure that the woman is relaxed before starting; perform the procedures as gently as possible to avoid unnecessary discomfort.

Table 30–2 Postpartal High-Risk Factors

Factor	Maternal Implication
Preeclampsia	↑ Blood pressure ↑ CNS irritability ↑ Need for bed rest → ↑ risk thrombophlebitis
Diabetes	Need for insulin regulation Episodes of hypoglycemia or hyperglycemia ↓ Healing
Cardiac disease	↑ Maternal exhaustion
Cesarean birth	↑ Healing needs ↑ Pain from incision ↑ Risk of infection ↑ Length of hospitalization
Overdistention of uterus (multiple gestation, hydramnios)	↑ Risk of hemorrhage ↑ Risk of thrombophlebitis (C/S risk) ↑ Risk of anemia ↑ Risk of breastfeeding problems (C/S risk) ↑ Stretching of abdominal muscles ↑ Incidence and severity of afterpains
Abruptio placentae, placenta previa	Hemorrhage → anemia ↓ Uterine contractility after birth → ↑ infection risk
Precipitous labor (less than 3 hours)	↑ Risk of lacerations to birth canal → hemorrhage
Prolonged labor (greater than 24 hours)	Exhaustion ↑ Risk of hemorrhage Nutritional and fluid depletion ↑ Bladder atony and/or trauma
Difficult birth	Exhaustion ↑ Risk of perineal lacerations ↑ Risk of hematomas ↑ Risk of hemorrhage → anemia
Extended period of time in stirrups at birth	↑ Risk of thrombophlebitis
Retained placenta	↑ Risk of hemorrhage ↑ Risk of infection

Table 30–3 Common Postpartal Concerns

Several postpartal occurrences cause special concern for mothers. The nurse will frequently be asked about the following events.

Source of Concern	Explanation
Gush of blood that sometimes occurs when she first arises	Because of normal pooling of blood in the vagina when the woman lies down to rest or sleep. Gravity causes blood to flow out when she stands.
Passing clots	Blood pools at the top of the vagina and forms clots that are passed upon rising or sitting on the toilet.
Night sweats	Normal physiologic occurrence that results as the body attempts to eliminate excess fluids that were present during pregnancy. May be aggravated by a plastic mattress pad.
Afterpains	More common in multiparas. Caused by contractions and relaxation of uterus. Increased by oxytocin, breastfeeding. Relieved with mild analgesics and time.
"Large stomach" after birth and failure to lose all weight gained during pregnancy	The baby, amniotic fluid, and placenta account for only a portion of the weight gained during pregnancy. The remainder takes approximately 6 weeks to lose. Abdomen also appears large because of decreased muscle tone. Postpartal exercises will help.

- Record and report the results as clearly as possible.
- Take appropriate precautions to prevent exposure to body fluids.

While performing the physical assessment, the nurse should also be teaching the woman. For example, when assessing the breasts of a lactating woman, the nurse can discuss breast care, breast milk production, the letdown reflex, and breast self-examination. A new mother may be very receptive to instruction on postpartal abdominal tightening exercises when the nurse assesses the woman's fundal height and diastasis. The assessment also provides an excellent time to provide information about the body's postpartal physical and anatomic changes as well as danger signs to report (Table 30–3). Because the time new mothers spend in the postpartum unit is limited, nurses need to use every available opportunity for client education about self-care. To assist nurses in recognizing these opportunities, examples of client teaching during the assessment are provided throughout the following discussion.

Vital Signs

The nurse may choose to organize the physical assessment in a variety of ways. Many nurses begin by assessing vital signs because the findings are more accurate when they are obtained with the woman at rest. In addition, establishing whether the vital signs are within the expected normal range will assist the nurse in determining if other assessments are needed. For instance, if the temperature is elevated, the nurse considers the time since birth and gathers information to determine whether the woman is dehydrated or whether an infection is developing.

Temperature elevations (less than 38°C [100.4°F]) caused by normal processes should last for only 24 hours. The nurse evaluates any elevation of temperature in light of associated signs and symptoms and carefully reviews the woman's history to identify other factors, such as premature rupture of membranes (PROM) or prolonged labor that might increase the incidence of infection in the genital tract.

(continued on page 768)

Assessment Guide

POSTPARTAL—FIRST 24 HOURS AFTER BIRTH

PHYSICAL ASSESSMENT/ NORMAL FINDINGS	ALTERATIONS AND POSSIBLE CAUSES*	NURSING RESPONSES TO DATA†
Vital Signs		
Blood pressure (BP): Should remain consistent with baseline BP during pregnancy.	High BP (preeclampsia, essential hypertension, renal disease, anxiety).	Evaluate history of preexisting disorders and check for other signs of preeclampsia (edema, proteinuria).
	Drop in BP (may be normal; uterine hemorrhage).	Assess for other signs of hemorrhage (↑ pulse, cool clammy skin).
Pulse: 50 to 90 beats/minute. May be bradycardia of 50 to 70 beats/minute.	Tachycardia (difficult labor and birth, hemorrhage).	Evaluate for other signs of hemorrhage (↓ BP, cool clammy skin).
Respirations: 16 to 24/minute.	Marked tachypnea (respiratory disease).	Assess for other signs of respiratory disease.
Temperature: 36.6°C to 38°C (98°F to 100.4°F).	After first 24 hours temperature of 38°C (100.4°F) or above suggests infection.	Assess for other signs of infection; notify physician/certified nurse-midwife.
Breasts		
General appearance: Smooth, even pigmentation, changes of pregnancy still apparent; one may appear larger.	Reddened area (mastitis).	Assess further for signs of infection.
Palpation: Depending on postpartal day, may be soft, filling, full, or engorged.	Palpable mass (caked breast, mastitis). Engorgement (venous stasis). Tenderness, heat, edema (engorgement, caked breast, mastitis).	Assess for other signs of infection: If blocked duct, consider heat, massage, position change for breastfeeding. Assess for further signs. Report mastitis to physician/certified nurse-midwife.
Nipples: Supple, pigmented, intact; become erect when stimulated.	Fissures, cracks, soreness (problems with breastfeeding), not erectile with stimulation (inverted nipples).	Reassess technique; recommend appropriate interventions.
Lungs		
Sounds: clear to bases bilaterally.	Diminished (fluid overload, asthma, pulmonary embolus, pulmonary edema).	Assess for other signs of respiratory distress.
Abdomen		
Musculature: Abdomen may be soft, have a "doughy" texture; rectus muscle intact.	Separation in musculature (diastasis recti abdominis).	Evaluate size of diastasis; teach appropriate exercises for decreasing the separation.
Fundus: Firm, midline; following expected process of involution.	Boggy (full bladder, uterine bleeding).	Massage until firm; assess bladder and have woman void if needed; attempt to express clots when firm. If bogginess remains or recurs, report to physician/certified nurse-midwife.
May be tender when palpated.	Constant tenderness (infection).	Assess for evidence of endometritis.
Cesarean section incision dressing; dry and intact.	Moderate to large amount of blood or serosanguineous drainage on dressing.	Assess for hemorrhage. Reinforce dressing and notify healthcare provider.
Lochia		
Scant to moderate amount, earthy odor; no clots.	Large amount, clots (hemorrhage).	Assess for firmness, express additional clots; begin peripad count.
	Foul-smelling lochia (infection).	Assess for other signs of infection; report to physician/certified nurse-midwife.
Normal progression: First 1 to 3 days: rubra.	Failure to progress normally or return to rubra from serosa (subinvolution).	Report to physician/certified nurse-midwife.
Following rubra: Days 3 to 10: serosa (alba seldom seen in hospital).		

Assessment Guide—continued

PHYSICAL ASSESSMENT/ NORMAL FINDINGS	ALTERATIONS AND POSSIBLE CAUSES*	NURSING RESPONSES TO DATA[†]
Perineum		
Slight edema and bruising in intact perineum.	Marked fullness, bruising, pain (vulvar hematoma).	Assess size; apply ice glove or ice pack; report to physician/certified nurse-midwife.
Episiotomy: No redness, edema, ecchymosis, or discharge; edges well approximated.	Redness, edema, ecchymosis, discharge, or gaping stitches (infection).	Encourage sitz baths; review perineal care, appropriate wiping techniques.
Hemorrhoids: None present; if present, should be small and nontender.	Full, tender, inflamed hemorrhoids.	Encourage sitz baths, side-lying position; Tucks pads, anesthetic ointments, manual replacement of hemorrhoids, stool softeners, increased fluid intake.
Costovertebral Angle (CVA) Tenderness		
None.	Present (kidney infection).	Assess for other symptoms of urinary tract infection (UTI); obtain clean-catch urine; report to physician/certified nurse-midwife.
Lower Extremities		
No pain with palpation; negative Homans' sign.	Positive findings (thrombophlebitis).	Report to physician/certified nurse-midwife.
Elimination		
Urinary output: Voiding in sufficient quantities at least every 4 to 6 hours; bladder not palpable.	Inability to void (urinary retention). Symptoms of urgency, frequency, dysuria (UTI).	Employ nursing interventions to promote voiding; if not successful, obtain order for catheterization. Report symptoms of UTI to physician/certified nurse-midwife.
Bowel elimination: Should have normal bowel movement by second or third day after birth.	Inability to pass feces (constipation caused by fear of pain from episiotomy, hemorrhoids, perineal trauma).	Encourage fluids, ambulation, roughage in diet; sitz baths to promote healing of perineum; obtain order for stool softener.

CULTURAL ASSESSMENT[‡]	VARIATIONS TO CONSIDER	NURSING RESPONSES TO DATA[†]
Determine customs and practices regarding postpartum care. Ask the mother whether she would like fluids, and ask what temperature she prefers.	Individual preference may include: Room-temperature or warmed fluids rather than iced drinks.	Provide for specific request if possible. If woman is unable to provide specific information, the nurse may draw from general information regarding cultural variation.
Ask the mother what foods or fluids she would like.	Special foods or fluids to hasten healing after childbirth.	Mexican women may want food and fluids that restore hot-cold balance to the body. Women of European background may ask for iced fluids.
Ask the mother whether she would prefer to be alone during breastfeeding.	Some women may be hesitant to have someone with them when their breast is exposed.	Provide privacy as desired by mother.

(continued)

Assessment Guide—continued

PSYCHOSOCIAL ASSESSMENT/ NORMAL FINDINGS	VARIATIONS TO CONSIDER*	NURSING RESPONSES TO DATA†
Psychologic Adaptation		
During first 24 hours: Passive; preoccupied with own needs; may talk about her labor and birth experience; may be talkative, elated, or very quiet.	Very quiet and passive; sleeps frequently (fatigue from long labor; feelings of disappointment about some aspect of the experience; may be following cultural expectation).	Provide opportunities for adequate rest; provide nutritious meals and snacks that are consistent with what the woman desires to eat and drink; provide opportunities to discuss birth experience in nonjudgmental atmosphere if the woman desires to do so.
Usually by 12 hours: Beginning to assume responsibility; some women eager to learn; easily feels overwhelmed.	Excessive weepiness, mood swings, pronounced irritability (postpartum blues; feelings of inadequacy; culturally proscribed behavior).	Explain postpartum blues; provide supportive atmosphere; determine support available for mother; consider referral for evidence of profound depression.
Attachment		
En face position; holds baby close; cuddles and soothes; calls by name; identifies characteristics of family members in infant; may be awkward in providing care.	Continued expressions of disappointment in sex, appearance of infant; refusal to care for infant; derogatory comments; lack of bonding behaviors (difficulty in attachment, following expectations of cultural/ethnic group).	Provide reinforcement and support for infant caretaking behaviors; maintain nonjudgmental approach and gather more information if caretaking behaviors are not evident.
Initially may express disappointment over sex or appearance of infant but within 1 to 2 days demonstrates attachment behaviors.		
Client Education		
Has basic understanding of self-care activities and infant care needs; can identify signs of complications that should be reported.	Unable to demonstrate basic self-care and infant care activities (knowledge deficit; postpartum blues; following prescribed cultural behavior and will be cared for by grandmother or other family member).	Identify predominate learning style. Determine whether woman understands English and provide interpreter if needed; provide reinforcement of information through conversation and through written material (remember that some women and their families may not be able to understand written materials because of language difficulties or inability to read); provide information regarding infant care skills that are culturally consistent; give woman opportunity to express her feelings; consider social service home referral for women who have no family or other support, are unable to take in information about self-care and infant care, and demonstrate no caretaking activities.

*Possible causes of alterations are identified in parentheses.
†This column provides guidelines for further assessment and initial nursing actions.
‡ These are only a few suggestions. It is not our intent to imply this is a comprehensive cultural assessment.

Alterations in vital signs may indicate complications, so the nurse assesses them at regular intervals. After an immediate, transient rise after birth, the blood pressure should remain stable. The pulse often shows a characteristic slowness that is no cause for alarm. Pulse rates return to prepregnant norms very quickly unless complications arise.

The nurse informs the woman of her vital signs and provides information about the normal changes in blood pressure and pulse. This may be an opportunity to determine whether the mother knows how to assess her own and her infant's temperature, how to read a thermometer, and how to select a thermometer from the wide variety now available.

Nursing Practice

An easy way to remember the components specific to the postpartal examination is to remember the term BUBBLEHE: B-breast, U-uterus, B-bladder, B-bowel, L-lochia, E-episiotomy/laceration/edema, H-Homans'/hemorrhoids, E-emotional.

Auscultation of Lungs

The breath sounds should be clear. Women who have been treated for preterm labor or preeclampsia are at higher risk for pulmonary edema (see "Care of the Woman with a Hypertensive Disorder" in Chapter 16∞ for further discussion).

Breasts

Before examining the breasts, the nurse dons gloves and then assesses the fit and support provided by the woman's bra and, if appropriate, offers information about how to select a supportive bra. A properly fitting bra supports the breasts and helps maintain breast shape by limiting stretching of supporting ligaments and connective tissue. If the mother is breastfeeding, the straps of the bra should be cloth, not elastic (because cloth has less stretch and provides more support), and easily adjustable. The back should be wide and have at least three rows of hooks to adjust for fit. Traditional nursing bras have a fixed inner cup and a separate half cup that can be unhooked for breastfeeding while the cup continues to support the breast. Purchasing a nursing bra one size larger than the prepregnant size will usually result in a good fit because the breasts increase in size with milk production.

The nurse can then ask the woman to remove her bra so the breasts can be examined. The nurse notes the size and shape of the breasts and any abnormalities, reddened or hot areas, or engorgement. The breasts are also lightly palpated for softness, slight firmness associated with filling, firmness associated with engorgement, warmth, and tenderness. The nipples are assessed for fissures, cracks, soreness, and inversion. The nurse teaches the woman the characteristics of the breast and explains how to recognize problems such as fissures and cracks in the nipples.

The nonbreastfeeding mother is assessed for evidence of breast discomfort, and relief measures are instituted if necessary. (See discussion of lactation suppression in the nonbreastfeeding mother in Chapter 31∞.) Breast assessment findings for a nonbreastfeeding woman may be recorded as follows: "Breasts soft, filling, no evidence of nipple tenderness or cracking, nipples everted."

Abdomen and Fundus

Before examination of the abdomen, the woman should void. This practice ensures that a full bladder is not displacing the uterus or causing any uterine atony; if atony is present, other causes (such as uterine relaxation associated with a regional block, overstretched uterus, or distended bladder) must be investigated.

The nurse determines the relationship of the fundus to the umbilicus and also assesses the firmness of the fundus. The top of the fundus is measured in finger breadths above, below, or at the umbilicus (Figure 30–6 ●). See Clinical Skills Manual: "Assessing the Status of the Uterine Fundus After Birth" SKILLS. The nurse notes whether the fundus is in the midline or displaced to either side of the abdomen. If not midline, the uterus position should be located. The most common cause of displacement is a full bladder; this finding requires further assessment. If the fundus is in midline but higher than expected, it is usually associated with clots within the uterus. The nurse should then record the results of the assessment.

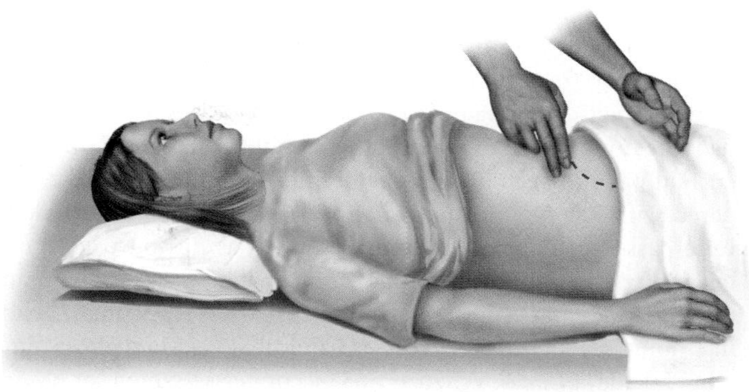

● **Figure 30–6** Measurement of descent of fundus for the woman with vaginal birth. The fundus is located two finger breadths below the umbilicus.

In the woman who has had a cesarean birth, the abdominal incision is extremely tender. The nurse should palpate the fundus with extreme care and inspect the abdominal incision for signs of healing, such as approximation (edges of incision appear "glued" together), bleeding, and any signs of infection, including drainage, foul odor, or redness. The nurse should document whether internal sutures, steri-strips, or staples are intact. The nurse can also review characteristics of normal healing, incision care, and discuss signs of infection.

Lochia

The nurse then evaluates the lochia, including character, amount, odor, and the presence of clots. Nurses must wear disposable gloves just before assessing the abdomen and fundus, or when they are ready to assess the perineum and lochia. During the first 1 to 3 days the lochia should be rubra. A few small clots are normal and occur as a result of blood pooling in the vagina. However, the passage of numerous or large clots is abnormal, and the cause should be investigated immediately. After 2 to 3 days, the lochia flow becomes serosa.

Nursing Practice

Assessing the status of the uterine fundus may cause discomfort for the mother. In addition to explaining the importance of the assessing fundal position and how to determine firmness to the mother, you can show her how to perform frequent light massage of the fundus herself to promote uterine involution. Involving her in her own care encourages her participation. In addition, having her massage her own uterus may lessen bleeding and reduce the need for more thorough massage.

MyNursingKit Case Study: Woman Recovering from Cesarean Birth

Lochia should never exceed a moderate amount, such as that needed to partially saturate perineal pads daily, with an average of six. However, because this number is influenced by an individual woman's pad-changing practices, as well as the absorbency of the pad, the nurse needs to question her about the length of time the current pad has been in use, whether the amount is normal compared with her typical menstrual period, and whether any clots were passed before this examination, such as during voiding. If heavy bleeding is reported but not seen, the nurse asks the woman to put on a clean perineal pad and then reassess the woman's pad in 1 hour (see Figure 30–7 ●). See Clinical Skills Manual: "Evaluating Lochia" SKILLS. When a more accurate assessment of blood loss is needed, the perineal pads can be weighed, with 1 g considered the approximate equivalent of 1 mL of blood.

Clots and heavy bleeding may be caused by uterine relaxation (atony), retained placental fragments, or rarely, an unknown cervical laceration, seen as heavy bleeding but with firm fundus, that may require further assessment (Table 30–4). Because of the evacuation of the uterine cavity during cesarean birth, women with such surgery usually have less lochia after the first 24 hours than mothers who give birth vaginally. If the woman is at increased risk for bleeding, or is actually experiencing heavy flow of lochia rubra, her blood pressure, pulse, and uterus need to be assessed frequently, and the physician/CNM may prescribe oxytocin (Pitocin) or methylergonovine maleate (Methergine). (See "Drug Guide: Methylergonovine Maleate [Methergine]," in Chapter 31.)

The odor of the lochia is nonoffensive and never foul. If a foul odor is present, so is an infection. When using narrative nursing notes, chart the amount of lochia first, followed by character. For example:

- Lochia: moderate rubra
- Lochia: small rubra/serosa

Client teaching that the nurse may address during assessment of the lochia may center on normal changes, effect of position changes, or what can be expected in the amount and color of the flow. Hygienic measures, such as wiping the perineum from front to back and washing her hands after toileting and changing pads, may be reviewed if appropriate. The nurse should approach the timing of teaching hygienic practices delicately, along with the content to be included. By establishing positive goals for the teaching—promoting comfort, enhancing tissue healing, and preventing infection—the nurse can avoid value-laden statements regarding personal beliefs about the need for cleanliness or control of body odor. The nurse should review with the mother the need to notify a healthcare professional if there is regression in the lochia flow pattern (e.g., color or amount).

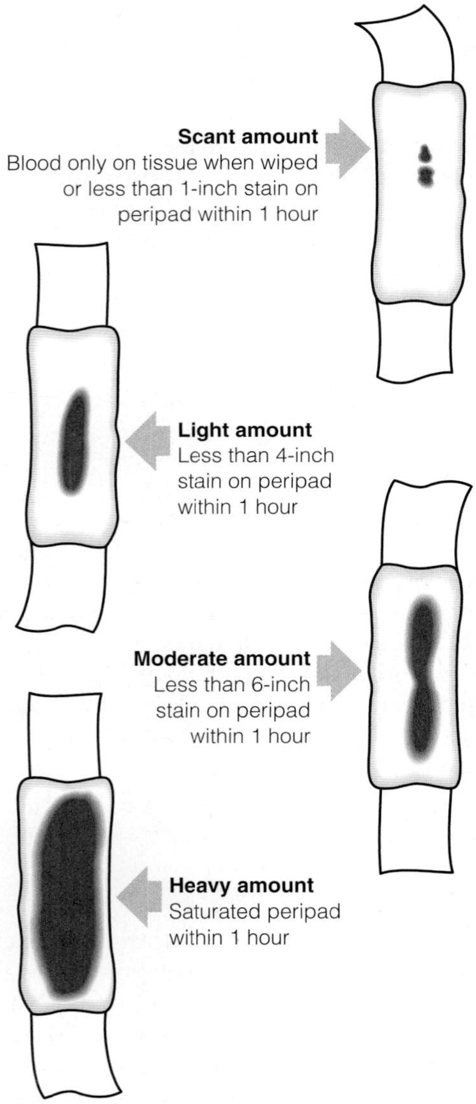

● **Figure 30–7** Suggested guideline for assessing lochia volume.

Source: Jacobson, H. (1985, May–June). A standard for assessing lochia volume. *Maternal-Child Nursing.*

Perineum

The perineum is inspected with the woman lying in a Sims' position. The nurse lifts the buttock to expose the perineum and anus.

If an episiotomy was done or a laceration required suturing, the nurse assesses the wound. To evaluate the state of healing, the nurse inspects the wound for redness, edema, ecchymosis, drainage, and approximation (REEDA scale). After 24 hours some edema may still be present, but the skin edges should be well approximated so that gentle pressure does not separate them. Gentle palpation should elicit minimal tenderness, and there should be no hardened areas suggesting infection. Ecchymosis interferes with normal healing, as does infection. Foul odors associated with drainage indicate infection. Hematomas sometimes occur, although these are considered abnormal.

The nurse next assesses whether hemorrhoids are present around the anus. If present, they are assessed for size, number, and pain or tenderness. (See Figure 30–8 ●.) See Clinical Skills Manual: "Postpartum Perineal Assessment" SKILLS.

During the assessment, the nurse talks with the woman to determine the effectiveness of comfort measures that have been used. The nurse provides teaching about the episiotomy or perineal laceration. Some women do not thoroughly understand what and where an episiotomy is, and they may believe that the stitches must be removed as with other types of surgery. Frequently, when women fear that the stitches must be removed manually, they are afraid to ask about them. While explaining the findings of the as-

Table 30–4 Changes in Lochia That Cause Concern

Change	Possible Problem	Nursing Action
Presence of clots	Inadequate uterine contractions that allow bleeding from vessels at the placental site.	Assess location and firmness of fundus. Assess voiding pattern. Record and report findings.
Persistent lochia rubra	Inadequate uterine contractions; retained placental fragments; infection; undetected cervical laceration.	Assess location and firmness of fundus. Assess activity pattern. Assess for signs of infection. Record and report findings.

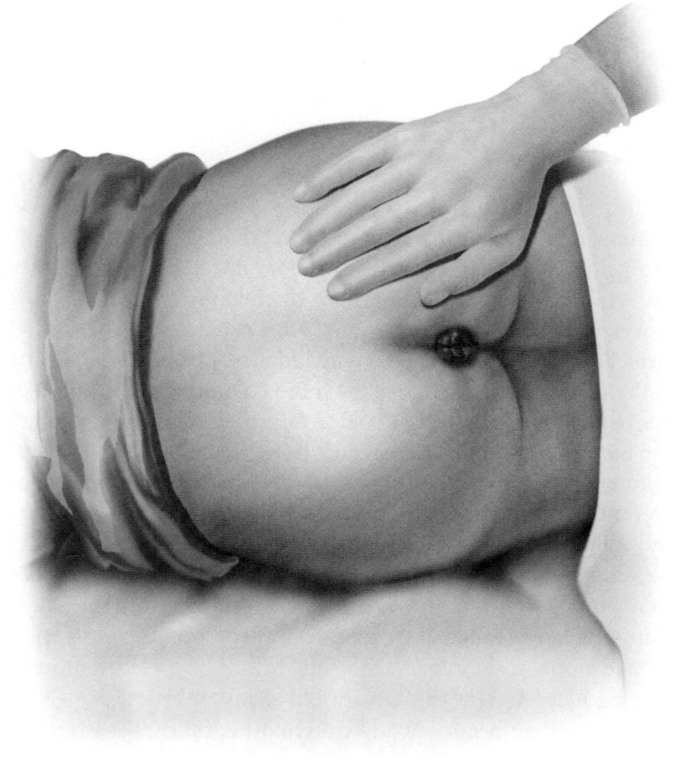

● **Figure 30–8** Intact perineum with hemorrhoids.

sessment, the nurse provides information about the episiotomy, its location, and the signs that are being assessed. In addition, the nurse can casually add that the sutures are special and will dissolve slowly over the next few weeks as the tissues heal. By the time the sutures are dissolved the tissues are strong and the incision edges will not separate. This is also an opportunity to teach comfort measures that may be used and reinforce the need to consult with the healthcare provider before using over-the-counter (OTC) medications/supplements if breastfeeding (see "Relief of Perineal Discomfort" in Chapter 31∞).

An example of documenting a perineal assessment might read: "Midline episiotomy; no edema, tenderness, or ecchymosis present. Skin edges well approximated"; or, if a perineal laceration repair, "Skin edges intact, no edema, tenderness, or ecchymosis, pain meds helpful. Woman reports sitz bath and Tucks pads or pain relief measures are controlling discomfort."

Nursing Practice

In evaluating the perineum, use the REEDA scale as a quick reminder of what to assess. Specifically:

R = redness

E = edema or swelling

E = ecchymosis or bruising

D = discharge

A = approximation (how well the edges of an incision—the episiotomy—or a repaired laceration seem to be holding together)

Lower Extremities

Postpartal women are at increased risk for *thrombophlebitis,* thrombus formation, and inflammation involving a vein (see Chapter 32∞). The most likely site of thrombophlebitis is in the woman's legs. Conditions that predispose a client for thrombophlebitis are hypercoagulability, severe anemia, obesity, and traumatic childbirth. To assess for thrombophlebitis, the nurse should have the woman stretch her legs out with the knees slightly flexed and the legs relaxed. The nurse then grasps the woman's foot and sharply dorsiflexes it. The second leg is assessed in the same way. No discomfort or pain should be present. If pain is elicited, the nurse notifies the physician/CNM that the woman has a positive Homans' sign (Figure 30–9 ●). The pain is caused by inflammation of the vessel. The nurse also evaluates the legs for edema by comparing both legs, because usually only one leg is involved. Any areas of redness, tenderness, and increased skin temperature are also noted.

Complementary Care

LYSINE FOLLOWING EPISIOTOMY

Lysine, an essential amino acid, has been identified as a supplement that decreases the incidence of pain following an episiotomy. Lysine is available as a supplement. The recommended adult dosage is 12 mg/kg of body weight per day. It is also present in dietary sources, including meat, cheese, fish, eggs, soybeans, and nuts.

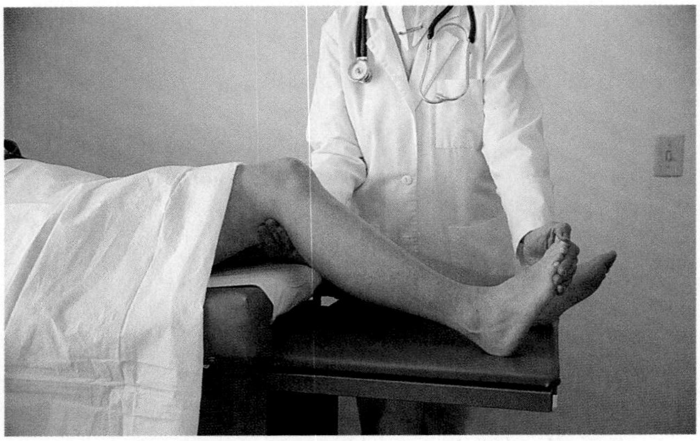

● **Figure 30–9** Homans' sign: With the woman's knee flexed, the nurse dorsiflexes the foot. Pain in the foot or leg is a positive Homans' sign.

Source: Photographer: Elena Dorfman.

Some facilities have discontinued performing a Homans' sign in the nursing assessment, stating it is not diagnostic and could lead to an emboli if the clot is dislodged during assessment. Although assessment of the Homans' sign is not diagnostic, supporters advocate its use as a screening tool. There are no published reports of an emboli occurring as a result of performing a Homans' sign. In the event of a positive Homans' sign, diagnosis is made by compression or duplex ultrasonography. Heparin therapy is used in postpartum women who do develop a deep vein thrombosis.

Early ambulation is an important aspect in the prevention of thrombophlebitis. Most women are able to be up shortly after birth or once they have fully recovered from the effects of regional anesthetic agents, if one has been used. The mother's legs should be assessed for return of sensation following regional anesthesia. The cesarean birth client requires range of motion exercises until she is ambulating more freely.

Client teaching associated with assessment of the lower extremities focuses on the signs and symptoms of thrombophlebitis. In addition, the nurse may review self-care measures to promote circulation and measures to prevent thrombophlebitis, such as leg exercises that may be performed in bed, dorsiflexion on an hourly basis while on bed rest, ambulation, and avoiding pressure behind the knees and crossing the legs.

Usually, the nurse records the results of the assessment on a flowsheet or a summary nursing note. If tenderness and warmth have been noted, they might be recorded as follows: "Tenderness, warmth, slight edema, and slight redness noted on posterior aspect of left calf—positive Homans'. Woman advised to avoid pressure to this area; lower leg elevated and moist heat applied per agency protocol. Call placed to Dr. Garcia to report findings."

Elimination

During the hours after birth the nurse carefully monitors a new mother's bladder status. A boggy uterus, a displaced uterus, or a palpable bladder are signs of bladder distention and require nursing intervention.

Following birth, the postpartal woman should be encouraged to void every 4 to 6 hours. The nurse should assess the bladder for distention until the woman demonstrates complete emptying of the bladder with each voiding. The nurse may employ techniques to facilitate voiding, such as helping the woman out of bed to void or pouring warm water on the vulva, running water in the sink, and encouraging the woman to relax and take deep breaths. The physician will order catheterization when the bladder is distended and the woman cannot void, when she is voiding small amounts (less than 100 mL) frequently, or when no voiding has occurred in 8 hours. Although many physicians or CNMs write orders stating that the woman can be catheterized in 8 hours if she has not voided, the nurse needs to assess the bladder and any voiding pattern frequently before the end of the 8-hour period. Some women require catheterization sooner. The cesarean birth mother may have an indwelling catheter inserted prophylactically. The same assessments should be made in evaluating bladder emptying once the catheter is removed.

During the physical assessment, the nurse elicits information from the woman about the adequacy of her fluid intake, whether she feels she is emptying her bladder completely when she voids, and any signs of urinary tract infection (UTI) she may be experiencing.

In the same way, the nurse obtains information about the new mother's intestinal elimination and any concerns she may have about it. Many mothers fear that the first bowel movement will be painful and possibly even damaging if an episiotomy has been done. Often, women have defecated during labor or childbirth; therefore, bowel movements normally return within 2 to 3 days after a vaginal childbirth. Stool softeners may be ordered to increase bulk and moisture in the fecal material and to allow more comfortable and complete evacuation. Constipation is avoided to prevent pressure on sutures and increase discomfort. To enhance bowel elimination and help the woman reestablish her normal bowel pattern, the nurse can encourage ambulation, increased fluid intake (up to 2000 mL/day or more), and additional fresh fruits and roughage in her diet.

During the assessment, the nurse may provide information about postpartal diuresis and explain why the woman may be emptying her bladder so frequently. Information about the need for additional fluid intake, with suggestions of specific amounts, may be helpful. The woman should drink at least eight (8 oz) glasses of water or juice in addition to other fluids. Breastfeeding mothers will have a higher requirement. The nurse discusses signs of urinary retention and overflow voiding and may review symptoms of UTI if it seems an appropriate moment for teaching. The nurse can also review methods of assisting bowel elimination and provide opportunities for the woman to ask questions.

Rest and Sleep Status

Physical fatigue often affects other adjustments and functions of the new mother. The mother requires energy to make the psychologic adjustments to a new infant and to assume new roles. Fatigue is often a highly significant factor in a new mother's apparent disinterest in her newborn. Frequently the woman is so tired from a long labor and birth that everything seems to be an effort. To avoid inadvertently classifying a very tired mother as one with a potential attachment problem, the nurse should do a psychologic assessment on more than one occasion. After a nap the new mother is often far more receptive to her baby and her surroundings. During the postpartal assessment, the nurse evaluates the amount of rest a new mother is getting. If the woman reports difficulty sleeping at night, the nurse

Developing Cultural Competence

POSTPARTUM PRACTICES

Rest, seclusion, and dietary restraint practices in many traditional non-Western cultures (African, traditional Mexico, Chinese, Japanese, South Asian groups) are designed to assist the woman and her baby during postpartum vulnerable periods. The period of postpartum vulnerability and seclusion varies between 7 and 40 days. In Ghana, new mothers are relieved from all chores, told to abstain from sex, and not allowed to leave the home (Holtz & Grisdale, 2008; Lauderdale, 2008). Decreased activity and seclusion practices are designed to decrease the influence of spirits or of spreading evil and misfortune. The time of seclusion coincides with the period of lochial flow or postpartum bleeding.

should try to determine the cause. If it is simply the strange environment, a warm drink and back rub may prove helpful. Appropriate nursing measures are indicated if the woman is bothered by normal postpartal discomforts such as afterpains, diaphoresis, or episiotomy or hemorrhoidal pain. The impact of rooming-in on the mother's ability to rest should be assessed. See Chapter 31∞ for more detailed discussion of comfort/pain relief measures.

The nurse should encourage a daily rest period and schedule hospital activities to allow time for napping. The nurse can also provide information about the fatigue a new mother experiences, strategies to promote rest/sleep at home, and the impact it can have on a woman's emotions and sense of control.

Nutritional Status

Determination of postpartal nutritional status is based primarily on information provided by the mother and on direct assessment. During pregnancy the daily recommended dietary allowances call for increases in calories, protein, and most vitamins and minerals. After birth, the nonbreastfeeding mother's dietary requirements return to prepregnancy levels, whereas the nursing mother's requirements increase.

Visiting the mother during mealtime provides an opportunity for unobtrusive nutritional assessment and counseling. The nonbreastfeeding mother should be advised about the need to reduce her caloric intake by about 300 kcal and to return to prepregnancy levels for other nutrients. The breastfeeding mother should increase her caloric intake by about 200 kcal over the pregnancy requirements, or a total of 500 kcal over the nonpregnant requirement. Basic discussion often proves helpful, followed by referral as needed. In all cases, literature on nutrition should be provided, so that the woman will have a source of information after discharge.

The nurse should inform the dietician of any mother who is a vegetarian, has food allergies or lactose intolerance, or whose cultural or religious beliefs require specific foods. Appropriate meals can then be prepared for her. Many women, especially those who gained more than the recommended number of pounds, are interested in losing weight after birth. The dietician can design weight-reduction diets to meet nutritional needs and food preferences. The nurse may also refer women with unusual eating habits or numerous questions about good nutrition to the dietician.

Table 30–5 Daily Eating to Encourage Healthful Nutrition during the Postpartal Period

2 to 3 servings of milk, yogurt, and cheese group
2 to 3 servings of meat or protein group
3 to 5 servings of vegetable group
4 servings of whole grain
2 to 4 servings of fruit group
6 to 11 servings of bread, cereal, rice, and pasta group
Fats, oils, and sweets sparingly

New mothers are advised that it is common practice to prescribe iron supplements for 3 months after birth. The hemoglobin and hematocrit values are then checked at the postpartal visit to detect any anemia.

As a part of the nutritional assessment, the nurse can provide teaching about the nutritional needs of the woman during the postpartal period. See Table 30–5 as well as the discussion in Chapter 12∞.

PSYCHOLOGIC ASSESSMENT

During the first several postpartal weeks, the woman must accomplish certain physical and developmental tasks:

- Restoring physical condition
- Developing competence in caring for and meeting the needs of her infant
- Establishing a relationship with her new child
- Adapting to altered lifestyles and family structure resulting from the addition of a new member

Adequate assessment of the mother's psychologic adjustment is an integral part of postpartal evaluation. This assessment focuses on the mother's general attitude, feelings of competence, available support systems, and caregiving skills. It also evaluates her fatigue level, sense of satisfaction, and ability to accomplish her developmental tasks.

Some new mothers have little or no experience with newborns and may feel totally overwhelmed. They may show these feelings by asking questions and reading all available material or by becoming passive and quiet because they simply cannot deal with their feelings of inadequacy. Unless a nurse questions the woman about her plans and previous experience in a supportive, nonjudgmental way, the nurse might conclude that the woman is disinterested, withdrawn, or depressed. Clues indicating adjustment difficulties include excessive continued fatigue, marked depression, excessive preoccupation with physical status or discomfort, evidence of low self-esteem, lack of support systems, marital problems, inability to care for or nurture the newborn, and current family crises (illness or unemployment). These characteristics frequently indicate a potential for maladaptive parenting, which may lead to child abuse or neglect (physical, emotional, intellectual) and cannot be ignored. Referrals to public health nurses or other available community resources may provide greatly needed assistance and alleviate potentially dangerous situations.

ASSESSMENT OF EARLY ATTACHMENT

A nurse in any of the various postpartal settings can periodically observe and note progress toward attachment. The assessment should include both parents when possible; however, in this section, these behaviors focus primarily on the mother's attachment process. As discussed previously, research shows that fathers experience similar attachment feelings to those experienced by mothers. The following questions can be addressed in the course of nurse-client interaction:

- Is the mother attracted to her newborn? To what extent does she seek face-to-face contact and eye contact? Has she progressed from fingertip touch, to palmar contact, to enfolding the infant close to her own body? Is attraction increasing or decreasing? If the mother does not exhibit increasing attraction, why not? Do the reasons lie primarily within her, in the baby, or in the environment?
- Is the mother inclined to nurture her infant? Is she progressing in her interactions with her infant?
- Does the mother act consistently? If not, is the source of unpredictability within her or her infant?
- Is her mothering consistently carried out? Does she seek information and evaluate it objectively? Does she develop solutions based on adequate knowledge of valid data? Does she evaluate the effectiveness of her maternal care and adjust appropriately?
- Is she sensitive to the newborn's needs as they arise? How quickly does she interpret her infant's behavior and react to cues? Does she seem happy and satisfied with the infant's responses to her efforts? Is she pleased with feeding behaviors? How much of this ability and willingness to respond is related to the baby's nature and how much to her own?
- Does she seem pleased with her baby's appearance and sex? Is she experiencing pleasure in interaction with her infant? What interferes with the enjoyment? Does she speak to the baby frequently and affectionately? Does she call him or her by name? Does she point out family traits or characteristics she sees in the newborn?
- Are there any cultural factors that might modify the mother's response? For instance, is it customary for the grandmother to assume most of the childcare responsibilities while the mother recovers from childbirth?

When the nurse has addressed these questions and assembled the facts, the nurse's intuition and knowledge should combine to answer three more questions: Is there a problem in attachment? What is the problem? What is its source? The nurse can then devise a creative approach to the problem as it presents itself in the context of a unique, developing mother-infant relationship.

DISCHARGE ASSESSMENT AND FOLLOW-UP

The final discharge assessment should include a physical examination and appropriate discharge teaching that includes both maternal and newborn care guidelines. The mother's laboratory values are examined. If the mother was nonimmune to rubella, a rubella vaccine is administered before discharge. Rh-negative mothers whose infants are Rh positive need RhoGAM before they go home. If either is given, the nurse should document this in the mother's chart. If referrals, such as social service programs, support groups, lactation consultant, or a pediatrician, are needed, they should be provided before the family leaves the facility.

Some obstetricians, certified nurse-midwives, and nurse practitioners see postpartal women 1 to 2 weeks after birth in addition to the routine 6-week checkup. These visits provide an opportunity for physical assessment as well as evaluation of the mother's psychologic and informational needs and needs of the family. The routine physical assessment, which can be made rapidly, focuses on the woman's general appearance, breasts, reproductive tract, bladder and bowel elimination, and any specific problems or complaints. In addition, the nurse should talk with the mother about her diet, fatigue level, family adjustment, and psychologic status. The nurse explores any problems with child care and refers the mother to a pediatric nurse practitioner or pediatrician if needed. Available community resources, including public health department follow-up visits, are mentioned when appropriate. If not already discussed, teaching about family planning is appropriate at this time, and the nurse provides information regarding birth control methods. Women who gave birth vaginally tend to abstain from resuming sexual intercourse for a longer period of time than those who had a cesarean birth. Women who breastfed resumed sexual relations later than those who did not breastfeed.

Postdischarge care for the postpartal woman may also be accomplished by home visits, follow-up phone calls, or both. The optimal time for a home visit or follow-up phone call is between 3 to 4 days after birth; this provides opportunities for further assessment of mothers and their infants and teaching. (See "Assessment Guide: Postpartal—First Home Visit and Anticipated Progress at 6 Weeks" in Chapter 31∞.) During this time period, infections, poor infant feeding, excessive weight loss, jaundice, and other problems become apparent (Simpson & James, 2005). The follow-up telephone call is often initiated by a nurse from the postpartal unit of the agency where the mother gave birth. It is made soon after discharge and is designed to provide assessment and care if necessary, to reinforce knowledge and provide additional teaching, and to make referrals if indicated. Alternatively, a follow-up phone call from a nurse at the physician's or nurse-midwife's office can provide new mothers with a source of support and an opportunity to ask questions. Women who appear to be having adjustment problems should be scheduled for an appointment for further evaluation.

In ideal situations, a family approach involving the father, infant, other siblings, and grandparents permits a total evaluation and provides an opportunity for all family members to ask questions and express concerns. In addition, a family approach can sometimes enable the nurse to identify disturbed family patterns more readily and suggest, or even institute, therapeutic measures to prevent future problems of neglect or abuse.

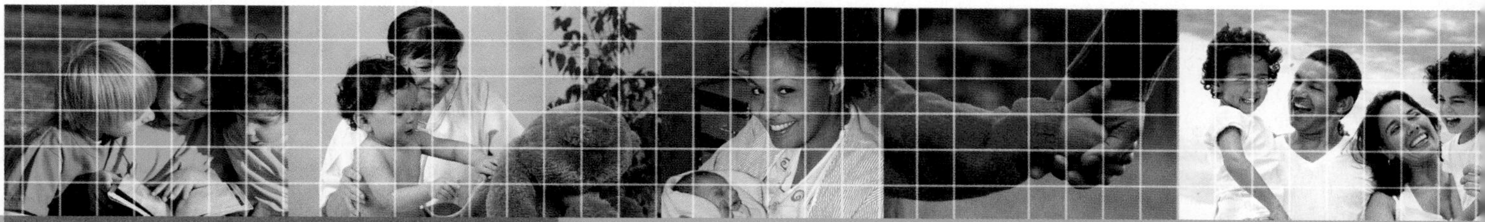

CRITICAL CONCEPT REVIEW

LEARNING OUTCOMES / CONCEPTS

30.1 Describe the basic physiologic changes that occur in the postpartal period as a woman's body returns to its prepregnant state.

1. Uterus is at the level of umbilicus within a few hours after childbirth. Decreases by about one finger breadth per day.
2. Placental site heals by a process of exfoliation, so no scar formation occurs.
3. Lochia flow progresses from rubra to serosa to alba.
4. Ovarian function and menstruation return in approximately 6–12 weeks in the nonlactating mother.
5. Breasts begin milk production.
6. Intestines are sluggish for a few days, leading to constipation, but return to prepregnant state within a week.
7. Postpartum diuresis occurs, bladder tone is decreased, and bladder takes approximately 6 weeks to return to prepregnant state.

A higher-than-usual boggy uterus, which deviates to the side, usually indicates a full bladder.

8. Bradycardia is normal for the first 6–10 days.
9. Hemostatic system reaches prepregnant state in 3–4 weeks. WBC count is often elevated. Activation of clotting factors predisposes to thrombus formation.

30.2 Discuss the psychologic adjustments that normally occur during the postpartal period.

1. Psychologic adjustment includes:
   - Taking-in.
   - Taking-hold.
   - Maternal role attainment.
   - Possibility of postpartum blues.

30.3 Explain the components and methods of a systematic postpartal assessment.

1. Systematic postpartal assessment includes:
   - Vital signs.
   - Breast examination.
   - Assessment of fundus, incision, episiotomy, and perineum.
   - Assessment of lochia in terms of type, quantity, and characteristics.
   - Assessment of bladder and bowels.
   - Assessment of lower extremities.
   - Psychologic assessment.
     - Expected phase of adjustment to parenthood.
     - Expected level of attachment to infant.
   - Client education concerning self-care.

30.4 Describe the normal characteristics and common concerns of the mother considered in a postpartal assessment.

1. The nurse will often be asked about these common postpartal concerns:
   - A gush of blood that sometimes occurs when the woman first arises.
   - Passing clots.
   - Night sweats.
   - After pains.
   - "Large stomach" after birth and failure to lose all the weight gained during pregnancy.
2. See Table 30–3 for explanations of these common postpartal concerns.

30.5 Examine the physical and developmental tasks that the mother must accomplish during the postpartal period.

1. The woman's physical condition returns to a nonpregnant state.
2. The woman gains competence and confidence in herself as a parent.

(continued)

LEARNING OUTCOMES — CONCEPTS

LEARNING OUTCOMES	CONCEPTS
30.6 Explain the factors that influence the development of parent-infant attachment.	1. Parent-infant attachment is influenced by: ■ Involvement with woman's own family. ■ Stability of relationships and home environment. ■ Mother's ability to trust. ■ Mother's level of self-esteem. ■ Mother's ability to enjoy herself. ■ Mother's knowledge of expectations of childbearing and child rearing. ■ Positive reaction to present pregnancy.

CRITICAL THINKING IN ACTION

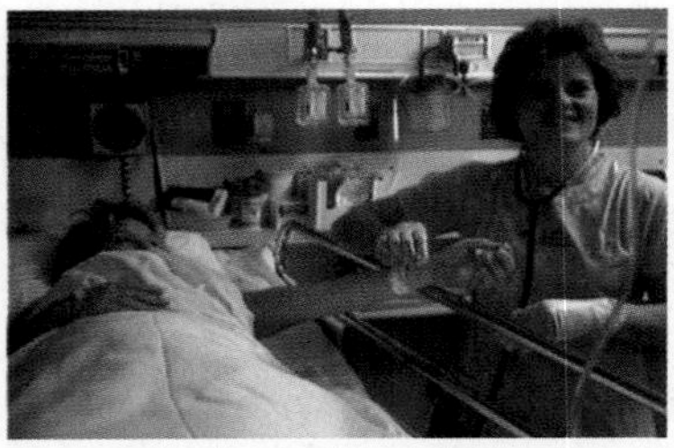

Janet Burns, a 25-year-old G3 P3, is 2 hours past a low forceps vaginal birth with a right medial lateral episiotomy of a live 8 pound baby boy. You obtain vital signs of BP 118/70, T 98.8°F, P 76, R 14. You observe the fundus is +1 finger above the umbilicus and slightly to the right. Her episiotomy is slightly ecchymotic and well approximated without edema or discharge. Ice has been applied to the episiotomy for the last 20 minutes. Lochia rubra is present and a pad was saturated in 90 minutes. Janet has an intravenous of Ringer's lactate with 10 units of Pitocin infusing at 100 mL/hr in her lower left arm and is complaining of moderate abdominal cramping. Janet's baby is sleeping peacefully in the bassinet next to her bed. She tells you that she is very tired and requests some pain medication so she can sleep for a while.

1. What nursing assessment is of immediate concern?
2. Discuss care of her episiotomy and perineum.
3. What other self-care measures could you advise?
4. Discuss postpartal occurrences that may cause special concern for the mother.
5. Janet expressed concern about her episiotomy healing. What information can you offer?

See MyNursingKit for possible responses.

REFERENCES

Alexander, J. M. (2005). Epidural anesthesia for labor pain and its relationship to fever. *Clinics in Perinatology, 32*(3), 777–787.

Al-Oballi Kridli, S. (2002). Health beliefs and practices among Arab women. *American Journal of Maternal Child Nursing, 27*(3), 178–182.

Beck, C. T. (2002). Revision of the postpartum depression predictors inventory. *Journal of Obstetric, Gynecologic, and Neonatal Nursing, 31*(4), 394–402.

Beck, C. T. (2008). *Postpartum mood and anxiety disorders: Case studies, research, and nursing care* (2nd ed.). Washington, DC: Association of Women's Health, Obstetric and Neonatal Nurses.

Blackburn, S. T. (2007). *Maternal, fetal, & neonatal physiology: A clinical perspective* (3rd ed.). St. Louis: Saunders.

Cunningham, F. G., Leveno, K. J., Bloom, S. L., Hauth, J. C., Rouse, D. J., & Spong, C. Y. (2010). *Williams obstetrics* (23rd ed.). New York: McGraw-Hill.

D'Avanzo, C. E., & Geissler, E. M. (2008). *Cultural health assessment* (4th ed.). St. Louis: Mosby.

Holtz, C. & Grisdale, S. (2008). Global health in reproduction and infants. In C. Holtz. *Global health care: Issues and policies* (1st ed., pp. 437–476). Boston: Jones & Bartlett.

James, D. C. (2008). Postpartum care. In K. R. Simpson & P. A. Creehan. *Perinatal nursing* (3rd ed., pp. 473–526). Philadelphia: Lippincott Williams & Wilkins.

Lauderdale, J. (2008). Transcultural perspectives in childbearing. In M. M. Andrews & J. S. Boyle, *Transcultural concepts in nursing care* (5th ed.). Philadelphia: Lippincott Williams & Wilkins.

Lipscomb, K., & Novy, M. J. (2007). The normal puerperium. In A. H. Decherney, L. Nathan, T. M. Goodwin, & N. Laufer (Eds.), *Current diagnosis and treatment: Obstetrics & gynecology* (10th ed.). Boston: McGraw-Hill.

Mercer, R. T. (1995). *Becoming a mother.* New York: Springer.

Mercer, R. T. (2004). Becoming a mother versus maternal role attainment. *Journal of Nursing Scholarship, 36*(3), 226–232.

Mercer, R. T. & Walker, L. O. (2006). A review of nursing interventions to foster becoming a mother. *Journal of Obstetrics, Gynecology, Neonatal Nurses. 35(5)*, 568–82.

Purnell, L. D., & Paulanka, B. J. (2008). *Transcultural health care: A culturally competent approach.* (3rd ed.). Philadelphia: Davis.

Rubin, R. (1961). Puerperal change. *Nursing Outlook, 9,* 753.

Rubin, R. (1984). *Maternal identity and the maternal experience.* New York: Springer.

Shehata, H. A., & Okosun, H. (2004). Neurological disorders in pregnancy. *Current Opinion in Obstetrics & Gynecology, 16*(2), 117–122.

Simpson, K. R., & James, D. C. (2005). *Postpartum care: Continuing education for registered nurses and certified nurse-midwives.* White Plains, NY: March of Dimes.

Tatum, W., Liporace, J., Benbadis, S., & Kaplan, P. (2004). Updates on the treatment of epilepsy in women. *Archives of Internal Medicine, 164*(2), 137–145.

Varney, H., Kriebs, J. M., & Gegor, C. L. (2004). *Varney's midwifery* (4th ed.). Sudbury, MA: Jones & Bartlett.

Zauderer, C. (2009). Maternity care for Orthodox Jewish couples: Implications for nurses in the obstetric setting. *Nursing for Women's Health, 13(2),* 112–131.

CHAPTER

31 The Postpartal Family: Early Care Needs and Home Care

More than anything else that happened after my baby was born, I was surprised by the fatigue I felt. In the first few weeks I spent every minute that my baby slept cleaning, doing laundry, and the like. Then, during my checkup, the nurse-midwife told me that I had to rest when my baby slept. What a difference that made. Suddenly I was less overwhelmed and more able to enjoy being a mother. —Mai Ling, 26

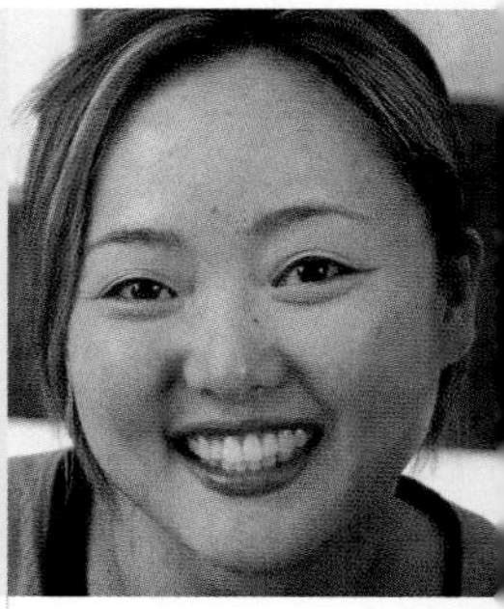

LEARNING OUTCOMES

31.1 Formulate nursing diagnoses and nursing care based on the findings of the "normal" postpartum assessment and teaching needs.

31.2 Discuss nursing interventions to promote postpartum maternal comfort, rest, and well-being.

31.3 Explain factors that affect postpartal family wellness in the provision of nursing care and client teaching.

31.4 Compare the postpartal nursing needs of the woman who experienced a cesarean birth with the needs of a woman who gave birth vaginally.

31.5 Examine the nursing needs of the childbearing adolescent during the postpartal period.

31.6 Describe possible approaches to sensitive, holistic nursing care for the woman who relinquishes her newborn.

31.7 Identify teaching topics related to postpartum discharge.

31.8 Identify the main purposes and components of home visits during the postpartal period.

31.9 Summarize actions a nurse should take to ensure personal safety as well as fostering a caring relationship during a home visit.

31.10 Discuss maternal and family assessment and anticipated progress after birth.

31.11 Delineate interventions to address the common concerns of breastfeeding mothers following discharge.

31.12 Describe the assessment and care of the newborn during postpartal home care.

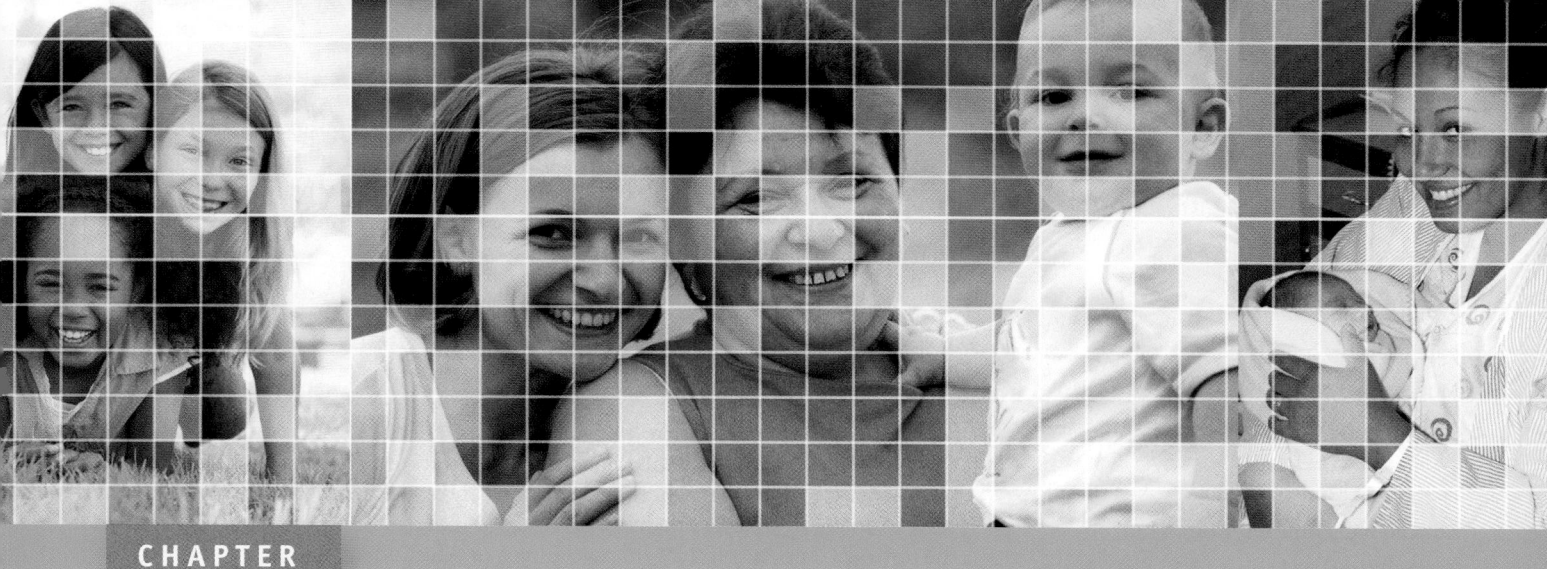

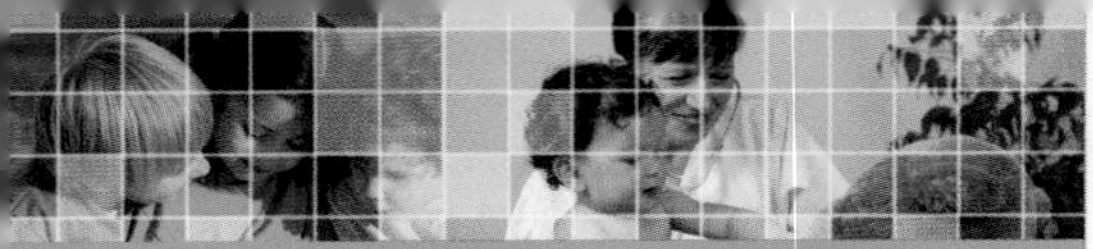

KEY TERMS

Continuous epidural infusion (CEI), 794

Cosleeping, 818

Couplet care, 792

Late preterm infant, 799

Mother-baby care, 792

Patient-controlled analgesia (PCA), 794

Postpartal home care, 800

Shaken baby injuries, 818

Tummy time, 813

Chapter 30∞ provides a thorough discussion of postpartal adaptation and nursing assessment. This chapter describes how the nurse can use the remaining steps of the nursing process effectively to plan and provide care. Specific nursing responses to the mother's physical needs and the family's psychosocial needs are described at length.

NURSING CARE DURING THE EARLY POSTPARTAL PERIOD

For most postpartal women, physical recovery goes smoothly and is considered a healthy process. Because of this perception, caregivers too often assume that the woman and her family have no real needs and that no care plan is needed. Nothing could be further from the truth. Every member of the family has needs, although the needs may not be obvious, especially if they are psychologic or educational.

NURSING DIAGNOSIS

The postpartal family's needs, which should be identified during assessment, are the basis for developing nursing diagnoses. Many nurses have suggested that nursing diagnoses are difficult to make in a wellness setting because of their emphasis on "problems." Nurses involved in the effort to formulate standardized diagnoses recognize this difficulty and continue working to develop nursing diagnoses that are more congruent with wellness settings.

Many agencies that use nursing diagnoses prefer to use only the NANDA list. Consequently, physiologic alterations form the basis of many postpartal diagnoses. Examples of such diagnoses include:

- *Ineffective Breastfeeding* related to postpartal pain from a cesarean birth or maternal fatigue
- *Constipation* related to fear of tearing stitches or pain
- *Acute Pain* related to perineal trauma secondary to episiotomy or birth

Diagnoses related to family coping or instructional needs are also used frequently. Examples of these diagnoses include:

- *Health-Seeking Behaviors: Information About Infant Care* related to an expressed desire to improve parenting skills
- *Anxiety* related to self and infant care secondary to lack of knowledge of appropriate care practices
- *Readiness for enhanced family coping* related to successful adjustment to new baby

NURSING PLAN AND IMPLEMENTATION

An important component of postpartal nursing care is client teaching, which must be individualized to the learning capability and readiness of the parent(s). As part of the teaching role, the nurse discusses desired outcomes and goals with the mother and family members as soon as possible following the birth. Interventions can then be designed to achieve optimal health promotion. Strategies for promoting effective parent learning are discussed shortly, and specific teaching content is provided throughout the rest of this chapter. Home care visits and phone contacts help ensure that new parents have the necessary skills and resources to care for their infant. A "Clinical Pathway: The Postpartal Period" begins on the next page.

PROMOTION OF MATERNAL COMFORT AND WELL-BEING

The nurse can promote and restore maternal physical well-being by monitoring uterine status, vital signs, cardiovascular status, elimination patterns, nutritional needs, sleep and rest, and learning needs. Some women also require medication to relieve pain, treat anemia, provide immunity to rubella, and prevent development of antibodies in the nonsensitized Rh-negative woman. Most postpartal women need nursing interventions to promote their comfort and relieve stress.

MONITORING UTERINE STATUS

The nurse completes an assessment of the uterus as discussed in Chapter 30. The assessment interval is usually every 15 minutes for the first hour after childbirth, every 30 minutes for the next hour, and then hourly for approximately 2 more hours. After that, the nurse monitors uterine status every 8 hours or more frequently if problems arise such as the following:

- Bogginess (uterus is not firm and is difficult to palpate because it lacks shape and consistency)
- Positioning out of midline
- Heavy lochia flow
- Presence of clots

Clinical Pathway

THE POSTPARTAL PERIOD

CATEGORY	FIRST 4 HOURS	4 TO 8 HOURS PAST BIRTH	8 TO 24 HOURS PAST BIRTH
Referral	Report from labor nurse if not continuing in an LDR room	Lactation consultation as needed	Home nursing, WIC referral if indicated **EXPECTED OUTCOMES** Referrals made
Assessments	Postpartum assessments q30min × 2, q1h × 2, then q4h. Includes: ■ Fundus firm, midline, at or below umbilicus ■ Lochia rubra less than 1 pad/h; no free flow or passage of clots with massage ■ Bladder: voids large amounts of urine spontaneously; bladder not palpable following voiding ■ Perineum: sutures intact; no bulging or marked swelling; no c/o severe pain. Minimal bruising may be present. If hemorrhoids present, no tenseness or marked engorgement; less than 2 cm diameter ■ Breasts: soft, colostrum present Vital Signs: ■ BP WNL; no hypotension; not > 30 mm systolic or 15 mm diastolic over baseline ■ Temperature: less than 38°C (100.4°F) ■ Pulse: bradycardia normal, consistent with baseline ■ Respirations: 16 to 24/min; quiet, easy Comfort level: less than 3 on scale of 1 to 10	Continue postpartum assessment q4h × 2, then q8h Breast: evaluate nipple status; should be no evidence of cracks or bruising Observe feeding technique with newborn Vital signs assessment q8h; all WNL; report temperature greater than 38°C (100.4°F) Assess Homans' sign q8h Continue assessment of comfort level	Continue postpartum assessment q8h Breasts: nipples should remain free of cracks, fissures, bruising Feeding technique with newborn: should be good or improving Vital signs assessment q8h; all WNL; report temperature greater than 38°C (100.4°F) Continue assessment of comfort level **EXPECTED OUTCOMES** Vital signs medically acceptable, voids qs, postpartum assessment WNL; comfort level: less than 3 on 1 to 10 scale, involution of uterus in process, demonstrates and verbalizes appropriate newborn feeding techniques

Information is included for both vaginal birth (VB) and cesarean birth (CB). However, because many of the nursing care interventions are the same for either, specific interventions or suggestions related to vaginal birth are designated VB, and those specific to cesarean are designated CB.

ADL, activities of daily living; BP, blood pressure; CB, cesarean birth; CNM, certified nurse-midwife; c/o, complaints of; D/C, discharge; DC, discontinue; LDR, labor, delivery, and recovery; LOC, level of consciousness; LOS, level of sensation; OOB, out of bed; OR, operating room; PCA, patient-controlled analgesia; PO, per oral; PP, postpartum; PRN, as needed; qs, quantity sufficient; s/s, signs and symptoms; TC & DB, turn-cough and deep breathe; VB, vaginal birth; VS, vital signs; WNL, within normal limits.

(continued on page 782)

Clinical Pathway—continued

THE POSTPARTAL PERIOD

CATEGORY	FIRST 4 HOURS	4 TO 8 HOURS PAST BIRTH	8 TO 24 HOURS PAST BIRTH
Teaching/ psychosocial	Explain postpartum assessments Teach self-massage of fundus and expected findings; rationale for fundal massage Instruct to call for assistance first time OOB and PRN Demonstrate pericare, surgigator, sitz bath PRN Explain comfort measures Begin newborn teaching; bulb suctioning, positioning, feeding, diaper change, cord care Orient to room if transferred from LDR room Provide information on early postpartal period Assess mother-infant attachment	Discuss psychologic changes of postpartum period; facilitate transition through tasks of taking on maternal role Discuss pericare/hygiene; encourage use of supportive brassiere for formula- or breastfeeding Stress need for frequent rest periods Continue newborn teaching: soothing/comforting techniques, swaddling; return demonstrations indicate woman's understanding Provide opportunities for questions and review; reinforce previous teaching Breastfeeding: nipple care: air-drying, lanolin; proper latch-on technique; tea bags Formula-feeding: supportive bra, ice bags, breast binder Assess mother-infant attachment	Reinforce previous teaching, complete teaching evaluation Discuss involution; anticipated physical changes in first 2 weeks postpartum; postpartal exercises; need to limit visitors Discuss postpartal nutrition; balanced diet Breastfeeding: ■ Increase calories by 500 kcal over nonpregnant state (200 kcal over pregnant intake) ■ Explain milk production, let-down reflex, use of supplements, breast pumping, and milk storage Formula feeding: ■ Return to nonpregnant caloric intake ■ Explain formula preparation and storage Discuss birth control options, sexuality Discuss sibling rivalry and plan for supporting siblings at home Discuss pets; suggestions for improving acceptance of infant by pets **EXPECTED OUTCOMES** Mother verbalizes teaching comprehension Positive bonding and emotional behaviors observed
Nursing care management and reports	Ice pack to perineum to decrease swelling and increase comfort Straight catheter PRN × 1 if distended or voiding small amounts If continues unable to void or voiding small amounts, insert Foley catheter and notify physician/CNM	Sitz baths PRN If woman Rh– and infant Rh+, RhoGAM workup; obtain consent; complete teaching Determine rubella status Obtain consent for rubella vaccine if indicated; explain purpose, procedure, implications of vaccine Obtain hematocrit	Continue sitz baths PRN May shower if ambulating without difficulty DC heparin lock if present Administer rubella vaccine as indicated **EXPECTED OUTCOMES** Using sitz bath; voids qs; lab work WNL; performs ADL without sequelae
Activity	Assistance when OOB first time, then PRN Ambulate ad lib Rests comfortably between assessments	Encourage rest periods Ambulate ad lib; may leave birthing unit after notifying staff of plan to ambulate off unit	Up ad lib **EXPECTED OUTCOMES** Ambulates ad lib

Clinical Pathway—continued

THE POSTPARTAL PERIOD

CATEGORY	FIRST 4 HOURS	4 TO 8 HOURS PAST BIRTH	8 TO 24 HOURS PAST BIRTH
Comfort	Institute comfort measures: ■ Perineal discomfort: pericare; sitz baths, topical analgesics ■ Hemorrhoids: sitz baths, topical analgesics, digital replacement of external hemorrhoids; side-lying or prone position ■ Afterpains: prone with small pillow under abdomen; warm shower or sitz baths; ambulation ■ Administer pain medication	Continue with pain management techniques Offer alternative pain management options: distraction with music, television, visitors; massage; warmed blankets or towels to affected area; using breathing techniques when infant latches on to breast and/or during cramping until medication's action is felt	Continue with pain management techniques **EXPECTED OUTCOMES** Comfort level less than 3 on 1 to 10 scale Verbalizes alternative pain management options
Nutrition	Regular diet Fluid of 2000 mL per day or more	Continue diet and fluids	Continue diet and fluids **EXPECTED OUTCOMES** Regular diet/fluids tolerated
Elimination	Voiding large amounts of straw-colored urine	Voiding large quantities May have bowel movement	Same **EXPECTED OUTCOMES** Voiding qs; passing flatus or bowel movement
Medications	Pain medications as ordered Methergine 0.2 mg q4h PO if ordered Stool softener Tucks pad PRN, perineal analgesic spray	Continue meds Lanolin to nipples PRN; tea bags to nipples if tender; heparin flush to heparin lock (if present) q8h or as ordered May take own prenatal vitamins	Continue medications RhoGAM and rubella vaccine administered if indicated **EXPECTED OUTCOMES** Vaccines administered; pain controlled
Discharge planning/home	Evaluate knowledge of normal postpartum and newborn care Evaluate support systems	Discuss typical newborn schedule; plan for periods of rest Birth certificate paperwork completed Evaluate plans for transporting newborn; car seat available	Review discharge instruction sheet/checklist Describe postpartum warning signs and when to call physician/CNM Provide prescriptions. Provide gift packs as appropriate for formula- or breastfeeding Arrangements for baby pictures as per agency protocol Postpartum and newborn visits scheduled **EXPECTED OUTCOMES** Discharged home; mother verbalizes postpartum warning s/s, follow-up appointment times/dates
Family involvement	Identify available support persons Assess family perceptions of birth experience Parenting: demonstrates culturally expected early parenting behaviors	Involve support persons in care, teaching; answer questions Evidence of parental bonding behaviors present	Continue to involve support persons in teaching, involve siblings as appropriate Plans made for providing support to mother following discharge **EXPECTED OUTCOMES** Evidence of parental bonding behavior; support persons verbalize understanding of woman's need for rest, good nutrition, fluids, and emotional support
Date			

Table 31–1 Position of the Uterine Fundus Following Birth

Time	Position of Fundus
Immediately after birth	Top of fundus is in the midline about midway between the symphysis pubis and umbilicus.
Six to twelve hours after birth	Top of fundus is in the midline and at the level of the umbilicus.
One day after birth	Top of fundus is in the midline and one finger-breadth below the umbilicus.
Second day after birth and thereafter	Top of fundus remains in the midline and descends about one finger-breadth per day.

See Table 31–1. Occasionally medications are needed to promote uterine contractions. These include oxytocin, discussed in Chapter 23∞, and methylergonovine maleate [Methergine] (see the accompanying Drug Guide and Table 32–1). The nurse also monitors the amount, consistency, color, and odor of the lochia on an ongoing basis. Continued assessment is warranted during the first 24 hours because early postpartum hemorrhage typically occurs in the 24 hours after birth and is most commonly related to uterine atony (AWHONN, 2006).

MyNursingKit Case Study: Perineal Discomfort

Evidence in Action

To reduce the incidence of postpartum hemorrhage, it is recommended that uterine massage occur every 10 minutes for the first hour after birth (Cochrane Review) (Hofmeyr, Abdel-Aleem, & Abdel-Aleem, 2008).

RELIEF OF PERINEAL DISCOMFORT

Before selecting a method to help relieve perineal discomfort, the nurse needs to assess the perineum to determine the degree of edema and other problems. It is also important to ask the woman if she believes any special measures will be particularly effective and to offer her choices when possible. The nurse uses disposable gloves while applying all relief measures and washes hands before and after using the gloves. At all times it is essential for the nurse

Drug Guide

METHYLERGONOVINE MALEATE (METHERGINE)

Overview of Action

Methylergonovine maleate (Methergine) is an ergot alkaloid that stimulates smooth muscle tissue. Because the smooth muscle of the uterus is especially sensitive to this drug, it is used postpartally to stimulate the uterus to contract in order to decrease blood loss by clamping off uterine blood vessels and to promote the involution process. In addition, the drug has a vasoconstrictive effect on all blood vessels, especially the larger arteries. This may result in hypertension, particularly in a woman whose blood pressure is already elevated.

Route, Dosage, and Frequency

Methergine has a rapid onset of action and may be given orally or intramuscularly.

Usual IM dose: 0.2 mg following expulsion of the placenta. The dose may be repeated every 2 to 4 hours if necessary.

Usual oral dose: 0.2 mg every 4 hours (six doses).

Maternal Contraindications

Pregnancy, hepatic or renal disease, cardiac disease, hypertension, or preeclampsia contraindicate this drug's use. Methylergonovine maleate must be used with caution during lactation (Wilson, Shannon, & Shields, 2010).

Maternal Side Effects

Hypertension, nausea, vomiting, headache, bradycardia, dizziness, tinnitus, abdominal cramps, palpitations, dyspnea, chest pain, and allergic reactions may be noted.

Effects on Fetus or Newborn

Because Methergine has a long duration (3 hours [Wilson et al., 2010]) and action and can thus produce tetanic contractions, it *should never be used during pregnancy or in labor*, when it may result in a sustained uterine contraction that may cause amniotic fluid embolism (increased pressure in uterus may allow entry of amniotic fluid under the edge of the placenta and thus entry into the maternal venous system), uterine rupture, cervical and perineal lacerations (resulting from tetanic contractions and rapid birth of the baby), and hypoxia and intracranial hemorrhage in the baby (because of tetanic contractions, which severely decrease the maternal-placental-fetal blood flow, or uterine rupture, which causes cessation of blood flow to the unborn baby) (Wilson et al., 2010).

Nursing Considerations

- Monitor fundal height and consistency and the amount and character of the lochia.
- Assess the blood pressure before and routinely throughout drug administration.
- Observe for adverse effects or symptoms of ergot toxicity (ergotism) such as nausea and vomiting, headache, muscle pain, cold or numb fingers and toes, chest pain, and general weakness (Wilson et al., 2010).
- Provide client and family teaching regarding importance of not smoking during Methergine administration (nicotine from cigarettes leads to constricted vessels and may lead to hypertension) and signs of toxicity.

to remember hygienic practices, such as moving from the front of the perineum (area of the symphysis pubis) to the back (area around the anus). Avoiding contamination between the anal area and the urethral/vaginal area is vital to the prevention of infection. It is important to remember that in some cultures or religions, such as Orthodox Judaism, women are prohibited to touch or change their own perineal pads and will require the nurse or a family member to do so.

Perineal Care

Perineal care after each elimination cleanses the perineum, prevents infection, and helps promote comfort. The woman should be instructed to wash her hands before and after changing peripads or performing pericare. The nurse demonstrates how to cleanse the perineum and assists the woman as necessary. Many agencies provide "peri bottles" that the woman can use to squirt warm tap water over her perineum following elimination. To cleanse her perineum, the woman should use moist antiseptic towelettes or toilet paper in a blotting (patting) motion and should be taught to start at the front and proceed toward the back to prevent contamination from the anal area.

Many women have never used perineal pads and will need teaching and assistance in using them during the postpartal period. To prevent contamination, the perineal pad should be applied from front to back (place the front portion against the perineum first) and changed when saturation occurs or after each perineal cleansing. The woman is advised to hold the pad on the sides to prevent contamination. The pad needs to be placed snugly against the perineum but should not produce pressure. If the pad is worn too loosely, it may rub back and forth, irritating perineal tissues and causing contamination between the anal and vaginal areas. The pad should be changed after urination and defecation. Women should be advised to cleanse the perineal area with soap and water at least one time per day in addition to using the peri bottle after each void or pad change (AWHONN, 2006). Advise the woman that the pad should be changed at least four times per day to prevent contamination from bacteria (AWHONN, 2006). Women should be advised that perineal pain is common and will decrease gradually each day. Most women note complete resolution within 8 weeks of birth (Andrews, Thakar, Sultan, et al., 2007). (For information regarding the care of the perineum following an episiotomy, see "Teaching Highlights: Episiotomy Care.")

Complementary Care

LAVENDER OIL FOR PERINEAL PAIN

For centuries, lavender oil has been infused into warm water for relief of perineal pain associated with childbirth. Lavender is grown in Africa, Russia, the Arabic peninsula, and the Mediterranean region. The fragrance of lavender is said to promote a calming effect. The anti-anxiety qualities, combined with its soothing properties when diffused in water, make it a popular alternative therapy modality for postpartum women. Lavender may also have some antibacterial effects that may prevent infection in postpartal women.

Teaching Highlights

EPISIOTOMY CARE

Describe the process of wound healing.

Discuss the risks of contamination of the episiotomy by bacteria from the anal area.

Describe techniques that are used to keep the episiotomy clean and promote healing:

- Sitz bath
- Use of peri-bottle following each voiding or defecation
- Pad change following each elimination and at regular intervals

Describe comfort measures:

- Ice pack or ice-filled glove to perineum immediately following childbirth
- Sitz bath
- Judicious use of analgesics or topical anesthetics
- Tightening buttocks before sitting

Identify signs of episiotomy infection (redness, edema, drainage, incomplete approximation of the edges).

Advise the woman to contact her caregiver if signs of infection develop.

Ice Pack

If an episiotomy is done at the time of birth, an ice pack is generally applied to the perineum to reduce edema and provide numbing of the tissues, which promotes comfort. In some agencies, chemical ice bags are used: These are usually activated by folding both ends toward the middle. The nurse can create inexpensive ice bags by filling a disposable glove with ice chips or crushed ice and then taping the top of the glove. To protect the perineum from burns caused by contact with such an ice pack, the glove needs to be rinsed under running water to remove any powder and then wrapped in an absorbent towel or washcloth before placing it against the perineum. To attain the maximum effect of this cold treatment, a pattern of applying the ice pack for approximately 20 minutes and then removing it for about 10 minutes should be followed during the first 2 hours to reduce edema. Usually ice packs are needed for the first 24 hours to reduce pain (AWHONN, 2006). The nurse provides information about the purpose of the ice pack, as well as anticipated effects, benefits, and possible problems, and explains how to prepare an ice pack for home use if edema is present and early discharge is planned.

Sitz Bath

The warmth of the water in the sitz bath provides comfort, decreases pain, and promotes circulation to the tissues, which promotes healing and reduces the incidence of infection (Figure 31–1 ●). In some facilities, the use of the sitz bath has declined and is reserved only for women who have third- and fourth-degree lacerations (see Chapter 32 ∞ for further discussion), whereas in other facilities, it is offered to all women who have edema or a laceration following birth. Sitz baths may be

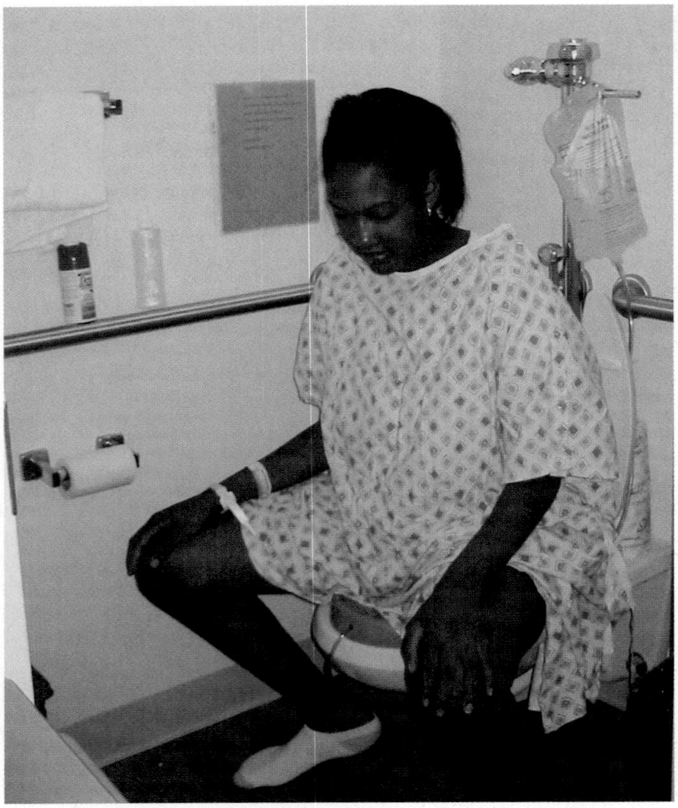

● **Figure 31–1** Sitz bath. A sitz bath promotes healing and provides relief from perineal discomfort during the initial weeks following birth.

Teaching Highlights

SELF-EVALUATION OF THE PERINEUM

After the mother completes the sitz bath, teach her to inspect the perineal area for burns (that could be related to using water that is too hot), edema, and approximation by using a handheld mirror. If the mother routinely inspects the area, she will be aware of changes that may indicate an infection, such as redness, poor approximation, drainage, or odor.

ordered three times a day (TID) and as needed (PRN). The nurse prepares the sitz bath by cleaning the equipment and adding water at 38.9°C to 40.6°C (102°F to 105°F). The woman is encouraged to remain in the sitz bath for about 20 minutes. It is important for the woman to have a clean, unused towel to pat dry her perineum after the sitz bath and to have a clean perineal pad to apply. Care needs to be taken during the first sitz bath because the moist heat may cause the woman to faint. The nurse places a call bell well within reach and asks the woman to use it if she feels dizzy or lightheaded or develops difficulty hearing. The nurse also checks on the woman at frequent intervals.

Cool sitz baths have been used because they are effective in reducing perineal edema and reducing the response of nerve endings that cause perineal discomfort (Tejirian & Abbas, 2005). However, many women are reluctant and voice discomfort while sitting in a cool tub of water (Steen, Briggs, & King, 2006). Because women may find the practice uncomfortable, nurses should ask the woman if she would prefer a warm or cool sitz bath based on personal choice (Steen et al., 2006). In administering a cool sitz bath, have the woman start with the water at room temperature and add ice according to the woman's comfort.

The nurse provides information about the purpose and use of the sitz bath; anticipated effects, benefits, and possible problems; and safety measures to prevent overheating, scalds, chills, or injury from fainting or slipping while getting into or out of the tub. Home use of sitz baths may be recommended for the woman with an extensive episiotomy. The woman may use a portable sitz bath or her bathtub. It is important for the nurse to emphasize that in using a bathtub, the woman draws only 4 to 6 in of water, assesses the temperature, and uses the water only for the sitz and not for bathing. If the woman takes a sitz bath, she should release the water, have a helper clean the tub, and draw new water before bathing to prevent infection.

Topical Agents

Topical anesthetics such as Dermoplast aerosol spray and Americaine spray may be used to relieve perineal discomfort. The woman is advised to apply the anesthetic after a sitz bath or perineal care. Witch hazel compresses may be used to relieve perineal discomfort and edema. Nupercainal ointment or Tucks or witch hazel pads may be ordered for relief of both hemorrhoidal and perineal pain. The nurse should emphasize the need for the woman to wash her hands before and after using the topical treatments.

The nurse provides information about the anesthetic spray or topical agent. The woman needs to understand the purpose, use, anticipated effects and benefits, and possible problems associated with the product. The nurse can combine a demonstration of application with teaching. A return demonstration is a useful method of evaluating the woman's understanding.

RELIEF OF HEMORRHOIDAL DISCOMFORT

Some mothers experience hemorrhoidal pain after giving birth. Relief measures include the use of sitz baths, topical anesthetic ointments, rectal suppositories, or witch hazel pads applied directly to the anal area. The woman may be taught to digitally replace external hemorrhoids in her rectum. Handwashing to prevent contamination to the vagina is essential. She may also find it helpful to maintain a side-lying position when possible and to avoid prolonged sitting. The mother is encouraged to maintain an adequate fluid intake, and stool softeners are administered to ensure greater comfort with bowel movements. Mothers should be advised to avoid straining with bowel movements because this can increase the severity and discomfort associated with hemorrhoids. The hemorrhoids usually disappear a few weeks after birth if the woman did not have them before her pregnancy.

RELIEF OF AFTERPAINS

Afterpains are the result of intermittent uterine contractions. A primipara may not experience afterpains because her uterus is able to maintain a contracted state. However, multiparous women and those who have had a multiple-gestation pregnancy or hydramnios frequently experience discomfort from afterpains as the uterus contracts intermittently. Breastfeeding women are also more likely to experience afterpains than formula-feeding women because of the release of oxytocin when the infant suckles.

The nurse can suggest that the woman lie prone, with a small pillow under her lower abdomen, and explain that the discomfort may feel intensified for about 5 minutes but then diminishes greatly if not completely. The prone position applies pressure to the uterus and therefore stimulates contractions. When the uterus maintains a constant contraction, the afterpains cease. Additional nursing interventions include a sitz bath (for warmth), positioning, ambulation, or administration of an analgesic agent. For breastfeeding mothers, an analgesic administered 30 minutes to an hour before nursing helps promote comfort and enhances maternal-infant interaction (Table 31–2).

The nurse provides information about the cause of afterpains and methods to decrease discomfort. She or he explains any medications that are ordered, including their expected effect, benefits, and possible side effects, and any special considerations such as the possibility of dizziness or sleepiness with particular medications.

RELIEF OF DISCOMFORT FROM IMMOBILITY AND MUSCLE STRAIN

Discomfort may be caused by immobility. The woman who has been in stirrups or has pulled back on her legs for an extended period of time may experience muscular aches from such extreme

Table 31–2 Essential Information for Common Postpartum Drugs

TYLENOL No. 3 (300 mg acetaminophen and 30 mg codeine)	
Drug Class: Narcotic analgesic. **Dose/Route:** Usual adult dose: 1 to 2 tablets PO every 4 hours PRN. **Indication:** For relief of mild to moderate pain. **Adverse Effects:** Respiratory depression, apnea, lightheadedness, dizziness, nausea, sweating, dry mouth, constipation, facial flushing, suppression of cough reflex, ureteral spasm, urinary retention, pruritus, hepatotoxicity (overdose). **Nursing Implications:** Determine whether woman is sensitive to acetaminophen or codeine; has history of impaired hepatic or renal function. Monitor bowel sounds, respirations, urine output. Administer with food or after meals if GI upset occurs; encourage woman to drink one full glass (240 mL) with the tablet to reduce the risk of the tablet lodging in the esophagus.	**Client Teaching:** Inform client about name of drug, expected action, possible side effects, that it is secreted in breast milk (*Note:* Some physicians/certified nurse-midwives may avoid ordering this medication for breastfeeding mothers), and review safety measures (assess for dizziness, use side rails, call for assistance when getting out of bed and ambulating, report to nurse any signs of adverse effects); ask if she has any questions. **Nursing Diagnoses Related to Drug Therapy:** *Health-Seeking Behavior* related to information regarding drug therapy *Risk for Injury* related to dizziness secondary to effect of drug *Constipation* related to slowed gastrointestinal activity secondary to effects of medications.
PERCOCET (325 mg acetaminophen and 5 mg oxycodone)	
Drug Class: Narcotic analgesic. **Dose/Route:** 1 to 2 tablets PO every 4 hours PRN. **Indication:** For moderate to moderately severe pain. Can be used in aspirin-sensitive women. **Adverse Effects:** Acetaminophen: Hepatotoxicity, headache, rash, hypoglycemia. Oxycodone: Respiratory depression, apnea, circulatory depression, euphoria, facial flushing, constipation, suppression of cough reflex, ureteral spasm, urinary retention. **Nursing Implications:** Determine whether woman is sensitive to acetaminophen or codeine; has bronchial asthma, respiratory depression, convulsive disorder. Observe woman carefully for respiratory depression if given with barbiturates or sedative/hypnotics. Consider that postcesarean-birth woman may have depressed cough reflex, so teaching and encouragement to deep breathe and cough are needed. Monitor bowel sounds, urine and bowel elimination.	**Client Teaching:** Teaching should include name of drug, expected effect, possible adverse effects, that drug is secreted in the breast milk, encouragement to report any signs of adverse effects immediately. **Nursing Diagnoses Related to Drug Therapy:** *Ineffective Breathing Pattern* related to respiratory depression *Constipation* related to slowed gastrointestinal activity secondary to the effects of medications.

(continued)

Table 31–2 Essential Information for Common Postpartum Drugs—continued

RUBELLA VIRUS VACCINE, LIVE (Meruvax 2)

Dose/Route:
Single-dose vial, inject subcutaneously in outer aspect of the upper arm.
Indication:
Stimulate active immunity against rubella virus. Rubella titer of less than 1:10 or antibody negative on ELISA test.
Adverse Effects:
Burning or stinging at the injection site; about 2 to 4 weeks later may have rash, malaise, sore throat, or headache.
Nursing Implications:
Obtain informed consent. Determine whether woman has sensitivity to neomycin (vaccine contains neomycin); is immunosuppressed, or has received blood transfusions (not to be administered within 3 months of blood transfusion, plasma transfusion, or serum immune globulin). To be given at discharge.

Client Teaching:
Name of drug, expected effect, possible adverse effects, possible comfort measures to use if adverse effects occur; rubella titer will be assessed in about 3 months. Instruct woman to AVOID PREGNANCY FOR 3 MONTHS following vaccination. Provide information regarding contraceptives and their use.
Nursing Diagnoses Related to Drug Therapy:
Deficient Knowledge regarding drug therapy
Health-Seeking Behavior related to information about postpartum contraception regarding an expressed desire to avoid pregnancy following rubella vaccination
Pain related to rash and malaise

RhoGAM (Rh immune globulin specific for D antigen)

Dose/Route:
Postpartum: One vial IM within 72 hours of birth. Antepartal: One vial microdose RhoGAM IM at 28 weeks in Rh-negative women; after amniocentesis, spontaneous or therapeutic abortion, or ectopic pregnancy.
Indication:
Prevention of sensitization to the Rh factor in Rh-negative women and to prevent hemolytic disease in the newborn in subsequent pregnancies (see Chapter 15). Mother must be Rh negative, not previously sensitized to Rh factor. Infant must be Rh positive, direct antiglobulin negative.
Adverse Effects:
Soreness at injection site.
Nursing Implications:
Confirm criteria for administration are present. Ensure correct vial is used for the client (each vial is cross-matched to the specific woman and must be carefully checked).
Inject entire contents of vial.

Client Teaching:
Name of drug, expected action, possible side effects; report soreness at injection site to nurse; woman should carry information regarding Rh status and dates of RhoGAM injections with her at all times; explain use of RhoGAM with subsequent pregnancies.
Nursing Diagnoses Related to Drug Therapy:
Health-Seeking Behavior related to information about future need for Rh immune globulin regarding an expressed desire to understand the long-term implications of her Rh-negative status
Pain related to soreness at injection site

AMBIEN (Zolpidem tartrate)

Drug Class:
Hypnotic, sedative.
Dose/Route:
5 to 10 mg PO at bedtime.
Indication:
Promote sleep.
Adverse Effects:
Dizziness, daytime drowsiness, diarrhea, drugged feelings, amnesia.
Nursing Implications:
Determine if woman has compromised respiratory function. Monitor respirations, blood pressure, pulse. Modify environment to increase relaxation and promote sleep. Monitor for drug interaction if woman is taking other CNS depressants.

Client Teaching:
Name of drug, expected effect, possible adverse effects, safety measures (siderails, use call bell, ask for assistance when out of bed); medication is secreted in breast milk.
Nursing Diagnoses Related to Drug Therapy:
Risk for Injury related to possible ataxia or vertigo
Altered Thought Processes related to drug-induced confusion
Health-Seeking Behavior related to information regarding drug therapy

positioning. It is not unusual for women to experience joint pains and muscular pain in both arms and legs, depending on the effort they exerted during the second stage of labor.

Early ambulation is encouraged to help reduce the incidence of complications such as constipation and thrombophlebitis. It also helps promote a feeling of general well-being. The nurse provides information about ambulation and the importance of monitoring any signs of dizziness or weakness. Assist the woman the first few times she gets up during the postpartal period. Fatigue, effects of medications, loss of blood, and lack of food intake may cause feelings of dizziness or faintness when the woman stands up. Because this may be a problem during the woman's first shower, the nurse should remain in the room, check the woman frequently, and have a chair close by in case she becomes faint. During this first shower the nurse instructs the woman in the use of the emergency call button in the bathroom; she is advised that, if she becomes faint during a future shower, she should sit down and press the call button for assistance immediately.

RELIEF OF DISCOMFORT FROM POSTPARTAL DIAPHORESIS

Postpartal diaphoresis (excessive perspiration) may cause discomfort for new mothers. The nurse can offer a fresh, dry gown and change bed linens to enhance the mother's comfort. Some women may feel refreshed by a shower. For women experiencing hot flashes as a result of changing hormones, a cool shower may be preferable over a warm or hot shower. It is necessary to consider cultural practices and realize that some Hispanic and Asian women prefer to delay showering. Nurses can offer these women a warm or cool washcloth to increase comfort. The nurse provides information about the normal physiologic changes that cause diaphoresis and methods to increase comfort.

Because diaphoresis may also increase thirst, the nurse can offer fluids as the woman desires. Again, the nurse needs to ask the woman about her preferred beverage. Women of western European background may prefer iced drinks, whereas Asian women may prefer hot tea or water at room temperature. It is important to ascertain the woman's wishes rather than operate from one's own values or cultural beliefs.

SUPPRESSION OF LACTATION IN THE NON-BREASTFEEDING MOTHER

For the woman who chooses not to breastfeed, lactation may be suppressed by mechanical inhibition. Although signs of engorgement do not usually appear until the second or third postpartum day, engorgement is best prevented by beginning mechanical methods of lactation suppression as soon as possible after birth. Ideally, this involves having the woman begin wearing a supportive, well-fitting bra within 6 hours after birth. A tight fitting sports bra may be preferred by some women. The bra is worn continuously until lactation is suppressed (usually about 5 to 7 days) and is removed only for showers. The bra provides support and eases the discomfort that can occur with tension on the breasts because of fullness. Ice packs should be applied over the axillary area of each breast for 20 minutes four times daily. This practice should begin soon after birth. In addition, ice is useful in relieving discomfort if engorgement occurs.

The mother is advised to avoid any stimulation of her breasts by her baby, herself, breast pumps, or her sexual partner until the sensation of fullness has passed (usually about 5 to 7 days). Such stimulation increases milk production and delays the suppression process. Heat is avoided for the same reason; therefore, the mother is encouraged to let shower water flow over her back rather than her breasts.

Some mothers may inquire about suppression medications used in the past for non-nursing mothers. Women should be informed that, because of concerns related to side effects, these medications are no longer used. Mechanical, rather than pharmacologic, methods are now employed.

RELIEF OF EMOTIONAL STRESS

The birth of a child, with the changes in role and the increased responsibilities it produces, is a time of emotional stress for the new mother. During the early postpartal period the mother may be emotionally labile, and mood swings and tearfulness are common. Initially the mother may repeatedly discuss her experiences of labor and birth. This allows the mother to integrate her experiences. If she believes that she did not cope well with labor, she may have feelings of inadequacy and may benefit from reassurance that she did well. Some women feel that they did not have any perception of time during the labor and birth and want to know how long it really lasted, or they may not remember the entire experience. In this case, it is helpful for the nurse to talk with the woman and provide the information that she is missing and desires.

During this time the new mother must also adjust to the loss of her fantasized child and accept the child she has borne. This task may be more difficult if the child is not of the desired sex or if he or she has birth defects (see Chapter 28∞). Women who deliver prematurely may experience guilt or have feelings of inadequacy. Immediately after the birth (the taking-in period) the mother is focused on bodily concerns and may not be fully ready to learn about personal and infant care. Following the initial dependent period, the mother becomes very concerned about her ability to be a successful parent (the taking-hold period). During this time the mother requires reassurance that she is effective. She also tends to be receptive to teaching and demonstration designed to assist her in mothering successfully. The depression, weepiness, and "letdown feeling" that characterize the postpartum blues are often a surprise for the new mother. She requires reassurance that these feelings are normal, an explanation of why they occur, and a supportive environment that permits her to cry without feeling guilty.

PROMOTION OF MATERNAL REST AND ACTIVITY

Following childbirth some women feel exhausted and in need of rest. Other women may be euphoric and full of psychic energy, ready to relive and recount the experience of birth repeatedly. The nurse can provide a period for airing of feelings and then encourage a period of rest. Nurses also promote rest by organizing their activities to avoid frequent interruptions for the woman.

RELIEF OF FATIGUE

Physical fatigue often affects other adjustments and functions of the new mother. For example, fatigue can reduce milk flow, thereby increasing problems with establishing breastfeeding. Energy is also needed to make the psychologic adjustments to a new infant and to assume new roles. It is helpful for the new mother to know that fatigue may persist for several weeks or even months. Persistent fatigue is especially common when mothers attempt to perform activities while the baby is napping, instead of resting themselves. Mothers who have other children may feel overwhelmed with trying to meet the needs of their other child(ren) (Hunter, Rychnovsky & Yount, 2009). The nurse teaches women that this practice can lead to chronic fatigue and should be

Developing Cultural Competency

POSTPARTAL RECUPERATION

Most mothers view the postpartal period as a time for recuperation. In many non-Western cultures, the 40 days following the birth are a time of recovery when female relatives or friends assist the new mother in her daily activities (Lin, Wang, & Chang, 2007). In Northern Africa, for example, the 40-day period after birth is considered a time of transition for the mother. The mother and infant are not separated during this time. This practice is known to prevent postpartum psychosis and facilitate bonding (Jones, 2006). This is also the custom in India, where it is believed that the mother and new baby need protection from evil spirits as well as from exposure to illness, because they are both considered vulnerable during this time period (Jones, 2006).

In Mexico, this period is briefer, lasting only 20 days. During the first 7 days, nonhousehold members are not permitted to visit or enter the home. The mother gradually increases activity after the first week. The end of the postpartum period is marked by a *sobada,* a massage performed by the midwife on the 20th day after birth (Spector, 2009).

avoided. Severe ongoing fatigue can also be a symptom of a thyroid disorder and should be evaluated by a clinician. Although most new mothers feel tired, if they have perceived the pregnancy and birth as a natural process, they tend to view themselves as healthy and well. Fatigue can also be a symptom of postpartum depression and should be discussed with the healthcare provider if symptoms continue or are accompanied by other signs of depression.

Specific groups of mothers are at a higher risk for postpartum fatigue. These include mothers of multiples, mothers with infants who are still hospitalized that engage in multiple trips to the hospital to visit their babies, mothers of infants with birth defects or special needs, mothers who lack social support, and mothers who return to work before the advised 6-week time period. A mother who has been on extended bed rest during the pregnancy may also be more at risk for fatigue. Because many families are now geographically separated and may be unable to come and spend time with the mother and new baby, fatigue may also be more common in these women when the mother is left to care for herself and baby in the early postpartum period.

RESUMPTION OF ACTIVITY

Ambulation and activity may gradually increase after birth. The new mother should avoid heavy lifting, excessive stair climbing, and strenuous activity. One or two daily naps are essential and are most easily achieved if the mother sleeps when her baby does. Women with older children often find it difficult to get adequate rest because they want to spend time with their older children when the infant is napping. The woman should be cautioned that fatigue and exhaustion can become a vicious cycle and should be avoided. Assistance in the household can help prevent this and can enable the mother to spend special time with older children while others take over household tasks.

By the second week at home, the woman may resume light housekeeping. Although it is customary to delay returning to work for 6 weeks, most women are physically able to resume practically all activities by 4 to 5 weeks. In some cases, if bleeding returns, it is often a sign that the mother is overdoing her activities and should decrease some activity. Delaying the return to work until after the final postpartal examination minimizes the possibility of problems.

Evidence-Based Nursing

AVOIDING SLEEP DISTURBANCE IN POSTPARTUM PERIOD

Clinical Question

What are the primary ways to avoid sleep disturbance in the postpartum period?

The Evidence

The postpartum period is a stressful and anxious time for the new family. Lack of sleep and fatigue are commonly reported by new parents. Hunter et al. (2009) conducted an integrative review of the literature to determine the current knowledge of postpartum sleep patterns, sleep disturbances, and known strategies for prevention. Qualitative and quantitative studies were reviewed to establish recommendations. Multiple studies from multiple sites provide the strongest level of evidence for practice. Women in the postpartum period slept on average 1.5 to 2 fewer hours per 24 hours than nonpregnant women. More frequent awakenings and a reduction in REM sleep were also reported. During the immediate postpartum period, the hospital provides a disruptive environment, as mothers are awakened for procedures such as vital signs. The most frequently cited cause of sleep disturbance was related to newborn sleep and feeding patterns.

Best Practice

Well postpartum women should be able to safely forego nighttime interruptions by nurses for vital signs and other noncritical procedures. Prenatal education should be provided about the need to plan for adequate rest, and couples should be encouraged to develop proactive strategies based on their individual circumstances. Such strategies might be alternating care of the newborn at night, plans to conserve energy, and realistic expectations of household chores. Recruiting assistance periodically to provide the parents an opportunity to sleep is also a strategy to avoid long-term sleep deprivation. Behavioral sleep interventions such as relaxation techniques and self-care measures can also improve sleep quality and quantity.

Critical Thinking

What are strategies that may be effective for single mothers who must care for their newborn without assistance?

See MyNursingKit for possible responses.

POSTPARTAL EXERCISES

The woman should be encouraged to begin simple exercises while in the birthing unit and to continue them at home. Kegel exercises should be reviewed and begun while the woman is still in the hospital. She is advised that increased lochia or pain means she should reevaluate her activity and make necessary alterations. Most agencies provide a booklet describing suggested postpartal exercises, such as those shown in Figure 31–2 ●. (Exercise routines vary for women undergoing cesarean birth or tubal ligation after childbirth.)

Exercise during the postpartum period has several health benefits for new mothers. Exercise can help maintain insulin and high-density lipoprotein (HDL) cholesterol levels, as well as improve aerobic fitness. The postpartal woman is more likely to have positive views of her well-being, more self-esteem, and less fatigue if she continues to do stretching and her own pattern of exercise after she is home. The addition of pelvic floor exercises can also decrease such problems as urinary leakage or urinary incontinence. Exercise also helps facilitate postpartum weight loss, reduces stress, and provides the mother with needed time alone.

SEXUAL ACTIVITY AND CONTRACEPTION

Typically, postpartum couples resume sexual intercourse once the episiotomy is healed and the lochial flow has stopped (AWHONN, 2006). Because this usually occurs by the end of the third week, before the 6-week check, it is important that the woman and her partner have information about what to expect. The nurse may inform the couple that, because the vaginal vault is "dry" (lacking estrogen), some form of water-soluble lubrication such as K-Y jelly or Astroglide may be necessary during intercourse. The female-superior and side-lying coital positions may be preferable because they allow the woman to control the depth of penile penetration. Couples should be counseled that intercourse may be uncomfortable for the woman for some time and that patience is imperative.

Breastfeeding couples should be forewarned that during orgasm milk may spurt from the nipples because of the release of oxytocin. Some couples find this spurt pleasurable or amusing, but others choose to have the woman wear a bra during sexual activity. Nursing the baby before lovemaking reduces the chance of milk release (Convery & Spatz, 2009).

Other factors may inhibit satisfactory sexual experiences: the baby's crying may "spoil the mood," the woman's changed body may seem unattractive to her or her partner, maternal sleep deprivation may reduce the woman's desire, and the woman's physiologic response to sexual stimulation may be altered because of hormonal changes. By 3 months postpartum, many couples have returned to prepregnant levels of sexual interest and activity; however, this is highly variable. It is not abnormal for women, especially when breastfeeding, to experience decreased libido for several months (Convery & Spatz, 2009). Decreased libido can be associated with hormonal changes, fatigue, stress, and lack of time because of family and work demands.

With anticipatory guidance during the prenatal and postpartal periods, the couple can be forewarned of potential temporary problems. Anticipatory guidance is enhanced if the couple can discuss their feelings and reactions as they are experienced. (See "Teaching Highlights: Resuming Sexual Activity After Childbirth.")

Information on contraception is often provided as part of discharge teaching if it is permissible within the healthcare agency. The nurse can also be an important resource for the woman and her partner during postpartum follow-up. Couples typically choose to use contraception to control the number of children they will have or to determine the spacing of future children. However, some religious-based hospital facilities prohibit nurses and other healthcare providers from discussing contraception. If the nurse is discussing birth control, it is important to emphasize that in choosing a specific method, consistency of use is essential. The nurse needs to identify the advantages, disadvantages, risks, and contraindications of the various methods to help the couple, or the single mother, make an informed choice about the most practical and compatible method. (For a more detailed discussion of contraceptive methods, see Chapter 5.) Breastfeeding women are commonly concerned that a contraceptive method will interfere with their ability to breastfeed. Breastfeeding women should be given available options and choose the method that best fits their lifestyle, financial situation, and personal preference.

Teaching Highlights

RESUMPTION OF SEXUAL ACTIVITY AFTER CHILDBIRTH

- Delay intercourse until no lochia is present because lochia indicates that healing is not yet complete.
- Tenderness of the vagina and perineum may cause discomfort. The partner may test the woman's level of comfort by slipping a lubricated finger inside her vagina. The female-superior and side-lying positions may be preferable because they let the woman control the depth of penetration of the penis.
- Vaginal dryness may occur because the vagina is "hormone poor." It can be avoided by using a water-soluble lubricant.
- Based on the amount of breast engorgement and tenderness present, the partner may need to avoid breast stimulation during foreplay or use a very gentle approach.
- Escape of milk during sexual activity can be minimized by breastfeeding immediately beforehand.
- Fatigue and the new baby's schedule may have a negative impact on the woman's feelings of desire. Napping when the baby sleeps helps decrease fatigue. However, fatigue may be a reality couples need to accept during the early postpartum months.
- Contraception is important even during the early postpartum period. The woman's body needs adequate time to heal and recover from the stress of pregnancy and childbirth. Couples opposed to contraception may choose abstinence at this time.

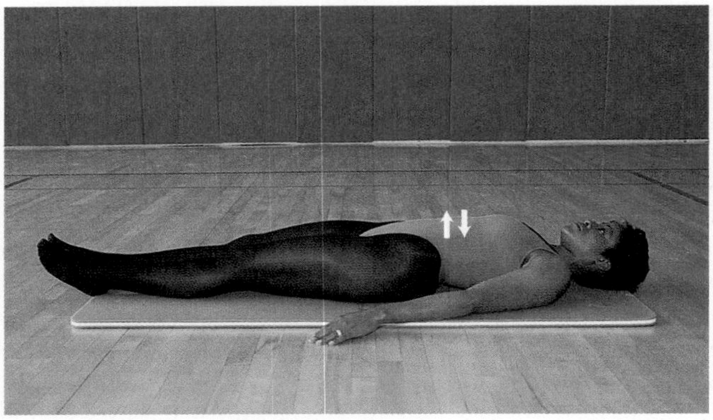

A

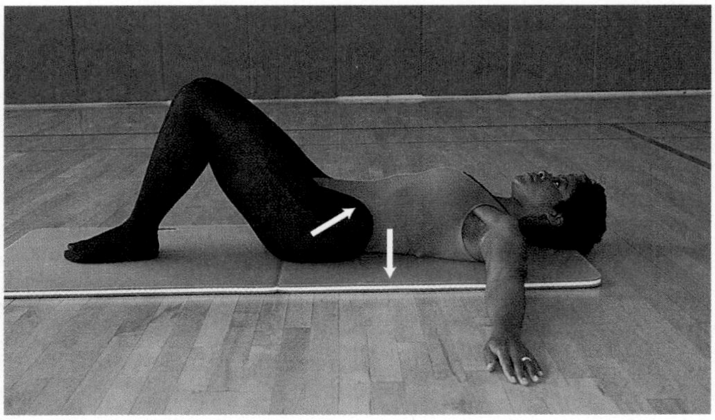

B

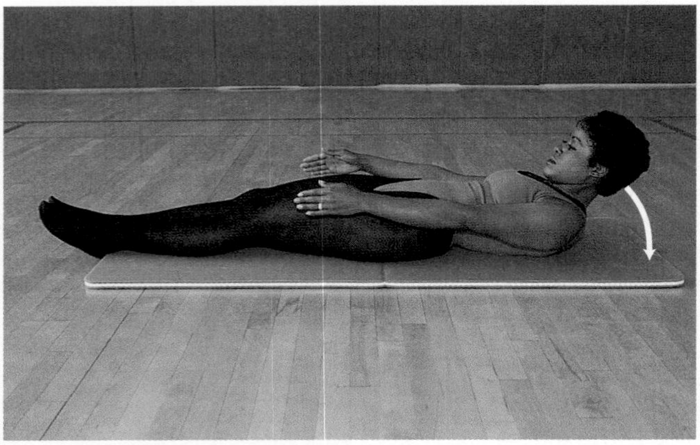

C

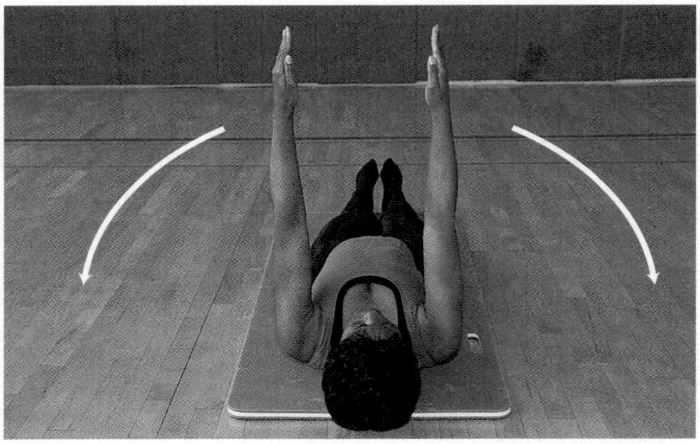

D

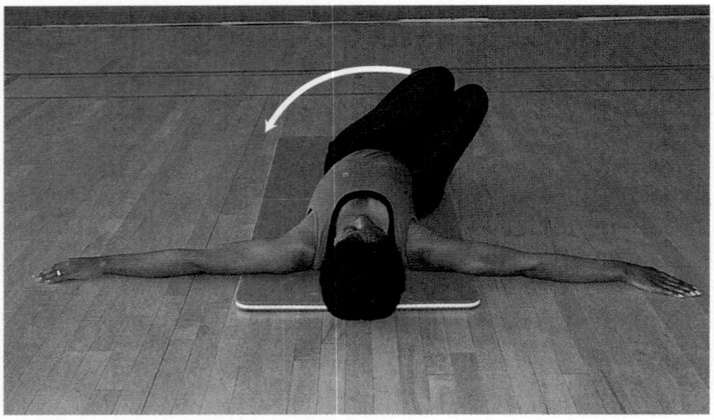

E

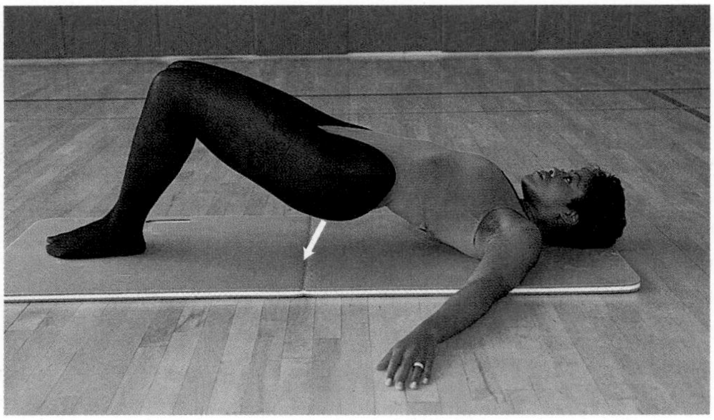

F

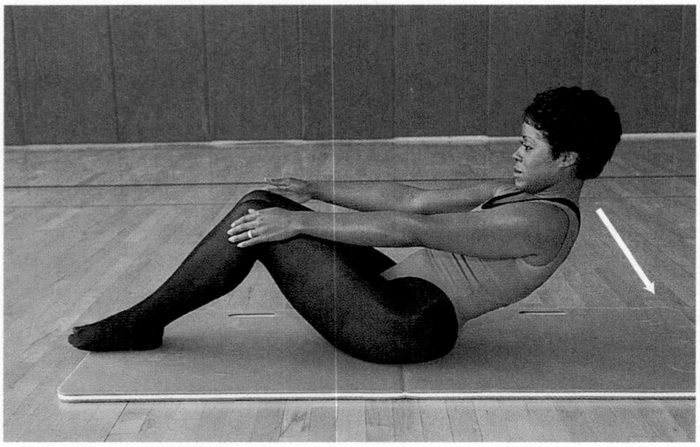

G

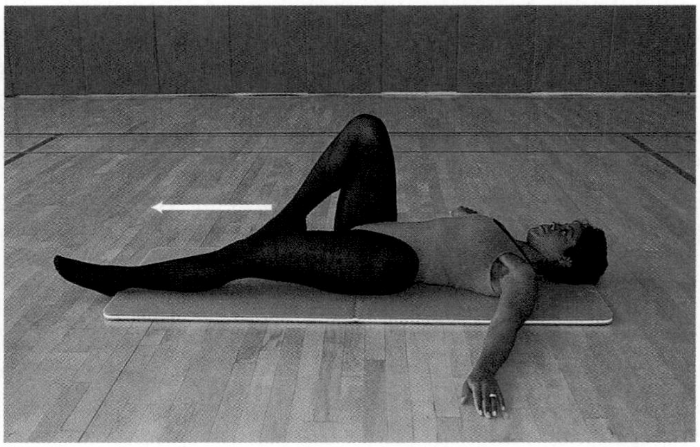

H

● **Figure 31–2** Postpartal exercises. Begin with five repetitions two or three times daily, and gradually increase to 10 repetitions. First day: ***A,*** Abdominal breathing. Lying supine, inhale deeply, using the abdominal muscles. The abdomen should expand. Then exhale slowly through pursed lips, tightening the abdominal muscles. ***B,*** Pelvic rocking. Lying supine with arms at sides, knees bent, and feet flat, tighten abdomen and buttocks, and attempt to flatten back on floor. Hold for a count of 10; then arch the back, causing the pelvis to "rock." On the second day, add ***C,*** Chin to chest. Lying supine with legs straight, raise head and attempt to touch chin to chest. Slowly lower head. ***D,*** Arm raises. Lying supine, arms extended at a 90-degree angle from body, raise arms so that they are perpendicular and hands touch. Lower slowly. On fourth day, add ***E,*** Knee rolls. Lying supine with knees bent, feet flat, arms extended to the side, roll knees slowly to one side, keeping shoulders flat. Return to original position, and roll to opposite side. ***F,*** Buttocks lift. Lying supine, arms at sides, knees bent, feet flat, slowly raise the buttocks, and arch the back. Return slowly to starting position. On sixth day, add ***G,*** Abdominal tighteners. Lying supine, knees bent, feet flat, slowly raise head toward knees. Arms should extend along either side of legs. Return slowly to original position. ***H,*** Knee to abdomen. Lying supine, arms at sides, bend one knee and thigh until foot touches buttocks. Straighten leg and lower it slowly. Repeat with other leg. After 2 to 3 weeks, more strenuous exercises, such as push-ups and side leg raises, may be added as tolerated. Kegel exercises, begun antepartally, should be done many times daily during postpartum to restore vaginal and perineal tone.

Evidence in Action

It is recommended by the Advisory Committee on Immunization Practices that postpartum women should receive Tdap (Reduced Diphtheria Toxoid, and Acellular Pertussis) vaccine if they have not received it earlier (Organizational guideline) (Advisory Committee on Immunization Practices, 2008).

PHARMACOLOGIC INTERVENTIONS

Pharmacologic preparations, including pain medications, vaccinations (rubella and Tdap), and Rh immune globulin, are frequently administered in the postpartal period (see Table 31–2).

PROMOTION OF EFFECTIVE PARENT LEARNING

Meeting the educational needs of the new mother and her family is a primary challenge facing the postpartum nurse. Each woman's educational needs vary based on her age, background, educational level, experience, and expectations. However, because the mother spends only a brief period of time in the postpartal area, identifying and addressing individual instructional needs can be difficult. Effective education provides the childbearing family with sufficient knowledge to meet many of their own health needs and to seek assistance if necessary.

The nurse first assesses the learning needs of the new mother through observation, sensitivity to nonverbal cues, and tactfully phrased questions. For example, "What plans have you made for handling things when you get home?" may elicit a response of several words and may provide the opportunity for some information sharing and guidance. Some agencies also use checklists of common concerns for new mothers. The woman can check the concerns that are of interest to her.

Teaching during the postpartum period is a continuous process in which the nurse takes opportunities throughout interactions with the new parents to identify learning opportunities and offer teaching interventions. The nurse can also plan and implement teaching in a logical, nonthreatening way based on knowledge and respect of the family's cultural values and beliefs. Unless the nurse believes a culturally related activity would be harmful, it can be supported and encouraged.

Nurses need to consider the mother's physical and psychosocial needs when conducting postpartum teaching. Initially, women may be exhausted from the birth experience and their concentration may be impaired. Later, the new mother may be preoccupied with visitors and phone calls. Information should be delivered a little at a time and repeated to make sure that the parents understand what the nurse has discussed with them. Repetition is a valuable tool in the postpartum environment. In addition, many women are discharged during the first 48 hours after birth, making postpartum education difficult (Bernstein, Spino, Finch, et al., 2007). When performing teaching sessions, the father's schedule must also be considered. If the father returns to work during the immediate postpartal period, he may be more likely to attend teaching sessions scheduled in the late afternoon or early evening (Figure 31–3 ●). In some cultures, such as the Hispanic culture, female relatives often assist the new mother and baby. It is important to include any care providers in the teaching session.

Postpartal units use a variety of instructional methods, including handouts, formal classes, videotapes, and individual interaction.

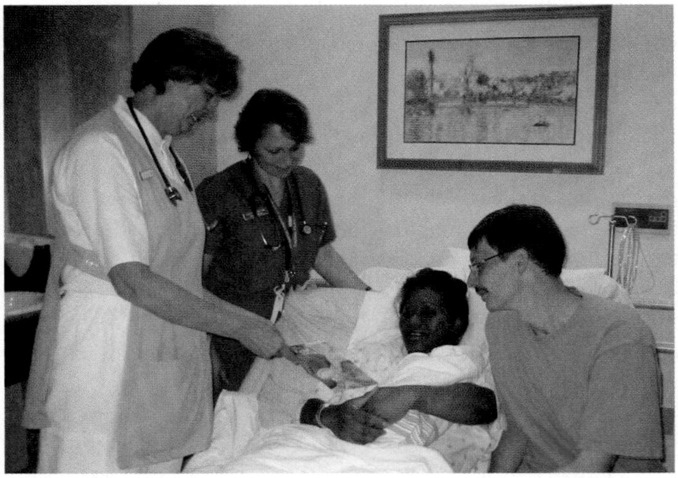

● **Figure 31–3** Postpartum teaching. The nurse provides educational information to both parents.

Printed materials are helpful for new mothers to consult if questions arise at home. Some facilities offer a hotline service that new mothers can call with questions or concerns. As the cultural diversity in the United States continues to grow, the need for culturally sensitive information is imperative. Along with culturally diverse material, teaching aid should be presented in the woman's native language when possible. Written materials should be available and translators or language lines should be utilized. Many clients are now accustomed to using the Internet and may prefer to use online support groups and access educational materials found online. As technology expands, the nurse must remain current with the changing technology and the resources it creates. Evaluation of learning may also take several forms: return demonstrations, question-and-answer sessions, and even formal evaluation tools. Follow-up phone calls after discharge provide additional evaluative information and continue the helping process for the family.

Teaching content should include information on role changes and psychologic adjustments as well as skills. Risk factors and signs of postpartum depression should be reviewed with all women. Information is also essential for women with specialized educational needs such as the mother who has had a cesarean birth, the parents of twins, the parents of an infant with congenital anomalies, parents with other young children, parents with a child that will require long-term hospitalization, and so on. Because more and more women with disabilities are now having children, they may require additional support and education. Anticipatory guidance can help prepare parents for the many changes they will experience with a new family member.

PROMOTION OF FAMILY WELLNESS

A positive maternity experience is likely to have a positive effect on the entire family. The family that receives appropriate information and has adequate time to interact with its newest member in a supportive environment will feel more comfortable and secure at home.

Today most facilities support *family-centered care* that is focused on keeping the mother and baby together as much as the mother desires. This type of care is called **mother-baby care**, or **couplet care**, and provides increased opportunities for parent-child interaction because the newborn shares the mother's room and they are cared for together. Mother-baby care enables the mother to have time to bond with her baby and learn to care for her or him in a supportive environment. It is especially conducive to a hunger-demand feeding schedule for both breast- and formula-feeding babies. This arrangement also allows the father, siblings, grandparents, and others to participate in the care of the new baby. Women who give birth in a facility that offers mother-baby care are often more satisfied with their postpartum experience than women who are cared for under different care models. The World Health Organization (WHO) advocates for a "rooming-in" model of care where the mother and infant remain together as much as possible (WHO, 2007).

Mother-baby unit policies must be flexible enough to permit the mother to return the baby to the nursery if she finds it necessary because of fatigue or physical discomfort. Some mother-baby units also return the newborns to a central nursery at night so the mothers can get more rest.

Nursing Practice

Because siblings may feel left out with the addition of a new family member, provide positive feedback to promote attachment. For example, pointing out to the older child that "Carlos is looking at you" or asking, "Do you think he knows you're his big sister?" can help make siblings feel accepted and valued. Also identify ways in which siblings can help the new mother, for example, by bringing her a cup of water or singing the baby a favorite lullaby.

REACTIONS OF SIBLINGS

Mother-baby care provides excellent opportunities for family bonds to grow when the mother, father/partner, newborn, and siblings begin functioning as a family unit immediately after the birth. When mother-baby care is not available, liberal sibling visitation policies can meet the family's needs. A visit to the mother-baby unit reassures children that their mother is well and still loves them. It also provides an opportunity for the children to become familiar with the new baby. For the mother, the pangs of separation are lessened as she interacts with her children and introduces them to the newest family member (Figure 31–4 ●). Even infants who require intensive care nursery admissions should be allowed to have sibling visits whenever possible. Although there is a valid concern to prevent preemies and other infants who require intensive care services from infection, policies that involve taking the child's temperature before each visit and documenting the child's health status can provide a safeguard that still promotes family bonding. Some of these infants may be hospitalized for weeks or months. Sibling visitation allows the early incorporation of the infant into the family unit for siblings.

Teach parents that, although they may have prepared their children for the presence of a new brother or sister, the actual

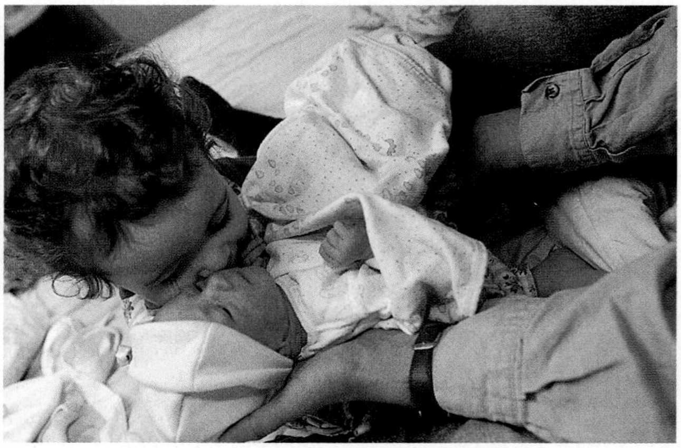

● **Figure 31–4** Siblings and the newborn. The sister of this newborn becomes acquainted with the new family member during a nursing assessment.

arrival of the infant in the home requires some adjustments. Although it may be more chaotic for the parents, allowing the children to come to the hospital to pick up mom and the new baby can signify their importance in the family process. If small children are waiting at home, it is helpful if the father carries the baby inside. This practice keeps the mother's arms free to hug and touch her older children. Many mothers bring a doll home with them for an older child. Caring for the doll alongside the mother or father helps the child to identify with the parents. This identification helps decrease anger and the need to regress for attention.

Parents may also provide supervised times when older children can hold the new baby and perhaps even help with a feeding or diapering. Many parents may have concerns about the children "hurting" the new baby, but with proper supervision, the siblings are more likely to develop an attachment to their new sibling. The other children feel a sense of accomplishment and learn tenderness and caring. The nurse also suggests that parents spend one-to-one quality time with each of their older children each day. This may require some careful planning, but it confirms the parents' continuing love for the other children and promotes their acceptance of the newborn.

PARENT-INFANT ATTACHMENT

Nursing interventions to enhance the quality of parent-infant attachment should be designed to promote feelings of well-being, comfort, and satisfaction. Certain groups of women are at higher risk for alterations in parent-infant attachment. These include women who have less than a ninth-grade education; are unemployed, single, or unmarried; have a previous history of depression or psychologic problems; gave birth to a female infant; or had an infant admission into the neonatal intensive care nursery (Conde, Figueiredo, Costa, et al., 2008). These mothers warrant additional assessment and support from the nurse to ensure proper bonding is taking place.

Some parents may lack any experience with babies and may feel overwhelmed by the infant. Bonding is a series of steps in which the mother and infant develop a realtionship. Although certain medical interruptions can delay bonding, such as when an extremely premature infant is hospitalized for a prolonged period of time, bonding still takes place.

Following are some suggestions for ways of promoting parent-infant attachment during the postpartal stay:

- Determine the parenting style and goals of the infant's mother and father/partner and adapt them when possible in planning nursing care for the family. This includes giving the parents choices about their initial time with their new infant.
- Provide time and as much privacy as possible for the new family to become acquainted. Allow siblings to visit throughout the postpartal stay if requested by the parents.
- Arrange the healthcare setting so that the individual nurse-client relationship can be developed. A primary nurse can develop rapport and assess the mother's strengths and needs.
- Use anticipatory guidance to prepare the parents for expected problems of adjustment. Model appropriate behaviors based on the infant's cues and behaviors.
- Include parents in any nursing intervention, planning, and evaluation. Give choices when possible.
- Initiate and support measures to alleviate fatigue in the parents.
- Help parents identify, understand, and accept both positive and negative feelings related to the overall parenting experience.
- Support and assist parents in determining the personality and unique needs of their infant.

The beginnings of parent-newborn attachment may be observed in the first few hours after birth. Continued assessments may occur during the postpartal stay and in home visits after discharge. As the nurse assesses attachment, it is important to remember that cultural values, beliefs, and practices will direct the childcare activities and self-care practices. For example, some women of Mexican American and Southeast Asian descent may deflect compliments directed toward their baby because of their belief that they may attract the attention of evil spirits. (See Table 31–3 for behaviors related to attachment.)

NURSING CARE FOLLOWING CESAREAN BIRTH

After a cesarean birth the new mother has postpartal needs similar to those of women who have given birth vaginally. Because she has undergone major abdominal surgery, however, the woman's nursing care needs are also similar to those of other surgical clients.

PROMOTION OF MATERNAL PHYSICAL WELL-BEING AFTER CESAREAN BIRTH

The chances of pulmonary infection are increased because of immobility after the use of narcotics and sedatives and because of the altered immune response in postoperative clients. Therefore, the woman is encouraged to cough and deep breathe every 2 to 4 hours while awake until she is ambulating frequently. Leg exercises are also encouraged every 2 hours until the woman is ambulating. These exercises increase circulation, help prevent thrombophlebitis, and also aid intestinal motility by tightening abdominal muscles.

Early ambulation, eating a low roughage diet shortly after birth, and breastfeeding or infant feeding soon after birth all enhance the recovery of the mother and decrease complications in the postoperative period. Even though a cesarean birth is an operative procedure, most women giving birth are relatively healthy and therefore are less likely to experience postoperative complications when compared with other surgical clients.

The nurse monitors and manages the woman's pain experience during the postpartum period. Sources of pain include incisional pain, gas pain, referred shoulder pain, periodic uterine

Table 31–3 Parent Attachment Behaviors

Assessment Area	Attachment	Behavior Requiring Assessment and Information
Caretaking	Talks with baby. Demonstrates and seeks eye-to-eye contact. Touches and holds baby. Changes diapers when needed. Baby is clean. Clothing is appropriate for room temperature. Feeds baby as needed and baby is gaining weight. Positions baby comfortably and checks on baby.	Does not refer to baby. Completes activities without addressing the baby or looking at the baby. Lack of interaction. Does not recognize need for or demonstrate concern for baby's comfort or needs. Feeding occurs intermittently. Baby does not gain weight. Waits for baby to cry and then hesitates to respond.
Perception of the baby	Has knowledge of expected child development. Understands that the baby is dependent and cannot meet parent's needs. Accepts sex of child and characteristics.	Has unrealistic expectations of the baby's abilities and behaviors. Expects love and interaction from the baby. Believes that the baby will fulfill parent's needs. Is strongly distressed over sex of baby or feels that some aspect of the baby is unacceptable.
Support	Has friends who are available for support. Seems to be comfortable with being a parent. Has realistic beliefs of parenting role.	Is alone or isolated. Is on edge, tense, anxious, and hesitant with the baby. Demonstrates difficulty incorporating parenting with own wants and needs.

Note: These are a few of the behaviors that may be associated with attachment. It is vitally important for the nurse to observe the parents on more than one occasion and to take into consideration individual characteristics, values, beliefs, and customs.

contractions (afterbirth pains), discomfort related to breastfeeding, and pain from voiding, defecation, or constipation.

Nursing interventions are oriented toward preventing or alleviating pain or helping the woman cope with pain. The nurse should undertake the following measures:

- Administer analgesics as needed, especially during the first 24 to 72 hours after childbirth. Use of analgesics relieves the woman's pain and enables her to be more mobile and active. Some facilities administer ibuprofen on a continuous basis in the early postpartum period to decrease swelling, reduce pain, and decrease the need for, or frequency of, narcotic agents.
- Promote comfort through proper positioning, frequent position changes, massage, back rubs, oral care, and the reduction of noxious stimuli such as noise and unpleasant odors.
- Encourage visits by significant others, including the newborn and older children. These visits distract the woman from the painful sensations and help reduce her fear and anxiety.
- Encourage the use of breathing, relaxation, guided imagery, and distraction (e.g., stimulation of cutaneous tissue) techniques taught in childbirth preparation class.

Epidural analgesia administered just after the cesarean birth is an effective method of pain relief for most women in the first 24 hours following birth (see "Drug Guide: Postpartum Epidural Morphine").

The physician may order **patient-controlled analgesia (PCA)**. With this approach the woman is given a bolus of analgesia, usually morphine or fentanyl, at the beginning of therapy. Using a special intravenous (IV) pump system, the woman presses a button to self-administer small doses of the medication as needed. For safety, the pump is preset with a time lockout so that the woman cannot deliver another dose until a specified period of time has elapsed. The use of a PCA helps women feel a greater sense of control and less dependence on nursing staff. The frequent, smaller doses help the woman experience rapid pain relief without grogginess and avoid the discomfort associated with injections.

Another technique of pain control that is sometimes used is the **continuous epidural infusion (CEI)** technique, in which the epidural catheter is left in place following the cesarean birth and medication is continually administered via an electric pump. The device also has a button that the woman can depress if additional pain relief is needed. Fentanyl is the most commonly used drug because it tends to provide good pain relief (Viscusi, 2008). Nursing assessments are hourly for women with a CEI in place and include vital signs, level of pain, amount of drug received, and amount of self-administration. The tubing is inspected to ensure connections are maintained because movement by the woman in bed could disrupt the line. The epidural site should also be assessed to ensure the catheter has not been displaced.

Another technique used for pain control for post-cesarean birth is the use of a continuous peripheral nerve block that delivers a local anesthetic through a tiny catheter that is positioned directly into the wound site. An external balloon allows medication to be delivered at a steady rate up to 5 days after the birth and creates a numbing effect at the incision site. After a specified time period, the catheter is displaced by gently pulling it from the site. Additional surgical intervention is not required to remove the device. The use of one of these devices can reduce the amount of

Drug Guide

POSTPARTUM EPIDURAL MORPHINE

Overview of Obstetric Action

Epidural morphine is used to provide relief of pain associated with cesarean birth, extensive episiotomies (mediolaterals), or third- and fourth-degree lacerations. Epidural morphine pain relief results directly from its effect on the opiate receptors in the spinal cord (it depresses pain impulse transmission). Morphine binds opiate receptors, thereby altering both the perception of and emotional response to pain. Women experience little or no discomfort or pain during recovery and for up to 24 hours afterward. There is no motor or sympathetic block or associated hypotension. Onset of analgesia is slower, but duration is longer.

Route, Dosage, and Frequency

Morphine (5 to 7.5 mg) is injected through a catheter into the epidural space, providing pain relief for about 24 hours (Wilson et al., 2010).

Maternal Contraindications

Allergy to morphine, narcotic addiction, chronic debilitating respiratory disease, infection at the injection site, or administration of parenteral corticosteroids in past 14 days (Wilson et al., 2010).

Maternal Side Effects

Late-onset respiratory depression (rare but may occur 8 to 12 hours after administration), nausea and vomiting (occurring between 4 and 7 hours after injection), itching (begins within 3 hours and lasts up to 10 hours), urinary retention, and rarely somnolence. Side effects can be managed with naloxone.

Neonatal Effects

No adverse effects because medication is injected after the birth of the baby.

Nursing Considerations

- Obtain history: sensitivity (allergy) to morphine, presence of any contraindications (Wilson et al., 2010).
- Assess orientation, reflexes, skin color, texture, breath sounds, presence of lesions or infection over area of lumbar spine, voiding pattern, urinary output within normal limits (Wilson et al., 2010).
- Monitor and evaluate analgesic effect. Ask client about comfort level and notify anesthesiologist of inadequate pain relief.
- Check catheter for obvious knots, breaks, and leakage at insertion site and catheter hub.
- Assess for pruritus (scratching and rubbing, especially around face and neck).
- Administer comfort measures for narcotic-induced pruritus, such as lotion, backrubs, cool/warm packs, or diversional activities. If the itching can be tolerated, naloxone should be avoided, especially because it counteracts the pain relief.
- If allergic reaction (urticaria, edema, or respiratory difficulties) occurs, administer naloxone or diphenhydramine per physician order.
- Provide comfort measures for nausea/vomiting, such as frequent oral hygiene or gradual increase of activity; administer naloxone, trimethobenzamide (Tigan), or metoclopramide HCl per physician order.
- Assess postural blood pressure and heart rate before ambulation.
- Assist client with her first ambulation and then as needed.
- Assess respiratory function every hour for 24 hours, then q2–8 hr as needed. Also assess level of consciousness and mucous membrane color. May need to monitor client via apnea monitor for 24 hours.
- Monitor urinary output and assess bladder for distention. Assist client to void.

systemic analgesia that is needed in the postpartum period (Gucev, Yasui, Chang, et al., 2008). Most recently, ultrasound guidance has been utilized to produce better pain relief results (Gucev et al., 2008). Although these devices are not widely used, they can be an option for a woman undergoing a cesarean birth.

Although the use of general anesthesia continues to decline, women who receive general anesthesia warrant additional assessments in the immediate postpartum period. Vital signs should be monitored continually until the woman has regained consciousness. Cardiopulmonary equipment should be in close range with cardiac monitoring available as needed. The pulse oximeter should be used to determine the woman's oxygen status.

If a general anesthetic was used, abdominal distention may produce marked discomfort for the woman during the first few postpartal days. Measures to prevent or minimize abdominal distention include leg exercises, abdominal tightening, ambulation, avoiding carbonated or very hot or cold beverages, and avoiding the use of straws. Women can be started on a low-residue diet within 6 hours of birth (Göçmen, Göçmen, & Saraoğlu, 2002). Medical intervention for gas pain includes using rectal suppositories and enemas to stimulate passage of flatus and stool and encouraging the woman to lie on her left side. Lying on the left side allows the gas to pass from the descending colon to the sigmoid colon so that it can be expelled more readily.

Many physicians also order a nonsteroidal anti-inflammatory drug (NSAID) in addition to the previously mentioned agents once the woman is tolerating oral fluids well. NSAIDs assist with decreasing inflammation and do not have the negative side effects associated with many narcotics, such as sedation and constipation. NSAIDs are often given in combination with narcotic agents in the immediate postpartum period and often result in a decreased intake of narcotic agents.

Sometimes women who have a cesarean birth have other discomforts that can be relieved with pharmacologic interventions.

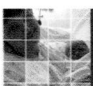

The nurse assesses the woman for other symptoms, such as nausea, itching (which is typically related to the morphine used in the epidural), and headache. If the woman is experiencing nausea, an antiemetic can be administered. Itching can also be relieved with pharmacologic interventions. NSAIDs are effective in managing headaches and other body aches.

The nurse can minimize discomfort and promote satisfaction as the mother assumes the activities of her new role. Instruction and assistance in assuming comfortable positions when holding or breastfeeding the infant will do much to increase the mother's sense of competence and comfort. The woman should be taught to splint her incision when she ambulates to decrease pulling on the incision and the discomfort created by contraction of the abdominal muscles.

Other measures are aimed at other needs that are unique to the woman who has had an operative birth. These include (AWHONN, 2006):

- Assessing the consistency of the abdomen. Women with a firm, distended abdomen may be having difficulty passing flatus or stool.
- Assessment of the intravenous (IV) site, flow rate, and patency of the IV tubing.
- Monitoring the condition of surgical dressings or the incision site using the REEDA scale (redness, edema, ecchymosis, discharge, and approximation of the suture line) along with skin temperature at and around the incision line.

The cesarean birth mother usually does extremely well postoperatively. Most women are ambulating by the day after the surgery. Usually by the second postpartal day the woman can shower, which seems to provide a mental as well as physical lift. Most women are discharged by the third day after birth.

PROMOTION OF PARENT-INFANT INTERACTION AFTER CESAREAN BIRTH

Many factors associated with cesarean birth may hinder successful and frequent parent-infant interaction. These factors include the physical condition of the mother and newborn and maternal reactions to stress, anesthesia, and medications. The father or significant other may be concerned about the mother and preoccupied with her condition, resulting in less interaction with the newborn. The mother and her infant may be separated after birth because of birthing unit routines, prematurity, or neonatal complications or a birth defect. A healthy infant born by uncomplicated cesarean is no more fragile than one born vaginally.

In some cases, signs of depression, anger, or withdrawal may indicate a grief response to the loss of the fantasized birth experience. Fathers as well as mothers may experience feelings of "missing out," guilt, or even jealousy toward another couple who had a vaginal birth. The cesarean birth couple may need the opportunity to tell their story repeatedly to work through these feelings. The nurse can provide factual information about their situation and support the couple's effective coping behaviors. The nurse should acknowledge their feelings while emphasizing the importance of a healthy birth outcome. Enhanced communication during the labor, birth, and in the immediate period along with specific teaching related to issues regarding a cesarean birth are associated with less maternal distress and improved satisfaction with the birth experience (Porter, van Teijlingen, Chi Ying Yip, et al., 2007). It is also important to remember that some women may feel more comfortable with a cesarean birth and may have requested a primary or repeat cesarean birth (Wiklund, Edman, & Andolf, 2007). During the initial taking-in phase, the new parents are processing their new role and may be nurturing themselves and each other. This is normal and expected.

By the second or third day the cesarean birth mother moves into the "taking-hold" period and is usually receptive to learning how to care for herself and her infant. During this period, the focus shifts from the mother and father/partner to the baby. Vulnerability can occur during this period and the parents may feel overwhelmed. The need for nursing intervention to guide the new parents is essential. Special emphasis should be given to home management. The nurse can encourage the mother to let others assume responsibility for housekeeping and cooking. Fatigue not only prolongs recovery but also interferes with breastfeeding and mother-infant interaction, increases the risk of prolonged postpartum blues, and leads to feelings of being overwhelmed.

The presence of the father or significant other during the birth process positively influences the woman's perception of the birth event. The partner's presence reduces the woman's fears, enhances her sense of control, and enables the couple to share feelings and respond to each other with touch and eye contact. Later, they have the opportunity to relive the experience and fill in any gaps or missing pieces. The presence of the father or significant other is especially valuable if the mother has had general anesthesia. The partner can take pictures, hold the baby, and foster the discovery process by directing the mother's attention to the details of the newborn. Sometimes, during the taking-hold phase, the father/partner can feel neglected or excluded. This will soon pass as the letting-go stage begins. During this transition, the family incorporates the baby into the family unit and other family members, such as grandparents and siblings, get to know the baby and be included in the new family routine.

The infant born by cesarean is typically removed from the operating room before the mother is able to hold the newborn. Separation of the family unit is not medically necessary unless the infant needs to be stabilized or there is a complication occurring in the operating room. The practice is typically historical in na-

Thinking Critically

REPEAT CESAREAN

You walk in and find Dana Sullivan, a 29-year-old G2P2, crying 48 hours after a repeat cesarean birth. She states, "I'm not ready to go home. With my first baby they made me go home after 2 days. Can they make me again?"

See MyNursingKit for possible responses.

ture. Agencies that embrace family-centered care can advocate to keep the mother-baby couple together as much as possible. The nurse can play a crucial role in facilitating interaction by encouraging the father or support person to stand beside the warmer and interact with the infant. Often, the infant can be given to the father or support person to hold. The father or support person can hold the infant close to the mother and place the infant against the mother's cheek so direct eye contact can occur. The nurse can also arrange for the infant to stay with the parents in the recovery area in the immediate postoperative period. This gives the family time to interact when the infant is in an alert state.

Often new parents perceive the parenting role as an extension of the childbearing role. Inability to fulfill expected childbearing behavior (vaginal birth) may lead to parental feelings of role failure and frustration. If the parents' attitude is more positive than negative, successful resolution of subsequent stressful events is more likely. The nurse can help families alter their negative definitions of cesarean birth and bolster and encourage positive perceptions.

NURSING CARE OF THE POSTPARTAL ADOLESCENT

The adolescent mother may have special postpartal needs, depending on her level of maturity and support system. The nurse needs to assess maternal-infant interaction, roles of support people, plans for discharge, knowledge of childrearing, and plans for follow-up care. It is imperative that a community health service contact the adolescent shortly after discharge.

Contraception counseling is an important part of teaching. The incidence of repeat pregnancies during adolescence is high. The younger the adolescent, the more likely she is to become pregnant again. Nurses should be aware of the state laws that govern their jurisdiction in order to determine if providing contraception without parental consent is allowed. In states where adolescents can obtain birth control without parental consent, it is often more comfortable for the adolescent to address these issues without others present (see Chapter 13∞). Adolescents may encounter obstacles when attempting to obtain contraceptives. These may include embarrassment about discussing the topic; concerns about confidentiality, such as not wanting their parents to know or having to give permission; and lack of knowledge regarding available methods (Lemay, Cashman, Elfenbein, et al., 2007). Nurses can play a key role in overcoming these obstacles by providing teaching and referrals that address these barriers.

The nurse has many opportunities for teaching the adolescent about her newborn in the postpartal unit. Because the nurse is a role model, the manner in which she handles the newborn greatly influences the young mother. If he is present, the father should be included in as much of the teaching as possible. If the grandparents are going to take an active role in caring for the infant, they should also be included in teaching *if* desired by the new mother.

As with older parents, a newborn examination done at the bedside gives adolescents information about their baby's health and shows possible positions for handling the baby. The nurse can also use this time to provide information about newborn and infant behavior. Parents who have some idea of what to expect from their infant are less frustrated with the newborn's behavior.

The adolescent mother appreciates positive feedback about her newborn and her developing maternal responses. Praise and encouragement will increase her confidence and self-esteem. Young mothers with low self-esteem, family conflict, and few social supports are more likely to encounter postpartum depression (Reid & Meadows-Oliver, 2007). Careful assessment of these factors should be made during the postpartum so appropriate referrals can be provided before discharge.

Group classes for adolescent mothers should include information about infant care skills, such as taking the baby's temperature, clearing the nose and mouth, monitoring growth and development, feeding the infant, providing well-baby care, and identifying danger signals in the ill newborn. These classes can also address unique needs of teen mothers, such as peer relationships, added responsibilities, and goal setting.

Ideally, teenage mothers should visit adolescent clinics for assessment of themselves and their newborn for several years after birth. In this way, the adolescent's enrollment in classes on parenting, need for vocational guidance, and school attendance can be supported and followed closely. School systems' classes for young mothers are an excellent way of helping adolescents finish school and learn how to parent at the same time. Some public high schools have on-site childcare centers to assist with childcare needs and to provide an opportunity for adolescents to learn important child development principles and childcare tasks.

NURSING CARE OF THE WOMAN WHO RELINQUISHES HER INFANT

Women who choose to give their infants up for adoption typically are single, white, never-married adolescents. It is much less common in black and Hispanic cultures to consider adoption. The majority of young women who relinquish their children have higher education and income levels, higher future educational or career goals, and mothers and fathers that favor adoption. Less than 1% of all births in the United States result in an adoption (Child Welfare Information Gateway, 2005). Still others may feel that they are not emotionally ready for the responsibilities of parenthood, or their partner may strongly disapprove of the pregnancy. These and many other reasons may prompt the woman to relinquish her baby.

Some mothers are forced to relinquish their infants because of lifestyle choices such as illicit drug use, past history of abusing children, and incarceration. The number of infants that are placed for adoption because of these circumstances is unknown. Many of these infants may be placed with relatives or in the foster care system. Several factors must be met, including clear evidence that the parent is unfit and that severing the parental rights are in the best interest of the child (Child Welfare Information Gateway, 2007a).

Starting in 1997, Infant Safe Haven Acts were enacted to protect newborns from death caused by abandonment; provide a means for a mother to place her baby up for adoption anonymously; and to ensure that relinquished babies are left with safe providers who can care for them and provide medical services. The relinquishing mother is protected from prosecution for neglect or abandonment under the law (Child Welfare Information Gateway, 2007b).

Surrogacy is also becoming more common in the United States, resulting in relinquishment agreements that may not show up in the adoption statistics. Even though the mother has entered a legal agreement to give up the child she is carrying, she still faces grief issues. The mother who chooses to let her child be adopted usually experiences intense ambivalence. Several factors contribute to this ambivalence. First, there are social pressures against giving up one's child. Additionally, the woman has usually made considerable adjustments in her lifestyle to carry and give birth to this child, and may be unaware of the growing bond between her and her child. Her attachment feelings may peak upon seeing her baby. At the same time, she may not have told friends and relatives about the pregnancy and so may lack a support system to help her work through her feelings and support her decision making. After childbirth, the mother needs to complete a grieving process to work through her loss and its accompanying grief, loneliness, guilt, and other feelings. Mothers who relinquish their infants and have open adoptions experience less grief than those who have closed adoptions (Henney, Ayers-Lopez, McCoy, et al., 2007).

When the relinquishing mother is admitted to the birthing unit, the nurse should be informed about the mother's decision to relinquish the baby. The nurse needs to respect any special requests for the birth and encourage the woman to express her emotions. After the birth the mother should have access to the baby; she will decide whether she wants to see the newborn. Seeing the newborn often aids the grieving process and provides an opportunity for the birthmother to say goodbye. When the mother sees her baby, she may feel strong attachment and love. The nurse needs to assure the woman that these feelings do not mean that her decision to relinquish the child is wrong; relinquishment is often a painful act of love (Henney et al., 2007).

Postpartal nursing care also includes arranging ongoing care for the relinquishing mother. Some mothers may request an early discharge or a transfer to another medical unit. When possible, the nurse supports these requests.

PREPARATION FOR DISCHARGE

In preparation for discharge, the nurse evaluates the mother and newborn's progress toward identified outcomes and provides discharge teaching.

MyNursingKit Discharge Teaching Checklist

DISCHARGE CRITERIA

Ideally, preparation for discharge begins the moment a woman is admitted to the birthing unit. Before discharge, the nurse assesses the mother's physical and psychologic condition, the newborn's adjustment to extrauterine life, the family's overall adjustment, and the need for outside resources. Nursing efforts should be directed toward assessing the parents' knowledge, expectations, and beliefs and then providing anticipatory guidance and teaching accordingly. Because teaching is one of the primary responsibilities of the postpartum nurse, many agencies have elaborate teaching programs and videos. The nurse should spend time with the parents to determine if they have any last-minute questions. A sample postpartal discharge teaching checklist is found on MyNursingKit. In general, the following criteria should be assessed and met before discharge:

- Normal vital signs
- Appropriate involution of the uterus
- Appropriate amount of lochia without evidence of infection
- Knowledge of signs of infection
- Episiotomy or laceration well approximated with a decrease in edema or bruising
- Ability to perform pericare and apply medications to perineal or anal area if ordered
- Ability to void and pass flatus (some facilities' criteria may include having a bowel movement before discharge)
- Ability to take fluids and foods without difficulty
- Ability to care for self and newborn
- Has received rubella vaccine or RhoGAM if indicated (see Table 31–2) (Bruhn & Tillett, 2009)

Additional outcomes for the cesarean birth mother include the following:

- States in own words the reason for the cesarean birth
- Maintains desired pain control
- Maintains moderate mobility level

Ensuring that the woman has met the criteria before discharge decreases the incidence of complications or readmission in the postpartum period.

DISCHARGE TEACHING

In general, discharge teaching includes at least the following information and maternal activities:

1. Review of literature and videos the woman has received or viewed that explains recommended postpartum exercises, the need for adequate rest, the need to avoid overexertion initially, and the recommendation to abstain from sexual intercourse until lochia has ceased. (If the family desires information about birth control methods, the nurse can provide such information at this time.)
2. Information geared to the specific nutritional needs of breastfeeding or formula-feeding mothers. (If the mother has been receiving vitamins and/or iron supplements, the nurse encourages her to continue until the first postpartal examination.) Demonstrates proper breastfeeding techniques and breast care or describes formula preparation, formula-feeding techniques, and nonlactating breast care.
3. How to provide basic care for the infant; when to anticipate that the cord will fall off; when the infant can have a tub bath; when the infant will need her or his first immunizations; and so on. (Parents should also be comfortable feeding and handling the baby, and should

practice basic principes of safety, including the need to use a car seat when the infant is in a car.) See more detailed discussion later in the home care section.

4. Procedure for obtaining copies of her infant's birth certificate.
5. When to schedule the first appointment for her postpartal examination and for her newborn's first well-baby examination.
6. Signs of possible complications (see Table 31–4) and encouragement for the woman to contact her caregiver if she develops any of them. Signs and symptoms that indicate possible problems in the infant and who the parents should contact about them.
7. Information on local agencies and/or support groups, such as La Leche League, Mothers of Twins, adolescent groups, or new mother support groups, that might be of particular assistance to the family. Displays appropriate interaction with baby. Identifies the symptoms of postpartum depression and available resources.
8. Phone number of the mother-baby unit or information hotline and encouragement to call if she has any questions or concerns. Plans for home care visits so that the parents know when to expect the visit and what it entails.

The nurse can also use this final opportunity to reassure the couple of their ability to be successful parents. The nurse can stress the infant's need to feel loved and secure and urge parents to talk to each other and work together to solve any problems that arise.

CONSIDERATIONS FOR FOLLOW-UP CARE

In 1998, the Newborns' and Mothers' Health Protection Act went into effect. This federal law ensures that all insurance companies cover a 48-hour stay for vaginal deliveries and a 96-hour stay for women who have undergone a cesarean birth (United States Department of Labor, 2009). In consideration of the risks associated with voluntary early discharge, more than half of all U.S. states have passed legislation mandating a home visit if the family was discharged before 48 hours. Discharge before 48 hours should occur only at the family's request. Research has demonstrated that extending the length of stay does not increase costs when death rates and readmission costs are considered and indicates that the 1998 legislation was effective (Burgos, Schmitt, Stevenson, et al., 2008).

Early discharges have implications for the mother. The risk of postpartum hemorrhage, difficulties with breastfeeding, and opportunities for the mother to become comfortable with her new baby may be compromised. The risk of postpartum depression commonly occurs in the first month following the birth. Women who receive some type of follow-up assessment from a nurse experience less depression than those who do not receive postpartum follow-up (Goulet, D'Amour, & Pineault, 2007). In addition, extended family members who live at a distance and have agreed to assist the new family in the first few weeks after birth may not have arrived yet. Furthermore, in the first 24 hours after childbirth, the mother may be too tired or may not be ready emotionally to participate in learning activities. In all cases of early discharge, a home visit by an experienced postpartal nurse can be invaluable.

These early discharges present a challenge to nurses because the time available for nursing assessments and client teaching is greatly reduced. In addition, many conditions in the newborn, such as jaundice, ductal-dependent cardiac lesions, and gastrointestinal obstructions, may take longer than 2 days to develop, and identification of these problems depends on a skilled, experienced professional (AAP Committee on Fetus and Newborn, 2004). Other experts contend that breastfeeding may not be well established before 48 hours and discharge before this time can lead to increased rates of dehydration and poor breastfeeding outcomes (de Almeida & Draque, 2007).

Special emphasis has also been placed on the needs of **late preterm infants**, born between 34 and 37 weeks (Engle, Tomashek, Wallman, & Committee on Fetus & Newborn 2007). These infants are at a greater risk for increases in mortality and morbidity because they are physically not mature and are more prone to have physiological and metabolic complications (Engle et al., 2007). Readmissions for infection and jaundice are more common in later preterm infants than in term infants (Engle et al., 2007). The American Academy of Pediatrics (AAP) has identified specific risk factors in late preterm infants that increase the likelihood of readmission and neonatal mortality. These include: being first born, breastfeeding at the time of discharge, having a mother who has had labor and childbirth complications, having public insurance as your source of payment, and being Asian/Pacific Islander (Engle et al., 2007). Special attention by the home health nurse is warranted for these infants to ensure a proper home transition and to identify possible early complications (Engle et al., 2007).

Following discharge, various services are available in most communities to meet the needs of the postpartal family. The goal is to help ensure that all family members have the opportunity to meet healthcare needs, regardless of their resources. Some types of follow-up care include telephone follow-up and home visits.

Table 31–4 When to Contact the Primary Care Provider

After discharge, a woman should contact her physician/CNM if any of the following develop:

- Sudden, persistent, or spiking fever
- Change in the character of the lochia—foul smell, return to bright-red bleeding, excessive amount, passage of large clots
- Pain at the site of a laceration, episiotomy, or abdominal incision
- Evidence of wound infection including redness, swelling, severe or worsening pain, or foul-smelling discharge
- Evidence of mastitis, such as breast tenderness, reddened areas, malaise
- Evidence of thrombophlebitis, such as calf pain, tenderness, redness
- Evidence of urinary tract infection, such as urgency, frequency, burning on urination
- Continued severe or incapacitating postpartal depression
- Inability to care for self or baby for any physical or psychologic reason

Telephone Follow-Up

Telephone follow-up is offered to families before discharge, and a mutually agreed upon time is set for the call. Typically the call is made within 3 days after discharge or earlier if desired, lasts about 20 minutes, and is goal directed. To perform effective telephone assessment, the nurse must be able to listen skillfully, ask open-ended questions, and project an attitude of caring. If the assessment reveals any signs of a postpartum complication, the nurse refers the woman to her healthcare provider for further evaluation. The plan of care developed and implemented during a telephone conversation is limited to supportive counseling, teaching, and referral.

It is also fairly common for a home care nurse to make a telephone follow-up call to a family a few days after a home visit to provide additional information, address questions or areas of confusion, and make referrals if indicated. The mother may have multiple questions, and is generally at a high level of learning readiness. Some women may prefer a telephone-based follow-up because it requires less preparation and time than a home visit.

In addition to these scheduled follow-up telephone calls, nurses in birthing, newborn, and postpartum units, as well as clinic nurses, often receive phone calls from postpartal families seeking advice or care. These calls must be triaged immediately. Calls with urgent or life-threatening implications should be referred appropriately, either by initiating an immediate call to the practitioner or, in rare circumstances, calling 911.

Finally, many communities have established 24-hour help lines for new parents to call when they have questions or need support. In areas where help lines are not available, parents may be directed to call the birthing center. In either case, the nurse provides the number so that it is readily accessible for the family.

Home Visit

If the mother, family, and physician/CNM have chosen discharge earlier than 48 hours after vaginal birth, in some states, the mother may request a total of three home visits. The home setting provides an opportunity for the nurse and family to interact in a more relaxed environment in which the family has control. In some instances, the challenges of assessing and enhancing self-care and infant care may be unique in the home, and the nurse will have many opportunities to exercise critical thinking to develop creative options with the family. The nurse should explain that, unlike community health visits, only one or two home visits are typically planned and spaced out over the next week, and long-term follow-up by the postpartal nurse is not anticipated. Occassionally the nurse may schedule additional home visits based on the findings of the first home visit and the follow-up phone call.

EVALUATION

Anticipated outcomes of comprehensive postpartal nursing care of the family include the following:

- The mother is reasonably comfortable and has learned pain relief measures.
- The mother is rested and understands how to add more activity over the next few days and weeks.
- The mother's physiologic and psychologic well-being have been supported.
- The mother verbalizes her understanding of self-care measures.
- The new parents demonstrate how to care for their baby.
- The new parents have had opportunities to form attachment with their baby.
- Follow-up care contacts have been initiated as needed.

CONSIDERATIONS FOR THE HOME VISIT

Before the home visit, the nurse (who is experienced in postpartal maternal and newborn care) prepares by identifying the purpose of the home visit and gathering needed materials and equipment. A personal contact while the woman is still in the birth setting or a previsit telephone call is used to arrange the appointment with the woman and her family. During the previsit contact, it is important for the nurse to clearly identify the purpose and goals of the visit and to begin establishing rapport.

PURPOSE AND TIMING OF THE HOME VISIT

Postpartal home care is focused more on assessment, teaching, facilitating learning, and counseling than on physical care. First, it provides an opportunity to assess the status of the mother and infant for signs of any complications. The established guidelines for discharge of the mother and baby mean the nurse can expect certain levels of health and wellness. However, because the status of the mother and newborn can change, the nurse should stay alert for deviations from the norm and identify conditions that may warrant further medical evaluation or rehospitalization. The nurse can also complete follow-up blood work if needed.

In addition, the nurse assesses adaptation of the family to the new baby and adjustment of any siblings. The nurse also assesses the parents' skill in bathing, dressing, handling, and comforting their newborn, and the appropriateness and safety of the home environment.

Another purpose of the home visit is to ascertain current informational needs, and to offer requested information, in a more relaxed setting. Postpartal home care provides opportunities for enhancing self- and infant-care techniques initially presented in the birth setting. Many times, questions and concerns arise at home that were not identified in the hospital.

In addition, the nurse answers questions about breastfeeding, provides support and encouragement, and addresses the need for referrals to clinics, classes, or postpartal support groups.

MAINTAINING SAFETY

In the past, nurses were perceived as a mainstay of communities and could move in most settings without fear or concern for safety. Today, some communities are not safe for visiting nurses. It is important for the nurse to follow basic safety rules when conducting a home visit. Obviously, the nurse needs to know the specific address and ask for directions during the previsit contact. If the area is not familiar, the nurse should trace out the route on a map or use an Internet program to provide directions before leaving for the visit and take a map along. Some vehicles are now equipped with a global positioning system (GPS). However, some newer areas may not be included or found within the system, so the nurse should always have a back-up plan in place. It is also wise for the nurse to wear a name tag and carry identification. The nurse should avoid wearing expensive jewelry or pins of a religious or political nature that might be seen as offensive. A fully charged cellular phone provides a means of contact and is advisable, as is a working flashlight, especially for night visits. The nurse should also notify an instructor or supervisor when leaving for a visit and check in as soon as the visit is completed.

Many agencies that provide home care services have established violence prevention programs to help ensure safety. Nurses in the community need to be aware of their environment and alert to environmental cues, whether overt or subtle. In addition, the following recommendations are important (McPhaul, Rosen, Bobb, et al., 2007).

- Invest time in personal safety by driving around a neighborhood before making an initial visit to identify potential cues to violence. Avoid walking through a crowd or staying in an elevator with others if it makes you uneasy.
- In high-risk areas, visit the family during daylight hours. Inform the family when you plan to arrive and advise them to call a supervisor if you do not arrive within 15 minutes of the arranged time. Provide them with a contact name and phone number.
- Do not park in deserted or unlit areas. Make sure your car is in good working order and has gas. Keep doors locked and windows closed.
- Before leaving for the visit, lock personal belongings in the trunk of the car, out of sight. Do not carry a purse, medications, or other items.
- In accordance with agency policy, wear scrubs, a lab coat, or other uniform that identifies you as a nurse.
- Be aware of personal body language and how it might be interpreted. (For example, avoid crossing arms or shoving hands in pockets, which may suggest hostility; remain calm and convey a sense of respect at all times.)
- Pay attention to the body language of anyone present during the visit, not just the client.
- Be alert for signs that a person is becoming enraged (reddened neck and/or face, clenched fists, pacing). If any family member is violent, or if drug or alcohol abuse is occurring, leave the home and report the incident to your supervisor.
- Leave the home immediately if a gun or knife is visible. Do not confront the client or family member.
- If a situation arises that feels unsafe, or a "gut feeling" tells you something is not right, terminate the visit immediately.

If the visit is in an area that seems unsafe, it may be wise for two nurses to go together. Nurses should avoid entering areas where violence is in progress. In such cases, they should return to the car and contact the police or dial 911. Most people are more comfortable in familiar neighborhoods and have some hesitation when entering homes in other residential areas. First home visits may feel uncomfortable because they are unfamiliar, but with experience comfort increases (Figure 31–5 ●).

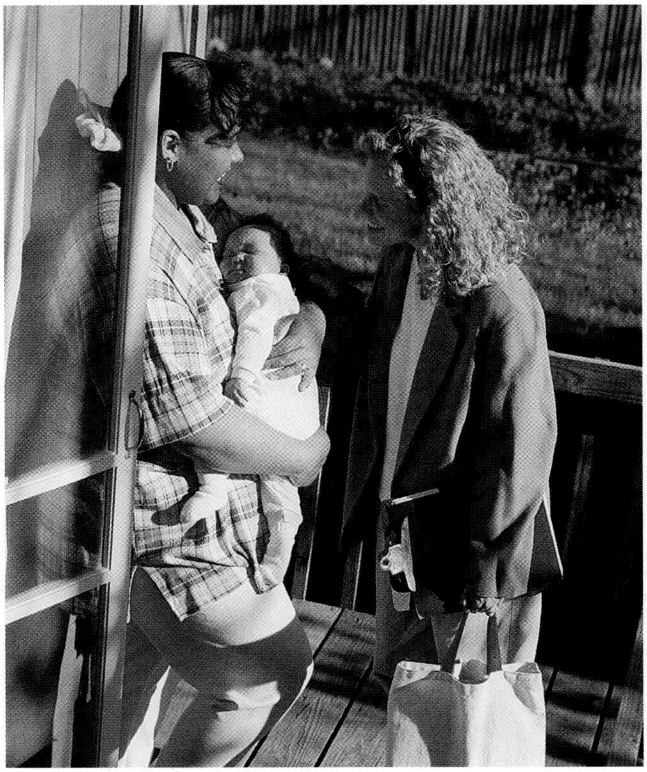

● **Figure 31–5** Nurse arriving for a home visit.

FOSTERING A CARING RELATIONSHIP WITH THE FAMILY

Although the nurse in the birthing center strives to enhance family autonomy and control, the atmosphere of the institutional environment may cause the new mother and family to feel disempowered. It is important for the professional nurse to recognize that the parameters of the home visit are different. In the home, the family members have control of their environment and the nurse is an invited visitor. The nurse can rely on the same characteristics of a caring relationship that have been integral to hospital-based practice—regard for clients, genuineness, empathy, and establishment of trust and rapport—when providing care in the home setting (Table 31–5). Evidence of these characteristics forms the foundation for a caring relationship.

When the door is answered, the nurse should introduce herself or himself and confirm that the location is correct. If a place to sit is not indicated, the nurse may inquire, "Where is the best place to sit so that we can talk for a while?" In some families, offering refreshments may be an important aspect of welcoming a visitor. In this case, it is beneficial to the relationship for the nurse to accept the refreshment graciously. Many cultures have strong

Table 31–5 Fostering a Caring Relationship

Demonstrated Goal	Approaches to Achieve Goal
Regard	Introduce yourself to the family. Call the family members by their surnames until you have been invited to use the given or a less formal name. Ask to be introduced to other members of the family who are present. Allow the mother or spokesperson to assume this role. Remember, in some cultures, it may be a male figure or a mother figure who assumes the primary role. Use active listening. Maintain objectiveness. Ask permission before sitting.
Genuineness	Mean what you say. Make sure that your verbal and nonverbal messages are congruent. Be nonjudgmental. Do not make assumptions about individuals or settings. Always strive to demonstrate caring behaviors. Be prepared for the visit, honestly answer questions and provide information, and be truthful. If you do not know the answer to a question, tell the client you will find the information and report back.
Empathy	Listen to the mother and family "where they are" without judgment. Be attentive to what the birthing experience is for them so that you will understand from their perspective. Remember that empathy denotes understanding, not sympathy.
Trust and rapport	Be prepared for the visit and be on time. Follow-up on any areas that are needed.

ties to certain foods and beverages during the postpartum period. Accepting the food or beverage conveys acceptance of cultural norms. It is helpful for the nurse to be familiar with various cultural norms and traditions (Spector, 2009).

The maternal psychologic assessment focuses on attachment, adjustment to the parental role, sibling adjustment, her perception of her new role and coping, and educational needs.

In ideal situations a family approach involving the presence of the father and any siblings provides an opportunity to observe family interactions and opportunities for all family members to ask questions and express concerns. In addition, any questionable family interaction pattern such as one suggestive of abuse or neglect may be evident and further referral could be considered if needed. (See "Assessment Guide: Postpartal—First Home Visit and Anticipated Progress at 6 Weeks.")

As discussed, the nurse completes planned assessments, provides direct care as necessary, carries out family and client teaching, mentions available community resources such as new mother support groups and makes referrals to community agencies as necessary, and schedules an additional home visit or telephone contact. The aspects assessed and addressed during the home visit are discussed in the following sections.

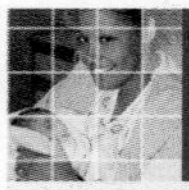

Developing Cultural Competence

ROLE OF EXTENDED FAMILY

In some cultures, extended family members such as grandmothers and aunts play a major role in the care of the postpartal woman and her family. Sometimes, these family members take full responsibility for running the household throughout the postpartum period. In other families, they concentrate entirely on the mother's or newborn's care. When culturally appropriate, include these extended family members in postpartum education sessions.

HOME CARE: THE MOTHER AND FAMILY

During the first home visit, the nurse completes a physical assessment of the mother and a psychosocial assessment of the family. Teaching for self-care is commonly required for new mothers, especially breastfeeding mothers with nipple soreness, engorgement, and other concerns. Family teaching related to resumption of sexual activity and contraception may also be required.

ASSESSMENT OF THE MOTHER AND FAMILY

Before performing the physical assessment, the nurse should ensure the mother's privacy. The physical assessment focuses on maternal physical adaptation, which is assessed by focusing on vital signs, breasts, abdominal musculature, elimination patterns, reproductive tract, and laboratory values. The nurse also talks with the mother about her diet, fatigue level, ability to rest and sleep, pain management, and signs of postpartal complications. In addition, for breastfeeding mothers, the nurse assesses the woman's feeding technique and presents information about possible problems that may occur.

Many new mothers are concerned about weight loss. Women who have gained excess weight during the pregnancy are at risk for obesity in later life. Counseling the mother about proper diet and exercise is an effective strategy to lose weight in the postpartum period. Nursing women should be counseled that extreme weight loss strategies are not advised, but that healthy food choices and exercise can aid in weight reduction. There are also weight loss programs designed specifically for nursing mothers that can offer counseling, group support, and monitoring in the postpartum period.

Assessment Guide

POSTPARTAL—FIRST HOME VISIT AND ANTICIPATED PROGRESS AT 6 WEEKS

PHYSICAL ASSESSMENT/ NORMAL FINDINGS	ALTERATIONS AND POSSIBLE CAUSES*	NURSING RESPONSES TO DATA†
Vital Signs		
Blood pressure: Return to normal prepregnant level.	Elevated blood pressure (anxiety, essential hypertension, renal disease), preeclampsia (can occur postpartum).	Review history, evaluate normal baseline; refer to physician/CNM if necessary.
Pulse: 60 to 90 beats/min (or prepregnant normal rate).	Increased pulse rate, tachycardia, chest pain (excitement, anxiety, cardiac disorders).	Count pulse for full minute, note irregularities; marked tachycardia or beat irregularities require additional assessment and possible physician/CNM referral.
Respirations: 16 to 24/min.	Marked tachypnea or abnormal patterns (respiratory disorders).	Evaluate for respiratory disease; refer to physician/CNM if necessary.
Temperature: 36.6°C to 37.6°C (98°F to 99.6°F).	Increased temperature (infection).	Assess for signs and symptoms of infection or disease state.
Weight		
2 days: Possible weight loss of 12 to 20+ lb.	Minimal weight loss (fluid retention, preeclampsia).	Evaluate for fluid retention, edema, deep tendon reflexes, and blood pressure elevation.
6 weeks: Returning to normal prepregnant weight.	Retained weight (excessive caloric intake).	Determine amount of daily exercise. Provide dietary teaching. Refer to dietician if necessary for additional dietary counseling.
	Extreme weight loss (excessive dieting, inadequate caloric intake).	Discuss appropriate diets, refer to dietician for additional counseling if necessary.
Breasts		
Nonbreastfeeding: 2 days: May have mild to moderate tenderness; small amount of milk may be expressed. 6 weeks: Soft, with no tenderness; return to prepregnant size.	Some engorgement (incomplete suppression of lactation). Redness; marked tenderness (mastitis). Palpable mass (tumor).	Engorgement may be seen in nonbreastfeeding mothers. Advise client to wear a supportive, well-fitted bra; avoid very warm showers; avoid pumping or any stimulation of breasts; use ice packs for comfort; evaluate for signs and symptoms of mastitis (rare in nonbreastfeeding mothers). Parcooked cabbage leaves can be placed against the breast to relieve engorgement.
Breastfeeding: Full, with prominent nipples; lactation established.	Cracked, fissured nipples (feeding problems). Redness, marked tenderness, or even abscess formation (mastitis). Palpable mass (full milk duct, tumor).	Counsel about nipple care. Observe infant feeding. Evaluate client condition, evidence of fever, redness, or tender area, refer to physician/CNM for initiation of antibiotic therapy, if indicated. Opinion varies as to value of breast examination for breastfeeding mothers; some feel a breastfeeding mother should examine her breasts monthly, after feeding, when breasts are empty; if palpable mass is felt, refer to physician for further evaluation. For breast inflammation instruct the mother to: 1. Keep breast empty by frequent feeding. 2. Rest when possible. 3. Take prescribed pain relief med. 4. Force fluids. 5. Take antibiotics if ordered. If symptoms are accompanied by fever, flulike symptoms, or redness, instruct woman to call her physician/CNM and take an analgesic.

(continued)

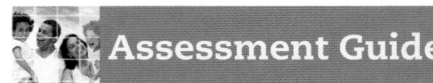

Assessment Guide—continued

POSTPARTAL—FIRST HOME VISIT AND ANTICIPATED PROGRESS AT 6 WEEKS

PHYSICAL ASSESSMENT/ NORMAL FINDINGS	ALTERATIONS AND POSSIBLE CAUSES*	NURSING RESPONSES TO DATA†
Abdominal Musculature		
2 days: Improved firmness, although "bread dough" consistency is not unusual, especially in multipara. Striae pink and obvious.	Marked relaxation of muscles.	Evaluate exercise level; provide information on appropriate exercise program.
Cesarean incision healing.	Use the REEDA scoring system which includes: redness, ecchymosis, edema, discharge from incision site, and approximation. Assess for tenderness and pain.	Evaluate for infection; refer to physician/CNM if necessary.
6 weeks: Muscle tone continues to improve; striae may be beginning to fade, may not achieve a silvery appearance for several more weeks; linea nigra fading.		
Elimination Pattern		
Urinary Tract: Return to prepregnant urinary elimination routine.	Urinary incontinence, especially when lifting, coughing, laughing, and so on (urethral trauma, cystocele).	Assess for cystocele; instruct in appropriate muscle tightening exercises; refer to physician/CNM.
	Pain or burning when voiding, urgency and/or frequency, pus, blood, or white blood cells (WBC) in urine, pathogenic organisms in culture (urinary tract infection).	Evaluate for urinary tract infection; obtain clean-catch urine; refer to physician/CNM for treatment if indicated.
Routine urinalysis within normal limits (proteinuria disappeared).	Sugar or ketone in urine—may be some lactose present in urine of breastfeeding mothers (diabetes).	Evaluate diet; assess for signs and symptoms of diabetes; refer to physician/CNM.
Bowel Habits: 2 days: May be some discomfort with defecation, especially if client had severe hemorrhoids or third- or fourth-degree extension.	Severe constipation or pain when defecating (trauma or hemorrhoids).	Discuss dietary patterns; encourage fluids and high fiber diet, adequate roughage. Counsel on the effects of medications. Continue use of stool softener if necessary to prevent pain associated with straining; continue sitz baths, periods of rest for severe hemorrhoids; assess healing of episiotomy and/or lacerations; severe constipation may require administration of laxatives, stool softeners, and an enema if not contraindicated (check with physician/CNM).
6 weeks: Return to normal prepregnancy bowel elimination.	Marked constipation (inadequate fluid/fiber intake).	See previous discussed interventions.
	Fecal incontinence or constipation (rectocele).	Assess for evidence of rectocele; instruct in muscle tightening exercises; refer to physician/CNM.
Reproductive Tract		
Lochia: 2 days: Lochia rubra or lochia serosa, scant amounts, fleshy odor.	Excessive amounts and/or large clots (nonfirm uterus), foul odor (infection), passing tissue (possible retained placenta).	Assess for evidence of infection and/or failure of the uterus to decrease in size; refer to physician/CNM.
6 weeks: No lochia, or return to normal menstruation pattern.	See above.	See above.

Assessment Guide—continued

POSTPARTAL—FIRST HOME VISIT AND ANTICIPATED PROGRESS AT 6 WEEKS

PHYSICAL ASSESSMENT/ NORMAL FINDINGS	ALTERATIONS AND POSSIBLE CAUSES*	NURSING RESPONSES TO DATA†
Fundus and Perineum: 2 days: Fundus is at least two finger breadths below the umbilicus; uterine muscles still somewhat lax; introitus of vagina lacks tone—gapes when intra-abdominal pressure is increased by coughing or straining.	Uterus not decreasing in size appropriately (infection).	Assess fundus for firmness and/or signs of infection; refer to physician/CNM if indicated.
Episiotomy and/or lacerations healing; no signs of infection; may have some bruising and tenderness.	Evidence of redness, severe pain, poor tissue approximation in episiotomy and/or laceration (wound infection).	Utilize cool or warm sitz baths, topical medications.
6 weeks: Uterus almost returned to prepregnant size with almost completely restored muscle tone.	Continued flow of lochia, failure to decrease appropriately in size (subinvolution).	Assess for evidence of subinvolution and/or infection; refer to physician for further evaluation and treatment if necessary.
Hemoglobin and Hematocrit Levels		
6 weeks: Hemoglobin (Hb) 12 g/dL; Hematocrit (Hct) 37% $\pm$ 5%	Hb less than 12 g/dL; Hct 32% (anemia)	Assess nutritional status, assess for signs or symptoms of anemia, begin (or continue) supplemental iron; for marked anemia (Hb less than or equal to 9 g/dL) additional assessment and/or physician/CNM referral may be necessary.
Attachment		
Bonding process demonstrated by soothing, cuddling, and talking to infant; appropriate feeding techniques; eye-to-eye contact; calling infant by name.	Failure to bond demonstrated by lack of behaviors associated with bonding process, calling infant by nickname that promotes ridicule, inadequate infant weight gain, infant is dirty, hygienic measures are not being maintained, severe diaper rash, failure to obtain adequate supplies to provide infant care (malattachment).	Provide counseling; talk with the woman about her feelings regarding the infant; provide support for the caretaking activities that are being performed; refer to public health nurse for continued home visits; refer if abuse or neglect is suspected.
Parent interacts with infant and provides soothing, caretaking activities.	Parent is unable to respond to infant needs (inability to recognize needs, inadequate education and support, fear, family stress).	Provide support for caretaking activities observed; provide information regarding caretaking activities, such as responding to infant cry; methods of wrapping infant; methods of soothing the infant such as swaddling, rocking, increasing stimuli by singing to the infant or decreasing stimuli by putting infant to rest in quiet room; methods of holding the infant; differences in the cry. Identify support system such as friends, neighbors; provide information regarding community resources and support groups.
Parents express feelings of comfort and success with the parent role.	Evidence of stress and anxiety (difficulty moving into or dealing with the parent role).	Provide support and encouragement; provide information regarding progression into parent role and assist parents in talking through their feelings; refer to community resources and support groups.
Woman is in the informal or personal stage of maternal role attainment.	Woman is still greatly influenced by others, has not developed an image or style of her own (woman remains in the anticipatory stage).	Provide role modeling for the woman in working through problem solving with the infant, provide encouragement as she thinks through decisions and develops her sense of problem solving; encourage her to make decisions regarding infant care.

(continued)

Assessment Guide—continued

POSTPARTAL—FIRST HOME VISIT AND ANTICIPATED PROGRESS AT 6 WEEKS

PHYSICAL ASSESSMENT/ NORMAL FINDINGS	ALTERATIONS AND POSSIBLE CAUSES*	NURSING RESPONSES TO DATA†
Adjustment to Parental Role		
Parents are coping with new roles in terms of division of labor, financial status, communication, readjustment of sexual relations, and adjusting to new daily tasks.	Inability to adjust to new roles (immaturity, inadequate education and preparation, ineffective communication patterns, inadequate support, current family crisis).	Provide counseling, refer to parent groups.
Education		
Mother understands self-care measures.	Inadequate knowledge of self-care (inadequate education).	Provide education and counseling.
Parents are knowledgeable regarding infant care.	Inadequate knowledge of infant care (inadequate education).	
Siblings are adjusting to new baby.	Excessive sibling rivalry.	
Parents have a method of contraception.	Birth control method not chosen.	

*Possible causes of alterations are identified in parentheses.
†This column provides guidelines for further assessment and initial nursing intervention.

BREASTFEEDING CONCERNS FOLLOWING DISCHARGE

Because mothers are discharged from the birthing unit before breastfeeding is well established, they are frequently alone when they encounter changes in the breastfeeding process. Many women stop nursing if the situations they encounter seem problematic. For this reason, the nurse providing a home visit is in a unique position to positively impact the success of breastfeeding (Association of Women's Health, Obstetric and Neonatal Nurses [AWHONN], 2006). Table 31–6 summarizes self-care measures the nurse can suggest to a woman with a breastfeeding problem.

Evidence-Based Nursing

POSTPARTUM WEIGHT MANAGEMENT

Clinical Questions
What are the most effective weight management interventions for postpartum women?

The Evidence
There is a high prevalence of obesity during childbearing. Excessive prepregnancy weight or weight gain during pregnancy, ethnicity, postpartum changes in roles, dietary changes during pregnancy, and changes in physical activity are all risk factors for weight retention after birth. The majority of women do not lose all of the weight gained during pregnancy, and this often contributes to later obesity. A team of expert advanced practice nurses, researchers, and a physician conducted a comprehensive, systematic review of published intervention studies to identify the best available evidence for guiding weight management interventions in postpartum women. Systematic reviews of multiple studies guided by content experts provide the highest level of evidence for practice.

Best Practice
Keller, Records, Ainsworth, et al. (2008) identified that interventions should target women early in their childbearing years so that they have the most significant long-term impact. Asbee, Jenkins, Butler, et al. (2009) found that intensive dietary and lifestyle counseling during the prenatal period can help prevent women from gaining too much weight during the pregnancy. Multilevel strategies were found to be the most effective in helping women manage their weight in the postpartum period. A multilevel approach is one in which individual strategies are enhanced by interpersonal efforts and community-based support. Teaching mothers about physical activity and appropriate nutrition is effective, whether delivered at the individual or group level. Effective interpersonal level activities included social support through group participation and engaging the family in healthy eating habits. At the community level, locating safe places to walk and exercise in their neighborhoods and helping mothers map walking routes to parks, schools, and other safe destinations is effective in increasing physical activity.

Critical Thinking
Is there a distinction between group and individual counseling in terms of effectiveness? Are these findings generalizable to all ethnic groups?

See MyNursingKit for possible responses.

Table 31–6 Common Breastfeeding Problems and Remedies

Problem	Possible Cause	Remedies
Nipples Not Graspable	Flat or inverted nipples	■ Use Hoffman technique to break adhesions. ■ Wear breast shells to encourage nipples to protrude. ■ Grasp nipples and roll gently between the fingers to increase protractility. ■ Form the nipple before breastfeeding by hand shaping, ice, or wearing nipple shells a half-hour before feeding. ■ Use a breast pump to draw nipples out so that the mother can then put the baby to the breast.
	Engorged breasts	■ Treat engorgement by feeding the baby more frequently. ■ A hand or electric pump or manual emptying of the breast can be done if the baby in unable to grasp the nipple.
	Large breasts	■ Support breast with opposite hand, or use rolled towel under breast to bring nipple to the level of baby's mouth. ■ Avoid having the nipple pointing downward because this makes latch-on more difficult. ■ Use C-hold to make nipple accessible to baby.
Engorgement	Missed or infrequent feedings	■ Breastfeed frequently (every 1 1/2 hours). ■ Massage and hand express or pump to empty breasts completely when feedings are missed or when a full feeling develops in breasts and baby is not available or willing to feed. ■ Avoid excessive stimulation or pumping between feedings because this will increase milk production. ■ Place warm compresses on breast just before feeding to soften breast. ■ Use cold applications between feedings to slow milk production (frozen bagged vegetables, ice packs, and par-cooked cabbage leaves (AWHONN, 2006).
	Breasts not emptied at feedings	■ Massage breasts and use warm cloths before feedings. ■ Breastfeed long enough to empty breasts (10 to 15 minutes on each side at each feeding). ■ If baby will not feed long enough to empty breasts, hand express or pump after feeding.
	Inadequate let-down	■ Use relaxation techniques, massage, and warm compresses before breastfeeding. ■ Relax in warm shower with water running from back over shoulders and breasts, hand expressing to relieve fullness. ■ Use hand or electric pump before placing baby on breast to encourage let-down. ■ Listen to soothing music, use visualization or breathing techniques. ■ If caused by anxiety, try to eliminate the source of tension.
	Baby sleepy or not eager to feed	■ Use rousing techniques (e.g., hold baby upright, unwrap blanket, change diaper). ■ Pre-express milk onto nipple or baby's lips to entice baby. ■ Avoid use of bottles of water or formula; these will decrease baby's willingness to suckle.
Inadequate Let-Down	Let-down not well established	■ Give the baby ample time at the breast (at least 15 minutes per side) to allow for let-down and complete emptying. ■ Breastfeed in a quiet spot away from distractions. ■ Massage breasts and apply warm compresses before breastfeeding. ■ Drink juice, water, or tea (no caffeine) before and during breastfeeding. ■ Condition let-down by setting up a routine for beginning feedings. ■ Use relaxation, visualization, and breathing techniques. ■ Stimulate the nipple manually before breastfeeding. ■ Concentrate thought on the baby and milk flow; turn on a faucet so that the sound of running water helps stimulate let-down. ■ Take a warm shower before feedings. ■ Use breast pump to stimulate the let-down. ■ Avoid waiting to put baby to breast until the baby is famished because this may increase maternal anxiety. ■ Assess for maternal pain, cold temperature, or anxiety before feeding.
	Mother overtired or overextended	■ Nap or rest when the baby rests. ■ Limit distractions, limit visitors, focus on personal needs. ■ Lie down to breastfeed. ■ Simplify daily chores; set priorities.

(continued)

Table 31–6 Common Breastfeeding Problems and Remedies—continued

Problem	Possible Cause	Remedies
	Mother tense, pressured	■ Identify the causes of tensions and eliminate or minimize them. ■ Decrease fatigue. ■ Have others assist with other household duties or tasks. ■ Use relaxation, visualization, and breathing exercises to promote relaxation and comfort.
	Mother caught in cycle of little milk, worry, less milk	■ Try all the actions above. ■ Counsel mother that most women do produce enough milk. ■ Have infant weighed to ensure adequate weight gain which is a reflection of milk supply. ■ Encourage frequent, uninterrupted feedings. ■ Consult a lactation consultant as needed.
Cracked Nipples	All causes of sore nipples carried to extreme	■ Refer to all actions for sore nipples. ■ Ensure infant is properly positioned. ■ Feed infant more frequently. ■ Avoid soaps, perfumes, or other cleaning products that can dry out nipples and predispose them to cracking. ■ Express milk post-feeding and rub into nipple allowing it to air dry. ■ Use emollients or lanolin as directed by physician/CNM/lactation consultant. ■ Consult doctor about using ibuprofen (Motrin), acetaminophen (Tylenol), or other painkiller. ■ Improve nutritional status, increasing protein, vitamin C, zinc.
	Local infection (baby with staph or other organism may have infected mother's nipples)	■ Refer to physician.
Plugged Ducts	Poor positioning	■ Try a variety of positions for complete emptying. ■ Alternate positions so that different areas of the nipple have different compression pressure. ■ Incomplete emptying of breast. ■ Breastfeed at least 10 minutes per side after let-down. ■ Alternate breastfeeding positions. ■ If baby does not empty breasts, pump or express milk after feedings.
	External pressure on breast	■ Use larger-size bra, insert bra extender, or go braless. ■ Wear a sports bra instead of a traditional bra. ■ Use nursing bra instead of pulling up conventional bra to breastfeed to avoid pressure on ducts. ■ Avoid bunching up sweater or nightgown under arm during breastfeeding.
Sore Nipples	Poor positioning	■ Alternate breastfeeding positions throughout the day. ■ Bring the baby close to feed so the baby does not pull on the breast. ■ Place the nipple and some of the areola in the baby's mouth. ■ Check to ensure the baby is put on and off the breast properly. ■ Check to ensure the nipple is back far enough in the baby's mouth. ■ Hold the baby closely during feeding so the nipple is not constantly being pulled. ■ Ensure that shoulder, hip, and knees are all properly aligned and facing the mother.
	Baby chewing or nuzzling onto nipple	■ Form the nipple for the baby. ■ Set up a pattern of getting the baby onto the breast using the rooting reflex.
	Baby sucking on end of nipple	■ Ensure the nipple is way back in the baby's mouth by getting the baby properly onto the breast. ■ Check for an inverted nipple. ■ Check for engorgement. ■ If baby is initially placed incorrectly on the end of the nipple, break the suction using a fish hook motion with your index finger and reposition baby on nipple properly. ■ Do not allow baby to nurse on end of nipple, reposition immediately.
	Baby chewing his or her way off the nipple (nipple being pulled out of baby's mouth at end of feeding)	■ Remove the baby from the breast by placing a finger between the baby's gums to ensure suction is broken. ■ End feeding when the baby's suckling slows, before he or she has a chance to chew on the nipple.

Table 31–6 Common Breastfeeding Problems and Remedies—continued

Problem	Possible Cause	Remedies
	Baby overly eager to nurse	■ Breastfeed more often. ■ Pre-express milk to hasten let-down, avoiding vigorous suckling.
	Dry colostrum or milk causing nipple to stick to bra or breast pads	■ Moisten bra or pads before taking off so as not to remove keratin. ■ Ensure that nipples are dry before replacing bra or clothing against nipples.
	Nipples not allowed to dry	■ Remove plastic liners from milk pads. ■ Air dry breast completely after nursing. ■ Change nursing pads frequently. ■ Switch to cotton nursing pads.
	Nipple skin not resistant to stress	■ Improve diet, especially adding fresh fruits and vegetables and vitamin supplements. ■ Eliminate or decrease use of sugary foods, alcohol, caffeine, cigarettes. ■ Check use of cleansing or drying agents.
	Natural oils removed or keratin layers broken down by drying agents (soap, alcohol, shampoo, deodorant)	■ Eliminate irritants. ■ Wash breasts with water only.

Newborn feeding is discussed in detail in Chapter 27. Regardless of feeding method, it is important for the nurse to assess the newborn's fluid and nutritional intake. As part of the physical assessment the newborn's nude weight is determined. If the weight loss since birth is 10% or more, the nurse assesses the baby for signs of dehydration such as loose skin with decreased skin turgor, dry mucous membranes, sunken anterior fontanelle, and decreased frequency and amount of voiding and stooling. Risk factors for suboptimal breastfeeding include maternal obesity, primiparity, young maternal age, use of formula supplementation, use of pacifiers, cesarean birth, second stage greater than 1 hour, low birth weight, breastfeeding difficulty, and flat or inverted nipples (Walker, 2007).

Nipple Soreness

Some discomfort often occurs initially with breastfeeding; it peaks between day 3 and 6 and then recedes. Breastfeeding difficulty and nipple soreness are often causes for women to discontinue breastfeeding. The nurse should counsel the mother not to switch to formula feeding or delay feedings because these measures cause engorgement and more soreness (Riordan & Wambach, 2010). Discomfort that lasts throughout the feeding or past the first week demands attention.

The baby's position at the breast is a critical factor in nipple soreness. The mother's hand should be off the areola, and the baby should be facing the mother's chest, with ear, shoulder, and hip aligned (see Figure 27–5). Because the area of greatest stress to the nipple is in line with the newborn's chin and nose, nipple soreness may be decreased by encouraging the mother to rotate positions when feeding the infant. Changing positions alters the focus of greatest stress and promotes more complete breast emptying.

Nipple soreness may also develop if the infant has faulty sucking habits. Nipples may have injured tips that are bruised, scabbed, or blistered from the nipple entering the baby's mouth at an upward angle and rubbing against the roof of the mouth or from poor latch-on (Riordan & Wambach, 2010). Soreness may also result from continuous negative pressure if the infant falls asleep with the breast in his or her mouth.

Chewed nipples, which result from improper positioning, are cracked or tender at or near the base. In these cases, the baby's jaws close only on the nipple instead of on the areola, or the baby's mouth is not opened wide enough or has slipped down to the nipple from the areola as a result of engorgement. Soreness on the underside of the nipple is caused by the infant nursing with her or his bottom lip tucked in rather than out, causing a friction burn. In such cases, even vigorous sucking produces little milk because the milk sinuses under the areola are not compressed. This situation results in a frustrated infant and marked soreness for the mother. The problem is overcome by manipulating the baby's bottom lip with a fingertip before beginning the feeding, positioning the infant with as much areola as possible in his or her mouth, and rotating the baby's positions at the breast.

Nipple soreness is especially pronounced during the first few minutes of a feeding. If the mother is not expecting this discomfort, she may become discouraged and quickly stop. The let-down reflex may take a few minutes to activate, and it may not occur if the mother stops nursing too quickly. The infant is unsatisfied, and the possibility of breast engorgement increases.

Nipple soreness can also result from the vigorous feeding of an overeager infant. Thus the mother may find it helpful to nurse more frequently. Again, promoting let-down just before feeding may help. Other self-care measures include applying ice to the nipples and areola for a few minutes before feeding to promote

Nursing Practice

If the mother continually has soreness because of a delay in let-down, encourage her to massage the breast in a circular pattern and apply warm compresses just before each breastfeeding session. These activities encourage let-down, increasing the chance that it will occur at the same time that the infant is placed on the breast.

Complementary Care

REMEDIES FOR NIPPLE SORENESS

Older remedies for nipple soreness are receiving renewed acceptance. For instance, tea bags may be moistened in warm water and applied to the nipples. The tannic acid seems to help toughen the nipples, and the warmth is soothing and promotes healing. Tannic acid also has anti-inflammatory properties that can help relieve discomfort. Other therapies have included warm compresses and heat applications (Morland-Schultz & Hill, 2005).

nipple erectness and numb the tissue initially. To promote dryness, the mother may leave her bra flaps down for a few minutes after feeding (Figure 31–6 ●) or expose her nipples to sunlight or ultraviolet light for 30 seconds at first, gradually increasing to 3 minutes. Drying the nipples with a hair dryer on a low heat setting also facilitates drying and promotes healing (Riordan & Wambach, 2010). The use of petroleum-based products such as Vaseline, A & D, cocoa butter, and baby oil to lubricate the nipples is discouraged because the petroleum interferes with skin respiration and may prolong soreness. Because of the risk of allergic reactions, Massé cream (risk of peanut allergy) is discouraged. In addition, products that are washed off before breastfeeding are avoided because of the irritation that washing produces. During bathing, mothers should be advised to only rinse their nipples with water and to avoid soap because this can dry the nipple out and lead to soreness.

Current research as to the effectiveness of nipple lubricants is inconclusive. Thus many lactation experts recommend that the mother's own milk be applied to the nipples and allowed to air dry. Breast milk is high in fat, fights infection, and will not irritate the nipples. Moreover, it is readily available at no cost to the mother. For some women with very dry or severely sore nipples, hypoallergenic medical-grade anhydrous lanolin cream or peppermint gel may help prevent or aid in healing cracked nipples (Melli, Rashidi, Nokhoodchi, et al., 2007). This product poses a low risk of allergy because the alcohols that contribute to the allergic response have been removed.

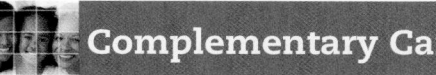

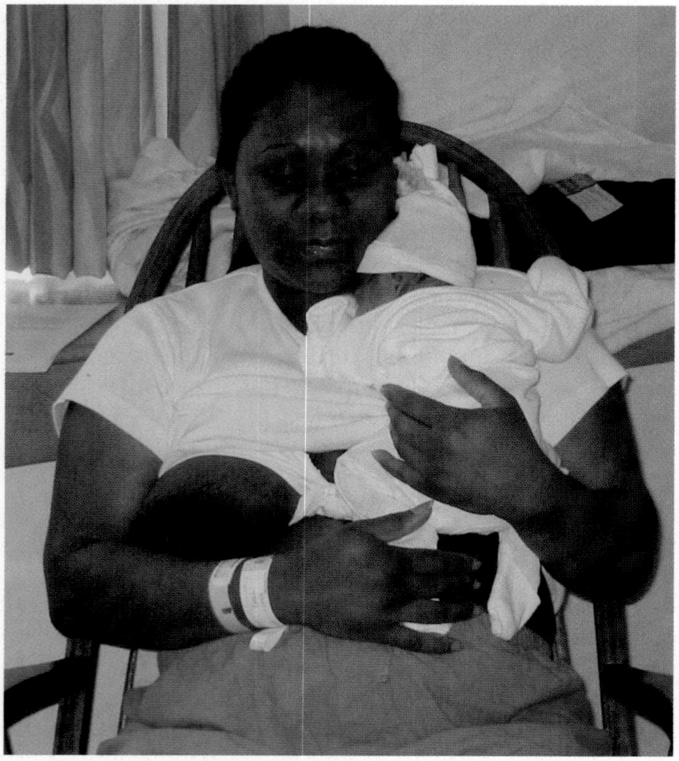

● **Figure 31–6** Mothers with sore nipples can leave bra flaps down after feedings to promote air drying and prevent chapping.

If the woman finds that her bra or clothing rubs against her nipples and adds to her discomfort, she may insert shells into her bra. Medela Shells relieve friction and promote air circulation. If a woman uses breast pads inside her bra to keep milk from leaking onto her clothes, she should change the pads frequently so the nipples remain dry. Some women may be sensitive to the plastic liner within the disposable pad, so the plastic can be removed or they can be encouraged to try cotton pads.

If nipple soreness persists, the woman should be advised to consult a certified lactation consultant to determine the etiology of the soreness. Nipple dermatitis, which causes swollen, reddened, burning nipples, is most commonly caused by thrush or by allergic response to breast cream preparations. If the nipple soreness has a sudden onset and is accompanied by burning or itching, shooting pains through the breast, and a deep pink coloration of the nipple, it may be caused by a thrush infection transmitted from the infant to the mother. White patches or streaks in the infant's mouth indicate a need for treatment of the mouth and nipple infection. The infection can be treated with a variety of antifungal preparations and does not preclude breastfeeding. It is important for both the mother and the infant to receive treatment to prevent cross-transferring of the fungus.

Cracked Nipples

When a breastfeeding mother complains of soreness, the nurse carefully examines the nipples for fissures or cracks and observes the mother during breastfeeding to see whether the infant is correctly positioned at the breast. If the positioning is correct and cracks exist, interventions are necessary. All the interventions described for sore nipples may be used. It may also help the mother to begin nursing on the breast that is less sore. This approach allows the let-down reflex to occur in the affected breast and permits the infant to do more vigorous sucking on the less tender breast, which decreases trauma to the cracked nipple. For the mother's comfort, analgesics may be taken approximately 1 hour before nursing.

Thinking Critically

DIFFICULTIES WITH BREASTFEEDING

Ann Nyembe calls you from home in tears on her third postpartum day. She states that, although breastfeeding was going well in the hospital, her breasts are now swollen, hard, and very painful, and her baby is refusing to suckle. Ann expresses extreme disappointment that "the breastfeeding didn't work" because she truly believes that breast milk is best for babies and she had enjoyed her breastfeeding experience in the hospital, especially nursing the baby immediately after birth. But she also states she has not been able to stop crying all day and can no longer tolerate her painful breasts. In addition she says that the baby "seems happier" with the bottle. What would you do?

See MyNursingKit for possible responses.

Breast Engorgement

A distinction exists between breast fullness and engorgement. All lactating women experience a transitional fullness at first, initially caused by venous congestion and later caused by accumulating milk. However, this fullness generally lasts only 24 hours, the breasts remain soft enough for the newborn to suckle, and there is no pain. Engorged breasts are hard, painful, and warm and appear taut and shiny. The consistency is like gravel.

The infant should suckle for an average of 15 minutes per feeding and should feed at least 8 to 12 times in 24 hours (Riordan & Wambach, 2010). If the baby is unable to nurse more frequently, the mother may express some milk manually or with a pump, taking care to avoid traumatizing the breast tissue. As just noted, warm compresses before nursing stimulate let-down and soften the breast so that the infant can grasp the areola more easily. Cool compresses after nursing can help slow refilling of the breasts and provide comfort to the mother. Ice packs may also be used as a comfort measure. The mother should wear a well-fitted nursing bra 24 hours a day to support the breasts and prevent discomfort from tension.

Plugged Ducts

Some mothers experience plugging of one or more ducts, especially in conjunction with or following engorgement. When breast milk pools within a duct and then dries, it forms a white, hardened plug that is typically visible at the outlet of the duct at the nipple surface. Because milk accumulates behind a plugged duct, women also experience an area of fullness, tenderness, and/or lumpiness in the associated region of the breast.

Self-care measures include the use of heat and massage. The nurse can encourage the mother to massage her breasts from her chest wall forward to the nipple while standing in a warm shower or following the application of moist heat to the breast. Warm compresses can be used and changed as temperature requires. The mother should then nurse her infant starting on the unaffected breast if the plugged breast is tender. Some lactation consultants advocate starting on the affected side because the more vigorous sucking may help dislodge the plug. A breast pump may also be effective in unplugging the duct.

Prevention of plugged ducts involves frequent nursing and the use of a variety of positions to ensure complete emptying. Some mothers discover that pressure from a shoulder strap on a purse, their infant sling, or a car seat belt causes recurring plugged ducts in the compressed area. Repositioning the device may help prevent plugged ducts in these women. Prevention and prompt correction of plugged ducts is important because it could lead to mastitis (discussed in Chapter 32).

Effect of Alcohol and Medications

Mothers may ask the home care nurse about the use of alcohol and medications when breastfeeding. According to the American Academy of Pediatrics (2005), alcohol consumption among breastfeeding women should be limited to occasional use. Breastfeeding mothers should not consume alcohol for at least 2 hours before nursing (O'Keefe, 2005). Alcohol levels in breast milk parallel those found in the maternal plasma, peaking 30 to 60 minutes after consumption. Mothers who do occasionally drink while lactating should be advised to consume the alcohol after breastfeeding rather than shortly before a feeding in order to minimize the amount the infant receives. Mothers with alcoholism who consume large quantities of alcohol daily may be advised not to breastfeed.

As discussed in Chapter 30, most medications pass into the breast milk. Women should consult their primary care provider or other practitioner before taking over-the-counter medications, prescription medications, or herbal supplements.

Breastfeeding and the Working Mother

The best preparation for maintaining lactation after returning to work is frequent, unlimited breastfeeding. Even when well planned, the first day back to work may be fraught with emotional and physical distress. Anticipatory guidance from the nurse may facilitate the transition from maternity leave to work. The earlier the breastfeeding mother returns to work, the more often she will need to pump her breasts to express the breast milk. Because milk production follows the principle of supply and demand, if breasts are not pumped, the milk supply will decrease.

An electric breast pump and double collection system are considered the optimal means of milk expression. However, this is not the only method; mechanical means may not suit some women. Sometimes a mother has a flexible schedule and can return home or have the baby brought to her to nurse at lunch time. If this is not possible, the infant may be fed expressed milk via bottle or spoon. (For proper storage of breast milk, see "Bottle-Feeding Breast Milk" in Chapter 27.) The mother should wait until lactation is well established before introducing the bottle. Most babies adjust to the bottle within 7 to 10 days.

To maintain a milk supply, the working mother must pay special attention to her fluid intake. She can ensure adequate intake by drinking extra fluid at each break and when possible during the day. It is also helpful to nurse more on weekends, nurse during the night, eat a nutritionally sound diet, and continue manual expression or pumping when not nursing.

Night nursing presents a dilemma: It may help a working mother maintain her milk supply, but it may also contribute to fatigue. Some women choose to have the infant sleep nearby so

Nursing Practice

Infants with special needs sometimes benefit from a longer duration of breastfeeding. Infants who are prone to allergies, gastrointestinal reflux, or impaired motility of the gastrointestinal tract may receive benefits from continued breastfeeding that the mother may be unaware of. These women should be counseled to discuss weaning with the pediatrician or infant specialist before weaning because the benefits of breastfeeding may influence the woman's choice of timing regarding weaning (see Chapter 34).

that breastfeeding is more easily accomplished; other women find it difficult to sleep soundly when the infant is in close proximity. For the mother who works long hours or has a rigid work schedule, the best alternative may be to limit breastfeeding to morning and evening feedings, with supplemental feedings at other times. This choice allows her to maintain a close relationship with the infant and provides some of the unique benefits of breast milk.

Generally the new mother has a final postpartum examination with her caregiver about 6 weeks after childbirth. However, if the nurse's assessment indicates a need, the nurse refers the woman to her healthcare provider for care before the 6-week check and for appropriate follow-up.

HOME CARE: THE NEWBORN

In the home, a newborn physical examination is performed as described in Chapter 25. The nurse also assesses and reinforces knowledge related to infant care as detailed in the following paragraphs.

HANDLING AND POSITIONING

Demonstrate methods of positioning and handling the newborn as needed. As the family members provide care, the nurse can instill confidence by giving them positive feedback. If a family member encounters problems, the nurse can suggest alternatives and serve as a role model.

When holding the newborn, one of the following positions can be used (Figure 31–7 ●). The *cradle hold* is frequently used during feeding. It provides a sense of warmth and closeness, permits eye contact, frees one of the adult's hands, and provides security because the cradling protects the newborn's body. Extra security is provided by gripping the baby's thigh with the hand while the arm supports the newborn's body. This grip is important to use when the infant is being carried. The *upright position* provides security and a sense of closeness and is ideal for burping the infant. One hand should support the neck and shoulders, while the other hand holds the buttocks or is placed between the newborn's legs. The newborn may also be held upright in a cloth sling carrier that gently holds the baby against the parent's chest and frees the hands for other tasks. The *football hold* frees one of the caregiver's hands and permits eye contact. This hold is ideal for shampooing, carrying, or breastfeeding. It frees the caregiver to talk on the telephone, answer the door, or do the myriad tasks that await attention at this busy time.

The infant's position should be changed periodically throughout the early months of life, because skull bones are soft, and permanently flattened areas may develop if the newborn consistently lies in one position. The awake newborn is frequently positioned on her or his side with the dependent arm forward to provide support and to prevent rolling. The side-lying position aids drainage of mucus and allows air to circulate around the cord. It is also comfortable for the newly circumcised male. After feeding, the newborn may be placed on the right side to aid diges-

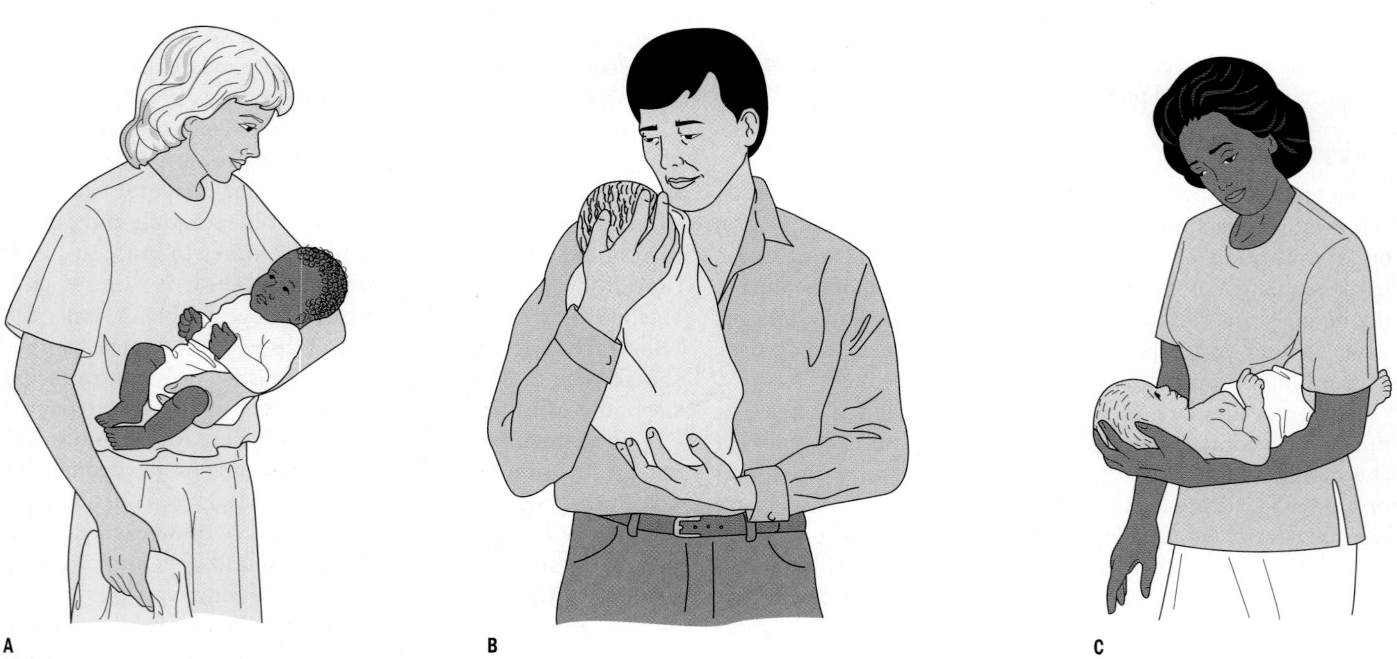

● **Figure 31–7** Various positions for holding an infant. ***A,*** Cradle hold. ***B,*** Upright position. ***C,*** Football hold.

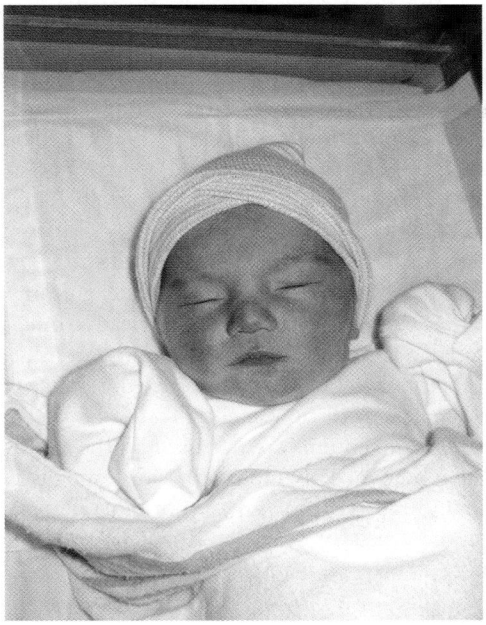

● **Figure 31–8** Infants should be placed on their backs when sleeping.

tion and to prevent aspiration of regurgitated feedings; this position also makes it easier to expel air bubbles from the stomach.

Although the side-lying position is appropriate when the infant is awake and under observation, infants should always sleep on their backs (Figure 31–8 ●). The American Academy of Pediatrics has recommended sleeping in nonprone positions since 1992 to reduce the risk of sudden infant death syndrome (SIDS). Since the initiation of the "Back to Sleep" campaign, there has been an increase in malformation of the skull caused by a decrease in tummy time. The syndrome is also known as *deformational plagiocephaly,* or positional plagiocephaly. These infants commonly have a flat spot on their skull, usually on the back or side, that is caused from continued placement in the same position. Infants who are not placed on their stomachs while awake at least three times daily are at risk for this skull malformation. Often these malformations will resolve on their own by one year of age, but sometimes infants need to wear a specially fitted helmet to correct the malformation (van Vlimmeren, van der Graaf, Boere-Boonekamp, et al., 2007).

Prone positioning while awake, also known as **tummy time**, is important for all babies because it assists them with learning developmentally appropriate skills; builds muscle strength for their shoulders, neck, and back; and prevents deformational plagiocephaly (National Institute of Child Health & Human Development, 2006). Infants should be placed on their tummies only when they are under direct supervision of a parent or adult.

Evidence in Action

Newborns should be placed in the supine position during sleep to reduce the risk of SIDS (Organization Guidelines) (American Academy of Pediatrics: Task force on Sudden Infant Death Syndrome, 2005).

BATHING

An actual bath demonstration is the best way for the nurse to provide information to parents. Because excess bathing and the use of soap remove natural skin oils and dry out the newborn's sensitive skin, bathing should be done every other day or twice a week. Sponge baths are recommended for the first 2 weeks or until the umbilical cord completely falls off and the umbilicus has healed. Some agencies use a tub bath for the bath demonstration.

At home, bath supplies can be kept in a plastic bag or some type of container to eliminate the necessity of hunting for them each time. For the baby's tub, the family may want to use a plastic dishpan, a clean kitchen or bathroom sink, or a large bowl. If using a sink, care should be taken to keep the infant away from faucets via which accidental burns could occur. Expensive baby tubs are not necessary, but some prefer to purchase them.

Before starting, if no one else is at home, the parent may want to take the phone off the hook and put a sign on the door to prevent being disturbed. Having someone home during the first few baths will be helpful, because that person can get forgotten items, attend to interruptions, and provide moral support. The room should be warm and free of drafts.

Sponge Baths

After the supplies are gathered, the tub (or any of the containers mentioned) is filled with water that is warm to the touch. Even though the newborn will not be placed in the tub, the bath giver carefully tests the water temperature with an elbow or forearm. Families may also choose to purchase a thermometer to help them determine when the bath water is at approximately 37.8°C (100°F) and safe to use. An unperfumed, mild soap such as Castile or Neutrogena should be used and kept on a soap dish or paper towel, not added to the water. Before the bath, the newborn should be wrapped in a blanket, with a T-shirt and diaper on, to keep her or him warm and secure.

To start the bath, the adult wraps a washcloth once around the index finger and wets it with water. *Soap is not used on the face.* Each eye is gently wiped from inner to outer corner. This direction prevents the potential for clogging the tear duct at the inner corner, where the eye naturally drains. A different portion of the washcloth is used for each eye to prevent cross contamination. Cotton balls can also be used for this purpose, a new one for each eye. Some swelling and drainage may be present the first few days after birth because of eye prophylaxis.

The bath giver washes the ears next by wrapping the washcloth once around an index finger and gently cleaning the external ear and behind the ear. Cotton swabs are never used in the ear canal because it is possible to put the swab too far into the ear and damage the ear drum. In addition, the swab may push any discharge farther down into the ear canal. The caregiver then wipes the remainder of the baby's face. Many babies start to cry at this point. The face should be washed every day and the mouth and chin wiped off after each feeding.

The neck is washed carefully but thoroughly with the washcloth. Soap may now be used. Formula or breast milk and lint collect in the skin folds of the neck, so it may be helpful to sit the newborn up, supporting the neck and shoulders with one hand while washing the neck with the other hand.

Next the bath giver unwraps the blanket, removes the T-shirt, and wets the chest, back, and arms with the washcloth. The bath giver may then lather the hands with soap and wash the baby's chest, back, and arms. The umbilical cord should be kept clean and dry. Wetting the cord is avoided, if possible, because it delays drying. The close proximity of the umbilical vessels makes the cord a possible entry area for infection. See Chapter 26 for care of umbilical cord and signs and symptoms of problems. Soap is rinsed off with the wet washcloth, and the upper part of the body is dried with a towel or blanket. The newborn's upper body is then wrapped with a clean, dry blanket to prevent a chill.

The bath giver then unwraps the newborn's legs, wets them with the washcloth, and lathers, rinses, and dries them well. If the newborn has dry skin, a small amount of unscented lotion or ointment (petroleum jelly or A & D ointment) may be used. Ointments are thought to be better than lotions for dry, cracked feet and hands. Baby oil is not recommended, because it clogs skin pores. Powders are not currently recommended. Families should be warned that baby powder can cause serious respiratory problems if inhaled. If parents want to use powder, they should be advised to use one that is talc free. The powder should be shaken into the hand and then placed on the newborn rather than shaken directly onto the baby.

The genital area is cleansed with soap and water daily and with water after each wet or dirty diaper. Females are washed from the front of the genital area toward the anus to prevent fecal contamination of the urethra and thus the bladder. Newborn females often have a thick, white mucous discharge or a slight bloody discharge from the vaginal area. This discharge is normal for the first 1 to 2 weeks after birth and should be wiped off with a damp cloth during diaper changes. The labia should be wiped, but the inner labial folds should not be aggressively cleaned.

Parents of uncircumcised males should cleanse the penis daily. Even minimal retraction of the foreskin is not advised (see in-depth discussion of care of uncircumcised male babies in Chapter 26). Males who have been circumcised also need daily gentle cleansing. Squeeze warm water over the baby's penis, letting the warm water run over the circumcision site. The area is rinsed off with warm water and lightly patted dry. A small amount of petroleum jelly, A & D ointment, or bactericidal ointment may be put on the circumcised area until the healing is complete, but excessive amounts may block the meatus and should be avoided. It is important to avoid using ointments if a Plastibell is in place because use of ointments may cause the Plastibell ring to slip off the penis too early. The Plastibell usually falls off within 5 to 8 days.

It is important to cleanse the diaper area with each diaper change to prevent diaper rash. Although this cleansing is done on a routine basis, a diaper rash may occasionally occur. Baby powder or cornstarch is not recommended for diaper rash. Baby powder may cake with urine and irritate the perineal area; cornstarch may promote fungal infection. Ointments that provide a barrier, such as zinc oxide, A & D ointment, and petroleum jelly, are more effective for diaper rash. If the ointment does not help the rash, families using single-use (disposable) diapers should try another brand. If they use cloth diapers, a different detergent or fabric softener, more thorough rinsing, and hanging them in the sun to dry may alleviate the problem. If the rash persists, parents should discuss the problem with their nurse practitioner or physician, because it may be caused by a fungal infection.

The last step in bathing is washing the hair (a step some suggest doing first). The newborn is swaddled in a dry blanket, leaving only the head exposed, and held in the football hold with the head tilted slightly downward to prevent water from running into the eyes. Water should be brought to the head by a cupped hand. The infant should never be placed under running water because extreme changes in temperature can lead to burns. The hair is moistened and lathered with a small amount of mild shampoo. A very soft brush may be used to massage the shampoo over the entire head, including the fontanelles. The hair is then rinsed and toweled dry. Oils or lotions are not used on the newborn's head unless there is evidence of cradle cap. Moistening the scaly area with lotion or mineral oil half an hour or more before shampooing softens the crusts or scales and makes it easier to remove them with a soft brush during the shampoo.

Tub Baths

The baby may be put in a small tub after the cord has fallen off and the circumcision site is healed (approximately 2 weeks) (Figure 31–9 ●). Newborns usually enjoy a tub bath more than a sponge bath, although some cry during either type. Only 3 or 4 inches of water is needed in the tub. To prevent slipping, a washcloth is placed in the bottom of the tub or sink. Some parents choose to bring the newborn into the tub with them.

The baby's face is washed in the same manner as for a sponge bath. The parent then places the newborn in the tub using the cradle hold and grasping the distal thigh. The neck is supported by the parent's elbow in the cradle position. An alternative hold

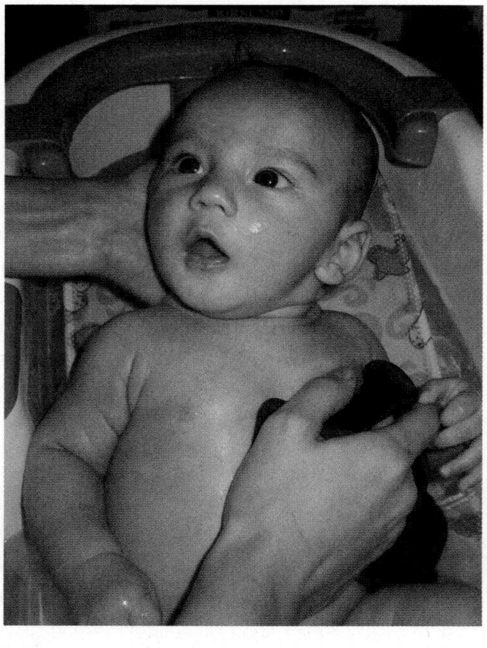

● **Figure 31–9** When bathing the newborn, the caregiver must support the head. Wet babies are very slippery.

is to support the newborn's head and neck with the forearm while grasping the distal shoulder and arm.

Because wet newborns are slippery, some parents pull a cotton sock (with holes cut out for the fingers) over the supporting arm to provide a "nonskid" surface. The newborn's body may be washed with a soapy washcloth or hand. To wash the back, the bath giver places his or her noncradling hand on the newborn's chest with the thumb under the newborn's arm closest to the adult. Gently tipping the newborn forward onto the supporting hand frees the cradling arm to wash the back. After the bath, the newborn is lifted out of the tub in the cradle position, dried well, and wrapped in a dry blanket. The hair is then washed in the same way as for a sponge bath.

NAIL CARE

The nails of the newborn are seldom cut in the birthing center. During the first days of life, the nails may adhere to the skin of the fingers, and cutting is contraindicated. Within a week the nails separate from the skin and frequently break off. If the nails are long or if the newborn is scratching his or her face, the nails may be trimmed. Trimming is most easily done while the infant is asleep. Nails should be cut straight across using adult cuticle scissors or blunt-ended infant cuticle scissors. Infant nails may also be filed.

DRESSING THE NEWBORN

Newborns need to wear a T-shirt, diaper (diaper cover or plastic pants if using cloth diapers), and a sleeper. On a fairly cool day, they should be wrapped in a light blanket while being fed. Newborns should be covered with a blanket in air-conditioned buildings. The blanket should be unwrapped or removed when inside a warm building. At home, the amount of clothing the newborn wears is determined by the temperature. Families who maintain their home at 15.5°C to 18.3°C (60°F to 65°F) should dress the infant more warmly than those who maintain a temperature of 21.1°C to 23.9°C (70°F to 75°F).

Newborns should wear head coverings outdoors to protect their sensitive ears from drafts. A blanket can be wrapped around the baby, leaving one corner free to place over the head while outdoors or in crowds for added protection. The nurse must advise families about the ease with which a newborn's skin can burn when exposed to the sun. To prevent sunburn, the newborn should remain shaded, wear a light layer of clothing, or be protected with sunscreen specifically formulated for infants.

Diaper shapes vary and are subject to personal preference (Figure 31–10 ●). Prefolded and disposable diapers are usually rectangular. Cloth diapers may also be triangular or kite folded. Extra material is placed in front for males and toward the back for females to increase absorbency. Cloth diapers, some of which now use velcro and highly absorbant materials, have been used more frequently in recent years because of the environmental concerns related to disposible diapers.

Baby clothing should be laundered separately with a mild soap or detergent. Diapers may be presoaked before washing. All clothing should be rinsed twice to remove soap and residue and to decrease the possibility of rash. Some newborns may not tolerate clothing treated with fabric softeners added to the washer or dryer.

TEMPERATURE ASSESSMENT

As the nurse prepares to teach parents about taking their baby's temperature, it is important to provide opportunities for discussion and demonstration. Families often need a review of how to take the baby's temperature and when to call their primary healthcare provider.

The nurse discusses the different types of thermometers available for home use. It is important that parents understand the differences and how to select the appropriate one. Tympanic membrane (ear) thermometers use infrared temperature scanning techniques to determine the infant's temperature. Infrared forehead thermometers are also available, but these devices may be less accurate than internal monitoring techniques (Pusnik & Drnovsek, 2005). Other parents elect to use a digital thermometer. The nurse reviews the correct procedure for using the chosen thermometer. The same digital thermometers should not be used for both oral and rectal temperature taking. Parents should label the thermometer and use it for only one route.

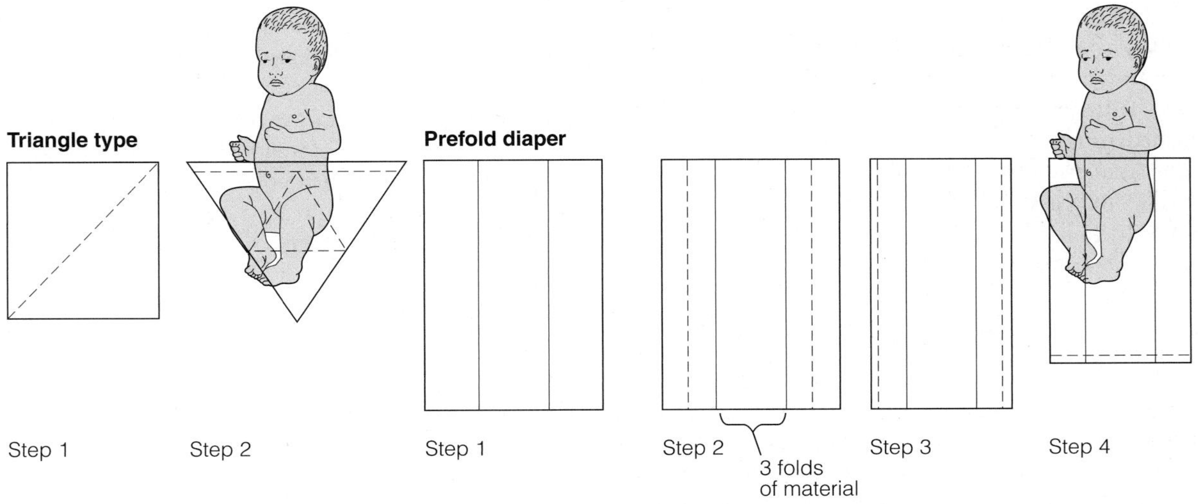

● **Figure 31–10** Two basic cloth diaper shapes. Dotted lines indicate folds.

Nursing Practice

Healthcare facilities no longer use glass thermometers because of the risks associated with resulting mercury spillage should one break. Parents should be advised not to use mercury thermometers and should be encouraged to discard them at a hazardous materials site specific to mercury thermometers. Before teaching families about temperature taking, you might find it helpful to visit a local pharmacy and review the types of thermometers available, the costs of the most commonly used methods, and the instructions provided. This will enable you to answer questions accurately when you work with parents or caregivers.

Parents need to take the newborn's temperature only when the signs of illness are present. They should call their pediatrician or pediatric nurse practitioner immediately if the temperature exceeds 38.4°C (101°F) rectally or 38°C (100.4°F) axillary. In premature infants, a low temperature may be a sign of infection; therefore, if the temperature is below 36.1°C (97°F) rectally or 36.6°C (97.8°F) axillary, the pediatrician should be notified.

Parents should discuss management of flu, colds, teething, constipation, diarrhea, gas discomfort, and other common ailments with their clinician before they occur. When analgesic or antipyretic medication is needed, clinicians frequently recommend acetaminophen or ibuprofen drops. Parents should not give any form of aspirin for an illness unless specifically directed to do so by their healthcare provider; use of aspirin in viral illnesses has been linked to Reye's syndrome in children.

STOOLS AND URINE

The appearance and frequency of a newborn's stools can cause concern for parents. The nurse prepares them by discussing and showing pictures of meconium stools and transitional stools and by describing the difference between breast milk and formula stools. Although each baby develops his or her own stooling patterns, parents can expect the following (see Figures 24–9 & 27–13∞).

- Breastfed newborns may have 6 to 10 small, semiliquid, yellow stools per day by the third or fourth day, when milk production is established, unless the mother is having problems with her milk supply. Once breastfeeding is well established, usually by 1 month, the newborn may have only one stool every few days because of the increased digestibility of breast milk. However, they may still have several daily. Constipation is unlikely to occur in newborns receiving only breast milk. Infrequent stooling in the first few weeks may indicate inadequate milk intake.
- Formula-fed babies may have only one or two stools a day; they are more formed and yellow or yellow-brown.

The parents may also be shown pictures of a constipated stool (small, pelletlike) and diarrhea (loose, green, or perhaps blood tinged). Families should understand that a green color is common in transitional stools, so that transitional stools are not confused with diarrhea during the first week of a newborn's life.

Nursing Practice

If parents using disposable diapers are unable to determine if the diaper is wet, advise them to tear off the top layer of the diaper and examine the cotton batting beneath the absorbent layer. It is easier for parents to see urine saturation and a change of color on this portion of the diaper in order to determine if the infant has voided.

Constipation may indicate that the newborn needs additional fluid intake. Parents may try offering additional water in an attempt to reverse the constipation. Parents should be counseled that each baby develops his or her own stooling pattern, and some babies may not pass a stool daily. As long as the infant appears comfortable and is not in distress, this can be normal for that infant and is not a cause for concern.

Babies normally void five to eight times per day. Fewer than six to eight wet diapers a day may indicate that the newborn needs more fluids. Frequency of voiding is easy to assess with cloth diapers. Parents who use superabsorbent single-use disposable diapers may have difficulty determining voiding patterns because the surface of the diaper feels dry. The liquid pools inside the filling of the diaper.

SLEEP AND ACTIVITY

The newborn demonstrates several different sleep–wake states after the initial periods of reactivity described in Chapter 24∞ and six newborn sleep–wake states have been identified (see Table 31–7): It is not uncommon for a newborn to sleep almost continuously for the first 2 to 3 days following birth, awakening only for feedings every few hours. Indeed, it is not uncommon to have difficulty feeding the infant during the first 24 to 48 hours because of this deep sleep. Some newborns bypass this stage and require only 12 to 16 hours of sleep. The parents need to know that this pattern is normal.

Infants typically do not sleep through the night until they are at least 3 months of age or weigh 12 to 13 lb (5443 gms to 5897 gms). Some infants sleep through the night as early as 8 weeks whereas others do not sleep through the night until 6 months of age or beyond. It is estimated that two-thirds of infants sleep through the night by the age of 6 months. Although newborns typically sleep up to 16 hours per day, they do so in short time intervals. Some parents may be tempted to try home remedies, such as giving infants cereal in their bottles or other additives that are said to assist their children in sleeping through the night. Parents should be counseled that these remedies are not recommended.

CRYING

For the newborn, crying is the only means of expressing needs vocally. Families learn to distinguish different tones and qualities of the newborn's cry. The amount of crying is highly individual. Some cry as little as 15 to 30 minutes in 24 hours, and others cry as long as 2 hours every 24 hours. When crying continues after causes such as discomfort and hunger are eliminated, the newborn may be comforted by swaddling or by rocking and other reassuring activities.

Table 31–7 Infant Sleep and Awake States*

Infant States	Physical Characteristics	Body Activity	Eye Movements	Facial Movements	Breathing Pattern	Responses	Caregiver Implications
SLEEP STATES							
Quiet sleep (also known as deep sleep)	Anabolic, restorative sleep, increased cell mitosis and replication, lowered oxygen consumption, release of growth hormone.	Typically still, may occasionally startle or twitch.	None.	None or may have occasional sucking movements.	Slow and regular.	Only intense or disturbing stimuli will arouse infant, threshold to stimuli is high.	Difficult to arouse for feedings. Teach parents to time feedings when infant is in a more responsive state. Infant may arouse slightly if an attempt is made to awaken but typically returns to the quiet sleep state.
Active sleep (also known as light sleep or rapid eye movement [REM] state)	Processing and recording information. Often linked to learning. Is the highest proportion of sleep and precedes awakening.	Some body movements.	REM, eyelids flutter beneath closed eyelids.	May smile or make fussing or crying noises.	Irregular.	More responsive to internal stimuli (hunger) and external stimuli (such as being picked up by caregiver). When stimulated may arouse, return to quiet sleep, or remain in active sleep.	Inexperienced care providers may attempt to feed when infant makes normal crying sounds.
AWAKE STATES							
Drowsy	May return to sleep or awaken further.	Smooth movements with variable activity level. May experience mild startles intermittently.	Eyes may open and close. May appear heavy-lidded, or eyes may appear like slits.	May have no facial movements and appear still, or may have some facial movements.	Irregular.	Usually reacts to stimuli but may be slowed. May change to other states such as quiet alert, active alert, or crying.	To stimulate infant, provide verbal, sight, or oral stimulation. If left alone, infant may return to a sleep state.
Quiet alert	Attentive to environment, focus attention on stimuli.	Minimal.	Eyes bright and wide.	Attentive appearance.	Regular.	Most attentive, focus attention on stimuli.	In the first hours after birth, may experience intense alertness before going into a long sleeping period. This state increases in intensity as the infant becomes older. Providing stimuli will help maintain an active alert state or a drowsy or active-alert state. Infant provides pleasure and positive feedback to care providers. Good time to feed infant.
Active alert	Infant's eyes are open, not as bright as in quiet alert. More body activity than in a quiet alert state.	Smooth movements may be interspersed with mild startles from time to time.	Eyes open with a gazed, dull appearance.	May be still with or without facial movements.	Irregular.	Reacts to stimuli with delayed responses to stimuli, or may change to quiet alert or crying state.	Infant may be fussy and become sensitive to stimuli, may become more and more active and start crying. If fatigue or caregiver interventions disturb this state, infant may return to a drowsy or sleep state.
Crying	Communication tool, response to unpleasant stimuli from environment or internal stimuli. Characterized by intense crying for more than 15 seconds.	Increased motor activity, skin color changes to darkened appearance, red, or ruddy.	Eyes may be tightly closed or open.	Grimaces.	More irregular than in other states.	Very responsive to internal or external unpleasant stimuli.	Indicates that the infant's limits have been reached. May be able to console himself or herself and return to an alert or sleep state, or may need intervention from caregiver.

Source: March of Dimes. (2003). *Understanding the behavior of term infants.* White Plains, NY: Author.

*A *state* is a group of characteristic behaviors and physiologic changes that occur together in a regular pattern.

There is some indication that newborns who are held more tend to be calmer and cry less when not being held. Some parents are afraid that holding may "spoil" the newborn and need reassurance that this is not the case. Picking babies up when they cry teaches them that adults are responsive to them. This helps build a sense of trust in humankind. Excessive crying should be noted and assessed, taking other factors into consideration. After the first 2 or 3 days, newborns settle into individual patterns.

Coping with prolonged crying may be a challenge for new parents, who may respond by withdrawing their affection from the newborn, providing routine care and feeding, but not becoming emotionally attached. Other parents may respond by neglecting, abandoning, or even hitting or shaking their newborn. Parents need to understand the serious, even life-threatening consequences of such behavior. For example, a neglected or abandoned newborn can quickly become dehydrated, and hitting can cause internal hemorrhage, bruising, and fractures. Shaking can cause brain hemorrhage, spinal cord injury, retinal hemorrhage or detachment, long-term developmental problems, mental retardation, or even death. This collection of symptoms that are caused by vigorously shaking an infant is known as **shaken baby injuries**. (For more information on child abuse, see Chapters 44 and 56.)

To increase parents' coping abilities, suggest that they initially respond to the baby's crying by checking for hunger, a wet or soiled diaper, excessive cold or heat, restrictive or chafing clothing or blankets, or other comfort concerns. If these are not present, suggest holding or rocking the infant as previously discussed. Other calming measures include burping the infant (which provides repetitive tactile stimulation and disperses air bubbles), placing the infant in a mechanized infant swing, or taking the infant for a ride in a stroller or car. Some infants are soothed by white noise such as the sound of a dryer or the static on an untuned radio, whereas others are soothed when bound "papoose style" on the mother's or father's chest, swaddled, bathed, or massaged.

Crying can also be associated with gastrointestinal upset in infants. The parents should discuss concerns with the physician or nurse practitioner to ensure the crying is not associated with a physical cause, such as acid reflux, ear infections, or other physical conditions. In addition, it is not uncommon for infants to cry after feedings because of pain from a buildup of air bubbles in the stomach and an inability to pass flatus. Some practitioners recommend simethicone after each feeding to decrease the incidence of flatus pain. Placing the infant in a prone position across the lap while burping the infant can also aid in passing flatus.

Nursing Practice

Advise parents that if they become frustrated with a crying baby, they should put the baby in the crib or in a safe location and allow themselves time to calm down. Sometimes going outside the door, counting to 10, doing deep breathing, or calling a friend can help. Remind parents that crying never hurts a baby, but shaking can seriously injure the baby. Reassure parents that all new parents have times when they feel frustrated and do not know what to do. This is a normal part of parenting a newborn.

SAFETY CONSIDERATIONS

Newborns should not have pillows, blankets, or stuffed animals in the crib while they sleep; these items could cause suffocation. Mattresses should fit snugly in a crib to prevent entrapment and suffocation, and the crib should be inspected regularly to determine whether it is in safe working order. Crib slats should be no more than 2 3/8 in. apart. Parents can be encouraged to attend infant cardiopulmonary resuscitation (CPR) classes, especially if there is a family history of SIDS or the infant requires special care.

Many families, especially breastfeeding families, practice **cosleeping**, in which the infant sleeps with the mother or both parents during the night. The American Academy of Pediatrics does not recommend cosleeping as it is considered a risk factor for SIDS. Some families and cultures, however, may still particiapte in this practice and thus warrant appropriate teaching measures.

Cosleeping families should be counseled to follow these safety guidelines:

- Place the infant on a firm mattress, never on comforters, pillows, or a waterbed.
- Never sleep with your infant if you have been using drugs, or have become intoxicated.
- Ensure that the infant is protected from rolling off the bed or becoming entrapped in bed rails or a space between the frame and the mattress.
- As with crib sleeping, remove all decorative pillows, stuffed animals, toys, or blankets that could impair the baby's breathing. Do not cover the baby with blankets, sheets, or down comforters.
- Make sure the baby is sleeping on his or her back.
- Ensure plenty of ventilation to the infant.
- Avoid overdressing the infant because the parent's body heat will reduce the need for excess clothing.
- Never smoke in bed with the infant. Family members should smoke outdoors and not in the household with the infant.
- If additional children are sleeping in the bed, make sure they are not sleeping directly next to the infant.

Smoking poses multiple risks to the newborn and any older children living in the household. Infants living in a household with a smoker have a higher rate of hospital admissions during the first year of life. They are more prone to ear infections, asthma, allergies, and other respiratory problems (see Chapter 48). The American Academy of Pediatrics (2005) recommends that the safest place for the infant to sleep is in the same room with the infant in a crib in close proximity to the parents for the first 6 months of life. The use of pacifiers has also been associated with a reduction in SIDS deaths (AAP, 2005).

Smoking also creates a fire hazard within the household. Smoking is the primary cause of household fires in the United States. The incidence of such fires increases dramatically when other intoxicating agents are ingested, such as alcohol or drugs. Parents should be counseled to smoke outdoors; use large, heavy ashtrays to avoid tipping; ensure that all cigarette butts are properly extinguished; and never smoke in bed.

POSTPARTAL CLASSES AND SUPPORT GROUPS

These services range from educational, such as classes on nutrition, exercise, infant care, and parenting, to specific healthcare programs, such as well-baby checks, immunization clinics, family-planning services, new mother support groups, and more.

Postpartal classes are becoming more common as caregivers recognize the continuing needs of the childbearing family. In many instances, classes are prepared to meet the specific needs of a variety of families so that, for example, single mothers and adolescent mothers can attend class with peers. A series of structured classes may focus on topics such as parenting, postpartal exercise, or nutrition, or there may be loosely structured group sessions that address mothers' concerns as they arise. Such classes offer chances for the new mother to socialize, share her concerns, and receive encouragement. Because baby-sitting arrangements may be difficult or expensive, it is desirable to provide child care for newborns and siblings; in some instances infants may remain with mothers in the class.

Many communities offer support groups through birthing centers, hospitals, or other facilities. La Leche League, an excellent support group for breastfeeding mothers, typically meets monthly and is open to all pregnant and breastfeeding mothers of infants and toddlers. Women who have children with special needs may need additional support. Referring them to peer counselors or support groups is an effective way to help them find both support and information. Once again, such groups provide an opportunity for parents to share information, advice, and experiences.

Many parents today look to the Internet for information on parenting and newborn care. Nurses have an opportunity to assist parents in evaluating the reliability of the information they find. Criteria that suggest that Internet information is reliable and of high quality include affiliation with a university medical or nursing school or a government agency; inclusion of authors' credentials, education, board certification, and affiliations; referencing of information; currency of information; similarity of information when compared with other sources; and easy accessibility.

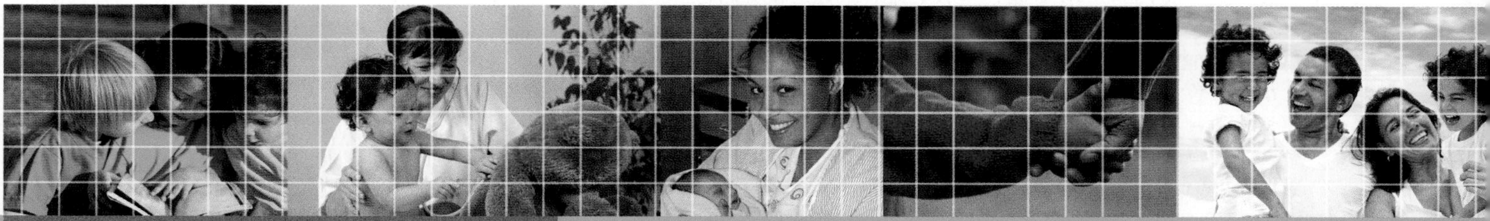

CRITICAL CONCEPT REVIEW

LEARNING OUTCOMES	CONCEPTS
31.1 Formulate nursing diagnoses and nursing care based on the findings of the "normal" postpartum assessment and teaching needs.	1. Nursing diagnoses focus on the normal and expected postpartal course. 2. Nursing diagnoses allow the nurse to identify expected outcomes and select nursing interventions that will help the family meet the expected outcomes and achieve optimal health promotion. 3. The nurse should discuss desired outcomes and goals with the mother and family members.
31.2 Discuss appropriate nursing interventions to promote maternal comfort, rest, and well-being.	1. The nurse can promote and restore maternal physical well-being by monitoring uterine status, vital signs, cardiovascular status, elimination patterns, nutritional needs, sleep and rest, and support and educational needs. 2. The nurse should: ■ Encourage the new mother to rest when the infant rests. ■ Counsel the new mother to resume activities gradually. ■ Recommend exercise to provide health benefits to the new mother. 3. In addition, the postpartum woman may need medications to promote comfort, treat anemia, provide immunity to rubella, and prevent development of antigens (in the nonsensitized Rh-negative woman).
31.3 Explain factors that affect postpartal family wellness in the provision of nursing care and client teaching.	1. Possible reactions of siblings. 2. Resumption of sexual activity: ■ Discuss possible temporary problems such as sleep deprivation, vaginal dryness, and lack of time together. 3. Contraception. 4. Parent-infant attachment: ■ Help parents realize there will be both positive and negative feelings about parenthood. ■ New parents need to understand that the infant is unique with a distinctive personality.

(continued)

LEARNING OUTCOMES	CONCEPTS
31.4 Compare the postpartal nursing needs of the woman who experienced a cesarean birth with the needs of a woman who gave birth vaginally.	1. Woman who experienced a cesarean birth has all the needs of the woman who had a vaginal birth: ■ Assessment of the fundus. ■ Assessment of breasts. ■ Perineal evaluation (may have varicose veins or hemorrhoids from pregnancy). ■ Assessment of lochia flow. ■ Assessment of bowel and bladder. 2. After a cesarean birth the woman needs assessment of the abdomen: ■ Incision. ■ Turn, cough, and deep breathe. ■ Bowel sounds. 3. After a cesarean birth the mother will have a greater need for pain medication. She will also have increased fatigue because of the surgical intervention. The mother may need encouragement to interact with the infant.
31.5 Examine the nursing needs of the childbearing adolescent during the postpartal period.	1. The nurse should evaluate the adolescent mother in terms of her level of maturity, available support systems, cultural background, and existing knowledge, and then plan care accordingly.
31.6 Describe possible approaches to sensitive, holistic nursing care for the woman who relinquishes her newborn.	1. The mother who decides to relinquish her baby needs emotional support. She should be able to decide whether to see and hold her baby, and any special requests regarding the birth should be honored.
31.7 Identify teaching topics related to postpartum discharge.	1. Prior to discharge the couple should be given any information necessary for the woman to provide appropriate self-care. 2. Parents should have a beginning skill in caring for their newborn and should be familiar with warning signs of possible complications for mother or baby. 3. Printed information is valuable in helping couples deal with questions that may arise at home. 4. Available types of follow-up care and community resources (telephone calls, home visits, baby care/postpartum classes, new mother support groups).
31.8 Identify the main purposes and components of home visits during the postpartal period.	The main purposes of the home visit: 1. Assess the status of the mother and infant. 2. Assess adaptation and adjustment of the family to the new baby. 3. Determine current informational needs. 4. Provide teaching as needed. 5. Use as an opportunity to answer additional questions related to infant care and feeding, and to provide emotional support to the mother and family. The components of the postpartal home visit include: 1. Establish contact with the mother prior to the visit. 2. Identify the purpose and goals of the visit. 3. Establish rapport with the mother. 4. Maintain safety during the visit. 5. Assess the status of the mother, newborn, and family. 6. Reinforce teaching concerning maternal and newborn care.
31.9 Summarize actions a nurse should take to ensure personal safety as well as fostering a caring relationship during a home visit.	Nurses need to act proactively to maintain their safety when making home visits by exercising reasonable caution and remaining alert to environmental cues. Fostering a caring relationship in the home involves: 1. Evidence of genuineness and empathy. 2. Establishment of trust and rapport. 3. Positive regard for the mother and family.
31.10 Discuss maternal and family assessment and anticipated progress after birth.	1. Expected maternal assessments: ■ Vital signs. (Should be at prepregnancy level.) ■ Weight. (Expect weight to be near prepregnancy level at 6 weeks postpartum.) ■ Condition of the breasts. ■ Condition of the abdomen, including a healing cesarean incision, if applicable. ■ Elimination pattern. (Should return to normal by 4 to 6 weeks postpartum.) ■ Lochia. (Should progress from lochia rubra to lochia serosa to lochia alba. If not breastfeeding, menstrual pattern should return at 6 weeks postpartum.) ■ Fundus. (Fundus should decrease in size one finger-breadth per day after the birth of the baby. Uterus should return to normal size by 6 weeks postpartum.) ■ Perineum. (Episiotomy and lacerations should show signs of healing.)

LEARNING OUTCOMES | CONCEPTS

2. Family assessment:
   - Bonding. (Appropriate demonstration of bonding should be apparent.)
   - Level of comfort. (Parents should display appropriate levels of comfort with the infant.)
   - Siblings are adjusting to new baby.
   - Parental role adjustment. (Parents should be working on division of labor, changes in financial status, communication changes, readjustment of sexual relations, and adjustment to new daily tasks.)
   - Contraception. (Parents understand need to choose and use a method of contraception.)

31.11 Delineate interventions to address the common concerns of breastfeeding mothers following discharge. →

Common concerns of the breastfeeding mother include:
1. Nipple soreness.
2. Cracked nipples.
3. Engorgement.
4. Plugged ducts.

Breastfeeding mothers are encouraged to:
1. Nurse frequently.
2. Change the infant's position regularly.
3. Allow nipples to air dry after breastfeeding.

31.12 Describe the assessment and care of the newborn during postpartal home care. →

1. Assess the infant's weight, length, heart rate, head circumference, and any signs of jaundice.
2. Watch the mother feed the baby and discuss any concerns she has about feeding.
3. Reinforce teaching in the following areas:
   - Position and handling.
   - Bathing.
   - Dressing.
   - Temperature assessment.
   - Stool and urine.
   - Sleep and activity.
   - Crying.
   - Safety considerations.
   - Newborn screening and necessary immunizations.

CRITICAL THINKING IN ACTION

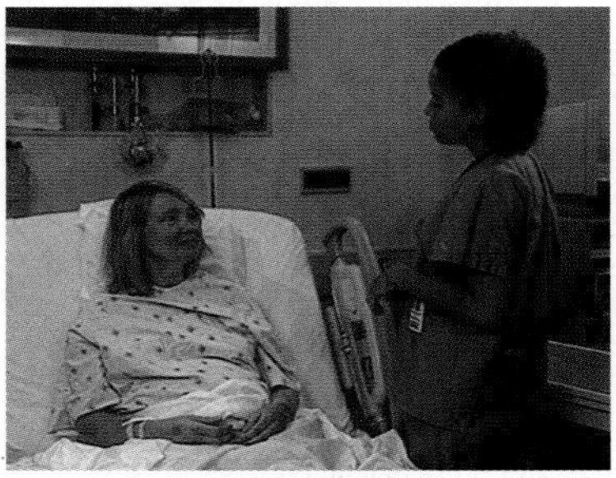

Wendy Calahan, a 31-year-old G3, P2, gave birth to an 8.5 pound baby boy by primary cesarean birth for failure to progress. The baby's Apgar scores were 9 and 9 at 1 and 5 minutes. The baby was admitted to the newborn nursery for transitional observation. Wendy was transferred to the postpartum unit, where you assume her care. You introduce yourself and orient her to the room, call bell, and safety measures. You perform an initial assessment, with all findings within normal limits. Wendy tells you she is very tired and would like to rest while her baby is in the nursery. Her husband and family have left the hospital after spending time with her in the recovery room but will return later. She admits she is disappointed that she could not give birth vaginally even though she pushed for 2 hours. She says, "This baby was just too big."

1. How would you discuss with Wendy the need for frequent assessments after birth?
2. Explain "maternity or baby blues."
3. Explore activities to minimize maternity blues.
4. Discuss concerns of a woman experiencing her second pregnancy.
5. Discuss behaviors that inhibit paternal attachment.

See MyNursingKit for possible responses.

REFERENCES

Advisory Committee on Immunization Practices (ACIP) Centers for Disease Control and Prevention. Prevention of pertussis, tetanus, and diphtheria among pregnant and postpartum women and their infants. Recommendations of the Advisory Committee on Immunization Practices (ACIP). *MMWR Recomm Rep* 2008 May 30; 57(RR-4), 1–51.

American Academy of Pediatrics, Committee on Fetus and Newborn. (2004). Hospital stay for healthy term newborns. *Pediatrics, 113*(5), 1434–1436.

American Academy of Pediatrics. (2005, November). Policy statement: The changing concept of sudden infant death syndrome: Diagnostic coding shifts, controversies regarding the sleeping environment, and new variables to consider in reducing risk. *Pediatrics, 116*(5), 1245–1255.

Andrews, V., Thakar, R., Sultan, A. H., & Jones, P. W. (2007). Evaluation of postpartum perineal pain and dyspareunia: A prospective study. *European Journal of Obstetrics, Gynecology, & Reproductive Biology* (2007 Aug 1) [Epub ahead of print].

Asbee, S. M., Jenkins, T. R., Butler, J. R., White, J., Elliot, M., Rutledge, A. (2009) Preventing excessive weight gain during pregnancy through dietary and lifestyle counseling. *Obstetrics and Gynecology, 113*, 305–312.

Association of Women's Health, Obstetrical, and Neonatal Nurses (AWHONN). (2006). *The compendium of postpartum care.* Washington, DC: AWHONN.

Bernstein, H. H., Spino, C., Finch, S., Wasserman, R., Slora, E., Lalama, C., et al. (2007).

Decision-making for postpartum discharge of 4300 mothers and their healthy infants: The Life Around Newborn Discharge study. *Pediatrics, 120*(2), e391–400 [Epub 2007 Jul 16].

Bruhn, K. & Tillett, J. (2009). Administration of vaccinations in pregnancy and postpartum. *The American Journal of Maternal/Child Nursing. 34*(2), 98–105.

Burgos, A. E., Schmitt, S. K., Stevenson, D. K., & Phibbs, C. S. (2008). Readmission for neonatal jaundice in California, 1991–2000: Trends and implications. *Pediatrics, 121*(4), e864–e869.

Child Welfare Information Gateway. (2005). Voluntary relinquishment for adoption. Retrieved August 10, 2009, from http://www.childwelfare.gov/pubs/s_place.cfm

Child Welfare Information Gateway. (2007a). Grounds for involuntary termination of parental rights. Retrieved August 10, 2009, from http://www.childwelfare.gov/systemwide/laws_policies/statutes/groundtermin.cfm

Child Welfare Information Gateway. (2007b). Infant safe haven laws. Retrieved August 10, 2009, from http://www.childwelfare.gov/systemwide/laws_policies/statutes/safehaven.cfm

Conde, A. A., Figueiredo, B., Costa, R., Pacheco, A., & Pais, A. (2008). Perception of the childbirth experience: Continuity and changes over the postpartum period. *Journal of Reproductive and Infant Psychology, 26*(2), 139–154.

Convery, K. M. & Spatz, D. L. (2009). Sexuality & breastfeeding: What do you know? *The American Journal of Maternal/Child Nursing. 34*(4), 218–223.

de Almeida, M. F. B., & Draque, C. M. (2007). Neonatal jaundice and breastfeeding. *Neonatal Reviews, 8*(7), e282. Retrieved August 10, 2009, from http://neoreviews.aappublications.org/cgi/content/short/8/7/e282.

Engle, W. A., Tomashek, K. M., Wallman, C., & Committee on Fetus & Newborn. (2007). Late preterm infants: A population at risk. *Pediatrics, 120*(6), 1390–1401.

Göçmen, A., Göçmen, M., & Saraoğlu, M. (2002). Early post-operative feeding after caesarean delivery. *Journal of Internal Medicine Research, 30*(5), 506–511.

Goulet, L., D'Amour, D., & Pineault, R. (2007). Type and timing of services following postnatal discharge: Do they make a difference? *Women's Health, 45*(4), 19–39.

Gucev, G., Yasui, G. M., Chang, T. Y., & Lee, J. (2008). Bilateral ultrasound-guided continuous ilioinguinal-iliohypogastric block for pain relief after cesarean delivery. *Anesthesia & Analgesia,106*, 1220–1222.

Henney, S. M., Ayers-Lopez, S., McCoy, R. G., & Grotevant, H. D. (2007). Evolution and revolution: Birthmothers' experiences with grief and loss at different levels of adoption openness. *Journal of Social and Personal Relationships, 24*(6), 875–889.

Hofmeyr, G. J., Abdel-Aleem, H., & Abdel-Aleem, M. A. (2008). Uterine massage for preventing postpartum haemorrhage. *Cochrane Database of Systematic Reviews,* Issue 3.

Hunter, L., Rychnovsky, J., & Yount, S. 2009. A selective review of maternal sleep characteristics in the postpartum period. *Journal of Obstetric, Gynecologic, and Neonatal Nursing, 38*(1), 60–68.

Jones, C. C. (2006). The functions of childbirth and postpartum henna traditions. Retrieved September 8, 2007, at http://www.hennapage.com/henna/encyclopedia/pregbirth/postpart.pdf.

Keller, C., Records, K., Ainsworth, B., Permana, P., & Coonrod, D. (2008). Interventions for weight management in postpartum women. *Journal of Obstetric, Gynecologic, and Neonatal Nursing, 37*, 71–79.

Lemay, C. A., Cashman, S. B., Elfenbein, D. S., & Felice, M. E. (2007). Adolescent mothers' attitudes toward contraceptive use before and after pregnancy. *Journal of Pediatric & Adolescent Gynecology, 20*(4), 233–240.

Lin, J. P., Wang, H. H., & Chang, H. H. (2007). "Doing the month" experiences of Vietnamese primipara in Taiwan. *Hu Li Za Zhi, 54*(2), 47–54.

McPhaul, K. M., Rosen, J., Bobb, S., Okechukwu, C., Geiger-Brown, J., Kauffman, K., Johnson, J. V., & Lipscomb, J. (2007). An exploratory study of mandated safety measures for home visiting case managers. *Canadian Journal of Nursing Research, 39*(4), 173–189.

Melli, M. S., Rashidi, M. R., Nokhoodchi, A., Tagavi, S., Farzadi, L., Sadaghat, K., et al. (2007). A randomized trial of peppermint gel, lanolin ointment, and placebo gel to prevent nipple crack in primiparous breastfeeding women. *Medical Science Monitor, 13*(9), CR406–CR411.

Morland-Schultz, K., & Hill, P. D. (2005). Prevention of and therapies for nipple pain: A systematic review. *Journal of Obstetric, Gynecologic, and Neonatal Nursing,* 34(4), 428–437.

National Institute of Child Health & Human Development. (2006). Tummy time. Retrieved on August 10, 2010, at http://www.nichd.nih.gov/health/topics/tummy_time.cfm

O'Keffe, K. (2005). Expanded AAP breastfeeding policy calls for support of nursing moms. *AAP News, 26*, 1–10.

Porter, M., van Teijlingen, E., Chi Ying Yip, L., & Bhattacharya, S. (2007). Satisfaction with cesarean section: Qualitative analysis of open-ended questions in a large postal survey. *Birth, 34*(2), 148–154.

Pusnik, I., & Drnovsek, J. (2005). Infrared ear thermometers—Parameters influencing their reading and accuracy. *Physiological Measurement, 26*(6), 1075–1084.

Reid, V., & Meadows-Oliver, M. (2007). Postpartum depression in adolescent mothers: An integrative review of the literature. *Journal of Pediatric Health Care, 21*(5), 289–298.

Riordan, J. & Wambach, K. (2010). *Breastfeeding and human lactation* (4th ed.). Boston: Jones & Bartlett.

Spector, R. E. (2009). *Cultural diversity in health and illness* (7th ed). Upper Saddle River, NJ: Prentice Hall Health.

Steen, M., Briggs, M., & King, D. (2006). Alleviating postpartal perineal trauma: To cool or not to cool? *British Journal of Nurse Midwifery, 14*(5), 305–306.

Tejirian, T., & Abbas, M. A. (2005). Sitz bath: Where is the evidence? Scientific basis of a common practice. *Disorders of the Colon & Rectum, 48*(12), 2336–2340.

United States Department of Labor. (2009). Fact sheet: Newborn & mother's health protection act. Retrieved on August 10, 2009, at http://www.dol.gov/ebsa/newsroom/fsnmhafs.html.

van Vlimmeren, L. A., van der Graaf, Y., Boere-Boonekamp, M. M., L'Hoir, M. P., Helders, P. J., & Engelbert, R. H. (2007). Risk factors for deformational plagiocephaly at birth and at 7 weeks of age: A prospective cohort study. *Pediatrics, 119*(2), e408–e418.

Viscusi, E. R. (2008). Patient-controlled drug delivery for acute postoperative pain management: A review of current and emerging technologies. *Regional Anesthesia Pain Medicine, 33*(2), 146–158.

Walker, M. (2007). International breastfeeding initiatives and their relevance to the current state of breastfeeding in the United States. *Journal of Nurse Midwifery & Women's Health, 52*(6), 549–555.

Wiklund, I., Edman, G., & Andolf, E. (2007). Cesarean section on maternal request: Reasons for the request, self-estimated health, expectations, experience of birth and signs of depression among first-time mothers. *Acta Obstetrics & Gynecology Scandanavia, 86*(4), 451–456.

Wilson, B. A., Shannon, M. T., & Shields, K. M. (2010). *Nurse's drug guide 2010.* Upper Saddle River, NJ: Pearson Education.

World Health Organization. (2007). Pospartum care of the mother and newborn: A practical guide. Retrieved on September 8, 2007, at http://www.who.int/reproductive-health/publications/msm_98_3/msm_98_3_11.html

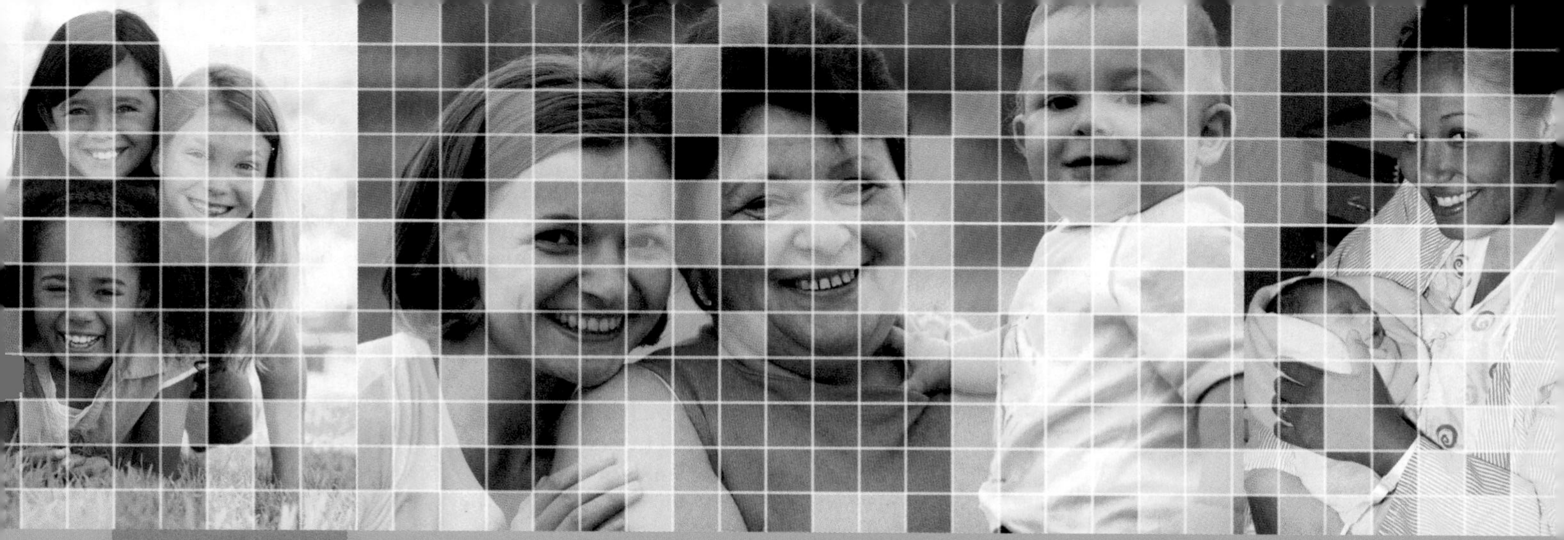

CHAPTER

32 The Postpartal Family at Risk

We are surviving. Maybe just. I was told that babies ate at six-ten-two-six-ten-two, but no one said that he would eat at five-seven-nine-eleven or so it seems. I am either getting ready to feed him or just finished feeding and changing him. But I love him without bounds. I feel a need to protect him from ever being hurt or wounded. During that first week, when I was tired and recovering from the emergency cesarean, I was afraid that I would not be able to shelter and help this young son grow up. —Kate, 34

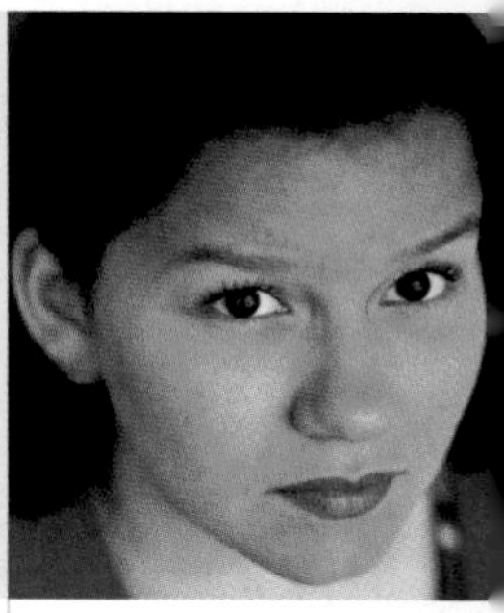

LEARNING OUTCOMES

32.1 Identify the causes of and appropriate nursing interventions for early and late hemorrhage during the postpartal period.

32.2 Develop a nursing care plan that reflects knowledge of etiology, pathophysiology, clinical therapy, nursing and preventive management for the woman experiencing postpartum hemorrhage, reproductive tract infection, urinary tract infection, mastitis, thromboembolic disease, or a postpartal psychiatric disorder.

32.3 Evaluate the woman's knowledge of self-care measures, signs of complications to be reported to the primary care provider, and measures to prevent recurrence of complications.

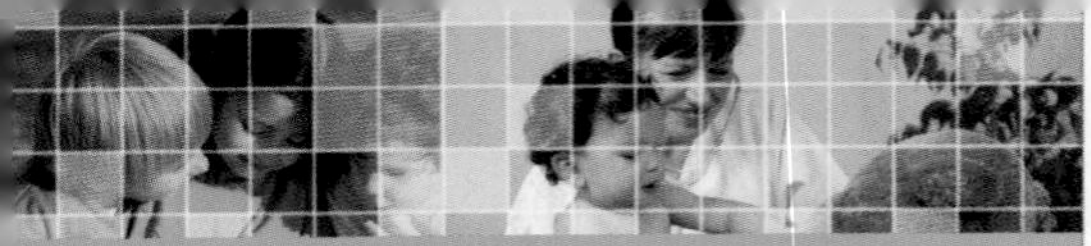

KEY TERMS

Early (primary) postpartal hemorrhage, 824

Endometritis (metritis), 832

Late (secondary) postpartal hemorrhage, 824

Mastitis, 839

Pelvic cellulitis (parametritis), 832

Peritonitis, 832

Postpartum blues (adjustment reaction with depressed mood), 849

Postpartum major mood disorder (postpartum depression), 849

Postpartum psychosis, 849

Puerperal infection, 831

Puerperal morbidity, 831

Subinvolution, 829

Thrombophlebitis, 842

Uterine atony, 825

The postpartal period is typically viewed as a smooth, uneventful transition time—and often it is, even with the challenges of new parenthood and the integration of a new person into the family. However, it is equally important for the nurse to be aware of physical or emotional complications that may develop postpartally. The nurse should teach the family the signs of postpartal complications, findings to report to the physician or certified nurse-midwife (CNM), and preventive measures, if available.

Written instructions to supplement any discussion will be of great value in the early weeks at home with a newborn when life can be chaotic and instructions may be forgotten. The family should have telephone numbers for postpartum follow-up services and other resources to answer questions. By communicating an attitude of willingness to answer questions and listen to concerns, the nurse enhances the parents' comfort in making calls later for what they might otherwise perceive as issues "too trivial to bother someone about."

When a telephone follow-up or an examination at the home visit provides evidence of a developing complication, the nurse shares these findings or impressions with the woman, and they mutually plan an appropriate next step. In the case of telephone follow-up, the nurse usually counsels the woman to notify her physician or certified nurse-midwife, being prepared to schedule an appointment immediately if risk assessment indicates. The nurse who identifies a complication at the home visit will need to communicate the clinical findings to the certified nurse-midwife or physician and document them, as well as any interventions, for the permanent record. (See Chapter 31 ∞ for a more detailed discussion of home care for the postpartal family.)

Complications, by their very nature, suggest the need for immediate collaborative management and are inherently stressful. Postpartum complications sometimes necessitate readmission of the postpartum client to the hospital, thereby disrupting the family and adding concerns not only about her health but the way in which infant care will be managed. The most common complications of the postpartal period are hemorrhage, infection, thromboembolic disease, and postpartal psychiatric disorders. This chapter will focus on these issues.

CARE OF THE WOMAN WITH POSTPARTAL HEMORRHAGE

Hemorrhage in the postpartum period is described as either early (immediate or primary) or late (delayed or secondary). **Early (primary) postpartal hemorrhage** occurs in the first 24 hours after childbirth. **Late (secondary) postpartal hemorrhage** occurs from 24 hours to 6 weeks after birth. Postpartal hemorrhage continues to be a cause of significant maternal mortality and morbidity and accounts for approximately one-sixth of all maternal deaths attributed to pregnancy-related hemorrhage in the United States (Poggi, 2007).

The traditional definition of postpartal hemorrhage has been a blood loss of greater than 500 mL following childbirth. That definition is currently being questioned, however, because careful quantification indicates that the average blood loss in a vaginal birth is actually greater than 500 mL, the average blood loss after a cesarean childbirth exceeds 1000 mL, and the average blood loss is more than 1500 mL during repeat cesarean birth (James, 2008; Poggi, 2007). Clinical estimates of blood loss tend to underestimate actual loss by up to 50%.

Some clinicians believe that postpartal hemorrhage can be objectively and reliably defined as a decrease in the hematocrit of 10% between the time of admission and the postbirth period. However, clinical estimation of blood loss at childbirth is difficult because blood mixes with amniotic fluid and is obscured as it oozes onto sterile drapes or is sponged away. Without vigilant watching, it may be difficult for the nurse to appreciate the significance of slow, steady blood loss over the next few hours. As the amount of blood loss increases, as in the case of hemorrhage, estimates are likely to be even less accurate. Moreover, postpartal hemorrhage may occur intra-abdominally, into the broad ligament, or into hematomas arising from genital tract trauma, wherein the blood loss is concealed. Given the increased blood volume of pregnancy, the clinical signs of hemorrhage—such as increasing pulse, decreased blood pressure, and decreasing urinary output—do not appear until as much as 1000 to 2000 mL has been lost, shortly before the woman becomes hemodynamically unstable (James, 2008).

EARLY (PRIMARY) POSTPARTAL HEMORRHAGE

At term, blood volume and cardiac output have increased so that 20% of cardiac output, or 600 mL per minute, perfuses the pregnant uterus, supporting the developing fetus. When the placenta separates from the uterine wall, the many uterine vessels that have carried blood to and from the placenta are severed abruptly. The normal mechanism for hemostasis after delivery of the placenta is contraction of the interlacing uterine muscles to occlude the open sinuses that previously brought blood into the placenta. Absence of prompt and sustained uterine contractions (uterine atony) can result in significant blood loss. Other causes of postpartal hemorrhage include laceration of the genital tract; episiotomy; retained placental fragments; vulvar, vaginal, or subperitoneal hematomas; uterine inversion; uterine rupture; problems of placental implantation; and coagulation disorders.

Uterine Atony

Uterine atony (relaxation of the uterus) is a common cause of early postpartal hemorrhage (Cunningham, Gant, Leveno, et al., 2010). As many as 1 in 20 new mothers will experience some degree of uterine atony. Although uterine atony can occur after any childbirth, its contributing factors include the following:

- Overdistention of the uterus caused by multiple gestation, hydramnios, or a large infant (macrosomia)
- Dysfunctional or prolonged labor, which indicates that the uterus is contracting abnormally
- Oxytocin augmentation or induction of labor
- Grand multiparity, because stretched uterine musculature contracts less vigorously
- Use of anesthesia (especially halothane) or other drugs, such as magnesium sulfate, calcium channel blockers such as nifedipine, or tocolytics, any of which cause the uterus to relax
- Prolonged third stage of labor—more than 30 minutes
- Preeclampsia
- Asian or Hispanic heritage
- Operative birth (includes vacuum extraction or forceps-assisted births)
- Retained placental fragments
- Placenta previa

Hemorrhage from uterine atony may be slow and steady rather than sudden and massive. The blood may escape the vagina or collect in the uterus, evident as large clots. The uterine cavity may distend with up to 1000 mL or more blood although the perineal pad and linen protectors remain suspiciously dry. A treacherous feature of postpartal hemorrhage is that maternal vital signs may not change until significant blood loss has occurred because of the increased blood volume associated with pregnancy. The woman with preeclampsia is an exception to this finding because she does not have the normal hypervolemia of pregnancy and cannot tolerate even normal postchildbirth blood loss (Cunningham et al., 2010).

Ideally, postpartal hemorrhage is prevented, beginning with adequate prenatal care, good nutrition, avoidance of traumatic procedures, risk assessment, early recognition, and management of complications as they arise. Any woman at risk should be typed and cross-matched for blood and have intravenous (IV) lines in place with needles suitable for blood transfusion (18-gauge minimum). Excellent labor management and childbirth techniques are imperative.

After expulsion of the placenta, the fundus is palpated to ensure that it is firmly contracted. If it is not firm (if it is boggy), fundal massage is performed until the uterus contracts. Fundal massage is painful for the woman who has not received regional anesthesia; consequently, the nurse will need to explain why this procedure is necessary and give verbal support as massage is initiated. If bleeding is excessive, the clinician will likely order intravenous (IV) oxytocin at a rapid infusion rate and may elect to do a bimanual massage (Figure 32–1A ●). Table 32–1 summarizes critical nursing information about the use of uterine stimulants. The need for intravenous fluid replacement and blood transfusion is determined on the basis of hemoglobin and hematocrit results as well as coagulation studies.

Conservative management includes uterine stimulants to contract the atonic musculature. Oxytocin, ergotamine, and prostaglandin are most often used. Misoprostol, best known to the obstetric community for its use in labor induction, is being used to prevent and treat uterine atony after failed attempts to control bleeding with oxytocics. Misoprostol used rectally is absorbed quickly and causes uterine contraction within minutes (Rebarker & Roman, 2003). When conservative measures do not successfully control bleeding, surgical intervention is required. In order of increasing invasiveness, surgical procedures include uterine balloon tamponade, selective radiographic-guided pelvic arterial embolization, uterine suturing techniques, ligation of the uterine or hypogastric arteries, and, as a last resort, hysterectomy, which clearly ends childbearing (AAP & ACOG, 2007; Poggi, 2007).

Uterine packing, common in the past for cases of postpartal hemorrhage, has been used less often out of concerns of concealed hemorrhage and uterine overdistention that might actually increase bleeding. Instead, physicians in many clinical settings are resorting to uterine balloon tamponade, using large Foley catheters or Sengstaken-Blakemore tubes to control bleeding. Both of these tubes have open tops, which permit any continuous drainage from the uterus to be visualized even as pressure tamponade is effectively controlling bleeding.

Lacerations of the Genital Tract

Early postpartum hemorrhage is associated with lacerations of the perineum, vagina, or cervix. Several factors predispose women to higher risk of reproductive tract lacerations:

- Nulliparity
- Epidural anesthesia
- Precipitous childbirth (less than 3 hours)

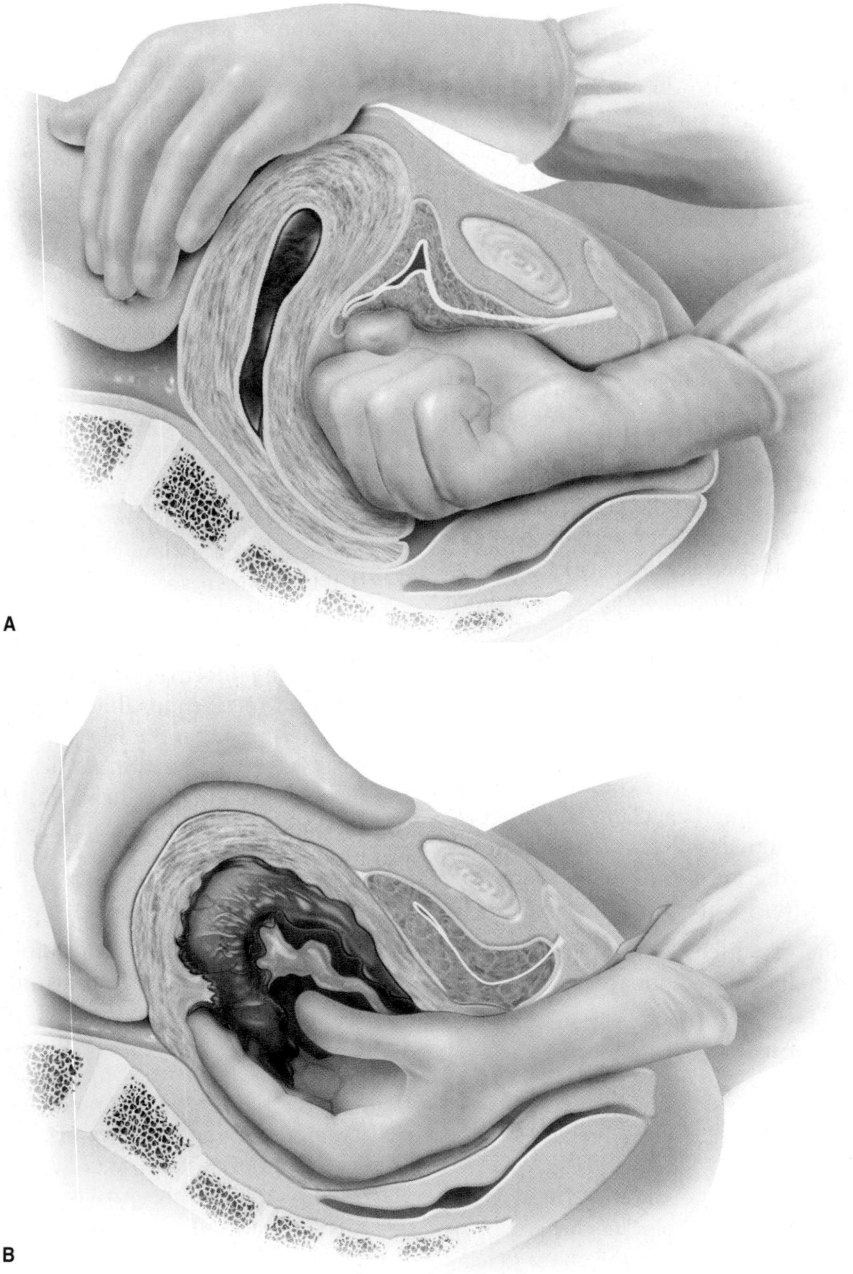

● **Figure 32–1** Manual compression of uterus and removal of placenta. ***A,*** Manual compression of the uterus and massage with the abdominal hand usually will effectively control hemorrhage from uterine atony. ***B,*** Manual removal of placenta. The fingers are alternately abducted, adducted, and advanced until the placenta is completely detached. Both procedures are performed only by the medical clinician.

Source: Adapted from Cunningham, F. G., MacDonald, P. C., & Gant, N. F. (Eds.). (1989). *Williams obstetrics* (18th ed., pp. 417–418). Norwalk, CT: Appleton & Lange.

- Forceps- or vacuum-assisted birth
- Macrosomia
- Use of oxytocin

Thorough inspection of the genital tract by the birth attendant facilitates recognition and timely repair of most lacerations. Genital tract lacerations should be suspected when vaginal bleeding persists in the presence of a firmly contracted uterus. The nurse who suspects a laceration should notify the clinician so that the laceration can be immediately sutured to control the hemorrhage and restore the integrity of the reproductive tract (AAP & ACOG, 2007).

Episiotomy is an often underappreciated source of postpartal blood loss because of slow, steady bleeding. The risk for bleeding is increased with mediolateral episiotomies. (See discussion in Chapter 23∞.)

Retained Placental Fragments

Retained placental fragments may be a cause of early postpartal hemorrhage and are also the most common cause of late hemorrhage.

Table 32–1	Uterine Stimulants Used to Prevent and Manage Uterine Atony			
Drug	**Dosing Information**	**Contraindications**	**Expected Effects**	**Side Effects**
Oxytocin (Pitocin, Syntocinon)	IV use: 10 to 40 units in 500 to 1000 mL crystalloid fluid at 50 milliunits/min administration rate. Onset: immediate. Duration: 1 h. ***IV bolus administration not recommended.*** IM use: 10 units. Onset: 3 to 5 min. Duration: 2 to 3 h.	None for use in postpartum hemorrhage. Avoid undiluted rapid IV infusion which causes hypotension.	Rhythmic uterine contractions that help to prevent or reverse postpartal hemorrhage caused by uterine atony.	Uterine hyperstimulation, mild transient hypertension, water intoxication rare in postpartum use.
Methylergonovine maleate (Methergine)	IM use: 0.2 mg q2–4h. Onset: 2 to 5 min. Duration: 3 h (for 5 dose maximum). PO use: 0.2 mg q4h (for 6 doses). Onset: 7 to 15 min. Duration: 3 h (for 1 week). ***IV administration not recommended.***	Women with labile or high blood pressure, known sensitivity to drug, or cardiac disease. Use with caution during lactation	Sustained uterine contractions that help to prevent or reverse postpartal hemorrhage caused by uterine atony; management of postpartal subinvolution.	Hypertension, dizziness, headache, flushing/hot flashes, tinnitus, nausea and vomiting, palpitations, chest pain. Overdose or hypersensitivity is recognized by seizures; tingling and numbness of fingers and toes.
Ergonovine maleate (Ergotrate Maleate)	IM use: 0.2 mg q2–4h. Onset: 7 min. Duration: 3 h (5 dose maximum). PO use: 0.2 mg q6–12h. Onset: 15 min. Duration: 3 h (for 2–7 days). ***IV administration not recommended.***	Women with labile or high blood pressure or known sensitivity to drug.	Sustained uterine contractions that help to prevent or reverse postpartal hemorrhage caused by uterine atony; management of postpartal subinvolution.	Hypertension, dizziness, headache, nausea and vomiting, chest pain. Hypersensitivity is noted by systemic vasoconstrictive effects: seizure, chest pain, general weakness, and tingling and numbness of fingers and toes that leads rarely to gangrene.
Prostaglandin (PGF_2, carboprost tromethamine [Hemabate], Prostin/15M)	IM use: 0.25 mg 15 to 90 minutes, repeated up to maximum 8 doses. Physician may elect to administer by direct intramyometrial injection.	Women with active cardiovascular, renal, liver disease, or asthma or with known hypersensitivity to drug.	Control of refractory cases of postpartal hemorrhage caused by uterine atony; generally used after failed attempts at control of hemorrhage with oxytocic agents.	Nausea, vomiting, diarrhea, headache, flushing, bradycardia, bronchospasm, wheezing, cough, chills, fever.
Misoprostol (Cytotec)	800 to 1000 microgram rectally.	History of allergies to prostaglandins.	Used to prevent and treat uterine atony after failed attempts to control bleeding with oxytocics.	Diarrhea, abdominal pain, headache.
Dinoprostone (Prostin E2)	Suppository (vaginally or rectally) 20 microgram every 2 hours. Store frozen—must be thawed to room temperature.	Avoid if woman is hypotensive, or has asthma or acute inflammatory disease.	Stimulate uterine contractions.	Fever is common and occurs within 15 to 45 min of insertion; bleeding, abdominal cramps, N/V.

Implications for Nursing Management of the Postpartal Woman Receiving Uterine Stimulants

- Assess fundus for evidence of contraction and amount of uterine bleeding at least q10–15 min × 1–2 h after administration, then q30–60 min until stable. ***More frequent assessments are determined by the woman's condition or by orders of the physician/CNM.***
- Assess blood loss by hematocrit and hemoglobin levels.
- Monitor pulse and blood pressure q15 min for at least 1 h after administration, then q30–60 min until stable.
  - Apply pulse oximeter and administer oxygen according to agency protocol.
  - Weigh peripads or Chux dressing.
- Note expected duration of action of drug being administered, and take care to recheck fundus at that time.
- When the drug is ineffective, the fundus remains atonic (boggy or uncontracted), and bleeding continues, massage the fundus. If massage fails to cause sustained contraction, notify the physician/CNM immediately.
- Monitor woman for signs of known side effects of the drug; report to physician/CNM if side effects occur.
  - Continuous EKG monitoring may be indicated for hypotension, continuous bleeding, tachycardia, or shock.
  - Elevate the legs to a 20- to 30-degree angle to increase venous return.
- Remind the woman and her support person that uterine cramping is an expected result of these drugs and that medication is available for discomfort. Administer analgesic medications as needed for pain relief. Provide nonpharmacologic comfort measures. If analgesic medication ordered is insufficient for pain relief, notify the physician/CNM. Provide information to client and family regarding importance of not smoking during Methergine administration (nicotine from cigarettes leads to constricted vessels and may lead to hypertension) and signs of toxicity.

When Prostaglandin Is Used

- Check temperature q1–2h and/or after chill. Administer antipyretic medication as ordered for prostaglandin-induced fever.
- Auscultate breath sounds frequently for signs of adverse respiratory effects.
- Assess for nausea, vomiting, and diarrhea. Administer antiemetic and antidiarrheal medications as ordered. (In some settings, women are premedicated with these drugs.)

Evidence-Based Nursing

UTERINE MASSAGE AND POSTPARTUM HEMORRHAGE

Clinical Question

Is uterine massage effective in preventing postpartum hemorrhage?

The Evidence

Postpartum hemorrhage is a major cause of maternal mortality and morbidity, particularly in areas that are under-resourced. Postpartum hemorrhage is most common in areas where access to health services is the poorest. In these settings, maternal risk factors may increase the risk of bleeding even more. There is a need for simple interventions that can reduce the rate of postpartum hemorrhage in areas with less technologically advanced obstetrical care. The most common cause of postpartum hemorrhage is uterine atony, and uterine massage is thought to stimulate uterine contraction. Hofmeyr, Abdel-Aleem, and Abdel-Aleen (2008) conducted a systematic review of the research relative to uterine massage as a preventive intervention. One large, well-designed randomized controlled trial met all of the quality criteria of the review. Large, multisite, randomized trials provide a strong level of evidence for practice.

Best Practice

Uterine massage involves placing a hand on the mother's lower abdomen and stimulating the uterus by massaging and squeezing the uterus. Uterine massage given every 10 minutes for 60 minutes after birth was effective in reducing blood loss. The need for additional drugs to reduce blood loss was also reduced by nearly 80%. Simple uterine massage can reduce the number of women who lose more than 500 ml of blood by more than half. Uterine massage also reduced the need for maternal blood transfusion, thus reducing the associated risks.

Critical Thinking

Should uterine massage be a routine part of postpartum care, or should it be applied only in under-resourced populations?

See MyNursingKit for possible responses.

Nursing Practice

Postpartal nurses are wise to appreciate that most deaths from postpartal hemorrhage are not caused by catastrophic bleeding episodes but by ineffective management of slow, steady blood loss.

Retention of fragments is usually attributable to partial separation of the placenta during massage of the fundus before spontaneous placental separation. Therefore, this practice should be avoided.

Following birth, the placenta should always be inspected for intactness and for evidence of missing fragments or cotyledons on the maternal side and for vessels that transverse to the edge of the placenta outward along the membranes of the fetal side, which may indicate succenturiate placenta and a retained lobe. Uterine exploration may be required to remove missing fragments. This cause should be immediately suspected if bleeding persists and no lacerations are noted (Figure 32–1B ●). Sonography may be used to diagnose retained placental fragments. Curettage, formerly standard treatment, is now thought by some to traumatize the implantation site, thereby increasing bleeding and the potential for uterine adhesions. However, it may be necessitated by the degree of hemorrhage (Cunningham et al., 2010).

Vulvar, Vaginal, and Pelvic Hematomas

Hematomas occur as a result of injury to a blood vessel from birth trauma, often without noticeable trauma to the superficial tissue, or from inadequate hemostasis at the site of repair of an incision or laceration. The soft tissue in the area offers no resistance, and hematomas containing 250 to 500 mL of blood may develop rapidly. Signs and symptoms vary somewhat with the type of hematoma. Hematomas may be vulvar (involving branches of the pudendal artery), vaginal (especially in the area of the ischial spines), vulvovaginal, or subperitoneal. The latter are rare; however, they are the most dangerous because of the large amount of blood loss that can occur without clinical symptoms until the woman becomes hemodynamically unstable. Subperitoneal hematomas involve the uterine artery branches or vessels in the broad ligaments.

Risk factors for hematomas include preeclampsia, use of pudendal anesthesia, first full-term birth, precipitous labor, prolonged second stage of labor, macrosomia, forceps- or vacuum-assisted births, and history of vulvar varicosities. Hematomas less than 5 cm (2 in.) in size and nonexpanding are managed expectantly with ice packs and analgesia. They usually resolve over several days. For larger hematomas and those that expand, surgical management is usually required; the hematoma is evacuated, the bleeding vessel ligated, and the wound closed, with or without vaginal packing. An indwelling urinary catheter may be necessary because voiding may be impossible with packing in place.

The hematoma site is an ideal medium for the growth of flora normally present in the genital tract. Consequently, broad-spectrum antibiotics are usually ordered to prevent infection or abscess.

The nurse can decrease the risk of vulvar or vaginal hematoma by applying an ice pack to the woman's perineum during the first hour after birth and intermittently for the next 8 to 12 hours. If a small hematoma develops despite preventive measures, a sitz bath after the first 12 hours will aid fluid absorption once bleeding has stopped and will promote comfort, as will the judicious use of analgesic agents.

Uterine Inversion

Uterine inversion—a prolapse of the fundus to or through the cervix so that the uterus is, in effect, turned inside out after birth—is a rare but life-threatening cause of postpartal hemorrhage. Although not always preventable, uterine inversion is often associated with factors such as: fundal implantation or abnormal adherence of the placenta, protracted labor, weakness of the uterine musculature, uterine relaxation secondary to anesthesia or

MyNursingKit Care Plan Activity: Postpartal Care Following Vaginal Birth drugs such as magnesium sulfate, and excess traction on the umbilical cord or vigorous manual removal of the placenta. Most cases of uterine inversion are managed by immediate repositioning of the uterus within the pelvis by the physician.

LATE (SECONDARY) POSTPARTAL HEMORRHAGE

Although early postpartal hemorrhage usually occurs within hours after birth, delayed hemorrhage generally occurs within 1 to 2 weeks after childbirth, most frequently as a result of **subinvolution** (failure to return to normal size) of the placental site or retention of placental fragments. Blood loss at this time may be excessive but rarely poses the same risk as that from immediate postpartal hemorrhage. Late postpartum hemorrhage is much less common but can be extremely stressful for the woman and her family who are at home by this time.

The site of placental implantation is always the last area of the uterus to regenerate after childbirth. In the case of subinvolution, adjacent endometrium and the decidua basalis fail to regenerate to cover the placental site. Deficiency of immunologic factors has been implicated as a cause. Faulty implantation in the less vascular lower uterine segment, retention of placental tissue, or infection may contribute to subinvolution. With subinvolution, the postpartum fundal height is greater than expected. In addition, lochia flow often fails to progress from rubra to serosa to alba normally. Lochia rubra that persists longer than 2 weeks postpartum is highly suggestive of subinvolution (Poggi, 2007). Some women report scant brown lochia or irregular heavy bleeding. Leukorrhea, backache, and foul lochia may occur if infection is a cause. There may be a history of heavy early postpartal bleeding or difficulty with expulsion of the placenta. When portions of the placenta have been retained in the uterus, bleeding continues because normal uterine contractions that constrict the bleeding site are prohibited. Presence of placental tissue within the uterus can be confirmed by pelvic ultrasound.

Subinvolution is most commonly diagnosed during the routine postpartal examination at 4 to 6 weeks. The woman may relate a history of irregular or excessive bleeding or describe the symptoms listed previously. An enlarged, softer-than-normal uterus palpated bimanually is an objective indication of subinvolution. Treatment includes oral administration of methylergonovine maleate [Methergine] 0.2 mg orally every 3 to 4 hours for 24 to 48 hours (see Table 32–1). When uterine infection is present, antibiotics are also administered. The woman is reevaluated in 2 weeks. If retained placenta is suspected or other treatment is ineffective, curettage may be indicated (Poggi, 2007).

NURSING MANAGEMENT

NURSING ASSESSMENT AND DIAGNOSIS

Careful and ongoing assessment of the woman during labor and birth and evaluation of her prenatal history will help identify factors that put her at risk for postpartal hemorrhage. Following birth, periodic assessment for evidence of vaginal bleeding is a major nursing responsibility. Regular and frequent assessment of fundal height and evidence of uterine tone or contractility will alert the nurse to the possible development or recurrence of hemorrhage. The nurse observes and documents vaginal bleeding to determine whether further medical intervention is needed. This assessment can be done visually, by pad counts, or by weighing the perineal pads. In cases of excessive bleeding, nurses should be alert for signs of impending hypovolemic shock and the development of coagulation problems, such as DIC.

When regional anesthesia is used, frequent assessment of the woman's perineum is important. Once the effects of anesthesia have subsided, vaginal and vulvar hematomas are generally associated with perineal pain. The pain is often intense, out of proportion or excessive, and usually from the woman's "stitches." If the hematoma is localized in the posterior vaginal area, rectal pressure may also be a presenting complaint. Hematomas that develop in the upper vagina may cause difficulty voiding because of pressure against the urinary meatus or urethra. Rather than automatically attributing complaints of perineal pain to the presence of an episiotomy, the nurse should examine the perineal area for signs of hematomas: ecchymosis; edema; tenseness of tissue overlying the hematomas; fluctuant, bulging mass at the introitus; and extreme tenderness to palpation. Estimating the size of the hematoma on first assessment of the perineum enables the nurse to better identify increases in size and the potential blood loss. The nurse notifies the physician/CNM if a hematoma is suspected.

Nursing diagnoses that may apply to a woman experiencing postpartal hemorrhage include the following:

- *Deficient Fluid Volume* related to blood loss secondary to uterine atony, lacerations, or retained placental fragments
- *Health-Seeking Behaviors* related to lack of information about signs of delayed postpartal hemorrhage

PLANNING AND IMPLEMENTATION

HOSPITAL-BASED NURSING CARE

If the nurse detects a soft, boggy uterus, it is massaged until firm. If the uterus is not contracting well and appears larger than anticipated, the nurse may express clots during fundal massage. Once clots are expressed, the uterus tends to contract more effectively.

If the woman seems to have a slow, steady, free flow of blood, the nurse should do pad counts and if possible begin to weigh the perineal pads (1 mL = 1 g) (James, 2008). The nurse monitors the woman's vital signs every 15 minutes, or more frequently if indicated. If the fundus is displaced upward or to one side because of a full bladder, the nurse encourages the woman to empty her bladder—or catheterizes her if she is unable to void—to allow for efficient uterine contractions.

When there are risk factors for postpartal hemorrhage or frequent fundal massage has been necessary to sustain uterine contractions, the nurse maintains any vascular access (IV) started during labor and anticipates the need for a second IV in case additional fluids, meds, or blood is necessary. Sometimes physicians and CNMs write orders that specify "discontinue IV after present bottle." The astute postpartum nurse will assess the consistency of the fundus and the presence of normal versus excessive lochia before

Nursing Practice

As has been mentioned, bogginess indicates that the uterus is not contracting well, which results in increased uterine bleeding. This blood may remain in the uterus and form clots or may result in increased flow. In assessing the amount of blood loss, first massage the uterus until it is firm and then express clots. Do not be misled by the fact that a woman has a firm uterus. Significant bleeding can occur from causes other than uterine atony. To accurately determine the amount of blood loss, it is not sufficient to assess only the peripads. You should also ask the woman to turn on her side so you can assess underneath her for pooling of blood.

discontinuing the infusion. If the assessments are not reassuring, the nurse continues the intravenous (IV) infusion and notifies the physician or CNM.

The nurse reviews postpartum hemoglobin and hematocrit values when available, compares them to the admission baseline, and notifies the physician or CNM if the hematocrit has decreased by 10 percentage points or more. In cases where there is risk of postpartal hemorrhage (e.g., women with prenatal anemia or labor and delivery complications) and blood has been crossmatched earlier, the nurse checks that blood is available in the blood bank.

The nurse assesses the woman for signs of anemia, such as fatigue, pallor, headache, thirst, and orthostatic changes in pulse or blood pressure, and reviews the results of all hematocrit determinations. All medical interventions, intravenous infusions, blood transfusions, oxygen therapy, and medications such as uterine stimulants are monitored as necessary and evaluated for effectiveness. The nurse also monitors urinary output to determine adequacy of fluid replacement and renal perfusion and reports amounts less than 30 mL/h to the physician (James, 2008). The nurse also helps the woman plan activities so that adequate rest is possible.

The woman who is experiencing anemia and fatigue related to hemorrhage may need assistance with self-care and progressive ambulation for several days. When she is able to be out of bed to shower, use of a shower chair permits independence while providing a measure of safety in case the woman experiences weakness or dizziness. The emergency call light should be easily accessible.

The mother may find it difficult to care for her baby because of the fatigue associated with blood loss. The nurse can often find ways to promote maternal-infant attachment while accommodating the mother's health needs. The mother may require additional assistance in caring for her infant. If she has intravenous lines in place, even carrying the newborn may be awkward. For the mother who feels compelled to do as much as possible, the nurse may also need to give the mother "permission" to return her infant to the nursery so she can have adequate periods of uninterrupted rest.

If the father of the child or partner is involved in the birth experience, including that person in the plan of care is a productive strategy. This person can support the mother's recovery by helping to meet her physical needs while encouraging her to rest. The mother is likely to feel less concern over her limited opportunities for the newborn's care if she can witness the father/partner interacting with and caring for the newborn. The extent to which the father/partner becomes involved with the care of the mother and baby must be carefully balanced with the need to be rested for the extra responsibilities the support person will assume when the mother and newborn child are discharged from the hospital.

TEACHING FOR SELF-CARE

The woman and her family or other support persons should receive clear, preferably written, explanations of the normal postpartum course, including changes in the lochia and fundus and signs of abnormal bleeding. Instructions for the prevention of bleeding should include fundal massage, ways to assess the fundal height and consistency, and inspection of any episiotomy and lacerations, if present. The woman should receive instruction in perineal care (see discussion on perineal care in Chapter 31∞). The mother and her family are advised to contact her caregiver if any of the signs of postpartal hemorrhage occur (Table 32–2). If iron supplementation is ordered, instructions for proper dosage should be provided along with client teaching to enhance absorption and avoid constipation and nausea (ACOG, 2006).

COMMUNITY-BASED NURSING CARE

For postpartal women, the usual discharge instructions include advice such as: "You take care of your baby, and let someone else care for you, the family, and the household." Because of her fatigue and weakened condition, the woman who experiences postpartal hemorrhage may be unable even to care for her newborn unassisted. The caregivers at home need clear, concise explanations of her condition and needs for recovery. For example, they should understand the woman's need to rest and to be given extra time to rest after any necessary activity.

To ensure her safety, the woman should be advised to rise slowly to minimize the likelihood of orthostatic hypotension. Until she regains strength, she should be seated when holding the newborn.

The person who assumes responsibility for grocery shopping and meal preparation needs advice about the importance of including foods high in iron in the daily menus. Having the

Table 32–2 Signs of Postpartal Hemorrhage

Excessive or bright-red bleeding (saturation of more than one pad per hour)
A boggy fundus that does not respond to massage
Abnormal clots
High temperature
Any unusual pelvic discomfort or backache
Persistent bleeding in the presence of a firmly contracted uterus
Rise in the level of the fundus of the uterus
Increased pulse or decreased BP
Hematoma formation or bulging/shiny skin in the perineal area
Decreased level of consciousness

woman indicate her preferences from a list of such foods will promote cooperation with the diet. The nurse also explains the rationale for continuing medications containing iron.

The woman should continue to count perineal pads for several days so that she can recognize any recurring problems with excessive blood loss. The debilitated condition and anemia associated with hemorrhage increase the woman's risk of puerperal infection. She and her caregivers should use good handwashing and minimize exposure to infection in the home. The nurse should give the woman's caregiver a list of the signs of infection and ensure that she or he understands the importance of alerting the physician immediately if signs occur.

A sense of emergency often accompanies late postpartal hemorrhage. Because it commonly occurs 1 to 2 weeks after birth, the couple is generally at home, involved in the day-to-day activities demanded by their new roles, when the unexpected, excessive bleeding begins. Quick decisions about childcare arrangements must often be made so that the mother can return to the hospital. Both mother and father are likely to be alarmed by the excessive bleeding and concerned about her prognosis. There may be additional worries about separation from the newborn, especially when the mother is breastfeeding. The father may find himself torn between the needs of the mother and those of the newborn. Ideally, arrangements can be made to minimize separation of the family members.

In addition to meeting the woman's physical needs, the nurse assesses the couple's coping strategies and resources for dealing with the impending crisis. Providing realistic information, offering to call those in their support network, and exploring effective coping strategies can be of immeasurable value as the family tries to maintain a sense of balance in this situation.

EVALUATION

Expected outcomes of nursing care include the following:

- Signs of postpartal hemorrhage are detected quickly and managed effectively.
- Maternal-infant attachment is maintained successfully.
- The woman is able to identify abnormal changes that might occur following discharge and understands the importance of notifying her caregiver if they develop.

CARE OF THE WOMAN WITH A REPRODUCTIVE TRACT INFECTION OR WOUND INFECTION

Puerperal infection is an infection of the reproductive tract associated with childbirth that occurs any time up to 6 weeks postpartum. The most common postpartal infection is endometritis (metritis), which is infection limited to the uterine lining. Indeed, the cause of postpartal fever is presumed to be metritis until proven otherwise. However, infection can be spread by way of the lymphatic and circulatory systems to become a progressive disease resulting in parametrial cellulitis and peritonitis. The woman's prognosis is directly related to the stage of the disease at the time of diagnosis, the causative organism, and the state of her health and immune system.

The standard definition of **puerperal morbidity**, established by the Joint Committee on Maternal Welfare, is a temperature of 38°C (100.4°F) or higher, with the temperature occurring on any 2 of the first 10 postpartum days, exclusive of the first 24 hours, and when taken by mouth by standard technique at least four times a day. However, serious infections can occur in the first 24 hours or may cause only persistent low-grade temperatures. Therefore, careful assessment of all postpartum women with elevated temperatures is essential.

The vagina and cervix of approximately 70% of all healthy pregnant women contain pathogenic bacteria that, alone or in combination, are sufficiently virulent to cause excessive infection. Although the uterus is considered a sterile cavity before rupture of the fetal membranes, bacterial contamination of amniotic fluid with membranes still intact at term is more common than previously believed and may contribute to premature labor. Following rupture of membranes and during labor, contamination of the uterine cavity by vaginal or cervical bacteria can easily occur. Other factors must also be present for infection to occur such as the change to an alkaline pH of the vagina postpartally that favors growth of aerobes. Uterine infections are relatively uncommon following uncomplicated vaginal births, but they continue to be a major source of morbidity for women who give birth by cesarean.

Routine antibiotic prophylaxis for cesarean childbirth has significantly reduced infection rates (AAP & ACOG, 2007). Antibiotic therapy alone has not caused the decrease in overall postpartal morbidity and mortality that is seen today. Aseptic technique, fewer traumatic operative births, a better understanding of labor dystocia, improved surgical intervention, and a population that is generally at less risk from malnutrition and chronic debilitative disease have also contributed to this reduction.

POSTPARTAL UTERINE INFECTION

Postpartal uterine infection is known variously as *metritis* and *endometritis*. Risk factors for postpartal uterine infection include the following:

- Cesarean birth—the single most significant risk (10 times greater than in vaginal births) (James, 2008)
- Prolonged premature rupture of the amniotic membranes (PPROM)
- Prolonged labor preceding cesarean birth
- Multiple vaginal examinations during labor
- Compromised health status (low socioeconomic status, poor nutritional intake, anemia, obesity, smoking, and use of illicit drugs or alcohol)
- Use of fetal scalp electrode or intrauterine pressure catheter for internal monitoring during labor
- Obstetric trauma—episiotomy and lacerations of perineum, vagina, or cervix
- Chorioamnionitis
- Diabetes (four times more common than in nondiabetic mothers) (Davies & Gibbs, 2008)

MyNursingKit Nursing Care Plan: Woman with a Puerperal Infection

- Preexisting bacterial vaginosis or *Chlamydia trachomatis* infection
- Instrument-assisted childbirth—vacuum or forceps
- Manual removal of the placenta
- Lapses in aseptic technique by surgical staff or prolonged duration of surgery

Endometritis (Metritis)

Endometritis (metritis), an inflammation of the endometrium portion of the uterine lining, may occur postpartally in 1% to 3% of women who give birth vaginally and ranges from 5% to 15% of those who give birth by cesarean (Duff, Sweet, & Edwards, 2009). After expulsion of the placenta, the placental site provides an excellent culture medium for bacterial growth. The site in the contracted uterus is a round, dark red, elevated area of 4 cm (1.6 in.), with a nodular surface composed of numerous veins, many of which may become occluded because of clot formation. The remaining portion of the decidua is also susceptible to pathogenic bacteria because of its thinness (approximately 2 mm) and its large blood supply. The cervix presents a bacterial breeding ground because of the multiple small lacerations attending normal labor and spontaneous birth.

Both aerobic and anaerobic organisms cause metritis, which is often polymicrobial (Duff et al., 2009). See Table 32–3 for a list of common causative organisms. Clinical findings of metritis in the initial 24 to 36 hours postpartally tend to be related to group B streptococcus (GBS). Late-onset postpartal metritis is most commonly associated with genital mycoplasmas and *Chlamydia trachomatis*. These microbes have a longer replication time and latency period than other bacteria and are not consistently eradicated by antibiotics used for early postpartal infections.

In mild cases of metritis, the woman generally has vaginal discharge that is bloody, foul smelling, and either scant or profuse. In more severe cases, she also has uterine tenderness; sawtooth temperature spikes, usually between 38.3°C (101°F) and 40°C (104°F); tachycardia; chills, and foul-smelling lochia are cited as a classic signs of endometritis (Duff et al., 2009).

Table 32–3	Common Causative Organisms in Metritis	

Aerobes	Anaerobes
■ Group A, B, D streptococcus	■ *Peptostreptococcus*
■ Enterococcus	■ *Clostridium* species
■ *Staphylococcus* species	■ *Bacteroides* species
■ *Escherichia coli*	■ *Chlamydia trachomatis*
■ *Klebsiella pneumoniae*	■ Genital *mycoplasma*
■ *Proteus mirabilis*	

Data from: Baxley, E. G. (2001). Postpartum biomedical concerns. Section B postpartum endometritis. In S. D. Ratcliffe, E. G. Baxley, J. E. Byrd, & E. L. Sakornbut (Eds.), *Family practice obstetrics* (2nd ed., pp. 602–607). Philadelphia: Hanley & Belfus; Duff, W. P., Sweet, R. L., & Edwards, R. K. (2009). Maternal and fetal infectious disorders. In R. K. Creasy & R. Resnik (Eds.), *Maternal-fetal medicine: Principles and practice* (6th ed., pp. 739–796). Philadelphia: Saunders; James, D. C. (2008). Postpartum care. In K. R. Simpson & P. A. Creehan, *AWHONN perinatal nursing* (3rd ed., pp. 473–526). Philadelphia: Lippincott Williams & Wilkins.

Pelvic Cellulitis (Parametritis)

Pelvic cellulitis (parametritis) is infection involving the connective tissue of the broad ligament or, in more severe forms, the connective tissue of all the pelvic structures. The infection generally ascends upward in the pelvis by way of the lymphatics in the uterine wall but may also occur if pathogenic organisms invade a cervical laceration that extends upward into the connective tissue of the broad ligament—a direct pathway into the pelvis. Infection involving the peritoneal cavity is **peritonitis**.

A pelvic abscess is most commonly found as a palpable mass in the uterine ligaments, the cul-de-sac of Douglas, and the subdiaphragmatic space. Parametritis may be a secondary result of pelvic vein thrombophlebitis. This condition occurs when the clot, usually in the right ovarian vein, becomes infected and the wall of the vein breaks down from necrosis, spilling the infection into the connective tissues of the pelvis.

A woman suffering from parametritis may demonstrate a variety of symptoms, including marked high temperature (38.9°C to 40°C [102°F to 104°F]), chills, malaise, lethargy, abdominal pain, subinvolution of the uterus, tachycardia, and local and referred rebound tenderness. If peritonitis develops, the woman becomes acutely ill, with severe pain, marked anxiety, high fever, rapid and shallow respirations, pronounced tachycardia, excessive thirst, abdominal distention, nausea, and vomiting.

PERINEAL WOUND INFECTIONS

Given the degree of bacterial contamination that occurs with normal vaginal birth, it is surprising that more women do not have infections of the episiotomy or repaired lacerations of the perineum, vagina, or vulva. Good aseptic technique is the likely rationale. When perineal wound infection occurs, it is recognized by the classic signs: redness, warmth, edema, purulent drainage, and, later, gaping of the wound that had previously been well approximated. Local pain may be severe. Infected perineal wounds, like other infected wounds, are treated by draining the purulent material. Sutures are removed, and the wound is left open. A regimen of broad-spectrum antibiotics is used. When the surface of the wound is free of infectious exudate and tissue granulation is evident, the mother returns for secondary closure of the wound under regional anesthesia.

CESAREAN WOUND INFECTIONS

The infection rate following cesarean births is 3% to 5%, with the highest rate occurring after emergency cesarean because there is more traumatization of the tissue (Duff et al., 2009). Predisposing factors to infection include obesity, diabetes mellitus, prolonged postpartal hospitalization, PROM, metritis, prolonged labor, anemia, steroid therapy, and immunosuppression. Signs of an abdominal wound infection, which may not be evident until after discharge, include erythema; warmth; skin discoloration; edema; tenderness; purulent drainage, sometimes mixed with sanguineous fluid; or gaping of the wound edges. Fever, pain, malodorous lochia, and other systemic signs are also common. Abdominal distention and decreased bowel sounds may be noted. Culture of the wound drainage commonly reveals mixed pathogens.

CLINICAL THERAPY

The infection site and causative organism are diagnosed by careful history and complete physical examination, blood tests, aerobic and anaerobic endometrial cultures (although cultures may be of limited value because multiple organisms are usually present), and urinalysis to rule out urinary tract infection (UTI). When a localized infection develops, it is treated with antibiotics, sitz baths, and analgesics as necessary for pain relief. If an abscess has developed or a stitch site is infected, the suture is removed and the area is allowed to drain. Packing the wound with saline gauze twice to three times daily, using aseptic technique, allows removal of necrotic debris when packing is removed. Broad-spectrum antibiotic coverage is used to treat postpartal wound infections. Cephalosporins, penicillinase-resistant penicillin, are commonly used with anaerobic coverage by clindamycin and gentamicin or ampicillin in refractory cases (Duff et al., 2009; James, 2008).

The incidence of metritis has been reduced by prophylactic administration of antibiotics to women undergoing cesarean childbirth. Metritis, once diagnosed, is treated by aggressive administration of antibiotics (Duff et al., 2009). With appropriate antibiotic coverage, improvement should occur within 48 to 72 hours (James, 2008). Antibiotics are generally continued until the woman is afebrile for 24 to 48 hours (James, 2008). The route and dosage are determined by the severity of the infection. Careful monitoring is also necessary to prevent the development of a more serious infection.

Parametritis and peritonitis are treated with intravenous antibiotics. Broad-spectrum antibiotics effective against the most commonly occurring causative organisms are chosen initially, until the results of culture and sensitivity reports are available. If multiple organisms are present, the approach to antibiotic therapy is continued unless no improvement is observed; then the antibiotic is changed. Antibiotics are generally continued until the woman has been afebrile for 48 hours. Oral antibiotics are rarely needed on discharge.

The woman with a severe systemic infection is acutely ill and may require care in an intensive care unit. Supportive therapy includes maintenance of adequate hydration with intravenous fluids, analgesic medications, ongoing assessment of the infection, and possibly continuous nasogastric suctioning if paralytic ileus develops.

NURSING MANAGEMENT

NURSING ASSESSMENT AND DIAGNOSIS

Inspect the woman's perineum every 8 to 12 hours for signs of early infection. The REEDA scale helps the nurse remember to consider *r*edness, *e*dema, *e*cchymosis, *d*ischarge, and *a*pproximation. Immediately report any degree of induration (hardening) to the clinician.

The nurse notes and reports the presence of fever, malaise, abdominal pain, foul-smelling lochia, larger than expected uterus, tachycardia, and other signs of infection so that treatment can begin. The white blood cell (WBC) count, a usual objective measure of infection, cannot be used reliably because of the normal increase in WBCs during the postpartum period; a WBC count of 14,000 to 16,000 mm^3 is not an unusual finding. An increase in WBC level of more than 30% in a 6-hour period, however, is indicative of infection.

Nursing diagnoses that may apply to the women with a puerperal infection include the following:

- *Risk for Injury* related to the spread of infection
- *Pain* related to the presence of infection
- *Risk for Impaired Parenting* related to delayed parent-infant attachment secondary to malaise and other symptoms of infection

PLANNING AND IMPLEMENTATION

HOSPITAL-BASED NURSING CARE

The nurse caring for a woman during the postpartal period is responsible for teaching the woman self-care measures that are helpful in preventing infection. The woman should understand the importance of perineal care, good hygiene practices to prevent contamination of the perineum (including wiping from front to back, changing perineal pads after voiding), and thorough handwashing. Careful attention to aseptic technique during labor, birth, and postpartum is essential. Once edema and perineal pain are under control, the nurse can also encourage sitz baths, which are cleansing and promote healing. Adequate fluid intake and a diet high in protein and vitamin C, which are necessary for wound healing, also help prevent infection (James, 2008).

If the woman has a draining wound or purulent lochia, it is especially important that those in contact with soiled items and linens practice good handwashing. Clear, concise instructions about wound care and how to discard soiled dressings appropriately must be provided to safeguard the woman and her caregivers. If the woman is seriously ill, ongoing assessment of urine-specific gravity, as well as intake and output, is necessary. It is also necessary to carefully administer antibiotics as ordered and regulate the intravenous fluid rate. Ongoing assessment of the woman's condition is vital to detect subtle changes in her health status. The nurse also addresses the woman's comfort needs related to hygiene, positioning, oral hygiene, and pain relief.

Promoting maternal-infant attachment can be difficult with the acutely ill woman. The nurse may provide pictures of the infant and keep the mother informed of the infant's well-being. Mementos, such as a footprint, a note written by the father "from the baby," or a videotape of the baby can be comforting to the mother during their separation. If she feels up to it, the new mother will also benefit from brief visits with her newborn. The woman who wishes to breastfeed when her condition allows can maintain lactation by pumping her breasts regularly. Understanding that the opportunity to breastfeed is simply delayed, not eliminated, by the infectious process may improve the woman's morale.

The partner of a seriously ill woman will be concerned about her condition and torn about spending time with her and with their newborn. Because maternal-infant bonding may be compromised, allow for privacy with limited interruptions to facilitate father-newborn bonding. See "Nursing Care Plan: The Woman with a Puerperal Perineal Wound Infection" on pages 834–837 for specific nursing care measures.

Nursing Care Plan

THE WOMAN WITH A PUERPERAL PERINEAL WOUND INFECTION

INTERVENTION	RATIONALE	EXPECTED OUTCOME
1. Nursing Diagnosis: Ineffective Tissue Perfusion: Peripheral related to interruption of venous blood flow secondary to complications of labor and birth		
NIC Intervention: **Embolus care: Peripheral:** Limitation of complications for a patient experiencing, or at risk for, occlusion of peripheral circulation		**NOC Outcome:** **Tissue perfusion: Peripheral:** Extent to which blood flows through the small vessels of the extremities and maintains tissue function
Goal: The patient's presenting signs and symptoms are relieved.		
■ Assess, record, and report signs of thrombophlebitis.	■ Early detection of developing thrombophlebitis permits prompt treatment. As the thrombus increases in size, signs of obstruction also increase.	■ Patient will have increased venous return from lower leg as evidenced by decreased edema in lower leg, negative Homans' sign, and no pain or tenderness in lower leg.
■ Assess leg for edema, peripheral pulse, temperature, color, and tenderness every 8 hours.	■ Assessment provides baseline data that may be used to monitor success of treatment. Edema/swelling, diminished or absent peripheral pulse, pallor, cool skin temperature, and tenderness are symptoms of DVT and indicate dysfunction of peripheral circulation in the lower extremities. Measure circumference of lower leg to monitor for swelling. Peripheral pulses in both legs should be palpated for pulse rate and pulse strength to allow for comparison. Lower extremities that are cool to the touch may be due to reflex arterial spasm.	
■ Assess Homans' sign every 8 hours.	■ Normally there is no pain or discomfort associated with this procedure. Pain is caused by inflammation of the vessel. If pain is elicited, the nurse documents the response as a positive Homans' sign and reports findings to the physician.	
■ Maintain bed rest during the acute phase.	■ Bed rest is ordered to decrease possibility that portion of clot will dislodge and result in pulmonary embolism.	
■ Provide warm, moist soaks as ordered.	■ Warmth promotes blood flow to affected area.	
■ Maintain limb in elevated position.	■ Elevation of affected limb promotes venous return and helps decrease edema.	
■ Initiate progressive ambulation following the acute phase and provide properly fitting elastic stockings prior to ambulation.	■ Elastic stockings or "Teds" help prevent pooling of venous blood in lower extremities. ■ Patient may begin to ambulate within a few days when symptoms subside.	
■ **Collaborative Activities:** Administer intravenous heparin as ordered, by continuous intravenous drip, heparin lock, or subcutaneously, including: 1. Monitor IV or heparin lock site for signs of infiltration.	■ Heparin does not dissolve blood clot but is administered to prevent further clotting and improve tissue perfusion. It is safe for breastfeeding mothers because heparin is not excreted in mother's milk.	

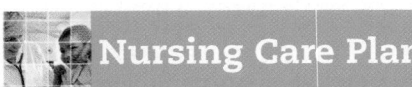

Nursing Care Plan—continued

THE WOMAN WITH A PUERPERAL PERINEAL WOUND INFECTION

INTERVENTION	RATIONALE	EXPECTED OUTCOME
2. Obtain international normalized ratio (INR) and partial thromboplastin time (PTT) per physician order and review prior to administering heparin.		
3. Observe for signs of anticoagulant overdose with resultant bleeding, including: a. Hematuria b. Epistaxis c. Ecchymosis d. Bleeding gums		
4. Provide protamine sulfate, per physician order, to combat bleeding problems related to heparin overdose.	■ Protamine sulfate is heparin antagonist, given intravenously, which is almost immediately effective in counteracting bleeding complications caused by heparin overdose.	
5. Monitor and report any signs of pulmonary embolism.	■ Pulmonary embolism is a major complication of DVT/thrombophlebitis.	
6. Initiate or support any emergency treatment.	■ Signs and symptoms may occur suddenly and require immediate emergency treatment; prognosis is related to size and location of embolism.	
7. Obtain prothrombin time (PT) and review prior to beginning warfarin. Repeat periodically per physician order.	■ PT is the test most commonly used to monitor the blood of clients receiving warfarin.	
2. Nursing Diagnosis: Pain related to tissue hypoxia and edema secondary to vascular obstruction		
NIC Intervention:		**NOC Outcome:**
Pain management: Alleviation of pain or a reduction in pain to a level of comfort that is acceptable to the patient		**Pain: Disruptive effects:** Observed or reported disruptive effects of pain on emotions and behavior
Goal: Patient will obtain relief of pain.		
■ Administer analgesics per physician order. Notify physician if pain is not relieved.	■ Analgesics act to relieve pain and enable the woman to rest. Aspirin or ibuprofen products are contraindicated because they inhibit platelet adhesiveness. Acetaminophen may be ordered by the physician.	■ Patient will have reduction in pain as evidenced by a pain level < 5 at all times.
■ Provide supportive nursing comfort measures such as back rubs, quiet time for sleep, and diversional activities.	■ Once pain decreases, patient is more likely to ambulate which will help increase venous return and decrease edema.	
3. Nursing Diagnosis: Risk for Impaired Parenting related to decreased maternal-infant interaction secondary to bed rest and IVs		
NIC Intervention:		**NOC Outcome:**
Attachment promotion: Facilitation of the development of the parent-infant relationship		**Parent-infant attachment:** Behavior that demonstrates an enduring affectionate bond between a parent and infant
Goal: Patient will demonstrate evidence of positive physical and social interaction with newborn.		

(continued)

Nursing Care Plan—continued

THE WOMAN WITH A PUERPERAL PERINEAL WOUND INFECTION

INTERVENTION	RATIONALE	EXPECTED OUTCOME
■ Maintain mother-infant attachment when mother is on bed rest: 1. Provide frequent contacts for mother and infant; modified rooming-in if possible by having the crib placed close to the mother's bed and nurse check often to help mother lift or move infant. 2. Encourage mother to continue feeding infant.	■ Maternal-infant attachment is enhanced by frequent contact and opportunities to interact.	■ Patient will develop attachment bonds as evidenced by physical interactions (good eye contact, touching the baby, holding baby close, attempting to comfort baby, kissing baby) and social interactions (calling baby by name, making positive comments about baby, asking questions about baby, asking questions about baby care, and talking to baby).

4. Nursing Diagnosis: Health-Seeking Behaviors related to lack of information about DVT/thrombophlebitis, its treatment, preventive measures, and the medication warfarin

NIC Intervention:
Health education: Development and provision of instruction and learning experiences to facilitate voluntary adaptation of behavior conducive to health in individuals, families, groups, or communities

NOC Outcome:
Knowledge: Health promotion: Extent of understanding conveyed about the promotion and protection of health

Goal: Patient will understand her condition, its treatment, and long-term implications.

INTERVENTION	RATIONALE	EXPECTED OUTCOME
■ Discuss ways of avoiding circulatory stasis such as avoiding prolonged standing, sitting, and crossing legs.	■ Such discussion is essential to help the woman understand the condition, her medication, and its implications. She must have a clear understanding to be able to provide effective self-care. ■ Prolonged sitting, standing, and crossing legs should be avoided as these activities decrease venous return.	■ Patient has health promotion knowledge as evidenced by: Woman verbalizes understanding of ways to avoid circulatory stasis, need to wear supportive stockings, medication's dosage and side effects, and the importance of a balanced diet which includes vitamin K foods. Woman verbalizes understanding of signs and symptoms of bleeding that need to be reported to healthcare provider.
■ Review need to wear support stockings and to plan for rest periods with legs elevated.		
■ In the presence of DVT, discuss the following: 1. The use of warfarin, its side effects, possible interactions with other medications, and the need to have dosage assessed through periodic checks of the prothrombin time. 2. Signs of bleeding, which may be associated with warfarin sodium and need to be reported immediately, include the following: hematuria, epistaxis, ecchymosis, bleeding gums, and rectal bleeding. 3. Monitor menstrual flow: bleeding may be heavier.	■ Patient placed on warfarin (Coumadin) therapy for 2–6 months at home.	
4. Review need for woman to eat a ***consistent*** amount of leafy green vegetables (lettuce, cabbage, brussels sprouts, broccoli) every day.	■ These foods are high in vitamin K and will affect balance between dose of warfarin and prothrombin time.	

Nursing Care Plan—continued

THE WOMAN WITH A PUERPERAL PERINEAL WOUND INFECTION

INTERVENTION	RATIONALE	EXPECTED OUTCOME
5. Instruct the woman to report ***any*** bleeding that continues more than 10 minutes.		
6. Instruct the woman to do the following: ■ Routinely inspect the body for bruising. ■ Carry MedicAlert card indicating she is on anticoagulant therapy. ■ Use electric razor to avoid scratching skin. ■ Use soft-bristle toothbrush. ■ Avoid binge alcohol intake or keep at minimum. ■ Avoid taking certain herbs such as ginger, garlic, and ginkgo and any other drugs without checking with the physician. ■ Note that stools may change color to pink, red, or black as a result of anticoagulant use. ■ Advise all health providers, including dentists, that she is taking anticoagulants.		

COMMUNITY-BASED NURSING CARE

The woman with a puerperal infection needs assistance when she is discharged from the hospital. If the family cannot provide this home assistance, a referral to home care services is needed. Home care services should be contacted as soon as puerperal infection is diagnosed so that the nurse can meet with the woman for a family and home assessment and development of a home care plan.

The family needs instruction in the care of a newborn, including feeding, bathing, cord care, immunizations, and significant observations that should be reported (see Chapter 31∞). A well-baby appointment should be scheduled. The woman who wishes to breastfeed when her condition allows can maintain lactation by pumping her breasts regularly. Breastfeeding mothers receiving antibiotics should be instructed to inspect the infant's mouth for signs of thrush and to report the finding to their physician.

The mother should be instructed regarding activity, rest, medications, diet, and signs and symptoms of complications. She should also be scheduled for a return medical visit. She needs to know the importance of taking the entire course of prescribed antibiotics even though she may begin to feel better before the bottle is empty. She also needs to be informed about the importance of pelvic rest; that is, she should not use tampons or douches nor have intercourse until she has been examined by the physician and told it is safe to resume those activities.

EVALUATION

Expected outcomes of nursing care include the following:

- The infection is quickly identified and treated successfully, without further complications.
- The woman understands the infection and the purpose of therapy; she cooperates with ongoing antibiotic therapy after discharge.
- Maternal-infant attachment is maintained.

CARE OF THE WOMAN WITH A URINARY TRACT INFECTION

The postpartal woman is at increased risk of developing urinary tract problems caused by the normal postpartal diuresis, increased bladder capacity, decreased bladder sensitivity from stretching or trauma, and possible inhibited neural control of the bladder following the use of general or regional anesthesia and contamination from catheterization. The number of catheterizations performed during labor has increased. It is essential that the mother empty the bladder completely with each voiding.

OVERDISTENTION OF THE BLADDER

Overdistention occurs postpartally when the woman is unable to empty her bladder, usually because of trauma or the effects of anesthesia. Women who have not sufficiently recovered from the effects of anesthesia cannot void spontaneously, and catheterization is necessary. After the effects of regional anesthesia have worn off, if the woman cannot void, postpartal urinary retention is highly indicative of UTI. Other risk factors for urinary retention after childbirth include nulliparity, instrumental childbirth, and prolonged labor (Yip, Shota, Pang, et al., 2005).

Clinical Therapy

Overdistention in the early postpartal period is often managed by draining the bladder with a straight catheter as a one-time measure. If the overdistention recurs or is diagnosed later in the postpartal period, an indwelling catheter is generally ordered for 24 hours. An alternative urinary retention protocol involves bladder ultrasound scans with intervention based on the amount of urine volume. For example, if the volume is greater than 400 mL, the bladder is drained and the catheter removed, whereas if the volume is 400 mL or less, a spontaneous void is awaited for 1 hour after which another scan is performed (Yip et al., 2005).

> **Nursing Practice**
>
> Postpartum urinary retention is often defined as "the absence of spontaneous urination within 6 hours of a vaginal delivery or within 6 hours after removal of an indwelling catheter post-Cesarean delivery." The astute nurse will watch the woman's bladder—not the clock!—for signs of retention. As urinary retention promotes uterine atony and a subsequent increase in bleeding and also contributes to the possibility of UTI, timely intervention is crucial.

NURSING MANAGEMENT

NURSING ASSESSMENT AND DIAGNOSIS

The overdistended bladder appears as a large mass, reaching sometimes to the umbilicus and displacing the uterine fundus upward. Increased vaginal bleeding occurs, the fundus is boggy, and the woman may complain of cramping as the uterus attempts to contract. Some women also experience backache and restlessness.

Nursing diagnoses that may apply when a woman has difficulties with overdistention of the bladder include the following:

- *Risk for Infection* related to urinary stasis secondary to overdistention
- *Urinary Retention* related to decreased bladder sensitivity and normal postpartal diuresis

PLANNING AND IMPLEMENTATION

Diligent monitoring of the bladder during the recovery period and preventive health measures greatly reduce the chances for overdistention of the bladder. The nurse should encourage the mother to void spontaneously and help her use the toilet, if possible, or the bedpan, if she has received conductive anesthesia, prevents overdistention in most cases. The woman should also be helped to a normal position for voiding (i.e., sitting with the legs and feet lower than the trunk) and provide privacy to encourage voiding. The woman should receive medication for whatever pain she may be having before she attempts to void, because pain may cause a reflex spasm of the urethra. Applying perineal ice packs after childbirth helps minimize edema, which may interfere with voiding. Pouring warm water over the perineum or having the woman void in the sitz bath may also be effective.

If catheterization becomes necessary, careful, meticulous aseptic technique is employed during catheter insertion. The vagina and vulva are traumatized to some degree by vaginal birth, and edema is common. This edema may obscure the urinary meatus; therefore, the nurse needs to be extremely careful in cleansing the vulva and inserting the catheter. It is imperative to discard a catheter that has inadvertently been introduced into the vagina and thus contaminated. Catheterization is an uncomfortable procedure because of the postpartal trauma and edema of the tissue, so the nurse should be careful and gentle not only in inserting the catheter but also in handling and cleaning the perineal area.

If the amount of urine drained from the bladder reaches 900 to 1000 mL, the catheter is clamped and taped firmly to the woman's leg. The nurse takes the woman's vital signs before and after the procedure and notes the woman's responses. After an hour, the catheter may be unclamped and placed on gravity drainage. This technique protects the bladder and prevents rapid intra-abdominal decompression. When the indwelling catheter is removed, a urine specimen is often sent to the laboratory. The tip of the catheter is also removed and may be sent for culture.

EVALUATION

Expected outcomes of nursing care include the following:

- The woman voids adequately to meet the demands of the increased fluid shifts during the postpartal period.
- The woman does not develop infection caused by stasis of urine.
- The woman actively incorporates self-care measures to decrease bladder overdistention.

CYSTITIS (LOWER URINARY TRACT INFECTION)

Retention of residual urine, bacteria introduced at the time of catheterization, and a bladder traumatized by birth combine to provide an excellent environment for the development of cystitis. *Escherichia coli* has been demonstrated to be the causative agent in most cases of postpartal cystitis and pyelonephritis (in both lower and upper UTI). Generally, the infection ascends the urinary tract from the urethra to the bladder and then to the kidneys because vesicoureteral reflux (backward flow of urine) forces contaminated urine into the renal pelvis.

Clinical Therapy

When cystitis is suspected, a clean-catch midstream urine sample is obtained for microscopic examination, culture, and sensitivity tests. The specimen may require collection by the nurse with the woman on a bedpan because few postpartal women can collect a true midstream, clean-catch specimen without contaminating the specimen with lochia. A catheterized specimen is avoided when possible because of the increased risk of infection. When the bacterial concentration is greater than 100,000 colonies of the same organism per milliliter of fresh urine, infection is generally present. Counts between 10,000 and 100,000 suggest infection, particularly if clinical symptoms are noted.

In the clinical setting, antibiotic therapy is often initiated before culture and sensitivity reports are available. Frequently used antibiotics include a preparation of trimethoprim-sulfamethoxazole—double strength (Bactrim DS, Septra DS), one of the short-acting sulfonamides, nitrofurantoin (Macrobid), and, in the case of sulfa allergy, ampicillin or amoxicillin–clavulanic acid (Augmentin). The antibiotic is changed later if indicated by the results of the sensitivity report (Duff et al., 2009; James, 2008). Antispasmodics or urinary analgesic agents, such as Pyridium, may be given to relieve discomfort.

NURSING MANAGEMENT

NURSING ASSESSMENT AND DIAGNOSIS

Symptoms of cystitis often appear 2 to 3 days after childbirth. The initial symptoms of cystitis may include frequency, urgency, dysuria, and nocturia. Hematuria and suprapubic pain may also be present. A slightly elevated temperature may occur, but systemic symptoms are often absent (James, 2008).

When a UTI progresses to pyelonephritis, systemic symptoms usually occur, and the woman becomes acutely ill. Symptoms include chills, high fever, flank pain (unilateral or bilateral), nausea, and vomiting, in addition to the signs of lower UTI. Costovertebral angle tenderness on palpation and pain may or may not be present. The nurse obtains a urine culture so that sensitivity can identify the causative organism.

Nursing diagnoses that may apply if a woman develops a postpartal UTI include the following:

- *Pain with Voiding* related to dysuria secondary to infection
- *Health-Seeking Behaviors* related to need for information about self-care measures to prevent UTI

PLANNING AND IMPLEMENTATION

Screening for asymptomatic bacteriuria in pregnancy should be routine. The nurse needs to encourage frequent emptying of the bladder during labor and postpartum to prevent overdistention and trauma to the bladder. Catheterization technique and nursing actions to prevent overdistention (previously discussed) also apply. The woman with pyelonephritis must understand the importance of follow-up care after discharge to prevent recurrence or further complications.

TEACHING FOR SELF-CARE

Advise the postpartal woman to continue good perineal hygiene after discharge. The nurse also advises the woman to maintain a good fluid intake (at least 8 to 10, 8-oz glasses daily), especially of water, and to empty her bladder whenever she feels the urge to void, but at least every 2 to 4 hours while awake. Once sexual intercourse is resumed, the new mother should void before (to prevent bladder trauma) and following intercourse (to wash contaminants from the vicinity of the urinary meatus). Wearing underwear with a cotton crotch to facilitate air circulation also reduces the risk of UTI.

Acidification of the urine is thought to aid in preventing and managing UTI. The nurse thus advises the woman to avoid carbonated beverages, which increase the alkalinity of urine, and to drink low sugar juices and take vitamin C or cranberry tablets, which increase the acidity of urine (Gilbert, 2007).

EVALUATION

Expected outcomes of nursing care include the following:

- The woman identifies the signs of UTI and her condition is treated successfully.
- The woman incorporates self-care measures to prevent the recurrence of UTI as part of her personal hygiene routine.
- The woman cooperates with any long-term therapy or follow-up.
- Maternal-infant attachment is maintained and the woman is able to care for her newborn effectively.

CARE OF THE WOMAN WITH MASTITIS

Mastitis is an infection of the breast connective tissue that occurs primarily in lactating women. The incidence of sporadic mastitis is 5% to 10% of breastfeeding mothers and less than 1% in nonlactating mothers (Duff et al., 2009; Newton, 2007). The usual causative organisms are *Staphylococcus aureus, Haemophilus parainfluenzae, H. influenzae, Escherichia coli,* and *Streptococcus* species. Infectious mastitis is a more serious infection, with fever, chills, headache, flulike muscle aches and malaise, and a warm, reddened, painful area of the breast, often wedge shaped because of the connective tissue septal divisions of the breast (Figure 32–2 ●). Because symptoms seldom occur before the second to fourth week postpartum, birthing unit nurses often are not fully aware of how uncomfortable and acutely ill the woman can be; they must ensure that all breastfeeding women are taught preventive techniques, ways of recognizing it, and the appropriate response of immediate notification of their physician/CNM.

The infection usually begins when bacteria invade the breast tissue after it has been traumatized in some way (see the factors

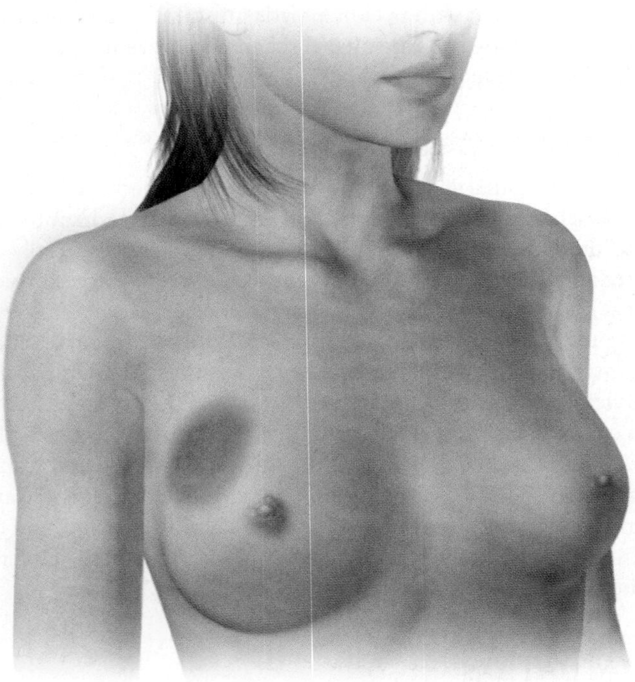

● **Figure 32–2** Mastitis. Erythema and swelling are present in the upper outer quadrant of the breast. Axillary lymph nodes are often enlarged and tender. The segmental anatomy of the breast accounts for the demarcated, often V-shaped wedge of inflammation.

Table 32–4 Factors Associated with Development of Mastitis

Milk Stasis
Failure to change infant position to allow emptying all lobes
Failure to alternate breasts at feedings
Poor suck
Poor letdown
Actions That Promote Access/Multiplication of Bacteria
Poor handwashing technique
Improper breast hygiene
Failure to air dry breasts after breastfeeding
Use of plastic-lined breast pads that trap moisture against nipple
Breast/Nipple Trauma
Incorrect positioning for breastfeeding
Poor latch-on
Failure to rotate position on nipple
Incorrect or aggressive pumping technique
Cracked nipples
Obstruction of Ducts
Restrictive clothing
Constricting bra
Underwire bra
Change in Number of Feedings/Failure to Empty Breasts
Attempted weaning
Missed feeding
Prolonged sleeping, including sleeping through night
Favoring side of nipple soreness
Lowered Maternal Defenses
Fatigue
Stress

commonly associated with mastitis in Table 32–4). Milk serves as a favorable medium for the invasive bacteria; thus milk stasis is another risk factor. The most common sources of pathogenic organisms are the infant's nose and throat, although other sources include the hands of the mother or birthing unit personnel and the woman's circulating blood. Infants of women with mastitis generally remain well.

In some cases, *Candida albicans* is the causative organism of mastitis, entering the breast through a small fissure or abrasion on the nipple; the baby will often have thrush, a candidal infection of the mouth. There may be a history of a recent course of antibiotics in the woman. Signs include late-onset nipple pain and burning pain of the nipple/areola, followed by stabbing pain of the breast during and between feedings, often radiating to the chest wall (Lawrence & Lawrence, 2009). Eventually, the skin of the affected breast becomes pink, shiny, flaking, and pruritic. Women may notice a yeasty odor to their milk. Unless the mother and her newborn are treated for *Candida*, recolonization will occur when breastfeeding is resumed. Pacifiers, bottles, and pump equipment in contact with *Candida* should be boiled for 20 minutes, and clothing in contact with the breast should be laundered in dilute bleach solution (Mass, 2004).

CLINICAL THERAPY

Diagnosis is usually based on history and physical examination; a culture and sensitivity testing of breast milk obtained by a midstream-type collection process may be done. The nipple is washed first; then the first 3 mL of breast milk are manually expressed and discarded, after which the actual specimen is collected. A leukocyte count of 1 million/mL and a bacterial count of greater than 10,000/mL are diagnostic (Newton, 2007).

Treatment of mastitis involves bed rest for at least 24 hours; increased fluid intake (at least 2 to 2.5 L/day); a supportive bra; frequent breastfeeding; local application of warm, moist-heat compresses; and analgesics that are compatible with breastfeeding (James, 2008). Nonsteroidal anti-inflammatory agents are recommended to treat both fever and inflammation. Also, a course of 7 to 10 days of antibiotics is appropriate, usually with a penicillinase-resistant penicillin or cephalosporin (Duff et al., 2009).

Candidal infections can be especially stubborn. Initial treatment generally involves antifungal (Nystatin [Mycostatin]), miconazole (Monistat-Derm), or clotrimazole (Lotrimin) creams or ointments once or twice daily. Treatment regimen must include the simultaneous treatment of the mother and baby dyad. Oral nys-

Complementary Care

PROBIOTICS

Probiotics are a category of dietary supplements consisting of beneficial microorganisms (*pro* means "for" and *biotic* means "life" versus *antibiotic,* which literally means "against life"). Probiotics compete with disease-causing microorganisms in the gastrointestinal tract. When antibiotics are taken, they kill many of the beneficial bacteria that exist naturally in the digestive tract. Supplementing with probiotics after a course of antibiotics is frequently prescribed by nutritionists and complementary practitioners. Commonly used probiotics include *Lactobacillus acidophilus* and *Bifidobacterium bifidum;* there are other species of *Lactobacillus* and *Bifidobacterium* that have been shown to be effective in such conditions as diarrhea and vaginal infections (Reid & Bocking, 2003). Bifidobacterium also competes against *Candida albicans.* Probiotics can be taken in the form of powder, capsules, and suppositories, or in fermented milk products such as yogurt or *kefir.*

tatin (Mycostatin suspension) is the most common treatment for the baby, followed by oral fluconazole (Diflucan) (Lawrence & Lawrence, 2009). Oral Diflucan for the mother is excreted in breast milk but is not considered toxic to the infant and can be used if other agents fail (Lawrence & Lawrence, 2009). Women should be instructed to cleanse their nipples with warm water and allow to air dry before application of the antifungal medication. For women who prefer to avoid medication, an alternative treatment is cleansing of the nipples with a solution of 1 tablespoon of vinegar in 1 cup of water or 1 teaspoon of baking soda in 1 cup of water, followed by air drying.

Improved outcome, decreased duration of symptoms, and decreased incidence of breast abscess result if the breasts continue to be emptied by either nursing or pumping. Thus continued breastfeeding is recommended in the presence of mastitis. The woman should be contacted within 24 hours of initiation of treatment to ensure that symptoms are subsiding.

Ten percent of cases will progress to abscess formation if mastitis remains untreated, treatment fails, or the infant is abruptly weaned. Abscess is more common when there is a lag of 24 hours or more between onset of symptoms and when the woman seeks care (Newton, 2007). Breast abscess may require incision and drainage, and intravenous antistaphylococcal antibiotics (Duff et al., 2009).

NURSING MANAGEMENT

NURSING ASSESSMENT AND DIAGNOSIS

Each day the nurse assesses the mother's breast consistency, skin color, surface temperature, nipple condition, and presence of pain to detect early signs of problems that may predispose her to mastitis. The mother should be observed breastfeeding her baby to ensure proper technique.

If an infection develops, the nurse assesses for contributing factors such as cracked nipples, poor hygiene, engorgement, supplemental feedings, change in routine or infant feeding pattern, abrupt weaning, and lack of proper breast support so that these factors can be corrected as part of the treatment plan.

Nursing diagnoses that may apply to the woman with mastitis include the following:

- *Health-Seeking Behaviors* related to lack of information about appropriate breastfeeding practices
- *Ineffective Breastfeeding* related to pain secondary to development of mastitis

PLANNING AND IMPLEMENTATION

Preventing mastitis is far simpler than treating it. Ideally mothers are instructed in proper breastfeeding technique prenatally. The nurse assists the mother to breastfeed soon after childbirth and reviews correct technique. Comanagement of breastfeeding between the nurse and a certified lactation specialist is often possible. Nurses need to encourage new mothers, even those not breastfeeding, to wear a good supportive bra at all times to prevent milk stasis, especially in the lower lobes.

Meticulous handwashing by the breastfeeding mother and all personnel is the primary measure in preventing epidemic nursery infections and subsequent maternal mastitis. Prompt attention to mothers who have blocked milk ducts eliminates stagnant milk as a growth medium for bacteria. If the mother finds that one area of her breast feels distended, she can rotate the position of her infant for nursing, manually express milk remaining in the breast after feeding (usually necessary only if the infant is not sucking well), or massage the caked area toward the nipple as the infant nurses. Mothers who develop mastitis can apply warm, moist compresses to the affected area before and during breastfeeding. The nurse encourages the mother to breastfeed frequently, starting with the unaffected breast until letdown occurs in the affected breast, then switching to the affected breast until it is emptied completely (James, 2008). After nursing, the mother can leave a small amount of milk on each nipple to prevent cracking and allow nipples to air dry. Early identification of and intervention for sore nipples are also essential, as is prompt assessment of the breastfeeding mother's breast when thrush is discovered in her newborn's mouth.

DISCHARGE PLANNING AND HOME CARE TEACHING

The nurse must stress to the breastfeeding woman the importance of adequate breast and nipple care to prevent the development of cracks and fissures, a common portal for bacterial entry. (For a detailed discussion of breastfeeding and breastfeeding home care issues, see Chapters 27 and 31∞.)

The woman should be aware of the importance of regular, complete emptying of the breasts to prevent engorgement and stasis. She should also understand the role of letdown in successful breastfeeding, correct positioning of the infant on the nipple, proper latch-on, and the principle of supply and demand. If the mother is

Table 32–5 Comparison of Findings of Engorgement, Plugged Duct, and Mastitis

Characteristics	Engorgement	Plugged Duct	Mastitis
Onset	Gradual, immediately postpartum	Gradual, after feedings	Sudden, after 10 days
Site	Bilateral	Unilateral	Usually unilateral
Swelling and heat	Generalized	May shift, little or no heat	Localized, red, hot, and swollen
Pain	Generalized	Mild but localized	Intense but localized
Body temperature	$< 38.4°C$ (101.1°F)	$< 38.4°C$ (101.1°F)	$> 38.4°C$ (101.1°F)
Systemic symptoms	Feels well	Feels well	Flulike symptoms

Source: Lawrence, R. A., & Lawrence, R. M. (1999). *Breastfeeding: A guide for the medical profession* (5th ed., p. 276). Mosby Inc., with permission from Elsevier Science.

taking antibiotics, she needs to understand the importance of completing the full course of antibiotics, even if the infection seems to clear quickly. Infants tolerate the small amount of antibiotics in breast milk without difficulty. The infant should also be checked for possible colonization with the same bacteria present in the mother's breast. Breastfeeding mothers who are returning to work outside the home need information on how to do so successfully. Because mastitis tends to develop after discharge, it is important to include information about signs and symptoms in the discharge teaching and printed materials (Table 32–5). All flulike symptoms should be considered a sign of mastitis until proven otherwise. If symptoms develop, the woman should contact her caregiver immediately because prompt treatment helps to prevent abscess formation.

COMMUNITY-BASED NURSING CARE

The home care nurse who suspects mastitis on the basis of assessment findings refers the woman to the physician. The nurse may be asked to obtain a sample of breast milk to be cultured for the causative organism.

If the mother feels too ill to breastfeed or develops an abscess that prevents nursing, the home care nurse can help the mother obtain a breast pump to help her maintain lactation and can provide opportunities for demonstration and return demonstration of pumping. The nurse can also assist the mother to deal with her feelings about temporarily being unable to breastfeed. Referral to a lactation consultant or to La Leche League can be invaluable to the woman's physical and emotional adjustment to mastitis.

EVALUATION

Expected outcomes of nursing care include the following:

- The woman is aware of the signs and symptoms of mastitis.
- The woman reports the mastitis signs and symptoms early and is treated successfully.
- The woman resumes breastfeeding if she chooses.
- The woman understands self-care measures she can employ to prevent the recurrence of the mastitis.

CARE OF THE WOMAN WITH POSTPARTAL THROMBOEMBOLIC DISEASE

Thromboembolic disease may occur antepartally, but it is generally considered a postpartal complication. *Venous thrombosis* refers to blood clot (thrombus formation) at an area of impeded blood flow in a superficial or deep vein, usually in the legs. When the thrombus is formed in response to inflammation in the vein wall, it is termed **thrombophlebitis**. Pulmonary embolism, a rare, life-threatening condition, occurs when thrombi formed in the deep leg veins are carried to the pulmonary artery, obstructing pulmonary blood flow to one or both lungs. These vascular occlusive processes—venous thrombosis, thrombophlebitis, septic pelvic thrombophlebitis, and pulmonary thromboembolism—are known as thromboembolic diseases (Krakow, 2008).

Three major causes of thromboembolic disease are hypercoagulability of blood, venous stasis, and injury to the epithelium of the blood vessel. Changes in the woman's coagulation system in pregnancy contribute to hypercoagulability and compression of the common iliac vein by the gravid uterus, which leads to venous stasis. These factors increase the risk of thromboembolic disease in pregnant and postpartal women approximately 2 to 6 times (Poggi, 2007). Superficial vein thrombophlebitis complicates the general childbearing period for 1 in 500 to 750 women. In contrast, deep vein thrombosis (DVT), which is more serious, occurs most commonly in postpartum women between postpartum days 10 to 20.

Risk factors associated with increased risk of thromboembolic disease include:

- Cesarean birth
- Immobility
- Obesity
- Cigarette smoking
- Previous thromboembolic disease
- Trauma to extremity (can include injury from incorrect positioning or prolonged interval in stirrups during labor)
- Varicose veins
- Diabetes mellitus

Table 32–6 Measures to Decrease Risk of Thromboembolic Disease in Childbearing Women

Antepartum Measures	Intrapartum Measures	Postpartum Measures
Advise woman to avoid sedentary lifestyle and to exercise as possible (walking is ideal). Recommend plenty of fluids to avoid dehydration. Advise to quit smoking. Teach to avoid prolonged standing or sitting in one position or sitting with legs crossed. Encourage elevation of legs when sitting. Teach to avoid tight knee-high hose or other constrictive garments. Encourage to take frequent breaks during long car trips to walk around, thereby preventing prolonged venous stasis.	Encourage ambulation unless contraindicated in early labor. Later, encourage leg exercises. Do not use pillows under knees. Pad stirrups. Ensure correct positioning in stirrups that minimizes pressure on the popliteal area. Limit time in stirrups as possible. After cesarean birth, initiate leg/foot exercises as soon as possible (in recovery). Use antiembolism stockings for women at risk for DVT.	Encourage early ambulation. For clients on bed rest, advise or assist with turning and leg exercises every 2 hours (woman may be encouraged to rotate ankles and to "write baby's name in the air with her toes"). Encourage fluids to avoid dehydration. Advise no smoking. Use antiembolism stockings with those at risk, including after cesarean birth. Advise against prolonged sitting and crossing legs. Encourage elevation of legs while sitting.

- Advanced maternal age
- Inherited coagulation disorders
- Multiparity
- Exogenous hormone use (oral contraceptives, hormone replacement therapy)
- Malignancy
- Anemia

Factors contributing directly to the development of thromboembolic disease postpartally include (1) increased amounts of certain blood-clotting factors; (2) postpartal thrombocytosis (increased quantity of circulating platelets and their increased adhesiveness); (3) release of thromboplastin substances from the tissue of the decidua, placenta, and fetal membranes; and (4) increased amounts of fibrinolysis inhibitors. Because all women are at risk for thromboembolic disease during the childbearing period, attention should be given to measures that might prevent this complication (Table 32–6).

SUPERFICIAL LEG VEIN DISEASE

Superficial thrombophlebitis is far more common postpartally than during pregnancy. Often the clot involves one of the saphenous veins. This disorder is more common in women with preexisting varices (enlarged veins), although it is not limited to these women. They may also occur as a sequelae to IV catheterization. Symptoms usually become apparent about postpartal day 3 or 4 and include tenderness in a portion of the vein, some local heat and redness, normal temperature or low-grade fever, and occasionally slight elevation of the pulse. A tender palpable cord may be noted along a portion of the veins. Treatment involves application of local heat, elevation of the affected limb, bed rest, analgesics, and the use of elastic support hose. Anticoagulants are usually not necessary unless complications develop. Pulmonary embolism is extremely rare.

DEEP VEIN THROMBOSIS

Deep vein thrombosis (DVT) is more frequently seen in women with a history of thrombosis. Obstetric complications, such as hydramnios, preeclampsia, and operative birth, are also associated with an increased incidence. After a clinical diagnosis of DVT, a woman's risk in a subsequent pregnancy increases.

Clinical manifestations may include edema of the ankle and leg and an initial low-grade fever often followed by high temperature and chills. Other findings include tenderness or pain, a palpable cord, changes in limb color, and difference in limb circumference of more than 2 cm (0.8 in.). Depending on the vein involved, the woman may complain of pain in the popliteal and lateral tibial areas (popliteal vein), pain in the entire lower leg and foot (anterior and posterior tibial veins), inguinal tenderness (femoral vein), or pain in the lower abdomen (iliofemoral vein). The Homans' sign (refer to Chapter 30, Figure 30–9) may or may not be positive. A positive Homans' sign is a specific finding but has low sensitivity for helping diagnose DVT (Chelmow, Aronson, & Wosu, 2007). Most DVTs occur in the left leg. Because of reflex arterial spasm, sometimes the limb is pale and cool to the touch—the so-called milk leg or *phlegmasia alba dolens*—and peripheral pulses may be decreased.

CLINICAL THERAPY

Because cases of thromboembolic disease are seldom clear-cut, diagnosis involves a variety of approaches, such as client history and physical examination, occlusive cuff impedance plethysmography (IPG), venous ultrasonography (VUS), and contrast

Thinking Critically

POSTPARTUM LEG PAIN

Wanda Sugiyama, G1P1, had a cesarean birth after a prolonged labor and failure to progress. As she is walking in the hallway with her husband, you notice that Wanda is limping slightly, and you comment on that observation. Wanda responds that she is having pain in her right lower leg. She says, "Maybe I pulled a muscle during labor." What would you do?

See MyNursingKit for possible responses.

venography (increased circumference of affected extremity). In questionable cases, venography provides the most accurate diagnosis of pelvic and calf DVT; however, it is not practical for multiple examinations or prospective screening and may itself induce phlebitis (Lockwood, 2009). Positive D-dimer has a high sensitivity in nonpregnant women but it is not a reliable marker because of the wide variation in normal lab valves in the pregnant and postpartum population (Lockwood, 2009).

Treatment involves the administration of intravenous heparin, using an infusion pump to permit continuous, accurate infusion of medication. Strict bed rest and elevation of the leg are required; analgesics are given as necessary to relieve discomfort. If fever is present, deep thrombophlebitis is suspected, and the woman is also given antibiotics. In most cases thrombectomy (surgical removal of the clot) is not necessary.

Once the symptoms have subsided (usually in several days), the woman may begin ambulation while wearing elastic support stockings. Intravenous heparin is continued until prothrombin time reaches 1.5 to 2, and treatment with sodium warfarin (Coumadin) is begun (James, 2008). The woman continues taking warfarin for 3 to 6 months at home (Lockward, 2009). While taking warfarin, prothrombin times are assessed periodically to maintain correct dosage levels.

NURSING MANAGEMENT

NURSING ASSESSMENT AND DIAGNOSIS

The nurse carefully assesses the woman's history for factors predisposing her to development of thrombosis or thrombophlebitis. In addition, as part of regular postpartal assessment, the nurse is alert to any complaints of pain in the legs, inguinal area, or lower abdomen because such pain may indicate DVT. The nurse also assesses the woman's legs for evidence of edema, temperature change, or pain with palpation.

Nursing diagnoses that may apply to a postpartal woman with a thrombotic disease include the following:

- *Ineffective Tissue Perfusion in Periphery* related to obstructed venous return
- *Pain* related to tissue hypoxia and edema secondary to vascular obstruction
- *Risk for Impaired Parenting* related to decreased maternal-infant interaction secondary to bed rest and intravenous lines
- *Deficient Knowledge* related to self-care after discharge on anticoagulant therapy

PLANNING AND IMPLEMENTATION

HOSPITAL-BASED NURSING CARE

The nurse evaluates the need for support hose for women with varicosities during labor and the postpartum period. Adequate fluid intake is necessary during labor to avoid dehydration. Because trauma is often a factor in the development of thrombophlebitis, avoid keeping the woman's legs elevated in stirrups for prolonged periods. If stirrups are used, they should be comfortably padded and adjusted to provide correct support and prevent pressure on popliteal vessels. Early ambulation is encouraged following birth, and the knee gatch on the bed should be avoided. Women confined to bed following a cesarean birth are encouraged to perform regular leg exercises to promote venous return.

Once DVT is diagnosed, the nurse maintains the heparin therapy, provides appropriate comfort measures, and monitors the woman closely for signs of pulmonary embolism. The nurse also assesses for evidence of bleeding related to heparin and keeps the antagonist for heparin, protamine sulfate, readily available.

DISCHARGE PLANNING

The nurse instructs the woman to avoid prolonged standing or sitting because these positions contribute to venous stasis. The nurse also advises the woman to avoid crossing her legs because of the pressure it causes. The nurse recommends that the woman take frequent breaks during car trips and while working if she sits most of the day. Walking is acceptable because it promotes venous return. The woman is reminded to mention her history of thrombosis or thrombophlebitis to her physician during subsequent pregnancies so that preventive measures can be instituted early (Lockwood, 2009).

Clients on warfarin need to be educated about foods high in vitamin K and the need to strive for consistent daily intake. When the dietary intake of these foods such as cauliflower, soybean and canola oil, mayonnaise. broccoli, green and black tea, peppers, spinach, collard greens and others decreases significantly, there is a risk of bleeding. Many multivitamins contain vitamin K; clients on warfarin may take them but should do so consistently. Vitamin C doses up to 500 mg per day and vitamin E doses up to 400 international units per day are considered safe; higher doses can affect coagulation.

Women who are discharged on warfarin must understand the purpose of the medication and be alert for signs of bleeding such as bleeding gums, epistaxis, petechiae or ecchymosis, and evidence of blood in the urine or stool. Certain medications such as aspirin and other nonsteroidal anti-inflammatory drugs increase anticoagulant activity and should be avoided; when she is taking warfarin the woman should check for possible medication interaction before taking *any* other medication. She should also have vitamin K available in case bleeding occurs.

While taking anticoagulants, the woman will be asked to undergo frequent coagulant tests to guide dosing. Point-of-care testing is now available to decrease the inconvenience of going to the laboratory. Home self-testing involves a single capillary finger stick (Coaguchek, ProTime, Avocet) to test thromboplastin-mediated clotting expressed as prothrombin time (PT) or international normalized ratio (INR). The risk of bleeding increases significantly when the INR is greater than 3 (Lockwood, 2009). Bleeding should be reported if it fails to stop within 10 minutes. Because careful monitoring is important, the woman should clearly understand the need to keep scheduled appointments for PT assessment. (See "Nursing Care Plan: The Woman with Thromboembolic Disease" on pages 845–848 for specific nursing care measures.)

Nursing Care Plan

THE WOMAN WITH THROMBOEMBOLIC DISEASE

INTERVENTION	RATIONALE	EXPECTED OUTCOME
1. Nursing Diagnosis: Ineffective Tissue Perfusion: Peripheral related to interruption of venous blood flow secondary to complications of labor and birth		
NIC Intervention: **Embolus care: Peripheral:** Limitation of complications for a patient experiencing, or at risk for, occlusion of peripheral circulation		**NOC Outcome:** **Tissue perfusion: Peripheral:** Extent to which blood flows through the small vessels of the extremities and maintains tissue function
Goal: The patient's presenting signs and symptoms are relieved.		
■ Assess, record, and report signs of thrombophlebitis.	■ Early detection of developing thrombophlebitis permits prompt treatment. As the thrombus increases in size, signs of obstruction also increase.	■ Patient will have increased venous return from lower leg as evidenced by decreased edema in lower leg, negative Homans' sign, and no pain or tenderness in lower leg.
■ Assess leg for edema, peripheral pulse, temperature, color, and tenderness every 8 hours.	■ Assessment provides baseline data that may be used to monitor success of treatment. Edema/swelling, diminished or absent peripheral pulse, pallor, cool skin temperature, and tenderness are symptoms of DVT and indicate dysfunction of peripheral circulation in the lower extremities. Measure circumference of lower leg to monitor for swelling. Peripheral pulses in both legs should be palpated for pulse rate and pulse strength to allow for comparison. Lower extremities that are cool to the touch may be due to reflex arterial spasm.	
■ Assess Homans' sign every 8 hours.	■ Normally there is no pain or discomfort associated with this procedure. Pain is caused by inflammation of the vessel. If pain is elicited, the nurse documents the response as a positive Homans' sign and reports findings to the physician.	
■ Maintain bed rest during the acute phase.	■ Bed rest is ordered to decrease possibility that portion of clot will dislodge and result in pulmonary embolism.	
■ Provide warm, moist soaks as ordered.	■ Warmth promotes blood flow to affected area.	
■ Maintain limb in elevated position.	■ Elevation of affected limb promotes venous return and helps decrease edema.	
■ Initiate progressive ambulation following the acute phase and provide properly fitting elastic stockings prior to ambulation.	■ Elastic stockings or "Teds" help prevent pooling of venous blood in lower extremities. ■ Patient may begin to ambulate within a few days when symptoms subside.	
■ **Collaborative Activities** Administer intravenous heparin as ordered, by continuous intravenous drip, heparin lock, or subcutaneously, including: 1. Monitor IV or heparin lock site for signs of infiltration.	■ Heparin does not dissolve blood clot but is administered to prevent further clotting and improve tissue perfusion. It is safe for breastfeeding mothers because heparin is not excreted in mother's milk.	

(continued)

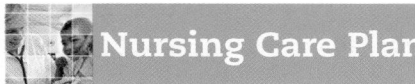

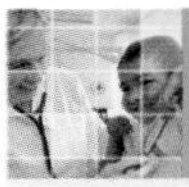

Nursing Care Plan—continued

THE WOMAN WITH THROMBOEMBOLIC DISEASE

INTERVENTION	RATIONALE	EXPECTED OUTCOME
2. Obtain international normalized ratio (INR) and partial thromboplastin time (PTT) per physician order and review prior to administering heparin.		
3. Observe for signs of anticoagulant overdose with resultant bleeding, including: a. Hematuria b. Epistaxis c. Ecchymosis d. Bleeding gums		
4. Provide protamine sulfate, per physician order, to combat bleeding problems related to heparin overdose.	■ Protamine sulfate is heparin antagonist, given intravenously, which is almost immediately effective in counteracting bleeding complications caused by heparin overdose.	
5. Monitor and report any signs of pulmonary embolism.	■ Pulmonary embolism is a major complication of DVT/thrombophlebitis.	
6. Initiate or support any emergency treatment.	■ Signs and symptoms may occur suddenly and require immediate emergency treatment; prognosis is related to size and location of embolism.	
7. Obtain prothrombin time (PT) and review prior to beginning warfarin. Repeat periodically per physician order.	■ PT is the test most commonly used to monitor the blood of clients receiving warfarin.	

2. Nursing Diagnosis: Pain related to tissue hypoxia and edema secondary to vascular obstruction

NIC Intervention:

Pain management: Alleviation of pain or a reduction in pain to a level of comfort that is acceptable to the patient

NOC Outcome:

Pain: Disruptive effects: Observed or reported disruptive effects of pain on emotions and behavior

Goal: Patient will obtain relief of pain.

INTERVENTION	RATIONALE	EXPECTED OUTCOME
■ Administer analgesics per physician order. Notify physician if pain is not relieved.	■ Analgesics act to relieve pain and enable the woman to rest. Aspirin or ibuprofen products are contraindicated because they inhibit platelet adhesiveness. Acetaminophen may be ordered by the physician.	■ Patient will have reduction in pain as evidenced by a pain level < 5 at all times.
■ Provide supportive nursing comfort measures such as back rubs, quiet time for sleep, and diversional activities.	■ Once pain decreases, client is more likely to ambulate which will help increase venous return and decrease edema.	

3. Nursing Diagnosis: Risk for Impaired Parenting related to decreased maternal-infant interaction secondary to bed rest and IVs

NIC Intervention:

Attachment promotion: Facilitation of the development of the parent-infant relationship

NOC Outcome:

Parent-infant attachment: Behavior that demonstrates an enduring affectionate bond between a parent and infant

Goal: Patient will demonstrate evidence of positive physical and social interaction with newborn.

Nursing Care Plan—continued

THE WOMAN WITH THROMBOEMBOLIC DISEASE

INTERVENTION	RATIONALE	EXPECTED OUTCOME
■ Maintain mother-infant attachment when mother is on bed rest: 1. Provide frequent contacts for mother and infant; modified rooming-in if possible by having the crib placed close to the mother's bed and nurse check often to help mother lift or move infant. 2. Encourage mother to continue feeding infant.	■ Maternal-infant attachment is enhanced by frequent contact and opportunities to interact.	■ Patient will develop attachment bonds as evidenced by physical interactions (good eye contact, touching the baby, holding baby close, attempting to comfort baby, kissing baby) and social interactions (calling baby by name, making positive comments about baby, asking questions about baby, asking questions about baby care, and talking to baby).

4. Nursing Diagnosis: Health-Seeking Behaviors related to lack of information about DVT/thrombophlebitis, its treatment, preventive measures, and the medication warfarin

NIC Intervention:	NOC Outcome:
Health education: Development and provision of instruction and learning experiences to facilitate voluntary adaptation of behavior conducive to health in individuals, families, groups, or communities	**Knowledge: Health promotion:** Extent of understanding conveyed about the promotion and protection of health

Goal: Patient will understand her condition, its treatment, and long-term implications.

■ Discuss ways of avoiding circulatory stasis such as avoiding prolonged standing, sitting, and crossing legs.	■ Such discussion is essential to help the woman understand the condition, her medication, and its implications. She must have a clear understanding to be able to provide effective self-care. ■ Prolonged sitting, standing, and crossing legs should be avoided as these activities decrease venous return.	■ Patient has health promotion knowledge as evidenced by: Woman verbalizes understanding of ways to avoid circulatory stasis, need to wear supportive stockings, medication's dosage and side effects, and the importance of a balanced diet, which includes vitamin K foods. Woman verbalizes understanding of signs and symptoms of bleeding that need to be reported to healthcare provider.
■ Review need to wear support stockings and to plan for rest periods with legs elevated.		
■ In the presence of DVT, discuss the following: 1. The use of warfarin, its side effects, possible interactions with other medications, and the need to have dosage assessed through periodic checks of the prothrombin time. 2. Signs of bleeding, which may be associated with warfarin sodium and need to be reported immediately, include the following: hematuria, epistaxis, ecchymosis, bleeding gums, and rectal bleeding. 3. Monitor menstrual flow: bleeding may be heavier.	■ Patient placed on warfarin (Coumadin) therapy for 2–6 months at home.	

(continued)

Nursing Care Plan—continued

INTERVENTION	RATIONALE	EXPECTED OUTCOME
4. Review need for woman to eat a *consistent* amount of leafy green vegetables (lettuce, cabbage, brussels sprouts, broccoli) every day.	■ These foods are high in vitamin K and will affect balance between dose of warfarin and prothrombin time.	
5. Instruct the woman to report *any* bleeding that continues more than 10 minutes.		
6. Instruct the woman to do the following: ■ Routinely inspect the body for bruising. ■ Carry MedicAlert card indicating she is on anticoagulant therapy. ■ Use electric razor to avoid scratching skin. ■ Use soft-bristle toothbrush. ■ Avoid binge alcohol intake or keep at minimum. ■ Avoid taking certain herbs such as ginger, garlic, and ginkgo and any other drugs without checking with the physician. ■ Note that stools may change color to pink, red, or black as a result of anticoagulant use. ■ Advise all health providers, including dentists, that she is taking anticoagulants.		

COMMUNITY-BASED NURSING CARE

Because the mother with postpartal thromboembolic disease will depend on others for much of her initial home care, it is helpful for the father of the newborn to be involved in preparations for discharge. The nurse should provide ample time to answer questions and clarify instructions, verbally and in writing. It is especially important to assess the couple's plans to ensure complete bed rest for the mother. They might explore ways for her to maintain bed rest and still spend quality time with her newborn and any other children. For example, young children can sit on the bed for storytelling or play quiet games, and the newborn's crib can be placed next to the mother's bed.

The father/partner may be assuming multiple roles in these circumstances—household manager, parent, worker, and caregiver. Fatigue is inevitable. There may also be financial concerns as a result of prolonged health care or his extended time away from work to care for the family. Many concerns will not surface until the couple actually returns home and fully comprehends the reality of their situation. For that reason, it is valuable to provide them with an accessible resource person and to plan telephone or home visit follow-up care.

Signs of postpartum thrombophlebitis may not occur until after discharge from the birthing unit. Consequently all couples must be taught to recognize its signs and symptoms and appreciate the importance of reporting them immediately and not massaging the affected leg. If signs and symptoms occur after discharge, a short readmission may be required. In that case every effort is made to allow mother, father, and newborn to remain together.

EVALUATION

Expected outcomes of nursing care include the following:

- The woman seeks treatment for her thrombophlebitis early and is managed successfully, without further complications.
- At discharge the woman is able to explain the purpose, dosage regimen, and necessary precautions associated with any prescribed medications such as anticoagulants.
- The woman can discuss the self-care measures and ongoing therapies (such as need for rest and the use of elastic stockings) that are indicated.
- The woman has bonded successfully with her newborn and is able to care for her baby effectively.

CARE OF THE WOMAN WITH A POSTPARTUM PSYCHIATRIC DISORDER

The relationship of affective disorders to childbirth is reflected in the fact that the rate of admission to a psychiatric hospital is greater during the year after childbirth than at any other time in a woman's life.

TYPES OF POSTPARTUM PSYCHIATRIC DISORDERS

The classification of postpartum psychiatric disorders is a subject of some controversy. The *Diagnostic and Statistical Manual of Mental Disorders* (APA, 2000) has added a postpartum onset specifier to the mood disorder diagnostic category of psychiatric disorders. It is proposed that postpartum psychiatric disorders be considered one diagnosable syndrome with three subclasses: (1) adjustment reaction with depressed mood, (2) postpartum psychosis, and (3) postpartum major mood disorder. The incidence, etiology, symptoms, treatment, and prognosis vary with each subclass.

Adjustment Reaction with Depressed Mood

Adjustment reaction with depressed mood is also known as **postpartum blues**, or as *maternal blues* or "*baby blues.*" It occurs in as many as 50% to 80% of mothers and is characterized by mild depression interspersed with happier feelings (Beck, 2006). Postpartum blues typically occur within a few days after the baby's birth and are self-limiting, lasting from a few hours to 10 days or longer. The depression is more severe in primiparas than in multiparas and seems related to the rapid alteration of estrogen, progesterone, and prolactin levels after birth. New mothers experiencing postpartum blues commonly report feeling overwhelmed, unable to cope, fatigued, anxious, irritable, and oversensitive. A key feature is episodic tearfulness, often without an identifiable reason. Often, when the woman is asked why she is crying, she will respond that she does not know. Cunningham et al. (2010) speculate that several factors contribute to the blues:

- Emotional letdown that follows labor and childbirth
- Physical discomfort typical in the early postpartum
- Fatigue
- Anxiety about caring for the newborn after discharge
- Fears about her physical attractiveness

Validating the existence of this phenomenon, labeling it as a real but normal adjustment reaction, and providing reassurance can offer a measure of relief. Assistance with self and infant care, rest, good nutrition, information, and family support aids recovery. The partner should be encouraged to watch for and report signs that the new mother is not returning to a more normal mood but slipping into a deeper depression. Most affected women reported that they did not seek help because they felt their depression was caused by the stress of becoming a mother, thought it was a normal reaction, and/or feared that they would be labeled mentally ill and considered unfit mothers (Driscoll, 2008).

Postpartum Psychosis

Postpartum psychosis, which has an incidence of 1 to 2 per 1000, usually becomes evident within the first 1 to 3 months postpartum (Doucet, Dennis, Letourneau, et al., 2009). Although relatively rare, new onset postpartum psychosis gains considerable national attention in the media when there is an incident of infanticide associated with it. Symptoms include agitation, hyperactivity, insomnia, mood lability, confusion, irrationality, difficulty remembering or concentrating, poor judgment, delusions, and hallucinations that tend to be related to the infant. With appropriate treatment, improvement is seen in 95% of women in 2 to 3 months. Surprisingly, it is not associated with depression during the antenatal period (Haessler & Rosenthal, 2007). Recurrence in subsequent pregnancies may be as high as 20% to 30% (Doucet et al., 2009). Postpartum psychosis is considered an emergency because of the risk of suicide and/or infanticide (Doucet et al., 2009).

Postpartum Major Mood Disorder

Postpartum major mood disorder, also known as **postpartum depression (PPD)**, develops in about 4.5% to 28% of postpartum women across studies (Doucet et al., 2009). Although it may occur at any time during the first postpartum year, the periods of greatest risk occur around the fourth week, just before the initiation of menses, and upon weaning.

Risk factors for postpartum depression include the following:

- Primiparity
- Ambivalence about maintaining the pregnancy
- History of postpartum depression or bipolar illness
- Lack of social support
- Lack of a stable and supportive relationship with parents or partner
- Lack of a supportive relationship with her parents, especially her father, as a child
- The woman's dissatisfaction with herself, including body image problems and eating disorders

Women with postpartum depression are at risk for suicide, most prominently as they enter or exit the deeply depressed state. In a deep depression, the woman is unlikely to be able to plan and carry out suicide. For that reason, signs of improvement in depression should be celebrated with some caution. Whereas the woman with postpartal psychosis may attempt suicide because of illogical thought processes, the woman with major depression attempts suicide because her suffering is so great that dying seems a more favorable option than continuing to live in such pain. She may also attempt suicide to save her newborn from some perceived or real threat—including the possibility that she herself might harm the baby.

CLINICAL THERAPY

Women with a history of postpartum psychosis or depression or other risk factors should be referred to a mental health professional for counseling and biweekly visits between the second and sixth week postpartum for evaluation. Medication, individual or group psychotherapy, and practical assistance with child care and other demands of daily life are common treatment measures for both disorders; however, the specific therapies used may vary.

Treatment of postpartum depression is not unlike treatment of any significant depression: psychotherapy and antidepression medications, usually the selective serotonin reuptake inhibitors. Based on an expert consensus guideline for breastfeeding mothers, it is recommended that sertraline (e.g., Zoloft, Lustral) be the first-line treatment for PPD and paroxetine (e.g., Paxil, Seroxat, Deroxat) as an alternative first-line treatment (Beck, 2008). It is recommended that a combination of antidepressants and psychosocial interventions be used regardless of whether the woman is breastfeeding. It is important to realize that many of the drugs used in treating postpartum psychiatric conditions may be contraindicated in breastfeeding women. Fluoxetine (e.g., Prozac, Sarafem) is not recommended for lactating women because of its long half-life (Beck, 2008). Some of the antidepressive drugs have been linked to an increase in congenital defects so birth control use should also be emphasized. The woman and her partner should be reminded that antidepressants may take several weeks to have an effect. Providers may prefer to start antidepressants before the birth of the baby (usually started at 36 weeks of gestation) so that a therapeutic blood level is achieved before the birth of the baby.

Support groups have proved to be successful adjuncts to such treatment. Within a support group of postpartal women and their partners, a couple may feel consolation that they are not alone in their experience. Moreover, the group provides a forum for exchanging information about postpartum depression, learning stress reduction measures, and experiencing renewed self-esteem and support. The most effective support groups provide for safe child care to facilitate attendance. If a support group is not available locally, the woman and her family may be encouraged to contact Depression after Delivery (DAD), now a national Web-based support network that provides education and volunteers, or Postpartum Support International. The Mills Depression and Anxiety Symptom-Feeling Checklist is also available online.

Treatment of postpartum psychosis is directed at the specific type of psychotic symptoms displayed and may include lithium, antipsychotics, or electroconvulsive therapy in combination with psychotherapy, removal of the infant, and social support. It is important for the nurse to realize that many of the drugs used in treating postpartum psychiatric conditions are contraindicated in breastfeeding women.

NURSING MANAGEMENT

NURSING ASSESSMENT AND DIAGNOSIS

Assessment for factors predisposing a client to postpartal depression or psychosis should begin prenatally (Beck, 2002). Questions designed to detect problems can be included as part of the routine prenatal history interview or questionnaire. Women with a personal or family history of psychiatric disease, particularly postpartum depression or psychosis, need prenatal instructions on the signs and symptoms of depression and may need additional emotional support. Ideally a depression assessment should be completed each trimester to update a pregnant woman's risk status (Beck, 2002).

If not done previously, the nurse assesses the woman for predisposing factors during labor and the postpartum stay. Several depression scales are available for assessing postpartum depression. The routine use of a screening tool in a matter-of-fact approach significantly increases the diagnosis. The Edinburgh Postnatal Depression Scale (Table 32–7) is the most widely used screening tool for postpartum depression in large populations of women. The tool has been validated, computerized, and used in telephone screening. Mothers who score above 12 on the Edinburgh Postpartum Depression Scale are likely to be suffering from postpartum depression. Another tool is Beck's (2002) revised Postpartum Depression Predictors Inventory (PDPI-revised). This tool is also a practical and simple screening checklist to use during routine care with all postpartum women to identify those who might be experiencing postpartum depression so that early management might be initiated (Table 32–8).

No matter what approach the nurse uses to assess for postpartum depression, enabling the woman's voice to be heard about her feelings of maternal role transition and how she is adjusting in this vulnerable time is of inestimable value (Beck, 2008). Listening to her story provides a critical emie (insider's) view of her circumstances as opposed to an etic (outsider's) view.

In providing daily care, the nurse observes the woman for objective signs of depression—anxiety, irritability, poor concentration, forgetfulness, sleep difficulties, appetite change, fatigue, and tearfulness—and listens for statements indicating feelings of failure and self-accusation. Severity and duration of symptoms should be noted. Behavior and verbalizations that are bizarre or seem to indicate a potential for violence against herself or others, including the infant, are reported as soon as possible for further evaluation.

The nurse needs to be aware that many normal physiologic changes of the puerperium are similar to symptoms of depression (lack of sexual interest, appetite change, fatigue). It is essential that observations be as specific and as objective as possible and that they are carefully documented. Anxiety was a prominent feature of illness for some women and suggested that women be assessed for their level of anxiety, particularly regarding infant care (Doucet et al., 2009). Because of the strong association of interrupted sleep and postpartum depression and the finding that severe fatigue was an excellent predictor of postpartum depression, assessing fatigue level at 2 weeks postpartum by telephone may be helpful in predicting depression risk early. Restorative sleep improves one's ability to cope and make decisions, thereby producing a sense of better self-control. A central challenge for nursing is identifying women at risk of suicide. Family members of the depressed woman should also be alert to signals that she may be intent on self-harm; they must be advised that threats should always be taken seriously. Family members should be told to be especially vigilant for suicide when the woman seems to be feeling better.

Possible nursing diagnoses that may apply to a woman with a postpartum psychiatric disorder include the following:

- *Ineffective Individual Coping* related to postpartum depression

Table 32–7 Edinburgh Postnatal Depression Scale

In the past 7 days:

1. I have been able to laugh and see the funny side of things.
   As much as I always could
   Not quite so much now
   Definitely not so much now
   Not at all
2. I have looked forward with enjoyment of things.
   As much as I ever did
   Rather less than I used to
   Definitely less than I used to
   Hardly at all

*3. I have blamed myself unnecessarily when things went wrong.
   Yes, most of the time
   Yes, some of the time
   Not very often
   No, never

4. I have been anxious or worried for no good reason.
   No, not at all
   Hardly ever
   Yes, sometimes
   Yes, very often

*5. I have felt scared or panicky for no very good reason.
   Yes, quite a lot
   Yes, sometimes
   No, not much
   No, not at all

*6. Things have been getting on top of me.
   Yes, most of the time I haven't been able to cope at all
   Yes, sometimes I haven't been coping as well as usual
   No, I have been coping quite well
   No, I have been coping as well as ever

*7. I have been so unhappy that I have had difficulty sleeping.
   Yes, most of the time
   Yes, sometimes
   Not very often
   No, not at all

*8. I have felt sad or miserable.
   Yes, most of the time
   Yes, quite often
   Not very often
   No, not at all

*9. I have been so unhappy that I have been crying.
   Yes, most of the time
   Yes, quite often
   Only occasionally
   No, never

*10. The thought of harming myself has occurred to me.
   Yes, quite often
   Sometimes
   Hardly ever
   Never

Note: Response categories are scored 0, 1, 2, and 3 according to increased severity of the symptoms. Items marked with an asterisk are reverse-scored (3, 2, 1, 0). The total score is calculated by adding together the scores for each of the 10 items. A score above the threshold of 12 to 13 out of 30 indicates with 86% sensitivity that the woman is suffering from postpartum depression.

Source: Cox, J. L., Holden, J. M., & Sagovsky, R. (1987). Detection of postnatal depression: Development of the 10-item Edinburgh Postnatal Depression Scale. *British Journal of Psychiatry, 150,* 782–786. Users may reproduce the scale without further permission provided they respect copyright by quoting the names of the authors, the title, and the source of the paper in all reproduced copies.

- *Risk for Altered Parenting* related to postpartal mental illness
- *Risk for Violence against self (suicide), newborn, and other children* related to depression

PLANNING AND IMPLEMENTATION

Nurses working in antepartal settings or teaching childbirth classes play indispensable roles in helping prospective parents appreciate the lifestyle changes and role demands associated with parenthood. Offering realistic information and anticipatory guidance and debunking myths about the perfect mother or perfect newborn may help prevent postpartum depression. Social support teaching guides are available for nurses to help postpartum women explore their needs (Sealy, Fraser, Simpson, et al., 2009).

The nurse should alert the mother, spouse, and other family members to the possibility of postpartum blues in the early days after birth and reassure them of the short-term nature of the condition. Symptoms of postpartum depression should be described and the mother encouraged to call her healthcare provider if symptoms become severe, if they fail to subside quickly, or if at any time she feels she is unable to function. Encouraging the mother to plan how she will manage at home and providing concrete suggestions on how to cope aid in her adjustment to motherhood. Table 32–9 on page 853 provides suggestions that serve as primary prevention measures for postpartum depression.

COMMUNITY-BASED NURSING CARE

Home visits, especially for early-discharge families, are essential to fostering positive adjustments for the new family constellation. Telephone follow-up at 2 to 3 weeks postpartum to ask whether the mother is experiencing difficulties is also helpful. If a mother calls with a seemingly innocuous question, she should be asked two or three open-ended questions about her general status (Katz, 2007). These questions allow the woman to open up if there is an underlying depression that she is too guilty/afraid to express initially; for example:

1. How do you feel things are going?
2. How are things going?
3. Are you feeling like you expected?

Monitoring for signs of depression or performing brief screening at well-child follow-ups also can be valuable for early identification and timely intervention (Katz, 2007).

In all women, the presence of three symptoms of depression on one day or one symptom for 3 days may signal serious

Table 32–8 Postpartum Depression Predictors Inventory (PDPI)—Revised, and Guide Questions for Its Use

During Pregnancy			
Marital status		**Check One**	
1. Single		☐	
2. Married/cohabitating		☐	
3. Separated		☐	
4. Divorced		☐	
5. Widowed		☐	
6. Partnered		☐	
Socioeconomic status			
Low		☐	
Middle		☐	
High		☐	
Self-esteem	**Yes**		**No**
Do you feel good about yourself as a person	☐		☐
Do you feel worthwhile	☐		☐
Do you feel you have a number of good qualities as a person	☐		☐
Prenatal depression			
1. Have you felt depressed during your pregnancy	☐		☐
If yes, when and how long have you been feeling this way?			
If yes, how mild or severe would you consider your depression?			
Prenatal anxiety			
Have you been feeling anxious during your pregnancy	☐		☐
If yes, how long have you been feeling this way			
Unplanned/unwanted pregnancy			
Was the pregnancy planned	☐		☐
Is the pregnancy unwanted	☐		☐
History of previous depression			
1. Before this pregnancy, have you ever been depressed	☐		☐
If yes, when did you experience this depression?			
If yes, have you been under a physician's care for this past depression?	☐		☐
If yes, did the physician prescribe any medication for your depression	☐		☐
Social support			
1. Do you feel you receive adequate emotional support from your partner	☐		☐
2. Do you feel you receive adequate instrumental support from your partner (e.g., help with household chores or babysitting)?	☐		☐
3. Do you feel you can rely on your partner when you need help?	☐		☐
4. Do you feel you can confide in your partner? (repeat same questions for family and again for friends)	☐		☐
Marital satisfaction			
1. Are you satisfied with your marriage (or living arrangement)?	☐		☐
2. Are you currently experiencing any marital problems?	☐		☐
3. Are things going well between you and your partner?	☐		☐
Life stress			
1. Are you currently experiencing any stressful events in your life such as:			
Financial problems	☐		☐
Marital problems	☐		☐
Death in the family	☐		☐
Serious illness in the family	☐		☐
Moving	☐		☐
Unemployment	☐		☐
Job change	☐		☐

Table 32–8 Postpartum Depression Predictors Inventory (PDPI)—Revised, and Guide Questions for Its Use—continued

After Delivery, Add the Following Items

Childcare stress	**Yes**	**No**
1. Is your infant experiencing any health problems?	☐	☐
2. Are you having problems with your baby feeding?	☐	☐
3. Are you having problems with your baby sleeping?	☐	☐
Infant temperament		
1. Would you consider your baby irritable or fussy?	☐	☐
2. Does your baby cry a lot?	☐	☐
3. Is your baby difficult to console or soothe?	☐	☐
Maternity blues		
1. Did you experience a brief period of tearfulness and mood swings during the first week after delivery?	☐	☐

Comments:

Source: AWHONN. (2002). Beck, C.T. Revision of the Postpartum Predictors Inventory. *Journal of Obstetric, Gynecologic, and Neonatal Nursing, 31*(4), 394–402 (Table 2 on PDPI, pp. 399–400). Washington, DC: Author.

Table 32–9 Primary Prevention Strategies for Postpartum Depression

1.	Celebrate childbirth but appreciate that it is a life-changing transition that can be stressful—at times it can seem overwhelming. Share your feelings with each other and/or others.
2.	Consider keeping a journal in which you write down feelings. Not only is it emotionally cathartic, it provides a great memory book.
3.	Appreciate that you do not have to know everything to be a good parent—it is okay to seek advice during this transition.
4.	Connect with others who are parents—use them as a support and information network.
5.	Set a daily schedule and follow it even if you do not feel like it. Structuring activity helps counteract inertia that comes with feeling sad or unsettled.
6.	Prioritize daily tasks. Decide what must be done and what can wait. Try to get one major thing done every day. Remember, you do not always have to look like a magazine fashion model.
7.	Remember that you do not have to entertain or care for everyone who drops by. Doing something for someone else, however, often tends to make you feel better.
8.	If someone volunteers to help you with tasks or baby care, take him or her up on it. While your volunteer is in action, do something pleasurable or get some rest.
9.	Maintain outside interests. Plan some time every day—even if it's just 15 minutes—to do something exclusively for "you" that is pleasurable.
10.	Eat a healthful diet. Limit alcohol. Quit smoking. Get some exercise. (All of these can positively affect the immune system.)
11.	Get as much sleep as possible. Rest whenever you can, such as when the baby is napping. If you have other young children, bring them onto your bed to read or play quietly while you lie down.
12.	Limit major changes (moves, job changes, etc.) the first year insofar as possible.
13.	Spend time with others.
14.	If things get overwhelming, and you feel yourself slipping into depression, reach out to someone for help.
15.	Attend a postpartum support group if one is available. Consider also an international program such as Postpartum Support International, 927 North Kellogg Avenue, Santa Barbara, CA 93111, 1-805-967-7636 or online at www.postpartum.net

depression and requires immediate referral to a mental health professional. Immediate referral should also be made if rejection of the infant or threatened or actual aggression against the infant has occurred. In such cases the newborn is never left unattended with the mother. Depression does appear to interfere with optimal mothering; there is less interaction between mother and child, an increased incidence of mood and cognitive development problems, and more visits to the doctor in these children (Beck, 2002).

Awareness of the term postpartum depression does not necessarily imply awareness of its symptoms or sources of assistance. Public education is needed to address this fact in order to provide social support and encourage treatment for symptomatic woman and their families (Sealy et al., 2009).

A diagnosis of postpartum depression or other psychiatric disorder poses major problems for the family, especially the father. The symptoms of these disorders are difficult to witness and may be harder to understand than physical problems such as hemorrhage and infection. The father may feel hurt by his partner's hostility, worry that she is becoming insane, or be baffled by her mood swings and lack of concern about herself, the newborn, or household responsibilities. He may be troubled by their lack of intimacy or deteriorating communication. Certainly, he has cause for concern about how the newborn and any other children are being affected. Very real practical matters—running the household; managing the children, including the totally dependent newborn; and caring for the mother—may be added to his usual routines and work responsibilities. It is not surprising that, even in the most supportive families, relationships may suffer in response to these circumstances. It is often the father or another close family member who in desperation makes contact with the healthcare agency. This is especially difficult when the mother is reluctant to admit she is suffering emotional difficulty or is too ill to recognize her own needs.

The integration of the newborn into the family and care of the newborn and other children can be further compromised by co-occurrent postpartum depression in fathers. An examination of research studies that cite incidences of paternal postpartum depression indicate 24% to 50% incidence of depression among men whose partners were experiencing postpartum depression (Goodman, 2004).

Information, emotional support, and assistance in providing or obtaining care for the infant may be needed. The nurse can assist family members by identifying community resources, making referrals to public health nursing services and social services, and providing a list of telephone numbers as well as emergency services that she may need. Postpartum follow-up is especially important, as well as visits from a psychiatric home health nurse.

EVALUATION

Expected outcomes of nursing care include the following:

- The woman's signs of depression are identified and she receives therapy quickly.
- The newborn is cared for effectively by the father or another support person until the mother is able to provide care.
- The mother and newborn will remain safe.
- The newborn is integrated into the family.

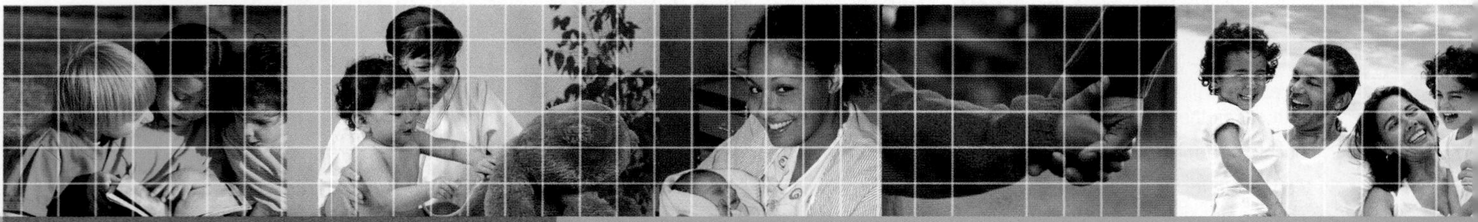

CRITICAL CONCEPT REVIEW

LEARNING OUTCOMES	CONCEPTS
32.1 Identify the causes of and appropriate nursing interventions for early and late hemorrhage during the postpartal period.	1. The main causes of postpartum hemorrhage and the appropriate nursing interventions include: ■ Uterine atony: perform fundal massage and check for clots. ■ Laceration of vagina and cervix (suspect if mother is bleeding heavily in presence of firmly contracted fundus): contact physician to suture the laceration. ■ Retained placental fragments (suspect if client is bleeding, fundus is firm and no lacerations are present): thoroughly inspect placenta. ■ Subinvolution (usually occurs 1–2 weeks after birth): provide mother with discharge instructions, including information about possible complications.
32.2 Develop a nursing care plan that reflects knowledge of etiology, pathophysiology, clinical therapy, nursing and preventive management for the woman experiencing postpartum hemorrhage, reproductive tract infection, urinary tract infection, mastitis, thromboembolic disease, or a postpartal psychiatric disorder.	1. Thorough nursing history for any predisposing factors for complications: ■ Overdistention of uterus due to a large baby, multiple gestation, or multiparity. ■ Rapid or prolonged labor. ■ Oxytocin induction of labor. ■ Precipitous delivery. ■ C-section. ■ PROM. ■ Urinary catheterization.

LEARNING OUTCOMES | CONCEPTS

2. Nursing assessments of all body systems include:
   - Frequent fundal checks and massage of fundus if bogginess is detected.
   - Frequent perineal pad checks.
   - Assessment for normal changes in lochia.
   - Prevention of overdistention of the bladder.
   - Frequent vital sign assessments.
   - Assessment for Homans' sign each shift.
   - Inspection of the perineum, all incisions, breasts and nipples each shift.
   - Assessment for signs of postpartum "blues" or depression.
3. Signs and symptoms:
   - Postpartum hemorrhage: excessive vaginal bleeding.
   - Infection: fever, purulent discharge from vagina or incision, burning during urination, redness and pain in the breast about fourth postpartum week.
   - Thrombophlebitis: pain and swelling in the lower extremities.
   - Postpartum depression: feelings of overwhelming sadness and lack of desire to care for infant.
4. To prevent complications the nurse will:
   - Assess fundus for signs of bogginess.
   - Assess perineal pads for excessive bleeding.
   - Assess incisions for signs of infection.
   - Assess bladder for signs of distention and encourage woman to void frequently.
   - Use good handwashing techniques to prevent transmission of infective material.
   - Assess breasts for cracking, plugged ducts, and signs of mastitis. Teach mother proper latching-on techniques and breast care.
   - Assess lower extremities for signs of thrombophlebitis, encourage early ambulation, and assess for pulmonary embolus.
   - Assess woman for signs of depression.
   - Assess the newborn's integration into the family.

32.3 Evaluate the woman's knowledge of self-care measures, signs of complications to be reported to the primary care provider, and measures to prevent recurrence of complications.

1. Teaching for self care includes:
   - Knowledge of progress of involution.
   - Care of the breasts.
   - Prevention of infection.
   - Expected emotional changes.
   - Need for extra rest.
   - Nutritional needs.
   - Knowledge of dosage regimens and side effects of prescribed medication.
   - Signs and symptoms of complications:
     - Increased vaginal bleeding.
     - Fever.
     - Foul-smelling vaginal discharge.
     - Pain and/or redness in an incision.
     - Pain, redness, or swelling in the breasts and/or legs.
     - Overwhelming feelings of sadness or inability to care for infant.

CRITICAL THINKING IN ACTION

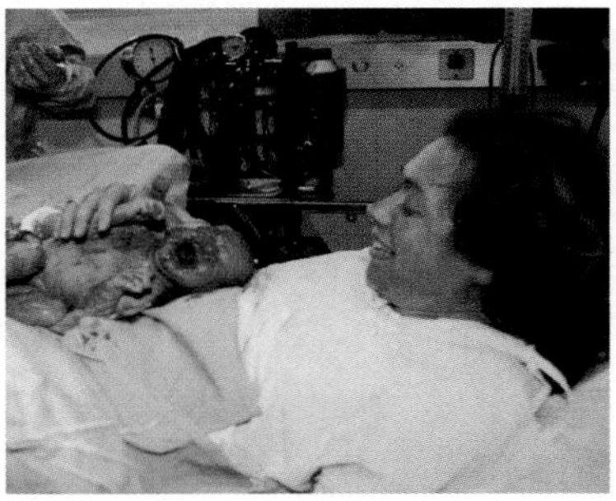

Betty Jones, a 32-year-old G4 P2012, is admitted to the postpartum unit after a precipitous birth of a preterm (35 weeks' gestation) 4-pound baby girl followed by a postpartum tubal ligation. Betty's vital signs and postpartum assessment are within normal limits. She has an abdominal dressing that is dry and intact and she is able to void. Her IV with 10 units of Pitocin is infusing well in her lower left arm. She admits to 3 on a pain scale of 10. Betty admits to active use of crack cocaine throughout her pregnancy, and smoked it most recently 5 hours before she gave birth. She is HIV positive with a CD_4 count of 726 cells/mm^3 and was treated with zidovudine during the pregnancy, labor, and birth. She also has a history of genital herpes and had been treated for chlamydia during the pregnancy. Her infant has been admitted to the special care nursery because of her preterm status. Betty anticipates her baby will be taken into foster care when discharged from the nursery. Wishing to establish as much of a relationship with her infant as possible before that happens, she asks if she can breastfeed the baby while she is in the hospital.

1. What is your response to Betty's request to breastfeed her infant?
2. Over the course of the first postpartum day, Betty appears lethargic and spends most of her time sleeping. After her evening visitors leave, you observe that she is highly energetic and excitable. Would urine testing be useful to help determine if Betty has used cocaine this evening?
3. Discuss supportive nursing care for infants born of HIV-positive mothers.
4. Betty wishes for an early discharge from the hospital. What physical criteria must be met before leaving the hospital?
5. Discuss when she should contact her physician/CNM after her discharge.

See MyNursingKit for possible responses.

REFERENCES

American Academy of Pediatrics (AAP), Committee on Fetus and Newborn, & American College of Obstetricians and Gynecolgists (ACOG), Committee on Obstetrics. (2007). *Guidelines for perinatal care* (6th ed.). Evanston, IL: Author.

American College of Obstetricians and Gynecologists. (2006). *Postpartum hemorrhage* (Practice Bulletin No. 76). Washington, DC: Author.

American Psychiatric Association (APA). (2000). *Diagnostic and statistical manual of mental disorders: DSM-IV-TR* (4th ed., text rev.). Washington, DC: Author.

Beck, C. T. (2002). Revision of the Postpartum Depression Predictors Inventory. *Journal of Obstetric, Gynecologic, and Neonatal Nursing, 31*(4), 394–402.

Beck, C. T. (2006). Postpartum depression: It isn't just the blues. *American Journal of Nursing, 106*(5), 40–51.

Beck, C. T. (2008). *Postpartum mood and anxiety disorders: Case studies, research, and nursing care.* (Practice Bulletin) (2nd ed.). Washington, DC: Association of Women's Health, Obstetric and Neonatal Nurses.

Chelmow, D., Aronson, M. P., & Wosu, U. (2007). Intraoperative and postoperative complications of gynecologic surgery. In A. H. DeCherney, L. Nathan, T. M. Goodwin, & N. Laufer (Eds.), *Current obstetric & gynecologic: Diagnosis & treatment* (10th ed., pp. 779–796). New York: Lange Medical Books/McGraw-Hill.

Cunningham, F. G., Leveno, K. J., Bloom, S. L., Haxth, J. C., Rouse, D. J., & Spong, C. Y. (2010). *Williams obstetrics* (23rd ed.). New York: McGraw-Hill.

Davies, J. K. & Gibbs, R. S. (2008). Obstetrics and perinatal infections. In R. S. Gibbs, B. Y. Karlan, A. F. Haney, & Nygaard, I. (Eds.), *Danforth's obstetrics and gynecology* (10th ed., pp. 340–364). Philadelphia: Lippincott Williams & Wilkins.

Doucet, S., Dennis, C. L., Letourneau, N. & Blackmore, E. R. (2009). Differentiation and clinical implications of postpartum depression and postpartum psychosis. *Journal of Obstetric, Gynecologic, and Neonatal Nursing, 38*(3), 269–279.

Driscoll, J. W. (2008). Psychosocial adaptation to pregnancy and postpartum. In K. R. Simpson & P. A. Creehan, *AWHONN perinatal nursing* (3rd ed., pp. 78–87). Philadelphia: Lippincott Williams & Wilkins.

Duff, P., Sweet, R. L., & Edwards, R. K. (2009). Maternal and fetal infectious disorders. In R. K. Creasy & R. Resnik (Eds.), *Maternal-fetal medicine: Principles and practice* (6th ed., pp. 739–795). Philadelphia: Saunders.

Gilbert, E. S. (2007). *Manual of high risk pregnancy and delivery* (4th ed.). St. Louis: Mosby.

Goodman, J. H. (2004). Paternal postpartum depression, its relationship to maternal postpartum depression, and implications for family health. *Journal of Advanced Nursing, 45*(1), 26–35.

Haessler, A., & Rosenthal, M. B. (2007). Psychological aspects of obstetrics & gynecology. In A. H. DeCherney, L. Nathan, T. M. Goodwin, & N. Laufer (Eds.), *Current obstetric & gynecologic: Diagnosis & treatment* (10th ed., pp. 1003–1024). New York: Lange Medical Books/McGraw-Hill.

Hofmeyr, G., Abdel-Aleem, H., & Abdel-Aleen, M. (2008) Uterine massage for preventing postpartum hemorrhage. *Cochrane Database of Systematic Reviews.* Issue 3, Art. No.: CD006431.

James, D. C. (2008). Postpartum care. In K. R. Simpson & P. A. Creehan, *AWHONN perinatal nursing* (3rd ed., pp. 473–526). Philadelphia: Lippincott Williams & Wilkins.

Katz, V. L. (2007). Postpartum care. In S. G. Gabbe, J. R. Niebyl, & J. L. Simpson (Eds.), *Obstetrics: Normal and problem pregnancies* (5th ed., pp. 566–585). Philadelphia: Churchill Livingston/Elsevier.

Krakow, D. (2008). Medical and surgical complications of pregnancy. In R. S. Gibbs, B. Y. Karlan, A. F. Haney, & Nygaard, I. (Eds.), *Danforth's obstetrics and gynecology* (10th ed., pp. 276–312). Philadelphia: Lippincott Williams & Wilkins.

Lawrence, R. M., & Lawrence, R. A. (2009). The breast and the physiology of lactation. In R. K. Creasy & R. Resnik (Eds.), *Maternal-fetal medicine: Principles and practice* (6th ed., pp. 125–142). Philadelphia: Saunders.

Lockwood, C. J. (2009). Thromboembolic disease in pregnancy. In R. K. Creasy & R. Resnik (Eds.), *Maternal-fetal medicine: Principles and practice* (6th ed., pp. 853–867). Philadelphia: Saunders.

Mass, S. (2004). Breast pain: Engorgement, nipple pain and mastitis. *Clinical Obstetrics and Gynecology, 47*(3), 676–682.

Newton, E. R. (2007). Breastfeeding. In S. G. Gabbe, J. R. Niebyl, & J. L. Simpson (Eds.), *Obstetrics: Normal and problem pregnancies* (5th ed., pp. 586–615). Philadelphia: Churchill Livingston/Elsevier.

Pettker, C. M., & Lockwood, C. J. (2007). Thromboembolic disorders. In S. G. Gabbe, J. R. Niebyl, & J. L. Simpson (Eds.), *Obstetrics: Normal and problem pregnancies* (5th ed., pp. 1064–1080). Philadelphia: Churchill Livingstone/Elsevier.

Poggi, S. B. H. (2007). Postpartum hemorrhage & the abnormal puerperium. In A. H. DeCherney, L. Nathan, T. M. Goodwin, & N. Laufer (Eds.), *Current obstetric & gynecologic: Diagnosis & treatment* (10th ed., pp. 477–497). New York: Lange Medical Books/McGraw-Hill.

Rebarker, A., & Roman, A. S. (2003, March). Seven ways to control postpartum hemorrhage. *Contemporary OB/GYN, 48*(3), 34–53.

Reid, G., & Bocking, A. (2003). The potential for probiotics to prevent bacterial vaginosis and preterm labor. *American Journal of Obstetrics & Gynecology, 189*(4), 1202–1208.

Sealy, P. A., Fraser, J., Simpson, J. P., Evans, M., & Hartford, A. (2009). Community awareness of postpartum depression. *Journal of Obstetric, Gynecologic, and Neonatal Nursing, 38*(2), 121–133.

Yip, S. K., Shota, D., Pang, M. W., & Day, L. (2005). Postpartum urinary retention. *Obstetrics and Gynecology, 106*(3), 602–606.

EXPLORE PEARSON **mynursingkit**™

MyNursingKit is your one stop for online chapter review materials and resources. Prepare for success with additional NCLEX®-style practice questions, interactive assignments and activities, web links, animations and videos, and more!

Register your access code from the front of your book at **www.mynursingkit.com**

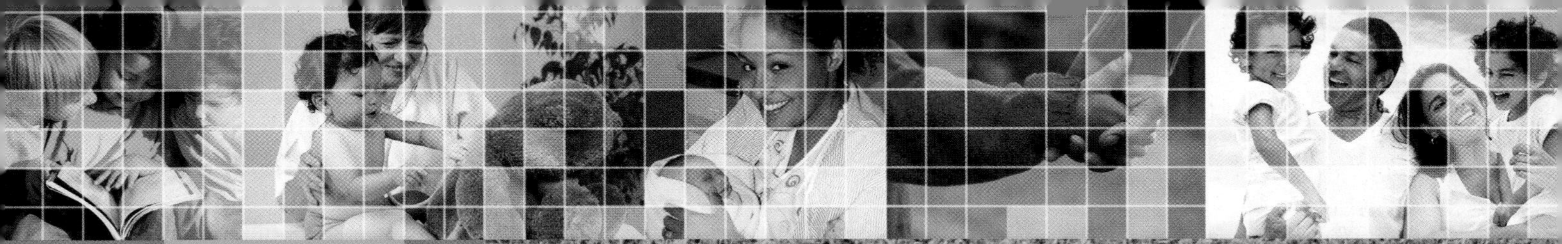

PART

6

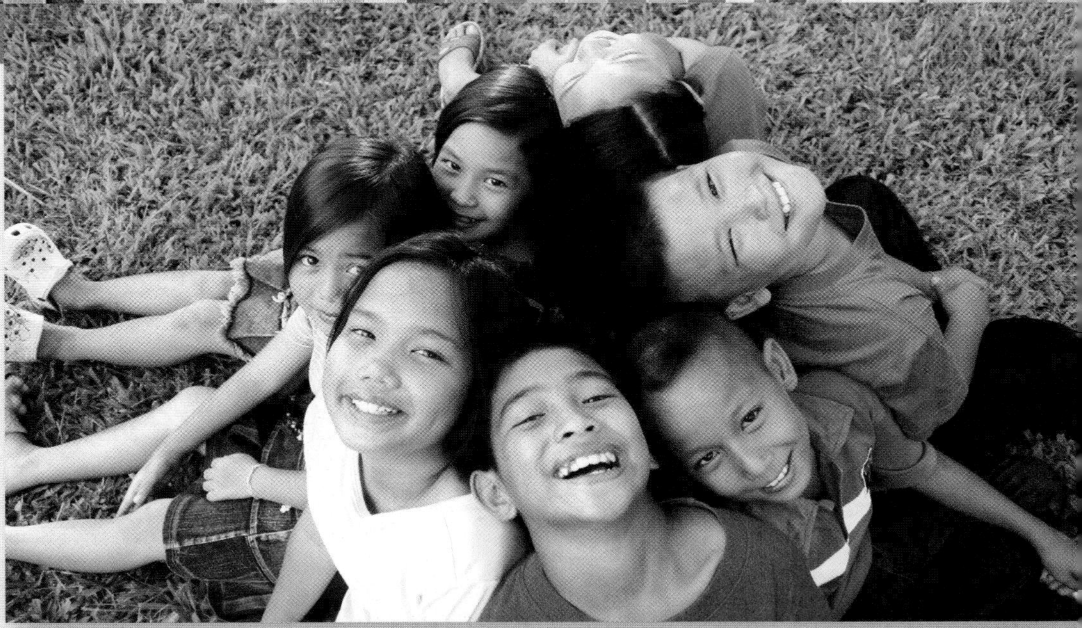

Care and Needs of Children

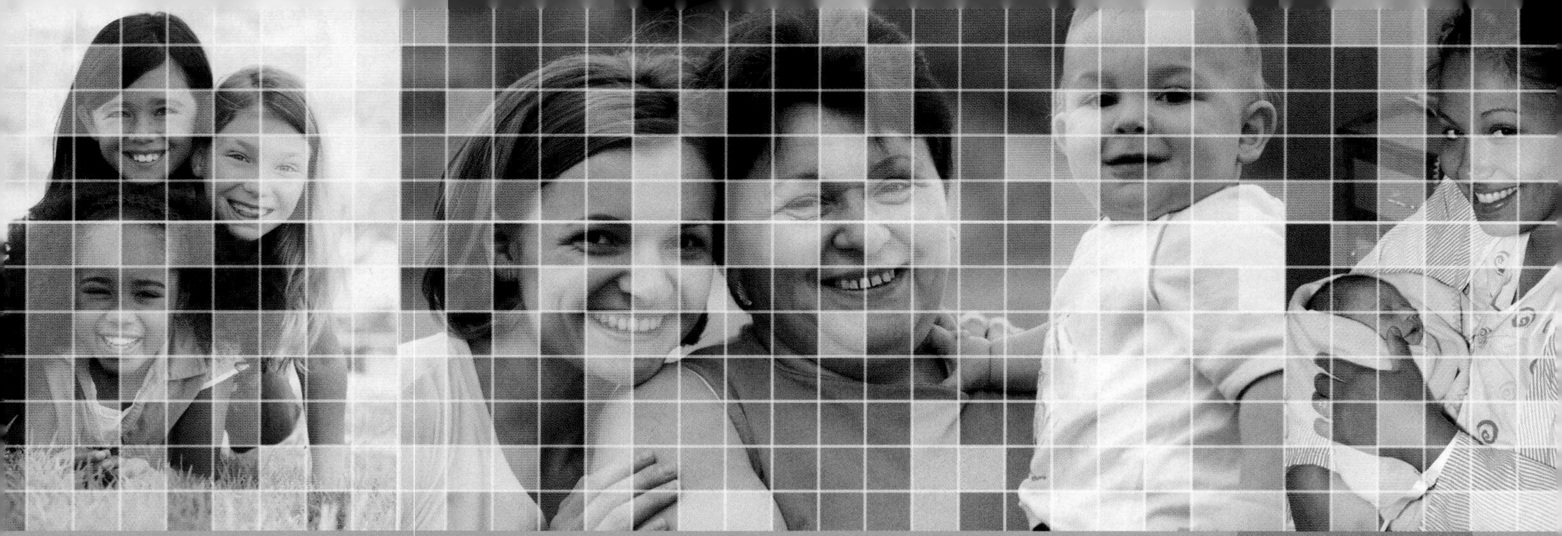

CHAPTER

Growth and Development 33

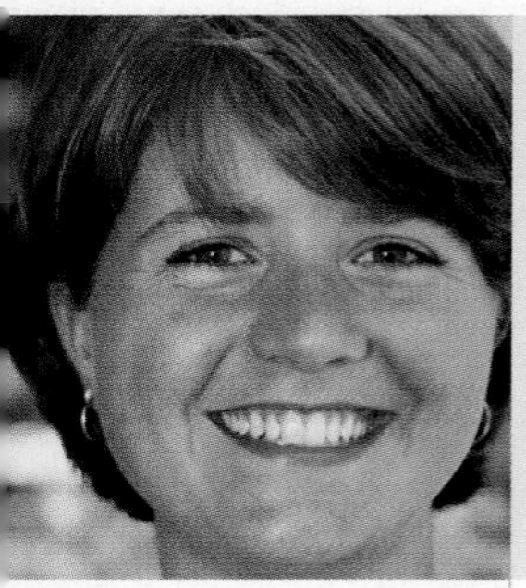

We want to help our adopted daughter Irena grow into a normal and special child. She had challenges in her short life in Romania that we can only imagine. We worry about how we can help her grow and develop. —Mother of Irena, 2

LEARNING OUTCOMES

33.1 Describe major theories of development as formulated by Freud, Erikson, Piaget, Kohlberg, social learning theorists, and behaviorists.

33.2 Recognize risks to developmental progression and factors that protect against those risks.

33.3 Plan nursing interventions for children that are appropriate for the child's developmental state, based on theoretical frameworks.

33.4 Explain contemporary developmental approaches such as temperament theory, ecologic theory, and the resilience framework.

33.5 Recognize major developmental milestones for infants, toddlers, preschoolers, school-age children, and adolescents.

33.6 Synthesize information from several theoretical approaches to plan assessments of the child's physical growth and developmental milestones.

33.7 Describe the role of play in the growth and development of children.

33.8 Use data collected during developmental assessments to implement activities that promote development of children and adolescents.

Children develop as they interact with their surroundings. They learn skills at different ages, but the order in which they learn them is universal. Development is affected by factors such as nutrition and cultural practices, as well as the social situation in the country or neighborhood. While each child will develop in a unique manner influenced by genetic makeup, life experiences, and the interactions among these factors, certain principles of development assist parents and the nurse in fostering positive adaptations for the child.

This chapter covers general principles of growth and development and explores several theories related to childhood development, as well as their nursing applications. Each age group, from infancy through adolescence, is described in detail. Developmental milestones, physical and cognitive characteristics, play patterns, and communication strategies are presented, as are conditions that interfere with usual developmental progression. The information provided helps guide developmentally appropriate care for children in each age group and in a variety of situations. These concepts can be applied when caring for all children, including those in special situations.

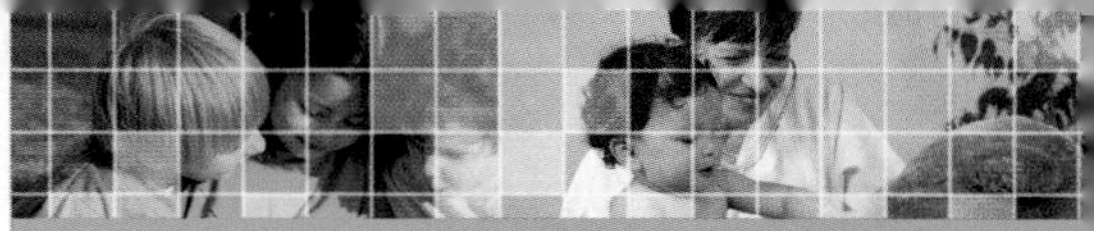

KEY TERMS

accommodation, 862
adaptation phase, 871
adjustment phase, 871
anticipatory guidance, 860
assimilation, 862
associative play, 883
cephalocaudal development, 859
conservation, 886
cooperative play, 887
defense mechanisms, 860
development, 859
dramatic play, 884
ecologic theory, 867
expressive jargon, 881
growth, 859
nature, 867
nurture, 867
object permanence, 865
parallel play, 879
protective factors, 870
proximodistal development, 859
puberty, 888
resilience, 870
risk factors, 870
solitary play, 877

PRINCIPLES OF GROWTH AND DEVELOPMENT

It is essential to understand the concepts of growth and development when learning to care for children. A skilled pediatric nurse integrates knowledge of physical growth and psychosocial development into each child healthcare encounter. **Growth** refers to an increase in physical size. Growth represents quantitative changes such as height, weight, blood pressure, and number of words in the child's vocabulary. **Development** refers to a qualitative increase in capability or function. Developmental skills, such as the ability to sit without support or to throw a ball overhand, unfold in a complex manner influenced by the relationship between the child's innate capabilities and the stimuli and support provided in the environment. The quantitative and qualitative changes in body organ functioning, ability to communicate, and performance of motor skills develop over time and are key components in the process of planning pediatric health care.

Each child displays a unique maturational pattern during the process of development. Although the exact age at which skills emerge differs, the sequence or order of skill performance is uniform among children. Skill development proceeds according to two processes: from the head downward; and from the center of the body outward.

- **Cephalocaudal development** (Figure 33–1 ●) proceeds from the head downward through the body and toward the feet. For example, at birth an infant's head is much larger proportionately than the trunk or extremities. Similarly, infants learn to hold up their heads before sitting and to sit before standing. Skills such as walking that involve the legs and feet develop last in infancy.
- **Proximodistal development** (see Figure 33–1) proceeds from the center of the body outward toward the extremities. For example, infants are first able to control the trunk, then the arms; only later are fine motor movements of the fingers possible. As the child grows, both physical and cognitive skills differentiate from general to more specific skills. Pediatric nurses use these concepts of predictable and sequential developmental direction to analyze the infant's and child's present state and to partner with parents to plan ways to encourage and support the next emerging developmental abilities.

During the childhood years, extraordinary changes occur in all aspects of development. Physical size, motor skills, cognitive ability, language, sensory ability, and psychosocial patterns all undergo major transformations. Nurses study normal patterns of development to identify children who demonstrate unexpected developmental findings. These assessments can guide the nurse in planning interventions for the child and family, such as referring the child for a diagnostic evaluation or rehabilitation, or

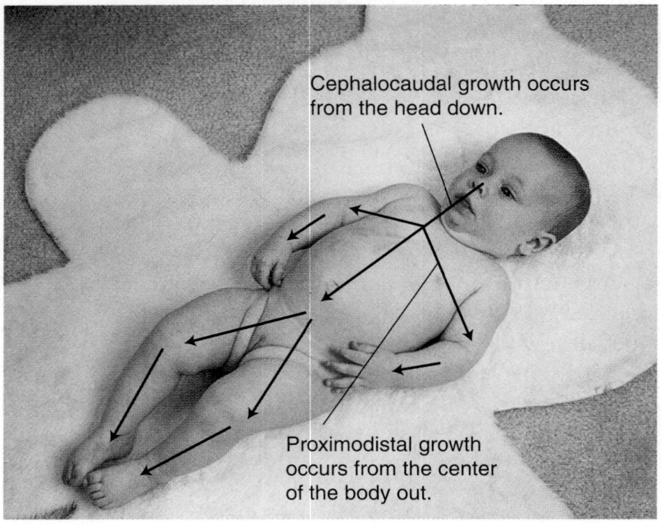

● **Figure 33–1** Cephalocaudal and proximodistal development. In normal cephalocaudal growth, the child gains control of the head and neck before the trunk and limbs. In normal proximodistal growth, the child controls arm movements before hand movements. For example, the child reaches for objects before being able to grasp them. Children gain control of their hands before their fingers; that is, they can hold things with the entire hand before they can pick something up with just their fingers.

teaching the parents how to provide adequate stimulation for the child. Nurses use **anticipatory guidance** to predict upcoming developmental tasks or needs of a child and to perform appropriate teaching related to them. When development is proceeding normally, the nurse uses his or her knowledge of these normal patterns to provide approaches based on the child's cognitive and language ability, to offer appropriate toys and activities during illness, and to respond therapeutically during interactions with the child. For situations with special challenges, such as in adoptions, additional interventions may be needed (see "Growth and Development").

Growth and Development

About 15% of annual adoptions in the United States, or 20,000, are international adoptions (Johnson, 2005). China, South Korea, Russia, Guatemala, and Ukraine are presently the most frequent countries of origin for orphans being adopted in the United States. While all adoptions can be stressful for the new parents and child, international adoptions pose a unique set of circumstances that influence the child's development.

Parents need to protect themselves and others from infectious diseases when traveling to bring home a child from another country. They should consult their local health district and healthcare providers for a list of recommended immunizations for the country they are visiting. They should also obtain a list of medications and supplies to carry for themselves and the child, such as antidiarrheal medicine, decongestants, analgesics, bandages, hand sanitizer (Barnett & Chen, 2005).

Parents require counseling to learn about cultural practices, language, and other differences they may encounter. Once they bring the child home, they will need support as the child grows to integrate the child's history and culture into their family. The moment when the child meets an adoptive parent may be seen as joyous by the parent but can be traumatic for the young child, who is separated from familiar adults. Parents need preparation for establishing trust with the child (Nickman, Rosenfeld, Fine, et al., 2005). Several agencies offer information to prepare new parents for their adoption experience (see MyNursingKit).

The adopted child should be examined once home for length, weight, and head circumference. If growth is delayed, continued monitoring and dietary interventions may be needed. The psychosocially based problem of eating disorder of infancy and childhood (also called failure to thrive) should also be considered. (See Chapter 34 ∞ for a thorough discussion of this condition.) Parasitic infection and chronic diseases are possible causes of continuing growth abnormalities. Perform developmental screening to provide a baseline for future developmental observations. Frequent physical and psychosocial assessments will be needed, and teaching is provided for parents to enhance development.

MAJOR THEORIES OF DEVELOPMENT

Child development is a complex process. Many theorists have attempted to organize their observations of behavior into a description of principles or a set of stages. Each theory focuses on a particular facet of development. Most developmental theorists separate children into age groups by common characteristics (Table 33–1).

FREUD'S THEORY OF PSYCHOSEXUAL DEVELOPMENT

Theoretical Framework

Sigmund Freud (1856–1939) was a physician in Vienna, Austria. His work with adults experiencing a variety of neurological disorders led him to develop the approach called psychoanalysis, which explored the driving forces of the unconscious mind. These psychoanalytic techniques led Freud to believe that early childhood experiences form the unconscious motivation for actions in later life. He believed that sexual energy is centered in specific parts of the body at certain ages. Unresolved conflict and unmet needs at a certain stage lead to a fixation of development at that stage (Craig & Dunn, 2007).

Freud viewed the personality as a structure with three parts: The *id* is the basic sexual energy that is present at birth and drives the individual to seek pleasure; the *ego* is the realistic part of the person, which develops during infancy and searches for acceptable methods of meeting impulses; and the *superego* is the moral/ethical system, which develops in childhood and contains a set of values and a conscience (Craig & Dunn, 2007). The ego diverts impulses and protects itself from excess anxiety by use of **defense mechanisms**, including regression to earlier stages and repression or forgetting of painful experiences such as child abuse (Table 33–2).

Table 33–1 Developmental Age Groups

Developmental Stage	Age Group	Characteristics
Infancy	Birth to 12 months	Includes infants or babies up to 1 year of age, all of whom require a high level of care in daily activities.
Toddlerhood	1–2 years	Characterized by increased motor ability and independent behavior.
Preschool	3–5 years	The preschooler refines gross and fine motor ability and language skills and often participates in a preschool learning program.
School age	6–12 years	Begins with entry into a school system and is characterized by growing intellectual skills, physical ability, and independence.
Adolescence	13–18 years	Begins with entry into the teen years. Mature cognitive thought, formation of identity, and influence of peers are important characteristics of adolescence.

Thinking Critically

INTERNATIONAL ADOPTION COUNSELING

Michael and Alyssa had tried for several years to have a biologic child. After an unsuccessful in vitro fertilization, they decided to try to adopt a child. They explored opportunities with adoption agencies and learned that international adoption would be possible for them. They adopted 2-year-old Irena from Romania several months ago. Irena appears small for her age, but she appears to be thriving in her new environment. She is learning to say a few English words and is responding appropriately to care and interactions.

Despite thorough investigation of Michael and Alyssa by the adoption agency, they received only scant information about Irena's history. They were told that she was left at an orphanage by her birth mother when she was about 7 months old; the birth mother stated that the pregnancy and birth were normal. According to reports, the birth mother had decided to relinquish the child because she had two older children to care for and her husband had left home nearly a year before and had not been heard from since.

How can you work with Michael and Alyssa to ensure special attention to Irena's growth and healthcare needs? Consider performing developmental screening and comparing her results with those expected at her age (see Chapter 37 ∞). What challenges in her early life may have influenced Irena's physical growth, her ability to interact with others, the timing of developmental milestones, and speech?

What will Irena's cultural needs be as she grows older? How can Michael and Alyssa prepare to tell her about her adoption and background someday? How can they learn about Irena's country of origin?

See MyNursingKit for possible responses.

Table 33–2 Common Defense Mechanisms Used by Children

Defense Mechanism	Definition	Example
Regression	Return to an earlier behavior	A previously toilet trained child becomes incontinent when a new infant is born into the family.
Repression	Involuntary forgetting of uncomfortable situations	An abused child cannot consciously recall episodes of abuse.
Rationalization	An attempt to make unacceptable feelings acceptable	A child explains hitting another because "he took my toy."
Fantasy	A creation of the mind to help deal with unacceptable fear	A hospitalized child who is weak pretends to be Superman.

STAGES

Oral (Birth to 1 Year). The infant derives pleasure largely from the mouth, with sucking and eating as primary desires.

Anal (1 to 3 Years). The young child's pleasure is centered in the anal area, with control over body secretions as a prime force in behavior.

Phallic (3 to 6 Years). Sexual energy becomes centered in the genitalia as the child works out relationships with parents of the same and opposite sexes.

Latency (6 to 12 Years). Sexual energy is at rest in the passage between earlier stages and adolescence.

Genital (12 Years to Adulthood). Mature sexuality is achieved as physical growth is completed and relationships with others occur.

Nursing Application

Freud emphasized the importance of meeting the needs of each stage in order to move successfully into future developmental stages. The crisis of illness can interfere with normal developmental processes and add challenges for the nurse striving to meet an ill child's needs. For example, the importance of sucking in infancy guides the nurse to provide a pacifier for the infant who cannot have oral fluids. The preschool child's concern about sexuality guides the nurse to provide privacy and clear explanations during any procedures involving the genital area. It may be necessary to teach parents that masturbation by the young child is normal and to help parents deal with it through distraction or refocusing. The adolescent's focus on relationships suggests that the nurse should include questions about significant friends during history taking. Table 33–3 summarizes techniques the nurse can use to apply these theoretical concepts to the care of children.

ERIKSON'S THEORY OF PSYCHOSOCIAL DEVELOPMENT

Theoretical Framework

Erik Erikson (1902–1994) studied Freud's theory of psychoanalysis under Freud's daughter, Anna. He later established his own developmental theory, which describes psychosocial stages during eight periods of human life. For each stage, Erikson identified a crisis, that is, a particular challenge that exists for healthy personality development to occur (Erikson, 1963, 1968). The word "crisis" in this context refers to normal maturational social needs rather than to a single critical event. Each developmental crisis has two possible outcomes. When needs are met, the consequence is healthy and the individual moves on to future stages with particular strengths. When needs are not met, an unhealthy outcome occurs that will influence future social relationships.

STAGES

Trust versus Mistrust (Birth to 1 Year). The task of the first year of life is to establish trust in the people providing care. Trust is fostered by provision of food, clean clothing, touch, and comfort. If basic needs are not met, the infant will eventually learn to mistrust others.

Autonomy versus Shame and Doubt (1 to 3 Years). The toddler's sense of autonomy or independence is shown by controlling body excretions, saying no when asked to do something, and directing motor activity and play. Children who are consistently criticized for expressions of autonomy or for lack of control—for example, during toilet training—will develop a sense of shame about themselves and doubt in their abilities.

Initiative versus Guilt (3 to 6 Years). The young child initiates new activities and considers new ideas. This interest in exploring the world creates a child who is involved and busy. Constant criticism, on the other hand, leads to feelings of guilt and a lack of purpose.

Industry versus Inferiority (6 to 12 Years). The middle years of childhood are characterized by development of new interests and by involvement in activities. The child takes pride in accomplishments in sports, school, home, and community. If the child cannot accomplish what is expected, however, the result will be a sense of inferiority.

Identity versus Role Confusion (12 to 18 Years). In adolescence, as the body matures and thought processes become more complex, a new sense of identity or self is established. The self, family, peer group, and community are all examined and redefined. The adolescent who is unable to establish a meaningful definition of self will experience confusion in one or more roles of life.

Nursing Application

Erikson's theory is directly applicable to the nursing care of children. Health promotion and health maintenance visits in the community provide opportunities for helping caregivers meet children's needs. Parents benefit from learning what the child's developmental tasks are at each stage and from discussing ideas about how to encourage healthy psychosocial development. Such discussions also may highlight parental concerns and provide a forum for reassurance about normal developmental characteristics, such as a child who does not follow through on each activity as a preschooler or tries different hairstyles each month as an adolescent. The child's usual support from family, peers, and others is interrupted by hospitalization. The challenge of hospitalization also adds a situational crisis to the normal developmental crisis a child is experiencing. Although the nurse may meet many of the hospitalized child's needs, continued parental involvement is necessary both during and after hospitalization to ensure progression through expected developmental stages (see Table 33–3).

PIAGET'S THEORY OF COGNITIVE DEVELOPMENT

Theoretical Framework

Jean Piaget (1896–1980) was a Swiss scientist who wrote detailed observations of the behavior of his own and other children. Based on these observations, Piaget formulated a theory of cognitive (or intellectual) development. He believed that the child's view of the world is influenced largely by age and maturational ability. Given nurturing experiences, the child's ability to think matures naturally (Ginsberg & Opper, 1988; Piaget, 1972; Zirkle, 2005). The child incorporates new experiences via **assimilation** and changes to deal with these experiences by the process of **accommodation**. An example of assimilation occurs when the infant uses reflexes to suck on objects that touch the lips. With more experience the infant accommodates to learn that not all objects are pleasant to suck and cognitive structures change to integrate and learn from the experiences.

Table 33–3 Nursing Applications of Theories of Freud, Erikson, and Piaget

Age Group	Theorist/Developmental Stage	Characteristics of Stage	Nursing Applications
Infant (birth to 1 year)	Freud: Oral stage.	The baby obtains pleasure and comfort through the mouth.	When a baby is not able to take foods or fluids, offer a pacifier if not contraindicated. After painful procedures, offer a baby a bottle or pacifier or have the mother breastfeed.
	Erikson: Trust versus mistrust stage.	The baby establishes a sense of trust when basic needs are met.	Hold the hospitalized baby often. (***A***) Offer comfort after painful procedures. Meet the baby's needs for food and hygiene.
			Encourage parents to room in.
			Manage pain effectively with use of pain medications and other measures.
	Piaget: Sensorimotor stage.	The baby learns from movement and sensory input.	Use crib mobiles, manipulative toys, wall murals, and bright colors to provide interesting stimuli and comfort.
			Use toys to distract the baby during procedures and assessments.
Toddler (1–3 years)	Freud: Anal stage.	The child derives gratification from control over body excretions.	Ask about toilet training and the child's rituals and words for elimination during admission history.
			Continue child's normal patterns of elimination in the hospital.
			Do not begin toilet training during illness or hospitalization.
			Accept regression in toileting during illness or hospitalization.
			Have potty chairs available in hospital and childcare centers.
	Erikson: Autonomy versus shame and doubt stage.	The child is increasingly independent in many spheres of life.	Allow self-feeding opportunities.
			Encourage child to remove and put on own clothes, brush teeth, or assist with hygiene. (***B***)
			If immobilization for a procedure is necessary, proceed quickly, providing explanations and comfort.
	Piaget: Sensorimotor stage (end); preoperational stage (beginning).	The child shows increasing curiosity and explorative behavior. Language skills improve.	Ensure safe surroundings to allow opportunities to manipulate objects.
			Name objects and give simple explanations.
Preschooler (3–6 years)	Freud: Phallic stage.	The child initially identifies with the parent of the opposite sex but by the end of this stage identifies with the same-sex parent.	Be alert for children who appear more comfortable with male or female nurses, and attempt to accommodate them.
			Encourage parental involvement in care.
			Plan for playtime and offer a variety of materials from which to choose.
	Erikson: Initiative versus guilt stage.	The child likes to initiate play activities.	Offer medical equipment for play to lessen anxiety about strange objects. (***C***)
			Assess children's concerns as expressed through their drawings.
			Accept the child's choices and expressions of feelings.

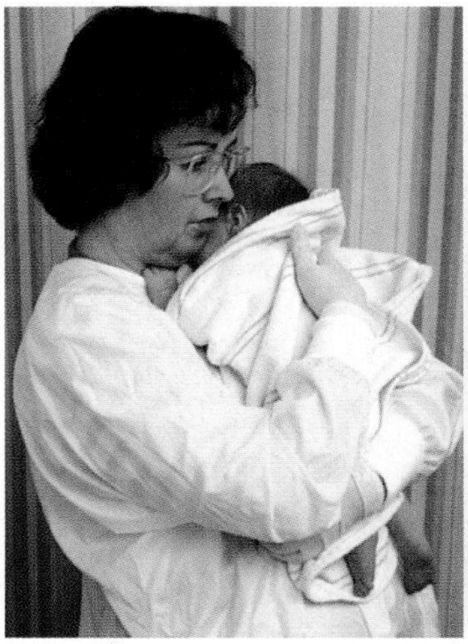

A

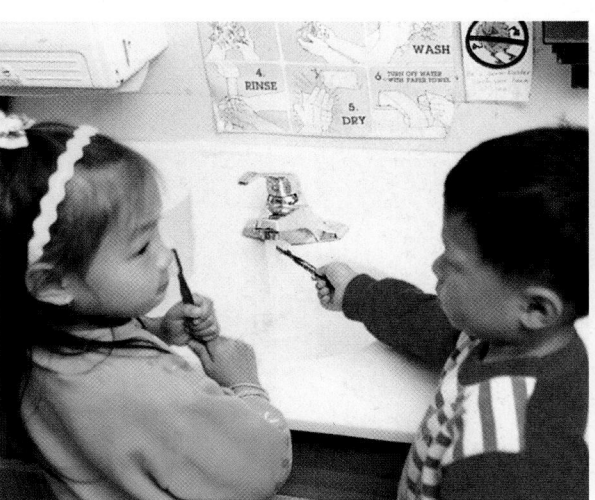

B

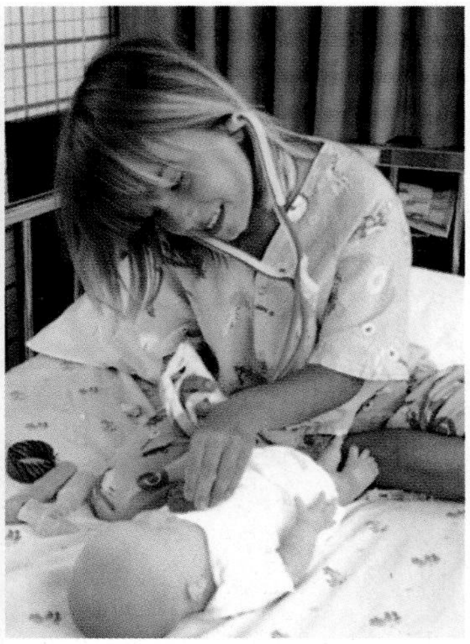

C

(continued)

Table 33–3 Nursing Applications of Theories of Freud, Erikson, and Piaget—continued

Age Group	Theorist/Developmental Stage	Characteristics of Stage	Nursing Applications
Preschooler (3–6 years)—*continued*	Piaget: Preoperational stage.	The child is increasingly verbal but has some limitations in thought processes. Causality is often confused, so the child may feel responsible for causing an illness.	Offer explanations about all procedures and treatments. Clearly explain that the child is not responsible for causing an illness in self or family member.
School age (6–12 years)	Freud: Latency stage.	The child places importance on privacy and understanding the body.	Provide gowns, covers, and underwear.
			Knock on door before entering.
			Explain treatments and procedures.
	Erikson: Industry versus inferiority stage.	The child gains a sense of self-worth from involvement in activities.	Encourage the child to continue school work while hospitalized.
			Encourage child to bring favorite pastimes to the hospital. (***D***)
			Help child adjust to limitations on favorite activities.
	Piaget: Concrete operational stage.	The child is capable of mature thought when allowed to manipulate and see objects.	Give clear instructions about details of treatment.
			Show the child equipment that will be used in treatment.
Adolescent (12–18 years)	Freud: Genital stage.	The adolescent's focus is on genital function and relationships.	Ensure access to gynecologic care for adolescent females and testicular examinations for adolescent males.
			Provide information on sexuality.
			Ensure privacy during healthcare.
			Have brochures and videos available for teaching about sexuality.
	Erikson: Identity versus role confusion stage.	The adolescent's search for self-identity leads to independence from parents and reliance on peers.	Provide a separate recreation room for teens who are hospitalized. (***E***)
			Take health history and perform examinations without parents present.
			Introduce adolescent to other teens with same health problem.
	Piaget: Formal operational stage.	The adolescent is capable of mature, abstract thought.	Give clear and complete information about healthcare and treatments.
			Offer both written and verbal instructions.
			Continue to provide education about the disease to the adolescent with a chronic illness, as mature thought now leads to greater understanding.

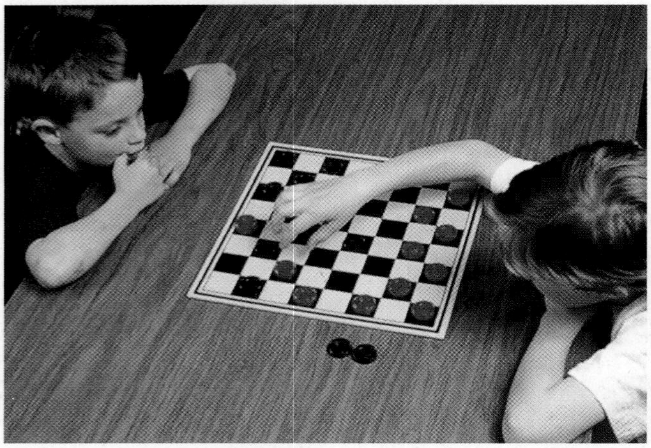

D

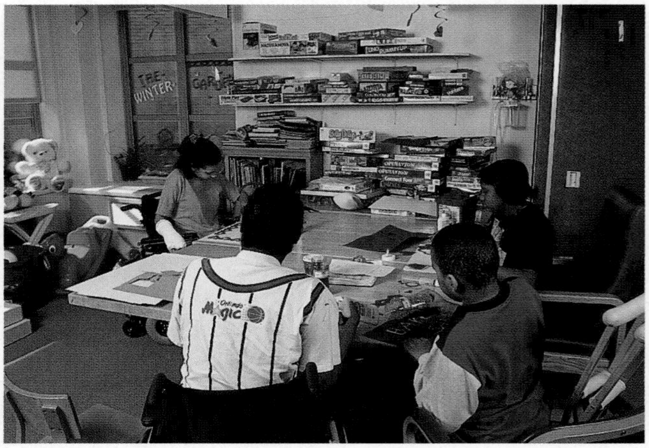

E

STAGES

Sensorimotor (Birth to 2 Years). Infants learn about the world by input obtained through the senses and by their motor activity. Six substages are characteristic of this stage.

Use of Reflexes (Birth to 1 Month). The infant begins life with a set of reflexes such as sucking, rooting, and grasping. By using these reflexes, the infant receives stimulation via touch, sound, smell, and vision. The reflexes thus pave the way for the first learning to occur.

Primary Circular Reactions (1 to 4 Months). Once the infant responds reflexively, the pleasure gained from that response causes repetition of the behavior. For example, if a toy grasped reflexively makes noise and is interesting to look at, the infant will grasp it again.

Secondary Circular Reactions (4 to 8 Months). Awareness of the environment grows as the infant begins to connect cause and effect. The sounds of bottle preparation will lead to excited behavior. If an object is partially hidden, the infant will attempt to uncover and retrieve it.

Coordination of Secondary Schemes (8 to 12 Months). Intentional behavior is observed as the infant uses learned behavior to obtain objects, create sounds, or engage in other pleasurable activity. **Object permanence** (the knowledge that something continues to exist even when out of sight) begins when the infant remembers where a hidden object is likely to be found; it is no longer "out of sight, out of mind." The concept of object permanence is not fully developed, however. The infant knows the parent well, objects to new people, and seems very worried when the parent leaves. Other caretakers may be rejected as the infant does not understand that the parent will return. This phase of "stranger anxiety" is quite common and heralds the infant's growing recognition of and desire to be cared for by the parent.

Tertiary Circular Reactions (12 to 18 Months). Curiosity, experimentation, and exploration predominate as the toddler tries out actions to learn results. The child turns objects in every direction, places them in the mouth, uses them for banging, and inserts them in containers as he or she explores their qualities and uses.

Mental Combinations (18 to 24 Months). Language provides a new tool for the toddler to use in understanding the world. Language enables the child to think about events and objects before or after they occur. Object permanence is now fully developed as the child actively searches for objects in various locations and out of view. The child who has had successful separations from the parents followed by return, such as hours spent in another's home or childcare center, begins to understand that the missing parent will return.

Preoperational (2 to 7 Years). The young child thinks by using words as symbols, but logic is not well developed.

- During the preconceptual substage (2 to 4 years), vocabulary and comprehension increase greatly but the child is egocentric (that is, unable to see things from the perspective of another).
- In the intuitive substage (4 to 7 years), the child relies on transductive reasoning (drawing conclusions from one general fact to another). For example, when a child disobeys a parent and then falls and breaks an arm that day, the child may ascribe the broken arm to bad behavior. Cause-and-effect relationships are often unrealistic or a result of magical thinking (the belief that events occur because of thoughts or wishes).

Additional characteristics noted in the thought of preschoolers include centration, or the ability to consider only one aspect of a situation at a time, and animism, or giving life to inanimate objects because they move, make noise, or have certain other qualities.

Concrete Operational (7 to 11 Years). Transductive reasoning has given way to a more accurate understanding of cause and effect. The child can reason quite well if concrete objects are used in teaching or experimentation. The concept of conservation (that matter does not change when its form is altered) is learned at this age.

Formal Operational (11 Years to Adulthood). Fully mature intellectual thought has now been attained. The adolescent can think abstractly about objects or concepts and consider different alternatives or outcomes.

Nursing Application

Piaget's theory is essential to pediatric nursing. The nurse must understand a child's thought processes in order to design stimulating activities and meaningful, appropriate teaching plans. What activities could be planned for a hospitalized child based on his or her expected cognitive level? How can cognitive development be encouraged in a school-age child receiving home health services? Understanding a child's concept of time suggests how far in advance to prepare that child for procedures. Similarly, decisions about offering manipulative toys, reading stories, drawing pictures, or giving the child reading matter to explain healthcare measures depend on the child's cognitive stage of development (see Table 33–3).

KOHLBERG'S THEORY OF MORAL DEVELOPMENT

Theoretical Framework

Lawrence Kohlberg (1927–1987) was a German theorist who used Piaget's cognitive theory as a basis for his theory of moral development. He presented stories involving moral dilemmas to children and adults and asked them to solve the dilemmas. Kohlberg then analyzed the motives they expressed when making decisions about the best course to take. Based on the explanations given, Kohlberg established three levels of moral reasoning. Although he provided age guidelines, he stated that they are approximate and that many people never reach the highest (postconventional) stage of development (Santrock, 2007).

MyNursingKit Video: Growth and Development

STAGES

Preconventional (4 to 7 Years). Decisions are based on the desire to please others and to avoid punishment.

Conventional (7 to 12 Years). Conscience or an internal set of standards becomes important. Rules are important and must be followed to please other people and "be good."

Postconventional (12 Years and Older). The individual has internalized ethical standards on which to base decisions. Social responsibility is recognized. The value in each of two differing moral approaches can be considered and a decision made.

Nursing Application

Decision making is required in many areas of health care. Children can be assisted to make decisions about health care and to consider alternatives when available. Keep in mind that young children may agree to participate in research simply because they want to comply with adults and appear cooperative. Guidelines for child participation in research are available (see Chapter 1).

Parents can be provided with information so that they can assist their children in moral judgments. Encourage talking with a child or adolescent about how a particular decision was made. Parents can then add information and help the child learn to integrate more factors into decision making. Talking about the process is important in helping children progress to higher moral development stages. Focusing on the feelings of others, using positive discipline techniques, and clearly identifying positive and negative behaviors are important.

SOCIAL LEARNING THEORY

Theoretical Framework

Originally from Canada, psychologist Albert Bandura (1925–) has conducted research at Stanford University for many years. He believes that children learn attitudes, beliefs, customs, and values through their social contacts with adults and other children. Children imitate (or model) the behavior they see; if the behavior is positively reinforced, they tend to repeat it. The external environment and the child's internal processes are key elements in social learning theory (Bandura, 1986, 1997a).

Bandura believes that an important determinant of behavior is self-efficacy, or the expectation that someone can produce a desired outcome. For example, if adolescents believe they can avoid use of drugs or alcohol, they are more likely to do so. A child who has confidence in his or her ability to exercise regularly or lose weight has a greater chance of success with these behavior changes. Parents who have confidence in their ability to care adequately for their infants are more likely to do so (Bandura, 1997b). See "Evidence-Based Nursing: Concept of Self-Sufficiency" below for further examples of application of the concept of self-efficacy.

Evidence-Based Nursing

CONCEPT OF SELF-EFFICACY

Clinical Question

How can nurses use the concept of self-efficacy when planning interventions for children and families?

Evidence

1. A federally funded study sought to measure the effectiveness of a preventive parent training program among low-income families with small children. The weekly sessions involved viewing a videotape and discussing positive and negative parenting skills observed. The researchers compared characteristics of the parents who chose to attend the sessions, including a measure of parental self-efficacy, or belief that they could manage a range of tasks and situations in caring for their young children. Parents with lower self-efficacy scores were significantly more likely to enroll in and attend the parenting training sessions (Garvey, Julion, Fogg, et al., 2006).
2. Mothers who have a greater degree of self-efficacy about ability to breast feed are significantly more likely to begin and to continue breastfeeding. A Breastfeeding Self Efficacy Scale has been developed to identify risk and protective factors that influence the self-efficacy of new mothers. Educational level, support from other women, quality of postpartum care, maternal anxiety, and plans made for feeding method all influence the breastfeeding self-efficacy scores of women (Dennis, 2006).

Best Practice

In addition to providing information about health behaviors, nurses need to integrate methods to increase self-efficacy in teaching projects with families. Assessments should be designed to identify self-efficacy of parents and children around health topics of interest. When planning interventions to encourage health behaviors in children and adolescents, assess the youth's belief that the new behaviors are important and that they can be adopted. Include interventions that demonstrate that others have adopted the health behaviors and plan approaches to enhance the child's belief in ability to change.

Critical Thinking Application

Plan a teaching project about the importance of physical activity for presentation to a group of 12-year-olds. What approaches will enhance the self-efficacy of the children? How would interventions to enhance self-efficacy differ for young elementary-school children from those in middle or high school? What theoretical approaches discussed earlier in this chapter help you to understand the cognitive abilities of children at various ages and suggest ways to influence their self-efficacy?

See MyNursingKit for possible responses.

Nursing Application

The importance of modeling behavior can readily be applied in health care. Children are more likely to cooperate if they see adults or other children performing a task willingly. A frightened child may watch another child perform vision screening or have blood drawn and then decide to allow the procedure to take place. Contact with positive role models is useful when teaching children and adolescents self-care for chronic diseases such as diabetes. Give positive reinforcement for desired performance.

Nurses can use the concept of self-efficacy to increase the chance of success with lifestyle behavior changes. For example, encouraging youth who are trying to quit smoking, providing them with role models, and pointing out parental successes with their children all demonstrate methods of fostering self-efficacy.

BEHAVIORISM

Theoretical Framework

John Watson (1878–1958) was an American scientist who applied the research of animal behaviorists like Pavlov and Skinner to children. Pavlov and, later, Skinner worked with animals, presenting a stimulus such as food and pairing it with another stimulus such as a ringing bell. Eventually the animal being fed began to salivate when the bell rang. As Skinner and then Watson began to apply these concepts to children, they showed that behaviors can be elicited by positive reinforcement, such as a food treat, or extinguished by negative reinforcement, such as scolding or withdrawal of attention. Watson believed that he could make a child into anyone he desired—from a professional to a thief or beggar—simply by reinforcing behavior in certain ways (Santrock, 2007).

Nursing Application

Behaviorism has been criticized for being simplistic and for its denial of people's inherent capacity to respond willfully to events in the environment. This theory does, however, have some use in health care. When particular behaviors are desired, healthcare providers can establish positive reinforcement to encourage these behaviors. Using behavioral techniques, nurses may influence behavior of children by giving a sticker to a child after physical examination or blood draw. Parents often use reinforcement in toilet training and other skills learned in childhood.

ECOLOGIC THEORY

Theoretical Framework

There is controversy among theorists concerning the relative importance of heredity versus environment—or nature versus nurture—in human development. **Nature** refers to the genetic or hereditary capability of an individual. **Nurture** refers to the effects of the environment on a person's performance (Figure 33–2 ●). Piaget believed in the importance of internal cognitive structures that unfold at their appointed times, given any environment that provides basic opportunities. He emphasized the strength of nature. The behaviorist John Watson, on the other hand, believed that behaviors are primarily shaped by environmental responses; he thus stressed the predominance of nurture.

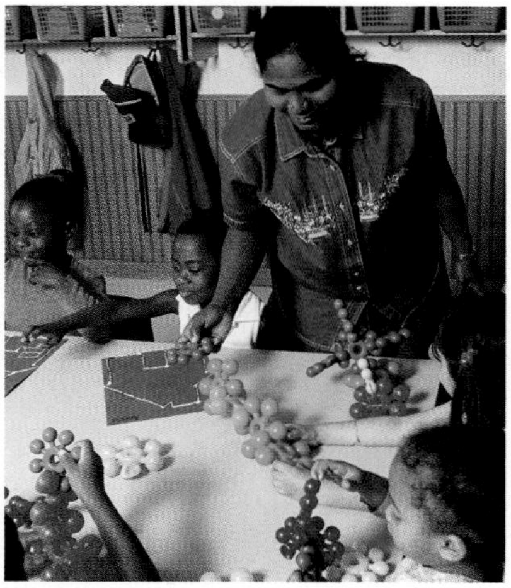

● **Figure 33–2** An example of nurturing. Children exposed to pleasant stimulation and who are supported by an adult will develop and refine their skills faster. Group activities such as these provide an opportunity for both motor skill and psychosocial development. Can you identify which skills are being developed?

Contemporary developmental theories increasingly recognize the interaction of nature and nurture in determining the child's development.

Urie Bronfenbrenner (1917–2005), a professor at Cornell University, formulated the ecologic theory of development to explain the unique relationship of the child with all of life's experiences or systems (Bronfenbrenner, 1986, 2005; Bronfenbrenner, McClelland, Ceci et al., 1996). **Ecologic theory** emphasizes the presence of mutual interactions between the child and these various settings or systems. Neither nature nor nurture is considered of more importance. Bronfenbrenner believes each child brings a unique set of genes—as well as specific attributes such as age, gender, health, and other characteristics—to his or her interactions with the environment. The child then interacts in many settings at different levels or systems (Figure 33–3 ●).

Levels/Systems

Microsystem. This level is defined as the daily, consistent, close relationships such as home, child care, school, friends, and neighbors. For the child with a chronic illness requiring regular care, the healthcare providers may even be part of the microsystem. In the ecologic model, the child influences each of the settings in the microsystem, in addition to being influenced by them, with reciprocal interactions.

Mesosystem. This level includes relationships of microsystems with one another. For example, two microsystems for most children are the home and the school. The relationships between these microsystems are shown by parents' involvement in their children's school. This involvement, in turn, influences the effects of the home and school settings on the children.

Exosystem. This level is composed of those settings that influence the child even though the child is not in close

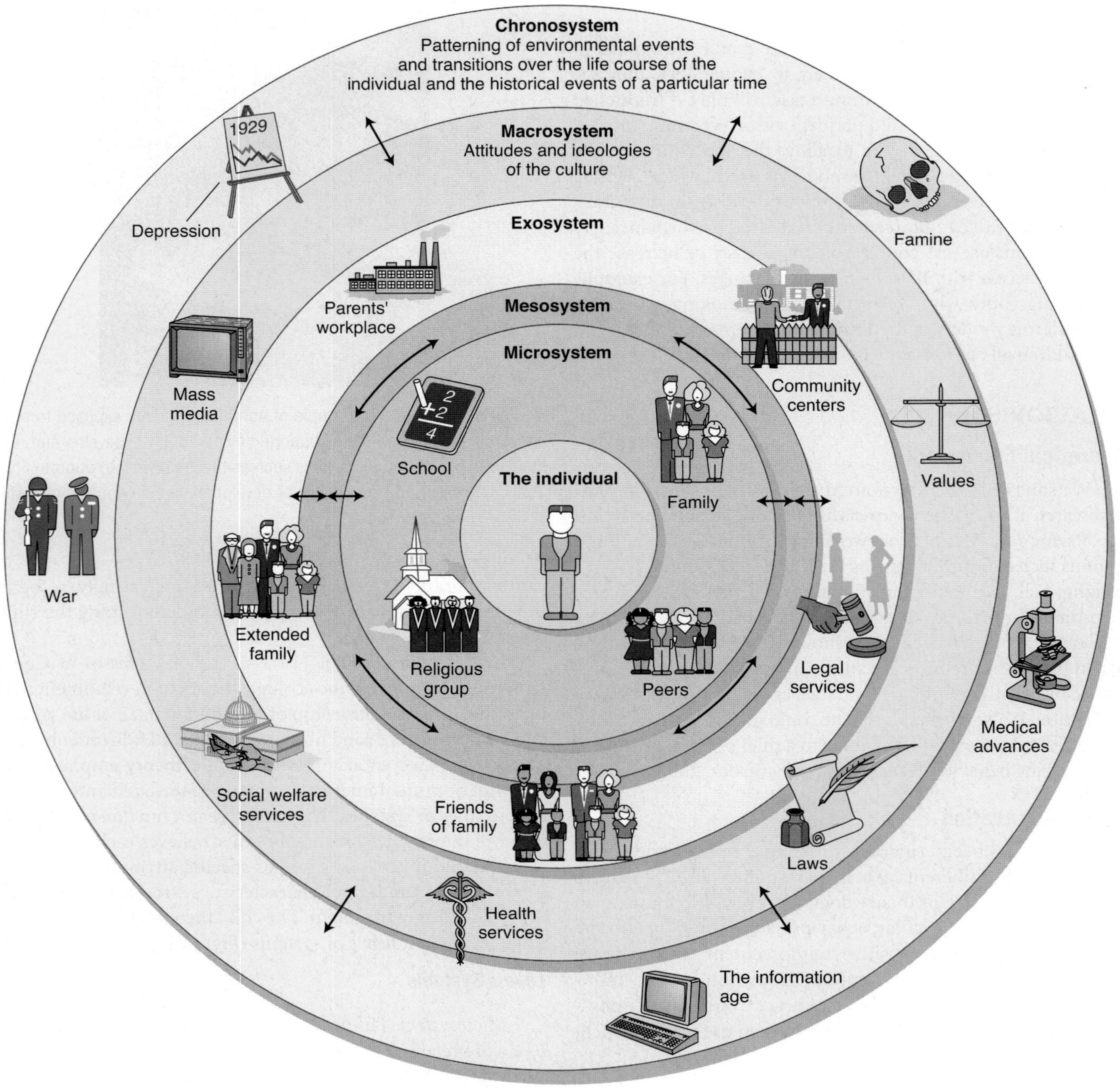

● **Figure 33–3** Ecologic theory. Bronfenbrenner's ecologic theory of development views the individual as interacting within five levels or systems.

Data from Santrock, J. W. (2007). *Life span development*. Madison, WI: Brown & Benchmark. Based on Bronfenbrenner's (1979, 1986) works in Contexts of child rearing: Problems and prospects. *American Psychologist, 34,* 844–850; Ecology of the family as a context for human development: Research perspectives. *Developmental Psychology, 22,* 723–742.

daily contact with the system. Examples include the parents' jobs and the governing board of the local school district. Although the child may not go to the parents' workplaces, he or she can be influenced by policies related to health care, sick leave, inflexible work hours, overtime, or travel, or even by the mood of the boss (through its impact on the parent). Likewise, when a local school board votes to ban certain books or to finance a field trip, the child is influenced by these decisions; the child, in turn, can help establish an atmosphere that will guide future school board decisions.

Macrosystem. This level includes the beliefs, values, and behaviors expressed in the child's environment. Culture is a powerful influence in the macrosystem, as is the political system. For instance, a democratic system creates different beliefs, values, and even eating practices than an anarchic system.

Table 33–4 Assessment of Ecologic Systems in Childhood—Bronfenbrenner

Microsystems	Mesosystems	Exosystems	Macrosystems	Chronosystems
Parents	Parents' involvement in childcare or school	Community centers	Cultural group membership	Child's and parents' ages
Significant others in close contact	Parents' involvement in community	Local political influences	Beliefs and values of group	Period in historical time
Childcare arrangements	Parents' relationships with significant others (e.g., grandparents, care providers)	Parents' work	Political structure	
School	Influences of religious community (e.g., church, synagogue, mosque) or parents and school	Parents' friends and activities		
Neighborhood contacts		Social services		
Clubs		Health care		
Friends, peers		Libraries		
Religious community (e.g., churches, synagogues, mosques)				

Chronosystem. This final level brings the perspective of time to the previous settings. The time period during which the child grows up influences views of health and illness. For example, the experiences of children with influenza in the 19th versus 20th centuries were quite different. The age of the parent, child, and other family members also influence views of health.

Nursing Application

Nurses use ecologic theory when they assess the child's settings to identify influences on development. Table 33–4 provides an assessment tool based on this theory. Interventions are planned to enhance the strengths of the child's settings and to improve on areas that are not supportive.

TEMPERAMENT THEORY

Theoretical Framework

In contrast to behaviorists such as Watson or maturational theorists such as Piaget, Stella Chess, and Alexander Thomas recognize the innate qualities of personality that each individual brings to the events of daily life. They, like Bronfenbrenner, believe the child is an individual who both influences and is influenced by the environment. However, Chess and Thomas focus on one specific aspect of development—the wide spectrum of behaviors possible in children—identifying nine parameters of response to daily events (Table 33–5). Their theory is based on a research study entitled the New York Longitudinal Study, which began with infants in 1956 and has continued

Table 33–5 Nine Parameters of Personality

Parameter	Description	Scoring
1. Activity level	The degree of motion during eating, playing, sleeping, bathing.	Scored as high, medium, or low.
2. Rhythmicity	The regularity of schedule maintained for sleep, hunger, elimination.	Scored as regular, variable, or irregular.
3. Approach or withdrawal	The response to a new stimulus such as a food, activity, or person.	Scored as approachable, variable, or withdrawn.
4. Adaptability	The degree of adaptation to new situations.	Scored as adaptive, variable, or nonadaptive.
5. Threshold of responsiveness	The intensity of stimulation needed to elicit a response to sensory input, objects in the environment, or people.	Scored as high, medium, or low.
6. Intensity of reaction	The degree of response to situations.	Scored as positive, variable, or negative.
7. Quality of mood	The predominant mood during daily activity and in response to stimuli.	Scored as positive, variable, or negative.
8. Distractibility	The ability of environmental stimuli to interfere with the child's activity.	Scored as distractible, variable, or nondistractible.
9. Attention span and persistence	The amount of time devoted to activities (compared with other children of the same age) and the degree of ability to stick with an activity in spite of obstacles.	Scored as persistent, variable, or nonpersistent.

Data from Chess, S., & Thomas, A. (1996). *Temperament: Theory and practice*. Philadelphia: Brunner/Mazel, division of Taylor & Francis.

Table 33–6 Patterns of Temperament

Pattern	Description	% of N.Y. Longitudinal Study Participants
The "easy" child	Generally moderate in activity Shows regularity in patterns of eating, sleeping, and elimination Usually positive in mood Adapts to new situations when subjected to new stimuli Able to accept rules Works well with others	Approximately 40%
The "difficult" child	Displays irregular schedules for eating, sleeping, and elimination Adapts slowly to new situations and persons Displays a predominantly negative mood Intense reactions to the environment common	Approximately 10%
The "slow-to-warm-up"	Initial withdrawal, followed by gradual, quiet, slow interaction with the environment Adapts slowly to new situations Mild reactions to environment	Approximately 15%
Mixed	Some of each personality type's characteristics apparent	Approximately 35%

Chess & Thomas, 1995.

into the adulthood of these participating individuals. By careful observations of responses to life events, Chess and Thomas identified characteristics of personality that provide the basis for the study on temperament. Infants generally display clusters of responses, which are classified into three major personality types (Table 33–6). Although most children do not demonstrate all behaviors described for a particular type, they usually show a grouping indicative of one personality type (Chess & Thomas, 1995, 1996).

Recent research demonstrates that personality characteristics displayed during infancy are often consistent with those seen later in life. Predicting future characteristics is not possible, however, because of the complex and dynamic interaction of personality traits and environmental reactions.

Many other researchers have expanded the work of Chess and Thomas, developing assessment tools for temperament types. The concept of "goodness of fit" is an outgrowth of this theory. Goodness of fit refers to whether parents' expectations of their child's behavior are consistent with the child's temperament type. There is a "good fit" when the properties of the environment are in accord with the child's capabilities, characteristics, and style of behavior (Chess & Thomas, 1999; Rettew, Stanger, McKee, et al., 2006). For example, an infant who is very active and reacts strongly to verbal stimuli may be unable to sleep well when placed in a room with older siblings. A child who is slow to warm up may not perform well in the first few months at a new school, much to the parents' disappointment. When parents understand a child's temperament characteristics, they are better able to shape the environment to meet the child's needs.

Nursing Application

The concept of personality type or temperament is a useful one for nurses. Nurses can assess the temperament of young children and alter the environment to meet their needs. This may involve moving a hospitalized child to a single room to ensure adequate rest if the child is easily stimulated, or allowing a shy child time to become accustomed to new surroundings and equipment before beginning procedures or treatments.

Parents are often relieved to learn about temperament characteristics. They learn to appreciate their children's qualities and to adapt the environment to meet the children's needs. A burden of guilt can also be lifted from parents who feel that they are responsible for their child's actions. Parents may be taught ways to enhance goodness of fit between the child's personality and the environment (Table 33–7).

RESILIENCY THEORY

Theoretical Framework

Why do some children coming from similar backgrounds have such different behavioral outcomes? The resiliency theory examines both the individual's characteristics as well as the interaction of these characteristics with the environment. **Resilience** is the ability to function with healthy responses, even when faced with significant stress and adversity (Henderson, Bernard, & Sharp-Light, 2007). In this model the individual or family members experience a crisis that provides a source of stress, and the family interprets or deals with the crisis based on resources available. Families and individuals have **protective factors**, which are characteristics that provide strength and assistance in dealing with crises, and **risk factors**, which are characteristics that promote or contribute to their

Table 33–7 Ways to Improve Goodness of Fit Between Parents and Child

Child's Behavior	Parents' Adaptations
Extremely active	Plan periods of active play several times a day. Have restful periods before bedtime to foster sleep.
Shy	Allow time to adapt at own pace to new people and situations.
Easily stimulated	Have quiet room for sleeping for an infant. Have quiet room for homework for a school-age child.
Short attention span	Provide projects that can be completed in a short period. Gradually encourage longer periods at activities.

Table 33–8 Components of Resiliency Model

Component	Meaning	Example
A = Crisis event or health challenge	Nature of healthcare challenge	Parent leaving home after domestic dispute
V = Vulnerability; risk factors	Stresses and risks related to dealing with the health challenge	Prior abandonment; financial instability; child's developmental understanding of abandonment
T = Typology	Family methods of functioning	Reliance on extended family; parent alcoholism
B = Protective factors	Strengths for dealing with challenge	Child's desire to succeed in school; positive role modeling of maternal grandparents
C = Appraisal	Family's interpretation of crisis event	Abandonment by loved one; inability to trust others
PS = Problem solving or coping techniques	Skills that help family work toward solution	Use of community resources; acceptance of school and community counselors; child's involvement in classroom activities
X = Response	Positive or negative response to tension created by the health challenge	Remaining parent using counseling available; child identifying with a teacher in school; establishment of sense of mutual interdependence among remaining family members

Data from Ahern, N. R. (2006). Adolescent resilience: An evolutionary concept analysis. *Journal of Pediatric Nursing, 21,* 175–185.

challenges (Aronowitz, 2005). Risk and protective factors can be identified in children, in their families, and in their communities (see Chapter 44 for further description of the interplay of social and environmental factors with individual characteristics). A crisis for a young child might be a transfer to a new childcare provider. Protective factors could involve past positive experiences with new people, an "easy" temperament, and the new childcare provider's awareness of adaptation needs of young children to new experiences. Risk factors for a similar child might be repeated moves to new care providers, limited close relationships with adults, and a "slow-to-warm-up" temperament.

Once confronted by a stress or crisis, the child and family first experience the **adjustment phase**, characterized by disorganization and unsuccessful attempts at meeting the crisis. In the **adaptation phase**, the child and family meet the challenge and use resources to deal with the crisis. Adaptation may lead to increasing resilience as well when the child and family learn about new resources and inner strengths and develop the ability to deal more effectively with future crises. The model and examples are described in Table 33–8.

Nursing Application

Nurses gather information about the individual characteristics, prior life experiences, and environmental factors that act as protective and risk factors for children. Table 33–9 lists questions that can be helpful as the nurse gathers information from a child or family members. Nurses then use concepts of resiliency theory in planning interventions for children and families. Nursing strategies can target risk factors, such as encouraging gun safety in families with firearms, and by teaching about use of gun trigger locks and locked gun cabinets. In addition, protective factors can be emphasized, such as encouraging holding and verbalization to parents of infants to provide an environment that meets needs for trust establishment and speech development.

Table 33–9 Assessment Questions to Determine Resilience Capability

Category	Questions
To determine risk factors, ask:	■ Describe the event that occurred and what it has been like for your family. ■ What other stressors do you have in your family right now? ■ Are there financial worries? ■ Are there things you think and worry about late at night? ■ Describe your job, your friends. ■ What is a typical day like? ■ Describe your neighborhood. ■ Do you have friends, people to call in emergencies?
To determine protective factors, ask:	■ What gives you strength? ■ How do you deal with this stress? ■ What do you think you do well in your family? ■ Who do you call when you need help? ■ Do you have a computer? Internet access? ■ Are you religious? Spiritual? ■ Do you exercise regularly? ■ How do you spend free time?

INFLUENCES ON DEVELOPMENT

Both nature and nurture are important in determining individual patterns of development. The interaction of these two forces can explain differences in time frames for acquisition of developmental skills, personality variations between identical twins, and other unique characteristics of individuals. Genetic and environmental factors interact and contribute to individual differences in rates and outcomes of child development.

Genetic inheritance plays an important part in the child's potential and the unfolding of developmental milestones. See Chapters 4 and 7 for a description of chromosomes and genes. Every chromosome carries many genes that determine physical characteristics, intellectual potential, personality type, and other traits. Children are born with the potential for certain features; however, their interaction with the environment influences how and to what extent particular traits are manifested.

Some Asian cultures calculate age from the time of conception. This practice acknowledges the profound influence of the prenatal period. The mother's nutrition and general state of health play a part in pregnancy outcome. Poor nutrition can lead to small infants and infants with compromised neurologic performance, slow development, or impaired immune status with resultant high disease rates. Low maternal stores of iron can result in anemia in the infant (American Academy of Pediatrics, 2004). Maternal smoking is associated with low-birth-weight infants. Ingestion of alcoholic beverages, including beer and wine, during pregnancy may lead to fetal alcohol syndrome (Figure 33–4 ●). Illicit drug use by the mother may result in neonatal addiction, convulsions, hyperirritability, poor social responsiveness, and other neurologic disturbances.

Even prescription or over-the-counter drugs may adversely affect the fetus. This was brought to general attention with the drug thalidomide, commonly used in Europe to treat nausea during the 1950s. This drug resulted in the birth of infants with limb abnormalities to women who used the drug during pregnancy. Differences in physiology related to gastric emptying, renal clearance, drug distribution, and other factors contribute to variations in pharmacokinetics during pregnancy. Drugs can cause teratogenesis (abnormal development of the fetus) or mutagenesis (permanent changes in the fetus' genetic material) (McCarter-Spaulding, 2005).

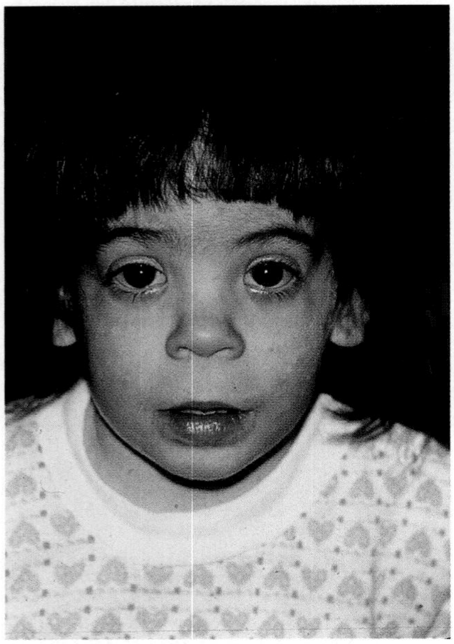

● **Figure 33–4** Fetal alcohol syndrome.

Used with permission from Dr. Sterling Clarren, Seattle, WA. Clarren, S. K., & Smith, D. W. (1978). The fetal alcohol syndrome. *New England Journal of Medicine, 298,* 1063–1067.

Table 33–10 FDA Pregnancy Categories for Drugs

Pregnancy Category	Description
A	Controlled studies with humans have not demonstrated a risk of the drug to the fetus.
B	Controlled studies with animals have not demonstrated a risk of the drug to the fetus.
C	Animal studies have found adverse effects of the drug on the fetus and there are no controlled studies with humans, or no animal or human studies are available; drug is used only if benefit justifies the potential risk.
D	There is evidence of risk to the fetus in humans; drug may be used in life-threatening situations or to treat a serious disease.
X	Animal and/or human studies have shown harm to the fetus from the drug that outweighs any potential benefit; drug is contraindicated in pregnancy.

The U.S. Food and Drug Administration (FDA) has established risk categories for drugs in pregnancy (Table 33–10).

Some maternal illnesses are harmful to the developing fetus. An example is rubella (German measles), which is rarely a serious disease for adults but which can cause deafness, vision defects, heart defects, and mental retardation in the fetus if it is acquired by a pregnant woman. A fetus can also acquire diseases such as acquired immunodeficiency syndrome (AIDS)/human immunodeficiency virus (HIV) infection or hepatitis B from the mother.

Radiation, chemicals, and other environmental hazards may adversely affect a fetus when the mother is exposed to these influences during her pregnancy. The best outcomes for infants occur when mothers eat well; exercise regularly; seek early prenatal care; refrain from use of drugs, alcohol, tobacco, and excessive caffeine; and follow general principles of good health.

As we have seen, both nature and nurture are important in determining individual patterns of development. These two forces interact in unique ways in each individual, explaining differences in time frames for acquisition of developmental skills among children, personality variations between identical twins, and other unique characteristics of individuals. An environmental factor that is extremely important in the development of children is the profile of family characteristics. The family is an important component in the lives of all children and plays an essential role in fostering the development of youth. A significant concept in families is that of parenting. How children are parented interacts with their individual characteristics to influence risk and protective factors, personality characteristics, and developmental outcomes. Chapter 2 discusses types of families, frameworks used to understand families, the roles of families in fostering the development of children, and types of parenting styles.

The families into which children are born influence them profoundly. Children are supported in different ways and acquire different world views depending on such factors as whether one or both parents work, how many siblings are present, and whether an extended family is close by. Note should be made of variations in family structure such as single parent, homosexual parents, extended family, and stepparents. How might a nontraditional "family" setting, such as an adoptive home with many children, influence a child's development?

Another factor that influences child development is that of culture. The traditional customs of the many cultural groups represented in North American society influence the development of the children in these groups. Foods commonly eaten vary among people with different cultural backgrounds and influence the incidence of health problems such as cardiovascular disease in these groups. The Native American practice of carrying infants on boards often delays walking when measured against the norm for walking on some developmental tests. Children who are carried by straddling the mother's hips or back for extended periods have a low incidence of developmental dysplasia of the hip since this keeps their hips in an abducted position. It is important for nurses to take cultural practices into account when performing developmental screening; some tests may not be culturally sensitive and can inaccurately label a child as delayed when the pattern of development is simply different in the group, perhaps due to childrearing practices in the family. In addition, certain ethnic or racial groups are more prone to develop certain diseases due to genetic variations. Examples include Hispanics, who have a high incidence of diabetes; African Americans, who more commonly have sickle cell disease; and northern European Americans, who have a higher incidence of phenylketonuria.

All cultural groups have rules regarding patterns of social interaction. Schedules of language acquisition are determined by the number of languages spoken and the amount of speech in the home. The particular social roles assumed by men and women in the culture affect school activities and ultimately career choices. Attitudes toward touching and other methods of encouraging developmental skills vary among cultures. Chapter 44 ∞ includes further description of other factors that influence child development such as school and child care, community services, and additional community and family factors.

INFANT (BIRTH TO 1 YEAR)

Imagine the experience of tripling body weight in 1 year, or becoming proficient in understanding fundamental words in a new language and even speaking a few. These and many more accomplishments take place in the first year of life. Starting the year as a mainly reflexive creature, the infant can walk and communicate by the year's end. Never again in life is development so rapid and profound.

PHYSICAL GROWTH AND DEVELOPMENT

The first year of life is one of rapid change for the infant. The birth weight usually doubles by about 5 months and triples by the end of the first year (Figure 33–5 ●). Height increases by about a foot during this year. Teeth begin to erupt at about 6 months, and by the end of the first year the infant has six to eight deciduous teeth (see Chapter 36 ∞). Physical growth is closely associated with type and quality of feeding (see Chapter 34 ∞ for a discussion of nutrition in infancy).

Body organs and systems, although not fully mature at 1 year, function differently than they did at birth. Kidney and liver maturation helps the 1-year-old excrete drugs or other toxic substances more readily than in the first weeks of life. The changing body proportions mirror changes in developing internal organs. Maturation of the nervous system is demonstrated by increased control over body movements with growing differentiation from general to specific skills, thus enabling the infant to sit, stand, and walk. Sensory function also increases as the infant begins to discriminate visual images, sounds, and tastes (Table 33–11).

COGNITIVE DEVELOPMENT

The brain continues to increase in complexity during the first year. Most of the growth involves maturation of cells, with only a small increase in number of cells. This growth of the brain is accompanied by development of its functions. One has only to compare the behavior of an infant shortly after birth with that of a 1-year-old to understand the incredible maturation of brain function. The

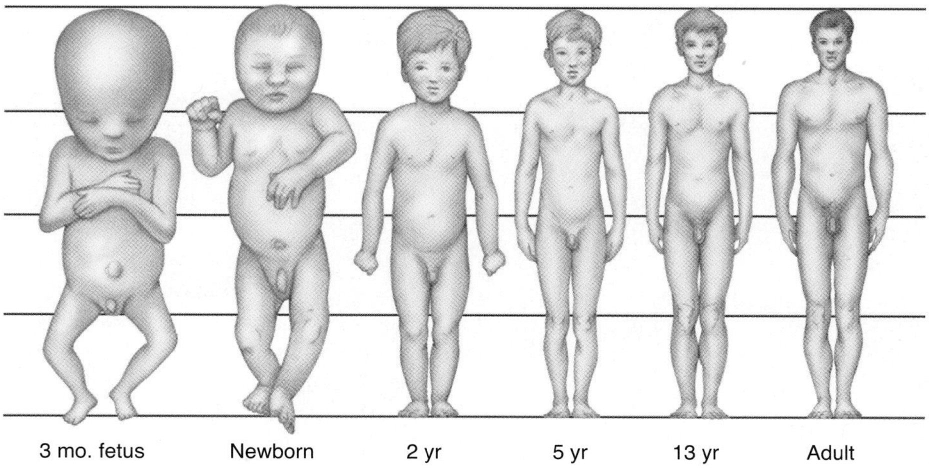

● **Figure 33–5** Body proportions at various ages.

Table 33–11 Physical Growth and Development Milestones during Infancy

Age	Physical Growth	Fine Motor Ability	Gross Motor Ability	Sensory Ability
Birth to 1 month	Gains 140–200 g (5–7 oz)/week Grows 1.5 cm (1/2 in.) in first month Head circumference increases 1.5 cm (1/2 in.)/month	Holds hand in fist (***A***) Draws arms and legs to body when crying	Inborn reflexes such as startle and rooting are predominant activity May lift head briefly if prone (***B***) Alerts to high-pitched voices Comforts with touch (***C***)	Prefers to look at faces and black-and-white geometric designs Follows objects in line of vision (***D***)

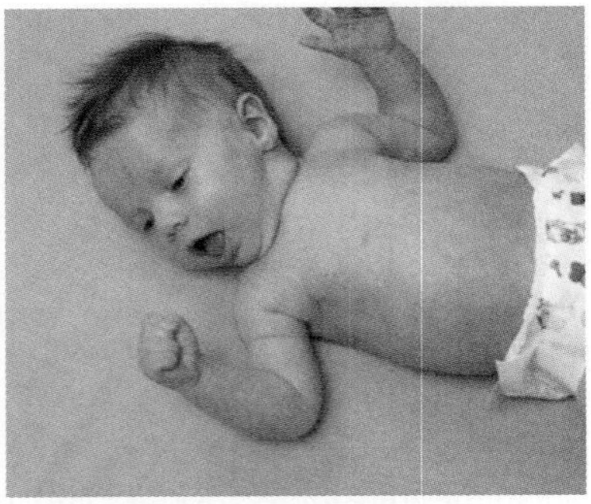

A Holds hand in fist

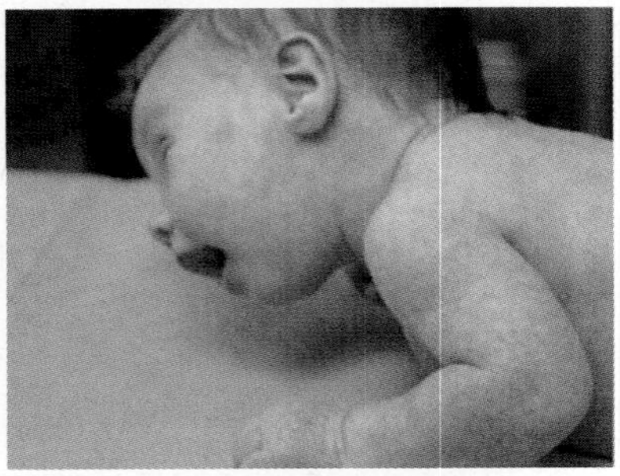

B May lift head

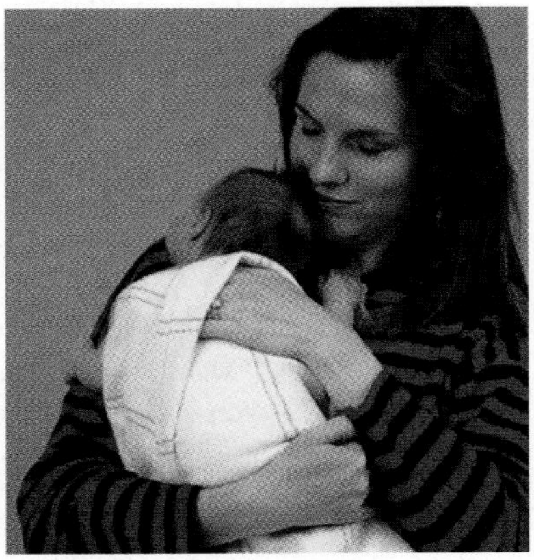

C Comforts with touch

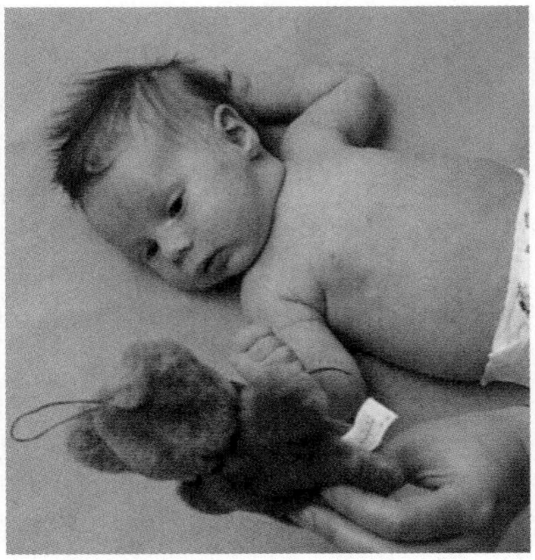

D Follows objects

2–4 months	Gains 140–200 g (5–7 oz)/week Grows 1.5 cm (1/2 in.)/month Head circumference increases 1.5 cm (1/2 in.)/month Posterior fontanelle closes Ingests 120 mL/kg/24 hr (2 oz/lb/24 hr)	Holds rattle when placed in hand (***E***) Looks at and plays with own fingers Brings hands to midline	Moro reflex fading in strength Can turn from side to back and then return (***F***) Decrease in head lag when pulled to sitting; sits with head held in midline with some bobbing When prone, holds head and supports weight on forearms (***G***)	Follows objects 180 degrees Turns head to look for voices and sounds

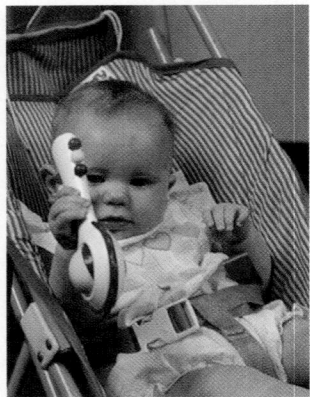

E Holds rattle

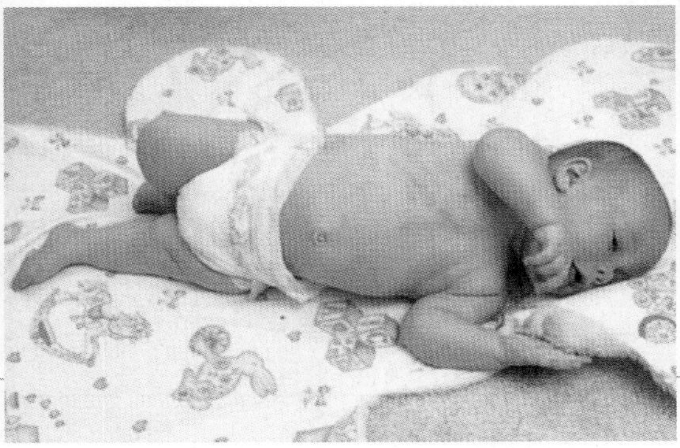

F Can turn from side to back

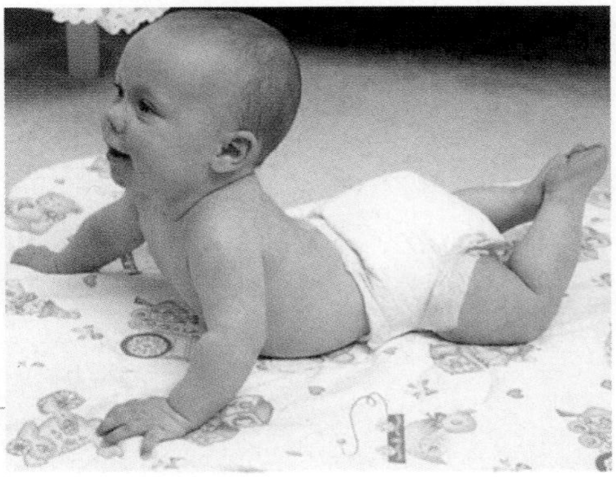

G Holds head up and supports weight with arms

Table 33–11 Physical Growth and Development Milestones during Infancy—continued

Age	Physical Growth	Fine Motor Ability	Gross Motor Ability	Sensory Ability
4–6 months	Gains 140–200 g (5–7 oz)/week Doubles birth weight at 5–6 months Grows 1.5 cm (1/2 in.)/month Head circumference increases 1.5 cm (1/2 in.)/month Teeth may begin erupting by 6 months Ingests 100 mL/kg/24 hr (1 1/2 oz/lb/24 hr)	Grasps rattles and other objects at will; drops them to pick up another offered object (***H***) Mouths objects Holds feet and pulls to mouth Holds bottle Grasps with whole hand (palmar grasp) Manipulates objects (***I***)	Head held steady when sitting No head lag when pulled to sitting Turns from abdomen to back by 4 months and then back to abdomen by 6 months When held standing supports much of own weight (***J***)	Examines complex visual images Watches the course of a falling object Responds readily to sounds 6–8 months

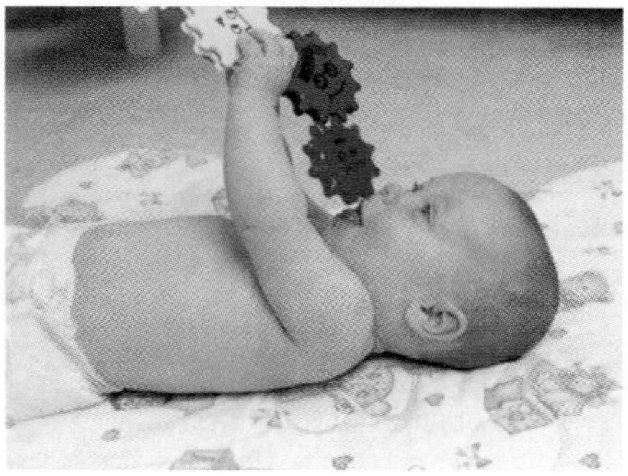

H Grasps objects at will

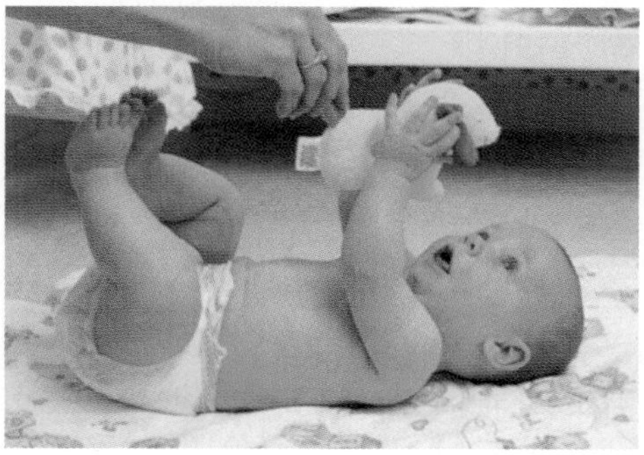

I Manipulates objects

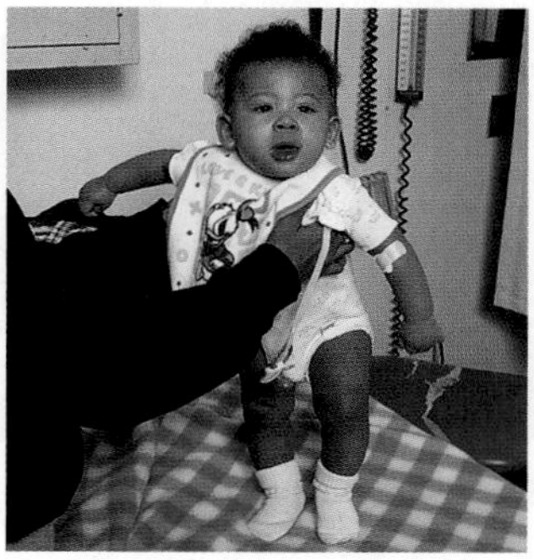

J Supports most of weight when held standing

Age	Physical Growth	Fine Motor Ability	Gross Motor Ability	Sensory Ability
6–8 months	Gains 85–140 g (3–5 oz)/week Grows 1 cm (3/8 in.)/month Growth rate slower than first 6 months	Bangs objects held in hands Transfers objects from one hand to the other Beginning pincer grasp at times	Most inborn reflexes extinguished Sits alone steadily without support by 8 months (***K***) Likes to bounce on legs when held in standing position	Recognizes own name and responds by looking and smiling Enjoys small and complex objects at play

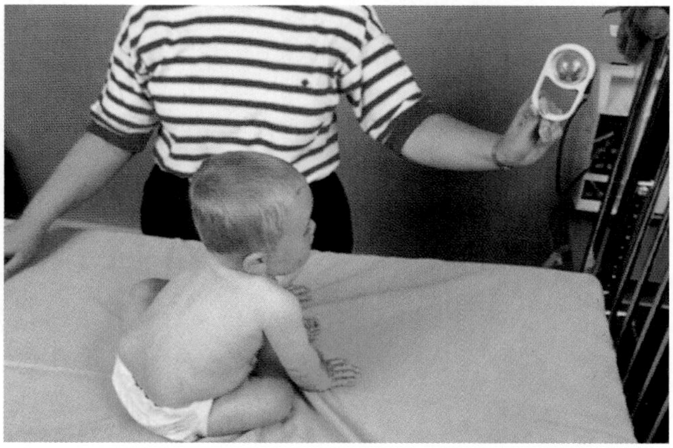

K Sits alone without support

(continued)

Table 33–11 Physical Growth and Development Milestones during Infancy—continued

Age	Physical Growth	Fine Motor Ability	Gross Motor Ability	Sensory Ability
8–10 months	Gains 85–140 g (3–5 oz)/week Grows 1 cm (3/8 in.)/month	Picks up small objects (***L***) Uses pincer grasp well (***M***)	Crawls or pulls whole body along floor by arms (***N***) Creeps by using hands and knees to keep trunk off floor Pulls self to standing and sitting by 10 months Recovers balance when sitting	Understands words such as "no" and "cracker" May say one word in addition to "mama" and "dada" Recognizes sound without difficulty 10–12 months
10–12 months	Gains 85–140 g (3–5 oz)/week Grows 1 cm (3/8 in.)/month Head circumference equals chest circumference Triples birth weight by 1 year	May hold crayon or pencil and make mark on paper Places objects into containers through holes (***O***)	Stands alone (***P***) Walks holding onto furniture Sits down from standing (***Q***)	Plays peek-a-boo and patty cake

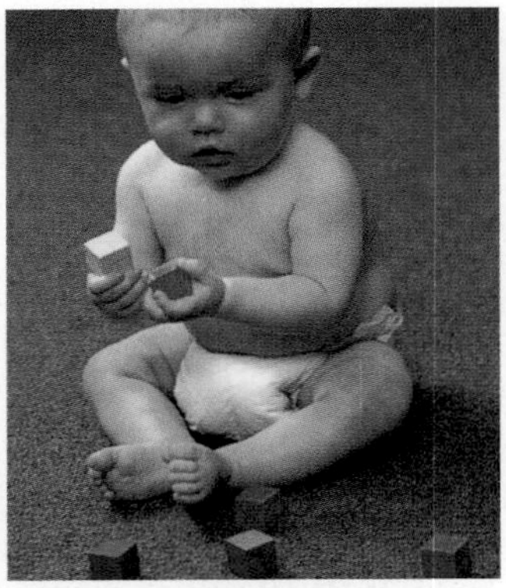

L Picks up small objects

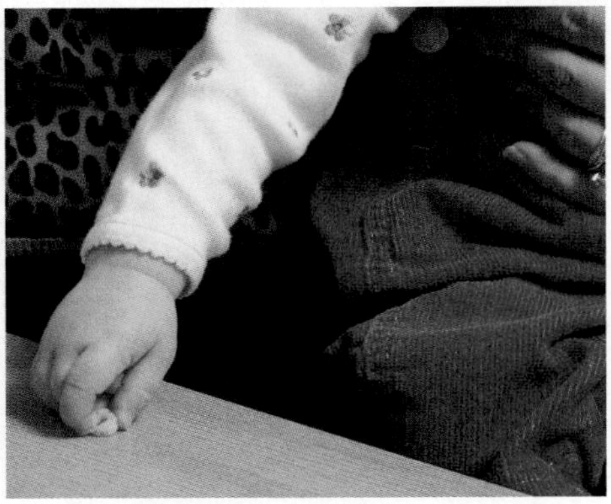

M Uses pincer grasp well

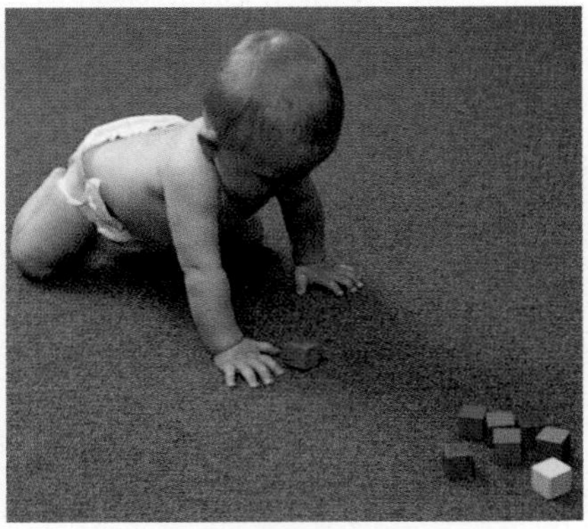

N Crawls or pulls body by arms

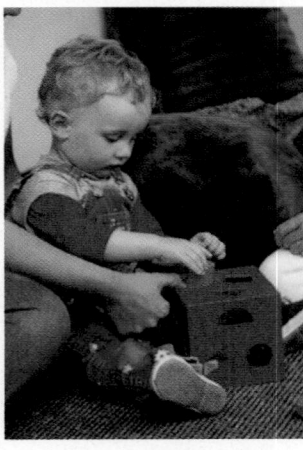

O Places objects in container through holes

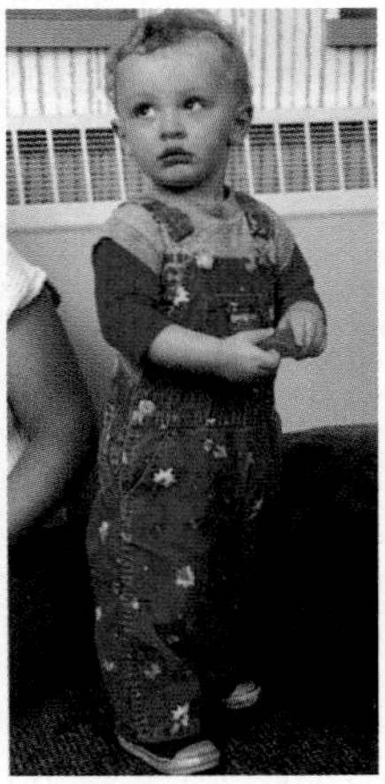

P Stands alone

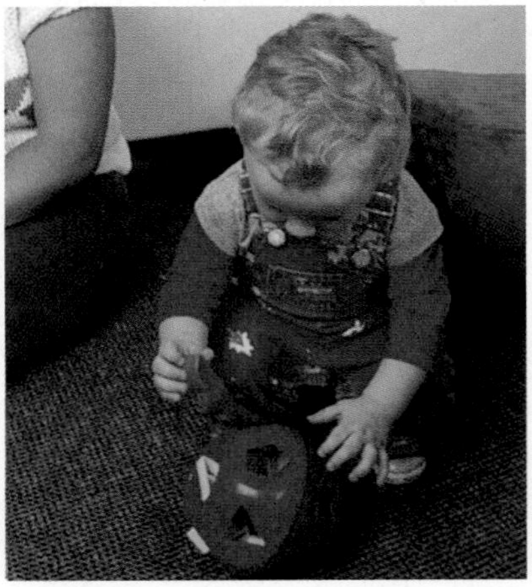

Q Sits down from standing

newborn's eyes widen in response to sound; the 1-year-old turns to the sound and recognizes its significance. The 2-month-old cries and coos; the 1-year-old says a few words and understands many more. The 6-week-old grasps a rattle for the first time; the 1-year-old reaches for toys and feeds himself or herself.

The infant's behaviors provide clues about thought processes. Piaget's work outlines the infant's actions in a set of rapidly progressing changes in the first year of life. The infant receives stimulation through sight, sound, and feeling, which the maturing brain interprets. This input from the environment interacts with internal cognitive abilities to enhance cognitive functioning.

PLAY

An 8-month-old infant is sitting on the floor, grasping blocks and banging them on the floor. Infants spend much of their time

Complementary Care

INFANT MASSAGE

Infant massage is a technique for communicating with and soothing infants. This technique has been used in many cultures throughout history, but it is not traditional within most families in the United States and Canada. It has many benefits for both infants and parents and can be taught to families who are interested. Some of the benefits for babies include improved sleep, soothability, decreased stress hormones, and positive parent-child interaction (Underdown, Barlow, Chung, et al., 2006). Premature infants are particularly benefited by this intervention. Massage periods of 10 to 15 minutes daily can be encouraged and facilitated. Such episodes will enhance bonding and attachment between parents and infant.

engaging in **solitary play**, or playing by themselves. When a parent walks by, the infant laughs and waves hands and feet wildly. Physical capabilities enable the infant to move toward and reach out for objects of interest. Cognitive ability is reflected in manipulation of the blocks to create different sounds. Social interaction enhances play. The presence of a parent or other person increases interest in surroundings and teaches the infant different ways to play.

The play of infants begins in a reflexive manner. When an infant moves extremities or grasps objects, the foundations of play are established. The feel and sound of these activities give pleasure to the infant, who gradually performs them purposefully. For example, when a parent places a rattle in the hand of a 6-week-old infant, the infant grasps it reflexively. As the hands move randomly, the rattle makes an enjoyable sound. The infant learns to move the rattle to create the sound and then finally to grasp the rattle at will to play with it.

The next phase of infant play focuses on manipulative behavior. The infant examines toys closely, looking at them, touching them, and placing them in the mouth. The infant learns a great deal about texture, qualities of objects, and all aspects of the surroundings. At the same time, interaction with others becomes an important part of play. The social nature of play is obvious as the infant plays with other children and adults.

Toward the end of the first year, the infant's ability to move in space enlarges the sphere of play (Table 33–11). Once the infant is crawling or walking, he or she can get to new places, find new toys, discover forgotten objects, or seek out other people for interaction. Play is a reflection of every aspect of development, as well as a method for enhancing learning and maturation.

PERSONALITY AND TEMPERAMENT

Why does one infant frequently awaken at night crying while another sleeps for 8 to 10 hours undisturbed? Why does one infant smile much of the time and react positively to interactions while another is withdrawn with unfamiliar people and frequently frowns and cries? Such differences in responses to the environment are believed to be inborn characteristics of temperament. Infants are born with a tendency to react in certain ways to noise and to interact differently with people. They may display varying degrees of regularity in activities of eating and sleeping, and manifest a capacity for concentrating on tasks for different amounts of time.

Nursing assessment identifies personality characteristics of the infant that the nurse can share with the parents. With this information the parents can appreciate more fully the uniqueness of their infant and design experiences to meet the infant's needs. Parents can learn to modify the environment to promote adaptation. For example, an infant who does not adapt easily to new situations may cry, withdraw, or develop another way of coping when adjusting to new people or places. Parents might be advised to use one or two babysitters rather than engaging new sitters frequently. If the infant is easily distracted when eating, parents can feed the infant in a quiet setting to encourage a focus on eating. Although the infant's temperament is unchanged, the ability to fit with the environment is enhanced. See Chapter 36 for further application of this information to health promotion of the infant.

COMMUNICATION

Even at a few weeks of age, infants communicate and engage in two-way interaction. Comfort is expressed by soft sounds, cuddling, and eye contact. The infant displays discomfort by thrashing the extremities, arching the back, and crying vigorously. From these rudimentary skills, communication ability continues to develop until the infant speaks several words at the end of the first year of life (Table 33–12).

Nurses assess communication to identify possible abnormalities or developmental delays. Language ability may be assessed with the Denver II Developmental Test and other specialized language screening tools (see Chapters 36 and 37). Normal infants understand (receptive speech) more words than they can speak (expressive speech). Abnormalities may be caused by a hearing deficit, developmental delay, or lack of verbal stimulation from caretakers. Further assessment may be required to pinpoint the cause of the abnormality.

Nursing interventions focus on providing a stimulating environment. Encourage parents to speak to infants and teach words. Hospital nurses should include the infant's known words when providing care.

Growth and Development

Strategies for communicating with infants include the following:

- Hold for feedings.
- Hold, rock, and talk to infant often.
- Talk and sing frequently during care.
- Tell names of objects.
- Use high-pitched voice with newborns.
- When the infant is upset, swaddle and hold securely.

Table 33–12 Psychosocial Development during Infancy

Age	Play and Toys	Communication
Birth–3 months 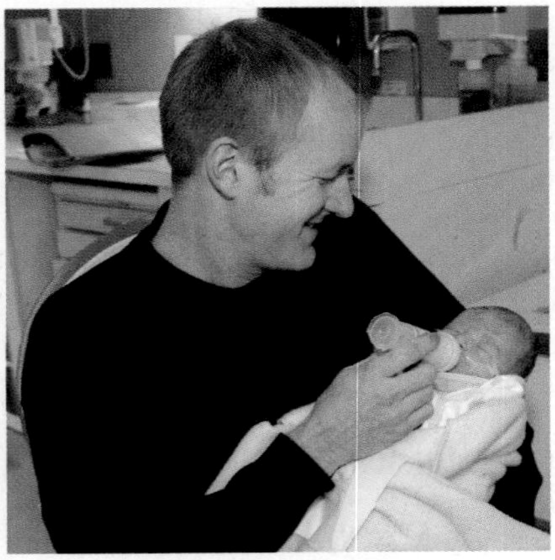	Prefers visual stimuli of mobiles, black-and-white patterns, mirrors Auditory stimuli are music boxes, tape players, soft voices Responds to rocking and cuddling Moves legs and arms while adult sings and talks Likes varying stimuli—different rooms, sounds, visual images	Coos Babbles Cries
3–6 months	Prefers noise-making objects that are easily grasped like rattles Enjoys stuffed animals and soft toys with contrasting colors	Vocalizes during play and with familiar people Laughs
6–9 months	Likes teething toys Increasingly desires social interaction with adults and other children Soft toys that can be manipulated and mouthed are favorites	Cries less Squeals and makes pleasure sounds Babbles multisyllabically (mamamamama) Increases vowel and consonant sounds Links syllables together Uses speechlike rhythm when vocalizing with others
9–12 months	Enjoys large blocks, toys that pop apart and go back together, nesting cups and other objects Laughs at surprise toys like jack-in-the-box Plays interactive games like peek-a-boo Uses push-and-pull toys	Understands "no" and other simple commands Says "dada" and "mama" to identify parents Learns one or two other words Receptive speech surpasses expressive speech

TODDLER (1 TO 3 YEARS)

Toddlerhood is sometimes called the first adolescence. An infant only months before, the child from 1 to 3 years is now displaying independence and negativism. Pride in newfound accomplishments emerges.

PHYSICAL GROWTH AND DEVELOPMENT

The rate of growth slows during the second year of life. Parents may become concerned because the child has a limited food intake, and need reassurance that this is normal (see Chapter 34 ∞ for further discussion of nutrition in toddlerhood). By age 2 years, the birth weight has usually quadrupled and the child is about one half of the adult height. Body proportions begin to change, with the legs longer and the head smaller in proportion to body size than during infancy (see Figure 33–5). The toddler has a pot-bellied appearance and stands with feet apart to provide a wide base of support. By approximately 33 months, eruption of deciduous teeth is complete, with 20 teeth present.

Gross motor activity develops rapidly (Table 33–13), as the toddler progresses from walking to running, kicking, and riding a Big Wheel tricycle (Figure 33–6 ●). As physical maturation occurs, the toddler develops the ability to control elimination patterns (Growth & Development and "Developing Cultural Competence").

COGNITIVE DEVELOPMENT

During the toddler years, the child moves from the sensorimotor to the preoperational stage of development. The early use of language awakens in the 1-year-old the ability to think about objects or people when they are absent. Object permanence is well developed.

Table 33–13 Growth and Development Milestones during Toddlerhood

Age	Physical Growth	Fine Motor Ability	Gross Motor Ability	Sensory Ability
1–2 years	Gains 227 g (8 oz) or more per month Grows 9–12 cm (3.5–5 in.) during this year Anterior fontanelle closes	By end of 2nd year, builds a tower of four blocks (***A***) Scribbles on paper (***B***) Can undress self (***C***) Throws a ball	Runs Shows growing ability to walk and finally walks with ease Walks up and down stairs a few months after learning to walk with ease (***E***) Likes push and pull toys (***F***)	Visual acuity 20/50
2–3 years	Gains 1.4–2.3 kg (3–5 lb)/year Grows 5–6.5 cm (2–2.5 in.)/year	Draws a circle and other rudimentary forms Learns to pour Learning to dress self (***D***)	Jumps Kicks ball Throws ball overhand	

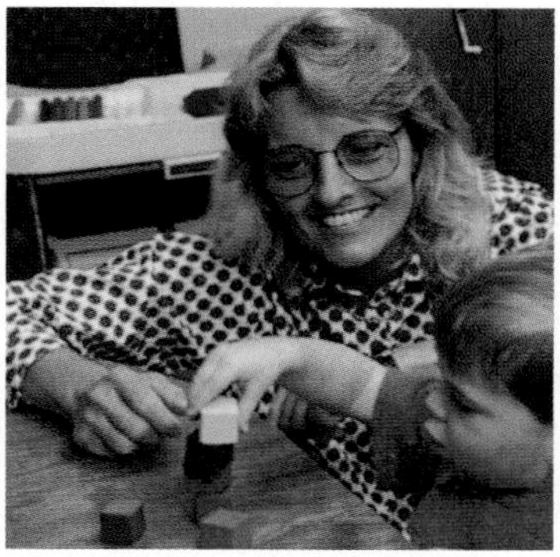

A Second year tower of four blocks

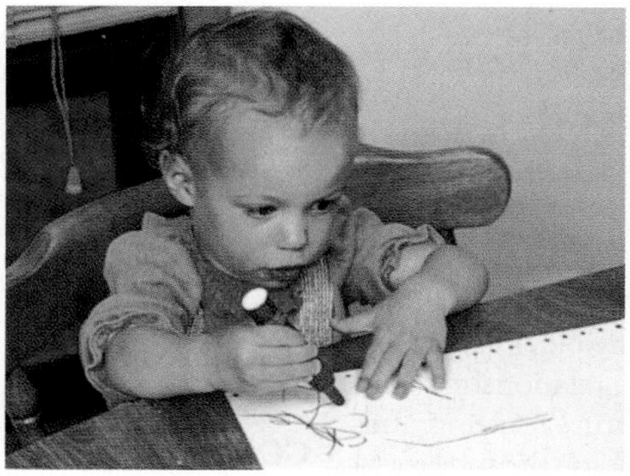

B Scribbles on paper

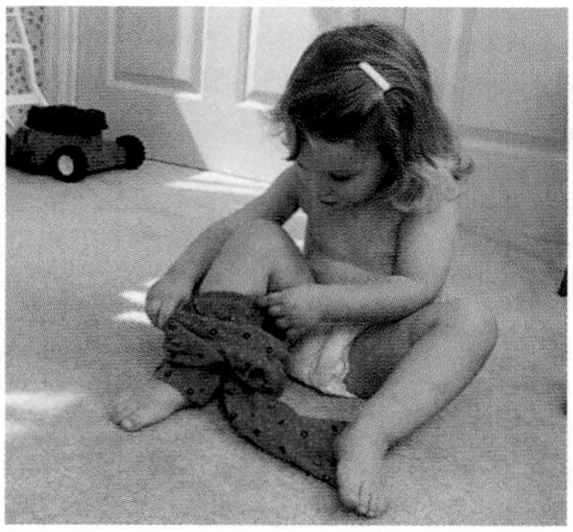

C Can undress self

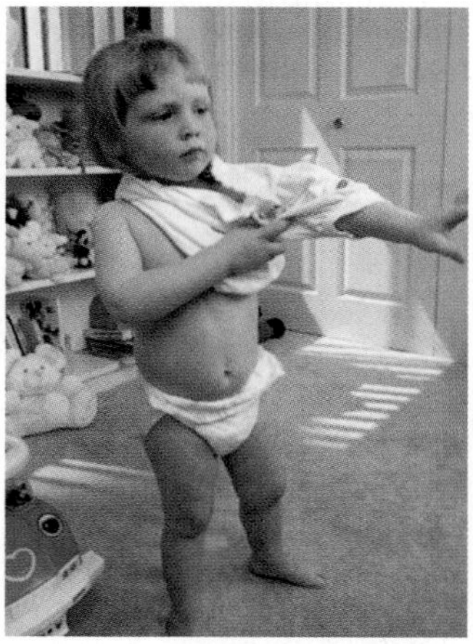

D Learning to dress self

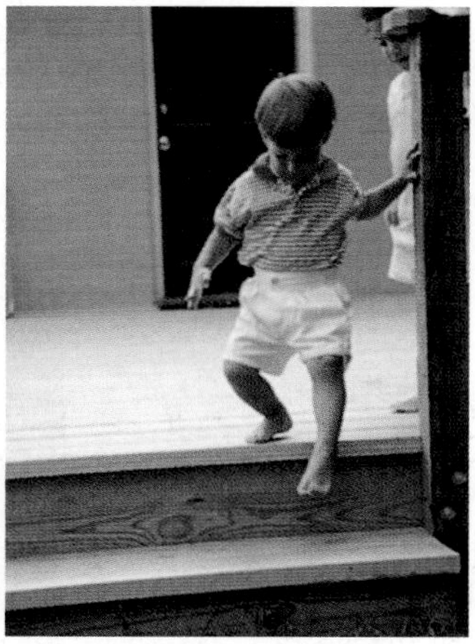

E Walks up and down stairs

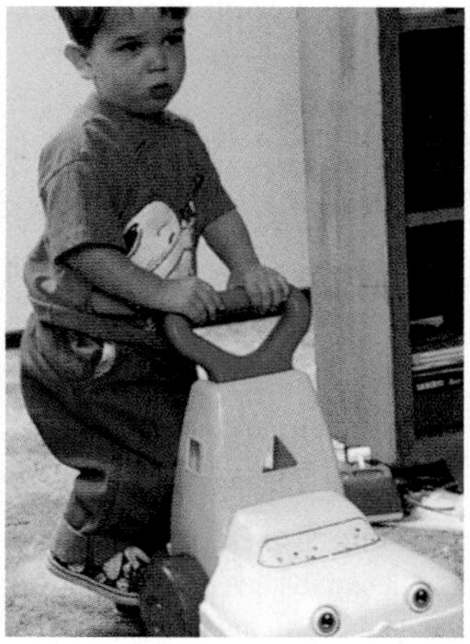

F Likes push and pull toys

At about 2 years of age, the increasing use of words as symbols enables the toddler to use preoperational thought. Rudimentary problem solving, creative thought, and an understanding of cause-and-effect relationships are now possible.

PLAY

Many changes in play patterns occur between infancy and toddlerhood. Developing motor skills enable toddlers to bang pegs into a pounding board with a hammer, for example. The social nature of toddler play is also readily seen. Toddlers find the company of other children pleasurable, even though socially interactive play may not occur. Two toddlers tend to play with similar objects side by side, occasionally trading toys and words. This is called **parallel play**. This playtime with other children helps toddlers develop social skills. Toddlers engage in play activities they have seen at home, such as pounding with a hammer and talking on the phone. This imitative behavior teaches them new actions and skills.

Physical skills are manifested in play as toddlers push and pull objects, climb in and out and up and down, run, ride a Big Wheel, turn the pages of books, and scribble with a pen. Both

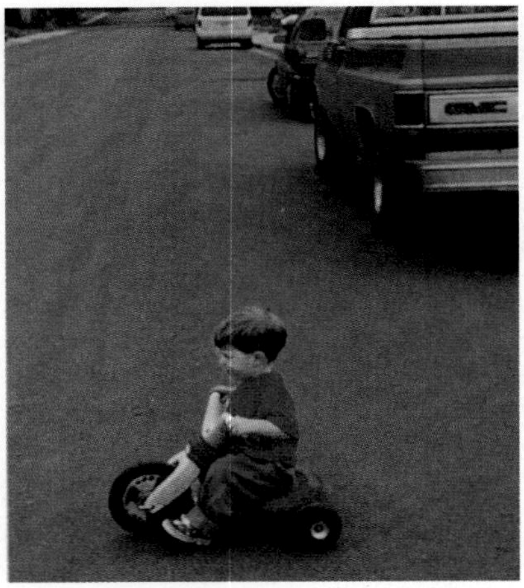

● **Figure 33–6** Gross motor activity. This toddler has learned to ride a Big Wheel, which he is doing right into the street. Toddlers must be closely watched to prevent injury.

gross motor and fine motor abilities are enhanced during this age period.

Cognitive understanding enables the toddler to manipulate objects and learn about their qualities. Stacking blocks and placing rings on a building tower teach spatial relationships and other lessons that provide a foundation for future learning. Various kinds of play objects should be provided for the toddler to meet play needs. These play needs can easily be met whether the child is hospitalized or at home (Table 33–14).

Developing Cultural Competence

CHILDREARING PRACTICES

In traditional Native American families, children are allowed to unfold and develop naturally at their own pace. Children thus wean and toilet train themselves with little interference or pressure from parents. In other groups, toilet training is accomplished at an early age. The nurse should be sensitive to the childrearing practices of the family and support them in these culturally accepted practices, rather than imposing a more structured approach to toilet training.

PERSONALITY AND TEMPERAMENT

The toddler retains most of the temperamental characteristics identified during infancy but may demonstrate some changes. The normal developmental progression of toddlerhood also plays a part in responses. For example, the infant who previously responded positively to stimuli, such as a new babysitter, may appear more negative in toddlerhood. The increasing independence characteristic of this age is shown by the toddler's use of the word "no." The parent and child constantly adapt their responses to each other and learn anew how to communicate with each other.

COMMUNICATION

Because of the phenomenal growth of language skills during the toddler period, adults should communicate frequently with chil-

Growth and Development

Strategies for toilet training include the following:

- When are children ready to learn toileting?
- Are parents responsible for the differences in ages at which toilet training is accomplished?
- Does toilet training provide clues to a child's intellectual ability?

We know that children are not ready for toilet training until several developmental capabilities exist: to stand and walk well, to pull pants up and down, to recognize the need to eliminate and then to be able to wait until in the bathroom. Once this readiness is apparent, the child can be given a small potty chair and the procedure explained.

Children often prefer their own chair on the floor to using the large toilet. The child should be placed on the chair at regular intervals for a few moments and can be given a reward or praise for successes. If the child seems not to understand or does not wish to cooperate, it is best to wait a few weeks and then try again. Just as all of development is subject to individual timetables, toilet training occurs with considerable variability from one child to another. Identify for parents the developmental characteristics of their child and encourage them to appreciate without anxiety the unfolding of skills. These timetables are not predictive of future development.

The child who is ill or hospitalized or has other stress often regresses in toilet-training activities. It is best to quietly reinstitute at-

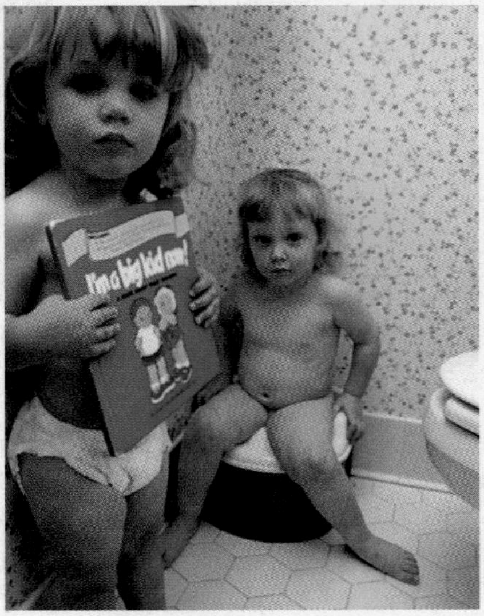

tempts at training after the trauma. Potty chairs should be available on pediatric units and toileting habits identified during initial assessment so that regular routines can be followed and the child's usual words for elimination can be used.

Table 33–14 Psychosocial Development during Toddlerhood

Age	Play and Toys	Communication
1–3 years	Refines fine motor skills by use of cloth books, large pencil and paper, wooden puzzles	Increasingly enjoys talking
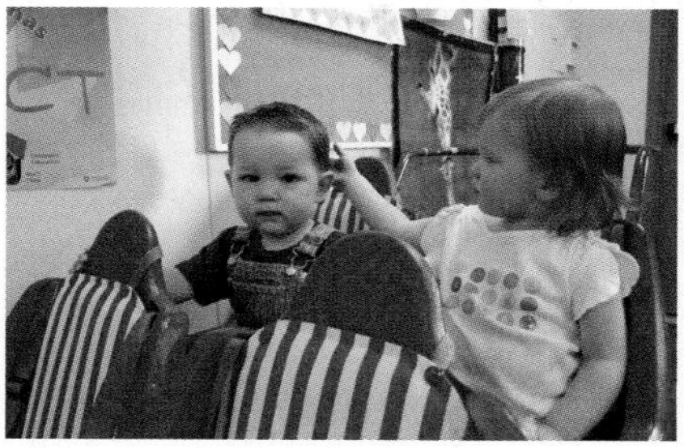	Facilitates imitative behavior by playing kitchen, grocery shopping, toy telephone	Exponential growth of vocabulary, especially when spoken and read to
	Learns gross motor activities by riding Big Wheel tricycle, playing with soft ball and bat, molding water and sand, tossing ball or bean bag	Needs to release stress by pounding board, frequent gross motor activities, and occasional temper tantrums
	Cognitive skills develop by educational television shows, music, stories, and books	Likes contact with other children and learns interpersonal skills

dren in this age group. Toddlers imitate words and speech intonations, as well as the social interactions they observe.

At the beginning of toddlerhood, the child may use four to six words in addition to "mama" and "dada." Receptive speech (the ability to understand words) far outpaces expressive speech. By the end of toddlerhood, however, the 3-year-old has a vocabulary of almost 1000 words and uses short sentences.

Communication occurs in many ways, some of which are nonverbal. Toddler communication includes pointing, pulling an adult over to a room or object, and speaking in expressive jargon. **Expressive jargon** is using unintelligible words with normal speech intonations as if truly communicating in words. Another communication method occurs when the toddler cries, pounds feet, displays a temper tantrum, or uses other means to illustrate dismay. These powerful communication methods can upset parents, who often need suggestions for handling them. It is best to verbalize the feelings shown by the toddler, for example, by saying, "You must be very upset that you cannot have that candy. When you stop crying you can come out of your room," and then to ignore further negative behavior. The toddler's search for autonomy and independence creates a need for such behavior. Sometimes an upset toddler responds well to holding, rocking, and stroking.

Growth and Development

Strategies for communicating with toddlers include the following:

- Give short, clear instructions.
- Do not give choices if none exist. For example, do not ask "Do you want to take your medicine now?" but rather say "What juice do you want after you take your medicine—apple or orange?"
- Offer a choice of two alternatives when possible.
- Approach positively and slowly, allowing time for the toddler to adjust.
- Tell toddler what you are doing, and say the names of objects.

Parents and nurses can promote a toddler's communication by speaking frequently, naming objects, explaining procedures in simple terms, expressing feelings that the toddler seems to be displaying, and encouraging speech. The toddler from a bilingual home is at an optimal age to learn two languages. If the parents do not speak English, the toddler will benefit from a daycare experience in which the providers do, so that he or she can learn both languages.

The nurse who understands the communication skills of toddlers is able to assess expressive and receptive language and communicate effectively, thereby promoting positive healthcare experiences for these children (Table 33–15).

Table 33–15 Communicating with a Toddler

Procedures such as drawing blood can be frightening for a toddler. Effective communication minimizes the trauma caused by such procedures:

- Avoid telling toddlers about the procedure too far in advance. They do not have an understanding of time and can become quite anxious.
- Use simple terminology. "We need to get a little blood from your arm. It will help us to find out if you are getting better." If the parent is willing, say, "Your mom will hold your arm still so we can do it quickly."
- Allow the toddler to cry. Acknowledge that it must be frightening and that you understand.
- Perform the procedure in a treatment room so that the toddler's bed and room are a safe haven.
- Be sure the toddler is restrained, with the joints above and below the procedure immobilized.
- Use a Band-Aid to cover up the site. This can reassure the toddler that the body is still intact.
- Allow the toddler to choose a reward such as a sticker after the procedure.
- Praise the toddler for cooperation and acknowledge that you know this was difficult.
- Comfort the toddler by rocking, offering a favorite drink, playing music, and holding. If parents are present, they can offer the comfort needed.

Table 33–16 Physical Growth and Development Milestones during the Preschool Years

Physical Growth

Gains 1.5–2.5 kg (3–5 lb)/year

Grows 4–6 cm (1 1/2–2 1/2 in.)/year

Fine Motor Ability

Uses scissors (***A***)

Draws circle, square, cross (***B***) Draws at least a six-part person

Enjoys art projects such as pasting, stringing beads, using clay

Learns to tie shoes at end of preschool years (***C***)

Buttons (***D***)

Brushes teeth (***E***)

Uses spoon, fork, knife

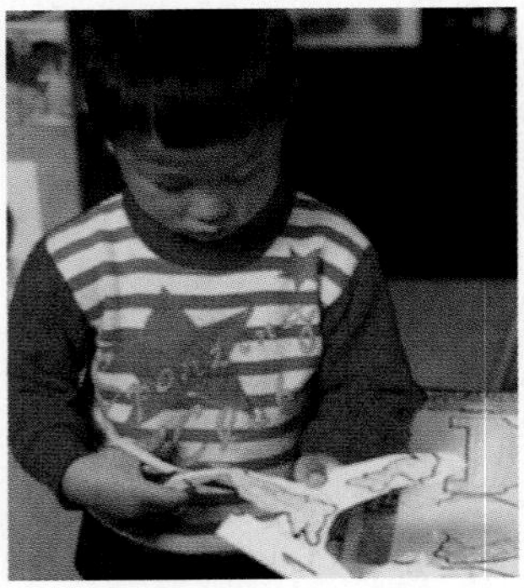

A Uses scissors

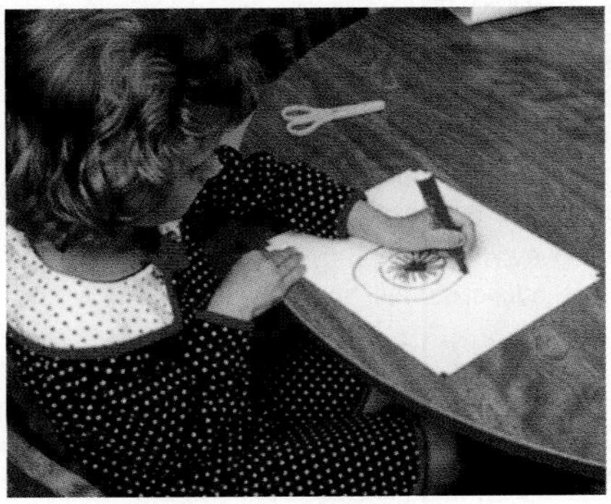

B Draws circle, square, cross

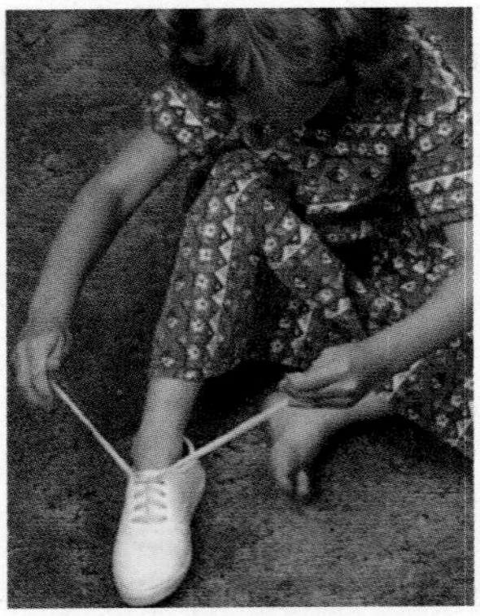

C Ties shoes

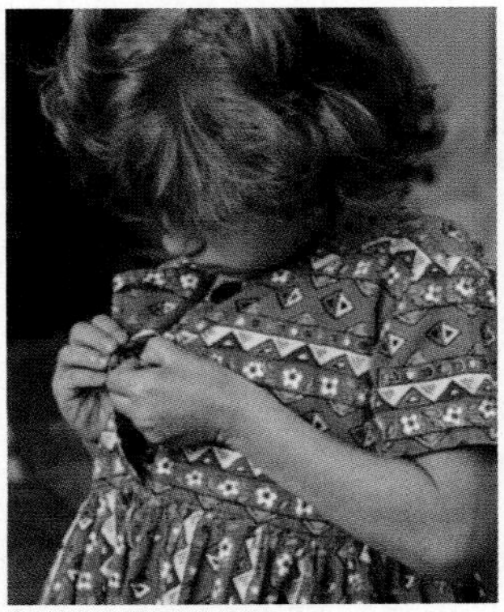

D Buttons clothes

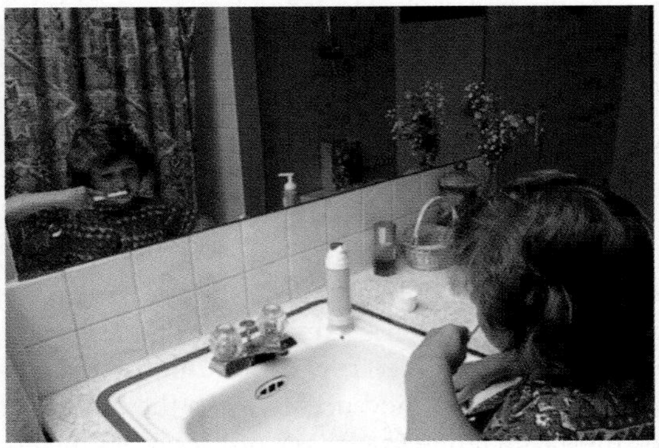

E Brushes teeth

Gross Motor Ability

Throws a ball overhand

Climbs well (***F***)

Rides bicycle (***G***)

Sensory Ability

Visual acuity continues to improve

Can focus on and learn letters and numbers (***H***)

Fine Motor Ability

Eats three meals with snacks

Uses spoon, fork, and knife

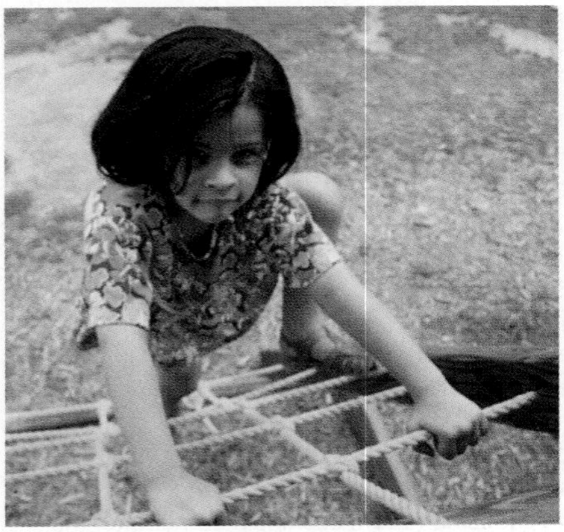

F Climbs well

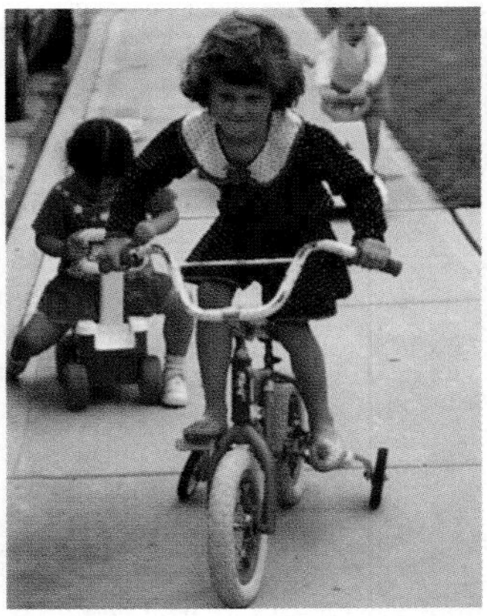

G Rides bicycle or bicycle with training wheels

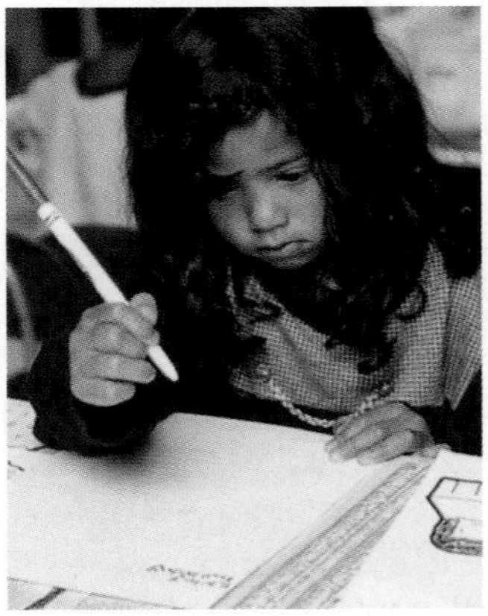

H Learns letters and numbers

PRESCHOOL CHILD (3 TO 6 YEARS)

The preschool years are a time of new initiative and independence. Most children are in a childcare center or school for part of the day and learn a great deal from this social contact. Language skills are well developed, and the child is able to understand and speak clearly. Endless projects characterize the world of busy preschoolers. They may work with play dough to form animals, then cut out and paste paper, then draw and color.

PHYSICAL GROWTH AND DEVELOPMENT

Preschoolers grow slowly and steadily, with most growth taking place in long bones of the arms and legs. The short, chubby toddler gradually gives way to a slender, long-legged preschooler (Table 33–16).

Physical skills continue to develop (Figure 33–7 ●). The preschooler runs with ease, holds a bat, and throws balls of various types. Writing ability increases, and the preschooler enjoys drawing and learning to write a few letters.

The preschool period is a good time to encourage good dental habits. Children can begin to brush their own teeth with parental supervision and help to reach all tooth surfaces. Parents should floss children's teeth, give fluoride as prescribed if the water supply is not fluoridated, and schedule the first dental visit so the child can become accustomed to the routine of periodic dental care.

COGNITIVE DEVELOPMENT

The preschooler exhibits characteristics of preoperational thought. Symbols or words are used to represent objects and people, enabling the young child to think about them. This is a milestone in intellectual development; however, the preschooler still has some limitations in thought (Table 33–17).

PLAY

The preschooler has begun playing in a new way. Toddlers simply play side by side with friends, each engaging in his or her own activities, but preschoolers interact with others during play. One child cuts out colored paper, for example, while her friend glues it on paper in a design. This new type of interaction is called

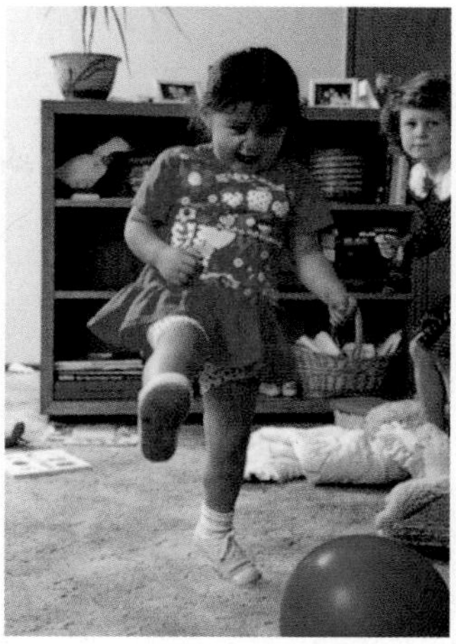

● **Figure 33–7** Development of physical skills in preschoolers. Preschoolers continue to develop more advanced skills such as kicking a ball without falling down.

associative play (Figure 33–8 ●). The child life therapist in hospital settings recognizes the therapeutic value of play in planning activities for children that enable them to work through feelings about procedures and separation, as well as facilitating the normal developmental need for interaction with other children.

In addition to this social dimension of play, other aspects of play also differ. The preschooler enjoys large motor activities such as swinging, riding a tricycle, and throwing a ball. Increasing manual dexterity is demonstrated in greater complexity of drawings and manipulation of blocks and modeling. These changes necessitate planning of playtime to include appropriate activities. Preschool programs and child life departments in hospitals help meet this important need.

Materials provided for play can be simple but should guide activities in which the child engages. Since fine motor activities are popular, paper, pens, scissors, glue, and a variety of other such objects should be available. The child can use them to create important images such as pictures of people, hospital beds, or friends. A collection of dolls, furniture, and clothing can be manipulated to represent parents and children, nurses and physicians, teachers, or other significant people. Because fantasy life is so powerful at this

Table 33–17 Characteristics of Preoperational Thought

Characteristic	Definition	Example
Egocentrism	Ability to see things only from one's own point of view	The child who cannot understand why parents may need to leave the hospital for work when the child wishes them to be present
Transductive reasoning	Connecting two events in a cause-effect relationship simply because they occur together in time	A child who, awakening after surgery and feeling pain, notices the intravenous infusion and believes that it is causing the pain
Centration	Focusing on only one particular aspect of a situation	The child who is concerned about breathing through an anesthesia mask and will not listen to any other aspects of preoperative teaching
Animism	Giving lifelike qualities to nonliving things	The child who views a monitoring machine as alive because it beeps

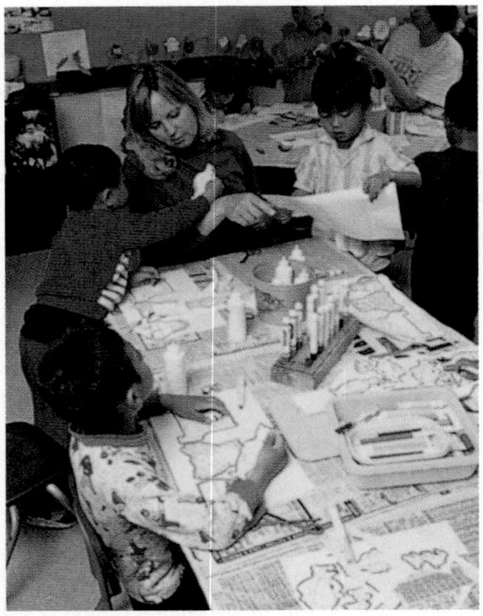

● **Figure 33–8** Associative play. These preschoolers are participating in associative play, which means they can interact. One child is cutting out shapes, and the other is gluing them in place.

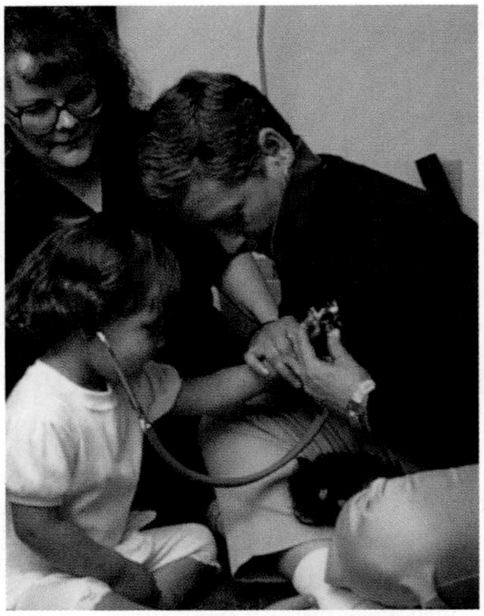

● **Figure 33–9** Dramatic play. Jasmine is participating in dramatic play with a nurse while her mother looks on. In dramatic play the child uses props to play out the drama of human life. It can be an excellent way for a nurse to assess the developmental level of children while talking to them. Notice that the child and the nurse are on the floor at the same level and the atmosphere is informal. Why is it important to be at the same level as the child?

age, the preschooler readily uses props to engage in **dramatic play**, that is, the living out of the drama of human life (Figure 33–9 ●).

The nurse can use playtime to assess the preschool child's developmental level, knowledge about health care, and emotions related to healthcare experiences. Observations about objects chosen for play, content of dramatic play, and pictures drawn can provide important assessment data. The nurse can also use play periods to teach the child about healthcare procedures and offer an outlet for expression of emotions (Table 33–18).

PERSONALITY AND TEMPERAMENT

Characteristics of personality observed in infancy tend to persist over time. The preschooler may need assistance as these characteristics are expressed in the new situations of preschool or nursery school. An excessively active child, for example, will need gentle, consistent handling to adjust to the structure of a classroom. Encourage parents to visit preschool programs to choose the one that would best foster growth in their child. Some preschoolers enjoy the structured learning of a program that focuses on cognitive skills, whereas others are happier and more open to learning in a small group that provides much time for free play. Nurses can help parents to identify their child's personality or temperament characteristics and to find the best environment for growth.

COMMUNICATION

Language skills blossom during the preschool years. The vocabulary grows to over 2000 words, and children speak in complete sentences of several words and use all parts of speech. They practice these newfound language skills by endlessly talking and asking questions.

The sophisticated speech of preschoolers mirrors the development occurring in their minds and helps them to learn about the world around them. However, this speech can be quite deceptive.

MyNursingKit Preparing a Preschooler for Surgery

Table 33–18 Psychosocial Development during the Preschool Years

Age	Play and Toys	Communication
3–6 years 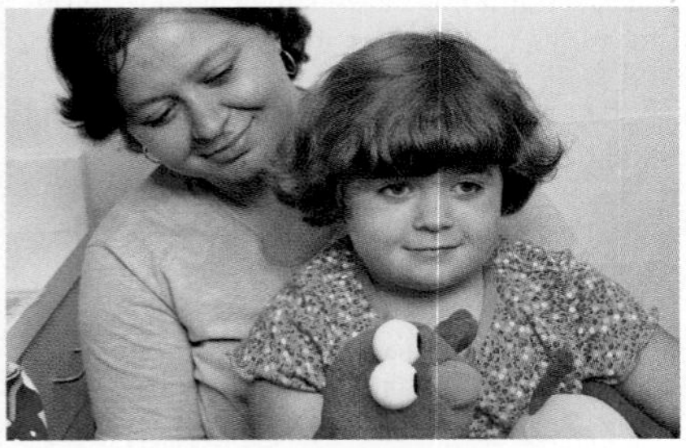	Associative play is facilitated by simple games, puzzles, nursery rhymes, songs Dramatic play is fostered by dolls and doll clothes, play houses and hospitals, dress-up clothes, puppets Stress is relieved by pens, paper, glue, scissors Cognitive growth is fostered by educational television shows, music, stories, and books	All parts of speech are developed and used, occasionally incorrectly Communicates with a widening array of people Play with other children is a favorite activity Health professionals can: ■ Verbalize and explain procedures to children ■ Use drawings and stories to explain care ■ Use accurate names for body functions ■ Allow the child to talk, ask questions, and make choices

Growth and Development

Strategies for communicating with preschoolers include the following:

- Allow time for child to integrate explanations.
- Verbalize frequently to the child.
- Use drawings and stories to explain care.
- Use accurate names for body functions.
- Allow choices.

Although preschoolers use many words, their grasp of meaning is usually literal and may not match that of adults. These literal interpretations have important implications for healthcare providers. For example, the preschooler who is told she will be "put to sleep" for surgery may think of a pet recently euthanized; the child who is told that a dye will be injected for a diagnostic test may think he is going to die; mention of "a little stick" in the arm can cause images of tree branches rather than of a simple immunization.

The child may also have difficulty focusing on the content of a conversation. The preschooler is egocentric and may be unable to move from individual thoughts to those the nurse is proposing in a teaching situation.

Concrete visual aids such as pictures of a child undergoing the same procedure or a book to read together enhance teaching by meeting the child's developmental needs. Handling medical equipment such as intravenous bags and stethoscopes increases interest and helps the child to focus. Teaching may have to be done in several short sessions rather than one long session.

SCHOOL-AGE CHILD (6 TO 12 YEARS)

Errol, 10 years old, arrives home from school shortly after 3 p.m. each day. He immediately calls his friends and goes to visit one of them. They are building models of cars and collecting baseball cards. Endless hours are spent on these projects and on discussions of events at school that day (Figure 33–10 ●).

Nine-year-old Karen practices soccer two afternoons a week and plays in games each weekend. She also is learning to play the flute and spends her free time at home practicing. Although practice time is not her favorite part of music, Karen enjoys the performances and wants to play well in front of her friends and teacher. Her parents now allow her to ride her bike unaccompanied to the store or to a friend's house.

These two school-age children demonstrate common characteristics of their age group. They are in a stage of industry in which it is important to the child to perform useful work. Meaningful activities take on great importance and are usually carried out in the company of peers. A sense of achievement in these activities is important to develop self-esteem and to prevent a sense of inferiority or poor self-worth.

PHYSICAL GROWTH AND DEVELOPMENT

School age is the last period in which girls and boys are close in size and body proportions. As the long bones continue to grow, leg length increases (see Figure 33–5). Fat gives way to muscle, and the child appears leaner. Jaw proportions change as the first deciduous tooth is lost at 6 years and permanent teeth begin to erupt. Body organs and the immune system mature, resulting in fewer illnesses among school-age children. Medications are less likely to cause serious side effects, since they can be metabolized more easily. The urinary system can adjust to changes in fluid status. Physical skills are also refined as children begin to play sports, and fine motor skills are well developed through school activities (Table 33–19 and Figure 33–11 ●).

Although it is commonly believed that the start of adolescence (age 12 years) heralds a growth spurt, the rapid increases in size commonly occur during school age. Girls may begin a growth spurt by 9 or 10 years and boys a year or so later. Nutritional needs increase dramatically with this spurt.

The loss of the first deciduous teeth and the eruption of permanent teeth usually occur at about age 6 years, or at the beginning of the school-age period. Of the 30 permanent teeth, 22 to 26 erupt

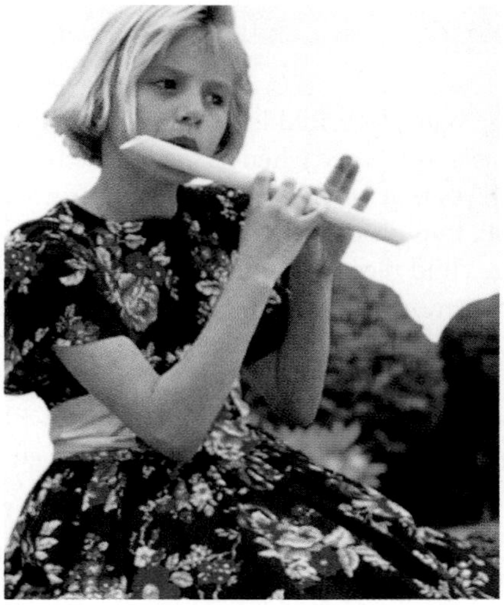

A

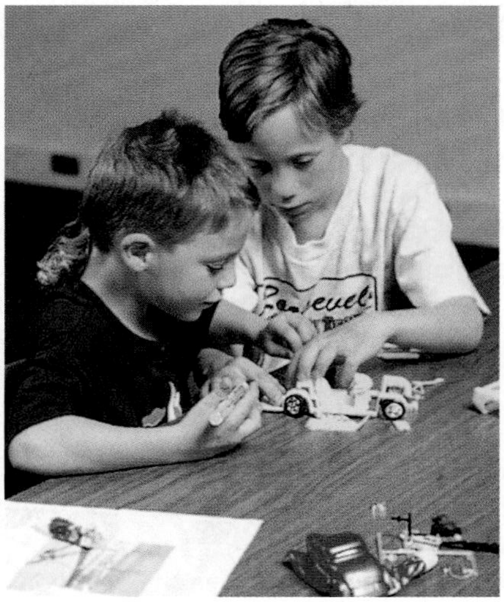

B

● **Figure 33–10** School-age children. ***A,*** School-age children may take part in activities that require practice. This is a consideration when children are hospitalized and unable to practice or perform. Why? ***B,*** School-age children enjoy spending time with others the same age on projects and discussing the activities of the day. This is an important consideration when they are in an acute care setting. When you are in the clinical setting, look for examples of this type of interaction taking place.

Table 33–19 Physical Growth and Development Milestones during the School-Age Years

Physical Growth	Fine Motor Ability	Gross Motor Ability	Sensory Ability
Gains 1.4–2.2 kg (3–5 lb)/year Grows 4–6 cm (1 1/2–2 1/2 in.)/year	Enjoys craft projects Plays card and board games	Rides two-wheeler (***A***) Jumps rope (***B***) Roller skates or ice skates	Can read Able to concentrate for longer periods on activities by filtering out surrounding sounds (***C***)

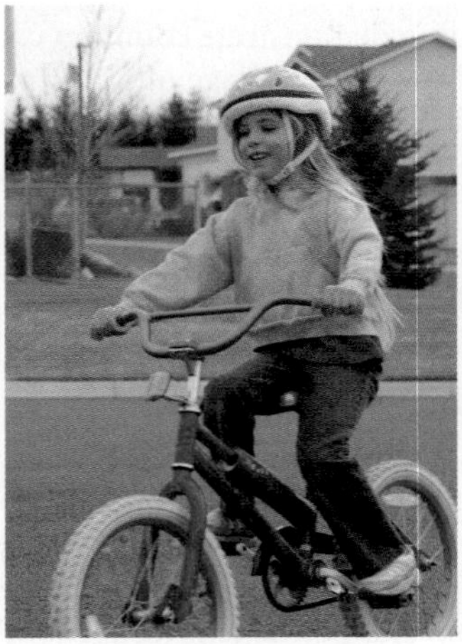

A Rides two-wheeler

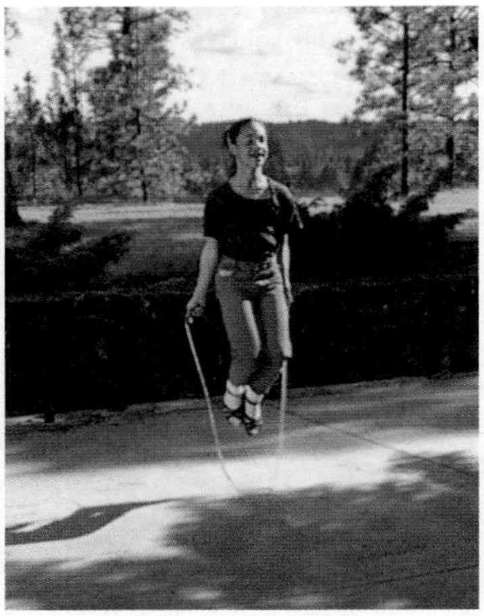

B Jumps rope

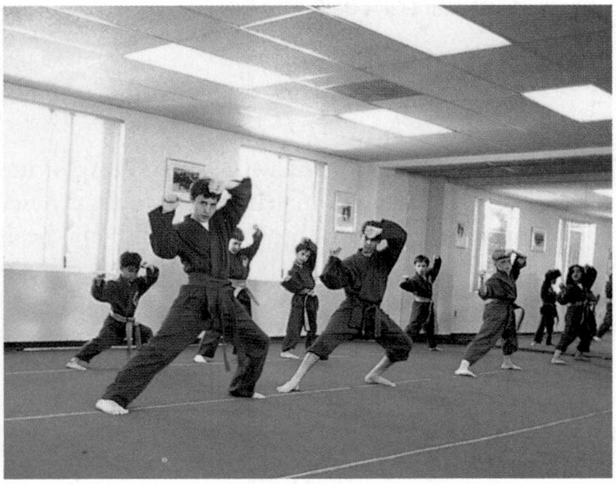

C Concentrates an activities for longer periods

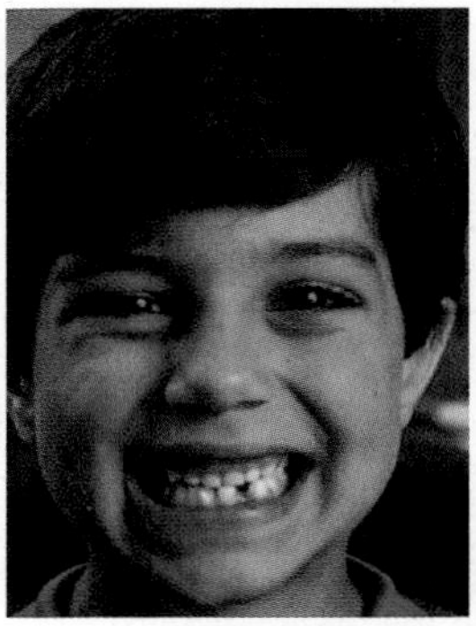

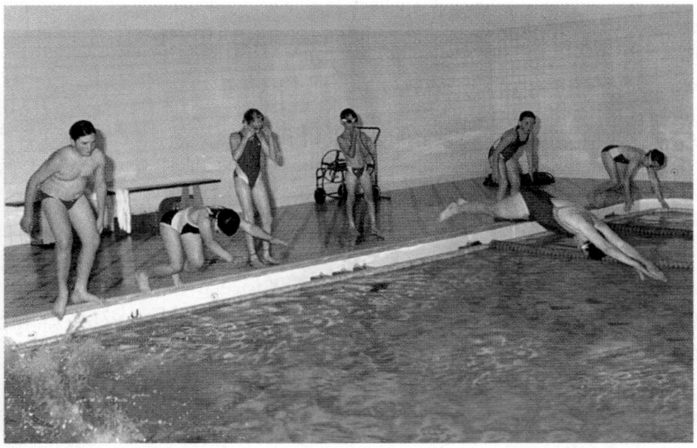

● **Figure 33–11** School-age children's physical development. *Left,* Front teeth are lost around age 6 years. The family may have rituals associated with the loss of teeth that could affect the child's behavior if he loses a tooth while in the hospital. *Right,* School-age girls and boys enjoy participating in sports. They begin to lose fat while developing their muscles, so they appear leaner than at earlier ages.

by age 12 years and the remaining molars follow during the teenage years. The school-age child should be closely monitored to ensure that brushing and flossing are adequate, that fluoride is taken if the water supply is not fluoridated, that dental care is obtained to provide for examination of teeth and alignment, and that loose teeth are identified before surgery or other events that may lead to loss of a tooth.

COGNITIVE DEVELOPMENT

The child enters the stage of concrete operational thought at about 7 years. This stage enables school-age children to consider alternative solutions and solve problems. However, school-age children continue to rely on concrete experiences and materials to form their thought content.

During the school-age years, the child learns the concept of **conservation** (that matter is not changed when its form is altered). At earlier ages a child believes that when water is poured from a short, wide glass into a tall, thin glass, there is more water in the taller glass. The school-age child recognizes that although it may look like the taller glass holds more water, the quantity is the same. The concept of conservation is helpful when the nurse explains medical treatments. The school-age child understands that an incision will heal, that a cast will be removed, and that an arm will look the same as before once the intravenous infusion is removed.

PLAY

When the preschool teacher tries to organize a game of baseball, both the teacher and the children become frustrated. Not only are

Table 33–20	Psychosocial Development during the School-Age Years	
Age	**Activities**	**Communication**
6–12 years 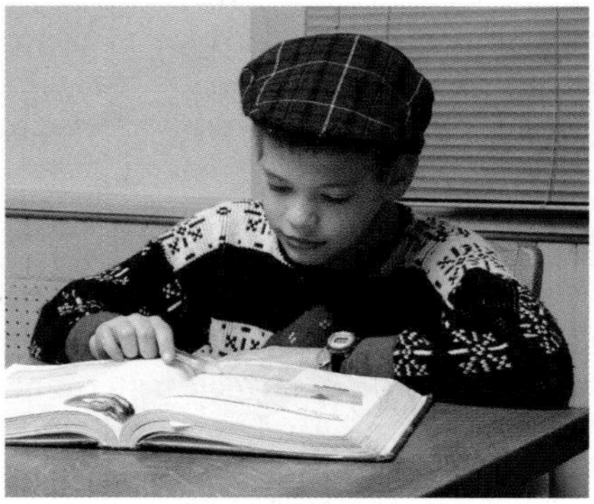	Gross motor development is fostered by ball sports, skating, dance lessons, water and snow skiing/boarding, biking A sense of industry is fostered by playing a musical instrument, gathering collections, starting hobbies, playing board and video games Cognitive growth is facilitated by reading, crafts, word puzzles, school work	Mature use of language Ability to converse and discuss topics for increasing lengths of time Spends many hours at school and with friends in sports or other activities Health professionals can: ■ Assess child's knowledge before teaching ■ Allow the child to select rewards following procedures ■ Teach techniques such as counting or visualization to manage difficult situations ■ Include both parent and child in healthcare decisions

the children physically unable to hold a bat and hit a ball, but they seem to have no understanding of the rules of the game and do not want to wait for their turn at bat. By 6 years of age, however, children have acquired the physical ability to hold the bat properly and may occasionally hit the ball. School-age children also understand that everyone has a role—the pitcher, the catcher, the batter, the outfielders. They cooperate with one another to form a team, are eager to learn the rules of the game, and want to ensure that these rules are followed exactly (Table 33–20).

The characteristics of play exhibited by the school-age child are cooperation with others and the ability to play a part in order to contribute to a unified whole. This type of play is called **cooperative play**. The concrete nature of cognitive thought leads to a reliance on rules to provide structure and security. Children have an increasing desire to spend much of playtime with friends, which demonstrates the social component of play. Play is an extremely important method of learning and living for the school-age child. Active physical play has decreased in recent years as television viewing and playing of computer games have increased, leading to poor nutritional status and a high rate of overweight among children. See Chapter 34 for further discussion of nutrition and physical activity in children.

When a child is hospitalized, the separation from playmates can lead to feelings of sadness and purposelessness. School-age children often feel better when placed in multibed units with other children. Games can be devised even when children are wheelchair bound (Figure 33–12 ●). Normal, rewarding parts of play should be integrated into care. Friends should be encouraged to visit or call a hospitalized child. Discharge planning for the child who has had a cast or brace applied should address the activities the child can engage in and those the child must avoid. Reinforce the importance of playing games with friends.

● **Figure 33–12** The hospitalized school-age child. The nurse can help the child and family accept and adjust to new circumstances. Encouraging the child in a wheelchair to participate in group activities can help build confidence in physical skills. Good self-esteem, goal attainment, personal satisfaction, and general health are the continued benefits.

PERSONALITY AND TEMPERAMENT

The enduring aspects of temperament continue to be manifested during the school years. The child classified as "difficult" at an earlier age may now have trouble in the classroom. Advise parents to provide a quiet setting for homework and to reward the child for concentration. For example, after homework is completed, the child can watch a television show. Creative efforts and alternative methods of learning should be valued. Encourage parents to see their children as individuals who may not all learn in the same way. The "slow-to-warm-up" child may need encouragement to try new activities and to share experiences with others, while the "easy" child will readily adapt to new schools, people, and experiences.

COMMUNICATION

During the school-age years, the child should learn how to correct any lingering pronunciation or grammatical errors. Vocabulary increases, and the child is taught about parts of speech in

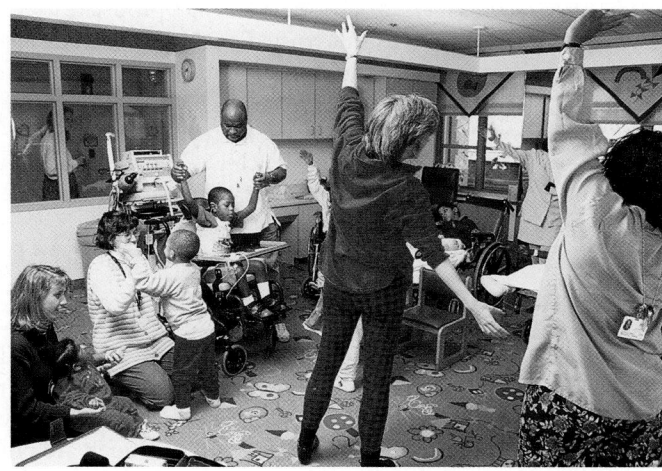

school. School-age children enjoy writing and can be encouraged to keep a journal of their experiences while in the hospital as a method of dealing with anxiety. It is uncommon for school-age children to understand words as literally as preschoolers.

SEXUALITY

While children become aware of sexual differences between genders during preschool years, they deal much more consciously with sexuality during school age. As children mature physically, they need information about their body changes so that they can develop a healthy self-image, and an understanding of the relationships between their bodies and sexuality. Children become interested in sexual issues and are often exposed to erroneous information on television shows, in magazines, or from friends and siblings. Schools and families need to use opportunities to teach school-age children factual information about sex, as well as fostering healthy concepts of self and others. It is advisable to ask occasional questions about sexual issues to learn how much the child knows and to provide correct information when answers demonstrate confusion. Both friends and the media are common sources of erroneous ideas. Appropriate and inappropriate touch should be discussed, with lists of trusted people who can be approached (teachers, clergy, school counselors, family members, neighbors) to discuss any episodes with which the child feels uncomfortable. Even these trusted people can be implicated in inappropriate episodes, so encourage the child to go to more than one person, an important approach if the child is uncomfortable about a relationship with any individual.

ADOLESCENT (12 TO 18 YEARS)

Adolescence is a time of passage signaling the end of childhood and the beginning of adulthood. Although adolescents differ in behaviors and accomplishments, they are in a period of identity formation. If a healthy identity and sense of self-worth are not developed in this period, role confusion and purposeless struggling will ensue. The adolescents encountered in nursing practice represent various degrees of identity formation, and each will offer unique challenges.

 Growth and Development

Strategies for communicating with school-age children include the following:

- Provide concrete examples of pictures or materials to accompany verbal descriptions.
- Assess knowledge before planning teaching.
- Allow child to select rewards following procedures.
- Teach techniques such as counting or visualization to manage difficult situations.
- Include child in discussions and history with parent.
- Be honest in explanations and all communications.

PHYSICAL GROWTH AND DEVELOPMENT

The physical changes ending in **puberty**, or sexual maturity, begin near the end of the school-age period. The prepubescent period is marked by a growth spurt at an average age of 10 years for girls and 13 years for boys. The increase in height and weight is generally remarkable and is completed in 2 to 3 years (Table 33–21). The growth spurt in girls is accompanied by an increase in breast size and growth of pubic hair. Menstruation occurs last and signals achievement of puberty. In boys the growth spurt is accompanied by growth in size of the penis and testes and by growth of pubic hair. Deepening of the voice and growth of facial hair occur later, at the time of puberty. See Chapter 35 ∞ for a description of the pubertal stages.

During adolescence children grow stronger and more muscular and establish characteristic male and female patterns of fat distribution. The apocrine and eccrine glands mature, leading to increased sweating and a distinct odor to perspiration. All body organs are now fully mature, enabling the adolescent to take adult doses of medications.

The adolescent must adapt to a rapidly changing body for several years. Height, weight, and body proportions increase. Such changes occur with great variability so an adolescent may be at different points of maturation than peers. These physical changes, hormonal variations, and differences in timing offer challenges to identity formation. The adolescent must incorporate the new body, its functions, and retain a healthy sense of self in relationship to peers. The formation of self identity is a psychological process but is necessarily closely connected with the bodily changes occurring.

COGNITIVE DEVELOPMENT

Adolescence marks the beginning of Piaget's last stage of cognitive development, the stage of formal operational thought. The adolescent no longer depends on concrete experiences as the basis of thought but develops the ability to reason abstractly. Such concepts as justice, truth, beauty, and power can be understood. The adolescent revels in this newfound ability and spends a great deal of time thinking, reading, and talking about abstract concepts.

The ability to think and act independently leads many adolescents to rebel against parental authority and experiment with risky behaviors. Through these actions, adolescents seek to establish their own identity and values.

ACTIVITIES

Maturity leads to new activities. Adolescents may drive, ride buses, or bike independently. They are less dependent on parents for transportation and spend more time with friends. Activities include participation in sports and extracurricular school activities, as well as "hanging out" and attending movies or concerts with friends (Table 33–22). The peer group becomes the focus of activities (Figure 33–13 ●), regardless of the teen's interests. Peers are important in establishing identity and providing meaning. Although same-sex interactions predominate, boy-girl relationships are more common than at earlier stages. Adolescents thus participate in and learn from social interactions fundamental to adult relationships.

Table 33–21 Physical Growth and Development Milestones during Adolescence

Physical Growth	Fine Motor Ability	Gross Motor Ability	Sensory Ability
Variation in age of growth spurt During growth spurt, girls gain 7–25 kg (15–55 lb) and grow 2.5–20 cm (2–8 in.); boys gain approximately 7–29.5 kg (15–65 lb) and grow 11–30 cm (4 1/2–12 in.)	Skills are well developed (***A***)	New sports activities attempted and muscle development continues (***B***) Some lack of coordination common during growth spurt	Fully developed

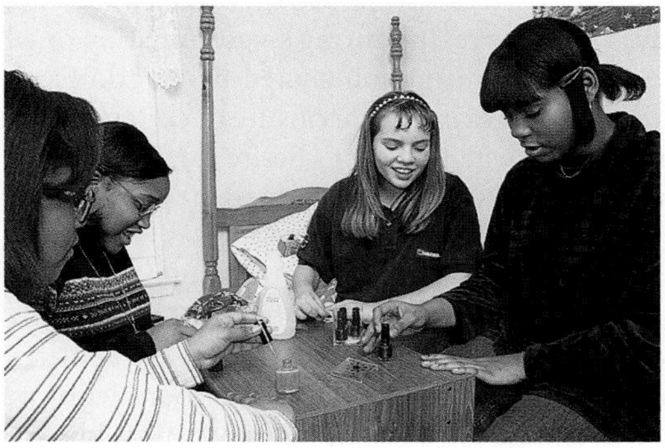

A Skills are well developed

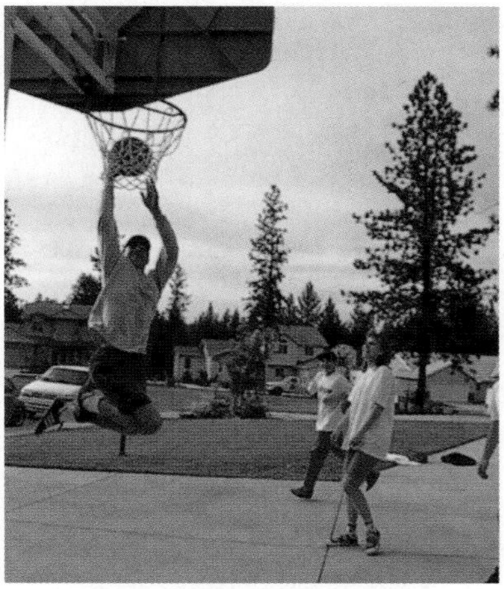

B New sports activities attempted

PERSONALITY AND TEMPERAMENT

Characteristics of temperament manifested during childhood usually remain stable in the teenage years. For instance, the adolescent who was a calm, scheduled infant and child often demonstrates initiative to regulate study times and other routines. Similarly the adolescent who was an easily stimulated infant may now have a messy room, a harried schedule with assignments always completed late, and an interest in many activities. It is also common for an adolescent who was an easy child to become more difficult because of the psychologic changes of adolescence and the need to assert independence.

As during the child's earlier ages, the nurse's role may be to inform parents of different personality types and to help them support the teen's uniqueness while providing necessary structure and feedback. Nurses can help parents understand their teen's personality type and work with the adolescent to meet expectations set by teachers and others in authority.

Table 33–22 Psychosocial Development during Adolescence

Age	Activities	Communication
12–18 years	Sports—ball games, gymnastics, water and snow skiing/boarding, swimming, school sports School activities—drama, yearbook, class office, club participation Quiet activities—reading, school work, television, computer, video games, music	Increasing communication and time with peer group—movies, dances, driving, eating out, attending sports events Applying abstract thought and analysis in conversations at home and school

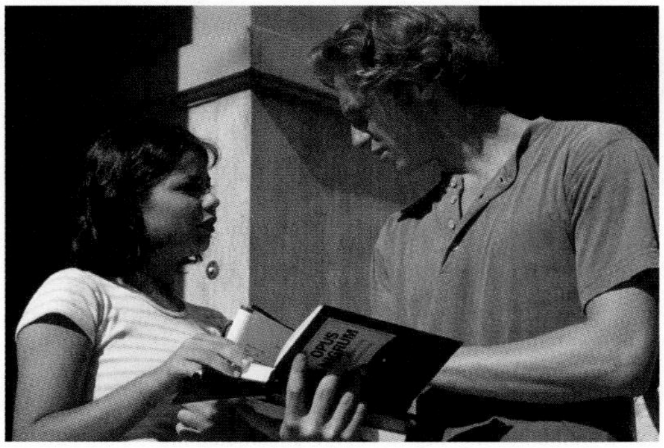

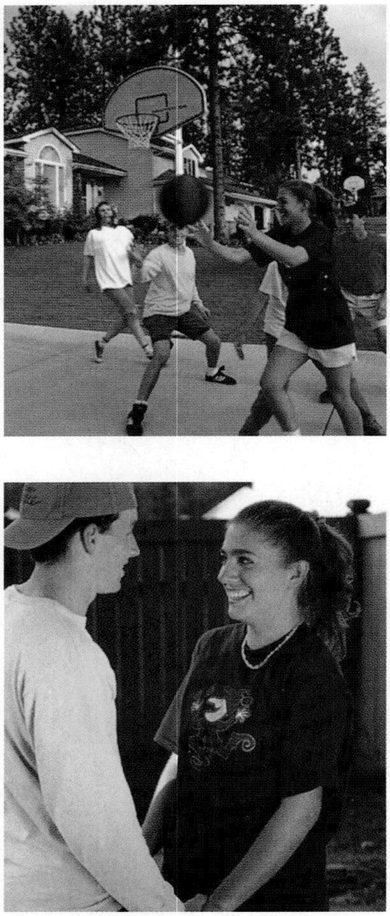

A

B

● **Figure 33–13** Peer group activities in adolescence. Social interaction between children of same and opposite sex is as important inside the acute care setting as it is outside. ***A,*** Teenagers enjoy playing together. ***B,*** Emotional relationships form during adolescence.

COMMUNICATION

The adolescent uses and understands all parts of speech. Colloquialisms and slang are commonly used with the peer group. The adolescent often studies a foreign language in school, having the ability to understand and analyze grammar and sentence structure.

The adolescent increasingly leaves the home base and establishes close ties with peers. These relationships become the basis for identity formation. There is generally a period of stress or crisis before a strong identity can emerge. The adolescent may try out new roles by learning a new sport or other skills, experimenting with drugs or alcohol, wearing different styles of clothing, or trying other activities. It is important to provide positive role models and a variety of experiences to help the adolescent make wise choices.

The adolescent also has a need to leave the past, to be different, and to change from former patterns to establish his or her own identity. Rules that are repeated constantly and dogmatically will probably be broken in the adolescent's quest for self-identity. This poses difficulties when the adolescent has a health problem, such as diabetes, or a heart problem that requires ongoing care. Introducing the adolescent to other teens who manage the same problem appropriately is usually more successful than telling the adolescent what to do.

Ensure privacy during the taking of health histories or interventions with teens. Even if a parent is present for part of a history or examination, the adolescent should be given the opportunity to relay information or ask questions alone with the healthcare provider. The adolescent should be given a choice of whether to have a parent present during an examination or while care is provided. Most information shared by an adolescent is confidential. Some states mandate disclosure of certain information to parents, such as an adolescent's desire for an abortion. In these cases the adolescent should be informed of what will be disclosed to the parent.

Setting up teen rooms (recreation rooms for use only by adolescents) or separate adolescent units in hospitals can provide necessary peer support during hospitalization. Most adolescents are not pleased when placed on a unit or in a room with young children. Choices should be allowed whenever possible. These might include preference for evening or morning bathing, the type of clothes to wear while hospitalized, timing of treatments, and who should be allowed to visit and for how long. Use of negotiations and agreements with adolescents may increase compliance. Firmness, gentleness, choices, and respect must all be balanced during care of adolescent patients.

SEXUALITY

With maturation of the body and increased secretion of hormones, the adolescent achieves sexual maturity. This complex process involves a growing interest in sexuality and romantic or sexual relationships, an interplay of the forces of society and family, and identity formation. The early adolescent progresses from dances and other social events with members of the opposite sex; the late adolescent is mature sexually and may have regular sexual encounters. About one-half of all high-school students in the United States have had intercourse, but only 63% of these youths

Growth and Development

Strategies for communicating with adolescents include the following:

- Provide written as well as verbal explanations.
- Direct history and explanations to teen alone; then include parent.
- Allow for safe exploration of topics by suggesting that teen is similar to other teens. ("Many teens with diabetes have questions about how to eat foods you and your friends like and still stay within your diet needs. How about you?")
- Arrange meetings for discussions with other teens.

used a condom at their last sexual encounter, putting this age group at high risk of acquiring sexually transmitted infections (Eaton, Kann, Kinchen, et al., 2006).

Teenagers need information about their bodies and emerging sexuality. To make informed decisions about their behavior, teenagers should understand the interests and forces they experience. Including sex education in school classes and healthcare encounters is important. Information on how to prevent sexually transmitted diseases is given, with most school districts now providing some teaching on AIDS. Far more common risks to teens, however, are diseases such as gonorrhea and herpes. Health histories should include questions on sexual activity, sexually transmitted diseases, and birth control use and understanding. Most hospitals routinely perform pregnancy screening on adolescent girls before elective procedures.

Adolescents benefit from clear information about sexuality, an opportunity to develop relationships with adolescents in various settings, an open atmosphere at home and school where problems and issues can be discussed, and previous experience in problem solving and self-decision making. Sexual issues should be among topics that adolescents can discuss openly in a variety of settings. Alternatives and support for their decisions should be available.

Some adolescents identify with a sexual minority group such as lesbian, gay, bisexual, or transgender. They are at particular risk of being stigmatized and harassed by other youth or adults. They are more likely to suffer a variety of problems such as isolation, rejection by family and friends, violence, suicide, and taking sexual risks (Rew, Whittaker, Taylor-Seehafer, et al., 2005). Nurses are instrumental in helping these youth by providing information for them and their parents, integrating sexual minority content into school sexual curricula, and providing referrals for health care and social care when needed. See Chapter 44 ∞ for further information about the health issues related to homosexuality and other sexual minority practices.

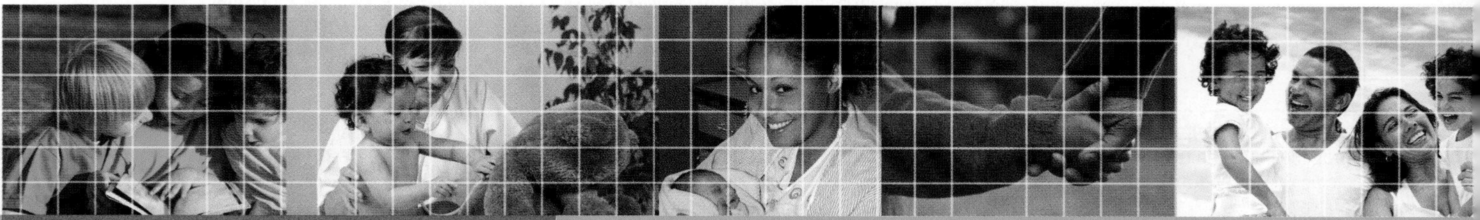

CRITICAL CONCEPT REVIEW

LEARNING OUTCOMES	CONCEPTS
33.1 Describe major theories of development as formulated by Freud, Erikson, Piaget, Kohlberg, social learning theorists, and behaviorists.	1. Freud: ■ Early childhood experiences form the unconscious motivation for action in later life. 2. Erikson: ■ There are eight periods that determine an individual's future social relationships. 3. Piaget: ■ Child's view of the world is influenced largely by age, experience, and maturational ability. 4. Kohlberg: ■ Moral decision making proceeds in a developmental fashion. 5. Social learning theorists: ■ Children learn attitudes, beliefs, and customs through social contact with adults and other children. 6. Behaviorists: ■ Behavior can be elicited by positive reinforcement and extinguished by negative reinforcement.
33.2 Recognize risk factors and factors that protect against those risks.	1. Risk Factors: ■ Financial problems ■ Stresses and worries ■ Family and job instability ■ Neighborhood and home hazards ■ Lack of resources 2. Protective Factors: ■ Coping mechanisms ■ Access to community, internet and other resources ■ Family and friend support ■ Religion, spirituality, and life meaning ■ Positive health behaviors

(continued)

LEARNING OUTCOMES	CONCEPTS
33.3 Plan nursing interventions for children that are appropriate for the child's developmental state, based on theoretical frameworks.	1. Infant: ■ Encourage parents to hold and stay with infant. ■ Provide opportunities for sucking. ■ Provide infant with toys that give comfort or stimulate interest. 2. Toddler: ■ Maintain toilet-training procedures. ■ Encourage appropriate independent behavior. ■ Give short explanations. ■ Provide rewards for appropriate behaviors. 3. Preschooler: ■ Encourage parents to be involved in care of child. ■ Provide safe versions of medical equipment for playtime. ■ Give clear explanations about procedures and illnesses. 4. School-age: ■ Provide for privacy and modesty. ■ Explain treatments and procedures clearly. ■ Encourage continuation of school work. 5. Adolescent: ■ Provide privacy. ■ Interview and examine adolescent without parents present, if possible. ■ Encourage adolescent participation in treatment and decision making. ■ Encourage visitation of peers.
33.4 Explain contemporary developmental approaches such as temperament theory, ecologic theory, and the resilience framework.	1. Ecologic theory: ■ Emphasizes the presence of mutual interactions between the child (who is unique) and various settings. 2. Temperament theory: ■ All children can be categorized into three patterns of temperament, which can be used to assist in adaptation of the child's environment and for a better understanding of the child. 3. Resiliency theory: ■ All individuals experience crises that lead to adaptation and development of inner strengths and the ability to handle future crises.
33.5 Recognize major developmental milestones for infants, toddlers, preschoolers, school-age children, and adolescents.	1. Infant: ■ Rolls over. ■ Sits up. ■ Stands. ■ Able to say one to two words. ■ Uses pincer grasp well. 2. Toddler: ■ Walks up and down stairs. ■ Undresses self. ■ Scribbles on paper. ■ Kicks a ball. ■ Has a vocabulary of 1000 words and uses short sentences. 3. Preschooler: ■ Uses scissors. ■ Rides bicycle with training wheels. ■ Throws a ball. ■ Writes a few letters. ■ All parts of speech well-developed. 4. School-age: ■ Possesses reading ability. ■ Rides a two-wheeled bike. ■ Jumps rope. ■ Plays organized sports. ■ Mature use of language. 5. Adolescent: ■ Fine motor skills well-developed. ■ Gross motor skills improve due to growth spurts.

LEARNING OUTCOMES / CONCEPTS

Learning Outcomes	Concepts
33.6 Synthesize information from several theoretical approaches to plan assessments of the child's physical growth and developmental milestones.	The nurse plans assessments of the child's: 1. Physical growth and development and prenatal influences. 2. Cognitive development. 3. Psychosocial development. 4. Personality and temperament. 5. Communication. 6. Sexuality.
33.7 Describe the role of play in the growth and development of children.	1. Infant: ■ Engages primarily in solitary play, although social interaction enhances play. ■ Learns and matures through feel and sound of activities and objects. ■ As the infant begins to crawl and walk, the sphere of play enlarges and the effect of play on growth and development increases. 2. Toddler: ■ Increased motor skills enable the toddler to engage in new ways of playing. ■ Play becomes more social, and often includes parallel play with other toddlers. ■ Engages in imitative behavior, which teaches them new actions and skills. ■ Increased cognitive abilities enable the toddler to manipulate objects and learn about their qualities. 3. Preschooler: ■ Interacts with others in associative play. ■ Enjoys large motor activities. ■ Increased manual dexterity is demonstrated in greater complexity of play activities. ■ Fantasy play enhances growth and development. 4. School-age: ■ Increased physical abilities allow greater range and complexity of activities. ■ Engages in cooperative play, which increases social and cognitive skills. 5. Adolescent: ■ Increased maturity leads to new activities and ways to play. ■ The peer group—as the focus of activities—plays an important role in establishing the adolescent's identity. ■ Participate in and learn from social interactions fundamental to adult relationships.
33.8 Use data collected during developmental assessments to implement activities that promote development of children and adolescents.	1. Discuss proper nutrition and feeding techniques. 2. Conduct health teachings and screenings that are appropriate for child's age. 3. Encourage family to discover child's personality characteristics and temperament. 4. Instruct parents in expected language skills and refer to appropriate providers for assistance. 5. Give parents information regarding appropriate and normal sexual behavior in young children. 6. Instruct school-age children concerning the expected body changes of puberty. 7. Give adolescent information concerning birth control and sexually transmitted diseases.

CRITICAL THINKING IN ACTION

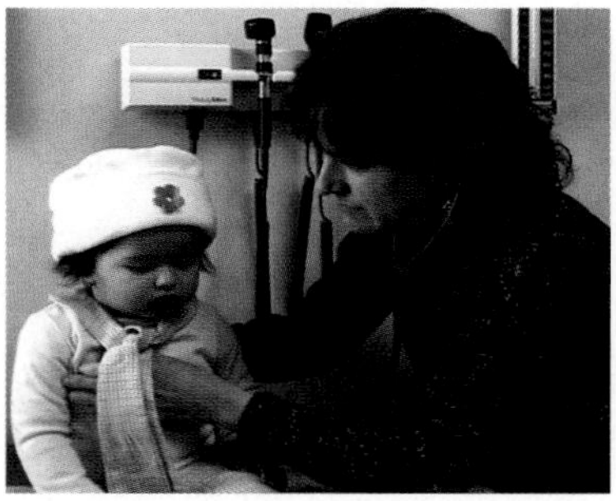

You encounter a 12-month-old child, Julia, while working in the developmental clinic. Her mother tells you that their family practice physician had concerns that Julia might have a developmental delay. She was a full-term baby and there were no complications throughout her mother's pregnancy or delivery. Julia's mother tells you that she has a generally shy and slow-to-warm-up temperament. She makes little eye contact with you and prefers to sit on her mother's lap and cling to her arms if a stranger gets close. She is able to pick up small objects, babble, crawl, and use her pincer grasp. She is not able to walk, hold a crayon, or speak any words. Julia clearly has a developmental delay.

1. What are some examples of toys you can suggest to Julia's parents based on her developmental level (not based on her age)?
2. What are some examples of hazards you can advise Julia's parents about avoiding based on her developmental level?
3. What is a suggestion you can give the parents about dealing with a child like Julia who has a shy or slow-to-warm-up temperament?

See MyNursingKit for possible responses.

REFERENCES

Ahern, N. R. (2006). Adolescent resilience: An evolutionary concept analysis. *Journal of Pediatric Nursing, 21*, 175–185.

American Academy of Pediatrics. (2004). *Pediatric nutrition handbook* (5th ed.). Elk Grove Village, IL: Author.

Aronowitz, T. (2005). The role of "envisioning the future" in the development of resilience among at-risk youth. *Public Health Nursing 22*, 200–208.

Bandura, A. (1986). *Social foundations of thought and actions: A social cognitive theory.* Englewood Cliffs, NJ: Prentice Hall.

Bandura, A. (1997a). *Self efficacy in changing societies.* New York: Cambridge University Press.

Bandura, A. (1997b). *Self efficacy: The exercise of control.* New York: Freeman.

Barnett, E. D., & Chen, L. H. (2005). Prevention of travel-related infectious diseases in families of internationally adopted children. *Pediatric Clinics of North America 52*, 1271–1286.

Bronfenbrenner, U. (1986). Ecology of the family as a context for human development: Research perspectives. *Developmental Psychology, 22*, 723–742.

Bronfenbrenner, U. (Ed.). (2005). *Making human beings human: Bioecological perspectives on human development.* Thousand Oaks, CA: Sage.

Bronfenbrenner, U., McClelland, P. D., Ceci, S. J., Moen, P., & Wethington, E. (1996). *The state of Americans.* New York: Free Press.

Chess, S., & Thomas, A. (1995). *Temperament in clinical practice.* New York: Guilford Press.

Chess, S., & Thomas, A. (1996). *Temperament: Theory and practice.* Philadelphia: Brunner/Mazel.

Chess, S., & Thomas, A. (1999). *Goodness of fit: Clinical applications from infancy through adult life.* Philadelphia: Brunner/Mazel.

Craig, G. J., & Dunn, W. L. (2007). Understanding human development. Upper Saddle River, NJ: Pearson Prentice Hall.

Dennis, C. L. (2006). Identifying predictors of breastfeeding self-efficacy in the immediate postpartum period. *Research in Nursing and Health, 28*, 256–268.

Eaton, D. K., Kann, L., Kinchen, S., Ross, J., Hawkins, J., Harris, W. A., et al., (2006). Youth Risk Behavior Surveillance–United States, 2005. *Morbidity and Mortality Weekly Report, 55*(SS05), 1–108.

Erikson, E. (1963). *Childhood and society.* New York: Norton.

Erikson, E. (1968). *Identity: Youth and crisis.* New York: Norton.

Garvey, C., Julion, S., Fogg, L., Kratovil., & Gross, D. (2006). Measuring participation in a prevention trial with parents of young children. *Research in Nursing & Health 29*, 212–222.

Ginsberg, H., & Opper, S. (1988). *Piaget's theory of intellectual development* (3rd ed.). Paramus, NJ: Prentice Hall.

Henderson, N., Benard, B., & Sharp-Light, M. (2007). *Resiliency in action.* Ojai, CA: Resiliency in Action, Inc.

Johnson, D. E. (2005). International adoption: What is fact, what is fiction, and what is the future? *Pediatric Clinics of North America, 52*, 1221–1246.

McCarter-Spaulding, D. E. (2005). Medications in pregnancy and lactation. *MCN. American Journal of Maternal Child Nursing, 30*, 10–17.

Nickman, S. L., Rosenfeld, A. A., Fine, P., MacIntyre, J. C., Pilowsky, D. J., Howe, R. A., et al. (2005). Children in adoptive families: Overview and update. *Journal of the American Academy of Child and Adolescent Psychiatry, 44*, 987–995.

Piaget, J. (1972). *The child's conception of the world.* Totowa, NJ: Littlefield, Adams.

Rettew, D. C., Stanger, C., McKee, L., Doyle, A., & Judziak, J. J. (2006). Interactions between child and parent temperament and child behavior problems. *Comprehensive Psychiatry, 47*, 412–420.

Rew, L., Whittaker, T. A., Taylor-Seehafer, M. A., & Smith, L. R. (2005). Sexual health risks and protective resources in gay, lesbian, bisexual, and heterosexual homeless youth. *Journal of Specialists in Pediatric Nursing, 10*, 11–19.

Santrock, J. (2007). *Life-span development* (10th ed.). Boston: McGraw-Hill.

Underdown, A., Barlow, J., Chung, V., & Stewart-Brown, S. (2006). Massage intervention for promoting mental and physical health in infants aged under 6 months. *Cochrane Review*, Issue 4, No CD005038.

Zirkle, D. L. (2005). Think First for Kids (TFFK): *A longitudinal analysis of a school-based injury prevention curriculum.* Unpublished doctoral dissertation, University of San Diego, California.

EXPLORE PEARSON **mynursingkit**™

MyNursingKit is your one stop for online chapter review materials and resources. Prepare for success with additional NCLEX®-style practice questions, interactive assignments and activities, web links, animations and videos, and more!

Register your access code from the front of your book at
www.mynursingkit.com

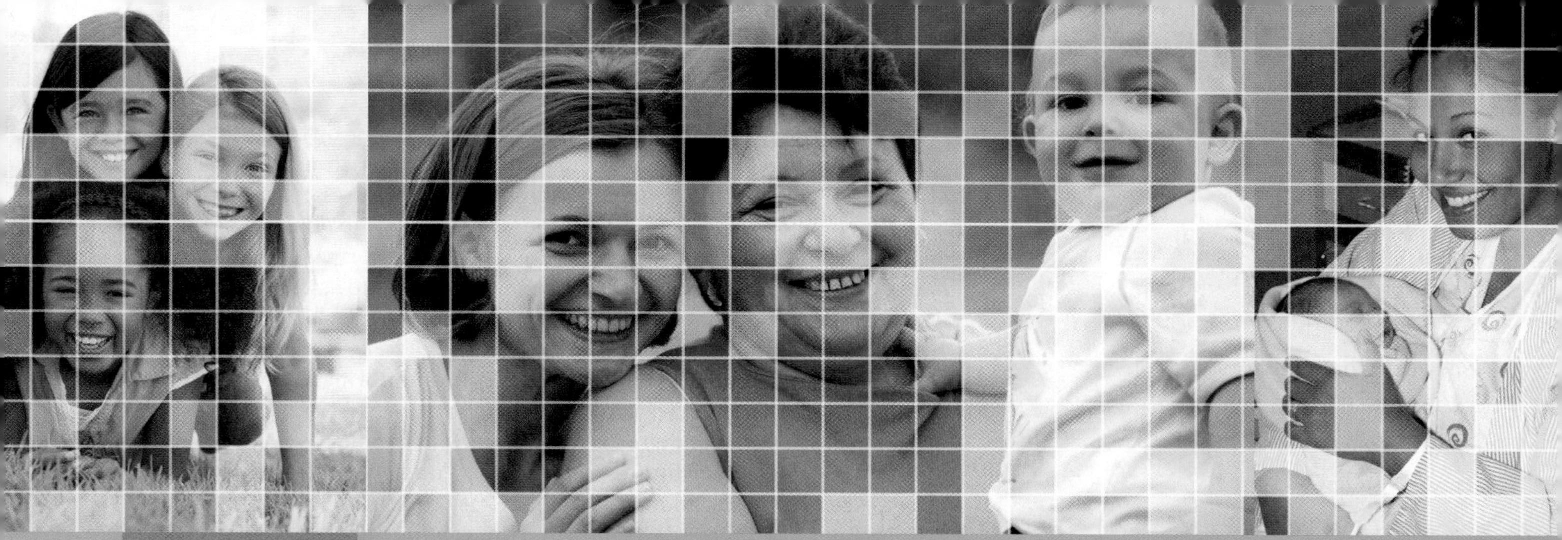

CHAPTER

34 Infant, Child, and Adolescent Nutrition

It is exciting to see Joey progressing into the school setting. Being with children his age will really help him develop in many ways. We're just worried because he needs to get only foods he can chew and swallow so he does not choke. He also needs his tube feedings during school to be sure he gets enough energy to do well. —Mother of Joey, 11 years old

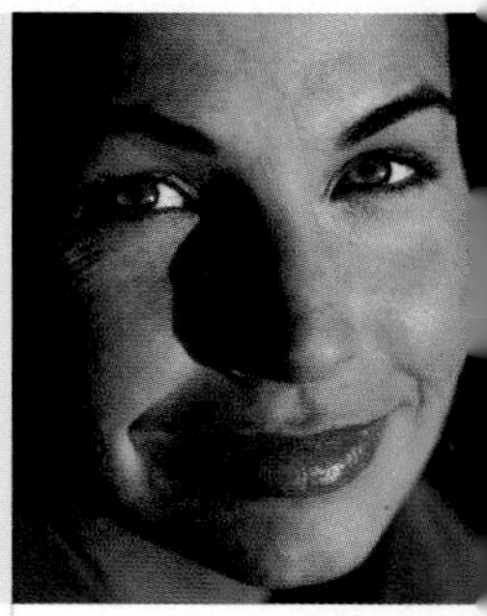

LEARNING OUTCOMES

34.1 Discuss major nutritional concepts pertaining to the growth and development of children.

34.2 Describe and plan nursing interventions to meet nutritional needs for all age groups from infancy through adolescence.

34.3 Integrate methods of nutritional assessment into nursing care of infants, children, and adolescents.

34.4 Discuss common nutritional problems of children growing up in developed countries.

34.5 Apply the nursing process to care for children with eating disorders.

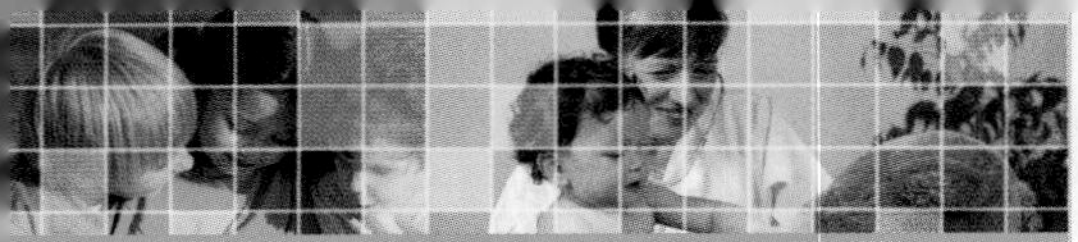

KEY TERMS

Anemia, 913
Anthropometric measurement, 904
Atopy, 920
Binge eating, 919
Body mass index (BMI), 904
Dietary Reference Intakes (DRIs), 896
Early childhood caries, 899
Enteral therapy, 923
Ergogenic aids, 921
Food allergy, 920
Food insecurity, 908
Food intolerance, 920
Food jags, 902
Food security, 908
Macronutrients, 896
Micronutrients, 896
Nutrition, 896
Physiologic anorexia, 901
Pica, 915
Probiotics, 922
Radioallergosorbent test (RAST), 920
Total parenteral nutrition (TPN), 923
Vegan, 922
Vegetarian, 922

MyNursingKit Dietary Reference Intakes

Adequate nutrition is an essential component of growth and development. The child's nutritional status begins before birth and is related to the mother's nutritional state. All children must be assessed for nutritional status and then followed by teaching or other interventions to enhance health. Nurses are instrumental in giving parents information about normal nutritional needs of infants, children, and adolescents. Common techniques to assess nutrition, such as measuring growth and monitoring hematocrit, provide needed information about whether intake of nutrients is adequate.

All children and their parents can benefit from information about nutritional needs, but some children have additional issues that must be considered. The nurse recognizes the special requirements of children with conditions such as feeding disorder, food allergies, cystic fibrosis, cerebral palsy, or diabetes. Nutrition monitoring is provided throughout childhood so that dietary counseling can be integrated with other teaching to promote development. How can the nurse bridge the various settings in which children's nutritional needs are met? These might include the home, childcare settings, schools, and hospitals. How can the nurse help the family prepare for meeting the nutritional needs of a child who has special needs during car or plane travel?

Some children have unique nutritional needs due to their social environments. Parents may not be knowledgeable about child nutritional requirements. Perhaps the family is vegetarian and needs extra help to ensure intake of essential nutrients. If finances are limited, the family may need resources such as food stamps, food banks, or budget planning. The nurse considers the high rate of childhood obesity and common nutritional deficits when applying concepts of health promotion with families. Whatever the nurse's setting, knowledge of nutrition must be integrated within nursing care.

GENERAL NUTRITION CONCEPTS

Nutrition refers to taking in food and assimilating it metabolically for use by the body. It is an essential component of life and therefore an important body of knowledge to consider in discussions of child growth and development. The body requires a wide array of nutrients. **Macronutrients**, or the major building blocks of the body, are carbohydrates, protein, and fat. Vitamins and minerals are **micronutrients**, or substances needed in small quantities for healthy body functioning. The need for nutrients is dependent on activity level, state of health, and presence of disease or other stress- and age-related requirements.

The **Dietary Reference Intakes (DRIs)** are a set of values established by the Food and Nutrition Board of the Institute of Medicine (2006) and the National Academy of Science that can be used to assess and plan intake for individuals of different ages. They commonly include Estimated Average Requirement, or EAR (intake needed to meet requirements of 50% of the population), Recommended Allowance, or RDA (intake needed to meet requirements of 97–98% of the population), Adequate Intake, or AI (used when data to support EAR is not available), and Upper Intake, or UI (maximum level unlikely to pose health risk). While the DRIs are the approach used in the United States, other countries have developed their own approaches to dietary standards. For example, Canada uses Adequate Intake and Reference Nutrient Intake, while the United Kingdom uses Recommended Daily Nutrient Intakes. The aims of these standards are to provide a method to evaluate individual and population diets and to plan nutrition programs and education. DRIs are generally specific to males and females in several age categories. See Appendix H ∞ for a list of DRIs for children and adolescents.

Although the DRIs provide useful information when evaluating diets, their use can be time consuming. What "quick check" can provide feedback about the daily diets of children? The nurse should be familiar with the U.S. MyPyramid Food Guide and hang it in schools, clinics, and hospitals. It is a fast way to examine children's intakes for one day and evaluate if they meet most requirements. Instead of calculating

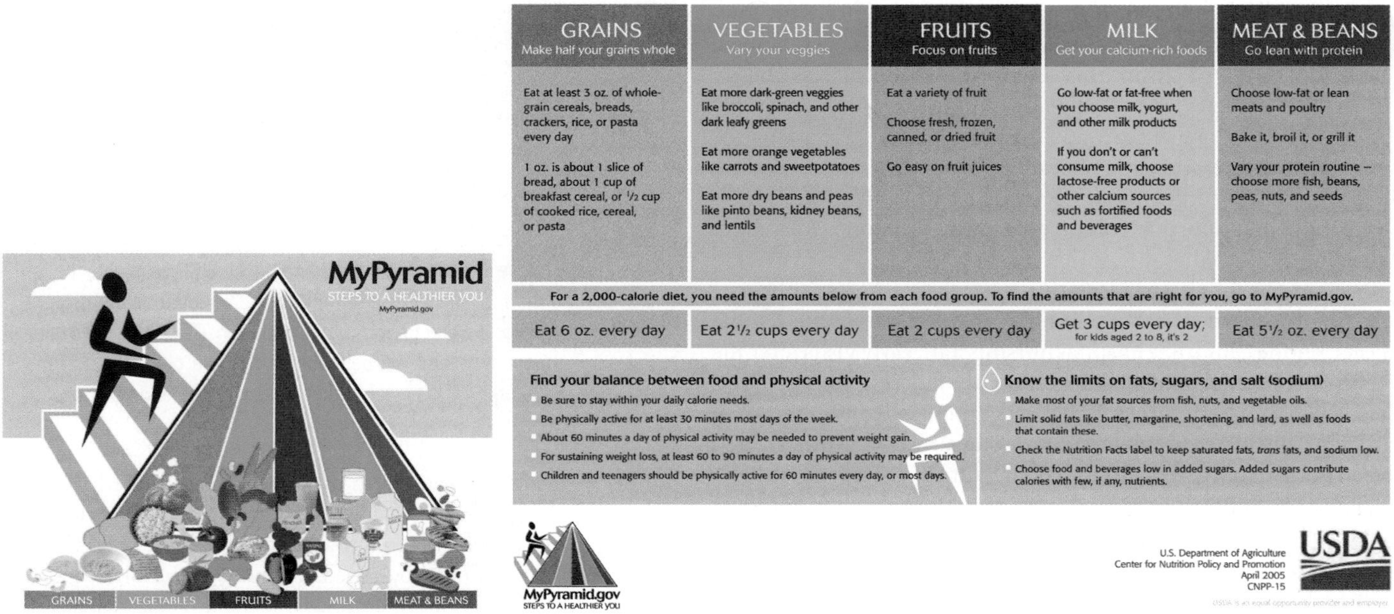

● **Figure 34–1** Food Guide Pyramid. The Food Guide Pyramid is used to provide teaching about amounts of foods recommended for daily intake.

Sources: Courtesy of the U.S. Department of Agriculture and U.S. Department of Health and Human Services (2005).

amounts of nutrients ingested, the pyramid focuses on categories of foods, which readily reflects the actual intake. The numbers of servings from various categories stay constant throughout childhood, while the serving sizes increase as the child gets older. See Figure 34–1● for the Food Guide Pyramid, and consult the USDA Web site for ethnic/cultural food guide pyramids for vegetarians and those from various ethnic groups, such as Hispanic and Native American (http://fnic.nal.usda.gov).

NUTRITIONAL NEEDS

Nutritional needs evolve during all of infancy and childhood. They support growth and development and influence the progression of the child along the developmental path. Nutritional intake helps to maintain the health of the child and fosters a state of maximal potential or health promotion. Specific needs during each developmental stage are discussed in this section. See further information about the newborn nutrition in Chapter 27∞.

INFANCY

Breast Milk and Formula-Feeding

From the first feeding of a few ounces of breast milk to a meal of soft table foods with the family at 1 year of age, the infant demonstrates an amazing growth in ability to ingest and digest a wide variety of foods. Never again will the child have such a high metabolic rate or high intake requirements in relation to size or such a change in the types of foods eaten. Infants have an extremely fast rate of growth, since birth weight is usually doubled by about 5 months of age and tripled by 1 year. Meeting nutritional needs is challenged by the small size of the infant's stomach and the immaturity of the digestive system. Their great amount of physical activity also necessitates high caloric intake. Nutrient demands for protein and vitamins must be met for the cells of the nervous system and body organs to develop properly. Both energy for metabolism and energy for growth are essential. The estimated energy requirement ranges from 300 kcal/d at one month to 800 kcal/day by 1 year (Institute of Medicine, 2005a). See Chapter 46∞ for descriptions of the water needs of infants and children.

The natural first food is breast milk and its intake should be encouraged for all infants. See Chapter 27∞ for a discussion of newborn nutrition and Chapter 28∞ for nutrition for the infant at risk. The American Academy of Pediatrics believes that breastfeeding is the best source of nutrition for babies through the first birthday and should be encouraged by health professionals (American Academy of Pediatrics [AAP], Committee on Nutrition, 2009; AAP Section on Breast-Feeding, 2005). The American Diabetes Association (2008) states that broad-based efforts are needed to break barriers to breastfeeding, citing that exclusive breastfeeding for 6 months, and breastfeeding with supplementary foods for at least 12 months, is the ideal feeding pattern for infants. The U.S. Preventive Services Task Force recommends breastfeeding education and behavioral counseling in 30- to 90-minute individual or group sessions with specially trained nurses or lactation specialists (www.preventiveservices.ahrq.gov). While breast milk is the best nutritional source for infants, babies may need some limited supplements.

Providing breastfeeding information and instruction positively influences the number of women who decide to breastfeed and increases the number of months they choose to continue breastfeeding. Teaching can emphasize the importance of breastfeeding to the child's well-being. Many advantages to breastfeeding are known, including excellent nutritional balance, promotion of

MyNursingKit Video: Breastfeedding and First Foods

gastrointestinal function, fostering immune defense with lowered allergy risk, lower incidence of otitis media, psychologic benefits, less risk of chronic diseases in adulthood such as obesity or type 2 diabetes and cardiovascular disease, and economic advantage (National Institutes of Health, 2008). Programs for encouraging breastfeeding should involve education and skill/problem-solving information provided by health professionals and trained supportive volunteers (Watt, McGlone, Russell, et al., 2006).

Some hospitals have lactation specialists who assist breastfeeding mothers; in others, nurses provide this service. Home visits, phone calls from hospital nursing staff, early visits after the birth to obstetric and pediatric offices, and resources such as LaLeche League can provide mothers with needed breastfeeding information and problem-solving suggestions. Mothers also need information on getting adequate nutritional intake and sufficient rest. Support programs are especially helpful to mothers who have difficulty breastfeeding, feel unsure how it will fit into family and work life, are very young, or have an infant with problems related to feeding.

The mother of a hospitalized infant needs special support to continue breastfeeding. The mother should be encouraged to come to the hospital to feed her baby on the same schedule she would use at home. If the infant cannot breastfeed, the hospital can provide an electric pump so the mother can maintain lactation. Often hospitals provide meals for the mother of a hospitalized baby so that she can maintain good nutrition and quality breast milk while her infant is in the hospital.

Some women decide not to breastfeed at all or are unable to breastfeed. And mothers who do breastfeed may, after the first few months, begin to use supplemental bottles of formula when the infant is away from them. Nurses support mothers in their decisions for infant feeding and provide them with information about formula preparation and feeding. Three types of formula are available—ready to feed, concentrate, and powder. All are nutritionally adequate for infants. Nurses can help parents decide which preparation of formula is best suited for their infants (see Table 34–1) and teach methods of preparation (see "Nursing Practice"). Most regular cow's milk and soy formulas contain about 20 calories/ounce, while higher caloric formula (24–25 calories/ounce) are available for preterm babies who have limited ability to ingest the high volume needed for growth. Healthcare providers assist the parents to choose a milk-based formula (e.g., Enfamil Lipil, Good Start, Similac) or soy-based formula (e.g., Isomil, Nursoy, Prosobee, Soyalac, or Good Start Soy). Some infants, such as those

Nursing Practice

Review type and preparation of formula at each healthcare visit. Concentrate or powder formula can be mixed with tap water but must be refrigerated once mixed. No water should be added to ready-to-feed formula. Formula that the infant does not drink should be discarded after use and not kept for future feedings. This minimizes the chance for bacteria to grow and to cause illness in the baby. When the family lives in older housing, caution them to run tap water for about 2 minutes before using it and to use only cold water for formula preparation. These practices minimize the chance that lead will be leached from the older pipes in the house (see Chapter 44 ∞ for further discussion of lead poisoning).

Teaching Highlights

SUPPLEMENTS FOR BREASTFED BABIES

1. Each baby receives a vitamin K injection after birth to promote adequate blood clotting. After that, no further vitamin K is needed since the child manufactures this vitamin in the gut once he or she begins eating.
2. Vitamin D is recommended at a minimum of 400 IU/day for all infants (Wagner, Greer, & Section on Breastfeeding, 2008).
3. Iron is not needed unless the infant is not eating food with iron by 4 to 6 months. The baby may need an iron source earlier if the mother was anemic during pregnancy or while breastfeeding.
4. Fluoride 0.25 mg is given after 6 months of age if water is not fluoridated to a level of 0.3 parts per million (ppm), or if the baby is not drinking any water.

Table 34–1 Advantages and Disadvantages of Formula Preparations

Formula Preparation	How Packaged	Advantages	Disadvantages
Ready to feed	Bottles or cans	No preparation needed	Most expensive type of formula
Concentrate	Cans of concentrated liquid	Easy to add equal amounts of formula concentrate and water directly into bottle and shake	Can be incorrectly measured, leading to inadequate or unsafe nutrition for infant; requires access to clean water supply such as city tap water or bottled water; well water may have too high a mineral concentration
Powder	Cans	Least expensive type of formula	Can be incorrectly measured, leading to inadequate or unsafe nutrition for infant; requires shaking to mix thoroughly; requires access to clean water supply such as city tap water or bottled water; well water may have too high a mineral concentration

with phenylketonuria or other metabolic disorders, require specialized formulas. Examples of these types of formula include low phenylalanine, casein hydrolysate, sodium caseinate, lactose free, and synthetic amino acid formulas (AAP, Committee on Nutrition, 2009). Breast- or bottle-feeding is discussed at each contact with health professionals to identify potential teaching needs.

Dental Health

Early childhood caries, the presence of one or more decayed, lost, or filled tooth surfaces in a primary tooth from birth to 6 years of age, can occur when a young child is allowed to breastfeed or drink from a bottle for long periods, especially when sleeping (Gussy, Waters, Walsh, et al., 2006) (Figure 34–2 ●). The milk, juice, or other fluid pools around the upper anterior teeth, salivary flow decreases, and acid buffering is decreased, resulting in tooth decay. Nurses should teach parents to avoid putting the child to bed with a bottle and encourage pacifier use or a bottle of water instead. The child should not walk around with a bottle during the day. Mothers who breastfeed should also be cautioned to limit feeding to specific times rather than letting the infant breastfeed every few minutes (sometimes done when infant and mother co-sleep) so that milk will not pool in the mouth during sleep. When sleepy the infant does not swallow well and the milk is in constant contact with the teeth where milk sugars can decay erupting teeth.

Parents can be taught beginning dental care for the infant, which includes wiping the teeth off daily once they erupt with a piece of moist gauze or a small infant toothbrush. Some pediatric dentists like to see the child for a first dental visit at about 1 year of age, while others wait until the child is older. The nurse should encourage the parents to select and establish contact with a dental provider when the child is nearing the end of infancy.

Weaning

The decision to wean the baby from the breast may be made for a variety of reasons, including family or cultural pressures, changes in the home situation, pressure from the woman's partner, or a personal opinion about when weaning should occur. Some infants wean themselves spontaneously, despite the wishes of the mother. For the woman who is comfortable with breastfeeding and well informed about the process, the appropriate time to wean her infant will become evident if she is sensitive to the child's cues. Often weaning falls between periods of great developmental activity for the child. Thus weaning commonly occurs at 8 to 9 months, 12 to 14 months, 18 months, 2 years, and 3 years of age. The infant who is weaned before 12 months should be given iron-fortified infant formula, not cow's milk. The ACOG recommends breastfeeding for a duration of at least 6 months, longer if feasible (American College of Obstetricians and Gynecologists, 2007).

If weaning is timed to respond to the child's cues, and if the mother is comfortable with the timing, it can be accomplished with less difficulty than if the process begins before mother and child are ready emotionally. Nevertheless, weaning is a time of emotional separation for mother and baby; it may be difficult for them to give up the closeness of their nursing sessions. The nurse who is understanding about this possibility can help the mother see that her infant is growing up and plan other comforting, consoling, and play activities to replace breastfeeding. A gradual approach is the easiest and most comforting way to wean the child from breastfeedings.

During weaning, the mother should substitute one cup feeding or bottle feeding for one breastfeeding session over a few days to a week so that her breasts gradually produce less milk. Eliminating the breastfeedings associated with meals first facilitates the mother's ability to wean the infant, because satiation with food lessens the desire for milk. Over a period of several weeks she can substitute more cup feedings or bottle feedings for breastfeedings. The slow method of weaning prevents breast engorgement, allows infants to alter their eating methods at their own rates, and provides time for psychologic adjustment.

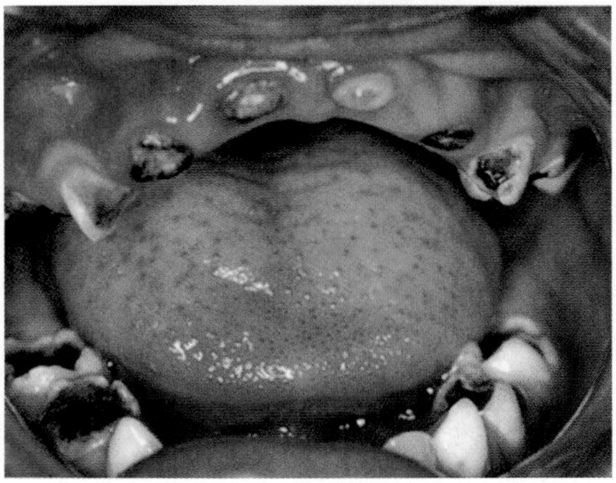

● **Figure 34–2** Early childhood caries. This child has had major tooth decay related to sleeping as an infant and toddler while sucking bottles of juice and milk.

Source: Courtesy of Dr. Lezley McIlveen, Department of Dentistry, Children's National Medical Center, Washington, DC.

Introduction of Complementary Foods

When should other foods be added to the infant's diet? Although some parents add other foods when the infant is only days or weeks old and such practices are often culturally derived, it is best to take cues from the infant's developmental milestones. The American Academy of Pediatrics recommends introducing semisolid food at 4 to 6 months (AAP, Committee on Nutrition, 2009). At this age the extrusion reflex (or tongue thrust) decreases and the infant can sit well with support. The infant is also developing the ability to appreciate texture and swallow nonliquid foods and can indicate desire for food or turn away when full. At 6–12 months, complementary foods are offered in addition to the intake of breast milk or formula, rather than replacing that essential nutrient (Hagan, Shaw & Duncan, 2008) (see Table 34–2).

The first complementary food added to the infant's diet is often rice cereal. The advantages of introducing cereal first is that it provides iron at an age when the infant's prenatal iron stores begin to decrease, it seldom causes allergy, and it is easy to digest. A tablespoon or two is fed to the infant once or twice daily just before formula or breastfeeding. The infant may appear to spit out food at first because of normal back-and-forth tongue movement. Parents should not interpret this early feeding behavior as

Table 34–2 Introduction of Solid Foods in Infancy

Recommendation	Rationale
Introduce rice cereal at 4–6 months.	Rice cereal is easy to digest, has low allergenic potential, and contains iron.
Introduce fruits or vegetables at 6–8 months. Some healthcare providers recommend vegetable introduction before fruits.	Fruits and vegetables provide needed vitamins. Vegetables are not as sweet as fruits; introducing them first may enhance acceptability to the infant.
Introduce meats at 8–10 months.	Meats are harder to digest, have high protein load, and should not be fed until close to 1 year of age.
Use single-food prepared baby foods rather than combination meals.	Combination meals usually contain more sugar, salt, and fillers.
Introduce one new food at a time, waiting at least 3–4 days to introduce another. Delay feeding eggs, strawberries, wheat, corn, fish, and nut products until close to 2–3 years of age.	If a food allergy or intolerance develops, it will be easy to identify. The foods listed are those most commonly associated with food allergy.
Avoid carrots, beets, and spinach before 4 months of age. Have well water evaluated for nitrates (the recommended level is less than 10 mg/L).	Nitrates in these foods and in water near agricultural runoff can be converted to nitrite by young infants, causing methemoglobinemia.
Infants can be fed mashed portions of table foods such as carrots, rice, and potatoes.	This is a less expensive alternative to jars of commercially prepared baby food; it allows parents of various cultural groups to feed ethnic foods to infants.
Avoid adding sugar, salt, and spices when preparing baby foods at home.	Infants need not become accustomed to these flavors; they may get too much sodium from salt or develop gastric distress from some spices.
Avoid honey until at least 1 year of age.	Infants cannot detoxify *Clostridium botulinum* spores sometimes present in honey and can develop botulism.

indicating dislike for the food. With a little practice the infant becomes adept at spoon feeding.

Once the infant eats 1/4 cup of cereal twice daily, usually at 6 to 8 months of age, vegetables or fruits can be introduced, at a rate of one new food every several days (Table 34–2). By 8 to 10 months of age, most fruits and vegetables have been introduced and strained meats or other protein (e.g., tofu, cheese, mashed cooked beans) can be added to the infant's diet. Finger foods are introduced during the second half of the first year as the infant's palmar and then finger grasp develops and as teeth begin to erupt (Figure 34–3 ●). Infants enjoy toast, O-shaped cereal, finely sliced meats, cheese and tofu, and small pieces of cooked, softened vegetables.

Certain foods are more commonly associated with development of food allergies, and avoiding them in infancy may decrease allergy incidence. Recommendations for infants at risk due to family history of allergy are to delay feeding of cow milk until 1 year, eggs until 2 years, and peanuts, nuts, fish, and shellfish until 3 years (AAP, 2009). As food and juice intake increase, formula- or breastfeedings decrease in amount and frequency (Table 34–3).

If breastfeeding is not chosen, or if supplemental feedings are given, only iron-fortified infant formula should be used during the first year of life. Cow's milk (including evaporated milk) can lead to bleeding and anemia (see content on iron and anemia on page 913 in this chapter), can interfere with absorption of some nutrients, and has a high solute load which immature kidneys can have diffi-

● **Figure 34–3** Introducing finger foods. The baby who has developed the ability to grasp with thumb and forefinger should receive some foods that can be held in the hand.

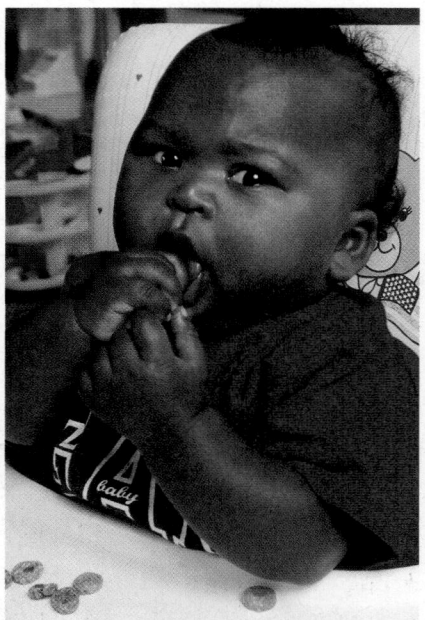

Table 34–3 Infant Nutritional Pattern

Age	Pattern
Birth–1 month	■ Eats every 2–3 hours, breast or bottle ■ 2–3 ounces (60–90 mL) per feeding
2–4 months	■ Has coordinated suck–swallow ■ Eats every 3–4 hours ■ 3–4 ounces (90–120 mL) per feeding
4–6 months	■ Begins baby food, usually rice cereal, 2–3 T, twice daily ■ Consumes breast milk or formula 4 or more times daily ■ 4–5 ounces (100–150 mL) per feeding
6–8 months	■ Eats baby food such as rice cereal, fruits, and vegetables, 2–5 T, three times daily ■ Consumes breast milk or formula 4 times daily ■ 6–8 ounces (160–225 mL) per feeding
8–10 months	■ Enjoys soft finger foods three times daily ■ Consumes breast milk or formula 4 times daily ■ 6 ounces (160 mL) per feeding ■ Uses cup with lid
10–12 months	■ Eats most soft table foods with family three times daily ■ Uses cup with or without lid ■ Attempts to feed self with spoon though spills often ■ Consumes breast milk or formula 4 times daily ■ 6–8 ounces (160–225 mL) per feeding

culty excreting. Iron-fortified formula should always be used when the infant under 12 months drinks formula. When breastfed babies are not eating foods with iron by 4 to 6 months, supplemental iron may need to be added. Careful dietary assessment and discussion of intake by the nurse at health visits helps the practitioner decide if supplemental iron is needed.

Weaning is the term used when babies give up breastfeeding or a bottle and obtain most fluids by cup. At about 8 to 9 months, a cup should be offered to the baby with assistance provided so that learning about drinking from a cup can begin. By about 1 year of age, babies are usually able to drink most liquids from a cup with a lid so bottles can be slowly withdrawn and replaced by cups. Breastfeeding may continue if the parent and infant desire, but introduction of other foods and a cup for drinking water or juice are still required. Older infants and toddlers should be offered cups with beverages other than water only at meal and snack times so they become accustomed to drinking with their meals rather than carrying a bottle or cup for much of the day. Drinking beverages other than water, such as fruit juices throughout the day, increases the risk of dental caries and excess calorie intake (AAP, Committee on Nutrition, 2009).

Parents who want to make baby foods at home can be encouraged and instructed to do so. Some commercially prepared foods have unnecessary additives such as salt, sugar, and food starch, and they may be costly for some families. Parents can easily blend fruits and vegetables the family is eating without adding salt, sugar, or seasoning. Prepared foods should be used promptly and stored in the refrigerator between feedings. Foods can also be placed into ice cube trays and frozen; a cube or two can be defrosted at mealtime. Nurses should caution parents not to use honey in foods for infants as it can lead to infant botulism since infants cannot detoxify *Clostridium botulinum* spores sometimes present in honey. If foods or fluids are microwaved, they should be shaken, stirred, and checked for temperature so that hot areas in the food do not burn the infant.

Nursing Practice

Advise parents to use caution when providing finger foods to the infant. Hard foods and some soft and malleable ones slip easily into the throat and may cause choking. Avoid hot dogs, hard vegetables, candy, and chunks of peanut butter. Infants and other young children should always be supervised while eating. Be sure parents are familiar with techniques for airway obstruction removal and have emergency numbers clearly listed on their phones.

TODDLERHOOD

MyNursingKit Typical Daily Intake at Various Ages

Why do parents of toddlers frequently become concerned about the small amount of food their children eat? Why do toddlers seem to survive and even thrive with minimal food intake? The toddler often displays the phenomenon of **physiologic anorexia**, caused when the extremely high metabolic demands of infancy slow to keep pace with the more moderate growth rate of toddlerhood. Although it can appear that the toddler eats nothing at times, intake over days or a week is generally sufficient and balanced enough to meet the body's demands for nutrients and energy.

Parents often need knowledge about the types of foods that constitute a healthy diet. Some easy-to-prepare foods are high in salt and other additives and can lead to exceeding the recommendation of *Healthy People 2010* for sodium intake (U.S. Department of Health and Human Services [USDHHS], 2006). The nurse can offer alternatives to hot dogs, microwave meals, or fast foods by providing information about easy preparation of sliced meats, cheese, tofu, fruits, and vegetables. Healthy snacks for young children include yogurt, cheese, milk, slices of bread with peanut butter, thinly sliced fruits, and soft vegetables.

Parents should be advised to offer a variety of nutritious foods several times daily (three meals and two snacks) and let the toddler make choices from the foods offered. They should offer foods only at mealtimes and have the child sit in a high chair or on a special seat at the table to eat (Figure 34–4 ●). Small portions are most appealing to the toddler. A general guideline for food quantity at a meal is one tablespoon of each food per year of age.

The toddler should drink 16 to 24 oz (1/2 to 3/4 L) of milk daily. Parents should be cautioned against giving the toddler more than a quart (one liter) of milk daily, since this interferes with the desire to eat other foods, leading to dietary deficiencies. Recall that the child should not be put to bed with a bottle or allowed to carry a bottle of milk or juice around during the day,

MyNursingKit | Plan a Nutrition Teaching Session

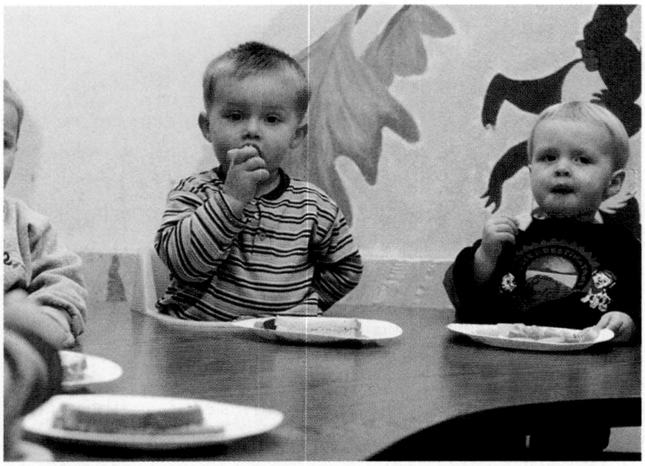

● **Figure 34–4** Fostering healthy eating habits. Toddlers should sit at a table or in a high chair to eat, to minimize the chance of choking and to foster positive eating patterns.

due to the risk of early childhood caries (see earlier discussion). In addition, parents should be advised to use only 100% fruit juice and to limit consumption of this juice to 4 to 6 ounces daily for children ages 1 to 6 years to decrease the opportunity for becoming overweight, or developing dental caries, and abdominal discomfort (O'Connor, Yang, & Hicklas, 2006). Unpasteurized juice should never be used since it may contain pathogens particularly harmful to young children (Centers for Disease Control and Prevention [CDC], 2005). Drinking water and eating whole fruits, which provide fiber, are healthier alternatives. Avoid more than one meal weekly from a fast food restaurant due to the generally high fat, high-sugar, and low fiber content of such meals.

Learning how to eat with others is an important task of toddlerhood. The toddler displays characteristic autonomy or independence during mealtime. Advise parents to provide opportunities for self-feeding of food with fingers and utensils and to allow some simple choices, such as type of liquid or cup to use. Young children should eat at a table with others, not be allowed to run and play while eating, and eat at specified meal and snack times. Toddlers should be taught to brush teeth after each meal and care providers should offer assistance and supervision. A dental visit should occur during toddlerhood.

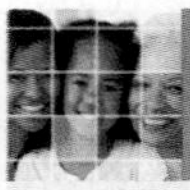

Growth and Development

MyNursingKit | Diet and Culture

Toddlers generally eat three meals and two to three snacks daily. Toddlers can drink 2% milk or "follow-up" formula starting at 2 years of age. Cups are recommended, and bottle use should be discontinued. Drinks should be consumed at mealtimes and for snacks while sitting at a table; carrying cups during the day while playing or at other activities is not recommended. The child is learning to use utensils but may prefer fingers and still needs small serving sizes.

Because social skills are developing, the hospitalized toddler may eat better if allowed to have meals with parents or other hospitalized children. See Chapter 41 ∞ for further suggestions about management of nutrition in hospitalized children.

PRESCHOOL

The diet of the preschooler is similar to that of the toddler, but mealtime is now a more social event. Preschoolers like the company of others while they eat, and they enjoy helping with food preparation and table setting (Figure 34–5 ●). Involving them in these tasks can provide a forum for teaching about nutritious foods and principles of preparation, such as the need for refrigeration, safety around stoves, and cleanliness. Visits to fast food restaurants should be limited to about once weekly, and parents can use the opportunity to assist the child in making wise choices of nutritionally adequate foods in that setting.

Although the rate of growth is slow and steady during the preschool years, the child may have periods of **food jags** (eating only a few foods for several days or weeks) and greater or lesser intake. Parents should be advised to assess food intake over a 1- or 2-week period rather than at each meal to obtain a more accurate impression of total intake. Food jags can be handled by providing the desired food along with other foods to foster choice. The child who chooses not to eat at snacktime or mealtime should not be given other foods in between. The child will become hungry and get accustomed to eating when food is provided. Three meals and two or three snacks daily are the norm. Fruit juice should be limited to 8 to 12 ounces daily, and begin teaching the "5-a-day" program that supports having five servings of fruits/vegetables each day.

The preschool period is a good time to continue encouraging good dental habits. Children can begin to brush their own teeth with parental supervision and help to reach all tooth surfaces. Fluoride supplements should be used when the water supply is not fluoridated. If the child has not yet visited a dentist, the first dental visit should be scheduled so the child can become accustomed to the routine of dental care.

SCHOOL AGE

The school-age years are a period of gradual growth when energy requirements remain at a steady level, although at some point during these years, most children experience a preadolescent growth spurt. Girls may begin a growth spurt by 10 or 11 years, and boys a year or so later. Nutritional needs increase dramatically with this spurt, with large numbers of calories and increased amounts of other nutrients required (see Appendix H for Dietary Reference Intakes ∞).

School-age children are increasingly responsible for preparing snacks, lunches, and even some other meals. These years are a good time to teach children how to choose nutritious foods and plan a well-balanced meal. Because school-age children operate at the concrete level of cognitive thought, nutrition teaching is best presented by using pictures, samples of foods, videotapes, handouts, and hands-on experience.

School-age children often prefer the types of food eaten at home and may be resistant to new food items. A hospitalized child may refuse to eat, slowing the recuperative process. Nurses should encourage family members to bring favorite foods from

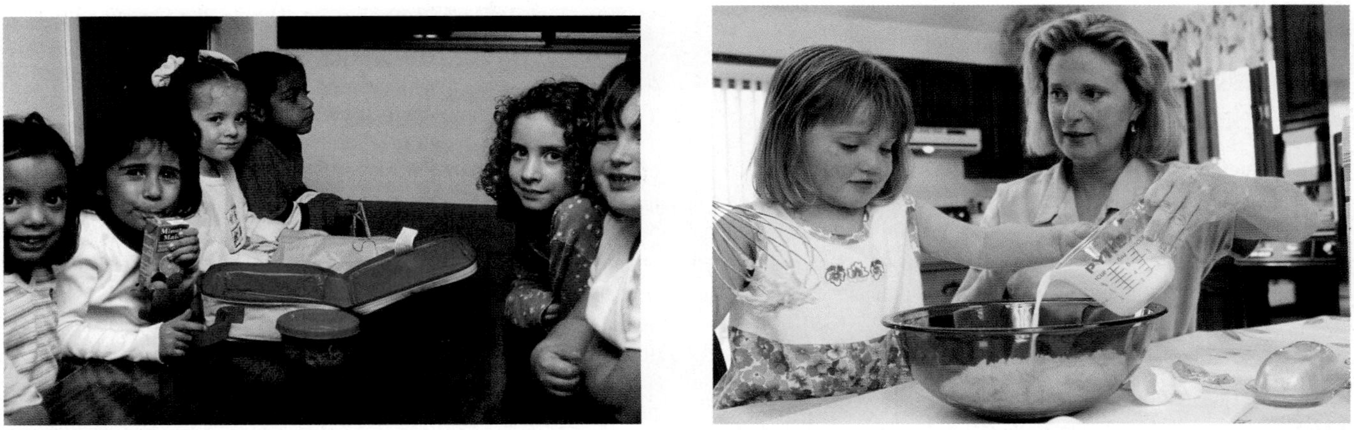

● **Figure 34–5** Preschool food habits. Preschoolers learn food habits by eating with others. Engaging them in food preparation enhances knowledge of food and promotes intake at meals.

home that meet nutritional requirements. This can be especially helpful when the hospital serves food only from the dominant cultural group. A child accustomed to a diet of rice, tofu, and vegetables may not enjoy a hospital meal of hamburger and fries. By school-age, food has become strongly associated with social interaction, so it is beneficial to have children eat together or to invite family members to take the child off the unit to eat or to bring in food from home and eat with the child. Many hospitals allow children to plan a pizza night or sponsor other events to encourage eating in a social atmosphere.

Most children consume at least one meal daily in school. While children may bring lunches to school, most participate in school lunch programs, and perhaps school breakfast programs. Nurses should become familiar with the policies of school districts in their areas for providing foods, snacks, and reduced-price food to students in need. Over the past decade, many school systems in the United States have allowed vending machines for carbonated sweetened beverages and snacks to be installed in public schools. Part of the profits from these machines has enabled revenue-strapped school districts to enhance their incomes. However, schools are increasingly challenged about the presence of the machines, especially in light of the growing problem of overweight among youth. Some school districts have now limited the number of machines or the hours during which they can be used by students. Nurses are able to provide information for districts about the problems of obesity and the need for healthy foods for youth.

The opening quote in this chapter is from the mother of Joey, a young boy with cerebral palsy who has a gastrostomy feeding tube to assist him in ingestion of adequate nutrients. Joey is attending school and the teacher has been taught to administer his tube feedings. Nurses often assist families who have children with special needs to integrate them into the school environment. How might the nurse plan for Joey to participate in school lunchtime with peers? Since he can eat some soft foods by mouth, what types of foods are commonly available at school that he might be able to enjoy?

The loss of the first deciduous teeth and the eruption of permanent teeth usually occur at about 6 years, or at the beginning of the school-age period. Of the 32 permanent teeth, 22 to 26 erupt by age 12 years, and the remaining molars follow in the teenage years. See Chapter 35 for the typical sequence of tooth eruption and Chapter 37 for dental care needs during childhood. The school-age child should be closely monitored to ensure that brushing and flossing are adequate, that fluoride is taken if the water supply is not fluoridated, that dental care is obtained to provide for examination of teeth and alignment, and that loose teeth are identified before surgery or sports participation.

ADOLESCENCE

MyNursingKit Fast Food Analysis

Most adolescents need well over 2000 calories daily to support the growth spurt, and some adolescent boys require nearly 3000 or more calories daily. When teenagers are active in a variety of sports, these requirements increase further. Because adolescents prepare much of their own food and often eat with friends, they need to be taught about good nutrition. Developing a diet that includes a large number of calories, meets vitamin and mineral requirements, and is acceptable to the teen may be a challenge.

The pregnant adolescent has even more challenging nutrient requirements. See Chapter 13 for details about needs during pregnancy. An adolescent who is hospitalized and does not like the hospital lunch sometimes has a friend who visits bring a soft drink and chips; however, the teen may be receptive to offers of juice and pizza, a more nutritious meal. Small improvements should be viewed positively as they may lead to further changes.

Fast food represents a significant intake for many adolescents. It is commonly high in fat, calories, and sodium while being low in essential nutrients such as calcium, folic acid, riboflavin, vitamins A and C, and fiber. Many schools are redesigning cafeterias and food programs to entice more teens to eat at school rather than nearby fast food restaurants. Adding fruits and salads and allowing choice can enhance quality of food intake. School nurses play a vital role in helping to tailor a healthy school nutrition program and teaching teens about the most healthy choices at their favorite fast food restaurants.

Peer group influence is important to teens, so group sessions in which adolescents eat lunch together can provide a forum for influencing food habits. What other methods might encourage positive nutritional habits among teens?

Evidence-Based Nursing

ADOLESCENTS AND NUTRITIONAL CHOICES

Clinical Question

Adolescents are largely independent in their food choices. They often eat "on the run" and are influenced by peers and the media. At the same time, rates of obesity are on an escalating upward trajectory. Nurses need to understand and apply evidence-based practices for influencing eating behaviors in adolescents.

Evidence

Jenkins and Horner (2005) conducted a literature review on adolescent nutrition publications in the last decade. Twenty-two articles on eating patterns, barriers, and nutrition interventions met their criteria for review and became the basis of their analysis. Important topics were family effects on adolescent eating, cultural and economic factors, school effects on diet, and community effects on adolescent eating behaviors. While the studies identified important influences on adolescent eating, the authors noted that there is a lack of information about ethnic minority group influences, socioeconomic factors, interventions that will assist adolescents to change unhealthy behaviors, and the role of parents in adolescent eating. In another study by several nurses in North Carolina, 10 adolescents made significantly healthier choices from a fast food menu after a short nutrition education session that focused on the food pyramid and food categories (Allen, Taylor, & Kuiper, 2007).

Best Practice

While adolescent nutritional intake is an important health concern, there is a limited body of knowledge to guide the health professional. Findings of importance are that child and adolescent eating patterns set an important example for life and that the family eating patterns, school setting, and community influences must all be examined to identify risk and protective factors in the adolescent diet. Important barriers to adolescent health eating include availability of "junk food" snacks, lack of parental involvement in the lives of teens, and the media messages about food consumption.

Critical Thinking

1. What developmental stages of the adolescent provide both challenges to healthy eating and ability to make wise food choices?
2. Construct a list of questions about family food patterns that will help you identify risk and protective factors of the family.
3. Visit a local high school and then travel 1/2 mile in each direction from the school. Record the number of fast food restaurants, billboards about foods, and any other food-related resources or media. Watch 2 hours of television at 3–5 p.m., when adolescents frequently arrive home. Record the number of food-related messages, what types of foods are advertised, and other observations.
4. How can you integrate knowledge about adolescent nutrition into your potential role as a school nurse at a high school?

See MyNursingKit for possible responses.

MyNursingKit Video: Nutritional Status

NUTRITIONAL ASSESSMENT

What is the best indication that the child's nutrition is adequate? Which data-collection methods provide the most accurate information about a child's dietary intake? The nurse plays an important role in assessing the diets of children and in seeking additional evaluation from dietitians and nutritionists in complex situations.

PHYSICAL AND BEHAVIORAL MEASUREMENT

Growth Measurement

A common method of evaluating the adequacy of diet is measurement of growth. **Anthropometric measurement** is the term used to refer to assessment of various parts of the body. Anthropometry of young children commonly includes weight, length, and head circumference. Standing height is substituted for length once the child can stand. Head circumference, also known as occipital-frontal circumference (OFC), is measured during infancy, and into early years when there are growth concerns. Additional measurements that may be included in special circumstances include chest circumference, mid-upper arm circumference, and skinfold measurement at sites such as triceps, abdomen, and subscapular regions. Grids are available for each measurement and assist in providing a thorough nutritional assessment when weight and height are abnormally high or low. Skills 9–1 through 9–6 in the accompanying Clinical Skills Manual SKILLS present techniques for accurate measurement of weight, length, height, chest circumference, and head circumference.

MyNursingKit Growth Chart Analysis

After collecting the measurements, the nurse plots them on the appropriate standardized growth curves for weight, length to height, head circumference, and body mass index (Figure 34–6 ●). **Body mass index (BMI)** is a calculation based on the child's weight and height, or length, and is calculated as kilograms of weight/m^2 of height. This is a useful calculation for determining if the child's height and weight are in proportion and identifies which percentile the child falls in for each measurement. Children normally fall between the 10th and 90th percentiles. A measurement below the 10th percentile, especially for BMI, may indicate undernutrition, while one over the 90th percentile can indicate overnutrition. However, it is important to look at the differences between measurements. An infant in the 90th percentile for length, weight, and head circumference is proportional and may be a naturally large baby. On the other hand, a child who is consistently in the 10th percentile for all measurements, but is growing steadily and is at a normal development level, may simply be a small child. Much cultural and individual variation exists in size. See Appendix C ∞ for standardized growth curves by gender and age for infants, children, and adolescents. See MyNursingKit to find out more about the growth curves and a course in accurate assessment techniques. Visit the Centers for Disease Control and Prevention (www.cdc.gov) to find specialized growth grids for children with conditions such as Down syndrome.

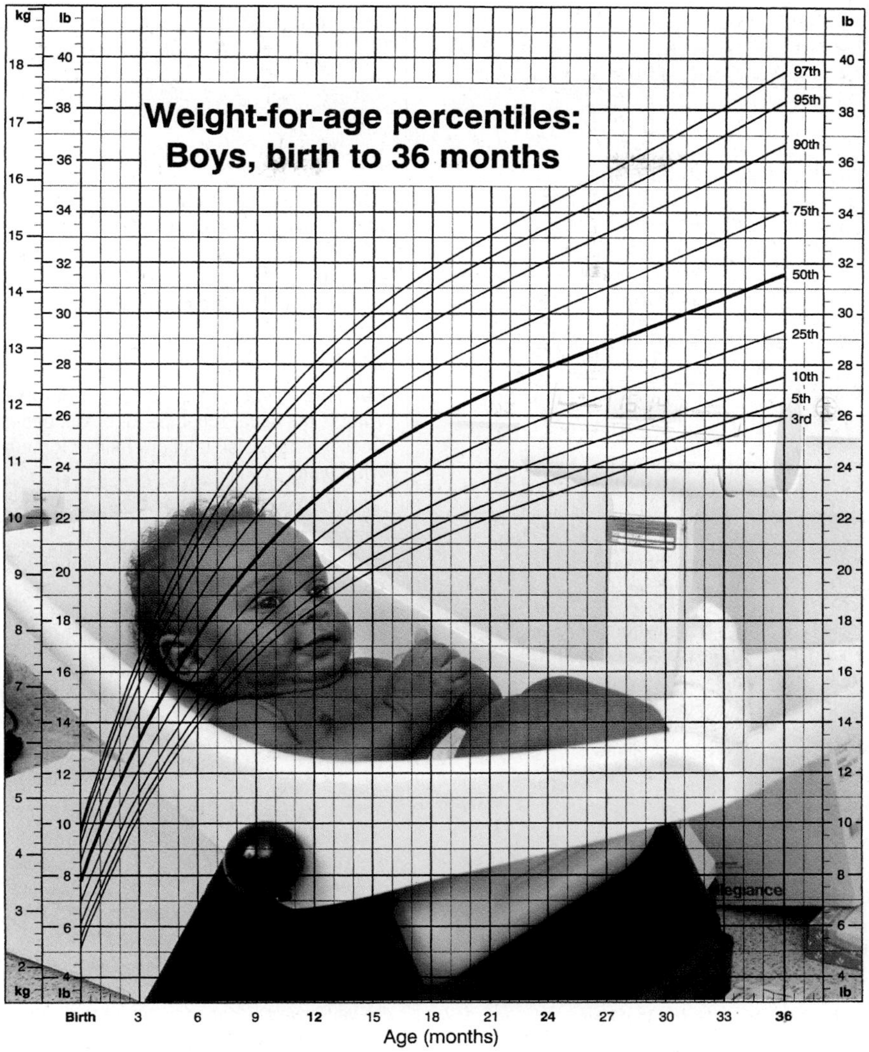

● **Figure 34–6** Plotting measurements on the growth curve. The nurse accurately measures the child and then places height and weight on appropriate growth grids for the child's age and gender.

The nurse should plot measurements on the same growth curve with earlier percentiles for the child. When measurements follow the same percentile over time, growth is generally normal for the child and nutrition is likely adequate. However, a sudden or sustained change in percentile may indicate a chronic disorder, emotional difficulty, or a nutritional intake problem. Further assessment of physical status and dietary intake will be needed.

Additional Physical Measurement

Many observations from the physical assessment provide clues to nutritional status. Dietary intake can affect every body system, and a combination of certain symptoms may suggest specific nutritional problems. Some common physical manifestations of nutritional status are outlined in Table 34–4.

Laboratory measurements can provide useful information when nutritional status is questionable. Some common studies include hematocrit and hemoglobin, serum glucose and fasting insulin, lipids and lipoproteins, and liver and renal function studies. Adding some further measurements such as chest circumference

Developing Cultural Competence

GROWTH PATTERNS AMONG IMMIGRANT CHILDREN

The revised growth grids now in use were standardized using a cross section of the U.S. population. However, children from some other countries or cultures may fall outside of these curves. For example, new immigrants or adoptees may be in lower percentiles and may "catch up" over several months or years. Children of immigrants from developing countries tend to be larger than their parents. Even when small, children should follow normal growth patterns. For example, a child who remains at the 10th or 25th percentile for height but continues to slowly grow does not fall to a lower percentile.

Table 34–4 Clinical Manifestations of Dietary Deficiencies/Excesses

Nutrient	Deficiency Manifestation	Excess Manifestation
Vitamin A	Night blindness Skin dryness and scaling	Headache Drowsiness Hepatomegaly Vomiting and diarrhea
Vitamin C	Abnormal hair (coiled shape) Skin abnormalities (dermatitis and lesions) Purpura Bleeding gums Joint tenderness Sudden heart failure	Usually none—excess is excreted in urine
Vitamin D	Rib deformity Bowed legs	Drowsiness
B vitamins	Weakness Decreased deep tendon reflexes Dermatitis	Usually none—excess is excreted in urine
Protein	Hepatomegaly Edema Scant, depigmented hair	Kidney failure
Carbohydrate	Emaciation Decreased energy Retarded growth and development	Overweight
Iron	Lethargy Slowed growth and developmental progression Pallor	Vomiting, diarrhea, abdominal pain Pallor Cyanosis Drowsiness Shock

Table 34–5 Dietary Screening History for Infants

Overview Questions

What was the infant's birth weight?
At what age did the birth weight double and triple?
Was the infant premature?
Does the infant have any feeding problems such as difficulty sucking and swallowing, spitting up, fatigue, or fussiness?

If Infant Is Breastfed

How long does the baby nurse at each breast?
What is the usual schedule for breastfeeding?
Does the baby also take any milk or formula? Amount and frequency? What type?

If Infant Is Formula Fed

What formula is used? Is it iron fortified?
How is it prepared?
Do you hold or prop the bottle for feedings?
How much formula is taken at each feeding?
How many bottles are taken each day?
Does the baby take a bottle to bed for naps or nighttime? What is in the bottle?

If Infant Is Fed Other Foods

At what age did the baby start eating other foods?

Cereal	Finger foods
Fruit/juices	Meats
Vegetables	Other protein sources

Do you use commercial baby food or make your own?
Does the baby eat any table foods?
How often does the baby take solid foods?
How is the baby's appetite?
Do you have any concerns about the baby's feeding habits?
Does the baby take a vitamin supplement? Fluoride?
Have there been any allergic reactions to foods? Which ones?
 Does the baby spit up frequently?
 Have there been any rashes?
What types of stools does the baby have? Frequency? Consistency?

and skinfolds (measurement of fat at certain body sites such as triceps, scapular, and abdominal areas) may also be useful (Lee & Nieman, 2006).

DIETARY INTAKE

The nurse should obtain detailed information about the child's dietary intake when there is a potential for nutritional deficiency due to disease, knowledge deficit, or socioeconomic status. The mother's dietary intake during pregnancy may provide information about the child's nutritional state and it can be assessed for pertinent information. After the information is collected, the dietary intake should be compared to the recommended levels for a child of that age and gender (see Figure 34–1 for the Food Guide Pyramid; see Appendix H for Recommended Dietary Allowances). The 24-hour recall of intake, a food frequency questionnaire, and a dietary screening history (Tables 34–5 and 34–6) provide a good overview of the infant's or child's intake and eating patterns. A food diary provides precise information about the child's food intake.

MyNursingKit Youth Adolescent Questionnaire

Twenty-Four-Hour Recall of Food Intake

The 24-hour diet recall is frequently used to assess the adequacy of the diet. People can generally remember their intake in the past day so results are fairly accurate, it is easy to gather the data and analyze results, and only a few minutes are needed. The nurse should ask the parent or child to list all foods eaten during the past 24 hours (Figure 34–7 ●). It is usually helpful to ask for a description of activities in the last day, then start with the most recent event and move backwards, integrating food intake into the daily schedule. For example, the nurse might begin by saying, "You mentioned you got up early to come to the clinic today. What did Sam eat at home before you left? Did he have a snack as you trav-

Table 34–6 Dietary Screening History for Children
What types of food or beverage does the child especially like?
What foods or beverages does the child dislike?
What is the child's typical eating schedule? Meals and snacks?
Does the child eat with the family or at separate times? Where does the child eat each meal?
Who prepares the food for the family? What methods of cooking are used? Baking? Frying? Broiling? Grilling? What ethnic foods are commonly eaten?
Does the family eat in a restaurant frequently? What type? What type of food does the child usually order?
Is the child on a special diet?
Does the child need to be fed, feed himself or herself, need assistance eating, or need any adaptive devices for eating?
What is the child's appetite like?
Does the child take any vitamin supplements (iron, fluoride)?
Does the child have any allergies? What types of symptoms?
What types of regular exercise does the child get?
Are there any concerns about the child's eating habits?

eled here or after you arrived?" While asking about the foods eaten, the nurse should inquire specifically about the following:

- All meals and snacks
- Amounts of each food item consumed (having various size measuring cups, bowls, and plates so accurate amounts can be indicated is helpful)
- Types of specific foods used, such as whole milk vs. nonfat or 2%, brand names of cereals, specific types of margarine or butter
- Additives used, such as condiments, table salt, spices, milk to mix formula

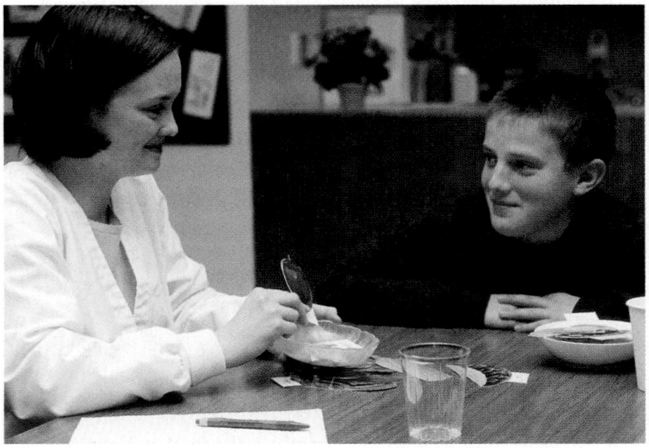

● **Figure 34–7** Twenty-four-hour diet recall. The nurse is interviewing a child about foods eaten in the last day. Note the models of food and dishes for accurate assessment of serving sizes.

- Food preparation methods, including adding fats to cook, removal or retention of fats on meats
- Vitamins and supplements, types and doses
- Whether the intake is typical (in situations such as illness or vacation, intake may be different than usual)

Once the 24-hour recall is obtained, the nurse needs to analyze the intake by first doing a quick check to compare servings of various food types with the Food Guide Pyramid, as described earlier. Next the nurse should do a detailed analysis to compute calories, carbohydrate, protein, and fat intake and compare them to recommended amounts. All major vitamins and minerals are also computed and comparisons made to the DRIs. This computation may be done by hand, using a book of nutrients in common foods, or may be done on the computer. Several computer programs are available, and the federal government has a Web site that provides intake levels and comparisons to the RDAs. It may be useful to compute a personal 24-hour recall or that of a child in the clinical setting with the Healthy Eating Index (www.cnpp.usda.gov/HealthyEatingIndex.htm).

Food Frequency Questionnaire

Food frequency questionnaires are available that can be easily administered to parents or children. Usually they ask about how often certain types of foods are eaten in a specified period such as a week. Long questionnaires can evaluate a total diet, while short ones focus on specific items such as fruit and vegetable intake. A short questionnaire about milk intake or fruit and vegetable intake may be helpful before planning a teaching project on nutrition to a class of school-age children. Knowing their usual intake of a food item can provide helpful information for planning the project. See MyNursingKit for one example of questions from a food frequency questionnaire.

MyNursingKit USDA Healthy Eating Index

Dietary Screening History

The nurse should ask the parent about the infant's or child's eating habits using questions in Tables 34–5 and 34–6. Responses provide information about the family's eating habits and food beliefs beyond that collected on a 24-hour dietary recall or food frequency questionnaire.

Developing Cultural Competence

DIETARY INTAKE VARIES AMONG CULTURES

Each culture has eating practices that influence dietary intake. It is important to understand the foods commonly eaten by each cultural group and their contribution to the total nutrition of the child. Depending on the populations nurses work with, they may need to ask about intake of freshly caught fish or wild game such as pheasants and elk. Home-prepared sausages and cheese may be part of diets. Berries and garden produce might be eaten. Foods from ethnic markets may include spices, dried mushrooms, and other products. Some groups do not eat meat or specific types of meats. Using open-ended questions in gathering data will increase the likelihood of obtaining an accurate evaluation of diet.

Food Diary

Parents are asked to keep a food diary when the child has a nutrition problem or disorder that requires dietary management, such as malnutrition, obesity, or diabetes. All meals and snacks, with food preparation method and quantities eaten over a 1- to 7-day period, are recorded. Eating patterns change significantly for holidays or family gatherings, so parents should be asked to select typical days for the food diary or to record specific events affecting food intake. Including one weekday and one weekend day may be helpful. Parents need to be reminded of all the places children might have eaten, such as the childcare center, school, friends' houses, or neighbors. Food diaries can provide a great deal of helpful information, but they take time and motivation to complete well (Lee & Nieman, 2006). The nurse should be sure instructions are complete and that the form has a place to record amounts, preparation, events occurring, and where food was eaten. The nurse or parent may need to obtain the school lunch menu and talk with the school lunch personnel to add accurate school intake. The nurse completes the nutritional assessment indicated for a child and may consult with or refer the family to a dietitian or nutritionist for additional assessment and teaching.

COMMON NUTRITIONAL CONCERNS

CHILDHOOD HUNGER

While most Americans live in a land of plenty, significant numbers of children periodically experience hunger. **Food security** is access at all times to enough nourishment for an active, healthy life. In contrast, **food insecurity** indicates an inability to acquire or consume adequate quality or quantity of foods in socially acceptable ways, or the uncertainty that one will be able to do so; about 18% of U.S. children live in households that periodically experience food insecurity (Federal Interagency Forum on Child and Family Statistics, 2005).

The major cause of hunger in children is poverty, and since 17.6%, or nearly one in five children, is poor, their families may be unable to provide sustainable nutrition at all times (Children's Defense Fund, 2007). Many single-income families have a head of household moving into the workforce, so incomes are often not sufficient to provide for family food needs (see Chapter 1 for a description of Temporary Assistance for Needy Families [TANF]). Families may be ineligible for food assistance programs even though they cannot afford enough food for all their members. Children with special nutritional needs are at particular risk since it may be more costly to buy and prepare formula or foods for a child with allergies, diabetes, or an immune disorder.

Children with insufficient dietary intake are at risk for a wide array of health problems. They may become anemic; have a high rate of infectious disease due to lowered immune response; have slowed developmental maturation, delayed or stunted physical growth, and learning disorders; and be at greater risk of overweight, cardiovascular disease, and diabetes in adulthood (AAP, 2009). Subsequently, the national and individual cost of childhood hunger is great.

Table 34–7 Food Insecurity Screening

1. Does your household ever run out of money to buy food to make a meal?
2. Do you or members of your household ever eat less than you feel you should because there is not enough money for food?
3. Do you or members of your household ever cut the size of meals or skip meals because there is not enough money for food?
4. Do your children ever eat less than you feel they should because there is not enough money for food?
5. Do you ever cut the size of your children's meals or do they skip meals because there is not enough money for food?
6. Do your children ever say they are hungry because there is not enough food in the house?
7. Do you ever rely on a limited number of foods to feed your children because you are running out of money to buy foods for a meal?
8. Do any of your children ever go to bed hungry because there is not enough money to buy food?

Scoring: 5–8 yes responses = hungry; 1–4 yes responses = risk of hunger. From Washington State Department of Health.

Nurses are well positioned to evaluate families for food insecurity in a variety of hospital, clinic, school, and home settings. In addition to the assessment of the individual child's nutritional status, further questions can determine families with potential problems. Nurses should administer the screening tool to identify risk in families (Table 34–7). Most parents go without food themselves in order to feed their children, so food insecurity may

Teaching Highlights

COMMUNITY RESOURCES FOR FOOD

Food Stamp Program—Eligibility based on household size and income; refer students and those with low incomes, especially when they have young children; education services often available

Child Nutrition Programs—School lunch, breakfast, and milk programs; free and lowered cost meals in schools; assist parents to apply

Special Child Programs—Summer programs, Head Start, childcare centers and homeless children programs may provide nutritional support in some communities

Women, Infants, and Children (WIC)—Supplemental foods and nutrition education to pregnant, breastfeeding, and postpartum women and to their young children; assessment of child growth often included

Nutrition Education and Training Program—Nutrition education for teachers and school food service personnel

Community Services—May include food banks, field gleaning (collecting produce from farmers' fields that will not be sold due to excess or small blemishes), and other programs

Find out what services are available to provide food and nutrition education in your community. Make a list to use in clinical settings with families.

Nursing Care Plan

THE CHILD WHO IS OVERWEIGHT

INTERVENTION	RATIONALE	EXPECTED OUTCOME
1. Nursing Diagnosis: Imbalanced Nutrition: More than Body Requirements related to excessive intake in comparison to metabolic needs		
NIC Priority Intervention: **Weight reduction assistance:** Facilitating loss of weight and body fat		**NOC Suggested Outcome:** **Weight control:** Personal actions resulting in achievement and maintenance of optimum body weight for health
Goal: The child will demonstrate adequate intake of all nutrients without excessive energy intake.		
■ Perform thorough nutritional assessment of child.	■ Assessment assists in identification of dietary risks and strengths as well as health conditions related to nutrition.	■ Child meets all dietary requirements while achieving weight and body mass index goal.
■ Share results of assessment with child and family by showing weight, height, and body mass index grids.	■ Many families do not consider their child overweight. Concrete information about the child's size in comparison with recommendations assists in establishing the importance of weight management.	
■ Assess access to sufficient nutritious foods for the family at all times.	■ Food insecurity promotes inadequate intake alternating with excess intake of high-caloric foods.	
■ Identify with the child and family 2–3 target areas to begin weight management. Examples might include: ■ Having fast food only once weekly ■ Switching to low-fat dairy products ■ Keeping two more fresh fruits and vegetables in the house and two less snack foods	■ Changing dietary patterns drastically is difficult and may lead to giving up the attempt at weight management. Partnering with the family to set goals enhances chances of success.	
■ Integrate nutrition information into each visit. Examples of topics include: ■ Dietary requirements for age group ■ Effects of simple sugar and fat intake on weight ■ Beneficial effects of fruits, vegetables, whole grains, and nonfat dairy ■ Reading food labels ■ Healthy choices in fast food restaurants ■ Calculation of fat content of foods	■ Nutrition information is best learned in an ongoing program.	
■ Use growth grids to help child and family establish a weight reduction or maintenance goal.	■ Goals motivate families to achieve desired health behaviors. The goal for a young child may be weight maintenance so that as the child grows in height, the correct proportion is reached, while weight reduction may be needed for older children or youth who are very obese.	
2. Nursing Diagnosis: Readiness for Enhanced Family Coping related to need to foster health of family member		
NIC Priority Intervention: **Health system guidance:** Facilitating child's use of appropriate nutrition and health services to foster weight control		**NOC Suggested Outcome:** **Health-promoting behavior:** Actions to promote, sustain, and increase wellness

(continued)

Nursing Care Plan—continued

THE CHILD WHO IS OVERWEIGHT

INTERVENTION	RATIONALE	EXPECTED OUTCOME
Goal: The family will assist child to manage stressors and to develop new strategies to support weight control goals.		
■ Include key family members in some of the counseling sessions with the overweight child.	■ Key members of the family are those who purchase foods, provide support for the child, and participate in decisions about health.	■ Child expresses satisfaction with family understanding and support of weight.
■ Encourage the family to eat together at least once daily if possible or to increase number of meals eaten together weekly.	■ The family is an important support system in weight loss programs. Eating as a family or in a social situation can provide a chance to promote healthy foods; intake is generally lower fat and calorie than when eating alone.	
■ Seek a resource for the child to be monitored about twice monthly; this may be a healthcare provider office, nutritionist, school nurse, or other person.	■ Provides opportunity to monitor the child's progress and to offer support, additional information, and problem-solving techniques.	

3. Nursing Diagnosis: Activity Intolerance related to sedentary lifestyle

NIC Priority Intervention:

Exercise promotion: Facilitating regular exercise to maintain and increase endurance and energy use

NOC Suggested Outcome:

Endurance: Extent that energy enables the child to sustain activity

INTERVENTION	RATIONALE	EXPECTED OUTCOME
Goal: The child will demonstrate activity tolerance by adequate oxygenation, respiratory effort, and ability to speak during brisk walking, biking, or other activity.		
■ Establish daily exercise routine beginning with 15–30 minutes daily of walking.	■ Starting with brief amounts of exercise makes the child feel comfortable and enhances potential for success.	■ Child demonstrates ability to engage in moderate activity for 60 minutes with minimal respiratory discomfort.
■ Gradually increase activity over 1–2 months until 60 minutes of daily exercise is maintained.	■ Gradual increase as the cardiovascular and respiratory systems adapt is generally comfortable for children; 60 minutes of moderate activity daily is recommended for children.	
■ Use activities enjoyed by the child and suggest options as necessary; refer the family to community resources such as swimming pools, organized sports, and biking groups.	■ Activities the child enjoys will be more likely to remain in usual activity patterns; exercising with others in groups increases motivation.	
■ Have families plan at least 1–2 activities they can do together weekly.	■ This fosters family relationships and provides support and motivation for the child.	
■ Limit screen activities to a maximum of 2 hours daily. Have child keep a log of hours of television, video games, computer, and other similar activities. Tell child never to snack while doing screen activities.	■ Increased use of screen activities is related to poor dietary habits and increased sedentary behaviors and excess weight.	

Nursing Care Plan—continued

THE CHILD WHO IS OVERWEIGHT

INTERVENTION	RATIONALE	EXPECTED OUTCOME
■ Ask about use of tobacco in children in 5th grade or higher. Inquire about exposure to environmental tobacco smoke at all ages. Perform teaching to discourage tobacco use or offer cessation programs as needed.	■ Most adults who smoke began the habit in childhood; middle school years are the most common age for smoking initiation. Smoking by others in the household can be harmful to children. Smoking decreases respiratory reserves and worsens several cardiovascular disease risks.	
4. Nursing Diagnosis: Chronic Low Self-Esteem related to weight		
NIC Priority Intervention: **Self-esteem enhancement:** Assisting the child to increase personal judgment of self-worth		**NOC Suggested Outcome:** **Quality of life and self-esteem:** Expressed satisfaction with life circumstances and positive judgment of self-worth
Goal: The child expresses positive perception of self-worth and confidence in ability to deal with issues related to weight.		
■ Facilitate development of a positive outlook by exposing child to others who have been successful with weight loss.	■ Increases motivation and feelings of self-efficacy.	■ Child speaks positively about accomplishments in weight control management.
■ Praise child for weight loss, weight maintenance, increased physical activity, and other achievements. Help the child establish rewards for meeting goals, such as purchase of new clothing.	■ Enhances judgment of self-worth and pride in accomplishments.	
■ Partner with parents so that they understand the value of praise and never label the child by derogatory words such as "fat."	■ Family members are usually the most intimate support system for the child.	

not have directly affected all children. However, anxiety over providing food can be very stressful for families, and diet quality deteriorates as insecurity increases. If families have experienced food insecurity or may be likely to at some time, nurses should be sure to provide them with access to community agencies and programs that can help. What resources are available locally to help families with food insecurity?

OVERWEIGHT AND OBESITY

The current incidence of overweight children in the United States is epidemic and is associated with a wide array of health problems, such as the appearance of type 2 diabetes in youth (Institute of Medicine, 2005b; Institute of Medicine, 2007). See Chapter 55 for a discussion of diabetes. Overweight can also influence self-image, dietary quality, and amount of physical activity. Prevalence of obesity (BMI $\geq$ 95th percentile) is 18.2% for males and 16% for females from 2 to 19 years (CDC, 2006a). When using the 85th percentile of BMI as a cutoff to indicate overweight, an additional 16% of males and females are affected. Thus, 33% of youth are overweight or obese (Institute of Medicine, 2007). Since overweight in childhood and adolescence frequently tracks into adulthood, the implications for health care are obvious.

Many reasons are cited for the increase in overweight children. The number of calories consumed is not increasing. However, children tend to exercise less, particularly in daily life. They infrequently walk or ride bikes, either because of the convenience of driving or due to unsafe neighborhoods. Television viewing is very high among youth; television and other screen activities account for an average of 5.5 hours daily. Even children under 6 years spend an average of 2 hours daily on screen activities, and 26% of those less than 2 years of age have television sets in their bedrooms (Rideout & Hamel, 2006). Inactive pursuits do not require high caloric energy, leading to an imbalance in intake and demand for calories. Additionally television viewing is often accompanied by ingestion of high-calorie foods and subjects children to media advertisements for unhealthy foods.

MyNursingKit Video: Children and Overweight

Developing Cultural Competence

OVERWEIGHT CAUSES HEALTH DISPARITIES AMONG CERTAIN GROUPS

Overweight is more common among some ethnic and socioeconomic groups. Lack of knowledge about foods and physical activity, limited access to fresh produce and safe places to exercise, and easy access to increasing numbers of fast foods may all constitute risk factors. Lower income, and Hispanic, black, or Native-American ethnic identity are all associated with higher incidence of overweight, especially among women. National goals to eliminate health disparities in income and ethnic groups have been set (*Healthy People 2010*, U.S. Department of Health and Human Services, 2006).

Growth and Development

When girls experience menarche before 11 years of age, they are more frequently overweight. A study of girls from the National Institute of Child Health and Human Development Study of Early Child Care and Youth Development found that higher body mass index (BMI) scores in girls, and higher rate of change in BMI from 3 to 6 years of age were associated with early puberty in childhood (Lee, Appugliese, Kaciroti, et al., 2007). Another longitudinal study found that rapid infancy weight gain was associated with increased risk of obesity at 5 and 8 years of age (Dunger, Ahmed, & Ong, 2006). Early weight monitoring, even at the very young ages of infancy, preschool and early school age is important. The nurse should also remain alert for signs of breast development in fourth or fifth grade girls and early menarche (grade 6). Such youth may already be overweight and should be identified for efforts directed at obesity prevention. Such prevention efforts are needed to decrease risks of obesity such as type 2 diabetes.

The percentage of calories from fat consumed in the United States is among the highest in the world. Although no more than 25–35% of calories should come from total dietary fat, and no more than 10% from saturated fat, about 35% of calories consumed in the United States are supplied by fat and 12% by saturated fat (Institute of Medicine, 2005a). Most fats should be supplied from polyunsaturated and monounsaturated fatty acids, but current diets contain low amounts of those fats and high amounts of trans-fatty acids (USDHHS, 2005). The high rate of dietary fat is related to the amount of fast food consumed, and influenced by snacking as well.

Goals of nursing management are to prevent new cases of overweight, identify children who are overweight, and to support youth and families to establish health lifestyles that promote weight loss and maintenance of recommended weight (Small, Anderson, & Melnyk, 2007). Perform assessment of height, weight, and BMI. Measure blood pressure and analyze if it is within normal limits. Evaluate amount of screen activities and physical activity levels.

Nurses can help parents and children build good nutritional and exercise habits throughout life, thus decreasing the incidence of overweight and its attendant health risks. Parents should be advised that television viewing should be limited to a maximum of 2 hours daily, and that television and video games should not be placed in children's bedrooms. Daily exercise routines of 30–60 minutes can be included in most families. Aim to meet the current recommendation of 60 minutes daily for children with some activity including muscle strengthening and flexibility. Also, nurses should teach about the Food Guide Pyramid and its integration into a healthy life. Healthy snacks include fruits, vegetables, grains, and nuts. "Super sizing" fast foods and eating out often should be avoided.

Risks for poor health often cluster together in individuals and families. Nurses need to be alert for situations in which parents are overweight and children have elevated blood pressure, exercise infrequently, or are in upper percentiles for weight, BMI, or skinfold. Be alert for early menarche which can help identify overweight girls who need intervention for obesity prevention. The presence of risk factors necessitates further dietary and risk assessment so that a management plan can be implemented. Visit the Companion Website for information that will be helpful to families in the clinical setting. See resources such as "Helping Your Overweight Child" and "Take Charge of Your Health: A Teenager's Guide to Better Health" (http://win.niddk.nih.gov/publications/).

Consult the "Nursing Care Plan" in this chapter for further interventions appropriate for the overweight child.

FOOD SAFETY

Every year in the United States, about 76 million people contract food-borne illnesses. Some are quite mild while others can be very severe. About 300,000 people are hospitalized and 5,000 die from these illnesses (CDC, 2007). Children are at greater risk of severe illness and death from food and water due to their immature gastrointestinal and immune systems. Children who are immunocompromised are at even greater risk. The most common pathogens are *Campylobacter, Salmonella, Shigella, Cryptosporidium, Listeria, Yersinia,* and *Escherichia coli*. Infants are at extremely high risk of *Campylobacter, Rotavirus*, and *Salmonella* illness (CDC, 2007). Worldwide over 3 million people die of illness related to unsafe drinking water each year, and most of those deaths are among children.

Foodborne illness transmission is associated with food preparation and storage practices, lack of adequate training of retail employees about foods and hygiene, and increasing amounts and types of foods being imported from other countries. Some examples of contaminated foods in the last few years include undercooked hamburger meat, cross-contamination of salad bar items from meats, unpasteurized apple cider, green onions, raw spinach, prepackaged salad and delicatessen meat, berries, and sprouts. While most infected persons experience acute diarrhea, some can develop complications such as hemolytic uremic syndrome (Chapter 54) or thrombocytic purpura (Chapter 51). Health personnel should integrate teaching regularly so that fami-

Teaching Highlights

FOOD SAFETY GUIDELINES

Four Key Food Safety Practices:

1. *Clean:* Wash hands and surfaces often
2. *Separate:* Don't cross-contaminate
3. *Cook:* Cook to proper temperature
4. *Chill:* Refrigerate promptly

(Data from Partnership for Food Safety Education, Safe Food Handling, Retrieved May 18, 2007, from http://www.fightbac.org/content/view/6/11/)

lies can decrease risks of food-borne illness. Recommend that families avoid consumption of unpasteurized milk, raw or undercooked oysters, raw or undercooked eggs, raw or undercooked ground beef, and undercooked poultry (CDC, 2007). Check the information regarding outbreaks at www.foodsafety.org.

Food may carry products other than microorganisms that can be harmful. An example is mercury, which may be concentrated in certain types of fish. This metal can cause harm to the developing nervous system of fetuses, infants, and young children when consumed regularly. The U.S. Food and Drug Administration (FDA) and Environmental Protection Agency (EPA) note that fish are an important part of a healthy diet, but that certain recommendations should be followed to lower risk of mercury's detrimental effects. Women who may become pregnant, are pregnant or breastfeeding, and young children should:

- Eliminate shellfish, shark, swordfish, king mackerel, and tilefish from the diet.
- Eat up to 12 ounces (two average meals) a week of a variety of low-mercury fish, such as shrimp, canned light tuna, salmon, pollock, and catfish. Albacore or white tuna has more mercury than light tuna, so limit white tuna to one meal weekly.

Check for local advisories about the safety of fish caught in local waters. In the absence of advice, up to 6 ounces (one meal) weekly may be eaten from local waters. Do not eat other fish during that week (Food and Drug Administration, 2004).

COMMON DIETARY DEFICIENCIES

Dietary deficiencies can occur in children and some are common in selected populations. While children can have deficits in nearly any nutrient, a number of nutrient deficits are more common in childhood. Limitations in the food supply or patterns of dietary intake cause most deficiencies, while children with certain disease processes, such as metabolic diseases, may have difficulty absorbing or using nutrients ingested (see Chapter 55 ∞ for a discussion of inborn errors of metabolism). The nutrient deficiencies of a population are a result of genetic factors, characteristics of the food supply, and intake patterns of particular groups.

Developing Cultural Competence

VITAMIN A DEFICIENCY

Vitamin A deficiency is common in developing countries. The vitamin is found in liver, dairy products, and fish. Provitamin A sources are yellow and dark green vegetables. The vitamin is fat soluble and stored in the liver. When deficient, children develop night blindness, vision loss, and high rates of infection. Public health efforts have been directed at identifying populations of children with low vitamin A status and providing the vitamin in capsule form or in commonly ingested foods.

Iron

Newborns have a store of iron obtained from their mothers in the uterus if the maternal nutritional state was satisfactory and the baby was of normal gestational age. Breast milk contains little iron, but the iron it does contain has high bioavailability. However, by 4 to 6 months of age, the baby's iron stores begin to decrease and a dietary source of iron must be added. Enriched rice cereal is commonly used to meet these initial iron needs. In babies who do not have adequate stores or do not take in enough iron, **anemia**, or a reduction in the number of red blood cells, can result (Figure 34–8 ●). Feeding cow's milk during infancy can also cause anemia by irritating the gut and leading to small but consistent loss of blood from the gastrointestinal tract; cow's milk should not be fed in the first year of life. When formulas are used, they should be iron fortified to help avoid iron deficiency anemia. Iron-fortified infant cereals are a good source of the mineral.

Adolescent females comprise another group commonly deficient in iron. Their deficiency is related to loss of blood in menses, metabolic need of the growth spurt, and poor dietary balance due to sporadic dieting. Further discussion of the symptoms and treatment of iron deficiency anemia can be found in Chapter 51 ∞. Encourage intake of good iron sources such as meats, eggs, dried fruits, iron-fortified cereal.

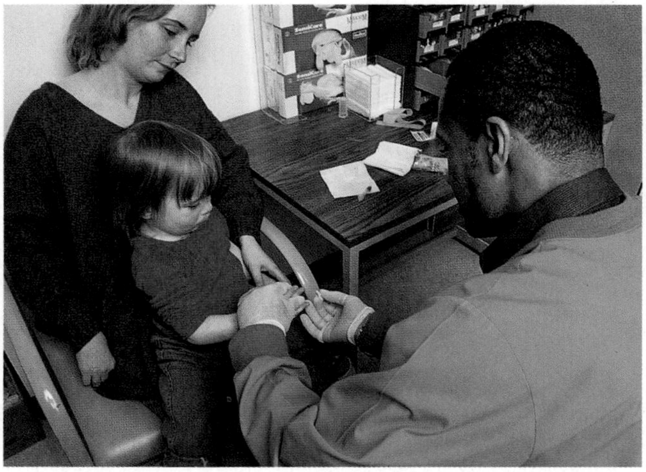

● **Figure 34–8** Screening for anemia. Most Head Start centers participate in screening programs to identify children at risk for anemia.

Calcium

Calcium is an essential nutrient for bone development during childhood and adolescence. An increased intake of soda pop and fruit juices is related to a decrease in calcium intake, especially among adolescents. During the adolescent growth spurt, almost 40% of the adult bone mass is accumulated (AAP, 2009). Inadequate intake puts the person at risk for osteoporosis later in life since it is not possible to make up for earlier deficits. Although genetic variables account for some of the influence on adult bone mass, increasing calcium intake has been shown to promote bone formation. While the recommended daily intake for adolescents is 1300 mg, the average intake for adolescent males is 1145 mg and for females is only 700–850 mg (only half of the recommended level) (Storey, Forshee, & Anderson, 2004). Nurses should encourage foods such as milk and milk products, egg yolks, grains, legumes, nuts, and fruit juice with added calcium.

Adolescents at highest risk for impaired bone development include female athletes and others who diet to a great degree to maintain slimness. Teens who exercise excessively may manifest the "female athlete triad" of disordered eating that leads to excessive thinness, excessive exercise, and amenorrhea (Waldrop, 2005). A high rate of fractures and osteomalacia can result, in addition to an extreme risk of osteoporosis in adulthood. Asking about menstrual patterns as well as exercise and diet can be combined with physical measurements of height and weight to obtain pertinent information about the teen athlete. See the discussion of the eating disorders anorexia nervosa and bulimia nervosa later in this chapter.

Vitamin D

Vitamin D is needed for bone mineralization. Vitamin D deficiencies were once believed to be rare; however, an increase in cases of vitamin D-deficient rickets has recently been observed. Although Vitamin D can be synthesized in the skin upon exposure to sunlight, the amount of sunlight needed for manufacture is variable and determined by the amount of skin exposed, the color of the skin, the latitude, and time of the year (Wagner, Greer, & Section on Breastfeeding, 2008). Because of this variability it is now recommended that all infants and children receive a minimum intake of 400 IU daily. This vitamin is needed to enhance absorption of calcium, so a lack of vitamin D can contribute to calcium deficiency

Drug Guide

IRON

Overview of Action

Iron is a necessary component of hemoglobin and is therefore essential in the oxygen transfer carried out by red blood cells. It is used in microcytic and hypochromic anemia, which result from iron deficiency. Supplements are frequently used during pregnancy when intake often does not meet iron needs, and in infants with decreased iron stores, such as with small-for-gestational-age and premature infants.

Route, Dosage, Frequency

Ferrous Fumarate: 3 mg/kg/day po elemental iron

Ferrous Gluconate: 8 mg/kg/day po—over 2 years elemental iron

Ferrous Sulfate: 5 mg/kg/day po elemental iron

Ferrous Sulfate Dried: 160 mg/day po elemental iron

Iron Dextran: up to 25 mg/day (under 5 kg weight); up to 50 mg/day (5–10 kg weight); up to 100 mg/day (over 10 kg)—IM, IV

RDAs for Iron

7–12 months: 11 mg

1–3 years: 7 mg

4–8 years: 10 mg

9–13 years: 8 mg

14–18 years: males 11 mg; females 15 mg

Pregnancy: 27 mg

Lactation: 9–10 mg

Nursing Considerations

Administer PO: The mg doses of various forms of iron are not equivalent; rather, the amount of elemental iron in various preparations is important. Administration with a snack decreases absorption but is often recommended, as GI irritation will be lessened. Accompanying iron with vitamin C may enhance iron absorption.

Liquid preparations should be given with fluid, such as juice, and by a dropper or straw because they can stain teeth. **IM:** Do not mix with other medications. Given to the upper outer buttock; therefore, this form is used only in older children and adults. Change needle after drawing up iron. Use long needle and **Z-track** injection technique. Permanent tissue staining can occur if not deep IM. Aspirate after inserting needle and inject slowly. **IV:** Given undiluted. Do not mix with other medications (known to be incompatible with some other medicines) and do not use the multidose bottle (latter only for IM injection). A small test dose is administered and if no reaction occurs, the remainder of the dose is slowly infused over 1–6 hours. Double check dose with another nurse and follow prescriber instructions carefully. Flush vein after infusion with normal saline.

Assess: Obtain a diet history. Be alert for elements that can decrease iron absorption, such as low-calcium or high-phosphate diet, infection, or decreased GI acid. Watch for signs of deficiency in infants after 4–6 months of age when maternal iron stores are depleted (earlier in premature infants). A CBC including hematocrit, hemoglobin, and reticulocytes is done to establish iron deficiency anemia. Before administering **parenteral** iron, a test dose of 0.5 mL is given.

Monitor: Epinephrine 1:1000 available for parenteral administration. Watch for hypersensitivity. Hemoglobin, hematocrit, other lab studies regularly.

Teaching: Take oral preparation between meals unless GI distress occurs. Teach food sources of iron. Take liquid forms with straw and water to decrease chance of teeth staining. Dairy products, eggs, whole grains, tea, and coffee decrease iron absorption.

Data from information in Bindler, R. M., & Howry, L. B. (2005). Pediatric drug guide. *Upper Saddle River, NJ: Prentice Hall-Health.*

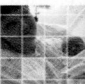

as well. Human milk contains little vitamin D, so breastfed infants should receive 400 IU of vitamin D/day. Formula fed infants and older children drinking milk should receive a 400 IU supplement/day if consuming less than 1000 mL of formula or milk/day (1000 mL of formula and of milk contain 400 IU of vitamin D). Likewise, adolescents who do not consume 400 IU via diet should receive the amount in a supplement (Wagner, Greer, & Section on Breastfeeding, 2008). Encourage parents to discuss vitamin D intake and recommendations with the care provider at health promotion visits so proper intake can be ensured.

Folic Acid

Epidemiologic evidence has linked increasing maternal folic acid (the most common form of folate in the human body) intake with decreased incidence of neural tube defects such as spina bifida in offspring. Folate levels are low among adolescents, putting them at particular risk of birth defects when they have babies (AAP, Committee on Nutrition, 2009). The FDA approved fortification of cereals and breads with folate to decrease the population risk of related congenital anomalies. All women from 15 to 45 years should consume 0.4 mg of folic acid daily and pregnant women should consume 0.6 mg. In addition to cereals and breads, other good sources of folate include spinach, avocado, green leafy vegetables, beans and peas, liver, and fruits such as oranges and grapefruits.

Protein-Energy Malnutrition

Although the micronutrient deficiencies described earlier are the most common problems in developed countries, macronutrient deficiencies are the most common nutritional problems worldwide. While kwashiorkor indicates protein deficiency, and marasmus is a lack of energy-producing calories, both deficiencies often occur together and are referred to as protein-energy malnutrition (PEM). Protein deficiency manifests with edema, leading to the large abdomens and rounded faces seen in severely malnourished children. Other symptoms include scant, depigmented hair, skin changes, and decreased serum proteins. It can occur following severe diarrhea or other infection in susceptible children. Caloric deficiency results in emaciation, decreased energy levels, and retarded development (see Table 34–4). PEM may occur when a child is weaned in order for the mother to provide breast milk to a new baby. Adoptees and immigrants to developed countries sometimes manifest with at least mild PEM, so careful nutritional assessment is needed to provide adequate nutrition.

FEEDING AND EATING DISORDERS

Deficiencies in food intake related to available nutrients and safety of the food supply were discussed in the previous section. In addition to these issues of availability, nutrient intake is affected by psychologic issues of individuals as well. Disorders of food intake span the entire developmental spectrum and can affect pregnant women, young children, and adolescents. Some of the most common feeding and eating disorders are discussed in the following sections.

Pica

Pica is an eating disorder characterized by ingestion of nonfood items or food items consumed in abnormal quantities or forms. Examples of ingested items include starch, peeling paint, paper, soil components, flour, and coffee grounds. Clinical manifestations include zinc and iron deficiencies as well as symptoms of lead or other heavy metal poisoning (see Chapter 44 ∞) if these substances are contained in peeling paint or other ingested material. Pica most commonly manifests in pregnancy when women have abnormal cravings for nonfood products, and this can seriously impair the developing fetus (see Chapter 14 ∞ for more information). Some children also ingest abnormal amounts of nonfood items and fail to take in adequate nutrients from food. Treatment for children involves removing them from the substances, ensuring an adequate and nutritious diet, and treating any dietary deficiencies noted.

Feeding Disorder of Infancy and Early Childhood (Failure to Thrive)

Feeding disorder of infancy and early childhood, or failure to thrive (FTT), describes a syndrome in which infants or young children fail to eat enough food to be adequately nourished. This disorder accounts for 5% to 10% of pediatric hospitalizations in children under 1 year of age, and many more children are managed in community settings (Stanton, Jenson, Behrman, et al., 2007).

Etiology and pathophysiology. The cause of feeding disorder can be organic, as in congenital acquired immunodeficiency syndrome (AIDS) (see Chapter 50 ∞), inborn errors of metabolism (see Chapter 55 ∞), congenital heart defect (see Chapter 49 ∞), neurologic disease (see Chapter 56 ∞), and esophageal reflux (see Chapter 53 ∞). However, most cases of FTT have no organic cause. FTT resulting from nonorganic causes is called *feeding disorder of infancy or early childhood.*

Infants and children whose parents or caretakers experience poverty, depression, substance abuse, mental retardation, or psychosis are at risk for this disorder. Parents may be socially and emotionally isolated, or may lack knowledge of infant nutritional and nurturing needs. A reciprocal interaction pattern may exist in which the parent does not offer enough food or is not responsive to the infant's hunger cues, and the infant is irritable, not soothed, and does not give clear cues about hunger. Parental neglect is a contributor to the condition. Preterm and small-for-gestational-age babies more commonly have eating disorders (Block, Krebs, and Committee on Child Abuse and Neglect, 2005).

Clinical manifestations. The characteristics of this feeding disorder are persistent failure to eat adequately with no weight gain or with weight loss in a child under 6 years of age that is not associated with other medical conditions or mental disorders, and is not caused by lack of or unavailability of food. Weight is generally below the 5th percentile, and weight-for-length is less than 80% of ideal weight (Block et al., 2005; Olsen, 2006). Infants with feeding disorder refuse food, may have erratic sleep patterns, are irritable and difficult to soothe, and are often developmentally delayed (Figure 34–9 ●).

Clinical therapy. A thorough history and physical examination are needed to rule out any chronic physical illness. The infant or

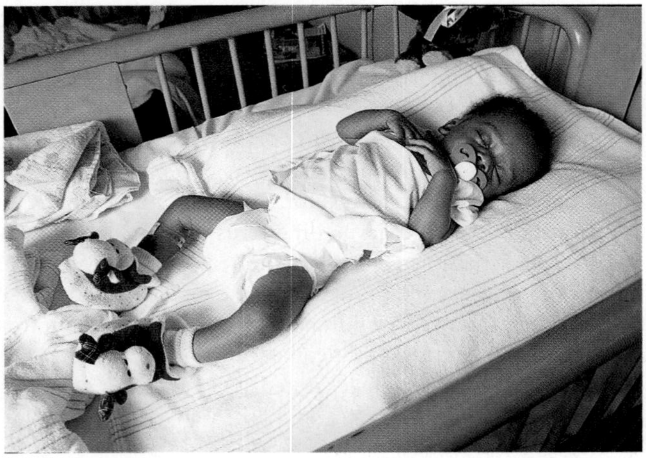

• **Figure 34–9** Feeding disorder of infancy or failure to thrive (FTT). Infants with failure to thrive may not look severely malnourished, but they fall well below the expected weight and height norms for their age. This infant, who appears to be about 4 months old, is actually 8 months old. He has been hospitalized for feeding disorder of infancy.

child may be hospitalized so that healthcare providers can establish a routine for feeding and sleeping. The goals of treatment are to provide adequate caloric and nutritional intake, promote normal growth and development, and assist parents in developing feeding routines and responding to the infant's cues of physical and psychologic hunger.

NURSING MANAGEMENT

NURSING ASSESSMENT AND DIAGNOSIS

Nursing assessment of the child is essential for establishing the best intervention plan for a child with FTT. Accurate weight and height each time any child is seen for health care provides an important record of growth patterns over time. This helps identify the child with an eating disorder. The child's activity level, developmental milestones, and interaction patterns provide important information. When feeding the child, observe how the child indicates hunger or satiety, the ability of the child to be soothed, and general interaction patterns such as eye contact, touch, and "cuddliness."

Developing Cultural Competence

HEIGHT AND WEIGHT GROWTH STANDARDS

Each child should maintain a height and weight growth pattern similar to the population standard. Asian-American children may normally be below the fifth percentile on growth charts and not have an eating disorder. Suspect an eating disorder when the infant or child falls one standard deviation below his or her own curve and either fails to gain weight or loses weight over several months.

Ask parents about stresses in their lives; these may prevent appropriate interaction with the child. Asking about the pregnancy and birth can elicit information about early disturbances in the child-parent relationship. Are there other children in the family and have eating problems occurred with them? Observe the child and parent behaviors while they feed the child; cues given by each person and interactional modes such as rocking, singing, talking, and body postures are important.

Some of the nursing diagnoses pertinent for the young child with an eating disorder include the following:

- *Imbalanced Nutrition: Less than Body Requirements* related to inability to ingest proper amounts of food
- *Delayed Growth and Development* related to inadequate food intake
- *Risk for Impaired Parenting* related to lack of knowledge about the child's nutritional needs
- *Fatigue* related to malnutrition

PLANNING AND IMPLEMENTATION

Nursing care centers on performing a thorough history and physical assessment, observing parent-child interactions during feeding times, and providing necessary teaching to enable parents to respond appropriately to their child's needs. The child is often hospitalized initially and evaluated for potential organic causes while staff members feed the child. Tube feedings may be needed temporarily until normal intake can be ensured. Accurate weights, nutritional assessments, and developmental evaluation should be done to see if the child grows more normally. Additional diagnostic tests may be carried out at this time to rule out organic causes of poor growth.

Once a diagnosis of nonorganic failure to thrive is confirmed, parents become involved in feeding the child. Observations of feeding and continued careful physical assessments are needed. Carefully record the child's intake at each meal or feeding. Teach parents how to understand and respond to the child's cues of hunger and satiety. Teach them to hold, rock, and touch the infant during feedings and establish eye contact with infants and older children.

Upon discharge, referral to an agency that can continue monitoring of the home situation is needed. This provides an opportunity to observe feeding during a home visit and evaluate stresses and behavior patterns among family members. Frequent growth measurement and development must be ensured so the child is adequately nourished. Parents may need referral to community resources to help them manage stressful situations in their lives and to enhance their parenting skills.

EVALUATION

Expected outcomes of nursing care include the following:

- Adequate growth and normal development of the infant is achieved.
- An improved parent-child relationship is established.

MyNursingKit Video: Anorexia Nervosa

Anorexia Nervosa

Anorexia nervosa is a potentially life-threatening eating disorder that occurs primarily in teenage girls and young women. An estimated 5% of young women and 1% of young men in the United States are affected by anorexia nervosa or a related eating disorder (American Dietetic Association [ADA], 2006). The typical patient is white and from a middle- to upper-middle-class family. Age at onset varies, and incidence peaks at 12 to 13 years and again at 17 to 18 years.

Etiology and pathophysiology. Many causes are believed to contribute to the onset of anorexia. Cultural overemphasis on thinness may contribute to the excessive concern with dieting, body image, and fear of becoming fat that is experienced by many adolescents. Chemical changes have been found in the brain and blood of individuals with anorexia, leading to theories about a biologic cause. Often a significant life stress, loss, or change precedes the onset of anorexia. Stress hormones are commonly elevated in adolescents with anorexia, and immune system function may be disturbed (Gluck, 2006).

Many experts view family issues as contributory to anorexia. Intrafamilial conflicts and dysfunctional family patterns may occur when parents are overly controlling and perfectionistic. The adolescent's eating behaviors may be an attempt to exercise independence and resolve internal psychologic conflicts.

The adolescent may engage in lengthy and vigorous exercise (up to 4 hours daily) to prevent weight gain. Laxatives or diuretics may be used to induce weight loss. As the disorder progresses, the adolescent perceives the ever-thinner body as becoming more beautiful. Youths may share weight loss techniques with friends who are anorectic and search out Internet sites that are positive about anorexia. The body responds to the abnormal eating behaviors as if starvation were occurring. Leukopenia, electrolyte imbalance, and hypoglycemia develop as a result of PEM. Once the body mass decreases below a critical level, menstruation ceases.

Clinical manifestations. Adolescents with anorexia are characterized by extreme weight loss accompanied by a preoccupation with weight and food, excessive compulsive exercising, peculiar patterns of eating and handling food, and distorted body image. They may prepare elaborate meals for others but eat only low-calorie foods. Characteristically, the fear of becoming fat does not decrease with continued weight loss. Accompanying signs and symptoms of depression, crying spells, feelings of isolation and loneliness, and suicidal thoughts and feelings are common. The disorder is often associated with mental illness such as obsessive-compulsive disorder, anxiety disorders (see Chapter 57 ∞), and history of abuse (ADA, 2006).

Physical findings include cold intolerance, dizziness, constipation, abdominal discomfort, bloating, irregular menses, and malnutrition (Figure 34–10 ●). Hypothalamic suppression can lead to disturbances of gynecologic function, osteoporosis, decreased bone density, and fractures. Lanugo (fine, downy body hair) may be present. Fluid and electrolyte imbalances, especially potassium imbalances, are common. The child or adolescent is usually energetic despite significant weight loss. Extreme weight loss often leads to cardiac arrhythmias (bradycardia).

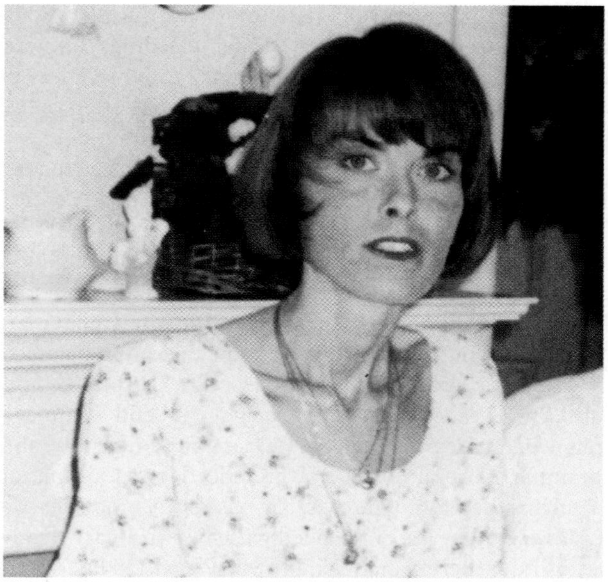

● **Figure 34–10** Anorexia nervosa. This young woman began to have symptoms of anorexia at age 12 years. Her parents obtained ongoing counseling for her and the family. She died of the disorder in her early 20s.

Clinical therapy. Diagnosis is based on a comprehensive history, physical examination revealing characteristic clinical manifestations, and the *DSM-IV* criteria included in Table 34–8. Diagnostic tests commonly include hematocrit and hemoglobin, serum electrolytes, and serum vitamins and vitamin-precursors. Bone density examination for females with lengthy amenorrhea is recommended (American Psychiatric Association [APA], 2006).

The goal of treatment is to address the physiologic problems associated with malnutrition, as well as the behavioral and cognitive components of the disorder. A firm focus is placed on reaching a targeted weight with a gradual weight gain of 0.1 to 0.2 kg/day (0.25 to 0.5 lb/day). Weight gain of 2–3 pounds/week

Table 34–8 DSM-IV Diagnostic Criteria for Anorexia Nervosa

A. Refusal to maintain body weight at or above a minimally normal weight for age and height (e.g., weight loss leading to maintenance of body weight less than 85% of that expected; or failure to make expected weight gain during period of growth, leading to body weight less than 85% of that expected).
B. Intense fear of gaining weight or becoming fat, even though underweight.
C. Disturbance in the way in which one's weight or shape is experienced, undue influence of body weight or shape on self-evaluation, or denial of the seriousness of the current body weight.
D. In postmenarchal females, amenorrhea, i.e., the absence of at least three consecutive menstrual cycles. (A woman is considered to have amenorrhea if her periods occur only following hormone, e.g., estrogen, administration).

Source: Used with permission from American Psychiatric Association. (2000). *Diagnostic and statistical manual of mental disorders* (4th ed., Text revision). Washington, DC. Copyright © American Psychiatric Association.

during hospitalization, or 0.5–1 pound/week during outpatient treatment is expected (APA, 2006). Enteral feedings or total parenteral nutrition (TPN) may be necessary to replace lost fluid, protein, and nutrients, although the adolescent often perceives these feedings as a punitive measure.

Individual treatment and family therapy are used to address dysfunctional family patterns and assist the family to accept and deal with the adolescent as an independent and less-than-perfect individual. Family involvement is crucial to effect a lasting change in the adolescent. Nurses, psychologists, family therapists, and dietitians commonly partner to plan and implement therapy.

Long-term outpatient treatment, in either an individual or a group setting, is frequently necessary. Counseling may be continued for 2 to 3 years to ensure that weight gain and self-image are maintained. Antidepressant drugs such as imipramine (Tofranil) or desipramine (Norpramin) may be prescribed for coexisting conditions such as depression, anxiety, or obsessive-compulsive disorders. However, they are not generally useful in primary treatment of the disorder (Berkman, Bulik, Brownley, et al., 2006).

Indications for hospitalization include loss of 25% to 30% of body weight or being at 85% or less of healthy weight, fluid and electrolyte imbalances, cardiac arrhythmias, hypotension, or the need to provide a more intense period of therapy if outpatient treatment fails to produce improvement. Behavior modification techniques are used extensively in combination with counseling and other methods in the care of the hospitalized adolescent with anorexia.

NURSING MANAGEMENT

NURSING ASSESSMENT AND DIAGNOSIS

Obtain a thorough individual and family history. Ask about usual eating patterns, daily caloric intake, exercise patterns, and menstrual history. Ask about medication use; include prescription, nonprescription, and herbal products. Is there a family history of eating disorders? Assess for signs of malnutrition. Obtain height and weight measurements and compare with norms for the general population. Because the anorectic patient often wears layers of clothes when being weighed, strive to obtain an accurate measurement.

Nursing diagnoses for the adolescent with anorexia nervosa include the following:

- *Imbalanced Nutrition: Less than Body Requirements* related to inadequate food intake
- *Risk for Deficient Fluid Volume* related to inadequate fluid intake or fluid volume loss from overuse of laxatives and diuretics
- *Risk for Imbalanced Body Temperature* related to excessive weight loss and absence of subcutaneous fat
- *Constipation* related to inadequate food intake and overuse of laxatives
- *Disturbed Body Image* related to distorted perception of body size and shape
- *Chronic Low Self-Esteem* related to dysfunctional family dynamics
- *Compromised Family Coping* related to parental tendency to be overly controlling and perfectionistic

PLANNING AND IMPLEMENTATION

Nursing care centers on meeting nutritional and fluid needs, preventing complications, administering medications, supporting psychologic interventions, and providing referral to appropriate resources. Specific treatment measures vary depending on physical complications, length and degree of illness, emotional symptoms accompanying the disorder, and family dynamics. Resistance to treatment is common, and nurses who care for adolescents with anorexia must deal with their own feelings of frustration and anger.

PROVIDE PSYCHOLOGICAL SUPPORT

Care for the adolescent with anorexia necessarily includes psychological support as an important component. The nurse will refer the family to a specialist who can counsel and recommend further treatment. Families should be involved in support groups with the anorectic youth, and should also receive information about the condition and the youth's plan of care. The adolescent is often treated in individual counseling and encouragement to participate is needed. Interventions that improve self-concept and lead to a realistic body image are needed. They may include encouragement for participation in sports, praise for participation in the treatment plan, and immediate referral for relapses as treatment progresses.

MEET NUTRITIONAL AND FLUID NEEDS

Monitor nutritional and fluid intake, encourage consumption of food, and observe eating behaviors at mealtime. Elimination patterns may be altered as a result of increased intake during hospitalization. Monitor for possible problems, including abdominal distention, constipation, or diarrhea. Daily monitoring of serum electrolytes is necessary.

If TPN is administered, watch for complications such as circulatory overload, hyperglycemia, or hypoglycemia. Use strict aseptic technique when changing tubing or dressings.

ADMINISTER MEDICATIONS

Monitor vital signs if the adolescent is receiving antidepressants. Watch for signs of hypertension and tachycardia. Administer medications after meals because it helps to prevent gastric irritation. Be alert for substance abuse. Anorectics often use products such as excess laxatives or ephedra (also known as ma huang) to induce weight loss. Changes in the central nervous system, vital signs, and other findings may indicate over-the-counter or herbal drug use.

PROVIDE REFERRAL TO APPROPRIATE RESOURCES

Refer parents and other family members to the American Anorexia and Bulimia Association, National Anorectic Aid Society, and National Association of Anorexia Nervosa & Associated Disorders for further information about the disorder and a list of support groups in their area.

EVALUATION

Expected outcomes for nursing care include recommended level of weight gain, maintenance of adequate fluid volume and balanced electrolytes, maintenance of normal blood pressure and heart rhythm, beginning of positive sense of self-esteem, intake of nutritionally balanced diet, and use of psychologic counseling to understand the disorder.

Bulimia Nervosa

Bulimia nervosa is an eating disorder characterized by **binge eating** (a compulsion to consume large quantities of food in a short period of time). Usually the episodes of bingeing are followed by various methods of weight control (purging), such as self-induced vomiting, large doses of laxatives or diuretics, or a combination of methods. Bulimia affects 1% of the general populations, but 5% or more of young women (Hoek, 2006). Like anorexia, it affects mainly adolescent girls and young women who are white and in the higher socioeconomic classes (Hoek, 2006). The disorder usually begins in middle to late adolescence, frequently emerging during college.

Etiology and pathophysiology. Causes of bulimia nervosa are similar to those of anorexia nervosa: sensitivity to social pressure for thinness, body image difficulties, and long-standing dysfunctional family patterns. Families may be chaotic and distant from the girl, rather than overinvolved as with the anorectic. Many bulimic individuals experience depression. It is not clear whether the depression is a cause or a result of the bulimic individual's inability to control the bingeing and purging cycles. An adolescent with bulimia often binges after any stressful event.

Bingeing usually occurs in secret for several hours until the individual is stopped by abdominal discomfort, by another person, or by vomiting. At first the episodes of binge eating are pleasurable. Immediately following the binge episode, however, feelings of guilt, shame, anger, depression, and fear of loss of control and weight gain arise. As these feelings intensify, the bulimic adolescent becomes increasingly anxious. This usually initiates the purge behaviors.

Purging eliminates the discomfort from bloating and also prevents weight gain. This relieves the feelings of depression and guilt, but only temporarily. Adolescents with bulimia commonly practice the binge-purge cycle many times a day, losing their ability to respond to normal cues of hunger and satiety.

Clinical manifestations. Bulimia is often a "silent" disorder since it is easily concealed from healthcare providers and families. Only about 6% of those with the condition are believed to receive treatment (Hoek, 2006). Adolescents with bulimia are preoccupied with body shape, size, and weight. They may appear overweight or thin and usually report a wide range of average body weight over the years. Physical findings depend on the degree of purging, starvation, dehydration, and electrolyte disturbance. Erosion of tooth enamel, increased dental caries, and gum recession, which result from vomiting of gastric acids, are common findings. The back of a hand can have calluses from inducing vomiting. Abdominal distention is often seen. Esophageal tears and esophagitis may also occur.

Table 34–9 DSM-IV Criteria for Bulimia Nervosa

A. Recurrent episodes of binge eating. An episode of binge eating is characterized by both of the following:
   1. Eating, in a discrete period of time (e.g., within any 2-hour period), an amount of food that is definitely larger than most people would eat during a similar period of time and under similar circumstances
   2. A sense of lack of control over eating during the episode (e.g., a feeling that one cannot stop eating or control what or how much one is eating)

B. Recurrent inappropriate compensatory behavior in order to prevent weight gain, such as self-induced vomiting; misuse of laxatives, diuretics, enemas, or other medications; fasting; or excessive exercise.

C. The binge eating and inappropriate compensatory behaviors both occur, on average, at least twice a week for 3 months.

D. Self-evaluation is unduly influenced by body weight and shape.

E. The disturbance does not occur exclusively during episodes of anorexia nervosa.

Source: Used with permission from the Diagnostic and Statistical Manual of Mental Disorders, 4th ed., © 2000. American Psychiatric Association.

Clinical therapy. A comprehensive history is necessary because most adolescents with bulimia appear normal in weight or only slightly underweight. Diagnostic tests include hematocrit, hemoglobin, and serum electrolytes; they may identify signs of altered electrolyte and hematologic status. Lowered potassium levels are related to repetitive vomiting since gastric contents have a high potassium level (APA, 2006). The diagnosis is confirmed by the presence of specific *DSM-IV* criteria (Table 34–9).

Treatment includes management of physiologic problems and cognitive-behavior therapy. Medications, such as gluoxetine 60 mg/day for adolesctnes, may be prescribed (Berkman et al., 2006). Management involves a variety of healthcare providers such as physicians, nurses, and therapists. Behavior modification focuses on modifying the dysfunctional eating patterns and restoring normal patterns. Until the episodes of bingeing and purging are under control, feelings of discouragement and hopelessness prevail. Thus, the focus early in treatment is on initiating an immediate behavioral change. Once initial interventions have been successful, group therapy sessions work well for persons with anorexia or bulimia. Specific treatment measures may include the following:

- Educating the adolescent about good nutrition (including food choice and caloric content)
- Encouraging the adolescent to keep a log or food journal and assisting the adolescent to make connections between emotional states, stress, and the impulse to binge or purge
- Setting up a daily dietary routine of three meals and three snacks a day (using the same foods for each meal and snack every day to change misconceptions about the weight-gaining potential of certain foods and to decrease anxiety about what food must be eaten at the next meal)

Once these initial measures have been taken, the underlying psychosocial issues are explored. The goals of therapy are to provide the bulimic adolescent with adaptive coping skills and to improve self-esteem.

Most adolescents with bulimia do not require hospitalization. Serious abnormalities in fluid and electrolyte levels caused by uncontrollable cycles of bingeing and vomiting, accompanied by depression or suicidal activity, are indications of the need for hospitalization. The prognosis is good with long-term therapy.

MyNursingKit Case Study: Peanut Allergy at School

NURSING MANAGEMENT

NURSING ASSESSMENT AND DIAGNOSIS

Obtain a thorough individual and family history, including daily dietary intake and weight fluctuations. Inquire about problems such as abdominal pain or distention, which may indicate an abnormal eating or elimination pattern. Assess the oral mucosa for signs of damage to tooth enamel caused by purging; examine hands for evidence of vomiting-induced calluses.

Following are nursing diagnoses that may be appropriate for the adolescent with bulimia nervosa:

- *Imbalanced Nutrition: Less than or More than Body Requirements* related to disordered food intake
- *Risk for Deficient Fluid Volume* related to fluid volume loss
- *Impaired Oral Mucous Membrane* related to chemical effects of vomited gastric acids
- *Deficient Knowledge (adolescent)* related to health risks of excessive use of laxatives and diuretics
- *Anxiety* related to discomfort with weight and eating patterns
- *Chronic Low Self-Esteem* related to dysfunctional family dynamics
- *Ineffective Individual Coping* related to life stressors

PLANNING AND IMPLEMENTATION

Nursing care includes monitoring nutritional intake and elimination patterns, preventing complications, and providing appropriate referrals.

During hospitalization the patient should keep a food diary. Be alert to the adolescent who hides, gives away, or discards food from the tray or who exits to use the bathroom after meals. The adolescent should be monitored for at least 30 minutes after meals by remaining in a central area in the company of the nurse or other responsible individuals. Withdrawal from laxatives and diuretics is managed with careful observation for alterations in fluid and electrolyte status. Cardiac monitoring may be necessary if potassium levels are seriously altered. Esophageal tearing or esophagitis is treated to promote mucosal healing. Medications such as antidepressants may be administered. Encourage continuation of group and other therapy sessions.

Bulimic adolescents and their families can be referred to organizations such as those listed earlier in the section on anorexia for assistance and information about the disorder.

EVALUATION

Expected outcomes for nursing care for the adolescent with bulimia include healthy mucous membranes and skin, adequate intake of fluids and food, balanced food intake, maintenance of normal weight, adequate support and healthy psychological balance, and absence of bingeing and purging.

FOOD REACTIONS

Food reaction encompasses any adverse reaction to foods or substances ingested in foods. The most common food reaction is **food intolerance**, an abnormal physiologic response to a food that is not immunoglobulin E (IgE)-mediated. Examples include indigestion or flatulence upon eating certain foods, a sweating reaction to some spices, rhinitis, and hives with urticaria (Burks & Ballmer-Weber, 2006). Milk and grain products are common causes of food intolerance. Chemical additives, antibiotics, preservatives, and food colorings also can cause food sensitivity reactions.

The most serious type of reaction is **food allergy**, an IgE-mediated reaction that is potentially systemic, characteristically rapid in onset, and may be manifested as swelling of the lips, mouth, uvula or glottis, generalized urticaria, and in severe reactions, anaphylaxis. Food allergies are the most common cause of anaphylaxis and are more prevalent in children with a family history of allergic reactions to various substances and foods (**atopy**). The foods that most commonly cause allergy are fish, shellfish, peanuts, tree nuts, eggs, soy, wheat, corn, strawberries, and cow's-milk products. About 1% of children have an allergy to peanuts and the incidence is increasing. A majority of the 150 deaths from food allergies that occur annually in the United States are due to peanut allergy (Palmer & Burks, 2006).

Children who have both food allergy and asthma are most at risk of death from anaphylaxis due to a food allergy. Allergic individuals need to be aware of hidden substances in prepared foods. For example, the child allergic to nuts will experience a reaction to a food if nut extracts are used in its preparation. Note that certain foods can cause either allergy or intolerance so accurate diagnosis is needed. An example is cow's milk that can cause an allergy with IgE-mediated systemic reaction, or an intolerance from gastrointestinal response to milk proteins (diarrhea, vomiting, abdominal pain) as a result of lack of the enzyme lactase in the gastrointestinal tract.

Delayed hypersensitivity reactions are attributed to digestive products of food and require a thorough diet history over several days to identify the offending food. These reactions are more difficult to diagnose, since the reaction can occur up to 24 hours after ingestion of the food. There may also be biphasic reactions that occur 1 to 30 hours after an initial anaphylaxis. Such reactions can be severe and life threatening. Therefore every child with a food allergy who ingests the allergen should be promptly treated with epinephrine and transported to an emergency facility for further management and monitoring.

Diagnostic tests to identify suspected food allergies include measurement of serum IgE levels, scratch tests, and the **radioallergosorbent test (RAST)**, in which radioimmunoassay measures IgE antibodies to specific allergens (see Chapter 50 ∞ for further information about these tests). In cases of

Developing Cultural Competence

LACTOSE INTOLERANCE

Some ethnic groups have a high incidence of lactose intolerance due to low amounts of the enzyme lactase in the gut. While most members of the group have adequate amounts of lactase in childhood to drink milk products, by adulthood 70% to 100% of some groups are lactose intolerant. Blacks, Native Americans, and Asians often have lactase deficiency, which may begin to emerge during childhood. When a child develops intolerance to milk products, suggest alternative sources of calcium and other nutrients found in milk.

Nursing Practice

Children with food allergies should wear an alert bracelet and carry an emergency medication such as EpiPen. Nurses in schools and offices must instruct families, schoolteachers, and others about the child's allergy and what to do in case of accidental ingestion of the food product. Assist them to set up prevention and emergency treatment plans.

past allergic response, the food is absolutely avoided. In food intolerance, a diet diary is kept, noting date, type of foods eaten, and reaction, if any. Foods should be eaten singly for several days to determine whether they cause a reaction.

Treatment consists of eliminating the offending foods from the child's diet.

Nursing Management

Prevention is the first step. Instruct parents of infants to introduce new foods at a rate of not more than one new food every 3 to 5 days. If a sensitivity is noted, the causative food can be easily identified. Discuss any changes in diet or preparation of formula. Reassure parents that the child's symptoms will disappear when the offending foods are removed from the diet.

Be alert for skin, respiratory, and other characteristic manifestations of sensitivity or allergy. Refer such cases to an allergist immediately for diagnosis. If an allergy is identified, help the family to identify and remove the offending foods. Emphasize the importance of reading food labels for hidden foods that can trigger an allergic reactions (Simons, Weiss, Furlong, et al., 2005). The child and school should have an EpiPen and other emergency treatment for the allergic child, accessible at all times. The child with a food allergy should wear a medical alert bracelet. Be sure that school personnel know about the allergy and know to avoid giving the child the food product. Ensure that a food allergy plan is in place in the school and within each additional setting where the child spends time.

Refer the family to the Food Allergy Network. Recognize that food allergies can be stressful for children and families, as they worry about exposure in daily life (www.foodallergy.org/).

The child with food intolerance needs to avoid the food to ensure comfort and an absence of the annoying symptoms associated with it. Although intolerance is not life threatening, unlike allergy, the family needs to learn about hidden sources of the food product so that it can be avoided and alternative foods can be suggested for their use.

NUTRITIONAL SUPPORT

SPORTS NUTRITION AND ERGOGENIC AGENTS

Regular physical activity should be encouraged for all children, with at least 60 minutes of activity recommended daily. However, during vigorous or prolonged exercise, or during hot weather, child and adolescent athletes may have special nutritional needs. A well-balanced diet, reflective of recommended foods, is needed. A wide variety of fresh fruits and vegetables, grains, and complex carbohydrates usually provides for adequate caloric intake. When the child is hungry, extra calories should come from the food groups listed here, rather than from increased intake of fat. When the child or teen is very active, sports bars or drinks can provide the additional needed calories in a nutritionally balanced manner. As always, the height, weight, and BMI percentiles are the best assurance that the child is growing adequately over time. Adequate energy to perform the sport as well as be attentive and productive at school and for other activities should also be considered.

Water should be increased during activity both to minimize chance of dehydration and also to maximize performance. About 1 hour before vigorous exercise, the child should drink 1 to 2 glasses (8 to 16 ounces) of water and should repeat the same amount of fluid just before the exercise begins. Young children may not feel thirsty and should be encouraged to drink 6 to 12 ounces of fluid every 15 to 20 minutes during exercise (AAP, Committee on Nutrition, 2009; Cotugna, Vickery, & McBee, 2005). Water is usually the best replacement, but during extended exercise, sports drinks may be a good alternative for some of the fluid intake. More water is needed after activity. Weight loss of 1 pound indicates a loss of about 1/2 quart of fluid. The nurse should be sure the child takes in fluid to replace all losses.

Some common nutrients that may be deficient in all teens, but even more often in the athlete are calcium and iron. The increased blood volume common in the well-conditioned person necessitates greater intake. Calcium-rich foods such as milk products and dark green vegetables, and iron-rich foods such as meats and grains can guard against deficiencies. While many adolescents believe that they need extra protein during athletic season, most Americans eat adequate protein to meet even the increased needs of sports. On the other hand, the vegetarian child or adolescent may need help to plan a diet with adequate protein.

Many teens take a wide variety of dietary supplements, believing that they act as **ergogenic aids**, or products that enhance performance during sports by influencing energy, alertness, or body composition. Most of the claims of these products are unproven, and their safety has not usually been investigated, especially in the young. Effects on youth whose bodies are still developing are particularly unknown and the risks are high for permanent interference with some normal growth patterns. Offer guidance and help the family and teen investigate claims before choosing to use a product. If youths use supplements, they should be instructed in doses, desired effects, and potential side effects of supplements. Some sports and coaches may encourage small size and dieting, or encourage use of dietary supplements to increase weight and muscle. Children and adolescents in activities such as ballet, wrestling, track or running, and horse racing may have health risks associated with inconsistent or inadequate intake.

Approximately 4% of U.S. high school students (4.8% of males and 3.2% of females) report taking illegal anabolic steroids; up to 6.5% in some communities report use. Interestingly, their use is higher among 9th and 10th graders than 11th and 12th graders (CDC, 2006b). These products can have a wide array of side effects.They may stop growth of long bones, lead to endocrine imbalance, and cause increased tendon rupture. They are also illegal in sporting events. Andro and DHEA are steroidal hormones used by some athletes. They cause masculinization of females, disruption of glucose balance and insulin sensitivity, and dyslipedia (Rosenfield, 2005).

Some common amino acid nutritional supplements include creatine, carnitine, and glutamine. Although the side effects of these substances are minimal, their possible enhancement of performance is temporary and outcomes of long-term use are unknown. Increasing protein intake to meet needs during high activity is a better alternative. Creatine has been studied more than most supplements; it is made by the body and is present in many protein sources. Supplemental creatine increases the creatine level in muscle and may help to increase performance in short bursts of activity, while not affecting endurance sports. The increase in muscle mass that can occur is actually due to water and is lost quickly when the supplement is discontinued (Williams, 2006).

Minerals such as chromium, iron, and calcium are used by some youths. The nurse should ask careful and sensitive questions such as "Many athletes take supplements to aid in performance in sports. What supplements do you take or are you considering?" Information should be provided to enhance the youth's understanding of nutrition and sports performance. Generally, a balanced diet with adequate carbohydrate, protein, and fat will meet the needs of most athletes and lead to maximal sport performance. School nurses can work with physical education teachers and coaches to plan appropriate programs for youth to prevent use of ergogenic aids (Rosenfield, 2005).

MyNursingKit Vegetarian Teens: Plan a 2-Day Menu

HEALTH-RELATED CONDITIONS

Many health conditions influence the child's nutritional state. Conversely, the child's nutritional state can influence the state of health. See "Pathophysiology Illustrated" for examples of some common conditions that influence nutritional needs. These conditions are discussed in various chapters throughout the text. When reading about them, discuss with classmates how to adjust normal nutritional assessment and teaching due to the presence of a healthcare concern. Which conditions influence absorption of nutrients? Which cause changes in nutritional intake requirements? Some children benefit from special dietary aids, such as eating utensils and cups that are easy to grasp. Therapists can evaluate and make recommendations about devices that can assist the child at meals.

Complementary Care

HERBS AND PROBIOTICS

Many families use food products to promote health and treat diseases. These include herbal products that may be acquired from health food stores or the Internet. Herbs are not tested nor regulated by the government, so amounts of ingredients are often not known. Ask families about what herbal products they use regularly or to treat disease. Learn about the herbs and any research that has been conducted with children.

Another type of food product is a **probiotic**, a live microorganism that improves the balance of gut microflora, thereby providing a health benefit. Common probiotics include *Lactobacillus* and *Bifidobacterium*, which are commonly found in the human gastrointestinal tract, are enhanced by eating yogurt with live cultures, and may be helpful in treating diarrhea or atopic dermatitis (Schuerman & Vezeau, 2007; Bowman & Russell, 2006). Inquire about the family's treatment for conditions such as diarrhea. Daily intake of pasteurized yogurt with live cultures can safely be encouraged for children.

VEGETARIANISM

Some families choose to eat vegetarian diets and can be helped and encouraged in their endeavors. Several variations in intake occur. **Vegetarians** eat no poultry, meat, or fish. Lacto-ovovegetarians eat eggs and dairy products, while lactovegetarians eat dairy products but not eggs. In contrast, **vegans** are strict vegetarians and eat no animal products. When someone says he or she is vegetarian, it is best if the nurse asks specific questions about what the individual will and will not eat.

The vegetarian can be very healthy, but may need some additional help to ensure nutritional adequacy. Some common deficiencies include vitamins D and B_{12}, zinc, iron, calories, protein, and fat. Completing a 24-hour diet recall for pregnant or lactating women and vegetarian children, with analysis for RDAs, can be helpful. The nurse should be sure to routinely assess growth and other nutritional measures, as well as provide ideas of various foods to meet nutritional needs and perform other general nutritional teaching. When a vegetarian child is hospitalized, the nurse should plan with the nutrition department and the child's family to meet intake needs.

Growth and Development

When a pregnant teen follows a vegetarian diet, she needs additional help to encourage adequate nutrition (Johnston & Sabate, 2006). A 24-hour or 2-day diet diary helps identify nutritional needs. Consider additional pregnancy needs for energy, protein, omega 3 fatty acids, iron, vitamin D, and calcium; note that Vitamin B_{12} is recommended as a supplement. Use the vegetarian Food Guide Pyramid available through the American Dietetic Association.

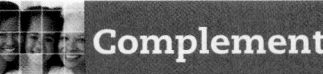

PATHOPHYSIOLOGY ILLUSTRATED

CONDITIONS THAT INFLUENCE NUTRITIONAL NEEDS

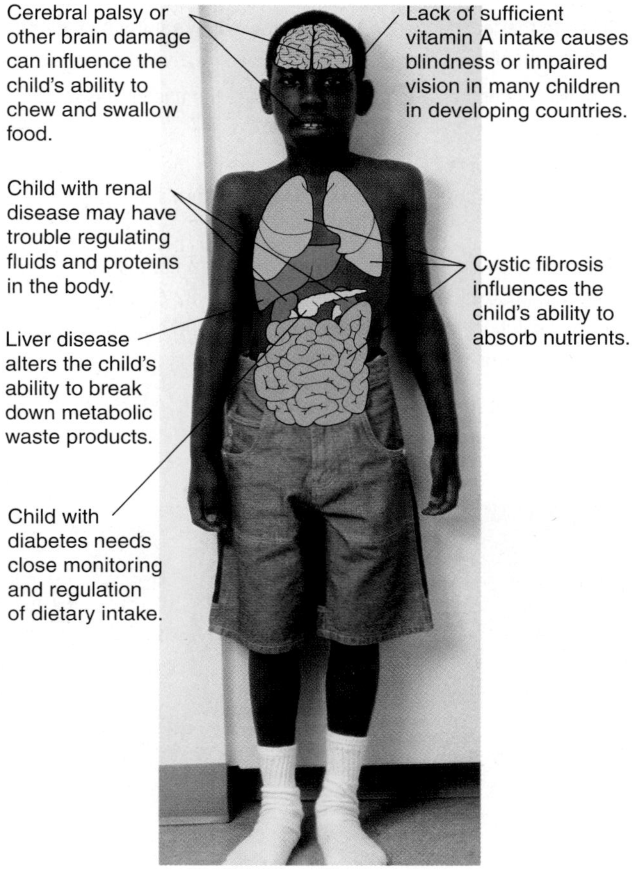

Cerebral palsy or other brain damage can influence the child's ability to chew and swallow food.
Lack of sufficient vitamin A intake causes blindness or impaired vision in many children in developing countries.
Child with renal disease may have trouble regulating fluids and proteins in the body.
Cystic fibrosis influences the child's ability to absorb nutrients.
Liver disease alters the child's ability to break down metabolic waste products.
Child with diabetes needs close monitoring and regulation of dietary intake.

ENTERAL THERAPY

Enteral therapy is a form of nutritional support provided when a child cannot take in enough food orally to sustain health. Since it is the closest form of nutritional support to the natural method of eating, it has the least untoward effects and greatest rate of success. Some children who use enteral therapy are those with cerebral palsy or other neurologic conditions which lead to weakness of the throat and mouth, those with neoplasm or immune dysfunction, and those in acute states of recovery from accidents or illness (Figure 34–11 ●).

Although a tube can be inserted into the nasal opening and placed through the esophagus into the stomach (nasogastric tube), a tube surgically placed into the stomach through an abdominal opening, a jejunal or gastric tube, is preferred for long-term use. As long as the child can absorb and use nutrients, enteral therapy can be successful in providing calories and essential nutrients. Commercially prepared formulas are available, and specially formulated solutions can be adapted for children with specific dietary needs. Nursing care includes care of the gastrostomy tube and entry site to prevent infection and

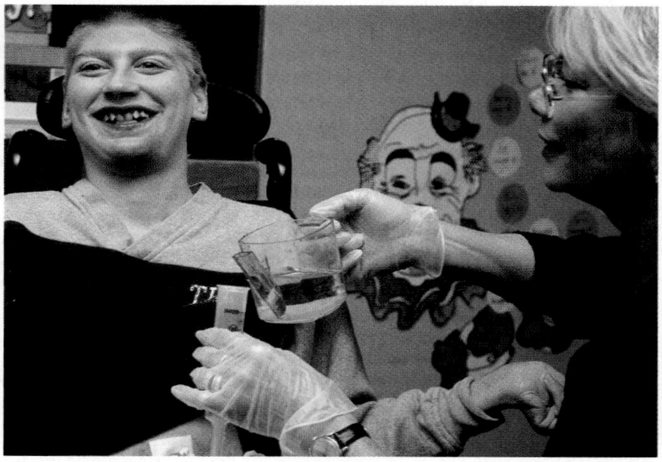

● **Figure 34–11** Enteral therapy. This child has returned to school following surgery. Due to cerebral palsy, he has difficulty chewing and swallowing food. The school nurse has taught his teacher to safely administer some enteral feedings during school hours.

skin breakdown. Ensure that a nasogastric tube is correctly placed before each tube feeding. For both nasogastric and gastric feedings an empty syringe is often used to check residuals or the amount of fluid not absorbed since the previous feeding. Teach families enteral feeding techniques when they will perform the process at home and arrange for periodic evaluation of technique. Perform regular nutritional assessments. See Chapter 53 ∞ for suggestions on management of nursing care during tube feedings. See also Skill 15–3 in the accompanying Clinical Skills Manual SKILLS.

TOTAL PARENTERAL NUTRITION (TPN)

Total parenteral nutrition (TPN) makes it possible to provide intravenous nutritional support for people who cannot eat or are unable to absorb nutrients from the intestinal tract in a normal manner and are at risk of severe malnutrition. Examples of children who benefit from this method of nutrition are those with congenital malformation of the gastrointestinal tract, brain injury, or severe burns; it may also be used for support after bone marrow transplant, sepsis, or other critical conditions.

A catheter is inserted so that a sterile nutrition solution is infused directly into the bloodstream. A central venous catheter is used to promote safe infusion. Fluids usually contain glucose; electrolytes such as sodium, potassium, calcium, magnesium, phosphate, and chloride; vitamins; and proteins. Lipid emulsions are another type of TPN used in some children. Meticulous care is needed, whether in the hospital or at home, to ensure safe TPN infusion and treatment. The nurse performs initial assessment, ongoing evaluation and monitoring of treatment, verifies the solution type and rate of administration, ensures that solution storage recommendations are followed, and administers the solutions in the hospital or other settings. See Skill 12–7 for the protocols for TPN management in the Clinical Skills Manual SKILLS.

MyNursingKit Nursing in Action: Administering a Gavage/Tube Feeding

Thinking Critically

THE CHILD WITH SPECIAL NUTRITIONAL NEEDS

Joey was diagnosed with cerebral palsy early in life. He is now 11 years old and has recently been enrolled in school. Part of the healthcare plan being implemented in the school involves fostering a positive nutritional state. Joey has limited ability to swallow, related to muscle weakness of cerebral palsy, and is therefore unable to ingest enough calories by mouth to ensure his optimal growth and development. Joey had a feeding tube inserted into his stomach at an early age and receives some of his nutrition by this method.

The school nurse has met with Joey's parents and his home health nurse to learn about the amount and type of tube feedings he receives, as well as the texture of oral feedings he can manage. The nurse will plan the feeding schedule at school to facilitate adequate nutrition in that setting. In addition, careful ongoing nutritional assessment will be needed to evaluate if Joey is getting the calories and other nutrients he needs for growth and development. The school nurse is also educating the classroom teachers and other school personnel about Joey's unique nutritional requirements.

- What do the teachers need to know about Joey's nutritional needs during school?
- How will you organize Joey's care if you are the case manager for his integration within the school system?
- How can the nurse help the family prepare for meeting nutritional needs of a child who has special needs like Joey's during travel by car or plane?
- If Joey's family plans to visit another state on a car trip this summer, what will they need to bring with them? Consider his feeding solution, tubing, and other supplies, and how to maintain refrigeration for enteral solutions.

See MyNursingKit for possible responses.

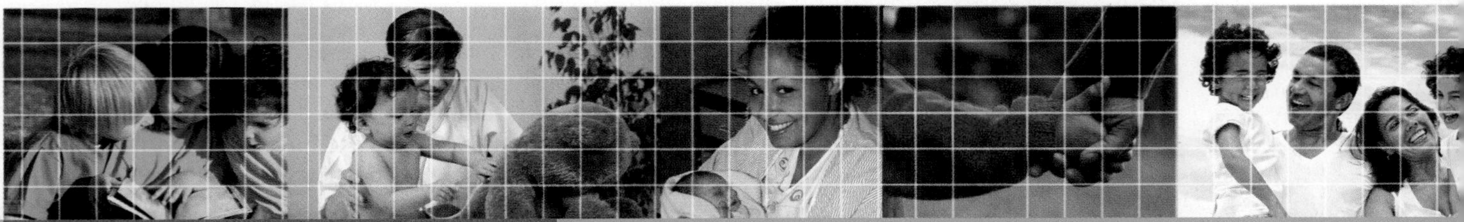

CRITICAL CONCEPT REVIEW

LEARNING OUTCOMES	CONCEPTS
34.1 Discuss major nutritional concepts pertaining to the growth and development of children.	Infancy: 1. Increased need for calories because of: ■ Rapid physical growth. ■ Increased physical activity. 2. Proper nutrition is needed for development of the nervous system and organs. 3. Should receive only breast milk or formula until tongue thrust has decreased and infant can sit well. 4. No cow's milk until 1 year of age. 5. Food introduction principles are needed by parents. Toddlerhood: 1. Development of physiologic anorexia. 2. Amount of milk and fruit juice should be limited so child will eat nutritious solid food. 3. Should begin to learn to eat in social situations. Preschool: 1. Should begin to help with simple food preparation. 2. May exhibit extreme food preferences (food jag). 3. Emphasize brushing of teeth and first dental visit. School-age: 1. Time of gradual growth with preadolescent growth spurt. 2. Increased need for calories during growth spurt. 3. May be resistant to trying new foods. 4. Expect loss of first deciduous teeth and eruption of permanent teeth. Adolescence: 1. Need for increased calories during growth spurt. 2. Increased physical activity (such as sports) will increase caloric needs. 3. Encourage balanced intake and minimize fast foods.

LEARNING OUTCOMES	CONCEPTS
34.2 Describe and plan nursing interventions to meet nutritional needs for all age groups from infancy through adolescence.	Infancy: 1. Encourage breastfeeding, if possible. 2. Assist mother to continue to breastfeed the hospitalized infant. 3. Discuss feeding during each contact with the mother. 4. To decrease occurrence of dental caries, teach parents that infant should not be given a bottle at bedtime. 5. Teach beginning dental care. 6. Supplemental foods begin with rice cereal and progress to vegetables and then fruit. 7. Begin use of cup for liquids at 8–9 months of age. Toddlerhood: 1. Encourage parents to provide health foods that are easily eaten: ■ Small portions. ■ Place 1 tablespoon of food per year of age on child's plate. 2. Limit milk to 1 quart per day. 3. Limit fruit juice to 6 ounces per day. 4. Parents should establish meal time rules. Preschool: 1. Encourage parents to use meal preparation as time for teaching about proper nutrition and kitchen safety. 2. Limit fruit juice to 12 ounces per day. 3. Encourage parents to limit fast food to once per week. School-age: 1. Present nutritional teaching to child by using pictures and providing hands-on experiences. 2. Encourage families to bring food from home for the hospitalized child. 3. Allow hospitalized children to eat together. 4. Become knowledgeable concerning nutritional assistance available to the child and family. Adolescence: 1. Encourage teen to drink fruit juice in place of soft drinks. 2. Provide healthy choices of food for teen. 4. Allow peer interaction during meals, if possible.
34.3 Integrate methods of nutritional assessment into nursing care of infants, children, and adolescents.	Nutritional assessments include: 1. Growth measurements: ■ Height (length). ■ Weight. ■ Head circumference. ■ Skinfold measurement. 2. Body mass index. 3. Laboratory tests: ■ Hemoglobin and hematocrit. ■ Lipid profile. ■ Liver function. ■ Renal function. ■ Serum glucose. 4. Mother's dietary intake during pregnancy. 5. 24-hour food recall. 6. Food frequency questionnaire. 7. Food diary.
34.4 Discuss common nutritional problems of children in developed countries.	Common nutritional problems include: 1. Hunger due to poverty. 2. Obesity. 3. Foodborne illness. 4. Dietary deficiencies.

(continued)

LEARNING OUTCOMES — CONCEPTS

34.5 Apply the nursing process to care for children with eating disorders.

1. Assessment:
   - Obtain individual and family history.
   - Obtain accurate height and weight.
   - Observe eating behaviors.
   - Investigate use of prescription and OTC medications.
2. Planning and implementation:
   - Monitor nutritional and fluid intake.
   - Encourage nutritious food consumption.
   - Monitor elimination pattern.
   - Administer medications as needed.
3. Evaluation:
   - Promote adequate food and fluid to establish healthy nutritional lifestyle.
   - Encourage positive self-esteem.

CRITICAL THINKING IN ACTION

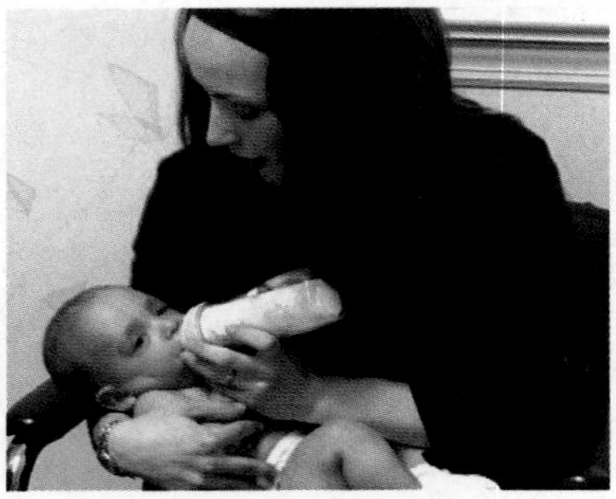

A mother is seeing the pediatric nurse practitioner you are working with for her son Jonathan's 3-month, well-baby checkup at the local community health clinic. The baby is in the 90th percentile for weight and in the 50th percentile for length and is fed Similac formula with Iron. According to the medical history, Jonathan had RSV when he was 1 month old and there are smokers in the house. The nurse practitioner has asked you to educate the mother about feeding her 3-month-old baby. The mother has raised concerns that the baby is not sleeping through the night and the baby's grandmother has suggested adding cereal to his bottle at night to help him sleep. Jonathan has met all developmental milestones and has not yet developed teeth.

1. What type of advice can you give the mother about adding cereal to the bottle?
2. Why is rice cereal recommended as the first food to introduce when Jonathan is able to start solid foods?
3. What is the reason only iron-fortified formula or breast milk is recommended the entire first year of life for Jonathan, rather than cow's milk?
4. Based on Jonathan's length and weight percentiles on the growth chart, his mother wonders if he should be put on a "diet." What would be the appropriate response to her concern?

See MyNursingKit for possible responses.

REFERENCES

Allen, K. N., Taylor, J. S., & Kuiper, R. A. (2007). Effectiveness of nutrition education on fast food choices in adolescents. *Journal of School Nursing, 23*, 337–341.

American Academy of Pediatrics, Committee on Nutrition. (2009). *Pediatric nutrition handbook* (6th ed.). Elk Grove Village, IL: American Academy of Pediatrics.

American Academy of Pediatrics, Section on Breastfeeding (2005). Breastfeeding and the use of human milk. *Pediatrics, 115*, 496–506.

American College of Obstetricians and Gynecologists. (2007). *Breastfeeding: Maternal and infant aspects* (ACOG Committee Opinion, No. 361). Washington, DC: Author.

American Diabetes Association (2008). Nutrition recommendations and interventions for diabetes. *Diabetes Care 31*, S61–S78.

American Dietetic Association. (2006). *Nutrition intervention in the treatment of anorexia nervosa, bulimia nervosa, and eating disorders not otherwise specified (EDNOS)*. Retrieved August 3, 2006, from http://www.eatright.org/cps/rde/xchg/ada/hs.xls/advocacy_adapo701_ENU_HTML.htm

American Psychiatric Association Working Group on Eating Disorders. (2006). *Practice guideline for the treatment of patients with eating disorders* (3rd ed.). Retrieved May 20, 2007, from http://www.psych_pract/treatg/pg/Eating Disorder3ePG_04-28-06.pdf

Berkman, N. D., Bulik, C. M., Brownley, K. A., Loh, K. N., Sedway, J. A., Rooks, A., et al. (2006). *Management of eating disorders*. Rockville, MD: Agency for Healthcare Research and Quality. AHRQ Pub No. 06.E010.

Bindler, R. M., & Howry, L. B. (2005). Pediatric drug guide. Upper Saddle River, NJ: Prentice Hall-Health.

Block, R. W., Krebs, N. F., and Committee on Child Abuse and Neglect and Committee on Nutrition (2005). Failure to thrive as a manifestation of child neglect. *Pediatrics 116*, 1234–1237.

Bowman, B. A., & Russell, R. M. (2006). *Present knowledge in nutrition* (9th ed.). Washington DC: International Life Sciences Institute.

Burks, W., & Ballmer-Weber, B. K. (2006). Food allergy. *Molecular Nutrition and Food Research, 50*, 595–603.

Centers for Disease Control and Prevention (2005a). Preventing dental caries with community programs. Retrieved May 3, 2007, from http://www.cdc.gov/OralHealth/factsheets/dental_caries.htm

Centers for Disease Control and Prevention (2006a). QuickStats: Prevalence of overweight among persons aged 2–19 years, by sex—National Health and Nutrition Examination Survey (NHANES), United States, 1999–2000 through 2003–2004. *Morbidity and Mortality Weekly Report (MMWR), 55*, 1229.

Centers for Disease Control and Prevention (2006b). Youth Risk Behavior Surveillance—United States, 2005. *MMWR, 55* (SS-5), 1–108.

Centers for Disease Control and Prevention (2007). Preliminary FoodNet data on the incidence of infection with pathogens transmitted commonly through food—10 states, 2006. *MMWR, 56*, 336–339.

Children's Defense Fund. (2007). *The state of America's children*. Washington, DC: Author.

Cotugna, N., Vickery, C. E., & McBee, S. (2005). Sports nutrition for young athletes. *Journal of School Nursing, 21*, 323–328.

Dunger, D. B., Ahmed, M. L., & Ong, K. K. (2006). Early and late weight gain and the timing of puberty. *Molecular and Cellular Endocrinology, 254–255*, 140–145.

Failla-Tommasino, J. (2002). E. coli 0157:H7: An emerging bacterial threat. *Clinician Reviews, 12*(7), 48–54.

Federal Interagency Forum on Child and Family Statistics. (2005). *America's children: Key national indicators of well-being, 2005*. Washington, DC: Author.

Food and Drug Administration. (2004). Backgrounder for the 2004 FDA/EPA consumer advisory: What you need to know about mercury in fish and shellfish. Washington, DC: U.S. Department of Health and Human Services. http://www.fda.gov/Food/FoodSafety/Product-SpecificInformation/Seafood/FoodbornePathogensContaminants/Methymercury/ucm115662.htm, accessed 7/30/09.

Gluck, M. E. (2006). Stress response and binge eating disorder. *Appetite 46*, 26–30.

Gussy, M. G., Waters, E. G., Walsh, O., & Kilpatrick, N. M. (2006). Early childhood caries: Current evidence for aetiology and prevention. *Journal of Paediatrics and Child Health 42*, 37–43.

Hagan, J. F., Shaw, J. S., & Duncan, P. M. (2008). *Bright futures: Guidelines for health supervision of infants, children and adolescents* (3rd ed.). Elk Grove Village, IL: American Academy of Pediatrics.

Hoek, J. W. (2006). Incidence, prevalence and mortality of anorexia nervosa and other eating disorders. *Current Opinion in Psychiatry 19*, 389–394.

Institute of Medicine (2005a). *Dietary reference intakes for energy, carbohydrate, fiber, fat, fatty acids, cholesterol, protein, and amino acids*. Washington DC: National Academies Press.

Institute of Medicine (2005b). *Preventing childhood obesity*. Washington DC: National Academies Press.

Institute of Medicine (2006). *Dietary reference intakes*. Washington DC: National Academies Press.

Institute of Medicine (2007). *Progress in preventing childhood obesity*. Washington DC: National Academies Press.

Jenkins, S., & Horner, S. D. (2005). Barriers that influence eating behaviors in adolescents. *Journal of Pediatric Nursing, 20*, 258–267.

Johnston, P. K., & Sabate, J. (2006). Nutritional implications of vegetarian diets. In M. E. Shils, M. Shike, A. C. Ross, B. Caballero, & R. J. Cousins (Eds). *Modern nutrition in health and disease*. Philadelphia: Lippincott Williams & Wilkins (10th ed., pp. 1638–1654).

Lee, J. M., Appugliese, D., Kaciroti, M., Corwyn, R. F., Bradley, R. H., & Lumeng, J. C. (2007). Weight status in young girls and the onset of puberty. *Pediatrics, 119*, e624–630.

Lee, R. D., & Nieman, D. C. (2006). *Nutrition assessment* (4th ed.). Boston: McGraw-Hill.

National Institutes of Health (2008). *Breastfeeding*. Retrieved May 6, 2009, from http://www.nlm.nih.gov/medlineplus/ency/article/002450.htm

O'Connor, T. M., Yang, S. J., & Nicklas, T. A. (2006). Beverage intake among preschool children and its effect on weight status. *Pediatrics, 118*, e1010–e1018.

Olsen, E. M. (2006). Failure to thrive: Still a problem of definition. *Clinical Pediatrics, 45*, 1–6.

Palmer, K., & Burks, W. (2006). Current developments in peanut allergy. *Current Opinion in Allergy and Clinical Immunology, 6*, 202–206.

Rideout, V., & Hamel, E. (2006). *The media family: Electronic media in the lives of infants, toddlers, preschoolers and their parents*. Menlo Park, CA: Henry J. Kaiser Family Foundation.

Rosenfield, C. (2005). The use of ergogenic agents in high school athletes. *Journal of School Nursing 21*, 333–339.

Schuerman, G., & Vezeau, T. (2007). All bugs aren't bad: Probiotics in the treatment of pediatric atopic dermatitis. *American Journal for Nurse Practitioners, 11*(4), 28–36.

Simons, E., Weiss, C. C., Furlong, T. J., & Sicherer, S. J. (2005). Impact of ingredient labeling practices on food allergic consumer. *Annals of Allergy, Asthma and Immunology, 95*, 426–428.

Small, L., Anderson, D., & Melnyk, B. M. (2007). Prevention and early treatment of overweight and obesity in young children: A critical review and appraisal of the evidence. *Pediatric Nursing, 33*, 127, 149–161.

Stanton, B. F., Jenson, H. B., Behrman, R. E., Kliegman, R. M., & Jenson, H. B. (2007). *Nelson textbook of pediatrics* (18th ed.). Philadelphia: Saunders.

Storey, M. L., Forshee, R. A., & Anderson, P. A. (2004). Associations of adequate intake of calcium with diet, beverage consumption, and demographic characteristics among children and adolescents. *Journal of the American College of Nutrition, 23*, 18–33.

United States Department of Health and Human Services (2006). *Healthy People 2010: Midcourse Review*. U.S. Government Printing Office or www.health.gov/healthypeople/document.html

United States Department of Health and Human Services and United States Department of Agriculture (2005). *Dietary Guidelines for Americans*. Washington DC: U.S. Government Printing Office or http://www.healthierus.gov/dietaryguidelines/

Wagner, C. L., Greer, F. R., & the Section on Breastfeeding and Committee on Nutrition (2008). Prevention of rickets and vitamin D deficiency in infants, children, and adolescents. *Pediatrics, 122*, 1142–1152.

Waldrop, J. (2005). Early identification and interventions for female athlete triad. *Journal of Pediatric Health Care, 19*, 213–220.

Watt, R. G., McGlone, P., Russell, J. J., Tull, K. I., & Dowler, E. (2006). The process of establishing, implementing and maintaining a social support infant feeding programme. *Public Health Nutrition, 9*, 714–721.

Williams, M. H. (2006). Sports nutrition. In M. E. Shils, M. Shike, A. C. Ross, B. Caballero, & R. J. Cousins (Eds.), *Modern nutrition in health and disease* (10th ed., pp. 1723–1740). Philadelphia: Lippincott Williams & Wilkins.

EXPLORE PEARSON **mynursingkit**™

MyNursingKit is your one stop for online chapter review materials and resources. Prepare for success with additional NCLEX®-style practice questions, interactive assignments and activities, web links, animations and videos, and more!

Register your access code from the front of your book at **www.mynursingkit.com**

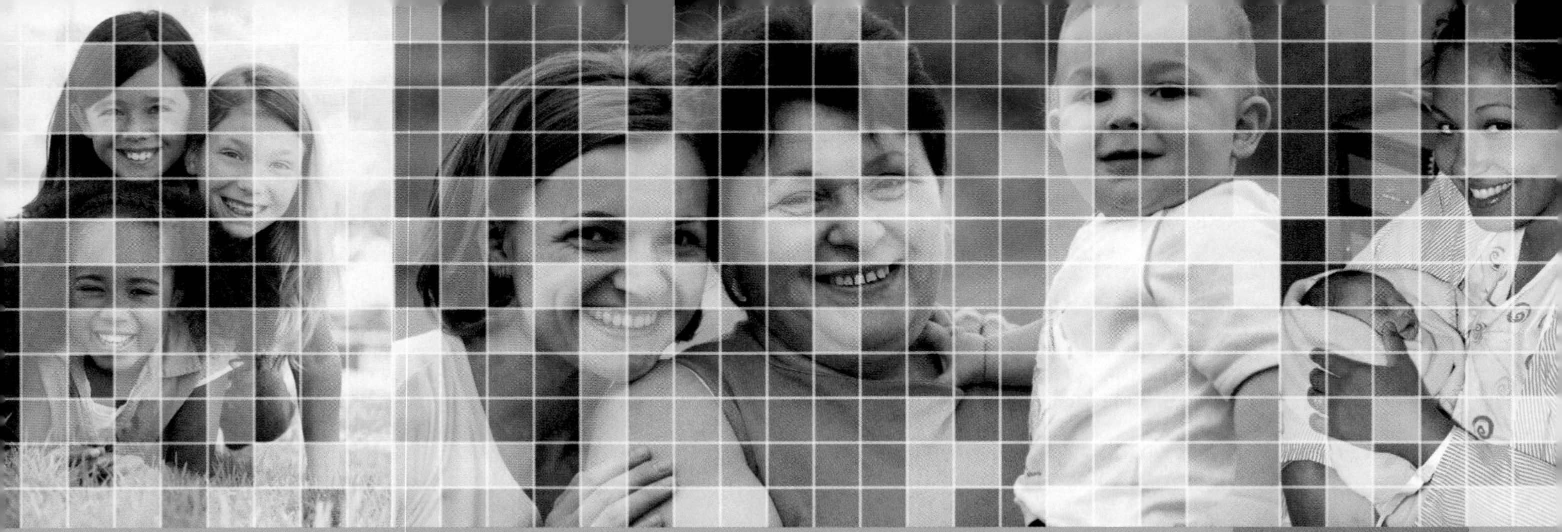

CHAPTER

Pediatric Assessment 35

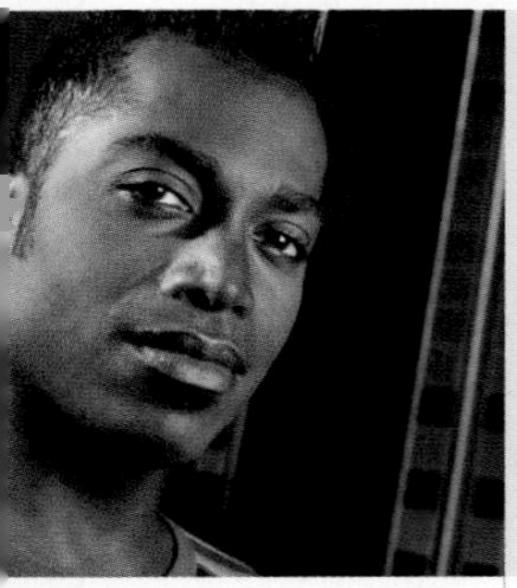

I was scared when we brought Latoya to the hospital. She looked helpless, afraid, and sick. The nurses and doctors took over when we got to the hospital, and I felt better because they seemed to know what to do. —*Father of Latoya, 6 months old*

LEARNING OUTCOMES

35.1 Describe the elements of a health history for infants and children of different ages.

35.2 Identify communication strategies to improve the quality of historical data collected.

35.3 Describe the strategies to gain cooperation of a young child for assessment.

35.4 Describe the differences in sequence of the physical assessment for infants, children, and adolescents.

35.5 Modify physical assessment techniques according to the age and developmental stage of the child.

35.6 List 5 normal variations in pediatric physical findings (such as a Mongolian spot in an infant) found during a physical assessment.

35.7 Determine the sexual maturity rating of males and females based upon physical signs of secondary sexual characteristics present.

35.8 Recognize at least five important signs of a serious alteration in health condition that require urgent nursing intervention.

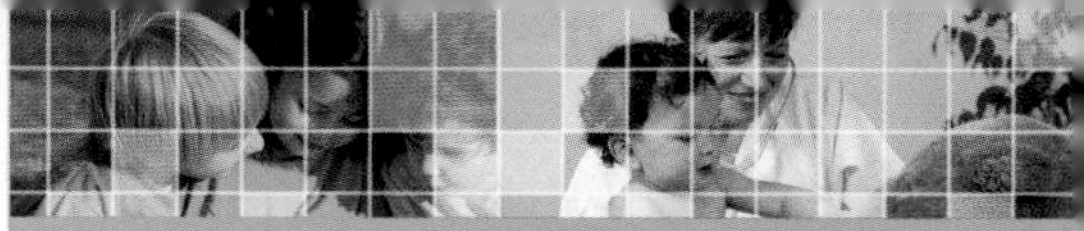

How do examination techniques vary by the age of the child? How does the nurse encourage infants and toddlers to cooperate with the examination? This chapter provides an overview of pediatric assessment, including history taking and examination techniques geared to the unique needs of pediatric patients. Strategies for obtaining the child's history are presented first. The remainder of the chapter then outlines a systematic process for physical examination of the child.

KEY TERMS

Apical impulse, 957
Auscultation, 936
Bronchophony, 956
Coloboma, 942
Crepitus, 955
Egophony, 956
Hypertelorism, 941
Inspection, 936
Nasal flaring, 947
Palpation, 936
Percussion, 936
Retractions, 953
Tactile fremitus, 955
Whispered pectoriloquy, 956

ANATOMIC AND PHYSIOLOGIC CHARACTERISTICS OF INFANTS AND CHILDREN

Children and infants are not only smaller than adults, but also significantly different physiologically. Knowledge of pediatric anatomic and physiologic differences will aid in recognizing normal variations found during the physical examination. It also assists with understanding the different physiologic responses children have to illness and injury. The illustration in "As Children Grow: Children Are Not Just Small Adults" provides an overview of important anatomic and physiologic differences between children and adults.

OBTAINING THE CHILD'S HISTORY

COMMUNICATION STRATEGIES

The health history interview is a very personal conversation with a parent, caretaker, or adolescent during which private concerns and feelings are shared. Try to ensure that both parties clearly understand this exchange of information and that it is an effective communication with the parent or the child. Effective communication is difficult to accomplish because parents and children often do not correctly interpret what the nurse says, just as the nurse may not understand completely what the parent or child says. People's interpretation of information is based on their life experiences, culture, and education.

Strategies to Build Rapport with the Family

When obtaining the history, make sure the parents understand the purpose of the interview and that the information will be used appropriately. To develop rapport, demonstrate interest in and concern for the child and family during the interview. This rapport forms the foundation for the collaborative relationship between the nurse and parent that will lead to the best nursing care for the child. The following strategies help to establish rapport with the child's family during the nursing history:

- Introduce yourself (name, title or position, and role in caring for the child). To demonstrate respect, ask all family members present what name they prefer you to use when talking with them.
- Explain the purpose of the interview and why the nursing history is different from the information collected by other health professionals. For example, "The nurses use this information to plan nursing care best suited for your child."
- Provide privacy and remove as many distractions as possible during the interview. If the patient's room does not offer privacy, attempt to find a vacant patient room or lounge. Assure the parents and the child that the information provided during the assessment is protected under the Health Insurance Portability and Accountability Act (HIPAA), a federal law that requires written consent to be provided before health information can be shared with healthcare providers outside the facility.
- Direct the focus of the interview with open-ended questions. Use close-ended questions or directing statements to clarify information. Open-ended questions are useful to initiate the interview, develop a rapport, and understand the parent's perceptions of the child's problem. For example: "What problems led to Roberto's admission to the hospital?" Close-ended

AS CHILDREN GROW

CHILDREN ARE NOT JUST SMALL ADULTS

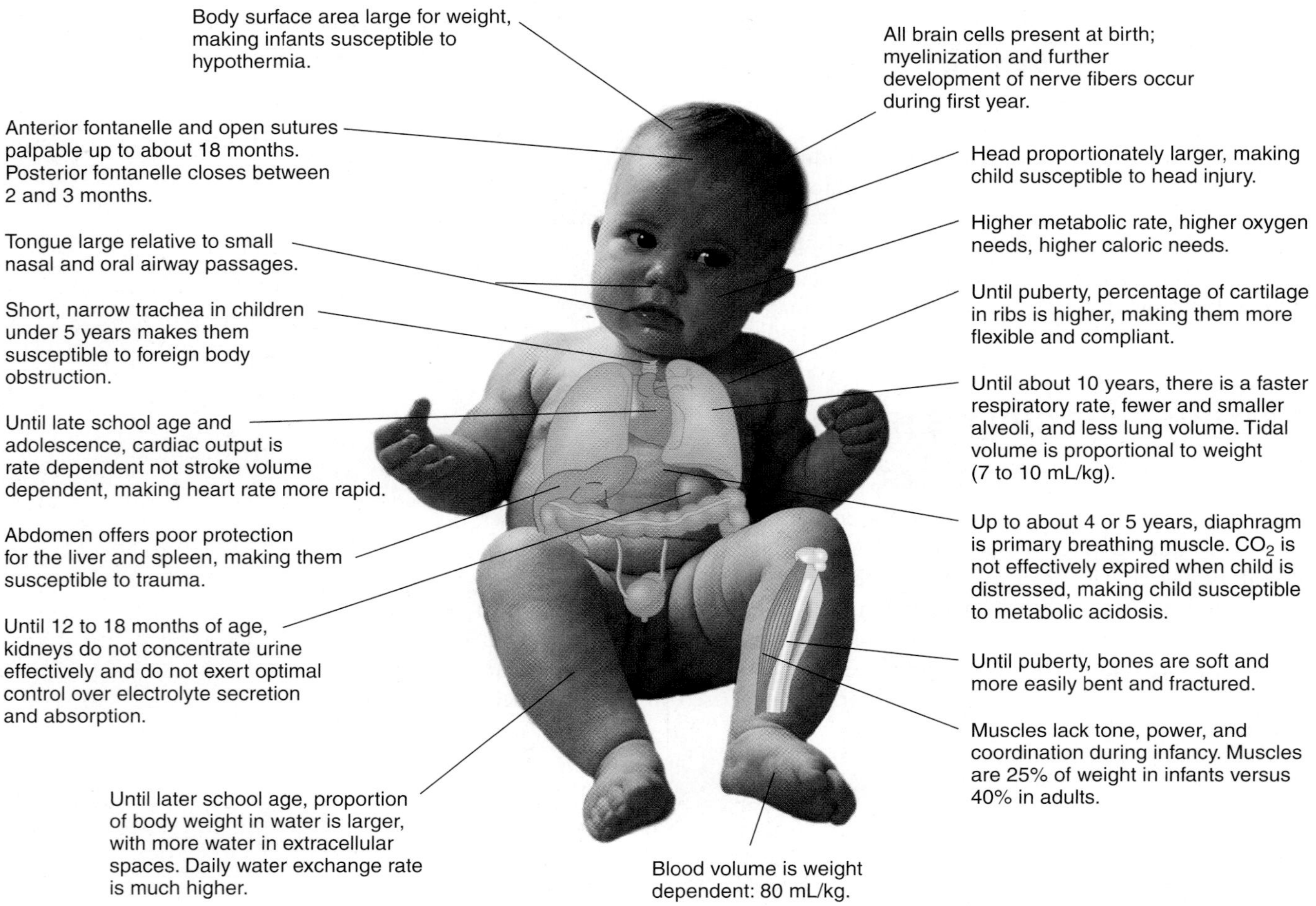

Body surface area large for weight, making infants susceptible to hypothermia.
Anterior fontanelle and open sutures palpable up to about 18 months. Posterior fontanelle closes between 2 and 3 months.
Tongue large relative to small nasal and oral airway passages.
Short, narrow trachea in children under 5 years makes them susceptible to foreign body obstruction.
Until late school age and adolescence, cardiac output is rate dependent not stroke volume dependent, making heart rate more rapid.
Abdomen offers poor protection for the liver and spleen, making them susceptible to trauma.
Until 12 to 18 months of age, kidneys do not concentrate urine effectively and do not exert optimal control over electrolyte secretion and absorption.
Until later school age, proportion of body weight in water is larger, with more water in extracellular spaces. Daily water exchange rate is much higher.
Blood volume is weight dependent: 80 mL/kg.
All brain cells present at birth; myelinization and further development of nerve fibers occur during first year.
Head proportionately larger, making child susceptible to head injury.
Higher metabolic rate, higher oxygen needs, higher caloric needs.
Until puberty, percentage of cartilage in ribs is higher, making them more flexible and compliant.
Until about 10 years, there is a faster respiratory rate, fewer and smaller alveoli, and less lung volume. Tidal volume is proportional to weight (7 to 10 mL/kg).
Up to about 4 or 5 years, diaphragm is primary breathing muscle. CO_2 is not effectively expired when child is distressed, making child susceptible to metabolic acidosis.
Until puberty, bones are soft and more easily bent and fractured.
Muscles lack tone, power, and coordination during infancy. Muscles are 25% of weight in infants versus 40% in adults.

Children are not just small adults. There are important anatomic and physiologic differences between children and adults that will change based on a child's growth and development.

questions are used to obtain detailed information. For example: "How high was Tommy's fever this morning?"

- Ask one question at a time so that the parent or child understands what piece of information is desired and so that it is clear which question the parent is answering. "Does any member of your family have diabetes, heart disease, or sickle cell anemia?" is a multiple question. Ask about each disease separately to ensure the most accurate response.
- Involve the child in the interview by asking age-appropriate questions. Young children can be asked, "What is your doll's name?" or "Where does it hurt?" Demonstrating an interest in the child initiates development of rapport with both child and parents. Ask older children and teens questions about their illness or injury. Offer them an opportunity to privately discuss their major concerns when their parents are not present.
- Be honest with the child when answering questions or when giving information about what will happen. Children need to learn that they can trust their nurse.
- Choose the language style best understood by the parent and child. Commonly used phrases or clinical terms can have different meanings to persons in various regions of the country or to different ethnic groups. To improve communication, request frequent feedback from the parents or child to ensure that their interpretation of phrases is accurate. For example, "You used the term hyperactivity. Would you explain the behavior a bit more for me?"
- Use an interpreter to improve communication when not fluent in the family's primary language. To ensure confidentiality of information for parents, avoid using a family member for history taking.

Developing Cultural Competence

PHRASING YOUR QUESTIONS

Some cultural groups, particularly Asians, try to anticipate the answers you want to hear, or say yes even if they do not understand the question. This is done in an effort to please you or as an expression of politeness. Remember to phrase your questions in a neutral manner.

Careful Listening

Complete attention is necessary to "hear" and accurately interpret information the parents and child give during the nursing history. Carefully listen to the information provided by the parent, as well as how it is expressed, and observe behavior during the interaction.

- Does the parent hesitate or avoid answering certain questions?
- Pay attention to the parent's attitude or tone of voice when the child's problems are discussed. Determine if it is consistent with the seriousness of the child's problem. The tone of voice can reveal anxiety, anger, or lack of concern.
- Be alert to any underlying themes. For example, the parent who talks about the child's diagnosis, but repeatedly refers to the impact of the illness on the family's finances or on meeting the needs of other family members, is requesting that these issues be addressed.
- Observe the parent's nonverbal behavior (posture, gestures, body movements, eye contact, and facial expression) for consistency with the words and tone of voice used. Is the parent interested in and appropriately concerned about the child's condition? Behaviors such as sitting up straight, making eye contact, and appearing apprehensive reflect appropriate concern for the child. Physical withdrawal, failure to make eye contact, or a happy expression could be inconsistent with the child's serious condition.

Developing Cultural Competence

INTERACTION PATTERNS

Certain cultures, including certain Asian and Native American groups, consider the use of silence during conversations as respectful. Avoid interruption of silence and allow the person time to reflect and formulate responses to questions. In other cultures silence may be noticed when the issue discussed is painful or sensitive. Be compassionate and recognize that parents and children will talk when they are ready (Seidel, Ball, Dains, et al., 2006).

Prolonged eye contact may be avoided by some cultural groups, such as persons of Native Americans, African American, Hindu, Japanese, and Chinese heritage, because it is considered impolite, aggressive, or a sign of disrespect. Other cultures such as persons of Arabic, European, and Russian heritage seek eye contact and some may look for a response or impact regarding what is said (Purnell, 2009).

Subtle nonverbal and verbal cues often indicate that the parent has not provided complete information about the child's problem. Observe for behaviors such as avoiding eye contact, change in voice pitch, or hesitation when responding to a question. Being supportive and asking clarifying questions encourage further description or the expression of information that is difficult for the parent or child to share. For example: "It sounds like that was a very difficult experience. How did Emily react?"

Encourage parents to share information, even if it is private or sensitive, especially when it influences nursing care planning. Often parents avoid sharing some information because they want to make a good impression, or they do not understand the value of the missing information. If parents hesitate to share information, briefly explain why the question was asked—for example, to make their child's hospital experience more pleasant or to begin planning for the child's discharge and home care.

In some cases the parent becomes too agitated, upset, or angry to continue responding to questions. When the information is not needed immediately, move on to another portion of the history to determine whether the parent is able to respond to other questions. Depending on the emotional status of the parent, it may be appropriate to collect the remaining historical data later.

DATA TO BE COLLECTED

Nurses collect and organize health, medical, and personal-social history to plan a child's nursing care. In addition, health status, psychosocial, and developmental data are organized to help develop the nursing diagnoses and the nursing care plan.

Patient Information

Obtain the child's name and nickname, age, sex, and ethnic origin. The child's birth date, race, religion, address, and phone number can be obtained from the admission form. Ask the parent for an emergency contact address and phone number, as well as a work phone number. Record the name of the person providing the patient history and that person's relationship to the patient.

Physiologic Data

Collect information about the child's health problems and diseases chronologically in a format similar to the traditional medical history.

Chief complaint. This is the child's primary problem or reason for hospital admission or visit to a healthcare setting, stated in the parent's or child's exact words.

History of the present illness or injury. A detailed description of the current health problem is obtained. This includes the onset and sequence of events, characteristics of and changes in symptoms over time, influencing factors, and the current status of the problem. Each problem is described separately. Table 35–1 lists the specific data to be collected about each illness and injury.

Past history. This more detailed description of the child's prior health problems includes all major past illnesses and injuries. Identify all major illnesses, including common communicable diseases. Identify major injuries, their cause or mechanism, and their severity. Obtain information about each prior surgery, its

Table 35–1 History of Present Illness or Injury

Characteristic	Defining Variables
Onset	Sudden or gradual, previous episodes, date and time began
Type of symptom	Pain, itching, cough, vomiting, runny nose, diarrhea, rash, etc.
Location	Generalized or localized—anatomically precise
Duration	Continuous or episodic symptoms, length of episodes
Severity	Effect on daily activities, e.g., interrupted sleep, decreased appetite, no interest in play
Influencing factors	What relieves or aggravates symptoms, what precipitated the problem, recent exposure to infection or allergen
Past evaluation for the problem	Laboratory studies, physician's office or hospital where done, results of past examinations
Previous and current treatment	Prescribed and over-the-counter drugs used, complementary therapies (e.g., heat, ice, rest), response to treatments

Table 35–2 Birth History

Prenatal condition	■ Mother's age, health during pregnancy, prenatal care, weight gained, special diet, expected date of birth ■ Details of illnesses, radiograph or sonogram findings, hospitalizations, medications, complications, and their timing during pregnancy ■ Prior obstetric history
Intrapartum—description of birth	■ Site of birth (hospital, home, birthing center) ■ Labor induced or spontaneous, length of labor, time/duration or rupture of membranes ■ Vaginal or cesarean birth, forceps or suction used, vertex or breech position ■ Length of pregnancy (weeks), single or multiple birth
Condition of baby at birth	■ Weight, Apgar score, cried immediately ■ Need for incubator, resuscitation, oxygen, ventilator ■ Any abnormalities detected, meconium staining
Postnatal condition	■ Difficulties in the nursery—feeding, respiratory difficulties, jaundice, cyanosis, rashes, seizures ■ Length of hospital stay, special nursery, home with mother ■ Breast- or bottle-fed, weight lost/gained in hospital ■ Medical care needed in first week—readmission to hospital

purpose, and if the surgery required hospitalization. For all hospitalizations, identify the reason and length of stay. Identify the circumstances for any prior transfusion (blood or blood products), type of transfusion, and reaction. Obtain information about each specific diagnosis, treatment, outcome, complication or residual problem, and the child's reaction to the event. Use the guidelines in Table 35–2 to obtain a *birth history* when the child's present problem may be related to problems during the pregnancy, birth, and newborn care.

Current health status. A detailed description of each aspect of the child's typical health status is obtained.

- Health maintenance—child's primary care provider, dentist, and other healthcare providers, timing of last visit to each.
- Medications—prescribed and over-the-counter medications (oral, topical, injectable) used daily or less frequently. Identify other medications and complementary therapies (herbs, plants, teas) used for the home management of fever, colds, coughs, cuts, and rashes.
- Allergies—to food, medication, animals, insect bites, or environmental exposure, and the type of reaction (e.g., respiratory difficulty, rash, hives, itching).
- Immunizations—review child's record for immunization status, vaccines and dates received, any unexpected reactions. See Chapter 45∞.
- Safety measures used—car restraint system, window guards, medication storage, sports protective gear, smoke detectors, bicycle helmet, firearm storage, and others.
- Activities and exercise—physical mobility and limitations, adaptive equipment used; play and/or sports activities.
- Nutrition—formula-fed or breastfed, if breastfed, for how long, type and amount of daily formula intake; when solid foods were introduced, enrollment in the WIC (Women, Infants, and Children) Program; eating and snacking habits, variety of foods consumed, "junk foods" eaten, appetite. See Chapter 34∞.
- Sleep—length and timing of naps and nighttime sleep; nightmares or night terrors, snoring, other sleep disturbances; where the child sleeps, and bedtime rituals.

Familial and hereditary diseases. Historical data should be collected for three generations of family members, including the parents, grandparents, aunts, uncles, cousins, child, and siblings. Collect information about the health status of each parent. Record information in either a pedigree (see Chapter 7∞) or a narrative format. Specific diseases to ask about are listed in Table 35–3.

Review of systems. A comprehensive overview of the child's health is collected during the review of systems. While this often helps to identify additional signs and symptoms associated with

Table 35–3	Familial or Hereditary Diseases
Infectious diseases	Tuberculosis, HIV, hepatitis, varicella, herpes
Heart disease	Heart defects, myocardial infarctions, hypertension, dyslipidemia, sudden childhood deaths
Allergic disorders	Eczema, hay fever
Eye disorders	Glaucoma, cataracts, vision loss
Ear disorders	Hearing loss, unusual shape or position of ears
Hematologic disorders	Sickle cell anemia, thalassemia, G6PD deficiency, leukemia
Respiratory disorders	Cystic fibrosis, asthma
Cancer	Type, early age of onset
Endocrine disorders	Diabetes mellitus type I and II, hypothyroidism, hyperthyroidism, Turner syndrome
Brain disorders	Mental retardation, epilepsy, Huntington chorea, psychiatric disorders
Musculoskeletal disorders	Arthritis, muscular dystrophy, scoliosis, spina bifida
Gastrointestinal disorders	Pyloric stenosis, ulcers, colitis, kidney disease
Problem pregnancies	Repeated miscarriages, stillbirths
Learning problems	Attention deficit disorder, Down syndrome

the child's condition, other problems may be revealed that have no direct relationship to the child's health problem but that could complicate nursing care or home care. For example, asking about any sleep problems might reveal sleep walking that must be planned for during a hospital admission. For each problem, obtain the treatment, outcomes, residual problems, and age at time of onset. Use the guidelines in Table 35–4 for data collection.

Psychosocial Data

Obtain information about family composition to establish a socioeconomic and sociologic context for planning the child's care in the hospital, community, and at home.

- Family composition, including family members living in the home, their relationship to the child, marital status of parents or other family structure, and people helping to care for the child
- Household members' employment status, health insurance coverage, agencies used such as Medicaid, unemployment, food stamps, or Temporary Assistance for Needy Families (TANF)
- Description of the housing and home environment (atmosphere, emotional stresses, family activities); safe play area; use of city or well water; sanitation; and availability of electricity, heat, and refrigeration
- School or childcare arrangements; description of the neighborhood, including playgrounds, transportation, and proximity to stores
- Changes in family or lifestyle since last seen; number of times the family has moved; how the child and family members have coped with the changes

Information about daily routines, psychosocial data, and other living patterns forms the basis for many nursing diagnoses as well as the nursing care plan. Collection of information should focus on issues that have an impact on the quality of daily living, even if some data seem to overlap with disease data (Table 35–5).

Newborns. The psychosocial history for parents of newborns should focus on readiness to care for the newborn at home. Inquire about support for the parent in the initial postpartum period, safe transport, and a home environment that provides heat, refrigeration, and safe water supplies.

Children. The psychosocial history for children should focus on the home environment, behaviors and progress in the childcare or school setting, family and peer relationships.

Adolescents. The psychosocial history for adolescents should focus on critical areas in their lives that may contribute to a less than optimal environment for normal growth and development. Key topics that should be addressed are included in the HEADS screening tool (Goldenring & Rosen, 2004):

- H–home environment
- E–employment, education, eating
- A–activities
- D–drugs (substance abuse)
- S–sexuality, suicidal thoughts, safety, savagery (exposure to violence)

Developmental Data

Information about the child's motor, cognitive, language, and social development will help to plan nursing care. Ask the parent about the child's milestones and current fine and gross motor skills. Obtain the age at which the child first used words appropriately and the current words used or language ability. For children in school, ask about academic performance to assess cognitive development. Ask the parent about the child's manner of interaction with other children, family members, and strangers. For adolescents, ask about school performance and activities indicating development of independence and autonomy. Guidelines for a nursing assessment of development can be found in Chapter 33∞.

DEVELOPMENTAL APPROACH TO THE EXAMINATION

The sequence and approach to the examination varies by age. Provide a comfortable atmosphere for the examination with privacy so that modesty is respected. Explain the procedures as you begin to perform them. In young children, a foot-to-head sequence is often used so that the least distressing parts of the examination are completed first. In older cooperative children, the head-to-toe approach is generally used.

Table 35–4 Review of Systems

Body Systems	Examples of Problems to Identify
General	General growth pattern, overall health status, ability to keep up with other children or tires easily with feeding or activity, fever, sleep patterns Allergies, type of reaction (hives, rash, respiratory difficulty, swelling, nausea), seasonal or with each exposure
Skin and lymph	Rashes, dry skin, itching, changes in skin color or texture, tendency for bruising, swollen or tender lymph glands
Hair and nails	Hair loss, changes in color or texture, use of dye or chemicals on hair Abnormalities of nail growth or color
Head	Headaches
Eyes	Vision problems, squinting, crossed eyes, lazy eye, wears glasses, eye infections, redness, tearing, burning, rubbing, swelling eyelids
Ears	Ear infections, frequent discharge from ears, or tubes in ears Hearing loss (no response to loud noises or questions, inattentiveness, was hearing test ever done?), hearing aids or cochlear implant
Nose and sinuses	Nosebleeds, nasal congestion, colds with runny nose, sinus pain or infections Nasal obstruction, difficulty breathing, snoring at night
Mouth and throat	Mouth breathing, difficulty swallowing, sore throats, strep infections, mouth odor Tooth eruption, cavities, braces Voice change, hoarseness, speech problems
Cardiac and hematologic	Heart murmur, anemia, hypertension, cyanosis, edema, rheumatic fever, chest pain, bruises easily
Chest and respiratory	Trouble breathing, choking episodes, cough, wheezing, cyanosis, exposure to tuberculosis, bronchiolitis, bronchitis, other infections
Gastrointestinal	Bowel movements, regularity or frequency, color, consistency, discomfort; constipation or diarrhea; abdominal pain; bleeding from rectum; flatulence; encopresis Nausea or vomiting, appetite
Urinary	Frequency, urgency, dysuria, foul smelling urine, dribbling, strength of urinary stream, undescended testicles Toilet trained—age when day and night dryness attained, enuresis
Reproductive	For pubescent children
Female	Menses onset, amount, duration, frequency, discomfort, problems; vaginal discharge, breast development
Male	Puberty onset, emissions, erections, pain or discharge from penis, swelling or pain in testicles
Both	Sexual activity, use of contraception, sexually transmitted infections
Musculoskeletal	Weakness, clumsiness, poor coordination, balance, tremors, abnormal gait, painful muscles or joints, swelling or redness of joints, fractures
Neurologic	Seizures, fainting spells, dizziness, numbness, brain injuries Learning problems, attention span, hyperactivity, memory problems

Newborns and Infants under 6 Months of Age

Infants are among the easiest children to examine, as they do not resist the examination procedure. Keep the parent present to provide comfort and security for the infant during the examination by feeding, using a pacifier, cuddling, or changing the diaper to keep the infant calm and quiet. Distraction such as rocking or clicking noises may help when the infant begins to get distressed. Observe the infant for general level of activity, overall mood, and responsiveness to handling.

Be flexible with the sequence of the examination to listen to lung, heart, and abdominal sounds when the infant is quiet or asleep. If the infant continues to be quiet, palpate the abdomen while the muscles are relaxed. The remainder of the examination can proceed in a head-to-toe sequence. Portions of the examination that are likely to disturb the infant, such as the examination of the hips, should be performed at the end.

Infants over 6 Months of Age

Because of developing separation and stranger anxiety, it is often best to examine the infant and toddler on the parent's lap and then held against the parent's chest for some steps, such as the ear examination (Figure 35–1 ●). The infant will not object to having clothing removed, but make sure the room is warm for the infant's comfort. Observe the infant's general level of activity, mood, and responsiveness to handling by the parent.

Table 35–5 Daily Living Patterns

Role relationships	■ Family relationships/alterations in family process ■ Social interactions: e.g., peer relationships, child care, preschool, school, neighborhood, participation in organized sports
Self-perception/ self-concept	■ Personal identity and role identity ■ Self-esteem, body image, presence of nonvisible disorder such as a brain injury
Coping/stress tolerance	■ Temperament, coping behaviors ■ Discipline methods used ■ Any substance abuse
Values and beliefs	■ Faith-based practice, religion, belong to any spiritual group or community ■ Any foods, drinks, medications, or treatments not allowed according to spiritual beliefs, special food preparation ■ Personal values/beliefs
Home care provided for child's condition	■ Resources needed/available, respite care available ■ Knowledge and skills of parents, other family members
Sensory/perceptual problems	■ Adaptations to daily living for any sensory loss (vision, hearing, cognitive, or motor)

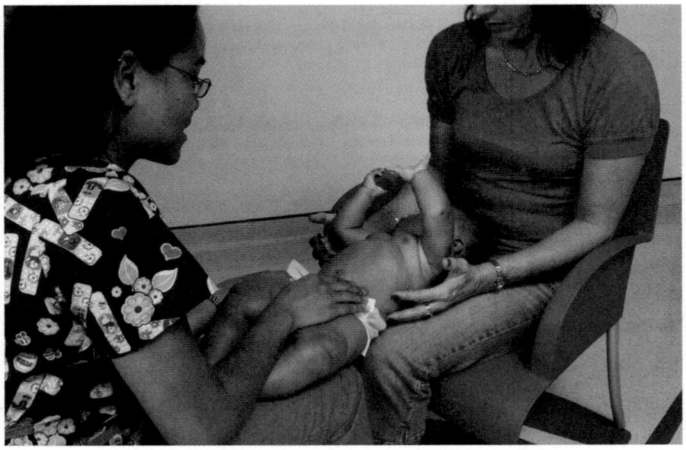

• **Figure 35–1** Facilitating physical examination cooperation. Infants and toddlers are often fearful of separation from the parent. With the legs of the nurse and mother put together knee-to-knee, this infant has a surface to lie on that facilitates the abdominal examination.

Smile and talk soothingly to the infant during the procedure. Use toys to distract the older infant. Use a pacifier or bottle to quiet the child when necessary. Because the infant may be fearful of being touched by a stranger, begin with the feet and hands before moving to the trunk. However, take advantage of opportunities to listen to heart, lung, and abdominal sounds when the infant is sleeping or quiet.

Toddlers

Toddlers may be active, curious, shy, cautious, or slow to warm up. Because of stranger anxiety, keep toddlers with their parents, often examining them on the parent's lap. It is possible to create a flat surface for the abdominal and genital examination by sitting knee-to-knee with the parent. For invasive procedures (ear and mouth exam) the parent can hold the child close to the chest with legs between the parent's legs. The cranial nerve assessment or developmental assessment can be used as a method to gain cooperation for other procedures. Much of the neurologic and musculoskeletal assessment can be conducted by observing the child play and walk around in the examining room.

Tell the child what you will do at each step of the examination, using a confident voice that expects cooperation rather than asking. When a choice is possible, let the child have some control. For example, let the toddler choose which ear to examine first or to stand or sit for a certain part of the examination. Let the child hold a security object if it helps. Attempt to reduce the child's anxiety by demonstrating the use of instruments on the parent or security object. Begin the examination by touching the feet and then moving gradually toward the body and head. Instruments to examine the ears, eyes, and mouth often cause anxiety and should be used at the end of the examination.

Preschoolers

Assess the willingness of the child to be separated from the parent. Younger children may prefer to be examined on the parent's lap, while older children will be comfortable on the examining table. Most children are willing to undress, but leave the underpants on until conducting the genital examination. Most children in this age group are cooperative during the physical examination. Some children will prefer to have the head, eyes, ears, and mouth examined first while others will prefer to postpone them to the end.

Allow the child to touch and play with the equipment. Give simple explanations about the assessment procedures, and offer choice when there is one during the examination. Use distraction to gain the child's cooperation during the examination, such as asking the child to count, name colors, or talk about a favorite activity. Give positive feedback when the child cooperates.

School-Age Children

School-age children willingly cooperate during the examination and sit on the examining table. Anticipate the development of modesty in school-age children and offer a patient gown to cover the underwear. Let the older school-age child determine if the examination will be conducted in privacy or with the parent or siblings present.

A head-to-toe sequence can be used in this age group. Demonstrate how the instruments are used and let the child handle them if they wish. During the examination, tell the child what you are doing and why. Offer as many choices as possible to help the child feel empowered. The examination is a good opportunity to teach the child about how the body works, such as letting the child listen to heart and breath sounds.

Adolescents

Protect the adolescent's modesty by providing a private place to undress and put on the patient gown, and then during the examination by covering the parts of the body not being assessed. Use the head-to-toe sequence and the same procedures used for adults. Perform the examination in private without parent or siblings unless the adolescent specifically requests the parent's presence. Have another health professional serve as a chaperone (preferably the same sex as the patient) during the examination when the parent or accompanying adult is not present.

Adolescents often have a lot of concerns regarding their developing bodies. When appropriate, provide reassurance about the normal progression of secondary sexual characteristic development and what further changes to expect.

GENERAL APPRAISAL

The examination begins upon first meeting the child (Figure 35–2 ●). Measure the infant's weight, length, and head circumference (see Skills 9–1 through 9–5 in the Clinical Skills Manual SKILLS). If the child is between 24 and 36 months of age and can stand, measure the child's height rather than length. Accurate measurement is important as medication dosages are based upon weight. Growth measurements are then plotted on growth charts throughout childhood to assure health or to identify the impact of disease on the child. Growth charts for all ages of boys and girls are provided in Appendix A∞.

Once the weight and height of children have been measured, calculate the body mass index and plot it on the growth curve to determine if the child's height and weight are proportional for age (see Chapter 34∞). The body mass index (BMI) is a formula used to assess total body fat and nutritional status. For children it helps determine if the child's height and weight are proportional for their age. Visit the CDC website and enter the child's height and weight for an automatic calculation of the BMI. A BMI for age under the 5th percentile indicates the child is underweight. The child is at risk for overweight when the BMI for age is greater than the 85th percentile, and the child is overweight when greater than the 95th percentile.

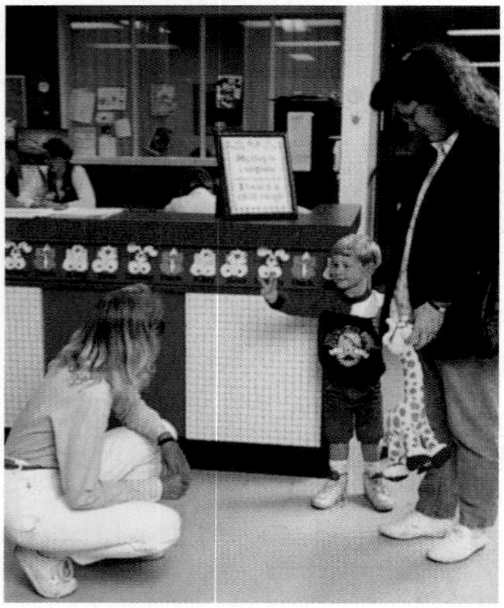

● **Figure 35–2** Initial assessment. Examination of the child begins from the first contact. Observe the behavior of the child and parent by using visual cues to make a proper assessment. Does the child appear well nourished? Does the child appear secure with the parent?

Nursing Practice

Following are the specific examination techniques:

Inspection. Purposeful observation of the child's physical features and behaviors. Physical feature characteristics include size, shape, color, movement, position, and location. Detection of odors is also a part of inspection.

Palpation. Use of touch to identify characteristics of the skin, internal organs, and masses. Characteristics include texture, moistness, tenderness, temperature, position, shape, consistency, and mobility of masses and organs. The palmar surface of the fingers and finger pads helps determine position, size, consistency, and masses. The ulnar surface of the hand is best to detect vibrations.

Auscultation. Listening to sounds produced by the airway, lungs, stomach, heart, and blood vessels to identify their characteristics. Auscultation is usually performed with a stethoscope to enhance the sounds heard.

Percussion. Striking the surface of the body, either directly or indirectly, to set up vibrations that reveal the density of underlying tissues and borders of internal organs.

Take the child's temperature, heart rate, respiratory rate, and blood pressure (see Skills 9–8 through 9–14 SKILLS).

Observe the child's general appearance and behavior. The child should appear well nourished and well developed. Infants and young children are often fearful and seek reassurance from their parents. The child may resist interacting with the nurse until rapport is established.

Observe the behavior and tone of voice used by the parent when he or she is talking to the child. Is the child encouraged to speak? Is the child appropriately reassured or supported by the parent? The child should feel secure with the parent and perceive permission to interact with the nurse.

ASSESSING SKIN AND HAIR CHARACTERISTICS

Examination of the skin requires good lighting to detect variations in skin color and to identify lesions. Daylight is preferred when available. Rather than inspecting the entire skin surface of the child at one time, examine the skin simultaneously with other body systems as each region of the body is exposed. Follow standard precautions by wearing gloves when palpating mucous membranes, open wounds, and lesions.

Developing Cultural Competence

SKIN TONE DIFFERENCES

The palms of the hands and soles of the feet are often lighter than the rest of the skin surface in darker-skinned children. In addition, their lips may appear slightly bluish.

INSPECTION OF THE SKIN

Skin Color

The color of the child's skin usually has an even distribution. Check for color variations—such as increased or decreased pigmentation, pallor, mottling, bruises, erythema, cyanosis, or jaundice—that may be associated with local or generalized conditions. Some variations in skin color are common and normal, such as freckles found in the white population and Mongolian spots found on dark-skinned infants. See "Newborn Skin" in Chapter 28 for more information.

Ecchymosis or bruising is common on the knees, shins, and lower arms as children stumble and fall. Bruises are uncommon in infants under 9 months of age before walking (Kaczor, Pierce, Makoroff, et al., 2006). Bruises on these infants or on children in other parts of the body, especially in various stages of healing, should raise a suspicion of child abuse. Bruises often go through various color changes as the body reabsorbs blood over several days. The transition of color often progresses through reddish blue, brownish blue, brownish green, greenish yellow, and yellow-brown before returning to normal skin color. Note any tattoos or body piercings.

When a skin color abnormality is suspected, inspect the buccal mucosa and tongue to confirm the color change. This is important in darker-skinned children because the mucous membranes are usually pink, regardless of skin color. Press the gums lightly for 1 to 2 seconds. Any residual color, such as that seen in jaundice or cyanosis, is more easily detected in blanched skin. Jaundice may also be noticed in the sclerae of the eyes and is associated with liver disorders. Generalized cyanosis is associated with respiratory and cardiac disorders.

PALPATION OF THE SKIN

Lightly touch or stroke the skin surface to palpate the skin and to evaluate the following characteristics:

- *Temperature*—normally feels cool to the touch when placing the wrist or dorsum of the hand against the child's skin. Excessively warm skin may indicate the presence of fever or inflammation, whereas abnormally cool skin may be a sign of shock or cold exposure.
- *Texture*—soft, smooth skin over the entire body. Identify any areas of roughness, thickening, or *induration* (area of extra firmness with a distinct border). Abnormalities in texture are associated with endocrine disorders, chronic irritation, and inflammation.

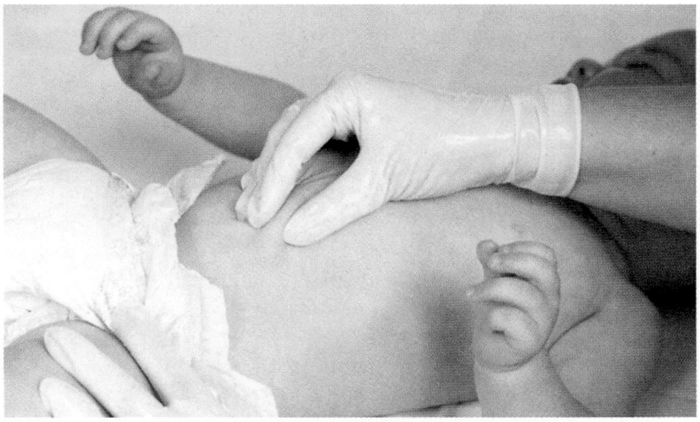

● **Figure 35–3** Tenting of the skin associated with poor skin turgor. Assess skin turgor on the abdomen, forearm, or thigh. Skin with normal turgor will return to a flat position quickly.

- *Moistness*—normally dry to the touch, but may feel slightly damp when the child has been exercising or crying. Excessive sweating without exertion is associated with a fever or with an uncorrected congenital heart defect.
- *Resilience*—taut, elastic, and mobile because of the balanced distribution of intracellular and extracellular fluids. To evaluate skin turgor, pinch a small amount of skin on the abdomen between the thumb and forefinger, release the skin, and watch the speed of recoil (Figure 35–3 ●). Skin with good turgor rapidly returns to its previous contour. Skin with poor turgor tents or stands up for 3 to 4 seconds before resuming its previous contour (Seidel, Ball, Dains, et al., 2006). Poor skin turgor is commonly associated with dehydration.

If *edema,* an accumulation of excess fluid in the interstitial spaces, is present, the skin feels doughy or boggy. To test for the degree of edema present, press for 5 seconds against a bone beneath the area of puffy skin, release the pressure, and observe how rapidly the indentation disappears. If the indentation disappears rapidly, the edema is "nonpitting." Slow disappearance of the indentation indicates "pitting" edema, which is commonly associated with kidney or heart disorders.

CAPILLARY REFILL TIME

One technique to evaluate the adequacy of tissue *perfusion* (oxygen circulating to the tissues) is the capillary refill time (Figure 35–4A and B ●). The capillary refill time is normally less than 2 seconds. When the time is prolonged, assess the child for dehydration, hypovolemic shock, or a physical constriction such as a cast or bandage that is too tight.

SKIN LESIONS

Skin lesions usually indicate an abnormal skin condition. Characteristics such as location, size, type of lesion, pattern, and discharge, if present, provide clues about the cause of the condition. Inspect and palpate the isolated or generalized skin color abnormalities, elevations, lesions, or injuries to describe all characteristics present.

A

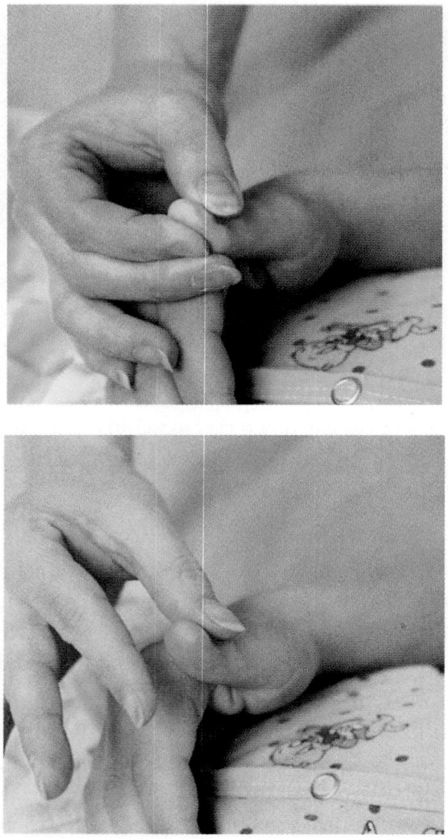

B

● **Figure 35–4** Capillary refill technique. ***A,*** Press on the end of a finger or toe for 2 to 3 seconds until the skin is blanched. ***B,*** Quickly release the finger and count the number of seconds it takes for the color or blood return to the veins. A capillary refill time of greater than 2 seconds could be related to dehydration, shock or constriction around a limb, such as a tight bandage or cast.

Primary lesions (such as macules, papules, and vesicles) are often the skin's initial response to injury or infection. Mongolian spots and freckles are normal findings also classified as primary lesions. The illustrations in "Pathophysiology Illustrated" on page 939 describe common primary lesions. Secondary lesions (such as scars, ulcers, and fissures) are the result of irritation, infection, and delayed healing of primary lesions (see "Pathophysiology Illustrated—Common Primary Skin Lesions and Associated Conditions" in Chapter 59).

Some common patterns of skin lesions include the following:

- Annular—circular, begins in center and spreads to periphery, e.g., ringworm; when annular lesions run together they are polycyclic
- Linear—in a row or stripe, e.g., poison ivy
- Herpetiform—grouped or clustered, e.g., herpes, chicken pox
- Reticulated—networked or lace-like, e.g., parvovirus B19

INSPECTION OF THE HAIR

Inspect the scalp hair for color, distribution, and cleanliness. The hair shafts should be evenly colored, shiny, and either curly or straight. Variation in hair color not caused by bleaching may be associated with a nutritional deficiency. Normally, hair is distributed evenly over the scalp. Investigate areas of hair loss. Hair loss in a child may result from tight braids or skin lesions such as ringworm (see "Fungal Infections" in Chapter 59). Notice any unusual hair growth patterns. An unusually low hairline on the neck or forehead may be associated with a congenital disorder such as hypothyroidism.

Children are frequently exposed to head lice. Inspect the individual hair shafts for small nits (lice eggs) that adhere to the hair (see Chapter 59). None should be present.

Observe the distribution of body hair as other skin surfaces are exposed during examination. Fine hair covers most areas of the body. Body hair in unexpected places should be noted. For example, a tuft of hair at the base of the spine often indicates a spinal defect.

Note the age at which pubic and axillary hair develops in the child. Pubic hair begins to develop in children between 8 and 12 years of age, and axillary hair develops about 6 months later. See pages 964–965. Facial hair is noted in boys shortly after axillary hair develops. Development at an unusually young age is associated with precocious puberty.

> **Developing Cultural Competence**
>
> **HAIR CHARACTERISTICS**
>
> Hair varies by genetic origin. Children of African origin often have hair that can appear curly, wavy, or coiled, and this hair more easily breaks. Children of Asian origin have hair that is coarse and straight. Children of Caucasian origin have hair with fine to medium coarseness that is straight or wavy.

PALPATION OF THE HAIR

Palpate the hair shafts for texture. Hair should feel soft or silky with fine or thick shafts. Endocrine conditions such as hypothyroidism may result in coarse, brittle hair. Part the hair in various spots over the head to inspect and palpate the scalp for crusting or other lesions. If lesions are present, describe them using the characteristics in "Pathophysiology Illustrated."

ASSESSING THE HEAD FOR SKULL CHARACTERISTICS AND FACIAL FEATURES

INSPECTION OF THE HEAD AND FACE

During early childhood the skull's sutures permit expansion for brain growth. Infants and young children normally have a rounded skull with a prominent occipital area. The shape of the head changes during childhood, and the occipital area becomes less prominent. An abnormal skull shape can result from premature closure of the sutures (see Chapter 56). Children who

PATHOPHYSIOLOGY ILLUSTRATED

COMMON PRIMARY SKIN LESIONS AND ASSOCIATED CONDITIONS

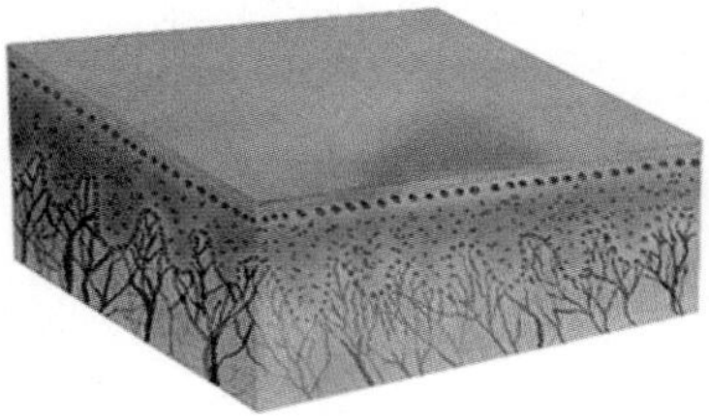

Lesion
Name: Macule
Description:
Flat, nonpalpable, diameter less than 1 cm (½ in.)
Example: Freckle, rubella, rubeola, petechiae

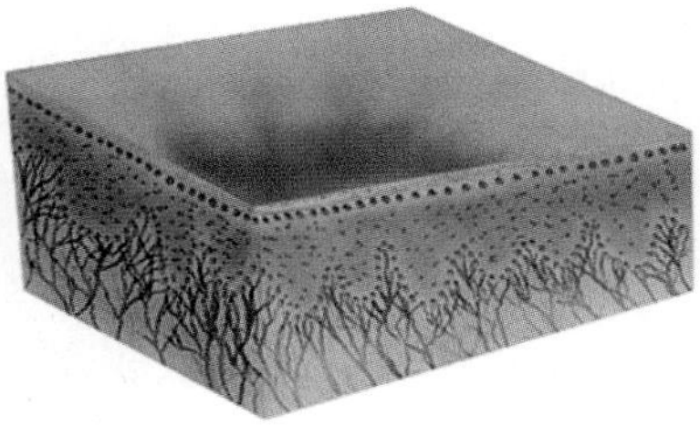

Lesion Name: Patch
Description:
Macule, diameter greater than 1 cm (½ in.)
Example: Vitiligo, Mongolian spot

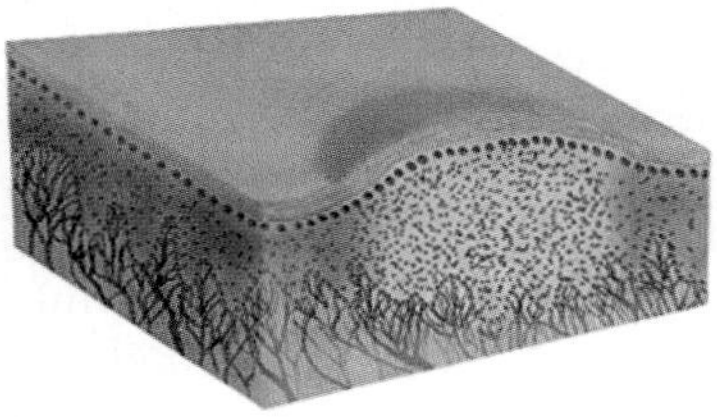

Lesion Name: Papule
Description:
Elevated, firm, diameter less than 1 cm (½ in.)
Example: Warts, pigmented nevi

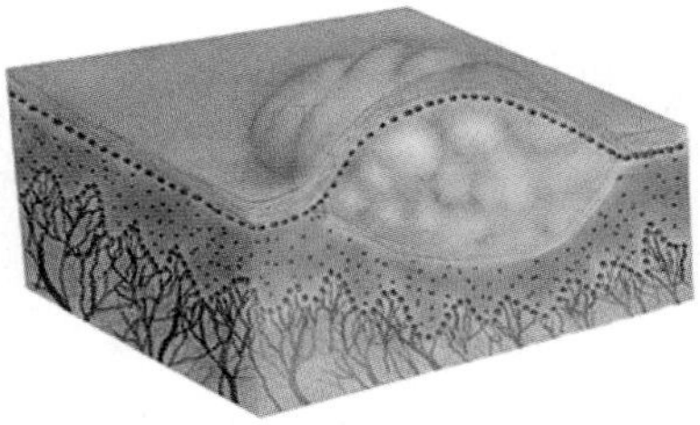

Lesion Name: Nodule
Description:
Elevated, firm, deeper in dermis than papule, diameter 1–2 cm (½ in.–1 in.)
Example: Erythema nodosum

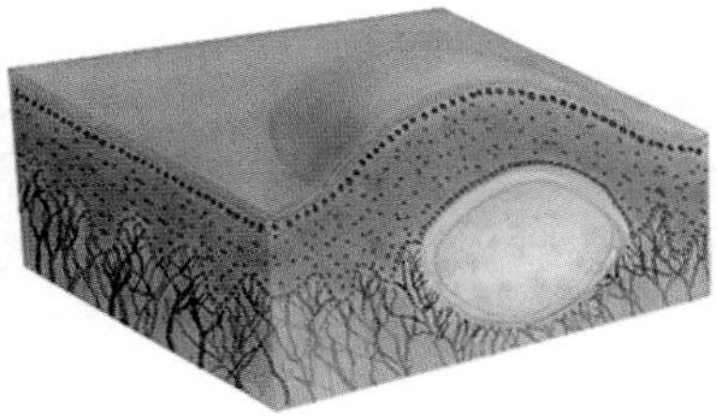

Lesion Name: Tumor
Description:
Elevated, solid, diameter greater than 2 cm (1 in.)
Example: Neoplasm, hemangioma

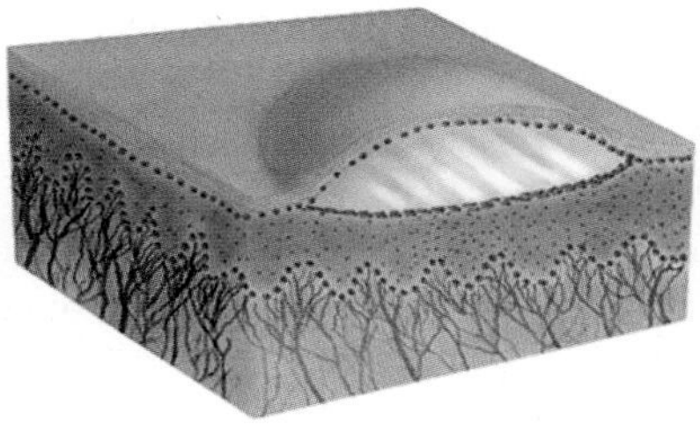

Lesion Name: Vesicle
Description:
Elevated, filled with fluid, diameter less than 1 cm (½ in.)
Example: Early chicken pox, herpes simplex

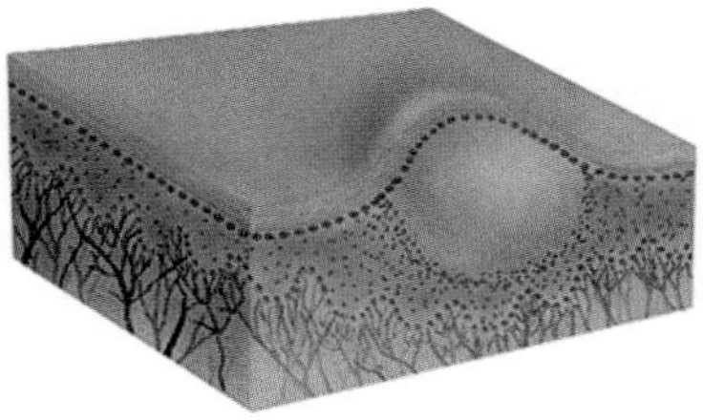

Lesion Name: Pustule
Description:
Vesicle filled with purulent fluid
Example: Impetigo, acne

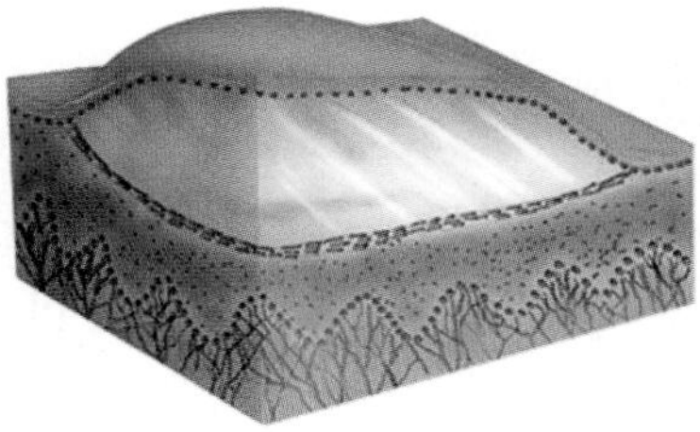

Name: Bulla
Description:
Vesicle diameter greater than 1 cm (½ in.)
Example: Burn blister

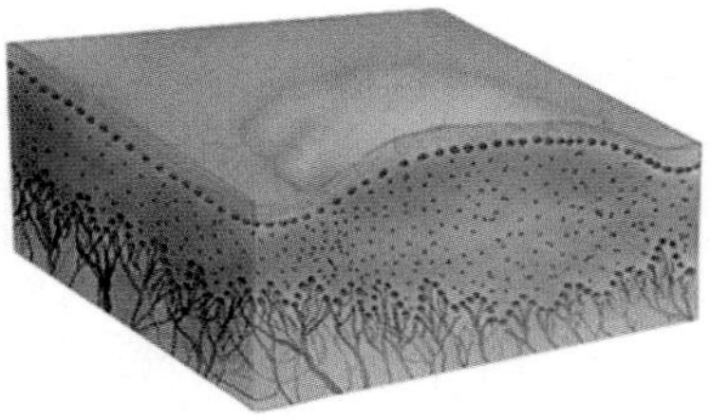

Lesion Name: Wheal
Description:
Irregular elevated solid area of edematous skin
Example: Urticaria, insect bite

were low-birth-weight infants often have a flat, elongated skull because the soft skull bones were flattened by the weight of the head early in infancy. Head flattening is also associated with the back-lying sleep positions in infants.

The head circumference of infants and young children is routinely measured until 3 years of age to ensure that adequate growth for brain development has occurred. The Clinical Skills Manual SKILLS describes the proper technique for use of the tape measure (see Skill 9–5). A larger-than-normal head is associated with hydrocephalus, and a smaller-than-normal head suggests microcephaly.

Inspect the child's face for symmetry during several facial expressions such as resting, smiling, talking, and crying (Figure 35–5 ●). Significant asymmetry may result from paralysis of trigeminal or facial nerves (cranial nerves V or VII), in utero positioning, and swelling from infection, allergy, or trauma.

Next inspect the face for unusual facial features such as coarseness, wide eye spacing, or disproportionate size. Tremors, tics, and twitching of facial muscles are often associated with seizures.

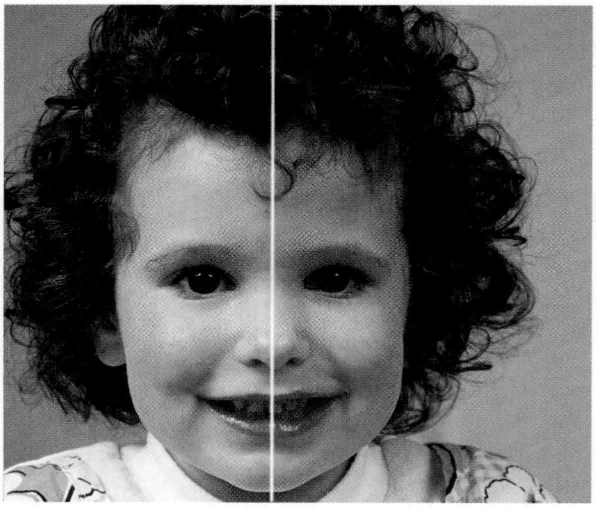

● **Figure 35–5** Inspecting for facial symmetry. Draw an imaginary line down the middle of the face over the nose and compare the features on each side. Significant asymmetry may be caused by paralysis of cranial nerve V or VII, in utero positioning, or swelling from infection, allergy, or trauma.

PALPATION OF THE SKULL

Palpate the skull in infants and young children to assess the sutures and fontanelles and to detect soft bones (see "As Children Grow: Sutures").

Sutures

Use your fingerpads to palpate each suture line. The edge of each bone in the suture line can be felt, but normally there is no separation of the two bones. If additional bone edges are felt, a skull fracture may be present. The suture lines of the skull are seldom palpated after 2 years of age. After that time the sutures rarely split.

AS CHILDREN GROW

SUTURES

The sutures are separations between the bones of the skull that have not yet joined. The fontanelles are formed at the intersection of these sutures where bone has not yet formed. Fontanelles are covered by tough membranous tissue that protects the brain. The posterior fontanelle closes between 2 and 3 months. The anterior fontanelle and sutures are palpable up to the age of 18 months.

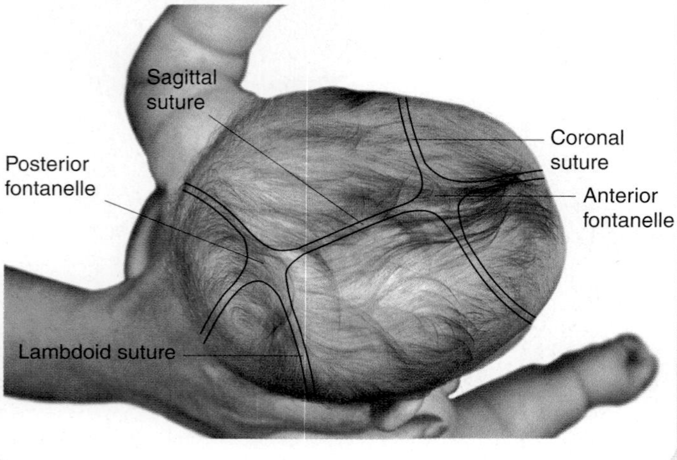

MyNursingKit Animation: 3D Eye

Fontanelles

At the intersection of the sutures, palpate the anterior and posterior fontanelles. The fontanelle should feel flat and firm inside the bony edges. The anterior fontanelle is normally smaller than 5 cm (2 in.) in diameter at 6 months of age and then becomes progressively smaller. It closes between 12 and 18 months of age. The posterior fontanelle closes between 2 and 3 months of age.

A tense fontanelle, bulging above the margin of the skull when the child is sitting, is an indication of increased intracranial pressure. A soft fontanelle, sunken below the margin of the skull, is associated with dehydration.

ASSESSING EYE STRUCTURES, FUNCTION, AND VISION

INSPECTION OF THE EXTERNAL EYE STRUCTURES

Inspect the external eye structures, including the eyeballs, eyelids, and eye muscles. Test the function of cranial nerves II, III, IV, and VI, which innervate the eye structures. Equipment needed for this examination includes an ophthalmoscope, vision chart, penlight, small toy, and an index card or paper cup.

Eye Size and Spacing

Inspect the eyes and surrounding tissues simultaneously when examining facial features (Figure 35–6 ●). The eyes should be the same size but not unusually large or small. Observe for eye bulging, which can be identified by retracted eyelids or a sunken

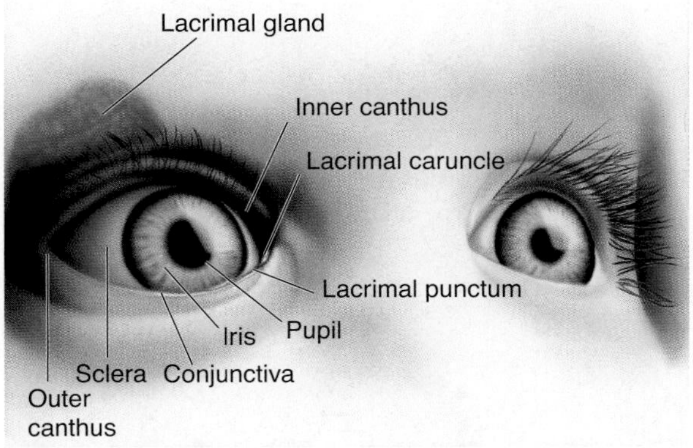

● **Figure 35–6** External structures of the eye. Notice that the light reflex is at the same location on each eye.

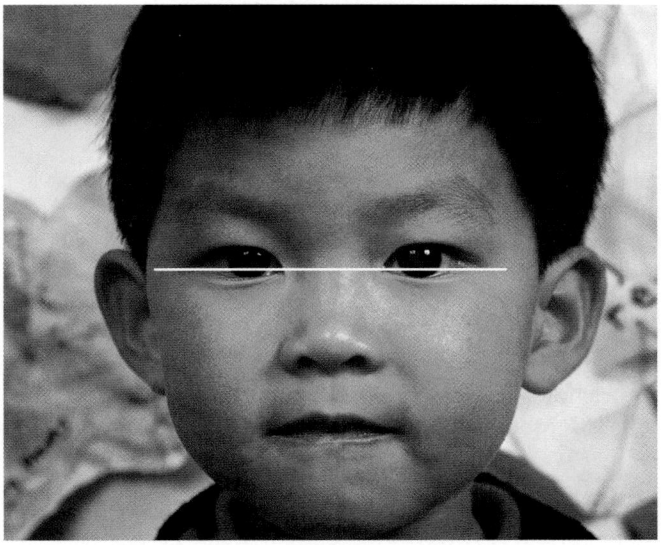

● **Figure 35–7** Inspecting for palpebral slant. Draw an imaginary line across the medial canthi and extend it to each side of the face to identify the slant of the palpebral fissures. When the line crosses the lateral canthi, the palpebral fissures are horizontal and no slant is present. When the lateral canthi fall above the imaginary line, the eyes have an upward or Mongolian slant. A downward or anti-Mongolian slant is present when the lateral canthi fall below the imaginary line. Epicanthal folds are present when an extra fold of skin partially or completely covers the caruncles in the medial canthi. Which type of slant does this child have?

appearance. Bulging may be associated with a tumor, and a sunken appearance may reflect dehydration.

Next inspect the eyes to see if they are appropriately distanced from each other. **Hypertelorism**, or widely spaced eyes, can be a normal variation in children.

Eyelids and Eyelashes

Inspect the eyelids for color, size, position, mobility, and condition of the eyelashes. Eyelids should be the same color as surrounding facial skin and free of swelling or inflammation along the edges. Sebaceous glands that look like yellow striations are often present near the hair follicles. Eyelashes curl away from the eye to prevent irritation of the conjunctivae.

Inspect the conjunctivae lining the eyelids by pulling down the lower lid and then everting the upper lid. The conjunctivae should be pink and glossy. The lacrimal punctum, the opening for the lacrimal gland on each lid, is located near the medial canthus. No redness or excess tearing should be present.

When the eyes are open, inspect the level at which the upper and lower lids cross the eye. Each lid normally covers part of the iris but not any portion of the pupil. The lids should also close completely over the iris and cornea. *Ptosis,* drooping of the lid over the pupil, is often associated with injury to the oculomotor nerve, cranial nerve III. Sunset sign, in which the sclera is seen between the upper lid and the iris, may indicate retracted eyelids or hydrocephalus.

Inspect the eyes for the palpebral slant (Figure 35–7 ●). The eyelids of most people open horizontally. Children of Asian descent often have an extra fold of skin, known as the epicanthal fold, covering all or part of the medial canthus of the eye. An upward slant is a normal finding in Asian children; however, children with Down syndrome also often have an upward slant (Figure 35–8 ●). A downward slant is seen in some children as a normal variation.

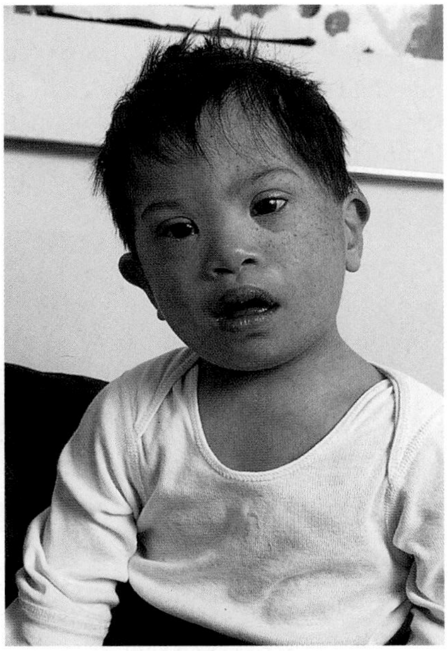

● **Figure 35–8** Upward palpebral slant. The eyes of this boy with Down syndrome show an upward slant.

Eye Color

Inspect the color of each sclera, iris, and bulbar conjunctiva. The sclera is normally white or ivory in darker-skinned children. Sclerae of another color suggest the presence of an underlying disease. For example, yellow sclerae indicate jaundice. Typically the iris is blue or light colored at birth and becomes pigmented within 6 months. Inspect the iris for the presence of *Brushfield spots,* white specks in a linear pattern around the iris circumference, which are often associated with Down syndrome. The bulbar conjunctivae, which cover the sclera to the edge of the cornea, are normally clear. Redness can indicate eyestrain, allergies, or irritation.

Pupils

Inspect the pupils for size and shape. Normally the pupils are round, clear, and equal in size. Some children have a **coloboma**, a keyhole-shaped pupil caused by a notch in the iris. This sign can indicate that the child has other congenital anomalies.

To test the pupillary response to light, shine a bright light into one eye. A brisk constriction of both the pupil exposed to direct light and the other pupil (consensual response) is a normal finding.

To test pupillary response to accommodation, ask the child to look first at a near object (e.g., a toy) and then at a distant object (e.g., a picture on the wall). The expected response is pupil constriction with near objects and pupil dilation with distant objects. This procedure tests cranial nerve II.

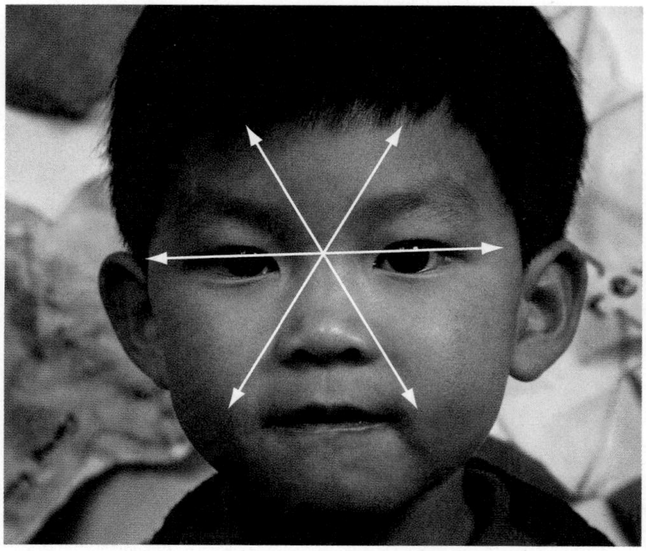

● **Figure 35–9** Assessing extraocular movements. Begin the eye muscle examination with inspection of the extraocular movements. Have the child sit at your eye level. Hold a toy or penlight about 30 cm (12 in.) from the child's eyes and move it through the six cardinal fields of gaze. Both eyes should move together, tracking the object. This procedure tests cranial nerves III, IV, and VI.

ASSESSMENT OF THE EYE MUSCLES

It is important to detect strabismus, or crossed eyes, because if it goes uncorrected vision impairment can occur. Use the following procedures to detect a muscle imbalance:

- *Extraocular movements.* Seat the child at eye level to evaluate the extraocular movements. Hold a toy or penlight 30 cm (12 in.) from the child's eyes and move it through the six cardinal fields of gaze. The child's head may need to be held still until fine-motor eye movement develops. Both eyes should move together, tracking the object. This procedure tests the oculomotor, trochlear, and abducens nerves (cranial nerves III, IV, and VI) (Figure 35–9 ●).
- *Corneal light reflex.* To test the corneal light reflex, shine a light on the child's nose, midway between the eyes. Identify the location where the light is reflected on each eye. The light reflection is normally symmetric, at the same spot on each cornea (see Figure 35–6). An asymmetric corneal light reflex indicates strabismus.
- *Cover-uncover test.* This test can be used to identify eye muscle weakness in older, cooperative children, starting at about 4 or 5 years. See Figure 35–10 ● for the technique. Because the eyes work together, no obvious movement of either eye is expected. Eye movement indicates a muscle imbalance.

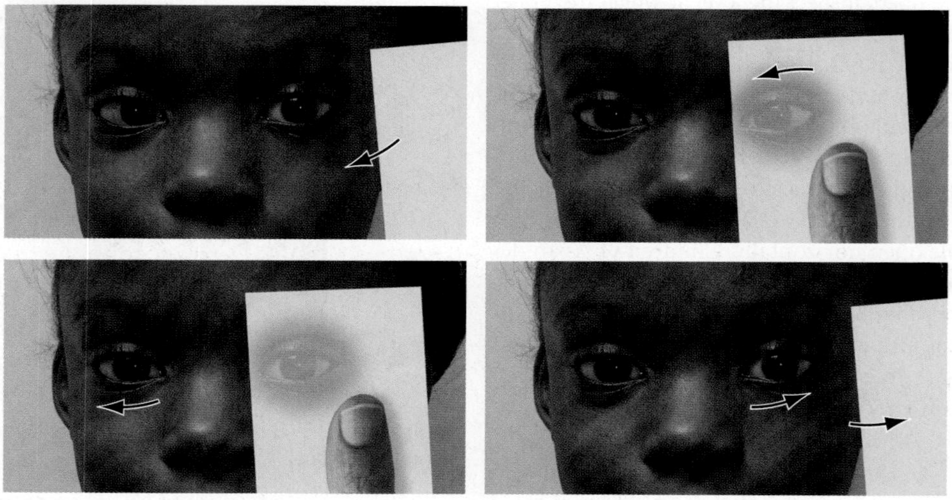

A Right, uncovered eye is weaker. **B** Left, covered eye is weaker.

● **Figure 35–10** The cover-uncover test. With the child at your eye level, ask the child to look at a picture on the wall. ***A,*** As you cover one eye with an index card or paper cup, simultaneously observe for any movement of the uncovered eye. If it jumps to fixate on the picture, the uncovered eye has a muscle weakness. ***B,*** As you remove the cover from the eye, simultaneously observe the covered eye for any movement to fixate on the picture. If the eye has a muscle weakness, it drifts to a relaxed position once covered.

VISION ASSESSMENT

Because vision is such an important sense for learning, assessment is essential to detect any serious problems. Vision is evaluated using an age-appropriate vision test, but no simple method exists. It is possible to assess vision in infants and children by observing their behavior in response to certain maneuvers and during play.

Infants and Toddlers

When the infant's eyes are open, test the blink reflex by moving your hand quickly toward the infant's eyes. A quick blink is the normal response. Absence of the blink reflex can indicate that the infant is blind.

To test an infant's ability to visually track an object, hold a light or toy about 15 cm (6 in.) from the infant's eyes. When the infant has fixated on or is staring at the object, move it slowly to each side. The infant should follow the object with the eyes and by moving the head. Once an infant has developed skills to reach for and then pick up objects, observe play behavior to evaluate vision. The ability to easily find and pick up small toys is a good indicator of vision in children under 3 years of age.

Standardized Vision Charts

Standardized vision charts cannot be used to test vision until the child can understand directions and can cooperate, usually at about 3 or 4 years of age. The HOTV, Snellen E, and Picture charts are used to test visual acuity of preschool-age children just as the Snellen Letter chart is used for school-age children and adolescents. For all screening tools used to test far vision, make sure the child is the appropriate distance from the chart, usually 10 or 20 feet. Cover one eye so each eye is evaluated separately before testing them together. See Skills 9–18 through 9–19 in the Clinical Skills Manual **SKILLS**, for the use of these charts.

Nursing Practice

Criteria for referral for further vision evaluation include:

- Newborn—not tracking an object or parent's face from midline to either side
- Age 3 to 5 years—20/40 or less in either eye
- Age 6 years and older—20/30 or less in either eye
- A difference in vision between the eyes of one line or more on the Snellen eye chart, for example, 20/30 in one eye and 20/40 in the other eye, even when one eye is within the expected range
- Any problems with ocular alignment
- Any other indication of vision impairment, regardless of acuity

Data from American Academy of Pediatrics Committee on Practice and Ambulatory Medicine and Section on Ophthalmology. (2003). Eye examination in infants, children, and young adults by pediatricians. *Pediatrics, 111*(4), 902–907.

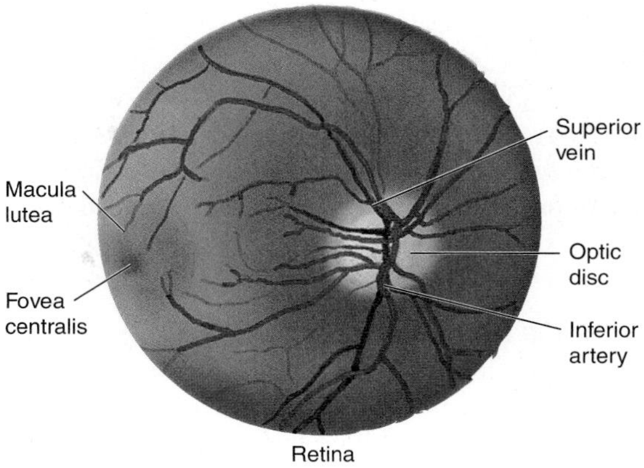

● **Figure 35–11** Normal fundus or retina. When using an ophthalmoscope, only a small portion of the fundus is seen at a time.

INSPECTION OF THE INTERNAL EYE STRUCTURES

The funduscopic examination is an inspection of the internal eye structures—the retina, optic disc, arteries and veins, and macula (Figure 35–11 ●). The ophthalmoscope is a complex instrument and requires practice to master. The examination is difficult to perform on uncooperative children, and most often it is performed by experienced examiners.

Darken the room so the child's pupils dilate. Encourage cooperation by explaining the procedure to the child. Have a picture on the wall or have the parent or assistant hold a toy for the child to stare at so that the child's eye will remain open.

Using the Ophthalmoscope

The ophthalmoscope has a lens-and-mirror system and a bright light for inspecting the structures of the internal eye. Turn the ophthalmoscope on and set the lens power at 0. Keep a forefinger on the disk to change the lens power as needed. Look through the lens of the ophthalmoscope, stabilizing it by resting the top against an eyebrow and the handle against a cheek. Use your right eye to examine the child's right eye and your left eye to examine the child's left eye. This position is best for visualizing the eye, and it reduces direct exposure to infection. Place a hand on the child's head for stabilization.

Red reflex. Shine the ophthalmoscope light at the child's eye from a distance of 30 cm (12 in.). The first image seen is the red reflex, the red glow of the vascular retina. When the red reflex is seen, the ophthalmoscope is being used correctly and the child's lens is clear. Keep the red reflex in view to make sure your head and the ophthalmoscope move as one unit. If you lose the red reflex when moving closer to the child, move back, find the red reflex, and start again.

The red reflexes should be an orange-red glow that is symmetric and uniform (Prentiss & Dorfman, 2008). Black spots or opacities within the red reflex are abnormal and may indicate congenital cataracts. If a white reflex is seen rather than a red reflex, a tumor or cataract may be present. The red reflex can also be tested by shining a small flashlight into the eye.

Nursing Practice

Keep the red reflex in view to make sure your head and the ophthalmoscope move as one unit as you move closer to the child's eye. If you lose the red reflex, move back, find the red reflex, and start again.

Visualizing the internal eye structures. Slowly move closer to the child. Deeper levels of the vitreous humor are inspected before the pink retina comes into view. The retina is a deeper pink in dark-skinned children. A blood vessel is the first retinal structure usually seen. Continue moving closer to the child's eye and adjust the plus or minus lenses to focus on this blood vessel. Retinal arteries appear smaller and brighter red than veins. The blood vessels branch to spread and cover the retina.

Inspect and follow the branching of the blood vessels toward the nose until they merge into the optic disc. Dark areas along the blood vessels may indicate retinal hemorrhages. Carefully inspect sites where arteries and veins cross. Notches and indentations at these sites are associated with hypertension.

The optic disc margin is normally sharply defined, round, and yellow to creamy pink. Blurring of the disc margins or bulging of the optic disc is a sign of increased intracranial pressure. Use the diameter of the optic disc to identify the location of other landmarks on the retina.

The macula is located approximately 2 disc diameters lateral to the optic disc. To see the macula, ask the child to look at the light. It appears as a yellow dot surrounded by deep pink. The macula is inspected last because the bright light causes the child to blink and look away.

ASSESSING THE EAR STRUCTURES AND HEARING

Equipment needed for this examination includes an otoscope, noisemakers (bell, rattle, tissue paper), and a tuning fork 500 to 1000 Hz.

INSPECTION OF THE EXTERNAL EAR STRUCTURES

MyNursingKit Animation: Otoscope Examination

The position and characteristics of the pinna, the external ear, are inspected as a continuation of the head and eye examination. The pinna is considered "low set" when the top lies completely below an imaginary line drawn through the medial and lateral canthi of the eye toward the ear. Low-set ears are often associated with congenital renal disorders (Figure 35–12 ●).

Inspect the pinna for any malformation. The pinna should be completely formed, with an open auditory canal. Next, inspect the tissue around the pinna for abnormalities. A pit or hole in front of the auditory canal may indicate the presence of a sinus. If the one pinna protrudes outward, there may be swelling behind the ear, a sign of mastoiditis, an infection of the mastoid process of the temporal bone of the skull.

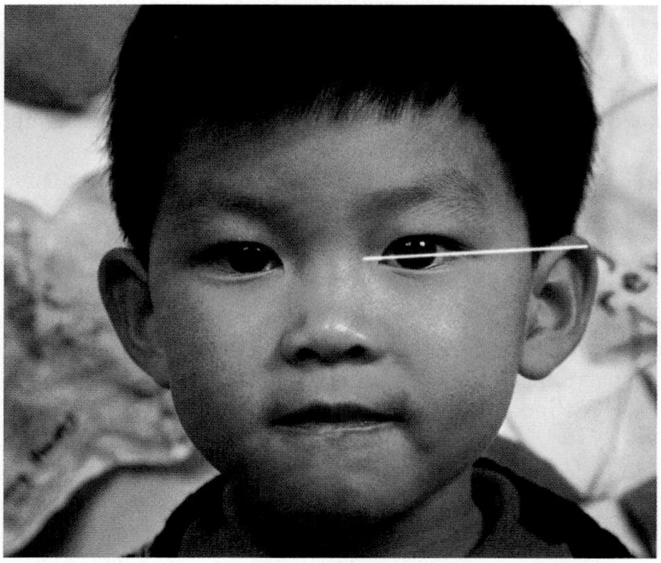

● **Figure 35–12** Ear placement. To detect the correct placement of the external ears, draw an imaginary line through the medial and lateral canthi of the eye toward the ear. This line normally passes through the upper portion of the pinna. The pinna is considered "low set" when the top lies completely below the imaginary line. Low-set ears are often associated with renal disorders.

Inspect the external auditory canal for any discharge. A foul-smelling, purulent discharge may indicate the presence of a foreign body or an infection in the external canal. Clear fluid or a blood-tinged discharge may indicate a cerebrospinal fluid leak caused by a basilar skull fracture.

INSPECTION OF THE TYMPANIC MEMBRANE

Examination of the tympanic membrane is important in infants and young children because they are prone to otitis media, a middle ear infection. The eustachian tubes are shorter, wider, and more horizontally positioned in infants and young children than in older children and adults. This positioning enables bacteria to move up the eustachian tube from the pharynx, causing an infection. See "As Children Grow: Eustachian Tube" in Chapter 47∞.

The otoscope, an instrument with a magnifying lens, bright light, and speculum, is used to examine the internal auditory canal and tympanic membrane. Infants and young children often resist having their ears inspected with the otoscope because of past painful experiences. For that reason it may be wise to delay the otoscopic examination until portions of the assessment requiring cooperation are completed. Use simple explanations to prepare the child. Let the child play with the otoscope or demonstrate how it is used on the parent or a doll. Figure 35–13 ● illustrates one method for restraining an uncooperative child. See also Skill 7–3 in the Clinical Skills Manual SKILLS.

Using the Otoscope

To begin the otoscopic examination, hold the handle of the otoscope in the palm with the thumb pointed toward the speculum. If using a pneumatic squeeze bulb, hold it between the index fin-

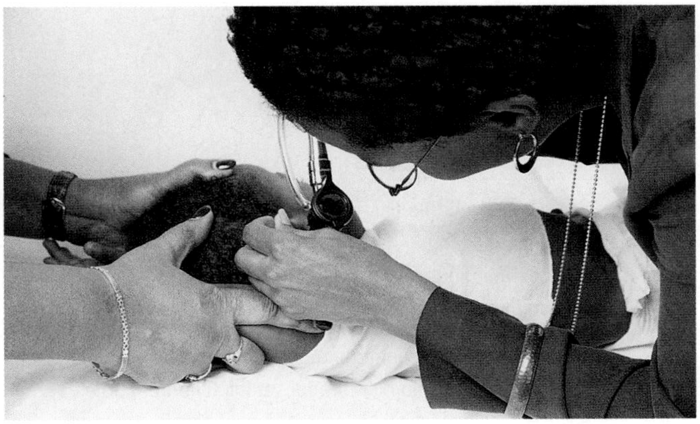

● **Figure 35–13** Inspecting the tympanic membrane. To restrain an uncooperative child, place the child prone on the examining table. Have an assistant hold the child's arms next to the head to restrain the child's head movements. Restrain the child's body movements by lying across the child's body. Keep your hands free to hold the otoscope and position the external ear.

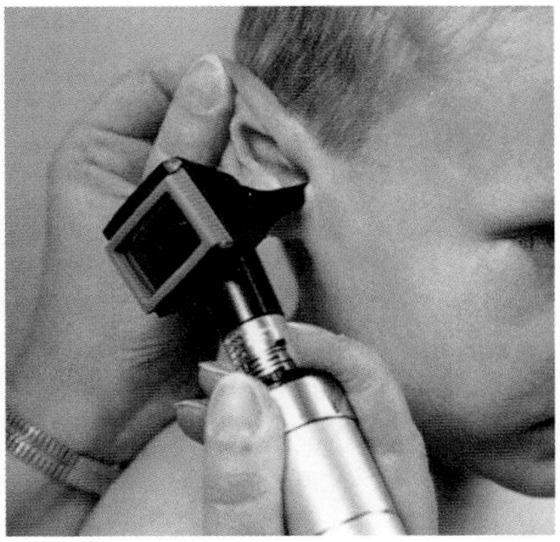

● **Figure 35–14** Otoscopic examination technique. To straighten the auditory canal, pull the pinna back and up for children over 3 years of age. Pull the pinna down and back for children under 3 years of age.

ger and the handle. Choose the largest ear speculum that fits into the auditory canal to form a seal for testing the movement of the tympanic membrane. A large speculum is also less likely to injure the auditory canal if the child moves suddenly.

Hold the otoscope in the hand closest to the child's face, and rest the back of the hand holding the otoscope against the child's head to stabilize it. The other hand is used to pull the pinna back and either up or down, to straighten the auditory canal and improve visibility of the tympanic membrane (Figure 35–14 ●).

Slowly insert the speculum into the auditory canal, inspecting the walls for signs of irritation, discharge, or a foreign body. The walls of the auditory canal are normally pink, and some cerumen is present. Children often put beads, peas, or other small objects into their ears. If the auditory canal is obstructed by cerumen or a foreign body, warm water irrigation can be used to clean the canal.

Nursing Practice

Never irrigate the ear canal if any discharge is present, as the tympanic membrane may be ruptured. Water could enter the middle ear and potentially worsen the infection.

The tympanic membrane, which separates the outer ear from the middle ear, is usually pearly gray and translucent. It reflects light, and the bones (ossicles) in the middle ear are normally visible (Figure 35–15 ●). When the pneumatic attachment is

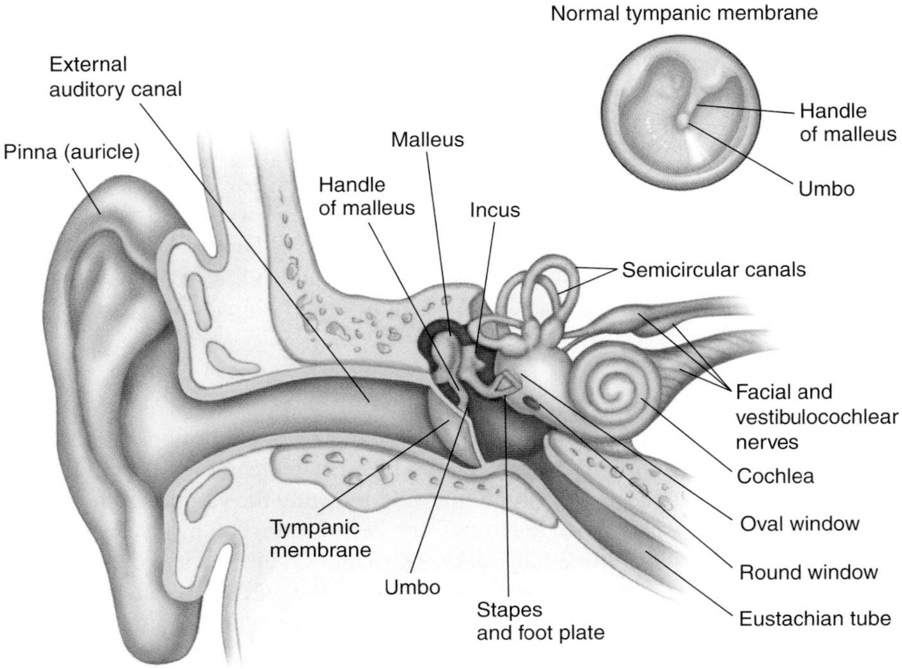

● **Figure 35–15** Cross-section of the ear. The tympanic membrane normally has a triangular light reflex with the base on the nasal side pointing toward the center. The bony landmarks, the umbo and handle of malleus, are seen through the tympanic membrane.

Table 35–6 Unexpected Findings on Examination of the Tympanic Membrane and Their Associated Conditions

Characteristics	Tympanic Membrane Unexpected Findings	Associated Conditions
Color	Redness	Infection in middle ear
	Slight redness	Prolonged crying
	Amber	Serous fluid in middle ear
	Deep red or blue	Blood in middle ear
Light reflex	Absent	Bulging tympanic membrane, infection in middle ear
	Distorted, loss of triangular shape	Retracted tympanic membrane, serous fluid in middle ear
Bony landmarks	Extra prominent	Retracted tympanic membrane, serous fluid in middle ear
Movement	No movement	Infection or fluid in middle ear
	Excessive movement	Healed perforation

squeezed and released, the tympanic membrane normally moves in and out in response to the positive and negative pressure applied. Table 35–6 lists the abnormal findings during examination of the tympanic membranes. See Figures 46–4 and 46–5 for the tympanic membrane appearance when otitis media is present.

HEARING ASSESSMENT

Hearing evaluation is important in children of all ages because hearing is essential for normal speech development and learning. Often hearing is evaluated by observing the child's responses to various auditory stimuli. Hearing loss may occur at any time during early childhood as the result of birth trauma, frequent otitis media, meningitis, or antibiotics that damage cranial nerve VIII. Hearing loss may also be associated with congenital anomalies and genetic syndromes.

Use hearing and speech articulation milestones as an initial hearing screen. Select an age-appropriate method to screen hearing. When a hearing deficiency is suspected as a result of screening, refer the child for audiometry or tympanometry to obtain the most accurate hearing evaluation. See Skills 9–20 and 9–21 in the Clinical Skills Manual **SKILLS**.

Growth and Development

Infant:

- No startle reaction to loud noises
- Does not turn toward sounds by 4 months of age
- Babbles as a young infant but does not keep babbling or develop speech sounds after 6 months of age

Young child:

- No speech by 2 years of age
- Inability to follow age-appropriate directions, such as "bring me the block"
- Speech sounds are not distinct at appropriate ages

Infants and Toddlers

Select noisemakers with different frequencies that will attract the child's attention, such as a rattle, bell, and tissue paper. Ask the parent or an assistant to entertain the infant with a quiet toy, such as a teddy bear. Stand behind the infant, about 2 feet (60 cm) away from the infant's ear but outside the infant's field of vision, and make a soft sound with the noisemaker. Have the parent or assistant observe the child for any of the following responses when the noisemaker is used: widening the eyes, briefly stopping all activity to listen, or turning the head toward the sound. Repeat the test in the other ear and with the other noisemakers.

Preschool and Older Children

Use whispered words to evaluate the hearing of children over 3 years of age. Position your head about 12 inches (30 cm) away from the child's ear, but out of the range of vision so the child cannot read your lips. Use words easily recognized by the child, such as Mickey Mouse, hot dog, and Popsicle, and ask the child to repeat the words. Repeat the test with different words in the opposite ear. The child should correctly repeat the whispered words. If the child will not repeat the whispered words, use a whisper to ask the child to point to different body parts or objects. Remember to stay out of the child's line of sight so lip reading is not possible. The child should point to the correct body part each time.

Bone and Air Conduction of Sound

Use a tuning fork to evaluate the hearing of school-age children who can follow directions. Lightly tap the tines of the tuning fork to begin the vibration. Avoid touching the vibrating tines, which will dampen the sound. Test bone conduction by placing the handle of the tuning fork on the child's skull. Test air conduction by holding the vibrating tines close to the child's ear (Figure 35–16 ●).

To perform the *Weber test*, place the vibrating tuning fork on top of the child's skull in the midline. Ask the child to say where

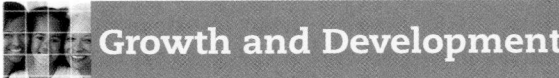

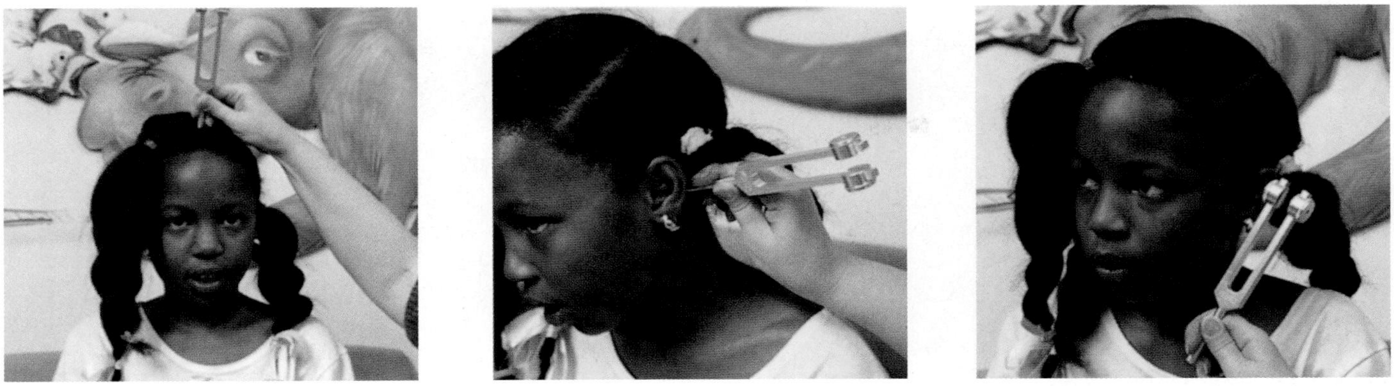

A B C

● **Figure 35–16** Testing bone and air conduction. ***A***, Weber test. Place vibrating tuning fork on midline of the child's head. ***B***, Rinne test, step 1. Place vibrating tuning fork on mastoid process. ***C***, Rinne test, step 2. Reposition still vibrating tines between 2.5 and 5 cm (1 and 2 in.) from ear.

the sound is heard best, either in both ears equally or in one ear. The sound should be heard equally in both ears. If the sound heard better in one ear (lateralized to affected ear), conductive hearing loss may be present.

To perform the *Rinne test,* place the vibrating tuning fork handle on the mastoid process behind an ear and begin counting the seconds. Ask the child to say when the sound is no longer heard. Immediately move the tuning fork, holding the vibrating tines about 2.5 to 5 cm (1 to 2 in.) from the same ear and begin counting the seconds. Again, ask the child to indicate when the sound is no longer heard. The child normally hears the air-conducted sound twice as long as the bone-conducted sound. Repeat the Rinne test on the other ear. When the sound is heard longer by bone conduction than air conduction, the affected ear may have conductive hearing loss. When sound is heard longer by air conduction than bone conduction, but less than twice as long, the affected ear may have sensorineural hearing loss.

ASSESSING THE NOSE AND SINUSES FOR AIRWAY PATENCY AND DISCHARGE

An otoscope with a nasal speculum or a penlight is needed for this examination.

INSPECTION OF THE EXTERNAL NOSE

Examine the external nose characteristics and placement on the face during the assessment of the facial features. Inspect the external nose for size, shape, symmetry, and midline placement on the face. The nose should be proportional in size to other facial features, have symmetric nasolabial folds, and be positioned in the middle of the face. Asymmetry of the nasolabial folds may be associated with injury to the facial nerve (cranial nerve VII). A flattened nasal bridge is the expected finding in Asian and black children. A saddle-shaped nose is associated with congenital defects such as cleft palate.

Inspect the external nose for unusual characteristics. For example, a crease across the nose between the cartilage and bone is often caused when an allergic child frequently wipes an itchy nose upward with a hand.

PALPATION OF THE EXTERNAL NOSE

When a deformity is noted, gently palpate the nose to detect any pain or break in contour. No tenderness or masses are expected. Pain and a contour deviation are usually the result of trauma.

Nasal Patency

The child's airway must be patent to ensure adequate oxygenation. To test for nasal patency, occlude one nostril and observe the child's effort to breathe through the open nostril with the mouth closed. Repeat on the other nostril. Breathing should be noiseless and effortless. **Nasal flaring**, an effort the child makes to widen the airway, is a sign of respiratory distress and should not be present.

If the child struggles to breathe, a nasal obstruction may be present. Nasal obstruction may be caused by a foreign body, congenital defect, dry mucus, discharge, polyp, or trauma. Newborns may have respiratory distress because of choanal atresia, a congenital membranous or bony obstruction between the nose and the nasopharynx. Young children commonly place objects up their nose, and unilateral nasal flaring is a sign of such an obstruction.

ASSESSMENT OF SMELL

The olfactory nerve (cranial nerve I) can be tested in school-age children and adolescents. When testing smell, choose scents the child will easily recognize such as orange, chocolate, and mint. When the child's eyes are closed, occlude one nostril and hold the scent under the nose. Ask the child to take a deep sniff and identify the scent. Alternate odors between the nares. The child can normally identify common scents.

Growth and Development

Infants under 6 months of age will not automatically open their mouths to breathe when their nose is occluded, such as by mucus.

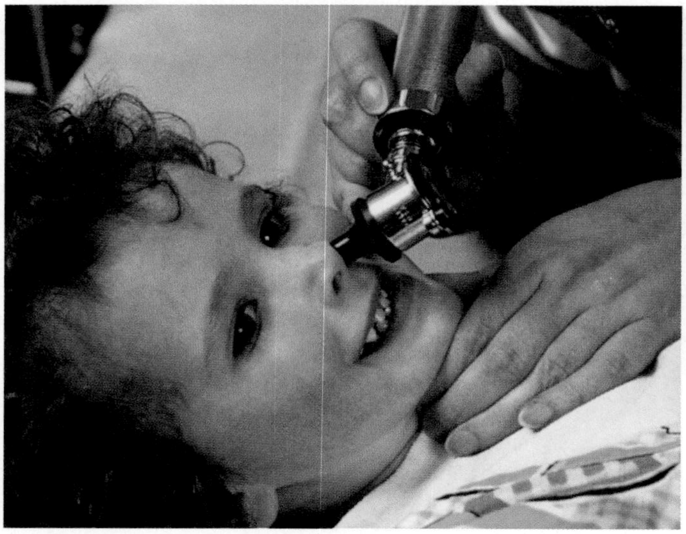

● **Figure 35–17** Technique for examining the nose.

INSPECTION OF THE INTERNAL NOSE

Inspect the internal nose for color of the mucous membranes and the presence of any discharge, swelling, lesions, or other abnormalities. Use a bright light, such as an otoscope light or penlight. For infants and young children, push the tip of the nose upward and shine the light at the end of the nose. The nasal speculum of the otoscope can be used in older children (Figure 35–17 ●). Avoid touching the septum of the nose with the speculum to prevent injury.

MyNursingKit Animation: Mouth and Throat Examination

Mucous Membranes and Nasal Septum

The mucous membranes should be dark pink and glistening. A film of clear discharge may also be present. Turbinates, if visible, should be the same color as the mucous membranes and have a firm consistency. When the turbinates are pale or bluish gray, the child may have allergies. A polyp, a rounded mass projecting from the turbinate, is also associated with allergies. The nasal septum should be straight without perforations, bleeding, or crusting. Crusting will be noted over the site of a nosebleed.

Discharge

Observe for the presence of nasal discharge, noting if it is unilateral or bilateral. Nasal discharge is not a normal finding unless the child is crying. Discharge may be watery, mucoid, purulent, or bloody, depending on the condition present. A foul-smelling discharge in only one nostril is often associated with a foreign body. Table 35–7 lists conditions associated with nasal discharge.

INSPECTION OF THE SINUSES

The illustration in "As Children Grow: Growth and Development of Sinuses" shows how the maxillary and ethmoid sinuses develop during early childhood. Sinus infections can occasionally occur in young children. Suspect a sinus problem when the child has a headache or pain and swelling around one or both eyes.

Table 35–7 Nasal Discharge Characteristics and Associated Condition

Discharge Description	Associated Condition
Watery	
Clear, bilateral	Allergy
Serous, unilateral	Spinal fluid from a basilar skull fracture
Mucoid or purulent	
Bilateral	Upper respiratory infection
Unilateral	Foreign body
Bloody	Nose bleed, trauma

Inspect the face for any puffiness and swelling around one or both eyes; normally, neither is present. To palpate over the maxillary sinuses, press up under both zygomatic arches with the thumbs. To palpate the ethmoid sinuses, press up against the bone above both eyes with the thumbs. No swelling or tenderness is expected. Tenderness may indicate sinusitis.

ASSESSING THE MOUTH AND THROAT FOR COLOR, FUNCTION, AND SIGNS OF ABNORMAL CONDITIONS

Equipment needed to examine the mouth and throat includes a tongue blade and penlight. Wear gloves when examining the mouth.

INSPECTION OF THE MOUTH

Young children often need coaxing and simple explanations before they will cooperate with the mouth and throat examination. Most children readily show their teeth. If the child resists by clenching the teeth, gently separate them with a tongue blade. Mouth structures for inspection are illustrated in Figure 35–18 ●.

Lips

Inspect the lips for color, shape, symmetry, moisture, and lesions. The lips are normally symmetric without drying, cracking, or other lesions. Lip color is normally pink in white children and more bluish in darker-skinned children. Pale, cyanotic, or cherry-red lips indicate poor tissue perfusion caused by various conditions. Note any clefts or edema.

Nursing Practice

Avoid examining the mouth if there are signs of respiratory distress, high fever, drooling, and intense apprehension. These may be signs of epiglottitis. Inspecting the mouth may trigger a total airway obstruction. See Table 48-3 in Chapter 48 ∞ for more information.

AS CHILDREN GROW

GROWTH AND DEVELOPMENT OF SINUSES

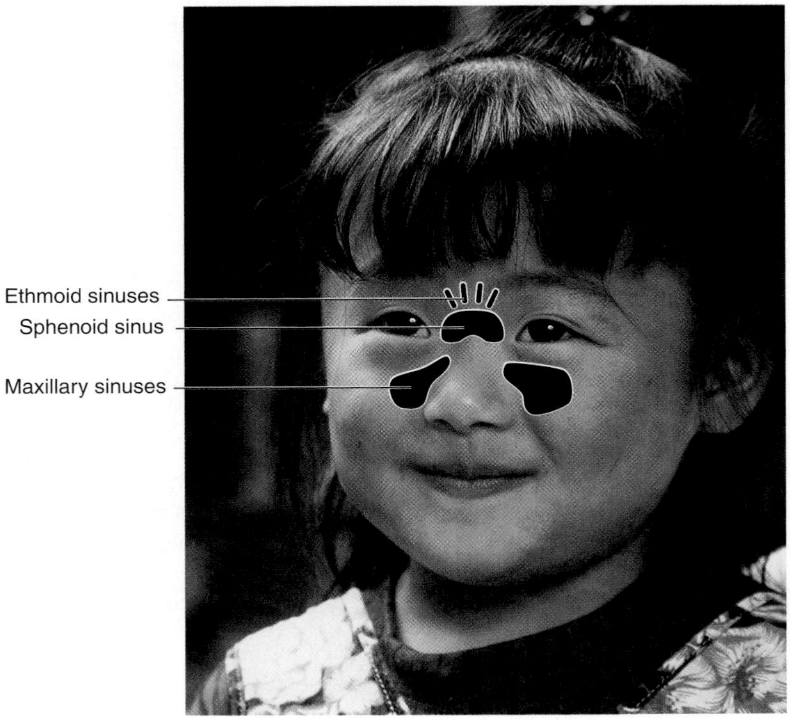

Sinuses grow and develop during childhood. Maxillary sinuses can be identified in 1-year-old children. Ethmoid sinuses have developed in children by 6 years of age. Sinus problems under 7 years occur infrequently.

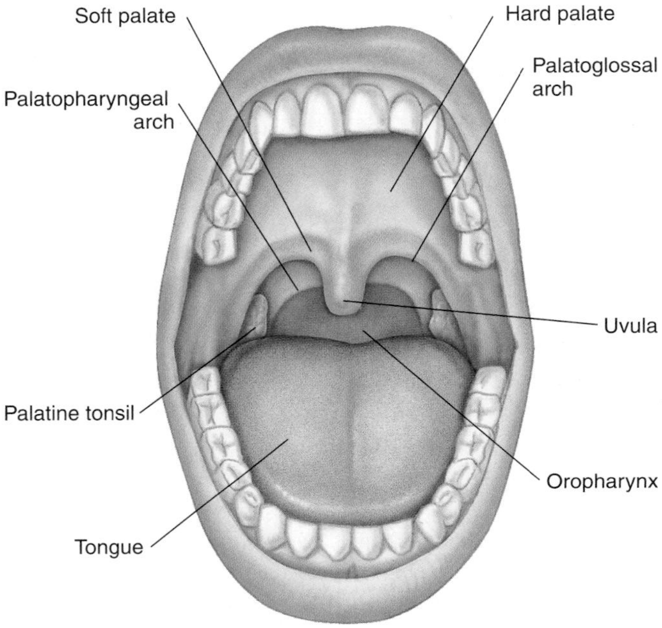

● **Figure 35–18** The structures of the mouth.

Teeth

Inspect and count the child's teeth. The timing of tooth eruption is often genetically determined, but it occurs in a regular sequence. Figure 35–19 ● presents the typical sequence of tooth eruption for both deciduous and permanent teeth.

Inspect the condition of the teeth, look for loose teeth, and note any spaces where teeth are missing. Compare empty tooth spaces with the child's developmental stage of tooth eruption. Once the permanent teeth have erupted, none should be missing. Teeth are normally white, without a flattened, mottled, or pitted appearance. Discolorations on the crown of a tooth may indicate caries. Discolorations on the tooth surface may be associated with some medications or fluorosis.

Mouth Odors

During inspection of the teeth, be alert to any abnormal odors that may indicate problems such as diabetic ketoacidosis, infection, or poor hygiene. Be alert for alcohol odors in older children that could signal substance abuse.

Gums

Inspect the gums for color and adherence to the teeth. The gums are normally pink, with a stippled or dotted appearance. Use a tongue blade to help visualize the gums around the upper and lower molars. No raised or receding gum areas should be apparent around

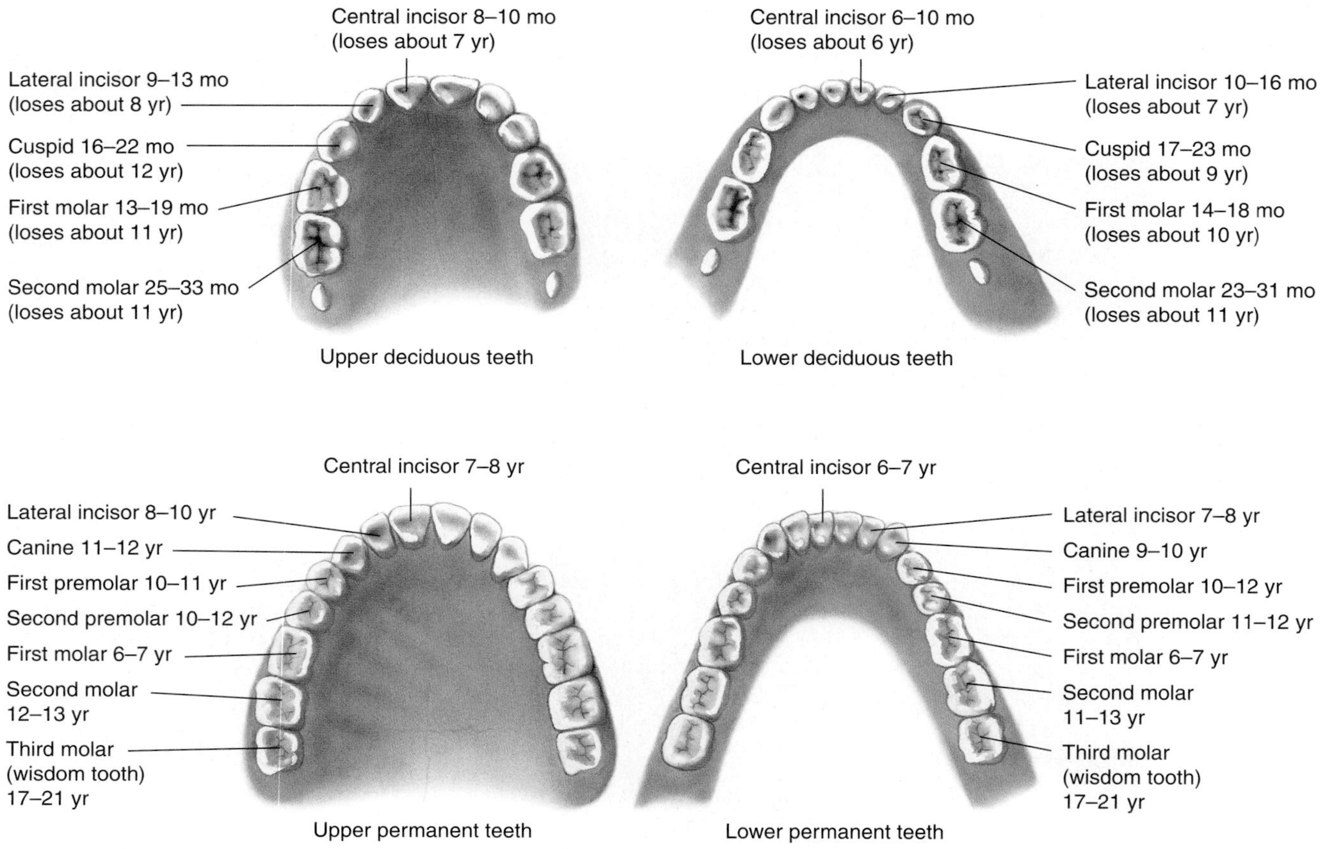

● **Figure 35–19** Typical sequence of tooth eruption for both deciduous and permanent teeth. The bottom deciduous teeth are shed before upper teeth, and bottom permanent teeth erupt first as well.

the teeth. When inflammation, swelling, or bleeding is observed, palpate the gums to detect tenderness. Inflammation and tenderness are associated with infection and poor nutrition.

Buccal Mucosa

Inspect the mucous membrane lining the cheeks for color and moisture. The mucous membrane is usually pink, but patches of hyperpigmentation are commonly seen in darker-skinned children. The Stensen duct, the parotid gland opening, is opposite the upper second molar bilaterally. Normally pink, the duct opening becomes red when the child is infected with mumps. Small pink sucking pads can be present in infants. No areas of redness, swelling, or ulcerative lesions should be present.

Tongue

Inspect the tongue for color, moistness, size, tremors, and lesions. The child's tongue is normally pink and moist, without a coating, and it fits easily into the mouth. A protuberant tongue is associated with various genetic conditions, such as Down syndrome. A pattern of gray, irregular borders that form a design (geographic tongue) is often normal, but it may be associated with fever, allergies, or drug reactions. Tremors are abnormal. A white adherent coating on an infant's tongue may be caused by thrush, a *Candida* infection (see Chapter 59∞).

Observe the mobility of the tongue. Ask the child to touch the gums above the upper teeth with the tongue. This tongue movement is adequate to enunciate all speech sounds clearly. Ask the child to stick out the tongue and lift it so the underside of the tongue and the floor of the mouth can be inspected for distended veins, an unexpected finding.

Palate

Inspect the hard and soft palate to detect any clefts or masses or an unusually high arch. The palate is normally pink, dome-shaped, and has no cleft. The uvula hangs freely from the soft palate. A high-arched palate can be associated with sucking difficulties in young infants.

PALPATION OF THE MOUTH STRUCTURES

Palpate any masses seen in the mouth to determine their characteristics, such as size, shape, firmness, and tenderness. No masses should be found.

To assess the tongue's strength, while simultaneously testing the hypoglossal nerve (cranial nerve XII), place the index finger against the child's cheek and ask the child to push against your finger with the tongue. Some pressure against the finger is normally felt.

To palpate the palate, insert the little finger, with the finger-pad upward, into the mouth. While the infant sucks against your finger, palpate the entire palate. This procedure also tests the strength of the sucking reflex, innervated by the hypoglossal nerve (cranial nerve XII). No clefts should be palpated.

INSPECTION OF THE THROAT

Use a flashlight to inspect the throat for color, swelling, lesions, and the condition of the tonsils. Ask the child to open the mouth wide and stick out the tongue, and use a tongue blade, if needed, to visualize the posterior pharynx. Moistening the tongue blade may decrease the child's tendency to gag. The throat is normally pink without lesions, drainage, or swelling. Swelling or bulging in the posterior pharynx may be associated with a peritonsillar abscess.

Tonsils

During childhood the tonsils are large in proportion to the size of the pharynx because lymphoid tissue grows fastest in early childhood. The tonsils should be pink without exudate, but crypts (fissures) may be present as a result of prior infections. The size of the tonsils can be graded as indicated in the "Pathophysiology Illustrated: Tonsil Size with Infection" diagram.

When using a tongue blade to see the throat and tonsils, the gag reflex may be triggered. A symmetric rising movement of the uvula should be observed as the child gags.

ASSESSING THE NECK FOR CHARACTERISTICS, RANGE OF MOTION, AND LYMPH NODES

INSPECTION OF THE NECK

Inspect the neck for size, symmetry, swelling, and any abnormalities such as webbing, an extra fold of skin on each side of the neck. A short neck with skin folds is normal for infants. The neck is normally symmetric with no swelling present. Swelling may be caused

PATHOPHYSIOLOGY ILLUSTRATED

TONSIL SIZE WITH INFECTION

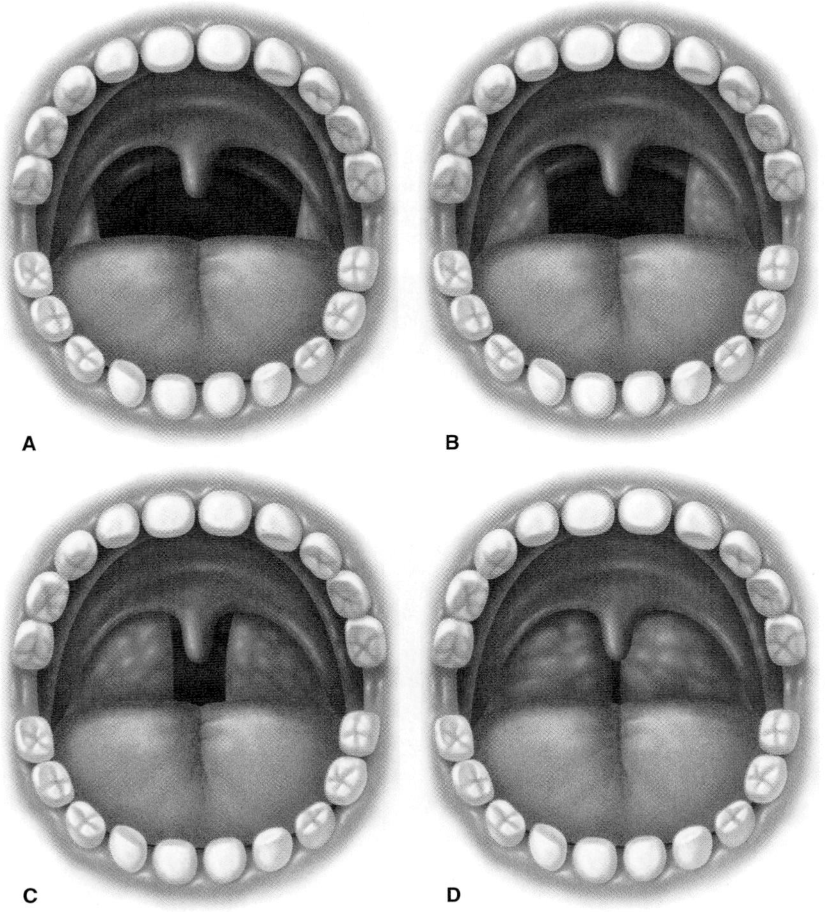

Tonsil size can be graded from 1+ to 4+ in relation to how much of the airway is obstructed. Tonsil size of 1+ and 2+ is normal. Tonsil size of 3+ is common with infections such as strep throat. Tonsils that "kiss" or nearly touch each other (4+) significantly reduce the size of the airway.

by local infections such as mumps or a congenital defect. The neck lengthens between 3 and 4 years of age. Webbing is commonly associated with Turner syndrome (see Chapter 55∞).

Infants develop head control by 2 months of age. By this age an infant can lift the head up and look around when lying on the stomach. A lack of head control can result from neurologic injury, such as an anoxic episode.

PALPATION OF THE NECK

Face the child and use your fingerpads to simultaneously palpate both sides of the neck for lymph nodes, as well as the trachea and thyroid.

Lymph Nodes

To palpate the lymph nodes, slide your fingerpads gently over the lymph node chains in the head and neck. One sequence is to palpate the lymph nodes in the occipital area, around the ears, under the jaw, and then the cervical chain in the neck (Figure 35–20 ●). Firm, clearly defined, nontender, movable lymph nodes up to 1 cm (1/2 in.) in diameter are common in young children. Enlarged, firm, warm, tender lymph nodes indicate a local infection.

Trachea

Palpate the trachea to determine its position and to detect the presence of any masses. The trachea is normally in the midline of the neck. It is difficult to palpate in children less than 3 years of age because of their short necks. To palpate the trachea, place your thumb and forefinger on each side of the child's trachea near the chin and slowly slide them down the trachea. Any shift to the right or left of midline may indicate a tumor or a collapsed lung.

Thyroid

As the fingers slide over the trachea in the lower neck, attempt to feel the isthmus of the thyroid, a band of glandular tissue crossing over the trachea. The lobes of the thyroid wrap behind the trachea and are normally covered by the sternocleidomastoid muscle. Because of the anatomic position of the thyroid, its lobes are not usually palpable in the child unless they are enlarged.

RANGE OF MOTION ASSESSMENT

To test the neck's range of motion, ask the child to touch the chin to each shoulder and to the chest and then to look at the ceiling. Move a light or toy in all four directions when assessing infants. Children should freely move the neck and head in all four directions without pain.

When the child is unable to move the head voluntarily in all directions, passively move the child's neck through the expected range of motion. Limited horizontal range of motion may be a sign of *torticollis,* persistent head tilting. Torticollis results from a birth injury to the sternocleidomastoid muscle or from unilateral vision or hearing impairment. Pain with flexion of the neck toward the chest (Brudzinski's sign) may indicate meningitis (see Chapter 56∞).

ASSESSING THE CHEST FOR SHAPE, MOVEMENT, RESPIRATORY EFFORT, AND LUNG FUNCTION

Examination of the chest includes the following procedures: inspecting the size and shape of the chest, palpating chest movement that occurs during respiration, observing the effort of breathing, and auscultating breath sounds. A stethoscope is needed.

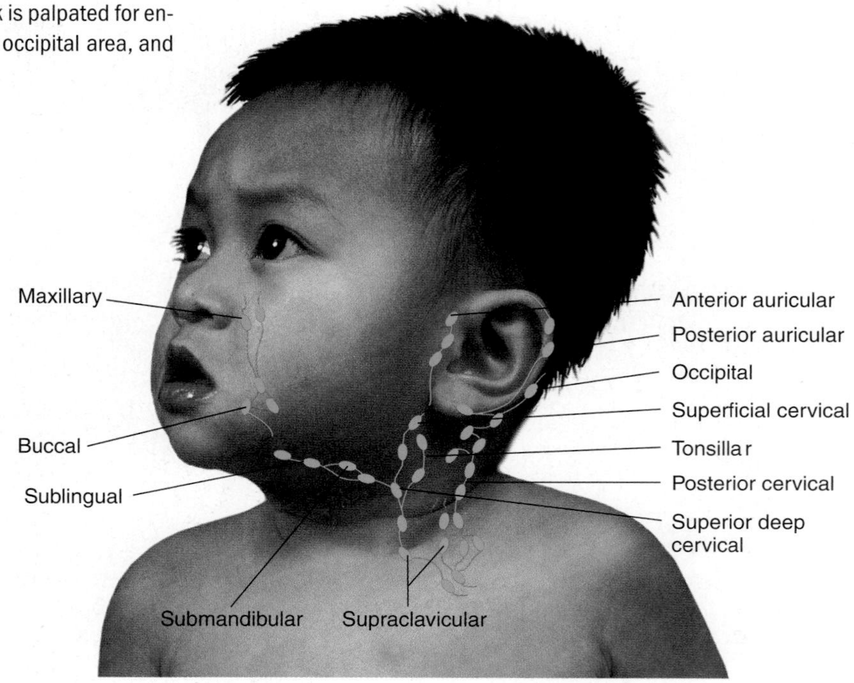

● **Figure 35–20** Palpating the lymph nodes. The neck is palpated for enlarged lymph nodes around the ears, under the jaw, in the occipital area, and in the cervical chain of the neck.

INSPECTION OF THE CHEST

The chest skeleton provides most of the landmarks used to describe the location of findings during examination of the chest, lungs, and heart. The intercostal spaces are the horizontal markers. The sternum and spine are the vertical landmarks. When both a horizontal and a vertical landmark are used, the location of findings can be precisely described on the right or left side of the patient's chest (Figures 35–21 ● and 35–22 ●).

Position the child on the parent's lap or on the examining table with all clothing above the waist removed to inspect the chest. The thoracic muscles and subcutaneous tissue are less developed in children than in adolescents and adults, so the chest wall is thinner and the rib cage is more prominent.

Size and Shape of the Chest

Inspect the chest for any irregularities in shape. A chest is considered rounded when the anteroposterior diameter is approximately equal to the lateral diameter. If a child over 2 years of age has a rounded chest, a chronic obstructive lung condition such as asthma or cystic fibrosis may be present.

An abnormal chest shape results from three structural deformities (Figure 35–23 ●). If the sternum protrudes, increasing the anteroposterior diameter, pigeon chest (pectus carinatum) may be present. If the lower portion of the sternum is depressed, decreasing the anteroposterior diameter, funnel chest (pectus excavatum) may be present. Scoliosis, curvature of the spine, causes a lateral deviation of the chest (see Chapter 58∞).

> **Growth and Development**
>
> In infants, the chest is rounded with the anteroposterior diameter approximately equal to the lateral diameter. The chest becomes more oval with growth. By 2 years of age the lateral diameter is greater than the anteroposterior diameter.

Chest Movement and Respiratory Effort

Chest movement with breathing is normally symmetric bilaterally. On inspiration the chest and abdomen should rise simultaneously and fall on expiration. The chest movement of infants and young children is less pronounced than the abdominal movement as the diaphragm is the primary breathing muscle in infants and children under 6 years old. The thoracic muscles are less developed and serve as accessory muscles in cases of respiratory distress. As the thoracic muscles develop, they become primarily responsible for ventilation. **Retractions**, depression of sections of the chest wall with each inspiration, are seen when the accessory

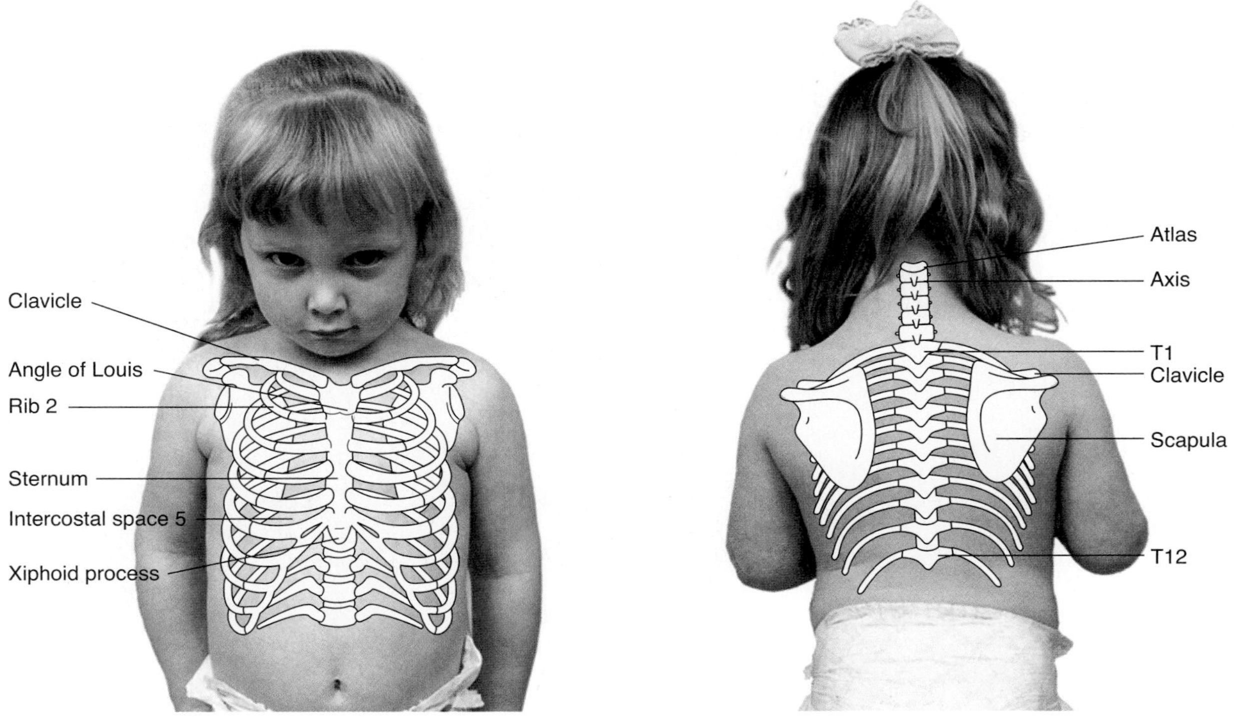

● **Figure 35–21** Landmarks of the chest. Intercostal spaces and ribs are numbered to describe the location of findings. ***A,*** To determine the rib number on the anterior chest, palpate down from the top of the sternum until a horizontal ridge, the angle of Louis, is felt. Directly to the right and left of that ridge is the second rib. The second intercostal space is immediately below the second rib. Ribs 3–12 and the corresponding intercostal spaces can be counted as the fingers move toward the abdomen. ***B,*** To determine the rib number on the posterior chest, find the protruding spinal process of the seventh cervical vertebra at the shoulder level. The next spinal process belongs to the first thoracic vertebra, which attaches to the first rib.

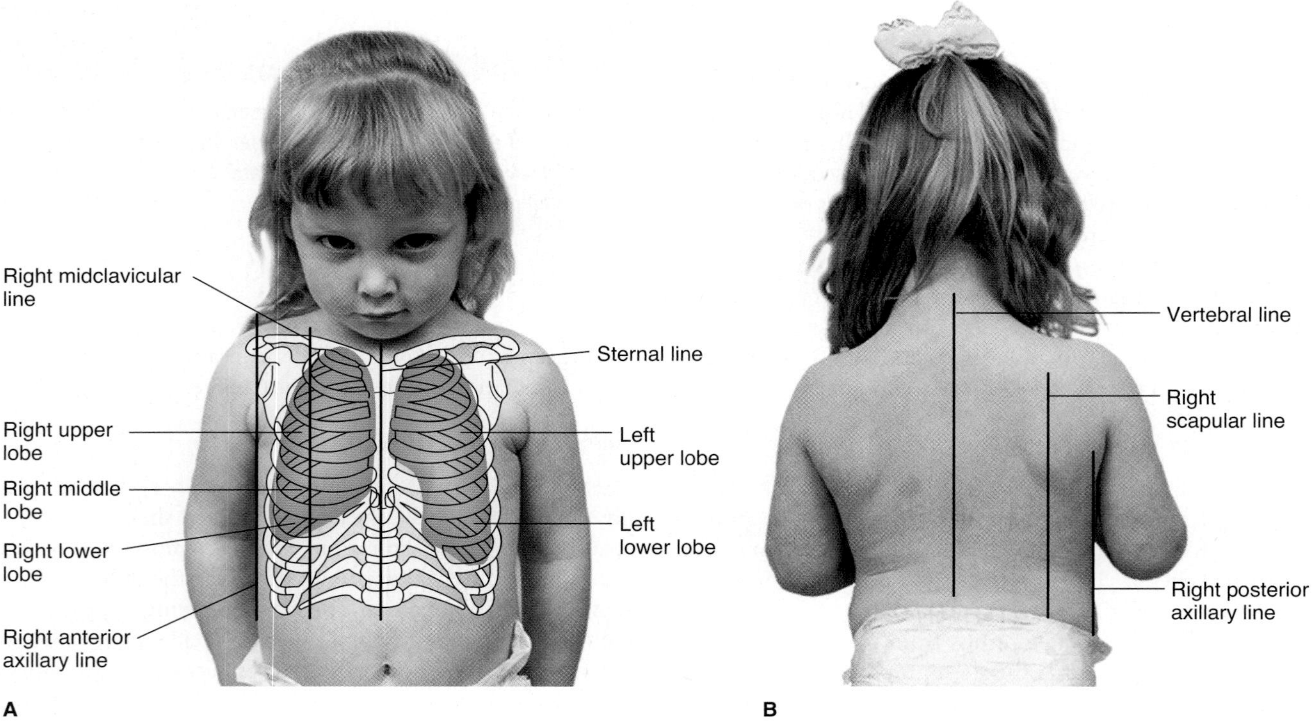

● **Figure 35–22** Vertical landmarks of the chest. The sternum and spine are the vertical landmarks used to describe the anatomic location of findings. The distance between the finding and the center of the sternum (midsternal line) or the spinal line can be measured with a ruler. Imaginary vertical lines, parallel to the midsternal and spinal lines, are used to further describe the location of findings. ***A,*** anterior vertical landmarks, ***B,*** posterior vertical landmarks.

● **Figure 35–23** Two types of abnormal chest shape. ***A***, Funnel chest (pectus excavatum). ***B***, Pigeon chest (pectus carinatum).

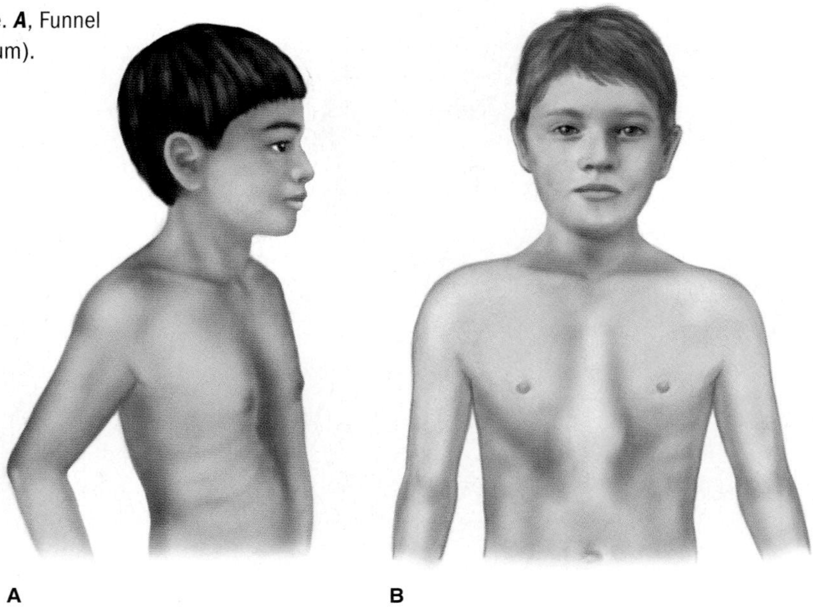

muscles are used for breathing in cases of respiratory distress. Asymmetric chest rise is associated with a collapsed lung.

Respiratory Rate

Because young children use the diaphragm as the primary breathing muscle, observe or feel the rise and fall of the abdomen to count the respiratory rate in children under age 6 years (see Skill 9–9 in the Clinical Skills Manual SKILLS). Table 35–8 gives the normal respiratory rates for each age group. Make every effort to count the respiratory rate when the child is quiet.

Infants and children have a faster respiratory rate than adults because their higher metabolic rate causes an increased

Table 35–8 Normal Respiratory Rate Ranges by Age

Age	Respiratory Rate per Minute
Newborn	30–55
1 year	25–40
3 years	20–30
6 years	16–22
10 years	16–20
17 years	12–20

Nursing Practice

To get the most accurate reading of a newborn's and young infant's respiratory rate, wait until the baby is sleeping or resting quietly. Use the stethoscope to auscultate the rate or place your hand on the abdomen. Count the number of breaths for an entire minute, because newborns and young infants can have irregular respirations.

need for oxygen. Young children are also unable to increase the depth of respirations because the intercostal muscles are inadequately developed to lift the chest wall and increase intrathoracic volume (Ralston, Hazinski, Zaritsky, et al., 2006, p. 40).

The respiratory rate rises in response to excitement, fear, respiratory distress, fever, and other conditions that increase oxygen needs. A sustained respiratory rate higher than normal for age is an important sign of respiratory distress. The child is at risk for developing hypoxemia if treatment is not started.

PALPATION OF THE CHEST

Use palpation to evaluate chest movement, respiratory effort, deformities of the chest wall, and tactile fremitus.

Chest Wall

To palpate the chest motion with respiration, place your palms and outspread fingers on each side of the child's chest. Confirm the bilateral symmetry of chest motion. Use your fingerpads to palpate any depressions, bulges, or unusual chest wall shape that might indicate abnormal findings such as tenderness, cysts, other growths, crepitus, or fractures. None should be found. **Crepitus**, a crinkly sensation palpated on the chest surface, is caused by air escaping into the subcutaneous tissues. It often indicates a serious injury to the upper or lower airway. Crepitus may also be felt when there is body movement near a fracture.

Tactile Fremitus

Crying and talking produce vibrations (**tactile fremitus**) that can be palpated on the chest. Place the palms of your hands on each side of the chest to evaluate the quality and distribution of these vibrations. Ask the child to repeat a series of words or numbers, such as Mickey Mouse or ice cream. As the child repeats the words, move your hands systematically over the anterior and posterior chest, comparing the quality of findings side to side. The vibration or tingling sensation is normally palpated over the entire chest. Decreased sensations indicate that air is trapped in the lungs, as occurs with asthma.

AUSCULTATION OF THE CHEST

Auscultate the chest with a stethoscope to assess the quality and characteristics of breath sounds, to identify abnormal breath sounds, and to evaluate vocal resonance. Use an infant or pediatric stethoscope when available to help localize any unexpected breath sounds. Use the stethoscope diaphragm because it transmits the high-pitched breath sounds better.

Breath Sounds

Evaluate the quality and characteristics of breath sounds over the entire chest, comparing sounds between the sides. Select a routine sequence for auscultating the entire chest so assessment of all lobes of the lungs will be consistently performed. Figure 35–24 ● shows one suggested chest auscultation sequence. Listen to an entire inspiratory and expiratory phase at each spot on the chest before moving to the next site.

Three types of normal breath sounds are usually heard when the chest is auscultated. *Vesicular breath sounds* are low-pitched, swishing, soft, short expiratory sounds. They are usually heard in older children but not in infants and young children. *Bronchovesicular breath sounds* are medium-pitched, hollow, blowing sounds heard equally on inspiration and expiration in all age groups. The location of these sounds on the chest is related to the child's developmental status. *Bronchial/tracheal breath sounds* are hollow and higher pitched than vesicular breath sounds.

Breath sounds normally have equal intensity, pitch, and rhythm bilaterally. Absent or diminished breath sounds may indicate a pneumothorax or airway obstruction.

Nursing Practice

Auscultation of breath sounds is difficult when an infant is crying. First, try to quiet the infant with a pacifier, bottle, or toy. If the infant continues to cry, assess breath sounds, vocal resonance, and tactile fremitus at the end of each cry as the infant takes a deep breath. Encourage toddlers and preschoolers to take deep breaths by providing a pinwheel or mobile to blow. This may enhance auscultation of subtle wheezes that occur at the end of expiration.

When trying to encourage the child to breathe normally while auscultating the chest, use suggestive language to increase cooperation: "You certainly are good at breathing slowly. Have you been practicing?" The child will often deepen and slow the breathing pattern as you draw attention to it and give praise.

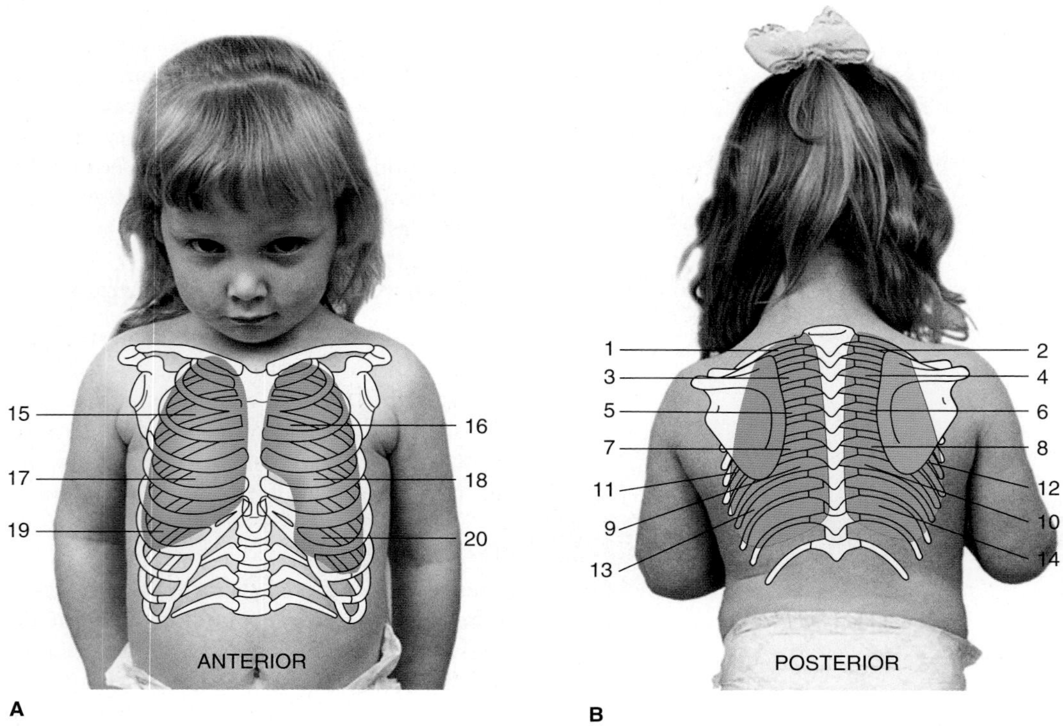

● **Figure 35–24** One sequence for auscultation of the chest.

Growth and Development

Infants and young children have a thin chest wall because of immature muscle development. The breath sounds of one lung are heard over the entire chest. It takes practice to accurately identify absent or diminished breath sounds in infants and young children. Because the distance between the lungs is greatest at the apices and midaxillary areas in young children, these sites are best for identifying absent or diminished breath sounds. Carefully auscultate, comparing the quality of breath sounds heard bilaterally.

Vocal Resonance

Auscultate the chest to evaluate how well voice sounds are transmitted. Have the child repeat a series of words, such as those used for evaluating tactile fremitus. Use the stethoscope to auscultate the chest, comparing the quality of sounds from side to side and over the entire chest. Voice sounds, with words and syllables muffled and indistinct, are normally heard throughout the chest.

If voice sounds are absent or more muffled than usual, an airway obstruction condition such as asthma may be present. When a lung consolidation condition such as pneumonia is present, the vocal resonance quality changes in characteristic ways. **Whispered pectoriloquy** is present when syllables are heard distinctly in a whisper. **Bronchophony** is the increased intensity and clarity of sounds while the words remain indistinct. **Egophony** is the transmission of the "eee" sound as a nasal "ay" sound.

Abnormal Breath Sounds

Abnormal breath sounds, also called adventitious sounds, generally indicate disease. Examples of abnormal breath sounds are crackles, rhonchi, and friction rubs. It takes practice to routinely identify these adventitious sounds. When assessing abnormal breath sounds, determine their location, the respiratory phase in which sounds are present, and whether sounds change or disappear when the child coughs or shifts position. Table 35–9 describes adventitious sounds.

Abnormal Voice Sounds

Observing the quality of the voice and other audible sounds is also important during an examination of the lungs. *Stridor* is a noise resulting from air moving through a narrowed trachea and larynx; it is associated with croup. *Wheezing* is a noise resulting from the passage of air through mucus or fluids in a narrowed lower airway, with sounds as described for sibilant rhonchi. It is associated with asthma. A cough is a reflexive clearing of the airway associated with a respiratory infection. Hoarseness is associated with inflammation of the larynx.

PERCUSSION OF THE CHEST

Percussion is a method sometimes used to assess the resonance of the lungs and the size of underlying organs, such as the heart and liver. Radiograph examination is now used more commonly for these evaluations.

Table 35–9 Description of Selected Adventitious Sounds and Their Cause

Type	Description	Cause
Fine crackles	High-pitched, discrete, noncontinuous sound heard at end of inspiration *(Rub pieces of hair together beside your ear to duplicate the sound.)*	Air passing through watery secretions in the smaller airways (alveoli and bronchioles)
Sibilant rhonchi	Musical, squeaking, or hissing noise heard during inspiration or expiration, but generally louder on expiration	Bronchospasm or an anatomic narrowing of the trachea, bronchi, or bronchioles
Sonorous rhonchi (coarse crackles)	Coarse, low-pitched sound like a snore, heard during inspiration or expiration; may clear with coughing	Air passing through thick secretions that partially obstruct the larger bronchi and trachea

Thinking Critically

ASSESSING A CHILD WITH BRONCHIOLITIS

Latoya, 6 months old, is brought by her mother and father to the emergency room. She is an emergency admission from the local pediatrician's office with a diagnosis of bronchiolitis. As Latoya's nurse, you are responsible for assessing her condition after she arrives on the pediatric nursing unit.

What historical information do you collect, and what approach do you take to examine Latoya? What procedures are used to perform a physical examination on a 6-month-old? Identify all the components of the physical assessment used to detect signs of respiratory difficulty and inadequate tissue perfusion. How do you organize your findings to make sense of them to plan nursing care?

See MyNursingKit for possible responses.

ASSESSING THE BREASTS

INSPECTION OF THE BREASTS

The nipples of prepubertal boys and girls are symmetrically located near the midclavicular line at the fourth to sixth ribs. The areola is normally round and more darkly pigmented than the surrounding skin. Inspect the anterior chest for other dark spots that may indicate supernumerary nipples, which are small, undeveloped nipples and areola that may be mistaken for moles. Their presence may be associated with congenital renal or cardiac anomalies.

See pages 964–965 for pubertal development.

PALPATION OF THE BREASTS

Palpate the developing breasts of adolescent females for abnormal masses or hard nodules while the child is supine. Use a concentric pattern covering all quadrants of each breast, including the axilla, all around the areola, and then around the nipple. Breast tissue normally feels dense, firm, and elastic. Any mass needs further evaluation.

The majority of boys have unilateral or bilateral breast enlargement during adolescence called gynecomastia. It is often most noticeable around 14 years of age and commonly disappears by the time of full sexual maturity. Palpate the tissue to differentiate actual breast tissue from fatty tissue in the pectoral area, and to detect any masses.

ASSESSING THE HEART FOR HEART SOUNDS AND FUNCTION

A stethoscope and sphygmomanometer are needed to assess the heart.

INSPECTION OF THE PRECORDIUM

Begin the heart examination by inspecting the precordium, or anterior chest. Place the child in reclining or semi-Fowler's position, either on the parent's lap or on the examining table. Inspect the shape and symmetry of the anterior chest from the front and side views. Asymmetry and bulging of the left side of the chest wall may indicate an enlarged heart.

Observe for any chest movement associated with the heart's contraction. The **apical impulse**, sometimes called the point of maximum intensity, is located where the left ventricle taps the chest wall during contraction. The apical impulse is usually seen in thin children. A heave, an obvious lifting of the chest wall during contraction, may indicate an enlarged heart.

PALPATION OF THE PRECORDIUM

Place the entire palmar surface of your fingers together on the chest wall to systematically palpate the precordium for any pulsations, heaves, or vibrations. Palpating with minimal pressure increases the chance of detecting abnormal findings.

The apical impulse is normally felt as a slight tap against one fingertip. Use the topographic landmarks of the chest to describe its location (see Figures 35–21 and 35–22). Any other sensation palpated is usually abnormal. A *lift* is the sensation of the heart lifting up against the chest wall. It may be associated with an enlarged heart or a heart contracting with extra force. A *thrill* is a rushing vibration that feels like a cat's purr. It is caused by turbulent blood flow from a defective heart valve and a heart murmur. If present, the thrill is palpated in the right or left second intercostal space. To describe a thrill's location, use the topographic landmarks of the chest (see Figures 35–21 and 35–22) and estimate the diameter of the thrill palpated.

Growth and Development

The location of the apical impulse changes as the child's rib cage grows. In children under 7 years old, it is located in the fourth intercostal space just medial to the left midclavicular line. In children over 7 years old, it is located in the fifth intercostal space at the left midclavicular line.

AUSCULTATION OF THE HEART

Auscultation is used to count the apical pulse, to assess the characteristics of the heart sounds, and to detect abnormal heart sounds. Use the bell of the stethoscope to detect these lower pitched sounds.

To assess heart sounds completely, auscultate the heart with the child in both sitting and reclining positions. Differences in heart sounds caused by a change in the child's position or by a change in the position of the heart near the chest wall can then be detected. If differences in heart sounds are detected with a position change, place the child in the left lateral recumbent position and auscultate again.

Heart Rate and Rhythm

The apical heart rate can be counted at the site of the apical impulse (Skill 9–8) **SKILLS** either by palpation or by auscultation. Count the apical rate for 1 minute in infants and in children who have an irregular rhythm. The brachial or radial pulse rate should be the same as the auscultated apical heart rate. Table 35–10 gives normal heart rates in children of different ages.

Listen carefully to the heart rate rhythm. Children often have a normal cycle of irregular rhythm associated with respiration called *sinus arrhythmia* in which the child's heart rate is faster on inspiration and slower on expiration. When any rhythm irregularity is detected, ask the child to take a breath and hold it while you listen to the heart rate. The rhythm should become regular during inspiration and expiration. Other rhythm irregularities are abnormal.

Table 35–10 Normal Heart Rates for Children of Different Ages

Age	Heart Rate Range (beats/min)	Average Heart Rate (beats/min)
Newborns	100–170	120
Infants to 2 years	80–130	110
2–6 years	70–120	100
6–10 years	70–110	90
10–16 years	60–100	85

Growth and Development

The child's heart rate varies with age, decreasing as the child grows older. The heart rate also increases in response to exercise, excitement, anxiety, and fever. Such stresses increase the child's metabolic rate, creating a simultaneous need for more oxygen. Children respond to the need for more oxygen by increasing their heart rate, a response called sinus tachycardia.

Differentiation of Heart Sounds

Heart sounds result from the closure of the valves and vibration or turbulence of blood produced by that valve closure. Two primary sounds, S_1 and S_2, are heard when the chest is auscultated.

S_1, the first heart sound, is produced by closure of the tricuspid and mitral valves at the beginning of ventricular contraction. The two valves close almost simultaneously, so only one sound is normally heard.

S_2, the second heart sound, is produced by the closure of the aortic and pulmonic valves. Once blood has reached the pulmonic and aortic arteries, the valves close to prevent leakage back into the ventricles during diastole. The timing of the valve closure varies with respirations. Sometimes S_2 is heard as a single sound and at other times as a split sound, that is, two sounds heard a fraction of a second apart.

Sound is easily transmitted in liquid, and it travels best in the direction of blood flow. Auscultate heart sounds at specific areas on the chest wall in the direction of blood flow, just beyond the valve (Figure 35–25 ●). The sounds produced by the heart valves or blood turbulence are heard throughout the chest in thin infants and children. Both S_1 and S_2 can be heard in all listening areas.

Auscultate heart sounds for quality (distinct versus muffled) and intensity (loud versus soft). First, distinguish between S_1 and S_2 in each listening area. Heart sounds are usually distinct and crisp in children because of their thin chest wall. Muffling or indistinct sounds may indicate a heart defect or congestive heart failure. Document the area where heart sounds are heard the best. Table 35–11 and Figure 35–25 review the location where each sound is normally best heard for assessment of quality and intensity. If the child has a potential murmur, auscultate the heart in the sitting, reclining, and standing positions to see if differences are noted by position change.

Nursing Practice

To distinguish between S_1 and S_2 heart sounds in each listening area, palpate the carotid pulse while auscultating the heart. The heart sound heard simultaneously with the pulsation is S_1.

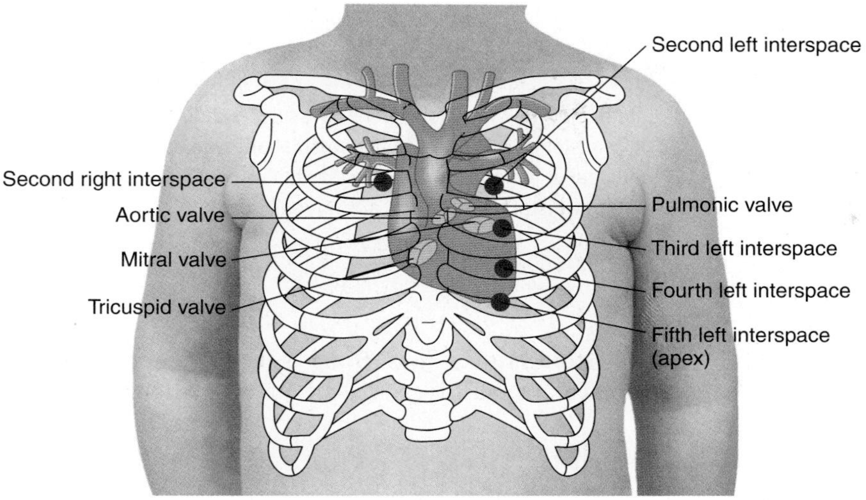

● **Figure 35–25** Auscultating heart sounds. Sound travels in the direction of blood flow. Rather than listen for heart sounds over each heart valve, auscultate heart sounds at specific areas on the chest wall away from the valve itself. These areas are named for the valve producing the sound. Aortic: Second right intercostal space near the sternum. Pulmonic: Second left intercostal space near the sternum. Tricuspid: Fifth right or left intercostal space near the sternum. Mitral (apical): In infants—third or fourth intercostal space, just left of the left midclavicular line. In children—fifth intercostal space at the left midclavicular line.

Table 35–11 Listening Sites for Auscultation of the Quality and Intensity of Heart Sounds

Heart Sound	Locations Best Heard	Where Heard Softly
S_1	Apex of the heart Tricuspid area Mitral area	Base of the heart Aortic area Pulmonic area
S_2	Base of the heart Aortic area Pulmonic area	Apex of the heart Tricuspid area Mitral area
Physiologic splitting	Pulmonic area	
S_3	Mitral area	

Splitting of the Heart Sounds

After distinguishing the first and second heart sounds, try to detect physiologic splitting. A split S_2 is more apparent during inspiration when the child takes a deep breath. More blood returns to the right ventricle, causing the pulmonic valve to close a fraction of a second later than the aortic valve. Auscultate over the pulmonic area while the child breathes normally and then while the child takes a deep breath. Splitting is normally more easily detected after a deep breath. The splitting returns to a single sound with regular breathing. If splitting does not vary with respiration, it is called fixed splitting, an abnormal finding associated with an atrial septal defect.

Third Heart Sound

A third heart sound, S_3, is occasionally heard in children as a normal finding. S_3 is caused when blood rushes through the mitral valve and splashes into the left ventricle. It is heard in diastole, just after S_2. It is distinguished from a split S_2 because it is louder in the mitral area than in the pulmonic area.

Murmurs

Occasionally, abnormal heart sounds are auscultated. These sounds are produced by blood passing through a defective valve, great vessel, or other heart structure.

To hear murmurs in children takes practice. Often, murmurs must be very loud to be detected. For softer murmurs, normal heart sounds must be distinguished before an extra sound is recognized. When a murmur is detected, define the characteristics of the extra sound, including:

- *Intensity.* How loud is it? Can a thrill also be palpated?
- *Location.* Where is the murmur the loudest? Identify the listening area and precise topographic landmarks. Is the child sitting or lying down? Do the murmur characteristics change when the child changes position?
- *Radiation.* Is the sound transmitted over a larger area of the chest, to the axilla, or to the back?
- *Timing.* Is the murmur heard best after S_1 or S_2? Is it heard during the entire phase between S_1 and S_2?
- *Quality.* Describe what the murmur sounds like—for example, machinelike, musical, or blowing.

Nursing Practice

Following are guidelines for grading the intensity of a murmur:

INTENSITY	DESCRIPTION
Grade I	Barely heard in a quiet room
Grade II	Quiet, but clearly heard
Grade III	Moderately loud, no thrill palpated
Grade IV	Loud, a thrill is usually palpated
Grade V	Very loud, heard when the stethoscope is barely on the chest wall, a thrill is palpated
Grade VI	Heard without the stethoscope in direct contact with the chest wall, a thrill is palpated

Auscultate for a venous hum over the supraclavicular fossa above the middle of the clavicle or over the upper anterior chest with the bell of the stethoscope. A venous hum is heard as a continuous low-pitched hum throughout the cardiac cycle. It may be loudest during diastole or when the child stands, and it does not change with respirations. It may be quieted by having the child turn the neck. A venous hum may be associated with anemia, but it has no pathologic significance.

COMPLETING THE HEART EXAMINATION

A complete assessment of cardiac function also includes measuring the blood pressure, palpating the pulses, and evaluating signs from other systems.

Blood Pressure

Assessing the blood pressure is important to detect hypertension. The child should be seated and quiet for 3 to 5 minutes before the blood pressure is taken in the right arm with a correctly sized cuff. With the cuff snugly wrapped around the arm, hold the arm with the antecubital fossa at the level of the heart. Use the bell of the stethoscope to hear softer Korotkoff sounds. The systolic reading is the onset of Korotkoff sounds. The diastolic reading is the fifth Korotkoff sound or the disappearance of Korotkoff sounds in children and adolescents (Cromwell, Munn, & Zolkowsky-Wynn, 2005). If the Korotkoff sounds can be heard to 0 mm Hg, even after repeating, record the diastolic reading as the fourth Korotkoff sound (Brady, Siberry, & Solomon, 2008). See Skill 9–10 for the technique for obtaining the blood pressure in children in the Clinical Skills Manual **SKILLS**.

Compare the systolic and diastolic readings with the standard blood pressure values by age, sex, and height in Appendix D. Use the child's height percentile for age and sex from the standard growth curves. A blood pressure value at the 50th percentile for the child's age, sex, and height percentile is considered the midpoint of the normal blood pressure range. A systolic or diastolic reading above the 95th percentile indicates hypertension.

Palpation of the Pulses

Palpate the characteristics of the pulses in the extremities to assess the circulation. The technique and sites for palpating the pulse are the same as those used for adults. Evaluate the pulsation for rate, regularity of rhythm, and strength in each extremity and compare your findings bilaterally.

Palpate the femoral arteries and compare their strength with the strength of the brachial pulse. The femoral pulsations are usually stronger than or as strong as the brachial pulsations. A weaker femoral pulse is associated with coarctation of the aorta.

Nursing Practice

In any child in which there is a concern about a heart condition, obtain a blood pressure reading in both an arm and a leg and compare the readings. The blood pressure in the leg should be the same or up to 10 mm Hg higher than the arm reading. If the reading in the leg is lower than the arm, coarctation of the aorta may be present.

Growth and Development

Infants have a low systolic blood pressure, and detecting the distal pulses is often difficult. Use the brachial artery in the arms and the popliteal or femoral artery in the legs to evaluate the pulses. The radial and distal tibial pulses are normally palpated easily in older children.

Other Signs

To assess the heart and tissue perfusion, consider other signs, including skin color, capillary refill, and respiratory distress. The mucous membranes are usually pink. Cyanosis is most commonly associated with a congenital heart defect in children. Capillary refill is normally less than 2 seconds, indicating good circulation and perfusion of the tissues. Signs of respiratory distress, such as tachypnea, flaring, and retractions, may be associated with the child's attempts to compensate for hypoxemia caused by a congenital heart defect.

ASSESSING THE ABDOMEN FOR SHAPE, BOWEL SOUNDS, AND UNDERLYING ORGANS

TOPOGRAPHIC LANDMARKS OF THE ABDOMEN

The location of underlying organs and structures of the abdomen must be considered when the abdomen is examined. The abdomen is commonly divided by imaginary lines into quadrants for the purpose of identifying underlying structures (Figure 35–26 ●).

INSPECTION OF THE ABDOMEN

Begin the examination of the abdomen by inspecting the shape and contour, condition of the umbilicus and rectus muscle, and abdominal movement. Inspect the child's abdomen from the front and side with good lighting. Perform inspection and auscultation before palpation and percussion because touching the abdomen may change the characteristics of bowel sounds.

Shape and Contour

Inspect the shape of the abdomen to identify an abnormal contour. The child's abdomen is normally symmetric and rounded or flat when the child is supine. A scaphoid or sunken abdomen is abnormal and may indicate dehydration.

See Chapter 28 ∞ for guidelines to assess the newborn's umbilical stump. After the stump falls off, inspect the umbilicus for continued drainage which may indicate an infection or a granuloma. Inspect the umbilicus in older infants and toddlers.

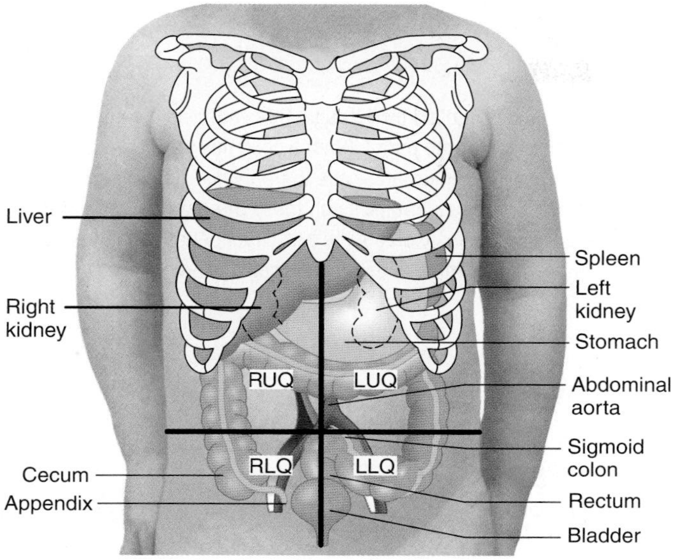

● **Figure 35–26** Topographic landmarks of the abdomen. The abdomen is commonly divided by imaginary lines into quadrants for the purpose of identifying underlying structures.

Children in these age groups often have an umbilical hernia, a protrusion of abdominal contents through an open umbilical muscle ring.

Inspect the abdominal wall for any depression or bulging at midline above or below the umbilicus, indicating separation of the rectus abdominis muscles. The depression may be up to 5 cm (2 in.) wide. Measure the width of the separation to monitor change over time. As abdominal muscle strength develops, the separation usually becomes less prominent. However, the splitting may persist if congenital muscle weakness is present.

Abdominal Movement

Infants and children up to 6 years of age breathe with the diaphragm. The abdomen rises with inspiration and falls with expiration, simultaneously with the chest rise and fall. When the abdomen does not rise as expected, peritonitis may be present.

Other abdominal movements such as peristaltic waves are abnormal. Peristaltic waves are visible rhythmic contractions of the intestinal wall smooth muscle, which move food through the digestive tract. Their presence generally indicates an intestinal obstruction, such as pyloric stenosis.

AUSCULTATION OF THE ABDOMEN

To evaluate bowel sounds, auscultate the abdomen with the diaphragm of the stethoscope. Bowel sounds normally occur every 10 to 30 seconds. They have a high-pitched, tinkling, metallic quality. Loud gurgling (borborygmi) is heard when the child is hungry. Listen in each quadrant long enough to hear at least one bowel sound. Before determining that bowel sounds are absent, auscultate at least 5 minutes in each quadrant. Absence of bowel sounds may indicate peritonitis or a paralytic ileus. Hyperactive bowel sounds may indicate gastroenteritis or a bowel obstruction.

Next auscultate over the abdominal aorta and the renal arteries for a vascular hum or murmur. No murmur should be heard. A murmur may indicate a narrowed or defective artery.

PERCUSSION OF THE ABDOMEN

Use indirect percussion when the child is supine to identify the borders of the liver, spleen, bladder, and any masses. To perform *indirect percussion,* lay your middle finger of the nondominant hand on the child's abdomen. Keep your other fingers off the abdomen. With a springlike motion, use the fingertip of the other hand to tap the finger in contact with the chest. Different tones are expected when the abdomen is percussed, depending on the underlying structures. Dullness is found over the liver, spleen, and full bladder. Tympany is found over the stomach or the intestines when an obstruction is present. Tympany may be found over areas beyond the stomach in infants because of air swallowing. A resonant tone may be heard over other areas.

PALPATION OF THE ABDOMEN

Both light and deep palpation are used to examine the abdomen's organs and to detect any masses. Light palpation evaluates the tenseness of the abdomen (how soft or hard it is), the liver, the presence of any tenderness or masses, and any defects in the abdominal wall. Deep palpation detects masses, defines their shape and consistency, and identifies tenderness in the abdomen.

Perform the abdominal examination when the child is calm and cooperative because the organs and other masses are more easily palpated when the abdominal wall is relaxed. Infants and toddlers often feel more secure lying supine across both the parent's and the examiner's laps. A bottle, pacifier, or toy may distract the child and improve cooperation for the examination. The abdomen is more relaxed when the child's knees are flexed.

Stand beside the child and place warmed fingertips across the child's abdomen. Palpate with the edge of your fingers, not just your fingerpads, and palpate using a sequence to examine the entire abdomen. Watch the child's face during palpation for a grimace or constriction of the pupils, which indicates pain.

Nursing Practice

Use suggestive words to help the child relax so you can palpate the abdomen. "How soft will your tummy get when my hand feels it? Does it get softer than this? Yes. See, it softens as you breathe out. Will it also be softer here?" In this way, the child learns to relax the abdomen and is challenged to do it better.

When children are ticklish, use a firm touch and do not pretend to tickle the child at any point in the examination. Alternatively, put the child's hand on the abdomen and place your hand over the child's. Let your fingertips slide over to touch the abdomen. The child has a sense of being in control, and you may be able to palpate directly.

Older children may need distraction, especially when there is a question of abdominal tenderness and guarding. Have the child perform a task that requires some concentration, such as pressing the hands together or pulling locked hands apart.

Light Palpation

For light palpation, use a superficial, gentle touch that slightly depresses the abdomen. Usually the abdomen feels soft and no tenderness is detected. Palpate any bulging along the abdominal wall, especially along the rectus muscle and umbilical ring, which could indicate a hernia. If an umbilical hernia is present, measure the diameter of the muscular ring, rather than the protrusion. The muscle ring normally becomes smaller and closes by 4 years of age.

To palpate the lower liver edge, place the fingerpads in the right midclavicular line at the level of the umbilicus. Lightly palpate and move the fingers closer to the costal margin with each expiration. As the liver edge descends with inspiration, a flat, narrow ridge is usually felt. The liver edge is normally palpated 2 to 3 cm (1 in.) below the right costal margin in infants and toddlers, but it may not be palpable in older children. If the liver edge is more than 3 cm (1 in.) below the right costal margin, the liver is enlarged, possibly due to congestive heart failure or hepatic disease.

Deep Palpation

To perform deep palpation, press the fingers of one hand (for small children) or two hands (for older children) more deeply into the abdomen. Because the abdominal muscles are most relaxed when the child takes a deep breath, ask the child to take regular deep breaths when palpating each area of the abdomen. The spleen tip may be felt at the left costal margin in the midclavicular line when the child takes a deep breath. If the spleen is more easily palpated below the left costal margin, it is enlarged. The kidneys are in a deep layer of abdominal muscles and intestines, and thus are rarely palpated except in newborns. If a kidney is actually palpated, an abnormal mass may be present and should have further evaluation. A tubular mass commonly palpated in the lower left or right quadrant is often an intestine filled with feces. A distended bladder is often palpated as a firm, central, dome-shaped mass above the symphysis pubis in young children. Any fixed mass that moves laterally, pulsates, or is located along the vertebral column may be a neoplasm.

ASSESSMENT OF THE INGUINAL AREA

The inguinal area is inspected and palpated during the abdominal examination to detect enlarged lymph nodes or masses. The femoral pulse, a part of the heart examination, may be assessed simultaneously with the abdominal examination.

Inspection

Inspect the inguinal area for any change in contour, comparing sides. A small bulging noted over the femoral canal in girls may be associated with a femoral hernia. A bulging in the inguinal area in boys may be associated with an inguinal hernia.

Palpation

Palpate the inguinal area for lymph nodes and other masses. Small lymph nodes, less than 1 cm (1/2 in.) in diameter, are often present in the inguinal area because of minor injuries on the legs. Any tenderness, heat, or inflammation in these palpated lymph nodes could be associated with a local infection.

Growth and Development

Preschool-age children are often taught that strangers are not permitted to touch their "private parts." When a child this age actively resists examination of the genital area, ask the parent to tell the child you have permission to look at and touch these parts of the body. Some children develop modesty during the preschool period. Briefly explain what you need to examine and why. Then calmly and efficiently examine the child.

ASSESSING THE GENITAL AND PERINEAL AREAS FOR EXTERNAL STRUCTURAL ABNORMALITIES

Nurses may perform an external genital examination or assist another healthcare provider. In younger children the genital and perineal examination is performed immediately after assessment of the abdomen. The genitals and perineum may be examined last in older children and adolescents. Gloves, lubricant, and a penlight are needed for the examination.

Examination of the genitalia and perineal area can cause stress in children because they sense their privacy has been invaded. To make young children feel more secure, position them on the parent's lap with their legs spread apart. Children can also be positioned on the examining table with their knees flexed and the legs spread apart like a frog.

INSPECTION OF THE FEMALE GENITALIA

Inspect the external genitalia of girls for color, size, and symmetry of the mons pubis, labia, urethra, and vaginal opening (Figure 35–27 ●). Simultaneously look for any abnormal findings such as swelling, inflammation, masses, lacerations, or discharge.

Inspect the mons pubis for pubic hair and its characteristics. See page 965 for guidelines to assess the stage of pubic hair development.

The labia minora are usually thin and pale in preadolescent girls but become dark pink and moist after puberty. In young infants the labia minora may be fused and cover the structures in the vestibule. These adhesions may need to be separated.

Use the thumb and forefinger of one gloved hand to separate the labia minora for viewing structures in the vestibule. Inspect the vestibule for lesions. No lesions or signs of inflammation are expected around the urethral or vaginal opening. Redness and excoriation are often associated with an irritant such as bubble bath. The hymen is just inside the vaginal opening. In preadolescents it is usually a thin membrane with a crescent-shaped opening. The vaginal opening is usually about 1 cm (1/2 in.) in adolescents when the hymen is intact. Sexually active adolescents may have a vaginal opening with irregular edges.

Preadolescent girls do not normally have a vaginal discharge. Adolescents often have a clear discharge without a foul

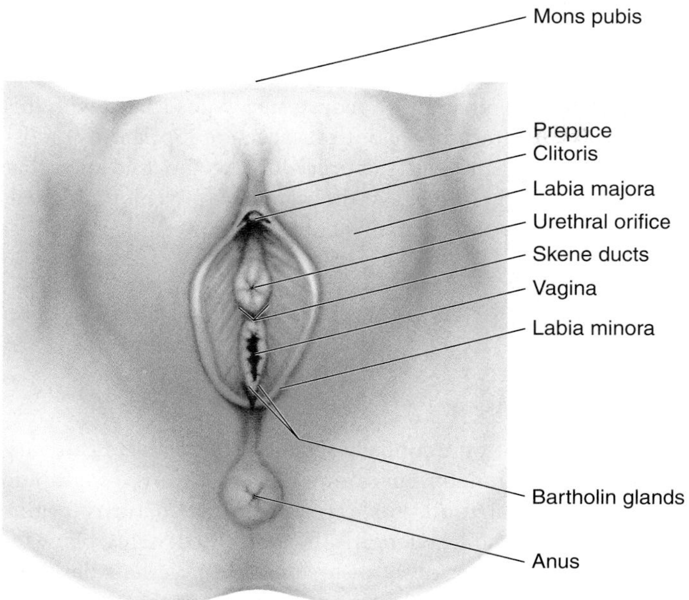

● **Figure 35–27** Anatomic structures of the female genital and perineal area.

odor. Menses generally begin approximately 2 years after breast bud development. A foul-smelling discharge in preschool-age children may be associated with a foreign body. Various organisms may cause a vaginal infection in older children.

An internal vaginal examination is indicated when abnormal findings such as a vaginal discharge or trauma to the external structures is noted. An experienced examiner should perform the vaginal examination of the child.

PALPATION OF THE FEMALE GENITALIA

Palpate the vaginal opening with a finger of your free, gloved hand. The Bartholin and Skene glands are not usually palpable. Palpation of these glands in preadolescent children indicates enlargement because of an infection such as gonorrhea.

INSPECTION OF THE MALE GENITALIA

Inspect the male genitalia for the structural and pubertal development of the penis, scrotum, and testicles. Place boys in tailor position, seated with their legs crossed in front of them. This position puts pressure on the abdominal wall to push the testicles into the scrotum. See page 965 for guidelines to assess the staging of pubic hair and external genital development.

Nursing Practice

Signs of sexual abuse in young children include bruising or swelling of the vulva, foul-smelling vaginal discharge, enlarged opening of the vagina, and rash or sores in the perineal area.

Penis

Inspect the penis for size, foreskin, hygiene, and position of the urethral meatus. The length of the nonerect penis in the newborn is normally 2 to 3 cm (1 in.). The penis enlarges in length and breadth during puberty. The penis is normally straight. A downward bowing of the penis may be caused by a chordee, a fibrous band of tissue associated with hypospadias.

The foreskin is usually not completely separated from the glans at birth. Separation of the preputial adhesions normally occurs between 3 to 6 years of age without any medical intervention (Pulsifer, 2005). When the boy is not circumcised, a foreskin opening large enough for a good urinary stream is normal, even when the foreskin does not fully retract. Avoid forcible retraction of the foreskin to prevent damage to the tissues and the formation of adhesions between the foreskin and glans (Horner, 2007). Use gentle traction to evaluate the degree of foreskin retraction and the meatal location and size. It is usually possible to visualize the meatus; however, a foreskin opening large enough for a good urinary stream is normal, even when the meatus cannot be seen. The foreskin of children over 6 years of age normally retracts past the corona easily. If the foreskin is tight and cannot be retracted, phimosis is present.

The glans penis is normally clean and smooth without inflammation or ulceration. The urethral meatus is a slit-shaped opening near the tip of the glans. No discharge should be present. A round, pinpoint urethral meatus may indicate meatal stenosis. Location of the urethral meatus at another site on the penis is abnormal, indicating hypospadias or epispadias. Inspect the urinary stream. The stream is normally strong without dribbling. Erythema and edema of the glans (balanitis) may result from infection or trauma. In the uncircumcised penis, purulent discharge and an edematous foreskin may be seen.

Scrotum

Inspect the scrotum for size, symmetry, presence of the testicles, and any abnormalities. The scrotum is normally loose and pendulous with rugae, or wrinkles. The scrotum of infants often appears large in comparison to the penis. A small, undeveloped scrotum that has no rugae indicates undescended testicles. Enlargement or swelling of the scrotum is abnormal. It may indicate an inguinal hernia, hydrocele, torsion of the spermatic cord, or testicular inflammation. A deep cleft in the scrotum may indicate ambiguous genitalia.

PALPATION OF THE MALE GENITALIA

Palpate the shaft of the penis for nodules and masses. None should be present.

Testicles

Palpate the scrotum for the presence of the testicles. Make sure your hands are warm to avoid stimulating the cremasteric reflex that causes the testicles to retract. Place your index finger and thumb over both inguinal canals on each side of the penis. This keeps the testicles from retracting into the abdomen (Figure 35–28 ●).

Gently palpate each testicle with only enough pressure to identify the shape and size. The testicles are normally smooth

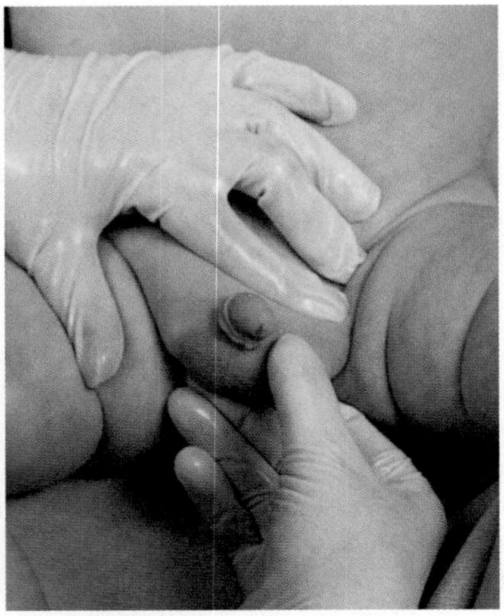

● **Figure 35–28** Palpating the scrotum for descended testicles and spermatic cords.

and equal in size. They are approximately 1 to 1.5 cm (1/2 in.) in diameter until puberty, when they increase in size. A hard, enlarged, painless testicle may indicate a tumor.

If a testicle is not palpated in the scrotum, the examiner palpates the inguinal canal for a soft mass. When the testicle is found in the inguinal canal, try to move it to the scrotum to palpate the size and shape. The testicle is descendable when it can be moved into the scrotum. An undescended testicle is one that does not descend into the scrotum or cannot be palpated in the inguinal canal.

Scrotum

Palpate the length of the spermatic cord between the thumb and forefinger from the testicle to the inguinal canal. It normally feels solid and smooth. No tenderness is expected.

When bulging or swelling of the scrotum is present, palpate the scrotum to identify the characteristics of the mass. Try to determine whether the mass is unilateral or bilateral. An experienced examiner may try to reduce the mass by pushing it back through the external inguinal ring. A mass that decreases may indicate an inguinal hernia. A mass that does not decrease may indicate a hydrocele or an incarcerated hernia. To distinguish between a hydrocele and an incarcerated hernia, place a bright penlight under the scrotum and look for a red glow or transillumination through the scrotum. A hydrocele transilluminates; a hernia does not.

ANUS AND RECTUM

Inspect the anus for sphincter control and any abnormal findings such as inflammation, fissures, or lesions. The external sphincter is usually closed. Inflammation and scratch marks around the anus may be associated with pinworms. A protrusion from the rectum may be associated with a rectal wall prolapse or a hemorrhoid.

Lightly touching the anal opening should stimulate an anal contraction or "wink." Absence of a contraction may indicate the presence of a lower spinal cord lesion. Passage of meconium by newborns indicates a patent anus.

A rectal examination is not routinely performed on children. It is indicated for symptoms of intra-abdominal, rectal, bowel, or stool abnormalities. Only an experienced examiner should perform a rectal examination. To reduce anxiety associated with this examination, distract the child with an age-appropriate toy or discussion when assisting with this procedure. Let the child know that the lubricant might feel cold. As the examiner's finger is positioned, help the child to relax the sphincter by "pushing out the poop."

ASSESSMENT OF PUBERTAL DEVELOPMENT AND SEXUAL MATURATION

The age of onset of secondary sexual characteristics can vary with race and ethnicity, environmental conditions, geographic location, and nutrition. For example, sexual maturity begins earlier in taller and heavier girls. In the United States, black females have an earlier onset of breast and pubic hair development, followed by Mexican American girls, and then white girls (Anderson & Must, 2005). Black males develop secondary sexual characteristics earlier than white males and Mexican American males (Graham, 2005).

FEMALES

Breast development in girls usually precedes other pubertal changes. Figure 35–29 ● shows the Tanner stages of breast development. *Thelarche* or breast budding is the first stage of pubertal development in the majority of girls, indicating breast Tanner stage II. Breast tissue is seen and palpated below a slightly enlarging areola (1 cm in diameter of palpable glandular tissue) (Kaplowitz, 2004). While breast budding normally occurs between 9 and 14 years of age, breast development may begin as early as 6 years in black girls and 7 years in white girls. Breast development before these ages is abnormal and needs further evaluation (Greydanus, Matytsina, & Gains, 2006).

Inspect the adolescent's breasts while she is sitting to determine the stage of development. A girl's breasts often develop at different rates and appear asymmetric, and most teens have one breast slightly larger than the other. Catch-up growth of the smaller breast often occurs during late adolescence (Greydanus, Matytsina, & Gains, 2006).

Preadolescent girls have no pubic hair. Initial pubic hair is lightly pigmented, sparse, and straight. Figure 35–30 ● illustrates the normal stages of female pubic hair development. Breast development usually precedes pubic hair development. The presence of pubic hair before 8 years of age is unusual and may indicate premature pubertal development.

MALES

Initial signs of pubertal development in males are enlargement of the testicles and thinning of the scrotum. Straight, downy pubic hair first appears at the base of the penis 6 months later. The hair becomes darker, dense, and curly, extending over the pubic area in a diamond pattern by the completion of puberty. The presence of pubic hair before 9 years of age may be an indication of pre-

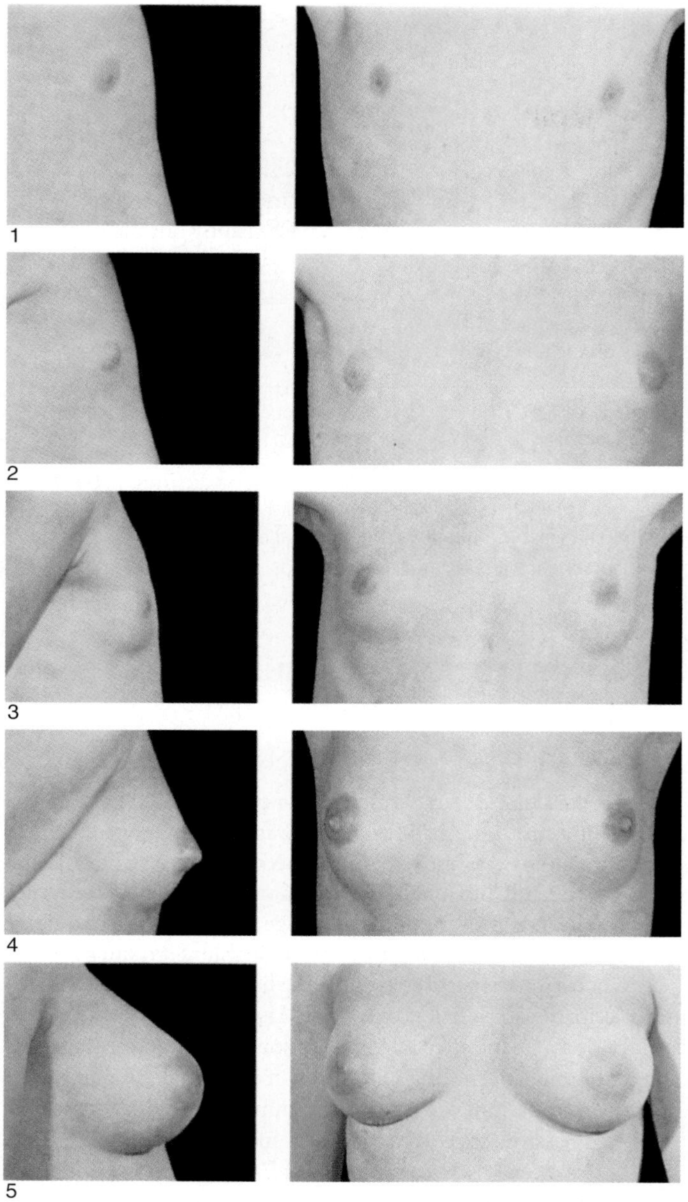

● **Figure 35–29** Normal stages of breast development.

Source: Used with permission from Van Wieringen et al. (1971). *Growth diagrams 1965* Netherlands, Groningen: Wolters-Noordhof.

mature pubertal development. Delayed onset of testicular enlargement after 14 years of age needs evaluation. Penile enlargement generally follows testicular enlargement about one year later in genitalia Tanner stage 3. Stages of pubic hair development follow a standard pattern, as seen in Figure 35–31 ●.

SEXUAL MATURITY RATING

The sexual maturity rating (SMR) is an average of the breast and pubic hair Tanner stages in females and of the genital and pubic hair Tanner stages in males. The rating is a number between 2 and 5, as stage 1 is prepubertal. The SMR is then related to other physiologic events that happen during puberty.

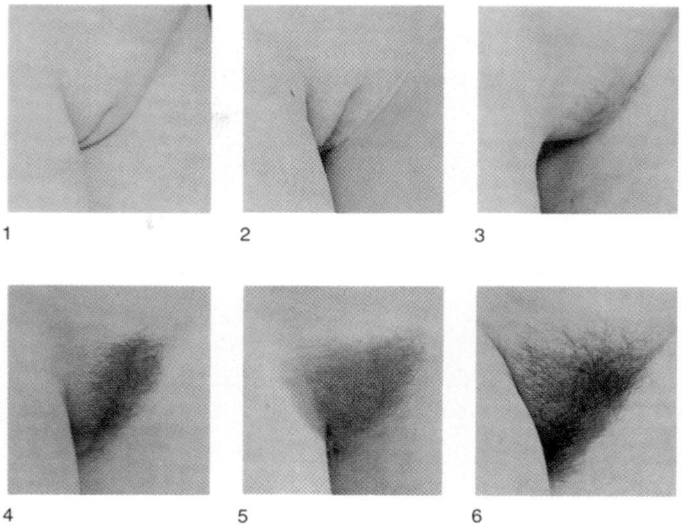

● **Figure 35–30** The stages of female pubic hair development with sexual maturation. Soft downy hair along the labia majora is an indication that sexual maturation is beginning. Hair grows progressively coarse and curly as development proceeds.

Source: Used with permission from Van Wieringen et al. (1971). *Growth diagrams 1965* Netherlands, Groningen: Wolters-Noordhof.

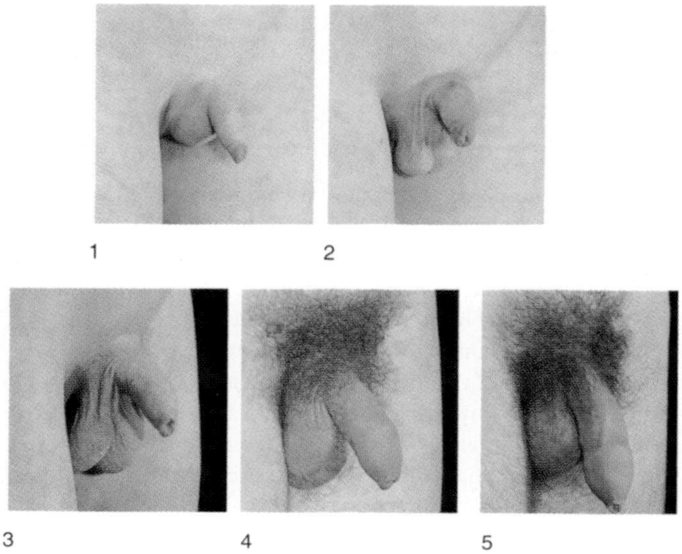

● **Figure 35–31** The stages of male pubic hair and external genital development with sexual maturation.

Source: Used with permission from Van Wieringen et al. (1971). *Growth diagrams 1965* Netherlands, Groningen: Wolters-Noordhof.

In females, menarche generally occurs in SMR 4 or breast stage 3 to 4. The peak height velocity usually occurs before menarche at a mean age of 11.5 years. In males, ejaculation usually occurs at SMR 3, with semen noted between SMR 3 and 4. The peak height velocity usually occurs in SMR 4 or genital stage 4 to 5, at about 13.5 years of age. Compare the stage of the child's secondary sexual characteristics with information in Figure 35–32 ●.

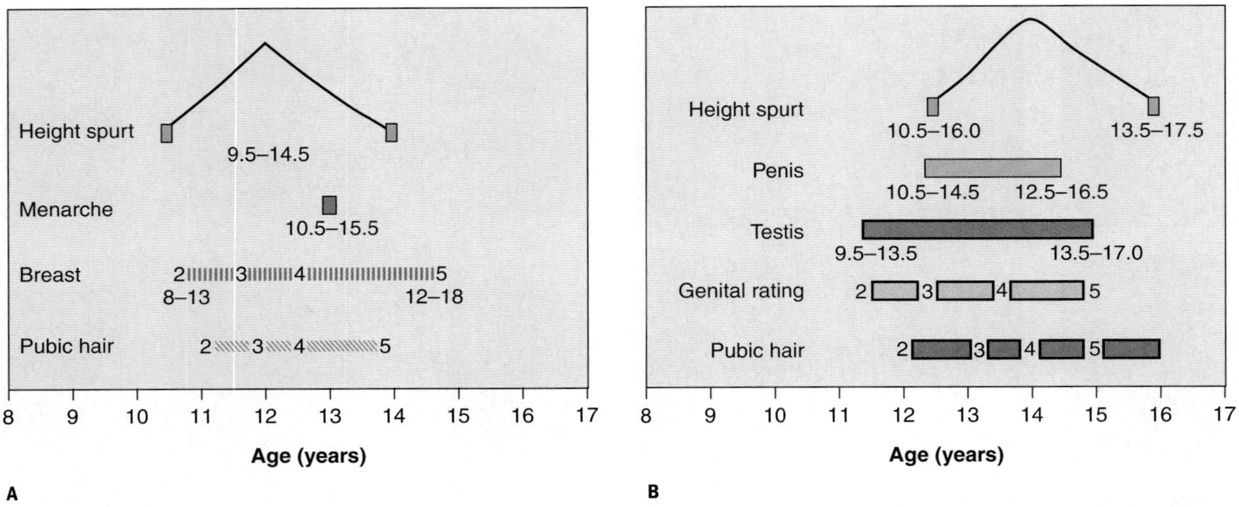

● **Figure 35–32** Sexual maturity rating—approximate timing of developmental changes. The numbers indicate stages of pubertal development. Range of ages during which some changes occur is indicated by the inclusive numbers for each characteristic. ***A,*** Females. ***B,*** Males.

Source: Used with permission from Marshall, W. A., & Tanner, J. M. (1969). *Archives of Disease in Childhood,* 44, 291.

MyNursingKit Animation: Movement of Joints

ASSESSING THE MUSCULOSKELETAL SYSTEM FOR BONE AND JOINT STRUCTURE, MOVEMENT, AND MUSCLE STRENGTH

INSPECTION OF THE BONES, MUSCLES, AND JOINTS

Inspect and compare the arms and then the legs for differences in alignment, contour, skin folds, length, and deformities. The extremities normally have equal length, circumference, and numbers of skin folds bilaterally. Extra skin folds and a larger circumference may indicate a shorter extremity.

Inspect and compare the joints bilaterally for size, discoloration, and ease of voluntary movement. Joints are normally the same color as surrounding skin, with no sign of swelling. Children should voluntarily flex and extend joints during normal activities without pain. Redness, swelling, and pain with movement may indicate injury or infection.

PALPATION OF THE BONES, MUSCLES, AND JOINTS

Palpate the bones and muscles in each extremity for muscle tone, masses, or tenderness. Muscles normally feel firm, and bony masses are not normally present. Doughy muscles may indicate poor muscle tone. Rigid muscles, or hypertonia, may be associated with an active seizure or cerebral palsy. A mass over a long bone may indicate a recent fracture or a bone tumor.

Palpate each joint and surrounding muscles to detect any swelling, masses, heat, or tenderness. None is expected when the joint is palpated. Tenderness, heat, swelling, and redness can result from injury or a chronic joint inflammation such as juvenile rheumatoid arthritis.

RANGE OF MOTION AND MUSCLE STRENGTH ASSESSMENT

Range of Motion

Observe the child during typical play activities, such as reaching for objects, climbing, and walking, to assess range of motion of all major joints. Children spontaneously move their joints through the full normal range of motion with play activities when no pain is present. Limited range of motion may indicate injury, inflammation of a joint, or a muscle abnormality.

When a joint is suspected of having limited active range of motion, perform passive range of motion. Flex and extend, abduct and adduct, or rotate the affected joint cautiously to avoid causing extra pain. Full range of motion without pain is normal. Limitations in movement may indicate injury, inflammation, or malformation. Increased passive range of motion may indicate muscle weakness.

Muscle Strength

Observe the child's ability to climb onto an examining table, throw a ball, clap the hands, or move around on the bed. The child's ability to perform age-appropriate play activities indicates good muscle tone and strength. Attainment of age-appropriate motor development is another indicator of good muscle strength (Table 35–12).

To assess the strength of specific muscles in the extremities, engage the child in some games. Compare muscle strength bilaterally to identify muscle weakness. For example, the child squeezes the examiner's fingers tightly with each hand; pushes against and pulls the examiner's hands with his or her hands, lower legs and feet; and resists extension of a flexed elbow or knee. Children normally have good muscle strength bilaterally. Unilateral muscle weakness may be associated with a nerve injury. Bilateral muscle weakness may result from hypoxemia or a congenital disorder such as Down syndrome. Asymmetric weakness may be associated with conditions such as cerebral palsy.

Table 35–12 Selected Gross Motor Milestones for Age

Gross Motor Milestones	Age Attained
Rolls over from prone to supine position	7 months
Sits without support	6 months
Pulls self to standing position	10 months
Creeps or crawls	10 months
Walks alone	15 months
Climbs on furniture	24 months
Walks up stairs, one step at a time	24 months
Rides tricycle	36 months

Sources: Data from: Feigelman, S. (2007). The first year, in R. M. Kliegman, R. E. Behrman, H. B. Jenson, & B. F. Stanton, *Nelson textbook of pediatrics* (18th ed., 43–48), Philadelphia: Saunders Elsevier; Feigelman, S. (2007). The second year, in R. M. Kliegman, R. E. Behrman, H. B. Jenson, & B. F. Stanton, *Nelson textbook of pediatrics* (18th ed., 48–54), Philadelphia: Saunders Elsevier.

When generalized muscle weakness is suspected in a preschool- or school-age child, ask the child to stand up from the supine position. Children are normally able to rise to a standing position without using their arms as levers. Children who push their body upright using the arms and hands may have generalized muscle weakness, known as a positive Gowers' sign. This may indicate muscular dystrophy (see Chapter 58∞).

POSTURE AND SPINAL ALIGNMENT

Posture

Inspect the child's posture when standing from a front, side, and back view. The shoulders and hips are normally level. The head is held erect without a tilt, and the shoulder contour is symmetric. After beginning to walk, young children often have a pot-bellied stance because of lumbar lordosis. The spine has normal thoracic convex and lumbar concave curves after 6 years of age. Table 35–13 describes normal posture and spinal curvature development.

Table 35–13 Normal Development of Posture and Spinal Curves

Age	Posture and Spinal Curves
2–3 months	Holds head erect when held upright; thoracic kyphosis when sitting.
6–8 months	Sits without support; spine is straight.
10–15 months	Walks independently; straight spine.
Toddler	Protruding abdomen; lumbar lordosis.
School-age child	Height of shoulders and hips is level; balanced thoracic convex and lumbar concave curves.

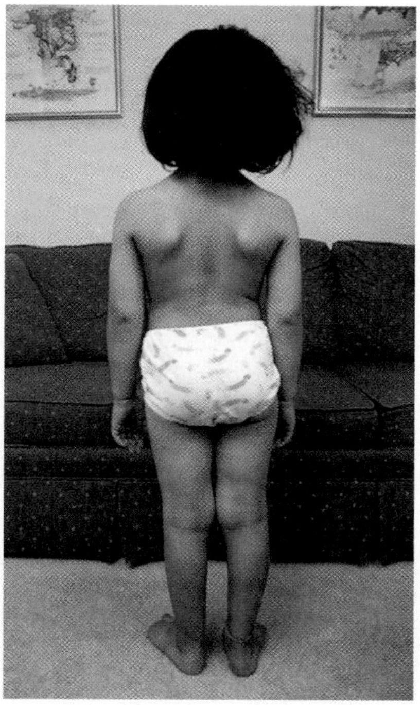

● **Figure 35–33** Evaluating spinal alignment. Does this child have legs of different lengths or scoliosis? Look at the level of the iliac crests and shoulders to see if they are level. See the more prominent crease at the waist on the right side? This child could have scoliosis.

Spinal Alignment

Assess the school-age child and adolescent for scoliosis, a lateral spine curvature. Stand behind the child, observing the height of the shoulders and hips (Figure 35–33 ●). Ask the child to bend forward slowly at the waist, with arms extended toward the floor. No lateral curve should be present in either position. The ribs normally stay flat bilaterally. The lumbar concave curve should flatten with forward flexion (Figure 35–34 ●). A lateral

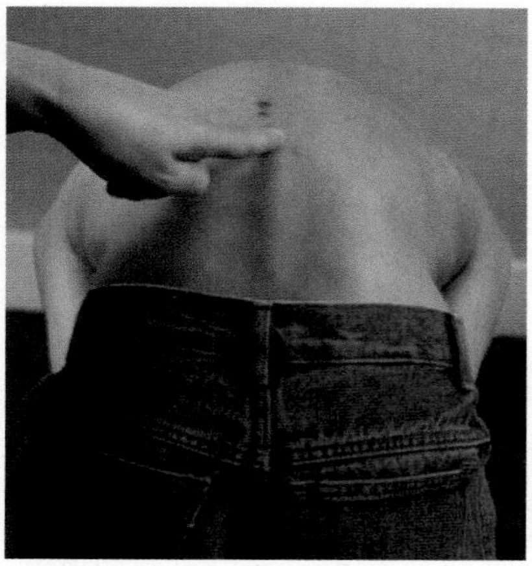

● **Figure 35–34** Inspection of the spine for scoliosis. Ask the child to slowly bend forward at the waist, with arms extended toward the floor. Run your forefinger down the spinal processes, palpating each vertebra for a change in alignment. A lateral curve to the spine or a one-sided rib hump is an indication of scoliosis.

curve to the spine or a one-sided rib hump is an indication of scoliosis (see Chapter 58).

INSPECTION OF THE UPPER EXTREMITIES

Arms

The alignment of the arms is normally straight, with a minimal angle at the elbows, where the bones articulate.

Hands

Count the fingers. Extra finger digits (polydactyly) or webbed fingers (syndactyly) are abnormal. Inspect the creases on the palmar surface of each hand. Multiple creases across the palm are normal. A single transverse crease across the entire palm of the hand is associated with Down syndrome (Figure 35–35 ●).

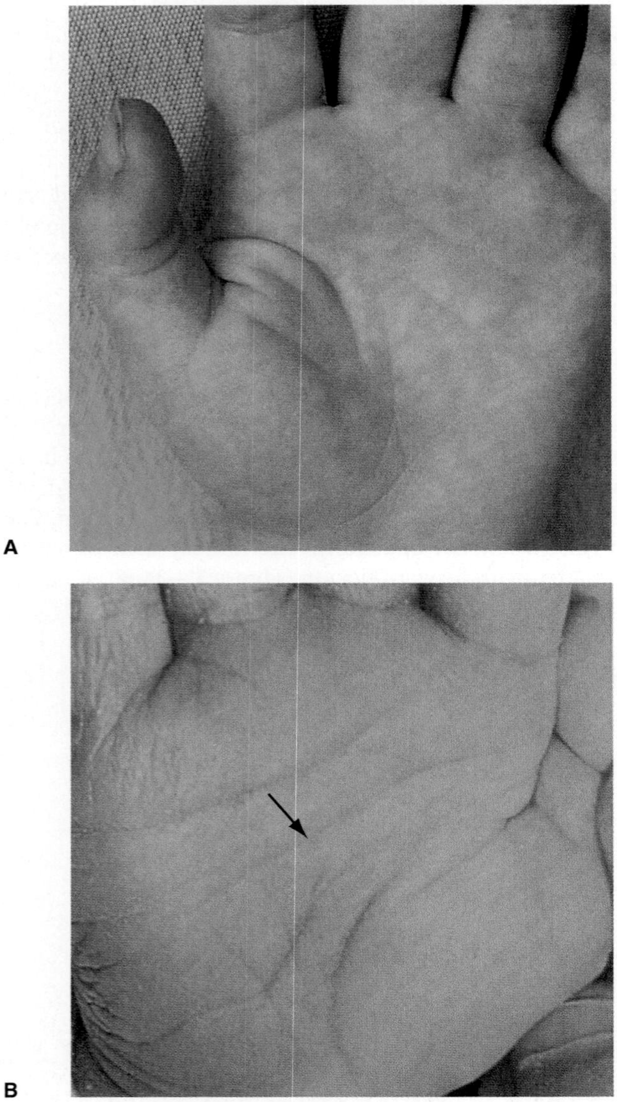

● **Figure 35–35** Inspection of the palms. ***A***, Normal palmar creases. ***B***, Transverse crease associated with Down syndrome.

Source: Used with permission from Zitelli, B. J., & Davis, H. W. (Eds.). (1997). *Atlas of pediatric physical diagnosis* (3rd ed.). St. Louis, MO: Mosby-Year Book.

Inspect the nails for size, shape, and color. Nails are normally convex, smooth, and pink. Clubbing, widening of the nailbed with an increased angle between the proximal nail fold and nail, is abnormal (see Figure 49–3 in Chapter 49). Clubbing is associated with chronic respiratory and cardiac conditions.

INSPECTION OF THE LOWER EXTREMITIES

Hips

Assess the hips of newborns and young infants for dislocation or subluxation. First inspect and compare the number of skin folds on the upper legs. An uneven number of skin folds may indicate a hip dislocation or difference in leg length. Then check for Allis' sign, a difference in knee height symmetry (Figure 35–36 ●). The Ortolani-Barlow maneuver is used to assess an infant's hips for dislocation or subluxation. See Figure 25–6 in Chapter 25.

View the child from behind and observe as the child stands on one leg and then the other. The iliac crests should stay level. If the iliac crest opposite the weight-bearing leg appears lower, the hip bearing weight may be dislocated.

Legs

Inspect the alignment of the legs. After a child is 4 years of age, the alignment of the long bones is straight, with minimal angle at the knees and feet where the bones articulate. Assess alignment of the lower extremities in infants and toddlers to ensure that normal changes are occurring. To evaluate the toddler with bowlegs, have the child stand on a firm surface. Measure the distance between the knees when the child's ankles are together. No more than 1.5 in. (3.5 cm) between the knees is normal. See Figure 35–37 ● for assessment of knock-knees.

Feet

Inspect the feet for alignment, the presence of all toes, and any deformities. The weight-bearing line of the feet is usually in alignment with the legs. Many newborns have a flexible forefoot inversion (metatarsus adductus) that results from uterine positioning. Any fixed deformity is abnormal.

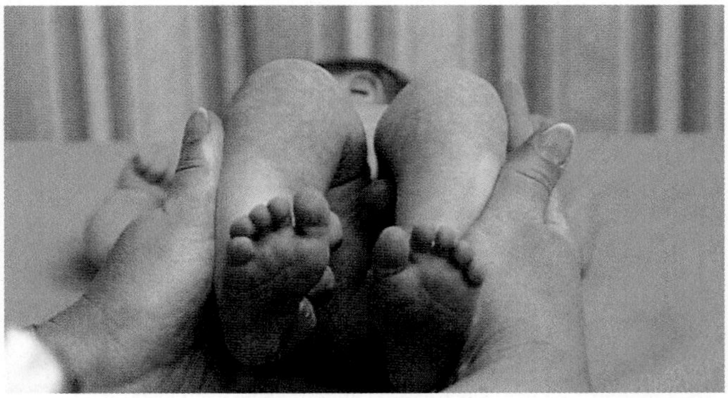

● **Figure 35–36** Checking knee height symmetry. Flex the infant's hips and knees so the heels are as close to the buttocks as possible. Place the feet flat on the examining table. The knees are usually the same height. A difference in knee height (Allis sign) is an indicator of hip dislocation (see also "Barlow-Ortolani Maneuver" in Chapter 25).

Source: Courtesy of Dee Corbett, RN, Children's National Medical Center, Washington, DC.

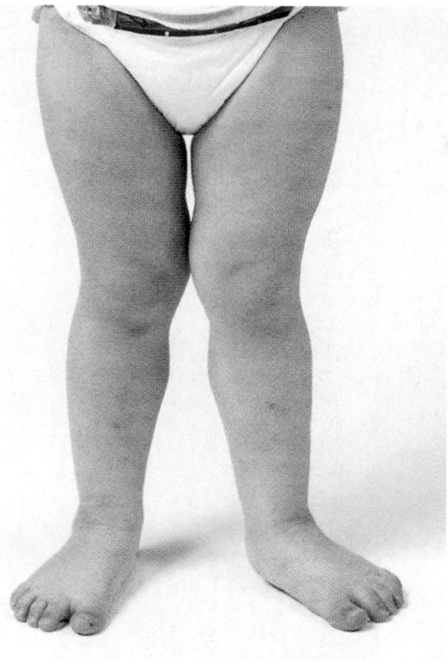

• **Figure 35–37** To evaluate the child with knock-knees, have the child stand on a firm surface. Measure the distance between the ankles when the child stands with the knees together. The normal distance is not more than 2 in. (5 cm) between the ankles.

Growth and Development

Infants are often born with a twisting of the tibia caused by positioning in utero (tibial torsion). The infant's toes turn in as a result of the tibial torsion. Toddlers go through a skeletal alignment sequence of bowlegs (genu varum) and knock-knees (genu valgum) before the legs assume a straight alignment.

Inspect the feet for the presence of an arch when the child is standing. Children up to 3 years of age normally have a fat pad over the arch, giving the appearance of flat feet. Older children normally have a longitudinal arch. The arch is usually seen when the child stands on tiptoe or is sitting. Inspect the nails of the feet as for the hands.

ASSESSING THE NERVOUS SYSTEM FOR COGNITIVE FUNCTION, BALANCE, COORDINATION, CRANIAL NERVE FUNCTION, SENSATION, AND REFLEXES

Equipment needed for this examination includes a reflex hammer, cotton balls, a penlight, and tongue blades.

COGNITIVE FUNCTION

Observe the child's behavior, facial expressions, gestures, communication skills, activity level, and level of consciousness to assess cognitive functioning. Match the neurologic examination to the child's stage of development. For example, cognitive function is evaluated much differently in infants than in older children because infants cannot use words to communicate.

Nursing Practice

The neurologic examination provides an opportunity to develop rapport with the child. Many of the procedures can be presented as games that young children enjoy. You can assess cognitive function by how well the child follows directions for tests of strength and coordination. As the assessment proceeds, the child develops trust and may be more cooperative with examination of other body systems.

Behavior

The behavior of infants and children during the assessment indicates their alertness. Infants and toddlers are curious but seek the security of the parent, either by clinging or by making frequent eye contact. Older children are often anxious and watch all of the examiner's actions. Lack of interest in assessment or treatment procedures may indicate a serious illness. Excessive activity or an unusually short attention span may be associated with an attention deficit hyperactivity disorder.

Communication Skills

Speech, language development, and social skills provide good clues to cognitive functioning. Listen to speech articulation and words used, comparing the child's performance with standards of social development and expected language development for age (Table 35–14). Toddlers can normally follow simple directions

Table 35–14 Expected Language Development for Age

Language Milestones	Age Attained
Babbles speech-like sounds, including p, b, and m	3-4 months
Has 1-2 words like "mama," "dada," "bye-bye"	12 months
Increases words each month, 2 word combinations (e.g., "Where baby?" and "Want cookie")	1-2 years
2 to 3 word sentences to ask for things or talk about things, large vocabulary, speech understood by family members	2-3 years
Sentences may have 4 or more words, speech understood by most people	3-4 years
Says most sounds correctly except a few like *l, s, r, v, z, ch, sh, th*. Tells stories and uses same grammar as rest of family	4-5 years

Source: Data from: American Speech and Language Association (2007). How does your child hear and talk? Retrieved January 23, 2008, from www.asha.org/public/speech/development/chart.htm

such as "Show me your mouth." By 3 years of age, the child's speech should be easily understood. Delay in language and social skill development may be associated with mental retardation or hearing loss.

Memory

Immediate, recent, and remote memory can be tested in children starting at approximately 4 years of age. Immediate memory can be tested by asking the child to repeat a series of words or numbers, such as the names of favorite characters from a book, television show, or movie. Children can remember more words or numbers with age: 3 words or numbers at age 4 years, 4 words or numbers at age 5 years, and 5 words or numbers at age 6 years.

To evaluate recent memory, ask the child to remember a special name or object. Then 5 to 10 minutes later during the examination, have the child recall the name or object. To evaluate remote memory, ask the child to repeat his or her address or birth date or a nursery rhyme. By 5 or 6 years of age, children are normally able to recall this information without difficulty.

Level of Consciousness

When approaching the infant or child, observe his or her level of consciousness and activity, including facial expressions, gestures, and interaction. Children are normally alert, and sleeping children arouse easily. The child who cannot be awakened is unconscious. A lowered level of consciousness may be associated with a number of neurologic conditions such as a brain injury, seizure, infection, or brain tumor.

CEREBELLAR FUNCTION

Observe the young child at play to assess coordination and balance. Development of fine-motor skills in infants and preschool children provides clues to cerebellar function.

Balance

Observe the child's balance during play activities such as walking, standing on one foot, and hopping. See Table 35–15 for milestones in balance for age. The Romberg procedure can also be used to test balance in children over 3 years of age (Figure 35–38 ●). Once balance and other motor skills are attained, children do not normally stumble or fall when tested. Poor balance may indicate cerebellar dysfunction or an inner ear disturbance.

Table 35–15 Expected Balance Development for Age

Balance Milestones	Age Attained
Stands without support briefly	12 months
Walks alone well	15 months
Walks backwards	2 years
Balances on 1 foot momentarily	3 years
Hops on 1 foot	4 years

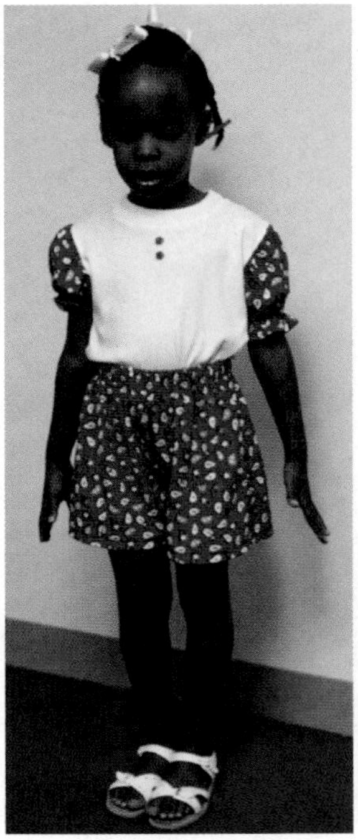

● **Figure 35–38** Romberg procedure. Ask the child to stand with feet together and eyes closed. Protect the child from falling by standing close. Preschool-age children may extend their arms to maintain balance, but older children can normally stand with their arms at their sides. Leaning or falling to one side is abnormal and indicates poor balance.

Coordination

Tests of coordination assess the smoothness and accuracy of movement. Development of fine-motor skills can be used to assess coordination in young children (Table 35–16). After 6 years of age, the tests for adults (finger-to-nose, finger-to-finger, heel-to-shin, and alternating motion) can be used (Figure 35–39 ●). Jerky movements or inaccurate pointing (past pointing) indicate

Table 35–16 Expected Fine-Motor Development for Age

Fine-Motor Milestones	Age Attained
Transfers objects between hands	5–6 months
Thumb finger grasp	8 months
Feeds self	18 months
Scribbles with crayon or pencil	18 months
Builds 2-block tower	15 months
Builds 4-block tower	18 months

Sources: Data from: Feigelman, S. (2007). The first year, in R. M. Kliegman, R. E. Behrman, H. B. Jenson, & B. F. Stanton, *Nelson textbook of pediatrics* (18th ed., 43–48), Philadelphia: Saunders Elsevier; Feigelman, S. (2007). The second year, in R. M. Kliegman, R. E. Behrman, H. B. Jenson, & B. F. Stanton, *Nelson textbook of pediatrics* (18th ed., 48–54), Philadelphia: Saunders Elsevier.

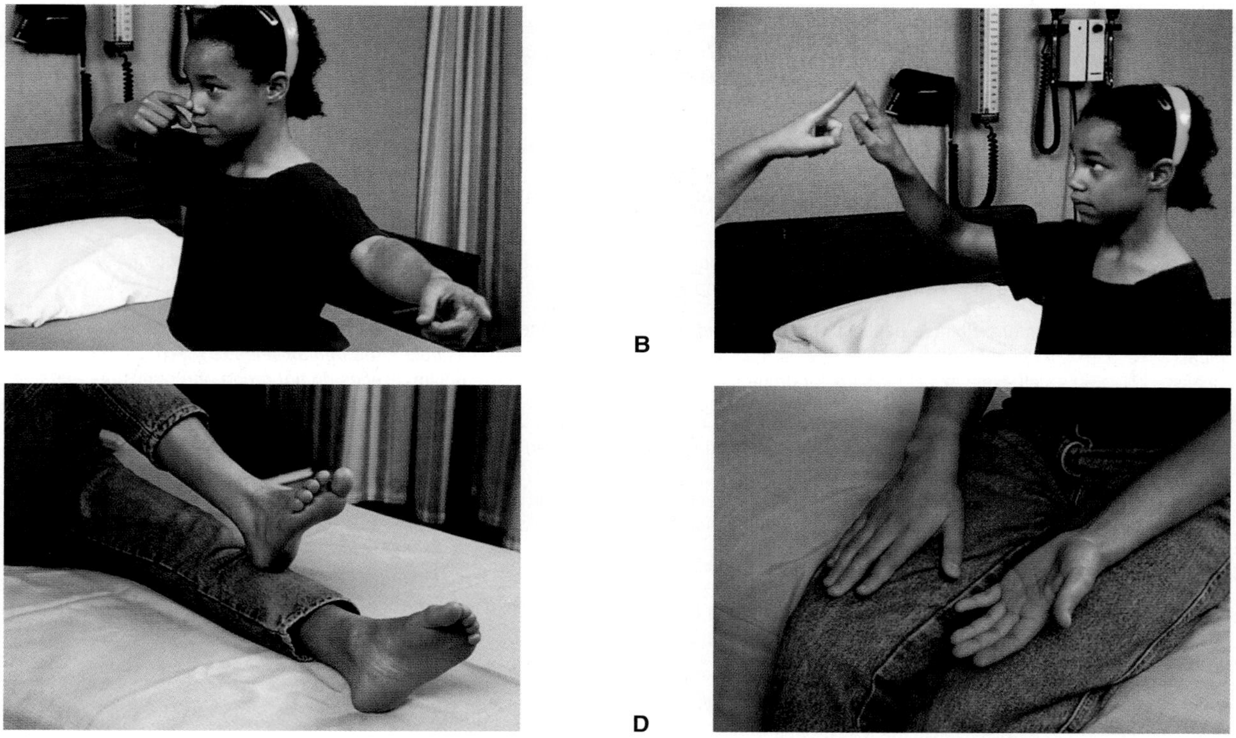

A B C D

● **Figure 35–39** Tests of coordination. ***A,*** Finger-to-nose test. Ask the child to close the eyes and touch his or her nose, alternating the index fingers of the hands. ***B,*** Finger-to-finger test. Ask the child to alternately touch his or her nose and your index finger with his or her index finger. Move your hand to several positions within the child's reach to test pointing accuracy. Repeat the test with the child's other hand. ***C,*** Heel-to-shin test. Ask the child to rub his or her leg from the knee to the ankle with the heel of the other foot. Repeat the test with the other foot. This test is normally performed without hesitation or inappropriate placement of the foot. ***D,*** Rapid alternating motion test. Ask the child to rapidly rotate his or her wrist so the palm and dorsum of the hand alternately pat the thigh. Repeat the test with the other hand. Hesitating movements are abnormal. Mirroring movements of the hand not being tested indicate a delay in coordination skill refinement.

poor coordination, which can be associated with delayed development or a cerebellar lesion.

Gait

A normal gait requires intact bones and joints, muscle strength, coordination, and balance. Gait is related to the motor development of the child. Toddlers beginning to walk have a wide-based gait and limited balance. With practice the toddler's balance improves and the gait develops a narrower base.

Inspect the child when walking from both a front and a rear view. The iliac crests are normally level during walking, and no limp is expected. A limp may indicate injury or joint disease. Staggering or falling may indicate cerebellar ataxia. Scissoring, in which the thighs tend to cross forward over each other with each step, may be associated with cerebral palsy or other spastic conditions.

CRANIAL NERVE FUNCTION

To assess the cranial nerves in infants and young children, modify the procedures used to assess school-age children and adults (Table 35–17). Abnormalities of cranial nerves may be associated with compression due to an injury, tumor, or infection in the brain.

SENSORY FUNCTION

To assess sensory function, compare the responses of the body to various types of stimulation. Bilateral equal responses are normal. Loss of sensation may indicate a brain or spinal cord lesion. Withdrawal responses to painful procedures indicate normal sensory function in an infant.

Superficial Tactile Sensation

Stroke the skin on the lower leg or arm with a cotton ball or a finger while the child's eyes are closed. Cooperative children over 2 years of age can normally point to the location touched.

Superficial Pain Sensation

Break a tongue blade to get a sharp point. After asking the child to close the eyes, touch the child in various places on each arm and leg, alternating the sharp and dull ends of the tongue blade. A paper clip may also be used. Children over 4 years of age can normally distinguish between a sharp and dull sensation each time. To improve the child's accuracy with the test, let the child practice describing the difference between the sharp and dull stimulation.

An inability to identify superficial touch and pain sensation may indicate sensory loss. Identify the extent of sensory loss, such

Table 35–17 Age-Specific Procedures for Assessment of Cranial Nerves in Infants and Children

Cranial Nerve[a]	Assessment Procedure and Normal Findings[b]
I Olfactory	Infant: Not tested. Child: Not routinely tested. Give familiar odors to child to sniff, one naris at a time. *Identifies odors such as orange, peanut butter, and chocolate.*
II Optic	Infant: Shine a bright light in eyes. *A quick blink reflex and dorsal head flexion indicates light perception.* Child: Test vision and visual fields if cooperative. *Visual acuity appropriate for age.*
III Oculomotor IV Trochlear VI Abducens	Infant: Shine a penlight at the eyes and move it side to side. *Focuses on and tracks the light to each side.* Child: Move an object through the six cardinal points of gaze. *Tracks object through all fields of gaze.* All ages: Inspect eyelids for drooping. Inspect pupillary response to light. *Eyelids do not droop and pupils are equal size and briskly respond to light.*
V Trigeminal	Infant: Stimulate the rooting and sucking reflex. *Turns head toward stimulation at side of mouth and sucking has good strength and pattern.* Child: Observe the child chewing a cracker. Touch forehead and cheeks with cotton ball when eyes are closed. *Bilateral jaw strength is good. Child points to location touched by cotton ball.*
VII Facial	All ages: Observe facial expressions when crying, smiling, frowning, etc. *Facial features stay symmetric bilaterally.*
VIII Acoustic	Infant: Produce a loud sound near the head. *Blinks in response to sound, moves head toward sound or freezes position.* Child: Use a noisemaker near each ear or whisper words to be repeated. *Turns head toward sound and repeats words correctly.*
IX Glossopharyngeal X Vagus	Infant: Observe swallowing during feeding. *Good swallowing pattern.* All ages: Elicit gag reflex. *Gags with stimulation.*
XI Spinal accessory	Infant: Not tested. Child: Ask child to raise the shoulders and turn the head side to side against resistance. *Good strength in neck and shoulders.*
XII Hypoglossal	Infant: Observe feeding. *Sucking and swallowing are coordinated.* Child: Tell the child to stick out the tongue. Listen to speech. *Tongue is midline with no tremors. Words are clearly articulated.*

[a]Bracketed nerves are tested together.

[b]Italic indicates normal findings.

as all areas below the knee. Other sensory function tests (temperature, vibratory, deep pressure pain, and position sense) are performed when sensory loss is found. Refer to other texts for a description of these procedures.

INFANT PRIMITIVE REFLEXES

Evaluate the movement and posture of newborns and young infants by the Moro, palmar grasp, plantar grasp, placing, stepping, and tonic neck primitive reflexes. These reflexes appear and disappear at expected intervals in the first few months of life as the central nervous system develops. Movements are normally equal bilaterally. An asymmetric response may indicate a serious neurologic problem on the less responsive side. See "Newborn Primitive Reflexes" in Chapter 25 for more information.

SUPERFICIAL AND DEEP TENDON REFLEXES

Evaluate the superficial and deep tendon reflexes to assess the function of specific segments of the spine.

Superficial Reflexes

Assess superficial reflexes by stroking a specific area of the body. The plantar reflex, testing spine levels L4 to S2, is routinely evaluated in children (Figure 35–40 ●).

Deep Tendon Reflexes

To assess the deep tendon reflexes, tap a tendon near specific joints with a reflex hammer (or with the index finger for infants), comparing responses bilaterally. The biceps, triceps, brachioradialis, patellar, and Achilles tendons are usually evaluated in children. Inspect for movement in the associated joint and palpate the strength of the expected muscle contraction. The numeric scoring of deep tendon reflexes is as follows:

Grade	Response Interpretation
0	No response
1+	Slow, minimal response
2+	Expected response, active
3+	More active or pronounced than expected
4+	Hyperactive, clonus may be present

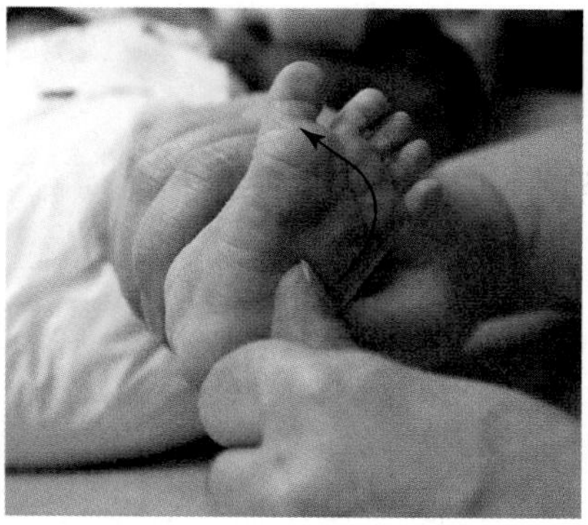

● **Figure 35–40** Assessing the plantar reflex. To assess, stroke the bottom of the infant's or child's foot in the direction of the arrow. Watch the toes for plantar flexion or the Babinski response, fanning and dorsiflexion of the big toe. The Babinski response is normal in children under 2 years of age. Plantar flexion of the toes is the normal response in older children. A Babinski response in children over 2 years of age can indicate neurologic disease.

Table 35–18 provides guidelines for assessment of the deep tendon reflexes. The best response to deep tendon reflex testing is achieved when the child is relaxed or distracted. Children often anticipate the knee jerk and either tighten up or exaggerate the response. Making the child focus on another set of muscles may provide a more accurate response. When testing the reflexes on the lower legs, have the child press his or her hands together or try to pull them apart when gripped together. Responses are normally symmetric bilaterally. The absence of a response is associated with decreased muscle tone and strength. Hyperactive responses are associated with muscle spasticity.

ANALYZING DATA FROM THE PHYSICAL EXAMINATION

Once the physical examination has been completed, group any abnormal findings for each system with those of other systems. Use clinical judgment to identify common patterns of physiologic responses associated with health conditions. Individual abnormal physiologic responses are also the basis of many nursing diagnoses. Be sure to record all findings from the physical assessment legibly, in detail, and in the format approved by your institution.

Table 35–18 Assessment of Deep Tendon Reflexes and the Associated Spinal Segment Tested

Deep Tendon Reflex	Technique and Normal Findings[a]	Spine Segment Tested
Biceps 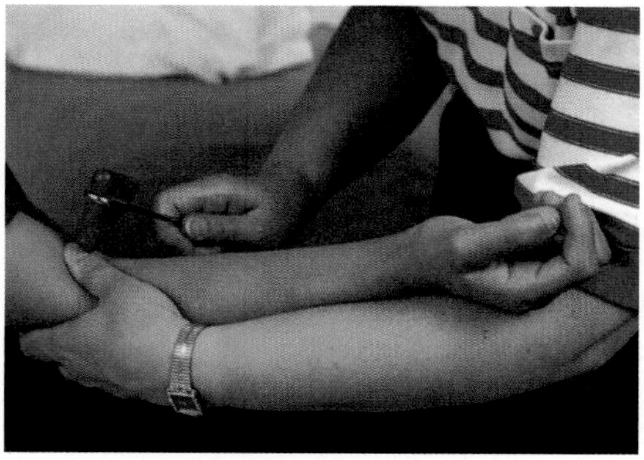	Flex the child's arm at the elbow, and place your thumb over the biceps tendon in the antecubital fossa. Tap your thumb. *Elbow flexes as the biceps muscle contracts.*	C5 and C6
Triceps 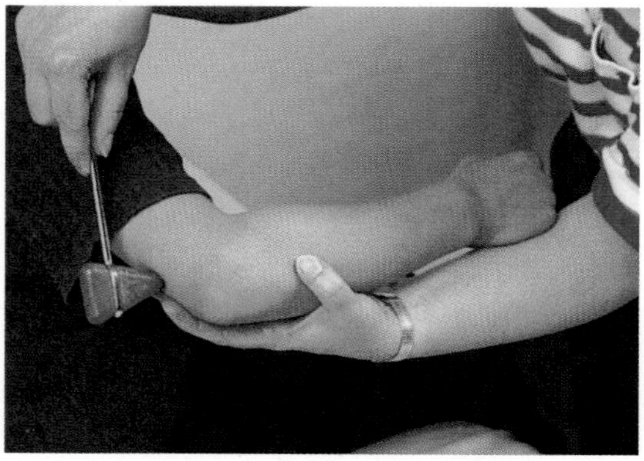	With the child's arm flexed, tap the triceps tendon above the elbow. *Elbow extends as the triceps muscle contracts.*	C6, C7, and C8

(continued)

Table 35–18 Assessment of Deep Tendon Reflexes and the Associated Spinal Segment Tested—continued

Deep Tendon Reflex	Technique and Normal Findings[a]	Spine Segment Tested
Brachioradialis 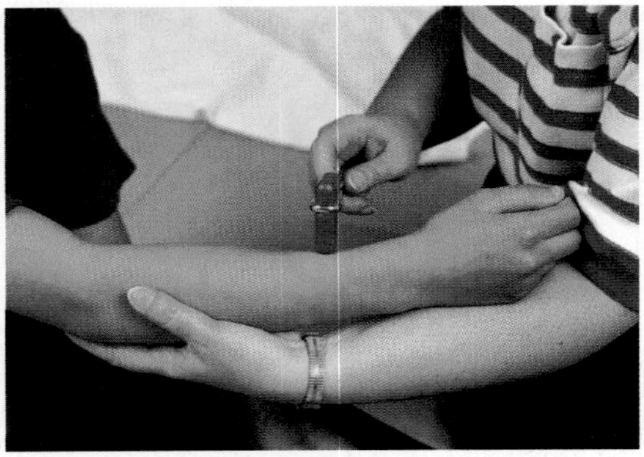	Lay the child's arm with the thumb upright over your arm. Tap the brachioradial tendon 2.5 cm (1 in) above the wrist. *Forearm pronates (palm facing downward) and elbow flexes.*	C5 and C6
Patellar 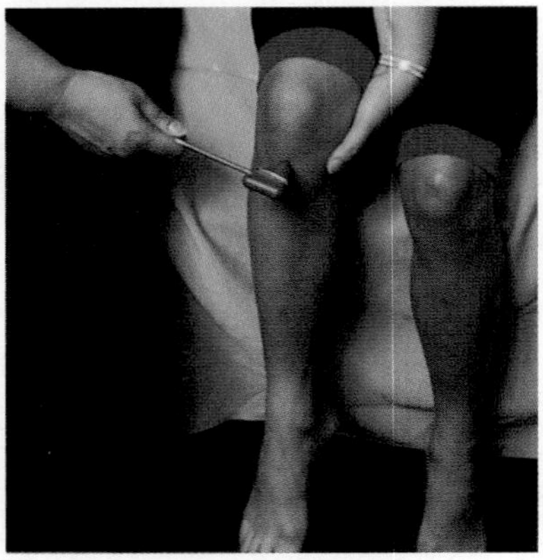	Flex the child's knees, and when the legs are relaxed, tap the patellar tendon just below the knee. *Knee extends (knee jerk) as the quadriceps muscle contracts.*	L2, L3, and L4
Achilles 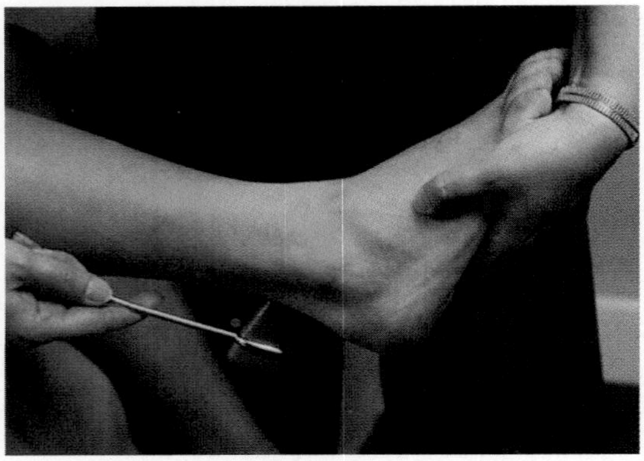	While the child's legs are flexed, support the foot and tap the Achilles' tendon. *Plantar flexion (ankle jerk) as the gastrocnemius muscle contracts.*	S1 and S2

[a]Italics indicate normal findings.

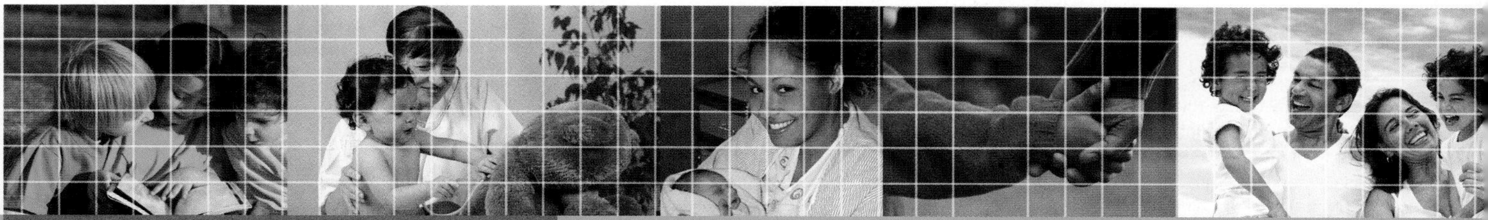

CRITICAL CONCEPT REVIEW

LEARNING OUTCOMES — CONCEPTS

35.1 Describe the elements of a health history for an infant or child of different ages.

Historical data to collect includes:
1. Chief complaint.
2. History of the present illness or injury.
3. Past history.
4. Current health status.
5. Review of systems.
6. Family history.
7. Psychosocial data.
8. Developmental data.

35.2 Identify communication strategies to improve the quality of historical data collected.

1. Introduce self, including purpose of interview.
2. Provide privacy, including confirmation confidentiality.
3. Use open-ended questions.
4. Ask one question at a time.
5. Direct question to the child when appropriate.
6. Be honest with the child and family.
7. Obtain feedback from parents to confirm understanding.

35.3 Describe strategies to gain cooperation of a young child for assessment.

1. Allow the young child to stay in caretaker's lap for most of the examination.
2. Allow the young child to hold and examine any equipment before it is used on the child.
3. Make a game out of tests for muscle strength, coordination, and developmental assessment.

35.4 Describe the differences in sequence of the physical assessment for infants, children, and adolescents.

1. Be flexible in the examination sequence to assess the heart, lungs, and abdomen when the infant is quiet or asleep.
2. Any procedures causing anxiety (examination of throat and ears) should be delayed until the end of the physical assessment of toddlers and young child.
3. Physical examination of the school-age child should proceed in a head-to-toe fashion, with the exception of the genitalia examination (should be done last).
4. The physical examination of the adolescent may be completed without the presence of the parent, especially the examination of the genitalia.

35.5 Modify physical assessment techniques according to the age and developmental stage of the child.

Infants and toddlers:
1. Head circumference is required until age 3 years.
2. Palpate fontanels until closure.
3. Assess vision and hearing response with the use of toys and familiar objects.
4. Perform the examination with the infant and toddler on the lap of the caregiver and use distraction.

Preschooler:
1. Ask young child to show teeth to begin assessment of the mouth and throat.
2. Use words or names easily recognized to assess hearing and memory.
3. Use play and activities to assess muscle strength and coordination.
4. Males should sit "tailor fashion" to assess genitalia.

Adolescent:
1. Ask if the adolescent wishes the parent to be present, and if not have a chaperone of the same sex present.
2. Assess stage of breast and pubic hair development in females. Assess stage of genital and pubic hair development in males.

(continued)

LEARNING OUTCOMES / CONCEPTS

LEARNING OUTCOMES	CONCEPTS
35.6 List five normal variations in pediatric physical findings (such as a Mongolian spot in an infant) found during a physical assessment.	1. Epicanthal folds of the eyes 2. Sucking pads in mouth of infant 3. Rounded chest in infants 4. Breath sounds heard over entire chest 5. Splitting of S2 with breathing 6. Abdominal movement with breathing 7. Bowlegs and knock knees 8. Pubertal development
35.7 Determine the sexual maturity rating of males and females based upon physical signs of secondary sexual characteristics present.	The sexual maturity rating (SMR) for: 1. Females: Average of breast development and pubic hair (Tanner stages). 2. Males: Average of genital development and pubic hair (Tanner stages).
35.8 Recognize at least five important signs of a serious alteration in health condition that require urgent nursing intervention.	1. Altered level of consciousness. 2. Bradycardia. 3. Tachypnea (greater than 60 breaths per minute). 4. Pain. 5. Signs of dehydration (no tears, dry mucous membranes, doughy skin turgor, sunken fontanelle, increased urine concentration). 6. Stridor. 7. Retractions. 8. Cyanosis.

CRITICAL THINKING IN ACTION

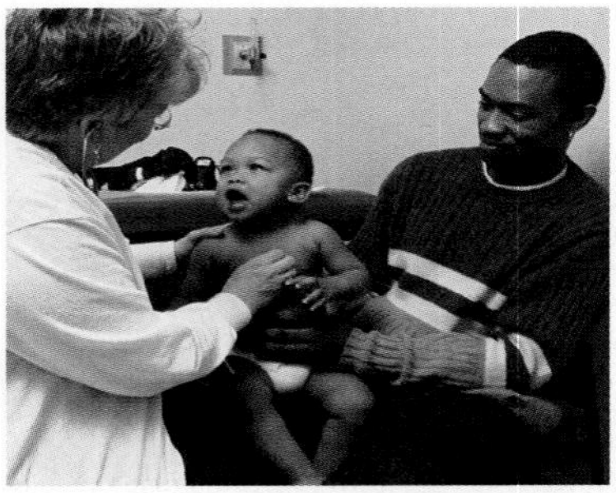

It is a relatively calm night in the Children's hospital emergency room when a 6-month-old infant named Colby is brought in by emergency personnel from an automobile crash. Colby was buckled in his infant, rear-facing, car safety seat, riding with his parents when another car rear-ended them. The parents were not hurt and did not need to go to the hospital. The father immediately called 911 on his cell phone after the crash. When the ambulance arrived at the emergency room, you were given this report by the EMT. Colby was alert and quiet in his father's arms when the ambulance arrived on the scene, and he did not have any obvious signs of trauma. Colby and his father were brought to the hospital to make sure Colby did not sustain any injuries from the crash. His vital signs are as follows: temperature—98.9°F, respirations—32, pulse—110 and blood pressure is 85/39. Colby is alert, quiet in his father's arms, and in no apparent distress. His pupils are equal, round, and reactive to light. His anterior fontanelle is flat and he has equal movements of extremities. His breath sounds are clear and equal bilaterally. His heart sounds have a regular rate and rhythm without murmur. He voided around 2 hours ago, before the accident.

1. The fontanelles are an important body part to examine in infants and toddlers. In the scenario with Colby, it can give an indication of increased intracranial pressure related to a brain injury. Describe the placement of the fontanelles, and when they should close and become unpalpable. Why is the head more likely to sustain injury in an infant like Colby versus an adult?
2. After reviewing the scenario, what can you tell the parents about Colby's vital signs at this time? What is the difference between adult vital signs and Colby's vital signs?
3. Describe what structures in the chest and abdominal area of Colby's body would be of concern after being in this automobile crash.
4. If a heart murmur were to be found on examination of Colby, what would be the five ways to describe it?

See MyNursingKit for possible responses.

REFERENCES

American Academy of Pediatrics Committee on Practice and Ambulatory Medicine and Section on Ophthalmology. (2003). Eye examination in infants, children, and young adults by pediatricians. *Pediatrics, 111*(4), 902–907.

American Speech and Language Association (2007). How does your child hear and talk? Retrieved January 23, 2008, from http://www.asha.org/public/speech/development/chart.htm

Anderson, S. E., & Must, A. (2005). Interpreting the continued decline in the average age at menarche: Results from two nationally representative surveys of U.S. girls studied 10 years apart. *Journal of Pediatrics, 147,* 753–760.

Brady, T., Siberry, G. K., & Solomon, B. (2008). Pediatric hypertension: A review of proper screening, diagnosis, evaluation, and treatment. *Contemporary Pediatrics, 25*(11), 46–56.

Cromwell, P. F., Munn, N., & Zolkowski-Wynn, J. (2005). Evaluation and management of hypertension in children and adolescents (Part one): Diagnosis. *Journal of Pediatric Health Care, 19*(3), 172–175.

Feigelman, S. (2007). The first year. In R. M. Kliegman, R. E. Behrman, H. B. Jenson, & B. F. Stanton, *Nelson textbook of pediatrics* (18th ed., 43–48). Philadelphia: Saunders Elsevier.

Feigelman, S. (2007). The second year. In R. M. Kliegman, R. E. Behrman, H. B. Jenson, & B. F. Stanton, *Nelson textbook of pediatrics* (18th ed., 48–54). Philadelphia: Saunders Elsevier.

Goldenring, J. M., & Rosen, D. S. (2004). Getting into adolescent heads: An essential update. *Contemporary Pediatrics, 21*(1), 64–90.

Graham, E. A. (2005). Economic, racial, and cultural influences on the growth and maturation of children. *Pediatrics in Review, 26*(8), 290–294.

Greydanus, D. E., Matytsina, L., & Gains, M. (2006). Breast disorders in children and adolescents. *Primary Care Clinics of North America, 33,* 455–502.

Horner, G. (2007). Genitourinary assessment: An integral part of the complete physical examination. *Journal of Pediatric Health Care, 21*(3), 162–170.

Kaczor, K., Pierce, M. C., Makoroff, K., & Corey, T. S. (2006). Bruising and physical child abuse. *Clinical Pediatric Emergency Medicine, 7,* 153–160.

Kaplowitz, P. (2004). Extensive personal experience: Clinical characteristics of 104 children referred for evaluation of precocious puberty. *Journal of Clinical Endocrinology and Metabolism, 89*(8), 3644–3650.

Prentiss, K. A., & Dorfman, D. H. (2008). Pediatric Ophthalmology in the Emergency Department. *Emergency Medical Clinics of North America, 26,* 181–198.

Pulsifer, A. (2005). Pediatric genitourinary examination: A clinician's reference. *Urologic Nursing, 25*(3), 163–168.

Purnell, L. D. (2009). *Guide to culturally competent care* (2nd ed.). Philadelphia: Davis.

Ralston, M., Hazinski, M. F., Zaritsky, A. L., Schexnayder, S. M., & Kleinman, M. E. (Eds.). (2006). *Pediatric Advanced Life Support Provider Manual*, Dallas, TX: American Heart Association.

Seidel, H. M., Ball, J. W., Dains, J., & Benedict, G. W. (2006). *Mosby's guide to physical examination* (6th ed.). St. Louis: Mosby Elsevier.

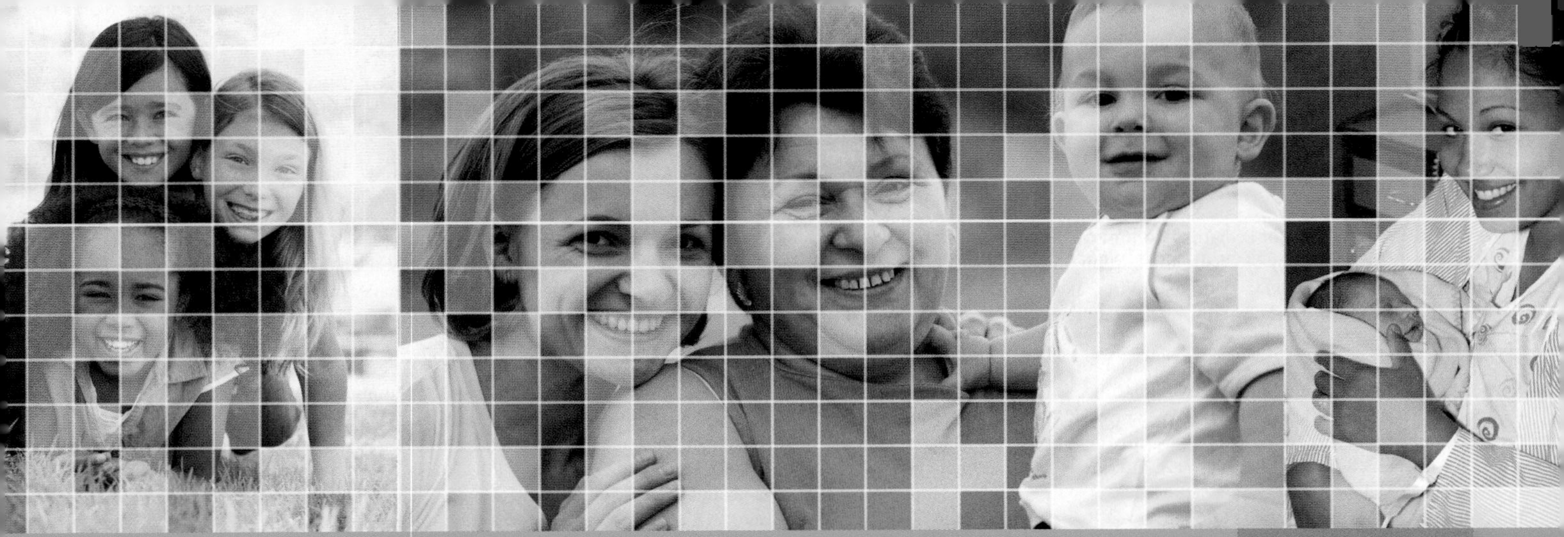

CHAPTER 36

Health Promotion and Maintenance: General Concepts, the Newborn, and the Infant

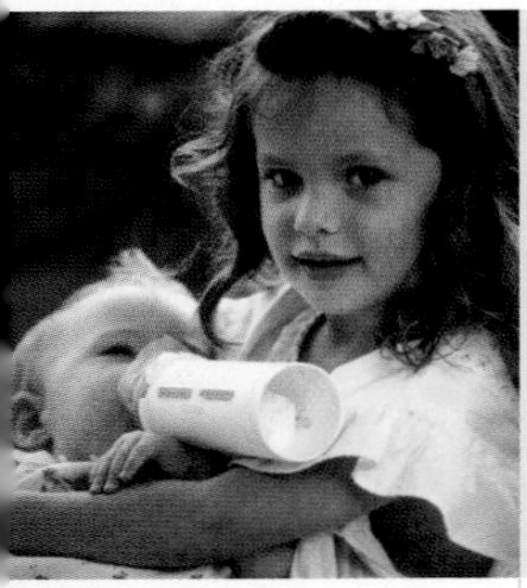

Mommy was really glad to go see the nurse today. She brought our baby and me. Grandma said that they would give us a card that would help us buy food. I'm glad because I'm tired of eating peanut butter. Mommy said we could get some milk and juice, and even some chicken.
—Melody, age 4, sister of 7-month-old Amanda

LEARNING OUTCOMES

36.1 Define health promotion and health maintenance.
36.2 Describe how health promotion and health maintenance are addressed by partnering with families during health supervision visits.
36.3 Describe the components of a health supervision visit.
36.4 Explore the nurse's role in providing health promotion and health maintenance for the newborn and infant.
36.5 Describe the general observations made of infants and their families as they come to the pediatric healthcare home for health supervision visits.
36.6 Describe the areas of assessment and intervention for health supervision visits of newborns and infants—growth and developmental surveillance, nutrition, physical activity, oral health, mental and spiritual health, family and social relations, disease prevention strategies, and injury prevention strategies.
36.7 Plan health promotion and health maintenance strategies employed during health supervision visits of newborns and infants.
36.8 Recognize the importance of family in newborn and infant healthcare, and include family assessment in each health supervision visit.
36.9 Integrate pertinent mental healthcare into health supervision visits for newborns and infants.
36.10 Synthesize data about the family and other social relationships to promote and maintain health of newborns and infants.

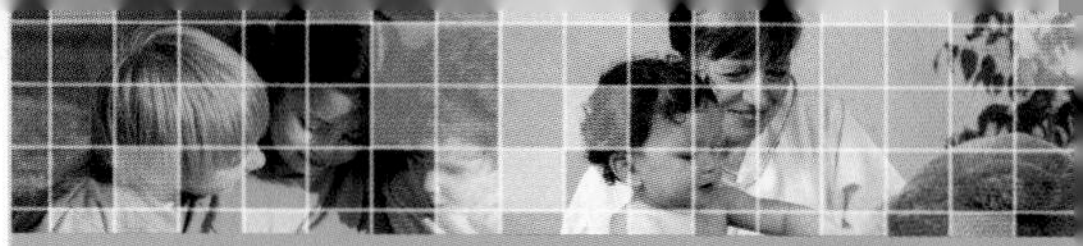

KEY TERMS

Anticipatory guidance, 979
Developmental delay, 989
Developmental surveillance, 982
Early childhood caries (ECC), 991
Health, 979
Health maintenance, 979
Health promotion, 979
Health supervision, 980
Partnership, 982
Pediatric healthcare home, 980
Postpartum, 987
Screening, 986
Self-regulation, 992
Separation anxiety, 991
Spiritual dimension, 986
Stranger anxiety, 991

MyNursingKit National Guidelines for Preventive Health Services

One of the two major goals of *Healthy People 2010* is to help individuals of all ages to increase life expectancy and improve their quality of life. The concepts of health promotion and health maintenance provide for nursing interventions that contribute to meeting this goal. Many students in health professions begin their studies with a strong interest in care of ill individuals. However, as time progresses, they learn that "well" people need care also. They need teaching to improve diet, reduce stress, and obtain immunizations. They may seek information about how to exercise properly or ensure a safe environment for their children. These examples of care and teaching are components of health promotion and health maintenance.

Nursing is a holistic profession that examines and works with all aspects of the lives of individuals, and has a strong focus on family and community as well. Nurses are uniquely positioned to provide health promotion and health maintenance activities, and indeed these activities should be a part of each encounter with families. What is the difference between health promotion and health maintenance? When should nurses engage in activities that focus on health? How are these activities integrated into health supervision visits for the infant and young child? How do nurses partner with other healthcare professionals to offer comprehensive health services in settings accessible to parents and young children? How can nurses help children and their families to maximize length and quality of life? These are some of the questions that will be explored in this chapter, with specific activities that target families with infants and young children.

GENERAL CONCEPTS

In order to understand health promotion and health maintenance it is important to develop a definition of health. The World Health Organization defines **health** as a state of complete physical, mental, and social well-being and not merely the absence of disease and infirmity (World Health Organization, 2001). Others view the quality of "complete well-being" impossible to attain, and view health as "a dynamic state of well-being characterized by a physical and mental potential, which satisfies the demands of the life commensurate with age, culture, and personal responsibility" (Bircher, 2005). Therefore, even individuals with chronic disease can be viewed as healthy if they are successfully adapting to their conditions. Health is viewed as dynamic, changing, and unfolding; it is the realization of a state of actualization or potential (Pender, Murdaugh, & Parsons, 2006). This basic human right is necessary for development of societies.

Health promotion refers to activities that increase well-being and enhance wellness or health (Pender et al., 2006). These activities lead to actualization of positive health potential for all individuals, even those with chronic or acute conditions. Examples include providing information and resources in order to:

- Enhance good nutrition at each developmental stage.
- Integrate physical activity into the child's daily events.
- Provide adequate housing.
- Promote oral health.
- Foster positive personality development.

Health promotion is concerned with development of strategies that seek to foster conditions that allow populations to be healthy and to make healthy choices (World Health Organization, 2001, 2005). Nurses engage in health promotion by partnering with children and families to promote family strengths in the areas of lifestyles, social development, coping, and family interactions. They also provide **anticipatory guidance** for families because they understand the child's upcoming developmental stages and teach families how to provide an environment to assist in meeting the milestones of the stages. This concept is explored more fully later in this chapter.

Health maintenance (or health protection) refers to activities that preserve an individual's present state of health and that prevent disease or injury occurrence. Examples of these activities include developmental screening or surveillance to identify early deviations from normal development, providing immunizations to prevent illnesses, and teaching about common childhood safety hazards. Health maintenance activities are commonly preventive in nature, and terminology common to community or public health nursing explains the levels and aims of preventive actions. Prevention levels are identified as primary prevention, secondary prevention, and tertiary prevention (Table 36–1).

While it is clear that health promotion and health maintenance activities are closely linked and often overlap, there are some differences. Health maintenance focuses on known potential health risks and seeks to prevent them or to identify them early so that intervention can occur. Health promotion looks at the strengths and goals of individuals, families, and populations, and seeks to use them to assist in reaching higher levels of wellness. It involves partnerships with the family as health goals are set, and with other health professionals and resources to provide for meeting the goals. Nurses apply both health promotion and health maintenance concepts when providing healthcare, recognizing that the concepts overlap. Health promotion and health maintenance are integrated into healthcare visits for children, with the care provider applying both knowledge of health maintenance concepts and adding information the family has identified that will assist in increasing health or wellness (health promotion). These activities commonly take place at "well child" or health supervision visits.

Health supervision for children is the provision of services that focus on disease and injury prevention (health maintenance), growth and developmental surveillance, and health promotion at key intervals during the child's life. What health promotion and health maintenance activities are parts of health supervision visits? How can these activities be integrated into all settings where care is provided for children? What are the recommended times for health visits to occur and what care is provided at certain times? How can health supervision visits be organized to accomplish the goals of the family and health professionals? These and other questions will be answered in this section and the following section focused on nursing management.

Table 36–1 Levels of Preventive Health Maintenance Activities

Level	Description	Example of Nursing Actions
Primary Prevention	Activities that decrease opportunity for illness or injury	Giving immunizations Teaching about car safety seats
Secondary Prevention	Early diagnosis and treatment of a condition to lessen its severity	Developmental screening Vision and hearing screening
Tertiary Prevention	Restoration to optimum function	Rehabilitation activities for child after a car crash

Data from Murray, Zentner, & Yakimo, 2009.

Nursing Practice

The American Academy of Pediatrics and the National Association of Pediatric Nurse Associates and Practitioners concur that a pediatric healthcare home should offer the following:

- Family-centered care and trusting partnership
- Sharing of unbiased and clear information
- Provision of primary care to include acute and chronic care, breastfeeding promotion, immunizations, growth and development, screenings, healthcare supervision, and counseling about health, nutrition, safety, parenting, and psychosocial issues
- Continuously accessible care
- Continuity of care
- Provision of compassionate, developmentally appropriate and culturally competent care
- Referral to early intervention and child care
- Coordination of services and collaboration of professionals
- Maintenance of a comprehensive central record
- Referral to specialists as needed

(Pan, 2006; American Academy of Family Physicians, 2007; NAPNAP, 2009)

All children need a medical home, where accessible, continuous, and coordinated health supervision is provided during the developmental years (Schoenbaum & Abrams, 2006). Accessibility refers to both financial and geographic access; continuous indicates that the care is ongoing with consistent care providers; coordination refers to the need for communication among health professionals to provide for the needs of the child. A medical home or **pediatric healthcare home** is therefore the site of comprehensive, continuous, culturally sensitive, coordinated, and compassionate healthcare by a pediatric healthcare professional focused on the overall well-being of children and families (National Association of Pediatric Nurse Associates and Practitioners [NAPNAP], 2009; American Academy of Family Physicians, 2007). When a family has an established partnership with a care provider, family-centered health services can be provided based on the family's risks and protective factors. These services may be provided in physicians' offices, community health clinics, the home, schools, childcare centers, shelters, or mobile vans (Figure 36–1 ●). The U.S. Department of Health and Human Services (DHHS), the American Academy of Pediatrics (AAP), and the American Medical Association have developed national guidelines for preventive health care services for infants, children, and adolescents. NAPNAP supports the list of comprehensive services of a pediatric healthcare home identified by the AAP.

The health supervision visit is individualized to the family and child. Standardized screenings and examinations are included, and time is provided for the family's specific concerns and questions about the child's health. Nurses play an integral

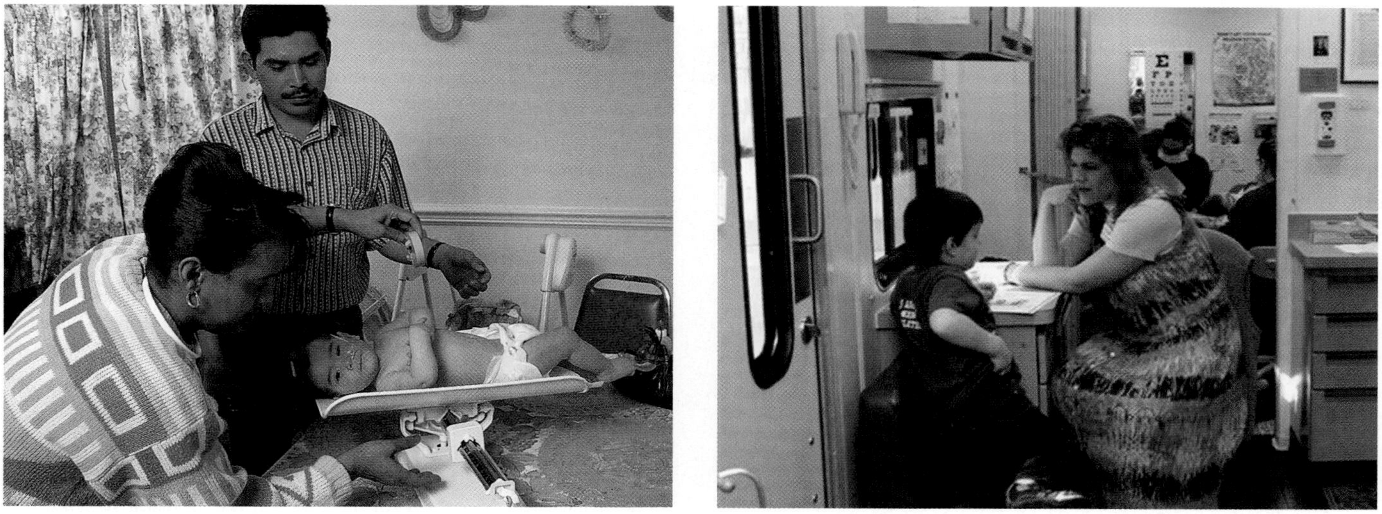

A B

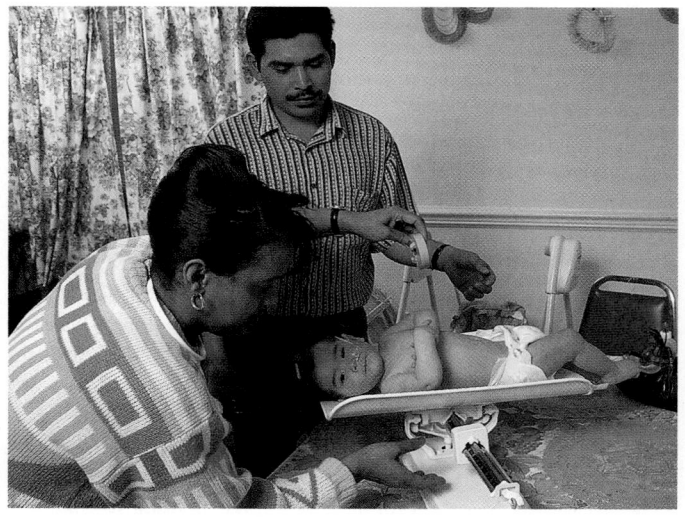

● **Figure 36–1** Delivery of health promotion services. ***A,*** The nurse is providing a health supervision visit in the child's home after discharge from the hospital for an acute illness. ***B,*** A nurse is providing information to a child visiting a mobile healthcare van.

part in these comprehensive visits, and they partner with other healthcare providers to accomplish health supervision.

A tracking system in the pediatric healthcare home site helps to identify appropriate health supervision activities for each child at every visit. Most often computers are used to list appropriate topics for visits at specific ages. If a child misses a visit, the family can be contacted by phone and encouraged to come in for the recommended care. A family may be called if their child is lacking some immunizations. Recognizing that not all families get into the healthcare home for each recommended visit, every health encounter, including an episodic illness visit or care for a chronic illness, is a potential time to complete health promotion and health maintenance activities. For example, immunizations may sometimes be given during a visit for an acute condition such as otitis media (ear infection) if the child has missed a prior health supervision visit. Even when children are seen in hospitals, emergency rooms, or other settings, it is important to ask about their pediatric healthcare home and when the last visit occurred. Identify children who need basic health supervision services and provide them or refer to other settings for meeting these needs at another time.

Nurses play an important role in managing health supervision visits. Depending on the setting, the nurse may provide all services or support other care providers by obtaining an updated health history, screening for diseases and other conditions, conducting a developmental assessment, and providing immunizations, anticipatory guidance, and health education. Nurses in all settings are instrumental in identifying children who need health supervision and are not obtaining recommended care (Figure 36–2 ●).

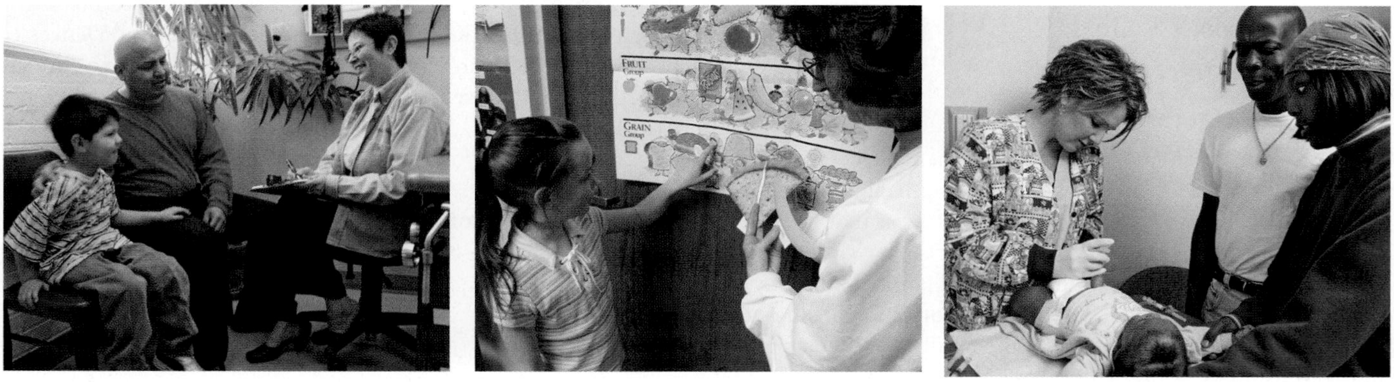

A B C

● **Figure 36–2** Identifying children who need healthcare. The nurse plays many roles in providing health promotion and health maintenance for children. ***A,*** Data are collected from the time a nurse calls the child and family to the examination room and during the history-taking phase. The nurse asks questions while observing the child's behaviors and the relationship between parent and child. The nurse also performs screening tests, including blood pressure, tuberculosis, vision and hearing, and developmental screening. ***B,*** Interventions that include teaching may take place. ***C,*** A nurse may administer immunizations as parents watch and assist by holding the child. Nurses also play important roles in teaching families information to enhance health.

While health supervision visits can address many health-related topics, there is generally a limited time in which to engage a child or family. The nurse needs to direct the encounters and have some ideas for pertinent agendas. *Bright Futures* booklets provide guidance about how the nurse can manage health supervision visits. Six concepts should be integrated into care:

1. The care provider *builds effective partnerships* with the family. A **partnership** is a relationship in which participants join together to ensure healthcare delivery in a way that recognizes the critical roles and contributions of each partner in promoting health and preventing illness. The partners in child health include the child, family, health professionals, and the community.
2. The nurse *fosters family-centered communication* by showing interest in the child and family, and effectively conveying information and understanding.
3. The nurse *focuses on health promotion and health maintenance topics during visits*, recognizing that families may not initiate these discussions.
4. The nurse *manages time well* to enable health promotion topics to be addressed during visits. This includes reviewing the child's health record and selecting topics pertinent for the child's age and the family's situation.
5. The nurse *educates the family during "teachable moments."* Large teaching plans are not always needed; children and families often learn best when presented with small bits of information based on the parent's questions or the nurse's observations.
6. The nurse *becomes an advocate for child health issues*. When an issue arises while caring for a child, seek additional data from various sources, talk with others, and strategize how the problem could be solved.

(Hagan, Shaw, & Duncan, 2008)

COMPONENTS OF HEALTH PROMOTION/HEALTH MAINTENANCE VISITS

The nurse identifies and addresses pertinent topics for health promotion and health maintenance during health supervision visits. Nurses also apply their knowledge of areas that need to be addressed with an infant or child of a particular age, and then make general observations of the child and family to identify additional topics for discussion. While categories to consider vary depending on the age of the child, the family's particular needs, and community resources, there are some common topics that generally require attention. Often, nurses start with the topics described as follows, integrating general observations as they progress with a visit, and further identifying assessment areas needed in particular situations.

Pediatric nurses make *general observations* of infants and their families whenever they encounter them. Nurses who are observant during the health supervision visit have many opportunities for assessing the family. These general observations begin when the family is called in and welcomed by the nurse to the facility. They continue as the infant or child is weighed and measured, and throughout the visit. Nurses observe the physical contact between the child and other family members, the developmental tasks displayed by the child, and parental level of stress or ease in conducting childcare activities.

Growth and developmental surveillance provide important clues about the child's condition and environment. The child's height, weight, and body mass index are calculated at each health supervision visit, and results are placed on percentile charts (see Chapter 33 and Chapter 34 for more information). Parents are given the information in written form and it is interpreted for them. Physical assessment is performed to be sure the child is growing as expected and has no abnormal or unexplained physical findings (see Chapter 35). **Developmental surveillance** is a flexible, continuous process of skilled observations that also provides data about the child's capabilities, allows for early identification of any neurologic problems, and helps to verify that the home environment is stimulating. Early development is important to later health and it must be evaluated consistently and systematically during healthcare visits (Fine & Mayer, 2006). Information may be collected from several sources, for instance, a questionnaire that the parent completes, questions asked during the interview, or observation of the child during the visit. Parents can also be interviewed to identify any developmental concerns they may have about the child or adolescent. When talking with parents, review physical, social, and communication milestones for infants, young children, older children, or adolescents. Detailed milestones for each age group are found in Chapter 33. Standardized developmental questionnaires are effective for developmental surveillance of most children, especially when time for health supervision visits is limited. Screening tests should be administered at the 9-, 18-, and the 24- or 30-month visits (Council on Children with Disabilities, 2006). A commonly used test is the Denver II, which can be applied as a developmental chart, like a growth curve, to monitor the child's developmental progress (Figure 36–3 ● and Figure 36–4 ●). When performing developmental screening with the Denver II or any other standardized screening tools, nurses make sure all directions are followed by:

- Choosing the proper test for the child's age and desired information.
- Reading directions thoroughly or using specific training tools available.
- Practicing as needed until proficient with the test.
- Calculating the infant's or child's age correctly, especially if premature.
- Attempting to develop rapport with the infant or child to get the best performance.
- Following directions for administration of items; in some cases, parents can be asked if a child demonstrates specific skills at home, especially if the child is not willing to perform an item during testing.

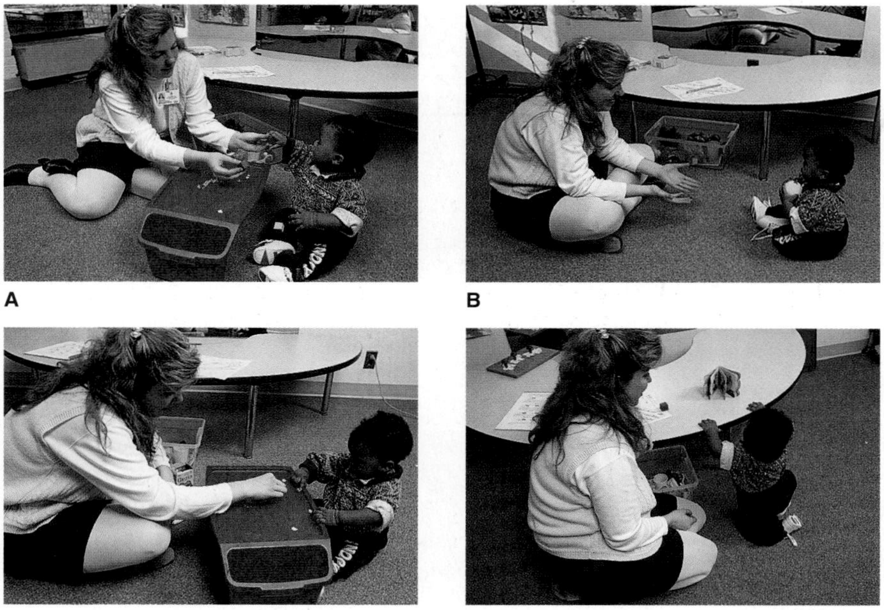

A B C D

● **Figure 36–3** The Denver II Assessment. Follow all directions for performing the Denver II assessment and for interpreting responses. Develop rapport with the child and approach the assessment as fun. This often helps the child participate more actively during the entire Denver II assessment. This 9-month-old boy is able to perform the following age-appropriate behaviors: ***A,*** Banging two cubes; ***B,*** playing ball with the examiner; ***C,*** using a thumb-finger grasp; ***D,*** pulling to stand.

- Noting the behavior and cooperativeness of the child during the screening process.
- Analyzing the findings using the test instructions to make the correct interpretation.

Failure to perform an item in a single domain does not mean the child has failed the test (see "Developing Cultural Competence"). The child should be reevaluated at a future visit. Schedule the appointment at a time of day when the child is awake and rested. Provide parents with guidance on specific methods for stimulating the child. Failure of multiple items within one domain or across multiple domains is of greatest concern. When poor development patterns in one or more domains are revealed, referral for diagnostic developmental assessment is needed.

Nutrition evaluation is a vital part of each health supervision visit. It makes important contributions to general health and fosters growth and development. Include observations and screening relevant to nutritional intake at each health supervision visit. Eating proper foods for age and activity ensures that children have the energy for proper growth, physical activity, cognition, and immune function. Nutrition is closely linked to both health promotion and health maintenance. See Chapter 34 for detailed nutritional assessments for each age group. Find out what questions parents have about feeding their children. Use the information gathered to provide both health promotion and health maintenance interventions.

Physical activity provides many physical and psychologic health benefits. However, there is growing disparity between recommendations and reality among most children. Research by the Centers for Disease Control and Prevention (CDC) has identified that about 23% of children from 9 to 13 years report no free-time physical activity. When schools do not offer daily physical education, many children have no regular activity. Participation in physical activity declines as youth get older, and females are considerably less active than males (Centers for Disease Control and Prevention [CDC], 2006a; CDC, 2006b). Inquire about activities the child prefers and amount of time for activity during the day. As the child grows older, include questions about sedentary activities such as number of hours spent watching television or playing computer games. See if the child plays sports at school or in the community. Ask about activities in a typical day to measure amount of activity. Once the nurse gathers data about physical activity, interventions are implemented to enhance activity patterns.

While *oral health* may seem to require the knowledge of a specialist, there are many implications that relate to general health care. Oral health is important because teeth assist in language development, impacted or infected teeth lead to systemic illness, and teeth are related to positive self-image formation. Dental caries is the most common chronic disease of children. Many youth in the United States are affected by tooth decay and pain that interfere with activities of daily living such as eating, sleeping, attending

Developing Cultural Competence

ENGLISH AS A SECOND LANGUAGE AND DEVELOPMENTAL TESTING

Children who have recently come from other countries and even some born in this country who live in families from minority ethnic groups may have difficulty with some items on developmental tests. For example, children who are not skilled in the English language may not understand some instructions or be able to answer questions about definitions of words. When parents do not speak English as a primary language and the examiner uses English, common terms might be misinterpreted. Parents might not understand what is meant if you ask, "Does your baby have a mobile over the crib at home?" or "Is she starting to be afraid of strangers?" How can you be alert for language differences and become sensitive to miscommunication?

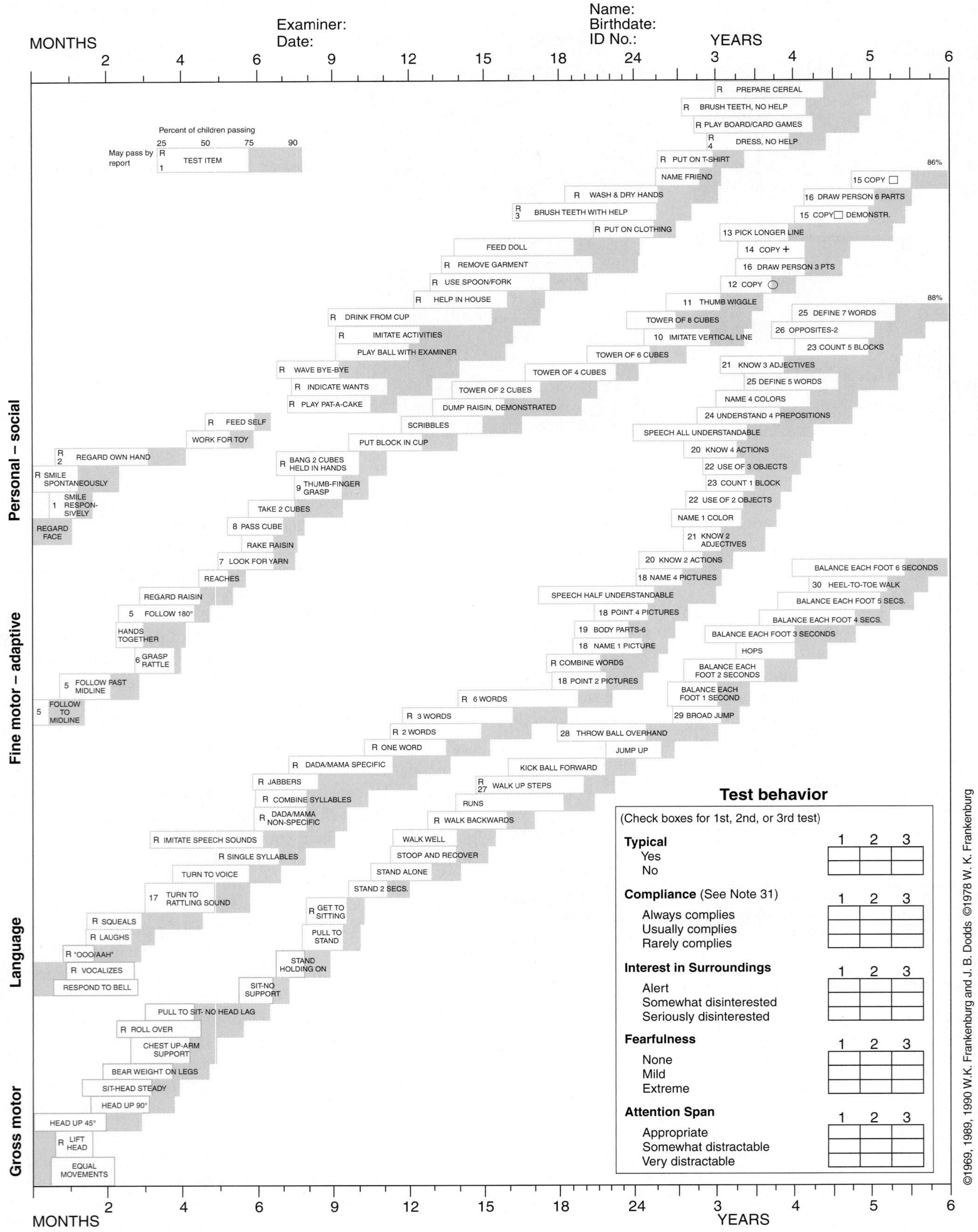

● **Figure 36–4** Denver II Assessment, front.

DIRECTIONS FOR ADMINISTRATION

1. Try to get child to smile by smiling, talking, or waving. Do not touch him/her.
2. Child must stare at hand several seconds.
3. Parent may help guide toothbrush and put toothpaste on brush.
4. Child does not have to be able to tie shoes or button/zip in the back.
5. Move yarn slowly in an arc from one side to the other, about 8" above child's face.
6. Pass if child grasps rattle when it is touched to the backs or tips of fingers.
7. Pass if child tries to see where yarn went. Yarn should be dropped quickly from sight from tester's hand without arm movement.
8. Child must transfer cube from hand to hand without help of body, mouth, or table.
9. Pass if child picks up raisin with any part of thumb and finger.
10. Line can vary only 30 degrees or less from tester's line.
11. Make a fist with thumb pointing upward and wiggle only the thumb. Pass if child imitates and does not move any fingers other than the thumb.

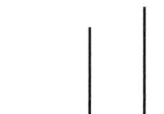

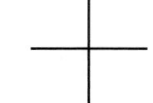

12. Pass any enclosed form. Fail continuous round motions.
13. Which line is longer? (Not bigger.) Turn paper upside down and repeat. (pass 3 of 3 or 5 of 6).
14. Pass any lines crossing near midpoint.
15. Have child copy first. If failed, demonstrate.

When giving items 12, 14, and 15, do not name the forms. Do not demonstrate 12 and 14.

16. When scoring, each pair (2 arms, 2 legs, etc.) counts as one part.
17. Place one cube in cup and shake gently near child's ear, but out of sight. Repeat for other ear.
18. Point to picture and have child name it. (No credit is given for sounds only.) If less than 4 pictures are named correctly, have child point to picture as each is named by tester.

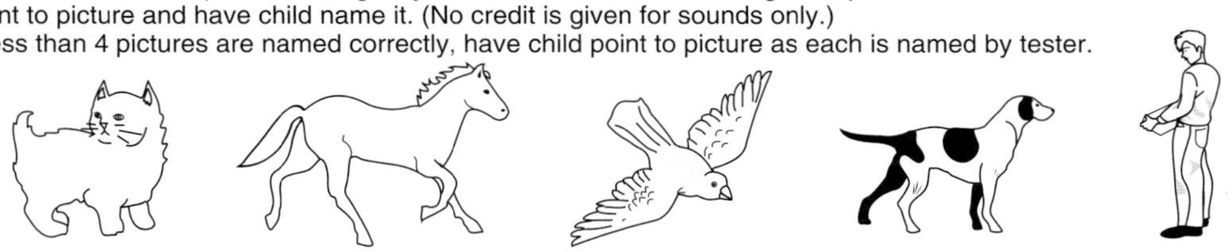

19. Using doll, tell child: Show me the nose, eyes, ears, mouth, hands, feet, tummy, hair. Pass 6 of 8.
20. Using pictures, ask child: Which one flies?... says meow?... talks?... barks?... gallops? Pass 2 of 5, 4 of 5.
21. Ask child: What do you do when you are cold?... tired?... hungry? Pass 2 of 3, 3 of 3.
22. Ask child: What do you do with a cup? What is a chair used for? What is a pencil used for? Action words must be included in answers.
23. Pass if child correctly places <u>and</u> says how many blocks are on paper. (1, 5).
24. Tell child: Put block **on** table; **under** table: **in front of** me, **behind** me. Pass 4 of 4. (Do not help child by pointing, moving head or eyes.)
25. Ask child: What is a ball?... lake?... desk?... house?... banana?... curtain?... fence?... ceiling? Pass if defined in terms of use, shape, what it is made of, or general category (such as banana is fruit, not just yellow). Pass 5 of 8, 7 of 8.
26. Ask child: If a horse is big, a mouse is_____? If fire is hot, ice is_____? If sun shines during the day, the moon shines during the ____? Pass 2 of 3.
27. Child may use wall or rail only, not person. May not crawl.
28. Child must throw ball overhand 3 feet to within arm's reach of tester.
29. Child must perform standing broad jump over width of test sheet (8 1/2 inches).
30. Tell child to walk forward, ⊂⊃⊂⊃⊂⊃⊂⊃ → heel within 1 inch of toe. Tester may demonstrate. Child must walk 4 consecutive steps.
31. In the second year, half of normal children are non-compliant.

OBSERVATIONS:

● **Figure 36–4** Denver II Assessment, back.

Used with permission from W. K. Frankenburg, Denver, CO.

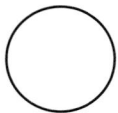

Nursing Practice

Over one-half of children from homes with low incomes have not received dental care in the last year; about 14% of them have unmet dental care needs. One-third of families who have difficulty paying for food or rent do not receive any preventive dental visits. Hispanic children are even more likely to have no or inadequate dental care. Low educational level of parents, and functional impairment of the child are additional risk factors for unmet dental needs (Kenney, McFeeters, & Yee, 2005). All children in the Medicaid program are eligible for dental coverage in the Early and Periodic Screening, Diagnostic, and Treatment Services (EPSDT). Private and public clinics in many communities provide low-cost or free care for families with limited financial resources. Many families do not realize their children could receive these services. Find out what resources are available in your state and community, and refer as needed. See Chapter 1 for further description of programs mentioned here.

MyNursingKit Case Study: Domestic Violence

school, and speaking (Dye, Tan, Smith, et al., 2007). The nurse applies health promotion to dental health by teaching about oral care and access to dental visits. Health maintenance activities relate to prevention of caries and illness related to dental disease.

Mental and spiritual health are important concepts to address in health promotion and health maintenance visits. Parents can be encouraged to keep a record of mental health issues to bring to health supervision visits. This helps them understand that the healthcare professional is willing to partner with them to assist in dealing with mental health. Suggest topics such as child and parental mood, child temperament, stresses and ways that family members manage stress, or sleep patterns. Make notes in the record as a reminder of questions to ask at the next visit (Jellinek, Patel, & Froehle, 2002). The child and family are both observed for appropriateness of affect and mood. Be alert for signs of depression, stress, anxiety, and child abuse or neglect. The nurse establishes both health promotion and health maintenance goals related to child and family mental health. Health promotion goals relate to adequate resources to meet family challenges, and protective factors such as involvement in extended family and the community. Teaching stress reduction techniques such as meditation, relaxation, and imagery, as well as providing resources for yoga or other techniques, is helpful. Health maintenance goals relate to prevention of mental health problems. Examples include providing resources when domestic violence occurs, or referring cases of suspected child abuse or neglect. The **spiritual dimension** is a connection with a greater power than that in the self, and guides a person to strive for inspiration, respect, meaning, and purpose in life (Murray, Zentner, & Yakimo, 2009). Spiritual health is seen in the large context as those entities that provide meaning in life. For some, this may be membership in a faith-based group; for others it may be feeling part of a society with a purpose of greater good, or setting goals for the future. Ask about the family's meaningful activities. Provide links to faith-based groups as needed.

The *relationships* that a child establishes with others begin at birth. The first and most important set of relationships develops with the family. The mother, father, siblings, and perhaps extended family are the contexts in which the baby learns to relate with others. With growth the world widens to encompass other children, friends of the family, peers, school, and the larger community network. Analyzing the child's relationships at all ages provides important clues to social interactions. From the moment the family is called in from a waiting area, be alert for clues to family interactions. Likewise, other social interactions are important to evaluate. Does the young infant interact in an age-appropriate manner with the healthcare provider or other children in the area? Ask the parents questions about family and social interactions. Once assessment has taken place, establish goals and interventions related to family and social relationships.

Disease prevention strategies focus mainly on health maintenance, or prevention of disease. Some health disruptions can be detected early and treatment for the condition can begin. **Screening** is a procedure used to detect the possible presence of a health condition before symptoms are apparent. It is usually conducted on large groups of individuals at risk for a condition and represents the secondary level of prevention (Figure 36–5 ●). Most screening tests are not diagnostic by themselves but are followed by further diagnostic tests if the screening result is positive. Once a screening test identifies the existence of a health condition, early intervention can begin, with the goal of reducing the severity or

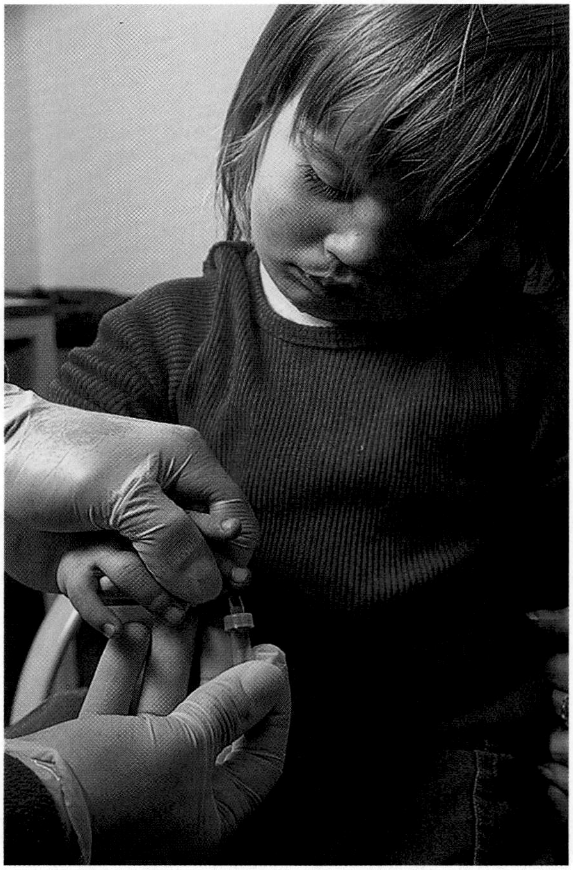

● **Figure 36–5** Blood screening test. This young child is having a blood screening test to detect iron deficiency anemia. Children are often screened for adequate levels of iron in later infancy and during toddlerhood.

complications of the condition (secondary prevention). Another way to prevent diseases is to immunize children against common communicable diseases (primary prevention). See Chapter 45∞ for the complete list of childhood immunizations and schedules for administration.

Most childhood mortality and hospitalization is related to injury (National Center for Health Statistics, 2007) (see Chapter 1∞ for more information). Therefore, it is important for the nurse to integrate *injury prevention* strategies in all health supervision visits. The family is constantly challenged to maintain a safe environment as the child grows older, reaches more advanced developmental levels, is exposed to a widening world outside of the family, and has less supervision. Safety teaching should be integrated with developmental progression. Asking parents to bring their questions about safety to each visit can be a good starting point for discussion. The nurse considers knowledge about the age of the child and information from the health supervision visit to plan health maintenance interventions related to injury. Teaching is performed, resources are made available, and parents and children who have experienced injury are invited to present their experiences.

Many other topics might be discussed during health supervision visits. They may relate to either health maintenance activities designed to preserve health, or health promotion activities designed to enhance or improve the state of wellness. They include topics such as extended family members and their role in the child's life, cultural variations or inclusion, or development of moral values and ethical behaviors.

HEALTH PROMOTION AND MAINTENANCE OF THE NEWBORN AND INFANT

The month following delivery is a time of huge transition for the new mother and her family. Not only is the mother coping with hormonal shifts and a **postpartum** (after giving birth) body, but roles and relationships are also changing. The role of the nurse is to assess knowledge about self-care and newborn care, teach health promotion and maintenance activities, promote parental confidence in newborn caregiving, and facilitate a partnership among healthcare professionals and the family.

Infancy is a major life transition for the baby and parents. The infant accomplishes phenomenal physical growth and many developmental milestones while the family adapts to the addition of a new member and establishes new goals for each of its existing members. Infant health supervision visits are very important to support the health of the baby and the family unit. These visits begin after the newborn period, at about 1 month of age. This is the time when parents establish an ongoing partnership with a healthcare provider. A "medical home" or "pediatric healthcare home" is identified to serve the baby's health needs. The goals of health supervision visits are to identify and address the health promotion and health maintenance needs of the infant.

Facilitating breastfeeding, helping parents to understand their newborn's and infant's temperament, and employing strategies to ensure adequate sleep by the baby and parents are examples of health promotion activities. Health maintenance activities focus on disease and injury prevention. Some examples of these interventions include administering immunizations and teaching about infant car seats.

An established relationship with a healthcare provider and agency is important so that trust develops and the family will feel comfortable about turning to the professionals for information and guidance as the baby grows. Nurses play a vital role in welcoming new families into office and clinic settings, establishing rapport, and applying principles of communication so that trust and positive partnerships develop between providers and families. Infancy is a time when the child grows in physical, psychologic, and cognitive ways; health supervision visits play a key role in fostering healthy growth and development. When should the infant be seen for health supervision visits? What are key components of these visits? How can the nurse best assess and intervene to ensure the infant's health and safety? These are some of the questions that will be answered in this section of the chapter.

EARLY CONTACTS WITH THE FAMILY

Most obstetrical care providers encourage the expectant mother to choose her newborn's care provider prior to the baby's birth (see "Thinking Critically"). Pediatric care providers usually welcome a short office visit, sometimes at no charge, to allow the expectant mother and care provider to assess their compatibility prior to initiating the care provider relationship. Many pediatric care providers have written information for expectant parents, explaining their professional philosophy of care as well as information about services.

Health promotion and maintenance for the newborn begin during the stay in the hospital or birthing center (see Chapters 27, 28, 29∞). Upon discharge referral may be indicated to a lactation consultant or followup healthcare visit. The American Academy of Pediatrics (2004) recommends that if the newborn is discharged from the hospital in less than 48 hours, an experienced healthcare professional who is competent in newborn assessment should examine the newborn in the clinic or home setting within 48 hours of discharge. For newborns discharged between 48 and 72 hours of age, the first follow-up visit should occur by 5 days of age. The purpose of this visit is to ensure that the newborn is continuing to progress normally and that no previously undiscovered problems have surfaced. At this initial contact, the nurse promotes

Thinking Critically

CHOOSING THE NEWBORN'S CARE PROVIDER

Parents are encouraged to visit the pediatric healthcare home before the baby is born. This will help the parents decide if the health care provider offers the type of care they want for their infant. Prepare a list of questions that parents could ask during an appointment to visit the provider they are interested in interviewing. Be sure this list addresses the availability of healthcare providers, frequency of well child supervision, cost and insurance information, and other pertinent topics.

See MyNursingKit for possible responses.

maternal confidence in caregiving and offers education and anticipatory guidance. Careful assessments are made for hyperbilirubinemia, feeding problems, or other abnormalities. Further visits are established as needed from 5 days to 1 month; the first scheduled health supervision of infancy is at 1 month of age.

Health promotion and maintenance for infancy occur in a series of health supervision visits during the first year of life. Schedules vary among facilities, but a common pattern includes visits at about 1 month, 2 months, 4 months, 6 months, 9 months, and 1 year of age. In addition, most children have some episodic illnesses such as gastrointestinal illness or otitis media and visit the facility at other times for treatment of these illnesses. A few children have chronic or serious healthcare problems during the first year, and have extensive contact with the healthcare home and other services.

During these first visits, assess the family for protective factors and risks. Protective factors might include knowledge level of infant needs, support from family and friends, and the mother's good health and nutritional state during pregnancy. Risk factors could include limited financial resources, lack of preparation for the baby, and illness or other stress among family members. Ask about how the family traveled to the visit, and if convenient times and transportation are available. Lack of access during times the family is not at work and other health system barriers sometimes interfere with attendance at health supervision visits (Garfield & Isacco, 2006). Knowledge of risk factors will shape the nursing interventions in the first health supervision in infancy. The nurse applies health promotion principles by building on strengths and fosters health maintenance by intervening to minimize risks.

GENERAL OBSERVATIONS

When the family comes to the clinic or office for care with a newborn or infant, general observations should begin at first contact (Figure 36–6 ●). Welcome the family warmly to the facility and comment on the baby. Ask how the family is doing with the baby and how the adjustment is going. Be alert for signs of fatigue or depression in the parents, as these can occur when caring for an infant and can interfere with bonding and positive transition. Look for clues about cultural orientation. The nurse gathers information in order to assess the needs of the family, to invite discussion, to validate positive parenting efforts, and to promote partnership between the family and the healthcare team. Upon entering the examination room, it is helpful to explain the plans for the visit, such as "I will weigh and measure Sarah now and show you how she is growing. Then I'll ask a few questions about her eating, sleeping, and other things. Then the nurse practitioner will be in to do Sarah's physical examination. Do you have any questions as we start? Will you undress Sarah now so we can weigh her accurately?"

GROWTH AND DEVELOPMENTAL SURVEILLANCE

Assessment of growth and development begins at birth and continues in newborn and infant health promotion and maintenance visits (see Chapter 33 for important background/theoreticical information about growth and development). Note the posture, flexion, reflexes, and physical attributes that help evaluate gestational age. Physical growth and meeting of developmental milestones provide important information about infants. The baby is measured for accurate length, weight, and head circumference. (See the Clinical Skills Manual SKILLS and Chapter 35 for more information; also see Figure 36–7 ●.) The mea-surements should be placed on growth grids and interpreted. Parents enjoy seeing how the baby is progressing and are usually eager to learn about the child's weight gain and growth percentiles. Be alert for an infant who demonstrates a change in percentile range. For example, if the baby was in the 75th percentile for length and weight at birth, but has fallen to below the 50th percentile for weight, additional assessment of the baby's

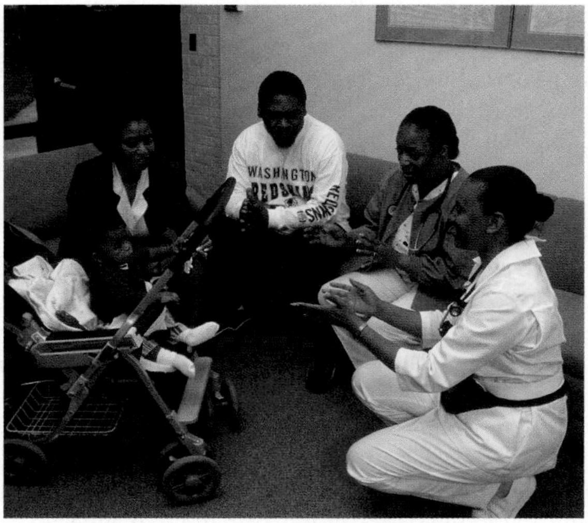

● **Figure 36–6** General observations. The nurse begins assessment of the infant's family when they are seen in the waiting room and called in for care. What observations can you make of the infant's general appearance? Developmental accomplishments? Interaction of parents with the baby?

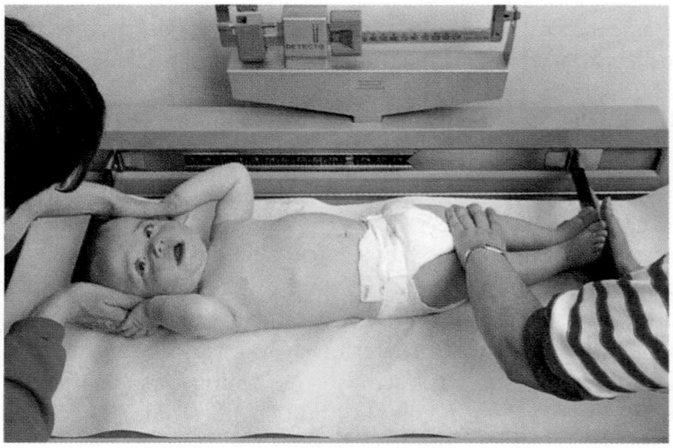

● **Figure 36–7** Measuring physical growth. Weighing and measuring length during health supervision visits provides important information about the child's nutrition and general development. This young infant was measured and then while the parents dressed the child the nurse placed the findings on the growth grid.

Developing Cultural Competence

CULTURAL INFLUENCES ON DEVELOPMENTAL TESTS

Be alert for differences in cultural practices and beliefs that may influence developmental milestones. For example, if a child is kept on a cradleboard for much of the time, the baby may be slow in learning to crawl. This baby may progress directly to standing by furniture without demonstrating as much creeping or crawling as other infants. If an item such as "waves good-bye" or "plays patty-cake" represents a practice not common in another culture, the child may not have had exposure to the skill. Be alert for cultural variations, allow the child time to learn a developmental skill, and retest during future healthcare visits.

feedings is needed. Likewise, if the head circumference is much lower or higher than the length and weight percentiles, further neurologic and developmental assessment should be done.

Growth measurement is followed by a physical assessment. The nurse may complete parts of the assessment, with the remainder performed by the physician, nurse practitioner, or other primary care provider. The assessment evaluates each body system, with particular attention paid to the heart, skin, musculoskeletal system, abdomen, and neurologic status. See Chapter 28 for assessment of the newborn and Chapter 35 for a thorough discussion of physical assessment throughout infancy and childhood.

Developmental surveillance is integrated into each infant healthcare visit by observing developmental milestones in the infant (see Chapter 33 for a summary of milestones expected at different ages). When there is no opportunity to observe a skill directly, ask parents about whether the infant performs the skill (see "Developing Cultural Competence"). In addition to direct observation, parents are usually requested to fill in a form that asks questions about common developmental tasks. Review the results and determine if additional questions should be asked. Signs of **developmental delay**—a delay in mastering functions, such as motor coordination and behavioral skills—in a full-term infant usually merit immediate investigation by a pediatrician, pediatric developmental specialist, pediatric neurologist, or a multidisciplinary team of professionals. Parents require additional emotional support, clear and honest communication, and resources to cope with the stress of this situation.

The nurse establishes health promotion and maintenance interventions related to growth and development assessment data. Anticipatory guidance related to development is a major component of health promotion. The nurse anticipates the next milestones the infant will be meeting, and recommends ways for the parents to support the infant in progression. Some health promotion activities include:

- Teaching about food introduction that will foster growth.
- Encouraging toys and activities that will assist in meeting the next developmental milestones.
- Demonstrating gross and fine motor skills that the infant has achieved.
- Demonstrating to parents how the child will focus on their faces and mimic their vocal sounds.

Other interventions are focused on health maintenance or disease and injury prevention. Safety hazards and ways to avoid them are discussed, and parents are given brochures, Web sites, or videotapes to enhance injury prevention information. Can you outline additional health promotion and health maintenance interventions that relate to the newborn's and infant's growth and development?

NUTRITION

The importance of nutrition during the newborn period and the first year of life cannot be overestimated. The baby will triple his or her birth weight by 1 year of age and has a great need for nutritional balance. From the first sips of breast milk or formula as a newborn, to eating the family meal at 1 year of age, the fast progression of nutritional intake patterns is obvious. See Chapter 30 for a thorough description of nutritional needs for the newborn, including detail on importance and support of breastfeeding, and Chapter 34 for information about nutritional needs in infancy.

During each visit the nurse seeks to learn what the baby is eating, and whether the family has any questions or concerns related to intake (Hagan, Shaw, & Duncan, 2008). Open-ended questions are a good way to begin, with more specific questions inserted after the parent's perceptions are known. Breastfeeding is encouraged and supported during the newborn and infancy periods with information about safe formula feeding provided when the family has chosen that method of feeding. Once the baby is in the second half of the first year, food patterns of the family become more important. Consider childcare settings as well.

Observations from other portions of the visit can provide clues about additional questions to ask. If an infant has not gained weight as expected and has fallen into a lower channel of weight percentile, more specific analysis of intake is needed. Ask for a recall of the baby's intake in the previous day. When the baby does not meet developmental milestones on schedule or is lethargic, intake may be inadequate for age. In these cases support may be needed to ensure adequate intake; a thorough description of

Evidence in Action

Healthy People 2010 set a goal for 75% of new mothers to initiate breastfeeding, and hospitals and birthing centers play a key role in encouraging breastfeeding. A recent study by the Centers for Disease Control and Prevention (CDC) found that the average score of hospitals and birth centers for providing breastfeeding support is 63% out of a possible 100%. Breast milk contains antibodies that protect the infant from infection; overweight and diabetes are less likely to develop later in the infant who is breastfed; and certain cancers are less common in persons who were breastfed. The CDC recommends that hospitals and birth centers actively assist, encourage, and support the new mother in breastfeeding. (CDC, 2008) feeding may be the first step in analyzing the problem and planning interventions. When the child's ability to take in nutrients or the parent's ability to feed the baby is questioned, an observation of a feeding might take place, either at the healthcare setting or during a home visit.

Additional nutritional assessment measures are used at certain points in the first year. A hematocrit or hemoglobin is generally performed between 9 and 12 months of age. Lead screening may be needed in certain population groups (see Chapter 44∞ for more information). Food security screening can be used when appropriate (see Chapter 34∞). Each visit includes nutritional teaching about important items. The topics for discussion vary according to age group. See Table 36–2 for suggested teaching topics at specific ages. Desired outcomes for nutrition in infancy include adequate growth, normal nutritional assessment findings, and knowledge by parents of the nutritional needs of the infant.

PHYSICAL ACTIVITY

Muscle development begins early in fetal life. The flexed position of the newborn demonstrates development of the flexor muscles and relaxation of the extensor muscles. This flexed position protects the newborn, conserves energy by reducing movement, and reduces heat loss (Blackburn, 2007). During the first month of life, the newborn gradually "unfolds" and the body straightens. Movements begin to change from reflexive to purposeful.

Physical activity is needed for adequate development of fine and gross motor skills in infancy. Unlike other times of life, the focus is on providing only the opportunities for activity, without a need to focus on motivation. As long as infants are meeting developmental milestones and have a stimulating environment that provides opportunity for fine and gross motor activity, they will use their motor skills, thus enhancing their performance. Time should be provided each day for the infant to reach for objects, freely exercise legs and arms, and increasingly use head control.

Playing with parents or others and being surrounded by toys and other stimulating items will encourage motor behavior in all body parts. Ask the parents for a description of the infant's typical day and listen for these types of play periods. While infants should sleep on their backs, they need supervised play periods when they are awake that are spent on the stomach. This encourages developmental skills and lessens flattening of the back of the head from excessive positioning on back (Graham, Kreutzman, Earl, et al., 2005).

Table 36–2 Nutrition Teaching for Health Promotion and Health Maintenance Visits

Age	Nutrition Teaching	
Newborn	Support breastfeeding efforts. Teach correct formula types and preparation if used. Teach burping and rate of feeding information.	Encourage families to view feedings as social interactions; emphasize importance of holding the infant and not propping bottles.
1 month	Continue teaching listed above. Suggest water during hot weather or if family wants to use a bottle at baby's bedtime.	
2 months	Continue teaching listed above. Review fluid needs of infants. Reinforce food safety for partially used bottles of breast milk or formula. Use warm water for heating bottles rather than microwave to avoid burning.	Warn against feeding honey in the first year of life due to risk of botulism. Begin daily cleaning of infant gums. Provide information about any supplements needed (for example, iron for premature infant, vitamin D for babies not exposed to adequate sunlight).
4 months	Continue teaching listed above. Discuss introduction of first foods between 4 and 6 months, and surveillance for symptoms of allergy or intolerance.	Discuss changing food patterns such as increasing amounts and decreasing numbers of daily milk feedings.
6 months	Continue teaching listed above. Reinforce proper introduction of new foods, to include rice cereal, vegetables, and fruits. Discuss any unusual food reactions observed. Introduce cup for drinking. Introduce soft finger foods.	Serve juice only in a cup and limit to no more than 6 ounces daily. Caution about common choking foods and items. Provide information about fluoride supplement if water supply is not fluoridated.
9 months	Continue teaching listed above. If mother does not continue to breastfeed, teach family to use iron-fortified formula for the first year of life. Encourage self-feeding of finger foods, integrating common foods for the family.	Introduce source of protein such as tofu, cheese, mashed beans, and slivers of meats.
12 months	Continue teaching listed above. Support mother who wishes to continue breastfeeding beyond 1 year of age.	Encourage cups for all feedings other than breast.

Table 36–3 Risk and Protective Factors Regarding Physical Activity in the Newborn Period and Infancy

Risk Factors	Protective Factors
■ Premature birth ■ Delayed developmental milestones ■ Limited stimulation by family or other care providers ■ Lack of knowledge by family about infant's physical activity needs ■ Limited community resources for families with infants	■ Meets developmental milestones at expected ages ■ Has contact with parents, siblings, and others for significant time each day ■ A supportive environment with room to play safely, stimulating surroundings ■ Physically active family ■ Family knowledge about infant's physical activity needs ■ Community programs that promote physical activity in infants and information for families

Data from Patrick, K., Spear, B., Holt, K., & Sofka, D. (Eds.). (2001). Bright futures in practice: Physical activity. Arlington, VA: National Center for Education in Maternal and Child Health.

Observe the physical skills of the infant (see Chapter 33) for motor developmental norms, ask questions about play periods provided, and compose a list of the family protective factors and risk factors in this area. Table 36–3 lists some risk and protective factors related to physical activity during newborn and infancy.

Based on the results of assessment and using the concept of anticipatory guidance, the nurse plans appropriate teaching for health promotion. Health maintenance deals with prevention of physical development delays. Examples of nursing activities are teaching parents to allow arms and legs of infants to be outside of covers for some period each day to enhance movement, and encouraging toys that encourage attention and movement, such as mobiles and music boxes. The nurse evaluates success of interventions by the child's progression in physical activity milestones at each health supervision visit. Adequate parental understanding of the importance of physical activity and the means of supporting the child's activities is an important outcome of care.

ORAL HEALTH

The first teeth begin to erupt about midway during infancy. Two front teeth are common at about 6 months of age. However, even before this, parents lay the foundation for good oral health. The mother's intake during pregnancy and breastfeeding are essential to ensuring adequate availability of calcium and other nutrients that will be used as the infant's teeth develop. The nurse in child health supervision settings ensures that the infant has adequate intake of these nutrients via breastfeeding and other foods. A dietary recall of the mother's intake, as well as the infant's, is one way of assessing for nutrients. When the water supply is not fluoridated, inquire about use of fluoride drops.

Help the family establish healthy dental habits. The parents should wipe the infant's gums with soft moist gauze once or twice daily. This helps to clean residues of food from the gums and gets the infant accustomed to having something wiping the gums, a practice that may assist when toothbrushing begins. Families are also cautioned to avoid having the infant breastfeed when sleeping, to avoid use of bottles in bed, and not to allow the infant to drink at will from a bottle during the day. These practices are linked to **early childhood caries** (see Chapter 34) and can lead to tooth decay. Nurses assess for the presence of teeth and whether patterns are similar to those expected (see Chapter 35 for additional information). It is wise to ask if the infant has had any difficulty with teeth eruption. Many infants have increased crying and disrupted sleep when teething. Suggest comfort measures such as offering cool beverages and safe "teething toys" for the infant. The American Academy of Pediatric Dentistry recommends an oral examination within 6 months of the eruption of the first tooth and no later than 12 months of age (CDC, 2006c).

MENTAL AND SPIRITUAL HEALTH

The infant's mental health is related to early experiences, inborn characteristics such as temperament and resilience, and relationships with caregivers. The first year of life provides many opportunities for the infant to develop positive mental health; interventions during this important period can enhance the child's future mental status.

One way to evaluate mental health is to look carefully at the growth and development surveillance data that were described earlier. Children who feel secure and have nurturing environments usually grow as expected and perform milestones at usual times. Slow growth and delayed development are sometimes related to feeding disorder of infancy and early childhood (see Chapter 34). In these cases a disturbed relationship with the primary caregiver influences the psychologic state of the infant and results in decreased food intake. Another way to assess mental health is to observe the child and parent interacting. Does the parent hold the newborn securely and does the infant cuddle and settle in to the parent's arms? (See Figure 36–8 ●.) Is there eye contact between parent and infant? Does the parent appear comfortable in holding and comforting the newborn? These interactions indicate bonding or positive attachment.

During the first year, the infant learns to identify the primary caregivers; beginning at about 6 months of age, infants may cry or protest when another person holds them. This is called **stranger anxiety** and indicates expected attachment to parents. Similarly, infants in the second half of the first year of life may exhibit **separation anxiety** by inconsolable crying and other signs of distress when parents are not present. These behaviors are normal, demonstrate healthy attachment to primary caregivers, and indicate mental health. Help parents to recognize them as expected occurrences. Provide them ideas of how to deal with this

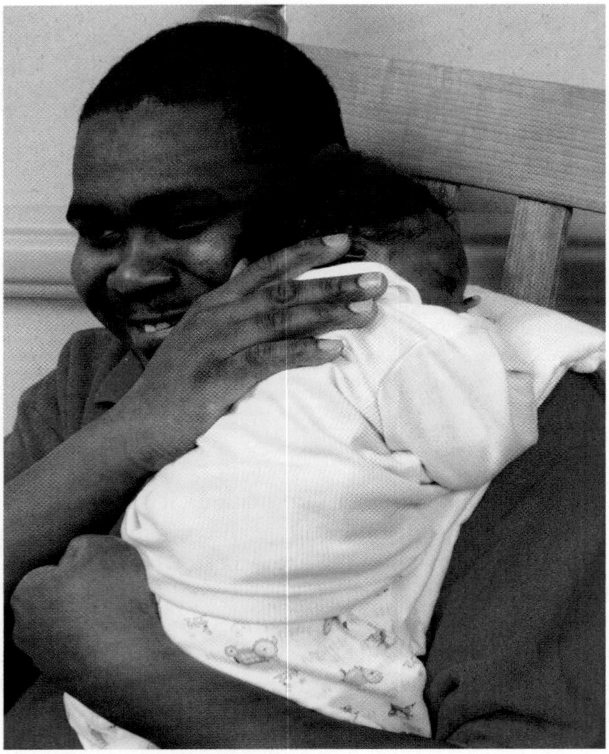

● **Figure 36–8** Assessing mental health. Interactions between the parent and infant provide clues to mental health. Do the adult and child appear comfortable with each other? Is eye contact and vocalization present? Are their bodies soft and relaxed or tense?

behavior. They can remain in sight and talk to the baby during health supervision examinations. They should be encouraged to hold and comfort the baby after painful procedures like immunizations. Once the infant has experienced that the parent leaves and returns, security in the care of others can emerge.

Another important indication of infant mental health is the ability to comfort oneself. **Self-regulation** is the process of dealing with feelings, learning to soothe self, and focusing on activities for increasing periods of time. Newborns learn how to comfort and calm themselves. Ask parents if the newborn or infant sucks a finger, softly rocks, or otherwise comforts self when distressed. Some infants prefer to be alone and quiet when tired or distressed; others calm better when held, rocked, or placed in an infant swing. Help the parents to identify and reinforce the baby's methods of self-soothing, and teach swaddling and rocking techniques. Self-regulation is needed by the baby when learning to go to sleep while tired and agitated. Nurses use health promotion principles to teach about sleep patterns in infants, and implement health maintenance when partnering with families to deal with problem sleep behaviors that lead to infant and parent fatigue (see "As Children Grow" and "Evidence-Based Nursing").

The newborn enters a family with spiritual strengths and limitations. The nurse assesses the family and provides additional resources when needed. Although the infant is not mature enough to understand the family's spiritual framework, the atmosphere in the family that relates to nurturing, valuing children, providing a safe and secure environment, and recognizing mental balance is conveyed readily to the infant. The infant's social and psychologic health are closely related to these factors. Assess the family's meaningful activities and practices and engagement in faith-based practices. Ask if they have needs or desires for referrals in the community such as to an organized religious body or other meaningful activities.

Many of the nurse's interventions are aimed at healthy mental health development in the infant. Health promotion activities focus on teaching parents the needs of infants for security and interaction. Suggest healthy sleep patterns starting with the newborn visit and explain how they can be achieved. Teach self-regulation skills so that the parents can help the infant become quiet and calm. Health maintenance seeks to identify infants with disruptions in mental health status, often manifested by growth or interaction abnormalities. When the infant has disturbed sleep patterns or difficulty calming self when upset, or the parents do not interpret infant cues related to hunger or discomfort, the nurse plans interventions to help prevent further problems. An expected outcome for these activities is the reestablishment of expected growth and development, and age-appropriate interactions of the infant with others.

RELATIONSHIPS

Family adaptation to a new baby begins in pregnancy, and evidence of initial family adaptation to pregnancy may be predictive of future parental coping (Hagan, Shaw, & Duncan, 2008). Upon birth, the family is the primary site where the infant learns to interact with other people. Therefore, family dynamics must be examined during health supervision visits. Strengths and needs of the family are identified during psychosocial screening (Commonwealth Fund, 2007). Some factors in the mental health of the parents directly affect the atmosphere in the home, and the resulting health of the newborn and infant. Depression in parents or other family members is an important condition that has the potential to influence the infant's health (see Chapter 26∞ for information about risks in the postpartum family). Interactions with parents who are depressed will be altered; caretaking, both physical and emotional, can be impaired. Another challenge to the mental health of families and the infants in these families is that of domestic violence, a situation in which parents or adult care providers commit violent acts toward one another. Another risk that occurs in some families with infants is child abuse or maltreatment. This problem is a serious issue that causes disturbed mental status in the baby. See Chapter 44∞ for a detailed description of child abuse and its effect on infants and older children. Suspected child abuse must be reported to legal authorities in order to protect children.

The infant's social interactions both within and outside the family display unbelievable growth in the first year. The role of the nurse related to infant social interactions in health supervision visits is to evaluate the social skills of the infant, learn what parents have noticed about the baby's temperament and how it fits with their lives, and make suggestions for positive social development. Desired outcomes for the infant include establishment of close relationships with parents and other family members, a stimulating

Evidence-Based Nursing

INFANT SLEEP

Clinical Question

Many babies have limited sleeping periods during the night, and their night awakenings disturb parents' sleep. Parents may have busy days and be unable to nap for adequate sleep to perform at a safe and productive level during the day. Parental stress and depression are associated with frequent child awakenings and strategies are needed to assist them in supporting the infant's sleep.

Evidence

Sleep of the infant is an important concern for many parents but there is little research-based evidence about what strategies really improve infant sleep. Parents have been advised to have the infant "cry it out" or to feed the child just before bedtime, strategies that have not been demonstrated to clearly improve sleep patterns. A group of nurse and pediatric researchers tested an intervention to assist parents in dealing with their infants' sleep problems. A 2-hour teaching session was offered to 39 families to discuss normal infant sleep and recommended comforting of the infant, followed by parental charts of infant sleep, and telephone support by the researchers. Parents were instructed to comfort their infants while leaving them in their cribs, and to increase the time between these comfort visits when the infant was crying, up to 10 minutes. Co-sleeping with the parent was discouraged. After the 16 weeks of the study, infant sleep had improved, co-sleeping had significantly decreased, breastfeeding had remained the same, and parents reported improved sleep quality, decreased fatigue and improved mood (Hall, Clauson, Carty, et al., 2006). In another study of 1,741 children, factors associated with poor sleep included parents staying with children while they fell asleep, responding to night awakenings by feeding, holding, rocking, or bringing the child to the adult bed (Touchette, Petit, Paquet, et al., 2005).

Best Practice

This evidence-based practice provides implications for nursing care. Ask parents of young newborns to record the infant sleep patterns. As the infant nears 3–4 months, patterns should demonstrate few night wakenings and feedings. Teach parents about how to minimize stimulation and interaction at night, as described above. Provide opportunities to review results at future health supervision visits, or offer telephone or other support to parents.

Critical Thinking

What reasons might working parents have for responding eagerly and interacting with an infant who awakens at night?

Do you think there are other reasons why infants awake at night? What clues help you to decide if an infant sleep problem exists?

See MyNursingKit for possible responses.

home environment that is responsive to the baby's temperament, and developmental progression in social interactions.

DISEASE PREVENTION STRATEGIES

Disease prevention in the newborn period includes metabolic screening, hearing screening, eye examination, immunization, prevention of environmental smoke exposure, sudden infant death syndrome (SIDS) risk reduction, formula safety, minimizing exposure to disease, and hand hygiene for the family.

Infants are prone to many infectious diseases, especially once passive immunity from the mother wanes at about 6 months of age (see Chapter 45 and Chapter 50). Recommended immunizations are administered on schedule to provide protection from some diseases. Recommended immunizations for newborn and infancy are listed in Table 36–4. Further details on immunizations can be found in Chapter 45. Instruct parents about coming immunizations and when the infant should be seen again. Be sure the parent understands the risks and benefits of each immunization. Answer their questions truthfully, and have resources on hand such as brochures and videotapes for interested parents.

During each health supervision visit in infancy, the nurse performs recommended screenings and counsels the parents about why such screening is important. Vision and hearing screenings are consistently performed. Screenings for anemia and lead poisoning are added at particular times or with certain groups. Families with certain genetic diseases such as sickle cell disease or cystic fibrosis may choose to have screening for the infant so that supportive care could begin early if the child has the disease. Parents benefit from teaching about common diseases and conditions of young children and measures for their prevention. Ask about secondhand smoke (environmental tobacco smoke [ETS]) and encourage smoking parents to quit. Teach parents to put infants to sleep on their backs to assist in lowering the chance of sudden infant death syndrome. Be sure parents have a phone number to call when they have

AS CHILDREN GROW

INFANT SLEEP PATTERNS

Birth–3 months

10–16 hours of sleep daily in about five sleep periods of 30 minutes to 4 hours; sleep spans day and night hours

3–6 months

14 hours of sleep daily with a longer sleep at night plus two to three naps daily

By 4–6 weeks, a consistent sleep pattern should emerge

6–12 months

12–14 hours of sleep daily with a longer sleep at night plus one to two naps daily

Data from Hoban, 2004.

Table 36–4 Routine Immunizations Recommended during Newborn and Infancy Periods

Immunization	Age Recommended
Hepatitis B	At birth (1st dose) 1–2 months (2nd dose) 6–18 months (3rd dose)
Diphtheria, tetanus, pertussis	2, 4, and 6 months (3 doses)
Rotavirus	2, 4, and 6 months (3 doses); first dose can be at 6 weeks but if doses are given at 2 and 4 months, the 6-month dose is not needed
Haemophilus influenzae type b	2, 4, and 6 months (3 doses; 3rd dose is not needed if PRP-OMP [Pedvax HIB or Comvax] are used for primary series)
Inactivated poliovirus	2, 4, and 6–18 months (3 doses)
Pneumococcal	2, 4, and 6 months (3 doses)
Influenza	6–23 months (1 dose annually)

Teaching Highlights

WHEN TO CONTACT THE HEALTHCARE PROVIDER

Instruct parents to contact a provider if the child has:

- Rectal temperature ≥ 100.4°F (38.0°C)
- Seizure
- Skin rash, purplish spots, petechiae
- Change in activity or behavior that makes the parent uncomfortable
- Unusual irritability, lethargy
- Failure to eat
- Vomiting
- Diarrhea
- Dehydration
- Cough

Data from Hagan, Shaw, & Duncan (2008).

questions about conditions or whether the baby should be seen by the healthcare provider (see "Teaching Highlights: When to Contact the Healthcare Provider"). Desired outcomes for disease prevention strategies include adequate management of health problems, integration of immunization and other preventive measures into care of the infant, and family understanding of preventive measures recommended for infants.

INJURY PREVENTION STRATEGIES

New parents are sometimes unaware of sources of potential injury for the newborn. Some aspects of injury prevention are pertinent to the newborn's immediate care and other topics promote discussion and provide opportunities for anticipatory guidance during all of infancy. In the immediate newborn period, the nurse should assess the parents' knowledge of injury prevention strategies, and promote healthy and safe behaviors. Injury prevention strategies include proper and consistent use of an infant car seat, and strategies to prevent falls, burns, choking, drowning, and suffocation.

During the first year of life, injury becomes an increasingly common cause of mortality. Strategies must be included in every health supervision visit to lower the risk of injury. Nurses should never assume that parents understand how to insert an infant car seat correctly or what types of toys and foods can lead to choking. Know the most common hazards at each age and teach parents methods of avoiding them (Tables 36–5 and 36–6).

Begin the conversation by asking parents what safety hazards they are aware of in the child's environment. Use this information as the starting point for discussion. Give positive feedback for their awareness of hazards and measures they have taken to prevent them. Consider using a home assessment survey that assists parents in identifying hazards that may be present in their homes. When infants visit friends, relatives, or neighbors, they may be exposed to other hazardous situations. Grandparents may not have a home that is "baby-proofed" and the infant could have access to electrical cords, machinery, medicines, or other hazards. Help the parents to evaluate the childcare home or center. Focus on car safety since this is a frequent cause of injury for infants. Provide brochures and other types of information about recommendations. Refer every family for a car seat examination at a certified examination center. Provide resources for car seats if the family is not able to afford one. Discuss other possible safety hazards such as extensions on the parent's bicycle and use of baby strollers in areas where cars are present.

NURSING MANAGEMENT

NURSING ASSESSMENT AND DIAGNOSIS

The nurse working in clinics, offices, and other settings that offer primary care for newborns and infants should be skillful in assessing health promotion and health maintenance. The infant's growth, developmental level, general physical health, and mental/social health are assessed. Family interactions and other settings where the infant spends time are evaluated for risks and protective factors that influence the child's development. Assess the health of siblings and patterns of integrating the infant into the rest of the family. Particular attention is directed at assessment of risk for diseases and injuries. The data-gathering phase always provides parents with the opportunity to ask questions and relay concerns. Further assessment may need to be directed at these areas.

Based on the assessment data, the nurse establishes nursing diagnoses that become the basis for nursing interventions. Both areas of strength and need are included; often the family's

Table 36–5 Injury Prevention in Infancy

Hazard	Development Characteristics	Preventive Measures
Falls	Mobility increases in first year of life, progressing from squirming movements to crawling, rolling, and standing.	Do not leave the newborn or infant unsecured in infant seat, even in newborn period. Do not place on high surfaces such as tables or beds unless holding child. ***(A)*** Once mobile by crawling, keep doors to stairways closed or use gates. Standing walkers have led to many injuries and are not recommended.
Burns	Infant is dependent on caretakers for environmental control. The second half of the first year is marked by crawling and increased mobility. Objects are explored by touching and placing in mouth.	Check temperature of bath water and food/liquids for drinking. Cover electrical outlets. Supervise infant so that play with electrical cords cannot occur.
Motor vehicle crashes	Infant is dependent on caretakers for placement in car. On impact with another motor vehicle, an infant held on a lap acts as a torpedo.	Use only approved restraint systems (according to federal Motor Vehicle Safety Standards). The seat must be used for every trip, even if very short. The seat must be properly buckled to the car's lap belt system. ***(B)***
Drowning	Infant cannot swim and is unable to lift head.	Never leave a newborn or infant alone in a bath of even 2.5 cm (1 in.) of water. Supervise when in water even when a life preserver is worn. Supervision should be provided by adults, not older children. Flotation devices such as arm inflatables are not certified life preservers.
Poisoning	Newborn and infant is dependent on caretakers to keep harmful substances out of reach.	Keep medicines out of reach. Teach proper dosage and administration of medicines to parents. Cleaning products and other harmful substances should not be stored where the infant can reach them. Remove plants from play areas. Have poison control center number by telephone.
Choking	The second half of infancy is marked by exploratory reaching and mouthing objects. Infant explores objects by placing them in the mouth. ***(C)***	Avoid foods that commonly cause choking. Keep small toys away from infants, especially toys labeled "not intended for use by those under 3 years."
Suffocation	The newborn and young infant has minimal head control and may be unable to move if vomiting or having difficulty breathing.	Position newborn and infant on back for sleep. ***(D)*** Do not place pillows, stuffed toys, or other objects near head. Do not use plastic in crib. Avoid latex balloons. Co-sleeping with the parent is discouraged due to danger of suffocation. Sleep with the baby near but not in the parental bed (American Academy of Pediatrics, 2005)
Strangulation	Infant is able to get head into railings or crib slats but cannot remove it.	Be sure older cribs have slats spaced 6 cm (2 3/8 in.) or less apart. The mattress must fit tightly against the crib rails.

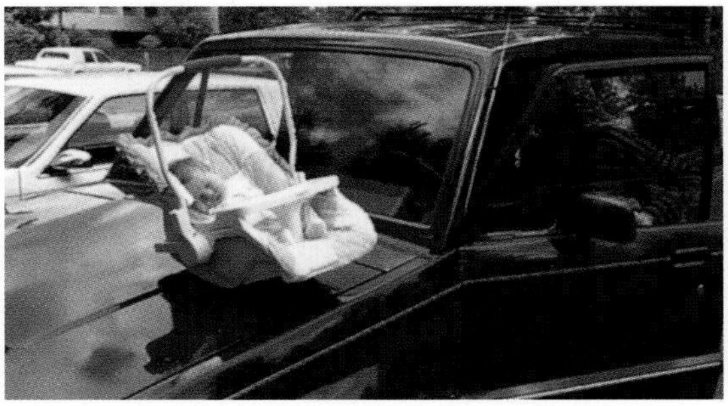

A Never leave infant unsecured or on high surface.

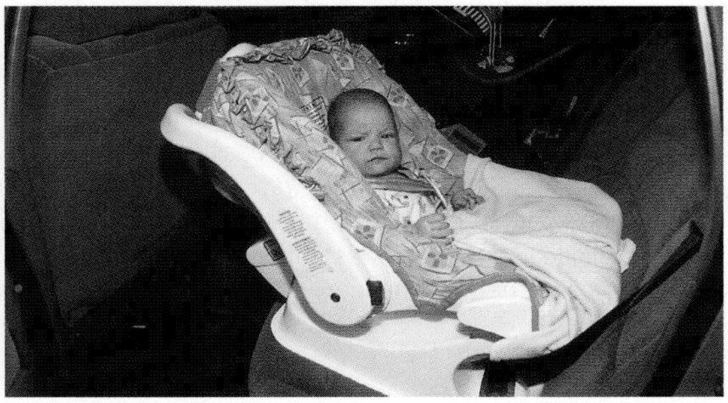

B Always use approved restraint system. Place infant in rear-facing seat in backseat of car

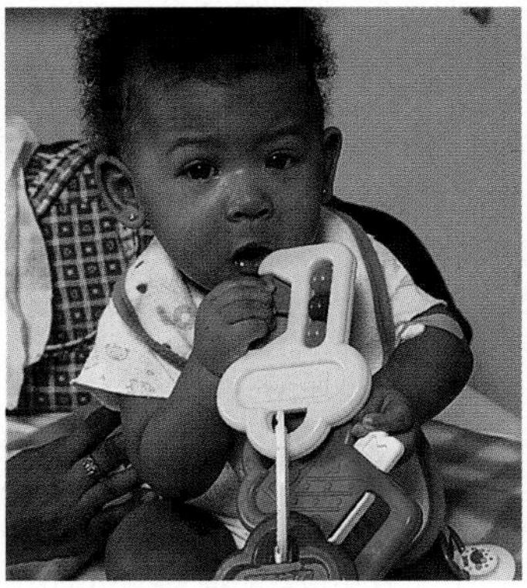

C Explores objects with mouth.

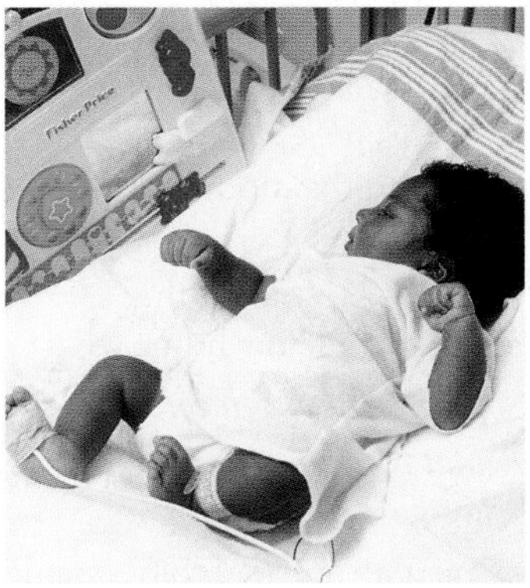

D Place infant on back for sleeping, keep toys clear.

Table 36–6 Injury Prevention Topics by Age

Age	Injury Prevention	Teaching Topics
Birth through 1 month	Use infant car safety seat. Put baby to sleep on back. Avoid loose bedding and toys in crib; avoid clothes and blankets with loose strings and do not tie a pacifier around the neck or with a string. Avoid tobacco use in the environment. Provide adult supervision of the baby at all times by trusted individuals. Test bath water temperature and never leave baby alone in bath.	Never place baby on high object such as counter, table, or bed; always keep one hand on the baby during activities like diaper changes to prevent falling. Wash hands correctly and often. Avoid contact with persons with communicable diseases. Have smoke alarms and avoid fire hazards. Learn infant CPR and airway obstruction removal. Never shake the baby. Have plans for emergency care.
2 months	Follow the above. Use only recommended playpens or cribs and keep sides up. Avoid moldy environments. Keep baby toys cleaned.	Avoid direct sunlight for the baby. Keep sharp and small objects out of baby's environment. Keep hot water heater lower than 120°F. Review emergency plan with all care providers.
4 months	Follow the above. Get all poisonous substances out of baby's view and reach; install locks to keep them inaccessible.	Do not use latex balloons or plastic bags near the baby.
6 months	Follow the above. If an infant-only car seat was used, switch to rear-facing convertible safety seat (intended for babies up to 40 lb) when baby is 20 to 30 lb or 26 inches. Empty containers of water immediately after use; be sure pools or other bodies of water are locked and not accessible to baby. Use sunscreen, hat, and long sleeves when baby is in the sun. Keep heavy and sharp objects out of reach; check that all poisons are locked away including in homes visited; keep pet food and cosmetics out of reach.	Do not drink hot liquids or eat soup while holding the baby. Have poison control number by phones and programmed into cell phones. Be alert for dangers of hot curling irons and other appliances. Have electrical cords out of reach and not hanging down. Have home and environment checked for lead hazards. Lower infant crib mattress if still in upper position. Install gates and guards on stairs and windows. Never use an infant walker.
9 months	Follow the above. Crawl on the floor and look for hazards at baby's eye level. Pad sharp corners on tables and other furniture.	Watch for tables, chairs, and other devices the baby may use for climbing to unsafe places.
12 months	Follow the above. Change to forward-facing car safety seat if baby is at least 20 lb; install correctly and have installation checked; place in back seat and never in front seat with a passenger air bag. Start teaching the child to wash hands frequently, showing how. Provide own personal items such as clothing and blankets to childcare providers; wash often. Change batteries in home smoke alarms and check system.	Turn handles to back of stove; use back rather than front burners; watch for hot liquids. Check care provider setting for safety hazards. Remember that responsible adults should always supervise your infant, not other children. Peruse home once again for hazards now that the child is more active, climbing, and walking. Check playgrounds for hazards and always supervise the child in a playground.

Data from Hagan, Shaw, & Duncan (2008).

strengths can be used to further promote health. Nursing diagnoses established during a health supervision visit of an infant might include the following:

- *Effective Breastfeeding* related to the mother's confidence and knowledge
- *Interrupted Breastfeeding* related to the mother's resumption of employment outside the home
- *Compromised Family Coping* related to recent role changes
- *Risk for Altered Parent/Child Attachment* related to anxiety associated with parenting role
- *Sleep Pattern Disturbance (infant)* related to frequently changing sleep routines and cycles
- *Impaired Skin Integrity (infant)* related to developmental factors
- *Risk for Infection (infant)* related to inadequate acquired immunity
- *Risk for Injury (infant)* related to design of environment
- *Risk for Altered Growth and Development* related to parental substance abuse

PLANNING AND IMPLEMENTATION

The nurse plays a vital role in successful health promotion and health maintenance activities. The newborn period is essential for building a relationship between parents and health care professionals that sets the stage for the months and years to come. Explain to the parents what procedures are being performed and their purpose. Encourage them to ask questions and share their perceptions of the infant's personality, development, and other traits. This will enhance their understanding that healthcare involves a partnership between them and the care providers. It will lead to trust that promotes their ability to share concerns honestly. The first year of the baby's life is a key time for establishing a trusting relationship with health professionals.

Recognize the importance of data provided by simple assessments such as length and weight. Analyze all findings to learn if the child is developing as expected. Much of the visit is spent in teaching parents about topics such as safety measures, providing anticipatory guidance related to development, assisting with integration of the newborn into the family, and relaying resources for support of the family in the community, on the Internet, or in other areas. Parenting classes, childcare facilities, and family planning resources are examples of common parental needs. Perform recommended physical and developmental assessment, administer screening tests, and give immunizations. Be sure parents understand the need for tests and treatments, and relay the results of tests to them.

Nurses who work in hospitals, emergency services, and other facilities are an important link in health supervision. Ask where and how often the child is seen for care. Check immunization schedules to be sure they are up-to-date. When the child is not being seen regularly, find out if the family does not know the importance of these visits or lacks resources to obtain the necessary care. Refer them to resources as needed so that they can identify a pediatric healthcare home. Some agencies that provide health supervision are equipped to perform home visits on a regular basis or in case of special need. When nurses make regular home visits to families with many risk factors, health outcomes are improved. Seeing the family in the natural setting enables the nurse to tailor interventions to the specific situation. Nutrition, safety, and other teaching is more effective when it matches the family's needs. For example, showing how to set up a stimulating environment with safe materials, even if toys are limited, is an effective nursing strategy. Ensure that home visits are performed whenever appropriate and available, either through the pediatric healthcare home or other community agency.

Before the family leaves the facility, be sure they have the next appointment scheduled. Summarize content of the present visit, emphasizing the family's strengths and the baby's newly acquired developmental skills. Sensitively list any areas that require work in the coming weeks, such as "baby-proofing" the home or encouraging the infant to reach for objects. Provide a journal or notebook in which the parents can record the infant's development and write down questions to ask in future visits. Suggest possible topics for the parents to think about, and provide books, brochures, and other printed material.

EVALUATION

Expected outcomes of nursing care for the infant and family in health promotion and health maintenance include the following:

- Parents state common safety hazards at the infant's present and upcoming ages.
- The newborn and infant demonstrate normal patterns of growth and progression in developmental milestones.
- The newborn and infant remains free of disease and injury.
- The newborn and infant are well adjusted, showing positive response to the environment and interactions with significant others.

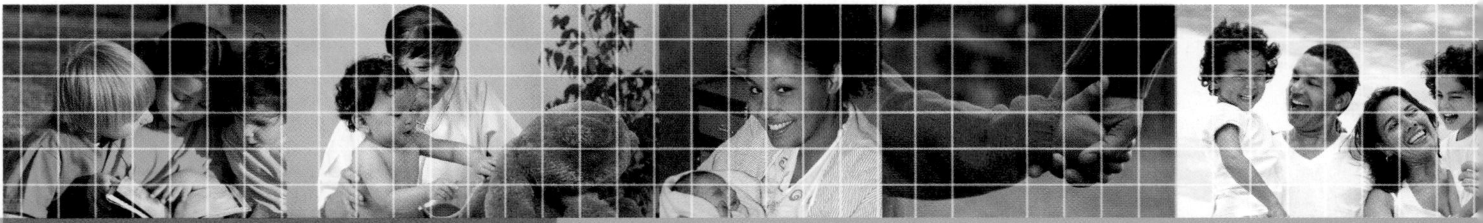

CRITICAL CONCEPT REVIEW

LEARNING OUTCOMES	CONCEPTS
36.1 Define health promotion and health maintenance.	1. Health promotion: ■ Activities that increase well-being and enhance wellness or health. 2. Health maintenance: ■ Activities that preserve an individual's present state of health and prevent disease or injury occurrence.
36.2 Describe how health promotion and health maintenance are addressed by partnering with families during health supervision visits.	1. Health promotion and health maintenance are integrated into healthcare visits. 2. Care provider adds identified information gathered at the visit which the nurse can then use to direct the activities.

(continued)

LEARNING OUTCOMES	CONCEPTS
36.3 Describe the components of a health supervision visit.	1. Assessment of: ■ Growth and development. ■ Amount and type of physical activity. ■ Oral health. ■ Nutrition. ■ Mental and spiritual health. ■ Relationships. 2. Conduct disease and injury prevention screenings.
36.4 Explore the nurse's role in providing health promotion and health maintenance for the newborn and infant.	1. Build effective partnerships with families. 2. Foster family-centered communication. 3. Address health promotion and health maintenance needs. 4. Manage time to provide for health promotion during routine healthcare visits. 5. Educate in family's teachable moments. 6. Advocate for children and their families.
36.5 Describe the general observations made of infants and their families as they come to the pediatric healthcare home for health supervision visits.	1. Do child and parent have close physical contact, eye contact, and vocalization during visit? 2. Do parents appear relaxed or stressed? 3. Does child behave as expected for age and situation? 4. Is parent able to effectively handle child being seen as well as any siblings present? 5. Does the baby respond to eye contact, movements, and vocalizations by the nurse?
36.6 Describe the areas of assessment and intervention for health supervision visits of newborns and infants—growth and developmental surveillance, nutrition, physical activity, oral health, mental and spiritual health, family and social relations, disease prevention strategies, and injury prevention strategies.	1. Growth and development: ■ Obtain length, weight, and head circumference. ■ Observe and interview family to determine if infant is reaching appropriate developmental milestones. 2. Nutrition: ■ Determine type of infant feeding family is using. ■ Instruct family concerning appropriate nutrition for infant's age. 3. Physical activity: ■ Assess daily routines and infant's ability to participate. ■ Provide instruction concerning appropriate toys. 4. Oral health: ■ Inspect infant's mouth. ■ Instruct parents concerning importance of toothbrushing. 5. Mental and spiritual health: ■ Instruct family concerning expected stranger anxiety and separation anxiety. ■ Explain need for infant to develop self-regulating (self-comforting) behaviors. 6. Family and social relations: ■ Encourage parents to play daily with infant and take a break when infant care becomes frustrating. 7. Disease prevention strategies: ■ Administer necessary immunizations. ■ Instruct parents concerning when to call the physician. 8. Injury prevention strategies: ■ Instruct parents in proper use of car seats and prevention of falls.
36.7 Plan health promotion and health maintenance strategies employed during health supervision visits of newborns and infants.	1. Explain procedures and the purpose of these procedures. 2. Encourage parents to ask questions and share general perceptions of the child.
36.8 Recognize the importance of family in newborn and infant health care, and include family assessment in each health supervision visit.	1. Health supervision visits begin with collaborative planning with the family. 2. Each visit should include: ■ Interview with family concerning developmental status of the child. ■ Observation of family interaction. ■ Discussion of parental concerns.

LEARNING OUTCOMES	CONCEPTS
36.9 Integrate pertinent mental healthcare into health supervision visits for newborns and infants.	1. Mental health issues to be addressed include: ■ Assessment of occurrence of common problems such as nightmares and temper tantrums. ■ Explanation of the promotion of a positive self-esteem. ■ Guidance in assisting infant in self-regulating behaviors. ■ Explanation of emergence of methods to assist child in handling daily stressors. ■ Instruction in normal developmental tasks such as toilet training.
36.10 Synthesize data about the family and other social relationships to promote and maintain health of newborns and infants.	1. Health promotion and maintenance activities related to social relationships focus on: ■ Increasing social skills with the people in the child's environment. ■ Successful management of temperament characteristics. ■ Adjusting to time away from home. ■ Improving language and communication skills.

CRITICAL THINKING IN ACTION

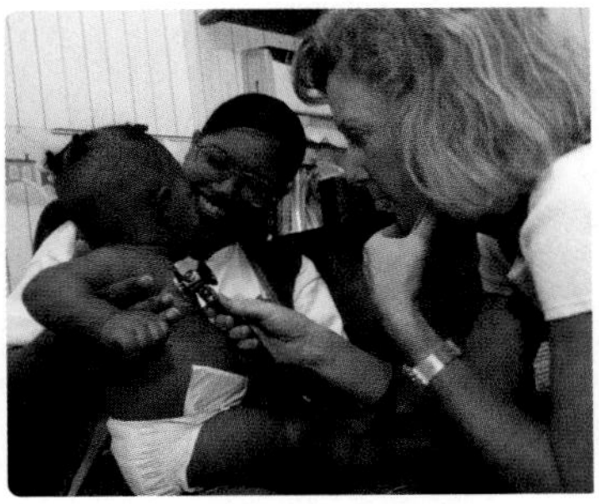

Sahil is a 6-month-old boy who is brought to the clinic by his mother, Clarisse, and his grandmother, who just moved into the home to help Clarisse. Sahil's father recently needed to leave the country on a prolonged work assignment. Clarisse is very nervous about being the main adult responsible for Sahil since her husband's departure. As you assess Sahil you find that he is smiling readily, is able to sit on his own with little support, and has length and weight at the 50th percentiles. His mother told you that she is breastfeeding and has been feeding Sahil some table food such as rice and tofu. She has returned to work so the grandmother will provide care during the day while Clarisse is at work. You review the immunization record and find that several immunizations are due at today's visit.

1. As Clarisse returns to work, Sahil will likely be consuming less breast milk and have more table foods and formula added to the diet. What questions will you ask Clarisse and Sahil's grandmother to evaluate their knowledge of dietary recommendations for infants? Compose a teaching plan that is appropriate for integration of increasing types of food into the diet of a 6-month-old child.
2. What immunizations are generally needed for 6-month-old infants? When should Sahil return for his next immunizations?
3. You have identified that Clarisse needs support and socialization with other young mothers. How will you locate community resources that are helpful to young families? Plan for the parenting information that would be helpful to build her confidence in caring for Sahil without her husband present. Suggest some ways that she, Sahil and the father can communicate with each other regularly.
4. The major health problem for infants is related to safety hazards. Sahil is becoming more mobile and curious. Write a teaching plan that includes topics and specific teaching requirements at his age.

See MyNursingKit for possible responses.

REFERENCES

American Academy of Family Physicians, American Academy of Pediatrics, American College of Physicians and American Osteopathic Association. *Joint principles of the patient-centered medical home*. (2007). Retrieved April 5, 2009, from www.acponline.org/hpp/approve_jp.pdf

American Academy of Pediatrics. (2004). Hospital stay for healthy term newborns. *Pediatrics, 113*(5), 1434–1436.

American Academy of Pediatrics. (2005). The Changing Concept of Sudden Infant Death Syndrome: Diagnostic Coding Shifts, Controversies Regarding the Sleeping Environment, and New Variables to Consider in Reducing Risk. *Pediatrics, 116*(5) 1245–1255.

Bircher, J. (2005). Toward a dynamic definition of health and disease. *Medical Health Care Philosophy 8*, 335–341.

Blackburn, S. T. (2007). *Maternal, fetal, and neonatal physiology: A clinical perspective*. St Louis: Saunders.

Centers for Disease Control and Prevention (2006a). Healthy Youth! Health Topics: Physical Activity. Retrieved May 28, 2007, from http://www.cdc.gov/HealthyYouth/physicalactivity/facts.htm

Centers for Disease Control and Prevention (2006b). Youth Risk Behavior Surveillance—United States, 2005. *Morbidity and Mortality Weekly Report 55*(SS-5), 1–108.

Centers for Disease Control and Prevention (2006c). Dental visits. Retrieved June 10, 2007, from http://www.cdc.gov.nohss/guideDV.htm

Centers for Disease Control and Prevention (2008). New CDC study finds gaps in breastfeeding support in U.S. hospitals and birth centers. Retrieved April 5, 2009, from www.cdc.gov/media/pressrel/2008/r080612.htm

Commonwealth Fund (2007). A practical guide for health development. Retrieved June 11, 2007, from http://www.commonwealthfun.org

Council on Children with Disabilities, Section on Developmental Pediatrics, Bright Futures Steering Committee and Medical Home Initiatives for Children with Special Needs Project Advisory Committee (2006). Identifying infants and young children with developmental disorders in the medical home: An algorithm for developmental surveillance and screening. *Pediatrics 118*, 405–420.

Dye, B. A., Tan, S., Smith, V., Lewis, B. G., Barker, L. K., Thornton-Evans, G., et al., (2007). Trends in oral health status: United States, 1988–1994 and 1999–2004. *U.S. Department of Health and Human*

Services, National Center for Health Statistics, Vital and Health Statistics, 11(248), 1–104.

Fine, A., & Mayer, R. (2006). *Beyond referral: Pediatric care linkages to improve developmental health.* The Commonwealth Fund. Publication no. 976.

Garfield, C. F., & Isacco, A. (2006). Fathers and the well-child visit. *Pediatrics, 117*, e637–e645.

Graham, J. M., Kreutzman, J., Earl, D., Halberg, A., Samayoa, C., & Guo, X. (2005). Deformational brachycephaly in supine-sleeping infants. *Journal of Pediatrics, 146*(2), 253–257.

Hagan, J. G., Shaw, J. S., & Duncan, P. M. (Eds.). (2008). *Bright futures: Guidelines for health supervision of infants, children, and adolescents* (3rd ed.). Elk Grove Village, IL: American Academy of Pediatrics.

Hall, W. A., Clauson, M., Carty, E. M., Janssen, P. A., & Saunders, R. A. (2006). Effects on parents of an intervention to resolve infant behavioral sleep problems. *Pediatric Nursing, 32*, 243–250.

Hoban, T. F. (2004). Sleep and its disorders in children. *Seminars in Neurology, 24*, 327–340.

Jellinek, M., Patel, B. P., & Froehle, M. C. (Eds.). (2002). *Bright futures in practice: Mental health* (Vols. I & II). Arlington, VA: National Center for Education in Maternal and Child Health.

Kenney, G. M., McFeeters, J. R., & Yee, J. Y. (2005). Preventive dental care and unmet dental needs among low-income children. *American Journal of Public Health, 95*, 1360–1366.

Murray, R. B., Zentner, J. P., & Yakimo, R. (2009). *Health promotion strategies through the life span* (8th ed.) Upper Saddle River, NJ: Prentice Hall.

National Association of Pediatric Nurse Associates and Practitioners (NAPNAP). (2009). *NAPNAP position statement on pediatric healthcare/medical home: Key issues on delivery, reimbursement, and leadership*. Retrieved April 5, 2009, from http://www.napnap.org/Docs/PediatricHealthcare.pdf

National Center for Health Statistics (2007). *Injury death and rates for children and teenagers by age, external cause, and intent*. Retrieved July 21, 2007, from http://webappa.cdc.gov/sasweb/ncipc/leadcause10.html

Pan, R. J. (2006). A Jacobian future: Can everyone have a medical home? *Pediatrics, 118*, 1254–1256.

Patrick, K., Spear, B., Holt, K., & Sofka, D. (Eds.). (2001). *Bright futures in practice: Physical activity*. Arlington, VA: National Center for Education in Maternal and Child Health.

Pender, N. J., Murdaugh, C. L., & Parsons, M. A. (2006). *Health promotion in nursing practice* (5th ed.). Upper Saddle River, NJ: Prentice Hall.

Schoenbaum, S. C., & Abrams, J. (2006). *No place like home*. New York: Commonwealth Fund.

Touchette, E., Petit, D., Paquet, J., Boivin, M., Japel, C., Tremblay, R. E., et al. (2005). Factors associated with fragmented sleep at night across early childhood. *Archives of Pediatrics & Adolescent Medicine, 159*, 242–249.

World Health Organization. (2001). *Background information about health promotion*. Retrieved June 6, 2003, from www.who.int/hpr/backgroundhp/

World Health Organization. (2005). From Bangkok, A new push for health promotion. *Newsletter of the PanAmerican Health Organization*. Retrieved July 11, 2006, from http://www.paho.org/English/DD/PIN/ptoday22_nov05.htm

CHAPTER

37 Health Promotion and Maintenance: The Toddler, the Preschooler, and the School-Age Child

Our school nurse is really great. She answers our questions about diabetes without making us feel like we're different than other kids. We can keep equipment like syringes in her office and she helps us to program our insulin pumps. —Jessalyn, 11 years old, child with diabetes

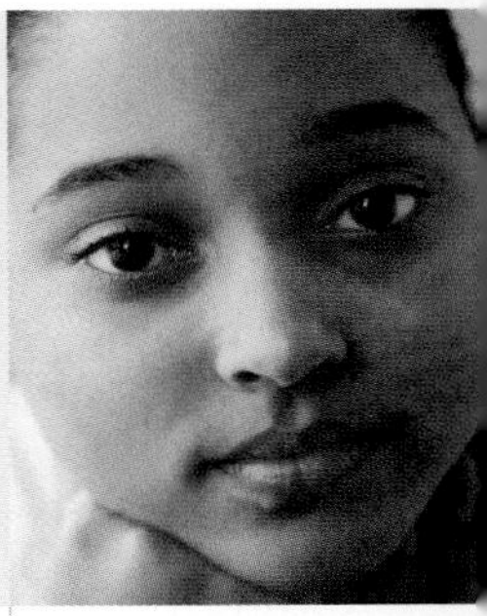

LEARNING OUTCOMES

37.1 Describe the areas of assessment and intervention for health supervision visits for children—growth and developmental surveillance, nutrition, physical activity, oral health, mental and spiritual health, family and social relations, disease prevention strategies, and injury prevention strategies.

37.2 State components of self-concept for preschool and school-age children.

37.3 Plan health promotion and health maintenance strategies employed during health supervision visits of children.

37.4 Discuss the importance of family in child health care, and include family assessment in each health supervision visit.

37.5 Integrate pertinent mental healthcare into health supervision visits for children.

37.6 Synthesize data about the family and other social relationships to promote and maintain health of children.

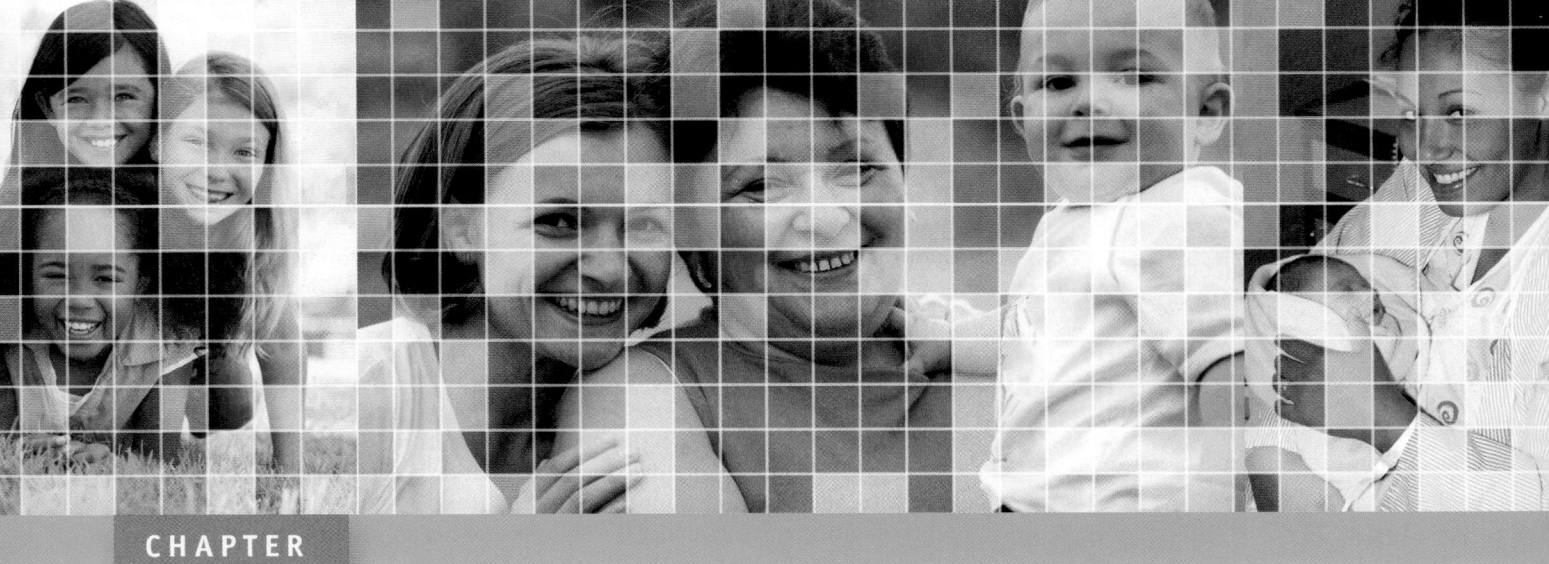

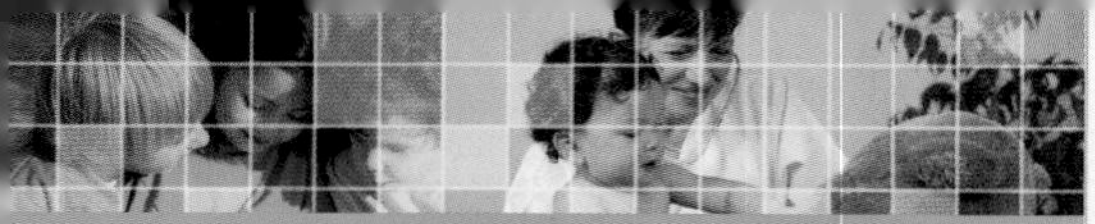

KEY TERMS

body image, 1018
deciduous teeth, 1006
early childhood caries (ECC), 1006
individualized approach, 1024
kinesthesia, 1005
night terrors, 1007
nightmares, 1007
population-based approach, 1024
self-concept, 1018
self-esteem, 1018
self-regulation, 1007
sexuality, 1018
sleep hygiene, 1020
spiritual health, 1021

HEALTH PROMOTION AND MAINTENANCE: THE TODDLER AND PRESCHOOLER

The years following infancy are challenging for parents as the child grows and acquires new developmental skills. The child progresses from the first tentative steps and words at a year of age through the "terrible twos" of toddlerhood and into preschool age when most children attend some type of education program, have well-developed verbal communication, and acquire many gross and fine-motor skills. Toddler and preschool ages are often grouped as "young childhood," since the family remains the primary system within which the child interacts. Care providers address common health concerns such as nutrition, sleep, and growing independence. Facing consistent changes in development, parents rely on the pediatric healthcare home (medical home) for advice and information. Regular visits are recommended for 12, 15, and 18 months, and at about 2, 3, 4, and 5 years of age. Nurses apply concepts of anticipatory guidance during visits for health promotion and health maintenance to assist parents in the transitions they face.

Health supervision of young children applies:

1. *Assessment*, using screening tests, evaluations, and observations.
2. *Education* that includes anticipatory guidance about coming developmental tasks.
3. *Intervention*, including parent counseling, home visits when appropriate, and scheduling future visits.
4. *Care coordination* among resources serving the family.

GENERAL OBSERVATIONS

The relationship with the family should be established as a partnership in care of the child. If, however, the family is new to this healthcare home, reach out to welcome them warmly and express interest in them as individuals and parents. Families often feel uncomfortable in healthcare settings, and it is important to establish positive rapport so they will be able to ask questions and bring up concerns about the child.

While calling the toddler in from the waiting room, it is wise to recall the child just 1 year before. It is amazing that this young child is now able to walk in, even if with a bit of help. Watch for the child's desire for independence or signs of continuing reliance on the parent. By preschool age, the child is totally independent in walking and usually engages in conversations easily. After welcoming the preschool child warmly, assess the child's social skills and motor activities. Direct greetings or questions to the child to evaluate stranger anxiety and ability to understand simple commands or questions. What verbal skills are observed? Observe the child's general appearance, nutrition, and state of health.

Health supervision visits are adapted for older toddlers and preschoolers to include observations of parental discipline and interaction style. Does the parent respond to the child's questions? Were age-appropriate toys or activities brought to the visit to help occupy the child while waiting? Is the child alert and observant of the environment?

GROWTH AND DEVELOPMENTAL SURVEILLANCE

An essential assessment integrated into the visit is measurement of growth. Weight and length are measured and compared to expected patterns of growth. Once the child can stand upright to be measured, sometime between 2 and 3 years of age, charts for standing height rather than recumbent length are used. Body mass index (BMI) is first calculated at 2 years of age and provides information about the relationship of height and weight (see Chapter 34 for additional information). Head circumference is usually measured until 1 to 2 years of age. (Consult growth grids in Appendix C.)

Growth continues to be a primary way of evaluating the child's nutritional status. It may also provide clues about conditions that have not yet been evaluated such as endocrine, cardiac, or other disorders. Depending on the results of growth measurement, the nurse may gather additional data. For a child under the 5th percentile for weight or BMI, detailed nutritional intake records should begin. Laboratory studies such as hematocrit and hemoglobin can be performed. Patterns of family growth can be examined. What size are the parents and siblings? Ask if the child has had any illness or hospitalization. For children above the 85th percentile for BMI, detailed dietary intake and physical activity history should be taken.

The physical assessment is performed, with some parts conducted by the nurse and others by the primary care provider such as a physician or nurse practitioner. See Chapter 35∞ for a thorough discussion of physical examination. The order of the examination and the approaches to the child are particularly important at this age. Leave intrusive procedures such as ear and eye examinations, and visualization of genitalia until the end of the examination. Integrate techniques such as allowing the child to play with the stethoscope, asking the child to "blow out" the light from the otoscope, or having the child make a game of pushing the legs against the examiner to measure symmetry of strength (Figure 37–1 ●). Preschoolers are generally interested in their bodies, and teaching about parts of the examination is helpful. During the physical examination, ask the parents pertinent questions. Consider the young child's expected developmental milestones (see information in Chapter 33∞) and ask questions related to these milestones. Developmental surveillance is integrated throughout the visit and developmental screening or testing is performed. Ask if the child has had developmental testing done at a childcare agency or another site.

Nurses generally have in-depth knowledge of child development, through growth and development courses and pediatric nursing curricula, and are thus well positioned to address parental concerns related to child development. Development is the key organizing principle of early childhood healthcare. Developmental screening and services should be integrated within healthcare, child care, and school settings, to include the multiple sites common for young children (Halfon, DuPlessls, & Inkelas, 2007). Topics pertinent at health supervision visits of young children include sleep patterns, discipline techniques, toilet training, learning and reading practices, communication, and parental issues and questions. Many children, especially by preschool age, are attending a childcare center. Ask about the experience and whether developmental skills are a focus of activity. Ask if the parent is pleased with childcare experience or needs further resources.

Health promotion growth and development issues for toddlers and preschoolers are addressed at each visit. Some common examples include:

- Explaining growth patterns and what is expected in the months ahead.
- Providing toys that encourage development of the coming developmental milestones.
- Showing parents the child's developmental progression on a screening tool.

Likewise, health maintenance activities are included in health supervision visits, with the primary purpose being prevention of disease and injury. Specific examples are included throughout the chapter, but some general areas addressed are:

- Connecting developmental skills with risks for injury such as drowning and car crashes.
- Recognizing the possibility of infectious diseases as the child begins a childcare experience and addressing recognition of and treatments for common diseases.

Expected outcomes for the child include normal growth and development patterns for motor, language, and social skills;

A B

● **Figure 37–1** Examining the toddler or preschooler. The approach to examination of the toddler or preschooler is important in order to elicit cooperation. ***A,*** The toddler may accept parts of the examination best when seated on the parent's lap such as shown in this photo of a boy with his father. ***B,*** The preschooler likes the opportunity to touch and become comfortable with equipment used, or in this case, holds a doll that receives the same examinations as the child.

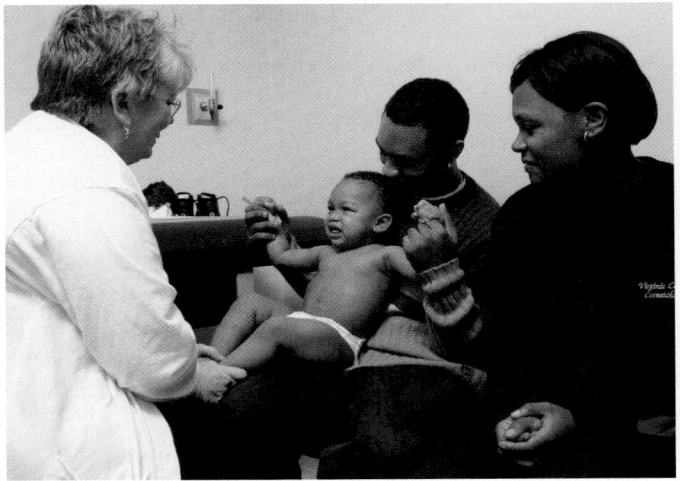

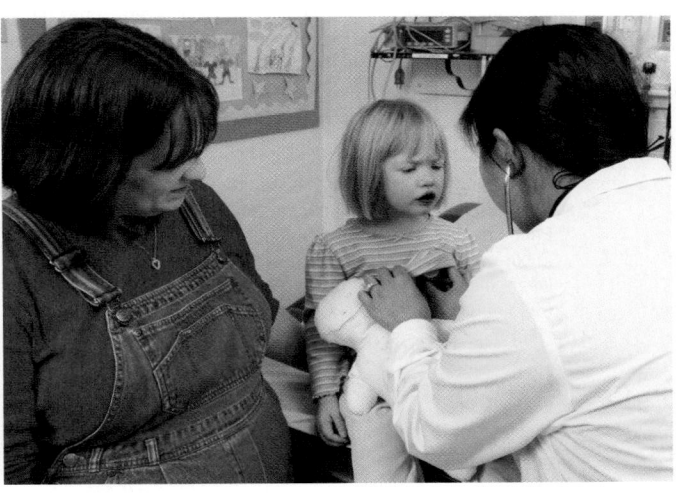

parental knowledge of stimulating activities for the child; awareness of the family about risks to growth and development; and healthy body systems for the child.

NUTRITION

The child's nutritional status continues to play an important part in promoting health and preventing health disruptions during toddler and preschooler years. Good nutrition fosters normal growth patterns, promotes developmental progression, and helps prevent disorders such as anemia, tooth decay, and immune dysfunction. Intake of food takes on an increasingly social dimension during early childhood as children interact more with adults and other children at mealtimes.

For toddlers, questions for the family focus on introduction of foods, the child's eating patterns, and transition from breast or bottle to other liquids. The toddler often consumes small amounts of foods, and parents consequently worry about the change in appetite. Showing them that the child is growing normally can help allay their anxiety about this common developmental variation. Preschoolers increasingly interact with others during food preparation and meal consumption. Questions focus on the child's likes and dislikes for particular foods, behavior at the table, and establishment of healthy family eating patterns. Ask how often the family eats out, especially at fast food restaurants. When parents are busy and older siblings are in activities, both toddlers and preschoolers may be eating foods such as french fries or milk shakes several times weekly. Suggest alternative approaches to the busy lifestyle, such as bringing fresh fruit slices along when an older sibling is at a sporting event, keeping a cooler in the car to maintain cool items, and limiting fast food meals to no more than one or two weekly. Obtain nutritional information about common fast food options in your community and share these with parents. Assist them to make healthy choices when eating out. Encourage the family to set times when they all eat together, even if only a few times weekly. If children help with preparations for this family meal, and then eat together, nutritional knowledge and intake can be positively enhanced. When the child is in a childcare center or home, encourage the parents to find out what food is provided for the child in that setting.

During the toddler and preschool years, children are gaining much more independence about food choices and patterns of eating. At the same time, their eating patterns depend mainly on the family and so assessment should involve the entire family unit (see "Developing Cultural Competence: Family Nutrition"). Parents can benefit from receiving information about nutrition in young children (Table 37–1).

Health promotion interventions include actions such as supporting breastfeeding for young toddlers and being sure preschoolers have a role in selecting foods for healthy snacks. Parental education is influential in shaping their young child's diet and should be integrated into all visits (Fuller, Keller, Olson, et al., 2005). Important health promotion teaching to include with every family is the importance of including "5 a day," or

Table 37–1 Nutrition Teaching for Health Promotion and Health Maintenance Visits

Age	Nutrition Teaching	
1 year	Support mother who continues to breastfeed. Wean child from bottle by substituting cup. If beginning to use cow's milk, use whole milk. Limit juice to 4–6 ounces daily; offer water several times daily; use plain water and avoid flavored water or sugared/electrolyte drinks. Encourage safety measures—use high chair with strap, secure child and use caution in grocery carts, do not allow foods to be eaten in car. Provide information on choking and airway obstruction removal training.	Provide food and water safety guidelines (see Chapter 34 ∞). Be sure all major food groups have been introduced. Limit high-fat and high-sugar foods. Review amounts of food commonly consumed and frequency of feedings. Review use of fluoride if water supply is not fluoridated.
2 years	Ask if the mother is still breastfeeding and support in the decision to continue or to wean child, as she desires. Encourage total removal of bottle if still in use. Ensure that all foods common to family have been offered. Offer child-sized eating utensils. Child can change to low-fat or skim milk if family desires. Limit milk to 2–3 servings daily.	Teach parents methods for dealing with temper tantrums over food—make food available at meal and snack times only, do not force intake, offer a variety of foods. Teach that child may have days of very low intake due to slowing growth rate.
3 years	Most children are weaned from breastfeeding and drink 1% or 2% milk. Teach normal intake and decreasing number of snacks. Engage child in food preparation and pouring liquids from small pitcher. Recognize that food jags (periods when only 1 or 2 foods are eaten) are common.	Recognize importance of social nature of eating; expect child to sit for a short period at meals with family. Meals and snacks should not be eaten while watching television.
4 years	Encourage involving child in snack selection and preparation. Start to teach food groups and importance of nutrition for the body.	Alter intake as appropriate depending on weight and BMI. Dairy products consumed should all be low or reduced fat.

Developing Cultural Competence

FAMILY NUTRITION

Each family integrates their own cultural backgrounds and past experiences into food preparation and choices. Ask what foods are common in the child's cultural group and help the family learn when to introduce each food. For example, rice may be a first food for an Asian baby, rather than rice cereal. Be sure the child also takes in adequate iron sources in the first foods offered. Tofu or bean paste may be a common protein source in some diets. A Native American child may eat fish or wild game, along with berries and roots. Ask and learn about each family's cultural patterns. Learn what you can about cultural groups in your community. Encourage the family to offer the young child their usual foods, as long as they meet needs for requirements, are prepared with minimal salt and seasoning, and are soft enough to avoid choking. Perform diet recalls and analyses to check for any specific teaching needs in all families.

5 servings of fruits and vegetables into the daily diet. Likewise, "3 a day of dairy" encourages families to provide at least three servings of dairy for children every day. Nurses and parents partner together to ensure that the young child establishes healthy eating habits at home and in other daily settings. Health maintenance activities focus primarily on disease and injury prevention, with examples of feeding practices that do not include common choking foods, and limiting daily fruit juice intake to prevent dental caries and excessive caloric intake. Desired outcomes related to nutrition include meeting normal growth and development milestones, maintenance of recommended weight, increasing understanding of healthy food patterns, and prevention of nutrition-related disorders.

PHYSICAL ACTIVITY

Both children and adults are commonly overweight and sedentary in today's society, so emphasis on physical activity should be a part of each health supervision visit. Nurses and parents are partners in planning activities for the young child; patterns set in motion at this early age are likely to continue into the rest of childhood and into adulthood.

The toddler and preschooler consistently show gains in fine and gross motor abilities. They move around independently and have more physical activity away from the home base. They commonly visit parks, swim, attend childcare centers, and help with some household tasks. These activities are important, both because they assist the child to continue to develop motor skills and because they limit the amount of time spent in sedentary behavior. The toddler and preschool years are an important time for setting the habits for physical activity during all of childhood.

During toddler years the main emphasis is on providing experiences that encourage further motor development. The child needs to walk, run, hop, push and pull objects, and throw balls. A minimum of 60 minutes per day of unstructured physical activity is needed (Gunner, Atkinson, Nichols, et al., 2005). Motor activity is a major component in all play times, and activities should engage the child's large and small muscle groups (Figure 37–2 ●). By the preschool years, coordination becomes increasingly important. Physical activity is important for all children, including those with developmental disabilities. The preschooler learns to balance, walk on one foot, skip, and throw and catch with greater accuracy. **Kinesthesia**, or the sense of one's body position and movement, develops during these years. Eye-hand coordination improves at the same time that visual acuity matures. The social component plays an important role as children learn to engage in games and activities cooperatively with others.

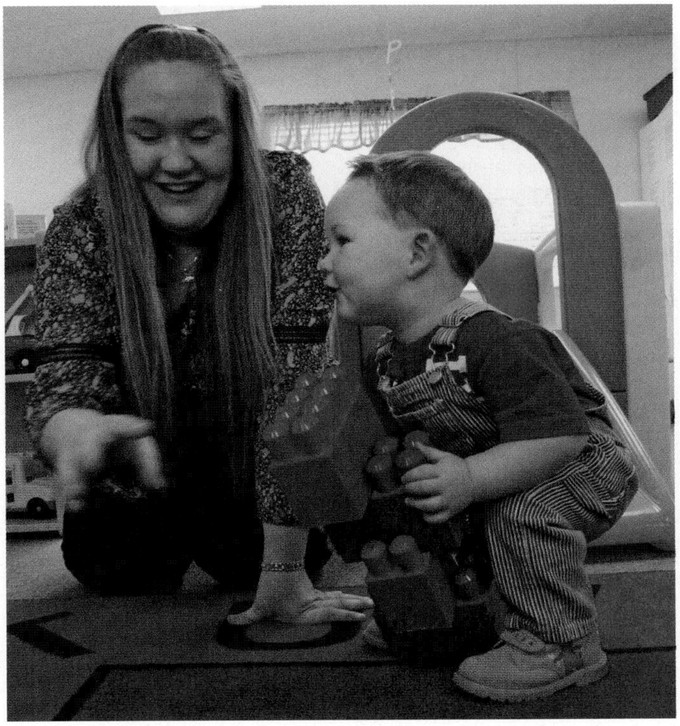

● **Figure 37–2** Motor activity. This toddler enjoys motor activity that uses large muscle groups. The preschooler begins to spend increasing amounts of time in coordination of both small and large muscle mass. List several physical activities that you can suggest for the parents of children in each of these age groups.

The nurse applies the concept of resilience by identifying both risk and protective factors related to physical activity (Table 37–2). The assessment becomes the basis for nursing interventions, both to reinforce positive physical activity and to make recommendations for changes where needed.

Since both children and adults are commonly overweight and sedentary in today's society, emphasis on physical activity should be a part of each health supervision visit. Nurses and parents are partners in planning activities for the young child; patterns set in motion at this early age will continue into the rest of childhood and into adulthood. Suggestions for the family may include setting guidelines to limit television and other screen activities to a maximum of 2 hours daily in order to facilitate adequate physical activity time. Children should not have television and computers in their bedrooms. Health promotion teaching imparts to parents the benefits of activity, such as a healthy immune and cardiovascular

Table 37–2 Risk and Protective Factors Regarding Physical Activity in Toddlerhood and Preschool

Risk Factors	Protective Factors
■ Developmental delay ■ Slow development of social skills	■ Expected developmental progression
■ Limited stimulation by family or other care providers ■ Limited social time with other children ■ Long work hours by parents	■ Easily engaged socially with others ■ Daily contact with other young children
■ Reluctance to try new physical activity ■ Limited access to balls, slides, balance beams, tricycles, and other materials that foster physical activity ■ Adequate safety gear for activities is not available	■ Eagerness to try new physical activity ■ Access to balls, slides, balance beams, tricycles, and other materials that foster physical activity ■ Adequate safety gear that properly fits child is available
■ Parents who have little physical activity on a daily basis ■ Lack of knowledge by family about child physical activity needs	■ Family members engage in daily physical activity ■ Family members spend time in physical activity with child ■ Family understands motor developmental milestones and importance of physical activity in childhood
■ Television or other screen activities are engaged in for more than 2 hours daily	■ Television and other screen activities are limited to no more than 2 hours daily
■ Limited community resources for childcare and physical activity ■ Unsafe neighborhood and lack of lawns, parks, and other facilities	■ Neighborhood contains access to childcare which integrates physical activity ■ Neighborhood is safe, and contains lawns, parks, and other facilities

MyNursingKit Video: Making the Pacifier Decision

system, positive self-concept of the child, and the child's learning of important motor skills. Health maintenance teaching focuses on disease prevention, such as avoidance of overweight, and injury prevention, with use of protective gear for sports.

Expected outcomes of health promotion and health supervision related to physical activity are daily inclusion of at least 60 minutes of activity into life patterns, normal developmental progression of the musculoskeletal system, growth in coordination, and appropriate balance between dietary intake and physical activity so that normal weight is maintained.

ORAL HEALTH

The early childhood years play an important part in the child's future oral health, and yet dental care remains one of the most preventable and common unmet healthcare needs for children in developed countries (Donahue, Waddel, Plough, et al., 2005). **Early childhood caries (ECC)** is defined as one or more decayed, missing, or filled tooth surfaces in a child 71 months of age or younger (American Academy of Pediatric Dentistry, 2005). This condition is promoted by inadequate preventive care, which can include diet, brushing, feeding habits, and lack of dental care. ECC is serious because young children with the condition are more likely to have continuing dental problems that can influence speech, cause pain, and delay development. Teaching prevention at an early age is key to preventing the problem.

MyNursingKit Video: Temper Tantrums

The nurse assists the family to ensure oral health for the young child. By 1 year of age, the child should have made a first visit to the dentist. By about 2 years of age, the toddler has a full set of 20 primary teeth, called **deciduous teeth**, that will be lost during childhood, beginning at about 6 years. Evaluate these teeth for condition and number. They help to maintain space for the permanent teeth, foster positive eating habits, and are needed for language development. Inquire about how the family cleans the teeth and ask them to demonstrate if the child has any dental decay. At the end of preschool, the first of these deciduous teeth are lost, an important developmental event for most children.

Based on the results of the assessment of the child's teeth, observation of language skills, and answers to questions directed at parents, plan interventions that will foster maintenance of oral health, thus preventing dental disease. (See Chapter 47 for emergency treatment of dental injury.) These may include referral to low-cost dental clinics, provision of toothbrush and toothpaste, demonstration to the parents and young child about proper brushing technique, and teaching about limiting sweet snacks and drinks. Remember to positively reinforce health promotion practices such as good oral hygiene for toddlers and preschoolers who brush, visit the dentist, and are careful to limit intake of sweets. Desired outcomes for oral health are eruption of a normal set of deciduous teeth, regular dental care, nutrition and hygiene practices that foster dental health, and knowledge of child and parent about oral health.

MENTAL AND SPIRITUAL HEALTH

The family plays a key role in fostering a positive self-image and setting the stage for the young child's mental health. As the family is called in for the visit, begin an assessment of the family's methods of influencing mental health. Observe communication and interactions in the family and the child's ability to interact with healthcare providers. Ask for a description of a typical day or what the child has recently begun to do. The child's sense of self and mental status are related to new accomplishments. Inquire about toilet training, tooth brushing, choosing clothes and getting dressed, using crayons, or other developmental tasks.

Toddlers and preschooler use **self-regulation** (the ability to soothe and comfort the self) to control anger, excessive desires for objects or foods, and other nonsocial behaviors. In order to assist the child in developing the ability to control and regulate self, parents often use discipline techniques. Ask about how the parent deals with the child who is having a temper tantrum or showing other undesirable behaviors. Reinforce positive ways of helping the child set limits for self and make suggestions when parents need assistance (see "Teaching Highlights: Positive Discipline"). The goal of discipline is to help the child develop a sense of right and wrong, and to learn acceptable ways of dealing with other people.

Adequate sleep and rest are needed for children to master self-regulation. Most toddlers have established regular sleeping patterns with occasional night awakenings. They sleep about 10 to 12 hours at night with one or two daytime naps (Murray, Zentner, & Yakimo, 2009). Parents have usually learned to establish clear routines such as reading a story, rubbing a back, and then leaving the child alone. Occasionally parents who work during the day may feel guilty about putting the child to sleep. Help them to spend quality time with the child after arriving home, and then to establish clear sleeping expectations. Transitional objects such as blankets or toys are important for the toddler and can be used during childcare experiences to provide comfort and help maintain normal routines. Some families prefer to have children sleep in the bed with parents. Advise against this pattern, but if this is the parents' decision, be sure they are aware of safety hazards such as suffocation in excessive bedding, injury related to falling between headboard and frame, parental smoking that could lead to a fire, or parental deep sleeping, or alcohol and drug use that can lead to such sound sleep that it is possible to roll onto and suffocate the child.

The preschooler sleeps about 9 to 11 hours and may have one or no naps each day (Murray et al., 2009). Some quiet playtime can be beneficial even for the preschooler who does not nap. At this age, some children develop awakenings at night and may need some assistance in falling back to sleep. **Nightmares** are frightening dreams that awaken the child, who is often crying and upset. Parents can reassure the child, rub the child's back, provide some repeat of a bedtime routine such as reading a story, and then allow the child to settle into sleep again. It is not advisable to bring children to the parental bed since they may start to awaken at night in order to continue this practice. **Night terrors** (or sleep terrors) are characterized by a child who cries out and appears frightened. However, in contrast to nightmares, the child having a night terror is not fully awake and may appear disoriented (Mason & Pack, 2005). Parents should quietly talk to and comfort the child, allowing the child to return to sleep. The child has no recollection of these events the next morning.

The toddler gains more independence in many aspects of life such as mobility and speech. The control over toileting is another milestone that signals greater independence and can lead to a sense of self-control. Ask parents if the toddler has shown interest in toilet training and how they intend to work with the child to attain control over bowel and bladder (see Chapter 33 for further discussion about toilet training). Preschoolers are

Teaching Highlights

POSITIVE DISCIPLINE

First, provide structure that enhances the possibility of desirable behaviors:

- Limit rules to those that are essential. It will be easier to enforce a few important rules than many that are nonessential.
- Provide an environment where the child is mainly free to explore safely in order to avoid constant cautions. For example, have adequate play space for toddlers with limited fragile glassware in the usual daily environment. It is easier for the toddler to learn not to touch a few objects when adequate objects are provided for play.
- Spend time interacting with the child several times each day. Praise positive behaviors frequently. Preschoolers often like to have charts with stars to record picking up toys, helping a parent, and other positive behaviors. Once a certain number of stars is reached, a reward, such as stickers or an outing with the parent, is earned.

When the child shows undesirable behaviors:

- Use distraction as the first approach and praise the child for selecting the new activity suggested by the parent.
- Tell the child one time that the behavior is unsatisfactory and what will happen if the behavior persists.
- Separate the child from a setting in which behavior is undesirable. Place the child in "time out," a separate place that is safe. Toddlers can be placed in a playpen or crib, while preschoolers are told to sit on a chair. One minute of time out per year of age is a good length of time. Once time out is over, provide a positive activity and move the child directly toward the activity.

When undesirable behaviors include other people, such as biting or hitting:

- Tell the child clearly that it is not okay to hurt another person. Encourage and role model proper language to explain feelings.
- Separate the child immediately from the situation and use time out.
- If there are repeated episodes, be sure the child is getting adequate sleep and food, has opportunities for active play that releases energy, and has positive attention from many people in the environment. Be sensitive to stresses such as a recent trauma or a new sibling.
- Encourage the child to "use words" instead of hitting or biting. Until able to do so on their own, parents can model this behavior. "You feel like saying, 'I am really upset that you took my toy away.' Let's use words instead of hitting so your sister knows that."

generally well trained for bowel and bladder with only occasional accidents. These should be treated with understanding rather than blame in order for healthy self-concept to develop.

Preschoolers are increasingly aware of gender and sexuality issues. They may ask questions about kissing, love, or their genitals. These questions should be truthfully answered, leaving the child with a positive sense of sexuality. Some exploration of genitals may occur, and children should be told simply that it is something that should occur in private, and then be offered other activities to engage them when with other people.

The family's spiritual orientation takes on additional meaning for the toddler and preschooler. They can participate in the family's faith-based practices, which enlarge their microsystem influences to include that of the religious group, thus reinforcing the child's learning about right and wrong. The nurse assesses the family's faith-based or spiritual beliefs and provides support for the family's approach, whether it is in established religious organizations or in the family's other meaningful activities.

Health promotion activities focus on development of a healthy self-concept in the toddler and young child by helping parents to set up successful play experiences, to praise the child for successes, to use effective limit-setting techniques, and to realize and appreciate the child's unique characteristics. Health maintenance seeks to avoid poor self-image that can occur with constant criticism or expectations not in alignment with the toddler or preschooler developmental capabilities. Further examples of the family interactions that can influence the child's self-concept are provided in the following section on relationships.

Desired outcomes for the child related to mental and spiritual health include emergence of a positive self-esteem, ability to self-regulate behaviors, emergence of methods to handle daily stressors, and normal developmental progression in tasks such as toilet training and sleep.

RELATIONSHIPS

Family members are part of the microsystem for the toddler and preschooler, and as such, form a vital part of the child's environment. Families with members who handle stress well and have healthy lifestyle patterns offer security for the young child. When parents are stressed or depressed, the mental status of all family members can be affected. Ask how things are going for the family in general. Inquire about siblings and whether there are any issues of concern that might influence the toddler or preschooler. Illness or behavior problems in a sibling can decrease the parent's ability to deal with other children. The focus on a sibling in need can be confusing to a toddler or preschooler. Be alert for signs of child abuse and for substance abuse in family members. Have the parents become separated or divorced? Is there a new stepparent?

During questions and observations, the nurse identifies family risk and protective factors. Reinforce strengths and provide services and referrals to deal with risks. Some strengths include the following:

- The family spends time together each day.
- Parents are proud of the child's accomplishments and knowledgeable about developmental progression.
- Childcare center personnel and family members interact regularly to plan consistent approaches for the toddler and preschooler.
- The teen mother of a toddler is enrolled in a high school continuation program with a childcare component.

Examples of risks to mental health include the following:

- Mother has been diagnosed with depression.
- Family member in home uses street drugs.
- Child awakens with night terrors.
- Child was recently in a serious car accident.
- Teen mother is estranged from own family and has few goals and resources.

Toddlers continue to grow in social abilities, while preschoolers demonstrate large strides in socializing with others. Expect that most toddlers will enjoy playing with other children, although they play "side by side" in a parallel manner and not cooperatively. They also engage in play with adults for short periods, such as throwing a ball. However, preschoolers begin to engage in activities that involve other children directly in cooperative play. They play "house" where one child plays the mother, and another the child. They engage in simple games where each plays a separate role. Their interactions with adults display similar maturity as they take on tasks such as setting the table for dinner or picking up books from the floor. Social skills involve getting along with others. Young children exhibit increasing skill in language development, a primary medium for social exchange. From just a few words at 1 year, the child has progressed to stating three-word sentences by 3 years of age. While all parts of speech are not in place, young children certainly have the ability to make needs and thoughts known. Assessment of language skills provides a mirror into this important means of socializing.

Successful social skills involve separating from the parent at times. During toddlerhood, most children spend some time away from parents. Initially they may be fearful and display crying, but gradually they learn to adapt to the new person and place. Preschoolers need to begin developing relationships with other adults and children in order to adapt to the school setting at about 5 years of age. Ask how many people the child has contact with each week and how they manage separation from the parent. Encourage parents to see separation as a skill the child is learning rather than something that is guilt-producing for them. When they leave the child in a secure setting, they should hug, provide a favorite object, and leave. Short periods initially will teach the child that the parent can be trusted to return.

Expected outcomes of health promotion and health maintenance activities with young children include increasing social skills with parents, siblings, and other children and adults; successful management of temperament characteristics; adjustment to time away from the home; and improving language/communication skills.

DISEASE PREVENTION STRATEGIES

Toddlers remain prone to many infectious diseases due to immature immune systems. By the preschool age, immune defenses are more mature and communicable diseases are less common. Some immunizations are given during this age period in order to complete a basic series. For the child who has not had all immunizations, extra visits to catch them up to recommended levels may be needed. At the end of the preschool period, the child has a complete review of the immunization record so any needed injections are given before school entry. See Table 37–3 for immunizations recommended during toddlerhood and preschool. Toddlers and preschoolers should be screened for health problems during health supervision visits, such as asthma, obesity, or other issues manifested by review of body systems. Earlier visits may have failed to identify a problem due to the child's young age, so areas such as vision, hearing, and developmental milestones are always included.

Recognize that the environment is a powerful influence on the health of children. Ask if parents or others in the home smoke. Discourage this practice and describe the health implications for the child. Is the neighborhood generally safe? Are there air, water, or other toxic exposures? Ask about lead exposure in the home (see Chapter 44 for more information). How much television and other screen time is common in the home? Older siblings who allow the preschooler to play violent video games or watch many hours of inappropriate television can be affecting the mental health of the young child. Do parents watch the evening news, even when it involves violence, in front of young children? Do they discuss television shows with the child?

Ask if the child has had any diseases, whether common ones such as middle ear infection, or less common ones such as a serious respiratory infection. Has the child been diagnosed with a chronic disorder such as cystic fibrosis or hemophilia? How has that affected their general health and family functioning?

Desired outcomes for disease prevention include integration of healthy lifestyle into the family's daily life, prompt treatment of acute diseases, and individualization of all health supervision topics for the child with a chronic condition or special healthcare need.

Table 37–3 Routine Immunizations Recommended During Toddlerhood and Preschool Age

Immunization	Age Recommended
Hepatitis B	6–18 months: Administer #3 if series not completed during infancy (usually #1 & 2 are administered in early infancy, with #3 from 6–18 months of age)
Hepatitis A	Series of two doses with first at 12 months and second at least 6 months later
Diphtheria, tetanus, acellular pertussis (Dtap)	15–18 months (#4) (first 3 administered in infancy) 4–6 years (#5)
Haemophilus influenzae type b	12–15 months (#4 or will be #3 for PRP-OMP type that requires only 3 doses for whole series) (first doses administered in infancy)
Inactivated poliovirus	4–6 years (#4) (first 3 doses administered in infancy)
Measles, mumps, rubella	12–15 months (#1)
Varicella	12–18 months (#1) 4–6 years (#2)
Pneumococcal	12–15 months (#4)
Influenza	Annually

Note: Schedule may need to be adapted if child did not receive all recommended immunizations during infancy. See Chapter 45 and the CDC and AAP Web sites for further information.

INJURY PREVENTION STRATEGIES

Injuries remain a common healthcare problem for children during the toddler and preschooler years. The child's mobility, physical skills, and lack of understanding of the presence of hazards put them at particular risk. In addition, children are sometimes left to play alone for short periods, and toddlers and preschoolers can quickly get into dangerous situations. Every healthcare visit needs to include an assessment of risks and teaching to prevent injuries. Tables 37–4 and 37–5 list injury hazards during these age periods.

Ask parents what they think the most common hazards are for the age of the child, and add other hazards to their awareness. Car safety always needs reinforcing as the types of seats recommended change as the child matures (Biagioli, 2005). Be certain that children from 20 to 40 lb:

- Use a convertible forward-facing seat that has been placed in the back seat.
- Have harness straps at or above the shoulders.

Toddlers and preschoolers over 40 lb should be placed in a belt-positioning booster seat:

- In the back seat.
- That uses both lap and shoulder belts.
- With the lap belt low and tight across the lap/upper thigh area and shoulder belt snug across the chest and shoulder.

Recommend that parents have their car seat checked by a childcare inspector. Give them the addresses of the closest inspection stations. These can be located by going through the National Highway Traffic Safety Administration (www.nhtsa.dot.gov). Check your particular state laws regulating car safety seats for children.

Other common and serious safety hazards are falls and drowning. In addition to providing general guidelines about safety, these most common injuries should be directly addressed. Children often fall down stairs, from counters where they have been placed or crawled, and from grocery carts. Drowning episodes occur when toddlers and preschoolers are not watched every moment while in the bathtub, near a pool or spa, at a lake or ocean, or when they fall from boats without personal flotation devices on. While all young children should begin to take swimming lessons, this does not guarantee their safety around water. Children

Table 37–4 Injury Prevention in Toddlerhood

	Hazard	Developmental Characteristics	Preventive Measures
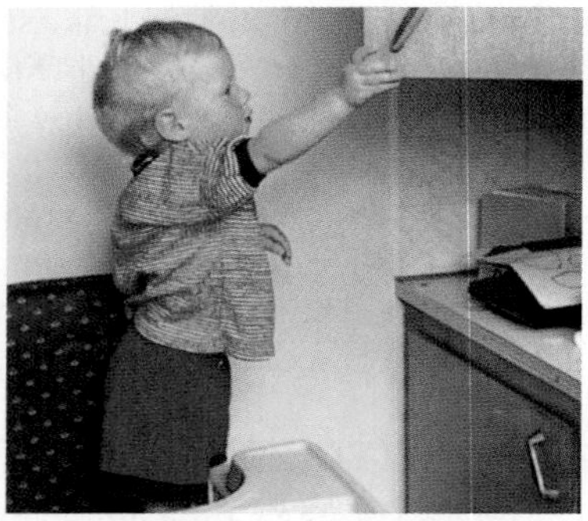	Falls	Gross motor skills improve: Toddler is able to move chairs to counters and can climb up ladders.	Supervise toddler closely. Provide safe climbing toys. Begin to teach acceptable places for climbing.
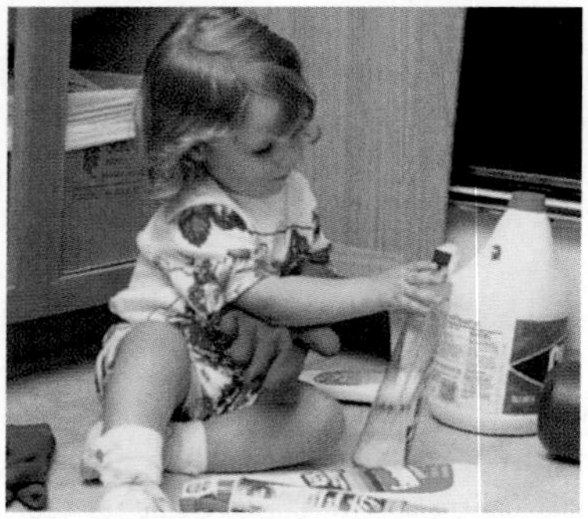	Poisoning	Gross motor skills enable toddler to climb onto chairs and then cabinets. Medicines, cosmetics, and other poisonous substances are easily reached.	Keep medicines and other poisonous material locked away. Use child-resistant containers and cupboard closures. Post the Poison Control Center number (1-800-222-1222) by telephone and tape it on cell phones and program the cell phone with the number.
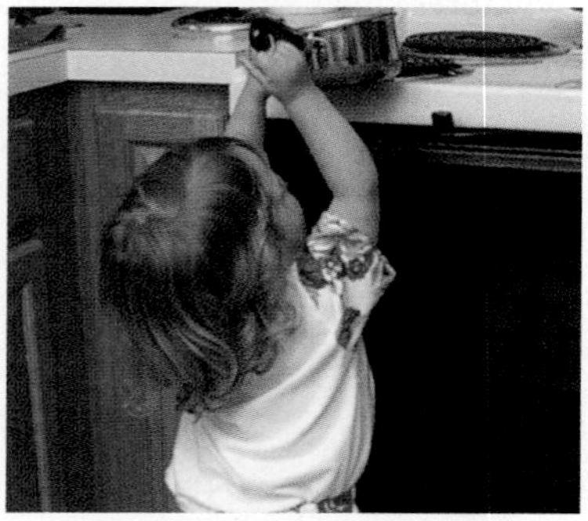	Burns	Toddler is tall enough to reach stove top. Toddler can walk to fireplace and may reach into fire. Electrical cords may be placed in mouth.	Keep pot handles turned inward on stove. Do not burn fires without close supervision. Use a fire screen. Supervise child during play and keep electrical cords, power strips, and other hazards out of reach or covered securely.
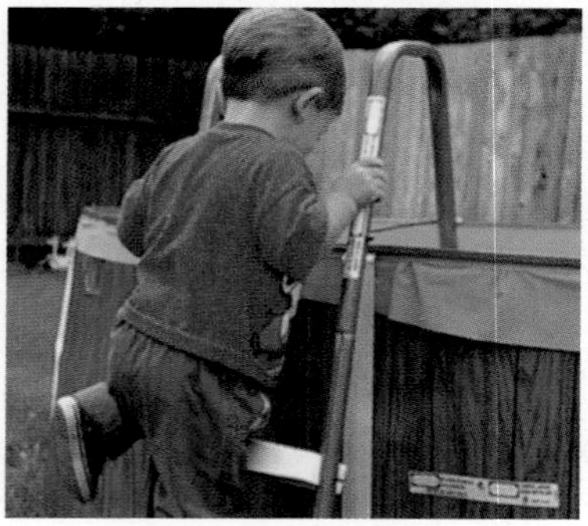	Drowning	Toddler can walk onto docks or pool decks. Toddler may stand on or climb seats on boat. Toddler may fall into buckets, toilets, and fish tanks and be unable to get top of body out.	Supervise any child near water. Swimming classes do not protect a toddler from drowning. Use child-resistant pool covers. Use approved child life jackets near water and on boats. Empty buckets when not in use.
	Motor vehicle crashes	Toddler may be able to undo seat belt, may resist using car seat, demonstrating characteristic negativism and autonomy.	Use approved safety only; toddler is not large enough to use car seat belts. Insist on safety seat use for all trips and position seat in rear seat of car. Verify that child is belted in properly before starting car. Keep the child in a rear-facing seat until at least 1 year of age and 20 pounds, but preferably longer, until achieving the highest weight or height recommended for the seat by the manufacturer.

Table 37–5 Injury Prevention in the Preschool Years

	Hazard	Developmental Characteristics	Preventive Measures
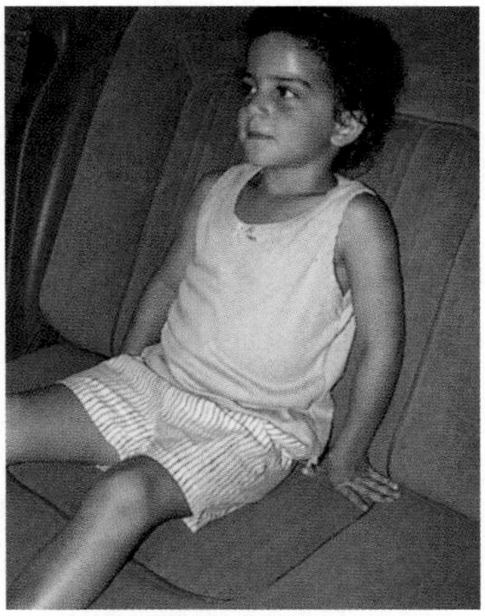	Motor vehicle crashes	Older preschooler independently gets into car and puts on seat belt. Child may forget to belt up or may do so incorrectly.	Verify that child is belted in properly before starting car. Keep the child in a rear-facing seat secured in the back seat until at least 1 year of age and 20 pounds, but preferably longer, until achieving the highest weight or height recommended for the seat by the manufacturer. Forward facing seats and booster seats are used in the back seat. These child restraint systems must be used until child weighs 18 kg (40 lb) and is 100 cm (40 in.) tall; the child who is 57 inches tall (8–12 years of age) can safely use regular car safety belts.
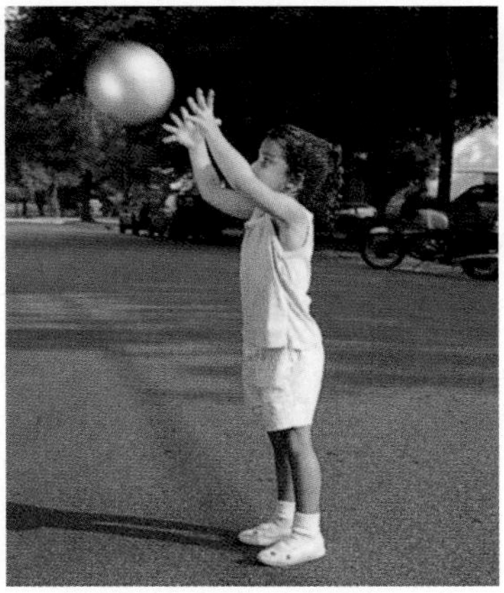	Motor vehicle and pedestrian accidents	Preschooler increasingly plays outside alone or with friends. Preschooler is unable to judge speed of moving car and assumes driver knows that he or she is present.	Teach child never to go into road. A safe, preferably enclosed, play yard is recommended. The child should be supervised by adults at all times.
	Drowning	Preschooler who has had swimming lessons may choose to go into a lake or pool.	Teach child never to go into water without an adult. Provide supervision whenever child is near water.
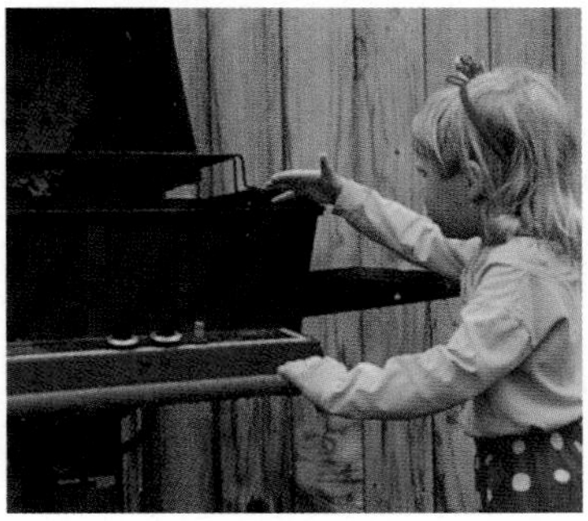	Burns	Preschooler can understand the hazards of fire.	Teach child to stop, drop, and roll if clothes are on fire. Practice escapes from home are useful. A visit to a fire station can reinforce learning. Teach child how to call 911.
	Needle sticks in hospital and home	Preschooler can ambulate and is interested in new objects.	Keep needles out of reach. Remove from hospital unit immediately after use. Instruct families on safe disposal if a family member uses needles at home (for example, a diabetic).
	Electrical injury in hospital and home	Preschooler is mobile and may trip over cords and equipment or may choose to examine them.	Avoid use of electrical cords if possible. Keep equipment out of major traffic areas. Cover any electrical outlets not being used for equipment. Monitor child closely.

also play with balls, and may follow them as they roll or are thrown into the street. Nursing interventions concentrate on relaying to parents the severity of the risk of falls, drowning, and other hazards for children. Teach them to be aware of the dangers and to avoid them, both at home and in other settings. Refer them to classes on first aid and cardiopulmonary resuscitation.

The child spends increasing time away from the parent. Childcare situations should provide the same supervision the child receives at home. Help parents to ask questions and feel confident in safety at other settings. For example, while parents may be cautious about gun safety at home, few of them inquire if a home the child is visiting has guns and how they are stored.

Preschool is a time when teaching can become directed both to the parents and to their children. Preschoolers are receptive to practicing street crossing and tricycle/bicycle riding skills. It may be helpful to have a place in the clinic or office where they can be taught basic skills such as handwashing or street crossing. Consider the time of year, climate, and geographic location and teach appropriately.

Nursing Practice

Young children die each year when they are left confined in parked vehicles. Occasionally children gain access to a vehicle and accidentally lock themselves inside. However in most cases, parents leave a child unattended, either forgetting the child is in the car, or remembering but underestimating the danger of heat effects (Guard & Gallagher, 2005). Nurses can be effective in instructing families to keep cars locked so young children cannot gain access, and to never leave a child in a parked car, either in or out of a car seat, even for a few moments.

Spring is often a good time to teach bicycle and water safety, while winter hazards may include wood stoves or other heating devices. See Table 37–6 for further information about toddler and preschooler hazards and safety teaching needed.

Desired outcomes for the child are integration of safe practices into car restraints and other daily activities, progression through toddlerhood and preschool with no serious injuries, prompt care for minor injuries, and increasing understanding by child, parent, and other care providers of the common safety hazards at this age.

NURSING MANAGEMENT

NURSING ASSESSMENT AND DIAGNOSIS

Nurses partner with other healthcare professionals such as physicians, nurse practitioners, and speech therapists to assess health promotion and health maintenance status of young children. The toddler and preschool years are characterized by much developmental progression, and strategies need to be constantly adapted to meet the particular needs of the child and family. It is

Table 37–6 Disease and Injury Prevention Topics by Age

Age	Injury Prevention Teaching Topics	
15 months	Wash adult and toddler hands frequently. Clean toys with soap and water regularly. Provide child's own bedding for childcare setting and wash weekly. Use forward-facing car safety seat if child is 20 lb; install correctly and have installation checked; place in back seat and never in front seat with a passenger air bag. Empty containers of water immediately after use; be sure pools or other bodies of water are locked and not accessible. Use sunscreen, hat, and long sleeves in the sun. Keep heavy and sharp objects out of reach; check that all poisons are locked away including in homes visited; keep pet food and cosmetics out of reach.	Have poison control number by phones and taped onto and programmed into cell phones. Be alert for dangers of hot curling irons and other appliances. Have electrical cords out of reach and not hanging down. Keep water temperature from 120–125°F. Have home environment checked for lead hazards. Secure the child in shopping carts. Do not let child have access to alcoholic drinks. Remember that responsible adults should always supervise your child, not other children. Know CPR, airway obstruction removal, and other first aid.
18 months	Follow the above. Bolt heavy objects securely to the wall to prevent them from being pulled down (such as bookcases and televisions). Be cautious of the toddler near machinery in the yard, such as lawn mowers and farm equipment.	Use a helmet on the child when taking the child on the back of a bicycle. Check batteries in home smoke alarms, CO or radon monitors, and check system monthly; change batteries on a scheduled basis as recommended by manufacturer. Ask care providers about discipline methods; do not allow corporal punishment.
2–3 years	Follow the above. When the child is 40 lb, switch to a belt-positioning booster seat, using vehicle lap and shoulder belt; continue to place booster seat in rear seat of the car. Teach hand hygiene after toileting and other activities. Clean potty chair thoroughly. Keep guns unloaded and locked away in a different locked place than ammunition; have trigger locks installed.	Teach how to cross streets. Provide a helmet for riding tricycles. Check playgrounds for safety hazards and hard surfaces under equipment; ensure cushioned surface.
3–4 years	Follow the above. Do not let child play unsupervised.	Know CPR, airway obstruction removal, and other first aid for the child who has become a preschooler.
4–5 years	Follow the above. Continue teaching safety skills to the child. Continue supervising when near streets or water sources.	Teach safety around strangers (never go with a stranger; find a trusted person such as a parent or police).

Data from Hagan, J. F., Shaw, J. S., & Duncan, P. M. (Eds.). (2008). *Bright futures: Guidelines for health supervision of infants, children, and adolescents* (3rd ed.). Elk Grove Village, IL: American Academy of Pediatrics.

important to realize that the parents are partners in the care of the child and that every health supervision visit should address their questions and concerns. Their observations of the child are an invaluable part of the process. As the preschooler becomes more verbal, he or she becomes another partner in the healthcare team. Ask preschoolers what they want to learn, what questions they have about staying well, and other pertinent questions.

Toddlers and preschoolers are examined for growth, physical health status, and mental/social characteristics. Development is an area that many pediatricians feel ill-prepared to address but which parents commonly want addressed. Additionally, developmental surveillance must occur at every healthcare visit, with standardized screening at 9, 18, and 24–30 months (Council on Children with Disabilities, 2006; Drotar, Stancin, & Dworkin, 2008). Nurses are adept at describing normal developmental milestones, evaluating the progression of children, and using anticipatory guidance to address parental developmental concerns.

Based on a thorough assessment, the nurse will establish nursing diagnoses that are appropriate for the young child and family. Potential nursing diagnoses established during a health supervision of a toddler or preschooler might include the following:

- *Anxiety* related to change of environment (new care provider)
- *Parental Role Conflict* related to lack of support from significant others
- *Risk for Delayed Growth and Development* related to lead exposure
- *Sleep Deprivation* related to nightmares and night terrors
- *Health-Seeking Behaviors* related to parental desire for safety information
- *Impaired Skin Integrity* related to hyperthermia (sunburn)

PLANNING AND IMPLEMENTATION

Based on the nursing diagnoses, the nurse works with other partners to plan strategies to meet the needs of the family. Explain that assessment questions are asked to provide a picture of the child that can be helpful in partnering with parents to plan health care. Reinforce the importance of the family coming to health supervision visits with their own list of issues. Work with other healthcare professionals to be sure all needs of a particular child and family are addressed.

Some teaching takes place as the examination occurs. Explain the height and weight measurements and what they mean. Relate them to questions about dietary intake and family food patterns. During the physical examination, insert information about common infections such as otitis media (middle ear infection) and share immunization information.

If the family has been reluctant to ask questions, reflect on the child's development. "Many children have trouble sleeping through the night; is that the case for Cassandra? What helps her to sleep? What is it like at her bedtime?" Developmental areas such as sleep, discipline, toilet training, and expected developmental milestones should be addressed. If the parents were provided in an earlier visit with a journal to record observations and questions, ask if they have brought it with them.

Health promotion activities are emphasized during the visit. Health promotion related to physical activity includes teaching about toys that encourage activity, such as balls, music, push toys, and tricycles (Gunner et al., 2005). Review nutritional intake and encourage introduction of new foods, healthy snack and meal choices, and positive eating for busy families (Fuller et al., 2005). Emphasize the importance of play to healthy child development (Ginsburg, and the Committee on Communications, 2007). Provide ideas for incorporating free play time each day. Apply concepts of anticipatory guidance as you address the child's approaching developmental progression. If the child will soon be toilet trained, provide information about possible approaches. If the child is learning to swim or has access to water, reinforce safety precautions near water. For the child going to a new childcare center, provide the parents with a list of questions they can ask the care provider, and tips to assist in the transition to a new setting.

Health maintenance activities are added to the visit as you give immunizations and screen for tuberculosis, lead screening, or problems with language, vision, or hearing. Provide instruction on use of nonprescription medications, including use of acetaminophen after immunizations. Precautions, safe dosing, and checking with the healthcare provider should be addressed. The focus of these activities is to prevent disease or to find it early before there are serious consequences. Whenever you find information that may indicate a problem, be sure to refer the child to the primary care provider, such as the physician or nurse practitioner. You may even recommend that the child be seen by another specialist such as a speech pathologist or dentist. Other health maintenance activities that must be part of each visit with a toddler or preschooler involve teaching about common hazards and how to avoid them. Emergency care in case of injury is also helpful information for parents, so first aid classes can be recommended.

Conclude the visit with some words of praise about both the parent's and child's accomplishments. Schedule the date for the next visit. List any resources helpful to the family, including the clinic/office contact information and emergency services.

EVALUATION

Parents should be asked occasionally to evaluate the care they are receiving at the health promotion and health maintenance site. Use these comments to monitor and adjust procedures as needed. The expected outcomes for nursing care of the toddler and preschooler include the following:

- The child demonstrates normal patterns of growth and progression in developmental milestones.
- The child remains free of disease and injury.
- Parents relay satisfaction with the pediatric healthcare home.
- The child manifests positive physical, social, and emotional adjustment.

Teaching Highlights

TOY AND PLAYGROUND SAFETY

Play is essential to the physical and cognitive growth of toddlers and preschoolers. However, toys can present hazards for young children and parents need to receive guidelines to follow in selecting toys. These include:

- Select toys intended for the age of your child, as indicated on the label. Some toys have small parts or can break into small parts, and should not be given to children under 3 years. They should not be too heavy for the child to manipulate them appropriately.
- Assemble toys as directed and check them frequently for breakage; remove all packing materials before providing toys for the child.
- Do not use older repainted toys unless certain that paint used contained no lead.
- Select cloth toys that are nonflammable, flame resistant, or flame retardant.
- Do not allow latex balloons and especially noninflated balloons to be used as toys.

C. S. Mott Children's Hospital 2006; Safe Kids USA, 2007.

Playgrounds provide a location for healthy development of children, but can also be responsible for child injuries. Home playgrounds are the site of most playground injuries. Some tips can be provided for parents:

- Surfaces should be composed of soft and loose material such as mulch or fine sand. The surface should be 12 inches deep and extend 6 feet around equipment.
- Equipment should not allow the child to be more than 5 feet off the surface.
- Strangulation poses a high risk so be sure to remove ties, ribbons, drawstrings, and other hanging items.
- Ensure that the equipment is intended for the age of the child.
- Consult the U.S. Consumer Product Safety Commission for playground equipment standards. Inspect equipment regularly.
- Always supervise the young child on a playground at all times.

National Safe Kids Campaign, 2004.

HEALTH PROMOTION AND MAINTENANCE: THE SCHOOL-AGE CHILD

The older childhood years span the time when most children enter kindergarten at about 5 years of age, and progress until about 12 to 13 years of age, when adolescence begins. Even though health promotion and health maintenance remain important during this time, less frequent visits to the pediatric healthcare home are recommended. In addition, most children are relatively healthy and need few immunizations, which may lead to only sporadic visits for care. Whenever older school-age children are seen in healthcare, even for illness or emergency care, it is wise to ask when the last "well-child" or health supervision visit was scheduled. Encourage the parents to make an appointment if the child is due for a visit. Visits are generally recommended at about 5 years of age, when most children are going to kindergarten, and then at 6 years, 8 years, and 10, 11, and 12 years. The visits during this time will focus on monitoring physical and developmental changes, establishing good health habits related to important issues such as nutrition, physical activity, and mental health; learning the importance of avoiding tobacco, alcohol, and drugs; ensuring success in school, family, and extracurricular activities; and fostering good decision-making and problem-solving skills.

GENERAL OBSERVATIONS

The first school-age visit usually occurs just before entry into kindergarten. During this visit the child has a thorough examination to be certain that physical development is normal, developmental milestones have been met for fine and gross motor skills, school readiness is displayed in social skills and language, and final sets of basic immunizations are completed. The child is often excited about the visit because it is associated with beginning school; some anxiety is often felt, as it may be the first time the child is aware of getting "shots." As with earlier visits, the nurse's observations begin as the child is called in for the visit. It is wise to speak to the child first, introducing yourself and welcoming the child and parents to the office or clinic. Many children of this age actively participate in conversations, making teaching and gathering data easy. For children who are quiet or look to the parents, allow more time for them to get to know the personnel, directing most initial questions to parents. This may be the first visit where the child is old enough to be a partner in the healthcare visit. Establishing positive rapport with the child will be more likely to enhance efforts designed to teach about health.

Notice whether the child brought a book, toy, or some other object to the visit. How are the parents interacting with the child? What types of speech tones are used? Is there mutual respect or are parents and child ignoring each other or having disagreements? The child should walk with symmetry and ease of movement, follow instructions about where to go and taking off shoes for weighing, and demonstrate clear language skills with parent or healthcare personnel.

By the time children come for the 6 year visit and 8 year visit, they are expected to be increasingly active in sports, school activities, music, or other interests. Look for clues about their interests as they arrive. Did they bring books or a CD player? What are the book topics or favorite types of music? Ask what they are doing during the summer, or what their two favorite after-school activities entail. Have them describe a typical day to obtain clues about their life.

Some children do not commonly come to clinics, offices, or other settings for health supervision visits. School nurses or nurse practitioners in school-based clinics sometimes offer health promotion/health maintenance activities in the school setting. A major focus of school nurses is making the environment conducive to health for groups of children. School nurses may:

- offer some parts of examination to individual children, such as growth and developmental surveillance.
- conduct health screening, such as vision, hearing, or scoliosis.
- work with food service personnel and administration to improve meal and snack quality and minimize unhealthy choices in vending machines.
- work with teachers to integrate concepts such as physical activity and self-esteem into classroom activities.

The nurse often links children with healthcare needs to other community services.

During health supervision visits, watch the parents' responses as children answer questions. Be alert for the parent who interrupts the child or constantly "corrects" what is said. Comments by the parent should involve praise of the child or looking to the child for opinions on certain topics. This indicates that a partnership is developing in the family and that family members work together and value each other. Direct some questions to the parents also. Ask if they came with specific questions or concerns that should be addressed. If the child has an individualized education or health plan (see Chapter 39∞), ask if the parent brought a copy, if the plan is still appropriate, or if it needs updating; facilitate a meeting with the school district about the plan if indicated. Allow the parent an opportunity to meet with the physician, nurse practitioner, or other professional in a private place and without the child present if desired. Be alert for family dynamics that can influence mental health status. Ask if there have been any important changes in the family and how they have influenced the child. During conversations, be alert for reports of separation, divorce, remarriages, ill parents or siblings or grandparents, recent or upcoming moves, parent job changes, substance abuse, incarceration of family members, custody disputes, or other issues. Integrate a family history of diseases into the examination. Such topics can be followed up with further questions, as described later in the mental health section, to learn how they influence the child.

GROWTH AND DEVELOPMENTAL SURVEILLANCE

As the child comes into the health supervision site, take height and weight measurements. Be sure to have the child remove shoes and coats. Ask the child and parents if they know the child's current height and weight, and if they have any questions. Plot the percentiles for these measurements, calculate body mass index (BMI) and its percentile, and explain the meaning of these findings later in the visit. Recognize that children do not grow uniformly; they have periods of slow growth followed by fast spurts. Similar to earlier ages, watch for children who have changed channels on a growth grid, and for those above the 85th percentile or below the 5th percentile for body mass index, and gather additional nutritional data in these cases (see Chapter 34∞).

School-age children are learning about their bodies, and so should be active participants in the physical examination. Explain what you are doing and why. Carry out a head-to-toe examination, paying particular attention to systems and skills that influence performance in school, such as vision, hearing, muscular strength, and coordination. See Chapter 35∞ for detailed information about the physical examination. Remember to provide feedback about the findings; families appreciate knowing that the child's vision is normal and strength is well developed. Tell them what findings are normal as well as areas that may need more assessment or intervention. Inquire about the child's sleep patterns. During the examination, ask for a description of any illnesses the child has had. Children of school age are generally healthy, with only a few upper respiratory infections or other minor illnesses annually. Unusual complaints may indicate a need for further testing, as discussed in the disease prevention section later in this chapter.

School-age children frequently have minor injuries. These might include falls from bicycles, skin rashes from exposure to plants on a hiking trip, bruises from a ball sport, and other minor mishaps. Be alert for more serious problems that may indicate a need for additional detailed data gathering and teaching (see the injury prevention section of this chapter for examples).

Developmental surveillance continues to be an important part of the examination for school-age children. Some milestones can be observed during the visit, while other information is obtained by report of parent and child. This information is combined with reports about school and other activities in order to establish that the child is developing as expected.

Desired outcomes for growth and developmental surveillance include normal progression with developmental tasks, absence of physical and psychosocial abnormalities or trauma, and integration of safe practices into daily life.

NUTRITION

Key concepts related to nutrition in school-age children are independence and formation of habits that influence the future. First, children are increasingly independent in food choices. They usually have strong likes and dislikes for certain foods. They may arrive home from school each day to an empty house and prepare their own snacks. During school, they choose what to eat from the school lunch or the sack lunch sent by family. They may even have access to vending machines or sales of snacks during school hours. While independence in food choices is growing, the child is greatly influenced in those choices by friends and the media. Foods that may be rejected often include fresh vegetables and fruits, since they get little media attention, and friends may not prefer them.

At a time when the child chooses many of the foods in the daily diet, habits are being formed that will affect nutrition and health in general in the years to come. Good choices will help to promote health—to maintain weight at a recommended level, provide nutrients for adequate growth and activity, and prevent onset of some chronic diseases. Conversely, poor choices can lead to overweight and its accompanying problems, lack of adequate calcium and resultant osteoporosis, eating disorders, or lack of energy for brain growth and optimal performance in school. The patterns established during this period are often influential in later nutritional status. Knowledge about foods, family participation in good nutritional practices, and access to healthy foods can all be enhanced by nursing intervention during this critical formative period.

Continue to perform height and weight measurement, body mass index calculation, and examination of percentiles for each measurement on growth grids. Slow, steady growth is the norm during the early school-age years; it will be followed by a growth spurt when the child nears puberty.

During the visit, observations provide information about nutritional status. What is the condition of the nails, skin, and hair? What is the energy level and reported physical activity? Does the child look lean or overweight? As the child nears puberty, there may be an increase in fat stores as a preparation for the pubertal growth spurt. Integrate some questions for the parent and child into the visit that provide clues about diet. While observing the child and family and asking dietary questions, list risks and protective factors related to nutrition. Examples of protective factors include adequate access to nutritious foods, a family garden, and weight and height within normal limits; risk factors may include inadequate access to nutritious foods, excess intake of calories during television viewing, and lack of vegetables in the daily diet. Reinforce the positive practices of the family and inform the child of how food choices relate to energy level, school performance, and general health. Risk factors become the basis for teaching and planning with the family for necessary change. It is difficult to tackle several nutritional changes at one time, so concentrate on those most needing attention, and on those the family agrees are important. Provide information about healthy snacks to keep at home, ways to improve calcium intake, the importance of getting at least five fruit/vegetable servings daily, limitation of soda pop to one serving daily, and the importance of family meals (Figure 37–3 ●). Desired outcomes for health maintenance include absence of overweight and other potential chronic diseases, adequate intake of all nutrients, and increasing child and family knowledge about nutrition.

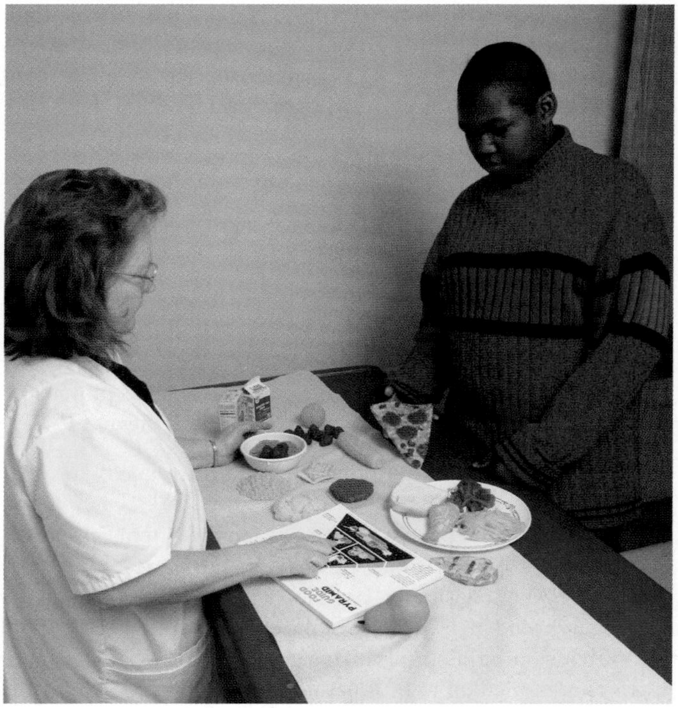

● **Figure 37–3** Food choices. This school-age child is receiving teaching from the nurse about food choices. What benefit do the food models provide in this situation? What other teaching techniques can you suggest?

PHYSICAL ACTIVITY

Just as food choices during the school-age years are likely to influence the child's future nutrition, physical activity during these years is often crucial to development of lifelong exercise. During these years, the child who is physically active continues to refine skills such as eye-hand coordination, muscular strength, agility, and speed. Some children become skilled at ball sports such as basketball, football, soccer, or baseball. Others focus on gymnastics, wrestling, horseback riding, or hockey (Figure 37–4 ●). Some do not like team or organized sports but choose roller blading, skateboarding, skiing, or biking. Whatever the interest, it is important that children identify some physical activity and continue to develop motor skills. The benefits include socialization, positive sense of accomplishment and self-esteem, weight control, and increasing physical ability (Figure 37–5 ●). Children who do not have an activity of importance often fall behind their peers in agility and skill, making future attempts at an activity very difficult and less likely to be successful.

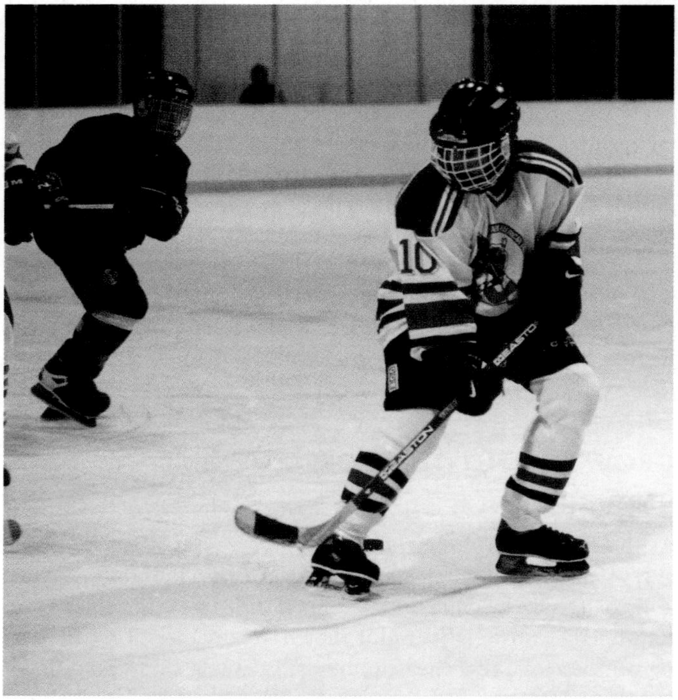

● **Figure 37–4** Physical activity. Everyone needs to be physically active. Some children participate in school sports. Others, such as these boys playing hockey, choose a sport that is available in the community. Other children prefer to walk, ride a bike, or engage in other more solitary activities. Determine what is enjoyable for a particular child and provide assistance in integrating desired activity into daily routines.

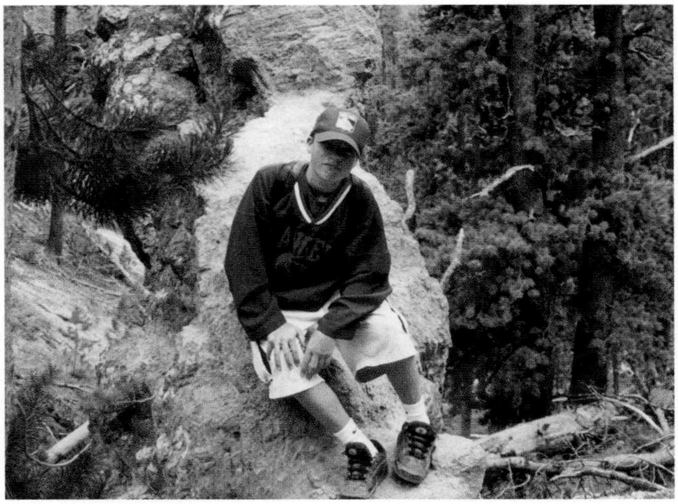

• **Figure 37–5** Benefits of physical activity. School-age children often enjoy hikes with family, clubs, or other groups. What are the physical and mental health benefits from this activity?

As in earlier periods in life, the nurse lists risk and protective factors related to school-age physical activity (Table 37–7). Families are often significant in promoting physical activity for children. Find out what the parents do for physical activity and how often. Do they attend a sports club after work or does the child see them engaging in exercise? Most families can include some walking, yard work, or other activity that is done together in order to engage the child. Do they walk to a neighbor's house or a nearby store rather than driving? Do they always take elevators, or choose the stairs in buildings? What is the activity level of siblings? When older siblings are involved in sports, the younger child often is encouraged to develop skills in the same sport.

The child spends much of the day in school, and so this setting is important to consider. In an effort to conserve financial resources, some schools have decreased physical education (PE) programs. Children may not have regular PE classes, and there may be few standards of performance. In addition, many states and provinces have established tests and standards for performance in certain cognitive areas. In an attempt to increase teaching time to meet standards, some schools have cut out recess and other breaks. Some schools are located in unsafe areas and outside recreation is not advisable.

It is unrealistic to expect children to sit for long periods without physical activity, and such practice reinforces the poor habits of inadequate exercise among children. Schools that offer a variety of activities, including intramural (rather than only organized competitive) sports, are more likely to encourage a wide variety of children to be active. At least half of the recommended 60 minutes of daily vigorous physical activity should be provided in school,

Table 37–7 Risk and Protective Factors Regarding Physical Activity in School-Age Children

Risk Factors	Protective Factors
■ Developmental delay and special needs	■ Expected developmental skill level
■ Limited role modeling of daily physical activity by parents and other family members	■ Parents exercise daily and exercise with the child some of this time in a setting the child can see ■ Parents set expectation that everyone in family will choose a physical activity and engage in it regularly
■ Limited facilities in the neighborhood to encourage activity, such as parks, skateboard facilities, rinks, ball courts	■ Neighborhood provides access to parks, skateboard facilities, rinks, ball courts, and other facilities
■ Inadequate financial resources to join clubs or pay for organized sports	■ Family has adequate financial resources to pay for health club or organized sports
■ Safety gear for activities chosen is not available due to cost, or child is reluctant to use the gear	■ Recommended safety gear that properly fits child is available ■ The child understands importance of safety gear and accepts using such equipment
■ School cuts to physical education programs and recess	■ Schools provide physical education each day with a variety of offerings; student gets to choose and set goals for some activities ■ Schools schedule recess or physical activity breaks twice daily
■ School tryouts for sports that eliminate all but the best players in certain sports	■ Sports teams are leveled so that all students desiring to play a particular sport, such as soccer, are able to do so
■ Reluctance to try new activity	■ Willing to try new activities
■ Worry about competence and physical appearance	■ Feels self-confident in ability and physical appearance ■ Sets goals for learning physical skills
■ Television viewing or other screen activities for more than 2 hours daily	■ Television viewing and other screen activities are limited to no more than 2 hours daily

Data from Hagan, J. F., Shaw, J. S., & Duncan, P. M.. (Eds.). (2008). *Bright futures* (3rd ed.). Elk Grove Village, IL: American Academy of Pediatrics.

along with an adequate amount of unstructured play time during recess (Institute of Medicine, 2005). Nurses are influential members of school committees and can encourage the integration of activity in the school day. They may be able to serve on a school or community committee, informing other committee members of the benefits of exercise to enhance cognitive performance and general health. Teachers and school administrators can be supplied with models of successful school activity programs. Nurses can often be influential in finding community volunteers to work with teams of students. Student nurses, physical education students, senior citizens, and others in the community may be able to help young children play baseball, tennis, or soccer. Other volunteers may teach stretching or warmup activities. Community partners such as businesses may provide protective gear or uniforms for school sports, especially if the business name can be displayed. In addition, schools can offer alternative activities that some children might prefer to traditional organized sports.

It is essential to consider physical activity for the child who has special healthcare needs. It may be difficult for schools to plan an activity for the child with cerebral palsy, visual impairment, or developmental delay. Search for other community resources and help the family to access them. There may be programs for children to ride horses, swim, ski, and engage in other physical activities. Search out the Special Olympics for children with disabilities [weblink www.specialolympics.org]. Imagine the thrill that awaits a child who has rarely moved quickly when riding a sled or sliding on skis.

To summarize, health promotion activities for the nurse includes teaching about activities that parents can do together, becoming active in fostering physical education programs in schools, acting as a positive role model, and helping interested children to partner with community resources for activity. Health maintenance outcomes include encouragement for use of safety gear and correct techniques to prevent injury from sport participation.

ORAL HEALTH

Many changes occur in the mouth during the school-age years, necessitating periodic examination. About 6 years of age, most children lose a tooth, usually in the front. Following that, all 20 of the deciduous or primary teeth will be lost, and the permanent teeth will simultaneously begin to erupt. See Chapter 35 for the schedule of deciduous tooth loss and permanent tooth eruption. In addition, the jaw line elongates and teeth move into new positions. Periodic dental visits focus on both the placement of teeth and oral hygiene.

During the health promotion visit, examine the teeth. Look to see how many deciduous and permanent teeth are present. Describe the child's oral hygiene. Ask how often the child brushes, flosses, and visits the dentist. The child should have learned how to brush and floss during preschool years but is now performing the skills independently. If dental caries or poor oral hygiene are apparent, ask the child to demonstrate brushing and flossing. Reinforce the need for brushing twice daily and flossing once daily. Provide toothpaste and toothbrushes as gifts during health supervision visits. Local dentists will often provide these supplies to encourage oral hygiene.

Thinking Critically

DENTAL HEALTH

The parents of 7-year-old Mario just moved to your city. You learn in a healthcare visit that Mario has never been to a dentist. You notice that several of his teeth are decayed. He has started to lose his primary teeth and has two permanent teeth in place. A dietary recall demonstrates that he drinks two to three sweetened beverages daily and likes to eat candy whenever possible.

Describe the daily dental hygiene that Mario should be practicing. Plan a teaching session for Mario and his parents. What other cues will you look for in his dietary recall in order to identify risk and protective factors for oral health? How will you locate resources in the community to recommend for the family so that Mario can receive dental care?

See MyNursingKit for possible responses.

Dental visits are recommended every 6 months. If the child is not visiting on that schedule, ask if finances or transportation is an issue, if the family needs a referral to a dentist, or if there is some other reason. If caries or malocclusion is present, stress the need for a dental appointment soon. Inquire about use of fluoride if the water supply is not fluoridated. Ask if the child has had sealants applied to the permanent teeth; these will help to prevent future caries. Offer to help parents locate resources to assist with dental care expenses if needed. State and community programs are often available to assist families and nurses should search out resources in their own communities and regions.

Many children have a high intake of sugared foods and snacks. If this is apparent from the nutritional assessment, discuss the importance of limiting these foods and brushing after their consumption. Frequent brushing is needed when the child has braces. Ask how they are caring for the braces and what the orthodontist has recommended.

The nurse's health promotion activities include positive reinforcement of good hygiene habits, and health maintenance involves teaching about the need for improved care and limiting food that furthers the formation of caries. Desired outcomes include proper oral hygiene, attendance at recommended dental visits, and absence of dental caries.

MENTAL AND SPIRITUAL HEALTH

Self-Esteem and Self-Concept

The school-age years are marked by the emergence of new cognitive skills and the development of self-esteem. **Self-esteem** reflects feelings of self-worth or value. **Self-concept** refers to evaluations of the self in certain specific areas, such as those related to academic achievement, athletic ability, physical appearance, and social interactions (Santrock, 2007). A child with a positive self-concept feels competent, is able to meet challenges, and applies lessons from successes and failures. Specific facets of self-concept include **body image**, the idea that one forms about one's body, and **sexuality**, the person's view of self as a sexual being. Together, self-concept and self-esteem include all

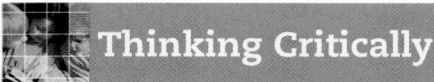

Teaching Highlights

EVALUATING AND FOSTERING SELF-ESTEEM

Parents play an important part in fostering the child's self-esteem. The nurse can ask them to evaluate the child and provide suggestions about positive actions.

EVALUATION QUESTIONS	POSITIVE ACTIONS
What does your child do well?	Build on the child's strengths and talents; point out the child's abilities.
How does your child respond to failure?	Assist the child to assess performance; help the child see that mistakes are expected and have lessons to teach.
Does your child have close friends?	Arrange structured play times such as going to a movie or cooking with a friend.
How does your child respond to new challenges?	Give the child responsibilities at home; encourage your child to try new experiences; help the child feel a sense of control over outcomes.
How does your own personality compare to your child's?	Recognize differences in style; appreciate the unique qualities of the child; tailor expectations to the child and not to self or other children.
Are you setting reasonable and attainable expectations for your child?	Ask the child what is attainable; establish goals for behaviors together.

Data from Spratt, E. (2002). Assessing and reinforcing your child's self-esteem. In M. Jellinek, B. P. Patel, & M. C. Froehle (Eds.), *Bright futures in practice: Mental health—Volume II. Tool kit* (p. 94). Arlington, VA: National Center for Education in Maternal and Child Health.

of the cognitive, emotional, spiritual, sexual, and physical aspects of the individual.

The child who believes in his or her ability to face good times and bad has a lowered chance of mental illness such as depression, eating disorder, and anxiety. Parents are encouraged to evaluate and help to build the child's sense of self-esteem (see "Teaching Highlights: Evaluating and Fostering Self-Esteem").

Many of the areas discussed already in this chapter provide clues to the child's self-concept. Does the child take part in sports or other physical activities? Such activity may reflect a positive self-concept and body image. However, if the child is forced to do these sports by parents and feels inadequate in their performance, these activities may promote a negative self-concept and body image. Ask about children's activities and how they feel about them. Do they enjoy them? How do they rate their performance?

Is the child increasingly independent and responsible for self? Success in achieving developmental milestones leads to a positive sense of self-esteem in the child. Parents are encouraged to evaluate and help to build the child's sense of self-esteem. A low sense of self-esteem is noted when the child states a disinterest in exercise, school clubs, and family activities. This can lead to loneliness, depression, and mental health problems such as eating disorders. When these feelings are noted during a health supervision visit, the nurse should recommend that the child see a counselor at school or another setting, and should recommend that parents be included in the sessions so that they can best help the child.

It is obvious that the family plays a critical part in the child's developing self-esteem and mental health. In order to understand the child, it is necessary to ask questions about and explore dynamics in the family. Several protective factors have been identified for families:

- Communication is open and clear.
- Parents use a variety of problem-solving skills.
- Members are encouraged, appreciated, and feel understood.
- Rules and expectations are consistent and fair.
- Family is committed to each other, including spending time together.
- Religious or spiritual orientation is present.
- Social connectedness, support, or extended family is available.
- Resilience or the ability to adapt to new situations and challenges is present (Cole, Clark, & Gable, 2007).

School-age children continue to develop their abilities to self-regulate activities and responses to situations. At this age the abilities to solve problems and assume more responsibility for self are important. Encourage parents to discuss issues with the child and to seek solutions together when appropriate. The child assumes more responsibility for assisting with meal preparation and home chores, coming home alone after school, and caring for younger siblings. Encourage the parents to praise the child for assuming more family responsibilities and recognize that the child will need some guidance when taking on new tasks.

Ask about and observe the family's relationships. Evaluate the effect of family interactions on the child. Model respectful interchanges by listening carefully to the child, as well as the parent. Gently speak directly to the child if parents answer for the child or seem to put him or her down. Provide brochures and examples of ways to show children their importance. Encourage both parents to come to child healthcare visits and support the involvement of both parents in childrearing. Ask about family stressors such as job changes, financial concerns, illness, substance abuse, and domestic violence. About one half of marriages end in divorce, so be prepared to offer suggestions to deal with this situation (see Chapter 36 for further discussion of effects of divorce on children). Ask about and identify risk factors and protective factors. The child's strengths are used to assist the family functioning and will, in turn, give the child a sense of accomplishment. Some examples include the following:

- A child who is able to act independently can be given responsibility for parts of the home or family function, such as planning the menu for dinner two evenings weekly.
- A creative child can be given the task of planning books and other activities for a younger sibling.
- A child with a talent for design can be asked to set the table for dinner guests.

Sexuality and Sexuality Education

The school-age child is developing a sense of body image and sexuality. Look at the child's appearance and dress. Some children may have poor posture, display a sense of insecurity, and seem uncomfortable with themselves. Others may dress as if they were much older, seem sophisticated, and are clearly assuming the role identification with their gender group. Ask the parents in a private setting what observations they have about the child's body image and sexuality. Inquire about friends in whom the child seems romantically or sexually interested, and whether the parent has concerns.

Questions related to sexuality will emerge during school years. They should be answered truthfully and fully. Even children who do not ask questions usually need information related to sexuality education. They may get information in school beginning in about fourth grade, but often still have misconceptions about the bodies of men and women, sexual intercourse, how babies are born, and other topics. Suggest that parents read books with their children that deal with these issues at a level children understand. If books are available at home, children will be likely to look at them and ask questions. They should be in the home from third grade on since many young girls have body changes as early as 9 or 10 years of age (see Chapter 35). This can often put both parent and child at ease and open the door to discussion. Parents should be advised to talk with teachers to learn what is presented in school and be able to supplement and clarify this information. Having discussions at a young age will help lead to further discussion as the child gets older. Nurses often perform sexuality education in schools or work with school districts in establishing policies regarding sexuality education plans. [Weblink to Sexuality Information and Education Council of the United States (SIECUS) www.siecus.org]

Suggest to parents that computers and other media provide information that can confuse children. Encourage them to watch movies with their children, encourage frank discussions related to sexuality observed, and answer questions truthfully. Children generally learn about topics such as sexual intercourse, homosexuality, and childbirth from school discussions and the media. It is better to learn from parents than from friends or the media. A few moments alone with parents and the child separately at healthcare visits may help to identify the concerns of each related to sexuality.

By about fourth to sixth grades, most girls have started to have prepubertal body changes and may have begun to menstruate. This is another opening to discussions about mature bodies of men and women and the transformation from childhood to greater maturity. Boys mature about 2 years later than girls. Without an event such as menstruation, parents may be less likely to start discussions with male children. Suggest that parents consciously begin conversations with boys periodically to explain changes they see in themselves and their peers. See Chapter 35 for further discussion of the body changes seen in the prepubertal period and during puberty.

Sleep

Sleep is still important for children in order to have the energy to perform well in school and other activities. They generally take charge of bedtime routines with reminders about the time to go to sleep, and they sleep through the night. Sleep time varies from 8 to 12 hours, depending on child and activity level. Busy schedules may interrupt this pattern, leading to irritability, lack of concentration, or even hyperactive behavior. Help children and families plan for healthy practices of **sleep hygiene**, or behaviors that foster a regular and sufficient sleep pattern, as well as daytime alertness (Edelman & Mandle, 2006; LeBourgeois, Giannotti, Cortesi, et al., 2005).

Sleepwalking and sleep talking sometimes occur at this age, but usually decrease as the child nears adolescence. Children who have

Teaching Highlights

SLEEP HYGIENE

Nurses should inquire about the sleep patterns and amount of sleep that children receive. Ask if they are frequently tired or have trouble sleeping. Some simple behaviors help to promote sleep and are referred to as sleep hygiene. They include:

- Go to bed and get up at approximately the same time each day, including weekends.
- Follow a bedtime routine to prepare for sleep.
- Recognize that we do not "make up" sleep that is "lost" by sleeping in.
- Avoid caffeine, including tea, coffee, and carbonated beverages for several hours before sleep.
- Avoid exposure to alcohol or tobacco for several hours before sleep.
- Gradually slow down activity about an hour or two before bedtime.
- Do not watch television, play games, text on the phone or conduct other activities in the sleep location.
- Avoid naps in the late afternoon or evening.
- Darken the room for sleep.

LeBourgeois et al., 2005.

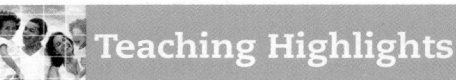

stress at home, such as parental fighting, ill family members, or inadequate food or shelter, may not get enough sleep and fall asleep at school. Ask the child if he or she is falling asleep in class, and seek additional information about family stressors. This can lead to interventions such as recommending family counseling or referring to resources to obtain better housing or more stable food sources.

School

School is a major microsystem influence in the lives of children, and it plays a role in self-concept and mental health formation. The child is usually ready for kindergarten when:

- communication and cognitive skills are sufficient to support learning.
- the child can successfully separate from parents.
- experiences with other children show ability to make friends and regulate own behavior.
- the child can follow rules and directions (Hagan et al., 2008).

Help parents learn ways that they can facilitate a healthy transition to school, such as ensuring good sleep and eating routines, reading with the child, showing interest in school activities, and finding a space in the home for the child's school-related work (American Academy of Pediatrics, 2007a).

When examining a school-age child ask for a description of a best friend. If the child is unable to provide this, isolation may be occurring. Inquire about what the three best and three worst things are about school. Children with low self-concepts often have trouble talking about and evaluating school. Find out where the child attends school, if the area is generally safe, and how the child gets to school. Encourage the parents to meet the child's teachers, to become active in school activities, and to be available to solve problems with school personnel when needed. Partner with the parents and child when interventions are needed. An office nurse may contact a school nurse when the child needs support in the school environment. This may occur if the child has become ill and missed school, has family stressors, does not get along well with a teacher, or has a condition such as attention deficit disorder. Identify the risk and protective factors in the school environment and plan interventions to support the child when risks are present.

Evaluating Mental Health and Spiritual Health

Certain mental health disorders are commonly seen during the school years. One example includes anxiety problems that result in worries, fears, physical symptoms, stress, and sleep disorders without significantly impairing daily functioning. However, some anxiety disorders affect functioning and have more striking characteristics such as clinging, abdominal pain and headache, and refusal to attend school. Posttraumatic stress syndrome and depression may also be seen. See Chapter 57∞ for further description of these disorders. Anxiety disorder, posttraumatic stress, and depression should be referred to a mental health specialist for treatment. However, all children worry at times and this type of anxiety can be helped by learning coping skills and relaxation techniques.

Spiritual health is the ability to develop a spiritual nature, including awareness of a life purpose or meaning, a sustaining power during times of stress, a feeling of harmony with the universe, and a sense of fulfillment (Pender, Murdaugh, & Parsons, 2006; Murray et al., 2009). School age is a time when children learn more about the people and the world around them, and begin to find their place in that world. Connection with faith-based groups assists some children and families in defining the purpose of life, while others may do so through social activity or a strong moral sense of responsibility. Ask children what brings happiness, how they help other people, or if they are members of a church, synagogue, or mosque. If families seem to have little purpose, parents are withdrawn or depressed, or the child has difficulty answering questions about meaningful activities, suggest methods of engagement in the community. Strategies might include providing contacts at local religious events, posting flyers about community events designed to bring unity to various cultural groups, or suggesting services needing volunteers in the community. Families who spend time together and find meaning in supporting each other nurture the spiritual health of their members. Suggest that every family plan a "family night" weekly when they play games, talk, eat, or engage in other activities together.

The nurse has an important role in fostering the mental and spiritual health of school-age children. Health promotion fosters strengths of families and children, leading to healthy self-concept and positive self-esteem. Health maintenance seeks to prevent mental health disruptions. Be alert for risk factors in families since they represent the need for intervention. Expected outcomes for health promotion and health maintenance activities with school-age children include formation of a positive sense of self-esteem and healthy body image, use of coping skills to deal with stress, sleep patterns that meet needs for rest, and a growing purpose and meaning in life.

RELATIONSHIPS

While the school-age child is gradually moving away from the family as the center of life, the family remains an important anchor. Ask about siblings, grandparents, and other extended family members. Sometimes these persons assist in the child's formation of a self-concept. Peers are increasingly important to the school-age child's self-identity. School age is a time of cooperative engagement with others. All children need to learn how to make and maintain friendships and work with others on projects and in recreation.

Inquire about the child's friends and activities at school. In private, ask parents if they are comfortable with the child's selection of friends. Find out if the parents facilitate friendships by allowing other children to come to the home and providing transportation as needed. When the child experiences a risk factor such as a move to a new town or school, role-play how to meet new children and how to make friends. If the child feels like an outcast or outsider among peers at school, explore how the family can create a safe and secure place for the child in extracurricular activities with children who have similar interests. When children are home schooled, the family should encourage social events and contacts after usual school hours.

Since peers are important to the school-age child, the child may feel pressure to appear like others, to fit in, and to do what others encourage. Although such pressures are often associated with teen years, they usually begin earlier, at least by 8 or 9 years of age. Ask children what kinds of things their friends try to get them to do that they know they should not do, or if friends have tried to get them to smoke. Middle school years are the most common age for beginning to smoke, so always ask if the child has tried smoking, being careful to do this when the parent is not present and the child is more likely to be honest. When parents are not in the room they may also tell you about other activities, such as playing with guns, trying alcohol or other substances, or other risky behavior. It is best to ask children what they do in these situations, what they want to do, and who they can talk to about these events. Offer information about the risks connected with behaviors that are described, and suggest people such as parents, teachers, counselors, or clergy who are possible resources. If the child's health is at risk, be sure to report the activity to the physician or other healthcare provider so that it can be pursued and the child's safety can be assured. Activities such as playing with firearms or visiting a friend whose parents are making methamphetamine, for example, place children in extreme danger.

Parents often need guidance to help them in setting limits for their school age children. The child is becoming more independent but unacceptable behaviors must still be managed by successful discipline techniques. Some guidelines that can help families include talking calmly while expressing clearly behaviors that are unacceptable, using techniques such as natural consequences or withholding privileges, modeling, and suggesting stress relief such as physical activity (American Academy of Pediatrics, 2007b; Barkin, Scheindlin, Ip, et al., 2007).

School age is often a time when children first experience violence in relationships with others. Some children are bullied, while others are the bullies. Anger and aggression can occur, and children may engage in violence with each other. Ask children to describe when they last had a disagreement with someone and how the problem was solved. Suggest people who can help, such as school nurses, teachers, and counselors, and be sure that children feel safe in schools, neighborhoods, and homes. Ask parents how they resolve arguments between children at home and what help they need to help children learn problem-solving skills. Find out what policies the local schools have to assist in decreasing harassment of and by children. Become active on school committees that help children learn how to solve problems peacefully and how to respond to episodes of violence. See Chapter 44∞ for further discussion of violence in children and a detailed discussion of bullying.

The child's temperament (see Chapter 33∞) still plays a part in response to situations and the ability to self-regulate. The "difficult" child may have trouble getting to sleep or being quiet in the classroom. Have parents plan more physical activity for this child. Teach the child that bedtime routines are helpful and that sitting near the front of the class can help with concentration. The "slow to warm up" child may need ideas about what to say when meeting new people. Parents can help the child prepare for a new school by visiting the school with the child, talking about it, and meeting with the teacher so that a warm welcome can occur. The "easy" child is usually adaptable in most situations and is regular in activities. However, this child may object when other children interrupt, fail to take turns, or otherwise "break the rules" of behavior. They might need help to understand differences in temperament in order to be more tolerant of classmates and their behaviors. Often nurses in schools address the issue of individual differences by speaking with classes or small groups of children.

The nurse takes an active role in promoting the child's health by anticipating developmental issues and preparing parents and child to deal with them. Health maintenance outcomes include prevention of problems such as bullying.

DISEASE PREVENTION STRATEGIES

School-age children are generally healthy. The immune system is mature (see Chapter 50∞), personal hygiene practices are more mature than at earlier ages, and immunizations are usually complete. Engage school-age children in active pursuit of their own health. Teach strategies that can enhance the prevention of diseases. Nurses in offices and schools can teach children how to wash hands effectively, how respiratory infections are transmitted, what can cause gastrointestinal illness, and how to best manage their own health problems (Figure 37–6 ●). Ask children in your settings what topics are of most interest to them and be prepared to suggest common areas of concern such as safety, skin care, athletics, and illnesses. Children can understand the connection between eating well and avoiding illness, maintaining normal weight and preventing type 2 diabetes, avoiding smoking to prevent cancer and other respiratory diseases, maintaining oral hygiene to promote oral health, and exercising to prevent hypertension.

School-age children are in the concrete stage of intellectual development, according to Piaget (see Chapter 33∞). This means that teaching is most effective when opportunities are provided to touch, feel, and otherwise become actively engaged in learning. When teaching about smoking, provide models of lungs and have the students breathe through a straw to demonstrate the effects of airway narrowing. These concrete activities will teach them concepts better than simple lecture or reading (Figure 37–7 ●). Concepts of health promotion tend to be abstract since they deal with

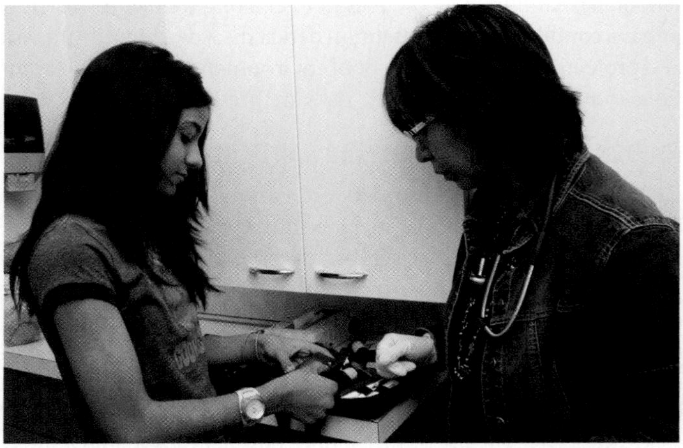

● **Figure 37–6** School nurse's role in managing health problems. A student with diabetes is showing the school nurse how she programs her insulin pump. The nurse has partnered with nurses in the endocrinology office to learn about the type of pump the student is using. Such collaboration contributes to the monitoring and management of diabetes.

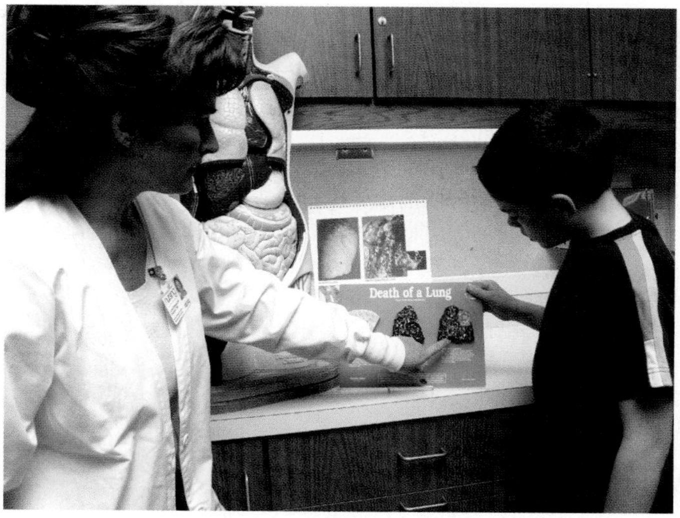

● **Figure 37–7** Concrete experiences for health teaching. This boy is learning about the effects of smoking on the body through the concrete experience of examining a model of the lungs. Why does this type of hands-on technique help school-age children to learn concepts?

supporting one's highest potential for wellness. Thus, it becomes even more important to provide concrete methods of learning.

Immunizations are generally up-to-date for school-age children. However, some children may have missed earlier doses due to illness or missed healthcare visits. Evaluate the immunization record to be sure it meets all recommendations. The most common immunization needs at this time include the following:

- Hepatitis B (whole series or a missed third dose)
- Hepatitis A (two doses if not previously administered)
- Polio, and measles-mumps-rubella (if booster doses of each were not given prior to school entry)
- Tetanus-diphtheria-acellular pertussis (Tdap) at the 11–12-year visit
- Varicella if not given earlier and the child has not had the disease
- Influenza annually
- Certain vaccines for children at high risk, such as pneumococcal, meningococcal, human papillomavirus (HPV) (see Chapter 45∞ for further information on immunizations)

Screening for health risks should occur during the visit. These include hearing and vision screening, blood pressure monitoring, tuberculin skin test, and in some cases screening for hyperlipidemia and lead exposure. Unusual complaints may indicate a need for further testing. Examples include the following:

- Pain other than brief discomfort after an injury
- Headaches
- Bruising
- Lack of coordination
- Repeated infections
- Decreasing vision or hearing
- Problems or changes in school performance or behavior

Children who have an identified health problem or developmental disability may have additional needs for screening and for interventions to assist with health maintenance. For example, the child with cystic fibrosis will need information to lessen risk of respiratory infection, and the child with diabetes may need additional blood studies. The child who has difficulty reading will need alternative approaches to teaching correct hand hygiene; demonstration with explanation may be the best approach. A family history of some diseases increases the child's risk and necessitates testing. For example, if a parent has had early cardiovascular disease (before age 55 years), a lipid profile should be performed on the child.

Inquire about any medications the child takes, including vitamins, fluoride, and nonprescription medications. Some families use complementary therapy for common conditions such as respiratory infections or gastrointestinal complaints. Complementary therapy is quite common in families where children have chronic conditions such as attention deficit hyperactivity disorder, autism, and skin conditions (Rosen & Breuner, 2007; Gardiner & Riley, 2007).

Parents should receive explanations about the screening tests performed and the results obtained. Inform them about vision and hearing results. Send home or call about results of blood tests when available. Be sure they understand the findings and have resources to assist in preventing or treating the specific disease in their children. Have them call with questions about health problems the child develops, and provide information about lowering risks of diseases. Be sure that families know when to keep children home from school (elevated temperature, active vomiting or diarrhea, coughing up brown or green mucus). Assist schools in setting guidelines for management of infectious diseases in that setting. Contact the local county and state health department for infectious disease guidelines for schools. Desired outcomes for the school-age child include prevention of infectious diseases, prompt treatment for acute infections, and careful management of existing health conditions in order to maximize health potential.

INJURY PREVENTION STRATEGIES

Injuries are a common cause of morbidity and mortality among school-age children, and each health maintenance encounter should include injury prevention strategies. Children of this age have more independence and may be harmed by activities they engage in without adults, such as playing with fire or firearms. They participate in many sports and other physical activities and may suffer related injuries. Some children unfortunately suffer harm due to physical abuse or other forms of violence (see Chapter 44∞).

Many common injuries are preventable with simple use of protective gear and following safety guidelines. More than 10% of youth rarely or never wear seat belts in automobiles (Centers for Disease Control and Prevention, 2006). Certain groups of children are more at risk than others of not taking protective measures. Many children ride bicycles, but only a fraction of them use helmets. Strategies to make helmet use more attractive and to ensure correct wearing of helmets are needed (see "Evidence-Based Nursing: Bicycle Helmet Effectiveness and Use").

Evidence-Based Nursing

BICYCLE HELMET EFFECTIVENESS AND USE

Clinical Question

About 900 children die of bicycle-related injuries annually in the United States (Royal, Kendrick, & Coleman, 2007). Although helmets can reduce injury, many times they are not worn or are worn incorrectly.

The Evidence

A review of 22 studies on helmet use among children provides insight into which strategies are most likely to encourage use of this important safety equipment. Community-based information appeared to be the most effective location for delivery of messages, while information provided in schools was found to be slightly less successful. Provision of free helmets was also a positive factor in helmet use, and was more effective than partially subsidized helmets (Royal et al., 2007).

Best Practice

Nurses should provide information about helmet use for bicycles and other vehicles. Engaging children at community events and in schools should be targeted. Inquire about helmet use at every healthcare visit. Reinforce proper fit and maintenance of helmets.

Critical Thinking

Where will you find information about helmet safety? What educational programs are available in your schools and communities? Are helmets made available for families that might not be able to afford their purchase? How do you determine if a child is wearing a helmet correctly? Plan educational materials and programs for children who bicycle, ride skate boards, or use scooters.

See MyNursingKit for possible responses.

Developing Cultural Competence

USE OF SAFETY PROTECTION

There are marked differences in behaviors that influence unintentional injuries. While only about 10% of children rarely or never wear a seatbelt in the car, almost 18% of black males, 13% of Hispanic males, and 12% of white males do not use seat belts (Centers for Disease Control and Prevention, 2006). Males of all races are therefore more likely to avoid seatbelt use than females, but black males are at highest risk. How will you inquire about seatbelt use in an open-ended manner during health promotion visits? Consider asking these questions:

- Tell me about where you sit when you ride in the car?
- Who do you usually ride with?
- Are there seat belts?
- How often do you use them?

Plan strategies to include for all children and families, especially those at high risk of not using seatbelts.

Identify youth engaging in risky activities and teach them safe practices. Join with schools and community groups to establish education programs. Provide information about adequate conditioning for sports in order to decrease chance of overuse injury (Committee on Sports Medicine and Fitness, and Council on School Health, American Academy of Pediatrics, 2006). Each visit should contain basic history questions related to injury prevention. Pursue topics that appear to indicate problems. Once information is collected during the visit, plan two or three health maintenance topics that seem most important for injury prevention in this family. When there is a history of injury in the child, partner with the family to plan ways to avoid repeated harm. Table 37–8 lists some common injury hazards during the school years, and Table 37–9 offers suggestions for injury prevention teaching.

NURSING MANAGEMENT

NURSING ASSESSMENT AND DIAGNOSIS

Assessment of health promotion and health maintenance topics occurs in many settings with school-age children. They may be seen in offices, clinics, or other settings designed to provide such care. They may come for episodic care for a fracture or infection when health promotion and health maintenance can be easily integrated. They may be seen in the home or neighborhood center, and are frequently encountered by nurses in schools. Opportunities for assessment and intervention should be used whenever they occur. The individual child is examined, and the family, friends, school, and community are addressed. In addition these visits provide an opportunity to identify early and intervene for health-related problems that emerge or become apparent in school age.

Assessment can be considered on two levels with school-age children. Individual children may be assessed for height and weight, for immunization status, and for use of protective gear during sports. Populations of children may also be assessed since school age is the first time that large numbers of children are together in certain settings. The findings from such assessments will become the basis of an **individualized approach** or a **population-based approach** to health promotion and health maintenance. For example, nurses commonly measure height and weight, calculate body mass index for *individual* children seen in a clinic, share results with the family, and address appropriate teaching about weight control and nutritious intake. In other settings, nurses may measure a *classroom* of children and use the collective data to plan appropriate interventions. If 40% of children in a school are classified as overweight by BMI percentile, much emphasis should be placed on teaching about dietary intake, physical activity, and the relationship of recommended weight levels to chronic disease risk. However, if only a small number of children are overweight, interventions may not be as extensive about this topic.

Table 37–8 Injury Hazards in the School-Age Years

	Hazard	Developmental Characteristics	Preventive Measures
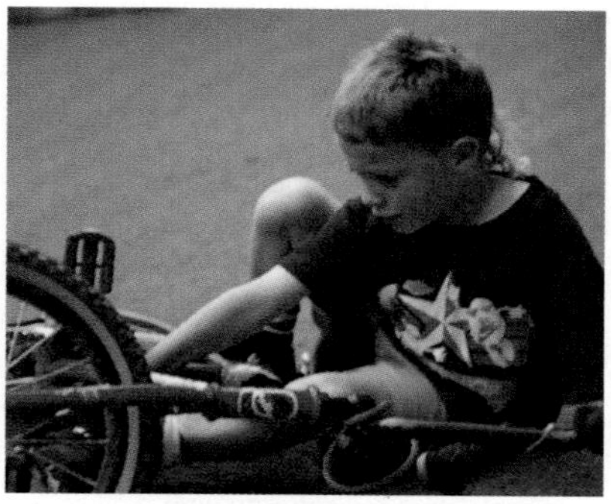	Motor vehicle/ pedestrian/ biking crashes	Child plays outside; may follow ball into road; rides two-wheeler.	Teach child safe outside play, especially near streets. Reinforce use of bike helmet. Teach biking safety rules and provide safe places for riding.
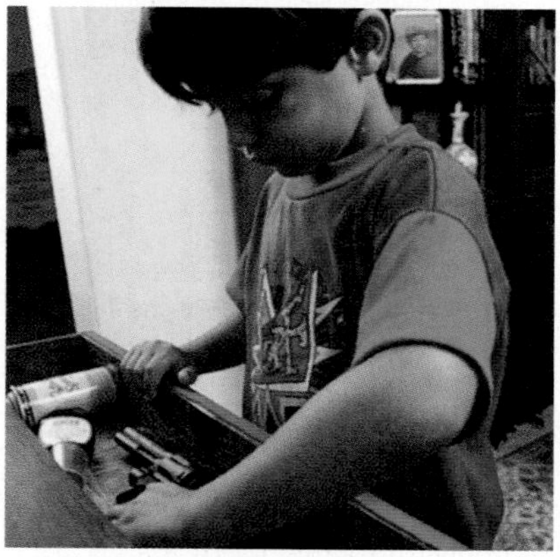	Firearms	Child may have been shown location of guns; is interested in showing them to friends.	Teach child never to touch guns without parent present. Guns should be kept unloaded and locked away. Guns and ammunition should be stored in different locations. Be sure guns have trigger locks.
	Burns	Child may perform experiments with flames or toxic substances.	Teach child what to do in case of fire or if toxic substances touch skin or eyes. Reinforce teaching about 911.
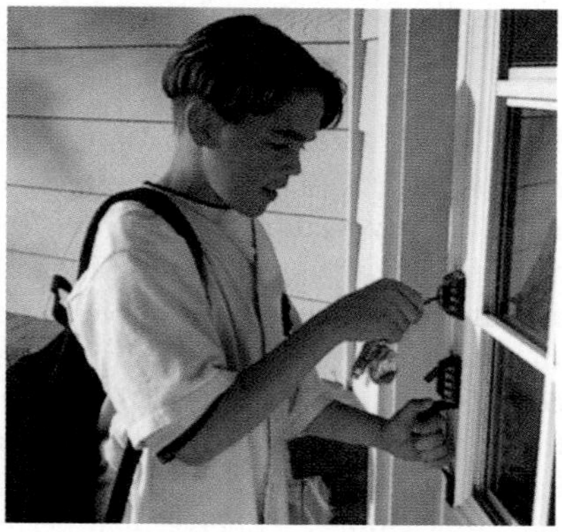	Assault	Child may be left alone after school and may walk, bike, or take public transportation alone.	Provide telephone numbers of people to contact in case of an emergency or if child feels lonely. Leave child alone for brief periods initially, and evaluate child's success in managing time. Teach child not to accept rides from or talk to or open doors to strangers. Teach child how to answer the phone.

Nurses perform assessment of growth in school-age children, look for achievement of developmental tasks, assess physical and mental health, and assess social characteristics. Based on the assessment of the individual child or populations of children, nursing diagnoses for children and families are established. Possible nursing diagnoses include the following:

- *Delayed Growth and Development* related to abuse
- *Impaired Parenting* related to lack of knowledge about child health maintenance
- *Sleep Deprivation* related to sleep terrors
- *Risk for Violence Directed at Others* related to history of witnessing family violence
- *Risk for Loneliness* related to long periods alone after school
- *Health-Seeking Behaviors* related to locating swimming classes

PLANNING AND IMPLEMENTATION

The nurse is instrumental in planning interventions to promote and maintain health in school-age children. These interventions may take place in offices, homes, or clinics with an individual

Table 37–9 Injury Prevention Topics by Age

Age	Injury Prevention Teaching	
5–8 years	Use a booster seat, properly positioned in the back seat of the car; use lap and shoulder belts. Never place the child in a front car seat with a passenger air bag. Be sure the child knows how to swim and works on these skills regularly. Teach safety precautions for bicycling and other activities, including protective gear. Protect the child with sunscreen when outside. Check smoke alarms and keep them in proper function. Have an escape plan in case of fire in the home. Keep poisons, electrical appliances, and fire starters locked. Keep firearms unloaded and locked; store ammunition in a separate locked location; have trigger locks installed on guns; keep dangerous knives locked. Provide protective gear for bicycling and other activities and insist that it be worn. Teach safety precautions for bicycling and other activities.	Teach safety with strangers. Provide a list of people a child can approach if feeling threatened by touch or other experience. Choose care providers carefully; occasionally pick up child earlier than expected; ask about policies regarding discipline and do not leave child with someone who uses corporal punishment. Be sure the child knows emergency numbers, names, and plans. Review carefully any hazardous event that has occurred with the child and summarize what was done correctly and how response could be improved. Limit screen time to 2 hours daily; do not allow violent games or viewing. Review behavior with strangers regularly such as not getting in cars, and not engaging in phone or Internet conversations.
8–10 years	Use car booster seat until child sits upright against back seat with bent knees over edge of seat; insist on use of lap and shoulder belts. Do not place child in front seat of car with a passenger air bag.	Do not allow child to operate power tools or machinery. Continue to reinforce other teaching described above, include child more fully, and enlarge responsibility to the child with increasing age.
10–12 years	Continue to reinforce teaching described above. Parents and child should attend class on cardiopulmonary resuscitation and airway obstruction removal.	Avoid high noise levels such as when listening to music through earphones.

Data from Hagan, Shaw, & Duncan (Eds.). (2008). *Bright futures: Guidelines for health supervision of infants, children, and adolescents* (3rd ed.). Elk Grove Village, IL: American Academy of Pediatrics.

child, or in schools and other community settings with groups of children.

When working with individuals, summarize the strengths and needs identified during the visit, and ask the child and family if they concur. Plan together with them to provide the needed information for topics developed during the visit. Be sure to emphasize those areas where the family excels. For example, positively reinforce use of car seat belts (see "Teaching Highlights: Car Safety for the School-Age Child"), use of protective sports gear, and being current with immunizations. Summarize the next expected developmental tasks, such as increasing independence and growing self-responsibility for choosing snacks and television shows. Then provide anticipatory guidance to assist with the child's growing independence. As peers are becoming more important, always focus some discussion on maintaining healthy social relationships through school peers, religious or community events, and sibling contacts.

Most families welcome a combination of discussion and reading material or pertinent Web sites for later exploration. Provide telephone numbers of resources for questions and community contacts. Tell the parents when the next health promotion/maintenance visit is recommended. If working with school children for episodic care, ask when the last health maintenance visit occurred. If a child is seen for health care after a bicycling accident, the family may be receptive to teaching about safety precautions. When the child is exposed to skin injuries, a review of the last tetanus booster may review health maintenance needs. Use every opportunity to work with individual children and insert appropriate health promotion/health maintenance topics.

When working with groups of children, health promotion focuses on known needs, interests, and risk areas. Nurses in school settings have used a variety of creative approaches to promote the health of youth. Nurses in schools can set up a program to train students in health topics; these students then become peer coaches or health advocates in working with other students. Another activity is evaluating the components of school health programs and making recommendations for additions as needed. In school settings, nurses have used a variety of creative approaches to promote the health of youth. Nurses in this setting can establish programs to train students in health topics; these students then become coaches or health advocates who can work with other students, especially those of younger ages. Nurses may also evaluate components of school health programs and offer recommendations for additions as needed. Bulletin boards, community newspapers, television, and community group membership may all be as effective as teaching in school classrooms. Stress reduction teaching should be provided on group and individual levels. Nurses can teach or assist in development of pro-

Teaching Highlights

CAR SAFETY FOR THE SCHOOL-AGE CHILD

Recommendations include the following:

- For children over 40 lb (generally 4 to 8 years of age), use a belt positioning, forward-facing booster seat located in the back seat. Always use both lap and shoulder belt. Make sure the lap belt fits low and tight across the lap/upper thigh area, and the shoulder belt is snug across the chest and shoulder to avoid abdominal injuries.
- Children 4 ft 9 in. and taller can sit in a regular car seat restrained with lap and shoulder belt that are snug and correctly located across the lap and chest. The back seat is preferred for all children and necessary for children 12 years and younger.

Note: ALL children 12 years and younger should ride in the back seat.

gressive relaxation, deep breathing, biofeedback, yoga, or meditation. Interventions will be most effective if they begin with an understanding of the population served.

EVALUATION

Seek evaluation from parents during visits for care. Were their questions answered? Do they know where to turn for advice? Do they know when the child should be seen again for health promotion/maintenance?

The expected outcomes for nursing care of individual school-age children include the following:

- The child demonstrates normal patterns of growth and development.
- The child, family, and community provide a supportive and nurturing environment for the child.
- The child shows growing independence in directing own health promotion activities.

Expected outcomes of nursing care for groups of children include the following:

- The children identify lifestyle decisions that influence their health status.
- The school and community offer resources that help to lessen risk factors related to health, and disease/injury prevention.

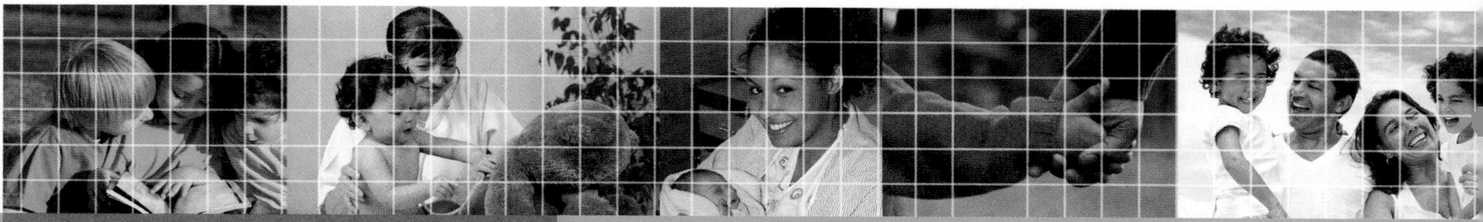

CRITICAL CONCEPT REVIEW

LEARNING OUTCOMES | CONCEPTS

37.1 Describe the areas of assessment and intervention for health supervision visits for children—growth and developmental surveillance, nutrition, physical activity, oral health, mental and spiritual health, family and social relations, disease prevention strategies, and injury prevention strategies.

1. Growth and development:
   - Obtain length, weight, and head circumference.
   - Observe and interview family to determine if infant is reaching appropriate developmental milestones.
2. Nutrition:
   - Determine type of infant feeding family is using.
   - Instruct family concerning appropriate nutrition for infant's age.
3. Physical activity:
   - Assess daily routines and infant's ability to participate.
   - Provide instruction concerning appropriate toys.
4. Oral health:
   - Inspect infant's mouth.
   - Instruct parents concerning importance of toothbrushing.
5. Mental and spiritual health:
   - Instruct family concerning expected stranger anxiety and separation anxiety.
   - Explain need for infant to develop self-regulating (self-comforting) behaviors.
6. Family and social relations:
   - Encourage parents to play daily with infant and take a break when infant care becomes frustrating.
7. Disease prevention strategies:
   - Administer necessary immunizations.
   - Instruct parents concerning when to call the physician.
8. Injury prevention strategies:
   - Instruct parents in proper use of car seats and prevention of falls.

(continued)

LEARNING OUTCOMES / CONCEPTS

LEARNING OUTCOMES	CONCEPTS
37.2 State components of self-concept for preschool and school-age children.	1. Self-concept refers to the evaluation of the self by the child. 2. Self-concept includes ideas about body image and sexuality. 3. Self-esteem reflects the child's feeling of self worth or value.
37.3 Plan health promotion and health maintenance strategies employed during health supervision visits of children.	1. Summarize the strengths and needs (risk and protective factors) of the child and family based on assessment during the health supervision visit. 2. Establish a nursing diagnosis list appropriate for the child and family. 3. Use a variety of approaches such as discussion, Web resources, and printed material to provide the information that children and families need regarding topics such as nutrition, physical activity, relationships, and safety.
37.4 Discuss the importance of family in child health care, and include family assessment in each health supervision visit.	1. Health supervision visits begin with collaborative planning with the family. 2. Each visit should include: ■ Interview with family concerning developmental status of the child. ■ Observation of family interaction. ■ Discussion of parental concerns.
37.5 Integrate pertinent mental health care into health supervision visits for children.	1. Mental health issues to be addressed include: ■ Assessment of occurrence of common problems such as nightmares and temper tantrums. ■ Explanation of the promotion of a positive self-image.
37.6 Synthesize data about the family and other social relationships to promote and maintain health of children.	1. Health promotion and maintenance activities related to social relationships focus on: ■ Increasing social skills with the people in the child's environment. ■ Successful management of temperament characteristics. ■ Adjusting to time away from home. ■ Improving language and communication skills.

CRITICAL THINKING IN ACTION

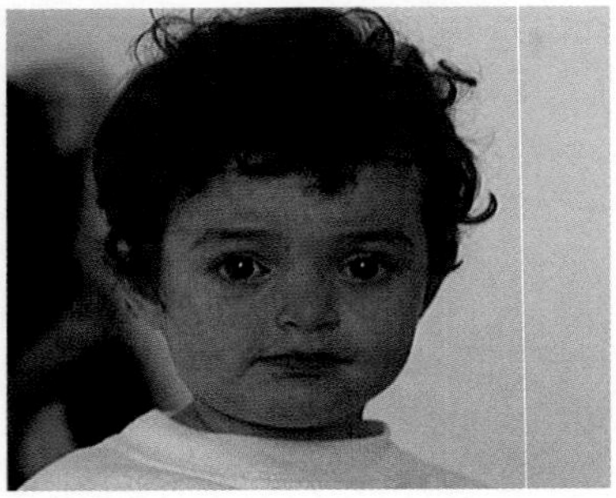

Quinton and his mother have come into the office for his 2-year-old well-child check-up. During the visit you learn that his mother stays home with him during the day and his father often works overtime. His only significant medical history incident was when he had stitches placed in his forehead for falling on the edge of a table when he was 15 months old. There is a family history of attention deficit disorder and Crohn's disease. His height is in the 75th percentile, weight is in the 50th percentile, and body mass index is between the 25th and 50th percentiles. His temperature is 98.9°F and his pulse is 80. He is described by his parents as a picky eater and tends to eat the same foods frequently. They also say he tends to eat well on some days and other days will hardly eat anything. On the days he is not eating well, his mother will often resort to giving him soda or a sugary snack just so he is "getting something." Quinton sleeps about 7 hours per night and his mother usually ends up sleeping with him because he continues to fight going to sleep after being put to bed. He does not have a regular bedtime or rest routine and he usually naps in the car during the day. His mother tells you that her only break during the day when she is at home with Quinton is when he is watching television in his bedroom, so he often watches 2-4 hours per day. Quinton has a soft stool every day and has not showed any interest in potty training at this time. He is developmentally able to go up and down stairs, kick a ball, scribble on paper, and is able to speak in 3-4 word sentences. During the visit at the office, it is obvious his parents have difficulty controlling him and frequently make threats and offer bribes to get him to behave properly. He starts screaming and kicking when his parents set limits on his behavior in the office and his parents say they are frequently exhausted and do not know what to do about his high energy level. They also are concerned because they feel like the discipline methods they have been using are not working, and he is getting into so many things in the home that they are concerned he may hurt himself. They have used spanking and time-outs, but they do not seem to improve his behavior. They think he may have some type of medical condition like attention deficit disorder considering it does run in their family.

1. At 2 years of age, a consistent routine will help a toddler behave more appropriately. What are some of the things you can tell Quinton's parents regarding his sleep and nutrition habits to help establish a better routine?
2. How can you advise Quinton's parents about positive approaches to disciplining him?
3. How can you advise Quinton's parents about disciplining him when it is needed?
4. What are some suggestions you can give Quinton's parents about handling his temper tantrums?

See MyNursingKit for possible responses.

REFERENCES

American Academy of Pediatric Dentistry (2005). *ADA statement on early childhood caries*. Retrieved November 23, 2008, from www.ada.org/prof/resources/positions/statements/caries.asp

American Academy of Pediatrics (2007a). *Healthy children: Back to school*. Retrieved 3/2/08 from www.aap.org

American Academy of Pediatrics (2007b). *Discipline*. Retrieved March 2, 2008, from www.aap.org

Barkin, S., Scheindlin, G., Ip, E. H., Richardson, I., & Finch, S. (2007). Determinants of parental discipline practices: A national sample from primary care practices. *Clinical Pediatrics 46*, 64–69.

Biagioli, F. (2005). Child safety seat counseling: Three keys to safety. *American Family Physician 72*(3), 1–6.

C. S. Mott Children's Hospital (2006). *Toy safety: Preschoolers*. Retrieved February 27, 2008, from www.med.unich.edu/1libr/pa/pa_plymatpr_pep.htm

Centers for Disease Control and Prevention (2006). Youth Risk Behavior Surveillance—United States, 2005. *Morbidity and Mortality Weekly Report 55*, 1–108.

Cole, K. A., Clark, J. A., & Gable, S. (2007). Promoting Family Strengths. In N. Henderson (ed.). *Resiliency in Action* (pp. 199–204). Ojai, CA: Resiliency in Action.

Committee on Sports Medicine and Fitness, and Council on School Health, American Academy of Pediatrics. (2006). *Active health living: Prevention of childhood obesity through increased physical activity*. Retrieved August 3, 2006, from www.aap.org/advocacy/releases/may06.physical activity.htm

Council on Children with Disabilities, Section on Developmental Behavioral Pediatrics, Bright Futures Steering Committee and Medical Home Initiatives for Children with Special Needs Project Advisory Committee (2006).

Donahue, G. J., Waddell, N., Plough, A. L., del Aguila, M. A., & Garland, T. E. (2005). The ABCDs of treating the most prevalent childhood disease. *American Journal of Public Health 95*, 1322–1329.

Drotar, D., Stancin, T., & Dworkin, P. (2008). Pediatric developmental screening: Understanding and selecting screening instruments. Washington, DC: The Commonwealth fund.

Edelman, C. L., & Mandle C. L. (2006). *Health promotion throughout the life span* (6th ed.). St. Louis: Mosby.

Fuller, C., Keller, L., Olson, J., & Plymale, A. (2005). Helping preschoolers become health eaters. *Journal of Pediatric Health Care 19*, 178–182.

Gardiner, P., & Riley, D. S. (2007). Herbs to homeopathy—Medicinal products for children. *Pediatric Clinics of North America 54*, 859–874.

Ginsburg, K. R., & the Committee on Communications & the Committee on Psychosocial Aspects of Child and Family Health (2007). *Pediatrics, 119*, 182–191.

Guard, A., & Gallagher, S. S. (2005). Heat related deaths to young children in parked cars: An analysis of 171 fatalities in the United States, 1995–2002. *Injury Prevention, 11*, 33–37.

Gunner, K. B., Atkinson, P. M., Nichols, J., & Eissa, M. A. (2005). Health promotion strategies to encourage physical activity in infants, toddlers, and preschoolers. *Journal of Pediatric Health Care, 19*, 253–258.

Hagan, J. F., Shaw, J. S., & Duncan, P. M. (2008). *Bright Futures: Guidelines for health supervision of infants, children, and adolescents*. Elk Grove Village, IL: American Academy of Pediatrics.

Halfon, N., DuPlessls, H., & Inkelas, M. (2007). Transforming the U.S. child health system. *Health Affairs 26*, 315–330.

Institute of Medicine (2005). *Preventing childhood obesity*. Washington DC: The National Academies Press.

Jellinek, M., Patel, B. P., & Froehle, M. C. (Eds.).(2002). *Bright futures in practice: Mental health* (Vols. I & II). Arlington, VA: National Center for Education in Maternal and Child Health.

LeBourgeois, M. K., Giannotti, F., Cortesi, F., et al., (2005). The relationship between reported sleep quality and sleep hygiene in Italian and American adolescents. *Pediatrics, 115*, 257–265.

Mason, T. B. A., & Pack, A. I. (2005). Sleep terrors in childhood. *Journal of Pediatrics, 147*, 388–392.

Murray, R. B., Zentner, J. P., & Yakimo, R. (2009). *Health promotion strategies through the life span* (8th ed.). Upper Saddle River, NJ: Prentice Hall.

National Safe Kids Campaign (2004). Playground injury fact sheet. Retrieved February 27, 2008, from www.usa.safekids.org/tier3_cd.cfm?folder_id=540&content_item_id=1151

Pender, N. J., Murdaugh, C. L., & Parsons, M. A. (2006). *Health promotion in nursing practice* (5th ed.). Upper Saddle River, NJ: Prentice Hall.

Rosen, L. D., & Breuner, C. C. (2007). Primary care from infancy to adolescence, *Pediatric Clinics of North America, 54*, 837–858.

Royal, S. T., Kendrick, D., & Coleman, T. (2005). Non-legislative interventions for the promotion of cycle helmet wearing by children. *Cochrane Database of Systematic Reviews, 2*, CD003985.

Safe Kids USA (2007). *Toy safety*. Retrieved February 28, 2008 from http://sk.convio.net/site/PageNavigator/Campaingns/ToySafety/campaignToySafetyTips

Santrock, J. W. (2007). *Child development* (11th ed.). Boston: McGraw-Hill.

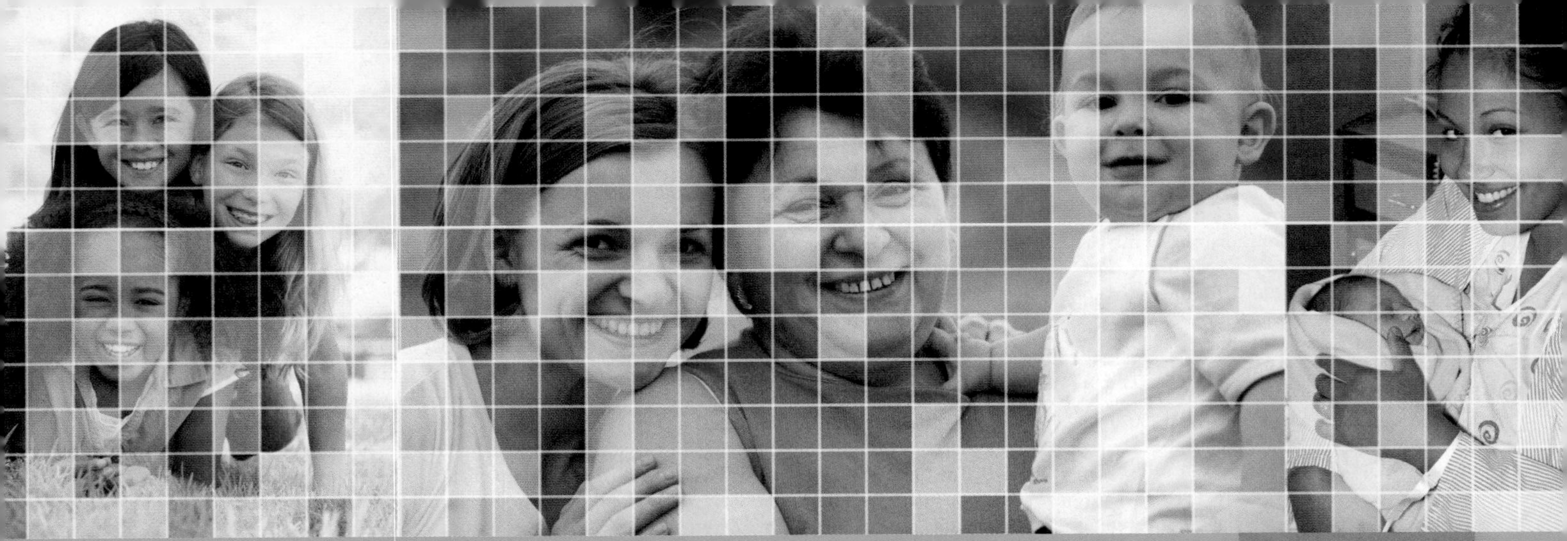

CHAPTER 38

Health Promotion and Maintenance: The Adolescent

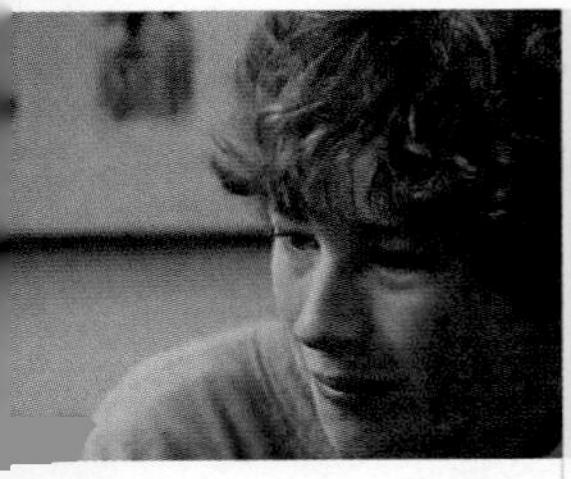

I know I should not be using chewing tobacco but a lot of my friends use it and I want to fit in with them. I would like to quit but I really don't know how. —*Jeremy, 16 years*

LEARNING OUTCOMES

38.1 Identify the major health concerns of the adolescent years.

38.2 Describe the general observations made of adolescents and their families as they come to the pediatric healthcare home for health supervision visits.

38.3 Apply communication skills to interactions with adolescents and their families.

38.4 Apply assessment skills to plan data-gathering methods for nutrition, physical activity, and mental health status of youth.

38.5 Synthesize data from history and examination of adolescent and family with knowledge of adolescent development to plan approaches useful with the family during health supervision visits.

38.6 Intervene with adolescents by integrating activities to promote health and to prevent disease and injury.

Adolescents are often seen only sporadically for health care, even though visits are recommended annually. They are usually healthy, may not need immunizations, and consequently do not often come for health care. If adolescents seek care for a minor illness, birth control, or a sports examination, the visit should be viewed as a health supervision opportunity.

While all components of the usual visit may not be performed, at least those parts most important are inserted into care. If time is limited, the nurse has to decide which topics to address during a healthcare visit. It is advisable to start with the topic of most interest to the teen and then to include injury prevention teaching, since injury is the greatest risk to teens. Health promotion topics such as dietary and exercise habits could be discussed if there is time.

Four lifestyle behaviors are responsible for most of the preventable diseases, and they all typically have origins in adolescent years. These four areas should be assessed: sedentary lifestyle, unhealthy diet, tobacco use, and risky drinking (Olson, Gaffney, Hedberg, et al., 2005). Mental health assessment and teaching are other areas of prime importance. If the teen is at immediate risk, such as considering suicide in response to depression, this must be dealt with immediately by collaborating with a mental health specialist.

What general principles can guide programs to promote health in adolescents? Some researchers have analyzed theory application and approaches of programs, and others have suggested key elements of programs (see "Thinking Critically"). Programs assist adolescents in taking on health promotion behaviors by fostering a sense of competence, promoting decision making, and increasing motivation for change toward healthy behaviors (Murray, Zenter, & Yakimo, 2009). When establishing youth programs, whether with individual adolescents or with groups, the nurse includes evaluation of the effectiveness of the plan, and uses methods to expand and sustain successful approaches.

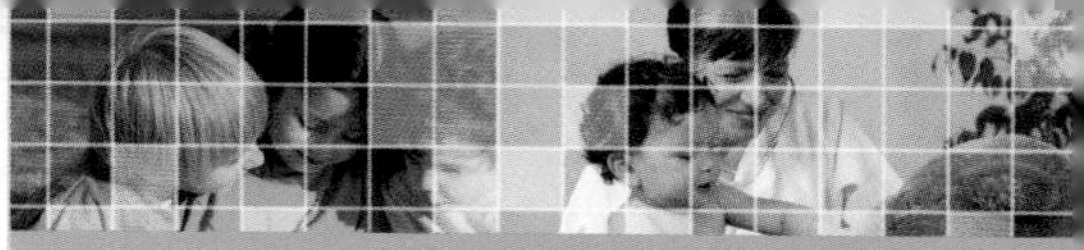

KEY TERMS

modeling, 1032

outcome expectancy, 1032

self-efficacy, 1032

GENERAL OBSERVATIONS

The beginning of the visit with an adolescent can be an important time to gather information, just as it is with younger children. However, the observations you make will relate to the adolescent's more advanced stage of development.

Ideally the facility has a waiting area that is designed for adolescents. Teens often dislike waiting for health care with either young children or older adults. Teen waiting areas are popular because they provide a special place, thereby relaying that the adolescent is important, and can use video and other popular methods to impart health information while the teen waits (Figure 38–1 ●). As you call the adolescent back for care, observe if parents or friends are present, or if the teen is alone. Young adolescents often come with parents to the facility, and parents often then wait in the waiting room during the examination. If the young adolescent comes in for a special problem, such as a skin lesion or other health concern, the parent may accompany the adolescent into the examination room. If someone comes with the teen, it may be necessary to provide some private time by asking the other person to wait outside for a moment. Reassure parents that there will be time to talk with them about any of their concerns and questions, and provide them with an opportunity to ask questions and obtain information.

Some teens are comfortable in healthcare settings and actively engage in conversation, while others are nervous and will need more explanations and reassurance during the first steps of measurement and blood pressure. By adolescence, boys and girls should be assuming more of a partnership role in their own health care. As the visit begins, greet adolescents warmly, ask what concerns and questions they have, and ask for their opinions and reactions throughout the visit. This will show that their thoughts are important and that they play an important role in guiding the healthcare visits. When adolescents are visiting the same office or clinic that they came to during childhood, they usually know and feel comfortable with the care providers. If the setting is new to them, explain procedures and introduce personnel so they feel more at ease.

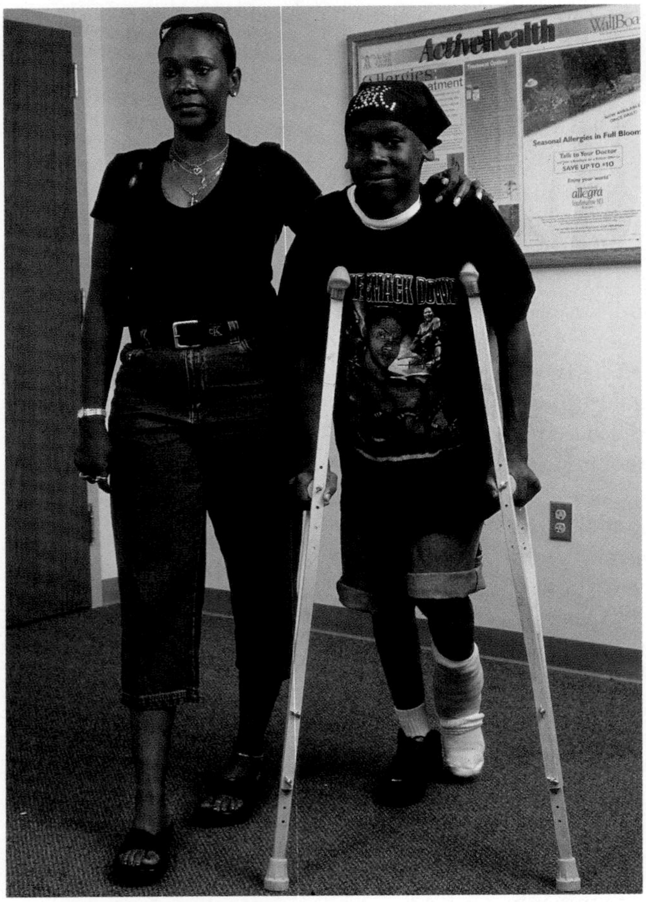

● **Figure 38–1** Healthcare visit with a teen. Parents often accompany teens with a healthcare problem in for the examination. Provide an opportunity to see both the teen and parent privately and integrate general health promotion and health maintenance into the visit. What questions can you ask this teen? What teaching might be needed?

> **Thinking Critically**
>
> **APPLYING THEORY TO PLAN FOR ADOLESCENT HEALTH**
>
> Several theories guide healthcare professionals in establishing health promotion programs for adolescents. These theories provide an organized approach to planning and suggest the strategies that will be most successful, based on the person's motivation and developmental age (Murray et al., 2009). One such theory that is commonly used in adolescent care is the *social cognitive theory*.
>
> This theory was developed by Walter Bandura, who is described in Chapter 33 ∞ (Bandura, 1986, 1997a, 1997b; Hortz & Petosa, 2008). The key components of his theory involve **self-efficacy** (the person's belief in the ability to perform a behavior) and **outcome expectancy** (what the person expects to get from performing a certain behavior). Learning a new behavior occurs through **modeling**, or imitating the behavior of someone else. Bandura believes that individuals make decisions about health behaviors based on thought about the consequences and outcomes of those behaviors. The *person's characteristics,* such as self-efficacy and outcome expectancy, interact with the external *environment* and the *behavioral choices* available. All of these components together determine health behaviors, and all can be influenced to promote health.
>
> When seeking to promote physical activity behaviors in youth, some essential components are:
>
> - Encouraging the youth to believe they could perform the activity (self-efficacy).
> - Pointing out the positive aspects of the behavior (outcome expectancy).
> - Showing the youth how to do the activity (modeling).
> - Providing a physical setting and opportunity for performing the behavior (environment).
> - Allowing trial and error, choice in time and extent of activity (behavioral choices).
>
> Compose a teaching plan to encourage increased physical activity for a teen, using all components of the social cognitive theory. List the outcome measures or goals for the teaching, the interventions, and methods of evaluation.
>
> See MyNursingKit for possible responses.

GROWTH AND DEVELOPMENTAL SURVEILLANCE

Adolescence spans several years, and growth and developmental issues vary throughout the period. For young adolescents, or those from about 12 to 13 years of age, growth measurement remains important. These youth are still growing, and use of percentile grids continues to be an important part of care. Growth should remain in the same percentile channel as during childhood, with girls reaching nearly adult height at this age, and boys still continuing to grow. As always, be alert for youth who have either increased or decreased percentiles, or are above the 85th percentile or below the 5th percentile for body mass index. They will need additional assessment of nutritional intake and physical activity.

By middle (14–16 years) and late adolescence (17–19 years), adult growth is nearly achieved, earlier for girls than boys. While measurement continues to be performed, nurses assess the BMI more carefully to be sure the height and weight indicate appropriate intake and exercise. Overweight at this age is likely to continue into adulthood, particularly if parents are overweight, so early intervention will be needed to decrease this potential. Other youth may have eating disorders and should be referred to a specialist for care. Children from homes without sufficient financial resources may be hungry and lack adequate food of high quality. Parents who were eligible for Women, Infants, and Children (WIC) Nutrition Program services when children were younger may not receive them once the child is an adolescent, so the increasing dietary intake needs of their teens cannot be met. If an adolescent is thin and has little energy, consider this possibility; administer the food security questionnaire found in Chapter 34 ∞. Even the child who is overweight may live in a family with insufficient resources since foods with high fat and caloric content are often less expensive than those with greater nutrient value. For example, a "dollar menu" at a fast food restaurant meets hunger needs faster and with less expense than a home-prepared meal of fresh fruits, vegetables, and grains. In addition, people who have experienced periods of hunger from inadequate food resources may overeat when food is available, a pattern that promotes weight gain (Olson, Bove, & Miller, 2007).

Few options exist for measuring the developmental competence of adolescents, but observations and questions during care provide information about the meeting of developmental milestones. Key tasks for adolescents involve separating from the parents and establishing positive relationships with peers. The young teen may come to an appointment with a parent and still rely on that parent to answer some questions during the examination. However, middle and late teens should be increasingly able to come alone, answer questions themselves, and assume responsibility for healthcare decisions. Offer older teens the option of coming into the room alone, stating, "Your mom can wait here and we can come and get her later. Does that sound all right?" During time with the adolescent, ask questions to learn about peer interactions and activities.

The adolescent may receive a physical examination from either the nurse practitioner or the physician. See Chapter 35∞ for components of the examination. Some particular parts of the examination to include for teens are scoliosis screening, sexual maturity rating (Tanner stages), breast exam, testicular exam, testing for sexually transmitted infections (among those sexually active), pelvic exam and pap smear (for sexually active females), annual hematocrit for anemia in menstruating adolescents, hearing screening (at 12, 15, and 18 years), annual blood pressure, lipid screening for those with family history of early heart disease or other risk factors, and tuberculosis screening for those in high-risk areas.

Most adolescents do not want their parents present during the examination, but occasionally will want a parent present for something like a first pelvic examination or a blood draw. Ask them their wishes in a confidential setting so they can freely make the choice. They also may choose to have a same-gender healthcare provider complete the genitourinary examination. Expected outcomes of care include screening and early identification for common health problems, normal patterns of growth, and meeting of developmental milestones.

NUTRITION

The young adolescent needs a well-balanced diet to support the growth of this period, and the late adolescent requires intake that supports physical activity and provides nutrients for metabolism and to promote the immune system. While nutritional intake is important, teens often do not eat well. They may be busy and do not want to plan meals, they like to eat foods that are popular with other teens (so high fat and sugar intake can be common), they may be dieting to achieve weight loss, and some do not have enough financial resources to access proper foods.

Combine the information from measurement of the adolescent with the answers to questions about diet to identify possible areas for intervention. Find out what questions the teen has about foods, diet, maintaining desired weight, and topics such as vegetarianism or supplements to enhance athletic performance. See Chapter 34∞ for further detail about these special nutritional topics. Health promotion plans focus on practices that lead to healthy growth and development. They may include teaching about:

- Getting five fruits and vegetables daily.
- Including whole grain products to replace refined products whenever possible.
- The importance of eating three meals each day, including breakfast and lunch.
- Eating together as a family several times weekly, which enhances quality food intake.
- How to plan menus and prepare foods for balanced intake.

Health maintenance plans center on those practices that prevent disease, including:

- Limiting refined sugar and high-fat intake (such as soft drinks and fried foods) to maintain weight at recommended level.
- Including two to three servings of dairy products daily to enhance bone formation and decrease chance of osteoporosis as an adult.
- Using resources for treatment of eating disorders if they are identified.

While much of nutrition teaching should be aimed directly at the adolescent, parents are also included. They can be effective contributors to healthy intake by providing plenty of fruits and vegetables for snacks, having foods attractively prepared and ready for consumption when the teen is hungry, planning several meals together as a family each week, encouraging milk or other forms of calcium intake, and setting a good example for food intake. Help parents to identify the youth with an eating disorder and provide resources for intervention in these cases. Consider as well the teen with a baby. The adolescent who is pregnant or breastfeeding has even more need for nutritional teaching and may need financial resources to access sufficient food (see Chapter 13∞). How can the nurse combine in the teaching plan the growth and developmental needs of an adolescent with those of her new baby?

PHYSICAL ACTIVITY

Many adolescents suffer from the effects of inadequate physical activity. As children get older and enter the teenage years, physical activity decreases, particularly in girls. Only about 36% of adolescents report daily vigorous activity for 5 days/week. The percentage is lower among some groups, with only 28% of females reporting that level of activity. Only about 15% of teens in 12th grade report exercise (Eaton, Kann, Kinchen, et al., 2006). The recommendation of *Healthy People 2010* (U.S. Department of Health & Human Services, 2006) is quite moderate, stating that adolescents should get at least 20 minutes of vigorous activity 3 days weekly. However, an expert panel now recommends 60 minutes of moderate or vigorous activity daily (Strong, Malina, Blimkie, et al., 2005). At a time when teens are not very active as a group, physical education requirements in school are also decreasing. Only 22% of 12th-grade students regularly attend a PE class (Eaton et al., 2006). Physical activity levels must therefore be assessed at each health supervision visit or in other contacts with adolescents. Apply resilience theory as discussed in Chapter 33∞, and assess youth, family, and community for risk and protective factors regarding physical activity (Table 38–1).

Table 38–1 Risk and Protective Factors Regarding Physical Activity in Adolescence

Risk Factors	Protective Factors
■ Lives in rural or other isolated setting with little opportunity for contact with other teens ■ Lives in urban area that is unsafe or provides little opportunity for outside physical activity ■ Presence of neighborhood hazards and unsafe areas ■ Lack of neighborhood programs for physical activity promotion	■ Has opportunities for participation in physical activity at home, at school, and in the community ■ School provides daily physical education classes ■ Neighborhood and community provide physical activity options ■ Has many friends living close who participate in physical activity ■ Public policies maintain parks, green spaces, biking trails, playgrounds
■ Has a developmental disability that impairs physical movement	■ Programs are available for adolescents with developmental disabilities or other healthcare needs
■ Does not like physical activity	■ Likes physical activity
■ Has a pattern and history of low activity levels ■ Is overweight ■ Does not feel competent in most sports	■ Has exercised during all of childhood, often with parents
■ Limited financial resources to pay registration fees or buy protective gear for sports	■ Availability of financial and other resources for sports gear and protective equipment
■ Family members who have little physical activity ■ Parents who are not active in school sports and committees ■ Parents who do not like physical activity and have had low levels while their teen was growing up ■ Parents who have little time or facilities for exercise, or always exercise at a club—out of view of their family	■ Parents participate in regular physical activity and encourage the adolescent to do so also ■ Youth and parents agree to a limit of 2 hours daily of screen time
■ Lack of youth and parent knowledge about physical activity needs and benefits	■ Knowledgeable about benefits of activity; committed to maintaining exercise patterns

Data from Hagan, Shaw, & Duncan, 2008.

Some youth have established regular physical activity programs, and their behaviors should be encouraged (Figure 38–2 ●). Be alert for adolescents who exercise but have other health problems. Some athletes try to eat very little to remain a certain weight for wrestling, running, or other sports. Integrate nutritional teaching that includes the importance of adequate intake for sports performance. Other athletes use nutritional supplements to enhance performance. While most are not harmful, few have proven benefits and their cost is not warranted. Some may actually be harmful to adolescents, such as prolonged use of creatinine and any use of steroids.

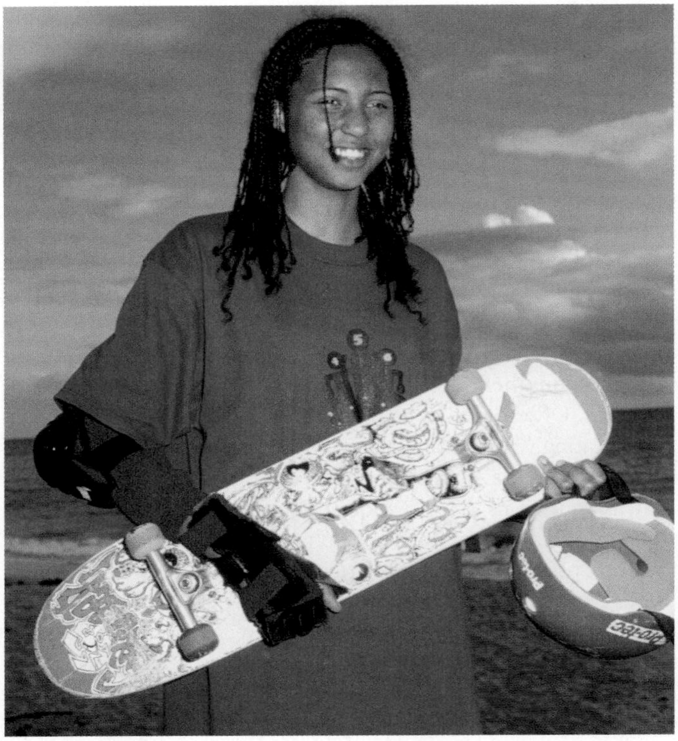

● **Figure 38–2** Teen use of safety measures. This teen girl is an avid "boarder." How can you encourage and praise her for this activity? What clues do you have that she is using adequate safety measures?

Other youth have very little physical activity and feel incompetent in performing many sports. Work with them to find at least one thing they can do on a daily basis—walking their dog in the neighborhood, riding a bike to the store, using stairs instead of elevators when possible, parking on the far side of the school lot and walking farther, swimming at a club their parents belong to or at a local YMCA or YWCA, or saving money to take lessons for something they have always dreamed of doing, such as horseback riding or golf. The community health nurse can form interest groups at schools and community centers that provide an outlet for adolescents who cannot "make the team" for school sports. Encourage parents and adolescents to set goals together to integrate some physical activity daily.

What risk and protective factors for physical activity exist in your community? Go to www.activelivingbydesign.org to examine the positive effect community planning can have on its members' exercise levels.

The nurse's activities for health promotion concentrate on teaching the health and mental benefits of physical activity such as increased energy, weight control, and a feeling of control and success. Health maintenance focuses on viewing physical activity as a method to prevent disease such as cardiovascular disease and diabetes. Youth who have family members with these diseases or meet adults who have them are more likely to understand the importance of their own activity. Desired outcomes include maintenance of weight within recommended level, daily exercise of 60 minutes, and establishment of lifetime exercise routines.

ORAL HEALTH

Continued dental care during the adolescent years can ensure oral health. The recommendations remain the same as those for young children. The adolescent should floss daily, brush twice daily with a small amount of fluoridated toothpaste, and visit a dental care provider every 6 months. By about 14 years of age, those adolescents who do not have fluoridated water and have been taking fluoride can stop this supplement. Even the molars have been formed by that age so fluoride tablets are no longer needed. Continue to examine the condition of the teeth and the number of erupted permanent teeth present. Be alert for any unusual growths and ulcers in the mouth and refer for care as needed.

Unavailability of dental insurance for the adolescent is a potential concern. The teen whose family does not have dental insurance needs referrals for care to affordable resources. Dental specialists clean off plaque that has formed, apply sealants to erupting molars, examine the teeth for caries, and perform restorative care. Certain groups are more at risk for inadequate dental care (see "Developing Cultural Competence"). When working with these populations, nurses can question access to care, and make recommendations that foster regular checkups.

Evaluate risk factors for threats to oral health such as tobacco use, particularly chewing tobacco (see quote from Jeremy in the opening scenario). A risk for oral injury exists with engagement in certain sports. Ask about physical activity and recommend that a mouth guard be worn during sports activities if the youth engages in hockey, football, or some other sports. Some teens may wish to whiten the teeth or obtain orthodontia to improve appearance. The nurse can help the youth and parents to find resources for needed care.

Expected outcomes for oral health include dental visits twice annually, daily positive oral health habits, absence of risk factors for poor oral health or injury, and obtaining recommended follow-up care for problems.

Developing Cultural Competence

DENTAL CARE

Analysis of several national surveys such as the National Health and Nutrition Examination Survey (NHANES) and National Survey of Children's Health (NSCH) shows marked disparity in oral health. The major factor in disparity of dental care is poverty. While 71% of children and adolescents from families living above the poverty line have dental care, only 36% of those below the poverty line receive such care. Black and Hispanic youth are also likely to have less access to dental services and more decayed teeth than white youth. The highest rates of families without dental insurance are foreign-born Hispanics (67% uninsured) and U.S.-born Hispanics (25% uninsured) (Liu, Probst, Martin, et al., 2007). Families in rural settings are less likely to have insurance than those in urban settings.

When working with adolescent populations from groups at high risk for lack of dental coverage or high incidence of caries, include dental assessment in health supervision visits, and have resources for care readily available to carry out referrals as needed.

MENTAL AND SPIRITUAL HEALTH

Adolescents have many challenges to their mental health and need support to emerge from adolescence with mental and spiritual strengths. Mental health topics must be addressed at each health supervision opportunity to promote mental health among teens. Mental health is closely linked to developmental tasks such as growing independence, formation of close relationships with peers, becoming confident in accomplishments, and setting goals for the future. Some chronic mental health disorders such as schizophrenia can emerge during adolescence, so mental health screening is important to perform with this age group.

As during other developmental stages, the self-concept continues to evolve, influencing how the adolescent reacts to the environment. Self-regulation—making decisions to govern oneself—becomes critically important. Self-esteem, or a positive feeling about the self, is key to meeting life's challenges. Ask what the teen is proud of and has accomplished and what disappointments have occurred as well. Provide resources to deal with disappointments and give praise for the teen's accomplishments.

The adolescent's self esteem is connected to perception of body image. Factors such as early or late maturation, overweight or underweight, or the role of the media can influence the teen's body image. A healthy image includes the realization that the body has positive and less positive attributes and that the individual can influence the body by healthy eating and physical activity. Be alert for the teen whose wish for a different body leads to eating disorders and excessive exercise or intake of nutritional supplements.

Sexuality involves both body changes that signal mature sexual development, and the mental concept of oneself as a sexual being. Body changes and mental concepts do not necessarily mature at the same time, and adolescents may not be ready for sexual maturity; decisions about sexual behavior are not necessarily equivalent to achieving sexual maturation. Most young adolescent girls have begun menstruating, and by early to middle adolescence, boys are having nocturnal emissions and ejaculations. Ask teens if they have received information about puberty, body changes, and sexuality. Tell young adolescents that most teens have questions and that they may ask about any areas of interest, including contraception and sexually transmitted infections. Ask older adolescents directly if they have had sexual intercourse and if so, what they are doing to protect against pregnancy and sexually transmitted infections. Provide support for adolescents who have decided not to have sexual intercourse, encouraging them to continue this plan, telling them that sexual feelings are normal, but that decisions about sexual intercourse are their right and privilege. Ask if the adolescent has ever experienced unwanted pressure for intercourse and if there has been help and support to deal with the situation. Intimate partner violence, date rape, and other trauma signals a need for referral to a mental health specialist. See Chapter 44 for further information.

MyNursingKit Video: Teen Mental and Spiritual Health

Ask if teens have confusion about their sexuality. If teens have self-identified as homosexual, let them know they are welcome and ask about decisions regarding sexual practices, reinforcing the

Nursing Practice

The nurse who works with adolescents dealing with sexuality issues may find that the values of some teens are very different from one's personal values. How do you react when a teen decides to have sexual intercourse or has become pregnant? Can you help teens to make wise decisions without telling them what they should do?

It is important for adolescents to learn the significance of sexual intercourse and the meaning of close relationships. Teaching them early about this will enable them to respect others at the time they do have intimate relations. Respect is also the key to working with teens. Nurses should treat them with respect, expecting them to consider options and make wise decisions. Nurses who cannot work with certain groups of teens because of moral values differing from their own have the obligation to refer the teens for care to resources where they can receive the information and services they are requesting.

need for protection against sexually transmitted infections. Provide community resources to support gay or lesbian teens so that they can develop a social group in which they feel comfortable. Some adolescents are seen for health care at the time they become sexually active. Use this opportunity to reinforce and correct prior knowledge about the body and protection against pregnancy and sexually transmitted infections (see "Nursing Practice: Sexuality").

Most adolescents still need discipline or guidance from parents at certain times. Rather than a constant battle over daily events, it is best if there are just a few important rules that parents have to enforce only rarely. When working with parents, nurses can assist them to set useful boundaries for teens and offer resources such as parenting groups and Web sites for assistance.

Sleep is necessary for anyone to function safely and at a level of one's potential. Unfortunately, many youth do not get the sleep needed for healthy functioning. Teens have an increased need for sleep due to their growth rates and activity levels. At the same time, their internal clocks change, making it more difficult to get to sleep at the usual time. It is thought that a decrease in secretion of melatonin occurs, so the teen does not feel tired in the late evening. However, they often do not have the number of hours of sleep needed by the time they wake up for school or work. The problem may be worsened if the student participates in sports or other activities. They may need to get to school before normal starting hours for music, sports, or other activities, or perhaps stay late into the evening for practices. Some adolescents then work weekends or evenings as well. And of course social activities usually fill much of their time. While about 9 hours of sleep is needed, most adolescents get about 6 hours (Mayo Clinic, 2007). The effects of sleep deprivation can be serious. Teens cannot perform to their potential in school or at work. Many parents state that adolescents are moody and difficult to communicate with when they are tired. There may be a connection between lack of sleep and substance abuse, and teens commonly use caffeinated beverages to stay awake. Some people tend to eat more when they are tired, and get less physical activity. Perhaps one of the most serious consequences deals with the danger of driving while sleepy; this is a common cause of accidents. Ask adolescents about what time they go to bed, when they awaken, and whether they are frequently tired. Provide suggestions for regular sleep schedules, avoiding caffeine products in the evening, making screen technology unavailable during sleep time, and planning a day of relaxation into every week.

School plays an increasingly important role in adolescent mental health. Peer support, meaningful activities, and a forum for learning time management and other skills are all provided by school. At the same time, some youth stress because of inability to fit in, worry about grades and their futures, and violent or unsupportive school situation. Discuss the elements of school that adolescents like and those they do not like. Evaluate presence of support in the schools. Ask the adolescent about future plans and how those are influencing choices for courses and friends in school.

Temperament or personality type characteristics continue into adolescence, but they generally do not change from earlier years. For example, the active infant and young child is usually an active teenager. The slow-to-warm-up baby may be the adolescent who needs more time to adjust to a new school or teachers. If the adolescent or parent has trouble with personality characteristics, it may be helpful to talk about these traits, help them to establish a positive sense about the attributes, and discuss ways to adapt the environment as needed. For example, parents should not expect a slow-to-warm-up teen to be interested in running for a class office. Someone with irregular sleep and eating habits will find it difficult to have a job at a set time and will need to set alarms and other reminders.

Spirituality offers comfort and support for the adolescent. Being a member of a teen group in a faith-based home can offer a peer group with similar values and bring meaning to life. Some adolescents reject the faith of their parents and seek a different group; others seek to leave religious practices totally while others become more committed to them. Ask them if they have the resources they need to bring meaning to their lives; provide them if needed. Realize that participation in community food kitchens, raising money for causes, and other activities also provide meaning for many adolescents (Figure 38–3 ●).

The nurse actively promotes the mental health of youth by understanding their developmental needs and providing information and resources. Gentle guidance and active partnership with youth help to provide the resources to ensure healthy self-concept, sexuality, and personality development. While most teenagers have many protective factors that can be identified and fostered, a few have risks that can harm mental health. It is important to identify the risks also, and to use health maintenance techniques to lessen the risk factors. Depression and substance use are two common risks to mental health. Depression is discussed in Chapter 57 ∞ and substance abuse is discussed in Chapter 44 ∞. See the quick checklists in Table 38–2 to help in identifying these problems during health supervision visits.

Although health promotion and health maintenance activities commonly occur in office or clinic settings, there are many other settings where nurses work with adolescents, and mental health activities are often integrated into these settings. Consider offering health promotion/maintenance wherever students might be found. Some nontraditional settings include correctional facilities, school-based

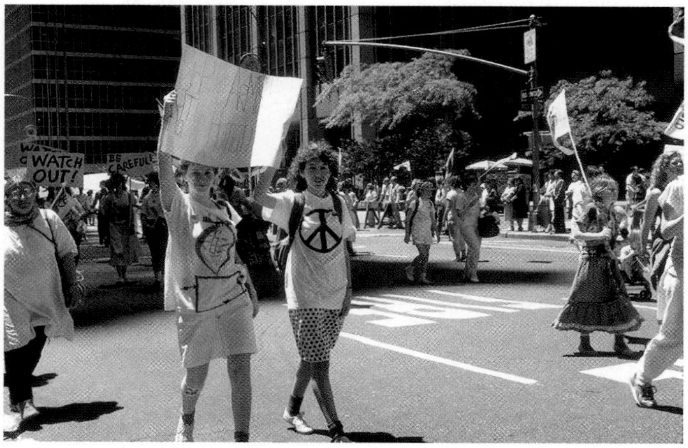

● **Figure 38–3** Spiritual health for teens. Teens often become associated with causes. This helps them to feel part of a social group and also provides the opportunities to examine belief systems and to make decisions about meaningful activities.

health centers, and programs for pregnant teens. Adolescents in these facilities can benefit from services to improve diet, physical activity, and lifestyle behaviors that influence mental health.

The desired outcomes for mental and spiritual health promotion and maintenance include meaningful activities in the adolescent's life, emerging independence, good choices about lifestyle behaviors, and development of successful coping skills.

RELATIONSHIPS

Adolescents form stronger bonds with friends than at any time earlier in development; at the same time they need their parents for guidance and reassurance as they become more independent. As teenagers strive for independence, they frequently strike out at parents, test limits, and have conflicts with parents. Interactions in the family provide consistent and important ties at the same time that social interactions become a central part of life. Health promotion helps teens to form strong friendships with peers and to continue to value and participate in the family. It helps parents to understand the developmental needs and their role in establishing a new type of relationship with the emerging young adult in the family. Partnerships with care providers are important to help families work together to achieve these outcomes.

When adolescents are seen for healthcare visits, assess relationships with others. Provide time alone with both the adolescent and the parents (if they are present) so that everyone has time to talk freely and to ask questions. Some areas already discussed, such as school performance and activities, provide information about the adolescent's friends and how time is spent. Ask teens to describe their best friends and what they do together. Ask parents their opinions of the youth's friends. Inquire about the youth's roles in the family. Does the teen have jobs and responsibilities? What freedom is allowed? What are relationships like with siblings and extended family members such as grandparents and cousins? What activities are done together as a family? Are there differences in the teen's and the parents' answers to these questions? What are the teen's and parents' desires for how the family unit functions together?

Provide an opportunity alone with the teen to talk about issues such as domestic violence. Is the youth abused or is there violence between adults in the family? Are there stressors such as lack of sufficient finances, an ill parent, or a lost job? How have these occurrences affected the adolescent? Minor adjustments can be helped by discussion, whereas some major problems will need referral to mental health specialists.

In their relationships with peers, adolescents often have many of the same issues that emerge with parents. They may have disagreements with friends or feel hurt by things that are said or done. Ask teens about how things are going with friends and what problems they have. Talk about negotiating, joining groups to form new friendships, and the importance of respecting and not making fun of others. Give them strategies for living up to their own standards even when friends are enticing them to do other things. Suggest that having friends one can trust and who have the same ideals can be very supportive and fun in adolescent years. Expected outcomes are the formation of strong relationships both within and outside of the family, along with independence in decision making.

Table 38–2 Signs of Depression and Substance Abuse

Depression	Substance Use
Changes in behavior, school performance, sleep, and appetite	Changes in behavior, school performance, sleep, and appetite
Physical complaints	Accidents and other unexplained events
Loss of interest in usual activities	Lack of responsibility
Difficulty in motivating self and setting goals	Labile (changeable) mood and behavior
Change in friends	Inability to set goals
Feelings of worthlessness	Hopelessness
Consideration of death or suicide	Depression
	Feelings of ambivalence
	A variety of physical changes depending on the substance

Data from Chang, Sherrit, & Knight (2005) and Jellinek, Patel, & Froehle (2002).

DISEASE PREVENTION STRATEGIES

Teenagers typically do not have many diseases and most are minor illnesses like respiratory and gastrointestinal illness. However, there are some diseases that occur and nurses must always be aware of signs of potential disease. Some common health issues that are described throughout this book include the following:

- Acne and skin infections (see Chapter 59)
- Body piercing and tattooing (see Chapter 44)
- Sports overuse injuries (see Chapter 58)
- Constipation and diarrhea (see Chapter 53)
- Dental problems (see Chapters 36 and 37)

MyNursingKit Case Study: Immunization Update

MyNursingKit Weblink Application: Smoking Education

Other observations may signal more serious health concerns and need to be referred for further evaluation. Some examples include the following:

- Scoliosis (see Chapter 58)
- Anemia (see Chapter 51)
- Excessive tiredness (see Chapter 52)
- Bruising (see Chapter 51)
- Sexually transmitted infections (see Chapter 54)
- Eating disorder (see Chapter 44)
- Abuse or severe bullying (see Chapter 44)

Several screening tests should be performed during health supervision visits with adolescents, including vision, hearing, smoking, depression, stress, alcohol or other substance use, blood pressure, urinalysis, sexually transmitted infection risk, and in some cases pap smears and breast examinations. Screening tests with abnormal results require follow-up and intervention. For example, if the adolescent is anemic, iron tablets may be needed and teaching about high-iron foods should be done. Vision impairment requires referral to an eye specialist. Presence of sexually transmitted infections requires teaching and medication treatment. History of sexual activity will guide the nurse to tests that should be included in the examination (see "Nursing Practice").

The adolescent should receive extensive information about ways to protect health and prevent disease. The hazardous outcomes of smoking are discussed, and smoking cessation programs are encouraged for smokers. Unprotected sexual activity is presented as a serious health threat. Use of sunscreens to prevent burns and future skin cancer is encouraged. Females are taught breast self-exam, and males are taught testicular exam. For youth who are overweight and sedentary, the possible outcomes such as type 2 diabetes and cardiovascular disease are mentioned. While it would not be advisable to threaten or frighten an adolescent with descriptions of diseases, an understanding of the potential serious outcomes can be motivators for behavior change.

In addition to teaching to prevent disease, the nurse also administers any needed immunizations. Many adolescents have not had immunizations since about school entry time, so their record should be carefully reviewed (See Chapter 45). When checking the adolescent's record, consider the following questions about some common immunizations that are needed:

- *When was the last tetanus-diphtheria (Td) booster?* It is recommended every 10 years if no wounds have required an update in the interim. If the child received it at age 5 years, a booster is needed at 15 years. A Tdap (tetanus-diphtheria and acellular pertussis) booster is given, with the preferred age of 11–12 years. If a dose of Td was given during adolescence, wait for at least 5 years, and administer one dose of Tdap.
- *Was a second measles-mumps-rubella administered?* A second dose may not have been routine when teens were younger so they may need it now.
- *Is hepatitis A common in your state?* If so, the teen needs to get that vaccine.
- *Has the youth had hepatitis B vaccine?* This is important for all youth, and some may not have received it as infants.
- *Did the youth have a clear history of varicella disease?* If not, the vaccine is needed.
- *Has the youth received meningococcal vaccine?* Meningococcal vaccine is now recommended for all youth.
- *Has the adolescent female received the human papillomavirus vaccine?* Human papillomavirus vaccine (3-dose series) is recommended for females from 11 to 12 years, or for those 13–26 years not previously immunized.
- *Has the youth received the annual influenza vaccine?* Annual influenza vaccine is now recommended for all children and adolescents.

The results of health screening are shared with the teen and with the parent as appropriate. Teaching and other interventions for disease prevention are examples of health maintenance activities. Expected outcomes are increasing knowledge of common diseases and methods of prevention among teen and parent, use of screening tests by the healthcare provider, and use of the healthcare home by the adolescent for treatment of diseases.

Nursing Practice

Sexually active teens should be screened annually for the following:

- Chlamydia
- Gonorrhea
- Trichomoniasis
- Human papillomavirus
- Herpes simplex virus
- Bacterial vaginosis

Individuals should be screened for syphilis and HIV/AIDS if requesting testing or meeting any of these criteria:

- History of sexually transmitted infection
- More than one sexual partner in past 6 months
- Intravenous drug use
- Sexual intercourse with a partner at risk
- Sex in exchange for drugs or money
- Homelessness
- Males—sex with other males
- Syphilis—residence in areas where disease is prevalent
- HIV/AIDS—blood or blood product transfusion before 1985

All individuals from 13 to 64 years should be offered a voluntary HIV test at each healthcare encounter. Those at high risk of infection ($<$ 20 years and sexually active, $>$ 20 years with inconsistent use of barrier protection and a new or more than one sex partner in last 3 months) should be retested annually (Branson, 2006).

See Chapter 54 for further information on screening procedures.

Data from Hagan, J. F., Shaw, J. S., & Shaw, P. M. (2008). *Bright futures: Guidelines for health supervision of infants, children, and adolescents* (3rd ed.). Elk Grove Village, IL: American Academy of Pediatrics; Branson, B. M. (2006). *Revised recommendations for HIV testing in health care settings in the United States.* Retrieved August 13, 2007, from www.cdc.gov/hiv/topics/testing/resources/slidesets/pdf/testing_healthcare.pdf

INJURY PREVENTION STRATEGIES

Injury is the greatest health hazard for adolescents, so injury prevention must be integrated into every health contact with youth. The major hazard is automobile crashes (see Chapter 1∞). Many teens learn to drive and have a license by 16 years of age. They often transport friends, get distracted by social interactions in the car, have little experience about what to do if a car slides or has mechanical problems, may drink and drive, talk or text on cell phones while driving, and are often tired when driving (Figure 38–4 ●). Several states have instituted graduated driving licensing to help decrease some risks. Commonly, the youth cannot drive other youth for the first few months, cannot drive during night hours, and has serious consequences for speeding or other infractions. Parents in states without these laws may wish to establish them for their own adolescents. Driving should always be presented as a privilege and a responsibility. Suggest that parents consider enforcing serious consequences such as losing the ability to drive for a time after any infraction (See "Nursing Practice: Parent Restrictions and Teen Driving"). Because of the great risk of injury and death from car crashes, ask at each health visit if the teen drives, rides with other teens, what rules parents have established about driving, and whether the teen ever drinks and drives or rides with someone who does. Reinforce the need to wear a lap and shoulder belt at all times and to never drink and drive.

Youth are at risk for injury with other motorized vehicles. Motorcycles, four-wheelers, boats, jet skis, farm machinery, and tools are other sources of injury. Ask about the youth's exposure to various machines and teach about avoiding alcohol and drug use, and safety gear and precautions to be used. Every health visit should include other questions that help to identify a wide variety of injury hazards. Be sure to discuss and provide written material to perform injury prevention teaching. Such measures are important health maintenance activities (Table 38–3 and Table 38–4). Desired outcomes for nursing care include absence of serious injury, the ability to state sources of risk for injury, and emergency plans for assistance when engaging in any risky activities.

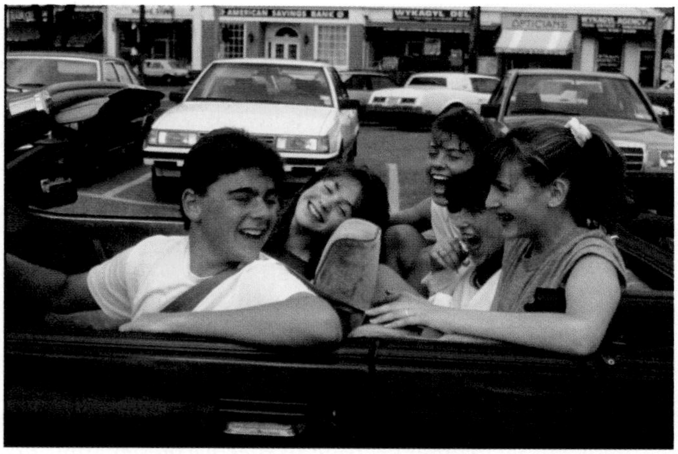

● **Figure 38–4** Injury prevention for teens. Adolescents often drive motorized vehicles and may be at risk for injury if not properly prepared or protected. What teaching and experience do these youth need for safe enjoyment of the experience of driving and riding with friends? Do schools in your area offer driver education classes? What are the state requirements for youth driver licensure?

Nursing Practice

Graduated driver licensing is an approach used to decrease motor vehicle crashes among novice teen drivers. Common approaches are to increase the period required for learner's permit, decrease driving after dark, and limit passengers in the car. Another method that has been suggested to improve safety records is to involve parents in practice driving times. Parents need support and information as they interact with the teen driver. Video presentation, newsletter, and a parent-teen driving agreement have all been helpful in supporting the family during the first year of a teen's driving experience (Simons-Morton & Ouimet, 2006). What financial and space resources would be needed to make this intervention more widely available? How could nurses be active in political discussions to promote graduated driver licensing and supports for parents of novice teen drivers?

NURSING MANAGEMENT

NURSING ASSESSMENT AND DIAGNOSIS

Nurses assess adolescents in a variety of settings, including offices, clinics, schools, home, correctional facilities, extended care facilities, sports-related endeavors, and family planning clinics. A wide array of health concerns should be included in these assessments. They include:

- measurement of growth
- presence of any unusual findings on physical examination
- lifestyle choices related to dietary intake, physical activity, and oral hygiene
- assessment of mental status, family interactions, and social connections with peers
- any risky behaviors the adolescent engages in such as smoking, unprotected sexual relations, alcohol or drug use, or unsafe driving practices

The people and organizations around the adolescent such as family, school, and neighborhood are all assessed. Remember to list both risks and protective factors. The protective factors can be used during implementation to enhance the youth's resilience.

Based on a thorough assessment, you will establish nursing diagnoses that are appropriate for the adolescent and family. Some possible nursing diagnoses might include the following:

- *Rape-Trauma Syndrome* related to date rape
- *Impaired Dentition* related to ineffective oral hygiene
- *Imbalanced Nutrition: More Than Body Requirements* related to lack of basic nutritional knowledge and obesity in both parents

Table 38–3 Injury Prevention in Adolescence

	Hazard	Developmental Characteristics	Preventive Measures
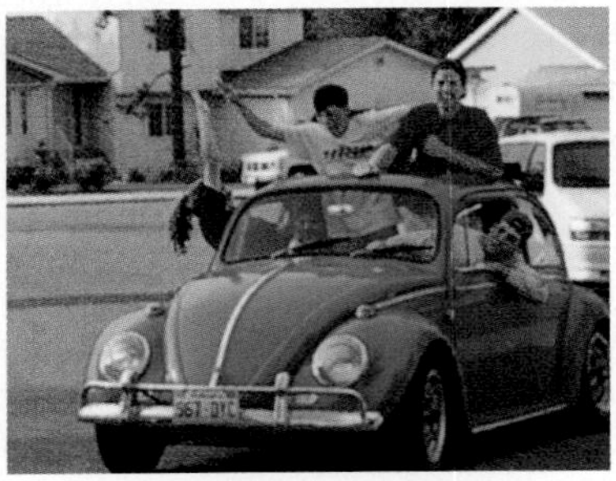	Motor vehicle crashes	Adolescents learn to drive, enjoy new independence, and often feel invulnerable.	Insist on driver's education classes. Enforce rules about safe driving. Seat belts should be used for every trip. Discourage drug and alcohol use. Get treatment for teenagers who are known substance abusers.
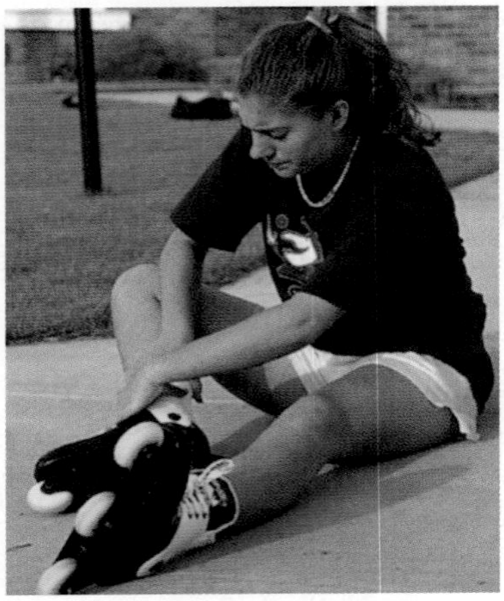	Sporting injuries	Adolescents may participate in physically challenging sports such as soccer, gymnastics, or football. They may be allowed to drive motorboats.	Encourage use of protective sporting gear. Teach safe boating practices. Perform teaching related to hazards of drug and alcohol use, especially when using motorized equipment.
	Drowning	Adolescents overestimate endurance when swimming. They take risks diving.	Encourage swimming only with friends. Reinforce rules and teach them about risks.

- *Readiness for Enhanced Nutrition* related to increasing interest in nutritional knowledge
- *Disturbed Sleep Pattern* related to frequently changing sleep/wake schedule
- *Low Self-Esteem* related to situational crisis of friends making fun of adolescent

PLANNING AND IMPLEMENTATION

Whatever the setting, the nurse partners with the adolescent, the parents, and other persons such as teachers or school counselors to plan appropriate goals and related interventions. Nurses work with individual adolescents in offices, schools, and other settings, and often work with groups of adolescents to perform teaching. Apply communication skills that are effective with teens, such as listening to concerns, allowing for discussion, and bringing peers who have had experiences related to the topic being discussed.

Many nursing interventions will involve teaching, so it is wise to develop a number of resources for working with teens. Consult the Web resources on this textbook's companion website, and visit agencies in your community to gather appropriate materials. Teaching topics should be directed both at health promotion (providing information to enhance the adolescent's state of health) and health maintenance (sharing tips about how to avoid disease and injury). A good starting point is to have the adolescent identify a personal health goal and begin teaching there. In addition to teaching, direct care is provided when administering immunizations, performing vision screening, and examining the spine and posture for scoliosis.

One of the challenges during health supervision for adolescents is including the right mix of teen and parent decision making and involvement. It is again important to apply communication skills by tactfully allowing time for both parent and adolescent to be seen alone. Realize that health supervision provides support and information for parents, such as useful discipline techniques, recognition of common parental feelings about teens, and the need for growing independence by their youth. When providing teaching to groups of teens in schools, there may be policies about what needs to be sent home to parents. For topics such as sexually transmitted diseases or substance use, some schools require that an outline be sent home for parents to read. Parents may call with questions about content and approach, or some may choose to attend and sit in on the presentation. In order to create an effective presentation, this obviously requires that partnering take place with the school administration, teachers, parents, and others. The ability to collaborate successfully with many individuals and agencies is an important skill for the nurse.

Wherever adolescents are seen, whether in offices or other private settings, schools, correction facilities, or other places with

Table 38–4 Injury Prevention Topics for Adolescents

Topic	Teaching
Driving	Always wear seat and shoulder belt. Do not drink alcohol or take drugs and drive or ride with others who do. Do not talk on a cell phone as you drive. Do not drive when you are tired. Drive with parents or other adults for several months in winter driving conditions if you live where there is snow, ice, or heavy rains. Keep your car in good repair.
Sun	Wear sunscreen. Limit direct exposure to the sun, especially early in the summer when the skin is most sensitive to burns. This can be achieved by wearing sunscreen, hats, and clothing that prevent sunburns.
Machinery	Learn how to use power tools correctly. Always have someone near when you use tools or machinery.
Emergency care	Learn first aid, CPR, and airway obstruction removal.
Water safety	Learn to swim well. If you supervise younger children near water, never leave them alone, even for a minute.
Fires	Do not play with fire. Follow guidelines to avoid igniting gasoline. Test smoke alarms in your house every 6 months and change batteries annually.
Firearms	Know and follow rules to keep firearms locked, with ammunition locked in a separate place. Never take out a gun to show a friend unless your parent is also present. Take firearm safety classes if you hunt or target shoot.
Hearing	Avoid loud music especially for long periods and through ear phones.
Sports	Wear protective gear recommended for your sport.
Abuse	Report any abuse to an adult you trust. Date with other couples whenever possible and report date rape. Do not drink or take drugs.

Data from Hagan, J. F., Shaw, J. S., & Duncan, P. M. (2008). *Bright futures: Guidelines for health supervision of infants, children and adolescents,* 3rd ed. Elk Grove Village, IL: American Academy of Pediatrics.

groups present, it is important to leave information about how to contact the nurse or another care provider. Provide brochures, referral numbers, names, and emails related to the topics discussed. Encourage annual visits for health supervision visits and suggest a variety of places to obtain this care. For example, if a youth will soon graduate from high school, find out if he or she will be working or attending college and provide links to health insurance or care providers in the new location.

Evidence-Based Nursing

FARM INJURY AND HAZARDS

Clinical Question

Injury is common in communities where children live and work on farms. Most injuries occur on weekends during the spring or summer. Before lunch and late afternoon are common times of the day for injury, likely due to being tired at those times.

Evidence

A study by nurses in Pennsylvania found that lacerations and musculoskeletal injuries caused by animals and equipment were common farm injuries among youth (Conway, McClune, & Nosel, 2007). Males of approximately 13 years have been found to have the highest rate of injury from equipment, with outcomes such as amputation, fractures, spinal injury, and death (Beer, Deboy, & Field, 2007). The rural lifestyle also presents other potential health hazards. Examples include exposure to pesticides and dusts, injury from the pastime of target shooting, drowning in unsupervised bodies of water or irrigation ditches, and contaminated water supplies (Cherry, Huggins, & Gilmore, 2007).

Best Practice

Nurses should intervene when working with families from rural areas to help them plan to promote safety for children on the farm. Realize that many rural families seek health care in urban areas, so even the nurse who works in a city may see rural families in the agency. Encourage parents to consult the North American Guidelines for Children's Agricultural Tasks to match the child's physical and mental abilities with the tasks on a farm. Then suggest that parents supervise children in farm tasks, know first aid to follow for injuries, realize that serious accidents can occur, have a cell phone to call for help, and know what facilities are available for phone advice and for emergency rescue. Help families plan ahead to keep rural children safe.

Critical Thinking

What items would you include on a checklist for parents of children on a farm? How might pesticides or other chemicals used on a farm injure youth who work near them? Plan educational materials and programs for families that live on farms.

See MyNursingKit for possible responses.

EVALUATION

Expected outcomes for care of adolescents and their families during health promotion and health maintenance include the following:

- Normal growth patterns and maintenance of healthy weight
- Physical activity of 60 minutes daily
- Absence of debris and plaque on dental surfaces
- Establishment of positive self-concept
- Positive relationships with peers, family members, teachers, and others
- Healthy lifestyle habits that promote prevention of disease and injury

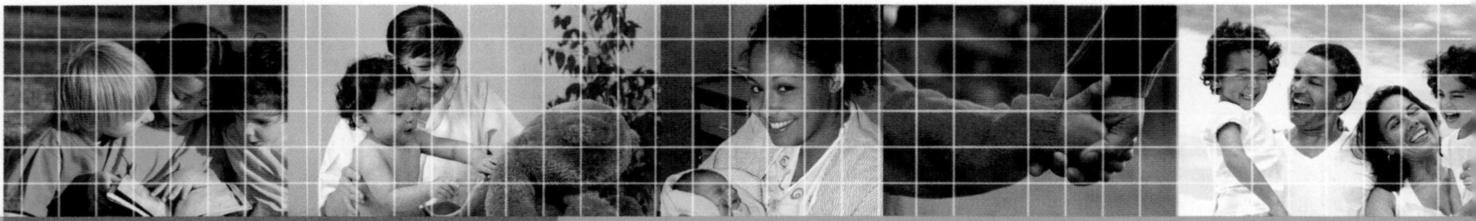

CRITICAL CONCEPT REVIEW

LEARNING OUTCOMES / CONCEPTS

38.1 Identify the major health concerns of the adolescent years.

1. School performance.
2. Sexual issues.
3. Body image issues.
4. The need for independence.

38.2 Describe the general observations made of adolescents and their families as they come to the pediatric healthcare home for health supervision visits.

1. Teen waiting areas.
2. Presence of parents.
3. Teen conversation.

38.3 Apply communication skills to interactions with adolescents and their families.

1. Assist parents to understand that the adolescent is striving to be independent.
2. Reassure adolescent that the parent is trying to provide guidance during a confusing time of life.
3. Encourage parents to reward positive behaviors.
4. Encourage adolescent to discuss specific issues rather than global subjects.

38.4 Apply assessment skills to plan data-gathering methods for nutrition, physical activity, and mental health status of youth.

1. Nutrition:
   - Discuss weight changes since last healthcare visit.
   - Discuss usual meal routines and favorite foods.
2. Physical activity:
   - Question adolescent regarding participation in sports, including amount of practice.
   - Discuss other forms of physical activity engaged in daily or weekly.
3. Mental health status:
   - Assess adolescent's perception of accomplishments and disappointments in life.
   - Ask adolescent about sexual activity.

38.5 Synthesize data from history and examination of adolescent and family with knowledge of adolescent development to plan approaches useful with the family during health supervision visits.

1. Partner with the adolescent, parents, and others to plan care.
2. Apply communication skills effective with teens.
3. Develop resources in order to apply effective teaching with adolescents.

38.6 Intervene with adolescents by integrating activities to promote health and to prevent disease and injury.

1. Screening tests:
   - Scoliosis.
   - Mental health status.
   - Anemia.
   - Sexually transmitted infections.
2. Review immunization status.
3. Review information concerning need for sun protection.
4. Discussion of birth control and prevention of sexually transmitted diseases.
5. Discussion of safe driving practices:
   - Seat belts.
   - Do not drink and drive.
6. Discussion of prevention of common sports injuries

CRITICAL THINKING IN ACTION

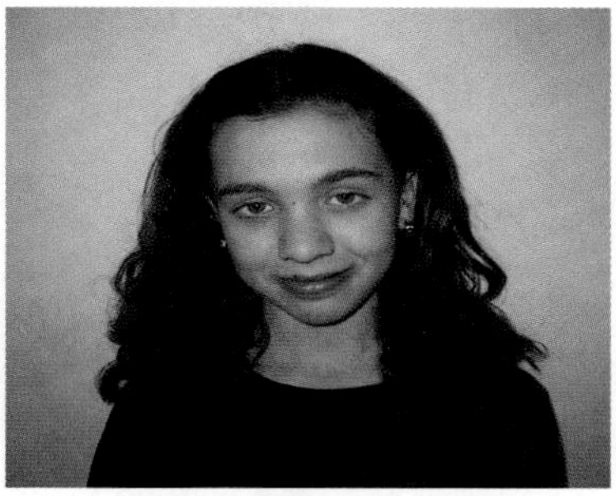

Tammy is a 13-year-old coming into the office for her yearly checkup and she has never been in the hospital or had surgery. She is a good student and is excited to start seventh grade next year. She has not had any immunizations since going into kindergarten. Tammy arrives with her mother, with whom she lives; she has no contact with her biological father. Her mother decides to stay in the waiting room, but did note on the written history form that there is a family history of high cholesterol and heart disease in family members under 50 years old. Tammy's mother is a single parent working full time with two other children at home. Tammy's body mass index is in the 85th percentile and she passed her hearing and vision tests. Her blood pressure is 115/70 and her urinalysis shows blood, but Tammy has her menses today. Tammy has a period every month and menarche started at 10 years old. Her menses lasts five to seven days and she denies experiencing cramping or excessively heavy menses. Tammy enjoys being a member of the volleyball team and is involved in a church youth group. She does not get to spend much time with her friends because she watches her two younger siblings in the afternoons while her mother is at work. When her mother is away, she admits to sitting and playing video games or watching TV most of the day. Tammy says she has had a boyfriend, but denies sexual activity. She also denies any experimentation with substance use.

1. What vaccines is Tammy due for at this age if she has not already had them?
2. Based on the information you collected about Tammy, what are some of the areas of recommended health teaching?
3. A dietary assessment demonstrates that Tammy frequently skips meals and eats fast food almost daily. What are some of the suggestions you can give Tammy to improve her nutritional status?
4. What are some of the injury prevention topics you can discuss with Tammy?

See MyNursingKit for possible responses.

REFERENCES

Bandura, A. (1977a). *Self-efficacy in changing societies*. New York: Cambridge University.

Bandura, A. (1977b). *Self-efficacy: The exercise of control*. New York: Freeman.

Bandura, A. (1986). *Social foundations of thought and actions: A social cognitive theory*. Englewood Cliffs, NJ: Prentice Hall.

Beer, S. R., Deboy, G. R., & Field, W. E. (2007). Analysis of 151 agricultural driveline-related incidents resulting in fatal and non-fatal injuries to U.S. children and adolescents under age 18 from 1970 through 2004. *Journal of Agricultural Safety and Health, 13,* 147–164.

Branson, B. M. (2006). Revised recommendations for HIV testing in health care settings in the United States. Retrieved August 13, 2007, from www.cdc.gov/hiv/topics/testing/resources/slidesets/pdf/testing_healthcare.pdf

Chang, G., Sherritt, L., & Knight, J. R. (2005). Adolescent cigarette smoking and mental health symptoms. *Journal of Adolescent Health, 36,* 517–522.

Cherry, D. C., Huggins, B., & Gilmore, K. (2007). Children's health in the rural environment. *Pediatric Clinics of North America, 54,* 121–133.

Conway, A. E., McClune, A. J., & Nosel, P. (2007). Down on the farm: Preventing farm accidents in children. *Pediatric Nursing, 33,* 45–48.

Eaton, D. K., Kann, L., Kinchen, S., Ross, J., Hawkins, J., Harris, W. A., et al. (2006). Youth Risk Behavior Surveillance—United States, 2005. *Morbidity and Mortality Weekly Report (MMWR), 55*(SS05), 1–108.

Hagan, J. F., Shaw, J. S., & Duncan, P. M. (Eds.). (2008). *Bright futures: Guidelines for health supervision of infants, children, and adolescents* (3rd ed.). Elk Grove Village, IL: American Academy of Pediatrics.

Hortz, B., & Petosa, R. L. (2008). Social cognitive theory variables mediation of moderate exercise. *American Journal of Health Behavior, 32,* 305–314.

Jellinek, M., Patel, B. P., & Froehle, M. C. (Eds.). (2002). *Bright futures in practice: Mental health* (Vols. I and II). Arlington, VA: National Center for Education in Maternal and Child Health.

Liu, J., Probst, J. C., Martin, A. B., Wang, J. Y., & Salinas, C.F. (2007). Disparities in dental insurance coverage and dental care among US children: The National Survey of Children's Health. *Pediatrics, 119,* S12–S21.

Mayo Clinic. (2007). Teen sleep: Why is your teen so tired? Retrieved August 13, 2007, from http://www.mayoclinic.com/health/teens-health/CC00019

Murray, R. B., Zentner, J. P., & Yakimo, R. (2009). *Health promotion strategies through the life span* (8th ed.). Upper Saddle River, NJ: Prentice Hall Health.

Olson, A. L., Gaffney, C. A., Hedberg, V. A., Gladstone, S., Dugan, S., Mathes, T., et al. (2005). The Health Teen Project: Tools to enhance adolescent health counseling. *Annals of Family Medicine, 3*(Suppl 2), 563–565.

Olson, C. M., Bove, C. F., & Miller, E. O. (2007). Growing up poor: Long-term implications for eating patterns and body weight. *Appetite, 49,* 198–207.

Simons-Morton, B., & Ouimet, M. C. (2006). Parent involvement in novice teen driving: A review of the literature. *Injury Prevention, 12,* 30–37.

Strong, W. B., Malina, R. M., Blimkie, C. J., Daniels, S. R., Dishman, R. K., Gutin, B., et al. (2005). Evidence-based physical activity for school-age youth. *Journal of Pediatrics, 146,* 732–737.

U.S. Department of Health and Human Services (2006). *Healthy People 2010: Midcourse Review*. Washington, DC: U.S. Department of Health and Human Services.

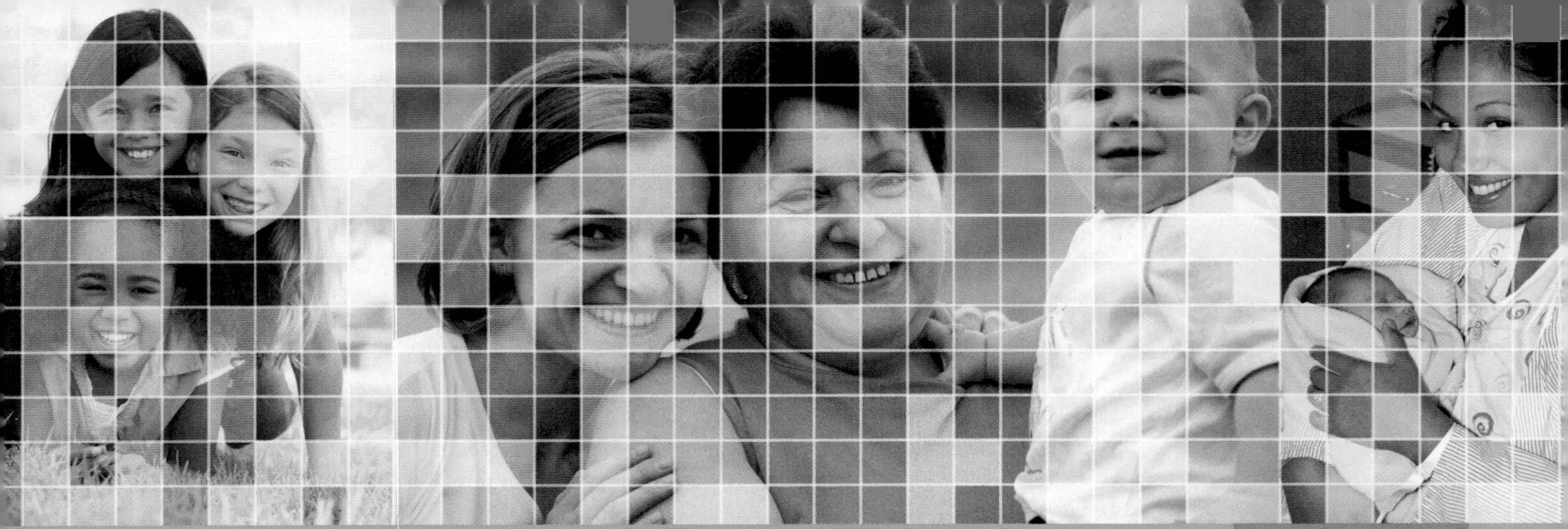

CHAPTER

39

Family Assessment and Concepts of Nursing Care in the Community

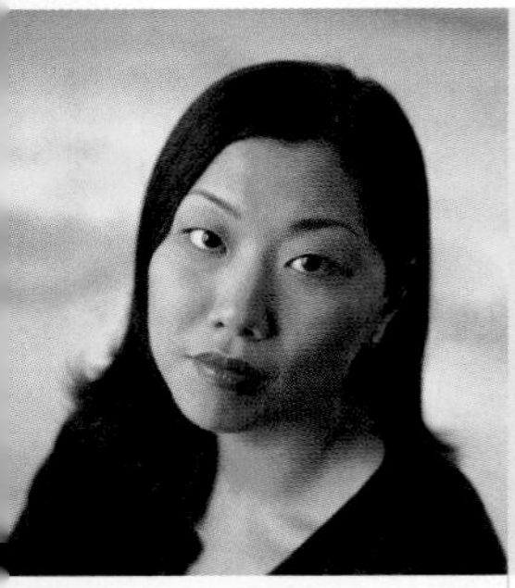

Sometimes Jessica's asthma attacks really frighten me because she struggles so hard to breathe. She has a lot of trouble with asthma in the summertime with all the heat. I am afraid to let her play outside with her friends for fear that she will have another attack. I would really like to know how to keep Jessica's asthma under control. —Mother of Jessica, 8 years old

LEARNING OUTCOMES

39.1 Categorize the family strengths that help families cope with stressors.

39.2 Describe the advantages of using a family assessment tool.

39.3 Identify a variety of family support services that might be available in a community.

39.4 List the variety of community healthcare settings where nurses provide health services to children.

39.5 Compare the roles of the nurse in each identified healthcare setting.

39.6 Contrast the emergency care planning that is important in each community setting.

Children receive most of their healthcare in community settings. Depending upon the community, healthcare resources, and age of the child, this care may be provided in a variety of settings. When providing health care to the child and family, it is important for the nurse to assess the family's strengths, be aware of community resources, and help families manage the complex healthcare that is often provided in the home.

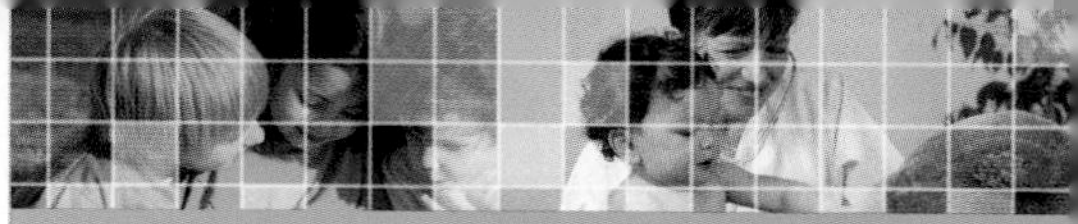

KEY TERMS

Emergency preparedness plan, 1052
Family, 1045
Family resilience, 1045
Family strengths, 1045
Medically fragile, 1053

FAMILY ASSESSMENT

The **family** is an interdependent network of individuals that mutually influence each other. Families must be understood in their own context. It is important to understand each family's strengths and uniqueness and how the family and its members respond to the complex and often conflicting demands for time and attention. Nurses need to be able to assess family strengths and support mechanisms, to identify coping strategies, and to determine when families have overextended their resources and need additional support. In some cases nurses can provide the additional support needed, and at other times referral to other health professionals is appropriate to address the family's needs.

Children and families live within a variety of home environments, and interactions within those settings directly or indirectly influence behaviors and learning. Because of these environmental influences on the family, it is important to consider the relationship of the family with the social networks within the community.

FAMILY STRESSORS

Family stressors come from many sources, such as work demands, school issues, extended family demands, achieving quality family time, and community roles. Many families live in a stressed state due to inadequate finances, healthcare concerns, relationship challenges, and other pressures. Most families have developed coping strategies to deal with daily routine stressors.

A child's illness or injury is a stressor that affects the entire family. The response by family members can lead to changes in the interactions among family members and with the environment. Unexpected events are often more stressful as the family has not had time to consider available resources and prepare a response. Identifying how families respond to the stress of an illness or injury of the child or of another family member is important because nursing interventions and support may reduce the impact on the entire family.

FAMILY STRENGTHS

Family strengths are the relationships and processes that support and protect families and family members during times of adversity and change. Nurses can identify and use a family's strengths when problem solving within the family (Wright & Leahey, 2005, p. 161). Four types of strengths that enable families to develop, adapt to change, and cope with challenges are (Tarko & Reed, 2004):

- Individual or family traits, such as optimism or resilience
- Individual or family assets, such as finances
- Individual or family capabilities, skills, and competencies, such as problem solving
- Another quality less permanent than a trait or asset, such as motivation

Identifying a **family's resilience**—the family's capacity to demonstrate a positive response to an adverse situation and to emerge from the situation feeling strengthened, more resourceful, and more confident—is an important focus for family assessment prior to planning nursing interventions (Simon, Murphy, &

Smith, 2005). Four significant characteristics of a resilient family include (Benard, 2004):

- Social competence, involving cultural flexibility, empathy, and caring
- Problem solving that involves planning, help-seeking, critical and creative thinking that enables the family to make decisions
- Autonomy for the family unit, involving flexibility and adaptation to change
- Having a sense of purpose that involves setting goals and having optimism and faith

Most families have the capacity to develop resilience. Nursing support may be needed to help family members learn new skills, make adaptations, and gain confidence in their abilities to manage the challenges of the child's health condition. Some potential resources to promote resilience include religious faith, finances, social support, physical health, family flexibility, and family coping mechanisms. Families with diminished resources will be more susceptible to disruption because of a healthcare crisis or event. Nurses can help families identify their strengths, and areas for improvement that can lead to increased resiliency. Resilience of children is discussed in Chapter 44.

Functional families use their strengths and a variety of coping strategies to successfully reduce stress. See "Nursing Practice" for family strengths that promote resilience and coping. Coping strategies of dysfunctional families are defensive (e.g., denial of family problems, exploiting a family member, use of threats or withdrawal of affection and support, dominance and submissive patterns, and family substance abuse).

Nurses can point out family strengths to develop a rapport and relationship with the family. Focus on family competence, and acknowledge and validate family members' emotions. Once the family recognizes the strengths it brings to the management of their child's healthcare problem, the more likely the family will become an effective partner in the process. The nurse can often help families recognize that strengths used in prior life experiences may transfer to the current healthcare experience.

Nursing Practice

MyNursingKit The HOME Inventory

Family strengths helpful in managing stressors include the following:

- *Communication skills*—the ability of family members to listen, gather information, and to discuss their concerns in an honest and open manner
- *Shared family values and beliefs*—the family's common perceptions of reality and willingness to have hope and to appreciate that change is possible; family celebrations; family traditions
- *Intrafamily support*—the provision of support and reinforcement by extended family members, to promote family cohesion and an atmosphere of belonging; family time and routines
- *Self-care abilities*—the family's ability to take responsibility for health problems and the demonstrated willingness of individual members to take good care of themselves
- *Problem-solving skill*—the family's use of negotiation in problem solving, using everyday experiences as resources, and focusing on the present rather than past events or disappointments; effective utilization of healthcare resources
- *Community linkages*—maintenance of active linkages with the community; reaching out to others in the social network including extended family and friends

COLLECTING DATA FOR FAMILY ASSESSMENT

To obtain an accurate and concise family assessment, the nurse needs to establish a trusting relationship with the child and family. Identify the greatest concern of the parent(s) and child, and expect their concerns to be different. Acknowledge these multiple concerns and demonstrate respect for the diversity of the family. The goal is to obtain family information that will be useful when planning nursing interventions that will help the family care for the child and improve the child's outcomes while valuing each family member.

Information about the family is collected continuously during the healthcare process, through interviews, observations of family interactions, reports from other healthcare providers or agencies working with the family, and with a family assessment tool (see "Nursing Practice").

See Chapter 35 for suggested data to collect about the psychosocial history and daily living patterns. Observation of the home and family members is recommended in some cases to obtain valuable information about family functioning.

FAMILY ASSESSMENT TOOLS

Family assessment tools help in obtaining information about the family's functioning, and some tools focus on family stresses, coping strategies, and family strengths. Information about the

Nursing Practice

Family assessment data to collect:

- Name, age, sex, and family relationship of all people residing in the household
- Family type, structure, values
- Cultural associations, including cultural norms and customs related to childrearing and infant feeding
- Family roles and interaction patterns; family decision making roles
- Support systems network, including extended family, friends, faith-based affiliations, and community associations
- Communication patterns, including language barriers
- Environmental data—place of residence, condition of housing, number of persons living in the residence, sleeping arrangements, play areas, neighborhood characteristics

way the family functions in nurturing its members, solving problems, and communicating may help identify strategies that can be effective for managing the child's health care. They may enable the nurse to work more effectively with the family, such as collaborating with the family in planning for health maintenance and health promotion strategies.

Family Ecomap

By illustrating the family's relationships and interactions with social networks in the community, an **ecomap** enables nurses and other healthcare providers to visualize the family's social network. Family participation in the preparation of the ecomap may reveal information about how the family perceives or receives social support, and the strength of family relationships with significant other persons and organizations. The ecomap provides an opportunity to identify the community resources being used by the family and to highlight any potential community resources that may help promote the family's health. Figure 39–1 ● shows a sample ecomap for Jessica's family.

Friedman Family Assessment Tool

This tool, developed by Marilyn Friedman, provides a method for nurses to assess the entire family in the context of the community where the family resides (Tarko & Reed, 2004; Friedman, Bowden, & Jones, 2003). Information collected contains data about a family's relationships, functioning, strengths, and problems. (See Appendix G for the short form.)

Calgary Family Assessment Model

This tool, developed by Lorraine Wright and Maureen Leahey (2009), has three categories of information (structural, developmental, and functional family data) for assessment of a family's strengths and problems. The complete model is available in their textbook *Nurses and Families: A Guide to Family Assessment and Intervention*. The model enables collection of extensive family information, and it can facilitate assessment of family challenges, such as problems integrating a treatment plan in family routines. A family genogram or ecomap may also be helpful in completing the assessment.

Home Observation for Measurement of the Environment (HOME)

The HOME Inventory is an assessment tool developed to measure the quality and quantity of stimulation and support available to the child in the home environment (Caldwell & Bradley, 1984). The tool is also used to identify relationships between the home environment and the child's development (Totsika & Sylva, 2004). Four age-specific scales are available (birth to 3 years, 3 to 6 years, 6 to 10 years, and 10 to 15 years). Examples of subscales contained in each age-specific HOME Inventory include parental

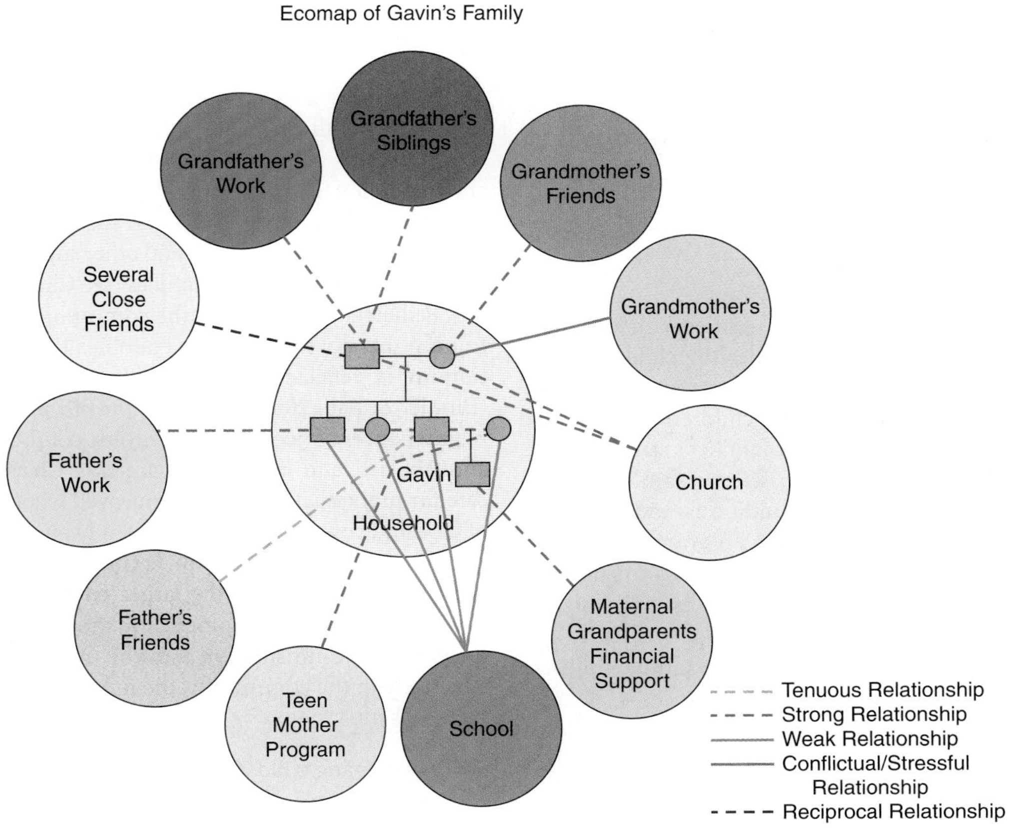

● **Figure 39–1** Ecomap. An ecomap illustrates the family's relationships and interactions with groups and individuals in the immediate external environment.

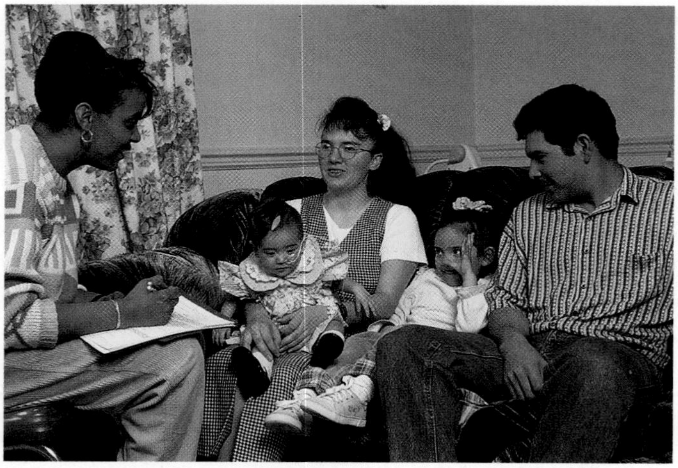

● **Figure 39–2** HOME Inventory. A visit to the home when all family members are present provides the best information for completion of an assessment tool such as the Home Observation for Measurement of the Environment (H.O.M.E.).

responsivity, acceptance of child, the physical environment, learning materials, variety in experience, and parental involvement. Data are collected during an informal, low-stress interview and observation over 45 to 90 minutes in the home setting (Figure 39–2 ●). The child's primary caregiver and the child must be present and awake during the interview as observation of their interaction is an essential part of the assessment. The intent is to allow family members to act normally. Assessment of the home environment may help to identify nursing interventions that promote the child's growth and development, such as items in the home that can be used for toys and strategies for parent interaction with the child to promote learning. See MyNursingKit for the Web site with more information about the HOME inventory.

FAMILY SUPPORT SERVICES IN THE COMMUNITY

Family support services exist in all communities with a purpose of supporting families in the rearing of healthy children. Contemporary lifestyles (e.g., divorced or single parents, both parents in the workforce and separated from children for long time periods, and separation from extended families) stress families trying to provide for their children's needs. Other family stressors include economic factors, poor living conditions, and homelessness. Many communities have developed programs to support the health and development of children, parental competencies, and positive family relationships. Most programs are designed with the premise that no family is entirely self-sufficient and most can benefit from some external support. Examples of these family support services include the following:

- Head Start and Early Head Start
- Before- and after-school programs for children of working parents
- School-based health and counseling services
- Play groups for preschool children
- Peer support groups
- Social service programs offered by the faith community
- Home visiting programs for high-risk children and parents
- Job skills training, adult education, and literacy programs
- Crisis care and respite care programs

Compile a list of the formal and informal family support services in your community. Nurses play an important role in linking families to the types of community support services they need after performing a family assessment and collaborating with families to identify and seek assistance most beneficial to their needs.

COMMUNITY-BASED HEALTH CARE

Health care for children has been rapidly shifting from the hospital to community settings over the past 15 years. Health plans and healthcare providers continue to explore options to provide safe, high-quality care with fewer hospitalizations or shorter stays when hospitalization is needed. Patterns of healthcare delivery are changing due to technologic developments and efforts to reduce healthcare costs, as these examples illustrate:

- Day surgery and invasive diagnostic procedures performed in outpatient surgical settings.
- Short-stay or observation units in emergency departments to reduce the number of hospital admissions.
- Intravenous antibiotic therapy provided in the home.
- Pediatric hospice and palliative care in the home setting.

The trend in out-of-hospital care has significantly increased for children with chronic health conditions and advanced disease states. Technologic advances, such as portable medical equipment, enable families to provide complex healthcare services in the home and other community settings, and such care in the community is less costly. Home care services and other support services have been developed to support these families (see Chapter 40∞).

Pediatric health care in the community occurs along a continuum that covers the entire child healthcare system. This continuum is reflected in the Continuum of Pediatric Health (Bindler & Ball, 2007), including health promotion and health maintenance services, care for chronic conditions, acute illnesses and injuries, and end-of-life care (see Chapter 1∞). Health care for individual children is improved when there is continuity of care and communication between healthcare settings.

The nurse working with families in a community setting uses knowledge of how the larger environment influences the child's health and development and the family's functioning, and integrates that information into the nursing care plan. To work effectively in the community, the nurse needs to gain experience and skills in:

- Conducting child and family assessments, working with families to plan individualized healthcare strategies, and implementing and evaluating nursing care strategies to match family economic, cultural, and social situation, and available resources.

- Working with community agencies (schools, faith-based groups, and other community-based resources) to assess, plan strategies, and implement and evaluate approaches addressed to the healthcare needs of the community's children.

COMMUNITY HEALTHCARE SETTINGS

Children receive most of their health care (health promotion and episodic health care for acute illnesses and injuries) in community settings. Depending on the community, healthcare resources, and age of the child, care may be received in all or only a few of the following settings:

- A healthcare center or a physician's office is the usual site for health promotion, health maintenance, episodic acute care, and health management of children with chronic conditions. See Chapters 36 through 38 for age-specific health promotion and health maintenance guidelines.
- A public health clinic may provide health promotion and health maintenance services. A homeless shelter may also have the capacity to offer such services.
- A hospital outpatient center may provide specialized services to children with chronic conditions or a full range of services similar to a health center.
- Schools usually provide health promotion and health maintenance services, plus first aid and emergency care as needed. School-based health centers may additionally provide counseling, health education, and care for acute conditions. Some school settings offer other services, such as preschool and after-school childcare services.
- Childcare centers provide first aid for emergencies and some health promotion services.
- The home is now a site for a child's acute condition or chronic condition management, rehabilitation, and end-of-life care when the family is supported by home health services.

Nurses may serve as a community health nurse, home health nurse, school nurse, pediatric nurse in an office setting, and nurse practitioner or advanced practice nurse in these settings. The nurse in any of the above settings has an important role in promoting the health and safety of the child, being a leader in setting policies in the center, and using the nursing process to help families meet the healthcare needs of their children. The nurse may assume the role of direct care provider, educator, advocate, or planner.

THE OFFICE OR HEALTHCARE CENTER SETTING NURSING ROLES

The nursing process is used when providing care for children in the health center. The range of assessment responsibilities may vary by setting as well as the preparation and experience of the nurse (Figure 39–3 ●). Specific functions of the pediatric nurse in this setting include the following:

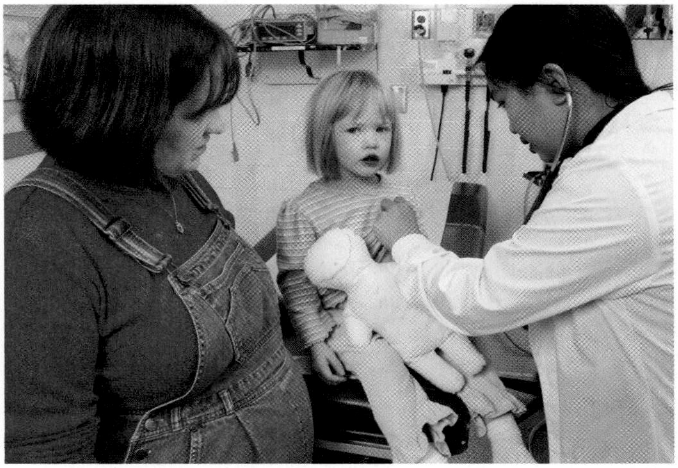

● **Figure 39–3** Assessment in an office setting. Nurses carefully assess children in the office setting who present with an acute care illness. It is important to identify how serious the child's illness is and to monitor the child for progression of symptoms during the visit. This is also a time to gather information about the child's illness and to identify health information that will be needed for the family to care for the child at home.

- Identifying children in need of urgent care or isolation
- Performing nursing assessments, including the health history, vital signs, growth and development, nutritional status, immunization status, family strengths and challenges
- Conducting physical examinations
- Performing age-appropriate screening tests to detect health problems such as vision or hearing loss, anemia, and lead poisoning to ensure that the child has access to all needed health services (see Chapters 36–38)
- Assisting with physician examinations and diagnostic tests
- Developing nursing diagnoses and implementing a plan of care
- Providing immunizations (see Chapter 45)
- Providing information about procedures and offering reassurance
- Providing patient education for health promotion or management of the health condition
- Linking families with community resources
- Ensuring that the healthcare setting is a safe environment and that infection control guidelines are followed. See the Clinical Skills Manual SKILLS for infection control methods.

An important goal is to develop a positive relationship with the child and family so that optimal health care is provided. This relationship is strengthened over time during future healthcare visits. (See "Nursing Practice.")

Identifying Severely Ill and Injured Children

Each child with an episodic illness or injury presenting to the health center must be assessed upon arrival to determine the urgency of care needed. A rapid assessment for changes in mental

Nursing Practice

It is as important to develop a relationship with the child and family in a community setting as it is in the hospital. The initial interaction often sets the stage for a long-term relationship with the family that returns to the same setting for health care over many years. As you approach the child and family, put aside the stressors you may be feeling. Take a few moments to play with the infant or child and to comment on a positive attribute of the child to the parents. The parent's, and perhaps the child's, stress level will also be reduced, facilitating the beginning of a long-term partnership with the child and family.

status, airway patency, breathing, and circulation is used to identify the child that needs immediate medical attention. The child with an urgent condition must be monitored frequently to detect any worsening of condition and need for emergency care.

Emergency Response Planning

The nurse collaborates with the physician to develop an emergency response plan for the health center. The nurse teaches office staff to recognize a child needing immediate assessment by the nurse. The nurse is often responsible for ensuring that all emergency care equipment, supplies, and medications are organized and readily available in a central treatment room (see "Nursing Practice"). The nurse may also coordinate mock drills so that all employees know and perform their designated role when a true emergency occurs.

Educating the Child and Family

Patient education regarding injury prevention, growth and development, nutrition, healthy lifestyles, and the home care of episodic illnesses and injuries are important nursing roles. The nurse may be responsible for selecting patient education materials for the waiting area and those specifically used to teach families about various conditions. Knowledge of the community and population served by the health center enables the nurse to select appropriate education materials.

Nurses teach families to provide the condition-specific care for the child at home. Examples of information provided include:

- Signs that the condition is not improving as expected and when to return to the physician.
- How and when to administer prescribed medications and their potential side effects.
- Modifications in diet and activity.
- Other supportive care for the child's condition.
- Education to help the child and family recognize the need to initiate care for a new episode of a chronic condition (i.e., asthma, sickle cell anemia, or hemophilia) that may prevent the need for a healthcare visit or reduce the severity of the episode.

Nursing Practice

Required emergency equipment for managing a pediatric emergency in a health center includes the following in various pediatric sizes (American Academy of Pediatrics Committee on Pediatric Emergency Medicine, 2007):

- Oxygen delivery system (bag-valve masks in 450 and 1000 mL sizes, clear oxygen face masks with and without reservoir)
- Airway equipment (oral and nasopharyngeal airways, suction devices, laryngoscope handle and blades, endotracheal tubes and stylet, end-tidal CO_2 detector, nasogastric tubes)
- Pulse oximeter, peak flow meter, a nebulizer or metered-dose inhaler with a spacer/mask
- Intravenous (IV) and intraosseous needles, IV tubing, and normal saline or lactated Ringer's IV solution
- A length-based resuscitation tape and preprinted drug dosage chart to quickly identify equipment sizes and drug dosages by the length or weight of the child
- Drugs (epinephrine 1:1000, albuterol for inhalation, activated charcoal, naloxone, and 5% dextrose)

Locate the emergency equipment in every clinical setting where you have assignments so that you can quickly take the child to it or bring the equipment to the child if an emergency occurs.

Identifying Community Resources

Nurses are often involved in identifying community resources needed by the child and family to help promote the child's health. Compiling a manual of community resources and regularly updating names and phone numbers of contacts will make it easier to provide information efficiently. Examples of community resources that might be included are early intervention programs, support groups, language and translation services, food banks, lead paint abatement services, social services, and mental health services.

Ensuring a Safe Environment for Children

The health center has many potential hazards such as equipment, cleaning supplies, sharps, medications, and laboratory materials from which the child needs to be protected. The child must be attended at all times when in the examination area. Guidelines for infection control must be developed and implemented to reduce the transmission of infectious diseases between child patients and between the healthcare providers and children.

SPECIALTY HEALTHCARE SETTING NURSING ROLES

Pediatric nurses also provide care for children with acute and chronic conditions within hospital outpatient or specialty care ambulatory settings. Children may be referred to physician specialists for diagnostic workups or for the long-term management of their chronic conditions. In some cases health promotion, health maintenance, and episodic illness care are provided to children with chronic conditions in these settings. With experience, pediatric nurses working in a hospital ambulatory setting develop specialized knowledge and skill to meet the specific needs of the population of children cared for in that setting. The roles for nurses in these settings are similar to those described for the health center.

SCHOOL SETTING NURSING ROLES

The role of school nurses has changed over the past decade as the population of children attending school has changed. School nursing is a specialized practice of professional nursing that advances the well-being, academic success, and lifelong achievement of students. School nurses address a wide range of physical and mental health challenges among the students in their school setting. They advocate for the students by becoming active in policy development that affects the school community. They are proactive in health promotion, health maintenance, and work to create a healthy school setting (Denehy, 2006). See MyNursingKit for the Web site of the National Association of School Nurses.

School nurses practice independently as the only licensed healthcare provider in the educational setting and, depending on the community, serve 750 to 2000 children in one or more schools (Guttu, Engelke, & Swanson, 2004). Health aides may be present in the school setting and need training and supervision by the school nurse. Healthcare needs of faculty and staff are also addressed. Many school nurses have obtained certification or advanced education to become a school nurse practitioner, enabling them to better manage this independent practice.

School nurses work to remove or minimize the health barriers to learning so students can improve school performance. School health services include preventive services, health promotion and health maintenance, health education, emergency care, and the referral and management of acute and chronic health problems. The traditional tasks of screening, first aid, and monitoring immunization status are still performed (Figure 39–4 ●). See "Nursing Practice" for the *Healthy People 2010* national health objectives that illustrate the breadth of school nursing.

The school nurse also plans, develops, manages, and evaluates healthcare services to all children in the educational setting. In many cases, the nurse works with families of the students to ensure that needed care is provided. Approximately 5% of children are administered daily medication at school (McCarthy, Kelly, Johnson, et al., 2006). Other roles of the nurse in the school setting include the following: maintaining infection control, participating on teams to develop student individualized education plans (IEP) and individualized health plans (IHP), updating health records, collecting data on services provided to students, consulting with health teachers about educational topics, advocating for better nutrition and physical activity, investigating environmental safety hazards, developing an emergency preparedness plan, and planning for crisis intervention and support services. See Chapter 40∞ for more information on IEPs and IHPs.

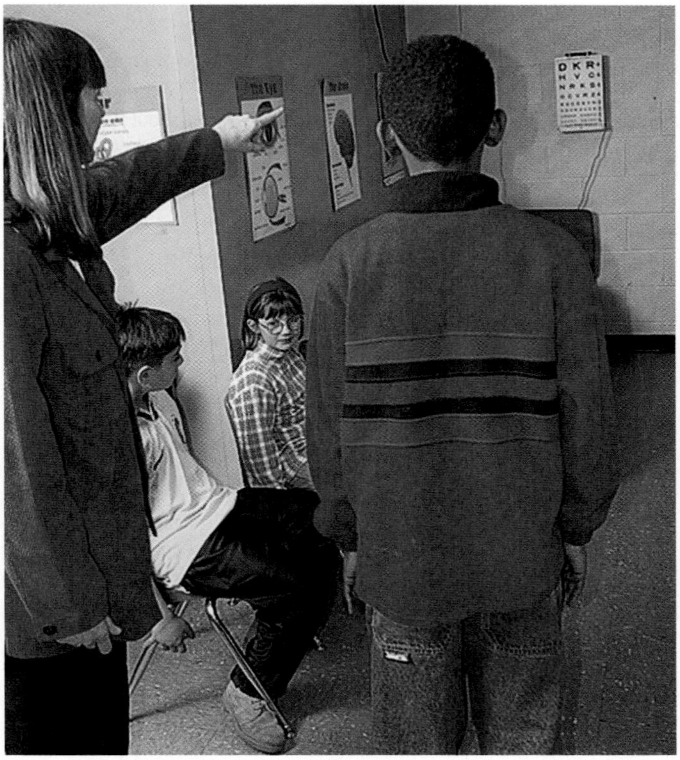

● **Figure 39–4** Screening in the school setting. The school is often the setting for screening tests of large groups of students to identify those that may have a problem that interferes with learning. Screening tests are often organized so all children in a particular grade are assessed, as in this vision screening test.

Collaboration with the other health professionals in the community is becoming increasingly important to promote health in the school setting, as the following examples illustrate:

- Partnering with the school physician consultant to discuss and update standing orders for the care of children. These standing orders usually address urgent and emergency care potentially needed by students and the variety of student healthcare problems that may occur.
- Working with the parent-teacher association and other community organizations to organize health fairs and injury prevention programs for students.
- Communicating with the child's primary healthcare provider or pediatric specialist about a child's specific health condition that needs to be effectively managed in the school setting. It is essential to have the parent's permission to obtain patient information and to follow confidentiality requirements. The school nurse has regular opportunities to monitor the child's health status and to provide information that may help the healthcare providers with the child's ongoing management.

Preparation for Emergencies

Every school needs a plan to ensure effective emergency care and transport for an acutely ill or injured child. The school is a

MyNursingKit School Policy Review

Nursing Practice

The *Healthy People 2010* objectives that relate to school health issues include the following:

- Increase high school completion rate.
- Increase the percentage of middle, junior high, and senior high schools that provide health education to prevent health problems in the following areas: unintentional injury, violence, suicide, tobacco use and addiction, alcohol and other drug use, unintended pregnancy, HIV/AIDS and sexually transmitted infection, unhealthy dietary patterns, inadequate physical activity, and environmental health.
- Increase the percentage of the nation's elementary, middle, junior high, and senior high schools that have a nurse-to-student ratio of at least 1 to 750.
- Increase the percentage of the nation's primary and secondary schools that have official school policies ensuring the safety of students and staff from environmental hazards, such as chemicals in special classrooms, poor indoor air quality, asbestos, and exposure to pesticides.
- Increase the percentage of public and private schools that require use of appropriate head, face, eye, and mouth protection for students participating in school-sponsored physical activities.
- Reduce weapon-carrying on school property.
- Increase the percentage of children and adolescents age 6 to 19 years whose intake of meals and snacks at school contributes to good overall dietary quality.
- Increase the percentage of school-based health centers with an oral health component.
- Increase the percentage of the nation's public and private schools that require daily physical education for all students.
- Increase the percentage of adolescents who participate in daily school physical education.
- Increase the percentage of adolescents who spend 50% of school physical education time being physically active.
- Increase the percentage of the nation's public and private schools that provide access to their physical activity spaces and facilities for all persons outside of normal school hours.
- Reduce the number of school or workdays missed by persons due to asthma.

Department of Health and Human Services, Office of Disease Prevention and Promotion. (2006). *Healthy People 2010 Midcourse Review.* Washington, DC: Author, Retrieved April 24, 2007 from http://www.healthypeople.gov/data/midcourse/pdf/FA14.pdf

common location for injury in children under age 17 years (Guttu et al., 2004). Acute illnesses can also occur during school hours. The school nurse often works with the school administrators, the physician consultant, and the local emergency medical services (EMS) agency to develop an emergency response plan. School personnel need training to identify an emergency that requires activation of the local EMS system and to provide emergency care until the EMS providers arrive. Because other potential emergencies can occur, such as natural and manmade disasters, and behavioral crises, each school needs an **emergency preparedness plan**, a community-based coordinated response plan for the incident. See page 1056 for more information.

Facilitating a Child's Return to School

The school nurse also helps the child return to the classroom following an acute illness or injury, especially when environmental adaptation is required or when a change in health status has occurred. The child's parents or the pediatric nurse in the hospital or community setting may initiate the request to coordinate the child's return to school. Educational materials about the child's condition can be recommended to educate students, faculty, and staff. The school nurse then begins to work with the family to prepare teachers and school administrators for the child's special needs, such as limited mobility or medications. The child's teacher and classmates can be prepared for the child's physical changes if appropriate. Sometimes the teacher's expectations of the child need to be modified, such as a child with a mild brain injury who may have decreased ability to concentrate for several weeks during recovery. Often an IHP must be developed or modified (see Chapter 40).

Thinking Critically

ASTHMA ATTACKS AT SCHOOL

Jessica, 8 years old, is anxious because her asthma attack is getting worse. Her teacher sees that she is having trouble breathing, so she sends her to the school health office for treatment. Jessica has a nebulizer at school, and this treatment often relieves her symptoms and permits her to return to classes. When the asthma attack does not respond to the treatment, the school contacts her mother to come pick her up from school. This means another visit to the emergency department for treatment. Jessica does not like to miss school or to worry her mother. Her mother wishes there were some way to reduce the number and severity of her asthma attacks.

What measures can Jessica take to control her asthma on a daily basis and reduce the number of attacks? What special arrangements are needed to permit a child to receive care for asthma or another chronic condition while at school? What education does the teacher need to make an assessment and decision for Jessica to go to get her treatment? See Chapter 48 for more information about asthma management.

See MyNursingKit for possible responses.

Evidence-Based Nursing

IMPROVING SCHOOL NURSE ACCESS TO STUDENT ASTHMA ACTION PLANS

Clinical Question

What methods work to increase the number of children with asthma who have an asthma action plan at school?

The Evidence

A pilot study explored ways to increase communication between physicians and school nurses and to empower nurses to implement an asthma education program. Participating physicians were given education on national asthma guidelines, baseline data to include in asthma action plans, a Medicaid reimbursement code for development of asthma action plans, and office support for development of plans. School nurses received similar education, support to provide asthma education in the school, and asthma action plans from participating physicians. Community organization representatives provided support to the project and facilitated communication. Study results revealed that 32 additional students (a 44% increase) had asthma action plans after the intervention (Frankowski, Keating, Rexroad, et al., 2006). Another study compared direct school nurse communication with a child's physician versus parent communication for the purpose of obtaining an asthma action plan for the child's management at school. Twenty children with asthma in grades 6 through 8 from four school districts met daily with the nurse for 2 weeks to learn correct peak flow meter technique and to track peak flow readings. The school nurse sent this information to the parents and the child's physician with a request for an asthma action plan. The control group consisted of 20 same-aged students with asthma in the same communities but different schools. School nurses continued a standard practice of requesting asthma action plans through the control group children's parents. Significantly more asthma action plans were obtained from the physicians who were directly approached and provided with data about the child's peak flow readings (Pulcini, DeSisto, & McIntyre, 2007).

Best Practice

Community collaboration may be one way to improve access to and use of asthma action plans. School nurses with access to asthma action plans report using them more than 90% of the time to manage a child's asthma episode (McLaughlin, Maljanian, Kornblum, et al., 2006). Children who receive appropriate asthma management at school are more likely to return to the classroom for learning than to go home or to the emergency department.

Critical Thinking

During a school clinical placement, identify the estimated number of children with asthma and contrast that to the number with an asthma action plan. What strategies has the school nurse used to obtain asthma action plans? How effective have the strategies been? What other strategies might increase the number of asthma action plans?

See MyNursingKit for possible responses.

Children with Complex Healthcare Conditions

Previously homebound children, who are **medically fragile**, needing skilled nursing care with or without medical equipment to support vital functions, now attend school. See Chapter 40 for a discussion of these children and their care in the community.

CHILDCARE SETTINGS NURSING ROLES

An estimated 13 million children under 6 years of age receive care in out-of-home childcare settings while parents are at work (Brady, 2005). Many types of childcare arrangements exist, such as in-home care by a family member or nanny, a babysitter cooperative, a licensed childcare family home setting for up to five children, or a licensed childcare center for six or more children.

States establish minimum licensure requirements and guidelines for the safe operation of childcare settings that address the staff qualifications, staff-child ratio, staff training requirements, safe food handling, safe health practices, and environmental safety. Guidelines for the safe operation of childcare centers are available through the National Resource Center for Health and Safety in Child Care. See MyNursingKit for this center's Web site.

Nurses can assume an important consultant role in the establishment of the childcare center's policies for health practices, teaching staff about safe health practices, and monitoring and promoting health practices in the setting. The nurse consultant can also teach staff to identify children with illnesses and to provide first aid for injured children. Nurses may provide health screening and direct care in childcare centers for ill children (Alkon, Farrer, & Bernzweig, 2004).

Evidence in Action

Nurses providing consultation services in childcare centers were found in one study to have the following outcomes: policies and practices were changed for medication administration, immunizations, and illness management; and staff had increased competence in meeting hygiene standards, handling injuries, and working with parents (Dellert, Gasalberti, Sternas, et al., 2006).

MyNursingKit National Resource Center for Health and Safety in Child Care

Reducing Disease Transmission

Children attending childcare centers are at increased risk for otitis media, upper respiratory infections, gastroenteritis, gastrointestinal infections, and bacterial meningitis (Brady, 2005). Children are close together in large numbers, put things in their mouths, may be contagious before symptoms occur, and are susceptible to most infectious agents. The nurse can educate and work with the childcare center manager and staff to reduce disease transmission in the following ways:

- Developing guidelines for review of each child's immunizations and plans for exclusion of unimmunized children when a vaccine-preventable disease occurs in the center (see Chapter 45)

- Checking each child daily for signs and symptoms of illness (e.g., behavior changes, rashes, fever, vomiting, diarrhea, and eye drainage) and developing guidelines for the exclusion and return of children with different infectious conditions. Visit MyNursingKit for the Web site with this information.
- Teaching staff when and how to perform hand hygiene, manage secretions, sanitize toys and surfaces, and manage cuts and scrapes
- Developing guidelines for diapering infants and toddlers to reduce disease transmission
- Caring for the sick child and reducing exposure to others until the child goes home

Health Promotion and Health Maintenance

Health promotion activities are those that further the child's highest level of functioning and development, such as activities to stimulate physical development, nutrition to foster growth and ability to perform at maximum level, and a well-rounded program to promote fine motor, gross motor, language development, emotional growth, cognition, and social skills. Nurses can design and offer health education programs for the children (e.g., toothbrushing, handwashing, and blowing the nose into a tissue) to promote healthy habits. Health maintenance activities are those that prevent injury or disease, such as immunization monitoring, infection control, and practices like putting infants on their back to sleep. See "Sudden Infant Death Syndrome" in Chapter 48 for additional information.

Environmental Safety

Ensure that the childcare center maintains a current list of family members who may take a child from the facility, and has guidelines for verifying identity when necessary.

The nurse should inspect the childcare environment to identify hazards that could cause injury to the children. Cleaning supplies and other toxins must be stored in a locked cabinet to prevent children from exposure. Inspect toys used by children to ensure that there are no sharp edges or points, small parts, or pinching parts. Playground equipment should also be checked for safety (Figure 39–5 ●).

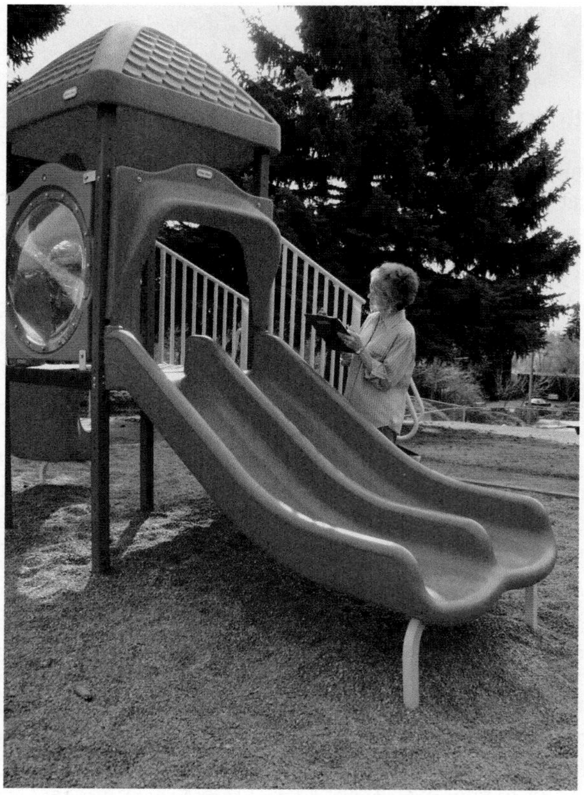

● **Figure 39–5** Childcare center safety assessment. Assess the childcare center's environment for safety hazards. Check the area around playground equipment, making sure there are wood chips or cushioned tiles under the equipment. Inspect the playground equipment for protruding screws, loose nuts and bolts, and instability at least monthly.

Emergency Care Planning

As in the school setting, guidelines for assessing and identifying the child with an emergency health condition and the development of an emergency care plan for an acutely ill or injured child is essential. This plan should include giving first aid, calling emergency medical services to transport the child to the emergency department, notifying the parent, and accompanying the child to the emergency department until the parent arrives.

HOME HEALTHCARE NURSING ROLES

Home healthcare is a component of the continuum of comprehensive health care provided to children and families. An estimated 500,000 children use home health services in the United States (American Academy of Pediatrics, 2006). Most children receive intermittent skilled nursing visits to assess the child and to see how family members are managing the child's healthcare needs. Home health services may be provided to children with complex health conditions, short-term acute care conditions, and even for terminal conditions. See Chapter 43 for more information about palliative and hospice care in the home setting.

Many children needing home health care are medically fragile, dependent upon a medical device for survival or prevention of further disability. Parents and other care providers without backgrounds in health care are given the responsibility of providing technology-assisted health care to their child. Technology-assisted care in the home may include any of the following: ventilators; tracheostomies; suctioning; nasogastric, gastrostomy, or parenteral feeding with feeding pumps; and intravenous fluids and medications with intravenous pumps. In some cases, families have created mini-intensive care units in their home.

The home environment is believed to be optimal for the long-term care of these children so they participate in family life and have their growth and development promoted. The family gains some control by having the child in the home rather than trying to fit visits to the child with maintenance of family life. However, these families are often stressed by trying to balance the child's constant care requirements and the needs of the remainder of the family.

Health insurers pay many of the costs associated with home care; however, the family may be financially burdened by paying some costs out-of-pocket, such as medications, supplies, and transportation. In some cases a parent must give up employment to provide care to the child and to qualify for Medicaid which is the major payer of home health services for children. Parents often feel like they have no choice about providing the ongoing care to their child (Carnevale, Alexander, Davis, et al., 2006). Healthcare systems (healthcare providers and insurers) are challenged to simultaneously address the child's illness and developmental needs while providing the support needed by these families so that children do well in their home environments.

Nurses need a variety of skills and knowledge to work in the home care setting, such as:

- Knowledge and experience in acute care practice with various medical technologies used with children. These skills enable nurses to provide direct care, teach the family and child self-care practices, and monitor the child's progress.
- Community assessment skills; an understanding of community resources, financing mechanisms, and multiagency collaboration; and good communication skills.
- An understanding of the community's health resources to better assist families to find the most supportive services to match the child's and family's needs.
- An understanding of the community's cultural diversity and the cultural values of the families served.
- Skill in educating family members to assume care of the child.

Nurses in the home care setting use the nursing process to assess the child, family, and home environment. Then the nurse assists the family to manage care of a child more independently while promoting the child's growth and development. A major goal of working with families in the home care setting includes promoting or restoring the child's health while attempting to minimize the effects of the disability and illness, including terminal illness (Figure 39–6 ●).

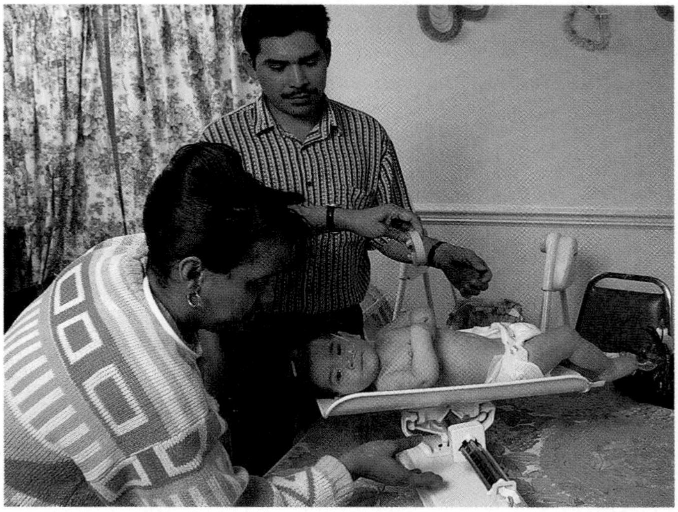

● **Figure 39–6** Nursing role in the home setting. Nurses provide both short-term and long-term services to families in the home setting. In some cases, families need support for a short time after the child is discharged from the hospital following an acute illness. In other cases, families need assistance with complex nursing care for the child dependent on technology for survival.

NURSING MANAGEMENT

NURSING ASSESSMENT AND DIAGNOSIS

Home health nurses assess the home, the child and the family during intermittent skilled nursing visits. Assessment of the home is focused on safety of the environment and the resources for the child's care. When working with the hospital discharge planner to initiate home health services, the following aspects of the home are assessed:

- Home readiness (safe sleeping arrangements, adequate supplies, ability to meet nutritional and fluid needs, telephone access, heat, electricity, refrigeration, lack of any communicable diseases in the home, and safe access into and out of the home).
- Potential hazards related to the child's age, condition and requirements for technology-assisted care (e.g., tripping hazard when extension cords are used to plug equipment into electrical outlets).
- Aspects of the home environment that could cause an acute illness, such as use of a woodstove or fireplace for heating that could cause respiratory distress or active renovation of a house built before 1960 that could expose the child to lead dust. The nurse may also identify family members who smoke.

Assessment of the child is focused on the current health status, growth, developmental progress, and social interaction with family members and health care providers. Observe for the potential for abuse and neglect as children with complex health conditions are at a higher risk.

Family strengths and coping abilities are evaluated. The family is assessed for parenting methods and skills in providing the child's needed medical procedures and monitoring the child's health status. The presence of siblings, their developmental and physical status, and their needs should also be assessed.

Examples of nursing diagnoses that could apply to the family as the child transitions from the hospital to home setting include the following:

- Impaired home maintenance related to insufficient family organization and planning
- Impaired adjustment (parents) related to multiple stressors in caring for a child with a complex health condition
- Ineffective therapeutic regimen management related to complexity of medical interventions
- Impaired social interaction related to therapeutic isolation

Developing Cultural Competence

ASSESSMENT

When assessing the child and family in the home, recognize when there are potential conflicts between recommended medical care and the family's preferences. Identify which family member is most influential in decisions about the child's care. Use open-ended questions to talk with families and understand the problem from their point of view. Ask the family to identify the problem, what caused the problem, their concerns about living with the problem, and the impact on their lives. Information obtained can be used to educate the family and to develop a nursing care plan that integrates the family's preferences for the child's care.

PLANNING AND IMPLEMENTATION

Nursing care should focus on promoting an environment within the home for the child to develop, learn social skills, and gain a sense of identity based on family values. Nurses help families in the home setting in the following ways:

- Assuring competent care to the child
- Educating parents about the child's condition and the physical signs and symptoms that may indicate a change in health status
- Educating parents and demonstrating methods to promote the child's development
- Linking families to community resources, including support groups, respite care, and therapeutic recreation
- Assisting families in time management skills and patient care management
- Advocating for increased insurance coverage or locating other sources of financial assistance

MyNursingKit Emergency Information Forum

MyNursingKit Disaster Preparedness Resources

COLLABORATING WITH THE FAMILY

The nurse works in partnership with the family in the home to promote the health of the child and of the family unit. Families lose privacy and often find it stressful to have home care nurses in the home for extended hours. When the home care nurse is ill or on vacation, the family may be stressed by providing the care or adjusting to a substitute nurse.

The home care nurse must acknowledge that the family has the control in the home care setting as the family employs the nurse. Therefore, it is essential that the nurse develops a respectful and trusting relationship with the family. Every interaction is a negotiation with the family, or between the family and child, if there are differences in what they want. The nurse must be flexible and set aside power. Conflicts may occur when differences in opinion about the child's care become apparent. Open communication is essential so the nurse can learn what is important to the child and family, and then modify the nursing care plan when appropriate. House rules for such things as parking, private areas in the home, and routines may need to be negotiated, but then rules must be followed. Role expectations of the nurse must be clearly understood to reduce stress in the family. The success of home care is also based upon effective cultural communication. For example, some Jewish families follow strict dietary guidelines that do not permit milk and meat to be mixed. The nurse needs to abide by the family's dietary guidelines and food preparation practices.

When nurses provide home care, it is important for a parent to be present and work in partnership with the nurse. Informed consent is needed for invasive treatments and decisions for provision of needed emergency care to prevent serious consequences. If parents must leave, a disclaimer protecting the home care nurse from liability may be necessary (Margolan, Fraser, & Lenton, 2004).

The range of nursing care activities in the home setting that may be included in a child's care plan include sensory stimulation, routines of daily living, positioning and skin care with gentle handling, respiratory care, nutrition and elimination, medications, and other supportive therapies. Other providers, such as physical therapists, speech-language therapists, occupational therapists, and social workers, may provide other health care services in collaboration with the home health nurse.

EMERGENCY PREPAREDNESS

The nurse should help the family develop an emergency care plan for any child whose condition could worsen rapidly and become life threatening (e.g., severe congenital heart defect, tracheostomy, or apnea), or be beyond the care that the parents or home health nurse can provide. Information should provide guidelines for when to call 9-1-1. The emergency care plan should include an essential medical history that provides the emergency care providers with enough information to understand the child's health condition, to prevent delays in disease-specific treatment, and to minimize unnecessary interventions until the child's personal physician can be consulted. See MyNursingKit for the American Academy of Pediatrics Web site with an emergency information form.

When the child is dependent on technology, the family should notify the power company so that the home is on the high priority list for service after power outages. Backup generators may be needed if electrical power for life-sustaining equipment is essential. Families need to develop a plan for safe evacuation of the home in case of fire or other emergency. This is very challenging when the child cannot mobilize independently and requires equipment for continued survival or quality of life. See Teaching Highlights for information to help families develop a plan for safe evacuation of the home. The child should also be registered for a disaster shelter that can accommodate the healthcare needs of the child and at least one caregiver.

EVALUATION

Expected outcomes of nursing care include the following:

- Care of the child's medical needs is integrated into the family's routines when possible.
- The family has an emergency care plan for the child in the event of a disaster, a weather emergency, or if the child's condition suddenly worsens.
- The home health nurse and family work in partnership to promote the child's health and growth and development.

Teaching Highlights

HAVING A FIRE ESCAPE PLAN

Developing a fire escape plan is important when the family has one or more children with special healthcare needs. Important steps to have families take in developing the plan include:

- Have working smoke detectors in the home and teach children what the alarm means.
- Draw a diagram of your house. Mark all windows and doors.
- Plan two routes out of every room.
- Think about an escape plan if the fire starts in the kitchen, bedroom, or basement.
- Figure out the best way to get infants and young children out of the house. Will you carry them? Is there more than one small child, and if so, how will you get them out if you are the only adult?
- Teach preschool and school-age children to follow the escape plan by crawling, touching doors, and going to the window if the door is hot. Show children how to cover their nose and mouth to reduce smoke inhalation.
- Prepare an alternate fire escape plan in case you are alone with the child when the fire begins.
- Keep home exits clear of toys and debris.
- Select a safe meeting place outside the home. Teach children not to go back inside the burning home.

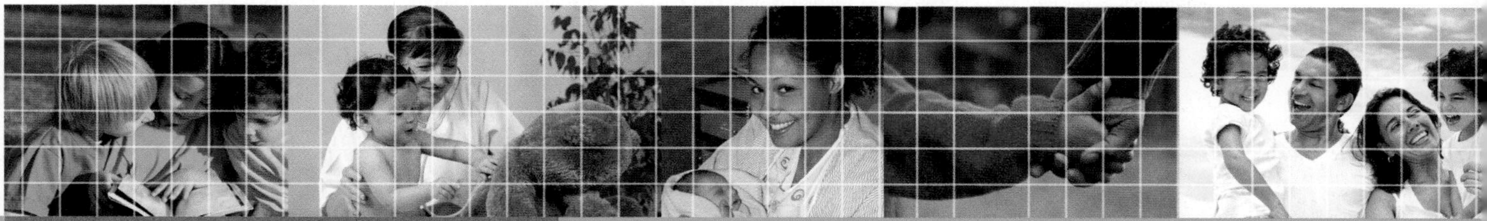

CRITICAL CONCEPT REVIEW

LEARNING OUTCOMES	CONCEPTS
39.1 Categorize the family strengths that help families cope with stressors.	1. Individual or family traits: ■ Optimism or resilience. 2. Individual or family assets: ■ Finances. 3. Individual or family capabilities, skills, or competencies: ■ Problem solving.
39.2 Describe the advantages of using a family assessment tool.	Family assessment tools can be used to collect information about: 1. The family's functioning. 2. Coping strategies. 3. Family strengths. 4. Problem solving and communication.
39.3 Identify a variety of family support services that might be available in a community.	1. School-based: Head Start, Early Head Start, before- and after-school programs for children of working parents, health and counseling services. 2. Play groups for preschool children. 3. Peer support groups, parenting programs. 4. Social service programs offered by the faith community. 5. Home visiting programs. 6. Job skills training, adult education, and literacy programs. 7. Crisis care and respite care programs.
39.4 List the variety of community healthcare settings where nurses provide health services to children.	1. Childcare centers. 2. Schools. 3. Health centers and physician offices. 4. Hospital out-patient clinic. 5. Public health clinic, homeless shelters. 6. The home.

(continued)

LEARNING OUTCOMES / CONCEPTS

39.5 Compare the roles of the nurse in each identified healthcare setting.

1. Nurses in childcare centers and schools triage emergent problems, maintain immunization records of each child, perform regular vision and hearing screenings, and refer children for other therapies.
2. Nurses in a health center or physician's office perform routine growth and development screenings, administer immunizations, care for children with acute illnesses, and arrange for referrals to other community services.
3. Nurses in specialty out-patient clinics care for children with chronic health conditions, provide health promotion and health maintenance care, and arrange referrals for other community services.
4. Nurses in public health clinics and homeless shelters assess children for developmental level, administer immunizations, and assist in arranging community services.
5. Nurses in the home assess the environment and coordinate and assist families to plan care for children with chronic conditions, acute illnesses, or terminal conditions.

39.6 Contrast the emergency care planning that is important in each community setting.

1. Health center and physician office: central availability of emergency equipment and medications, mock drills to practice the emergency care response.
2. School: emergency response plan for the child with an emergency condition; emergency preparedness plan for a disaster or behavioral crisis.
3. Childcare center: emergency response plan for the child with an emergency condition.
4. Home: emergency care plan, safe evacuation plan, registering the child assisted by technology for a disaster shelter.

CRITICAL THINKING IN ACTION

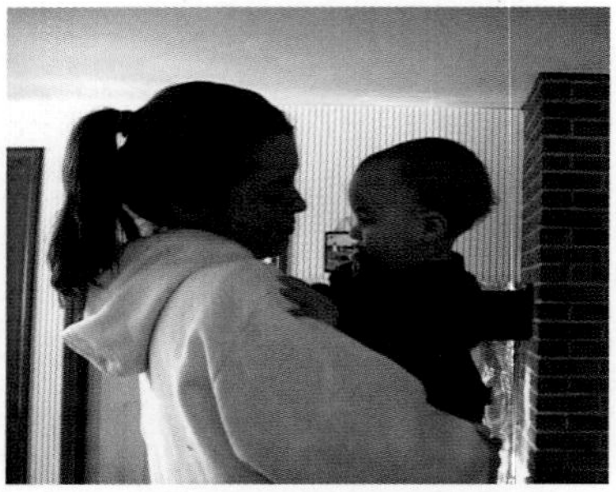

Gavin is a 1-year-old coming into the clinic for his well-child check. The clinic is set up to see teen mothers and their babies for well-child visits and immunizations. Diane, his mother, has been bringing him there since he was born. Gavin qualifies for healthcare coverage through the Medicaid system in their state. He was born full term and has never been in the hospital or had surgery. Diane is still attending high school and plans to graduate this year. She and Gavin are living with her boyfriend's (Gavin's father) parents until they can raise enough money to live on their own. Gavin's father does not come to the well-baby visits. Gavin attends daycare while his mother is at school. He is up-to-date on immunizations so far and there is no significant family medical history, but there is smoking in the home. Gavin has been walking since he was 9 months old. He is able to point, wave, clap, and has 2 words. He is able to drink from a cup and put objects into a cup. He has been growing and thriving at an appropriate pace. Diane describes him as a good eater and tells you that he is currently on whole milk. He has soft stools daily and 5-6 wet diapers per day. He sleeps through the night and takes 2 naps per day. Diane describes him as an extremely active child and has worked on childproofing everything in the house.

1. What is the role of the nurse in caring for Gavin and his parents in the clinic?
2. What data does the nurse collect to perform a family assessment?
3. What strengths and stressors are likely to be present in this family?
4. What are the elements of a healthcare or medical home?

See MyNursingKit for possible responses.

REFERENCES

Alkon, A., Farrer, J., & Bernzweig, J. (2004). Child care health consultants' roles and responsibilities: Focus group findings. *Pediatric Nursing, 30*(4), 315–321.

American Academy of Pediatrics, Committee on Child Health Financing, Section on Home Care. (2006). Financing of pediatric home health care. *Pediatrics, 118*(2), 834–838.

American Academy of Pediatrics, Committee on Pediatric Emergency Medicine. (2007). Preparation for emergencies in the offices of pediatricians and pediatric primary care providers. *Pediatrics, 120*(1), 200–212.

Benard, B. (2004). *Resiliency: What We Have Learned.* San Francisco: WestEd.

Bindler, R. C., & Ball, J. W. (2007). The Bindler-Ball heatlhcare model: A new paradigm for health promotion. *Pediatric Nursing, 32*(2), 121–126.

Brady, M. T (2005). Infectious disease in pediatric out-of-home child care. *American Journal of Infection Control, 33*(5), 276–285.

Caldwell, B. M., & Bradley, R. H. (1984). *The Home Observation for Measurement of the Environment.* Little Rock: University of Arkansas.

Carnevale, F. A., Alexander, E., Davis, M., Rennick, J., & Troini, R. (2006). Daily living with distress and enrichment: The moral experience of families with ventilator-assisted children at home. *Pediatrics, 117*(1), e48–e60.

Deheny, J. (2006). Just what do school nurses do? *Journal of School Nursing, 22*(4), 191–192.

Dellert, J. C., Galsalberti, D., Sternas, K., Lucarelli, P., & Hall, J. (2006). Outcomes of child care health consultation services for child care providers in New Jersey: A pilot study. *Pediatric Nursing, 32*(6), 530–535.

Department of Health and Human Services, Office of Disease Prevention and Promotion. (2006). *Healthy People 2010 Midcourse Review.*

Washington, DC: Author. Retrieved April 24, 2007, from http://www.healthypeople.gov/data/midcourse/pdf/FA14.pdf

Frankowski, B. L., Keating, K., Rexroad, A., Delaney, T., McEwing, S. M., et al. (2006). Community collaboration: Concurrent physician and school nurse education and cooperation increases the use of asthma action plans. *Journal of School Health*, *76*(6), 303–306.

Friedman, M. M., Bowden, V. R., & Jones, E. G. (2003). *Family nursing: Research, theory, and practice* (5th ed.). Upper Saddle River, NJ: Prentice Hall.

Guttu, M., Engleke, M. K., & Swanson, M. (2004). Does the school nurse-to-student ratio make a difference? *Journal of School Health*, *74*(1), 6–9.

Margolan, H., Fraser, J., & Lenton, S. (2004). Parental experiences of services when their child requires long-term ventilation. Implications for commissioning and providing services. *Child Care, Health & Development*, *30*(3), 257–264.

McCarthy, A. M., Kelly, M. W., Johnson, S., Roman, J., & Zimmerman, M. B. (2006). Changes in medications administered in schools. *Journal of School Nursing*, *22*(2), 102–107.

McLaughlin, T., Maljanian, R., Kornblum, R., Clark, P., Simpson, J., & McCormack, K. (2006). Evaluating the availability and use of asthma action plans for school-based asthma care: A case study in Hartford, Connecticut. *Journal of School Health*, *76*(6), 325–328.

Pulcini, J., DeSisto, M. C., & McIntyre, C. L. (2007). An intervention to increase the use of asthma action plans in schools: A MASNRN study. *Journal of School Nursing*, *23*(3), 170–176.

Simon, J. B., Murphy, J. J., & Smith, S. M. (2005). Understanding and fostering family resilience. *The Family Journal: Counseling and Therapy for Couples and Families*, *13*(4), 427–436.

Tarko, M. A., & Reed, K. (2004). Family assessment and intervention. In P. J. Bomar, *Promoting health in families* (3rd ed., pp. 274–298). Philadelphia: Saunders.

Totsika, V., & Sylva, K. (2004). The home observation for measurement of the environment revisited. *Child Psychology and Psychiatry*, *9*(1), 25–35.

Wright, L., & Leahy, M. (2009). *Nurses and families: A guide to family assessment and intervention* (5th ed.). Philadelphia: Davis.

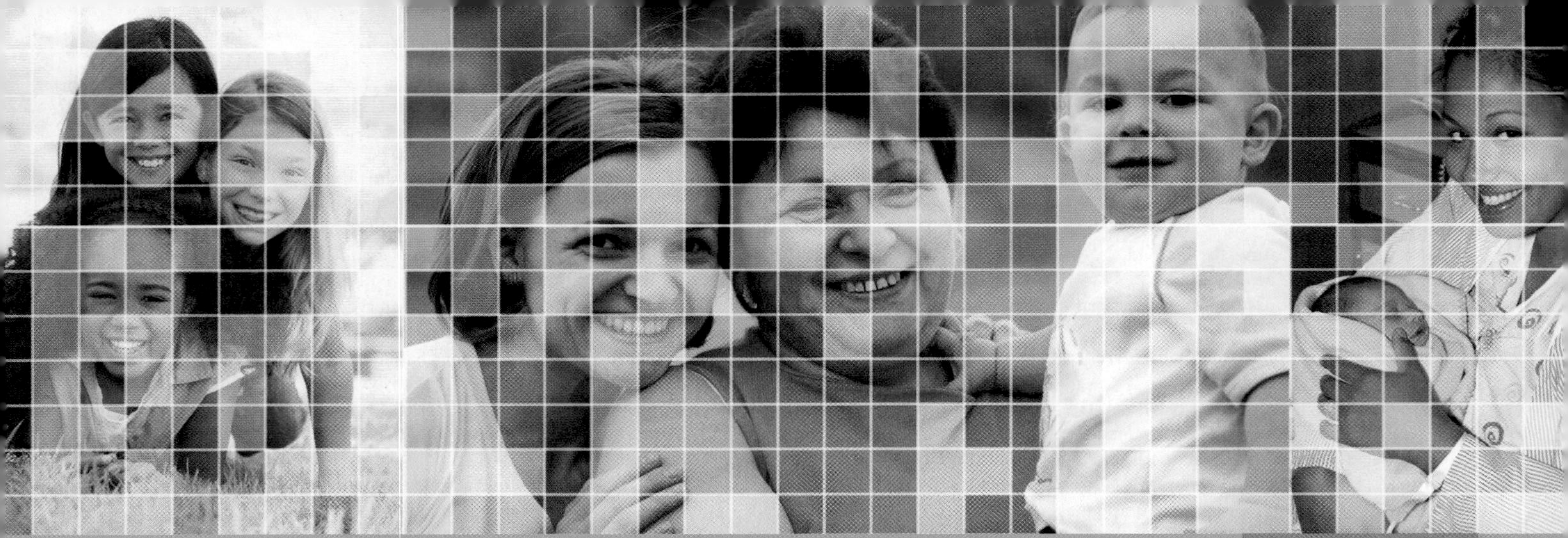

CHAPTER 40

Nursing Considerations for the Child and Family with a Chronic Condition

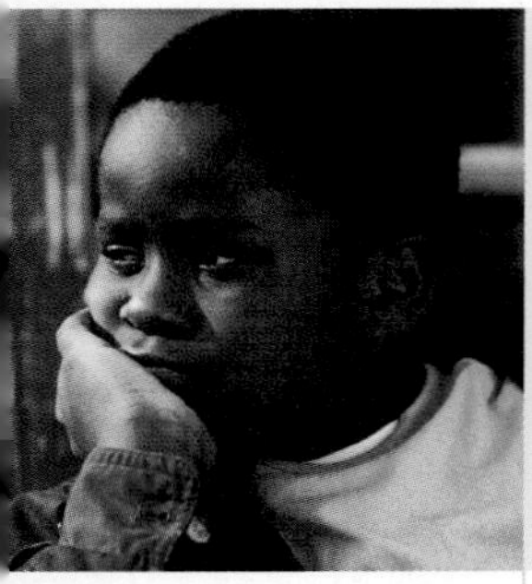

I am nervous about going to school for the first time since my diabetes was diagnosed. I am worried that my friends will make fun of me because I have to check my blood and give myself a shot at lunchtime. I wish this would just go away, but I know it is something I will have for the rest of my life. My parents had to learn how to check my blood and give shots too. My mom and dad were really upset, but they are getting used to the idea now and will do anything to make sure I am doing okay. —*Mark, 10 years old*

LEARNING OUTCOMES

40.1 Discuss causes of chronic conditions in children.

40.2 Describe the categories of chronic conditions in children.

40.3 Describe the nurse's role in caring for a child with a chronic condition.

40.4 Assess the family of a child with a chronic condition and discuss the impact of the child's condition on the family.

40.5 Describe nursing interventions for the child with a chronic condition to support transition to school and adult living.

40.6 Discuss the family's role in care coordination.

OVERVIEW OF CHRONIC CONDITIONS

A **chronic condition** is generally thought of as one that is long term, ongoing, may or may not be considered terminal, and requires some adaptation to daily living (Coffey, 2006). Others have defined a chronic condition as one that is expected to last at least 3 months (Allen, 2004). An estimated 10 million children under the age of 18 in the United States have some type of chronic condition (Goble, 2004). Chronic conditions vary in etiology, manifestations, severity, and their effect on the child's physical, psychosocial, and cognitive development. Chronic conditions develop from multiple causes.

- Genetic or inheritable conditions may manifest as a chronic condition. Examples include muscular dystrophy, hemophilia, sickle cell disease, and cystic fibrosis.
- Conditions may result from a congenital defect or insult to the infant during fetal development, such as neural tube defect, maternal substance abuse, cleft palate, and cerebral palsy.
- Insult or injury may be associated with birth and care following birth (sepsis, prematurity, intraventricular hemorrhage) that lead to conditions such as bronchopulmonary dysplasia, attention deficit disorder, and vision or hearing impairment.
- Conditions can be acquired through injury or acute medical condition such as brain injury, cancer, HIV infection, drowning, and mental health problems.

In most cases, these chronic conditions become lifelong disorders, but the impact on the affected child varies according to the severity of the condition, the stage of growth and development when the condition occurs, and the child's and family's responses to the condition. While some conditions require intense monitoring and technological support for survival, other conditions cause few limitations and minimal effect on quality of life (Figure 40–1 ●).

Chronic conditions have often been defined by diagnostic categories or by functional or social limitations. Examples of categories of chronic conditions include the following (Allen, 2004):

- Limitations in function that would typically be expected for the child's age and development
- Disfigurement
- Dependency on medications or a special diet for control of the condition
- Dependency on medical technology for functioning
- Need for more medical care and related services than typically used by a healthy child of the same age
- Special ongoing treatments at home or school

See Table 40–1 for examples of chronic conditions that fall into some of these categories. Many children with chronic conditions have special healthcare needs that fall into several of these areas. In the majority of cases, the more severe the chronic condition, the greater the number of categories of special healthcare needs. Many of these children have a **disability**, a limitation that interferes with a child's ability to fully participate in society, which can be related to medical impairment (chronic health condition), functional limitation (mobility, self-care, communication, or learning behavior impairment), or a mental condition that interferes with social interactions.

Many children with a chronic condition and children dependent on technology require specialized healthcare: The term **children with special healthcare needs (CSHCN)** is applied to "those who have or are at increased risk for a chronic physical, developmental, behavioral, or emotional condition and who also require health and related services of a type or amount beyond that required by children generally" (Inkelas & Garro, 2005, p. 207).

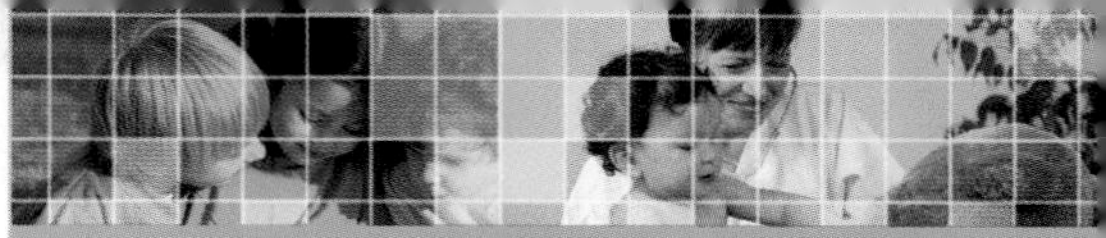

KEY TERMS

Accommodations, 1068
Care coordination, 1067
Caregiver burden, 1071
Case manager, 1067
Children with special healthcare needs (CSHCN), 1061
Chronic condition, 1061
Disability, 1061
Early intervention, 1068
Healthcare home, 1067
Individualized education plan, 1069
Individualized family service plan, 1069
Individualized health plan, 1069
Individualized transition plan, 1070
Medical home, 1067
Medically fragile, 1062
Respite care, 1071
Technology-assisted, 1062

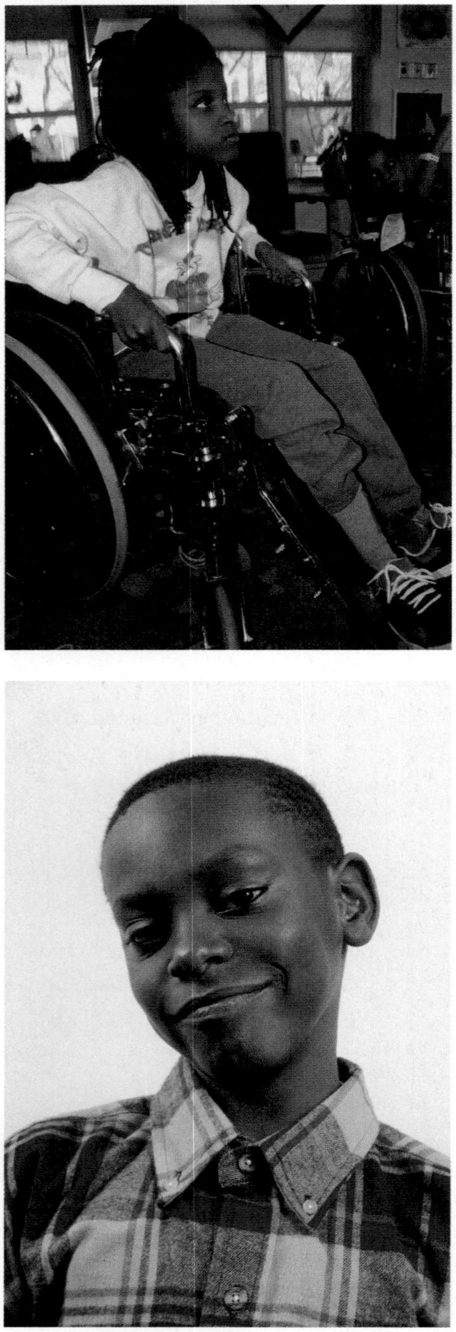

A

B

● **Figure 40–1** Visible and nonvisible health conditions. Children with chronic conditions may have a visible or nonvisible health condition, or nonvisible until an acute episode of their condition makes the condition visible. ***A,*** The child in a wheelchair has a visible disability. ***B,*** The child with a seizure disorder may have no visible signs of the condition unless a seizure is witnessed.

As mentioned earlier, children with special healthcare needs use significantly more healthcare resources than those without special healthcare needs, including more visits to clinics, emergency departments, dental visits, inpatient hospital days, and prescription medications. In 2000, children with special healthcare needs represented 15.6% of the nation's children, but they used 33.6% of the total child health expenditures, including dental care (Newacheck & Kim, 2005). Efforts to reduce health costs have resulted in fewer hospitalizations and more care in the community. Families may need considerable assistance for care coordination to ensure that their children have access to care. The Nursing Practice feature in this section lists the national health objectives in *Healthy People 2010* that are focused on the health status and healthcare delivery to children with special healthcare needs.

The child with a life-threatening illness or a chronic condition as the result of a complex illness, prematurity or a congenital defect may be considered **medically fragile** (Lee, Miles, & Holditch-Davis, 2006). Some of these children are **technology-assisted**, depending on a medical device that is required to sustain life (me-

Table 40–1 Examples of Conditions by Special Healthcare Need Category

Special Healthcare Need Category	Chronic Health Condition Examples
Dependent on medications or special diet	Diabetes mellitus, asthma, seizures, phenylketonuria, organ transplantation, cystic fibrosis, celiac disease
Dependent on medical technology	Renal failure, bronchopulmonary dysplasia
Increased use of healthcare services	Cancer, sickle cell disease, cystic fibrosis
Functional limitations	Down syndrome, brain injury, autism, myelodysplasia, cerebral palsy

Nursing Practice

The *Healthy People 2010* objectives for children with special healthcare needs are as follows:

- All children with special healthcare needs will have access to a medical home.
- All children with special healthcare needs will receive their care in family-centered, comprehensive, and coordinated systems.
- All families with CSHCN will have adequate private and/or public insurance to pay for the services they need.
- Services for CSHCN and their families will be organized in ways that families can use them easily.
- Families of CSHCN will participate in decision making at all levels and will be satisfied with the services they receive.

Source: U.S. Department of Health and Human Services. (2006). *Healthy People 2010 Midcourse Review,* Washington, DC: U.S. Government Printing Office. Retrieved November 4, 2007, from www.healthypeople.gov/data/midcourse/default.htm#pubs

chanical ventilators, intravenous nutrition or drugs, tracheostomy, suctioning, oxygen, or nutritional support with tube feedings) (Figure 40–2 ●). Other children depend on medical devices that compensate for vital body functions and require nursing care management such as renal dialysis, urinary catheters, and colostomies.

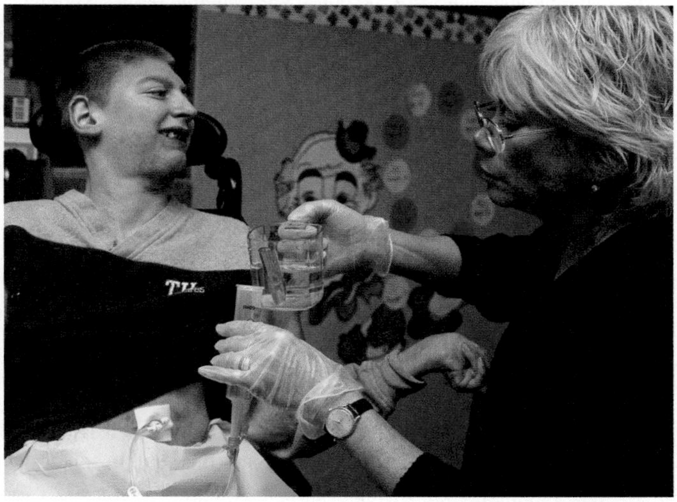

● **Figure 40–2** A technology-assisted child. This child needs a gastrostomy tube to ensure adequate nutrition is obtained to support growth and promote resistance to infection.

Children assisted by technology can be cared for at home because equipment has been manufactured that is small enough to be portable. Home-based equipment used for the child with a chronic condition may include ventilators, enteral feeding tubes, intravenous catheters, infusion pumps, dialysis equipment, and oxygen. With the support of home health services parents can learn to manage the child's care. The benefit to the child is support of physical, emotional, and cognitive growth and development within the home care setting, in a more normal environment.

All families with children experiencing a chronic condition need to make lifestyle adjustments, ensuring a baseline of care that helps maintain the child's health status and promotes growth and development. In many cases, the child has a baseline level of home management with episodic exacerbations that require the family to make sudden adjustments in family routines, such as may occur with the child who has seizures or an infection. These exacerbations often cause stress and disrupt family routines. In other cases, the chronic condition requires the family to learn and provide care that is complex and time-intensive, such as cystic fibrosis, diabetes mellitus, bronchopulmonary dysplasia, and significant cognitive impairment. These more severe chronic conditions often impact the child's physical and psychologic development. Table 40–2 outlines healthcare needs of these children and families and the nursing implications related to planning health services delivery to children and their families.

Table 40–2 Healthcare Needs of Children with Chronic Conditions

Healthcare Need	Definition	Nursing Actions
Access to care	Availability and accessibility to providers with knowledge as well as ancillary services needed by children and their families	Assist the family in obtaining transportation assistance if required Assist the family in identifying healthcare providers that provide health promotion and other services to address the child's specific healthcare needs
Appropriateness of care	Services and care delivered by individuals with expertise and experience that are developmentally and culturally appropriate for the child and family	Support the family by outlining educational and health services needed when developing an individualized education plan (IEP) and individualized health plan (IHP)
Comprehensiveness	Coverage of the preventive, primary, and tertiary care needs of children, and linkages with other service systems, such as education, social services, and family support systems	Provide the family with resource contacts such as social services, family support groups, and other systems to help the family manage the child's condition Assist the family in identifying a care coordinator or developing the skills to take on the care coordination role themselves
Coordination	Families linked to medical care, financial health resources, educational and community-based services; information is centralized	Provide guidance and resources if the family decides to assume the role of care coordinator Encourage the family to partner with the healthcare team to ensure continuity of care
Continuity	Through a medical home or pediatric healthcare home; linkages between primary, specialty, therapeutic, and home care exist throughout childhood	Facilitate communication between all the child's healthcare providers Include the family and older child in all decision making
Degree to which services and the service system are family centered	Importance of the family reflected in the way services are planned and delivered, building on individual and family strengths, and respecting the diversity of each family Assist the family in identifying local and specialized healthcare providers	Determine the needs of the child and the family to ensure they are being addressed Recognize and respect the culture and cultural practices of the child and family

ROLE OF THE NURSE

The nurse's role in caring for the child with a chronic condition includes the following:

- providing health supervision from infancy to transition into adulthood
- collaborating with the multidisciplinary healthcare team
- partnering with parents or caregivers to manage the child's care at home
- referring the family to appropriate community services
- assisting with planning for education services
- promoting positive parenting behaviors and psychosocial adaptation and well-being of the child and family
- promoting growth and development of siblings.

Assess individual family members' level of understanding of the condition, treatment, and anticipated outcome of the condition. Determine the family's stage of acceptance of the child's chronic illness, and how well the child's care is integrated into family routines. Evaluate the child's home care environment to determine the potential for abuse, lack of adequate care, or neglect, or for opportunities to enhance care provided. Assess the family's strengths, stressors, risk factors, and coping strategies. See the "Nursing Care Plan: The Child with a Chronic Condition" on page 1065. See Chapter 43 for stages that the family might progress through when faced with a diagnosis of a life-threatening illness or injury in their child.

THE CHILD WITH A NEWLY DIAGNOSED CHRONIC CONDITION

Informing the child of a newly acquired chronic condition is individualized and is based on the child's developmental level and age. Questions the child may ask vary, but often focus on the cause of the condition, how to make it better, and how it will affect daily life. Provide information tailored to the child's level of understanding and answer questions honestly. The nurse should also address the fears and concerns of the family. Provide condition-specific education to help prepare the family for care at home and begin discharge planning. The manner in which parents are informed of their child's condition and their ability to understand the information influences their ability to cope with the diagnosis (Nuutila & Salanterä, 2006). See Teaching Highlights: Discussing a Child's Condition and Teaching Highlights: Informing Parents of Their Child's Chronic Illness or Disability. The parents' heightened anxiety level may reduce the comprehension of information heard. See Developing Cultural Competence: Providing Information and Support.

Siblings of children with a chronic condition are also affected. They demonstrate emotional responses that range from a variety of responses from negative to positive (Ballard, 2004).

Teaching Highlights

DISCUSSING A CHILD'S CONDITION

When discussing a child's chronic condition with the family, use the child's name. Avoid labeling the child with a condition, such as "diabetic child"; instead refer to the situation as "the child with diabetes." This places the emphasis on the *child* rather than the *condition*.

Teaching Highlights

INFORMING PARENTS OF THEIR CHILD'S CHRONIC ILLNESS OR DISABILITY

The following guidelines may be considered when informing parents of the diagnosis of a chronic illness or disability in their child:

1. Inform parents of their child's diagnosis in person, in a private setting, and free from interruptions. Tell both parents together. Offer parents the opportunity to have a relative or friend as a support person during the discussion.
2. Present information in small amounts at a time and at the level of the parents' understanding.
3. Plan and organize the information to be provided. Use simple, direct language without medical jargon. Individualize the pace of the interview and approaches taken to present the explanation, taking into consideration a family's culture and the family's response to the information.
4. Share accurate, up-to-date information about the diagnosis, treatment options, specialty referrals, and community resources.
5. Talk about the strengths and positive attributes of the child, as well as the child's limitations and characteristics due to the illness or disability.
6. Evaluate the discussion to assess whether the family's needs were met and to determine the type of support and/or additional information that should be provided.
7. Plan a follow-up discussion to repeat and clarify the information provided, and to give the parents a chance to get additional questions answered.

Developing Cultural Competence

PROVIDING INFORMATION AND SUPPORT

Findings of the National Survey of Children with Special Health Care Needs indicated that Latino parents of CSHCN were less likely to indicate that they had received the information that they needed about their child's condition. In addition, parents of CSHCN who are African American and Hispanic CSHCN were not as likely as parents of non-Hispanic white CSHCN to report that healthcare providers spend adequate time with their child (Inkelas & Garro, 2005). To best meet the informational needs of all parents, start each visit assessing parental needs, and then plan the visit to include assessments and interventions to meet parental expectations.

Nursing Care Plan

THE CHILD WITH A CHRONIC CONDITION

GOAL	INTERVENTION	RATIONALE	EXPECTED OUTCOME
1. Deficient Knowledge (child) related to learning self-care skills			
	NIC Priority Intervention: *Individual Teaching:* Planning, implementation, and evaluating a teaching program designed to address a patient's particular need.		**NOC Suggested Outcomes** *Knowledge:* Extent of understanding conveyed about treatment regimen.
The child will acquire self-care skills for lifetime management.	■ Assess the child's developmental level and select an educational approach and self-care activities to match.	■ Learning goals for the child must match knowledge and skill expectations appropriate for developmental stage.	The child demonstrates the proper technique in the self-care skill and is able to assume responsibility for that skill with supervision by the parent. Responsibility for self-care increases as new skills are learned.
	■ Review with the child all steps involved in the self-care skill and how to perform the skill.	■ The child may have watched the routine used by parents many times, and asking the child to list each step helps the nurse identify extra training needed.	
	■ Use demonstration/return demonstration until the child is comfortable with procedures.	■ Evaluation permits positive reinforcement and guidance for modification of techniques.	
	■ Help parents develop a planned sequence of self-care skills to teach the child.	■ Parents need guidance to identify appropriate self-care skills that the child is developmentally ready to learn.	
	■ Discuss a plan for increased responsibility for self-care with the child and parents.	■ Parents often need encouragement to transition responsibility to the child, becoming a supervisor rather than the person controlling care.	
2. Interrupted Family Processes related to management of a chronic disease			
	NIC Priority Intervention: *Normalization Promotion:* Assisting parents and other family members of children with chronic illnesses or disabilities in providing normal life experiences for their children and families.		**NOC Suggested Outcomes** *Family Health Status:* Overall health status and social competence of family unit.
The child and family will manage the required treatments, monitoring, and medication regimen for the child's condition while maintaining family routines and functioning.	■ Assess the child's and family's lifestyle and attempt to fit the child's care needs into those schedules.	■ Fitting the child's care to the child's and family's lifestyle promotes adherence to regimen and healthier family processes.	The child and family maintain important family routines and successfully manage the child's condition.
	■ Discuss the family's routines for special occasions and vacations and any activities important to the child. Identify ways to modify the child's management for these occasions and activities.	■ It is important for the child to participate in special events with the family and peers as a normal child to promote psychologic development.	

(continued)

Nursing Care Plan—continued

THE CHILD WITH A CHRONIC CONDITION

GOAL	INTERVENTION	RATIONALE	EXPECTED OUTCOME
3. Individual Readiness for Enhanced Coping related to self-care management of chronic condition			
	NIC Priority Intervention: *Resiliency Promotion*: Assisting individuals, families, and communities in development, use, and strengthening of protective factors to be used in coping with environmental and societal stressors.		**NOC Suggested Outcomes** *Health-Seeking Behavior:* Actions to promote optimal wellness, recovery, and rehabilitation.
The child will develop a support system network.	■ Talk with the child about how to tell friends, teachers, and other important people about the chronic condition. ■ Discuss ways to explain the condition to important people and how to answer questions. ■ Role-play ways to talk about the condition with friends and teachers. ■ Encourage the child to attend peer support groups or camps specific to the child's condition.	■ These important people can assist the child in an emergency if they have enough information to assess the problem. ■ Having an opportunity to plan and role-play the conversation will reduce the child's anxiety about condition disclosure. ■ Sharing information about the condition helps others understand changes in lifestyle needed by the child. ■ Learning and support networks developed at camp can promote development of problem-solving skills that increase coping abilities.	The child identifies the friends, teachers, and other important persons informed about the chronic condition who can provide support when needed.

Negative responses predominate and include feelings of jealousy, resentment, anger, depression, and guilt (Ballard, 2004; Fanos, Fahrner, Jelveh, et al., 2004). Siblings of a child with a chronic condition need support from their parents to help with their coping and adjustment. Chapter 41∞ provides additional information related to siblings of ill children.

DISCHARGE PLANNING AND HOME CARE TEACHING

As the child with a newly diagnosed chronic condition transitions to the home, parents often feel overwhelmed with preparations for home care, the anxiety of caring for a child with special healthcare needs, and supporting the child's growth and development needs. Work with the parents to ensure a smooth transition from hospital to the home environment. Assist the family in the initial discussions with the multidisciplinary team that participates in developing the child's care plan. Ensure that the family understands the role of each care provider.

Education to provide care of the child at home may be initiated by the hospital nursing staff, and then transitioned to special nurse educators or the home health nurses. Care is taken to ensure that all aspects of management are discussed with the family and that they demonstrate an understanding of and ability to perform the care required.

During discharge planning it may be helpful to identify a parent peer or peer support group to provide support to the family. Parent peers who have had similar experiences may be very helpful in identifying strategies for the initial care transition in the home and additional issues that arise over time. If the family has a computer that family members frequently use, Internet resources for information and family support should be provided.

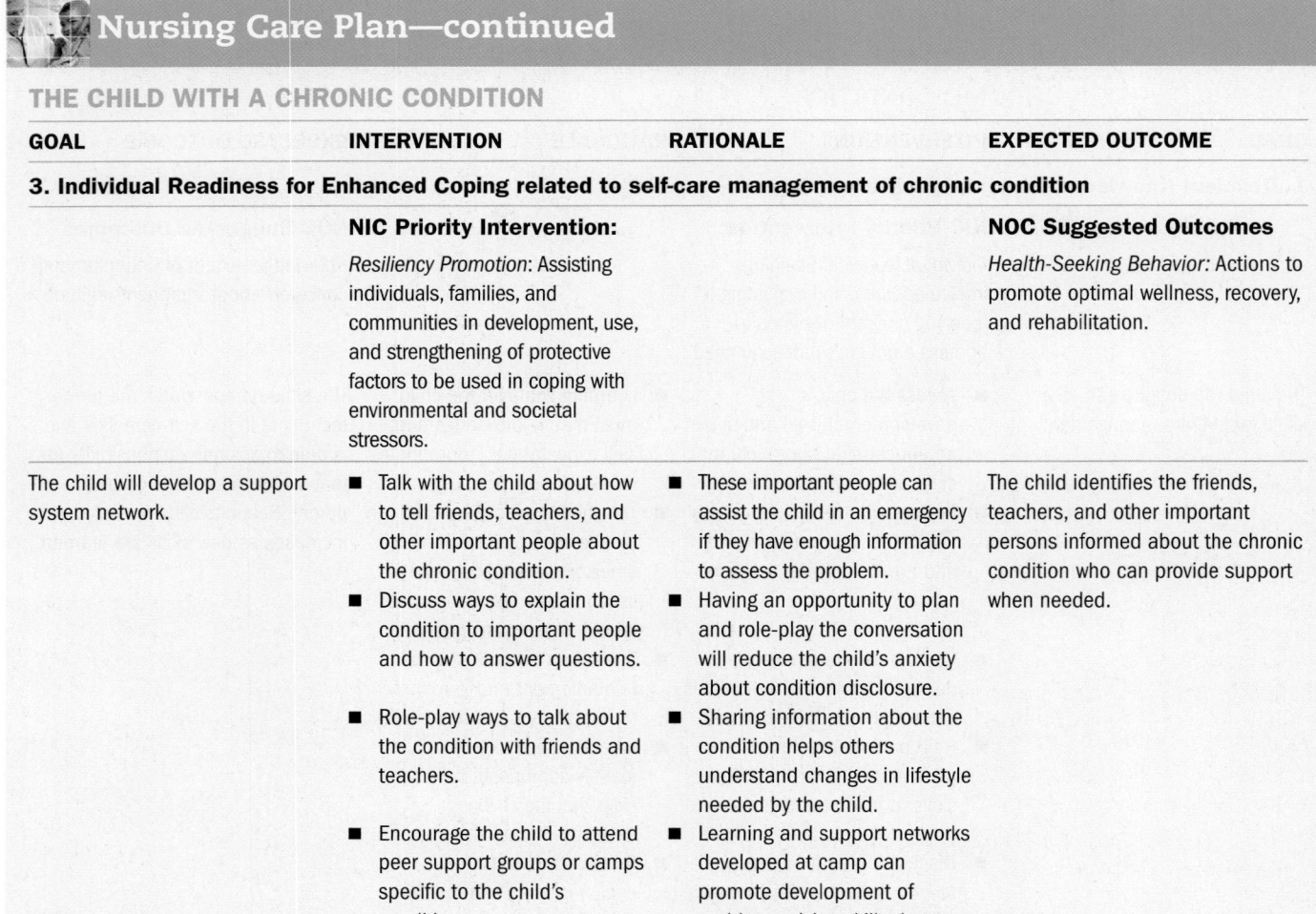

Collaborate with the family and healthcare team to ensure that the child has a medical or healthcare home in the local community to provide health promotion and maintenance and to assist with the coordination of local community resources. Promote communication and joint planning of care between the specialty care provider and local healthcare provider. Nurses working in hospital specialty clinics and other community settings can help ensure that children with chronic conditions receive multidisciplinary referrals and have appointments scheduled. Social services may be called to assist the family with identifying financial resources and other community resources for home management. Ongoing assistance may be required to help families deal with financial issues, time management, and other challenges.

COORDINATION OF CARE

Care coordination is the process of planning and integrating healthcare services among providers in an effort to achieve and promote good health in the child (American Academy of Pediatrics [AAP], 2005; Kruger, 2004). Because numerous healthcare providers and healthcare agencies are often involved in the care of the child with a chronic illness or injury requiring long-term care, coordination of health services is important to prevent gaps and overlaps, reduce healthcare costs, and improve family satisfaction (AAP, 2005). A **case manager**, often a nurse or social worker, may be given responsibility to help the family with care coordination. Case managers are often paid by a healthcare insurer to reduce healthcare costs by coordinating the healthcare team, determining family needs, identifying financial and local support resources, and arranging for needed healthcare services.

The goals of care coordination include (AAP, 2005):

- Gaining access to and integrating services and resources on behalf of the child
- Facilitating communication among multiple professionals
- Preventing duplication of services and unnecessary expenditures
- Advocating for improved individual outcomes
- Improving the child's and family's quality of life

Care coordination may also include helping the family modify the home to support required technology, such as mechanical ventilation or wheelchair use. Assistance may be required in purchasing or leasing ventilators, infusion pumps, or other specialized equipment. The coordination plan also includes determining the potential need for home health nursing, physical therapy, or other home health services.

Families become very well educated about their child's condition and the services that would make managing the condition easier. Once management goals are established by the multidisciplinary team, the case manager partners with the family to help in the decision making process regarding how goals will be met. An important role is helping the family to determine cost-effective strategies to meet healthcare goals and to delay the time when the child reaches the cap on health insurance benefits.

Some families assume the role of care coordinator for their child. It is essential for the family to understand that care coordination is time-consuming and requires ongoing assessment and evaluation of the child's status and anticipated outcomes. Support family members in their decision to lead the care coordination process by helping the parents to become knowledgeable about the child's condition and treatment regimen. Support the parents in taking an active role in the treatment planning and decision-making process so that they gain confidence in their abilities. Many hospitals have workshops for parents who are managing the complex care of their children. Parent-to-parent support groups can be valuable to the family by providing advice, support, and suggestions for referrals. Review the care coordination to ensure that the child has access to the most appropriate care and resources. Provide positive feedback to the parents as their advocacy skills increase.

Suggest that the family maintain a log of the healthcare team members, their roles, when the child was seen and any interventions, the results of interventions, and future planned interventions or treatments. The family can use this information when communicating with the healthcare providers, particularly in an emergency, and it may also help eliminate unnecessary duplication of procedures.

COMMUNITY SITES OF CARE

Most children with chronic conditions are cared for in the home without home nursing or other health services. The healthcare provider for children with chronic conditions varies by the type of condition, type of health insurance coverage, preferences of the family, and availability of pediatric specialty resources.

OFFICE OR HEALTH CENTER

Every child should have a **healthcare home** or **medical home**, a consistent, continuous, comprehensive, family-centered, and compassionate source of primary health care. A healthcare home or medical home for these children is especially important as children with chronic conditions need regular preventive health care just as healthy children do. Health promotion, disease prevention, and anticipatory guidance have greater significance for the child with special healthcare needs. This child already has a condition that places him or her at higher risk for additional problems, such as infectious diseases, injury, or developmental delay. Information about community resources that may help the child and family is usually more extensive when the child's healthcare home is in the local community. The goal is for the child to have as normal a childhood as possible.

Ideally this healthcare provider is located in the community where the family resides, making it more convenient for the family to obtain routine health care as well as care for episodic illnesses. Having a regular healthcare provider has many advantages for the family.

- Because the child and family are seen more frequently, a trusting, family-centered relationship can develop. The healthcare provider learns about the family's strengths and coping abilities.
- The healthcare provider sees the child and family when things are going well and during exacerbations. This may enable the healthcare provider to identify strategies that help the family to better coordinate the child's care.
- When the provider is based in the same community as the child, it is likely that information about community resources is known; this will reduce the efforts that families must make to identify appropriate services needed by the child.

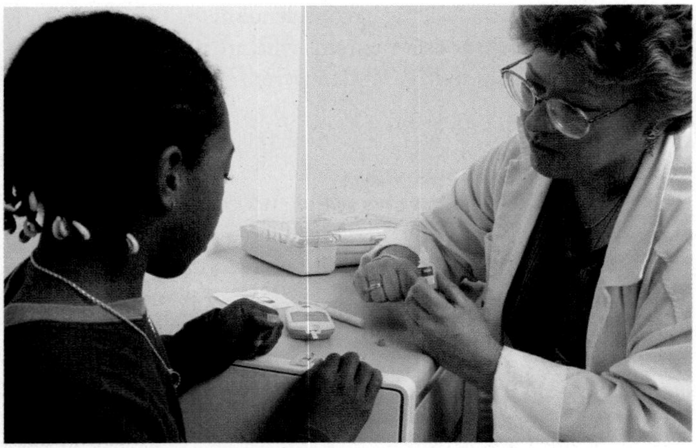

● **Figure 40–3** The nurse's role in the hospital ambulatory setting. Nurses often assume a larger role in working with children and families with a chronic health condition in the ambulatory setting. Developing a care plan and educating the family to manage diabetes type 1 is an important role of this pediatric nurse, who is also a certified diabetes educator.

SPECIALTY REFERRAL CENTERS

An optimal healthcare arrangement for the child with a chronic condition exists when the medical or healthcare home provider collaborates with a pediatric team or specialist that specializes in the care of children with a specific chronic condition. Pediatric specialists, advanced practice nurses, and other healthcare providers (e.g., physical therapists, social workers, and nutritionists) often function as a team providing coordinated care to the family and child with a chronic condition, such as spina bifida, cystic fibrosis, or diabetes. These specialty teams are often found in major medical centers, requiring travel to the facility. When communication flows from the team to the child's healthcare provider and back to the team, new treatments can be monitored by the child's physician, and consultation can be sought if the child's health status changes (Figure 40–3 ●).

Nurses working in hospital specialty clinics and other community settings can help ensure that these children receive the appropriate health promotion services. The nurse in a tertiary care facility needs to identify appropriate resources and to help the family connect with local community resources. This is a greater challenge if the child and family have traveled a distance to obtain the specialty services supporting the need for a primary care provider in the home community to provide regular care and to help coordinate local community resources.

SCHOOLS

All children, including those with chronic conditions and special healthcare needs, are entitled by federal law to a free education that is matched to their developmental and functional capabilities (Individual with Disabilities Education Act and Section 504 of the Rehabilitation Act of 1973). **Early intervention**, special services for infants and toddlers up to age 3 years who have developmental delay or are at risk for developmental delay, is provided through state and local education programs in the hopes that these children will have a lowered total cost of educational services (Blann, 2005). Provisions for adolescent transitional planning for adult living, including vocational training and independent living are also included in the Individual with Disabilities Education Act.

Attending school is an important transition for children with chronic conditions and their families. Sending the child to school has several benefits for the child and family. Children have an opportunity for socialization with children and adults beyond the immediate family (Rehm & Bradley, 2006). School attendance promotes a feeling of normalcy in the family and provides a break for the primary care provider. Integration into the school system requires collaboration of family, school personnel, the nurse, and other members of the healthcare team.

Nursing Practice

Federal laws for providing education services for children with special healthcare needs include:

- Rehabilitation Act PL 93-112 of 1973 prohibited discrimination against people with a disability. Section 504 specifies that each student who has a disability is entitled to **accommodations**—services or special assistance provided in the school setting to ensure that a student with a physical or mental impairment has access to an appropriate education, such as additional time to take a test, strategies that decrease an allergic child's exposure to peanuts, or frequent bathroom visits for the child needing intermittent catheterization—needed to attend school and participate as fully as possible in school activities (Moses, Gilchrest, & Schwab, 2005). This act covers many chronic conditions not covered under other education laws.
- The Education for All Handicapped Children Act, PL 94-142 of 1975 mandated that all children, even those with handicaps, be provided with public education and related services.
- Education for All Handicapped Children Amendments, PL 99-457 of 1986 expanded the scope of PL 94-142 to include appropriate services for infants and toddlers with disabilities and their families. The name of this legislation is now referred to as IDEA and newer amendments are described below.
- Individuals with Disabilities Education Act (IDEA), PL 105-17 of 1997 and the Individuals with Disabilities Education Act of 2004, PL 108-446 (reauthorization of the 1997 legislation) ensures that all children with disabilities have available to them a free appropriate public education that emphasizes special education and related services designed to meet their unique needs and prepare them for employment and independent living. Every child with a disability must have a written individualized education plan (IEP), and parents have the right to question placement decisions and to due process when settling differences.

Data from: U.S. Department of Education (2006a) http://idea.ed.gov/explore/home. Retrieved November 3, 2007; Moses, M., Gilchrest, C., & Schwab, N. C. (2005). Section 504 of the Rehabilitation Act: Determining eligibility and implications for school districts. *Journal of School Nursing, 21*(1), 48–58.

Educational System Planning

Careful planning is needed when a child with special needs attends school or receives other education services. Many children have chronic medical conditions that require management during the day in the school environment, such as asthma, diabetes, and attention deficit disorder. Some children simply need medications administered regularly or episodically. Other children require more extensive interventions integrated into the school day, such as blood glucose monitoring or intermittent self-catheterization. The education system is obligated to provide reasonable accommodations to ensure that the child's medical needs are met during the school day. The education system's obligation is negotiated with the family in formalized plans. The school nurse is an active participant on the team that collaborates with the family to develop these formalized plans.

- An **individualized family service plan (IFSP)** is developed for the early intervention process for infants with special healthcare needs and their families. The IFSP contains information about the services required to support a child's development and enhance the family's capacity to facilitate the child's development. The family and education service providers work as a team to plan, implement, and evaluate services specific to the family's unique concerns, priorities, and resources.
- An **individualized education plan (IEP)** is developed for a child with cognitive, motor, social, and communication impairments who needs special education services. The IEP is jointly planned with the school administrator, teacher, parents, and other special support professionals as appropriate for the child's condition (Figure 40–4 ●). The child is also included in the process when possible. The plan is developed after an assessment of the child's abilities and specific functional limitations.

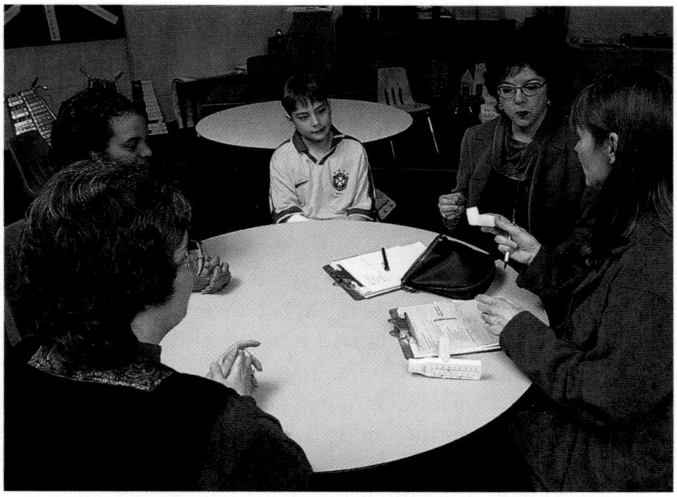

● **Figure 40–4** Managing chronic conditions during school hours. Because some children need medications or other therapies during school hours, the parents and child, school nurse, teacher, and school administrators develop a plan to manage the child's condition during school hours. This document is the child's individual school health plan.

Nursing Practice

The elements of an IEP are the following:

- Student's name
- Date of meeting to develop or review the IEP
- Statement of transition service needs of student beginning at age 14 years
- Present level of assessments and education performance, including how the child's disability affects the child's involvement and progress in a general curriculum or participation in appropriate activities
- Measurable annual goals that include benchmarks or short-term objectives in meeting the child's needs that enable the child to be involved in or progress in the general curriculum or participate in appropriate activities
- Special education and related services, supplementary aids and services, and program modifications or supports for school personnel needed to enable the child to make advancements toward attaining annual goals
- Explanation of the extent that the child will or will not participate with nondisabled children
- Any specific modification in the administration of state or districtwide assessments of achievement that are needed for the child to participate in the assessment, or reasons for excluding the child from assessment
- An explanation of how the child's progress toward annual goals will be measured
- An explanation of how the child's parents will be regularly informed of the child's progress toward annual goals and the extent to which the child's progress is sufficient to meet goals by the end of the year

Data from: U.S. Department of Education. (2006b). Individualized Education Programs, http://idea.ed.gov/explore/view/p/%2Croot%2Cdynamic%2CTopicalBrief%2C10%2C. Retrieved September 21, 2008.

- An **individualized health plan (IHP)** is developed for the child with medical conditions that need to be managed within the school setting. An IHP may be developed simultaneously with the IEP for the child with a health problem and a coexisting functional impairment. Some children only need an IHP for management of their chronic medical condition at school, such as daily medication administration or for glucose monitoring and insulin injection. An order from a licensed healthcare provider is required for medication administration and special treatments. Learning may be challenged when the child has frequent acute illness episodes that result in missed days of school, and the IHP often integrates methods to prevent the child from being penalized for those absences.
- An Individualized Section 504 Accommodation Plan may be used rather than an IHP for children with physical or

mental impairments. The same process is used for development of the plan.

- An **individualized transition plan (ITP)** is included in the development of an IEP for each child with a chronic disability who is 14 years or older. The ITP focuses on assisting the individual to receive vocational training and in moving successfully from the home into other community living settings as they grow older.

Parents have an important role in advocating for their child to ensure that the child receives the most appropriate educational services. School systems must provide a full range of educational services for the children with special healthcare needs, including services that support cognitive development, self-care skills, mobility, improved communication, and social skills. Because each child's severity and combination of impairments is unique, identifying and matching the specific services for each child requires discussion and negotiation. Parents should make an effort to learn about the different types of educational services that address a child's specific disability in preparation for the IEP meeting. Parents often need a mentor or experienced parent to help with the development of the IEP the first few times. In this way, the parents are better prepared to participate in the educational planning and development of the child's IEP. School nurses are employees of the school system and may be limited in their advocacy role on behalf of individual students. However, school nurses are in a good position to educate the IEP team about specific interventions needed by children with medical conditions and ways to integrate those interventions into the school day.

Teachers will need to learn to identify specific health problems, such as increased respiratory effort in a child with asthma or sweating, and pallor and loss of concentration in a child with diabetes. The child's teachers become part of the child's safety net for rapid access to needed healthcare intervention. With support from the school administration and school nurse, teachers can learn about the child's condition and special care that may be needed during the school day, such as a snack for the child with diabetes, management of the child who has a seizure, and ways to reduce the spread of infection within the classroom.

The Child's Response to Entering School

Children with chronic conditions—whether the conditions cause minimal interference in the child's daily life or significant interference, such as dependence on technology—face certain challenges in the school setting. They may for the first time recognize differences between themselves and other children, such as appearance, abilities, social skills, or special treatment needs. They may be teased and may experience social stigma for the first time (Rehm & Bradley, 2006). Some children, particularly adolescents, may attempt to hide their condition or fail to adhere to necessary recommendations, such as dietary restrictions, to appear like their peers.

MyNursingKit Healthy Ready to Work Resources

Education for Children Who Are Medically Fragile

Children who are medically fragile or technology-assisted are also entitled to education and education services in the school setting. The parents and the school system must carefully consider the child's need for skilled supportive nursing care. Parents are often anxious about how well the child will be cared for by others during the school day. Risks for the child in the school setting include safety issues related to ventilators, tracheostomy, and medication therapy, as well as exposure to infectious diseases. The school administration must provide the personnel resources and equipment needed to ensure that care and a care provider are consistently available. Modifications to the school setting for the child, such as wheelchair ramps or an elevator, may be needed. Sometimes the child is placed in a classroom with healthy children, and the teacher is expected to monitor the child with a chronic condition and provide care as needed. Health aides may be assigned to provide care for one or more children with school nurse supervision. Some children are placed in classes composed of children with special healthcare needs where health aides are more available to provide needed care.

Nurses play a key role in assisting the family to understand that a teacher's primary responsibility is to teach, not to provide health care. The teacher is responsible for the health and safety of all children in the classroom. Parents need to have realistic expectations about the level of skilled support services that can be provided to a child who is medically fragile in a classroom. Teachers and education leaders are often challenged to meet the obligations for the child's special education services in balance with the needs of all other children in the classroom.

Home Schooling

The family of a child who is medically fragile or technology dependent may choose the option of home schooling the child, with resources provided through the school system. Home schooling may be used for all of the child's education or for periods when the child is experiencing exacerbations or more complications from the condition. The benefits of home schooling include continuity of education when the child would otherwise be unable to attend school and reducing the child's stress and fatigue. Potential negative effects of home schooling include lack of peer and social interaction and decreased opportunity to develop social skills. The family that chooses home schooling needs to establish a routine for the education process.

Transition to Adulthood

Approximately 21% of adolescents have special healthcare needs resulting from improved survival rates for children with chronic conditions (Scal & Ireland, 2005). When their chronic condition could affect their future ability to work and live independently, customized transition planning is needed in preparation for adulthood and self-determination. A transition plan is developed in collaboration with the family based on the needs that have been identified in relation to the adolescent's goals for health care, employment, and community living. The adolescent should be involved in this process. Friends can also be involved and frequently provide valuable support to the teen in times of transition (Betz, 2007). Healthy & Ready to Work services may be particularly helpful to adolescents and families in planning for the transition to adulthood (www.hrtw.org/).

Adolescents need continuous access to health care as young adults to maximize lifelong functioning and potential. Transition planning needs to focus on identifying and moving the adolescent or young adult to adult-oriented healthcare services. Challenges in finding and establishing a healthcare relationship with an adult healthcare provider include the following (Lotstein, McPherson, Strickland, et al., 2005):

- The adolescent and parents may be unwilling to end a long-term relationship with present healthcare providers.
- High rates of uninsurance or underinsurance exist (once the young adult reaches 21 years, previous eligibility to the state's child health insurance program [SCHIP] and Medicaid may terminate).
- Adult providers may not be available or willing to see young adults with chronic conditions.

Adolescents with severe developmental or cognitive disabilities may have additional challenges because of their reliance on parents or other caregivers for healthcare decisions (Telfair, Alleman-Velez, Dickens, et al., 2005). A *Healthy People 2010* goal is to facilitate healthcare transition for adolescents, and the federal government is working to increase access to resources for this planning (Scal & Ireland, 2005).

HOME CARE

Many families become the primary caregiver for the child with a chronic condition, assuming responsibility for assessment and treatment despite the level of skill and complexity involved in that care. Numerous benefits to home care include the promotion of health, well-being, and development for the child, decreased financial costs to health insurance companies and the healthcare system, and a sense of satisfaction to families when they are able to care for their child at home. However, because of the burden of care, parent caregivers may experience depression, social isolation, poor physical health, and a high degree of stress associated with caring for the medically fragile child (Kuster, Badr, Chang, et al., 2004).

The family faces numerous challenges for home care, including modification of the home. Management of the condition involves technological support, medications, and treatment regimens, all potential necessities to maintain the child in the home. Family members must decide who has responsibility for different aspects of the child's care. Many families must also decide whether both spouses will continue to work or if one parent will stay home to care for the child. Home health nursing care may be needed if both parents continue to work or to cover the night shift so parents can sleep.

Moving the child who is chronically ill, or a technology-assisted child, to the home setting is a life-changing decision for the family and it must be done with collaboration between the family and the healthcare team. Preparation for the child's transition to the home requires that the family receive extensive training and instructions on the child's care. Management of the condition involves technological support, medications and treatment regimens, and all potential necessities to maintain the child in the home.

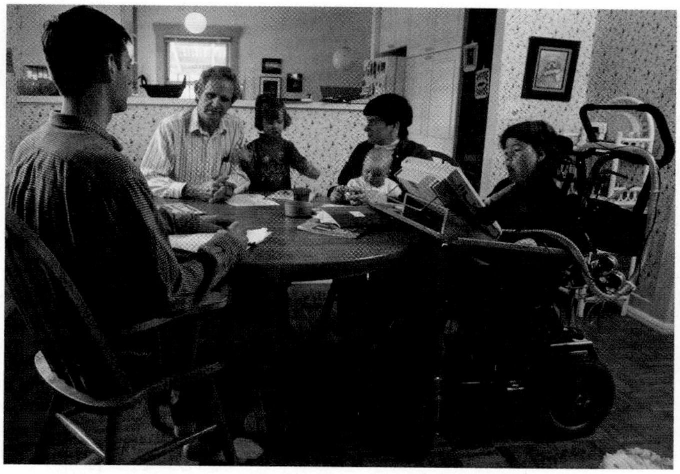

● **Figure 40–5** Avoiding caregiver burden. Daily caregiving demands of the child who is medically fragile continue 24 hours a day, 7 days a week. Parents need to identify ways to share the care of the child and other family care management. When the child lives with a single parent, additional healthcare resources are needed so the parent can sleep.

This transition is often challenging and intimidating for the family who now must assume the role of independent caregiver for a child who may have been hospitalized for several months. Family members often feel unprepared to handle the complex situation of the chronic condition and/or technological supports. They are at risk to develop **caregiver burden**, the unrelenting pressure and anxiety related to providing daily care to a child with disabilities while meeting other family obligations. Parents have greater personal strain and caregiver distress when the child has poor functional status, needs extensive care, and the parents have an existing financial burden (Kuster et al., 2004). The family needs to be highly motivated and possess strength and resiliency factors to overcome the obstacles that will arise. These characteristics will help them be successful in assuming management responsibility for the child's care (Figure 40–5 ●).

Respite Care

Respite care is an important support service to care for the child with a chronic condition while the parents take a short break away from the daily care. Respite allows parents an opportunity for rest so they may sustain their role as a caregiver. Care may be provided by extended family, friends, or an agency. The length of time may vary from a few hours to several days (MacDonald & Callery, 2004). An example of respite might be skilled nursing care in a facility or the home so the family can have a weekend away. Assist the family in identifying respite care that meets the individual family's needs from the services available in the community. Many states have passed legislation for in-home family support services that include respite care. Because many respite services charge for their assistance, the family may require help in identifying respite waiver subsidies available to them. Reliable childcare and enrollment in school are other mechanisms for families to obtain respite care. See "Evidence-Based Nursing: Identifying and Responding to Unmet Needs."

Evidence-Based Nursing

IDENTIFYING AND RESPONDING TO UNMET NEEDS

Clinical Question

What are the unmet needs of parents of children with complex healthcare conditions?

The Evidence

Parents who have a child with complex healthcare conditions have reported difficulties in obtaining the support needed to manage the child's care. Needs of families vary and depend on the diagnosis, prognosis, and specific needs of the child (Hummelinck & Pollock, 2006).

Interviews with 9 families (9 mothers and 2 fathers) having a child who had been diagnosed at least 1 year with a long-term illness helped illustrate the experiences that parents have in managing their children's health care and how healthcare providers affect their experiences. A specific need identified in this study included the need for healthcare professionals to show care toward the child. While some parents remember times that their child was treated with care, others recalled episodes when their child was treated in an unconcerned manner. The parents in this study also identified receiving information as an important need. While some parents reported they actually received too much information to comprehend, others reported either receiving inadequate or conflicting information (Nuutila & Salanterä, 2006).

A study of lower income mothers of 83 children with complex health problems treated in primary care offices revealed that 93% of mothers had at least one unmet need (Farmer, Marien, Clark, et al., 2004). The most frequently identified need was information about services for the child and ways to promote the child's health and development. More than 50% of parents also reported a need for caregiver supports, community services, help with family relationships, and financial costs. A greater number of unmet needs were reported when the child functioned at a lower level, and by mothers from minority groups or those who had perceptions of lower social support.

Additional studies have focused specifically on informational needs of parents of children with chronic illness. Hummelinck and Pollock (2006) interviewed 27 parents who had varying needs for information. While some of these parents actively sought information, resisting information was noted as a coping strategy among some of these parents. Most parents in this study perceived the information they received as inadequate. Jackson, Baird, Davis-Reynolds, Blackburn, and Allsebrook (2007) conducted in-depth interviews with 10 parents of children with healthcare needs and found that they had a particular preference for how information was presented. Most preferred that information be presented one-on-one by a professional with additional written information made available to them. These parents also expressed the importance of having access to a contact person for follow up questions and support.

Best Practice

These studies revealed that families with children who have special healthcare needs seek information, but the type of information sought varies by the type of condition, level of function, or special healthcare need. However, nearly all of these families need information about ways to promote the child's growth and development and community services that match the child's needs. Nurses are in a position to assist families by assessing their needs for information and then attempting to provide that information.

The need for care and support from healthcare professionals was also identified as a potentially unmet need. Nurses should always treat the child and family with care, compassion and a nonjudgmental attitude. Current listings of community services and contact information of healthcare professionals should also be provided to these families.

Critical Thinking

Select a specific pediatric chronic condition that usually requires parents to follow a complex routine to care for the child. Construct a series of questions to ask the family in order to learn about their perceived needs. Consider the potential supports and services such a family might need, and compile a list of local resources that could be recommended to the family.

See MyNursingKit for possible responses.

Emergency Preparedness

Advance planning is needed to ensure that medically fragile children who require technology for survival or have the potential for life-threatening episodes have the necessary resources in the event of a disaster. The designated shelter for such children, with health professionals and electrical power for the needed equipment, should be identified and known to the family. In the meantime, battery packs for power backup should be available at all times. Additionally, parents need to arrange for durable power of attorney so that consent for emergency medical care can be available as needed. The child and parents may become separated during the disaster, or the parents may become injured and unable to care for the child. Refer to Chapter 15 for more information related to emergency preparedness.

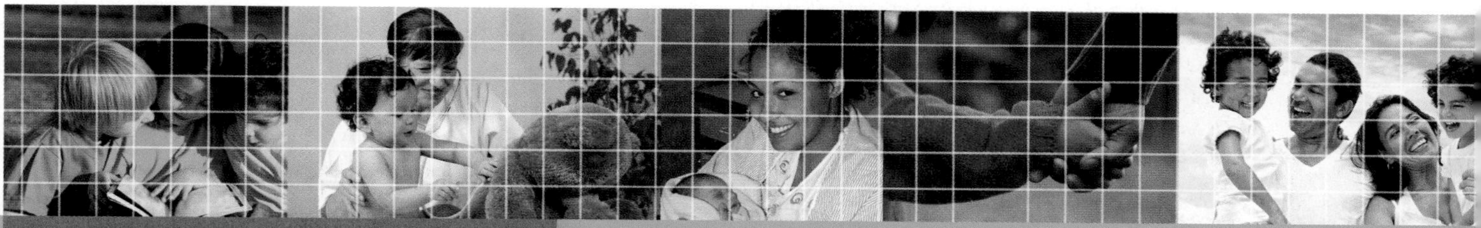

CRITICAL CONCEPT REVIEW

LEARNING OUTCOMES	CONCEPTS
40.1 Discuss causes of chronic conditions in children.	1. Genetic or inheritable conditions may be manifested as a chronic condition. 2. Conditions may result from a congenital defect or insult to the infant during fetal development. 3. Insult or injury may be associated with birth and care following birth that lead to chronic conditions. 4. Conditions can be acquired through injury or acute medical conditions such as brain injury, cancer, HIV infection, drowning, and mental health problems.
40.2 Describe the categories of chronic conditions in children.	1. Limitations in function that would typically be expected for the child's age and development. 2. Disfigurement. 3. Dependency on medications or a special diet for control of the condition. 4. Dependency on medical technology for functioning. 5. Need for more medical care and related services than typically used by a healthy child of the same age. 6. Special ongoing treatments at home or school.
40.3 Describe the nurse's role in caring for a child with a chronic condition.	1. Provide health supervision from infancy to transition into adulthood. 2. Collaborate with the multidisciplinary healthcare team. 3. Partner with parents or caregivers to manage the child's care at home. 4. Refer the family to appropriate community services, assisting with planning for education services. 5. Promote positive parenting behaviors and psychosocial adaptation and well-being of the child and family, and promote growth and development of siblings.
40.4 Assess the family of a child with a chronic condition and discuss the impact of the child's condition on the family.	1. Assess individual family members' level of understanding of the condition, treatment, and anticipated outcome of the condition. 2. Determine the family's stage of acceptance of the child's chronic illness, and how well the child's care is integrated into family routines. 3. Address the fears and concerns of the family. 4. Provide condition-specific education to help prepare the family for care at home and begin discharge planning.
40.5 Describe nursing interventions for the child with a chronic condition to support transition to school and adult living.	1. Assist the family to understand the educational role of the teacher. 2. Educate teachers and staff about the unique needs of the child. 3. Provide instruction concerning medical equipment needed by the child. 4. Supervise the healthcare aides attending the child at school. 5. Identify adult-oriented healthcare services for the adolescent or young adult. 6. Assist the family to identify and select alternative living arrangements. 7. Provide referrals to agencies that can assist in the acquisition of workplace skills.
40.6 Discuss the family's role in care coordination.	1. Family decides who has responsibility for different aspects of the child's care. 2. Family assumes responsibility for many expenses of the child. 3. Family becomes the primary caregiver of the child. 4. Family may become the child's case manager.

CRITICAL THINKING IN ACTION

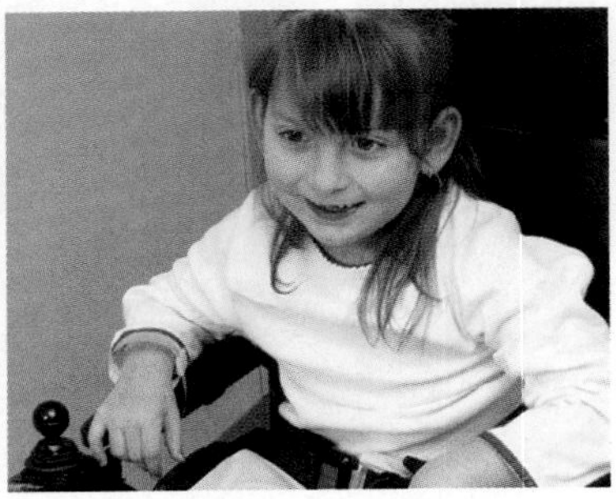

Haley is an 8-year-old child with cerebral palsy who will be attending school for the first time. Her mother had initially preferred home schooling for Haley, and now wants to support her social development with other children. A case manager is asked to assist with facilitating Haley's entry into school. The case manager coordinates a multidisciplinary meeting of the clinic nurse, physical therapist, physician, and Haley's family to review her health status and to discuss the transition to school. They also discuss potential accommodations needed for Haley's mobility limitations. The multidisciplinary team assists the parents in developing a plan for Haley's transition to school.

1. What role will the clinic nurse and case manager have in helping develop Haley's IEP and IHP?
2. What role will the school nurse have with the child, caregivers, teacher, and classmates during the facilitation of school entry?
3. What actions will the mother need to take in preparing the school personnel for Haley's health needs?
4. Haley's 10-year-old sister attends the same school. What effects of Haley's entry into school might the sibling experience?

See MyNursingKit for possible responses.

REFERENCES

Allen, P. J. (2004). The primary care provider and children with chronic conditions. In P. J. Allen & J. A. Vessey, *Primary care of the child with a chronic condition* (4th ed., pp. 3–22). St. Louis: Mosby.

American Academy of Pediatrics. (2005). Care coordination in the medical home: Integrating health and related systems of care for children with special health care needs. *Pediatrics, 116*(5), 1238–1244.

Ballard, K. L. (2004). Meeting the needs of siblings of children with cancer. *Pediatric Nursing, 30*(5), 394–401.

Betz, C.L. (2007). Facilitating the transition of adolescents with developmental disabilities: Nursing practice issues and care. *Journal of Pediatric Nursing, 22*(2), 103–115.

Blann, L. E. (2005). Early intervention for children and families with special needs. *MCN, 30*(4), 263–267.

Coffey, J. S. (2006). Parenting a child with chronic illness: A metasynthesis. *Pediatric Nursing, 32*(1), 51–59.

Fanos, J. H., Fahrner, K., Jelveh, M., King, R., & Tejeda, D. (2004). The sibling center: A pilot program for siblings of children and adolescents with a serious medical condition. *Journal of Pediatrics, 146*, 831–835.

Farmer, J. E., Marien, W. E., Clark, M. J., Sherman, A., & Selva, T. J. (2004). Primary care supports for children with chronic health conditions: Identifying and predicting unmet family needs. *Journal of Pediatric Psychology, 29*(5), 355–367.

Goble, L. A. (2004). The impact of a child's chronic illness on fathers. *Issues in Comprehensive Pediatric Nursing, 27*(3), 153–162.

Hummelinck, A., & Pollock, K. (2006).Parents' information needs about the treatment of their chronically ill child: A qualitative study. *Patient Education and Counseling, 62*, 228–234.

Inkelas, M., & Garro, N. (2005). A picture of needs for children with special health care needs: What we are learning from the national survey. *Journal of Pediatric Nursing, 20*(3), 207–210.

Jackson, R., Baird, W., Davis-Reynolds, L., Smith, C., Blackburn, S., & Allsebrook, J. (2007). Qualitative analysis of parents' information needs and psychosocial experiences when supporting children with health care needs. *Health Information and Libraries Journal, 25*, 31–37.

Kruger, B. J. (2004). Care Coordination. In P. J. Allen & J. A. Vessey (Eds.), *Primary care of the child with a chronic condition* (4th ed., pp. 102–119). St. Louis: Mosby.

Kuster, P. A., Badr, L. K., Chang, B. L., Wuerker, A. K., & Benjamin, A. E. (2004). Factors influencing health promoting activities of mothers caring for ventilator-assisted children. *Journal of Pediatric Nursing, 19*(4), 276–287.

Lee, Tzu-Ying, Miles, M. S., & Holditch-Davis, D. (2006). Fathers' support to mothers of medically fragile infants. *JOGNN, 35*(1), 46–55.

Lotstein, D. S., McPherson, M., Strickland, B., & Newacheck, P. W. (2005). Transition planning for youth with special health care needs: Results from the national survey of children with special health care needs. *Pediatrics, 115*(6), 1562–1568.

MacDonald, H., & Callery, P. (2004). Different meanings of respite: A study of parents, nurses and social workers caring for children with complex needs. *Child: Care, Health & Development, 30*(3), 279–288.

Moses, M., Gilchrest, C., & Schwab, N. C. (2005). Section 504 of the Rehabilitation Act: Determining eligibility and implications for school districts. *Journal of School Nursing, 21*(1), 48–58.

Newacheck, P. W., & Kim, S. E. (2005). A national profile of health care utilization and expenditures for children with special health care needs. *Archives of Pediatric and Adolescent Medicine, 159*, 10–17.

Nuutila, L., & Salanterä, S. (2006). Children with a long-term illness: Parents' experiences of care. *Journal of Pediatric Nursing, 21*(2), 153–160.

Rehm, R. S., & Bradley, J. F. (2006). Social interactions at school of children who are medically fragile and developmentally delayed. *Journal of Pediatric Nursing, 21*(4), 299–307.

Scal, P., & Ireland, M. (2005). Addressing transition to adult health care for adolescents with special health care needs. *Pediatrics, 115*(6), 1607–1612.

Telfair, J., Alleman-Velez, P. L., Dickens, P., & Loosier, P. S. (2005). Quality health care for adolescents with special health care needs: Issues and clinical implications. *Journal of Pediatric Nursing, 20*(1), 15–24.

U.S. Department of Education. (2006). Individualized Education Programs. Retrieved November 3, 2007, from http://idea.ed.gov/explore/view/p/%2Croot%2Cdynamic%2CTopicalBrief%2C10%2C

U.S. Department of Education (2006). Retrieved November 10, 2007, from http://idea.ed.gov/explore/home

U.S. Department of Health and Human Services. (2006). *Healthy People 2010 Midcourse Review.* Retrieved November 4, 2007, from http://www.healthypeople.gov/data/midcourse/default.htm#pubs

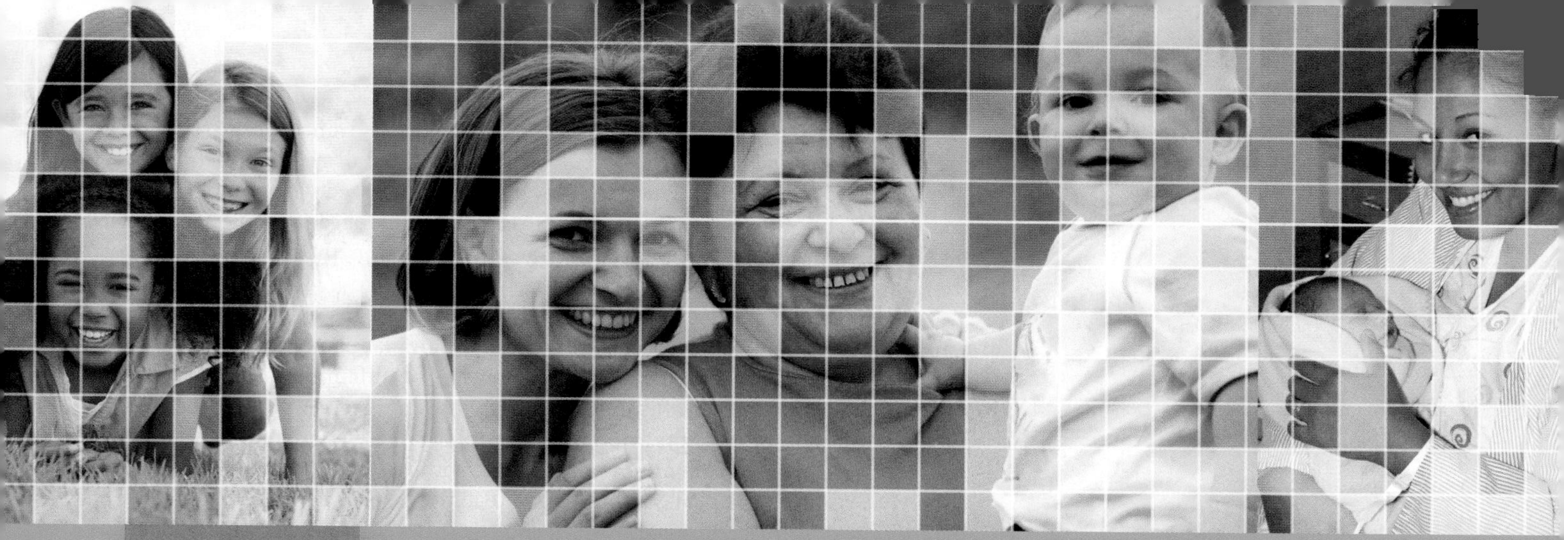

CHAPTER

41 Nursing Considerations for the Hospitalized Child

We live 50 miles from the hospital, and have three other children. We were worried about how we were going to be able to stay with Sabrina. She's only 4, and it's her first time in the hospital. Fortunately, they have beds for parents, so one of us can always be by her side throughout her procedure and recuperation. —Mother of Sabrina, 4 years old

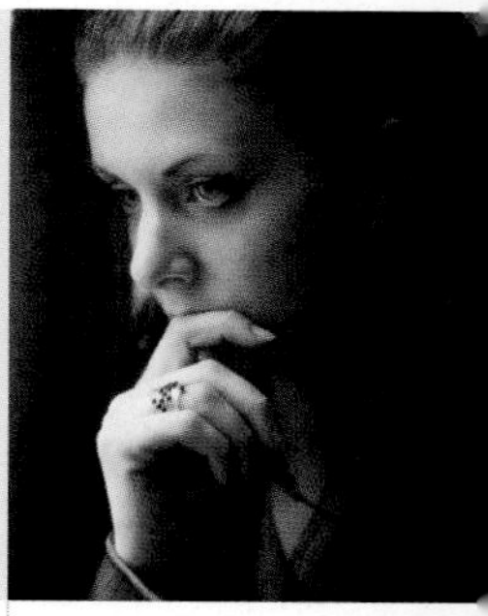

LEARNING OUTCOMES

41.1 Discuss the child's understanding of health and illness according to the child's psychosocial and developmental level.

41.2 Recognize the effect of hospitalization on the child and family.

41.3 Identify methods that the child and family use to adapt to hospitalization.

41.4 Apply family-centered care principles to the hospital setting.

41.5 Identify nursing strategies to minimize the stressors related to hospitalization.

41.6 Discuss family presence during procedures and nursing strategies used to prepare the family.

41.7 Discuss strategies for preparing children and families for discharge from the hospital setting.

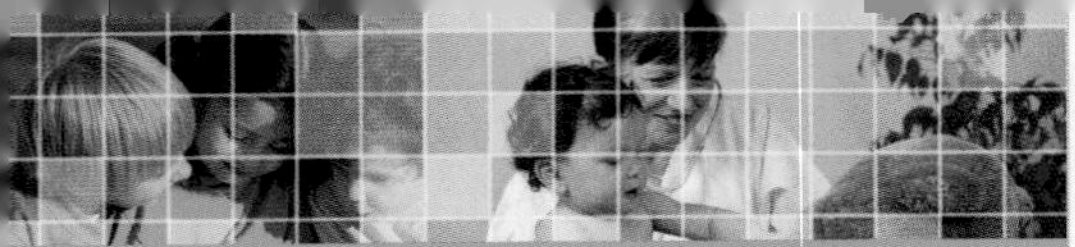

KEY TERMS

Animal-assisted therapy, 1094
Case manager, 1098
Child life specialist, 1090
Dramatic play, 1093
Rehabilitation, 1085
Rooming in, 1090
Separation anxiety, 1077
Stranger anxiety, 1078
Therapeutic play, 1091
Treatment room, 1087

Hospitalization, whether it is elective, planned in advance, or the result of an emergency or trauma, is stressful for children of all ages and their families. Because most pediatric conditions can be managed within the home and community, hospitalization is not always required to manage the child with an illness. However, while fewer children require hospitalization, those who are hospitalized usually have a high level of illness acuity.

Hospitalized children experience a variety of emotions as they are in an unknown environment, surrounded by strangers, unfamiliar equipment, and frightening sights and sounds. These children are subjected to unfamiliar procedures, some of which are invasive or painful and may even require surgery. For both children and families, routines are disrupted and normal coping strategies are tested.

Nurses today are challenged to provide individualized care for the hospitalized child with complex medical conditions, acute illnesses, or injury. As a key aspect of that role, nurses must address the psychosocial and developmental concerns that accompany hospitalization. (Developmental theorists and stages are presented in Chapter 33∞.)To minimize the stress of hospitalization, nurses provide support and education to children and their families before, during, and after hospitalization.

During hospitalization, nurses use a family-centered approach and work collaboratively with parents to implement various strategies that promote coping and adaptation and to prepare children for necessary procedures. Nurses also collaborate with members of a multidisciplinary team and partner with families to assist them in preparing for discharge home or transfer to a long-term care or rehabilitation facility.

EFFECTS OF HOSPITALIZATION ON CHILDREN AND THEIR FAMILIES

CHILDREN'S UNDERSTANDING OF HEALTH AND ILLNESS

Can you remember as a child thinking that yelling at your mother caused your strep throat? Young children have limited knowledge about the body and its relation to health and illness. They do not have the ability to understand how organs work and how they can be affected by illness (Koopman, Baars, Chaplin, et al., 2004). Their understanding is based primarily on their cognitive ability at various developmental stages and on previous experiences with healthcare professionals. As children become older they move from having no concept of illness to being able to understand multiple factors related to illness (Koopman et al., 2004). For example, perhaps as an adolescent you believed that you would never become ill or have an accident; or maybe you feared being in a car crash like that of a friend. Knowledge of a child's understanding of health and illness is essential in assisting a child to adapt to the hospital experience.

Hospitalization and the accompanying medical procedures are very stressful for children, especially very young children such as toddlers and preschoolers. The child's attempts to deal with these stressors impact both the psychological and physiological well-being of the child (Ryan-Wenger, Sharrer, & Campbell, 2005). Infants, toddlers, and preschoolers lack the cognitive skills to understand hospitalization and are the age groups most likely to exhibit regressive behaviors. Young children have fears and anxieties related to things such as the dark, strangers, and monsters. A hospital's unfamiliar environment can exacerbate those anxieties. In addition to these stressors, the hospitalized child may experience an emotional and physical threat to his or her well-being (Lau, 2002).

Significant stressors for hospitalized children of all ages include (Lau, 2002):

- Separation from parents, the primary caretaker, or peers
- Loss of self-control, autonomy, and privacy
- Painful and/or invasive procedures
- Fear of bodily injury and disfigurement

Nursing care of the hospitalized child focuses on minimizing the child's fears, anxieties, and disruption of the child's usual routine, and supporting the family through the stressful experience. Strategies include minimizing separation anxiety, loss of control, pain related to procedures, and fear. Table 41–1 highlights key stressors of hospitalization for children at each developmental stage.

Infant

By about 6 months of age, infants have developed an awareness of themselves as separate from their mothers or fathers. They are able to identify primary caretakers and to feel anxious when in contact with strangers. Hospitalization can be a traumatic time for an infant, particularly if the parents are not staying with the child. Infants can sense the anxiety their parents are experiencing during a hospitalization.

Common stressors to the infant include painful procedures, immobilization of extremities, and the sleep deprivation caused by the disruption of the infant's normal sleep patterns and routines. However, the most common stressor of hospitalization for the infant is separation from parents, which is manifested by **separation anxiety**. Bowlby and Robertson identified three phases of separation anxiety exhibited in young children who were separated from their mothers for long periods of time (Alsop-Shields & Mohay,

Table 41–1 Stressors of Hospitalization for Children at Various Developmental Stages

Developmental Stages and Stressors	Responses	Nursing Implications
INFANT		
Separation anxiety Stranger anxiety Painful, invasive procedures Immobilization Sleep deprivation, sensory overload	Sleep–awake cycle disrupted Feeding routines disrupted Displays excessive irritability	Encourage parental presence Adhere to infant's home routine as much as possible Utilize topical anesthetics or preprocedural sedation as prescribed Promote a quiet environment and reduce excess stimuli
TODDLER		
Separation anxiety Loss of self-control Immobilization Painful, invasive procedures Bodily injury or mutilation Fear of the dark	Cries if parents leave the bedside Is frightened if forced to lie supine Wonders why parents don't come to the rescue Associates pain with punishment	Encourage parental presence Allow parents to hold child in their lap for examinations and procedures when possible Allow choices when possible Utilize topical anesthetics or preprocedural sedation as prescribed Explain all procedures using simple developmentally appropriate language Provide a night-light
PRESCHOOLER		
Separation anxiety and fear of abandonment Loss of self-control Bodily injury or mutilation Painful, invasive procedures Fear of the dark and monsters	Displays difficulty separating reality from fantasy Fears ghosts and monsters Fears body parts will leak out when skin is not intact Fears that tubes are permanent Demonstrates withdrawal, projection, aggression, regression	Encourage parental presence Allow choices when possible Utilize topical anesthetics or preprocedural sedation as prescribed Explain all procedures Provide a night-light or flashlight
SCHOOL-AGE CHILD		
Loss of control Loss of privacy and control over bodily functions Bodily injury Separation from family and friends Painful, invasive procedures Fear of death	Displays increased sensitivity to the environment Demonstrates detailed recall of events to self and other patients	Encourage parental participation Allow the child choices when possible Explain all procedures and offer reassurance Utilize topical anesthetics or preprocedural sedation as prescribed Encourage peer interaction via internet, phone calls, and other methods of communication
ADOLESCENT		
Loss of control Fear of altered body image, disfigurement, disability, and death Separation from peer group Loss of privacy and identity	Displays denial, regression, withdrawal, intellectualization, projection, displacement	Include the adolescent in the plan of care Encourage discussion of fears and anxieties Explain all procedures Ask the adolescent his or her desire for parental involvement Encourage peer interaction

Table 41–2 Stages of Separation Anxiety

Protest	Despair	Denial (detachment)
Screaming, crying	Sadness	Lack of protest when parents leave
Clinging to parents	Quiet, appear to have "settled in"	Appearance of being happy and content with everyone
May resist attempts by other adults to comfort them	Withdrawal or compliant behavior	Show interest in surroundings
	Crying when parents return	Close relationships not established

Source: Data from Alsop-Shields, L., & Mohay, H. (2001). John Bowlby & James Robertson: Theorists, scientists and crusaders for improvements in the care of children in hospitals. *Journal of Advanced Nursing, 35*(1), 50–58.

Nursing Practice

Children encounter many members of the healthcare team, in addition to other hospital personnel when hospitalized. Children ages 6–18 months perceive these people as strangers and may cry when someone new enters the room. As the child sees a person over and over again, the stranger anxiety for that person subsides. Providing consistent caregivers as much as possible will limit the number of "strangers" that the child encounters while hospitalized.

2001). Characteristic behaviors of children in the three phases of separation anxiety are listed in Table 41–2. Infants and toddlers who are hospitalized often display some of these behaviors, particularly if parents are unable to remain with the child. In addition to separation anxiety, children between 6 and 18 months of age may display **stranger anxiety** (wariness of strangers) when confronted with unfamiliar healthcare professionals.

Encourage family members to be active participants in the care of the hospitalized infant through touch, sight, and sound. Infants get satisfaction from meeting their oral needs, so parents and nurses should provide sources for oral stimulation, such as pacifiers and age-appropriate teething toys. The infant should be rocked and touched with light stroking to provide tactile stimulation for developmental growth. However, minimize excessive noise and prolonged stimuli to allow the infant periods of rest.

Encourage parents to stay with the hospitalized infant. If family members are unable to remain at the hospital, encourage them to visit their infant as often as possible. Explain and emphasize the importance of parent–newborn attachment and bonding to the parents.

Toddler

Toddlers are the group most at risk for a stressful experience as a result of illness and hospitalization. These children are old enough to understand that their routine has been disrupted but they lack the cognitive ability to understand why the disruption has occurred. Separation from parents is the major stressor and toddlers protest vigorously when their parents depart. When one or both parents cannot be present, they can leave mementos to comfort the child. These might include an object belonging to a parent, a picture, or an audiotape or videotape with messages from the parents.

Disruption of routine also causes stress for the toddler. The nurse encourages parents to remain present as much as possible for important rituals such as toileting, carrying out bedtime routines, and singing favorite nursery rhymes. Autonomy is a developmental characteristic of the toddler (see Chapter 33). Having their activities limited and being confined especially threaten children in this age group. When possible, maintain the toddler's normal home routines for bathing and other activities. Offer the toddler choices when possible, such as choosing the color of Jell-O or which gown/pajamas to wear.

Preschooler

The greatest stressors for preschoolers are their fears: fear of being alone, fear of being in the dark, fear of abandonment, fear of loss of self-control related to the body and emotions, and fear of bodily injury or mutilation. Preschoolers may also feel guilty about being sick, or they may view illness and hospitalization as punishment.

Similar to the toddler, preschoolers desire a normal routine, and the nurse can partner with the family to maintain routines as much as possible. Developmentally, preschoolers exhibit a sense of initiative (see Chapter 33) as they explore the world around them. To promote that initiative, the nurse can encourage the preschool child's independence by offering choices such as "Do you want to take the red medicine or the purple medicine first?"

Parents should be encouraged to stay with the child if possible. For those who cannot stay, preschoolers need to know when to expect their parents to return to the hospital. Because most

Nursing Practice

Toddlers may challenge a nurse by refusing to cooperate with treatments and procedures, including physical assessments. To diffuse such confrontations, encourage cooperation by offering the toddler some sense of control. For example, a nurse might comment, "Once I have listened to your heart, lungs, and stomach you can choose whether you want to ride in the wagon or be pushed in the big buggy to the play room."

preschoolers lack a conception of time measurements like "two hours," "half-past four," or "three o'clock," respond with simpler statements of time, such as "after supper" or "before breakfast." Encourage parents to make telephone calls to the preschooler if possible. Some parents are able to make calls from work. Preschoolers get a sense of security from hearing their parent's voice confirming that the parent will return to the hospital.

Parents often believe it is better to leave the hospital room after their child has fallen asleep, as their departure won't stress the child. In fact, the opposite is true. If a child awakens to find the parent gone unexpectedly, he or she may become anxious and may develop a lack of trust. Instead, encourage parents to tell their child when they need to leave and why (e.g., has to go to work or go home). By providing honest information to the child, parents or caregivers demonstrate that they can be trusted.

School-Age Child

The school-age child relies on parents and others for support and understanding during stressful events and procedures. Although school-age children attempt to maintain their composure during painful or invasive procedures, generally they still require a great deal of support. Major sources of stress for hospitalized school-age children include:

- loss of control related to bodily functions,
- privacy issues,
- fear of bodily injury, pain, and concerns related to death, and
- separation anxiety from family and friends.

School-age children understand concepts, so parents who cannot remain at the bedside are encouraged to tell the child when they will return. Also encourage parents to be available for telephone calls to provide support and comfort to their child. Stressful procedures can lead to regression or other behavioral changes, although this is less likely than with younger patients. Inform the parents that this behavior is normal during stressful situations.

Developmentally, school-age children exhibit a sense of industry (see Chapter 33), taking pride in their achievements at home, at school, and in sports. To foster that sense of industry, allow the child to participate in their care as much as possible.

Growth and Development

School-age children between the ages of 5 and 8 years believe that the internal body consists mainly of a heart and bones. They view the digestive system as having two parts, the mouth and the stomach. Showing them how parts of the body are related can be helpful to enhance their understanding. However, young adolescents, ages 11 to 13 years, can describe the location and function of major body parts such as the brain, nose, eyes, heart, and stomach. They usually have gaps in understanding and may have misconceptions, however, so evaluating their knowledge is a part of the nursing plan in order to plan teaching to meet their knowledge needs.

Encourage them to continue with school work and engage in creative outlets such as art or crafts.

Adolescent

Preoccupation with appearance and body image are paramount in this age group. By offering education and explanations that focus on these issues, nurses can provide significant reassurance to the adolescent. Nevertheless, adolescents often try to maintain independence and rigid self-control when undergoing painful and invasive procedures. Because hospitalization may increase dependence on their parents, adolescents may respond with frustration and anger. The nurse who respects the adolescent's desire for privacy and independence is often successful in establishing a trusting relationship and assisting the adolescent to cope with the hospitalization and illness. Encourage the adolescent to discuss thoughts and feelings about experiences. Careful listening by the nurse is essential in establishing a positive rapport.

Major stressors for hospitalized adolescents include:

- Loss of independence, control, and privacy,
- Fear of bodily injury or changes in body image,
- Fear of disability, pain, and even death,
- Separation from peers, home, and school.

Adolescents are in the process of establishing their identity and becoming independent of their parents' influence, so control over aspects of their care is important. Partner with the family and multidisciplinary team to ensure that the adolescent is an active participant in decisions and the plan of care. Privacy and modesty are major concerns, as adolescents' physical characteristics are rapidly changing. To demonstrate respect for their feelings, knock on the door before entering and ask permission before conducting assessments or other procedures.

Nurses can assist the hospitalized adolescent by fostering appropriate social and coping skills through activities such as role playing and relaxation training (Pinckney & Stuart, 2004). By allowing choices in clothing, hair, and music, the nurse can acknowledge the importance of the adolescent's self-image.

The peer group is a major influence in adolescents' lives. Allowing flexible visiting hours for friends helps teens maintain their social network and provides needed support. When friends are not able to visit, providing teens with Internet access provides a means of accessing their friends for support. Encouraging participation in recreation and teen lounge facilities available during hospitalization provides the adolescent with additional peer group support opportunities.

FAMILY RESPONSES TO HOSPITALIZATION

The illness and hospitalization of a child disrupt a family's usual routines. Parental roles change when the child is hospitalized and care is being provided by nursing staff (Sarajärvi, Haapamäki, & Paavilainen, 2006). Roles may be altered as one parent stays at the hospital with the child while the other parent, or siblings, take on additional tasks at home. Family members may experience anxiety and fear, especially when the outcome is unknown or a potentially serious health condition prompted the hospitalization.

Parents who perceive their child is in pain find the experience difficult and require support. Family members' ability to cope can be challenged by a serious emergency, lengthy illness, chronic condition, poor prognosis, lack of family support, and lack of financial or community services. The stress on parents can be compounded by the burden of missed work, additional expenses, and concerns about feeding and caring for children at home. (See Chapter 43 for a description of nursing support for the child with life-threatening illness or injury.) It is essential that nurses assess parental needs and attend to those needs in order to establish a trusting relationship. Needs frequently identified by parents of hospitalized children include:

- the need to receive information about their child's condition, prognosis, and treatment on a regular basis,
- the need to receive help, encouragement, and support from nursing staff, and
- the need to have a trusting, confidential relationship with the nursing staff (Hopia, Tomlinson, Paavilainen, et al., 2005).

Parents who have support from nursing staff have less anxiety and more self-confidence, and are better equipped to make decisions and participate in their child's care.

Nurses also need to be alert to family members' cultural views about health, illness, and the causation of illness, which can influence their response to hospitalization and the family's management of the experience. Cultural influences may also determine which family member is the decision maker regarding healthcare practices, and provide guidelines for acceptable treatments (Spector, 2009).

The siblings of a hospitalized child may receive little attention from the parents who are overwhelmed and anxious about their hospitalized child's health. A sibling's response depends on a variety of factors including age, family size, severity of the illness, prior experience, and information received about the illness (Gursky, 2007).

Younger siblings who do not understand the causes of illness and hospitalization may feel guilty about fighting with or being mean to their brother or sister in the past. Some siblings may fear becoming ill themselves. Some may believe that they played a role in the child's illness and need reassurance that they did not cause the illness or injury. If the child did in some way contribute to the child's illness or injury, help them to cope with their guilt by providing them an opportunity to discuss their feelings. Siblings often have nightmares about the illness or injury their brother or sister has sustained and about the ill child dying (see Chapter 43).

As hospitalization causes family roles and routines to change, siblings may feel insecure and anxious. It is essential that siblings receive information about their brother's or sister's condition and hospitalization using language and concepts appropriate to their ages and developmental levels (Gursky, 2007). Providing information and support to siblings promotes coping and adaptation to a sibling's illness (Lobato, Kao, & Plante, 2006).

As appropriate, encourage siblings to visit. Such a visit is especially encouraged if the child could potentially die, as it allows the sibling the opportunity to say good-bye. (See Chapter 43 for further discussion of the dying child.) These visits often help to improve the mood of the hospitalized child and assist the sibling to overcome misconceptions or negative emotions. Because children's fantasies are often worse than reality, unfounded fears may be relieved by a visit.

Before the visit, prepare the siblings by explaining what they will likely encounter. Describe the hospital environment, including equipment, sounds, and smells. Describe how the brother or sister will appear. If the hospitalized child acts, moves, talks, or appears differently than before the hospitalization, provide an explanation beforehand. Consider using a doll, drawing pictures, or showing an actual photograph of the child to help prepare the siblings. (See "Teaching Highlights: Strategies for Working with the Sibling of a Hospitalized Child.")

During the visit, demonstrate how to talk to and touch the ill child and encourage the siblings to do the same. After the visit, discuss with siblings what they saw and felt, and answer any questions they may have. When a sibling cannot visit, contact with the hospitalized child can be maintained by sending pictures, drawings, cards, and messages recorded on audiotapes or videotapes, and through e-mail or instant messaging. Partner with the family to determine the most appropriate and effective method of communicating if the sibling is unable to visit. If parents are staying at the hospital with the hospitalized child, partner with them to help establish communication routines for the well siblings. For example, encourage the parents to call the siblings at home at

Teaching Highlights

STRATEGIES FOR WORKING WITH THE SIBLING OF A HOSPITALIZED CHILD

The nurse working with siblings of a hospitalized child can implement the following strategies to assist the siblings in understanding what is happening to their brother or sister:

- *Be truthful.* Explain why the child is hospitalized, what the treatment involves, and how long the hospitalization is expected to last.
- *Assure siblings that they did not cause the illness and that the hospitalized child did nothing wrong.* If a sibling had some involvement in or responsibility for the health crisis, referral for mental health counseling may be needed.
- *Allow siblings to ask questions and discuss fears and other feelings.*
- *Encourage siblings to visit if possible.* Cover tubes and wires with a sheet. Wash off blood or cover bloody bandages if possible. Prepare the siblings for any equipment, dressing, and procedures they might see and any sounds they might hear.
- *Warn siblings if the hospitalized child is not speaking.* Say something like, "John can't talk now. He seems to be sleeping deeply. He may be able to hear, though, so you can touch him and talk to him."
- *Encourage siblings to express their feelings related to the disruptive effect of the child's hospitalization on family life.*

a regular time each night. Allowing the siblings at home the opportunity to share their day, and to receive an update on the hospitalized child, provides a feeling of connectedness and may minimize feelings of worry and resentment. The phone call offers siblings a consistent link to the parent and the reassurance that they are important and loved.

FAMILY ASSESSMENT

To support the hospitalized child and provide family-centered care, nurses develop an understanding of the family dynamics and individualize the nursing care according to the needs of the child and family. To develop a plan of care that involves all family members, the nurse assesses the impact of the child's illness or hospitalization on the family. Table 41–3 provides a list of questions to guide the nurse in determining the roles of family, knowledge of family, support systems, and effects on siblings. (See Chapter 2∞ for further discussion of family assessment.)

Collaborate with the family to determine their resources, such as:

- coping strategies of family members,
- financial resources,
- access to health care, and
- availability of community services.

One family with limited financial support may manage quite well because they have effective coping strategies, whereas another family with greater financial resources may have difficulty if their coping strategies are ineffective. Staying with a hospitalized child can be a financial drain for parents if one or both must take a leave of absence from work, miss scheduled workdays, or travel to the hospital. Additional expenses may include hotel rooms, meals, parking fees, and childcare for other children. Assess the family's ability to manage these additional expenses. To evaluate the burden of hospitalization, use a multidisciplinary approach, which may lead to increased access to community resources and support for families.

Assess the family dynamics by evaluating:

- the quality of communication,
- methods of coping with stress,
- risk factors, and
- sources of strength.

Common sources of strength and support include friends and relatives, religious leaders, hospital chaplains and social workers.

Examine how the family has dealt with the health needs of the child if the child has been hospitalized or required home care in the past. (See "Developing Cultural Competence: Supporting Alternative Health Practices.") Determine the family members' level of understanding related to the child's hospitalization and anticipated therapy. Collaborate with family members to determine their desired role in the child's care. Assess the family's needs for referral to family service agencies or other community organizations that may be required. Evaluate the need for support groups or agencies that provide medical equipment or other assistance.

Table 41–3 Family Assessment

FAMILY ROLES

- What changes will the child's illness create in the family?
- Will household tasks need to be reallocated?
- What specific burdens will be placed on family members?
- Will one parent stay with the child or spend a great deal of time in the hospital?
- Will one parent or guardian be primarily responsible for communicating with other family members?

KNOWLEDGE

- What knowledge does the family have about the child's condition and treatment? Does the family need further information?
- How quickly can discharge planning and teaching begin?

SUPPORT SYSTEMS

- Does the child or family have health insurance? What percentage of costs will it cover? Will other financial support be needed? Will costs continue for ongoing care after hospitalization? If so, will existing health insurance cover those costs?
- Are close friends or family available to provide care for other children, assist with family tasks, or help in other ways?
- Are there community services such as support groups, camps for children with disabilities, education sessions, or equipment and financial resources to which the nurses can refer the family?

SIBLINGS

- Have siblings been informed of the ill child's condition and the expected outcome?
- Have they been reassured that they did not cause the illness?
- Do they understand the change in roles and family routines?
- Are they able to visit the ill child?
- Have their teachers been informed of the family stress?
- If the hospitalized child's life is threatened, are the siblings involved in a plan to promote coping?

Developing Cultural Competence

SUPPORTING ALTERNATIVE HEALTH PRACTICES

Many cultural groups, such as Asians, Blacks, Europeans, Hispanics, and Native Americans may continue to use traditional health care practices (Spector, 2009). This information may not be shared with nurses or physicians, both out of respect and in fear that they will be told not to use these methods. Recognizing and supporting use of traditional practices along with Western medicine can promote health and provide comfort for children and families. Ask the families about the use of traditional, complementary, or alternative therapies.

Teaching the child and family, providing support, and referring them to community resources are key elements in providing family-centered care. Additional resources available for the child and family include social workers, child and family mental health professionals, and advanced practice nurses. Additionally, hospital programs and parent support groups are available to assist families in coping with a child's illness.

NURSE'S ROLE IN THE CHILD'S ADAPTATION TO HOSPITALIZATION

MyNursingKit Preparing a Toddler for Venipuncture

Hospitalization of the child may be planned or unexpected. A child may be hospitalized for any of the following reasons:

- The child develops an acute illness or exacerbation of chronic illness.
- The child requires diagnostic or treatment procedures or requires elective surgery.
- The child who was previously healthy suffers an injury, necessitating unexpected hospitalization.

PLANNED HOSPITALIZATION

When hospitalization is planned, both children and their parents have time to prepare for the experience. Assess the family's knowledge and expectations and then provide information about likely experiences. A variety of approaches can be used to provide information and allay fears.

- Offer tours of the hospital unit or surgical area. This activity assists the child and family to become familiar with the environment they will encounter. During tours, preschoolers and school-age children can see and handle items with which they will come in contact. If a tour is not possible, photographs or a videotape or DVD can be used to demonstrate the medical setting and procedures.
- Let the child play with the surgical team's attire. The child may overcome fear of surgical attire by trying it on and engaging in play while wearing it (Figure 41–1 ●).

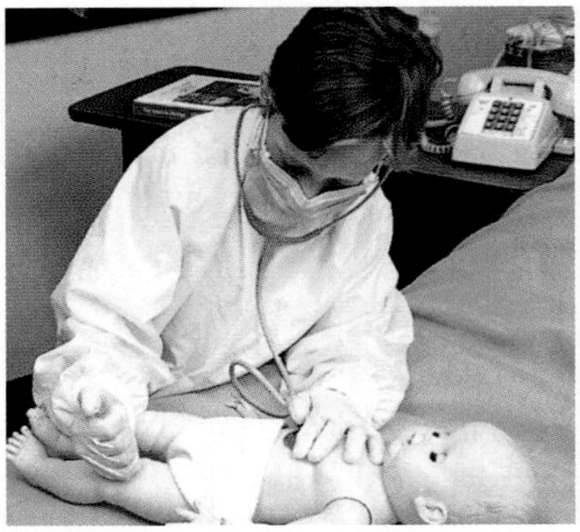

● **Figure 41–1** Allowing the child to dress up as a doctor or a nurse helps prepare the child for hospitalization. This helps the child adjust to treatment care and the recovery process. Why? What might the child's concerns be? Can you think of any concerns that could be related to a child's cultural background?

- Teach the child about medical equipment—what it does and how it is used—perhaps through demonstration on a doll (Figure 41–2 ●).
- Use puppets and skits to help explain procedures to children.
- Offer health fairs, as many hospitals do, to explain health procedures to children. During a tour, while hospitalized, or at home, the child can be exposed to books or films that explain in age-appropriate terms what to expect during various procedures.
- Reinforce teaching through coloring books or other educational materials.

Different approaches may be more effective in helping adolescents prepare for hospitalization. In addition to written materials, models, and videotapes, adolescents also learn from talking with peers who have had similar experiences. To demonstrate respect for their sense of independence and privacy, offer adolescents an opportunity for asking questions without their parents present.

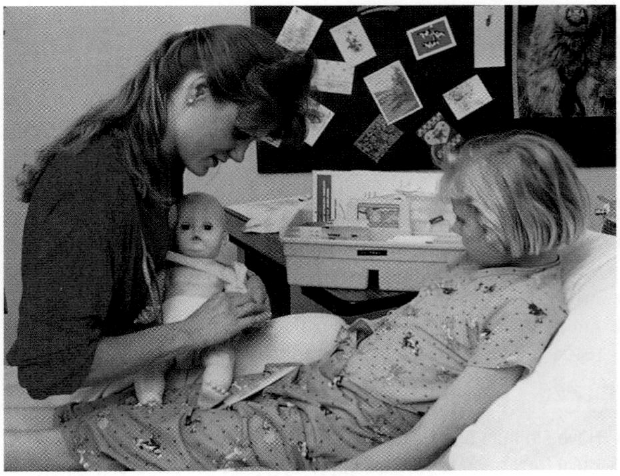

● **Figure 41–2** The child's anxiety and fear often will be reduced if the nurse explains what is going to happen and demonstrates how the procedure will be done by using a doll. Based on your experience, can you list five things you can do to prepare a school-age child for hospitalization?

Table 41–4 Parental Preparation of Children for Hospitalization

The nurse can assist the parents in preparing the child for hospitalization by suggesting the following interventions:

- Read stories to the child about the experience. Numerous books and pamphlets are available (see Table 41–5).
- Talk about going to the hospital, what it will be like. Talk about coming home.
- Encourage the child to ask questions about the hospital and surgery.
- Encourage the child to draw pictures of what the hospital will be like.
- Visit the hospital unit before hospitalization if possible.
- Let the child touch or see equipment if possible.
- Provide a doctor or nurse kit for the child to play with.
- Provide clothing so the child can dress up like a nurse or doctor if desired.
- Plan for support via parents' presence, telephone calls, special items belonging to the parents that child can keep during the stay.
- Be honest.

Include the family in preparing the child of any age for hospitalization. Parents can be instrumental in preparing a child for hospitalization by reviewing material presented, being available to answer questions, and being truthful and supportive (Table 41–4, Table 41–5).

UNEXPECTED HOSPITALIZATION

An unanticipated admission places the child at emotional risk for several reasons, including:

- the lack of preparation for the experience,
- the uncertainty and unpredictability of events that follow,
- the unfamiliarity of the environment, and
- the heightened anxiety of the child's parents.

For children with existing conditions, an admission for exacerbation of a disease, such as cystic fibrosis or leukemia, can provoke feelings of depression or hopelessness.

Assist the child and family who are not prepared for hospital admission to adapt to the experience by orienting them to the environment, providing an opportunity for questions, offering truthful responses, and explaining all procedures and expectations. Discuss the anticipated plan of care for the child and involve the family in the child's care. Give the family an opportunity to express their fears and concerns. Refer to social services and/or parent support groups if additional support is needed.

NURSING CARE OF THE HOSPITALIZED CHILD

Family-centered nursing care of the hospitalized child focuses on promoting the child's and family's coping strategies to deal with the stressors of hospitalization, promoting optimal development and safety and minimizing disruption of the child's usual routine as much as possible.

Table 41–5 Examples of Books for Children Regarding Hospitalization and Health Care

Barney Is Best, by N. W. Carlstrom	HarperCollins
Barney and Baby Bop Go to the Doctor, by M. Larsen	Scholastic, Inc.
The Berenstain Bears Go to the Doctor, by S. Berenstain & B. Berenstain	Random House
Clifford Visits the Hospital, by N. Bridwell	Scholastic, Inc.
Corduroy Goes to the Doctor, by D. Freeman & L. McCue	Viking Penguin, Inc.
Curious George Goes to the Hospital, by M. Rey & H. A. Rey	Houghton Mifflin Company
Franklin Goes to the Hospital, by P. Bourgeois & B. Clark	Scholastic, Inc.
The Fall of Freddie the Leaf, by L. Buscaglia	Henry Holt & Co.
Going to the Hospital, by F. Rogers	Putnam Juvenile
The Hospital Book, by J. Howe	Harper Collins Publishers
Let's Talk About Going to the Hospital, by M. Johnston	Rosen Publishing Group
A Night Without Stars, by J. Howe	Aladdin Paperbacks
A Visit to the Sesame Street Hospital, by D. Hautzig	Random House
When Molly Was in the Hospital: A Book for Brothers and Sisters of Hospitalized Children, by D. Duncan	Rayve Productions

SPECIAL UNITS AND TYPES OF CARE

Children admitted to a hospital may be cared for in one or more of the following units: general pediatric unit, short-stay unit, outpatient unit, ambulatory surgical unit, emergency department, or pediatric intensive care unit. Hospitalized children may require surgical treatment involving preoperative and postoperative care. Children with infectious diseases require isolation precautions. Other children may need rehabilitative care to achieve or restore maximum potential.

General Pediatric Care Unit

Smaller facilities typically incorporate all pediatric care specialties in one unit or area, whereas larger medical centers and children's hospitals have separate medical units for different specialties. Specialized units may include medical and/or surgical units, orthopedic units, oncology units, mental health units, and units specific to developmental levels (e.g., adolescent unit). Admission to a specialized unit may be the result of an acute condition, such as pneumonia or trauma, or as the result of an exacerbation of a chronic condition, such as asthma. Other causes for admission include surgical procedures requiring longer than a 24-hour stay and the need for inpatient treatments and services. Nursing care for regular hospital admission includes orienting the child and family to the unit and procedures, adhering to the child's normal routine as much as possible, including both the child and the family in the decision-making process, providing direct care to the child, promoting a safe environment for the child, and promoting the child's growth and developmental needs.

Short-Stay, Outpatient, and Ambulatory Surgical Units

Hospital stays for children have generally become short, with many procedures performed in outpatient units such as minor surgery (in ambulatory surgical centers), diagnostic tests (such as cardiac catheterizations), radiology studies requiring sedation, and treatments (such as chemotherapy). The child may be admitted in the morning and discharged that afternoon. In addition, children who have potentially serious illnesses may be placed on a short-stay or 23-hour observation unit for monitoring or limited treatment, after which medical staff decide either to hospitalize the child for additional treatment or, if improvement occurs, to discharge the child. These short stays are considered beneficial primarily because they cause minimal disruption of family patterns and are cost effective for the institution, health insurance company, and family. Nurses assist parents to prepare the child properly for planned admissions, monitor the child during the procedures, encourage family participation in care, and keep families well informed (Table 41–6).

Nursing care of the child in short-stay, outpatient, and ambulatory surgical units is the same as for regular hospital admission. However, time for teaching is compressed, requiring the nurse to implement teaching methods in a minimal amount of time to ensure the family understands discharge instructions. Effective teaching methods on this accelerated schedule include demonstration, videos, pamphlets with verbal review, and informal teaching sessions.

Table 41–6 Nursing Considerations in Preparing Parents and Child for Planned Short-Stay Admission

- Are there special requirements prior to arrival, such as not being permitted food or drink or needing extra fluid intake?
- What time and where must the child appear?
- Are any special forms, insurance numbers, or previous records needed?
- How long will the child stay in the hospital?
- Can the child bring something familiar from home such as a blanket or stuffed animal?
- Are parents expected or encouraged to be with the child or stay in the health facility?
- Is there a chance the child may need to remain longer than expected?
- What will the child's condition be for discharge home?
- Will special equipment or care be needed?
- What symptoms can indicate problems?
- Where can the family go or whom can they call in case of problems or questions?

Thinking Critically

PREPARING CHILDREN FOR HOSPITALIZATION OR SHORT-STAY SURGERY

Six-year-old Kate has had several nosebleeds and fainting spells recently. After examination by her physician and a number of diagnostic studies such as chest x-ray examination, echocardiography, and electrocardiography, coarctation of the aorta is diagnosed. Kate will come in this week for a cardiac catheterization. She is scheduled to have open heart surgery in 2 weeks.

Kate has had few health problems, and her experiences with healthcare professionals are limited. Her parents, who are anxious about the heart surgery, are concerned about how their daughter will adapt to hospitalization.

How should you prepare Kate for the cardiac catheterization and later for the surgery? Include knowledge of her developmental stages and cognitive understanding in your planned intervention approaches. How far in advance should teaching take place? What teaching aids are helpful? How can Kate's parents be involved in and reinforce the teaching? What kind of support do her parents, siblings, and friends need during hospitalization?

See MyNursingKit for possible responses.

Emergency Care

When a child is brought to an emergency department, the parents are usually frightened and insecure and may even be in a state of shock. The fast pace and critical nature of the unit creates an atmosphere in which parents are hesitant to ask questions and are anxious about the outcome. Many factors can contribute to the parents' anxiety and stress (see Chapter 43), including the unexpected nature of the situation, uncertainties in the emergency environment, the necessity for quick decision making, the need for numerous procedures, tests, and treatments, and fear of pain. The nurse keeps both the child and the family informed about what is being done and when more news may be available. The parents and child are encouraged to remain together as much as possible. Parents who wish to remain with a child even during invasive procedures or resuscitation efforts should be allowed to do so, and this option is supported by the Emergency Nurses Association (2005). The nurse collaborates with the family members to determine their desired presence in critical situations and keeps them informed about the health care provided. (See Chapter 43.)

Intensive Care Unit

Intensive care units provide specialized medical care to infants, and children requiring advanced technical support and interventions and continuous monitoring. (See Chapter 43.) Parents of a child in a pediatric intensive care unit (PICU) are likely to be anxious, particularly since the child's illness may be severe and the prognosis may be guarded. The unfamiliar equipment may create an atmosphere of fear or anxiety. Numerous healthcare professionals work in the intensive care environment, and without effective and open communication, parents may not know whom to question or even what questions to ask. Partner with the family and encourage them to write down their questions and direct them to the appropriate source if you're unable to answer the question.

Isolation

Children who require isolation to prevent spread of infection may experience lack of stimulation due to limited contact with other children and visitors. Frequent family visits are important and should be encouraged. Family members may be reluctant to wear protective garments either out of fear of using them incorrectly or a belief that they are unnecessary. Ensure that the family understands the reason for isolation and any special procedures. Having contact with and holding the child are encouraged when possible.

Rehabilitation

Rehabilitation is the process of assisting a child with physical or mental challenges to reach full potential through therapy and education. Rehabilitation units provide children with ongoing care and support to continue recovery beyond the initial period of illness or injury (Figure 41–3 ●). These may be separate units within a hospital or independent centers. The objective of rehabilitation is to assist the child with physical, psychosocial, or educational challenges to reach his or her fullest potential and to promote achievement of developmentally appropriate skills. Collaboration with a multidisciplinary team including parental involvement is essential.

PARENTAL INVOLVEMENT AND PARENTAL PRESENCE

Family members are essential to the child's care during illness. Families who feel supported by nursing staff during their child's hospitalization are more confident and better equipped to cope with the crisis and thus be open to participating in their child's care and developing skills to provide care for the child after discharge (Sarajärvi et al., 2006). The nurse should partner with the family and multidisciplinary team to determine the extent to which the parents desire to be involved in the child's care (Power & Franck, 2008; Sarajärvi et al., 2006).

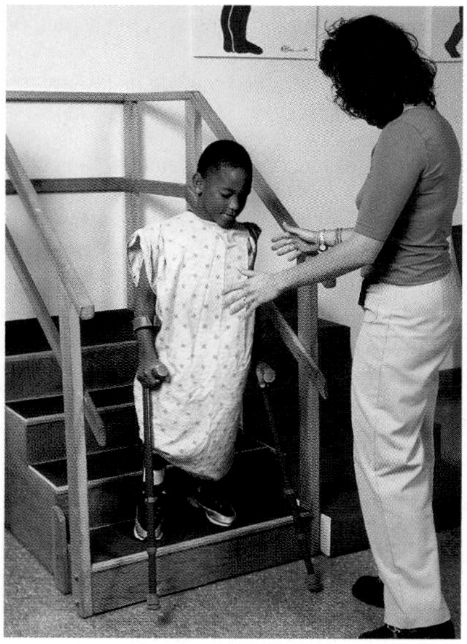

● **Figure 41–3** Rehabilitation units provide an opportunity for the child to relearn tasks like walking and climbing stairs. They provide an important transition from hospital to home community.

> **Developing Cultural Competence**
>
> **SUPPORT SYSTEMS**
>
> There are many cultural influences on health beliefs and practices. For example, Mexican Americans view family as a strong support. Extended family and godparents (compadres) may want to be with a hospitalized child. The father of the child is often the spokesperson, and mothers commonly are influential in decisions regarding child health care. Hawaiian families also often wish to have many family members present with a hospitalized child, and may value playing native music and use of aromatherapy (Lassetter & Baldwin, 2005). The nurse should incorporate all people the family wishes to have present in the hospital and include them in explanations about health care.

Integrity of the family unit is fostered through parental involvement during the child's hospital stay. For the parents, involvement provides them with controls and feelings as active participants in their child's progress. It also prepares the family for care that will be required when the child goes home. The child benefits greatly from parental presence and participation (see "Developing Cultural Competence: Support Systems") and experiences less emotional distress and anxiety if the parents are present. If the parent-child attachment remains uninterrupted, the child experiences fewer behavioral maladjustments.

Parents of hospitalized children may come in daily contact with numerous healthcare providers. The nurse partners with the healthcare team and the family to ensure that everyone is on the same page, with accurate and consistent information given related to hospital care and discharge planning. Providing both emotional support and education to families enhances their ability to care for the child at home (Sarajärvi et al., 2006).

PREPARATION FOR PROCEDURES

Hospitalized children may experience numerous procedures during hospitalization, from collection of urine or blood specimens to lumbar punctures and surgery. Maintain a positive attitude when preparing the child and reassure the child that it is normal to be frightened of unknown experiences. Special techniques can help the child to understand and cope with feelings about these procedures. To prepare the child, nurses choose techniques based on the child's developmental age, coping abilities, and previous experience.

Psychological Preparation

Preparation may begin a few moments to several days before the procedure, depending on the child's age and developmental level. In providing sensitive care to the child, nurses assume that a procedure can potentially be traumatic for the child. Even

MyNursingKit Case Study: Preparing an Adolescent for Surgery providing urine in a specimen cup or undergoing radiologic examination can be frightening if the child does not understand the reason for the procedure or know what to expect. Administration of medication can also make the child frustrated or anxious. When preparing the child for medication administration using techniques appropriate to the developmental level of the child, the nurse assures that the medication is safely given (see Table 41–7).

Use developmentally appropriate techniques to assess the child's knowledge and feelings about an upcoming procedure. With a school-age child, for example, the nurse might explain the procedure using drawings, stories, body outline dolls, anatomically

Table 41–7 Variations in Medication Administration to Children

Route	Developmental Considerations	Techniques
Oral	Children under 5 years cannot generally swallow pills and capsules.	■ Medications are usually given in liquid form (elixir, syrup, or suspension). ■ Avoid putting medications in a bottle of formula since it will be impossible to determine how much medication the child has taken, if some of the formula is left in the bottle. ■ Sometimes tablets are crushed or capsules are opened and mixed with a liquid flavoring or small amount of food. Check with pharmacy to be sure this does not inactivate the drug. Never crush enteric-coated or timed-release medicine. ■ When choosing a vehicle for crushed tablets, use only one spoonful of applesauce, pudding, jelly, or similar food or 1–2 mL of liquid. ■ Use a 1 mL oral syringe for amounts less than 1 mL to increase accuracy.
	Children may not want to take medicine.	■ Position young children upright to avoid choking and aspiration. ■ Give liquid medicines slowly by oral syringe (for infants) aimed at the inside of the cheek. ■ A preschooler may prefer to drink the medicine from a medicine cup, but the medication must first be measured using a syringe to ensure accuracy. ■ Have the expectation that the medicine will be taken. Let children choose the type of fluid to drink after, but do not ask if they will take their medicine now.
Rectal	Colon is small.	■ For children younger than 3 years, the nurse's gloved fifth finger is used for insertion. After this age, the index finger can usually be used. ■ Lubricate the tip of the suppository. The nurse may need to hold the buttocks together for a few minutes to keep the medication from being expelled.
Ophthalmic and otic	Young children may be fearful of medicines placed in the eyes or ears.	■ Adequate immobilization is needed to avoid injury. ■ The nurse's hand can be stabilized by resting the wrist on the child's head. ■ Explanations and therapeutic play can be used with children old enough to explain the process of administration. ■ Have medication at room temperature.
Topical	Skin of infants is thin and fragile.	■ Only prescribed doses and medicines appropriate for young children should be used on the skin. ■ Covering the area or keeping the child's hands occupied may be necessary to ensure adequate contact of medication with the skin.
Intramuscular	Anatomy and physiology of children differ from those of adults.	■ Gluteus maximus muscle (dorsal gluteal site) must not be used until the child has been walking for at least 1 year and has well-developed muscle mass. ■ Vastus lateralis (anterior thigh) site is preferred for young children because it is the largest muscle mass in children younger than 3 years. ■ Amounts to be administered should be limited to no more than 1–2 mL for ventrogluteal site depending on muscle size. Refer to Clinical Skills Manual for illustrations SKILLS. ■ The deltoid muscle is rarely used in young children except for the small amounts injected in some vaccines.
Intravenous	Veins are small and fragile.	■ Careful maintenance of sites is needed. ■ Common infusion sites include hands and feet, although scalp veins are sometimes used in infants. ■ Infusion pumps require frequent monitoring.
	Fluid balance is critical.	■ Syringe pumps are often used when minimal fluid is to be given over an extended period of time. ■ Central lines are commonly used for long-term intravenous medication therapy.

Note: See *Clinical Skills Manual for Maternal and Child Nursing Care, Third Edition,* for further medication administration techniques. See Appendix E for information related to how drug dosages are determined for children.

Source: Data from Bindler, R., & Howry, L. (2005). *Pediatric Drug Guide*. Upper Saddle River, NJ: Prentice Hall Health.

correct dolls, and conversation. When assessing the child's perception about procedures the nurse should consider the following:

- Does the child know the purpose of the procedure?
- Has the child experienced this procedure before? Was the experience painful, frightening, or reassuring?
- What does the child think will happen? Are the child's beliefs accurate?
- Is the procedure painful?
- What techniques does the child use to gain control in challenging situations?
- Will the parents or other caregiver be present to provide support?

When explaining procedures, use words that the child understands to describe the procedure and its purpose. Older children require explanations geared to their cognitive level and previous experiences. They will want to know what is happening, why, and what they can do to cope during the procedure (see Table 41–8).

For adolescents, provide written information, videos, and other available media. Schedule time for questions and discussions. Adolescents can make many choices about their own healthcare. When possible, ask them to make those choices with questions such as "Do you want your hand numbed for the IV start?" Maintain a positive attitude when preparing the adolescent and reassure them that it is normal to be frightened of unknown experiences.

Parental presence can provide comfort and support to the child during procedures. Parents should be allowed to choose whether they want to stay for the procedure (Figure 41–4 ●). Some parents may feel that they will be too upset to support the child; many choose to stay. Some adolescents want their parents to be involved in their care; others prefer to minimize their parents' roles. Partner with the adolescent to ensure that his or her wishes are known regarding parental presence.

Physical Preparation

Physical preparation depends on the age of the child and the procedure. Preprocedural sedation may be required. If sedation is required the child will not be able to have anything by mouth (NPO) for a period of time. Young infants might be provided sucrose for procedures (see Chapter 42∞ for pain management). Procedural checklists are often utilized.

PERFORMING THE PROCEDURE

Procedures on young children are generally performed in a **treatment room** (a room designated for performing treatments

MyNursingKit Video: Treatment Room

MyNursingKit Care Plan: Preparing a School-Age Child for Surgery

Table 41–8 Assisting Children through Procedures

Developmental Stage	Before Procedure	During Procedure
Infant	None for infant. Explain to parents the procedure, the reason for it, and their role. Allow parents the option of being present for procedures.	Nursing staff should immobilize the infant securely and gently. Parents should not be asked to hold the child down. Perform procedure quickly. Use touch, voice, pacifier, and bottle as distractions. Ask parent to hold, rock, and sing to infant after procedure.
Toddler	Give explanation just before procedure, since toddler's concept of time is limited. Explain that child did nothing wrong; the procedure is simply necessary.	Perform in treatment room. Nursing staff should immobilize the child securely. Give short explanations and directions in a positive manner. Avoid giving choices when none are available. For example, "We are going to do this now" is better than "Is it okay to do this now?" Allow child to cry or scream. Comfort child after procedure. Give child a choice of favorite drink if allowed or special sticker.
Preschool child	Give simple explanations of procedure. Basic drawings may be useful. While providing supervision, allow the child to touch and play with equipment to be used if possible. Since any entry into the body is viewed as a threat, state that the child's body will remain the same, and use adhesive bandages to reassure the child that the body is intact and parts will not "fall out."	Perform in treatment room. Nursing staff should immobilize the child securely. Give short explanations and directions in a positive manner. Encourage control by having the child count to 10 or spell name. Allow child to cry. Give positive feedback for cooperation and getting through procedure. Encourage the child to draw afterward to explore the experience.
School-age child	Clear, thorough explanations are helpful. Use drawings, pictures, books, and contact with equipment. Teach stress-reduction techniques such as deep breathing and visualization. Offer a choice of reward after procedure is completed.	Be ready to immobilize the child if needed. Allow child to remain in position by self if child is able to be still. Explain throughout procedure what is happening. Facilitate use of stress-control techniques. Praise cooperative efforts.
Adolescent	Give clear explanations orally and in writing. Teach stress-reduction techniques. Explore fear of certain procedures, such as staple removal or venipuncture.	Assist adolescent in self-control. Assist with use of stress-control techniques. Explain expected outcome and tell when results of test will be completed.

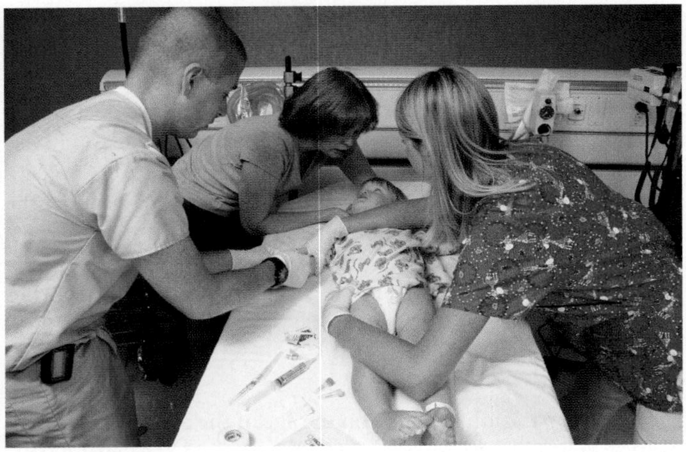

● **Figure 41–4** Health facility policies that permit parents to be present during a procedure performed on their child are an example of a family-centered care policy. The parent plays an important role in providing security and comfort to this child who is having blood drawn.

such as intravenous starts, blood drawing, and lumbar punctures) to promote the child's sense of security that his or her own room is a "safe" and relatively pain-free site unless this is contraindicated, such as in the presence of skeletal traction or isolation. Older children can be given the option of having a procedure performed in the treatment room or in their own hospital room. Older school-age children and adolescents may prefer to remain in their room for the procedure.

Perform the procedure as quickly and efficiently as possible. If the parents wish to participate, ask them to hold the child's hand or stand close by for comfort. Utilize nursing staff instead of parents to immobilize the child as needed. The parents, or another nurse, can be designated to support the child by means of a gentle touch, talking, singing, giving reassurance, or illustrating stress-reduction techniques.

After the procedure, no matter how the child responded, the child should be praised. A choice of reward often soothes the young child. If the procedure is performed in a treatment room, the child is returned to his or her room for comfort and reassurance.

Refer to Chapter 42 ∞ for discussion of pain management and sedation for procedures.

PREPARATION FOR SURGERY

A child's surgical experience may be elective, planned in advance, or the result of an emergency or trauma. How a child responds to the experience is related to the psychologic and physical preparation he or she receives. The accompanying nursing care plan, beginning on page 1092, provides information related to care of the child undergoing surgery. Additional nursing diagnoses include:

- risk for infection and injury related to exposure to nosocomial infection and use of preoperative medication,
- impaired skin integrity related to disruption of skin surface,
- risk for constipation related to surgical procedure and anesthetics,
- risk for fluid volume imbalance related to intravenous infusion and NPO status,
- impaired gas exchange related to anesthetics and pain,
- risk for impaired skin integrity related to limited mobility after surgery, and
- anxiety (child and family) related to change in health status and environments.

Preoperative Care

Preoperative care of the child includes both psychosocial and physical preparation for surgery. The goal of preoperative teaching is to reduce the fear associated with the unknown and decrease stress and anxiety associated with surgery.

Psychosocial preparation. Preoperative teaching is geared to the child's developmental level. If child life specialists (discussed on page 1090) are available, they can play an important role in preparing the child for surgery. When the child will be transferred to an intensive care unit or recovery room after surgery, a visit to the area before surgery can reduce the fear and anxiety associated with waking up in a strange environment filled with frightening sights, sounds, and smells. The use of videotapes or DVDs, anatomically correct puppets and dolls, drawings, and models is encouraged to teach the child about the surgical procedure (Figure 41–5 ●). Playing with stethoscopes, gowns, masks, and syringes without needles also helps the child feel more in control (see discussion about dramatic play on page 1093). Children are reassured that their parents can accompany them to the operating room floor and will be waiting when they awaken from surgery. Parents should be allowed to carry infants and young toddlers to the pediatric holding area or have them ride in one parent's lap in a wheelchair. Older toddlers and preschoolers should be allowed to ride in a special wagon if possible. Special teddy bears and blankets are generally allowed in the pre-op holding area and provide comfort to the child. The nurse should make sure that the item is labeled with the child's name. Prepare

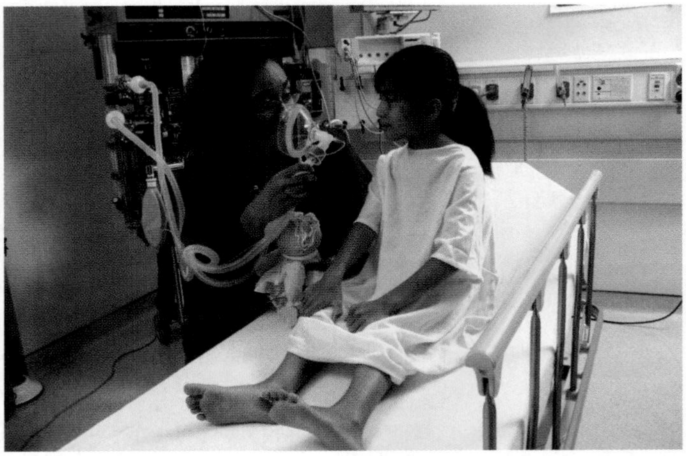

● **Figure 41–5** Showing young school-age children equipment that will be used in surgery will help to decrease anxiety related to the unknown. What are other methods the nurse can use to teach young school-age children about surgery?

family members for what to anticipate and what is expected of them. Explain the purpose of special equipment such as intravenous setups and monitoring devices. In some hospitals, only one or two immediate family members are allowed to visit the child at one time. Visitors may be required to wear special gowns, shoes, or hats, and they may be restricted to certain areas.

Parental presence during anesthesia induction. Many hospitals now allow parents to be present with their child during anesthesia induction and again in the post-anesthesia recovery area. Parents often want to support their child before and immediately after a surgical procedure, and their presence offers reassurance and comfort to the child. The decision to allow parents to be present during anesthesia induction must be made on an individual basis. Nurses should be open to change in practice and realize that incorporating the option of parental presence during anesthesia induction supports the principles of family-centered care (Romino, Keatley, Secrest, et al., 2005). The nurse explains expectations, such as surgical gown, cap, shoe covers, and the parent's role during induction. The nurse offers the parents an opportunity to ask questions and voice concerns.

Physical preparation. Preparation for surgery may occur in designated preoperative areas. Procedures generally conducted in preoperative areas include premedication, intravenous start (if not performed following general anesthesia), and preparation of the surgical site. If urinary catheterization is necessary, it is usually not performed until the child has been anesthetized.

Preoperative procedures and guidelines vary among hospitals and outpatient surgical centers. Preoperative checklists, such as the sample shown in Table 41–9, are used in ambulatory and acute care settings to ensure proper physical preparation of patients for surgery. Weigh the preoperative child accurately, measure vital signs, and ask about last fluid intake amount and type. Monitor urinary output. Reinforce teaching regarding necessary NPO status and provide support to the family as needed.

Nursing management during the preoperative period includes establishing accurate baseline data, administering prescribed fluids, and performing assessments of fluid status. When an intravenous infusion is prescribed, start the infusion (see the Clinical Skills Manual SKILLS), ensuring that the type of fluid and flow rate match those that are ordered and that would be expected for the weight of the child.

Of necessity, the young child who undergoes surgery usually is restricted from consuming oral foods and fluids just before, during, and for a period after surgery, thus creating a risk of fluid imbalance. The length of time the child is kept without oral intake before surgery varies. Recommendations from the American Society of Anesthesiologists indicate that clear liquids may be given up until 2 hours before surgery, breast milk until 4 hours before surgery and infant formula 6 hours before. Milk and a light meal may be consumed up until 6 hours before surgery. In general, older children will have a longer time without intake, infants much shorter (Crenshaw & Winslow, 2002). Infants will generally have very specific orders related to what time they should be made NPO for breast milk, formula, and clear liquids. This time will depend on what time the infant is scheduled for surgery. Because children beyond infancy do not usually eat or drink during the night, orders are usually written for NPO after midnight. If surgery is not scheduled for the morning, however, more specific orders should be written, especially for the toddler and preschool-age child, who will not be as tolerant of an extended NPO status. The ultimate decision on how long the child is NPO lies with the anesthesiologist.

Table 41–9 Preoperative Checklist

- ___ Check that consent forms are witnessed and signed and in the patient's chart.
- ___ Be sure the child's name band is in place.
- ___ Be sure any allergies are prominently noted in the child's chart and on a special name band.
- ___ Remove any prosthetic devices, including orthodontic appliances and body piercings.
- ___ Check the child's mouth for loose teeth and tongue piercings.
- ___ Remove eyeglasses, jewelry, and nail polish.
- ___ Bathe and cleanse the operative site if ordered.
- ___ Put the child in a hospital gown, allowing the child to wear underwear.
- ___ Check that all special tests have been completed and the results are in the child's chart.
- ___ Have the child void before surgery.
- ___ Keep the child NPO before surgery.
- ___ Give the child prescribed medications.
- ___ Check vital signs and record on chart.
- ___ Transport the child safely to the operating room.

Postoperative Care

Postoperative care of the child includes both physical and psychologic care. In the immediate postoperative period the nurse should: perform baseline monitoring of vital signs according to hospital protocol; maintain effective airway clearance and monitor for evidence of respiratory depression or distress (see Chapter 48∞); evaluate the child's level of consciousness; evaluate the surgical site for evidence of drainage or bleeding; and record urine output and output from drainage tubes. The nurse should also examine the postoperative orders and ensure that the child receives the correct type and amount of intravenous fluid prescribed. In addition the nurse should provide comfort and pain relief. See Chapter 42∞.

Resumption of oral intake depends on the surgical procedure, the child's condition, and surgeon protocol. Once oral fluids are resumed the nurse should monitor for emesis. When the child is consuming adequate fluids, the rate of intravenous fluids should be decreased or discontinued according to physician orders.

Parents are encouraged to visit with the child as soon after surgery as possible (Figure 41–6 ●). In some facilities, children are brought to postoperative anesthesia care units (PACUs) after surgery, where they recover from anesthesia. Depending on the child's condition, he or she may be discharged home directly

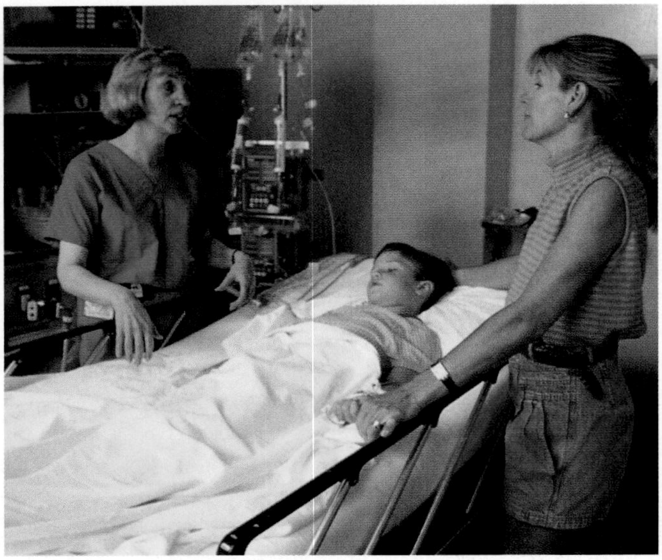

● **Figure 41–6** This child has just undergone surgery and is in the postanesthesia care unit (PACU). Although the child's physical care is immediate and important, remember that both the child and the family have strong psychosocial needs that must be addressed concurrently. It is important to reunite the family as soon as possible after surgery.

from an outpatient surgical procedure, or admitted to a short-stay, general pediatric, or intensive care unit.

Postoperative Home Care Instructions

Routine postoperative instructions for the family of the child undergoing outpatient or one-day-stay surgical procedures include monitoring for signs of infection such as drainage, redness, or swelling of the surgical incision, fever, and change in behavior. Instructions for follow-up visit, medications, other treatments, wound care, and signs and symptoms that require medical attention are also provided. Additional instructions are tailored according to the surgical procedure and the child's condition. The nurse ensures the family understands home care instructions through their return demonstration statement of understanding.

STRATEGIES TO PROMOTE COPING AND NORMAL DEVELOPMENT OF THE HOSPITALIZED CHILD

During hospitalization, care of the child focuses not only on meeting physiologic needs, but also on meeting psychosocial and developmental needs. Nurses can employ several strategies to help children adapt to the hospital environment, promote effective coping, and provide developmentally appropriate activities: child life programs, rooming in, therapeutic play, and therapeutic recreation.

ROOMING IN

The practice of **rooming in** involves a parent staying in the child's hospital room during the course of the child's hospitalization. Some hospitals provide cots, others have special built-in beds on pediatric units, and in some institutions a parent is provided a separate room on the unit. Parents who stay at the bedside usually want to help care for their child (Power & Franck, 2008). Communication between the nurse and family is important so that the parent's desire for involvement is understood and supported.

Rooming in provides the child with the comfort and security of parental presence. Some parents may feel more comfortable staying with their child and participating in care, others may experience more stress if they are missing work and are away from home and other children. Partner with the parent to assist them in establishing a rooming-in plan that is beneficial to both the child and family. For example, in longer hospital stays, parents may alternate turns staying with the child. Grandparents, aunts and uncles, and grown siblings may be included in the plan.

Some facilities offer free or reduced-cost meals to the parent rooming in. The parent who does not receive these meals may often skip many meals because of the financial impact on an already overburdened budget related to illness and hospitalization. The nurse should be alert to the parent who never leaves the bedside and make sure the parent is eating. Emphasize the importance of the child's need for a healthy parent. Social services or other departments may be able to assist the family in obtaining meals while rooming in with the hospitalized child.

Parents rooming in with their child for an extended hospitalization can be encouraged to take advantage of facilities such as the Ronald McDonald House or Ronald McDonald Family Room or other areas available for parents, at some point during the stay, as a respite for a few hours. This break will provide them with an opportunity for needed rest and privacy.

CHILD LIFE PROGRAMS

Many hospitals have child life programs that focus on the psychosocial needs of hospitalized children. Professional child life specialists, paraprofessionals, and volunteers staff these departments (Figure 41–7 ●, A and B). A **child life specialist** plans activities to provide age-appropriate playtime for children either in the child's room or in a specialized playroom. Some of the planned activities, designed to assist children in working through feelings about illness, may include playing with medical equipment, acting out procedures or treatments on dolls, using games to act out feelings, or drawing pictures about hospital treatments (Figure 41–8 ●).

THERAPEUTIC PLAY

Play is a significant component of childhood, and the stress of illness and hospitalization increases the value of play. Yet because of the need to contain costs, hospitals may minimize their play programs. Therefore, nurses should document the need for and benefits of play. Beyond facilitating normal development, play sessions can provide a means for the child to:

- learn about health care,
- express anxieties,
- work through feelings, and
- achieve a sense of mastery or control over frightening or little-understood situations.

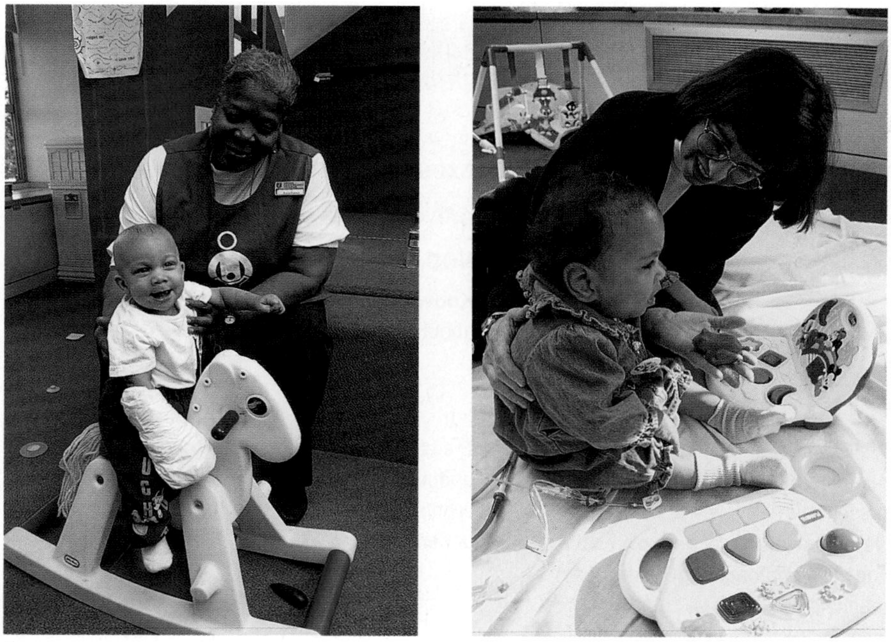

A B

● **Figure 41–7** ***A,*** Volunteers such as this grandmother can provide stimulation and nurturing to help young children adapt to lengthy hospitalizations. ***B,*** Child life specialists plan activities for young children in the hospital to facilitate play and stress reduction.

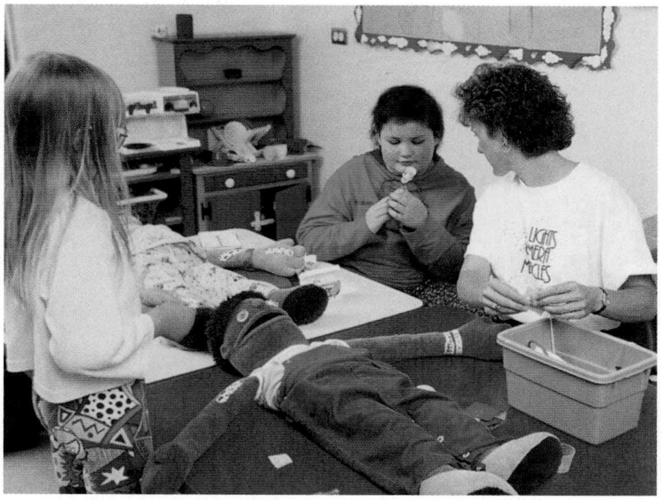

● **Figure 41–8** A child life specialist works with children being treated for cancer. Special dolls are used to familiarize children with the procedures that they will undergo.

Play that presents an opportunity to deal with the fears, concerns, and stressors of health experiences is called **therapeutic play**. Therapeutic play has many benefits for both the child and the health professional. It allows the child an opportunity to relive, understand, and integrate fearful healthcare experiences. Children can achieve a sense of mastery by being in control of the occurrences during play. Such control helps to reduce the child's stress and anxiety about the events. At the same time, the healthcare professional can observe the child's play to learn more about the type of events that make the child anxious. The child's coping methods can be observed and additional techniques offered to the child. *Play therapy* is a mental health technique used to treat children with mental health problems, rather than normal life events that have caused anxiety. This technique is discussed in Chapter 57∞.

Through therapeutic play, the child's knowledge of his or her illness or injury can be assessed. A common technique involves using an outline drawing of the body (Figure 41–9 ●) or having the child draw a picture about the hospitalization. Drawings can be used to determine what the child knows and understands about the hospitalization. They can also give an indication regarding the anxiety and stress the child is feeling (Tielsch &

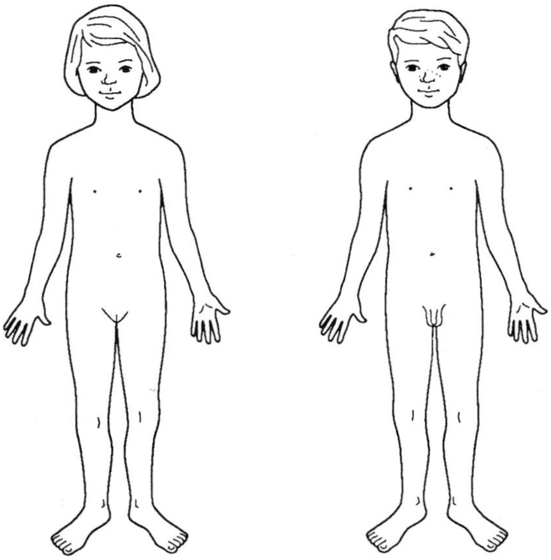

● **Figure 41–9** The nurse can use a simple gender-specific outline drawing of a child's body to encourage children to draw what they think about their medical problem. Such drawings reveal a child's interpretation, which the nurse can work with to provide appropriate care.

Nursing Care Plan

THE CHILD UNDERGOING SURGERY

INTERVENTION	RATIONALE	EXPECTED OUTCOME
1. Nursing Diagnosis: Deficient knowledge related to preoperative and postoperative events		
NIC Priority Intervention: **Teaching, preoperative:** Assisting the parent and child to understand and mentally prepare for surgery and postoperative recovery		**NOC Suggested Outcome:** **Knowledge:** Extent of understanding conveyed about treatment regimen
Goal: The child and family will acquire knowledge related to the operation.		
■ Ask questions of the parent and child about surgery.	■ Prior knowledge and understanding can be reinforced and used to guide your presentation.	The child and family are able to verbalize details about expected preoperative and postoperative events. They ask questions that demonstrate understanding.
■ Teach about preoperative and post-operative events using appropriate developmental methods such as dolls, drawings, stories, and tours.	■ Developmental level determines the cognitive approach that works best for teaching.	
■ Reinforce information the family has received about the purpose of surgery.	■ The physician may have explained operation.	
■ Have the child demonstrate postoperative events that pertain to his or her care such as deep breathing, putting bandage on doll, taping intravenous line on doll, and pressing patient-controlled analgesia button.	■ Concrete experience promotes learning.	The child demonstrates skills needed in the postoperative period.
■ Allow the parents and child to ask questions.	■ Learners must have opportunity to ask questions.	
2. Nursing Diagnosis: Anxiety related to change in health status		
NIC Priority Intervention: **Anxiety reduction:** Minimizing apprehension, dread, foreboding, or uneasiness related to an unidentified source of anticipated danger.		**NOC Suggested Outcome:** **Coping:** Actions to manage stressors that tax an individual's resources.
Goal: The child and family will show decreased behavior indicating anxiety.		
■ Question the child about expectations of hospitalization and previous experiences.	■ Previous experiences can influence present anxiety level.	
■ Orient the child to the hospital setting, routines, staff, and other patients.	■ Familiarity with the setting and people can decrease anxiety by removing unknown factors.	
■ Institute age-appropriate play and interactions with the child.	■ Play can increase trust level and decrease anxiety.	
■ Explain procedures and prepare for those that might cause trauma. Encourage parents to support the child.	■ The child is more likely to trust caregivers if they are truthful and if parents are present.	The child and family demonstrate less anxiety. They verbalize understanding and comfort in hospital routines. Parents support the child for traumatic procedures.
■ Allow the parents and child to ask questions.	■ Questioning provides an opportunity to explain the unknown, which decreases anxiety.	
3. Nursing Diagnosis: Pain related to surgical procedure		
NIC Priority Intervention: **Pain management:** Alleviation of pain or a reduction in pain to a level of comfort that is acceptable to the patient.		**NOC Suggested Outcome:** **Pain control behavior:** Personal actions to control pain.

Nursing Care Plan—continued

THE CHILD UNDERGOING SURGERY

INTERVENTION	RATIONALE	EXPECTED OUTCOME
Goal: The child will maintain an adequate comfort level.		
■ Assess behavioral cues (e.g., crying, movement, guarding ability to participate in activities of daily living).	■ Behavior of preverbal children provides clues to pain experience.	The child's pain is controlled as demonstrated by a low number on the pain assessment tool (behavioral or verbal).
■ Use an appropriate pain assessment tool for verbal and nonverbal children.	■ An age-appropriate pain assessment tool allows verbal children to quantify the amount of pain. Pain assessment tools designed for nonverbal children allow the nurse to quantify the amount of pain when the child cannot provide a self report. (See Chapter 42 for descriptions of a variety of pain assessment tools.)	
■ Administer prescribed pain medications around the clock.	■ Narcotics and nonnarcotic analgesics alter pain perception	
■ Use age-appropriate nonpharmacologic methods of pain control (e.g., distraction, repositioning, massage).	■ Nonpharmacologic interventions interfere with pain perception and may decrease the child's anxiety.	
4. Nursing Diagnosis: Therapeutic Regimen Management, Effective		
NIC Priority Intervention: Facilitating family participation in the emotional and physical care of the patient		**NOC Suggested Outcome:** **Treatment Regimen:** Extent of understanding conveyed about a specific treatment regimen
Goal: The child and family will verbalize self-care required at home.		
■ Provide oral and written home care instructions regarding surgical wound care, medications, activities, and diet.	■ Teaching regarding home care is necessary early in hospitalization.	The child and family demonstrate skills needed for home care following discharge. They verbalize plans for future care.
■ Provide a number to call for questions or concerns. Instruct on follow-up visits.	■ Parents need to know emergency information and that follow-up care is required.	

Allen, 2005). In addition to assessment, drawing can be used as a nursing intervention. Demonstrate to the child on a drawing what will occur during surgery or a treatment. The child's drawings of healthcare experiences allow him or her to express fears and gain mastery over the situation.

Dramatic play, in which medical situations encountered are reenacted by the child, often helps the child cope with painful treatments and intrusive procedures. Play using safe medical equipment such as bandages and syringes without needles, and providing scrubs and uniforms for dress-up are effective materials for encouraging dramatic play. Dramatic play offers an outlet for anxiety in children trying to deal with stressful and confusing situations. At the same time, these activities allow the nurse to observe and assess the child's perception of the illness and procedures. The nurse is then able to clarify any of the child's misconceptions.

A variety of techniques may be used to promote therapeutic and dramatic play (Table 41–10), depending on the child's developmental stage. The nurse can ensure that a selection of age-appropriate toys, distraction materials (stress balls, bubbles, music), and "prizes" are available.

Many hospitals, particularly children's hospitals, provide playrooms on each of the units to allow children a place to play and socialize with same-age peers. These rooms are generally brightly decorated in children's themes, and provide numerous opportunities for play, such as board games, video games, supplies for painting or drawing, and age-appropriate toys for each developmental level. For younger children, families may be encouraged to bring the child's favorite age-appropriate toys from home. For older children, there may be options for computer communication with children in other hospitals. Portable electronic gaming equipment may be available to children in isolation or those unable to come

Table 41–10 Therapeutic Play Techniques

Technique	Assessment	Interventions
Stories	Have the child make up a story about a picture. Analyze content and emotional clues in the story. Have child tell a story about an important experience in a group of other children.	Read or make up stories to explain illness, hospitalization, or other specific aspects of health care. Emotions such as fear can be included.
Drawings	Ask the child to draw a picture about being in the hospital. Consider subject matter, size, and placement of items in drawings, colors used, presence or absence of physical barriers, and general emotional feeling.	Use the child's drawings or outlines of the body to explain care, procedures, or conditions. Provide an opportunity for the child to draw pictures of his or her choice or directed topics such as a picture of the child's family or healthcare encounter. Ask the child: "Tell me about your picture." Be alert to the child's emotions: "This child must be frightened by the big x-ray machine."
Music	Observe types of music chosen and effects of played music on behavior.	Encourage parents and children to bring favorite tapes to the hospital for stress relief. Have tapes playing during tests and procedures. Parents can tape their voices to play for infants and young children during separations. During longer hospitalizations children can tape messages for siblings or classmates, who are then encouraged to retape their responses. Playtime can include the opportunity to play instruments and sing.
Puppets	The puppets can ask questions of young children, who are often more likely to answer the puppet than a person.	Perform short skits to teach children necessary healthcare information. Include emotional content when appropriate.
Dramatic play	Provide dolls and medical equipment, and analyze the roles assigned to dolls by the child, the behavior demonstrated by the dolls in the child's play, and the apparent emotions. Dolls with health problems like those of the child are especially helpful.	Provide dolls and equipment for play sessions. To ensure safety, supervise closely when actual equipment is used. Respond to emotions and behavior shown. Use dolls and equipment such as casts, nebulizer, intravenous apparatus, and stethoscope to explain care. Use dolls with problems or handicaps similar to those of the child when available. Provide toys that foster expression of emotion, such as a pounding board and indoor darts.
Pets	Provide animal-assisted therapy. Watch the interaction between child and animal.	Respond to emotions the child shows. Facilitate touch and stroking of animals.

Note: Additional techniques, such as sand or water play, may be appropriate in specific situations.

to the playroom or teen lounge. Specific interventions according to developmental level are discussed in the pages that follow.

Infant

Infants require external stimuli for growth. The use of mobiles, music, mirrors, and other methods promotes stimulation and offers comfort to the newborn or infant. Parents and family are encouraged to cuddle or rock the infant and sing lullabies. Talking to the infant encourages interaction and play.

Toddler

Approach toddlers slowly and make the initial approach in their parents' presence, if possible, to decrease feelings of stranger anxiety. Playing a variation of peek-a-boo or hide-and-seek using the curtain surrounding the toddler's crib or bed helps promote the realization that objects out of sight, such as parents, do return. Transitional objects, such as a familiar blanket or stuffed animal, can temporarily substitute for the security of parents. The toddler can be read familiar stories. Repetition of stories promotes a sense of stability in the unfamiliar hospital environment.

A doll is a familiar toy that can be used to recreate a stressful environment, thereby providing an opportunity for the child to express and work through feelings. Other developmentally appropriate toys for toddlers include familiar objects from home such as measuring cups or spoons, wooden puzzles, building blocks, and push-and-pull toys. Playing with safe hospital equipment helps toddlers overcome the anxiety associated with these items. Supervise these play sessions and remove hospital equipment when you leave.

Preschooler

The nurse can intervene to reduce the stress produced by preschoolers' fears through the use of some kinds of play. A simple outline of the body or a doll can be used to address the child's fantasies and fears of bodily harm. Playing with safe hospital equipment may help preschoolers to work through feelings such as aggression (Figure 41–10 ●).

Preschoolers prefer crayons and coloring books, puppets, felt and magnetic boards, play dough, books, and recorded stories. Preschoolers and older children often enjoy **animal-assisted therapy**. Children's hospitals and units may have visits from pets, most commonly dogs, to provide diversion and relaxation (McDowell, 2005) (Figure 41–11 ●).

School-Age Child

Although play begins to lose its importance in the school-age years, the nurse can still use some techniques of therapeutic play

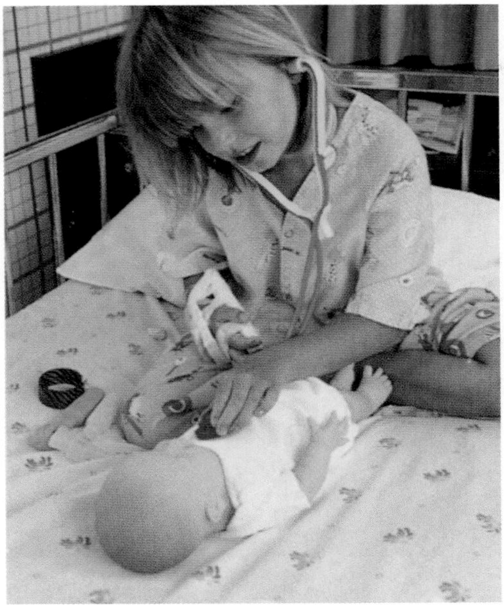

● **Figure 41–10** Age-appropriate play will help the child adjust to hospitalization and care.

to help the hospitalized child deal with stress. School-age children often regress developmentally during hospitalization, demonstrating behaviors characteristic of an earlier state, such as separation anxiety and fear of body injury. Outlines of the body and anatomically correct dolls or condition specific dolls can be used to illustrate the cause and treatment of the child's illness (Figure 41–12 ●). Use terms for body parts that are suitable for older children. Drawings provide an outlet for expression of fears and anger.

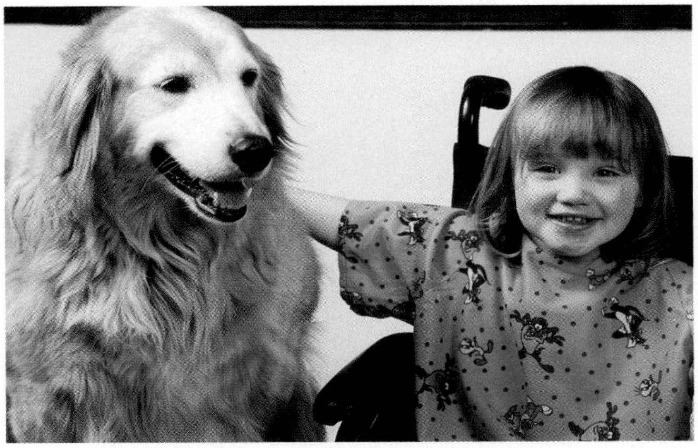

● **Figure 41–11** Hospitals may have animal-assisted therapy from specially trained animals to provide comfort and distraction during health care. Both the child and the dog seem to be smiling.

School-age children enjoy collecting and organizing objects and often ask to keep disposable equipment that has been used in their care. They may use these items later to relive the experience with their friends. Games, books, puzzles, school work, crafts, tape recordings, and computers provide an outlet for aggression and increase self-esteem in the school-age child. The type of play used should promote a sense of mastery and achievement.

THERAPEUTIC RECREATION

Many of the special play techniques used with younger children are not suitable for adolescents, but adolescents do need a planned recreation program to help them meet developmental needs during hospitalization. Peers are important, and the isolation of

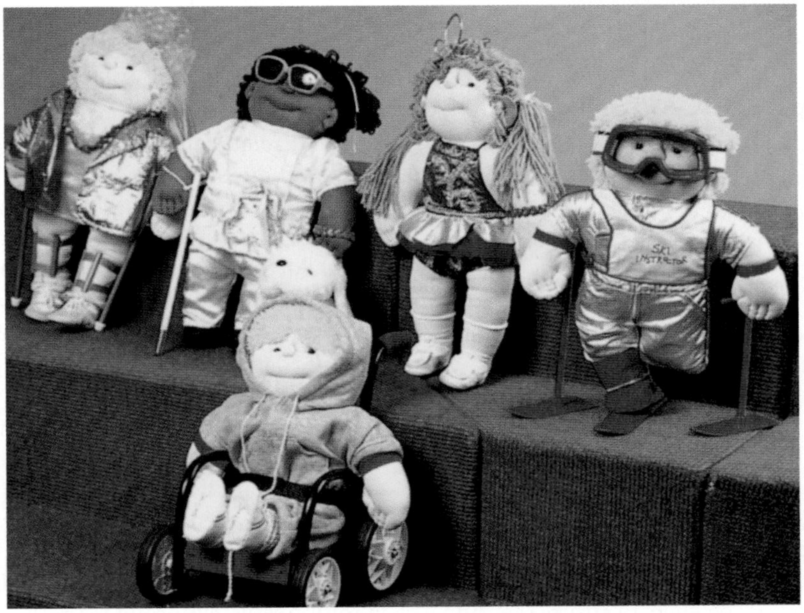

● **Figure 41–12** Having the child play with dolls that have "disabilities" similar to his or her own will help the child adjust. Such play helps the child realize what activities are possible.

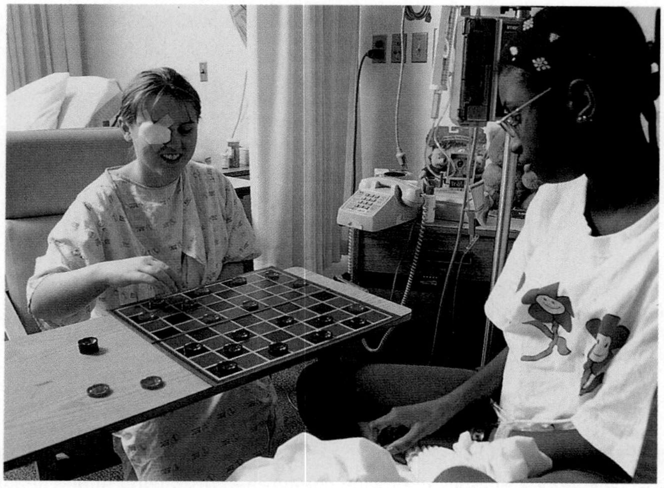

● **Figure 41–13** Having interaction with other hospitalized adolescents and maintaining contact with friends outside the hospital are very important so that the teenager does not feel isolated and alone. A friendly yet competitive checkers game helps to stimulate these teenagers and allows for self-expression. What are the other benefits?

hospitalization can be difficult. Telephone contact with other teenagers and visits from friends should be encouraged. Interactions with other teenagers at a pizza party, video game, or movie night or during other activities can help adolescents feel normal (Figure 41–13 ●). Physical activities that provide an outlet for stress are recommended. Even adolescents on bed rest or in wheelchairs can play a modified form of basketball. Some hospitals provide a teen room or teen lounge with age-appropriate activities such as a pool table, video games, and computers.

The independence of adolescence is interrupted by illness. Nurses can provide choices for teenagers to assist them in regaining control. Providing adolescents options and encouraging them to choose an evening recreational activity can promote their feelings of independence.

STRATEGIES TO MEET EDUCATIONAL NEEDS

Some hospitalizations are so short that the absence of the child or adolescent from school and peers is of minimal concern. However, if hospitalization is expected to last longer than a few days or if the child's condition will change so that he or she needs special school arrangements, the nurse should assess the effects of hospitalization on the child's education.

When an elective procedure occurs, encourage families to assist in the arrangement of the extended school absence with teachers. The child can then be provided with schoolwork to complete in the hospital or at home when capable. This minimizes educational deficits and future problems for the child. Pencils, paper, comfortable work areas, computers, and quiet work times are provided to meet the child's educational needs. Telephone calls, Internet connections, and live video conferencing with teachers can be arranged as needed. The hospital teachers collaborate with the child's school teachers to ensure the child is meeting the educational objectives to avoid deficits upon return to school.

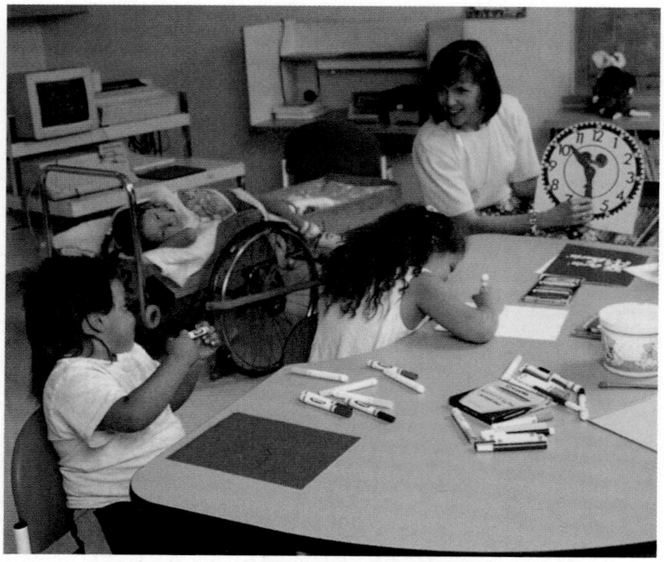

● **Figure 41–14** Shriners Hospital in Spokane, Washington, has a special classroom and teacher for children undergoing a lengthy hospital stay, enabling them to remain current with their schoolwork. The child who falls behind other students might not fit in when he or she returns to school or might be required to repeat a grade. What are the potential consequences of these situations?

Nurses should also consider the social aspects of school and peers. Peers can be encouraged to visit a hospitalized classmate, send cards and letters, call on the phone, or communicate via the Internet. Classmates may even videotape a class session, allowing everyone the opportunity to send messages to the hospitalized child. When the child returns to school, information may be shared about the child's special needs. Maintain the child's and family's privacy by discussing with them the information needed by others, and obtaining written permission before disclosing any information. The hospital and school nurse often collaborate with each other, as well as the child and family, to plan for the child's needs. The child with chronic health problems or who requires long-term hospitalization has additional needs with regard to school. Hospitals or rehabilitation units may have classrooms, teachers, and facilities to promote learning (Figure 41–14 ●). Many school districts provide tutors or computer connections for students who are hospitalized or receiving home care for extended periods. Teachers can visit children at the hospital or at home. Parents are often pivotal in making arrangements to meet the child's educational needs, since they interact with the child, the school, and the healthcare team.

Child and Family Teaching

Teaching is an essential part of the nurse's role in care of hospitalized children and their families and begins with the initial contact of the family with healthcare providers. Teaching may be informal, as when the nurse integrates an explanation during routine care, or structured, as when the nurse plans and implements a formal teaching program. However, with shorter hospitalization stays, few group interactions are possible, necessitating that most teaching be conducted during conversations and patient care (London, 2004).

Growth and Development

For children who can hear, touch, see a model or equipment, read, look at pictures, or even smell things like alcohol swabs, learning is more complete. This is particularly important for the school-age child in the stage of concrete operational thought, who must be able to manipulate material in order to learn.

Nurses emphasize to the family that most teaching will occur in informal sessions rather than in formalized programs. The family should be aware of the teaching process to encourage active listening and participation. Essential to ensuring the family's understanding is to actively involve them in the learning process. The nurse and family partner together to identify the family's learning needs and appropriate teaching method to best convey the information. Recall that family members may be at various cognitive and anxiety levels and therefore have needs for different types of teaching. Develop a plan with both the family and other healthcare professionals to facilitate learning among the child and family members.

Teaching directed at children that takes into account their developmental level, cognitive abilities, and perception will facilitate a deeper understanding of the illness (Koopman et al., 2004). Teaching directed at parents must be geared to their level of understanding. If English is not spoken or is the parents' second language, then an interpreter may be necessary. If interpreters are needed to facilitate understanding, be sure they are contacted and are available for teaching sessions.

Depending on the information to be presented, teaching may use the cognitive, psychomotor, or affective domains of learning. Teaching that includes all three domains is more effective. Explanations or reading materials, including pamphlets, booklets, videos, and models, are tailored to a level the parent can understand. The choice of tools used varies depending on the child's diagnosis and available materials.

Timing is a critical factor in teaching. Parents and children are less receptive to teaching when they are preoccupied with stress or activities. Collaborating with the parents in scheduling specific times for teaching sessions may be helpful.

Teaching Plans

A teaching plan is a written plan that includes goals and expected outcomes, interventions needed to achieve the specified goals, and a method and time for evaluation of the expected outcomes. The teaching plan may also specify teaching methods and types of materials to be used. By developing a teaching plan, a nurse helps to ensure that all the necessary information is included and taught efficiently. Additionally, this written documentation of teaching allows for continuity of care between nurses and other disciplines. Multidisciplinary teaching plans provide clear communication for all health team members in the teaching process.

The child's primary caretaker should be an active participant in the development of the teaching plan as well as its implementation. The primary caretaker is most often a parent but may be a close family member (uncle, aunt, or grandparent). Before establishing a teaching plan the nurse should assess the child's or parent's knowledge, skills, and feelings by considering the following questions:

- What does the parent/caretaker or child know about the health issue?
- What are the expectations of the child and family?
- What is the cognitive level or ability to learn?
- Is there a desire to learn?
- What previous experiences affect the learning experience, either positively or negatively?
- What previous interventions have been the most useful for the child and family?
- What resources are available to the parents, child, and nurse that enhance understanding of the health condition?
- Are there feelings or beliefs that might interfere with the learning process?
- What complementary care does the family use, and how does this relate to the teaching plan?

After these questions are answered the nurse decides what knowledge, skill, or change in attitude is desired, and then establishes outcome criteria or objectives with the parent and child. The nurse then explores possible teaching methods and materials. A variety of sources, including written materials (books, pamphlets, handouts, and stories), computer software, audiovisual presentations, dolls, and body models are available to encourage interest from the child and family. Refer to Chapter 1∞ for information on reading level of patient education materials. In some settings, audiovisual and computer resources may be limited. Small group teaching sessions (e.g., for children with recently diagnosed diabetes or cystic fibrosis) may be another option and provide the child with an opportunity to interact and learn from peers experiencing the same condition. Gathering two or three parents together on a unit to learn and share experiences may also be helpful. For some conditions, standardized teaching plans are available in books and from healthcare agencies. These plans can serve as a guide in developing an individualized teaching plan.

Teaching for Children with Special Healthcare Needs

Children who have disabilities may have special learning needs (Allen & Vessey, 2004). If the child has a visual impairment or perceptual difficulty, material is presented in auditory and tactile ways. Children who have hearing deficits require visual and tactile presentations. Children who have learning disabilities may require more frequent reinforcement and shorter teaching sessions. These children are evaluated often for comprehension in order to adjust teaching as necessary.

Children who have chronic conditions or special healthcare needs may have been hospitalized numerous times and have received other health care at home and in the community. They usually have adapted coping mechanisms that help them deal with their illness. Nurses can talk with the child to determine what has helped in the past, provide information about what to expect during the current hospitalization, assign staff members who are familiar when possible, and follow each child's lead in assisting his or her coping.

Do not assume that the child with a history of numerous hospitalizations understands all activities since each hospitalization is different. Explain even the most routine activities. Regularly review the updated plan of care with the parents and child. Provide the child with opportunities to ask questions and express concerns and fears. Assess the child's individual learning needs. Older children can be asked how they best like to learn. Determine the necessity for special equipment or teaching methods.

PREPARATION FOR HOME CARE

Nurses play an important role in preparing the child and family for discharge home; this preparation starts early during the hospitalization. The nurse works with the social service department, home care agencies, and the family to plan for equipment, procedures, and other home care needs. Home care nurses collaborate with the hospital nurse and assist families to meet the child's healthcare needs.

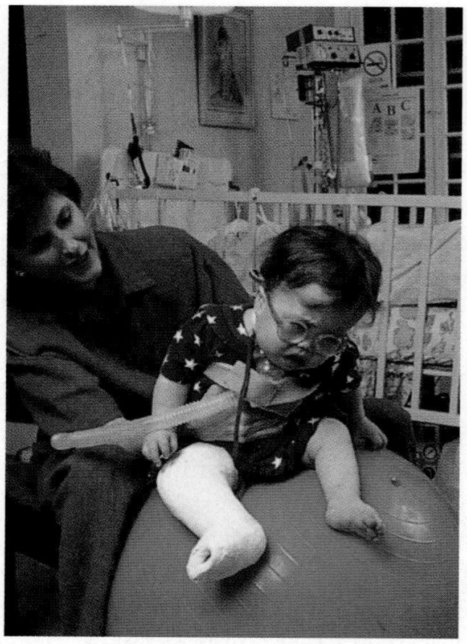

● **Figure 41–15** This child with chronic medical problems is being cared for at home. Are there any legal implications for the hospital and the nurse associated with the preparation of the child and family for home care?

ASSESSING THE CHILD AND FAMILY IN PREPARATION FOR DISCHARGE

Preparations for the discharge process are best started upon admission to the hospital. The healthcare team, including the primary healthcare provider, nurse, social worker, and discharge planner partner with the family to ensure a smooth transition. Assess the family's ability to manage the child's care and if any special adaptation to the home environment is necessary.

When a child who has been hospitalized for an extended time is to be discharged home, the school district is contacted by the hospital school teacher (if available) or social worker, and plans for education or reentry into school are made. This involves an assessment of the child by the school district and formulation of an individualized education plan (IEP). The IEP may include home tutors, specialized services from persons such as physical or speech therapists, or arrangements for transport of the child with a disability to the school and provisions for special medical care as needed. An individualized health plan (IHP) may also be required. See Chapter 40∞ for definitions and a detailed discussion on individualized education plans and individualized health plans.

Some common problems that interfere with successful discharge planning include financial concerns, the family's unavailability for teaching and planning, lack of equipment, and lack of teamwork among involved healthcare disciplines. Nurses who assess for these potential problems from the initial contact with the child and family can intervene and assist the family to resolve these problems as soon as possible.

PREPARING THE FAMILY FOR HOME CARE

The family may need to learn physical and rehabilitative procedures for the child's care. Short-term care may be necessary until the child regains full function. In other situations, care may be required throughout the child's life. This may involve measuring vital signs or assessing blood glucose levels.

For the child requiring complex long-term care, parents may need to learn about intravenous lines, medications, oxygen administration, or ventilators (Figure 41–15 ●). See Chapter 40∞ for discussion of the child with a chronic condition.

Parents need to be taught how to use the equipment needed for the child's care and must show that they can use it correctly. They must be able to identify symptoms of distress and report them immediately to the healthcare provider. The education provided and the parents' ability to perform care are discussed with a visiting nurse or individual who manages the home care program. Parents should be encouraged to learn cardiopulmonary resuscitation. Refer to Chapter 39∞.

Help parents explore options for respite. If they cannot provide daily care or need a break, they should be able to rely on others for a short period. Some agencies are available to provide respite care. Ongoing assistance may be needed to help families deal with financial, time, and other challenges. If parents must take a leave of absence from work to provide care for the child, inform them about the coverage provided by the Family Medical Leave Act (U.S. Department of Labor, 2008).

PREPARING PARENTS TO ACT AS CASE MANAGERS

The family is an integral part of the plan of care for an ill or hospitalized child. The child with a chronic illness or an injury requiring long-term care will probably require the services of numerous healthcare personnel or healthcare agencies. One person needs to be identified as a **case manager** to coordinate healthcare and to prevent gaps and overlaps. In some hospitals nurses act as case managers. They may organize a patient care conference while the child with a chronic condition is hospital-

Evidence-Based Nursing

PREPARING FAMILIES TO PROVIDE HEALTH CARE FOR CHILDREN AT HOME

Clinical Question

What preparation do families need to provide health care for children at home?

Evidence

Children are often discharged from hospitals while still requiring complicated healthcare procedures, so parents need to learn how to perform these procedures safely. Parents may not be able to be in the hospital consistently during the hospitalization or they may not be as involved in the child's care as would be helpful for learning the needed skills. Using a qualitative approach, researchers interviewed families of 14 children hospitalized for a variety of chronic illnesses. Parents identified a lack of support by personnel when they were present in the hospital; they often felt in the way and did not want to disturb the routines of the unit. Parents reported that they were frequently not included in decision making about the child, and yet felt responsibility for managing the multiple needs of the child's condition once they returned home (Ygge & Arnetz, 2004).

A survey method was used by Sarajärvi et al. (2006) to describe support that families received during their child's illness from both the families and the nurse's point of view. Questionnaires were collected from 344 families of children who either visited an outpatient clinic or were hospitalized during the time of the study and from 60 pediatric nurses working in these settings. Forty-one percent reported that they had been supported by the nursing staff, 21 percent felt they were not supported at all, and 37 percent did not answer. Families stated that they received support via "discussion (37%), listening (34%), information (12%), and time given to the families (11%)" (p. 207). Nurses identified that they had provided support primarily via listening and discussion. They also indicated that they had given the most information about diagnostic testing and treatment and less about the illness itself. Some nurses reported that they had not provided any information to the families. Only one-third of the nurses felt that they had provided adequate information related to care of the child at home. Families reported the need for more support, including the need for more information about their child's illness and care at home.

Best Practice

For home care to be successful, informational support is essential (Sarajärvi et al., 2006). Preparing families for care of their children is a complex task and the situation in the hospital is sometimes not conducive to teaching and learning. Nurses can support parents during rooming in by making them comfortable and integrating them into discussions and decisions about the child's care; they are collaborators in all of the care involved.

Teaching families is often viewed as a short-term task, but in reality it is ongoing and needs to be integrated into all interactions in order to adequately prepare the family for discharge (London, 2004). Nurses should view every interaction as a teachable moment and constantly include teaching whenever a parent is present. Explain medications, what assessments are being performed, and how this will be adapted in the home situation. Provide resources for the responsibility the parent takes on as the child returns home, including phone numbers, parent support groups, reading material, and Internet sources. Ask parents what care they feel comfortable with and what they need more assistance to perform. Involve them in the decision about referral to home health care or school nurse.

Critical Thinking

- What conditions in the hospital will assist parents to feel welcome and part of the hospital routine?
- How can you help parents feel that they are adequately supported through the information that they are given about the child's illness and follow-up care?
- How can you adapt your teaching plan to include integration of home care into every interaction with the parents?
- How can you record the teaching needs of parents so that other nurses can continue with needed information, demonstrations, and assessments?
- What techniques need to be part of discharge care so that parents leave with resources to get future questions answered as they take over total care of the child?

See MyNursingKit for possible responses.

ized. Management goals are set and decisions are made about which healthcare provider or agency is responsible for helping the child meet each goal.

Parents can also be case managers. The parent as case manager coordinates medical care, hospital stays, and visits to specialists; meets with school district representatives to plan the individualized education program for the child; finds equipment, personnel, and other services for home care; and manages the child's overall care.

Nurses should strongly encourage parents who want to take over case management to do so. Help them learn the management skills required. Many community agencies such as social service or home health agencies hold workshops for parents managing the complex care of their children.

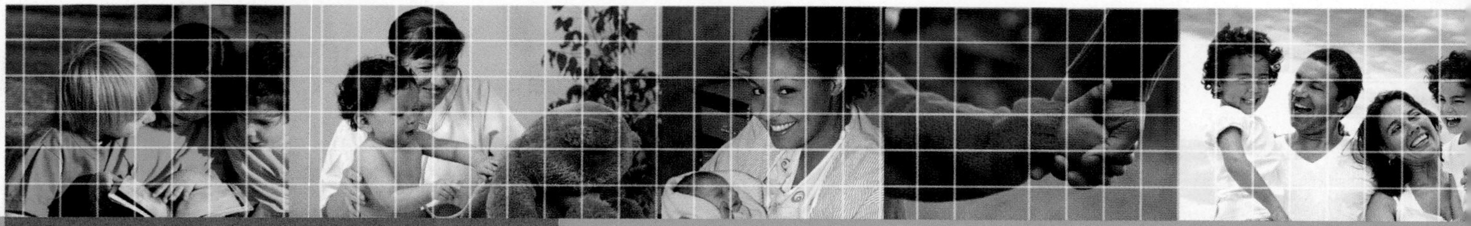

CRITICAL CONCEPT REVIEW

LEARNING OUTCOMES / CONCEPTS

41.1 Discuss the child's understanding of health and illness according to the child's psychosocial and developmental level.

1. Infant:
   - Has no concept of illness. Distressed by separation from parent.
2. Toddler:
   - Age group most at risk for stressful experience.
   - Separation from parent is the major stressor.
   - Old enough to understand routine disruption, but not old enough to understand why.
3. Preschooler:
   - Distressed by parental separation and their fears, especially fear of body injury or mutilation.
   - May view illness as punishment.
4. School-age child:
   - Understands basic reason for illness. Also understands body parts and functions. Fear their body will not return to normal after an illness.
5. Adolescent:
   - Understands cause of illness. Concerned with the effect of illness on body image. Concerned about privacy.

41.2 Recognize the effect of hospitalization on the child and family.

1. Disruption of usual routines.
2. Anxiety and fear:
   - Unknown or serious outcome.
   - Financial difficulties.
   - Lack of family support.
   - Lack of community support.
3. Parents report increased satisfaction when family needs and preferences are considered.
4. Sibling difficulties:
   - Lack of parental attention.
   - Jealousy over attention given to sick child.
   - Lack of information about child who is ill.
   - Guilt over role in illness.
   - Anxiety and insecurity over changing roles.

41.3 Identify methods that the child and family use to adapt to hospitalization.

1. Preparation for planned hospitalization
   - Tours.
   - Therapeutic play.
   - Health fairs.
   - Books.
2. For unplanned admission
   - Orientation to environment.
   - Explanation of procedures and expectations.
3. Child life programs

41.4 Apply family-centered care principles to the hospital setting.

1. Rooming in.
2. Promoting development and safety.
3. Minimizing disruption of routines.
4. Orientation to special units and expectations.

41.5 Identify nursing strategies to minimize the stressors related to hospitalization.

1. Promote parental involvement in care.
2. Orient child and family to hospital setting, routines, staff.
3. Age-appropriate play.
4. Age-appropriate explanations of procedures.
5. Encourage parents to support child.

41.6 Discuss family presence during procedures and nursing strategies used to prepare the family.

1. Determine extent to which parents desire to be involved in child's care.
2. Support parents' desires related to presence during procedures.

41.7 Discuss strategies for preparing children and families for discharge from the hospital setting.

1. Collaborate with multidisciplinary team and family to plan for home care as needed.
2. Assess the family's ability to manage care at home.
3. Teach family any special skills they need to care for the child at home.

CRITICAL THINKING IN ACTION

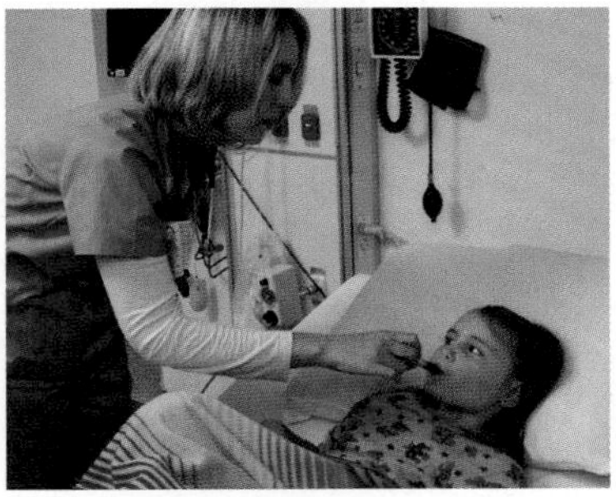

Five-year-old Tiona has a history of obstructive sleep apnea and was scheduled for a tonsillectomy and adenoidectomy (T&A). Because of her history of sleep apnea, Tiona was scheduled to spend the night in the hospital to monitor her for any potential respiratory complications. Following the operation, Tiona refused to drink liquids because she was afraid it would hurt when she swallowed. After receiving intravenous pain medication, Tiona realized that she could swallow without too much pain and began to eat popsicles and drink liquids. She was then switched to oral pain medication. The next morning Tiona is drinking liquids well enough that she is to be discharged home.

1. What information should the nurse include in the discharge teaching plan for Tiona's mother?
2. As Tiona and her mother are preparing to leave the hospital, Tiona states "I am going to be good so I do not have to come to the hospital anymore!" How should the nurse respond?
3. Tiona's mother states that she is worried that her daughter will not drink enough at home. What can the nurse suggest to Tiona's mother to encourage her to drink fluids?
4. Children Tiona's age have many fears and stressors related to hospital and surgery. How can Tiona's mother assist her daughter to express her feelings about the hospital experience once she is home?

See MyNursingKit for possible responses.

REFERENCES

Allen, P. J., & Vessey, J. A. (2004). *Primary care of the child with a chronic condition* (4th ed.). St. Louis: Mosby.

Alsop-Shields, L., & Mohay, H. (2001). John Bowlby and James Robertson: Theorists, scientists, and crusaders for improvements in the care of children in hospitals. *Journal of Advanced Nursing, 35*(1) 50–58.

Crenshaw, J. T., & Winslow, Elizabeth (2002). Preoperative fasting: Old habits die hard: Research and published guidelines no longer support the routine use of 'NPO after midnight,' but the practice persists. *American Journal of Nursing, 102*(5), 36–44.

Emergency Nurses Association. (2005). Position statement: Family presence at the bedside during invasive procedures and/or resuscitation. Retrieved April 1, 2007, from *www.ena.org/about/position/pdfs/family%20presence%20at%20the%20bedside%20during%20invasive%20procedures.pdf*

Gursky, B. (2007). The effect of educational interventions with siblings of hospitalized children. *Journal of Developmental & Behavioral Pediatrics, 28*(5), 392–398.

Hopia, H., Tomlinson, P. S., Paavilainen, E., & Astedt-Kurki (2005). Child in hospital: family experiences and expectations of how nurses can promote family health. *Journal of Clinical Nursing, 14*(2), 212–222.

Koopman, H. M., Baars, R. M., Chaplin, J., & Zwinderman, K. H. (2004). Illness through the eyes of the child: The development of children's understanding of the causes of illness. *Patient Education and Counseling, 55,* 363–370.

Lassetter, J. H., & Baldwin, J. H. (2005). Improving the experience of hospitalization for Hawaiian children on the mainland through cultural sensitivity to Hawaiian ways of healing. *Journal of Pediatric Nursing, 20,* 170–176.

Lau, W. K. (2002). Stress in children: Can nurses help? *Pediatric Nursing, 28*(1), 13–19.

Lobato, D., Kao, B., & Plante, W. (2006). Siblink: Meeting the needs of siblings of children with chronic illness and disability. *The Brown University Child and Adolescent Behavior Letter, 22*(9), 1, 5–6.

London, F. (2004). How to prepare families for discharge in the limited time available. *Pediatric Nursing, 30,* 212–214, 227.

McDowell, B. M. (2005). Non-traditional therapies for the PICU – Part 2. *Journal for Specialist in Pediatric Nursing, 10*(2), 81–85.

Pinckney, R. B., & Stuart, G. W. (2004). Adjustment difficulties of adolescents with sickle cell disease. *Journal of Child and Adolescent Psychiatric Nursing, 17*(1), 5–12.

Power, N., & Franck, L. (2008). Parent participation in the care of hospitalized children: A systematic review. *Journal of Advanced Nursing, 62*(2), 622–641.

Romino, S. L., Keatley, V. M., Secrest, J., & Good, K. (2005). Parental presence during anesthesia induction in children. *AORN Journal, 81*(4), 780–792.

Ryan-Wenger, N. A., Sharrer, V. W., & Campbell, K. K. (2005). Changes in children's stressors over the past 30 years. *Pediatric Nursing, 31*(4), 282–291.

Sarajärvi, A., Haapamäki, M. L., & Paavilainen, E. (2006). Emotional and information support for families during their child's illness. *International Nursing Review, 53,* 205–210.

Spector, R. E. (2009). *Cultural diversity in health and illness* (7th ed.). Upper Saddle River, NJ: Prentice Hall.

Tielsch, A. H., & Allen, P. J. (2005). Listen to them draw: Screening children in primary care through the use of human figure drawings. *Pediatric Nursing, 31*(4), 320–327.

U.S. Department of Labor. (2008). *Family and Medical Leave Act.* Retrieved October 19, 2008, from *www.dol.gov/esa/whd/fmla/*

Ygge, B. M., & Arnetz, J. E. (2004). A study of parental involvement in pediatric hospital care: Implications for clinical practice. *Journal of Pediatric Nursing, 19,* 217–223.

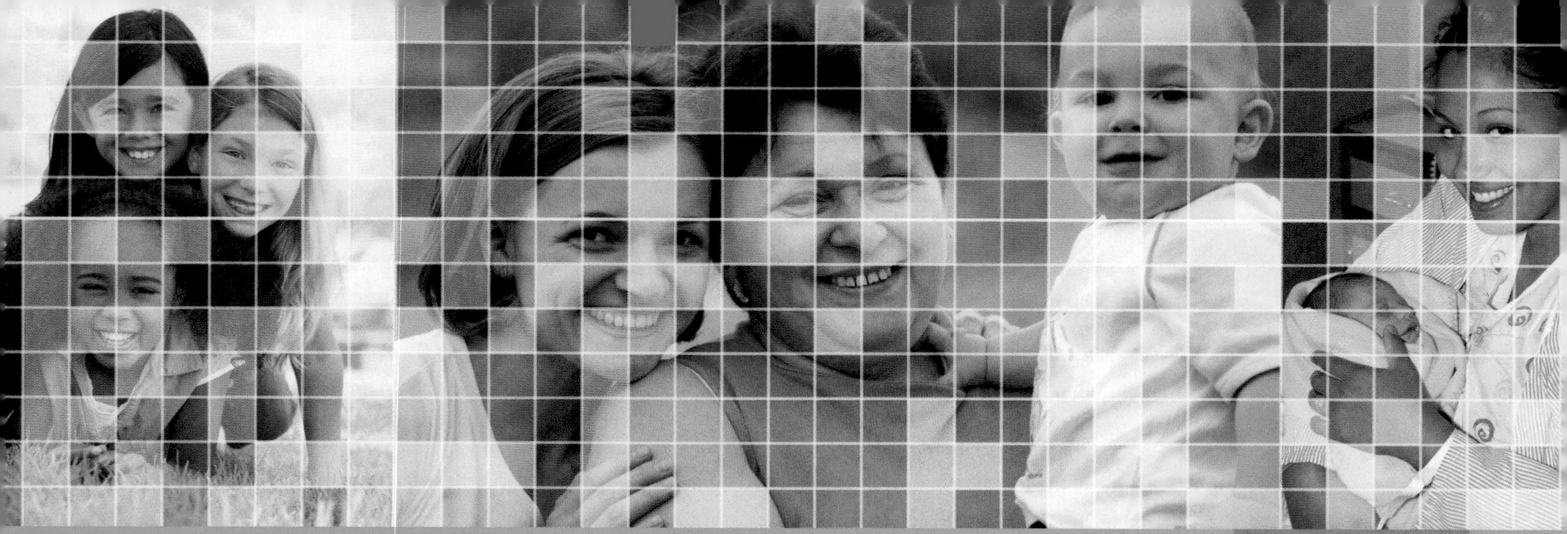

CHAPTER

Pain Assessment and Management in Children

42

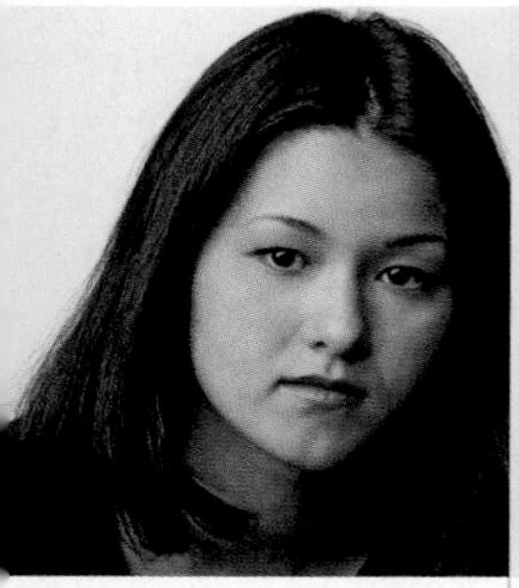

Felicia must be in pain so soon after her surgery. I know I would have pain if it were me. Can she get pain medicine without getting another needle? —Mother of Felicia, 5 years old

LEARNING OUTCOMES

42.1 Identify the physiologic and behavioral consequences of pain in infants and children.

42.2 Assess the developmental abilities of children to perform a self-assessment of pain intensity.

42.3 Describe the nursing assessment and management for a child receiving an opioid analgesic.

42.4 Explain the physiology that enables nonpharmacologic (complementary) methods of pain control to be effective.

42.5 Assess children of different ages with acute pain and develop a nursing care plan that integrates pharmacologic interventions and developmentally appropriate nonpharmacologic (complementary) therapies.

42.6 Develop a nursing care plan for assessing and monitoring the child having sedation and analgesia for a medical procedure.

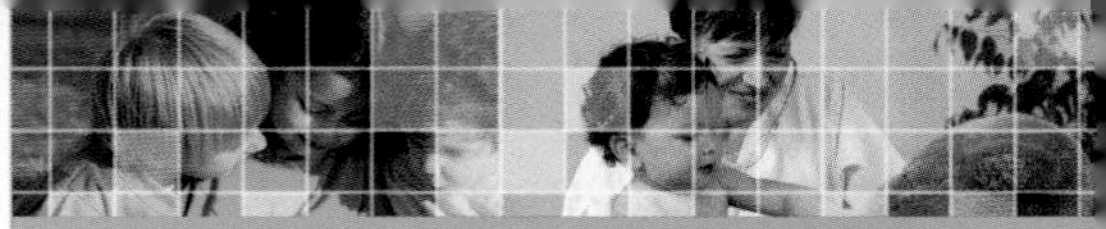

KEY TERMS

Acute pain, 1103
Anxiolysis, 1122
Chronic pain, 1104
Deep sedation, 1122
Distraction, 1115
Electroanalgesia, 1115
Equianalgesic dose, 1111
Moderate sedation, 1122
Neuropathic pain, 1104
Nonsteroidal anti-inflammatory drugs (NSAIDs), 1112
Opioids, 1111
Pain, 1103
Patient-controlled analgesia (PCA), 1113
Physical dependence, 1112
Tolerance, 1112
Withdrawal, 1112

Every child has his or her own perception of pain. A neurological response to tissue injury, **pain** is an unpleasant sensory and emotional experience associated with actual or potential tissue damage (Young, 2005). Effective pain management is every child's right.

PAIN

Pain may be either acute or chronic. **Acute pain** is sudden and of short duration that may be associated with a single event, such as surgery, or an acute exacerbation of a condition such as a sickle cell crisis. An immediate pain response occurs immediately at the time of tissue damage, and the inflammatory response that follows the initial injury causes a sustained pain response (see Pathophysiology Illustrated).

Due to a two-way control of nociceptive transmission within the spinal tracts, pain perception can be inhibited or changed when a competing nonpain impulse is sent along the same nerve pathways, a simple explanation of the pain Gate Control Theory. Stimulation of the larger A-delta fibers by ice or massage causes the substantia gelatinosa in the dorsal horn of the spinal cord to "close the gate" and decrease the transmission of pain impulses to the brain. The brain cortex also has bi-directional control of nociceptive transmission and can inhibit some pain stimuli (Huether & Defriez, 2006, p. 453). *Endorphins,* endogenous opioids produced by the brain in response to painful stimuli, help inhibit pain impulses in the spinal cord and the brain (Huether & Defriez, 2006, p. 454).

MyNursingKit Video: Pain Perception

PATHOPHYSIOLOGY ILLUSTRATED

PAIN PERCEPTION

① *Nociceptors* (free nerve endings at the site of tissue damage) transmit information via specialized nerve fibers to the spinal cord.
② Unmyelinated C fibers slowly transmit dull, burning, diffuse pain as well as chronic pain. Large, myelinated A-delta fibers quickly transmit sharp, well-localized pain. Nociceptors are stimulated by mechanical, thermal, and chemical injury. Biochemical mediators (bradykinin, prostaglandin, leukotrienes, serotonin, histamine, catecholamines, and substance P) are produced in response to tissue damage. These substances help move the pain impulse from the nerve endings to the spinal cord.
③ After the sensory information reaches the substantia gelatinosa in the dorsal horn of the spinal cord, the pain signal may be modified depending on the presence of other stimuli, from either the brain or the periphery.
④ The pain signal is then transmitted through the lateral spinothalamic tract, to the thalamus of the brain where perception occurs.
⑤ Once the sensation reaches the brain, interpretation of pain occurs, and emotional responses may increase or decrease the intensity of the pain perceived.

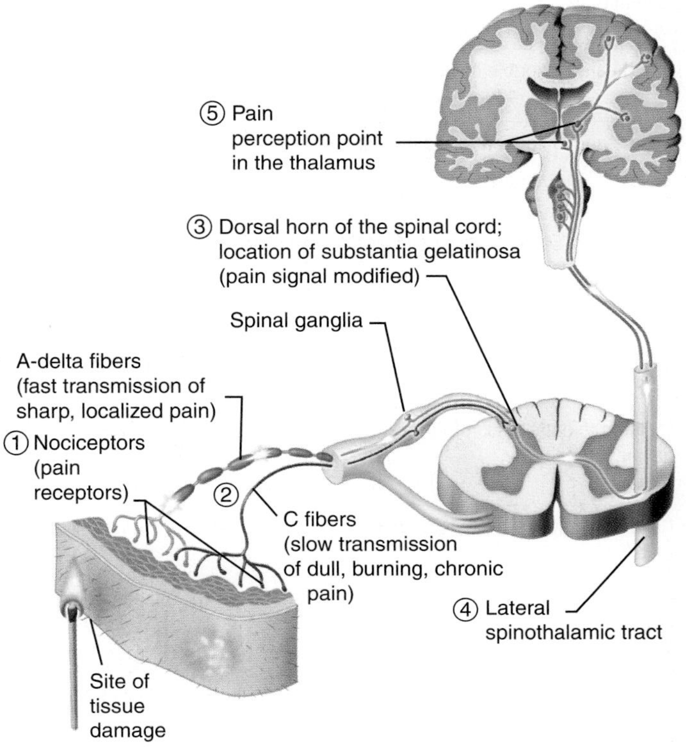

Chronic pain is a persistent pattern of pain, lasting longer than 6 months; it is generally associated with a prolonged disease process such as juvenile rheumatoid arthritis. Chronic pain may be nociceptive or **neuropathic pain**, initiated or caused by a primary lesion or dysfunction of the nervous system. It does not arouse the sympathetic nervous system in the same way as acute pain. Ongoing stimulation of nociceptors can sensitize the peripheral and central nervous systems leading to neuroanatomical, neurochemical, and neurophysiological changes.

MISCONCEPTIONS ABOUT PAIN IN CHILDREN

Healthcare professionals once believed that children feel less pain than adults. Undertreatment of pain was based on these attitudes about pain and the difficulty and complexity of pain assessment in children. Research has shown that past beliefs about children's perception of pain were incorrect. Even the smallest infants do feel and remember pain. Effective pain treatment is the right of every infant and child. In 2001, the Joint Commission introduced standards for assessing and managing the pain of all patients (Joint Commission, 2008). For a review of past myths and the contrasting reality, see Table 42–1.

MyNursingKit JCAHO

DEVELOPMENTAL ASPECTS OF PAIN PERCEPTION, MEMORY, AND RESPONSE

A number of factors influence the pain perceived by the child, including maturation of the nervous system, the child's developmental stage, and previous pain experiences (see Table 42–2). Newborns and infants develop a memory of pain. Preschool-age children demonstrate pain memory by making efforts to delay a painful procedure.

A child's responses to acute or chronic pain are also influenced by other factors such as their understanding of the pain source, their ability to control what will happen, their use of a pain control strategy such as distraction, as well as emotions like fear, anxiety, frustration, and anger (Anthony & Schanberg, 2005). Children also report more pain intensity when recalling a past painful experience than when they rated it the time of its occurrence (von Baeyer, Marche, Rocha, et al., 2004).

Table 42–1 Misconceptions about Pain in Infants and Children

Myth	Reality
Newborns and infants are incapable of feeling pain. Children do not feel pain with the same intensity as adults because a child's nervous system is immature.	The anatomic and functional requirements for pain processing are present early in fetal life. Preterm and full-term newborns may be more sensitive to pain stimuli because of immature spinal cord descending pain control mechanisms (von Baeyer, Marche, Rocha, et al., 2004).
Infants are incapable of expressing pain.	Infants express pain with both behavioral and physiologic cues that can be assessed.
Infants and children have no memory of pain.	Preterm infants have been noticed to associate the smell of alcohol with heel sticks and to try to pull the foot away to avoid the pain. Infants cry in anticipation of immunizations (Young, 2005).
Parents exaggerate or aggravate their child's pain.	Parents know their child and are able to identify when the child is in pain.
Children are not in pain if they can be distracted or if they are sleeping.	Children use distraction to cope with pain, but they soon become exhausted when coping with pain and fall asleep.
Repeated experience with pain teaches the child to be more tolerant of pain and cope with it better.	Children who have more experience with pain respond more vigorously to pain. Experience with pain teaches how severe the pain can become.
Children tolerate discomfort well. They become accustomed to pain after having it for a while.	Children do not tolerate pain any better than adults. Infants may develop pain sensitivity with repeated exposure and have a higher pain reaction (von Baeyer, Marche, Rocha, et al., 2004).
Children recover more quickly than adults from painful experiences such as surgery.	Children heal quickly from surgery, but they have the same amount of pain from surgery as an adult.
Children tell you if they are in pain. They do not need medication unless they appear to be in pain.	Children may be too young to express pain or afraid to tell anyone other than a parent about the pain. The child fears the treatment for pain may be worse than the pain itself.
Children without obvious physical reasons for pain are not likely to have pain.	The cause of pain cannot always be determined. The feeling of pain is subjective and should be accepted by nurses.
Children run the risk of becoming addicted to pain medication when used for pain management.	Addiction is extremely rare when the child is treated for an acute condition (less than 1%) (Plaisance & Logan, 2006).

Table 42–2 The Child's Understanding of Pain, Behavioral Responses, and Verbal Descriptions by Developmental Stage

Age Group	Understanding of Pain	Behavioral Response	Verbal Description
		Infants	
6 months	No understanding of pain; is responsive to parental anxiety	Generalized body movements, chin quivering, facial grimacing, poor feeding	Cries
6–12 months	Has a pain memory; is responsive to parental anxiety	Reflex withdrawal to stimulus, facial grimacing, disturbed sleep, irritability, restlessness	Cries
		Toddlers	
1–3 years	Does not understand what causes pain and why they might be experiencing it	Localized withdrawal, resistance of entire body, aggressive behavior, disturbed sleep	Cries and screams, cannot describe intensity or type of pain Use common words for pain such as *owie* and *boo-boo*
		Preschoolers	
3–6 years (preoperational)	Pain is a *hurt* Does not relate pain to illness; may relate pain to an injury Often believes pain is punishment Unable to understand why a painful procedure will help them feel better or why an injection takes the pain away	Active physical resistance, directed aggressive behavior, strikes out physically and verbally when hurt, low frustration level	Has the language skills to express pain on a sensory level Can identify location and intensity of pain, denies pain, may believe his or her pain is obvious to others
		School-Age Children	
7–9 years (concrete operations)	Does not understand the cause of pain, but understands simple relationships between pain and disease Understands the need for painful procedures to monitor or treat disease May associate pain with feeling bad or angry May recognize psychologic pain related to grief and hurt feelings	Passive resistance, clenches fists, holds body rigidly still, suffers emotional withdrawal, engages in plea bargaining	Can specify location and intensity of pain and describes pain physical characteristics in relation to body parts
10–12 years (transitional)	Better understanding of the relationship between an event and pain Has a more complex awareness of physical and psychologic pain, such as moral dilemmas and mental pain	May pretend comfort to project bravery, may regress with stress and anxiety	Able to describe intensity and location with more characteristics, able to describe psychologic pain
		Adolescents	
13–18 years (formal operations)	Has a capacity for sophisticated and complex understanding of the causes of physical and mental pain Recognizes that pain has both qualitative and quantitative characteristics Can relate to the pain experienced by others	Want to behave in a socially acceptable manner (like adults), show a controlled behavioral response May not complain about pain if given cues that nurses and other healthcare providers believe it should be tolerated	More sophisticated descriptions as experience is gained; may think nurses are in tune with their thoughts, so they don't need to tell the nurse about their pain

Young children are unable to give a detailed description of their pain because of their limited vocabulary and pain experiences. Depending on their developmental stage, children use different coping strategies, such as escape, postponement or avoidance, diversion, and imagery, to deal with pain. Children may not complain of pain for several reasons:

- Some children believe they need to be brave.
- Preschoolers and adolescents may assume the nurse knows they have pain.
- Some children are afraid that it will hurt more to have the pain treated.

Developing Cultural Competence

EXAMINE YOUR OWN EXPERIENCE

Think about your childhood pain experiences and how your family encouraged you to be stoic or to express pain. Such childhood experiences often contribute to a health professional's attitudes about the pain experienced by children. For example, some healthcare providers may believe that being in pain for a little while is not so bad, that pain helps build character, or that using pain medication is a sign of a weak character. However, all nurses need to acknowledge the child's right to pain management, and it is the standard of care.

CULTURAL INFLUENCES ON PAIN

Culture and social learning greatly influence the child's expression of pain. Children are able to perceive pain in the facial expression of others by 5 to 6 years (Deyo, Prkachin, & Mercer, 2004). They observe family members in pain and try to imitate their responses. Through the process of parental approval and disapproval they learn how to behave when in pain, how much pain should be tolerated, how much discomfort justifies a complaint, how to express a complaint of pain, and who to approach for pain relief. See "Developing Cultural Competence: Examine Your Own Experience."

Some cultural groups (people of Italian and Jewish descent) use verbal and nonverbal methods to express pain freely while others (Anglo-Saxon–Germanic, Irish, Amish, and Appalachian) encourage a more stoic response with a diminished expression of pain. However, not all members of a cultural group will demonstrate the same pain response. Children will have individualized responses to pain based on their past experiences.

CONSEQUENCES OF PAIN

Unrelieved pain is stressful and has many undesirable physiologic consequences (Table 42–3). For example, the child with acute postoperative pain takes shallow breaths and suppresses coughing to avoid more pain. These self-protective actions increase the potential for respiratory complications. Unrelieved pain may also delay the return of normal gastric and bowel functions and cause a stress ulcer. Anorexia associated with pain may delay the healing process. Pain drains energy resources needed for healing and growth.

Table 42–3 Physiologic Consequences of Unrelieved Pain in Children

Responses to Pain	Potential Physiologic Consequences
Respiratory Changes	
Rapid shallow breathing	Alkalosis
Inadequate lung expansion	Decreased oxygen saturation, atelectasis
Inadequate cough	Retention of secretions
Neurologic Changes	
Increased sympathetic nervous system activity and release of catecholamines	Tachycardia, elevated blood pressure, change in sleep patterns, irritability
Metabolic Changes	
Increased metabolic rate with increased perspiration	Increased fluid and electrolyte losses
Increased cortisol production	Increased cortisol and blood glucose levels
Immune System Changes	
Depressed immune and inflammatory responses	Increased risk of infection, delayed wound healing
Gastrointestinal Changes	
Increased intestinal secretions and smooth muscle sphincter tone, nausea, anorexia	Impaired gastrointestinal functioning, poor nutritional intake, ileus
Altered Pain Response	
Increased pain sensitivity	Hyperalgesia, decreased pain threshold, exaggerated memory of painful experiences

Source: Data from Mitchell, A., & Boss, B. J. (2002). Adverse effects of pain on the nervous systems of newborns and young children: A review of the literature. *Journal of Neuroscience Nursing, 34*(5), 228–236; Walden, M. (2007). Pain in the newborn and infant. In C. Kenner & J. W. Lott, *Comprehensive neonatal nursing: An interdisciplinary approach* (4th ed., pp. 360–371), Philadelphia: Elsevier Saunders; McCance, K. L., Forshee, B. A., & Shelby, J. (2006). Stress and disease. In K. L. McCance & S. E. Huether (Eds.), *Pathophysiology: The biologic basis for disease in adults and children* (5th ed., pp. 447–462), St. Louis: Elsevier Mosby.

Growth and Development

Children slowly acquire words for pain over the first 6 years of life. The pain words used spontaneously by children in one study were as follows: "ouch" as early as 17 months, "hurt" and "ow" by 18 months of age, "boo-boo" by 21 months, "ache" by 36 months, "sore" by 45 months, and "pain" by 72 months (Stanford, Chambers, & Craig, 2005). Other pain words include "owie," "stinging," "sore," "cutting," "burning," "itching," "hot," and "tight."

PAIN ASSESSMENT

The goal of pain assessment is to provide accurate information about the location and intensity of pain and its effects on the child's functioning.

PAIN HISTORY

Parents can provide a great deal of information about the child's response to pain, such as the following:

- How the child typically expresses pain. Children and parents use similar terms to describe pain, such as a *hurt, owie, boo-boo, stinging, sore, cutting, burning, itching, hot,* and *tight*. Knowing the appropriate word to use makes communicating with the child easier. The parent can often inform the healthcare team about signs that will help to recognize the child's pain.
- The child's previous experiences with painful situations and reactions.
- How the child copes with and manages pain. The child with several past pain experiences may not exhibit the same types of stressful behaviors as the child with few pain experiences.
- What works best to reduce the child's pain?
- The parent's and child's preferences for analgesic use and other pain interventions.

Ask older children to give a history of painful procedures, but recognize that they may modify their pain descriptions depending on the type of questions asked and what they expect will happen as a result of their response. Examples of questions to ask include the following:

- What kinds of things made you hurt in the past and what made it feel better?
- Do you tell others about being in pain and what do you want them to do for the pain?
- What do you not want done when you are hurting? What would you like the nurse to do for the hurt?
- Where is the hurt, and what does it feel like? What could be causing the hurting?

PAIN ASSESSMENT SCALES

Various pain scales are used to assess pain in children.

Pain Behavior Scales for Nonverbal Children

Physical and behavioral indicators are used to quantify pain in infants and nonverbal children. For example, the Neonatal Infant Pain Scale (NIPS) and the FLACC Behavioral Pain Assessment Scale rely on the nurse's observation of the child's behavior.

The NIPS is designed to measure procedural pain in preterm and full-term newborns up to 6 weeks after birth. The newborn facial expression, cry quality, breathing patterns, arm and leg position, and state of arousal are observed. This tool has high interrater reliability and validity. See Table 42–4.

The FLACC is designed to measure acute pain in infants and young children following surgery, and it can be used until the child is able to self-report pain with another pain scale. FLACC is an acronym for the five categories that are assessed: Face, Legs, Activity, Cry, and Consolability. The tool has validity and reliability for evaluation of postoperative pain (Manworren & Hynan, 2003; Willis, Merkel, Voepel-Lewis, et al., 2003). See Table 42–5.

Young children (3 years and older) can localize pain if given an outline of the front and back of the body. The child can mark where the pain is located or color the area of pain with crayons. The child should use one color for the place where it hurts the most, and another color for areas with less pain. See MyNursingKit for body outlines to use for pain assessment.

Self-Report Pain Scales

Other scales depend on the child's self-report of pain intensity (see Skill 13–1 SKILLS). To use pain scales, the child must be developmentally ready and understand the concept of a little or a lot of pain well enough to tell the nurse. Children 2 to 3 years of age are usually able to understand the concept of "more or less." This child cannot be given more than three choices on a pain scale (none, some, a lot) when assessing pain. When the child can understand rank order, such as by placing several blocks of different sizes in a row from biggest to smallest, the child is developmentally ready for a numeric scale (Young, 2005). Examples of self-report pain scales for young children include the Faces Pain Scale and the Oucher Scale.

Faces pain rating scale. This scale has a series of six or seven cartoon-like faces with expressions from smiling (or neutral) to tearful, depending upon the model selected. The Wong-Baker scale is commonly used for children from 3 years through adolescence (Figure 42–1 ●). After explanations about the meaning for each face, the child selects the face that is the closest match to the pain felt. Older children can use the words associated with the tool to provide a pain rating. The Faces Pain Rating Scale has good validity and reliability for measuring pain intensity (O'Rourke, 2004). The nurse should not use this tool or the Oucher Scale to compare with the child's facial expression to determine pain level.

Oucher scale. The Oucher Scale presents a series of six photographs of a child expressing increased intensity of pain in combination with

Table 42–4 Neonatal Infant Pain Scale (NIPS)

Characteristic	Scoring Criteria
FACIAL EXPRESSION	
0 = Relaxed muscles	■ Restful face with neutral expression
1 = Grimace	■ Tight facial muscles; furrowed brow, chin, and jaw (Note: At low gestational ages, infants may have no facial expression)
CRY	
0 = No cry	■ Quiet, not crying
1 = Whimper	■ Mild moaning, intermittent cry
2 = Vigorous cry	■ Loud screaming, rising, shrill, and continuous (Note: Silent cry may be scored if infant is intubated, as indicated by obvious facial movements)
BREATHING PATTERNS	
0 = Relaxed	■ Relaxed, usual breathing pattern maintained
1 = Change in breathing	■ Change in drawing breath; irregular, faster than usual, gagging, or holding breath
ARM MOVEMENTS	
0 = Relaxed/restrained (with soft restraints)	■ Relaxed, no muscle rigidity, random movements of arms
1 = Flexed/extended	■ Tense, straight arms; rigid; or rapid extension and flexion
LEG MOVEMENTS	
0 = Relaxed/restrained (with soft restraints)	■ Relaxed, no muscle rigidity, occasional random movements of legs
1 = Flexed/extended	■ Tense, straight legs; rigid; or rapid extension and flexion
STATE OF AROUSAL	
0 = Sleeping/awake	■ Quiet, peaceful, sleeping; or alert and settled
1 = Fussy	■ Alert and restless or thrashing; fussy

Source: From Lawrence, J., Alcock, D., Mcgrath, D. P., et al. (1993). The development of a tool to assess neonatal pain. *Neonatal network, 12*(6), 61; and Taylor, B. J., Robbins, J. M., Gold, J. I., Logsdon, T. R., Bird, T. M., & Anand, K. J. S. (2006). Assessing postoperative pain in neonates: a multicenter observational study, *Pediatrics, 118*(4), e992–e1000.

Table 42–5 FLACC Behavioral Pain Assessment Scale

	SCORING		
Categories	**0**	**1**	**2**
Face	No particular expression or smile	Occasional grimace or frown; withdrawn, disinterested	Frequent to constant frown, clenched jaw, quivering chin
Legs	Normal position or relaxed	Uneasy, restless, tense	Kicking or legs drawn up
Activity	Lying quietly, normal position, moves easily	Squirming, shifting back and forth, tense	Arched, rigid, or jerking
Cry	No cry (awake or asleep)	Moans or whimpers, occasional complaint	Crying steadily, screams or sobs; frequent complaints
Consolability	Content, relaxed	Reassured by occasional touching, hugging, or being talked to; distractible	Difficult to console or comfort

Instructions: Observe the child for 5 minutes or longer. Observe the legs and body uncovered. Reposition the patient or observe activity. Assess body for tenseness and tone. Initiate consoling interventions if needed. Each of the five categories is scored from 0 to 2, resulting in a total score between 0 and 10. A total score of 0 = relaxed and comfortable; 1–3 = mild discomfort; 4–6 = moderate pain; 7–10 = severe discomfort or pain.

Source: Used with permission from Merkel, S. I., Voepel-Lewis, T., Shayevitz, J. R., & Malviya, S. (1997). The FLACC: A behavioral scale for scoring post-operative pain in young children. *Pediatric Nursing, 23*(3), 293–297; and Voepel-Lewis, T., Malviya, S., & Tait, A. (2005). Validity of parent ratings as proxy measures of pain in children with cognitive impairment. *Pain Management Nursing, I6*(4), 168–174.

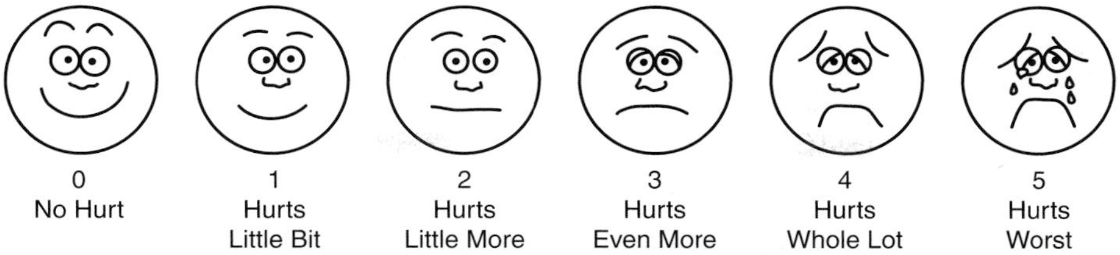

● **Figure 42–1** The Faces Pain Rating Scale. The Faces Pain Rating Scale is valid and reliable in helping children to report their level of pain. Make sure the child has an understanding of number concepts and then teach the child to use the scale. Point to each face and use the words under the picture to describe the amount of pain the child feels. Then ask the child to select the face that comes closest to the amount of pain felt. Use the number under the face to score the pain.

Source: Used with permission from Wong, D. L., & Baker, C. M. (1988). Pain in children: Comparison of assessment scales. Pediatric Nursing, *14, 9–16.*

a vertical Visual Analogue Scale (Figure 42–2 ●). The tool has been developed and tested in three cultural groups: Caucasian, African American, and Hispanic. The tools have good validity and reliability for children over 3 years of age (O'Rourke, 2004).

Poker chip tool. This tool uses four checkers or poker chips to quantify pain. The child is asked to pick the number of chips that best match the pain felt, with one chip being a little pain and four being the most pain he or she could have.

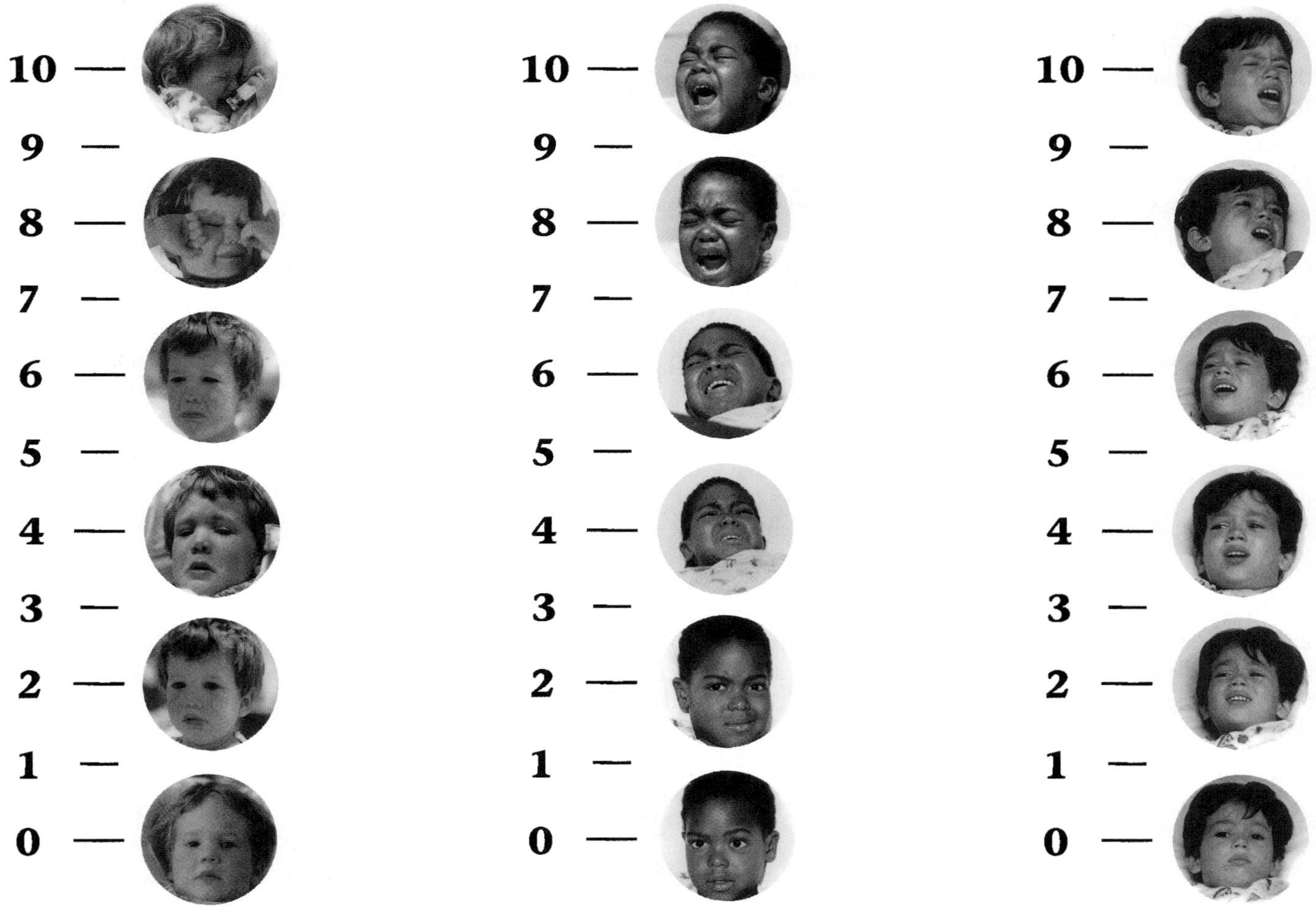

● **Figure 42–2** The Oucher Scale. Use the Oucher Scale that is the best match for the ethnicity of the child. After determining that the child has an understanding of number concepts, teach the child to use the scale. Point to each photo and explain that the bottom picture is "no hurt," the second picture is a "little hurt," the third picture is "a little more hurt," the fourth picture is "even more hurt," the fifth picture is "a lot of hurt," and the sixth picture is the "biggest or most hurt you could ever have." The numbers beside the photos can be used to score the amount of pain the child reports.

Source: The Caucasian version of the Oucher used with permission from Judith E. Beyer, RN, PhD, 1983. The African-American version of the Oucher used with permission from Mary J. Denyes, RN, PhD, and Antonia M. Villarruel, RN, PhD, 1990. The Hispanic version of the Oucher used with permission from Antonia M. Villarruel, RN, PhD, 1990.

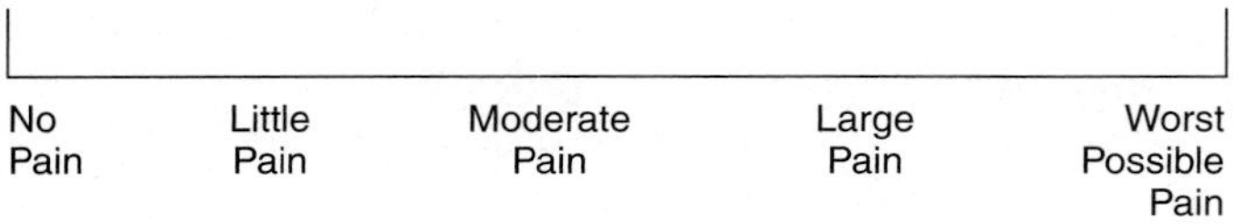

● **Figure 42–3** The Word-Graphic Rating Scale. Word-Graphic Rating Scale has words rather than numbers under the line. It may be used by itself or with the Adolescent Pediatric Pain tool. Teach the child to use the tool by pointing to the side of the line that is no pain. Then run your finger along the line and tell the child that this location is the worst possible pain. If the child has some pain, ask the child to make a mark along the line that is the best match for the amount of pain felt. Use a millimeter ruler to measure from the "no pain" end of the line to the marked location to identify the pain score. Make sure the line is the same length each time pain is assessed so comparisons can be made.

Source: Used with permission from Sinkin-Feldman, L., Tesler, M., & Savedra, M. (1997). Word placement on the Word-Graphic Rating Scale by pediatric patients. Pediatric Nursing, *23, 31–34.*

School-age children and adolescents have better number concepts and language skills, so additional tools can be used to assess their pain. The nurse should ask the child to describe the pain and give its location. Providing some words such as sharp, dull, aching, pounding, cold, hot, burning, throbbing, stinging, tingling, or cutting can help children describe their pain.

Numeric pain scale. This tool, also called the Visual Analog Scale, is a single 10-cm horizontal or vertical line that has descriptors of pain at each end (no pain, worst possible pain). Marks and numbers are placed at each cm on the line. The child marks the amount of pain felt, and the numbers on the line are used to score the pain.

Word-graphic-rating scale. This tool has words rather than numbers describing increasing pain intensity across a 10-cm Visual Analog Scale without numbers. The child marks the line that is closest to the level of pain felt. A millimeter ruler can be used to quantify the pain and record the pain score (Figure 42–3 ●).

Adolescent pediatric pain tool. This tool includes a human figure drawing, the Word-Graphic Rating Scale, and a choice of descriptive words, e.g., burning, ache, sharp, and dull. Adolescents indicate pain sites on the human figure outline, use the Word-Graphic-Rating Scale as described, and use the word choices to characterize the pain felt. See MyNursingKit for the human figure outline.

ACUTE PAIN

Children experience acute pain related to a variety of illnesses and injuries, surgery, and invasive procedures. Just as with adults, children must have their pain assessed and managed.

CLINICAL MANIFESTATIONS

Children have both physiologic and behavioral indicators of pain.

Physiologic Indicators

Acute pain stimulates the adrenergic nervous system and results in physiologic changes, including tachycardia, tachypnea, hypertension, pupil dilation, pallor, increased perspiration, and increased secretion of catecholamines and adrenocorticoid hormones (Huether & Defriez, 2006). These signs demonstrate a complex stress response. The body adapts physiologically to acute pain; the vital signs return to near normal, and perspiration decreases after several minutes, so these signs cannot be used for monitoring pain.

Behavioral Indicators

Newborns and infants demonstrate knitted brows, squinted eyes with cheeks raised, eyes closed, crying, jerky or flailing movements, and stiff posture in response to pain (Stevens, McGrath, Yamada, et al., 2006). See Figure 42–4 ●. Children in acute pain may be distressed and anxious, especially if they have experienced pain previously (Huether & Defriez, 2006; Young, 2005). Behaviors that could indicate pain or anxiety in infants and toddlers include restlessness or agitation, hyperalertness or vigilance, sleep disturbances, and irritability. Children and adolescents may demonstrate the following additional behaviors:

- Short attention span (child is difficult to distract)
- Facial grimacing, biting or pursing lips

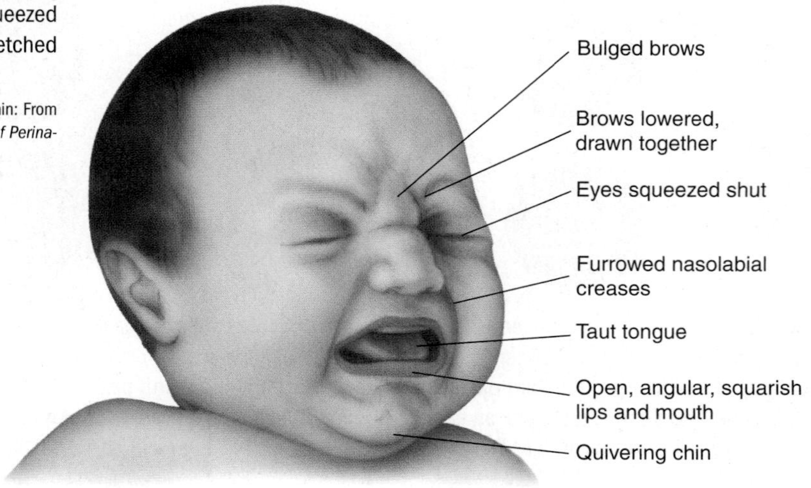

● **Figure 42–4** Neonatal pain facial expression. Neonatal characteristic facial responses to pain include bulged brow, eyes squeezed shut, furrowed nasolabial creases, open lips, pursed lips, stretched mouth, taut tongue, and a quivering chin.

Source: Adapted from Carlson, K. L., Clement, B. A., & Nash, P. (1996). Neonatal pain: From concept to research questions and the role of the advanced practice nurse. *Journal of Perinatal Neonatal Nursing, 10*(1), 64–71.

- Posturing (guarding a painful joint by avoiding movement), remaining immobile, or protecting the painful area
- Drawing up knees, flexing limbs, massaging affected area
- Lethargy, remaining quiet, or withdrawal
- Sleep disturbances

CLINICAL THERAPY

Pain management includes both drug and nondrug measures. Children need adequate pain medication, but complementary therapies can enhance pain management and ultimately reduce the amount of pain medication needed.

Opioids

Opioids are analgesics commonly given for severe pain, such as after surgery or a severe injury. Opioids (e.g., morphine and codeine) may be administered by oral, subcutaneous, intramuscular, and intravenous routes. Administration of opioids by an oral route is as effective as by intramuscular and intravenous routes when the drug is given in an **equianalgesic dose** (the amount of drug, whether given by oral or parenteral routes, needed to produce the same analgesic effect) (see Drug Guide 42–1). Oral and intravenous routes are preferred for children. Rectal preparations of some opioids are also available. The intramuscular and subcutaneous routes cause pain and stress at the time of injection, and titration of the dosage to achieve a desired response level that can occur with intravenous administration is not possible (Zempsky, Cravero, et al., 2004). The optimal analgesic dose varies widely among patients in all age groups (American Pain Society, 2005). Meperidine is rarely used in children because its metabolite has the potential to cause seizures (Brislin & Rose, 2005).

Common side effects include sedation, nausea, vomiting, constipation, urinary retention, and itching, and these should be treated by rotating the opioids used or with specific therapies as follows:

- Sedation – supplement lower opioid dose with nonsedating analgesia (Greco & Berde, 2005)
- Nausea and vomiting – antiemetic, use alternate opioid

Drug Guide

OPIOID ANALGESICS AND RECOMMENDED DOSES FOR CHILDREN AND ADOLESCENTS*

DRUG	APPROXIMATE EQUIANALGESIC ORAL DOSE	APPROXIMATE EQUIANALGESIC PARENTERAL DOSE	RECOMMENDED STARTING DOSE (ADULTS GREATER THAN 50 KG)		RECOMMENDED STARTING DOSE (CHILDREN & ADULTS LESS THAN 50 KG)	
			ORAL	PARENTERAL	ORAL	PARENTERAL
Morphine	30 mg	10 mg	15–30 mg every 3–4 hr	10 mg every 3–4 hr	0.3 mg/kg every 3–4 hr	50–100 mcg/kg every 3–4 hr
Codeine	120 mg	75 mg IM or Subcutaneous	30–60 mg every 3–4 hr	60 mg every 2 hr	0.5–1 mg every 3–4 hr[a]	NR
Hydromorphone (Dilaudid)	7.5 mg	1.5 mg	4–8 mg every 3–4 hr	1.5 mg every 3–4 hr	0.1–0.2 mg/kg every 3–4 hr	10–20 mcg/kg every 3–4 hr
Levorphanol (Levo-Dromoran)	4 mg (acute) 1 mg (chronic)	2 mg (acute) 1 mg (chronic)	2–4 mg every 6–8 hr	2 mg every 6–8 hr	0.04 mg/kg every 6–8 hr	0.02 mg/kg every 6–8 hr
Meperidine (Demerol)	300 mg	75 mg	NR	75 mg every 3 hr	NR	NR
Methadone (Dolophine, others)	10 mg (acute) 2–4 mg (chronic)	5 mg (acute) 2–4 mg (chronic)	5–10 mg every 4–8 hr	10 mg every 4–8 hr	0.1–0.2 mg/kg every 12–36 hr	0.1–0.2 mg/kg every 12–36 hr
Oxycodone (Roxicodone)	20 mg	NA	5 mg every 3–4 hr	NA	0.1–0.2 mg/kg every 3–4 hr[a]	NA
Fentanyl	NA	0.01 mg	5 mcg/kg Lozenge	50–100 mcg every 1–2 hr	5–15 mcg/kg Oralet[b]	1 mcg/kg every 1–2 hr

NR = Not recommended; NA = Not available

*For all parenteral opioids, start with the low dose and titrate to effective pain control.

[a] Caution: Doses of aspirin and acetaminophen in combination with opioid/NSAID preparation must also be adjusted to the patient's body weight.

[b] The Oralet is not widely used because of nausea and vomiting side effects.

Source: Data from: American Pain Society (2008). *Principles of analgesic use in the treatment of acute pain and cancer pain* (6th ed., pp. 19–21), Glenview, IL: Author; and Greco, C., & Berde, C. (2005). Pain management for the hospitalized pediatric patient. *Pediatric Clinics of North America*, *52*(4), 995–1027.

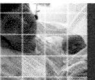

Nursing Practice

Respiratory depression (unresponsiveness and a respiratory rate less than 12 breaths/min in young children) may progress to respiratory arrest and is the major life-threatening complication of opioid administration. Clinical signs that predict the development of respiratory depression include sleepiness, small pupils, and shallow breathing. Children at particular risk for respiratory depression induced by an opioid are those with an altered level of consciousness, an unstable circulatory status, a history of apnea, or a known airway problem such as obstructive sleep apnea. Some hospitals use continuous pulse oximetry when children receiving opioids are at risk for respiratory depression.

Respiratory depression is most likely to occur when the child is sleeping, a state that augments the depressant effect on the respiratory center and potential airway obstruction by the tongue (American Pain Society, 2008). Identify the time interval before drug-specific peak respiratory depression occurs, and then carefully monitor the child's vital signs during that period to detect respiratory depression. Naloxone is the drug used for reversal of opioids' adverse effects at a dosage titrated to gradually reduce the effects of the opioids without causing withdrawal symptoms (American Pain Society, 2005, p.71).

- Constipation – stool softener, stimulant laxative, increased fluids and dietary fiber
- Urinary retention – bethanechol, catheterization
- Pruritus – antihistamine, use alternate opioids, or naloxone 0.1–0.2 mcg/kg/hr continuous IV infusion (given simultaneously with opioid) (Greco & Berde, 2005)

When given opioids over an extended period of time, children develop **physical dependence**, the physiologic adaptation to an analgesic or sedative drug at the peripheral and central neurons. These children may experience **withdrawal**, the physical signs and symptoms that occur when a sedative or pain drug is stopped suddenly. Severe withdrawal may be seen when children with a physical dependence are given naloxone to treat respiratory depression (Brislin & Rose, 2005). **Tolerance** is an adaptation to an opioid dosage that results in a shorter duration of drug effectiveness over time. For example, a child might develop physical dependence or tolerance after being in an intensive care setting long term with pain management for life-threatening injuries, multiple surgeries, and invasive procedures. See Table 42–6 for signs and symptoms of withdrawal. Children should be slowly weaned off of opioids over 2 to 4 weeks to prevent withdrawal symptoms. One plan is to reduce the daily dose by 10% to 20% over several days. Clonidine may reduce some symptoms of opioid withdrawal.

Acetaminophen and Nonsteroidal Anti-inflammatory Drugs

Nonsteroidal anti-inflammatory drugs (NSAIDs) such as aspirin, primarily given orally, are effective for the relief of mild to moderate pain and chronic pain. Drug Guide 42–2 presents recommended dosages of these drugs. They are most commonly used for bone, inflammatory, and connective tissue conditions. An NSAID may be prescribed in combination with an opioid to increase the effectiveness of the narcotic drug, which may ultimately reduce the amount of opioids needed. Acetaminophen is a nonnarcotic analgesic that is used like an NSAID (see Drug Guide 42–3).

Drug Administration

Pain from surgery, major trauma, or cancer is present for predictable periods because of the effects of tissue damage. Pain relief should be provided around the clock. Every effort should be made to give the child analgesics without causing more pain. The preferred routes of administration are intravenous, local nerve block, and oral.

Continuous infusion analgesia is recommended for children with persistent severe pain, since it eliminates peaks and valleys in pain control. Analgesics may also be given intravenously on a scheduled basis (e.g., every 3 to 4 hours). Delays in analgesia administration increase the chances of *breakthrough pain* (pain that emerges as the pain medication wears off resulting in the loss of pain control) and the subsequent anticipation of pain. Giving analgesics on an as-needed basis for acute pain results in the loss of pain control. More medication is often needed to restore pain control than would have been required for continuous infusion analgesia.

Table 42–6 Clinical Manifestations of Opioid or Sedative Withdrawal

System	Signs and Symptoms
Central nervous system	Irritability, increased wakefulness, tremulousness, hyperactive deep tendon reflexes, clonus, inability to concentrate, frequent yawning, sneezing, delirium, hypertonicity, visual or auditory hallucinations
Gastrointestinal system	Feeding intolerance with vomiting, diarrhea, uncoordinated suck and swallow
Sympathetic nervous system	Tachycardia, tachypnea, increased blood pressure, nasal stuffiness, sweating, lacrimation, chills alternating with hot flashes, sweating, fever, salivation

Source: Data from American Pain Society (2008). *Principles of analgesic use in the treatment of acute pain and cancer pain* (6th ed.). Glenview, IL: Author; American Pain Society (2005). Guideline for the management of cancer pain in adults and children, Glenview, IL: Author.

Drug Guide

ACETAMINOPHEN, NSAIDS AND RECOMMENDED DOSES FOR CHILDREN AND ADOLESCENTS

ORAL PEAK ACTION TIME	USUAL ADULT DOSE	USUAL PEDIATRIC DOSE	COMMENTS
Nonopioid Analgesic			
Acetaminophen 0.5–2 hr	650–1000 mg every 4 hr	10–15 mg/kg every 4–6 hr	Lacks the peripheral anti-inflammatory activity of other NSAIDs; rectal suppository available
NSAIDs			
Aspirin 1–2 hr	650–975 mg every 4–6 hr	10–15 mg/kg every 4–6 hr	Do not use in children under 19 years with possible viral illness (National Reyes Syndrome Foundation, 2005); may cause gastric upset and bleeding; rectal suppository available
Choline magnesium trisalicylate (Trilisate) 2 hr	1000–1500 mg every 12 hr	25 mg/kg every 12 hr	Does not increase bleeding time like other NSAIDs; available as oral liquid
Ibuprofen (Motrin, others) 0.5 hr	200–400 mg every 4–6 hr	6–10 mg/kg every 6–8 hr	Available as oral suspension
Naproxen (Naprosyn) 2–4 hr	250–500 mg every 6–8 hr	5–10 mg/kg every 12 hr	Available as oral liquid
Ketorolac 0.75–1 hr	30–60 mg IV loading dose, then 15–30 mg every 6 hours	1 mg/kg IV loading dose, up to 60 mg, then 0.5 mg/kg IV or IM every 6 hours	IV or IM use only in children less than 50 kg; should not be used for children with bleeding disorder or at risk for bleeding complications; do not use longer than 5 days (Brislin & Rose, 2005)

Source: Data from: American Pain Society (2008). *Principles of analgesic use in the treatment of acute pain and cancer pain* (6th ed., pp. 6–10), Glenview, IL: Author; Greco, C., & Berde, C. (2005). Pain management for the hospitalized pediatric patient. *Pediatric Clinics of North America, 52*(4), 995–1027; and Bindler, R., & Howry, L. (2005). *Pediatric drug guide with nursing implications*, Upper Saddle River, NJ: Prentice Hall.

Evidence in Action

Analgesics were often withheld from children with acute abdominal pain until surgeons could complete an assessment, as it was believed that analgesia would interfere with diagnosis. Recent studies have revealed that children receiving an opioid prior to surgical consultation had lower pain intensity and the clinical signs of an acute abdomen were not obscured (Green, Bulloch, Kabani, et al., 2005; Kokki, Lintula, Vanamo, et al., 2005).

Patient-controlled analgesia. **Patient-controlled analgesia (PCA)** is a method of administering an intravenous analgesic, such as morphine, using a computerized pump programmed by the healthcare professional and controlled by the child (Skill 13–2 **SKILLS**). After initial pain control has been achieved with a continuous IV infusion of morphine (basal dose), the child presses a button to receive a smaller analgesic dose (bolus dose) for episodic pain relief. This method of pain management is especially useful for pain control in the first 48 hours after surgery when oral pain management is not possible. Safety features to prevent overdoses include the ability to set the maximum number of bolus infusions per hour and the maximum amount of drug received in a specific time period. Children and adolescents benefit from PCA by receiving continuous pain control and having the ability to control their comfort level with no trauma from injections. Once children can take oral analgesics, PCA is discontinued.

Children (often 5 years and older) selected for PCA should be able to self-report pain with a pain scale and understand that pushing the button will give them medication to relieve pain. Parents are sometimes given responsibility for pushing the injection button for younger children or those with disabilities, but concerns about potential overmedication of children with parent-controlled analgesia have been reported (Greco & Berde, 2005). Careful documentation of bolus doses by a family member are important to prevent overmedication. See "Teaching Highlights: Teaching About Patient-Controlled Analgesia."

Regional Pain Management

Epidural pain control provides selective analgesia for a body region, and it has become more common for postoperative pain

Drug Guide

ACETAMINOPHEN

Overview of Action

Produces analgesia by unknown mechanism; acts centrally in the central nervous system by increasing the pain threshold by inhibiting cyclooxygenase. Acts in the hypothalamus to cause antipyresis. Used in treatment of mild to moderate pain and of fever. Does not have anti-inflammatory effects. Does not affect bleeding time.

Routes, Dosage, Frequency

Oral or rectal: 10 to 15 mg/kg/dose every 4 to 6 hours, as needed. Do not exceed 120 mg/day in child 2 to 5 years, or 2.6 g/day in child 6 to 12 years. If not prescribed by healthcare provider, seek medical advice after use for 5 days for pain.

Contraindications: Previous hypersensitivity to the drug. Use cautiously in children with G6PD deficiency, renal or hepatic dysfunction, rheumatoid arthritis, poor nutrition, immunosuppression, or bone marrow depression.

Drug interactions: Chronic coadministration with carbamazepine, phenytoin, barbiturates, and rifampin may increase potential for chronic hepatotoxicity. Cholestyramine may decrease acetaminophen absorption.

Side effects: Liver damage with overdose.

Nursing Implications

- *Assess:* Note hepatic and renal function. Assess pain level or actual temperature prior to administration.
- *Administer:* Follow dosage directions carefully for different liquid preparations, which have different concentrations. Make sure the parent has the correct dispensing spoon or syringe for liquid preparations. Do not give preparations with aspartame to children with phenylketonuria. Plain or chewable tablets may be crushed and given with fluid; avoid giving with high-carbohydrate meals, which can decrease drug absorption.
- *Monitor:* Evaluate the response to medication. Periodic renal and hepatic studies may be ordered for patients on long-term therapy.
- *Patient teaching:* Do not give with other over-the-counter medications such as cold medications which may also contain acetaminophen or aspirin; the dosage will need to be adjusted to prevent overdose. Consult a physician if pain relief is not obtained. Store out of the child's reach as this medication is a frequent cause of childhood poisoning.

Data from: Wilson, B. A., Shannon, M. T., & Shields, K. M. (2009). *Prentice Hall nurse's drug guide.* Upper Saddle River, NJ: Prentice Hall; Dlugosz, C. K., Chater, R. W., & Engle, J. P. (2006). Appropriate use of nonprescription analgesics in pediatric patients. *Journal of Pediatric Health Care, 20*(5), 316–325.

Teaching Highlights

PATIENT-CONTROLLED ANALGESIA (PCA)

- What is PCA? Analgesia means pain relief: you get to control the amount of medicine you receive by using the machine.
- The machine gives the medicine by passing it through the tube that is connected to your intravenous line. When you push the button, the machine pumps pain medicine into the intravenous line to make you feel better.
- The machine limits the amount of medicine you can get to what the doctor orders. You can get any amount up to the maximum by pushing the button repeatedly. The push button will not let you make a mistake if you drop it or roll on it.
- Whenever you feel pain, hurt, or discomfort, push the button to get more medicine. You should be the only one to push the button. Do not let another family member push the button.
- No needles for pain shots are needed as long as the intravenous line is in place.
- The PCA may not relieve all of your pain, but it should make you feel comfortable. Let the nurse know if you think your PCA is not working.
- The PCA will be used until you can take pills or drink liquid pain medicine.

management. A catheter is inserted into either the lumbar or the caudal space. Small doses of drugs are needed for sedation and analgesia. Local nerve blocks, such as a popliteal block for the lower leg or interscalene block (in a muscle of the cervical vertebrae) for the upper extremity are used for anesthesia and analgesia frequently for pain control after surgery.

The regional block is most often performed when the child is anesthetized. A subcutaneous catheter is inserted into the local area for infusion of the analgesia. Pain control is achieved without systemic side effects from the medication. A single dose of local anesthetic agent may be used, or a continuous infusion may be given using a pump (Brislin & Rose, 2005). Tingling felt in the fingers or toes of the affected extremity is the first sign that the nerve block is receding.

NONPHARMACOLOGIC METHODS OF PAIN MANAGEMENT

Complementary therapies are nonpharmacologic methods used for pain management that can be used with analgesics, such as cognitive and behavioral strategies. See "Complementary Care: Complementary Therapies for Pain Control." One or more of these methods may provide adequate pain relief when the child has low levels of pain. When used with analgesics, complementary therapies often enhance the effectiveness of the analgesic or reduce the dosage required.

Complementary Care

COMPLEMENTARY THERAPIES FOR PAIN CONTROL

Cutaneous Stimulation

Gently rub the painful area, massage the skin gently, and hold or rock the child. Touching competes with the pain stimuli that are transmitted from the peripheral nerves to the spinal cord and brain and may reduce the pain felt by the child. Swaddling and containment in fetal position are both methods to reduce the pain responses of neonates (Huang, Tung, Kuo, et al., 2004).

Sucrose Solution

Concentrated sucrose solutions (2 ml of 24% solution) may be used as a pain relief measure in preterm and term newborns up to 1 month of age. Sucrose in contact with the oral mucosa promotes natural pain relief by activating endogenous opioids (Morash & Fowler, 2004). Give the solution 2 minutes before the procedure, and the analgesic effect of sucrose lasts approximately 3 to 5 minutes. Allow the infant to continue sucking on a pacifier or to breastfeed during the procedure to reduce distress and enhance the effectiveness of the sucrose solution.

Distraction

Distraction involves engaging a child in a wide variety of pleasant activities that help focus attention on something other than pain and the anxiety. Examples of distraction activities are listening to music, singing a song, blowing bubbles, playing a game, watching television or a video, and focusing on a picture while counting. Guided imagery and breathing techniques may be forms of distraction for school-age children and adolescents. Virtual reality games were found to be effective distractions for children with acute burn injuries (Das, Grimmer, Sparnon, et al., 2005). Teach parents how to be distraction coaches and suggest developmentally appropriate distraction activities for the child. Children in severe pain cannot be distracted; but do not assume the pain is gone if a child can be distracted.

Guided Imagery

Imagery is a cognitive behavioral process that encourages the child to relax (often with progressive muscle relaxation techniques) and focus on vivid mental images as if they were real, and to ignore things, such as a painful procedure. For example, help the child to visualize and explore a favorite place, do a fun activity, remember a funny story, or be a superhero. Ask the child to think about all the sights, sounds, smells, tastes, and feelings that will help enhance the image and experience. Imagery has been used successfully by school-age children and adolescents to reduce pain and anxiety associated with surgery (Huth, Van Kuiken, & Broome, 2006).

Relaxation Techniques

Relaxation techniques are used to reduce muscle tension that may aggravate pain. Progressive muscle relaxation is one relaxation technique. Teach children to tense and relax different muscle groups, starting with the hands and feet, and then moving to more central muscles. Ask the child to tense a muscle group for 10 seconds and notice how it feels, and then ask the child to relax the muscle group for 10 seconds and compare the feelings. With practice, the child should be able to detect the difference between tense and relaxed muscles and then to reduce the tension. Relaxation techniques may be combined with rhythmic breathing.

Breathing Techniques

Rhythmic deep breaths can be used with distraction or muscle relaxation during a painful procedure, or as a mechanism to reduce stress. Encourage the child or adolescent to take a deep breath, hold it for 5 seconds, and blow out through the mouth, as if to push the tension out or the needle away. Another breathing technique is patterned, shallow breathing. The child is encouraged to take shallow breaths in through the nose and blow out through the mouth while thinking of a particular image. The image could be a train and short breaths could be the "toot, toot" of the train engine.

Hypnosis

Hypnosis is an altered state of awareness facilitating heightened concentration, decreased awareness of external stimuli, increased relaxation, and increased suggestibility. In most cases a therapist uses images and the language of the child to induce relaxation and give posthypnotic suggestions for the relief of anxiety, tension, and pain. Children more easily respond to hypnosis than adults because of their imaginative powers for fun and fantasy. Hypnosis has been successful in assisting children to control acute postoperative pain, procedural pain and stress, and acute pain associated with conditions such as migraine headaches, hemophilia and sickle-cell anemia. Children can be taught self-hypnosis to give them a sense of mastery and control over pain and distress (Richardson, Smith, McCall, et al., 2006).

Application of Heat and Cold

Heat application promotes dilation of blood vessels. The increased blood circulation permits the removal of cell breakdown debris from the site. Heat also promotes muscle relaxation, breaking the pain-spasm-pain cycle. To reduce edema, do not apply heat in the first 24 hours after an injury.

The application of cold is believed to slow the ability of pain fibers to transmit pain impulses. Cold also controls pain by decreasing edema and inflammation, and by causing partial or complete anesthesia or numbness of the skin. When cold is applied, assess the skin for redness or signs of irritation. Take care to prevent thermal injury. Discontinue cold applications immediately if the skin alternately blanches and reddens afterwards.

Electroanalgesia

Also known as transcutaneous electrical nerve stimulation (TENS), **electroanalgesia** delivers small amounts of electrical stimulation to the skin by electrodes. This electronic stimulation is stronger than the pain impulses and is thought to interfere with the transmission of pain impulses from the peripheral nerves to the spinal cord and brain. TENS may be used for both acute and chronic pain management. The only known side effect is skin irritation at the electrode site.

Acupuncture

A traditional Chinese treatment for pain relief, acupuncture has been gaining greater acceptance in Western medicine. Acupuncture is based on the theory that energy, or chi, flows along channels through the body (meridians) that are connected by acupuncture points. Pain occurs with obstruction of the energy flow, and inserting needles at the appropriate acupuncture points restores the energy flow (Kundu & Berman, 2007). Limited research has been conducted about the use and effectiveness of acupuncture in children. Because of the use of needles, few children under 10 years will cooperate with the procedure.

NURSING MANAGEMENT

NURSING ASSESSMENT AND DIAGNOSIS

Nurses have an ethical obligation to relieve a child's suffering not only because of the consequences of unrelieved pain but also because appropriate pain management may have benefits such as earlier mobilization, shortened hospital stays, and reduced costs. To provide effective nursing management of children in pain, anticipate the presence of pain and recognize the child's right to pain control.

When assessing pain in children, keep the following questions in mind:

- What is happening in tissues that might cause pain? Assume that children who have had surgery, injury, vaso-occlusive episode, or illness are experiencing pain, since these events also cause pain in adults.
- What external factors could be causing pain? For example, is the cast too tight or is the child poorly positioned in bed?
- Are there any indicators of pain, either physiologic or behavioral?
- How is the child responding emotionally?
- How does the child or parent rate the pain?

Physiologic symptoms such as nausea, fatigue, dyspnea, bladder and bowel distention, and fever may influence the intensity of pain felt by a child. The child's behavior or responses to pain stimuli may also be affected by fear, anxiety, separation from parents, anger, culture, age, or a previous pain experience.

When working with an infant or child, determine which pain scale is the most appropriate for the circumstance and developmental stage. When using a self-report pain assessment tool, *use the same tool each time* you assess for pain or for the evaluation of pain management. This makes comparison of assessment results possible. A chronologic record of the child's pain assessments must be documented along with actions taken to relieve pain, in addition to the follow-up assessments to determine the effectiveness of those actions.

Remember that surgery and trauma can result in multiple sites of pain (incision or laceration, cut or bruised muscles, interrupted blood supply, nasogastric tube placement, insertion sites of intravenous lines). When using pain scales in the assessment of a verbal child, attempt to identify all sites of pain. Then evaluate the intensity of pain at each site.

Examples of nursing diagnoses for children in pain include the following:

- *Acute Pain (abdominal)* related to injury and surgery
- *Anxiety* related to anticipation of pain from an invasive procedure
- *Impaired Physical Mobility* related to pain
- *Nausea* related to opioid pain medication

Other nursing diagnoses are included in the nursing care plan for the child with postoperative pain.

PLANNING AND IMPLEMENTATION

Nursing management involves the following actions to increase and maintain patient comfort: pharmacologic intervention; complementary therapy; monitoring, evaluating, and documenting the effectiveness of pain-control measures to provide optimal comfort; and patient education.

PHARMACOLOGIC INTERVENTION

Give analgesics as ordered by the physician, ensuring that the dose is appropriate for the child's weight. When administering an opioid by intravenous infusion or PCA, monitor the flow rate and the site for infiltration. Follow institutional guidelines for monitoring vital signs, and use a pulse oximeter or cardiorespiratory monitor in children at risk for respiratory depression. Vital signs (heart rate and blood pressure) may not change in response to effective analgesia when infection, trauma, or other stressors keep them elevated. Make sure analgesic antagonists such as naloxone are available should complications develop. Check for the presence of other side effects of analgesics, such as sedation, nausea, vomiting, itching, urinary retention, and constipation. An alternative opioid or medications to treat the side effects may be ordered when analgesia is needed long term.

Oral NSAIDs are generally ordered for less severe pain or chronic pain. These drugs may mask fever. Be alert to the potential complication of gastrointestinal hemorrhage in critically ill children who have increased gastric acids as a physiologic stress response to pain.

Assess the child for pain 15 to 30 minutes following intravenous pain medication and 1 hour after oral pain medication to determine if adequate pain control was achieved. Evaluate the child's level of pain frequently to identify any increase in pain intensity. Use information collected from the child and parent, as well as from an appropriate pain scale. Dramatic reductions in pain should occur, although not all pain may disappear. Be certain to record results of pain-control measures to guide future nursing actions. Use a flowsheet to document assessments and medication administration during the postoperative period.

Many children sleep after receiving an analgesic. This sleep is not a side effect of the drug or a sign of an overdose, but the result of pain relief. Pain interrupts sleep, and once pain is relieved, the child can sleep comfortably. However, sleep does not always indicate pain control. A child in pain may fall asleep in exhaustion. Look for other symptoms of pain, such as excess movement or moaning.

Nursing Practice

Naloxone may be used to treat respiratory depression caused by an opioid drug at a dose and slow infusion rate that does not reverse the pain-control effects of the narcotic. A continuous infusion or repeated doses may be needed for severe overdoses.

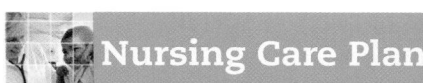

Nursing Care Plan

THE CHILD WITH POSTOPERATIVE PAIN

INTERVENTION	RATIONALE	EXPECTED OUTCOME
1. Nursing Diagnosis: Severe Abdominal Pain related to surgery and injury		
NIC Priority Intervention: **Pain management:** Alleviation of pain or a reduction in pain to a level of comfort that is acceptable to the patient		**NOC Suggested Outcome:** Comfort level: Feelings of physical and psychologic ease
Goal: The child will report relief (to a level acceptable to the child on a pain scale).		
■ Give analgesic by a pain-free method.	■ The child may deny pain to avoid analgesia by painful route.	The child reports pain relief after administration of analgesia.
■ Have the child select a pain scale and rate the amount of pain perceived before and 30–60 minutes after analgesia is given to ensure pain relief.	■ The child's pain rating is the best indicator of pain. Maintenance of pain control requires less analgesia than treating each acute pain episode.	
■ Assess pain control each hour to ensure that the child's pain is relieved.	■ Frequent monitoring identifies inadequate pain control before it becomes significant.	
■ Reposition the child every 2 hr to maintain good body alignment.	■ New positions decrease muscle cramping and skin pressure.	
■ Provide therapeutic touch or massage. Encourage the parents to read a story or play favorite music.	■ Complementary therapy reduces stress and enhances the analgesic action.	
2. Nursing Diagnosis: Disturbed Sleep Pattern related to inadequate pain control		
NIC Priority Intervention: **Sleep enhancement:** Facilitation of regular sleep/awake cycles		**NOC Suggested Outcome:** **Sleep:** Extent and pattern of sleep for mental and physical rejuvenation
Goal: The child will experience fewer disruptions of sleep by pain.		
■ Give analgesia by continuous infusion or every 3–4 hr around the clock.	■ Pain breakthrough occurs even during sleep and disturbs the healing effects of sleep.	The child's sleep is undisturbed by pain. Child sleeps for age-appropriate number of hours per day.
3. Nursing Diagnosis: Ineffective Individual Therapeutic Regimen Management related to self-management of pain control and use of nondrug pain-control measures		
NIC Priority Intervention: **Self-modification assistance:** Reinforcement of self-directed change initiated by the patient to achieve personally important goals		**NOC Suggested Outcome:** **Treatment behavior pain control:** Personal actions to palliate or eliminate pain
Goal: The child and family will effectively use patient-controlled analgesia (PCA) and complementary therapy pain-control measures.		
■ Teach the child how the PCA works and when to push the button.	■ The child must know that pain can be relieved by pushing the PCA button and how the button works.	The child's pain rating stays low.
■ Teach the family and the child how to use age-appropriate imagery, distraction, relaxation techniques, and other complementary therapy pain-control measures.	■ Complementary therapy pain-control measures reduce the amount of analgesia needed.	The child and family independently use complementary therapies for pain control.

(continued)

Nursing Care Plan—continued

THE CHILD WITH POSTOPERATIVE PAIN

INTERVENTION	RATIONALE	EXPECTED OUTCOME
Goal: The child and family will use appropriate analgesia after discharge.		
■ Discuss appropriate pain control to use at home after discharge.	■ The family and child may be anxious about pain management at home.	The family understands pain-relief measures for use at home and knows where to call if help is needed.
4. Nursing Diagnosis: Risk for Ineffective Breathing Pattern related to opioid overdose		
NIC Priority Intervention:		**NOC Suggested Outcome:**
Respiratory monitoring: Collection and analysis of patient data to ensure airway patency and adequate gas exchange		**Vital signs status:** Temperature, pulse, respirations, and blood pressure within expected range for the individual
Goal: The child will maintain adequate ventilations.		
■ Verify that correct dose of opioid analgesia is given for the child's weight.	■ Respiratory depression is a significant complication of opioid analgesia when too much analgesia is given.	There is no episode of respiratory depression associated with analgesia.
■ Monitor vital signs and depth of inspirations before analgesic is administered and at time of peak drug action.	■ Respiratory depression episode must not progress to respiratory arrest. All opioids act on brainstem center, which decreases responsiveness to CO_2 tension.	
■ Calculate agonist dose ordered by physician to be sure it will reverse respiratory depression, but not counteract effect of analgesia.	■ Valuable time will be saved if agonist is needed for episode of respiratory depression. Complete reversal of analgesia will cause the child to have significant pain.	
5. Nursing Diagnosis: Constipation related to opioid administration and decreased motility of gastrointestinal tract		
NIC Priority Intervention:		**NOC Suggested Outcome:**
Constipation management: Prevention and alleviation of constipation		**Bowel elimination:** Ability of gastrointestinal tract to form and evacuate stool effectively.
Goal: The child will have minimal constipation.		
■ Palpate the abdomen, and assess bowel sounds and abdominal distention.	■ Signs of constipation must be anticipated and identified.	The child has bowel movements at least every 2 days while on opioid pain control.
■ Request physician order for stimulating laxative and stool softener.	■ Opioids increase the transit time of feces and interfere with bile enzymes needed for evacuation.	
■ Provide fluids of choice to increase fluid intake when IV fluids are decreased.	■ Extra fluids will counteract opioid action of increasing the absorption of water from the large intestine.	
■ Inform family and child that constipation is a side effect of pain medication.	■ Parents can become partners in managing fluid intake and monitoring bowel movements.	

Become an advocate for the child when the dose or type of analgesic ordered is inadequate. When the child with severe pain has been taking opioids for several days, an increasing amount of the opioid may be needed to produce or maintain the same level of pain relief. The duration of effective analgesia becomes shorter than expected, and breakthrough pain occurs. Review the child's record to verify that the opioid was given at the appropriate dose and frequency before asking the physician to modify the child's pain medication.

Thinking Critically

DETERMINING WHEN A CHILD IS IN PAIN

Felicia, who is 5 years old, was struck by a car. Six hours ago, she had surgery to repair a liver laceration, but she also has numerous bruises and abrasions on her body. After spending 3 hours in the postanesthesia unit, she was moved to the pediatric inpatient unit. She has an intravenous line in place, as well as a nasogastric tube attached to low suction. Her abdominal dressing is clean and dry. Felicia has orders for morphine IV every 3 hours around the clock for the first 24 hours.

Felicia's mother is rooming in with her during her hospital stay. Twelve hours after surgery, Felicia is dozing but is responsive to verbal stimuli. Her most recent IV morphine was given 2 hours ago. The nurse attempts to determine how well Felicia's pain is managed. Her facial expression indicates that she is not in pain. Felicia's mother feels that she is resting comfortably.

How do you know whether Felicia is in pain? Can you expect her to tell you if she feels pain? What other pain relief measures could reduce or help to control her pain in the first 24 hours? What is the appropriate dose of IV morphine for Felicia, who weighs 25 kg? What is the timing of assessments of response to pain and potential side effects? What signs of respiratory distress indicate a need for naloxone administration?

See MyNursingKit for possible responses.

Evidence-Based Nursing

CHALLENGES TO ADEQUATE PAIN MANAGEMENT

Clinical Question

Why does adequate management of children with acute pain continue to be a problem despite the increased knowledge about children's needs for pain relief?

Evidence

In the past decade, numerous studies have reported that many children reporting moderate to severe levels of pain were undermedicated. A study conducted in 10 NICUs investigated the pain assessment and management of 250 neonates. Surgery or painful procedures were performed on 96% of the neonates during the 72-hour study period. Wide variability in pain assessment and management was noted in these NICUs. Nurses documented a numeric pain assessment in 88% of neonates while physicians and neonatal nurse practitioners documented a pain assessment for only 36% of the neonates. Study findings revealed the best predictor of neonatal pain management in the 72 hours after surgery was physician pain assessment. In actual practice after major surgery, 84% of neonates received opioids and 35% received nonopioid analgesia, but 7% of neonates received no analgesia. After minor surgery 60% received opioids, 60% received nonopioid analgesia, but 12% received no analgesia (Taylor, Robbins, Gold, et al., 2008).

A university hospital planned a 4-phase organizational change to improve pain management for children by targeting nurse and physician knowledge, attitudes, beliefs, and behaviors. Interventions included an attitude survey, education on individualizing interventions to individual children, nonpharmacologic pain management strategies, interdisciplinary patient care rounds, development of interdisciplinary pain management plans, changing policy to allow nurses to give IV morphine, and to have the anesthesiologist write all pediatric postoperative pain orders. Results demonstrated a progressive increase in pediatric pain assessments, increased doses of pain medication administered, and increased documentation of treatment effectiveness. Nurses valued their role in the decision-making process (Jordan-Marsh, Hubbard, Watson, et al., 2004).

Best Practices

The hospital environment is as important as individual nursing decisions to provide adequate pain management for children. Pediatric nurses need to know how to assess pain in children of all ages, how to select and administer pain medication, and how to use complementary therapies to enhance pain management. Serious gaps in knowledge were found when nursing students were surveyed about their knowledge of pain management (Plaisance & Logan, 2006). A supportive hospital environment is important in helping nursing graduates to complete their learning and to set expectations for the pain management of children.

Critical Thinking

In the clinical setting, identify the infrastructure supports to promote pain management of children, such as pain assessment tools, pain flow sheets, pain management policies and guidelines, educational opportunities, and resources for complementary therapies. Identify additional supports that would help you as an inexperienced nurse to gain competence in pediatric pain management.

See MyNursingKit for possible responses.

COMPLEMENTARY THERAPY

Complementary therapies are the nonpharmacologic methods of pain control that can be used with or without analgesics. One or more of these methods may provide adequate relief of low levels of pain. When used with analgesics, nonpharmacologic techniques often increase the effectiveness of the analgesic or reduce the dosage required. See the "Complementary Therapies for Pain Management" on page 1115. See the "Teaching Highlights: Helping a Child Cope with Pain," to help parents participate in complementary therapies for their child.

Teaching Highlights

HELPING A CHILD COPE WITH PAIN

Parents provide security and help reduce the child's anxiety associated with pain and hospitalization. Children often feel more secure telling their parents about their pain and anxiety. When parents are actively participating in the child's care during hospitalization, teach them about how complementary therapies can be used to enhance the child's pain management. Help the parent select the age-appropriate complementary therapy for the child:

- Infants: holding, cuddling, sucking a pacifier, massage
- Toddlers: massage, stories, bubbles, touch, holding and rocking, music (Figure 42-5 ●)
- Preschoolers: engaging in play, stories, music, imagining being a superhero, watching television or a video
- School-age children: rhythmic breathing, muscle relaxation, guided imagery, talking about pleasant experiences, playing games, listening to radio, watching television or a video
- Adolescents: rhythmic breathing, muscle relaxation, guided imagery, having visitors, playing games, watching television, listening to radio or CD player

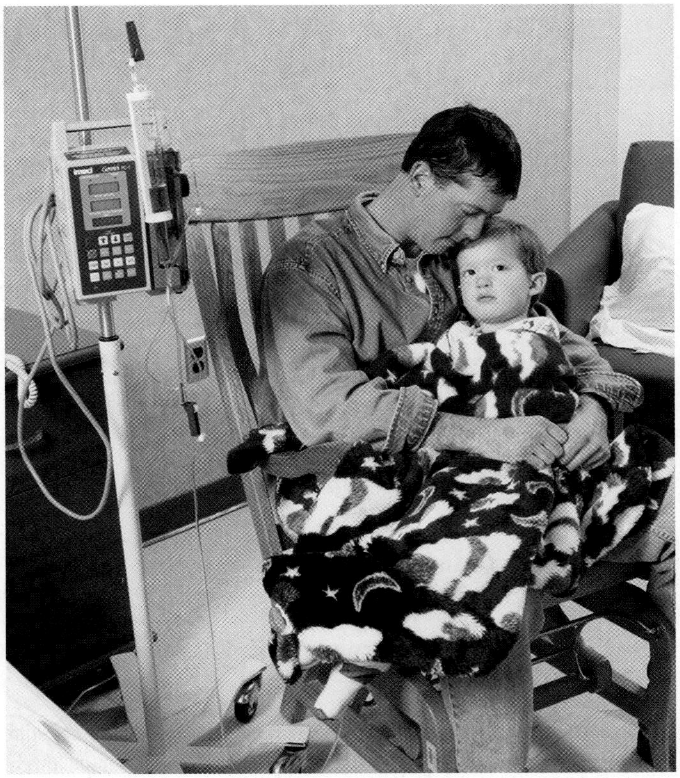

● **Figure 42–5** Parent's role in pain management. The presence of the parent is an important part of pain management. Children often feel more secure telling their parents about their pain and anxiety.

MEASURES TO INCREASE COMFORT DURING PAINFUL PROCEDURES

Make every effort to increase the child's comfort during painful procedures. Topical anesthetics can be used to reduce the pain associated with an immunization, other injection, intravenous insertion, or venipuncture, or the first needle stick of another procedure. Give time for the medication to become effective. Mechanisms for administration of topical anesthetics include the following:

- Vapocoolant sprays can be used for injections.
- EMLA (eutectic mixture of local anesthetics) cream, an emulsion of 2.5% lidocaine and 2.5% prilocaine, is effective if applied 1 to 2 hours before a needle stick procedure on intact skin in children and infants as young as 3 months of age (Weise & Nahata, 2005). See Figure 42–6 ●.
- L-M-X4, 4%, liposomal lidocaine (formerly called ELA-MAX), is effective if applied 30 minutes before needle stick (Fein & Gorelick, 2006).
- With iontophoresis, a patch containing 10% lidocaine hydrochloride and 0.1% epinephrine is placed over the site of the planned needle stick, and a small machine generates electric current to transport anesthetic into the skin. In about 10 minutes anesthesia reaches a depth of about 10.7 mm (Pasero, 2006).
- The Synera anesthetic patch, containing 70 mg of lidocaine and 70 mg of tetracaine, can be applied for 20 to 30 minutes prior to a procedure to anesthetize the skin for superficial venous access and dermatologic procedures in children older than 3 years (Endo Pharmaceuticals, 2006).
- LET (lidocaine, epinephrine, and tetracaine) is a topical anesthetic for laceration repair. The LET liquid is applied to a cotton ball and taped to the skin and the LET gel is applied to the skin and covered with an occlusive dressing. The anesthetic works in 20 to 30 minutes (Hatfield, Messner, & Lingg, 2006).

A local anesthetic such as lidocaine buffered by sodium bicarbonate or bupivacaine is often injected subcutaneously to provide analgesia for emergent invasive procedures.

Assemble a pain management kit to promote distraction, imagery, and relaxation in children. Include items such as magic wands, pinwheels, bubble liquid, a slinky spring toy, a foam ball, party noisemakers, and pop-up books. It may also be helpful to include items for therapeutic play such as syringes, adhesive bandages, alcohol swabs, and other supplies from a medical kit. The pain management kit may be especially helpful for distracting children who are being prepared for medical procedures.

DISCHARGE PLANNING AND HOME CARE TEACHING

Children are frequently discharged from the hospital with oral analgesics following surgery, injury, or treatment of acute medical conditions. The child usually leaves the hospital or surgical center pain-free, and the parents may not anticipate pain. Provide information about the child's need for pain medication

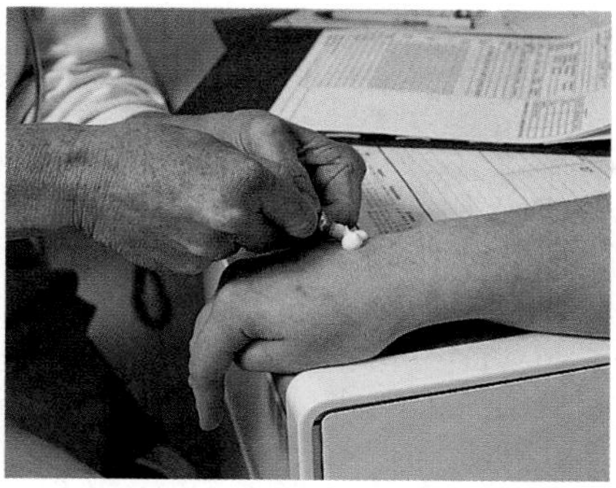

A

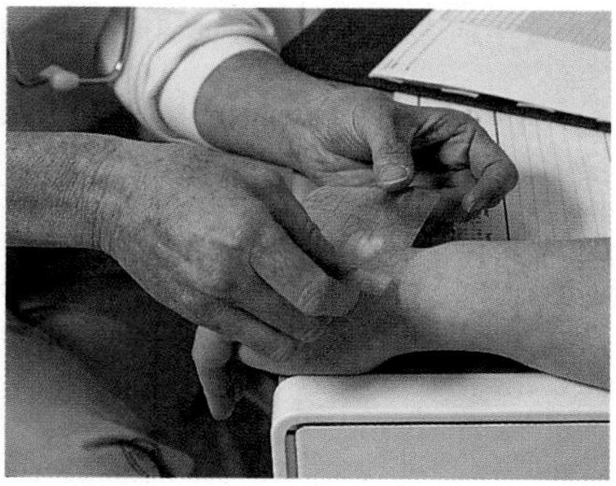

B

● **Figure 42–6** Technique for applying EMLA cream. When painful procedures are planned, use EMLA cream to anesthetize the skin where the painful stick will be made. ***A***, Apply a thick layer of cream over intact skin (one half of a 5-g tube). ***B***, Cover the cream with a transparent adhesive dressing, sealing all the sides. The cream anesthetizes the dermal surface in 45 to 60 minutes.

around the clock for the first 1 to 2 days to prevent the child from feeling pain, and the benefits of pain management in promoting the child's healing.

Provide guidance to help parents assess their child's pain, and for school-age children and adolescents to assess their own pain. Teach parents and children about the dosage and frequency of administration and the side effects of the analgesic ordered. Review complementary therapies and encourage children and parents to use the techniques that work best for them.

Remember that many common health problems (otitis media, pharyngitis, and urinary tract infection) have pain as one of the presenting symptoms. Often the only medication prescribed is an antibiotic to clear the infection. This may leave the child in pain for 48 to 72 hours until the antibiotic brings the infection under control. Give parents recommendations for pain control and comfort measures during this period. Review the dose, dosing device, and formulation of acetaminophen used by parents to identify any risk for overdose. See page 1224.

EVALUATION

Expected outcomes of nursing care include the following:

- The child's pain level is assessed frequently and pain management is effective in improving the child's comfort.
- The child successfully uses a PCA pump to control acute pain.
- Age-appropriate complementary therapies enhance the comfort provided by medications.
- Parents maintain the child's pain management after discharge.

CHRONIC PAIN

Some children have medical conditions that cause chronic pain and episodic acute pain, such as rheumatoid arthritis, cancer, headaches, recurrent abdominal pain, and HIV infection. Children and adolescents have reported that chronic and recurrent pain has an impact on the quality of their life and restricts daily living activities such as school attendance, sleep, appetite, social interactions, and recreation (Roth-Isigkeit, Theyen, Stöven, et al., 2005).

CLINICAL MANIFESTATIONS

Physical and psychologic signs and symptoms should be viewed together. The child may perceive pain but not appear to be in pain. Chronic pain of long duration that is persistent or continuous permits physiologic adaptation so normal heart rate, respiratory rate, and blood pressure levels are often seen (Huether & Defriez, 2006). Behavioral indicators of chronic pain may include inactivity, posturing, depression, and difficulty concentrating and sleeping. Chronic pain may be associated with vague and nonspecific symptoms without an easily identifiable cause.

CLINICAL THERAPY

No tools have been developed to assess chronic pain for any child age group. It may be valuable to use multiple tools to assess pain, including a body outline where all pain sites can be marked, a self-report pain scale, and a list of words that describe pain characteristics.

Children with chronic pain need an individualized pain treatment plan with a primary focus on improved function and comfort. Analgesic medications are prescribed, including NSAIDs, acetaminophen, and opioids, often in combination. Complete pain relief may not be possible, and the child may need additional pain medication for acute flare-ups of their condition. Tricyclic antidepressants may be prescribed for their analgesic properties and because depression may be a co-existing condition. Gabapentin, an anti-seizure medication, has efficacy in treating neuropathic pain (Hollan, 2007). Exercise and physical therapy are important to help promote improved function. Complementary therapies are also used.

Nursing Management

When assessing chronic pain in the child, approach pain as if it is the primary problem for attention. View the physical, behavioral, and psychological signs and symptoms together.

- Obtain the history of pain onset, its development over time, intensity, duration, location, what makes it worse or relieves it, and its impact on daily life (sleeping, appetite, school, and social interactions).
- Identify past and other current pain problems in the family. The child may have some learned pain behaviors, such as using pain for attention.

- Identify how much distress the child and family experience with pain, including anxiety, depression, and hopelessness.
- Determine what the family and child believe causes the pain, their response to it, and current methods to treat the pain, including complementary therapies.
- Observe the child's appearance, posture, gait, emotional, and cognitive state. Perform a complete neurologic examination. Assess muscle spasms, trigger points, and areas sensitive to light touch (American Pain Society, 2003).

Monitor pain intensity at each office visit and frequently during hospitalizations. Encourage older school-age children and adolescents with recurrent episodes to keep a pain diary to describe the characteristics, timing, activities, and potential triggers of their pain, as well as their response to pain treatment measures. A pain assessment scale should be used to rate the pain intensity before and after medications and other pain-control measures are used. This record can help improve pain management.

Work with the physician or pain management team to individualize the pain management plan to meet the child's needs, family's beliefs and values, and their cultural preferences for care. Assist the child and family to identify age-appropriate and acceptable complementary therapies to help cope with discomfort. Encourage daily exercise to promote function.

Work with the family to proactively manage constipation when the child takes opioids for pain. Constipation is a side effect that does not improve over time (Anghelescu, Oakes, & Hinds, 2006). Fluids and fiber should be added to the diet, and the child should also take a stimulating laxative and potentially a stool softener.

SEDATION AND PAIN MANAGEMENT FOR MEDICAL PROCEDURES

Children undergo a wide variety of painful diagnostic and treatment procedures in the hospital and in outpatient settings. Procedures such as chest tube insertion, arterial puncture, lumbar puncture, bone marrow aspiration, fracture reduction, laceration repair, insertion of a central or peripheral intravenous line, and burn debridement cause significant pain in children. The anticipation of these procedures causes anxiety and emotional distress that can lead to greater pain intensity. Children who have previously experienced severe pain may be unwilling to cooperate with healthcare personnel (Young, 2005).

CLINICAL THERAPY

Sedation

Sedation is a medically controlled state of depressed consciousness used for painful diagnostic and therapeutic procedures. **Anxiolysis** is minimal sedation in which cognitive and motor functions may be impaired. **Moderate sedation** (formerly called conscious sedation) occurs with lower doses of sedatives and enables the child to maintain protective reflexes independently, continuously maintain a patent airway, and make an appropriate response to physical stimuli or verbal command. **Deep sedation** is a controlled state of depressed consciousness or unconsciousness in which protective airway reflexes are lost, but the child can respond to painful stimuli. Ventilation is affected in deep sedation (Doyle & Collett, 2006). See Table 42–7. Sedation may be used alone for nonpainful procedures such as a radiographic study. Analgesia must be given in association with sedation for invasive procedures as the sedated child can still feel pain but cannot communicate its presence.

Drugs for sedation include the following (Boswinkel & Litman, 2005):

- Benzodiazepines: diazepam (Valium), midazolam (Versed), and lorazepam (Ativan)
- Hypnotics or barbiturates: thiopental, pentobarbital, methohexital
- Ketamine
- Propofol (Diprivan) or Etomidate
- Analgesics: Fentanyl, Alfentanil

Every healthcare facility should have guidelines for the use of sedation to ensure safe healthcare practices. Health professionals monitoring the child should have specific qualifications, such as training in pediatric advanced life support. The child must be carefully monitored for respiratory depression and signs of deep sedation, so the airway can be protected and ventilatory support can be provided if needed. Antagonist agents must be available for opioids and benzodiazepines when the effects of sedation and respiratory depression need to be reversed (Coté, 2005).

Table 42–7 Characteristics of Minimal, Moderate, and Deep Sedation

Assessment Factors	Minimal Sedation	Moderate Sedation	Deep Sedation
Airway	Maintains airway independently and continuously	Maintains airway independently and continuously	Unable to maintain airway
Cough and gag reflexes	Reflexes intact	Reflexes intact	Partial or complete loss of reflexes
Level of consciousness	Responds to verbal stimuli	Easily aroused with verbal or gentle physical stimulation	Not easily aroused, responds to repeated or painful stimuli

Source: Adapted from: Doyle, L., & Colletti, J. E. (2006). Pediatric procedural sedation and analgesia. *Pediatric Clinics of North America, 53*, 279–292.

Nursing Practice

Whenever sedation is given, be prepared to monitor the child's vital signs and provide advanced life support if the child should progress to deep sedation. The following equipment should be immediately available: suction apparatus, a bag-valve mask for assisted ventilation with capability of 90% to 100% oxygen delivery, and an oxygen supply (5 L/min for more than 60 minutes). Antagonists to sedative medication must be premeasured and ready to administer.

Nursing Management

When the child receives sedation, nursing assessments to monitor the child's status include visual confirmation of respiratory effort, color, and vital signs. Pulse oximetry and other technology may be used for monitoring, but the equipment must not replace visual assessment. Vital signs must be checked every 15 minutes until the child regains full consciousness and level of functioning. If light sedation progresses to deep sedation, maintain a patent airway, and check vital signs every 5 minutes.

Criteria for discharging the child after sedation include the following:

- Satisfactory and stable cardiovascular function and airway patency.
- Easily arousable, with protective reflexes intact.
- Adequate hydration.
- Able to stand and walk without assistance, or the infant holds the head up and sits up unassisted if old enough to do so.
- Discharge status is the same as admission status.

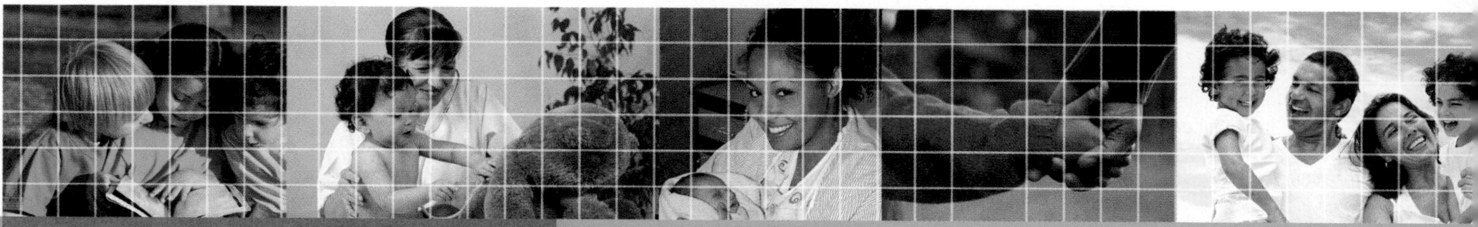

CRITICAL CONCEPT REVIEW

LEARNING OUTCOMES	CONCEPTS
42.1 Identify the physiologic and behavioral consequences of pain in children.	1. Physiologic consequences of acute pain: ■ Tachycardia and rapid shallow breathing. ■ Inadequate cough. ■ Inadequate lung expansion. ■ Depressed immune response. ■ Increased perspiration and loss of electrolytes and fluids. ■ Increased intestinal secretions. 2. Behavioral consequences of acute pain: ■ Short attention span. ■ Irritability. ■ Facial grimacing. ■ Posturing, protecting painful area, immobility. ■ Lethargy or withdrawal. ■ Sleep disturbance.
42.2 Assess the developmental abilities of preschool children to perform a self-assessment of pain intensity.	1. An understanding of more and less. 2. Identifying a number larger than another. 3. Placing pieces of paper of different sizes in sequential order by size.
42.3 Describe the nursing assessment and management for a child receiving an opioid analgesic.	1. Use oral and intravenous route, if possible. 2. Identify the time of peak drug effect and monitor child's vital signs to detect respiratory depression. 3. Observe for nausea, constipation, and itching. 4. Have naloxone (Narcan) available for treatment of respiratory distress.
42.4 Explain the physiology that enables nonpharmacologic (complementary) methods of pain control to be effective.	Nonpharmacologic methods of pain control are effective in children due to the Gate Control Theory and decrease the transmission of pain impulses to the brain. The use of methods such as nonpainful touch and massage stimulate the larger A-delta fibers and cause the substantia gelatinosa in the dorsal horn of the spinal cord to "close the gate." Nonpharmacologic methods compete with the transmission of pain impulses to the brain.

(continued)

LEARNING OUTCOMES / CONCEPTS

Learning Outcomes	Concepts
42.5 Assess children of different ages with acute pain and develop a nursing care plan that integrates pharmacologic interventions and developmentally appropriate nonpharmacologic (complementary) therapies.	Interventions common to all ages: 1. Assess pain frequently. 2. Anticipate need for pain medication. 3. Monitor vital signs. Pharmacologic and nonpharmacologic interventions by age group: 1. Infants and toddlers: ■ Administer oral or intravenous medications around the clock. ■ Hold, swaddle, rock, or provide nonnutritive sucking. ■ Allow infant to suck sucrose solution. ■ Have toddler blow bubbles. 2. Preschooler: ■ Use distraction techniques such as a magic wand, pinwheel, or noise maker. ■ Allow child to watch appropriate TV shows or videos. 3. School-age child and adolescent: ■ Instruct in use of PCA or epidural until able to take oral medications. ■ Use hypnotherapy if child is able to cooperate. ■ Engage child in breathing techniques for relaxation. ■ Use guided imagery, visitors, TV, radio, tapes, or CDs for distraction.
42.6 Develop a nursing care plan for assessing and monitoring the child having sedation and analgesia for a medical procedure.	1. Explain procedure to the child and parents. 2. Employ nonpharmacologic methods such as distraction and guided imagery to decrease anxiety. 3. Ensure that emergency equipment and agonist medications are available. 4. Monitor the depth of sedation during the procedure; be prepared to open the child's airway and assist ventilations if deep sedation occurs. 5. Use pulse oximetry and a cardiorespiratory monitor during procedure; visually monitor vital signs. 6. After procedure is completed, visually monitor vital signs and level of consciousness until child is stable and awake.

CRITICAL THINKING IN ACTION

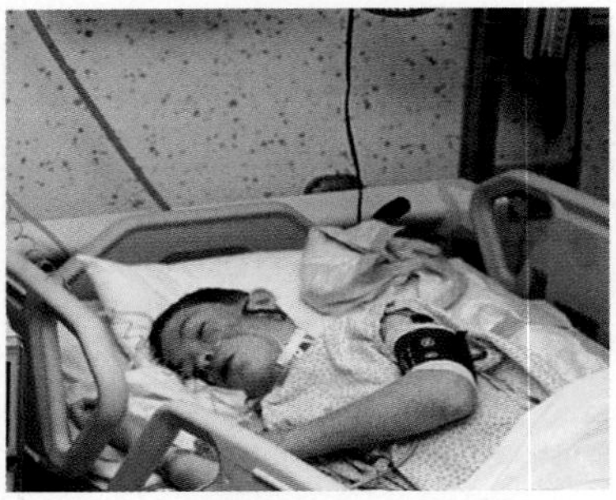

A 12-year-old boy, Kevin, is recovering from a 4-wheeler crash at a local children's hospital. He was riding the 4-wheeler unsupervised and without permission while his parents were at work. He suffered three broken bones, several lacerations, and an abdominal injury that required surgery. His parents are very worried about his injuries and at the same time angry with him for not following the rules. Kevin appears expressionless in his hospital bed, but cries and grimaces at any slight movement. When asked on a scale of 1–10 (10 being the most pain) how much pain he is feeling, he says a 10. His parents are reluctant to let him have any pain medications because they fear he may become dependent on the medication. His father states that Kevin should be a man and tolerate the pain, and he thinks enduring the pain will teach him a lesson about responsibility. The nurse explains that pain management is necessary to improve Kevin's healing, help him mobilize sooner, and potentially shorten his hospital stay. She explains the physiologic consequences of ineffective pain management and discusses how the medication will help him sleep and rest. She explains that some of the pain medications can be addicting, but the chances of Kevin becoming addicted to pain medications for this injury are extremely rare. She also reviews the nonpharmacological methods of relieving pain. The parents are still reluctant to the medications, but agree to conform to the doctor's orders.

1. What are some of the potential physiological consequences to letting Kevin suffer pain?
2. What are some examples of opioid analgesics appropriate for Kevin?
3. What are some examples of NSAIDs available to Kevin?
4. What are the signs of tolerance to the prescribed opioid?

See MyNursingKit for possible responses.

REFERENCES

American Pain Society. (2008). *Principles of analgesic use in the treatment of acute pain and cancer pain* (6th ed.). Glenview, IL: Author.

American Pain Society. (2003). *Pediatric chronic pain: A position statement from the American Pain Society*. Retrieved October 22, 2003, from www.ampainsoc.org/cgi-bin/print/print/pl

American Pain Society. (2005). *Guidelines for the management of cancer pain in adults and children*. Glenview, IL: Author.

Anghelescu, D., Oakes, L., & Hinds, P. S. (2006). Palliative care and pediatrics. *Anesthesiology Clinics of North America, 24*, 145–161.

Anthony, K. K., & Schanberg, L. E. (2005). Pediatric pain syndromes and management of pain in children and adolescents with rheumatic disease. *Pediatric Clinics of North America, 52*, 611–639.

Boswinkel, J. P., & Litman, R. S. (2005). The pharmacology of sedation. *Pediatric Annals, 34*(8), 607–611.

Brislin, R. P., & Rose, J. B. (2005). Pediatric acute pain management. *Anesthesiology Clinics of North America, 23*, 789–814.

Coté, C. J. (2005). Strategies for preventing sedation accidents. *Pediatric Annals, 34*(8), 625–633.

Das, D. A., Grimmer, K. A., Sparnon, A. L., McRae, S. E., Thomas, B. H. (2005). The efficacy of playing a virtual reality game in modulating pain for children with acute burn injuries: A randomized controlled trial. *BMC Pediatrics, 5*(1). Retrieved July 25, 2007, from *http://www.biomedcentral.com/1471-2431/5/1*

Deyo, K. S., Prkachin, K. M., & Mercer, S. R. (2004). Development of sensitivity to facial expression of pain. *Pain, 107*, 16–21.

Doyle, L., & Colletti, J. E. (2006). Pediatric procedural sedation and analgesia. *Pediatric Clinics of North America, 53*, 279–292.

Endo Pharmaceuticals Inc. (2006). Synera prescribing information. Chadds Ford, PA: Author.

Fein, J. A., & Gorelick, M. H. (2006). The decision to use topical anesthetic for intravenous insertion in the pediatric emergency department. *Academic Emergency Medicine, 13*(3), 264–268.

Greco, C., & Berde, C. (2005). Pain management for the hospitalized pediatric patient. *Pediatric Clinics of North America, 52*(4), 995–1027.

Green, R., Bulloch, B., Kabani, A., Hancock, B. J., & Tenenbein, M. (2005). Early analgesia for children with acute abdominal pain. *Pediatrics, 116*(4), 978–983.

Hatfield, L., Messner, E. R., & Lingg, K. (2006). Evidence-based strategies for the pharmacological management of pediatric pain during minor procedures in the emergency department. *Topics in Emergency Medicine, 28*(2), 129–137.

Hollan, M. (2007). A practical way to manage chronic pain. *Clinical Advisor, 10*(1), 51–59.

Huang, C., Tung, W., Kuo, L., & Chang, Y. (2004). Comparison of pain responses of premature infants to the heelstick between containment and swaddling. *Journal of Nursing Research, 12*(1), 31–40.

Huether, S. E., & Defriez, C. B. (2006). Pain, temperature regulation, sleep, and sensory function. In K. L. McCance & S. E. Huether (Eds.), *Pathophysiology: The biologic basis for disease in adults and children* (5th ed., pp. 447–462). St. Louis: Mosby–Year Book.

Huth, M. M., Van Kuiken, D. M., & Broome, M. E. (2006). Playing in the park: What school-age children tell us about imagery. *Journal of Pediatric Nursing, 21*(2), 115–125.

Joint Commission. (2008). *Health care issues.* Retrieved November 25, 2008, from *http://www.jointcommission.org/NewsRoom/health_care_issues.htm#9*

Jordan-Marsh, M., Hubbard, J., Watson, R., Hall, R. D., Miller, P., & Mohan, O. (2004). The social ecology of changing pain management: Do I need to cry? *Journal of Pediatric Nursing, 19*(3), 193–203.

Kokki, H., Lintula, H., Vanamo, K., Heiskanen, J., & Eskelinen, M. (2005, April). Oxycodone vs placebo in children with undifferentiated abdominal pain. *Archives of Pediatric and Adolescent Medicine, 159*, 320–325.

Kundu, A., & Berman, B. (2007). Acupuncture for pediatric pain and symptom management. *Pediatric Clinics of North America, 53*, 885–899.

Manworren, R. C. B., & Hynan, L. S. (2003). Clinical validation of FLACC: Preverbal patient pain scale. *Pediatric Nursing, 29*(2), 140–146.

McCance, K. L., Forshee, B. A., & Shelby, J. (2006). Stress and disease. In K. L. McCance & S. E. Huether (Eds.), *Pathophysiology: The biologic basis for disease in adults and children* (5th ed., pp. 447–462), St. Louis: Elsevier Mosby

Merkel, S. I., Voepel-Lewis, T., Shayevitz, J. R., & Malviya, S. (1997). The FLACC: A behavioral scale for scoring post-operative pain in young children. *Pediatric Nursing, 23*(3), 293–297.

Mitchell, A., & Boss, B. J. (2002). Adverse effects of pain on the nervous systems of newborns and young children: A review of the literature. *Journal of Neuroscience Nursing, 34*(5), 228–236.

Morash, D., & Fowler, K. (2004). An evidence-based approach to changing practice: Using sucrose for infant analgesia. *Journal of Pediatric Nursing, 19*(5), 366–370.

National Reyes Syndrome Foundation. (2005). What is the role of aspirin, retrieved March 1, 2008, from *http://www.reyessyndrome.org/aspirin.htm*

O'Rourke, D. (2004). The measurement of pain in infants, children and adolescents: From policy to practice. *Physical Therapy, 84*(6), 560–570.

Pasero, C. (2006). Lidocaine iontophoresis for dermal procedure analgesia. *Journal of PeriAnesthesia Nursing, 21*(1), 48–52.

Plaisance, L., & Logan, C. (2006). Nursing students' knowledge and attitudes regarding pain. *Pain Management Nursing, 7*(4), 167–175.

Richardson, J., Smith, J. E., McCall, G., Pilkington, K. (2006). Hypnosis for procedure-related pain and distress in pediatric cancer patients: A systematic review of effectiveness and methodology related to hypnosis interventions. *Journal of Pain and Symptom Management, 31*(1), 70–84.

Roth-Isigkeit, A., Theyen, U., Stöven, H., Schwarzenberger, J., & Schmucker, P. (2005). Pain among children and adolescents: Restrictions in daily living and triggering factors, *Pediatrics, 115*(2), e152–e162.

Stanford, E. A., Chambers, C. T., & Craig, K. D. (2005). A normative analysis of the development of pain-related vocabulary in children. *Pain, 114*, 278–284.

Stevens, B., McGrath, P., Yamada, J., Gibbins, S., Beyene, J., et al. (2006). Identification of pain indicators for infants at risk for neurological impairment: A Delphi consensus study. *BMC Pediatrics, 6*(1). Retrieved July 25, 2007, from *http://www.bioimedcentral.com/147-2431/6/1*

Taylor, B. J., Robbins, J. M., Gold, J. I., Logsdon, T., R., Bird, T. M., & Anand, K. J. S. (2006). Assessing postoperative pain in neonates: A multicenter observational study, *Pediatrics, 118*(4), e992–e1000.

Voepel-Lewis, T., Malviya, S., & Tait, A. (2005). Validity of parent ratings as proxy measures of pain in children with cognitive impairment, *Pain Management Nursing, 16*(4), 168–174.

Von Baeyer, C. L., Marche, T. A., Rocha, E. M., & Salmon, K. (2004). Children's memory for pain: Overview and implications for practice. *Journal of Pain, 5*(5), 241–249.

Walden, M. (2007). Pain in the newborn and infant. In C. Kenner & J. W. Lott, *Comprehensive neonatal nursing: An interdisciplinary approach*, (4th ed., pp. 360–371), Philadelphia: Elsevier Saunders.

Weise, K. L., & Nahata, M. C. (2005). EMLA for painful procedures in infants. *Journal of Pediatric Health Care, 19*(10), 42–47.

Willis, M. H. W., Merkel, S. I., Voepel-Lewis, T., & Malviya, S. (2003). FLACC behavioral pain assessment scale: A comparison with the child's self-report. *Pediatric Nursing, 29*(3), 195–198.

Wilson, B. A., Shannon, M. T., & Shields, K. M. (2009). *Prentice Hall nurse's drug guide.* Upper Saddle River, NJ: Prentice Hall.

Young, K. D. (2005). Pediatric procedural pain. *Annals of Emergency Medicine, 45*(2), 160–171.

Zempsky, W. T., Cravero, J. P., and the Committee on Pediatric Emergency Medicine and Section on Anesthesiology and Pain Medicine. (2004). Relief of pain and anxiety in the pediatric patients in emergency medical systems. *Pediatrics, 114*(5), 1348–1356.

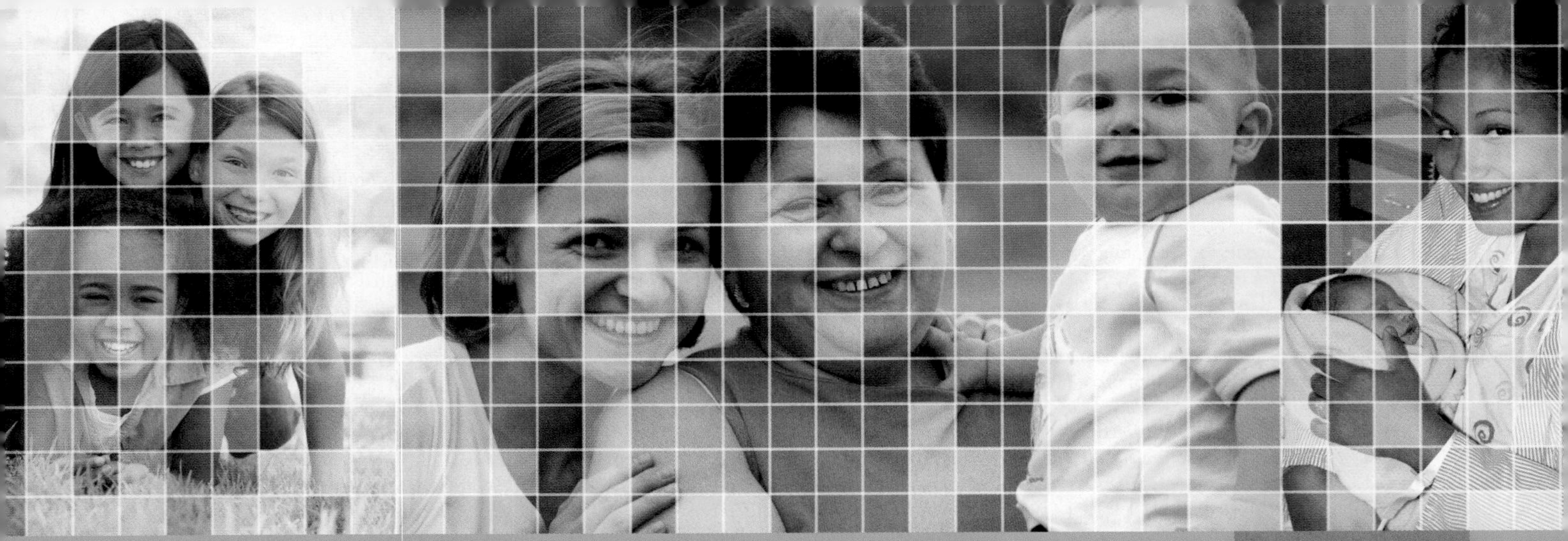

CHAPTER

43 The Child with a Life-Threatening Condition and End-of-Life Care

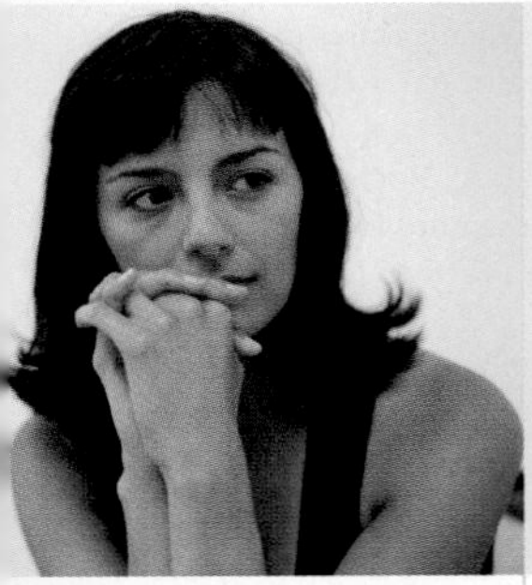

It all happened so fast. No one saw the car coming. Next thing I knew, we were in the emergency room talking about abdominal and head injuries. Now Alexa is in the intensive care unit, and I'm worried because she is still unconscious and on a ventilator. It was helpful for the nurse to tell me that even though Alexa couldn't respond it was good to talk to her, because she will probably hear me and be comforted. —Mother of Alexa, 6 years old

LEARNING OUTCOMES

43.1 Describe the child's experiences with life-threatening illness or injury according to developmental level.

43.2 Discuss the family's experience and reactions to having a child with a life-threatening illness or injury.

43.3 Describe the coping mechanisms used by the child and family in response to stress.

43.4 Develop a nursing care plan for the child with a life-threatening illness or injury.

43.5 Apply assessment skills to identify the physiologic changes that occur in the dying child.

43.6 Develop a nursing care plan to provide family-centered care for the dying child and family.

43.7 Implement strategies for bereavement support of the parents and siblings after the death of a child.

43.8 Describe strategies to support nurses who care for children who die.

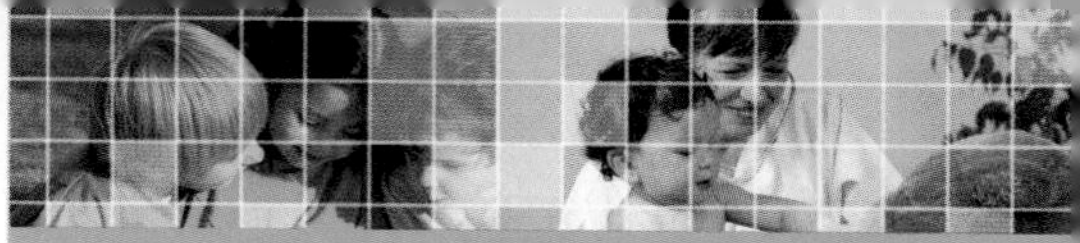

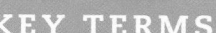

KEY TERMS

Air hunger, 1141
Brain death, 1138
Coping, 1128
Death anxiety, 1140
Death imagery, 1142
Family crisis, 1132
Life-threatening condition, 1127
Hospice care, 1137
Palliative care, 1137
Regression, 1128
Repression, 1128
Support systems, 1128

The intense emotional and physical demands placed on the critically ill or injured child present a challenge to nurses' attempts to provide developmentally appropriate care. The child's parents and siblings are confronted with a stressful situation. A family-centered model of nursing practice offers a framework for performing interventions that help to minimize stress and enhance coping by the ill or injured child, parents, and siblings.

LIFE-THREATENING ILLNESS OR INJURY

A **life-threatening condition** is one in which there is a considerable likelihood of death even though treatment may prolong the child's life or the child may have a complete recovery from the illness or injury (Institute of Medicine, 2003a; Watters, Sayre, Silbergleit, 2005). A threat to a child's life may be expected, as in a chronic illness or progressive disabling disease. More often the death is unexpected due to an unintentional injury, the leading cause of death in children, or an acute illness. How children, parents, and siblings cope with the threat will depend on the anticipated or unanticipated nature of the event and the conditions surrounding the child's admission to the hospital.

When death results from a chronic disease or terminal illness, the child and family have time to adjust to episodes of life-threatening crisis and impending death. Parents can become involved in the child's therapy as integral members of the treatment team. Emergency admission for an acute illness or unintentional injury, in contrast, brings with it sudden stressors as the child and family are thrust into an unfamiliar environment, confronted with frightening or invasive procedures, and faced with an uncertain outcome.

Nursing care of children and families coping with specific chronic diseases or terminal illnesses such as cancer, cystic fibrosis, or muscular dystrophy is discussed elsewhere in this book. The following discussion focuses on care of children with life-threatening illnesses or injuries and care of the dying child.

CHILD'S EXPERIENCE

Admission to the hospital, emergency department, or pediatric intensive care unit (PICU) is one of the most frightening experiences a child can have. The critically ill child may appear extremely anxious and fearful, or withdrawn, solemn, and preoccupied with his or her physical condition. The illness or injury often brings pain, decreased energy, and changes the child's level of consciousness.

Young children admitted to the PICU may be unable to understand what is happening to them. The PICU environment appears overwhelming, fast paced, and frightening. The child's normal sleep patterns can be disrupted because of the lack of day–night patterns in many intensive care units (Figure 43–1 ●). Being cared for by strangers contributes to the child's anxiety. The child's limited ability to move intensifies feelings of powerlessness and vulnerability.

Children's responses to stress are influenced by their developmental levels, past experiences, types of illness, coping mechanisms, and available emotional support. Nurses must consider how the child's developmental level and coping skills will influence his or her ability to deal with the emergency department or PICU experience. Successful coping can provide the child with the skills to handle difficult situations in the future.

An emergency admission places the child at emotional risk due to the lack of preparation for the experience, the uncertainty and unpredictability of events that follow, the unfamiliarity of the environment, and the heightened anxiety of parents. An admission for exacerbation of a disease such as cystic fibrosis or leukemia can provoke feelings of depression or hopelessness. Chapter 41 describes the stressors and responses to hospitalization of children by age group.

The child cared for in the PICU will experience the same stressors as any child who is hospitalized, but children in the PICU are likely to be at greater risk for short- and long-term psychological and behavioral problems (Board, 2005). These children

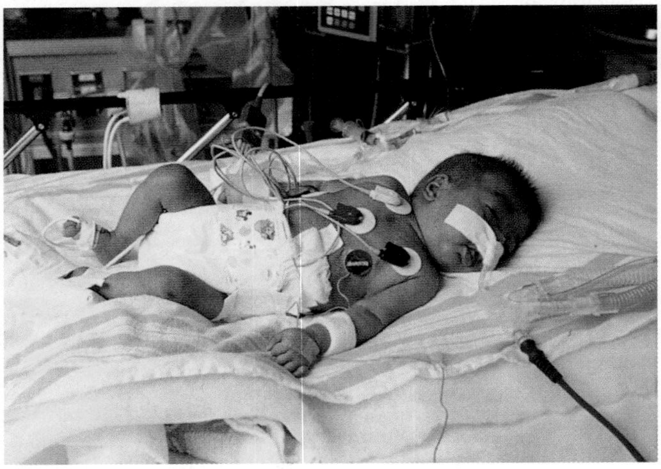

● **Figure 43–1** Child's experience of hospitalization. Jooti feels pain, hears noises, has her sleep disrupted, and has limited mobility because of all the equipment attached to her.

are sicker and experience more invasive procedures. They are restricted to their bed and attached to equipment and monitors associated with their care. However, they are also more often treated with sedation and analgesia, and this may lessen memories of stressful experiences (Board, 2005).

COPING MECHANISMS

Coping refers to the cognitive and behavioral responses that help a person manage specific internal and external demands that exceed personal resources, enabling the person to solve problems and to respond appropriately. The child may mirror the parents' behaviors and responses, which may help or hinder the child's response to stress. The child's temperament, previous coping experiences, and availability of **support systems** (extended network of family, friends, and religious and community contacts that provide nurturance, emotional support, and direct assistance to parents) all combine to influence his or her ability to cope with the current experience.

The nature and severity of the illness and an emergency admission to the hospital stress a child's coping capabilities. Defense mechanisms displayed by children in these situations include **regression**, or return to an earlier behavior (a common reaction to stress), denial, **repression** (involuntary forgetting), postponement, and bargaining.

Nursing Practice

Injured children and adolescents requiring hospitalization for a serious injury are at risk for acute stress disorder (ASD) and posttraumatic stress disorder (PTSD). A recent study revealed that variables associated with ASD in children after a motor vehicle crash included being injured and receiving medical treatment (Winston, Baxt, Kassam-Adams, et al., 2005). In adolescents, perceived threat to life, violence-related injury, no control over the event leading to the injury, and death of a family member at the scene increased the risk of developing PTSD (Holbrook, Hoyt, Coimbra, et al., 2005).

Thinking Critically

PICU STRESSORS

The PICU receives a call from a community hospital requesting transport for an unstable 12-year-old boy who is in status epilepticus. Jeremiah has a seizure disorder controlled with medications, but several days ago he decided to stop taking his medications. So many seizure medications have been given in the community hospital emergency department to stop Jeremiah's seizures that he is now unconscious and must be intubated to maintain his airway until the medications wear off.

The transport team is in the air within minutes and arrives at the rural community hospital 25 minutes later. The team stabilizes Jeremiah, receives reports from the medical and nursing teams, meets briefly with his parents, answers a few questions, and is back in the air.

Jeremiah is admitted directly to the PICU and connected to cardiorespiratory and noninvasive blood pressure monitors. His existing intravenous lines and endotracheal tube are evaluated for patency as team members quickly complete a head-to-toe assessment. When Jeremiah's parents arrive, his nurse meets them and prepares them for what they will see.

What stressors do children like Jeremiah face after sudden admission to the PICU? What age-specific strategies can you use to help him cope with the experience when he regains consciousness? What stressors will parents face during the initial period when you work with them? How can you intervene to help them in this crisis?

See MyNursingKit for possible responses.

NURSING MANAGEMENT

Nursing care of the child with a life-threatening illness or injury and his or her family includes assessing the child's physical and psychosocial needs, assessing the family's psychosocial needs, providing physical and psychosocial care for the child, and providing support for parental physical and emotional needs.

NURSING ASSESSMENT AND DIAGNOSIS

Nursing assessment involves physiologic parameters, plus skilled observation of the child's psychosocial and emotional needs. An understanding of normal psychosocial and cognitive development is important to plan developmentally appropriate interventions. Assessment should include the child's response to illness, the environment, coping strategies, and the need for information and support.

The accompanying "Nursing Care Plan" includes common nursing diagnoses for the child with a life-threatening illness or injury. The following nursing diagnoses may also be appropriate:

- *Impaired Verbal Communication* related to the effects of endotracheal intubation and mechanical ventilation
- *Spiritual Distress* related to the crisis of illness or suffering

Nursing Care Plan

THE CHILD COPING WITH A LIFE-THREATENING ILLNESS OR INJURY

INTERVENTION | **RATIONALE** | **EXPECTED OUTCOME**

1. Nursing Diagnosis: Anxiety (Child) related to separation from parents, foreign environment, strangers as caretakers, invasive procedures

NIC Priority Intervention:

Anxiety reduction: Minimizing apprehension, dread, foreboding, or uneasiness related to an unidentified source of anticipated danger

NOC Suggested Outcome:

Anxiety control: Ability to eliminate or reduce feelings of apprehension and tension from unidentified source

Goal: The child will exhibit or express an increased sense of security.

INTERVENTION	RATIONALE	EXPECTED OUTCOME
■ Encourage parents to remain at the bedside (open visitation) and to participate in the child's care by touching, talking to, reading to, and singing to the child.	■ Presence of the parents is comforting to the child.	The child appears more relaxed and acknowledges parents' presence. Behavioral manifestations of anxiety are absent. Restful periods of sleep are noted.
■ Talk with the child. Avoid discussions at bedside that the child should not overhear.	■ The child may overhear and remember, even if unconscious.	
■ Offer to arrange a visit from the chaplain or other spiritual support.	■ Spiritual support often provides comfort and sustenance in a time of crisis.	
■ Provide the child with developmentally appropriate explanations when possible. Encourage the child to ask questions and express concerns.	■ Information reduces anxiety and builds trust.	
■ Make the child's bedside more personal and familiar by encouraging parents to bring in security objects, family photos, and favorite toys from home.	■ Security objects decrease foreignness of hospital environment. The child derives comfort from presence of personal items.	
■ Involve the child in play appropriate to developmental age (see Chapter 33).	■ Play provides familiarity, decreases fantasy, and provides motor activity.	
■ Provide care using a primary nursing care model.	■ Consistency in caregivers helps to build the child's trust. Caregiver learns child's cues.	

2. Nursing Diagnosis: Powerlessness (Moderate) related to inability to communicate, and control relinquished to the healthcare team

NIC Priority Intervention:

Self-Esteem Facilitation: Encouraging a patient to assume more responsibility for own behavior.

NOC Suggested Outcome:

Health Beliefs: Perceived Control: Personal conviction that one can influence an outcome.

Goal: The child or adolescent will have an increased sense of control over the situation.

INTERVENTION	RATIONALE	EXPECTED OUTCOME
■ Provide opportunities for choices when possible. Encourage participation in self-care.	■ Such opportunities provide sense of control and autonomy through decision making.	The child or adolescent expresses satisfaction over ability to control some elements of situation.
■ Prepare the child or adolescent in advance (timing dependent on developmental level) for procedures. Describe the sensations that will be experienced. Allow some choice in timing or method of pain relief.	■ Information provides anticipatory guidance and a sense of involvement and value to the child.	The child or adolescent participates in self-care and decision making.

(continued)

Nursing Care Plan—continued

THE CHILD COPING WITH A LIFE-THREATENING ILLNESS OR INJURY

INTERVENTION	RATIONALE	EXPECTED OUTCOME
■ Provide routines for the child both within a 24-hour period and for scheduled care. Tell the child before the procedure (timing dependent upon developmental level), repeat explanation of why procedure is necessary, complete procedure in a consistent manner, and offer praise or a special story when completed. When possible, incorporate rituals from home.	■ Self-control is maintained through rituals.	
■ Provide other means of communication to the intubated child (e.g., a word board or finger board).	■ Maintaining communication provides autonomy and independence for the child.	
■ For the child requiring restraints or immobilizers, use as seldom as possible, provide appropriate explanations, and release at regular intervals. Wrapping IV lines well and using armboards can help maintain lines and avoid the need for restraints.	■ Release from restraints or immobilizers helps diminish the sense of powerlessness that accompanies their use.	

3. Nursing Diagnosis: Acute Pain related to injuries, invasive procedures, surgery

NIC Priority Intervention:

Pain management: Alleviation of pain or a reduction in pain to a level of comfort that is acceptable to the patient

NOC Suggested Outcome:

Comfort level: Feelings of physical and psychologic ease

Goal: The child will experience reduced pain and improved comfort.

INTERVENTION	RATIONALE	EXPECTED OUTCOME
■ Assess the child's pain: location, intensity, what makes it better or worse.	■ Assessment provides baseline information from which a plan of care can be developed.	The child experiences a perceived or actual improvement in comfort level.
■ If appropriate, use pain assessment scale (see Chapter 42 ∞).	■ Use of scale provides continuity and consistency in monitoring of the child's pain.	
■ Provide optimal pain relief with prescribed analgesics. Provide comfort measures—position changes, back rubs, etc. Provide diversional activities as appropriate or possible. Incorporate the family in pain relief modality.	■ Physiologic and psychologic methods of pain control can be used in combination to maximally improve outcomes.	

- *Disturbed Sleep Pattern* related to circadian asynchrony, excessive stimulation, pain, and anxiety caused by the critical care unit environment
- *Deficient Diversional Activity* related to forced inactivity
- *Anticipatory Grieving* related to potential loss of body function or impending death of self

PLANNING AND IMPLEMENTATION

Nursing care focuses on promoting a sense of trust, providing education about the illness or injury, preparing the child for procedures, facilitating the use of play, and promoting a sense of control.

Physiologic care for the child in the PICU may include the following: frequent physiologic assessment, pain and sedation management, nutritional support, medication administration, managing multiple IV lines and pumps, maintaining ventilatory and hemodynamic monitoring equipment, and wound care.

PROVIDE PSYCHOSOCIAL CARE FOR THE CHILD

Children admitted to a PICU need support for the stressful experience. Children often feel and hear even when unconscious, so touch and verbal interchanges are important. Nurses play a key

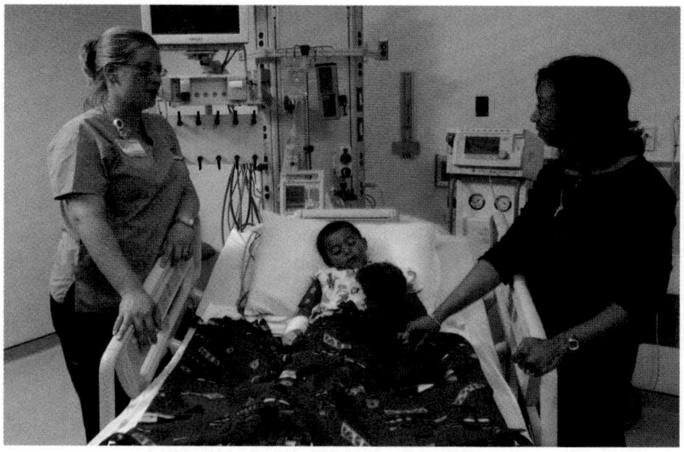

● **Figure 43–2** Personalizing the child's bedside. By their very nature, PICUs are ominous and sterile. To lessen this effect, it can help to personalize the child's space. Being there with the child and parent, answering questions, or just talking can be a comfort to both.

role in providing developmentally appropriate support to the child. Nursing interventions are directed at building a trusting relationship, minimizing the stressors experienced by the child, and promoting coping. Ongoing reassessment of progress in meeting the child's needs is critical.

PROMOTE A SENSE OF SECURITY

For children of all ages, feeling secure depends on a sense of physical and psychologic safety. A sense of physical security is difficult to attain within the PICU because frequent procedures are part of the child's treatment plan. Parental presence at the bedside is one of the best ways to decrease anxiety and promote a sense of security. Including parents as partners in the child's care provides comfort and reassurance to the child. Children whose parents have high anxiety levels pick up their parents' emotional cues and become more anxious. Consistency of staff is invaluable in developing familiarity and a trusting relationship with the child.

Personalizing the child's bedside can promote comfort and a sense of security. Pictures from home, a favorite blanket or toy, music tapes, or posters can make the environment friendlier and more familiar to the child (Figure 43–2 ●). Religious or spiritual icons may also provide psychologic support.

PROVIDE EDUCATION AND PREPARE THE CHILD FOR PROCEDURES

A child's ability to understand the cause of the illness and its therapy depends on his or her cognitive abilities. Help younger children to understand that illness and hospitalization are not a punishment.

Preparation for procedures is important at all ages, even for the unconscious or sedated child. Toddlers will benefit from being talked to, soothed, and touched during and after the procedure. Provide preschoolers, school-age children, and adolescents with an explanation of the sensations they can expect to experience (temperature, vibrations, sounds, smells, tastes, sight). (See Chapter 41∞.)

FACILITATE THE USE OF PLAY

Play can be used to alleviate stress and to help prepare children for procedures. The nurse can also use play to assess the child's developmental level. Even within the PICU, therapeutic play diminishes negative fantasies, provides motor activity, and helps the child cope with stressors (see Chapter 41∞). Children with limited mobility due to tubes and immobilizers can still feel a sense of accomplishment, for example, by completing a puzzle, even if the nurse points and moves each piece as the child responds through nods and gestures, where it should be placed. Play can help children work through a painful situation, making it more tolerable.

PROMOTE A SENSE OF CONTROL

Children between toddlerhood and adolescence experience a loss of control during a life-threatening illness. This loss of control may be related to the body, emotions, normal routines, or privacy. Nursing interventions should promote a sense of control over these areas.

Children hospitalized in an intensive care unit experience a heightened sense of loss of control, secondary to the many machines, noises, and limits on mobility. These children often self-remove or threaten to self-remove technological equipment or devices employed in their care, such as an endotracheal tube, peripheral intravenous line or central line, nasogastric tube, or arterial line. The child's actions are often referred to as treatment interference. Treatment interference may be conscious or unconscious (Snyder, 2004).

Physical immobilizers are sometimes used in children with altered consciousness to prevent the unintentional removal of technologic devices or equipment. While immobilizers are sometimes necessary, they contribute to the child's sense of powerlessness. The Joint Commission requires that hospitals have policies and procedures for the use of restraints or immobilizers, and a plan to regularly release them for short periods. Restrain all children as little as possible, and explain the rationale for immobilizers, emphasizing that they are not a punishment (see Skills 7–1 to 7–6 SKILLS). Nurses should also position devices in a way that maintains comfort as much as possible (Snyder, 2004).

Enhance the child's coping skills by teaching the child and family a combination of relaxation, visual imagery, or distraction techniques, and comforting self-talk phrases, such as "This will be over soon. If I stay calm, it will be all right. It will be over faster and then I can do something fun." Help the parents become the child's coping coaches.

EVALUATION

Expected outcomes of nursing care include the following:

- A trusting relationship is developed with the child and family.
- The child is given preparation and support for procedures.
- The child's coping is promoted by family presence and therapeutic play.

Nursing Practice

In addition to dealing with the child's life-threatening condition, parents may need to quickly arrange for the care of other children. For example, the sibling may be at band practice and a ride home must be planned. Parents must decide if one of them will leave the hospital to pick up the child and inform him or her about the sibling's illness/injury, or whether a family member or friend will do it for them. This decision may not be easy and will depend in part on the condition of the hospitalized child. The parents may need assistance to make these arrangements when they are in a state of crisis.

PARENTS' EXPERIENCE OF A CHILD'S LIFE-THREATENING ILLNESS OR INJURY

The uncertainty and unpredictability of a child's life-threatening illness or injury challenge a family's stability. The sudden loss of the parenting role with the child's emergency admission causes stress. Families display many different reactions and coping strategies. The needs of the family must be met if the child with a life-threatening condition is to be adequately cared for. Parents can transmit their anxiety to the child, who then becomes even more anxious. Family-centered care must be provided to meet the needs of parents with a variety of personalities, coping mechanisms, and responses to the crisis. Clear, concise communication is imperative.

THE FAMILY IN CRISIS

The critical care environment and the implications of a child's life-threatening illness or injury are far removed from the everyday experiences of most families. The unfamiliar environment and the uncertainty and seriousness of the illness or injury create a **family crisis**, which occurs when the family encounters a problem that seems insurmountable and usual coping skills are not effective.

Since families have little time to prepare for the experience, a sudden admission threatens family integrity, causing enormous stress and separation from loved ones. The interruption of the unique parent-child relationship can be more stressful to parents than the physical PICU environment. Siblings are also affected; see discussion on page 1136. In addition, extended family members such as grandparents must be considered. Grandparents are concerned both for the grandchild and their child, one of the parents of the ill or injured child (Hall, 2004). Stresses are further intensified in the case of divorce, separation, and stepparenting. Financial problems, a long distance from home to hospital, or another ill or injured family member can compound the crisis.

PARENTAL REACTIONS TO LIFE-THREATENING ILLNESS OR INJURY

When faced with a threat to their child's life, parents typically progress through stages that might include shock and disbelief; anger and guilt; deprivation and loss; anticipatory waiting; and readjustment or mourning. Some families progress through these stages in a linear fashion, while others go back and forth between stages, especially if the child's condition improves and then worsens.

Shock and Disbelief

The universal reaction to a child's life-threatening condition is shock and disbelief. As the familiar is disrupted, parents experience a loss of control, an inability to regain their bearings, and feelings of immobility. The hospital environment, emergency department, or PICU may seem unreal. The emotions parents experience initially are intensified by the physical appearance of their child (particularly after a major injury); the presence of monitors, tubing, and equipment; and the actual injury or illness.

Shock and disbelief begin in the first few moments after hearing the "news" and can last for days. The shock helps postpone the full impact of the crisis. During this period, parents search for answers and explanations about the illness or injury. Information must be repeated many times to parents, since in this stage they are often unable to assimilate information easily.

Anger and Guilt

Anger and guilt surface as parents become more aware of their child's illness or injury. Their anger may be directed toward themselves or each other because they could not protect the child. Other individuals may be blamed such as the driver of a motor vehicle who injured the child. Parents may also be angry with their child. This anger may be a result of injuries the child sustained when breaking known rules such as drinking and driving, playing with matches, or riding a bike without a helmet. Lastly, the anger may not be directed at anyone specifically. Injuries caused by natural disasters such as an earthquake, flood, or hurricane provoke just as much anger as those that result from the actions of people, and they may pose a challenge to the parents' spiritual beliefs.

Parents typically react to their child's illness or injury with some degree of guilt. This reaction may be magnified in the PICU environment. The fact that the guilt usually has no basis in real events does not lessen the feeling. A question parents frequently ask at this stage is, "Why not me instead of my child?" Parents' feelings of guilt may have one of two causes:

1. They may feel responsible for causing the illness or injury. Statements such as, "If only I hadn't sent him to the store on his bike, this wouldn't have happened," reflect feelings of guilt for causing or failing to prevent the injury.
2. They may feel guilty about not noticing the onset of an illness or disregarding earlier illness symptoms. The mother of a 1-year-old with meningitis repeatedly said, "I shouldn't have waited so long to take her to the doctor!"

Deprivation and Loss

As the shock associated with the child's life-threatening condition slowly recedes, new stressors emerge. Within minutes or hours, parents are deprived of their familiar role as the parent of a healthy child and find themselves in the unexpected and unfamiliar role as the parent of a critically ill child.

The difficulty and ambivalence in giving over part of their responsibility as the child's primary caretakers can threaten their self-esteem and self-control. If parents cannot participate in the child's care, they may feel helpless or worthless.

Anticipatory Waiting

Once the child's condition is stabilized and survival seems likely, parents often move into a period of anticipatory waiting. This stage is characterized as "life suspended in time." Parents spend a great deal of time waiting: for test results, for explanations, for their child to become conscious, or for surgery to be over. Parents may fear leaving the area because they may miss an important procedure, physician visit, or decisions or changes in treatment. Lack of mobility decreases the parents' use of typical coping mechanisms, so anxiety and the sense of powerlessness may increase. If the parents have a cell phone, write down the number and ensure them that they will be called for any change in the child's condition. This allows parents to feel like they can leave at least for a few minutes. If the parents do not have a cell phone, provide a pager if available.

Parents may have a preoccupation with medical details. During this period, they may ask questions about the long-term effects of the illness or injury on the child, about the potential for brain damage, or about the need for additional surgeries. Parents may place demands on staff and be frustrated when the child's progress is slow.

Readjustment or Mourning

The last stage that parents experience is readjustment or mourning. Readjustment is experienced as the child recovers, improves steadily, and prepares for transfer and discharge. In contrast, parents of the child who dies reenter the cycle of emotions characteristic of grief. Parents also mourn when the child remains seriously ill or unresponsive, when the outcome remains uncertain for an extended period, or when long-term care is required.

Table 43–1 lists the most important needs of parents when a child is hospitalized with a life-threatening illness or injury.

NURSING MANAGEMENT

Nursing care of the family includes assessing the family's psychosocial needs and providing support for parental physical and emotional needs.

NURSING ASSESSMENT AND DIAGNOSIS

Nurses who work with families of critically ill children have a unique opportunity to help them adapt and to promote family functioning. Begin by assessing the family's reaction to the illness,

Table 43–1 Nursing Interventions to Meet Parental Needs When the Child Is Hospitalized with a Life-Threatening Illness or Injury

Parental Needs	Nursing Interventions
Information	■ Provide information and frequent updates about the child's condition using terminology that parents can understand. ■ Repeat the information and provide other materials frequently as parents forget or cannot concentrate on details with all their stress. ■ Explain the child's condition, equipment being used, and procedures of care. ■ Facilitate a discussion with the physician at least daily. ■ Provide general information about unit policies, team members, and phone numbers.
Proximity to their child	■ Provide permission for the parents to remain at the bedside. ■ Encourage parents to touch and speak with the child and demonstrate ways if parents are hesitant. ■ Work within the unit to provide open, flexible visiting hours.
Reestablishment of their parental role and control	■ Implement family-centered care so parents feel recognized as important to their child's recovery and as the decision maker for the child's treatment options.
Participation in their child's care	■ Encourage parents to participate in care (e.g., bathing and hair care, diaper changes, feeding, range of motion exercises, massages). ■ Encourage parents to help with diversional activity (e.g., reading, singing, telling stories). ■ Encourage parents to explain equipment and procedures to the child to reduce the child's fears.
Confidence in the treatment plan and caregivers	■ Try to maintain continuity in staffing and healthcare contacts. ■ Demonstrate caring for the child. ■ Provide assurance that the child is receiving appropriate treatment and pain management.
Psychologic support	■ Acknowledge that the situation is difficult. ■ Help parents to focus on the positive or unchanged aspects of the child's appearance. ■ Encourage parents to get rest and nutrition to help them maintain physical resources necessary for coping. ■ Provide space and privacy as needed. ■ Give hope if realistic—an essential component of coping. ■ Offer the choice of other family members to be present. ■ Discuss the possible responses of siblings and the long-term emotional responses of the patient.

coping skills, stressors, and needs. See Chapter 39∞. This initial assessment provides a baseline of information for developing a care plan and strategies to meet the psychosocial as well as physiologic needs of families.

Several nursing diagnoses may apply to parents who are dealing with their child's life-threatening condition. Examples include the following:

- *Interrupted Family Processes* related to the impact of a critically ill child on the family system
- *Spiritual Distress* related to the child's life-threatening condition, suffering, or death
- *Fatigue* related to extreme stress, sleep deprivation, and crisis
- *Hopelessness* in parents related to the child's deteriorating physical condition
- *Anticipatory Grieving* related to potential death of the child or loss of body functions
- *Parental Coping: Compromised* related to the severity of the illness or injury in the child

PLANNING AND IMPLEMENTATION

Nursing care focuses on providing family-centered care to help meet the needs of families, minimize stress, and enhance family coping. See Table 1–1 in Chapter 1∞. Nurses are challenged to blend and balance technology with caring.

PROVIDE INFORMATION AND BUILD TRUST

Orienting parents to the hospital, as well as to the unit routines, helps them to adapt to their surroundings. Parents will gain a sense of control and independence if they know where to get supplies, and how to find the lounge, cafeteria, and restrooms.

Provide frequent and accurate information. Deliver information on the child's illness, condition, and plan of care in a manner and language readily understandable to parents. Upon admission, provide the parents with an idea of what to expect in the days ahead and to be prepared for special procedures or major changes in therapy. Parents also need to be prepared before they see the child the first time. Explain the tubes and monitors that are present and how the child will look and react.

Honesty in discussions is extremely important. If parents feel misled or that information is being withheld, a trusting relationship will be impossible. Informed parents, however, will feel that they are active participants in decision making and care planning for their child. Trust is facilitated when parents believe that the staff truly cares about the child and sees the child as a special individual. Trust is especially important when difficult decisions must be made, such as withdrawal of life support, or to reduce the risk for conflict.

Parents also need a sense of hope regarding their child's condition to help them cope. Focus on the positives as the child progresses through the different phases of the life-threatening condition.

FACILITATE POSITIVE STAFF–PARENT RELATIONSHIPS AND COMMUNICATION

Given the intensity of the parents' experience when their child is critically ill, it is easy to see how problems can arise between staff and parents. Each healthcare team member must be aware of the child's current status so that parents receive consistent information from all staff. A consistent message can instill confidence. Provide explanations geared to the parents' level of understanding, using language the parents can understand.

Introduce the parents to the nurse and physician with overall responsibility for the child's care. This is especially important in teaching hospitals that have rotating interns and residents. The attending physician with the overall responsibility should meet with parents as often as necessary to talk about changes in the child's condition or treatment plan and to allow time for parents to ask questions (Figure 43–3 ●). Encourage parents to keep a daily log or notebook to record information on the child's care, progress, and needs, as well as questions they want to ask. Family care conferences can be helpful when a large number of team members provide care. Arrange for daily visits by an interpreter if the family does not speak or understand English. Have information about the child's condition and care summarized for communication at that time.

Nursing Practice

Explain to the child and parents, in easy-to-understand terms, the purpose of equipment that is being used. Answer alarms quickly. Follow with an explanation of why alarms sound, including the fact that many times monitor alarms will sound when the child moves, if the monitor becomes disconnected, or if the monitor patches are loose.

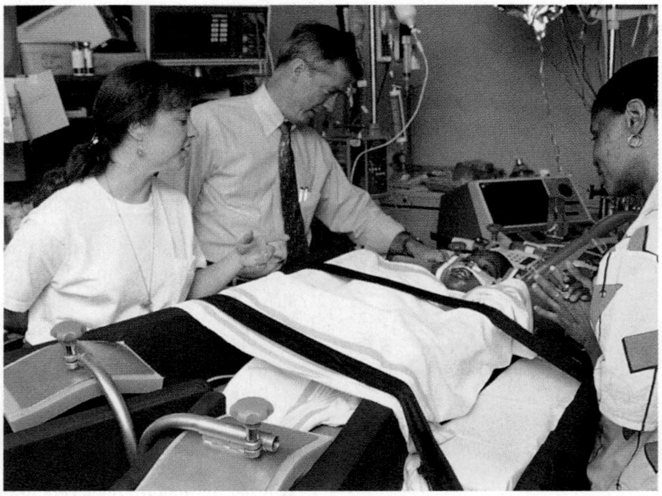

● **Figure 43–3** Communicating with parents about care. In times of crisis, everyone likes to know that someone is in charge and who that person is. The parents should meet and talk with the staff physician in charge and the nurses as often as possible. Parents need to know that someone is responsible, even if different people are providing care.

PROMOTE PARENTAL INVOLVEMENT

An important role of nurses is to encourage and support parents in their parenting role. The parents' place when possible is at the bedside—their very presence can comfort the child, minimize fears, and reduce the child's distress during invasive procedures. Being at the child's bedside in the pediatric intensive care unit has also been shown to decrease parental stress (Smith, Hefley, Anand, et al., 2007). Parents provide continuity and may notice subtle condition changes that a newly assigned nurse may miss. Throughout the child's hospitalization, parents will continue to need reassurance and encouragement.

Participation in care of the child is an integral aspect of family-centered care and enhances the family's ability to cope with the child's illness or injury. Providing information about behaviors and emotions the child is likely to exhibit as well as guidelines about what physical care they can provide helps the parents gain a sense of control over the situation and a sense of empowerment (Melnyk, Alpert-Gillis, Feinstein, et al., 2004). Encourage parents to take a role at the bedside, such as providing personal care. Parents who are unable to remain at the child's bedside may feel that they are not an important team member. When parents are unable to remain at the bedside they should be allowed to call the unit at any time to check on their child.

FAMILY PRESENCE DURING RESUSCITATION AND INVASIVE PROCEDURES

Many hospitals are implementing policies that permit families to be present during resuscitation and invasive procedures. Healthcare professionals have expressed concern that parents who are allowed to witness resuscitation efforts might lose control and interfere. Another concern is that medical staff, especially those in training, might feel uncomfortable, and that there is an increased risk for litigation (Mangurten, Scott, Guzzetta, et al., 2006). However, reports related to family presence during resuscitation have failed to demonstrate any increase in litigation and family satisfaction is higher when being allowed at the bedside (ENA, 2005).

Parents and other family members (e.g., grandparents) may wish to be present during invasive procedures (such as lumbar puncture) or resuscitation of the child. The nurse partners with the family to determine their needs at the time. To better facilitate the needs of the family, the following is determined:

- Who desires to be present during resuscitation or invasive procedures?
- What role will they play during the procedure (e.g., snuggle child for comfort)?

Healthcare agencies should have established protocols for family presence during invasive procedures or resuscitation (ENA, 2005). Care must be family-centered and individualized to each situation, according to the child's and family's needs. The nurse ensures that a support person from the multidisciplinary team (e.g., another nurse, social worker) is available to stay with the family members during resuscitation. If parents choose not to witness the resuscitation, regular updates (5–10 minute intervals) should be provided to the parents as they wait in a private area. A hospital chaplain or other family support team member should support the parents while they wait.

Evidence in Action

Studies show that family presence does not interrupt care or interfere with the healthcare providers' ability to intervene in the care of the child (ENA, 2005). The Emergency Nurses Association (ENA, 2005) supports the option of family presence during invasive procedures and resuscitation. In addition the AAP supports family presence during all aspects of care in the emergency department (O'Malley, Brown, Krug and The Committee on Pediatric Emergency Medicine, 2008).

PROVIDE FOR PARENTAL PHYSICAL AND EMOTIONAL NEEDS

The experience of having a child with a life-threatening condition drains the parents' physical and emotional reserves. Parents often need encouragement to take care of themselves and to take a break periodically. A statement such as "It is important for you to eat and rest because Alexa is really going to need you when she wakes up" helps parents to realize that becoming exhausted benefits neither them nor the child.

Many communities have a residence for families of hospitalized children, supported in many cases by Ronald McDonald Children's Charities. This is often an inexpensive but warm and supportive environment for parents of ill children. A Ronald

Nursing Practice

1. Prior to entering the room where the child is being resuscitated, inform the parents about the environment–the equipment they will see in, on, and near their child and its purpose. Tell them who is in the room (e.g., she is a doctor, he is a nurse, she is a respiratory therapist) working on the child.
2. Inform the parents that if they feel uncomfortable or if they get in the way of the resuscitation team's work, they will be escorted out.
3. Have the parents sit so that they are able to look at the child's face, holding his or her hand. The parents can be given duties (e.g., "Sit near Jeff s face, and let him know how much you love him").
4. If the parents are looking around, explain what is being done for the child and why. Parents need to know that their child did not endure unnecessary suffering. Attention to procedure-related pain management is important.
5. If the child is declared dead in the ED, reassure the parents that they were there at the last moment and that their child (use the child's name) felt loved.

Adapted from: Levetown, M. (2004, p. 38). Breaking bad news in the emergency department: When seconds count. *Topics in Emergency Medicine, 26*(1), 35–43.

McDonald Family Room may be found in some hospitals and is provided as a comfortable setting where families of hospitalized children can get away from the high-tech hospital atmosphere while remaining close to the child. Computer resources in one of these locations or in a Family Resource Center may make it possible for parents to stay in contact with concerned family and friends. When financial burdens are a consideration, parents may need family support and social service referrals.

The ill child's parents are often at different levels of coping during a crisis. The severity of the child's illness or injury may foster cohesion between the parents and build a stronger relationship. Unfortunately, the reverse may also be true—differences in styles or levels of coping may foster a sense of isolation, placing a strain on the couple's relationship. Nurses should be alert to family dynamics and refer the family for counseling or therapy, if indicated.

MAINTAIN OR STRENGTHEN FAMILY SUPPORT SYSTEMS

Support systems enable parents to cope with overwhelming problems and crises. Most parents indicate that having family or friends nearby is crucial as a support system. See "Complementary Care: Prayer."

Extended family, especially grandparents and friends, frequently offer the family assistance, but parents may need to be reassured that it is all right to ask for help as well. Some parents are uncomfortable asking for help, instead attempting to handle multiple responsibilities themselves, often to the point of exhaustion. Some parents are unable to respond to offers of help because it requires too great a mental effort on their part. The nurse should assist the parents in responding to these offers for assistance.

Nurses may need to intervene on parents' behalf when they have inadequate support. Parents may be frustrated by people who come to visit unannounced, stay too long, or visit too often. They may find it difficult to tell well-meaning but insensitive friends that they cannot deal with visitors right now. In these situations, it may be helpful for the nurse to offer to serve as a gatekeeper. Suggest that parents inform family and friends about specific times for visits or phone calls to allow for rest periods. An extended family member may be given the responsibility of relaying information to others.

> **Complementary Care**
>
> **PRAYER**
>
> In the United States, prayer has been reported as the most frequently used form of complementary therapy (National Center for Complementary and Alternative Medicine, 2005). A national survey of 2055 households explored the use of prayer and other complementary therapies. Results revealed that 35% of respondents used prayer for health concerns. Prayer was often directed toward wellness, but it was also used in conjunction with conventional medical care (McCaffrey, Eisenberg, Legedza, et al., 2004).

Families of children with a life-threatening illness or injury often have emotional needs beyond the support capabilities of the nurse caring for the child. Referrals to family and support services or pastoral care may be beneficial in these instances.

EVALUATION

Expected outcomes of nursing care include the following:

- The nurse establishes a trusting relationship and effective communication with the family.
- Parents participate in their child's care as much as desired.
- Parents and extended family members receive emotional support and nurturance needed to sustain them through the child's illness.

THE SIBLINGS' EXPERIENCE

As the parents' focus shifts to the critically ill child, they may need support in dealing with the healthy siblings. Siblings also need care and may feel left out when everyone's attention is focused on the ill child. Siblings of critically ill children may demonstrate behaviors ranging from jealousy or envy to resentment, guilt, hostility, anger, insecurity, regression, fear and anxiety. Nurses should recognize that siblings may fear becoming ill themselves or believe that they played a role in the child's illness. Siblings often have nightmares about the illness or injury their brother or sister has sustained and about the ill child dying.

Inform siblings about their brother or sister's condition using language and concepts appropriate to their ages and developmental levels. As appropriate, siblings should be allowed to visit. Such a visit should be encouraged if the child could potentially die, to allow the sibling to say good-bye. Because children's fantasies are often worse than reality, unfounded fears may be relieved by a visit. These visits often help to lift the spirits of the ill child and provide comfort for the siblings and the parents (Mauer, 2008).

Preparation for the visit is important. Before the visit, talk with the siblings about what to expect and describe how their brother or sister will look. If the ill child acts, moves, talks, or looks different than usual, provide an explanation beforehand. Describe the hospital environment, including equipment, sounds, and smells. Use a doll, draw pictures, or show an actual picture of the child to prepare the siblings. See Chapter 41∞, "Teaching Highlights: Strategies for Working with the Sibling of a Hospitalized Child."

During the visit the nurse should demonstrate how to talk to and touch the ill child and encourage the siblings to do the same (Figure 43–4 ●). The length of the visit should be relatively short and based on the child's developmental age. After the visit the nurse should talk with siblings about what they saw and felt, and answer their questions. When a sibling cannot visit, contact with the ill child can be maintained by sending pictures, drawings, cards, and messages recorded on audiotapes or cell phones if allowed (Figure 43–5 ●).

If parents are staying at the hospital with the ill child, encourage them to call the siblings at home daily. This allows the siblings at home to feel connected by the opportunity to share

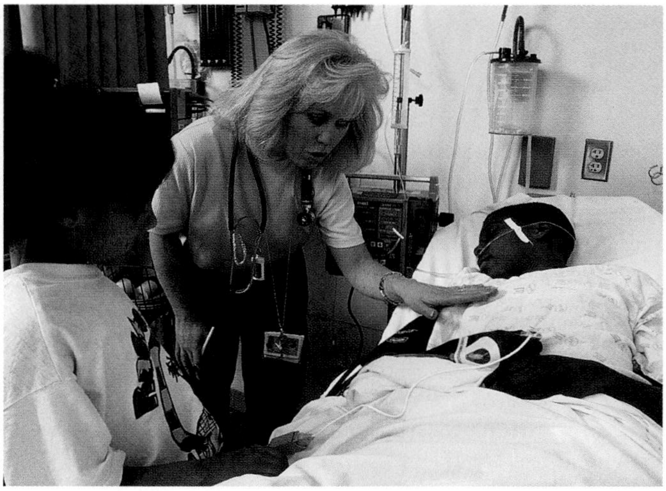

● **Figure 43–4** Sibling visits. During the sibling's visit to the ill child, it is important to talk with the sibling and answer any questions in an honest manner at a level the child can understand.

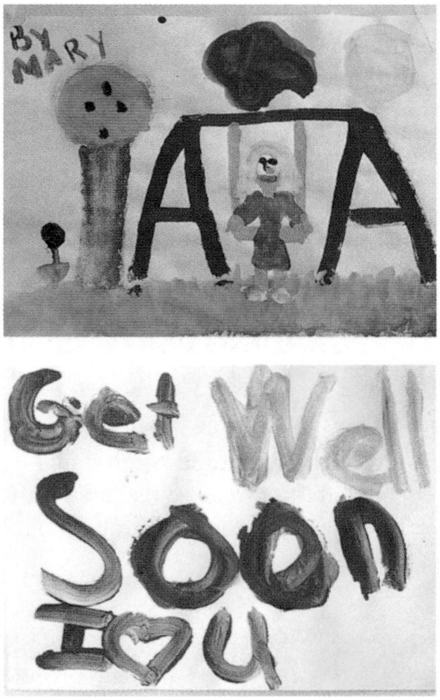

● **Figure 43–5** Alternatives to sibling visits. It is important that parents and siblings feel comfortable communicating with the seriously ill child. If siblings cannot visit, they should be encouraged to paint or record messages. They need to be able to express themselves and to feel that they are helping.

their day and to receive an update on the ill child. The phone call offers siblings a consistent link to the parents and the reassurance that they are important and loved. Internet contact or text messaging may be another way to communicate with older siblings. Arrange for parents to access a computer, if possible, for families who might find this contact supportive.

EVALUATION

Expected outcomes of nursing care include:

- Siblings are prepared for visits to the child with a life-threatening illness or injury.
- Siblings receive emotional support and assistance to cope with the unfamiliar environment.

END-OF-LIFE CARE

When the family is faced with end-of-life decision making and care because of a child's chronic condition or multiple acute care episodes, the family needs honest information about various treatment options and potential outcomes. Depending on cognitive abilities, developmental stage, physical and mental status, and prior experiences with healthcare, the child may also participate in the decision-making process (Beale, Baile, & Aaron, 2005). The family may need to consider issues such as **palliative care**, hospice care, do-not-resuscitate requests, continuation of schooling, organ/tissue donation, and autopsy.

PALLIATIVE CARE

Pediatric palliative care is a multidisciplinary care strategy designed to relieve the physical, social, emotional, and spiritual suffering in children and their families by managing symptoms and monitoring all aspects of suffering during the course of the child's illness (Korones, 2007). Pain, sleep disturbances, anxiety, seizures, dyspnea, pruritus, and constipation are symptoms that may require management (Himelstein, 2005). Palliative care should be offered and integrated with the curative or life-prolonging care (Korones, 2007). Palliative care may occur in the home, hospital, or other facility.

Approximately 8600 children die each year from conditions such as cancer, congenital defects, cystic fibrosis, and HIV infection who could benefit from palliative care (Rushton, 2005). Palliative care is also an option for very preterm neonates and children with lethal genetic anomalies. Children may require these services for many years.

HOSPICE CARE

Hospice is a philosophy of care for a terminally ill child that is focused exclusively on comfort and ensuring that the remaining time for the child is lived as comfortably and fully as possible. The terminally ill child is maintained as alert as possible without pain, and the family is provided with choices about health care and death with dignity (Korones, 2007). Care may be provided in the home, a special hospital unit, or a free-standing facility. Families and children receive emotional, spiritual, and medical support from the care team that may include nurses, physicians, religious and faith leaders, social workers, and mental health professionals. Hospice also provides grief counseling and support to parents for 1 year following the death of the child.

It is estimated that less than 1% of dying children receive hospice services (Himelstein, Hidon, Boldt, et al., 2004). However, an estimated 5000 children in their last 6 months of life could potentially benefit from hospice care on any given day (Institute of Medicine, 2003).

When a child receives palliative or hospice care, the family and healthcare providers collaborate to determine which treatments are appropriate to continue with the child's end-of-life care, such as intravenous fluids, gastrostomy feedings, and certain medications. Health plan coverage for pediatric palliative/hospice care services or alternative financial assistance is investigated.

ETHICAL ISSUES SURROUNDING A CHILD'S DEATH

Because the death of a child is so emotionally charged, many potential misunderstandings and conflicts can develop between families and healthcare providers. The more common ethical issues that need to be addressed include withdrawing or withholding treatment, parental treatment refusal, and do-not-resuscitate orders.

BRAIN DEATH CRITERIA

Brain death is the irreversible cessation of all functions of the brain, including the cerebral cortex and brainstem. Brain death criteria may be used when determining if withdrawal of life-supporting equipment is appropriate or when organ transplantation is planned. See Table 43–2. The timing of the two examinations for brain death is determined by the age of the child and circumstances of brain injury.

WITHDRAWAL OF OR WITHHOLDING TREATMENT

The decision to withdraw or withhold life-sustaining treatments from the dying child is very difficult and emotional for parents. Some parents feel that this is a form of abandonment, and it may make them feel as though they contributed to the child's death (Baergen, 2006). Withholding nutrition and hydration may be especially difficult because parents often associate food with nurturing and love, or they fear that death will be hastened. Other treatments such as medications, mechanical ventilation, and dialysis may be withdrawn if death is inevitable and continuing treatment causes more suffering than benefit. See "Evidence-Based Nursing: Improving the Quality of Pediatric End-of-Life Care in the PICU."

The nurse may feel conflicted when parents are unable to discontinue aggressive therapies that the nurse feels are extending the child's suffering. Consultation with a member of the hospital ethics committee can help clarify the issues involved and reduce the emotions of health professionals associated with the conflict. During the consultation an unbiased professional collects facts about the child's condition, clarifies the beliefs and values of parents and health professionals, and improves communication while investigating options for compromise (Rushton, 2004).

Nursing Practice

Care must be used when asking parents if they are willing to withdraw or forego therapies. An effective communication strategy is to inform parents that an intervention was initiated to give the child the best chance at recovery, but it has not been effective and is not beneficial for the child. When asking to withhold therapy such as cardiopulmonary resuscitation, it is helpful to indicate that the therapy is not effective in reversing the overwhelming illness or brain damage (Levetown, 2004).

CONFLICTS REGARDING PARENTS' REFUSAL OF TREATMENT

Parents and healthcare providers sometimes disagree over what, if any, medical interventions should be provided when the child is dying. Parents may refuse treatments based on religious convictions or because they wish to avoid prolonging the child's life

Table 43–2 Brain Death Criteria

Brain Functioning	Clinical Signs
Coma	Unconscious, no vocalization
Absent clinical functions of the brain	No purposeful movement No increase in heart rate with pressure on eyeballs
Absent brainstem function	Pupils midposition or dilated, nonresponsive to light No blink response to corneal stimulation No spontaneous eye movements with abrupt rotation of head or ice water irrigation in each ear No gag reflex when to oropharynx stimulation or cough to tracheal suctioning No respiratory movement when removed from ventilator

Adapted from Mathers, L. H., & Frankel, L. R. (2007). Brain death. In R. M. Kliegman, R. E. Behrman, H. B. Jenson, B. F. Stanton, *Nelson textbook of pediatrics* (18th ed., pp. 411–413). Philadelphia: Elsevier Saunders.

Evidence-Based Nursing

IMPROVING THE QUALITY OF PEDIATRIC END-OF-LIFE CARE IN THE PICU

Clinical Question

What improvements to quality of care matter most to parents of children who die in the PICU?

Evidence

A study involving 56 parents of children who had died in the PICU 1 to 4 years previously focused on their priorities for improving end-of-life care and communication in the PICU. The six priorities identified were honest and complete information, ready access to staff, coordination of communication and care, emotional expression and support by staff as it conveys caring for the child and family, preservation of the integrity of the parent-child relationship, and faith (Meyer, Ritholz, Burns, et al., 2006). In another study 36 parents of children who had died in three hospitals were interviewed to identify what mattered to parents of children with life-threatening conditions. Continuity of care was valued: it resulted in relationships and improved communication between healthcare providers and parents and the feeling that they and their children were known as individuals. Parents had greater confidence in the quality of care their child received (Heller & Solomon, 2005).

Best Practice

Knowing what parents value during this time is important for planning nursing care and multidisciplinary palliative care. Facilitating opportunities for regular communication that includes full disclosure about the child's condition by a single familiar person may help reduce amount of conflicting information parents hear, and it may assist with decision making. Other communication options such as family conferences or office hours at the bedside may help improve communication. Ensure that family-centered care integrates values important to the family during nursing care planning and communications with them.

Critical Thinking

Consider the special needs of the parents of a newborn with a cardiac congenital anomaly that cannot be corrected by surgery. Identify the most common patterns of communication with family members in the NICU and evaluate their effectiveness in promoting family-centered care and decision making. Suggest two other communication methods that could improve communication with family members and improve the family's perception of care that their newborn receives.

See MyNursingKit for possible responses.

in order to provide a peaceful death (IOM, 2003). Initiating highly technical, but possibly futile, interventions may cause emotional and financial stress that overwhelms parents.

Consultation with the hospital's ethics committee should be obtained to help resolve the conflict. The healthcare team may seek to have a surrogate legal guardian appointed in certain situations when recommended care is refused. The conflict sometimes makes it difficult for the nurse to have a supportive relationship with the parents, but proper concern for and care of the child in these cases should be provided.

DO-NOT-RESUSCITATE ORDERS

Parents faced with a child's end-stage, irreversible life-limiting condition may be asked to consider a do-not-resuscitate (DNR), do-not-intubate, or allow natural death order, and decide if a resuscitation attempt would be in the child's best interest. Parents must consider allowing the child to die with dignity and the possibility of causing more harm and suffering if resuscitation is implemented. Parents may feel they are "giving up" on their child and need ongoing support. When the patient is an adolescent, he or she should be involved in discussions and have a role in decision making. Provide honest information and help the family understand that the child will still receive pain management, comfort care, oxygen, suctioning, and other supportive nursing care while complying with a DNR order.

SCHOOL CONSIDERATIONS

The Americans with Disabilities Act of 1990 and the Education for All Handicapped Children Act mandate that all children with disabilities—including those with terminal illnesses—are entitled to the same education as other students. Children with a chronic or terminal illness may be at high risk of dying while at school. Concerns of school officials about accepting a DNR order include the effect of a student's death on a classmate and liability issues. Most school districts have no policy regarding DNR orders (Hone-Warren, 2007).

Collaboration between the child, family, nurse and other healthcare providers, school officials, and social workers or other personnel with knowledge or expertise in DNR requests at school may lead to an agreement regarding the DNR request that respects the rights and interests of the dying child.

CARE OF THE DYING CHILD

Caring for a dying child is challenging and requires the utmost sensitivity and compassion. Children as young as 5 years of age can sense when they are seriously ill. A child's awareness of death develops more rapidly when he or she is experiencing the progression of a disease and related medical treatment. Children with life-limiting illnesses often learn about death and their own illness from exposure to other seriously ill and dying children during hospitalization or clinic visits.

AWARENESS OF DYING BY DEVELOPMENTAL AGE

Infants and toddlers are not actually aware of death, but they are aware of and react to changes in normal routines and the behavior of parents. Toddlers know they feel bad, but they do

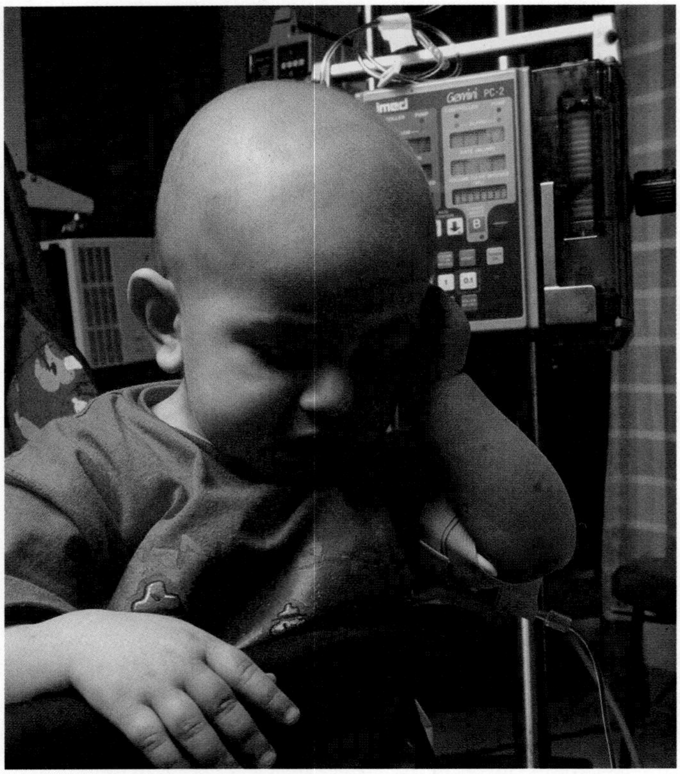

● **Figure 43–6** Toddlers' reactions to impending death. The toddler with a life-limiting condition recognizes that he feels bad and that routines are different. His anxiety may increase due to the concern and feelings of sadness exhibited by his parents.

not understand that their physical symptoms are associated with impending death. (See Figure 43–6 ●.)

Preschool children can see their bodies deteriorate and feel the effects of medications used during disease progression and treatment. Changes in self-concept occur as they perceive these body changes. They often describe their illness in terms of mutilation to their body. These physical changes may make them realize that they are dying.

School-age children also have subtle fears about body integrity and anxieties about the seriousness of their illness. This greater preoccupation with illness is considered by many professionals as the child's version of **death anxiety**, a feeling of apprehension or fear of death. Children may express death anxiety as a concern with treatments that invade the body or interfere with normal body functions.

Adolescents have a mature understanding of death, but the normal developmental milestones of adolescence add to their problems in facing a terminal illness. They are struggling to establish their own identity and plans for the future. At a time when body image is extremely important, they may be faced with the possibility of mutilation and disfigurement. Dying adolescents are often isolated from their peers during a period when peers are the most essential social group. Adolescents with terminal illnesses may be angry because they recognize that their loss is occurring at a time when the whole world is opening up to them.

Do not expect adolescents to handle feelings in the same way that adults do. Adolescents often avoid expressing anger against the family, seeking to control and direct these feelings elsewhere. They may become angry at changes in treatment procedures, lack of explanations, and threats to their independence. As death nears, the adolescent may permit comforting and support and may accept care from warm and loving family members, as long as he or she is not treated condescendingly.

NURSING MANAGEMENT

Nursing care of the dying child and family focuses on providing family-centered support for their physical and psychosocial needs.

NURSING ASSESSMENT AND DIAGNOSIS

Assess the child's physiologic status and comfort level. Physiologic changes in the dying child may be directly related to the child's disease process or injury. Signs and symptoms of approaching death are provided in "Clinical Manifestations: The Dying Child."

Assess the child's awareness of impending death. Examples of questions the child may ask include: "What will death be like? What happens after I die? Will I be with [a deceased person whom the child was close to] again? Will my parents be all right? Will you remember me?" Assess the ability of the parents to talk with the child about dying.

Assess the family for coping skills and need for social supports. Identify any cultural or spiritual traditions, rituals, and beliefs related to loss and grieving.

Examples of nursing diagnoses that apply to the dying child and family include the following:

- *Fear (Child)* related to unanswered questions and concerns of abandonment
- *Death Anxiety (Child)* related to own impending death
- *Anticipatory Grieving (Parents)* related to imminent death of child
- *Hopelessness (Parents)* related to failure of therapies to prolong life

PLANNING AND IMPLEMENTATION

Nursing care for the dying child and the family includes providing comfort, assisting the child in a peaceful death, assisting the child and family with coping strategies, and facilitating grief.

PHYSIOLOGIC CARE

A major goal in care of the dying child is to promote comfort and keep the child pain-free. Provide analgesia to promote optimal pain relief. Oral, transdermal, or rectal analgesia is available for families who choose to withhold intravenous fluids. Complementary care for comfort and pain management can be used by the nurse and family members (see Chapter 42).

Clinical Manifestations

THE DYING CHILD

SYSTEM	CLINICAL MANIFESTATIONS
Cardiovascular System	■ The heart rate may initially increase as hypoxia develops, then the heart rate and blood pressure decrease, resulting in decreased cardiac output. ■ A change in pulse pressure and a decrease in the volume of Korotkoff's sounds indicate imminent death. ■ Peripheral circulation decreases, leading to diaphoresis, clammy cool skin, and changes in skin coloring (mottled to cyanotic). Mottling is a sign of imminent death.
Respiratory System	■ Impaired cardiac function leads to pulmonary congestion, tachypnea, diminished breath sounds, and hypoxia. ■ Dyspnea; **air hunger**, the most severe form of dyspnea, may cause the child to look panicked, gasp for breath, and sit upright. ■ Cheyne-Stokes breathing (periods of shallow breathing alternating with apnea) is a sign of imminent death. ■ Parenteral fluids may cause edema and increased respiratory secretions leading to shortness of breath and cough. ■ As muscles relax, secretions accumulate in the oropharynx and bronchi causing noisy breathing as air passes through the secretions. ■ Moaning or grunting with breathing is common.
Neurologic System	■ Decreased cerebral perfusion, hypoxemia, metabolic acidosis, the influences of disease-related factors, and an accumulation of toxins from renal and liver failure lead to neurologic dysfunction. ■ Agitation or restlessness, withdrawal, increasing drowsiness, confusion; may be unconscious during final hours. ■ The child may speak of visions (persons or objects) not visible to others. ■ Hearing and vision acuity may deteriorate. Remember that hearing is one of the last senses to diminish before death.
Musculoskeletal System	■ Extreme muscle weakness and fatigue, difficulty with swallowing. ■ May be unable to reposition self, toilet self, or effectively cough and clear secretions.
Renal System	■ Decreased kidney function and urine production. ■ Sphincters relax and incontinence can occur.
Gastrointestinal System	■ Decreased oral fluid intake and anorexia are common. ■ Sphincters relax and bowel incontinence can occur.

If dyspnea or air hunger occurs, elevate the head of the bed, open a window, or use a circulating fan. An opioid may be prescribed for air hunger or tachypnea as its action dilates the pulmonary vessels, reduces oxygen consumption, and decreases pulmonary congestion.

Other physiologic care includes keeping the airway clear of secretions, bathing and keeping the skin dry and intact, changing the child's position frequently, and encouraging favorite foods and liquids as tolerated. Involve the parents in physical care and encourage them to hold and comfort the child.

COMMUNICATING WITH THE CHILD ABOUT HIS OR HER IMPENDING DEATH

Parents may prefer not to talk with the child about the seriousness of the illness and potential for death for several reasons: because of a desire to protect the child from bad news, because they fear it might take away the child's hope, or because they may feel incapable of answering the child's questions about dying. They may also fear that they will be unable to cope with their own feelings during a frank discussion of the possibility of the child's imminent death.

Evidence in Action

Investigators in Sweden asked 449 parents whose child had died from cancer if they had talked with their child about death. Of the 147 parents who had, none regretted having the discussion. In contrast, 26% of parents who did not talk with their child regretted not having a discussion. Parents were more likely to talk with their child if they sensed that the child was aware of his or her imminent death, if they were religious, or if the child was 9 years or older at the time of diagnosis and death (Kreicbergs, Valdimarsdóttir, Onelöv, et al., 2004).

Even when children are not told they are dying, they know their condition is worsening. They are undergoing treatments, not feeling well, and picking up cues from their parents. Some children keep most of their thoughts about death to themselves. If they have not been told that they are dying, they may feel isolated and get the message not to discuss their condition. They may fear that the family members will abandon them emotionally. Children often avoid displaying anger, since they fear desertion more than death. They may also believe that expressing their awareness of death and their fears will place added emotional burdens on family members that could be unbearable to the family.

The child may ask if he or she is dying. Offer to set up a meeting with the parents and the healthcare team to discuss their fears and concerns about telling their child the truth. Some parents may prefer that the child's questions be answered honestly by a member of the healthcare team. If the family chooses to talk with the child, assist them with possible developmentally appropriate words they can use to talk with their child.

Provide the child with opportunities for fantasy play, drawing, and storytelling, without emphasizing or reinforcing death themes. Listen to what children tell you about themselves and their lives. **Death imagery**, references to death or death-related topics (going away, separation, funerals) may be themes of their stories. Strategies for talking with a dying child are described in Table 43–3.

When caring for adolescents, remember that outbursts of anger are common but not personally directed at the nurse. Provide activities to help adolescents channel their feelings. Continue providing support in spite of their behavior. This approach may encourage adolescents to accept comforting without losing face. Be available to listen when the adolescent wants to talk and express feelings and frustrations. Promote friendships with other adolescents who have similar interests or problems.

Parents may not recognize the child's death anxiety because of their own fears, concerns, and feelings of helplessness. Depending on the family's cultural and religious beliefs, a chaplain or other healthcare professional who specializes in working with terminally ill children and families may help reduce a child's spiritual fears and promote peace and comfort among family members.

Developing Cultural Competence

DIVERSE PERSPECTIVES ON DEATH

Consider cultural differences when working with families dealing with the death of a loved one, for example (Dratler, Burns, & Dratler, 2006):

- African Americans often place great importance on their families being present and the expression of emotions. They value shared decision making between the patient and family members. Suffering as a meaningful spiritual experience is valued by many.
- Asian families often desire to protect the terminally ill from knowledge of their condition, so decisions are usually made by family members. They often prefer aggressive treatments.
- In some Filipino cultures words are considered so powerful that talking about the patient's death will make it happen, and as a result they may refuse to discuss any medical options.
- Hispanics generally believe the family should be responsible for making health care decisions. Faith is very important in times of death. They also believe death is a natural part of life, and the anniversary of a loved one's death is celebrated every year.

FAMILY SUPPORT

Parents need to be present when possible during the child's actual dying as it is a pivotal event in their parent-child relationship. Their presence helps fulfill their parenting role, their last time to be a good parent (Woodgate, 2006). Parents also prefer to have a familiar nurse provide the care as the child is dying.

Work closely with the family when the child's death is imminent, because they will remember the experience and words spoken for the rest of their lives. Prepare the family for changes in the child's appearance and behavior. Providing the parents with a room to be alone with the child ensures privacy at this extremely personal time.

Ask the family what is important to them in the final moments and hours of their child's life and what will be important to them in the grief process. Certain religious or cultural practices may need to be planned and should be accommodated

Table 43–3 Strategies for Communicating with the Dying Child

- Be open when the child initiates a conversation. Disruptive behavior, withdrawal, anger, hyperalert state, or sleeping more than usual may indicate the child's struggle with emotions and be an opportunity to engage the child in discussion.
- Assess how much the child knows and how much he or she wants to know. Identify any fantasies and concerns, and provide correct information. Be honest with the child when a clear question is asked.
- Allow the child to express his or her feelings and to be upset. Empathize with the child.
- Reassure the child that you will be available to listen and give support.
- Recognize that some children communicate best through nonverbal means, e.g., art, play, music, and writing. The child may be willing to talk through a puppet or a stuffed animal.
- Acknowledge the importance of the child's life. Let dying children know that they will never be forgotten.
- Allow the child to participate in decisions concerning their death as much as possible.

Data from Beale, E. A., Baile, W. F., & Aaron, J. (2005). Silence is not golden: Communicating with children dying from cancer. *Journal of Clinical Oncology, 23*(15), 3629–3631; Dunlop, S. (2008). The dying child: should we tell the truth? *Paediatric Nursing, 20*(6), 28–31; Kersun, L. S., & Shemesh, E. (2007). Depression and Anxiety in Children at the End of Life. *Pediatric Clinics of North America, 54,* 691–708; McSherry, M., Carroll, J. M., & Rourke, M. T. (2007). Psychosocial and Spiritual Needs of Children Living with a Life-Limiting Illness. *Pediatric Clinics of North America, 54,* 609–629.

when possible. Holding the child is a universal request and should be permitted, along with touching, stroking, kissing, and talking soothingly.

Many families find that saying good-bye as a group is helpful. Families need to cry together and to tell each other how much they will miss each other. Assure them that the vigil with the child prevents the child from feeling isolated or abandoned as death approaches. The dying child should never be left alone when dying is imminent.

TISSUE AND ORGAN DONATION

Families may be asked about making an anatomic gift. Nurses can become better prepared to serve the family of the dying child and potential organ recipients by becoming familiar with the healthcare facility's criteria for organ and tissue procurement. Generally, an organ procurement organization coordinator will work in collaboration with the nurses and other members of the healthcare team to help explain the process of organ donation and to ensure families are not coerced to make an anatomic gift (DeVeaux, 2006).

NEED FOR AUTOPSY

When the exact cause of death is unclear, an autopsy may be suggested. An autopsy may be required by state law for an unnatural or unexpected death, such as suicide, homicide, or sudden infant death syndrome. When parents have a choice, they may be hesitant to consent to autopsy because it further invades the child's body. Support the family during decision making by explaining that the autopsy will likely reveal the cause of death. This information may be valuable if the death is potentially due to a genetic disorder, affecting future childbearing decisions.

POSTMORTEM CARE AND FAMILY SUPPORT

Offer ongoing support after the child dies. Questions like the following may help begin the conversation: "I am sorry for your loss. How can I help?" "What are your traditions when an infant or child dies?" "Is there someone I can call for you?" Although crying with families was once considered unprofessional, it is now recognized as an expression of caring and empathy. Nurses should feel free to express their sorrow and grief for the child and family. See Table 43–4 for more common mourning and after-death rituals.

Table 43–4 Cultural Traditions in Mourning and After-Death Rites

Religious Group	Rituals You Might Observe
American Indians	■ Beliefs and practices vary widely among tribes
Buddhism	■ Last-rite chanting at bedside ■ Cremation common
Catholicism	■ Sacrament of the sick, baptism of newborn ■ Obligated to take ordinary but not extraordinary means to prolong life ■ Burial is common
Christian Science	■ No medical help is sought to prolong life ■ No donation of body parts. Disposal of body and parts decided by family
Hinduism	■ Death is seen as a passage, expect rebirth ■ Religious prayers chanted before and after death ■ Cremation common ■ Men and women display outward grief ■ Thread tied around wrist signifies a blessing, do not remove
Islam	■ Organ donation is acceptable ■ Autopsy only for medical or legal reasons ■ Body is washed only by Muslim of same gender
Jehovah's Witness	■ Donation of body parts is forbidden ■ Autopsy acceptable for legal reasons ■ Burial determined by family preference
Judaism	■ Autopsy and organ donation is not acceptable ■ Life support is not mandated ■ Body ritually washed, and burial occurs as soon as possible with all body parts buried together ■ Seven-day mourning period
Mormonism	■ If death inevitable, promote a peaceful and dignified death ■ Organ donation is an individual choice ■ Burial in "temple clothes"
Protestantism	■ Organ donation, autopsy, and burial or cremation is individual decision ■ Prolonging life may have restrictions
Seventh Day Adventist	■ Prefer prolonging life ■ Organ donation and autopsy are individual decisions ■ Disposal of body and burial are individual decisions

Adapted from Spector, R. E. (2009). *Cultural diversity in health and illness* (7th ed., pp. 141–142). Upper Saddle River, NJ: Prentice Hall Health, and Lipson, J. G.; Dibble, S. L.; Minarik, P. A. Cultural Traditions in Mourning and After Death Rituals, Table 5–8. *Culture and Nursing Care: A Pocket Guide.* San Francisco: UCSF Nursing Press.

Nursing Practice

When a sudden violence-related death of a child or adolescent occurs, forensic evidence is collected. Removal of medical equipment may not be permitted. Follow facility guidelines for evidence collection and the chain of possession prior to giving evidence to law enforcement authorities. The family may not be permitted to have as much physical contact with the child's body in these circumstances.

Identify the family's wishes for postmortem care before performing any care. Ask before removing any jewelry or other item from the child because cultural and spiritual practices may specify that the article remain on the child after death. Follow the healthcare facility's guidelines for postmortem care. Position the child according to guidelines or cultural/religious practices, clean the room, and remove medical equipment.

After the child's death, allow the family to spend as much time as they need with the child's body. Never rush family members who are saying good-bye to the child. Save all of the child's personal items—especially in the case of an infant. A lock of hair, hand- or footprints, the infant's identification band, the child's weight and height, or a picture of the infant can be sources of comfort and remembrance for families. Ask for permission before cutting a lock of hair as some cultural and religious groups prohibit it, such as Native Americans. Seal the last clothes or patient gown worn by the child in a plastic bag to retain the child's scent. When possible, use a special remembrance box or container for this purpose. If parents refuse to take the items, give them to another family member or retain them. Document the collection of the mementos and who received them in case parents ask for them at a later time (Foresman-Capuzzi, 2007).

When a newborn or young infant has died, wrap the baby in a blanket and offer the mother and other family members the opportunity to hold the baby. Parents may want to bathe and dress the infant. The family experiencing the death of a newborn may appreciate an offer to take pictures of the baby and family together, if picture taking is not prohibited by religious or cultural traditions. Some families may feel uncomfortable taking pictures and refuse the offer. The nurse should question the family about baptism or other ritual requests for the newborn, and facilitate arrangements for a religious or spiritual leader at the family's request. The mother experiencing the death of a newborn requires instructions on lactation suppression or milk donation options if she has been breastfeeding or pumping the breasts (Gale, 2006).

A bereavement folder should be provided to parents with information that includes resources available to help with a memorial service or funeral and potential sibling responses. Inform parents that certain dates, such as the day of the week the child died, the child's birthday, or family holidays, will be difficult and may trigger intense sadness. Parents may benefit from keeping a journal of their thoughts and memories, or writing letters or poems to or about their child.

EVALUATION

Expected outcomes of caring for the dying child and family may include the following:

- The child is pain-free and comfortable, and the child's physiologic needs are met.
- The cultural and spiritual needs of the dying child and family are met.
- The dying child and family receive support during the dying process.
- The family receives continued support after the child's death.

BEREAVEMENT

PARENTS' REACTIONS

The death of one's child is likely the most traumatic event a parent will experience. Grief, an individual's feelings and behaviors in response to death or loss, is painful, individualized, and exhausting. Many factors influence the parents' grief responses, including their perception of the preventability of the illness or injury, the suddenness and other circumstances of the death, the nature of their attachment to the child, previous losses, spiritual or religious orientation, and culture.

SUDDEN DEATH OF A CHILD

Although many children die because of chronic or terminal illness, more than half of child deaths between 1 and 19 years of age are caused by unexpected injuries (Miniño, Heron, Murphy, et al., 2007). A sudden or unexpected death that results from sudden infant death syndrome, injury, illness, suicide, or violence can place parents at risk for complicated grief (Truog, Christ, Browning, et al., 2006) because they have not had time to prepare for the child's death. Parents need support to deal with the death of the child and with their surviving children.

DEATH OF A NEWBORN OR YOUNG INFANT

In 2005, 28,440 infants died either shortly after birth or during the first year of life often because of low birth weight, severe congenital conditions and sudden infant death syndrome (Kung, Hoyert, Xu, et al., 2008). The death of a newborn forces parents to experience their child's entire life in a short period of time, and they are faced with overwhelming grief at the time when they anticipated the experience of joy. Unique experiences may occur with multiple birth, such as the death of one or more of the infants, leading to conflicting emotions for the parents. While they mourn the death of one child, they must parent and bond with the survivor(s). Refer parents to a perinatal bereavement program or support group.

GRIEF AND BEREAVEMENT

Although parents progress through distinct stages of grief, as described on page 1132, the time line and nature of the grief process differ for each individual. The intense pain and shock initially felt

Nursing Practice

Several strategies for working with parents whose child dies suddenly can help parents cope with this tragedy and improve their perception of care received (Knapp, Mulligan-Smith, and the Committee of Pediatric Emergency Medicine, 2005):

- Identify a spokesperson for the medical team to keep the family informed during resuscitation efforts. Have both parents present if possible.
- Provide private space with telephone access.
- Create time for families to assimilate the child's worsening status by providing several updates during the resuscitation. Prepare them for what is to come.
- Offer to telephone clergy, family, and friends.
- After the death, prepare the body for viewing.
- Provide time and a place for the family to say good-bye.
- Sit close and make eye contact. Share your emotions with the family. Accept whatever emotions family members express.
- Convey information to the family about the cause of death, autopsy, funeral preparations, and the normal grief process.
- Arrange for family follow-up to see how they are responding to the child's loss and to review autopsy findings.

by parents gradually give way to feelings of anger, guilt, depression, and loneliness. Very slowly, and with much support, energy returns and parents again begin to enjoy life experiences. Parents may experience friction due to differing rates and intensity of grief. Additional support may be needed to prevent a sense of loneliness and isolation.

The nurse should emphasize to parents that although the period surrounding their child's death is difficult, caring for themselves physically and mentally is important. The nurse can give a list of appropriate support groups, books, and articles to parents for later use. Parents can be referred to the organizations such as Compassionate Friends, First Candle, and SHARE Pregnancy and Infant Loss Support as well as to local support groups for bereaved parents or siblings. Some facilities have formal follow-up programs for bereaved parents to encourage a healthy progression through the grieving process. See MyNursingKit for Web sites of these organizations.

SIBLINGS' REACTIONS

Siblings experiencing the death of a brother or sister require supportive and compassionate care. In the course of the child's illness, the siblings probably will have received less attention from parents. Siblings have reported feeling loneliness, anxiety, anger, and jealousy during the dying process (Nolbris & Hellstrom, 2005). Depending on their development, they may fear that they caused their brother or sister to be injured or become ill, or worry that their bad thoughts caused the illness. Nurses and other support personnel can assist the surviving children to adapt to their parents' distraction, grief, and increased protectiveness of them. The siblings need to hear that the parents' grief in no way diminishes the love felt for them. Table 43–5 highlights children's understanding of death at different developmental stages, some of the possible behavioral responses, and nursing considerations for family education.

When talking to the siblings of a child who has died, be honest and answer questions truthfully. Provide explanations in developmentally appropriate terms, such as "Adam's heart will never beat again," "He will never get cold or hungry," and "He will never come home again." Reassure siblings that they did not cause their brother or sister to die (unless they did contribute to the child's death) and that death was not a punishment for wrongdoing. The nurse should allow the siblings to ask questions and acknowledge the emotions they are feeling by emphasizing that it is all right for them to be sad, angry, frightened, or tearful. The nurse should use the same amount of energy and concern in acknowledging the grief of the siblings and the adults.

As appropriate and comfortable for the family, siblings should be permitted to participate in planning the child's memorial or funeral service. Being able to grieve as a family provides siblings with a sense of connectedness to parents and provides security at a vulnerable time. If siblings attend the funeral, they should be prepared for what to expect, such as an open casket and the behaviors of mourners. The nurse can suggest designating a support person, such as a family member or close friend, who can monitor the siblings' needs while the parents attend to other matters. It is important to keep the family together as much as possible.

As with parental bereavement, sibling bereavement is a lifelong process. The nurse should encourage parents to make sure other caregivers and teachers know about the sibling's loss. Books for the family that might help children with grief include *It's OK to Cry: A Parent's Guide to Helping Children Through the Losses of Life* by H. Norman Wright, *Helping Children Grieve* by Ruth Arent, or *When Children Grieve* by John James.

STAFF REACTIONS TO THE DEATH OF A CHILD

Caring for dying children is especially stressful and demanding for healthcare professionals. Health professionals caring for the dying child may feel a sense of helplessness that they have failed the child, and sadness for the child's shortened life (Beale, Baile, & Aaron, 2005). Nurses involved in long-term relationships with children experience grief when these children die. Some nurses cope by distancing themselves socially from the dying child and family to maintain composure and a professional demeanor.

Caring for the dying child may be especially difficult for nurses who have young children. They tend to identify with the child, making it more difficult to recognize the dying child's anxiety and fears because of their own personal defenses against their sense of helplessness to alter the course of the child's disease.

Nurses who work with terminally ill children and their families need special preparation to meet the needs of these individuals and to manage personal stress simultaneously. Mentorship with experienced hospice nurses, as well as additional educational experiences, may help promote professional nursing care.

Table 43–5 Children's Understanding of Death and Possible Behavioral Responses

Understanding of Death	Potential Behaviors	Nursing Management
	Infant	
Cognitive stage: sensorimotor Senses tenseness of caregivers, and altered routines Senses separation	Resists cuddling and eats less Cries excessively, clingy Sleeps more than usual	Provide a sense of security, by holding and hugging Use a soothing voice Try to return to usual routines
	Toddler	
Cognitive stage: preoperational No understanding of true concept of death Aware someone is missing—separation anxiety Unable to distinguish death from temporary separation or abandonment	Regresses to younger stage of development Clingy, refuses to let parent out of sight Shows distress by biting, hitting, tears Problems eating and sleeping Sleep disturbances Fearfulness	Encourage parents to hold and cuddle the toddler to help reduce the fear of separation Follow familiar routines Be tolerant of regressive behaviors Talk and answer questions in terms the child will understand
	Preschooler	
Cognitive stage: preoperational Believes death is temporary Magical thinking—believes the dead person can be brought back to life Believes bad thoughts cause death Has beginning experience with death of animals and plants	Regression to earlier developmental stage, problems with bowel and bladder control, tantrums May fear going to sleep, has nightmares, afraid of the dark Crying spells Seems morbidly fascinated with death Asks many questions Complaints of abdominal pain	Listen to the child and answer questions honestly, reassure the child that his thoughts did not cause the death Try to follow usual routines Be tolerant of regressive behaviors, provide play activities. Keep memories alive with pictures and items that remind the child of the loved one Participate in rituals, e.g., going to the cemetery, releasing helium balloons, and planting flowers
	School-Age child	
Cognitive stage: concrete operations Has a more realistic understanding of death By 8–10 years, understands the permanence and irreversibility of death May have guilt or assume blame for the death May not realize that death can occur at any age	Crying, moody, may become more withdrawn and distant, or may deny sadness by hiding tears and acting more like adults Decreased concentration for school work, may refuse to go to school Psychosomatic complaints—stomachache or headache Angry outbursts, disruptive behaviors, aggression May try to comfort parents by taking over tasks May fear another loved person will die	Listen to the child and answer questions honestly Return to usual routines and activities Keep memories alive through activities such as art, music, creating a memory book, sewing a quilt, and planting a garden Share Internet resources Use coping support groups Encourage the family to seek faith-based support
	Adolescent	
Cognitive stage: formal operations Intellectually capable of understanding death Recognizes all people and self must die Better understands the association between illness and death Sense of invincibility conflicts with fear of death Able to recognize effect of death on others	May have severe depression, mood swings, withdrawal from friends May feel angry or guilty Acting-out or risk-taking behavior, delinquency, suicide attempts, promiscuity, drug or alcohol use Uses abstract and philosophical reasoning Girls may seek comfort from friends Eating and sleeping problems	Be available and encourage open communication Share your own grief and feelings with the adolescent Keep memories alive with pictures and items that remind the teen of the loved one Access counseling and support groups Encourage the child to seek support from his or her faith group Share Internet resources

Data from: Hinds, P. S., Oakes, L. L., Hicks, J., & Anghelescu, D. L. (2005). End-of-life care for children and adolescents. *Seminars in Oncologic Nursing, 21*(1), 53–62; Kirwin, K. M., & Havrin, V. (2005). Decreasing the risk of complicated bereavement and future psychiatric disorders in children. *Journal of Child and Adolescent Psychiatric Nursing, 18*(2), 62–78; Auman, M. J. (2007). Bereavement support for children. *Journal of School Nursing, 23*(1), 34–39; and Korones, D. N. (2007). Pediatric palliative care, *Pediatrics in Review, 28*(8), e46–e56.

Nurses who work with dying children and their families must learn to cope effectively with grief and develop empathy, competence, and confidence in their ability to provide more humane and effective nursing care. Nurses should feel free to express their sorrow and grief for the child and family. Some nurses attend funeral and memorial services when invited by the patient's family.

Nurses working in emergency departments caring for children who die suddenly or in hospice settings and hospital units that care for terminally ill children need support systems to help balance the stresses of working with dying children. Support systems may include discussions with peers or debriefing group sessions with mental health professionals that provide an opportunity for nurses to discuss their feelings and concerns (Figure 43–7 ●). Educational seminars on compassion fatigue may help nurses identify coping strategies for personal care (Meadors & Lamson, 2008).

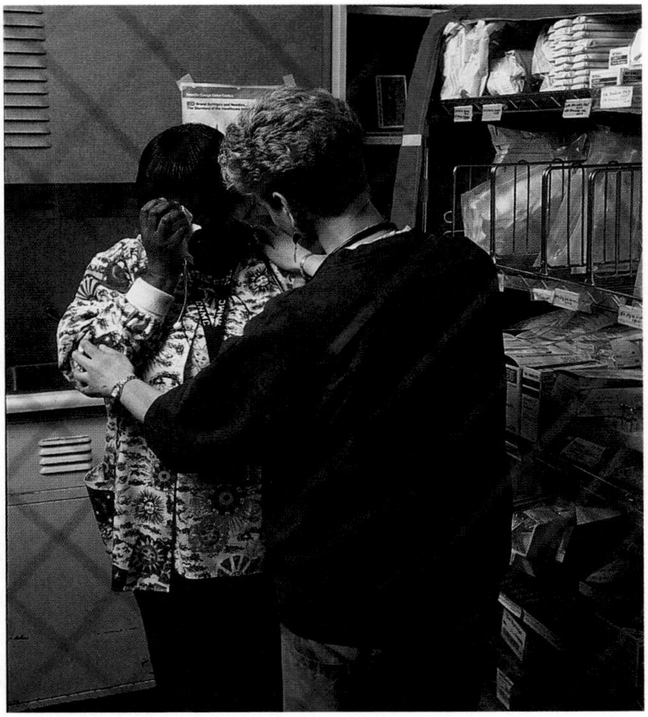

● **Figure 43–7** Nurses' need for support. Nurses need to express grief in a supportive environment after a child's death. Sharing the sadness and grief or futility of resuscitation efforts with colleagues can often help nurses continue to provide supportive care to the next families who need compassionate care.

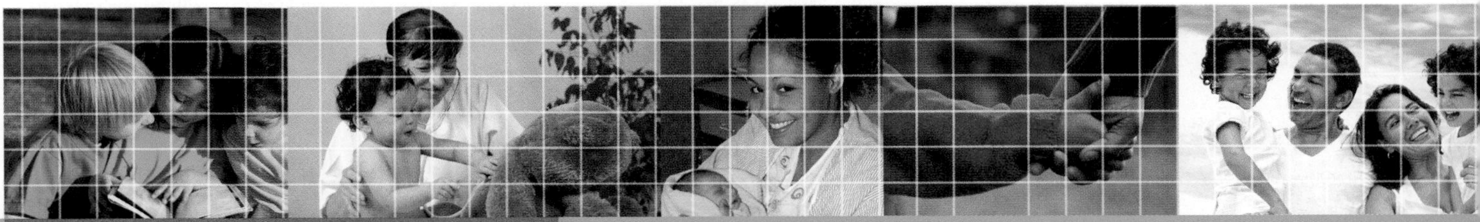

CRITICAL CONCEPT REVIEW

LEARNING OUTCOMES	CONCEPTS
43.1 Describe the child's experiences with life-threatening illness or injury according to developmental level.	1. Infant: ■ Sleep-wake cycle and feeding routine are disrupted. ■ Excessive irritability. 2. Toddler: ■ Frightened by immobilizers. ■ Associates pain with punishment. 3. Preschooler: ■ Fears mutilation. ■ Easily regresses to earlier stages. 4. School-age child: ■ Fears body injury and death. ■ Fears loss of control. 5. Adolescent: ■ Displays anger, rebellion, and withdrawal.
43.2 Discuss the family's experience and reactions to having a child with a life-threatening illness or injury.	1. Parents go through different stages: ■ Shock and disbelief. ■ Anger and guilt. ■ Deprivation and loss. ■ Anticipatory waiting. ■ Readjustment or mourning.

(continued)

LEARNING OUTCOMES | CONCEPTS

2. Siblings:
   - Insecurity and anxiety.
   - Jealousy or envy of attention given to sick child.
   - Resentment, fear, and anger.

43.3 Describe the coping mechanisms used by the child and family in response to stress.

Child:
1. Regression.
2. Denial.
3. Repression.
4. Postponement.
5. Bargaining.

Family:
1. Participation in care.
2. Participation in decision making.
3. Family support.
4. Anger and hostility.

43.4 Develop a nursing care plan for the child with a life-threatening illness or injury.

1. Encourage parents to stay at bedside.
2. Provide developmentally appropriate explanations about all procedures and equipment.
3. Provide opportunities for play where possible.
4. Provide opportunities for choice where appropriate.
5. Provide routines for scheduled care.
6. Treat the child's pain.

43.5 Apply assessment skills to identify the physiologic changes that occur in the dying child.

1. Decrease in peripheral circulation—cool and mottled skin.
2. Cheyne-Stokes respirations.
3. Secretions increase in the back of the throat.
4. Decreased perfusion to the brain—restlessness, agitation, less awareness of surroundings, coma.
5. Kidney function decreases—decreased urine output.
6. Incontinence as death approaches.

43.6 Develop a nursing care plan to provide family-centered care for the dying child and family.

1. Provide physical comfort for the child.
   - Treat pain effectively.
   - Instruct parents in nonpharmacologic pain relief.
2. Provide emotional comfort.
   - Encourage family to stay with child.
3. Establish homelike routines for child and family.
   - Allow child to take part in decision making.
   - Refer parents to support groups.
4. Maintain family functioning.
   - Encourage parents to take breaks.
   - Provide time for sibling interaction.
5. Promote cultural and spiritual values.
   - Incorporate family rituals in care of child.
6. Prepare family and child for impending death.

43.7 Implement strategies for bereavement support of the parents and siblings after the death of a child.

1. Parents
   - After the death, allow the family to stay with the dead child as long as they want.
   - Provide items used by the child, foot- or handprints, and lock of hair to parents.
   - Provide information and resources to support their own grieving and that of other children.
   - Make referrals for support as necessary. Contact parents on the anniversary of the child's death.
2. Siblings
   - Explain that they did not cause the child's death and the death was not a punishment.
   - Allow children to participate in planning the child's memorial and to attend.
   - Encourage parents to find a support program for children to participate in.
   - Encourage children to express their feelings and grief through art, stories, and writing.
   - Help children develop a keepsake box or album of photographs.

43.8 Describe the responses of nurses caring for children who die.

1. Grieving after caring for child over a long period of time.
2. Feelings of helplessness to change the end results.
3. Reluctance to form connections with other terminally ill children.
4. Identification with terminally ill child if own child is near same age.

CRITICAL THINKING IN ACTION

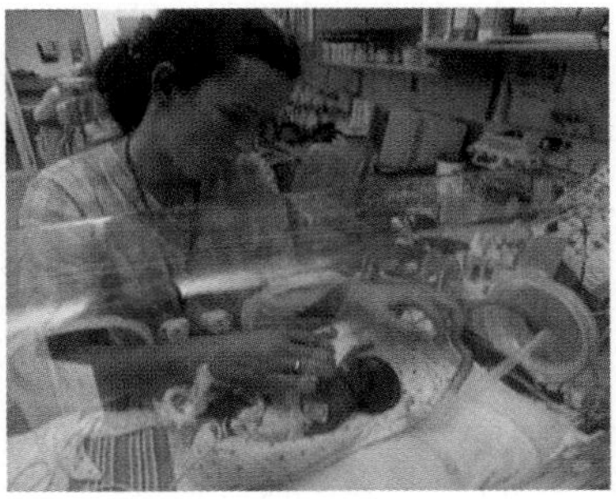

Kelly is a premature baby weighing 500 grams when born at 24 weeks gestation after her mother had premature rupture of membranes. Her parents, Shawn and Lori, are of Navajo Indian descent. Kelly's condition is extremely critical and she is on life support. You know that any amount of touch can be extremely stressful for infants this small and in critical condition. The mother has been pumping and freezing breast milk for future use. The parents are encouraged to assist the nurse in any way they can, but they are not able to touch Kelly. While the parents know how critical Kelly's condition is and have learned about the machines and medications being used, they are still confused and uncertain about the situation. They have not left the hospital at all. The grandparents have been helping care for Roseanne, Kelly's 7-year-old sister and she has visited her sister once. On the third day of life, Kelly gained weight and started to show an increase in activity. The parents thought this could be a positive sign, but the nurse explained that swelling caused the weight gain and the increased activity was from agitation as Kelly struggled to breathe. When the parents were at the bedside, Kelly started to become cyanotic and her oxygen saturation level dropped to the 60s. The healthcare team tried to save her but were unsuccessful. This was a devastating loss for the family and all the medical personnel involved.

1. What are some of the stressors Kelly experienced while in the hospital?
2. What are the stages of grief Kelly's family is likely to experience?
3. What are some strategies that can be used to help Roseanne deal with the loss of her sister?
4. What are some of the strategies for supporting Kelly's parents?

See MyNursingKit for possible responses.

REFERENCES

Auman, M. J. (2007). Bereavement support for children. *Journal of School Nursing, 23*(1), 34–39.

Baergen, R. (2006). How hopeful is too hopeful? Responding to unreasonably optimistic parents. *Pediatric Nursing, 32*(5), 482–486.

Beale, E. A., Baile, W. F., & Aaron, J. (2005). Silence is not golden: Communicating with children dying from cancer. *Journal of Clinical Oncology, 23*(15), 3629–3631.

Board, R. (2005). School-age children's perceptions of their PICU hospitalization. *Pediatric Nursing, 31*(3), 166–175.

DeVeaux, T. E. (2006). Non-heart-beating organ donation: Issues and ethics for the critical care nurse. *Journal of Vascular Nursing, 24*, 17–21.

Dratler, M. B., Burns, M. K., & Dratler, H. L. (2006). Conveying adverse news in end-of-life situations. *Gastroenterology Clinics of North America, 35*, 41–52.

ENA (2005). Emergency nurses association position statement: family presence at the bedside during invasive procedures and cardiopulmonary resuscitation. Retrieved September 19, 2009, from www.ena.org/SiteCollectionDocuments/Position%20Statements/Family_Presence_-_ENA_PS.pdf

Foresman-Capuzzi, J. (2007). Grief telling: Death of a child in the emergency department. *Journal of Emergency Nursing, 33*(5), 505–508.

Gale, G. (2006). Implementing a palliative care program in a newborn intensive care unit. *Advances in Neonatal Care, 6*(1), e1–e37.

Hall, E. O. C. (2004). A double concern: Grandmothers' experiences when a small grandchild is critically ill. *Journal of Pediatric Nursing, 19*(1), 61–69.

Heller, K. S., & Solomon, M. Z. (2005). Continuity of care and caring: What matters to parents of children with life-threatening conditions. *Journal of Pediatric Nursing, 20*(5), 335–346.

Himelstein, B. P. (2005). Palliative care in pediatrics. *Anesthesiology Clinics of North America, 23*, 837–856.

Himelstein, B. P., Hilden, J. M., Boldt, A. M., & Weissman, D. (2004). Pediatric palliative care. *New England Journal of Medicine, 350*(17), 1752–1762.

Hinds, P. S., Oakes, L. L., Hicks, J., & Anghelescu, D. L. (2005). End-of-life care for children and adolescents. *Seminars in Oncologic Nursing, 21*(1), 53–62

Holbrook, T. L., Hoyt, D. B., Coimbra, R., Potenza, B., Sise, M., & Anderson, J. P. (2005). Long-term posttraumatic stress disorder persists after majory trauma in adolescents: New data on risk factors and functional outcomes, *Journal of Trauma, Injury, Infection, and Critical Care, 58*(4), 764–771.

Hone-Warren, M. (2007). Exploration of school administrator attitudes regarding do not resuscitate policies in the school setting. *Journal of School Nursing, 23*(2), 98–103.

Institute of Medicine. (2003). Patterns of childhood death in America. In *When children die: Improving palliative and end-of-life care for children and their families* (pp. 41–71). Washington, DC: National Academy Press.

Kirwin, K. M., & Havrin, V. (2005). Decreasing the risk of complicated bereavement and future psychiatric disorders in children. *Journal of Child and Adolescent Psychiatric Nursing, 18*(2), 62–78

Knapp, J., Mulligan-Smith, D., and the Committee of Pediatric Emergency Medicine. (2005). Death of a child in the emergency department. *Pediatrics, 115*(5), 1432–1437.

Korones, D. N. (2007). Pediatric palliative care. *Pediatrics in Review, 28*(8), e46–e56.

Kreicbergs, U., Valdimarsdóttir, U., Onelöv, E., Henter, J. I., & Steineck, G. (2004). Talking about death with children who have severe malignant disease. *New England Journal of Medicine, 351*(12), 1251–1253.

Kung, H., Hoyert, D. L., Xu, J., & Murphy, S. L. (2008). Deaths: Final Data for 2005, *National Vital Statistics Reports, 56*(10), 11–12.

Levetown, M. (2004). Breaking bad news in the emergency department: When seconds count. *Topics in Emergency Medicine, 26*(1), 35–43.

Mangurten, J., Scott, S. H., Guzzetta, C. E., Clark, A. P., Vinson, L., Sperry, J., Hicks, B., Voelmeck, W. (2006). Effect of family presence during resuscitation and invasive procedures in a pediatric emergency department. *Journal of Emergency Nursing, 32*(3), 225–233.

Mauer, S. (2008). A family affair. *Advance for Nurses, 10*(8), 33–34.

McCaffrey, A. M., Eisenberg, D. M., Legedza, A. T. R., Davis, R. B., & Phillips, R. S. (2004, April 26). Prayer for health concerns: Results of a national survey on prevalence and patterns of use. *Archives of Internal Medicine, 164*, 858–862.

Meadors, P., & Lamson, A. (2008). Compassion fatigue and secondary traumatization: Provider self care on intensive care units for children. *Journal of Pediatric Health Care, 22*(1), 24–34.

Melnyk, B. M., Alpert-Gillis, L., Feinstein, N. F., Crean, H. F., Johnson, J., Fairbanks, E., et al. (2004). Creating opportunities for parent empowerment: Program effects on the mental health/coping outcomes of critically ill young children and their mothers. *Pediatrics, 113*(6), e597–e607.

Meyer, E. C., Ritholz, M. D., Burns, J. P., & Truog, R. D. (2006). Improving the quality of end-of-life care in the pediatric intensive care unit: Parents' priorities and recommendations. *Pediatrics, 117*(3), 649–657.

Miniño, A. M., Heron, M. P., Murphy, S. L., & Kochanek, K. D. (2007). Deaths: Final data for 2004. *National Vital Statistics Reports, 55*(19), 21.

National Center for Complementary and Alternative Medicine. (2005). Prayer and Spirituality in Health: Ancient Practices, Modern Science. *CAM at the NIH: Focus on Complementary and Alternative Therapy, 12*(1), 1–4.

Nolbris, M., & Hellstrom, A. L. (2005). Siblings' needs and issues when a brother or sister dies of cancer. *Journal of Pediatric Oncology Nursing, 22*(4), 227–233.

O'Malley, P. J., Brown, K., Krug, S. E., and The Committee on Pediatric Emergency Medicine (2008). Patient- and Family-Centered Care of Children in the Emergency Department. *Pediatrics, 122*(2), e511–e521.

Rushton, C. H. (2004). Ethics and palliative care in pediatrics. *American Journal of Nursing, 104*(4), 54–63.

Rushton, C. H. (2005). A framework for integrated pediatric palliative care: Being with dying. *Journal of Pediatric Nursing, 20*(5), 311–325.

Smith, A. B., Hefley, G. C., & Anand, K. J. S. (2007). Parent bed spaces in the PICU: Effect on parental stress. *Pediatric Nursing, 33*(3), 215–221.

Snyder, B. S. (2004). Preventing treatment interference: Nurses' and parents' intervention strategies. *Pediatric Nursing, 30*(1), 31–40.

Spector, R. E. (2009). *Cultural diversity in health and illness* (7th ed., pp. 141–142). Upper Saddle River, NJ: Prentice Hall Health.

Truog, R. D., Christ, G., Browning, D. M., & Meyer, E. C. (2006). Sudden traumatic death in children: "We did everything, but your child didn't survive." *Journal of American Medical Association, 295*(22), 2646–2654.

Watters, D., Sayre, M. R., & Silbergleit, R. (2005). Research Conditions That Qualify for Emergency Exception from Informed Consent. *Academic Emergency Medicine, 12*(11), 1040–1044.

Winston, F. K., Baxt, C., Kassam-Adams, N. L., Elliott, M. R., & Kallan, M. J. (2005). Acute traumatic stress symptoms in child occupants and their parent drivers after crash involvement. *Archives of Pediatric and Adolescent Medicine, 159*(11), 1074–1079.

Woodgate, R. L. (2006). Living in a work without closure: Reality for parents who have experienced the death of a child. *Journal of Palliative Care, 22*(2), 75–83.

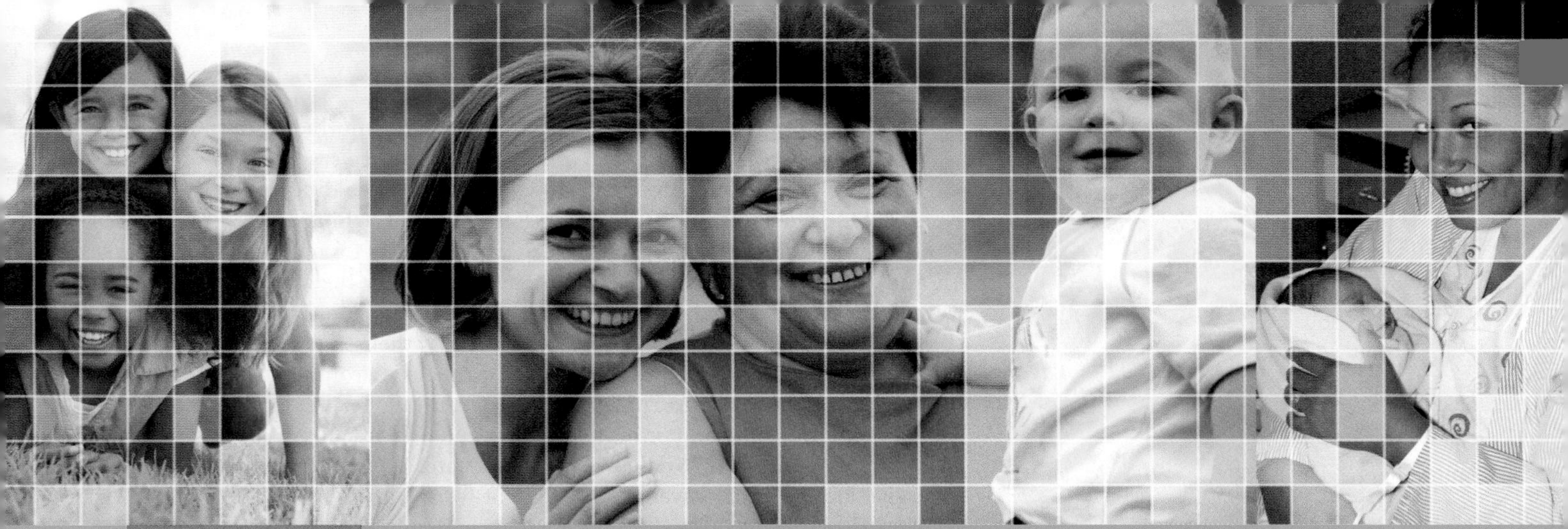

CHAPTER

44 Social and Environmental Influences on the Child

Amy has always been a challenge. She has already left home a couple of times and lived on the streets. Lately she has been more interested in school and is at home and trying to do well. We want her to succeed and learn the skills she needs in her life. I wish she would not have all of these body piercings, but we don't want to make too big an issue of it as long as she is doing well in school. —Mother of Amy, 15 years old

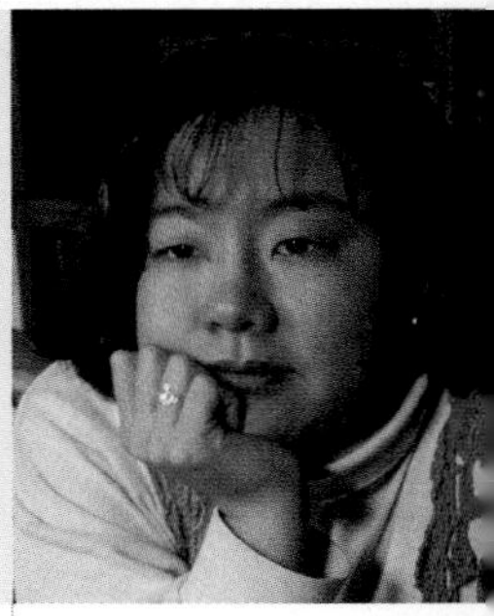

LEARNING OUTCOMES

44.1 Identify major social and environmental factors that influence the health of children and adolescents.

44.2 List external influences that influence child and adolescent health.

44.3 Apply the ecologic model and resiliency theory to assessment of the social and environmental factors in children's lives.

44.4 Examine the effects of substance use, physical activity, and other lifestyle patterns on health.

44.5 Plan nursing interventions for children who experience violence.

44.6 Evaluate the environment for hazards to children, such as exposure to substances and potential for poisoning.

44.7 Explore the nursing role in prevention and treatment of child abuse and neglect, and other forms of violence.

44.8 Plan nursing interventions for children related to social and environmental situations.

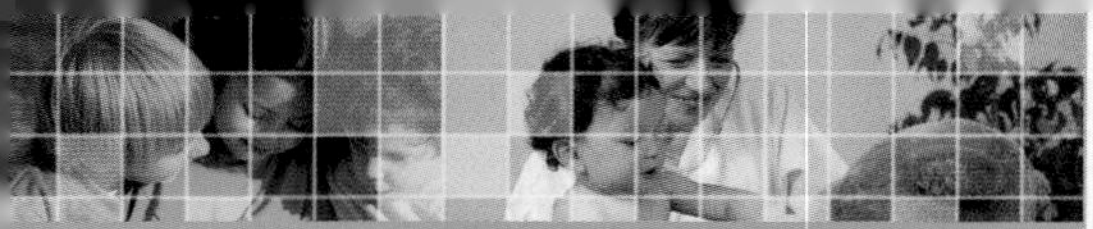

KEY TERMS

Bisexual, 1168
Bullying, 1170
Chelation, 1188
Child sexual abuse, 1176
Cyberbullying, 1170
Disaster, 1181
Emotional abuse, 1176
Emotional neglect, 1176
Gay, 1168
Hazing, 1171
Homosexuality, 1168
Incest, 1176
Lesbian, 1168
Physical abuse, 1175
Physical neglect, 1176
Protective factors, 1152
Resiliency theory, 1152
Risk factors, 1152
Toxins, 1183
Toxicants, 1183
Transgendered, 1168
Violence, 1169

Many of the major causes of mortality and morbidity in children are closely linked with social influences in the child's world. The social contexts for young children growing up today are different from those of even a decade ago. Examining the social contexts in which children live and grow can provide insights into behavior, and present opportunities for nursing interventions. All nurses must examine the social influences and apply the knowledge gained to plan health care that will benefit youth as they grow into adulthood.

Children and adolescents are also influenced by their environments. The physical setting, exposure to chemical agents, and other environmental factors are increasingly identified as instrumental in determining health. Nurses assess the environment for its risk and protective factors, and then use this information to plan nursing care appropriate to enhance the heath status of children and adolescents.

What are the settings where nurses might work with youth in the community? What are the challenges of today's society that children must often face at very young ages? How can nurses help children face these challenges, and emerge as healthy and contributing members of society? What roles do nurses play in identifying and using the protective factors and in minimizing the risk factors of youth? This chapter will examine and apply these social and environmental concepts in a variety of nursing settings.

Examine again the major causes of death for children from 1 year of age through adolescence that are presented on the Companion Website. See Chapter 1 for more discussion. Notice that most morbidity is related to preventable causes linked to present-day lifestyles. Car crashes, fires, drowning, and homicides are a few examples of common causes of death in children.

Now examine the major reasons for hospitalization on the Companion Website. By the time children are 5 years of age, injuries rank as the second cause, and by 10 years, mental disorders are the major cause of hospitalization. By the teen years, pregnancy and mental disorders are the most common admitting diagnoses to hospitals. All of these conditions are related, at least in part, to the social and environmental settings in which children live. These settings and their influences must be examined to understand how best to intervene with children.

BASIC CONCEPTS

In this chapter, two main theories provide a framework for examining societal influences on children. The ecologic model and resiliency theory are discussed in Chapter 33, and should be reviewed now to assist in evaluating the environmental settings that influence children.

The ecologic theory views the child and the environment as interacting forces, with children influencing systems around them, even while they are influenced by these systems (Bronfenbrenner, 2005). Close (meaning nearby) systems providing daily contact are microsystems, but other systems such as parental work and political or cultural environments are also important. Understanding these systems, or the forces in which children function, can provide information that guides care providers. For example, if the parents' employers do not provide healthcare insurance, their children may not get needed healthcare such as immunizations, treatment for diseases, and growth monitoring.

Resiliency theory examines risk and protective factors in the child's environment as they influence the child's adaptation to stressful events, and can be modified to lead to more productive and healthy outcomes. Resilience is the ability to exhibit healthy responses, even when faced with significant stress and adversity (see Chapter 33 for a further description of resiliency theory) (Henderson, Bernard, & Sharp-Light, 2007). Families may have protective factors that provide strength and assistance in dealing with crises, and risk factors that promote or contribute to healthcare challenges (Aronowitz, 2005). For example, if a young child is hospitalized for treatment of an acute infectious illness, some **protective factors** might include the ability of one parent to stay with the child at all times, the ability of a grandmother to care for siblings at home during this time, and the child's ability to adapt to new situations and communicate readily with staff members. On the other hand, **risk factors** might include lack of comprehensive health insurance to pay for the hospitalization, lack of an identified healthcare "home" (consistent care provider) for the child, and incomplete immunizations. The concepts of resiliency theory can be applied to Amy's family as described in the opening quotation. She experienced disruption in family stability. The risk and protective factors interacted with her own personality in ways that resulted in her desire to appear as an independent person, establishing her identity through body art, and finally, a desire to return to school.

The National Longitudinal Study of Adolescent Health (ADD Health Study, 2005) was conducted with over 100,000 adolescents in the United States, and found that parent-family connectedness, school connectedness, a belief in a higher being, and academic success were predictive of youth having lower health risks. Interviews are presently being carried out with the participants who are now young adults; the resulting longitudinal data will show what characteristics and influences persist into adult life (ADD Health Study, 2005). Nurses can assist adolescents and their families in establishing a sense of attachment to each other. Encourage families to include adolescents in activities, attend their sports and other school events, have meals together regularly, and attend faith-based activities or other community events as a family.

Theoretical frameworks are discussed in Chapter 33∞ and are useful when examining social and environmental influences on children because they guide us to examine certain factors that can be altered or understood. They suggest the assessment data to collect and pertinent nursing interventions to use. They also foster partnerships with other care providers who use these and similar theories to plan social, psychologic, and other care for children and their families.

SOCIAL INFLUENCES ON CHILD HEALTH

POVERTY

An important risk factor that influences the health of children is poverty. Conversely, basic financial stability is a protective factor that contributes to the general health and well-being of children. Eighteen percent of children are poor (Forum on Child and Family Statistics, 2007) and in a family earning less than $20,650 annually for a family of three persons or less than $18,104 for a family of four (Federal Interagency Forum on Child and Family Statistics, 2007; Inglehart, 2007).

Children who are poor are more likely to have unmet health needs, to have difficulty in school, to become teen parents, and to experience multiple health problems, including stunted growth and lead poisoning. Inadequate, unsafe housing, food insecurity, and poor dietary quality are more common (Federal Interagency Forum, 2007). What is the face of poverty? Some statistics that may prove surprising include the following:

- The children most likely to be living in poor households are those below 5 years of age.
- About 43% of children living in a single-headed household are poor, while only 9% in married-couple households are poor.
- Ethnic variations are startling; 5% of white, 20% of Hispanic, and 13% of black children in married couple families live in poverty; 33% of white, 50% of Hispanic, and 50% of black children in female-headed families live in poverty.
- Poverty rates are higher in suburban and rural areas than in central cities.
- Nearly 80% of poor children have at least one parent working full time (Federal Interagency Forum on Child and Family Statistics, 2007).

Poverty leads to homelessness for some children. Children consititute 25% of the homeless population, and families represent 39% (Mullin & Ambrosia, 2005). Families with children are the fastest growing group of homeless people. Each year, from 0.9 to 1.6 million children experience homelessness (Committee on Community Health Services, 2005). The reasons for homelessness are also common risks for a number of the other challenges to health discussed in this chapter, including poor finances, abuse or other violence, and mental instability.

Children who experience homelessness often have multiple physical and mental health problems, and lack health insurance to provide care for these problems. Some of the common problems faced by homeless children and families include trauma, substance use, respiratory and skin infections, tuberculosis and HIV, and nutritional disorders. Children may have developmental delays, learning problems, or growth disruptions (Yousey & Carr, 2005). Teens who have been homeless are more likely to engage in other risky behavior, such as unprotected sex, sex with multiple partners, and substance abuse. They are more likely to need emergency care, to be depressed or have other mental illness, and to become pregnant than other teens (Kidd & Davidson, 2006).

Health problems related to homelessness, and other family characteristics, continue even after finding a place to live. Even after families leave homeless shelters, children frequently become separated from their mothers due to parent stress, lack of access to resources, and inability of parents to provide adequate homes

> **Thinking Critically**
>
> **DEMOGRAPHICS AND NURSING CARE**
>
> Nurses should understand the demographics in the areas where they work. What is the poverty rate in your community? What ethnic groups are overrepresented among the poor? Locate the resources such as food services, health care for the underserved, and enhanced school programs in order to refer poor families. Recognize that health promotion services may not be high priority when a family does not have adequate housing or food. When children are seen in any setting, such as in school or in an emergency room or hospital for acute care, perform needed assessments and intervention. Measure growth, assess vision and hearing, evaluate dietary intake, and check immunization status. Find out the stresses the family experiences and what resources they need to meet basic necessities. Construct a nursing care plan for a family living in poverty with two young children.
>
> See MyNursingKit for possible responses.

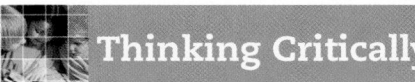

for the children. Complex, ongoing care is needed. This may begin in a shelter for the homeless, but should continue while the family obtains a place to live, accesses other community services, gets the children safely enrolled in school, and has financial and mental stability. Nursing management for families with children that are poor or homeless focuses on identification of poverty, careful assessment of health risks, and linking the family to resources that can assist with stability and health. There is often no way to identify a poor child from appearance, and they may hide their status when they are in school or come to a healthcare facility. Addresses given may not be accurate, or the address of a shelter might be used. Children living at shelters or in cars and on the street usually do not take the school bus but prefer to walk to avoid stigma. Be alert for children who have multiple health problems and repeated infectious diseases. They may be hungry and without adequate nutrition either at times or consistently. Degrees of personal hygiene may vary depending on access to laundry and bathing facilities. See Table 44–1 for examples of nursing care needs for homeless children and families.

STRESS

The adverse effect of stress on adults is well documented and the impact of stress on children has also been recognized. Stress can be acute, such as when a child has an argument with a friend, a test in school, or a family crisis. Stress can also become chronic

Table 44–1 Common Health Problems and Nursing Management of Children Who Are Poor and/or Homeless

Common Health Problems	Nursing Management
Lack of immunizations	Check immunization records Provide immunizations at schools and in homeless shelters
Common infectious diseases	Facilitate free clinics in shelters, schools, community settings Teach hygiene measures Provide information about resources for bathing, hygiene Provide resources for disease management Arrange for medications when needed
Sleep deficits	Inform parents about respite facilities Arrange for children to have quiet sleep time in school if possible
Vision and hearing deficits	Perform screening for deficits Provide resources for eyeglasses, hearing aids, care for ear infections (Service organizations such as Lion's Club are good options)
Nutritional deficits	Perform height and weight checks and nutritional assessment Evaluate family for food security (see Chapter 31∞) Be sure child is registered for school breakfast and lunch programs if available Ensure that children are linked to summer food programs at end of academic year Link to Women, Infants, and Children (WIC) Nutrition Program Inform about resources for meals and field gleaning in the community
Dental care problems	Teach oral hygiene Provide toothbrushes and toothpaste Provide bottled water if child lives in a car or on the street Perform oral assessment Refer to dental programs for people with low incomes
Injuries	Teach basic safety precautions Visit the living situation if possible to assess for safety hazards Provide helmets, car seats, or other gear as needed Teach "street safe" skills Provide resources for violence prevention and intervention
Adolescent pregnancy and sexually transmitted infections	Provide sexuality teaching Inform about access to family planning services Assess for child abuse and prostitution
Mental illness	Assess for depression Evaluate for suicide potential Provide links to services Plan programs to foster self-esteem Arrange for a "Big Brother" or "Big Sister" Refer to extracurricular activities in the school and community Arrange for a school bus stop away from a shelter so other students do not stigmatize the homeless child

Evidence-Based Nursing

HOMELESSNESS FROM THE VIEWPOINT OF MOTHERS AND CHILDREN

Clinical Question

Children are the age group showing the fastest growth in homelessness. Due to their ages, children are vulnerable to developmental delays, mental health problems, and effects of violence. Mothers are the main support for young children but when they are homeless they may not be able to provide the care children need for healthy growth and development. Most nurses have not been homeless and do not understand the experience of homelessness for children.

Evidence

A qualitative study of 28 homeless women with young children used interviews to learn about the experience of homelessness. Violence was a frequent experience in their lives. The women described stress, but often a feeling of respite provided by the shelter. Poor mental health and a lack of resources were major stresses, both of which directly influenced the mothering ability of the women (Tischler, Rademeyer, & Vostanis, 2007).

Another qualitative research study was conducted by nurses, using interviews with 10 youth, to learn about their experiences of homelessness. The interviews were carried out at a community agency serving the youth. As they described their encounters with healthcare services several themes emerged. Youth felt marginalized and labeled as troublemakers or psychotics. They described lack of explanations for care, and scant time being spent with them in healthcare agencies. The teens felt like they had little control over their care, and there was lack of coordination throughout care received. On the other hand, some youth reported feeling listened to, felt they were not judged, and felt that they mattered in some of the healthcare settings (Darbyshire, Muir-Cochrane, Fereday, et al., 2006). A study by four nurses sought to describe the homeless experience from the perspective of children (DeForge, Zehnder, Minick, et al., 2001). They interviewed 14 children with an average age of 10 years who were located in shelters in a metropolitan area. The children had been in the shelters from 2 weeks to 6 months, and most had prior periods living in shelters, hotels, or with relatives. The researchers identified five themes common to the children:

- "I'm not homeless." The children viewed homelessness as having no resources, and having to live outside. They felt that they had resources and felt they might be ridiculed if people thought they were homeless.
- "I like living in a shelter sometimes." While the children had mixed feelings about living in shelters, most were glad to have food, a place to sleep, and a feeling of safety. They described friends in the shelter and were glad to have those relationships.
- "Living in a shelter is hard." The children complained about rules and rigid schedules in the shelters. They missed freedom of movement, play space, and privacy.
- "Stop the violence." All children described living in violent neighborhoods and the wish that violence would stop. Fighting back was perceived as important to protecting oneself.
- "I need approval." Children frequently described how important it was to be noticed and praised by teachers and other adults.

Best Practice

Although these studies were small, there were important findings for nurses. Mothers of young children experience stresses that interfere with their ability to parent young children. The youth had multiple healthcare and social needs. Positive experiences were noted when care providers took time to discuss their health and explain care. Trust was promoted when a sense of self-worth was enhanced. Clear information was appreciated, and coordinated care resulted in more positive and comprehensive health care.

Critical Thinking

Find at least two agencies that provide health care for persons who are homeless in your community. What are some of the common health problems treated? How are youth engaged in care? What explanations are provided? Are mothers of young children offered parenting classes and stress reduction interventions? What links are available to other community resources? What is the nursing role in the community agencies you located?

See MyNursingKit for possible responses.

when the family frequently does not have enough food, when fighting or abuse is frequent, or when the child is overscheduled and feels under constant pressure to perform (Sparrow, 2007). Children manifest stress in a variety of ways, including regressive behavior, interrupted sleep, hyperactive behavior, gastrointestinal symptoms, crying, and withdrawal from normal events. Common stressful events for children include moving to a new home or school, marital difficulties in the family, abuse, one or both parents deployed in the military (Figure 44–1 ●), and being expected to achieve at an extremely high level in school or sports. The busy pace of today's lifestyles and the media's encouragement of early development in children may put undue stress upon some children and preteens (Elkind, 2007). Adolescents may be stressed by fulfilling many roles, such as student, part-time worker, and active member of a family. They may be in school all day, be in sport or music practice for 2 to 3 hours after school, and then have a job for several additional hours. Lack of adequate sleep is common and adds further to stress, in addition to putting the teen at risk for car crashes and poor school performance. For poor families, commonly reported stressors are related to food, shelter, transportation, medical care, and personal-time needs.

The child experiencing stress has more frequent respiratory and gastrointestinal illnesses and is more likely to be the victim of an injury. The negative long-term effects of stress on body organs and systems suggest that children under stress are more likely to develop illnesses such as strokes, hypertension, and heart attacks later in life.

Nurses help children manage stress by encouraging good coping strategies. Emphasize health lifestyles with all children, including good nutrition, exercise, and plenty of sleep. Encourage parents to provide youth with activities that foster self-esteem, and to avoid unrealistic expectations about performance in sports

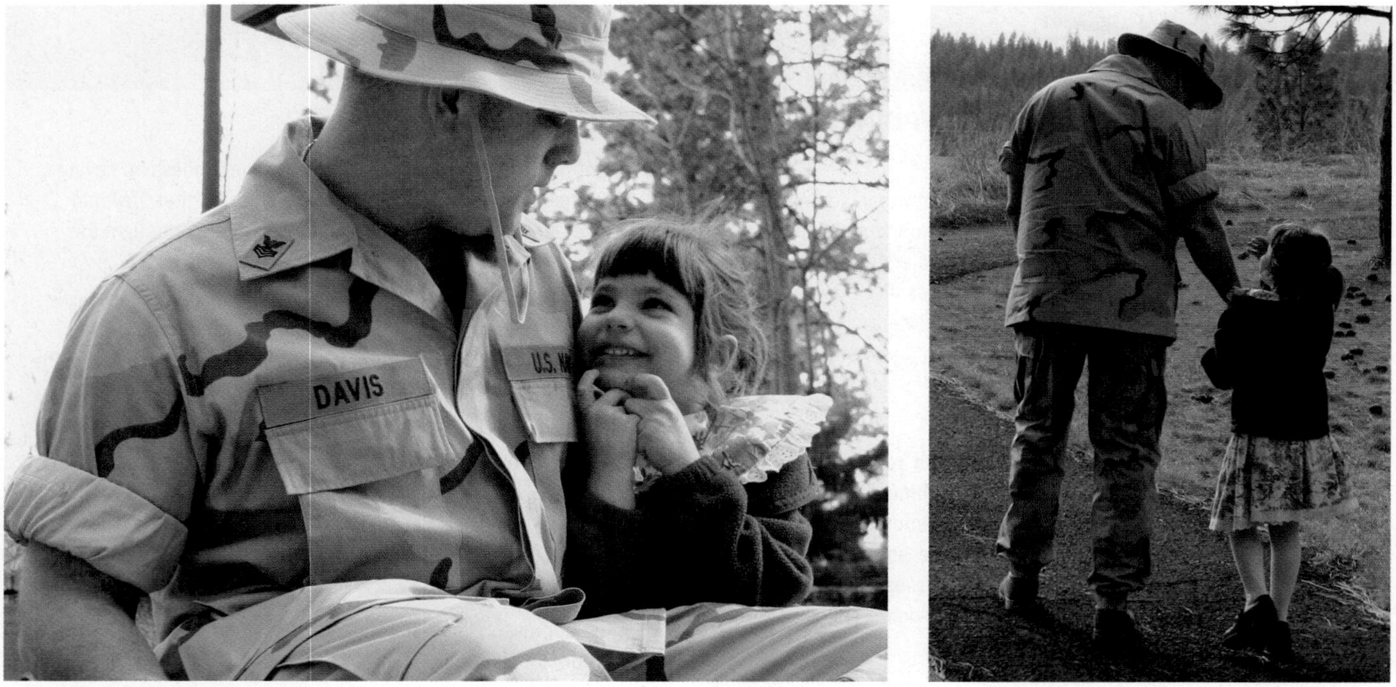

● **Figure 44–1** Stress from military deployment. The special relationship between a father about to be deployed in the military and his young daughter is clear. This father has two other children and is spending time with each of them, as well as with the family together, before leaving. The cycle of leaving and returning home can be stressful for families. Nurses can assist military families in making plans for health care, finances, and communication while gone and providing resources for emotional support for the entire family.

and other activities. Provide resources to help with food acquisition, shelter, transportation, and medical care for families needing them. Adolescents may benefit from various approaches for stress management such as massage, rest, physical activity, and yoga.

Partner with military families to assist them as one or both parents are deployed for duty in a remote location. Connect parents with resources for childcare, mental health services, and arrangements that need to be made to prepare for the absence. Due to frequent moves, the family may not be strongly connected to resources in the community. During deployment the remaining parent may return to the home of origin; some family support may then be present. Help families explain to children why and where the parents are going, and how they will keep in touch during absence. Children need to know who they will stay with, whether they will attend the same school, and how food and other needs will be provided. Parents need family, mental health, and financial support, whether they are being deployed or are the parent remaining at home (Chartrand & Siegel, 2007; Rentz, Marshall, Loomis, et al., 2007).

Complementary Care

YOUTH AND YOGA

The health benefits of yoga have been described previously with adults, and more recently yoga has been introduced to a younger population. In a study with 25 adolescents who had irritable bowel syndrome, half were randomly assigned to a yoga group, while half had usual care with no yoga intervention. Youth in the yoga group had less anxiety, less gastrointestinal symptoms, and lower levels of disability than youth in the usual-care group (Kuttner, Changers, Hardial, et al., 2006). In another study that tested a 12-week program for children that included yoga in its physical activity component, body composition and other health markers were improved (Slawta, Bentley, Smith, et al., 2006). Yoga may be a valuable tool for increasing physical activity and enhancing stress reduction among children and adolescents.

FAMILIES

The families into which children are born influence them greatly. Children are supported in different ways and acquire different world views depending on such factors as whether one or both parents work, how many siblings are present, and whether an extended family is close by. Note variations in family structure such as single parent, adolescent parent, homosexual parents, extended family, grandparents raising grandchildren, and stepparents. Societal changes have impacted family life and the needs of children in profound ways. Working parents often raise children with little time for quality relationships and without the financial resources needed for optimum development (Annie E. Casey Foundation, 2007). All of these factors influence the physical and mental health of children, and can determine their needs for nursing intervention.

According to data from the U.S. Census Bureau, approximately 1.5 million children's parents divorced in 2000 (Kreider & Fields, 2005). Children are affected in many ways when the family experiences a divorce, even if the divorce was preceded by many periods of stress and tension in the home. Children vary in their responses to the parents' divorce, depending on their own individual characteristics, the situation that led to the divorce, and the developmental stage of the child. Some of the developmental responses include:

- 3–5 years – fear, anxiety, worry, sorrow, grief, regression, searching and questioning, temper tantrums, loneliness, unhappiness, aggression
- 6–8 years – worry, anxiety, fantasy, self-blame, difficulty in school, anger, aggression
- 9–10 years – anger, anxiety, manipulation of parents, withdrawal from friends and activities
- 11–13 years – panic, risk taking, loneliness, fear of abandonment, denial
- 14–17 years – anger, truancy, use of substances, sexual acting out, struggles with morality (Wallerstein & Blakeslee, 2003)

Both risk factors of the family (e.g., recent separation, parental stress, and limited healthcare coverage) and their strengths (e.g., loving relationships, influential grandparents or other extended family members, and general good health) should be identified and used in planning care. Parents who are divorced can be assisted to plan strategies to ensure that the child does not feel responsible for the divorce and is able to form strong relationships with both parents. See Chapter 2 for a thorough discussion of family factors as they relate to family-centered care, and a description of strategies for assessment and intervention with families.

SCHOOL AND CHILD CARE

Once a child is 5 or 6 years of age, several hours daily are spent in a school setting. Children develop physical skills through participation in education and sports. Psychosocial stages are met as the child interacts with children and adults and achieves social interaction patterns and pride in accomplishments. The presentation of concepts that challenge thought processes enhances cognitive development.

Although the primary role of schools is educational, they also perform several health-related functions. School health screening programs play an important role in identifying children with such health problems as hearing loss, visual impairment, and scoliosis. Nurses provide assessment, teaching, and clinical management related to some health problems. Some schools have clinics that examine and provide even more complete health care for children. Many schools teach good nutrition, healthful living, safe sexual practices, and other health-related subjects. A school nurse may be present, at least part time, to plan these classes or to work with teachers. Nurses assist school districts in providing plans for emergency health care when needed. With the increase in mainstreaming, school staff now have the responsibility for administering medications, maintaining urinary catheters, and providing respiratory care and other treatments to ensure the child's proper growth and development. See Chapter 39 for further discussion of school nurse activities.

Some children spend part or nearly all of their days in childcare settings (Figure 44–2 ●). Over 60% of children under 6 years receive some type of childcare regularly. About 19% of children are in childcare up to 9 hours each week, 38% for 10–19 hours each week, 36% for 30–45 hours each week, and 10% over 45 hours each week. The closeness of the parent-child relationship, the quality of care, and the length of the childcare day are important in determining childcare effects on children. The mother's sensitivity to her child is the best indicator of child behavior regardless of childcare arrangements (Federal Interagency Forum on Child and Family Statistics, 2007; National Institute of Child Health and Human Development, 2007).

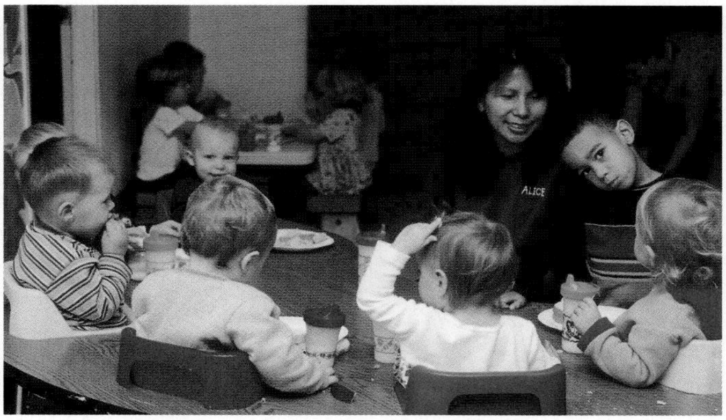

● **Figure 44–2** Childcare settings. Most children will spend time in childcare settings. It is important to explore options and find the best fit for the child's needs.

Nursing management involves helping parents to explore types of daycare options available and to evaluate programs in their communities (Table 44–2). Care options for young school-age children, either before or after school, can also be shared with parents. When available, recommend early intervention programs with at-risk children, such as the Zero to Three Project and Head Start, which contribute to children's health and welfare. Nurses frequently manage the health programs in early intervention, providing screening, doing health evaluations, and establishing early intervention education plans. Nurses assist families in evaluation of childcare centers and share information about accreditation. The National Association for the Education of Young Children (2007) has established childcare criteria.

COMMUNITY

The community in which a child lives may support the child's development or, conversely, expose the child to hazards. Social programs such as Head Start preschools, sports activities, after-school programs, and child abuse treatment centers offer valuable services that improve the experience of growing children. On the other hand, an economically depressed community with scant services and a high homicide rate is unsupportive and hazardous for growing children.

The physical environment is supportive when the child has sidewalks on which to walk to school, open spaces in which to learn and play, and clean air to breathe. Children who must walk to school on unsafe roads, have access to contaminated drinking supplies, or live near polluting manufacturing companies or in crowded housing or old structures are at risk for injuries and health problems such as lead poisoning (see discussion of poisoning later in this chapter).

Teaching Highlights

EVALUATION OF CHILDCARE

The nurse can help parents to evaluate childcare options and make decisions about placement for their children. Parents should always be welcomed to visit an agency or home childcare—this is essential so they can see the routines in action. Some questions they can ask are suggested as follows:

Administration

Is the facility licensed?

Who are the administrators? What is their training and experience?

How many staff are employed? What is their training?

Is there a parent board? What part do they play in administering the center?

Physical Environment, Health, and Safety

What is the neighborhood like? Is transportation to the center convenient?

What is the condition of lighting, heat, cooling, ventilation system, play spaces (inside and out), and the building's general condition?

Is playground equipment safe?

Is there a soft material such as bark, sand, or rubber tiles under climbing equipment?

Is there always supervision for the children?

Are there emergency medical forms and signed forms for field trips?

Who may pick up children? How are they signed in and out?

What is the immunization policy and how are records examined and maintained?

Are criminal background checks of staff done for potential child abuse and other problems?

What is the policy for children with infectious diseases and other illness?

How are foods prepared? Are staff licensed in food handling?

What is the state of general cleanliness?

Who changes diapers? Are recommendations for standard precautions to prevent pathogen transfer followed?

What arrangements and routines are made for naps and quiet times?

Developmental Approaches

Is the curriculum appropriate for different age groups?

Are there materials and plans for gross motor, fine motor, language, and social development?

How much time do children spend in structured time? Free time?

How is discipline handled?

Do the children appear occupied and happy?

What reading materials are available?

What type and quantity of field trips are planned?

What is the educational level and longevity of the childcare workers?

Is there a diversity among the children's backgrounds and experiences?

(Adapted from the National Association for the Education of Young Children, 2007)

Table 44–2 Types of Child Care

Type of Care/Description	Advantages	Disadvantages
In home/ Caretaker comes to home of the child	Child can remain at home Little exposure to infectious diseases No need for alternative care when child is ill	Limited contact with other children to encourage development Limited ability to rapidly locate alternate when provider is ill Most costly
Family child care/ Parent brings child to home of a caretaker	Limited number of children Family type atmosphere Some exposure to other children and encouragement of development	Little governmental regulation or examination Care provider may be distracted by activities in the home
Parent brings child to a center where many children receive care	A learning curriculum plan is in place Contact with other children can enhance development Subject to regulation and licensing Care providers are focused solely on the children	Exposure to multiple children increases infectious disease risk Demands of multiple children may distract or tire care providers

CULTURE

The child's cultural group may influence the use of traditional and contemporary healthcare practices. If the parents or children are recent immigrants, they may still be learning the English language and finding out about healthcare resources. Children and adolescents of immigrants may feel stress as they combine their family's traditional culture with the new culture in which the family now lives. They may also have a great deal of responsibility to interpret for the family since they often can speak two languages and understand practices in the new culture.

Recent immigrants may experience culture shock, a state of crisis related to the difference in values and lifestyle between the two cultures they have experienced. This can lead to stress-related symptoms, and create a need for healthcare intervention. Children whose parents emigrated from another country may feel different from peers and develop conflict with their parents, particularly during adolescence.

All cultural groups have rules about patterns of social interaction. Schedules of language acquisition are determined by the number of languages spoken and the amount of speech in the home. The particular social roles assumed by men and women in the culture affect school activities and ultimately career choices. Attitudes toward touching and other methods of encouraging developmental skills vary among cultures.

Nurses must become aware of common characteristics of the cultural groups they serve so that they can provide culturally competent nursing care. Arrange for interpreters when needed. Be aware that families often accept and use both traditional and Westernized health care, and remain nonjudgmental about traditional healing practices. Provide ethnic foods in healthcare facilities. Evaluate youth in immigrant families for conflict between family and societal expectations.

LIFESTYLE ACTIVITIES AND THEIR INFLUENCE ON CHILD HEALTH

Many patterns of daily life play a part in determining the length and quality of one's life. The child's use of tobacco products and controlled substances influences both physical and mental health. Patterns of exercise and use of protective gear protect against early disabilities. The use of decorative patterns that affect the skin and can introduce pathogens is an example of a lifestyle pattern that influences mental health, body image, and the body's physical health.

TOBACCO USE

Tobacco use is the most preventable cause of adult death in the United States. It leads to 438,000 premature deaths annually, and will be responsible for the premature death of 5 million of today's youth as they reach adult years (U.S. Department of Health & Human Services (DHHS), 2006). Major health problems linked to tobacco use include cardiovascular disease, cancer, chronic lung disease, increased prevalence of car crashes, low birth weight, and other maternal problems. Even passive smoking (secondhand smoke) or environmental tobacco smoke (ETS) is linked to increased heart disease, blood pressure, respiratory problems, and decreased youth academic performance (Collins, Wileyto, Murphy, et al., 2007; Reardon, 2007). Cigarette use is most common; however, chewing tobacco, snuff, cigars, and bidis (small, brown, hand-rolled cigarettes) also pose significant health hazards.

Many nurses view tobacco use as an adult issue, but each day 3000 youths try their first cigarette, and the major age for trying tobacco is 9 to 14 years (Figure 44–3 ●). Nicotine is highly addictive, and most people become addicted to the substance in adolescent years. Early initiation of smoking is an extremely risky behavior because 80% of current adult smokers began smoking before 18 years of age (MMWR, 2006a). Although sale of tobacco products to children and advertisements aimed at this age group are forbidden by federal law, many youths obtain and use tobacco. After steadily increasing rates of youth smoking for many years, rates began to decrease in 1997. However, a significant number of youth still continue to use tobacco, making this an important health topic. About 30% of high school students and 13% of middle school students in the United States have smoked within the last 30 days (MMWR, 2006c). Significant numbers of youth also report using chewing tobacco and cigars in the month prior to being surveyed. Approximately 7.8% of females and 14.8% of males from 13 to 15 years living in the Americas report current use of tobacco other than cigarettes (MMWR, 2006b).

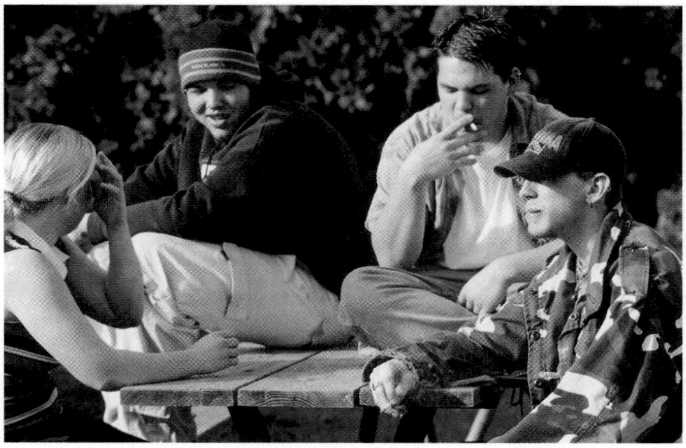

● **Figure 44–3** Childhood smoking. Approximately 70% of children have tried smoking by their high school years. Early intervention can begin with discussions about smoking starting at 9 or 10 years of age.

Certain characteristics contribute to the likelihood of tobacco use. They include increasing age, male gender, ethnic group, ease of obtaining tobacco products, and smoking among family members. Low socioeconomic group membership, access to tobacco products, low price of products, advertising, and lack of parental involvement in the youths' lives are associated with tobacco use (U. S. Department of Health and Human Services, 2006). Gender differences may exist for youth who are beginning or seeking to quit smoking. For example, girls may be more worried about the smell and effect of tobacco on clothing and appearance, while boys more commonly express concern about smoking's effect of sports or activities (Amos & Bostock, 2006).

Developing Cultural Competence

SMOKING RATES AMONG YOUTH

Among youth in the United States, white youth are significantly more likely to smoke than either Hispanic or black peers. About 26% of white students reported smoking in the previous month, while 22% of Hispanic and 13% of black students report this behavior (MMWR, 2006a). American Indian and Alaska Natives also have high smoking rates, while Asian Americans have low rates (DHHS, 2006).

Several programs have been developed to encourage youth to avoid tobacco use. In addition, smoking cessation programs are available to assist youth who are already regular smokers, and successfully achieve the goals of cessation or decrease in tobacco use. Use of incentives, and counselor-based, individually tailored telephone interventions have been effective (Backinger, Michaels, Jefferson, et al., 2007; Liu, Peterson, Kealey, et al., 2007). Once a teen is identified as a smoker, using a biologic marker such as urine cotinine (a by-product of tobacco) levels can help to identify the frequency of smoking. This information can be used to make suggestions to the teen about the potential outcomes of the behavior and the cessation program that is most likely to be helpful.

NURSING MANAGEMENT

NURSING ASSESSMENT AND DIAGNOSIS

Nurses are in a unique position to inquire about the incidence of smoking and other tobacco use among youth. Insert questions into all well-child visits, beginning at about 9 to 10 years of age. Inquire about whether family members (especially parents and siblings) smoke or chew, and ask if some of the child's friends have tried smoking. Try to find out the child's knowledge and beliefs about the benefits and risks of tobacco use. As the child gets older, ask more direct and detailed questions. A nonjudgmental and collegial approach will be best to obtain a truthful response. School nurses can make observations about numbers of teens smoking and general attitudes about tobacco use. When children come to hospitals and other health facilities for care, use of tobacco should be part of general admission questions.

Some nursing diagnoses that may apply to youth who smoke or show potential for this behavior include the following:

- *Activity Intolerance* related to lowered oxygen supply
- *Impaired Gas Exchange* related to ventilation-perfusion imbalance
- *Chronic Low Self-Esteem* related to negative self-appraisal
- *Deficient Knowledge* regarding dangers of tobacco use related to developmental focus on present
- *Imbalanced Nutrition, Less than Body Requirements* related to effects of chemical dependence

PLANNING AND IMPLEMENTATION

The roles of nurses in preventing and intervening in youth smoking are to inform youth, identify smokers, and implement programs (Table 44–3). Provide developmentally appropriate information about the hazards of tobacco use in all settings where youth are present. Addicted teens who share their stories of difficult withdrawal from tobacco, and adults who have had cancer of the lungs or larynx may be effective speakers. Offer information on prevention and cessation programs to youths and families in clinics, outpatient surgery centers, community activities, and hospitals. Use opportunities such as adolescent pregnancy and illness to reinforce the hazardous effects of tobacco on the individual and on those around. Adolescent mothers should understand the risks for small-for-gestational age babies when they smoke in pregnancy and the increased risk of sudden infant death syndrome (SIDS) when infants are exposed to secondhand smoke (see Chapter 48∞). Speak to young athletes about the effects of tobacco on athletic performance. Show youth the ways this product can interfere with meeting life goals. Role-play how to tell other youth "no" when tobacco is offered. Establish programs that increase the sense of self-esteem without tobacco use. Be sure to include parents in the programs so that they see and acknowledge their role in setting an example about tobacco use, and in providing guidelines for the child. Provide information on the influence of environmental tobacco smoke (secondhand smoke).

Adopt a nonjudgmental attitude when asking questions about smoking so that youth using tobacco can be identified. Ask questions without parents present and assure youth that the information will not be shared. Encourage youth to cut back and to quit use of tobacco products. Offer assistance to them in these efforts. Encourage positive coping techniques for youth who are engaged in cessation. Such techniques include keeping busy, avoiding smoking situations, using oral stimulation such as a toothpick or gum, exercising, relaxing, and using nicotine replacement approaches (Jannone & O'Connell, 2007).

Work with the schools and school districts to help establish preventive and cessation programs. There should be clear guidelines about school policies regarding smoking on school grounds. Keeping occasional youth smokers from becoming regular users should be a goal in order to avoid nicotine addiction. Find out what positive incentives can be offered to youth who are successful in quitting smoking. Contract with them to achieve their goals.

Table 44–3 Nursing Role in Youth Smoking Prevention

Inform

- Hang posters, provide brochures, and facilitate presentations about smoking risks in all settings where youth are present.
- Target smokers with special information about the effects of nicotine on their bodies.

Identify

- Ask questions about smoking and other tobacco use at every health encounter beginning at about 9 to 10 years of age.
- For users, ask amount and type of tobacco.
- Find resources where youth obtain tobacco in the community and become proactive in stopping sales.

Implement

- Encourage youth tobacco users to quit.
- Facilitate referral to cessation programs.
- Arrange positive rewards for youth successful in cessation.

EVALUATION

Expected outcomes of nursing interventions regarding tobacco use are lowered rates of regular use, delayed initiation of use, and success of cessation programs. Use the *Healthy People 2010* (DHHS, 2006) objectives as guidelines:

- Reduce the proportion of children who are regularly exposed to tobacco smoke at home to 6%.
- Increase smoke-free and tobacco-free environments in schools, including all school facilities, property, vehicles, and school events, to 100%.
- Eliminate tobacco advertising and promotions that influence adolescents and young adults.
- Increase adolescents' disapproval of smoking to 95%.
- Reduce tobacco use by adolescents to 21%.
- Increase the average age of first use of tobacco products from 12 years to 14 years.

ALCOHOL USE

Alcohol use by the young is common. An estimated 75% have tried alcohol, which is the drug of choice and convenience for youth. Each day, 7000 children take their first drink by 12th grade, and 83% have had alcoholic drinks. Current use is also common with 45% of high school students admitting to drinking within the last month, and 28% having engaged in binge drinking, or having five or more drinks within a 2-hour period. Even young children are affected since 44% of eighth graders and 66% of 10th graders have tried alcohol, while 20% of eighth graders and 35% of 10th graders have had alcohol in the last month. Alcohol use frequently starts at an early age since 25.6% of high school students report that their first drink was before age 13 years. Binge drinking is also a problem, as 25.5% of high school students report at least one incidence of having five or more drinks within 2 hours in the 30 days prior to the survey (MMWR, 2006c).

Many factors influence the child and adolescent who drink alcohol. Patterns in the family, media advertisements, and social environments in high school and college that honor or expect drinking all contribute to the problem. Access to alcohol is easy for most youth as older siblings or classmates often obtain drinks for them. It is a "rite of passage" for many at teen birthday parties or college events. Alcohol is the most common and accepted drug in today's society and, as such, youth are exposed and often experience its effects without understanding or considering the implications of its use. A significant risk factor for initiation of alcohol use is a transition time, such as change from middle to high school, or a major family stress, such as parental separation or divorce (Loveland-Cherry, 2006).

SUBSTANCE USE

Substance use occurs in children and adolescents of all socioeconomic levels and is a growing health problem. The use of any drug can pose a serious psychologic and physical risk to children and adolescents.

In addition to alcohol, a variety of other drugs are used by youth. Almost 40% of students have used marijuana and 20% have used it in the last month; about 7% have used cocaine, with over 3% having used it in the last month. Inhalant use of glue, paints, or other substances is more common, with 12% reporting use and 4% having used in the last month. Approximately 6% report methamphetamine use (see Figure 44–4 ●); and 2.4% used heroin (MMWR, 2006c). Synthetic drugs such as phencyclidine (PCP) (commonly referred to as "designer" drugs), mimic other narcotics, stimulants, and hallucinogens and are also dangerous.

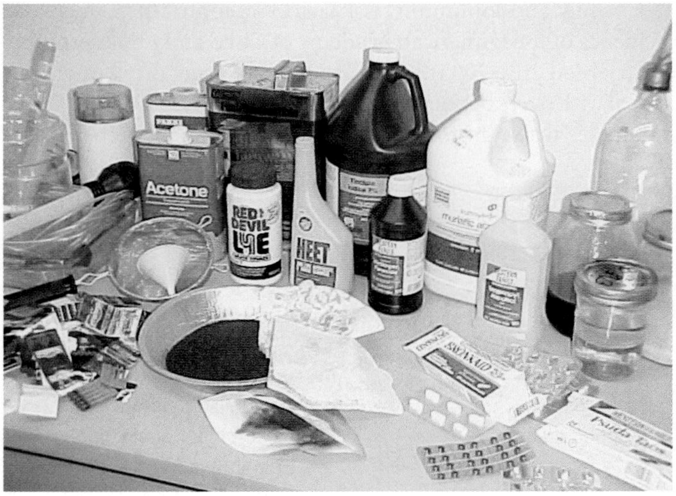

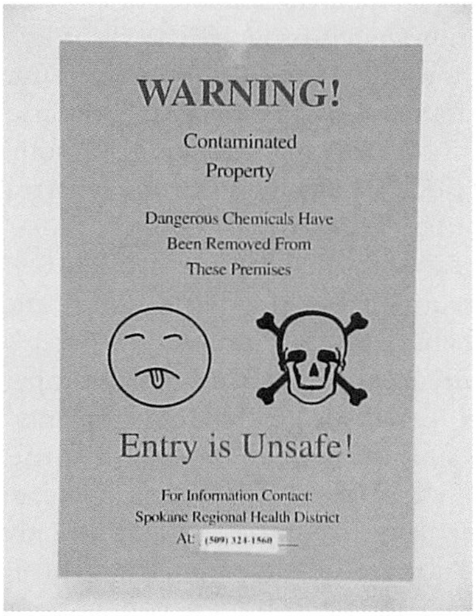

● **Figure 44–4** Methamphetamine use. Methamphetamine is a popular drug because it can be manufactured with items that are available to the lay public. Manufacture of the substance in homes has become a concern of health departments and communities at large. Children can be harmed by the chemicals produced and may experience neglect and abuse. They may suffer even after the home is found and adults are apprehended as they must be placed in foster homes.

Courtesy of Spokane Regional Health District, Spokane, WA

Table 44–4 Common Contemporary Club Drugs, Street Names, and Drug Information

Drug	Action	Street Names	Route	Time of Action
Methylenedioxymethamphetamine (MDMA)	Stimulant; appetite suppressant; increased pulse, BP, temperature, overhydration, hyponatremia, memory loss	Ecstasy, XTC, X, Adam, Clarity, Lover's speed, E	PO (tablets, capsules)	3–6 hours
Gamma-hydroxybutyrate (GHB)	CNS depressant, euphoria, growth hormone release, hypersalivation, hypotonia	Grievous Bodily Harm, G., Liquid Ecstasy, Georgia Home Boy, Date-rape drug	PO (liquid, powder, tablets, capsules)	4 hours
Ketamine	Anesthetic; decreased memory, attention, learning; increased BP; respiratory collapse	Special K, K, Vitamin K, Cat Valiums	IV, respiratory (injected, snorted or smoked; liquid or powder)	1–2 hours
Rohypnol (benzodiazepine)	Amnesia, sedative; decreased BP, urinary retention; given prior to sexual assault	Roffies, Rophies, Roche, Forget-me Pill	PO, respiratory (snorted; tablets)	8–12 hours
Methamphetamine	Stimulant; highly addictive; memory loss, violence, psychosis; cardiac and neurologic damage	Speed, Ice, Chalk, Meth, Crystal, Crank, Fire, Glass, Tina, Tweak, Yaba (meth and caffeine)	PO, respiratory, IV (smoked, snorted, injected)	Several hours; long-term permanent effects
Lysergic acid diethylamide (LSD)	Hallucinogen; increased pulse, BP, temperature; psychosis, flashbacks	Acid, Boomers, Yellow Sunshines	PO (liquid, tablets, capsules)	1–2 hours; possible flashbacks later

Data from National Institute on Drug Abuse. 2004. *NIDA Community Drug Alert Bulletin—Club Drugs.* Bethesda, MD: U.S. Department of Health and Human Services; Reitman, D. S. (May, 2005). "Club Drugs 101": Substance use and abuse for 21st century pediatricians. *Consultant for Pediatricians,* 207–211.

Some common contemporary drugs and street names are listed in Table 44–4.

Prescription drugs are sometimes used for nonmedical purposes. For example, methylphenidate (Ritalin) is used for treatment of attention deficit/hyperactivity disorder (ADHD), and generally acts as a stimulant. Its unprescribed use among youth has increased dramatically over the past few years (Arria & Wish, 2006). Prescription pain medications are another example of drugs that are easily abused by youth who are treated with them after surgery or other procedures.

Over-the-counter medications are legal, but frequently abused. Easily obtainable at grocery stores and drug stores, these drugs include antihistamines, atropine, bromides, caffeine, ephedrine, pseudoephedrine, phenylpropanolamine, and amphetamine-like substitutes. Volatile inhalants, such as glues, are dangerous substances of abuse, and their use appears to be rising among school-age children and adolescents. Anabolic steroids are the drugs of abuse most commonly used by athletes; about 4% of students report use of illegal steroids (MMWR, 2006c). Some common contemporary drugs and street names are listed in Table 44–4. Adolescents and young adults most commonly use "club drugs" to achieve greater satisfaction during nights of dancing, drinking, and attending clubs. Use of these drugs with alcohol can lead to deadly consequences. (See Nursing Practice.)

Etiology and Pathophysiology

In most cases substance abuse represents a maladaptive coping response to the stressors of childhood and adolescence. Individual, peer, family, and community risk factors all contribute to increased incidence of use (American Academy of Child and Adolescent Psychiatry [AACAP], 2005). A child may begin using drugs or alcohol to deal with stress because family members or peers do so. Children in families with a history of substance abuse are at higher risk of

Nursing Practice

Following are common inhalant agents:

AEROSOLS	SOLVENTS
Cooking spray	Nail polish remover
Whipped cream	Paint thinner or cleaner
Spray paint	Lighter fluid
Cosmetic sprays	Degreaser
ADHESIVES	**OTHER**
Model glues	Gasoline
Rubber cements	Helium

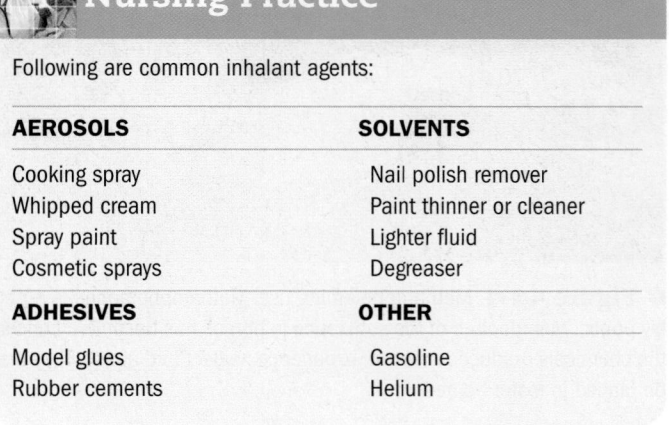

abusing drugs and alcohol. Other risk factors include rebelliousness, aggressiveness, low self-esteem, dysfunctional parental relationships, lack of adequate support systems, academic underachievement, poor judgment, and poor impulse control.

Initial experimentation with alcohol or drugs may be unpleasant. With continued use, however, the adolescent learns to "achieve the high," an illusion of power and well-being. The adolescent wants the high more frequently and actively seeks alcohol or drugs. Tolerance to the substance occurs with continued use, and ever-increasing amounts are required to achieve a pleasurable high. Physical and psychologic dependence ensues as the body's tissues require the substance to function properly. Withdrawal symptoms occur when the child or adolescent is deprived of the substance.

Clinical Manifestations

Substance abuse in children and adolescents is commonly overlooked and underdiagnosed by healthcare providers, due in part to the wide range of clinical presentations, which vary according

Clinical Manifestations

COMMONLY ABUSED DRUGS

DRUG	POTENTIAL FOR DEPENDENCE	CLINICAL MANIFESTATIONS
Depressants		
Alcohol, barbiturates (amobarbital, pentobarbital, secobarbital)	*Physical and psychologic:* High; varies somewhat among drugs	*Physical:* Decreased muscle tone and coordination, tremors *Psychologic:* Impaired speech, memory, and judgment, confusion; decreased attention span; emotional lability
Stimulants		
Amphetamines (e.g., Benzedrine), caffeine, cocaine	*Physical:* Low to moderate *Psychologic:* High; withdrawal from amphetamines and cocaine can lead to severe depression	*Physical:* Dilated pupils, increased pulse and blood pressure, flushing, nausea, loss of appetite, tremors *Psychologic:* Euphoria; increased alertness, agitation, or irritability; hallucinations; insomnia
Opiates		
Codeine, heroin, meperidine (Demerol), methadone, morphine, opium, oxycodone (Percodan)	*Physical and psychologic:* High; varies somewhat among drugs; withdrawal effects are uncomfortable but rarely life threatening	*Physical:* Analgesia, depressed respirations and muscle tone (may lead to coma or death), nausea, constricted pupils *Psychologic:* Changes in mood (usually euphoria), drowsiness, impaired attention or memory, sense of tranquility
Hallucinogens		
Lysergic acid diethylamide (LSD), mescaline, phencyclidine (PCP)	*Physical:* None *Psychologic:* Unknown	*Physical:* Lack of coordination, dilated pupils, hypertension, elevated temperature; severe PCP intoxication can result in seizures, respiratory depression, coma, and death *Psychologic:* Visual illusions and hallucinations, altered perceptions of time and space, emotional lability, psychosis
Volatile Inhalants		
Glues, typing correction fluid, acrylic paints, spot removers, lighter fluid, gasoline, butane	*Physical and psychologic:* Varies with drug used	*Physical:* Impaired coordination, liver damage (in some cases) *Psychologic:* Impaired judgment, delirium
Marijuana	*Physical:* Low *Psychologic:* Usually low; occasionally moderate to high	*Physical:* Tachycardia, reddened conjunctiva, dry mouth, increased appetite *Psychologic:* Initial anxiety followed by euphoria; giddiness; impaired attention, judgment, and memory

to type of drug abused, amount, frequency, time of last use, and severity of drug dependence.

Common physical manifestations include alterations in vital signs, weight loss, chronic fatigue, chronic cough, respiratory congestion, red eyes, and general apathy and malaise. Withdrawal may be shown by anxiety, headache, tremors, nausea and vomiting, malaise, weakness, insomnia, depressed mood or irritability, and hallucinations. The mental status examination (refer to Chapter 35∞) may reveal alterations in level of consciousness, impaired attention and concentration, impaired thought processes, delusions, and hallucinations. Low self-esteem, feelings of guilt or worthlessness, and suicidal or homicidal thoughts are also common.

Poor school performance and changes in mood, sleep habits, appetite, dress, and social relationships are nonspecific characteristics of the substance-abusing child.

Clinical Therapy

Multiple psychiatric diagnostic criteria exist for each drug class. Children and adolescents who have other psychosocial disorders commonly use or abuse drugs or alcohol. Treatment should therefore focus not only on the substance use or abuse, but also on the issues underlying the problem. Intervention includes the family as well as the substance-abusing child or adolescent.

The primary goal of treatment is to teach the child and other family members to develop and sustain positive coping patterns, and to support them during this process. Most treatment programs offer inpatient and outpatient services, as well as after-care programs. These programs usually consist of peer support that focuses on developing a drug- and alcohol-free lifestyle, healthy family relationships, and positive coping skills. Family involvement is strongly encouraged. Hospitalization is required if the physical dependence is significant and withdrawal places the child at risk for complications such as seizures, depression, or suicidal behavior.

Teaching Highlights

IDENTIFYING THE YOUTH WHO IS ABUSING SUBSTANCES

Families are often confused about the behavior of adolescents and unsure whether it represents normal development or abuse of substances. Some characteristics of normal development that help to differentiate these occurrences are listed as follows. When concerned about possible substance use, the parent can confront the child or talk with school nurses or counselors.

- Many youth are periodically distant with parents but remain involved with peers in school sports and other activities. Withdrawal from all activities and friends may indicate substance abuse.
- Adolescents often complain about school, but when teachers report the student meets expectations and is consistently performing in the classroom, this is normal behavior.
- Teens may be weepy on occasion when having a difficult time with friends or not performing as desired. Continued, consistent weepiness is more likely to indicate depression or substance abuse.
- Teens like to stay up late and are frequently tired in the morning, whereas abusing teens may "nod off" frequently during the day.
- Many adolescents like to achieve a disheveled look in clothing, but the teen who frequently neglects basic hygiene or does not seem to have the energy to wash and dress may be depressed or be abusing substances.
- All teens get some infections, but abusing teens may have reddened eyes, oral sores, and constant respiratory discomfort from "snorting" substances.

NURSING MANAGEMENT

NURSING ASSESSMENT AND DIAGNOSIS

Mental health assessment of all older children and adolescents requires screening for alcohol and other substances. Maintaining a confidential approach will increase the ability to obtain truthful information about use of substances (AACAP, 2005). Assessment tools provide useful information for the healthcare provider.

Nurses may encounter the substance-abusing child or adolescent in the emergency department or outpatient clinic, in schools and other community settings, or during hospitalization for an injury or other acute problem. Diagnosis includes assessment of both the family and the substance-abusing child or adolescent. Nursing assessment includes taking a thorough history from the parents and child, observing the child's behavior, and performing a physical examination. The history should include the age at which drug use began, pattern of use, length of time the drug has been used, amount of drug used, and psychologic state while on drugs. A history of parental drug use and noninvolvement in parenting the child puts the child at higher risk for substance abuse, reflecting the combined effects of genetic and environmental influences. Environmental factors such as access to the substance, use with other teens or adults, and resources for treatment are important to consider. Evaluate the home, education, alcohol, drugs, smoking, and sex practices of the teen.

PHYSIOLOGIC ASSESSMENT

Look for physical signs and symptoms of substance abuse, including bloodshot eyes, dilated pupils, slurred speech, and weight loss. Blood and urine levels of substances and metabolite are sometimes measured. The adolescent may appear sleepy or restless, or may show signs of clumsiness or inconsistent behavior. Consider all types of substance abuse, including model glue, gasoline, and other sources. Consider signs of withdrawal as well as current intoxication.

PSYCHOLOGIC ASSESSMENT

Changes in social habits may indicate substance abuse. Parents may report a drop in the school-age child's or adolescent's grades or decreased interest in school activities. The adolescent does not introduce new friends to parents, and has less contact with parents, teachers, and other adults who were previously important. The youth may appear more energetic than usual, always "on a high," or exhibit weight loss. Note the child's current drug use, potential for violence, and motivation to make changes. Assess the degree of family support available.

FAMILY ASSESSMENT

In families with substance-using adults, children may experience neglect and abuse, as well as exposure to drugs. When family members are substance users, young children may experience periods when adults cannot provide supervision, cannot encourage healthy activities, or when they are exposed to potentially unsafe or violent episodes. When parents are manufacturing products such as methamphetamine, young children are exposed to toxic chemicals and run the risk of suffering burns and other sequellae from home laboratory production and explosions. Be alert for unusual injuries, signs of inconsistent parenting, and delays in or disturbed growth and development. Be prepared to refer parents for care and for following protocols for child abuse prevention (see section on abuse and neglect later in this chapter).

Nursing diagnoses for children and adolescents who abuse drugs or alcohol might include the following:

Impaired Social Interaction related to altered thought processes

Chronic Low Self-Esteem related to dysfunctional family and social relationships

Risk for Injury related to altered perceptions and sensorium

Risk for Violence: Self-Directed or Other-Directed related to physiologic dependence on drugs, alcohol, and other substances

PLANNING AND IMPLEMENTATION

Care of children and adolescents who abuse drugs, alcohol, and other substances is challenging and often frustrating. Long-term mental health counseling may be necessary to resolve underlying issues and foster lifestyle and behavioral changes.

Prevention is the most desirable intervention. The nurse can play a major role in teaching children and their families about substance abuse. Education should begin in primary school, and continue with intensification during middle school and high school. Nurses also can play a major role in community education. Various prevention programs have been developed by federal and private organizations. Referral to support organizations may be beneficial for the child, parents, and other family members. Self-help groups, available in most communities, include Alcoholics Anonymous, Narcotics Anonymous, Al-Anon, Nar-Anon, and Ala-Teen. Parents may receive support from a group such as Parents Anonymous.

The youth's protective factors can be identified and used in planning appropriate interventions. For example, a child with goals for a future career can be helped to see how substance use will interfere with goal attainment. Identifying a strong role model through a program like Big Brothers or Big Sisters can assist children who lack that strength in their families.

The child who has begun to use and abuse drugs needs an intensive intervention program. Referral to a psychiatric health specialist is needed for diagnosis and intervention. Group programs and those that integrate the family are most effective. Find out what resources are present in your community to treat youth who are using alcohol or other drugs. Nurses are active in treatment programs as well as sustaining treatment effects and avoiding relapse during visits to community agencies once the youth returns to family, school, and other surroundings.

EVALUATION

Expected outcomes of nursing interventions include abstention from alcohol and street drugs, successful participation in substance abuse programs, and developmentally appropriate social and cognitive skills.

PHYSICAL INACTIVITY/ SEDENTARY BEHAVIOR

In the past few decades, children have become increasingly sedentary. This change is a reflection of lifestyles in which car travel is valued, computers and televisions are part of daily life, neighborhoods are sometimes unsafe places for play, and schools do not routinely require daily physical education classes (Figure 44–5 ●). Children and adolescents spend an average of about 3 hours per day watching television, and an additional 2 hours on the computer (Chernin & Linebarger, 2005). This is 20 to 30 hours weekly for most children, and significantly more for some. About 37% of high school students watch television over 3 hours each day and about 21% use computer or video games over 3 hours daily (MMWR, 2006a). Excessive screen time influences behavior because there is physical inactivity during viewing, a lack of social interaction and cognition, and a tendency to eat high-fat snacks with high calorie content.

Physical inactivity leads to many health concerns. A primary outcome is overweight or obesity (see Chapter 34∞). Other outcomes can be an increased rate of type 2 diabetes (see Chapter 55∞), increased exposure to television/computer game violence and sexual activity at early ages, and early progression of cardiovascular disease (see Chapter 49∞).

However, patterns of physical activity established in childhood can lead to increased exercise behaviors in adulthood, contributing to lower rates of low back pain, overweight, osteoporosis, heart disease, diabetes, colon cancer, and high blood pressure; and lead to a more positive self-image.

Although many children demonstrate low levels of physical activity, a profound decrease in vigorous activity is common in grades 9 through 12. Boys more commonly participate in team sports than girls. Although about 54% of students attend physical education (PE) classes at least once a week, only 33% have daily PE classes (MMWR, 2006c).

Health professionals can integrate assessment of physical activity into all health care, and make recommendations to children and families that will help to increase opportunities for physical activity. Nurses can assess height, weight, and body mass index to look for signs of overweight (see Chapter 34∞). Children should

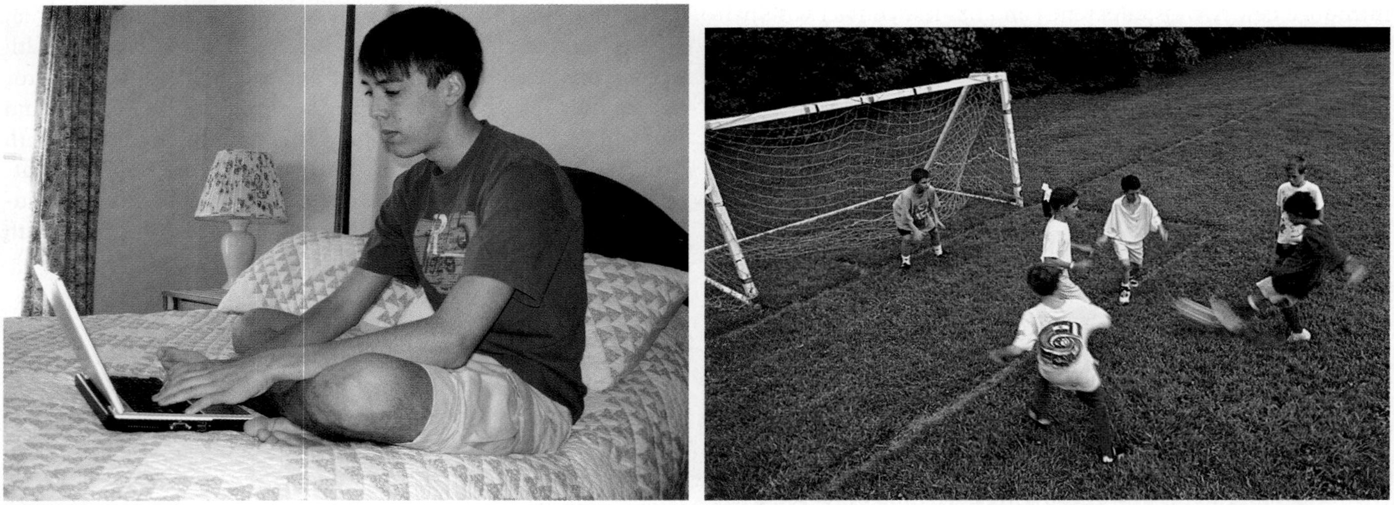

● **Figure 44–5** Role of sports in development. Physical inactivity is a growing problem among children and can contribute to poor health. It is important to balance sedentary activities, such as playing computer games, with physical and social activities. Sports are an excellent way for children to develop their psychosocial, cognitive, and motor skills.

Soccer photo courtesy of Rebecca Scheirer, Kensington, Maryland.

be asked about how they like to spend free time. Community and school activities should be encouraged and rewarded. Examples include fun runs, walks of benefit causes, aerobics classes, team sports, roadside cleanups, fairs, and carnivals. Help parents and children learn what they can do for physical fitness. Work with school physical education personnel to plan activities both in and out of physical education class that promote lifelong exercise routines. Work toward the goal of 60 minutes of daily moderate intensity physical activity for all children (U. S. Department of Health and Human Services, 2008). During health promotion visits, help children identify ways to gradually increase physical activity and decrease sedentary time.

INJURY AND PROTECTIVE EQUIPMENT

In the discussion of causes of childhood and adolescent morbidities and mortalities in Chapter 1∞, unintentional injuries are listed as a common problem. In fact, 71% of all deaths from age 10 years onward result from four causes—motor-vehicle crashes, other unintentional injury, homicide, and suicide (MMWR, 2004). Chapters 36, 37, and Chapter 38∞ discuss the frequent injuries seen in children at different developmental ages, and safety precautions to avoid injuries from car crashes, falls, poisonings, and other developmentally related injuries. Many common injuries are preventable with simple use of protective gear and following of safety guidelines (Figure 44–6 ●). Some sports and activities that require safety gear include rollerblading, skateboarding, roller hockey, ice hockey, football, soccer, baseball, scooters, all-terrain vehicles, and skiing or snowboarding fast or using jumps.

Over 10% of youths rarely or never wear car safety belts in automobiles; 37% of those who ride motorcycles do not wear helmets (MMWR, 2006a). Emphasize safe automobile and motorcycle behaviors in adolescence, with the recognition that risks increase if driving is combined with use of alcohol and controlled substances. Adolescents sometimes engage in practices that put them at particular risk, and nurses should be alert for such activities in their communities. Examples include car surfing (standing on the trunk, hood, or roof of a moving vehicle) or street racing (racing cars down a street at extremely high speed), or "extreme" sports.

About 44 million U.S. children ride bicycles, a beneficial physical activity. However, only about 15% are protected by helmet use, even though bicycling is the most common activity as-

Teaching Highlights

PHYSICAL ACTIVITY GUIDELINES FOR YOUTH

- Engage in moderate to vigorous physical activity (bike riding, walking, baseball, rollerblading, soccer, running, ice hockey) at least 60 minutes daily (on at least 3 days/week this should be vigorous activity) (DHHS, 2008).
- Engage in muscle strengthening activity at least 3 times weekly.
- Engage in bone strengthening activity at least 3 times weekly.
- Encourage schools to offer physical education to all students, and have students sign up when this is an elective.
- Encourage walking and bike riding to friends' homes and stores whenever safe.
- Plan physical activities together as a family.
- Get a pet and plan to walk the pet together daily.
- Limit television and other similar sedentary activities to no more than 2 hours daily.
- On days home, allow the child to watch television for up to 1 hour, and then insist on 1 hour of reading, 1 hour of physical activity, and 1 hour of socializing with others before returning to more television.

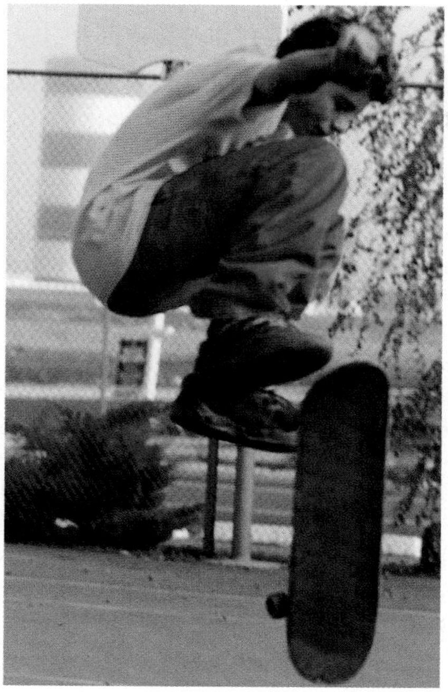

● **Figure 44–6** Use of protective gear. What protective gear should children use for skateboarding? How would you convince them to use the protection?

sociated with injury (MMWR, 2006a). Bike helmets could prevent up to 88% of serious brain injuries from bicycle crashes (National Safe Kids, 2008). Strategies to make helmet use more attractive to children and adolescents are needed. Nurses can play a major role in programs to educate and reward children for helmet use, and can assist families to find affordable helmets. Nurses can be active in identifying behaviors in youths in specific communities and working with schools and other community groups to support legislation for helmet use, evaluate proper fits of helmets, and work to locate sources for incentives and low-cost helmets (Rezendes, 2006). Efforts should also include adequate conditioning for sports, proper treatment of injuries, and prevention of overuse injuries.

A growing number of children engage in "extreme" sports, those that carry a high degree of risk and have not traditionally been common. Some examples are mountain biking, three-wheeling, ski racing, snowboarding through trees and on courses with pikes and other challenges, ice climbing, rock climbing, and wake boarding. While the nurse is probably unable to dissuade youth from engaging in these activities, safety measures should be emphasized. Find out what protective gear the youth wears and what is recommended. Provide examples of stories of youth who have been saved by use of such gear. Encourage the youth to engage in sports activities only when others are present and to have a plan for emergencies, including a working cell phone, leaving information with an adult about plans and expected return, and planning for harsh weather with items such as emergency blankets, gear, and food. Encourage the youth to talk with parents and other adults about the risks and responsibilities of the activities.

Developing Cultural Competence

ETHNIC DISPARITY IN UNINTENTIONAL CHILDHOOD INJURIES

Striking ethnic disparity rates exist in the rates of unintentional injury among children. These differences are due mainly to living in impoverished communities rather than any innate biologic variations. Although the unintentional injury rate in children under 14 years declined 39% from 1987 to 2000, the smallest reductions were among American Indian/Alaskan Natives (20% decline) and African-American children (36% decline), while higher reductions were seen in Asian/Pacific Islanders (52% decline) and white children (39% decline). African Americans and Native Americans have rates of injury 1.5 times those of white children (National Safe Kids Campaign, 2008). What are the major causes of unintentional injury in your community and state? What ethnic and age groups are at greatest risk? How can you integrate teaching in your practice that is specific to the findings in your community?

BODY ART

Body art in the form of painting, tattooing, and piercing has been used by humans throughout history. In recent years, there has been a resurgence of interest in this decorative art among teens. Many adolescents have multiple body piercings and tattoos and may even resort to performing these decorations on themselves or friends.

Approximately 20% of adolescents and young adults have tattoos, and even more have at least one body piercing (Armstrong, 2005; Gold, Schorzman, Murray, et al., 2005). In some states, teens must be 18 years of age or have parental permission to obtain body art, but students often report that it is easy to have an adult present who signs and claims to be a parent. Amy, described at the opening of this chapter, had her piercing done by a friend. In some states, tattoo and body piercing businesses must be licensed and comply with certain regulations, while in others there are no regulations. Amy demonstrates some common characteristics of teens that choose to use body art. It may be seen as a way to establish individualism and independence, and helps some teens to feel part of a peer group. Multiple tattoos and piercings are common, as is the case with Amy (Figure 44–7 ●).

Body art is a common source of infections with skin pathogens, as well as hepatitis B and C. Body piercing is a major method of transmission of hepatitis C, a disease that may not even become manifested until years later (see Chapter 53). It can be a source of HIV if proper techniques are not followed. Piercings in parts of the body such as the mouth or navel are most prone to bacterial infection and continued redness and irritation. Serious systemic infections such as endocarditis have occurred after some piercings (Leman & Plattner, 2007). The pierced site may not appear infected, but transfer of organisms causes serious infection and heart damage. Common infective agents include *Neisseria*, *Staphylococcus*, *Pseudomonas*, and *Streptococcus* (Larzo & Poe, 2006). When noting signs of systemic infection such as fever,

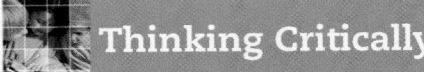

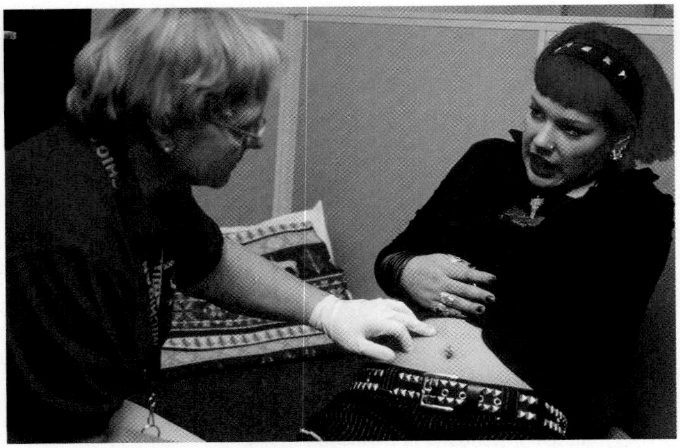

● **Figure 44–7** Health risks to adolescents. Talk openly with adolescents about their health and teach them to avoid health risks connected with tattoos and piercing.

weakness, malaise, and arthralgia (see Chapter 49 for full discussion of endocarditis), gather history about body piercings and refer for care to the primary healthcare provider. Pierced tongues can lead to chipped teeth or even be the cause of choking if dislodged from the site.

Another issue that the teen should consider is the relationship of the tattoos to future lifestyle changes. Advise teens to avoid tattooing the name of a person or musical group since relationships change and tastes in music evolve. Be sure they know the meaning of phrases, foreign words, or Asian symbols. Consider the visibility of the tattoo and its effect on future employment. Tattoos on the face, neck, or other readily visible places may be a detriment during employment interviews. Tattoos should always be considered permanent. Methods for removal may be costly, painful, and unsuccessful.

Another form of body art that is regarded as disfigurement is *branding* or scarification. In this process, the skin is burned to result in a scar. Commonly a desired sign, symbol, or word is inscribed. Results are usually not precise and do not adhere to expected designs. This procedure is done on the self or friend, using common household metal implements heated in fires or stoves. Others cut themselves in the form of a desired design, a process called *cutting*. This type of self-harm or self-injury is performed with razor blades, knives, scissors, broken glass, needles, or sharp pencils (Aguirre & Smith, 2007). These practices can result in infection, often do not yield the desired result, and may indicate underlying problems. They should be discouraged, and the youth involved should be referred for further assessment by primary care providers or counselors.

Since teens may choose to obtain body art even if parents object and if there are state laws to prohibit or make it difficult, nursing care must focus on providing information for the teen, assessing sites, identifying infections, and referring if needed. Care is almost always provided in community settings such as clinics or schools. Consider asking teens if they are thinking about body art since they often do not seek advice before obtaining the art and may not get adequate teaching.

Thinking Critically

THE ADOLESCENT WITH BODY PIERCINGS

Amy is 15 years old and attends an alternative high school. She recently had an ear piercing and it is sore. She comes to the health room to ask the advice of the school nurse. The area around the piercing is inflamed and mildly edematous. After asking some questions, the nurse learns that Amy's ear was pierced by a friend, using a needle that had been "sterilized" by passing it through a match flame. She has had a slight fever, but otherwise feels fine.

In her home state, adolescents under 18 years of age must have the signature of a parent for body piercings and tattoos, so Amy chose to have the procedure done by a friend. She believes this is safe since her friend has done many piercings on others. She admits that her parents are not very pleased with her body art, but that they allow her to do it as long as she agrees to stay in high school. She had previously run away and spent several weeks living on the streets.

- What healthcare and social needs does Amy have?
- How can you support both Amy and her parents?
- What physical care does Amy need to treat potential infection at her piercing site?
- What systemic infectious diseases is Amy at risk of acquiring due to repeated body piercings with unsterile technique?

See MyNursingKit for possible responses.

SEXUAL ORIENTATION

Adolescence is a time of identifying emerging sexuality. Most teens establish relationships with members of the opposite sex and learn how to interact in ways guided by their peer group, family, and culture. For some youth, the transition into adult sexuality is more challenging, as they feel emotional and sexual attraction to people of the same sex (**homosexuality**). The term **gay** is often used for homosexual males and **lesbian** for homosexual females. Other youth are **bisexual**, or attracted to both men and women, and some are **transgendered**, or are attracted to dress and act like members of the opposite sex. The abbreviation LGBT is sometimes used to refer collectively to these minority sexuality choices. About 3% of high school youth report same-sex experience (Remafedi, 2006).

Sexual attractions and practices different than the mainstream are not deviant nor symptoms of a mental disorder but should be viewed as part of a continuum of sexual expression. No gene, early life experience, or other event causes homosexuality.

LGBT youth are at risk for a variety of problems related to emotional and physical health. These include rejection by family members and peers, verbal harassment, sexual abuse and physical assault, a high rate of suicide, substance abuse, high rate of homelessness, and sexual risks of HIV and other sexually transmitted diseases. Their health risks need to be identified and appropriate care provided in welcoming and nonjudgmental healthcare facilities (Meckler, Elliot, Kanouse, et al., 2006).

Nurses can provide health care for LGBT youth in a variety of settings. School nurses and clinics can display a sign to demon-

Teaching Highlights

CARE FOR TATTOOS AND BODY PIERCINGS

Before the Procedure

- Does the studio look clean?
- Visit several studios to make comparisons of techniques, quality, and cleanliness.
- Ask to watch a tattoo or piercing done on someone else.
- What are the artist's sterilization and hygiene practices?
- Is the artist licensed? Trained?
- Look at pictures of completed art and talk with former clients.
- Insist that new, sterile equipment be opened in front of the person to be decorated.
- Consider if this permanent body decoration is desired for a lifetime.
- Consider what the tattoo or piercing will look like in several years.
- Consider the possible side effects such as infection, future dislike for the art, and allergy to dyes or metals.
- Be sure that hepatitis B vaccination is completed before the procedure.
- Be aware that no immunization is available to protect against the health risks of hepatitis C and HIV.

Care after the Procedure

- Touch the area only after carefully washing your hands.
- Keep the area elevated and use ice for the first 2 days to minimize swelling.
- Avoid contact with another person's body fluids until well healed.
- Turn the piercing jewelry gently several times daily using washed hands.
- Use antibacterial mouthwash or cleaner or ointment as recommended.
- Avoid pressure and rubbing on the site (such as belts on navel piercings).
- Watch carefully for signs of infection and report them to a healthcare provider:
  - Increased redness
  - Swelling
  - Pain
  - Hot feeling
  - Discharge
- Ask the artist how long healing will take. It varies from 2 months in the mouth or up to 6 or 8 months for a navel.
- Metal is dangerous during some medical procedures such as magnetic resonance imaging (MRI) or during surgery. Be sure to tell doctors and nurses about your piercings when you are hospitalized or receiving medical care, especially if they are in a part of the body not readily visible.
- If you decide to remove a piece of jewelry soon after it is placed, the skin may heal with only a slight scar.

strate that they are accepting of persons with minority sexual preferences. These signs are rainbows or triangles with several colors shown and can be obtained from local "gay pride" or other groups. Terminology in assessment should be gender-free. Ask "Do you have one or more sexual partners?" rather than "Do you have a boyfriend?" When youth identify as LGBT, provide usual care of all kinds. This includes preventive care such as immunizations, sports assessments, and injury prevention teaching. Be alert that the youth may have additional health challenges. Ask about peer and parental support; refer to support groups if needed. Provide resources for homelessness and when the teen is depressed or suicidal (see Chapter 57). Perform testing for sexually transmitted infections if the teen is having sexual contact, and teach preventive measures. Foster a positive sense of self-esteem through encouraging positive activities such as sports, music, and friendships with peers.

EFFECTS OF VIOLENCE

Violence is a threatened or actual use of physical force that leads to actual or potential physical or emotional trauma. In the past several years, adults and children alike have been shocked by the violent episodes in schools. Although these incidents had much media coverage, they are just one type of violence to which children may be regularly exposed. Children can be the recipients of violence during child abuse and homicides, and they themselves can perform acts of violence on others. They may be touched by violence when parents, siblings, or other family members are killed in gang conflicts, in terrorist attacks, or in wars. The effects of violence are far-reaching and ongoing; they permeate the victim's entire lifetime. This section explores some types of violence affecting children.

SCHOOLS AND COMMUNITIES

At a time when firearm deaths are decreasing overall, unintentional deaths and suicides have increased among children. Many of these deaths are committed with firearms found in the home: About 10% of deaths in children are due to firearm injury (Baxley & Miller, 2006). Forty percent of households with children have guns, and in 25% of those homes the firearms are stored loaded or are not secured under lock. Parents often report that children do not know firearm locations when the children are actually able to state the locations and have handled the guns (Baxley & Miller, 2006).

Homicide in children has gained attention in the last several years due to several shootings at schools and universities. While homicide is an extreme example, there are other types of violence.

Nursing Practice

When a group of children is attacked or killed in a school shooting, this tragic occurrence has the attention of the media. Little do many realize that this tragedy is really part of daily life across the country. About 8 children are killed by a firearm every day in the United States, or about 56 per week. An additional 200 to 300 children suffer from nonfatal firearm injuries (Children's Defense Fund, 2008). Nurses must intervene in this national tragedy. Become familiar with firearm injury statistics in your community. Teach families about the dangers of firearms. Urge safe storage. Teach children and youth about the danger of firearms. Help schools establish programs to ensure safety for students.

Children report being threatened verbally and with guns or knives at home, in schools, and in their neighborhoods. They may be beaten up or bullied or harassed. An estimated 3 million children are exposed to acts of domestic violence by adults in their homes (Kolar & Davey, 2007). They may be subjected to dangerous situations in their neighborhoods or during times of homelessness. Date rape or other sexual violence is reported by up to 9% of teens (MMWR, 2006c).

Risk factors more commonly seen in situations where violence has been committed against children have been identified (see Table 44–5). In addition, children who commit violence more commonly have ready access to firearms, are exposed to violence in the home or community, watch violent media, and have poor self-esteem or depression.

Another type of violence is terrorism and effects of war. The events of September 11, 2001, in the United States, and other examples in various countries take a large toll on the mental health of children and adolescents. Likewise, children who live through wars or have a parent or sibling die in war can be permanently affected by these events. Depression and mental health problems are common among youth who have experienced war (Bayer, Klassen, & Adam, 2007; Bolton, Bass, Betancourt, et al., 2007). The response of children to terrorism is not well studied. Disasters such as the World Trade Center attack can lead to sleep and eating problems, fears of entering tall buildings, regression in school performance and other behaviors, and posttraumatic stress disorder (see Chapter 57). Most children and adolescents experience profound sadness, cling to adults who provide security, and have a variety of somatic complaints. Several resources have been developed to help families and health professionals help children deal with war and violence. See the resources on the National Center for Children Exposed to Violence, Society of Pediatric Nurses, and American Academy of Child and Adolescent Psychiatry.

Table 44–5 Risk Factors Common in Families with Child Victims of Violence

- History of mental illness, domestic violence, incarceration, or substance abuse in the home
- Family stresses
- Inadequate child care or supervision
- Inadequate family social support
- Use of corporal punishment and other inappropriate discipline methods for the child
- Child abuse
- Access to firearms
- Gang membership in family or neighborhood
- High exposure to media violence
- Child hyperactivity and other developmental behavioral disorders

Data from Elders, J. (2003). The role of the pediatrician in violence in the school. Retrieved June 30, 2004, from www.schoolhealth.org/reduviol.html

BULLYING

One type of violence that frequently occurs in schools is **bullying**, or aggressive behavior that is intended to cause harm, exists in a relationship with imbalance of power, and occurs repeatedly. Bullies are aggressive, impulsive, and need to dominate others. Bullying behaviors include verbal abuse (taunting, teasing), name calling, threats, spreading rumors, social exclusion, and physical abuse (hitting, shoving, kicking, tripping). About 16% of children in a large national survey had suffered bullying, most commonly in grades 6 through 8, and more frequently among males. Almost 30% of 11- to 15-year-olds have been either victims or perpetrators of bullying; 75% of children from 6 to 13 years report being bullied and 34% report bullying others in the last year. Up to 160,000 U.S. children may miss school every day in efforts to avoid bullying (Bauer, Hermekohl, Lozano, et al., 2006). Although bullying is most commonly reported in schools, it can occur in neighborhoods as children go to and from school, on school buses, on sports teams, and in other settings.

Bullying can also occur using the internet (McColgan & Giardino, 2005). **Cyberbullying** occurs when a child or adolescent is targeted by another via Internet posting or other digital technology, and threatened, tormented, harassed, humiliated, or embarrassed. Personal information may be disclosed or fabricated, persons are excluded, offensive messages sent, or harmful messages sent out under the target person's name. Such attacks are socially aggressive and often anonymous (Willard, 2007).

Bullies are more likely to smoke, drink alcohol, and perform poorly in school, and one in four bullies has a criminal record by age 30 years (Health Resources and Services Administration, 2007). Bullies are more likely to bring weapons to school, putting other children at risk (Stein, Dukes, & Warren, 2007). Bullying is associated with future delinquent behavior, depression, low self-esteem, loneliness, suicidal ideation, and suicide attempts (Brunstein, Marrocco, Kleinman, et al., 2007).

Children who are bullied are more commonly socially isolated and anxious. Health problems such as migraines, stomach pains, suicidal thoughts, and other problems can result. Academic performance commonly deteriorates and rates of school absenteeism increase (Fekkes, Pijpers & Verloove-Vanhorick, 2006). Realizing the serious effects of such behaviors, a number of states have now passed legislation that reiterates the rights of all children to attend school in a safe and peaceful manner. Some state education departments mandate school district programs for students about bullying, and clear school policies about dealing with the behavior. See the Health Resources and Services Administration (HRSA) Maternal and Child Health Bureau Web site www.stopbullyingnow.hrsa.gov.

Nurses can be active in setting up school policies about bullying and integrating assessment and interventions related to bullying into health promotion visits. School programs should:

- Inform all students that bullying is not tolerated.
- Train teachers and other personnel about signs of bullying.
- Ensure adult supervision in hallways and on playgrounds, sites where bullying is most common.
- Teach children to promptly report bullying that is experienced or observed.
- Set up peer support for those who are bullied.
- Arrange therapeutic treatment through school counselors and other resources for those who bully; involve parents in the treatment plan.
- Measure incidence of bullying, monitor outcomes of policies, and use data to evaluate policies in schools.

Nurses who are in clinics, offices, and other health promotion settings can:

- Be alert for children with behavior changes (irritability, anxiety, poor self-concept).
- Consider bullying as a potential cause when fear or refusal to attend school is reported by child or parents.
- Ask questions during visits, such as "Have you ever been afraid to go to school?" or "What are the best and worst things about going to your school?" "What are the other kids in your neighborhood like?"
- Ask parents what they have done about any situations identified. Partner with the parent to act as liaison to the school or other agency.
- Refer identified bullies and victims of bullying to mental health specialists.

INCARCERATION

A growing number of children are entering the judicial system, and many are admitted at young ages. Juveniles were responsible for 12% of arrests for violent crimes, and their lifestyles and environments place them at high risk of death (Teplin, McClelland, Abram, et al., 2005). Children in detention, courts, and other facilities have frequently been victims as well as perpetrators of violence. They often have multiple risks such as substance abuse, early sexual activity, multiple sexual partners, sexual abuse, lack of a healthcare home, and mental health problems (Dixon, Howie, & Starling, 2005). Nurses may work within the juvenile justice system to provide episodic care for children or to partner with others to establish health-related programs within facilities. Youth who are incarcerated need the following:

- Basic physical care such as immunizations, vision, and hearing screening
- Nutrition assessment and teaching
- Skin assessment and hygiene practice teaching
- Information about sexuality, sexual practices, and sexually transmitted infections
- Assessment for substance abuse
- Teaching about hazards of substance use and assistance with quitting
- Mental health services
- Developmental assessment
- Individualized education plans to meet cognitive needs

HAZING

Hazing is an activity that is forced upon an individual, which causes humiliation and is required for membership in an organization or group. It can sometimes be potentially harmful. About 20 to 40 students die annually of events linked to hazing, and even middle and high school athletes engage in hazing activity (Campo, Poulos, & Sipple, 2005). Activities might include removing clothes, drinking large amounts of alcohol, using snuff or other substances, being locked in small places, being beaten, and many other behaviors. In spite of its common practice, many coaches are not aware of it, and many students do not know what to do about hazing practices. Ask during health visits if the student has ever had to do something to belong to the group or team. Ask about "scary" things others have had them do. Assist schools and colleges in setting up antihazing policies. Encourage students to report hazing. Be aware of the possibility of hazing when seeing children with traumatic injuries.

DOMESTIC VIOLENCE

Domestic violence or intimate partner abuse is that which occurs between adult partners in a family. It may involve the parents of a child, or one parent and the significant other. This type of abuse injures the child or adolescent either by witnessing a loved one being abused, or by being the victim. About 3.3 million children annually in the United States are exposed to violence against their mothers or other female care providers; children who live in homes where intimate partner abuse occurs are significantly more likely to be abused themselves (Casanueva & Martin, 2007).

DATING VIOLENCE

Dating violence is another type of intimate partner abuse; this type occurs in relationships among youth. Most dating violence is directed at females, and studies have focused largely on girls. Over 9% of adolescent girls report being victims of dating violence. African-American girls more commonly report dating violence than Hispanic or white girls (MMWR, 2006c). Girls who report dating violence were also more likely to report other risk behaviors, such as feeling sad, having attempted suicide, or having used substances such as tobacco and drugs. Early sexual activity, having a higher number of sex partners, and being less likely to use birth control are also associated with higher incidence of dating violence. A cluster risk profile may therefore put adolescents more at risk for dating violence.

Date rape is a term used when dating violence takes the form of rape. This can be particularly harmful to females who often do not want to share the event or press charges against the attacker.

Nurses should screen for violence at each health promotion visit, including gynecologic visits and prenatal care. Ask what is going well and not going well in intimate relationships, and whether the person ever feels unsafe or is forced to do things she does not wish to do. Recognize that while not as common, males may even be victims of violence in close relationships. Recognize that alcohol and other drugs are often connected with violence in relationships so ask about their use. Organize peer discussion groups about intimacy in order to help youth develop a sense of self-confidence and self-efficacy that will empower them to refuse activities in relationships in which they do not wish to engage.

NURSING MANAGEMENT

NURSING ASSESSMENT AND DIAGNOSIS

Nurses are in key positions to identify children at risk of being recipients and victims of violence. The ecologic framework can be used to assess children. Some questions that can be asked are listed in Table 44–6. It is important to detect both the risks that lead to vulnerability and the protective factors that can promote resilience and safety. Adapt questions to each age group and insert them in every healthcare encounter.

Table 44–6 Assessment Questions to Identify Violence Risk and Protective Factors

Microsystem

- Have you been hurt by your parents or anyone else at home?
- When was the last time you were made fun of or bullied at school? What did you do?
- Have you ever brought a gun or knife or other weapon to school?
- Do you have access to guns and knives at home? At friends' houses?
- What stresses are there in your family now?
- Tell me about school—what you like and don't like.

Mesosystem

- Do your parents attend school meetings? Talk with your teachers?
- Do you participate in any church, synagogue, or mosque services?
- Do you participate in any community activities?

Exosystem

- What stresses do your parents have at work, in their families, with their health or finances?
- Do you feel like your school helps to keep you safe?
- Are there plans for handling violent episodes at your school if they were to occur?
- Do you feel safe in your neighborhood?
- Where would you go or who would you call if you felt unsafe or were hurt and no one was at home?

Nursing care for violence is discussed in the Nursing Care Plan on pages 1173–1174. The following nursing diagnoses may be appropriate:

Risk for Violence: Self-Directed related to history of violence

Chronic Low Self-Esteem related to history of abuse

Dysfunctional Family Processes related to situational crises

Delayed Growth and Development related to environmental deficiencies

PLANNING AND INTERVENTION

Nurses intervene with individual children, with families, and in schools and communities to increase safety and decrease violence. Help children and families meet basic needs and access resources to assist with finances, respite care, domestic violence, and other issues. Education is a key element of intervention.

PROVIDING INFORMATION

Teach the family the dangers of firearms and the necessity for using gun locks and locked cabinets, storing guns unloaded, and storing guns and ammunition in separate places. Suggest alternative activities to minimize child exposure to violence in the media. Inform parents about rating systems for television and other media, and about lockout mechanisms for televisions and computers. Discuss the harmful effects of verbal and physical abuse to the child or other family members and explore alternatives.

Present the school-age child and adolescent with information about bullying and strategies for dealing with it. Provide school and community resources where the child can go if there are threats of any kind. Discuss date rape and violence with all teens and encourage them to report it.

NURSING CARE IN THE COMMUNITY

Both in schools and in community settings, nurses can plan peer mentoring to provide assistance to children at high risk of experiencing violence. Nurses can link and coordinate school and community programs for children to provide for parent involvement and child support. Discuss safety issues, both risks and protective actions, in schools and community groups. Report children who are at risk. Work to establish extended programs for children so that they are safe after school. Help children learn behaviors that will help them to be safe in their communities and at home. Teach positive problem-solving and conflict-management techniques to children and parents.

Youth with special needs are a special concern of nurses. Jails and detention centers often have a nurse who visits youth on a regular basis or when health problems occur. Health teaching

Nursing Care Plan

THE CHILD AND VIOLENT BEHAVIOR

INTERVENTION	RATIONALE	EXPECTED OUTCOME
1. Nursing Diagnosis: Risk for Violence: Other-Directed related to history of family violence		
NIC Priority Intervention: **Environmental management:** Violence prevention: Monitoring and manipulation of the environment to decrease the potential for violent behavior directed toward self, others, or the environment		**NOC Suggested Outcome:** **Impulse control:** Ability to restrain compulsive or impulsive behavior in child and others
Goal: The child demonstrates impulse control.		
■ Identify violent behaviors in the child.	■ Violence in the child usually develops over time.	The child expresses the ability to manage problems in acceptable ways.
■ Provide a safe place for exploration of feelings by referral to school or other counseling, support groups, and other resources.	■ The child needs an opportunity to explore feelings and vulnerability.	
■ Provide strategies for managing anger and alternative ways for coping with problems.	■ Coping strategies can be learned from others and can help in dealing with a stressful home situation.	
Goal: The child is secure in a safe environment.		
■ Perform a thorough assessment of hazards to the physical and emotional state in the child's home, neighborhood, and school.	■ Hazards to physical and emotional health promote violence to and from the child.	The child expresses a sense of physical and emotional safety in daily life.
■ Institute actions that will result in removal of child from unsafe situations.	■ Removal from family, community, or school may be needed to ensure child safety.	
■ Use community resources to provide respite care, teaching for families, and safety instructions for the child.	■ Stress reduction measures may help to decrease violent behaviors.	
2. Nursing Diagnosis: Risk for Injury related to physical or psychological conditions in the environment		
NIC Priority Intervention: **Safety behavior:** Family actions to minimize risk of physical or emotional trauma		**NOC Suggested Outcome:** **Parenting:** Social safety: Parental actions to avoid social relationships that might cause harm or injury **Risk control:** Actions to eliminate or reduce actual, personal, and modifiable health risks
Goal: Risk for physical and emotional injury to the child is decreased.		
■ Identify physical and psychologic factors that affect the child's safety. ■ Assist family to deal with issues such as mental status challenges, fatigue, financial concern, substance abuse, lack of adequate childcare resources, and other factors.	■ Multiple factors in the family can contribute to risk of violence and lack of safety for the child.	The child is not injured in physical or emotional ways in the home or other immediate settings.
■ Instruct family on methods of keeping the child safe.	■ Families need information about the impact of unsafe settings on the child and methods that can decrease risk of injury.	

(continued)

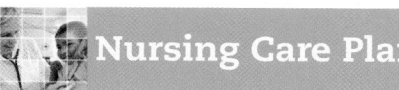

Nursing Care Plan—continued

THE CHILD AND VIOLENT BEHAVIOR

INTERVENTION	RATIONALE	EXPECTED OUTCOME
3. Nursing Diagnosis: Posttrauma Syndrome related to physical or psychosocial abuse		
NIC Priority Intervention: **Counseling:** Use of an interactive helping process focusing on the needs, problems, and feelings of the child who is a victim of abuse or other violence		**NOC Suggested Outcome:** **Abuse/violence recovery:** Healing of psychologic and physical wounds of abuse or violence
Goal: The child demonstrates abuse or violence recovery.		
■ Assess the child's affect and behaviors. ■ Evaluate social interactions and sense of trust in others.	■ Disturbed child behaviors can demonstrate a sense of mistrust and insecurity.	The child identifies feelings related to violent episode(s) and expresses healing of the self.
■ Assist the child in identifying feelings and coping strategies by providing counseling, art therapy, and other strategies.	■ Establishment of close interactions with others demonstrates reestablishment of a sense of trust. ■ A child who has experienced abuse or other violence needs a therapeutic relationship with a counselor to deal with the trauma and begin to rebuild trust and respect, and to learn coping mechanisms.	

may be provided in some facilities. Halfway houses and homeless shelters are examples of settings where violence prevention and intervention can occur with youth. Mental health centers and other programs have nurses that work with children who are victims of violence (for example, have witnessed domestic violence, have witnessed or had a family member murdered, have been abused at home or school) or perpetrators of violence. See Chapter 57 for a discussion of posttraumatic stress disorder and its effects on the child and adolescent.

Partner with families to assist them in dealing with children about war and terrorism. Recognize that youth who have experienced such events themselves are more at risk for mental health disruptions with future events. Answer questions from children honestly but reassure them that many people are trying to make the situation safe. Other suggestions for parents include the following:

- Limit television viewing and other media exposure because of its constant replaying of the events of terrorism or war. Preschoolers may think the events continue to happen, rather than being a onetime occurrence. Watch with children and talk with them about what is happening.
- Continue with structured family events such as meals, recreation, and faith-based activities. Spend time with your child.
- Take cues from the child about how much to discuss. Use words the child or adolescent can understand.
- Partner with the school so teachers know what parents have discussed and parents are aware of how events are discussed at school.
- If youth decide to become active by writing letters or joining campaigns, allow them to participate in this way.
- Be alert for regression in behavior, sleep and eating problems, or other indications of stress. Consider talking with the healthcare provider or a counselor in such situations.
- Expect that even after the child has adjusted, there may be delayed reactions. Anniversaries of events, holidays, and birthdays often bring renewed pain and sadness.
- Realize that adults must care for themselves, obtain stress relief, and talk with others in order to have strength and resources available for children.

EVALUATION

The expected outcomes of nursing care for violence prevention include a decrease in incidents of homicides, firearm injuries, abuse, date rape, and other violence among children. Additional outcomes are establishment of programs to decrease violence, and verbalization by all children of what to do if violence occurs and how to solve problems without becoming violent.

CHILD ABUSE

One of the most common types of violence against children is child abuse. Children from all socioeconomic groups and both genders are victims of abuse. This type of violence can have implications for both the physical and mental health of children, and can influence their health status even long after the abuse has occurred. Awareness of the problem of child abuse is increasing. More cases are being reported; however, these are probably only a small percentage of the total. Nearly 1 million U.S. children are maltreated annually, nearly 100,000 of them infants under 1 year of age (Brodowski, Nolan, Gaudiosi, et al., 2008). More than four children daily (about 1500 children annually) die from child abuse in the United States (Childhelp, 2005). Children under 2 years are more likely to die from abuse than those of older ages (Kellogg & Committee on Child Abuse, 2007). Infants are at greatest risk with 19% of maltreatment fatalities occurring in that young age group (Brodowski et al., 2008).

Physical abuse is only one part of a larger problem. The definition of child abuse has expanded over the past 10 years and includes physical neglect, emotional abuse and neglect, verbal abuse, and sexual abuse, as well as physical abuse. Abuse generally involves an act of commission, that is, actively doing something to a child physically, emotionally, or sexually, such as hitting, belittling, or molesting. Neglect more often involves an act of omission, such as not providing adequate nutrition, emotional contact, or necessary physical care, or abandoning a child. Because the evidence is often not visible, emotional abuse and neglect are more difficult to identify and prove than physical abuse or neglect. Risk factors for abuse and neglect are listed in Table 44–7.

Table 44–7 Risk Factors for Child Abuse and Neglect

Factors Increasing Risk for Physical Abuse

- Poverty
- Violence in the family
- Prematurity or low birth weight
- Unrelated male primary caretaker
- Parents who were abused as children
- Age less than 3 years
- Child disability or condition that requires a great deal of care (e.g., mental retardation, attention deficit hyperactivity disorder)
- Parental substance abuse or social isolation

Factors Increasing Risk for Sexual Abuse

- Absence of natural father or having a stepfather
- Being female
- Mother's employment outside the home
- Poor relationship with parent
- Parental relationship characterized by conflict
- Parental substance abuse or social isolation

PHYSICAL ABUSE

Physical abuse is the deliberate maltreatment of another individual that inflicts pain or injury and may result in permanent or temporary disfigurement or even death. Common methods of physical abuse in children are listed in Table 44–8.

Table 44–8 Methods of Physical Abuse in Children

Hitting, slapping, kicking, or punching
Whipping with belts, shoes, or electrical cords (***B***)
Inflicting burns with a lit cigarette or lighter (***A***)
Immersing child or body part in scalding water (commonly legs, perineal area, hands, or feet; see Figure 59-15)
Shaking the child violently ("shaken child" syndrome)
Tying the child to a fence, bed, tree, or other object
Throwing the child against a wall, down stairs, or against a window
Choking or gagging the child
Fracturing the legs, arms, ribs, or skull
Deliberately administering excessive doses of prescribed or nonprescribed drugs
Deliberately withholding prescribed medication

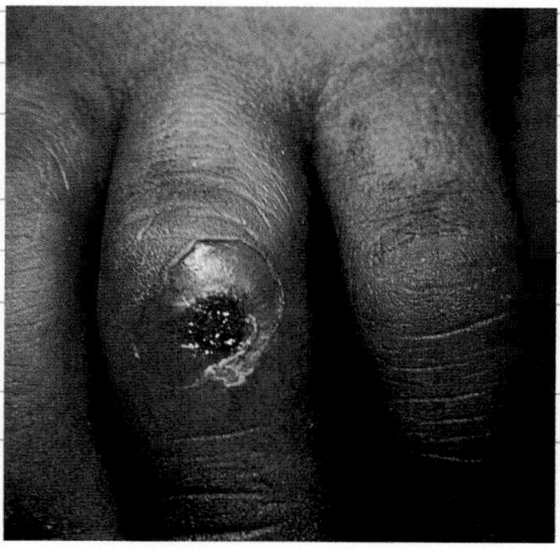

A

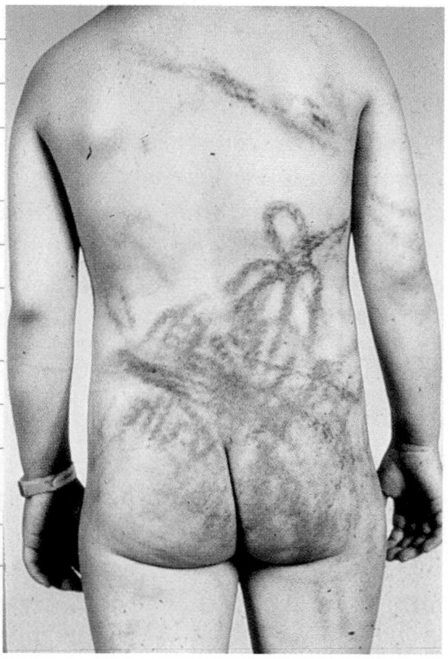

B

PHYSICAL NEGLECT

Physical neglect is the deliberate withholding of or failure to provide the necessary and available resources to the child. Behaviors constituting physical neglect include failure to provide for the following basic needs: supervision appropriate for child's age, adequate nutrition and hydration, hygiene (e.g., clean diapers and clothes, bathing and toileting facilities), shelter (e.g., warmth in winter), and appropriate health care (e.g., immunizations, dental care, medications, eyeglasses).

ABANDONED BABIES

There are no accurate statistics on numbers of babies that are abandoned in dumpsters, on doorsteps, and in other locations. This tragedy has been addressed by "Safe Haven" laws in some states that allow women to drop unwanted babies at certain locations such as hospitals and fire stations without legal recrimination. In spite of these laws, babies continue to be abandoned, perhaps because mothers do not know about the laws or because they do not believe they will not be found guilty. Young teen mothers may not want others to know they had a baby. In addition, placement of these babies in adoptive homes is difficult because of paternity suits. Nurses should know their state's "Safe Haven" law details. Inform adolescents and young women about the law and post information in community sites frequented by women. Partner with young pregnant women to link them to resources such as adoption agencies when they might not want to keep a baby.

EMOTIONAL ABUSE

Emotional abuse usually involves shaming, ridiculing, embarrassing, or insulting the child. It can also include the destruction of a child's personal property, such as tearing up the child's favorite family photographs or letters or harming, killing, or giving away the child's pet. These actions are frequently used as a means of frightening or controlling the child.

Verbal abuse is a common method of emotional abuse. Words can be a violent and volatile weapon against a child, eroding the child's fragile sense of self and destroying self-esteem. Common examples of verbal abuse include yelling obscenities at the child, calling the child names, threatening to "put the child away" or to give away or kill the child's pet, telling the child "I wish you were never born" or "You're worthless," and using words to humiliate, shame, or degrade the child.

EMOTIONAL NEGLECT

Emotional neglect is characterized by the caretaker's emotional unavailability to the child. The usual style of interaction is cold and lacking in sensitive personal attention. The child suffers from a lack of nurturance and failure of the parent or caretaker to meet basic dependency needs. An example of emotional neglect is the parent who is mentally ill, abusing alcohol or other substances, and cannot respond adequately to the child's developmental needs.

SEXUAL ABUSE

Child sexual abuse is the exploitation of a child for the sexual gratification of an adult. About 1.2 per 1000 children (almost 100,000) children in the United States are sexually abused each year. Approximately 10% of school children report that they have been sexually abused. Many children who are sexually abused are under the age of 5 years, some as young as 3 months. The average age for sexual molestation is 4 years. The perpetrator is usually the parent (80% of the time) or another person legally responsible who does the following:

- Inflicts or allows another to inflict physical or emotional pain or injury
- Creates or allows another to create a significant risk of serious physical or emotional pain or injury
- Commits or allows another to commit an act of sexual abuse, as defined by law, against the child

Between 100,000 and 500,000 children in the United States are sexually abused each year. Of child sexual abusers, 75% to 80% are immediate family members, other relatives, friends, or neighbors (U. S. Department of Health and Human Services, 2005).

The word "child" in sexual abuse and molestation refers to anyone who has not reached the age of consent, even if a teenager. **Incest** is sexual activity between close family members, so that marriage would be legally or culturally prohibited. Abusers often threaten to harm or kill the child or another family member if the child discloses the abuse. Some abusers are pedophiles, people who have sexual impulses toward preadolescent children. The pedophile is at least 16 years of age and is at least 5 years older than the victim, and the victim is 13 years of age or younger. Another form of sexual abuse is exhibitionism, or obtaining sexual arousal by exposing one's genitals to a stranger. Some children are victims of prostitution, forced to offer themselves for money or the pleasures of others, either in person or through videotapes and Internet sources.

Nursing Practice

Following are common forms of sexual abuse:

- Oral-genital contact
- Fondling and caressing the genitals
- Anal intercourse
- Sexual intercourse
- Rape
- Sodomy
- Prostitution
- Forcing viewing of or participation in pornography such as sexually explicit or nude photographs
- Encouraging nude photos or sexual activity via Internet or videotape

Clinical Manifestations

CHILD ABUSE

- Multiple bruises in various stages of healing
- Scald burns with clear lines of demarcation and in a glove or stocking distribution (see Figure 59–15 in Chapter 59)
- Rope, belt, or cord marks, usually seen on the mouth, buttocks, back, legs, and arms (see Figure A in Table 44–8)
- Burn scars in various stages of healing
- Multiple fractures in various stages of healing, spiral fractures not explained by accident
- Shortness of breath and distress upon being moved, indicating chest contusions and possible rib fractures
- Sedation from overmedication
- Exacerbation of chronic illness (such as diabetes or asthma) because of withholding of medication
- Cranial and abdominal injuries
- Change in behavior or school performance
- Fear and avoidance of certain people or situations

Etiology and Pathophysiology

Regardless of the type of abuse, the most common abuser is the child's parent or guardian or a male friend of the child's mother. Substance abuse is a major contributor to the problem, with half of cases related to parental alcohol or drug abuse (Childhelp, 2005). Risk factors associated with abusive behavior in adults include the following:

- Psychopathology, such as drug addiction or alcoholism, low self-esteem, poor impulse control, and other personality disorders
- Poor parenting experiences, such as abuse in the abuser's own childhood, rejection by the abuser's own parent(s), lack of knowledge of alternative methods of discipline, strong belief in or family tradition of harsh discipline, and lack of parental affection
- Marital stressors and problems with partners, such as hostile-dependent, abusive, or nonsupportive relationships, and one-sided decision making
- Environmental stressors, such as legal, financial, medical, or housing problems
- Social isolation, such as few friends and limited use of sitters, family, or other resources
- Inappropriate expectations for the developmental level of the child

Clinical Manifestations

Clinical manifestations of physical abuse are listed above. Behaviors inconsistent with developmental stage may be apparent. For example, the toddler or preschool child may be indiscriminately friendly with unfamiliar adults, including healthcare providers, rather than demonstrating shyness or anxiety. For the infant or young child with "shaken baby syndrome" or "shaken child syndrome," the symptoms are those of central nervous system injury from repeated coup and contrecoup injury (see Chapter 56). These may include vomiting, irritability, fatigue, poor feeding, bradycardia, apnea, enlarged fontanelle, and seizures. Bruises are usually not present, but computerized tomography (CT) is often definitive for the diagnosis (Hymel & Hall, 2005).

Manifestations of physical neglect include undernourishment (evidenced by constantly feeling hungry, hoarding or stealing food, and being underweight), unclean clothes and body, poor dental health (extensive cavities or generally poor condition of teeth), and inappropriate clothing for the season.

Manifestations of emotional abuse, verbal abuse, and emotional neglect include fear, poor physical growth, and failure to meet appropriate developmental milestones. The child may have difficulty relating to adults, impaired communication skills, and developmental delays. Behavioral manifestations include anxiety, fear, shame, aggression, delinquency, and depression.

Children who have been sexually abused may exhibit a variety of physical and behavioral signs and symptoms. Bruising, bleeding, and laceration of the genital area are obvious signs of trauma (Johnson, 2006). However, sexual abuse does not always result in apparent injury. Among the many long-term consequences of child sexual abuse are ongoing feelings of shame, guilt, anger, and hostility; decreased self-esteem, which leads to increased self-destructive behavior, risk of suicide, and decreased ability to establish positive relationships in adulthood; recurrence of victimization experiences; substance abuse; and eating disorders. The results can be long-lasting, with children experiencing posttraumatic stress disorder (PTSD) or substance abuse in adulthood. Factors associated with greater psychologic harm to the child include (1) a long period of abuse, (2) use of violent force or threat of violence, (3) abuse involving penetration (intercourse or oral–genital sex), and (4) abuse involving family members, especially the father or stepfather.

Clinical Therapy

Diagnosis of abuse is made on the basis of a careful history and thorough physical examination. X-ray, CT, and MRI studies may be ordered to identify signs of recurrent abuse (e.g., healed fractures). Laboratory studies may involve urine culture for signs of infection or screening for sexually transmitted infections; they can also rule out other causes of bleeding such as hemophilia. Genitourinary examination may be performed if sexual abuse is suspected. Some children are admitted directly to the hospital with the diagnosis of suspected abuse or neglect. Less obvious as a victim of abuse is the child admitted with a skull fracture who "fell off a chair."

Clinical Manifestations

SEXUAL ABUSE IN CHILDREN AND ADOLESCENTS

- Vaginal discharge
- Blood-stained underpants or diaper
- Genital redness, pain, itching, or bruising
- Difficulty walking or sitting
- Urinary tract infection
- Sexually transmitted infection
- Somatic complaints, such as headaches or stomachaches
- Sleeping problems, such as nightmares or night terrors
- Bed-wetting
- Unwillingness to go to babysitter, family member, neighbor, or other person
- New or excessive sexual curiosity or play
- Fear of strangers
- Constant masturbation
- Curling into fetal position
- Phobias about particular places, people, or things
- Abrupt changes in school performance and attendance
- Changes in eating habits
- Abrupt changes in behavior (especially withdrawal)
- Child or adolescent female acts like a wife or mother
- Excessively seductive behavior

Neglect, which is more difficult to define and identify, frequently requires hospitalization with a comprehensive medical, social, and psychiatric evaluation. Five basic categories must be considered when attempting to diagnose neglect: (1) medical care neglect (lack of necessary medical care), (2) gross safety neglect (lack of appropriate supervision), (3) physical neglect (lack of food and shelter), (4) emotional neglect, and (5) educational neglect.

All 50 states have extensive, complex statutes about reporting child abuse and neglect. A specialist must be consulted, especially if the child's testimony will be used in court.

Children do not routinely make false allegations of abuse. If indeed there is reason to believe the allegations are false, a child and adolescent therapist (psychiatrist, psychologist, psychiatric clinical nurse specialist, or social worker) with special expertise should be consulted to determine the truth. Keep in mind that children who withdraw their accusations have often been threatened or coerced into doing so. Because children who have been physically, emotionally, or sexually abused are at risk for major depression, they require skilled care by mental health professionals who are specially trained in this area. Initially the treatment goals include prevention of self-destructive or other dangerous acts. Children must be encouraged to express their fears and feelings in a safe and supportive environment. Equally important is the child's need to build coping skills and self-esteem. The child must be reassured and convinced that he or she is in no way responsible or to blame for what happened.

Individual treatment with art therapy is used initially because it is the least threatening method in the early stages of treatment, it can easily be tailored to meet the child's individual needs, and it prepares the child for other forms of treatment such as family and group therapy (Figure 44–8 ●). Family or group therapy may be of benefit in exploring the child's concerns and feelings. Anger is common, especially in children who were abused by a trusted adult such as the father or stepfather.

Nursing Practice

Every state has a child abuse law specifying the particular behaviors that define every type of abuse. Any professional who works with children and reasonably suspects that a child has been abused is required to report his or her suspicions to the local agency for child protective services. Reports made in good faith are not liable to countersuits. However, professionals who suspect abuse and do not report it may be held responsible by the judicial system. See U.S. Department of Health and Human Services for state laws (www.childwelfare.gov/systemwide/laws_policies/search/index/cfm).

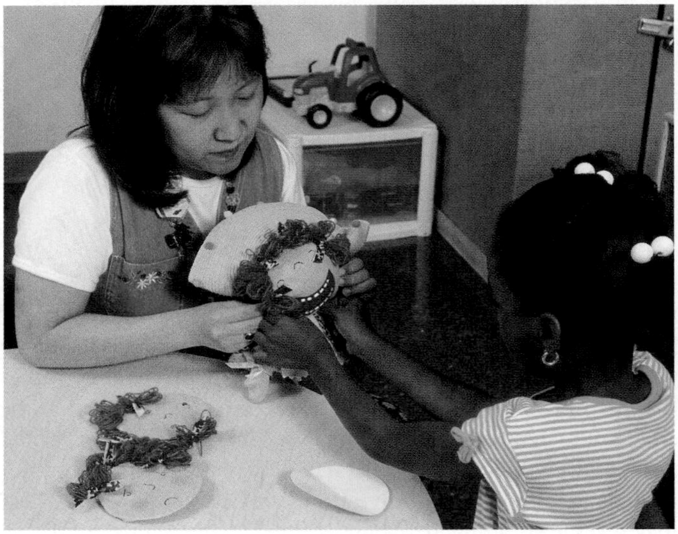

● **Figure 44–8** Clinical interventions with children. Therapeutic strategies with young children involve various methods of communication, such as dramatic play and art.

NURSING MANAGEMENT

NURSING ASSESSMENT AND DIAGNOSIS

Nursing assessment in instances of suspected child abuse or neglect requires a comprehensive history and physical examination, with documentation of findings. Consultation with social service agencies in the community is important if the family is receiving services.

Obtaining the history can be stressful for both the nurse and the parent. Use of therapeutic communication techniques and a quiet, unhurried environment are helpful. Be open, nonjudgmental, and calm. A statement such as "Hello, Mr. S. My name is Joan T. I'm Jonathan's nurse, and I will be asking you some questions about his overall health" may be a good start. It is important to differentiate true child abuse from cultural variations that might inaccurately be assumed to indicate abuse (Figure 44–9 ● A and B). Obtaining information about abusive and neglectful behaviors requires a trusting relationship with parents, who are often afraid to trust any professional.

The health history sequence should include (1) parental concerns, (2) general family history, and (3) specific child history. This sequence begins with nonthreatening topics and allows the nurse to demonstrate concern before asking about abuse-related concerns. Obtain details about how injuries occurred. Document the parents' and child's own words verbatim using quotation marks. Compare reports obtained from each family member for lack of consistency and details that change over time.

It is desirable to interview the parent and child separately as well as together. Parent-child interaction during an intensive history-taking session provides an opportunity to observe the child's behavior and the parent's method of handling and responding to the child.

Data gathered during history taking are particularly important in light of physical findings. Are there discrepancies between the history and physical assessment data? Do the parents give a history of an uncontrollable, inattentive toddler when the nurse observes a child who is attentive throughout a 15-minute examination? Assess the child's general appearance, including dress and behavior during the assessment. How do the child's affect, behavior, and development compare with those of other children the same age? Be alert for the signs of shaken child syndrome; this most often appears as a subtle neurologic condition. Measure head circumference and perform a neurologic examination (see Chapter 56∞).

Documentation of findings is important in all situations but is essential in cases of suspected child abuse and neglect. Each person who handles a laboratory specimen or other item (e.g.,

Developing Cultural Competence

CUPPING AND CAO GIO

Traditional treatment practices are sometimes mistaken for signs of physical abuse. The Chinese practice of cupping, which involves heating a bamboo cup and placing it on the skin, is a traditional treatment for headaches or abdominal pain. The Vietnamese practice of cao gio (rubbing out the wind), in which a coin or the fingers are forcefully rubbed on the chest, back, or neck, is used to treat minor ailments. Ask about marks on the skin, how they occurred, and what health practices the family uses.

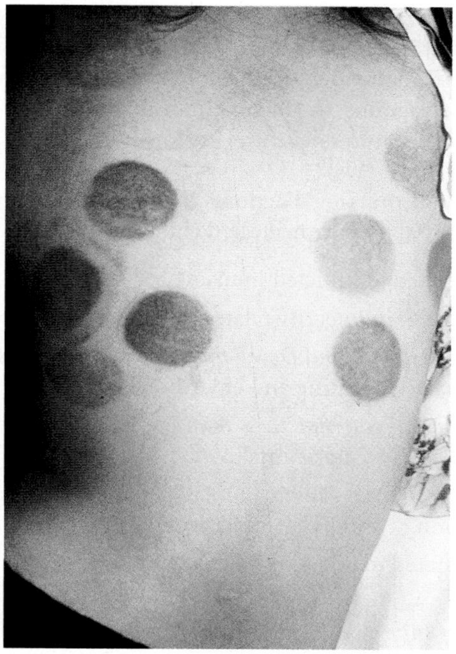

A

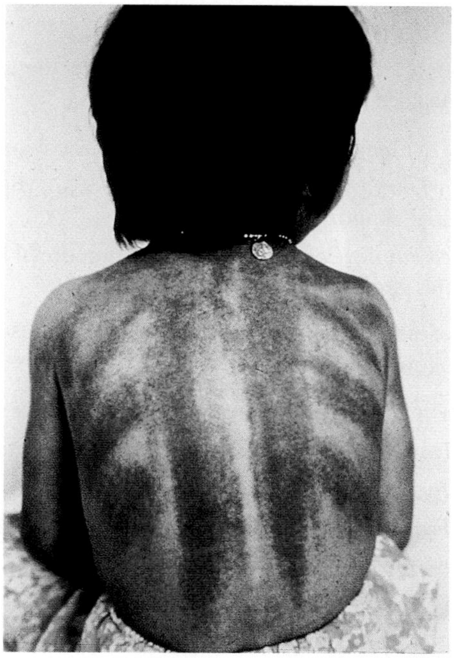

B

● **Figure 44–9** Cultural practices that may be mistaken for child abuse. It is important to differentiate cultural practices, such as ***A***, cupping, and ***B***, coining, from signs of child abuse.

Used with permission of the American Academy of Pediatrics, Visual Diagnosis of Child Physical Abuse Slide Kit. *Photographs copyright © AAP/Kempe.*

clothing soiled with semen) in cases of suspected child abuse must be identified in the patient's record, and the specimen must never be left unattended. Record physical findings as observed. Use figure diagrams to document skin injuries. Take photographs as directed to document the location, nature, and extent of injuries.

Among the nursing diagnoses that might be appropriate for the physically abused or neglected child are the following:

- *Pain* related to inflicted injuries
- *Impaired Skin Integrity* related to inflicted injuries
- *Delayed Growth and Development* related to lack of supportive parenting and environment
- *Imbalanced Nutrition: Less than Body Requirements* related to inadequate caloric intake
- *Impaired Health Maintenance* related to lack of parental provision of child's essential needs
- *Fear* related to actual physical harm or repeated risk of injury
- *Risk for Injury* related to physical abuse
- *Risk for Other-Directed Violence (Parent)* related to inability to manage anger

Additional diagnoses that might apply to the emotionally abused or neglected child include the following:

- *Defensive Coping* related to psychologic impairment
- *Chronic Low Self-Esteem* related to lack of appropriate emotional support from parents
- *Disabled Family Coping* related to dysfunctional family dynamics and pattern of physical abuse

Diagnoses that might apply to the sexually abused child include the following:

- *Anxiety* related to potential separation from parent
- *Rape-Trauma Syndrome* related to sexual exploitation
- *Ineffective Role Performance* related to domestic violence
- *Disturbed Personal Identity* related to disturbance of usual activities of childhood

PLANNING AND IMPLEMENTATION

Nursing care focuses on helping to remove the child from an abusive environment, preventing further injury, providing supportive care, and reinforcing the importance of follow-up care and counseling.

PREVENT FURTHER INJURY

Work with social services and community agencies to assess the child's home environment, individuals living in the home, and the actions surrounding the abuse. Assist in removing the child from the home to temporary custody of the court or foster care of another relative, if indicated. Counsel family members about abuse and refer them for appropriate therapy.

PROVIDE SUPPORTIVE CARE

Protect and treat the child's injuries (e.g., fractures, burns). Include parents in the child's treatment plan, and keep them informed about the child's progress. Even if suspected of inflicting injuries to the child, the parent is still the child's primary caretaker. Talk with the parent as you would with any parent. Be supportive of any guilt expressed. Encourage the parent to assist with the child's care. Observe parent-child interactions and document supportive behaviors and the child's response to the parent versus other care providers.

Interacting nonjudgmentally with a parent suspected of abusing his or her child can be difficult. Nurses should talk with a colleague about any anger they feel toward the parents or about the child's injuries or specific actions surrounding the abuse. Use team meetings to develop strategies that enable healthcare professionals to work with the parents and child.

HOME CARE TEACHING

If there is any question about the child returning to a potentially dangerous situation, support the child's removal from the situation. The child may receive supervised care in the home by court order. Day care, home nursing, and social worker visits may be arranged. Parents should be referred to parent effectiveness classes, family therapy, and support groups as necessary. When a neighbor or friend is the abuser, the family may need support and legal advice when a term of incarceration is finished and the perpetrator returns to the community. Some states and communities have sexual offender laws that publicize the presence of an offender on parole within neighborhoods.

Encourage the family to inform other care providers when the child's abuse history may affect a response to care. They should be alert to signs of PTSD so they can seek assistance if the child has continuing problems (see Chapter 57∞).

EVALUATION

Expected outcomes of nursing care for the child who has been abused or neglected include the following:

- Maintenance of normal growth and development
- Establishment of a positive sense of self-esteem
- Provision of parenting information and stress relief for parents

Nursing Practice

When children have been abused, they are often frightened in new situations. Sexually abused children may resist removing clothes for a physical examination or medical test. They may want to wear undergarments to the surgical suite. They may distrust members of the gender that abused. When aware of a history of abuse, ask the parents or guardians how to best facilitate the child's health care. Be sensitive to fears and allow the child to wear clothing, have a support person present, or whatever may provide a sense of security. Stability of nurses assigned to the child and the presence of a counselor may help to increase rapport and trust.

- Provision of a nurturing environment for the child
- Absence of episodes of abuse

MÜNCHHAUSEN SYNDROME BY PROXY

Münchhausen syndrome by proxy is a potentially deadly form of child abuse that involves the fabrication of signs and symptoms of a health condition in a child. In 94 to 99% of cases, the mother creates these fictitious signs in her child (the proxy). The victim is usually under 6 years, and commonly under 1 year of age. Frequently the child's symptoms of illness are used to gain entry into the medical system to meet the abuser's own psychologic needs for attention. The perpetrator may induce illness by giving the child medications (Cyr, 2007).

The issues of abuse are multidimensional. The child is a victim of the feigned illness, repeated hospitalizations, and invasive procedures. Equally disruptive is the deprivation of the child's daily routine caused by the periodic medical crises.

Münchhausen syndrome by proxy should be suspected when unexplained, recurrent, or extremely rare conditions occur; illness is unresponsive to treatment; and the history and clinical findings are inconsistent. The most commonly reported signs and symptoms are central nervous system dysfunction, apnea, diarrhea, vomiting, fever, seizures, signs of bleeding (in urine or stool), and rashes. The parent may overdose the child on medications, such as nonprescription drugs and even syrup of ipecac, causing a variety of side effects. The symptoms occur in the presence of the same caretaker and disappear when the child is separated from that caretaker.

The child often appears uncooperative, extremely anxious, fearful, and negative. The caretaker, who in contrast appears very cooperative, competent, and loving, often expresses a desire for the child to recover. The caretaker may even suggest diagnostic procedures to try to determine "what's wrong." Characteristically the caretaker thrives in the healthcare environment.

The cause of Münchhausen syndrome by proxy is often complex and rooted in the caretaker's own abusive or neglectful childhood. The disorder occurs in all socioeconomic classes. Often the perpetrator has some type of healthcare background, such as nursing or another allied health profession. The abuser is often young, married, from the middle socioeconomic class, and has a history of insecure attachment (Adshead & Bluglass, 2005).

A suspicion of Münchhausen syndrome by proxy requires a coordinated evaluation by an interdisciplinary team. Members of the team must organize and communicate a strategic plan regarding collection of evidence, confrontation of the abuser, and management of the hospitalized child. The child's safety is the ultimate concern. The case must also be reported to the appropriate child protective services.

Nursing Management

Take special care to maintain a trusting relationship with the caretaker so that he or she does not become suspicious and leave the hospital. Often the best person on the team to function in the role of "trusted other" is a member of the psychiatric consultation team.

Careful documentation of parent-child interactions, presence or absence of symptoms, and other pertinent observations is essential. The child must be closely monitored. If blood is present in the child's urine, stool, or vomitus, carefully document whether the nurse was present or whether the sample was provided by the parent. Covert video surveillance may be ordered by the hospital when the syndrome is highly suspected in a particular situation. Expert consultants may be needed to ensure legal requirements for investigation are met. When enough evidence is collected to prove Münchhausen syndrome by proxy, the caretaker is confronted by the physician or a member of the psychiatric team in planning with law enforcement officials.

ENVIRONMENTAL INFLUENCES ON CHILD HEALTH

DISASTERS

Disasters, serious and massive events that impact many people and are beyond the community's ability to manage, are experienced by people in all countries and cultures. Natural disasters include floods, ice storms, hurricanes, earthquakes, volcano eruptions, tornados, and wild fires. Trains or trucks carrying toxic chemicals and nuclear waste that crash or explode may also cause a disaster. Terrorism is another potential cause of disasters with the use of infectious organisms, toxic chemicals, or radioactive agents. (See Chapter 45∞ for information about infectious agents used for bioterrorism.) Disasters may cause death, injury, physical damage, psychological trauma, and economic disruption.

Children have special vulnerabilities during a disaster that impacts their mental health. They have limited understanding due to their cognitive development, and fewer coping skills to help deal with the impact of witnessing injuries. The disruption of normal life patterns (reliability, cohesion, and predictability) may be prolonged and cause stress. Fear and anxiety are heightened after the disaster, and the child often worries that it will happen again. They worry that someone will be injured or killed,

Growth and Development

Children, especially at young ages, are at an elevated risk of injury from environmental hazards during a disaster, such as the following:

- They are unable to flee or take evasive action to escape danger.
- Smaller size places them closer to the ground increasing skin and inhalation exposures. Their thinner skin may allow toxins to be absorbed more rapidly.
- Hand-to-mouth behaviors increase ingestion exposure in young children.
- Developing body organs may decrease detoxification and elimination of toxic substances.
- The higher metabolic rate and associated higher respiratory and heart rates increase poisoning dangers from carbon monoxide and other aerosol substances (Etzel, 2004).

they will be separated from their family, or they will be left alone. Children may believe that repeated television broadcasts of mass casualty events are additional events.

Children have unique responses to disasters, depending on prior life experiences; support of significant others, and their developmental stages. Some general reactions at different ages may include (Centers for Disease Control and Prevention, 2005):

- *Infancy to 6 years* – Increased crying and need for comforting; fear of separation from parents and other caregivers; clinging behaviors; regression in developmental tasks, may have returned to bed wetting or difficulty sleeping.
- *7 to 10 years* – Feelings of sadness and/or anger; afraid the event will happen again; decreased attention span and concentration that can lead to decreased school performance; peers may provide incorrect information that will need correction.
- *11 years and older* – Decreased contact with peers and usual activities; increased risk-taking behaviors or fear of leaving home; emotions related to the event may overwhelm them and may be unable to talk about them; emotional responses may lead to increased arguments and irritability with siblings and family members.

As the impact of the event becomes known, grief and depressive symptoms may emerge and children may have difficulty being engaged in other normal life activities. Some children develop posttraumatic stress disorder (PTSD), which involves symptoms that interfere with daily living months or years after the event. See Chapter 57∞ for a discussion of PTSD.

NURSING MANAGEMENT

EMERGENCY RESPONSE

Nurses are important first responders during disasters—providing emergency health care for rescued victims, first aid for the walking wounded, working in disaster shelters, and general public health interventions (e.g., vaccines, sanitation, food and water). While physical care is essential, psychological trauma is also addressed. Nurses with knowledge of child and adolescent development can meet the needs of youth in disasters. Nurses can provide a safe place for children, away from media and unfolding traumatic events, such as the rescue of dead and injured. Do not allow children to leave a scene unaccompanied by a parent or other responsible adult. Assess for panic reactions, unexpected behaviors, and changing conditions.

PSYCHOLOGIC SUPPORT

Once the initial disaster is managed and children return to home or other settings, mental health interventions appropriate for various age groups include:

- *Infancy to 6 years*—Children need support and care by primary caretakers whenever possible. Encourage parents to hold, cuddle, and provide reassurance that they are together and will deal with any losses together. The child's clinging behaviors should be accepted and supported. Television and media coverage should be limited to prevent the child's repeated exposure to the event.
- *7 to 10 years*—Explain the disaster and answer the child's questions and encourage the parents to do the same. Children may ask for information about such topics as how dead bodies are managed, how it feels to die in a mine, or what happens when someone bleeds to death. Help parents and schools to plan for accepting responses and answers to such questions. Techniques such as storytelling, drawing, and dramatic play may enable the child to express emotions and to understand the event (see Chapters 41 and 57∞ for more details on these techniques). Let children know that feelings of being upset, sad, or angry are normal; allow them to cry and express feelings, and be patient for a return to normal sleep and eating patterns. Parents should arrange for increased contact with parents or other significant adults, while the child gradually returns to peers and normal life activities.
- *11 years and older*—Older children may want to discuss the event with peers although many want increased contact with family members for a while. Help schools and other community agencies arrange for mental health specialists to assist children to explore and express their feelings in safe settings. Provide grief counseling for youth who have lost peers or family members (CDC, 2005; Speier, 2005).

As time passes nurses should remain vigilant for children and families who have not returned to normal life patterns. Behaviors such as inability to carry out normal life tasks such as eating, working, or attending school; reliving the event; changes in school performance, outbursts, and isolation are important signs that the child should be referred for mental health services. Encourage families to communicate with school personnel and to bring concerns about the child's status to healthcare visits. Realize that parents need ongoing support in order to assist the child (Lieberman & Knorr, 2007).

PREPARING FOR DISASTERS

Pediatric nurses have a significant role in working with families in preparing for a disaster, and in preventing exposure to a disaster (e.g., evacuating for a hurricane). Nurses can help families use developmentally appropriate information to talk with their children about disaster planning and information about disasters when they occur. They can help the family develop a disaster plan. Families sheltering in the home must prepare to manage on their own for 72 hours, as it will take this long for governmental resources to reach the site of the disaster and get set up. This means the family should have a 3-day supply of nonperishable food and bottled water, flashlights and batteries, battery-powered radio, and over-the-counter medications, and many other resources. Formula, diapers, bottles, powdered milk, moist towelettes, diaper rash ointment should be available for infants and children. Refer to the Federal Emergency Management Web site for most current recommendations for family supplies to have on hand [www.Ready.gov/].

Advance planning is needed to ensure that children assisted by technology have the resources needed in the event of a disaster. The family should register with the designated shelter for such children in the community. In the meantime, battery packs for power backup should be fully charged at all times. Additionally, parents need to arrange for durable power of attorney so that consent for emergency medical care can be available as needed should the child and parents become separated.

ENVIRONMENTAL CONTAMINANTS

Contaminants are **toxins**, harmful or poisonous chemicals produced by metabolism or an organism (e.g., ricin), or **toxicants**, harmful natural or synthetic chemicals not metabolically produced by an organism (Belson, Schier, & Patel, 2005). These products are commonly produced during industrial manufacture, but could be released as a form of terrorism. Children are generally more vulnerable than adults to such exposures because of their developing bodies. They consume high amounts of food, water, and air per unit of body weight. Consequences to the neurological system are particularly important to developmental and behavioral outcomes (Graff, Murphy, Ekvall, et al., 2006).

Knowledge of environmental contaminants and their effects on children is limited. A U.S. federal initiative has formed the National Children's Study and Centers, co-sponsored by the National Institute for Environmental Health Sciences and the Environmental Protection Agency, to study health and safety risks to children (Kimmel, Collman, Fields, et al., 2005). It is important to examine what is known and to urge families to use some general cautions to minimize potential risks to children.

Contaminants in the environment can influence children in complex ways. Prenatal exposure can affect the developing fetus. Exposure during lactation may bring contaminants to the breastfed baby. Environmental effects may occur as the child grows through skin contact, inhalation, or food and water ingestion. Since children are exposed to many chemicals on a daily basis, harmful exposures are often difficult to identify. One example of a known harmful agent is environmental tobacco smoke (ETS). The mother who smokes or is exposed to ETS runs an increased risk of having a baby that is small for gestational age or who dies of sudden infant death syndrome (SIDS, Chapter 48∞). The child exposed to ETS has an increased risk of occurrence and severity of asthma and other respiratory diseases.

The children of migrant farm workers constitute a group that is at particular health risk. From 3–5 million persons live in families that travel to work in various locations during the year. Exact numbers are unknown and only estimates are available (Committee on Community Health Services, 2005; McCauley, Anger, Keifer, et al., 2006). There are many environmental health risks, including exposure to pesticides, unsanitary drinking water, overcrowding, insect exposure, equipment hazards, poor transportation, social isolation, and poverty. Children living in migrant farm worker families are more likely to have respiratory and ear infections, gastroenteritis, intestinal parasites, skin infections, unmet dental needs, poor nutrition and anemia, delayed development, and occupation injury (Committee on Community Services, 2005). Families travel frequently so provision of coordinated health care is difficult, leading to low immunization rates, and academic challenges. Adolescents may even travel alone, lacking supervision by parents or other adults.

Some potentially harmful environmental exposures across various settings include:

- Pesticides such as organophosphates, organochlorine, chlorpyrifos, dialkylphosphates, carbamates, pyrethroids; children may be exposed through home use, parents who work in pesticide manufacturing, garden/farm/agricultural use, and ingestion through food treated with pesticide
- Outdoor air pollution from automobiles, power plants, and other sources; children spend time outside and therefore have increased exposure
- Indoor air pollution from dust mites, molds, lead particles from old housing, wood smoke, and other sources
- Heavy metal exposure, including lead, mercury, arsenic, chlorine
- Substances such as polychlorinated biphenyls (PCBs) stored in fatty tissues of the mother and causing fetal exposure, or in animal fats; also present in electrical wiring (de Burbure, Buchet, Leroyer, et al., 2006; Meadows-Oliver, 2006).

Nursing Management

Nurses are instrumental in identifying exposure to environmental toxic agents. Inquire about:

- Parental work with harmful substances such as dust and chemicals
- Age of home (homes built before 1978 or renovated in the last 6 months are at risk for contamination with chemicals)
- Safety items in home such as radon, carbon monoxide, and smoke alarms
- Child and family member with hobby requiring use of toxic materials, such as lead with stained glass work, glue with model building
- Child's consumption of non-food products

Nurses in public health agencies often coordinate care for migrant farm workers. Evaluating living conditions and hazards through home visits is necessary. Provision of care and electronic and paper records can enhance care with distant sites where the family spends part of the year. Screening for health and developmental progression should be carried out whenever children are evaluated. In some northern U.S. communities, Head Start or other day care centers open additional facilities during summer months when migrant families need such care while adults work in fields.

For children in all settings, consider the possibility of environmental exposure and refer for blood testing and further evaluation whenever delayed development or behavioral problems are evident. Test blood levels for contaminants such as lead (see next section). Hair, urine, and other testing may be possible as well. Identification of the toxic exposure and its removal from the environment are critical. Removal from the body by drug treatment is possible for some substances. Instruct the family in prevention of further exposure. Perform periodic growth and developmental measurements on the child and ensure return for further blood tests and other monitoring (Moya, Bearer, & Etzel, 2004).

POISONING

Young children are at risk for ingestion of foreign substances because of their characteristic behaviors, which involve exploration of the environment. Poisonings are the second leading cause of unintentional home-injury death and account for nearly one-third of all unintentional home injuries (Home Safety Council, 2004). Over 4 million poisonings occur annually in the United States, with the majority of these in private residences (Bronstein, Spyker, Cantilena, et al., 2007). About 38% of poisonings occur in children under 3 years of age and 51% in children under 6 years (Bronstein et al., 2007; Madden, 2005). In 2006, there were over 100 poisoning fatalities of children in the United States (Bronstein et al., 2007).

Infants and toddlers commonly place objects in their mouths. Some household items are nontoxic and cause little harm; however, items that contain caustic agents or toxic chemicals can cause irreversible damage or death. The Poison Prevention Packaging Act of 1970 mandates child protective devices for all potentially toxic substances, such as household cleansers and medications. However, many are still ingested by children. Most common causes of pediatric poisonings include cosmetics and personal care products, cleaning agents, analgesics and other medications, foreign bodies, topical agents, and cough/cold preparations. Agents most commonly causing death are analgesics and psychotropic medications (Watson, Litovitz, Klein-Schwartz, et al. 2004). Poisoning ingestion among adolescents is most commonly associated with suicide attempts (Bronstein et al., 2007).

Many other items commonly found in the home are less obvious sources of toxins. The leaves, stems, or flowers of many common household and garden plants are poisonous. Examples include Boston ivy, poinsettia, philodendron, lily of the valley, daffodil (bulbs), azalea, and rhododendron. Nail care products, mothballs, weed and bug killers, and rodent killers are other potential poisons. Although most poisons are ingested, other routes of contamination include dermal, inhalation, and ocular.

Parents who suspect that their child has ingested a poison should immediately call the Poison Control Center (PCC). The PCC will advise parents about treatment to begin at home, and if the child needs treatment in the emergency department. If the child has vomited, the vomitus should be brought to the emergency department. With older children, the possibility of intentional ingestion needs to be considered.

See "Clinical Manifestations: Commonly Ingested Toxic Agents" on page 1186. Blood and urine toxicology screens, as well as arterial blood gas and electrolyte testing, are performed. Testing of vomitus for the presence of medication or other poisonings may be helpful in determining the amount ingested.

In the emergency department the child's airway, breathing, circulation, and level of consciousness are assessed (see Appendix G). Specific information about the poison is obtained from the parent to guide medical management. Table 44–9 summarizes emergency management for poisoning.

Evidence in Action

After numerous years of syrup of ipecac serving as a mainstay in home treatment of poisonings, the American Academy of Pediatrics recommended that "syrup of ipecac should no longer be used routinely as a poison treatment intervention in the home" (American Academy of Pediatrics, 2003). However, the drug is still present in many homes and is a cause of poisoning for some children. The nurse should inform families to avoid the use of ipecac and encourage disposal of ipecac kept in the home. The family should be instructed to pour the ipecac down the drain or toilet and to discard the empty bottle. Syrup of ipecac is also used as a drug of abuse in some cases of Münchhausen syndrome by proxy (Eldridge, Van Eyk, & Komegay, 2007).

NURSING MANAGEMENT

Nursing care focuses on initial emergent care and stabilization of the child with poisoning, followed by family education to reduce the risk of repeated poisoning.

NURSING ASSESSMENT AND DIAGNOSIS

Take a history from the family about the child's suspected ingestion substance, time, amount, and symptoms. Initial assessment focuses on airway, vital signs, and neurological status. Assess drooling, diaphoresis, and increased or depressed respirations. Assess for wheezing, respiratory distress, or stridor. Assess for decreased responsiveness and seizure activity. Assess heart rate, skin color, capillary refill, peripheral and central pulses, and blood pressure. Assess pupils (abnormally large or pinpoint pupils may be observed). Assess mouth, lips, and tongue for corrosive burns or edema. Assess breath for unusual odor. Assess the child for vomiting and diarrhea. Assess vomitus for presence of medication or other ingested substances. Determine the child's height and weight or use a length-based tape to determine medication dosages and equipment sizes.

Nursing diagnoses for the child with ingestion of a toxic substance may include:

- *Risk for Ineffective Airway Clearance* related to excessive secretion effect of toxic substance
- *Risk for Impaired Gas Exchange* related to depressed neurologic status
- *Risk for Aspiration* related to depressed neurological status and vomiting
- *Risk for Decreased Cardiac Output* related to effects of toxic substance
- *Risk for Injury* related to repeated occurrence of poisoning
- *Interrupted Family Processes* related to poisoning of a family member

Table 44–9 Emergency Management for Poisoning in a Medical Facility

1. Stabilize the child. Assess ABCs (airway, breathing, and circulation). Provide ventilatory support and supplemental oxygen.
2. Perform a rapid physical examination, start an IV infusion, draw blood for toxicology screen, and apply a cardiac monitor.
3. Obtain a history of the ingestion, including substance ingested, where child was found, by whom, position, when, how long unsupervised, history of depression or suicide, allergies, and any other medical problems.
4. Reverse or eliminate the toxic substance using the appropriate method:
   a. Antidotes and agonists
      - Mucomyst (for acetaminophen poisoning)
      - Digibind (for digoxin poisoning)
      - Narcan (for opioid overdose)
      - Romazicon (for benzodiazepine overdose)

   b. Gastric lavage
      - A gastric tube is inserted through the mouth; nasal insertion may be needed in some cases.
      - Normal saline solution is instilled and aspirated until the return is clear. This is considered a less effective method of removing ingested substances from the stomach than vomiting. It is reserved for children with central nervous system depression, diminished or absent gag reflex, or unwillingness to cooperate with other measures.
      - This method is contraindicated in children who have ingested alkaline corrosive substances, as insertion of the tube may cause esophageal perforation.
      - Used in children who have ingested acids to decrease continued damage and potential perforation of the stomach and intestines.

   c. Activated charcoal
      - Given to absorb and remove any remaining particles of toxic substances.
      - Usual dosage administration is 1 g/kg of body weight.
      - A commercial preparation of activated charcoal is administered orally or through a gastric tube.
      - Available as a ready-to-drink solution in an opaque container.
      - May be mixed with apple juice or soda if protocol allows to encourage consumption.
      - Use a covered cup and straw when giving orally to prevent the child from seeing the black liquid and to minimize spillage.
      - Administer activated charcoal only after the child has stopped vomiting, because aspiration of charcoal is damaging to lung tissue.
      - Should not be administered for ingestion of caustic substances or hydrocarbons.

   d. Cathartics
      - Hastens excretion of a toxic substance and minimizes absorption. The most commonly used cathartic is magnesium sulfate.
5. Perform other measures depending on the child's condition, the nature of the ingested substance, and the time since ingestion. They may include diuresis, fluid loading, cooling or warming measures, anticonvulsive measures, antiarrhythmic therapy, hemodialysis, or exchange transfusions.
6. Constantly evaluate the child's total condition to maintain airway, breathing, and circulation. Therapeutic management is adjusted as needed to treat the evolving condition.
7. Consider the family's emotional status. Provide information about the child, involve them in care when possible, and arrange for support persons and services to be available to them.

PLANNING AND IMPLEMENTATION

Emergency care focuses on airway and hemodynamic stability, removal of toxic agents, and support of the family. See Table 44–9 for a summary of emergency management for poisoning.

Once immediate care has been provided, nursing care shifts to providing emotional support and preventing recurrence.

PROVIDE EMOTIONAL SUPPORT

Wait until the child is out of immediate danger before questioning parents in detail about the incident. Encourage parents to express feelings of anger, guilt, or fear about the incident.

PREVENT RECURRENCE

Discuss with parents the need to supervise infants and young children at all times. Ask parents how medicines and cleaning agents are stored and whether the house contains any plants. Teach parents proper methods of childproofing the home. Have the PCC number readily available. Suggest measures for preventing recurrence of poisoning. (See "Teaching Highlights: Avoiding Childhood Poisoning.")

The toll-free number for the American Association of Poison Control Centers (AAPCC) is 1-800-222-1222. The number can be accessed from anywhere in the United States and Puerto Rico, and the caller will be connected to the nearest poison control center.

EVALUATION

Expected outcomes for nursing care of the child with poisoning include:

- The child maintains an open airway, effective gas exchange, and ventilatory function.
- The child is free from wheezing, coughing, pneumonia, or other signs indicating aspiration.
- The child's heart rate and blood pressure remain stable and appropriate for age.
- Neurological status is appropriate for age.
- The family and child (if older) verbalize understanding of preventive measures and demonstrate measures to improve home environment safety.

Clinical Manifestations

COMMONLY INGESTED TOXIC AGENTS

TYPE	SOURCES	CLINICAL MANIFESTATIONS	CLINICAL THERAPY
Corrosives (strong acids and alkaline products that cause chemical burns of mucosal surfaces)	Batteries Household cleaners Clinitest tablets Denture cleaners Bleach Toilet bowl cleaners	Severe burning pain in mouth, throat, or stomach Swelling of mucous membranes; edema of lips, tongue, and pharynx (respiratory obstruction) Violent vomiting; hemoptysis Drooling; inability to clear secretions Signs of shock Anxiety Agitation	Do not induce vomiting! Dilute toxin with water to prevent further damage Give activated charcoal
Hydrocarbons (organic compounds that contain carbon and hydrogen; most are distillates of petroleum)	Gasoline Kerosene Furniture polish Lighter fluid Paint thinners	Gagging Choking Coughing Nausea Vomiting Alteration in sensorium (lethargy) Weakness Respiratory symptoms of pulmonary involvement, tachypnea, cyanosis, retractions, grunting	Do not induce vomiting! (Aspiration of hydrocarbons places child at high risk for pneumonia.) Use gastric lavage if severe central nervous system and respiratory impairment are present Use of activated charcoal is controversial Provide supportive care Decontaminate skin by removing clothing and cleansing skin
Acetaminophen	Many over-the-counter products	Nausea Vomiting Sweating Pallor Hepatic involvement (pain in upper right quadrant, jaundice, confusion, stupor, coagulation abnormalities)	Induce vomiting or perform gastric lavage, depending on amount ingested Administer charcoal or NAC (concentrated form of Mucomyst), which binds with the metabolite, preventing absorption and protecting the liver
Salicylate	Products containing aspirin	Nausea Disorientation Vomiting Dehydration Diaphoresis Hyperpnea Hyperpyrexia Bleeding tendencies Oliguria Tinnitus Convulsions Coma	Depends on amount ingested Induce vomiting Administer intravenous sodium bicarbonate, fluids, and vitamin K
Mercury	Broken thermometers Chemicals Paints Pesticides Fungicides	Tremors Memory loss Insomnia Weight loss Diarrhea Anorexia Gingivitis	Similar to that for lead poisoning (see text discussion)
Iron	Multiple vitamin supplements and therapeutic iron tablets	Vomiting Hematemesis Diarrhea Bloody stools Abdominal pain Metabolic acidosis Shock Seizures Coma	Induce vomiting Administer intravenous fluids and sodium bicarbonate Deferoxamine chelation therapy

Teaching Highlights

AVOIDING CHILDHOOD POISONING

Families with children require instructions for avoiding childhood poisoning. Teach family members these interventions to help avoid childhood poisonings:

- Place household cleaners, medications, vitamins, and other potentially poisonous substances out of the reach of children or in locked cabinets.
- Use warning stickers such as Mr. Yuk on all containers.
- Buy products with child-resistant caps.
- Store products in their original containers.
- Never place household cleansers or other products in food or beverage containers.
- Remove all houseplants from the child's play areas.
- Put the Poison Control Center phone number by every phone in the house.
- Use caution when visiting other settings that are not childproofed (e.g., grandparents' homes). Remember that visitors may have pills in their purses or pockets that are easily reached by children.

INGESTION OF FOREIGN OBJECTS

There are about 100,000 cases of ingestion of foreign objects annually in the United States, and approximately 80% of cases of ingestion of foreign objects occur in childhood. The majority of cases present in children between 6 and 36 months of age (Kay & Wyllie, 2005). The most common objects ingested are coins, accounting for 27–70% of cases. Pins, parts of toys, batteries, and bones from foods are some other commonly ingested objects. Adults often witness infants and young children ingesting foreign bodies, and older children will usually report swallowing a foreign object. Most small, round, smooth objects may not cause any clinical distress. However, if the foreign body is lodged in the esophagus, children may present with substernal pain, drooling, and dysphagia. Some children may exhibit respiratory symptoms including wheezing or coughing.

Serious complications can occur following foreign body ingestion. These complications include perforation of the intestinal tract, the most serious sequelae of foreign body ingestion. Sharp objects are associated with a higher perforation rate than dull objects. Approximately 75% of perforations occur in the region of the ileocecal valve. Development of strictures at the site of a retained foreign body may also occur. Respiratory complications arise if the object becomes lodged in the trachea, bronchi, or lungs. See Chapter 48 for care of the child with a foreign body airway obstruction.

Since approximately 60–90% of foreign bodies ingested in children are radio-opaque (Kay & Wyllie, 2005), radiographs of the neck, chest, esophagus, and abdomen are useful tools in verifying ingestion and to identify the location of the object. Endoscopic examination and retrieval of the ingested foreign body may be necessary. Approximately 5–10% of children will have the foreign body lodged in the oropharynx, 20% of foreign bodies will be located in the esophagus, 60% will be located in the stomach, and 10% will be located distal to the stomach, usually in the small intestine (Kay & Wyllie, 2005).

Most (80–90%) foreign bodies pass spontaneously through the gastrointestinal system and are eliminated through stool. However, foreign bodies may become lodged in the esophagus and pose a significant risk to the child. Smooth, small, round objects that have passed into the stomach are generally allowed to pass through the bowel without intervention. Esophageal foreign bodies are removed or advanced into the stomach due to the risk for mucosal erosion and catastrophic perforation (Uyemura, 2006). Potentially harmful objects such as batteries, sharp objects, and magnets are removed surgically.

Nursing Management

Nursing care centers on supporting the child, collaborative assistance in the identification and removal of the foreign body, and teaching the child and family measures to reduce reoccurrence. Assess the child for drooling, wheezing, substernal pain, dysphagia, and coughing. Obtain a thorough history from family. Determine, if possible, what was ingested, when the ingestion occurred, and any symptoms that the child experienced. Assess breath sounds.

Prepare the child for radiologic studies. Explain the procedures and reassure the child and family during the studies. Prepare for endoscopic examination and/or retrieval, if necessary. If the foreign object is in the stomach and the child is to be observed for natural excretion of the object, explain monitoring of stools to parents. Suggest the use of tongue blades to examine stools for presence of the foreign body and to report if the object has not been passed within the expected time frame (generally 48 hours). Encourage the family to return for further radiologic examinations to determine the foreign object's progress of passage.

Partner with the family and assist them in establishing a safe home environment for the child. Encourage the family to keep all small items out of the child's reach and to ensure the child is monitored at all times. Expected outcomes for nursing care of the child with ingested foreign body include removal of the foreign body, reduction in risk, and family verbalization of preventative measures to reduce risk of ingestion of foreign bodies.

LEAD POISONING

Lead poisoning has been successfully prevented in many areas of the United States, with a substantial decline in lead levels from the mid-1970s. The average serum lead level for children is now 0.6 micrograms/dL, down from 15 micrograms/dL in 1976. About 2.2% of children (434,000) from 1 to 5 years have levels above the recommended upper level of 10 micrograms/dL. Many of these children are poor and live in older houses in inner cities with dust and paint exposure (Whitehead & Leiker, 2007). Even children with levels below 10 micrograms/dL may experience cognitive defects due to lead exposure since there is no known safe level (Advisory Committee on Childhood Lead Poisoning Prevention, 2007; Bellinger, 2004). Lead in paint is the most common source of lead exposure for preschool children. Children are also exposed to lead when they ingest contaminated food, water, and soil or when they inhale dust contaminated with lead. Paints on toys and crafts from some foreign countries may contain lead; unless such products are certified safe they should not be used by children.

Children are at greater risk for lead poisoning because they absorb and retain more lead in proportion to their weight than adults do. Lead is particularly harmful to children under the age of 7 years.

Lead interferes with normal cell function, primarily of the nervous system, blood cells, and kidneys, and adversely affects the metabolism of vitamin D and calcium. Clinical manifestations depend on the degree of toxicity. Neurologic effects include decreased IQ scores, cognitive deficits, impaired hearing, and growth delays. Impaired mental function can occur with blood levels even lower than 10 micrograms/dL. Lead ingestion by a woman during pregnancy can result in fetal malformations, reduced birth weight, and premature birth. Severe lead poisoning, which can result in encephalopathy, coma, and death, is now rare.

Once in the body, lead accumulates in the blood, soft tissues (kidney, bone marrow, liver, and brain), bones, and teeth. Lead that is absorbed by the bones and teeth is released slowly; thus, exposure to even small doses, over time, can result in dangerously high levels of lead in the body. See "Clinical Manifestations: Lead Poisoning" below.

The Centers for Disease Control and Prevention now recommend screening children enrolled in Medicaid and those at risk for elevated lead levels. Screening occurs at 12 and 24 months, as well as for children in these groups who are 36–72 months but not previously screened. Follow-up at 1 and 2 years of age is recommended since children are then walking and may have exposure to reaching other sources of lead in the home. Some local health departments recommend more frequent screening due to the risk in the area (Advisory Committee on Childhood Lead Poisoning Prevention, 2007; Woolf, Goldman, & Bellinger, 2007). A blood lead (Pb-B) level is the most useful screening and diagnostic test for lead exposure.

A Pb-B below 10 micrograms/dL is considered acceptable, although it may still not screen out all children with impaired development due to lead. An environmental history should be obtained for children with Pb-B levels between 10 and 19 micrograms/dL to identify removable sources of lead. Follow-up testing is required. Children with Pb-B levels between 20 and 69 micrograms/dL require a full medical evaluation, including a detailed environmental and behavioral history, physical examination, and tests for iron deficiency. Interventions to remove sources of lead from the child's environment are necessary. For levels above 45 micrograms/dL, chelation therapy is considered for administration. Children with Pb-B levels greater than 70 micrograms/dL are critically ill from lead poisoning and require immediate chelation therapy and interventions to provide a lead-free environment.

Chelation is a reaction in which an organic compound, containing carbonyl (CO) and hydroxyl (OH) groups, coordinates with a metal to form a firmly bound ring-like structure. Chelation therapy for lead poisoning involves the administration of an agent that binds with lead, decreasing its effects and increasing its rate of excretion from the body. Calcium disodium ethylenediamine tetraacetate ($CaNa_2$ EDTA) IM or IV, dimercaprol (BAL) deep IM, d-penicillamine PO, or succimer (DMSA) PO may be used. Children with Pb-B levels between 25 and 69 micrograms/dL receive $CaNa_2$ EDTA for 5 to 7 days, followed by a rest period and then a second chelation treatment. Children with Pb-B levels greater than 70 micrograms/dL are given both BAL and $CaNa_2$ EDTA, followed by a rest period and a second chelation treatment using $CaNa_2$ EDTA alone. Chelation therapy has

Clinical Manifestations

LEAD POISONING

Class I (less than 9 micrograms/dL)	Generally asymptomatic although subtle neurological effects may be present with any exposure
Class IIA (10–14 micrograms/dL) and IIB (15–19 micrograms/dL)	Mild impairment in growth, fine motor skills, and cognition Anemia
Class III (20–44 micrograms/dL)	General fatigue and motor impairment Difficulty concentrating Paresis or paralysis, tremor Headache Diffuse abdominal pain, vomiting, weight loss, constipation Anemia
Class IV (45–69 micrograms/dL)	Colic (intermittent, severe abdominal cramps), anorexia, vomiting Hyperirritability Increased lethargy Lead line (blue-black) on gingival tissue
Class V (over 70 micrograms/dL)	Encephalopathy, which may lead abruptly to seizures, changes in consciousness, coma, and death Ataxia

Adapted from Agency for Toxic Substances & Disease Registry (2006). *Lead toxicity clinical evaluation*. Atlanta: Author.

the potential for serious side effects. $CaNa_2$ EDTA can cause tubular necrosis and cardiac arrhythmia; IM administration is painful. BAL can lead to hypertension, tachycardia, headache, fever, or nephrotoxicity. Penicillamine is used only when treatment with other drugs is not effective due to multisystem side effects. Succimer is associated with GI side effects, rash, headache, and neurologic symptoms. Long-term follow-up of children receiving chelation therapy is essential. The child should never be discharged unless a lead-free home environment has been ensured.

Nursing Management

Nursing care centers on screening, education, and follow-up. Nurses often work with state and local health officials to plan screening for children at high risk of lead exposure. Ask parents about the child's development and eating habits and be alert for risk of lead exposure. Educate parents about sources of lead in the environment and techniques to reduce exposure. Make home visits to evaluate exposure to lead and to perform individualized teaching (Whitehead & Leiker, 2007). Emphasize the importance of housekeeping interventions to reduce exposure to lead dust. These interventions include damp mopping of hard surfaces, floors, window sills, and baseboards; washing the child's hands and face before meals; and frequent washing of toys and pacifiers. Be alert that home renovation can significantly increase the levels of lead in dust.

Teach parents the importance of including foods high in iron and calcium in the child's diet to counteract losses of these minerals associated with lead exposure. The child should eat meals at regular intervals, as lead is absorbed more readily on an empty stomach.

Be sure that parents understand the importance of follow-up testing of lead levels. If the child is developmentally delayed, refer the family to an infant stimulation or early intervention program. Referral to social services and either a visiting nurse or home healthcare nurse may also be appropriate.

> **Evidence in Action**
>
> Na_2 EDTA is *not* the same as $CaNa_2$ EDTA. Na_2 EDTA should never be administered for child lead poisoning treatment because it can lead to hypocalcemia and cardiac arrest (Brown, Willis, Omalu, et al., 2006; MMWR, 2006d). Nurses must double-check labels and have another licensed care provider verify that the correct drug is being used.

Nurses who administer chelating drugs are challenged by the complexity of treatment and required care. Chelation should always be managed by experts in such care, and in consultation with the Lead Poisoning Prevention Branch of the National Center for Environmental Health of the Centers for Disease Control and Prevention. (See Evidence in Action.) Careful monitoring of liver and kidney function, cardiac, GI, and neurologic systems are needed for all chelating drugs. Administration for some drugs is via IM route and is painful; children will need skilled nursing and child life specialist care.

Expected outcomes of nursing care for the child with lead or other poisoning include the following:

- The child exhibits normal growth and development, including cognition.
- Adequate nutritional intake is ensured for the child.
- Lead or other poisons are removed from the child's environment.
- The family expresses understanding of measures to establish a safe environment for the child.

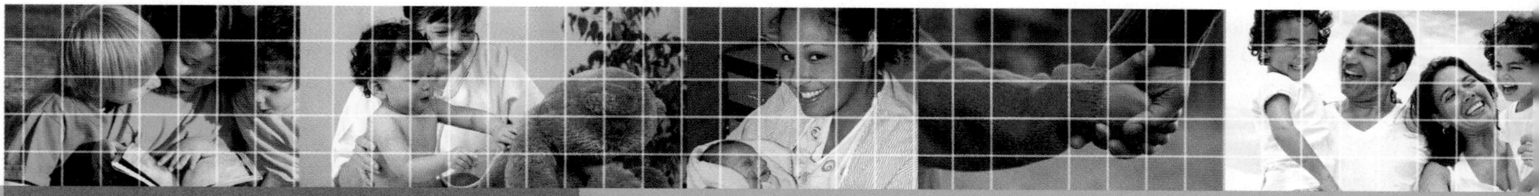

CRITICAL CONCEPT REVIEW

LEARNING OUTCOMES	CONCEPTS
44.1 Identify major social and environmental factors that influence the health of children and adolescents.	1. Present-day lifestyles: ■ Availability of firearms. ■ Availability of alcohol. 2. Importance of "fitting in" with a group. 3. Need for two incomes in the household. 4. Early sexual involvement.
44.2 List external influences that influence child and adolescent health.	1. Poverty. 2. Homelessness. 3. Stress. 4. Family structure. 5. School and child care. 6. Community. 7. Culture.

(continued)

LEARNING OUTCOMES	CONCEPTS
44.3 Apply the ecological model and resiliency theory to assessment of the social and environmental factors in children's lives.	1. The theory of ecologic development provides a framework to use in assessing the interactions of children with the environment. 2. The theory of resilience examines risk and protective factors of children in order to formulate interventions to assist the child dealing with health problems.
44.4 Examine the effects of substance use, physical activity, and other lifestyle patterns on health.	1. Children and adolescents are more vulnerable to addiction and negative effects due to developing cognition, organ, and body systems. 2. Increased use of computers, televisions, and video games has led to decreased physical activity, which may contribute to obesity. 3. Body art and piercing may lead to a variety of health concerns. 4. Concerns over sexual orientation are normal during adolescence. Homosexual orientation may sometimes be associated with higher rates of rejection by family, abuse and harassment, suicide, and sexually transmitted diseases.
44.5 Plan nursing interventions for children who experience violence.	1. Assist family in dealing with issues such as mental status challenges, fatigue, financial concerns, and substance abuse. 2. Instruct family in methods to help child feel safe. 3. Assess child's behaviors. 4. Evaluate social interactions and trust in others. 5. Assist child in identifying feelings and coping strategies by providing counseling and other therapies.
44.6 Evaluate the environment for hazards to children, such as exposure to substances and potential for poisoning.	1. Disasters require preparation plans, emergency response, assessment of unique child risks due to developmental stage, and psychologic support of those involved. 2. Contaminants in the environment necessitate assessment for toxins, understanding of poisons and their emergency management and ongoing treatment, application of safety precautions for lead poisoning, and measures to avoid ingestion of objects.
44.7 Explore the nursing role in prevention and treatment of child abuse and neglect, and other forms of violence.	1. All nurses have the responsibility to report suspected abuse and neglect. 2. Teach children that no one has the right to touch and feel certain places in the body. 3. Teach children the importance of reporting any incidence of abuse. 4. Assist in the interview and examination of the abused child. 5. Help to remove the child from the abusive environment, prevent further injury, and ensure that supportive care and counseling are provided.
44.8 Plan nursing interventions for children related to social and environmental situations.	1. Assess the child and the social settings and environment for risk and protective factors. 2. Understand and apply risks for behaviors of youth at various developmental stages (e.g., ingestion of poisons for young children and exposure to tobacco and other substances for adolescents). 3. Perform teaching to prevent social and environmental risk. Intervene when children and adolescents are in health situations caused by social and environmental issues. 4. Become familiar with community resources, refer youth and families as needed, and coordinate care among resources.

CRITICAL THINKING IN ACTION

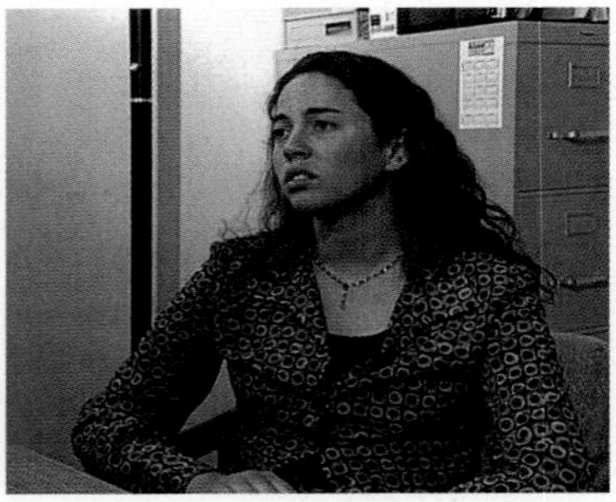

You are working at the inpatient adolescent psychiatric unit where there are approximately 20 teens between the ages of 12 and 17 years old. The teens are admitted for several different diagnoses, including depression, suicide attempts, bipolar disorders, and eating disorders. The nurses are in charge of medication administration, vital signs, unit safety issues, physical assessments, and basic therapeutic interventions. You are working with a client named Cindy, 15 years old, who was admitted due to a suicide attempt and has been given a dual diagnosis of bulimia nervosa and depression. She has had extreme weight loss and gain over the past year and is currently 67 inches tall and weighs 140 pounds. She has stated she tried to commit suicide with a knife because she was upset over the loss of her boyfriend. She thought she was fat and was trying to lose weight by using laxatives and vomiting after meals. There is a family history of depression and substance abuse, but Cindy denies any substance use. She lives with her mother and has no contact with her father. She does not feel she has anyone to discuss her feelings with and states her mother is gone from the house frequently. Cindy admits to often eating fast food and snacking on other junk food and soda. She has been in the hospital for 2 weeks and was resistant to treatment at first, but seems to be improving with therapy and medication. She has lost 3 pounds while she has been hospitalized and her vital signs are usually: temperature 98.7°F, pulse 70, respirations 12, and blood pressure 110/70. (Review the content on bulimia in Chapter 34 to answer the following questions.)

1. What are some of the signs of bulimia Cindy may exhibit?
2. What can you tell the mother about Cindy's vital signs and stability at this time? How can you explain the weight loss?
3. What behavioral signs of bulimia should be part of your nursing assessment of Cindy while she was hospitalized?
4. What are the treatment recommendations for Cindy?

See MyNursingKit for possible responses.

REFERENCES

ADD Health Study (2005). ADD Health. The National Longitudinal Study of Adolescent Health. Retrieved September 26, 2007, from www.cpc.unc.edu/addhealth

Adshead, G., & Bluglass, K. (2005). Attachment representations in mothers with abnormal illness behavior by proxy. *British Journal of Psychiatry, 187*, 328–333.

Advisory Committee on Childhood Lead Poisoning Prevention (2007). Interpreting and managing blood lead levels <10 μg/dL in children and reducing childhood exposures to lead. *Morbidity and Mortality Weekly Report, 56*(RR08), 1–14, 16.

Aguirre, B., & Smith, B. D. (2007). Handling young patients who cut themselves. *The Clinical Advisor*. August, 64–69.

American Academy of Child and Adolescent Psychiatry. (2005). Practice parameter for the assessment and treatment of children and adolescents with substance use disorders. *Journal of the American Academy of Child and Adolescent Psychiatry, 44*, 609–621.

American Academy of Pediatrics. (2003). *Poison treatment in the home*. Retrieved August 22, 2006, from www.dap.org/policy/s0/0120.html

Amos, A., & Bostock, Y. (2006). Young people, smoking and gender – a qualitative exploration. *Health Education Research*, doi:10.1093/her/cy075

Annie E. Casey Foundation (2007). *Kids Count 2007*. Retrieved September 20, 2007, from www.aecf.org/kidscount.org/sld/databook.jsp

Armstrong, M. L. (2005). Tattooing, body piercing, and permanent cosmetics: A historical and current view of state regulations, with continuing concerns. *Journal of Environmental Health, 68*(8), 38–45.

Aronowitz, T. (2005). The role of "envisioning the future" in the development of resilience among at-risk youth. *Public Health Nursing, 22*, 200–208.

Arria, A. M., & Wish, E. D. (2006). Nonmedical use of prescription stimulants among students. *Pediatric Annals 35*, 565–571.

Backinger, C. L., Michaels, C. M., Jefferson, A. M., Fagan, P., Hurd, A. L., & Grana, R. (2007). Factors associated with recruitment and retention of youth into smoking cessation intervention studies: A review of the literature. *Health Education Research, 19*, doi:10.1093/her/cym053

Bauer, N. S., Herrenkohl, T. I., Lozano, P. L., Rivara, F. P., Hill, K. G., & Hawkins, J. D. (2006). Childhood bullying involvement and exposure to intimate partner violence. *Pediatrics, 118*, 235–242.

Baxley, F., & Miller, M. (2006). Parental misperceptions about children and firearms. *Archives of Pediatric and Adolescent Medicine, 160*, 542–547.

Bayer, C. P., Klasen, F., & Adam, H. (2007). Association of trauma and PTSD symptoms with openness to reconciliation and feelings of revenge among former Ugandan and Congolese child soldiers. *JAMA, 298*, 555–559.

Bellinger, D. C. (2004). Lead. *Pediatrics, 113*(Suppl), 1016–1022.

Belson, M. G., Schier, J. G., & Patel, M. M. (2005). Case definitions for chemical poisoning. *Morbidity and Mortality Reports, 54*(RR-1), 1–24.

Bolton, P., Bass, J., Betancourt, T., Speelman, L., Onyango, G., Clougherty, K., et al. (2007). Interventions for depression symptoms among adolescent survivors of war and displacement in Northern Uganda: A randomized control trial. *JAMA, 298*, 519–527.

Brodowski, M. L., Nolan, C. M., Gaudiosi, J. A., Yuan, Y. Y., Zikratova, L., Oritz, M. J., et al. (2008). Nonfatal maltreatment of infants – United States, October 2005–September 2006. *Morbidity and Mortality Weekly Report, 57*, 336–339.

Bronfenbrenner, U. (2005). *Making human being human: Bioecologic perspectives*. Thousand Oaks, CA: Sage.

Bronstein, A. C., Spyker, D. A., Cantilena, L. R., Green, J., Rumack, B. H., Heard, S. E. (2007). 2006 annual report of the American Association of Poison Control Centers' National Poisoning Data System. *Clinical Toxicology, 45*, 815–917.

Brown, M. J., Willis, T., Omalu, B., & Leiker, R. (2006). Deaths resulting from hypocalcemia after administration of edentate disodium: 2003–2005. *Pediatrics, 118*, e534–536.

Brunstein, K. A., Marrocco, F., Kleinman, M., Schonfeld, I. S., & Gould, M. S. (2007). Bullying, depression, and suicidality in adolescents. *Journal of the American Academy of Child and Adolescent Psychiatry, 46*, 40–49.

Campo, S., Poulos, G., & Sipple, J. W. (2005). Prevalence and profiling: Hazing among college students and points of intervention. *American Journal of Health Behavior, 29*, 137–149.

Casanueva, C. E., & Martin, S. L. (2007). Intimate partner violence during pregnancy and mother's child abuse potential. *Journal of Interpersonal Violence, 22*, 603–622.

Centers for Disease Control and Prevention. (2005). Maintaining a healthy state of mind for parents and caregivers. Retrieved from http://www.redcross.org

Chartrand, M. M., & Siegel, B. (2007). At war in Iraq and Afghanistan: Children in US military families. *Ambulatory Pediatrics, 7*, 1–2.

Chernin, A. R., & Linebarger, D. L. (2005). The relationship between children's television viewing and academic performance. *Archives of Pediatrics & Adolescent Medicine, 159*, 687–689.

Childhelp. (2005). *National child abuse statistics*. Scottsdale, AZ: Author.

Children's Defense Fund. (2008). *Data each day in America*. Retrieved October 20, 2008, from www.childrensdefense.org/site/pageServer?pagename=research_national_data_each_day

Collins, B. N., Wileyto, E. P., Murphy, J. F., & Munafo, M. R. (2007). Adolescent environmental tobacco smoke exposure predicts academic achievement test failure. *Journal of Adolescent Health, 41*, 363–370.

Committee on Community Health Services (2005). Providing care for immigrant, homeless, and migrant children. *Pediatrics, 115*, 1095–1100.

Cyr, A. M. (2007). What is Münchhausen syndrome by proxy? *Nursing, 37*, 30.

Darbyshire, P., Muir-Cochrane, E., Fereday, J., Jureidini, J., & Drummond, A. (2006). Engagement with health and social care services: Perceptions of homeless young people with mental health problems. *Health and Social Care in the Community, 14*, 553–562.

De Burbure, C., Buchet, J. P., Leroyer, A., Nisse, C., Haguenoer, J. M. Smerhovsky, et al. (2006). Renal and neurologic effects of cadmium, lead, mercury, and arsenic in children: Evidence of early effects and multiple interactions at the environmental exposure level. *Environmental Health Perspectives, 114*, 584–590.

DeForge, V., Zehnder, S., Minick, P., & Carmon, M. (2001). Children's perspectives of homelessness. *Pediatric Nursing 27*, 377–383.

Dixon, A., Howie, P., & Starling, J. (2005). Psychopathology of female juvenile offenders. *Journal of Child Psychology and Psychiatry 45*, 1150–1158.

Eldridge, D. L., Van Eyk, J., & Komegay, C. (2007). Pediatric toxicology. *Emergency Medical Clinics of North America 25*, 283–308.

Elkind, D. (2007). *The hurried child: 25th anniversary edition*. Cambridge, MA: Da Capo Lifelong Publishing.

Etzel, R. A. (2004). Environmental risks in childhood. *Pediatric Annals, 33*, 431–436.

Federal Interagency Forum on Child and Family Statistics. (2007). *American's children: Key national indicators of well-being 2007*. Washington, DC: U.S. Government Printing Office.

Fekkes, M., Pijpers, F. I., & Verloove-Vanhorick, S. P. (2006). Effects of antibullying school program on bullying and health complaints. *Archives of Pediatric and Adolescent Medicine, 160*, 638–644.

Gold, M. A., Schorzman, C. M., Murray, P. J., Downs, J., & Tolentino, G. (2005). Body piercing practices and attitudes among urban adolescents. *Journal of Adolescent Health, 36*, 352, e17–e24.

Graff, J. C., Murphy, L., Ekvall, S., & Gagnon, M. (2006). In-home toxic chemical exposures and children with intellectual and development disabilities. *Pediatric Nursing, 32*, 596–603.

Henderson, N., Bernard, B., & Sharp-Light, N. (2007). *Resiliency in action*. Ojai, CA: Resiliency in Action, Inc.

Home Safety Council. (2004). Retrieved July 4, 2004, from hwww.homesafetycouncil. org/resource_center/resourcecenter.aspx

HRSA. (2007). *The national bullying prevention campaign*. Washington, DC: Author.

Hymel, K. P., & Hall, C. A. (2005). Diagnosing pediatric head trauma. *Pediatric Annals, 34*, 358–370.

Inglehart, J. K. (2007). Insuring all children – the new political imperative. *New England Journal of Medicine, 357*, 70–76.

Jannone, L., & O'Connell, K. A. (2007). Coping strategies used by adolescents during smoking cessation. *Journal of School Nursing 23*, 177–184.

Johnson, C. F. (2006). Sexual abuse in children. *Pediatrics in Review, 27*, 17–26.

Kay, M., & Wyllie, R. (2005). Pediatric foreign bodies and their management. *Current Gastroenterology Reports, 7*, 212–218.

Kellogg, N. D., & the Committee on Child Abuse and Neglect (2007). Evaluation of suspected child physical abuse. *Pediatrics, 119*, 1232–1241.

Kidd, S. A., & Davidson, L. (2006). Youth homelessness: A call for partnerships between research and policy. *Canadian Journal of Public Health, 97*, 445–447.

Kimmel, C. A., Collman, G. W., Fields, N., & Eskenazi, B. (2005). Lessons learned for the National Children's Study from the National Institute of Environmental Health Sciences/U.S. Environmental Protection Agency Centers for children's environmental health and disease prevention research. *Environmental Health Perspectives, 113*, 1414–1418.

Kolar, K. R., & Davey, D. (2007). Silent victims: Children exposed to family violence. *Journal of School Nursing, 23*, 86–91.

Kreider, R. M., & Fields, J. (2005). Living arrangements of children: 2001. *Current Population Reports, 27-104*, Washington, DC: U.S. Census Bureau.

Kuttner, L., Chambers, C. T., Hardial, J., Israel, D. M., Jacobsen, K. & Evans, K. (2006). A randomized trial of yoga for adolescents with irritable bowel syndrome. *Pain Research and Management, 11*, 217–123.

Larzo, M. R., & Poe, S. G. (2006). Adverse consequences of tattoos and body piercings. *Pediatric Annals, 35*, 187–192.

Leman, S. K., & Plattner, M. (2007). When beautification of the body turns ugly. *The Clinical Advisor February*, 27–33.

Lieberman, A. F., & Knorr, K. (2007). The impact of trauma: A developmental framework for infancy and early childhood. *Pediatric Annals, 36*, 209–215.

Liu, J., Peterson, A. V., Kealey, K. A., Mann, S. L., Bricker, J. B., & Marek, P. M. (2007). Addressing challenges in adolescent smoking cessation: Design and baseline characteristics of the HS group-randomized trial. *Preventive Medicine, 45*, 215–225.

Loveland-Cherry, C. J. (2006). Alcohol, children and adolescents. In J. J. Fitzpatrick (Ed.), *Alcohol use, misuse, abuse, and dependence* (pp. 135–177). New York: Springer.

Madden, M. A. (2005). Pediatric poisonings: Recognition, assessment, and management. *Critical Care Nursing Clinics of North America 17*, 395–404.

McCauley, L. A., Anger, W. K., Keifer, M., Langley, R., Robson, M. G., Rohlman, D. (2006). Studying health outcomes in farmworker populations exposed to pesticides. *Environmental Health Perspectives, 114*, 953–960.

McColgan, M. D., & Giardino, A. P. (2005). Internet poses multiple risks to children and adolescents. *Pediatric Annals, 34*, 405–414.

Meadows-Oliver, M. (2006). Environmental toxins. *Journal of Pediatric Health Care, 20*, 350–352.

Meckler, G. D., Elliot, M. N., Kanouse, D. E., Beals, K., Schuster, M. A. (2006). Nondisclosure of sexual orientation to a physician among a sample of gay, lesbian, and bisexual youth. *Archives of Pediatrics and Adolescent Medicine, 160*, 1248–1254.

MMWR. (2004). Youth risk behavior surveillance—United States, 2003. *Morbidity and Mortality Weekly Report, 53* (SS-2), 1–95.

MMWR. (2006a). Cigarette use among high school students—United States, 1991–2005. *Morbidity and Mortality Weekly Report, 55*, 724–726.

MMWR. (2006b). Use of cigarettes and other tobacco products among students aged 13–15 years—worldwide, 1999–2005. *Morbidity and Mortality Weekly Report, 55*, 553–556.

MMWR. (2006c). Youth risk behavior surveillance—United States, 2005. *Morbidity and Mortality Weekly Report, 55*(SS05), 1–108.

MMWR. (2006d). Deaths associated with hypocalcemia from chelation therapy—Texas, Pennsylvania, and Oregon, 2003–2005. *Morbidity and Mortality Weekly Report, 55*(08), 2004–2007.

Morris, R. I., & Strong, L. (2004). The impact of homelessness on the health of families. *Journal of School Nursing, 20*, 221–227.

Moya, J., Bearer, C. F., & Etzel, R. A. (2004). Children's behavior and physiology and how it affects exposure to environmental contaminants. *Pediatrics, 113*, 996–1006.

Mullin, K. A., & Ambrosia, T. (2005). Role of the nurse practitioner in providing health care for the homeless. *American Journal for Nurse Practitioners, 9*(9), 37–44.

National Association for the Education of Young Children (2007). Introduction to the NAEYC early childhood program standards and accreditation criteria; Program standards. Retrieved September 20, 2007, from www.naeyc.org/academy/IntroNewCriteria.asp

National Institute of Child Health & Human Development (2007). Add Health Study. Retrieved September 25, 2007, from www.nichd.nih.gov/health/topics/add_health_study.cfm?renderforprint=1

National Institute on Alcohol Abuse and Alcoholism (NIAAA). (2005). The effects of alcohol on physiological processes and biological development. *Alcohol Research and Health, 28*, 125–132.

National Safe Kids (2007). *Injury facts*. Retrieved September 26, 2007, from http://usa.safekids.org

Reardon, J. Z. (2007). Environmental tobacco smoke: Respiratory and other health effects. *Clinical Chest Medicine, 28*, 559–573.

Remafedi, G. (2006). Adolescent homosexuality. *Archives of Pediatrics and Adolescent Medicine, 160*, 1303–1304.

Rentz, E. D., Marshall, S. W., Loomis, D., Casteel, C., Martin, S. L., & Gibbs, D. A. (2007). Effect of deployment on the occurrence of child maltreatment in military and nonmilitary families. *American Journal of Epidemiology, 165*, 1199–1206.

Rezendes, J. L. (2006). Bicycle helmets: Overcoming barriers to use and increasing effectiveness. *Journal of Pediatric Nursing, 21*, 35–44.

Slawta, J., Bentley, J., Smith, J., Kelly, J., & Syman-Degler, L. (2006). Promoting healthy lifestyles in children: A pilot program for Be a Fit Kid. *Health Promotion Practice, 7*, 1–8.

Sparrow, J. D. (2007). Understanding stress in children. *Pediatric Annals, 36*, 187–195.

Speier, A. H. (2005). *Psychosocial issues for children and adolescents in disasters* (2nd ed.). Washington DC: SAMHSA's National Mental Health Information Center.

Stein, J. A., Dukes, R. L., & Warren, J. I. (2007). Adolescent male bullies, victims and bully-victims: A comparison of psychosocial and behavioral characteristics. *Journal of Pediatric Psychology, 32*, 273–282.

Teplin, L. A., McClelland, C. M., Abram, K. M., & Mileusnic, D. (2005). Early violent death among delinquent youth: A prospective longitudinal study. *Pediatrics, 115*, 1586–1593.

Tischler, V., Rademeyer, A., & Vostanis, P. (2007). Mothers experiencing homelessness: Mental health, support and social care needs. *Health and Social Care in the Community, 15*, 246–253.

U.S. Department of Health and Human Services. (2005). Summary: Child Maltreatment. Retrieved from http://www.acf.hhs/gov/programs; cb/pubs/cm03/summary.htm

U.S. Department of Health and Human Services. (2006). *Healthy People 2010: Midcourse Review*. Washington, DC: Author.

U.S. Department of Health and Human Services (2008). 2008 Physical Activity Guidelines for Americans. Retrieved October 20, 2008, from www.health.gov/PAguidelines/guidelines/default/aspx

Uyemura, M. C. (2006). Foreign body ingestion in children. *American Family Physician, 72*, 287–291.

Wallerstein, J. S., & Blakeslee, S. (2003). *What about the kids? Raising your children before, during, and after divorce*. New York: Hyperion.

Watson, W. A., Litovitz, T. L., Klein-Schwartz, W., Rodgers, G. C., Youniss, J., Redi, N., et al. (2004). 2003 annual report of the American Association of Poison Control Center toxic exposure surveillance. *American Journal of Emergency Medicine, 22*, 335–404.

Whitehead, N. S., & Leiker, R. (2007). Case management protocol and declining blood lead concentrations among children. *Preventing Chronic Disease, 4*. Retrieved September 20, 2007, from www.cdc.gov/pcd/issues/2007/jan/06_0023.htm

Willard, N. E. (2007). *Cyberbullying and Cyberthreats: Responding to the challenge of online social aggression, threats, and distress* (2nd ed.). Champaign, IL: Research Press.

Woolf, A. D., Goldman, R., & Bellinger, D. C. (2007). Update on the clinical management of childhood lead poisoning. *Pediatric Clinics of North America, 54*, 271–294.

Yousey, Y., & Carr, M. (2005). A health care program for homeless children using Health People 2010 objectives. *Nursing Clinics of North America, 40*, 791–801.

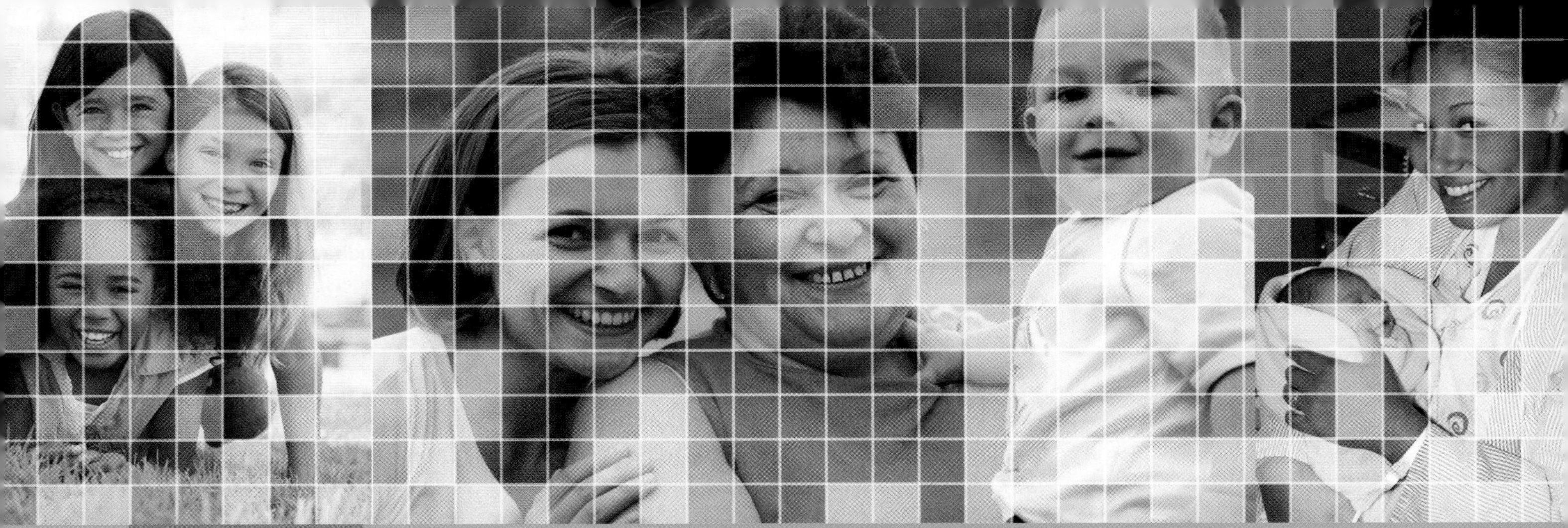

CHAPTER

45 Immunizations and Communicable Diseases

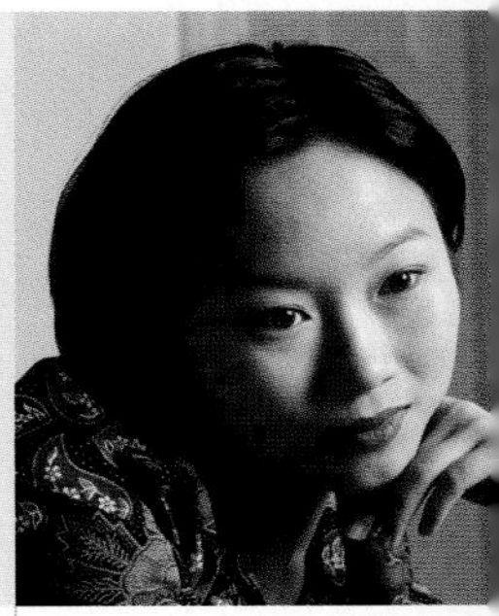

We came in today because Chang has a fever. I know Lian and Chang need immunizations. Lian will be going to kindergarten in the fall, so it is very important for her to get all of the immunizations she needs now. —Mother of Lian, 5 years old, and Chang, 2 years old

LEARNING OUTCOMES

45.1 Describe the reasons why children are more vulnerable than adults to contracting communicable diseases.

45.2 Describe the process of infection and modes of transmission.

45.3 Explain the role that vaccines play in reducing and eliminating communicable diseases.

45.4 Develop a nursing care plan for children of all ages needing immunizations.

45.5 Outline a plan to maintain the potency of vaccines.

45.6 Recognize common infectious and communicable diseases.

45.7 Develop a nursing care plan for a child with a common communicable disease.

KEY TERMS

Acellular pertussis vaccine, 1196
Active immunity, 1194
Antibodies, 1194
Antigen, 1195
Asplenia, 1196
Communicable disease, 1194
Conjugated forms, 1196
Direct transmission, 1194
Endogenous pyrogens, 1222
Herd immunity, 1204
Incubation period, 1209
Indirect transmission, 1194
Infectious disease, 1194
Killed virus vaccine, 1195
Live virus vaccine, 1196
Nosocomial infection, 1223
Opisthotonos, 1218
Orchitis, 1214
Pandemic flu, 1224
Passive immunity, 1194
Prodrome, 1221
Prostration, 1213
Recombinant forms, 1196
Toxic appearance, 1222
Toxoid, 1196
Transplacental immunity, 1196

An **infectious disease** is any communicable disease caused by microorganisms that are commonly transmitted from one person to another or from an animal to a person. A **communicable disease** is an infection often caused by **direct transmission**, acquired from a person or animal through contact with body fluids, such as through kissing, sneezing, or coughing. With **indirect transmission** infection is acquired through contact with contaminated objects, or by vectors (ticks, mosquitoes, other insects), for example Lyme disease. For a communicable disease to occur three factors need to be in place:

1. an infectious agent or pathogen
2. an effective means of transmission
3. susceptible host needs to be present (see "Pathophysiology Illustrated: The Chain of Infection").

Communicable diseases are a major cause of morbidity in infants and children in the United States, and can sometimes result in death.

SPECIAL VULNERABILITY OF INFANTS AND CHILDREN

Infants and young children are often susceptible hosts. Infants in particular are susceptible because the immune system is not fully mature at birth and disease protection through immunization is incomplete. **Passive immunity** to infections for which the mother has developed **antibodies** (proteins capable of responding to specific infectious agents) may be acquired via the placenta or breast milk. These antibodies provide limited protection for some infections, but this protection decreases over several months after birth. Immunodeficiency and poor health may also increase a child's risk of contracting an infectious disease.

As infants and children grow, they develop **active immunity** with antibodies developing for specific infections through immunization or exposure to the natural disease. As children interact more frequently with other children and adults, their exposure to infectious agents increases (Figure 45–1 ●). As healthy children are exposed to more infections, they naturally develop antibodies. Thus, subsequent infections with the same type of organism may be less severe or avoided. (Refer to Chapter 50, "Anatomy and Physiology of Pediatric Differences of the Immune System.")

The poor hygiene behaviors of young children facilitate transmission of infectious diseases in child care and other close environments. The fecal-oral and respiratory routes are the most common sources of transmission in children. Children usually do not wash their hands after toileting unless they are closely supervised. They put toys and their hands in their mouths, and then rub their nose and eyes. They often are unable to care for a runny nose without help. Diapers may leak stool and provide the fecal exposure to organisms. In addition, the staff in childcare centers or other people caring for children may not use proper hand hygiene techniques. All of these behaviors promote the transmission of infection. (See "Teaching Highlights: Reducing the Transmission of Infection.")

Reducing the number of preventable childhood illnesses is a major national focus, and nurses are important partners in this effort. Because of the significance of these preventable diseases as a public health problem, objectives have been developed to target the reduction or elimination of the following infectious diseases (Department of Health and Human Services [DHHS], 2006):

- Elimination—rubella and congenital rubella syndrome, diphtheria, *Haemophilus influenza* type b, measles, mumps, polio, and tetanus
- Reduction—pertussis, hepatitis B, varicella, foodborne pathogens, and HIV infections

Nurses have an important health promotion role in reducing the transmission of infectious diseases by immunization and in educating families to interrupt the transmission of infection in other ways, such as quarantine or hand hygiene, isolating ill children, implementing standard and transmission precautions, promoting immunizations, and sanitizing toys and contact surfaces.

PATHOPHYSIOLOGY ILLUSTRATED

THE CHAIN OF INFECTION TRANSMISSION

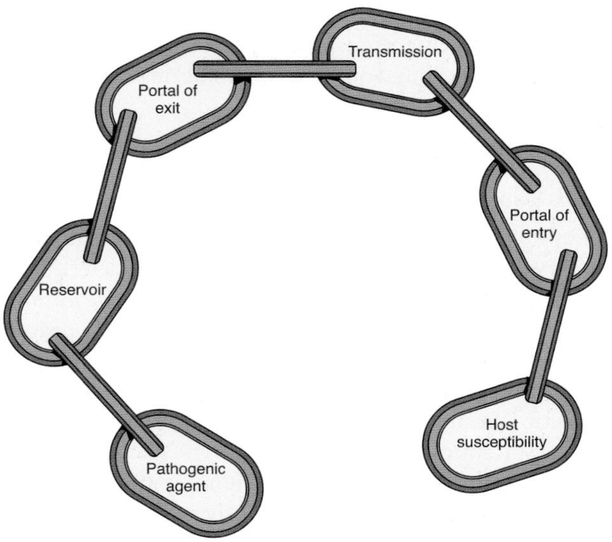

An effective chain of infection transmission requires a suitable habitat or reservoir for the pathogen. To prevent or control the spread of infection, one of the links in the chain must be broken, such as eliminating one or more of the habitats or reservoirs (e.g., insecticide spraying to kill mosquitoes that carry malaria). Isolating an infected individual interferes with disease transmission, and killing the pathogen eliminates the causal agent.

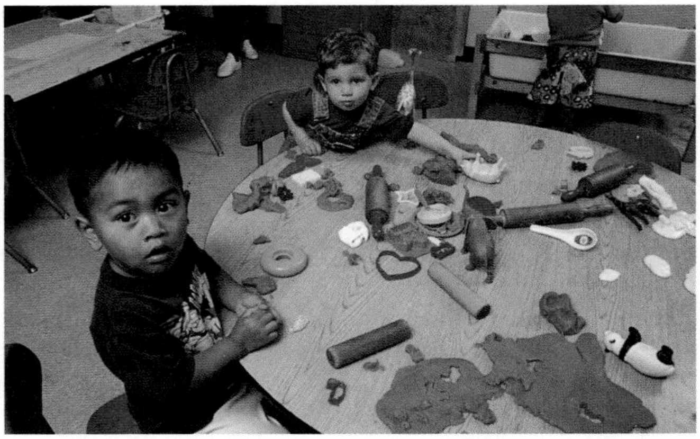

● **Figure 45–1** Transmission of infectious disease. Infectious diseases are easily transmitted in settings such as childcare centers where multiple children handle common objects and then put fingers in the mouth.

IMMUNIZATION

The development and use of immunizations has been one of the many significant breakthroughs of modern medicine. Immunization introduces an **antigen** (a foreign substance that triggers an immune system response) into the body, so that the person produces antibodies and immunity against a disease.

Teaching Highlights

REDUCING THE TRANSMISSION OF INFECTION

Teach families to reduce transmission of infection among family members with the following practices:

- Use disposable tissues and discard immediately after use.
- Wash hands thoroughly with soap and water or cleansing gels after all contact with the child's diaper, runny nose, and mucous membranes.
- Teach children to cough or sneeze into their elbow rather than their hands.
- Teach children to wash their hands with soap and water after toileting and before eating.
- Do not allow children to share dishes and utensils.
- Wash hands before preparing food, and again several times during the food preparation process. Follow guidelines for safe food preparation and storage. Wash dishes and cutting boards in warm soapy water or use the sanitizing cycle on the dishwasher.
- Wipe counters and surfaces that are used for diaper change or that the child touches with a disinfectant such as bleach solution, Lysol, or isopropyl alcohol. Make sure the diaper changing area is well away from food preparation areas.
- Dispose of diapers in closed containers.

MyNursingKit Vaccine Administration Record

In active immunity resulting from the antigen in a vaccine, antibody production is stimulated without causing clinical disease. When a child needs antibodies faster than the body can develop them, passive immunity may be provided with antibodies produced by another human or animal host (e.g., immune globulin) and given to the child. This approach is also used with at-risk children after disease exposure to prevent the disease from occurring or to reduce its severity. For example, if an unimmunized toddler with cancer is receiving chemotherapy and is exposed to chicken pox, the child needs immediate protection (passive immunity). Varicella immune globulin is given to reduce the child's risk for developing chicken pox, a potentially fatal infection for this child. Passive immunity does not confer lasting immunity, so the child should get the varicella vaccine at a later time to develop active immunity.

Since the first vaccines were developed in the late 1800s, the incidence of many diseases has decreased dramatically. The average infant born in 2009 receives immunizations for 14 childhood diseases by age 6 years. Vaccines have also been developed for older children, adolescents, and adults to protect against pertussis, meningococcus, human papillomavirus, and herpes zoster. Vaccines improve the health of children and reduce the parents' burden of caring for ill children.

The following lists the types of vaccines against childhood illnesses used in the United States:

- **Killed virus vaccine**. A microorganism has been killed but is still capable of inducing the human body to produce antibodies. Example: inactivated poliovirus vaccine.

MyNursingKit Immunizations and Older Children

- **Toxoid**. A toxin has been treated (by heat or chemical) to weaken its toxic effects but retain its antigenicity. Example: tetanus toxoid.
- **Live virus vaccine**. A microorganism is in a live but attenuated, or weakened, form. Example: measles and varicella vaccines.
- **Recombinant forms**. An organism has been genetically altered for use in vaccines. Examples: hepatitis B and **acellular pertussis vaccine** (a vaccine that uses pertussis proteins rather than the whole cell to stimulate active immunity).
- **Conjugated forms**. An altered organism is joined with another substance to increase the immune response. Examples: The *Haemophilus influenzae* type b (Hib) vaccine is conjugated with a protein-carrier like tetanus toxoid; but no immunity to tetanus develops when it is the protein carrier.

Today's vaccines are often produced synthetically with recombinant DNA technology or genetic engineering to improve vaccine safety and efficacy, and to reduce side effects. See the "Drug Guide: Recommended Pediatric Immunizations" on pages 1199–1203.

CLINICAL MANIFESTATIONS

Children can have a variety of responses to vaccines as the body responds to the administered antigen. Vaccine recipients commonly have a local reaction that includes erythema, swelling, pain, and induration at the site of the injection. Systemic reactions such as fever, fussiness or irritability, malaise, and anorexia may occur. Other systemic reactions (rash and arthralgia) are associated with some vaccines.

Allergic reactions to vaccines occur occasionally, such as a wheal and urticaria, within minutes to hours after the injection. A severe local allergic reaction is manifested by warmth, erythema, edema, petechiae, or ulceration occurring 2 to 8 hours after vaccination. A non-life-threatening systemic allergic reaction, such as generalized urticaria or transient petechiae, may occur within minutes. Anaphylaxis is a life-threatening reaction that is manifested by hypotension, generalized urticaria, angioedema, and laryngeal edema that may rarely occur with any vaccine. The reactions to specific vaccines can be found on the Drug Guide on pages 1199–1203.

Nursing Practice

Thimerosol, a bacteriostatic agent that contains ethyl mercury, was previously used to prevent contamination of vaccines in multidose vials. Because of the possible association between mercury poisoning and nerve and brain damage, vaccine manufacturers worked to remove thimerosol from vaccines. Influenza is the only vaccine given to children that still contains trace amounts of thimerosal (American Academy of Pediatrics, 2009).

COLLABORATIVE CARE

Immunization Schedules

Vaccines are recommended for administration at specific ages and intervals. Timing for first immunizations is determined by the age at which **transplacental immunity** (passive immunity transferred from mother to infant) decreases or disappears, and the infant or child develops the ability to make antibodies in response to the vaccine. Scientists continue to study the duration of protection from vaccines. Many vaccines are repeated at a later age to boost immunity.

The recommended schedule for immunization is updated at least annually to reflect new vaccines and the need for repeat immunization. The Advisory Committee on Immunization Practices (ACIP) of the Centers for Disease Control (CDC), the American Academy of Pediatrics (AAP), and the American Academy of Family Practitioners (AAFP) collaborate to provide a uniform recommended schedule. See Figure 45–2 ● for the 2010 recommendations for vaccines that all children should receive. Schedules and recommendations vary for children who begin immunizations later in childhood or need catch-up doses. See MyNursingKit for the most current immunization schedule for children and adolescents.

Supplemental immunizations for meningococcal and pneumococcal infections are recommended for certain children with chronic conditions, as noted in Table 45–1.

Improving Immunization Rates

Efforts to increase the numbers of children protected from vaccine-preventable diseases and to monitor immunization status is a national public health initiative. *Healthy People 2010* states important goals for reduction of vaccine preventable diseases (DHHS, 2006). The reported level of full immunization (greater than 95%) for children entering kindergarten and first grade has been achieved in 75% of the states, based on state requirements required for

(continues on page 1204)

Table 45–1 Supplemental Immunizations

Vaccine	Recommendation
Meningococcal (MPSV4)	This alternate meningococcal vaccine is for children 2 to 10 years of age with **asplenia** (absent or dysfunctional spleen). It can be given concurrently with other vaccines in a different site. In school-age children, protection is thought to last 3 to 5 years (American Academy of Pediatrics, 2009, p. 461). The MCV4 vaccine can also be used for this age group (see p. 1202).
23-valent Pneumococcal	For children older than 2 years of age with sickle-cell disease, asplenia, chronic cardiovascular and pulmonary disorders, diabetes mellitus, nephrotic syndrome, renal failure, HIV infection, cochlear implant, cerebrospinal fluid leaks, or other immune compromised status. It is also recommended for American Indian and Alaska Native children residing in areas with high rates of invasive pneumococcal disease. An additional dose may be given 5 years after the first dose (American Academy of Pediatrics, 2009, p. 533).

Recommended Immunization Schedule for Persons Aged 0 Through 6 Years—United States • 2010

For those who fall behind or start late, see the catch-up schedule

Vaccine ▼ Age ►	Birth	1 month	2 months	4 months	6 months	12 months	15 months	18 months	19–23 months	2–3 years	4–6 years
Hepatitis B[1]	HepB	HepB				HepB					
Rotavirus[2]			RV	RV	RV[2]						
Diphtheria, Tetanus, Pertussis[3]			DTaP	DTaP	DTaP	*see footnote*[3]	DTaP				DTaP
Haemophilus influenzae type b[4]			Hib	Hib	Hib[4]	Hib					
Pneumococcal[5]			PCV	PCV	PCV	PCV				PPSV	
Inactivated Poliovirus[6]			IPV	IPV		IPV					IPV
Influenza[7]								Influenza (Yearly)			
Measles, Mumps, Rubella[8]						MMR			*see footnote*[8]		MMR
Varicella[9]						Varicella			*see footnote*[9]		Varicella
Hepatitis A[10]							HepA (2 doses)			HepA Series	
Meningococcal[11]										MCV	

Range of recommended ages for all children except certain high-risk groups

Range of recommended ages for certain high-risk groups

This schedule includes recommendations in effect as of December 15, 2009. Any dose not administered at the recommended age should be administered at a subsequent visit, when indicated and feasible. The use of a combination vaccine generally is preferred over separate injections of its equivalent component vaccines. Considerations should include provider assessment, patient preference, and the potential for adverse events. Providers should consult the relevant Advisory Committee on Immunization Practices statement for detailed recommendations: **http://www.cdc.gov/vaccines/pubs/acip-list.htm**. Clinically significant adverse events that follow immunization should be reported to the Vaccine Adverse Event Reporting System (VAERS) at **http://www.vaers.hhs.gov** or by telephone, **800-822-7967**.

1. **Hepatitis B vaccine (HepB).** (Minimum age: birth)
   At birth:
   - Administer monovalent HepB to all newborns before hospital discharge.
   - If mother is hepatitis B surface antigen (HBsAg)-positive, administer HepB and 0.5 mL of hepatitis B immune globulin (HBIG) within 12 hours of birth.
   - If mother's HBsAg status is unknown, administer HepB within 12 hours of birth. Determine mother's HBsAg status as soon as possible and, if HBsAg-positive, administer HBIG (no later than age 1 week).

   After the birth dose:
   - The HepB series should be completed with either monovalent HepB or a combination vaccine containing HepB. The second dose should be administered at age 1 or 2 months. Monovalent HepB vaccine should be used for doses administered before age 6 weeks. The final dose should be administered no earlier than age 24 weeks.
   - Infants born to HBsAg-positive mothers should be tested for HBsAg and antibody to HBsAg 1 to 2 months after completion of at least 3 doses of the HepB series, at age 9 through 18 months (generally at the next well-child visit).
   - Administration of 4 doses of HepB to infants is permissible when a combination vaccine containing HepB is administered after the birth dose. The fourth dose should be administered no earlier than age 24 weeks.
2. **Rotavirus vaccine (RV).** (Minimum age: 6 weeks)
   - Administer the first dose at age 6 through 14 weeks (maximum age: 14 weeks 6 days). Vaccination should not be initiated for infants aged 15 weeks 0 days or older.
   - The maximum age for the final dose in the series is 8 months 0 days
   - If Rotarix is administered at ages 2 and 4 months, a dose at 6 months is not indicated.
3. **Diphtheria and tetanus toxoids and acellular pertussis vaccine (DTaP).** (Minimum age: 6 weeks)
   - The fourth dose may be administered as early as age 12 months, provided at least 6 months have elapsed since the third dose.
   - Administer the final dose in the series at age 4 through 6 years.
4. ***Haemophilus influenzae* type b conjugate vaccine (Hib).** (Minimum age: 6 weeks)
   - If PRP-OMP (PedvaxHIB or Comvax [HepB-Hib]) is administered at ages 2 and 4 months, a dose at age 6 months is not indicated.
   - TriHiBit (DTaP/Hib) and Hiberix (PRP-T) should not be used for doses at ages 2, 4, or 6 months for the primary series but can be used as the final dose in children aged 12 months through 4 years.
5. **Pneumococcal vaccine.** (Minimum age: 6 weeks for pneumococcal conjugate vaccine [PCV]; 2 years for pneumococcal polysaccharide vaccine [PPSV])
   - PCV is recommended for all children aged younger than 5 years. Administer 1 dose of PCV to all healthy children aged 24 through 59 months who are not completely vaccinated for their age.
   - Administer PPSV 2 or more months after last dose of PCV to children aged 2 years or older with certain underlying medical conditions, including a cochlear implant. See *MMWR* 1997;46(No. RR-8).
6. **Inactivated poliovirus vaccine (IPV)** (Minimum age: 6 weeks)
   - The final dose in the series should be administered on or after the fourth birthday and at least 6 months following the previous dose.
   - If 4 doses are administered prior to age 4 years a fifth dose should be administered at age 4 through 6 years. See *MMWR* 2009;58(30):829–30.
7. **Influenza vaccine (seasonal).** (Minimum age: 6 months for trivalent inactivated influenza vaccine [TIV]; 2 years for live, attenuated influenza vaccine [LAIV])
   - Administer annually to children aged 6 months through 18 years.
   - For healthy children aged 2 through 6 years (i.e., those who do not have underlying medical conditions that predispose them to influenza complications), either LAIV or TIV may be used, except LAIV should not be given to children aged 2 through 4 years who have had wheezing in the past 12 months.
   - Children receiving TIV should receive 0.25 mL if aged 6 through 35 months or 0.5 mL if aged 3 years or older.
   - Administer 2 doses (separated by at least 4 weeks) to children aged younger than 9 years who are receiving influenza vaccine for the first time or who were vaccinated for the first time during the previous influenza season but only received 1 dose.
   - For recommendations for use of influenza A (H1N1) 2009 monovalent vaccine see *MMWR* 2009;58(No. RR-10).
8. **Measles, mumps, and rubella vaccine (MMR).** (Minimum age: 12 months)
   - Administer the second dose routinely at age 4 through 6 years. However, the second dose may be administered before age 4, provided at least 28 days have elapsed since the first dose.
9. **Varicella vaccine.** (Minimum age: 12 months)
   - Administer the second dose routinely at age 4 through 6 years. However, the second dose may be administered before age 4, provided at least 3 months have elapsed since the first dose.
   - For children aged 12 months through 12 years the minimum interval between doses is 3 months. However, if the second dose was administered at least 28 days after the first dose, it can be accepted as valid.
10. **Hepatitis A vaccine (HepA).** (Minimum age: 12 months)
    - Administer to all children aged 1 year (i.e., aged 12 through 23 months). Administer 2 doses at least 6 months apart.
    - Children not fully vaccinated by age 2 years can be vaccinated at subsequent visits
    - HepA also is recommended for older children who live in areas where vaccination programs target older children, who are at increased risk for infection, or for whom immunity against hepatitis A is desired.
11. **Meningococcal vaccine.** (Minimum age: 2 years for meningococcal conjugate vaccine [MCV4] and for meningococcal polysaccharide vaccine [MPSV4])
    - Administer MCV4 to children aged 2 through 10 years with persistent complement component deficiency, anatomic or functional asplenia, and certain other conditions placing tham at high risk.
    - Administer MCV4 to children previously vaccinated with MCV4 or MPSV4 after 3 years if first dose administered at age 2 through 6 years. See *MMWR* 2009;58:1042–3.

CS207330-A

The Recommended Immunization Schedules for Persons Aged 0 through 18 Years are approved by the Advisory Committee on Immunization Practices (**http://www.cdc.gov/vaccines/recs/acip**), the American Academy of Pediatrics (**http://www.aap.org**), and the American Academy of Family Physicians (**http://www.aafp.org**).

Department of Health and Human Services • Centers for Disease Control and Prevention

Figure 45–2 Recommended immunization schedule for children 0 to 6 years, United States, 2008.

From: www.cdc.gov/vaccines/recs/schedules/child-schedule.htm#printable

Recommended Immunization Schedule for Persons Aged 7 Through 18 Years—United States • 2010

For those who fall behind or start late, see the schedule below and the catch-up schedule

Vaccine ▼ Age ►	7–10 years	11–12 years	13–18 years
Tetanus, Diphtheria, Pertussis[1]		Tdap	Tdap
Human Papillomavirus[2]	see footnote 2	HPV (3 doses)	HPV series
Meningococcal[3]	MCV	MCV	MCV
Influenza[4]		Influenza (Yearly)	
Pneumococcal[5]		PPSV	
Hepatitis A[6]		HepA Series	
Hepatitis B[7]		Hep B Series	
Inactivated Poliovirus[8]		IPV Series	
Measles, Mumps, Rubella[9]		MMR Series	
Varicella[10]		Varicella Series	

Range of recommended ages for all children except certain high-risk groups

Range of recommended ages for catch-up immunization

Range of recommended ages for certain high-risk groups

This schedule includes recommendations in effect as of December 15, 2009. Any dose not administered at the recommended age should be administered at a subsequent visit, when indicated and feasible. The use of a combination vaccine generally is preferred over separate injections of its equivalent component vaccines. Considerations should include provider assessment, patient preference, and the potential for adverse events. Providers should consult the relevant Advisory Committee on Immunization Practices statement for detailed recommendations: **http://www.cdc.gov/vaccines/pubs/acip-list.htm**. Clinically significant adverse events that follow immunization should be reported to the Vaccine Adverse Event Reporting System (VAERS) at **http://www.vaers.hhs.gov** or by telephone, **800-822-7967**.

1. **Tetanus and diphtheria toxoids and acellular pertussis vaccine (Tdap).** (Minimum age: 10 years for Boostrix and 11 years for Adacel)
   - Administer at age 11 or 12 years for those who have completed the recommended childhood DTP/DTaP vaccination series and have not received a tetanus and diphtheria toxoid (Td) booster dose.
   - Persons aged 13 through 18 years who have not received Tdap should receive a dose.
   - A 5-year interval from the last Td dose is encouraged when Tdap is used as a booster dose; however, a shorter interval may be used if pertussis immunity is needed.
2. **Human papillomavirus vaccine (HPV).** (Minimum age: 9 years)
   - Two HPV vaccines are licensed: a quadrivalent vaccine (HPV4) for the prevention of cervical, vaginal and vulvar cancers (in females) and genital warts (in females and males), and a bivalent vaccine (HPV2) for the prevention of cervical cancers in females.
   - HPV vaccines are most effective for both males and females when given before exposure to HPV through sexual contact.
   - HPV4 or HPV2 is recommended for the prevention of cervical precancers and cancers in females.
   - HPV4 is recommended for the prevention of cervical, vaginal and vulvar precancers and cancers and genital warts in females.
   - Administer the first dose to females at age 11 or 12 years.
   - Administer the second dose 1 to 2 months after the first dose and the third dose 6 months after the first dose (at least 24 weeks after the first dose).
   - Administer the series to females at age 13 through 18 years if not previously vaccinated.
   - HPV4 may be administered in a 3-dose series to males aged 9 through 18 years to reduce their likelihood of acquiring genital warts.
3. **Meningococcal conjugate vaccine (MCV4).**
   - Administer at age 11 or 12 years, or at age 13 through 18 years if not previously vaccinated.
   - Administer to previously unvaccinated college freshmen living in a dormitory.
   - Administer MCV4 to children aged 2 through 10 years with persistent complement component deficiency, anatomic or functional asplenia, or certain other conditions placing them at high risk.
   - Administer to children previously vaccinated with MCV4 or MPSV4 who remain at increased risk after 3 years (if first dose administered at age 2 through 6 years) or after 5 years (if first dose administered at age 7 years or older). Persons whose only risk factor is living in on-campus housing are not recommended to receive an additional dose. See *MMWR* 2009;58:1042–3.
4. **Influenza vaccine (seasonal).**
   - Administer annually to children aged 6 months through 18 years.
   - For healthy nonpregnant persons aged 7 through 18 years (i.e., those who do not have underlying medical conditions that predispose them to influenza complications), either LAIV or TIV may be used.
   - Administer 2 doses (separated by at least 4 weeks) to children aged younger than 9 years who are receiving influenza vaccine for the first time or who were vaccinated for the first time during the previous influenza season but only received 1 dose.
   - For recommendations for use of influenza A (H1N1) 2009 monovalent vaccine. See *MMWR* 2009;58(No. RR-10).
5. **Pneumococcal polysaccharide vaccine (PPSV).**
   - Administer to children with certain underlying medical conditions, including a cochlear implant. A single revaccination should be administered after 5 years to children with functional or anatomic asplenia or an immunocompromising condition. See *MMWR* 1997;46(No. RR-8).
6. **Hepatitis A vaccine (HepA).**
   - Administer 2 doses at least 6 months apart.
   - HepA is recommended for children aged older than 23 months who live in areas where vaccination programs target older children, who are at increased risk for infection, or for whom immunity against hepatitis A is desired.
7. **Hepatitis B vaccine (HepB).**
   - Administer the 3-dose series to those not previously vaccinated.
   - A 2-dose series (separated by at least 4 months) of adult formulation Recombivax HB is licensed for children aged 11 through 15 years.
8. **Inactivated poliovirus vaccine (IPV).**
   - The final dose in the series should be administered on or after the fourth birthday and at least 6 months following the previous dose.
   - If both OPV and IPV were administered as part of a series, a total of 4 doses should be administered, regardless of the child's current age.
9. **Measles, mumps, and rubella vaccine (MMR).**
   - If not previously vaccinated, administer 2 doses or the second dose for those who have received only 1 dose, with at least 28 days between doses.
10. **Varicella vaccine.**
    - For persons aged 7 through 18 years without evidence of immunity (see *MMWR* 2007;56[No. RR-4]), administer 2 doses if not previously vaccinated or the second dose if only 1 dose has been administered.
    - For persons aged 7 through 12 years, the minimum interval between doses is 3 months. However, if the second dose was administered at least 28 days after the first dose, it can be accepted as valid.
    - For persons aged 13 years and older, the minimum interval between doses is 28 days.

CS207330-A

The Recommended Immunization Schedules for Persons Aged 0 through 18 Years are approved by the Advisory Committee on Immunization Practices (**http://www.cdc.gov/vaccines/recs/acip**), the American Academy of Pediatrics (**http://www.aap.org**), and the American Academy of Family Physicians (**http://www.aafp.org**).

Department of Health and Human Services • Centers for Disease Control and Prevention

Figure 45–2 Continued.

From: www.cdc.gov/vaccines/recs/schedules/child-schedule.htm#printable

Drug Guide

RECOMMENDED PEDIATRIC IMMUNIZATIONS

IMMUNIZATION TYPE	SIDE EFFECTS	CONTRAINDICATIONS	NURSING CONSIDERATIONS
Diphtheria, Pertussis, and Tetanus Toxoid (DTaP, Tdap)			
Type: Inactivated *Route:* Intramuscular *Dosage:* 0.5 mL *Age(s) given:* 2, 4, 6, 15–18 months; 4–6 years (5 doses); 11–12 years (Tdap) May give at same time as all other vaccines, in a separate site. *Storage:* Refrigerate, do not freeze. A Tdap vaccine for adolescents became part of the vaccine schedule starting in 2006.	*Common:* Redness, pain, swelling, nodule at injection site; fever—38.3°C (101°F); drowsiness, irritability, fussiness; anorexia within 2 days of injection. Increase in frequency and magnitude of local reactions with 4th and 5th doses (e.g., entire limb swelling). *Serious:* Allergic reaction, anaphylaxis; shock or collapse (hypotonic-hyperresponsive episode—sudden loss of muscle tone, pallor, fever, and unresponsiveness), fever above 38.8°C (102°F); febrile seizure; persistent inconsolable crying; coma or permanent brain damage.	Gelatin allergy (do not use Tripedia). Serious side effects after a prior dose: e.g., anaphylaxis, encephalopathy within 7 days, or a progressive neurologic disorder (e.g., uncontrolled epilepsy). Adolescents with a history of coma or prolonged seizures within 7 days of a pertussis vaccine should not get Tdap. *Precautions*: If the child had the following reactions within 48 hours of the previous dose: —Fever of 40.5°C (105°F) or higher —Inconsolable crying for 3 hours or longer —Pale or limp episode or collapse —Guillain-Barré syndrome less than 6 weeks after previous dose —Seizure within 3 days of dose. Delay administration until moderate to severe febrile illnesses have resolved. Defer the vaccine when the child has a progressive neurologic problem until the child is stable.	Use same brand for all doses where feasible. Prior to immunization, ask about previous reactions. DTaP may coincide with or hasten the recognition of a seizure disorder. In children with a history of seizures with or without fever, give acetaminophen with vaccine and every 4 hours for 24 hours. Shake vaccine before withdrawing. Solution will be cloudy. If it contains clumps that cannot be resuspended, do not use. Daptacel stopper vial contains latex. Pediarix stopper vial is latex-free. When required, simultaneous administration of tetanus immune globulin or diphtheria antitoxin should be given in separate sites. Inform parents of the potential for an increased reaction to the 4th and 5th doses. DT is given to children younger than 7 years with a prior serious reaction to the pertussis component of the vaccine. Do not restart the series, no matter how long since the previous dose was given. A tetanus booster may be given for a contaminated wound or burn, if 5 or more years since the last dose (American Academy of Pediatrics, 2009. p. 657).
Haemophilus influenza Type B (Hib)			
Type: Inactivated *Route:* Intramuscular *Dosage:* 0.5 mL *Age(s) given:* 2, 4, 6, 12–15 months; (4 doses for HbOC[a] [HibTITER] and PRP-T[a] [ActHIB]) *or* 2, 4, 12–15 months (3 doses for PRP-OMP[a] [PedvaxHIB]) May give at same time as all other vaccines in a separate site. *Storage:* Refrigerate, do not freeze.	*Common:* Pain, redness, or swelling at site *Serious:* Anaphylaxis (extremely rare); fever	Prior anaphylactic reaction *Precautions*: Moderate or severe acute illness with or without fever	Ask if child is immunosuppressed before administration. Solution is clear and colorless. Refrigerate reconstituted PedvaxHIB and discard within 24 hours. Use or discard reconstituted ActHIP and OmniHIB within 30 minutes. Use the same vaccine preparation for all doses of the primary series if possible since schedules vary for different products.

(continued)

Drug Guide—continued

RECOMMENDED PEDIATRIC IMMUNIZATIONS

IMMUNIZATION TYPE	SIDE EFFECTS	CONTRAINDICATIONS	NURSING CONSIDERATIONS
Hepatitis A			
Type: inactivated *Route*: Intramuscular *Dosage*: 0.5 mL, (1.0 mL over 18 years) *Age(s) given*: 12 months; second dose 6–12 months after first dose. May give at same time as all other vaccines in a separate site. *Storage*: Refrigerate, do not freeze; do not use if it has been frozen.	*Common*: pain, tenderness, soreness, redness, swelling, and warmth at injection site; rash, fever. *Serious:* Rare reports of anaphylaxis/anaphylactoid reactions	Known hypersensitivity to any component of vaccine, including neomycin. Anaphylactic reaction to prior vaccine dose. *Precautions:* Pregnancy Moderate or severe acute illness with or without fever	Shake well, slightly opaque white suspension. No reconstitution is needed. Vaqta vials have a latex stopper. Can be given for post-exposure prophylaxis against hepatitis A (Victor, Monto, Surdina, et al., 2007). Immune globulin and vaccine can be given at the same time in different sites. Do not restart the series, no matter how long since the previous dose.
Hepatitis B (HB)			
Type: Inactivated *Route*: Intramuscular *Dosage*: Engerix-B[a]: 10 mcg or Recombivax HB[a]: 5 mcg *Age(s) given*: Birth, 1 month after first dose; 6 months after first dose; three doses May give at same time as all other vaccines in a separate site. *Storage*: Refrigerate, do not freeze. Vaccine brands can be interchanged for 3-dose series. Newborn dose should be monovalent (single vaccine) preparation.	*Common*: pain or redness at injection site; *Serious:* Allergic reaction or anaphylaxis; fever	Serious hypersensitivity such as anaphylaxis reaction to prior dose or vaccine component (e.g., yeast). Pregnancy *Precautions*: Infant weighing less than 2000 grams Moderate or severe acute illness with or without fever	Prior to immunization, check status of mother's hepatitis B test and presence of other liver disease. If mother has HBsAg+ or unknown status, give vaccine to infant within 12 hours of birth along with hepatitis B immune globulin in another site. Shake vaccine before withdrawing. Solution will appear cloudy. Formulations (pediatric, adult, dialysis) have different strengths. Read package insert to determine the proper dosage for the formulation used. A 3-dose series can be started at any age. Do not restart the series, no matter how long since the previous dose was given. Review guidelines for timing of subsequent doses for the child's age. Check the anti-HB levels in infants of HBsAG+ mothers at age 9–18 months, after series completion. (American Academy of Pediatrics, 2009, p. 345).
Human Papillomavirus (HPV) (Quadravalent)			
Type: Recombinant *Route*: Intramuscular *Dosage*: 0.5 mL	*Common:* Pain, swelling, erythema at the injection site, pruritus, fever, and fainting.	Severe allergic reaction to prior dose or hypersensitivity to any vaccine components (e.g. yeast).	Shake well before use. Solution is a white cloudy liquid. No dilution or reconstitution.

Drug Guide—continued

RECOMMENDED PEDIATRIC IMMUNIZATIONS

IMMUNIZATION TYPE	SIDE EFFECTS	CONTRAINDICATIONS	NURSING CONSIDERATIONS
Human Papillomavirus (HPV) (Quadravalent)—continued			
Age(s) given: girls 11–12 years, second dose 2 months later, third dose 6 months after the first dose. May be administered with hepatitis B vaccine in separate site. *Storage:* Refrigerate, do not freeze.	*Potential Serious Reactions:* Headache, gastroenteritis, bronchospasm, asthma, arthritis.	Pregnancy. Bleeding disorder. *Precautions:* Lactating women—It is not known if the vaccine is excreted in human milk. Moderate to severe acute illness with or without fever. Can be given when mild acute illness is present.	Protect vaccine from light to protect its potency. Administer vaccine before onset of sexual activity; may be given to girls as young as 9 years (Moore & Seybold, 2007). Educate parents and adolescents about this vaccine's potential to prevent cervical cancer and human papilloma virus infections. Educate adolescents that this vaccine prevents only one sexually transmitted infection.
Influenza			
Type: Inactivated (TIV), or live attenuated for intranasal use (LAIV) *Route:* Intramuscular (all ages), intranasal (2 years and older) *Dosage:* 0.25 mL in infants 6–35 months, 0.5 mL beginning at 3 years *Age(s) given:* Annually in the fall, beginning at 6 months of age; then annually to all children (Fiore, Shay, Broder, et al., 2008). May give at same time as all other vaccines in a separate site. *TIV Storage:* Refrigerate, do not freeze; do not use if frozen. *LAIV Storage:* Keep frozen. May be thawed and refrigerated for up to 24 hours before use.	*Common after TIV:* Soreness or swelling at injection site, fever, aches. Life-threatening allergic reactions are rare. *Common after LAIV:* Runny nose or nasal congestion, fever, headache or muscle aches, abdominal pain and occasional vomiting. No life-threatening problems were detected during clinical trials.	Severe allergic reaction such as anaphylaxis to prior vaccine dose or vaccine component (e.g., history of anaphylaxis to chicken or egg protein, known sensitivity to gentamycin or other aminoglycosides). LAIV is contraindicated in children with immune deficiency disorders or immunocompromised (e.g., receiving chemotherapy, long term immunosuppression, HIV); pregnancy, previous history of Guillain-Barré syndrome. *Precaution:* Postpone vaccine when child has acute febrile illness; may be given with minor illness, with or without fever. Delay vaccine in presence of active neurologic disease.	Thawed LAIV is pale yellow, clear to slightly cloudy. LAIV dose is split (0.25 mL) with a dose divider clip. Administer in each nostril while child is sitting in an upright position. Insert the tip of the sprayer inside the nose and depress the plunger to spray. Children between 6 months and 9 years who are receiving the influenza vaccine for the first time should get 2 doses separated by at least 4 weeks (TIV) and 6 weeks (LAIV). Reimmunize with one dose each year as immunity wanes, and vaccines are modified to include the new season's viruses. Children under 9 years immunized for the first time in the prior year, but only receiving one dose, should get a second dose, like previously unimmunized children.
Measles, Mumps, Rubella (MMR)			
Type: Live attenuated *Route:* Subcutaneous *Dosage:* 0.5 mL *Age(s) given:* 12–15 months; 4–6 years (2 doses) May give at same time as all other vaccines in a separate site. Give MMR and varicella vaccines on the same day or at least 4 weeks apart.	*Common:* Elevated temperature 1–2 weeks after immunization; redness or pain at injection site; noncontagious rash; joint pain. *Serious:* Allergic reaction or anaphylaxis; febrile seizure; meningitis (usually mild); encephalopathy; immune	Prior severe allergic reaction, e.g., anaphylaxis, to vaccine or vaccine component (eggs, neomycin or gelatin). Pregnancy. Malignancy, immune deficiency disease, immunosuppressive therapy, *Precautions*: History of thrombocytopenia or thrombocytopenic purpura	Inquire about immunosuppression. Reconstituted vaccine is a clear, yellow solution. Give entire contents of reconstituted vial even if more than 0.5 mL. Observe child with an egg allergy for 90 minutes after injection (Cox, 2006). Recommended for children infected with HIV unless severely immunocompromised.

(continued)

Drug Guide—continued

RECOMMENDED PEDIATRIC IMMUNIZATIONS

IMMUNIZATION TYPE	SIDE EFFECTS	CONTRAINDICATIONS	NURSING CONSIDERATIONS
Measles, Mumps, Rubella (MMR)—continued			
Storage: Refrigerate, do not freeze. When reconstituted, keep refrigerated and away from light; discard if unused within 8 hours.	thrombocytopenia purpura; and rare cases of coma and permanent brain damage.	Moderate or severe acute illness with or without fever. A slight increased risk of febrile seizures 7–10 days after MMRV vaccine has been noted in children aged 12–23 months (Centers for Disease Control and Prevention, 2008b).	Follow guidelines for timing of vaccine if child received immune globulin or blood product in past 3 to 11 months (Kroger, Atkinson, Marcuse, et al., 2006, p. 8). Educate adolescent girls to avoid pregnancy for 3 months after immunization. Give tuberculosis (TB) test at same time as MMR or 4–6 weeks later.
Meningococcal Tetravalent Conjugate (MCV4)			
Type: Conjugate *Route*: Intramuscular *Dosage*: 0.5 mL in children 11–12 years, and those about to enter high school, boarding school, or college, if not vaccinated May be given at same time as typhoid, Tdap, or Td vaccine. *Storage*: Refrigerate until used, do not freeze.	*Common:* swelling and pain at injection site, malaise, headache, and fatigue. Less than 5% experience a severe systemic reaction (Bilukha & Rosenstein, 2005). Guillain Barré syndrome occurring within 6 weeks after MCV4 vaccine has had a very low incidence rate (17 cases among 1.25 million doses), a rate that could have occurred by chance (Asch-Goodkin, 2006; Dempsey, & Freed, 2006).	Severe allergic reaction (e.g., anaphylaxis) after prior dose or to a vaccine component (e.g., diphtheria toxoid). Previous history of Guillain-Barré syndrome, unless at high risk for meningococcal disease.	Protect vaccine from light. Vial stopper contains latex. May be given to children aged 2 to 10 years when immunosuppressed by disease or medication. Alternate vaccine (MPSV4) may also be used (see Table 45–1). Until adequate supply exists, preadolescents and adolescents going to boarding school or college have highest priority for the vaccine. Duration of protection is unknown, but expected to exceed 3 years (Dempsey, & Freed, 2006).
Pneumococcal Conjugate (PCV7) (Heptavalent)			
Type: Conjugate *Route:* Intramuscular *Dosage:* 0.5 mL *Age(s) given:* 2, 4, 6, 12–15 months *Storage:* Refrigerate, do not freeze.	*Common:* Soreness, swelling, redness at injection site; mild to moderate fever; irritability, drowsiness, restless sleep, decreased appetite, vomiting and diarrhea, rash or hives. *Severe:* Allergic reaction or anaphylaxis	Severe allergic reaction, e.g., anaphylaxis, after a prior dose or to a vaccine component (e.g., diphtheria toxoid). *Precaution:* Moderate or severe acute illness with or without fever.	Clear, colorless, or slightly opalescent liquid. Give 1 dose to children aged 24–59 months with any missing dose. Use PPV23 for children 2 years and older at high risk for acquiring pneumococcal infection (see Table 45–1). Do not restart the series, no matter how long since the previous dose was given.
Poliovirus Vaccine (IPV)			
Type: Inactivated *Route:* Subcutaneous or intramuscular depending upon vaccine used *Dosage:* 0.5 mL *Age(s) given:* 2, 4, 12–18 months; 4–6 years (4 doses)	*Common:* Swelling and tenderness, irritability, tiredness. *Serious:* Allergic reaction or anaphylaxis.	Severe allergic reaction, e.g., anaphylaxis, after prior dose or to vaccine components (neomycin, streptomycin, polymyxin B). *Precautions*: Pregnancy	Prior to immunization, ask if the child has an allergy to one of the vaccine components (whichever of the antibiotics the specific vaccine to be used contains). Clear, colorless suspension. Do not use if it contains particulate matter, becomes cloudy, or changes color.

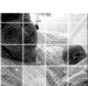

Drug Guide—continued

RECOMMENDED PEDIATRIC IMMUNIZATIONS

IMMUNIZATION TYPE	SIDE EFFECTS	CONTRAINDICATIONS	NURSING CONSIDERATIONS
Poliovirus Vaccine (IPV)—continued			
May give at same time as all other vaccines in a separate site. *Storage:* Refrigerate, do not freeze.		Moderate or severe acute illness with or without fever.	All doses must be separated by at least 4 weeks. Do not restart the series, no matter how long since the previous dose was given.
Rotavirus Vaccine (PRV)			
Type: Live *Route*: Oral *Dosage*: 2 mL *Age(s) given*: 2, 4, and 6 months (3 doses); all 3 doses of vaccine should be completed by 32 months of age. May give at same time as all other vaccines *Storage*: Refrigerate, do not freeze.	*Common:* vomiting, diarrhea, irritability *Potential serious adverse reactions*: seizures, bronchiolitis, gastroenteritis, pneumonia, fever, urinary tract infection.	Severe allergic reaction to a previous dose or to a vaccine component. *Precautions*: Moderate or severe acute illness with or without fever. Pre-existing gastrointestinal disease. Previous history of intussusception. Immunosuppression Receipt of a blood product within 6 weeks, unless this will delay the first dose until the child is 13 weeks or older (Kroger, Atkinson, Marcuse, et al., 2006, p. 7).	Pale yellow clear liquid. Protect vaccine from light. Squeeze the liquid into the infant's mouth toward the inner cheek until the dosing tube is empty. Do not repeat the dose if the infant spits out, vomits, or regurgitates during or after the dose (Parashar, Alexander, & Glass, 2006). No restrictions on the infant's intake of formula, breast milk, or food before or after vaccine. Discard the empty tube and cap into approved biological waste container.
Varicella Virus Vaccine			
Type: Live attenuated *Route:* Subcutaneous *Dosage:* 0.5 mL *Age(s) given:* 12–18 months; or any time up to 12 years of age (1 dose); 13 years or older (2 doses 4–8 weeks apart) *Storage:* Keep frozen at 5°F or colder. May refrigerate up to 72 hours before reconstitution. Once reconstituted, use vaccine within 30 minutes or discard. Do not refreeze. Diluents kept at room temperature.	*Common:* Pain or redness at injection site; fever up to 38.8°C (102°F) in children or up to 37.7°C (100°F) in adults. Less commonly a vaccine-related rash (mild exanthem of 6 to 10 lesions that last for 2 to 3 days) may occur during first month after the injection. *Severe:* Allergic reaction or anaphylaxis; thrombocytopenia; febrile seizure; CNS manifestations.	Severe allergic reaction (e.g., anaphylaxis) after a prior dose or to a vaccine component (e.g., neomycin or gelatin). Substantial suppression of cellular immunity. Pregnancy *Precautions:* Receipt of blood products or immune globulin within past 3 to 11 months. Moderate or severe acute illness with or without fever.	Prior to immunization, ask if child is immunodeficient or on immunosuppression treatment or has an allergy to a vaccine component. Clear, colorless to pale yellow liquid when reconstituted. Give the entire contents of the vial even if more than 0.5 mL. Give MMR and varicella vaccines on the same day or at least 4 weeks apart (Kroger, Atkinson, Marcuse, et al., 2006, p. 13). Instruct adolescent girls of childbearing age to avoid pregnancy for 3 months after immunization. Give vaccine to unimmunized child exposed to varicella within 3 days to help build immunity quickly.

Data from American Academy of Pediatrics. (2009). *Red Book: Report of the Committee on Infectious Disease.* (27th ed.). Elk Grove Village, IL: Author; Bindler, R. M., & Howry, L. B. (2005). *Pediatric drugs and nursing implications* (3rd ed.). Upper Saddle River, NJ: Prentice Hall Health; Merck & Co. Inc. (2006). *Gardisil,* retrieved June 13, 2006, from www.fda.gov/cber/label/hpvmer060806LB.pdf; Kroger, A. T., Atkinson, W. L., Marcuse, E. K., & Pickering, L. K. (2006). General recommendations on immunization: Recommendations of the Advisory Committee on Immunization Practices (ACIP). *Morbidity and Mortality Weekly Report, 55*(RR-15), 1–48; and Centers for Disease Control and Prevention (2008a). Summary of Recommendations for Childhood and Adolescent Immunization, retrieved March 9, 2008, from www.immunize.org/catg.d/p2010.pdf

kindergarten entrance, thereby achieving a *Healthy People 2010* objective (Stanwyck & Jain, 2007). However the objectives for full immunization of 90% of adolescents have not been achieved for any vaccine (Centers for Disease Control and Prevention, 2008d).

Lower immunization rates are often associated with economic factors, limited access to health care, lack of primary care at hours convenient for working parents, inadequate education about the importance of immunization, and religious prohibitions. The estimated cost of fully immunizing a child through the adolescent years in 2007 was $1,170 for all approved vaccines (Lee, Santoli, Hannan, et al., 2007). The federal Vaccines for Children program provides free vaccines for qualified children and adolescents up to 19 years of age, and it has resolved some of the economic factors associated with vaccine coverage.

MyNursingKit Catch-Up Schedule for Immunizations

However, an increasing number of parents are choosing not to immunize their children for philosophical or other reasons such as (Benin, Wisler-Scher, Colson, et al., 2006; Salmon, Moulton, Omer, et al., 2005):

- Disagreement with government regulation and monitoring of immunizations.
- Increasing public awareness that the number of vaccine adverse events exceeds the number of cases of vaccine-preventable diseases.
- Belief that they can control their child's susceptibility to disease and the outcome if they become infected.

Common misconceptions about vaccines and communicable diseases that may influence parent decision making are provided in Table 45–2 along with factual information. See also Evidence-Based Nursing for information on parental decision making about vaccines.

Vaccine Injury Compensation

Serious reactions to vaccines may occur in rare instances. When a link between a child's immunization and a serious adverse reaction is identified, the National Vaccine Injury Compensation Program provides compensation for the family. The Vaccine Adverse Event Reporting System (VAERS) was established in 1988 to track serious vaccine reactions. See Table 45–3 for the serious reactions and disabilities tracked by vaccine. See MyNursingKit for the Web site with updated VAERS reporting guidelines.

NURSING MANAGEMENT

NURSING ASSESSMENT AND DIAGNOSIS

Nurses are responsible for reviewing a child's health record to determine whether the child needs vaccinations. Identify any potential contraindications to vaccines by asking the following:

- Have there been previous reactions to any immunizations?
- Are there allergies to any vaccine components (e.g., eggs, neomycin, gelatin, or yeast)?

Table 45–2 Common Misconceptions about Vaccines and Correct Information

Common Misconceptions	Correct Vaccine Information
Vaccine-preventable diseases have been eliminated.	While the incidence of vaccine-preventable diseases is low in the United States, most diseases are never completely eliminated. Travelers may reintroduce the disease from a country or a community where the disease still exists. Recent outbreaks of measles, mumps, and pertussis have been linked to groups of children not immunized because of religious and personal beliefs (Nield & Kamat, 2006; Omer, Pan, Halsey, et al., 2006). If numerous parents in one community decide not to immunize their children, the **herd immunity** (immunization of healthy children so that pathogens do not have hosts to reproduce and survive, indirectly protecting unimmunized infants) level drops and children in that community are at higher risk of infection.
Immunization weakens the immune system. Multiple vaccines overload the immune system and cause harmful effects.	A small amount of an inactivated or attenuated virus or bacteria is given to the child. The child's immune system recognizes the foreign substance and develops antibodies to protect against it. The immune system of infants is capable of generating protective immune responses to multiple vaccines given simultaneously (Nield & Kamat, 2006).
Thimerosal use in vaccines may cause mercury poisoning.	Thimerosal, a bacteriostatic agent that contains ethyl mercury, was used to sterilize vaccines in multidose vials. Because of the possible association between mercury poisoning and nerve and brain damage, thimerosal has been eliminated from the majority of vaccines while maintaining their sterility. Of vaccines manufactured in the United States, only the influenza vaccine has trace amounts (Nield & Kamat, 2006).
It would be better to let the child get the disease than get immunized.	Many parents do not understand the dangers inherent in some of these diseases, such as suffering, permanent disability, and even death. Unimmunized children are at a greater risk of getting the disease and of spreading it to pregnant women and to infants and children with serious medical conditions. Risks of getting the disease need to be considered along with the low risks associated with immunizations.
Vaccines do not work; children still get the disease.	No vaccine is 100% effective, and immunity does wane over time, leading to the need for a second immunization.

Table 45–3 National Vaccine Injury Compensation Program—Vaccine Injury Table, Effective November 10, 2008

Vaccine	Adverse Event Covered	Time Period for First Symptom or Manifestation of Onset—for Compensation
Tetanus toxoid-containing vaccines (e.g., DTaP, Tdap, DTP-Hib, DT, Td, or TT)	Anaphylaxis or anaphylactic shock Bacterial neuritis Any acute complication or sequela (including death) of above events.	0–4 hours 2–28 days Not applicable
Pertussis antigen-containing vaccines (e.g., DTaP, Tdap, DTP, P, DTP-Hib)	Anaphylaxis or anaphylactic shock Encephalopathy (or encephalitis) Any acute complication or sequela (including death) of above events.	0–4 hours 0–72 hours Not applicable
Measles, mumps, rubella virus-containing vaccines in any combination (e.g., MMR, MR, M, R)	Anaphylaxis or anaphylactic shock Encephalopathy (or encephalitis) Any acute complication or sequela (including death) of above events.	0–4 hours 5–15 days Not applicable
Rubella virus-containing vaccines (e.g., MMR, MR, R)	Chronic arthritis Any acute complication or sequela (including death) of above events.	7–42 days Not applicable
Measles virus-containing vaccines (e.g., MMR, MR, M)	Thrombocytopenia purpura Vaccine strain measles viral infection in an immunodeficient recipient. Any acute complication or sequela (including death) of above events.	7–30 days 0–6 months Not applicable
Polio inactivated virus-containing vaccines (e.g., IPV)	Anaphylaxis or anaphylactic shock Any acute complication or sequela (including death) of above events.	0–4 hours No limit
Hepatitis B antigen-containing vaccines	Anaphylaxis or anaphylactic shock Any acute complication or sequela (including death) of above events.	0–4 hours No limit
Haemophilus influenzae type B polysaccharide conjugate vaccines	No condition specified for compensation	Not applicable
Varicella vaccine	No condition specified for compensation	Not applicable
Rotavirus vaccine	No condition specified for compensation	Not applicable
Pneumococcal conjugate vaccine	No condition specified for compensation	Not applicable
Any new vaccine recommended by the Centers for Disease Control and Prevention for routine administration to children after publication by Secretary, HHS of notice of coverage[a]	No condition specified for compensation	Not applicable

From: Health Resources and Services Administration. (2008). *Vaccine Injury Table,* Accessed May 11, 2009, from www.hrsa.gov/vaccinecompensation/table.htm

[a]As of December 1, 2004, hepatitis A vaccines were added to the Vaccine Injury Table under this category. As of July 1, 2005, *trivalent* influenza vaccines were added to the Table under this category. As of February 1, 2007, meningococcal (conjugate and polysaccharide) and human papillomavirus (HPV) vaccines have been added to the Table under this category. See the following Web site for aids for interpretation of defined conditions: www.hrsa.gov/vaccinecompensation

- Does the child have a serious medical condition (seizures, cancer, HIV infection, immune diseases)?
- Has the child received any blood products or immune globulin in the past year, or had any vaccines in the last 4 weeks?
- If the patient is a female, is there a possibility of pregnancy?

Healthcare providers miss many opportunities to immunize children. Children (and siblings present) should have their immunization status assessed during all healthcare visits and hospitalizations, and in schools. If the child has not received all appropriate immunizations for his or her age, determine the best combination of vaccines to give at this visit to better protect the child. However, make sure the appropriate interval has passed for additional dosages.

To reduce the number of missed opportunities for full immunization of children, use the following guidelines (American Academy of Pediatrics [AAP], 2009):

- Place a reminder in the child's health record to alert health professionals about the child's need for immunizations. Establish a system to send parents a reminder when the child's immunizations are due or overdue.
- Give immunizations when the child has a minor illness, even with a low-grade fever and antibiotic treatment, or has a recent exposure to an infectious disease.

Evidence-Based Nursing

PARENT DECISION MAKING ABOUT VACCINATING THEIR CHILDREN

Clinical Question

Why are parents choosing not to vaccinate their infants and young children?

The Evidence

In one qualitative study 33 mothers in the postpartum period and again 3 to 6 months after the child's birth were interviewed. Mothers were poorly informed about the vaccines their infant would or did receive. Some mothers accepted or refused vaccines for their infants. Some mothers were hesitant to vaccinate their infants or chose selected vaccines for their infant, but they were willing to discuss or hear additional information about vaccines. Mothers seeking more information were not sure how to get their questions answered or who to trust. They gained trust when information could be answered satisfactorily. Mothers who chose not to vaccinate were concerned about potential permanent adverse effects of vaccines and financial rewards pediatricians received for getting patients fully immunized (Benin, Wisler-Scher, Colson, et al., 2006).

In another study, 23 mothers of children younger than 3 years were interviewed regarding the MMR vaccine. These mothers made their immunization decision in terms of their child's vulnerability to the disease (the strength of the child's immunity) or that the three-in-one vaccine was too much for the child's immune system. Vaccine decisions were related to social relationships with other mothers, families, and friends; interactions with health professionals; and prior medical experiences that led to trust or suspicion about immunization recommendations (Poltorak, Leach, Fairhead, et al., 2004; Cheater, 2006).

A study investigated the decisions of 69 parents regarding a second MMR vaccine for their children. A parent's exposure to a child either with autism or measles, mumps, or rubella was a primary factor in the decision made. Parents who knew or had a child with autism felt the consequences of the vaccine were worse than a relatively treatable disease. When parents had exposure to negative consequences of measles, mumps, or rubella, they decided to vaccinate their child. Physicians were seen as trusted sources of vaccine information, but parents were concerned about physician bonus payments when children were vaccinated. Parents also indicated that vaccine information reported in the mass media was more interesting than the information provided by their healthcare providers (MacDonald, 2005; McMurray, Cheater, Weighall, et al., 2004).

Best Practice

Identifying why parents choose not to immunize their child can be helpful in developing education for parents and other strategies to improve immunization rates. Parents do want to protect their children, either from diseases or from the potential harm of vaccines. Work to develop a trusting relationship with parents as this is important in their decision-making process. Listen to the parents' questions and concerns. Be fully informed about vaccine schedules, why vaccines are given at specific ages, and vaccine safety information in preparation for these discussions.

Critical Thinking

Use the vaccine information in the Drug Guide and information in Table 45–2 to develop a convincing explanation about the value and relative safety of vaccines for discussions with parents.

See MyNursingKit for possible responses.

Nursing Practice

Immune globulin, blood products, and immunosuppressive agents inhibit the child's response to live virus vaccines, so ask parents about any recent administration of these products. Refer to the most current guidelines from the Centers for Disease Control and Prevention's Advisory Committee on Immunization Practices (ACIP) to identify the correct interval (3 to 11 months) between the administration of the blood product, immune globulin, or completion of immunosuppresion therapy and administration of a life virus vaccine (Kroger, Atkinson, Marcuse, et al., 2006).

If immune globulin is given within 14 days after a live virus vaccine, readminister the vaccine after the period specified, unless serologic testing determines that the child developed adequate serum antibodies (American Academy of Pediatrics, 2009, p. 37).

- Give multiple vaccines at the same visit. Two injections can be given in different sites in the same extremity. Use combination vaccines such as the DTaP-HepB-IPV vaccine to reduce the number of overall injections.
- Give medically stable low-birth-weight infants the same immunizations as full-term infants, according to chronological age with full-dose vaccine, and regardless of most postnatal steroids (Gad & Shah, 2007).
- Give immunization even when a prior dose caused a local reaction or a family member had an adverse response.

The accompanying Nursing Care Plan explores two potential nursing diagnoses that apply to the child needing immunizations. Additional nursing diagnoses may include the following:

- *Risk for Impaired Skin Integrity* related to vaccine response
- *Ineffective Health Maintenance* related to cultural beliefs regarding routine immunization
- *Risk for Injury* related to vaccine reaction

The Nursing Care Plan also emphasizes that nursing management focuses on protecting the potency of vaccines, being a strong advocate for immunization, educating parents about immunizations and possible side effects, addressing their fears about possible reactions, obtaining consent, and reporting adverse reactions.

Nursing Care Plan

THE CHILD NEEDING IMMUNIZATIONS

INTERVENTION	RATIONALE	EXPECTED OUTCOME
1. Nursing Diagnosis: Risk for Infection related to incomplete immunization series		
NIC Priority Interventions: **Immunization Vaccination Management: Administration:** Monitoring immunization status, facilitating access to immunizations, and provision of immunizations to prevent communicable disease.		**NOC Suggested Outcome:** **Immune Status:** Adequacy of natural and acquired appropriately targeted resistance to internal and external antigens.
Goal: The child will become adequately protected from disease-preventable illnesses.		
■ Review the child's immunization record for needed vaccines at each healthcare visit.	■ Assessment identifies the children who have missed needed immunizations.	The child is adequately protected from vaccine-preventable illnesses.
■ Identify all due vaccines that can be provided simultaneously.	■ Multiple vaccines given at the same visit more adequately protects the child.	
■ Identify potential contraindications to needed vaccines. Review past reactions to vaccines.	■ Reduces the risk for the child and other caretakers to have adverse reactions to vaccines.	
2. Nursing Diagnosis: Effective Therapeutic Regimen Management		
NIC Priority Interventions: **Decision-Making Support:** Providing information and support for a patient who is making a decision regarding health care.		**NOC Suggested Outcome:** **Knowledge Treatment: Regimen:** Extent of understanding conveyed about a specific treatment regimen.
Goal: Parents will sign consent for vaccines to be given.		
■ Educate the parents and adolescents about the need for specific vaccines and the risk if not given. Obtain signed consent before giving vaccines.	■ Informed consent is required for all treatments.	The parent(s) complete(s) consent form, which is placed in the child's file.
Goal: Parents and adolescents will state the side effects of vaccines given.		
■ Review past reactions to vaccines and describe common potential reactions and why they occur.	■ Parents should expect common reactions and know they indicate the child's body is building protection to the illness.	Parents report all serious side effects to the healthcare provider.
■ Describe serious side effects that should be reported to the healthcare provider.	■ Parents need to be prepared for potential serious side effects so they can obtain care if needed.	
Goal: Parents will manage common side effects of vaccines.		
■ Teach parents general comfort measures for common side effects; for example: ■ Cool pack to tender leg ■ Acetaminophen or ibuprofen for fever and discomfort ■ Rocking and holding the infant ■ Gentle movement of affected extremity	■ Parents will know how to make the child more comfortable during the 24–48 hours after the vaccine is given.	The child is given comfort measures after vaccine administration.

MyNursingKit Develop Immunization Schedules

MyNursingKit Immunization FAQ

PLANNING AND IMPLEMENTATION

Nursing management focuses on protecting the potency of vaccines, being a strong advocate for immunization, educating parents about immunizations and possible side effects, addressing their fears about possible reactions, obtaining consent, and reporting adverse reactions.

PROTECT VACCINE POTENCY

Take special care to ensure vaccine potency in the following ways:

- Store vaccines properly in the refrigerator or freezer (i.e., separate doors for refrigerator and freezer, storage conditions should be adequate: Refrigeration: 35°F to 46°F [2°C to 8°C]; Freezer: 5°F [−15°C] or lower as stated in vaccine package inserts.
- Keep jugs of water in the refrigerator and trays of ice in the freezer to help maintain a consistent temperature.
- Store the vaccines in the middle of the units; place the older vaccines in the front.
- Check the temperature of each unit twice daily and record the temperatures on a log.
- Review the temperature log weekly, and keep the logs on file for 3 years or use an automatic temperature measurement system (Veraas, 2006).
- Make sure the facility has an emergency plan for safe storage of vaccines in case of a power outage or natural disaster.

OBTAIN CONSENT

Federal legislation requires consent before administering a vaccine. It is often the nurse's responsibility to obtain consent after informing the parents or the child's legal guardian about the needed vaccines and supplying the most current Vaccine Information Statement (VIS) for the vaccines to be given (a requirement of the National Vaccine Injury Act). See MyNursingKit for the Web site with current VIS for each vaccine.

Explain the risks and benefits of each immunization, as well as common local reactions using the information in the VIS. In order for parents to provide informed consent, the nurse needs to be able to answer questions to their satisfaction. If the parent chooses not to accept a particular vaccine, document the informed refusal. If there is a disease outbreak, the nonimmunized child must be kept out of school. Local, city, or state courts decide how to settle any conflicts.

The nurse is required to record the following:

1. month, day, and year of administration
2. vaccine given
3. manufacturer
4. lot number and expiration date of the immunization given
5. site and route of administration
6. name, title, and address of the person who administers the vaccine. In addition, the nurse ensures that any severe immunization reaction is reported to the National Vaccine Injury Compensation Program.

> **Thinking Critically**
>
> **IMMUNIZATIONS**
>
> A 5-year-old girl, Lian, has accompanied her mother and 2-year-old brother Chang to the pediatric clinic. Lian's mother is concerned because Chang has had a fever of 38.3°C (101°F) for the past 3 days. Although Chang has visited this clinic several times in the past few months for health care, this is the first time Lian has come along.
>
> When asked, Lian's mother says Lian had a healthcare visit about 2 years ago, but she does not know if she had all of her shots. In checking Lian's health records, the nurse notes that she needs DTaP, polio, varicella, and hepatitis B vaccines. Chang needs polio, MMR, and Hib vaccines.
>
> Should Lian be given any of these immunizations today, even though her brother is ill? Which immunizations could be given during one visit? Should Chang receive any immunizations today?
>
> See MyNursingKit for possible responses.

ADMINISTER VACCINES

Check the expiration of vaccines before use. Follow the manufacturer's directions for reconstituting vaccines and use the solution provided. Write the date and time on the bottle if it is a multidose vial. Some reconstituted vaccines (varicella and MMR) have a short shelf life and are available only in single-dose vials.

Use of longer needles (25 mm rather than 16 mm) reduces the rate of local reactions and tenderness in infant immunizations. A recent study concluded that 25 mm needles reduced local reactions to the 5th DTaP vaccine, whether the deltoid or vastis lateralis muscle was used (Jackson, Starkovich, Dunstan, et al., 2008). Stretch the skin to decrease the amount of subcutaneous tissue the needle must go through to ensure that the vaccine is given deeply in the muscle mass. Some vaccines are given subcutaneously; for these immunizations, select a 5/8-inch 23- to 25-gauge needle (Kroger, Atkinson, Marcuse, et al., 2006, pp. 16–17).

REDUCE PAIN AND ANXIETY

Make an effort to reduce the pain associated with vaccine injections, especially since infants and children must return for more injections. Give the appropriate immunizations to the child as efficiently as possible, while providing support to the child (Figure 45–3 ●). Suggestions for pain management include the following techniques:

- Coach the parent to hold and talk with the child during the injections. Funny faces, a toy, or other distraction might also help. Provide comfort measures after the injection.
- Give infants up to 4 months of age, 25% sucrose water to drink (mix 1 packet of table sugar with 10 mL of tap water) prior to the injection (see Chapter 42 ∞). Then allow the infant to suck on a pacifier or breastfeed during the injections.
- Apply pressure at the site for 10 seconds before the injection.

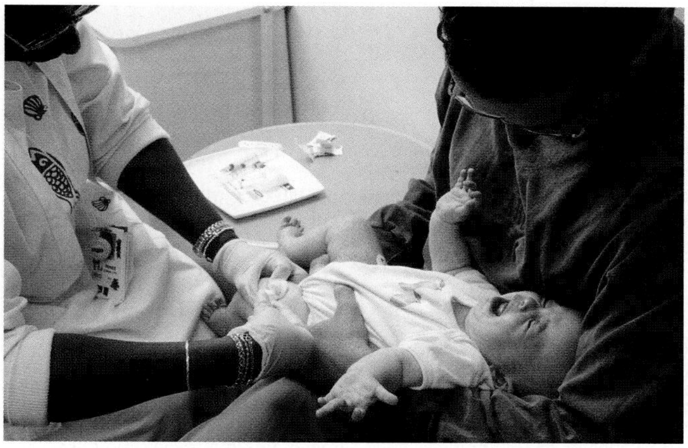

● **Figure 45–3** Giving immunizations. Give immunizations quickly and efficiently. Do not prolong the wait and let fear grow. The child will be anxious, especially if more than one injection must be given.

- Instruct parent how to apply EMLA cream to one or more sites 1 hour before the injection. A prescription can be given at the end of the visit for EMLA, for use at the next visit. See Chapter 42 for information regarding use of EMLA cream.
- Spray vapocoolant spray immediately before the injection on the planned injection site, or spray it on a cotton ball that is then held against the skin.
- Two providers can give two injections simultaneously in different extremities.
- Do not prolong the process of giving immunizations, and give the child honest answers that the needles will cause some pain.
- Let the child select the arm or leg for the injection and forms of distraction to promote coping. After the injections are completed, let the parent comfort the child.

Parents also need guidance for care of the child after immunizations (see the Teaching Highlights).

PREPARE FOR EMERGENCIES

Be prepared for potential vaccine anaphylaxis. Keep epinephrine and resuscitation equipment immediately available. The dose for epinephrine (aqueous 1:1000) is 0.01 mL/kg per dose up to 0.5 mL intramuscularly. The dose can be repeated every 10 to 20 minutes for up to a total of 3 doses until symptoms subside or other emergency care interventions are initiated (AAP, 2009, p. 66).

Remember to report certain severe reactions following immunization to the Vaccine Compensation Injury Program. See Table 45–3.

EVALUATION

Expected outcomes of nursing care include the following:

- Parents are fully informed and give consent for immunizations.

Teaching Highlights

CARE OF THE CHILD AFTER IMMUNIZATIONS

When a child receives an immunization, educate parents to observe for any reactions that might occur.

- Local pain, redness, and swelling are common. Use ice on the sites to help reduce swelling and pain. Acetaminophen or ibuprofen may be given to reduce a fever and pain. The symptoms should disappear in a day or two.
- The child may have a fever, joint pain, muscle aches, or fatigue within hours to days after the vaccine is given. Give acetaminophen or ibuprofen for pain.
- A few hives around the injection site may indicate a mild allergic reaction to the vaccine.
- Call the child's healthcare provider if there is concern about any of the above symptoms.
- A severe allergic reaction is indicated by a flushed face; swelling of the face, mouth, or throat; wheezing or other difficulty breathing; shock (confusion, lack of movement or response, or unconsciousness); and abdominal cramping. Call 911 for emergency treatment. Have the child lie down and raise his or her legs until the ambulance arrives to promote blood return to the vital organs.

- All immunizations appropriate for the child's age are given at each health visit.
- The parents are prepared to manage mild reactions to immunizations at home.

INFECTIOUS AND COMMUNICABLE DISEASES IN CHILDREN

Infectious and communicable diseases cause acute illnesses resulting from bacterial, viral, protozoan, or fungal organisms. Infants and children develop infectious and communicable diseases more frequently than adults do and frequently become symptomatic after exposure. Antibodies are then developed. The epidemiology, clinical manifestations, treatment, prevention, and nursing care of selected infectious and communicable diseases of childhood are described in detail in Table 45–4. Infectious diseases transmitted by animal vectors are detailed in Table 45–5. See Chapter 6 for information on sexually transmitted infections; Chapter 47 for information about conjunctivitis; Chapter 48 for information on tuberculosis; and Chapter 53 for information on hepatitis and parasites.

CLINICAL MANIFESTATIONS

The child with an infectious or communicable disease has a cluster of symptoms specific to the disease that appear at the end of the **incubation period**, the time interval between exposure and

(continues on page 1221)

MyNursingKit Case Study: Reporting an Adverse Vaccine Event

MyNursingKit Immunization Safety Research

Table 45–4 Selected Infectious and Communicable Diseases in Children

Disease	Clinical Manifestations	Clinical Therapy	Nursing Management
		Chickenpox (Varicella)*§	
Causal agent: Varicella-zoster, human herpesvirus 3. *Epidemiology:* Humans are the source of infection. Peak occurrence is in the late fall, winter, and spring. Maternal antibodies disappear 2–3 months after birth. *Transmission:* Direct contact of the virus to the mucous membranes or conjunctiva primarily through airborne secretions and occasionally with lesion contact. *Incubation period:* 14–21 days *Period of communicability:* As long as 5 days before the onset of the rash to a maximum of 6 days after the appearance of vesicles, when all lesions have crusted over. This period may be prolonged after passive immunization or in immunodeficient children. 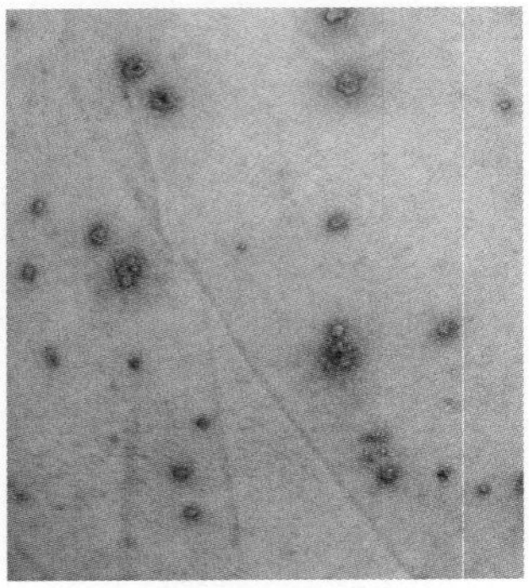	Acute onset of mild fever, malaise, anorexia, headache, mild abdominal pain, and irritability occurs before and with eruption. Macular rash for a few hours that progresses to pruritic vesicular lesions for 1 to 5 days, and then to crusts. Up to 250 to 500 lesions of all stages may be present at any one time (see figure). Crusts may remain for 1–3 weeks. The lesions begin on the trunk, scalp, and face, and then spread to the rest of the body. Ulcerative lesions may be seen in the mucous membranes. Mouth lesions may lead to decreased fluid intake and dehydration. *Complications:* Complications are rare but can include secondary infection (cellulitis, local abscesses, sepsis, meningitis, encephalitis, pneumonia), thrombocytopenia, and Reye syndrome. Chickenpox can be fatal in newborns of infected mothers and immunocompromised children. Monitor children carefully who are undergoing chemotherapy, steroid treatment, or transplant therapy after exposure to the disease.	Fluid from vesicle or scab can be tested using polymerase chain reaction for diagnosis. Medical management is supportive. Oral and IV acyclovir is used for immunocompromised patients, children treated with chronic salicylate therapy, and oral or aerosol corticosteroids (American Academy of Pediatrics, 2009, p. 716). Varicella-zoster immune globulin is given as soon as possible to newborns of infected mothers, premature neonates exposed postnatally, and exposed immunocompromised, unimmunized children up to 4 days after exposure (Marin, Güris, Chaves, et al., 2007). *Prognosis:* Most children recover fully. Children who are immunocompromised or who were treated with corticosteroids during the incubation period must be treated aggressively. *Prevention:* Varicella is vaccine-preventable. See the Drug Guide. The vaccine may be given within 72 hours after exposure to prevent or to significantly modify the disease. Wild virus cases occur in vaccinated children.	■ Use airborne and contact precautions. ■ Isolate all hospitalized children with a recent exposure to varicella to protect newborns and immunocompromised patients. Nurses caring for the child should have documented immunity. ■ At home, isolate the child from susceptible individuals (medically fragile and immunocompromised children or adults, and women early in pregnancy). Notify the school or childcare facility of the child's illness. ■ Secondary cases are often more severe than the primary case. The child with atopic eczema or sunburn may have a more severe rash. ■ Give acetaminophen or ibuprofen to control fever. ■ Control itching with oral antihistamines, soothing oatmeal and Aveeno baths, or Caladryl lotion. ■ Trim the child's fingernails and keep them clean. Place soft cotton mittens over the hands of young children when itching cannot be controlled. ■ Change bed linens frequently. ■ Reassure the child that the lesions are temporary and will go away. ■ Observe the child for signs of complications (e.g., drowsiness, meningeal signs, respiratory distress, and dehydration). Disorientation and restlessness may indicate viral encephalitis. ■ Monitor for acyclovir side effects (e.g., nausea, vomiting, diarrhea, abdominal pain, allergic skin reactions, headache). Monitor renal function if the child has renal insufficiency.
		Coxsackievirus	
Causal Agent: Coxsackievirus A16 and Enterovirus 71 *Epidemiology*: Occurs worldwide, most commonly in summer and early fall. Sporadic outbreaks are seen, especially among children in out-of-home settings. Immunity probably occurs after clinical or subclinical infection, but duration of the immunity is unknown. *Transmission*: Fecal-oral and respiratory routes. *Incubation period*: 3–6 days. *Period of communicability*: 2 days before rash to 2 days after it disappears.	Each of the coxsackieviruses causes a different set of manifestations. Herpangina is characterized by the sudden onset of fever, sore throat, and small, discrete grayish papulovesicular ulcerative pharyngeal lesions that gradually increase in size. In hand, foot, and mouth disease, lesions are more diffuse and may occur on the buccal surfaces of the cheeks, gums, and sides of the tongue. Papulovesicular lesions occur on the hands and feet and last for 7–10 days. Children may be irritable; experience fever, anorexia, dysphagia, malaise, and a sore throat. *Complications*: Children with immune deficiencies may have persistent central nervous system infections (American Academy of Pediatrics, 2009, p. 287).	Diagnosis usually based on clinical signs. Diagnostic tests include a cell culture to detect the virus. Medical care is supportive. Immune globulin IV may be used in life threatening neonatal infections and in immunodeficient children with chronic meningoencephalitis (American Academy of Pediatrics, 2009, p. 288). *Prognosis*: Recovery is generally good with supportive care. Children with central nervous system and cardiopulmonary failure may have delayed neurodevelopment and reduced cognitive functioning (Chang, Huang, Gau, et al., 2007). *Prevention*: Avoid contact with infected persons early in the disease.	■ Isolate the child while contagious. Use standard and contact precautions if the child is hospitalized. ■ Apply topical lotions and give systemic medications as ordered to lessen the pain and relieve the irritation. ■ Offer cool drinks and soft, bland foods (no citrus, salty, or spicy foods). Swallowing may be painful. Observe for dehydration. ■ Offer warm saline mouth rinses. ■ Provide reassurance and support to parents. ■ Give nonaspirin antipyretics for fever. Keep the child out of school or child care while the child is febrile.

Table 45–4 Selected Infectious and Communicable Diseases in Children—continued

Disease	Clinical Manifestations	Clinical Therapy	Nursing Management
		Diphtheria*§	
Causal agent: Corynebacterium diphtheriae *Epidemiology:* Occurs mostly in colder months in unimmunized, partially immunized, and immunized children with waning immunity. Cases of cutaneous and wound diphtheria occur sporadically in the tropics. Maternal immunity lasts up to 6 months after birth. The disease is endemic in areas where immunization is no longer routine. *Transmission:* Contact with nasal or eye discharge, or skin lesion; or less commonly by indirect contact with contaminated items. Unpasteurized milk has served as a vehicle. *Incubation period:* 2–7 days or longer. *Period of communicability:* Usually 2–4 weeks or until 4 days after antibiotics are started.	Symptoms can be mild or severe with a gradual onset over 1–2 days. Low-grade fever, anorexia, malaise, rhinorrhea with a foul odor, cough, sore throat, hoarseness, stridor or noisy breathing, cervical lymphadenitis, and pharyngitis may be present. In more severe cases a membranous lesion (thick, bluish-white to grayish-black patch that covers the tonsils) can spread to cover the soft and hard palates and the posterior portion of the pharynx. Attempts at removing the membrane causes bleeding. *Complications:* Produces an endotoxin that causes myocarditis and peripheral neuropathy (diplopia, slurred speech, difficulty swallowing, or paralysis of the palate) or ascending paralysis similar to Guillain-Barré syndrome.	Diagnostic tests include a culture from any mucosal or cutaneous lesion. Antitoxin and antibiotics (penicillin G or erythromycin) are administered IV within 3 days of symptom onset, without waiting for laboratory results. Test the child for sensitivity to horse serum before giving the antitoxin. The membrane may need to be removed to treat airway obstruction. *Prognosis:* With treatment, prognosis is good. If untreated, death may occur due to airway obstruction. *Prevention:* Diphtheria is a vaccine-preventable disease. See the Drug Guide. This is a reportable disease.	■ Use droplet precautions for pharyngeal disease and contact precautions for cutaneous disease. ■ Monitor closely for signs of increasing respiratory distress, as well as cardiac and neurologic complications. Provide humidified oxygen as necessary. ■ Have emergency airway equipment available. ■ Administer antibiotics. Give no medications containing caffeine or other stimulants. ■ Use oral suction gently as necessary. ■ Allow children to use mouthwash if desired. Gargling is not permitted because it can irritate the pharyngeal surfaces. ■ Encourage liquids as tolerated. Intravenous fluids may be necessary. ■ Provide emotional support to the family. ■ Initiate the search for patient contacts to give antibiotics and immunization boosters.
		Erythema Infectiosum (Fifth Disease)	
Causal agent: Human parvovirus B19 *Epidemiology:* Occurs worldwide, most often in winter and spring. Also occurs in epidemics, with peak activity every 6 years. The incidence is highest in children between the ages of 5 and 14 years. *Transmission:* Respiratory secretions and blood, as well as mother to fetus (Dyer, 2007). *Incubation period:* 6–21 days *Period of communicability:* Believed to be the highest the week before symptom onset. 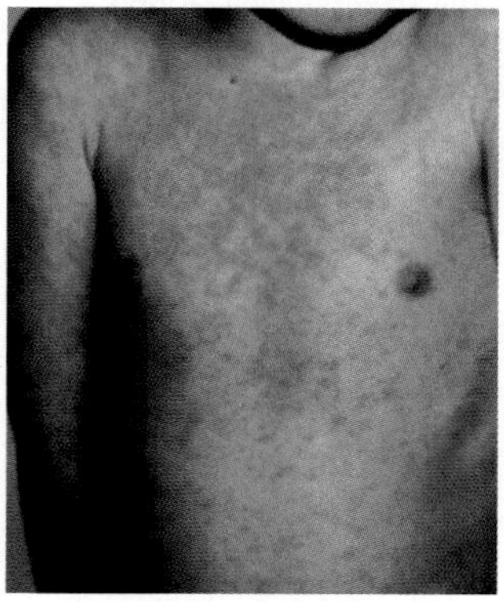	Stage 1 begins as a flulike illness (headache, chills, malaise, nausea, body ache) lasting 2–3 days, followed by a symptom-free period of 1–7 days. Stage 2: a fiery-red rash on the cheeks giving a "slapped face" appearance and circumoral pallor. In 1–4 days a lace-like symmetric, erythematous, maculopapular rash appears on the trunk and limbs, spreading proximal to distal but sparing the palms and soles (see figure). Stage 3 lasts 1–3 weeks as the rash fades, but can reappear if the skin is irritated or exposed to sunlight. The rash may be mildly pruritic. *Complications:* Children with hemolytic conditions may have transient aplastic crisis. Arthritis and arthralgia may occur.	Diagnosis by physical signs, or a serologic test for immunoglobulin (Ig) M parvovirus B19-specific antibody (important when exposure to a pregnant woman is likely). Treatment is supportive and recovery is usually spontaneous. Children with hemolytic conditions may need blood transfusions if an aplastic crisis occurs. Immunodeficient patients may develop a chronic infection for which IV immune globulin therapy is often effective (American Academy of Pediatrics, 2009, p. 493). *Prognosis:* Fetal infection may occur resulting in fetal hydrops or spontaneous abortion. *Prevention:* Avoid contact with infected persons. Exposed pregnant women should promptly seek medical attention.	■ Children with aplastic crisis are often hospitalized. ■ Use standard and droplet precautions. Isolation is needed only for children with aplastic crisis or when immunosuppressed. ■ Give acetaminophen or ibuprofen to control fever. ■ Use soothing oatmeal or Aveeno baths if the rash is pruritic. Antipruritics may also help to relieve itching. ■ Encourage rest and offer frequent fluids. ■ Keep children out of direct sunlight if possible. Provide protective, light, loose clothing if exposure to sunlight cannot be avoided. ■ Provide quiet diversionary activity. ■ There is no reason to keep the immune competent child out of school or day care. ■ Explain the three stages of rash development to parents.

(continued)

Table 45–4 Selected Infectious and Communicable Diseases in Children—continued

Disease	Clinical Manifestations	Clinical Therapy	Nursing Management
		***Haemophilus Influenzae*, Type B§**	
Causal agent: Coccobacilli *H. influenzae* bacteria (several serotypes, encapsulated or nonencapsulated). *Epidemiology:* Occurs most often in the spring and summer. Most commonly affected are infants and young children in childcare centers. Low-birth-weight children and children with chronic illnesses have an increased susceptibility. *Transmission:* Direct contact or droplet inhalation. Asymptomatic colonization in the respiratory tract is common. *Incubation period:* Unknown. *Period of communicability:* 3 days from onset of symptoms.	Begins with a viral upper respiratory infection. The organism passes through the mucosal barrier to directly invade the bloodstream. It can cause several severe invasive illnesses, including meningitis, epiglottitis, pneumonia, septic arthritis, and cellulitis. It is also a cause of sepsis in infants, and other illnesses such as sinusitis, otitis media, bronchitis, and pericarditis. Each disease has specific clinical manifestations. Invasive disease has decreased 99% since introduction of the vaccine (American Academy of Pediatrics, 2009, p. 315). *Complications:* If untreated by antibiotics, severe sequelae and death can occur from conditions such as meningitis, epiglottitis, sinusitis, pneumonitis, and cellulitis, especially in young infants.	Diagnosed by culture of blood, cerebrospinal fluid, or middle ear aspirate. Treatment consists of antibiotic therapy. Rifampin may be given to unprotected household contacts (not pregnant women), if another child has not completed immunizations, within 1 week after diagnosis. *Prognosis:* With rapid diagnosis and treatment, recovery is good but highly dependent on the disease the organism has caused. When treatment is delayed, the prognosis for full recovery becomes much more guarded. *Prevention:* Immunization is now available for *H. influenzae* type B. See the Drug Guide.	■ Use droplet precautions until 24 hours after the initiation of antibiotics. ■ Antibiotic therapy is administered intravenously for severe infections. Infections such as otitis media can be managed with oral antibiotics. ■ Unimmunized children younger than 4 years are at increased risk for developing disease from *H. influenzae.* Specific prophylactic measures for susceptible children may be ordered by the physician. ■ Administer acetaminophen or ibuprofen to increase the child's comfort. ■ Perform nursing care measures specific to the illness. ■ Inform family members that rifampin turns urine and other body fluids orange, and it will cause stains.
		Influenza§	
Causal agent: Orthomyxoviridae, types A and B. *Epidemiology:* Prevalent in the United States from October to March, but the virus is active in other parts of the world year-round. During annual epidemics, 10% to 40% of healthy children can be infected (American Academy of Pediatrics, 2009, p. 401). *Transmission:* Spreads by aerosolized particles and direct contact with respiratory secretions. *Incubation period:* 1 to 4 days. *Period of communicability:* One day before symptoms until 5 days after onset of illness.	Abrupt onset of fever (38°C to 40°C), chills, cough, runny nose, sore throat, malaise, aches, headache, and anorexia. Children may have nausea and vomiting, diarrhea, and abdominal pain. Children may also present with croup, bronchiolitis, conjunctivitis, or other nonspecific febrile illness. *Complications:* Otitis media, exacerbations of chronic lung conditions such as asthma and cystic fibrosis. Pneumonia, croup, bronchiolitis, and wheezing may occur in up to 25% of children. Myositis, myocarditis, encephalitis, transverse myelitis, Reye syndrome, and Guillain-Barré syndrome are all potential complications.	Diagnostic tests may include viral culture, rapid antigen testing from throat or nasopharynx, polymerase chain reaction, and immuno-fluorescence. Influenza rapid antigen detection tests are available (Grijalva, Poehling, Edwards, et al., 2007). Treatment is supportive. Antiviral agents are given to children at high risk for severe infection (American Academy of Pediatrics, 2007). Oseltamivir, and zanamivir are approved for children 1 year of age or older, and relenza is approved for children 5 years and older (Food and Drug Administration, 2006a). When antiviral medication is initiated within 2 days of symptoms the duration of symptoms may be reduced by 1 to 1½ days. *Prevention:* Influenza vaccine is now recommended for children between 6 and 59 months of age. See the Drug Guide.	■ Use droplet and contact precautions for hospitalized infants and children. ■ The child is usually cared for at home. Encourage parents to wash hands frequently and to reduce exposure of other family members to the infected child. ■ Provide fluids to keep nasal secretions moist and to prevent dehydration. ■ Provide acetaminophen or ibuprofen for fever management and mild pain. ■ If antiviral medications are given, be alert for nausea and vomiting. Zanamivir can exacerbate asthma. Oseltamivir (Tamiflu) is being monitored for cases of delirium and self-injury in children (Food and Drug Administration, 2006b). ■ Provide rest and quiet diversional activities. ■ Teach parents to be alert to signs of complications from the viral infection.
		Measles (Rubeola)*§	
Causal agent: Morbillivirus, a member of the paramyxovirus group. *Epidemiology:* Occurrence peaks in the late winter and early spring. Cases continue to occur in the US, primarily in unimmunized children and adolescents (Centers for Disease Control, 2008c). Many	Children are quite ill in the 3–5 day prodromal phase, with symptoms including high fever, conjunctivitis, coryza, cough, anorexia, and malaise. Koplik spots (small, irregular, bluish white spots on a red background) appear on the buccal mucosa about 2 days before and after the rash appears.	Diagnosis can be made by a serologic test for immunoglobulin (Ig) M measles antibody. Treatment is supportive. No antiviral therapy is available. Antibiotics are used for secondary bacterial infections. *Prognosis:* Recovery is generally good with supportive care.	■ If the child is hospitalized, maintain airborne precautions during the contagious period. ■ Use a cool-mist vaporizer to help clear respiratory passages. ■ Suction nose and oral cavity gently as necessary. ■ Give nonaspirin antipyretics for fever and antipruritics for itching.

Table 45–4 Selected Infectious and Communicable Diseases in Children—continued

Disease	Clinical Manifestations	Clinical Therapy	Nursing Management
cases are imported from developing countries without routine immunization. Maternal immunity is active until the infant is age 12–15 months. *Transmission:* Airborne, respiratory droplets and contact with infected persons. *Incubation period:* About 8–12 days. *Period of communicability:* Begins during the prodromal phase and ends 2–4 days after the rash appears.	The characteristic red, blotchy, maculopapular rash that becomes confluent usually appears 2–4 days after onset of prodromal phase. The rash begins on the face and spreads to the trunk and extremities (see figure). Symptoms gradually subside in 4–7 days. Other symptoms include anorexia, malaise, fatigue, and generalized lymphadenopathy. *Complications:* Diarrhea, otitis media, bronchopneumonia, bronchitis, laryngotracheobronchitis, and encephalitis. Complications and sequelae occur most often in children who are malnourished, medically fragile, and immunosuppressed. The younger the child, the greater the risk for complications.	*Prevention:* Measles is a vaccine-preventable disease. See the Drug Guide. Immune globulin, administered up to 6 days after exposure, may be helpful in preventing the disease in susceptible persons (immunocompromised children, infants less than 1 year of age, pregnant women). All healthcare workers should have documented immunity. This is a reportable disease. 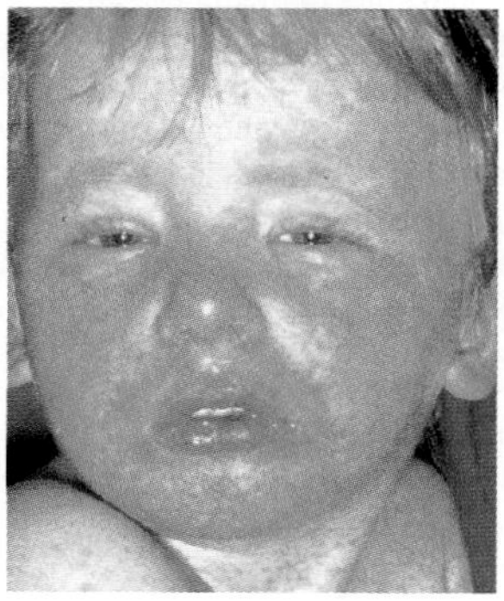	■ Assess lungs carefully, especially in young children, in whom pneumonias are a common complication. ■ Antitussives may be ordered to control coughing. ■ Keep lights dim, and cover windows if the child has photophobia. ■ Elevate the head of the bed. Keep the room cool with good air circulation. Provide light, nonirritating blankets. ■ Keep skin clean and dry. No soaps. ■ Maintain fluid intake. Offer cool liquids frequently in small amounts. Blended, pureed, and mashed foods are most easily tolerated. ■ Maintain bed rest. Visitors should be immune to measles. ■ Provide diversions such as music, stories, and favorite toys.
Meningococcus			
Causal Agent: Neisseria meningitides, a gram-negative diplococcus. *Epidemiology:* Often occurs in winter or early spring. Majority of infections in the U.S. are caused by serogroups B, C, and Y. Highest rates are in children under 2 years and in 11 years and older (Bilukha & Rosenstein, 2005). Outbreaks have occurred in child care centers, college dormitories, and military recruit camps. Groups at risk for invasive disease include those with asplenia (Gardner, 2006). *Transmission:* Direct contact with droplet respiratory secretions. *Incubation period:* 1 to 10 days *Period of communicability:* until 24 hours after antibiotic started.	Abrupt onset of flu-like symptoms of fever, chills, malaise, muscle aches, stiff neck, vomiting, and **prostration** (extreme exhaustion). Meningitis is the most common invasive disease with neurologic signs of drowsiness, disorientation, hallucinations, and convulsions (Kaplan, Schutze, Leake, et al., 2007). Meningococcemia: An urticarial, maculopapular or petechial rash appears that may progress to purpura. The condition may further deteriorate to shock, hypotension, disseminated intravascular coagulation (DIC), and coma. *Complications:* Approximately 10% to 20% of patients have severe morbidities such as limb amputations and hearing loss (Milonovich, 2007).	Diagnostic tests include cultures of the blood and cerebrospinal fluid culture, and a Gram stain of petechial skin scrapings. Treatment is with penicillin G given IV (cefotaxime, ceftriaxone, and ampicillin are alternate antibiotics); chloramphenicol for children allergic to penicillin. The child is managed aggressively in the ICU to provide respiratory support and manage shock with IV fluids and vasopressers. Plasma, blood or platelets are used to treat DIC. *Prognosis*: About 8% of all patients with invasive disease die, but the mortality rate is higher for children 11 years and older (21.2%) (Kaplan, Schutze, Leake, et al., 2007). *Prevention*: A vaccine has been approved for adolescents 11 years and older. Vaccine available for children older than 2 years with asplenia and other high risk conditions. Neither vaccine protects against serogroup B which causes 50% of illnesses in infants and young children (Gardner, 2006). This is a reportable disease.	■ Use standard precautions and droplet precautions until antibiotic has been administered for 24 hours. Disease onset is abrupt and rapidly progresses to life threatening. Be alert for development of shock and respiratory compromise. Have emergency equipment available and be prepared to perform resuscitation. ■ When giving IV fluids and blood products, make sure the child does not get overloaded with fluids, and monitor for evidence of increased intracranial pressure. ■ Keep the family informed of the child's status and treatment as the disease progresses. Help the family to mobilize its support system. ■ The surviving child will likely need rehabilitation. Work with the social worker or case manager to transition the child to long-term care. ■ Help identify close contacts that should receive prophylactic antibiotics, preferably within 24 hours, and educate them about the expected side effects (i.e., orange urine with rifampin). ■ Teach close contacts to be observant for signs of illness and to seek health care promptly if they occur.

(continued)

Table 45–4 Selected Infectious and Communicable Diseases in Children—continued

Disease	Clinical Manifestations	Clinical Therapy	Nursing Management
	Mononucleosis		
Causal agent: Epstein-Barr virus (EBV), a member of the herpesvirus group. *Epidemiology:* Occurs worldwide in no seasonal pattern. Infection commonly occurs early in life, and spread among family members is common. Infection during adolescence is common in the U.S. (Junker, 2005). *Transmission:* Direct contact with infected oropharyngeal and genital tract secretions. EBV can survive for several hours outside the body. EBV can also be transmitted by blood transfusion. *Incubation period:* 30–50 days. *Period of communicability:* Infected individuals may become asymptomatic carriers (American Academy of Pediatrics, 2009, p. 290).	Very young children may have irritability, but be otherwise asymptomatic. A maculopapular rash may be seen. Disease characteristics in other children include malaise, headache, anorexia, abdominal pain, fatigue, and fever for 2–3 days, followed by lymphadenopathy and a sore throat. Hepatosplenomegaly may occur. Pain from swelling of the tonsils and lymph nodes may be significant. The self-limited syndrome typically lasts 2–3 weeks. Weakness and lethargy may continue for several months. *Complications:* Rare side effects include central nervous system symptoms such as encephalitis, aseptic meningitis, and Guillain-Barré syndrome. Splenic rupture, respiratory failure, and thrombocytopenia can also occur. In immunodeficient children, fatal infections or lymphomas can develop.	Diagnostic tests include the serologic monospot test or a heterophil antibody response test. Greater than 10% atypical lymphocytes and a positive heterophil antibody response test are diagnostic (American Academy of Pediatrics, 2009, p. 290). Treatment is supportive. Corticosteroids may be used to control tonsillar swelling and pain when there is impending airway obstruction, massive splenomegaly, myocarditis, or hemolytic anemia. Antibiotics (ampicillin and amoxicillin) should be avoided as a nonallergic rash often develops (American Academy of Pediatrics, 2009, p. 291). *Prognosis:* After recovery, the virus remains latent in the lymphoid system. It can be reactivated during periods of immunosuppression. *Prevention:* No known prevention.	■ Children are usually treated at home. Standard precautions should be used. ■ Give antipyretics and analgesics for fever and sore throat. Offer warm salt water for gargling. Offer soft foods and encourage fluids. ■ Maintain bed rest during acute phase. ■ Give adolescents a sense of responsibility by involving them in decisions about care whenever possible. Be sure to include parents and adolescents in discussions. ■ Reassure adolescents that they can return to school when the fever is gone and swallowing is normal. ■ Teens should avoid kissing until the fever has been gone several days. ■ Contact sports should be avoided until the liver and spleen are normal, usually in about 4 weeks. ■ If splenomegaly is present, alcohol should be avoided for 3 months after liver function test results return to normal.
	Mumps (Parotitis)§		
Causal agent: Rubulavirus in the Paramyxoviridae family. *Epidemiology:* Occurs worldwide in unvaccinated children, most often in winter and spring. Infection and vaccination induce lifelong immunity. Maternal antibodies begin to disappear in infants at the age of 12–15 months. The majority of U.S. cases occur in persons aged 18 to 24 years (Reef, Dayan, Bellini, et al., 2006). *Transmission:* Contact with respiratory tract secretions. *Incubation period:* 12–25 days. *Period of communicability:* 1–2 days before parotid swelling until 9 days after swelling subsides.	Malaise; low-grade fever; and earache, headache, pain with chewing, decreased appetite and activity; followed by bilateral or unilateral parotid gland swelling (see figure). Swelling peaks around the third day. Meningeal signs (stiff neck, headache, and photophobia) occur in about 15% of patients. *Complications:* **Orchitis** (inflammation of the epididymis, pain on testicular palpation, and scrotal swelling—most often unilateral) may occur in postpubertal males; sterility is relatively rare (American Academy of Pediatrics, 2009, p. 468). Oophoritis, pancreatitis, aseptic meningoencephalitis, and unilateral permanent deafness are sometimes seen. 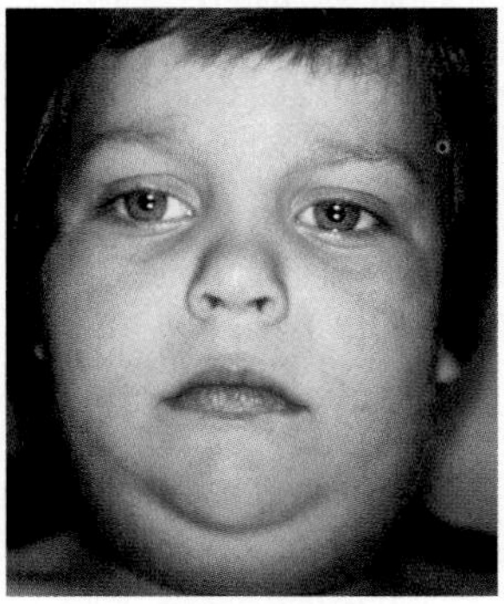	Diagnostic tests include a viral culture from a throat washing, urine, or cerebrospinal fluid. Serum mumps immunoglobulin (Ig) G antibody titer may also be performed. Therapy is supportive, focused on symptom relief. *Prognosis:* Mumps is usually self-limiting. *Prevention:* Mumps is a vaccine-preventable disease. See the Drug Guide. This is a reportable disease. In 2006, an outbreak of nearly 2,600 cases occurred in 11 states after infection case was imported from Britain (Centers for Disease Control, 2006).	■ Use standard and droplet precautions for hospitalized children while contagious. ■ Children are usually cared for at home. They are generally uncomfortable but are rarely very ill. ■ Avoid exposure to immunocompromised or susceptible individuals. ■ Give acetaminophen or ibuprofen to control fever and pain. ■ Encourage fluid intake. Swallowing and chewing may be painful. Offer soft and blended foods. Avoid foods and beverages that increase salivary flow (citrus, spices, and candies) and cause pain. ■ Apply warm or cool compresses, whichever is preferred, to the parotid area. ■ Be alert for signs of complications. Provide scrotal supports if testicular swelling occurs. ■ Keep children out of school or childcare until 9 days after parotid swelling occurs. Encourage diversional activities.

Table 45–4 Selected Infectious and Communicable Diseases in Children—continued

Disease	Clinical Manifestations	Clinical Therapy	Nursing Management
	Pertussis (Whooping Cough)§		
Causal agent: Bordetella pertussis. *Epidemiology:* Occurs worldwide. Rates have increased due to waning immunity: among children 5 to 14 years, adolescents, and adults (Wilson, 2006). This group can spread the disease to unimmunized children. Immunity by infection or vaccine does not last long (Cherry, 2005). *Transmission:* Respiratory droplets and direct contact with respiratory membrane discharge. *Incubation period:* 7–21 days (commonly 7–10 days). *Period of communicability:* 1 week after exposure. Communicable for 5–7 days post beginning antibiotic therapy, and most contagious before the paroxysmal cough stage.	The onset is insidious. *Catarrhal stage:* begins with nasal congestion, a runny nose, low-grade fever, and a mild nonproductive cough, lasting about 2 weeks. *Paroxysmal stage:* The cough is more severe at night and becomes paroxysmal when the child attempts to expel a thick mucoid plug. The child then takes a forceful inspiration through a narrowed glottis causing the "whooping." (Young infants do not "whoop," rather they present with frequent apnea.) Sucking on a bottle may trigger coughing. Coughing may be accompanied by flushing; cyanosis; vomiting; and profuse drainage from the nose, eyes, and mouth. Dehydration may result from decreased oral intake. *Convalescent stage:* Up to 6 weeks when paroxysms gradually subside. Adolescents and adults have upper respiratory infection symptoms with persistent coughing spasms lasting longer than 7 days. *Complications:* Pneumonia, atelectasis, otitis media, encephalopathy, seizures, and death.	Diagnostic tests: culture and polymerase chain reaction (PCR) testing. Treatment with macrolide antibiotics (erythromycin, azithromycin and clarithromycin); corticosteroids, if ordered; and supportive care. *Prognosis:* The disease is most severe in infants younger than 1 year, and most deaths occur in this age group. *Prevention:* Pertussis is a vaccine-preventable disease. See the Drug Guide. A new vaccine is approved for adolescents and adults. Close contacts should be treated with macrolide antibiotics for prophylaxis (Tiwari, Murphy, & Moran, 2005). Vaccine protection wanes after 5 to 10 years. This is a reportable disease. An estimated 800,000 to 3.3 million cases occur in the U.S. per year in a cyclic pattern (Cherry, 2005).	■ Use droplet precautions until 5–7 days after antibiotics are initiated. Most hospitalized cases occur in children younger than age 5. ■ Use a cardiac monitor and pulse oximetry to continuously assess respirations and oxygen saturation. The smaller the child, the greater the risk for respiratory distress and apnea. ■ Remain with the child during coughing spells, when hypoxic and apneic episodes are most likely. Give oxygen if ordered. Have emergency equipment available. ■ Provide humidification. Gentle suctioning may be necessary. ■ Give nonaspirin antipyretics as needed for fever. ■ Encourage frequent rest periods. ■ Allow the child to eat desired foods in small frequent feedings. ■ Encourage the child to take fluids. The child may need IV hydration if oral intake is not tolerated. ■ Provide emotional support to parents. ■ Teach parents to watch for signs of respiratory failure and dehydration if the child is managed at home.
	Pneumococcal infection§		
Causative agent: Streptococcus pneumoniae, a gram-positive diplococcus. *Epidemiology:* Found in the pharynx of healthy people. Outbreaks occur in winter and spring In temperate climates, 8 of 90 serotypes account for most of the invasive pediatric infections. Most common in African Americans, American Indians, and Alaska Natives. Of particular concern is the development of penicillin and multiantibiotic-resistant strains. *Transmission:* Respiratory secretions, and droplets. *Incubation period:* 1–3 days. *Period of communicability:* Unknown. Probably less than 24 hours after effective antibiotic therapy is initiated.	The signs and symptoms are related to the focal area of infection. The organism causes otitis media, sinusitis, pharyngitis, laryngotracheobronchitis, pneumonia, meningitis, and bacteremia. Otitis media—upper respiratory infection, fever, ear pain, and decreased appetite. Bacteremia—unexplained fever and no localized infection site. Pneumonia—fever, chills, chest pain, dyspnea, malaise, and a productive cough. Meningitis—inconsolable crying, increased irritability, lethargy, refusal to eat, nausea, vomiting, diarrhea, myalgia, photophobia, and seizures. *Complications:* Prior to the introduction of a vaccine, this was a major cause of otitis media, sinusitis, meningitis, bacteremia, and pneumonia. Other complications include septic arthritis, osteomyelitis, endocarditis, and brain abscess.	Diagnostic test is a bacterial culture from the site of infection. Symptomatic care is provided. Antibiotic selection is based on susceptibility of organism to penicillin, macrolides, and others. Up to 50% of pneumococcal strains are penicillin resistant. Third generation cephalosporins (cefotaxime or ceftriaxone) may be used. Vancomycin and rifampin may be used in combination when strains are resistant to antibiotics listed above (American Academy of Pediatrics, 2009, p. 528). *Prevention:* Many serotypes are preventable with immunization. See the Drug Guide and Table 45–1. Significant reduction in invasive disease and antibiotic resistant strains caused by serotypes in the vaccine have occurred since initiation vaccination of infants. However strains not in the vaccine are emerging to cause invasive disease (Pichichero & Casey, 2007).	■ If the child is hospitalized, maintain standard precautions. ■ Provide nonaspirin antipyretics for control of fever and comfort. ■ Encourage fluids, and monitor intake and output. ■ Monitor vital signs and level of consciousness to identify signs of worsening condition. ■ Educate parents about the need for the vaccine, as the unimmunized child could become infected repeatedly with different serotypes. ■ Many children with mild disease will be treated at home. Educate parents about signs indicating a need to seek additional medical care, the need for proper medication administration, and comfort measures for the child. ■ Individuals with congenital asplenia, traumatic splenectomy, malignancy, sickle cell disease, and nephrotic syndrome are at higher risk for invasive disease. ■ Additional factors that increase risk of pneumococcal disease include poverty, crowded housing, homelessness, and exposure to tobacco smoke.

(continued)

Table 45–4 Selected Infectious and Communicable Diseases in Children—continued

Disease	Clinical Manifestations	Clinical Therapy	Nursing Management
		Poliomyelitis§	
Causal agent: Poliovirus is an enterovirus with three serotypes. *Epidemiology:* Occurs worldwide. Primarily affects children and immunocompromised or unimmunized adults caring for infants who received live poliovirus vaccine. Since live poliovirus vaccine was discontinued in the United States, no vaccine-associated paralytic poliomyelitis have been reported since 2000 (American Academy of Pediatrics, 2009, p. 541). *Transmission:* Primarily by the fecal-oral route, but also the respiratory route. *Incubation period:* Usually 7–10 days (range 3–36 days). *Period of communicability:* Greatest shortly before and with onset of clinical symptoms when the virus is in the throat. Excreted in the feces for several weeks.	Affects the central nervous system. Less severe cases may be limited to fever and stiffness in the neck and back, headache, vomiting, and sore throat. In more severe cases, fever, headache, stiff neck, Kernig or Brudzinski sign, decreased deep tendon reflexes, and progressive weakness occur. Respiratory difficulty occurs with cranial nerve involvement and may interfere with the ability to talk because frequent pauses are needed. Onset of paralysis may be sudden, in hours, or gradual over 3–5 days. Paralysis results from damage to motor neurons. *Complications:* Permanent motor paralysis, respiratory arrest, myocardial failure, aseptic meningitis, and postpolio syndrome.	Diagnosis is made by cell culture from stool or throat swabs. Treatment is supportive. No chemotherapeutic agents that directly kill the poliovirus are available. *Prognosis:* Respiratory paralysis may lead to death. Motor paralysis may result in long-term disability. *Prevention:* Poliomyelitis is a vaccine-preventable disease. See the Drug Guide. This is a reportable disease.	■ Use standard and droplet precautions in the hospital and keep the child on strict bed rest. ■ Observe closely for respiratory paralysis (ineffective cough, talking with frequent pauses, shallow and rapid respiratory rate). Have emergency equipment at bedside. Assist ventilations as needed until mechanical ventilation is set up. ■ Administer sedatives and nonaspirin analgesics as ordered to allow for rest and comfort. Moist hot packs may relieve discomfort. ■ Encourage fluids. ■ Position the child to promote body alignment. ■ Perform range of motion exercises to prevent contractures after the acute phase. ■ Provide emotional support. ■ Patients are alert and aware. Tell them what is happening to them. ■ Long-term orthopedic (physical therapy) support may be needed by some children.
		Roseola (Exanthem Subitum, 6th Disease)	
Causal agent: Herpesvirus type 6. *Epidemiology:* Occurs worldwide, primarily in children 6–24 months of age (after maternal antibodies decline). Intrauterine transmission may also occur (Moore & Kalvaitis, 2007). *Transmission:* Likely to be from respiratory secretions of healthy individuals. *Incubation period:* Appears to be 5–15 days. *Period of communicability:* Asymptomatic virus shedding in healthy individuals (American Academy of Pediatrics, 2009, p. 378).	Prodrome: sudden, high fever up to 40.5°C (105°F) for 3–8 days, during which the child has a normal appetite and behavior. The fever phase is followed by a characteristic pale pink, discrete, maculopapular rash, lasting 1 to 2 days, starting on the trunk and spreading to the face, neck, and extremities. The child may have mild upper respiratory symptoms, tympanic membrane redness, and cervical/occipital lymphadenopathy (Dyer, 2007). *Complications:* Children may have febrile seizures during high fever stage. Encephalopathy may develop in rare cases.	Roseola is self-limiting, and treatment is supportive. *Prognosis:* Roseola is benign in most cases. Nearly all children older than 4 years have an antibody titer to HHV-6 (American Academy of Pediatrics, 2009, p. 379).	■ Children are rarely hospitalized, but if they are, use standard precautions. ■ Give nonaspirin antipyretics to control fever. ■ Observe closely for any seizure activity, especially during the acute febrile periods. ■ Encourage fluids. ■ Reassure parents that the rash will disappear in a few days.
		Rotavirus§	
Causal agent: Reoviridae family of rotaviruses *Epidemiology:* Occurs during late fall to early spring in yearly diarrhea epidemics in the U.S. Most common cause of severe diarrhea in children younger than 5 years. *Transmission:* Fecal-oral route *Incubation:* 1 to 3 days *Period of communicability:* Virus is present in stool before onset and may persist for 21 days after symptom onset.	Acute onset of fever (in some cases higher than 39°C [102° F]) and vomiting followed by watery diarrhea 1 to 2 days later. Up to 10–20 diarrheal stools a day. Symptoms lasting 3 to 8 days. *Complications*: Dehydration and electrolyte disturbances. It is a major cause of childhood death in developing countries (Parashar, Alexander, & Glass, 2006).	Diagnosis by enzyme immunoassay or latex agglutination assay of a stool specimen. Treatment involves adequate amounts of oral rehydration solution. Introducing a regular diet within a few hours of rehydration shortens the duration of the disease (Dennehy, 2005). If severely dehydrated, IV fluid resuscitation is performed. No antiviral therapy is available.	■ Use standard and contact precautions. Rotavirus is an important cause of nosocomial gastroenteritis (Parashar, Alexander, & Glass, 2006). ■ Hand hygiene with soap and water removes 75% of virus from contaminated hands. Use of alcohol-based hand sanitizers after washing with soap and water increases effectiveness (Dennehy, 2005). ■ Clean contaminated surfaces and follow by disinfecting with an alcohol-containing disinfectant (Dennehy, 2005).

Table 45–4 Selected Infectious and Communicable Diseases in Children—continued

Disease	Clinical Manifestations	Clinical Therapy	Nursing Management
Rotavirus§—continued			
		Prevention: A vaccine is approved for regular administration to infants. See the Drug Guide.	■ Assess hydration status frequently. ■ Continue breastfeeding during oral rehydration therapy. Formula feeding can begin 12 to 24 hours after starting oral rehydration therapy. ■ Feed older children complex carbohydrates and lean meats, yogurt, fruits, and vegetables 12 to 24 hours after starting oral rehydration therapy.
Rubella (German Measles)§			
Causal agent: An RNA virus, member of the family Togaviridae, genus *Rubivirus.* *Epidemiology:* Occurs worldwide. Most prevalent in winter and spring. Maternal antibodies disappear 6–9 months after birth. Most U.S. cases occur among unimmunized foreign-born Hispanic adults. Congenital rubella syndrome is most likely the result of lack of immunization. Four cases were reported from 2001 to 2004 in the U.S. (Centers for Disease Control, 2005a). *Transmission:* Droplet spread, direct contact with infected persons, or contact with articles soiled by nasal secretions. *Incubation period:* 14–21 days (most commonly 16–18 days). *Period of communicability:* 7 days before until 4 days after rash onset. Infants with congenital rubella may shed the virus for months after birth.	Rubella has a characteristic pink, nonconfluent, maculopapular rash that appears on the face, progresses to the neck, trunk, and legs, and disappears in the same order. Prodromal symptoms (low-grade fever, headache, malaise, coryza, sore throat, and anorexia) occur 1–5 days before the rash. Forscheimer spots (discrete, erythematous pinpoint or larger lesions on the soft palate) are seen. Enlarged postauricular, suboccipital, and posterior cervical lymph nodes are common up to 7 days before the rash. Some cases are asymptomatic. Neonatal signs of congenital rubella syndrome include growth retardation, radiolucent bone disease, hepatosplenomegaly, thrombocytopenia, and purpuric skin lesions ("blueberry muffin" appearance) (see figure). *Complications:* Rare complications include arthritis in adolescents, encephalitis, and congenital rubella syndrome.	Diagnostic tests include cell culture from a nasal swab, and detection of IgM or IgG antibodies. Treatment is supportive. Rubella is generally self-limiting in children. *Prognosis:* Disease is usually mild and benign. Major risk is for fetus if the mother is infected in the first trimester. Congenital rubella syndrome is associated with ophthalmologic, cardiac, auditory, and neurologic anomalies. *Prevention:* Rubella is a vaccine-preventable disease. See the Drug Guide. Females of childbearing age need to be immunized to reduce the risk for congenital rubella syndrome. All healthcare workers should have documented immunity. 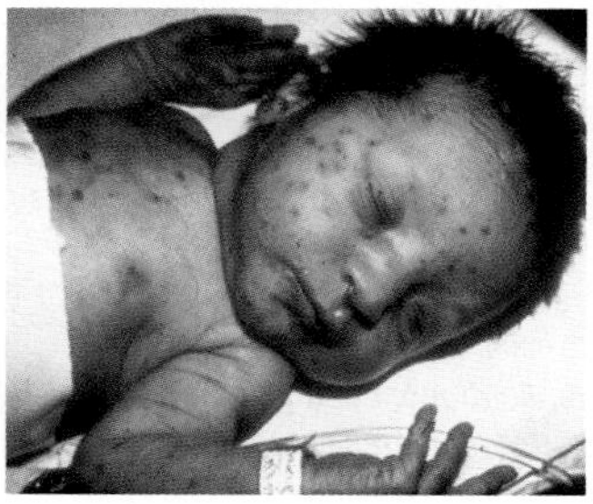	■ Maintain standard and droplet precautions for contagious children. ■ Maintain contact precautions for infants with congenital rubella syndrome until 1 year of age unless nasopharyngeal and urine cultures are repeatedly negative after 3 months of age (American Academy of Pediatrics, 2009, p. 581). ■ Children are usually treated at home. They should be isolated from pregnant women. ■ Give nonaspirin analgesics and antipyretics for any pain and fever. ■ Allow children to choose what they would like to eat and drink. Encourage fluids. ■ Provide quiet activities. ■ Exclude children from childcare or school for 7 days after onset of rash. School and childcare facilities should be notified of the child's illness.
Streptococcus A			
Causal agent: Group A streptococci (GAS). *Epidemiology:* The illness is caused by various M-protein groups of group A alpha- and beta-hemolytic streptococci. Different serotypes are associated with pharyngeal and pyodermal infections; also rheumatic fever and acute glomerulonephritis (American Academy of Pediatrics, 2009, p. 616). Pharyngeal infections occur more often in late fall, winter, and spring. Pyodermal infections occur in warmer seasons in association with minor skin injuries and insect bites.	*Pharyngeal:* Abrupt onset with a sore throat, dysphagia, malaise, high fever, chills, headache, abdominal pain, anorexia, and vomiting. A beefy red pharynx with exudate (strep throat) and tender cervical nodes are seen. Palatal petechiae may be seen. *GAS respiratory tract infection:* Children younger than 3 years may have serous rhinitis and a respiratory illness with moderate fever, irritability, and anorexia rather than pharyngitis. *Scarlet fever:* A characteristic erythematous, sandpaper rash appears in some cases 12–48 hours after onset of symptoms, starting on	Diagnosis can be made by a rapid strep test or a culture of secretions from the pharynx and tonsils. Cultures of skin lesions are not indicated (American Academy of Pediatrics, 2009, p. 620). Prompt antibiotic treatment is effective. Oral penicillin V is the drug of choice, or erythromycin if the child is allergic to penicillin. Uncomplicated impetigo is treated with mupirocin ointment. Invasive strains causing necrotizing fasciitis or myositis need surgical intervention (exploration and debridement of dead tissue).	■ Children with uncomplicated infections are usually cared for at home. ■ Promote bed rest during the febrile stage. ■ Give nonaspirin antipyretics to control fever. Teach parents important signs of a worsening condition. ■ For pharyngeal infections, offer warm salt water for gargling, a soft diet, and nonacidic beverages. Encourage fluids. Provide cool, clear liquids. Swallowing may be difficult. ■ Explain to parents the importance of giving the child the full course of antibiotics.

(continued)

Table 45–4 Selected Infectious and Communicable Diseases in Children—continued

Disease	Clinical Manifestations	Clinical Therapy	Nursing Management
	***Streptococcus A*—continued**		
Transmission: Contact with respiratory secretions for pharyngitis or skin lesions for pyoderma. *Incubation period:* Pharyngeal: usually 2–5 days. Pyodermal: usually 7–10 days. *Period of communicability:* For weeks in untreated pharyngeal infections. Noncontagious within 24 hours of starting antibiotics.	the neck and spreading to the trunk and extremities. In 3–4 days, the rash begins to fade and the tips of the toes and fingers begin to peel. The classic strawberry tongue is seen on days 4–5. *Pyodermal:* Lesions (impetigo) are honey-colored crusts at the site of open lesions (see figure). *Complications:* If untreated, acute otitis media, sinusitis, peritonsillar or retropharyngeal abscess, cervical lymphadenitis, acute rheumatic fever, and acute glomerulonephritis. Invasive disease with toxic shock syndrome, bacteremia, necrotizing fasciitis or myositis can be fatal.	*Prognosis:* Recovery is usually good with antibiotic therapy. Children can become long-term carriers (American Academy of Pediatrics, 2009, p. 622). *Prevention:* None. 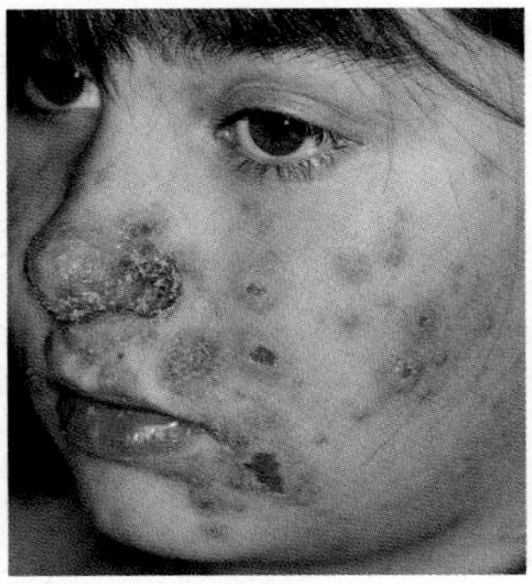	■ Encourage other family members with sore throats to have throat cultures taken. ■ For impetigo, teach the parents to wash the skin, remove crusts, and apply antibiotic ointment. ■ If the child is hospitalized, maintain droplet precautions for pharyngeal infections and contact precautions for skin lesions for 24 hours after beginning antibiotics. Monitor vital signs, especially temperature. Administer antibiotics as ordered. ■ If the child develops invasive streptococcal infection, use standard precautions. The child with toxic shock syndrome will need intensive care to manage shock and fluid and electrolyte imbalances.
	Tetanus*§		
Causal agent: Clostridium tetani or tetanus bacillus. *Epidemiology:* Bacillus is common and exists as a spore in soil, dust, and animal excretions. The organism produces an endotoxin that affects the central nervous system. *Transmission:* The organism is transmitted to humans through puncture wounds or broken skin. Newborns can acquire tetanus if a contaminated implement is used to cut the cord, or clay is applied to the umbilical cord as a ritual in some Middle Eastern cultures. *Incubation period:* 3 days–3 weeks (average 8 days). *Period of communicability:* Not communicable from person to person.	Headache, stiffness of the neck and jaw, with painful facial spasms and difficulty chewing and swallowing occur over a few days. Noise or sudden movement may stimulate spasms. Facial muscle spasms may produce a grinning expression (risus sardonicus). Localized prolonged and painful muscle contraction may occur at the site of the wound. Eventually rigidity of the abdomen and trunk produce **opisthotonos** (rigid hypertextension of the entire body). Affected respiratory muscles may cause airway obstruction and suffocation. Newborns have increasing difficulty with sucking, irritability, and neck stiffness. *Complications:* Laryngospasm, respiratory distress, death.	Tetanus immune globulin and tetanus toxoid are given in separate sites to unimmunized persons as soon as possible. Medications are given to treat muscle spasms. Intensive care is provided with assisted ventilation, IV metronidazole or penicillin G, nutrition, and supportive care. The wound is cleaned and debrided. Complete recovery may take weeks. *Prognosis:* 30% mortality; much higher in newborns. Intensive care has improved survival. *Prevention:* Tetanus is a vaccine preventable disease. See the Drug Guide. Tetanus boosters are updated every 10 years, or, if a potentially contaminated wound occurs, in 5 years. Proper surgical debridement of wounds decreases the chance of infection.	■ Prevent disease by checking immunization records and administering immunizations as necessary. ■ Assist with wound debridement. ■ The child with tetanus is hospitalized. Use standard precautions. ■ Monitor the child's condition. Handle as little as possible. Reduce stimulation by placing child in a quiet, darkened room. ■ Offer skin and respiratory care. The child may need an endotracheal tube, suctioning, and supplemental oxygen for airway support. ■ Provide feedings via total parenteral nutrition or feeding tube. ■ Maintain hydration with IV fluids and electrolytes. ■ Try to reduce the child's anxiety, as mental status may be unaffected by disease process. ■ Prepare the family for a possible poor prognosis.

*Indicates that a vaccine or antitoxin is available for use in high-risk or as-needed situations.
§Indicates that the disease has a safe and effective vaccine.

Table 45–5 Selected Infectious Diseases Transmitted by Insect or Animal Hosts (Zoonosis)

Disease	Clinical Manifestations	Clinical Therapy	Nursing Management
Lyme Disease			
Causal agent: Borrelia *burgdorferi,* a spirochete, which is transmitted by ixodid ticks. *Epidemiology:* It occurs in 49 states and the District of Columbia. Most cases occur in the Northeastern, Mid-Atlantic, and North Central states (American Academy of Pediatrics, 2009, p. 431). Exposure occurs in any outdoor setting where ticks are endemic. Lyme disease occurs year round, with the highest risk of infection in the summer. Incidence is highest among children in the U.S. between 5 and 19 years. *Transmission:* The tick transmits the infection after feeding for 24 to 36 hours. Lyme disease is the most common vectorborne illness in North America. *Incubation period:* 1–55 days after an infected tick bite. A rash in 48 hours is an allergic reaction or infection, not Lyme disease. *Period of communicability:* The infection is not communicable from person to person. 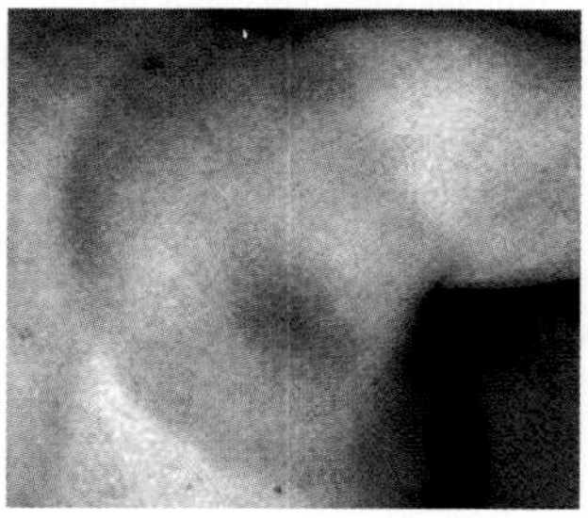	Stage 1 (localized): malaise, fatigue, headache, stiff neck, mild fever, and muscle and joint aches. Erythema migrans starts as a red macule or papule that expands over days or weeks to become a large annular red area, sometimes with partial central clearing; usually at least 5 cm in diameter (see figure). The rash may look like a bruise in dark-skinned patients. Only 50% of patients have the rash (Savely, 2006). Stage 2 (early disseminated) occurs 1–4 months after the bite in untreated children. The most common symptoms are multiple erythema migrans, cranial nerve palsies, arthralgia, headache, fatigue, and meningitis. Stage 3 (late disseminated) occurs months later and includes recurrent Lyme arthritis and central nervous system changes that may become chronic problems. *Complications*: Left untreated, Lyme disease can cause significant neurologic deficits, including arm and leg weakness, Bell's palsy, encephalopathy, optic neuropathy, meningitis, severe headaches, and cognitive and behavioral changes as well as chronic arthritis, and disorders of the peripheral nerves.	Diagnostic tests include the enzyme-linked immunosorbent assay (ELISA) plus the Western blot test. Treatment for localized disease is a 2–3 week course of oral antibiotics (amoxicillin or cefuroxime in children 8 years and younger, doxycycline or tetracycline in children older than 8 years). For disseminated disease oral or IV antibiotics (depending upon body system involved) may be given for up to 4 weeks. *Prognosis:* Lyme disease does not cause acute life-threatening illness, but it may result in significant morbidity, especially when chronic. *Prevention:* Avoid areas that are heavily tick infested, and wear protective clothing. Check for ticks (especially hidden in hair) after every outing. Check pets because they can carry home ticks that are then transferred to the child. Remove ticks as soon as possible. There is no acquired immunity. No vaccine is currently available.	■ Tell parents to mark the date of tick bite on the calendar and monitor the child for flu-like symptoms for the next 30 days. If symptoms develop seek medical attention promptly. ■ If children are hospitalized, use standard precautions. ■ Educate parents about the need to complete the long course of medications, informing them that the spirochete can go dormant. ■ Have the child avoid sun exposure when taking doxycycline. ■ Provide nonaspirin analgesics and antipyretics for relief of fever and discomfort. ■ Children with Lyme disease may tire easily. Promote rest and avoid vigorous activities. ■ Teach parents to safely remove ticks. To remove a tick, grasp it gently but firmly with fine-point tweezers where the mouthparts are attached. Pull gently until the tick releases. Clean the area with soap and water.
Malaria			
Causal agent: Plasmodium, four species (*P. falciparum, P. vivax, P. ovale, P. malariae*) *Epidemiology:* Occurs in tropical and subtropical regions on four continents (Africa, Americas, Asia, and Oceana). Children have the highest mortality. The disease is acquired during travel to an endemic area. *P. falciparum* causes the most serious disease. Approximately 20% of cases reported in the U.S. occurred in children under 18 years (Maples, 2006). *Transmission:* The saliva of an infected female Anopheles mosquito introduces the parasite to the person when feeding between dusk and dawn. The parasite infects the hepatic cells	Nonspecific signs such as high fever alternating with chills, profuse diaphoresis, fatigue. Periods of symptomatic improvement may be seen between cycles lasting 48 or 72 hours depending upon type of infection. Children may also have fever, anorexia, vomiting, splenomegaly, and anemia. Additional symptoms include myalgia, malaise, headache, abdominal pain, back pain, pallor, diarrhea, nausea and vomiting. Attacks may recur over the course of the year after infection, but the parasites die out gradually if reinfection does not occur. Children who live in endemic areas and survive the first 5 years of life develop immunity to the severe	Diagnostic tests include examining blood smears for parasites, or a plasmodium HRP2 antigen enzyme-linked immunosorbent assay (ELISA). Laboratory tests often reveal anemia and thrombocytopenia. Treatment includes fluid replacement, anemia management, and antipyretics. The blood is monitored for parasite density. ICU care is needed in severe disease to monitor for mental status changes, severe anemia, renal failure, and pulmonary edema. Children may need blood transfusions. Antimalarial medications are chloroquine, quinine sulfate and tetracycline, clindamycin, doxycycline, mefloquine, and atova-quone-poguanil, selected based	■ Use standard precautions for the hospitalized patient. ■ Maintain fluid intake. Monitor intake and output. ■ Monitor blood glucose level and be prepared to respond to sudden hypoglycemia. ■ Observe for signs of increasing illness severity such as confusion, seizures, and shock. Be prepared to protect the patient from injury and provide emergency support with airways and oxygen until the child can be transferred to the ICU. ■ Monitor the hematocrit and hemoglobin levels. ■ Administer antipyretics to control the fever and promote comfort. ■ Provide education and emotional support to parents.

(continued)

Table 45–5 Selected Infectious Diseases Transmitted by Insect or Animal Hosts (Zoonosis)—continued

Disease	Clinical Manifestations	Clinical Therapy	Nursing Management
Malaria—continued			
and reproduces. When the hepatic cell ruptures, parasites are released and infect the red blood cells. Transmission can occur by blood transfusion or transplacentally *Incubation period:* Varies by type. *P. falciparum* in 7–10 days, up to 1 year for the other types. *Period of communicability:* Communicable by blood or blood product transfusion, or the transplantation of organs from an infected person.	effects of the disease as long as they have frequent re-exposure to the infection. *Complications*: Severe anemia in young children. Cerebral malaria occurs in children 3 to 6 years of age. Older children and adolescents more commonly have pulmonary edema, respiratory failure, renal failure, spontaneous bleeding, and shock. Children with asplenia are at high risk for death. Causes 1–2 million deaths worldwide annually (Agrawal & Teach, 2006).	upon drug-resistance of the Plasmodium species. Medications may be given orally or by IV. Hypoglycemia may result from quinine treatment. *Prevention*: While in endemic areas use DEET insect repellent, screened rooms, DEET-treated mosquito netting, and cover the body with light-colored clothing. Begin antimalarial chemoprophylaxis prior to travel in an endemic region. A vaccine is being tested.	■ Educate families traveling to endemic areas about taking antimalarial drugs and the need to take it correctly despite the nausea and vomiting side effects. Discuss protecting children during mosquitoes' nocturnal feeding times with protective clothing, mosquito repellent, and mosquito netting around the bed.
Rabies (Hydrophobia)			
Causal agent: Rhabdoviridae, two types (urban, in dogs; wild, in wildlife). *Epidemiology:* Occurs worldwide. Urban rabies is generally controlled by vaccination of dogs and cats. Rabies can occur in many wild animals, particularly bats, foxes, skunks, and raccoons. *Transmission:* Infected saliva from bite of rabid animal. Virus enters the wound and travels along the nerves from point of entry to the brain where it multiplies and migrates along the efferent nerves to the salivary glands. Human-to-human transmission is rare with corneal or other organ transplant (Mani & Murray, 2006). *Incubation period:* Highly variable; average 30 to 90 days. This period depends on the amount of virus in the saliva, how close to the brain or major nerves the bite occurred, and how deeply the saliva penetrated the skin.	Children may be free of symptoms during the long incubation period. Illness may begin with mild respiratory or gastrointestinal symptoms, fever, headache, chills, and malaise. Initial acute symptoms may also include pain or paresthesia at the site of exposure. Acute neurologic signs include furious rabies (anxiety, agitation, hallucinations, and other bizarre behavior) or paralytic rabies (paresthesia or weakness that progresses to paralysis and complete respiratory paralysis) (Mani & Murray, 2006). Painful contractures in the muscles used for swallowing lead to hydrophobia (50% of patients), a reflex contraction at the sight of liquid. The patient progresses to coma and respiratory failure. *Complications*: Usually results in death.	No diagnosis is possible during incubation. Diagnosis is confirmed by fluorescent antibody staining of the dead animal's brain tissue or patient saliva or reverse transcriptase-polymerase chain reaction of saliva or brain tissue (Mani & Murphy, 2006). Immediately wash animal bites thoroughly with soap and water and irrigate well with a virucidal agent such as povidene iodine (Mani & Murphy, 2006). Avoid suturing if possible. Give postexposure prophylaxis with human rabies immune globulin (HRIG) and human diploid cell rabies vaccine (HDCV) to all persons bitten by animals potentially rabid. Half of the HRIG is infiltrated around the wound and the remainder is given IM. HDCV is repeated on days 3, 7, 14, and 28 after the bite (5 doses), but the HDCV series may be stopped if the animal is found free of rabies. The vaccine is of no value once rabies symptoms are present. *Prognosis:* If symptoms develop, no drug improves the prognosis. *Prevention:* Immunize all domestic animals against rabies.	■ Work with the family and animal control to quarantine the animal for observation, if possible. ■ Administer HRIG and HDCV as ordered. Inject vaccine into the muscle to prevent vaccine failure. ■ Support the family while reinforcing the urgency for the vaccine and series of injections. ■ Educate parents about the vaccine side effects—irritation at the injection site, itching, headache, muscle aches, nausea, and dizziness. ■ If the child acquires rabies, he or she will be hospitalized. ■ Institute standard and contact precautions. The virus is transmitted primarily in the saliva and cerebrospinal fluid. ■ Make the child as comfortable as possible. ■ Keep liquids out of sight of the hydrophobic child. ■ Provide emotional support to the family of the dying child. ■ Teach children to avoid contact with all unknown animals, dead or alive.
Rocky Mountain Spotted Fever (Tickborne Typhus Fever, Sao Paulo Typhus)			
Causal agent: Rickettsia rickettsii *Epidemiology:* Rocky Mountain spotted fever (RMSF) occurs in most of the U.S., southwestern Canada, and Mexico. More than half of all U.S. cases occur in Oklahoma, North Carolina, South	Onset may be gradual or rapid with vague signs. Children may be very ill. Sudden onset is characterized by a moderate to high fever (40°C [104°F]) that ordinarily lasts for 2–3 weeks, significant malaise, abdominal pain, nausea, vomiting,	Diagnostic tests are immunofluorescent or immunoperoxidase staining of biopsied lesions, but they are not always reliable (Cohen, 2004). Treatment of choice is doxycycline regardless of patient age for 5–7 days	■ Use standard precautions. ■ Children may require prolonged hospitalization, including monitoring in the intensive care unit. ■ Have hemodynamic monitoring equipment and emergency supplies readily available.

Table 45–5 Selected Infectious Diseases Transmitted by Insect or Animal Hosts (Zoonosis)—continued

Disease	Clinical Manifestations	Clinical Therapy	Nursing Management
Rocky Mountain Spotted Fever (Tickborne Typhus Fever, Sao Paulo Typhus)—continued			
Carolina, and Tennessee. Generally occurs between April and September. Most infections occur in children who are younger than 15 years of age. Infection induces immunity. *Transmission:* Transmitted by bites of ticks, principally dog and wood ticks. *Incubation period:* 2–14 days (most commonly 7 days) after bite of an infected tick. *Period of communicability:* There is no evidence of person-to-person transmission. 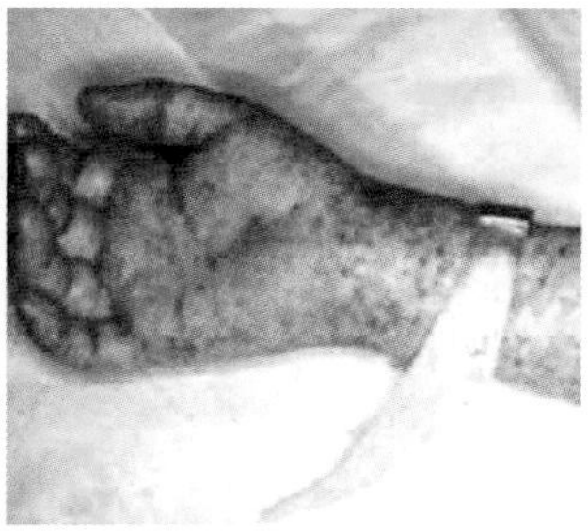	deep muscle pain, persistent headache, chills, and conjunctival injection. The characteristic rash, red macules and papules that blanche usually appears on the palms and soles between the 2nd and 5th days, and may become widely disseminated (see figure). The rash may not be easily seen in children with dark skin. The rash becomes petechial on the 5th or 6th day, and purpura may occur. It is rarely pruritic. Up to 10% of children do not develop a rash (Cohen, 2004). The child may have splenomegaly, hepatomegaly, and jaundice. *Complications:* Gastrointestinal bleeding, disseminated intravascular coagulation, pneumonitis, pulmonary edema, respiratory distress, encephalitis, cardiac and renal complications can occur.	or until the child is afebrile for 3 days (Chapman, 2006). Hospitalization is often necessary. *Prognosis:* Delay in treatment can cause a more severe disease. A mortality rate of 2% to 4% is associated with delayed treatment (Razzaq & Schutze, 2005). *Prevention:* Avoid areas that are heavily tick infested, and wear protective clothing. Check for ticks and if found remove promptly. Infected ticks must be attached and feeding for 4–6 hours to transmit the disease. Seek medical attention promptly for a child who has been bitten and becomes symptomatic.	■ Administer antibiotics as ordered. ■ Observe for any abnormal bleeding. ■ Make the child as comfortable as possible. If the child is unconscious, support the extremities and keep the eyes closed and lubricated. ■ Provide quiet diversion activities. ■ Provide emotional support, and keep parents informed about the child's condition.

development of symptoms. Some diseases have a **prodrome**, the phase of early manifestations of the infection until the development of the overt clinical syndrome. In some cases communicable diseases have nonspecific signs such as fatigue, malaise, weakness, and decreased responsiveness or inability to concentrate. Skin rash, poor appetite, vomiting, diarrhea, and body aches are other common signs and symptoms. Fever is the most common sign of infectious disease in infants and children.

Physiology of Fever

The hypothalamus is the body's thermostat or control center for the regulation of body temperature (see "Pathophysiology Illustrated: Fever"). As blood circulates through the hypothalamus, the body is directed to conserve or release heat, depending on the temperature of the blood.

CLINICAL THERAPY

Diagnostic tests include cultures from sites of potential infection (skin, pharynx, blood, urine, feces, cerebrospinal fluid, etc.). (See Skills 10–4 to 10–18 in the Clinical Skills Manual **SKILLS** for guidelines for collecting specimens.) Blood may be obtained to perform tests for condition-specific immunoglobulin antibodies. In some cases, radiographs or special imaging may be used to identify localized infection in an organ, such as the lungs.

A fever can be a beneficial physiologic response to infection, because it signifies that the body is fighting organisms that thrive at lower body temperatures. A fever also helps to mobilize the immune response by increasing neutrophil production and T-cell proliferation (Crocetti & Serwint, 2005). Medical management may include postponing treatment of low-grade fevers (under 38.9°C [102°F]) to promote the body's natural defenses against an infection; fever is not inherently harmful until it reaches 41°C (105.9°F).

Developing Cultural Competence

DISEASE CAUSATION

In some cultures, infectious diseases are seen as punishment or the result of curses or evil spirits. For example, American Indians traditionally view illnesses as the result of disharmony or displeasing the spirits. They may not believe in the germ theory of disease causation.

PATHOPHYSIOLOGY ILLUSTRATED

FEVER

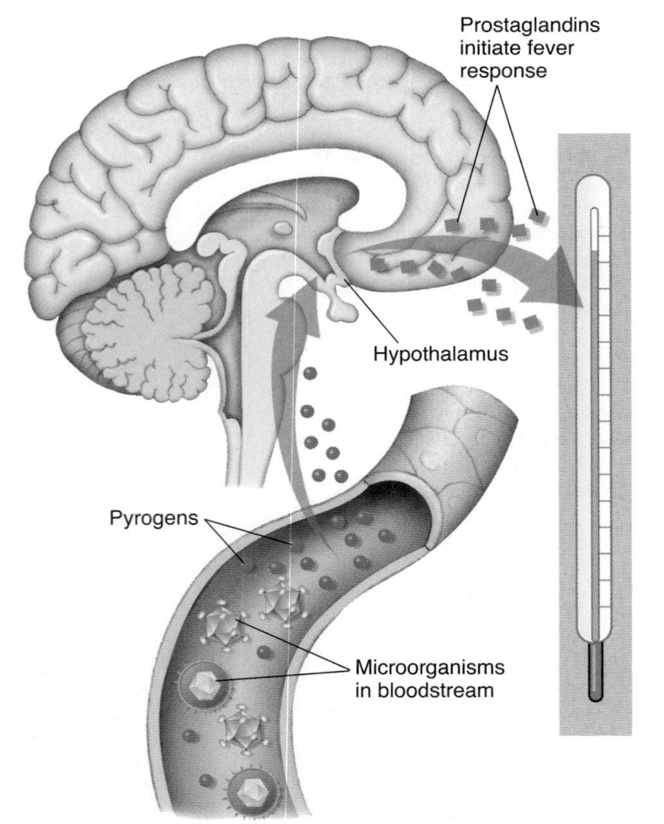

The hypothalamus functions as the body's thermostat, directing the body to conserve or dissipate heat. When microorganisms invade the body, **endogenous pyrogens** (interleukins, interferons, and tumor necrosis factor) are released by macrophages into the bloodstream. These substances travel to the hypothalamus, where they trigger the production and release of prostaglandins. Prostaglandins are believed to raise the body's thermoregulatory set point, thus causing the fever to occur (Crocetti & Serwint, 2005). A rise in the hypothalamus's set point leads to a cold response with shivering and chills, vasoconstriction, and decreased peripheral perfusion. Blood is diverted from the extremities to more central vessels. This helps increase the core body temperature by decreasing heat loss. Shivering increases both metabolic action and heat production. The hypothalamus then maintains the temperature at the new set point. When the temperature is elevated, the heart rate, respiratory rate, and metabolic rate increase. Vasodilation occurs and the skin flushes, becoming warm to the touch.

Fevers are often treated, especially if associated with discomfort, with acetaminophen or ibuprofen. Aspirin is no longer recommended because of its association with Reye's syndrome. Antipyretics inhibit prostaglandin synthesis, which results in lowering of the body's temperature set point and reducing the fever. See "Complementary Therapy: Fever Treatment."

Complementary Care

FEVER TREATMENT

Many Latino and Asian cultures subscribe to the hot and cold theory of disease causation. "Hot" and "cold" do not refer to temperature, but to categories. Fever, a hot condition, is treated by giving the patient cold substances (either foods or medicines). Cold foods include vegetables, fruits, and fish. Cold medicines include orange flower water, linden, and sage. See Table 2–2 "Hot and Cold Conditions and Foods" in Chapter 2 ∞.

Nursing Practice

Community-acquired methicillin-resistant *Staphylococcus aureus* (CA-MRSA) causes aggressive infection in healthy children and adolescents. Necrotizing fasciitis (an advancing soft tissue infection), abscess formation, scalded skin syndrome, and toxic shock–like syndrome may develop. Some cases have been fatal. Risk factors include participation in contact team sports, crowded living conditions, childcare center attendance, recurrent skin infections, and similar lesions in a family member. CA-MRSA colonizes in the anterior nares, a primary reservoir. Transmission occurs by direct contact with an infected person or contact with contaminated objects (Tufts & Hardman, 2006; Le, 2006). Mupiricin ointment applied intranasally twice a day for 5 days with or without chlorhexidine baths helps reduce MRSA colonization and prevents recurrent infection (Fergie & Purcell, 2007).

Antibiotics are often prescribed to treat bacterial infectious diseases; however, strains of bacteria have developed resistance to many antibiotics. One example is community-acquired methicillin-resistant *Staphylococcus aureus*. Children with chronic conditions may be more susceptible to infection by drug-resistant pathogens. Many specialty organizations and medical centers are developing best practice guidelines for the use of antibiotics in treating common infections, such as acute otitis media. See Chapter 47 ∞.

Antiviral medications may be prescribed for viral infections, such as chickenpox, herpes simplex virus type I, and influenza. When the child is immunocompromised, antiviral medication should be started early to minimize the potential life-threatening consequences of the infection.

Cases of many communicable diseases must be reported to the state health department, using standardized state forms or on a designated website.

NURSING MANAGEMENT

NURSING ASSESSMENT AND DIAGNOSIS

Assess the child's hydration status and fluid intake, vital signs, comfort level, and appetite. Observe for seizures and for a **toxic**

appearance (lethargy, poor perfusion, hypoventilation or hyperventilation, and cyanosis). The child with a fever may be irritable and restless, sleep fitfully, and have nonspecific muscular pain. Identify febrile children who may be at higher risk for a serious illness, in particular:

- Infants and children having a toxic appearance.
- Newborns less than 28 days of age with a temperature over 38°C (100.4°F).
- Children less than 4 years of age with a temperature over 41°C (105.8°F).
- Children with conditions such as a congenital heart disease, ventriculoperitoneal shunt, asplenia, and sickle cell disease.

Observe the child for other signs of infection, such as a rash, nausea and vomiting, or diarrhea, as well as generalized symptoms of a poor appetite, myalgias, and malaise.

The following nursing diagnoses may be appropriate for children with infectious and communicable diseases:

- *Hyperthermia* related to infectious disease process
- *Impaired Skin Integrity* related to hyperthermia and scratching skin lesions
- *Impaired Oral Mucous Membranes* related to infectious disease process
- *Deficient Fluid Volume* related to repeated episodes of vomiting and diarrhea
- *Ineffective Therapeutic Regimen Management (Family)* related to complexity of care required by child

PLANNING AND IMPLEMENTATION

Most children with communicable diseases are cared for at home; however, infected children are seen in all healthcare settings. Nursing care includes treating infection, administering antibiotics on schedule, monitoring antibiotic blood levels if indicated to ensure appropriate results, promoting the child's comfort, and educating parents.

PREVENT DISEASE TRANSMISSION

Children are often admitted to the hospital for treatment of severe infections. In addition, countless numbers of **nosocomial** (hospital-acquired) **infections** occur each year. All items with which the infected child comes into contact are contaminated (linens, toys, medical equipment, etc.). Follow the facility's standard and transmission-based precautions to reduce the spread of infectious diseases to staff and other children. Discuss any concerns to the hospital's infection control nurse. (See the "Infection Control" chapter in the Clinical Skills Manual **SKILLS** for more detailed information.)

Recall that the fecal-oral and respiratory routes are the most common sources of infections in children. In health centers, isolate children with suspicious rashes and respiratory infections from other children. Wipe down the hard surfaces and toys in the examining room with antiseptic solution before another child uses the room. Dispose of linens in appropriately marked linen bags.

Evidence in Action

Two recent studies evaluated alternating acetaminophen and ibuprofen for fever treatment. Results revealed that the children achieved a lower temperature when receiving an alternating medication regimen versus a single antipyretic, demonstrating the synergistic effect of the two medications (Nabulsi, Tamim, Mahfoud, et al., 2006; Sarrell, Wielunsky, & Cohen, 2006). Overdose may be a risk if the administration schedule and dose are not strictly followed. The potentially synergistic effects of the two medications on the kidneys can cause renal tubular toxicity when used repeatedly for an illness (Miller, 2007). This practice should *not* be recommended to families for home care of fever.

FEVER MANAGEMENT

Nursing care for treatment of fever includes administering antipyretics, removing unnecessary clothing, and encouraging increased fluid intake. Identify clear fluids the child prefers to drink, and encourage the intake of extra fluids.

EDUCATING THE FAMILY

Teach parents to care for their child at home. This includes how and when to give antipyretics and antibiotics if ordered, appropriate foods and beverages to provide, and the care of rashes and other symptoms. Parents often fear fever, believing it is a disease rather than a symptom of an illness. See the Teaching Highlights to provide information and reassurance. Help them to recognize signs that the child's condition is worsening.

Teach parents to give all the antibiotic doses for the full number of days prescribed and help develop a schedule that matches the family's routines. Make sure they know whether to give the antibiotic with or without food. Inform them to discard the antibiotic when all doses have been given, and not to share the antibiotic with any other family member.

Educate parents about methods to reduce disease transmission in the home, including the following:

- Limit exposure to the ill child by elderly family members and infants.
- Use hot soapy water or the dishwasher to clean the ill child's dishes and utensils.
- Disinfect hard surfaces touched by the ill child and all diaper-changing areas.
- Place dressings with drainage in a plastic bag for disposal.
- Encourage good hand hygiene.
- Make sure all children are immunized.

To prevent CA-MRSA, encourage adolescent athletes to shower with soap and water after practice and competitions, avoid sharing towels and personal items, and cover all wounds and appropriately dispose of bandages. Encourage athletes to care for wounds and report those that are potentially infected. Shared athletic equipment should be regularly disinfected, and trainers who care for wounds should practice good hand hygiene. See MyNursingKit for a Web site regarding CA-MRSA.

Nursing Practice

Acetaminophen and ibuprofen preparations are available as infant drops, liquid syrup, chewable tablets, and adult-strength tablets or capsules. Identify the preparation used in the home to recommend the correct dosage for the child. The dose of acetaminophen is 10-15 mg/kg/dose and of ibuprofen is 4-10 mg/kg/dose.

ACETAMINOPHEN	IBUPROFEN
Infant drops–80 mg/ per dropper in package	Infant drops–50 mg/1.25 ml, using package dropper
Children's liquid–160 mg/ 5 mL	Children's liquid–100 mg/5 mL
Chewable tablets–80 mg or 160 mg	Chewable and junior tablets– 50 mg and 100 mg
Adult tablets or caplets– 325 mg and 500 mg	Adult tablets or caplets–200 mg

EVALUATION

Expected outcomes of nursing care include the following:

- Opportunities for spread of infection between patients and family members are minimized.
- The child's fever is effectively managed with antipyretics.
- The full treatment with antibiotics, if ordered, is completed.

EMERGING INFECTION CONTROL THREATS

Public health officials are conducting disease surveillance to identify emerging infections, such as **pandemic flu**, a worldwide influenza epidemic, or for potential weapons of terrorists (anthrax, smallpox, plague, botulism, hemorrhagic fever, or tularemia). See Table 45–4 for influenza information. See Table 45–6 for the signs and symptoms of biologic agents that could potentially be used for terrorism and appropriate clinical therapy. Early recognition of these infections is essential so

Teaching Highlights

GUIDELINES FOR EVALUATING AND TREATING FEVER IN CHILDREN

Facts about fevers:

- A fever is not a disease; it is the body's response to an infection. It means the child's body is using natural defenses to fight an infection.
- If the child has a fever and does not look sick, it may be better to let the child use his or her natural defenses to fight off the virus or bacteria causing the fever.

Treating the fever:

- Use a thermometer to check the child's temperature.
- Give acetaminophen or ibuprofen (do not use aspirin) using the correct dose and preparation for the child's weight (drops are 3 times as concentrated as syrup). Follow guidelines on the bottle for the maximum number of doses allowed per day, and do not alternate the medications to prevent a possible overdose.
- Remove all but a light layer of the child's clothing.
- Monitor the child's behavior and response to fever medication. The medication will reduce the child's temperature, but the temperature may rise again in 4 to 6 hours. The temperature will not return to normal until the child is recovering from the illness. Check the temperature and give another dose of fever medicine. The main goal of fever medication is to improve the child's comfort.
  - If sponging the child, give fever medication first, and then use tepid water to sponge the child. Cool water may increase shivering and discomfort. Alcohol should not be used.
  - Provide generous amounts of fluids for the child to drink and allow the child to rest.

Contact your healthcare provider immediately if:

- The infant is under 2 months old and has a fever over 38.0°C (100.4°F).
- The child has a fever over 40.1°C (104.2°F) and any of the following symptoms are present in the child:
  - The child acts or looks very sick.
  - Inconsolable crying or whimpering. The child cries when moved or otherwise touched by the parent or other family members.
- Difficult to awaken.
- A stiff neck.
- Purple spots on the skin.
- Difficulty breathing that does not improve after the nose is cleared.
- Unable to swallow and drooling saliva.
- The child has a convulsion.

Call your healthcare provider within 24 hours if:

- The child is 2 to 4 months old (unless fever occurs within 48 hours of a DTaP shot and the infant has no other serious symptoms).
- The child's fever is higher than 40.1°C (104.2°F), especially if the child is younger than age 3 years.
- The child complains of burning or pain with urination.
- The fever has been present more than 24 hours without an obvious cause or location of infection.
- The fever subsided for more than 24 hours and then returned, or the fever has been present for more than 72 hours.

that public health measures can be initiated to reduce disease transmission and to prepare the mass casualty response needed to care for large numbers of ill adults and children.

NURSING MANAGEMENT

Maintain a high level of suspicion when greater than the expected number of individuals with similar signs and symptoms are present in a school or seek care in any healthcare facility. Initiating airborne and contact precautions and instituting isolation before a definitive diagnosis is appropriate when the level of suspicion is high. Assess children and provide supportive nursing care for the identified infection. See MyNursingKit for the Web site with regularly updated guidelines for the management of specific health threats.

Table 45–6 Clinical Manifestations of Aerosolized Organisms That Are Potential Biologic Weapons of Terrorists

Organisms	Aerosol Transmission Clinical Manifestations	Clinical Therapy
Anthrax *Causal agent: Bacillus anthracis*	■ Cutaneous—papule that progresses to a vesicle then to a skin ulcer with a depressed black scab in the center. Not painful. Child may have fever, malaise, headache, and regional lymphadenopathy. ■ Gastrointestinal—nausea, loss of appetite, bloody diarrhea, hematemesis, fever, stomach pain, severe abdominal pain followed by fever and septicemia. ■ Inhalation—brief prodrome with symptoms like a sore throat, mild fever, malaise, muscle aches; followed by development of dyspnea, cough, chest pain, shortness of breath, and systemic symptoms. Shock, pleural effusion, and meningitis may develop and death may occur without treatment.	■ IV ciprofloxacin or doxycycline for patients older than 12 years. For children younger than 12 years, IV ciprofloxacin plus clindamycin. ■ For postexposure prophylaxis: vaccine approved for those older than 18 years (3 doses at 0, 2, and 4 weeks) and oral ciprofloxacin or amoxicillin for 30 days (Markenson, 2005).
Botulism *Causal agent: Clostridium botulinum*	■ Ptosis, diplopia, blurred vision. Sluggishly reactive pupils. ■ Speech and swallowing problems, loss of gag reflex. ■ Acute, afebrile symmetric descending flaccid paralysis, progressing to loss of head control, hypotonia, generalized weakness, deep tendon reflexes diminish or disappear. Constipation. ■ May be preceded by abdominal cramps, nausea, vomiting, or diarrhea. ■ May become confused or obtunded.	■ Slow IV infusion of equine antitoxin diluted in normal saline. ■ Epinephrine and diphenhydramine for serum sickness or urticaria.
Hemorrhagic Fever *Causal agent: Ebola or Marburg virus*	■ Abrupt onset of fever, myalgia, headache, nausea, vomiting, abdominal pain, photophobia, diarrhea, chest pain, cough, pharyngitis. ■ Maculopapular rash prominent on trunk soon after fever, bleeding into skin (petechiae, ecchymosis, subconjunctival hemorrhages), shock and circulatory collapse in short period. ■ Ghostlike appearance, looks critically ill.	■ Management of hypotension and shock and maintenance of fluid and electrolyte balance. ■ Replacement of blood, platelets, and plasma for severe hemorrhage.
Plague *Causal agent: Yersinia pestis* Pneumonic plague with aerosol route of transmission	■ Severe respiratory illness with high fever, chills, headache, cough, breathing difficulty. ■ Rapidly developing pneumonia, bloody or watery sputum. ■ May lead to respiratory failure and shock.	■ Streptomycin IM or gentamicin IV. Alternate antibiotics include IV chloramphenicol or doxycycline. ■ Oral doxycycline and ciprofloxacin for mass casualty events (Leggiadro, 2007).
Smallpox *Causal agent: Variola major virus* 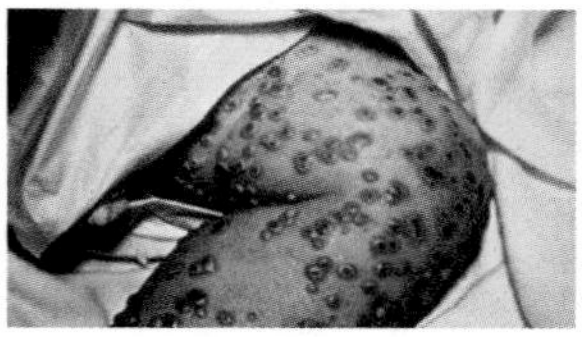	■ Prodrome 2 to 4 days before rash: abrupt onset with fever (101°F or higher), malaise, headache, muscle pain, prostration, nausea and vomiting, and backache. ■ Rash begins with red spots in mouth and on tongue that break open, followed by few macules on the forehead, face, and extremities. A generalized rash begins as macules, progressing to papules, to tense vesicles, to tense deep umbilicated pustules. Most cases have discrete, semiconfluent to confluent vesicles. Lesions are firm, all in same stage of development, more concentrated on the extremities than the trunk. The temperature usually falls and the patient feels better. ■ The pustules form scabs by the end of the second week, and the scabs fall off after 3–4 weeks.	■ Supportive care ■ Antibiotics for secondary infection.

(continued)

Table 45–6 Clinical Manifestations of Aerosolized Organisms That Are Potential Biologic Weapons of Terrorists—continued

Organisms	Aerosol Transmission Clinical Manifestations	Clinical Therapy
Tularemia *Causal agent: Francisella tularensis*	■ Febrile illness, fatigue, chills, headache, malaise, dyspnea, chest pain. ■ May develop hemorrhagic inflammation of airways that progresses to pneumonia, pleuritis, and hilar lymphadenopathy. ■ May also have pharyngitis, bronchiolitis, and pneumonia with systemic symptoms.	■ Streptomycin IM or gentamicin IV, alternate drug is IV ciprofloxacin. For children use gentamicin IV, alternate drugs are doxycycline and chloramphenicol. ■ Supportive care in the intensive care unit. ■ Postexposure prophylaxis for 14 days with ciprofloxacin, for children use doxycycline.

Data from: Markenson, D. (2005). The treatment of children exposed to pathogens linked to bioterrorism. *Infectious Disease Clinics of North America, 19,* 731–745; Stocker, J. T. (2006). Clinical and pathological differential diagnosis of selected potential bioterrorism agents of interest to pediatric health care providers, *Clinics in Laboratory Medicine, 26*, 329–344; Koirala, J. (2006). Plague: Disease, management, and recognition of act of terrorism. *Infectious Disease Clinics of North America, 20,* 273–287; Centers of Disease Control (2008a), Bioterrorism, retrieved November 15, 2008, from www.bt.cdc.gov/bioterrorism

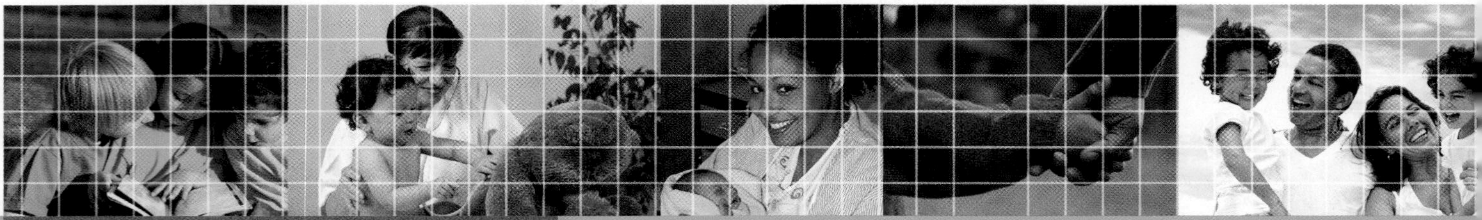

CRITICAL CONCEPT REVIEW

LEARNING OUTCOMES — CONCEPTS

45.1 Describe the reasons why children are more vulnerable than adults to contracting communicable diseases. →

1. Infants and children have immature immune systems.
2. Infants' protection from maternal antibodies decrease with age.
3. Incomplete immunization status.
4. Lack of prior exposure to infectious agents.
5. Poor hygiene practices of infants and children.

45.2 Describe the process of infection and modes of transmission. →

1. Process of infection requires:
   - An infectious agent.
   - Effective means of transmission.
   - Susceptible host.
2. Modes of transmission:
   - Direct: requires physical contact between source of infection and new host.
   - Indirect: pathogens survive outside host (contaminated object or vector) before causing disease.

45.3 Explain the role that vaccines play in reducing and eliminating communicable diseases. →

1. Vaccines keep children from acquiring common childhood diseases.
2. When large numbers of children are immunized, herd immunity protects unimmunized infants.
3. Immunizations have made many communicable diseases very rare in developed countries.

45.4 Develop a nursing care plan for children of all ages needing immunizations. →

1. Teach the importance of immunization during the prenatal period, including immunizations the infant will receive in the nursery.
2. Review immunization schedule with parents before newborn leaves hospital.
3. Provide written materials about immunizations.
4. Review immunization status of infant and child at every visit with healthcare provider.
5. Assess child for potential contraindications to vaccines prior to administration.
6. Review expected side effects of immunizations with parents and teach methods to improve the child's comfort.

LEARNING OUTCOMES / CONCEPTS

45.5 Outline a plan to maintain the potency of vaccines.

1. Maintain the refrigerator and freezer at the consistent recommended temperature.
2. Store vaccines in the center of the unit.
3. Check and record the temperature of each unit daily.
4. Have a plan for vaccine protection when power outages occur.

45.6 Recognize common infectious and communicable diseases.

1. Chickenpox (Varicella):
   - Causes fluid-filled vesicles with elevated temperature and itching.
2. Coxsackieviruses:
   - May cause respiratory symptoms or skin and mucous membrane lesions.
3. Diphtheria:
   - Seen in countries with low immunization rates.
   - May cause severe respiratory symptoms.
4. Erythema Infectiosum (Fifth disease):
   - Begins with mild, flu-like illness and ends with a red rash on the cheeks and lace-like rash on body.
5. Haemophilus Influenza, Type B:
   - Begins with respiratory symptoms, but may progress to meningitis, cellulitis, or pneumonia.
6. Influenza:
   - Sudden onset of respiratory symptoms, headache, nausea, vomiting, and diarrhea.
7. Measles (Rubeola):
   - High fever, red rash.
   - Koplik spots on buccal mucosa.
8. Mononucleosis:
   - Symptoms begin with high fever, sore throat, and malaise.
   - Severe cervical lymphadenopathy and possible liver and spleen enlargement.
9. Mumps (Parotitis):
   - Begins with fever and pain while chewing.
   - Swelling of parotid glands.
10. Pertussis (Whooping Cough):
    - Begins with vague respiratory symptoms.
    - Paroxysmal cough that sounds like a "whoop."
11. Pneumococcal infection:
    - Signs are related to location of infection.
12. Poliomyelitis:
    - Begins with fever, sore throat, and stiff neck.
    - Affects central nervous system, may progress to paralysis.
13. Roseola (Exanthem subitum):
    - Sudden high fever in child 6 months to 2 years of age, no toxic symptoms.
    - Following fever phase, child develops a maculopapular rash over most of body.
14. Rotavirus:
    - Fever, vomiting, and diarrhea.
15. Rubella:
    - Mild disease causing low grade fever and rash.
    - Prenatal exposure causes birth defects.
16. Streptococcus A:
    - Rapid onset of severe sore throat with high fever.
    - May progress to scarlet fever.
    - Pyodermal skin lesions with honey crust.
17. Tetanus:
    - Headache, stiffness of the neck and jaw, painful facial spasms, and difficulty chewing and swallowing.
    - Muscle spasms, oposthotonis.

45.7 Develop a nursing care plan for a child with a common communicable disease.

1. Isolate child from others as much as possible.
2. Treat high fever and other symptoms with non-aspirin antipyretic medications.
3. Discourage scratching by trimming fingernails or putting mitts over hands.
4. Encourage use of tepid baths with Aveeno or oatmeal, to relieve itching.
5. Medicate with antihistamines to assist with complaints of itching.
6. Encourage fluids to promote hydration.
7. Educate and support the parents for home care of the child.

CRITICAL THINKING IN ACTION

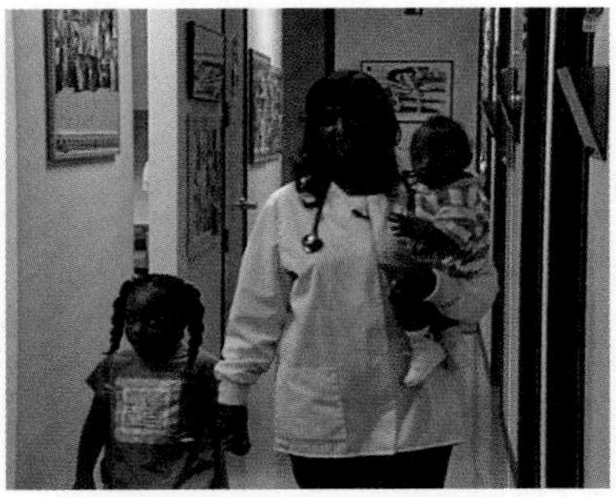

Keisha, 7 years old, and Brandon, 1 year old, are brought to the pediatric clinic, needing immunizations. Even though Brandon is sick today, their mother would still like Keisha to have her immunizations, and she would also like both children to have a complete check-up before their vaccines to make sure they are healthy.

You examine Keisha's vital signs as: 80th percentile in height, 40th percentile in weight, temperature 98.9°F, blood pressure 105/62, urinalysis with a trace of leukocytes, and she passes her hearing and vision screening. She seems extremely anxious about having to get a needle. There is evidence of eczema and allergic rhinitis.

You examine Brandon as a sick visit while he clings to his mother. His vital signs are: temperature 102°F, respiratory rate of 30 breaths per minute, and heart rate of 90 beats per minute. Brandon's exam exhibits evidence of a coxsackievirus, evidenced by grayish, papulovesicular, ulcerative lesions in his mouth. This type of illness does not respond to antibiotics. You advise the mother to avoid exposing other persons because it is contagious and to offer cool drinks and bland foods. She is also told warm saline mouth rinses would be helpful, to observe for dehydration, and to give ibuprofen or acetaminophen as needed.

1. Since Brandon has been into the office several times for various infections, what education can be given to his mother to reduce the chances of future infections?
2. Keisha has eczema and allergic rhinitis. Would this be a contraindication to giving vaccines?
3. What are questions the nurse should ask the mother before administering vaccines to Keisha to make sure there are no contraindications to giving them?
4. What should the mother be told about caring for Keisha after her vaccines?
5. How should the mother be told to manage Brandon's fever?

See MyNursingKit for possible responses.

REFERENCES

Agrawal, D., & Teach, S. J. (2006). Evaluation and management of a child with suspected malaria. *Pediatric Emergency Care, 22*(2), 127–133.

American Academy of Pediatrics Committee on Infectious Disease. (2007). Antiviral therapy and prophylaxis for influenza in children. *Pediatrics, 119*(4), 852–860.

American Academy of Pediatrics Committee on Infectious Disease. (2009). *Red book: Report of the Committee on Infectious Disease* (28th ed.). Elk Grove Village, IL: Author.

Asch-Goodkin, J. (2006). What's new on the immunization front: Influenza and meningococcal vaccines. *Contemporary Pediatrics, 23*(12), 17.

Benin, A. L., Wisler-Scher, D. J., Colson, E., Shapiro, E. D., & Holmboe, E. S. (2006). Qualitative analysis of mothers' decision-making about vaccines for infants: The importance of trust. *Pediatrics, 117*(5), 1532–1541.

Bilukha, O. O., & Rosenstein, N. (2005). Prevention and control of meningococcal disease. *Morbidity and Mortality Weekly Report, 54*(RR07), 1–21.

Centers for Disease Control and Prevention. (2005a). Achievements in public health: Elimination of rubella and congenital rubella syndrome—United States, 1969–2004. *Morbidity and Mortality Weekly Report, 54*(11), 279–282.

Centers for Disease Control and Prevention. (2006, May 18). Update: Multistate outbreak of mumps–United States, January 1–May 2, 2006. *Morbidity and Mortality Weekly Report, 55*, 1–5.

Centers for Disease Control and Prevention. (2008a). *Bioterrorism.* Retrieved November 15, 2008, from www.bt.cdc.gov/bioterrorism

Centers for Disease Control and Prevention. (2008b). Update: Recommendations from the Advisory Committee on Immunization Practices (ACIP) regarding administration of combination MMRV vaccine. *Morbidity and Mortality Weekly Report, 57*(10), 258–260.

Centers for Disease Control and Prevention. (2008c). Update: Measles–United States, January–July, 2008. *Morbidity and Mortality Weekly Report, 57*(33), 893–896.

Centers for Disease Control and Prevention. (2008d). Vaccination coverage among adolescents aged 13–17 years—United States, 2007, *Morbidity and Mortality Weekly Report, 57*(40), 1100–1103.

Chang, L., Huang, L., Gau, S. S., Wu, Y., Hsia, S., Fan, T., et al. (2007). Neurodevelopment and cognition in children after enterovirus 71 infection. *New England Journal of Medicine, 356*(12), 1226–1234.

Chapman, A. S. (2006). Diagnosis and management of tickborne rickettsial diseases: Rocky Mountain spotted fever, ehrlichioses, and anaplasmosis – United States, *Morbidity and Mortality Weekly Report, 55*(RR-4), 1–27.

Cheater, F. M. (2006). Mothers' decisions about MMR vaccination were framed by their child's vulnerabilities and wider social trends. *Evidence Based Nursing, 9*(1), 27.

Cherry, J. D. (2005). The epidemiology of pertussis: A comparison of the epidemiology of the disease pertussis with the epidemiology of *Bordatella pertussis* infection. *Pediatrics, 115*(5), 1422–1427.

Cohen, B. A. (2004). Papular rash on hands and feet after 3 days' fever and headache. *Contemporary Pediatrics, 21*(7), 15–17.

Cox, J. E. (2006). Egg-based vaccines. *Pediatrics in Review, 27*(3), 118–119.

Crocetti, M. T., & Serwint, J. R. (2005). Fever: Separating fact from fiction. *Contemporary Pediatrics, 22*(1), 34–41.

Dempsey, A. F., & Freed, G. L. (2006). A new day in preventing meningococcal disease: Sizing up available vaccines. *Contemporary Pediatrics, 23*(10), 31–39.

Dennehy, P. H. (2005). Update on a high morbidity infection: Rotavirus. *Contemporary Pediatrics, 22*(12), 34–40.

Department of Health and Human Services, Office of Disease Prevention and Promotion. (2006). *Healthy People 2010 Midcourse Review.* Washington, DC: Author. Retrieved April 24, 2007, from www.healthypeople.gov/data/midcourse/pdf/FA14.pdf

Dyer, J. A. (2007). Childhood viral exanthems. *Pediatric Annals, 36*(1), 21–29.

Fergie, J., & Purcell, K. (2007). The epidemic of methicillin-resistant *Staphylococcus aureus* colonization and infection in children: Effects on the community, health systems, and physician practices, *Pediatric Annals, 36*(7), 404–412.

Fiore, A. E., Shay, D. K., Broder, K., Iskander, J. K., Uyeki, T. M., Mootrey, G., et al., (2008). Prevention and control of influenza: Recommendations of the Advisory Committee on Immunization Practices (ACIP), 2008. *Morbidity and Mortality Weekly report, 57*(RR-7), 26–27.

Food and Drug Administration. (2006a). *FDA approves a second drug for prevention of influenza A and B in adults and children.* Retrieved April 3, 2006, from www.fda/gov/bbs/topics/news/2006/new01231.html

Food and Drug Administration. (2006b). *Tamiflu.* Retrieved April 30, 2007, from www.fda.gov/medwatch/safety/2006/safety2006.htm#tamiflu

Gad, A., & Shah, S. (2007). Special immunization considerations of the preterm infant. *Journal of Pediatric health Care, 21*(6), 385–391.

Gardner, P. (2006). Prevention of meningococcal disease. *New England Journal of Medicine, 355*(14), 1466–1473.

Grijalva, C. G., Poehling, K. A., Edwards, K. M., Weinberg, G. A., Staat, M. A., et al. (2007). Accuracy and interpretation of rapid influenza tests in children. *Pediatrics, 119*(1), e6–e11.

Health Resources and Services Administration. (2008). *Vaccine injury table.* Retrieved November 1, 2008, from www.hrsa.gov/vaccinecompensation/table.htm

Jackson, L. A., Starkovich, P., Dunstan, M., Yu, O., Nelson, J., et al., (2008). Prospective assessment of the effect of needle length and injection site on the risk of local reactions to the fifth diphtheria-tetanus-acellular pertussis vaccination. *Pediatrics, 121*(3), e646–e652.

Junker, A. K. (2005). Epstein-Barr virus. *Pediatrics in Review, 26*(3), 79–84.

Kaplan, S. L., Schutze, G. E., Leake, J. A. D., Barson, W. J., Halasa, N. B., et al. (2007). Multicenter surveillance of invasive meningococcal infections in children. *Pediatrics, 118*(4), e979–e984.

Koirala, J. (2006). Plague: Disease, management, and recognition of act of terrorism. *Infectious Disease Clinics of North America, 20,* 273–287

Kroger, A. T., Atkinson, W. L., Marcuse, E. K., & Pickering, L. K. (2006). General recommendations on immunization: Recommendations of the Advisory Committee on Immunization Practices (ACIP). *Morbidity and Mortality Weekly Report, 55*(RR-15), 1–48.

Le, J. (2006). Management of community-acquired methicillin-resistant *Staphylcoccus aureus* infections in children. *Pharmacotherapy, 26*(12), 1758–1770.

Lee, G. M., Santoli, J. M., Hannan, C., Messonnier, M. L., Sabin, J. E., et al., (2007). Gaps in vaccine financing for underinsured children in the United States, *Journal of the American Medical Association, 298*(6), 680–682.

Leggiadro, R. J. (2007). Bioterrorism: A clinical reality. *Pediatric Annals, 36*(6), 352–358.

MacDonald, M. (2005). Parents' decisions on MMR vaccination for their children were based on personal experience rather than scientific evidence. *Evidence-Based Nursing, 8,* 60.

Mani, C. S., & Murray, D. L. (2006). Rabies. *Pediatrics in Review, 27*(4), 129–135.

Maples, H. D. (2006). Malaria prophylaxis in children. *Pediatrics in Review, 27*(9), 346–349.

Marin, M., Güris, D., Chaves, S., Schmid, S., & Seward, J. F. (2007). Prevention of varicella: Recommendations of the Advisory Committee on Immunization Practices (ACIP), *Morbidity and Mortality Weekly Report, 56*(RR-4), 1–38.

Markenson, D. (2005). The treatment of children exposed to pathogens linked to bioterrorism. *Infectious Disease Clinics of North America, 19,* 731–745.

McMurray, R., Cheater, F. M., Weighall, A., et al. (2004). Managing controversy through consultation: A qualitative study of communication and trust around MMR vaccination decisions. *British Journal for General Practitioners, 54,* 520–525.

Miller, A. A. (2007). Alternating acetaminophen with ibuprofen for fever: Is this a problem? *Pediatric Annals, 36*(7), 384–388.

Milonovich, L. M. (2007). Meningococcemia: Epidemiology, pathophysiology, and management. *Journal of Pediatric Health Care, 21*(2), 75–80.

Moore, J., & Kalvaitis, K. (2007). HHV-6 primarily causes febrile illness. *Infectious Diseases in Children, 20*(2), 63.

Moore, S. L., & Seybold, V. K. (2007). HPV vaccine. *Clinician Reviews, 17*(1), 36–41.

Nabulsi, M. M., Tamim, H., Mahfoud, Z., Itani, M., Sabra, R., et al. (2006). Alternating ibuprofen and acetaminophen in the treatment of febrile children: a pilot study. *BMC Medicine, 4*(4). Retrieved April 24, 2007, from www.biomedcentral.com/1741-7015/4/4

Nield, L. S., & Kamat, D. M. (2006). Vaccine refusal: When parents just say "no." *Consultant for Pediatricians, 5*(10), S5–S8.

Omer, S. B., Pan, W. K. Y., Halsey, N. A., Stokley, S., Moulton, L. H., et al. (2006). Nonmedical exemptions to school immunization requirements. *Journal of American Medical Association, 296,* 1757–1762.

Parashar, U. D., Alexander, J. P., & Glass, R. I. (2006). Prevention of rotavirus gastroenteritis among infants and children: Recommendations of the Advisory Committee on Immunization Practices (ACIP). *Morbidity and Mortality Weekly Report, 55*(RR-12), 1–13.

Pichichero, M. E., & Casey, J. R. (2007). Emergency of a multiresistant serotype 19a pneumococcal strain not included in the 7-valent conjugate vaccine as an otopathogen in children. *Journal of the American Medical Association, 298*(15), 1772–1778.

Poltorak, M., Leach, M., Fairhead, J., & Cassell, J. (2004). MMR Talk and vaccination choices: An ethnographic study in Brighton. *Social Science and Medicine, 61,* 709–719.

Razzaq, S., & Schutze, G. E. (2005). Rocky Mountain spotted fever: A physician's challenge, *Pediatrics in Review, 26*(4), 125–129.

Reef, S., Dayan, G., Bellini, W., Barsky, A., Redd, S., et al. (2006). Update: Mumps activity—United States, January 1–October 7, 2006. *Morbidity and Mortality Weekly Report, 55*(42), 1152–1153.

Salmon, D. A., Moulton, L. H., Omer, S. B., deHart, M. P., Stokley, S., & Halsey, N. A. (2005). Factors associated with refusal of childhood vaccines among parents of school-aged children. *Archives of Pediatric and Adolescent Medicine, 159*(5), 470–476.

Sarrell, E. M., Wiielunsky, E., & Cohen, H. A. (2006, February). Antipyretic treatment in young children with fever: Acetaminophen, ibuprofen, or both alternating in a randomized, double-blind study. *Archives in Pediatric and Adolescent Medicine, 160,* 197–202.

Savely, G. R. (2006). Update on Lyme disease. *Clinician Reviews, 16*(4), 45–50.

Stanwyck, C., & Jain, N. (2007). Vaccination coverage among children in kindergarten–United States, 2006–2007 school year. *Morbidity and Mortality Weekly Report, 56*(32), 819–821.

Stocker, J. T. (2006). Clinical and pathological differential diagnosis of selected potential bioterrorism agents of interest to pediatric health care providers, *Clinics in Laboratory Medicine, 26,* 329–344

Tiwari, T., Murphy, T. V., & Moran, J. (2005). Recommended antimicrobial agents for the treatment and postexposure prophylaxis of pertussis: 2005 CDC guidelines. *Morbidity and Mortality Weekly Report, 54*(RR-14), 1–16.

Tufts, G., & Hardman, M. E. C. (2006). Community-acquired methicillin-resistant *Staphylococcus aureus. Clinician Reviews, 16*(1), 52–57.

Veraas, K. (2006). Nursing and other medical staff issues in vaccine administration. *Pediatric Annals, 35*(7), 519–521.

Victor, J. C., Monto, A. S., Surdina, T. Y., Suleimenova, S. Z., Vaughan, G., et al., (2007). Hepatits A vaccine versus immune globulin for postexposure prophylaxis, *New England Journal of Medicine, 357*(17), 1685–1694.

Wilson, T. R. (2006). Update on adolescent immunization: Review of pertussis and the efficacy, safety, and clinical use of vaccines that contain tetanus-diphtheria-acellular pertussis. *Journal of Pediatric Health Care, 20*(4), 229–237.

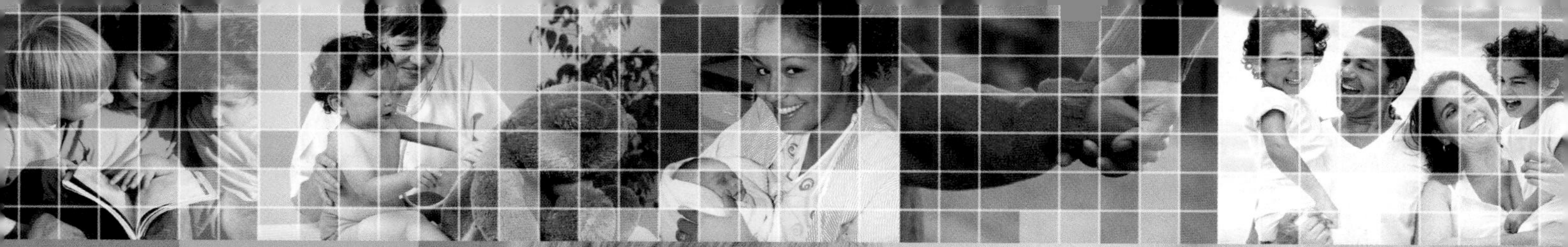

PART

7

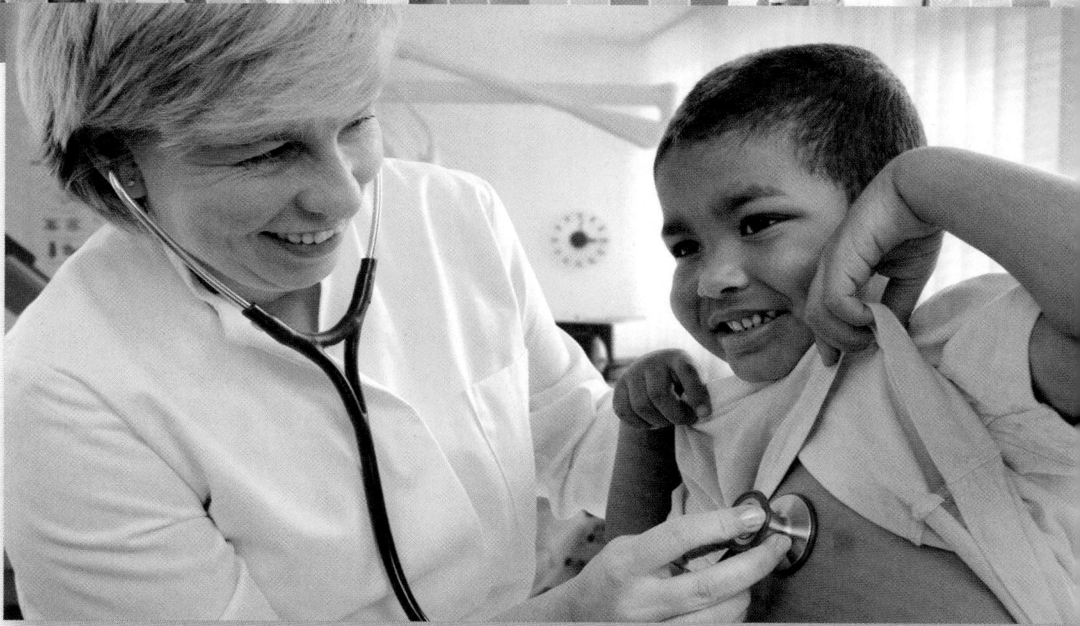

Caring for Children with Alterations in Health Status

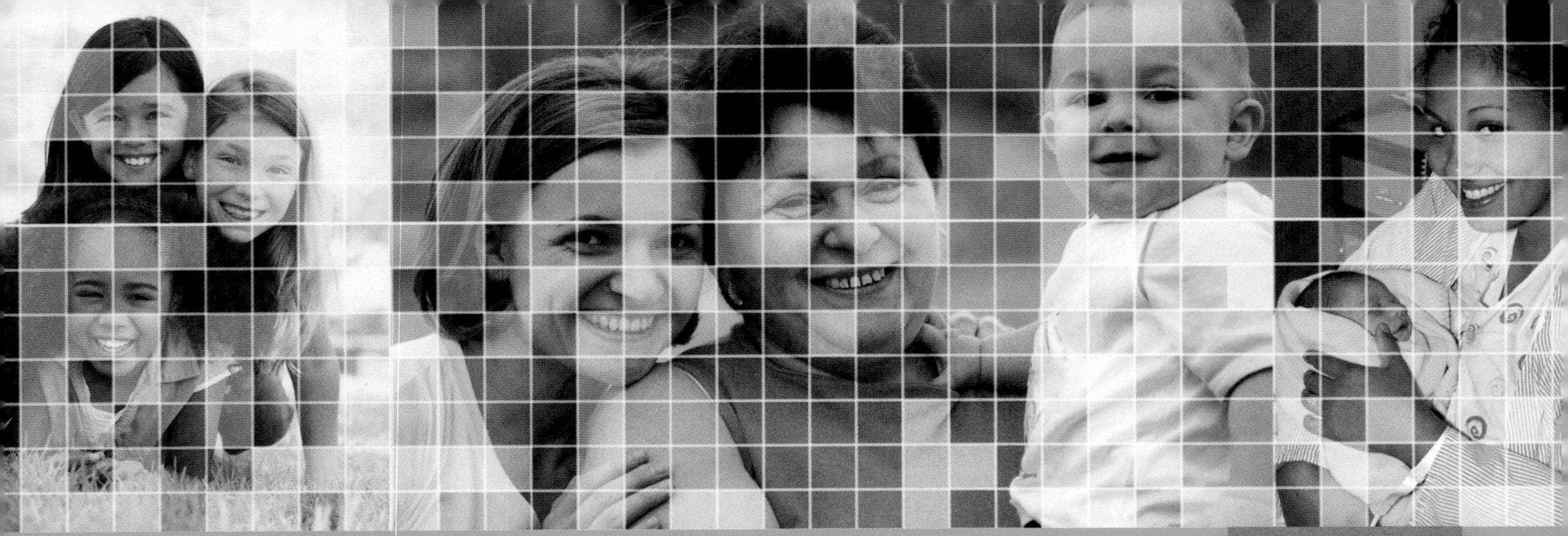

CHAPTER

46

The Child with Alterations in Fluid, Electrolyte, and Acid-Base Balance

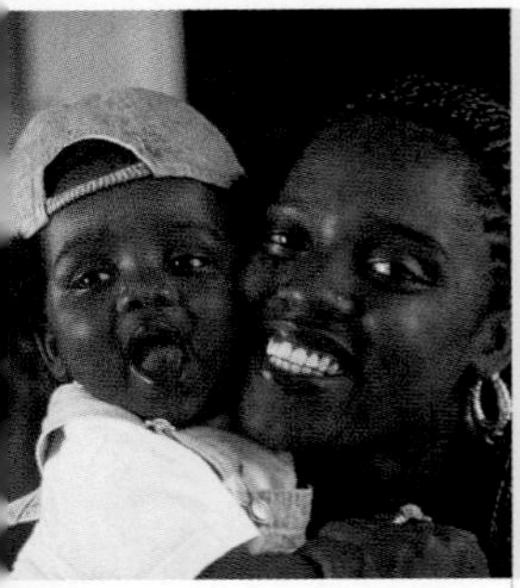

LeShan always likes to eat, so when he won't even drink I know he is sick. We just didn't know how sick he was or that he had gotten dehydrated. I wonder if we should have done something else for him at home. —*Mother of LeShan, 18 months old*

LEARNING OUTCOMES

46.1 Describe normal fluid and electrolyte status for children at various ages.

46.2 Identify regulatory mechanisms for fluid and electrolyte balance.

46.3 Recognize threats to fluid and electrolyte balance in children.

46.4 Describe acid-base balance and recognize disruptions common in children.

46.5 Analyze assessment findings to recognize fluid-electrolyte problems and acid-base imbalance in children.

46.6 Describe appropriate nursing interventions for children experiencing fluid-electrolyte problems and acid-base imbalance.

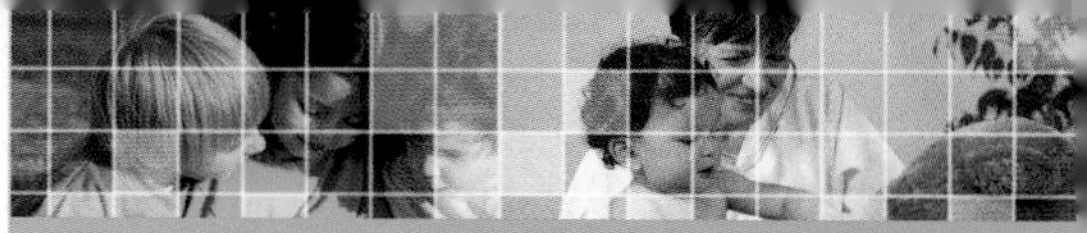

KEY TERMS

Acidemia, 1261
Acidosis, 1263
Alkalemia, 1261
Alkalosis, 1263
Body fluid, 1233
Buffer, 1262
Dehydration, 1235
Diffusion, 1233
Electrolytes, 1233
Extracellular fluid, 1233
Filtration, 1245
Hypertonic dehydration (or hypernatremic dehydration), 1235
Hypertonic saline, 1250
Hypotonic dehydration (or hyponatremic dehydration), 1235
Hypotonic fluid, 1248
Insensible water loss, 1233
Interstitial fluid, 1233
Intracellular fluid, 1233
Intravascular fluid, 1233
Isotonic dehydration (or isonatremic dehydration), 1235
Isotonic fluid, 1248
Kussmaul respirations, 1268
Oncotic pressure, 1245
Osmolality, 1247
Osmosis, 1247
pH, 1260
Pitting edema, 1246
Saline, 1243
Sensible water loss, 1233

A thorough understanding of fluid, electrolyte, and acid-base homeostasis and imbalances is essential when providing nursing care to children like LeShan in the chapter opener. This chapter presents information about the processes that maintain fluid and electrolyte balance and describes the common imbalances that may occur in children. It also describes how the body regulates acid-base status and explains the management of acid-base imbalances.

Many health conditions cause changes in body fluids that must be regulated and managed. Sometimes management of fluid status in the home or in a short-term ambulatory facility can prevent more serious illness or hospitalization.

ANATOMY AND PHYSIOLOGY OF PEDIATRIC DIFFERENCES

Infants and young children differ physiologically from adults in ways that make them vulnerable to fluid, electrolyte, and acid-base imbalances.

Fluid in the body is in a dynamic state. Much of the human body is composed of water. **Body fluid** is body water that has solutes dissolved in it. Some of the solutes are **electrolytes**, or charged particles (ions). Electrolytes such as sodium (Na^+), potassium (K^+), calcium (Ca^{++}), magnesium (Mg^{++}), chloride (Cl^-), and inorganic phosphorus (Pi) ions must be present in the proper concentrations for cells to function effectively. In people of all ages, fluid continuously leaves the body through the skin, in feces and urine, and during respiration. **Sensible water loss** is that which is measurable and observable, such as urine. **Insensible water loss** cannot be directly measured or observed, such as that lost through the skin and respirations. For adults and children, intake of oral fluid is approximately equivalent to urinary output in normal circumstances. Likewise, water provided in food and by the body's metabolic processes is approximately the same as insensible loss from feces, skin, and respirations.

In people of all ages, body fluid is located in several compartments. The two major fluid compartments contain the **intracellular fluid** (fluid inside the cells) and the **extracellular fluid** (outside the cells). The extracellular fluid is made up of **intravascular fluid** (within the blood vessels) and **interstitial fluid** (between the cells and outside the blood and lymphatic vessels) (Figure 46–1 ●). Extracellular fluid accounts for about one third of total body water, and intracellular fluid for about two thirds. The concentrations of electrolytes in the fluid differ depending on the fluid compartment. For example, extracellular fluid is rich in sodium ions; intracellular fluid, by contrast, is low in sodium ions but rich in potassium ions (Table 46–1).

Fluid moves between the intravascular and interstitial compartments by a process called filtration. Water moves into and out of the cells by the process of osmosis. These processes are discussed later in the chapter. Electrolytes move across cell membranes both by **diffusion** of particles from a location of greater to less concentration and by active transport that is effective even against the concentration gradient.

The percentage of body weight composed of water varies with age. The percentage of total body water is highest at birth (and higher in premature than in full-term infants) and decreases with age (see "As Children Grow: Fluid and Electrolyte Differences"). Newborns and young infants also have a proportionately larger extracellular fluid volume than older children and adults because their brain and skin (both rich in interstitial fluid) occupy a greater proportion of their body weight. Much of the body's extracellular fluid is exchanged each day. Infants have a high daily fluid requirement with little fluid volume reserve; this makes the infant vulnerable to dehydration. As an infant grows, the proportion of water inside the cells increases (Bindler & Howry, 2005).

Infants and children under 2 years of age lose a greater proportion of fluid each day than older children and adults and are thus more dependent on adequate intake. They have a greater amount of skin surface or body surface area (BSA) and thus have greater insensible water losses through the skin. Because of this relatively large BSA,

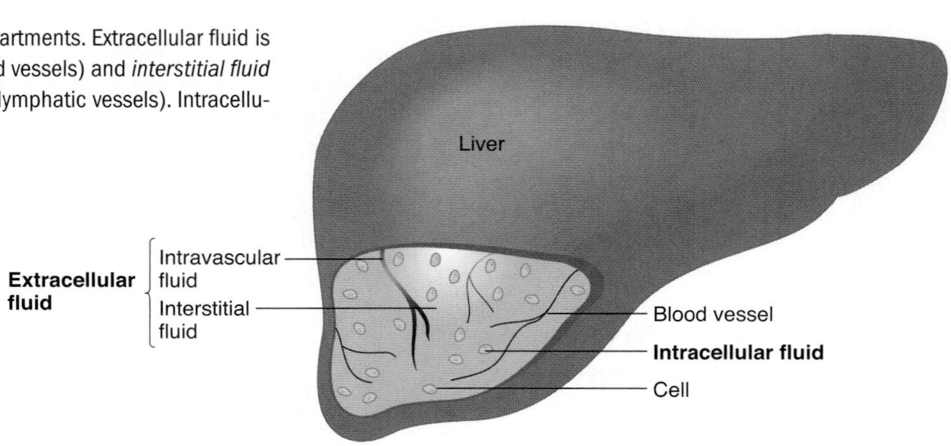

● **Figure 46–1** The major body fluid compartments. Extracellular fluid is composed mainly of *vascular fluid* (fluid in blood vessels) and *interstitial fluid* (fluid between cells and outside the blood and lymphatic vessels). Intracellular fluid is that within cells.

Table 46–1 Electrolyte Concentrations in Body Fluid Compartments

	Extracellular Fluid (ECF)		
Components	**Vascular**	**Interstitial**	**Intracellular Fluid**
Na^+	High	High	Low
K^+	Low	Low	High
Ca^{++}	Low	Low	Low (higher than ECF)
Mg^{++}	Low	Low	High
Pi	Low	Low	High
Cl^-	High	High	Low
Proteins	High	Low	High

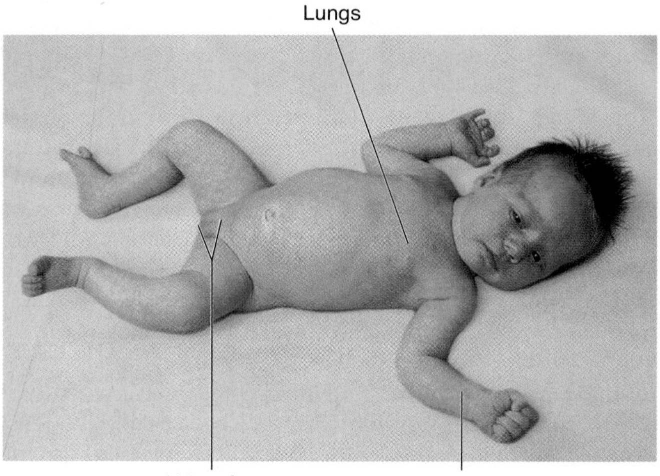

● **Figure 46–2** Normal routes of fluid excretion from infants and children.

they are also at greater risk when skin is affected, such as in burns. In addition, respiratory and metabolic rates are high during early childhood, so children have greater water loss from the lungs and greater water demand to fuel the body's metabolic processes (Figure 46–2 ●). Due to these factors, the exercising child dehydrates easily and must consume more fluid during physical activity, particularly during hot weather (Mayo Clinic, 2007).

When fluid status is compromised, a number of body mechanisms are activated to help restore balance. Several of these mechanisms occur in the kidney. The kidneys conserve water and needed electrolytes while excreting waste products and drug metabolites. In children under 2 years of age, however, the glomeruli, tubules, and nephrons of the kidneys are immature. They are thus unable to conserve or excrete water and solutes effectively (see Chapter 54∞). Because more water is generally excreted, the infant and young child can become dehydrated quickly or develop electrolyte imbalances. In addition, infants have a weaker transport system for ions and bicarbonate, placing them at greater risk for acidosis and acid-base imbalances. Children under 2 years of age also have difficulty regulating electrolytes such as sodium and calcium. Renal response to high solute loads is slower and less developed, with function improving gradually during the first year of life.

Finally, in addition to the immaturity of physiologic processes, many health conditions make young children more vulnerable to fluid deficit. Examples include water loss due to phototherapy used to treat newborns with hyperbilirubinemia; water loss with increased respiratory rate during illness, fever, vomiting, and diarrhea; and drainage from blood loss or drainage tubes.

FLUID VOLUME IMBALANCES

When fluid excretion and losses are balanced by the proper volume and type of fluid intake, fluid balance will be maintained. If, however, fluid output and intake are not matched, fluid imbalance may occur rapidly. The major types of fluid imbalances are:

- extracellular fluid volume deficit (dehydration);
- extracellular fluid volume excess; and
- interstitial fluid volume excess (edema).

AS CHILDREN GROW

FLUID AND ELECTROLYTE DIFFERENCES

The newborn and infant have a high percentage of body weight composed of water, especially extracellular fluid, which is lost from the body easily. Note the small stomach size which limits ability to rehydrate quickly.

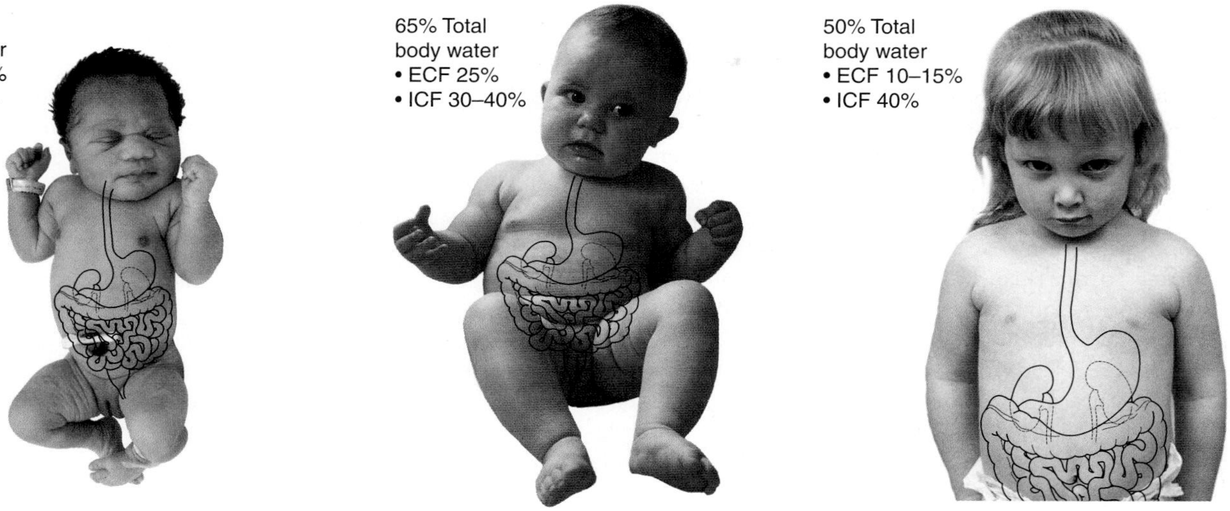

Newborn

75% Total body water
- ECF 45%
- ICF 30%

Brain and skin occupy a greater proportion of body weight and are high in interstitial fluid

Infant

65% Total body water
- ECF 25%
- ICF 30–40%

High BSA promotes fluid loss

Little fluid reserve in intracellular fluid

5–6x greater fluid exchange daily

High metabolic rate requires generous fluid intake

Child/Adolescent

50% Total body water
- ECF 10–15%
- ICF 40%

Kidneys are immature until 2 years and unable to conserve water and electrolytes or fully assist in acid–base balance

EXTRACELLULAR FLUID VOLUME IMBALANCES

EXTRACELLULAR FLUID VOLUME DEFICIT (DEHYDRATION)

Extracellular fluid volume deficit occurs when there is not enough fluid in the extracellular compartment (vascular and interstitial). Depending on the cause of dehydration, sodium may be at normal, low, or elevated levels. (Hyponatremia and hypernatremia are described later in the chapter, on pages 1247–1250.) The state of body water deficit is called **dehydration**. There are three major types of dehydration:

- **Isotonic dehydration** (or **isonatremic dehydration**) occurs when fluid loss is not balanced by intake, and the loss of water and sodium are in proportion. The serum sodium is therefore within normal limits or slighty low, even though the circulating blood volume is lowered. Most of the fluid lost is from the extracellular component. This type of dehydration is commonly manifested in the illnesses of young children such as vomiting and diarrhea.
- **Hypotonic dehydration** (or **hyponatremic dehydration**) occurs when fluid loss is characterized by a proportionately greater loss of sodium than water. Serum sodium is below normal levels. Compensatory fluid shifts occur from the extracellular to intracellular components in an attempt to establish normal proportions, thus leading to even greater extracellular dehydration. Severe and prolonged vomiting and diarrhea, burns, and renal disease can lead to this condition, as well as administration of intravenous fluid without electrolytes in treatment of dehydration.
- **Hypertonic dehydration** (or **hypernatremic dehydration**) occurs when fluid loss is characterized by a proportionately greater loss of water than sodium. Serum sodium is above normal levels. Compensatory fluid shifts occur from the intracellular to extracellular components in an attempt to establish normal proportions. The extracellular component therefore remains fairly normal, delaying the onset of signs and symptoms of dehydration until the condition is quite serious. Neurologic symptoms reflecting intracellular imbalance may occur simultaneously with more common symptoms of dehydration. The condition may be caused by health

problems such as diabetes insipidus (see Chapter 55) or administration of intravenous fluid or tube feedings with high electrolyte levels.

The body continuously attempts to compensate for fluid and electrolyte imbalance by shifting fluid and electrolytes from one component to another. Therefore, it is rare for only one type of dehydration to occur; the child's fluid and electrolyte status and symptoms are constantly changing. Ongoing assessment and management are needed.

Etiology and Pathophysiology

Extracellular fluid volume deficit is usually caused by the loss of sodium-containing fluid from the body. Vomiting, diarrhea, nasogastric suction, hemorrhage, and burns most often cause loss of fluid containing sodium. Vomiting and diarrhea are common manifestations of disease in children throughout the world, and each year up to 5 million children die from dehydration related to diarrhea. In the United States, about 300 to 500 die annually from this problem, about 220,000 are hospitalized, and 1.5 million receive outpatient care (Dale, 2004; Dennehy, 2005).

Another cause of extracellular fluid volume deficit in infants is increased water loss in low-birth-weight infants kept under radiant warmers to maintain heat (Figure 46–3 ●). Less frequently, adrenal insufficiency, accumulation of extracellular fluid in a "third space" such as the peritoneal cavity, and overuse of diuretics may be the cause. The latter etiology is most often seen in adolescents with bulimia (see Chapter 34).

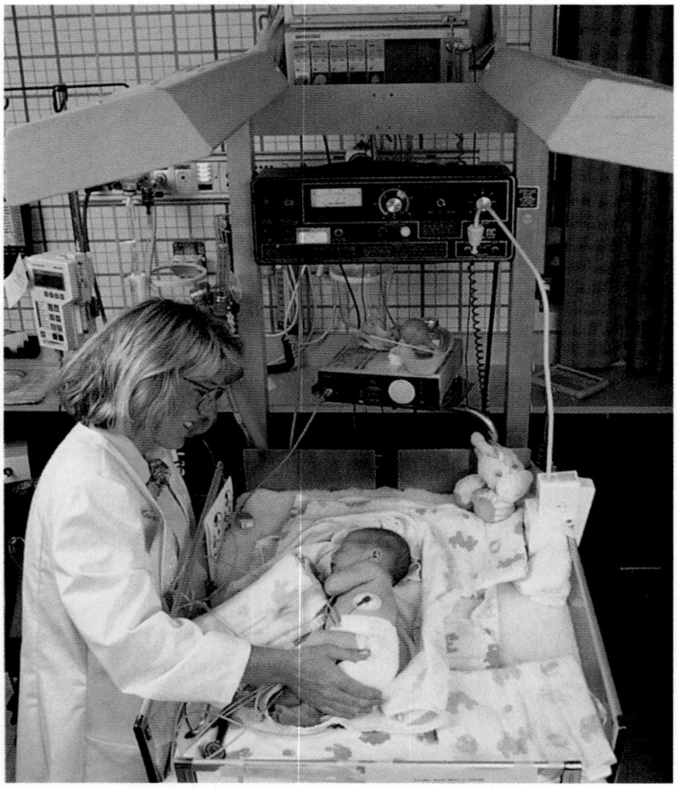

● **Figure 46–3** Fluid loss from overhead warming. Use of an overhead warmer or phototherapy increases insensible fluid excretion through the skin, thus increasing the fluid intake needed.

MyNursingKit Identifying Intravenous Fluids

Excessive exercise during very hot weather without sufficient fluid replacement can lead to fluid and electrolyte imbalance. Children are more prone than adults to imbalance from exercise, as a result of several of the physiologic differences described in the pediatric variations section earlier. Since children have a greater BSA, they can gain more heat from the environment when it is hot and lose more when it is cold. The high metabolic rate of children is further increased during exercise so that fluid lost in metabolism is significant. Young children do not sweat effectively and may be unable to eliminate heat by this method. Children may not feel thirsty and so fail to drink even when dehydrated (Armstrong, Casa, Millard-Stafford, et al., 2007; Mayo Clinic, 2007).

Burns and gastroenteritis are characterized by initial dehydration in the first 3 days due to a high loss of extracellular fluid. About 80% of the fluid loss is extracellular, and only about 20% intracellular. However, with time, the relationship begins to change, so that in illnesses over 3 days, about 60% of fluid loss is extracellular while 40% is intracellular (Custer & Rau, 2009). Since the electrolyte composition of extracellular and intracellular fluids differs (see Table 46–1), electrolyte management will need to change for long-term conditions.

Clinical Manifestations

The signs of dehydration relate to the severity or degree of the body water deficit (Table 46–2). They are a result of both the decreased fluid (e.g., diminished turgor and mucous membrane moisture) and the body's response to the fluid deficit (e.g., pulse and blood pressure changes).

Mild dehydration is hard to detect, because children appear alert and have moist mucous membranes. Infants may be irritable and older children are thirsty. In moderate dehydration the child is often lethargic and sleepy, but there may be periods of restlessness and irritability, especially in infants. Skin turgor is diminished, mucous membranes appear dry, and urine is dark in color and diminished in amount. Pulse rate is usually increased, and blood pressure can be normal or low. Severe dehydration is manifested by increasing lethargy or nonresponsiveness, markedly decreased blood pressure, rapid pulse, non-elastic skin turgor, dry mucous membranes, sunken and dry eyes, and markedly decreased or absent urinary output.

Clinical Therapy

Diagnosis of dehydration is best accomplished by clinical observations. Medical management depends on accurate identification of the degree of dehydration. In addition to physical signs and symptoms (see Table 46–2), elevated blood urea nitrogen (BUN) (>17 mg/dL) and low serum bicarbonate (≤16–17 mEq/L) are useful to identify dehydration from moderate and severe diarrhea (Madati & Bachur, 2008). The treatment of extracellular fluid volume deficit is administration of fluid containing sodium, by oral rehydration therapy or by intravenous fluids.

Table 46–2 Severity of Clinical Dehydration

	Mild	Moderate	Severe
Percent of body weight lost	Up to 5% (40–50 mL/kg)	6–9% (60–90 mL/kg)	10% or more (100 mL/kg)
Level of consciousness	Alert, restless, thirsty	Irritable or lethargic (infants and very young children); alert, thirsty, restless (older children and adolescents)	Lethargic to comatose (infants and young children); often conscious, apprehensive (older children and adolescents)
Blood pressure	Normal	Normal or low; postural hypotension (older children and adolescents)	Low to undetectable
Pulse	Normal	Rapid	Rapid, weak to nonpalpable
Skin turgor	Normal	Poor	Very poor
Mucous membranes	Moist	Dry	Parched
Urine	May appear normal	Decreased output (<1 mL/kg/hr); dark color; increased specific gravity	Very decreased or absent output
Thirst	Slightly increased	Moderately increased	Greatly increased unless lethargic
Fontanel	Normal	Sunken	Sunken
Extremities	Warm; normal capillary refill	Delayed capillary refill (>2 sec)	Cool, discolored; delayed capillary refill (> 3–4 sec)
Respirations	Normal	Normal or rapid	Changing rate and pattern
Eyes	Normal	Slightly sunken, decreased tears	Deeply sunken, absent tears

Clinical Manifestations

EXTRACELLULAR FLUID VOLUME DEFICIT

CLINICAL MANIFESTATIONS	ETIOLOGY
Weight loss	Decreased fluid volume; 1 L of fluid weighs 1 kg
Postural blood pressure drop (older children)	Inadequate circulating blood volume to offset the force of gravity when in upright position
Increased small vein filling time	Decreased vascular volume
Delayed capillary refill time	Decreased vascular volume
Flat neck veins when supine (older children)	Decreased vascular volume
Dizziness, syncope	Inadequate circulation to brain
Oliguria	Inadequate circulation to kidneys
Thready, rapid pulse	Cardiac reflex response to decreased vascular volume
Sunken fontanel (infants)	Decreased fluid volume
Decreased skin turgor	Decreased interstitial fluid volume

Growth and Development

Urine specific gravity may increase in older children who are dehydrated, but children under 2 years of age are not able to concentrate urine effectively. A rising specific gravity may not be seen in the younger dehydrated child.

Oral rehydration therapy has been used for years in developing countries without an accessible supply of intravenous fluids. More recently, experts have recognized the benefits of its early use to prevent severe dehydration and to treat mild and moderate dehydration in children in developed countries. The therapy successfully treats the dehydration caused by many gastrointestinal illnesses and prevents hospitalization for many infants and young children. It is the treatment of choice for

Table 46–3 Common Intravenous Solutions, Uses, and Components

		Components							
IV Solution	Uses	CHO (g/100 mL)	Protein (g/100 mL)	Cal/L	NA^{+} (mEq/L)	K^{+} (mEq/L)	Cl^{-} (mEq/L)	HCO_3 (mEq/L)	Ca^{++} (mEq/L)
D_5W	Restores water loss, plasma volume, and calories; lowers sodium levels	5	–	170	–	–	–	–	–
Normal saline (0.9% NaCl)	Restores water and sodium loss; maintains sodium and chloride at present levels	–	–	–	154	–	154	–	–
Ringer's solution	Expands intracellular fluid; replaces extracellular losses	0–10	–	0–340	147	4	155.5	–	4
Lactated Ringer's solution	Replaces fluid loss from burns, bleeding, and severe diarrhea	0–10	–	0–340	130	4	109	28	3
Albumin 25% (salt poor albumin)	Restores major plasma protein in blood loss that has been treated with NS (plasma expander)	–	25	1000	100–160	–	<120	–	–

Note: A normal saline solution is a salt solution that has the same percentage of salt as the human body. This is a 0.9% solution of sodium chloride. The term normal indicates that there is the same weight, in grams, of sodium and chloride in the solution. Variations and combinations are available to tailor intake to needs of the child. For example, 1/2 NS (0.45% NaCl) or 1/4 NS (0.225% NaCl) are often used in young children; the lower sodium content helps to avoid inadvertent hypernatremia. D5 1/2 NS and D5 1/4 NS are combinations of D5W and NS; they provide both carbohydrate and sodium (Holliday, Ray, & Friedman, 2007).

Adapted from Custer, J. W., & Rau, R. E. (eds.). (2009). The Harriet Lane handbook (18th ed.). Johns Hopkins University Press; and LeMone, P., & Burke, K. M. (2008). Medical surgical nursing (4th ed.). Upper Saddle River, NJ: Prentice Hall Health.

children with diarrhea who have mild to moderate dehydration (Fontaine, Garner & Bhan, 2007; Hartling, Bellemare, Wieve, et al., 2006). Commercially available solutions contain water, carbohydrate (sugar), sodium, potassium, chloride, and lactate. Examples include Pedialyte, Infalyte, Rehydralate, Ricelyte, Resol, Nutralyte, Hydralyte, and Lytren. Some clinicians allow lactose-free milk, breast milk, or half-strength milk to be given in addition to oral rehydration therapy solution. When the child is severely dehydrated, electrolytes are measured by laboratory analysis, and intravenous fluid is given, often accompanied by oral rehydration. The intravenous fluid is commonly Ringer's lactate or dilute saline, such as one half or one quarter normal saline (see Table 46–3 for types of intravenous fluids and their uses). The fluid combination replenishes the extracellular fluid volume and adds solutes to return the body fluid back to normal. The child may be hospitalized or treated with intravenous fluids in a short-stay unit until the dehydration is controlled. Once hydrated, the child resumes an age-appropriate diet.

NURSING MANAGEMENT

NURSING ASSESSMENT AND DIAGNOSIS

Weigh the child daily with the same scale and without clothing. Compare to past weights and calculate weight loss. Carefully measure intake and output, urine specific gravity, level of consciousness, pulse rate and quality, skin turgor, mucous membrane moisture, quality and rate of respirations, and blood pressure. Compare the blood pressure when the child is supine with the pressure when the child is sitting with legs hanging down or standing. If the child is dehydrated, the sit-

Thinking Critically

THE DEHYDRATED CHILD

LeShan is 18 months old. Several days ago he developed vomiting and diarrhea. His parents tried to get him to eat, but he had little appetite. He drank a little water and a few sips of juice, but the next morning he was listless and would not drink anything. The diarrhea continued.

His mother has brought him to the urgent care center. LeShan is irritable on arrival, and his mother reports that he has been alternately irritable and lethargic. His mucous membranes and tongue appear dry, and skin turgor over the abdomen is slightly decreased. His mother notes that LeShan has had only two wet diapers today and says the urine in his diaper was dark in color. She also reports that he weighed 12 kg (26 lb) at the clinic last week. However, when the nurse weighs him, the scale reads only 11 kg (24 1/2 lb). What do LeShan's symptoms suggest about his degree of dehydration? What nursing interventions should be planned?

See MyNursingKit for possible responses.

Nursing Practice

To obtain urine from an infant for testing specific gravity, place two cotton balls in the diaper. When they are wet, push them into a 10-mL syringe and squeeze out the urine with the plunger. Remember to use gloves for this procedure.

ting or standing blood pressure will be lower than the supine blood pressure, because blood accumulates in the dependent legs. Obtain samples of urine and blood as needed for dehydration evaluation.

The nursing diagnosis *Deficient Fluid Volume* applies to all children who have an extracellular fluid volume deficit. Other diagnoses depend on the severity of the condition and the age of the child. Several nursing diagnoses that might be appropriate for the mildly to severely dehydrated child are included in the accompanying Nursing Care Plans. Additional care of the child with dehydration from gastroenteritis can be found in Chapter 53∞. Nursing diagnoses might include the following:

- *Deficient Fluid Volume* related to active fluid volume loss or failure of regulatory mechanisms
- *Risk for Ineffective Peripheral Tissue Perfusion* related to hypovolemia
- *Risk for Injury* related to postural hypotension

PLANNING AND IMPLEMENTATION

Nursing care of the dehydrated child focuses first on prevention of the problem, and then on providing oral rehydration fluids, teaching parents oral rehydration methods, and, if necessary, administering intravenous fluids to restore fluid balance. The accompanying Nursing Care Plans summarize care of the child with mild to severe dehydration.

PREVENT DEHYDRATION

Nursing care can often prevent dehydration. Carefully monitor temperature probes in radiant warmers and isolettes for newborns to prevent overheating and resulting dehydration. Teach parents proper clothing for infants to prevent overheating. Nurses play an important role in educating parents, youth, school personnel, and coaches about the dangers of heat-related illness. Prevention is essential, so that children can exercise safely (National Federation of State High School Associations, 2005). Prior to a new exercise regimen, assessment for risk factors is performed. This includes medical conditions that put the child at high risk, such as cystic fibrosis, diabetes, obesity, or mental retardation. Prior history of heat-related illness or recent change from a cooler to hotter environment increases risk. Long exercise periods increase the stress upon the body. The major nursing interventions are partnering with families and athletic coaches to prevent problems and to recognize and treat them promptly.

PROVIDE ORAL REHYDRATION FLUIDS

In mild or moderate dehydration, oral rehydration fluid is the first intervention. It is given in frequent small amounts; for example, 1 to 3 teaspoons of fluid every 10 to 15 minutes is a useful guideline for starting oral rehydration. For the first 2 to 4 hours of treatment, 50 mL of fluid for each kg of the child's weight should be the target intake (Spandorfer, Alessandrini, Joffe, et al., 2005). Instruct parents to continue to administer 1 teaspoon every 2 to 3 minutes even if the child vomits, as small amounts of the fluid may still be absorbed. Table 46–4 outlines guidelines for oral rehydration therapy.

MyNursingKit Case Study: Dehydration and Fluid Calculation

Table 46–4 Oral Rehydration Therapy Guidelines

Child's Condition	Recommendation
No diarrhea, no dehydration	■ Continue on age-appropriate diet.
Minimal dehydration	■ If the child weighs <10 kg, give 60–120 mL oral rehydration solution (ORS) for each diarrheal stool or vomiting episode; if over 10 kg in weight, give 120–240 mL ORS for each diarrheal stool or vomiting episode. Meanwhile, continue breastfeeding, or resume age-appropriate diet after initial hydration. ■ Start slowly, administering 3–5 mL in a small cup or spoon every few minutes. Increase amounts gradually if no vomiting occurs. ■ Recommend or provide samples of ORS; suggest ready-to-feed or powdered forms to use by parents.
Moderate dehydration	Give 50–100 mL/kg ORS in 3–4 hours in addition to replacing fluids lost as described above.
Severe dehydration	The child is hospitalized and treated with intravenous fluids. When hydrated adequately or concurrently with intravenous rehydration, begin oral rehydration therapy with 100 mL/kg of fluid in 4 hours and stool replacement as described above.
Rehydration complete	Resume normal diet.

Data from Managing acute gastroenteritis among children: Oral rehydration, maintenance, and nutritional therapy (2004). *Pediatrics, 114,* 507; Morbidity and Mortality Weekly Reports (2003), 52, (RR-16), 1–16.

Nursing Care Plan

THE CHILD WITH MILD OR MODERATE DEHYDRATION

INTERVENTION	RATIONALE	EXPECTED OUTCOME
1. Nursing Diagnosis: Ineffective Management of Therapeutic Regimen related to knowledge deficit about diarrhea and vomiting		
NIC Priority Intervention: **Family involvement:** Facilitate family participation in care of the child		**NOC Suggested Outcome:** Effective therapeutic regimen management
Goal: Parents will describe appropriate home management of fluid replacement for diarrhea and vomiting.		
■ Explain how to replace body fluid with an oral rehydration solution. Encourage parents to keep the solution at home and begin use with the first sign of diarrhea.	■ Use of an oral rehydration solution can enable successful treatment of vomiting and diarrhea at home.	Parents are successfully able to treat the child's diarrhea and vomiting at home.
■ Teach parents to continue the child's normal diet in addition to providing replacement fluids for diarrhea.	■ Diet plus fluid supplementation leads to faster recovery.	
■ Provide verbal and written instructions to parents at each well-child visit.	■ Parents are provided with a reference for later use.	
2. Nursing Diagnosis: Deficient Knowledge (Parent) related to causes of dehydration		
NIC Priority Intervention: **Teaching:** Teach causes of dehydration		**NOC Suggested Outcome:** **Knowledge:** Treatment regimen
Goal: Parents will state common causes of childhood dehydration.		
■ Teach parents childhood conditions that commonly lead to dehydration.	■ If parents recognize situations that can lead to dehydration, they will be more alert to its appearance.	Parents recognize conditions of risk for dehydration in children.
3. Nursing Diagnosis: Risk for Deficient Fluid Volume related to worsening of child's condition		
NIC Priority Intervention: **Fluid management:** Promote fluid balance		**NOC Suggested Outcome:** **Fluid balance:** Balance of water in extra- and intracellular compartments of body
Goal: Parents will seek health care for the child's worsening condition.		
■ Teach parents to seek care when the child's vomiting or diarrhea worsens, or the child's mental alertness changes.	■ Severe dehydration may occur if milder forms are not successfully treated.	Parents seek prompt attention for the child's worsening condition, preventing the development of severe dehydration.

TEACH PARENTS ORAL REHYDRATION METHODS

Instruct parents about the types of fluids and amounts to be given. Begin teaching with parents of all newborns and reinforce teaching at each well-child visit. Advise parents to continue the child's normal diet in addition to providing the rehydration solution. Cereal, starches, soup, fruits, and vegetables are all allowed. Tell parents to avoid simple sugars, which can worsen diarrhea because of osmotic effects. This includes soft drinks (if used, they should be diluted with equal parts of water), undiluted juice, Jell-O, and sweetened cereal.

Repeated vomiting of large volumes of fluid, increasing diarrhea, or a worsening of the child's condition can indicate the

Nursing Practice

Encourage parents to keep an oral rehydration solution in liquid or powder form on hand at all times and to use these solutions rather than juice, soda, or other drinks when the child first develops diarrhea.

If an oral rehydration solution is too concentrated, it can make diarrhea worse. Juice, cola, and many sports drinks are very concentrated and should be diluted to half strength if they are the only fluids available to be given to a child who has diarrhea. Sugar facilitates the absorption of sodium in oral rehydration fluids. In addition, tell parents not to give diet beverages for oral rehydration because they contain no sugar and will not be effectively absorbed.

Nursing Care Plan

THE CHILD WITH SEVERE DEHYDRATION

INTERVENTION	RATIONALE	EXPECTED OUTCOME
1. Nursing Diagnosis: Deficient Fluid Volume related to excess losses and inadequate intake		
NIC Priority Intervention: **Fluid management:** Promote fluid balance		**NOC Suggested Outcome:** **Fluid balance:** Balance of water in extra- and intracellular components of the body
Goal: The child will return to normal hydration status and will not develop hypovolemic shock.		
■ Monitor weight daily. Assess intake and output every shift. Assess heart rate, postural blood pressure, skin turgor, small vein filling time, capillary refill time, fontanelle (infant), and urine specific gravity every 4 hours or more frequently as indicated.	■ Frequent assessment of hydration status facilitates rapid intervention and evaluation of the effectiveness of fluid replacement.	The child has signs of normal hydration.
■ Administer intravenous fluid as ordered. Monitor for crackles in dependent portions of the lungs.	■ Replace fluid lost from the body. Excessive replacement of sodium-containing fluids could cause extracellular fluid volume excess.	
2. Nursing Diagnosis: Risk for Injury related to decreased level of consciousness		
NIC Priority Intervention: **Fall prevention:** Institute special precautions		**NOC Suggested Outcome:** **Fall prevention:** Minimize risk factors that precipitate falls
Goal: The child will not experience injury.		
■ Raise the side rails of the bed. Ensure that a small child does not become tangled in bed covers.	■ Safety measures protect the child.	The child does not fall or suffer other injuries
■ Monitor level of consciousness every 2–4 hours or more often as indicated.	■ Frequent assessment provides evidence of the need for safety interventions and of the effectiveness of therapy.	
■ Monitor serum sodium concentration daily or more often.	■ Elevated serum sodium concentration causes brain cell shrinkage and decreased level of consciousness.	
■ Have the child sit before rising from bed and assist to stand slowly.	■ Slow adjustment to upright posture reduces light-headedness from decreased blood volume.	
3. Nursing Diagnosis: Activity Intolerance related to bed rest immobility		
NIC Priority Intervention: **Activity therapy:** Plan activities to meet child's developmental needs		**NOC Suggested Outcome:** **Energy conservation:** Manage energy to sustain activity
Goal: The child will engage in normal activity for age.		
■ Plan activities appropriate for the age of the child that can be done in bed.	■ Activities will provide distraction and promote recovery.	The child engages in normal developmental activities and receives adequate rest.
■ Group nursing interventions to provide time for the child to rest.	■ The child will require more rest than usual.	
■ Provide assistance during meals and other activities as needed.	■ Prevention of overexertion will conserve body fluid and promote healing.	

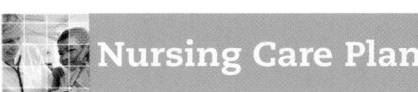

MyNursingKit Care Plan: Hyponatremic Dehydration in Breastfeeding

need for intravenous therapy. Teach parents when to seek further medical care. If the child's condition worsens or does not improve after 4 hours of oral rehydration therapy, parents should contact a healthcare professional. Dizziness or lethargy are symptoms that can be manifestations of dehydration and indicate need for further healthcare.

MONITOR INTRAVENOUS FLUID ADMINISTRATION

The hospitalized child usually requires intravenous fluids. Use volume control devices for measuring and monitoring intake. Be sure that the amount of fluid administered corresponds with the diagnosed dehydration state of the child (Table 46–5). Usually, about one half of the 24-hour total maintenance and replacement needs are given in the first 6 to 8 hours, with a slower rate infused for the remainder of the 24 hours. During the first 1 to 3 hours, the infusion rate may be highest to rapidly expand the vascular space. Electrolytes, such as potassium, are not added until the child has voided a sufficient quantity of urine for age, in order to avoid hyperkalemia. Rapid infusion of 20 to 30 mL/kg over 1 to 2 hours is sometimes used in outpatient settings, followed by oral fluids. Careful monitoring of intake and output is needed to ensure that the intravenous line remains in place until the child is tolerating oral fluids and taking in enough to maintain hydration. Verify that the type of fluid described is being administered. When oral fluids are maintained, the child may be discharged and hospitalization avoided.

Maintain the intravenous line carefully so fluid infusion can be kept on schedule (refer to the Clinical Skills Manual **SKILLS**). Use a pump to prevent inadvertent, rapid infusion, which can lead to fluid overload and electrolyte imbalance (Figure 46–4 ●). Play with the toddler and preschool child frequently and use diversionary methods as necessary to distract the child from the intravenous line. Monitor the child carefully and implement safety precautions as necessary. Once the child begins to tolerate some oral fluids, substitute oral rehydration therapy for intravenous fluids. Frequent administration of appropriate fluids is needed.

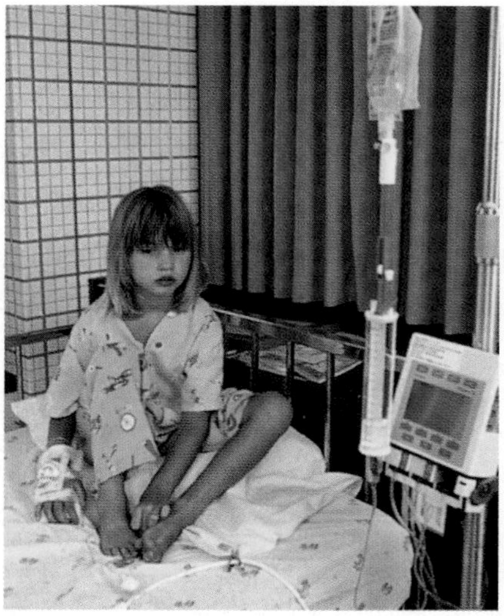

● **Figure 46–4** Volume control device. The use of a volume control device with an intravenous saline solution is important to prevent a sudden extracellular fluid volume overload.

Table 46–5 Calculation of Intravenous Fluid Needs

Step	Calculation	
Calculate the maintenance fluid needs of the child, using guidelines at right.	Usual Weight	Maintenance Amount
	Up to 10 kg	100 mL/kg/24 hr
	11–20 kg	1000 mL + (50 mL/kg for weight above 10 kg)/24 hr
	>20 kg	1500 mL + (20 mL/kg for weight above 20 kg)/24 hr
Calculate replacement fluid for that loss, using formula at right to obtain mL/kg/24 hr required.	Percentage of body weight loss × 10 × normal weight = mL/kg/24 hr required	
Calculate continued losses; add them to total of maintenance and replacement needs.		

DISCHARGE PLANNING AND HOME CARE TEACHING

Prior to discharge, parents need instructions about types of fluids and amounts to encourage. Teach the signs of dehydration (see Table 46–2) so that if the child does not take in adequate fluids, parents can seek help immediately. Instruct them to begin the child's normal diet once hydration is completed, determined by adequate urinary output and normal behaviors. Review methods of minimizing the child's chance of acquiring gastrointestinal infections (e.g., avoiding contact with other children who are infected; using careful handwashing and dishwashing procedures when another child in the home is sick). During well-child visits, encourage all parents to keep oral rehydration fluids at home in case they are needed; they are available in most grocery stores and pharmacies. Address the needs for increasing fluids in hot weather and when the child is exercising.

EVALUATION

Expected outcomes of nursing care include the following:

- Balance of water and electrolytes in intracellular and extracellular compartments
- Normal urinary output
- Adequate fluid intake for maintenance needs
- Vital signs within normal limits

Evidence-Based Nursing

HOME CARE FOR CONDITIONS CAUSING DEHYDRATION

Clinical Question

Rotavirus gastroenteritis (RGE) is a common and potentially serious cause of childhood vomiting and diarrhea, and can lead to dehydration among young children.

The Evidence

It is estimated that RGE causes 3.5 million cases of diarrhea, 50,000 hospitalizations, and 20 deaths annually in the United States. RGE can generally be successfully treated at home, but parents must be aware of assessment and treatment guidelines (Koslap-Petraco, 2006).

Best Practice

RGE carries a major risk of dehydration in children. While it may begin as a mild illness, it can quickly progress to severe diarrhea and vomiting. Most children are cared for at home with RGE but often call in to healthcare facilities. It is important to ask parents about duration and severity of symptoms, review proper administration of oral rehydration therapy, and teach them what symptoms require immediate emergency care.

Critical Thinking

What questions can you ask on the phone that will help to establish the degree of dehydration of a child at home? What symptoms require immediate medical care? A vaccine for rotavirus was recently implemented in healthcare practice. Plan the information you need to provide to all parents about this preventive measure (see Chapter 45 for further detail).

See MyNursingKit for possible responses.

EXTRACELLULAR FLUID VOLUME EXCESS

Extracellular fluid volume excess occurs when there is too much fluid in the vascular and interstitial compartment. This imbalance may also be called saline excess or extracellular volume overload. If this disorder occurs by itself (without saline disturbance), the serum sodium concentration is normal. There is simply too much extracellular fluid, even though it has a normal concentration.

Infants and children who develop an extracellular fluid volume excess have a condition that causes them to retain **saline** (sodium and water) or have been given an overload of sodium-containing isotonic intravenous fluid (Figure 46–5 ●). What conditions cause retention of saline? The hormone aldosterone is secreted by the adrenal cortex. One of its normal functions is to cause the kidneys to retain saline in the body (see "Pathophysiology Illustrated: Aldosterone Effects"). Saline excess can be caused by any condition that results in excessive aldosterone secretion, such as adrenal tumors that secrete aldosterone, congestive heart failure, liver cirrhosis, and chronic renal failure. Most glucocorticoid medications (such as prednisone) have a mild saline-retaining effect when taken on a long-term basis. Intravenous fluid volume regulation is important, especially in young children. Either inaccurate calculation of needed fluid or inadvertent infusion of excess fluids can cause overload.

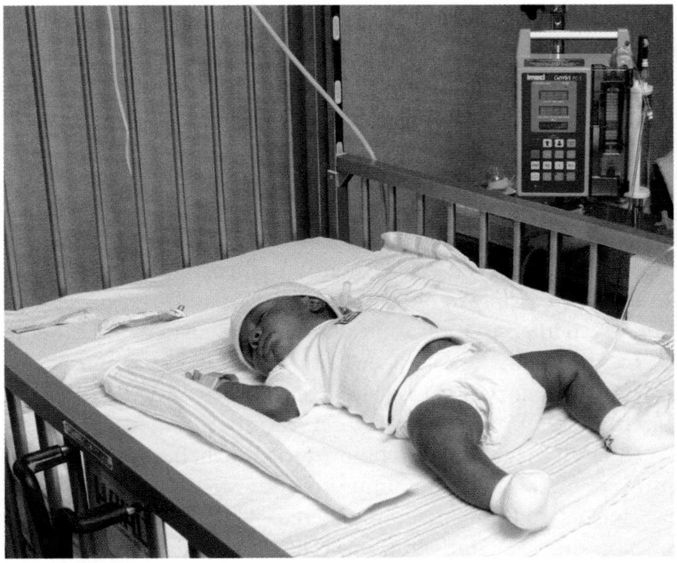

● **Figure 46–5** Preventing extracellular fluid volume overload. If isotonic fluid containing sodium is given too rapidly or in too great an amount, an extracellular fluid volume excess will develop. Carefully monitor fluid intake, excretion, and retention in infants and children.

Extracellular fluid volume excess is characterized by sudden weight gain. A gain of 0.5 kg (1 lb) in a day is related to fluid, and represents 500 mL of saline. An overload of fluid in the blood vessels and interstitial spaces can cause clinical manifestations such as bounding pulse, distended neck veins in children (not usually evident in infants), periorbital edema, hepatomegaly, dyspnea, orthopnea, and lung crackles. Edema is the sign of overload of the interstitial fluid compartment. In an infant, edema is often generalized (Figure 46–6 ●). Edema in children with extracellular fluid volume excess occurs in the dependent parts of the body, that is, in the parts closest to the ground. Thus, edema is evident in sacral areas in a child supine in bed. Scrotum or labia may be edematous. (Edema that develops from other causes is described in the next section of this chapter.)

The clinical therapy for extracellular fluid volume excess focuses on treating the underlying cause of the disorder. For example, a child who has congestive heart failure is given medications to strengthen the heart's ability to contract. Managing the cause also helps to reduce the extracellular fluid volume excess. Diuretics may be given to remove fluid from the body, thus reducing the extracellular fluid volume directly.

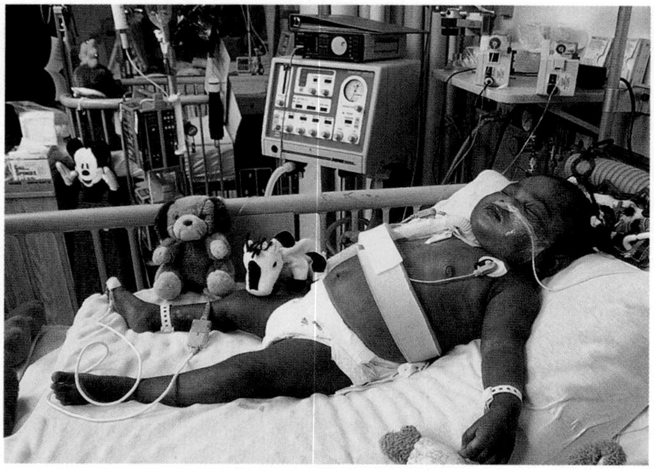

● **Figure 46–6** Signs of generalized edema. This infant with cong ital heart disease has signs of generalized edema. Note the fluid retent in the face and abdomen.

Nursing Management

Rapid weight gain is the most sensitive index of extracellular fluid volume excess. Therefore, daily weighing with the same scale and articles of clothing is an important nursing assessment. Measure the child's intake and output. For babies in diapers, a diaper is weighed dry and then wet, with grams of weight increase equal to urine volume in milliliters. When treatment is successful, output is greater than intake. Assess the character of the pulse and observe for neck vein distention when the child is sitting (usually visible only in older children). Monitor for signs of pulmonary edema (an indication of severe imbalance) by listening to lung sounds in the dependent lung fields (crackles) and assessing for respiratory distress (rapid respiratory rate, use of accessory muscles of respiration). Observe for edema.

A child may develop a fluid overload whenever an isotonic intravenous solution containing sodium, such as normal saline or Ringer's solution, is administered. Therefore, monitor the infusion rate frequently and carefully and use a volume control device and pump whenever possible to aid in accurate administration. Use only small bags (e.g., 250 or 500 mL) for infants and young children, and check pumps frequently. If an excess of fluid has already developed, administer the medical therapy as prescribed and monitor for any complications of the medical therapy. For example, many diuretics increase potassium excretion in the urine, which may lead to an abnormally low plasma potassium concentration unless potassium intake is increased. (Refer to the discussion of hypokalemia later in this chapter.) It is also important to monitor for the development of extracellular fluid volume deficit as a result of diuretic therapy.

If edema is present, provide careful skin care and protection for edematous areas. Teach parents how to provide skin care and perform position changes at home. See the following section for additional interventions related to edema.

If a child has a long-term condition such as chronic renal failure that predisposes to extracellular fluid volume excess, a dietary sodium restriction may be prescribed (see Chapter 54 for further detail). Teach parents how to manage sodium restriction. Plan low-sodium meals that fit the family's cultural practices. If the child is old enough to participate, incorporate games into the teaching. If a scale is available, teach parents to take and record an accurate daily weight.

Desired outcomes include electrolyte balance, maintenance of intact skin, and dietary intake as prescribed.

PATHOPHYSIOLOGY ILLUSTRATED

ALDOSTERONE EFFECTS

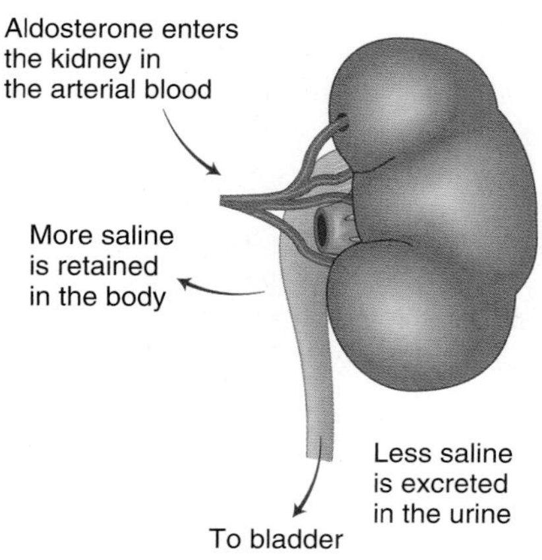

Aldosterone enters the kidney in the arterial blood
More saline is retained in the body
Less saline is excreted in the urine
To bladder

Aldosterone has a saline-retaining effect. Increased aldosterone secretion can be caused by adrenal tumors or congestive heart failure.

Developing Cultural Competence

LOW-SODIUM DIETS

To adapt teaching about low-sodium diets to the cultural practices of a family, ask clients what types of food they usually eat. Help them to choose low-sodium foods from their diets and to avoid high-sodium foods. This approach is more effective than giving the same list of restricted foods to each family.

For example, some Asians may use monosodium glutamate to flavor foods and can be encouraged to add this at the table for family members who can have extra sodium rather than during cooking. Many Hispanic groups use large amounts of cheese, which can provide significant sodium. Encourage them to look for low-sodium cheese and substitute cottage cheese for other types since it is lower in sodium.

Canned foods tend to have high sodium, so teach all families to use fresh or frozen produce rather than canned when possible. Low-sodium milk is available and is a good option for young children. Teach families how to read and interpret food labels to identify salt (sodium) content.

INTERSTITIAL FLUID VOLUME EXCESS (EDEMA)

Edema is an abnormal increase in the volume of the interstitial fluid. It may be caused by an extracellular fluid volume excess or it may result from other causes.

The causes of edema are best understood in the context of normal capillary dynamics. Fluid moves between the vascular and interstitial compartment by the process of **filtration**. Filtration is the net result of forces that tend to move fluid in opposing directions. The strongest forces determine the direction of fluid movement.

At the capillary level, two forces (blood hydrostatic pressure and interstitial osmotic pressure) tend to move fluid from the capillaries into the interstitial fluid, while two other forces (blood colloid osmotic pressure and interstitial fluid hydrostatic pressure) tend to move fluid in the opposite direction (from the interstitial fluid into the capillaries). The net result of these forces usually moves fluid from the capillaries into the interstitial compartment at the arterial end of the capillaries, and fluid from the interstitial compartment back into the capillaries at the venous end of the capillaries. This process brings oxygen and nutrients to the cells and removes carbon dioxide and other waste products.

Edema occurs if the balance of these four forces is altered so that excess fluid either enters or leaves the interstitial compartment (see "Pathophysiology Illustrated: Capillary Dynamics and Edema"). This may occur through:

1. increased blood hydrostatic pressure
2. decreased blood colloid osmotic pressure
3. increased interstitial fluid osmotic pressure
4. blocked lymphatic drainage

Many clinical conditions are associated with these altered forces (Table 46–6), as described in the following list:

Table 46–6 Clinical Conditions That Cause Edema

Condition	Resulting Hemodynamic Change	Result
Increased blood hydrostatic pressure	Increased capillary blood flow	Inflammation Local infection
	Venous congestion	Extracellular fluid volume excess Right heart failure Venous thrombosis External pressure on vein Muscle paralysis
Decreased blood osmotic pressure	Increased albumin excretion	Nephrotic syndrome (albumin leaks into urine) Protein-losing enteropathies (excess albumin in feces)
	Decreased albumin synthesis	Kwashiorkor (low-protein, high-carbohydrate starvation diet provides too few amino acids for liver to make albumin) Liver cirrhosis (diseased liver unable to make enough albumin)
Increased interstitial fluid osmotic pressure	Increased capillary permeability	Inflammation Toxins Hypersensitivity reactions Burns
Blocked lymphatic drainage	Venous congestion	Tumors Goiter Parasites that obstruct lymph nodes Surgery that removes lymph nodes

1. *Increased blood hydrostatic pressure.* When extracellular fluid volume excess occurs, the increased fluid volume in the vascular compartment congests the veins. The pressure against the sides of the capillary is increased and more fluid then enters the interstitial compartment.
2. *Decreased blood colloid osmotic pressure.* Much of the osmotic pressure that pulls fluid into the capillaries is a result of the presence of albumin and other plasma proteins made by the liver. The part of the blood osmotic pressure that results from plasma proteins is often called **oncotic pressure**, or blood colloid osmotic pressure. Any condition that decreases plasma proteins will decrease blood colloid osmotic pressure and cause edema. For example, if a clinical condition causes large amounts of albumin to leak into the urine, the liver will not be able to make albumin fast enough to replace it. As a result the plasma protein level will fall, decreasing the blood osmotic pressure. Without this pulling force to return fluid to the capillaries, edema will occur. This is the cause of edema in children who have nephrotic syndrome (see Chapter 54∞).
3. *Increased interstitial fluid osmotic pressure.* Ordinarily, only a few small proteins enter the interstitial fluid, and the interstitial fluid osmotic pressure is small. If the capillary becomes abnormally permeable to proteins, however, the influx of large amounts of proteins into the interstitial fluid causes a dramatic increase in interstitial fluid osmotic pressure. The increased pulling force keeps an abnormal amount of fluid in the interstitial compartment. This mechanism plays an important part in the edema caused by a bee sting or a sprained ankle. It occurs to a greater extent in burns, leading to swelling at the same time that there is a great loss of fluid volume through the burned skin (see Chapter 57∞).
4. *Blocked lymphatic drainage.* The lymph vessels normally drain small proteins and excess fluid from the interstitial compartment and return them to the blood vessels. If lymph vessels are blocked, fluid accumulates in the interstitial compartment. This may occur when a tumor blocks lymphatic drainage.

Edema causes localized or generalized swelling, which may cause pain and restrict motion. Edema due to extracellular fluid volume excess or right-sided heart failure usually occurs in the

PATHOPHYSIOLOGY ILLUSTRATED

CAPILLARY DYNAMICS AND EDEMA

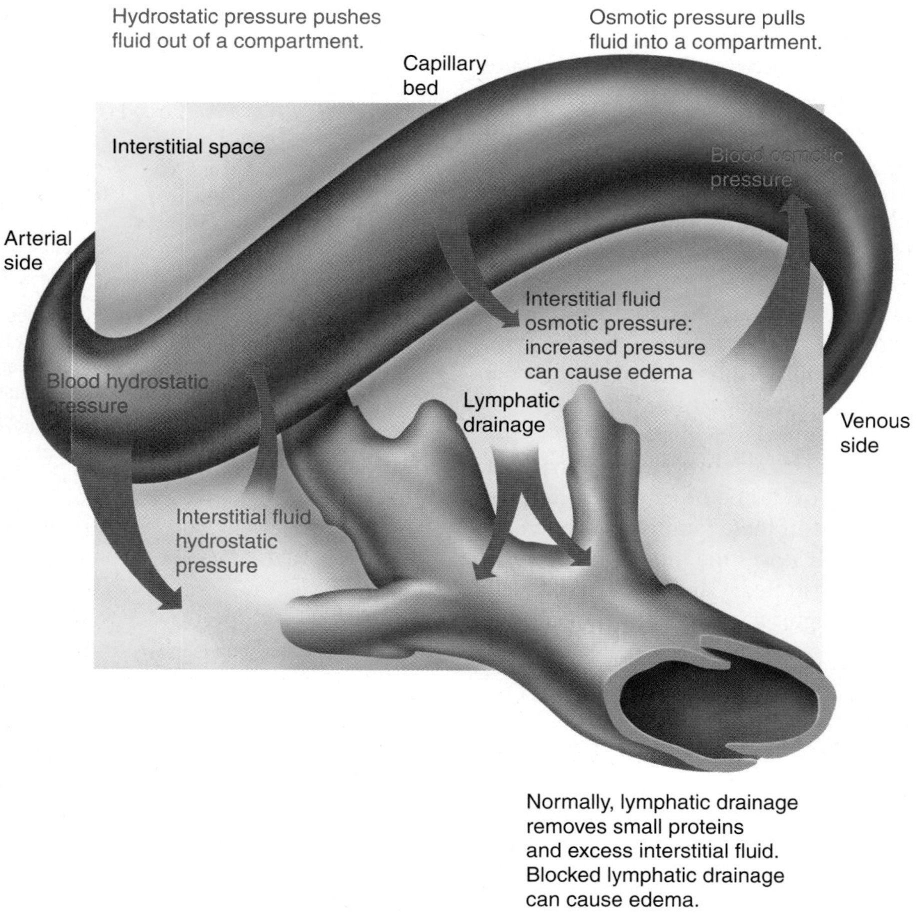
Hydrostatic pressure pushes fluid out of a compartment.
Osmotic pressure pulls fluid into a compartment.
Capillary bed
Interstitial space
Blood osmotic pressure
Arterial side
Interstitial fluid osmotic pressure: increased pressure can cause edema
Blood hydrostatic pressure
Lymphatic drainage
Venous side
Interstitial fluid hydrostatic pressure
Normally, lymphatic drainage removes small proteins and excess interstitial fluid. Blocked lymphatic drainage can cause edema.

With normal capillary dynamics, fluid moves out of the compartment by the force of hydrostatic pressure in the blood vessel and is pulled out by interstitial osmotic pressure. Fluid is forced into the compartment by interstitial hydrostatic pressure and pulled in by compartment osmotic pressure. Abnormal capillary dynamics can cause edema.

dependent portion of the body. In a child who is walking, dependent edema is observed in the ankles; in a bedfast, supine child, it is seen in the sacral area. The skin over an edematous area often appears thin and shiny.

The main focus of clinical therapy for edema is to treat the underlying condition that caused the edema. Such conditions are discussed throughout this book. The edema from inflammation of an injury is initially treated with cold to reduce capillary blood flow and thus reduce blood hydrostatic pressure.

Nursing Management

A child or parent may make comments that alert the nurse to the development of edema. Shoes may become tight by the end of the day (dependent edema); the waistband of pants or a skirt may be "outgrown" suddenly (generalized edema or ascites [accumulation of fluid in the peritoneal cavity]); the eyes may be puffy (periorbital edema); a ring may be too tight; fingers may "feel like sausages." In many cases visual inspection is sufficient to recognize edema. Observe for **pitting edema**, a "pit" or concave indentation that remains after an edematous area is pressed downward by the examiner's fingers. To detect changes in the amount of swelling, measure around the edematous part. If the edema is caused by extracellular fluid volume excess, daily measurements of weight and intake and output are a necessary part of the daily assessment. Nursing assessment should also focus on the integrity of the skin, presence of pain, restricted motion, and alterations in the child's body image.

Elevation of an area of localized edema helps to reduce the swelling. The skin over an edematous area needs extra care because it is fragile and prone to breakdown (Figure 46–7 ●). Care-

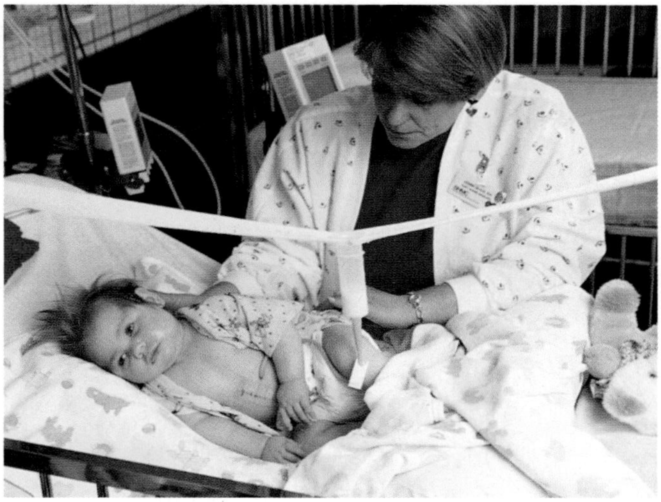

● **Figure 46–7** Care of edematous tissue. Edematous tissue is easily damaged. It must be kept clean and dry and free of pressure.

fully position an infant or child on bed rest and turn frequently to prevent pressure sores. Perform turning carefully to avoid skin abrasion by rubbing against the sheets. Pat the skin dry after cleansing rather than rubbing it. Trim the child's fingernails smooth to prevent scratching. Teach parents skin care for the child at home. Teach older children to inspect their skin carefully to identify areas needing special care.

If restricted mobility is a problem, make specific plans to help the child manage activities. For example, if an edematous finger restricts the motion of a hand, food can be cut into bite-sized portions before the meal is served, so that the child can still eat independently.

Discomfort from edema may require creative nursing interventions. Distraction with toys or activities appropriate to the child's developmental level can be useful. Interventions to treat the underlying problem can also reduce the edema and its accompanying discomfort. Interventions for edema should be added to the nursing management of the underlying condition that causes the edema. Administration of the prescribed medical therapy and observation for the complications of therapy are nursing responsibilities.

Discuss with school-age children and adolescents feelings of embarrassment about the edematous appearance. They need to understand the reason for edema and be able to explain it to peers. Arrange for the child to meet other children with similar concerns.

Desired outcomes of care include maintenance of intact skin, normal respiratory sounds and effort, and normal weight patterns.

ELECTROLYTE IMBALANCES

All body fluids contain electrolytes, although the concentration of those electrolytes varies depending on the type and location of the fluid. When a serum electrolyte value is reported from the laboratory, it provides information about the concentration of that electrolyte in the blood. It may not necessarily reflect the concentration of the electrolyte in other body compartments. Refer to Table 46–1 to see which electrolytes have the highest and lowest concentrations in the blood and other fluid compartments.

Electrolytes are normally gained and lost in relatively equal amounts so that the body remains in balance. However, when a child has an abnormal route of loss, such as vomiting, wound drainage, or nasogastric suction, electrolyte balance can be disturbed. In addition, supplementation with electrolytes via intravenous fluids in proportions different than body fluids can also cause electrolyte imbalance. Children with disease states that interfere with normal mechanisms of electrolyte regulation, such as renal disease, also have disturbance in electrolyte levels. Monitoring for signs of imbalance becomes important in all of these situations.

SODIUM IMBALANCES

The serum sodium concentration reflects the **osmolality** of body fluids; that is, their degree of concentration or dilution. It refers to the number of moles of the substance per kilogram of water in the solution. Serum sodium concentration reflects the proportion of water and sodium in the extracellular compartment. When the osmolality of body fluids becomes abnormal, the cells swell or shrink. These cell size changes are due to **osmosis**, the movement of water across a semipermeable membrane into an area of higher particle concentration. Sodium levels are maintained at high extracellular and low intracellular levels by the sodium-potassium pump, which moves these electrolytes against their expected concentration gradients (Figure 46–8 ●).

HYPERNATREMIA

Hypernatremia is a condition of increased osmolality of the blood. The body fluids are too concentrated, containing excess sodium relative to water. Sodium level generally falls between 132–141 mmol/L and a serum sodium level above 146 mmol/L in children (146 mmol/L in newborns) is diagnostic of hypernatremia (Robertson & Shilkofski, 2005) (Table 46–7).

Hypernatremia is caused by conditions that cause the body to lose relatively more water than sodium or to gain relatively more sodium than water (Table 46–8). Special circumstances in which a high solute intake may occur without adequate water include an infant formula that is too concentrated or one that is prepared with salt instead of sugar. A breastfed baby not receiving adequate breast milk who has normal water loss may develop hypernatremic dehydration. This is a risk at 2 to 3 days of age, when babies generally have a diuresis, if the baby does not feed well or the mother does not yet produce an adequate amount of breast milk (Moritz, Manole, Bogen, et al. 2005; Shrof, Hignett, Pierce, et al., 2007).

An infant or child who has hypernatremia is generally thirsty. The urine output is small unless the hypernatremia is caused by diabetes insipidus. A decreased level of consciousness manifested by confusion, lethargy, or coma results from shrinking of the brain cells. Seizures can occur when hypernatremia occurs rapidly or is severe. Severe hypernatremia can be fatal.

Serum sodium, specific gravity of urine, antidiuretic hormone (ADH) and 24-hour urine are common diagnostic tests.

MyNursingKit Care Plan: Infant Feeding

MyNursingKit Formula Preparation at a Home Visit

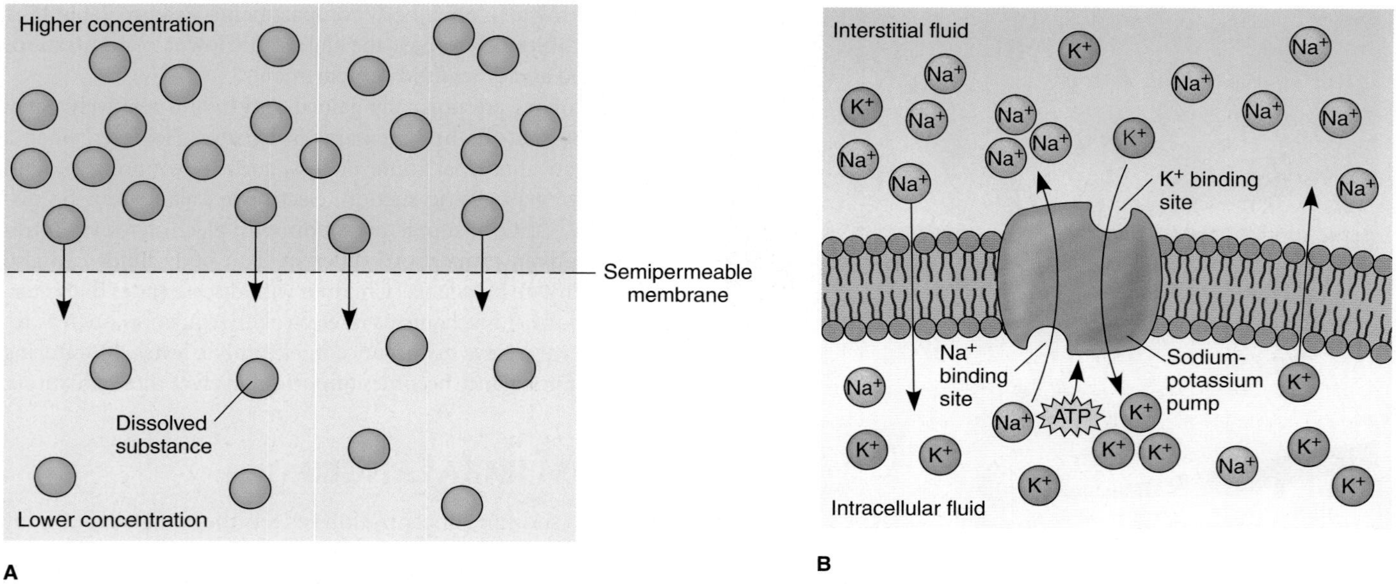

● **Figure 46–8** The sodium-potassium pump. ***A,*** Water balance is maintained by the simple passage of molecules from greater to lesser concentration across cell membranes. ***B,*** Sodium levels are maintained by an active transport system, the sodium-potassium pump, which moves these electrolytes across cell membranes in spite of their concentration.

Table 46–7 Normal Serum Values

Blood Component	Values
Sodium	Newborn: 131–144 mmol/L Children: 132–141 mmol/L
Potassium	Premature infants: 4.5–7.2 mmol/L Full-term infants: 3.2–5.7 mmol/L Children: 3.3–4.7 mmol/L
Calcium (total)	Premature infants: 1.7–2.3 mmol/L Full-term infants: 2.10–2.64 mmol/L (8.4–10.6 mg/dL) Children: 2.12–2.64 mmol/L (8.5–10.6 mg/dL)
Magnesium	Infants: 0.65–1.02 mmol/L or 1.6–2.5 mg/dL Children: 0.7–1.1 mmol/L or 1.6–2.7 mg/dL
Arterial pH	Infants: 7.18–7.5 Children: 7.27–7.49 Adolescents: 7.35–7.41
Arterial Po_2	Infants: 60–70 mm Hg (8–9.3 pKa) Children: 80–108 mm Hg (10.7–14.4 pKa) Adolescents: 80–100 mm Hg (4.3–6.4 pKa)
Arterial Pco_2	Infants: 27–41 mm Hg (3.6–5.5 pKa) Children and adolescents: 32–48 mm Hg (4.3–6.4 pKa)
Arterial bicarbonate	Infants: 19–24 mmol/L Children: 18–25 mmol/L Adolescents: 20–29 mmol/L

From Soldin, S. J., Brugnara, C., & Wong, E. C. (2005). *Pediatric Reference Ranges* (5th ed.). Washington, DC: AACC Press.

Note: Laboratories may have slightly different levels for normal depending on assays performed. Always consult the normal values for your particular laboratory.

Table 46–8 Causes of Hypernatremia

Loss of Relatively More Water than Sodium	Gain of Relatively More Sodium than Water
Inadequate breastfeeding intake with normal output	Inability to communicate thirst
Diabetes insipidus (not enough antidiuretic hormone)	Limited or no access to water
Diarrhea or vomiting without fluid replacement	High solute intake without adequate water (e.g., tube feedings)
Excessive sweating without fluid replacement	Intravenous hypertonic saline
High solute intake without adequate water (causes kidneys to excrete water)	Improper formula preparation leading to excessive concentration
Increased aldosterone	

Hypernatremia is treated by intravenous administration of **hypotonic fluid**, or fluid that is more dilute than normal body fluid. This therapy dilutes the body fluids back to normal concentration. If a child is dehydrated, **isotonic fluids** (those with the osmolality of body fluids) may be administered first to replenish the volume, followed by hypotonic fluid to correct the osmolality. The underlying cause of the disorder is also treated.

Nursing Management

Monitor serum sodium level and measure intake and output and urine specific gravity. Normal specific gravity under 2 years is 1.001 to 1.015, while in children over 2 years 1.010 to 1.030 is the normal range. Specific gravity changes toward normal levels as therapy progresses. Frequently assess responsiveness to monitor the effect of hypernatremia on brain cells. As the concentration of body fluids returns to normal, the child will become more alert and responsive. Watch for rebound hyponatremia while monitoring the fluid replacement. Implement safety interventions such as raised bed rails for protection. Ensure adequate rest and introduce developmentally appropriate activities when the child is alert.

Water deprivation is a form of child neglect or abuse. In neglect, the parents simply do not provide adequate water for the child. A form of child abuse that sometimes includes water deprivation is Munchausen syndrome by proxy (see Chapter 44∞). A small child who is hospitalized with hypernatremia that does not have a detectable cause may be subject to water deprivation. Assess the child's general condition, developmental tasks, the family dynamics, and the parents' understanding of formula preparation and the child's fluid intake needs.

Teaching can prevent many cases of hypernatremia. Be sure the breastfeeding mother has instruction and resources about lactation before discharge after birth. If the infant is discharged soon after birth, be sure to schedule an appointment to check weight within the first few days, and alert the parents to expected output of at least six wet diapers daily. By about 10 days, infants should have regained the birth weight.

When an infant is sick or developing slowly, parents sometimes want to feed the infant more concentrated formula to make him or her stronger. Parents and caregivers of bottle-fed babies should be taught never to give undiluted formula concentrate or evaporated milk. Parents should be cautioned to keep salt out of reach, since eating handfuls of salt has caused hypernatremia. Teach parents to offer extra fluids during hot weather. Teach oral rehydration therapy for use at home during mild vomiting and diarrhea (see page 1239).

Nurses can prevent hypernatremia in hospitalized infants and children by administering water between tube feedings, keeping water available, and offering it frequently. Offering frequent small amounts and using Popsicles and other creative interventions can increase children's intake.

Teaching Highlights

PREPARING INFANT FORMULA

Careful teaching about how to mix powdered formula is needed so that it is not too concentrated; this can help to prevent hypernatremia in the infant. Demonstrate the technique so that parents are well informed. Pictures are an important teaching tool if the parents are not able to read labels or instructions. When families use concentrated formula, equal amounts of concentrate and water should be mixed. Caution parents that even if an infant is premature or small, they should mix the formula as instructed. A useful strategy is to have the parents bring the formula being used to a healthcare visit and ask them to mix it as you watch. Any errors in technique can easily be corrected.

Desired outcomes of treatment for hypernatremia include balance of electrolytes and fluid in the intracellular and extracellular compartments, and alert level of consciousness.

HYPONATREMIA

In hyponatremia the osmolality of the blood is decreased. The body fluids are too dilute, containing excess water relative to sodium. Hyponatremia is the most common sodium imbalance in children (Kliegman, Behrman, Jenson, et. al., 2007). A serum sodium level below 132 mmol/L in children (131 mmol/L in newborns) is diagnostic of hyponatremia.

Etiology and Pathophysiology

Hyponatremia is caused by conditions that cause gain of relatively more water than sodium or loss of relatively more sodium than water (Table 46–9). Oral intake of water causes hyponatremia in unusual conditions such as forced fluid intake. More commonly, parents feed an infant only water or dilute formula to save money instead of regular-strength formula or breast milk. Excessive swallowing of swimming pool water by an infant can have the same effect. Infants are vulnerable to the type of hyponatremia caused by water intoxication since they have a poorly developed thirst mechanism and may continue to drink, and then are unable to excrete excess water quickly due to immature kidney function (Chamley, Carson, Randall, et al., 2005). Forced water intake is another cause and form of child abuse. Exercise-induced hyponatremia can occur when people in prolonged physical activity such as marathon running consume hypotonic fluids in the form of water or sports drinks above the levels lost in respiratory, gastrointestinal, skin, and urinary routes (Exercise-Associated Hyponatremia Consensus Panel, 2005).

CLINICAL MANIFESTATIONS

The child with hyponatremia has a decreased level of consciousness, which results from swelling of brain cells. This can

Table 46–9 Causes of Hyponatremia

Gain of Relatively More Water than Sodium	Loss of Relatively More Sodium than Water
Excessive intravenous D_5W (5% dextrose in water)	Diarrhea or vomiting with replacement by tap water only instead of fluid containing sodium
Excessive tap water enemas	Excessive sweating
Irrigation of body cavities with distilled water	Diuretics, especially thiazides
Excessive antidiuretic hormone	
Forced excessive oral intake of tap water	
Congestive heart failure	

be manifested as anorexia, nausea, vomiting, headache, muscle weakness, decreased deep tendon reflexes, agitation, lethargy, or confusion. The condition can progress to respiratory arrest, dilated pupils, decorticate posturing, and coma. If hyponatremia arises rapidly or is extreme, seizures may occur. Hyponatremia is a frequent cause of seizures in infants under 6 months of age. Severe hyponatremia can be fatal.

Clinical Therapy

Laboratory studies are the same as those used to diagnose hypernatremia. In most cases, hyponatremia is treated by restricting the intake of water. This therapy allows the kidneys to correct the imbalance by excreting excess water from the body. If a child is having seizures from hyponatremia, intravenous **hypertonic saline** (more concentrated than body fluid) may be administered. Use of this concentrated fluid is a way to rapidly increase body fluid concentration, but it must be monitored carefully because it can easily cause rebound hypernatremia. For exercise-associated hyponatremia, intravenous access is established at the first-aid site, hypertonic saline is administered, and oxygen is delivered (Exercise-Associated, 2005). In cases of diabetes insipidus, treatment for the condition is needed (see Chapter 55∞).

NURSING MANAGEMENT

NURSING ASSESSMENT AND DIAGNOSIS

Hyponatremia should be prevented in hospitalized children receiving intravenous solutions (particularly postoperatively) by administering isotonic rather than hypotonic solutions. Monitor serum sodium level and measure intake and output. If an infant with hyponatremia has normal antidiuretic hormone (ADH) levels, and other causes have been ruled out, carefully question parents about proper preparation of formula and feeding practices. A toddler or school-age child may be subjected to forced fluid intake as a form of child abuse. Sensitive interviewing and a caring manner can help identify such problems in a family.

Since hyponatremia is characterized by decreased level of consciousness, frequently assess responsiveness to monitor the response to therapy. The child will become more alert and responsive as the concentration of body fluids returns to normal.

The highest priority nursing diagnosis for hyponatremia addresses the *Risk for Injury* related to the child's decreased level of consciousness. The following diagnoses might also apply:

- *Self-Care Deficit* related to weakness and tiredness
- *Altered Health Maintenance* related to parental misinterpretation about infant formula preparation
- *Ineffective Breastfeeding* related to inadequate sucking by infant or inadequate milk production

PLANNING AND IMPLEMENTATION

Nurses can prevent hyponatremia in hospitalized children by using normal saline instead of distilled water for irrigations and by avoiding tap water enemas. Verify intravenous types and amounts and question use of hypotonic fluids in a child with no intake of sodium. Help the child comply with any prescribed fluid restrictions. Allow the child to choose favorite fluids to drink. Teach parents to replace body fluids lost through diarrhea or vomiting with oral electrolyte solutions (see pp. 1239–1242).

Expected outcomes are maintenance of safety, balance of fluid and electrolytes, and establishment of adequate formula or breastfeeding intake.

POTASSIUM IMBALANCES

Potassium, an essential electrolyte, performs many necessary functions in the body such as muscle contraction and enzymatic reactions. Potassium intake in healthy children comes from potassium-rich foods such as fruits and vegetables. Potassium is absorbed easily from the intestine. A normal potassium distribution is important for proper function.

A potassium imbalance arises when the serum potassium concentration rises or falls outside the normal range. Potassium imbalances are caused by alterations in potassium intake, distribution, or excretion; or by loss of potassium through an abnormal route such as burns, emesis, or renal failure.

Most potassium ions in the body are found inside the cells. The sodium-potassium pump in cell membranes moves potassium ions into cells to maintain the high intracellular potassium concentration. Potassium ions can be shifted into or out of cells by various physiologic factors (see "Pathophysiology Illustrated: Potassium Ions"). Potassium is excreted from the body through urine, feces, and sweat. The hormone aldosterone increases potassium excretion in the urine.

HYPERKALEMIA

Hyperkalemia is an excess of potassium in the blood. Potassium levels generally range from 3.2 to 5.7 mmol/L for newborns, and 3.3 to 4.7 mmol/L for infants and children. Hyperkalemia is reflected by a level above 5.7 mmol/L in newborns or above 5.5 mmol/L in children (see Table 46–7).

PATHOPHYSIOLOGY ILLUSTRATED

POTASSIUM IONS

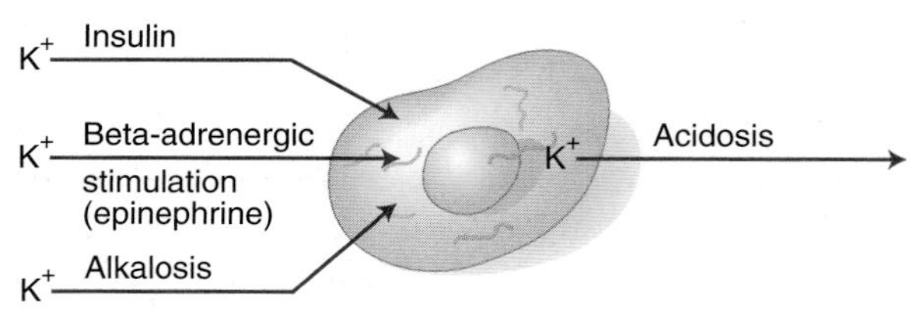

Factors that shift potassium ions into or out of cells.

Etiology and Pathophysiology

Hyperkalemia is caused by conditions that include increased potassium intake, shift of potassium from cells into the extracellular fluid, and decreased potassium excretion. Renal insufficiency is a primary cause of hyperkalemia (Custer & Rau, 2009). Premature infants commonly have low systemic blood flow and resultant poor renal function, leading to hyperkalemia. Increased potassium intake is frequently due to intravenous potassium overload. Excessive or too rapid intravenous administration of potassium-containing solutions can occur if the potassium requirement is overestimated or if the intravenous infusion runs in too fast.

Blood transfusion is another source of potassium intake that may cause hyperkalemia. Potassium ions leak out of red blood cells that are stored in a blood bank. The longer the blood is stored, the more potassium leaks out of cells and accumulates in the fluid portion of the transfusion. Hyperkalemia from administration of stored blood arises when multiple units are transfused, as when infants receive exchange transfusions or children receive multiple blood transfusions after a serious injury or in surgery.

Shift of potassium from cells into the extracellular fluid occurs when there is massive cell death, as with a crush injury, in sickle cell anemia (hemolytic crisis), or when chemotherapy for a malignancy is rapidly effective (tumor lysis syndrome). In these situations the dead cells release their high-potassium contents into the extracellular fluid. Potassium ions also shift out of cells in metabolic acidosis caused by diarrhea and in diabetes mellitus when insulin levels are low.

Decreased potassium excretion occurs with acute or chronic oliguria during renal failure, severe hypovolemia, and conditions that decrease the secretion of aldosterone by the adrenal cortex (lead poisoning, Addison's disease, hypoaldosteronism). Several medications can cause hyperkalemia, including some cancer chemotherapies, potassium-sparing diuretics, angiotensin-converting enzyme inhibitors, and nonsteroidal anti-inflammatories.

Clinical Manifestations

The clinical manifestations of hyperkalemia are all related to muscle dysfunction since potassium plays a vital role in muscle activity. Hyperactivity of gastrointestinal smooth muscle causes intestinal cramping and diarrhea in some children. The skeletal muscles become weak, beginning typically with leg weakness and ascending. Weakness can progress to flaccid paralysis. The child is often lethargic. Dysfunction of cardiac muscle causes cardiac arrhythmias such as tachycardia and may result in heart failure and cardiac arrest. Abnormalities in the electrocardiogram include a prolonged QRS complex, a peak in T waves, atrioventricular block, and ventricular dysrhythmia (Custer & Rau, 2009).

Clinical Therapy

The major diagnostic test is serum potassium. Hyperkalemia is treated by management of the underlying condition that caused the imbalance. If the serum potassium concentration is very high or is causing dangerous cardiac arrhythmias, treatment to decrease the serum potassium level may be ordered. These treatments may remove potassium from the body or drive it from the extracellular fluid into the cells. Potassium is removed from the body by peritoneal dialysis or hemodialysis, by potassium-wasting diuretics, or with a cation exchange resin (Kayexalate) administered orally or rectally. Medical treatments that drive potassium ions into cells are intravenous sodium bicarbonate, intravenous insulin, glucose, and calcium gluconate.

NURSING MANAGEMENT

NURSING ASSESSMENT AND DIAGNOSIS

Monitor serum potassium levels with prescribed laboratory analysis. Ongoing assessment of muscle strength is important because the muscle weakness may progress to flaccid paralysis. (This paralysis is reversible on correction of the potassium imbalance.) Diarrhea can occur in infants and children. An older child may complain of intestinal cramping. Monitor the pulse rate carefully.

Nursing diagnoses for a child who has hyperkalemia depend on the severity of the clinical manifestations. The cause of the imbalance may also lead to useful diagnoses that guide teaching for the child and the parents. The following nursing diagnoses may apply:

- *Activity Intolerance* related to decreased cardiac output secondary to cardiac arrhythmias
- *Risk for Injury* related to muscle weakness
- *Self-Care Deficit: Hygiene and Dressing* related to neuromuscular impairment
- *Anxiety* related to change in health status
- *Ineffective Health Maintenance* related to parental lack of exposure about potassium intake in chronic renal failure
- *Ineffective Management of Therapeutic Regimen by Family* related to complexity of therapy

PLANNING AND IMPLEMENTATION

Nursing care includes measures to prevent hyperkalemia from developing in hospitalized children. If hyperkalemia does develop, care shifts to administering intravenous solutions, monitoring cardiopulmonary status, ensuring safety, promoting adequate nutrition, and preparing the child and family for discharge.

Growth and Development

The nursing diagnoses for hyperkalemic children will prompt a nurse to provide safety measures appropriate to the child's developmental level and to assist the child with activities that muscle weakness makes difficult. It is important to provide play and diversional activities that take into account the child's degree of muscle strength as well as the appropriate developmental level.

PREVENT HYPERKALEMIA

Any child receiving an intravenous infusion that contains potassium is at risk for hyperkalemia. Check that urine output is normal (1–2 mL/kg/hr) before administering intravenous potassium solutions. Turn over intravenous solutions to which potassium has been added several times to mix the contents thoroughly before connecting them to the infusion tubing. Double-check the potassium order and intravenous dosage with another nurse. Observe the child closely and perform cardiorespiratory monitoring.

Be sure blood or packed red blood cells are fresh, especially for the child receiving multiple transfusions, and for all newborns. Use a cardiac monitor during infusion of these products to watch for arrhythmias.

ADMINISTER INTRAVENOUS SOLUTIONS

Once a child is diagnosed as hyperkalemic, ensure that any infusions with added potassium are stopped. Several infusions may need to be managed, including glucose, sodium bicarbonate, and calcium gluconate. Maintain the infusion at the prescribed rate and monitor the child's condition frequently.

MONITOR CARDIOPULMONARY STATUS

Upon diagnosis of hyperkalemia, an electrocardiogram is performed and a cardiac monitor applied. Monitor for any changes in cardiac status and for cardiac arrhythmias. Report abnormal rate and character of pulse as well as shortness of breath.

ENSURE SAFETY

Since the child is weak, raise side rails. Position the child carefully. Assist the child with activities requiring leg muscle strength, such as climbing into bed or pushing up in bed. Encourage quiet activities with frequent rest periods. Document and report any change in muscle weakness.

PROMOTE ADEQUATE NUTRITIONAL INTAKE

Adequate caloric intake is necessary to prevent tissue breakdown and the resultant potassium release from cells. Offer the child nourishing snacks if his or her appetite is decreased. Restrict potassium-rich foods.

DISCHARGE PLANNING AND HOME CARE TEACHING

If the child has chronic renal failure or another condition that decreases aldosterone secretion, teach parents and children to restrict foods high in potassium. Most oral rehydration solutions, including Pedialyte, contain potassium and should not be used to provide fluid for the child. Instruct the family not to use salt substitutes, which commonly contain potassium. Parents should check with the care provider and pharmacist before giving even over-the-counter products to the child, as some of these medications contain potassium. Management of renal failure at home with frequent visits for dialysis and other treatments can be challenging. Refer to Chapter 54∞ for further suggestions to help parents handle this condition.

EVALUATION

Expected outcomes for the child with hyperkalemia include the following:

- Return to a state of fluid and electrolyte balance
- Maintenance of safety
- Adequate nutritional intake to provide essential potassium
- Normal cardiac rate and rhythm

HYPOKALEMIA

Hypokalemia occurs when the serum potassium concentration is too low. Total body potassium may be decreased, normal, or even increased when the serum level is low, depending on the cause of the imbalance. Serum potassium levels below 3.3 mmol/L in children (3.2 mmol/L for newborns) are diagnostic of hypokalemia.

Etiology and Pathophysiology

Hypokalemia is caused by conditions that include increased potassium excretion, decreased potassium intake, shift of potassium from the extracellular fluid into cells, and loss of potassium by an abnormal route.

Increased potassium excretion through the gastrointestinal tract is the major cause of hypokalemia in children. In addition to diuretics and other medications, causes of increased urinary potassium excretion are osmotic diuresis (glucose present in urine), hypomagnesemia, increased aldosterone (hyperaldosteronism, congestive heart failure, nephrotic syndrome, cirrhosis), and increased cortisol (Cushing's disease and syndrome) (Custer & Rau, 2009). Eating large amounts of black licorice increases renal excretion of potassium.

Decreased potassium intake will lead to hypokalemia slowly, or more rapidly if combined with increased excretion or loss of potassium. Hospitalized children that are placed on NPO status and receive prolonged intravenous therapy should have added potassium. Adolescents concerned about weight loss or those with anorexia nervosa may embark on fad diets low in potassium.

Shift of potassium from the extracellular fluid into cells occurs in alkalosis and hypothermia (unintentional or induced for surgery). Hyperalimentation often causes hypersecretion of insulin, which also shifts potassium into cells.

Vomiting is a route for the loss of potassium; self-induced vomiting in bulimia, for example, can cause hypokalemia. Nasogastric suctioning (Figure 46–9 ●) and intestinal decompression can cause potassium loss. Hypokalemia can also be caused by several medications (Table 46–10).

Clinical Manifestations

Since the ratio of intracellular to extracellular potassium determines the responsiveness of muscle cells to neural stimuli, it is not surprising that the clinical manifestations of hypokalemia involve muscle dysfunction. Gastrointestinal smooth muscle activity is slowed, leading to abdominal distention, constipation, or paralytic ileus. Skeletal muscles are weak and unresponsive to

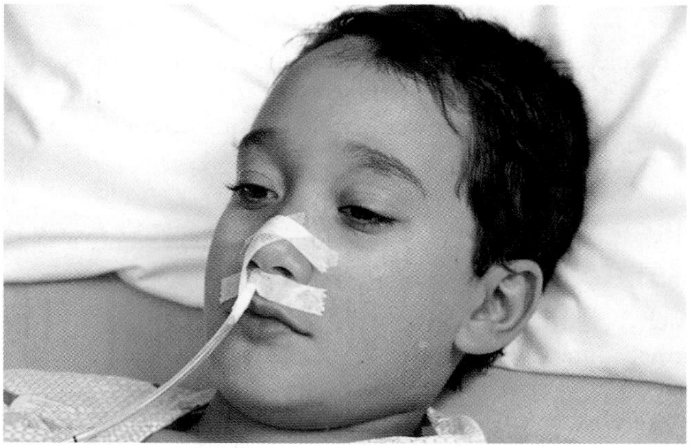

• **Figure 46–9** Nasogastric tubes and potassium levels. Because this child has a nasogastric tube in place, it is important to monitor his potassium levels.

stimuli, and weakness may progress to flaccid paralysis. The respiratory muscles may be impaired. Cardiac arrhythmias can occur. Symptoms may range from mild fatigue to flat or absent T waves (Custer & Rau, 2009). Polyuria results from changes in the kidney caused by hypokalemia.

Clinical Therapy

Serum measurement of potassium is the major diagnostic tool, and electrocardiograph may be used. Medical management of hypokalemia focuses on replacement of potassium while treating the cause of the imbalance. Potassium replacement may be given intravenously or orally.

NURSING MANAGEMENT

NURSING ASSESSMENT AND DIAGNOSIS

Monitor serum potassium levels. Observe for muscle weakness, which is frequently detected first in the legs. Parents may report that muscle weakness restricts the child's activities and impairs interactions with peers. Skeletal muscle strength can be difficult to assess if the child is lethargic.

Muscle weakness may affect the respiratory muscles. Assess the child frequently to determine the need for assisted ventilation. Cardiac monitoring is important for continued assessment of hypokalemia-associated arrhythmias. Apical pulse rate should be monitored.

Assess for diminished bowel sounds. Ask the parents if the child has recently been awakening to use the toilet at night or has begun bed-wetting after previously being dry at night. These may be symptoms of polyuria associated with chronic hypokalemia.

The most important nursing diagnoses in the child with severe hypokalemia relate to cardiac arrhythmias and respiratory muscle weakness. The following nursing diagnoses may apply:

- *Risk for Activity Intolerance* related to decreased cardiac output secondary to cardiac arrhythmia
- *Ineffective Breathing Pattern* related to respiratory musculoskeletal impairment
- *Risk for Injury* related to muscle weakness
- *Self-Care Deficit: Hygiene and Dressing* related to neuromuscular impairment
- *Constipation* related to decreased motility
- *Anxiety* related to change in health status
- *Ineffective Health Maintenance* related to management of potassium supplements or high-potassium diet
- *Ineffective Management of Therapeutic Regimen* related to complexity of potassium therapy
- *Imbalanced Nutrition: Less than Body Requirements* related to lack of basic nutritional knowledge regarding safe weight-loss diet

PLANNING AND IMPLEMENTATION

Nursing care of the child with hypokalemia focuses on ensuring adequate potassium intake, monitoring cardiopulmonary status, promoting normal bowel function, ensuring safety, providing dietary counseling, and preparing the child and family for discharge.

ENSURE ADEQUATE POTASSIUM INTAKE

Since potassium is excreted from the body every day, daily potassium intake is necessary to prevent hypokalemia. A hypokalemic child

Table 46–10 Drugs That May Cause Electrolyte Disturbance

Hyperkalemia	Hypokalemia	Hypocalcemia	Hypermagnesemia	Hypomagnesemia
Potassium-containing medications Potassium-sparing diuretics Angiotensin-converting enzyme inhibitors Cytotoxic agents	Beta-adrenergic agonists Insulin Potassium-wasting diuretics Parenteral penicillins Glucocorticoids Aminoglycoside antimicrobials Systemic antifungals Antineoplastics Laxatives	Antacids (if overused) Laxatives (if overused) Oil-based bowel lubricants Anticonvulsants Phosphate-containing preparations Protein-type plasma expanders during rapid infusion Antineoplastics	Magnesium antacids Magnesium-containing cathartics	Magnesium-wasting diuretics Antineoplastics Systemic antifungals Aminoglycoside antimicrobials Laxatives

Growth and Development

Bradycardia occurs at a different level for children of various ages. For infants, a pulse rate below 100 is considered bradycardia. For young children, 80 may be the identified number, whereas for adolescents, a pulse below 60 is bradycardia. Look at the child's age and normal pulse range to find changes that indicate bradycardia.

who is able to eat should be given a high-potassium diet. Teach parents (and the child if old enough) which foods are high in potassium and how to incorporate them into the daily diet (Table 46–11).

Children who have no oral intake for a period of time should receive intravenous fluids that contain potassium. Calculate the dosage to be sure it is accurate. Ensure that the infusion runs on schedule. Sometimes the child will complain of burning along the vein when potassium is infused. The infusion may need to be slowed temporarily to allow it to continue. Check serum potassium to watch for high or low potassium levels. Monitor urine output. An oliguric child can develop hyperkalemia when receiving supplements.

MONITOR CARDIOPULMONARY STATUS

Hypokalemia potentiates digitalis toxicity. A hypokalemic child receiving digitalis needs careful surveillance for digitalis toxicity, which is manifested as anorexia, nausea, vomiting, and bradycardia. Observe for these effects. Take the pulse rate and rhythm regularly. Monitor respirations and ease of breathing to watch for decreased respiratory muscle activity.

PROMOTE NORMAL BOWEL FUNCTION

Ensure adequate fluids and fiber in the diet. Monitor and record the number of stools and report inadequate stools.

ENSURE SAFETY

Keep bed side rails up. Assist the child as needed to move into and out of bed. Reposition the child frequently to preserve skin integrity of limbs that are not moved regularly. Perform passive range of motion if the child is not moving. Use supportive pillows to position the child properly.

PROVIDE DIETARY COUNSELING

The adolescent trying to lose weight and not consuming a nutritious diet needs dietary teaching. More intensive treatment will be needed for teens who are anorexic or bulimic (see Chapter 36 for interventions).

DISCHARGE PLANNING AND HOME CARE TEACHING

Teach parents how to give potassium supplements, if prescribed. Liquid or powdered potassium supplements can be mixed with juice or sherbet to improve the bitter taste. The parent should call the mixture "medicine" so that the child does not learn to dislike all juices. Teach the parents signs of hypokalemia and hyperkalemia and whom to call to report these symptoms. These signs must be reported promptly so medications can be adjusted.

EVALUATION

Expected outcomes for the child with potassium imbalance include normal rate and rhythm of heart and respiratory system, regular bowel movements, maintenance of safety, and knowledge of child and family regarding food sources of potassium.

CALCIUM IMBALANCES

A normal serum calcium concentration is important for many physiologic functions, including muscle and nerve function, secretion of hormones, bone formation and strength, and clotting of the blood. Calcium is the most abundant mineral in the body, with about 98% of it being present in bones (Roberts, 2005). There are three forms of calcium in plasma—calcium bound to protein, calcium bound to small organic ions (e.g., citrate), and free ionized calcium (CA^{++}), which is phsiologically active. A discussion of dietary calcium intake and its importance in bone formation can be found in Chapter 34 (also see "Developing Cultural Competence: Calcium Intake and Osteoporosis").

Calcium imbalances are caused by alterations in calcium intake, absorption, distribution, or excretion. Calcium absorption requires vitamin D for maximum efficiency and is greatest in the

Table 46–11 Food Sources of Electrolytes

Potassium-Rich Foods		Calcium-Rich Foods		Magnesium-Rich Foods
Apricots	Orange juice	Milk	Legumes	Whole-grain cereal
Bananas	Peaches	Cheese	Nuts	Dark green vegetables
Cantaloupe	Potatoes	Yogurt	Figs	Soy
Cherries	Prunes	Pudding	Chicken	Almonds
Dates	Raisins	Egg yolks	Salmon (canned with bones)	Peanut butter
Figs	Strawberries	Grains (cream of wheat, farina, bran muffins)	Tofu	Bananas
Molasses	Tomato juice	Sardines (canned)	Fruit drinks with added calcium	Egg yolk

Developing Cultural Competence

CALCIUM INTAKE AND OSTEOPOROSIS

Ingestion and absorption of calcium is important in the growing child to ensure formation of strong bones. Adolescents who ingest more calcium have less risk of osteoporosis later in life. It has been noted that black women have less bone loss and fewer fractures than white women. Studies with black and white individuals have demonstrated that blacks absorb more calcium from the diet, and lost less in their urine, leading to increased bone density (Heaney, 2006). Nurses should recognize this difference and monitor intake of all adolescents. Recognize the high risk of developing osteoporosis in those who are white and consuming little calcium. Interventions should focus on ways of increasing intake.

duodenum. Calcium distribution involves calcium entry into and exit from bones and the distribution of different forms of calcium in the plasma. Ionized calcium is the only physiologically active form; additional calcium is bound to protein or ions. Calcium is excreted in urine, feces, and sweat (see "Pathophysiology Illustrated: Calcium Imbalances").

Parathyroid hormone is the major regulator of the plasma calcium concentration. It increases the plasma calcium concentration by increasing calcium absorption, increasing calcium withdrawal from bones, and decreasing calcium excretion in the urine. The plasma calcium concentration has an important influence on cell membrane permeability and influences the threshold potential of excitable cells. For this reason, calcium imbalances alter neuromuscular irritability.

HYPERCALCEMIA

Hypercalcemia refers to a plasma excess of total calcium (above 2.64 mmol/L in infants and children) (see Table 46–7). Because so much calcium is stored in the bones, however, the serum levels of calcium may not reflect body stores.

Etiology and Pathophysiology

Hypercalcemia is caused by conditions that include increased calcium intake or absorption, shift of calcium from bones into the extracellular fluid, and decreased calcium excretion. Hypercalcemia due to increased calcium intake or absorption may occur if an infant is fed large amounts of chicken liver (source of vitamin A) or is given megadoses of vitamin D or vitamin A, or if a child or adolescent consumes large amounts of calcium-rich foods concurrently with antacids (milk-alkali syndrome). Infants with very low birth weight can develop hypercalcemia if they have inadequate phosphorus intake, as bone phosphorus and calcium will be resorbed. Hypercalcemia may also occur when children receiving total parenteral nutrition are given excessive doses of calcium.

PATHOPHYSIOLOGY ILLUSTRATED

CALCIUM IMBALANCES

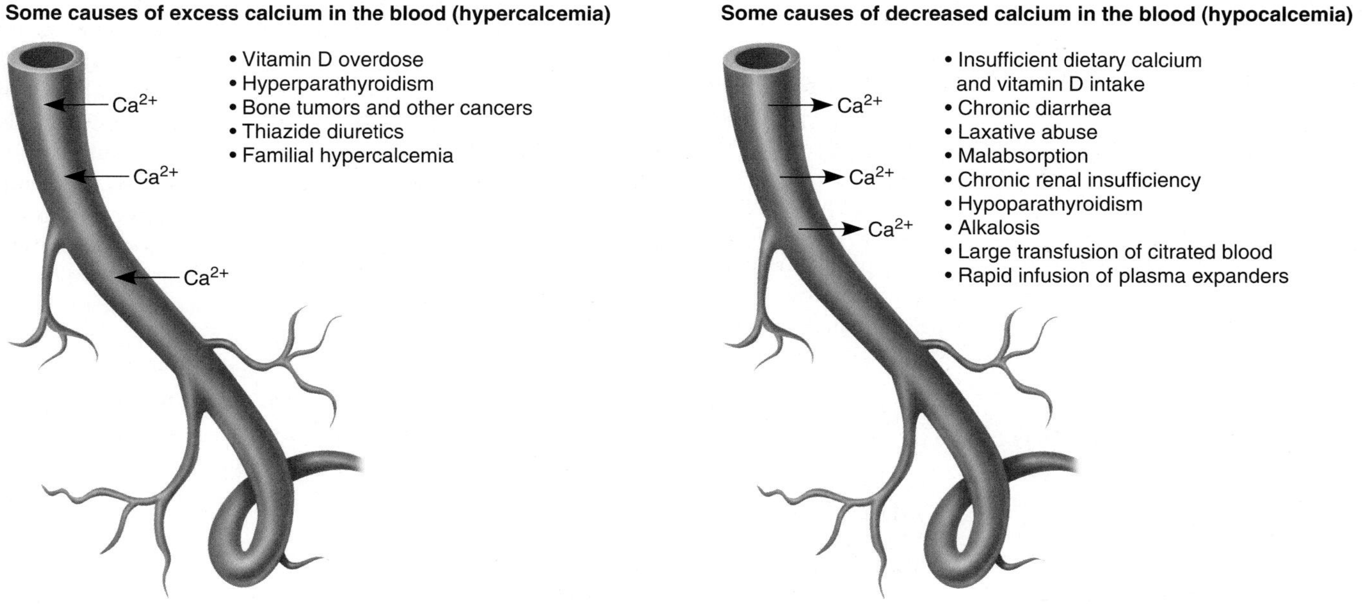

Some causes of excess calcium in the blood (hypercalcemia)
Ca2+
Ca2+
Ca2+
• Vitamin D overdose
• Hyperparathyroidism
• Bone tumors and other cancers
• Thiazide diuretics
• Familial hypercalcemia
Some causes of decreased calcium in the blood (hypocalcemia)
Ca2+
Ca2+
Ca2+
• Insufficient dietary calcium and vitamin D intake
• Chronic diarrhea
• Laxative abuse
• Malabsorption
• Chronic renal insufficiency
• Hypoparathyroidism
• Alkalosis
• Large transfusion of citrated blood
• Rapid infusion of plasma expanders

A variety of conditions can lead to hypercalcemia and hypocalcemia.

Most cases of hypercalcemia in children are due to a shift of calcium from bones into the extracellular fluid. The excessive amounts of parathyroid hormone produced in hyperparathyroidism cause calcium withdrawal from bones. Prolonged immobilization also causes withdrawal of calcium from bones. Often, the excess calcium ions are excreted in the urine. However, if calcium is withdrawn from bones faster than the kidneys can excrete it, hypercalcemia results. Hypercalcemia also occurs with many types of malignancies, such as leukemias. The malignant cells produce substances that circulate in the blood to the bones and cause bone resorption. The calcium from the bones then enters the extracellular fluid, causing hypercalcemia. Bone tumors destroy bone directly, leading to the release of calcium. Familial hypercalcemia and infantile hypercalcemia are rare congenital disorders.

Thiazide diuretics (e.g., thiazide and hydrochlorthiazide) decrease calcium excretion in the urine and may contribute to development of hypercalcemia. Lithium and theophylline can induce hypercalcemia.

Clinical Manifestations

Hypercalcemia may have nonspecific symptoms, making diagnosis difficult. Many signs and symptoms of hypercalcemia are manifestations of decreased neuromuscular excitability. Constipation, anorexia, nausea, and vomiting can occur. Fatigue and skeletal muscle weakness predominate. Confusion, lethargy, and decreased attention span are common. Polyuria develops. Severe hypercalcemia may cause cardiac arrhythmias and arrest. Newborns with hypercalcemia have flaccid muscles and exhibit failure to thrive. Hypercalcemia increases sodium and potassium excretion by the kidneys and can lead to polyuria and polydipsia.

Clinical Therapy

Serum calcium is tested although the blood level may not accurately reflect bone stores. Additional laboratory tests include serum albumin, phosphate, magnesium, alkaline phosphate, electrolytes, blood urea nitrogen, creatinine, and parathyroid hormone. Hypercalcemia is treated by increasing fluids and administering the diuretic furosemide (Lasix) to increase excretion of calcium in the urine. Treatment to decrease intestinal absorption of calcium involves effective use of glucocorticoids. Bone resorption can be decreased by administration of glucocorticoids and calcitonin. Phosphate is sometimes given to treat hypercalcemia, but it may cause dangerous precipitation of calcium phosphate salts in body tissues. Dialysis may be used, if necessary. The underlying condition causing the imbalance is treated.

NURSING MANAGEMENT

NURSING ASSESSMENT AND DIAGNOSIS

Nursing assessment of a child with hypercalcemia includes monitoring serum calcium levels, level of consciousness, gastrointestinal function, urine volume, specific gravity, cardiac rhythm, and pH. With chronic hypercalcemia, assessment of activity tolerance and developmental level becomes important.

Many nursing diagnoses are appropriate for children who have hypercalcemia. Diagnoses that address cardiac and neuromuscular manifestation are especially important. The following nursing diagnoses may apply:

- *Risk for Activity Intolerance* related to decreased cardiac output secondary to cardiac arrhythmia
- *Risk for Injury* related to decreased level of consciousness
- *Risk for Injury* related to neuromuscular impairment
- *Risk for Injury* related to possibility of spontaneous fractures
- *Self-Care Deficit: Hygiene and Dressing* related to neuromuscular impairment
- *Anxiety* related to change in health status
- *Constipation* related to decreased motility
- *Risk for Imbalanced Nutrition: Less than Body Requirements* related to anorexia and nausea
- *Risk for Impaired Urinary Elimination* related to renal calculi

PLANNING AND INTERVENTION

Carefully calculate calcium in total parenteral nutrition and other solutions, administer these solutions with caution, and use cardiac monitoring to prevent hypercalcemia in hospitalized children.

Interventions to increase fluid intake are important for children with hypercalcemia or those who are immobilized. An increased fluid intake, appropriate to the child's age, is necessary to keep the urine dilute and to help reduce constipation (a common symptom of hypercalcemia). An acidic urine helps to keep calcium from forming stones. Because urinary tract infections may cause the urine to be alkaline, institute nursing interventions to prevent urinary tract infection. Thiazide diuretics, which decrease calcium excretion, should not be given to the hypercalcemic child. Provide a high-fiber diet to help reduce constipation.

Increasing mobility through assisted weight bearing helps decrease the withdrawal of calcium from bones that is caused by immobility. If the hypercalcemia is caused by withdrawal of calcium from bones, the child is at risk for fractures with minor trauma and must be handled with special care. See Chapter 55 for further discussion of care following fractures and prolonged casting.

Teach parents to avoid giving calcium-rich foods (such as dairy products) and calcium antacids (e.g., Tums) to children with hypercalcemia. Vitamin D supplements should be avoided as they increase calcium absorption from the gastrointestinal tract.

Expected outcomes include cardiac pump effectiveness, safety, normal bowel excretion, and adequate nutritional status.

HYPOCALCEMIA

Hypocalcemia is a serum deficit of calcium (below 2.1 mmol/L in infants and children) (Soldin et al., 2005). Recall that serum calcium levels may not reflect body stores of this mineral, as most of the body's calcium is stored in bone.

Etiology and Pathophysiology

Hypocalcemia is caused by conditions that include decreased calcium intake or absorption, shift of calcium to a physiologically unavailable form, increased calcium excretion, and loss of calcium by an abnormal route.

Decreased calcium intake or absorption causes hypocalcemia in children with chronic generalized malnutrition, or with a diet low in vitamin D and calcium. Female adolescents trying to lose weight or maintain a low weight often decrease foods that contain calcium and may develop chronic hypocalcemia. They may have premature bone loss and inadequate bone. (See Chapter 34 for further discussion of calcium intake during adolescence.) This deficit cannot be made up later in life, increasing the risk of osteoporosis.

Even with a normal calcium intake, hypocalcemia occurs if the mineral is not absorbed. If a child does not have enough vitamin D, calcium is not absorbed efficiently from the duodenum. Sunlight speeds formation of vitamin D in the skin. Children institutionalized without access to sunlight (e.g., severely developmentally delayed children, those with very dark skin, or children kept well covered when outside) may become hypocalcemic because of the lack of vitamin D (see Chapter 34). Uremic syndrome is another cause of vitamin D deficiency. It interferes with the kidney's ability to activate vitamin D. High phosphate intake can cause hypocalcemia. Chronic diarrhea and steatorrhea (fatty stools) also reduce calcium absorption from the gastrointestinal tract.

About 40% of calcium is bound to proteins and not available for interactions, 10% is bound to small organic ions such as citrate, and 50% is ionized and physiologically active. Calcium becomes physiologically unavailable when calcium shifts into bone or free ionized calcium in plasma binds to proteins or small organic ions in the plasma. Excessive calcium shifts into bones in various types of hypoparathyroidism, including DiGeorge syndrome (congenital absence of the parathyroid glands). Hypomagnesemia impairs parathyroid hormone function and may cause hypocalcemia. Some types of neonatal hypocalcemia are associated with delayed parathyroid hormone function or hypomagnesemia. Calcium shifts rapidly into bone when rickets is treated. A high plasma phosphate concentration causes plasma calcium to decrease. Ionized hypocalcemia, due to an increased binding of plasma ionized calcium, occurs very rapidly. The ionized hypocalcemia persists until the alkalosis resolves or the citrate is metabolized by the liver. Children who receive liver transplants are hypocalcemic for several days because of impaired citrate metabolism.

Increased calcium excretion occurs in steatorrhea, when calcium secreted into the gastrointestinal fluid binds to the fecal fat in addition to the dietary calcium that is bound in the feces. A similar situation occurs in acute pancreatitis.

Loss of calcium by an abnormal route may contribute to hypocalcemia; calcium is lost through burn or wound drainage or sequestered in acute pancreatitis. Many medications can cause hypocalcemia (see Table 46–10).

Clinical Manifestations

The signs and symptoms of hypocalcemia are manifestations of increased muscular excitability (tetany). In children they include twitching and cramping, tingling around the mouth or in the fingers, carpal spasm, and pedal spasm. Laryngospasm, seizures, and cardiac arrhythmias are more severe manifestations of hypocalcemia and may be fatal. Hypocalcemia may cause congestive heart failure, especially in newborns.

Although these symptoms are diagnostic of acute calcium deficiency, a more common state in children and adolescents is chronic low intake of calcium. This may be manifested by spontaneous fractures in infants and in adolescents who exercise excessively.

> **Growth and Development**
>
> Hypocalcemia in infants is more often seen as tremors, muscle twitches, and brief tonic-clonic seizures. Perform careful neurologic assessments on infants at risk of electrolyte imbalance.

Clinical Therapy

Laboratory measurement of serum calcium and cardiac monitoring are used for diagnosis. Hypocalcemia is treated by oral or intravenous administration of calcium (see "Drug Guide: Calcium Gluconate"). The original cause of the imbalance is also treated. If the hypocalcemia is due to hypomagnesemia, the magnesium must be replenished before the calcium replacement can be successful. When the cause is chronic low dietary intake, counseling is needed about high-calcium foods, and perhaps the necessity for vitamin D intake or supplements.

NURSING MANAGEMENT

NURSING ASSESSMENT AND DIAGNOSIS

Carefully assess growth in the young female who is trying to diet. Whenever an adolescent female is very thin, be sure to ask about excessive sports and other activities, and about regularity of menstrual periods. If periods are irregular or not occurring, collect additional dietary information to help determine whether the girl is lacking in intake of calcium, calories, and other nutrients. These assessments are needed even if serum calcium values are normal. Look for signs of inadequate nutrition such as fat and muscle wasting, dry hair, and cold hands and feet. Assess for muscle cramps, stiffness, and clumsiness; grimacing caused by spasms of facial muscles and twitching of arm muscles; and laryngospasm. Increased neuromuscular excitability may be detected by testing for Trousseau's sign or Chvostek's sign. Many healthy newborns have a positive Chvostek's sign; however, this assessment should be reserved for children over several months of age. Monitor serum calcium levels and perform cardiac monitoring to observe for cardiac arrhythmias.

The effects of increased neuromuscular excitability in the child with hypocalcemia are the basis for several nursing diagnoses. These include the following:

- *Risk for Injury* related to potential for fractures
- *Risk for Injury* related to increased neuromuscular excitability

MyNursingKit Understanding School-Age Athletes and Fluid Needs

Drug Guide

CALCIUM GLUCONATE

Overview of Action

Calcium is a normal body electrolyte and may need to be infused in infants or young children with health problems leading to low calcium. It is also used during exchange transfusion in newborns since citrate in the blood transfusion can bind body calcium. In the form of CaCl, calcium may be used during resuscitation. Calcium regulates excitability of muscles and nerves, and therefore affects cardiac function (inotropic effect); is necessary for blood clotting; plays a role in storage and release of neurotransmitters, in renal function, and in maintaining cell membranes; and is an antidote to excessive magnesium infusion.

Routes, Dosage, Frequency

Hypocalcemia

Neonate: IV 200–800 mg/kg/day divided into doses given every 6 hrs

Infant: PO 400–800 mg/kg/day divided into doses given every 6 hrs

IV: 200–500 mg/kg/day divided into doses given every 6 hrs

Child: PO or IV 200–500 mg/kg/day divided into doses given every 6 hrs

Adolescent: PO or IV 5–15 g/day divided into doses given every 6 hrs

Cardiac Arrest

Infant/Child: IV 100 mg/kg/dose (or 1 mL/kg/dose) every 10 minutes as needed for resuscitation

Adolescent: IV 500–800 mg/dose (or 5–8 mL/dose) every 10 minutes as needed for resuscitation (maximum of 3 g/dose)

Contraindications

Ventricular fibrillation, metastatic bone disease, renal calculi, hypercalcemia, pregnancy (category B); not to be injected into myocardium or given by SC or IM routes

Side Effects

Tingling, heat sensation, fainting, hypotension, bradycardia, cardiac arrhythmias, cardiac arrest, pain at IV infusion site, venous thrombosis; with PO administration, constipation, increased gastric acid secretion

Nursing Implications

- Verify dose carefully with the prescriber and another nurse.
- Monitor heart rate and rhythm—hypotension and bradycardia can occur.
- Use extreme caution if given in cardiac or renal disease.
- Maintain IV carefully to avoid extravasation; do **not** administer by peripheral infusion, scalp vein, IM, or SC.
- Precipitates when given in infusion with bicarbonate.

Data from Bindler, R., & Howry, L. (2005). *Pediatric Drug Guide.* Upper Saddle River, NJ: Prentice Hall Health, pp. 223–226.

- *Risk for Ineffective Breathing Pattern* related to laryngospasm
- *Activity Intolerance* related to decreased cardiac output secondary to cardiac arrhythmias
- *Disturbed Sensory Perception* related to electrolyte imbalance
- *Anxiety* related to change in health status
- *Imbalanced Nutrition: Less than Body Requirement* related to lack of basic nutritional knowledge of sources and recommended amounts of calcium intake

PLANNING AND IMPLEMENTATION

To correct calcium deficiency in the hospitalized child, give oral or intravenous calcium as prescribed. Monitor for complications of calcium supplementation. Monitor for the side effect of constipation with oral supplements; or for tissue sloughing, elevated serum calcium, or decreased serum phosphate with intravenous supplementation. Calcium is never given intramuscularly because it causes tissue necrosis. A 10% calcium gluconate intravenous solution should be readily available for emergency use in severe hypocalcemia.

Take measures to ensure safety for the child who is hospitalized with hypocalcemia. Seizure precautions may be necessary. Explain the cause of muscle cramps to parents and older children.

Counsel the family about dairy products and nondairy foods rich in calcium (see Table 46–11). For the adolescent female whose weight and menstrual patterns show irregularities, total calories and calcium intake should be increased. Teaching may also be needed about proper calcium intake and its importance both to athletic performance and to the prevention of osteoporosis. Encourage three glasses of nonfat milk per day. Teach ways to use milk in the diet. For example, sprinkle nonfat dry milk on cereal and other foods. If the child is lactose-intolerant, emphasize nondairy sources of calcium and advise parents to purchase special milk treated with lactase. This milk is more costly, and inadequate family finances may prevent its use. If a child has a health condition leading to chronic diarrhea, encourage increased intake of calcium-rich foods. Calcium supplements in the form of calcium carbonate tablets may be used.

EVALUATION

Expected outcomes of nursing care include ingestion of recommended dietary allowances for calcium, absence of discomfort related to calcium imbalance, and freedom from injury.

MAGNESIUM IMBALANCES

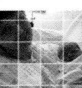

Magnesium is necessary for enzyme function in cells, acetylcholine release, glycolysis, stimulation of ATPases, and bone formation. Since magnesium is a component of chlorophyll, dark green leafy vegetables are a good dietary source of magnesium. Nuts and grains are also good sources of magnesium. Magnesium is absorbed primarily from the terminal ileum. It is distributed among the extracellular fluid (small amounts), the cells (larger amounts), and the bones (large amounts). Magnesium is excreted in urine, feces, and sweat.

Magnesium imbalances are caused by alterations in magnesium intake, distribution, or excretion; by loss of magnesium through an abnormal route; or by a combination of these factors. The plasma magnesium concentration influences the release of acetylcholine at neuromuscular junctions. Thus, magnesium imbalances are characterized by alterations in neuromuscular irritability.

HYPERMAGNESEMIA

Hypermagnesemia occurs when the plasma magnesium concentration is too high (above 2.7 mg/dL [1.1 mmol/L]) (see Table 46–7). Keep in mind that the serum levels measured in the laboratory may not reflect body magnesium stores, because most magnesium in the body is located in the bones and inside the cells.

Hypermagnesemia is caused by conditions that involve increased magnesium intake and decreased magnesium excretion. Impaired renal function leading to decreased magnesium excretion is the most common cause of hypermagnesemia in children. In both oliguric renal failure and adrenal insufficiency, magnesium ions that cannot be excreted in the urine accumulate in the extracellular fluid.

Less frequently, increased magnesium intake may cause hypermagnesemia. Magnesium sulfate ($MgSo_4$) given to treat eclampsia in the mother before birth causes hypermagnesemia in the newborn. Abnormally high amounts may also be taken in magnesium-containing enemas, laxatives, antacids, and intravenous fluids. Epsom salt is a readily available product that is a nearly pure magnesium sulfate preparation; its use as an enema has caused death in children (Tofil, Benner & Winkler, 2005) (see Table 46–10). Aspiration of seawater, as in near-drowning, is an uncommon but potentially serious source of excessive magnesium intake. Children with Addison's disease can have abnormally high magnesium levels.

Clinical manifestations of hypermagnesemia include decreased muscle irritability, hypotension, bradycardia, drowsiness, lethargy, and weak or absent deep tendon reflexes. In severe hypermagnesemia, flaccid muscle paralysis, fatal respiratory depression, cardiac arrhythmias, and cardiac arrest occur.

Hypermagnesemia is managed primarily by increasing the urinary excretion of magnesium. This is usually accomplished by increasing fluid intake (except in oliguric renal failure) and by the administration of diuretics. Dialysis may sometimes be necessary.

Nursing Management

Monitor serum magnesium levels. Take the child's blood pressure (to watch for hypotension), heart rate and rhythm (to monitor for bradycardia and cardiac arrhythmias), respiratory rate and depth (to observe for respiratory depression), and deep tendon reflexes (to assess muscle tone and paralysis or movement). Keep the side rails of the bed raised. Children with hypermagnesemia or oliguria should not be given magnesium-containing medications or sea salt.

> **Nursing Practice**
>
> Instruct parents of a child with chronic renal failure to read labels to detect magnesium in antacids and cathartics. Encourage them to check with their pharmacist and other healthcare providers before administering any over-the-counter medication to the child.

Teach parents of children with chronic renal failure that these children should never be given milk of magnesia, antacids that contain magnesium, or other sources of magnesium. When hypermagnesemia is treated with diuretics, monitor potassium levels to watch for hypokalemia.

Expected outcomes of nursing care include maintenance of electrolyte balance, normal neuromuscular tone, safety, and regular heart rate and rhythm.

HYPOMAGNESEMIA

Hypomagnesemia refers to a plasma magnesium concentration that is too low (below 1.5 to 1.7 mg/dL [0.62 to 0.70 mmol/L]). Remember that the serum levels of magnesium may not reflect body stores, since most of the magnesium in the body is found in cells and bones.

Hypomagnesemia is caused by conditions that include decreased magnesium intake or absorption, shift of magnesium to a physiologically unavailable form, increased magnesium excretion, and loss of magnesium by an abnormal route.

Decreased magnesium intake or absorption can occur if a child who is not eating has prolonged intravenous therapy without magnesium. Chronic malnutrition is another cause of decreased magnesium intake. Magnesium absorption is decreased in chronic diarrhea, short bowel syndrome, malabsorption syndromes, and steatorrhea.

Magnesium may shift to a physiologically unavailable form after transfusion of many units of citrated blood products; magnesium bound to the citrate is not physiologically active. Such transfusions cause prolonged hypomagnesemia in liver transplant patients, who have impaired citrate metabolism. Magnesium shifts rapidly into bones that have been deprived of adequate stores.

Increased magnesium excretion in the urine occurs with diuretic therapy, the diuretic phase of acute renal failure, diabetic ketoacidosis, and hyperaldosteronism. Chronic alcoholism, occasionally seen in adolescents, increases urinary magnesium excretion. Magnesium contained in gastrointestinal secretions is bound to fat and excreted in the stool.

Loss of magnesium by an abnormal route occurs with prolonged nasogastric suction and through sequestration of magnesium in acute pancreatitis. Several medications may cause hypomagnesemia (see Table 46–10).

Hypomagnesemia is characterized by increased neuromuscular excitability (tetany). The clinical manifestations are hyperactive reflexes, skeletal muscle cramps, twitching, tremors, and cardiac arrhythmias. Seizures can occur with severe hypomagnesemia.

Hypomagnesemia is managed by administering magnesium and treating the underlying cause of the imbalance.

Nursing Management

In addition to monitoring serum magnesium levels, nursing assessment of hypomagnesemia includes monitoring deep tendon reflexes, testing for Trousseau's and Chvostek's signs, monitoring cardiac function, and observing for muscle twitching. Children who are able to talk may report muscle cramping. Because magnesium levels are not routinely measured in many settings, request the test for any child who has risk factors and early manifestations of hypomagnesemia. When intramuscular or intravenous magnesium is ordered, administer carefully as directed and monitor vital signs. Electrocardiogram and renal studies may precede drug administration. Have resuscitative drugs and equipment readily available during drug administration.

Teach parents of a child with hypomagnesemia or continuing risk factors such as chronic diarrhea to include magnesium-rich foods in the diet (see Table 46–11). Before administering magnesium supplements, verify that the child's urine output is adequate. Monitor deep tendon reflexes if intravenous magnesium is given, and observe for complications of magnesium supplementation. Oral magnesium may lead to diarrhea, and intravenous magnesium can cause flushing, elevated serum magnesium, cardiac arrhythmias, or decreased deep tendon reflexes.

Expected outcomes of nursing care for the child with an imbalance in magnesium are restoration and maintenance of electrolyte balance.

CLINICAL ASSESSMENT OF FLUID AND ELECTROLYTE IMBALANCE

How can a nurse assess children appropriately for fluid and electrolyte imbalance without thinking through the clinical manifestations of every possible disorder one after the other? First, perform a rapid risk factor assessment on each child to see which factors are present (Tables 46–12 and 46–13).

Table 46–12 Risk Factor Assessment for Fluid Imbalances

Type of Fluid	Factors to Assess
Isotonic fluid (extracellular fluid volume imbalances)	Source of increased intake? Aldosterone secretion increased or decreased? Source of loss from the body?
Water	Source of increased intake? Antidiuretic hormone secretion increased or decreased? Source of unusual loss from the body?

Table 46–13 Risk Factor Assessment for Electrolyte Imbalances

Potential Electrolyte Imbalance	Assessment Finding
Electrolyte intake and absorption	Increased? Decreased?
Electrolyte shifts	From electrolyte pool to plasma? From plasma to electrolyte pool?
Electrolyte excretion	Increased? Decreased?
Electrolyte loss by abnormal route	Vomiting? Diarrhea? Nasogastric suction? Wound? Burn? Excessive sweating?

A risk factor assessment may be performed mentally while providing care. Look for factors that alter the intake, retention, and loss of isotonic fluid and water. Use this information to evaluate which fluid imbalance is most likely to occur in a particular child. Next, look for factors that alter electrolyte intake and absorption, distribution between plasma and other electrolyte pools, excretion, and abnormal routes of electrolyte loss. Use this information to evaluate which electrolyte imbalances are most likely to occur in the child. A review of pathophysiology is important to understand the role of the other electrolytes and substances, such as phosphorus, in the body.

After evaluating possible imbalances for the child, perform a clinical assessment. Assess for fluid imbalances by assessing weight changes, vascular volume, interstitial volume, and cerebral function (Table 46–14). Assess for electrolyte imbalances by assessing serum electrolyte levels, skeletal muscle strength, neuromuscular excitability, gastrointestinal tract function, and cardiac rhythm (Table 46–15). Next, check for other manifestations specific to a particular high-risk imbalance (e.g., polyuria in hypokalemia). Evaluate any serum laboratory values available. This method of risk factor assessment followed by clinical assessment provides a rapid yet thorough approach to assessment for fluid and electrolyte imbalances.

PHYSIOLOGY OF ACID-BASE BALANCE

Normal acid-base balance is necessary for proper function of the cells and the body. The number of hydrogen ions (H^+) present in a fluid determines how acidic it is. Increasing the hydrogen ion concentration makes a solution more acidic. Because the hydrogen ion concentration in body fluids is very small, acidity is expressed as **pH** (the negative logarithm of the hydrogen ion concentration) rather than as the hydrogen ion concentration itself. The range of possible pH values is 1 to 14. A pH of 7 is neutral. The lower the pH, the more acidic the solution. A pH above

Table 46–14 Summary of Clinical Assessment of Fluid Imbalances

Assessment Category	Specific Assessments	Changes with Fluid Imbalances
Rapid changes in weight	Daily weights	Weight gain—extracellular volume excess Weight loss—extracellular volume deficit; clinical dehydration
Vascular volume	Small vein filling time	Increased—extracellular volume deficit; clinical dehydration
	Capillary refill time	Increased—extracellular volume deficit; clinical dehydration
	Character of pulse	Bounding—extracellular volume excess Thready—extracellular volume deficit; clinical dehydration
	Postural blood pressure measurements	Postural drop—extracellular volume deficit; clinical dehydration
	Lung sounds in dependent portions	Crackles—extracellular volume excess
	Central venous pressure	Increased—extracellular volume excess Decreased—extracellular volume deficit; clinical dehydration
	Tenseness of fontanelle (infants)	Bulging—extracellular volume excess Sunken—extracellular volume deficit; clinical dehydration
	Neck vein filling (older children)	Full when upright—extracellular volume excess Flat when supine—extracellular volume deficit; clinical dehydration
Interstitial volume	Skin turgor	Skin tents—extracellular volume deficit; clinical dehydration
	Presence or absence of edema	Edema—extracellular volume excess
Cerebral function	Level of consciousness	Decreased—clinical dehydration

7 is basic. The higher the pH, the more basic the solution. Body fluids are normally slightly basic (see Table 46–7).

The pH of body fluids is regulated carefully to provide a suitable environment for cell function. The pH of the blood influences the pH inside the cells. **Acidemia** refers to a decreased blood pH below normal levels, while **alkalemia** is an increased blood pH. Normal arterial blood pH ranges are 7.36 to 7.42 for infants, 7.37 to 7.43 for children, and 7.35 to 7.41 for adolescents. For the enzymes outside the cells to function optimally, the pH must be in the normal range. If the pH inside the cells becomes too high or too low, then the speed of chemical reactions becomes inappropriate for proper cell function. Cell protein function relies on the correct level of hydrogen ions. Thus, acid-base imbalances result in clinical signs and symptoms, and, in severe cases, they may cause death.

In the course of their normal function, all cells in the body produce acids. Cells produce two kinds of acids: carbonic acid (H_2CO_3) and metabolic (noncarbonic) acids. Carbonic acid is formed from carbon dioxide and water, while common metabolic acids are pyruvic, sulfuric, lactic, and hydrochloric acids. These acids are released

Table 46–15 Summary of Clinical Assessment of Electrolyte Imbalances

Assessment Category	Specific Assessments	Changes with Electrolyte Imbalances
Skeletal muscle function	Muscle strength	Weakness, flaccid paralysis—hyperkalemia; hypokalemia
Neuromuscular excitability	Deep tendon reflexes	Depressed—hypercalcemia; hypermagnesemia Hyperactive—hypocalcemia; hypomagnesemia
	Chvostek's sign (not seen in infants)	Positive—hypocalcemia; hypomagnesemia
	Trousseau's sign	Positive—hypocalcemia; hypomagnesemia
	Paresthesias	Digital or perioral—hypocalcemia
	Muscle cramping or twitching	Present—hypocalcemia; hypomagnesemia
Gastrointestinal tract function	Bowel sounds	Decreased or absent—hypokalemia
	Elimination pattern	Constipation—hypokalemia; hypercalcemia Diarrhea—hyperkalemia
Cardiac rhythm	Arrhythmia	Irregular—hyperkalemia; hypokalemia; hypercalcemia; hypocalcemia; hypermagnesemia; hypomagnesemia
	Electrocardiogram	Abnormal—hyperkalemia; hypokalemia; hypercalcemia; hypocalcemia; hypermagnesemia; hypomagnesemia
Cerebral function	Level of consciousness	Decreased—hyponatremia; hypernatremia

PATHOPHYSIOLOGY ILLUSTRATED

BUFFER RESPONSES TO ACID AND BASE

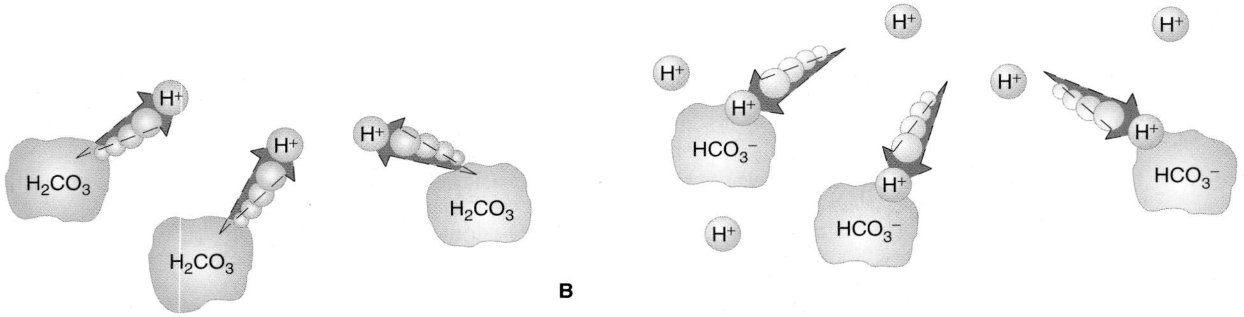
H+
H2CO3
H+
H2CO3
H+
H2CO3
H+
H2CO3
H+
H+
HCO3−
H+
HCO3−
H+
H+
H+
HCO3−
H+

A

B

A, How buffers respond to an excess of base. If the blood has too much base, the acid portion of a buffer pair (e.g., H_2CO_3 of the bicarbonate buffer system) releases hydrogen ions (H^+) to help return the pH to normal.

B, How buffers respond to an excess of acid. If the blood has too much acid, the base portion of a buffer pair (e.g., HCO_3^- of the bicarbonate buffer system) takes up hydrogen ions (H^+) to help return the pH to normal.

into the extracellular fluid and must be neutralized or excreted from the body to prevent dangerous accumulation. They can be neutralized to some degree by the buffers in body fluids. The lungs excrete carbonic acid in the form of carbon dioxide and water. Metabolic acids are excreted by the kidneys.

BUFFERS

The maintenance of hydrogen ions within normal range relies heavily on buffers. A **buffer** is a compound that binds hydrogen ions when their concentration rises and releases them when the concentration falls (see "Pathophysiology Illustrated: Buffer Responses to Acid and Base"). Several kinds of buffers are present in the body, such as bicarbonate, protein, hemoglobin, and phosphate. Various body fluids have buffers to meet their special needs. The bicarbonate buffer system neutralizes metabolic acids (see "Pathophysiology Illustrated: The Bicarbonate Buffer System"); however, it cannot neutralize carbonic acid.

All buffer systems have limits. For example, if there are too many metabolic acids, the bicarbonate buffers become depleted. The acids then accumulate in the body until they are excreted by the kidneys. Clinically, this is seen as a decreased serum bicarbonate concentration and decreased blood pH.

PATHOPHYSIOLOGY ILLUSTRATED

THE BICARBONATE BUFFER SYSTEM

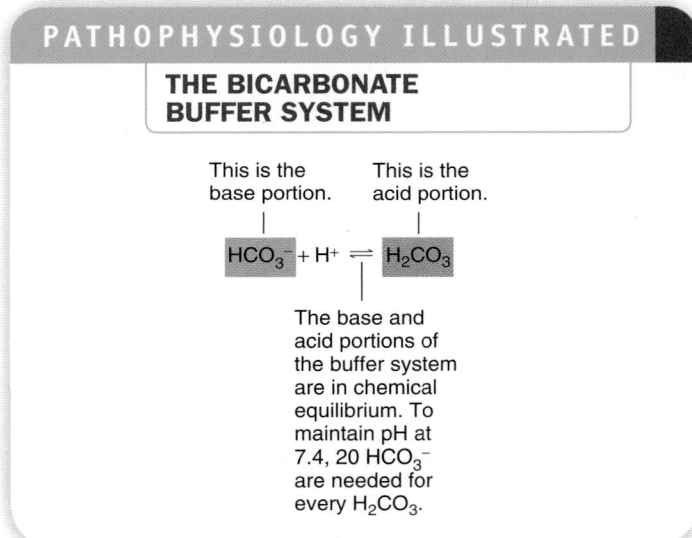

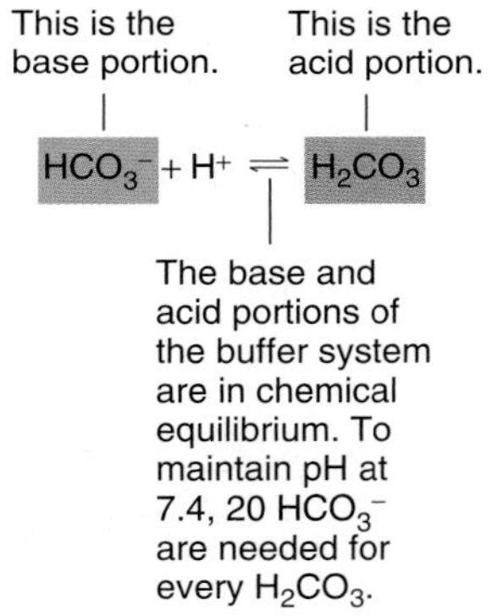
This is the base portion.
This is the acid portion.
HCO3− + H+ ⇌ H2CO3
The base and acid portions of the buffer system are in chemical equilibrium. To maintain pH at 7.4, 20 HCO3− are needed for every H2CO3.

ROLE OF THE LUNGS

The lungs are responsible for excreting excess carbonic acid from the body. A child breathes out carbon dioxide and water, the components of carbonic acid, with each breath. With faster and deeper breaths, more carbonic acid is excreted. Since carbonic acid is converted in the body to carbon dioxide and water by the enzyme carbonic anhydrase, an indirect laboratory measurement of carbonic acid is PCO_2 (see Table 46–7).

Although a child can voluntarily increase or decrease the rate and depth of respirations, they are usually involuntarily controlled. Chemoreceptors in the hypothalamus of the brain and in the aorta and carotid arteries monitor the PCO_2 and pH of the blood. These arteries also monitor the PO_2 of the blood. The input from the chemoreceptors is combined with other neural input to change breathing according to needs. Rate and depth increase or decrease according to the amount of carbonic acid that needs to be excreted.

If a child has a condition that decreases the excretion of carbonic acid or causes breathing to be too slow or shallow (such as overmedication following surgery), carbonic acid accumulates in the blood. Clinically, this is seen as an increased blood PCO_2. The reverse will also be true.

PATHOPHYSIOLOGY ILLUSTRATED

THE KIDNEYS AND METABOLIC ACIDS

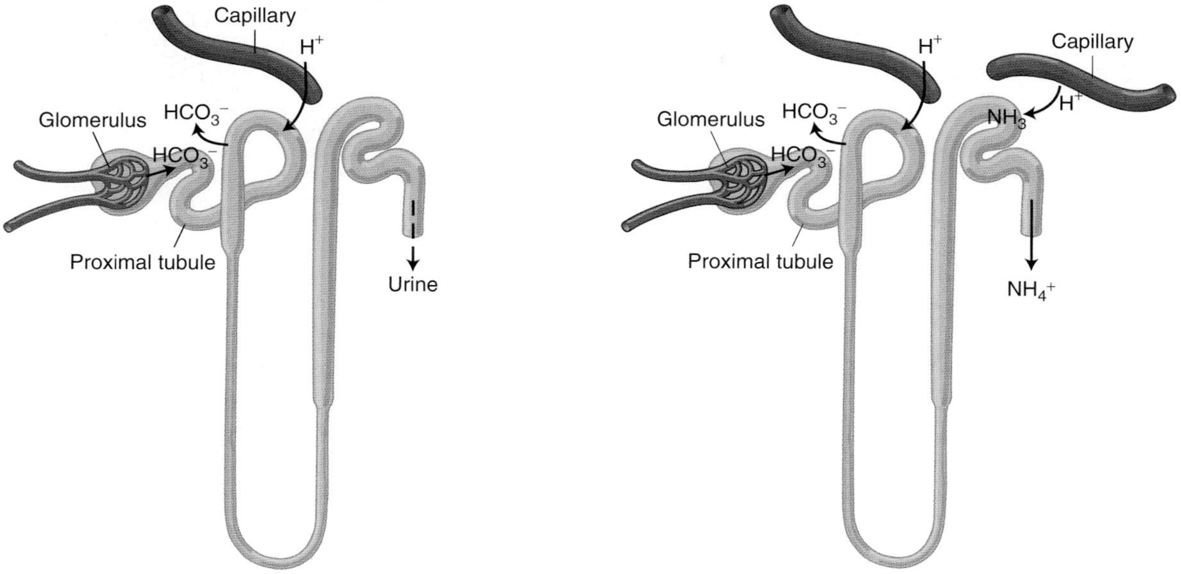

A

B

A, Recycling of bicarbonate by the kidneys. Bicarbonate ions that are in the blood are filtered into the renal tubules at the glomerulus. In the proximal tubules, bicarbonate ions are reabsorbed into the blood at the same time that hydrogen ions are transported from the blood into the renal tubular fluid.

B, Secretion and buffering of hydrogen ions in the kidneys. If the urine is too acidic, the cells that line the urinary tract could be damaged. To prevent this problem, hydrogen ions secreted into the distal tubules are neutralized by phosphate buffers or bound to ammonia and excreted in the form of ammonium ions.

ROLE OF THE KIDNEYS

The kidneys excrete metabolic acids from the body in two ways. They reabsorb filtered bicarbonate and form bicarbonate when needed to restore balance. Bicarbonate is formed when acids and ammonium combine with extra ions. The blood bicarbonate concentration is an indicator of the amount of metabolic acids present, since bicarbonate is used in buffering the acids (see Table 46–7). When the concentration is normal, metabolic acids are present in usual amounts (see "Pathophysiology Illustrated: The Kidneys and Metabolic Acids").

In a healthy child, the result of these renal processes is excretion of metabolic acids and maintenance of blood bicarbonate concentration within normal limits. However, a child whose kidneys are not producing enough urine may be unable to excrete metabolic acids effectively. Accumulation of these acids uses up many of the available bicarbonate buffers, resulting in a decreased serum bicarbonate concentration.

ROLE OF THE LIVER

The liver also plays a role in maintaining acid-base balance by metabolizing protein, which produces hydrogen ions. It also synthesizes proteins needed to maintain osmotic pressures in the fluid compartments.

ACID-BASE IMBALANCES

There are four acid-base imbalances. Two are the result of processes that cause too much acid in the body and are referred to as **acidosis**. The other two are the result of processes that cause too little acid in the body and are called **alkalosis**. An acid-base disorder caused by too much or too little carbonic acid is called a respiratory acid-base imbalance. A disorder caused by too much or too little metabolic acid is called a metabolic acid-base imbalance.

Nursing Practice

Acidosis: Relatively too much acid in the body

Respiratory acidosis: Relatively too much carbonic acid

Metabolic acidosis: Relatively too much metabolic acid

Alkalosis: Relatively too little acid in the body

Respiratory alkalosis: Relatively too little carbonic acid

Metabolic alkalosis: Relatively too little metabolic acid

Arterial blood gas measurements (ABGs) provide a laboratory evaluation of a child's current acid-base status. In addition, oxygen saturation, or the percentage of hemoglobin saturated with arterial blood, is normally 95–100%. Table 46–16 provides a method that can help interpret the pH, P_{CO_2}, and bicarbonate concentrations, the most important acid-base measures. End-tidal CO_2 can provide a continuous noninvasive measurement. (Remember that P_{CO_2} reflects carbonic acid status, and bicarbonate concentration reflects the metabolic acid status.)

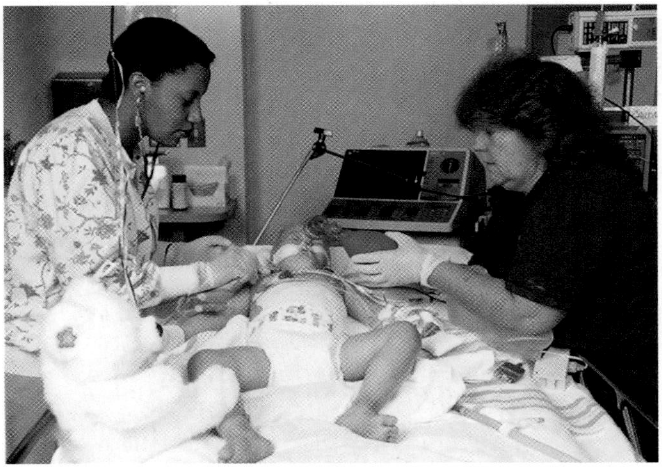

● **Figure 46–10** Respiratory acidosis/alkalosis and mechanical ventilation. This child may develop respiratory acidosis or respiratory alkalosis. If the tidal volume is set too low during mechanical ventilation, carbon dioxide (carbonic acid) will accumulate in the body (respiratory acidosis) because it is not being excreted by the lungs. If the tidal volume is set too high, carbon dioxide will be depleted in the body (respiratory alkalosis) because it is being excreted in great quantities.

RESPIRATORY ACIDOSIS

Respiratory acidosis is caused by the accumulation of carbon dioxide in the blood. Since carbon dioxide and water can be combined into carbonic acid, respiratory acidosis is sometimes called carbonic acid excess. The condition can be acute or chronic. It is controlled by the lungs.

Etiology and Pathophysiology

Any factor that interferes with the ability of the lungs to excrete carbon dioxide can cause respiratory acidosis. These factors may interfere with the gaseous exchange within the lungs, may impair the neuromuscular pump that moves air in and out of the lungs, or may depress the respiratory rate (Table 46–17; Figure 46–10 ●).

As the P_{CO_2} begins to increase, the pH of the blood begins to decrease. Compensatory mechanisms begin to act in the form of nonbicarbonate buffers, additional hydrogen ion excretion by the kidneys, and formation and decreased bicarbonate excretion by the kidneys. These compensatory mechanisms take several days to become active so the child manifests a changing clinical situation, depending on the underlying cause and the amount of compensation occurring (Table 46–18).

Table 46–16 Questions to Ask to Interpret Arterial Blood Gas Measurements

Question to Ask	Conclusion
What is the pH?	■ If the pH is normal, the child has no imbalance or has compensated for an imbalance. ■ If the pH is below normal, the child has acidosis. ■ If the pH is above normal, the child has alkalosis.
What is the P_{CO_2}?	■ If the P_{CO_2} is normal, the child does not have an acid-base imbalance. ■ If the P_{CO_2} is above normal, the child has respiratory acidosis. This may be the primary disorder or may be a compensatory response to metabolic alkalosis. Looking at the bicarbonate concentration helps you decide. ■ If the P_{CO_2} is below normal, the child has respiratory alkalosis. Again, this can be the primary disorder or may be a compensatory response to metabolic acidosis.
What is the bicarbonate concentration?	■ If the bicarbonate concentration is within normal range, the child does not have a metabolic acid-base imbalance. ■ If the bicarbonate is above normal, the child has metabolic alkalosis. This can be a primary disorder or can be compensatory in respiratory acidosis. ■ If bicarbonate is below normal, the child has metabolic acidosis, either as a direct disorder or as a compensatory response to respiratory alkalosis.
What do the results together tell you?	■ If the pH is abnormal and either the P_{CO_2} or bicarbonate concentration is normal, there is an uncompensated acid-base disorder. ■ If all three values are abnormal, the child has a partially compensated disorder and the pH will provide the definitive answer. ■ If P_{CO_2}, pH, and bicarbonate are all decreased, then partially compensated metabolic acidosis is most likely. ■ If pH is normal and P_{CO_2} and bicarbonate are abnormal, there is a fully compensated acid-base disorder.
What are the child's history and clinical signs?	■ Does your interpretation fit with what you know about the child's medical condition and with assessments you are making? ■ This last step helps you to integrate laboratory data with the clinical picture to strengthen your nursing care of the child with an acid-base imbalance.

Table 46–17 Causes of Respiratory Acidosis

Factors Affecting the Lungs	Factors Affecting the Neuromuscular Pump	Factors Affecting Central Control of Respiration
Aspiration	Flail chest	Sedative overdose
Spasm of the airways	Pneumothorax or hemothorax	General anesthesia
Laryngeal edema	Mechanical underventilation	Head injury
Epiglottitis	Hypokalemic muscle weakness	Brain tumor
Croup	High cervical spinal cord injury	Central sleep apnea
Pulmonary edema	Botulism	
Atelectasis	Tetanus	
Severe pneumonia	Kyphoscoliosis	
Cystic fibrosis	Poliomyelitis	
Bronchopulmonary dysplasia	Muscular dystrophy	
Pulmonary embolism	Congenital diaphragmatic hernia	
	Guillain-Barré syndrome	

Table 46–18 Laboratory Values in Uncompensated and Compensated Respiratory Acidosis

Type of Respiratory Acidosis	Pco_2	pH	HCO_3^-
Uncompensated	Increased	Decreased	Normal
Partially compensated	Increased	Decreasing but moving toward normal	Increasing
Fully compensated	Increased	Normal	Increased

Clinical Manifestations

Acidosis in the brain cells causes central nervous system depression, manifested by confusion, lethargy, headache, increased intracranial pressure, and even coma. Acute respiratory acidosis can lead to tachycardia and cardiac arrhythmias. The child's arterial blood gases always show an increased Pco_2, the laboratory sign of increased carbonic acid. Serum pH can be decreased or normal.

Clinical Therapy

Treatment of respiratory acidosis requires correction of the underlying cause. For example, treatment may include bronchodilators for bronchospasm, mechanical ventilation for neuromuscular defects, decreasing sedative use, or surgery for kyphoscoliosis.

NURSING MANAGEMENT

NURSING ASSESSMENT AND DIAGNOSIS

Nursing assessment plays a pivotal role in decisions about interventions for respiratory acidosis. This is especially true in chronic conditions such as cystic fibrosis and kyphoscoliosis. Assess respiratory rate, rhythm, and depth carefully. Take the apical pulse and be alert for tachycardia or arrhythmia. A cardiac monitor may be used. Obtain serial arterial blood gas measurements in acute conditions to evaluate changing status. Assess the level of consciousness and energy. Observe for chronic fatigue, headache, or decreased level of consciousness.

Several nursing diagnoses may apply to the child with respiratory acidosis. The most important addresses the child's *Risk for Injury.* Other nursing diagnoses depend on the specific clinical manifestation and the particular cause of the acidosis. Examples include the following:

- *Risk for Injury* related to decreased level of consciousness
- *Activity Intolerance* related to decreased cardiac output secondary to cardiac dysrhythmias
- *Ineffective Breathing Pattern (Hypoventilation)* related to neuromuscular impairment
- *Pain (Headache)* related to cerebral vasodilation
- *Ineffective Family Management of Therapeutic Regimen* related to complexity of bronchodilator therapy

PLANNING AND INTERVENTION

NURSING CARE IN THE COMMUNITY

Teach children at risk for respiratory acidosis and their parents preventive measures to use at home. For the child with a chronic condition such as cystic fibrosis, muscular dystrophy, or kyphoscoliosis, demonstrate deep breathing and encourage its use several times each day. Teach the family signs of infection—including fever, increased respiratory secretions, and discomfort with breathing—so that these problems can be treated promptly, preventing further respiratory involvement. Position the child to facilitate chest expansion. Teach parents about proper administration of any necessary medications. For

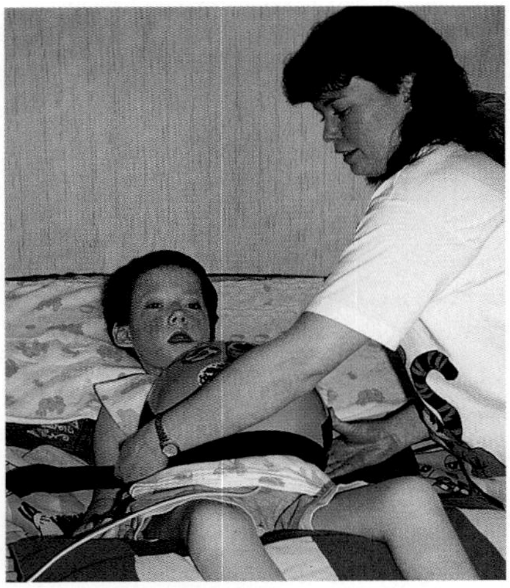

● **Figure 46–11** Home respirator use. This child, who has muscular dystrophy, uses a "turtle" respirator at home to assist with breathing. His parents required instructions from the nurse on use of the respirator. The family has a generator to provide electricity for the respirator during power outages.

example, the child with cystic fibrosis may receive antibiotics to prevent respiratory infections. Teach parents and older children about home respirator use (Figure 46–11 ●).

HOSPITAL-BASED NURSING CARE

For the hospitalized child, the focus is on ensuring safety. Keep bed side rails raised, and turn and position the child frequently. Evaluate mental status and document and report any changes in alertness. When laboratory values of blood pH and P_{CO_2} are available, evaluate them promptly and report any changes or abnormalities. Administer medications as ordered. Carefully monitor the doses of sedatives to avoid further respiratory depression. Provide suctioning and encourage deep breathing.

EVALUATION

Expected outcomes of nursing care for the child with respiratory acidosis include maintenance of safety, adequate rate and rhythm of respirations, and management of causative disorders.

Growth and Development

It is usually difficult to get a young child to do deep breathing or to use the "blow bottle" that is often given to older children and adults. To make deep breathing fun, use a pinwheel and have the child turn it during play. Alternatively, give a child a straw and have him or her blow bubbles in a glass of water, or have the child use the straw to blow scraps of paper across the bedside table.

RESPIRATORY ALKALOSIS

Respiratory alkalosis occurs when the blood contains too little carbon dioxide. It is sometimes called carbonic acid deficit.

Excess carbon dioxide loss is caused by hyperventilation, in which more air than normal is moved into and out of the lungs. Some common causes of hyperventilation are hypoxia due to severe asthma, salicylate poisoning, and sepsis. Other causes are anxiety, fear, pain, meningitis, septicemia, and mechanical overventilation.

In many cases, respiratory alkalosis lasts for several hours only. Renal compensation does not occur, as these compensatory mechanisms take several days to begin action. An example is the hyperventilation that occurs with acute anxiety. If the condition persists, however, the kidneys will begin to retain more acid and excrete more bicarbonate. Hydrogen ions will be released from body buffers to decrease plasma bicarbonate. While the imbalance continues, cellular function is thus protected by returning pH to normal levels (Table 46–19).

Arterial blood gas measurements show a decreased P_{CO_2} in respiratory alkalosis. Blood pH is generally elevated. The lack of carbon dioxide causes neuromuscular irritability and paresthesias in the extremities and around the mouth. Muscle cramping and carpal or pedal spasms can occur. The child may be dizzy or confused.

Medical management focuses on correcting the condition that caused the hyperventilation so that the body's compensatory mechanisms can return carbon dioxide levels to normal.

NURSING MANAGEMENT

Assess the child's level of consciousness and ask if the child feels light-headed or has tingling sensations or numbness in the fingers or toes, or around the mouth. Assess the rate and depth of respirations. Monitor the hospitalized child's P_{O_2} with serial arterial blood gas measurements to evaluate changes in status. Make a careful assessment about the cause of hyperventilation. Did an occurrence cause anxiety for the child? Is the child in pain? (See Chapter 42∞.) Has the child received salicylates in any form? Is the child mechanically ventilated? Is there a central nervous system infection such as meningitis?

Table 46–19 Laboratory Values in Uncompensated and Compensated Respiratory Alkalosis

Type of Respiratory Alkalosis	P_{CO_2}	pH	HCO_3^-
Uncompensated	Decreased	Increased	Normal
Partially compensated	Decreased	Increasing but moving toward normal	Decreasing
Fully compensated	Decreased	Normal	Decreased

Nursing Practice

Check the Po_2 before any therapy for respiratory alkalosis is started, because it is dangerous to stop hyperventilation if oxygenation is poor.

PLANNING AND IMPLEMENTATION

Nursing care for the child with respiratory alkalosis centers on preventing injury, teaching stress management techniques, maintaining pain control, promoting respiratory function, ensuring safety, maintaining fluid status, and providing health supervision and home care.

TEACH STRESS MANAGEMENT TECHNIQUES

When anxiety is the cause of respiratory alkalosis, instruct the child to breathe slowly; demonstrate the rhythm. Use a calm voice, stuffed toys, and supportive reassurance. Teach stress-control techniques such as relaxation and imagery for situations that cause anxiety.

MAINTAIN PAIN CONTROL

Use medications, imagery, distraction, positioning, massage, and other techniques to decrease pain and maintain pain management. See Chapter 42∞ for a description of these and other measures to assist with pain control.

PROMOTE RESPIRATORY FUNCTION

Have the child cough, or suction as needed. Be certain that mechanical ventilation systems are working properly.

ENSURE SAFETY

Provide a safe environment for the child who has a decreased level of consciousness. Be sure the child is supervised when sitting or standing up. Keep bed rails up.

REGULATE FLUID STATUS

Renal compensation to manage ongoing respiratory alkalosis requires adequate urinary output. Regulate fluid intake to ensure urine output unless fluids are restricted due to medical condition.

NURSING CARE IN THE COMMUNITY

Teach parents to keep aspirin and other salicylate products out of reach of children, preferably in a locked medicine box. Provide stickers with the number of the Poison Control Center.

EVALUATION

Expected outcomes of nursing care for the child with respiratory alkalosis include normal respiratory rate and rhythm, maintenance of safety, and regulation of fluid status.

METABOLIC ACIDOSIS

Metabolic acidosis is a condition in which there is an excess of any acid other than carbonic acid. For this reason, it is sometimes called noncarbonic acid excess.

Etiology and Pathophysiology

Metabolic acidosis is caused by an imbalance in production and excretion of acid or by excess loss of bicarbonate. Excess accumulation occurs by one of two mechanisms. First, a child can eat or drink acids or substances that are converted to acid in the body. Examples include aspirin, boric acid, and antifreeze. Second, cells can make abnormally high amounts of acid that cannot be excreted. This is the case in ketoacidosis of untreated diabetes mellitus, untreated growth hormone deficiency, bladder construction that uses part of the bowel, or the starvation that can occur in anorexia or bulimia. A disorder of excretion occurs in conditions such as oliguric renal failure (Figure 46–12 ●).

The body can lose bicarbonate through the urine or through excessive loss of intestinal fluid. Diarrhea, fistulas, and ileal drainage are all possible sources. Carbonic anhydrase inhibitors can cause loss of excess bicarbonate in the urine.

Below-normal pH of the blood stimulates the chemoreceptors in the brain and arteries and respiratory compensation begins. The child's rate and depth of breathing increase and carbonic acid is removed from the body. The blood pH shifts to a more normal range even though the cause is not corrected. The underlying condition and the degree of compensation alter the clinical laboratory values observed (Table 46–20).

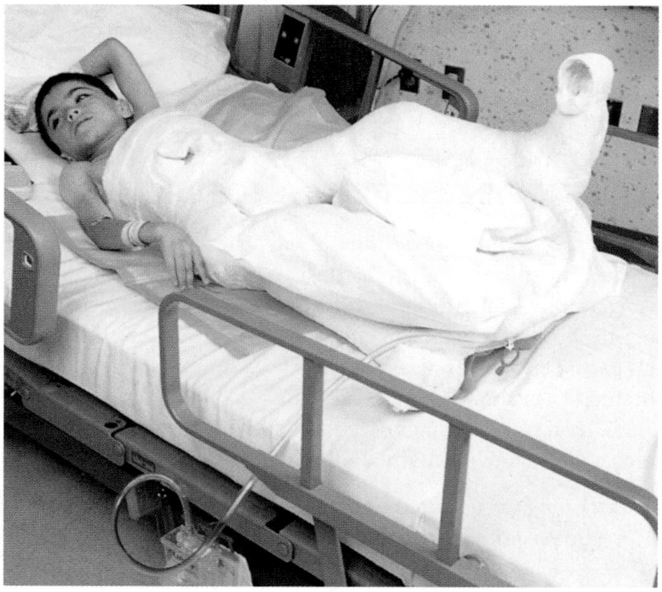

● **Figure 46–12** Disorders of excretion. With any postoperative or immobilized child, it is important to monitor urine output to detect oliguria. If the kidneys do not produce sufficient urine, the metabolic acids accumulate in the body and cause metabolic acidosis. Inadequate fluid intake in the postoperative or immobilized child can lead to oliguria and, potentially, metabolic acidosis.

Table 46–20 Laboratory Values in Uncompensated and Compensated Metabolic Acidosis

Type of Metabolic Acidosis	HCO_3^-	pH	Pco_2
Uncompensated	Decreased	Decreased	Normal
Partially compensated	Decreased	Decreasing but moving	Decreasing

Clinical Manifestations

Laboratory values show decreased blood pH and decreased HCO_3 and Pco_2. An attempt at respiratory compensation causes one of the most important signs of metabolic acidosis, increased rate and depth of respirations (hyperventilation) or **Kussmaul respirations**. Severe acidosis can cause decreased peripheral vascular resistance and resultant cardiac arrhythmias, hypotension, pulmonary edema, and tissue hypoxia. Confusion or drowsiness may result, as well as headache or abdominal pain.

Clinical Therapy

Treatment of metabolic acidosis depends on identification and treatment of the underlying cause. In severe metabolic acidosis, intravenous sodium bicarbonate may be used to increase the pH and to prevent cardiac arrhythmias. This treatment is difficult to manage, because renal excretion can cause excess retention of bicarbonate; therefore, intravenous sodium bicarbonate is used only in severe situations, such as prolonged cardiac arrest.

NURSING MANAGEMENT

NURSING ASSESSMENT AND DIAGNOSIS

Teach prevention of poisoning at each health promotion visit. For the child admitted with acidosis, assess the rate and depth of respirations. Evaluate the child's level of consciousness frequently. Be alert for signs or complaints of headache and abdominal pain. Serial arterial blood gas measurements will usually be obtained to evaluate changes in status.

Several nursing diagnoses can apply to the child with metabolic acidosis, including the following:

- *Risk for Injury* related to confusion/drowsiness or decreased responsiveness
- *Risk for Decreased Cardiac Output* related to cardiac arrhythmias
- *Altered Tissue Perfusion: Cerebral* related to tissue hypoxia
- *Ineffective Family Management of Therapeutic Regimen* related to complexity of management of diabetes mellitus

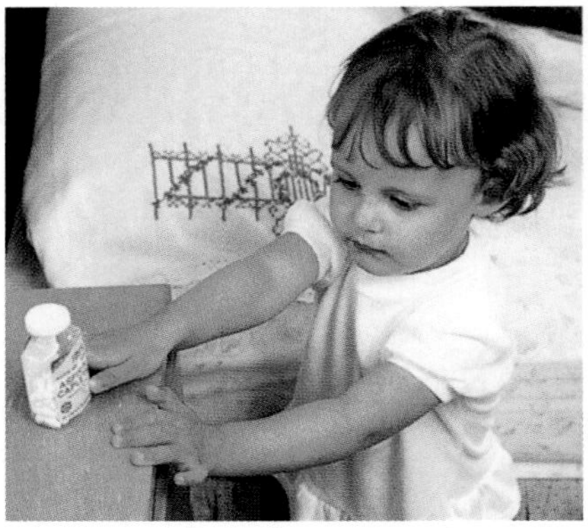

● **Figure 46–13** Preventing metabolic acidosis from poisoning. Teaching parents to use safety latches on cabinets to keep aspirin away from small children can help prevent one cause of metabolic acidosis.

PLANNING AND IMPLEMENTATION

Ensure safety, taking into account the child's level of consciousness and alertness. Turn the child and change his or her position to prevent pressure on the skin. Limit the child's activities to decrease cardiac workload.

Position the child to facilitate chest expansion. Provide oral care during rapid respirations since the mouth may become dry.

Monitor intravenous solutions and laboratory values indicating acid-base balance. Report changes promptly.

Once the child is stabilized, provide teaching to compensate for knowledge deficits. Teach parents of young children to keep medications and acids locked up and out of reach to prevent poisoning (Figure 46–13 ●). This includes medicines with aspirin as well as substances commonly kept in the garage for car maintenance. Teach about home management of diabetes and about early identification and treatment to avoid diabetic ketoacidosis. Expected outcomes of nursing care relate to prevention of acidosis and restoration of normal body balance during disease processes.

METABOLIC ALKALOSIS

Metabolic alkalosis occurs when there are too few metabolic acids. It is sometimes called noncarbonic acid deficit.

A gain in bicarbonate or a loss of metabolic acid can cause metabolic alkalosis. Bicarbonate is gained through excessive intake of bicarbonate antacids or baking soda or through metabolism of bicarbonate precursors such as the citrate contained in blood transfusions. Increased renal absorption of bicarbonate can occur in profound hypokalemia, primary hyperaldosteronism, or extreme deficit in extracellular fluid volume. Acid can be lost through severe vomiting, such as that seen in infants with pyloric stenosis, and through continued removal of gastric contents through suction.

When the chemoreceptors in the brain and arteries detect the rising pH of metabolic alkalosis and respirations decrease, the body retains carbonic acid. This carbonic acid can neutralize the bicarbonate and return pH toward normal.

Blood pH, bicarbonate, and Pco_2 are usually elevated in metabolic alkalosis (Table 46–21). Hypokalemia often occurs si-

Table 46–21 Laboratory Values in Uncompensated and Compensated Metabolic Alkalosis

Type of Metabolic Alkalosis	HCO_3^-	pH	Pco_2
Acute condition; uncompensated	Increased	Increased	Normal
Partially compensated	Increased	Increased but moving toward normal	Increasing
Fully compensated	The need for oxygen drives respirations and limits full compensation for metabolic alkalosis.		

multaneously (refer to pages 1252–1254 to review signs of hypokalemia). Respiratory rate and depth usually decrease. Increased neuromuscular irritability, cramping, paresthesia, tetany, seizures, and excitation can occur. Finally, this state can progress to weakness, confusion, lethargy, and coma.

Clinical therapy is directed at treating the underlying cause of the condition. Increasing the extracellular fluid volume with intravenous normal saline facilitates renal excretion of bicarbonate.

Nursing Management

Assess the child's level of consciousness frequently. Alertness may decrease after an initial period of excitement, so regular assessments are needed. Monitor neuromuscular irritability. Observe for nausea and vomiting. Assess the rate and depth of respirations carefully. Obtain serial arterial blood gas measurements as ordered.

Facilitate ease of respirations. Ensure safety by keeping bed rails elevated and by turning the child frequently. Position the child on the side to avoid aspiration of vomitus.

If antacids were the cause of the alkalosis, teach the child and parents about correct use of these medications.

MIXED ACID-BASE IMBALANCES

It is possible for two acid-base imbalances to occur at the same time. For example, a child with cystic fibrosis can develop respiratory acidosis from lung problems and concurrent metabolic alkalosis from vomiting during an illness. Treatment with diuretics may cause concurrent metabolic alkalosis resulting from extracellular volume depletion and hypokalemia in a child with congestive heart failure and chronic respiratory acidosis. In these cases, all underlying causes must be identified and treated. Care of children with mixed acid-base imbalances is often complicated, requiring hospitalization and careful management. Upon discharge the nurse can teach parents about signs of imbalance that need to be reported and treated to prevent further complications. Evaluation of care is based on outcomes of adequate respiratory ventilation and metabolic balance.

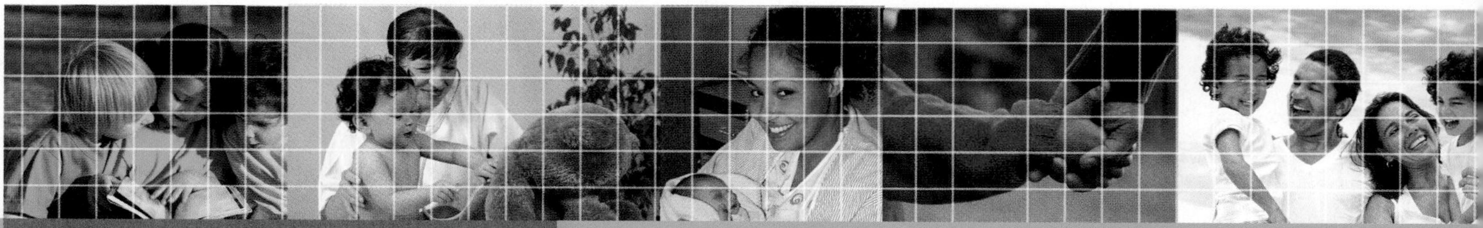

CRITICAL CONCEPT REVIEW

LEARNING OUTCOMES	CONCEPTS
46.1 Describe normal fluid and electrolyte status for children at various ages.	1. Newborn: ■ Basal metabolic rate is double that of children. ■ Approximately four to five times greater water intake needs per kilogram of body weight. ■ Only 10% of ability to excrete sodium. 2. Infants: ■ Larger extracellular fluid volume than older children and adults. ■ High daily fluid requirement with little fluid volume reserve. 3. Child/adolescent: ■ Total body water is 50% of total body weight. ■ Kidneys unable to conserve water and electrolytes until after age 2 years. ■ Children under 2 years have a greater proportion of skin surface.

(continued)

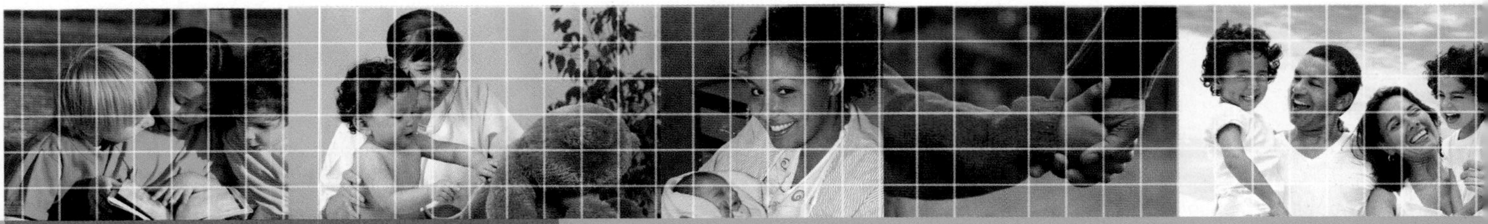

CRITICAL CONCEPT REVIEW

LEARNING OUTCOMES / CONCEPTS

46.2 Identify regulatory mechanisms for fluid and electrolyte balance.

1. Kidneys conserve water and electrolytes while excreting waste products and drug metabolites:
   - Children under 2 years of age have immature glomeruli, tubules, and nephrons.

46.3 Recognize threats to fluid and electrolyte balance in children.

1. Higher respiratory and metabolic rates increase water demands and water loss:
   - Allow dehydration to occur more quickly in children.
2. Immature kidneys lead to greater water and electrolyte loss.
3. Higher body surface area (BSA) increases insensible water loss through the skin.
4. Young child unable to communicate thirst.
5. Young child may not cooperate with oral rehydration.

46.4 Describe acid-base balance and recognize disruptions common in children.

Acid-base balance:

1. Lungs:
   - Responsible for excreting excess carbonic acid from body.
2. Kidneys:
   - Reabsorb filtered bicarbonate.
   - Form bicarbonate if needed to restore balance.
3. Liver:
   - Metabolizes protein, which produces hydrogen ions.
   - Synthesizes proteins needed to maintain osmotic pressure in the fluid compartments.

Disruptions in acid-base balance:

1. Respiratory acidosis:
   - Associated with chronic diseases that decrease respiratory effort.
2. Respiratory alkalosis:
   - Often seen with severe infections, anxiety, pain, and lowered levels of oxygen.
3. Metabolic acidosis:
   - May be seen in diabetic ketoacidosis or severe anorexia.
4. Metabolic alkalosis:
   - Seen in chronic metabolic conditions and with prolonged vomiting.

46.5 Analyze assessment findings to recognize fluid-electrolyte problems and acid-base imbalance in children.

1. Laboratory assessments:
   - Serum electrolyte levels.
   - Serum creatinine.
   - Serum glucose.
   - Pco_2.
   - pH.
   - HCO_3^-.
2. Physical assessments:
   - Daily weights.
   - Vital signs.
   - Tenseness of anterior fontanel (infant only).
   - Skin turgor.
   - Bowel sounds.
   - Cardiac rhythm.
   - Level of consciousness.
   - Respiratory function.
   - Intake and output measurement.
   - Observation for neck vein distention.

LEARNING OUTCOMES / CONCEPTS

LEARNING OUTCOMES	CONCEPTS
46.6 Describe appropriate nursing interventions for children experiencing fluid-electrolyte problems and acid-base imbalance.	1. Weigh child daily. 2. Carefully assess skin for any breakdown from diarrhea or edema. 3. Turn and position child carefully to prevent skin breakdown. 4. Administer IV fluids as ordered. 5. Monitor oxygen saturation. 6. Maintain oxygen therapy as ordered. 7. Provide age-appropriate activities. 8. Instruct parents in signs and symptoms of dehydration. 9. Instruct parents in the use of oral rehydration methods.

CRITICAL THINKING IN ACTION

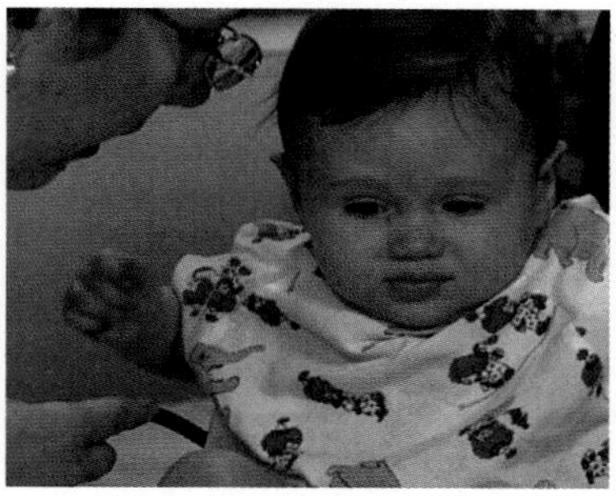

A 10-month-old named Devin comes to the emergency room by ambulance at 3:00 A.M. for respiratory distress. His parents state that he was experiencing a cough for the past week and developed a fever over 103 degrees Fahrenheit tonight. He woke up crying with a frightening cough and could barely catch his breath; the parents called 9-1-1. Devin's respiratory rate is 55 times per minute with moderate retractions, his temperature is 104.2 degrees Fahrenheit, and his heart has a regular rhythm with a rate of 120 beats per minute. His breath sounds demonstrate wheezing and rhonchi throughout all lung fields. At the hospital, he is given a breathing treatment with albuterol 0.5 mL and 2 mL of normal saline per nebulizer. His respiratory rate decreases to 40 and retractions improve. The arterial blood gas measurements show an increased Pco_2, a decreased pH, and a normal HCO_3. A diagnosis of croup syndrome and resultant respiratory acidosis is made. Devin is admitted for monitoring.

1. What are some of the other possible causes of respiratory acidosis in children such as Devin?
2. What are some of the signs and symptoms of respiratory distress and the central nervous system problems associated with Devin's particular acid-base imbalance?
3. Devin's heart rate and rhythm are monitored closely in the hospital. What is the reason for these assessments?
4. What is the treatment for Devin's acid-base imbalance?
5. What are some of the measures taken in the hospital to ensure Devin's safety?

See MyNursingKit for possible responses.

REFERENCES

Armstrong, L. E., Casa, D. J., Millard-Stafford, M., Moran, D. S., Pyne, S. W., & Roberts, W. O. (2007). Exertional heat illness during training and competition. *Medicine & Science in Sports & Exercise, 39*, 556–572.

Bindler, R., & Howry, L. (2005). *Pediatric Drug Guide.* Upper Saddle River, NJ: Prentice Hall.

Chamley, C. A., Carson, P., Randall, D., & Sandwell, M. (2005). *Developmental anatomy and physiology of children*. Edinburgh: Elsevier.

Custer, J. W., & Rau, R. E. (2009). *The Harriet Lane Handbook* (18th ed.). Philadelphia: Elsevier Mosby.

Dale, J. (2004). Oral rehydration solutions in the management of acute gastroenteritis among children. *Journal of Pediatric Health Care, 18*, 211–212.

Dennehy, P. H. (2005). Acute diarrheal disease in children: Epidemiology, prevention, and treatment. *Infectious Disease Clinics of North America, 19*, 585–602.

Exercise-Associated Hyponatremia Consensus Panel (2005). Consensus statement of the 1st international exercise-associated hyponatremia consensus development conference, Cape Town, South Africa 2005. *Clinical Journal of Sports Medicine, 15*, 208–213.

Fontaine, O., Garner, P., & Bhan, M. K. (2007). Oral rehydration therapy: The simple solution for saving lives. *British Medical Journal, 334*, 2–3.

Hartling, L., Bellemare, S., Wiebe, N., Russell, K., Klassen, T. P., & Craig, W. (2006). Oral versus intravenous rehydration for treating dehydration due to gastroenteritis in children. *Cochrane Database Systematic Reviews*, CD004390.

Heaney, R. P. (2006). Low calcium intake among African Americans: Effects on bones and body weight. *Journal of Nutrition 136*, 1095–1098.

Holliday, M. A., Ray, P. E., & Friedman, A. L. (2007). Fluid therapy for children: Facts, fashions, and questions. *Archives of Disease in Childhood, 92*, 546–550.

Kliegman, R. M., Behrman, R. E., Jenson, H. B., & Stanton, B. F. (2007). *Nelson textbook of pediatrics* (18th ed.). Philadelphia: Saunders Elsevier.

Koslap-Petraco, M. B. (2006). Homecare issues in rotavirus gastroenteritis. *Journal of the American Academy of Nurse Practitioners, 18*, 422–428.

Madati, P. J., & Bachur, R. (2008). Development of an emergency department triage tool to predict acidosis among children with gastroenteritis. *Pediatric Emergency Care, 24*(12), 822–830.

Mayo Clinic (2007). *Dehydration and youth sports: Curb the risk*. Retrieved September 10, 2007, from www.mayoclinic.com/health/dehydration/SM00037

Moritz, M. L., Manole, J. D., Bogen, D. L., & Ayus, J. C. (2005). Breastfeeding-associated hypernatremia: Are we missing the diagnosis? *Pediatrics, 116*, 3343–3347.

National Federation of State High School Associations (NFHS) (2005). *Heat stress and athletic participation*. Retrieved August 28, 2007, from www.nfhs.org/web/2005/03/sports_medicine_heat_stress_and_athletic_participation

Roberts, K. E. (2005). Pediatric fluid and electrolyte balance: Critical care case studies. *Critical Care Nursing Clinics of North America, 17*, 361–373.

Robertson, J., & Shilkofski, N. (2005). *The Harriet Lane Handbook*. Philadelphia: Elsevier Mosby.

Shrof, R., Hignett, R., Pierce, C., Marks, S., & van't Hoff, W. (2007). Life-threatening hypernatremic dehydration in breastfed babies. *Archives of Disease in Childhood, 91*, 1025–1026.

Soldin, S. J., Brugnara, C., & Wong, E. C. (2005). Pediatric Reference Ranges (5th ed.). Washington, D. C.: AACC Press.

Spandorfer, P. R., Alessandrini, E. A., Joffe, J. D., Localio, R., & Shaw, K. N. (2005). Oral versus intravenous rehydration of moderately dehydrated children: A randomized, controlled trial. *Pediatrics, 115*, 295–301.

Tofil, N. M., Benner, K. W., & Winkler, M. K. (2005). Fatal hypermagnesemia caused by an Epsom salt enema: A case illustration. *Southern Medical Journal, 98*, 253–256.

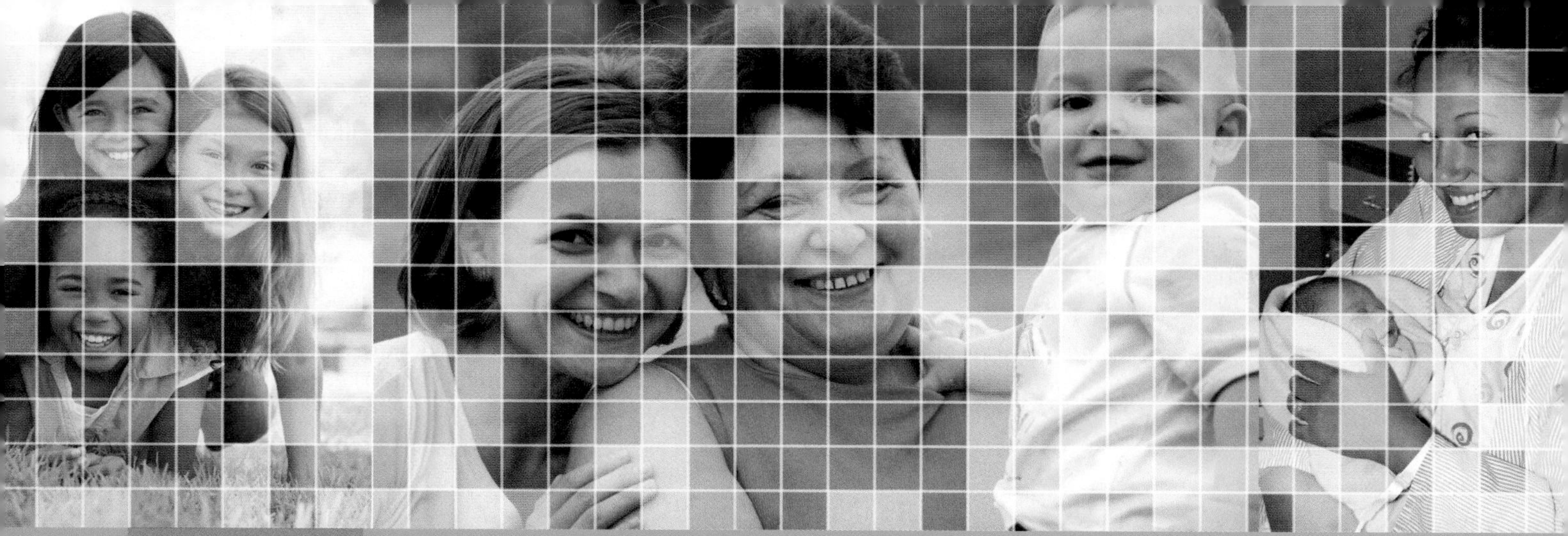

CHAPTER

47 The Child with Alterations in Eye, Ear, Nose, and Throat Function

The early intervention program that Raeanne attended to help her deal with her visual impairment really helped her to prepare for preschool. We learned a lot too about how to help her. We are still really nervous about her starting at preschool and being with a lot of other children. We want it to go well for her. —Mother of Raeanne, 3 years old

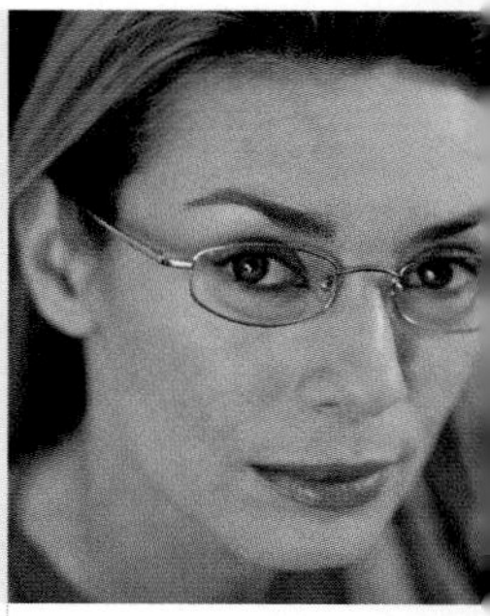

LEARNING OUTCOMES

47.1 Identify anatomy, physiology, and pediatric differences in the eye, ear, nose, and throat of children and adolescents.

47.2 Describe abnormalities of the eyes, ears, nose, throat, and mouth in children.

47.3 Plan for screening programs and identification of children with vision and hearing abnormalities.

47.4 Plan nursing care for children with vision or hearing impairments.

47.5 Use latest recommendations when implementing care and teaching for children with abnormalities of eyes, ears, nose, throat, and mouth.

47.6 Integrate preventive and treatment principles when implementing care for children related to eyes, ears, nose, and throat.

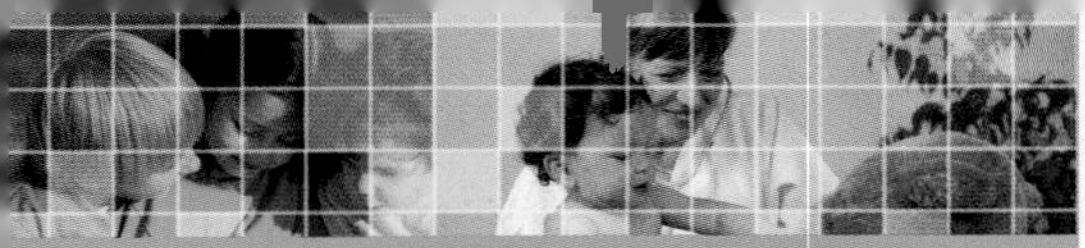

KEY TERMS

Audiography, 1296
Binocularity, 1277
Conductive hearing loss, 1294
Decibels, 1294
Mixed hearing loss, 1294
Myringotomy, 1291
Sensorineural hearing loss, 1294
Tinnitus, 1295
Tympanogram, 1296
Tympanostomy tubes, 1291
Vision, 1274
Visual acuity, 1274

The eye, ear, nose, and throat are connected, so a malformation, infection, or other condition in one of these structures may affect them all. Intact sensory structures enable children to reach developmental milestones; thus alterations, especially to the eye and ear, may delay a child's development. Most children with eye, ear, nose, and throat disorders are treated at home or in the community rather than in the hospital. How are conditions of the eye, ear, nose, and throat related? Which conditions have the potential to affect a child's growth, development, and behavior? In what settings do children with eye, ear, nose, and throat conditions receive care? How can parents be helped to foster development in their children when they have a visual or hearing disorder?

ANATOMY AND PHYSIOLOGY OF PEDIATRIC DIFFERENCES

EYE

How are the eyes of children different from those of adults? Chapter 35 provides a detailed discussion of the assessment of the eyes and **visual acuity**, the ability to discriminate letters or other objects. The eyes of newborns differ from the eyes of adults in several ways. Visual acuity in newborns ranges between 20/100 and 20/400. The lens is more spherical and cannot accommodate to both near and far objects, which means that the newborn sees best at a distance of about 8 inches (20 cm). Since the optic nerve is not yet completely myelinated, the ability to distinguish color and other details is decreased. If the infant is preterm, especially less than 32 weeks' gestation, retinal vascularization, particularly in the periphery of the retina, may be incomplete (O'Connor, Wilson, & Fiedler, 2007). The rectus muscles that control binocular vision may be somewhat uncoordinated at birth. The eyes should be aligned and movement coordinated by the age of 3 months.

The cornea of the infant and young child occupies a larger portion of the orbit than in the adult; the eyeball is about 3/4 of its adult size (Chamley, Carson, Randall, et al., 2005). Since the eyeball is relatively unprotected laterally, it is more easily injured. The sclera of the newborn is thin and translucent with a bluish tinge, and the iris is blue or gray. Eye color changes during the first 6 months of life. Infants produce tears to nourish and oxygenate the outer layers of the cornea. Parents do not see tears when a young infant cries because the infant's lacrimal system drains them efficiently into the nasal cavity.

As infants grow, their eyes mature and their vision improves. By the age of 2 or 3 years, most children have a visual acuity of 20/50, and by the age of 6 or 7 years, it is 20/20. Visual acuity is measured using standardized letter or picture charts. (See Chapter 35.) **Vision** refers to the complex process of acquiring meaning from what is seen, involving the eye, brain, and related neurologic and physiologic structures. Development interacts with a child's maturing physiologic system to bring increasing meaning to objects in sight (Table 47–1).

EAR

Why do infants and young children have more ear problems than adults? The eustachian tube, which connects the nasopharynx to the middle ear, is proportionately shorter, wider, and more horizontal in infants than in older children or adults (see "As Children Grow: Eustachian Tube"). During sucking, yawning, and other movements, the tube opens for milliseconds, allowing free passage of air between the nasopharynx and the middle ear. This predisposes young children to development of otitis media or middle ear infection.

The external ear canal is small at birth, although the internal ear and middle ear are relatively large. As a result the tympanic membrane is close to the surface and can be easily injured. Babies can hear at about 20 weeks' gestation, and the auditory nerve function is mature at about 5 months of age in the infant. Before 34 weeks' gestation, the exterior ear is soft with little cartilage apparent. When the ear of a

MyNursingKit Video: 3E Ear/Ear Anatomy

Table 47–1 Visually Related Developmental Milestones

Age	Milestone
Term neonate	Demonstrates alertness to light and visual stimulus presented 8–12 in. (20–30 cm) from eyes
1 month	Follows an object 60 degrees horizontally and 30 degrees vertically; blinks at an approaching object
2 months	Follows a person or moving object for 180 degrees from 6 ft (2 m) away; smiles in response to a face; raises head 30 degrees from prone
3 months	Tracks an object through 180 degrees; regards own hand; begins visual-motor coordination
4–5 months	Social smile; reaches for a cube 12 in. (30 cm) away; notices a raisin 12 in. (30 cm) away; stares at own hand
7–8 months	Reaches and grasps an object, picks up a raisin by raking, transfers objects from hand to hand
8–9 months	Pokes at holes in a peg board; well-developed pincer grasp; crawls; uncovers toy after seeing it hidden
12–14 months	Stacks blocks; places a peg in a round hole; stands and walks

Source: Data from C. D. Rudolph, A. M. Rudolph, M. K. Hostetter, G. E. Lister, & M. J. Siegel (eds.). *Rudolph's pediatrics* (21st ed.). New York: McGraw-Hill; Frigelman, S. (2007). The First Year. In R. M. Kliegman, R. E. Behrman, H. B. Jenson, & B. F. Stanton. (2007). *Nelson textbook of pediatrics* (18th ed.). Philadelphia: Saunders.

preterm is folded forward and released, its recoil is slow, while with term newborns the recoil is strong and fast.

NOSE, THROAT, AND MOUTH

Up to the age of 6 months, infants breathe primarily through the nose and not through the mouth. Edema and nasal discharge may interfere with adequate air intake and feeding. Mucosal swelling and exudate may block the small nasal passages of young children.

The palatine tonsils, visible on oral examination, are located on each side of the oropharynx. The method for examining a child's throat is discussed in Chapter 35. Although tonsils vary in size considerably during childhood, they are normally large, especially in school-age children. Lymph tissue decreases in size by about 10 years, so its appearance after this age can indicate abnormality. The nasopharyngeal tonsils (adenoids) lie in the posterior wall of the nasopharynx, just above the oropharynx. In children the adenoids may become enlarged, harboring bacteria and interfering with breathing.

The mucosal membranes of the mouth are expected to be intact and without lesions at all ages. The first teeth commonly erupt at about 6 months of age, and the first loss of teeth begins at about 6 years. See Chapter 35 for thorough descriptions of assessment of the oral cavity in infants and children.

AS CHILDREN GROW

EUSTACHIAN TUBE

Of the three anatomic differences in the eustachian tube between adults and small children (shorter, wider, more horizontal), which do you think could cause more problems for the child and why?

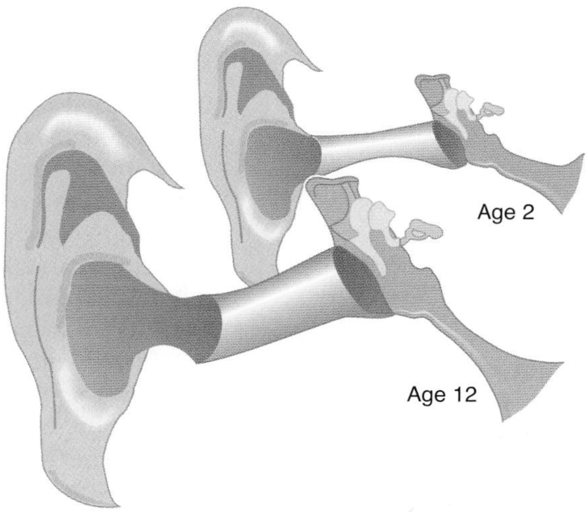

Position of eustachian tube is at less of an angle in the young child, resulting in decreased drainage. (more horizontal)

End of eustachian tube in nasal pharynx opens during sucking.

Eustachian tube equalizes air pressure between the middle ear and the outside environment and allows for drainage of secretions from middle ear mucosa.

DISORDERS OF THE EYE

INFECTIOUS CONJUNCTIVITIS

Conjunctivitis is an inflammation of the conjunctiva, the clear membrane that lines the inside of the lid and sclera. Bacteria, viruses, allergies, trauma, or irritants cause the conjunctiva to become swollen and red with a yellow or white discharge (Figure 47–1 ●). Parents commonly refer to all conjunctivitis as "pink eye."

Conjunctivitis in an infant under 30 days of age is called *ophthalmia neonatorum*. These infections are usually acquired from the mother during vaginal birth as a result of contact with infected vaginal discharge containing organisms such as *Chlamydia trachomatis* and *Neisseria gonorrhoeae*. See Chapter 29 for information on prophylactic eye treatment. Newborns occasionally get chemical conjunctivitis in response to prophylactic eye treatment. This may be a cause when the conjunctivitis develops within 24 to 48 hours after instillation of the medication.

Another cause of infection in infants is herpesvirus, which requires prompt and vigorous treatment to prevent eye injury or blindness. Infants with herpesvirus infections of the eye are treated with intravenous acyclovir as well as topical drops.

In infants who have frequent tearing and "mattering" (eyelid discharge that has formed a crust) on awakening, a plugged lacrimal duct may mimic conjunctivitis. Treatment involves massaging the tear duct every 4 hours when the infant is awake. Lacrimal ducts that remain plugged after the age of 1 year may have to be opened surgically.

Bacterial conjunctivitis can occur in children of any age. It is characterized by edema of the eyelid, red conjunctiva, and enlarged preauricular lymph glands. There is usually mucopurulent exudate that causes matting, making the eyes difficult to open upon awakening. Older children with conjunctivitis complain of itching or burning, mild photophobia, and a feeling of scratching under the lids. Parents may notice increased tearing or a mucoid or mucopurulent discharge, redness and swelling of the conjunctiva, a pink sclera, and crusty eyelids, especially in the morning. There is no change in vision. Common infectious organisms include *Staphylococcus aureus, Haemophilus influenzae, Streptococcus pneumoniae, Moraxella catarrhalis,* and *Escherichia coli* (Mah, 2006). Most cases are caused by hand-to-eye contact, and the disease can rapidly spread whenever groups of youth spend time together, such as among young children and adolescents in schools and childcare centers, and even among college students in dormitories, sororities, fraternities, and on sports teams. Although bacterial conjunctivitis can be bilateral, it is more commonly unilateral.

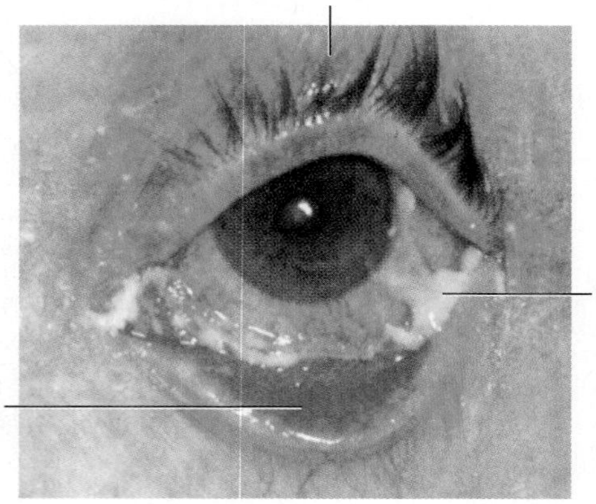

● **Figure 47–1** Acute conjunctivitis. The major difference between bacterial and viral conjunctivitis is that bacterial conjunctivitis has a purulent discharge that may result in crusting whereas the discharge from viral conjunctivitis is serous (watery). Allergic conjunctivitis produces watery to thick drainage and is characterized by itching.

Source: Used with permission from Newell, F. W. (1996). *Ophthalmology: Principles and concepts* (8th ed.). St. Louis, MO: Mosby-Year Book.

Other infections in newborns and children can be caused by viruses. *Viral conjunctivitis* is more often bilateral than unilateral. Adenovirus is a common cause and spreads from respiratory adenovirus infection in hand-to-eye transmission. Signs and symptoms are similar to those of bacterial conjunctivitis, although they are sometimes milder in severity and slower in onset.

Herpes simplex virus (HSV) can also cause infection, either by transfer from a herpes-infected mother to her baby during birth or by contact with an infected person in infants or children of any age. Ophthalmic herpes infection is often accompanied by characteristic vesicular lesions on the skin of the face. A culture of the lesions is performed for diagnosis, and any accompanying conjunctivitis is assumed to be caused by herpes virus. For the infection caused by HSV, prompt and vigorous treatment is needed to prevent eye injury or blindness, which can occur in children with recurrent herpes virus infections as a result of antibody reaction to the viral antigen. Herpes virus infections commonly recur so periodic treatment and sometimes prophylaxis may be needed.

Allergic conjunctivitis is a common cause of eye discomfort (Abelson & Granet, 2006). When conjunctivitis is caused by an allergy, the child complains of intense itching. Eyes are red with watery discharge, and the conjunctivae have a "cobblestone" appearance.

In most cases a diagnosis of the cause of conjunctivitis is made based on the history and symptoms. Cultures can be taken, especially in infants or in cases suspected of being unusual bacterial illness or herpes viruses. A Gram stain of discharge and conjunctival scraping for potential *Chlamydia* or herpes are performed. Infants and children must be promptly referred to primary care providers or eye specialists for treatment of possible eye infections. When diagnosed in the neonatal intensive care unit, the infant is isolated to prevent spread to other infants.

Antibiotic eye medication is prescribed in droplet or ointment form if a bacterial infection is suspected. Treatment may be started after a laboratory sample is obtained but before the results are known. Fluoroquinolones are now frequently used to treat bacterial conjunctivitis; drops or ointment can be used (Brunell, Wagner, Cuming, et al., 2006; Lichtenstein, Dorfman, Kennedy, et al., 2006). When gonococcal conjunctivitis occurs in newborns, ceftriaxone is recommended; the disease is resistant to penicillin. Chlamydial infections are treated with oral erythromycin or tetracycline. Careful total evaluation of the newborn with any conjunctivitis is also performed to watch for other signs of infection. Instructions for instilling eye medication are provided in the Clinical Skills Manual (see Skill 11–6 SKILLS).

Viral conjunctivitis may be treated with comfort measures such as cleaning drainage away with a warm clean cloth, and avoiding bright lights and reading. Ophthalmic antibiotics may sometimes be given to prevent bacterial invasion due to frequent rubbing of the eyes. Herpes simplex virus infections of the eye are treated promptly by an ophthalmologist, neonatologist, or others who are trained in this serious disease. Topical drugs are used, and often are combined with a systemic antiviral agent such as acyclovir. Neonatal herpes simplex virus is treated vigorously with parenteral acyclovir for 14 days (or longer if central nervous system involvement is found upon lumbar puncture), and with topical ophthalmic medication (trifluridine, iododeoxyuridine, or vidarabine). Recurrent lesions may necessitate suppressive or prophylactic treatment with oral acyclovir (American Academy of Pediatrics, 2006).

If an allergen is diagnosed as the cause of conjunctivitis, systemic or topical antihistamines may be prescribed. Topical steroids and vasoconstrictors may also be used (Abelson & Granet, 2006). Decongestants can be combined with systemic antihistamines for short-term therapy. Mast-cell stabilizers may be used to decrease the activation of mast cells that accompanies allergic reactions; their use is safe in children 3 years of age and older.

Nursing Management

Nurses routinely instill antibiotics into the eyes of newborns after birth. Perform a careful examination so that any cases of ophthalmia neonatorum can be referred promptly to an ophthalmologist. Women infected with gonococcus or chlamydia should be identified so their babies can receive attention and medication at birth to prevent infection. Babies born at home should have ocular examinations soon after birth.

In suspected conjunctivitis, gentle pressure for several seconds with a gloved index finger placed next to the inner corner of the eye may cause a discharge of mucopurulent drainage. Refer for care and report the findings. Since infectious conjunctivitis is extremely contagious, tell parents that children should not return to child care or school until they have been taking an antibiotic for 24 hours. Teach parents the importance of careful hand hygiene and the avoidance of shared towels. Tell parents that children should not rub their eyes. Mittens may help prevent infants from rubbing their eyes. Toddlers may be distracted by activities that keep their hands busy. Teach parents the proper techniques for instilling eye medications. For children with allergies, alert parents to signs of infection so if the child gets an eye infection, they will seek prompt treatment.

Teaching Highlights

INSTILLING EYE MEDICATIONS

It can be challenging to safely instill eye medication into young children. Give parents the following suggestions:

- Wash your hands well.
- Be sure the medicine is warmed at least to room temperature.
- Remove any drainage from the eye with a clean or sterile moist, warm cloth or gauze.
- Wash your hands again.
- Have the child lying on the back with eyes closed.
- Gently pull the lower lid down to form a small pocket.
- Apply a thin string (for ointment) or drops of the medicine.
- Allow the eyelid to return to normal position.
- Have the child keep the eye closed for several seconds.
- Help prevent spread of the infection by keeping the child's hands clean.
- Enhance comfort by keeping the head elevated to decrease swelling and avoid exposure to bright light.

PERIORBITAL CELLULITIS

Periorbital cellulitis is an infection of the eyelid and surrounding tissues that is usually caused by bacteria and is an uncommon complication of sinusitis. Children present with swollen, tender, red or purple eyelids; restricted, painful movement of the area around the eye; and fever. Periorbital cellulitis should be treated promptly to prevent the spread of the infection to the posterior orbit. Orbital cellulitis is a serious outcome that can lead to bacterial meningitis (Nageswaran, Woods, Benjamin, et al., 2006). Management includes hospitalization for intravenous antibiotics and the application of hot packs. Children usually respond favorably within 48 to 72 hours.

VISUAL DISORDERS

Vision, the complex process of acquiring meaning from what is seen, depends on many factors. The eyes must move quickly and in a coordinated manner. (See Chapter 35∞ for discussion of eye movement assessment.) They must function together for clear, single vision to occur. If this ability, called **binocularity**, is not present (perhaps due to strabismus or amblyopia), the child may have double vision and the brain cannot make sense of the images it receives. Normally, perceptions of objects seen are integrated with other senses through eye–hand coordination, and with the brain through visual imagery and discrimination of objects seen. Although visual acuity is essential, the child's movements, mental processes, and other senses all interact to give meaning to objects that are viewed. Vision therefore influences learning and school performance (U.S. Preventive Services Task Force, 2005).

Visual disturbances must be diagnosed and treated promptly to prevent impairment or loss of visual acuity (U.S. Department of Health and Human Services, 2006). Most children undergo a simple test for visual acuity during healthcare visits as soon as they can cooperate with the examiner. Once in school, children's visual acuity is screened every 2 to 3 years during the elementary years. Nurses often organize vision screening programs for children. Table 47–2 provides a series of questions that can be used to identify visual disturbances in children. A child who does not pass vision screening is referred to an ophthalmologist or optometrist for more detailed examination of near and far vision, eye structure and movement, and color discrimination.

Table 47–2 Assessment Questions for Identifying Visual Disturbances in Children

Young Child

Ask the parents:
- Does your child follow you with his or her eyes as you come into a room?
- Are other objects followed with ease?
- Do both eyes work together or does one seem to wander off?
- At what age did your baby sit, stand, walk?
- Does your child have any difficulty picking up objects?

School-Age Child

Ask the parents:
- Does your child like to look at pictures and read?
- Does your child hold toys or books close, or sit very close to the television?
- Does your child squint or rub the eyes?
- Is he or she at grade level in all subjects?
- Has your child demonstrated any learning difficulties?
- Does he or she use a computer, watch television, or play computer games?
- Does your child play sports and games at the same level of ability as peers?

Some of the common visual disorders in children are:

- *Hyperopia (farsightedness):* Light rays focus posterior to the retina, resulting in an inability to focus on nearby objects. All children have some degree of hyperopia until 9 to 10 years of age. However, their eyes can accommodate sufficiently to enable them to see near objects clearly. Blurring of vision occurs only in children with excessive hyperopia, or a difference in accommodation between the two eyes. Amblyopia, or a weakening of the poorer eye, can occur in these children if treatment is not obtained.
- *Myopia (nearsightedness):* Light rays focus anterior to the retina, resulting in an inability to see far-off objects. Although children of any age can manifest myopia, it most commonly develops at about 8 years of age. The child may complain of headaches and often squints to improve distance vision.
- *Astigmatism:* Light rays are refracted differently depending on their place of entry to the eye. The curvature of the cornea or lens is not uniformly spherical, causing blurred images. The child with astigmatism often holds pages very close to the face to obtain the best visual image.

For the description and management of four disorders that can significantly affect vision—strabismus, amblyopia, cataracts, and glaucoma—see "Clinical Manifestations: Visual Disorders."

Compensatory lenses are prescribed for most visual disorders. A significant difference in visual acuity between the eyes is often a result of amblyopia or strabismus, and further treatment may be needed. The visual acuity of a child with compensatory lenses should be reevaluated every 1 to 2 years. More frequent visits to an eye specialist are needed when a child is being treated for amblyopia or strabismus.

Nursing Management

The nurse plays an important role in identifying eye disorders in children and performing careful eye examinations of newborns and children. Observe for symmetry of placement and movement, ability to follow objects with each eye, and any abnormalities in appearance. The light reflex, cover-uncover test, and visual acuity testing are essential tests for every child. See Chapter 35∞ for a description of eye examination and the Clinical Skills Manual for visual acuity tests (Skills 9–18 and 9–19 SKILLS).

Nurses in schools plan and carry out visual acuity screening on children. Generally certain grades (such as kindergarten, 2, 4, 6, and 8) are screened annually along with any children new to a district. The nurse performs and records the screening results and informs the school and families of any children with abnormal results, who are then referred to an eye specialist for care. An important part of the screening process is following up on referrals to be certain that children receive the diagnostic care they need.

When abnormalities are found on screening, nurses refer families to the care of an eye specialist. When prescriptive lenses are used, the nurse instructs the parent and child on correct wear practices and care. If surgery is needed, surgical and postoperative follow-up are needed. This will include pain control, observing for signs of infection (ophthalmic or systemic), and administering needed eye medications. Sterile technique is used postoperatively to provide eye care. Promptly report deviations from normal such as increased pain, redness, discharge, or edema of the eye; increased temperature or pulse, which may indicate infection; increased sensitivity to light; or other abnormalities. Children are usually discharged home with instructions to minimize certain vigorous activities for a certain period of time. Perform postoperative and discharge teaching and emphasize the importance of follow-up visits.

COLOR BLINDNESS

Color blindness is an X-linked recessive disorder found in 10% of males and very rarely in females; it is more common in White than Black males. The most common form affects the ability to distinguish between the colors red and green; blue-yellow discrimination and other colors can also be involved (Subramanian, 2007). Preschool boys are tested for color blindness in some clinics to identify those with the disorder. Color blindness is not treatable, and management focuses on issues of safety (e.g., problems in distinguishing between red and green traffic signals) and techniques to improve discrimination of colors in the affected color groups.

RETINOPATHY OF PREMATURITY

Retinopathy of prematurity (ROP) occurs when immature blood vessels in the retina constrict and become necrotic. This condition, which may occur in infants of low birth weight or of short gestation, can heal completely or lead to mild myopia or retinal detachment and blindness.

Clinical Manifestations

VISUAL DISORDERS

ETIOLOGY	CLINICAL MANIFESTATIONS	CLINICAL THERAPY
Strabismus		
Can be congenital or acquired. Seen in up to 4% of all children; 30–50% of children with strabismus develop amblyopia Most common types: **Esotropia:** inward deviation of eyes ("crossed eyes") **Exotropia:** outward deviation of eyes ("wall-eyes") 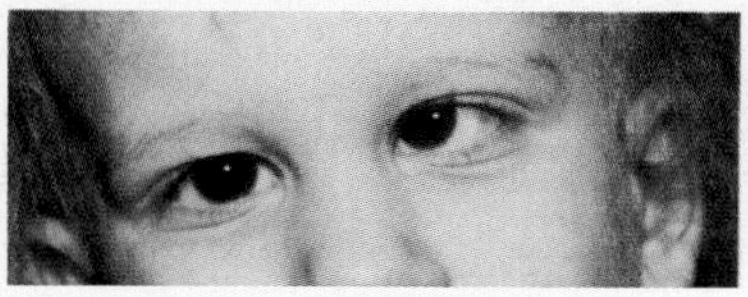 Strabismus. *Used with permission from Paediatrics, 2e, Thomas & Harvey, p. 130, 1997, by permission of the publisher Churchill Livingstone.*	Eyes appear misaligned to observer. May occur only when child is tired. Symptoms include squinting and frowning when reading; closing one eye to see; having trouble picking up objects; dizziness and headache. Corneal light reflex and cover-uncover tests confirm diagnosis. Child may have no other abnormalities but certain conditions such as cerebral palsy, hydrocephalus, Down syndrome, and seizure disorder are more commonly accompanied by strabismus.	Occlusion therapy (patching the fixating or good eye for 1–2 hours daily to force use of the weak eye) Compensatory lenses Surgery of the rectus muscles to correct muscle imbalance Eye drops to cause blurring of the good eye Prisms Vision therapy (eye exercises) If treatment is begun before 24 months of age, amblyopia (reduced vision in one or both eyes) may be prevented.
Amblyopia ("lazy eye")		
Reduced vision in one or both eyes; affects up to 4% of children. Amblyopia can result from anything which causes visual deprivation to one eye. The most common causes are untreated strabismus, with the child "tuning out" the image in deviating eye, congenital cataract, or uncorrected refractive errors causing visual differences between eyes.	Symptoms are the same as for strabismus. Vision testing can be used to diagnose condition.	Compensatory lenses Occlusion therapy for 2–6 hours daily through patching the eye or eye glass Occasionally vision therapy (eye exercises) is used in an attempt to improve the weaker eye. Atropine 1% 1 drop/day in unaffected eye. Treatment is discontinued when visual acuity no longer improves; 20/20 acuity rarely attained. Treatment is most successful if received by 5–6 years of age.
Cataracts		
Occurs when all or part of lens of eye becomes opaque, which prevents refraction of light rays onto retina Seen in 2/10,000 newborns 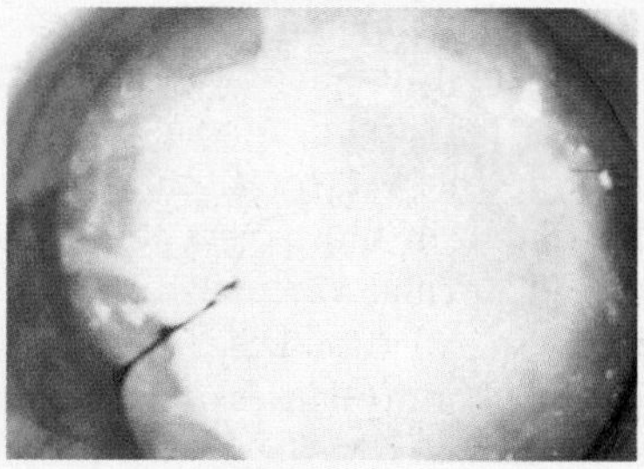 Congenital cataract. *Used with permission from Vaughan, D., Asbury, T., & Riordan-Eva, P. (1992) General ophthalmology (13th ed., p. 172). New York: McGraw-Hill Companies*	Can affect one or both eyes and may be congenital or acquired. Clouding of lens indicates presence of cataract; however, cataracts are not always visible to naked eye. Symptoms included distorted red reflex, symptoms of vision loss (see strabismus), white pupil. May be present alone but sometimes associated with other conditions such as fetal alcohol syndrome, Down syndrome, and Turner syndrome.	Must be diagnosed at a young age for successful treatment; many cases are missed. Specific treatment depends on whether one or both eyes are affected, extent of clouding and presence of other ocular abnormalities. Surgical removal of lens and corrective lenses; contact lenses frequently used; results of surgery are good; surgery before the age of 2 months is associated with the best results; visual acuity in 55% of children is 20/40 or better. Lens implant may be used. Eye protectors and restraints are used postoperatively to prevent injury; antibiotic or steroid drops may be used for several weeks; treatment for amblyopia may be necessary.

(continued)

Clinical Manifestations—continued

VISUAL DISORDERS

ETIOLOGY	CLINICAL MANIFESTATIONS	CLINICAL THERAPY
Glaucoma		
Increased intraocular pressure damages eye and impairs visual function; ciliary body of eye produces aqueous fluid that flows between iris and lens into anterior chamber; if enough fluid accumulates, blindness results; affects 1 in 100,000 newborns. May be congenital (occurring in first 3 years of life) or juvenile (occurring from 3–30 years) and affect one or both eyes. Primary glaucoma (50% of cases) is an isolated anomaly of drainage; secondary glaucoma (50% of cases) is associated with other ocular or systemic abnormalities	Symptoms of congenital glaucoma include tearing, blinking, corneal clouding, eyelid spasms, and progressive enlargement of eye; photophobia (extreme sensitivity to light). Symptoms of juvenile glaucoma include constant bumping into objects in child's periphery (painless visual field loss); seeing halos around objects. Diagnosis is made using tonometer, which measures intraocular pressure.	Surgery to reduce intraocular pressure is treatment of choice, since medications used to combat glaucoma in adults are not as effective in children. Compensatory lenses used following surgery. Treatment is not always successful, especially if the child has congenital glaucoma, so parents' feelings regarding care of a visually impaired child should be explored.

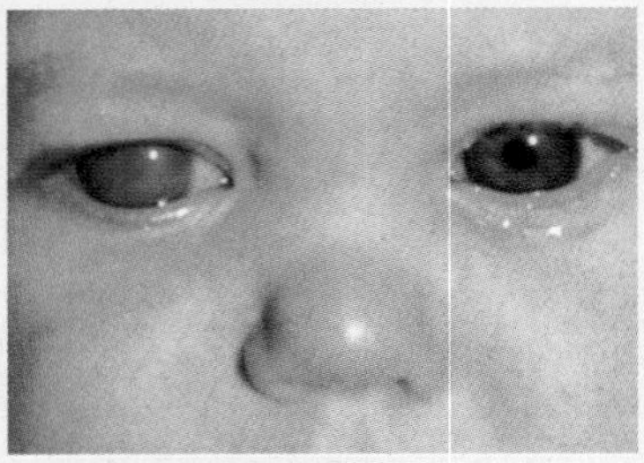

Congenital glaucoma.

Used with permission from Vaughan, D., Asbury, T., & Riordan-Eva, P. (1992). General ophthalmology (13th ed., p. 172). New York: McGraw-Hill Companies

Data from Donahue, S. P. (2007). Pediatric strabismus. *New England Journal of Medicine 356*, 1040–1047; Nield, L. S., Mangano, L. M., & Kamat, D. (2008, January). Strabismus: A close-up look. *Consultant for Pediatricians*, 17–25; Doshi, N. R., & Rodriguez, L. F. (2007). Amblyopia. *American Family Physician 75*, 361–368; Kliegman, R. M., Behrman, R. E. Jenson, H. B., et al., (2007). *Nelson textbook of pediatrics* (18th ed.). Philadelphia: Saunders (Part XXVIII, Disorders of the Eye, pp. 2569–2615).

ETIOLOGY AND PATHOPHYSIOLOGY

Retinopathy of prematurity results from injury to the developing capillaries of the retina. Oxygen therapy is associated with the development of retinopathy of prematurity (Figure 47–2 ●), but other factors such as respiratory distress, artificial ventilation, apnea, cerebral palsy, bradycardia, heart disease, multiple blood transfusions, infection, hypoxia, hypercarbia, acidosis, shock, and sepsis have also been linked with the disorder. It is most common in male infants born before 28 weeks of gestation and weighing under 1600 g (3 lb, 8 oz) at birth. A genetic link may be present as white infants are more commonly affected than those of African heritage, and Alaskan Natives have a high rate of the disorder. In developed countries ROP is the second most common cause of blindness, occurring in 12.5% of infants born from 23 to 26 weeks' gestation (Tasman, Patz, McNamara, et al., 2006; Yang, Donovan, & Wagge, 2006).

The retina is normally vascularized by about 8 months' gestation. For the premature infant, however, this process must continue after birth, and the environmental and other conditions listed in the preceding paragraph appear to affect its course. Arteriole constriction, followed by vascular proliferation of abnormal vessels, occurs. In most cases the abnormal vessels gradually regress and normal vascularization occurs. Sometimes, however, the abnormal vascularization continues into the vitreous cavity, causing abnormalities of the retina, optic disc, and macula. It is not known why the disease progresses in some cases, but progression is directly linked to lower birth weight, greater prematurity, and duration (not necessarily concentration) of oxygen therapy. Raeanne, the child described in the scenario at the beginning of this chapter, developed retinopathy of prematurity after receiving oxygen therapy to aid her underdeveloped lungs.

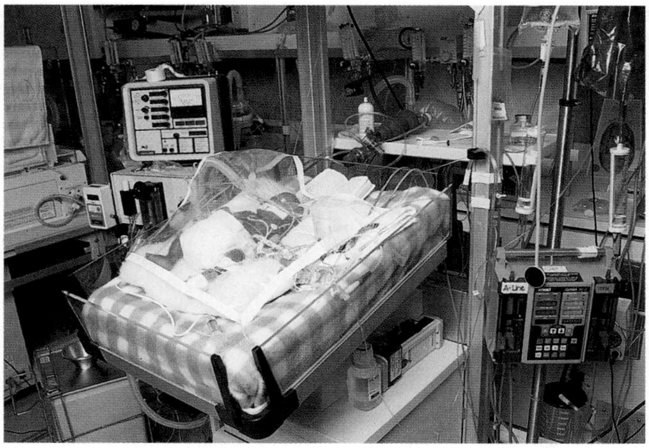

● **Figure 47–2** Artificial ventilation and risk for retinopathy of prematurity. This premature infant in the neonatal intensive care unit is receiving artificial ventilation—a risk factor for retinopathy of prematurity. The infant will need careful management of oxygen exposure and periodic eye examinations.

Although the developing capillaries are lost, in up to 90% of cases some degree of revascularization occurs later (Tasman et al., 2006). The degree of visual loss, varying from slight to total, is determined by the degree of revascularization.

CLINICAL MANIFESTATIONS

Retinopathy of prematurity is characterized by progressive changes in the retinal blood vessels, and in severe disease, by retinal detachment. Premature and low-birth-weight infants at risk for the disease are given frequent ocular examinations to ensure early detection of these changes. For infants who do not receive ophthalmologic examinations, resulting visual impairment may be detected only later in infancy when the child progresses slowly in meeting developmental milestones, fails to reach for objects, and does not follow objects or faces with the eyes. When visual impairment is present, the child usually manifests myopia. Total loss of vision can occur in the child who suffers a retinal detachment.

CLINICAL THERAPY

Diagnosis is made by ophthalmologic examination. A classification system that includes zone (area of retina with abnormal vasculature), stage (severity of disease), and plus disease (vascular dilation and tortuosity in posterior pole near optic nerve) is used to describe the location, extent, and severity of the disease (International Committee for the Classification of Retinopathy of Prematurity, 2005). All infants at risk, namely those born before 32 weeks of gestation and under 1500 g (3 lb, 7 oz) or; those born after 32 weeks gestation with birth weight from 1500 to 2000 g (3 lb, 7 oz to 4 lb, 3 oz), are assessed frequently using binocular ophthalmoscopy, by an ophthalmologist experienced with the condition. The disease is not manifested before 4 to 6 weeks after birth, so it is important that the infant receive regular eye examinations until the risk is discounted. Eye examinations continue every 1 to 3 weeks, with the frequency determined by the location of disease, progress of disease, and the

PATHOPHYSIOLOGY ILLUSTRATED

VISUAL ABNORMALITIES

A, In hyperopia light rays focus behind the retina, making it difficult to focus on objects at close range. ***B,*** In myopia light rays focus in front of the retina, making it difficult to focus on objects that are far away. ***C,*** In astigmatism light rays do not uniformly focus on the eye due to abnormal curvature of cornea or lens.

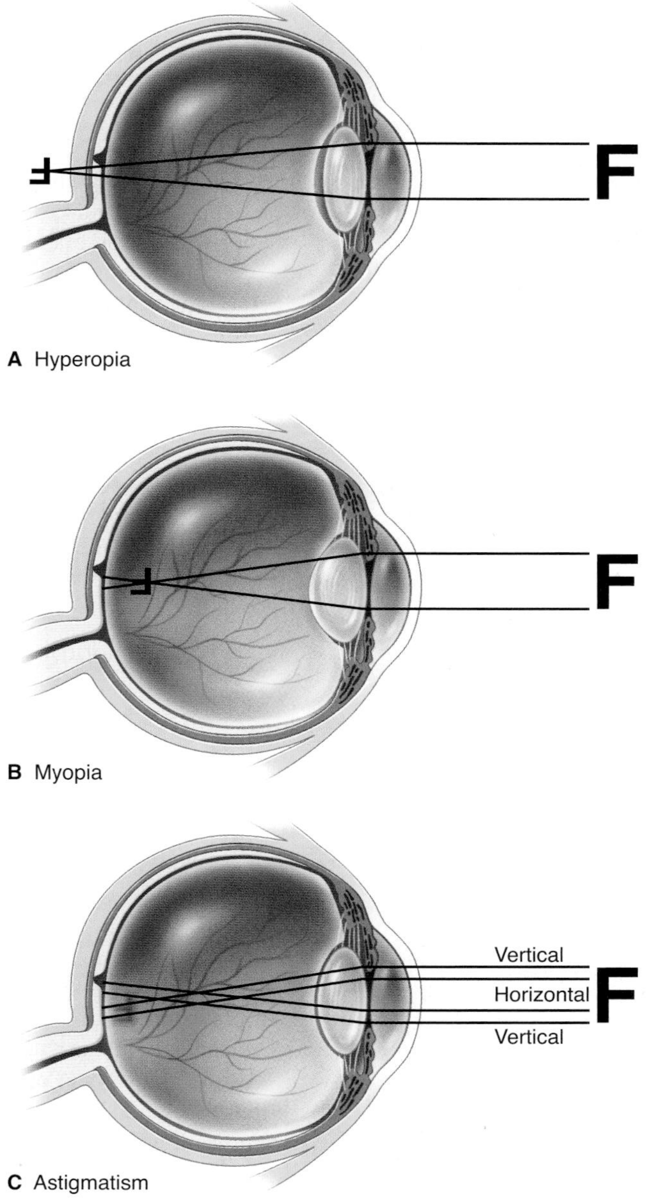

A Hyperopia

B Myopia

C Astigmatism

infant's degree of immature vascularization. Involvement of blood vessels in the periphery of the retina rarely leads to visual impairment. With involvement in other areas of the retina, risk of visual problems is more common (Quinn, 2005).

Treatment of infants with severe retinopathy of prematurity often involves laser therapy to stop progression of the disease process. Other surgical procedures such as a scleral buckle procedure and vitrectomy have been used in retinal detachments. Prompt treatment of accompanying problems such as strabismus, amblyopia, and myopia can promote maximal development.

NURSING MANAGEMENT

NURSING ASSESSMENT AND DIAGNOSIS

Assessment of the infant at risk for retinopathy of prematurity begins at birth by identifying infants who may require oxygen therapy and/or assisted ventilation. Look for risk factors such as prematurity and low birth weight. Assess the infant's breathing efforts and report any changes. Be certain the ventilation equipment is properly set to deliver the correct ventilatory pressure and amount of oxygen (see Skill 14–1 SKILLS). Note the cumulative risks in a particular case and suggest the need for a referral to an ophthalmologist, as necessary.

"Nursing Care Plan: The Child with a Visual Impairment Secondary to Retinopathy of Prematurity" outlines several nursing diagnoses. Other nursing diagnoses may be appropriate for an infant with the potential to develop retinopathy of prematurity or a child with resulting visual impairment. They include the following:

- *Altered Visual Sensory Perception* related to abnormal transmission of impulses
- *Potential Impaired Gas Exchange* related to ventilation-perfusion imbalance
- *Delayed Growth and Development* related to effects of visual impairment
- *Altered Family Processes* related to a child with a visual impairment

PLANNING AND IMPLEMENTATION

The nurse plays an important role in preventing retinopathy of prematurity. Encourage early and regular prenatal care to prevent unnecessary premature births. Administer oxygen only to newborns who need it, and in the amount specified by the physician to maintain prescribed oxygen saturation. Ensure that the proper ventilatory settings are used. Shield newborns from excessive exposure to light, since that may decrease susceptibility to retinopathy of prematurity. Be alert for infants with multiple risk factors and refer them, when appropriate, for ophthalmologic examination. Parents of infants at risk for retinopathy of prematurity require information about the disorder, as well as support, as the long-term effects on the child's vision are often identified only after subsequent examinations as the child grows.

Thinking Critically

THE CHILD WITH ROP

Raeanne, 3 years old, has a severe visual impairment. Born prematurely at 25 weeks of gestation, she received oxygen therapy, which damaged her retinal blood vessels. As a result, Raeanne developed retinopathy of prematurity (ROP). While in the hospital, Raeanne was given frequent ophthalmoscopic examinations. She received cryotherapy to the retinal vessels—a treatment designed to prevent detached retinae and the resulting total vision loss. Although this treatment halted progression of the disorder, Raeanne was left severely myopic (nearsighted).

For the first 3 years of life, Raeanne and her mother attended an early-intervention program, which provided stimulation for Raeanne and helped teach her mother techniques for enhancing her developmental progress. Raeanne will soon begin attending preschool. Her speech is well developed for a 3-year-old; she is socially mature, converses readily, and shows no developmental delays. However, she has had little contact with other children.

As the nurse in the preschool Raeanne will be attending, how will you assist both her parents and the preschool staff in helping Raeanne adapt to the preschool experience?

See MyNursingKit for possible responses.

The accompanying Nursing Care Plan summarizes care for the child with a visual impairment resulting from retinopathy of prematurity. The nurse is instrumental in case management for such children. Reinforce to parents the importance of follow-up eye examinations. Teach methods of stimulating development for the visually impaired child (refer to the next section).

EVALUATION

Expected outcomes of nursing care for the child with retinopathy of prematurity include the following:

- Early identification of visual impairment
- Normal developmental milestone achievement
- Positive management of child's visual condition by the family

VISUAL IMPAIRMENT

Visual impairment accounts for 11% of chronic medical conditions in children. Overall, 2.5% of children have visual impairment or blindness; the rate rises to 3.3% for children from 6 to 17 years of age. Low vision, or the inability to correct vision to a normal level, is present in 1.2 to 1.3 children per 1000, or 13.5 million children in the United States. Amblyopia is the most common cause of low vision in children, affecting 2% to 3% of children (Center for Health and Health Care in Schools, 2007; Hartmann, Bradford, Chaplin, et al., 2006).

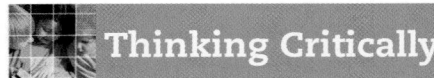

Nursing Care Plan

THE CHILD WITH A VISUAL IMPAIRMENT SECONDARY TO RETINOPATHY OF PREMATURITY

INTERVENTION	RATIONALE	EXPECTED OUTCOME
1. Nursing Diagnosis: Disturbed Visual Sensory Perception related to altered reception, transmission, and integration resulting of visual images		
NIC Priority Intervention: **Visual deficit enhancement:** Assistance in accepting and learning alternate methods for living with diminished vision		**NOC Suggested Outcome:** **Developmental progression:** Compensate for sensory deficits by maximizing use of impaired senses
Goal: The child will receive adequate sensory input.		
■ Provide kinesthetic, tactile, and auditory stimulation during play and in daily care (e.g., talking and playing). Provide music while bathing an infant, using bells and other noises on each side of infant. Verbally describe to a child all actions being carried out by adult.	■ Because visual sensory input is not present, the child needs input from all other senses to compensate and provide adequate sensory stimulation.	The child demonstrates minimal signs of sensory deprivation.
2. Nursing Diagnosis: Risk for injury related to impaired vision		
NIC Priority Intervention: **Fall prevention:** Instituting special precautions with patients at risk for injury		**NOC Suggested Outcome:** **Risk control:** Actions to eliminate or reduce modifiable health threats
Goal: The child will be protected from safety hazards that can lead to injury.		
■ Evaluate environment for potential safety hazards based on age of child and degree of impairment. Be particularly alert to objects that give visual cues to their dangers (e.g., stairs, stoves, fireplaces, candles). Eliminate safety hazards and protect the child from exposure. Take the child on a tour of new rooms, explaining safety hazards (e.g., schools, hotel room, hospital room).	■ The child may be at risk for injury related both to developmental stage and to inability to visualize hazards.	The child will experience no injuries.
3. Nursing Diagnosis: Risk for Delayed Growth and Development related to impaired vision		
NIC Priority Intervention: **Developmental enhancement:** Facilitating or teaching parents/caregivers to facilitate optimal growth and development of children		**NOC Suggested Outcome:** **Child growth and development:** Milestones of developmental progression
Goal: The child has experiences necessary to foster normal growth and development.		
■ Help parents plan early, regular social activities with other children.	■ The visually impaired child benefits developmentally from contact with other children.	The child demonstrates normal growth and development milestones.
■ Provide opportunities and encourage self-feeding activities.	■ To obtain adequate nutrients, the child needs to feel comfortable feeding self.	
■ Provide an environment rich in sensory input.	■ Sensory input is needed for normal development to occur.	
■ Assess growth and development during regular examinations to identify the child's strengths and needs.	■ Regular examinations aid in early identification of growth problems or developmental delays, so that appropriate interventions can be planned.	

(continued)

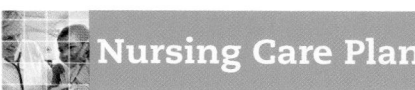

Nursing Care Plan—continued

THE CHILD WITH A VISUAL IMPAIRMENT SECONDARY TO RETINOPATHY OF PREMATURITY

INTERVENTION	RATIONALE	EXPECTED OUTCOME
4. Nursing Diagnosis: Risk for Compromised Family Coping related to child's prolonged disability from sensory impairment		
NIC Priority Intervention: **Family mobilization:** Utilization of family strengths to influence child's health positively		**NOC Suggested Outcome:** **Positive coping:** Extent to which family can mobilize resources to deal with the child's needs
Goal: The family identifies methods for coping with their visually impaired child.		
■ Provide explanation of visual impairment as appropriate.	■ The parents may feel guilt about the child's visual impairment, which can be allayed by knowledge of the cause.	The family successfully copes with the experience of having a visually impaired child.
■ Refer parents to organizations, early intervention programs, and other parents of visually impaired children.	■ The parents will receive needed information and support from others.	
■ Assist parents to plan for meeting developmental, educational, and safety needs of their visually impaired child. Offer resources for changing home environment to assist visually impaired child.	■ The child may require an enhanced environment in order to foster developmental progress.	

Many conditions discussed earlier in this chapter lead to temporary or permanent visual impairment. Infants who are premature; whose mothers were infected prenatally with rubella, toxoplasmosis, or other viruses; and who have certain congenital and hereditary conditions have a high risk of visual problems (Table 47–3). Fetal alcohol syndrome (FAS) is a major cause of visual disturbance; 90% of children with FAS have eye abnormalities. See Chapter 57∞ for further description of FAS.

Table 47–3 Common Causes of Visual Impairment in Children

Congenital or Hereditary	Acquired
Cataracts	Injury to eye or head
Glaucoma	Infections
Tay-Sachs disease	Rubella
Marfan syndrome	Measles
Down syndrome	Chickenpox
Fetal alcohol syndrome	Brain tumor
Prenatal infections (maternal infection)	Retinopathy of prematurity
Rubella	Cerebral palsy
Toxoplasmosis	
Herpes simplex	
Retinoblastoma	

The signs of visual impairment depend on the cause and degree of the problem and the age of the child (Table 47–4). The child's eyes may appear crossed or watery, and the lids may be crusty. Verbal children may complain of itching, dizziness, headache, or blurred, double, or poor vision.

The American Optometric Association and American Public Health Association recommend comprehensive vision examination starting at 6 months of age, while the American Academy of Ophthalmology and American Academy of Pediatrics recommend screening by 3 years of age (Center for Health and Health Care in Schools, 2007). The U.S. Preventive Services Task Force (USPSTF) recommends screening to detect amblyopia, strabismus, and defects in visual acuity in children younger than 5 years (U.S. Preventive Services Task Force, 2005). In spite of this differ-

Table 47–4 Signs of Visual Impairment

Infants	Toddlers and Older Children
May be unable to follow lights or objects	May rub, shut, or cover eyes
Do not make eye contact	Tilt or thrust head forward
Have a dull, vacant stare	Blink frequently
Do not imitate facial expressions	Hold objects close
	Bump into objects
	Squint

Growth and Development

Infants with visual impairment use kinesthesia, touch, and language to socialize. They appreciate and use touch more than other children and respond to verbal explanations when others use nonverbal communication. Vision affects both fine and gross motor skills, so skills such as hand-to-mouth coordination and walking may be delayed in children who are visually impaired.

ence in timing, it is clear that all young children should have vision examinations to identify vision problems early in life.

Clinical therapy depends on the child's condition and may include surgery, medication, and supportive aids. In the case of a disorder that results in permanent visual impairment, an interdisciplinary team of specialists works with the child and family. Nurses have an important role in this team to ensure developmental progression for the child and ongoing support for the family.

NURSING MANAGEMENT

NURSING ASSESSMENT AND DIAGNOSIS

Prevent visual deficits by teaching safety in activities that can injure the eye, engage in activities for early identification of the condition, and enhance development of children with low vision. Vision screening facilitates early detection and treatment of conditions that can lead to vision loss. Visual testing can be done at any age, including immediately after birth. Developmental milestones that require vision, such as following bright lights, reaching for objects, or looking at pictures in a book, can be used to assess vision. For children over the age of 3 years, visual acuity is most frequently measured by means of an age-appropriate acuity test (see Skills 9–18 and 9–19 SKILLS). Vision screening should begin at 3 years of age and take place during annual heathcare visits. Most states mandate school screening of vision. (See Chapter 35.) The photo screener, a device that can be used to take a photo of the child's eyes, is useful for infants, toddlers, and

Evidence-Based Nursing

NURSING ROLE IN VISION SCREENING AND FOLLOW-UP

Clinical Question

Screening for visual ability is important in order to identify children with impairments. The American Academy of Pediatrics recommends that children be screened at every well-child visit, beginning in the newborn period. Screenings should include vision history, vision assessment, external inspection of the eyes and lids, eye movement assessment, pupil examination, and elicitation of red reflex. Once the child can cooperate, usually by about 3 years, a vision test such as HOTV or tumbling E, along with ophthalmoscopic examination, should be added to the examination (U.S. Preventive Services Task Force, 2005). Nurses are often the health professionals that conduct vision examinations, evaluate results, and provide follow-up care. They participate in well-child health visits and often perform assessments of vision in schools.

The Evidence

A study of 1677 children in preschool, kindergarten, and first grade applied the HOTV acuity test and two types of photoscreening devices. (See the Clinical Skills Manual SKILLS for a further description of these types of screening.) Photoscreening was found to be significantly more effective than HOTV in identifying children with visual impairment, and was faster to perform (Leman, Clausen, Bates, et al., 2006).

Once visual impairment is identified, an essential nursing role is to refer for appropriate care and to follow up to determine if that care is received. A study attempted to determine the contributing factors to lack of follow-up care after a failed vision screening, and an interview was conducted with 66 families who had a child referred for eye examination after school screening. The researchers found that 85% of the families had low incomes. The barriers to eye care they identified included financial reasons, logistical problems (no ability to get to appointments), social or family issues (large family with adults all working or recent change in residence), and perceptual barriers (did not believe results or perceive the importance of the referral) (Kimel, 2006).

Another study focused on the school nurse-to-student ratio and its influence on care for students. While the National Association of School Nurses recommends a ratio of 1 nurse for 750 students, many schools do not achieve that recommendation. The schools in the study had ratios of 1:451 to 1:7440. While student vision screening and referral rates were similar for all of the schools, the schools with lower ratios (less students served per nurse) had significantly greater numbers of referred students who received further care (Guttu, Engelke, & Swanson, 2004).

Best Practice

Nurses play a vital role in ensuring that children receive early, periodic, and regular visual and eye screening. Evidence that suggests the most accurate methods should be closely examined. Photoscreening machines represent an important new addition to the tools that nurses can use. While identification of problems is important, the nursing roles of referral for care, identifying barriers to care, and ensuring that follow-up care has been received are also integral to vision care.

Critical Thinking

What vision screening methods are available in the offices, clinics, and schools in your community? How could you perform vision screening in the hospital setting if a child did not demonstrate expected visual ability for age? Design a follow-up program for a school that screens all kindergarten and first graders for visual acuity. What questions will you ask parents during a well-child visit for a 2-year-old to determine if vision is normal? How will you combine your knowledge of developmental milestones with screening for vision?

See MyNursingKit for possible responses.

preschoolers. The photo can be used to diagnose refraction errors, eye opacities, and misalignment (Donahue, Baker, Scott, et al., 2006). Visual fields and the ability to discriminate colors are tested at school age, when children can cooperate.

Children who are visually impaired may lag in development of cognitive and other skills. Sighted children learn the word *cup* using four senses—sight, touch, hearing, and taste—to obtain the information necessary to connect words with the objects they represent. In contrast, children with visual impairments rely on only three senses—touch, hearing, and taste. They learn concepts through differences in sounds, textures, and shapes.

Many visual disorders are linked with conditions that influence development. Thus, a child with cerebral palsy or fetal alcohol syndrome should be assessed frequently to identify a visual disorder, as well as to evaluate normal developmental milestones.

Nursing diagnoses for the child with impaired vision might include the following:

- *Disturbed Sensory/Perceptual Alteration (Visual)* related to altered sensory perception
- *Risk for Injury* related to poor vision
- *Risk for Delayed Growth and Development* related to visual impairment
- *Risk for Ineffective Family Coping* related to demands of a child with a sensory impairment

PLANNING AND IMPLEMENTATION

Promote safety in sports and other activities to prevent visual impairment when possible. Nursing care for a child with a visual impairment focuses on encouraging the child's use of all senses, promoting socialization, helping parents to meet the child's developmental and educational needs, and providing emotional support to parents. Refer the parents to an early intervention program as soon as the diagnosis is made. Nearly all care occurs in community and home settings.

ENCOURAGE USE OF ALL SENSES

Children who are partially sighted or blind use other senses to a great extent. Encouraging the use of the eyes as much as possible is important even if a child has poor vision (Figure 47–3 ●).

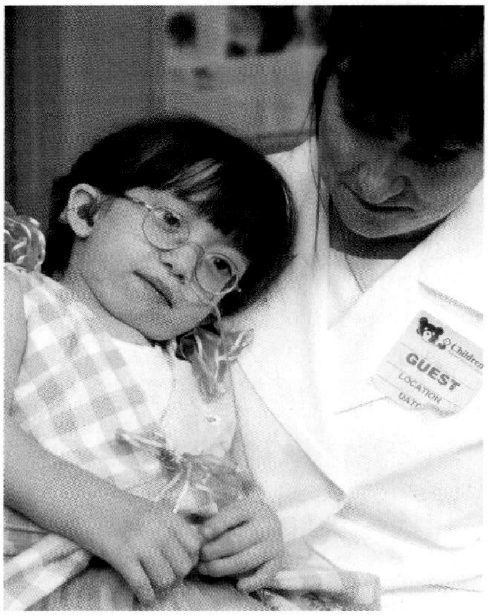

● **Figure 47–3** Encouraging use of the senses. This child needs ongoing developmental assessment and a comprehensive individualized education plan. Since she has impaired vision, the nurse uses touch and speaks with her throughout procedures to ensure sensory input.

Teaching Highlights

ENHANCING DEVELOPMENT OF THE VISUALLY IMPAIRED CHILD

- Encourage a toddler or preschooler who is visually impaired to look at pictures in well-lit settings. Have a school-age child read large-print books. Computers designed for the visually impaired are also available. The Optacon (a device that raises print so it can be felt by the child) and View Scan (which magnifies print) improve reading ability.
- Expose the infant and child to everyday sounds.
- Encourage the infant to use the sense of touch to explore people and objects. Have the parents purchase toys with sound and texture in mind. Directional concepts can be taught using games. Responding to the infant's and child's vocalizations encourages the use of speech.
- Teach specific techniques for toileting, dressing, bathing, eating, and safety.
- When the child becomes mobile, furniture and other objects in the environment should be kept in the same positions so the child can safely move around independently. Extra care must be taken to prevent injuries when a child does not see.
- Emphasize the child's abilities. Adolescents can use seeing-eye dogs or a white cane to function independently.
- Encourage the child to function independently within normal developmental parameters.
- If the child goes to a hospital or another strange environment, orient the child to the placement of objects and do not rearrange them.
- Teach those around the child to:
  - Announce their presence to the child when approaching.
  - Walk slightly ahead of the child so he or she can sense their movements.
  - Let the child hold the seeing person's arm rather than the reverse.
  - Identify the contents of meals and encourage the child to feed self.

PROMOTE SOCIALIZATION

The child's interactions and socializations should be as normal as possible (similar to those of sighted children of the same age and development).

- Stroke, rock, and hug infants and children who are visually impaired. Sing and talk to them. These infants do not make eye contact and have rather blank expressions.
- Call the child's name and speak before touching the child. Tell the child when the nurse and others are leaving the room. Describe locations of foods on the plate and tray to orient the child.
- Teach parents to read body language and vocalization as expressions of emotion. Facial expressions give a great deal of information, but infants and children with poor vision do not have the ability to learn by visual imitation. Show parents how to use tactile means to teach appropriate facial expressions. For example, a touch on the arm can be soft and stroking to indicate a smile, but firmer to indicate dismay or frown.
- Describe procedures such as blood pressure, ear examination, or cast application so the child knows what they will feel like. Let the child touch the equipment.
- Explain to parents that discipline and rewards for children with poor vision should be the same as those for other children in the family. The child should be given age-appropriate tasks.
- Encourage contact with peers as the child grows older. Teach the child to look directly at persons who are talking to him or her. Play, sports, and other activities can be modified to give the visually impaired child the same social experiences as a sighted child.

NURSING CARE IN THE COMMUNITY

Public laws require that each state provide educational and related services for children with disabilities (see Chapter 1). Parents and professionals should develop an individual education plan (as discussed in Chapter 39) that maximizes the child's learning ability. If possible, the child with a vision problem should attend child care and preschool with children who have normal visual acuity. What nursing actions are needed to help a child with a visual impairment adjust to child care or school?

- Provide parents with information about educational options before their child reaches school age. Education should take place in a setting that allows the child to have contact with other children and to participate in social activities.
- The child may be mainstreamed with a tutor, be partially mainstreamed in a resource room, attend special classes, or be tutored at home. If the child is to attend public school, suggest to parents that they contact the school well before enrollment to ensure that school personnel understand the child's disability.
- Make sure that equipment such as large-print books, Braille materials, audio equipment, or an Optacon (described in "Teaching Highlights: Enhancing Development of the Visually Impaired Child" on page 1286) is available. Ensure that frequent eye examinations are performed and assist with proper use and care of prescribed glasses or contact lenses, as necessary. Clean glasses daily with warm water and dry with a clean, soft cloth. Follow family directions for cleaning contact lenses.
- Familiarize the child with the new environment.

> **Growth and Development**
>
> Children with visual impairment may take longer to master self-help skills such as feeding and dressing. Perform regular developmental assessments and suggest adaptive ways that parents can help the child learn these skills.

PROVIDE EMOTIONAL SUPPORT

The family often needs help to understand the child's abilities and disabilities. Support them as they learn about their child's visual problems, tell friends and family, and then adjust to supporting the child.

- Encourage habilitation as soon as realistically possible. Make the adjustment easier by providing information about the child's specific type of visual impairment, available community services, and groups or associations for children with similar vision conditions.
- Suggest resources to families of children with visual disorders.
- Be supportive and listen to the family's concerns about the child's visual deficit.
- Make sure the parents meet their own physical and emotional needs so they are better able to care for and provide support to their child.

EVALUATION

Expected outcomes of nursing care for the child with a visual impairment include the following:

- Prevention of injury
- Growth and development to maximum potential
- Establishment of successful individualized education plan

INJURIES OF THE EYE

In the United States, eye injuries are common in all children aged 9 to 11 years, particularly in males. Boys from 11 to 15 years have four times more eye injuries than girls. About 42,000 sports injuries occur annually with about half of these in children (Committee on Sports Medicine and Fitness, 2004). Sports, darts, fireworks, air-powered BB guns, blunt and sharp objects, chemical and thermal burns, physical irritants, and abuse may cause eye trauma (Kliegman et al., 2007). Older children may be injured by chemicals in school science laboratories.

Promoting prevention of injury is an important nursing intervention. Protective eyewear should be used by participants in all sports with a risk of eye injury, with extreme caution in those with diminished vision or only one functional eye. Common injuries occur in baseball, basketball, swimming, bicycling, and football so preventive measures should be taken such as proper training and use of protective gear. Chemicals and objects such as scissors and knives should be placed out of reach.

Some injuries can be treated at home but many require emergency care or hospitalization. The nurse will document the history of the injury, perform an assessment of the eye, and measure the visual acuity. If a tetanus booster has not been given in the last 5 years, the child is reimmunized. Table 47–5 summarizes emergency treatment of common eye injuries.

DISORDERS OF THE EAR

OTITIS MEDIA

Otitis media, or inflammation of the middle ear, is sometimes accompanied by infection. This condition is one of the most common childhood illnesses. About 70% of infants have at least one case of acute otitis media during the first year of life, and 93% have been diagnosed with the problem by age 7 years. Peak incidence is in the first 2 years of life, particularly from 6 to 20 months of age (Bernius & Perlin, 2006). Otitis media occurs more frequently among boys and is most common during the winter months. Children with conditions such as cleft lip and palate or Down syndrome more often experience otitis media. Breastfeeding appears to be protective against otitis media. In the past decade, an increased number of cases have been observed, and recent changes have been made in recommendations for treatment (Pelton, 2005).

ETIOLOGY AND PATHOPHYSIOLOGY

The specific cause of otitis media is unknown, but it appears to be related to eustachian tube dysfunction. Often an upper respiratory infection precedes otitis media. This infection causes the mucous membranes of the eustachian tube to become edematous. As a result, air that normally flows to the middle ear is blocked, and the air in the middle ear is reabsorbed into the bloodstream. Fluid is pulled from the mucosal lining into the former air space, providing a medium for the rapid growth of pathogens. The tympanic membrane and fluid behind it become infected. The most common causative organisms are *Streptococcus pneumoniae, Haemophilus influenzae,* and *Moraxella catarrhalis* (Pelton, 2005).

Table 47–5 Emergency Treatment of Eye Injuries

Injury	Treatment
Subconjunctival hemorrhage (caused by coughing, mild trauma, or increased physical activity)	Usually heals spontaneously; child should see ophthalmologist if most of sclera is covered or if condition does not clear up in 1–2 weeks
Periorbital ecchymosis ("black eye")	Apply ice to eye area (both eyes) for 5–15 minutes every hour for the first 1–2 days after injury (even if only one eye is affected, both eyes may discolor); then apply warm compresses
Foreign body on conjunctiva	Do not let child rub eye; remove material on surface of eye by closing upper lid over lower lid, irrigating or everting upper lid, visualizing material, and removing it with slightly damp handkerchief; patch eye and transport child to emergency department if foreign body cannot be removed
Corneal abrasion	Superficial corneal abrasions are diagnosed by touching sterile fluorescein strip to lower conjunctiva; dye remains where corneal epithelial cells are disrupted; most corneal abrasions heal spontaneously although antibiotic ointment may be prescribed and eyes patched in some children
Burns (alkaline burns readily penetrate cornea and are more serious than acid burns)	For child with chemical burn, irrigate eye for 15–30 minutes; transport child to emergency department where irrigation should continue (see Clinical Skills Manual **SKILLS**); pupils are dilated to reduce pain and prevent adhesions; after irrigation is complete, eyes are patched and antibiotics are prescribed
Penetrating and perforating injuries	Obtain medical assistance immediately; never try to remove an object that has penetrated the child's eye; such objects should be removed by an ophthalmologist; prevent the child from rubbing injured eye; cover both eyes with shield before transportation to emergency department
Eye injuries caused by severe blows to head and eye (blunt trauma can seriously injure all eye structures, including orbit, which can be fractured)	Transport immediately to ophthalmologist's office or emergency department for evaluation and treatment

Growth and Development

Fluid accumulation in the middle ear prevents the efficient transmission of sound and can result in hearing loss over time, potentially delaying speech and language development. These delays may manifest as cognitive deficits or behavior problems. Motor development has been found to be impaired in children with chronic ear infections.

Conditions such as enlarged adenoids or edema from allergic rhinitis can also obstruct the eustachian tube and lead to otitis media. Pacifier use raises the soft palate and may alter dynamics in the Eustachian tube, providing for entry of microorganisms from the nasopharynx, especially in children with chronic otitis media (Marter & Agruss, 2007). Recurrent otitis media has an increased frequency in children of parents who smoke (Brook & Gober, 2005). Children with multiple siblings and those who attend child-care centers have increased rates of recurrent acute otitis media (Harrison, 2005). Ethnicity appears to be a factor (see "Developing Cultural Competence: Otitis Media").

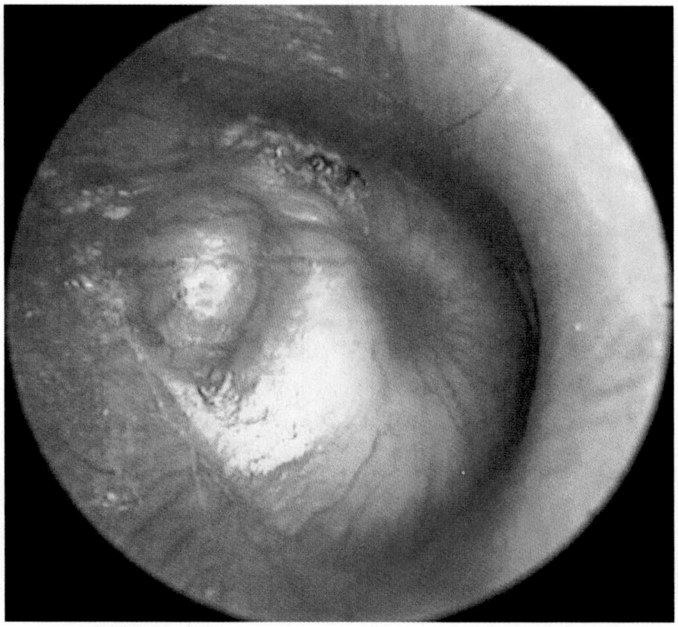

● **Figure 47–4** Acute otitis media. Acute otitis media is characterized by pain and a red, bulging, nonmobile tympanic membrane.

Source: Courtesy of Kevin Kavanagh, MD, FACS.

CLINICAL MANIFESTATIONS

Otitis media is the general term for inflammation of the middle ear. *Acute otitis media (AOM)* is diagnosed when the child has acute onset of ear pain, marked redness of the tympanic membrane upon otoscopy, and middle ear effusion (Figure 47–4 ●). Recurrent acute otitis media indicates repeated bouts of AOM, such as three in 6 months, or four in 12 months. *Otitis media with effusion (OME)* is evidence of fluid in the middle ear without inflammation (Figure 47–5 ●). OME sometimes becomes chronic in nature (continuing more than 3 months) and is more commonly associated with hearing loss.

Infants and young children have characteristic behaviors that indicate otitis media may be present. Pulling at the ear is a sign of ear pain (Figure 47–6 ●). Diarrhea, vomiting, and fever are typical of otitis media. Irritability and "acting out" may be signs of a related hearing impairment. The child with otitis media often has night awakenings with crying due to increased pressure when prone or supine. Some children with otitis media are asymptomatic; therefore, an ear examination should be performed at every healthcare visit (see Chapter 35∞). See the Clinical Manifestations table.

Developing Cultural Competence

OTITIS MEDIA

American Indian and Alaska Native (AI/AN) children have a very high rate of otitis media, perhaps due to culturally related bony structures of the ear, nose, and mouth. AI/AN children are seen about three times more frequently in outpatient clinics for otitis media than are other U.S. children (Hunter, Davey, Kohtz, et al., 2007). Black children have a higher incidence of the condition than White children (Centers for Disease Control and Prevention, 2008). Be alert for the common incidence in these population groups, plan prevention programs, and ensure prompt care and teaching about treatments for families of children affected. *What prevention measures would you emphasize with these families?* See the following Nursing Management section for suggestions of preventive approaches.

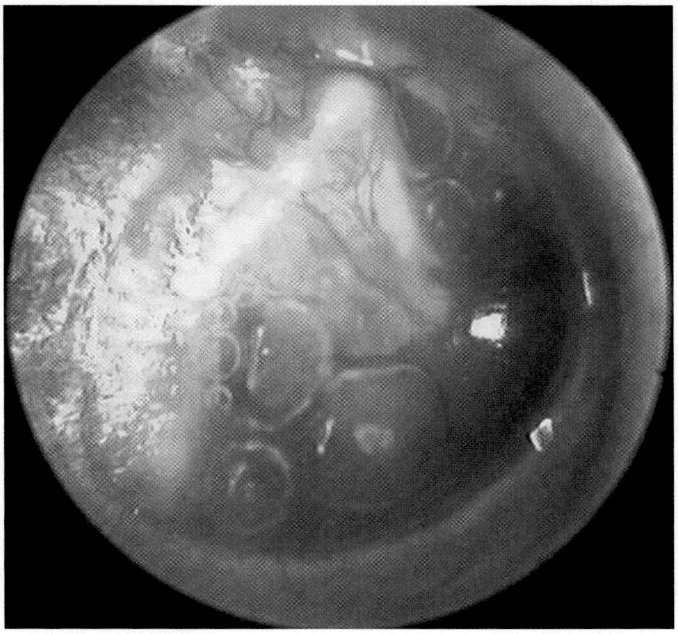

● **Figure 47–5** Otitis media with effusion. Otitis media with effusion is noted on otoscopy by fluid line or air bubbles.

Source: Courtesy of Kevin Kavanagh, MD, FACS.

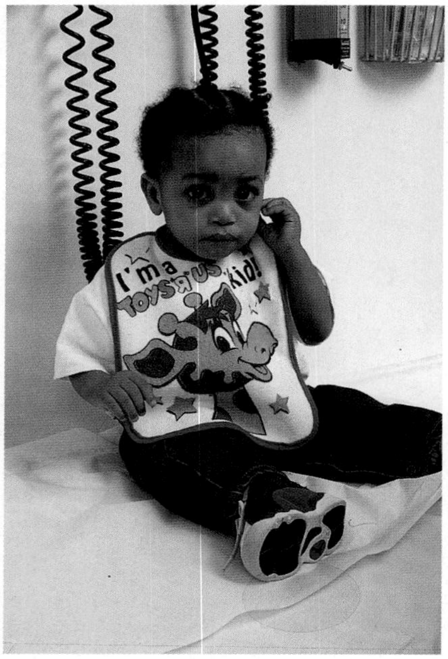

● **Figure 47–6** Signs of otitis media. This young child is pulling at the ear, an important sign of otitis media. Ask the parents about fussiness, presence of fever and night awakenings, additional signs that are often observed in children with this condition.

CLINICAL THERAPY

Diagnosis is based on otoscopic examination. Acute otitis media is diagnosed with certainty when there is a history of acute onset, presence of middle ear effusion (bulging or decreased mobility of the tympanic membrane, air fluid behind the membrane or otorrhea or discharge), and signs and symptoms of inflammation (erythema of tympanic membrane or discomfort that makes sleep and other activities difficult for the child) (American Academy of Pediatrics, Subcommittee on Management of Acute Otitis Media, 2004). Otoscopic examination includes visualization and pneumatic otoscopy. The trained clinician can perform pneumatic otoscopy in which positive air pressure in the external canal is used to measure the movement of the tympanic membrane. Special gradient acoustic reflectometry (SGAR) measures the condition of the middle ear by introducing a sound and measuring the tympanic membrane response (Windmill & Windmill, 2006). A "flat" tympanogram is also suggestive of otitis media. (The tympanogram is described in the next section, on hearing impairment.)

Since otitis media with effusion may only involve fluid in the middle ear, it is best diagnosed by pneumatic otoscopy and tympanometry. Since this type of otitis media is most commonly associated with hearing loss, audiologic testing should be performed in the pediatric healthcare home (medical home) (see Chapter 36∞) if the effusion persists for 3 months or longer.

Concern has developed about the increasing appearance of drug-resistant microbials as causative agents in otitis media. These organisms may explain the increase in otitis media observed in the last decade. Based on current knowledge, the American Academy of Pediatrics and the American Academy of Family Physicians joined to establish recommendations in 2004 (AAP, Subcommittee on Management of Acute Otitis Media, 2004; Leach & Morris, 2007). Acute otitis media is now treated

Clinical Manifestations

ACUTE OTITIS MEDIA AND OTITIS MEDIA WITH EFFUSION

ETIOLOGY	CLINICAL MANIFESTATIONS	CLINICAL THERAPY
Acute otitis media—bacterial infection in the middle ear from pathogens transferred from the nasopharynx; most common infectious agents are *S. pneumoniae, H. influenzae, M. catarrhalis*	*Behavioral*—ear pain, pulling at ear, rapid onset, irritability, malaise, poor feeding *Examination*—bulging tympanic membrane, air or fluid bubbles present behind tympanic membrane; immobile or poorly mobile tympanic membrane, red (or other color change such as white, gray, or yellow as long as bulging is present) tympanic membrane, reduced visibility of tympanic membrane landmarks with displaced light reflex	Treat ear pain with anesthetic ear drops, herbal pain products instilled into the auditory canal, or systemic acetaminophen or ibuprofen Verify that the tympanic membrane is intact before inserting ear drops Observe child's condition for 48–72 hours and, if not improved, treat with course of antibiotics
Otitis media with effusion—collection of fluid in the middle ear behind the tympanic membrane which is not infected with bacteria	*Behavioral*—difficulty hearing or responding as expected to sounds *Examination*—signs of acute inflammation are NOT present; tympanic membrane is retracted or neutral; immobile or partly mobile tympanic membrane; yellow or gray tympanic membrane; opaque or thickened tympanic membrane with visibility of landmarks reduced	Symptomatic treatment and pain relief Careful assessment of hearing acuity over several months Speech assessment if loss of hearing acuity occurs Developmental assessment

Drug Guide

AMOXICILLIN

Overview of Action

Bactericidal action inhibits cell-wall synthesis, a broader spectrum of activities than penicillin G. Effective on some gram-positive and gram-negative organisms, such as *Haemophilus influenzae, Escherichia coli, Proteus mirabilis, Neisseria gonorrhoeae,* meningococci, enterococci, and *Salmonella.* Used to treat infections of the ear, upper respiratory tract, GU system, skin, and soft tissue and as a prophylaxis against bacterial endocarditis. Topical forms may be used for eye infections.

Routes, Dosage, Frequency

PO

- Under 20 kg: 20 to 40 mg/kg/day in equally divided doses every 6 to 12 hours
- Over 20 kg: 250 to 500 mg every 8 hours (maximum dose 2 to 3 g)

For prophylaxis against bacterial endocarditis in susceptible children who are undergoing procedures:

Child: 25–50 mg/kg/day divided into doses and given every 8–12 hours; commonly for otitis media dose is 80–90 mg/kg/day divided into 2 doses and given every 12 hours (maximum dose 875 mg b.i.d.)

Adolescents: 250–500 mg every 8 hours

Nursing Implications

Assess: Assess previous allergy to this drug, penicillins, cephalosporins, other drugs, asthma, or family history of allergies. Obtain culture and sensitivity before treatment when ordered, but can start treatment before results.

Administer PO: Stable in gastric acid, give without regard to meals. Shake suspension well. Capsules may be taken apart or tablets crushed; mixed in small amount of food or fluid. Chewable tablets should be chewed thoroughly or crushed and followed with fluids.

Side Effects: Nausea, vomiting, diarrhea, pruritus, urticaria, anaphylaxis.

Monitor: Monitor child for hypersensitivity (especially within first 20 minutes following dose), rash (onset and characteristics), and side effects. Monitor blood counts, renal and hepatic function with prolonged or high-dose therapy or with premature infants and newborn. Maintain fluid intake. Watch for signs of superinfection; diarrhea (may indicate pseudomembranous colitis, which can occur while on drug or 4 to 6 weeks after drug is discontinued). If given for β-hemolytic streptococcal infection, 10-day course is needed to prevent risk of acute rheumatic fever or glomerulonephritis. If ampicillin rash occurs, it usually subsides in 6 to 14 days; however, rash can become severe, requiring drug discontinuance. Rash then usually resolves in 1 to 7 days.

Teaching: Child must take the medicine for the recommended time. If a revisit is scheduled, such as one for evaluation of treatment success in otitis media, parents are encouraged to keep this appointment. Report diarrhea, nausea, rash, or other side effects. Report if the child seems to have continued symptoms of infection (fever, irritability, pain, discharge from infected site, fatigue, or lethargy). Encourage generous fluid intake for age. Store medication out of reach of children.

Adapted from Bindler, R. M., & Howry, L. B. (2005). *Pediatric Drug Guide.* Upper Saddle River, NJ: Prentice Hall-Health.

with antibiotic therapy for 10 days in children under 6 years, and 5 to 7 days for children 6 years and over. Consistent with current guidelines, acute otitis media treatment is delayed for 48 to 72 hours after diagnosis in children 6 months to 2 years with nonsevere illness at presentation AND uncertain diagnosis, or in children 2 years and older without severe symptoms OR with uncertain diagnosis.

When prescribed, the choice of antibiotic depends on the probable organism, ease of administration, cost, previous effectiveness, and any history of allergies. First-line therapy is amoxicillin at a dose of 80 to 90 mg/kg/day. Amoxicillin with clavulanate or cefuroxime are second-line drugs. If an intramuscular drug is preferred, cefdinir at 14 mg/kg/day, cefpodoxime at 10 mg/kg/day, or cefuroxime at 30 mg/kg/day can be prescribed (Zacharyczuk, 2004). (See "Drug Guide: Amoxicillin.")

OME is not treated with antibiotics but is evaluated periodically to be sure there is not an additional AOM that needs treatment. Children with OME generally improve within 3 months. Since this type of otitis is more commonly associated with hearing loss and cochlear damage, follow-up with audiology is essential. If hearing is abnormal, speech testing should be performed (Otitis Media with Effusion, 2004).

Neither decongestants nor antihistamines have been shown to be effective in the treatment of otitis media with or without effusion. If infection recurs in spite of antibiotic treatment, **myringotomy** (surgical incision of the tympanic membrane) may be performed and **tympanostomy tubes** (pressure equalizing tubes) inserted to drain fluid from the middle ear. (See "Teaching Highlights: Care of the Child with Tympanostomy Tubes.")

NURSING MANAGEMENT

MyNursingKit Case Study: Otitis Media

NURSING ASSESSMENT AND DIAGNOSIS

Assess the tympanic membrane for color, transparency, mobility, presence of landmarks, and light reflex. Ask the parents whether the child has had a fever, been fussy, or been pulling at the ears. Observe for signs of impaired hearing.

Inquire about what the family has done at home to treat the ear infection and its associate pain. Some home remedies, such as rocking and singing to the child, are safe. Some other practices may be harmful (see "Complementary Care: Ear Wicking").

Teaching Highlights

CARE OF THE CHILD WITH TYMPANOSTOMY TUBES

After Surgery

- Encourage the child to drink generous amounts of fluids.
- Reestablish a regular diet as tolerated.
- Give pain medication (acetaminophen) as ordered for discomfort and at bedtime.
- Place drops in child's ears if prescribed.
- Restrict the child to quiet activities.

Following Postoperative Period

- Follow the care provider's instructions regarding swimming and water (some caution against swimming and other activities that might get water in ears; others do not).
- Ear plugs can be used to prevent water from getting into ears.
- Be alert for tubes becoming dislodged and falling out and alert care provider (they usually fall out within 1 year).
- Report purulent discharge from the ear, which may indicate a new ear infection. Contact the care provider.

Several nursing diagnoses that may apply are included in "Nursing Care Plan: The Child with Otitis Media." Additional nursing diagnoses might include the following:

- *Risk for Imbalanced Body Temperature: Hyperthermia* related to infectious process
- *Fatigue (Child and Parent)* related to sleep deprivation
- *Sensory/Perceptual Alteration Auditory* related to chronic ear infections and altered sensory reception

PLANNING AND IMPLEMENTATION

Most children with otitis media are not hospitalized; therefore, nursing management centers on care of the child in the home. The child having tympanostomy tubes inserted is generally treated in a day surgery setting. Occasionally, children admitted to the hospital for other problems have a concurrent ear infection. The accompanying Nursing Care Plan summarizes nursing care for the child with otitis media.

Emphasize preventive measures. Exposure to secondhand smoke in the home increases the incidence of otitis media in children, so encourage parents who smoke to avoid smoking near the child or in the home. If young children are in child care with fewer than 10 children, incidence decreases. Breastfeeding provides some protection from the disease. Placing babies to sleep with a pacifier may increase incidence and should be avoided in the infant with prior infections (Pelton, 2005). Many cases of otitis media are related to microbials such as *Haemophilus influenzae* and *Pneumococcal pneumoniae,* so immunization against these pathogens (see Chapter 45) can be effective preventive measures.

Help parents understand why there is a waiting period before prescriptions for antibiotics. When antibiotics are prescribed, review administration techniques, side effects, and the need for a repeat appointment when the medication is completed.

Chronic otitis media can create problems for the family. The child's waking at night with ear pain results in lack of sleep and parental fatigue. Parents often become frustrated and disillusioned by the healthcare system's inability to cure the child and may fear a permanent hearing impairment. Reassure parents that as the child grows older, the recurrent infections eventually cease. Teach them that asking for courses of antibiotics for every infection may not be the best treatment.

Provide pain relief techniques such as teaching correct administration of ear drops, oral administration of acetaminophen, and positioning the baby with the head slightly elevated. (See "Complementary Care: Naturopathic Extract for Ear Pain in Otitis Media.")

Provide hearing and language examinations at regular intervals, inform parents of results, and refer to an audiology specialist if hearing problems are identified. Make sure parents of children with tympanostomy tubes know how to care for the child and what symptoms to report. For the child with some hearing loss due to otitis media with effusion, a home environment that fosters cognitive skills can overcome the effects of lowered hearing during the time of infection. Focus interventions on helping parents to read and talk with children frequently who have otitis media with effusion.

Complementary Care

EAR WICKING

Some parents engage in a home treatment called "ear wicking" in which a specially designed candle with a narrow end is placed in the ear canal. The larger end remains outside the ear and is lit. As the candle burns slowly it is thought to "melt" ear wax so that it is easily removed. Dangers include burning of hair or skin, especially in young children who move during the procedure, and melting of candle wax into the ear which blocks the canal and must be surgically removed. Ear wicking should be discouraged for all, but especially in children.

Complementary Care

NATUROPATHIC EXTRACT FOR EAR PAIN IN OTITIS MEDIA

Since many children with otitis media experience ear pain that can disrupt their sleep and that of family members, anesthetic ear drops have been used for their analgesic effect on the tympanic membrane. Some families might prefer use of natural remedies for ear pain, such as Otikon (a naturopathic herbal extract of *Allium sativum, Verbascum thapsus, Calendula flores,* and *Hypericum peroforatum*) with a local anesthetic of ametocaine and phenazone. The naturopathic agent appears to be similar in effectiveness to anesthetic ear drops (Foxlee, Johansson, Wejfalk, et al., 2006; Sarrell, Mandelbery, & Cohen, 2003).

Nursing Care Plan

THE CHILD WITH OTITIS MEDIA

INTERVENTION	RATIONALE	EXPECTED OUTCOME
1. Nursing Diagnosis: Acute Pain related to inflammation and pressure on tympanic membrane		
NIC Priority Intervention: **Pain management:** Alleviation or reduction in pain to a level of comfort acceptable to patient and family		**NOC Suggested Outcome:** **Pain level:** Amount of reported or demonstrated pain
Goal: The child or parent will indicate absence of pain.		
■ Give analgesic such as acetaminophen. Use analgesic eardrops.	■ Analgesics alter perception or response to pain.	Verbal child states that pain is relieved. Nonverbal child has improved disposition and comfort.
■ Have the child sit up, raise head on pillows, or lie on unaffected ear.	■ Elevation decreases pressure from fluid.	
■ Apply warmth to the ear.	■ Heat increases blood supply and reduces discomfort.	
■ Have the child chew gum or blow on balloon to relieve pressure in ear.	■ Attempts to open the eustachian tube may help aerate the middle ear.	
2. Nursing Diagnosis: Infection related to presence of pathogens		
NIC Priority Intervention: **Infection control:** Minimizing the acquisition and transmission of infectious agents		**NOC Suggested Outcome:** **Risk control:** Actions to eliminate or reduce health threats
Goal: The child will be free of infection.		
■ Encourage breastfeeding of infants.	■ Breastfeeding affords natural immunity to infectious agents.	The child's temperature is normal, symptoms have disappeared, and tympanic membrane shows no signs of infection.
■ Instruct the parents to administer antibiotics exactly as directed and to complete prescribed course of medication.	■ Taking antibiotics as prescribed minimizes chance for overgrowth of pathogens.	
■ Telephone the parents 2 or 3 days after initial examination.	■ If symptoms have not improved in 36 hours, treatment should be evaluated.	
■ Examine ear 3 or 4 days after completion of antibiotic treatment, or if symptoms worsen in child on symptomatic treatment.	■ Checkup determines whether treatment is effective.	
3. Nursing Diagnosis: Risk for Delayed Growth and Development related to hearing loss		
NIC Priority Intervention: **Developmental enhancement:** Facilitating optimal growth and development of the child		**NOC Suggested Outcome:** **Growth and development:** Milestones of developmental progression
Goal: The child will have normal hearing.		
■ Assess hearing ability frequently.	■ Monitoring detects hearing loss early.	The child's general health and hearing improve, and incidence of condition decreases.
Goal: The child will have normal motor and language development.		
■ Assess motor and language development at each healthcare visit.	■ Early detection of developmental delays can lead to appropriate intervention.	The child has language and motor development within norms for age group.

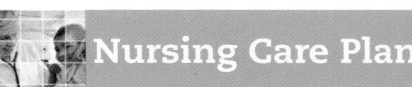

EVALUATION

Expected outcomes of nursing care for the child with otitis media include the following:

- Return to normal sleep and feeding patterns
- Maintenance of normal hearing and speech development
- Effective pain and temperature management
- Parental understanding of treatment regimen

OTITIS EXTERNA

Otitis externa is an inflammation of the skin and surrounding soft tissue of the ear canal. It is sometimes called "swimmer's ear" because it is common in children who swim frequently, especially during hot and muggy weather. The ear canal can also be injured by use of cotton-tipped applicators, foreign objects, or sprays used near the face. If the tympanic membrane is not intact because of tympanostomy tubes or breakage of the membrane, there may be drainage visible in the canal; this drainage may irritate the canal and lead to otitis externa. Any irritation of the canal can become infected with bacteria, virus, or fungi; sometimes it represents an allergic reaction. The child usually complains of pain and itching, and may have intense pain when the examiner presses on the tragus, or skin tab in front of the ear. Sometimes the ear appears swollen, and redness or drainage of the canal may be seen upon otoscopic examination.

Treatment of otitis externa requires removing the dried and flaking epithelium and cerumen. Burrows solutions or normal saline are used to irrigate and clean the canal if the tympanic membrane is intact. Steroid eardrops are used to decrease inflammation, and antibiotic drops are also used if a bacterial infection is suspected. If the child has tympanostomy tubes or a perforated tympanic membrane, non-ototoxic ear antibiotic such as quinolone antibiotic eardrops are used (Rosenfeld, Brown, Cannon, et al., 2006). Ibuprofen or acetaminophen may be helpful for pain control. The ear canal should then be kept dry by using ear plugs or a swim cap for swimming and gently blow-drying the canal after bathing. The child should not return to swimming for about 5 days. Cotton-tipped applicators or other objects should not be placed in the ear canal so that the skin in the canal can heal. If hair sprays or other solutions are irritating, they should not be used by the child or adolescent.

Nurses should be aware of the signs of otitis externa such as a painful ear, drainage, and irritated canal. Verify that the tympanic membrane is intact during otoscopic examination. Teach families to avoid the irritants identified such as cotton-tipped applicators, sprays, and frequent swimming. Demonstrate proper instillation of drops (see Clinical Skills Manual **SKILLS**) and give instructions for use of acetaminophen for pain relief in the acute period.

HEARING IMPAIRMENT

Approximately 1 million children (2 of every 100 births) in the United States have some form of hearing impairment (Moore, 2006; Yaeger, McCallum, Lewis, et al., 2006). Hearing impairment is expressed in terms of **decibels** (dB), which are units of loudness, and rated according to severity (Table 47–6). Children who have only a mild hearing loss (35 to 40 dB) may miss 50% of everyday conversation and are considered at high risk for school failure. Children with a hearing loss of more than 90 dB are considered legally deaf.

Table 47–6 Severity of Hearing Loss

Type of Loss	Hearing Ability
Slight/mild (20–40 dB)	Some speech sounds are difficult to perceive, particularly unvoiced consonant sounds
Moderate (41–60 dB)	Most normal conversational speech sounds are missed
Severe (61–80 dB)	Speech sounds cannot be heard at a normal conversational level
Profound (81–90 dB)	No speech sounds can be heard; considered legally deaf
Deaf (over 90 dB)	No sound at all can be heard

Source: Data from American Speech-Language-Hearing Association (2008). Type, degree, and configuration of hearing loss. Retrieved from www.asha.org/public/hearing/disorders/types.htm

Hearing disorders can be classified according to the location of the deficit. **Conductive hearing loss** occurs when conditions in the external auditory canal or tympanic membrane prevent sound from reaching the middle ear. **Sensorineural hearing loss** occurs when the hair cells in the cochlea or along the vestibulocochlear (acoustic) nerve (cranial nerve VIII) are damaged. This leads to permanent hearing loss. A **mixed hearing loss** indicates a hearing loss having a combination of conductive and sensorineural causes.

ETIOLOGY AND PATHOPHYSIOLOGY

About 50% of hearing loss is genetically caused, generally in a recessive inheritance pattern with GJB2 gene abnormalities (Yaeger et al., 2006). Another 25% is due to environmental causes around the time of birth (Weichbold, Nekahm-Heis, & Welzl-Mueller, 2006); the remainder is due to unknown causes. Infants at risk for hearing loss include those with:

- Family history of congenital hearing loss.
- Positive titer for TORCH infections (toxoplasmosis, rubella, cytomegalovirus, syphilis, herpes).
- Craniofacial abnormalities.
- Very low birth weight (less than 1500 g).
- Neonatal intensive care unit for over 5 days, or need for ECMO, assisted ventilation, administration of ototoxic medications (e.g., gentamycin, tobranycin) or loop diuretics (e.g., furosemide), or hyperbilirubinemia that requires exchange transfusion.

- Chemotherapy, particularly with aminoglycoside medications over 5 days.
- Low Apgar score at 1 or 5 minutes.
- Bacterial or viral meningitis.
- Head trauma, especially basal skull/temporal bone fractures requiring hospitalization.
- Caregiver concern regarding speech, language, hearing, developmental delay.
- Presence of syndromes associated with hearing loss (Down syndrome, Pierre Robin syndrome, Arnold-Chiari malformation) (Joint Committee on Infant Hearing, 2007).

Common causes of conductive hearing loss include impacted cerumen, the most frequent reason for conductive loss; outer ear infection ("swimmer's ear"); trauma; or a foreign body. Conductive loss also occurs if the tympanic membrane does not fully vibrate, as in otitis media. In these cases hearing loss may be restored after the infection clears. Chronic and untreated ear infections may lead to ear structural changes and permanent hearing impairment. The loss of acuity may be gradual or rapid and results in diminished hearing in all ranges.

Conditions leading to sensorineural hearing loss may be congenital (maternal rubella), genetic (Tay-Sachs disease), or acquired (such as from ototoxic drugs, bacterial meningitis, or loud noise). In sensorineural hearing loss, high-frequency sounds are most affected. Such hearing loss may be preceded by **tinnitus** or ringing in the ears. Teenagers who use earphones at high volumes or attend many rock concerts are at risk for hearing loss (Figure 47–7 ●). Other noise hazards include firecrackers, guns, and power and farm equipment.

Table 47–7 Behaviors Suggestive of Hearing Impairment

Age	Behavior
Infant	Has a diminished or absent startle reflex to loud sound Does not awaken when environment is very noisy Awakens only to touch Does not turn head to sound at 3–4 months Does not localize sound at 6–10 months Babbles little or not at all
Toddler and preschooler	Speaks unintelligibly, in a monotone, or not at all Communicates needs through gestures Appears developmentally delayed Appears emotionally immature, yells inappropriately Does not respond to doorbell or telephone Appears more interested in objects than people and prefers to play alone Focuses on facial expressions rather than verbal communications
School-age child and adolescent	Asks to have statements repeated Answers questions inappropriately, except when able to view speaker's face Daydreams and is inattentive Performs poorly at school or is truant Has speech abnormalities or speaks in a monotone Sits close to or turns television or radio up loudly Prefers to play alone

CLINICAL MANIFESTATIONS

Hearing is both an innate and a learned behavior. Infants and children who are hearing impaired exhibit a range of behaviors, depending on their age and the severity of the deficit. Infants who hear normally respond to sound in both obvious and subtle ways that do not occur in those who are hearing impaired (Table 47–7). As children mature, their hearing impairments affect their language skills. Hearing loss is often manifested as a cognitive deficit, a behavioral problem, or both.

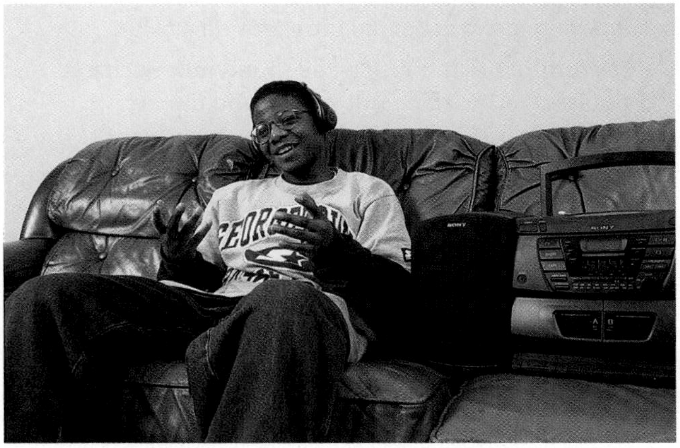

● **Figure 47–7** A frequent cause of hearing loss. Listening to loud music with headphones or at rock concerts is a frequent cause of hearing loss among teenagers and young adults. This adolescent needs to be informed about the possible outcomes of this activity.

CLINICAL THERAPY

Early identification of hearing loss is a key element in successful treatment (see "Growth and Development: Hearing Loss"). Detection of hearing loss in infants is important to ensure optimal development. Universal screening of all infants is recommended before 1 month of age, with diagnostic audiologic evaluation before 3 months, and beginning of early intervention programs by 6 months of age for those with hearing impairment (Connolly, Carron, & Roark, 2005; Windmill & Windmill, 2006). Many state laws now mandate screening of newborns. Observations of response to noise in all newborns should be accompanied by more sophisticated testing such as auditory brain stem response or transient evoked otoacoustic emissions, especially in those at high risk of deficits (Figure 47–8 ●). See Table 47–8.

An otoscopic examination with a tympanogram can be performed on an older infant to determine conductive hearing loss.

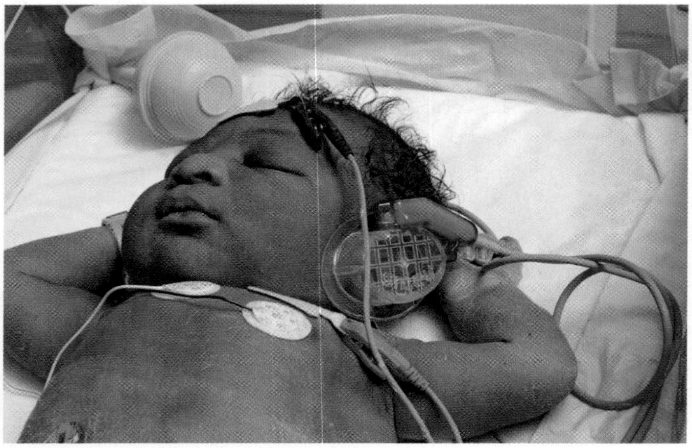

● **Figure 47–8** Newborn hearing screening. Newborn hearing screening is an effective tool in diagnosing some causes of hearing impairment very early in life.

Table 47–8 Screening Tests for Newborn Hearing

Test	Mechanism of Action
Otoacoustive emission (OAE) (either transient-evoked [TEOAE] or distortion-product [DPOAE])	A measure of low-intensity sounds from the cochlear hair cells in response to clicks from a probe placed in the ear canal Sensitive in frequency range above 1500 Hz May show false negative for loss below 1000–1500 Hz Detects inner ear hearing loss by evaluating cochlear and hair cell function Does not detect neural damage to 8th cranial nerve Can be sensitive to outer ear canal obstruction or middle ear effusion, leading to false positive result
Auditory brainstem response (ABR)	Electrical response to auditory stimuli from three surface scalp electrodes Reflects activity of cochlea, cranial nerve VIII, and auditory brainstem pathways Detects hearing loss from 1000 to 8000 Hz May show false negative results for losses in the 500–2000 Hz levels Will give a positive result if there is damage to cranial nerve VIII or brainstem pathways even if cochlear loss is not present

The **tympanogram** is a test that provides a graph of the ability of the middle ear to transmit sound. An airtight probe is inserted into the external ear canal and a tone is emitted. The probe measures the pressure, which is plotted on a graph. A "flat" tympanogram suggests conductive hearing loss. **Audiography** can be used with cooperative children over 3 years of age. Sounds of various frequencies and intensities are presented to the child through earphones, and the child is instructed to raise his or her hand when the sound is heard. Audiography cannot detect hearing loss caused by middle ear effusion but can indicate sensorineural loss.

Growth and Development

Children with hearing loss can easily fall behind their peers in language milestones since they cannot hear and speak in the same manner as other children. Without interventions to enable them to learn language, they can also fail to develop reading, literacy skills, related cognitive processes, and social-emotional development (Joint Committee on Infant Hearing, 2007). Carefully evaluate hearing and all developmental milestones during each regularly scheduled healthcare visit. Refer infants and children with abnormalities for further evaluation. When hearing loss is identified as a cause of delayed development, interventions guided by healthcare professionals with expertise in hearing loss are needed.

The hearing of preschool and school-age children is tested by asking them to repeat whispered words. Hearing of school-age children and adolescents also is assessed with the Weber and Rinne tests (see Chapter 35).

If a hearing loss is uncorrectable, a multidisciplinary team composed of pediatrician, audiologist, otolaryngologist, speech–language pathologist, nurse, teacher, and social worker should help the child and family adapt to the disability. If the deficit is due to recurrent ear infections, tympanostomy tube insertion may improve hearing.

A hearing aid may be prescribed for a conductive loss. A sensorineural loss is more difficult to treat, but cochlear implants and bone conduction hearing aids have been used in some children. A cochlear implant is a small electronic device that helps to provide sound for those who are deaf or profoundly hard of hearing (National Institutes of Health, 2006; National Institutes of Health, 2007). It consists of the following:

1. A microphone to pick up sound that is located outside of the body; worn as a headpiece behind the ear
2. A speech processor which organizes sound from the microphone; worn behind the ear or on a belt
3. A transmitter that transfers the sound into electrical impulses; part of the headpiece behind the ear
4. Electrodes that send the signals to the brain; this receiver is implanted in the skin behind the ear with a wire leading to the cochlear fluid in the middle ear

Growth and Development

Infants and young children respond automatically with a blink or the startle reflex to unexpected or loud noises. As they mature, they localize the sound source, then understand speech, and then communicate verbally.

Table 47–9 Communication Techniques for Children Who Are Hearing Impaired

Technique	Description
Cued speech	Supplement to lipreading; eight hand shapes represent groups of consonant sounds and four positions about the face represent groups of vowel sounds; based on the sounds the letters make, not the letters themselves; child can "see-hear" every spoken syllable a hearing person hears
Oral approach	Uses only spoken language for face-to-face communication; avoids use of formal signs; uses hearing aids and residual hearing
Total communication	Uses speech and sign, fingerspelling, lipreading, and residual hearing simultaneously; child selects communication technique depending on the situation

For children with uncorrectable hearing loss, several approaches are used to enhance communication (Table 47–9). Children with hearing impairment may receive speech therapy and instructions in lipreading, sign language, cuing, and fingerspelling.

NURSING MANAGEMENT

NURSING ASSESSMENT AND DIAGNOSIS

Nurses conduct newborn hearing tests soon after birth and make observations of the infant's responses to sound. As the child grows, assess hearing at every well-child visit. The best judges of hearing are parents; ask them if they have any concerns about their child's hearing. An infant's reaction to rattles, bells, or handclapping (about 12 in. [30 cm] from the ear) is an important observation. Evaluate language milestones when examining the older infant and child. Language development is a major area of focus in deaf children. Deaf infants begin to babble at about 5 to 6 months of age, the same age as hearing infants. However, this babbling ceases several months later in the hearing-impaired child.

School nurses use audiometers to evaluate hearing during screening programs in schools, and refer children who do not pass the screening test (see Skills 9–20 and 9–21 SKILLS). Measures to promote speech and communication development as well as safety are implemented.

Common nursing diagnoses for the child with impaired hearing include the following:

- *Disturbed Sensory/Perception (Auditory)* related to abnormal sound transmission
- *Risk for Impaired Verbal Communication* related to hearing loss
- *Risk for Delayed Growth and Development* related to communication impairment
- *Readiness for Enhanced Family Coping* related to caring for a child with a hearing impairment

PLANNING AND IMPLEMENTATION

Nurses can encourage prevention of hearing loss from exposure to loud noises such as loud music and power and farm equipment. Music should be turned down and ear protection worn for other activities. School nurses should be active in hearing conservation education programs in school. Several programs are available to assist the school nurse in teaching children at targeted ages about noise-induced hearing loss. The nurse should develop and deliver hearing conservation curricula to children at elementary, middle, and high school levels; inform teachers and other professionals about noise-induced hearing loss; and train volunteers to assist with school programs.

Newborn screening, developmental assessment, and childhood hearing screening facilitate identification of hearing loss in infants and children. Infants should be tested for hearing loss by 1 month of age. In cases of loss, intervention should begin before 6 months of age (Joint Committee on Infant Hearing, 2007).

Nursing care of the child with a hearing impairment focuses on facilitating the child's ability to receive spoken language and to send information, helping parents meet the child's schooling needs, and providing emotional support to parents. Refer the parents to an early intervention program as soon as the diagnosis of hearing impairment is made, in order to foster the child's development. If a cochlear implant is planned, the child needs surgical care and follow-up to monitor results and integrate sound gradually into the child's life. Pneumococcal and meningococcal vaccines and ongoing speech therapy are needed (Wilson-Clark, Squires, & Deeks, 2006).

FACILITATE ABILITY TO RECEIVE SPOKEN LANGUAGE

Be aware of how the child compensates for hearing loss and use these strategies in communication.

- If hearing loss is mild or temporary or if the child reads lips, first obtain the child's visual attention by lightly touching the child or saying the child's name.
- Position your face 3 to 6 ft (1 to 2 m) from the child's face and make sure that the child's eyes are focused on your face and lips. Make sure the room is well lit, with no backlighting. Speak at a normal rate and tone, and use facial expressions that show caring or concern. If the child does not understand, rephrase the information in shorter, simpler sentences. Use specific, concrete explanations, and give the child time to comprehend. Watch for subtle signs of misinterpretations and give consistent and immediate feedback since only 30% of the English language is visible on the lips.
- Be familiar with the different types of hearing aids. Hearing aids, which are microphones that amplify all sounds, can be worn in or behind the ear, in the frame of glasses, or on the

body with a wire attached to the ear. Place the hearing aid in the ear with the volume off, then slowly turn up to half volume. Adjust as needed. When talking to a child with a hearing aid, speak slowly within 6 to 18 inches (15 to 45 cm) from the microphone using a normal conversational tone. Talk to the child even if the child is not looking at you. Make sure the batteries are fresh for the best reception. Since all sound is amplified, reduce background noise as much as possible. Clean the hearing aid daily with a damp cloth. Change the batteries as needed, usually about once a week. The child's growth necessitates a new fitting, usually about once annually.

Acoustic feedback, an audible whistling sound that cannot always be heard by the child, is one of the most common problems with hearing aids. To eliminate this sound, readjust the hearing aid to make sure that it is inserted properly and that no hair or ear wax is caught between the ear mold and canal. Turning down the volume may also help. (See "Health Promotion: The Child with a Hearing Impairment.")

A remote microphone system is another type of device designed to improve hearing. This is often used in the classroom situation because it eliminates background noise. The speaker wears a transmitter that picks up the voice and transmits it to a receiver worn by the child.

FACILITATE ABILITY TO SEND INFORMATION

Maintain the child's hearing aid in proper condition. Many children with impaired hearing communicate using speech, which is

HEALTH PROMOTION

THE CHILD WITH A HEARING IMPAIRMENT

Growth and Developmental Surveillance

- Ensure that the child receives all immunizations at scheduled times. All children with cochlear implants should have pneumococcal vaccine (PCV7 for under 5 years or PPV23 for over 5 years). The immunization should be completed 2 weeks before surgery for cochlear implant. Children should be up to date on all immunizations, but rubella, mumps, and measles are especially important since infections with the diseases could cause further hearing loss.
- Complete developmental assessment, including receptive and expressive verbal skills at each visit.
- Teach about safety precautions for those with hearing impairment, such as inability to hear announcements at school, fire alarms at home, or sirens when in travel. Assist the family to install visual stimuli for fire alarms and other safety needs.

Communication

- Review the type of communication used by the child and the family's satisfaction.
- Ask about relationships with other children, both hearing impaired and those with normal hearing.

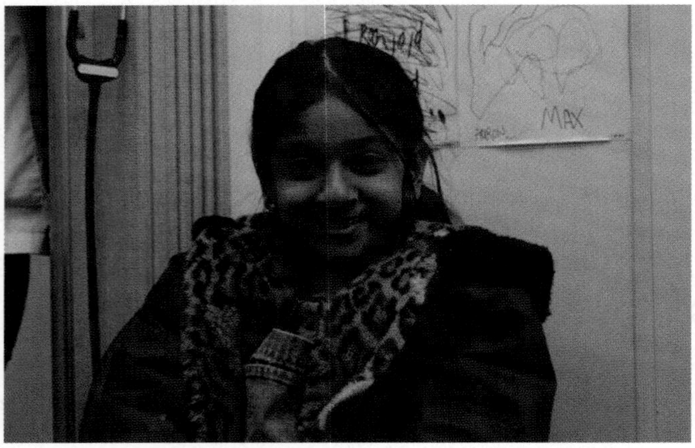

- Review discipline techniques used by the parents and consistency of limit setting.

Nutrition and Physical Activity

- Complete 24-hour diet recall and be sure the child receives adequate nutrition appropriate in energy for activities.
- Review the child's exercise patterns since some children with hearing impairment may avoid interactions with other children in sports.
- Refer the family to community activity programs as needed.

Mental Health

- Find out stressors parents may feel.
- Locate community resources for early intervention and ongoing programs.
- Assist the youth and family to plan for moves to new schools and communities, and for plans related to transition to young adulthood, including college, trade schools, or work in the community.

Disease Prevention Strategies

- Be sure signs of ear infection such as fever, irritability, disturbed sleep, rubbing ear, or ear drainage are promptly evaluated in the pediatric healthcare home.
- Teach parents to administer antibiotics for ear infections exactly as prescribed.
- Encourage breastfeeding of infants and avoiding smoking to minimize incidence of ear infections.
- Be sure the child has all recommended immunizations.

Injury Prevention Strategies

- Encourage family to preserve any hearing the child may have by avoiding exposure to loud sounds; when children are old enough to understand, be sure they safeguard against exposure to loud music, guns, and other risks.
- Teach the child and family to plan for safety when crossing streets, driving cars, escaping house fires, and other situations that normally rely on hearing.

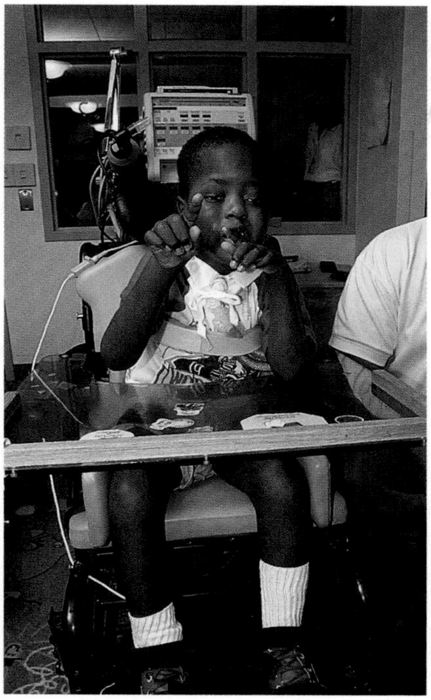

● **Figure 47–9** Communicating with American Sign Language (ASL). This child with a hearing impairment and tracheostomy is communicating by means of American Sign Language.

enhanced through speech therapy. In addition they are taught to sign, fingerspell, or use cued speech (Figure 47–9 ●). Articulation may be difficult, and understanding what the child is trying to say may be frustrating for both the nurse and the child. Taking time to listen carefully is important.

Take measures to promote speech and communication development as well as safety. Ask the parents to explain the child's communication techniques and to help interpret words. Have younger children point to pictures. Use assisted technologies such as a computer or picture board as well as drawings or gestures if necessary. This is especially helpful for communicating feelings of pain and hunger during hospitalization. If the child signs or fingerspells, make sure that you understand the signs for important functions. Give older children a pad of paper and pencil to write requests. People other than parents should be able to understand what the child is trying to communicate. Have an interpreter available if the child uses American Sign Language. Learn some common signs to communicate simple words or phrases. Orient the child carefully to new settings such as the hospital room or a new school.

HELP PARENTS TO MEET CHILD'S EDUCATIONAL NEEDS

Public laws apply to the education of children who are hearing impaired (see Chapter 1∞). After diagnosis, the parents and professionals together agree on an individualized education plan (see discussion in Chapter 39∞). Day care and preschool are recommended for children with hearing problems.

- Give parents information about adjustments that may have to be made for the hearing-impaired child who attends public school. By sitting at the front of the classroom, the child can hear and see more clearly. The teacher should always face the child when speaking, and background noise should be reduced.
- Tell parents that children who are hearing impaired have the same intelligence quotient (IQ) distribution as children without hearing impairment. However, communication and learning can be difficult, and extra support is needed.
- Children with hearing impairment should reach their intellectual potential, although development in certain areas may take place more slowly than it does in non-hearing-impaired children.

PROVIDE EMOTIONAL SUPPORT

By recognizing the effects of the diagnosis on the family, the nurse can help the family deal with their reaction to the child's hearing loss. Supporting healthy coping is an important intervention to help the parents carry on with their lives.

- Help the parents understand the child's disability and its effect on speech and language development. Provide accurate information about their concerns. Work jointly with other healthcare professionals and social service workers if necessary.
- Tell the family about the community services available for medical, nursing, psychologic, and financial assistance.

EVALUATION

Expected outcomes of nursing care for a child with hearing impairment include the following:

- Successful establishment of communication method
- Growth and development to maximum potential
- Establishment of successful individualized education plan
- Positive family coping

INJURIES OF THE EAR

Ear injuries of many types commonly occur in children. Lacerations, infections, and hematomas may occur in the external ear structures, especially the pinna. Children may place foreign objects in the ear, and insects may enter the ear canal. Rupture of the tympanic membrane may result from head injuries, blows to the ear, or insertion of objects into the ear canal. Caution children and parents not to place anything into the ear, including cotton swabs for cleaning.

See Table 47–10 for information on the emergency treatment of ear injuries. Any injury resulting in earache, decreased hearing, persistent bleeding, or other discharge should be seen by a physician.

Table 47–10 Emergency Treatment of Ear Injuries

Injury	Treatment
PINNA	
Minor cuts or abrasions	Wash thoroughly with soap and water and rinse well; leave exposed to air if possible or apply adhesive bandage; monitor for infection.
Hematomas	Needle aspiration should be performed and pressure dressing applied; undrained hematomas may become fibrotic; "cauliflower ear" deformity may develop.
Cellulitis or abscesses	Apply moist heat intermittently; make sure that prescribed antibiotic is taken; minor surgery may be performed for an abscess.
Deep lacerations	Apply pressure to stop bleeding; transport to physician's office or emergency department for suturing.
EAR CANAL	
Foreign bodies	Have child lie on back and turn head over edge of bed, with affected side down; wiggle earlobe and have child shake head; foreign object may fall out as result of gravity; if object remains in ear, call physician; do not try to remove foreign body with tweezers since this may push the object further into the ear.
Insects	Shine flashlights into ear to try to attract insect; instilling a few drops of mineral oil, olive oil, or alcohol kills insect, and irrigating ear canal gently may remove dead insect. See Skill 11–9 SKILLS.
TYMPANIC MEMBRANE	
Ruptures	Call physician if child has persistent ear pain after blow, blast injury, or insertion of foreign object; cover external ear loosely with piece of sterile cotton or gauze; if tympanic membrane has been ruptured, systemic antibiotics are prescribed.

DISORDERS OF THE NOSE, THROAT, AND MOUTH

EPISTAXIS

Epistaxis, or nosebleed, is common in school-age children, especially boys. Kiesselbach's plexus, an area of plentiful veins located in the anterior nares, is the most common source of bleeding. The most common cause is irritation from nosepicking, foreign bodies, or low humidity. Other causes include forceful coughing, allergies, or infections resulting in congestion of the nasal mucosa. Posterior nosebleeds have a variety of causes, some of which may indicate systemic disease (i.e., bleeding disorder) or injury. Bleeding from the posterior septum is more serious and may be life threatening. Hospitalization may be necessary.

Nursing Management

Children with nosebleeds are sometimes brought to the emergency department by a parent who has been unable to stop the flow of blood within a few minutes. Both parent and child may be frightened. Ask the parent briefly about any history of nosebleeds and other contributing factors, including medications. Take the child's pulse and blood pressure to assess for excessive blood loss. Carefully examine the nasal mucosa by asking the child to blow any clots out gently, if possible. Suctioning may be necessary.

Observing the flow may help determine whether the blood is coming from an anterior or a posterior location. A nosebleed confined to one side of the nose is almost always anterior, but posterior bleeding can flow on one or both sides. If blood cannot be seen, the child may be swallowing it and may become nauseated. Suspect posterior bleeding in children who have sustained blunt trauma to the head.

The child with anterior bleeding should sit upright quietly. The head should be tilted forward to prevent blood from trickling down the throat, which can lead to vomiting. The nares should be squeezed just below the nasal bone and held for 10 to 15 minutes while the child breathes through the mouth. If the bleeding does not stop, a cotton ball or swab soaked with Neo-Synephrine, epinephrine, thrombin, or lidocaine may be inserted into the affected nostril to promote topical vasoconstriction or anesthesia. Once the bleeding has stopped, the nostril may have to be cauterized with silver nitrate or electrocautery. If the bleeding cannot be stopped, absorbable packing may be used.

Posterior bleeding must also be stopped by packing, and the child must be monitored carefully. Arterial ligation is occasionally needed. Repeated or severe nosebleeds need further evaluation (Bernius & Perlin, 2006).

Assess the child's hematocrit or hemoglobin if significant bleeding has occurred. Take a complete history and do a physical examination of children with frequent epistaxis to rule out systemic disease. (See "Teaching Highlights: Prevention and Home Management of Epistaxis.")

After the nosebleed has stopped, the child is more vulnerable to recurrent bleeding and should avoid bending over, stooping, strenuous exercise, hot drinks, and hot baths or showers for the next 3 to 4 days. Sleeping with the head elevated on two or three pillows and humidifying the air with a vaporizer may also prevent a recurrence. Give parents suggestions for prevention and home management of epistaxis.

Teaching Highlights

PREVENTION AND HOME MANAGEMENT OF EPISTAXIS

Prevention

- Humidify the child's room, especially during the winter.
- Discourage the child from picking or rubbing the nose or inserting foreign objects in the nose.
- Instruct the child to blow the nose gently and release sneezes through the mouth.

Home Management

- Keep the child calm.
- Sit the child upright with head tilted slightly forward so blood does not run down the throat.
- Press a roll of cotton under the upper lip to compress the labial artery.
- Apply steady pressure to both nostrils just below the nasal bone with the thumb and forefinger for 15 to 20 minutes. Time by the clock.
- Apply an ice pack or cold compress to the bridge of the nose or the back of the neck.
- Call healthcare provider if the bleeding does not stop.
- Avoid vigorous exercise and aspirin or other noncoagulant drugs during the first few days after an episode of epistaxis.

Data from Health Care Guide, 2006

NASOPHARYNGITIS

Nasopharyngitis, also known as upper respiratory infection (URI) or the "common cold," causes inflammation and infection of the nose and throat and is a common illness of infancy and childhood. More than 200 viruses and numerous bacteria can cause this condition. The most common viruses include rhinovirus and coronavirus, and the most frequently occurring bacterium is group A *Streptococcus*. See Chapter 48 for a discussion of respiratory syncytial virus (RSV), a common cause of both upper and lower respiratory illness. The organisms incubate in 1 to 3 days, and the infection is communicable several hours before symptoms develop and for 1 to 2 days after they begin. Symptoms may last 4 to 10 days or longer. The pathogens spread when the infected person touches the hand of an uninfected person, who then touches his or her mouth or nose, resulting in self-inoculation with infected droplets.

A red nasal mucosa with clear nasal discharge and an infected throat with enlarged tonsils may be apparent in children with nasopharyngitis. Vesicles may be present on the soft palate and in the pharynx. Accompanying symptoms may vary, depending on the child's age (Table 47–11).

Between episodes of nasopharyngitis, the child should be asymptomatic. If a child continues to have upper respiratory infections, an underlying condition such as allergy, asthma, or polyps should be ruled out.

Table 47–11 Manifestations of Nasopharyngitis

Infants Younger Than 3 Months of Age	
Lethargy	Feeding poorly
Irritability	Fever (may be absent)
Infants 3 Months of Age or Older	
Fever	Anorexia
Vomiting	Irritability
Diarrhea	Restlessness
Sneezing	
Older Children	
Dry, irritated nose and throat	
Chills, fever	
Generalized muscle aches	
Headache	
Malaise	
Anorexia	
Thin nasal discharge, which may later become thick and purulent	
Sneezing	

Nursing Management

For infants who cannot breathe through the mouth, normal saline nose drops can be administered every 3 to 4 hours, especially before feeding (see Skill 11–10 SKILLS). For infants over 9 months of age, nasal stuffiness can be treated with normal saline nose. Children over 6 years of age can use nasal sprays.

Decongestant nose drops and sprays should not be used for more than 4 or 5 days or more often than recommended. Antihistamines may be helpful for children with allergic rhinitis or profuse nasal drainage. Long-acting nasal sprays and medications with several ingredients are not recommended. (See "Teaching Highlights: Over-the-Counter Cough and Cold Medications.")

Room humidification may help prevent drying of nasal secretions. Antipyretics such as acetaminophen reduce fever and make the child more comfortable. Aspirin is not recommended because of its association with Reye syndrome (refer to Chapter 56).

Children should avoid strenuous physical activity and engage in quiet play such as reading, listening to music or stories, or watching television or videotapes. Children should not be forced to eat. Encourage the intake of favorite fluids to liquify secretions. Tell parents that no medicine or vaccine can prevent the common cold, but eliminating contact with infected persons can reduce the spread of infection. Proper hand hygiene and disposal of tissues helps to decrease the spread of the infection. Cleaning counters, toys, door knobs, and other surfaces on a daily basis can decrease the spread of infections. Discourage sharing of food, dishes, and utensils at meals.

Teaching Highlights

OVER-THE-COUNTER COUGH AND COLD MEDICATIONS

Parents may try to treat children who have upper respiratory infections with the same medications they are accustomed to taking for a cold. Work with parents during a health promotion visit and help them plan for how to handle medications for the child. Guidelines are as follows:

- Do NOT use cough and cold products in children under 2 years unless given specific directions to do so by a healthcare provider.
- Read the label to be sure the medication is recommended for the child's age and condition. Give only the dose recommended for the age and weight of the child. Do NOT use products packaged for adults.
- Be sure you know how to measure the medication. Tablespoon and teaspoon are *not* the same, and using household spoons may lead to incorrect dosing. Use the measuring device that is provided with liquid medications for greatest accuracy. If one is not provided, purchase one at the pharmacy that is precisely labeled. Use only a measuring device with the precise marking to match the dose you need to give.
- Consult the pharmacist, nurse, or doctor if you have questions, if the child is taking other medicines, if the medication is not recommended for the age of your child, if the child's condition does not improve, or if other symptoms appear.
- Use the child-resistant cap after each opening of the bottle. Store the medication out of reach of all children, preferably in a locked location.
- Inspect containers and do not buy those that may have tears, imperfections, or tampering. Review all of the information in the "Drug Facts" box on the package label.
- If you use home remedies or other herbal products to treat colds, be sure to check on their safety with your healthcare provider first.

If the child becomes more ill or does not improve, stop the medicine and contact the healthcare provider. If you do not understand instructions on the package contact a healthcare provider before using it.

Adapted from U.S. Food and Drug Administration. *Got a sick kid?* Retrieved from www.fda.gov/cder/consumerinfo/sickkids.htm; and U.S. Food and Drug Administration. *Public Health Advisory—Nonprescription Cough and Cold Medicine Use in Children.* Retrieved from www.fda.gov/cder/drug/advisory/cough_cold.htm

Developing Cultural Competence

HOT AND COLD DISEASE THEORY

Many Hispanic and Asian cultural groups believe in the "hot and cold theory" of disease, in which health problems are viewed as the result of imbalance. For example, some Mexican Americans traditionally treat a "cold disease" such as an earache or common cold with "hot" substances. Ask families if they prefer to eat certain foods or use complementary treatments during an illness. Incorporating such preferences may help the child and increase the confidence of the family in healthcare providers.

SINUSITIS

Sinusitis is an inflammation of one or more of the paranasal sinuses. These sinuses, which have respiratory epithelium and are continuous with the respiratory tract, include the maxillary, ethmoid, frontal, and sphenoid sinuses. The sinuses may become infected with bacteria following a viral upper respiratory infection. Of the 6–8 respiratory infections children get annually, 5% to 10% of them are followed by sinusitis (Demetroulakos, 2007; Taylor, 2006). In most cases, the child's history reveals a cold for several days, followed by improvement in the cold symptoms but an increase in purulent nasal drainage. There is accompanying facial pain, headache, and fever. Chronic sinusitis may occur in children with uncontrolled allergies and asthma.

Signs and symptoms of sinusitis in children are sometimes nonspecific. A history of recent upper respiratory infection is common, persistent cough from postnasal drip can occur, and nasal discharge or swelling can be apparent. Malodorous breath, fever, mouth breathing, hyponasal speech, and cervical lymphadenopathy may be present (Bernius & Perlin, 2006). Young children may be anorexic or have difficulty feeding, and older children may complain of headache.

Diagnosis of sinusitis is usually based on history and physical examination findings. Percussion and illumination of sinuses are not generally useful in children. Computed tomography (CT), magnetic resonance imaging (MRI), and x-rays may be done but they can be costly and require sedation of young children and results may not be conclusive. For the child with repeated sinusitis or who appears toxic, aspiration of sinus aspirate may be performed for culture by an otolaryngologist.

Although most primary care providers treat suspected sinusitis with antibiotics, many cases will clear spontaneously without treatment. Amoxicillin is the first choice for therapy; amoxicillin/clavulanate, cephalosporins, azithromycin, and clindamycin are also sometimes used (Bernius & Perlin, 2006). Children with recurrent sinusitis should be referred for further care by an otolaryngologist and allergy specialist.

Parents whose child has persistent and purulent nasal drainage should be told to see a healthcare provider, particularly if the drainage is accompanied by facial pain, headache, and fever. Nurses should teach parents to correctly administer antibiotics (e.g., to take medications for the full course) if prescribed, and to use saline nose drops if needed for comfort. Infants may need their noses cleared with nose drops and a bulb syringe prior to feedings. (Refer to the Clinical Skills Manual **SKILLS** for correct use of a bulb syringe.) Antipyretics can be given for fever and to relieve pain.

PHARYNGITIS

Acute pharyngitis is an infection that primarily affects the pharynx, including the tonsils. It is seen most frequently in children 4 to 7 years of age and is rare in children less than 1 year of age. Approximately 80% of these infections are caused by viruses; the rest are caused by bacteria. Bacterial pharyngitis is commonly known as "strep throat," since in many cases it is caused by group A beta-hemolytic streptococcus (GABHS) (Armengol, Hendley, & Schlare, 2006).

The major complaint is a sore throat. See "Clinical Manifestations: Viral Pharyngitis, Strep Throat, Peritonsillar Abscess, and Retropharyngeal Abscess." Children with symptoms of strep throat who have minimal throat redness and pain, exudate, mild lymphadenopathy, and a low-grade fever, and who have been exposed to someone who has strep pharyngitis should have a throat culture. The classic signs of purulent drainage and white patches are not present in all cases of strep throat.

A child who finds swallowing difficult or extremely painful, who drools, or who exhibits signs of dehydration or respiratory distress should be seen by a physician immediately. These signs could be indicators of serious conditions such as peritonsillar or retropharyngeal abscess, epiglottitis (Chapter 48∞), or diphtheria (Chapter 45∞).

Peritonsillar abscess (a tonsil infection that spreads into surrounding tissues and causes cellulites) or retropharyngeal abscess (an infection of the lymph nodes that drain the adenoids, nasopharynx, and paranasal sinuses) are serious conditions. These conditions may have additional symptoms such as decreased neck movement, neck edema or pain, and respiratory distress (Dudas, 2006). CT scan or MRI may be helpful in diagnosis of abscess. See the Clinical Manifestations table below for manifestations of viral pharyngitis, strep throat, peritonsillar abscess, and retropharyngeal abscess.

The diagnosis of strep throat is made by throat culture, using the rapid or traditional strep tests (see Skill 10–5 **SKILLS**). Results of the rapid strep test may be available within minutes; those for the traditional test are available in 24 to 48 hours. A negative rapid test is followed by a traditional test in order to verify results. (See "Nursing Practice: Throat Cultures.")

Streptococcus pharyngitis is treated with oral penicillin for 10 days or with long-acting penicillin given in one injection. If the child is allergic to penicillin, erythromycin, azithromycin, or clarithromycin is given. Acute symptoms should resolve within 24 hours of therapy, at which time the child is no longer contagious. For viral pharyngitis, symptomatic treatment alone is used.

Peritonsillar abscess is treated by draining the abscess, providing antibiotics effective in treating the fluid cultured from the abscess, and hydration. Commonly administered antibiotics include ampicillin/sulbactam, penicillin G, and clindamycin. Once treatment has been achieved, the child is evaluated for possible tonsillectomy (Galito, 2008). Retrophyarngeal abscess is also frequently treated by drainage of the

MyNursingKit Nursing in Action: Child with a Sore Throat

Nursing Practice

Throat cultures must be properly performed for accurate diagnosis. Swab a sterile cotton-tip applicator across the tonsils, posterior edge of the soft palate, and uvula. Ask cooperative children to put their hands under their buttocks, open their mouth, and laugh or pant like a dog. Quickly swab the throat. You can place uncooperative and young children on their backs with their hands next to their heads and have a parent or an assistant hold them. Depress the tongue gently with a tongue blade and swab the throat and both tonsils.

Clinical Manifestations

VIRAL PHARYNGITIS, STREP THROAT (GROUP A BETA-HEMOLYTIC STREPTOCOCCUS [GABHS]),[a] PERITONSILLAR ABSCESS, AND RETROPHARYNGEAL ABSCESS

VIRAL PHARYNGITIS	STREP THROAT	PERITONSILLAR ABSCESS	RETROPHARYNGEAL ABSCESS
Nasal congestion	Abrupt onset	Fever	Fever
Mild sore throat	Tonsillar exudate[b]	Malaise	Sore throat
Conjunctivitis	Painful cervical lymphadenopathy[b]	Sore throat, more severe on one side	Inability to eat
Cough	Anorexia, nausea, vomiting, abdominal pain	Marked erythema and edema, especially of one side of throat and soft palate	Neck pain and edema
Hoarseness	Severe sore throat	Mouth odor	Pharyngitis
Mild pharyngeal redness	Headache, malaise	Difficulty speaking	Respiratory distress and stridor
Minimal tonsillar exudate	Fever > 38.3°C (101°F)	Difficulty opening mouth wide	
Mildly tender anterior cervical lymphadenopathy	Petechial mottling of soft palate	Cervical lymphadenitis	
Fever < 38.3°C (101°F)		Ear pain	

[a]Children 6 months to 3 years of age may have streptococcus with symptoms that resemble those of viral pharyngitis. Children with scarlet fever have the symptoms of strep throat plus a sandpaper-textured erythematous generalized rash and pallor around the lips.
[b]Classic signs of strep throat.
Data from Galito, N. J. (2008). Peritonsillar Abscess. *American Family Physician, 77*, 199–202, 209; Dudas, R. (2006). Retrophyarngeal Abscess. *Pediatrics in Review, 27*, 345–346.

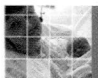

abscess, although intravenous antibiotics alone are effective in some cases. Ampicillin/sulbactam, clindamycin, cephalosporin, and penicillin are common antibiotics. Respiratory management may be needed (Dudas, 2006; Page, Bauer, & Lieu, 2008).

Nursing Management

Nursing care focuses on symptomatic relief. Acetaminophen reduces throat pain and generalized fever. Cool, nonacidic fluids and soft foods, ice chips, or frozen juice pops given frequently in small amounts facilitate swallowing and prevent dehydration. Humidification, chewing gum, and gargling with warm salt water (1 teaspoon [5 g] salt to 8 oz [250 mL] water) soothe an irritated throat. Alternatively, the salt water can be placed in a spray bottle and sprayed gently toward the throat. Commercial throat sprays or throat lozenges are not generally more effective than these home remedies. Encourage the child to rest, to conserve energy and promote recovery.

Teach parents the importance of completing the 10-day course of antibiotics if prescribed for bacterial pharyngitis. Reinforce to parents the importance of treating streptococcal infections, as untreated infections may lead to rheumatic fever, cervical adenitis, sinusitis, glomerulonephritis, or meningitis.

TONSILLITIS AND ADENOIDITIS

Tonsillitis is an infection or inflammation (hypertrophy) of the palatine tonsils. Although most children with pharyngitis may have infected tonsils, they do not necessarily have tonsillitis. The adenoids are lymphatic tissue located on the posterior pharyngeal wall and are sometimes called the pharyngeal tonsils; they can manifest with acute or chronic infection (Bahadori & Schwartz, 2006).

ETIOLOGY AND PATHOPHYSIOLOGY

Like pharyngitis, tonsillitis and adenoiditis may be caused by a virus or bacterium. The primary site of infection is the tonsils.

CLINICAL MANIFESTATIONS

Symptoms suggestive of tonsillitis include frequent throat infections with breathing and swallowing difficulties, persistent redness of the anterior pillars, and enlargement of the cervical lymph nodes. If children breathe through their mouths continuously, the mucous membranes may become dry and irritated. Adenoiditis is characterized by nasal stuffiness, discharge, and postnasal drip, which result in coughing or excessive clearing of the throat.

CLINICAL THERAPY

Diagnosis is made on the basis of visual inspection and clinical manifestations. Tonsils appear large and inflamed. Enlarged adenoids are diagnosed by radiologic studies.

Symptomatic treatment for tonsillitis is the same as for pharyngitis. Surgical removal of tonsils (tonsillectomy) is often recommended when children have recurrent throat infections (about three per year for 3 years), chronic tonsillitis, obstructive sleep apnea, or malformations causing nasal speech or a facial growth abnormality. If the child is under 3 years of age, the surgery is postponed if possible because it may stimulate growth of other lymphoid tissue in the nasopharynx. If the pharyngeal tonsils (adenoids) are enlarged, as suggested by mouth breathing, cough, impaired taste and smell, a muffled quality to the voice, and chronic otitis media, they may be removed at the same time.

A technique used to treat children from 4 to 13 years who have sleep obstruction due to large tonsillar size is temperature-controlled radiofrequency (TCRF), which decreases the size of tonsils (Coticchia, Yun, Nelson, et al., 2006). The target tissue is heated through a submucosal electrode; surgical time and recovery time are lower than in usual tonsillectomy procedures. Children had increased comfort, decreased snoring and other sleep problems, and very quick recovery from the procedure.

NURSING MANAGEMENT

NURSING ASSESSMENT AND DIAGNOSIS

Assess the throat carefully during each physical examination. Observe for tonsils that are simply large (a common finding in childhood) and those that are inflamed. Look for the degree of redness and presence of any exudate. Ask if the child has pain or difficulty swallowing. Ask about the history of past tonsillar infections and the length of time of the present discomfort.

If surgery is indicated, take a complete history of the child preoperatively. Monitor vital signs and observe for respiratory distress, hemorrhage, and dehydration postoperatively.

Several nursing diagnoses may apply to the child with tonsillitis. They include the following:

- *Pain* related to inflammation of the pharynx
- *Risk for Deficient Fluid Volume* related to inadequate intake
- *Risk for Ineffective Breathing Pattern* related to obstruction by enlarged tonsils
- *Impaired Swallowing* related to inflammation and pain
- *Health-Seeking Behaviors (Parents)* related to home care following discharge

PLANNING AND IMPLEMENTATION

The nurse provides general supportive care and, if medication is prescribed, encourages completion of the full course of treatment. The nursing management of children with tonsillitis is similar to that of children with pharyngitis (see earlier discussion).

If surgery is indicated, help the parents prepare their child for a short-term surgical procedure with a possible overnight

Teaching Highlights

CARE AFTER TONSILLECTOMY

After tonsillectomy the parent can take measures to increase the child's comfort.

- Have the child drink adequate cool fluids or chew gum, as this reduces spasms in the muscles surrounding the throat.
- Give acetaminophen elixir, or other analgesic as prescribed.
- Apply an ice collar around the child's neck.
- Have the child gargle with a solution of 1/2 teaspoon (2.5 g) each of baking soda and salt in a glass of water.
- Have the child rinse the mouth well with viscous lidocaine and then swallow the solution.

stay in the hospital (see Chapter 41). Children should be free of sore throat, fever, or upper respiratory infection for at least 1 week before surgery. They should not be given aspirin or ibuprofen for 2 weeks before surgery, since these medications can increase postoperative bleeding. Check if any herbal medications are taken and report them to the physician and anesthesiologist since some may interfere with anesthetic drugs used in surgery.

DISCHARGE PLANNING AND HOME CARE TEACHING

Discharge planning includes teaching parents about pain management, fluid and nutrition intake, activity restrictions, and possible complications in the postoperative period. Most children have a sore throat for 7 to 10 days after tonsillectomy. Advise parents how to relieve the child's throat pain. (See "Teaching Highlights: Care after Tonsillectomy.")

Children may experience ear pain, especially when swallowing, between 4 and 8 days after tonsillectomy. Advise parents that this pain is referred from the tonsillar area and does not indicate an ear infection.

Emphasize to parents the importance of adequate fluid intake. Children should be given any liquid they prefer for the first week, except citrus juices, which may produce a burning sensation in the throat. Soft foods such as gelatin, applesauce, frozen juice pops, and mashed potatoes can be added as tolerated.

Children do not need to be confined to bed, but they should avoid vigorous exercise for the first week after surgery. Advise parents that the child may return to school approximately 10 days after tonsillectomy.

Any surgery carries the risk of postoperative complications. Teach parents the normal signs of healing in the postoperative period, as well as signs of complications. (See "Teaching Highlights: Complications of Tonsillectomy and Adenoidectomy.")

Teaching Highlights

COMPLICATIONS OF TONSILLECTOMY AND ADENOIDECTOMY

Bleeding

- To prevent bleeding, aspirin or ibuprofen should not be given for pain for the first postoperative week. Use acetaminophen instead.
- Bleeding is most likely to occur within the first 24 hours or 7 to 10 days after the tonsillectomy, when the scar is forming. Report any trickle of bright red blood or increased swallowing to the physician immediately.

Infection

- The back of the throat will look white and have an odor for the first 7 to 8 days after the surgery. The child may also have a low-grade fever. These are not signs of infection.
- For temperatures over 38.3°C (101°F), acetaminophen may be used.
- Call the health care provider if the child develops a fever above 38.8°C (102°F).

Pain

- Administer acetaminophen as ordered.
- Offer frequent small amounts of cool liquids. Avoid citrus juice.
- Provide for rest and quiet activities for several days.

EVALUATION

Expected outcomes of nursing care for the child with tonsillitis include the following:

- Adequate intake of food and fluids
- Management of pain and fever
- Absence of postoperative complications such as bleeding, hemorrhage, and dehydration
- Healing without impairment following tonsillectomy

DISORDERS OF THE MOUTH

The mouth is an important structure that is directly linked to both the gastrointestinal and respiratory systems. Structural problems can occur in the mouth, often in conjunction with other defects such as tracheoesophageal fistula or cleft lip and palate (see Chapter 53). A second type of mouth disorder in children is ulceration. Children sometimes have changes in the mucous membranes of the mouth, associated with illnesses, infections, or as a side effect of drug treatments. Trauma is a third cause for mouth disorders in children. Accidents can cause fractures of the jaw, dental emergencies, or other trauma.

Nursing Management

Most mouth ulcers are treated symptomatically. Since the oral mucosa is fast growing, the cells can rapidly heal. Keeping the mouth clean and administering systemic or topical analgesics can assist with comfort. Foods should be mild and nonirritating. Acyclovir may be administered for treatment of herpes infections. Antibiotics are needed for bacterial infection of oral lesions. Stevens-Johnson syndrome necessitates removing the drug that causes the reaction, and treating the child with oral antihistamines and supportive therapy.

Nurses inform parents of proper treatment for injuries and may provide emergency treatment in schools and other community settings. Injury prevention is encouraged through use of protective gear during sports. Mouth guards can be helpful to prevent dental damage. See Chapter 44∞ for a discussion of protective sporting gear and of body piercing which may include the oral cavity. Because the mouth has a profuse blood supply, bleeding may be extensive for even minor injuries. It is best to use clean cloths to absorb the blood and prevent choking on it, and get the child to an emergency facility to have the lesion examined.

Dental injuries may involve fracture of a tooth, luxation (partial extrusion), or avulsion (complete removal). The periodontal ligament holds the tooth in the socket but its attachment is torn during a tooth avulsion (Krause-Parello, 2005). The child should be transported immediately to an emergency facility. (See "Teaching Highlights: Care of a Tooth Avulsion.")

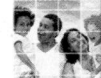

Teaching Highlights

CARE OF A TOOTH AVULSION

When a tooth is removed during an injury, prompt treatment may improve the chance that it can be reimplanted. If the child's condition is stable, try to reimplant the tooth and then transfer to an emergency dental facility.

- Handle the tooth only by the crown (its top) rather than the root to avoid further damage.
- Gently rinse the tooth with a stream of sterile saline. Do NOT place it under running water.
- Insert into the socket.
- Have the child provide gentle pressure by biting a piece of gauze or a moistened tea bag. If the child is unstable or has other injuries, enlist emergency medical transportation (call 9-1-1). In this case the tooth is transported with the child.
- If a dental aid kit is available it may contain a transport liquid such as Viaspan or Hank's Balanced Salt Solution. If these are not available, alternatives include cold milk, saline, saliva, or water. Place the tooth in one of these transfer liquids to keep it moist and send it with the child to the healthcare facility.

Data from Krause-Parello, C. A. (2005). Tooth avulsion in the school setting. *Journal of School Nursing 21,* 279–282.

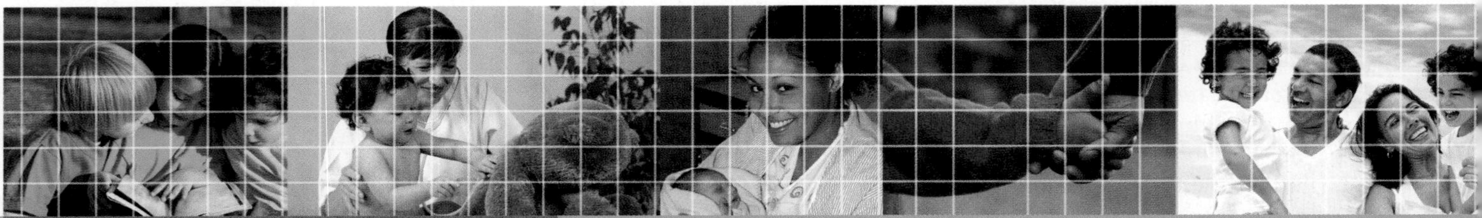

CRITICAL CONCEPT REVIEW

LEARNING OUTCOMES	CONCEPTS
47.1 Identify anatomy, physiology, and pediatric differences in the eye, ear, nose and throat of children and adolescents.	1. Eyes: ■ Visual Acuity. ■ Eye movement. 2. Ears: ■ Structure. 3. Mouth: ■ Tonsillar size. ■ Tooth eruption.

LEARNING OUTCOMES	CONCEPTS
47.2 Describe abnormalities of the eyes, ears, nose, throat, and mouth in children.	Eyes: 1. Conjunctivitis: ■ Inflammation of the conjunctiva. ■ Caused by viruses, bacteria, allergy, trauma, or irritants. 2. Cellulitis: ■ Infection of the eyelid and the surrounding tissues. 3. Visual disorders: ■ Errors of refraction. ■ Abnormal musculature. ■ Malignancies of the eye. ■ Glaucoma and cataracts. ■ Retinopathy of prematurity. 4. Injuries to the eye. Ears: 1. Otitis media: ■ Inflammation of the middle ear. 2. Otitis externa: ■ Inflammation of the skin and tissue of the ear canal. 3. Hearing impairment: ■ Genetic. ■ Environmental. ■ Unknown causes. Nose, throat, and mouth: 1. Epistaxis: ■ Caused by low humidity or irritation. 2. Nasopharyngitis: ■ Inflammation or infection of the nose and throat. 3. Sinusitis: ■ Inflammation of one or more of the paranasal sinuses. 4. Pharyngitis: ■ Infection primarily of the tonsils. 5. Tonsillitis: ■ Infection and hypertrophy of the palatine tonsils. 6. Mouth ulcers. 7. Trauma to the mouth and teeth.
47.3 Plan for screening programs and identification of children with vision and hearing abnormalities.	Vision: 1. Assess for eye symmetry and movement, for ability to follow objects with each eye, and for any abnormalities in appearance of eyes at each well-child visit. 2. Visual acuity screenings should be performed annually beginning at age 5. Hearing: 1. All newborns should be screened for hearing abnormalities while in the newborn nursery. 2. Hearing and speech development should be assessed at each well-child visit.
47.4 Plan nursing care for children with vision or hearing impairments.	Vision impairment: 1. Call the child's name and identify self upon entering the room and inform the child before leaving the room. 2. Describe all procedures before they are done. 3. Allow child to touch the equipment if possible. 4. Describe the foods and their location when food trays are delivered. Hearing impairment: 1. Touch the child to get his or her attention. 2. Stand in front of the child and speak normally. 3. Keep room well-lit. 4. Be familiar with the child's hearing amplification system so that it is placed correctly. 5. Provide a picture board to aid in communication. 6. Have an interpreter available if child understands only American Sign Language.
47.5 Use latest recommendations when implementing care and teaching for children with abnormalities of eyes, ears, nose, throat, and mouth.	1. Prevention of vision and hearing impairment and loss depends on early diagnosis and treatment. ■ Screen for visual and hearing acuity at every well-child visit and every 2–3 years during elementary school. ■ Instruct parents in the correct use of a child's adaptive devices (lenses and aides) and use of medication. ■ Inform parents about risks and benefits of cochlear implant surgery.

(continued)

LEARNING OUTCOMES / CONCEPTS

47.6 Integrate preventive and treatment principles when implementing care for children related to eyes, ears, nose, and throat.

Eyes:
1. Prevent eye injuries by teaching safety in activities that can injure the eye.
2. Encourage the use of protective eye wear for sports, school projects, and yard work.

Ears:
1. Instruct parents and child concerning the dangers of listening to loud music with and without headphones.
2. Encourage the use of ear protection when child is exposed to loud noise.

Nose, throat, and mouth:
1. Instruct parents concerning the importance of completing the entire course of antibiotics when treating a throat infection.
2. Stress the importance of the use of mouth guards when playing sports.

CRITICAL THINKING IN ACTION

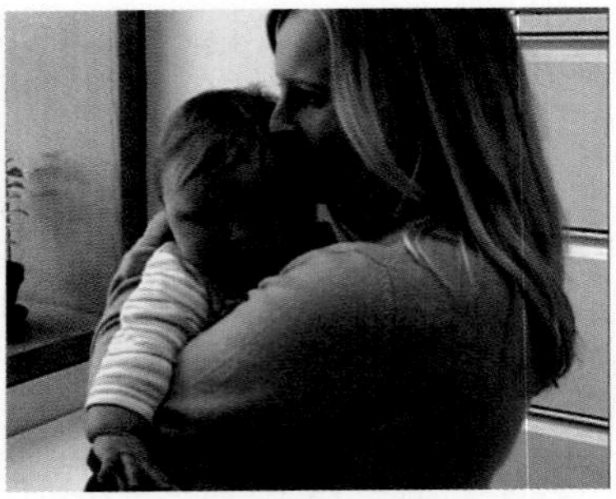

You are working at a local children's urgent care facility when a couple comes in carrying their screaming 9-month-old child, Becky. The parents are worried, as Becky has been crying steadily for the past 2 hours. You ask about recent illnesses or injuries and they tell you that she has had only two colds in her life and the most recent was about a week ago.

You assess Becky's vital signs as follows: weight 19 pounds (8.6 kilograms), temperature 101 degrees F, respirations 60 breaths per minute without retractions, and heart rate 120 beats per minute. She does not have any rashes or evidence of injuries, and upon examination she appears well nourished but clearly in distress. Her heart rate is regular and rhythm and breath sounds are equal bilaterally and clear to auscultation. Both tympanic membranes are red and bulging. Her abdomen is soft and without organomegaly. The doctor diagnoses bilateral acute otitis media and administers analgesic ear drops and ibuprofen in the office. Within 15 minutes, Becky has settled down, stopped crying, and is resting in her father's arms. The family is sent home with instructions to administer analgesics and return within 48 hours for further assessment.

1. What are the three main organisms that may have caused Becky's otitis media?
2. What are some of the guidelines you can give Becky's parents about otitis media treatment?
3. The mother says she has family members who have had tubes placed in their ears because of ear infections and wants to know if this is something that Becky will need to have done.
4. What are some methods parents can use to prevent future otitis media episodes?

See MyNursingKit for possible responses.

REFERENCES

Abelson, M. B., & Granet, D. (2006). Ocular allergy in pediatric practice. *Current Allergy and Asthma Reports, 6,* 306–311.

American Academy of Pediatrics, Committee on Infectious Diseases. (2006). *Red book* (27th ed.). Elk Grove Village, IL: Author.

American Academy of Pediatrics, Subcommittee on management of acute otitis media (2004). Diagnosis and management of acute otitis media. *Pediatrics, 113,* 1451–1465.

Armengol, C. E., Hendley, O., & Schlager, T. A. (2006). An office-based guide to diagnosing streptococcal pharyngitis. *Contemporary Pediatrics, 23*(5), 64–78.

Bahadori, R. A., & Schwartz, R. H. (2006). The adenoid in children: Out of sight, out of mind? *Infectious Diseases in Children, 19*(8), 11–12.

Bernius, M., & Perlin, D. (2006). Pediatric ear, nose, and throat emergencies. *Pediatric Clinics of North America, 53,* 195–214.

Bindler, R. M., & Howry, L. B. (2005). Pediatric drug guide. Upper Saddle River, NJ: Prentice Hall-Health.

Brook, I., & Gober, A. (2005). Recovery of potential pathogens and interfering bacteria in the nasopharynx of otitis media-prone children and their smoking and non-smoking patients. *Archives of Otolaryngology and Head & Neck Surgery, 131,* 509–512.

Brunell, P. A., Wagner, R. S., Cuming, G. S., Dorfman, M. S., & Murphey, D. K. (2006). Bacterial conjunctivitis in children: Containing the infection *Infectious Diseases in Children Supplement 1,* 1–19.

Center for Health and Health Care in Schools. (2007). Childhood vision: Public challenges and opportunities Retrieved from www.healthinschools.org

Centers for Disease Control and Prevention (2008). Streptococcus pneumoniae disease. Retrieved from www.cdc.gov/ncidod/dbmd/diseaseinfo/streppneum_t.htm

Chamley, C. A., Carson, P., Randall, D., & Sandwell, M. (2005). *Developmental anatomy and physiology of children.* St. Louis: Elsevier.

Committee on Sports Medicine and Fitness. (2004). Protective eyewear for young athletes. *Pediatrics, 113,* 619–622.

Connolly, J. L., Carron, J. D., & Roark, S. D. (2005). Universal newborn hearing screening: Are we achieving the Joint Committee on Infant (JCIH) objectives? *Laryngoscope, 115,* 232–236.

Coticchia, J. M., Yun, R. D., Nelson, L., & Koempel, J. (2006). Temperature-controlled radiofrequency treatment of tonsillar hypertrophy for reduction of upper airway obstruction in pediatric patients. *Archives of Otolaryngology and Head and Neck Surgery 132,* 425–430.

Demetroulakos, J. L. (2007). Sinusitis. MedlinePlus. Retrieved from www.nih.gov

Donahue, S. P. (2007). Pediatric strabismus. *New England Journal of Medicine, 356,* 1040–1047.

Donahue, S. P., Baker, J. D., Scott, W. E., Rychwalski, P., Neely, D. E., Tong, P., et al. (2006). Lions Clubs International Foundation Core Four Photoscreening: Results from 17 programs and 400,000 preschool children. *Journal of the American Association of Ophthalmology and Strabismus, 10,* 44–48.

Doshi, N. R., & Rodriguez, L. F. (2007). Amblyopia. *American Family Physician, 75,* 361–368.

Dudas, R. (2006). Retropharyngeal abscess. *Pediatrics in Review, 27,* 45–46.

Foxlee, R., Johansson, A., Wejfalk, J., Dawkins, J., Dooley, L., & Del Mar, C. (2006). Topical analgesia for acute otitis media. *Cochrane Database Systematic Review, 19,* CD005657.

Galito, N. J. (2008). Peritonsillar Abscess. *American Family Physician, 77,* 199–202, 209.

Guttu, M., Engelke, M. K., & Swanson, M. (2004). Does the school nurse-to-student ratio make a difference? *Journal of School Health, 74,* 6–9.

Harrison, C. J. (2005). The microbiology of acute otitis media: Past, present, and future. *Contemporary Pediatrics, 22*(12), 8–16.

Hartmann, E. E., Bradford, G. E., Chaplin, P. K. N., Johnson, T., Kemper, A. R., Kim, S., & Marsh-Tootle, W. (2006). Project universal preschool vision screening: A demonstration project. *Pediatrics, 117,* e226–e237. Retrieved from http://pediatrics.aappublications.org/cgi/content/full/117/2/3226

Health Care Guide. (2006). *Epistaxis.* Retrieved from www.health-care-guide.org/epistaxis.htm

Hunter, L. L., Davey, C. S., Kohtz, A., & Daly, K. A. (2007). Hearing screening and middle ear measure in American Indian infants and toddlers. *International Journal of Pediatric Otorhinolaryngology, 71,* 1429–1438.

International Committee for the Classification of Retinopathy of Prematurity (2005). The international classification of retinopathy of prematurity revisited. *Archives of Ophthalmology, 123,* 991–999.

Joint Committee on Infant Hearing (2007). Year 2007 position statement: Principles and guidelines for early hearing detection and intervention programs. *Pediatrics, 120,* 898–921.

Kimel, L. S. (2006). Lack of follow-up exams after failed school vision screenings: An investigation of contributing factors. *Journal of School Nursing, 22,* 156–162.

Kliegman, R. M., Behrman, R. E., Jenson, H. B., & Stanton, B. F. (2007). *Nelson textbook of pediatrics* (18th ed.). Philadelphia: Saunders.

Krause-Parello, C. A. (2005). Tooth avulsion in the school setting. *Journal of School Nursing, 21,* 279–282.

Leach, A. J., & Morris, P. S. (2007). Antibiotics for the prevention of acute and chronic uppurative otitis media in children. *Cochrane Reviews, 2,* 697–760.

Leman, R., Clausen, M. M., Bates, J., Stark, L., Arnold, K. K., & Arnold, R. W. (2006). A comparison of patched HOTV visual acuity and photoscreening. *Journal of School Nursing, 22,* 237–243.

Lichtenstein, S. J., Dorfman, J., Kennedy, R., & Stroman, D. (2006). Controlling contagious bacterial conjunctivitis. *Journal of Pediatric Ophthalmology & Strabismus, 43,* 19–26.

Mah, F. (2006). Bacterial conjunctivitis. *Pediatric Clinics of North America, 53*(Suppl. 1), 7–10.

Marter, A., & Agruss, J. C. (2007). Pacifiers: an update on use and misuse. *Journal for Specialists in Pediatric Nursing 12*(4), 278–285.

Moore, J. (2006). Pediatricians need greater awareness of hearing disorders. *Infectious Diseases in Children, 19*(8), 53–54.

Nageswaran, S., Woods, C. R., Benjamin, D. K., & Shetty, L. (2006). Orvital cellulitis in children. *Pediatric Infectious Disease Journal, 25,* 695–699.

National Institutes of Health (2006). *Cochlear implants fact sheet.* Washington, DC; Author.

National Institutes of Health (2007). *Cochlear implants.* Washington, D.C.: Author.

Nield, L. S., Mangano, L. M., & Kamat, D. (2008). Strabismus: A close-up look. *Consultant for Pediatricians,* January, 17–25

O'Connor, A. R., Wilson, C. M., & Fielder, A. R. (2007). Ophthalmological problems associated with preterm birth. *Eye, 21,* 1254–1260.

Otitis Media with Effusion. (2004). Clinical practice guideline. *Pediatrics, 113,* 1412–1429.

Page, N. C., Bauer, E. M., & Lieu, J. E. C. (2008). Clinical features and treatment of retropharyngeal abscess in children. *Otolaryngology—Head and Neck Surgery, 138,* 300–306.

Pelton, S. I. (2005). Otitis media: Re-evaluation of diagnosis and treatment in the era of antimicrobial resistance, pneumococcal conjugate vaccine, and evolving morbidity. *Pediatric Clinics of North America, 52,* 711–728.

Quinn, G. E. (2005). The "ideal" management of retinopathy of prematurity. *Eye, 19,* 1044–1049.

Rosenfeld, R. M., Brown, L., Cannon, C. R., Dolor, R. J., Ganiats, T. G., Hannley, M., et. al., (2006). Clinical practice guideline: Acute otitis externa. *Otolaryngology—Head & Neck Surgery, 134*(4Suppl), S4–23.

Rudolph, C. D., Rudolph, A. M., Hostetter, M. K., Lister, G. E., & Siegel, M. J. (Eds.). *Rudolph's pediatrics* (21st ed.). New York: McGraw-Hill.

Sarrell, E. M., Cohen, H. A., & Kahan, E. (2003). Naturopathic treatment for ear pain in children. *Pediatrics, 111,* e574–579.

Subramanian, M. (2007). Color blindness. Medline Plus, National Institutes of Health. U.S. Department of Health and Human Services. (2000). *Healthy People 2010* (2nd ed.). Washington, DC: U.S. Government Printing Office. www.healthypeople.gov.

Tasman, W., Patz, A., McNamara, J. A., Kaiser, R. S., Trese, M. T., & Smith, B. T. (2006). Retinopathy of prematurity: The life of a lifetime disease. *American Journal of Ophthalmology, 141,* 167–174.

Taylor, A. (2006). Sinusitis. *Pediatrics in Review, 27,* 395–397.

U.S. Department of Health and Human Services (2006). *Healthy People 2010: Midcourse review.* Washington, D.C.: Author.

U.S. Food and Drug Administration. (2006). *Got a sick kid?* Retrieved from www.fda.gov/cder/consumerinfo/sickkids.htm

U.S. Food and Drug Administration (2007). Public Health Advisory. *Nonprescription cough and cold medicine use in children.* Retrieved from www.fda.gov.cder/drug/advisory/cough_cold.htm

U.S. Preventive Services Task Force. (2005). Screening for visual impairment in children younger than five years: Recommendation statement. *American Family Physician, 71,* 333–336.

Weichbold, V., Nekahm-Heis, D. & Welzl-Mueller, K. (2006). Universal newborn hearing screening and postnatal hearing loss. *Pediatrics 117*(4), e631–e636.

Wilson-Clark, S. D., Squires, S., & Deeks, S. (2006). Bacterial meningitis among cochlear implant recipients—Canada, 2002. *MMWR, 55*(Sup01), 20–24.

Windmill, S., & Windmill, I. M. (2006). The status of diagnostic testing following referral from universal newborn hearing screening. *Journal of the American Academy of Audiology, 17,* 367–378.

Yaeger, D., McCallum, J., Lewis, K., Soslow, L., Shah, U., Potsic, W., et al. (2006). Outcomes of clinical examination and genetic testing of 500 individuals with hearing loss evaluated through a genetics of hearing loss clinic. *American Journal of Medical Genetics, 140,* 827–836.

Yang, M. B., Donovan, E. F., & Wagge, J. R. (2006). Race, gender, and clinical risk index for babies (CRIB) score as predictors of severe retinopathy of prematurity. *Journal of American Association for Pediatric Ophthalmology and Strabismus, 10,* 253–261.

Zacharyczuk, C. (2004, April). New guidelines outline AOM management options. *Infectious Diseases in Children,* 24.

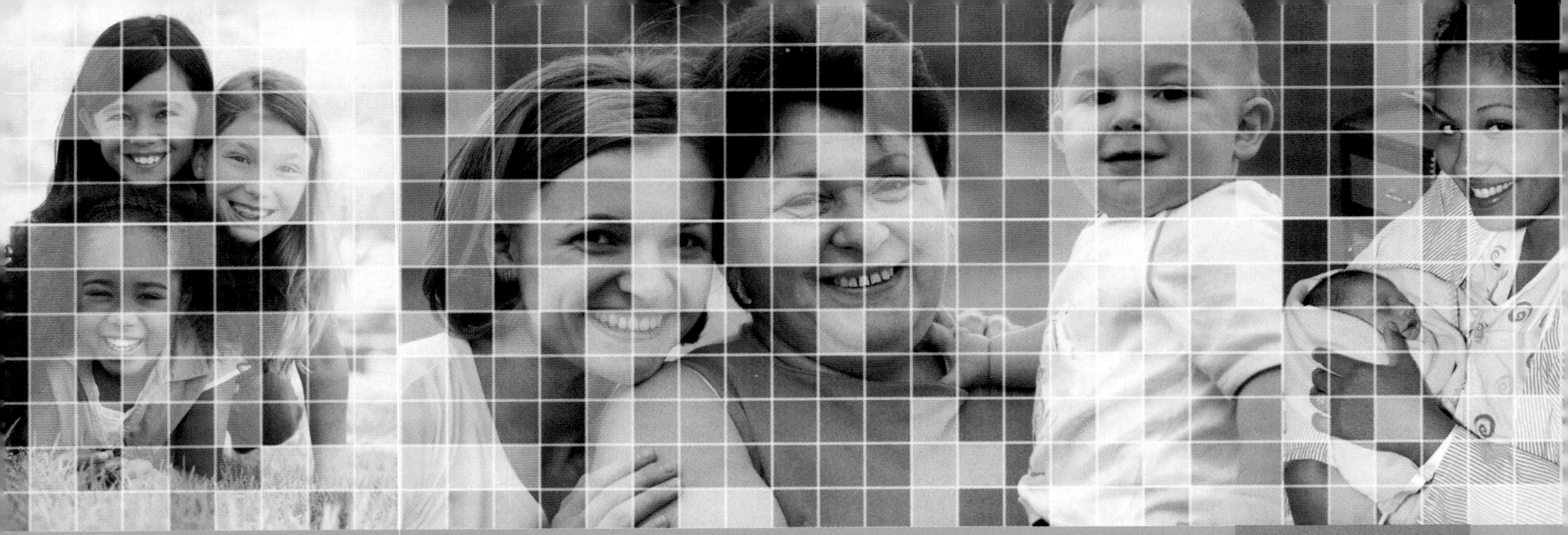

CHAPTER

48 The Child with Alterations in Respiratory Function

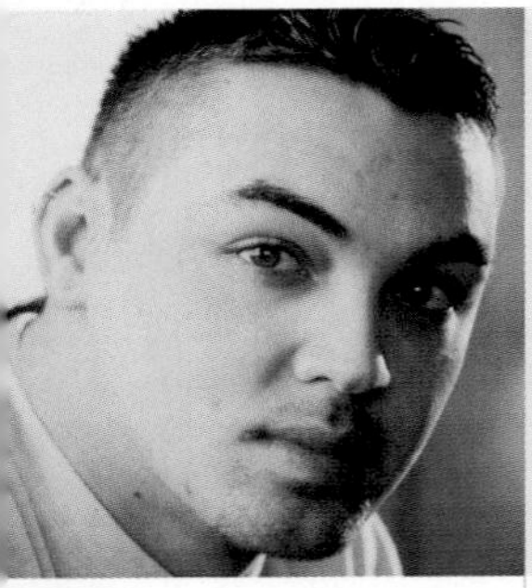

Emily gets sick so much faster than my other children. I guess the bronchopulmonary dysplasia and her tracheostomy make her more susceptible to infections. I really get concerned because she struggles so hard to breathe when she gets an infection. I have learned to suction and change her tracheostomy, but I am afraid that one day her tracheostomy tube will get completely blocked. I just hope I remember all the things I've learned if that happens, and that the emergency medical personnel come quickly. —Father of Emily, 8 months old

LEARNING OUTCOMES

48.1 Describe unique characteristics of the pediatric respiratory system anatomy and physiology and apply that information to the care of children with respiratory conditions.

48.2 Identify the assessment guidelines for a child with a respiratory condition.

48.3 List the different respiratory conditions and injuries that can cause respiratory distress in infants and children.

48.4 Assess the child's respiratory signs and symptoms to distinguish between respiratory distress and respiratory failure and describe the appropriate nursing care.

48.5 Distinguish between conditions of the upper respiratory tract that cause respiratory distress.

48.6 Distinguish between conditions of the lower respiratory tract that cause illness in children.

48.7 Develop a hospital-based nursing care plan for a child with a common acute respiratory condition.

48.8 Develop a school-based nursing care plan for the child with asthma.

48.9 Develop a home nursing care plan for the child with cystic fibrosis.

Respiratory problems may result from structural problems, functional problems, or a combination of both. Structural problems involve alterations in the size and shape of parts of the respiratory tract. Functional problems involve alterations in gas exchange and threats to this normal process from irritants (such as large particles and chemicals) or infectious organisms. Alterations in the immune and neurologic systems may also threaten respiratory function. See Chapter 47 for upper respiratory conditions such as colds, otitis media, sinusitis, and pharyngitis.

Most respiratory problems in children produce mild symptoms, last a short time, and can be managed at home. However, acute respiratory problems cause 25% of all hospitalization in children under 15 years of age, most often due to pneumonia, asthma, acute bronchitis, and bronchiolitis (DeFrances & Hall, 2007). Some respiratory conditions are chronic and have a significant impact on the child's growth and development.

ANATOMY AND PHYSIOLOGY OF PEDIATRIC DIFFERENCES

The child's respiratory tract constantly grows and changes until about 12 years of age. The young child's neck is shorter than an adult's, resulting in airway structures that are closer together.

UPPER AIRWAY DIFFERENCES

The child's airway is shorter and narrower than an adult's. These differences create a greater potential for obstruction (see "As Children Grow: Airway Development"). The infant's airway is approximately 4 mm in diameter, about the width of a drinking straw, in contrast to the adult's airway diameter of 20 mm. The trachea primarily increases in length rather than diameter during the first 5 years of life. The child's little finger is a good estimate of the child's tracheal diameter. The bronchial division of the trachea in a child is higher and at a different angle than the adult's (see "As Children Grow: Trachea Position"). The child's narrower airway causes an increase in **airway resistance**, the effort or force needed to move oxygen through the trachea to the lungs (see "Pathophysiology Illustrated: Airway Diameter").

Until 4 weeks of age, newborns are obligatory nose breathers. The coordination of mouth breathing is controlled by maturing neurologic pathways; thus, infants up to 2 to 3 months of age do not automatically open the mouth to breathe when the nose is obstructed. The only time a newborn breathes through the mouth is when he or she is crying. Nasal patency in newborns is therefore essential for such activities as breathing and eating. Infants, children, and adults can breathe through either the nose or the mouth.

LOWER AIRWAY DIFFERENCES

The tracheobronchial tree is complete at birth, but the distal (peripheral) bronchioles that extend to the alveoli are narrow and fewer in number than in an adult. Most neonates have sufficient alveoli by 32 to 36 weeks gestation to maintain gas exchange (Cifuentes & Carlo, 2007). Full-term newborns have only 25 million alveoli at birth, but they are not fully developed. Alveoli begin increasing in size and complexity after 8 years of age. The number of alveoli increases to 300 million by adulthood (Brashers, 2006b).

The bronchi and bronchioles are lined with smooth muscle. The newborn does not have enough smooth muscle bundles to help trap airway invaders. By 5 months of age, however, an infant has enough muscles to react to irritants by bronchospasm and muscle contraction.

Children under age 6 years use the diaphragm to breathe as the intercostal muscles are immature. The negative pressure caused by the downward movement of the diaphragm draws in air. By 6 years of age, the child uses the intercostal muscles more

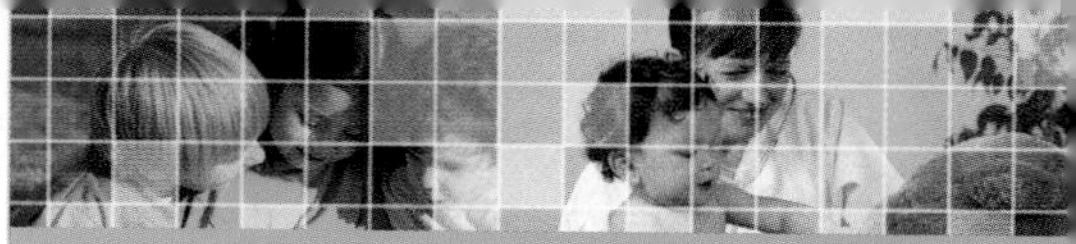

KEY TERMS

Adventitious sounds, 1315
Airway remodeling, 1335
Airway resistance, 1311
Alveolar hypoventilation, 1316
Apnea, 1317
Cor pulmonale, 1319
Dysphagia, 1324
Dysphonia, 1314
Dyspnea, 1314
Hypercapnia, 1316
Hypoxemia, 1316
Hypoxia, 1316
Laryngospasm, 1322
Paradoxical breathing, 1315
Periodic breathing, 1317
Polysomnography, 1319
Retractions, 1314
Stridor, 1321
Tachypnea, 1315
Trigger, 1335
Tripod position, 1315

MyNursingKit Animation: CO_2 and O_2 Transport

AS CHILDREN GROW

AIRWAY DEVELOPMENT

It is easy to see that a child's airway is smaller and less developed than an adult's airway, but why is this important? An upper respiratory tract infection, allergic reaction, positioning of the head and neck during sleep, and the small objects children play with can have serious consequences in the child.

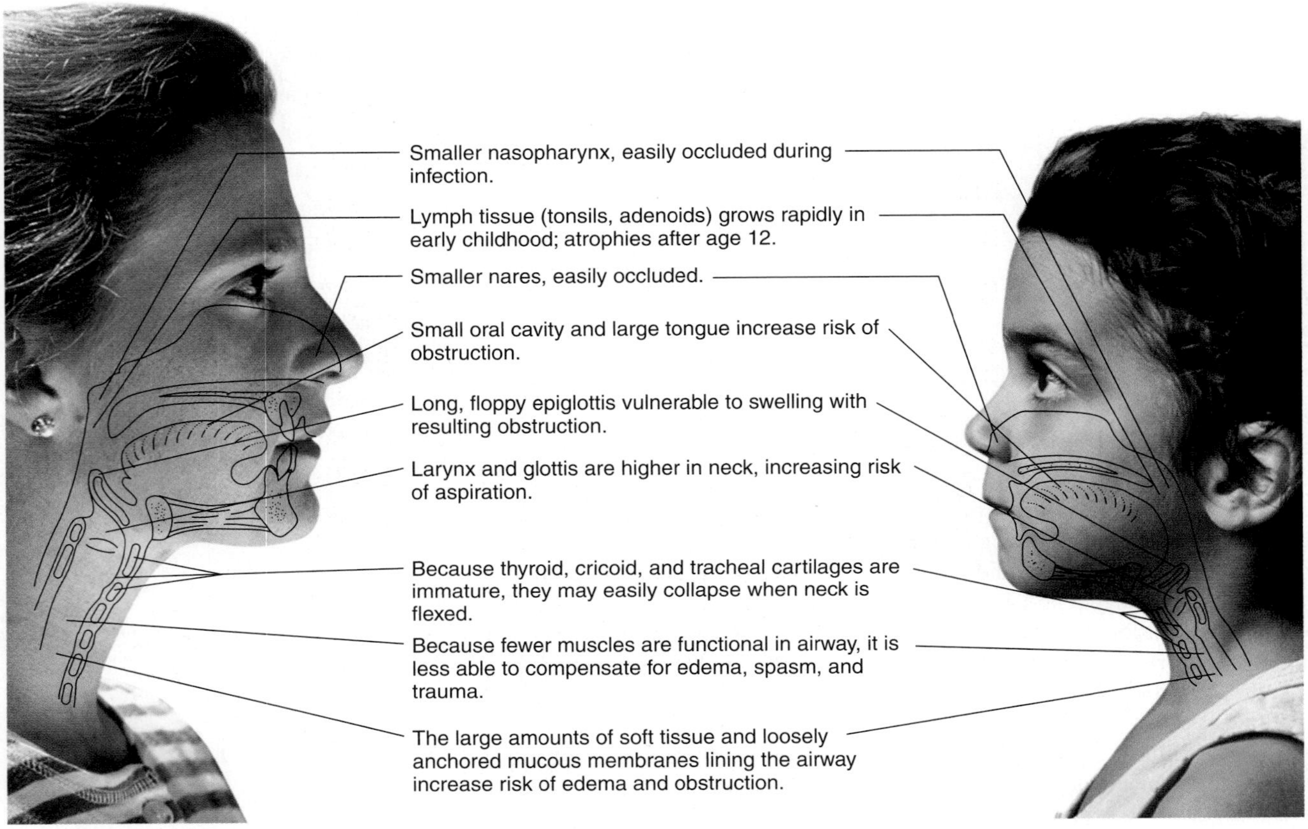
Smaller nasopharynx, easily occluded during infection.
Lymph tissue (tonsils, adenoids) grows rapidly in early childhood; atrophies after age 12.
Smaller nares, easily occluded.
Small oral cavity and large tongue increase risk of obstruction.
Long, floppy epiglottis vulnerable to swelling with resulting obstruction.
Larynx and glottis are higher in neck, increasing risk of aspiration.
Because thyroid, cricoid, and tracheal cartilages are immature, they may easily collapse when neck is flexed.
Because fewer muscles are functional in airway, it is less able to compensate for edema, spasm, and trauma.
The large amounts of soft tissue and loosely anchored mucous membranes lining the airway increase risk of edema and obstruction.

effectively. The ribs are primarily cartilage and very flexible, and in cases of respiratory distress, retractions may be seen (see "Pathophysiology Illustrated: Retraction Sites").

Oxygen consumption is higher in children than adults because of a higher metabolic rate. The rate of oxygen consumption increases when the child is in respiratory distress. The child also has fewer glycogen reserves, leading to more rapid muscle fatigue when accessory muscles must be used for breathing (Froh, 2006).

RESPIRATORY DISTRESS AND RESPIRATORY FAILURE

Many respiratory conditions associated with breathing difficulty can progress to respiratory distress. If the condition is not managed effectively, it can progress to respiratory failure. Foreign-body aspiration is a common cause of airway obstruction and respiratory distress.

FOREIGN-BODY ASPIRATION

Foreign-body aspiration is the inhalation of any object (solid or liquid, food or nonfood) into the respiratory tract. It is a major health threat for infants and young toddlers because of their increasing mobility and tendency to put objects into their mouths. Aspiration occurs most often during feeding and reaching activities, while crawling, or during playtime. However, aspiration may occur in children of any age. Foreign-body aspiration causes 7% of deaths to children under age 4 years (Arnold, 2006).

Etiology and Pathophysiology

In infants over 6 months of age and young children, any number of small objects that enter the child's mouth may cause aspiration.

AS CHILDREN GROW

TRACHEA POSITION

In children, the trachea is shorter and the angle of the right bronchus at bifurcation is more acute than in the adult. When you are resuscitating or suctioning, you must allow for the differences. Do you think that this difference is significant in respiratory infection? Why?

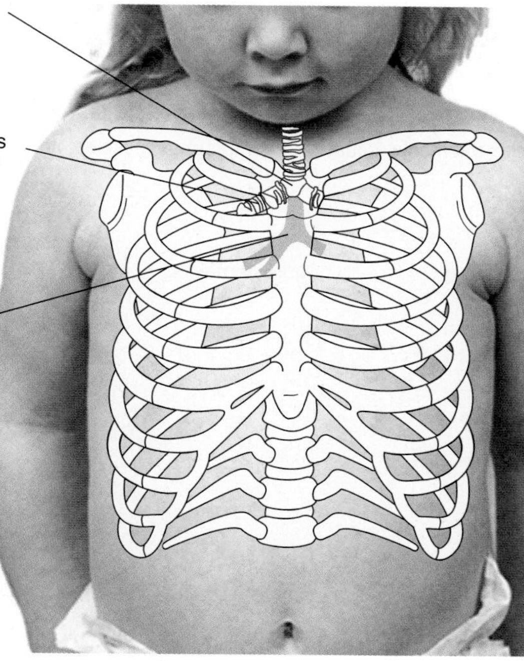
Bifurcation of trachea in children is at T3 level.
Right mainstem bronchus in children has a steeper slope than in adults.
Bifurcation in adults is at T6 level.

PATHOPHYSIOLOGY ILLUSTRATED

AIRWAY DIAMETER

An infant's airway diameter is approximately 4 mm, in contrast to the adult's 20 mm airway diameter. An inflammatory process in the airway causes swelling that narrows the airway, and airway resistance increases. Note that swelling of 1 mm reduces the infant's airway diameter to 2 mm, but the adult's airway diameter is only narrowed to 18 mm. Air must move more quickly in the infant's narrowed airway to get the same amount of air to the lungs. The friction of the quickly moving air against the side of the airway increases airway resistance. The infant must use more effort to breathe and breathe faster to get adequate oxygen.

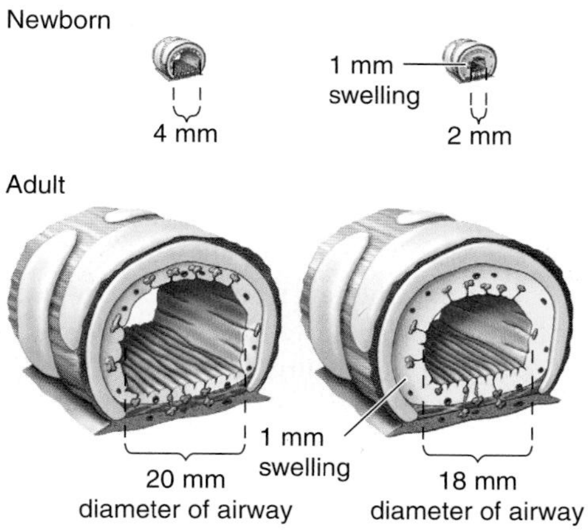
Newborn
4 mm
1 mm swelling
2 mm
Adult
20 mm diameter of airway
1 mm swelling
18 mm diameter of airway

Foods such as nuts, popcorn, or small pieces of raw vegetables or hot dog; small, loose toy parts such as small wheels and bells; or household objects and substances such as beads, safety pins, coins, buttons, latex balloon pieces, and colorful liquids (mouthwash, perfume) in enticing packages (screw-top bottles) are frequent causes of airway obstruction. Partial and sometimes complete airway obstruction can occur.

The severity of the obstruction depends on the size and composition of the object or substance and its location within the respiratory tract. Most aspirated foreign bodies (AFBs) usually cause

PATHOPHYSIOLOGY ILLUSTRATED

RETRACTION SITES

Infants and young children have immature chest muscles and cartilaginous ribs making the chest wall very flexible. The negative pressure created by the downward movement of the diaphragm is increased in cases of respiratory distress, and the chest wall is pulled inward, causing **retractions**. Intercostal retractions are seen in mild respiratory distress. As respiratory distress severity increases, substernal and subcostal retractions are seen. In cases of severe distress, supraclavicular and suprasternal retractions occur as the accessory muscles (sternocleidomastoid and trapezius muscles) are used.

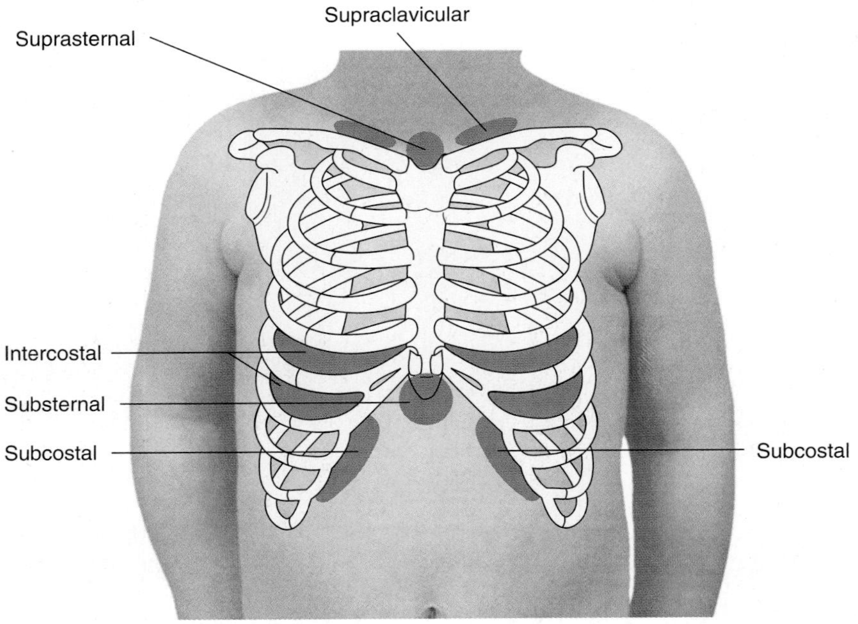

bronchial, not tracheal, obstruction. An object lodged high in the airway above the vocal cords is more easily removed by coughing or by back blows and chest thrusts.

The right lung is the most common site of the AFB in the lower airway because of the sloped angle of its bronchus (see page 1313). Objects may migrate from higher to lower airway locations. An object may also move back up to the trachea, creating extreme respiratory difficulty. If the AFB is lodged in the trachea, it becomes life-threatening.

Clinical Manifestations

Coughing, choking, gagging, **dysphonia** (muffled, hoarse, or absent voice sounds), and wheezing may be brief or may persist for several hours if the object drops below the trachea into one of the mainstem bronchi. In some cases the child may become asymptomatic after coughing for 15 to 30 minutes. The child may have signs of increased respiratory effort such as **dyspnea** (difficulty breathing), tachypnea, nasal flaring, and retractions. If the child cannot say the "P" in words like *Pluto* or *Peter Pan,* the child has diminished expiratory effort. If respiratory distress progresses, the child may have a concentrated focus on breathing, an anxious expression, and an upright position with the neck extended. As hypoxia increases behavior changes such as irritability and decreased responsiveness are seen.

If the AFB drops into the lower airway and is not removed, the child may present weeks later with a chronic cough, persistent or recurrent pneumonia, or a lung abscess.

Clinical Therapy

Clinical therapy focuses on taking a careful history to determine whether aspiration could have occurred. Witnessed coughing, gagging, or choking associated with feeding or crawling on the floor may confirm the aspiration. Decreased breath sounds, stridor, and respiratory distress increases suspicion in the child without a witnessed aspiration. A chest radiograph is performed however, only 15% of objects are radiopaque (Gibson, 2007). See Figure 48–1 ●. A special radiograph, called a forced expiratory film, may show local hyperinflation (air trapping) and a mediastinal shift away from the affected side, abnormalities that an AFB may cause.

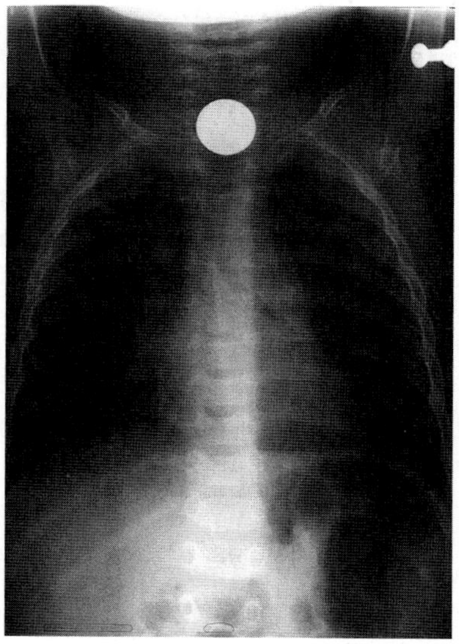

● **Figure 48–1** Aspirated foreign body. An aspirated foreign body (coin) is clearly visible in the child's trachea on this chest x-ray.
Courtesy of Rockwood Clinic, Spokane, WA.

An object lodged in the trachea is a life-threatening situation. Back blows and chest thrusts or abdominal thrusts are used to remove an object from an obstructed airway. (See Skill 14–14 SKILLS.) Fluoroscopy and fiberoptic bronchoscopy may be used to identify, locate, and extract the AFB. See the section on pneumonia, page 1330, for care of the child with complications of aspiration.

NURSING MANAGEMENT

NURSING ASSESSMENT AND DIAGNOSIS

PHYSIOLOGIC ASSESSMENT

The child will be in respiratory distress, and constant monitoring is essential. Perform the respiratory assessment following guidelines in Table 48–1. If the object remains lodged, observe the child for increasing signs of respiratory distress, especially vital signs, audible wheezing on auscultation, and retractions. Note changes in breath sounds, from noisy to decreasing to absent, on the affected side. Promptly document and report any subtle changes in the child's respiratory status. This can indicate that the object is moving and blocking a mainstem bronchus.

Attach the child to a cardiorespiratory monitor and pulse oximeter to assess the child for subtle signs of increasing hypoxia. A pulse oximetry reading (SpO_2) less than 95% indicates hypoxemia.

PSYCHOSOCIAL ASSESSMENT

The unexpected and acute nature of the event creates anxiety for both parents and child. The child will be fearful because of difficulty breathing. Assess the family's level of distress and coping ability.

Table 48–1 Assessment Guidelines for a Child in Respiratory Distress[a]

Position of Comfort
Is the child comfortable lying down? Does the child prefer to sit up or in **tripod position** (sitting forward with arms on knees for support and extending the neck)?
Vital Signs
Assess the rate, depth, and ease of respirations. See Table 35–8 for age-related respiratory rates. Assess the pulse for rate and rhythm.
Lung Auscultation
Are breath sounds bilateral, diminished or absent? Are **adventitious sounds** (wheezes, crackles, or rhonchi) present?
Respiratory Effort (work of breathing)
Are there audible inspiratory and expiratory breath sounds or stridor? Is there grunting with expiration? Is breathing labored? Are retractions present or are accessory muscles used to breathe? Is nasal flaring present? Is **tachypnea** (abnormally rapid rate of respirations) present? Can the child say a full sentence or is a breath needed every few words? Is the cry strong or weak? Do the chest and abdominal rise simultaneously with inspiration or is **paradoxical breathing** present in which the chest and abdomen do not rise simultaneously?
Color
What is the color of the mucous membranes or skin (pink, pale, cyanotic, or mottled)? Does crying improve or worsen the color?
Cough
Is the cough dry (nonproductive), wet (productive, mucousy), brassy (noisy, musical), or croupy (barking, seal-like)? Is the coughing effort forceful or weak?
Behavior Change
Is irritability, restlessness, or change in level of responsiveness present?

[a]Refer to Chapter 35 for the assessment techniques mentioned in this table.

DEVELOPMENTAL ASSESSMENT

As the child's condition stabilizes, observe how well the child's abilities match the parents' understanding of age-appropriate behaviors. See Chapters 36 and 37.

Common nursing diagnoses for a child with an AFB include the following:

- *Ineffective Airway Clearance* related to obstruction by a foreign body
- *Impaired Spontaneous Ventilations* related to respiratory muscle fatigue

MyNursingKit Video: Pediatric Respiratory Emergency Management

Nursing Practice

To increase the accuracy of pulse oximetry readings (SpO_2), avoid placing the sensor probe over sites with nail polish. Bright light or sunshine may falsely increase the reading. If the child has anemia, a normal pulse oximetry reading may not reflect good oxygen transport to the tissues. Check the SpO_2 when the child is still, as motion can cause false readings. Make sure the heart rate detected by the pulse oximeter matches the child's heart rate by direct assessment for accuracy. An inaccurate reading may occur if peripheral blood flow is decreased due to vasoconstriction, arrhythmias, or shock (Clark, Giuliano, & Chen, 2006; Popovich, Richiuso, & Danek, 2004).

- *Anxiety (Child)* related to difficulty breathing, unfamiliar surroundings, and procedures
- *Risk for Injury* related to small objects in environment

PLANNING AND IMPLEMENTATION

Be prepared to perform back blows and chest thrusts for an infant or abdominal thrusts for the child with complete obstruction. (See Skill 14–9 SKILLS.) When the child has a partial obstruction remain with the child and have resuscitation equipment at the bedside. Permit the child to stay in a position of comfort. Avoid performing procedures that increase the child's anxiety as sudden movements and increased respiratory efforts may cause the obstruction to move and completely obstruct the airway.

After the AFB is removed, the child is stabilized and observed for a few hours in a short-stay unit to ensure that there are no respiratory complications.

DISCHARGE PLANNING AND HOME CARE TEACHING

Discharge planning focuses on educating the family about potential safety hazards in the home and prevention of future aspirations. Encourage the parents to learn rescue breathing, back blows, chest thrusts, or abdominal thrusts.

EVALUATION

Expected outcomes of nursing care include the following:

- The child breathes spontaneously after removal of the foreign body.
- Parents complete a home safety check to prevent future aspiration incidents.

MyNursingKit Animation: Gas Exchange

RESPIRATORY FAILURE

Respiratory failure occurs when the body can no longer maintain effective gas exchange. **Alveolar hypoventilation** (poor ventilation of the alveoli) initiates the process that leads to respiratory failure. Hypoventilation occurs when oxygen need exceeds oxygen intake, the airway is partially occluded, or the transfer of oxygen and carbon dioxide in the alveoli is disrupted. This disruption may occur because of a malfunction of respiratory center stimulation (the alveoli do not receive the message to diffuse, e.g., a narcotic overdose), muscles of ventilation are fatigued and do not work effectively (e.g., status asthmaticus), or the relationship between ventilation and blood flow to the alveoli is impaired. Alveolar hypoventilation results in **hypoxemia** (lower than normal blood oxygen level) and **hypercapnia** (an excess of carbon dioxide in the blood). When the blood levels of oxygen and carbon dioxide reach abnormal levels, **hypoxia** (lower than normal oxygen in the tissues) occurs and respiratory failure begins.

Signs of impending respiratory failure include irritability, lethargy, cyanosis, and increased respiratory effort such as dyspnea, tachypnea, nasal flaring, and intercostal retractions. Grunting, a neonatal process to slow expiratory flow and prevent alveolar collapse during expiration, is a sign of disease severity and may be associated with the onset of respiratory failure (Cifuentes & Carlo, 2007). *Hypoxemia that persists when supplemental oxygen is given is a sign of respiratory failure.* See Clinical Manifestations.

Clinical Manifestations

Respiratory Failure and Imminent Respiratory Arrest

PHYSIOLOGIC CAUSE	CLINICAL MANIFESTATIONS
Respiratory failure The child is trying to compensate for oxygen deficit and airway blockage. Oxygen supply is inadequate; behavior and vital signs reflect compensation and beginning hypoxia.	*Initial signs* Restlessness Tachypnea Tachycardia Diaphoresis
The child tries to use accessory muscles to assist oxygen intake; hypoxia persists and efforts now waste more oxygen than is obtained.	*Early decompensation* Nasal flaring Retractions Grunting Wheezing Anxiety, irritability Mood changes Headache Hypertension Confusion
Imminent respiratory arrest The oxygen deficit is overwhelming and beyond spontaneous recovery. Cerebral oxygenation is dramatically affected; central nervous system changes are ominous.	*Severe hypoxia* Dyspnea Bradycardia Cyanosis Stupor and coma

Clinical Therapy

Pulse oximetry and arterial blood gases are used to assess respiratory failure. See Appendix B for expected laboratory values by age and Skill 10–6 SKILLS. Refer to Chapter 46 for interpretation of acidosis and alkalosis that must be considered simultaneously.

Medical management is focused on treating the cause of respiratory failure and reversing the severe hypoxemia with oxygen, mechanical ventilation, and positive end expiratory pressure (PEEP) to increase functional residual capacity. These children are admitted to the intensive care unit (ICU) for monitoring and ventilatory support.

The child's ability to maintain an open airway decreases as the level of responsiveness deteriorates. Endotracheal (ET) intubation is a short-term, emergency measure to stabilize the airway by placing a tube in the trachea. The ET tube must be protected and stabilized to prevent its displacement. End-tidal CO_2 monitoring is helpful to ensure that the tube is appropriately positioned in the trachea (see Skills 14–8 and 14–9 SKILLS). A tracheostomy is the creation of a surgical opening into the trachea through the anterior neck at the cricoid cartilage when longer term airway management is needed. The child may be sedated to optimize ventilation. Continuous positive airway pressure is one form of PEEP used to improve oxygenation and lung compliance. Death results if respiratory failure cannot be successfully managed.

Nursing Management

Early recognition of impending respiratory failure is the most important aspect of care for a child with any signs of respiratory compromise. Assess the child using guidelines in Table 48–1. Monitor the child for changes in vital signs, respiratory status, SpO_2, level of responsiveness. When the child has a chronic respiratory condition, development of respiratory failure may be gradual and signs will be subtle. Be particularly alert to behavior changes in addition to respiratory signs. Serial blood gases may be needed to monitor the child.

Place a child who has respiratory compromise in an upright position (elevate the head of the bed). Respiratory distress, anxiety, excessive crying, and even fever can deplete metabolic reserves and increase the child's need for oxygen. Administer oxygen as ordered and keep emergency equipment at the child's bedside. Be prepared to assist ventilations if the respiratory status deteriorates. (See Skills 9–8 to 9–10 SKILLS).

Because endotracheal and tracheostomy tubes prevent vocal cord vibration, intubated children cannot cry or talk. Infants and young children often express initial frustration when they realize they cannot communicate verbally. When the child is alert, give suggestions for ways to make noise and gain attention, such as striking the mattress. A communication board can be used with older children. Suction airway secretions as needed and provide tracheostomy care if present. See Skills 14–20 to 14–24 in the Clinical Skills Manual SKILLS.

Many children are discharged from the hospital and cared for at home for an extended period with a tracheostomy tube in place. Parents must demonstrate competence in all aspects of tracheostomy care (how to maintain and suction the airway, clean the tracheostomy site, and change the tube), as well as emergency resuscitation skills adapted to the tracheostomy. A home healthcare nurse can provide follow-up care and support for the child and family. (See Skill 14–11 SKILLS.)

> **Nursing Practice**
>
> As the child tires from the prolonged effort of breathing, the respiratory rate may begin to decrease. This is an ominous sign and may progress to respiratory arrest without intervention.

> **Thinking Critically**
>
> **OXYGEN DELIVERY DEVICES**
>
> Oxygen delivery devices are selected to match the concentration of oxygen needed by the child. In respiratory failure, a higher concentration of oxygen is needed to reverse the hypoxemia. Which oxygen delivery device should be used? Are there any contraindications to oxygen use in a child who is hypoxic?
>
> See MyNursingKit for possible responses.

APNEA

Infants commonly have **periodic breathing**, an irregular rhythm, and may have pauses of up to 20 seconds between breaths. This breathing pattern is not apnea. **Apnea** is the cessation of respiration lasting longer than 20 seconds, or any pause in respiration associated with cyanosis, marked pallor, hypotonia, or bradycardia. Apnea may be the first major sign of respiratory dysfunction in the newborn (see "Care of the Newborn with Respiratory Distress" in Chapter 29).

APPARENT LIFE-THREATENING EVENT (ALTE)

Apparent life-threatening event (ALTE) is defined as an episode of apnea accompanied by a color change (cyanosis, pallor, or occasionally ruddiness), limp muscle tone, choking, or gagging in a near-term or term infant who is greater than 37 weeks' gestation. These events are more common in infants between 1 and 8 weeks of age (Hall & Zalman, 2005). These episodes may occur during sleep, wakefulness, or feeding. ALTE should not be confused with sudden infant death syndrome (SIDS) (see page 1319). ALTE and SIDS have different clinical and epidemiologic factors; however, approximately 7% of infants who die from SIDS have an ALTE history (Hall & Zalman, 2005).

Potential causes of ALTE include gastroesophageal reflux, seizures or breath-holding episodes, neuromuscular disorders, respiratory disorders (e.g., pertussis, bronchiolitis, foreign body aspiration), congenital heart defect, cardiac arrhythmias, a small mandible leading to airway obstruction, obstructive sleep apnea, metabolic and endocrine problems, and child maltreatment. When a cause cannot be determined, it is called idiopathic ALTE.

MyNursingKit Teaching Plan: Discharge Instructions for a Child with a Tracheostomy Tube

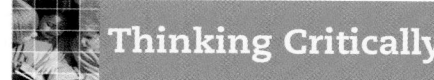

If repeated episodes of ALTE occur without identifiable cause, child abuse (Munchausen's syndrome by proxy) may be investigated (DeWolfe, 2005). (See Chapter 44.)

No minimum set of diagnostic tests has been identified for evaluation of these infants. Physical stimulation or emergency resuscitation may be required to revive the infant. Treatment is targeted at the underlying condition.

Nursing Management

After ALTE, infants are usually admitted to the hospital for evaluation and cardiorespiratory monitoring. Nursing care includes collecting a detailed history of the event, observing and monitoring cardiorespiratory status, providing supportive care to the infant and family, and anticipating the need for emergency resuscitation and for the diagnostic process.

Monitor cardiorespiratory status. Cardiorespiratory monitoring records heart rate and respiratory rate while the infant is awake and asleep. Pulse oximetry provides a noninvasive continuous evaluation of the infant's oxygenation status.

Anticipate emergency resuscitation. Because the infant who has had ALTE continues to be at risk for cardiopulmonary arrest, keep emergency resuscitation equipment and drugs readily accessible at all times.

Provide emotional support. Establishing rapport and open communication with the parents is essential for creating a sense of trust. To obtain further information about the episode, use open-ended questions and active listening skills. Parents are fearful and anxious about the infant's prognosis. Explanations of tests and treatment help to decrease their anxiety and increase their understanding of the situation.

During hospitalization the infant should be held and cuddled to provide a sense of security and well-being. Encouraging parents' participation in the infant's care helps to meet these needs and promotes family bonding. Often parents are afraid to touch the infant because they might disconnect the monitoring cable. Wrapping the cable inside the infant's blanket helps secure the wires, increasing parents' feelings of confidence in handling the infant.

Support the mother to continue breastfeeding and maintaining a supply of breast milk by pumping, if necessary. Ensure that the mother gets adequate fluids and nutrition. Provide privacy for breast pumping, and store breast milk for future feedings.

Discharge planning and home care teaching. Address home care needs in advance of the infant's discharge. Some infants are discharged with a cardiorespiratory monitor. Teach parents how to operate the monitor, what to do when the infant has an apneic episode, and how to perform cardiopulmonary resuscitation (CPR) and choking-intervention techniques (see Skill 14–13 SKILLS).

Teaching Highlights

HOME CARE INSTRUCTIONS FOR THE INFANT REQUIRING A CARDIORESPIRATORY MONITOR

Apnea Equipment

- Understand monitor type, lead wires, placement of skin electrodes and pulse oximetry sensor, and how to set the event recorder. Keep the battery fully charged, and keep the manual for troubleshooting handy.

Emergency Preparation

- Notify telephone company, electric company, local rescue squad, local emergency department (establishes priority status).
- Post in at least 2 places in the home the following information: phone numbers for emergency response, physician, equipment company, and power company, neighbor, parents' work and cell phone numbers, and cardiopulmonary resuscitation (CPR) guidelines.

Safety Precautions

- Place monitor on firm surface; keep away from other appliances (television, microwave oven) and water.
- Ensure that alarms are audible from all locations.
- Double-check that the monitor and event recorder are on before putting the infant down for a nap or at bedtime.
- Thread cable and wires through lower end of infant's clothes.
- Ensure integrity of leads, monitor cable, and power cord (replace if frayed).

Routine Care

- Understand reasons for apnea monitor. It should be used all the time, but if removed periodically, do so only when the infant is awake.
- Evaluate skin for irritation or breakdown from electrode placement and give skin care (no oils or lotion; move patches correctly).

Emergency Care

- Develop plan for respiratory failure and power failure.
- Demonstrate CPR and back blows and chest thrusts for airway obstruction.
- Understand how to respond to alarms for apnea, bradycardia, or loose lead.

Response to an Alarm

- Observe infant's respiratory movement first to determine if this is a real event.
- If respiration is absent, bradycardia is present, or infant is lethargic, stimulate by calling name and gently touching, proceeding to vigorous touch if needed.
- If no response, proceed with CPR.
- If a loose lead is suspected, determine if electrode patches are loose. Check the wires from electrode or monitor cable. Check the power supply. Is the monitor malfunctioning?

OBSTRUCTIVE SLEEP APNEA

Obstructive sleep apnea syndrome (OSAS) is a disorder of breathing during sleep that involves recurrent episodes of partial and complete upper airway obstruction that disrupts normal ventilation and sleep patterns (Bandla, Brooks, Trimarchi, et al., 2005). This results in labored breathing and snoring when the child tries to move air past the obstruction. The estimated prevalence of OSAS in children is 2% (Peeke, Hershberger, & Marriner, 2006).

The upper airway contains about 30 muscles that permit the pharynx to collapse, enabling the child to talk and swallow, but also maintain airway patency. When the child is awake, muscle tone is maintained and the airway remains patent even when obstructions such as enlarged adenoids and tonsils, craniofacial anomalies, or obesity are present. During sleep, the airway muscles relax, airway resistance increases, and the pharynx becomes obstructed. Reduced upper airway tone and obstruction then results in apnea episodes that lead to hypoventilation, hypoxemia, hypercapnia, and an elevated blood pressure. Hypertrophy of the adenoids and tonsils is the most common cause of OSAS, followed by craniofacial abnormalities, obesity, and neuromuscular disorders (e.g., cerebral palsy, muscular dystrophy).

Children with OSAS snore and have signs of labored breathing during sleep such as retractions and paradoxical breathing. After snoring or breathing pauses, the child may snort, gasp, choke, move, or arouse to take a breath. Sleep is restless and the child may sleep in unusual positions to hyperextend the neck and airway. Symptoms of sleep deprivation (poor attention, aggression, acting-out behavior, and poor school performance) may be noted. Physical findings may be normal, but mouth breathing and enlarged tonsils and adenoids may be present.

Diagnosis is made by **polysomnography**, a sleep study that simultaneously records the sleep state, gas exchange, breathing efforts, cardiac rhythm, and muscle activity and movement. Adenotonsillectomy is the most common treatment for OSAS, and the condition resolves in the majority of children. Continuous positive airway pressure (CPAP) is used for children with surgical contraindications or those with persistent OSAS (craniofacial anomalies, Down syndrome, or neuromuscular disorders) after adenotonsillectomy. Weight loss strategies may be implemented for obese children. OSAS may recur in children with obesity and rapid weight gain after adenotonsillectomy (Amin, Anthony, Somers, et al., 2008). Without treatment, complications can include failure to thrive, pulmonary hypertension, **cor pulmonale** (obstruction of pulmonary blood flow that leads to right ventricular hypertrophy and heart failure), systemic hypertension, and cognitive impairment.

Nursing Management

In the community setting, all children should be screened for snoring as part of their routine health care. When snoring is present, encourage the family to keep a sleep diary. Assess the child for signs of nasal obstruction, mouth breathing, and enlarged tonsils. Determine if the child has symptoms of sleep deprivation or if a condition is present that places the child at high risk for OSAS. Coordinate referral to a sleep center for polysomnogram evaluation. Discuss how to prepare the child for the strange setting and wires that will be attached during the sleep study. Most pediatric centers will allow the parent to stay with the child during the study.

Following adenotonsillectomy, the hospital nurse monitors the child for bleeding and respiratory distress, such as obstructive sleep apnea and pulmonary edema. Continuous pulse oximetry is used to detect oxygen desaturation. See Chapter 47 for care of the child having adenotonsillectomy.

Sleep center nurses provide education and support to families of children who need to use CPAP to treat the OSAS. The nurse helps identify the best fitting mask or nasal prong system for CPAP delivery. Parents may need guidance about helping children to go to sleep wearing the mask until they are accustomed to it.

SUDDEN INFANT DEATH SYNDROME (SIDS)

MyNursingKit Video: SIDS

Sudden infant death syndrome (SIDS) is defined as the sudden unexpected death during sleep of an infant under 1 year of age that remains unexplained after a thorough investigation, including an autopsy, a review of the circumstances of death, and the clinical history. SIDS is the third leading cause of infant mortality in the United States. Most SIDS deaths occur in infants between 2 and 4 months of age (Centers for Disease Control and Prevention, 2006). It is currently unpredictable and in some cases unpreventable.

SIDS is referred to as a "syndrome" because of the many and varied autopsy and clinical findings that characterize most infants who die of the disorder. The autopsy typically does not identify a disease process that caused the death. Infants in the prone and side-lying position are vulnerable because a brainstem abnormality (one that controls respiratory and autonomic responses to stressors) compromises their protective reflexes, such as arousal and head turning when experiencing asphyxia (Paterson, Trachtenberg, Thompson, et al., 2006). Homicide may be associated with 1% to 5% of suspected SIDS cases (Hymel & Committee on Child Abuse and Neglect, 2006). Other proposed causes include respiratory infection and long QT syndrome, a cardiac arrhythmia (Daley, 2004). (See Chapter 49.) SIDS is not associated with newborn apnea or immunizations (American Academy of Pediatrics [AAP] Task Force on Sudden Infant Death Syndrome, 2005). See Table 48–2 for factors that place infants at risk for SIDS.

The first symptom is a cardiopulmonary arrest. Clinical findings include evidence of a struggle or change in position during sleep and the presence of frothy, blood-tinged secretions from the mouth and nose. Typically parents find the infant dead in the crib in the morning or after a nap and report having heard no cries or disturbances during the night.

Nursing Management

The sudden, unexpected nature of the infant's death is confirmed in the emergency department. The nurse's role is to be empathetic and provide support during one of the greatest crises a family must face. The focus is on supporting the family during the communication of bad news and the shock of the infant's death. See Chapter 43.

Reassure the parents that they are not responsible for the infant's death and help them contact other family members and mobilize support. Older children may need reassurance that SIDS will not happen to them. They may also believe that bad thoughts or

Table 48–2 Risk Factors for Sudden Infant Death Syndrome (SIDS)

Infant Risk Factors

- Preterm or low birth weight
- Race (in decreasing order of frequency): most common in American Indian and Alaska Native infants, followed by non-Hispanic Blacks, non-Hispanic Whites, and Asian or Pacific Islanders, and Hispanics
- Gender: more common in males than females
- Age: most common in infants between 2 and 4 months of age
- Sleeping in prone or side-lying position; bed sharing, especially with people who smoke or are under the influence of alcohol or drugs

Environmental Risk Factors

- Exposure to environmental tobacco smoke, or mother smoked during pregnancy
- Loose bedding, use of pillows, comforters, quilts, blankets, stuffed animals
- Sleeping on soft surfaces (waterbed, sofa, pillows)
- Overheating (e.g., overdressing or excessive bedcovers)

Adapted from: Centers for Disease Control and Prevention. (2006). October 2006 is SIDS (sudden infant death syndrome) awareness month. Retrieved December 22, 2008 from http://www.cdc.gov/omh/Highlights/2006/HOct06SIDS.htm

wishes about their baby brother or sister caused the death. Support groups can help parents, siblings, and other family members express these fears and work through their feelings about the infant's death. The First Candle organization can help families locate a support group in their area. See MyNursingKit for this website.

Evidence in Action

A review of several studies has revealed that pacifier use when placing an infant down for a nap or sleep has a protective effect against SIDS. The American Academy of Pediatrics now recommends pacifier use for bedtime and naptime, but the pacifier should not be reinserted once the infant falls asleep (AAP Task Force on Sudden Infant Death Syndrome, 2005).

Nurses play an important role in SIDS prevention. Educate the parents of all newborns and infants about the recommended infant sleep position—on the back. The Back to Sleep Campaign, encouraging the placement of infants in supine position for sleeping was initiated in 1992 to reduce the incidence of SIDS. The 53% decrease in SIDS deaths and the decreased percentage of infants sleeping in prone sleep position (70% to 11.3%) between 1992 and 2004 demonstrates the success of this campaign (AAP Task Force on Sudden Infant Death Syndrome, 2005). Ask parents to make sure this position is used when the infant is cared for by another family member or childcare provider. Parents should also use a firm mattress and avoid the use of loose bedding, toys, and pillows. A sleeper rather than a blanket should be used to keep the infant warm while sleeping. See Chapter 56∞ for issues related to infant skull flattening from sleeping on the back.

Place hospitalized infants to sleep in supine position rather than side-lying or prone. See "Evidence-Based Nursing: Infant Sleep Positioning."

Evidence-Based Nursing

INFANT SLEEP POSITIONING

Clinical Question

In spite of evidence that supine position for newborns and infants reduces the risk for SIDS, why is this position not consistently used by nurses in hospitals?

Evidence

A survey conducted in 58 Missouri hospitals examined nurses' knowledge, attitude, and practice in positioning healthy newborns for sleep in the hospital. While nurses no longer used prone positioning for newborns, 75% of 528 responding nurses used side-lying or a mixture of side-lying and supine positioning. Almost all nurses (96%) reported awareness of guidelines for supine positioning of newborns. Reasons nurses used for the side-lying sleep position included fear of aspiration, increasing the infant's comfort, and improving the infant's sleep. The majority of nurses reported having found an infant in supine position that was in distress at some time (Bullock, Mickey, Green, et al. 2004). Another survey was conducted in 8 California hospitals with respondents including 96 newborn nursery staff (predominantly nurses) and 579 mothers. The majority of nurses (68.4%) reported placing infants on their side and 65.3% of nurses advised mothers to use either the side or supine position for sleep. Aspiration was the primary reason given for side-lying position. Most nursery staff (72%) reported awareness of guidelines for infant positioning for sleep. The majority of mothers (72%) reported seeing their newborn placed in a nonsupine position by nursery staff, and 44% of mothers were not given recommendations for a sleep position for their newborn. Mothers receiving a recommendation for newborn sleep position were told to use the side or back (Stastny, Ichinose, Thayer, et al., 2004).

Best Practices

The Back to Sleep campaign has successfully increased awareness of the importance of using the supine position for infant sleeping. Nurses may feel that side-lying position is safer to prevent aspiration, and not be aware that this position also increases the infant's risk for SIDS, especially if the infant rolls to prone position. Up to 80% of mothers were more likely to place their infant in supine position when nurses gave that advice and modeled the position in the hospital (Stastny et al., 2004). Nurses have an important opportunity to model appropriate sleep positioning for newborns and to educate parents about reducing the risk for SIDS.

Critical Thinking in Action

Identify methods to increase the use of supine positioning for newborns and infants who are hospitalized and to promote safe sleep for newborns and infants in the home.

See MyNursingKit for possible responses.

CROUP SYNDROMES

Croup is a term applied to a broad classification of upper airway illnesses that result from swelling of the epiglottis and larynx. The swelling usually extends into the trachea and bronchi. Included under the classification of croup syndromes are viral syndromes, such as spasmodic laryngitis (spasmodic croup), laryngotracheitis or laryngotracheobronchitis (LTB), and bacterial syndromes, such as bacterial tracheitis and epiglottitis (see "Pathophysiology Illustrated: Airway Changes with Croup").

LTB and bacterial tracheitis affect a large number of children across all age groups in both sexes. Epiglottitis, previously a common serious respiratory illness, is rare in the United States due to the Haemophilus influenza type B immunization. The initial symptoms of all three conditions include inspiratory **stridor** (a high-pitched, musical sound that is created by narrowing of the airway), a "seal-like" barking cough, and hoarseness. LTB is the most common disorder, but epiglottitis and bacterial tracheitis are more serious.

LARYNGOTRACHEOBRONCHITIS

Although the term *croup* is applied to several viral and bacterial syndromes, it most often refers to LTB, a viral invasion of the upper airway that extends throughout the larynx, trachea, and bronchi. Table 48–3 compares LTB and other croup syndromes.

Etiology and Pathophysiology

Acute viral LTB is most common in children 6 months to 6 years of age, with a peak age of 2 to 3 years (Dykes, 2005). Boys are affected more often than girls. LTB is of greatest concern in infants and children under the age of 6 years, because of potential airway obstruction. The causative organism is usually parainfluenza virus type I, II, or III, that appears during fall and winter months. Other viruses causing LTB include influenza, respiratory syncytial virus, and *Mycoplasma pneumoniae* (Rafei & Lichtenstein, 2006).

Airway tissues respond to the invading virus with inflammation and edema. Copious, tenacious secretions further increase the child's respiratory distress. The laryngeal inflammation causes the airway diameter to narrow in the subglottic area, site of the smallest upper airway diameter. Even small amounts of mucus or edema can quickly obstruct the airway. During inspiration, the walls of the inner airway are pulled together, causing further respiratory distress.

Clinical Manifestations

Most children brought to the emergency department with LTB have been ill for a couple of days with upper respiratory symptoms. These symptoms progress to a cough and hoarseness. Fever may or may not be present. Common presenting signs are

PATHOPHYSIOLOGY ILLUSTRATED

AIRWAY CHANGES WITH CROUP

Two important changes occur in the upper airway with croup: the epiglottis swells, thereby occluding the airway, and the trachea swells against the cricoid cartilage, causing restriction.

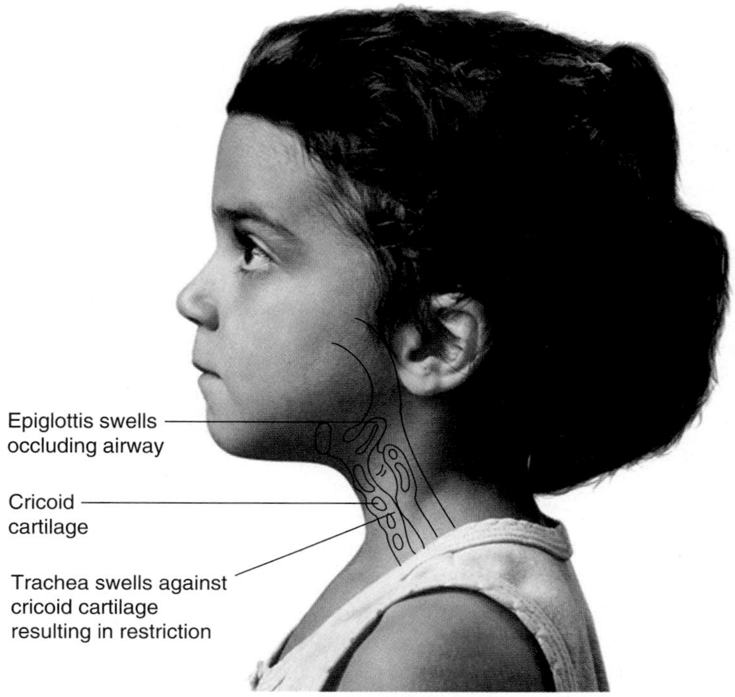

Table 48–3 Summary of Croup Syndromes

	Viral Syndromes		Bacterial Syndromes	
	Acute Spasmodic Laryngitis (Spasmodic Croup)	**Laryngotracheitis/ Laryngotracheobronchitis**	**Bacterial Tracheitis**	**Epiglottitis (Supraglottitis)**
Severity	Least serious	Serious; progresses if untreated	Guarded; requires close observation	Most life threatening (medical emergency)[a]
Age affected	3 months to 3 years	3 months to 8 years	1 month to 13 years[a]	2 years to 8 years
Onset	Abrupt onset; peaks at night, resolves by morning (recurs)[a]	Gradual onset; starts as URI, progresses to symptoms of respiratory distress; symptoms worse at night	Progressive from URI (1–2 days)	Progresses rapidly (hours)[a]; may progress to complete airway obstruction
Clinical manifestations	Afebrile; mild respiratory distress; barking-seal cough	*Early:* mild fever [less than 40°C (102.2°F)]; barking-seal, brassy, croupy cough; rhinorrhea; sore throat; stridor (inspiratory); apprehension; restless or irritable *Progressing to* retractions (progressive); increasing stridor; cyanosis	High fever [higher than 39°C (102.2°F)]; URI appears as viral croupy cough and croup initially; stridor (tracheal); purulent secretions; often prefers to lie flat	High fever [higher than 39°C (102.2°F)]; URI; intense sore throat; dysphagia[a]; drooling[a]; increased pulse and respiratory rate; prefers upright position (tripod position with chin thrust)[a]; cherry red epiglottis
Etiology	Unknown; allergic response to viral antigens rather than a direct infection is suspected; emotional influences	Parainfluenza, types I and II, RSV, or influenza; may develop a bacterial superinfection	Staphylococcus, Moraxella catarrhalis, and no-typeable Haemophilus influenza; may follow viral LTB	*Haemophilus influenzae*, streptococcus, staphylococcus

[a]Classic parameter or key point (distinguishes condition)

tachypnea, inspiratory stridor, and a seal-like barking cough. The presence of expiratory stridor, severe tachypnea, retractions, and a low SpO_2 are associated with a more severe airway inflammation and swelling. Changes in mental status may indicate hypoxemia and potential respiratory failure. See Table 48–3 to see clinical manifestations distinguishing these croup syndromes.

Clinical Therapy

Diagnosis is often made by history and clinical signs. Pulse oximetry is used to detect hypoxemia. If the diagnosis of LTB is in question, anteroposterior (AP) and lateral radiographs of the upper airway may be taken; these may show symmetric subglottic narrowing called a "steeple sign."

Management consists of maintaining and improving respiratory effort with medications and supplemental oxygen when the SpO_2 level is less than 92%. (See the Drug Guide.) Children who respond well to medications are often sent home from the emergency department after an observation period. Children with moderate to severe symptoms after nebulizer medications are admitted for further observation and treatment. Airway obstruction is a potential complication of LTB. The child may require intubation and transfer to the ICU to maintain airway patency if obstruction is imminent. Most children, however, respond positively to the medications and oxygen therapy and are discharged within 48 to 72 hours.

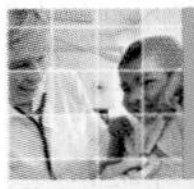

Nursing Practice

Throat cultures and visual inspection of the inner mouth and throat are contraindicated in children with LTB and epiglottitis. These procedures can cause **laryngospasms** (spasmodic vibrations that close the larynx) as a result of the child's anxiety or of probing this reactive and already compromised area. A complete airway obstruction may result.

NURSING MANAGEMENT

NURSING ASSESSMENT AND DIAGNOSIS

The initial and ongoing physical assessment of the child with LTB focuses on adequacy of respiratory functioning. Attach a cardiorespiratory monitor and pulse oximeter. Use a stridor assessment scale every 2 to 4 hours, or more frequently if respiratory distress increases (Table 48–4). Have the child in an area where continuous visual monitoring is possible to identify changes in airway patency.

Pay particular attention to the child's respiratory effort, breath sounds, preferred position, and responsiveness. Physical exhaustion can diminish the intensity of retractions and stridor. As the child uses the remaining energy reserve to maintain ventilation, breath sounds may actually diminish. Noisy breathing

Drug Guide

MEDICATIONS USED FOR TREATMENT OF LARYNGOTRACHEOBRONCHITIS

MEDICATION AND ACTION	NURSING MANAGEMENT
Beta-agonists and beta-adrenergics (e.g., albuterol, racemic epinephrine): aerosolized through face mask Rapid-acting bronchodilator, decreases bronchial and tracheal secretions and mucosal edema. Used until dexamethasone begins working.	■ Provides temporary relief in about 30 minutes, lasting about 2 hours; provides time for the corticosteroid to work; ■ May cause tachycardia (160–200 beats/min) and hypertension; dizziness, headache, and nausea may necessitate stopping medication; reduces the need for artificial airway
Corticosteroids (e.g., dexamethasone): IM, PO, nebulized budesonide Anti-inflammatory, used to decrease edema; has a long half-life of 36–54 hours	■ May cause cardiovascular symptoms (hypertension): closely observe for individual response; ■ Stridor resolves faster, child less frequently needs an emergency airway

Table 48–4 Clinical Scoring System for Assessing Children with Stridor

Sign	0	1	2	3
Stridor	None	With agitation	Mild at rest	Severe at rest
Retraction	None	Mild	Moderate	Severe
Air entry	Normal	Normal	Decreased	Severe decrease
Color	Normal	Normal	Cyanotic with agitation	Cyanotic with rest
Level of consciousness	Normal	Restless if disturbed	Restless if undisturbed	Lethargic

Source: From Perkin, R. M., & Swift, J. D. (2002). Infectious causes of upper airway obstruction in children. *Pediatric Emergency Medicine Reports, 7*(11), 120.
Scoring: To quantify the severity of stridor, add the individual scores for each of the sign categories. A score between 0 and 15 is possible. A rating of severity based on total score is as follows: less than 6 is mild, 7–8 is moderate, greater than 8 is severe.

(audible airway congestion, coarse breath sounds) in this situation verifies adequate energy stores. Responsiveness decreases as hypoxemia increases.

The following nursing diagnoses might be appropriate for the child with acute LTB:

- *Ineffective Breathing Pattern* related to tracheobronchial obstruction, decreased energy, and fatigue
- *Risk for Deficient Fluid Volume* related to inadequate fluid intake prior to admission
- *Fear (Child)* related to dyspnea, unfamiliar surroundings, procedures, and separation from support system

PLANNING AND IMPLEMENTATION

MAINTAIN AIRWAY PATENCY

Supplemental oxygen with humidity may be needed for hypoxemia. Allow the child to assume a comfortable position. Be immediately available to attend to the child's respiratory needs, and keep resuscitation equipment at the bedside. Administer medications. Ensure that a means of communication (sign language or simple word cues) is established so the older child can alert nursing staff to respiratory difficulty.

MEET FLUID AND NUTRITIONAL NEEDS

The illness preceding the emergency department visit may have compromised the child's fluid status. Recognize the potential fluid deficit and monitor the child's hydration and nutritional status. Fluids help liquefy secretions and provide calories for energy and metabolism.

Children with LTB usually prefer cool, noncarbonated, nonacidic drinks such as oral rehydration fluids or fruit-flavored drinks, gelatin, and popsicles. Encourage the parents to gain the child's cooperation in taking oral fluids. An intravenous infusion may be necessary to rehydrate the child, maintain fluid balance, or provide emergency access. Observe the child closely for difficulty in swallowing or drooling, which may be an early sign of epiglottitis.

DISCHARGE PLANNING AND HOME CARE TEACHING

During the child's observation period, take every opportunity to assess the parents' knowledge of symptoms of LTB and discuss actions to take if symptoms recur. For example, instruct parents to call the child's healthcare provider if:

- Mild symptoms do not improve after 1 hour of exposure to cool outdoor air or air conditioning.

Evidence in Action

High humidity has been a mainstay of treatment for croup and LTB; however, a recent study comparing the use of high and low humidity mist therapy in 140 children with moderately severe croup revealed that mist therapy is not beneficial. No differences in croup scores were found within 1 hour of mist therapy (Scolnik, Coates, Stephens, et al., 2006).

- The child's breathing is rapid and labored.
- The child does not drink adequate fluids and the urine output is reduced.

EVALUATION

Expected outcomes of nursing care include the following:

- The child responds to medications with decreased respiratory distress.
- The child's fear and anxiety is managed with family support and explanations about care.

EPIGLOTTITIS (SUPRAGLOTTITIS)

Epiglottitis is an inflammation of the epiglottis, the long narrow structure that closes off the glottis during swallowing. Because edema in this area can rapidly (within minutes or hours) obstruct the airway by occluding the trachea, epiglottitis is considered a potentially life-threatening condition. (Table 48–3 compares epiglottitis and other croup syndromes.)

Epiglottitis is caused by bacterial invasion of the soft tissue of the larynx by streptococcus, staphylococcus, or by *Haemophilus influenzae* type B (Hib) in unimmunized children. The resulting inflammation and edema in the tissues and surrounding the epiglottis lead to airway obstruction. Since the widespread use of the Hib vaccination, a tenfold decrease in the incidence of epiglottitis has occurred (Faden, 2006).

A previously healthy child suddenly becomes very ill with a high fever (greater than 39°C [102.2°F]) and sore throat. Four classic signs include dysphonia, **dysphagia** (difficulty in swallowing), drooling, and distressed respiratory effort with inspiratory stridor. The child sits up and leans forward with the jaw thrust forward to fully open the airway ("sniffing" or tripod position) and refuses to lie down. The child's anxiety increases as it becomes more difficult to breathe.

Diagnosis is often based on a lateral neck radiograph (Figure 48–2 ●), which reveals a narrowed airway and an enlarged, rounded epiglottis, seen as a mass at the base of the tongue. Laryngospasm and airway obstruction can occur as a result of the severe irritation and hypersensitivity of the airway muscles. For this reason, *visual inspection of the mouth and throat is contraindicated in children with suspected epiglottitis.*

Immediate clinical therapy usually involves insertion of an ET tube to maintain the airway. At the same time, a culture of the epiglottis is taken. Antibiotics effective for gram-positive organisms and *H. influenzae* are given until culture sensitivities are available, after which the antibiotic may be changed. Racemic epinephrine and corticosteroids are not effective. Rifampin prophylaxis (once a day for 4 days) should be given to any child contact that is immunocompromised or under age 48 months with incomplete Hib immunization. Antipyretics (acetaminophen, ibuprofen) may be useful in managing fever and sore throat pain.

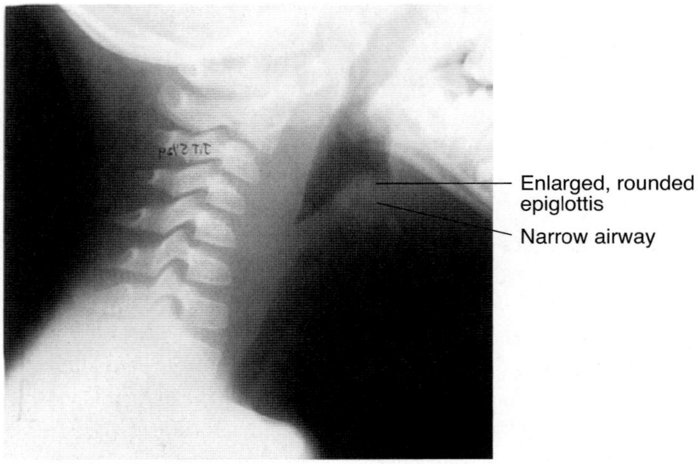

● **Figure 48–2** Epiglottitis. The phrase "thumb sign" has been used to describe this enlargement of the epiglottis. Recall the trachea's usual "little finger" size. Do you see the stiff, enlarged "thumb" above it in this lateral neck x-ray?

Nursing Management

Nursing management consists of airway management, drug therapy, hydration, and emotional and psychosocial support of the child and parents.

Until the child is intubated, the child is not left unattended. Allow the child to stay in the position of comfort. Observe the child's respiratory and airway status closely and often. Note any change in level of consciousness. Postpone anxiety-provoking procedures until the airway is stabilized. Crying stimulates the airway, increases oxygen consumption, and can precipitate laryngospasm. Supplemental humidified oxygen may be used initially to reverse hypoxemia.

Until the ET tube is removed, the child is managed in the PICU to ensure continual observation (see Skill 14–12 **SKILLS**). Reassure the child and parents that the inability to create sounds is temporary. Explain the need for various pieces of equipment to help reduce the child's stress. Administer antibiotics to treat the infection and IV fluids to provide hydration. Because the child was febrile with a sore throat before admission, fluid intake may have been compromised.

Most children show rapid improvement once oxygen, antibiotics, and fluid therapy are started. The ET tube can usually be removed within 1 to 2 days, and home care may involve completing the course of antibiotics. Parents need instructions on proper administration and potential side effects of drug therapy.

Nursing Practice

Observe the child continuously for inability to swallow, absence of voice sounds, increasing degree of respiratory distress, and acute onset of drooling. If any of these signs occur, get medical assistance immediately. The quieter the child, the greater the cause for concern.

BACTERIAL TRACHEITIS

Bacterial tracheitis is a secondary infection of the upper trachea following a viral LTB, often caused by *Staphylococcus aureus,* group A *streptococcus, Moraxella catarrhalis,* or *Haemophilus influenzae.* Characteristic signs include a cough, retractions, stridor, hoarseness, fever, and a toxic appearance. Drooling is rarely present, and the child may prefer to lie flat (Hopkins, Lahiri, Salerno, et al., 2006). Table 48–3 compares bacterial tracheitis and other croup syndromes.

Because of the similarity of symptoms, bacterial tracheitis is often misdiagnosed initially as LTB. Instead of improving with therapy, however, the child's condition becomes worse. Diagnosis is often made by blood cultures after the child is found unresponsive to usual LTB management. The subglottis is edematous with ulceration, and thick mucopurulent exudate may obstruct the airway. Antibiotics are given for a full 10- to 14-day course. Most children need intubation until swelling diminishes.

Nursing Management

The child with bacterial tracheitis is frequently cared for in the PICU after intubation. Mechanical suctioning of the thick tracheal secretions that pool high in the upper airway helps maintain a patent airway. Provide humidified air or oxygen. Antibiotics are administered as ordered. The previous section on epiglottitis discusses other nursing care interventions that may also be appropriate for the child with bacterial tracheitis.

LOWER AIRWAY DISORDERS

Lower airway disorders occur because a structural or functional problem interferes with the lungs' ability to complete the respiratory cycle. Disorders of the lower airway include bronchitis, bronchiolitis, pneumonia, and tuberculosis.

BRONCHITIS

Acute bronchitis, inflammation of the trachea and bronchi, is commonly the result of a viral upper respiratory tract infection. The bronchi can be affected simultaneously with adjacent respiratory structures during a respiratory illness. Bronchitis occurs most commonly in the winter months.

The classic symptom of bronchitis is a dry, hacking cough, which increases in severity at night. The cough may or may not be productive. The child may swallow sputum and vomit as a result. The chest and ribs may be sore because of the deep and frequent coughing. Over several days breath sounds may become coarse with fine crackles, and some scattered high-pitched wheezing may be heard. Treatment is palliative unless a secondary bacterial infection occurs that needs antibiotic therapy.

Nursing Management

Nursing management includes supporting respiratory function through rest, humidification, hydration, and symptomatic treatment. Refer to the sections on asthma and pneumonia for detailed information on treatment measures.

Home care should emphasize the self-limiting nature of the disorder. Advise parents who smoke that quitting or refraining from smoking in the child's presence may benefit the child.

BRONCHIOLITIS AND RESPIRATORY SYNCYTIAL VIRUS

Bronchiolitis is a lower respiratory tract illness that occurs when a viral or bacterial organism causes inflammation and obstruction of the bronchioles. Bronchiolitis is associated with a hospital admission rate of 30 per 1000 infants under age 1 year, and a mortality rate of 2 per 100,000 (Smyth & Openshaw, 2006). Children with bronchiolitis have an increased incidence of reactive airway disease and asthma later in childhood (Willis, 2007).

Etiology and Pathophysiology

Respiratory syncytial virus (RSV) is the most common cause, but adenovirus, parainfluenza virus, and human metapneumovirus may also be responsible. RSV occurs in annual epidemics from October to March. It is transmitted through direct contact with respiratory secretions or indirectly through contaminated surfaces. The virus is shed by the infected child for 3 to 8 days, and the incubation period is 2 to 8 days (AAP, 2009, pp. 560–561). Nearly all children have been infected with RSV by 2 years of age, and reinfection throughout life is common (AAP Subcommittee on Diagnosis and Management of Bronchiolitis, 2006). Infants at risk for severe infection with RSV include those under 24 months of age with chronic lung disease who have required medical therapy within 6 months of RSV season onset, those with significant congenital heart disease, and preterm infants under 35 weeks gestation (Fowlkes & Fry, 2006).

Viruses are able to invade the mucosal cells that line the small bronchi and bronchioles. The invaded cells die when the virus bursts from inside the cell to invade adjacent cells. The membranes of the infected cells fuse with adjacent cells, creating large masses of cells or "syncytia." The resulting cell debris clogs and obstructs the bronchioles and irritates the airway. In response, the airway lining swells and produces excessive mucus. Despite this protective effort by the bronchioles, the actual effect is partial airway obstruction and bronchospasms.

The cycle is repeated throughout both lungs as the airway cells are invaded by the virus. The partially obstructed airways allow air in, but the mucus and airway swelling block expulsion of the air. This creates the wheezing and crackles in the airways. Air trapped below the obstruction also interferes with normal gas exchange, leading to hypoxemia. The child with RSV is therefore at risk for respiratory failure as the oxygen level decreases and the carbon dioxide level increases. Apnea and pulmonary edema may occur.

Clinical Manifestations

Some children have mild symptoms such as rhinitis, cough, low grade fever, wheezing, tachypnea, poor feeding, vomiting, and diarrhea. Dehydration may be present if the child has been sick for several days. Parents report that the infant or child is acting more ill—appearing sicker, less playful, and less interested in eating.

Infants, especially, may refuse to feed or may spit up what they eat along with thick, clear mucus.

The infant or child with a more severe infection has tachypnea greater than 70 breaths per minute, grunting, increased wheezing, retractions, nasal flaring, irritability, lethargy, poor fluid intake, and a distended abdomen from overexpanded lungs. As hypoxia develops the infant becomes cyanotic and has decreasing mental status. As the airflow continues to decrease, breath sounds diminish. Thus the noisier the lungs, the better, as this indicates that the child is still able to move air in and out of the lungs. While RSV bronchiolitis resolves in 5 to 7 days, increased airway resistance and airway hypersensitivity may persist for weeks or even months.

Clinical Therapy

The history and physical examination provide the data needed to diagnose bronchiolitis. Chest radiographs show hyperinflation, patchy atelectasis, and other signs of inflammation. Enzyme-linked immunoabsorbent assay (ELISA) or immunofluorescent assay performed on a posterior nasopharyngeal specimen are laboratory tests used to identify the virus causing bronchiolitis (see Skills 10–13 and 10–14 SKILLS).

No effective therapy for RSV exists. Children who test positive for RSV are isolated or roomed together to minimize the spread of the virus to other hospitalized children. Humidified oxygen is provided to maintain the SpO_2 at readings greater than 90% (Willis, 2007). Other supportive care includes hydration with oral or IV fluids and nasal suctioning. Chest physiotherapy may have no benefit (AAP Subcommittee on the Diagnosis and Management of Bronchiolitis, 2006). CPAP may be used in the child with moderate to severe bronchiolitis. The child with apnea or respiratory failure will be cared for in the critical care unit, usually intubated and ventilated when too fatigued to breathe effectively (see Skill 11–20 SKILLS).

Few medications are prescribed for RSV and bronchiolitis. Antipyretics may be used. The use of inhaled bronchodilators have not demonstrated improvement in symptoms over time (AAP Subcommittee, 2006). Dexamethasone also has no documented benefit (Corneli, Zorc, Mahajan, et al., 2007). Antibiotics are not used routinely unless a bacterial infection is present. Ribavirin, an antiviral drug specifically available for RSV treatment, is reserved for cases of severe disease such as infants with complicated congenital heart disease or who are immunocompromised (AAP Subcommittee, 2006). Ribavirin is expensive with marginal benefit, and it is cumbersome to administer, and has potential health risks for caregivers.

Prevention of RSV is a focus for children at high risk for severe bronchiolitis, including the following groups of children (AAP, 2009, pp. 564–568):

- child under age 24 months with chronic lung disease of prematurity who have needed medical therapy within 6 months of the start of RSV season
- child under age 24 months with significant congenital heart disease, such as congestive heart failure, pulmonary hypertension, and cyanotic heart disease
- infants born at less than 28 weeks gestation or less during their first 12 months of life
- infants born at 29 to 32 weeks gestation up to 6 months of age
- infants born at 32 to 35 weeks gestation with 2 or more of the following risk factors: childcare attendance, exposure to environmental air pollutants, school-age siblings, congenital abnormalities of the airway, or severe neuromuscular disease

Prophylaxis with intramuscular palivizumab (Synagis) is used for the preceding groups of children as it is associated with reduced hospitalizations of high-risk infants. Palivizumab is expensive, but less costly than hospitalization for an infant with RSV. Monthly injections for 5 months are initiated in October or November, at the onset of the RSV season, and terminated at the end of the RSV season. Palivizumab does not interfere with administration of normal recommended childhood vaccines (AAP, 2006, p. 565).

NURSING MANAGEMENT

NURSING ASSESSMENT AND DIAGNOSIS

PHYSIOLOGIC ASSESSMENT

Assess airway and respiratory function carefully. Good observation skills are important to ensure timely interventions for worsening respiratory symptoms and prevention of respiratory distress (see Table 48–1 and the clinical manifestations of respiratory failure on page 1316). Assess the child's hydration status, weigh the child daily, and monitor the intake and output. Attach a cardiorespiratory monitor and pulse oximeter. An oxygen saturation level below 90% is the best indicator of the condition severity.

PSYCHOSOCIAL ASSESSMENT

Observe children and their parents for signs of fear and anxiety. The unfamiliar hospital environment and procedures can increase stress. Parents' questions, as well as their nonverbal cues, help direct nursing interventions during admission and throughout hospitalization.

The accompanying Nursing Care Plan: The Child with Bronchiolitis lists common nursing diagnoses for the child with bronchiolitis. Others that might also be appropriate include:

- *Ineffective Airway Clearance* related to increased airway secretions in bronchioles
- *Activity Intolerance* related to imbalance between oxygen supply and demand
- *Interrupted Family Processes* related to sudden acute illness of the infant

Nursing Practice

RSV bronchiolitis often increases in severity before beginning to resolve. Stay alert for signs of increased respiratory distress, and a greater need for oxygen. Inform the physician immediately of any significant changes in respiratory status.

Nursing Care Plan

THE CHILD WITH BRONCHIOLITIS

INTERVENTION	RATIONALE	EXPECTED OUTCOME
1. Nursing Diagnosis: Ineffective Breathing Pattern related to increased work of breathing		
NIC Priority Intervention: **Respiratory monitoring:** Collection and analysis of patient data to ensure airway patency and adequate gas exchange		**NOC Suggested Outcome:** **Vital signs status:** Temperature, pulse, respiration, and blood pressure within expected range for the child's age
Goal: The child will return to respiratory baseline. The child will not experience respiratory failure.		
■ Assess respiratory status (Table 48-1) when child is calm and not crying at least every 2–4 hours, or more often as indicated for an increasing or decreasing respiratory rate and episodes of apnea.	■ Changes in breathing pattern may occur quickly as the child's energy reserves are depleted. Baseline assessment provides data about the rate and quality of air exchange. Frequent assessment helps detect changes in the quality of respiratory effort.	The child returns to respiratory baseline within 48–72 hours.
■ Attach a cardiorespiratory monitor and pulse oximeter with alarms set. Record and report changes promptly to physician.	■ The alarm can alert the nurse to any sudden respiratory changes and lead to more rapid interventions.	
Goal: The child's oxygenation status will return to baseline.		
■ Administer humidified oxygen via mask, nasal cannula, hood, or tent.	■ Humidified oxygen loosens secretions, helps maintain oxygenation status, and eases respiratory distress.	The child's respiratory effort eases. The SpO_2 level remains at 95% or higher during treatment.
■ Assess and compare the child's SpO_2 level on room air and when on supplemental oxygen.	■ Comparison of SpO_2 levels provides information about improvement status.	
■ Note child's response to ordered medications.	■ Medications act systemically to improve oxygenation and decrease inflammation.	The child tolerates therapeutic measures with no adverse effects.
■ Position head of bed up or place child in position of comfort on parent's lap, if crying or struggling in crib or bed.	■ Position facilitates improved aeration and promotes decrease in anxiety (especially in toddlers) and energy expenditure.	The child rests quietly in position of comfort.
■ Assess tolerance to feeding and activities.	■ Provides an assessment of condition improvement.	
2. Nursing Diagnosis: Risk for Deficient Fluid Volume related to inability to meet body requirements and increased metabolic demand.		
NIC Priority Intervention: **Fluid management:** Promotion of fluid balance and prevention of complications resulting from abnormal or undesired fluid levels		**NOC Suggested Outcome:** **Hydration:** Amount of water in intracellular and extracellular compartments of body
Goal: Child's immediate fluid deficit is corrected.		
■ Evaluate need for intravenous fluids. Maintain IV, if ordered.	■ Previous fluid loss may require immediate replacement.	Child's hydration status is maintained during acute phase of illness as demonstrated by appropriate urine output and moist mucous membranes.
Goal: Child will be adequately hydrated, be able to tolerate oral fluids, and progress to normal diet.		
■ Calculate maintenance fluid requirements and give oral fluids, IV fluids, or both.	■ Assessment of fluid requirements enables the child to maintain hydration while transitioning to oral fluids.	Child takes adequate oral fluids after 24–48 hours to maintain hydration.

(continued)

Nursing Care Plan—continued

THE CHILD WITH BRONCHIOLITIS

INTERVENTION	RATIONALE	EXPECTED OUTCOME
■ Offer clear fluids and incorporate parent in care. Offer fluid choice when tolerated.	■ Choice of fluid offered by parent gains the child's cooperation.	The child accepts beverage of choice from parent or nursing staff.
■ Maintain strict intake and output monitoring and evaluate specific gravity at least every 8 hours.	■ Monitoring provides objective evidence of fluid loss and ongoing hydration status.	
■ Perform daily weight measurement on the same scale at the same time of day. Evaluate skin turgor.	■ Further evidence of improvement of hydration status.	Child's weight stabilizes after 24–48 hours; skin turgor is supple.
■ Assess mucous membranes and presence of tears.	■ Moist mucous membranes and tears are signs of adequate hydration.	Child shows evidence of improved hydration.

3. Nursing Diagnosis: Anxiety (Child and Parent) related to acute illness, hospitalization, uncertain course of illness and treatment, and home care needs

NIC Priority Intervention:

Anxiety reduction: Minimizing apprehension, dread, foreboding, or uneasiness related to an unidentified source of anticipated danger

NOC Suggested Outcome:

Anxiety control: Ability to eliminate or reduce feelings of apprehension and tension from an unidentifiable source

Goal: Child and parents will demonstrate behaviors that indicate less anxiety.

INTERVENTION	RATIONALE	EXPECTED OUTCOME
■ Encourage parents to express fears and ask questions; provide direct answers and discuss care, procedures, and condition changes.	■ Parents have the opportunity to vent feelings and receive timely, relevant information. This helps reduce parents' anxiety and increase trust in nursing staff.	Parents and child show less anxiety as symptoms improve and as child and parents feel more secure in hospital environment. *Parent* freely asks questions and participates in the child's care. The *child* cries less and allows staff to hold or touch him or her.
■ Incorporate parents in the child's care. Encourage parents to bring familiar objects from home. Ask about and incorporate in care plan the home routines for feeding and sleeping.	■ Familiar people, routines, and objects decrease the child's anxiety and increase parents' sense of control over an unexpected, uncertain situation.	

Goal: Parents will verbalize knowledge of bronchiolitis symptoms and use of home care methods before the child's discharge from the hospital.

INTERVENTION	RATIONALE	EXPECTED OUTCOME
■ Explain symptoms, treatment, and home care of bronchiolitis.	■ Anticipating the potential for recurrence assists the family to be prepared should respiratory symptoms recur after discharge.	Parent accurately describes respiratory symptoms and initial home care actions.
■ Provide written instructions for follow-up care arrangements, as needed.	■ Written and verbal instructions reinforce knowledge. Parents may not "hear" and remember details if only given verbally.	
■ Make sure parents can read the instructions, provide in family's primary language.	■ Many families have reading difficulty or may read a language other than English.	

PLANNING AND IMPLEMENTATION

Nursing management focuses on maintaining respiratory function, supporting overall physiologic function and hydration, reducing the child's and family's anxiety, and preparing the family for home care.

MAINTAIN RESPIRATORY FUNCTION

Close monitoring is essential to evaluate the child's improvement or to spot early signs of deterioration. Supplemental oxygen with humidity may be provided via nasal cannula, mask, hood, or tent. When the child resists or is frightened by the oxygen apparatus, engage the parent to soothe the child and promote acceptance of the therapy. Patent nares are important to promote oxygen intake. A bulb syringe and saline nose drops can be used to quickly clear the nasal passages. Elevate the head of the bed to ease the work of breathing and drain mucus from the upper airways.

SUPPORT PHYSIOLOGIC FUNCTION

Grouping nursing tasks decreases stress and promotes rest. Medications may be administered to control temperature and promote comfort as needed. Infants may have feeding difficulty and are at risk for aspiration. Smaller volumes and frequent feedings will help conserve energy in infants who are formula- or breastfed. When the risk of aspiration is high, nasogastric tube feedings may be used to provide nutrition. An IV infusion may be ordered to rehydrate the child and maintain fluid balance until oral fluid intake is adequate.

REDUCE ANXIETY

The need for hospitalization and assistive therapies creates anxiety and fear in the child and parents. The parents may be frightened by the child's continued respiratory difficulty and the assistive equipment at the bedside. Infants may respond to their parents' anxiety and be more irritable. Provide parents with thorough explanations and daily updates, and encourage their participation in the child's care. Reassure them that holding or touching the child will not dislodge wires or tubing, and that their presence will calm and support the child.

If the child has been ill for a few days before admission, the parents are likely to be tired. Acknowledging parents' physical and emotional needs creates a spirit of caring and enhances communication between staff and family. Encourage the parents to take turns at the child's bedside and to take breaks for meals and rest.

DISCHARGE PLANNING AND HOME CARE TEACHING

Children are discharged once they show sufficient stability in maintaining adequate oxygenation (as evidenced by easing of respiratory effort and decreased mucus production). In most children, symptoms decrease within 24 to 72 hours; however, resolution of all symptoms may take weeks. Coughing may continue for a few weeks after discharge.

Teach the parents proper administration of medications. Acetaminophen may be prescribed for persistent low-grade fevers and general discomfort. Advise parents that RSV infection can recur; therefore, they need to know how to recognize symptoms and when to call the physician.

EVALUATION

Expected outcomes of nursing care for the child with bronchiolitis are provided in the Nursing Care Plan.

Teaching Highlights

DISCHARGE TEACHING FOR BRONCHIOLITIS

General care instructions:

- Use the bulb syringe to suction the nares of an infant under age 1 year.
- Give fluids to help keep secretions thick and provide calories for energy.
- Encourage active toddlers to rest and take naps during recovery.

Advise parents to call the physician if:

- Respiratory symptoms interfere with sleep or eating.
- Breathing is rapid or difficult.
- Symptoms persist in a child who is less than 1 year old, has heart or lung disease, or was premature and had lung disease after birth.
- The child acts sicker—appears tired, less playful, and less interested in food (parents just "feel" the child is not improving).

PNEUMONIA

Pneumonia, an inflammation or infection of the bronchioles and alveolar spaces of the lungs, occurs most often in infants and young children. The incidence of pneumonia in the United States is 35 to 40 cases per 1000 children under age 5 years, and 16 to 22 cases per 1000 children 5 years and older (Sandora & Harper, 2005).

Pneumonia may be viral, mycoplasmal, or bacterial in origin. Children under 5 years most often have viral pneumonia due to RSV, human metapneumovirus, influenza, parainfluenza virus, adenovirus, rhinovirus, and enterovirus. While bacterial pneumonia is more common in children over 5 years, it occurs in all age groups. Common bacterial organisms include Group B streptococcus and *Escherichia coli* in newborns, *Chlamydia trachomatis* in infants, *Mycoplasma pneumonia* in school-age children, and *Streptococcus pneumonia* in all age groups. Children with cystic fibrosis or immunosuppression are susceptible to other bacterial, parasitic, or fungal infections.

Bacterial and viral invaders act differently within the lungs:

- Bacterial invaders circulate through the bloodstream to the lungs, where they damage cells and cause inflammation and edema. Cellular debris and mucus cause airway obstruction. Bacteria tend to be distributed evenly throughout one or more lobes of a single lung, a pattern termed *unilateral lobar pneumonia.*
- Viruses enter through the upper respiratory tract, infiltrating the alveoli nearest the bronchi of one or both lungs. Viruses invade the cells, replicating and bursting out forcefully, killing the cells and sending out cell debris. Adjacent areas are invaded, distributed in a scattered, patchy pattern referred to as bronchopneumonia.

MyNursingKit Interpreting Tuberculin Skin Test Results in Infants, Children, and Adolescents

- Aspiration of food, emesis, gastric reflux, or hydrocarbons causes a chemical injury and inflammatory response, which sets the stage for bacterial invasion.

Pneumonia is often preceded by an upper respiratory tract infection including rhinitis and a cough. Other symptoms include fever, rhonchi, crackles, wheezes, cough, dyspnea, tachypnea, restlessness, and decreased breath sounds if consolidation exists. Newborns and infants may have grunting, nasal flaring, irritability, lethargy, and a diminished appetite. Diminished breath sounds may be noted. Children with bacterial pneumonia may have chest pain and try to splint the chest when coughing.

Diagnosis is based upon history and physical findings. A chest radiograph sometimes helps distinguish the type of pneumonia. A white blood cell count greater than 20,000 may indicate bacterial pneumonia.

Clinical management for all types of pneumonia includes pain and fever control, and supportive care through airway management, fluids, and rest. Antibiotics are used to treat bacterial pneumonias. Some children with severe pneumonia need supplemental oxygen and IV fluids to maintain hydration. Complications such as an empyema (a collection of pus in the pleural space) or a pleural effusion are treated by drainage with a thoracostomy tube SKILLS.

Nursing Management

Most children with pneumonia are cared for at home. When children are hospitalized, assess the child, paying particular attention to respiratory rate, heart rate, and temperature, and observe color for pallor or cyanosis. Attach a pulse oximeter to monitor the SpO_2 level. Assess hydration status. Assess for the presence of pain with coughing.

Nursing measures used for the child with bronchiolitis are generally applicable (see page 1326). Provide ongoing respiratory assessments and supportive therapies (chest physiotherapy, antibiotics, hydration). Teach the child and parent how to splint the chest by hugging a small pillow or teddy bear to make coughing less painful. Pain medication (acetaminophen or ibuprofen) can also help with temperature control and may aid sleep. Promote hydration and nutrition by encouraging the intake of preferred clear liquids and small servings of soft foods.

Teach parents about administering prescribed antibiotics, any potential side effects, and the need to give the full course. Educate parents about signs that the child's condition may be worsening (increased breathing difficulty or refusal to take fluids). Follow-up may include a chest radiograph to see if the lungs are clear. Symptoms of pneumonia usually disappear long before the lungs are completely healed. Most children recover uneventfully, but some continue to have worsening reactive airway problems or abnormal results on pulmonary function tests.

Preventive measures are limited. The Haemophilus influenza type B (Hib) and pneumococcal conjugate (PCV7) vaccines protect against some causes of pneumonia. The 23-valent pneumococcal vaccine is recommended for children over 2 years of age with immunosuppression or some chronic conditions (see Chapter 45).

TUBERCULOSIS

Tuberculosis (TB) is an infection caused by *Mycobacterium tuberculosis,* which is transmitted through the air in infectious particles called droplet nuclei. In 2005, 863 children under age 15 years in the United States acquired TB. Nearly 25% of these children were foreign born, and 75% were Hispanic or non-Hispanic black (Starke, 2007).

Etiology and Pathophysiology

Children usually acquire a TB infection from infected adults who cough, sneeze, speak, or sing, and send out tiny droplets containing the bacillus. When inhaled, the bacillus is small enough to travel directly to the alveoli and cause infection. When the organism reaches the alveoli, an immune response is initiated, and macrophages surround and wall off the bacillus in small hard capsules, called tubercles. The bacillus can remain dormant (inactive) indefinitely, or it can progress to active TB by growing slowly and dividing within the macrophage. When the organisms number 1000 to 10,000 after 2 to 12 weeks, a cellular immune response to TB can be elicited with the TB skin test.

In persons with intact cell-mediated immunity, activated T cells and macrophages form granulomas that limit multiplication. The proliferation of TB is arrested, but small numbers of viable bacilli may remain in the granuloma. These individuals have latent tuberculosis infection (LTBI), a positive tuberculin skin test, and no clinical or radiographic signs of disease. They are not infectious and cannot transmit the disease.

The risk of transitioning from LTBI to active TB is greatest in children under age 5 years. Factors that increase that risk include immunosuppressive therapy, HIV co-infection, malnutrition, chronic medical conditions, TB infection in the past 2 years, and viral infections such as measles (Feja & Saiman, 2005). Up to 40% of untreated infants with LTBI develop active TB within 2 to 12 months after initial infection (Reznick & Ozuah, 2005). Active TB may develop within 4 to 6 weeks, before a tuberculin skin test becomes positive (Taylor, Nolan, & Blumberg, 2005). Children under age 10 years with active TB are rarely contagious, because they have small pulmonary lesions, an unproductive cough, and few or no bacilli are expelled (AAP, 2006, p. 680).

Extrapulmonary TB occurs in 10% to 20% of children, and more commonly in children under age 6 years (Feja & Saiman, 2005; Peredo-Pinto & Jacobs, 2008). Systemic disease, which can lead to serious illness or death, occurs if the tubercle extends into a blood vessel, spreading to the liver, spleen, kidney, bone marrow, or meninges (miliary TB).

Clinical Manifestations

Children with LTBI are asymptomatic. Children with pulmonary TB may have a persistent cough, weight loss or failure to gain weight, fever, fatigue, wheezing, and decreased breath sounds. Adolescents may have fever, weight loss, productive cough, hemoptysis, and night sweats (Feja & Saiman, 2005). When TB spreads outside the pulmonary system, additional signs are specific to the system invaded:

- superficial lymphadenitis: firm, nontender, matted lymph nodes

- miliary: high fever, vomiting, lethargy, headache, seizures, nuchal rigidity, and irritability; also hepatosplenomegaly and generalized lymphadenopathy
- osteoarticular: inflammation, pain, swelling, fever, and limited range of motion of the affected bone or joint

Clinical Therapy

Screening to identify a child's risk for LTBI should occur during health visits every 6 months until age 2 years, and then annually. Administer an intradermal tuberculin skin test (PPD) if one or more of these risk factors are present (AAP, 2009, p. 685):

- The child was born in any country or region except the United States, Canada, Australia, New Zealand, or Western Europe.
- The child traveled outside the United States and had contact with the resident population for more than a week in any country or region except those listed above.
- The child has a family member or contact with TB.
- A family member had a positive tuberculin skin test.

A positive test indicates that the child has been exposed to and infected with TB, and antibodies have been produced against the bacillus.

An enzyme-linked immunosorbent assay QuantiFERON-TB Gold (QFT-G) may have greater specificity than the PPD in identifying LTBI and active TB. Results can be available in 24 hours. The test may be more specific for children vaccinated with bacille Calmette-Guérin (BCG) (Todd, 2006). Other diagnostic tests include acid-fast stains of blood, gastric aspirate, and sputum cultures and a chest radiograph.

Active and latent TB are treated with antitubercular drugs, including isoniazid, rifampicin, pyrazinamide, and ethambutol. Therapy for active TB usually involves a 6-month regimen consisting of isoniazid, rifampin, and pyrazinamide for the first 2 months and isoniazid and rifampin for the remaining 4 months. LTBI is treated with a single daily dose of isoniazid for 9 months (or rifampin for 6 months if TB is drug resistant to isoniazid). To improve treatment adherence for both active TB and LTBI direct-observed drug therapy administered by a nurse or other healthcare provider twice a week for the duration of treatment is recommended to ensure the drug is being taken (Reznik & Ozuah, 2005).

Cases of active TB are reported to the public health department so that disease contacts can be found. A child diagnosed with TB is considered a sentinel case, and the adult contact with active TB must be identified.

Nursing Management

Assessment focuses on identifying children at high risk of TB exposure and infection and performing tuberculin skin testing as appropriate. Infant and young children with a tuberculin skin test conversion are at greater risk to develop active TB over the next few months, so assess them carefully for weight loss, fever, fatigue, coughing, and respiratory status. If TB is suspected, implement airborne isolation precautions until the infection status is known.

Nursing care focuses on administering medications and providing supportive care. Teach parents about the disease process, medications, possible side effects, and the importance of completing long-term therapy. Emphasize the importance of taking medications as prescribed on an empty stomach. Initiate direct-observed drug therapy twice a week.

Encourage proper nutrition and rest to promote normal growth and development. The child can return to school or child care when effective therapy has been instituted, adherence to therapy has been documented, and clinical symptoms have diminished substantially (AAP, 2009, p. 699). Most children with TB can lead essentially normal lives. See the discussion of pneumonia on page 1329 and of tubercular meningitis in Chapter 56∞ for other nursing care measures.

CHRONIC LUNG DISEASES

MyNursingKit Nursing Care Plan: The Child with BPD

BRONCHOPULMONARY DYSPLASIA

Bronchopulmonary dysplasia (BPD), also called chronic lung disease, is the persistence of lung disease following premature birth and respiratory support provided in the neonatal period. It is the most serious chronic respiratory disorder that begins during infancy. BPD usually occurs in infants born at less than 30 weeks gestation with a birth weight less than 1500 g (Baraldi & Filippone, 2007). Antenatal corticosteroids and surfactant replacement therapy have reduced the risk for BPD in more mature premature infants (Ehrenkranz, Walsh, Vohr, et al., 2005).

Etiology and Pathophysiology

BPD results from positive-pressure ventilation and oxygen treatment for respiratory failure and respiratory distress syndrome (see newborn respiratory distress information in Chapter 31∞). Provision of oxygen and ventilation at birth in which tidal volume and inspiratory pressure are not monitored is thought to damage the developing alveolar sacs in the immature lungs. Fewer and larger alveoli with less functional surface area result, and reduced capillary growth in the alveolar region leads to ventilation-perfusion mismatch. Pulmonary hypertension, interstitial fibrosis and smooth muscle hypertrophy may also develop (Froh, 2006). Pneumonia, sepsis, meconium aspiration syndrome, diaphragmatic hernia, and lung hypoplasia are causes of BPD in term or near-term newborns (Baraldi & Filippone, 2007).

Clinical Manifestations

The infant with BPD has persistent signs of respiratory distress: tachypnea, nasal flaring, grunting, retractions, wheezing, crackles, and irritability. Normal activities, such as feeding, can create increased oxygen demands and fatigue that lead to failure to thrive. The infant has intermittent bronchospasms, mucous plugging, and air trapping which may lead to a barrel-shaped chest (see "Pathophysiology Illustrated: Barrel Chest"). Cyanosis may be seen in severe cases.

Clinical Therapy

Diagnosis is made by the neonate's dependence on supplemental oxygen for at least 28 days after birth, and severity is increased if CPAP or mechanical ventilation is also needed. A chest radiograph often shows hyperexpansion, atelectasis, and interstitial thickening (Capper-Michel, 2004).

PATHOPHYSIOLOGY ILLUSTRATED

BARREL CHEST

A barrel chest may result from chronic respiratory conditions such as asthma or bronchopulmonary dysplasia, in which air trapping or hyperinflation of the alveoli occurs.

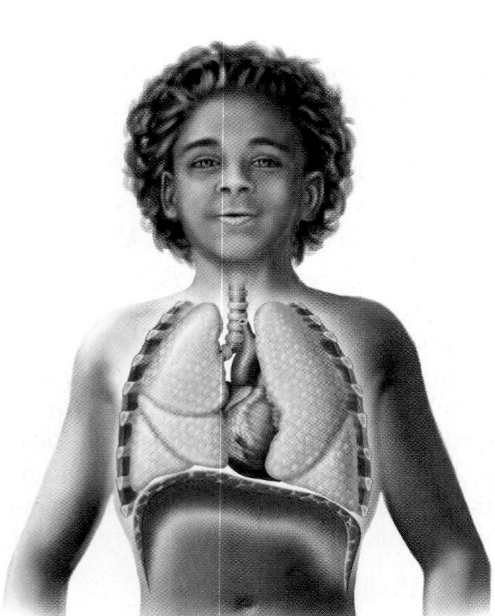

Medical management involves symptomatic treatment that supports respiratory function and good nutrition, which helps to accelerate lung maturity. Supplemental oxygen with humidity is used. A tracheostomy may be needed for long-term airway management to prevent narrowing of the trachea. Infants with severe BPD are carefully weaned off of assisted ventilation. Some children need gastrostomy or nasogastric tube feeding to get adequate calories.

Chest physiotherapy and medications (diuretics, bronchodilators, antiinflammatories, and methylxanthines) are used (see Drug Guide 48–2). Corticosteroids are not recommended for routine use (Baraldi & Filippone, 2007). Antibiotics are used to aggressively treat infections. Palivizumab is given monthly to prevent respiratory syncytial virus during RSV season. With improvement and adequate weight gain, the child is weaned off oxygen, diuretics, and bronchodilators. Some infants die due to respiratory failure and infection. Long-term sequelae include asthma and respiratory disease in adult life (Baraldi & Filippino, 2007).

NURSING MANAGEMENT

Nursing management focuses on assessing and managing the infant's acute episodes, ensuring adequate nutrition, and promoting growth and development.

NURSING ASSESSMENT AND DIAGNOSIS

Infants with BPD may become acutely ill at any time, so observe for signs of infection. During hospitalization for acute infections, a cardiorespiratory monitor and pulse oximeter are used. Assess airway and respiratory function, vital signs, color, and behavior changes to identify signs of worsening respiratory symptoms, even when oxygen is provided. Observe for airway obstruction when the infant has a tracheostomy and suction as needed. See the Clinical Skills Manual for tracheostomy care. For the infant with BPD cared for at home, monitor respiratory status and growth as the infant often experiences poor weight gain.

Nursing diagnoses that may be appropriate include:

- *Impaired Gas Exchange* related to ventilation-perfusions imbalance
- *Caregiver Role Strain* related to 24 hour responsibility for infant with BPD
- *Imbalanced Nutrition: Less than Body Requirements* related to high metabolic needs and fatigue associated with feeding
- *Risk for Delayed Development* related to chronic condition and limited opportunities to practice motor skills

PLANNING AND IMPLEMENTATION

Organize care for the hospitalized child to reduce unnecessary physical stimulation. Position the infant to facilitate breathing.

Administer medications as prescribed. Provide fluids and nutrition to meet energy needs. Fluid management is essential as excess fluids can lead to pulmonary edema. Support the mother who desires to breastfeed. A high-calorie formula (24 to 30 calories/oz) may be given to promote weight gain. Some children need nasogastric or gastrostomy tube feedings to get adequate calories for growth.

Once home, many infants need ventilation therapy, oxygen, tracheostomy care, multiple medications, fluid restrictions, and high-calorie feedings (Figure 48–3 ●). Make referrals for needed oxygen, respiratory supplies, medications, an early intervention program, and follow-up care well in advance of the infant's discharge. Some families need home health nursing assistance, espe-

Thinking Critically

INFANT WITH BPD

Emily is an 8-month-old infant with BPD cared for at home by her parents. She has a tracheostomy and receives humidification. Emily has periodic infections and episodes of respiratory distress that require hospitalization. When she develops a fever, more secretions than usual collect in the trachea. Suctioning is needed to ease Emily's breathing. What signs indicate that Emily needs to be suctioned? How do you select the correct-sized suction catheter? How do you suction Emily without causing hypoxia? When is it necessary to change Emily's tracheostomy tube?

See MyNursingKit for possible responses.

Drug Guide

MEDICATIONS USED TO TREAT BRONCHOPULMONARY DYSPLASIA

MEDICATION AND ACTION	NURSING MANAGEMENT
Bronchodilators (beta$_2$-adrenergics, anticholinergics, theophylline, albuterol nebulizer) Decreases airway resistance; increases expiratory flow in small airways; stimulates mucous clearance	Monitor vital signs and for signs of toxicity Administer medications at same time each day Encourage fluid intake
Anti-inflammatories (cromolyn sodium) Decreases inhibition of inflammatory mediators from mast cells	Ensure parents use proper technique for inhaler and spacer. Clean inhaler daily, rinsing and drying parts
Diuretics (furosemide, chlorothiazide, spironolactone) Remove excess fluid from lungs; decreases pulmonary resistance and increases pulmonary compliance; may cause electrolyte imbalances	Follow guidelines for allowable fluid intake Monitor serum potassium and sodium levels Teach families about sodium- and potassium-rich foods to eat or avoid, depending upon diuretic prescribed
Potassium chloride Prevents electrolyte imbalances associated with diuretics	Monitor serum potassium level Teach families about potassium-rich foods to avoid or use in moderation
Methylxanthines (caffeine, theophylline) Increases respiratory drive, decreases apnea, and relaxes muscle bundles that constrict airways	Monitor vital signs and respiratory status Monitor for adverse effects such as irritability, tremor, tachycardia, nausea and vomiting

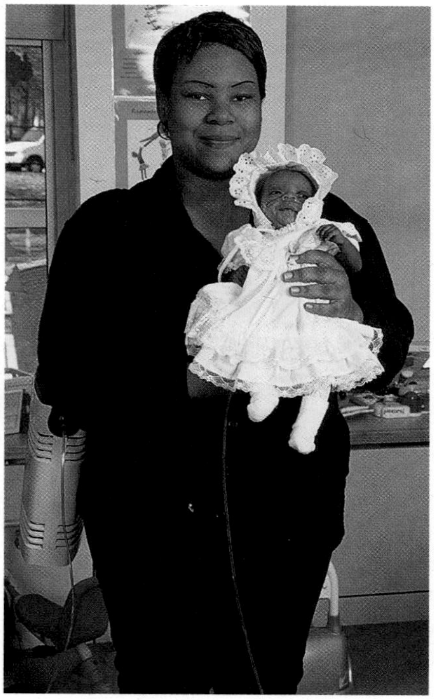

• **Figure 48–3** Home care for BPD. Many children with BPD are cared for at home, with the support of a home care program to monitor the family's ability to provide airway management, oxygen, and ventilator support. This premature infant girl, who is now 4 months old but weighs only about 5 pounds, still requires supplemental oxygen.

cially during the initial transition period. Teach parents to provide the complex care needed by the infant and to identify the signs of respiratory compromise indicating a need for rapid intervention.

Suggest ways to provide for the infant's normal development through rest, nutrition, stimulation, and family support (see "Health Promotion and Maintenance" overview).

EVALUATION

Expected outcomes of nursing care may include:

- The infant receives adequate calories to sustain growth.
- The family identifies acute illness episodes rapidly and seeks appropriate care.
- The infant's acute respiratory decompensation episodes are effectively managed.

ASTHMA

Asthma is a common chronic disorder of the airways that is complex and characterized by variable and recurring symptoms, airflow obstruction, bronchial hyperresponsiveness, and an underlying inflammation (National Asthma Education and Prevention Program, 2007, p. 12). In 2005, 9 million (12.7% of) children had been diagnosed with asthma, and 70% had had an asthma episode in the prior 12 months. These children missed an estimated 12.8 million days of school due to asthma.

MyNursingKit Asthma Guidelines for Children Under 5

HEALTH PROMOTION

THE CHILD WITH BRONCHOPULMONARY DYSPLASIA

Health Supervision

- Assess blood pressure to detect abnormal findings associated with pulmonary hypertension.
- Coordinate vision screening by an ophthalmologist every 2–3 months during the first year of life. Myopia and strabismus are common resulting from oxygen therapy as a premie.
- Coordinate pulmonary function tests annually or as needed for clinical condition.
- Perform hearing and other screening tests as recommended for age.

Growth and Developmental Surveillance

- Assess growth and plot measurements on a growth chart corrected for gestational age. Even if length and weight are lower than normal, monitor for continued growth following the growth curves.

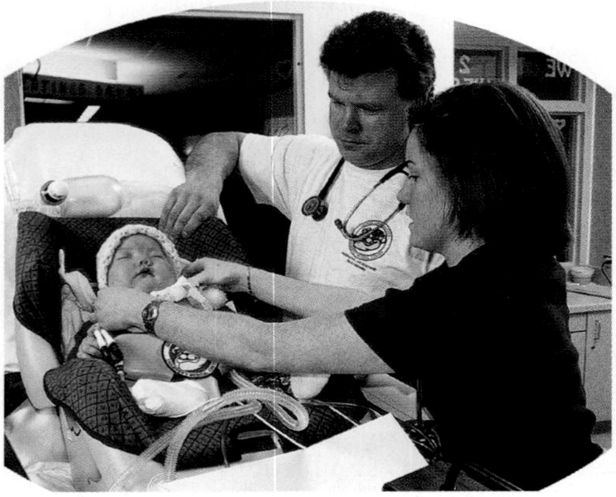

- Perform the Denver II and record the developmental assessment corrected for gestational age.

Nutrition

- Review fluid and caloric intake. Ensure that increased calories are provided to support growth while limiting fluids to prevent pulmonary edema. Assess difficulties with feeding related to oral motor function. Refer to a nutritionist as necessary.

Physical Activity

- Organize care to provide rest periods during the day.
- Provide developmentally appropriate toys and activities.
- Give parents ideas for promoting the infant's motor development, such as reaching for and moving toward toys and objects of interest.

Family Interactions

- Identify ways to coordinate night time care to reduce child and family sleep disturbances.
- Provide discipline appropriate for developmental age.

Disease Prevention Strategies

- Reduce exposure to infections. Encourage selection of a childcare provider who cares for a small number of children, if one is used. If possible, avoid the use of childcare centers during RSV season.
- Immunize the child with the routine schedule based on chronologic age.
- Administer the 23-valent pneumococcal vaccine at 2 years of age.
- Provide monthly injections of palivizumab throughout the RSV season.

Condition-Specific Guidance

- Develop an emergency care plan for times when the infant's condition rapidly worsens.

Asthma accounts for about 2.8% of all emergency department visits and 3% of all hospitalizations among children (Akinbami, 2006). Most children with asthma experience their first symptoms before the age of 5 years. See MyNursingKit for Web sites with more asthma statistics. See Developing Cultural Competence.

Etiology and Pathophysiology

Asthma is a chronic inflammatory disease of the lungs caused by the interplay of multiple factors (such as environmental exposures, viral illnesses, allergens, and a genetic predisposition) that occur at a crucial time in the immune system's development. More than 20 genes are associated with the susceptibility and pathology of asthma (Brashers, 2006a). Risk factors for asthma include passive smoke exposure, indoor air contaminants (for example, pet dander, cockroach feces), outdoor air pollutants, recurrent

Developing Cultural Competence

ASTHMA PREVALENCE

Non-Hispanic black children have an asthma prevalence rate of 15.8%, and 7.45% had an asthma episode in the past year. Non-Hispanic white children have an asthma prevalence of 12.7%, and 5.8% had an asthma episode in the past year. Hispanic children have an asthma prevalence rate of 12.4%, and 5.1% had an asthma episode in the past 12 months. Of Hispanic children, Puerto Ricans have the highest prevalence rate (26%), and 11.8% had asthma episodes in the past year. Cuban and Dominican children had prevalence rates similar to non-Hispanic black children, while Mexican children had the lowest prevalence rates of all groups (Lara, Akinbami, Flores, et al., 2006).

respiratory viral infections, and allergic disease (atopic eczema, food allergies). Protective factors include a large family size, later birth order, childcare attendance, dog in the family, and living on a farm. These factors increase exposure to infections early in life, enabling the child's immune system to develop along a nonallergic pathway (National Asthma Education and Prevention Program, 2007, p. 23).

Inflammation causes the normal protective mechanisms of the lungs (mucous formation, mucosal swelling, and airway muscle contraction) to overreact in response to a stimulus. Airway responsiveness is enhanced through inflammatory mechanisms. A **trigger**, an inflammatory or noninflammatory stimulus that initiates an asthma episode, increases the frequency and severity of smooth muscle contraction. Triggers include exercise, infectious agents, allergens, fragrances, food additives, pollutants, weather changes, and emotions.

The trigger may activate IgE and sensitized mast cells, leading to the release of inflammatory mediators (e.g., histamines, prostaglandins, and leukotrienes). These mediators initiate acute bronchospasm, vascular congestion, increased vascular permeability, edema formation, mucus production, impaired mucociliary function, and airway wall thickening. Epithelial cell damage is caused by eosinophil infiltration leading to airway hyperresponsiveness and obstruction. The reactive airway responses to stimuli are present before the trigger initiates the physiologic sequence that results in an asthma episode.

Airway narrowing results from bronchial constriction, airway swelling and production of copious amounts of mucus. Mucus clogs small airways, trapping air below the plugs (See "Pathophysiology Illustrated: Asthma"). Decreased perfusion of the alveolar capillaries results from hypoxic vasoconstriction and increased pressure due to hyperinflation of the alveoli.

The inflammatory mediators release pro-inflammatory cytokines causing chronic airway inflammation that may be associated with permanent **airway remodeling** (thickening of the sub-basement membrane, subepithelial fibrosis, airway smooth muscle hypertrophy and hyperplasia, blood vessel proliferation and dilation, and mucous gland hyperplasia and hypersecretion). Decreased airway elasticity and decreased lung function result (Brashers, 2006a).

Clinical Manifestations

The sudden appearance of breathing difficulty (cough, wheeze, or shortness of breath) is often referred to as an asthma episode or flare. The infant or child who has had episodes of frequent coughing or frequent respiratory infections should also be evaluated for asthma. Frequent coughing, especially at night, is the warning signal that the child's airway is very sensitive to stimuli, and it may be a sign of "silent" asthma.

During an acute episode, respirations are rapid and labored and the child often appears tired because of the ongoing effort to breathe. Nasal flaring and intercostal retractions may be visible. The child exhibits a productive cough and expiratory wheezing, a prolonged expiratory phase, decreased air movement, and respiratory fatigue. The child may complain of chest tightness. Anxiety is associated with respiratory distress, and it intensifies the child's physical responses.

In cases of severe obstruction, wheezing may not be heard because of the lack of airflow. Head bobbing may be seen in young children with the use of accessory muscles (sternocleidomastoids) to breathe. Hypoxia and the cumulative effect of administered

PATHOPHYSIOLOGY ILLUSTRATED

ASTHMA

Some asthma triggers are exercise, infection, and allergies. Asthma obstructs airflow through constriction and narrowing of the airway, along with increased production of mucus.

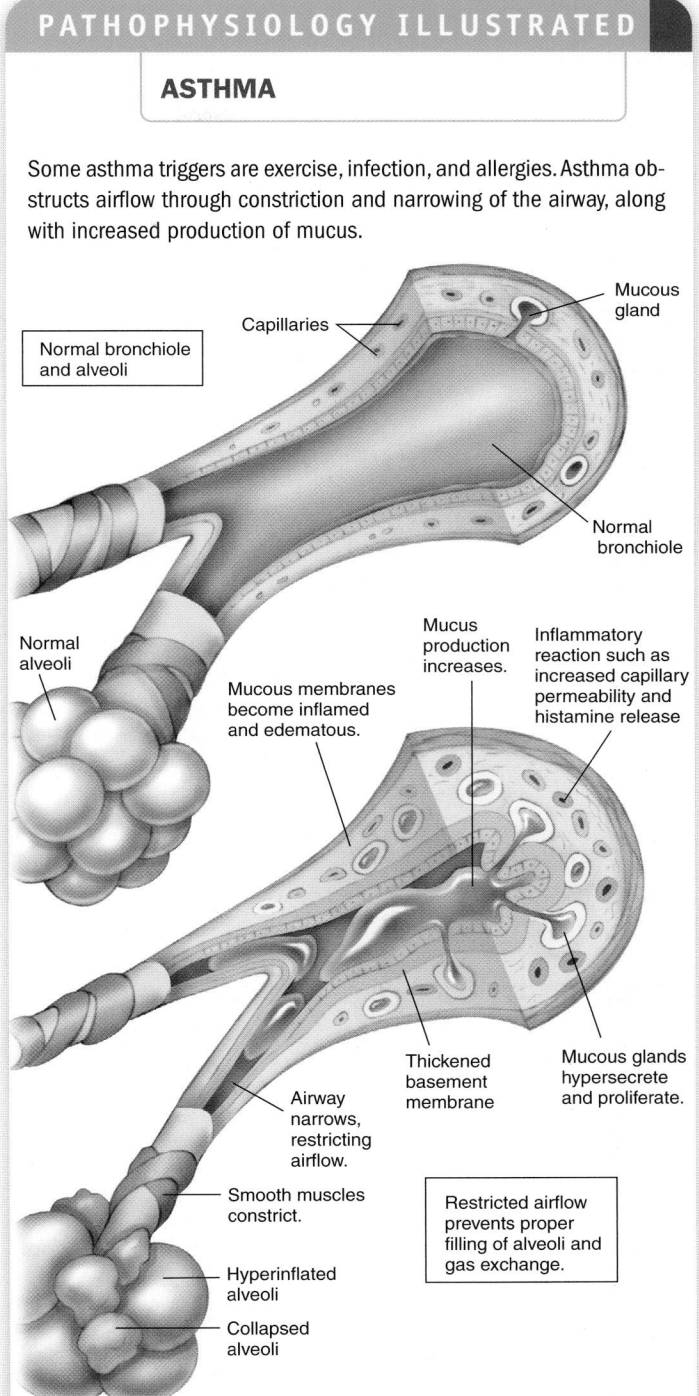

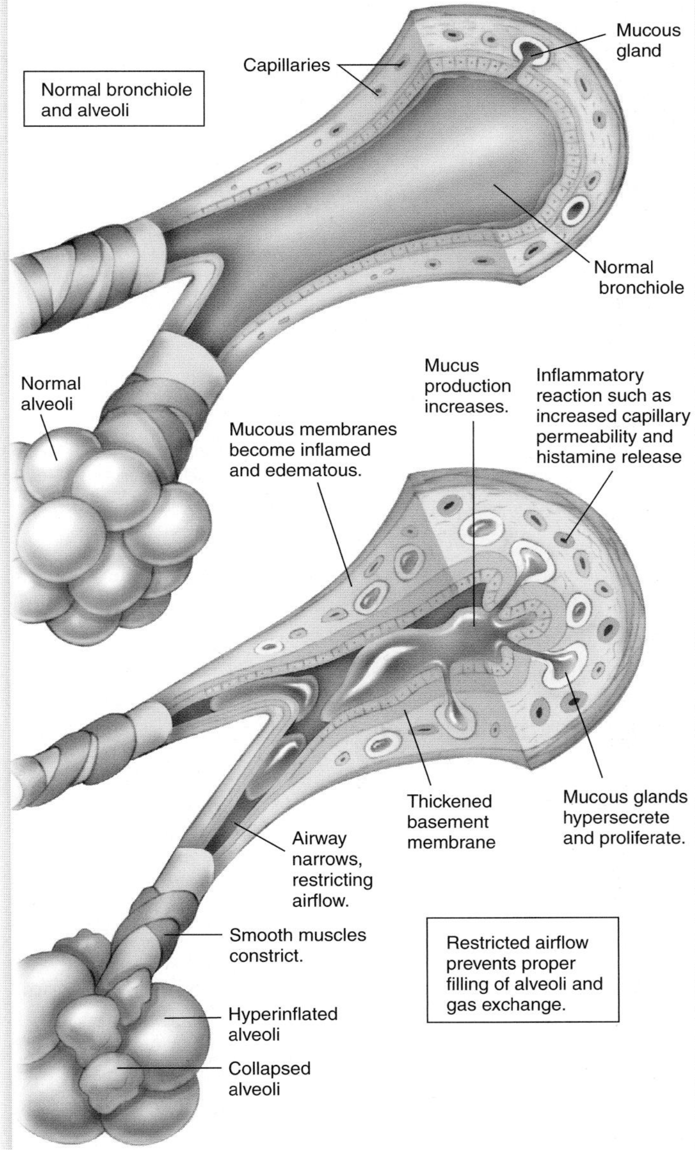

Table 48–5 Classification of Asthma Severity for Children Birth to 4 Years of Age

Components of Severity		Classification of Asthma Severity (0 to 4 Years of Age)			
		Intermittent	Persistent Mild	Moderate	Severe
Impairment	Symptoms	2 or fewer days a week	Greater than 2 days a week, but not daily	Daily	Throughout the day
	Nighttime awakenings	0	1 to 2 times a month	3 to 4 times a month	Greater than 1 time a week
	SABA use for symptom control (not prevention of exercise-induced bronchospasm)	2 or fewer days a week	Greater than 2 times a week, but not daily	Daily	Several times a day
	Interference with normal activity	None	Minor limitation	Some limitation	Extremely limited
Risk	Exacerbations requiring oral systemic corticosteroids	0 to 1 time a year	← 2 or more times a year →		
		← consider severity and interval since last exacerbation →			
		Frequency and severity may fluctuate over time for patients in any severity category.			
Recommended step for initiating therapy (see Figure 48–4)		Step 1	Step 2	Step 3 and consider short course of oral systemic corticosteroids	
		In 2 to 6 weeks, depending on severity, evaluate level of asthma control that is achieved. If no clear benefit is observed in 4 to 6 weeks, consider adjusting therapy or alternative diagnoses.			

SABA = short-acting $beta_2$ agonist

From: National Asthma Education and Prevention Program. (2007). *Expert panel report 3: Guidelines for the diagnosis and management of asthma* (p. 307), Bethesda, MD: National Heart Lung and Blood Institute, National Institutes of Health. Retrieved January 10, 2009 from http://www.nhlbi.nih.gov/guidelines/asthma/

medications may cause behaviors ranging from wide-eyed agitation to lethargic irritability. In children who have repeated acute exacerbations, a barrel chest and the use of accessory muscles of respiration are common findings.

Clinical Therapy

Diagnosis is made by history, physical examination, and spirometry or pulmonary function testing that shows evidence of episodic airflow obstruction (that is at least partially reversible) and airway hyperresponsiveness. Spirometry readings are most commonly measured as forced expiratory volume in 1 second (FEV_1) and expressed as a percentage of predicted FEV_1 for the child's height, age, gender, and race. A chest radiograph may help determine if a foreign body could account for symptoms. Skin testing may be used to identify allergens (asthma triggers).

Asthma may go into remission or increase in severity over time. Asthma severity is categorized by the child's amount of impairment and risk (or the number of episodes needing oral system corticosteroid therapy). See Tables 48–5 and 48–6 for the classification of asthma severity in children of different age groups. Recommended therapy is tied to this asthma severity classification. While current asthma treatment is effective in controlling symptoms, reducing airflow limitations, and preventing exacerbations, the underlying severity of asthma is not prevented (National Asthma Education and Prevention Program, 2007, p. 28).

Clinical therapy includes medications, hydration, education, and support of parents and child. Pharmacologic treatment is matched to the severity of asthma for daily control and for management of acute episodes. See the Drug Guide for medications used to treat asthma. The goal is to maintain asthma control long term, using the least amount of medication and reducing the risk for adverse effects.

A stepwise approach to medication therapy is recommended that matches the child's asthma severity, adding and changing specific medications if the severity progresses or diminishes while maintaining control (National Asthma Education and Prevention Program, 2007, p. 284). The child's response to therapy after 2 to 6 weeks guides the need to further step up the medications to better control symptoms. See Figures 48–4 ●, 48–5 ●, and 48–6 ● for the nationally recommended stepwise approach by age group (see pages 1340–1342). Recommendations for children with persistent asthma include the use of daily inhaled corticosteroids and additional long-term control medications as severity increases. Children with intermittent asthma may only need short-acting $beta_2$-agonists. If asthma control is difficult to achieve, refer the child to an asthma specialist.

Nursing Practice

When spirometry testing is performed, coach the child to give the best effort each time. Encourage the child to seal the lips tightly around the mouthpiece. Then, instruct the child to breathe out as hard as possible, and then to breathe in deeply.

Table 48–6 Classification of Asthma Severity in Children 5 Years to Adulthood

Components of Severity		Classification of Asthma Severity (5 to 11 Years of Age and 12 Years to Adulthood)			
		Intermittent	Persistent Mild	Moderate	Severe
Impairment	Symptoms	2 or fewer days a week	Greater than 2 days a week, but not daily	Daily	Throughout the day
	Nighttime awakenings	2 times or less per month	3 to 4 times a month	Greater than 1 time a week, but not nightly	Often 7 times a week
	SABA for symptom control (not prevention of exercise-induced bronchospasm)	2 or fewer days a week	Greater than 2 times a week, but not daily	Daily	Several times a day
	Interference with normal activity	None	Minor limitation	Some limitation	Extremely limited
	Lung function (5 to 11 years)	■ Normal FEV_1 between exacerbations ■ FEV_1 greater than 80% predicted ■ FEV_1 / FVC greater than 85%	■ FEV_1 greater than 80% predicted ■ FEV_1 / FVC greater than 80%	■ FEV_1 equals 60% to 80% predicted ■ FEV_1 / FVC equals 70% to 80%	■ FEV_1 less than 60% predicted ■ FEV_1 / FVC less than 75%
Normal FEV_1 / FVC: 8–19 yr 85%	Lung function (12 years to adulthood)	■ Normal FEV_1 between exacerbations ■ FEV_1 greater than 80% predicted ■ FEV_1 / FVC normal	■ FEV_1 greater than 80% predicted ■ FEV_1 / FVC normal	■ FEV_1 equals 60% to 80% predicted ■ FEV_1 / FVC reduced 5%	■ FEV_1 less than 60% predicted ■ FEV_1 / FVC reduced more than 5%
Risk	Exacerbations requiring oral systemic corticosteroids	0 to 1 time a year	← 2 or more times a year →		
		← consider severity and interval since last exacerbation → Frequency and severity may fluctuate over time for patients in any severity category.			
Recommended step for initiating therapy (**5 to 11 years**) (see Figure 48–5)		Step 1	Step 2	Step 3, medium dose ICS option Consider short course of oral system corticosteroids	Step 3, medium dose ICS option, or step 4
Recommended step for initiating therapy (**12 years to adulthood**) (see Figure 48–6)		Step 1	Step 2	Step 3 Consider short course of oral system corticosteroids	Step 4 or 5
		Evaluate level of asthma control achieved in 2–6 weeks and adjust therapy accordingly.			

* FEV_1 = forced expiratory volume in 1 second; FVC = forced vital capacity; SABA = short-acting $Beta_2$-agonist; ICS = inhaled corticosteroids

Adapted from: National Asthma Education and Prevention Program. (2007). *Expert panel report 3: Guidelines for the diagnosis and management of asthma* (pp. 308 and 344), Bethesda, MD: National Heart Lung and Blood Institute, National Institutes of Health. Retrieved January 10, 2009 from http://www.nhlbi.nih.gov/guidelines/asthma/

Nursing Practice

Signs of well-controlled asthma in children under age 12 years include symptoms 2 or fewer days a week; no more than one nighttime awakening a month; no interference with normal activity, school, or exercise; use of a short acting $beta_2$-agonist for symptom control 2 or fewer days a week; greater than 80% of predicted peak flow (in children 5 years and older); and no more than 1 asthma episode a year requiring oral corticosteroids (National Asthma Education and Prevention Program, 2007, pp. 309, 310, 345).

Most children with acute exacerbations respond to aggressive management in the emergency department. Children who do not respond or who are already being managed at home on corticosteroids have a greater chance of being admitted. Some children need mechanical ventilation. See "Status Asthmaticus" on page 1347.

Children with exercise-induced asthma have a history of coughing, breathlessness, chest pain, or wheezing that occurs during and after exercise. A spirometry or PEFR indicating a 15% decrease with exertion is diagnostic. Treatment is a short-acting $beta_2$-agonist 5 to 60 minutes before exercise or long-acting $beta_2$-agonist 30 to 60 minutes before exercise (Banasiak, 2007).

Drug Guide

QUICK RELIEF AND DAILY CONTROL MEDICATIONS USED TO TREAT ASTHMA

DAILY RELIEF MEDICATIONS, ROUTE, AND ACTION	NURSING MANAGEMENT
Short-acting Beta$_2$-agonists (SABA) Albuterol, levalbuterol, pirbuterol Metered Dose Inhaler or Nebulizer Relaxes smooth muscle in airway leading to rapid bronchodilation (within 5 to 10 minutes) and mucus clearing Drug of choice for acute therapy	■ Use before inhaled steroid, wait 1–2 minutes between puffs, wait 15 minutes to give inhaled steroid. Child should hold breath 10 seconds after inspiring. Then rinse mouth and avoid swallowing medication. Use a spacer. ■ Differences in potency exist, but all products are comparable on a per puff basis. ■ Some dose-related side effects include tachycardia, nervousness, nausea and vomiting, headaches. ■ Regular use more than 2 days a week for symptom control indicates a loss of control and need for additional therapy.
Corticosteroids Methylprednisolone, prednisone, prednisolone Oral Diminishes airway inflammation and obstruction, enhances bronchodilating effect of Beta$_2$-agonists. Used for short courses to establish control when initiating therapy or during periods of deterioration	■ Short-term therapy should continue until child achieves 80% peak expiratory flow personal best or symptoms resolve. ■ Give with food to reduce gastric irritation. ■ Give oral dose in early morning to mimic normal peak corticosteroid blood level. ■ Assess for potential adverse effects of long-term therapy, such as decreased growth, unstable blood sugar, immunosuppression.
Anticholinergic Ipratropium Metered dose inhaler or Nebulizer Inhibits bronchoconstriction and decreases mucus production	■ Not for primary emergency treatment because of delayed onset. ■ Rinse mouth afterwards to get rid of bitter taste. ■ Side effects include increased wheezing, cough, nervousness, dry mouth, tachycardia, dizziness, headache, palpitations. ■ Prevent medication contact with eyes.
DAILY CONTROL MEDICATIONS, ROUTE, AND ACTION	**NURSING MANAGEMENT**
Long-acting Beta$_2$-agonists (LABA) Salmeterol, formoterol Dry powder inhaler Relaxes smooth muscle in airway, used for nocturnal symptoms and prevention of exercise-induced bronchospasm	■ Should not be used for acute asthma flare. ■ Take pre-exercise dose 30 to 60 minutes before activity. Do not use additional dose before exercise if already using twice daily doses which should be 12 hours apart. ■ Caution against overdosage as side effects such as tachycardia, tremor, irritability, insomnia will last 8 to 12 hours. ■ Report failure to respond to usual dose as this may indicate need for stepped up therapy.
Inhaled Corticosteroids (ICS) Beclomethasone, budesonide, flunisolide, fluticasone, mometasone, triamcinolone Metered dose inhaler or Nebulizer Anti-inflammatory, controls seasonal, allergic, and exercise-induced asthma; effectively reduces mucosal edema in airways; effective for control of asthma, but ICS does not prevent development of chronic asthma (Guilbert, Morgan, Zeiger, et al., 2006).	■ Administer with spacer or holding chamber. ■ Rinse mouth and gargle following treatment to remove drug from oropharynx to reduce chance of cough, thrush, and dysphonia. ■ Separate parts and clean inhaler daily. ■ Monitor growth, however, recommended doses do not have long-term, or irreversible effects on vertical growth (Fong & Levin, 2007). ■ Prevent eye exposure through proper MDI, nebulizer, or DPI administration. ■ Monitor for headache, gastrointestinal upset, dizziness, infection. ■ Use exactly as prescribed.

Drug Guide—continued

QUICK RELIEF AND DAILY CONTROL MEDICATIONS USED TO TREAT ASTHMA

DAILY CONTROL MEDICATIONS, ROUTE, AND ACTION	NURSING MANAGEMENT
Methylxanthines Theophylline Oral Relaxes muscle bundles that constrict airways; dilates airway; provides continuous airway relaxation; sustained release for prevention of nocturnal symptoms.	■ Tablet should not be crushed or chewed. ■ Used for long-term control; works best when a therapeutic serum level (10–20 mcg/L) is maintained; give at the same time each day. ■ Requires serum level checks and dose adjustment. ■ Limit caffeine intake. ■ Side effects include tachycardia, dysrhythmias, restlessness, tremors, seizures, insomnia, hypotension, severe headaches, vomiting, and diarrhea.
Mast Cell Inhibitors Cromolyn sodium, nedocromil Metered dose inhaler or nebulizer Anti-inflammatory, inhibits early and late phase asthma response to allergens and exercise-induced bronchospasm; may be used for unavoidable allergen exposure	■ Not used at time of symptom development or acute exacerbation ■ Must be used up to 4 times a day to be effective ■ Therapeutic response seen in 2 weeks, maximum benefit may not be seen for 4 to 6 weeks. ■ Adverse reactions include wheezing, bronchospasm, throat irritation, nasal congestion, and anaphylaxis. Immediately report these symptoms to physician
Leukotriene Receptor Antagonist (LTRA) Montelukast, zafirlukast Oral Reduces inflammation cascade responsible for airway inflammation; improves lung function and diminishes symptoms and need for quick relief medications.	■ Available in granules for infants and chewable tablets for young children ■ Administer montelukast in the evening, may be given with food or without ■ Make sure child chews montelukast chewable tablet rather than swallowing whole; granules may be mixed in applesauce or ice cream, do not mix in liquid ■ Administer zafirlukast 1 hour before or 2 hours after meal. ■ Report fever, acute asthma episodes, flu-like symptoms, severe headaches or lethargy ■ Take as prescribed, do not withdraw abruptly
Immunotherapy Omalizumab A therapeutic antibody that targets IgE, blocking it from causing reactions leading to asthma symptoms	■ Approved for children 12 years and older with moderate or severe persistent asthma ■ Injections required every 2 to 4 weeks based on serum IgE levels.
Other Hyposensitization (allergy shots), subcutaneous Series of injections with gradual dose increase that can increase the child's tolerance of unavoidable allergens (e.g., mold, pollen)	■ May be of value for child with persistent asthma having allergies that can be addressed by immune therapy.

Data from: Banasiak, N. C. (2007). Childhood asthma: Part two: Management update. *Journal of Pediatric Health Care, 21*(3), 184–191; Bindler, R. & Howry, L. (2005). *Prentice Hall pediatric drug guide with nursing implications,* Upper Saddle River, NJ: Pearson Prentice Hall; Fong, E. W. & Levin, R. H. (2007). Inhaled corticosteroids for asthma, *Pediatrics in Review, 28*(6), e30–e35; National Asthma Education and Prevention Program. (2007). *Expert panel report 3: Guidelines for the diagnosis and management of asthma.* (pp. 311–318), Bethesda, MD: National Heart Lung and Blood Institute, Retrieved January 10, 2009 from http://www.nhlib.nih.gov/guidelines/asthma/

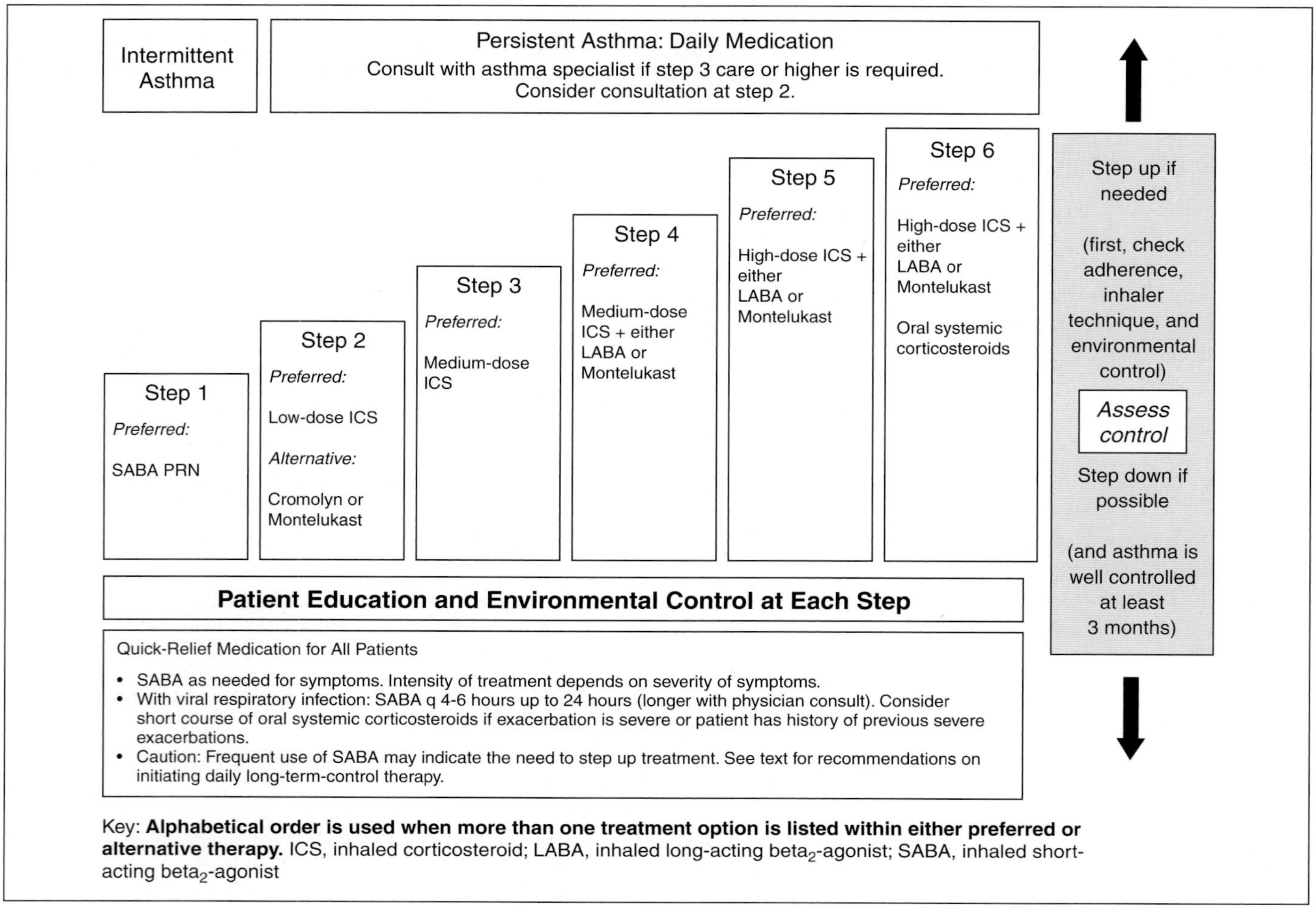

Intermittent Asthma
Persistent Asthma: Daily Medication
Consult with asthma specialist if step 3 care or higher is required.
Consider consultation at step 2.
Step 1
Preferred:
SABA PRN
Step 2
Preferred:
Low-dose ICS
Alternative:
Cromolyn or Montelukast
Step 3
Preferred:
Medium-dose ICS
Step 4
Preferred:
Medium-dose ICS + either LABA or Montelukast
Step 5
Preferred:
High-dose ICS + either LABA or Montelukast
Step 6
Preferred:
High-dose ICS + either LABA or Montelukast
Oral systemic corticosteroids
Step up if needed
(first, check adherence, inhaler technique, and environmental control)
Assess control
Step down if possible
(and asthma is well controlled at least 3 months)
Patient Education and Environmental Control at Each Step
Quick-Relief Medication for All Patients
• SABA as needed for symptoms. Intensity of treatment depends on severity of symptoms.
• With viral respiratory infection: SABA q 4-6 hours up to 24 hours (longer with physician consult). Consider short course of oral systemic corticosteroids if exacerbation is severe or patient has history of previous severe exacerbations.
• Caution: Frequent use of SABA may indicate the need to step up treatment. See text for recommendations on initiating daily long-term-control therapy.
Key: Alphabetical order is used when more than one treatment option is listed within either preferred or alternative therapy. ICS, inhaled corticosteroid; LABA, inhaled long-acting beta2-agonist; SABA, inhaled short-acting beta2-agonist

● **Figure 48–4** Stepwise approach to managing asthma in children 0 to 4 years of age.

Source: From National Asthma Education and Prevention Program. (2007). *Expert Panel Report 3: Guidelines for the Diagnosis and Management of Asthma* (p. 305). Bethesda, MD: National Institutes of Health, National Heart Lung and Blood Institute. Retrieved January 10, 2009, from http://www.nhlbi.nih.gov/guidelines/asthma/

NURSING MANAGEMENT

NURSING ASSESSMENT AND DIAGNOSIS

The nurse usually encounters the child and family in the emergency department or nursing unit. In these settings, acute care has become necessary because the child's level of respiratory compromise cannot be managed at home.

PHYSIOLOGIC ASSESSMENT

Identify the child's current respiratory status first by assessing the ABCs—airway, breathing, and circulation—to make sure the child's condition is not life threatening. If the child is moving air or talking, assess the quality of breathing. Assess the respiratory rate. Inspect the chest for retractions to assess the severity of respiratory distress. Auscultate the lungs for the quality of breath sounds and for the presence or absence of wheezing. Note whether a cough or stridor is present. Observe the child's color and assess the heart rate. Move on to other aspects of assessment only after finding no life-threatening respiratory distress.

Attach a pulse oximeter to monitor the SpO_2. Assess peak expiratory flow rate (PEFR), skin turgor, intake and output, and urine specific gravity. Because asthma can be a symptom of another illness, perform a head-to-toe assessment to identify other associated problems. See Table 48–1 for assessment guidelines.

The infant or child who has had episodes of frequent coughing or frequent respiratory infections (especially pneumonia or bronchitis) should also be evaluated for asthma. The cough indicates that the child's airway is sensitive to stimuli and may be a sign of silent asthma.

ASSESS ASTHMA MANAGEMENT

Key questions to consider asking parents and older children or adolescents include the following (National Asthma Education and Prevention Program, 2007, p. 332):

- Which medicines is the child currently taking? How often?
- How is the medication administered?
- How many times a week is a medication dose missed?
- Have you had problems related to giving the medicine (cost, time, lack of perceived need)?

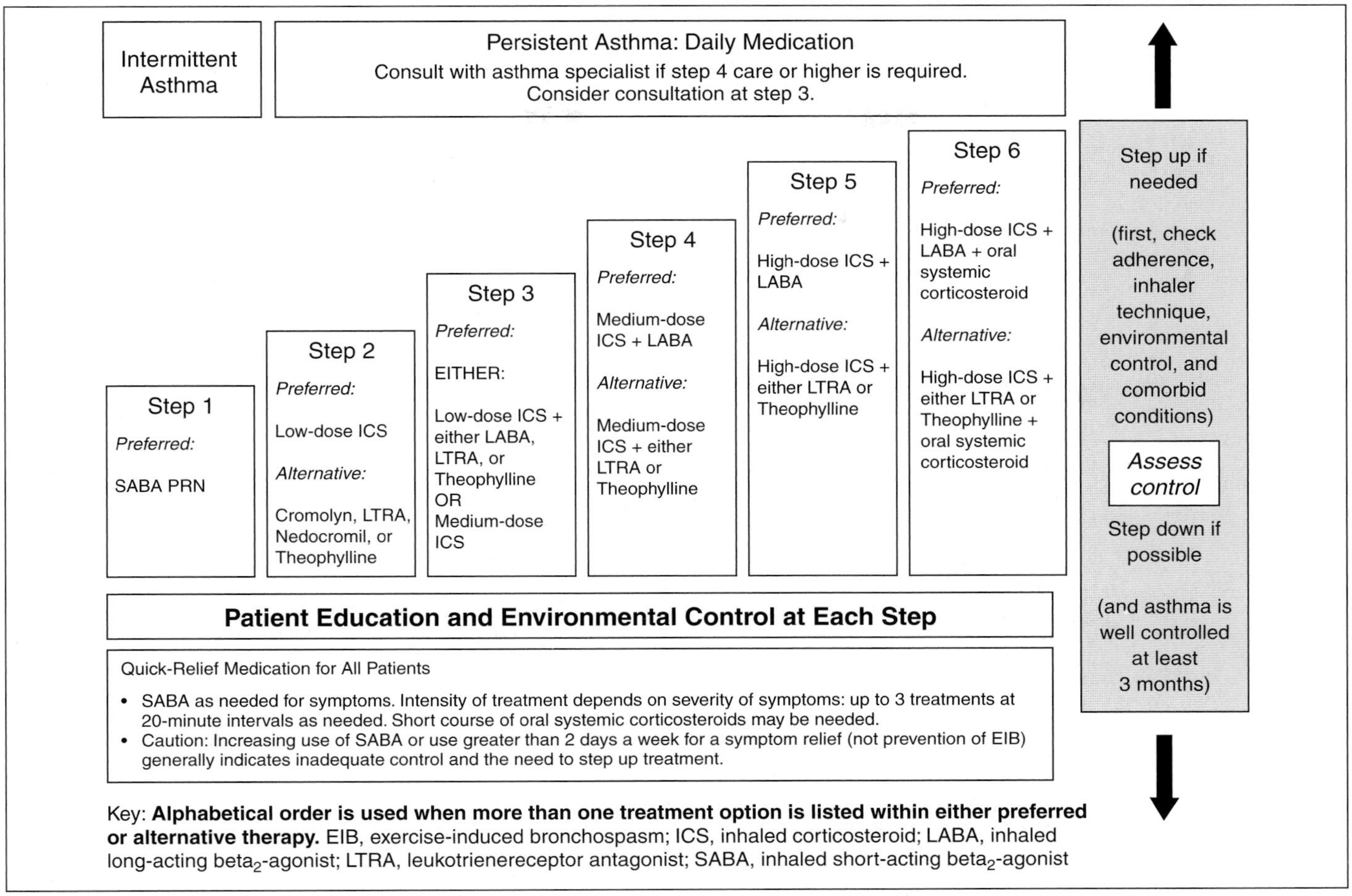

• **Figure 48–5** Stepwise approach to managing asthma in children 5 to 11 years of age.

Source: From National Asthma Education and Prevention Program. (2007). *Expert Panel Report 3: Guidelines for the Diagnosis and Management of Asthma* (p. 306). Bethesda, MD: National Institutes of Health, National Heart Lung and Blood Institute. Retrieved January 10, 2009, from http://www.nhlbi.nih.gov/guidelines/asthma/

- What concerns you about the prescribed asthma medication?
- What other treatments for asthma are you using (e.g., complementary therapies)?

PSYCHOSOCIAL ASSESSMENT

Assess the child's anxiety or fear related to the asthma episode or hospitalization. How are parents responding to the latest episode? Are they anxious, concerned, or frustrated? Do they potentially have concerns about finances, missing work, or other family members at home? Assess whether the child thinks this episode could have been avoided if medications had been used.

Examples of nursing diagnoses for the child experiencing an acute asthma episode include the following:

- *Ineffective Airway Clearance* related to airway compromise, copious mucous secretions, and coughing
- *Impaired Gas Exchange* related to airway obstruction
- *Risk for Deficient Fluid Volume* related to inability to drink adequate fluids when in respiratory distress
- *Anxiety/Fear (child and parents)* related to difficulty breathing
- *Ineffective Management of Therapeutic Regimen (Family)* related to lack of understanding about the need for daily management of a chronic disease

PLANNING AND IMPLEMENTATION

Pharmacologic and supportive therapies are used to reverse the airway obstruction and promote respiratory function. Nursing interventions focus on maintaining airway patency, meeting fluid needs, promoting rest and stress reduction for the child and parents, supporting the family's participation in care, and providing the family with information to enable them to manage the child's disease.

MAINTAIN AIRWAY PATENCY

If the child is exhibiting breathing difficulty, give supplemental oxygen by nasal cannula or face mask. Humidified oxygen should be used to prevent drying and thickening of mucus secretions. Place the child in a sitting (semi-Fowler's) or upright position to promote and ease respiratory effort. Evaluate the effectiveness of positioning and oxygen administration by pulse oximeter and by observing for improved respiratory status. (See Skill 14–1 SKILLS.)

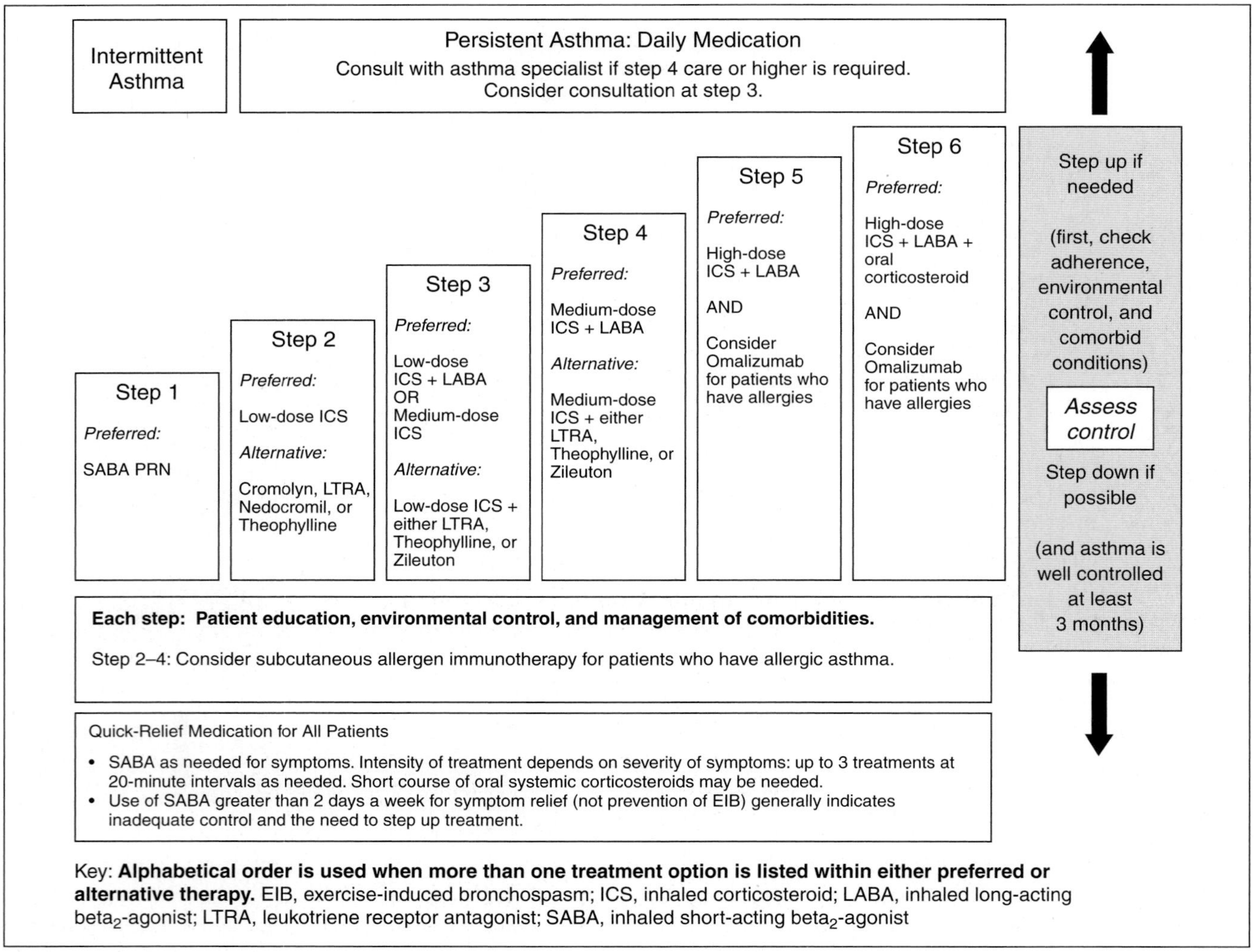

● **Figure 48–6** Stepwise approach to managing asthma in children 12 years of age and older.

Source: From National Asthma Education and Prevention Program. (2007). *Expert Panel Report 3: Guidelines for the Diagnosis and Management of Asthma* (p. 343). Bethesda, MD: National Institutes of Health, National Heart Lung and Blood Institute. Retrieved January 10, 2009, from http://www.nhlbi.nih.gov/guidelines/asthma/

The respiratory distress and need for supplemental oxygen can be stressful for parents and child alike (Figure 48–7 ●). Encouraging the parents' presence can be reassuring for the child. Keep the parents informed of procedures and results, and get their input when developing the treatment plan.

Most medications are given by inhalation (Figure 48–8 ●). This route of administration enables the pulmonary blood vessels to rapidly absorb the inhaled medication while minimizing the systemic effects. (See Skill 11–11 **SKILLS**.) The inhaled droplets provide the added benefit of moisture. Continuous inhalation treatments may be used for some children with severe exacerbations. See Growth and Development section box for considerations in administering medications with inhalation devices. Monitor the child for medication side effects. The frequency of vital sign assessment is determined by the severity of symptoms.

MEET FLUID NEEDS

Fluid therapy is often necessary to restore and maintain adequate fluid balance. Adequate hydration is essential to thin and break up trapped mucous plugs in the narrowed airways. An adequate oral intake may not be possible with the child's compromised respiratory status. An intravenous infusion may be needed, and this route also may be used for administering medications and providing glucose. Monitor the child's intake, output, and specific gravity to avoid overhydration that could lead to pulmonary edema in severe asthma episodes.

As respiratory difficulty diminishes, offer oral fluids slowly. The child's fluid preferences should be determined and choices given where possible. Involve parents to help gain the child's cooperation in taking oral fluids.

Nursing Practice

Iced beverages precipitate bronchospasms in some children with asthma. It is safest to offer room-temperature or slightly cooled fluids without ice to children with asthma.

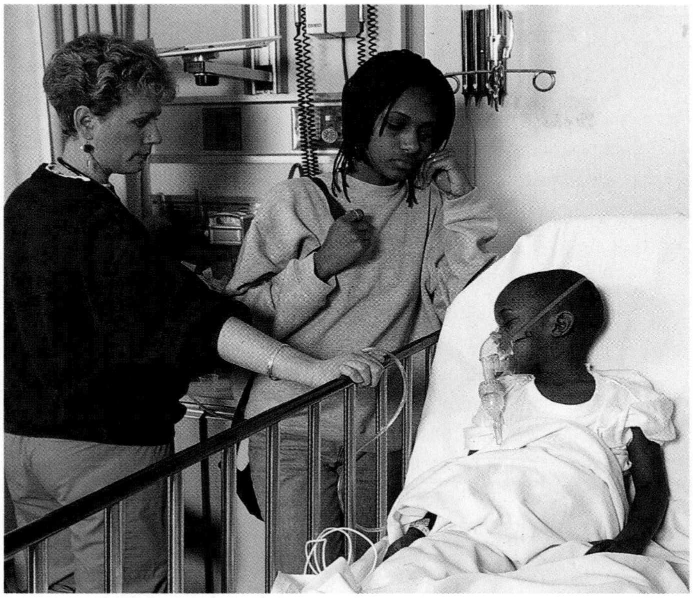

● **Figure 48–7** Treatment of acute asthma. Acute exacerbations of asthma may require management in the emergency department. The child is placed in a semisitting position to facilitate respiratory effort. Providing support to both the child and parent is an important part of nursing care during these acute episodes. This mother is exhausted after a sleepless night of caring for her son.

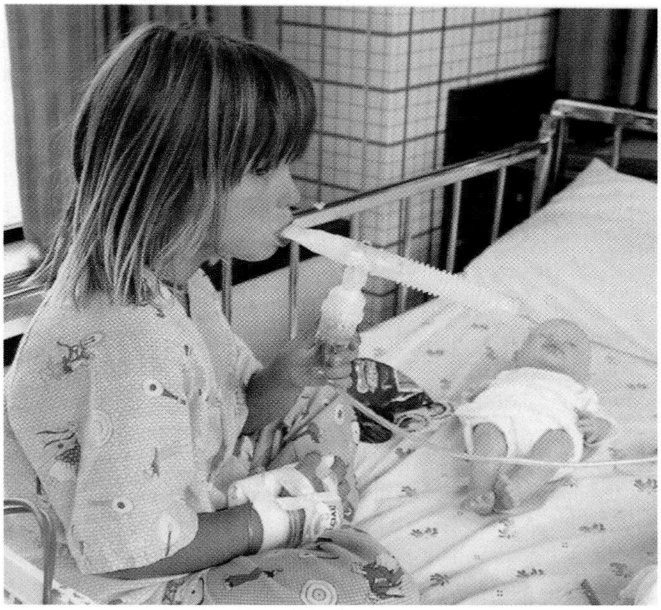

● **Figure 48–8** Administration of medication by inhalation. Medications given by aerosol therapy allow children the freedom to play and entertain themselves.

PROMOTE REST AND STRESS REDUCTION

The child who has had an acute asthmatic episode is usually very tired when admitted to the nursing unit. Labored breathing and hypoxemia have left the child exhausted. Put the child in a quiet room that is accessible for frequent monitoring to promote relaxation and rest. Group tasks to avoid repeatedly disturbing the child.

SUPPORT FAMILY PARTICIPATION

The parents may stay with the child, but may be exhausted after spending hours with their child in respiratory distress. Give parents the *option* of assisting with the child's treatments, rather than *expecting* them to assist with treatment in addition to comforting the child. Provide frequent updates about the child's condition and encourage the parents to take breaks as needed.

Length of hospitalization depends on the child's response to therapy. Any underlying or accompanying health problem, such as preexisting lung disease or pneumonia, can complicate and extend the child's hospital stay. Communicate with the family of the hospitalized child frequently about the child's condition.

DISCHARGE PLANNING AND HOME CARE TEACHING

Parents need a thorough understanding of asthma—how to prevent asthma episodes and how to follow the asthma action plan to manage the child's episodes earlier to avoid unnecessary hospitalization. When possible, educate parents when they are rested, but refer the child to a healthcare provider for more comprehensive education. Make sure the child receives an appointment with an allergist or asthma specialist if moderate to severe persistent asthma exists. Support of parents and the child should focus on helping them to understand and cope with the diagnosis and the need for daily management to promote near-normal respiratory function while the child continues to grow and develop normally. See "Developing Cultural Competence: Asthma Control."

Discharge planning for the asthmatic child focuses on increasing the family's knowledge about the disease, medication therapy, and the need for follow-up care according to guidelines of the National Asthma Education and Prevention Program. The required lifestyle changes may be difficult for the child and parents. The need to modify the home to remove allergens, removing a loved pet, or have family members stop smoking in the

Developing Cultural Competence

ASTHMA CONTROL

The benefits of efforts made by health practices to provide more culturally competent asthma care to children who were enrolled in Medicaid were evaluated. The health practices used a diversity of health professionals, offered cross-cultural or diversity training, made interpreters available, used culturally appropriate printed materials, promoted self-management skills, and provided reminders to health professionals about asthma guidelines. The health practices with the highest cultural competence scores had child patients less likely to be underusing asthma control medications (Lieu, Finkelstein, Lozano, et al., 2004).

Growth and Development

Metered-dose inhalers (MDI), nebulizers, and dry powder inhalers (DPI) are the devices used for inhalation therapy. These devices are relatively inefficient, and have special challenges for infants and young children. Many devices require cooperation, coordination, and appropriate technique that is taught and reinforced frequently. Clean all devices regularly and wash the child's face when a face mask is used for administration.

- Children over 5 years usually have the ability to use an MDI, coordinating medication release and inspiration; however they may prefer to use a holding chamber or spacer with a valve. With proper technique 10% to 15% of the dose may reach the lower airways (Virchow, 2005). Spacers can double the amount of drug delivered to the lungs (Bell, 2006). They also trap larger particles preventing them from reaching the mouth and being swallowed, which can cause local and systemic side effects. Wash the plastic spacer with household detergent and permit it to air dry. This reduces the electrostatic charge and frees more of the drug for delivery (Meadows-Oliver & Banasiak, 2005).
- Spacers have a mouthpiece or mask attachment. When selecting a spacer for infants and young children, choose one with a mask sized to fit the child's face that has a flexible seal to prevent an air leak. Masks may also increase the dead space and reduce the amount of drug delivered. The Aerochamber had the lowest volume of dead space (Shah, Berlinski, & Rubin, 2006). It may be difficult to maintain a seal when the child is uncooperative. Crying leads to prolonged exhalation and short inspiration, reducing lung deposition. Try to improve cooperation for medication delivery with play and distraction.
- Steps in using a metered-dose inhaler include: shake the canister and put the spacer on if used, breathe out, actuate the MDI (release a puff), put the mouthpiece between the lips and teeth (or the mask over the face), inhale deeply over 4 to 5 seconds (with mask child should take 4 to 6 breaths), and remove the mouthpiece and hold the breath 10 seconds. Teach the child to use an MDI without spacer, by breathing slowly through a straw.
- Some inhalers have a whistle. In some it warns that the inhaled breath is too fast or too shallow, but in other devices it indicates that an adequate breath has been taken. Be sure to inform the child and family about what the whistle on the child's inhaler indicates.
- Nebulizers change liquid medication into aerosol particles. No coordination of breathing is required, making them easier for young children to use. Nebulizers are not more efficient than MDIs with a spacer, but they may lead to better outcomes because the child only needs to breathe normally. The nebulizer mouthpiece should be in the mouth and breathing through the mouth is important for drug delivery. A face mask can be used for children who cannot coordinate mouth breathing. Nebulizers take 8 to 10 minutes for the treatment, and it may be difficult for infants and young children to cooperate for that duration.
- Dry powder inhalers are activated when the patient takes a breath, so puffs do not need to be coordinated with inhalation. No spacer is required and no propellant is used. Children must be able to take rapid, deep, and sustained breaths to effectively use the device (Fong & Levin, 2007). Drug delivery to the lower airway varies between 15% and 30% dependent upon the type of inhaler. Children less than 6 years of age who are wheezing may not be able to inspire at a rate fast enough to obtain the optimal amount of medication.
- Essential steps for using DPI include: remove the lid, load the dose (puncturing the blister or capsule), blow out away from the device, put the mouthpiece between the lips and teeth, and breathe in deeply and forcefully.

Data from: Brand, P. L. P. (2005). Key issues in inhalation therapy in children. *Current Medical Research and Opinion, 21*(Suppl 4), S27–S32; Dolovich, M. B., Ahrens, T. C., Hess, D. R., et al. (2005). Device selection and outcomes of aerosol therapy: Evidence-based guidelines. *Chest, 127,* 335–371; Everard, M. L. (2006). Aerosol delivery to children. *Pediatric Annals, 35*(9), 630–636; Marshik, P. L. (2004). Pharmacologic treatment of pediatric asthma. *Advance for Nurse Practitioners, 12*(3), 35–36, 41–46; Meadows-Oliver, M., & Banasiak, N. C. (2005). Asthma medication delivery devices, *Journal of Pediatric Health Care, 19*(2), 121–123; Virchow, J. C. (2005). What plays a role in the choice of inhaler device for asthma therapy? *Current Medical Research and Opinion, 21*(Suppl 4), S19–S25.

home may create stress and resistance. The nurse can facilitate discussion and clarification of ways to prevent asthma episodes. Teach the family how to measure and interpret peak expiratory flow readings (see "Teaching Highlights: Using a Peak Expiratory Flow Meter"). Discuss quick relief medications to manage asthma episodes, as well as control medications for daily management. Reassure the family that most children with asthma can lead a normal life with some modifications.

NURSING CARE IN THE COMMUNITY

Nurses provide care to children with asthma in pediatricians' offices, specialty asthma clinics, schools, and summer camps. Review the family's daily plan for monitoring the child's respiratory status. Encourage the school-aged child or parent of younger children to use a symptom diary for 2 weeks prior to a health visit to record all daytime and nighttime symptoms and PEFR measurements. Assess the parent's ability to identify the timing and type of stepped-up care needed to manage worsening symptoms. The goal is to bring asthma episodes under control with stepped-up care before emergency care is needed. See MyNursingKit for the Web site with a symptom diary and asthma action plan.

Health Maintenance

Provide routine health promotion and maintenance care, including immunizations; however live virus vaccines may need to be postponed if the child has used oral corticosteroids recently. Assess the child's growth pattern if the child is treated with inhaled corticosteroids (ICS) and courses of oral corticosteroid as these medications may affect overall growth.

Teaching Highlights

USING A PEAK EXPIRATORY FLOW METER

Use of a peak expiratory flow meter can help assess the severity of asthma. This device measures the child's ability to push air forcefully out of the lungs. Changes in the peak expiratory flow rate (PEFR) signal worsening lung function and the beginning of an asthma episode. To use a peak expiratory flow meter:

- Set the device at zero or the base level.
- Stand up and take as deep a breath as possible.
- Put the mouthpiece of the meter in the mouth and firmly close the lips around it. Do not cough or let your tongue block the mouthpiece. Blow out as hard and fast as possible over 1 to 2 seconds.
- Write down the reading.
- Repeat the process 2 times and record the highest of 3 numbers on the chart.
- Measure and record the best PEFR reading twice a day for 2 weeks so the physician can determine the child's personal best reading. (The child should be optimally treated with medications during the day so the best reading is obtained.)
- The physician will use the child's personal best average readings to individualize the color zones to guide treatment in the child's asthma action plan.

ZONE	PEFR	ACTION NEEDED
Green	80–100%	Good asthma control. Relatively symptom-free. Maintain usual treatment medications.
Yellow	50–80%	Caution! Asthma is worsening. Contact the healthcare provider to get guidance on additional medications.
Red	Less than 50%	Danger! Severe asthma episode. Use quick relief medications. Call healthcare provider or go to emergency department if PEFR does not return to yellow or green zone after quick relief medications.

Assess the amount of activity and exercise the child gets, as well as any symptoms experienced such as chest tightening, wheezing, or shortness of breath. Exercise-induced bronchospasm typically occurs 5 to 10 minutes after stopping the activity and resolves in another 20 to 30 minutes. Children who have symptoms with usual play activities should get a step up in medication management (National Asthma Education and Prevention Program, 2007, p. 297). First determine that the child gets some exercise. Then identify how frequently the child has exercise-induced symptoms, and compare that to the classification of asthma severity in Tables 48–5 or 48–6. For example, daily exercise-induced symptom indicates *moderate persistent* asthma. Make sure the daily control and quick relief medication asthma action plan is used by the child. See "Complementary Care: Exercise and Asthma."

Complementary Care

EXERCISE AND ASTHMA

Although exercise is a frequent trigger of asthma symptoms, routine exercise, such as swimming, has benefits for children and adults with asthma (Chiang, 2005). Children with asthma may need to learn correct swimming breathing techniques before learning strokes and to modify the breathing stroke ratio. The benefits of swimming were found by one program to increase the child's involvement in other sport and non-sport activities, reduce absences from school, and reduce hospitalizations. Children felt less disadvantaged because of asthma (Wardell, Huang, & Isbister, 2006). Improved cardiovascular fitness and self-esteem were added benefits.

Child and Family Education

Once the stress of the acute episode has passed, take advantage of opportunities to provide more extensive education at each health visit. See "Teaching Highlights: Home Care for the Child with Asthma" for a guide to topics that should be discussed in asthma education.

Engage the child in learning about asthma and to begin steps toward self-management as appropriate. An activity or coloring book may be a good teaching tool. Encourage the child to ask questions about his or her asthma. Provide printed educational materials and referral to a local support group to help parents gain additional knowledge and confidence that will enable them to help their child lead a normal life. Many hospitals have family resource centers that can assist the parents to find helpful information on the Internet. See MyNursingKit for educational resources.

Teach the child and family about the importance of the daily control medication program and collaborate with the physician to develop a written asthma action plan for the child and family. The plan should include the daily control medications, quick relief medications to take once symptoms of an asthma episode are identified, and when to call the health professional. School-age children

Teaching Highlights

HOME CARE FOR THE CHILD WITH ASTHMA

Identify current knowledge about the condition and its impact on the child:

- What happens in the lungs during an asthma episode?
- What are the child's early warning signs of an asthma episode?
- What are the child's symptoms (wake up at night, cough a lot)? How does the child respond to them?
- Is the child involved in any exercise activity? If no, why not? Do asthma symptoms occur?
- Does asthma interfere with social activities or activities with friends?
- What are the child's personal asthma triggers? (Suggest keeping a log of symptoms that occur during the day and night, including when and where, to help identify triggers.)
- Where do most asthma episodes begin—home, school, outdoors, with exercise?

Set up a schedule for parents to learn asthma management:

- Promote understanding that asthma is a chronic condition, rather than an episodic illness, that needs for daily management and environmental control to reduce or prevent asthma episodes.
- Review the asthma action plan for daily management, quick relief, and when to call the physician or to seek emergency care.
- Assess the child's technique when using a peak expiratory flow meter, and correct technique as needed. Discuss when to use the peak flow meter and how to interpret and use the results for asthma control. Keep a record of peak flow readings for 2 weeks prior to each health visit.

Review parents' understanding of medication therapy:

- Provide information about medications: name, type of drug, dose, method of administration, expected effect, possible side effects. Make sure families understand that control medications help prevent asthma episodes, and unlike with quick relief medications, the child will not feel their effect. Address any concerns about the use of "steroid" medication, and describe how they differ from the anabolic steroids abused by athletes.
- Assess the child's technique for the use of an MDI or DPI and correct as needed.
- When parents use a nebulizer to treat an infant or young child, suggest diversions that might help the child cooperate during the 8 to 10 minute treatment.

Address associated issues:

- What are the financial considerations of medication cost and lifestyle changes?
- Have arrangements been made for the child to use medications at childcare or school?
- Does the child have a medical identification bracelet or tag?
- Would a self-help group or camp experience be helpful for the child?

should be encouraged to assume more responsibility for care, including avoidance of known triggers, early symptom recognition, relaxation breathing, and the proper use of inhaled medication. Help the child learn the early signs of an asthma episode (coughing, breathlessness) so that treatment can be obtained before signs become more serious. Determine if the family uses any complementary and alternative therapies for asthma management.

Assess family support systems and family response to the chronic illness. Establish a partnership with the child and family that supports their ability to manage daily control medication regimens. Reasons middle school-age children give for nonadherence include the following: treatment is time consuming and annoying, they forget to carry medication with them, and medications taste bad (Ayala, Miller, Zagami, et al., 2006). Suggest that the child use a fanny pack to carry the inhaler and rinse the mouth with water or flavored mouthwash after the inhaler treatment.

Evidence in Action

One study of 63 children (mean age 9 years) with the onset of asthma investigated their needs for psychosocial support and satisfaction with care received. Half of the children reported a need for more information about asthma from their health professionals, especially about handling future asthma episodes. Many children wanted to talk with other children their age with asthma and handling asthma at school. Several of these children were worried about having another asthma episode and being sick with their asthma (McNelis, Musick, Austin, et al., 2007).

Preventing Asthma Episodes

Environmental control is an important part of asthma management. When possible, pets and plants should not be kept in the home (and never in the child's bedroom). Dust mites live in the carpets, mattresses, upholstered furniture, bedcovers, soft toys, and clothes. An effort should be directed at controlling dust mites in the child's bed and bedroom. The child's mattress and pillow should be encased in plastic covers. Pets should be bathed frequently to reduce pet dander. Cockroach eradication should be initiated. Smoke from cigarettes, wood stoves, and fireplaces should be eliminated.

School Management

Guide parents to have an individual health plan (that includes an asthma action plan) developed so that medications are given as needed at school, even in preparation for exercise. Provide a physician order so the child's asthma symptoms can be treated at school. Make sure the child has a supply of medications at school or child care as well as at home. Exercise is beneficial and should be included in the individual health plan. Make sure teachers of young children can help recognize signs of an asthma episode and reduce a child's anxiety about going to the nurse for quick relief medications. Many schools are attempting to become "asthma friendly" by improving the environment to reduce asthma triggers, providing awareness programs for students and staff, and coordinating with families to better manage asthma and reduce absenteeism (Centers for Disease Control and Prevention, Division of Adolescent and School Health, 2004).

EVALUATION

Expected outcomes of nursing care include the following:

- The child recognizes early asthma symptoms and promptly uses quick relief medications, hydration, and relaxation breathing before severe respiratory distress occurs.
- The child learns to avoid asthma triggers.
- The child and family implement a daily treatment plan for asthma and reduce the number of asthma episodes the child has.
- The child with a serious asthma episode responds to oxygen, fluids, and medication therapy, avoiding hospital admission.

STATUS ASTHMATICUS

Status asthmaticus is unrelenting, severe respiratory distress and bronchospasm in an asthmatic child, which persists despite pharmacologic and supportive interventions. These children are in acute respiratory distress. Clinical manifestations include the following: use of accessory muscles, restlessness and anxiety, altered mental status, cannot say more than a word or two without gasping for a breath, diaphoresis, and cyanosis. The child cannot lie down and often has diminished or absent breath sounds with increased respiratory effort, indicating the onset of respiratory failure (Mannix & Bachur, 2007).

Laboratory findings for the child who needs admission to an intensive care unit may include hypoxemia (may be masked by supplemental oxygen), hypercarbia, respiratory alkalosis that converts to respiratory acidosis, and sometimes metabolic acidosis (Marcoux, 2005). The PEFR of less than 30% to 50% of the predicted level indicates severe airway obstruction.

Without aggressive and immediate intervention the child with status asthmaticus may progress to respiratory failure and die. The child is placed on a cardiorespiratory monitor and pulse oximetry. Continuous nebulized albuterol, inhaled ipratropium, intravenous corticosteroids, magnesium, and aminophylline may be implemented (Mannix & Bachur, 2007). Electrolytes should be monitored. If the child's condition progresses to respiratory failure, noninvasive positive pressure ventilation or intubation may be performed. See nursing management of respiratory failure on page 1316 for more information.

CYSTIC FIBROSIS

Cystic fibrosis (CF) is a common inherited autosomal recessive disorder of the exocrine glands that results in physiologic alterations in the respiratory, gastrointestinal, and reproductive systems. The incidence of CF varies by race—1:3200 in whites, 1:15,000 in blacks, 1:7000 in Hispanics, and 1:31,000 in Asian Americans (Kaye and the Committee on Genetics, 2006; Strausbaugh & Davis, 2007). Gender is not a factor in disease incidence. Approximately 30,000 children and adults have CF in the United States, and approximately 40% are older than age 18 years. The median life span for individuals with cystic fibrosis is 35 years (Christian & D'Auria, 2006; Cystic Fibrosis Foundation, 2007a). (Figure 48–9 ●.)

Etiology and Pathophysiology

A gene isolated on the long arm of chromosome 7 directs the function of the transmembrane conductance regulator (CFTR) protein that regulates ion flux at epithelial surfaces (Kaye and the Committee on Genetics, 2006). More than 1500 mutations of the CFTR gene on chromosome 7 can cause cystic fibrosis (Strausbaugh & Davis, 2007). An estimated 1 in 29 Caucasians in the United States is a carrier of a defective CFTR gene, and carriers are healthy (Froh, 2006).

Chloride-ion transport across the exocrine and epithelial cells is impaired due to the defective CFTR protein. Decreased chloride secretion and increased sodium absorption results, causing the body to produce unusually thick, sticky mucus that clogs the lungs leading to infections, and obstructs the pancreas secretion of natural enzymes that enable the body to digest and absorb food (Strausbaugh & Davis, 2007; Cystic Fibrosis Foundation, 2007a).

In infants with CF, the usual viral illnesses from which healthy children normally recover often progress to bacterial pneumonias instead. Children develop a classic cough because the respiratory cilia in the lungs cannot clear the thick mucus. Air becomes trapped in the small airways, leading to hyperinflation, atelectasis and secondary respiratory infections. Even with antibiotics and a good response, bacteria and fungi colonize in the airways over time because the thick secretions encourage bacterial growth. Lung inflammation persists damaging the lungs even after antibiotic therapy clears

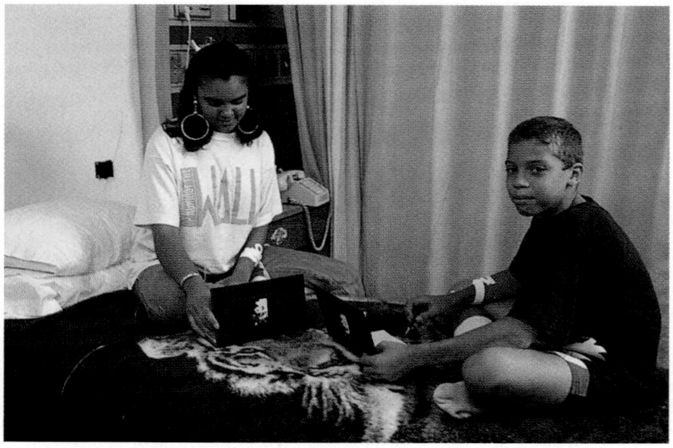

● **Figure 48–9** Siblings with cystic fibrosis. Cystic fibrosis is an inherited autosomal recessive disorder of the exocrine glands, so it is not uncommon to see siblings with it such as this brother and sister.

the infection (Rao & Grigg, 2006). Chronic infection and inflammation lead to bronchiectasis (a persistent abnormal dilation of the bronchi). Pneumothorax and hemothorax may occur in older children. The rate of progression is variable among affected children. Respiratory failure is the leading cause of mortality.

Failure of the obstructed pancreatic ducts to secrete the natural enzymes needed to digest fats and proteins results in poor digestion, and nutritional deficits may cause failure to thrive. The pancreas may stop producing sufficient insulin in some older children, leading to the development of cystic fibrosis–related diabetes mellitus.

Failure to secrete enough chloride and fluid into intestines causes meconium ileus (a small bowel obstruction in newborns), affecting 11% to 20% of newborns with cystic fibrosis (Strausbaugh & Davis, 2007). Older children may have intermittent and recurrent episodes of partial small bowel obstruction. Chronic inflammation may lead to the development of Crohn's disease. Some children develop liver disease (Strausbaugh & Davis, 2007). Nearly all males with CF are sterile because of blocked or absent vas deferens. Females have difficulty conceiving because of chronic illness and thickened mucous secretions in the reproductive tract.

Clinical Manifestations

One of the first signs of CF noticed by the parents is a salty taste to the skin. A meconium ileus may be found in the newborn. Stools of the child with CF characteristically may have the following characteristics: steatorrhea (fat or greasy), frothy (bulky and large quantity), foul smelling, and floating. Constipation is common and intestinal obstruction may occur in older children. Rectal prolapse, resulting from the large, bulky, difficult-to-pass stools, may occur.

Respiratory signs and symptoms include a chronic moist, productive cough and frequent respiratory infections. The child often has wheezing and shortness of breath. Frontal headaches, facial tenderness, and purulent nasal discharge are signs of a chronic sinus infection. Nasal polyps are found in 10% of children with CF (McMullen & Bryson, 2004). Clubbing and a barrel chest develop over time (Figure 48–10 ●).

Most children have difficulty maintaining and gaining weight despite a voracious appetite because of malabsorption and an increased metabolic rate associated with frequent infections. Infants and children may have a delayed bone age, short stature, and delayed onset of puberty.

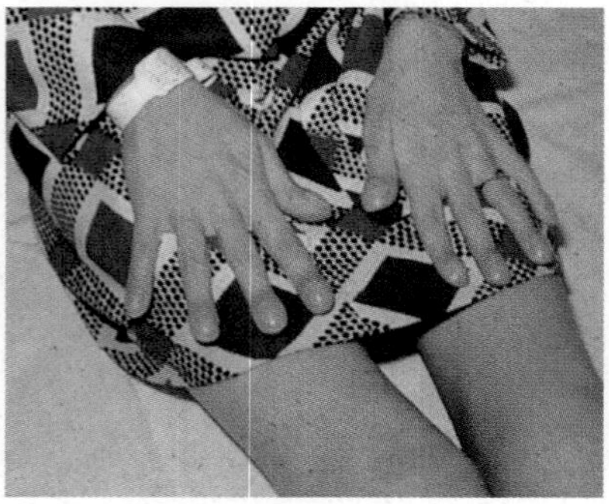

● **Figure 48–10** Digital clubbing. Enlargement of the distal phalanges, known as digital clubbing, occurs in children with cystic fibrosis due to chronic fibrotic changes within the lungs.

Clinical Therapy

CF is usually diagnosed in infancy or early childhood with one of four major presentations: newborn meconium ileus, malabsorption or failure to thrive, chronic recurrent respiratory infections, or fecal impaction and intussusception (see Chapter 53∞).

Newborn screening can be performed on dried blood samples to detect immunoreactive trypsinogen (IRT) concentrations which are high in newborns with CF. If the reading is high, a chromosome mutation analysis can be performed on the dried blood spot, or a second IRT test can be performed in 2 to 3 weeks. If the level is still high, a more extensive chromosome analysis can be performed to identify less common mutations causing CF. A sweat test is often performed to confirm the diagnosis (Kaye & Committee on Genetics, 2006). Newborn screening for CF is performed in 46 states and the District of Columbia (Cystic Fibrosis Foundation, 2009). Newborn screening shortens the interval to diagnosis by more than a year for 50% of cases (Baussano, Tardivo, Bellezza-Fontana, et al., 2006). Genetic testing is also available to identify carriers of CF gene mutations.

A sweat chloride test by pilocarpine iontophoresis is considered the gold standard for diagnosis of CF. A sweat chloride concentration of 50 to 60 mEq/L is suspicious. If the chloride concentration is greater than 60 mEq/L, it is diagnostic with other signs (meconium ileus, high IRT level, or positive family history). The test is often repeated to confirm the diagnosis (Figure 48–11 ●).

A spirometer is used on children older than 6 years to monitor pulmonary function. Sputum cultures are obtained to identify infectious organisms and antibiotic sensitivities.

Clinical therapy focuses on maintaining respiratory function, managing infection, promoting optimal nutrition and exercise, and preventing gastrointestinal blockage (Table 48–7). Newly diagnosed children without symptomatic lung disease are

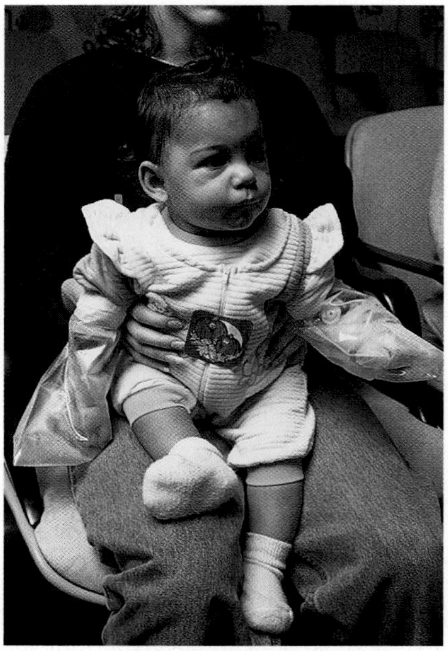

● **Figure 48–11** Sweat test. This 6-month-old girl is being evaluated for cystic fibrosis using the sweat test.

Table 48–7 Clinical Therapy for Cystic Fibrosis

Clinical Therapy	Rationale
RESPIRATORY THERAPY	
Exercise and physical fitness	Promotes maintenance of lung function
Chest physiotherapy twice a day for all lung segments (percussion or vibration with the child positioned to promote sputum drainage)	In association with coughing and breathing techniques secretions move to bronchi from lung areas
Immunizations	Prevention of viral and some bacterial infections
Chest tube drainage of air leaks	Resolves pneumothorax
Thoracoscopy to sew over ruptured alveoli	Repairs area of recurrent pneumothorax and prevents future episode in same location
Lung transplantation	Reversal of respiratory failure
GASTROINTESTINAL TRACT THERAPY	
Acid suppression preparation	Gastroesophageal reflux worsens lung function; enteric coating of enzyme supplements is affected by high acid content in duodenum
Hyperosmolar enemas, isotonic fluid lavage of the intestines (oral or by nasogastric tube)	Enema relieves meconium ileus in most infants; fluid lavage reduces distal intestinal obstruction
NUTRITION	
Well-balanced diet with 120–150% of recommended daily allowance (RDA) for calories and 200% of RDA for protein and moderate fat	Promotes essential nutrient balance for health, growth, and weight maintenance; nutritional counseling to support high-caloric intake (cultural-socioeconomic issues are important)
Pancreatic enzyme supplements	Assists in digestion of nutrients and decreasing fat and bulk

aggressively treated to slow the development of chronic respiratory infections and reduction in pulmonary function, and to improve nutrition and support growth.

Treatment is focused on controlling infection and inflammation, and on reducing mucus accumulation. Various forms of bronchial hygiene therapy are used regularly to reduce the accumulation of mucus in the lungs.

Frequent prolonged courses of antibiotics for infections may be prescribed to improve pulmonary function, exercise tolerance, and quality of life. Sputum culture results and sensitivities are also important in selection of the specific antibiotics used. Children who have evidence of *Pseudomonas aeruginosa* or *Burkholderia cepacia* infections have a poorer outcome. Medications are used to reduce sputum viscosity and to dilate the airways. Anti-inflammatory treatment is sometimes prescribed. Vitamins and pancreatic enzymes are also provided to improve the child's nutritional status.

Collaborative care with physicians, nurses, respiratory therapists, and nutritionists has led to improvements in medical management and optimal nutrition that have prolonged the lives of children and adults with CF. However, new complications such as CF-related diabetes must be carefully managed along with the progression of the disease. CF-related diabetes is difficult to manage because the child needs a large caloric intake that must be balanced by insulin dosage.

Lung transplantation is occasionally performed, and approximately 50% of cases survive for the first 5 years; however, there has been little improvement in survival and long-term outcomes over the past 20 years (Visner & Goldfarb, 2007). Immunosuppressive medications can cause significant problems in individuals infected with *Pseudomonas* or *Burkholderia cepacia*. End-stage lung disease is the cause of death in 80% of patients with CF (Liou, Woo, & Cahill, 2006).

NURSING MANAGEMENT

Care of the child with previously diagnosed CF is the focus of the following discussion.

NURSING ASSESSMENT AND DIAGNOSIS

PHYSIOLOGIC ASSESSMENT

Physical assessment of the child focuses on adequacy of respiratory function. Inquire about the frequency and character of the child's cough and sputum characteristics. Compare this information with the child's baseline. Changes in the cough may be more important than its presence or absence related to the development of a new infection. Auscultate the chest for breath sounds, crackles, and wheezes. Note any cyanosis or clubbing of the extremities. Obtain oxygen saturation and spirometry readings if changes in respiratory status are suspected.

Evaluate the child's growth, plotting the weight and height on a growth curve. Determine whether the child is maintaining an appropriate growth pattern. Children with significantly lower percentiles for height and weight should be considered malnourished. Inquire about the child's appetite and dietary intake. Ask how nutritional supplements, pancreatic enzymes, and vitamins are used.

Drug Guide

MEDICATIONS USED TO TREAT CYSTIC FIBROSIS

MEDICATIONS	ACTIONS
$Beta_2$-adrenergic receptor agonist bronchodilators, aerosol	Opens large and small airways; use before chest physiotherapy; and with symptoms; few studies exist to demonstrate their effectiveness
Dornase alpha (DNAse or Pulmozyme), aerosol	Loosens, liquefies, and thins pulmonary secretions in children with moderate to severe disease; decreases risk of developing pulmonary infections (Flume, O'Sullivan, Robinson, et al., 2007)
Hypertonic saline (7%), aerosol	Used following a bronchodilator, this solution potentially improves mucus clearance by increasing hydration of the airway, leading to fewer exacerbations of infection (Elkins, Robinson, Rose, et al., 2006)
Ibuprofen	Ibuprofen administered twice daily slows the rate of pulmonary function decline (Flume et al., 2007)
Antibiotics (aerosol, oral, IV)	Used to treat infections and selected based upon culture and sensitivities. Higher doses than normal and prolonged courses may be needed. Tobramycin is given to children with chronic *Pseudomonas aeruginosa* infection to suppress bacterial growth, given in alternating 28 day cycles (Bell, 2006).
Pancreatic enzyme supplements (Cotazym-S, Pancrease, Viokase)	Assists in digestion of nutrients decreasing fat and bulk; given prior to food ingestion, taken with meals and snacks
Multivitamins and vitamin E in water-soluble form, vitamins A, D, and K given when deficient, iron supplementation	Cystic fibrosis interferes with vitamin production; supplements are required in water-soluble form for better absorption (vitamins A, D, E, and K are naturally fat soluble); iron deficiency results from malabsorption syndrome
Ursodeoxycholate	May slow progression of hepatic lesion in cystic fibrosis. Given when patient has elevated liver enzymes or evidence of portal hypertension.
Lactulose	May abort early distal intestinal obstruction syndrome and prevent recurrences.

Observe the adolescent for the appearance of secondary sex characteristics, which are often delayed due to nutritional status.

Assess the child's stooling pattern. Identify whether the child has problems with abdominal pain or bloating, and whether these problems can be related to eating, stooling, or other activities. Palpate the abdomen for liver size, fecal masses, and evidence of pain.

PSYCHOSOCIAL ASSESSMENT

The emotional stress of this chronic disease may not be readily apparent, particularly if the child's symptoms are mild and not imminently life threatening. Ongoing observation of the child's and parents' behavior helps direct nursing interventions throughout hospitalization. Parents may feel guilt as carriers of the disease. Siblings may also show signs of difficulty in dealing with the illness, particularly if not affected by the disease. Siblings with CF may be affected if the child is showing signs of significant deterioration, being forced to acknowledge their own future course with the disease.

Ask parents how the child's illness has affected day-to-day functioning, potential conflicts with family activities, and how they have adapted to the child's plan of care. Investigate the need and options for respite care. Ask what the parents have told the child and siblings about the disease. What questions have the child and siblings asked about CF, and how have parents answered them? Has the child ever asked about his or her life expectancy? If not, what would parents say if asked?

Common nursing diagnoses for the child with cystic fibrosis include the following:

- *Ineffective Airway Clearance* related to thick mucus in lungs
- *Risk for Infection* related to the presence of mucous secretions conducive to bacterial growth
- *Imbalanced Nutrition: Less than Body Requirements* related to need for increased calories to meet metabolic needs
- *Parental Role Conflict* related to interruptions in family life due to the home care regimen and child's frequent exacerbations

PLANNING AND IMPLEMENTATION

Nursing management involves supporting the child and family initially, when the diagnosis is made, during subsequent hospitalizations, and during visits to specialty and primary healthcare providers. The nurse's role begins with implementing specific medical therapies and providing nursing care to meet the child's physiologic and psychosocial needs. Respiratory therapy, medications, and nutrition must be coordinated to promote optimal body function. Psychosocial support and reinforcement of the child's daily care needs are important in preparation for home care.

Children with CF require periodic hospitalization when a severe infection occurs or for a pulmonary and nutritional assessment. The child is often placed in a private room with standard precautions to reduce the spread of infectious organisms. Children with CF are not co-roomed to reduce the risk for transmission of *Pseudomonas aeruginosa* and *Burkholderia cepacia.*

Respect the parents' experiences as the child's primary care provider and include them in the child's routine care as much as possible. However, parents may view the hospital stay as a break from the rigorous daily pulmonary routine at home and need support in taking advantage of the respite. While the family is often proficient at providing physical care to the child, the nurse should take the opportunity to review basic and new information about respiratory care, medications, and nutrition. This is especially important as the child matures and begins to assume some self-care responsibilities.

PROVIDE RESPIRATORY THERAPY

Chest physiotherapy, to facilitate the removal of secretions from the lungs, is usually performed one to three times per day, before meals as coughing may stimulate vomiting (Figure 48–12 ●). Aerosol treatments with a bronchodilator, as well as DNAse and hypertonic saline to help thin respiratory secretions, may precede chest physiotherapy. Respiratory therapists and nurses often collaborate in teaching parents and other family members the skills for these necessary treatments. Some children use an oscillating vest for 30 minutes twice a day rather than chest physiotherapy. Exercise therapy is often utilized to increase endurance, and it is as beneficial as chest physiotherapy in secretion removal (Baker & Wideman, 2006). (See Skill 14–25 SKILLS.)

ADMINISTER MEDICATIONS AND MEET NUTRITIONAL NEEDS

Antibiotics for acute exacerbation are provided by oral, inhalation, and intravenous routes. They are continued until the child achieves the best possible lung function, often for at least 14 days. Children with CF have an increased clearance of most antibiotics, so they need higher doses and long treatment courses. Serum antibiotic drug levels may be ordered to ensure therapeutic dosing. In some cases, IV antibiotics are given at home to enable an earlier discharge. A portacath or central line may be placed for home IV therapy.

Digestive problems can be eased with pancreatic enzymes and dietary modification. Pancreatic enzyme supplements come in powder sprinkles and capsule form and are taken orally with all meals and large snacks. The amount needed is individualized based on the child's nutritional needs and digestive response to these supplements. Families need to learn which foods if any to avoid that contribute to a child's gastrointestinal problems. The goal is to achieve near-normal, well-formed stools and adequate weight gain.

Fat-soluble vitamins (A, D, E, and K) are not completely absorbed from food; therefore, they must be taken in water-soluble form. Multivitamins taken twice daily usually are sufficient to prevent deficiency.

Because of the child's high metabolic rate, some children need nutritional supplements or supplemental nasogastric or gastrostomy feedings to gain and maintain weight. The diet should be well balanced, with an emphasis on high caloric value. Fats and salt are both necessary in the diet.

PROVIDE PSYCHOSOCIAL SUPPORT

Help the parents and child learn what they must do to maintain health after discharge. Emotional support is essential because the diagnosis of this disorder creates anxiety and fear in both the parents and the child. They need assistance with emotional and psychosocial issues relating to discipline, body image (stooling odor, barrel chest), frequent rehospitalization, the potential fatal nature of the illness, the child's feeling of being different from friends, and overall financial, social, and family concerns. Because the disorder is inherited, families may have more than one child with CF. Refer families to genetic counseling and support groups. See My Nursing Kit for the Web site of the Cystic Fibrosis Foundation and other educational resources.

DISCHARGE PLANNING AND HOME CARE TEACHING

The financial burden of medications, supplies, and medical follow-up may not be recognized immediately by a family overwhelmed by the diagnosis. Initially, parents need assistance in

MyNursingKit Bronchial Hygiene Therapy

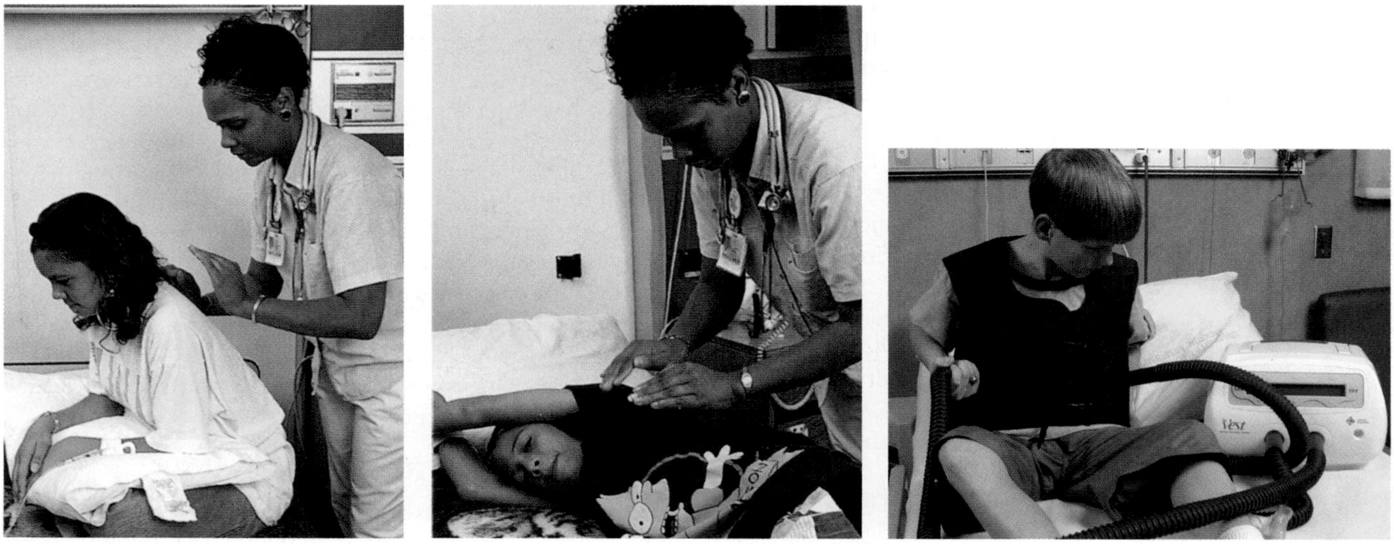

A B C

● **Figure 48–12** Chest physiotherapy. Postural drainage can be achieved by clapping with a cupped hand on the chest wall over the segment to be drained to create vibrations that are transmitted to the bronchi to dislodge secretions. ***A,*** If the obstruction is in the posterior apical segment of the lung, the nurse can do this with the child sitting up. ***B,*** If the obstruction is in the left posterior segment, the child should be lying on the right side. Several other positions can be used depending on the location of the obstruction. ***C,*** A high-frequency chest wall oscillation vest is another option for chest physiotherapy that the child can independently manage.

obtaining necessary equipment. If the family requires financial assistance, they should be referred to social services. Home care of the child with cystic fibrosis is expensive and can be draining on the family's finances.

NURSING CARE IN THE COMMUNITY

Nurses may encounter the child with CF in specialty clinics, health centers, and schools. Assess the child as described on page 1349. Observe the child's physical appearance, noting overall body proportions and any changes characteristic of CF. Respiratory function tests are usually performed every 6 months during CF visits. Assess hearing acuity on a regular basis, especially if the antibiotic tobramycin is used.

A psychosocial assessment is especially important when the child is going through major developmental stages. School-age children and adolescents are often embarrassed at being viewed as different from peers. Ask how the child or adolescent feels about the need for a special diet, medications, and the daily routine of respiratory management.

Review the child's use of bronchodilators and airway clearance techniques. If additional short-term therapies are prescribed to help improve pulmonary status, educate the child and family about the techniques to use and help them identify the best time to fit the additional treatment into the daily schedule. The chest physiotherapy three or four times a day regimen is a significant impact on family time. Alternate bronchial hygiene therapy techniques, such as a vest, may be more easily accepted by the family, especially since the parent does not have to physically perform the percussion and vibration. A regular vigorous exercise regimen is also beneficial in improving lung function, respiratory muscle strength, endurance, and airway clearance.

Parents often have difficulty encouraging the child with CF to eat the extra calories needed for optimal nutrition, setting the stage for a potential mealtime battleground. Parents need guidance about managing negative mealtime behaviors, in addition to guidelines for preparing nutritional calorie-dense foods. Increase calorie intake by offering high calorie snacks between meals and before bed.

Children with CF lose more than normal amounts of salt in their sweat. This loss can become intensified during hot weather, strenuous exercise, and fever. During periods of exercise and increased sweating, the child should be encouraged to drink more fluids and increase salt intake. Parents should allow the child to add extra salt to food and should permit some salty snacks (pretzels with salt, pickles, carbonated soda). Teach parents to recognize early symptoms of salt depletion, including fatigue, weakness, abdominal pain, and vomiting, and to contact the child's healthcare provider if these symptoms occur.

> **Nursing Practice**
>
> Use of cream or half and half added to soups, casseroles, and puddings; cream cheese spread on breads, muffins, and crackers; sour cream added to casseroles, and powdered milk added to regular milk, meatloaf, and custards are all ways to increase the calories in food eaten.

Adolescents with CF need special assistance in coping with their disorder, especially since the median survival is now more than 35 years. Help them identify normal adolescent changes versus those related to CF. Adolescents must learn how to cope with the difference they know exists between themselves and peers. Provide information about potential infertility along with guidelines for safe sexual practices to reduce the risk for sexually transmitted infections. Females with CF may be able to conceive and should be offered contraception.

Gradual assumption of responsibility for daily disease management is necessary. Adherence with the daily disease management may be a problem during adolescence. Individualized planning to achieve their daily care regimen while enabling them to interact with peers and participate in school activities may be most helpful. Link adolescents to services to assist with planning appropriate educational and occupational goals for their future. Palliative care planning should be initiated as the disease progresses to respiratory failure.

EVALUATION

Expected outcomes of nursing care include the following:

- The child and family develop proficiency in providing the daily pulmonary care and reducing the incidence of respiratory infections.
- The child and family develop a schedule and routine for daily pulmonary care that fits into family and school activities.
- The child consumes adequate calories and pancreatic enzymes to support growth and to stay within desirable weight ranges.

INJURIES OF THE RESPIRATORY SYSTEM

Airway compromise after an unintentional injury can cause death if not managed quickly and effectively. Children are vulnerable to changes in respiratory function after injury. A child's airway can become easily obstructed because of its small size. The airway may be obstructed by the tongue, small amounts of blood, mucus, or foreign debris, as well as swelling in the respiratory tract or adjacent neck tissue, leading to hypoxia. If the child's neck is flexed or hyperextended, the soft laryngeal cartilage may also compress and obstruct the airway.

SMOKE-INHALATION INJURY

Exposure of the child's face and airway to fire or thermal conditions leads to dramatic responses in the child's respiratory tract. Smoke and heat inhalation injury increases the child's risk for airway obstruction, carbon monoxide poisoning, acute respiratory distress syndrome, and late complications such as pneumonia and pulmonary embolism (Antoon & Donovan, 2007). The child's higher respiratory rate also increases his or her exposure to noxious chemicals.

The severity of the smoke-inhalation injury is influenced by the type of material burned and is more severe if the child was found in a closed space. The composition of materials determines how easily they ignite, how fast they burn, and how much heat they release. Smoke, a product of the burning process that is composed of gases and particles, is generated in varying volumes and density. The type and concentration of toxic gases, which are usually invisible, affect the severity of pulmonary damage. The duration of exposure to the smoke and toxic gases contribute significantly to the child's prognosis.

Exposure to extreme heat, common in house fires, leads to surface injury and upper airway damage. The upper airway normally removes heat from inhaled gases, sparing the lower airway from thermal damage. Airway edema develops rapidly over a few hours and places the small child at risk for airway obstruction and potentially for acute respiratory distress syndrome.

Carbon monoxide (CO) is a clear, colorless, odorless gas present in all fire conditions as the fire consumes oxygen. The CO molecule binds more firmly to hemoglobin than does oxygen. As a result, it replaces oxygen in the circulation and rapidly produces hypoxia in the child. The brain receives inadequate oxygen, resulting in confusion. This accounts for the inability of fire victims to escape as confusion progresses to loss of consciousness. The process can be rapidly reversed by the timely administration of 100% oxygen or hyperbaric oxygen treatment, if provided before hypoxia becomes too severe (Kao & Nañagas, 2004).

Damage to the lower airway often results from chemicals or toxic gas inhalation. Soot carried deeply into the lungs combines with water to deposit acid-producing chemicals on the lung tissue. These acids burn the tissue and destroy the cilia and surfactant. Tissue destruction, pulmonary edema, and disrupted gas exchange are the initial lung insult to the lungs. Days later, the damaged tissue sloughs off, obstructing the airways. The lungs become a breeding ground for microorganisms, leading to pneumonia. Healing leaves scars in the damaged alveoli, and this can greatly reduce future lung function.

Clinical manifestations of inhalation injury include burns of the face and neck, singed nasal hairs, soot around the mouth or nose, and hoarseness with stridor or voice change, even when the child initially has no respiratory distress. Edema develops rapidly over a few hours and may lead to airway obstruction with signs such as tachypnea, stridor, coughing, and wheezing. Respiratory distress develops and can lead to respiratory failure. If carbon monoxide poisoning is present the child will be confused or unconscious, and have cardiac arrhythmias.

Nursing Management

Most children who survive smoke-inhalation injury are admitted for close observation, airway management, and ventilatory support, if indicated. Initial treatment is 100% humidified oxygen administered through a nonrebreather mask. Carefully assess the child for respiratory function, and assess the level of consciousness for behavior changes that can indicate increasing hypoxia. Provide oxygen as ordered. Position the child to promote respiratory function. If respiratory distress develops, aggressive airway management with an endotracheal tube, mechanical ventilation, and monitoring are usually provided in an intensive care unit. Care is provided as described for the child with respiratory failure (see page 1316).

BLUNT CHEST TRAUMA

Blunt chest trauma in infants and toddlers is most often due to motor vehicle crashes and abuse. Bicycles, scooters, skateboards, and skates are more commonly associated with blunt chest trauma in school-age children. Injuries from high-energy motor vehicle crashes and hitting the steering column in a vehicle without an airbag occur more commonly in adolescents (Pitetti & Walker, 2005). Chest injuries may not be obvious and can be extremely difficult to evaluate.

Most children who die after sustaining severe blunt chest trauma were hypoxic because of poor airway and ventilatory control. A child's elastic, pliable chest wall and thin abdominal muscles provide minimal protection to underlying organs. This elasticity often prevents rib fractures, but the energy from blunt trauma is transferred directly from an external force to the internal organs, often causing a pulmonary contusion or pneumothorax. A rib fracture in children under 12 years old indicates trauma of significant force.

PULMONARY CONTUSION

A pulmonary contusion is defined as bruising damage to the tissues of the lung that often occurs without bony injury to the thorax. This causes bleeding from the capillaries into the alveoli, which may lead to capillary rupture in the air sacs. Pulmonary edema develops in the lower airways as blood and fluid from damaged tissues accumulate. The lower airway becomes obstructed, leading to a poor perfusion of the alveoli, poor compliance, hypoxemia, and hypoventilation (Pitetti & Walker, 2005).

Initially the child may appear asymptomatic. Respiratory distress, along with fever, wheezing, hemoptysis, and crackles, often develops over several hours. Careful observation is required during the first 12 hours after the injury to detect decreased perfusion related to ventilatory impairment.

The child with severe injury will need mechanical ventilation with low airway pressures, fluid restriction, supplemental oxygen, pain control, incentive spirometry, and avoiding prolonged immobilization. Pneumonia is a potential complication that can progress to respiratory failure (Pitetti & Walker, 2005).

Nursing Management

Nursing care centers on providing necessary physiologic support, such as oxygen therapy, positioning, positive pressure ventilation, fluid management, and comfort measures. When monitoring the status of a child who has a pulmonary contusion, do not rely on the child's color as an indicator of adequate oxygenation. Agitation and lethargy can signal increasing hypoxia. Cyanosis in children is often a late indicator of respiratory distress. Observe for hemoptysis (fresh blood in the emesis), dyspnea, decreased breath sounds, wheezes, crackles, and a transient temperature elevation. Inspect the thorax for symmetric chest wall movement and equal presence of breath sounds in both lungs. The child may initially appear well but requires careful and thorough monitoring to detect signs of deterioration. Children

PATHOPHYSIOLOGY ILLUSTRATED

PNEUMOTHORAX

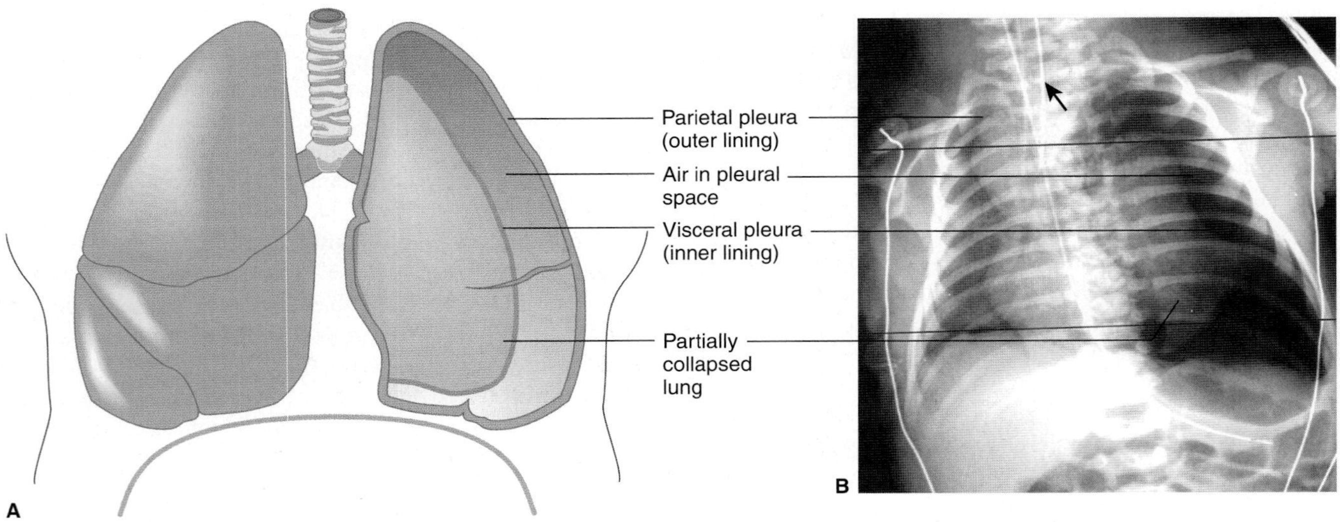

A, A pneumothorax is air in the pleural space that causes a lung to collapse. Whether the air results from an open injury or from bursting of alveoli due to a blunt injury, it is important to focus on airway management and maintain lung inflation. ***B,*** Tension pneumothorax, note the collapsed lung on the patient's left side and the deviation of the child's heart and trachea to the right side of the chest (see arrow).

Courtesy of Dorothy Bulas, M.D., Professor of Radiology and Pediatrics, Children's National Medical Center, Washington, DC.

with significant injuries are cared for in the ICU. Some children require ventilator support as the pulmonary tissues heal.

PNEUMOTHORAX

A pneumothorax occurs when air enters the pleural space because of tears in the tracheobronchial tree, the esophagus, or the chest wall. If blood collects in the pleural space, it is called a *hemothorax,* and if blood and air collect, it is called a *pneumohemothorax.*

There are three types of pneumothorax: open, closed, and tension. An open pneumothorax, sometimes referred to as a sucking chest wound, results from any penetrating injury that exposes the pleural space to atmospheric pressure, thereby collapsing the lung. A sucking sound may be heard as the air moves through the opening on the chest wall.

A closed pneumothorax is sometimes caused by blunt chest trauma with no evidence of rib fracture (see "Pathophysiology Illustrated: Pneumothorax"). The chest may be compressed against a closed glottis (such as may occur with breath holding), causing a sudden increase in pressure within the thoracic cavity. The pressure increase is transferred to the alveoli, causing them to burst. A single burst alveolus may be able to seal itself off, but with the destruction of many alveoli the lung collapses. Breath sounds are decreased or absent on the injured side, and the child is in respiratory distress. A thoracostomy is performed and a chest tube inserted (see Skill 14–15 **SKILLS**). A closed drainage system is attached to help remove the air and reinflate the lung by reestablishing negative pressure.

A tension pneumothorax is a life-threatening emergency that results when the air leaks into the chest during inspiration but cannot escape during expiration. Internal pressure continues to build, compressing the chest contents and collapsing the lung. Venous return to the heart is impaired as the trachea, heart, vena cava, and esophagus are compressed toward the unaffected lung when the mediastinum shifts, leading to decreased cardiac output. Signs of tension pneumothorax include increasing respiratory distress, decreased breath sounds, and paradoxical breathing.

Nursing Management

Nursing management focuses on airway management and maintaining lung inflation. The child arrives on the nursing unit with a chest tube and drainage system in place. Continued close observation for respiratory distress is essential. Carefully monitor vital signs. When the chest tube is removed, the site is covered with an occlusive dressing and the child's respiratory status is monitored for signs of respiratory distress. Complications include hemothorax (if the thoracostomy and chest tube are improperly placed), lung tissue injury, and scarring from poor tube placement (especially if the tube is placed too near the breast in girls).

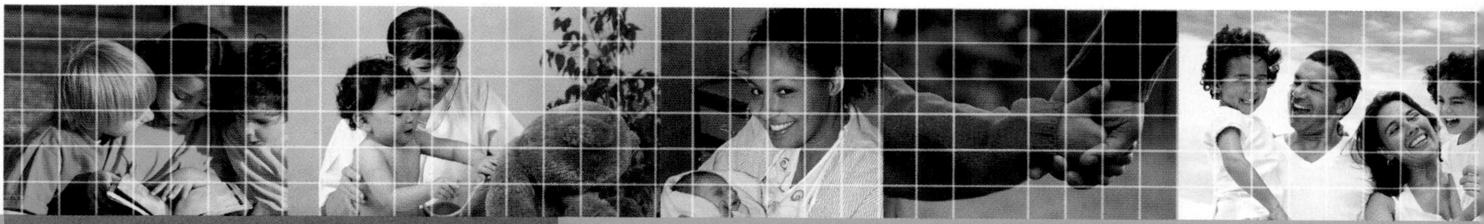

CRITICAL CONCEPT REVIEW

LEARNING OUTCOMES / CONCEPTS

48.1 Describe unique characteristics of the pediatric respiratory system anatomy and physiology and apply that information to the care of children with respiratory conditions.

1. A child's airway is shorter and narrower than an adult's:
   - Increased potential for obstruction.
2. Trachea is higher and at a different angle:
   - Increased risk for right mainstem aspiration and obstruction.
3. Newborns are obligatory nose breathers, they do not open mouth if nose is obstructed.
4. Newborn has inadequate smooth muscle bundles to help trap airway invaders:
   - Increased possibility of upper respiratory infection.
5. Until age 6 the child uses the diaphragm for breathing, so observe the abdomen to count respirations.

48.2 Identify the assessment guidelines for a child with a respiratory condition.

1. Assess the following:
   - Position of comfort
   - Vital signs
   - Respiratory effort
   - Color
   - Cough
   - Behavior change
   - Family history

48.3 List the different respiratory conditions and injuries that can cause respiratory distress in infants and children.

1. Respiratory conditions and injuries that can cause respiratory distress include:
   - Foreign body aspiration.
   - Obstructive sleep apnea.
   - Croup syndrome.
   - Epiglottitis.
   - Viral and bacterial respiratory infections.
   - Asthma.
   - Smoke inhalation.
   - Blunt chest trauma.
   - Pulmonary contusion.
   - Pneumothorax.

48.4 Assess the child's respiratory signs and symptoms to distinguish between respiratory distress and respiratory failure and describe the appropriate nursing care.

1. Signs of respiratory distress:
   - Tachypnea and tachycardia
   - Retractions
   - Nasal flaring
   - Inspiratory stridor
   - Pallor or mottled color
   - Labored breathing (dyspnea)
2. Signs of impending respiratory failure include:
   - Irritability, anxiety, mood changes
   - Lethargy or decreased responsiveness
   - Cyanosis
   - Wheezing
   - Nasal flaring
   - Retractions and accessory muscle use
   - Grunting
3. Nursing care includes:
   - Elevate head of the bed.
   - Monitor vital signs and level of responsiveness frequently for any changes.
   - Monitor oxygen saturation.
   - Give oxygen as ordered.
   - Keep emergency equipment at the bedside to assist ventilations if necessary.
   - Keep child from crying, if possible.

(continued)

LEARNING OUTCOMES	CONCEPTS
48.5 Distinguish between conditions of the upper respiratory tract that cause respiratory distress.	Foreign body aspiration ■ Spasmodic coughing or gagging, no fever or other signs of illness, dyspnea Spasmodic croup ■ Abrupt onset, usually at night and resolves by morning, afebrile, hoarseness, barking seal cough, mild respiratory distress, noisy inspiration Laryngotracheobronchitis ■ Gradual onset, upper respiratory infection, mild fever, barking seal or croupy cough, sore throat, hoarseness, stridor Epiglottitis ■ Rapid onset and progression, high fever, dysphagia, drooling, tripod positioning, intense sore throat, cherry red epiglottis Bacterial tracheitis ■ Gradual onset, high fever, croupy cough, stridor, thick purulent secretions, can lie flat, no drooling or dysphagia
48.6 Distinguish between conditions of the lower respiratory tract that cause illness in children.	Bronchitis ■ Dry hacking cough, increases in severity at night, painful chest and ribs Bronchiolitis ■ Mild respiratory symptoms that progress to tachypnea, wheezing, retractions, nasal flaring, irritability, poor fluid intake, hypoxia, cyanosis, and decreased mental status Pneumonia ■ Initial rhinitis and cough, followed by fever, crackles, wheezes, dyspnea, tachypnea, restlessness, diminished breath sounds Active pulmonary tuberculosis ■ Persistent cough, decreased appetite, weight loss or failure to gain weight, low-grade fever, night sweats, chills, enlarged lymph nodes.
48.7 Develop a hospital-based nursing care plan for a child with a common acute respiratory condition.	1. Maintain airway patency. 2. Frequently assess vital signs, respiratory effort, color, breath sounds, and for behavior change. 3. Allow child to assume position of comfort. 4. Meet fluid needs. 5. Promote rest and stress reduction for the child and parents. 6. Support the family's participation in care. 7. Give the family members information that lets them learn to manage the child's disease.
48.8 Develop a school-based nursing care plan for the child with asthma.	1. Develop an individual health plan. Include quick relief medications, exercise, and avoidance of known asthma triggers. 2. Maintain a log of PEFRs and quick relief medication administration. Give the family a copy for the child's healthcare provider. 3. Monitor child after giving quick relief medications for response. Call parents if little or no response. 4. Assess for signs of exercise-induced bronchospasm and report. 5. Coordinate an education and support group for children with asthma.
48.9 Develop a home nursing care plan for the child with cystic fibrosis.	1. Instruct parents in daily medications and set up an administration schedule. 2. Teach respiratory therapy techniques and help the family identify a workable schedule. 3. Discuss specific nutritional needs of the child. 4. Review the potential need for financial assistance. 5. Encourage child to exercise and to participate in physical activities to the level of child's respiratory condition. 6. Link family to appropriate support groups. 7. Ensure that child gets immunizations and has other health promotion needs addressed.

CRITICAL THINKING IN ACTION

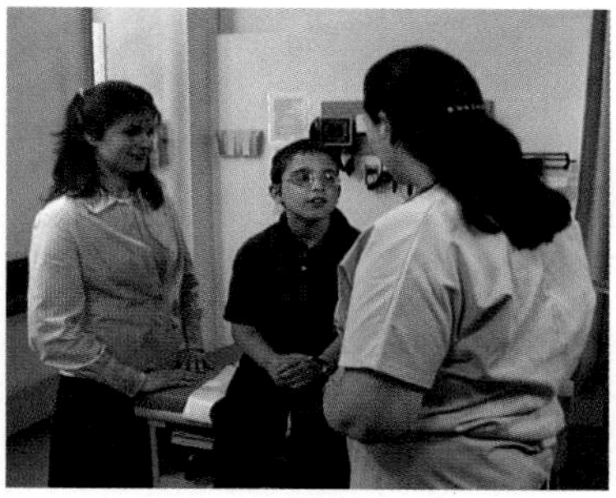

Adam and his mother have come to the health center in follow up of his hospitalization to get an asthma action plan and to discuss how to reduce his asthma episodes. Adam, who is 7 years old, has a history of episodic wheezing and nebulizer treatments, but he had never been hospitalized for asthma until last week. During his 2-day hospitalization, his parents were given initial education about how to manage his moderate persistent asthma.

His mother has brought along Adam's medications (inhaled corticosteroid MDI and salmeterol DPI for daily control, and an albuterol MDI for quick relief), his peak flow meter, spacer, and his asthma action plan. She tells you that he is also completing a dose of oral corticosteroids. You discuss the peak flow meter, the guidelines, and what type of action to take as needed. Based on his height of 48 inches, his peak flow meter green zone is 160–128, his yellow zone is 128–80, and his red zone is 80 or below. Adam is to use his daily control medications twice a day. If he has symptoms, he is to take his albuterol MDI with spacer, two puffs every 4–6 hours as needed.

1. What are some of the side effects associated with Adam's albuterol MDI?
2. What is the benefit to using a spacer on Adam's albuterol and inhaled corticosteroid MDI?
3. Address the concerns of Adam's mother about the daily use of inhaled corticosteroids.
4. What are the signs of respiratory distress to observe for with Adam?

See MyNursingKit for possible responses.

REFERENCES

Akinbami, L. J. (2006). The state of childhood asthma, United States, 1980–2005, *Advance Data from Vital and Health Statistics,* no. 381, Hyattstown, MD: National Center for Health Statistics.

American Academy of Allergy, Asthma, and Immunology (AAAAI). (2009). *Peak flow meter.* Retrieved November 19, 2009 from www.aaaai.org

American Academy of Pediatrics Task Force on Sudden Infant Death Syndrome. (2005). The changing concept of sudden infant death syndrome: Diagnostic coding shifts, controversies regarding the sleeping environment, and new variables to consider in reducing risk. *Pediatrics, 116*(5), 1245–1255.

American Academy of Pediatrics Subcommittee on Diagnosis and Management of Bronchiolitis. (2006). Diagnosis and management of bronchiolitis. *Pediatrics, 118*(4), 1774–1793.

American Academies of Pediatrics. (2009). *Red Book: 2009 Report of the Committee on Infectious Diseases* (28th ed.). Elk Grove Village, IL: Author.

Amin, R., Anthony, L., Somers, V., Fenchel, M., McConnel, K., Jefferies, J., et al. (2008). Growth velocity predicts recurrence of sleep-disordered breathing one year after adenotonsillectomy. *American Journal of Respiratory and Critical Care Medicine, 177*(6), 654–659.

Antoon, A. Y., & Donovan, M. K. (2007). Burn injuries. In R. M. Kliegman, R. E. Behrman, H. B. Jenson, & B. F. Stanton, *Nelson textbook of pediatrics* (18th ed., pp. 450–458). Philadelphia: Elsevier Saunders.

Arnold, L. D. (2006). Ingested and aspirated foreign bodies: Making sure what went in comes out. *Contemporary Pediatrics, 23*(11), 32–44.

Ayala, G. X., Miller, D., Zagami, E., Riddle, C., Willis, S., & King, D. (2006). Asthma in middle schools: What students have to say about their asthma. *Journal of School Health, 76*(6), 208–214.

Baker, C. F., & Wideman, L. (2006). Attitudes toward physical activity in adolescents with cystic fibrosis: Sex differences after training: A pilot study. *Journal of Pediatric Nursing, 21*(3), 197–210.

Banasiak, N. C. (2007). Childhood asthma: Part two: Management update. *Journal of Pediatric Health Care, 21*(3), 184–191.

Bandla, P., Brooks, L. J., Trimarchi, T., & Helfaer, M. (2005). Obstructive sleep apnea syndrome in children. *Anesthesiology Clinics of North America, 23,* 535–549.

Baraldi, E., & Filippone, M. (2007). Chronic lung disease after premature birth. *New England Journal of Medicine, 357*(19), 1946–1955.

Baussano, I., Tardivo, I., Bellezza-Fontana, R., Forneris, M. P., Lezo, A., Anfossi, L., et al. (2006). Neonatal screening for cystic fibrosis does not affect time to first infection with *Pseudomonas aeruginosa. Pediatrics, 118*(3), 888–895.

Bell, E. (2006). Pulmonary pharmacotherapy options changing for cystic fibrosis patients. *Infectious Diseases in Children, 19*(10), 12–13.

Bindler, R. M., & Howry, L. B. (2005). *Pediatric drugs and nursing implications* (3rd ed.). Upper Saddle River, NJ: Prentice Hall-Health.

Brand, P. L. P. (2005). Key issues in inhalation therapy in children. *Current Medical Research and Opinion, 21*(Suppl 4), S27–S32.

Brashers, V. L. (2006a). Alterations in pulmonary function. In K. L. McCance & S. E. Huether, *Pathophysiology: the biologic basis for disease in adults and children* (5th ed., pp. 1205–1248). St. Louis: Elsevier Mosby.

Brashers, V. L. (2006b). Structure and function of the pulmonary system. In K. L. McCance & S. E. Huether, *Pathophysiology: the biologic basis for disease in adults and children* (5th ed., pp. 1181–1204). St. Louis: Elsevier Mosby.

Bullock, L. F. C., Mickey, K., Green, J., & Heine, A. (2004). Are nurses acting as role models for the prevention of SIDS? *Maternal Child Nursing, 29*(3), 172–177.

Capper-Michel, B. (2004). Bronchopulmonary dysplasia. In P. J. Allen & J. A. Vessey, *Primary care of the child with a chronic condition* (4th ed., pp. 282–298). St. Louis: Mosby.

Centers for Disease Control and Prevention. (2006). *October 2006 is SIDS (sudden infant death syndrome) awareness month.* Retrieved December 22, 2008 from http://www.cdc.gov/omh/Highlights/2006/HOct06SIDS.htm

Centers for Disease Control and Prevention, Division of Adolescent and School Health. (2004). *Addressing asthma in schools.* Retrieved November 13, 2006 from http://www.cdc.gov/HealthyYouth/asthma/facts.htm

Chiang, L. (2005). Exploring the health related quality of life among children with moderate asthma. *Journal of Nursing Research, 13*(1), 31–39.

Christian, B. J., & D'Auria, J. P. (2006). Building life skills for children with cystic fibrosis. *Nursing Research, 55*(5), 300–307.

Cifuentes, J., & Carlo, W. A. (2007). Respiratory system. In C. Kenner & J. W. Lott, *Comprehensive neonatal care: An interdisciplinary approach* (4th ed., pp. 1–17). St. Louis: Elsevier Saunders.

Clark, A. P., Giuliano, K., & Chen, H-M. (2006). Pulse oximetry revisited: "But his O_2 was normal!" *Clinical Nurse Specialist, 20*(6), 268–272.

Corneli, H. M., Zorc, J. J., Mahajan, P., Shaw, K., Holubkov, R., Reeves, S. D., et al. (2007). A multicenter, randomized controlled trial of dexamethasone for bronchiolitis. *New England Journal of Medicine, 357*(4), 331–339.

Cystic Fibrosis Foundation. (2007a). *About cystic fibrosis: What you need to know.* Retrieved January 10, 2009, from http://www.cff.org/AboutCF/

Cystic Fibrosis Foundation. (2009). Newborn screening for cystic fibrosis. Retrieved January 10, 2009, from http://www.cff.org/GetInvolved/Advocate/WhyAdvocate/NewbornScreening/

Daley, K. C. (2004). Update on sudden infant death syndrome. *Current Opinion in Pediatrics, 16,* 227–232.

DeFrances, C. J., & Hall, M. J. (2007). *2005 National Hospital Discharge Survey. Advance data from vital and health statistics,* no. 385, Hyattsville, MD: U.S. Department of Health and Human Services, Centers for Disease Control, National Center for Health Statistics.

DeWolfe, C. C. (2005). Apparent life-threatening event: A review. *Pediatric Clinics of North America, 52,* 1127–1146.

Dolovich, M. B., Ahrens, T. C., Hess, D. R., Anderson, P., Dhand, R., Rau, J. L., et al. (2005).

Device selection and outcomes of aerosol therapy: Evidence-based guidelines. *Chest, 127*, 335–371.

Dykes, J. (2005). Managing children with croup in emergency departments. *Emergency Nurse, 13*(6), 14–19.

Ehrenkranz, R. A., Walsh, M. C., Vohr, B. R., Jobe, A. H., Wright, L. L., Fanaroff, A. A., et al., (2005). Validation of the National Institutes of Health consensus definition of bronchopulmonary dysplasia. *Pediatrics, 116*(6), 1353–1360.

Elkins, M. R., Robinson, M., Rose, B. R., Harbour, C., Moriarty, C. P., Marks, G. B., et al., (2006). A controlled trial of long-term inhaled hypertonic saline in patients with cystic fibrosis. *New England Journal of Medicine, 354*(3), 229–240.

Everard, M. L. (2006). Aerosol delivery to children. *Pediatric Annals, 35*(9), 630–636.

Faden, H. (2006). The dramatic change in the epidemiology of pediatric epiglottitis. *Pediatric Emergency Care, 22*(6), 443–444.

Feja, K., & Saiman, L. (2005). Tuberculosis in children. *Clinics of Chest Medicine, 26*, 295–312.

Flume, P. A., O'Sullivan, B. P., Robinson, K. A., Goss, C. H., Mogayzel, P. J., Willey-Courand, D. B., et al. (2007). Cystic fibrosis pulmonary guidelines: Chronic medications for maintenance of lung health. *American Journal of Respiratory and Critical Care Medicine, 176*, 957–969.

Fong, E. W., & Levin, R. H. (2007). Inhaled corticosteroids for asthma. *Pediatrics in Review, 28*(6), e30–e35.

Fowlkes, A. L., & Fry, A. M. (2006). Respiratory syncytial virus activity—United States, 2005-2006. *Morbidity and Mortality Weekly Report, 55*(47), 1277–1279.

Froh, D. L. (2006). Alterations in pulmonary function in children. In K. L. McCance & S. E. Huether (Eds.), *Pathophysiology: The biologic basis for disease in adults and children* (5th ed., pp. 1249–1278). St. Louis: Elsevier Mosby.

Gibson, W. A. (2007). Choking: Strategies for evaluation and management. *Consultant for Pediatricians, 6*(12), 640–644.

Guilbert, T. W., Morgan, W. J., Zeiger, R. S., Mauger, D. T., Boehmer, S. J., Szefler, S. J., et al. (2006). Long-term inhaled corticosteroids in preschool children at high risk for asthma. *New England Journal of Medicine, 354*(19), 1985–1997.

Hall, K. L., & Zalman, B. (2005). Evaluation and management of apparent life-threatening events in children. *American Family Physician, 71*(12), 2301–2308.

Hopkins, A., Lahiri, T., Salerno, R., & Heath, B. (2006). Changing epidemiology of the life-threatening upper airway infections: The reemergence of bacterial tracheitis. *Pediatrics, 118*(4), 1418–1421.

Hymel, K. P., and Committee on Child Abuse and Neglect. (2006). Distinguishing sudden infant death syndrome from child abuse fatalities. *Pediatrics, 118*(1), 421–427.

Kao, L. W., & Nañagas, K. A. (2004). Carbon monoxide poisoning. *Emergency Medical Clinics of North America, 22*(4), 985–1018.

Kaye, C. I., and the Committee on Genetics, American Academy of Pediatrics. (2006). Newborn screening fact sheets. *Pediatrics, 118*(3), e934–e963.

Lara, M., Akinbami, L., Flores, G., & Morgenstern, H. (2006). Heterogeneity of childhood asthma among Hispanic children: Puerto Rican children bear a disproportionate burden. *Pediatrics, 117*(1), 43–53.

Lieu, T. A., Finkelstien, J. A., Lozano, P., Capra, A. M., Chi, F. W., Jensvold, N., et al., (2004). Cultural competence policies and other predictors of asthma care quality for Medicaid-insured children. *Pediatrics, 114*(1), e102–e110.

Liou, T. G., Woo, M. S., & Cahill, B. C. (2006). Lung transplantation for cystic fibrosis. *Current Opinion in Pulmonary Medicine, 12*(6), 459–463.

Mannix, R., & Bachur, R. (2007). Status asthmaticus in children. *Current Opinion in Pediatrics, 19*, 281–287.

Marcoux, K. K. (2005). Current management of status asthmaticus in the pediatric ICU. *Critical Care Nursing Clinics of North America, 17*, 463–479.

Marshik, P. L. (2004). Pharmacologic treatment of pediatric asthma. *Advance for Nurse Practitioners, 12*(3), 35–36, 41–46.

McMullen, A. H., & Bryson, E. A. (2004). Cystic fibrosis. In P. J. Allen & J. A. Vessey, *Primary care of the child with a chronic condition* (4th ed., pp. 404–425). St. Louis: Mosby.

McNelis, A. M., Musick, B., Austin, J. K., Larson, P., & Dunn, D. W. (2007). Psychosocial care needs of children with recent-onset asthma. *Journal for Specialists in Pediatric Nursing, 12*(1), 3–12.

Meadows-Oliver, M., & Banasiak, N. C. (2005). Asthma medication delivery devices. *Journal of Pediatric Health Care, 19*(2), 121–123.

National Asthma Education and Prevention Program. (2007). *Expert Panel Report 3: Guidelines for the Diagnosis and Management of Asthma*, Bethesda, MD: National Institutes of Health, National Heart Lung and Blood Institute. Retrieved January 10, 2009 from http://www.nhlbi.nih.gov/guidelines/asthma/

Paterson, D. S., Trachtenberg, F. L., Thompson, E. G., Belliveau, R. A., Beggs, A. H., Darnall, R., et al. (2006). Multiple serotonergic brainstem abnormalities in sudden infant death syndrome. *Journal of American Medical Association, 296*(17), 2124–2132.

Peeke, K., Hershberger, M., & Marriner, J. (2006). Obstructive sleep apnea syndrome in children. *Pediatric Nursing, 32*(5), 489–494.

Peredo-Pinto, H., & Jacobs, N. M. (2008). A 17-month infant with a calf lesion and generalized hypotonia. *Pediatric Annals, 37*(2), 96–98.

Perkin, R. M., & Swift, J. D. (2002). Infectious causes of upper airway obstruction in children. *Pediatric Emergency Medicine Reports, 7*(11), 117–128.

Pitetti, R. D., & Walker, S. (2005). Life-threatening chest injuries in children. *Clinical Pediatric Emergency Medicine, 6*, 16–22.

Popovich, D. M., Richiuso, N., & Danek, G. (2004). Pediatric health care provider' knowledge of pulse oximetry. *Pediatric Nursing, 30*(1), 14–20.

Rafei, K., & Lichtenstein, R. (2006). Airway infectious disease emergencies. *Pediatric Clinics of North America, 53*, 215–242.

Rao, S., & Grigg, J. (2006). New insights into pulmonary inflammation in cystic fibrosis. *Archives of Diseases of Childhood, 91*, 786–788.

Reznik, M., & Ozuah, P. O. (2005). A prudent approach to screening for and treating tuberculosis. *Contemporary Pediatrics, 22*(11), 73–88.

Sandora, T. J., & Harper, M. B. (2005). Pneumonia in hospitalized children. *Pediatric Clinics of North America, 52*, 1059–1081.

Scolnik, D., Coates, A. L., Stephens, D., Da Silva, Z., Lavine, E., & Schum, S. (2006). Controlled delivery of high vs. low humidity vs. mist therapy for croup in emergency departments. *Journal of American Medical Association, 295*(11), 1274–1280.

Shah, S. A., Berlinksi, A. B., & Rubin, B. K. (2006). Force-dependent static dead space of face masks used with holding chambers. *Respiratory Care, 5*(2), 140–144.

Smyth, R. L., & Openshaw, P. J. M. (2006). Bronchiolitis. *Lancet, 368*, 312–322.

Starke, J. R. (2007). New concepts in childhood tuberculosis. *Current Opinion in Pediatrics, 19*(3), 306–313.

Stastny, P. F., Ichinose, T. Y., Thayer, S. D., Olson, R. J., & Keens, T. G. (2004). Infant sleep positioning by nursery staff and mothers in newborn hospital nurseries. *Nursing Research, 53*(2), 122–129.

Strausbaugh, S. D., & Davis, P. B. (2007). Cystic fibrosis: A review of epidemiology and pathobiology. *Clinics of Chest Medicine, 28*, 279–288.

Taylor, Z., Nolan, C. M., & Blumberg, H. M. (2005). Controlling tuberculosis in the United States: Recommendations from the American Thoracic Society, CDC, and the Infectious Diseases Society of America. *Morbidity and Mortality Weekly Report, 54*(RR-12), 43–45.

Todd, B. (2006). The QuantiFERON-TB gold test. *American Journal of Nursing, 106*(6), 33–37.

Virchow, J. C. (2005). What plays a role in the choice of inhaler device for asthma therapy? *Current Medical Research and Opinion, 21*(Suppl 4), S19–S25.

Visner, G. A., & Goldfarb, S. B. (2007). Posttransplant monitoring of pediatric lung transplant recipients. *Current Opinion in Pediatrics, 19*(3), 321–326.

Wardell, C., Huang, S., & Isbister, C. (2006). When children with asthma go swimming, the benefits can be many and long-lasting. *Contemporary Pediatrics, 23*(10), 89–96.

Willis, K. C. (2007). Bronchiolitis: Advanced practice focus in the emergency department. *Journal of Emergency Nursing, 33*(4), 346–351.

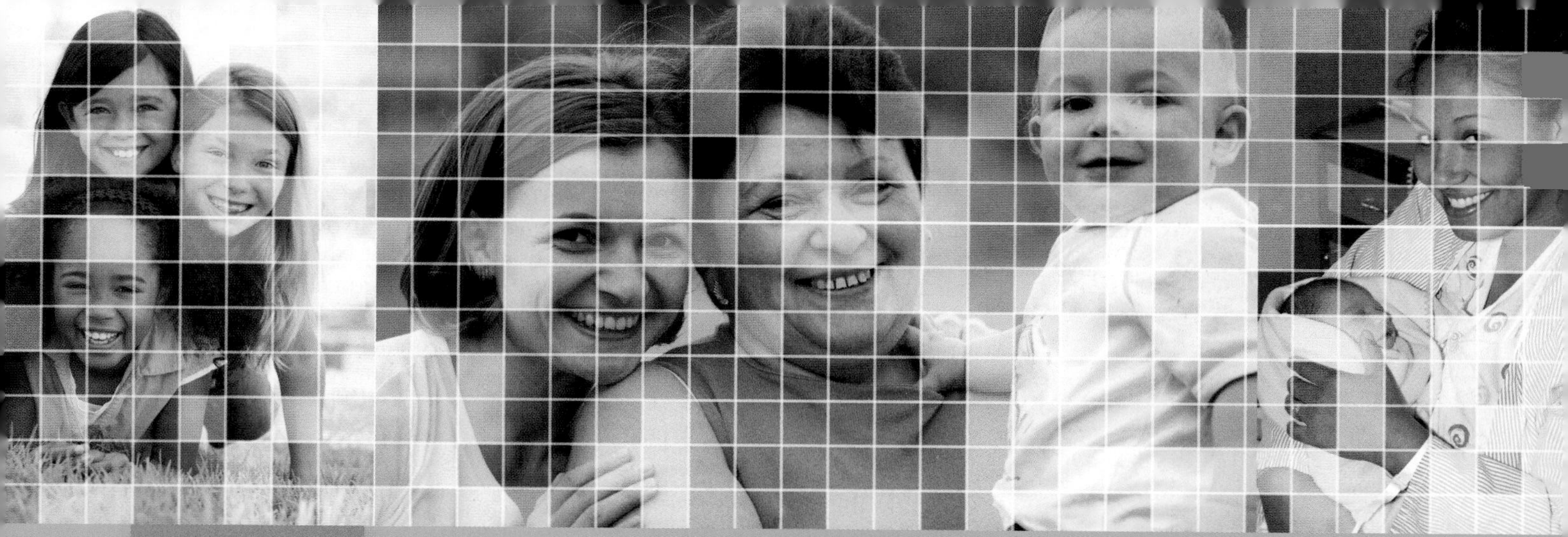

CHAPTER

49 The Child with Alterations in Cardiovascular Function

Brandy got sick so fast. Look how hard she is working to breathe. She gets tired before she can finish her formula. We didn't expect her to have to have heart surgery when she was still so small. We were told her chances for successful surgery would improve if she grew some more. I just want her to get stronger and have the chance to grow up to be like other kids. —Mother of Brandy, 1 month old

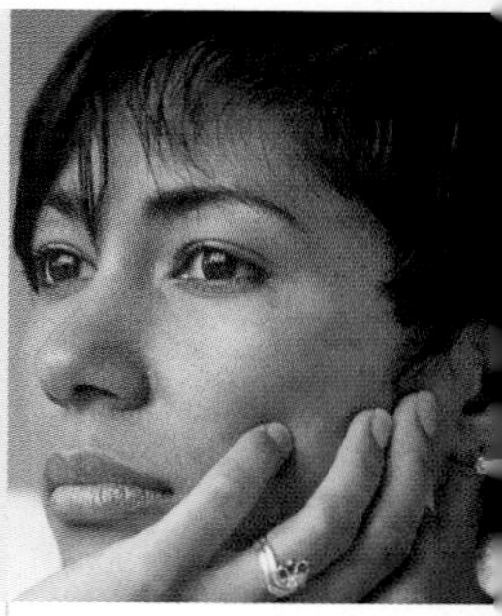

LEARNING OUTCOMES

49.1 Describe the anatomy and physiology of the cardiovascular system, focusing on the flow of blood and the action of heart valves.

49.2 Describe the pathophysiology associated with congenital heart defects with increased pulmonary circulation, decreased pulmonary circulation, mixed defects, and obstructed systemic blood flow.

49.3 Develop a nursing care plan for the infant with a congenital heart defect cared for at home prior to corrective surgery.

49.4 Develop a nursing care plan for the child undergoing open heart surgery.

49.5 Recognize the signs and symptoms of congestive heart failure in an infant and child.

49.6 Develop a nursing care plan for a child with congestive heart failure.

49.7 Differentiate among the acquired heart diseases that occur during childhood.

49.8 List strategies to reduce the child's risk of adult onset cardiovascular disease.

49.9 Describe the development of hypovolemic shock and nursing management of the condition.

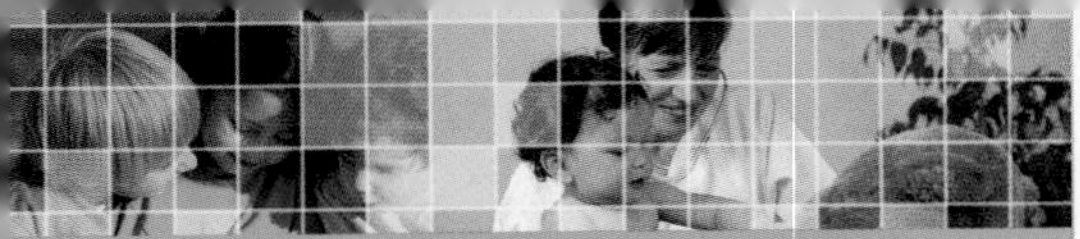

KEY TERMS

Arrhythmias, 1395
Cardiac output, 1360
Cardiomegaly, 1383
Desaturated blood, 1360
Digitalization, 1388
Heaving, 1368
Hemodynamics, 1361
Hypoxemia, 1360
Palliative procedure, 1362
Polycythemia, 1371
Preload, 1401
Radiofrequency ablation, 1396
Shock, 1398
Shunt, 1361
Stenosis, 1373
Syncope, 1372

MyNursingKit Animation: Congenital Heart Defects

Alterations in cardiovascular function may be a result of a congenital defect, acquired infection, or injury. Annually approximately 20 per 100,000 newborns are born with cardiac defects that require surgical correction (Schultz & Kreutzer, 2006, p. 56). Approximately one third of children born with congenital heart disease die as a result of their cardiac disease and about a third of those deaths occur in the first year of life (Connor, 2006). More than 35 types of heart defects have been documented. The frequency of occurrence is increasing, possibly due to better detection. Rapid advances in the treatment of congenital heart defects allow children to have surgery at younger ages, and most children survive to adulthood.

ANATOMY AND PHYSIOLOGY OF PEDIATRIC DIFFERENCES

The transition from fetal to pulmonary circulation is described in Chapter 27∞. Systemic vascular resistance increases after the umbilical cord is cut. The increased blood and pressure in the left side of the heart stimulates the closure of the foramen ovale. The ductus arteriosus normally constricts and closes within 10 to 15 hours after birth in response to higher oxygen saturation levels. The ventricles are equal in size at birth, but by 2 months of age the left ventricle is twice as large as the right ventricle. The higher systemic vascular pressures force the left ventricle to develop quickly.

Infants have a greater risk of heart failure than older children because the immature heart is more sensitive to volume or pressure overload. Infants have limited functional capacity because the undeveloped muscle fibers in the myocardium are unable to expand their stretch to increase the ventricular volume and stroke volume. The heart muscle fibers develop during early childhood and by 9 years of age, the weight of the heart has increased by 6 times (Connor, 2006). The systolic blood pressure also rises during childhood, reaching adult levels by puberty.

OXYGENATION

Oxygen bound to hemoglobin is transported to the tissues by the systemic circulation. Hematocrit and hemoglobin concentrations appropriate for the child's age are necessary for adequate oxygen transport (see Chapter 51∞). The oxygen arterial saturation is the amount of oxygen that can potentially be delivered to the tissues. **Desaturated blood** results when oxygenated and unoxygenated blood mix because of a congenital heart defect. Cyanosis is seen with arterial saturations less than 88% when the adult hemoglobin concentration is 12 gm/dL. In neonates, cyanosis is seen when arterial saturations are less than 79% (Schultz & Kreutzer, 2006, p. 52).

The child's bone marrow responds to chronic **hypoxemia** (a lower than normal level of oxygen in the blood) by producing more red blood cells to increase the amount of hemoglobin available for oxygenation. A hematocrit value of 50% or higher is common in children with cyanotic heart defects. Hemoglobin greater than 20 g/dL and a hematocrit greater than 55% to 60% are dangerous and put the child at risk for a thromboembolism, especially if dehydration occurs (Schultz & Kreutzer, 2006, p. 53).

CARDIAC FUNCTIONING

The infant's metabolic rate and oxygen requirements double at birth, so the heart rate is high to maintain a high cardiac output and adequate oxygen transport. The infant has little cardiac output reserve capacity until oxygen requirements begin to decrease. **Cardiac output**, the volume of blood ejected from the left ventricle each minute, depends almost completely on heart rate until the heart muscle is fully developed at 5 years of age. Stress, exercise, fever, or respiratory distress cause tachycardia, which increases cardiac output and oxygen transport.

CONGENITAL HEART DISEASE

Congenital heart disease refers to a defect in the heart or great vessels, or persistence of a fetal structure after birth. Congenital heart defects are one of the most common birth defects. More than 40% of infants born with a congenital heart defect have a critical heart

Nursing Practice

A pulse oximeter provides a noninvasive estimate of the percutaneous arterial oxygen saturation level (SpO_2). A reading of 95% to 98% is normal in children. A reading less than 94% in a quiet infant or child is abnormal (Sivarajan, Vetter, & Gleason, 2006, p. 3). An SpO_2 of less than 85% for more than 30 seconds is a major hypoxic event (Popovich, Richiuso, & Danek, 2004).

lesion that requires surgery or interventional catheterization in the first 6 months of life (Marino, Ostrow, & Cohen, 2006, p. 277).

ETIOLOGY AND PATHOPHYSIOLOGY

Most congenital heart defects develop during the first 8 weeks of gestation. They can develop as the result of a combined or interactive effect of genetic and environmental factors, such as:

- Fetal exposure to drugs (e.g., phenytoin, lithium), alcohol, and secondary tobacco smoke.
- Maternal viral infections such as rubella or coxsackie B5.
- Maternal metabolic disorders such as phenylketonuria, diabetes mellitus, and hypercalcemia.
- Increased maternal age.
- Genetic factors (family recurrence patterns).
- Chromosomal abnormalities are associated with at least 25% of children with congenital heart defects. Turner syndrome, Noonan syndrome, Marfan syndrome, DiGeorge syndrome, cri du chat syndrome, Down syndrome, and trisomy syndromes 13, 15, 18, and 21 are associated with specific congenital heart defects (Connor, 2006). Because of the genetic component, the incidence of congenital heart defects is expected to slowly rise as these children survive and have children of their own.

Congenital heart defects are generally categorized by pathophysiology and **hemodynamics**, the pressures generated by blood and the pathways blood takes through the heart and pulmonary system. These categories include the following:

- Increased pulmonary blood flow (see page 1364)
- Decreased pulmonary blood flow (see page 1371)
- Obstructed systemic blood flow (see page 1379)
- Mixed defects (with combined defects that increase and decrease pulmonary blood flow) have similar clinical characteristics, clinical therapy, and nursing management to those with decreased pulmonary blood flow, and will be discussed in that section (see page 1371).

CLINICAL MANIFESTATIONS

The presence of a heart murmur is often the first indication of a congenital heart defect. A murmur indicates blood is flowing with higher pressure than normal to get through a narrowed valve or vessel, or through a **shunt** (an abnormal anatomic opening between the systemic and pulmonary circulation). Other clinical manifestations and the timing of their appearance vary by the pathophysiology and severity of the defect. See "Clinical Manifestations: Heart Defects by Pathophysiology." Newborns may become symptomatic as soon as the umbilical cord is cut or within the first few days of life. Some children may be asymptomatic except for a heart murmur. Signs and symptoms in older children may include exercise intolerance, chest pain, arrhythmias, syncope, and sudden death.

CLINICAL THERAPY

Multiple tests are used to diagnose cardiac defects. See Table 49–1. Blood tests such as a hematocrit and hemoglobin are taken to assess for anemia or polycythemia. Arterial blood gases may be obtained, especially when cyanosis or a complex heart defect is suspected.

Clinical Manifestations

HEART DEFECTS BY PATHOPHYSIOLOGY

PATHOPHYSIOLOGY AND TYPE OF DEFECT	CLINICAL MANIFESTATIONS
Increased pulmonary blood flow (PDA, ASD, VSD, AV canal)	Tachypnea, tachycardia, murmur, congestive heart failure (CHF), poor weight gain, diaphoresis, periorbital edema, frequent respiratory infections
Decreased pulmonary blood flow (PS, TOF, pulmonary or tricuspid atresia, TGA)	Cyanosis, hypercyanotic spells, poor weight gain, polycythemia
Obstruction to systemic blood flow (COA, AS, HLHS, MS, interrupted aortic arch)	Diminished pulses, poor color, delayed capillary refill time, decreased urine output, CHF with pulmonary edema
Mixed defects—postnatal survival is dependent upon mixing of systemic and pulmonary blood (TGA, TAPVR, truncus arteriosus, double outlet right ventricle)	Cyanosis, poor weight gain, pulmonary congestion, CHF may occur with increased shunting

*AS—aortic stenosis, ASD—atrial septal defect, AV—atrioventricular, COA—coarctation of aorta, HLHS—hypoplastic left heart syndrome, MS—mitral stenosis, PDA—patent ductus arteriosus, PS—pulmonic stenosis, TAPVR—total anomalous pulmonary venous return, TOF—tetralogy of Fallot, TGA—transposition of great arteries, VSD—ventricular septal defect

Table 49–1 Diagnostic Tests Used in Children with Congenital Heart Disease

Diagnostic Test	Purpose
Radiographic studies (chest radiograph, computed tomography, magnetic resonance imaging)	Reveals size and contour of the heart and characteristics of pulmonary vascular markings, anatomic characteristics of the heart
Electrocardiogram (ECG)	Records quality of major electrical activity in the heart, identifies arrhythmias. A Holter monitor allows 24 to 48 hour ECG recording
Echocardiogram (two-dimensional and transesophageal)	Identifies heart's structures, the pattern of movement, hemodynamics, and the presence of defects
Cardiac catheterization	Allows precise measurement of oxygen saturation, cardiac output, and pressures in each chamber and heart vessel; also identifies anatomic alterations
Exercise testing	Enables ECG recording with controlled increase in activity to identify significant cardiac compensation or inadequate cardiac output
Hyperoxia test	Measures differences in arterial blood gas level when child is on room air and on 100% oxygen

One third of infants born with congenital heart defects develop life-threatening symptoms in the first few days of life. Treatment for congenital heart defects depends on the severity of symptoms and whether the condition is imminently life threatening. Interventional catheterization or surgical correction with restoration of normal hemodynamics and physiology is the treatment of choice for many defects. A **palliative procedure** (a surgical procedure that does not create normal anatomic or hemodynamic results) may be performed in children with a potentially fatal or lethal condition. It may also be performed as an initial procedure, allowing an infant to grow before definitive corrective surgery. Table 49–2 lists the types of interventions during cardiac catheterization and surgical procedures performed on children with congenital heart defects.

MyNursingKit Animation: Digoxin

Cardiac Catheterization

Interventional cardiac catheterization is performed to correct some congenital heart defects. A balloon may be used to create a larger opening in the atrial septum (atrial septostomy), to dilate a narrowed pulmonic or aortic valve, and to expand a coarctation of the aorta. A stent can be inserted to keep the ductus arteriosus patent as an alternative to long-term prostaglandin E_1 (PGE_1) infusion. A coil can be used to occlude a patent ductus arteriosus or other vessels, and a septal closing device is used for some atrial and ventricular septal defects. Anticoagulant therapy may be ordered during the procedure and for several months following the placement of the occlusion device.

MyNursingKit Case Study: Newborn after Heart Surgery

Nursing Practice

Children respond to severe hypoxemia with bradycardia. Cardiac arrest in children generally results from prolonged hypoxemia related to respiratory failure or shock rather than from a primary cardiac insult as in adults. Bradycardia is therefore a significant warning sign of cardiac arrest. Appropriate management of hypoxemia reverses bradycardia and prevents cardiac arrest.

NURSING MANAGEMENT FOR CARDIAC CATHETERIZATION

Cardiac catheterization is often an outpatient procedure, but some children will be admitted for observation. The child is NPO for several hours, except for medications, and arrives at the catheterization laboratory 1 to 2 hours before the procedure. Before entering the laboratory, the child is asked to void and is given an oral sedative.

NURSING ASSESSMENT AND DIAGNOSIS

Before the procedure, assess the child's vital signs, hematocrit and hemoglobin concentrations, and capillary refill time. Collect baseline data on skin temperature, color, and strength of pedal and popliteal pulses for comparison with postcatheterization assessments.

After the procedure, monitor the child for potential complications such as arrhythmia, bleeding, hematoma development, thrombus formation, and infection for several hours. No bleeding should occur at the catheterization site. Assess vital signs, perfusion of the lower extremities (pulses, temperature, color, capillary refill, and sensation) and compare to precatheterization status. Assess the pressure dressing over the catheterization site every 5 minutes for 15 minutes, every 15 minutes for 1 hour, and hourly, or as directed by the physician. Check under the buttocks to make sure blood does not ooze out and run under the child. The child's temperature and vital signs should remain stable. Seek immediate medical intervention if reduced limb warmth

Table 49–2 Clinical Interventions for Congenital Heart Defects

Cardiac Catheterization Interventions and Therapeutic Use	Purpose
Balloon Atrial Septostomy—Rashkind, or with Transatrial Needle Puncture and Balloon Dilation	
Palliative for TGA	Creation of larger defect (at the foramen ovale) between atria to increase blood mixing, performed during cardiac catheterization.
Balloon Dilation Procedure	
Corrective for PS and MS, palliative for AS, COA	A balloon is inserted and inflated to stretch the opening of a narrowed valve or blood vessel. A stent may be inserted to keep the vessel open.
Device Closure	
Corrective for PDA, ASD, VSD	Closure of ductus arteriosus by an umbrella or coil device, and closure of a septal defect by a septal occluder.

Surgical Procedures	Purpose
Aorta End-to-End Anastomosis	
Corrective, COA	Resection of the narrowed section of the aorta and reattachment of the proximal and distal sections.
Blalock-Taussig Shunt, Modified	
Palliative, TOF, single ventricle lesions with pulmonary outflow obstruction	Creation of aorto-pulmonary conduit (from the brachicephalic artery to pulmonary artery) to increase pulmonary blood flow.
Brock	
Corrective, PS	Blind incision of pulmonary valve.
Damus-Kaye-Stansel	
Corrective, TGA, complex single ventricle defects	Pulmonary artery is cut in two with the proximal section attached to the ascending aorta and the distal section to the right ventricle.
Fontan	
Palliative, HLHS, single ventricle defects	Creation of conduit between inferior vena cava and pulmonary artery to increase pulmonary blood flow—total right heart bypass. This permits the right ventricle to assume the responsibility for the systemic circulation and eject blood into the aorta.
Glenn, Bi-directional Glenn	
Palliative, HLHS, single ventricle defects	Superior vena cava connected to right pulmonary artery along with closure of aortopulmonary shunt. Systemic venous blood from the head is sent to the lungs directly without ventricular pumping.
Jatene (Arterial Switch)	
Corrective, TGA	Aorta and pulmonary arteries are transected and reattached to opposite stumps, coronary arteries are moved to new aorta area.
Norwood	
Palliative, aortic hypoplasia, single ventricle defects, e.g., HLHS	Atrial septectomy, anastomosis of the main pulmonary artery to the aorta, and an arterial-pulmonary shunt.
Norwood with Sano Modification	
Palliative, HLHS	Creation of a right ventricle to pulmonary artery conduit so that both the direct pulmonary and aorta blood flow originates in the right ventricle.
Patch Aortoplasty	
Corrective, COA	Insertion of a Dacron patch or opened left subclavian vein to expand the lumen of the aorta.
Pulmonary Artery Banding	
Palliative, VSD, AV canal, single ventricle defects	Placement of constricting band around pulmonary artery to reduce pulmonary blood flow and pressure.

(continued)

Table 49–2 Clinical Interventions for Congenital Heart Defects—continued

Cardiac Catheterization Interventions and Therapeutic Use	Purpose
Rastelli	
Corrective, TGA with pulmonic stenosis, TOF, tricuspid atresia, truncus arteriosus, and double outlet right ventricle	Creation of a conduit between the right ventricle to pulmonary artery with closure of the ventricular septal defect. In the case of truncus arteriosus, the pulmonary arteries are removed from the truncus.
Ross	
Corrective, AS	The diseased aortic valve is replaced with the patient's pulmonic valve (pulmonary autograft), and a homograft (valve from a human donor) replaces the pulmonic valve.
Subclavian flap aortoplasty	
Corrective, COA	Division of the distal subclavian artery and inserting a flap into the aorta through the coarcted segment.
Transplant	
Corrective, HLHS, complex defects, cardiomyopathies	Replacement of diseased heart with donor heart.

AS—aortic stenosis, ASD—atrial septal defect, AV—atrioventricular, COA—coarctation of aorta, HLHS—hypoplastic left heart syndrome, PDA—patent ductus arteriosus, PS—pulmonic stenosis, TOF—tetralogy of Fallot, TGA—transposition of great arteries, VSD—ventricular septal defect

and decreased perfusion in the extremity or bleeding is noted. Monitor intake and output because the contrast medium may cause diuresis.

The following nursing diagnoses may apply to the child who undergoes cardiac catheterization:

- *Fear* related to separation from support system in a stressful situation
- *Risk for Imbalanced Fluid Volume* related to inadequate fluid intake due to NPO status and diuretic effect of contrast medium
- *Ineffective Tissue Perfusion (Cardiopulmonary)* related to mechanical reduction of arterial and venous blood flow

PLANNING AND IMPLEMENTATION

Prepare the child for cardiac catheterization with age-appropriate information. A tour of the catheterization laboratory may reduce the child's fears about the large equipment. Because the child will be sedated but arousable for the procedure, explain the sensations that he or she will experience.

Nursing care during a cardiac catheterization focuses on monitoring the child's vital signs, reassuring the child, and providing emergency care if necessary. After the catheters and guidewires are removed at the end of the procedure, direct pressure must be applied for 15 minutes. A pressure dressing is then placed over the site for several hours.

The child is kept on bed rest for 4 to 6 hours with an effort to keep the leg straight for several hours. Avoid elevating the head of the bed as flexion of the hips is not permitted during this period. Limit activity for 24 hours and provide quiet diversional activities.

Encourage the child to drink small amounts of clear liquids initially, and then progress to other fluids and food as the child tolerates them. Provide adequate fluids to maintain hydration status, especially if the child takes diuretics. The child's intake and output should be balanced.

DISCHARGE PLANNING AND HOME CARE TEACHING

Children are routinely discharged several hours after the cardiac catheterization. Teach the parents to watch the child for signs of complications and make sure they know when to notify the physician. See Teaching Highlights.

EVALUATION

Expected outcomes of nursing care include the following:

- Any potential complications (thrombosis or hemorrhage) following cardiac catheterization are rapidly identified and cared for.
- The child maintains fluid balance.

CONGENITAL HEART DEFECTS THAT INCREASE PULMONARY BLOOD FLOW

ETIOLOGY AND PATHOPHYSIOLOGY

The most common congenital heart defects result from a connection between the left and right side of the heart (septal defect) or between the great arteries (patent ductus arteriosus) that allows blood to flow between the left and right side of the heart. The pressures on the left side of the heart are higher, so blood shunts from the left to the right side of the heart and increases the

Teaching Highlights

HOME CARE AFTER CARDIAC CATHETERIZATION

- Check for signs of complications several times in the first 24 hours after catheterization and notify the physician immediately if any of these signs are noted:
  - Bleeding or a bruise increasing in size at the catheterization site
  - Foot on side of catheterization site is cooler than other foot
  - Loss of feeling in foot on side of catheterization
  - Fever
- If the child is treated with diuretics, observe for signs of dehydration (dry mucous membranes, absence of tears, and strong urine).
- Encourage fluids to help flush the dye out of the body and to prevent dehydration.
- Permit quiet play such as games, puzzles, and videos for the first 24 hours after the procedure.

amount of blood pumped to the lungs. The size of the connection and how much blood passes through it determine how quickly the child develops signs of CHF (see page 1379). The increased blood flow to the lungs causes increased pulmonary vascular resistance (constriction of the pulmonary vascular bed) in an effort to reduce the blood flow, and pulmonary artery hypertension (see page 1392). Right ventricular hypertrophy (RVH) develops to overcome the increasing pulmonary vascular resistance and deliver the blood to the lungs.

CLINICAL MANIFESTATIONS

The infant's heart rate, respiratory rate, and metabolic rate are increased due to the high pulmonary blood flow. Sucking takes energy and diaphoresis often occurs with feeding. The infant may be unable to take in enough calories to support the metabolic rate and growth, so poor weight gain is noted. If CHF develops, signs include dyspnea, tachypnea, intercostal retractions, and periorbital edema. Frequent respiratory infections occur as the wet environment in the lungs supports bacterial growth. See Table 49–3 for the pathophysiology, clinical manifestations, and clinical therapy for the specific congenital heart defects with increased pulmonary blood flow.

CLINICAL THERAPY

See Table 49–2 for tests used to diagnose the condition. Coagulation studies, platelet counts, and serum electrolytes are often obtained for children having open heart surgery, in addition to a chest radiograph, complete blood count, and urinalysis.

Surgery to correct or manage defects that cause significant increased pulmonary blood flow is performed early in infancy to prevent irreversible pulmonary vascular disease. Unless complications develop before surgery, the child should make a complete recovery without limitations. The major complication of these defects is pulmonary artery hypertension.

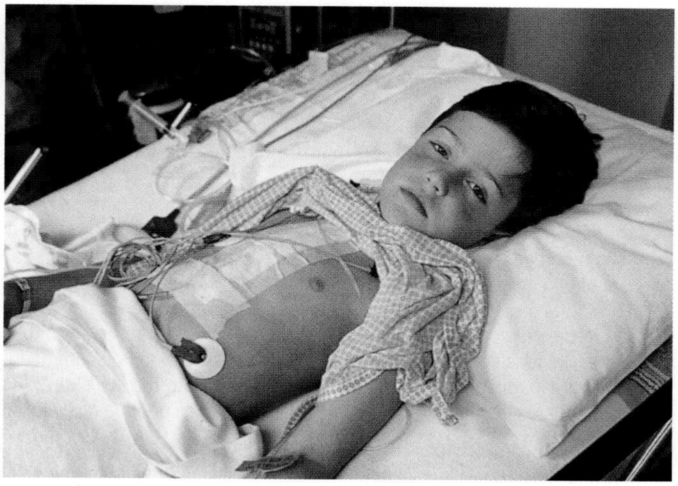

● **Figure 49–1** A child with atrial septal defect repair. Surgery is performed with this type of defect to prevent pulmonary artery hypertension.

Conservative treatment, such as waiting until the child is symptomatic or older, may be selected for some children with these defects. See Figure 49–1 ●. For example, a small ventricular septal defect may close spontaneously, or repair of an atrial septal defect is postponed until preschool or early school-age years. Indomethacin may be given to preterm infants with a patent ductus arteriosus when immediate closure of the ductus is needed. Interventional cardiac catheterization may be performed for defects. See Table 49–3.

Postpericardiotomy syndrome occurs as a complication in approximately 30% of children when surgery involves an incision through the pericardium, leading to pericardial and pleural inflammation (Tsai & Klein, 2005). The cause is unknown, but it results from an autoimmune response to blood or other tissue in the pericardium. The syndrome generally develops within a few weeks to a few months after surgery, more often in children over 2 years than in infants. It is characterized by a high fever up to 40°C (104°F) and severe chest pain that worsens with deep inspiration and in the supine position. The median duration of the condition is 2 to 3 weeks. Mild cases are treated with bed rest and NSAIDs. Severe cases may need hospitalization and more aggressive treatment with pericardiocentesis, diuretics, and corticosteroids (Park, 2008).

NURSING MANAGEMENT PRIOR TO SURGERY

NURSING ASSESSMENT AND DIAGNOSIS

PHYSIOLOGIC ASSESSMENT

Prior to surgery the infant or child is seen regularly to assess growth and for signs of worsening CHF. See Table 49–4 for assessment

(continues on page 1368)

Table 49–3 Pathophysiology, Clinical Manifestations, and Clinical Therapy for Heart Defects That Increase Pulmonary Blood Flow

Pathophysiology, Clinical Manifestations, and Clinical Therapy | **Anatomy**

Patent Ductus Arteriosus (PDA)

Pathophysiology
A common congenital defect caused by persistent fetal circulation that accounts for 5% to 10% of all congenital heart defects (Park, 2008). When pulmonary circulation is established and systemic vascular resistance increases at birth, pressures in the aorta become greater than in the pulmonary arteries. Blood is then shunted from the aorta to the pulmonary arteries, increasing circulation to the pulmonary system. It is a common problem of preterm infants as the ductus arteriosus is not as responsive to the increased oxygen after conversion to pulmonary circulation, and it is less likely to close spontaneously (Joshi & Sekhavat, 2006).

Clinical Manifestations
Dyspnea; tachypnea; tachycardia; full, bounding pulses; widened pulse pressure; hypotension may be noted when cardiac output is low. May be asymptomatic.
CHF, intercostal retractions, hepatomegaly, and poor growth when a large PDA exists.
A continuous "machinery" murmur during systole and diastole, and a thrill in the pulmonic area.
High risk for frequent respiratory infections and pneumonia.

Diagnostic Tests
The chest radiograph and ECG show left ventricular hypertrophy.
The PDA can be visualized, and left-to-right shunt can be measured on echocardiogram.

Clinical Therapy
Surgical ligation of PDA is the treatment of choice. Transcatheter closure by obstructive device is attempted in some older children.
Intravenous indomethacin often stimulates closure of the ductus arteriosus in premature infants, but cannot be used if CHF is present.
Prophylaxis for infective endocarditis is required until the PDA is closed.

Prognosis
No long-term sequelae occur if treated before pulmonary vascular disease develops. If PDA is not treated, child's life span is shortened because pulmonary artery hypertension and pulmonary vascular obstructive disease develop.

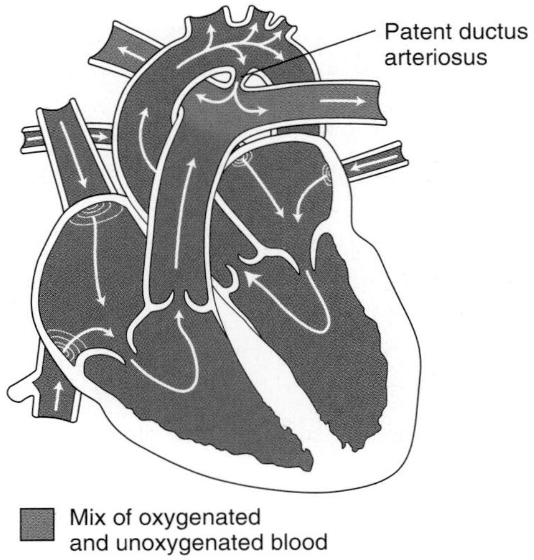

Atrial Septal Defect (ASD)

Pathophysiology
The opening in the atrial septum that permits left-to-right shunting of blood. This defect occurs frequently, either in isolation (5% to 10% of cases) or as a part of a cardiac defect (in 30% to 50% of children with a congenital heart defect) (Park, 2008). The opening may be small, as when the foramen ovale fails to close, or large, as when the septum may be completely absent.

Clinical Manifestations
Infants and young children usually have no symptoms. Small and moderate-size ASDs may not be diagnosed until preschool years or later.
CHF, easy tiring, and poor growth occur with a large ASD.
A soft systolic ejection murmur in the pulmonic area with wide fixed splitting of S_2 through all phases of respiration.

Diagnostic Procedures
Echocardiogram identifies a dilated right ventricle due to blood overload and the shunt size.
The chest radiograph and ECG reveal little information unless the ASD is large, has excessive shunting, and right ventricular hypertrophy is present.

Clinical Therapy
Spontaneous closure of some ASDs occurs within the first 4 years of life. No activity limitations are needed.
Surgery to close or patch the ASD is performed when significant increased pulmonary blood flow causes CHF, or when spontaneous closure has not occurred by 4 years of age.
Secundum ASDs may be closed by a septal occluder during cardiac catheterization.

Prognosis
Many persons with uncorrected small and moderate-size ASDs have lived to middle age without symptoms, but a risk for embolism exists. CHF and pulmonary artery hypertension may develop in untreated adults. Atrial arrhythmias may also occur in adults.

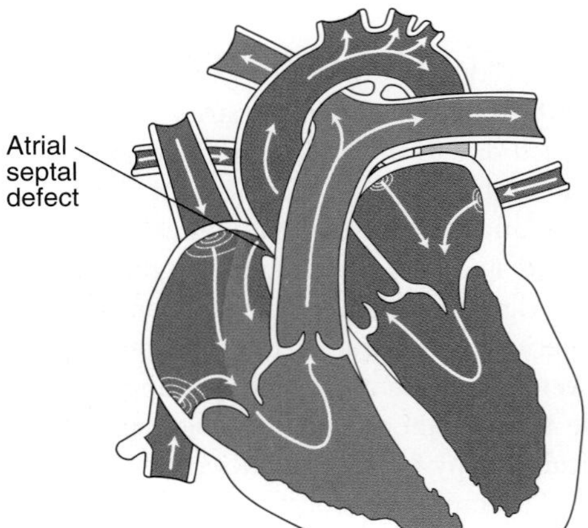

Table 49–3 Pathophysiology, Clinical Manifestations, and Clinical Therapy for Heart Defects That Increase Pulmonary Blood Flow—continued

Pathophysiology, Clinical Manifestations, and Clinical Therapy	Anatomy

Ventricular Septal Defect (VSD)

Pathophysiology
An opening in the ventricular septum results in increased pulmonary blood flow. Blood is shunted from the left ventricle directly across the open septum into the pulmonary artery. This is the most common congenital heart defect, occurring in isolation in 15% to 20% of cases, or in combination with other defects (Park, 2008).

Clinical Manifestations
Only 15% of VSDs are large enough to cause CHF, or an increased number of pulmonary infections, and pulmonary hypertension.
A systolic murmur is auscultated at the third or fourth left intercostal space at the sternal border.

Diagnostic Procedures
A chest radiograph and ECG reveal little when VSDs are small. An enlarged heart and pulmonary vascular markings on chest radiograph occur in cases of large VSDs with shunting. Right and left ventricular hypertrophy may be seen on ECG.
Echocardiogram establishes the diagnosis if shunting is present.
Cardiac catheterization may be used in preparation for surgery. Findings reveal increased oxygen in the right ventricle and increased systolic pressure in the right ventricle and pulmonary artery.

Clinical Therapy
Most small VSDs close spontaneously within the first 6 months of life. Treatment is conservative when no signs of CHF or pulmonary artery hypertension are present.

Surgical patching of VSD during infancy is performed when poor growth is evident.
Device closure of VSD during cardiac catheterization may be attempted for some defects (Gillespie, Schneider, & Rome, 2006).

Prognosis
Highest risk associated with surgical repair is in the first few months of life. Children respond well to surgery and experience substantial catch-up growth. Tachyarrhythmias and right bundle branch block are possible complications.

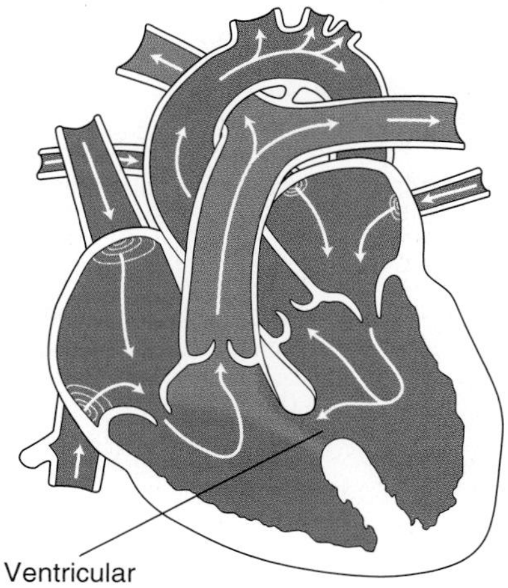

Atrioventricular Canal (Endocardial Cushion) Defect (AV Canal)

Pathophysiology
Endocardial cushions are fetal growth centers for mitral and tricuspid valves and atrioventricular (AV) septum. The most complex AV canal defect results in one AV valve and large septal defects between both atria and ventricles. A total or partial AV canal defect occurs in about 2% of congenital heart defect cases (Park, 2008). This defect is associated with Down syndrome.

Clinical Manifestations
Severity of symptoms depends on amount of left to right shunting of blood across the septum. May be asymptomatic.
Infants may develop CHF, tachypnea, tachycardia, poor growth, recurrent respiratory infections, and repeated respiratory failure.
A holosystolic murmur is loudest at the left lower sternal border, and the intensity reflects the amount of mitral regurgitation. S_1 is accentuated and S_2 is split.

Diagnostic Procedures
On chest radiograph, cardiomegaly and pulmonary vascular markings are present.
On ECG, atrial enlargement, right ventricular hypertrophy, and an incomplete right bundle branch block are noted.
Echocardiogram reveals dilation of the ventricles, septal defects, and details of valve malformation.
Cardiac catheterization reveals increased oxygen in the right atrium, increased right ventricle and/or pulmonary artery pressure.

Clinical Therapy
Surgery is performed during infancy to prevent pulmonary vascular disease. Patches are placed over septal defects, and valve tissue is used to form functioning valves. The mitral valve may be replaced.

CHF is treated (see page 1383). Oxygen may be required until surgery, but it may increase pulmonary blood flow and worsen CHF.
Infective endocarditis prophylaxis required until 6 months after corrective surgery.

Prognosis
Long-term survival following successful surgery is unknown. Arrhythmias and mitral valve insufficiency occur postoperatively. Infants with and without Down syndrome have similar short-term survival rates.

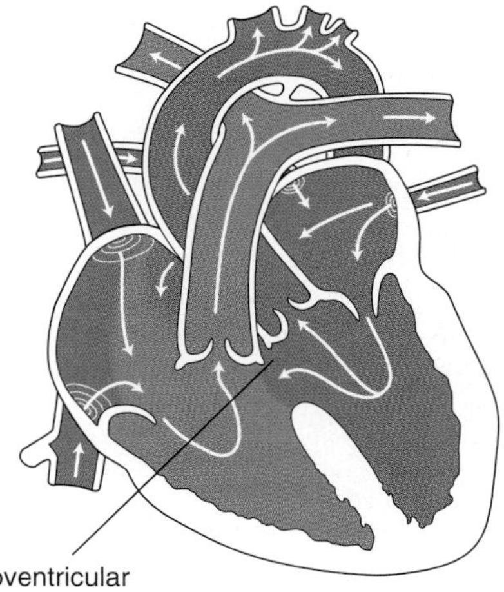

Table 49–4 Guidelines for Assessment of the Child with a Cardiac Condition[a]

Assessment Focus	Assessment Guidelines
Respirations	■ What is the respiratory rate and depth? ■ Is a cough present? ■ Are there signs of increased respiratory effort such as tachypnea, dyspnea, retractions, nasal flaring, expiratory grunting? ■ Auscultate breath sounds. Are any adventitious sounds present (wheezes, crackles)?
Pulse characteristics	■ Assess the pulse rate, rhythm, and quality. ■ Compare the apical, brachial, and radial pulse rates. ■ Compare the brachial and femoral pulses for strength.
Blood pressure	■ Compare the blood pressure to expected value for age, sex, and height percentile. (See Appendix D.) ■ Compare blood pressure values between upper and lower extremities.
Color	■ Observe overall color: Note pallor, dusky color, or cyanosis. ■ Compare the color in peripheral and central locations (e.g., nail beds to mucous membranes). Does crying improve or worsen the color? ■ Assess pulse oximetry.
Chest	■ Inspect the anterior chest for bulging or **heaving** (lifting of the chest wall during contraction). ■ Palpate the chest wall over the heart for pulsations, heaves, or vibrations. ■ Locate the point of maximum intensity.
Heart auscultation	■ Auscultate the heart for the heart sounds and their quality (loud versus weak, distinct versus muffled). ■ Are any extra heart sounds or murmurs present? Describe murmurs by their intensity, location, radiation, timing, and quality. ■ Auscultate the heart with reclining positions to detect differences in heart sounds.
Fluid status	■ Observe for signs of periorbital, facial, or peripheral edema. ■ Observe for abdominal distention. ■ Palpate the liver to detect hepatomegaly. ■ Assess capillary refill.
Activity and behavior	■ Is exercise tolerance present? Does the child tire with feeding? ■ Note presence of diaphoresis and when it occurs. ■ Identify changes in activity level or behavior (lethargy, restlessness, irritability, and decreased responsiveness).
General	■ Assess pattern of growth.

[a]See Chapter 35 for assessment techniques.

guidelines. Failure to gain weight is an indication of an increased metabolic rate and inability to consume adequate calories for both metabolic function and growth. Assessment of length and head circumference helps to determine the full impact of the condition on growth.

PSYCHOSOCIAL ASSESSMENT

Assess the ability of the parents to cope with the infant's diagnosis. Parents may initially feel shock, guilt, or anxiety. Parents need an opportunity to express their feelings and to begin learning to manage the child's illness. The initial period of diagnosis, hospitalization, and early care of the infant at home are very stressful. Parents need special support if their infant has a life-threatening heart defect.

Examples of nursing diagnoses associated with heart defects having increased pulmonary blood flow and their complications include the following:

- *Excess Fluid Volume* related to heart failure and pulmonary vasculature overload
- *Ineffective Infant Feeding Pattern* related to shortness of breath and fatigue
- *Risk for Infection* related to pulmonary vascular congestion and chronic illness
- *Interrupted family processes* related to crisis of child's serious illness

PLANNING AND IMPLEMENTATION

When the child has a large defect, CHF may be present. See page 1384 for care guidelines.

FAMILY EDUCATION

Participate with members of the cardiology team to provide information and educate the family about the child's condition. Information may include the following:

- General information about the congenital heart disease, including a description of the heart's anatomy and physiology and the defect

Nursing Practice

Following are some valuable resources for parents of a child with a congenital heart defect:

- *It's My Heart* by the Children's Heart Foundation
- *The Parent's Guide to Children's Congenital Heart Defects* by Gerri Freid Kramer and Shari Maurer, Three Rivers Press
- *The Heart of a Child: What Families Need to Know about Heart Disorders in Children* by C. A. Neill, E. A. Clark, and C. Clark, Johns Hopkins Press

- Information about genetic and environmental influences associated with congenital heart disease
- Overview of the child's prognosis and timing of medical and surgical interventions

See MyNursingKit for Web sites with patient education resources.

PSYCHOSOCIAL SUPPORT

Parents are often anxious about an uncertain surgical outcome. Determine if parents have a support system as they learn about the infant's diagnosis and make difficult decisions about the child's surgery. Some parents may be concerned that signing consent for surgery places the child in even more danger of illness or even death. Identify some resources for support, such as social services, pastoral services, or a parent of a child with a similar heart defect.

Parents should be offered genetic counseling if planning a future pregnancy.

HOME CARE

Children are often managed at home until surgery. Parents should encourage feeding to promote growth, but allow the infant to feed only for 20 to 30 minutes, as directed by health professionals who assess how tiring feeding is for the infant. Breastfeeding is encouraged because of its beneficial effects for the infant. If the breastfed infant has difficulty gaining weight, pumping the breasts and supplementing breast milk with calorie fortification may be encouraged. Transpyloric, nasogastric, or gastrostomy tube feedings may also be given at night or 24 hours a day to ensure that adequate calories are ingested. See Figure 49–2 ●. When tube feedings are used, encourage the infant to take some formula orally to provide positive oral stimulation. See feeding suggestions for the infant with CHF on page 1385.

Reduce the infant's exposure to infectious diseases, and encourage frequent hand hygiene. Respiratory infections increase hypoxemia in children with cyanosis. Fever increases the metabolic rates and oxygen demands. Vomiting and diarrhea may cause an electrolyte disturbance and digoxin toxicity (Cook & Higgins, 2004). Notify the physician about fever, poor feeding, vomiting, and diarrhea.

Health promotion visits are important and all immunizations are provided according to the recommended schedule. Monthly prophylaxis for respiratory syncytial virus (RSV) with Palivizumab should be provided during the peak season. See Chapter 48∞.

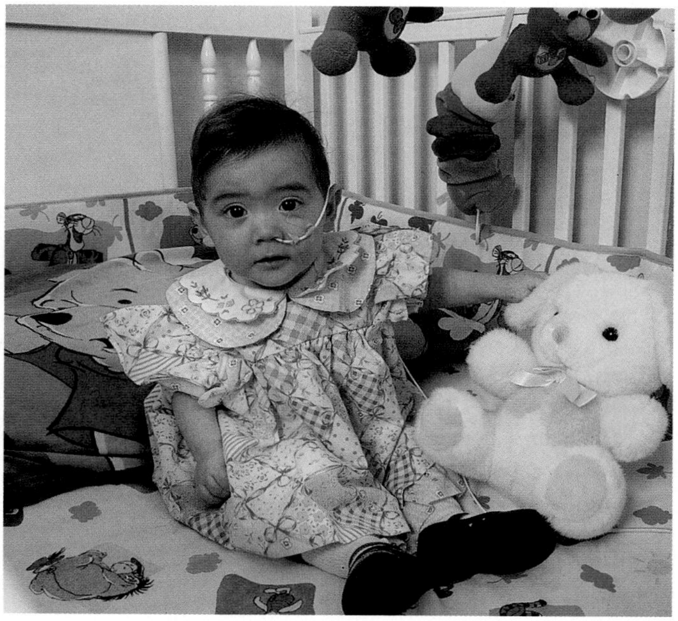

● **Figure 49–2** Infant feeding. Infants with cardiac conditions often require supplemental feedings to provide sufficient nutrients for growth and development. The parents of this infant girl have been taught how to give her nasogastric feedings at home.

PREPARATION FOR SURGERY

When the child is preschool age or older, prepare the child for the settings, equipment, and experiences to expect before and after surgery. Follow guidelines for preoperative treatment described in Chapter 41∞. If an infant or toddler is having surgery, inform the parents about how the child will look, equipment that will be used, and what care will be provided in the immediate postoperative period.

EVALUATION

- Nutritional intake is adequate with oral and supplemental tube feeding as necessary.
- The child maintains a growth pattern that follows the established growth curve percentile.
- The child receives all immunizations and RSV prophylaxis to reduce the potential for acute illnesses.

NURSING MANAGEMENT AT THE TIME OF SURGERY

The goal of nursing management is to perform assessments, provide supportive care to the family, and meet the child's nursing care needs before and after surgery.

NURSING ASSESSMENT AND DIAGNOSIS

At the time of surgery, the child needs a careful history and physical examination to detect any acute illnesses as well as the child's physiologic status. See Table 49–4.

In the immediate postoperative period, the child will be cared for in the intensive care unit. When the child returns to the general nursing unit, assessment focuses on signs of surgical complications such as infection, arrhythmias, and impaired tissue perfusion. Monitor the child's temperature and inspect the surgical incision site. Fever, excessive incisional pain, spreading erythema around the incision, and wound drainage beginning 3 to 4 days postoperatively may be early signs of infection. Assess the chest and lungs for breath sounds, respiratory effort, and signs of distress that may indicate pneumonia or fluid in the pleural space.

Monitor the vital signs, including blood pressure. The child may not be on a cardiac monitor, so auscultation of the apical pulse to detect an irregular heart rate or bradycardia is essential, signs of reduced cardiac output that require immediate intervention. Check pulse oximetry, capillary refill, extremity warmth, pedal pulses, level of consciousness, and urine output to assess tissue perfusion. Reduced urine output is a sign of decreased cardiac output. Continue to assess the child's pain.

Examples of nursing diagnoses following cardiac surgery include the following:

- *Ineffective Breathing Pattern* related to respiratory muscle fatigue
- *Acute Pain* related to surgical incision and expansion of chest with coughing and deep breathing exercises
- *Risk for Imbalanced Fluid Volume* related to impact of surgery on heart's pumping action
- *Risk for Infection* related to surgery and chronic disease status

PLANNING AND IMPLEMENTATION

PAIN MANAGEMENT

Pain management with 24-hour intravenous opioids should be provided for 1–2 days postoperatively or until the child is taking fluids. Then oral analgesics should be given around the clock. Follow the guidelines for pain management provided in Chapter 42∞. Teach parents and caregivers to lift and move the child so that stress on the incision and potential pain is reduced. Do not lift the child under the arms.

PROMOTE RESPIRATORY FUNCTION

Encourage the child to take deep breaths and cough or to perform spirometry exercises regularly to promote full lung expansion (see Skill 14–26 SKILLS). Provide tips for splinting the chest (a pillow or stuffed animal) to reduce the pain from coughing and deep breathing. Chest physiotherapy may be performed in children under 3 years of age. Inspect the child's incision regularly for signs of infection.

MANAGE FLUIDS AND NUTRITION

Encourage the infant or child to begin oral fluids and nutrition when permitted. Although oral fluids are rarely limited following surgery for defects with increased pulmonary blood flow, intake and output should be assessed carefully. Promote bowel elimination following surgery and opioids.

Parents may be encouraged to bring in favorite foods for the child when they can be tolerated. Administer antibiotics as prescribed. If intravenous antibiotics are continued after the child's oral intake is established, the line can be converted to a heparin or saline lock.

ACTIVITY

Encourage the child to increase activity gradually with longer periods out of bed every day, but ensure adequate rest periods to promote healing. Provide diversional activities and opportunities for therapeutic play so the child can better manage the stresses associated with pain and frightening procedures.

DISCHARGE PLANNING AND HOME CARE TEACHING

Infants and children may be discharged from the hospital within a few days of surgery. Parents need information spread over several days to prepare for care of the child at home. See "Teaching Highlights: Care of the Child after Cardiac Surgery."

Prepare parents for potential behavior problems of young children that may result from the stress of hospitalization, such as nightmares, separation anxiety, and overdependence on parents. Encourage parents to reassure children about their security, and to promote play and other means to deal with their feelings. If the child's behavioral symptoms continue for several weeks, referral for psychological assessment and support may be needed for posttraumatic stress disorder. See Chapter 57∞.

Reassure parents of children with a complete correction of the cardiac defect that there should be no further cardiovascular problems. Provide parents with full information about the child's defect and the surgery performed to share with the child's current and future healthcare providers. Encourage parents to allow the child to live a normal and active life.

EVALUATION

Examples of expected outcomes of nursing care include the following:

- The child's pain is effectively managed.
- Full lung expansion is achieved with spirometry exercises or chest physiotherapy.
- The child's incision heals without infection.
- Catch-up growth occurs over the next few months to years.

Teaching Highlights

CARE OF THE CHILD AFTER CARDIAC SURGERY

- Place infants and children in car safety seats for travel home from the hospital. Place a small blanket over the incision to prevent the straps from rubbing.
- Sponge bathe the infant or use a tub bath with a low water level. Avoid soaking the incision until sutures are out and the incision is healed. Clean the incision daily with gentle baby or pH-balanced soap. Do not use oils, creams, lotions, or ointments on the incision. Cover the incision with a clean shirt or bib to keep it clean and dry.
- Pick up infants and young children by placing one hand under the head and the other hand under the hips. Avoid picking up the child by grasping under the arms.
- Encourage a nutritious diet and snacks so the infant or child has an opportunity to catch up for previous growth deficits.
- Allow the child to increase activity gradually as tolerated. Report increased fatigue or decreased activity tolerance to the physician. Postpone rough play, bike riding, and climbing for 6 weeks until the sternum incision has healed completely. The child can return to school in about 3 weeks but should not carry books or a backpack for several weeks.
- Report any signs of wound infection, fever over 40.3°C (101°F), flulike symptoms, chest pain, increased respiratory rate or respiratory distress, appetite change, or irritability to the physician.
- Acetaminophen or ibuprofen can be given for pain control. Use the recommended dose for the child's weight.
- Antibiotic prophylaxis for infective endocarditis should be given for dental and invasive respiratory procedures as directed for 6 months after corrective surgery. See the Drug Guide on page 1393. Report any unexplained fever or illness during the first 2 months following surgery as the child is at higher risk for infective endocarditis during that time.

DEFECTS CAUSING DECREASED PULMONARY BLOOD FLOW AND MIXED DEFECTS

Information about these defect categories is combined in this section because the clinical therapy and nursing interventions are similar.

ETIOLOGY AND PATHOPHYSIOLOGY

Defects Causing Decreased Pulmonary Blood Flow

Defects that obstruct the pulmonary blood flow result in little or no blood reaching the lungs to get oxygenated. If an atrial or ventricular septal opening exists, right-sided pressures exceed those on the left because of the obstructed pulmonary blood flow, resulting in right to left shunting.

The bone marrow is stimulated to produce more red blood cells to increase the hemoglobin available to carry oxygen. **Polycythemia**, an above-normal increase in the number of red blood cells, may result and place the child at risk for thromboembolism. Over time platelet survival is reduced and clotting factors are impaired, increasing the infant's risk of bleeding with surgery. Brain abscesses are more common in cases of polycythemia and septal defects; bacteria in the systemic circulation do not get filtered out by the lung capillaries (Park, 2008, p. 145).

When infants and children with cyanosis rise in the morning, they may experience an abrupt decrease in systemic resistance and pulmonary blood flow. This physiologic change can trigger a hypercyanotic (hypoxic or "tet") episode when combined with a sudden increase in cardiac output and venous return associated with crying, feeding, exercise, a warm bath, and straining with defecation. The partial pressure of oxygen (PO_2) is lowered, and the partial pressure of carbon dioxide (PCO_2) rises. Hypoxemia becomes progressively worse as the respiratory center in the brain overreacts, increasing the respiratory effort. The extra respiratory effort further increases the cardiac output and contributes to a life-threatening decline unless rapid intervention is successful.

Mixed Defects

Many complex congenital heart defects involve a combination of defects that increase and decrease pulmonary blood flow, making the newborn dependent upon the mixing of the pulmonary and systemic circulations for survival during the postnatal period. This mixing of oxygen-saturated and desaturated blood results in a general desaturated systemic blood flow and cyanosis. Pulmonary congestion occurs because of increased pulmonary blood flow and obstruction of systemic flow.

CLINICAL MANIFESTATIONS

Defects Causing Decreased Pulmonary Blood Flow

Clinical manifestations in infants initially include cyanosis shortly after birth, dyspnea, and a loud murmur. The skin may initially be ruddy or mottled before cyanosis is observed. Cyanosis that does not respond as expected to oxygen is a classic sign of decreased pulmonary blood flow. Signs and symptoms of chronic hypoxemia include fatigue, clubbing of the fingers and toes, exertional dyspnea, and delayed developmental milestones (Figure 49–3 ●). Infants may need to stop sucking periodically during feedings to breathe, and diaphoresis may be seen with the increased work of feeding. These infants have a higher metabolic rate, and inadequate calories may be consumed resulting in poor

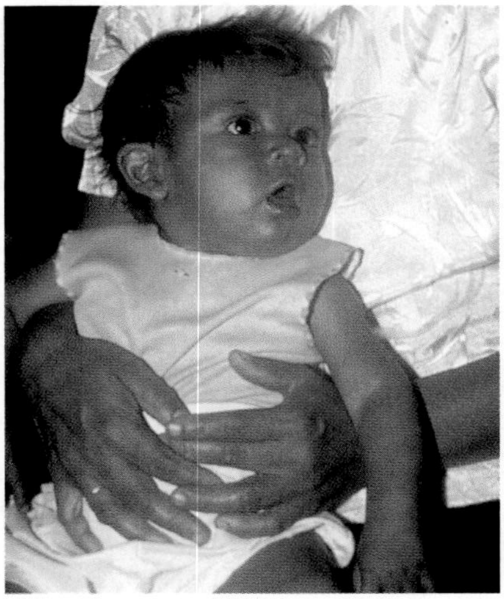
A

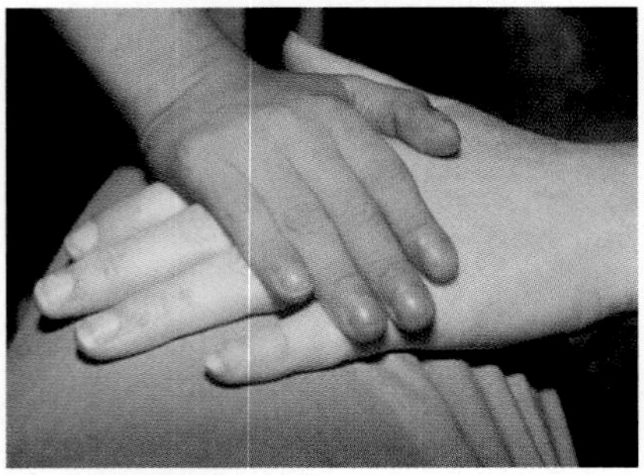
B

● **Figure 49–3** Signs of reduced pulmonary blood flow. ***A,*** This infant is cyanotic due to a heart defect that reduces pulmonary blood flow. ***B,*** Clubbing of the fingers in an older child is one manifestation of a heart defect that reduces pulmonary blood flow.

weight gain. See Table 49–5 for the pathophysiology, clinical manifestations, and clinical therapy for these defects.

When the infant or child has severe obstruction to pulmonary blood flow, hypercyanotic episodes can occur suddenly. Toddlers with uncorrected cyanotic heart disease often squat to relieve dyspnea (Figure 49–4 ●). The knee–chest position reduces the cardiac output by decreasing the venous return from the lower extremities and by increasing the systemic vascular resistance. Hypercyanotic episodes usually appear between 2 months and 2 years of age. Signs include increased rate and depth of respirations; increased heart rate; increased cyanosis, pallor, and poor tissue perfusion; diaphoresis; irritability and crying; and seizures and loss of consciousness.

Older children may have additional symptoms such as exercise-induced dizziness and **syncope** (transient loss of consciousness and muscle tone), which are serious signs indicating a need for medical evaluation.

Mixed Defects

These complex congenital heart defects cause varying degrees of cyanosis and CHF. See Table 49–6 for the pathophysiology, clinical manifestations, and clinical therapy for these complex mixed defects.

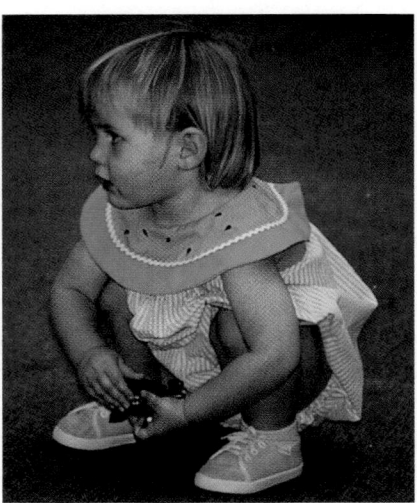

● **Figure 49–4** Children compensate for inadequate blood flow. A young child with an uncorrected or partially corrected defect that reduces pulmonary blood flow may squat (assumes a knee-chest position) to reduce systemic blood flow return to the heart.

CLINICAL THERAPY

Early management of these defects is important to prevent secondary damage to the heart, lungs, and brain, including the adverse effects of hypoxemia on the child's cognitive and psychomotor development. Surgery is performed during the newborn period or early infancy; corrective surgery is performed when possible. A palliative procedure may be performed first to preserve life in children with potentially lethal heart defects and complications (see Table 49–1). With some defects, corrective surgery can be postponed with a palliative procedure, giving the infant an opportunity to grow and improve the success of corrective surgery. See Figure 49–5 ● for various palliative shunts (surgically created

(continues on page 1374)

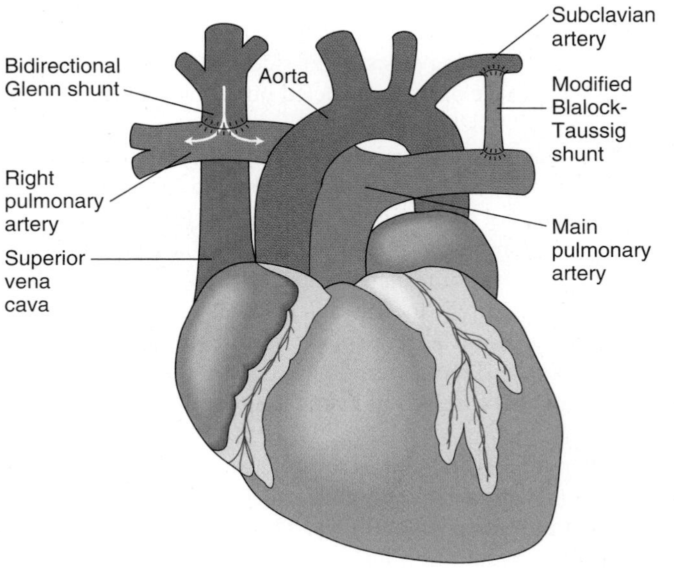

● **Figure 49–5** Anatomic location of the modified Blalock-Taussig and Glenn shunts for palliative procedures.

Table 49–5 Pathophysiology, Clinical Manifestations, and Clinical Therapy for Defects with Decreased Pulmonary Blood Flow

Defect Pathophysiology, Clinical Manifestations, and Clinical Therapy | **Anatomy**

Pulmonic Stenosis (PS)

Pathophysiology

Stenosis (narrowing of valve or valve area) can be above valve, below valve, or at valve. Stenosis obstructs blood flow into the pulmonary artery, which increases preload and results in right ventricular hypertrophy. Isolated PS accounts for 8% to 12% of all congenital heart defects, but it also is associated with tetralogy of Fallot (Park, 2008). Stenosis in the subvalvular area may develop as the heart muscle grows.

Clinical Manifestations

Children with mild stenosis may have no symptoms and grow normally.
In moderate stenosis, dyspnea and fatigue occur on exertion. Signs of CHF and hepatosplenomegaly are rare but may result from chronic pressure overload. Heart failure and chest pain on exertion occur in severe cases.
A loud systolic ejection murmur with a widely split S_2 and thrill may be found in the pulmonic listening area.

Diagnostic Tests

The chest radiograph may show an enlarged pulmonary artery with normal heart size and normal pulmonary vascularity.
The ECG may show right atrial enlargement and right ventricular hypertrophy.
An echocardiogram provides information about the pressure gradient across valve and size of valve ring.
Cardiac catheterization findings include increased right ventricular pressure and a normal or slightly lowered pulmonary artery pressure.

Clinical Therapy

Balloon dilation of the valve, performed during cardiac catheterization, treats simple pulmonic stenosis.
Surgical valvotomy may be used when other defects such as VSD are present.
Surgical resection may be needed for narrowing above the valve area.
Pulmonary regurgitation may result, but is not a significant problem.

Prognosis

Pulmonic stenosis does not typically increase in severity. Lifelong infective endocarditis prophylaxis may be needed.

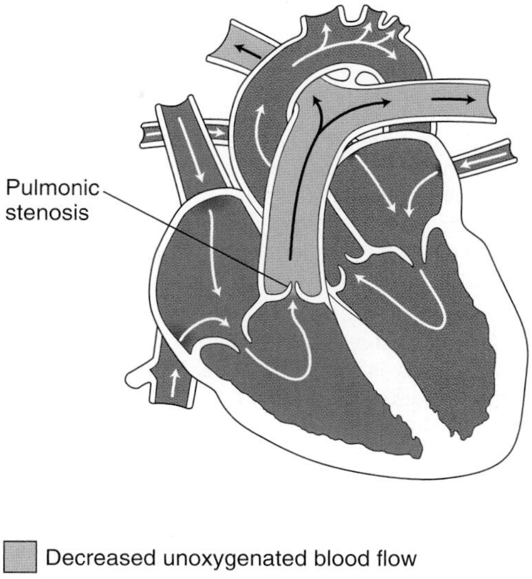

Tetralogy of Fallot (TOF)

Pathophysiology

Four defects are involved: pulmonic stenosis, right ventricular hypertrophy, ventricular septal defect (VSD), and overriding of aorta. Some children have a fifth defect, an ASD. TOF occurs in about 5% to 10% of congenital heart defects (Park, 2008). Elevated pressures in the right side of the heart cause a right-to-left shunt.

Clinical Manifestations

The infant becomes hypoxic and cyanotic as the ductus arteriosus closes. The degree of pulmonary stenosis determines severity of symptoms.
A systolic murmur is heard in the pulmonic area and transmitted to the suprasternal notch. A thrill may be palpated in the pulmonic area.
Polycythemia, hypercyanotic spells, metabolic acidosis, poor growth, clubbing, and exercise intolerance may develop.
Toddlers with uncorrected defects instinctively squat (assume a knee-chest position) to decrease the return of systemic venous blood to the heart. See Figure 49–5.

Diagnostic Tests

A chest x-ray shows the boot-shaped heart due to the large right ventricle, decreased pulmonary vascular markings, and a prominent aorta.
The ECG shows right ventricular hypertrophy.
The echocardiogram shows the VSD, obstruction of pulmonary outflow, an overriding aorta, and the size of the pulmonary arteries. The condition may be detected by fetal echocardiography.
Cardiac catheterization provides details about the anatomic defects.
Blood tests reveal an elevated hematocrit and hemoglobin and an increased clotting time.

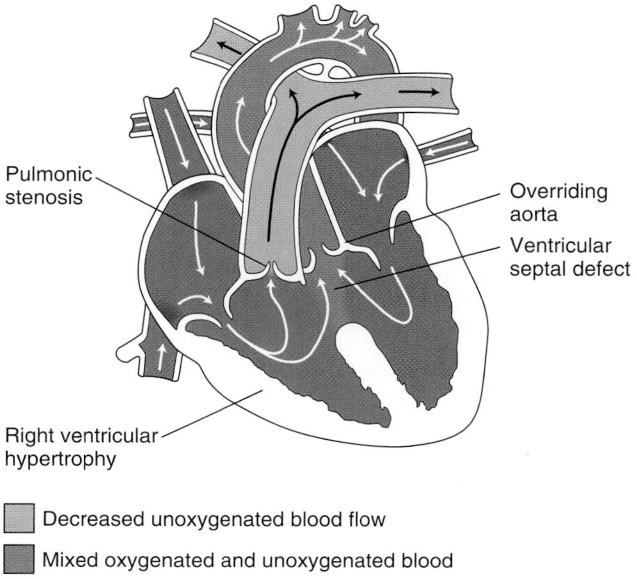

(continued)

Table 49–5 Pathophysiology, Clinical Manifestations, and Clinical Therapy for Defects with Decreased Pulmonary Blood Flow—continued

Defect Pathophysiology, Clinical Manifestations, and Clinical Therapy	Anatomy
Tetralogy of Fallot (TOF)—continued	
Clinical Therapy Hypercyanotic episodes are managed (see below). Monitoring the child for metabolic acidosis or prolonged unconsciousness is critical. Some children need palliative surgery (modified Blalock-Taussig shunt) to delay total correction surgery. A total repair is often performed before 6 months of age when the infant has a hypercyanotic episode. **Prognosis** Not all children are cured by surgery, but most have improved quality of life and improved longevity. Arrhythmias may result from surgery. Ventricular arrhythmias may occur more than 20 years after surgery and may cause sudden death. Right ventricular dysfunction may also occur (Schultz & Kreutzer, 2006).	
Pulmonary or Tricuspid Atresia	
Pulmonary atresia is the absence of communication between the right ventricle and the pulmonary artery, either at the site of the pulmonary valve or in the main pulmonary artery. In tricuspid atresia, the tricuspid valve is absent resulting in no communication between the right atrium and ventricle. Blood flows to the left side of the heart through the foramen ovale. The ductus arteriosus provides the only flow of blood to the pulmonary arteries. Other congenital defects are often present such as a VSD or TGA. **Clinical Manifestations** Cyanosis is present at birth. Tachypnea, CHF, pulmonary edema, hepatomegaly, acidosis, hypoxic spells, clubbing, polycythemia, and growth delays occur. A continuous murmur from the PDA is heard in the pulmonic area. A single S_2 is heard in the aortic area, and a harsh systolic murmur may be heard in the tricuspid area. **Diagnostic Tests** The chest radiograph may reveal a normal size or slightly enlarged heart. The ECG may reveal right atrial hypertrophy. The echocardiogram shows a small hypoplastic right ventricular cavity and tricuspid valve, an absent right ventricular outflow tract, a dilated right atrium, and right-to-left shunting across the atrial septum. **Clinical Therapy** Prostaglandin E_1 is given immediately to maintain a patent ductus arteriosus. Digoxin and diuretics are also used. The Rastelli balloon atrial septostomy is performed to increase the atrial opening. A Rastelli or modified Fontan procedure results in improved survival. **Prognosis** Outcome depends upon the size of the pulmonary outflow tract developed by surgery and the fibrosis in the right ventricle. The child has increased risk for arrhythmia and right ventricular dysfunction.	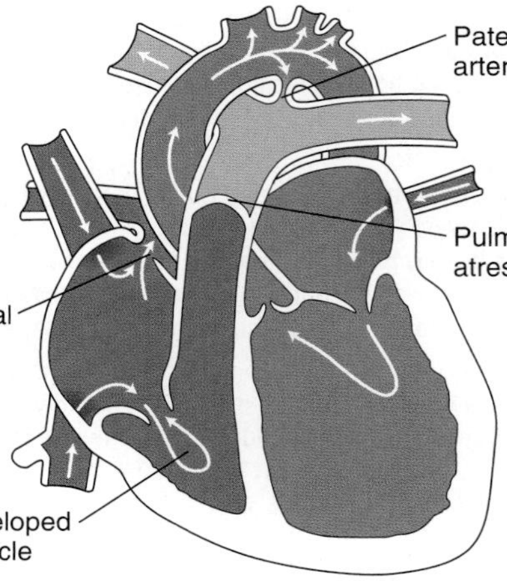

channels for blood flow) that may be performed. See Tables 49–5 and 49–6 for clinical therapy for specific congenital heart defects.

If closure of the ductus arteriosus causes life-threatening cyanosis in newborns, prostaglandin E_1 (PGE_1) is given to reopen the ductus arteriosus and improve pulmonary or systemic blood flow. Treatment with PGE_1 provides time to transfer the newborn to a cardiac center for diagnostic evaluation and surgical intervention. Adverse effects include respiratory depression and apnea, so the infant must be closely monitored and sometimes ventilation must be assisted.

The child's hemoglobin and hematocrit values are monitored for polycythemia or anemia. If the blood viscosity becomes too high, red cell pheresis may be performed. These infants also do not tolerate anemia well with less oxygen-carrying hemoglobin.

Hypercyanotic Episodes

Hypercyanotic episodes are treated aggressively. To decrease the pulmonary vascular resistance, the initial treatment involves calming the child, giving oxygen, and administering morphine and propranolol intravenously. Packed red blood cells may be administered

Table 49–6 Pathophysiology, Clinical Manifestations, and Clinical Therapy for Mixed Defects

Defect Pathophysiology, Clinical Manifestations, and Clinical Therapy | **Anatomy**

Transposition of the Great Arteries (TGA)

The pulmonary artery is the outflow tract for the left ventricle, and the aorta is the outflow tract for the right ventricle, creating parallel circulations. The condition is life threatening at birth, and survival initially depends on an open ductus arteriosus and foramen ovale. This condition accounts for 5% to 7% of congenital heart defects (Park, 2008). An ASD or VSD may also be present with TGA.

Clinical Manifestations

Cyanosis, apparent soon after birth, progresses to hypoxia and acidosis. Cyanosis does not improve with oxygen administration. Cyanosis may be less apparent when a large VSD is present.

CHF may develop immediately or over days or weeks. Tachypnea (60 breaths/min) is often present without retractions or other signs of dyspnea.

A systolic murmur is present if a VSD is present; no other murmur is generally heard. S_2 is loud.

Infants take a long time to feed and need frequent rest periods because of rapid respiratory rate and fatigue.

Growth failure may be evident as early as 2 weeks of age if corrective surgery is not performed.

Diagnostic Tests

A chest radiograph may reveal a classic egg-shaped heart on a string with enlarged ventricles and increased pulmonary vascular markings.

The ECG reveals right ventricular hypertrophy.

The echocardiogram often shows the abnormal position of the great arteries rising from the ventricles.

Cardiac catheterization shows increased right ventricular pressure, and the catheter can enter the aorta through the right ventricle.

Blood tests reveal an increased hematocrit and hemoglobin or polycythemia.

Clinical Therapy

Prostaglandin E_1 is ordered to maintain a patent ductus arteriosus until a palliative procedure can be performed.

Corrective surgery (arterial switch) is usually performed before 1 week of age.

Balloon atrial septostomy may be performed during cardiac catheterization in newborns as a first stage to permit oxygenated and unoxygenated blood to mix until surgery is performed.

Prognosis

Survival without surgery is impossible. The initial survival following surgery is approaching 100% (Connor, 2006). Arrhythmias (sick sinus syndrome, atrial flutter, and atrial fibrillation), right ventricular failure, and tricuspid regurgitation are common complications. A pacemaker may be needed to manage arrhythmias.

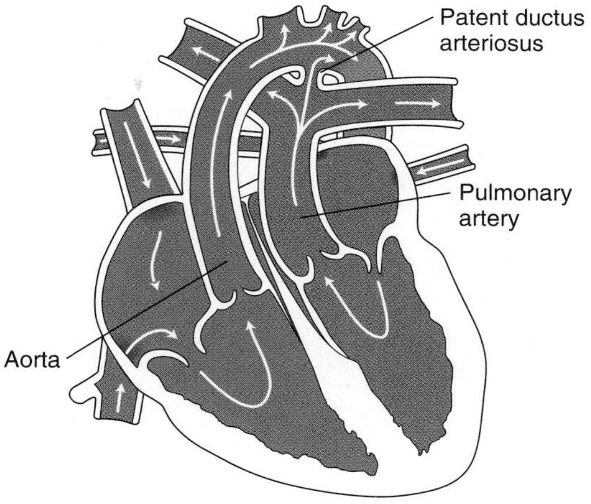

Truncus Arteriosus

A single large vessel empties both ventricles and provides circulation for the pulmonary, systemic, and coronary circulations. A VSD is usually present. This occurs in less than 1% of congenital heart defects (Park, 2008).

Clinical Manifestations

Cyanosis develops soon after birth; however, this is also a condition of increased pulmonary blood flow. Severe CHF, dyspnea, retractions, fatigue, poor feeding, poor growth, polycythemia, clubbing, increased pulse pressure, bounding peripheral pulses, a widened pulse pressure, frequent respiratory infections, and cardiomegaly occur.

The VSD produces a harsh systolic murmur in the lower sternal border. A systolic click may be heard in the apex and pulmonic area.

Diagnostic Tests

The chest radiograph shows cardiomegaly, a large aorta, and increased pulmonary vascular markings.

The ECG reveals right and left ventricular hypertrophy.

The echocardiogram shows the absence of two semilunar valves.

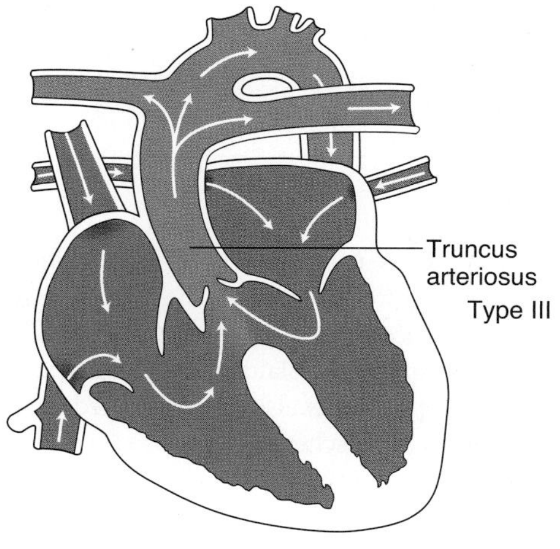

Mixed oxygenated and unoxygenated blood

(continued)

Table 49–6 Pathophysiology, Clinical Manifestations, and Clinical Therapy for Mixed Defects—continued

Defect Pathophysiology, Clinical Manifestations, and Clinical Therapy	Anatomy

Truncus Arteriosus—continued

Cardiac catheterization documents a left-to-right shunt at the level of the ventricle, and equal pressure in the ventricles, the truncus, and pulmonary arteries.

Clinical Therapy

A Rastelli procedure is performed to close the VSD and create a passage to the pulmonary arteries. Repeated surgery is necessary to enlarge the pulmonary artery conduit.

Digoxin and diuretics are given.

Prognosis

Complete heart block occurs in up to 5% of patients (Marino, Ostrow, & Cohen, 2006). The long-term prognosis is based on presence of other anomalies.

Total Anomalous Pulmonary Venous Return

The pulmonary veins empty into the right atrium or veins leading to the right atrium rather than into the left atrium. Mixed blood must pass through the foramen ovale or an ASD to provide the systemic circulation. Any obstruction of the pulmonary veins increases the condition's severity. This accounts for 1% of congenital heart defects (Park, 2008).

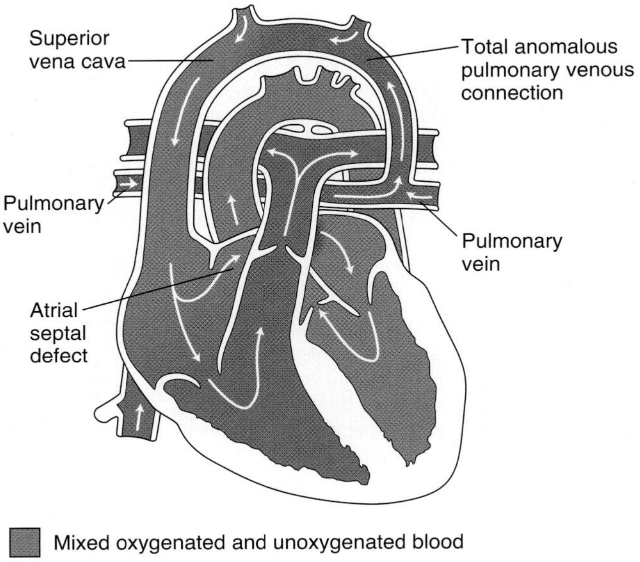

Clinical Manifestations

Mild cyanosis and frequent respiratory infections occur. Increased cyanosis may occur with feedings as the filled esophagus compresses the common pulmonary vein, leading to increased pulmonary blood flow and signs of CHF. A precordial bulge may be palpated. The S_2 has a wide, fixed split when there is no pulmonary vein obstruction. An ejection murmur and gallop rhythm may be heard in the pulmonic area.

Diagnostic Tests

The chest radiograph shows cardiac enlargement, a large pulmonary artery, and increased pulmonary blood flow.

The ECG reveals hypertrophy of the right atrium and ventricle.

The echocardiogram shows enlargement of the right atrium, a patent foramen ovale, and lack of connection between the pulmonary veins and left atrium.

Cardiac catheterization shows a higher oxygen level in the right atrium and the abnormal circulation.

Clinical Therapy

Prostaglandin E_1 is given to maintain patent ductus arteriosus.

Hypoxemia and CHF are treated.

Balloon atrial septostomy may be performed to promote better mixing of blood so surgery can be delayed until the infant is stabilized.

Surgery to reconnect or baffle the pulmonary veins to the left atrium is performed.

Prognosis

Survivors have lived more than 20 years after correction. Atrial arrhythmias may develop after surgery.

MyNursingKit Teaching Plan: Infective Endocarditis Prophylaxis

to improve oxygen delivery to the tissues when the child is anemic. Postpone all unpleasant procedures. To increase the systemic vascular resistance, the infant is placed in the knee–chest position and given intravenous fluids to expand circulatory volume. Dopamine or phenylephrine (Neo-Synephrine) is also given. Immediate palliative or corrective surgery is often scheduled.

Infective Endocarditis

Prophylactic antibiotics for infective endocarditis are required for most children with complex cardiac defects prior to surgery and for 6 months after surgery. See the Drug Guide on page 1393. Children whose surgery involved prosthetic patches or devices and those who have unrepaired cyanotic congenital heart disease, including palliative shunts and conduits, need life-long infective endocarditis prophylaxis (Wilson, Taubert, Gewitz, et al., 2007).

Outcomes and Prognosis

Children with complex congenital heart defects need multiple stages of surgery, revisions of previous surgeries, valve replacements, or interventional catheterization to reopen valves or vessels that have become stenotic. An implanted pacemaker may be needed for arrhythmias associated with anomalies of the con-

Evidence-Based Nursing

NEURODEVELOPMENTAL OUTCOMES IN CHILDREN WITH COMPLEX CONGENITAL HEART DISEASE

Clinical Question

What information do parents and school officials need to plan for educational supports for children who have had surgery for complex congenital heart defects?

Evidence

In the last decade, surgery for infants with complex congenital heart defects has been performed at younger ages, reducing the time infants have severe pathophysiology (prolonged hypoxemia, profound acidosis, and low cardiac output). Children with congenital heart defects have more central nervous system abnormalities than the general population (Brown, Wernovsky, Mussatto, et al., 2005). A group of 94 infants with complex heart defects having open heart surgery were followed and evaluated at school age to assess functional (motor and neurologic) outcomes. As toddlers, many were found to have microcephaly (30%), gross and fine motor delays (42%), global delays (23%), and behavioral difficulties (35%) (Limperopoulos, Majnemer, Shevell, et al., 2000). At school age, mild fine and gross motor impairments were still present, but few children had severe impairments. An association between increasing surgical circulatory arrest time and fine and gross motor function delays was present (Majnemer, Limperopoulos, Shevell, et al., 2006). A group of 74 school-age children having had arterial switch surgery for TGA were found to have mild neurologic abnormalities, and speech, expressive language, and behavior problems when compared with controls (Karl, Hall, Ford, et al. 2004). A study evaluating the outcome of 26 children, ages 3.5 to 6 years of age, who had had surgery for TGA and HLHS found that children with HLHS had more problems with visual-motor skills, expressive language, attention, and behavior than the children with TGA (Brosig, Mussatto, Kuhn, et al., 2007).

Best Practice

Congenital heart defects and treatment regimens are associated with motor problems in some children or difficulties in coordination and balance, handwriting, participation in recreation and peer activities, and development of self-esteem. Children may need special educational assessment and developmental screening to identify the specific neurodevelopmental problems. Children may need to have an individualized education plan developed when disabilities affect learning.

Critical Thinking

Develop an outline of important information for a parent of a child with a complex congenital heart defect to discuss with the child's teacher and school officials when the child enters school.

See MyNursingKit for possible responses.

duction system or unavoidable surgical incisions in areas of the sinoatrial node or sinoventricular node (such as the Fontan procedure and repair of tetralogy of Fallot) (Kaltman, Madan, Vetter, et al., 2006).

Although most children with congenital heart disease have normal IQ scores, and children with corrected simple defects can lead normal lives, neurologic insults can occur for many reasons. CHF, prolonged hypoxemia, profound acidosis, and low cardiac output increase the infant's risk for neurologic sequelae. Inadequate nutrition during rapid brain growth in the first year, intraventricular hemorrhage, hypoxic-ischemic injury, or periventricular leukomalacia (focal necrotic lesions in the periventricular white matter) can cause neurologic problems (Zeltser & Tabbutt, 2006, pp. 38–39). Cardiopulmonary bypass and deep hypothermic circulatory arrest used during most surgeries are other potential causes of neurologic insults.

Children with complex defects are at risk for visuospatial, visual motor, and speech deficits even when IQ scores fall within normal ranges (Brosig, Mussatto, Kuhn, et al., 2007). Children with hypoplastic left heart syndrome (HLHS) are at higher risk for neurocognitive impairment because of a higher incidence of congenital brain abnormalities, ductal-dependent systemic blood flow, severe acidosis at diagnosis, deep hypothermic cardiac arrest during surgery, and postoperative challenges of maintaining adequate systemic blood flow and cerebral perfusion. It is thought that some infants with complex congenital defects have abnormal brain development (Miller, McQuillen, Hamrick, et al., 2007).

NURSING MANAGEMENT

Nursing management of the hospitalized child focuses on monitoring PGE_1 therapy for newborns, treating hypercyanotic episodes, supporting families to care for the child at home, and providing postsurgical care.

NURSING ASSESSMENT AND DIAGNOSIS

PHYSIOLOGIC ASSESSMENT BEFORE SURGERY

Infants receiving PGE_1 therapy are cared for in an intensive care nursery where their cardiovascular status can be closely monitored until palliative procedures are performed.

Prior to or between stages of surgery, the infant or child is seen regularly to assess growth, and monitor for signs of CHF (tachycardia, tachypnea, crackles, frothy secretions, low urine output, and pulmonary edema). The child's poor growth may affect height, weight, and head circumference, so plot serial measurements on the same growth curve to monitor the significance of the growth problems. Monitor physiologic status using the guidelines in Table 49–4.

The child needs careful observation for signs of increased cyanosis in the morning or at other high-risk times. Observe for neurologic signs of thromboembolism due to polycythemia such as headache, dizziness, excessive irritability, and paralysis.

Older children with cyanotic defects may have clubbing of the fingers and toes.

ASSESSMENT FOLLOWING SURGERY

Children are admitted to the ICU following surgery. Once the child returns to the general nursing unit, monitor the child's heart functioning. Assess vital signs, pulse oximetry, skin color, and perfusion of the skin by capillary refill and distal pulses. Monitoring fluid intake and output following surgery is critical. A sudden sustained increase in pulse and respirations and a decrease in peripheral perfusion may be early signs of hemorrhage. Signs of respiratory distress may indicate the development of a pneumothorax or CHF. See page 1370 for other nursing assessment guidelines in the postoperative period.

PSYCHOSOCIAL ASSESSMENT

Assess the parents' need for information and emotional support. In many cases, the infant's condition is first identified at birth; however, a defect could have been identified by fetal sonogram. The parents will be grieving the loss of a perfect newborn and be extremely anxious about the infant's condition and prognosis.

Examples of nursing diagnoses that may apply to a child with decreased pulmonary blood flow include the following:

- *Decreased Cardiac Output* related to ventricular restriction and an obstructed outflow tract
- *Risk for Infection* related to unfiltered bacteria in the blood and sites of blood shunting that promote bacterial growth
- *Ineffective Family Therapeutic Regimen Management* related to complexity of therapeutic regimen: assessment and management of cyanotic spells, which are unpredictable events
- *Activity Intolerance* related to cyanosis and dyspnea on exertion
- *Delayed Growth and Development* related to congenital anomaly and hypoxemia

PLANNING AND IMPLEMENTATION

HOME CARE OF THE CHILD BEFORE SURGERY

Infants with tetralogy of Fallot and other serious defects are often managed at home to grow and potentially improve surgical outcome. Parents are usually anxious during the wait for surgery. They may fear that the infant will not survive until surgery or that they will be unable to manage any problems the infant may have. Provide information and teach parents how to care for the infant at home. Arrange for home health nursing and other community services that may be required. Many of these children require supplemental nutrition and oxygen for emergencies. Because unoxygenated and oxygenated blood mix, supplemental oxygen does not improve the child's usual oxygen saturation (SpO_2) level.

Cyanosis with or without CHF often results in delayed gross motor skills. Make referrals to community-based early intervention programs to help parents learn about realistic developmental goals and to promote the child's development. Encourage parents to treat the infant as normally as possible. Children with mild cyanotic lesions do not need to adjust activity. The child with moderate to severe disease should be able to tolerate crying for a few minutes without difficulty. Prolonged crying should not be permitted because it causes fatigue and further hypoxia.

Hypercyanotic episodes become life threatening if not treated immediately. The child becomes progressively more hypoxic and limp, loses consciousness, is likely to have a seizure or cerebrovascular accident, and may die. Teach parents to observe for signs of worsening cyanosis, particularly in the morning, that could signal the beginning of a hypercyanotic episode. Some families use a pulse oximeter daily and need to know the child's typical SpO_2 and change that may indicate an emergency.

Develop an emergency plan for the infant in anticipation of acute problems such as a hypercyanotic episode or respiratory distress. The parents should learn cardiopulmonary resuscitation. Provide the parents with a card or brief history form with information about the child's condition, medications, necessary emergency care, and the physician's name so emergency care providers have vital information for initial medical care. See My Nursing Kit for the Web site for an emergency information form.

Teach parents to report signs of illness to the physician. Vomiting and diarrhea may lead to dehydration, a particular risk in children with polycythemia because the blood can become more viscous and lead to thrombus formation. Fever increases the metabolic rate and causes further stress on the heart. Aggressive management with antipyretic medication and fluid volume replacement is necessary.

Signs of infective endocarditis (low-grade fever, fatigue, and malaise) occurring within 2 months of surgery or a high-risk procedure should be reported. Parents should be taught about the need to request antibiotic prophylaxis for the child.

Although parents may travel with cyanotic children, they should talk with the physician before taking them to areas of high altitude. Supplemental oxygen when traveling on an airplane may be necessary.

Nursing Practice

Provide guidelines for the initial care of a hypercyanotic episode. The parents should call for an ambulance and try to calm and reassure the infant. The infant should be placed in a knee–chest position by holding the infant facing the parent's chest, placing one arm under the knees, and folding the legs upward toward the infant's chest. Use the other arm to support the infant's back. Alternatively, the infant can be placed supine with knees bent up to the chest. If oxygen is available, provide it in a manner that does not further upset the infant. If none is available in the home, it will be administered in the ambulance during transport to the emergency department.

HOSPITAL-BASED CARE OF THE INFANT AND CHILD

The newborn receiving continuous infusion of PGE_1 is cared for in the NICU. Side effects of prostaglandin E_1 treatment such as cutaneous vasodilation, bradycardia, tachycardia, hypotension, seizure activity, fever, and apnea are monitored and managed.

Avoid any unpleasant or anxiety-provoking procedures in an effort to prevent a hypercyanotic episode. If a hypercyanotic episode occurs in an infant or toddler prior to surgery, follow guidelines for treatment on pages 1374–1376.

Following surgery, the child is initially cared for in the ICU until heart function has stabilized. Once the child returns to the general nursing unit, nursing care is the same as described for the child having surgery for increased pulmonary blood flow (see page 1374).

EVALUATION

Examples of expected nursing care outcomes include the following:

- The parents recognize a hypercyanotic episode and initiate appropriate emergency treatment.
- The parents manage fever and medical illnesses to prevent dehydration and thromboembolism.
- The child becomes stable following surgery and has no complications.
- The child attains expected development following surgical repair of the congenital heart defect.

DEFECTS OBSTRUCTING SYSTEMIC BLOOD FLOW

ETIOLOGY AND PATHOPHYSIOLOGY

An anatomic stenosis (narrowing of a valve, of the area around the valve, or in the great artery above the valve) causes obstruction to blood flow and results in a pressure load on the left ventricle and decreased cardiac output. The greater the narrowing, the more obstructed blood flow is to the circulation. This results in higher pressure in the ventricle and decreased cardiac output. Newborns with severe left outflow obstruction or left ventricular dysfunction may develop decreased cardiac output and shock.

CLINICAL MANIFESTATIONS

Low cardiac output is responsible for the clinical manifestations: diminished pulses, poor color, delayed capillary refill time, and decreased urinary output. The blood cannot move past the obstruction, so it backs up into the left atrium and then the lungs, causing CHF and pulmonary edema. The child with mild obstructions may have leg cramps, cooler feet than hands, and stronger pulses in the upper extremities than the lower extremities. The blood pressure, usually 10 to 15 mm Hg higher in the legs than the arms, may be lower in the legs than expected. Decreased blood supply to the gastrointestinal tract may lead to necrotizing enterocolitis. See Chapter 53. See Table 49–7 for the pathophysiology, clinical manifestations, and clinical therapy for the congenital heart defects that obstruct systemic blood flow.

> ## Complementary Care
>
> **HERBAL PRODUCTS TO AVOID**
>
> Caution parents of children with congenital heart defects to avoid using herbal products that may interfere with the medications prescribed to manage the child's heart condition. For example, products containing ginkgo interact with warfarin, of particular concern for any child on anticoagulant therapy.

CLINICAL THERAPY

Neonates with severe systemic outflow obstruction or left ventricular dysfunction may develop decreased cardiac output and shock. PGE_1 and inotrope medications may be required to support the systemic circulation until the obstruction is relieved or ventricular function improves.

Nursing Management

Provide nursing care to children with aortic stenosis and coarctation of the aorta as described for "Congenital Defects that Increase Pulmonary Blood Flow" on page 1365. Provide nursing care to infants with hypoplastic left heart syndrome (HLHS) as described for "Defects Causing Decreased Pulmonary Blood Flow and Mixed Defects" on page 1377.

Parents of children with life-threatening defects such as HLHS must make decisions about their child's treatment very quickly, choosing what is best for their individual situation (palliative care, Norwood procedure, or heart transplant). Parents are faced with the potential death of the newborn before having an opportunity to grieve the loss of a normal infant. Nurses play an important role in supporting parents through this difficult decision-making period. Ensure that parents are fully informed about each treatment option and their associated mortality, the intense care needed by the surviving infant, potential neurocognitive and neurodevelopmental outcomes, and unknown long-term survival. If parents choose comfort or palliative care, interventions such as PGE_1 are discontinued and the infant is given appropriate analgesia and comfort care. Seek the support of clergy, social workers, or other supportive individuals in the family's life to assist them through this period. Reassure parents that they are good parents, no matter what decision they make. See Chapter 43.

CONGESTIVE HEART FAILURE

Congestive heart failure (CHF) is a disorder of circulation in which cardiac output is inadequate to support the body's circulatory and metabolic needs. It may result from a congenital heart defect that increases pulmonary blood flow or obstructs the systemic blood

(continues on page 1383)

HEALTH PROMOTION

THE ADOLESCENT WITH CONGENITAL HEART DISEASE

Preventive Care

- Encourage regular visits to the primary care provider for general health and illness care. Perform health screening according to recommended schedules (see Chapter 38). Give all recommended immunizations, including the influenza vaccine.
- Encourage routine dental visits twice a year. Make sure the adolescent knows that regular dental care and antibiotic prophylaxis help reduce endocarditis risk.
- Encourage female adolescents to initiate gynecologic care to ensure that appropriate contraception and other gynecologic care needs are addressed. Educate the adolescent about the risks associated with pregnancy and the potential need for special care during pregnancy.
- Provide counseling about health risks associated with tobacco use, alcohol and drug use, and unprotected sex.

Exercise and Nutrition

- Inquire about the adolescent's preferred exercise and activity level. An individualized assessment with graded exercise testing on a treadmill or bicycle may be performed in children with complex congenital heart defects to determine specific exercise and activity limitations for the adolescent's condition (Paridon, Alpert, Boas, et al., 2006). Decreasing exercise performance with age has been found in children with HLHS treated with the Fontan procedure and transplantation (Jenkins, Chinnock, Jenkins, et al., 2008). Participation in competitive sports and strenuous work may be limited for some adolescents. Those who have had a complete repair can participate in team sports. Adolescents taking anticoagulants may have activity limitations because of the risk for bleeding.
- Encourage adolescents to participate in normal gym activities and other recreational and sports activities to the best of their physical abilities.

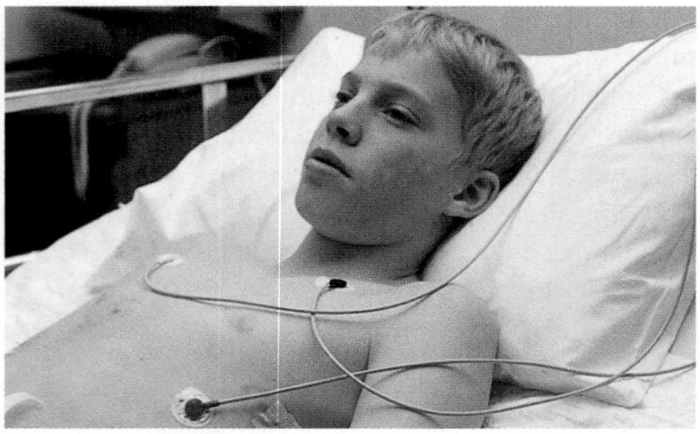

- Encourage the adolescent to eat nutritious meals and snacks, and to avoid excess weight gain that could stress the heart function.

Mental and Spiritual Health

- Discuss the adolescent's concerns for the future, as there may be significant uncertainty about the disease course and outcome.
- Identify and refer adolescents as needed for counseling or to a support group of adolescents of similar age with congenital heart disease.

Education for Self-Care

- Begin the process of transitioning the adolescent to adult health care. Provide education about the congenital heart defect, surgeries that have been performed, and the types of symptoms resulting. Remember that previous education has been targeted to the parents. Correct any misperceptions that the successful cardiac surgery has resulted in a normal heart if that is not the case.
- Provide a written succinct summary of the adolescent's condition and medical management that can be shared with other health professionals. Include the diagnosis, surgeries or other interventions, medications and their side effects, laboratory values, information on the functional status, and expectations regarding disease progression (Knauth, Verstappen, Reiss, et al., 2006).
- Discuss the medications needed and why, and develop plans for the adolescent to assume responsibility for self-administration.
- Discuss the genetic aspects of the condition and provide resources for genetic counseling if desired.
- Discuss any activity or other limitations, such as strenuous work or sports participation.
- Discuss the danger signs of the condition (such as arrhythmias, or the potential of dehydration in an adolescent with cyanosis) and how to seek urgent or emergency care.

Vocational Education

- Reassure adolescents who have had complete repairs of the congenital heart defect and have no disabilities that they have no limitations in their career or vocational selection.
- Refer adolescents with cardiac disabilities to career and vocational counseling in an effort to match their interests and physical limitations. These adolescents should be informed about their rights under the Americans with Disabilities Act of 1990.
- Families and patients should be informed to identify health insurance options, and to identify those policies that have fewer restrictions. Adolescents should be informed that healthcare coverage is an important benefit to investigate when considering any future job change.

Table 49–7 Pathophysiology, Clinical Manifestations, and Clinical Therapy for Defects that Obstruct the Systemic Blood Flow

Defect Pathophysiology, Clinical Manifestations, and Clinical Therapy	Anatomy
Aortic Stenosis (AS)	
Narrowing of the aortic valve obstructs blood flow to systemic circulation. The valve often has two valve leaflets (bicuspid) rather than three. The pressure gradient across the valve usually increases as the child grows and cardiac output increases. Aortic stenosis accounts for up to 10% of congenital heart defects (Park, 2008). **Clinical Manifestations** Most infants and children are asymptomatic with normal growth and development. Life-threatening aortic stenosis occurs in some newborns. CHF develops in infants with significant stenosis. The blood pressure is normal, but a narrow pulse pressure may be noted. Peripheral pulses may be weak. The child may complain of chest pain after exercise, but exercise intolerance is uncommon. Fainting and dizziness are serious signs that require intervention. A systolic heart murmur and thrill may be detected in the aortic or pulmonic areas with transmission to the neck. An ejection click may be heard. Splitting of the S_2 may be noted with severe aortic stenosis. Interventions may result in aortic insufficiency causing a high-pitched diastolic decrescendo murmur along the left sternal border near the mitral area. **Diagnostic Tests** The chest radiograph may reveal a slight prominence of the left ventricle and aorta with increased severity. The ECG may show mild left ventricular hypertrophy and inverted T waves with increased severity. An echocardiogram reveals the number of the valve leaflets, pressure gradient across valve, and size of the aorta. Exercise testing may be used in asymptomatic children to determine the amount of obstruction present. **Clinical Therapy** Newborns with life-threatening aortic stenosis need PGE_1 to maintain a patent ductus arteriosus until the aortic valve can be dilated. Treatment involves balloon dilation during cardiac catheterization or surgical valvotomy. Surgical treatment is palliative rather than curative. Aortic valve replacement (sometimes with the pulmonary valve) is performed when stenosis is severe or if significant regurgitation results from other interventions. **Prognosis** Chest pain, syncope, and sudden death can occur in symptomatic children, particularly during vigorous exercise. Increasing left side obstruction or aortic insufficiency may develop as the child ages. Stenosis is usually progressive during childhood as the valve calcifies. Valve replacement may be necessary once the child reaches adulthood, requiring lifelong anticoagulant therapy.	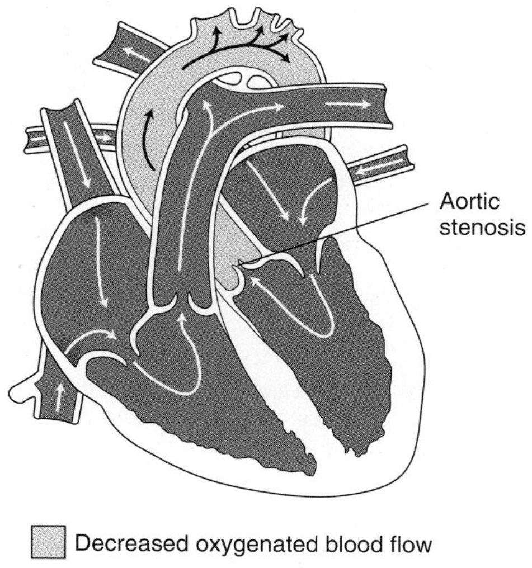
Coarctation of the Aorta (COA)	
Narrowing or constriction in the descending aorta, often near the ductus arteriosus or left subclavian artery, obstructs the systemic blood outflow. This defect occurs in 8% to 10% of congenital heart defects and is common in children with Turner syndrome (Park, 2008; Schneider & Goldmuntz, 2006). **Clinical Manifestations** Many children are asymptomatic and grow normally. Infants with severe constriction may have cyanosis in the lower extremities, heart failure, and shock as the ductus arteriosus closes. Renal failure and necrotizing enterocolitis may develop. Infants with moderate constriction may have poor feeding, failure to thrive, increased respiratory effort, and CHF. Blood pressure in the legs is lower than in the arms. Brachial and radial pulses are typically bounding, but femoral pulses are weak or absent. Older children may complain of weakness and pain in the legs after exercise. S_2 is loud and single on auscultation. A systolic ejection murmur may be heard at the upper right and middle or lower left sternal border. A thrill may be palpated in the suprasternal notch.	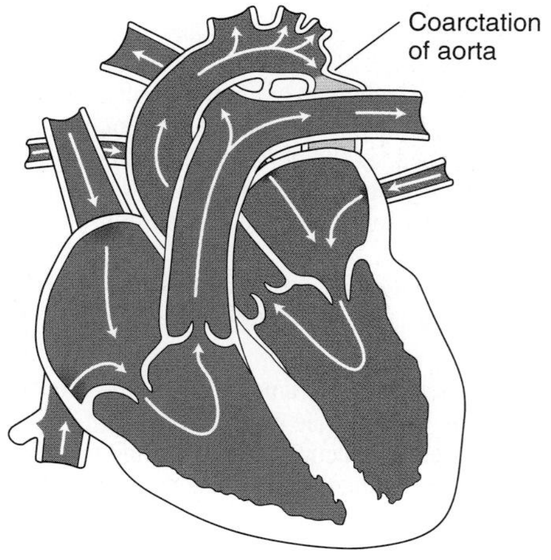

(continued)

Table 49–7 Pathophysiology, Clinical Manifestations, and Clinical Therapy for Defects that Obstruct the Systemic Blood Flow—continued

Defect Pathophysiology, Clinical Manifestations, and Clinical Therapy | **Anatomy**

Coarctation of the Aorta (COA)—continued

Diagnostic Procedures

The chest radiograph may reveal cardiomegaly, pulmonary venous congestion, and indentation of the descending aorta. Rib notching is rarely seen before 10 years of age.

CT scan and MRI shows the aortic arch and site of coarctation.

ECG shows left ventricular hypertrophy, and right ventricular hypertrophy may be seen in severe cases.

Echocardiogram shows the size of the aorta, the actual coarctation, and functioning of the aortic valve and left ventricle.

Clinical Therapy

In symptomatic newborns, PGE_1 is given to reopen the ductus arteriosus and promote blood flow to the lower extremities. Treatment to prevent CHF may be initiated with inotropic medications, diuretics, and oxygen (Park, 2008).

Surgical resection is often preferred to balloon dilation during cardiac catheterization, to reduce the risk for recoarctation. Balloon dilation may be performed for recoarctation (Park, 2008).

Balloon dilation and surgical resection are palliative, as coarctation may recur.

Prognosis

Chronic systemic hypertension is more likely to occur in children older than 1 year at the time of repair (Marino, Ostrow, & Cohen, 2006).

Hypoplastic Left Heart Syndrome (HLHS)

The mitral and aortic valves are absent or stenosed along with an abnormally small left ventricle and small aorta. It accounts for about 1% of congenital heart defects and 9% of defects in critically ill newborns. Up to 29% of infants have a brain abnormality (Park, 2008).

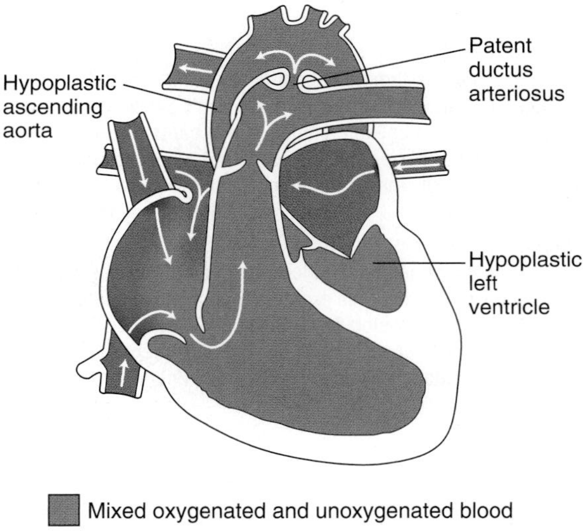

Clinical Manifestations

With closure of the ductus arteriosus, the newborn has progressive cyanosis, tachycardia, tachypnea, dyspnea, retractions, and decreased peripheral pulses.

Poor peripheral perfusion, pulmonary edema, and CHF lead to shock, acidosis, and sometimes death.

A single loud heart sound is present and often no murmur is present.

Diagnostic Procedures

The chest radiograph shows cardiomegaly and increased pulmonary vascularity.

The echocardiogram shows the small left ventricle. This condition may be diagnosed prenatally.

Clinical Therapy

Prostaglandin E_1 is given immediately to maintain a patent ductus arteriosus.

Supplemental oxygen is avoided.

Three treatment options include the Norwood and Sano procedures, a heart and lung transplant (see page 1389), and comfort or palliative care.

The Norwood procedure is performed in the first week of life, followed by the Glenn procedure at about 3 to 8 months of age, and the Fontan procedure between 18 months and 3 years of age (Khairy, Poirer, & Mercier, 2007).

Heart transplantation outcomes are not as good as with the Norwood. Few infant hearts are available for transplantation. Each heart transplant is likely to last 10 to 15 years (Kon, 2005).

Up to 50% of parents choose nonsurgical comfort care when fully informed about treatment options and condition morbidity (Kon, 2005).

Prognosis:

Without surgery, the median survival time is 3 days. The surgical 5-year survival rate is estimated to be 50% to 70%, but life expectancy cannot be predicted (Kon, 2005). The single ventricle causes physical activity limitations and fails over time. A heart transplant may be required during adolescence or adulthood. Many children have significant neurocognitive and neurodevelopmental impairment regardless of surgical intervention (Mahle, Visconti, Freier, et al., 2006). Arrhythmias and thromboemboli are other potential complications (Khairy et al., 2007).

outflow tract. Other causes include problems with heart contractility, pathologic conditions that require high cardiac output (e.g., severe anemia, acidosis, or respiratory disease), acquired heart disease (e.g., cardiomyopathy, rheumatic heart disease, and Kawasaki disease) or disorders such as Duchenne muscular dystrophy.

ETIOLOGY AND PATHOPHYSIOLOGY

Pulmonary blood volume overload associated with congenital heart defects is the most common cause of CHF in infants. Up to 90% of infants with uncorrected heart defects develop CHF within the first 6 to 12 months of life (Connor, 2006). Some defects allow blood to flow from the left side of the heart to the right increasing the blood pumped to the pulmonary system. This overloads the pulmonary system, and if prolonged can lead to pulmonary artery hypertension (see page 1392). Obstructive congenital defects (i.e., abnormally small pulmonary vessels) restrict the flow of blood, so the heart muscle hypertrophies to work harder to force blood through these structures.

When cardiac output remains insufficient, the body's organs and tissues receive inadequate oxygen. A sympathetic nervous system response increases the heart rate, heart muscle contractility, and peripheral vascular resistance. The kidneys respond to the lowered circulating volume by activating the renin-angiotensin mechanism to retain salt and water. The heart muscle fibers stretch to accommodate the increased blood volume and the myocardium hypertrophies to manage the increased ventricular pressure. These responses increase cardiac output to the vital organs. The compensatory mechanisms increase their intensity and further compromise the heart. Progressive systemic edema and pulmonary congestion occur leading to right- or left-sided heart failure, and eventually bilateral failure.

CLINICAL MANIFESTATIONS

Initial signs of congestive heart failure may be subtle and not immediately recognized. The infant tires easily, especially during feeding. Weight loss or lack of normal weight gain, diaphoresis, irritability, and frequent respiratory infections may be evident. Older children may have exercise intolerance, dyspnea, abdominal pain or distention, and peripheral edema.

As the disease progresses, symptoms such as tachypnea, tachycardia, pallor or cyanosis, nasal flaring, grunting, retractions, cough, or crackles may occur. A third heart sound may be auscultated. Generalized fluid volume overload is seen more commonly in toddlers and older children. Periorbital and facial edema and hepatomegaly are signs of fluid volume excess. Jugular vein distention is seen in older children. See "Clinical Manifestations: Congestive Heart Failure."

Cardiomegaly, enlargement (hypertrophy) of the heart muscle, occurs in an effort to maintain cardiac output. Cyanosis, weak peripheral pulses, cool extremities, hypotension, and heart murmur are precursors of cardiogenic shock, which can occur if CHF is not adequately treated (see page 1402.)

CLINICAL THERAPY

Diagnosis is based primarily on clinical manifestations such as tachycardia, respiratory distress, and crackles. A chest radiograph reveals cardiac enlargement and venous congestion or signs of pulmonary edema. Echocardiography may reveal specific cardiac defects or dysfunction. An electrocardiogram may show tachycardia, bradycardia, or ventricular hypertrophy. Electrolytes, lactic acid, arterial blood gases, and a complete blood count are obtained.

The goals of medical management are to make the heart work more efficiently and to remove excess fluid. This decreases the work of the heart and improves systemic circulation without flooding the pulmonary system. Diuretics, such as furosemide, bumetanide, chlorothiazide, and spironolactone, are given to promote fluid excretion. Inotropic medicines and afterload-reducing agents (angiotensin-converting enzyme inhibitors) are sometimes prescribed. Digoxin is the drug most commonly used to improve the heart's ability to contract and therefore increase its output. Beta-blockers, such as propranolol and carvedilol, are being evaluated for safety and effectiveness for children with CHF (Menteer, Hogarty, & Chrisant, 2006). See "Drug Guide: Drugs Used to Treat Congestive Heart Failure" for medications used to treat CHF.

Surgery or interventional cardiac catheterization for a congenital heart defect may become the treatment of choice. Cardiac transplantation may be performed for children with end-stage cardiomyopathy or complex congenital heart defects such as hypoplastic left heart syndrome.

Clinical Manifestations

CONGESTIVE HEART FAILURE

PATHOPHYSIOLOGY	CLINICAL MANIFESTATIONS
Pulmonary venous congestion	Tachypnea, wheezing, crackles, retractions, cough, grunting, nasal flaring, irritability, tiring with play, increased tachypnea and diaphoresis with feeding
Systemic venous congestion	Hepatomegaly, ascites, periorbital edema, fluid retention weight gain Jugular venous distention and dependent edema in older children
Impaired cardiac output	Tachycardia, weak pulses, hypotension, capillary refill time greater than 2 seconds, pallor, cool extremities, oliguria
High metabolic rate	Failure to thrive or slow weight gain, diaphoresis

Drug Guide

DRUGS USED TO TREAT CONGESTIVE HEART FAILURE

DRUG AND ACTIONS	NURSING MANAGEMENT
Digoxin (Lanoxin) Increases myocardial contractility to improve systemic circulation	Assess the heart rate for bradycardia for 1 minute prior to giving a dose or for changes in heart rhythm or quality. Monitor the child for digitoxicity. See page 1388 for more nursing management.
Furosemide (Lasix) Rapid diuresis; blocks reabsorption of sodium and water in renal tubules	Monitor patients during rapid diuresis for vital signs, intake and output, and fluid and electrolyte imbalances.
Thiazides (Diuril) Chlorothiazide (suspension) Hydrochlorothiazide (tablets) Maintenance diuresis, decreases absorption of sodium, water, potassium, chloride, and bicarbonate in rensal tubules	Monitor blood pressure and intake and output rates and patterns. Monitor lab values for hypokalemia. Assess for digitoxicity if hypokalemia is present.
Spironolactone (Aldactone) Maintenance diuresis (potassium-sparing)	Assess for signs of fluid and electrolyte imbalance, and digitoxicity.
ACEi (angiotensin converting enzyme inhibitor) (e.g., Captopril, Enalopril) Promotes vascular relaxation and reduced peripheral vascular resistance, reduces afterload	Assess for common side effects such as cough, hyperkalemia, and worsening renal function.
Propranolol (Inderal) Increases contractility	Monitor vital signs and peripheral perfusion. Monitor intake and output ratio and daily weight. Dietary sodium is usually restricted.
Carvedilol (Coreg) Improves left ventricular function, promotes vasodilation of systemic circulation, used for chronic heart failure and dilated cardiomyopathy	Monitor for signs of CHF improvement. Monitor for dizziness and hypotension. Monitor digoxin levels as drug may increase plasma digoxin concentration. Monitor liver function periodically.

Data from: Bindler, R. M., & Howry, L. B. (2005). *Pediatric drug guide*. Upper Saddle River, NJ: Prentice Hall; and Wilson, B. A., Shannon, M. T., & Shields, K. M. (2009). *Nurses' drug guide 2009*. Upper Saddle River, NJ: Prentice Hall.

Supportive medical therapies (airway management, ventilatory support, oxygen, rest, and fluid and dietary management) are part of the treatment plan. Most children improve rapidly after medication is administered.

NURSING MANAGEMENT

NURSING ASSESSMENT AND DIAGNOSIS

PHYSIOLOGIC ASSESSMENT

The diagnosis of CHF depends primarily on physical symptoms. Assess the child's vital signs, behavioral patterns, cardiac function, respiratory function, and fluid status using guidelines in Table 49–4. Use the age-specific heart and respiratory rates in Chapter 35 (see pages 955 and 958) to identify tachycardia and tachypnea. Obtain a detailed history of the onset of symptoms from the parents, as CHF often develops slowly.

Measure intake and output carefully. Weigh the infant's diapers before use and after changing. Each 1 gm difference in weight equates to 1 mL urine. Weigh the child at the same time each day. If ascites is present, take serial abdominal measurements to monitor changes (see Skill 9–7, Abdominal Girth in the Clinical Skills Manual SKILLS for guidelines). Observe for changes in peripheral edema and circulation. Turn the child frequently and assess the skin for redness and breakdown.

FAMILY ASSESSMENT

Review the child's previous hospitalizations and assess the family's knowledge about the child's condition. Families of children with CHF are anxious about the potential deterioration of the child's condition and their ability to provide ongoing care. Assess the family's anxiety level and coping strategies. Evaluate the family's economic status. Medication is crucial to treatment, and a family's inability to obtain the necessary medications jeopardizes the child's outcome. Identify the parent's ability to recognize changes in the child's condition and to provide needed care. Determine if another family member is available who could assist young parents or provide respite care.

DEVELOPMENTAL ASSESSMENT

Since fatigue limits the activities of the child with CHF, the opportunity to practice the skills needed to attain normal developmental milestones is more limited. Assess development with a tool such as the Denver II (see Chapter 36), and ask parents when the child attained expected developmental milestones such as sitting, manipulating objects, standing, or walking. Ask parents about contact and play with other children and a typical day's activity schedule. Parents may limit the child's contact with other children because of frequent infections and exercise intolerance. When CHF is well controlled, the child's energy level increases and developmental skills often improve. Repeating assessments every 2 to 3 months in infants and toddlers provides useful information about development and disease management.

Several nursing diagnoses that may apply to the child with CHF can be found in the accompanying Nursing Care Plans. The primary nursing diagnosis is *Decreased Cardiac Output* related to cardiac anomaly.

PLANNING AND IMPLEMENTATION

Nursing care for the child with congestive heart failure focuses on administering and monitoring effects of medications, maintaining adequate oxygenation and myocardial function, promoting rest, fostering development, providing adequate nutrition, and providing emotional support to the child and family (Figure 49–6 ●). (See "Nursing Care Plan: The Child Hospitalized with Congestive Heart Failure.")

ADMINISTER AND MONITOR PRESCRIBED MEDICATIONS

Children with CHF usually receive digoxin and furosemide. These medications are potent and must be administered correctly. See "Drug Guide: Digoxin" on page 1388.

MAINTAIN OXYGENATION AND MYOCARDIAL FUNCTION

Oxygen therapy may be ordered. Make sure that tubing is patent, the oxygen flow rate is correct, the oxygen delivery device is working properly, and humidification is provided. Keep the child calm and quiet. Position the child in a semi-Fowler's or 45-degree angle position to promote maximum oxygenation.

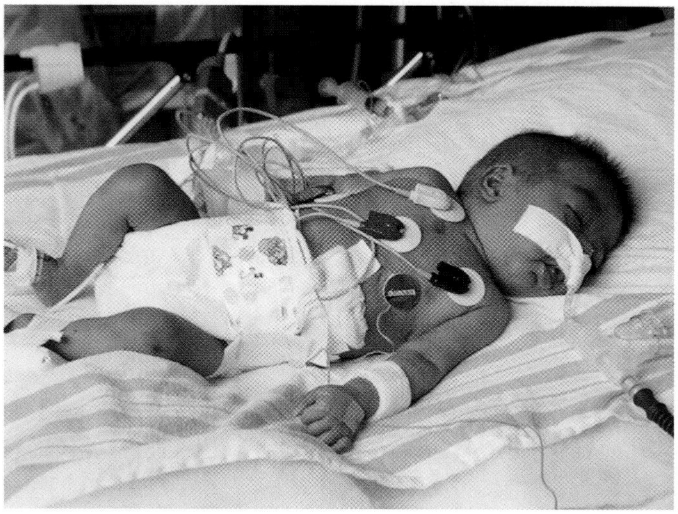

● **Figure 49–6** Jooti is receiving intravenous fluids and oxygen. Her condition is being continuously monitored for congestive heart failure.

PROMOTE REST

Group assessments and interventions together to ensure that the child has some uninterrupted rest each hour. Rocking is restful for infants. Encourage older children to engage in quiet activities such as playing board games or watching television.

FOSTER DEVELOPMENT

Encourage parents to play with the child, using toys to stimulate eye-hand coordination and fine motor movements. Such toys include rattles, blocks, and stuffed animals for infants, and books, paper and crayons, and dolls for older children. Encourage sitting, standing, or walking for short periods with adequate rest afterward to promote the development of large muscles. Singing, talking, and playing music facilitate cognitive and language skills.

PROVIDE ADEQUATE NUTRITION

Teach parents about feeding techniques. Encourage the mother who chooses to breastfeed the infant. The antibodies in breast milk reduce infections, and the milk is naturally low in sodium. However, the sucking involved in breast- or bottle-feeding may cause dyspnea that forces the infant to rest frequently during feeding. Feedings should last no more than 20 to 30 minutes. Frequent small feedings generally work best, with burping after every half ounce of intake to minimize vomiting. Holding or positioning the baby in an

Nursing Practice

Digoxin and digitoxin are both digitalis preparations, but not the same drug. Digoxin is the drug of choice in pediatrics. Digitoxin is 10 times more powerful than digoxin, and is rarely used in children. Read labels carefully and double-check doses to ensure that you give the child the right dose of the right drug.

Nursing Care Plan

THE CHILD HOSPITALIZED WITH CONGESTIVE HEART FAILURE

INTERVENTION	RATIONALE	EXPECTED OUTCOME
1. Nursing Diagnosis: Decreased Cardiac Output related to cardiac anomaly (VSD)		
NIC Priority Intervention: **Hemodynamic regulation:** Optimization of heart rate, preload, afterload, and contractility		**NOC Suggested Outcome:** **Cardiac pump effectiveness:** Extent to which blood is ejected from the left ventricle per minute to support systemic perfusion pressure
Goal: The child's cardiac output will be sufficient to meet the body's metabolic demands.		
■ Administer digoxin as ordered.	■ Digoxin increases contractility of the heart and force of contraction.	The child's cardiac output is sufficient as indicated by increased energy, adequate feeding intake, and decreased edema.
■ Regularly count the apical pulse and listen to heart sounds, especially before each dose of digoxin. Record the apical pulse rate with each dose of digoxin.	■ Digoxin may cause bradycardia. Pulse and heart sounds provide information about heart functioning.	
■ Use cardiac monitor if prescribed.	■ Monitor notes bradycardia and arrhythmias.	
■ Monitor serum potassium level and for digitoxicity.	■ Hypokalemia increases risk of digoxin toxicity.	The child maintains normal serum potassium levels and therapeutic levels of digoxin.
■ Provide for rest periods each hour.	■ Rest decreases need for high cardiac output.	The child rests hourly and has adequate energy to eat and play.
Goal: The child will manifest adequate oxygenation		
■ Evaluate respiratory rate and sounds. Use pulse oximetry to determine oxygen saturation readings.	■ Provides information about oxygenation and ease of respiration.	The child maintains a normal SpO_2 level and respiratory rate for age without evidence of adventitious sounds or diaphoresis.
■ Provide oxygen and humidification if prescribed. Observe for diaphoresis, a sign of increased respiratory effort.	■ Supplemental oxygen decreases tachypnea, and humidification moistens secretions to keep airway clear.	
■ Place child in semi-Fowler's position.	■ Position facilitates lung expansion.	
2. Nursing Diagnosis: Excess Fluid Volume related to heart failure		
NIC Priority Intervention: **Fluid management:** Promotion of fluid balance and prevention of complications resulting from abnormal or undesired fluid levels		**NOC Suggested Outcome:** **Fluid balance:** Balance of water in the intracellular and extracellular compartments of the body
Goal: The child's peripheral and central edema will decrease. Intake and output will be balanced once excess fluid is excreted.		
■ Administer diuretics as ordered.	■ Diuretics mobilize fluids and facilitate excretion.	The child's intake and output are proportional, and electrolyte levels remain within normal ranges.
■ Measure intake and output carefully. Weigh diapers to assess output of infants. Weigh daily. Measure abdominal girth daily. Observe for peripheral edema.	■ Adequate output is a good indicator of renal perfusion. Assessments demonstrate effectiveness of treatment.	
■ Monitor electrolytes.	■ Electrolyte imbalance is common when diuretics are given.	

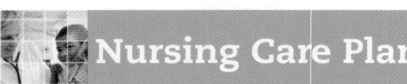

Nursing Care Plan—continued

THE CHILD HOSPITALIZED WITH CONGESTIVE HEART FAILURE

INTERVENTION	RATIONALE	EXPECTED OUTCOME
Goal: The child's peripheral and central edema will decrease.		
■ Change child's position frequently.	■ Position change promotes circulation to skin over pressure points.	The child has no skin breakdown after edema resolves.
■ Inspect skin frequently for redness and skin breakdown over pressure points.	■ Inspection identifies earliest stages of skin breakdown.	
3. Nursing Diagnosis: Imbalanced Nutrition: Less than Body Requirements related to high metabolic needs and rapid tiring while feeding.		
NIC Priority Intervention: **Nutrition Management:** Assistance with or provision of a balanced dietary intake of food and fluids		**NOC Suggested Outcome:** **Nutrition Status:** Extent to which nutrients are available to meet metabolic needs
■ Hold infant at 45-degree angle for feeding.	■ Position facilitates breathing while eating.	The infant or child gains recommended weight according to growth grids. All dietary requirements are met, and mealtimes are pleasant.
■ Record intake carefully.	■ Evaluation of intake indicates whether caloric and other nutritional needs are met.	
■ Weigh child daily.	■ Weight indicates growth (in absence of fluid retention).	
■ Give frequent small meals with rest periods in between.	■ Digesting small meals requires less energy.	
■ Use high-calorie formula or give high-calorie snacks.	■ High-calorie formulas and snacks provide calories efficiently.	
■ Use soothing approaches such as holding infants for feeding and having parents eat with older child.	■ Restful approach facilitates intake with minimum cardiac work.	
■ Transition to supplemental tube feedings if the infant is not able to gain weight.	■ Tube feedings provide added calories without taxing the infant's energy.	

infant seat at a 45-degree angle decreases venous return to the heart and decreases its metabolic demand. This is a favorable position for feeding and other activities (Cook & Higgins, 2004). Make sure parents understand that changes in feeding habits (decreased intake, vomiting, sleeping through feedings, and increased perspiration with feedings) may indicate deteriorating cardiac status.

The infant needs adequate nutrition to support growth. Some infants need a higher caloric formula (24 to 30 calories per ounce) to obtain adequate nutrition. Infants with significant heart problems often develop failure to thrive due to feeding difficulties. (See Chapter 34. ∞) When infants have significant dyspnea with feeding, nutritional supplementation by nasogastric, transpyloric, or gastrostomy tube may be prescribed. Parents are often advised to give the infant a chance to feed normally for a specific period to promote oral stimulation and bonding. The remainder of the formula is then given by tube feeding. (See Skills 15–2 and 15–3 SKILLS.)

PROVIDE EMOTIONAL SUPPORT

The family is often anxious about the condition of the child hospitalized with CHF. Give parents a chance to express concerns about their child's condition. Explain the child's treatment regimen, and make sure family members understand the child's need for nutrition and rest. Refer parents to the appropriate support groups; talking with parents of children with cardiac conditions may be a source of emotional support.

DISCHARGE PLANNING AND HOME CARE TEACHING

Identify and address home care needs well in advance of discharge. Show parents how to feed the child to maximize nutritional intake. While the child is hospitalized, teach the family about the administration of medications and signs of a worsening condition (e.g., increased feeding difficulty, irritability,

Drug Guide

DIGOXIN

Action

Digoxin increases the force of the myocardial systolic contraction, decreasing the degree of activation of the sympathetic nervous system and renin-angiotensin system, slowing the heart rate, and reducing the conduction velocity through the atrioventricular node. Digoxin is used in the treatment of CHF and for ventricular rate control in chronic atrial fibrillation.

Routes, Dosage, Frequency

Dosage varies by age and whether giving a digitalizing or maintenance dose.

Dose for Digitalization

Digitalization (dosing to more rapidly achieve maximum pharmacologic value without toxicity) may be given in divided dosages:

AGE	PO DOSE	IM/IV DOSE
Premature neonates	20 mcg/kg	15 mcg/kg
Neonate	30 mcg/kg	20 mcg/kg
1 to 24 months	40 to 50 mcg/kg	30 to 40 mcg/kg
2 to 10 years	30 to 40 mcg/kg	20 to 30 mcg/kg
Over 10 years and	10 to 15 mcg/kg	8 to 12 mcg/kg under 100 kg
Adult	10 to 15 mcg/kg (1 mg)	10 to 15 mcg/kg (1 mg)

Dose for Maintenance

AGE	PO DOSE	IM/IV DOSE
Premature neonates	5 mcg/kg	3 to 4 mcg/kg
Neonate	8 to 10 mcg/kg	6 to 8 mcg/kg
1 to 24 months	10 to 12 mcg/kg	7.5 to 9 mcg/kg
2 to 10 years	8 to 10 mcg/kg	6 to 8 mcg/kg
Over 10 years and	2.5 to 5 mcg/kg	2 to 3 mcg/kg under 100 kg
Adult	0.1 to 0.375 mg/day	0.1 to 0.375 mg/day

Doses are reduced in renal dysfunction, especially if creatinine clearance is under 10 mL/minute.

Nursing Management

Assessment: Before giving digitalizing dose, establish baseline vital signs, quality of peripheral pulses, clinical symptoms, and run an ECG strip. Check serum electrolytes, and hepatic and renal function. Assess hydration status, and hydrate if hypovolemic.

Administration: Digoxin is given intravenously or orally in extremely small doses. Carefully measure and verify the dose calculation and appropriateness of dose for weight of the child. Verification of the dose and calculation by another nurse is usually required.

PO: Give at same times daily without regard for food. Food will slow absorption, but it does not decrease total absorption. Use the provided calibrated dropper for the elixir. Be certain to administer digoxin, *not digitoxin,* tablets. Tablet may be crushed and mixed with fluid or food if patient cannot swallow it whole.

IV: Give undiluted or diluted in 4 mL of sterile water, D5W, or saline, and administer over at least 5 minutes. Use immediately after dilution. Do not mix with other medications. Patients are changed from IV to PO form as soon as possible.

Monitor

- *Before giving any dose, take apical pulse for 1 minute.* Withhold medication and call for a physician's advice before administering the drug if bradycardia is detected (less than 60 to 100 beats/min in children, dependent upon age, less than 60 beats/min in adolescents, or below a guideline noted in the physician's order) or changes in heart rhythm or quality are noted.
- Observe the child carefully for digitoxicity. Early signs include cardiac arrhythmias in children. Nausea, vomiting, anorexia, diarrhea, restlessness, drowsiness, fatigue, and visual disturbance are seen in older children (Park, 2008).
- Serum digoxin levels are taken 6 to 8 hours after a dose. A therapeutic serum level ranges from 0.8 to 2 ng/mL. Levels over 2 ng/mL are toxic.
- Monitor hepatic and renal functions. Dosage will be reduced if creatinine clearance is 50 mL/minute or less. Check serum electrolytes, particularly potassium, calcium, and magnesium; closely monitor children also on diuretics. Careful monitoring of intake and output is required, especially in cases of impaired renal function.
- Some antibiotics (e.g., tetracycline, erythromycin, clarithromycin, and beta-lactams) are associated with an antibiotic-digoxin interaction. Monitor serum digoxin levels closely during antibiotic therapy as altered intestinal flora may precipitate digitoxicity.
- If a child taking digoxin orally is NPO or vomiting, seek a physician's order regarding the course of action; the drug must not be omitted.
- If routes of administration (tablet, elixir, parenteral) are changed, absorption of digoxin may be altered. Generally, tablets and elixir dosages will need to be decreased by 20% to 25% when changing to IV or capsule preparations.

Patient Education

- Take the pulse prior to giving medication. When the pulse rate falls below or rises above guidelines provided, contact the physician. Administer the medication exactly as prescribed.
- Do not administer over-the-counter medications or herbal products for colds, coughs, allergies, GI upset, or obesity without approval.
- Keep the medication locked and out of reach of children.

Data from Bindler, R. M. & Howry, L. B. (2005). Pediatric drug guide. *Upper Saddle River, NJ: Prentice Hall.*

lethargy, breathing difficulty, and puffiness around the eyes or extremities). Arrange for home care nursing visits to reinforce the education provided, to monitor the child's condition, and to assess the family's ability to manage the child's care. Ensure that the family has a phone contact for emergency assistance. (See "Nursing Care Plan: The Child with Congestive Heart Failure Being Cared for at Home.")

Parents are frequently taught to take the child's pulse and to report any significant change to the physician. An increase in pulse rate can signal CHF, and a decrease can indicate digoxin toxicity. Teach parents to identify signs of dehydration when the child is managed on diuretics. An acute illness could lead to dehydration more quickly when the child takes these medications.

Demonstrate administration of drugs, and then supervise while the parents measure and administer medications. Teach parents about the toxic effects of digoxin and other drugs. Advise them to notify the physician immediately if any of these side effects occur. Teach parents about the potential interaction between digoxin and certain antibiotics so they can remind the primary care provider to prescribe safe antibiotics when they are needed. Because digoxin is a potential poison, encourage parents to keep it locked up at home and away from children. In case of accidental ingestion, immediate medical care is needed. Be sure parents keep the poison control number on all phones.

EVALUATION

Expected outcomes of nursing care can be found in the Nursing Care Plans.

Thinking Critically

THE INFANT WITH VENTRICULAR SEPTAL DEFECT

Brandy, who is 1 month old, was diagnosed with a ventricular septal defect (VSD) at birth and started developing signs of respiratory distress and difficulty with feeding.

Brandy's mother had been alerted to watch for these signs as a possible indication of congestive heart failure (CHF). Brandy was quickly hospitalized so her CHF could be treated with digoxin, furosemide (Lasix), and potassium. Over the next 2 days, she lost the weight she had gained due to fluid retention.

Corrective surgery was performed to place a patch over the septal opening. Brandy was cared for in the intensive care unit before being transferred to another unit.

- Why did Brandy develop congestive heart failure?
- Why was corrective surgery performed so soon?
- Is Brandy at risk to develop congestive heart failure after having had surgery?
- What teaching and support do Brandy's parents need to care for her at home after the heart surgery?

See MyNursingKit for possible responses.

CARDIOMYOPATHY

Cardiomyopathy is a serious disorder of the heart's muscle that affects the ventricular systolic function, diastolic function, or both (Towbin, Lowe, Colan, et al., 2006). The highest incidence of cardiomyopathy in the pediatric population occurs during the first year of life. Males have a higher incidence than females. Almost 40% of children with symptoms of cardiomyopathy die of the condition within 2 years or receive a heart transplant (Cox, Sleeper, Lowe, et al., 2006).

Dilated cardiomyopathy is the most common form, in which the four chambers dilate and systolic contraction is weakened. Myocarditis and neuromuscular disorders, such as muscular dystrophy, are the most common identified causes of this type of cardiomyopathy; however, 66% of cases have no known cause (Towbin et al., 2006). The child usually presents in CHF with tachypnea, wheezing, and poor cardiac output. Arrhythmias may develop that can cause cardiac arrest. Treatment involves digoxin, an ACE inhibitor, diuretics, antiarrhythmics, anticoagulants, and carvedilol or metoprolol, and ultimately a heart transplant may be considered.

In hypertrophic cardiomyopathy, the heart muscle is thickened and one or more chambers are small or normal in size. About 50% of hypertrophic cardiomyopathy cases are genetically transmitted as an autosomal dominant trait (Park, 2008). Palpitations may occur because of atrial or ventricular arrhythmia. Symptoms include exertional dyspnea, fatigue, dizziness, fainting, and chest pain; sudden unexpected death may occur. Treatment involves beta-blockers, calcium channel blockers, and antiarrhythmics. A heart transplant may be considered. Sudden death may be associated with sports or vigorous exercise (Park, 2008).

Nursing Management

Nursing management for dilated cardiomyopathy is the same as for children with CHF unless or until a heart transplant is performed. Nursing management for hypertrophic cardiomyopathy involves frequent visits to assess the child's condition and to review progress with antiarrhythmic medications.

HEART TRANSPLANTATION

Approximately 260 heart transplants are performed each year for children with end-stage cardiac failure or complex congenital heart defects with ventricular failure such as hypoplastic left heart syndrome or end-stage cardiomyopathy (Gabrys, 2005). Ventricular assist devices and extracorporeal membrane oxygenation (ECMO) use prior to and following transplantation improves the child's recovery from end-organ failure and enhances transplantation outcome (Blume, Naftel, Bastardi, et al., 2006). Up to 75% of children are surviving after 5 to 8 years (Morales, Dreyer, Denfield, et al., 2007).

Rejection and infection are the major causes of mortality and morbidity. The immunosuppression regimen usually includes calcineurin inhibitors (cyclosporin or tacrolimus), cell toxins (azathioprine), and corticosteroids. Signs of acute organ rejection include low-grade fever, increasing resting heart rate, fatigue, abdominal pain, nausea, vomiting, and decreasing exercise tolerance. As some children may be asymptomatic, endomyocardial biopsy is

MyNursingKit Care Plan: Pediatric Heart Transplant

Nursing Care Plan

THE CHILD WITH CONGESTIVE HEART FAILURE BEING CARED FOR AT HOME

INTERVENTION	RATIONALE	EXPECTED OUTCOME
1. Nursing Diagnosis: Delayed Growth and Development related to effects of physical disability		
NIC Priority Intervention: **Developmental enhancement:** Teaching parents to facilitate optimal gross motor, fine motor, language, cognitive, social, and emotional growth of preschool children		**NOC Suggested Outcome:** **Child development** (2 years): Milestones of physical, cognitive, and psychosocial progression by 2 years of age
Goal: The child will meet developmental milestones for age group.		
■ Perform baseline developmental assessment.	■ Assessment provides comparison for later assessments and basis for planning specific games, toys, and activities.	The child displays normal language, fine motor, and gross motor activity.
■ Plan for short play periods after rest.	■ Short play periods maintain energy and facilitate play.	
■ Introduce age-appropriate toys and activities such as rattles and blocks for infants and art projects for older children.	■ Play activities facilitate learning and mastery of developmental tasks.	
■ Plan for interactions with healthy children.	■ Social skills are learned through contact with others.	
2. Nursing Diagnosis: Ineffective Therapeutic Regimen Management related to complexity of therapeutic regimen		
NIC Priority Intervention: **Mutual goal setting:** Collaborating with the family to identify and prioritize care goals, and then developing a plan for achieving those goals		**NOC Suggested Outcome:** **Compliance behavior:** Actions taken on the basis of professional advice to promote wellness, recovery, and rehabilitation
Goal: Parents will demonstrate correct administration of medications.		
■ Have parents prepare the medication dosages and administer the digoxin, diuretics, and other medications to the child under the supervision of the home health nurse.	■ Demonstrating techniques used to administer medications provides opportunities to identify dosage errors and to suggest methods to help ensure the child gets all needed medications.	Parents report that child continues to demonstrate improvement and adequate cardiac output without signs of congestive heart failure.
Goal: Parents will state side effects of medications and symptoms of congestive heart failure.		
■ Describe side effects of medications. Give parents handouts with telephone number to call to ask questions or report side effects.	■ If side effects are understood, serious complications can be avoided.	
■ Describe subtle onset of CHF and its symptoms (increasing weakness, exhaustion, irritability, difficulty feeding, cough or difficult respirations, edema).	■ Parents can evaluate child regularly and note subtle changes requiring medical management.	
3. Nursing Diagnosis: Imbalanced Nutrition: Less than Body Requirements related to chronic illness and tiring while feeding		
NIC Priority Intervention: **Weight gain assistance:** Facilitation of body weight gain		**NOC Suggested Outcome:** **Nutritional status: Food and fluid intake:** Amount of food and fluid taken into the body over a 24-hour period

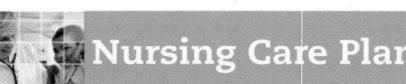

Nursing Care Plan—continued

THE CHILD WITH CONGESTIVE HEART FAILURE BEING CARED FOR AT HOME

INTERVENTION	RATIONALE	EXPECTED OUTCOME
Goal: The infant or child will demonstrate normal weight gain for age.		
■ Teach parents methods to promote food intake related to positioning, size of feedings, food choices.	■ Positioning, frequency of feedings, size of feedings, and use of high-caloric foods can enhance nutritional intake.	The infant or child shows normal weight gain.
■ Observe feeding during home visit.	■ Feedback can assist parents in integrating positive feeding techniques.	Parents report and demonstrate successful feedings of child.
4. Nursing Diagnosis: Activity Intolerance (Child) related to poor cardiac output		
NIC Priority Intervention: **Energy management:** Regulating energy use to treat or prevent fatigue and optimize function		**NOC Suggested Outcome:** **Energy conservation:** Extent of active management of energy to initiate or sustain activity
Goal: The child will perform all necessary activities of daily living without undue tiring.		
■ Help parents alternate activities and rest throughout the child's day.	■ Activities to promote development must be alternated with rest due to decreased cardiac output.	The child performs necessary activities and rests frequently each day.
■ Have parents limit child's exposure to persons with contagious disease.	■ When the child is ill and tired, the immune system can be compromised.	
■ Help family plan quiet surroundings to provide for child's rest.	■ Home setting may need to be altered to promote rest.	
5. Nursing Diagnosis: Caregiver Role Strain (Parent) related to 24-hour responsibility for child's care		
NIC Priority Intervention: **Caregiver support:** Provision of the necessary information, advocacy, and support to facilitate primary patient care by someone other than a healthcare professional		**NOC Suggested Outcome:** **Caregiver endurance potential:** Factors that promote family care provider continuance over an extended period of time
Goal: Parents will express ability to meet own needs.		
■ Assess family and community supports. Provide information related to respite care.	■ Variable family and community supports are available.	Parents report some time away from the child and report renewal in caring for the child.
■ Encourage parents to seek activities to meet personal needs.	■ Parents need time for own personal needs to successfully care for child.	

performed during cardiac catheterization frequently during the first year after transplant to detect rejection, and then annually if no rejection occurs. Statin medications are prescribed to control hyperlipidemia, and hypertension is treated with calcium channel blockers. Hyperlipidemia and blood vessel thickening in the transplanted heart that increase the risk of arrhythmia and heart dysfunction may cause death 3 or more years after the transplant (Schowengerdt, 2006).

Bacterial, fungal, and viral (i.e., cytomegalovirus) infections cause the most problems; however, some common childhood illnesses (acute otitis, colds) may be well tolerated. Certain antibiotics interact with cyclosporine and tacrolimus (elevating serum levels) and should be avoided to prevent renal failure (Gabrys, 2005).

Nursing Management

Depending upon the age at time of transplant, the child may not have had all immunizations (see Chapter 45). Live virus vaccines are contraindicated in children with heart transplants. Help parents arrange for schools and childcare centers to provide early notification of cases of measles, mumps, rubella, and chickenpox. Preventive treatment for the child can be provided as necessary. Good hand hygiene to reduce the spread of infection should be encouraged at home and at school.

After recovery from surgery, children may have near-normal exercise capabilities, normal heart function, and return to school and other activities. Immunosuppressive medications will be continued long term and can cause a variety of physical side effects such as hair growth, gum hyperplasia, weight gain, moon face, acne, and rashes. Children and adolescents may need support to develop positive self-esteem.

Organ rejection is a major concern of families. Provide education for the parents and child to recognize the signs and to seek treatment promptly. Adolescents need special attention to promote adherence to the immunosuppression protocol.

PULMONARY ARTERY HYPERTENSION

Pulmonary artery hypertension (PAH), increased pressure in the pulmonary artery, is a complication of congenital heart defects that increase pulmonary blood flow, pulmonary conditions, and congenital diaphragmatic hernia. Right ventricular hypertrophy and pulmonary vascular resistance develops if increased pulmonary blood flow is sustained. The pulmonary vascular bed reduces this excessive pulmonary blood flow by vasoconstriction. Pulmonary vascular disease develops if the smooth muscle in the small pulmonary arteries hypertrophies to sustain the vasoconstriction. The pulmonary artery pressure increases to push blood across the constricted vascular bed, causing pulmonary artery hypertension. Inflammation, hypertrophy of pulmonary vessels, and fibrosis develop. The right heart function becomes impaired (Rosenzweig & Barst, 2005). The condition is progressive and can become life threatening (Berger, 2007).

Hypoxemia results from pulmonary hypertension and helps maintain the vasoconstriction. The infant displays tachypnea, cyanosis, retractions, and fatigue. Feeding is difficult, and weight loss with fluid and electrolyte imbalance is likely. Older children have exertional dyspnea, increased fatigue, chest pain, and syncope.

Clinical therapy involves surgery to correct an obstructive lesion or close a defect. Therapy for pulmonary artery hypertension related to noncardiac conditions involves bronchodilators, calcium channel blockers, prostaglandins, antibiotics, anticoagulants, corticosteroids, and low-flow oxygen. In some cases heart transplantation is considered (Rosenzweig & Barst, 2005). No cure is available, but life can be prolonged with these measures.

Nursing Management

Nursing care focuses on promoting rest for oxygen conservation, monitoring fluid intake and output carefully, and administering medications and oxygen. Airplane travel may be possible with supplemental oxygen. Exercise should be tailored to avoid dyspnea. Give parents needed support and information about their child.

ACQUIRED HEART DISEASES

INFECTIVE ENDOCARDITIS

Infective endocarditis is an inflammation of the lining, valves, and arterial vessels of the heart caused by bacterial, enterococci, and fungal infections. Up to 90% of pediatric cases occur in children with congenital heart defects, and not all cases are preventable (Hoyer & Silberbach, 2005). Infectious endocarditis is also associated with rheumatic heart disease, a central venous catheter or heart surgery, or intravenous drug abuse. The endocardium is injured by a high velocity or turbulent blood flow due to a heart defect or an indwelling catheter in the right side of the heart. Infectious organisms introduced into the blood stream by dental or medical procedures adhere to the injury site, colonize, and in some cases form a vegetation. The time between bacteremia and development of symptoms is estimated to be 7 to 14 days (Wilson et al., 2007).

Symptoms can be mild and develop slowly, or they can be severe and develop rapidly. Common symptoms are fever, fatigue, joint and muscle aches, weight loss, headache, and diaphoresis. Other signs may include a heart murmur, hepatosplenomegaly, and congestive heart failure. Children with indwelling catheters may initially have pulmonary signs related to septic pulmonary embolism.

Infective endocarditis is diagnosed primarily by blood culture; however, urine and cerebrospinal fluid also may be cultured. Elevated erythrocyte sedimentation rate, anemia, elevated C-reactive protein level, increased white blood cell count, alterations in the electrocardiogram, and changes in heart sounds and murmurs are indicators of the condition. Transesophageal and transthoracic echocardiography is used to identify vegetation or infective lesions in the heart, the extent of valve damage, and cardiac function.

Clinical therapy consists of intravenous antibiotics such as penicillin G, ceftriaxone, vancomycin, nafcillin, oxacillin, gentamicin, ciprofloxacin, cefazolin for 2 to 8 weeks until the infective organism is eradicated. Serum levels of antibiotics are monitored to maintain a therapeutic range. Surgery may be necessary to replace a heart valve or because of risk of embolism. If CHF occurs, bed rest and medications such as digoxin and furosemide are prescribed. The majority of patients are cured with appropriate medical and surgical treatment (Baddour, Wilson, Bayer, et al., 2005).

Prevention of infective endocarditis is preferred, and antibiotic prophylaxis is recommended for dental procedures and invasive respiratory procedures for selected individuals at highest risk for adverse outcomes from infective endocarditis (see page 1376). See "Drug Guide: Medications Used for Infective Endocarditis Prophylaxis for Dental and Invasive Respiratory Procedures."

Nursing Management

Nursing care focuses on assessing the child's respiratory and cardiovascular status, administering medications, and teaching the parents about the child's care. Take the child's vital signs. Assess oxygen saturation and level of consciousness as CHF and embolism may occur. The parents will be anxious about the child's condition, especially if this occurs following surgery for a congenital heart defect or in a critically ill child or newborn. Monitor the parents' coping skills and need for information.

Administer medications as ordered and monitor serum antibiotic levels. Monitor for side effects of antibiotics and for infiltration at the infusion site. Keep invasive procedures to a

Drug Guide

MEDICATIONS USED FOR INFECTIVE ENDOCARDITIS PROPHYLAXIS FOR DENTAL AND INVASIVE RESPIRATORY PROCEDURES

ANTIBIOTIC RECOMMENDATIONS	NURSING MANAGEMENT
Amoxicillin for Oral Use Ampicillin OR Cefazolin or ceftriaxone IM or IV when unable to take oral medication Cephalexin OR clindamycin OR azithromycin or clarithromycin when allergic to penicillin or ampicillin Cefazolin or ceftriaxone OR clindamycin IV or IM when allergic to penicillin or ampicillin and unable to take oral medication	■ One large dose is given 30 to 60 minutes before the procedures. If the preprocedure dose is not taken, the dose may be taken up to 2 hours postprocedure. ■ Teach parents and the child to keep at least one dose in the home to take before dental visits or for dental emergencies. ■ Have parents inform each healthcare provider of the child's need for prophylaxis. ■ Dentists and physicians can write the prescription.

Modified from Wilson, W., Taubert, K. A., Gewitz, M., Lockhart, P. B., Baddour, L. M., Levinson, M., et al. (2007). Prevention of infective endocarditis: Guidelines from the American Heart Association Rheumatic Fever, Endocarditis, and Kawasaki Disease Committee, Council on Cardiovascular Disease in the Young, and the Council on Clinical Cardiology, Council on Cardiovascular Surgery and Anesthesia, and the Quality of Care and Outcomes Research Interdisciplinary Working Group. *Circulation, 116*, 1736–1754.

minimum. Use careful aseptic technique when managing central lines and venous access devices.

The child is often lethargic and on bed rest. Encourage parents to participate in the child's care and plan quiet age-appropriate activities. Home infusion therapy is often ordered so care can continue on an outpatient basis. Instruct parents about care procedures and reinforce the importance of follow-up visits. Home schooling may be needed during the recovery period.

Nursing care also focuses on prevention of endocarditis. Good oral hygiene and regular dental care are important preventive measures. Stress the importance of telling future healthcare providers, including dentists and surgeons, about the child's infective endocarditis history so prophylactic antibiotics can be given for invasive dental and respiratory procedures (Wilson et al., 2007).

RHEUMATIC FEVER

Rheumatic fever is an inflammatory disorder of connective tissue that that results from an autoimmune response to some strains of group A beta-hemolytic streptococci. This disorder may cause long-term damage to heart valves, and affects the joints, brain, and skin tissues. Although rheumatic fever is not common, children between 5 years and early adolescence are most commonly infected, and recurrent episodes can occur (Carapetis, McDonald, & Wilson, 2005). Rheumatic heart disease develops in approximately 10% of individuals who have rheumatic fever (Connor, 2006).

One to 3 weeks after an untreated streptococcal infection, the hallmark signs of rheumatic fever may occur. Carditis involving the mitral or aortic valve may be detected by the development of a new murmur. Chest pain may be caused by pericardial inflammation. Two or more large joints become inflamed with pain, swelling, tenderness, erythema, and heat. The signs may migrate from joint to joint (migratory polyarthritis). Subcutaneous nodules may be palpated over bony prominences and along extensor tendons. A nonpruritic skin rash (erythema marginatum) with pink macules and blanching in the middle of the lesions appears on the trunk, but never on the face and hands. If the central nervous system is affected, Sydenham chorea (St. Vitus dance), characterized by aimless movements of the extremities and facial grimacing, is present.

Diagnosis is based on the Jones Criteria, the presence of two or more of the major signs noted above and evidence of a recent streptococcal infection, such as a positive throat culture or ASLO titer of 320 Todd units. When one major sign, evidence of a recent streptococcal infection, and one or more minor signs (arthralgia, fever, elevated erythrocyte sedimentation rate or C-reactive protein, or a prolonged PR interval on electrocardiogram) are present, rheumatic fever is suspected (Ferrieri, 2002).

Clinical therapy includes antibiotics (penicillin, sulfadiazine, or erythromycin) to eradicate the streptococcal infection. Aspirin is used for fever, arthritis, and arthralgias. Corticosteroids may be used to reduce the inflammation and for severe carditis causing CHF (Carapetis et al., 2005). Most children recover fully, but they are at risk for subsequent episodes of rheumatic fever. Children should be monitored carefully by echocardiogram for potential cardiac complications. Long-term antibiotic prophylaxis to reduce the risk for recurrent episodes is given well into adulthood.

Nursing Management

The most important role of the nurse is prevention of rheumatic fever. Nurses in clinics, offices, and schools need to ensure that all children with possible streptococcal infections have a throat culture taken. Even if the sore throat is mild, a culture is needed if family members or other contacts have had a streptococcal infection. Emphasize to the family the importance of giving all doses of the antibiotic prescribed when a culture is positive.

The child with rheumatic fever is hospitalized for a period of time. During the acute inflammatory phase, take the child's temperature at least every 4 hours and monitor vital signs. The child is on bed rest while monitoring for the onset of carditis, and for 4 weeks if carditis develops. Auscultate the child's heart and note any unusual sounds. Observe the child for changes in skin, joints, or behavior. Be sure family members have throat cultures done to identify possible asymptomatic streptococcal carriers.

Administer antibiotics and aspirin as ordered. The child is usually lethargic and often has joint pain. Aspirin often relieves pain dramatically after a few doses. Position and handle the child's joints carefully. Provide quiet activities, and encourage visits or telephone calls from family members and friends. Provide emotional support for the child with chorea; the purposeless involuntary movements can last for 5 to 15 weeks and are disturbing. Encourage the family to participate in the child's hospital care.

The child is generally cared for at home during the recovery phase. Activities may be limited, especially if heart damage is suspected. Help parents plan quiet activities, such as playing board games or computer games, watching videos, or reading. Arrange rest periods after the child returns to school. Reassure the child and parents that the effects of chorea will eventually subside.

On discharge a daily oral low-dose antibiotic is prescribed or a monthly long-acting antibiotic injection is given. Make sure the child and parents understand the importance of taking prescribed medication until adulthood to prevent future infection and possible heart damage from recurrent rheumatic fever. Make sure the parents understand that the child's future sore throats may be streptococcal and that a throat culture should be taken even when the child is taking daily antibiotics. The child may need a different antibiotic for the infection. Emphasize the importance of follow-up care to prevent new infections and to monitor heart function.

KAWASAKI DISEASE

Kawasaki disease is an acute febrile, systemic vascular inflammatory disorder that affects small and midsize arteries, including the coronary arteries. It is the leading cause of acquired heart disease in children in the United States (Vetter, 2006). Children under 4 years of age account for 80% of cases, and 50% of cases occur in children under 2 years. Although this disorder is most common in children of Asian and Pacific Islander origin, it is seen in all racial and ethnic groups (Park, 2008).

Etiology and Pathophysiology

The etiology of Kawasaki disease is unknown; it is thought to be caused by an infectious agent that has not yet been identified. The disorder appears to result in an exaggerated immune response in a genetically susceptible child (Vetter, 2006). This multisystem inflammatory disease involving the small and midsize arteries sometimes causes aneurysms in the coronary arteries as well as other arteries. As the coronary arteries heal, they can become stenotic, leading to reduced blood flow and potential infarcts (Milana & Chandran, 2006).

Clinical Manifestations

The three stages of the disease are acute, subacute, and convalescent.

- The acute stage of Kawasaki disease, lasting 1 to 2 weeks, is characterized by irritability, high fever that persists for more than 5 days, hyperemic conjunctivae, red throat, swollen hands and feet, maculopapular or erythema multiforme-like rash on the trunk and perineal area, unilateral enlargement of the cervical lymph nodes, diarrhea, and hepatic dysfunction.
- The subacute stage, lasting 2 to 4 weeks, is characterized by cracking lips and fissures, desquamation of the skin on the tips of the fingers and toes, joint pain, cardiac disease, and thrombocytosis (Figure 49–7 ●).
- In the convalescent stage, 6 to 8 weeks after disease onset, the child appears normal but lingering signs of inflammation may be present.

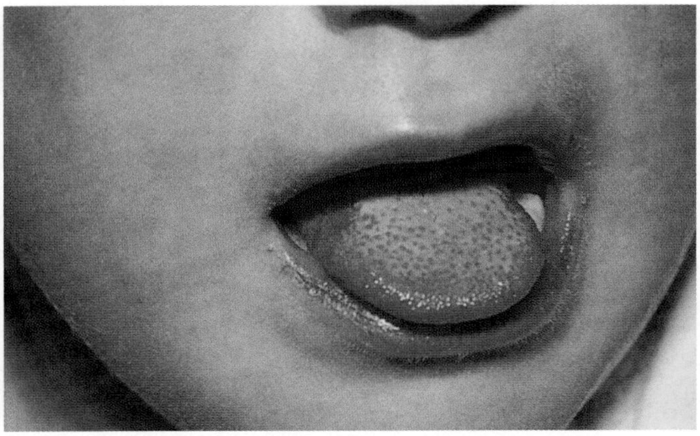

● **Figure 49–7** This child shows many of the signs of the acute stage of Kawasaki disease: strawberry tongue, dry cracking lips, buccal mucosa erythema.

Other clinical manifestations may occur during the acute phase, such as arthralgias, abdominal pain with diarrhea, liver dysfunction, gallbladder hydrops, and aseptic meningitis.

Clinical Therapy

Diagnosis is based on clinical signs using the criteria given in Table 49–8 as there is no specific diagnostic test. Blood studies may reveal elevations of the erythrocyte sedimentation rate, white blood cell count, and alanine aminotransferase level, mild anemia, hypoalbuminemia, and white blood cells in the urine (Milana & Chandran, 2006). Initial and repeat echocardiography is used to identify specific vascular changes in the heart and coronary arteries.

Kawasaki disease is treated with intravenous immunoglobulin (2 g/kg given in a single infusion) and aspirin. High doses of aspirin (80 to 100 mg/kg/day in 4 divided doses) are given while the fever is high. The dose is decreased to 3 to 5 mg/kg/day or less once the fever has dropped because it has antiplatelet activity. High doses of immune globulin given before the 10th day of fever reduce the incidence of coronary artery lesions and aneurysms, as well as decrease inflammatory signs (Milana & Chandran, 2006). When the fever persists after the first administration of immune globulin, a second dose may be given. When the second dose of immune globulin is ineffective, corticosteroids may be administered.

Children are usually hospitalized for 3 or more days, depending upon the presence of cardiac lesions and how long the

Table 49–8 Diagnostic Criteria for Kawasaki Disease

Kawasaki disease is diagnosed when a high spiking fever over 39°C (102.2°F) for 5 days or longer is present along with four of the following five principal features not explained by another disease process. When fewer than four criteria are present, but echocardiography or angiography reveals coronary artery abnormalities, Kawasaki disease is also diagnosed.

Body Part Affected	Principal Features
Eyes	Bilateral bulbar conjunctivitis without exudate
Skin	Intense erythema of the buccal and pharyngeal surfaces with dry, swollen, cracked, and fissuring lips and a strawberry tongue Erythema of the palms and soles, edema of the hands and feet, and then desquamation after 2 or more weeks of symptoms Dermatitis of the trunk with an erythematous maculopapular rash
Lymph nodes	Cervical lymphadenopathy, frequently unilateral, with a lymph node over 1.5 cm in diameter found early in the disease

Modified from Vetter, V. L. (2006). Kawasaki disease. In V. L. Vetter, *Pediatric cardiology: The requisites in pediatrics* (p. 132), St. Louis: Elsevier Mosby.

fever persists. Most children recover fully. Careful monitoring for cardiac disease continues for several weeks or months. Coronary aneurysms may develop in 5% of children treated with intravenous immune globulin (Newberger, Sleeper, McCrindle, et al., 2007). Many smaller coronary aneurysms resolve spontaneously in 1 to 2 years after treatment (Milano & Chandran, 2006). Some children with stenosed coronary arteries may need angioplasty or coronary artery bypass grafts.

Nursing Management

Nursing care focuses on promoting comfort, monitoring for early signs of complications or disease progression, and supporting the family.

Assessment is important in identifying signs of Kawasaki disease, as the acute phase of this disorder is commonly confused with other diseases. When the child is hospitalized, take the temperature every 4 hours and before each dose of aspirin. Carefully assess the extremities for edema, redness, and desquamation every 8 hours. Examine the eyes and the mucous membranes for inflammation. Monitor the child's dietary and fluid intake and weigh the child daily. Carefully assess heart sounds and rhythm.

Administer aspirin and monitor for side effects of aspirin such as bleeding and gastrointestinal upset. Administer intravenous immune globulin as a blood product, carefully regulating the infusion rate to run slowly according to the physician's orders, and observing for any reactions to the infusion. The infusion rate should not be over 1 mL/min. If a reaction occurs, stop the infusion immediately (see Chapter 50∞).

Promote the child's comfort. Keep the child's skin clean and dry, and lubricate the lips. Use cool compresses and tepid sponges to make the feverish child more comfortable. Change the child's clothes and bed linens frequently. Give the child frequent small feedings of soft foods and liquids that are neither too hot nor too cold.

Use passive range of motion exercises to facilitate joint movement. Because the child with Kawasaki disease is often lethargic and irritable, plan rest periods and quiet age-appropriate activities. Encourage the parents to participate in their child's care. This comforts and reassures the child. Give the parents information about the disease and the child's treatment.

Before the child is discharged, teach the parents to administer aspirin as ordered and to watch for side effects. Advise the parents that the child may need to avoid contact sports or other activities that could cause bleeding. Limitation of strenuous activity is recommended for all children with coronary aneurysms or stenoses. Emphasize the need for follow-up care to monitor for cardiac complications.

Inform the parents of a child with Kawasaki disease to postpone needed live virus vaccines (measles and varicella) for 11 months after immune globulin administration, but other immunizations may be given on schedule.

CARDIAC ARRHYTHMIAS

Cardiac **arrhythmias** (abnormal heart rhythms or dysrhythmias) occur frequently in children, but less often than in adults. These include tachyarrhythmias (sinus tachycardia) and bradyarrhythmias (sinus bradycardia) that occur with acute conditions such as hypoxia, acidosis, increased intracranial pressure, hypothermia, and hypoglycemia. Most of these arrhythmias resolve once the condition is treated. Less common arrhythmias are often associated with congenital heart disease, including atrial fibrillation, atrial flutter, ventricular fibrillation, and heart block. Arrhythmias must be recognized because they cause decreased cardiac output and CHF, or an even more serious arrhythmia may develop that could result in sudden death.

Bradycardia

Bradycardia is a heart rate less than the lower limit of normal for the child' age, usually a rate less than 80 beats per minute in infants and less than 60 beats per minute in children and adolescents (Doniger & Sharieff, 2006). Some athletes may normally have a heart rate of 60.

For sinus bradycardia due to an acute condition, oxygen, ventilation, and medications such as epinephrine or atropine are used until the condition resolves. Other chronic bradycardias due to heart block often require a pacemaker.

Supraventricular Tachycardia

Supraventricular tachycardia (SVT), the most common pathologic tachycardia, is the abrupt onset of a rapid, regular heart rate, often too fast to count. Prolonged episodes of continuous SVT for more than 24 hours may lead to CHF. Cardiac output is affected because diastolic filling cannot occur with such a rapid heart rate. Prolonged episodes of SVT are life threatening and can progress to CHF or cardiogenic shock if untreated.

MyNursingKit Heart Sounds

Early signs in infants include poor feeding, irritability, and pallor. Older children may have episodes of altered consciousness (dizziness or syncope). The presenting heart rate with SVT will be greater than 220 beats/min in infants and greater than 180 beats/min in children.

Electrocardiography, including a 24-hour rhythm recording, confirms the diagnosis. Vagal stimulation such as applying ice or iced saline solution to the face or rectal stimulation with a thermometer may reduce the heart rate. An older child can perform the Valsalva maneuver (e.g., holding the breath and straining, or blowing forcefully on the thumb) to increase intrathoracic and venous pressures and thus slow the heart rate. Adenosine may be administered when vagal stimulation does not work. Digoxin, amiodarone, or propranolol may also be administered during acute episodes if more aggressive therapy is needed. For life-threatening episodes unresponsive to medications, the child may be sedated for invasive procedures such as synchronized cardioversion or esophageal overdrive pacing. Recurrent attacks are common, and digoxin and beta blockers may be given to reduce the frequency of episodes (Kaltman, et al., 2006). **Radiofrequency ablation** may be performed during cardiac catheterization. Radiofrequency energy is transmitted to the site of the accessory conduction system pathway triggering the tachycardia. If the procedure is successful, medications to control the tachycardia can be discontinued. In some cases, a cardioverter-defibrillator may need to be implanted.

Long QT Syndrome

Long QT syndrome (LQTS) is a rhythm disturbance of autosomal dominant and autosomal recessive inheritance that puts children at risk for ventricular fibrillation and sudden death. The ventricular tachycardia with a prolonged QT interval impairs cardiac output leading to syncope or seizures. Electrolyte abnormalities (hypokalemia, hypocalcemia, and hypomagnesemia) and medications may also cause the disorder. LQTS may cause 3000 to 4000 sudden deaths each year and some cases of sudden infant death syndrome (Doniger & Sharieff, 2006). Males younger than 15 years are at higher risk for sudden death due to the syndrome (Hobbs, Peterson, Moss, et al., 2006).

The arrhythmia may be triggered by demanding physical exercise, extreme emotional stress, or an abrupt loud noise (e.g., doorbell, alarm clock). Arrhythmia may occur without warning and result in sudden death. Presenting signs include syncope, seizure, cardiac arrest, or palpitation during exercise or with emotion.

If the child is resuscitated or evaluated because of presenting signs, the arrhythmia is commonly detected by electrocardiogram. The disorder is treated by beta-blockers (propranolol) in doses that lessen the chance of drug-induced bradycardia (Park, 2008). A cardiac pacemaker or implantable cardioverter-defibrillator may be used in patients considered at high risk for sudden death. The child should not participate in competitive sports and should be observed when swimming.

Nursing Management

Nursing care of children with SVT or long QT syndrome focuses on assessing the child's condition, administering medications, and providing emotional support to the child and parents. Children are treated in the emergency department or intensive care unit. The child is placed on a cardiac monitor, and frequent assessment is critical. Report continued abnormal rates or rhythms to the physician. Carefully observe and record changes in level of consciousness, color, weakness, irritability, and feeding pattern. Administer medications as ordered. Have emergency drugs and resuscitation equipment available at the bedside. Provide for rest and adequate nutrition.

Episodes of arrhythmia are frightening for both the child and parents. Carefully explain the treatment plan and home care. Teach parents to take the child's apical pulse. Make sure parents are trained in cardiopulmonary resuscitation and know how to seek emergency care. Emphasize that prescribed medications help prevent or reduce the frequency of the episodes. Help the child and family recognize and avoid medications that can trigger another episode. The child with SVT should not use cardiac stimulant drugs such as decongestants. For the child with LQTS, teach the parents and adolescents to remind the primary care provider not to prescribe medications that prolong the QT interval (e.g., antihistamines, antidepressants, and macrolide antibiotics). An updated list of these medications can be found online. See My Nursing Kit.

DYSLIPIDEMIA

Hyperlipidemia is a condition in which one or more lipids (total cholesterol, low-density lipoproteins [LDL], triglycerides, high-density lipoproteins [HDL]) have an abnormal level in the blood. It is important to identify children who have a genetic history or lifestyle that makes them more susceptible to future coronary heart disease and to implement preventive health measures to reduce the child's risk of disease and premature death as an adult. A high LDL, a low HDL, elevated blood pressure, type 1 or 2 diabetes mellitus, cigarette smoking, and obesity are major risk factors (Daniels, Greer, and the Committee on Nutrition, 2008).

Abnormalities in the lipid levels may be the result of excessive production, lack of clearance of the lipoprotein particles, a genetic defect in lipid metabolism, or other defects such as enzyme deficiencies. Some children have primary dyslipidemia due to familial hypercholesterolemia. Obesity is the leading secondary cause of dyslipidemia. Examples of secondary causes include hypothyroidism, diabetes, nephritic syndrome and certain drugs such as corticosteroids, beta blockers, and isotretinoin (Belay, Belamarich, & Racine, 2004). Most commonly, children have lipid abnormalities due to a combination of heredity and lifestyle factors.

A blood test for total cholesterol, HDL, and triglycerides identifies hyperlipidemia. See Table 49–9. The LDL level is calculated from the triglyceride, HDL, and total cholesterol levels. Children over 2 years of age should be screened for hyperlipidemia with a fasting lipid panel with the following risk factors: a positive family history of dyslipidemia or cardiovascular disease before 55 years in men or 65 years in women, the family history is unknown, or the child has cardiovascular risk factors, such as overweight or obesity (body mass index greater than 85th percentile), hypertension (blood pressure greater than 95th percentile), cigarette smoking, or diabetes mellitus (Daniels, Greer, and the Committee on Nutrition, 2008).

Table 49–9 Laboratory Values for Assessment of Dyslipidemia in Children Between 2 and 19 Years Old

Test	Recommended Level	Levels of Higher Risk
Total Cholesterol	Under 170 mg/dL	Borderline: 170–199 mg/dL Abnormal: 200 mg/dL or higher
LDL-C	Under 100 mg/dL	Borderline: 100–129 mg/dL Abnormal: 130 mg/dL or higher
Triglyceride	Under 200 mg/dL	Abnormal: 200 mg/dL or higher
HDL-C	40 mg/dL or higher	Abnormal: Under 40 mg/dL

Adapted from Giddings, S., Dennison, B. A., Birch, L. L., et al. (2005). Dietary guidelines for children and adolescents: A guide for practitioners. Consensus statement from the American Heart Association. *Circulation, 112*, 2061–2075.

Evidence in Action

The cardiovascular risk of children (obesity, blood pressure, dyslipidemia, hyperglycemia, and metabolic syndrome) is highly correlated to their parents' cardiovascular risk factors (Reis, Kip, Marroquin, et al., 2006). Identifying these risks in children may provide an important education opportunity to encourage parents to seek health care for their own cardiovascular risk factors.

The primary management of dyslipidemia in most children includes dietary modifications, exercise, and other changes in lifestyle. The child's diet is carefully analyzed and changes are made to satisfy the dietary guidelines so that saturated fats are less than 7% of total caloric intake, and cholesterol intake is less than 200 mg per day for treatment of elevated LDL levels (Giddings, Dennison, Birch et al., 2005). A healthy total fat intake is 20% to 35% of daily calories. If the child is obese, weight loss is encouraged. However, intensive dietary and exercise programs have resulted in modest reductions in LDL-C (Belay, Belamarich, & Tom-Revzon, 2007).

If the child continues to have high serum lipid levels, pharmacologic treatment may be initiated for children 8 years and older. Cholestyramine or colestipol, which bind bile acid in the intestine, niacin, and statins may be prescribed. The initial goal is to lower LDL concentration to less than 160 mg/dL. However, target LDL concentration may be as low as 130 mg/dL or even 110 mg/dL when there is a strong family history of cardiovascular disease and other risk factors such as obesity and diabetes mellitus (Daniels, Greer, and the Committee on Nutrition, 2008).

Nursing Management

Nursing care focuses on identifying children at risk for dyslipidemia, providing education about diet and exercise, and monitoring eating patterns. Identification and management of dyslipidemia takes place in many community settings. Office and clinic nurses identify children who need to have serum lipid measured. Nurses in schools provide education on ways to reduce risk factors. The child's history of exercise patterns, weight percentile, and dietary intake provides important information. Obtain information on familial heart disease, hypertension, diabetes, and smoking to determine risk factors.

Work with nutritionists to provide dietary teaching and monitor family eating patterns. The food plan for the child and entire family should consist primarily of fruit, vegetables, whole grains, low-fat and nonfat dairy products, lean meat and fish, legumes, and nuts. Help parents understand that modeling food choices helps children learn to select and eat better food choices and reduce lipid levels. For children with familial hypercholesterolemia, lifelong dietary control is essential.

Help the child select an enjoyable moderate to intense activity for daily participation, and then obtain 30 minutes of aerobic exercise (e.g., jogging, swimming, biking, roller blading, soccer) at least 3 to 4 times a week to promote cardiovascular fitness. Discourage smoking by the child or the parents as it increases the risk for cardiovascular disease.

Educate children and adolescents taking statin medications to report any adverse effects to their healthcare provider: myalgia, muscle soreness, weakness, tenderness, or dark-colored urine. Include the entire family in the treatment plan; it is difficult for a single family member to change eating and exercise patterns.

HYPERTENSION

Hypertension in children and adolescents is defined as a systolic or diastolic blood pressure reading that is equal to or greater than 95th percentile for age, sex, and height. Normal blood pressure is defined as a systolic or diastolic reading that falls below the 90th percentile for age, sex, and height. Persistent hypertension has previously been estimated to occur in 1% to 3% of the pediatric population, however, blood pressure levels are increasing in children due to increased incidence of obesity, increased high salt food intake, and decreased physical activity (Mitsnefes, 2006). Increasing rates of hypertension in childhood is a significant concern because it is a major risk factor for heart disease and stroke during adulthood.

The most common causes of secondary hypertension in children under 6 years are coarctation of the aorta and renal disorders, and renal disorders accounts for most secondary hypertension in children between 6 and 10 years (Mitsnefes, 2006).

Children rarely have symptoms of hypertension and the condition is usually detected during a health examination. Symptoms of severe hypertension may include headaches, dizziness, and visual changes.

Developing Cultural Competence

BLOOD PRESSURE

A recent study contrasted the blood pressure of 1740 children aged 13 to 14 years in three states with the following racial and ethnic heritage: White (14.3%), Black (22%), Hispanic (50%), American Indian (2%), and mixed heritage (11.7%). No significant differences in blood pressure were related to racial or ethnic origin; however, 23.9% of the children had a higher blood pressure than expected from other national studies. High blood pressure was most often attributable to higher body mass index (BMI) (Jago, Harrell, McMurray, et al., 2006).

Clinical Therapy

The diagnosis of hypertension is based on three or more separate readings a week apart in which the systolic or diastolic reading is greater than or equal to the 95th percentile for sex, age, and height (Feld & Corey, 2007). Blood chemistry (BUN, creatinine, and electrolytes), complete blood count, urinalysis, and urine culture tests should be performed to detect secondary causes of hypertension. Serum lipid studies and a fasting glucose should be performed to identify dyslipidemia or diabetes. Polysomnography may be performed to identify a sleep disorder as obstructive sleep apnea is associated with hypertension. A drug screen may be appropriate to identify substances that could cause hypertension (National High Blood Pressure Education Program Working Group on High Blood Pressure in Children and Adolescents, 2004).

Nonpharmacologic measures for reduction of blood pressure include weight reduction and increased exercise. Dietary modification involves reduced sodium and saturated fats, three to five fruit servings daily, and an adequate intake of calcium and dietary fiber. Smoking, alcohol, and drugs should be strongly discouraged. Children also need 30 to 60 minutes of physical activity each day.

Medications are used for children with persistent, severe hypertension that is not resolved with nonpharmacologic therapies. Angiotensin-converting enzyme (ACE) inhibitors and calcium channel blockers are most commonly prescribed for children because of their low side effects (Mitsnefes, 2006).

Nursing Management

A complete history is taken to evaluate the child with persistent high blood pressure, identifying potential risk factors such as family history for hypertension, smoking, or a systemic disease. Is the child obese? How many servings of fruits does the child eat daily? What is the daily number of dairy product servings? What is the child's daily salt intake? What are the child's daily exercise routines? Review any medications or other potential agents used by the child or adolescent.

Assess the child's blood pressure and consistently use the right arm and appropriately sized cuff (see Skill 9–10 SKILLS). Compare the leg blood pressure to that in the arm. Compare readings to the blood pressure values for gender, age, and height percentile (see Appendix D ∞). Monitor the child with borderline hypertension every 3 to 6 months. Take at least two readings during the visit and average them if they differ.

MyNursingKit Animation: Blood Pressure

Complementary Care

TRANSCENDENTAL MEDITATION FOR STRESS MANAGEMENT AND BLOOD PRESSURE CONTROL

Meditation has been demonstrated to reduce cardiovascular reactivity to acute stress. A study was conducted with 78 normotensive students, average age 12 years, randomly assigned by classroom to either a meditation or health education control group. Participants in the transcendental meditation group were taught to close their eyes and focus on the movement of their diaphragm while breathing in a slow, deep, relaxed manner. Meditation was practiced 4 minutes a day (20 minutes a week) with a teacher, and students were asked to practice meditation at home. Control group students had weekly 20 minute sessions on high blood pressure prevention and cardiovascular disease risk factor reduction. They were asked to do 20-minute daily walks. Resting and 24-hour ambulatory blood pressure measurements were obtained before and after the intervention period. Study results revealed that the meditation group had greater decreases in resting systolic blood pressure than the control group. Daytime ambulatory blood pressure measurements after school revealed significantly lower systolic and diastolic readings in the meditation group. No significant differences between the groups were seen by ethnicity, gender, or anthropometric measurements. Transcendental meditation shows promise as a potential complementary therapy to help normotensive children maintain their blood pressure within normal ranges, and to potentially help treat hypertension in children and adolescents (Barnes, Davis, Murzynowski, et al., 2004).

Teach both the child and the parents how to improve the diet and develop exercise routines. Provide suggestions about substitute seasonings for salt and a list of salty foods to avoid. Increasing intake of low-fat dairy products and fruits can contribute to blood pressure control.

Emphasize the importance of avoiding smoking. Discuss ways to increase activity and reduce time watching television or playing computer games. Provide suggestions for the management of stress and stressful situations. Teaching that involves the entire family is usually the most effective. Instruct the family on correct administration of prescribed medications when used.

INJURIES OF THE CARDIOVASCULAR SYSTEM

SHOCK

Shock is an acute, complex state of circulatory dysfunction resulting in failure to deliver sufficient oxygen and other nutrients to meet cell and tissue demands. It can be caused by a variety of conditions such as hemorrhage, dehydration, sepsis, obstruction of blood flow, and cardiac pump failure.

PATHOPHYSIOLOGY ILLUSTRATED

HYPOVOLEMIC SHOCK

If hemorrhage reduces the circulating blood volume sufficiently, vasoconstriction occurs, shifting blood to maintain the perfusion of vital organs. When the blood loss exceeds 20% to 25%, the child's body can no longer compensate and hypovolemic shock ensues.

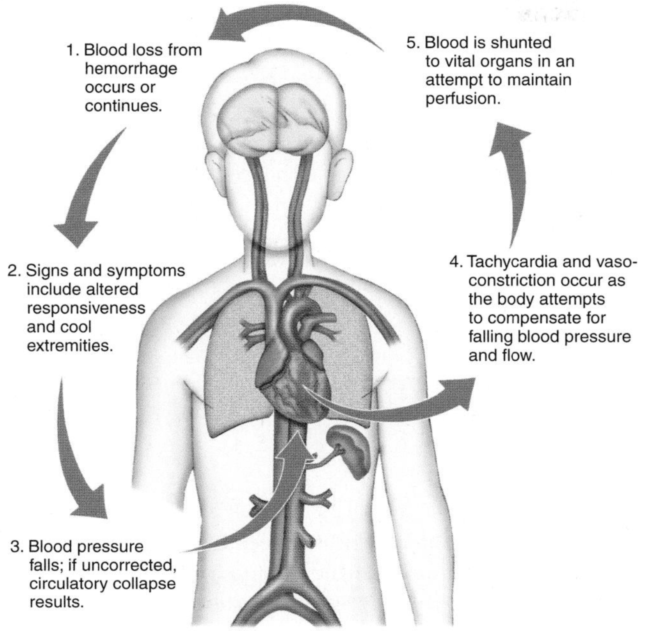

1. Blood loss from hemorrhage occurs or continues.
2. Signs and symptoms include altered responsiveness and cool extremities.
3. Blood pressure falls; if uncorrected, circulatory collapse results.
4. Tachycardia and vasoconstriction occur as the body attempts to compensate for falling blood pressure and flow.
5. Blood is shunted to vital organs in an attempt to maintain perfusion.

HYPOVOLEMIC SHOCK

Hypovolemic shock is a clinical state of inadequate tissue and organ perfusion resulting from the movement of blood or plasma out of the intravascular compartment leading to inadequate intravascular volume (see "Pathophysiology Illustrated: Hypovolemic Shock"). The blood or plasma in the vascular space may be decreased because of hemorrhage or fluid movement into the interstitial spaces.

Etiology and Pathophysiology

Major causes of decreased intravascular blood volume include the following:

- Hemorrhage from significant injury
- Plasma loss from burns, nephrotic syndrome, and sepsis
- Fluid and electrolyte loss associated with dehydration, diabetic ketoacidosis, and diabetes insipidus

Decreased intravascular blood volume results in inadequate delivery of oxygen and nutrients to cells and accumulation of toxic wastes in the capillaries and can cause a decrease in cardiac output and mean arterial pressure. Cellular hypoxia and acidosis develop simultaneously. The accumulation of toxins and inadequate tissue oxygenation cause cellular damage.

The child's body attempts to compensate by the following measures:

- The renin-angiotensin-aldosterone system is stimulated to retain sodium and water when perfusion of the kidneys is decreased.
- The antidiuretic hormone is secreted when the atria have reduced blood volume leading to water retention.
- The heart rate and myocardial contractility increase to improve cardiac output.
- The respiratory rate increases to improve oxygenation and decrease waste accumulation in the cells.
- The hydrostatic pressure falls, permitting fluid to shift into the vascular space and increasing the circulating blood volume.
- The peripheral vasculature constricts to maintain the systemic vascular resistance and to increase perfusion to the vital organs as long as possible.

The child can compensate until 20% to 25% of volume loss occurs, and then life-threatening hypotension results.

Clinical Manifestations

Signs of early hypovolemic shock in children are nonspecific but need to be recognized before hypotension occurs. Signs that the child is compensating for a decreased blood volume are tachycardia, usually sustained at a rate greater than 130 beats per minute; increased respiratory effort; delayed capillary refill (greater than 2 seconds); weak peripheral pulses; pallor; and cold extremities (signs of decreased perfusion). Urine output decreases (less than 0.5–1 mL/kg/hr in infants and young children) when renal blood flow drops. In cases of dehydration, dry mucous membranes and poor skin turgor are also present.

When hypovolemic shock is not treated in early stages, the condition progresses until the child can no longer compensate; the systolic blood pressure drops and the pulse pressure narrows. Reduced cerebral blood flow ultimately results in a decreased level of consciousness. The condition may progress to cardiopulmonary failure if not reversed. See "Clinical Manifestations: Hypovolemic Shock."

Clinical Therapy

No laboratory tests can be used to evaluate the volume deficit rapidly enough to diagnose hypovolemic shock. The child is examined for characteristic signs to confirm the diagnosis. Laboratory tests commonly performed after hypovolemic shock is diagnosed include hematocrit and hemoglobin, arterial blood gases, serum electrolytes, glucose, osmolality, blood urea nitrogen, and urinalysis.

Emergency care focuses on improving tissue perfusion. An open airway is established, oxygen is administered, and ventilation is assisted if necessary. Bleeding is controlled, and an intravenous or intraosseous line is started to provide large volumes of crystalloid fluids.

Ringer's lactate solution is the preferred fluid for initial resuscitation because it contains buffers that counteract the effects

Clinical Manifestations

HYPOVOLEMIC SHOCK

SYSTEM	EARLY SHOCK	UNCOMPENSATED SHOCK	PROFOUND SHOCK
Cardiac	Mild tachycardia, weak distal pulses, strong central pulses	Moderate tachycardia, thready distal pulses, weak central pulses, decreasing systolic blood pressure	Frank hypotension, absent distal pulses, thready central pulses, severe tachycardia or bradycardia
Respiratory	Mild tachypnea	Moderate tachypnea	Severe tachypnea
Neurologic	Normal, anxious, irritable, or combative behavior	Confusion, agitation, lethargy, decreased pain response	Comatose state
Skin	Mottled appearance; capillary refill time greater than 2 seconds; cool, clammy extremities	Pallor, capillary refill time greater than 3 seconds, cold, dry extremities, sunken eyes	Pale, cold skin, cyanosis, capillary refill greater than 5 seconds
Renal	Decreased urine output, increased specific gravity in older infants and children (newborns cannot concentrate urine)	Oliguria, increased specific gravity	No urine output

Data from: Markenson, D. S., (2002). *Pediatric prehospital care* (pp. 174–175). Upper Saddle River, NJ: Brady; McKiernan, C. A., & Lieberman, S. A. (2005). Circulatory shock in children: An overview. *Pediatrics in Review* 26(12), 451–459; and Ralston, M., Hazinski, M. F., Zaritsky, A. L., Schexnayder, S. M., & Kleinman, M. E. (2006). *Pediatric advanced life support: Provider manual*, (p. 100), Dallas, TX: American Heart Association.

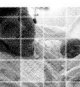

Nursing Practice

Initial signs that a child with hypovolemic shock is responding to fluid resuscitation include slowing of the heart rate, improved color, improved responsiveness, increased warmth of the extremities, and a faster capillary refill time. The systolic blood pressure should be increased.

of acidosis (Ecklund & Ecklund, 2007). A fluid volume of 20 mL/kg is administered rapidly over 5 minutes. The same amount of fluid is given in 5 minutes if the child's physiologic condition does not improve after fluid is first administered. If no improvement is seen after the second fluid bolus, blood or albumin is usually ordered. Once the child's physiologic condition is stabilized, the cause of the hypovolemic shock becomes the focus of examination and treatment.

NURSING MANAGEMENT

NURSING ASSESSMENT AND DIAGNOSIS

Ask the parent (or child, if appropriate) about possible injuries or the duration and severity of acute illnesses. If no external bleeding is evident, determine whether an injury may be causing internal bleeding. For example, the liver and spleen are highly vascular organs that have little protection from direct blunt forces. Significant bleeding from injury to one of these organs can cause hypovolemic shock without evidence of bleeding. An acute illness such as gastroenteritis with prolonged vomiting and diarrhea can also result in dehydration and hypovolemic shock.

If external bleeding is apparent, determine the amount of blood lost. Although children lose the same amount of blood from a laceration as adults, the total volume of blood lost is proportional to their weight.

Frequently assess the child's heart rate, respiratory rate, blood pressure, capillary refill time, level of consciousness with the Glasgow Coma Scale (see Chapter 56), color, and skin temperature to identify any changes that indicate improvement or deterioration in the child's condition. Monitor urine output and specific gravity hourly. Signs of the child's improved status include:

- A decrease in heart rate, respiratory rate, and capillary refill time.
- An increase in systolic blood pressure and urine output.
- Improved color, level of consciousness, and skin temperature.
- Regaining of lost weight.

Assess the parents' response and coping mechanisms to the child's potentially life-threatening injury. Families are unprepared for the abrupt change in the child's condition because of the unpredictability of the injury. See Chapter 43.

Several nursing diagnoses may apply to the child with hypovolemic shock. They include the following:

- *Decreased Cardiac Output* related to hypovolemia
- *Deficient Fluid Volume* related to active fluid volume loss

Growth and Development

The child's total blood volume varies by weight. The child has approximately 80 mL of blood for every kilogram of body weight.

- Newborn: 3 kg × 80 mL = 240 mL (1 cup)
- 5-year-old child: 25 kg × 80 mL = 2000 mL (2 quarts)
- 13-year-old child: 50 kg × 80 mL = 4000 mL (1 gallon)

- *Ineffective Tissue Perfusion (Cardiopulmonary, Renal, and Cerebral)* related to impaired transport of oxygen across alveolar and capillary membrane
- *Compromised Family Coping* related to life-threatening condition of the child

PLANNING AND INTERVENTION

Nurses in the emergency department operating room and intensive care unit more commonly participate in the resuscitation of the child in hypovolemic shock, often using guidelines or protocols for nursing actions. Assist with the child's assessment and the establishment of intravenous access. Calculate and prepare the amount of intravenous fluid needed for administration according to the child's weight (20 mL/kg). Ensure rapid fluid administration by intravenous push or pressure bag. Monitor the child's physiologic response to the fluid bolus within 5 minutes. Prepare a second and third fluid bolus. Use warmed intravenous fluids for resuscitation because hypothermia may interfere with the child's response to treatment. Keep the child covered or use heat lamps to reduce body-heat loss.

When packed red blood cells are administered, verify that the correct blood has been obtained for the child. Change the intravenous fluid to normal saline to prevent clotting during blood administration (see Skill 12–6 SKILLS). Assess the child carefully for a transfusion reaction (see Chapter 51). Monitor the child's physiologic circulatory responses for improvement or deterioration in status. Notify the physician of any deterioration.

Provide support to the child and family during the acute phase of treatment. Parents and children with hypovolemic shock resulting from injury are usually apprehensive. The child may be fearful because of the sudden hospitalization or agitated because of an altered level of consciousness. As parents often fear for the child's life in cases of severe injury, update them about the child's condition frequently. Explain the care being provided and how it helps the child. Listen to their concerns and correct any misconceptions (see Chapter 43).

EVALUATION

Examples of expected nursing care outcomes include the following:

- The child receives adequate fluid resuscitation to prevent progression to uncompensated shock.
- The family copes with the stress of the child's injury.

DISTRIBUTIVE SHOCK

Distributive shock is an abnormal distribution of blood volume, usually resulting from a decrease in systemic vascular resistance. The blood accumulates in the extremities because of vasodilation and capillary permeability. Less blood is returned to the heart, so **preload** (amount of blood in the ventricle at the end of diastole that stretches the heart muscle before contraction) drops and cardiac output falls. Causes of distributive shock include anaphylaxis, sepsis, and spinal cord injury.

Septic Shock

Immunodeficient children are at high risk for septic shock. Septic shock begins as an infection and progresses to sepsis with a bacterial toxin. Once the toxin enters the circulatory system, the body's inflammatory processes over-respond. Mediators along with procoagulation factors initiate inflammation, coagulation, and inhibit fibrinolysis. White blood cells multiply throughout the body and macrophages produce cytokines, which dilate the blood vessels and increase permeability. Fibrin deposits impede blood flow. Congestion occurs in some tissue beds reducing the delivery of oxygen and nutrients to the cells, and bacteria may be trapped and multiply unchecked. Interstitial edema and hypovolemia may be followed by multiple organ dysfunction and failure (Moloney-Harmon, 2005). (see "Pathophysiology Illustrated: Septic Shock"). Toxic shock syndrome is one form of septic shock that may rapidly progress and cause death.

Septic shock has three phases: compensated, uncompensated, and refractory.

- *Compensated phase.* The child has a fever, tachycardia, tachypnea, warm extremities, bounding pulses, brisk capillary refill, and normal urine output. Responsiveness may be altered. Perfusion appears adequate; however, because of high metabolic demands with infection and fever, perfusion is really inadequate. Cardiac output is high but systemic vascular resistance is low, leading to an uneven flow and pooling in the extremities. Blood moves sluggishly, and anaerobic metabolism and lactic acidosis occur in tissue beds where oxygen no longer circulates. Microvascular thrombi may cause further blood flow obstruction.
- *Uncompensated phase.* Hypotension and inadequate oxygen and nutrient delivery to the tissues occurs, leading to progressive mental status changes, prolonged capillary refill time, mottled cool extremities, weak pulses, hypotension, and decreasing urine output. Fever or hypothermia may be present (Moloney-Harmon, 2005). Cellular damage from the infection becomes so significant that the metabolic processes cannot be supported even when adequate fluids have been given to maintain intravascular volume. Poor tissue perfusion to vital organs initiates multiple organ failure.

PATHOPHYSIOLOGY ILLUSTRATED

SEPTIC SHOCK

In septic shock, blood pools in the extremities. Blood flow is sluggish and the tissues receive amounts of oxygen inadequate for cell metabolism.

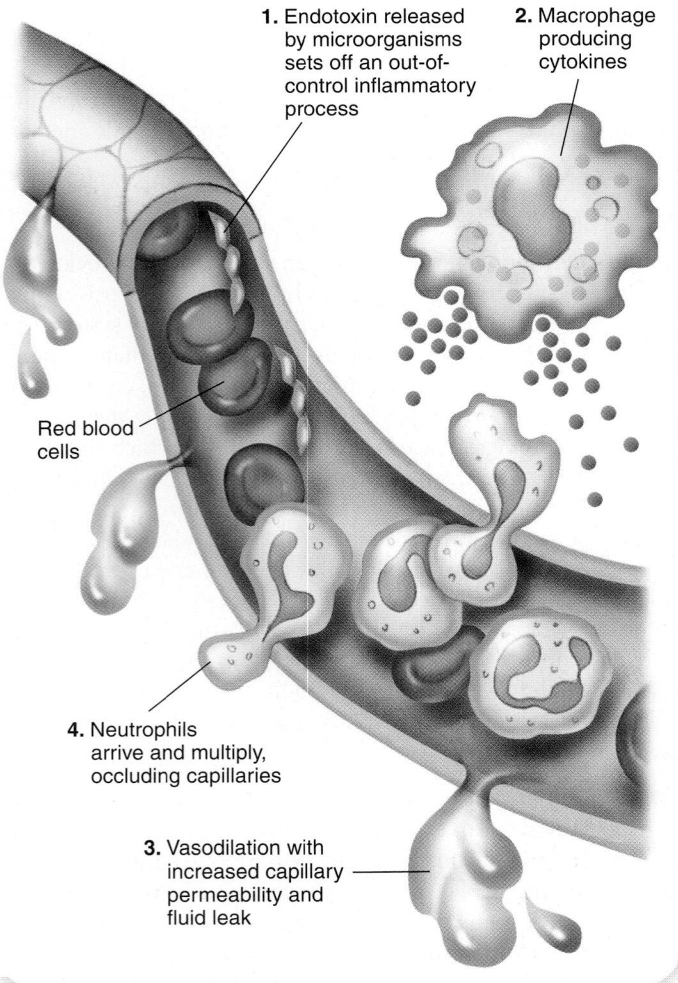
1. Endotoxin released by microorganisms sets off an out-of-control inflammatory process
2. Macrophage producing cytokines
Red blood cells
4. Neutrophils arrive and multiply, occluding capillaries
3. Vasodilation with increased capillary permeability and fluid leak

- *Refractory phase.* The shock becomes irreversible. Cardiac output falls as the myocardium becomes unresponsive. Cardiac arrest soon occurs.

Treatment for septic shock is initiated with appropriate antibiotics effective for the suspected organism causing sepsis. Fluid resuscitation is used to stabilize the circulation and ensure adequate tissue perfusion. Vasopressors are given during the hypodynamic phase. Metabolic acidosis is treated. Enteral or parenteral nutritional support may be initiated early. Morbidity and mortality are high even when treatment is initiated early. A major complication is disseminated intravascular coagulation (see Chapter 51).

PATHOPHYSIOLOGY ILLUSTRATED

OBSTRUCTIVE SHOCK DUE TO MEDIASTINAL SHIFT

Obstructive shock can occur when a tension pneumothorax obstructs blood flow to and from the heart. Here, the great vessels are compressed during the mediastinal shift.

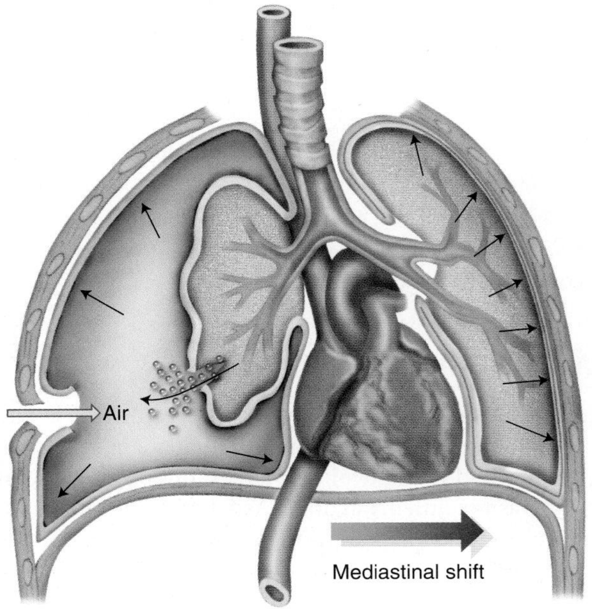
Air
Mediastinal shift

Nursing Management

The child with septic shock is cared for in an intensive care unit. Nursing care focuses on detecting and managing subtle changes in the child's condition that improve the child's chances for survival.

OBSTRUCTIVE SHOCK

Obstructive shock occurs when a blockage of the main bloodstream interferes with tissue perfusion (see "Pathophysiology Illustrated: Mediastinal Shift"). Causes in children include compression of the vena cava, pericardial tamponade, pulmonary embolism, tension pneumothorax, pleural effusion, and congenital heart defects with outflow obstruction (e.g., coarctation of the aorta). Management is focused on treatment of the underlying condition.

Nursing Management

The child is usually cared for in the intensive care unit with nursing care focused on supporting the child's respiratory and cardiovascular functioning. See Chapter 48, page 1354 for care of the child with a tension pneumothorax.

CARDIOGENIC SHOCK

Cardiogenic shock is an abnormality of myocardial function in which the heart fails to maintain adequate cardiac output and tis-

PATHOPHYSIOLOGY ILLUSTRATED

CARDIOGENIC SHOCK

When the heart fails, cardiac output and blood pressure decrease. Blood backs up into the lungs, causing pulmonary edema. Inadequate amounts of oxygen reach the myocardium, further impairing the heart's pumping action. The result is cardiogenic shock.

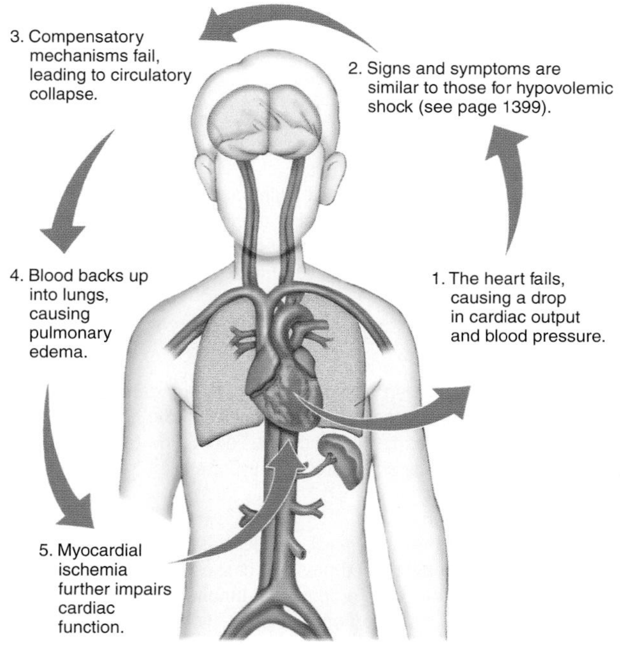
3. Compensatory mechanisms fail, leading to circulatory collapse.
2. Signs and symptoms are similar to those for hypovolemic shock (see page 1399).
4. Blood backs up into lungs, causing pulmonary edema.
1. The heart fails, causing a drop in cardiac output and blood pressure.
5. Myocardial ischemia further impairs cardiac function.

sue perfusion (see "Pathophysiology Illustrated: Cardiogenic Shock"). Causes of cardiogenic shock in children may include pump failure, severe obstructive congenital heart disease such as hypoplastic left heart syndrome, cardiomyopathy, arrhythmias, sepsis, poisoning, or myocardial injury (Ralston, Hazinski, Zaritsky, et al., 2006, p. 76).

Clinically, cardiogenic shock resembles hypovolemic shock with low cardiac output. Tachycardia, tachypnea, decreased oxygen saturation, hypotension, diminished peripheral pulses, and cool, pale extremities are common signs. Disorientation and restlessness occur as the compensatory mechanisms fail. Compensatory responses divert blood to the heart and brain; however, reduced blood flow to the kidneys, liver, and intestines can lead to ischemia and end-organ failure. Increased systemic vascular resistance puts more stress on the failing heart. Each contraction causes more blood to accumulate in the heart and pulmonary vessels, eventually leading to CHF, metabolic acidosis, and circulatory collapse. Signs of respiratory distress are seen as CHF develops.

The goals of medical treatment are rapid restoration of myocardial function with adequate ventilation, resolution of the initial metabolic insult, correction of arrhythmias, fluid management, and administration of diuretics and inotropic drugs.

Nursing Management

The child will be cared for in the intensive care unit. Nursing care focuses on monitoring and supporting the respiratory and cardiovascular status, fluid management, and medication administration. See Chapter 43 for care of the child with a life-threatening condition.

MYOCARDIAL CONTUSION

Myocardial contusion, a rare injury in children, results from a strong, blunt force against the chest wall that injures the heart muscle. Blood flow to areas of the heart muscle is disrupted, or myocardial cells are directly destroyed. This potentially life-threatening condition most often occurs in adolescents who have struck the steering wheel of a motor vehicle during a crash or in children who have been struck in the chest with a baseball.

A myocardial contusion should be suspected in cases of injury to the anterior chest. The child has chest discomfort because of fractured ribs or chest wall contusion. An electrocardiogram reveals arrhythmias or signs of myocardial infarct. A two-dimensional echocardiogram may show an abnormality in heart wall movement. Cardiac troponin I levels and cardiac isoenzyme concentrations may be monitored for elevation. Long-term sequelae are unknown, but could potentially include aneurysm, myocardial rupture, and cardiac tamponade (Roddy, Lange, & Klein, 2005).

Nursing Management

The child will be cared for in the intensive care unit and carefully monitored for arrhythmias and cardiac functioning.

COMMOTIO CORDIS

Commotio cordis, also known as a cardiac concussion, is a blunt, nonpenetrating blow to the precordium that causes ventricular fibrillation and sudden death. The impact timing on the precordium is believed to coincide with the period of vulnerable cardiac repolarization. It is estimated to cause 20% of sudden deaths in young athletes participating in sports such as baseball, softball, ice hockey, and lacrosse (Singh & Silberbach, 2006). In some cases the event is triggered by physical contact with another person, such as a fist, elbow, knee, or head.

The most common arrhythmias recorded after the victim's collapse include ventricular fibrillation and ventricular tachycardia. Survival improves if prompt cardiopulmonary resuscitation or defibrillation is provided.

Nursing Management

The role of the nurse is to implement rapid cardiopulmonary resuscitation and to facilitate defibrillation. Nursing care is then focused on monitoring for cardiac arryhthmias, often in the intensive care unit.

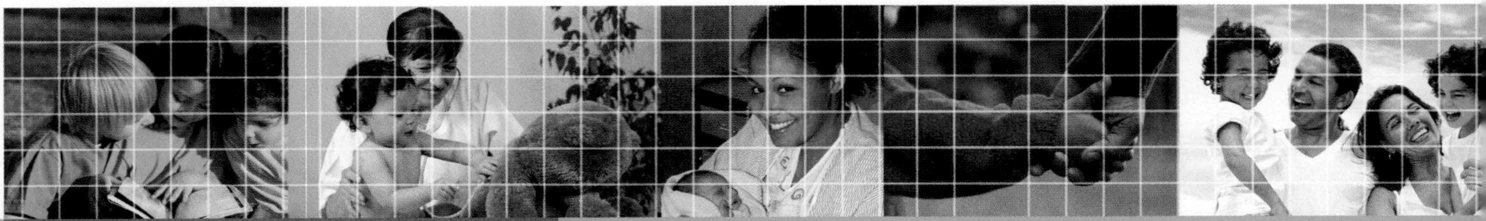

CRITICAL CONCEPT REVIEW

LEARNING OUTCOMES / CONCEPTS

49.1 Describe the anatomy and physiology of the cardiovascular system, focusing on the flow of blood and the action of heart valves.

1. Unoxygenated blood enters the right atrium from the superior and inferior vena cavae.
2. Blood flows through the tricuspid valve into the right ventricle.
3. The blood then moves through the pulmonary valve into the pulmonary artery to the lungs.
4. The blood receives oxygen in the lungs and then enters the left atrium by the pulmonary veins.
5. The blood then travels through the mitral valve and enters the left ventricle.
6. Blood is pumped from the left ventricle through the aortic valve into the aorta and the systemic circulation.

49.2 Describe the pathophysiology associated with congenital heart defects with increased pulmonary circulation, decreased pulmonary circulation, mixed defects, and obstructed systemic blood flow.

1. Defects with increased pulmonary circulation:
   - A connection occurs between the right and left side of the heart, or between the great arteries, which allows blood to flow between the right and left sides of the heart.
   - Blood is shunted to the right side of the heart, which increases blood flow to the lungs.
   - This causes increased pulmonary resistance and pulmonary hypertension.
   - Right ventricular hypertrophy develops.
2. Defects with decreased pulmonary circulation:
   - Structural defects decrease blood flow to the lungs, which decreases systemic oxygen content.
   - If a septal opening is present, increased right-sided pressure causes right-to-left shunting.
   - Decreased oxygen content causes the kidneys to produce a hormonal response, which increases the number of red blood cells leading to polycythemia, increasing the risk for thromboembolism.
   - Abrupt decreases in pulmonary blood flow and systemic vascular resistance combined with activity may cause hypercyanotic episodes.
3. Mixed defects:
   - Complex congenital heart defects involve a combination of defects that increase and decrease pulmonary blood flow.
   - Newborn is dependent upon the mixing of the pulmonary and systemic circulations for survival during the postnatal period.
4. Defects with obstructed blood flow:
   - Decreased cardiac output results from the increased pressure load on the ventricle caused by the obstructed blood flow.

49.3 Develop a nursing care plan for the infant with a congenital heart defect cared for at home prior to corrective surgery.

1. Instruct parents in the administration of necessary medications.
2. Instruct parents concerning the need for frequent small feedings.
3. Instruct parents concerning the signs and symptoms of congestive heart failure.
4. Instruct parents concerning the management of hypercyanotic episodes.

49.4 Develop a nursing care plan for the child undergoing open heart surgery.

Prior to surgery:

1. Give parents and child a tour of the special care area.
2. Prepare the child for anesthesia and equipment that will be used after surgery.
3. Reassure the child that someone will always be near.

After surgery:

1. Frequent assessment of:
   - Arterial and venous pressures.
   - Vital signs.
   - Oxygen saturation.
   - Core body temperature.
   - Level of consciousness.
2. Auscultate heart and lungs:
   - Observe and monitor for arrhythmias.
3. Monitor cardiac output.

LEARNING OUTCOMES	CONCEPTS
	4. Monitor intake and output: ■ Urine. ■ Chest tube bleeding and draining. 5. Assess pain level and treat accordingly. 6. Observe for signs and symptoms of infection.
49.5 Recognize the signs and symptoms of congestive heart failure in an infant and child.	1. Infant: ■ Tires easily, especially during feedings. ■ Weight loss or lack of weight gain. ■ Diaphoresis. ■ Irritability. ■ Frequent infections. ■ Tachycardia and tachypnea. ■ Pallor or cyanosis. ■ Nasal flaring. ■ Grunting. ■ Retractions. 2. Child: ■ Exercise intolerance. ■ Abdominal pain. ■ Peripheral edema. ■ Mottling or pallor. ■ Periorbital or facial edema. ■ Jugular vein distention. ■ Hepatomegaly.
49.6 Develop a nursing care plan for a child with congestive heart failure.	1. Obtain a detailed history of onset of symptoms. 2. Assess vital signs. 3. Assess heart by observation, palpation, and auscultation. 4. Monitor intake and output. 5. Weigh child daily. 6. Turn child frequently and assess skin. 7. Organize nursing actions to provide rest periods. 8. Provide small, frequent feedings.
49.7 Differentiate among the acquired heart diseases that occur during childhood.	1. Infective endocarditis. ■ Inflammation of the lining, valves, and arterial vessels of the heart caused by bacterial, enterococci, and fungal infections. Often associated with defective heart structures or injury to the endocardium from a central line. 2. Rheumatic fever. ■ Inflammatory disorder of connective tissue that results from an autoimmune response to some strains of group A beta-hemolytic streptococci. 3. Kawasaki syndrome. ■ Acute febrile, systemic vascular inflammatory disorder that affects small and midsize arteries, including the coronary arteries.
49.8 List strategies to reduce the child's risk of adult onset cardiovascular disease.	1. Educate parents to promote nutritional intake that ■ helps maintain a normal weight, ■ limits fat intake to 20% to 35% of intake, and saturated fats to less than 10% of intake ■ includes fruits, vegetables, whole grains, low-fat dairy products, lean meat and fish, legumes, and nuts 2. Encourage the child to participate in vigorous exercise for at least 30 minutes, 3 to 4 times a week. Encourage the child to reduce time with screen activities (television, computer). 3. Encourage families and children not to smoke. 4. Screen children for dyslipidemia and hypertension. Monitor fasting glucose

(continued)

LEARNING OUTCOMES / CONCEPTS

49.9 Describe the pathophysiology of hypovolemic shock and nursing management of the condition.

Pathophysiology
- Acute, complex state of circulatory dysfunction resulting in failure to deliver sufficient oxygen and other nutrients to meet cell and tissue demands.
- Caused by severely depleted blood volume or dehydration.

Nursing management
1. Assess vital signs, capillary refill, level of consciousness, skin temperature, urine output, specific gravity. Estimate blood loss.
2. Calculate, prepare and rapidly administer warmed crystalloid intravenous fluids.
3. Assess physiologic response to fluid boluses. Repeat fluid boluses if no improvement.
4. Keep child warm.
5. Administer blood if no response to crystalloid IV fluids.

CRITICAL THINKING IN ACTION

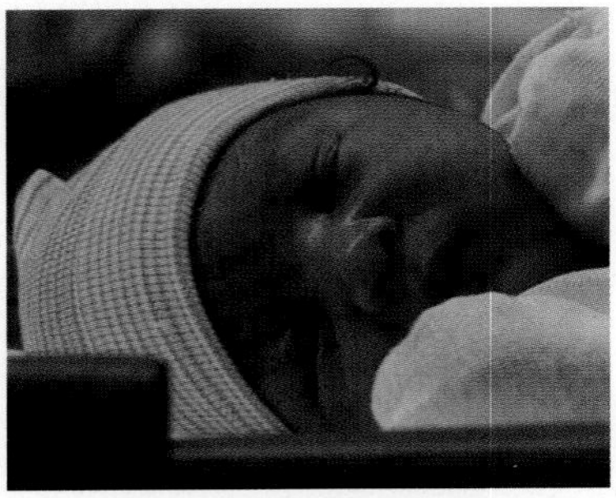

You are working in the hospital when Samantha, a 2-day-old infant, is diagnosed with a continuous, systolic, grade 3, heart murmur in the pulmonic area of the chest. This is the parents' first child and they are extremely worried about their 6-week-premature baby. Samantha has full, bounding pulses and weighed 5 pounds 6 ounces at birth, but has lost 3 ounces in the past 2 days. The mother's pregnancy was healthy until her water broke suddenly. The day after Samantha was born, the parents were told about the heart murmur and that an echocardiogram, ECG, and chest x-ray are needed to determine the cause. The tests show that she has a patent ductus arteriosus (PDA). The physician has prescribed 3 doses of a medication to aid in the closure of the duct. You explain that her vital signs and urine output will need to be monitored closely for decreases while she is on this medicine.

Several days later the heart murmur is still heard; the medicine did not work. The parents want to avoid surgery if possible and the doctor explains that if the ductus closes by the time she is 9–12 months old, and she is without symptoms, surgery could be avoided. If the PDA is not corrected, her life span will be shortened. She is discharged from the hospital, thriving and breastfeeding well, and the doctor advises about watching for poor weight gain, swelling, intercostal retractions, and breathing more than 60 times per minute. A follow-up appointment is made for 1 week later.

1. How would you explain a PDA to the parents?
2. What was the most likely cause of Samantha's weight loss? Is it the PDA that caused the weight loss?
3. What is the physiologic reason Samantha's life span would be shortened if she does not get surgical correction of her PDA?
4. How would you describe congestive heart failure to the parents?

See MyNursingKit for possible responses.

REFERENCES

Baddour, L. M., Wilson, W. R., Bayer, A. S., Fowler, V. B., Bolger, A. F., Levison, M. E., et al. (2005). Infective endocarditis: Diagnosis, antimicrobial therapy, and management of complications. *Circulation, 111,* e394–2433.

Barnes, V. A., Davis, H. C., Murzynowski, J. B., & Treiber, F. A. (2004). Impact of meditation on resting and ambulatory blood pressure and heart rate in youth. *Psychosomatic Medicine, 66,* 909–914.

Belay, B., Belamarich, P., & Racine, A. D. (2004). Pediatric precursors of adult atherosclerosis. *Pediatrics in Review, 25*(1), 4–13.

Belay, B., Belamarich, P. F., & Tom-Revzon, C. (2007). The use of statins in pediatrics: Knowledge base, limitations, and future directions. *Pediatrics, 119*(2), 370–380.

Berger, J. (2007). Pulmonary hypertension in congenital heart disease. *Medscape Cardiology.* Retrieved from http://www.medscape.com/viewarticle/551739_print

Bindler, R. M., & Howry, L. B. (2005). *Pediatric drug guide.* Upper Saddle River, NJ: Prentice Hall.

Blume, E. D., Naftel, D. C., Bastardi, H. J., Duncan, B. W., Kirklin, J. K., Webber, S. A., et al. (2006). Outcomes of children bridged to heart transplantation with ventricular assist devices: A multi-institutional study. *Circulation, 113,* 2313–2319.

Brosig, C. L., Mussatto, K. A., Kuhn, E. M., & Tweddel, J. S. (2007). Neurodevelopmental outcome in preschool survivors of complex congenital heart disease: Implications for clinical practice. *Journal of Pediatric Health Care, 21*(1), 3–12.

Brown, M. D., Wernovsky, G., Mussatto, K. A., & Berger, S. (2005). Long-term and developmental outcomes of children with complex congenital heart disease. *Clinics in Perinatalogy, 32,* 1043–1057.

Carapetis, J. R., McDonald, M., & Wilson, N. J. (2005). Acute rheumatic fever. *The Lancet, 366*(9480), 155–168.

Connor, J. A. (2006). Alterations in cardiovascular function in children. In K. L. McCance & S. E. Huether (Eds.), *Pathophysiology: The biologic basis for disease in adults and children* (5th ed., pp. 1147–1180). St. Louis: Mosby.

Cook, E. H., & Higgins, S. S. (2004). Congenital heart disease. In P. J. Allen & J. A. Vessey, *Primary care of the child with a chronic condition* (4th ed., pp. 382–403). St. Louis: Mosby.

Cox, G. F., Sleeper, L. A., Lowe, A. M., Towbin, J. A., Colan, S. D., Orav, E. J., et al., (2006). Factors associated with establishing a causal diagnosis for children with cardiomyopathy. *Pediatrics, 118*(4), 1519–1531.

Daniels, S. R., Greer, F. R., and the Committee on Nutrition. (2008). Lipid screening and cardiovascular health in childhood, *Pediatrics, 122,* 198–208.

Doniger, S. J., & Shariefff, G. Q. (2006). Pediatric dysrhythmias. *Pediatric Clinics of North America, 53,* 85–105.

Ecklund, M. M., & Ecklund, C. R. (2007). How to recognize and respond to hypovolemic shock. *American Nurse Today, 2*(4), 28–31.

Feld, L. G., & Corey, H. (2007). Hypertension in childhood. *Pediatrics in Review, 28*(8), 283–297.

Ferrieri, P. (2002). Proceedings of the Jones Criteria workshop. *Circulation, 106,* 2521–2523.

Gabrys, C. A. (2005). Pediatric cardiac transplants: A clinical update. *Journal of Pediatric Nursing, 20*(2), 139–143.

Giddings, S., Dennison, B. A., Birch, L. L., Daniels, S. R., Gilman, M. W., Lichtenstein, A. H., et al. (2005). Dietary guidelines for children and adolescents: A guide for practitioners. Consensus statement from the American Heart Association. *Circulation, 112*, 2061–2075.

Gillespie, M. J., Schneider, H. E., & Rome, J. (2006). The use of cardiac catheterization to diagnose and treat heart diseases in pediatric patients. In V. L. Vetter, *Pediatric cardiology: The requisites in pediatrics* (pp. 195–221), St. Louis: Elsevier Mosby.

Hobbs, J. B., Peterson, D. R., Moss, A. J., McNitt, S., Zareba, W., Goldenberg, I., et al. (2006). Risk of aborted cardiac arrest or sudden cardiac death during adolescence in the Long-QT Syndrome. *Journal of the American Medical Association, 296*(10), 1249–1254.

Hoyer, A. & Silverbach, M. (2005). Infective endocarditis. *Pediatrics in Review, 26*(11), 394–399.

Jago, R., Harrell, J. S., McMurray, R. G., Edelstein, S., El Ghornli, L, & Bassin, S. (2006). Prevalence of abnormal lipid and blood pressure values among ethnically diverse population of eighth-grade adolescents and screening implications. *Pediatrics, 117*(6), 2065–2073.

Jenkins, P. C., Chinnock, R. E., Jenkins, K. J., Mahle, W. T., Mulla, N., Sharkey, A. M., et al. (2008). Decreased exercise performance with age in children with hypoplastic left heart syndrome. *Journal of Pediatrics, 152*(4), 507–512.

Joshi, V. M., & Sekhavat, S. (2006). Acyanotic congenital heart defects. In V. L. Vetter, *Pediatric cardiology: The requisites in pediatrics* (pp. 79–96.), St. Louis: Elsevier Mosby.

Kaltman, J. R., Madan, N., Vetter, V. L., & Rhodes, L. A. (2006). Arrhythmias and sudden cardiac death. In V. L. Vetter, *Pediatric cardiology: The requisites in pediatrics* (pp. 79–96.), St. Louis: Elsevier Mosby.

Karl, T. R., Hall, S., Ford, G., Kelly, E. A., Brizard, C. P., Mee, R. B., et al. (2004). Arterial switch with full-flow cardiopulmonary bypass and limited circulatory arrest: neurodevelopmental outcome. *Journal of Thoracic and Cardiovascular Surgery, 127*, 213–222.

Khairy, P., Poirer, N., & Mercier, L. (2007). Univentricular heart. *Circulation, 115*, 800–812.

Knauth, A., Verstappen, A., Reiss, J., & Webb, G. D. (2006). Transition and transfer from pediatric to adult care of the young adult with complex congenital heart disease. *Cardiology Clinics, 24*, 619–629.

Kon, A. A. (2005). Discussing nonsurgical care with parents of newborns with hypoplastic left heart syndrome. *Newborn and Infant Reviews, 5*(2), 60–68.

Limperopoulos, C., Majnemer, A., Shevell, M. I., Rosenblatt, B., Rohlicek, C. & Tchervenkov, C. (2000). Functional limitations in young children with congenital heart defects after cardiac surgery. *Journal of Pediatrics. 108*(6), 1325–1331.

Mahle, W. T., Visconti, K. J., Freier, M. C., Kanne, S. M., Hamilton, W. G., Sharkey, A. M., et al. (2006). Relationship of surgical approach to neurodevelopmental outcomes in hypoplastic left heart syndrome. *Pediatrics, 117*(1), e90–e97.

Majnemer, A., Limperopoulos, C., Shevell, M., Rosenblatt, B., Rohlicek, C., et al., (2006). Long-term neuromotor outcome at school entry of infants with congenital heart defects requiring open-heart surgery. *Journal of Pediatrics, 148*(1), 72–77.

Marino, B. S., Ostrow, A. M., & Cohen, M. S. (2006). Surgery for congenital heart disease. In V. L. Vetter, *Pediatric cardiology: The requisites in pediatrics*, (pp. 277–320), St. Louis: Elsevier Mosby.

Menteer, J., Hogarty, A. N., & Chrisant, M. R., K. (2006). Heart failure in pediatrics. In V. L. Vetter, *Pediatric cardiology: The requisites in pediatrics* (pp. 159–169), St. Louis: Elsevier Mosby.

Milana, C., & Chandran, L. (2006). What's new in Kawasaki disease? *Contemporary Pediatrics, 23*(7), 40–47.

Miller, S. P., McQuillen, P. S., Hamrick, S., Xu, D., Glidden, D. V., Charlton, N., et al. (2007). Abnormal brain development in newborns with congenital heart disease. *New England Journal of Medicine, 357*(19), 1928–1938.

Mitsnefes, M. M. (2006). Hypertension in children and adolescents. *Pediatric Clinics of North America, 53*, 493–512.

Moloney-Harmon, P. A. (2005). Pediatric sepsis: The infection unto death. *Critical Care Nursing Clinics of North America, 17*, 417–429.

Morales, D. L. S., Dreyer, W. J., Denfield, S. W., Heinle, J. S., McKenzie, E. D., Graves, D. E., et al. (2007). Over two decades of pediatric heart transplantation: How has survival changed? *The Journal of Thoracic and Cardiovascular Surgery, 133*(3), 632–639.

National High Blood Pressure Education Program Working Group on High Blood Pressure in Children and Adolescents. (2004). The fourth report on the diagnosis, evaluation, and treatment of high blood pressure in children and adolescents. *Pediatrics, 114*(2), 555–576.

Newberger, J. W., Sleeper, L. A., McCrindle, B. W., Minich, L. L., Gersony, W., Vetter, V. L., et al. (2007). Randomized trial of pulsed corticosteroid therapy for primary treatment of Kawasaki disease. *New England Journal of Medicine, 356*(7), 663–675.

Paridon, S. M., Alpert, B. S., Boas, S. R., Cabrera, M. E., Caldarera, L. L., Daniels, S. R., et al. (2006). Clinical stress testing in the pediatric age group: A statement from the American Heart Association Council on Cardiovascular Disease in the Young, Committee on Atherosclerosis, Hypertension, and Obesity in Youth. *Circulation, 113*, 1905–1920.

Park, M. K. (2008). *Pediatric cardiology for practitioners* (5th ed.). St. Louis: Mosby.

Popovich, D. M., Richiuso, N., & Danek, G. (2004). Pediatric health care providers' knowledge of pulse oximetry. *Pediatric Nursing, 30*(1), 14–20.

Ralston, M., Hazinski, M. F., Zaritsky, A. L., Schexnayder, S. & Kleinman, M. E. (2006). *Pediatric advanced life support: Provider manual.* Dallas, TX: American Heart Association.

Reis, E. C., Kip, K. E., Marroquin, O. C., Kiesau, M., Hipps, L, & Peters, R. E. (2006). Screening children to identify families at increased risk for cardiovascular disease. *Pediatrics, 118*(6), e1789–e1797.

Roddy, M. G., Lange, P. A., & Klein, B. L. (2005). Cardiac trauma in children. *Clinical Pediatric Emergency Medicine, 6*, 234–243.

Rosenzweig, E. B., & Barst, R. J. (2005). Idiopathic pulmonary arterial hypertension in children. *Current Opinion in Pediatrics, 17*, 372–380.

Schneider, H. E., & Goldmuntz, E. (2006). The genetics of congenital heart disease. In V. L. Vetter, *Pediatric cardiology: The requisites in pediatrics* (pp. 145–157), St. Louis: Elsevier Mosby.

Schowengerdt, K. O. (2006). Advances in pediatric heart transplantation. *Current Opinion in Pediatrics, 18*, 512–517.

Schultz, A. H., & Kreutzer, J. (2006). Cyanotic heart disease. In V. L. Vetter, *Pediatric cardiology: The requisites in pediatrics* (pp. 51–78), St. Louis: Elsevier Mosby.

Singh, A., & Silberbach, M. (2006). Cardiovascular preparticipation sports screening. *Pediatrics in Review, 27*(11), 418–423.

Sivarajan, V. B., Vetter, V. L., & Gleason, M. M. (2006). Pediatric evaluation of the cardiac patient. In V. L. Vetter, *Pediatric cardiology: The requisites in pediatrics*, (pp. 1–30), St. Louis: Elsevier Mosby.

Towbin, J. A., Lowe, A. M., Colan, S. D., Sleeper, L. A., Orav, E. J., Clunie, S., et al. (2006). Incidence, causes, and outcomes of dilated cardiomyopathy in children. *Journal of the American Medical Association, 296*(15), 1867–1876.

Tsai, W., & Klein, B. L. (2005). The postoperative cardiac patient. *Clinical Pediatric Emergency Medicine, 6*, 216–221.

Vetter, V. L. (2006). Kawasaki disease. In V. L. Vetter, *Pediatric cardiology: The requisites in pediatrics* (pp. 131–144), St. Louis: Elsevier Mosby.

Wilson, B. A., Shannon, M. T., & Shields, K. M. (2009). *Nurses' drug guide 2009.* Upper Saddle River, NJ: Prentice Hall.

Wilson, W., Taubert, K. A., Gewitz, M., Lockhart, P. B., Baddour, L. M., Levinson, M., et al. (2007). Prevention of infective endocarditis: Guidelines from the American Heart Association Rheumatic Fever, Endocarditis, and Kawasaki Disease Committee, Council on Cardiovascular Disease in the Young, and the Council on Clinical Cardiology, Council on Cardiovascular Surgery and Anesthesia, and the Quality of Care and Outcomes Research Interdisciplinary Working Group. *Circulation, 116*, 1736–1754.

Zeltser, I., & Tabbutt, S. (2006). Critical heart disease in the newborn. In V. L. Vetter, *Pediatric cardiology: The requisites in pediatrics* (pp. 31–50), St. Louis: Elsevier Mosby.

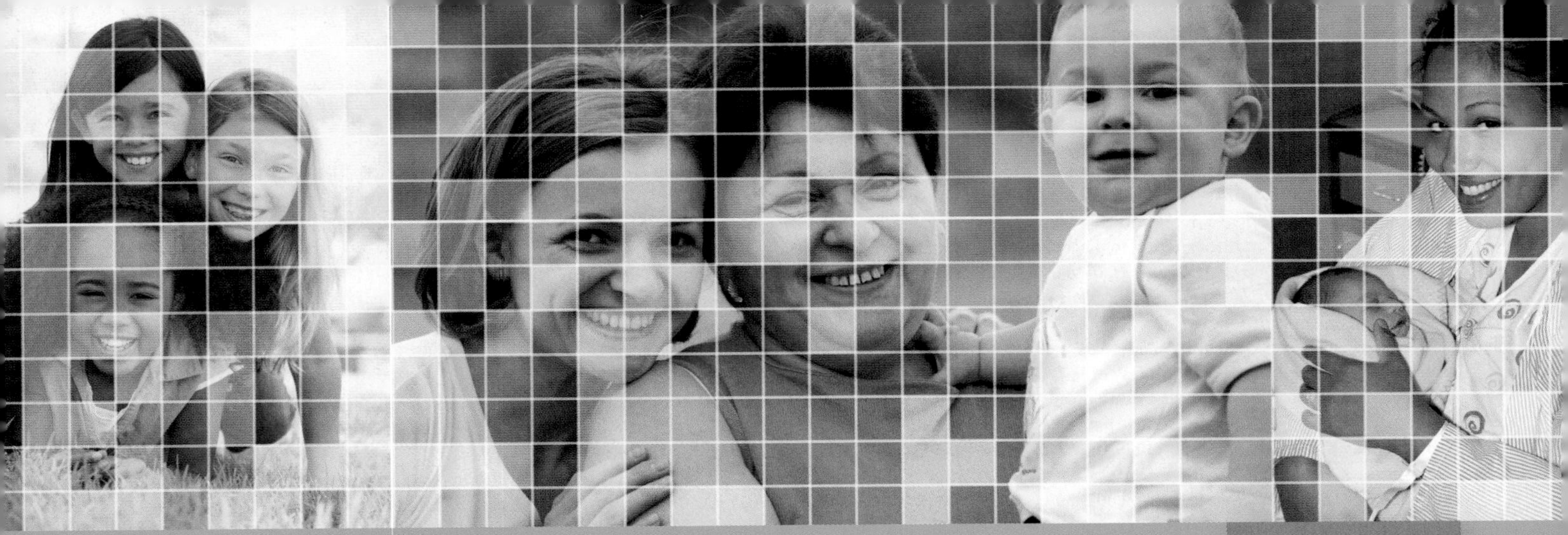

CHAPTER 50

The Child with Alterations in Immune Function

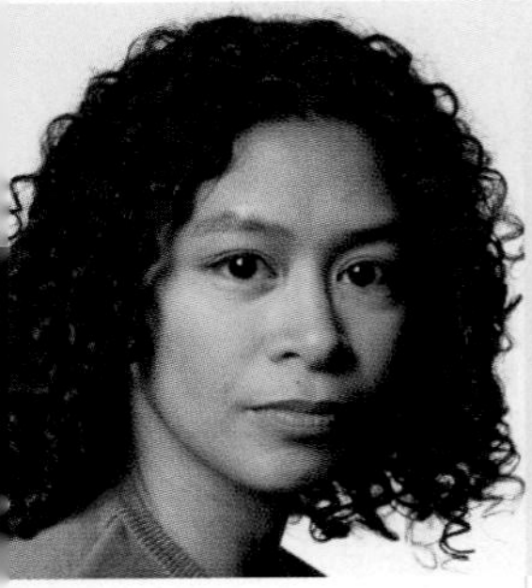

We knew that Raymond might have AIDS—my sister was HIV positive. But we have taken him in as our own child and cared for him. Somehow we thought he would be fine. Now, to find out that he does have AIDS is devastating, especially since my sister is also very ill. We need to learn a lot about how to help him. Can we send him to a preschool next year as we had planned? How will we get money to pay for his medicines? What do we tell other people? How do we get him to eat better? We just don't know where to turn right now. —*Aunt of Raymond, 2 years old*

LEARNING OUTCOMES

50.1 Describe the structure and function of the immune system and apply that knowledge to the care of children with immunologic disorders.

50.2 Identify infection control measures to prevent the spread of infection in children with an immunodeficiency.

50.3 Develop a nursing care plan in partnership with the family for a child with human immunodeficiency virus (HIV infection).

50.4 Describe nursing management for the child with systemic lupus erythematosus or juvenile arthritis.

50.5 Describe exposure prevention measures for the child with latex allergy.

50.6 Apply nursing interventions and prevention measures for the child experiencing other hypersensitivity reactions.

Signs and symptoms of immunologic disorders in children are often nonspecific. The immune system is one of the few body systems that regulate, either directly or indirectly, all other body functions. Thus, a problem with the immune system can result in multisystem consequences and may be life threatening. The child with recurring infections may have an undiagnosed immunologic disorder. Congenital abnormalities sometimes signal a defect in cellular immunity. This chapter will examine some of the more common disorders of immune function and discuss nursing care of children and families who have these diseases.

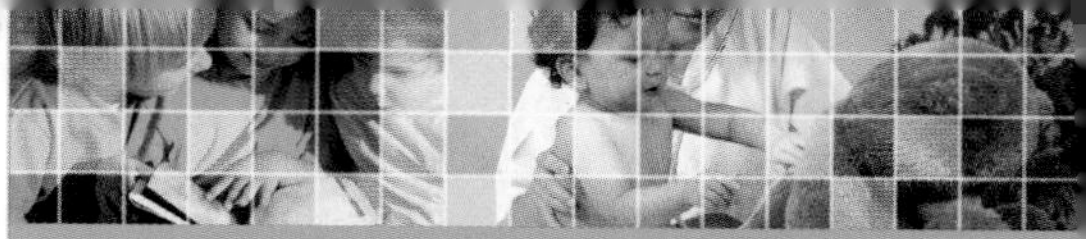

KEY TERMS

Acquired immunity, 1409
Allergens, 1431
Allergy, 1431
Antibodies, 1409
Antigens, 1409
Graft-versus-host disease, 1411
Hypersensitivity response, 1431
Immunodeficiency, 1411
Immunoglobulin, 1409
Natural immunity, 1409
Opportunistic infection, 1413
Primary immunodeficiency, 1411
Primary immune response, 1409
Secondary immunodeficiency, 1411
Secondary immune response, 1409
Vertical transmission, 1415

ANATOMY AND PHYSIOLOGY OF PEDIATRIC DIFFERENCES

The function of the immune system is to recognize any foreign substances within the body—in simple terms, to distinguish "nonself" from "self"—and to eliminate foreign substances as efficiently as possible. Whenever the body recognizes the presence of a substance that it cannot identify as part of itself, the body protects itself through the immune response. Normally, the immune system responds to an invasion of foreign substances, or antigens, in numerous ways. It produces **antibodies**, or proteins that work against **antigens**, the foreign substances that trigger the immune response. There are many types of antibodies, described later in this section. The immune system also produces other types of cells, such as T lymphocytes and natural killer (NK) cells.

Immunity is either natural or acquired. **Natural immunity** comprises the defenses present at birth, such as intact skin, body pH, natural antibodies from the mother, and inflammatory and phagocytic properties. **Acquired immunity** consists of humoral (antibody-mediated) and cell-mediated immunity and is not fully developed until a child is about 6 years of age.

Humoral immunity is responsible for destroying bacterial antigens. B lymphocytes, produced in the bone marrow, gut, and other lymphoid tissue, are the central factors in humoral immunity and develop into plasma cells that produce antibodies. Antibodies are a type of protein called **immunoglobulins** of which there are five types: IgM, IgG, IgA, IgD, and IgE (Table 50–1). IgM, IgG, and IgA act to control a number of body infections, whereas IgE is useful in combating parasitic infections and is part of the allergic response (Petry, Mathur, & Kamat, 2004). The role of IgD is not known.

Antibodies are found in serum, body fluids, and certain tissues. When a child is first exposed to an antigen, the B lymphocyte system begins to produce antibodies that react specifically to that antigen (see "Pathophysiology Illustrated: Primary Immune Response"). It takes approximately 3 days for this process, known as **primary immune response**, to occur. Subsequent encounters with the antigen trigger memory cells, resulting in a **secondary immune response** within 24 hours.

Infants and children have differing amounts of some immunoglobulins. IgG is the only immunoglobulin that crosses the placenta; as a result, a newborn's levels are similar to those of the mother (Buckley, 2007). This maternal IgG disappears by 6 to 8 months of age. The infant's IgG then increases gradually until mature levels are reached at 7 to 8 years. IgM levels are low at birth, rise markedly at 1 week of age, and continue to increase until adult levels are reached at about 1 year. IgA and IgE are not present at birth. Manufacture of these immunoglobulins begins by 2 weeks of age; however, normal values are not achieved until 6 to 7 years. It is thus easy to see why children under 6 years of age become ill so often—they do not have a full complement of immunoglobulins.

In contrast, cell-mediated immunity achieves full function early in life. The thymus begins producing T lymphocytes in the fetus and by birth many of these cells are present. The thymus is large at birth, grows during childhood and adolescence, and decreases in size in adulthood (Chamley, Carson, Randall, et al., 2005). Other lymphoid tissue such as the spleen and tonsils are also comparatively large in young

Table 50–1 Classes of Immunoglobulins

Immunoglobulin	Location	Action
IgM	Present in intravascular spaces (blood and lymph)	Mediates cytotoxic response and activates complement First antibody produced with primary immune response
IgG	Present in all body fluids	Active against bacteria, bacterial toxins, and viruses Activates complement The only immunoglobulin to cross the placenta
IgA	Present in secretions of gastrointestinal, respiratory, and genitourinary tracts	Prevents binding of viruses to cells of the respiratory and gastrointestinal tracts
IgD	Present in blood, lymph, and surfaces of B cells	Function not fully understood
IgE	Present in internal and external body fluids	Releases chemical mediators responsible for immediate hypersensitivity response

PATHOPHYSIOLOGY ILLUSTRATED

PRIMARY IMMUNE RESPONSE

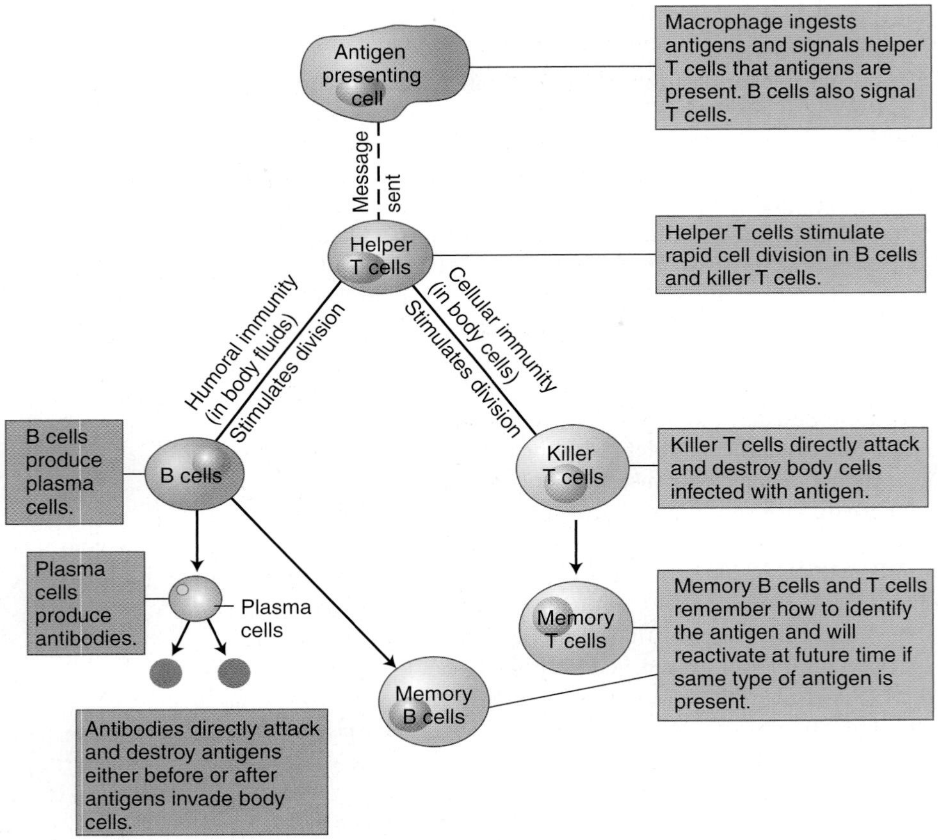

Growth and Development

Newborns are most prone to development of infection, particularly when born premature, since they have lower levels of their own immune protections, as well as less IgG obtained from the mother. Feeding of human milk is protective against newborn infections (Heird, 2007).

children. Because of this well-developed cellular immunity, any blood infused into newborns is generally irradiated to prevent **graft-versus-host disease** (a series of immunologic reactions in response to transplanted cells) from transfused lymphocytes.

Specialized types of T lymphocytes include killer T cells, suppressor T cells, and helper T cells. Suppressor T cells inhibit B lymphocytes from differentiating into plasma cells. Helper T cells aid in the proliferation and immunologic function of other cells. T lymphocytes have proteins on their surfaces that attract and trap receptors; these proteins can be used to measure the immune activity of these cells.

Natural killer cells (also known as non-B/non-T lymphocytes) originate in the bone marrow and thymus and migrate to the blood and spleen. They play a role in control of viral infection, tumors, and autoimmune disease. Newborns have somewhat lower numbers of NK cells than do older children and adults, decreasing their ability to respond to certain antigens.

Complement is a component of blood serum consisting of 11 protein compounds. It is an inactive enzyme that activates in response to antigen–antibody functions, resulting in a generalized inflammatory reaction that kills foreign cells. It also plays a role in causing some autoimmune diseases. The levels of some of the complement proteins are lower in newborns than in older children and adults, thus delaying and hampering response to certain infections.

IMMUNODEFICIENCY DISORDERS

Immunodeficiency, a state of decreased responsiveness of the immune system, can occur to varying degrees in response to any number of events. Children with congenital immune deficiency, or **primary immunodeficiency**, are born with a failure of humoral antibody formation (B-cell disorder), a deficient cellular immune system (T-cell disorder), or a combination of both defects. In congenital disorders, the immune deficiency is not caused by another condition. However, immunodeficiency may also be acquired, as in human immunodeficiency virus (HIV) infection. Acquired immunodeficiency is also called **secondary immunodeficiency**.

B-CELL AND T-CELL DISORDERS

In B-cell disorders, immunoglobulins may be present in inadequate numbers or nearly absent. X-linked hypogammaglobulinemia, selective IgA deficiency, and common variable immunodeficiency are examples of such disorders (Michaels & Green, 2007). Because newborns are protected from infection by maternal antibodies in the first months after birth, symptoms of B-cell disorders usually become apparent after 3 months of age once the infant loses maternal antibodies. Infants with these disorders have frequent recurrent bacterial infections and failure to thrive. With treatment, consisting of intravenous immunoglobulins and antibiotics, most children survive into adulthood. Prognosis depends on the degree of antibody deficiency.

T-cell disorders are characterized by inadequate numbers of T lymphocytes or absence of T-cell functions. Isolated T-cell disorders are rare and may be associated with congenital abnormalities (as in DiGeorge syndrome) or of unknown cause. DiGeorge syndrome is most often accompanied by abnormalities in chromosome 22, and is usually diagnosed soon after birth. The syndrome is characterized by absence (complete DiGeorge) or hypoplasia (partial DiGeorge) of parathyroid or thymus glands, hypocalcemia with tetany within 24–48 hours after birth, cardiac defects, low-set ears, hypertelorism (widely set eyes), and viral and bacterial infections in the neonatal period (Buckley, 2007; Goldmuntz, 2005). There is generally a mild to moderate decrease in T-lymphocyte counts (McLean-Tooke, Spickett, & Gennery, 2007). Prophylatic antibiotics are used to prevent bacterial infections. Children with partial DiGeorge are treated with calcium and vitamin D supplements. Those with complete DiGeorge need thymus transplantation in order to survive (Buckley, 2008).

Immunodeficiency with hyper-IgM is a T-cell disorder that primarily affects males and causes decreased T-cell function, variable abnormal levels of immunoglobulins, and high titers of some antibodies. It is usually X-linked but may be autosomal in some cases. Pulmonary and sinus bacterial infections generally occur in the first 2 years of life (Cleary, Insel, & Lewis, 2005; National Center for Biotechnology Information, 2007). Treatment with intravenous immune globulin (IVIG) therapy is helpful although later malignancies and liver disease can occur (Nagaraj, Egwim, & Adler, 2007). Hematopoietic cell transplantation decreases the morbidity and mortality associated with this disorder (Cleary et al., 2005). Table 50–2 compares laboratory values for selected congenital immunodeficiency disorders.

SEVERE COMBINED IMMUNODEFICIENCY DISEASE

Severe combined immunodeficiency disease (SCID) is a congenital condition characterized by severely impaired humoral and cellular immunity that is manifested by lack of appropriately functioning T cells and B cells (Davies, 2005; Tezcan, Ersoy, Sanal, et al., 2005). SCID occurs in X-linked recessive and autosomal recessive forms. In some cases, SCID may be the result of chromosomal abnormalities. The disorder is much more common in males than females and is estimated to occur in 1 per 50,000 live births. Without appropriate treatment, children born with SCID usually do not survive more than 1 year (Cleary et al., 2005; Davies, 2005; Kobrynski, 2006).

Etiology and Pathophysiology

Severe combined immunodeficiency disease is caused by genetic mutations that lead to impaired lymphoid development

Table 50–2 Laboratory Findings for Selected Congenital Immunodeficiency Disorders

Disorders	Laboratory Findings
B CELL	
X-linked hypogammaglobulinemia	Reduced IgA, IgM, IgE, IgG (< 100 mg/dL), absence of B cells in peripheral blood, normal T cells
Selective IgA deficiency	IgA < 10 mg/dL
Common variable immunodeficiency	IgA, IgM reduced; IgG <250 mg/dL
T CELL	
DiGeorge syndrome	Lymphopenia; absent T-cell functions, decreased T cells, normal B cells
X-linked immunodeficiency with hyper-IgM	Reduced IgG, IgA; elevated IgM; mutations in T-cell surface proteins
COMBINED	
Severe combined immunodeficiency syndrome (SCID)	Complete absence of T- and B-cell and NK immunity
Wiskott-Aldrich syndrome	Thrombocytopenia, low platelet volume, nonfunctional B-cells, normal IgG, decreased IgM, increased IgA, increased IgE; inability to respond to polysaccharide antigens

in children with low T and NK cells. The B lymphocytes may appear normal in number but their function is compromised due to the severe T-cell deficiency (Buckley, 2007; Cleary et al., 2005).

Clinical Manifestations

Symptoms of SCID develop early in life. The infant often demonstrates a susceptibility to infection, presenting during the first few months of life with persistent respiratory infections and diarrhea (Tezcan et al, 2005). Recurrent oral candidiasis, failure to thrive, and skin infections are also frequently seen in children. Additionally, failure to completely recover from infection, frequent reinfection, and infection with viruses such as cytomegalovirus and the bacterium *Pneumocystis carinii* (*jiroveci*) are common to the child with severe combined immunodeficiency disease (Buckley, 2007; Kobrynski, 2006). Children are also highly susceptible to serious infections such as meningitis, skin or organ infection, osteomyelitis, or sepsis.

Clinical Therapy

A marked reduction in lymphocyte counts indicates SCID. Patients with SCID generally have very few T-cells and NK cells (Davies, 2005). The B lymphocyte count may be decreased, elevated, or normal, although these cells do not function normally. Immunoglobulin levels are significantly reduced (Davies, 2005; Kobrynski, 2006). Refer to Table 50–2 for laboratory findings in SCID. Diagnosis is usually made only after extensive laboratory testing. In addition to a complete blood count, erythrocyte sedimentation rate, and B- and T-cell lymphocyte counts, other studies including IgA, IgG, and IgM antibody titers to immunizations received, and neutrophil count, may be performed (Table 50–3). A chest radiograph is conducted to assess thymus size.

The standard therapy for severe combined immunodeficiency disease is the administration of intravenous immune globulin (IVIG), which is administered to provide protection until humoral immunity is established. Hematopoietic stem cell transplantation (see Chapter 51∞) offers the best hope for children with SCID. T-cell function is restored with the transplantation, and new cells appear 3 to 4 months after infusion of the donor stem cell. Prognosis for the child is poor without aggressive therapy and transplant.

With the identification of the genetic defect for SCID in recent years, gene therapy has been successfully attempted to treat a small number of children. Due to the subsequent development of leukemia in a few of these patients, this form of treatment is under review (Bonilla & Geha, 2006; Puck & Malech, 2006).

Prevention and prompt treatment of infection are essential. Antibiotic therapy is targeted at infectious agents. Antibiotic prophylaxis and special immunization recommendations are needed. Children with T-cell deficiencies should receive cytomegalovirus-negative irradiated blood products due to the risk of infection and graft-versus-host disease from lymphocytes in the donor blood (Kobrynski, 2006).

NURSING MANAGEMENT

NURSING ASSESSMENT AND DIAGNOSIS

Obtain a thorough history of infections, including age of onset, type of causal organism, frequency, and severity. Assess family history, and determine if the child has had any unusual reactions to vaccines, medications, or foods. Measure the child's height and weight accurately to identify failure to thrive. Assess the child's nutritional intake and fluid and electrolyte balance. Assess for evidence of infections involving the skin, subcutaneous tissues, respiratory system, and mucous membranes. Palpate the abdomen for hepatomegaly and the lymph nodes for lymphadenopathy. Perform a developmental assessment and assess for delays in achievement of developmental milestones. Assess family support systems and coping mechanisms when a child is diagnosed with the disorder.

The primary nursing diagnosis for a child with SCID is *Risk for Infection* related to immunodeficiency. Other nursing diagnoses may include the following:

- *Imbalanced Nutrition: Less than Body Requirements* related to illness
- *Risk for Impaired Skin Integrity* related to immunologic deficit
- *Risk for Caregiver Role Strain* related to a child with a chronic, life-threatening illness
- *Risk for Delayed Growth and Development* related to physical disability and chronic illness

Table 50–3 Cells Evaluated in Laboratory Studies for Immune Conditions

Test and Type of Cell Evaluated	Action	Implication of Increased or Decreased Levels
WHITE BLOOD CELL (WBC) COUNT		
Neutrophil (54–62%)	Phagocytic cell that defends against bacteria	Increased in bacterial infection, inflammatory processes, and some malignancies
Eosinophil (1–3%)	Associated with antigen-antibody reaction	Increased in allergic reaction; decreased in children receiving corticosteroids
Basophils (0–3%)	Phagocytic cell; involved in immediate hypersensitivity reaction; stores histamine and has receptor sites for IgE	Increased in leukemia; decreased in allergy, acute infection, collagen and chronic diseases
Monocytes (4–9%)	Phagocytic cell active in chronic infection	Increased in tuberculosis, protozoan infection, monocytic leukemia
Lymphocytes (T, B, non-B/non-T [NK]) (25–33%)	Major components of immune system	Increased in many infections; decreased in children with immune deficiency
IMMUNOGLOBULINS		
(IgM, IgG, IgA, IgD, IgE) (See appendix for age-specific values.)	Many roles in a number of immunologic reactions	Increased in presence of infection or allergic response; decreased in children with immune deficiency

PLANNING AND IMPLEMENTATION

Nursing care of the immunodeficient child focuses on preventing infection (see "Teaching Highlights: Reducing Risk of Infection in the Child with Immunodeficiency Disease"). However, even with the use of environmental controls, such as keeping children inside special units (positive pressure rooms) to maintain a sterile environment, these children are prone to **opportunistic infections** (those caused by normally nonpathogenic organisms in persons who lack normal immunity).

Teaching Highlights

REDUCING RISK OF INFECTION IN THE CHILD WITH IMMUNODEFICIENCY DISEASE

Teach family members the following practices to reduce the risk of transmission of infection:

- Wash all bottles, nipples, and pacifiers with hot water and soap, or in the dishwasher.
- Do not allow child to share utensils, cups, bottles, or pacifiers.
- Use safe food preparation practices such as peeling fruit and vegetables and using different surfaces and utensils for preparing meats vs. other foods.
- Change diapers frequently and cleanse skin with mild soap and dry thoroughly.
- Wash hands before handling child, after changing diapers, and before feeding child.
- Maintain clean pets and keep the pet's environment clean.
- Avoid exposing the child to other family members' illnesses, such as colds.

PREVENT SYSTEMIC INFECTION

Frequent and thorough handwashing is important. Standard precautions are always used and transmission-based precautions are established when indicated. **SKILLS** Implement sterile aseptic technique when caring for all sites where needles, catheters, central lines, endotracheal tubes, pressure-monitoring lines, and peripheral intravenous lines, or other invasive equipment enter the child's body. Food and other items entering the hospital room may require special treatment. The child should be placed in a positive pressure isolation room, and contact with infectious individuals should be avoided. Inform parents that because of the risk of infection to the child, live vaccines are avoided for the child as well as siblings, parents, and other household members. Refer to the current recommendations for immunizations for the immunocompromised child. (See Chapter 45.)

PROMOTE SKIN INTEGRITY

The skin is the only intact defense that many immunodeficient children have. Provide thorough and frequent skin care, and observe all possible pressure areas closely for signs of breakdown or infection. Reposition the child frequently and encourage range of motion exercises.

PROMOTE NUTRITIONAL BALANCE

Encourage adequate fluid and nutritional intake. Provide foods that the child prefers and those with high nutritional value. Offer small frequent feedings of high-calorie, protein-rich foods. Refer to a dietitian as needed to plan with parents for the best individualized diet for the child.

MANAGE MEDICATION THERAPY

Many medications used long term in the treatment of children with SCID have numerous side effects. Monitor closely for side

Drug Guide

IMMUNE GLOBULIN

MEDICATION AND ACTION/INDICATION	NURSING IMPLICATIONS
Immune Globulin Contains globulin protein from large pools of normal human plasma of venous or placental origin. Intramuscular formulation used to provide passive immunity or to modify severity of certain specific infectious diseases, such as measles, varicella-zoster, hepatitis A, and hepatitis B. Intravenous formulation used as maintenance therapy in those unable to manufacture sufficient quantities of IgG antibodies, such as in immunodeficiency diseases, idiopathic thrombocytopenia purpura, and Kawasaki disease.	Consult package insert for IM formulations for specific diseases and inform family of the expected length of time for passive immunity. Active immunization to diseases may be needed following that time period. Monitor vital signs before, during, and after intravenous infusion. Have emergency drugs and equipment readily available; hypersensitivity reactions are most common with large or repeated doses. Stop infusion immediately and report hypersensitivity reactions.

Adapted from Bindler, R. M., & Howry, L. B. (2005). Pediatric drug guide. Upper Saddle River, NJ: Prentice Hall Health.

effects of antibiotics, such as overgrowth of resistant organisms (e.g., thrush infections in the mouth, *Clostridium difficile* infections of the gastrointestinal tract) and administer IVIG safely (see "Drug Guide: Immune Globulin").

PROVIDE EMOTIONAL SUPPORT AND REFERRAL TO APPROPRIATE SUPPORT GROUPS AND SERVICES

SCID is a life-threatening and devastating disease. Even with aggressive therapy, the prognosis is poor. Evaluate the family's knowledge about the disease and provide education about infection control measures and signs of infection. The parents may feel guilt because of the genetic nature of the disease and the difficulties of treatment. Listen closely to their concerns and encourage them to discuss their fears. Refer them to an appropriate support group or counselor if needed. Encourage genetic counseling if the parents plan to have more children. Evaluate the family's ability to care for the child at home. Offer financial resource information and other referrals as needed.

The family of a child who undergoes hematopoietic stem cell transplantation requires additional support and referrals. The transplantation procedure involves surgery for both the ill child and the donor, often another child in the family. After the transplant the ill child will be hospitalized for several months until T lymphocyte levels are sufficient to provide resistance to infection. During this period, parents may need to rely on social services to help manage the family situation, particularly if the child is hospitalized at a medical center far from the family's home. Assess the family's situation and make appropriate referrals to social services and support groups. Introduce parents to other families undergoing hematopoietic stem cell transplantation. (See Chapter 51 for discussion of hematopoietic stem cell transplantation.)

EVALUATION

The success of nursing care for the child with SCID is measured by outcomes such as the following:

- Absence of infection
- Adequate nutritional status as determined by normal growth patterns
- Maintenance of intact skin
- Adaptive coping by family to demands of a chronic illness
- Developmental performance within normal level for age

WISKOTT–ALDRICH SYNDROME

A combined congenital immunodeficiency syndrome, Wiskott–Aldrich syndrome is an X-linked disorder that causes mutation in the WAS gene and changes in WAS protein. The gene resides on Xp11.22 (Kobrynski, 2006). The incidence is 4 in 1 million live male births (Dibbern & Routes, 2007). The IgG and IgA levels are normal, IgM levels are decreased, and IgE levels may be increased (Kobrynski, 2006).

The diagnosis is made in the early neonatal period on the basis of the thrombocytopenia, which leads to bleeding as evidenced by petechiae, hematuria, bloody diarrhea, and hematemesis. In addition to thrombocytopenia and related symptoms, Wiskott–Aldrich syndrome is characterized by eczema and recurrent infections in infancy and childhood. Infections including otitis media, bacterial pneumonia, and skin infections are common (Ochs & Thrasher, 2006).

Treatment is supportive and includes antibiotic prophylaxis, platelet transfusions, and intravenous gamma globulin. Hypersplenism is a complication that may necessitate a splenectomy; however, this is done sparingly because of the risk of life-threatening infection following the procedure. The treatment of choice and the only cure for Wiskott–Aldrich Syndrome is hematopoietic stem cell transplantation (HSCT). Following HSCT, the child is at risk for both rejection and graft-versus host disease (see page 1435) (Kobrynski, 2006; Ochs & Thrasher, 2006).

Nursing Management

Nursing care is similar to that for the child with SCID. Refer the parents for genetic counseling to help them understand the transmission of the disease and the probability of having another child with the same disorder. Arrange for psychologic support for parents overwhelmed with guilt from learning that the illness is inherited.

Help the parents and family cope with the knowledge that the child has a chronic and potentially fatal illness. Referral to family counseling may be appropriate. Expected outcomes are the child's return to normal immunologic function, absence of hemorrhage, and successful coping with a life-threatening illness.

HUMAN IMMUNODEFICIENCY VIRUS AND ACQUIRED IMMUNE DEFICIENCY SYNDROME

Acquired immune deficiency syndrome (AIDS) is caused by the human immunodeficiency virus (HIV-1 primarily; HIV-2 less commonly) (AAP, 2006). As HIV destroys the body's ability to fight infection, opportunistic infections that would normally not affect healthy people destroy the immune system. AIDS, the advanced stages of HIV infection, may result if treatment is not initiated.

Most cases of HIV in children are the result of perinatal transmission. The Centers for Disease Control (CDC) estimates that approximately 240 infants are born with HIV infection each year in the United States compared with the peak incidence of 1650 in 1991 (CDC, 2006a). This change is primarily due to more effective identification and treatment of HIV-infected mothers and HIV-exposed infants. The leading cause of newly acquired HIV infection in teens is unprotected sexual intercourse, while use of injectable drugs is responsible for most other cases. In many cases, both of these factors are involved.

The virus affects multiple systems and eventually destroys the ability of the child's immune system to respond to infection. An understanding of the natural history of HIV disease is still evolving, and there are several important differences in the disease progression and clinical manifestations of pediatric and adult HIV infection.

Etiology and Pathophysiology

Children can acquire HIV in a form of **vertical transmission** from their mothers transplacentally or during delivery. Transmission can occur during birth from blood, amniotic fluid, and exposure to genital tract secretions, and after birth through breast milk from HIV-infected mothers. However, risk for perinatal transmission has been significantly reduced since mothers identified as infected receive antiretroviral medications (ART) during pregnancy, are delivered by cesarean section, and do not breastfeed. If the mother is not treated, there is a 25% chance that the newborn will be infected compared with a 2% or less chance if the mother is treated (CDC, 2007a). Prenatal testing is essential to further reducing the incidence of HIV infection in children.

HIV selectively targets and destroys T cells, thereby decreasing and eventually eliminating cellular immunity. HIV destroys the CD4 T cells (helper cells), which are crucial to normal function of the immune system. HIV selectively targets T cells, decreasing cellular immunity, and affecting humoral immunity as well. Thus, the child is left unprotected against a myriad of bacterial, viral, fungal, and opportunistic infections, which are ultimately fatal. Every organ system can be affected. (See "Pathophysiology Illustrated: Human Immunodeficiency Virus.")

Clinical Manifestations

The interval from HIV infection to the onset of overt AIDS is shorter in children than in adults, and shorter in children infected perinatally than in those infected through transfusion. Most children with AIDS have nonspecific findings, including lymphadenopathy, hepatosplenomegaly, nephropathy, oral candidiasis, failure to thrive and weight loss, diarrhea, chronic eczema and dermatitis, and fever. Raymond, described at the beginning of this chapter, had several of these findings, as well as a history of recurrent, acute infections (bronchitis, otitis media, and colds).

The neonate is asymptomatic at birth. The time period for the development of opportunistic infections varies; however, the interval from HIV infection to the onset of overt AIDS is shorter in children than in adults.

Most children with HIV infection have nonspecific findings, including lymphadenopathy, hepatosplenomegaly, nephropathy, oral candidiasis, failure to thrive and weight loss, delayed development, chronic diarrhea, chronic eczema and dermatitis, and fever of unknown origin (FUO). Specific symptoms usually appear within 2 years in children who acquire HIV infection perinatally and include conjunctivitis (pink eye), ear infections, and tonsillitis, bacterial and opportunistic infections, such as *Streptococcus*, *Haemophilus influenzae*, Salmonella, and *Pneumocystis jiroveci* pneumonia (formerly known as *Pneumocystis carinii*), and malignancies such as lymphomas, frequently occur as the disease progresses. Lymphoid interstitial pneumonitis (LIP) is a common manifestation of pediatric AIDS. Frequently children develop encephalopathy resulting in developmental delay or a deterioration of motor skills and intellectual functioning (Kline, 2006; Plowfield, 2007). See "Clinical Manifestations: Human Immunodeficiency Virus in Children."

MyNursingKit Video: AIDS/HIV

Clinical Therapy

There is no cure for HIV or AIDS. Care focuses on the prevention of HIV transmission, the detection of the presence of HIV, aggressive therapy to reduce progression to AIDS, and promoting the infant or child's growth and development and survival.

Most children with HIV infection are diagnosed early in life. Serologic tests for detection of the virus are monitored in infants born to HIV-infected mothers. These tests are performed within 48 hours of birth. Infants with initially negative tests should be retested at 1 to 2 months; tests are repeated at 3 and 6 months, and then again between 12 and 18 months. Because an infant born to an HIV-infected mother may have maternal antibodies up to 18 months of age, routine antibody tests are not helpful for diagnosing HIV infection in infants (Alvarez & Rathore, 2007).

MyNursingKit Animation: HIV Infection/Transmission

PATHOPHYSIOLOGY ILLUSTRATED

HUMAN IMMUNODEFICIENCY VIRUS

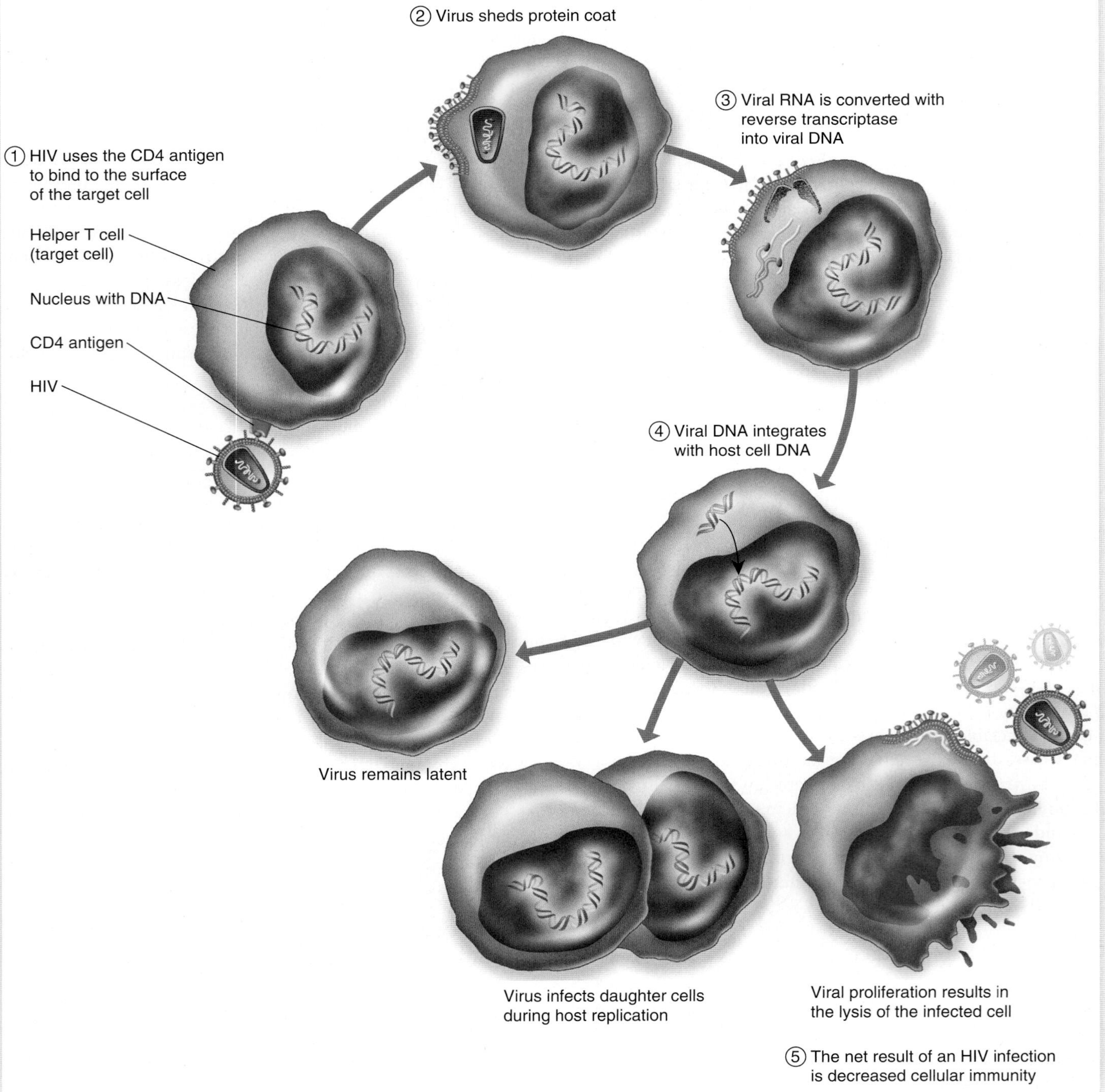
② Virus sheds protein coat
③ Viral RNA is converted with reverse transcriptase into viral DNA
① HIV uses the CD4 antigen to bind to the surface of the target cell
Helper T cell (target cell)
Nucleus with DNA
CD4 antigen
HIV
④ Viral DNA integrates with host cell DNA
Virus remains latent
Virus infects daughter cells during host replication
Viral proliferation results in the lysis of the infected cell
⑤ The net result of an HIV infection is decreased cellular immunity

Clinical Manifestations

HUMAN IMMUNODEFICIENCY VIRUS IN CHILDREN

ETIOLOGY	CLINICAL MANIFESTATIONS	CLINICAL THERAPY
Frequent, chronic, or unusual infections due to poor immune response	Chronic bilateral otitis media Oral candidiasis *Pneumocystis jiroveci* pneumonia (PCP) Skin disorders Fever	Antimicrobial therapy for treatment of infections Recommended immunizations Limit exposure to groups of people or to individuals with known infections of any kind
Poor nutritional intake due to lack of appetite caused by disease and medications	Failure to thrive (eating disorder of childhood) Weight and body mass index below 10th percentile Chronic diarrhea Skin irritation	Monitor growth Supplemental intake such as enteral feedings at night, and TPN if needed Meticulous skin care to prevent breakdown
Immune system overgrowth to compensate for lack of proper immune response	Hepatosplenomegaly and lymphadenopathy	Assess abdomen frequently Teach about safe transport to avoid injury to liver and spleen

Note: Be alert for the possibility of HIV infection in infants with combinations of listed clinical manifestations, especially in infants known to be at risk.

The preferred tests are the HIV DNA polymerase chain reaction (PCR) or the HIV RNA assay (viral load). Any positive result is confirmed by retesting. In addition, CD4+ percentage or counts should be performed at least every 3 to 4 months to evaluate the child's immune status (U.S. Department of Health and Human Services [DHHS], 2008a).

An antibody test to see if the maternal HIV antibodies have disappeared should be performed at 12 months of age. If the test is still positive it should be repeated at 15 to 18 months of age (DHHS, 2008a). If the antibody test is still positive at 18 months of age the child is considered to be infected with HIV. Antibody tests that are used include ELISA (enzyme-linked immunosorbent assay) or EIA (enzyme immunoassay). These tests are confirmed with the western blot test or the indirect immunofluorescence assay (IFA) (Alvarez & Rathore, 2007). The CDC considers children less than 13 years of age to be infected if their symptoms meet the CDC criteria for HIV infection. The CDC criteria address two issues: the diagnosis of HIV and the clinical classification of children infected with HIV (AAP, 2006) (Table 50–4).

Nursing Practice

Many people who are at risk of HIV infection may not have HIV testing readily available. To reduce barriers to early detection of the virus, rapid HIV tests have been made available. Specimens are obtained from saliva or fingerstick for blood sample. Oral fluids are obtained by gently swabbing both the upper and lower outer gums of the mouth. Results are available in one hour or less and some do not require blood draws. Some FDA approved options include OraQuick Rapid HIV-1/2 Antibody Test, Reveal Rapid HIV-1 Antibody Test, Uni-Gold Recombigen HIV Test, and Multispot HIV-1/HIV-2 Rapid Test. Health professionals must be prepared to offer counseling during the same visit as when the test is administered. Traditional laboratory tests are used to confirm positive rapid HIV tests (Delaney, Branson, Uniyal, et al., 2006; Greenwald, Burstein, Pincus, et al., 2006).

Table 50–4 Clinical Staging of Pediatric HIV Infection

Diagnosis of HIV infection in children

- HIV infected (two or more positive tests for HIV or clinical signs and symptoms of HIV infection or an AIDS-defining illness)
- Perinatally exposed (born to a mother known to be infected with HIV)
- Seroconverter (born to a mother known to be infected with HIV but has had two negative HIV tests)

When infected, the child with HIV is classified as:

- Category N (not symptomatic)
- Category A (mildly symptomatic)
- Category B (moderately symptomatic)
- Category C (severely symptomatic; multiple, recurrent serious bacterial infection)

Adapted from: American Academy of Pediatrics (2006). *Red Book: 2006 Report of the Committee on Infectious Diseases* (27th ed., pp. 380–381). Elk Grove Village, IL: AAP.

Medical management begins with prevention of the spread of HIV from mother to newborn. Due to the rapidity of disease progression in perinatally transmitted HIV infection, early identification of infected infants is important to ensure the most effective treatment. HIV-infected mothers should be identified during pregnancy, and their infants should undergo periodic laboratory testing, as described earlier. All infected mothers should receive combination antiretroviral therapy after the first trimester of pregnancy. Monotherapy is no longer recommended in the United States; however, if a mother with HIV infection is in labor and has not been on an antiretroviral regimen, this type of treatment may be used (Cibulka, 2006).

All infants of infected mothers with indeterminate HIV infection status should start prophylaxis against PCP by the age of 4 to 6 weeks and continue to one year of age unless the diagnosis of HIV infection is excluded. Prompt therapy with antiinfectives is used for bacterial and viral opportunistic infections. The need for prophylaxis after one year of age is dependent on the child's degree of immunosuppression (AAP, 2006; Baker, 2007).

Treatment for the child diagnosed with HIV involves highly active antiretroviral therapy (HAART). Initial medication therapy should include a combination of several antiretroviral (AVR) drugs. At least 3 drugs from a minimum of 2 different categories should be used. Twenty-five AVRs have been approved for use in adults and adolescents in the United States. Of these, fourteen have been approved for use in children as of February 2008 (see "Drug Guide: Medications Used to Treat Human Immunodeficiency Virus in Children") (DHHS, 2008 a & b; Alvarez & Rathore,

Drug Guide

MEDICATIONS USED TO TREAT HUMAN IMMUNODEFICIENCY VIRUS IN CHILDREN

MEDICATION AND ACTION/INDICATION	NURSING IMPLICATIONS
NUCLEOSIDE/NUCLEOTIDE REVERSE TRANSCRIPTASE INHIBITORS (NRTIS)	
Inhibits action of viral reverse transcriptase, an enzyme in the conversion of RNA to DNA Abacavir Didanosine Emtricitabine Lamivudine Stavudine Zidovudine (AZT)	Baseline data include physical assessment, laboratory studies (especially measurement of white and red blood cell counts); monitored at least monthly for changes. Common side effects include fever, headache, insomnia, myalgia, nausea, vomiting, diarrhea, anorexia, bone marrow suppression with resulting granulocytopenia and anemia, dyspnea, cough, skin rash. Teach signs and symptoms of infection.
PROTEASE INHIBITORS	
Blocks the function of the enzyme protease needed for viral formation and growth Atazanavir Fosamprenavir Lopinavir/Ritonavir Nelfinavir Ritonavir	Baseline data include physical assessment and laboratory studies (such as serum electrolytes, CBC, liver function studies, blood glucose, hemoglobin A_{1c}, serum amylase, CPK); monitored at least monthly for changes. Side effects include CNS, CV changes, life-threatening hematologic changes, respiratory distress, and allergy; monitor for specific side effects of the particular drug administered. Oral forms taken within 2 hours of a full meal.
NONNUCLEOSIDE REVERSE TRANSCRIPTASE INHIBITORS (NNRTIS)	
Bind to viral reverse transcriptase and disrupt the conversion of RNA to DNA Efavirenz Nevirapine	Baseline data include physical assessment and laboratory studies (such as liver and kidney function tests, CBC and differential); monitored at least monthly for changes. Side effects include fever, headache, nausea, diarrhea, hepatitis, altered liver function, anemia, neutropenia, drowsiness and fatigue, altered mental status, rash, Stevens-Johnson syndrome. Teach the family to notify healthcare provider immediately if rash appears.
FUSION INHIBITORS	
Prevents viral entry Enfuvirtide	Requires subcutaneous injection twice a day. There is a high incidence of local reaction at the injection site, limiting the use of this medication in children.

Data from U.S. Department of Health and Human Service (2008a). *Guidelines for the Use of Antiretroviral Agents in Pediatric HIV Infection.* Retrieved December 6, 2008 from http://aidsinfo.nih.gov/contentfiles/PediatricGuidelines.pdf; U.S. Department of Health and Human Service (2008b) Pediatric Antiretroviral Drug Information. Retrieved December 5, 2008 from http://aidsinfo.nih.gov/contentfiles/PediatricGL_Supl.pdf; Alvarez, A. M., & Rathore, M. H. (2007). Hot topics in Pediatric HIV/AIDS. *Pediatric Annals*, 36 (7), 423–432.

Note: The cost of antiretroviral therapy has decreased over the years as more generic drugs have become available. Worldwide, however, only about 24% of individuals who need ART are actually able to receive it (Alvarez & Rathore, 2007). What can be done to improve access to these drugs for children worldwide?

2007). Families should be advised that these drugs neither cure HIV nor prevent transfer from the person infected to others.

Children on antiretroviral therapy should be monitored closely for side effects and toxicity related to the medications. A complete blood count and blood chemistry along with a clinical history should be evaluated prior to beginning treatment, 4 to 8 weeks later, and then every 3 to 4 months. In addition, CD4+ cell counts and HIV RNA levels are recommended at the same time intervals to evaluate compliance with the medication regimen and effectiveness of the treatment. A lipid panel is also recommended every 6 to 12 months to monitor for signs of elevated cholesterol and triglyceride levels (DHHS, 2008a).

The earlier the child develops AIDS, the poorer the prognosis. However, as treatment improves, more children are living longer with the disease. An estimated 20% of children with HIV infection develop AIDS in the first year of life and most of them die by 4 years of age. The other 80%, however, may not develop serious disease until adolescence (NIAID, 2004). With rapid advances in the treatment of HIV infection ongoing, the lifespan of children and adolescents cannot be predicted as these treatments are significantly extending their lives (Plowfield, 2007).

NURSING MANAGEMENT

NURSING ASSESSMENT AND DIAGNOSIS

For infants at risk of HIV infection, obtain the HIV test results of the mother if available. When the mother's results are positive, the infant will need to be screened for HIV infection according to CDC guidelines as described in the previous section. Facilitate the screening and explain its necessity to the family.

PHYSIOLOGIC ASSESSMENT

Assessment centers on observation and evaluation of potential sites of infection. Assess breath sounds, respiratory status, arterial blood gases, level of consciousness, and mental status. Report any evidence of lymphocytic interstitial pneumonitis or neurologic abnormalities. Assess the child's height and weight frequently. Observe for signs of failure to thrive and assess for anemia. Assess for *Candida* infections in the mouth and the diaper area. Note any developmental delays in motor skills or intellectual functioning, which could result from encephalopathy and poor nutrition, and can signal an increasing severity in symptom level. These findings should be reported immediately so that further medical evaluation can be implemented.

PSYCHOSOCIAL ASSESSMENT

Assess family support systems and coping mechanisms, as the stress of caring for a child with HIV infection may overwhelm the parents. Assess the family's ability to care for the child. Inquire about the extended family's ability to provide daily care as well as emotional support. Support the family when they decide to inform a school-age child or adolescent of the diagnosis. When assessing an adolescent with HIV infection, evaluate the teen's understanding of how HIV is transmitted and the response to the diagnosis.

The accompanying Nursing Care Plan includes common nursing diagnoses that may apply to a child hospitalized with HIV infection. Other nursing diagnoses may include the following:

- *Diarrhea* related to gastrointestinal infection, malignancy, or drug reactions
- *Pain* related to infections
- *Impaired oral mucous membranes* related to infection
- *Delayed Growth and Development* related to chronic infection and poor nutrition
- *Risk for Compromised Family Coping* related to life-threatening illness
- *Caregiver Role Strain* related to anxiety about child's condition and demands of providing care

PLANNING AND IMPLEMENTATION

The first step in managing HIV infection is prevention. Nurses must be active in evaluating test results and instituting measures to prevent vertical transmission of HIV to the infants of infected mothers. Measures advised include adequate testing, prophylaxis for HIV exposed infants and opportunistic infections, and follow-up visits for evaluation of general health and development for all infants at risk of the disease.

Education related to HIV infection, transmission of the disease, and testing should be a routine part of anticipatory guidance provided to adolescents. Adolescents who are sexually active should be offered HIV testing. Many states have provisions that allow teens to be tested for HIV without parental knowledge (CDC, 2006b).There are also recommendations for inclusion of HIV education into comprehensive health education for students from kindergarten through 12th grade (Committee on Pediatric AIDS, 1998). Nurses can implement these policies and counsel teens about the dangers and prevention measures for HIV.

MyNursingKit Case Study: Toddler with HIV

If the child is diagnosed with HIV, close health supervision is needed to ensure that medications are taken and examinations are carried out. When HIV progresses to clinical AIDS, nursing care is similar to that of a child with any serious, chronic, life-threatening disease. Nursing care centers on preventing infection, managing pain, promoting respiratory and other organ function, promoting adequate nutritional intake, and providing emotional support to the parents and child, while promoting the child's growth and development. The accompanying Nursing Care Plan summarizes nursing care for the child hospitalized with AIDS.

PREVENT INFECTION

Immunosuppressed children become infected with bacteria as well as other organisms that are common in the environment. Protect the neonate from HIV-infected maternal secretions. Bathe the newborn as soon as possible after delivery and wash the eyes and face before administering prophylactic eye drops or ointment. Avoid invasive procedures in the newborn and encourage the mother to formula feed the baby rather than breast

Nursing Practice

Older school age children and adolescents with HIV should be informed of their diagnosis and counseled appropriately regarding sexual transmission (AAP, 2006). Telling the child is difficult for parents and they often avoid doing so. Because parents usually want to be the ones to tell the child, they need help to plan how to discuss the issue and ongoing support in the process of communication. Nurses can assist in the following ways:

- Help parents understand the need to discuss the diagnosis with the child.
- Provide information about how to tell the child. Role play with the parents how to tell the child and use information at the child's developmental understanding to assist parents to be honest.
- Provide sources of hope—the success of treatment, children living with HIV, and maintaining an active life.
- Assist the family to join support groups or Web-based groups.
- Help the family plan for respite care as needed.
- Provide emotional support for this difficult task and allow for ongoing opportunities to express concerns, fears, and anxieties.

Nursing Practice

The American Academy of Pediatrics recommends that HIV and AIDS education be part of health education in grades kindergarten through 12. School nurses should be educated about HIV infection, ethics, testing, and counseling. The particular roles defined for nurses in school settings include:

1. Participate in education programs for teachers.
2. Assist schools and other organizations to develop education programs.
3. Review, adapt, and develop educational materials.
4. Participate in public discussions about HIV infection.
5. Take part in meetings with school administrators, staff, and parents.
6. Facilitate networking among parents and HIV community groups support groups (Committee on Pediatric AIDS, 1998).

feed (Luxner, 2003, National Institute of Allergy and Infectious Diseases, 2004).

Proper disposal of needles and contaminated materials or equipment is essential to reduce the transmission of HIV (Figure 50–1 ●). Standard precautions (see Clinical Skills Manual **SKILLS**) are implemented to prevent exposure to HIV.

Frequent hand hygiene and limiting exposure of the child to individuals with upper respiratory or other infections are the best interventions to protect the child with HIV from acquiring other infections. Because the risk of serious outcomes for measles disease is great, a live measles-mumps-rubella vaccine is used unless the child is severely immunosuppressed. Vaccination with the live varicella vaccine is considered safe and effective in children with no or mild symptoms of HIV infection. The benefits and risks of the vaccine are weighed and the child should receive the immunization if appropriate (AAP, 2006). Tuberculosis is more common in children with HIV infection than in those who are not infected; therefore, annual skin tests that are performed and read by health professionals are recommended (AAP, 2006). Educate sexually active adolescents on the importance of practicing safe sex and the ramifications of high-risk sexual behaviors and intravenous drug abuse.

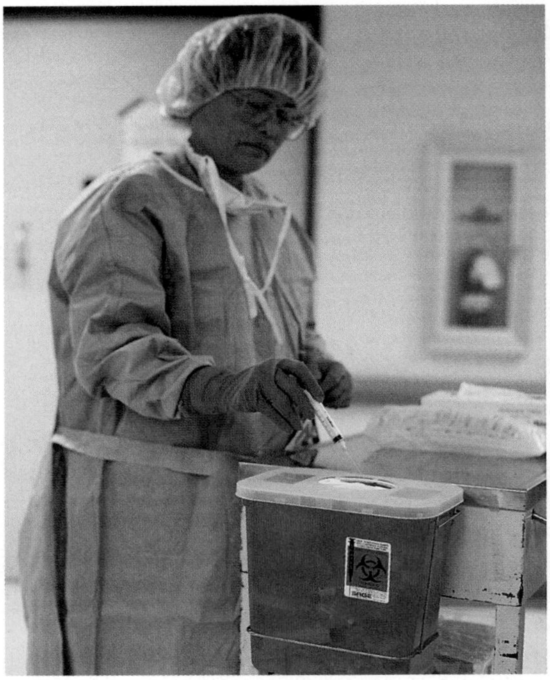

● **Figure 50–1** Biohazard disposal. This nurse is disposing of a needle and syringe in a biohazard container, a necessary practice to avoid the transmission of HIV through needle sticks with contaminated needles. This universal precaution provides protection even when the immune status of the patient is not known.

PROMOTE MEDICATION REGIMEN ADHERENCE

The treatment regimen with the use of antiretroviral therapies for the child with HIV infection may be complex, time consuming, and costly, presenting an overwhelming challenge to the child and the family. Adherence to the prescribed antiretroviral regimen is imperative as nonadherence will likely result in increased morbidity and mortality. Some common reasons for nonadherence include frequent dosing, child's or caregiver's inability or unwillingness to follow the prescribed regimen, child's displeasure with medication (pill size, number of pills or amount of liquid, bad taste), and caregiver's lack of knowledge related to the disease

MyNursingKit Case Study: Postexposure Management for Needlestick Injuries

Nursing Care Plan

THE CHILD WITH ACQUIRED IMMUNODEFICIENCY SYNDROME

INTERVENTION	RATIONALE	EXPECTED OUTCOME
1. Nursing Diagnosis: Risk for Infection related to immunosuppression		
NIC Priority Intervention: **Infection control:** Minimizing the acquisition and transmission of infectious agents		**NOC Suggested Outcome:** **Risk control:** Answers to eliminate or reduce actual, personal, and modifiable health threats
Goal: Risk Factors for Infection will be reduced as evidenced by absence of signs of infection.		
■ Assess the child every 2–4 hours for fever; lesions in the mouth; and redness, inflammation, soreness, and lesions on the skin or around intravenous lines.	■ Fever is one of the few signs of infection in the immunosuppressed child who does not have a sufficient number of white blood cells.	The child has no fever and shows no other signs of infection.
■ Auscultate for changes in breath sounds every 2 hours. Perform pulmonary toilet (coughing, deep breathing, incentive spirometry) every 2–4 hours.	■ Pneumonia is a likely infection in the child HIV infection.	
■ Enforce good hand hygiene. Allow no fresh flowers, fruits, or vegetables in child's room. Screen visitors for colds or recent exposure to varicella. Use blood and body fluid precautions (refer to Clinical Skills Manual SKILLS). Practice strict asepsis for dressing changes and suctioning.	■ Control of environmental factors helps prevent infection.	
■ Coordinate patient care assignments to avoid exposing the child to individuals with recent infections or immunizations.	■ Planning minimizes chances for infection.	
■ Organize patient care activities to allow for adequate periods of rest.	■ Rest periods allow the child to regain energy.	
■ Follow recommendations of CDC and AAP for immunizing immunosuppressed children. Avoid varicella vaccine. Perform annual TB testing.	■ Special recommendations consider the child's decreased immune response and the danger of acquiring disease from certain live virus vaccines.	

INTERVENTION	RATIONALE	EXPECTED OUTCOME
2. Nursing Diagnosis: Imbalanced Nutrition: Less than Body Requirements related to loss of appetite and decreased absorption of nutrients		
NIC Priority Intervention: **Nutrition management:** Assistance with or provision of a balanced dietary intake of food and fluids		**NOC Suggested Outcome:** **Nutritional status:** Extent to which nutrients are available to meet metabolic needs
Goal: The child will demonstrate adequate nutritional status to meet metabolic needs as evidenced by adequate weight gain for age.		
■ Encourage frequent small meals to promote nutritional and fluid intake.	■ Additional nutrition is required to rebuild the immune system.	The child eats frequent meals of adequate nutritional content. Periodic weight evaluation.
■ Maintain nasogastric tube feeding, if ordered. Total parenteral nutrition may be necessary to ensure adequate nutrition.	■ Supplementation may be needed to assure adequate calories.	
■ Eliminate unpleasant stimuli and odors from the environment during meals.	■ Unpleasant stimuli decrease the desire for food.	
■ Monitor skin turgor every shift.	■ Skin turgor reflects hydration status.	
■ Weigh daily.	■ It is important to monitor weight status.	
■ Involve a nutritionist in planning a diet for the child that includes favorite foods.	■ Including favorite food encourages intake.	

(continued)

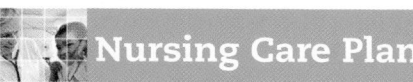

Nursing Care Plan—continued

THE CHILD WITH ACQUIRED IMMUNODEFICIENCY SYNDROME

INTERVENTION	RATIONALE	EXPECTED OUTCOME
3. Nursing Diagnosis: Risk for Impaired Skin Integrity related to skin infection, immobility, or diarrhea		
NIC Priority Intervention: **Skin surveillance:** Collection and analysis of patient data to maintain skin integrity		**NOC Suggested Outcome:** **Tissue Integrity:** Skin and Mucous Membranes: Structural intactness and normal physiological function of skin and mucous membranes
Goal: The child will have intact skin.		
■ Observe all pressure areas closely for signs of infection or breakdown.	■ Skin care is important in the immunocompromised child. The skin may be the only intact defense the child has.	The child is free of preventable skin breakdown.
■ Keep skin clean and dry. Provide perineal care to minimize irritation from diarrhea.	■ Prevents breaking or cracking of skin.	
4. Nursing Diagnosis: Deficient Knowledge (Parent) related to home care of child with AIDS		
NIC Priority Intervention: **Teaching, treatment:** Preparing a patient and family to understand and mentally prepare for a treatment		**NOC Suggested Outcome:** **Knowledge, treatment regimen:** Extent of understanding conveyed about treatment of HIV infection
Goal: The parent(s) will demonstrate knowledge about home care including medication regimen, measures to prevent infection, and signs and symptoms to report to healthcare providers.		
■ Explain the importance of optimizing the child's health status and reducing risk of complications through diet, rest, and meticulous personal hygiene. Be sure that parents and other family members understand how HIV infection is spread and take appropriate precautions.	■ Knowledge about the disorder and preventive measures is necessary to provide safe and effective home care for the child.	The parent describes appropriate home care and preventive measures for a child with AIDS.
■ Be sure that parents understand the need for adherence to the medication regimen and understand how to administer medications.	■ Knowledge of rationale increases compliance.	
■ Inform the family about signs and symptoms of infection that should be reported promptly to the physician or nurse (fever, chills, cough, mild erythema).	■ Prompt treatment increases outcome.	

(Plowfield, 2007). Strategies for achieving optimal management of the treatment regimen include educating the parent or care provider, and child when doing so is developmentally appropriate, about the purpose of the medication, the benefits of adhering to the regimen, and the potential consequences of failure to adhere to the regimen. Behavior modification techniques, using positive reinforcement, can be very effective in promoting the child's adherence. Provide support to the family, and tailor the medication regimen to the family's routine when possible. Offer praise to the child and parent for adhering to the regimen. If problems exist in managing the treatment regimen, carefully listen to the family to help determine the cause. Collaborate with the family in establishing goals to help meet the prescribed treatment regimen. If further intervention is required, options include direct observational therapy or home visits. Consider the effect of cultural beliefs on medication adherence (see "Developing Cultural Competence: HIV/AIDS and Blacks" and "Evidence-Based Nursing: Adolescents with HIV Infection and Medication Regimen Adherence"). If further intervention is required, other options include direct observational therapy or home visits.

Developing Cultural Competence

HIV/AIDS AND BLACKS

Nurses need to be aware of the incidence of HIV infection and AIDS in the black population and focus on opportunities for education and prevention. Blacks make up approximately 13% of the total U.S. population; however, 2005 statistics indicated that they accounted for 49% of the new HIV/AIDS diagnoses in the 33 states with long-term HIV reporting. In addition, between 2001 and 2004, 65% of infants infected perinatally with HIV infection were black, as were 61% of individuals under the age of 25 with a diagnosis of HIV/AIDS. The CDC has established the African American HIV/AIDS work group to address this concern (CDC, 2008).

PROMOTE RESPIRATORY FUNCTION

Because many children with HIV infection develop pneumonia, encourage the child to cough and deep breathe every 2 to 4 hours. In the community, regular physical activity encourages lung aeration. When in the hospital, blowing cotton balls with a straw, blowing bubbles, or other games may engage the interest of a younger child. Reposition infants frequently so all areas of the lungs can aerate. The plan of care should include rest periods to conserve energy and lower the body's demand for oxygen.

PROMOTE ADEQUATE NUTRITIONAL INTAKE

Because many children with HIV infection have failure to thrive, nutrition is an important part of their care. (See Chapter 34∞ for information to include in a detailed nutritional assessment.) A nutritionist should be involved in planning an appropriate diet for the child that provides necessary calories, protein, and other nutrients. Vitamins may be especially lacking in the diets of infected children. Antioxidants (vitamin A, vitamin E, zinc, and selenium) are known to enhance general immune system function; children consume these nutrients at recommended levels. Periodic dietary analysis and teaching are needed. Adequate nutrition is sometimes provided through total parenteral nutrition, or through nasogastric or gavage feeding.

Diarrhea resulting from gastrointestinal infection and lactose intolerance is a common finding in children with HIV infection, and it complicates other nutritional disturbances. Alternative formulas may be recommended. Although antidiarrheal medications are not generally used in infants, they may be prescribed for older children. Carefully monitor hydration status, skin turgor, and urine output. Provide careful perineal skin care to prevent infection.

The frequency of *Candida* infections lead to blisters, cracking, and discharge involving the oral mucous membranes. To keep the child's lips and mouth moist, mouth care should be performed every 2 to 4 hours with a non-alcohol-based solution such as normal saline.

PROVIDE EMOTIONAL SUPPORT

The family of the child with HIV infection is under emotional stress, and this is compounded if others in the family are infected.

Nursing Practice

Disclosure of patient information is a breach of confidentiality that may subject the nurse to legal action. Disclosure of confidential information occurs whenever a patient's condition—for example, a diagnosis of HIV infection—is discussed inappropriately with any third party.

The infected teen may see progression of disease in the parent and lose hope. Integrate social services and support groups into the care of the child as soon as the diagnosis is made. Spend time talking with the family to provide them with an opportunity to discuss their fears and feelings. In many parts of the United States, HIV infection still carries a tremendous stigma, and the family may not be able to discuss their feelings outside the healthcare environment. Safeguard the family's wishes about the privacy of the diagnosis.

Clarify any misconceptions the older child with HIV infection may have about transmission of the disease. Routes of transmission and the need for safe sexual practices must be discussed openly and clearly with adolescents. Providing support for adolescents is particularly important, as the dependence on family or other caregivers that this chronic and terminal disease brings can make it difficult to meet the developmental task of independence. Adolescents may benefit from contact with other infected peers.

DISCHARGE PLANNING

The diagnosis of HIV infection is surrounded by strong emotions and fears. Be honest and direct. Education is essential. Explain that there is no evidence that casual contact among family members can spread the infection. For the child who has been hospitalized, home care needs should be identified in advance of discharge.

Discuss the family's finances as well as health insurance coverage for the child's care. Assess the family's ability to provide nutritious food, required medications, and a supportive

Thinking Critically

THE TODDLER WITH HIV INFECTION

Raymond, a 2-year-old child, has had recurrent infections since he was born. After a recent illness with fever, vomiting, and diarrhea, blood tests were done to evaluate his immune function. He was diagnosed with HIV infection and admitted to the hospital for children.

- What physical needs does Raymond have at this time?
- He manifests failure to thrive, a frequent occurrence with HIV infection. How can the nurse and dietitian work together to plan a diet for him to enable him to grow?
- What information does Raymond's family need?
- What can you do to provide emotional support for them?
- What community and Internet resources could be helpful?

See MyNursingKit for possible responses.

Evidence-Based Nursing

ADOLESCENTS WITH HIV INFECTION AND MEDICATION REGIMEN ADHERENCE

Clinical Question

What factors are associated with medication adherence in the HIV-infected adolescent?

The Evidence

HIV infection is a significant health problem among adolescents in the United States (Flynn, Rudy, Douglas, et al., 2004). Adherence to highly active antiretroviral therapy (HAART) has been shown to decrease morbidity and mortality; however, medication adherence in this age group is not adequate (Naar-King, Templin, Wright, et al., 2006). Medication adherence is a major challenge in the care of the adolescent with HIV infection.

A study of 65 adolescents and young adults ages 16–25 years examined three psychosocial factors that affect adherence to a HAART regimen: self-efficacy, social support, and psychological distress. The study found that rates of adherence were inadequate for effective disease management. Psychological distress and self-efficacy were associated with nonadherence. Social support was not associated with adherence to the medication regimen but was associated with self-efficacy (Naar-King et al., 2006).

Another study examined predictors of adherence to an antiretroviral medication regimen over the past 3 days. The study examined 2088 children and adolescents ages 3–18 years enrolled in the Pediatric Aids Clinical Trials Group (PACTG). While adherence rates were 84% overall, the rate for adolescents ages 15–18 years was the lowest at 76%, compared with 83–89% for younger children. In addition to age, other factors that were related to nonadherence included stress, repeating a grade in school, and a diagnosis of anxiety or depression (Williams, Storm, Montepiedra, et al., 2006).

Best Practice

Adherence to the HAART regimen is problematic in the adolescent population. In addition to age, factors associated with nonadherence include lack of self-efficacy, stress, depression, and anxiety. Research indicates that adherence to the HAART regimen significantly improves outcomes. It is essential that adolescents receive comprehensive education related to the importance of adherence to their medication regimen. Discuss strategies with adolescents that will assist them in remembering to take their medication. Referrals for counseling and stress management along with treatment for depression are indicated in some cases.

Critical Thinking

What barriers may lead to medication nonadherence in the HIV-infected adolescent? What support does the adolescent need to improve medication adherence? What measures can the nurse take to improve medication adherence in the adolescent?

See MyNursingKit for possible responses.

environment. Refer to services as needed to ensure provision of quality care after discharge.

Support groups, home healthcare nursing services, financial assistance, and psychologic counseling are usually needed at some point during the child's illness, and the family should be aware that such services are available. Assist the family with coping mechanisms to deal with feelings of guilt about the child's condition.

NURSING CARE IN THE COMMUNITY

Much of the care of the child with HIV infection takes place in the community. With the continued success of aggressive therapy, the majority of HIV-infected children can be expected to attend childcare and school. Additionally, a substantial number of these children will reach adolescence, and some will reach adulthood. Evaluate the family and community support systems and provide resources and referrals as needed. Many children with HIV infection are placed in foster homes, and these families need careful instruction to manage this multifaceted illness.

School attendance guidelines recommend unrestricted school attendance and/or childcare center attendance for children with HIV infection. In addition, children should be allowed to participate in all activities to the extent that their health and other recommendations for management of infectious diseases permit (AAP, 2006). Contraindications to school attendance include lack of control of body secretions, biting, and open wounds that cannot be covered. Since it is not required that the school or childcare center be notified of a child's HIV status, the nurse should prepare the school personnel with training related to care for children with known and unknown cases of HIV. CDC guidelines for standard precautions should always be followed in the school, childcare, and home settings (Kukka, 2004). The nurse also may be responsible for providing medicines or other care for the HIV-infected child at school (Plowfield, 2007).

Assist the family in altering the home environment to provide standard precautions during care. Make sure the child and family understand that HIV is transmitted through blood, urine, stool, and other body fluids. Educate family members on the importance of hygiene measures. Encourage careful hand hygiene and instruct parents to use recommended precautions when handling body fluids. Explain that they should wear gloves when changing diapers; disposing of urine, stool, and emesis; or treating the child's cuts and scrapes. In addition, teach them to wash their hands immediately after contact with blood or other body fluids. Instruct parents to use a bleach solution for disinfection of objects when necessary and to avoid contact with people with infectious illnesses.

Precautions to guard against foodborne illness are particularly important for the HIV-infected child. Parents also need instruction on correct administration and side effects of any medications the child is taking. Giving a child a complicated combination of drugs can be challenging for all families; therefore, teaching should be tailored to the particular family and should be followed by repeated evaluation of the family's success with medication administration.

Nursing Practice

When a child has been diagnosed with HIV, even common childhood infections are a cause for concern. Conditions such as respiratory infection, fever, chickenpox, or gastrointestinal illness can progress rapidly to a life-threatening stage. Teach families to seek prompt treatment at the first sign of illness.

The parent's close observation and feeling that something is not right should be cause for concern and medical evaluation.

Teaching Highlights

FOOD SAFETY

The child with HIV infection has an increased susceptibility to foodborne disease. Instruct parents to practice the following:

1. Use a separate cutting board for meats, and wash it with hot soapy water after use.
2. Wash all utensils with hot soapy water between any uses.
3. Wash and peel fresh fruits and vegetables. Consider use of canned varieties to limit exposure to microorganisms.
4. Use a disposable cloth or cloth that is washed after each meal to clean dishes. A sponge can harbor microorganisms and should not be used.
5. If well water is the source of drinking water, have it checked for contaminants regularly.
6. Do not allow the child to eat raw or undercooked meats, fish, eggs, or cookie dough. Avoid natural honey.
7. Bleach solution (2 tablespoons liquid chlorine bleach added to 1 quart cold water) is a good low-cost sanitizer for cleaning surfaces in the kitchen.

Emphasize the importance of promoting the child's development. Perform frequent developmental screenings. Teach the parents how to support the child in achieving developmental milestones. Encourage contact with other children and adults, provide for appropriate toys, teach parents how to encourage the child's communication, and praise the family for what the child has already accomplished. Children who manifest decreasing developmental milestones or other neurologic symptoms should be assessed by the primary care provider for HIV-induced encephalopathy. The nurse's record of development will be of great importance in this situation. The child needs regular health maintenance care, such as child health supervision visits, immunizations, and care for any other health conditions.

EVALUATION

There are many desired outcomes of care for the child with HIV infection or AIDS. Expected outcomes of nursing care include the following:

- Decreased numbers of cases of pediatric HIV due to vertical transmission from known infected mothers
- Prevention of infectious diseases in children with HIV infection
- Adequate respiratory function and perfusion
- Nutritional intake to support normal growth patterns and prevent malnutrition
- Adequate family coping with the stress of chronic disease
- School attendance and support in the educational process

AUTOIMMUNE DISORDERS

In an immune system damaged by pathologic changes, an immune response may occur to some of the body's own proteins, resulting in the production of autoantibodies. These pathologic conditions in which the body directs the immune response against itself—identifying "self" as "nonself"—are called *autoimmune disorders.*

The primary feature of autoimmune disorders is tissue injury caused by a probable immunologic reaction of the host with its own tissues. Structural or functional changes occur as immune cells attack other cells in the body. Autoimmune disorders are grouped into systemic and organ-specific diseases. Systemic diseases, which generally involve more than one organ, include systemic lupus erythematosus and juvenile arthritis, which are discussed in this chapter. Organ-specific diseases, which primarily affect a single organ, include insulin-dependent diabetes mellitus type 1 (see Chapter 55 ∞) and thyroiditis. Idiopathic (or immune) thrombocytic purpura is an immune disease affecting blood platelets and clotting and is discussed in Chapter 51 ∞.

SYSTEMIC LUPUS ERYTHEMATOSUS

Systemic lupus erythematosus (SLE) is a chronic inflammatory, autoimmune disease of unknown origin that involves many organ systems. SLE is characterized by the presence of antinuclear antibodies (ANA) (Gottlieb & Ilowite, 2006). While it is primarily diagnosed in adulthood, approximately 15–20% of cases are diagnosed in childhood, usually in adolescence (Marinescu & Illowite, 2007; Stichweh, Arce, & Pascual, 2004). Systemic lupus erythematosus is more common among Native Americans, African Americans, Hispanics, and Asians than Caucasians. More severe disease is seen in African Americans and Hispanics (Gottlieb & Ilowite, 2006). Prior to puberty, females are affected more often than males, with a 3:1 ratio; after puberty, the ratio increases to 9:1 (Marinescu & Illowite, 2007; Gottlieb & Ilowite, 2006).

Etiology and Pathophysiology

The exact etiology of SLE is unknown. A genetic component is suspected, as the disease is often more prevalent in members of the same family. It is believed that in those genetically predisposed, an outside environmental agent causes the body to initiate an abnormal immune system response to its own tissues (Lupus Foundation of America, 2008; Pongmarutani, Alpert, & Miller, 2006). The body produces autoantibodies and combines with antigens to form immune complexes. These antigen–antibody complexes are deposited in the connective tissue, triggering an inflammatory response. The chronic inflammation then destroys connective tissue. The tissue damage varies according to the organ involvement, though the tissues most likely to be affected are the small blood vessels, glomeruli, joints, spleen, and heart valves. Because many systems can be affected simultaneously, organ damage with subsequent multisystem failure may occur.

Clinical Manifestations

Manifestations of SLE may be acute, with onset of nephritis, arthritis, or vasculitis, or may be noted as a gradual onset with nonspecific symptoms. Symptoms depend on the organ involved and the amount of tissue damage that has occurred. Initial nonspecific symptoms include fever, chills, fatigue, oral ulcers, malaise, and weight loss. The most common symptoms are rash, fever, mucositis, and arthritis. A butterfly rash on the face, consisting of a pink or red rash over the bridge of the nose extending to the cheeks, is a characteristic finding (Gottlieb & Ilowite, 2006). Children with SLE may have anemia, leukopenia, and thrombocytopenia. See "Clinical Manifestations: Systemic Lupus Erythematosus."

Systemic lupus erythematosus is characterized by periods of remission and exacerbation (flares). Flares are triggered by a variety of causes, including sun exposure, an upper respiratory infection or other infection, and stress. The child or family may be able to identify other triggers to flares, such as particular events, activities, or situations.

Clinical Therapy

Blood tests reveal anemia, an elevated blood urea nitrogen (BUN), abnormal plasma proteins, abnormal erythrocyte sedimentation rate (ESR), presence of antinuclear antibodies, and a positive LE (lupus erythematosus) cell reaction, which indicates nonspecific inflammation. The Coombs' test is positive. Radiologic examinations include chest radiographs and CT scans, as well as MRI of affected joints. A 24-hour urine collection and imaging studies, as well as renal biopsies, may be performed to evaluate lupus nephritis. Urinalysis may reveal proteinuria.

The goals of medical management are to create a remission of symptoms and to prevent complications. Corticosteroids, such as prednisone or methylprednisolone, are prescribed to control inflammation. Antimalarial preparations, such as hydroxychloroquine, are used to treat symptoms associated with skin lesions and renal and arthritic problems. Although the exact action of these drugs on SLE is not known, they often permit continued remission with a lowered dose of steroids. Nonsteroidal antiinflammatory drugs (ibuprofen, naproxen) are used to relieve muscle and joint pain. Immunosuppressant drugs, such as cyclophosphamide, azathioprine, mycophenolate mofetil, cyclosporine, and methotrexate, have been used to help control SLE (Buka & Cunningham, 2005; Gottlieb & Ilowite, 2006; Marinescu & Ilowite, 2007). Diet may be restricted if the child has excessive weight gain or fluid retention from steroids and renal damage. Prognosis depends on the severity of the internal organ involvement. Whereas systemic lupus erythematosus was once considered a fatal disease, the 5-year survival rate for juvenile onset SLE is 92% and the 10 year survival rate is 85% (Gottlieb &

Clinical Manifestations

SYSTEMIC LUPUS ERYTHEMATOSUS

SYSTEM	CLINICAL MANIFESTATIONS
Integumentary	A butterfly rash on the face, consisting of a pink or red rash over the bridge of the nose extending to the cheeks, is a characteristic finding Photosensitivity Alopecia Mouth or nose ulcers
Hematologic	Fatigue Fever Easy bruising Bloody stools Nosebleeds Fever
Musculoskeletal	Joint pain Swollen inflamed joints Myalgias Muscle weakness
Neurologic	Headache Peripheral neuropathy Psychosis Seizures Mood disorder Cognitive disorder Stroke
Pulmonary	Chest Pain Dyspnea Pulmonary hypertension Pulmonary embolism
Cardiac	Arrhythmias Chest pain Friction rub Raynaud's phenomenon (fingers turning white and/or blue in the cold)
Renal	Hematuria Hypertension Proteinuria Edema
Gastrointestinal	Abdominal pain (may radiate to the shoulder)

Adapted from: Gottlieb, B. S., & Ilowite, N. T. (2006). Systemic Lupus Erythematosus in Children and Adolescents. *Pediatric In Review, 27*(9), 323–328; Petty, R. E., & Laxer, R. M. (2005). Systemic Lupus Erythematosus in Cassidy, J. T., Petty, R. E., Laxer, R. M., & Lindsley, C. B. *Textbook of Pediatric Rheumatology* (5th ed), pp. 342–391. Philadelphia: Elsevier Saunders; Stichweh, D., Arce, E., & Pascual, V. (2004). Update on Pediatric Systemic Lupus Erythematosus. *Current Opinion In Rheumatology, 16,* 577–587.

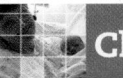

Growth and Development

The side effects of the corticosteroids, immunosuppressants, and antimalarial drugs used in the treatment of children with SLE are significant and include hair loss, susceptibility to infection, "moon face," retinal damage, and bone loss. These are significant side effects for the adolescent, who is commonly concerned about appearance. Teens with SLE may need special teaching, guidance, and support. Support groups or Internet chat rooms may be helpful.

Ilowite, 2006). Kidney failure is managed by hemodialysis or peritoneal dialysis. Renal transplantation has been very successful for treatment of renal failure secondary to lupus nephritis.

NURSING MANAGEMENT

NURSING ASSESSMENT AND DIAGNOSIS

PHYSIOLOGIC ASSESSMENT

Assess the child's nutritional status, including baseline weight and history of recent weight loss or weight gain. Assess the skin for rashes, ulcers, photosensitivity, ecchymosis, petechiae, cyanosis, and hair loss. Respiratory assessment includes breath sounds, respiratory rate, and pleural effusion or pleuritis. Cardiovascular assessment includes vital signs, heart sounds, and symptoms of pericarditis or friction rub. Musculoskeletal assessment includes joint pain, joint deformity, pain, weakness, and ability to perform activities of daily living. Assess the neurologic system for changes in affect or cognitive abilities and seizure activity. Palpate the spleen to detect splenomegaly.

PSYCHOSOCIAL ASSESSMENT

Because SLE is a chronic disease that primarily affects adolescents, psychosocial assessment is indicated. Assess family interactions, exploring stressful situations such as divorce or trauma. Treatment-related restrictions associated with medications and changes in appearance such as weight gain, cushingoid appearance, and skin rashes can lead to withdrawal, depression, and suicidal tendencies. Perform psychosocial assessments periodically as the child grows and adapts to the disorder or faces new developmental challenges with a chronic disease.

Several nursing diagnoses may apply to the child with SLE. These include the following:

- *Risk for Ineffective Management of Therapeutic Regimen, Family,* related to complexity of therapeutic regimen
- *Risk for Ineffective Tissue Perfusion (Renal)* related to interrupted blood flow in kidneys
- *Risk for Impaired Skin Integrity* related to photosensitivity
- *Risk for Activity Intolerance* related to joint pain and fatigue
- *Risk for Disturbed Body Image* related to side effects of medications and skin alterations
- *Risk for Infection* related to immunosuppressive medications
- *Acute Pain* related to joint inflammation and injury

PLANNING AND IMPLEMENTATION

The goals of nursing care are to assist the child to manage and cope with a chronic disease, prevent infection, maintain fluid balance, promote adequate nutrition, promote skin integrity, promote rest and comfort, manage side effects of medication, avoid triggers for disease flares, and provide emotional support.

PREVENT INFECTION

Infections are a leading cause of death for patients with systemic lupus erythematosus. Prophylactic antibiotics may be required for dental work and surgical procedures. Instruct the patient and family to inform all healthcare providers of the disease to plan for prophylactic measures. Emphasize the importance of receiving recommended immunizations and of obtaining a yearly influenza vaccine to prevent infection. Instruct the family on hand hygiene and infection control measures in the home. Warn adolescents about the dangers of tattooing and body piercing because of the risk of infection.

MAINTAIN FLUID BALANCE

Because most children with SLE have renal involvement, nursing care includes maintaining accurate intake and output measurements and frequent evaluation of the child's fluid and electrolyte status and weight.

PROMOTE ADEQUATE NUTRITION

Currently, there are no specific dietary plans for the child with SLE; however, the diet may be restricted according to renal involvement, weight gain, weight loss, or other complications. The child is at risk for weight gain associated with treatment with steroids and a decreased activity level during exacerbations of this disease. A well-balanced, nutritious diet with calcium and vitamin D supplements to support bone density as well as appropriate fluid intake for age should be encouraged.

PROMOTE SKIN INTEGRITY

Presence of ulcers on mucous membranes can cause weakening of the tissues, placing the child at increased risk for infection. Provide instructions on oral care to maintain intact oral mucosa. Encourage the use of good hygienic measures and a mild soap for the skin. Recommend that adolescents limit their use of cosmetics, especially oil-based. Reinforce the importance of avoiding sunlight as much as possible and the use of sun protection factor (SPF) of 30 or higher at all times when in the sun. Encourage the child to wear protective clothing to limit exposure to sunlight (see Chapter 59 for discussion of sun exposure). Additionally, avoidance of unprotected fluorescent lighting is recommended, since exacerbations of systemic lupus erythematosus have been reported following this exposure. Educate adolescents that the use of tanning beds will cause the same reaction as sun exposure (Lupus Foundation of America, 2008). Provide instructions on oral care to maintain intact oral mucosa. Provide instructions on the care of the head if alopecia occurs.

PROMOTE REST AND COMFORT

The child with SLE experiences fatigue and joint pain, leaving little energy reserve during acute episodes of the disease. Encourage frequent rest periods and a nutritious diet to maximize energy stores. A physical therapist can plan a program to encourage mobility and increase muscle strength. Implement measures such as application of heat to painful areas.

MANAGE SIDE EFFECTS OF MEDICATIONS

Observe for side effects of medications used for treatment, and teach the child and family about these effects. For example, immunosuppressant drugs can promote infection anywhere in the body, and nonsteroidal antiinflammatory drugs commonly cause gastric distress and bleeding of the gastrointestinal tract. The antimalarial drug hydroxychloroquine increases the risk of retinopathy and blindness; therefore, eye examinations should be performed every 6 months (Laxer, 2005). Corticosteroid side effects include cushingoid effects, weight gain, and hypertension. Sulfa drugs should be avoided because they increase photosensitivity.

MyNursingKit Animation: Methotrexate

AVOID TRIGGERS FOR DISEASE FLARES

Many children and their parents can recognize the signs of an impending flare and the triggers that precede them. Partner with the parents and child to implement measures to avoid these triggers. Discuss preventive behaviors such as avoiding sun exposure and avoiding stressors. Adolescents should be warned that alcohol, smoking, and drugs also pose an increased risk due to the potential to stimulate flares. Female adolescents who are sexually active should avoid birth control pills that contain the hormone estrogen, since the extra estrogen may exacerbate symptoms. Alternative birth control methods should be discussed with the adolescent. See "Complementary Care: SLE and Stress" for a discussion of stress reduction.

PROVIDE EMOTIONAL SUPPORT

Adolescents may have an altered body image as a result of rash, alopecia, arthritic changes in the joints, and chronic disease. Referral to a lupus support group, social services, or counseling may be helpful. The American Lupus Society and the Lupus Foundation of America can provide information to help parents and children adjust to the disease. The Arthritis Foundation also publishes a useful pamphlet, "Meeting the Challenge: A Young Person's Guide to Living with Lupus."

Numerous Internet support groups are also available for those with systemic lupus erythematosus.

EVALUATION

Successful outcomes of nursing care involve management of this chronic disease. Expected outcomes of nursing care include the following:

- Absence of pain
- Absence of infection
- Adequate intake and output levels, with demonstrated fluid and electrolyte balance and renal function
- Maintenance of intact skin
- Positive body image

> **Complementary Care**
>
> **SLE AND STRESS**
>
> Systemic lupus erythematosus exacerbations have been linked to stress. Stress-reducing techniques such as guided imagery, reading, yoga, and quiet games can benefit the child or adolescent and reduce exacerbations of SLE. The nurse can review the child's activities and partner with the child and family to evaluate the need for stress reductions. It may be necessary to discontinue a sport or music lesson or other activity temporarily to provide a chance for the child to relax each day. What stressors are common to children, and how can they be reduced in the child with SLE?

JUVENILE ARTHRITIS

Arthritis in children has been referred to as juvenile rheumatoid arthritis, or JRA, for many years. However, positive rheumatoid factor (RF) is rare in children under 7 years of age, so the term JRA may be misleading (Cassidy & Petty, 2005). Although some authors continue to refer to arthritis in children as JRA, many now use the term *juvenile idiopathic arthritis (JIA)* to more appropriately describe the disease. Some authors even use a third name, *juvenile chronic arthritis*. Because there is inconsistency with the terminology, the discussion here will focus on juvenile arthritis.

Juvenile arthritis refers to chronic joint inflammation diagnosed prior to 16 years of age. This disease results in decreased mobility, swelling, and pain. The peak age of onset for juvenile arthritis is between 1 and 3 years of age, with the illness occurring twice as often in females as in males (Cassidy & Petty, 2005). Approximately 18 of every 100,000 children develop juvenile arthritis each year and the prevalence is estimated to be up to 150 of every 100,000 children (Bernatsky, Duffy, Malleson, et al., 2007).

Juvenile arthritis affects joints and surrounding tissues in addition to potential effects on other organs such as the heart, lungs, liver, and eyes. During its course, the child may experience pain, impaired mobility, and interference with normal growth and development. Children may enter remission or manifest continued symptoms of a chronic disease. Remission may last for months, years, or a lifetime. Of children with juvenile arthritis, 70% experience permanent remission of the disease by adulthood. Rarely, the disease is unresponsive to treatment or the child may suffer lasting impairment such as bone and joint changes. Children with early onset have a better prognosis for complete recovery.

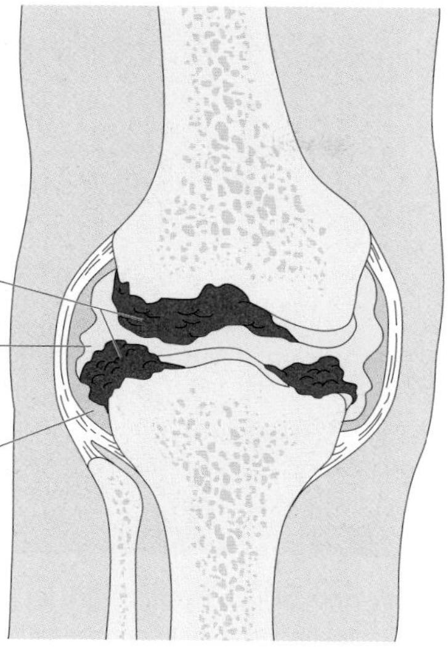

● **Figure 50–2** Joint inflammation and destruction in juvenile arthritis.

Etiology and Pathophysiology

The cause of juvenile arthritis is unknown, but it is thought to have an autoimmune basis. Inflammation begins in the joint and leads to pain and swelling (Figure 50–2 ●). Scar tissue eventually develops, resulting in limited range of motion. Although terminology varies among the different classifications, according to the most current classification the three major types of juvenile arthritis are polyarthritis, oligoarthritis arthritis (formerly known as pauciarticular arthritis), and systemic arthritis (Cassidy & Petty, 2005).

- *Polyarthritis* involves 5 or more joints during the first 6 months after diagnosis, particularly the knee, wrist, elbow, and ankle joints. This type of arthritis affects approximately 30% of the children with juvenile arthritis. This classificaition is further identified as RF positive or RF negative. Only 3–5% of these children are RF positive (Petty & Cassidy, 2005a).
- *Oligoarthritis arthritis* primarily affects the knees, ankles, and elbows, and occurs more frequently in females. Approximately 50–60% of children with juvenile arthritis have oligoarthritis. Four or fewer joints are affected in this type of juvenile arthritis. Uveitis occurs in 15–20 % of children with oligoarthritis (Petty & Cassidy, 2005b).
- *Systemic arthritis* affects males and females equally and is characteristically manifested by high fever, polyarthritis, and rheumatoid rash. Systemic arthritis affects internal organs and joints. Approximately 10–15% of children with juvenile arthritis have systemic arthritis with no peak age of onset reported (Petty & Cassidy, 2005c).

Clinical Manifestations

Juvenile arthritis may be restricted to a few joints or be systemic with involvement of multiple joints. Symptoms can include fever, rash, lymphadenopathy, splenomegaly, and hepatomegaly. The child may develop a limp or obviously favor one extremity over the other. A slow rate of growth or uneven growth of extremities may also be noted. Pain, stiffness, loss of motion, and swelling occur in the large joints such as the knees. Older children may develop symmetric involvement of the small joints of the hand. The disease is frequently chronic, extending over several years after an initial manifestation with pain and other symptoms. Remissions and exacerbations are characteristic.

Clinical Therapy

Diagnosis is made primarily on the basis of the history and assessment findings, in particular, arthritis having an onset before 16 years of age and persisting for at least 6 weeks, with no other identifiable cause (Marinescu & Ilowite, 2007). There are no specific laboratory tests to confirm the diagnosis although there are tests to help support the diagnosis. In some children, test results are positive for rheumatoid factor, human leukocyte antigen (HLA) B27, and antinuclear antibody (ANA). Erythrocyte sedimentation rate (ESR) and C-reactive protein (CRP) tests may be helpful in determining the amount of inflammation (Cassidy & Petty, 2005). Radiographs are generally performed to exclude other causes, such as fractures, rather than as a definitive diagnosis, though the radiographs are useful in monitoring for joint damage and bone development.

The goals of treatment are to relieve pain, control inflammation, manage systemic complications, preserve joint function and range of motion, and promote normal physical, psychosocial, behavioral, and vocational development (Cassidy & Petty, 2005; Emery, 2004). Nonsteroidal anti-inflammatory (NSAIDs) drugs such as aspirin, ibuprofen, and naproxen are used to reduce inflammation and pain. Children who do not respond to NSAIDs may be treated with disease-modifying antirheumatic drugs such as sulfasalazine and methotrexate. Steroids such as prednisone and methylprednisolone may be used with children with more severe forms of juvenile arthritis. Biologic response modifiers such as Etanercept have also been used to treat juvenile arthritis (Cassidy & Petty 2005; Emery, 2004; Marinescu & Ilowite, 2007). Physical and/or occupational therapy are performed to increase strength and mobility of joints while protecting them from injury. The physical therapist and/or occupational therapist tailors an exercise regimen specifically to the child. Range of motion exercises are essential to maintain joint mobility. Surgery is occasionally performed to relieve pain and maintain or improve joint function in children with joint contractures.

Complications such as chronic uveitis, which results from chronic inflammation, may occur in children with juvenile arthritis. Children less than 6 years of age with oligoarthritis or polyarthritis who have a positive ANA test should have an eye exam every 3–4 months. Children 7 or older or those with a negative

Nursing Practice

Infants and children with juvenile arthritis who are receiving aspirin therapy are at risk of developing Reye syndrome if they contract influenza or chickenpox. These children should be immunized with varicella vaccine and should receive influenza vaccine in the fall of each year. See Chapter 56 for further information about Reye syndrome.

ANA test need an exam every 6 months. Because uveitis is very rare in children with systemic arthritis, the recommended frequency for eye exams is every 12 months (Marinescu & Ilowite, 2007).

Growth interference for the child with juvenile rheumatoid arthritis is a potential complication. The specific disorder may result in bone growth disturbance such as contractures or effusions. The administration of corticosteroids can also inhibit growth.

NURSING MANAGEMENT

NURSING ASSESSMENT AND DIAGNOSIS

A careful history is important, as it is sometimes the primary mode of diagnosis. Assess for joint swelling and deformities, pain, decreased mobility, morning stiffness, fever, nodules under the skin, growth delays, and enlarged lymph nodes. The following nursing diagnoses may apply to the child with juvenile arthritis.

- *Activity Intolerance* related to chronic pain
- *Impaired Physical Mobility* related to joint stiffness and inflammation
- *Pain* related to joint inflammation
- *Disturbed Body Image* related to condition and physical appearance

PLANNING AND IMPLEMENTATION

Nursing care focuses on promoting mobility, encouraging adequate nutrition, and teaching the parents and child about the disease and its management. Most care will occur in the community, including physical therapy, with only occasional hospitalizations at the time of an exacerbation of the disease.

PROMOTE IMPROVED MOBILITY

The goals of physical therapy are to maintain joint function, strengthen muscles, increase tone, maintain body alignment, and prevent permanent deformities such as contractures. Range of motion exercises, stretching, hydrotherapy, and swimming exercises help to prevent deformities (Figure 50–3 ●). Encourage the child to perform activities of daily living. Exercise may be painful or even difficult for the child, but it is important because it strengthens and stretches the muscles and prevents potential contractures. Emphasize the importance of establishing a regular exercise and activity routine. Encourage periods of rest during exacerbations, as the child fatigues more easily.

PROMOTE ADEQUATE NUTRITION

Promote general health by encouraging a well-balanced diet. Children with decreased mobility may have reduced metabolic needs, and excess weight causes additional muscle strain. Periodically perform diet recalls and nutritional assessments. Plot growth carefully and watch for changes in growth percentiles (see Chapter 34∞ for additional information regarding nutrition assessment).

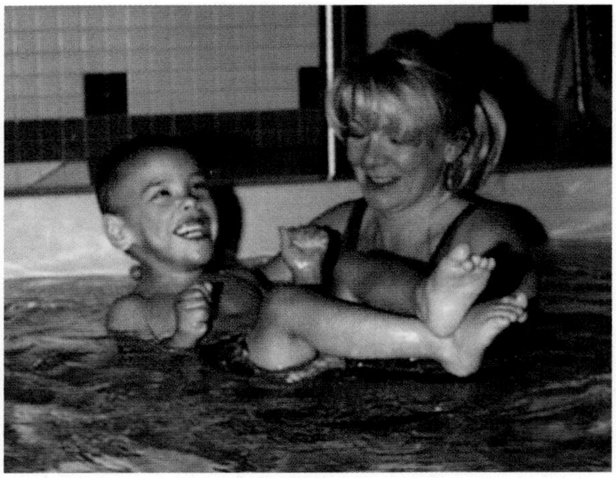

● **Figure 50–3** Hydrotherapy for joint function. The physical therapist uses hydrotherapy to help maintain joint function in a child who has juvenile arthritis.

NURSING CARE IN THE COMMUNITY

The child with juvenile arthritis may never, or rarely, be hospitalized. Most care takes place during visits to healthcare offices, clinics, and physical therapy. Educate parents on the child's condition and prognosis, and answer their questions about the child's treatment. The child may need support to adjust to the diagnosis of a chronic illness. Allow the child to express anger and frustration about the diagnosis of arthritis. Allow the opportunity for the child and parents to express feelings regarding the crippling effects of the disease. Social services, a child life specialist, or a psychologist may be consulted as needed.

Encourage the child to maintain contact with peers and to attend school whenever possible. Explain to the child and parents that overexertion may exacerbate the disease. Inform parents about possible complications of juvenile arthritis, such as altered growth related to early closure of epiphyseal plates, small joint contractures, and synovitis. Partner with the family and school officials to meet the child's needs. Accommodations at school may include providing a set of books for the home so that the child is not required to carry the books home daily. Additional time may be required for the child to move from class to class. Adaptive computers and tutors during exacerbations may be helpful. School nurses work with the child, family, and school personnel to establish the child's Individualized Education Plan (IEP) (Rettig, Merhar, & Cron, 2004). Refer parents and children to the Arthritis Foundation and the American Juvenile Arthritis Organization for further information and support.

EVALUATION

Expected outcomes of nursing care for the child with juvenile arthritis include the following:

- Maintenance of joint mobility and absence of joint deformity
- Absence of pain
- Positive body image

- Absence of infection
- Parental understanding and support of the therapeutic process

ALLERGIC REACTIONS

For unclear reasons, there continues to be a rise in the number of children diagnosed with some types of allergy, such as allergic rhinitis and asthma. Why are some children allergic to cats, for instance, while no one else in the family has allergies? To answer this question, the nurse needs a basic understanding of the mechanisms of allergy.

Allergy is an abnormal or altered reaction to an antigen. Antigens responsible for clinical manifestations of allergy are called **allergens**. Allergens can be ingested in food or drugs, injected or absorbed through contact with unbroken skin, and inhaled. Common allergens in children include:

- medications (such as penicillin)
- animal dander
- dust, mites, and mold
- plant pollens
- foods (such as nuts, seafood, or egg white)

An allergic reaction is an antigen–antibody reaction and can manifest itself as anaphylaxis, atopic disease, serum sickness, or contact dermatitis. Therefore, the symptoms can be mild to severe or life threatening, and they can be localized or systemic. Characteristic findings in children with allergies are summarized in Table 50–5.

The **hypersensitivity response**, an overreaction of the immune system, is responsible for allergic reactions. Hypersensitivity reactions have been classified into four types (see "Clinical Manifestations: Types of Hypersensitivity Reactions"). Type I hypersensitivity reactions are immediate, occurring within seconds or minutes of exposure to the antigen. The release of chemical substances such as histamine is responsible for the signs and symptoms. The first time a child is exposed to the allergen, there is no reaction. With every exposure thereafter, however, the allergic child may have a reaction to the allergen.

Nursing Practice

Anaphylaxis is a potentially life-threatening systemic reaction to an allergen that may manifest with itching; localized or generalized hives on the hands, feet, or mucosa; soft-tissue swelling; cough; dyspnea; pallor; sweating; and tachycardia. Symptoms can occur within minutes or up to 2 hours after exposure to an allergy-causing substance. The disorder is rare in children, and annual incidence of anaphylactic reactions is approximately 30 per 100,000 individuals (including adults) (Sampson & Leung, 2004).

Type II sensitivity reactions occur within 15 to 30 minutes after exposure to the antigen. Type III hypersensitivity reaction may be difficult to distinguish from type II reaction. Hypersensitivity reactions generally peak within 6 hours.

Type IV reactions are delayed responses that do not appear until several hours after exposure and require 24 to 72 hours to fully develop. A type IV reaction, which is not confined to any specific tissue, is elicited by relatively complex antigens such as those of bacteria and viruses and by simple antigens such as drugs and metals.

Assessment of the child with an allergy includes a complete physical examination; laboratory, x-ray, and pulmonary function studies; tests of nasal function; and skin testing. Treatment generally involves avoidance of the allergen, such as substitution of a different drug when the child has a drug allergy. Desensitization may sometimes be used with increasing doses of

Table 50–5 Characteristic Findings in Children with Allergies

System/Organ	Findings
Respiratory system	Wheezing, rhinitis (seasonal and perennial), cough, adventitious breath sounds, inspiratory stridor, edema of glottis, nasal congestion or discharge
Gastrointestinal system	Abdominal pain and colic, mouth sores, constipation, diarrhea, bloody stools, geographic tongue, vomiting
Skin	Angioedema, urticaria, eczema, atopic dermatitis, erythema multiforme, purpura, drug and food rashes, contact dermatitis
Nervous system	Headache, tension, fatigue, seizures, Ménière syndrome, tremor, irritability, sleep disorders, decreased concentration
Eye	Conjunctivitis, cataract, ciliary spasm, iritis, itching of eyes, tearing
Blood	Thrombocytopenic purpura, hemolytic anemia, leukopenia, agranulocytosis
Musculoskeletal system	Arthralgia, myalgia, torticollis
Genitourinary system	Dysuria, vulvovaginitis, enuresis
Miscellaneous	Anaphylactic shock, serum sickness

Clinical Manifestations

TYPES OF HYPERSENSITIVITY REACTIONS

TYPE	ETIOLOGY	CLINICAL MANIFESTATIONS	EXAMPLES
Type I Localized or systemic reactions (anaphylaxis)	Antibodies bind to certain cells, causing release of chemical substances such as histamine that produce an inflammatory reaction.	Hypotension, wheezing, spasm of smooth muscle; stridor, wheal, urticaria edema, wheezing, vomiting, diarrhea	Anaphylaxis Extrinsic asthma
Type II Tissue-specific reactions	Antibodies cause activation of complement system, which leads to tissue damage.	Variable; may include dyspnea or fever	Transfusion reaction ABO incompatibility Hemolytic anemia
Type III Immune-complex reactions	Immune complexes are deposited in tissues, where they activate complement, which results in a generalized inflammatory reaction.	Urticaria, fever, joint pain	Acute glomerulonephritis Serum sickness
Type IV Delayed reactions	Antigens stimulate T cells that release lymphokines, which cause inflammation and tissue damage.	Variable; may include fever, erythema, pruritus, contact dermatitis, blistering	Contact dermatitis Tuberculin skin test Graft-versus-host disease Stevens Johnson Syndrome Allograft rejection

the allergen administered subcutaneously in an office where resuscitation is readily available. This treatment is useful for allergy to bees or some pollens. For skin allergies, the allergen is avoided, skin is kept well lubricated, and topical steroids may be used. Oral antihistamines are sometimes used to treat allergy. Emergency medical care may be required to treat anaphylaxis.

Nursing Management

The child with allergies requires a thorough assessment, including a complete past medical history, family history, personal and social history, and review of symptoms. The history focuses on the following areas:

- What symptoms does the child experience? Encourage the child to describe the difficulty in his or her own words.
- Are the symptoms continuous or intermittent? What are the frequency and duration of episodes?
- When did the child first begin to experience symptoms? Did the child have eczema/atopic dermatitis or a feeding problem in infancy or childhood? Did the infant have frequent bouts of colic or skin problems when new foods were introduced? Was there a change in symptoms at puberty? Are the symptoms becoming worse or spontaneously improving?
- What known agents in the environment cause difficulties?
- Are there seasonal variations in symptoms? At what time of the day or night do symptoms usually occur?

The nurse may be responsible for performing intradermal skin tests for allergies (Figure 50–4 ●). Nursing care focuses on treating the symptoms, alleviating the anxiety of the child and parents, and identifying the allergens. Educating the child and family on methods to minimize or avoid exposure to allergens is important. Teach parents of children who have had severe reactions to bee or wasp stings how to take precautions and how to provide emergency treatment if the child is stung.

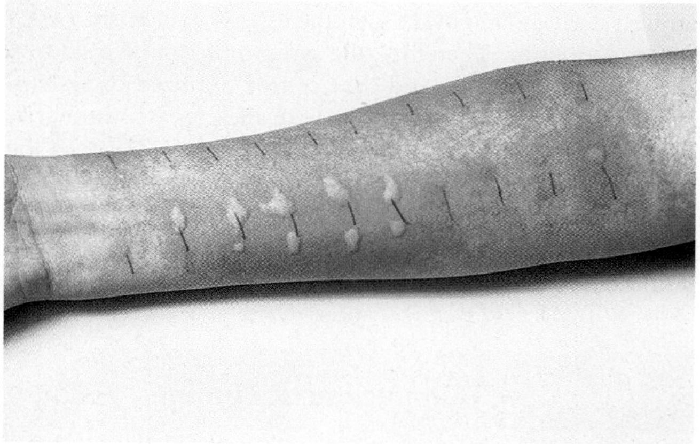

● **Figure 50–4** Results of intradermal skin testing on the forearm. Injections are given on each side of the markings. Note the positive results marked by induration and erythema in response to certain antigens.

Used with permission from VU/Southern Illinois University/Visuals Unlimited.

Families may need instructions on allergy-proofing the home. Pets, dust, carpets, fabrics, feather pillows and bedding, and cigarette smoke can all cause allergic reactions. If families are reluctant to give up pets, frequent baths can reduce dander,

Nursing Practice

If the child has had a severe or systemic reaction in the past to a bee or wasp sting, ensure that the parents know how to handle an anaphylactic reaction if the child is stung again. Kits with syringes of premeasured epinephrine are available by prescription. Instruct family members on how to use the kit. Make sure that the kit is properly stored without exposure to sun or high temperature. Have the family check the expiration date of the adrenaline frequently. The child should wear a medical alert bracelet. A kit should be readily available at school, child care, or other settings, with someone instructed in its use. An allergy specialist should be consulted to determine whether desensitization injections would be helpful for the child.

which is the usual allergen. Instruct the family on proper use of epinephrine (Figure 50–5 ●).

When the child has type I reactions to an environmental substance, avoidance of the allergen is most critical. In addition, care providers, families, and school personnel must be able to treat anaphylaxis if exposure to the allergen occurs. When the child is hospitalized, be sure to label the child's chart and bed and apply a red armband to alert others to allergies. School nurses keep records about children's allergies and inform school personnel about the allergies and cautions that need to be followed. See Chapter 34 ∞ for more information about serious reactions to food, such as peanut allergy. Nurses must be aware of the resuscitation procedures and equipment in all facilities such as hospital units, offices, childcare centers, and schools. See Chapter 47 ∞ for airway maintenance.

LATEX ALLERGY

Latex allergy is caused by an IgE-mediated response that develops after repeated exposure to latex. Latex is a sap from the rubber tree. A reaction to latex products can be manifested as an irritant reaction of the skin, a type IV delayed hypersensitivity with redness, inflammation, and blisters on the skin, or as a type I hypersensitivity, which is immediate and often has systemic manifestations (itchy eyes, asthma, or anaphylaxis) (Paskawicz, 2005).

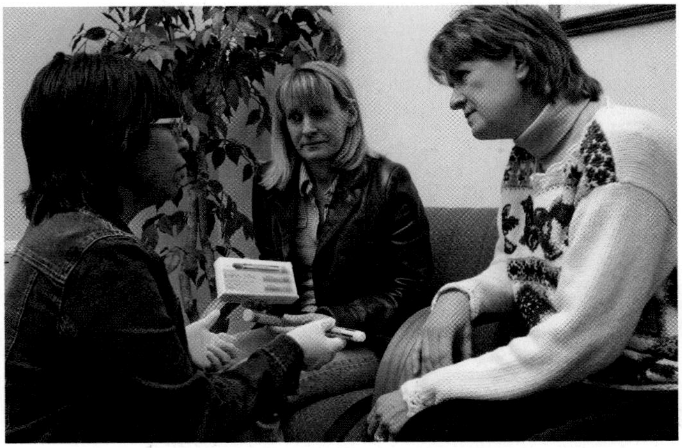

● **Figure 50–5** Instruction on epinephrine use. The school nurse is teaching a parent and a teacher about the correct use of the EpiPen, which is being maintained at home and at school in case of allergic reaction in a child who has a peanut allergy.

Teaching Highlights

REMOVING COMMON ALLERGENS FROM THE HOME

Preventing exposure to the known allergens in the home setting is important. Families can take several measures to minimize contact with allergens. These include:

- Keep pets out of the child's bedroom.
- Clean frequently with moist cloths and mops to remove dust.
- Use plastic covers on mattresses and pillows.
- Avoid using carpeting whenever possible; hard-surface floors are preferable.
- Avoid toys that collect dust (plastic and wood toys are better alternatives than stuffed fabric toys).
- Use high-efficiency air filters.
- Repair homes to prevent entry of water and subsequent molds.
- Consider dehumidification in moist climates, especially in the child's bedroom.

Latex allergy is a common finding among certain occupations, including healthcare workers, and in specific types of patients. An estimated 10% to 17% of healthcare workers, 40–65% of children with spina bifida and congenital genitourinary defects, and approximately one-third of children with three or more surgeries are sensitive to latex (Paskawicz, 2005). Latex-containing healthcare products may include gloves, drains, catheters, and intravenous ports. In some cases, intraoperative deaths have occurred when allergic individuals were exposed to latex products during surgery.

Children and adolescents at high risk should receive allergy testing for latex; the radioallergosorbent test (RAST) is most often used. This test measures circulating IgE antibodies to many allergens, and generally correlates well with specific skin test results. Healthcare personnel should use alternative products when caring for those persons at risk.

When a positive skin test has occurred or when the person has had a reaction to latex, all latex products must be removed

Nursing Practice

Starting in September 1998, the U.S. Food and Drug Administration ordered that warning labels be placed on any medical products that contain natural rubber and that a human is likely to come in contact with, advising that use of the product might cause an allergic reaction (Paskawicz, 2005). Check product labels in your healthcare facility for this warning. What products should have a label?

from the allergic individual's environment. Alternative products, such as nonlatex gloves and catheters, must be used when providing health care. People allergic to latex should also wear a medical identification bracelet at all times and should have an epinephrine kit readily available at home and school. Nurses should be alert for any signs of hypersensitivity when the child is receiving health care, and be prepared with drugs and equipment to treat anaphylaxis. This is especially important in operative settings when acute anaphylaxis is often life threatening. Nurses should emphasize to parents and children that many everyday products contain latex, including latex balloons and condoms (Table 50–6).

Table 50–6 Sources of Latex in the Home and Community with Recommended Alternatives

Frequently Contain Latex	Examples of Latex-Safe Alternatives/Barriers
Art supplies: paints, glue, erasers, fabric paints	Elmer's (School Glue, Glue-All, GluColors, Carpenters Wood Glue, Sno-Drift paste), FaberCastel erasers, Crayola (except stamps, erasers), Liquitex paints, DickBlick Tempera, acrylic paints & soap erasers, Play-Doh, Pro-Craft, Clic Eraser, Pentel erasers, pens, and pencils.
Balloons	Mylar balloons, self-sealing Myloons, Mister Balloon
Balls: Koosh balls, tennis balls, bowling balls, ball pits	PVC (Hedstrom Sports Ball), Nerf Foam Balls
Carpet backing, gym floor, gum mats	Broadloom carpets contain no NRL. For other products, provide barrier cloth or mat
Chewing gum	Bubblicious, Trident (Warner-Lambert), Wrigley gums (check new products)
Clothes: liquid appliques on tee-shirts, elastic on socks, underwear, sneakers, sandals	Cloth-covered elastic, neoprene (Decent Exposures, NO-LATEX Industries) Buster Brown elastic-free socks (Vermont Country Store)
Condoms, contraceptive sponges, diaphragm	Polyurethane (Avanti), female condom (Reality), Wide-seal Silicone Diaphragms (Milex), Trojan Supra Condom, FemCaps
	Cover with cloth, tape
CPR mannequins and medical training aids	Most Laerdal products
Crutches: tips, axillary pads, hand grips	Cover with cloth, tape
Dental dams, cups, bands, root canal material, orthodontic rubber bands	PURO/M27 intraoral elastics (Midwest Orthodontic), wire springs, sealant (Delton) dams (Meer Dental, Hygenic Corp), John O. Butler, Earloop masks (Richmond)
Diapers, incontinence pads, rubber pants	Huggies, First Quality, Gold Seal, Tranquility, Always, *some* Attends, Drypers Diapers (not training pants), Confidence (Paper-Pak), Pampers, Luvs
Feeding nipples	Silicone, vinyl (selected Gerber, Evenflo, MAM, Ross, Mead Johnson)
Latex gloves for food handling	Synthetic gloves for food handling
Handles on racquets, tools, bicycles	Vinyl, leather handles, or cover with cloth or tape
Kitchen cleaning gloves	PVC MYPLEX (Magla), cotton liners (Allerderm)
Mattress/pressure relief	Check each one for Latex content
Miscellaneous items	Some medical stickers by MediBadge, UAL, Cushie Tushie Potty Seat
Newsprint, ads, coupons, lottery scratch tickets	None
Pacifiers (check labels)	Soothies (Children's Med Ventures), selected Binky, Gerber, Infa, Kip, MAM
Paints, sealants, stains, etc.	There is no natural rubber in latex paint, though it may be present in some waterproof paints and sealants
Play pits, playground surfaces	Natural rubber latex may be a component of surfaces
Rubber bands, bungee cords	Plasti bands
Toothbrushes/infant massager	Soft bristle brush or cloth, Gerber/NUK, all Oral B products
Toys-Stretch Armstrong, old Barbies	Jurassic Park figures (Kenner), 1993 Barbie, Disney dolls (Mattel), many toys by Fisher Price, Little Tikes, Playskool, Discovery, Trolls (Norfin), Silly-putty
Water toys & equipment: beach thongs, masks, bathing suits, caps, scuba gear, goggles	PVC, plastic, nylon, Suits Me Swimwear
Wheelchair cushions	Jay, ROHO cushions, Sof Care bed/chair cushions (Gay-mar)
Wheelchair tires	Recommend using leather gloves
Zippered plastic storage bags	Waxed paper, plain plastic bags, Ziploc bags

From *Spina Bifida Association (2007) "Latex (Natural Rubber) in the Hospital Environment and Latex (Natural Rubber) in Home and Community" Retrieved December 5, 2008 from www.spinabifidaassociation.org/atf/cf/{EED435C8-F1A0-4A16-B4D8-A713BBCD9CE4}/2007%20Latex%20Lists.pdf*
Note: Associated allergies: Foods include banana, avocado, chestnut, kiwi, pear. Plants include poinsettia and milkweed pods.

Nursing Practice

Healthcare personnel are at high risk of developing latex allergy because of intense exposure to products containing latex. Nurses can protect themselves by using the following measures:

- Decrease exposure by using alternative products whenever available (use synthetic rubbers, polyethylene, nitrile, neoprene, vinyl gloves).
- Use powder-free gloves if using latex gloves (the powder has high amounts of latex, which are inhaled).
- Avoid oil-based hand creams and lotions before putting on latex gloves, as these preparations break down the latex.
- When symptoms of sensitivity to latex occur on exposure (rash, hives, nasal congestion, conjunctivitis, cough, or wheeze), contact the Employee Health Department of your facility.
- If diagnosed as latex allergic, avoid all contact and wear a medical identification bracelet.

GRAFT-VERSUS-HOST DISEASE

Graft-versus-host disease can occur when organs are transplanted or when bone marrow or stem cells are transfused into a recipient, typically as treatment for leukemia or severe combined immunodeficiency disease. The donated cells attach to the recipient child's bone marrow and begin production. The child's lymphocyte production increases and immune response develops. However, despite blood and tissue typing, sometimes the donor cells are incompatible with the recipient cells and the new cells begin to mount an immunologic response in the child who has received the transplant. The incidence of the disease is lower in matched siblings than in matched nonsibling transplants (Velardi & Locatelli, 2007).

Graft-versus-host disease may be either acute or chronic. Acute disease occurs in the first 100 days after transplant. The skin is most commonly affected, and the condition manifests as a pruritic and macular-papular rash that begins on the ears, palms, and soles, progressing to the trunk. Blistering and a burning sensation may occur. Gastrointestinal effects may include nausea, vomiting, anorexia, diarrhea, cramping, and abdominal pain. Impaired liver function is evident from jaundice and abnormal liver function tests (Velardi & Locatelli, 2007).

Chronic graft-versus-host disease occurs after 100 days posttransplant, but can appear within two months. This reaction is similar to an autoimmune reaction in the recipient's body. Recurrent infections, skin reactions, and thrombocytopenia are frequent occurrences. Mouth, throat, and esophageal ulcers, gastrointestinal disorders, cholestasis, and dry, irritated eyes can occur (Higman & Vogelsang, 2004).

Careful physical examination and laboratory tests assist in determining presence of the disease and stage of reaction. Early identification is key to beginning therapy and stopping progression of this life-threatening condition. Several drugs are used in treatment, commonly cyclosporine, tacrolimus, and prednisone (Velardi & Locatelli, 2007).

Nursing care focuses on careful physical assessment of all children who have received transplants to assist in early identification of the disease process. All body systems can be involved, especially in chronic disease, so frequent and thorough assessments are needed. Place particular emphasis on skin examination and report rashes that occur. Monitor gastrointestinal functioning by asking about nausea, vomiting, diarrhea, abdominal pain, bloody stools, and dietary intake. Weigh and measure the child and compare to earlier findings. Auscultate the lungs and be alert for signs of infection. Inquire about pain in joints or other body parts. Perform regular eye examinations and ask about burning or itching of eyes. Perform prescribed blood tests to monitor for liver and bone marrow function.

Nursing care for the child who has had a bone marrow or stem cell transplant is complex. Emphasize the need for regular examinations to identify any signs of disease. Children and their families need information and support about this immune system complication of transplantation of bone marrow or stem cells.

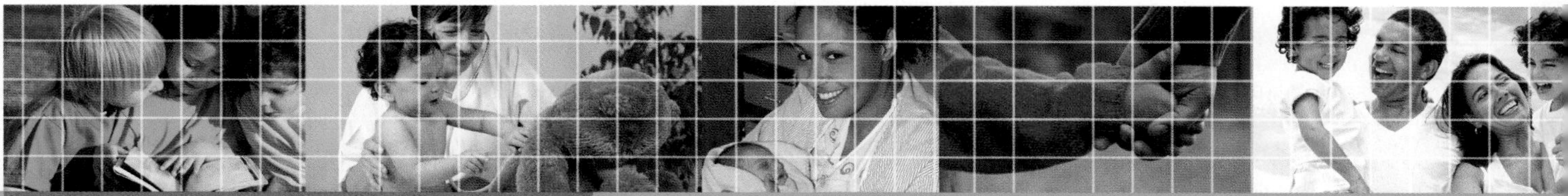

CRITICAL CONCEPT REVIEW

LEARNING OUTCOMES	CONCEPTS
50.1 Describe the structure and function of the immune system and apply that knowledge to the care of children with immunologic disorders.	1. Structure: ■ The immune system is composed of antibodies, leukocytes (white blood cells), and lymphoid tissue. ■ A child's immune system is not fully developed until age 6. 2. Function: ■ Recognizes any foreign substances within the body and eliminates them as efficiently as possible. 3. Immune system disorders may result in multisystem consequences because the immune system is involved in the regulation of all body functions.

(continued)

LEARNING OUTCOMES	CONCEPTS
50.2 Identify infection control measures to prevent the spread of infection in children with an immunodeficiency.	1. Perform frequent handwashing, standard precautions, and strict asepsis for invasive procedures. 2. Place the child in a positive-pressure room. 3. Avoid contact with persons with infectious disorders. 4. Avoid immunizations with live vaccines for child, siblings, and family members. 5. Food and items entering the child's room should receive special treatment.
50.3 Develop a nursing care plan in partnership with the family for a child with human immunodeficiency virus (HIV infection).	1. Prevent infection: ■ Perform frequent handwashing. ■ Prevent child's exposure to people with infections of any kind. ■ Instruct parents to follow modified immunization schedule. 2. Promote medication regimen adherence: ■ Instruct parents concerning the importance of compliance with medication regimen. 3. Promote respiratory function: ■ Inform parents of importance of deep breathing exercises for the prevention of pneumonia. ■ Instruct parents to include rest periods in the child's daily activities. 4. Promote adequate nutritional intake: ■ Encourage parents to provide nutritious meals. ■ Instruct parents concerning the importance of administering necessary vitamins to the child. 5. Provide emotional support: ■ Allow family to discuss fears and feelings about diagnosis. ■ Assist the family and child with the child's integration into the school environment.
50.4 Describe nursing management for the child with systemic lupus erythematosus or juvenile arthritis.	1. Nursing interventions common to both disorders include: ■ Promote adequate nutrition. ■ Assist in avoidance of flare-ups. ■ Manage side effects of medication. ■ Promote rest and comfort. ■ Provide emotional support. 2. Nursing interventions specific to SLE include: ■ Promote skin integrity. ■ Prevent infection. ■ Maintain fluid balance. 3. Nursing interventions specific to juvenile arthritis include: ■ Promote improved mobility.
50.5 Describe exposure prevention measures for the child with latex allergy.	1. Products that come in contact with child must be free of latex. 2. Encourage parents to place a medical alert identification bracelet on the child. 3. Instruct parents to keep an epinephrine kit available at home and at school. 4. Instruct parents concerning everyday products that contain latex.
50.6 Apply nursing interventions and prevention measures for the child experiencing other hypersensitivity reactions.	1. Careful physical assessment: ■ Monitor for early signs and symptoms of hypersensitivity reactions. ■ Careful attention must be given to assessment of the skin and GI system. 2. Instruct the family in proper immunization schedule for the child. 3. Instruct the family concerning signs and symptoms of infection. 4. Teach the family the importance of protecting the child from contact with individuals with infections: ■ Child should avoid all crowded areas. 5. Assist families to follow proper medication schedule: ■ Inform parents of possible side effects of medication.

CRITICAL THINKING IN ACTION

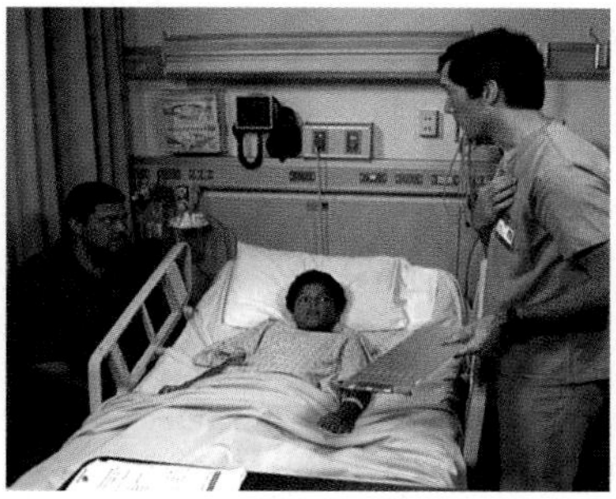

You are working at a pediatrician's office when 11-year-old Nirah and his parents come in. The husband, wife, and Nirah are all human immunodeficiency virus (HIV) infected. Nirah does not know he is HIV infected, but he has been very compliant with taking his antiretroviral medications. However, he has recently developed a cough and his parents decided to visit the pediatrician's office.

The pediatrician finds that Nirah has a fever of 102°F, respiratory rate of 60 breaths per minute, no visible retractions during respiration, and a pulse of 120 beats per minute. The physician decides to admit him to the hospital.

After the laboratory tests and radiographs are completed in the hospital, the physician tells the family that Nirah has pneumonia and strep throat. Nirah is started on IV antibiotics and shows improvement after three days of treatment. You monitor Nirah frequently and have him deep breathe. You also teach the parents how to encourage deep-breathing exercises.

1. How does HIV interfere with normal function of the child's immune system?
2. What are some of the measures of infection control for Nirah while he is hospitalized with HIV?
3. How can you promote Nirah's respiratory function?
4. When children, especially those with an immune system problem, are on antibiotics, they can develop thrush (Candida in the mouth). What is the treatment to prevent this side effect?

See MyNursingKit for possible responses.

REFERENCES

Alvarez, A. M., & Rathore, M. H. (2007). Hot topics in Pediatric HIV/AIDS. *Pediatric Annals, 36*(7), 423–432.

American Academy of Pediatrics (2006). *Red Book: Report of the committee on infectious diseases* (27th ed.). Elk Grove Village, IL: AAP.

Baker, C. J. (2007). *Red Book atlas of pediatric infectious diseases.* Elk Grove Village, Illinois: AAP.

Bernatsky, S., Duffy, C., Malleson, P., Feldman, D. E., St. Pierre, Y., & Clarke, A. E. (2007). Economic impact of juvenile idiopathic arthritis. *Arthritis & Rheumatism, 57*(1), 44–48.

Bindler, R. M., & Howry, L. B. (2005). *Pediatric drug guide with nursing implications.* Upper Saddle River, NJ: Pearson/Prentice Hall.

Bonilla, F. A., & Geha, R. S. (2006). Update on primary immunodeficiency diseases. *Journal of Allergy and Clinical Immunology, 117*(2), S435–S440.

Buckley, R. H. (2007). The T-, B-, and NK-Cell Systems. In R. M. Kliegman, R. E. Behrman, H. B. Jenson, & B. F. Stanton (Eds.), *Nelson textbook of pediatrics* (18th ed., pp. 873–879). Philadelphia: Saunders Elsevier.

Buckley, R. H. (2008). DiGeorge. In *Merck Manual Online*. Whitehouse Station, NJ: Merck Research Laboratories. Retrieved August 29, 2009 from http://www.merck.com.go.libproxy.wfubmc.edu/mmpe/sec13/ch164/ch164h.html?qt=DiGeorge&alt=sh

Buka, R. L., & Cunningham, B. B. (2005). Connective tissue disease in children. *Pediatric Annals, 34*(3), 225–238.

Cassidy, J. T., & Petty, R. E. (2005). Chronic arthritis in childhood. In J. T. Cassidy, R. E. Petty, R. M. Laxer, & C. B. Lindsley (Eds.), *Textbook of pediatric rheumatology* (5th ed., pp. 206–260). Philadelphia: Elsevier Saunders.

Centers for Disease Control and Prevention. (2006a). *CDC recommends routine, voluntary HIV screening in health care settings.* Retrieved August 7, 2007 from www.cdc.gov/od/oc/media/pressrel/r060921.htm

Centers for Disease Control and Prevention. (2006b). Revised recommendations for HIV testing of adults, adolescents, and pregnant women in health-care settings. *MMWR, 2006, 55* (No. RR-14), 1–24.

Centers for Disease Control and Prevention (2007a). *Mother to child (perinatal) HIV transmission and prevention.* Retrieved April 20, 2008 from www.cdc.gov/hiv/topics/perinatal/resources/factsheets/pdf/perinatal.pdf

Centers for Disease Control and Prevention. (2008). HIV/Aids among African Americans. Retrieved August 29, 2009 from www.cdc.gov/hiv/topics/aa/resources/factsheets/pdf/aa.pdf.

Chamley, C. A., Carson, P., Randall, D., & Sandwell, M. (2005). *Developmental anatomy and physiology of children*. St Louis: Elsevier.

Cibulka, N. J. (2006). Mother-to-child transmission of HIV in the United States. *American Journal of Nursing, 106*(7), 56–63.

Cleary, A. M., Insel, R. A., & Lewis, D. B. (2005). Disorders of lymphocyte function. In R. Hoffman, E. J. Benz, S. J. Shattil, B. Furie, H. J. Cohen, L. E. Silberstein, & P. McGlave (Eds.), *Hematology: Basic Principles and Practice* (4th ed. pp. 831–855). St. Louis: Elsevier.

Committee on Pediatric AIDS. (1998). Human immunodeficiency virus/acquired immunodeficiency syndrome education in schools. *Pediatrics, 101*(5), 933–935.

Davies, S. M. (2005). Hematopoietic stem cell transplantation for immunodeficiencies and genetic diseases. In R. Hoffman, E. J. Benz, S. J. Shattil, B. Furie, H. J. Cohen, L. E. Silberstein, & P. McGlave (Eds.), *Hematology: Basic Principles and Practice* (4th ed., pp. 1703–1712). St. Louis: Elsievier.

Delaney, K. P., Branson, B. M., Uniyal, A., Kerndt, P. R., Keenan, P. A., Jafa, K., et al. (2006). Performance of an oral fluid rapid HIV-1/2 test: Experience from four CDC studies. *AIDS, 20*, 1655–1660.

Dibbern, D. A., & Routes, J. M. (2007). *Wiscott–Aldrich syndrome.* Retrieved June 20, 2004, from www.emedicine.com/med/topic1162.htm

Emery, H. (2004). Pediatric rheumatology: What does the future hold? *Archives of Physical Medicine and Rehabilitation, 85*, 1382–1384.

Flynn, P. M., Rudy, B. J., Douglas, S. O., Lathey, J., Spector, S. A., Martinez, J., et al. (2004). Virologic and immunologic outcomes after 24 weeks in HIV type 1-infected adolescents receiving highly active antiretroviral therapy. *Journal of Infectious Diseases, 190*, 271–279.

Goldmuntz, E. (2005). DiGeorge Syndrome: New Insights. *Clinics in Perinatology, 32*, 963–978.

Gottlieb, B. S., & Ilowite, N. T. (2006). Systemic lupus erythematosus in children and adolescents. *Pediatrics in Review, 27*(9), 323–328.

Greenwald, J. L., Burstein, G. R., Pincus, J., & Branson, B. (2006). A rapid review of rapid HIV antibody tests. *Current Infectious Disease Reports, 8*, 125–131.

Heird, W. C. (2007). The feeding of infants and children. In R. M. Kliegman, R. E. Behrman, H. B. Jenson, & B. F. Stanton (Eds.), *Nelson textbook of pediatrics* (18th ed., pp. 214–224). Philadelphia: Saunders Elsevier.

Higman, M. A., & Vogelsang, G. B. (2004). Chronic graft-versus-host disease. *British Journal of Haematology, 125*, 435–454.

Kline, M. W. (2006). Perspectives on the pediatric HIV/AIDS pandemic: Catalyzing access of children to care and treatment. *Pediatrics, 117*, 1388–1393.

Kobrynski, L. J. (2006). Combined immune deficiencies in children. *Journal of Infusion Nursing, 29*(4), 213.

Kukka, C. (2004). Bloodborne infections: Should they be disclosed? Is differential treatment necessary? *Journal of School Nursing, 20*, 324–330.

Laxer, R. M. (2005). Pharmacology and drug therapy. In J. T. Cassidy, R. E. Petty, R. M. Laxer, & C. B. Lindsley (Eds.), *Textbook of pediatric rheumatology* (5th ed., pp. 76–141). Philadelphia: Elsevier Saunders.

Lupus Foundation of America. (2008). *About lupus*. Retrieved December 5, 2008 from www.lupus.org/webmodules/webarticlesnet/templates/new_aboutintroduction.aspx?articleid=311&zoneid=9

Luxner, K. L. (2003). The complicated prenatal experience. In M. H. Hogan & R. S. Glazebrook (Eds.), *Maternal-newborn nursing.* Upper Saddle River, NJ: Prentice-Hall.

Marinescu, L. M., & Ilowite, N. T. (July, 2007). Update on pediatric rheumatology: Growth spurt in the knowledge base. *Consultant for Pediatricians,* 397–404.

McLean-Tooke, A., Spickett, G. P., & Gennery, A. R. (2007). Immunodeficiency and autoimmunity in 22q11.2 deletion syndrome. *Scandinavian Journal of Immunology, 66*, 1–7.

Michaels, M. G., & Green, M. (2007). Infections in immunocompromised persons. In R. M. Kliegman, R. E. Behrman, H. B. Jenson, & B. F. Stanton (Eds.), *Nelson textbook of pediatrics* (18th ed., pp. 1100–1107). Philadelphia: Saunders Elsevier.

Naar-King, S., Templin, T., Wright, K., Frey, M., Parsons, J. T., & Lam, P. (2006). Psychosocial factors and medication adherence in HIV-positive youth. *AIDS Patient Care and STDs. 20*(1), 44–47.

Nagaraj, N., Egwim, C., & Adler, D. G. (2007, April). X-linked hyper-IgM syndrome associated with poorly differentiated neuroendocrine tumor presenting as obstructive jaundice secondary to extensive adenopathy. *Digestive Diseases and Sciences. 52*(9), 2312–2316.

National Center for Biotechnology Information (NCBI). (2007). Diseases of the immune system. *Genes and Diseases.* Retrieved August 7, 2007 from http://www.ncbi.nlm.nih.gov/

National Institute of Allergy and Infectious Diseases (2004). *HIV infection in infants and children.* Retrieved August 8, 2007 from www.niaid.nih.gov/factsheets/hivchildren.htm

Ochs, H. D., & Thrasher, A. J. (2006). The Wiskott–Aldrich syndrome. *Journal of Allergy and Clinical Immunology, 117*(4), 725–738.

Paskawicz, J. (2005). Latex allergy revisited. *Clinician Reviews 15*(11), 66–75.

Petry, L., Mathur, A., Kamat, D. M. (2004, May). Immunodeficiency disorders: What should primary care providers know? *Consultant for Pediatricians,* 228–232.

Petty, R. E., & Cassidy, J. T. (2005a). Polyarthritis. In J. T. Cassidy, R. E. Petty, R. M. Laxer, & C. B. Lindsley (Eds.), *Textbook of Pediatric Rheumatology* (5th ed., pp. 261–273). Philadelphia: Elsevier Saunders.

Petty, R. E., & Cassidy, J. T. (2005b). Oligoarthritis. In J. T. Cassidy, R. E. Petty, R. M. Laxer, & C. B. Lindsley (Eds.), *Textbook of Pediatric Rheumatology* (5th ed., pp. 274–290). Philadelphia: Elsevier Saunders.

Petty, R. E., & Cassidy, J. T. (2005c). Systemic Arthritis. In J. T. Cassidy, R. E. Petty, R. M. Laxer, & C. B. Lindsley (Eds.), *Textbook of pediatric rheumatology* (5th ed., pp. 291–303). Philadelphia: Elsevier Saunders.

Petty, R. E., & Laxer, R. M. (2005). Systemic lupus erythematosus. In Cassidy, J. T., Petty, R. E., Laxer, R. M., & Lindsley, C. B. (Eds.), *Textbook of pediatric rheumatology* (5th ed., pp. 342–391). Philadelphia: Elsevier Saunders.

Plowfield, L. A. (2007). HIV disease in children 25 years later. *Pediatric Nursing, 33*(3), 274–278, 273.

Pongmarutani, T., Alpert, P. T., & Miller, S. K. (2006). Pediatric systemic lupus erythematosus: Management issues in primary practice. *Journal of the American Academy of Nurse Practitioners, 18*, 258–267.

Puck, J. M., & Malech, H. L. (2006). Gene therapy for immune disorders: Good news tempered by bad news. *Journal of Allergy and Clinical Immunology, 117*(4), 865–869.

Rettig, P. A., Merhar, S. L., & Cron, R. Q. (2004). Juvenile rheumatoid arthritis and juvenile spondifoarthropathy. In P. J. Allen & J. A. Vessey (Eds.), *Primary care of the child with a chronic condition* (4th ed., pp. 582–600). St. Louis: Mosby.

Sampson, H. A., & Leung, D. Y. M. (2007). Anaphylaxis. In R. M. Kliegman, R. E. Behrman, H. B. Jenson, & B. F. Stanton (Eds.), *Nelson textbook of pediatrics* (18th ed., pp. 983–985). Philadelphia: Saunders Elsevier.

Spina Bifida Association (2007). *Latex (natural rubber) in the hospital environment and Latex (natural rubber) in home and community.* Retrieved December 5, 2008 from www.spinabifidaassociation.org/atf/cf/%7BEED435C8-F1A0-4A16-B4D8-A713BBCD9CE4%7D/2007%20Latex%20Lists.pdf

Stichweh, D., Arce, E., & Pascual, V. (2004). Update on pediatric systemic lupus erythematosus. *Current Opinion in Rheumatology 16*, 577–587.

Tezcan, I., Ersoy, F., Sanal, O., Turul, T., Uckan, D., Balci, S. et al. (2005). Long-term survival in severe combined immune deficiency: The role of persistent maternal engraftment. *The Journal of Pediatrics, 146*, 137–140.

U.S. Department of Health and Human Services. (2008a). *Guidelines for the use of antiretroviral agents in pediatric HIV infection.* Retrieved December 5, 2008 from http://aidsinfo.nih.gov/contentfiles/PediatricGuidelines.pdf

U.S. Department of Health and Human Services. (2008b). *Pediatric antiretroviral drug information.* Retrieved December 5, 2008 from http://aidsinfo.nih.gov/contentfiles/PediatricGL_SupI.pdf

Velardi, A., & Locatelli, F. (2007). Graft versus host disease (GVHD) and rejection. In R. M. Kliegman, R. E. Behrman, H. B. Jenson, & B. F. Stanton (Eds.), *Nelson textbook of pediatrics* (18th ed., pp. 930–931). Philadelphia: Saunders Elsevier.

Williams, P. L., Storm, D., Montepiedra, G., Nichols, S., Kammerer, B., Sirois, P. A., et al. (2006). Predictors of adherence to antiretroviral medications in children and adolescents with HIV infections. *Pediatrics, 118*(6), e1745–e1757.

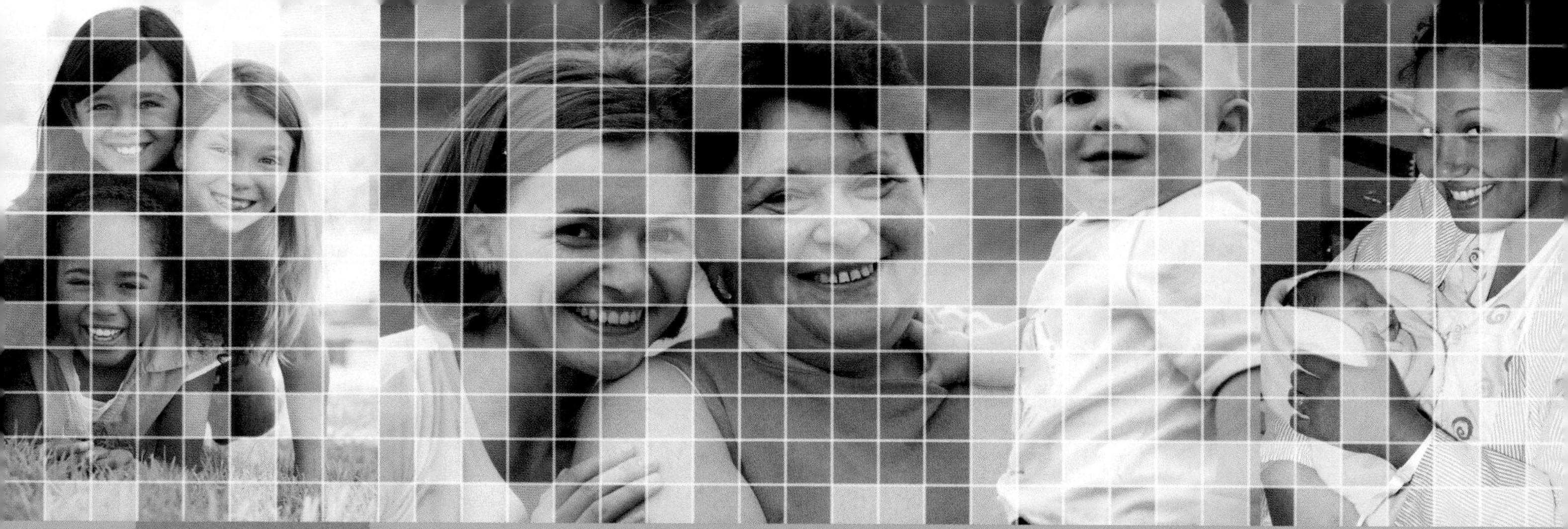

CHAPTER

51 The Child with Alterations in Hematologic Function

Having a child with sickle cell disease is very difficult for us. We know this is a genetic disease, and we feel responsible for Michael's pain. We also never seem to expect the bad times when they come. He'll be doing well and we almost forget . . . then he gets sick or doesn't drink enough and we're in the hospital again. His older sister has started talking about how she worries that sometime she'll have a child with sickle cell disease and we don't know what to tell her. —Father of Michael, 12 years old

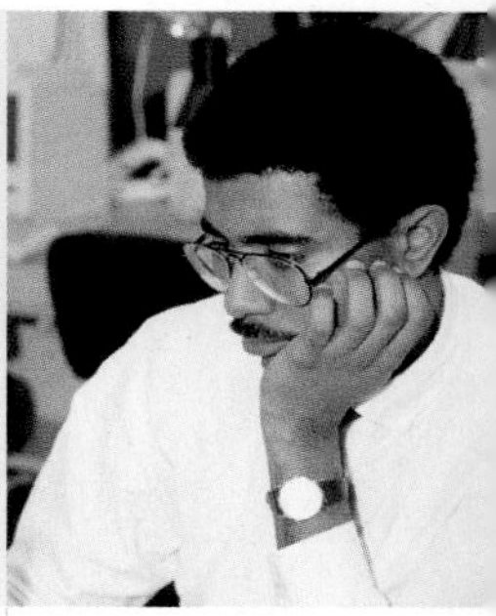

LEARNING OUTCOMES

51.1 Describe the function of red blood cells, white blood cells, and platelets.

51.2 Discuss the pathophysiology and clinical manifestations of the major disorders of red blood cells affecting the pediatric population.

51.3 Discuss the pathophysiology and clinical manifestations of the selected disorders of white blood cells affecting the pediatric population.

51.4 Discuss the pathophysiology and clinical manifestations of the major bleeding disorders affecting the pediatric population.

51.5 Describe the nursing management and collaborative care of a child with a hematologic disorder.

51.6 Discuss nursing implications for a child receiving hematopoietic stem cell transplantation (HSCT).

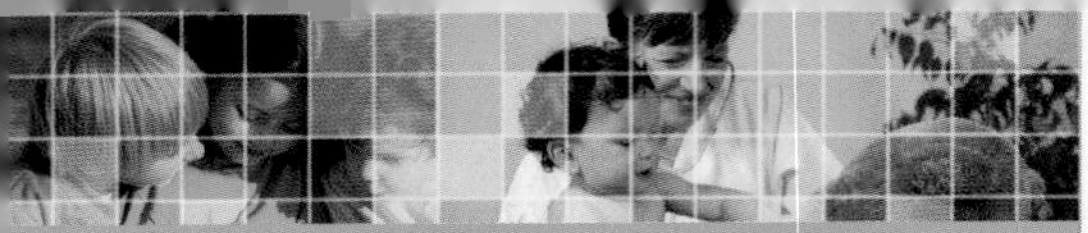

KEY TERMS

Anemia, 1441
Allogeneic transplantation, 1458
Autologous transplantation, 1458
Ecchymosis, 1454
Erythropoiesis, 1441
Hemarthrosis, 1454
Hematopoiesis, 1441
Hemoglobinopathy, 1443
Hemosiderosis, 1447
Hypersplenism, 1441
Leukopenia, 1441
Menorrhagia, 1442
Pancytopenia, 1453
Petechiae, 1453
Polycythemia, 1441
Purpura, 1453
Thrombocytopenia, 1441
Vaso-occlusion, 1444

MyNursingKit Animation: Circulatory System

The hematologic system is one of a few body systems that regulate, directly or indirectly, all other body functions. Because blood is involved in the function of all tissues and organs, changes in the blood may result in altered functioning of many body organs and structures. This chapter discusses the most common disorders of the blood and blood-forming organs in children. (See Chapter 52 for a discussion of leukemia.)

ANATOMY AND PHYSIOLOGY OF PEDIATRIC DIFFERENCES

Blood has two components: a fluid portion called plasma and a cellular portion known as the formed elements of the blood. The cellular elements are red blood cells (erythrocytes), white blood cells (leukocytes), and platelets (thrombocytes) (Figure 51–1 ●). Table 51–1 gives normal values for these blood components in children.

Production of *red blood cells* begins in the embryo by the second week of gestation. White blood cell and platelet production begins at 8 weeks. Most of this early production occurs first in the embryonic yolk sac and then in the liver; however, by 20 to 24 week's gestation, liver production decreases as bone marrow production be-

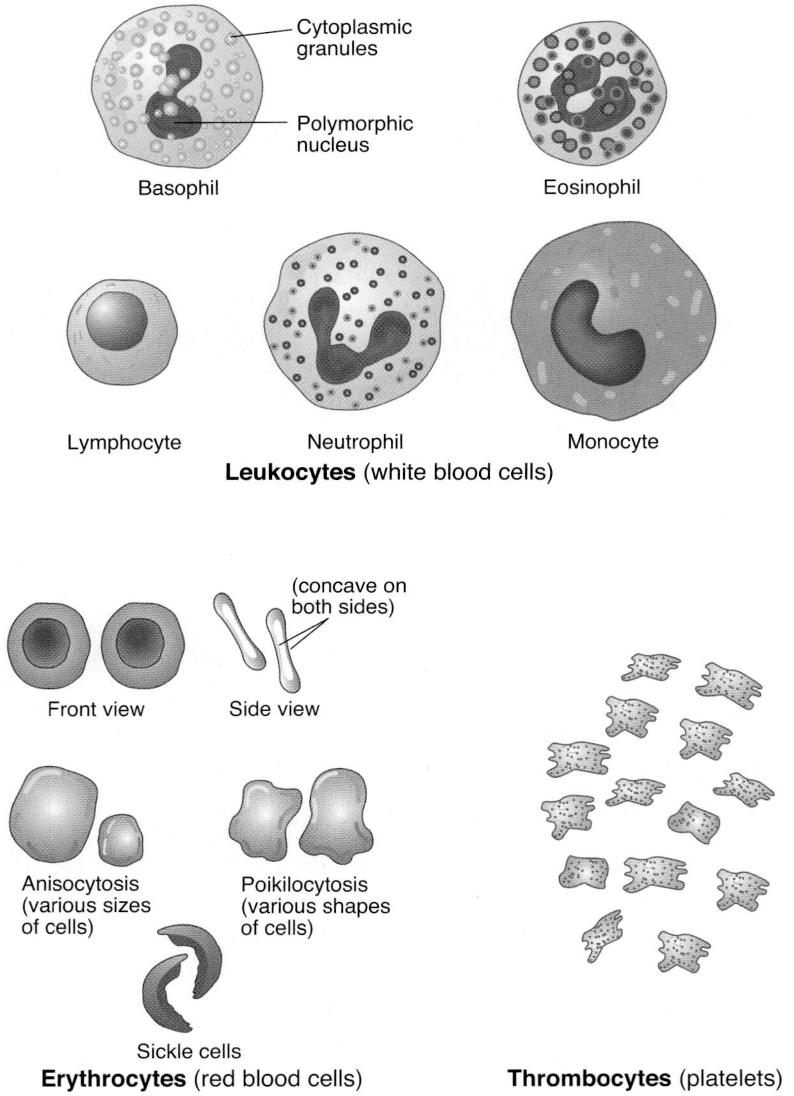

● **Figure 51–1** Types of blood cells.

Table 51–1 Mean Values for Common Hematology Tests in Children

Test*	Mean Value
Red blood cell (RBC)	3.8–4.9 × 10^{12}/L
Hemoglobin (Hb)	11.5–14.5 g/dL
Hematocrit (HCT)	35–43%
White blood cell (WBC)	7.8–12.2 × 10^{9}/L
Platelets	150–400 × 10^{9}/L

Adapted from: Hay, W. W., Levin, M. J., Sondheimer, J. M., Deterding, R. R., and Associate Authors (2005). *Current pediatric diagnosis and treatment* (17th ed.), New York: Lange Medical Books/McGraw-Hill; Pesce, M. A. (2007). Reference ranges for laboratory tests and procedures. In R. M. Kliegman, R. E. Behrman, H. B. Jenson, & B. F. Stanton, *Nelson textbook of pediatrics* (18th ed., pp. 2943–2949). Philadelphia: Elsevier Saunders. *See additional blood values in Appendix B.

Table 51–2 White Blood Cells and Their Functions

Type	Function
Neutrophils	Phagocytosis
Eosinophils	Allergic reactions
Basophils	Inflammatory reactions
Monocytes (macrophages)	Phagocytosis, antigen processing
Lymphocytes	Humoral immunity (B cell), cellular immunity (T cell)

gins to predominate (Chamley, Carson, Randall, et al., 2005; Ohls & Christensen, 2007). At birth, **hematopoiesis**, or blood cell production, occurs in the marrow of almost every bone. The flat bones, such as the sternum, ribs, pelvic and shoulder girdles, vertebrae, and hips, retain most of their hematopoietic activity throughout life.

RED BLOOD CELLS

Red blood cells, or erythrocytes, are the most abundant of the cellular elements of blood. They are formed through a process called **erythropoiesis**. The primary function of red blood cells is to transport oxygen from the lungs to the tissues. These cells also help to carry carbon dioxide from the tissues back to the lungs. Hemoglobin, a red pigment composed of protein and iron, is essential to this function.

Polycythemia is an above-average increase in the number of red cells in the blood. **Anemia** is a reduction in the number of red blood cells; the various types of anemia will be discussed in the following section.

At birth the newborn has a naturally occurring elevation in red blood cells (RBCs) due to a high level of erythropoietin, which stimulates red cell production. Once the newborn begins breathing air and the oxygen level in the blood increases, this production slows (Polin, Fox, & Abman, 2004). Levels of RBCs fall until about 2 to 3 months of age (to about 9 to 11 g/dL) and then begin increasing. Adult levels are reached during adolescence. Teenage males have RBC levels slightly higher than teenage females (see Appendix B).

WHITE BLOOD CELLS

White blood cells, or leukocytes, are the mobile units of the body's protective system. They are formed in bone marrow and lymph tissue. The white blood cell count is highest at birth, although levels vary greatly among infants. By 1 week of age, white blood cell values stabilize. Throughout childhood, there is a very slow decrease in white blood cell count (Boxer, 2007).

There are five types of white blood cells, each with a distinct function (Table 51–2). A differential blood count indicates the percentages of the different types of white cells in the blood and is sometimes useful in identifying the cause of an illness. For example, infections cause an increase in neutrophils; and allergies are related to an increase in eosinophils. The role of lymphocytes is discussed with acquired immunodeficiency syndrome in Chapter 50. A decrease in the number of white blood cells is called **leukopenia**, and can be caused by immune or bone marrow disorders.

PLATELETS

Platelets, or thrombocytes, are cell fragments that can form hemostatic plugs to stop bleeding. They are synthesized from components in the red bone marrow and are stored in the spleen. Platelet levels in newborns are lower than in older children and adults. Levels of many clotting factors, particularly those requiring vitamin K for activation (factors II, VII, IX, X, and anticoagulant factors—proteins C and S), are also lower in infants. For this reason, all newborns receive a prophylactic injection of vitamin K at birth. Values of platelets and other coagulation products soon reach normal childhood levels (Scott & Montgomery, 2007). A deficiency of platelets can lead to bleeding disorder and is termed **thrombocytopenia**. See Table 51–3 for guidelines for assessment of a child with a hematologic condition.

MyNursingKit | Animation: Types of Blood Cells

ANEMIAS

Anemia is defined as a reduction in the number of RBCs, the quantity of hemoglobin, and the volume of packed red cells to below-normal levels. This condition can be caused by loss or destruction of existing RBCs or by an impaired or decreased rate of red cell production. Anemia also can be a clinical manifestation of an underlying disorder, such as lead poisoning or **hypersplenism** (a syndrome characterized by splenomegaly and blood cell deficiencies). Common childhood anemias are discussed in this section.

Table 51–3 Guidelines for Assessment of a Child with a Hematologic Condition

Assessment Focus	Assessment Guidelines
Family History	Does a family member have sickle cell anemia/trait or other blood disorder? Does a family member have hemophilia or other inherited clotting alteration?
Growth and Development	Measure height and weight on a regular basis and plot on standardized growth charts. Perform nutritional assessment to see if child is getting enough calories. Assess child for attainment of developmental milestones.
Skin	Assess for pallor, flushing, rashes, ecchymosis. Observe for prolonged bleeding/clotting time, easy bruising, frequent nosebleeds.
Joints	Observe for edema, pain, inflammation, and range of motion.
Additional Assessments	Assess pain in various body parts. Identify frequency of infections. Assess for history of fatigue and lethargy.

IRON DEFICIENCY ANEMIA

Iron deficiency anemia is the most common type of anemia and the most common nutritional deficiency in children. Iron deficiency anemia can occur secondary to blood loss, malabsorption, or poor nutritional intake. See Chapter 34 for a discussion of iron deficiency anemia due to deficits in nutritional intake. Increased physiologic demands (such as rapid growth periods) for blood production can also lead to anemia.

Rapidly growing adolescents whose diets are high in fat and low in vitamins and minerals are particularly susceptible to iron deficiency anemia. Infants who do not consume adequate solid foods after 6 months of age and are fed only breast milk or formula that is not fortified with iron are also at risk for iron deficiency because neonatal iron stores have been depleted by this time and their iron needs are not being met. In addition, if the mother's nutritional status during pregnancy was inadequate, or the infant was born prematurely or as part of a multiple birth, insufficient iron may have been stored in the latter part of pregnancy, placing the infant at higher risk for anemia in the first months of life.

Chronic blood loss is always a potential cause of iron deficiency anemia. Those at risk of anemia include the infant who has had bleeding in the neonatal period; the child who loses blood as a result of conditions such as hemophilia or parasitic gastrointestinal illness; and the adolescent female who has **menorrhagia** (heavy menstrual bleeding).

Clinical manifestations and severity of symptoms are directly related to the amount of iron deficiency anemia. Pallor, fatigue, and irritability are characteristic findings. With prolonged anemia, nailbed deformities, growth retardation, developmental delay, tachycardia, and systolic heart murmur can occur. Pica, or consumption of nonfood items, is also associated with iron deficiency anemia.

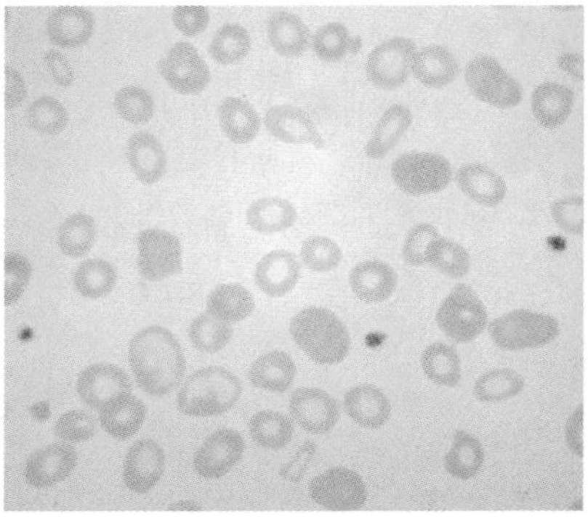

● **Figure 51–2** Iron deficiency anemia. Red blood cells appear hypochromic as a result of decreased hemoglobin synthesis.

Source: Courtesy of Dr. Ed Wong, Laboratory Medicine, Children's National Medical Center, Washington, DC.

Diagnosis is made on the basis of clinical presentation and laboratory studies. The hemoglobin, hematocrit, mean corpuscular volume, RBC count, and the reticulocyte count are evaluated to confirm the diagnosis and help determine the cause of the anemia (Coyer, 2005). (See "Developing Cultural Competence: Chi.") Microscopic analysis (Figure 51–2 ●) reveals RBCs are microcytic (small) in size and hypochromic (pale) in appearance (Borgna-Pignatti & Marsella, 2008). A diet history and analysis can provide information about food intake; see Chapter 34 for guidelines about diet history.

Treatment involves correction of the iron deficiency with oral elemental iron preparations and a diet high in iron. Ferrous sulfate at a dose of 2 to 6 mg/kg/day for about 4 weeks is a common treatment, followed by evaluation for its effectiveness. If the anemia is improving, treatment usually continues for about 2 months (Committee on Nutrition, 2004; Coyer, 2005). Because oral iron preparations cause several side effects such as constipation and gastrointestinal discomfort, the child may receive iron medications (to restore blood levels of iron) while the iron content of the diet is increased above the recommended dietary allowances (RDAs). Oral iron medications can then be tapered off once the child's food intake can supply the needed iron; the child is evaluated in about 6 months for recurring anemia.

Developing Cultural Competence

CHI

According to traditional Chinese beliefs, a person who does not feel well is lacking in chi (inner energy) and blood. Chinese Americans who follow traditional practices may be hesitant to have blood drawn for laboratory studies for fear of causing bodily weakness.

Nursing Management

The child with iron deficiency anemia is usually identified and treated in the community unless he or she has another serious illness. Nursing care focuses on screening for the disorder and educating the parents and child about the causes of iron deficiency anemia, dietary management, and the importance of complying with the medication regimen.

Screening for anemia is recommended at 9 to 12 months of age, at 15 to 18 months, and again at adolescence (see Chapters 36 and 38∞) (Committee on Nutrition, 2004). A hematocrit or hemoglobin level is obtained for screening. More detailed tests are performed if the blood test is abnormal. Children at high risk for nutritional deficiencies, such as those in low-income groups and WIC programs, may require additional tests. Most children in Head Start are screened annually by nurses. In addition, children showing signs of anemia such as low energy and pallor should be screened. Height and weight measurements are obtained at each healthcare visit, plotted on growth charts, and compared percentiles obtained at previous visits. Slow downward trends in percentiles are of concern and require further nutritional analysis (see Chapter 34∞). Perform developmental screening tests to assess for developmental delays (see Chapter 33∞).

Dietary management is the preferred long-term treatment for iron deficiency anemia. Teach child and family to plan for foods that are rich in iron. The infant over 6 months of age should have a diet that includes breast milk or iron-fortified formula and baby cereals with iron fortification. Avoid cow's milk in the first year of life since it can cause bleeding from the gastrointestinal tract, contributing to anemia. If the older infant or toddler consumes large quantities of milk and refuses to eat solid food, restriction on milk intake may be required. Older infants and toddlers can eat finger foods such as thinly sliced meats. Adolescents are encouraged to eat foods with high iron content and vitamin C such as lean meats and dried fruits.

Oral iron preparations are given to correct anemia (see Drug Guide, Chapter 34∞). Instruct the family about side effects such as black stools, constipation, and a foul aftertaste. Emphasize the importance of drinking fluids and eating foods high in dietary fiber to minimize constipation. The medicine should be stored safely to avoid accidental poisoning. Expected outcomes of care are intake of recommended levels of iron and return to normal hematocrit level.

NORMOCYTIC ANEMIA

In normocytic anemia, there is an increase in the destruction of red blood cells or decreased production of red blood cells. This type of anemia may be related to chronic hemolytic anemia, pancytopenia, disseminated intravascular coagulation (DIC; see the discussion later in this chapter), G6PD (glucose-6-phosphate dehydrogenase) deficiency, hemolytic uremic syndrome (see Chapter 54∞), some autoimmune diseases, or several other conditions (Coyer, 2005). Normocytic anemia can be caused by an infection such as septic arthritis or meningitis. It may also be found in a child with an inflammatory illness such as juvenile arthritis or chronic liver disease. Clinical manifestations of normocytic anemia are similar to those seen in iron deficiency anemia, with the possible occurrence of hepatomegaly and splenomegaly.

Clinical manifestations are similar to those seen in iron deficiency anemia, with the possible occurrence of hepatomegaly and splenomegaly, as well.

Treatment of normocytic anemia depends on the underlying cause. When the anemia is associated with inflammation or infection, the underlying condition is treated. For anemia caused by renal failure, recombinant human erythropoietin is administered. When hemorrhage is the underlying cause, the source of the bleeding is identified and treated. In acute emergencies, blood products are infused to make up for some of the losses.

Nursing management of normocytic anemia depends on the cause of the decreased RBCs. Children with inflammatory or infectious diseases require careful assessment and management of medication and other treatment regimens. Administer blood products and other intravenous fluids as ordered to restore blood volume. Follow-up and home visits to assess hematocrit, hemoglobin, and dietary intake. (Refer to the discussion later in this chapter for management of DIC, to Chapter 53∞ for management of intestinal infections, and to Chapter 54∞ for management of hemolytic uremic syndrome.)

SICKLE CELL DISEASE

Sickle cell disease is a hereditary **hemoglobinopathy** characterized by the partial or complete replacement of normal hemoglobin with abnormal hemoglobin S (Hgb S) in red blood cells (Table 51–4). This causes occlusion of small blood vessels, ischemia, and damage to affected organs. Sickle cell trait (carrying one gene for the disease) affects 1 in 12 African Americans and 1 in 16 Hispanic Americans (American Sickle Cell Anemia Association, 2005). Approximately 2 million Americans carry the sickle cell gene (Hb SA). Individuals with sickle cell trait have one sickle cell hemoglobin gene and one normal hemoglobin gene. They are carriers of the disease and generally do not have symptoms, although they have been known to occur when the body is under severe stress (Platt & Eckman, 2006).

MyNursingKit Administering Blood or Blood Products

Etiology and Pathophysiology

Sickle cell anemia is an autosomal recessive disorder. If both parents have the trait, with each pregnancy the risk of having a child with the disease is 25%. (See Chapter 3∞ for a discussion of recessive gene transmission.)

In sickle cell anemia, the hemoglobin in the RBC acquires an elongated crescent or sickle shape (Figure 51–3 ●). The sickled cells are rigid and obstruct capillary blood flow. Microscopic obstructions lead to engorgement and tissue ischemia. This local tissue hypoxia causes further sickling and ultimately large infarctions. Organ tissues become damaged by infarctions leading to scarring and impaired function. The spleen is the first organ affected by sickling. Ninety percent of children with HbSS disease have functional asplenia by 6 years of age (Driscoll, 2007). Children with sickle cell anemia can suffer from splenic sequestration when blood is trapped in the spleen, a life-threatening complication. Many children must undergo splenectomy in early childhood, leading to severely compromised immunity. Infection rate

MyNursingKit Animation: Sickle Cell Anemia

Table 51–4 Types of Sickle Cell Disease

Disorder	Characteristics
Sickle Cell Anemia (Hb SS)	Most common type of sickle cell disease (65% of SCD cases)
	RBCs are crescent shaped
	Homozygous condition (child has two sickle hemoglobin genes)
	Child is subject to sickle cell crises
	Average life span 45 years of age
Sickle C disease (Hb SC)	Child inherits one HbS gene and one HbC gene (25% of SCD cases)
	RBCs are C shaped
	Anemia is generally milder than in Hb SS disease
	Painful crises occur about 50% as often as in Hb SS disease
	Average life span 65 years of age
Sickle beta + thalassemia disease (Hb+ Sβ) and Sickle beta 0 thalassemia disease (Hb0 Sβ)	Combination of sickle cell trait and thalassemia trait. In sickle cell beta+ there is a reduced amount of Hemoglobin A, and life span is near normal. In sickle cell beta 0 there is no Hemoglobin A and the life span is mid-50s.

Data from: DeBaun, M. R., & Vichinsky, E. (2007). Hemoglobinopathies. In R. M. Kliegman, R. E. Behrman, H. B. Jenson, & B. F. Stanton (Eds.), *Nelson textbook of pediatrics* (18th ed., pp. 2025–2038). Philadelphia: Saunders Elsevier; Wang, W. (2007). Central nervous system complications sickle cell disease in children: An overview. *Child Neuropsychology, 13*, 103–119; Saunthararajah, Y., Vichinsky, E. P., Embury, S. H. (2005). Sickle cell disease. In R. Hoffman, E. J. Benz, S. J. Shattil, B. Furie, H. J. Cohen, L. E. Silberstein, & P. McGlave (Eds.), *Hematology: Basic principles and practice* (4th ed. pp. 605–644). St. Louis: Elsevier; Ioli, J., & Gilday, M. (September, 2004). Sickle cell signs. *Advance for Nurses*, 39–41; Mehta, S. R., Afenyi-Annan, A., Byrns, P. F., Lottenberg, R. (2006). Opportunities to improve outcomes in sickle cell disease. *American Family Physician, 74*(2), 303–310; Driscoll, M. C. (2007). Sickle cell disease. *Pediatrics in Review, 28*(7), 259–268.

is high due to impaired immunity. Bacterial infections are the leading cause of death in young children with sickle-cell disease.

Stroke is a significant risk to children with sickle cell anemia and can lead to developmental delay, mental retardation, and other neurologic deficits (Lindsey, Watts-Tate, Southwood, et al., 2005).

Sickling may be triggered by fever, hypoxia, emotional stress, or physical stress. Precipitating factors for sickle-cell crisis include increased blood viscosity (such as from a low fluid intake or fever) and hypoxia or low oxygen tension. Potential causes of hypoxia or low oxygen tension include high altitudes, poorly pressurized airplanes, hypoventilation, vasoconstriction when cold, or an emotionally stressful event. Any condition that increases the body's need for oxygen or alters the transport of oxygen (such as infection, trauma, or dehydration) may result in sickle cell crisis.

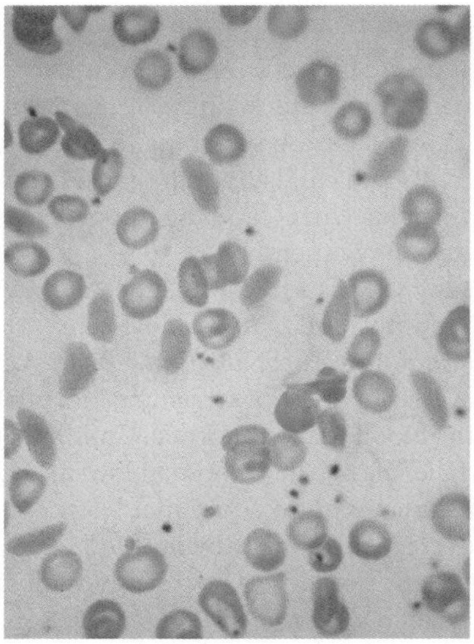

• **Figure 51–3** Sickle cell anemia. Many of these red blood cells show an elongated crescent shape characteristic of sickle cell anemia.

Source: Courtesy of Dr. Ed Wong, Laboratory Medicine, Children's National Medical Center, Washington, DC.

Sickled cells can resume a normal shape when rehydrated and reoxygenated. The membrane of these cells becomes more fragile, however, and cell life is shortened to about 15 days rather than the usual 120 days. In response, bone marrow spaces enlarge to produce more RBCs. Continuous formation and destruction of the child's RBCs contributes to the severe hemolytic anemia that is characteristic of sickle cell anemia (Platt & Eckman, 2006). (See "Pathophysiology Illustrated: Sickle Cell Anemia.")

Clinical Manifestations

Affected children are usually asymptomatic until 4 to 6 months of age because sickling is inhibited by high levels of fetal hemoglobin. Clinical manifestations are directly related to the shortened life span of blood cells (hemolytic anemia) and tissue destruction resulting from **vaso-occlusion** (blockage of a blood vessel). Illness results from recurrent vaso-occlusive events that involve painful crises and chronic organ damage. Pathologic changes happen in most body systems, resulting in multiple signs and symptoms. Examples of common organs affected include the following:

- Brain—cerebrovascular accident, often manifested by headache, aphasia, convulsions, visual changes
- Eyes—retinopathy, retinal detachment, diminished vision
- Bones—chronic ischemia of bones with susceptibility to infection and bone degeneration, manifested by osteoporosis, osteomyelitis, spinal deformities, or aseptic necrosis of the femoral head
- Liver—impaired blood flow from capillary obstruction leads to enlargement and scarring of the liver, manifested by hepatomegaly or cirrhosis
- Spleen—splenic infarct leads to fibrosis and increased rates of infection

PATHOPHYSIOLOGY ILLUSTRATED

SICKLE CELL ANEMIA

The clinical manifestations of sickle cell anemia result from pathologic changes to structures and systems throughout the body.

Hemoglobin S and Red Blood Cell Sickling

Sickle cell anemia is caused by an inherited autosomal recessive defect in Hb synthesis. Sickle cell hemoglobin (HbS) differs from normal hemoglobin only in the substitution of the amino acid valine for glutamine in both beta chains of the hemoglobin molecule.

When HbS is oxygenated, it has the same globular shape as normal hemoglobin. However, when HbS loses its oxygen, it becomes insoluble in intracellular fluid and crystallizes into rodlike structures. Clusters of rods form polymers (long chains) that bend the erythrocyte into the characteristic crescent shape of the sickle cell.

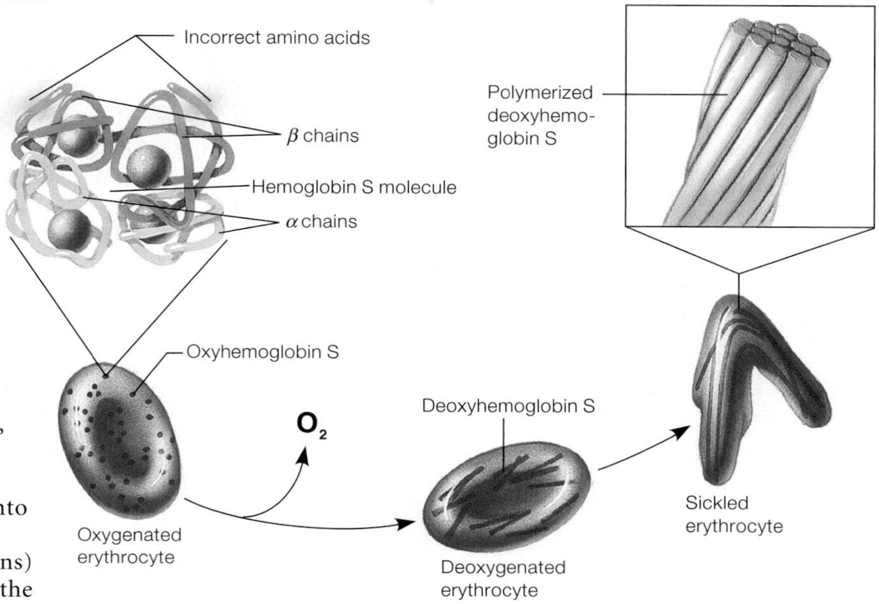

The Sickle Cell Disease Process

Sickle cell disease is characterized by episodes of acute painful crises. Sickling crises are triggered by conditions causing high tissue oxygen demands or that affect cellular pH. As the crisis begins, sickled erythrocytes adhere to capillary walls and to each other, obstructing blood flow and causing cellular hypoxia. The crisis accelerates as tissue hypoxia and acidic metabolic waste products cause further sickling and cell damage.

Sickle cell crises cause microinfarcts in joints and organs, and repeated crises slowly destroy organs and tissues. The spleen and kidneys are especially prone to sickling damage.

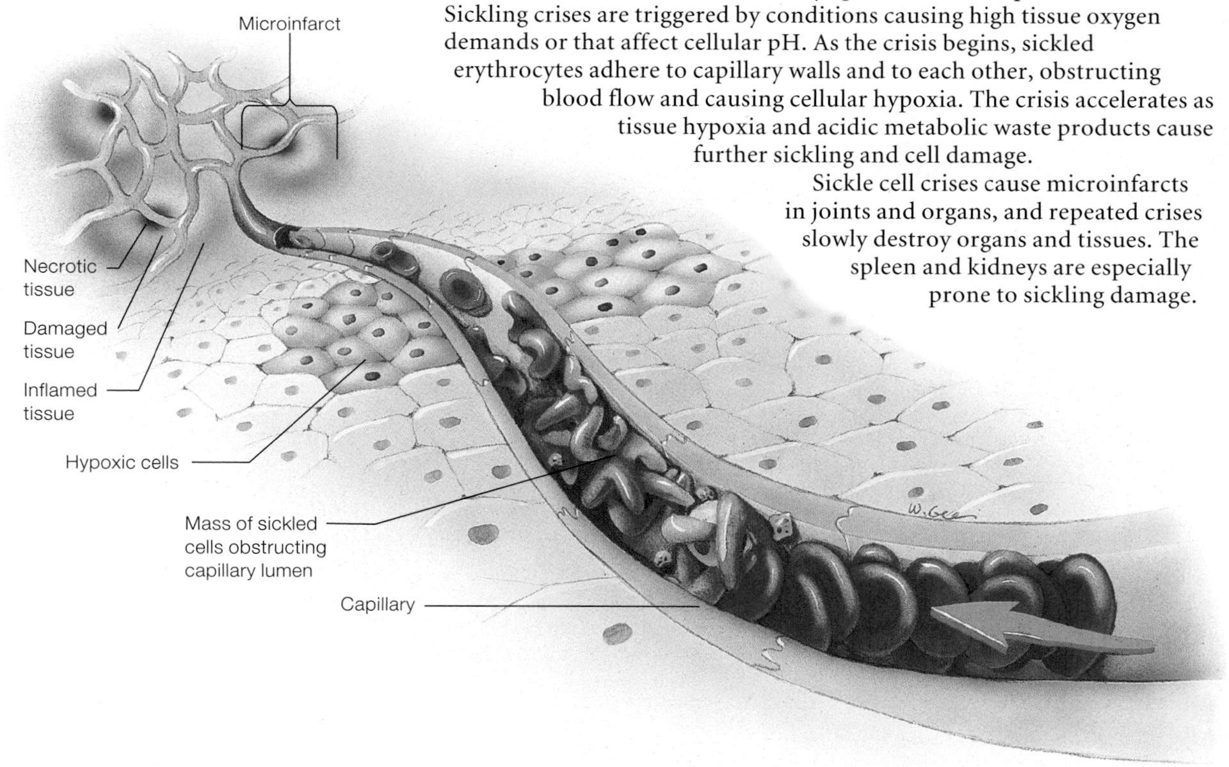

- Kidneys—ischemia of kidneys causes enuresis, hematuria, inability to concentrate urine
- Penis—microcirculatory obstruction and engorgement (priapism)
- Extremities—vaso-occlusion and chronic ischemia manifests as peripheral neuropathy, weakness, or arthralgia
- Skin—decreased peripheral circulation causes ulcerations

Sickle cell crises are acute exacerbations of the disease that vary markedly in severity and frequency. Table 51–5 outlines the most common types of crises affecting children with sickle cell disease. The most common reason for hospitalization of the child with sickle cell anemia is acute painful episodes (Beyer & Simmons, 2004). The sickled RBCs cause vaso-oclusion, microinfarction, and tissue ischemia. Pain results from avascular necrosis of the bone marrow and tissue ischemia. Pain is typically experienced in the back, abdomen, chest, and joints. Children with sickle cell anemia can also develop acute chest syndrome (ACS), a life-threatening complication of sickle cell disease. ACS is the second most common reason for hospitalization in children with SCD, occurring most frequently in children 2–4 years of age (Bryant, 2005).

Clinical Therapy

The initial diagnosis of sickle cell disease in newborns is often made by testing cord blood using hemoglobin electrophoresis. The sickle-turbidity test (Sickledex) may be used for quick screening in children over 6 months of age, once the fetal hemoglobin levels have fallen. Hemoglobin electrophoresis verifies positive Sickledex test results. Newborn screening of infants for hemoglobinopathies now occurs in most states. (See "Developing Cultural Competence: Sickle Cell Disease.")

Developing Cultural Competence

SICKLE CELL DISEASE

Historically, sickle cell disease has been thought of as occurring only in the African American population. In recent years, the disease has been diagnosed in those of Mediterranean, South American, Arabian, and East Indian descent. It is now recommended that all newborns be screened for sickle cell disease (Kral, Brown, Connelly, et al., 2006). While African American families may be familiar with the need for screening, parents of children from other cultures may question this practice. Explain the importance of early diagnosis of sickle cell disease and reinforce the fact that heritage cannot be predicted from appearance or name alone.

Management focuses on pain control, hydration, oxygenation, prevention of infection, and prevention of associated complications. Treatment of crises involves aggressive hydration, oxygen, pain management, and bed rest to reduce energy expenditure. Parenteral analgesics, such as Dilaudid and morphine are generally administered around the clock or via patient-controlled analgesia. In addition to parenteral narcotics the child may also receive intravenous Ketoralac (Toradol) or oral ibuprofen (Motrin) every six hours around the clock as adjunctive therapy. Oral and intravenous fluid replacement also promotes pain relief since dehydration is often a cause of crisis. Fluids also reduce the viscosity of the blood. Oxygen is usually administered to provide comfort and decrease the incidence of pulmonary complications.

Infection in a child with sickle cell anemia is a serious condition regarding immediate attention. When an infection is suspected, cultures (blood, urine, and throat) are obtained to

Table 51–5 Types of Sickle Cell Crises

Type	Cause/Precipitating Events	Clinical Manifestations	Severity
Vaso-occlusive crisis (pain crisis); most common type of crisis.	Stasis of blood with clumping of cells in the microcirculation, ischemia, and infarction Precipitated by: ■ Dehydration ■ Temperature extremes ■ Infection ■ Localized hypoxemia ■ Physical or emotional stress	Extremely painful Symptoms include: ■ Fever ■ Tissue engorgement ■ Painful swelling of joints in hands and feet ■ Priapism ■ Severe abdominal pain	Thrombosis and infarction of local tissue may occur if the crisis is not reversed Cerebral occlusion can result in stroke, manifested by paralysis and/or other central nervous system complications
Splenic sequestration	Pooling of blood in the spleen	Profound anemia, hypovolemia, and shock	Life-threatening crisis—death can occur within hours
Aplastic crises	Triggered by viral infection or depletion of folic acid	Diminished production and increased destruction of red blood cells Signs include profound anemia, pallor	Life-threatening

Data from: Day, S. (2004). Development and evaluation of a sickle cell disease assessment instrument. *Pediatric Nursing, 30*(6), 451–458; Jacob, E., Miaskowski, C., Savedra, M., Beyer, J. E., Treadwell, M., & Styles, L (2005). Trends in complete blood count values during acute painful episodes in children with sickle cell disease. *Journal of Pediatric Oncology Nursing, 22*(3), 152–159; Inati, A., Koussa, S., Taher, A., & Perrine, S. (2008). Sickle cell disease: New insights into pathophyisology and treatment. *Pediatric Annals, 37*(5), 311–321.

identify source of infection and the offending organism. Aggressive antibiotic therapy is implemented immediately.

Penicillin prophylaxis is recommended for children from 2 months to 5 years of age to prevent a potentially life-threatening infection with the *Streptococcus pneumoniae* (S. pneumoniae) bacteria. The medication may be continued past 5 years of age if the child has had a splenectomy or the healthcare provider feels the child is still at high risk for infection caused by *S. pneumoniae* (Sauntharrajah et al., 2005).

To prevent life-threatening infection in the child with sickle cell disease it is essential that the child receive recommended immunizations (Chapter 45∞). In addition, the child should also have the 23-valent pneumococcal vaccine (Pneumovax) at 2 and 5 years of age (Quinn, Rogers, & Buchanan, 2004). Children with SCD who are 6 months of age and older should receive an annual influenzae vaccine and children two years of age and older should receive the meningococcal vaccine (Mehta, Afenyi-Annan, Byrns, et al., 2007).

Blood transfusions improve tissue oxygenation, reduce sickling, and temporarily reduce the percentage of Hb S. Chronic transfusions may be indicated in the child with sickle cell anemia who has had a stroke (Lindsey et al., 2005; Platt & Eckman, 2006). However, frequent transfusions may result in an overload of iron in the body. The iron is stored in tissues and organs (**hemosiderosis**) because the body has no way of excreting it. For this reason, an iron-chelating drug such as deferoxamine (Desferal) which binds excess iron so it can be excreted by the kidneys is administered. An oral chelator, deferasirox (Exjade), is under investigation and may provide similar efficacy to deferoxamine infusion. Exjade could potentially simplify treatment by use of daily oral administration for patients with sickle cell anemia and thalassemia (Cappellini, Bejaoui, Agaoglu, et al., 2007; Piga, Galanello, Foni, et al., 2006). Treatment with hydroxyurea has been helpful in adults, and is being used frequently in children. This cytotoxic medication improves fetal hemoglobin levels. The presence of fetal hemoglobin reduces sickling and subsequently the frequency of painful crisis secondary to vaso-occlusion. In the pediatric population, hydroxyurea has been used most in adolescents, but recent studies have shown it to also be effective in children as young as 6 months of age (Anderson, 2006).

Hematopoietic stem cell transplantation (HSCT) is the only known cure for sickle cell anemia and has been used in children younger than 16 years with complications related to the disease. The treatment, however, is limited to children who have a family donor who is genotypically identical. The survival rate for children who have been able to receive an HLA-identical sibling donor stem cell transplant is 93% (Platt & Eckman, 2006). (See discussion regarding HSCT later in this chapter.)

Prognosis depends on the severity of the child's disease; children with more frequent exacerbations and hospitalization have poorer prognosis. Neonatal screening, early intervention, prophylactic antibiotics, and parent education have extended life spans in individuals with sickle cell disease with the median survival age of 45 for those with HbSS disease and 65 for those with HbSC (Driscoll, 2007).

Nursing Practice

It is important for all health facilities to have current guidelines for transfusion protocols. Become familiar with the policies and procedures where you work. For example, the child's blood type and patient identification needs to be checked by two registered nurses before starting the infusion. See the Clinical Skills Manual **SKILLS** for further information on blood transfusions.

NURSING MANAGEMENT

NURSING ASSESSMENT AND DIAGNOSIS

The nurse may be involved in sickle cell gene testing to identify carriers and children who have the disease. Once a child is diagnosed with the disease, a comprehensive physical assessment is essential because sickle cell anemia can affect any body system.

PHYSIOLOGIC ASSESSMENT

In children who are known to have sickle cell anemia, obtain a detailed history from the parents or child about past crises, precipitating events, medical treatment, and home management. Measure the child's height and weight accurately and compare to past measurements, since failure to thrive is common. Ask about chronic or acute pain that the child is experiencing. Pain may occur in nearly any body part, but most commonly manifests as headache, extremity pain, or abdominal discomfort. The ill child with sickle cell disease should receive a careful multisystem assessment. Fever, neurological changes such as decreased alertness or behavioral changes, and respiratory symptoms are emergency conditions that necessitate prompt treatment. When the child is in crisis, assess pain and note the presence of any signs of inflammation or infection. Carefully monitor the child for signs of shock (see Chapter 49∞).

PSYCHOSOCIAL ASSESSMENT

The family of a child with sickle cell disease requires a thorough psychosocial assessment. Ask if other family members have the diagnosis. If the child is newly diagnosed with the disorder, the

Thinking Critically

SICKLE CELL ANEMIA

Michael is a 12-year-old black child with sickle cell disease who is admitted to the hospital with severe abdominal pain. Which organ is likely filled with sickled cells and causing his pain? Michael is receiving oxygen by nasal cannula; why would he need this? What are the most important nursing assessments and interventions to integrate within Michael's care?

See MyNursingKit for possible responses.

family needs assistance to deal with feelings related to the serious, life-threatening nature of the disease. Assess parents' understanding of the disease transmission and ask whether genetic counseling has been obtained. Determine whether the family has adequate healthcare coverage to pay for the child's medical expenses and whether the child qualifies for assistance due to the disease disability. Ask older children about their knowledge of the disease, and explore their feelings related to the management of a chronic condition. When siblings or other family members are carriers, periodic counseling is needed so they can understand implications for dating, marriage, and having children.

Several nursing diagnoses that might apply to the child with sickle cell anemia are presented in the accompanying Nursing Care Plan. Other nursing diagnoses might include the following:

- *Caregiver Role Strain* related to illness chronicity
- *Risk for Impaired Parenting* related to having a child with a physical illness
- *Delayed Growth and Development* related to effects of physical disability
- *Impaired Physical Mobility* related to pain
- *Deficient Knowledge (child and parents)* related to lack of exposure about cause and treatment of sickle cell anemia

PLANNING AND IMPLEMENTATION

The accompanying Nursing Care Plan summarizes nursing care for the child with sickle cell anemia. Nursing management for the child in crisis focuses on increasing tissue perfusion, promoting hydration, controlling pain, preventing infection, ensuring adequate nutrition, preventing complications, and providing emotional support to the child and family.

INCREASE TISSUE PERFUSION

Administer blood transfusions and oxygen as ordered. To prevent hemolysis, the intravenous fluid used before and after a blood transfusion must be saline rather than D5W. Monitor for transfusion reactions (see Clinical Manifestations). Encourage

Nursing Practice

When giving a transfusion, never infuse cold blood since it may increase sickling. Use a blood-warming coil to bring blood to room temperature.

the child to rest. Work with the child and family to avoid emotional stress. Any activities that increase cellular metabolism also result in tissue hypoxia. Schedule caregiving activities and play to allow for optimal rest.

PROMOTE HYDRATION

The child with sickle cell anemia is adversely affected by dehydration. Calculate the child's fluid maintenance requirements (minimum daily fluid intake) (see Chapter 46) and monitor the child's oral fluid intake. Administer intravenous fluids as ordered. Adjust oral intake as necessary to keep the child well hydrated.

CONTROL PAIN

Administer prescribed analgesics around the clock during crises. If patient-controlled analgesia is used, be sure that the constant infusions run as ordered and that the parent or child understands the use of the button for bolus infusions, when needed (see

Nursing Practice

Blood reactions can occur as soon as the blood transfusion begins. Administer the first 20 mL of blood slowly and observe the child carefully for a reaction. Repeatedly assess the child according to agency policy and promptly report changes in condition. If a reaction occurs stop the transfusion immediately, call the physician, monitor vital signs, keep intravenous line open with normal saline, check for hematuria, and administer antihistamines, antipyretics, and diuretics if ordered.

Clinical Manifestations

BLOOD TRANSFUSION REACTIONS

TYPE OF REACTION AND ETIOLOGY	CLINICAL MANIFESTATIONS
Allergic reaction related to immune response to protein in the blood	Urticaria, itching, respiratory distress
Hemolytic reaction related to mismatched blood, history of multiple transfusions, or infusion with a solution containing dextrose or other additives	Fever, chills, hematuria, headache, chest pain; can progress to shock
Febrile or septic related to contamination of blood; may also be caused by idiopathic conditions	Chills, fever, headache, decreased blood pressure, nausea or vomiting, and leg and back pain
Circulatory overload related to infusions of excessive amounts of fluid or too rapid administration	Labored breathing, chest or low back pain, productive cough, rales upon auscultation, distended neck veins, increased central venous pressure

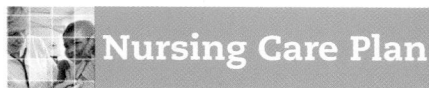

Nursing Care Plan

THE CHILD WITH SICKLE CELL ANEMIA

INTERVENTION	RATIONALE	EXPECTED OUTCOME
1. Nursing Diagnosis: Ineffective Tissue Perfusion related to affinity of hemoglobin for oxygen		
NIC Priority Intervention: **Circulatory care:** Promotion of arterial and venous circulation		**NOC Suggested Outcome:** **Tissue perfusion, peripheral:** Extent to which blood flows through the small vessels of the extremities and maintains tissue function
Goal: The child will show few signs and symptoms of tissue hypoxia.		
■ Instruct child to avoid physical exertion, emotional stress, low-oxygen environments (e.g., airplanes, high altitudes), and known sources of infection.	■ Decreased activity and exposure reduce the body's need for oxygen.	The child has no shortness of breath and shows no signs of hypoxia.
Goal: Repeated cerebrovascular accidents will be avoided.		
■ Administer blood transfusions as ordered.	■ Packed cells increase number of red blood cells available to carry oxygen to tissue cells. Transfusions promote circulation.	The child does not suffer a cerebrovascular accident.
■ Perform several caregiving activities together whenever possible.	■ Grouping activities allows for optimum rest.	
■ Give oxygen as ordered.	■ High concentration of oxygen in alveoli increases diffusion of gas across membranes.	
■ Administer and teach the family about prophylactic transfusions for the child who has had a cerebrovascular accident.	■ Lowers potential for a future cerebrovascular accident.	
2. Nursing Diagnosis: Risk for Deficient Fluid Volume related to inadequate fluid intake and dehydration		
NIC Priority Intervention: **Fluid management:** Promotion of electrolyte balance and prevention of complications resulting from abnormal or undesired fluid levels		**NOC Suggested Outcome:** **Hydration:** Amount of water in the intracellular and extracellular compartments of the body
Goal: The child will maintain or be restored to adequate hydration.		
■ Calculate the child's daily fluid requirements. Monitor the child's usual fluid consumption and make necessary adjustments. Encourage the child to take fluids. Observe for signs of dehydration.	■ Optimizing fluid intake ensures that the child gets needed fluid. Dehydration exacerbates crises.	The child shows signs of adequate hydration.
■ Record intake and output.	■ Early intervention can be effective in minimizing complications from dehydration. Child may need oral or intravenous rehydration therapy.	
3. Nursing Diagnosis: Pain related to chronic physical disability		
NIC Priority Intervention: **Pain management:** Alleviation of pain or a reduction in pain to a level of comfort acceptable to the patient		**NOC Suggested Outcome:** **Comfort level:** Feelings of physical and psychologic ease
Goal: The child will verbalize that pain is controlled.		
■ Administer analgesics, such as morphine or hydromorphone (Dilaudid), as ordered. Continuous intravenous infusion is used for the duration of a painful crisis.	■ Pain of sickle cell crises is excruciating.	The child is pain-free or pain control is significantly improved.
■ Position carefully.	■ Joints and extremities can be extremely painful.	

(continued)

Nursing Care Plan—continued

THE CHILD WITH SICKLE CELL ANEMIA—continued

INTERVENTION	RATIONALE	EXPECTED OUTCOME
4. Nursing Diagnosis: Risk for Infection related to chronic disease and splenic malfunction		
NIC Priority Intervention: **Infectious control:** Minimizing the acquisition and transmission of infectious agents		**NOC Suggested Outcome:** **Risk control:** Actions to eliminate or reduce actual, personal, and modifiable health threats
Goal: The child will not develop infection.		
■ Ensure adequate nutrition by providing high-calorie, high-protein diet. Make sure that the child's immunizations are up to date and that children less than age 5 years are receiving prophylactic antibiotics. Report any signs of infection to physician immediately.	■ Children with a chronic illness are at greater risk of infection.	The child is free of infection.
■ Isolate the child from possible sources of infection. Instruct parents about signs of infection and encourage them to seek prompt healthcare.	■ Restriction of persons with infection decreases the child's contact with infectious agents. Prompt care for infection reduces the chance of sickle cell crisis.	

Chapter 42∞). Help the child assume a comfortable position. Avoid putting stress on painful joints. See "Evidence-Based Nursing: Sickle Cell Anemia and Pain Management."

PREVENT INFECTION

Infection makes the child more susceptible to a crisis, and the crisis, in turn, increases susceptibility to infection. Teach the parents how to administer antibiotics for prophylaxis or treatment of infection. Because infections are particularly virulent in these children, tell parents to get immediate care when the child is ill. Emphasize the importance of immunizations. See earlier discus-

Growth and Development

To encourage fluid intake in a small child:

- Use a favorite cup or glass.
- Use straws.
- Take advantage of times the child is thirsty, such as on awakening or after play.
- Leave a cup within easy reach of the child.
- Offer frozen juice pops, crushed ice drinks, and flavored ice chips.

Complementary Care

PAIN AND SICKLE CELL ANEMIA

Pain management for children with sickle cell disease is a major challenge, both for healthcare providers and families. A nursing study that determined effectiveness of pain control and types of comfort measures used by families provides information that can be applied in caring for children with sickle cell disease in the hospital and home (Beyer & Simmons, 2004). The mothers in this study described a combination of traditional medicine and complementary approaches. They emphasized the importance of keeping the child healthy, in order to avoid crisis, by avoiding overheating or chilling. Regular medical checkups, adequate hydration, and immunizations were considered important. Being alert to early signs of pain was important so that the families could begin pharmacologic treatment as well as complementary therapies such as applying heat via baths and hot towels to decrease pain and increase relaxation; touching, holding, and massaging the extremities or chest and back; praying together; and distraction and diversionary activities such as playing games and taking drives. Nurses can learn from and apply these approaches with families. Ask them what they do to identify pain early and alleviate it. Add to the list of interventions the family can try and then partner with them to evaluate results. Continue to emphasize medical care while integrating the other comfort measures the family and child find helpful into nursing care plans.

Evidence-Based Nursing

SICKLE CELL ANEMIA AND PAIN MANAGEMENT

Clinical Question

What are the most effective pain management strategies for children with sickle cell disease? How can nurses facilitate the integration of pain measures used at home into care of the child when hospitalized?

The Evidence

Severe episodes of sickle cell crisis require hospitalization for pain management. Relief of pain is the primary goal for healthcare providers and is most significant to the child experiencing pain.

Research has found that this goal is not always met (Jacob, Miaskowski, Savedra, et al., 2006). Nurse researchers conducted a descriptive longitudinal study with 27 children to evaluate the pain management strategies used in sickle cell disease when they experienced pain during a vaso-occlusive episode. The children ranged in age from 5 to 19 years; there were 40 hospital admissions during the 9-month study. The researchers noted several surprising findings from the study. First, they found that children on average self-administered only 35% of the pain medication that was prescribed. The second finding was that the children did not report significant pain relief. It is surmised that adequate pain relief was not achieved during hospitalization because the dose of analgesics administered was too low (Jacob, Miaskowski, Savedra, et al., 2003).

As part of the larger study mentioned above, the researchers also evaluated the effect of pain on sleep, food intake, and activity levels. Children hospitalized in pain crisis reported disruption in their nighttime sleep, but sleeping more during the day. Food intake was markedly decreased throughout the hospitalization. Activity levels also remained relatively low throughout the hospitalization (Jacob et al., 2006).

In another study in which 21 female caretakers of children with sickle cell disease were interviewed, a variety of techniques were used to manage pain at home. Oral medications, massage, warmth to painful body parts, and other techniques were considered helpful (Beyer & Simmons, 2004).

Best Practice

Hospitalized children who self-administered their medication consistently undermedicated themselves and failed to achieve pain relief. The inability to achieve pain relief affected the child's ability to sleep and their desire to eat and remain active.

Children may not be taught how to use the PCA device properly or they may interpret that they should use the button as little as possible. If the child has pain, consider whether a higher dosage in the continuous infusion would help pain control. Thus, healthcare provider practices influence the child's pain management. In addition, children and families have developed many effective pain relief measures at home that may not be included in hospital care. More information is needed about methods of integrating these techniques into hospital care.

Recommendations include the need to evaluate whether increasing analgesic use to at least the amount prescribed would increase the amount of pain relief and in turn improve the child's sleeping, eating, and exercise patterns. Additional research is needed to determine the effectiveness of different PCA regimens and to evaluate the effectiveness of pain management algorithms. Effective evaluation tools are needed to measure effectiveness of the child self-medication by patient controlled analgesia. Tools for evaluating home care pain management are needed. Nurses must be willing to integrate the family's measures into care while the child is hospitalized.

Critical Thinking

How will you determine if the child in sickle cell crisis is obtaining adequate pain relief (consult Chapter 42 ∞ for ideas)? What personal beliefs of healthcare providers may influence effective pain management? How can these beliefs be addressed? If the primary healthcare provider has prescribed a subtherapeutic dosage of pain medication for a child in sickle cell crisis, what action could you take?

See MyNursingKit for possible responses.

sion on pages 1446–1447 and Chapter 45 ∞ for further information about recommended and supplemental immunizations.

ENSURE ADEQUATE NUTRITION

Emphasize the importance of adequate nutrition to promote growth. Encourage the child to eat a high-protein, high-calorie diet. Emphasize the importance of folic acid and vitamin C as supplements as prescribed. Perform regular growth measurements and if slow growth is apparent, perform 24-hour recalls and other nutritional assessments.

PREVENT COMPLICATIONS OF CRISES

Observe the child for signs of increasing anemia, infection, and shock (mental status change, pallor, vital sign changes). Maintain ongoing monitoring of the child's neurologic status for evidence of altered cerebral function. Assess for an enlarged spleen by gentle palpation. Administer blood transfusions and observe the child for any adverse reaction. Assess growth and developmental milestones.

PROVIDE EMOTIONAL SUPPORT

Sickle cell anemia is a chronic disease accompanied by life-threatening episodic crises. Family members often need support to help them deal with their feelings about the diagnosis and its implications. Explore resources in the home and community to see if parents will be able to administer medications and fluids and to provide adequate nutrition. Assess their knowledge of signs of infection and of sickle cell crisis and when to seek medical care for the child. Refer the parents for genetic counseling, particularly if they plan to have more children. Encourage adolescents and young adults in the family to receive genetic counseling and testing, as well. Referrals to support groups and contact with others with the disease can be helpful.

MyNursingKit Sickle Cell Resources

DISCHARGE PLANNING AND HOME CARE TEACHING

Identify and address home care needs well in advance of discharge. Give parents information about sickle cell disease and the child's treatment. Even parents of a child previously diagnosed with the disorder may benefit from information about the disease process and its management. Explain the basic effect of tissue hypoxia and the effects of sickling on circulation. Assist the family to explore resources in the home and community and determine if parents will be able to administer medications and fluids and to provide adequate nutrition.

Teach parents to look for signs of dehydration, such as dry mucous membranes, weight loss, and sunken fontanelles in infants. Give specific instructions about how many ounces of liquid the child needs to drink each day. Emphasize that increased fluid intake is needed to replace the fluids lost from overheating or exposure to hot weather. Make sure both the child and family understand the triggers and precipitating factors for sickle cell crises. Encourage them to avoid situations that cause crises. Instruct the child and parents about signs and symptoms of crises that should be reported to their healthcare provider.

When regular blood infusions are used, the resulting iron overload is damaging to body organs. Provide the family with instructions about the treatment for iron overload.

Tell parents that it is important to inform all treating physicians and dentists of the child's medical condition. The child should also wear medical identification (e.g., a medical identification bracelet). Special precautions are necessary when the child undergoes surgery of any kind, as hypoxia resulting from anesthesia is a major surgical risk.

Family members need ongoing support to deal with the stress of having a child with a chronic condition. Provide resources, respite care for parents, and information as needed for siblings.

Encourage older children with sickle cell anemia to participate in activities with other children between crises but to avoid strenuous physical exertion and contact sports. Play and social interactions that promote learning and development are important.

Teaching Highlights

HOME CARE CONSIDERATIONS FOR THE CHILD WITH SICKLE CELL ANEMIA

- Follow recommended schedules for well-child care visits and keep scheduled appointments with the child's hematologist.
- Be sure the child is up to date with immunizations, including hepatitis B, annual influenza, pneumococcal vaccine, and tuberculosis skin test.
- Special testing, such as heart and eye examinations, may be needed periodically to check for sequelae of the disease.
- Special medications, such as antibiotics, may be needed; pain relief medicine and blood transfusions may be administered.
- Dehydration can lead to crisis. Be sure the child gets extra fluids in hot weather, when ill, during physical activity, and during travel.
- As the child develops, provide information about the disease and encourage self-care. Be sure the school personnel understand the child's diagnosis and any care required during school hours.
- Contact your healthcare provider if the child has a high fever, a common illness that lasts more than one day, seizures, change in behavior, severe pain, abnormal skin color or breathing pattern, or any other symptoms that concern you.

EVALUATION

Expected outcomes of nursing care for the child with sickle cell anemia include the following:

- Management of pain to facilitate comfort level
- Maintenance of adequate hydration state to prevent cell sickling
- Absence of side effects of disease in respiratory system, central nervous system, and body organs
- Maintenance of normal immune status and prevention of infection
- Prompt recognition and treatment of complications of the disease
- Maintenance of normal growth and development for the child
- Provision of necessary services and resources for the parents and other family members
- Knowledge of disease and treatment by family

THALASSEMIAS

The thalassemias are a group of inherited blood disorders of hemoglobin synthesis characterized by anemia that can be mild or severe. There are three types of β-thalassemia: thalassemia minor, or thalassemia trait (produces mild anemia); thalassemia intermedia (produces moderate anemia and may require transfusions); and thalassemia major, also known as Cooley's anemia (produces anemia requiring transfusion). Clinical manifestations of β-thalassemia are caused by the defective synthesis of hemoglobin, structurally impaired RBCs (Figure 51–4 ●), and the shortened life span of the RBCs. The infant with β-thalassemia major manifests pallor, failure to thrive, hepatosplenomegaly, and severe anemia that leads to chronic hypoxemia (Richardson, 2007). In alpha-thalassemia the child may have a one gene defect (alpha thalassemia silent carrier) and generally be symptom free, have a two gene defect (alpha thalassemia trait) and have mild anemia or have alpha-thalassemia major, which results in hydrops fetalis, intrauterine congestive heart failure, cardiomegaly, hepatomegaly, and death (DeBaun & Vichinsky, 2007; Richardson, 2007).

Diagnosis is made by hemoglobin electrophoresis, which reveals a decreased production of one of the globin chains in hemoglobin and an elevated F and A hemoglobin. A complete blood

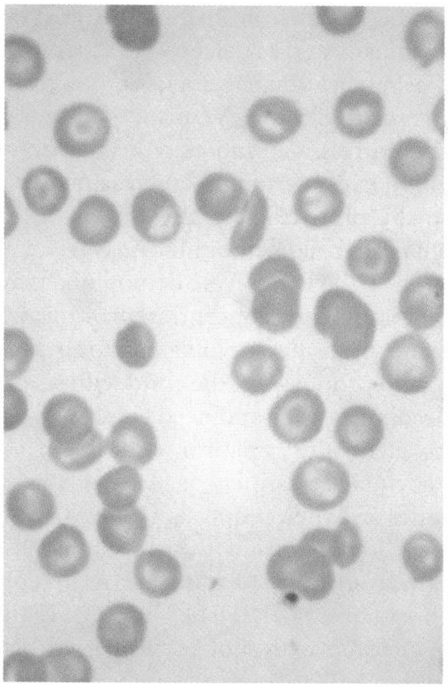

● **Figure 51–4** Red blood cell appearance in β-thalassemia. What characteristic abnormalities can be seen on this microscopic view?
Courtesy of Dr. Ed Wong, Laboratory Medicine, Children's National Medical Center, Washington, DC.

count shows a decreased hemoglobin, hematocrit, and reticulocyte count. Prenatal testing using chorionic villi sampling or amniocentesis can detect the disease in the fetus. Treatment is supportive. The goal of medical management is to maintain normal hemoglobin levels. Blood transfusion is the conventional therapy used to treat children with severe disease. Since iron overload is a side effect of this treatment, children may need to receive an iron-chelating drug such as deferoxamine or Exjade. (See previous discussion on page 1447.) A splenectomy may be required for the child with splenomegaly. Hematopoietic stem cell transplantation (HSCT) may be offered as an alternative therapy for children newly diagnosed with the disorder.

Nursing Management

Nursing care focuses on observing for complications of transfusion therapy, supporting the child and family in dealing with a chronic life-threatening illness, and referring the family for genetic counseling. Encourage parents to take an active role in the child's treatment regimen. Teach parents the technique for subcutaneous infusion of deferoxamine if that route is to be used for therapy at home.

Compliance with transfusion therapy often becomes an issue as children reach adolescence. Offering the adolescent treatment options, such as when to undergo transfusion, can help improve compliance. Adolescents with β-thalassemia and parents of newly diagnosed children can be referred to the Thalassemia Action Group, a national organization for patients, or to the Cooley's Anemia Foundation. Expected outcomes of nursing care include maintenance of normal hemoglobin and hematocrit, safe transfusion of blood products, maintenance of recommended body iron levels, and family understanding about the genetic transmission of the disease.

APLASTIC ANEMIA

Aplastic anemia is a deficiency in the number of the blood cells resulting from failure of the bone marrow to produce adequate numbers of all types of circulating blood cells. The condition may be congenital or acquired. Most aplastic anemia is immune-mediated and results from a combination of environmental exposure and an individual's genetically-determined response to the causative environmental agent (Corbeel, 2005; Young, Calado, & Scheinberg, 2006).

Congenital aplastic anemia (Fanconi anemia) is a rare autosomal recessive syndrome consisting of multiple congenital anomalies. Children with congenital aplastic anemia are at risk for developing malignancies such as acute nonlymphocytic leukemia (Freedman, 2007).

Acquired aplastic anemia in children can be idiopathic or occur from exposure to drugs or other substances. It can develop after exposure to ionizing radiation or insecticides or after ingestion of drugs such as sulfonamides, chloramphenicol, quinacrine, benzene solvents in model airplane glue, and lead. This type of anemia can also be a result of an infectious process such as viral hepatitis, or mononucleosis.

Symptoms are related to the degree of bone marrow failure and include **petechiae** (small pinpoint red or purple spots on the mucous membranes or skin), **purpura** (irregular bluish purple areas of bleeding into the tissues), bloody stools, epistaxis, or retinal bleeding. Other symptoms include weakness and tachycardia. Symptoms associated with anemia include pallor, fatigue, tachycardia, and congestive heart failure. Symptoms related to neutropenia include fever and bacterial infections. Death can result from complications associated with hemorrhage, sepsis, and malignancy.

Diagnosis is made by complete blood count studies, which reveal leukopenia with marked neutropenia, thrombocytopenia, and **pancytopenia** (decreased number of blood cell components); and by bone marrow aspiration, which reveals yellow, fatty bone marrow instead of red bone marrow.

Supportive treatment includes transfusions of packed cells, platelets, or both. Immunosuppressive drug therapy is effective for many children because it is believed the child's immune system is attacking the bone marrow. Immunosuppressive agents include antithymocyte globulin (ATG) and cyclosporine (Corbeel, 2005). The treatment of choice is hematopoietic stem cell transplantation (HSCT) from a compatible sibling or family member donor.

Nursing Management

Nursing care is similar to that for the child with leukemia (see Chapter 52∞). Nursing actions focus on preventing bleeding, administering and monitoring blood transfusions, preventing infection, encouraging mobility as tolerated, educating the parents and child about the disorder, and providing emotional support. Families need support in dealing with a child who has a life-threatening disease. Refer them to support groups for counseling, if indicated, and to social services. Expected outcomes of nursing care include absence of infection, no bleeding, and parental education related to the disease and treatment.

MyNursingKit Anemia Resources

BLEEDING DISORDERS

HEMOPHILIA

Hemophilia refers to a group of hereditary bleeding disorders that result from a deficiency in specific clotting factors. Hemophilia A, or classic hemophilia, is caused by a deficiency of factor VIII in the blood and accounts for 85% of persons with hemophilia. Hemophilia B, also known as Christmas disease (named for the first person diagnosed with the disorder), is caused by a deficiency of factor IX (Kumar, Abbas, Fausto, et al., 2010). Of people with hemophilia, 10–15% have hemophilia B (Ohls & Christensen, 2007).

Etiology and Pathophysiology

Hemophilia is an X-linked recessive disorder, which manifests almost exclusively as affected males and carrier females. Genes for clotting factors VIII and IX are located near the terminal long arm of the X chromosome (Scott & Montgomery, 2007). A daughter who inherits the gene from her father has a 50% chance at each pregnancy of transmitting it to her sons (see Chapter 7∞ for a description of genetic transmission). However, in as many as one third of children with hemophilia there is no family history and the disorder is caused by a new mutation. The degree of bleeding is related to the amount of clotting factor and the severity of the injury.

Clinical Manifestations

Hemophilia is manifested in different children by bleeding tendencies that range from mild to moderate or severe. Children with hemophilia often do not manifest symptoms until after 6 months of age as they become more mobile and incur injuries and bleeding from falls or from tooth eruption. Spontaneous bleeding, **hemarthrosis** (bleeding into a joint space), and deep tissue hemorrhage occur. Affected children frequently experience bleeding into the joint spaces of the knees, ankles, and elbows. Bleeding into joint spaces or bursae causes the child to have limited motion because of pain, tenderness, and swelling. Bone changes, contractures, and disabling deformities can result from immobility and from the effects of blood in the joint structures.

Children may have bleeding after circumcision, frequent bruising (**ecchymosis**), epistaxis, hematuria, and bleeding after tooth extraction, minor trauma, or minor surgical procedures. Large subcutaneous and intramuscular hemorrhages sometimes occur. Bleeding into the tissues of the neck, mouth, or chest is particularly serious because of the potential for airway obstruction. Intracranial bleeding may also occur and can be life threatening (Revel-Vilk, Golomb, Achonu, et al., 2004).

Females who carry the trait for hemophilia do not usually manifest symptoms of the disease. However, they may have prolonged bleeding during dental work, surgery, or trauma.

MyNursingKit Care Plan: A School-Age Child with Hemophilia

Clinical Therapy

Affected people and carriers can be diagnosed before birth through chorionic villus sampling or amniocentesis. Genetic testing of family members is increasingly being used to identify carriers. Diagnosis can also be made on the basis of the history, physical examination, and laboratory data. Laboratory tests show low levels of factor VIII or IX, and prolonged activated partial prothrombin time (APPT). Prothrombin time (PT), thrombin time (TT), fibrinogen, and platelet count are normal.

The goal of medical management is to control bleeding by replacing the missing clotting factor. Desmopressin (DDAVP), an analog of vasopressin, stimulates the release of factor VIII stored in the blood vessels, thereby increasing the percentage of available factor by approximately threefold. DDAVP is effective in some patients with mild hemophilia A (Curry, 2004; Manno & Larson, 2005).The child with severe hemophilia may be on a prophylactic regimen of factor concentrate therapy, while the child with mild to moderate hemophilia may only receive episodic therapy. Even with prophylaxis, the child with severe hemophilia may have a bleeding episode and need episodic treatment as well (Manco-Johnson, Abshire, Shapiro, et al., 2007; Miller, 2004). Prompt and adequate treatment is needed to prevent serious bleeding episodes and their sequelae.

The outlook for children with hemophilia has been greatly improved by the availability of transfusion therapy. In the past, many children with factor VIII deficiency died in the first 5 years of life. Today, children with moderate or mild hemophilia can lead normal lives. Gene therapy is being explored for treatment of hemophilia. Efforts in animal models such as dogs are underway. These research approaches offer the promise of new treatment options in the future (Warrington & Herzog, 2006).

NURSING MANAGEMENT

NURSING ASSESSMENT AND DIAGNOSIS

PHYSIOLOGIC ASSESSMENT

Obtain a complete medical history from the parents or child. In particular, ask about previous episodes of bleeding and the occurrence of hemophilia or any other bleeding disorders in family members. The history of bleeding will vary, depending on the severity of the disease.

Assess the child for any joint pain, swelling, or permanent deformity, particularly around the knees, elbows, ankles, and shoulders. Observe for prolonged bleeding or oozing of blood. Note the presence of hematuria and mild flank pain. Conduct a neurologic assessment, as the risk for intracranial hemorrhage and bleeding can lead to peripheral neuropathies.

PSYCHOSOCIAL ASSESSMENT

It is difficult for families to manage care of the child with hemophilia, especially if the disease is severe. Assess the family's coping mechanisms and support systems. Determine the ability of the family's resources to manage procedures and treatments; the factor concentrates and infusion equipment are costly. Assess older children's understanding of the disease, limitations, and their adaptation to the disease.

DEVELOPMENTAL ASSESSMENT

Because the child with hemophilia may have physical activity restrictions, physical skills may be delayed. Perform frequent developmental assessments, being particularly attentive to fine and gross motor skills.

The most important nursing diagnosis for the child with hemophilia is *Risk for Injury* related to bleeding disorder. Some of the other nursing diagnoses that might apply include the following:

- *Pain* related to bleeding episodes
- *Impaired Physical Mobility* related to joint stiffness or contractures
- *Impaired Home Maintenance Management* related to challenges of hemophilia
- *Interrupted Family Processes* related to family role shift required to care for a child with a chronic illness
- *Delayed Growth and Development* related to effects of physical disability

Nursing Practice

Take the following precautions when caring for children with bleeding disorders:

- Avoid taking temperatures rectally or giving suppositories.
- Check blood pressure by cuff as infrequently as possible.
- Avoid intramuscular or subcutaneous injections.
- Use only paper or silk tape for dressings.
- Except for factor replacement therapy, avoid all venipunctures.
- Use a peripheral finger stick to obtain blood samples.
- Do not give aspirin, ibuprofen, or other drugs that affect bleeding time.

PLANNING AND IMPLEMENTATION

Nursing care focuses on preventing and controlling bleeding episodes, limiting joint involvement and managing pain, and providing emotional support. Both short-term interventions and long-term management are necessary.

PREVENT AND CONTROL BLEEDING EPISODES

Bleeding problems are rare in infants with hemophilia. As children learn to walk and develop other motor skills, however, they often fall and suffer cuts and bruises. The risk of injury can be reduced by emphasizing to parents the need for close supervision and a safe environment. Parents should encourage children to play with safe, age-appropriate toys.

When the child is hospitalized, use nursing approaches to minimize the possibility of bleeding. Ensure that the hospital environment is safe by orienting the child to the room and keeping the floor and room clear of hazards as much as possible. If significant bleeding does occur, offer supportive measures and assist with factor replacement therapy. Carefully monitor the child's condition for any side effects when factor replacement therapy is administered. Control any superficial bleeding by applying pressure to the area for at least 15 minutes. Immobilize and elevate the affected area, and apply ice packs to promote vasoconstriction.

LIMIT JOINT INVOLVEMENT AND MANAGE PAIN

During bleeding episodes, hemarthrosis is managed by elevating and immobilizing the joint and applying ice packs. Administer analgesics as ordered. Once bleeding has been controlled, range of motion exercises strengthen muscles and joints and prevent flexion contractures. Physical therapy may be needed. Because excessive weight can place an added stress on joints, encourage the child to maintain an appropriate weight.

Nursing Practice

Use the acronym RICE (Rest, Ice, Compression, Elevation) to help you remember important measures to control a bleeding episode (Curry, 2004).

PROVIDE EMOTIONAL SUPPORT

The needs of families with hemophiliac children are best met through a comprehensive team approach. Refer the parents for genetic counseling as soon as possible after diagnosis. It is important to identify family members who carry the trait, as they may suffer excessive bleeding during surgery.

Encourage the parents to verbalize their feelings. Be understanding and sensitive to their needs. Teach the parents about hemophilia and explain how the disorder affects both the child and other family members. Refer the parents and child to organizations such as the National Hemophilia Foundation for further information.

DISCHARGE PLANNING AND HOME CARE TEACHING

The child may be hospitalized briefly during the first manifestation of bleeding for diagnosis and management. After that, most care takes place in the home. Identify and address home care needs well in advance of discharge. Advise parents to have the child wear a medical identification bracelet. Explain the cause of bleeding so both the child and parents understand the disease process. Teach the child and family how to identify internal bleeding. Signs and symptoms such as joint pain, abdominal pain, and obvious bleeding are indicators for immediate factor infusion. Make sure the child and parents know what situations could cause bleeding to occur. Teach parents to give acetaminophen instead of aspirin to relieve pain (Curry, 2004).

Instruct the parents and the child, when appropriate, to prepare and administer factor concentrate. If infusion of the missing factor is scheduled regularly, bleeding episodes can be controlled or avoided. Have the parents demonstrate the procedure and make sure they can administer the product correctly.

MyNursingKit Ethical Considerations: Hemophilia

Growth and Development

Encourage adolescents with hemophilia to participate in leisure activities such as computer games, reading clubs, and crafts. They should use knee pads, elbow pads, and helmets when participating in any physical sports. Swimming and other noncontact sports are good choices for physical activity. Activities important to development can be encouraged when coaches, teachers, and others know how to treat bleeding episodes. Advise adolescents to shave only with an electric razor.

The parents need to be familiar with properties of the factor concentrate to prepare the mixture correctly.

The child will need an individualized school health plan (see Chapter 39). Members of the school staff should be instructed in management of emergencies, and infusion equipment should be readily available. The nurse can identify key staff members in the school and teach them the actions that need to be taken.

Help the family and school plan an appropriate schedule of activities without overprotecting the child. Children with hemophilia should not engage in contact sports such as football and soccer, which may result in injury and trauma. Instead, encourage sports such as swimming, hiking, and bicycling.

Explain how the parents can coordinate their child's care with a number of health professionals. Provide ongoing case management, assisting the family to take on this task if able.

Hemophilia is not only a debilitating disorder for the child, but it also can be financially draining for the family. Frequent outpatient visits, emergency department visits, hospital admissions, and the cost of factor concentrate can exhaust a family's resources. If indicated, refer families to appropriate social services (e.g., the state's maternal and child health program for children with special healthcare needs) and organizations such as the National Hemophilia Foundation. Sharing experiences with other families of children with hemophilia can provide support.

EVALUATION

Expected outcomes of nursing care include the following:

- Prevention of injury to the child
- Management of pain to promote comfort level
- Promotion of normal growth and development
- Adequate knowledge of child and family for disease management, including recognition of bleeding and prompt initiation of infusions

VON WILLEBRAND DISEASE

Von Willebrand disease is the most common hereditary bleeding disorder occurring in up to 3% of the world's population. There are a variety of subtypes of this disorder that are classified based on the amount and functionality of the von Willebrand factor (vWF), a plasma protein and the carrier for clotting factor VIII. The most common form of the disorder is transmitted as an autosomal dominant trait, and can occur in both males and females. The gene for the disease is located on chromosome 12 (Curry, 2004).

The characteristic manifestations are easy bruising and epistaxis. Children with von Willebrand disease frequently have gingival bleeding and increased bleeding with lacerations or during surgery. Affected teenage girls may have menorrhagia (increased menstrual bleeding).

Diagnosis of von Willebrand disease is made after laboratory studies reveal decreased von Willebrand factor levels, von Willebrand factor antigen levels, and factor VIII activity; reduced platelet agglutination; prolonged bleeding time; and prolonged or normal activated partial thromboplastin time (APTT). Treatment is similar to that for the child with hemophilia and involves infusion of von Willebrand protein concentrate. Desmopressin (DDAVP) is administered to promote release of stored vWF and to prevent bleeding associated with dental or surgical procedures. Locally administered medications such as aminocaproic acid are sometimes used to manage bleeding in the mucous membranes.

Nursing Management

Teach parents about the disorder and instruct them not to give the child any aspirin or other drugs that can cause bleeding or inhibit platelet function. Teach management of bleeding episodes and intravenous infusion techniques, as for hemophilia. The prognosis is good, and children with von Willebrand disease usually have a normal life expectancy. Expected outcomes of nursing care include prompt management of bleeding and prevention of disease complications.

DISSEMINATED INTRAVASCULAR COAGULATION

Disseminated intravascular coagulation (DIC) is a life-threatening, acquired pathologic process in which the clotting system is abnormally activated, resulting in widespread clot formation in the small vessels throughout the body. Excess thrombin is generated, followed by deposition of fibrin strands in body tissues. These changes cause tissue hypoxia, resulting in eventual tissue necrosis. The circulating fibrin fragments later begin to interfere with platelet aggregation and other aspects of the clotting mechanism, resulting in bleeding or hemorrhage.

The most common cause of DIC is sepsis. Infections caused by gram-negative and gram-positive bacteria, fungi, viruses, and protozoa may lead to DIC (LeMone & Burke, 2008). Symptoms can include diffuse bleeding manifested by hematuria, petechiae, or purpura; an injection site that continues to ooze; circulatory collapse; and major vessel thrombosis. The prothrombin time and partial thromboplastin time are prolonged and the platelet count is decreased (Scott & Montgomery, 2007).

Medical management is supportive and includes identification and treatment of the underlying disorder; replacement of depleted coagulation factors, fibrinogen, and platelets; and anticoagulant therapy (heparin).

Nursing Management

DIC is a complex disorder managed by a critical care team. Nursing care focuses on assessing the bleeding, preventing further injury, and administering prescribed therapies. Observe for petechiae, ecchymoses, and oozing every 1 to 2 hours. Be sure to check dependent areas (those lower than other body parts), as blood pools in these areas. Intravenous sites are particularly prone to oozing and should be assessed every 15 minutes. Examine stool for the presence of blood, and measure blood loss as accurately as possible. Measure intake and output.

Because all body systems can be involved, careful, continuous assessment of all systems is needed. Institute bleeding control precautions, monitor prescribed therapy (transfusion, anticoagulant therapy), and report any signs of complications. Desired outcomes of nursing care are management of bleeding and adequate function of all body systems. Adequate family support in this life-threatening situation is a focus of nursing care.

IDIOPATHIC THROMBOCYTOPENIC PURPURA

Idiopathic thrombocytopenic purpura (ITP), also known as immune thrombocytopenic purpura, is a disorder characterized by increased destruction of platelets, even though platelet production in the bone marrow is normal. When the rate of platelet destruction exceeds the rate of platelet production, the number of circulating platelets decreases and blood clotting slows.

ITP is the most common bleeding disorder in children. The cause of ITP is unknown but it usually follows a viral infection (Panepinto & Brousseau, 2005).

Symptoms include multiple ecchymoses and petechiae, and mucosal bleeding in the mouth or nose. Diagnosis is made by history and through physical and laboratory findings, which show a decreased platelet count (less than 20,000 mm^3/dL). The child has normal hemoglobin and white blood cell counts. If the presentation is atypical, further laboratory testing involves a bone marrow aspiration to rule out other diagnoses (Buchanan, 2005).

Modalities of treatment vary among healthcare providers and may include corticosteroids, intravenous immune globulin (IVIG) and anti-Rh (D) immune globulin (Wang, Wiley, Luddy, et al., 2005). Platelet administration is not usually indicated unless intracranial hemorrhaging occurs since the administered platelets will be destroyed. Sixty to 80% of patients with ITP will recover completely; however, others will develop chronic disease (Wang et al., 2005). For children who do not respond to drug therapy over a period of 6 months to 1 year, splenectomy may be the treatment of choice since the platelets are destroyed in the spleen.

Nursing Management

Nursing care focuses on controlling and reducing the number of bleeding episodes. Preventive measures are similar to those for the child with hemophilia. Teach parents to use acetaminophen, rather than aspirin, to control pain. Provide emotional support to the family. Have the child avoid contact sports. Perform careful assessments of bleeding and take vital signs. Expected outcomes of care are prevention of bleeding and restoration of normal coagulation patterns.

MENINGOCOCCEMIA

Meningococcemia is a virulent disease process that develops in some individuals infected with the *Neisseria meningitidis. N. meningitidis* is a gram-negative bacteria that is transmitted primarily via the respiratory route (Woods, 2007). Onset is sudden. Often, a respiratory infection is followed by fever, myalgias, weakness, headache, diarrhea, and vomiting. The petechial rash, characteristic of this disease may develop before other serious symptoms and progresses rapidly (Milonovich, 2007; Woods, 2007). The child's condition may deteriorate rapidly within a period of a few hours. The clotting cascade is initiated, resulting in bleeding and thrombosis in the tissues (Milonovich, 2007). The child is critically ill and demonstrates multisystem disease. Frequently the skin is pink and then black as the tissues are damaged from reduced oxygen delivery.

Treatment consists of antibiotics, removal from sources of infection, and multisystem shock management (refer to Chapter 49∞ for a description of distributive shock). Prompt administration of antibiotics to the child who manifests fever with purpura can decrease the severity of outcome. Depending on the child's condition, total parenteral nutrition, sedation and pain relief, dialysis, or amputation may be required. Close contacts of the child should receive prophylactic antibiotics.

Nursing Management

Nursing care of the child with meningococcemia is complex. Treatment must begin quickly and the child generally has a lengthy hospitalization in a pediatric intensive care unit followed by years of care that may involve plastic surgery or prosthetic adaptation. Thorough assessments of all body systems are performed. Ongoing assessment of vital signs is essential.

Administer intravenous infusions when ordered to ensure correct and timely administration of antibiotics and other therapies. Measure urinary output to evaluate kidney function. Meticulous skin care is necessary to preserve the integrity of tissues. Take care to prevent further infections. Nutritional support in the form of total parenteral nutrition is common. The family needs support to deal with the changing critical nature of the child's illness and the possibility that death or permanent, severe deformities will result. When the child improves, continuing comprehensive care in the hospital and then in the community is needed to manage complex issues related to growth, development, nutrition, amputations, and prosthetics. Expected outcomes of nursing care include prevention of further infection, maintenance of body systems during acute phase of illness, and positive adjustment to amputations and deformities resulting from the disease.

HEMATOPOIETIC STEM CELL TRANSPLANTATION (HSCT)

MyNursingKit Hematopoietic Stem Cell Transplantation

Hematopoietic stem cell transplantation is a treatment used for diseases such as severe combined immunodeficiency disease, severe and unresponsive aplastic anemia, and leukemia (refer to Chapters 50 and 52∞). Sources of stem cells include bone marrow, peripheral blood, and cord blood. Hematopoietic stem cells exist primarily in the bone marrow but also circulate in the peripheral blood. These cells can grow into new body cells, and have become useful in treatment of immune and hematologic diseases when restoration of normal cells is needed (Trigg, 2004).

Hematopoietic stem cell transplants are either autologous, or allogenic. In **autologous transplantation**, the child's own marrow is taken, treated, stored, and reinfused after the child has received chemotherapy. **Allogeneic transplantation** may be syngeneic (from an identical twin), related, or unrelated. In allogeneic transplantation, the donor, often a sibling (related), has a compatible human leukocyte antigen (HLA). Human leukocyte antigens are proteins found on the surface of nearly all nucleated cells within the body, and they are responsible for regulating the immune response. When no relative is found to match the child, a histocompatible donor (unrelated) may be sought from the National Marrow Donor Program or a cord blood bank (Moore, 2005). With the development of this registry, bone marrow transplantation from HLA-matched unrelated donors has become possible for some children

The transplantation procedure begins with chemotherapy and, sometimes, total body irradiation directed at destroying circulating blood cells and the diseased bone marrow in the ill child. Following this treatment, the child is transfused with the donor stem cells. If the transplantation is successful, the cells implant themselves in the bone and begin to grow. Healthy bone marrow, capable of making blood cells, is the result.

The chemotherapy program for destruction of bone marrow takes 4 to 12 days. During this time, the child is cared for in strict isolation in a special unit that provides a germ-free environment (Figure 51–5 ●). Side effects of chemotherapy provide challenges for care in addition to those of preventing infection (see Chapter 52∞). The child is without any immunity for a minimum of 10 days after transplantation. It takes 2 to 4 weeks for the donor cells to begin proliferation and maturation. Medications to stimulate the production of red and white blood cells are administered during this period.

Pancytopenia (marked decrease in RBCs, WBCs, and platelets) lasts for several weeks following the transplant. Major risks during this period are anemia, infections, and bleeding. Once the bone marrow begins to produce new cells, graft-versus-host disease (rejection) is the major threat. Refer to Chapter 50∞ for a discussion of graft-versus-host disease.

Monitor the child undergoing HSCT by assessing the skin, mucous membranes, gastrointestinal function, respiratory function, cardiac function, and hydration status. Because graft-versus-host disease may occur at any time, even after the child returns home, frequent thorough assessments are necessary after discharge.

Supportive care after the transplantation procedure focuses on preventing infection, controlling bleeding, maintaining a nutritious diet and hydration, monitoring for signs of rejection, and providing psychosocial support. The treatment is lengthy, the child is often critically ill, and parents may have traveled to a medical center many miles from home for the procedure. Ask parents about other family members and how they are managing. Provide information about inexpensive housing available near the medical center. Encourage parents to discuss their feelings with other parents of children receiving bone marrow transplantation. Organizations such as the Bone Marrow Transplant Family Support Network can serve as resources for families.

When the child is ready for discharge, be sure the family is prepared to administer medications, recognize signs of graft-versus-host disease, provide adequate nutrition for the child, and perform other necessary care. Arrange for follow-up visits and provide the names of local healthcare contact people who can offer support and provide information. The child may need tutors or other educational assistance to promote integration back into the school setting. The major expected outcome of nursing care is the proper activity of bone marrow in the child with resulting normal levels and function of blood cells. Other outcomes are provision of family support, ongoing care and education for the child, adequate nutrition, and prevention of infection. See "Health Promotion: The Child with Hematopoietic Stem Cell Transplantation (HSCT)."

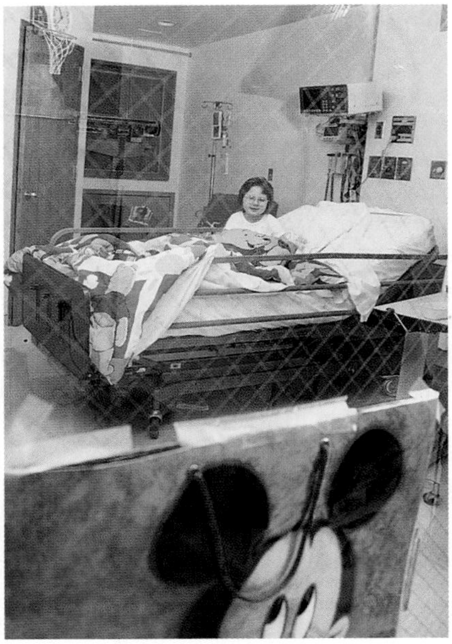

● **Figure 51–5** Bone marrow transplantation. The child undergoing bone marrow transplantation is hospitalized in a special unit while receiving chemotherapy before the transfusion. The child remains in the unit for several weeks afterward until the new marrow produces enough cells to maintain immunity.

HEALTH PROMOTION

THE CHILD WITH HEMATOPOIETIC STEM CELL TRANSPLANTATION (HSCT)

Growth and Development

- Measure and plot height and weight at each visit using standard growth curve charts.
- Measure onset and progression of puberty using Tanner staging.
- An individualized education plan (IEP) should be performed yearly to identify learning problems.
- Routine hearing screening is advised since hearing loss may occur as a result of ototoxic drug therapy.
- Vision should be screened at each primary care visit since corticosteroid use can cause cataracts, Graft versus host disease (GVHD) can result in keratoconjunctivitis, and cytomegalovirus (CMV) can cause retinitis.
- Blood pressure should be monitored each visit since children are commonly placed on medication for hypertension after HSCT because of nephrotoxic medications.
- Instruct parents to measure and record blood pressure at home if necessary.

Nutrition

- Teach family to avoid foods with potential vectors for infection, such as unpasteurized products and undercooked meats.
- A low-sodium diet may be required if the child has hypertension.
- Calcium supplements may be administered to reduce the risk of osteopenia.

Physical Activity

- If the child has thrombocytopenia, physical activity may be restricted.
- The child may experience fatigue. Ask about activity tolerance.

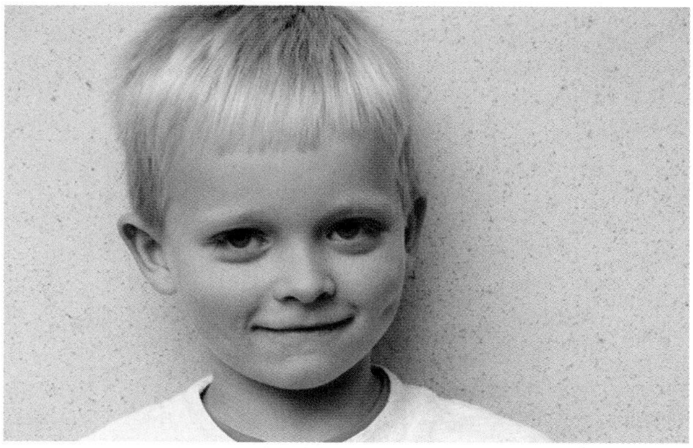

Oral Health

- Dental screening and any required restorative care should be done before transplant to reduce potential sources of infection.
- Routine dental care is resumed once the child's immune system is restored. Ask the family about the child's routine dental care.

Mental and Spiritual Health

- Apply developmental approaches to assess the child's feelings after a HSCT.
- Ask the child about coping with being in the hospital and at home rather than attending school.
- Many physical changes occur with treatment that may interfere with body image. Assess the child's or adolescent's body image in a manner appropriate to age.

Relationships

- In-hospital or in-home schooling is required after HSCT for 6 to 12 months until immune function has been obtained to reduce the risk of infection.
- Encourage peer contact, telephone calls, e-mail, and letters to reduce the child's feelings of isolation.
- On returning to school, the child is encouraged to participate fully in school activities.
- For the adolescent, sex education is important, especially to avoid sexually transmitted infections.

Disease Prevention Strategies

- Teach the family that hand hygiene is essential to prevent the spread of infection.
- Dishes should be washed in a dishwasher. Teach safe food preparation techniques.
- In-home child care is recommended because of the risk of infection in other childcare settings.
- Teach the family that the child should have minimal direct contact with animals to avoid infections.
- Determine the child's need for an altered immunization schedule after HSTC.
- Encourage the family to obtain an influenza vaccine annually for the child and all household or close contacts.
- Teach signs and symptoms of infection and stress the importance of prompt reporting.

Injury Prevention Strategies

- Review safe medication storage with the family.
- Help the family develop a plan for the safe disposal of used needles and syringes.

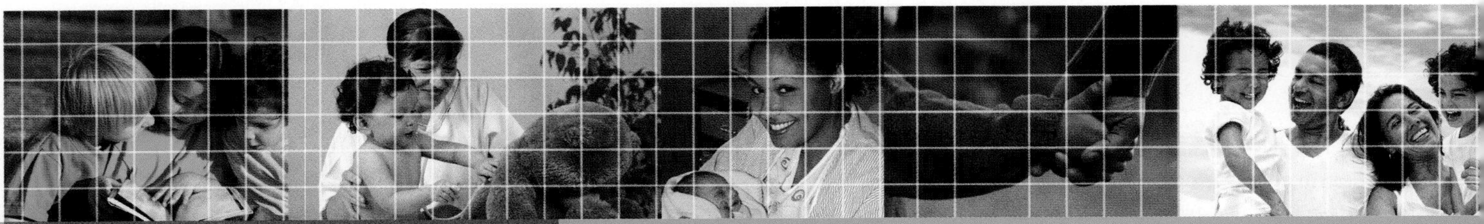

CRITICAL CONCEPT REVIEW

LEARNING OUTCOMES / CONCEPTS

51.1 Describe the function of red blood cells, white blood cells, and platelets.

1. Red blood cells:
   - Transport oxygen from the lungs to the tissues.
   - Transport carbon dioxide back to the lungs.
2. White blood cells:
   - Protect the body against bacterial invaders.
3. Platelets:
   - Form hemostatic plugs to stop bleeding.

51.2 Discuss the pathophysiology and clinical manifestations of the major disorders of red blood cells affecting the pediatric population.

Iron deficiency anemia:

1. Pathophysiology:
   - Lower than average number of red blood cells caused by blood loss, insufficient oral intake of iron, and increased internal demands due to rapid growth.
2. Clinical manifestations:
   - Pallor.
   - Fatigue.
   - Irritability.

Normocytic anemia:

1. Pathophysiology:
   - Increase in the destruction of red blood cells or decreased production of red blood cells.
   - Occurs because of hemorrhage, disease-induced inflammation, DIC, G6PD deficiency, and hemolytic uremic syndrome.
2. Clinical manifestations:
   - Same as iron deficiency anemia.
   - Hepatomegaly and splenomegaly.

Sickle cell anemia:

1. Pathophysiology:
   - Some or all normal hemoglobin is replaced with sickle-shaped cells.
   - Sickle shape is rigid, fragile, and breaks down faster.
   - Rigidity of cells causes clumping and obstruction of capillary blood flow.
2. Clinical manifestations:
   - Pain.
   - Splenic sequestration.
   - Febrile illnesses.
   - Tissue destruction.
   - Anemia.
   - Vaso-occlusive crisis.

Thalassemias:

1. Pathophysiology:
   - Production of beta chain of hemoglobin is impaired.
   - Red blood cells are fragile and have a decreased life span.
   - Increased hemolysis leads to hemosiderin and hemochromatosis.
2. Clinical manifestations:
   - Pallor.
   - Failure to thrive in the infant.
   - Hepatosplenomegaly.
   - Severe anemia.

LEARNING OUTCOMES	CONCEPTS
51.3 Discuss the pathophysiology and clinical manifestations of selected disorders of white blood cells affecting the pediatric population.	Aplastic anemia: 1. Pathophysiology: ■ Failure of the bone marrow stem cells to produce all types of blood cells. 2. Clinical manifestations: ■ Anemia. ■ Neutropenia. ■ Infection. ■ Thrombocytopenia. ■ Fever. ■ Fatigue. ■ Congestive heart failure. ■ Tachycardia.
51.4 Discuss the pathophysiology and clinical manifestations of the major bleeding disorders affecting the pediatric population.	Hemophilia: 1. Pathophysiology: ■ A group of genetic disorders that occurs primarily in males and causes a deficiency of specific clotting factors. 2. Clinical manifestations: ■ Mild to severe bleeding tendencies. ■ Bleeding usually occurs from minor trauma. ■ Hemarthrosis frequently occurs. von Willebrand disease: 1. Pathophysiology: ■ A genetic bleeding disorder that occurs in both men and women, and results in a deficiency of the plasma protein that carries clotting factor VIII. 2. Clinical manifestations: ■ Frequent bruising (ecchymosis). ■ Epistaxis. ■ Increased bleeding with surgery, lacerations, and dental extractions. ■ Teenage girls have increased menstrual bleeding. Disseminated intravascular coagulation: 1. Pathophysiology: ■ An acquired, abnormal activation of the clotting system resulting in widespread clot formation throughout the body. ■ Results from excessive thrombin formation caused by severe physiologic stress to the body. 2. Clinical manifestations: ■ Diffuse bleeding and oozing. ■ Shock. ■ Hypotension. ■ Impaired tissue perfusion. Idiopathic thrombocytopenia purpura: 1. Pathophysiology: ■ Increased destruction of platelets in the spleen with normal platelet production. ■ Usually follows a viral illness. 2. Clinical manifestations: ■ Multiple ecchymoses. ■ Petechiae. ■ Bleeding from gums. ■ Epistaxis. ■ Blood in urine and stool.
51.5 Describe the nursing management and collaborative care of a child with a hematologic disorder.	1. Prepare child for frequent blood tests. 2. Monitor child for transfusion reactions. 3. Prevent infection: ■ Perform frequent handwashing. ■ Limit child's contact with anyone with signs and symptoms of infection. 4. Provide for periods of rest. 5. Encourage intake of foods high in iron content. 6. Limit invasive procedures to prevent bleeding. 7. Teach family and/or child to avoid the use of aspirin products.

(continued)

LEARNING OUTCOMES — CONCEPTS

51.6 Discuss nursing implications for a child receiving hematopoietic stem cell transplantation (HSCT).

1. Prevent infection:
   - Child may be placed in protective isolation.
   - Avoid fresh fruit and flowers.
2. Control bleeding:
   - Limit invasive procedures.
   - No intramuscular injections or rectal temperature assessment.
   - Maintain pressure on any injection site for at least five minutes.
   - Transfuse with red blood cells or platelets as needed.
3. Maintain adequate nutrients and hydration:
   - Implement total parenteral nutrition (TPN) as needed.
   - Provide frequent, small meals.
4. Monitor for signs of rejection:
   - Assess temperature frequently.
   - Assess skin and GI system for signs and symptoms for graft-versus-host disease (GVHD).
5. Provide emotional support to the child and family.

CRITICAL THINKING IN ACTION

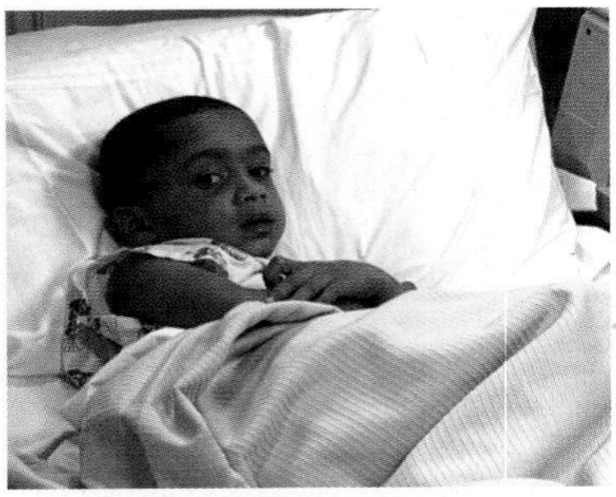

Frederick is admitted to the hospital with severe abdominal pain. He has been hospitalized for his sickle cell anemia several times in the past and now, as an 8-year-old, he and his mother are very familiar with the routine. The disease is stable most of the time, but about twice annually he is admitted to the hospital for complications of the disorder. His mother expresses how upsetting it is to watch her son suffering pain from this disease.

In the hospital a priority of nursing intervention is to control Frederick's pain. The doctor diagnoses that the abdominal pain is caused by sickled cells in his spleen. Frederick's hemoglobin is 6 g/dL, so a blood transfusion is ordered. Fluids and oxygen are also administered. Frequent vital signs and other monitoring are performed to identify any infections.

1. Besides correcting the anemia, what is another reason Frederick would be given a transfusion?
2. How would you explain what is happening to Frederick's spleen so that it is causing the abdominal pain?
3. In what way does sickle cell anemia affect the various systems of the body?
4. When giving a blood transfusion to Frederick, should warm or cold blood be given? What is the reason for your answer?

See MyNursingKit for possible responses.

REFERENCES

American Sickle Cell Anemia Association. (2005). *How common is sickle cell anemia?* Retrieved September 1, 2007 from www.ascaa.org/comm.htm

Anderson, N. (2006). Hydroxyurea therapy: Improving the lives of patients with sickle cell disease. *Pediatric Nursing, 32*(6), 541–543.

Beyer, J. E., & Simmons, L. E. (2004). Home treatment of pain for children and adolescents with sickle cell disease. *Pain Management Nursing, 5*, 126–135.

Borgna-Pignatti, C., & Marsella, M. (2008). Iron deficiency in infancy and childhood. *Pediatric Annals, 37*(5), 329–337.

Boxer, L. A. (2007). Leukopenia. In R. M. Kliegman, R. E. Behrman, H. B. Jenson, & B. F. Stanton (Eds.), *Nelson textbook of pediatrics* (18th ed., pp. 909–915). Philadelphia: Saunders Elsevier.

Bryant, R. (2005). Asthma in the pediatric sickle cell patient with acute chest syndrome. *Journal of Pediatric Health Care, 19*, 157–162.

Buchanan, G. R. (2005). Thrombocytopenia during childhood: What the pediatrician needs to know. *Pediatrics in Review, 26*, 401–409.

Cappellini, M. C., Bejaoui, M., Agaoglu, L., Porter, J., Coates, T., Jeng M., et al. (2007). Prospective evaluation of patient-reported outcomes during treatment with deferasirox or deferoxamine for iron overload in patients with β-thalassemia. *Clinical Therapeutics, 29*(5), 909–917.

Chamley, C., Carson, P., Randall, D., & Sandwell, W. (2005). *Developmental anatomy and physiology of children*. St Louis: Elsevier.

Committee on Nutrition, American Academy of Pediatrics. (2004). *Pediatric nutrition handbook* (5th ed.). Elk Grove Village, IL: American Academy of Pediatrics.

Corbeel, L. (2005). Immune-mediated aplastic anemia. *European Journal of Pediatrics 164*, 698–699.

Coyer, S. M. (2005). Anemia: Diagnosis and management. *Journal of Pediatric Health Care, 19*(6), 380–385.

Curry, Heather. (2004). Bleeding disorder basics. *Pediatric Nursing, 30*, 402–429.

Day, S. (2004). Development and evaluation of a sickle cell disease assessment instrument. *Pediatric Nursing, 30*(6), 451–458.

DeBaun, M. R., & Vichinsky, E. (2007). Hemoglobinopathies. In R. M. Kliegman, R. E. Behrman, H. B. Jenson, & B. F. Stanton (Eds.), *Nelson textbook of pediatrics* (18th ed., pp. 2025–2038). Philadelphia: Saunders Elsevier.

Driscoll, M. C. (2007). Sickle Cell Disease. *Pediatrics in Review, 28*(7), 259–268.

Freedman, M. H. (2007). The pancytopenias. In R. M. Kliegman, R. E. Behrman, H. B. Jenson, & B. F. Stanton (Eds.), *Nelson textbook of pediatrics* (18th ed., pp. 2047–2053). Philadelphia: Saunders Elsevier.

Hay, W. W., Levin, M. J., Sondheimer, J. M., Deterding, R. R., and Associate Authors (2005). *Current pediatric diagnosis and treatment* (17th ed.), New York: Lange Medical Books/McGraw Hill.

Inati, A., Koussa, S., Taher, A., & Perrine, S. (2008). Sickle Cell Disease: New insights into pathophysiology and treatment. *Pediatric Annals, 37*(5), 311–321

Ioli, J., & Gilday, M. (2004, September). Sickle cell signs. *Advance for nurses,* 39–41.

Jacob, E., Miaskowski, C., Savedra, M., Beyer, J. E., Treadwell, M., & Styles, L. (2003). Management of vaso-occlusive pain in children with sickle cell disease. *Journal of Pediatric Hematology/Oncology, 25,* 307–311.

Jacob, E., Miaskowski, C., Savedra, M., Beyer, J. E., Treadwell, M., & Styles, L. (2005). Trends in complete blood count values during acute painful episodes in children with sickle cell disease. *Journal of Pediatric Oncology Nursing, 22*(3), 152–159.

Jacob, E., Miaskowski, C., Savedra, M., Beyer, J. E., Treadwell, M., & Styles, L. (2006). Changes in sleep, food intake, and activity levels during acute painful episodes in children with sickle cell disease. *Journal of Pediatric Nursing, 21*(1), 23–34.

Kral, M. C., Brown, R. T., Connelly, M., Cure, J. K., Besenski, N., Jackson, S. M., & Abboud, M. R. (2006). Radiographic predictors of neurocognitive functioning in pediatric sickle cell disease. *Journal of Child Neurology, 21,* 37–44.

Kumar, V., Abbas, A. K., Fausto, N., Aster, J. C. (2010). Red blood cell and bleeding disorders. In V. Kumar, A. K. Abbas, N. Fausto, & J. C. Aster. Robbins and Cotran Pathologic Basis of Disease (8th ed.). St Louis: Saunders.

LeMone, P., & Burke, K. M. (2008). Nursing care of clients with hematologic disorders. In P. LeMone & K. Burke (Eds.), *Medical surgical nursing: Critical thinking in client care* (4th ed.). Upper Saddle River, NJ: Prentice Hall.

Lindsey, T., Watts-Tate, N., Southwood, E., Routhieaux, J., Beatty, J., Calamaras, D., et al (2005). Chronic blood transfusion therapy practices to treat strokes in children with sickle cell disease. *Journal of the American Academy of Nurse Practitioners, 17,* 277–282.

Manco-Johnson, M. J., Abshire, T. C., Shapiro, A. D., Riske, B., Hacker, M. R., Kilcoyne, R., et al. (2007). Episodic Treatment to Prevent Joint Disease in Boys with Severe Hemophilia, *The New England Journal of Medicine*, 357 (6), 535–544.

Manno, C. S., & Larson, P. J. (2005). Transfusion therapy for coagulation factor deficiencies. In R. Hoffman, E. J. Benz, S. J. Shattil, B. Furie, H. J. Cohen, L. E. Silberstein, & P. McGlave (Eds.), *Hematology: Basic principles and practice* (4th ed. pp. 2469–2480). St. Louis: Elsevier

Mehta, S. R., Afenyi-Annan, A., Byrns, P. F., & Lottenberg, R. (2006). Opportunities to improve outcomes in sickle cell disease. *American Family Physician, 74*(2), 303–310.

Miller, K. L. (2004). Factor products in the treatment of hemophilia. *Journal of Pediatric Health Care*, 18, 156–157.

Milonovich, L. M. (2007). Meningococcemia: Epidemiology, pathophysiology, and management. *Journal of Pediatric Health Care, 21*(2), 75–80.

Moore, T. (2005). *Bone marrow transplantation.* Retrieved September 10, 2007 from *www.emedicine.com/ped/topic2909.htm*

Ohls, R. K., & Christensen, R. D. (2007). Development of the hematopoietic system. In R. M. Kliegman, R. E. Behrman, H. B. Jenson, & B. F. Stanton (Eds.), *Nelson textbook of pediatrics* (18th ed., pp. 1997–2003). Philadelphia: Saunders Elsevier.

Panepinto, J. A., & Brousseau, D. C. (2005). Acute idiopathic thrombocytopenic purpura of childhood—Diagnosis and therapy. *Pediatric Emergency Care, 21,* 691–695.

Pesce, M. A. (2007). Reference ranges for laboratory tests and procedures. In R. M. Kliegman, R. E. Behrman, H. B. Jenson, & B. F. Stanton, *Nelson textbook of pediatrics* (18th ed., pp. 2943–2949). Philadelphia: Elsevier Saunders.

Piga, A., Galanello, R., Forni, G. L., Cappellini, M. D., Origa, R., Zappu, A., et al. (2006). Randomized phase II trial of deferasirox (Exjade, ICL670), a once-daily, orally-administered iron chelator, in comparison to deferoxamine in thalassemia patients with transfusional iron overload. *Haematologica, 91,* 873–880.

Platt, A. F., & Eckman, J. (2006, February). Relieving the symptoms of sickle cell disease. *The Clinical Advisor, 54,* 59–62, 67.

Polin, R. A., Fox, W. W., & Abman, S. H. (2004). *Fetal and neonatal physiology* (3rd ed.). Philadelphia: Saunders.

Quinn, C. T., Rogers, Z. R., & Buchanan, G. R. (2004). Survival of children with sickle cell disease. *Blood, 103*(11), 4023–4027.

Revel-Vilk, S., Golomb, M. R., Achonu, C., Stain, A. M., Armstrong, D., Barnes, M. A., et al. (2004). Effect of intracranial bleeds on the health and quality of life of boys with hemophilia. *The Journal of Pediatrics,* 144, 490–495.

Richardson, M. (2007). Microcytic Anemia. *Pediatrics in Review, 28*(1), 5–14.

Saunthararajah, Y., Vichinsky, E. P., Embury, S. H. (2005). Sickle cell disease. In R. Hoffman, E. J. Benz, S. J. Shattil, B. Furie, H. J. Cohen, L. E. Silberstein, & P. McGlave (Eds.), *Hematology: Basic principles and practice* (4th ed., pp. 605–644). St. Louis: Elsevier

Scott, J. P., & Montgomery, R. R. (2007). Hemorrhagic and thrombotic diseases. In R. M. Kliegman, R. E. Behrman, H. B. Jenson, & B. F. Stanton (Eds.), *Nelson textbook of pediatrics* (18th ed., pp. 2060–2089). Philadelphia: Elsevier Saunders.

Trigg, M. E. (2004). Hematopoietic stem cells. *Pediatrics, 13,* 1051–1057.

Wang, W. (2007). Central nervous system complications sickle cell disease in children: An overview. *Child Neuropsychology, 13,* 103–119.

Wang, J., Wiley, J. M., Luddy, R., Greenberg, J., Feuerstein, M., & Bussel, J. B. (2005). Chronic immune thrombocytopenic purpura in children: assessment of Rituximab treatment. *The Journal of Pediatrics, 146,* 217–221.

Warrington, K. H., & Herzog, R. W. (2006). Treatment of human disease by adeno-associated viral gene transfer. *Human Genetics, 119*(6), 571–603.

Woods, C. R. (2007). Neisseria meningitidis. In R. M. Kliegman, R. E. Behrman, H. B. Jenson, & B. F. Stanton (Eds.), *Nelson textbook of pediatrics* (18th ed., pp. 1164–1169). Philadelphia: Saunders Elsevier.

Young, N. S., Calado, R. T., & Scheinberg, P. (2006). Current concepts in pathophysiology and treatment of aplastic anemia. *Blood, 108*(8), 2509–2519.

PEARSON

EXPLORE mynursingkit™

MyNursingKit is your one stop for online chapter review materials and resources. Prepare for success with additional NCLEX®-style practice questions, interactive assignments and activities, web links, animations and videos, and more!

Register your access code from the front of your book at **www.mynursingkit.com**

CHAPTER 52

The Child with Cancer

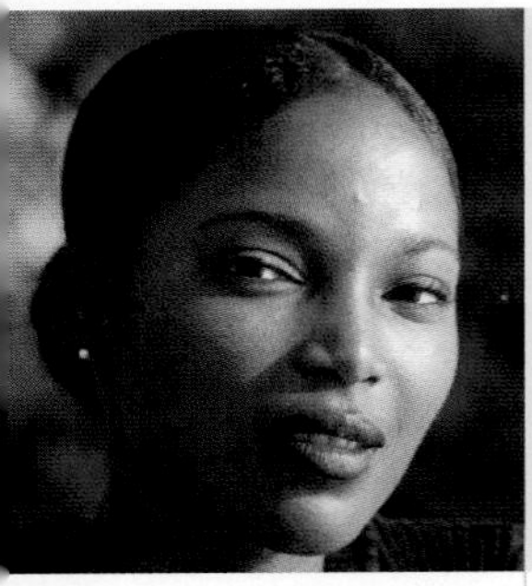

Rasheed was just diagnosed with leukemia seven months ago, but already he has been in the hospital five times. This time he had enterocolitis, an infection of the intestines. But he has now improved and is determined to fight the disease. It is his will and strength that help us all to be strong and to know that he will do well after his treatment is finished. —Mother of Rasheed, 12 years old

LEARNING OUTCOMES

52.1 Describe the incidence, known etiologies, and common clinical manifestations of cancer.

52.2 Synthesize information about diagnostic tests and clinical therapy for cancer to plan comprehensive care for children undergoing these procedures.

52.3 Integrate information about oncologic emergencies into plans for monitoring all children with cancer.

52.4 Recognize the most common solid tumors in children, describe their treatment, and plan comprehensive nursing care.

52.5 Plan care for children and adolescents of all ages who have a diagnosis of leukemia.

52.6 Recognize the most common soft-tissue tumors in children, describe their treatment, and plan comprehensive care.

52.7 Describe the impact of cancer survival on children and use this information to plan for ongoing physiologic and psychosocial care in the children's futures.

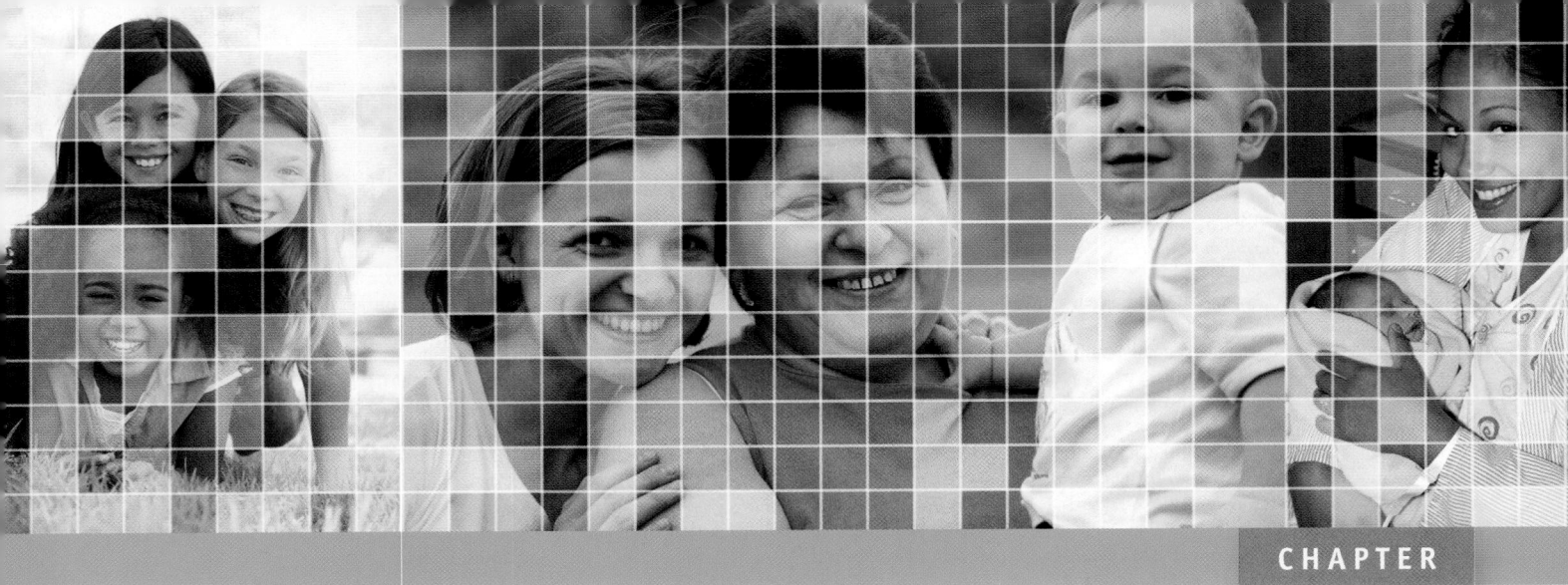

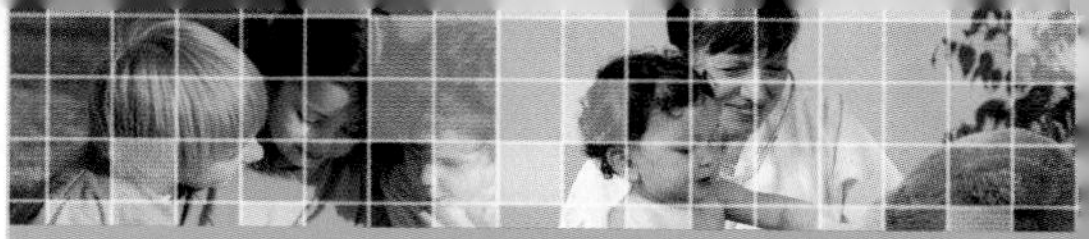

KEY TERMS

Apoptosis, 1465
Benign, 1465
Biotherapy, 1470
Carcinogens, 1467
Chemotherapy, 1470
Complementary therapy, 1475
Extravasation, 1482
Intrathecal, 1470
Leukocytosis, 1496
Leukopenia, 1496
Malignant, 1465
Metastasis, 1465
Myelosuppression, 1482
Nadir, 1477
Neoplasms, 1465
Neutropenia, 1482
Oncogene, 1467
Pancytopenia, 1496
Polypharmacy, 1482
Protocol, 1470
Proto-oncogene, 1467
Radiation, 1473
Secondary cancers, 1481
Thrombocytopenia, 1502
Tumor suppressor genes, 1467

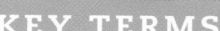

MyNursingKit Video: Cancer Overview

Cancer is a daunting diagnosis at any age, but in children it seems even more profound. The diagnosis and treatment are met with shock and disbelief, they require a change in the roles of everyone in the family, and challenge all children and families involved in many ways. Nurses who work in pediatric oncology have unique opportunities to assist children and families in mobilizing resources and learning about maximizing physical, emotional, and developmental health while dealing with the challenges of the illness and treatment.

Why do children develop different types of cancers than adults? Cancers in children often have different etiology than those in adults. Most adult cancers are epithelial in origin, whereas in children, nonepithelial or embryonal cell types predominate (Twombly, 2007). While many adult cancers are slow-growing and result from exposure to carcinogens over time, most childhood cancers are fast-growing, and a child who appears healthy may suddenly appear ill over a period of days or weeks. Cancer in adults is often the result of dietary practices or habits such as smoking. Some adult-onset cancers are the result of oncogenic responses to stimuli—that is, responses that stimulate cancerous changes in cells. Other cancers that occur in adults result from prolonged exposure to toxins such as coal dust and asbestos. Some cancers are known to be related to genetic causes. In adults, prevention through general lifestyle changes is a major focus of interventions. However, in children, cancer is usually embryonic (occurring during development of the fetus) or oncogenic in origin. Thus, lifestyle changes that begin in childhood have little effect on the incidence of childhood cancer, although they may help reduce the incidence of later cancer or other diseases. Occasionally, an environmental exposure is linked to the incidence of cancer in children.

Abnormal cellular growth can occur in any area of the body. Why are some growths called cancer and others not? Changes in cellular growth within the body are called **neoplasms** (meaning new growth). A neoplasm is further classified as benign or malignant. **Benign** means that a growth does not endanger life or health; it tends not to recur after treatment. **Malignant** means that if not treated a tumor will continue to grow, and will spread to other sites in the body (**metastasis**), ending in death. The common term for this type of cellular growth is cancer.

ANATOMY AND PHYSIOLOGY OF PEDIATRIC DIFFERENCES

The major physiologic difference between adults and children that affects cellular growth involves the immune system and how well it defends the body. The rate of cell growth in children also can play a role in the rapid progression of some childhood cancers. The continuing presence of fetal cells in small children is related to some cancers.

The immune system defends the body against foreign organisms and substances through two responses: nonspecific and specific. In a nonspecific response, the components of the immune system attack a variety of targets. Nonspecific components include phagocytic (cell-destroying) cells such as mononuclear leukocytes, polymorphonuclear (PMN) leukocytes, natural killer (NK) cells, and complements (noncellular proteins) that work together to destroy invading cells and substances. During the first month of a child's life, the nonspecific response is immature, so phagocytic cells have little ability to move toward cancer cells and fulfill their function. The nonspecific response is also impaired in premature and small-for-gestational-age (SGA) infants.

In a specific response, T lymphocytes and various proteins called immunoglobulin (Ig) attack only one type of invader. The specific response capability also is immature in infants. B-cell production of immunoglobulins (IgM, IgG, and IgA) is below adult levels, so that the infant is vulnerable to bacterial and viral infections. (For a discussion of immune function, see Chapter 50∞.)

In children, many cells are growing quickly. This fast growth can lead to the proliferation of cancerous as well as normal cells. Cell division that is out of control may normally trigger a mechanism called **apoptosis**, whereby the cell "realizes" something is wrong and destroys itself. The process of apoptosis or physiologic cell death may not be well developed in young children.

CHILDHOOD CANCER

The care of children who have cancer is a challenging specialty in pediatric nursing. For several years the child undergoes aggressive treatments that may be life threatening and cause serious illness. Treatments for cancer have improved prognosis in many cases, but in some, the prognosis still requires that the family deal with a life-threatening illness (see Chapter 43∞). The child is often cared for at home with outpatient visits for treatment and occasional hospitalization when needed. The periods of hospitalization are times of intense physical vulnerability for the child and intense emotional vulnerability for both the child and the family. To monitor the child closely, nurses need a sound knowledge of physiologic and psychologic responses, medical interventions, and nursing care. Integration of developmental knowledge into assessment and intervention is essential. Effective communication skills are necessary to support the child and family and promote realistic hope. See the Nursing Management section and the Nursing Care Plan for specific interventions required.

INCIDENCE

In the United States, cancer is diagnosed in approximately 11,000 children under 15 years of age. In children under 15 years of age, cancer is the leading cause of disease-related death, and the fourth leading cause of overall death, following unintentional injury, homicide, and suicide (National Cancer Institute, 2008a; Pollack, Stewart, Thompson, et al., 2007). About 1500 U.S. children die from cancer annually; one-third of the deaths are from leukemia, with brain and other nervous system neoplasms as the next most common cause (American Cancer Society, 2006a). However, mortality rates have declined by more than 47% since 1975. The overall five-year survival rate is 80% for childhood cancer, and 75% for 10 years (National Cancer Institute, 2008a). Survival rates vary for different types of cancer, ranging from 66% for neuroblastoma to 95% for Hodgkin disease (American Cancer Society, 2006a; Pollack et al., 2007). Figure 52–1 ● shows the most common forms of childhood cancers among children in different age groups.

ETIOLOGY AND PATHOPHYSIOLOGY

Alterations in cellular growth occur in response to external and internal stimuli. Neoplasms are caused by one or any combination of three factors: (1) external stimuli that cause genetic mutations, (2) immune system and gene abnormalities, and (3) chromosomal abnormalities.

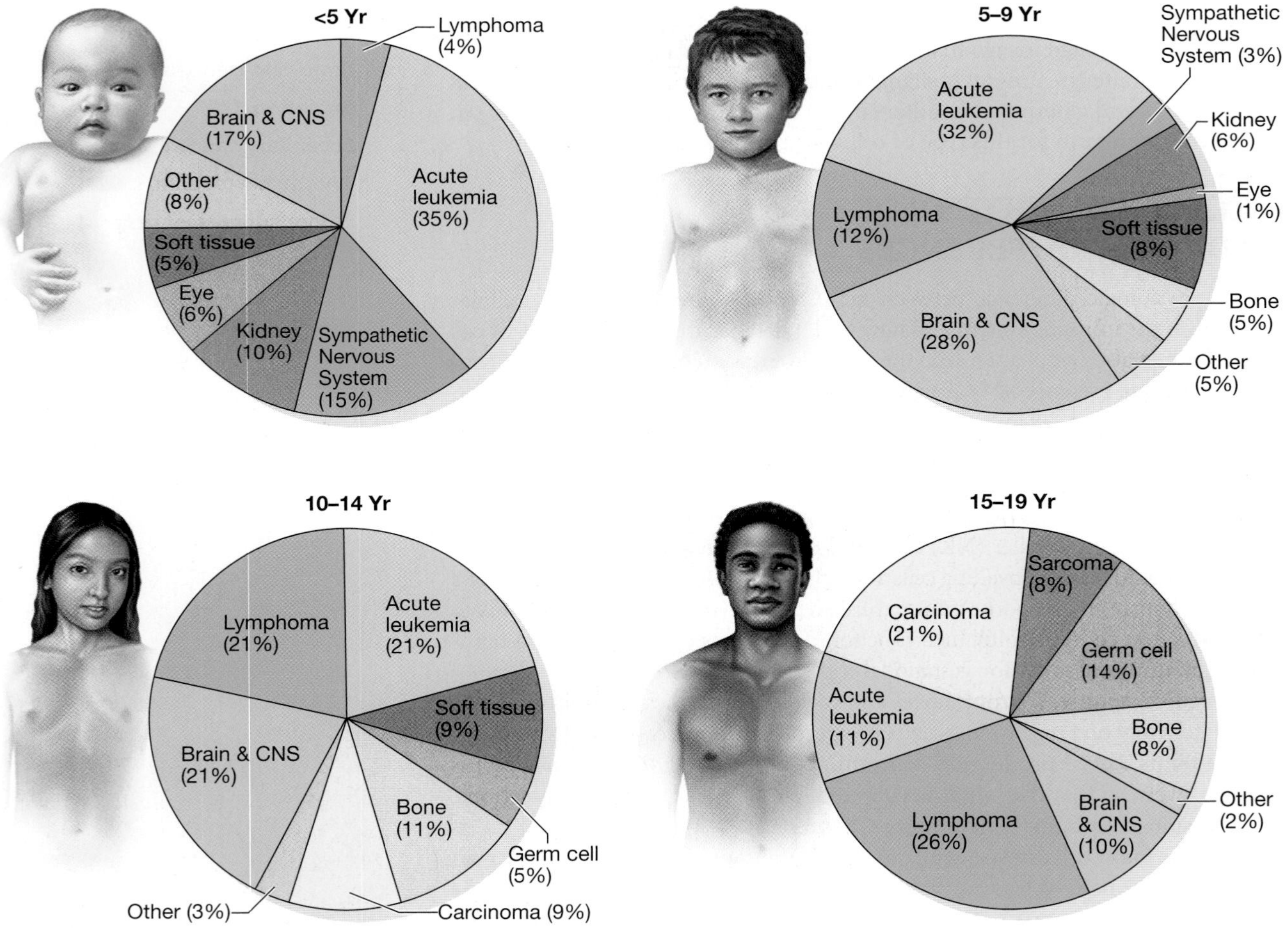

● **Figure 52–1** Percentage of primary tumors by site of origin for different age groups.

Data from Gurney, J. G., & Bondy, M. L. Cancer and benign tumors. In R. E. Behrman & H. B. Jenson (Eds.) (2007), *Nelson textbook of pediatrics* (18th ed., p. 1680). Philadelphia: Saunders.

External Stimuli

External stimuli may affect the child's general health and cause mutations in body cells. **Carcinogens** are chemicals or industrial processes that, when combined with genetic traits and in interaction with one another, result in cancer. Several carcinogens cause cancers that are diagnosed during childhood. Others cause cancers that begin in childhood but are not identified until adulthood. Some chemicals suspected of causing childhood cancer include diethylstilbestrol (maternal use of therapeutic estrogen hormones), anabolic androgenic steroids, alkylating chemotherapy agents, and immunosuppressants used for organ transplantation. Radiation exposure has been known to cause cancers such as leukemia and thyroid tumors in children exposed to nuclear fallout from atomic bombs, other nuclear accidents, and other excessive radiation sources.

External stimuli may also lead to secondary cancers in children, or those occurring after treatment for a primary cancer and of a different cellular type than the primary cancer. Secondary cancers can result when the child is treated for a primary cancer with high doses of radiation. Excessive exposure to ultraviolet radiation from the sun predisposes children to development of skin cancer in adolescence and adulthood (see Chapter 59).

Immune System and Gene Abnormalities

One critical function of a normal immune system is immune surveillance, in which phagocytic cells circulate throughout the body, detecting and destroying abnormal and cancerous cells. Children with congenital immune deficiencies, such as Wiskott–Aldrich syndrome, in which immune surveillance may fail, are at high risk for cancer. A form of non-Hodgkin lymphoma develops in some children treated with immune system–suppressing drugs. Children with acquired immunodeficiency syndrome (AIDS) may also be at higher risk of certain types of cancer, such as lymphoma, Kaposi sarcoma, and leiomyosarcoma (Stanescu, Foarfa, Georgescu, et al., 2007).

Viruses and other substances may alter the immune system, thereby allowing cancer to occur (see "Pathophysiology Illustrated: Proto-oncogene Alteration"). Their action is based on changing certain genes that normally regulate cellular growth and development (called **proto-oncogenes**) to related genes that allow unregulated cell division and cancerous growth (called **oncogenes**). Among the cancers thought to be linked to virus action and the change of proto-oncogenes to oncogenes are certain leukemias, rhabdomyosarcoma, Burkitt lymphoma, and some forms of Hodgkin disease.

Genetic changes can include autosomal dominant, autosomal recessive, and x-linked transfer. In these cases, the resulting cancers often occur relatively early in life. Cancers of these types are typically aggressive since the child has inherited the abnormal gene and it is within each cell, rather than a single mutation of one gene in a specific cell. Due to progress that is being made in the Human Genome Project, there is increasing ability to perform genetic testing for certain familial cancers. Examples of cancers that are sometimes caused by genetic abnormalities within families include retinoblastoma and Wilms' tumor (described later in this chapter), multiple endocrine neoplasia, type 2 (thyroid cancer), and familial adenomatous polyposis (invasive colon cancer). Not all cases of these cancers are familial, but their incidence suggests the need for careful history taking to identify any other cases in the family. Providing recommendations for referral to genetic counseling services and following up with further education and psychologic support are important nursing roles.

Tumor suppressor genes counteract the effect of oncogenes, keeping cellular growth within normal limits. When tumor suppressor genes are missing, unstemmed cellular growth can occur. These genes are commonly missing in children with retinoblastoma and Wilms' tumor.

Chromosomal Abnormalities

Normal chromosomes undergo change as a part of the genetic process. Most changes are not harmful. However, some result in chromosomal abnormalities such as hyperploidy (more than the normal number of chromosomes), deletion, translocation, and breakage.

Some chromosomal abnormalities have been linked to an increased incidence of cancer. Children with Down syndrome have a 20 to 30 times higher incidence of leukemia than nonaffected children (Ahga, Williams, Marrett, et al., 2005; Ross, Spector, Robison, et al., 2005). Children missing a band of genetic material on chromosome 13 often have retinoblastoma. Similarly, a Wilms' tumor often develops in children missing part of the genetic material from chromosome 11.

Teaching Highlights

WAYS TO DECREASE THE INCIDENCE OF CANCER IN CHILDREN

Many parents ask what they can do to decrease the incidence of cancer in children as they grow into adulthood. The three major teaching areas to address are:

Have children increase intake of fruits and vegetables. Most children do not eat enough of these foods (at least five servings/day are recommended), and increased intake is associated with lower rates of many cancers (Stan, Kar, Stoner, et al., 2008).

Protect skin with sunscreen. Early excessive exposure to sun and having one or repeated sunburns during childhood increase chances of skin cancers developing in adulthood (National Cancer Institute, 2007a).

Discourage smoking among children and be sure children are not exposed to environmental tobacco smoke. This will decrease the future chance of developing lung cancer.

When there is a history of cancer in the family, particularly if a type associated with familial incidence such as some breast or ovarian cancers, encourage the family to learn more about the cancer and teach the child to receive regular surveillance as they enter young adulthood.

Inform youth in all families about screening such as the Papanicolaou test, breast self-examination, and testicular examination that can lead to early detection. Encourage all females at age 9 years to receive the human papillomavirus, quadrivalent vaccine, recombinant (Gardasil) to prevent cervical cancers and other health problems caused by human papillomavirus (HPV). (See Chapter 45 for further information.)

PATHOPHYSIOLOGY ILLUSTRATED

PROTO-ONCOGENE ALTERATION

A proto-oncogene normally regulates cellular growth and development. When altered by a virus or other external cause, it can change to an oncogene, which allows unregulated genetic activity and tumor growth. Tumor-suppressor genes regulate the effects of oncogenes to decrease wildly proliferating cellular growth.

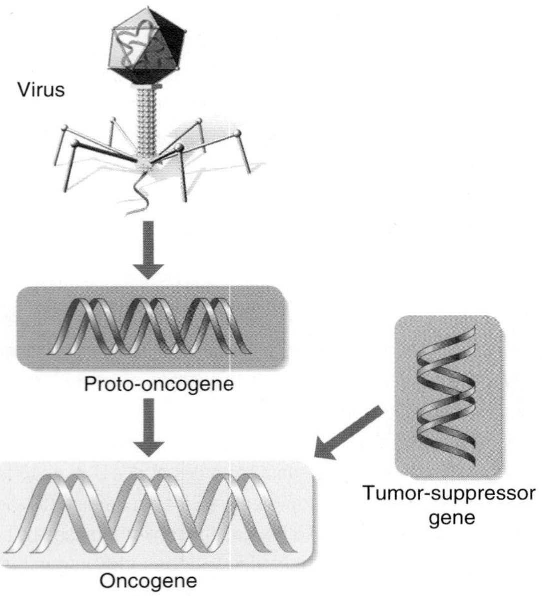

Regardless of the location and cause of abnormal cellular growth, the pathophysiologic process of cancer is similar. The altered cell begins to multiply as directed by the altered genetic structure of its DNA and the absence or inactivation of tumor suppressor genes. Each new cell transmits the new or altered pattern to the next generation. As the abnormal cells replicate, they form a growing neoplastic mass. Normal cells usually die as the increased metabolic rate of the neoplastic cells depletes available nutrition. The altered DNA in the tumor cells may also cause the abnormal cells to invade adjoining tissue. Through continued growth the mass expands until it enters and disrupts a major vessel or a vital organ.

CLINICAL MANIFESTATIONS

Each type of childhood cancer signals its presence differently. Because many of the presenting signs and symptoms of cancer are typical of common childhood illnesses, diagnosis may be delayed. In some cases, no symptoms are noted until the cancer is advanced. Some of the common presenting symptoms of cancer follow.

- *Pain* may be the result of a neoplasm either directly or indirectly affecting nerve receptors through obstruction, inflammation, tissue damage, stretching of visceral tissue, or invasion of susceptible tissue.
- *Cachexia* is a syndrome characterized by anorexia, weight loss, anemia, asthenia (weakness), and early satiety (feeling of being full).
- *Anemia* may be experienced during times of chronic bleeding or iron deficiency. In chronic illness the body uses iron poorly. Anemia is also present in cancers of the bone marrow when the number of red blood cells (RBCs) is reduced, in part because of the presence of large numbers of other bone marrow products. Treatment of cancer often promotes further anemia.
- *Infection* is usually a result of an altered or immature immune system. In addition, infection occurs when bone marrow cancers inhibit maturation of normal immune system cells. Infection may also occur in children treated with corticosteroids. Because their immune response is altered, the normal signs of infection may not appear.
- *Bruising* can occur if the bone marrow cannot produce enough platelets; bleeding after even minor trauma can lead to ecchymosis.
- *Neurologic symptoms* may result from impingement on the brain or nervous system. Signs of increased intracranial pressure, decreased or altered consciousness, eye abnormalities, or other neurologic or behavior changes may be evident.
- *Palpable mass* may be present for certain cancers. This is most commonly abdominal but may be mediastinal, in the neck, or at other sites.

A variety of other symptoms can occur depending on the location of the cancer. Subcutaneous nodules may appear if leukocytosis is present. Superior vena cava syndrome or respiratory difficulty can occur with mediastinal tumors (such as neuroblastoma), and enlarged lymph nodes are common with lymphomas (Hon, Leung, Chik, et al., 2005).

COLLABORATIVE CARE

Diagnostic Tests

The most common diagnostic tests performed on children with cancer are complete blood counts with differential, bone marrow aspiration (BMA) (Table 52–1), bone marrow biopsy (BMBX), lumbar puncture (LP), peripheral blood studies, radiographic examination, magnetic resonance imaging (MRI), computed tomography (CT; Figure 52–2 ●), ultrasound, and biopsy of tumor.

Additional studies helpful for certain cancers are nuclear medicine scans with radioactive isotopes such as gallium or iodine, bone scan with technetium 99m, or positron emission tomography (PET) and single photon emission computed tomography (SPECT) that combine nuclear medicine with CT (Yang, Kim, & Inoue, 2006). Specific tests such as pulmonary function tests and echocardiograms may be used in certain situations. Urine analysis is also performed.

The blood work is very detailed and includes RBC, WBC, platelets, hematocrit and hemoglobin, serum electrolytes, liver studies, and markers that are elevated in specific types of tumors. Absolute neutrophil count (ANC) is important; it uses both the

Table 52–1 Selected Diagnostic Tests for Childhood Cancer

Test	Purpose	Normal Laboratory Values	Diagnostic Values
Bone marrow aspiration	Examines bone marrow	Less than 5% blast cells (immature)	Greater than 25% blast cells in acute lymphoblastic leukemia, most with hypercellular marrow
Lumbar puncture	Examines cerebrospinal fluid	Cell count (microliters) Polymorphonuclear leukocytes 0 Monocytes 0–5 RBCs 0–5	Presence of malignant cells indicates central nervous system involvement
Complete blood count and differential	Examines cellular components of blood	WBC less than10,000/microLiter Platelets 150,000–400,000/microLiter Hemoglobin 12–16 g/dL	WBC greater than 10,000/microLiter Platelets 20,000–100,000/mL Hemoglobin 7–10 g/dL
Absolute Neutrophil Count (ANC)	Blood component ratio: % of segmental neutrophils times % of bands (immature neutrophils) times WBC count	ANC greater than 1000	ANC less than 500 = risk of infection

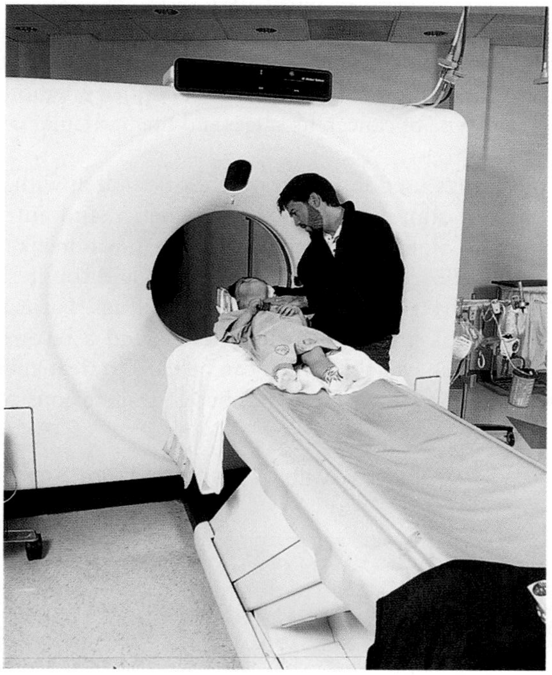

• **Figure 52–2** Computed tomography. CT can be a frightening procedure for children. This 2-year-old boy is comforted by his father before the procedure.

segmented (mature) and bands (immature neutrophils) as a measure of the body's infection-fighting capability. ANC is calculated by adding percent of segmented neutrophils to percent of bands, and then multiplying this percentage by the WBC count.

The tests are aimed at identifying the source of the cancer and any metastases to additional sites. This enables the oncology specialist to stage the cancer. Staging refers to the process of labeling the type of cancer cells, severity, and spread, which will determine the recommended treatment and assist in teaching the family about treatment and prognosis. Stage number 1 indicates less severe cancer without spread to other parts of the body, and higher numbers indicate both greater severity and spread to other sites.

Nursing Practice

Remove all jewelry and clothes with metal snaps from the child before an MRI scan. Ask about and remove body piercings; they may not always be visible. Some metallic objects implanted in the body are compatible with MRI but others contraindicate the use of MRI. Metallic objects include orthodontic braces, metal dental bridgework, cochlear implants, surgical clips or plates, and orthopedic rods. Ask about tattoos. When there are metal objects in the body on tattoos, be certain to report them to the managing health care provider and radiology technician so they can determine if MRI is safe.

Clinical Therapy

Clinical therapy for cancer is extremely complex and is managed by a specialist in pediatric oncology. Recommendations from the National Action Plan for Childhood Cancer include the following:

- Ensure that all children and adolescents suspected of having cancer are referred initially to a pediatric cancer center and have their care coordinated by the center.
- Establish national standards of quality care for children and adolescents with cancer, both medical and psychosocial, as defined by healthcare professionals and patient advocates.
- Quantify current patterns, quality, and outcomes of all phases of childhood and adolescent cancer care.
- Increase participation of children and adolescents in all phases of approved clinical trials (American Cancer Society, 2003).

Cancer itself has many effects on the body, such as altering nutrition and impeding circulation, all of which must be managed carefully. Cancer is treated with one or a combination of therapies: surgery, chemotherapy, radiation, **biotherapy**, and bone marrow transplantation. The choice of treatment is determined by the type of cancer, its location, and staging. Treatments all have side effects and these will also require clinical management. Many families also choose to use some type of complementary therapy, in addition to traditional medical approaches.

The goal of treatment may be curative, supportive, or provision of end-of-life care. Curative treatment rids the child's body of the cancer. Supportive treatment includes transfusions, pain management, antibiotics, and other interventions to assist the body's defenses and increase the child's comfort. End-of-life treatment is designed to make the child as comfortable as possible when no curative treatment is possible (see Chapter 43 for a detailed discussion of end-of-life care for children). Whatever combination of treatment is used, families have many questions and need resources for information.

Surgery. Surgery is used to remove or debulk (reduce the size of) a solid tumor. An example of a cancer that is commonly treated with surgery is a Wilms' tumor. Surgery may also determine the stage and type of cancer.

Chemotherapy. **Chemotherapy** is the administration of specific drugs that kill both normal and cancerous cells. The administration of various chemotherapeutic drugs is timed to achieve the greatest cellular destruction. The cell's cycle of replication determines the schedule (see "Pathophysiology Illustrated: Chemotherapy Drug Action"). Several chemotherapeutic drugs are administered simultaneously to maximize their lethal impact on cells at all stages of activity (see Table 52–2). Medications are most commonly oral, intravenous, or **intrathecal** (into spinal canal). Whereas DNA in a normal cell can repair itself after chemotherapy, the DNA in a neoplastic cell cannot. The particular chemotherapy treatment protocol used is based on research into different types of cancer cells. A **protocol** is a plan of action for chemotherapy based on the type of cancer, its stage, and the particular cell type (Figure 52–3 ●).

Other drugs used in the treatment of children with cancer include colony-stimulating factors, antiemetics, and nutritional supplements. Colony-stimulating factors are hormonelike glycoproteins that enhance blood cell production and counteract the myelosuppressive effects of chemotherapy drugs. For example, erythropoietin is produced in the kidney, and a recombinant form (epoetin) is available which can be used to treat anemia of cancer, thereby decreasing the number of transfusions needed.

MyNursingKit Chemotherapy Drug Combinations

Teaching Highlights

CANCER THERAPY

Most parents are not aware of the effects of cancer treatment and how they can help children through this experience. Depending on the stage and type of treatment, there are several ways to help:

- Children in radiation and chemotherapy are fatigued due to cancer and treatment effects. Provide extra rest periods with shorter activity periods between them.
- Have a suitcase ready in case the child develops a complication and needs to be taken to stay in the hospital for a few days. Several hospital stays of a few days are normal during treatment.
- When concerned about a symptom in the child, ask the care provider. Parents are often key in identifying problems early.
- Parents are usually concerned about central line care but feel more comfortable after a few days of caring for the line.
- Children may not feel hungry due to anorexia from the disease and as a side effect of treatment. When they are ready to eat, intake should be nutritious.
- Remember that the child is still at the normal developmental age. Treat them appropriately for their age, not as if they are older or younger. Utilize the child life specialist in the hospital to assist with planning activities appropriate to the child's developmental age.
- Try to maintain contact with the child's peer group and family members. When school attendance or direct contact is not possible due to immune suppression, arrange for phone calls, videocam exchanges, and other methods of communication.
- Seek information from other parents and resources on cancer care.
- Many families use complementary approaches to deal with the child's cancer. Most of these approaches are not contraindicated. However, be sure to tell the oncologist about what treatments you are choosing to use to be sure none of them will injure your child.
- Take time to get away and relax so that you have enough energy and are better able to deal with your child's therapy.

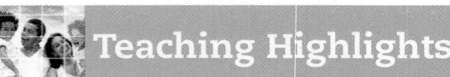

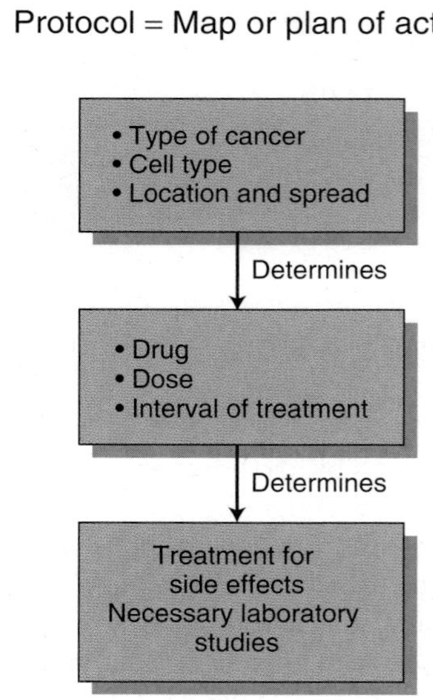

● **Figure 52–3** Chemotherapy protocol. A protocol is a map or plan of action that directs therapy by identifying the drug and its accompanying treatment.

PATHOPHYSIOLOGY ILLUSTRATED

CHEMOTHERAPY DRUG ACTION

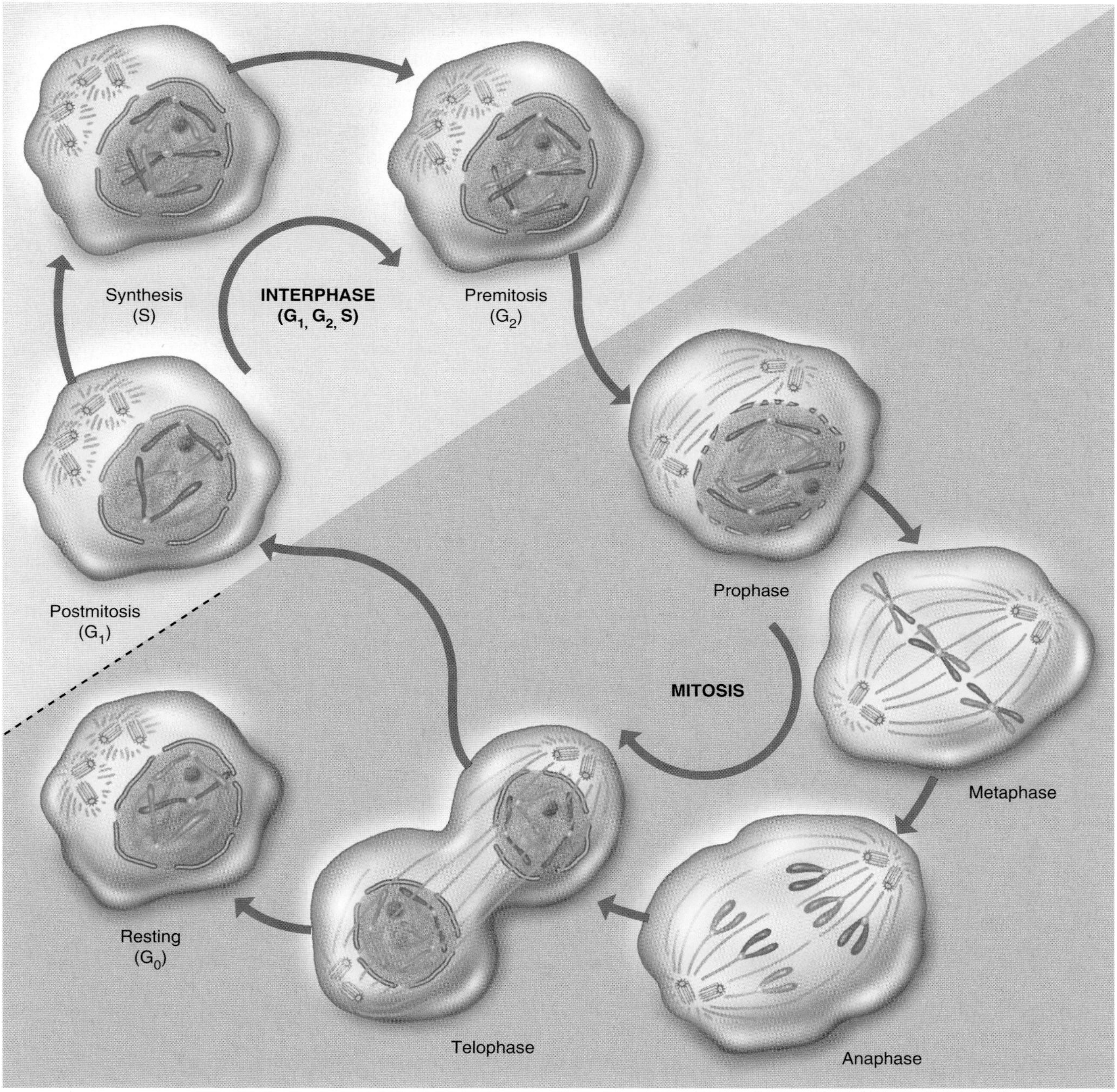

Chemotherapy drugs either act at specific parts of the cell cycle or are nonspecific for action (act throughout all cell phases). See Table 52–2 for further information about specific drugs and their site of action in the cell cycle.

Table 52–2 Medications Used for Cancer Chemotherapy

Medication and Action/Indication	Nursing Implications
CELL CYCLE SPECIFIC AGENTS	
Antimetabolites ■ 5-Azacytidine ■ 5-Fluorouracil ■ 6-Mercaptopurine ■ 6-Thioguanine ■ Cytosine arabinoside (cytarabine) ■ Hydroxyurea ■ Methotrexate The antimetabolites work at synthesis phase of cell division; interfere with function of nucleic acid; inhibit DNA or RNA synthesis.	Various routes are used for individual agents, such as oral, intravenous, and intrathecal. Most common side effects are nausea and vomiting, myelosuppression, stomatitis. Specific agents such as methotrexate and cytarabine can cause neurologic toxicity with high doses. Consult drug books and package inserts for detailed list of side effects. Obtain baseline CBC, liver function, renal function. Monitor intake & output and body weight. Ensure hydration and output levels ordered by oncologist. Monitor vital signs and cardiovascular and respiratory function. Watch for bleeding and signs of infection. Monitor carefully during administration for signs of anaphylaxis.
Vinca alkaloids ■ Etoposide ■ Teniposide ■ Irinotecan ■ Paclitaxel ■ Vinblastine ■ Vincristine Act during mitosis; bind with cell proteins to inhibit nucleic acid and protein synthesis.	Most are given intravenously with some drugs also available for oral route. Common side effects include nausea and vomiting, abdominal cramping and diarrhea, constipation, paralytic ileus, hair loss, hypotension or hypertension, peripheral neuropathy and neurologic toxicity (latter especially with vinblastine and vincristine). Obtain baseline blood work. Consult specific drug information for period of maximum myelosuppressive effect. Be alert for bruising, infection, and other signs of myelosuppression. Monitor carefully during administration for signs of anaphylaxis.
Miscellaneous—G_1 phase activity ■ L-asparaginase Causes depletion of asparagine, needed by cancer cells; makes cell in G_1 phase vulnerable to other agents; interferes with synthesis. Used in combination with other agents in leukemia and other cancers.	Administered intravenously or intramuscularly. Major side effects are severe nausea and vomiting, hypersensitivity, renal failure, myelosuppression, acid–base imbalance. Because of the risk of life-threatening hypersensitivity reactions, emergency medications and care must be immediately available. CBC, serum amylase, glucose, coagulation factors, bone marrow function, liver function tests performed before therapy and twice weekly. Monitor intake & output, neurologic status, gastrointestinal symptoms, abdominal pain.
Miscellaneous—G_2 phase activity ■ Etoposide Works at G_2 phase; binds cellular proteins to cause metaphase arrest; also acts on S phase of DNA synthesis. Used with other agents, particularly in recurrent disease.	Administered orally and intravenously. Common side effects are nausea and vomiting, myelosuppression, hair loss, diarrhea. Can cause anaphylaxis; hypotension and IV site pain with rapid infusion. Perform baseline CBC, liver, and renal function tests. Check IV site frequently since extravasation can cause necrosis. Monitor vital signs during infusion and stop drug if hypotension occurs. Keep emergency drugs and equipment readily available.
CELL CYCLE NONSPECIFIC AGENTS	
Alkylating agents ■ Cyclophosphamide ■ Carboplatin ■ Cisplatin ■ Busulfan ■ Chlorambucil ■ Ifosfamide ■ Thiotepa ■ Mechlorethamine ■ Melphalan ■ Procarbazine ■ Dacarbazine Substitute an alkyl group for a hydrogen atom, leading to blockage of DNA replication. Used for treatment of many cancers, either alone or in conjunction with other agents.	Most are administered orally and/or intravenously. Array of side effects depending on specific drug. Some common side effects are nausea and vomiting, diarrhea, myelosuppression, hair loss, neuropathies, pulmonary toxicity, renal damage; secondary tumors later in life associated with some agents. Obtain CBC and full blood work before and during treatment. Monitor for side effects of the specific agents administered. Ensure generous hydration and monitor Intake & Output. Teach family the importance of long-term monitoring for secondary tumors.

Table 52–2 Medications Used for Cancer Chemotherapy—continued

Medication and Action/Indication	Nursing Implications
CELL CYCLE NONSPECIFIC AGENTS, *continued*	
Antibiotics ■ Doxorubicin ■ Mitomycin-C ■ Dactinomycin ■ Bleomycin ■ Daunorubicin ■ Idarubicin ■ Mitoxantrone Interfere with nucleic acid, inhibiting DNA or RNA synthesis. Used in combination with other agents to treat leukemia and other childhood cancers.	Most are administered intravenously. Common side effects include nausea and vomiting, myelosuppression, oral ulcers, skin and pulmonary toxicity. Several have cumulative dose toxicity, such as cardiac abnormalities (doxorubicin) and skin/pulmonary (bleomycin); total dose the child has received must be monitored. Obtain baseline CBC and other blood studies and monitor throughout therapy. Monitor vital signs, lung function, cardiac function, neurologic status throughout and following therapy. Be alert for signs of myelosuppression and mucosal ulcers.
Nitrosoureas ■ Carmustine ■ Lomustine Cross-breakage in DNA strands so that DNA and RNA replication cannot occur. Used in lymphomas and other childhood cancers. Can cross blood-brain barrier.	Administered orally (lomustine) or intravenously (carmustine). Major side effect is myelosuppression. Others include pulmonary fibrosis, eye infarction, skin changes, hair loss, nausea, and vomiting. Obtain baseline and periodic CBC and other studies. Monitor pulmonary function, skin, and signs of infection or bleeding.
Hormones ■ Prednisone ■ Prednisolone ■ Dexamethasone Analog of hydrocortisone; anti-inflammatory; delayed and depressed immune response. Used in conjunction with other agents for many types of childhood cancer.	Often administered orally. Numerous side effects including edema, moon face, mood lability, increased appetite, disturbed sleep, immunosuppression, disturbed glucose control, osteoporosis. Teach child and family the effects of the drug. Minimize exposure to persons with infection. Monitor for infections in all systems. Monitor weight regularly. Take vital signs. Teach to take as directed. Drug must be tapered slowly at end of therapy.
Topoisomerase I inhibitor ■ Irinotecan ■ Mitoxantrone ■ Topotecan Inhibit the enzyme topoisomerase I in the cell nucleus, relaxing DNA and preventing its duplication. Used in conjunction with other agents to treat acute lymphocytic leukemia and other childhood cancers.	Administered intravenously: topotecan can be given intrathecally. Common side effects include nausea and vomiting, diarrhea, fever, dehydration, myelosuppression. Can alter liver function and cause skin changes. Obtain baseline and periodic CBC and other studies, including liver function. Monitor for signs of myelosuppression, gastrointestinal distress, change in liver function.

Filgrastim (Neupogen) increases production of neutrophils by the bone marrow (see Table 52–3). Antiemetics, such as ondansetron (Zofran), can be used to treat the nausea and vomiting that are common side effects of therapy. Nutritional supplements help maintain nutritional status.

Radiation. **Radiation** therapy involves unstable isotopes that release varying levels of energy to cause breaks in the DNA molecule and thereby destroy cells. Radiation has been used as a treatment method since the early 1900s, shortly after its discovery. It is often used for the local and regional control of cancer, and in combination with surgery and chemotherapy; it may be curative or palliative.

The area to be irradiated (treatment field) includes the tumor site and sometimes other involved areas, such as lymph glands. The goal is to irradiate the tumor but not healthy adjacent tissue. The total dose of radiation is divided (or fractionated) and given over several weeks. A common course of radiation treatment might be once daily 4 or 5 days per week for a period of 2 to 7 weeks.

Examples of cancers treated with radiation include Hodgkin disease, Wilms' tumor, retinoblastoma, rhabdomyosarcoma, and central nervous system disease in leukemia. Tumors that have a low sensitivity to radiation, such as osteosarcoma and soft-tissue sarcomas, require higher doses of radiation, or other treatments may be preferred.

Nursing Practice

Nurses who care for a child receiving implant radiation or who work in a radiation department need to wear a dosimeter film badge at all times to measure their radiation exposure.

Table 52–3 Medications Used to Treat Cancer: Colony-Stimulating Factors

Medication and Action/Indication	Nursing Implications
Epoetin alfa (human recombinant erythropoietin) This glycoprotein stimulates the bone marrow in RBC formation; useful when numbers of RBCs are low due to chemotherapy effects.	Give subcutaneously or intravenously. Do not shake and do not use if discolored or particles are present. Single-dose vials only, so discard any solution that is not used. Obtain red blood cell tests before therapy and periodically after; improvement in hematocrit should be seen in 7–14 days. Monitor blood pressure before and during therapy as hypertension can result. Monitor for change in neurologic response and headache; both seizures and strokes are possible side effects.
Filgrastim (Neupogen) and pegfilgrastim (Neulasta) These human granulocyte colony-stimulating factor preparations (G-CSF) increase the bone marrow's production of neutrophils.	Administered subcutaneously and intravenously; prepare as directed for IV infusion to prevent its absorption by IV tubing. Single-dose vials only so discard any solution that is not used. Incompatible with many medications; check package insert; do not give within 24 hours before or after chemotherapy drugs or their effect may be decreased. Obtain baseline and twice weekly CBC. Monitor for side effects such as bone pain and heart arrhythmias; report fevers and be alert for other signs of infection when neutrophil count is low.
Oprelvekin (Neumega) A hematopoietic growth factor, interleukin-11, that increases platelet count; useful in low platelet count due to chemotherapy effects on bone marrow.	Administered subcutaneously. Single-dose vials only, so discard any solution that is not used. Obtain baseline CBC and platelet count; monitor platelets throughout treatment. Monitor for side effects such as edema, fever, CNS changes, tachycardia, respiratory problems, and skin rash. Take daily weights and monitor for fluid retention.

MyNursingKit Stem Cell Transplantation

Biotherapy. Biotherapy is the use of biologic retooling and molecular intervention to produce targeted cancer therapy. Biologic retooling uses parts of the human body that are programmed to destroy cells, and applies them to the cancer cells. An example of this technique includes development of antibodies that are tumor-specific to certain cancers, and produced by the body in response to antigens of cancer cells (Henderson, Mossman, Nairn, et al., 2005). These antibodies promote apoptosis or death of the cancerous cells. Another example is the group of drugs that stimulate the body's own immune response. Cancer vaccines are under development that may work to help the body fight cancers; already developed is human papilloma virus vaccine (see Chapter 45). The actions of many of these agents are not completely understood, and some agents have more than one effect. For example, interferon has both antiviral and antiproliferative effects on some malignant cells. Interferon and tumor necrosis factor (TNF) are undergoing clinical trials to study their effectiveness and to develop protocols for their safe use against selected cancers.

Molecular targeting involves interference with metabolic pathways (for example, through enzyme disruption) in the tumor cells. It may therefore disturb the cell's growth and development and thereby depress proliferation.

An additional type of biological therapy is gene therapy, or attempting to replace a faulty gene with one that is normal. Genetic technology is growing rapidly and shows promise for future treatment of cancer and other childhood diseases. This complex field includes research to identify genes that lead to disease, recombinant techniques to enable genetic engineering, and studies of enzymes active in DNA and RNA formation. Nurses need to have enhanced knowledge of this important work as technologies are increasingly applied in cancer treatment (Loescher & Merkle, 2005).

Bone marrow and hematopoietic stem cell transplantation. Bone marrow and hematopoietic stem cell transplantation (HSCT) are used to treat leukemia, neuroblastoma, and some noncancerous conditions such as aplastic anemia. The goal of therapy is to administer a lethal dose of chemotherapy and radiation that will kill the cancer, and then to resupply the body with stem cells either from the child's own bone marrow that was previously removed (autologous transplant) and stored or from a compatible donor (allogeneic transplant). Umbilical cord blood is a potential source of stem cells used for transplant, as are peripheral blood stem cells (obtained from the donor's circulating blood rather than from bone marrow). The donor, whether autologous or allogeneic, can be given growth factors prior to donation to stimulate production of stem cells. An advantage of peripheral stem cells is that they can be easily collected rather than by the painful and invasive procedure of a bone marrow aspiration (Elfenbein, 2005).

Transplantation has become the treatment of choice for some cancers when a relapse occurs while the child is receiving another form of cancer therapy and for primary treatment of certain cancers. First, a histocompatible donor must be located. The child then receives intensive chemotherapy, often followed by total body irradiation. Beginning 7 to 10 days before the transplant, this treatment kills all circulating blood cells and bone marrow contents. Following this treatment, the child is intravenously transfused with the donor bone marrow or other source of stem cells. New blood cells usually form within 2 to 8 weeks. (See Chapter 50 for a description of care for the child undergoing transplantation.)

Stem cells that become established in the host child's bone marrow can also be obtained from newborn umbilical cord blood. For some children this has become a better option than waiting for a matching bone marrow donor. Cord blood can be easily collected at birth from a sibling of the ill child, as histocompatible matches often occur in siblings, or cord blood banks may offer a match. The umbilical cord blood is then infused into the child undergoing treatment, and the same mechanism occurs as in transplantation of bone marrow—implantation of the stem cells into the child's bone marrow and production of normal blood cells over about 2 to 6 weeks. Advantages of umbilical cord blood are that, unlike bone marrow collection, it is not painful for the donor and does not require anesthesia, there is an opportunity to easily collect samples from many ethnic groups that are underrepresented in bone marrow donor registries, graft-versus-host disease after treatment is less prevalent, and storage of umbilical cord blood for use later in life is possible. A variety of federally funded and private blood banks are available to store and provide umbilical blood.

Complementary therapies. Many families use **complementary therapies** in treatment of a child's cancer. These approaches to care are also referred to as alternative or unconventional, and may involve nutritional supplements, oral herbal supplements, touch therapy, and mind/body interventions. Very little research has been done on complementary therapies, although up to 80% of children have used at least one such therapeutic approach (Post-White & Hawks, 2005). Healthcare providers should be aware of these practices, inquire in a nonjudgmental manner about the therapies, and attempt to learn about specific therapies and practices. Although some herbs and nutritional products such as St. John's wort may decrease serum concentration of chemotherapeutic agents, or some may act as hormones in the body, most are not known to negatively affect contemporary medical treatment. The families should be assisted in seeking information and supported in use of their chosen therapies. Eating fruits and vegetables is associated with lower cancer incidence in adults, and some foods such as garlic and oranges may slow cancer growth or enhance medical chemotherapy. Some individuals use herbal supplements to treat cancer; these include cat's claw (bark of a tree root), mistletoe, and shark cartilage. The U.S. Food and Drug Administration has allowed testing of the efficacy of some herbal treatments for cancer. Some herbs can decrease nausea and vomiting, and others can boost the immune system's function. Several cancer drugs such as vincristine and paclitaxel are obtained from plant products.

Complementary Care

CANCER TREATMENT

Complementary therapy use in the treatment of cancer is widespread within families. However, in different countries the rates vary significantly. Even in the United States, rates vary from 84% use reported in New York City, 65% use in Florida, 59% use in Minnesota, 47% use in North Carolina, and 46% use in Boston (Post-White & Hawks, 2005). Cultural groups have different rates of complementary care use. What does this mean for nurses? It should indicate that no assumptions can be made about the use of complementary therapies within population groups, ethnic or racial groups, or by individuals. Questions should be asked of each family about what therapies are being used, what the expectations are for the therapy, and any effects seen. Offer to provide information about therapies in which the family has interest. Examples of complementary therapy include massage, prayer, nutritional supplements, herbs, and music.

Palliative care. In spite of modern medicinal practices and complementary therapies, some children do not survive childhood cancer. In these cases the focus of health care is to provide comfort and emotional support for the child and family. Too often, healthcare providers feel uncomfortable when a child is expected to die and may withdraw from close contact with the child or family, fail to provide adequate comfort measures, and leave the family without access to needed resources. When recognition of prognosis is delayed, children suffer more and end-of-life care is less integrated. Some symptoms for which children are commonly undertreated include pain, dyspnea, nutrition, elimination, and fatigue. Additionally, care may be required by a wide array of specialists and this can lead to fragmentation of care and lack of integrated palliative approaches (Himmelstein, Hilden, Boldt, et al., 2004). Care for the dying child can be enhanced by a palliative care team; an integrated plan of care; collaboration among families, primary care provider, and other practitioners; and a focus on the child's developmental level and family needs (Hurwitz, Duncan, & Wolfe, 2004 Rushton, 2005). Parents state that an advanced care directive that outlines the medical care plans for the child is helpful in preserving the child's quality of life and increases the child's comfort (Hammes, Klevan, Kempf, et al., 2005). See Chapter 43 for a detailed description of terminal care for children with terminal disease.

SPECIAL ISSUES IN CHILDHOOD CANCER

ONCOLOGIC EMERGENCIES

Oncologic emergencies can be organized into three groups: metabolic, hematologic, and those involving space-occupying lesions. The most common metabolic emergencies include tumor lysis syndrome and septic shock, while common hematologic emergencies include bone marrow suppression, gastrointestinal and central nervous system bleeding, and disseminated intravascular coagulation. The most common emergencies involving space-occupying lesions include brain herniation, spinal cord compression, and superior vena cava compression from a superior mediastinal mass. The next sections describe these and other oncologic emergencies in more detail.

Metabolic Emergencies

Metabolic emergencies result from the lysis (dissolving or decomposing) of tumor cells, a process called tumor lysis syndrome. This cell destruction releases high levels of uric acid, potassium, phosphates, and calcium into the blood and can lower serum sodium levels. It is seen most commonly in children with non-Hodgkin lymphoma (especially the sub-type Burkitt lymphoma) and acute lymphocytic leukemia (Alavi, Arzanian, Abbasian, et al., 2006; Rheingold & Lange, 2006; Spinazze & Schrijvers, 2006). (See "Clinical Manifestations: Management of Tumor Lysis Syndrome.") The nurse collects laboratory studies, including CBC, absolute neutrophil count (ANF), serum electrolytes, bicarbonate, uric acid, blood urea nitrogen (BUN) and creatinine, and urinalysis. The emergency can be life threatening, and the family will need ongoing support and explanations about care.

A second type of metabolic emergency is septic shock. During periods of immune suppression, the child is vulnerable to overwhelming infection, resulting in circulatory failure, inadequate tissue perfusion, and hypotension. Septic shock can be fatal (see Chapter 49 for a description of septic shock). But early and aggressive treatment improves outcome (Haut, 2005). Factors contributing to massive infection include inadequate neutrophil production, abnormal granulocytes (not able to be actively phagocytic), erosions through normal barriers such as blood vessels and mucous membranes, and altered bone marrow production caused by chemotherapy and some forms of radiation. Such infections may manifest with hyperthermia or hypothermia, tachycardia, tachypnea, hypotension, mental changes, and peripheral cyanosis and coolness, and must be vigorously treated with antimicrobial therapy and hydration management.

A third type of metabolic emergency occurs when treatment destroys large amounts of bone, resulting in hypercalcemia (elevated calcium in the serum). Hypercalcemia is most common in children with acute lymphocytic leukemia and rhabdomyosarcoma. Treatment includes hydration and adequate oral phosphate supplement (Spinazze & Schrijvers, 2006).

Another emergency occurs when some children develop syndrome of inappropriate antidiuretic hormone (SIADH) and

Evidence in Action

Septic shock is a serious complication of cancer and has a high mortality rate. Prognosis and treatment are improved when children are diagnosed and treated for septic shock early using aggressive interventions (Haut, 2005). The number of organs involved and especially the presence of respiratory infections influence outcomes (da Silva, Koch Nogueira, Russo Zamataro, et al., 2008). Prompt identification and reporting of signs of respiratory and other infections is important for nurses, families, and all healthcare providers.

Clinical Manifestations

MANAGEMENT OF TUMOR LYSIS SYNDROME

ETIOLOGY	CLINICAL MANIFESTATIONS	CLINICAL THERAPY	NURSING IMPLICATIONS
Breakdown of malignant cells releases intracellular components into blood	Hyperuricemia Hyperkalemia Hyperphosphatemia Hypocalcemia	■ Vigorous hydration with 2–4 times maintenance fluid ■ Correction of electrolyte imbalances ■ Administration of allopurinol or urate oxidase (Rasburicase) to reduce conversion of metabolic by-products to uric acid	■ Administration of fluids, beginning before therapy ■ Careful intake and output measures ■ Daily weight ■ Urine specific gravity (should remain less than 1.010) ■ Monitoring for desired and side effects of drug therapy
Electrolyte imbalance causes metabolic acidosis and serious abnormalities	Cardiac arrhythmias Impaired renal function Tetany, neurologic and mental status changes	■ ECG monitoring ■ Medications such as furosemide to facilitate potassium excretion ■ Dialysis may be needed	■ Administration of electrolytes and medications ■ Urine pH (should remain 7.0 to 7.5) ■ Perform Trousseau's and Chvostek's signs for tetany monitoring and assess neurologic function ■ Perform mental status examination ■ Obtain laboratory specimens as needed

have excessive release of ADH. The resulting decreased urinary output leads to water intoxication. See Chapter 54 for a detailed description of SIADH.

Hematologic Emergencies

Hematologic emergencies result from bone marrow suppression or infiltration of brain and respiratory tissue with high numbers of leukemic blast cells (hyperleukocytosis). Bone marrow suppression results in anemia and thrombocytopenia with resultant hemorrhage. Gastrointestinal and central nervous system bleeding (strokes) are common. Disseminated intravascular coagulation (DIC) occurs in some children and is a life-threatening complication. See Chapter 51 for a thorough description of this condition. Disruption of normal WBC production and resulting hyperleukocytosis can lead to obstruction of small blood vessels throughout the body.

Treatment involves infusion of packed red blood cells for anemia; and platelet transfusion, vitamin K, and fresh frozen plasma for thrombocytopenia and hemorrhage. Hyperleukocytosis is treated by hydration, bicarbonate infusion, and allopurinol (Rheingold & Lange, 2006; Haut, 2005).

Space-Occupying Lesion

Extensive tumor growth may result in spinal cord compression, increased intracranial pressure, brain herniation, seizures, massive hepatomegaly, and superior vena cava syndrome (obstruction of the superior vena cava by tumor). These emergencies are often caused by neuroblastoma, medulloblastoma, astrocytoma, Hodgkin disease, or lymphoma. After biopsy of the mass, treatment involves radiation therapy, chemotherapy, and corticosteroids.

PSYCHOSOCIAL NEEDS

The diagnosis of cancer is devastating for families. They cannot believe that their vibrant, young child or adolescent has a potentially life-threatening disease. Families are in a state of crisis when the diagnosis is made, with the first response being one of shock. At the same time that they are in a state of shock about the diagnosis, parents must gather resources to support the child, make treatment decisions, and adjust family life to integrate the needs of the child with cancer. Some families need to travel a great distance for the child's treatments, and others may have financial constraints that make healthcare costs a major concern. For nearly everyone, parental work schedules as well as arrangements for other children must be adjusted. Most cancer treatment will last for a minimum of several months up to several years, necessitating nearly constant adaptation. Parents, siblings, and extended families should all be included in plans of care (Brody & Simmons, 2007).

The child reacts to the diagnosis based on age. Infants and toddlers are unaware of the severity of the disease, but react to a change in routine and to the anxiety of the care providers. Preschoolers are beginning to understand illness; however, they may think they caused their illness and are confused about why the parent cannot make the illness go away. School-age children can understand a diagnosis of cancer and benefit from opportunities to talk about the experience. Adolescents find contact with others who have gone through their experience reassuring and supportive. Nearly all children are hospitalized after diagnosis, and care should include close proximity to parents, involvement in self-care appropriate for age, positive relationships with staff, and emotional care (Bjork, Nordstrom, & Hallstrom, 2006). Programs such as group therapy sessions, computer programs about cancer and treatment, and school reintegration all show potential for assisting youth who are adjusting to cancer. Children with cancer are commonly anxious about the treatments and disturbed schedules and routines (Kersun & Elia, 2007).

NURSING MANAGEMENT

NURSING ASSESSMENT AND DIAGNOSIS

HISTORY

During health promotion visits of all children, nurses are aware of the importance of a history of cancer in the family. Particularly when more than one person has had cancer, and when young children in the extended family have been affected, complete a genogram to isolate cases in the family (see Chapter 7 for examples of genograms). A history of exposure to known carcinogens is also important. Does a parent work in an industry with substances like chemicals or asbestos that might remain on clothing worn home? Was the child treated with radiation or chemotherapy for a previous cancer? Does the child have an identified condition with a high incidence of some type of cancer, such as Down syndrome? Does the child have any recognized congenital anomalies? A number of conditions are more commonly associated with certain types of cancer.

PHYSIOLOGIC ASSESSMENT

When performing any physiologic assessment on children, consider the possible signs and symptoms of cancer. These include anemia, frequent infections, bleeding disorders, loss of weight, fatigue, pain, and changes in mental health and neurologic status. Assessment of children with the most significant types of childhood cancers is presented later in the chapter.

Once cancer has been diagnosed, a thorough physical assessment of all systems is needed to help identify the presence and extent of cancer (see Chapter 35). Systems needing particularly thorough assessments are neurologic, respiratory, cardiac, and gastrointestinal. Assess hydration status and the tumor site if it is visible. Carefully measure height and weight, and compare with prior findings for the child. Observe gait and coordination, as well as any changes in mental status. Evaluate immunization status, pain, nutritional intake, fatigue, infections, bruising, shortness of breath, and elimination problems. Periodic laboratory studies will be performed. Tailor assessments to the side effects of particular treatments. For example, the child on chemotherapy is likely to experience a **nadir** (lowest point) of WBC count about 10 days after drug administration so blood counts are needed then.

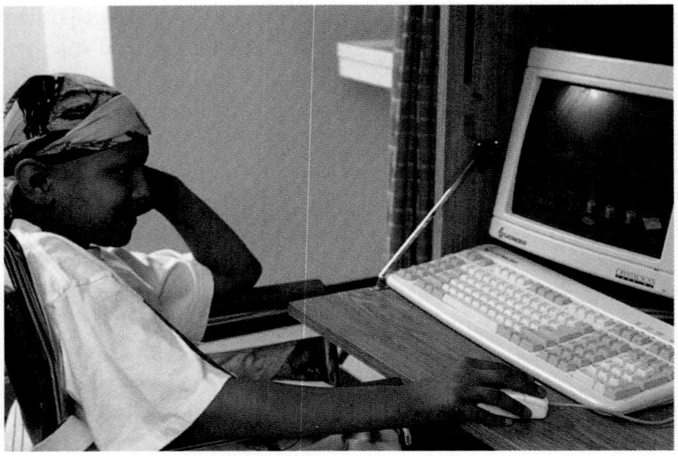

● **Figure 52–4** Hair loss. One of the most common threats to a child's body image at any age is hair loss induced by chemotherapy. Use of hats can improve self-concept.

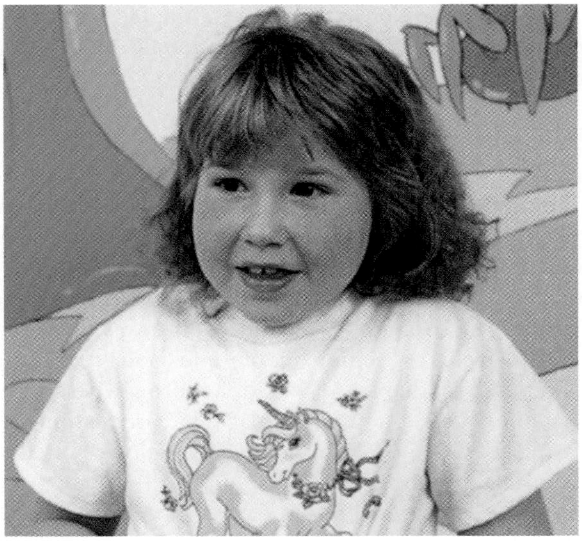

● **Figure 52–5** Cushingoid features. The child with cushingoid changes frequently has a rounded face and prominent cheeks.

PSYCHOSOCIAL ASSESSMENT

Assessment of body image, stress and coping abilities, knowledge of the condition and cognitive level, support systems, and developmental level provides data that help determine the appropriate nursing interventions for the child with cancer and the family.

Body Image

Hair loss, surgical scars, and cushingoid changes are three common treatment-induced threats to body image. Most children being treated for cancer experience hair loss (Figure 52–4 ●). Children who have cranial surgery lose hair as part of the surgical preparation. Chemotherapy frequently results in some degree of hair loss. The speed of hair loss is unique to the child and can be as rapid as overnight or slower, with hair left on the pillow and in the hairbrush.

A second challenge to the child's body image is surgery. The scars of cranial and neck surgery are obvious, as are amputation and limb salvaging. Abdominal surgery for lymphoma is more easily concealed but is still a threat to the child's body image.

A third source of altered body image is the cushingoid features such as round and flushed face, prominent cheeks, double chin, and generalized obesity (Figure 52–5 ●) that result from the use of corticosteroids. As the child's weight increases, stretch marks similar to those of pregnancy may occur. These stretch marks often remain after the corticosteroids are decreased.

Body image disturbances occur when a child cannot integrate changes and continues to cling to old images despite their inconsistency with reality. Common means for assessing body image are drawings, colored pictures cut out by the child to form a collage, discussion, and observation (Rollins, 2005). See

AS CHILDREN GROW

CHILDREN NEED HELP IN COPING WITH PHYSICAL EFFECTS OF CANCER TREATMENT

Children of different ages experience differing threats to body image as a result of cancer treatment. A preschool girl may be most upset at hair loss, since she now looks like a boy. For many parents, especially of daughters, the loss of the child's hair can be devastating. Ask the parents and the child what the loss is like for them. Prepare them for the fact that it can be rapid or slow. Find out how they will plan to cope. Some children want the hair cut very short so its loss will not be as traumatic. Offer resources for wigs, hats, or other ideas. Put them in touch with children who have lost hair and with those who have now regrown it.

A school-age child has the most difficult time with changes that interfere with the developmental task of industry. Amputation, which decreases the child's ability to participate in activities such as sports, dancing, and school work, can be a major challenge during the school-age years. Assist children to adapt to new sports when they are able to do so. Partner with schools, coaches, and families to facilitate children's participation in activities they choose.

Teenagers are often most worried about changes like hair loss and cushingoid features, which cause them to look different from peers. Introducing adolescents to others of their own age who are coping with similar conditions can assist them in their developmental tasks.

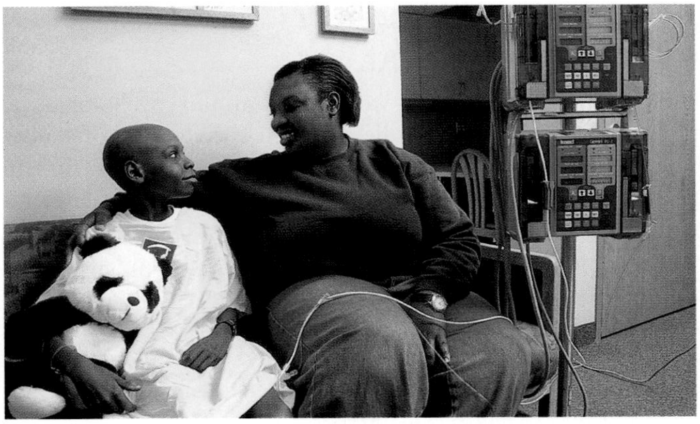

● **Figure 52–6** Family support. The child with cancer depends on parents and family members to provide support. Nurses can assist families and draw upon their strengths to help the child.

Chapter 41 for further discussion of these and other assessment techniques that can be used with children.

Stress and Coping

The diagnosis of cancer is a major stressor for both the child and the family. Although each child's prognosis and each family's coping mechanisms are unique, most families deal with the diagnosis in a manner similar to that of other families who have a child with a life-threatening illness (see Chapter 43). Assess the family (and child if old enough) for their understanding and acceptance of the diagnosis. Find out if the family has told the child and siblings about the diagnosis and if they need assistance in deciding how to do this (Packman, Greenhalgh, Chesterman, et al., 2005). Assess the level of anxiety during healthcare visits and scheduled treatments (Figure 52–6 ●). Evaluate the family's methods of coping, such as the ability to integrate relaxing and meaningful activities into family life, the use of support systems in the extended family and community, and the ability to alter expectations to take into account the child's health status. Some families demonstrate resilience and the ability to assist the child and all of their members. Other families, however, may be experiencing multiple stresses, making adaptation to the new diagnosis particularly difficult (Kazak, Rourke, Alderfer, et al., 2007). Concurrent stressors increase the difficulty of coping with childhood cancer. Evaluate the family for stressors such as illness or death of another family member, occupational changes, financial problems, relocation, and change in vacation plans. Evaluate the family's knowledge of the U.S. Family and Medical Leave Act benefits, which enable parents to use sick time, vacation, and leave without pay to care for an ill family member while safeguarding employment.

Knowledge

Anxious people tend to narrow their scope of attention and may read unintended messages into the behaviors of healthcare personnel. Anxiety also limits a person's ability to retain information.

Assess the child's knowledge of cancer and its treatment throughout the treatment period. As the child matures cognitively, reevaluate knowledge. Cancer and its treatment are complex topics. Parents are exposed to information in various forms, including written material, news reports, and Internet Web sites and resources. Evaluate their knowledge and information sources and provide them with opportunities to ask questions. Evaluate the learning style of the child and family in order to adapt approaches to meet their needs.

Support Systems

Cancer treatment generally occurs over a long time. The extended family is crucial in providing necessary support to the child, parents, and siblings. Identify key people in the family. They may be the parents, grandparents, or aunts and uncles. Support groups for children or other family members often help individuals and the family unit to meet the challenges of the disease. Thoroughly assess the coping strategies the family uses to meet the various challenges posed by the child's illness. This information helps to predict the success of interventions, such as home care with intravenous medications, and to decide when referrals for other supportive therapies are needed.

The return to school may pose difficulties for the child with cancer or it may be a source of support to be connected again to peers. The child is encouraged to go to school, even if only for half a day per week, to stay connected to peers. Evaluate the school's ability to accept a medically vulnerable child into the classroom. Assess whether the other children and teachers have been prepared for the appearance and needs of the child with cancer. Nurses who work in the oncology department of the hospital or clinic can ask if the family would give consent to visit the school, meet with the school nurse, and plan together to meet the child's educational needs. Help the teacher devise a plan to prepare the children, and offer to visit the classroom to explain what the child with cancer is experiencing. Arrangements can be made for tutors to help the child keep up with schoolwork if he or she cannot attend school. An individualized education plan is needed. Parents need information about the legal right to home schooling and a specialized plan since the child is newly ill and they will likely not have been exposed to this in the past.

Assess family resources to identify support systems available to help the family during crises and if a child is expected to die. Extended supports include friends, jobs, insurance coverage, religious affiliations, cultural support systems, and the school system. Parents commonly lose contact with close friends after the diagnosis of cancer in a child. This is an additional stressor for the family. Jobs are often a source of support because coworkers may have gone through the same experience. It may also be comforting for a parent to return to a job where he or she can feel a sense of security in tangible accomplishments. However, jobs can also be a source of stress if employers are unsympathetic to the demands of the child's hospitalization and clinic or office visits. The nurse caring for a child and family in the end-of-life care phase can best support family members by helping them to view the child's unique characteristics, conveying care and concern for the family, and continuing to have close contact with the dying child. Faith-based affiliations can be an important source of support. Evaluate whether such affiliations are meaningful for the family and, if so, plan for visits from the appropriate clergy. In some cultures, spiritual leaders are an important part of the family's support. Enable a healer to visit the child and conduct a healing ceremony if that will be supportive to the family and child.

DEVELOPMENTAL ASSESSMENT

Developmental assessment of children should be performed regularly during treatment for cancer at times when the child is feeling well so that results are accurate. Assessment of the child's physical and neurologic development helps determine the progress made during treatment and provides a baseline for evaluating the long-term effects of treatment. Children under 6 years of age who have cancer should receive regular developmental assessment with a standardized tool such as the Denver II Developmental Screening Test (see Chapter 36∞). A home healthcare nurse can perform such testing, or it can be done by a nurse in the pediatric healthcare home (medical home) who sees the child for a general health supervision visit. Recommend referral to a neuropsychologist for testing early in treatment and if changes in developmental performance are noted. Children who have received cranial radiation and intrathecal chemotherapy need regular scholastic evaluations. Impaired neurocognitive performance may be a long-term effect of treatment. Observe developmental milestones at each contact with the child and refer for further assessment if regression has occurred. Performance in school and social activities with friends provides important information about expected developmental milestones in older children. If the parents have signed up for a clinical trial (research) treatment for the child, children should also give verbal or written assent when they have the cognitive maturity to do so.

ASSESSMENT FOR IMPACT OF CANCER SURVIVAL

Children with cancer have a variety of common psychologic and physiologic problems, regardless of their specific type of cancer. They and their families are dealing with a complex illness that influences their lives for years. The impact of this experience extends into all areas of function. Over the past 20 to 30 years, treatment for childhood cancers has been increasingly successful. About 1 in 1000 young adults is a survivor of childhood cancer, and by 2010, 1 in 250 adults will be a cancer survivor (Florin & Hinkle, 2005). The success of new modalities and treatment combinations has, however, created special healthcare needs for many survivors (Figure 52–7 ●).

Surgery can have many results. Body organs may be removed and manipulated, leading to adhesions, intestinal obstruction, visual impairment, neurologic disruption, and sterility. Removal of the spleen can lead to serious infections. Amputation necessitates the need for prosthetic devices and physical rehabilitation.

Radiation has several long-term effects. It can impair the growth of bones and teeth, leading to conditions such as scoliosis, leg length discrepancy, or poor dental health. Chronic pain can result from skeletal toxicity (Kaste, 2008). Hypothyroidism can be observed in those who have had head and neck radiation (Skinner, Hamish, Wallace, et al., 2006). Cardiotoxicity and pulmonary toxicity can result from mediastinal radiation. Delayed puberty and sterility can result from radiation effects to the cranium and spinal regions. Impaired neurocognitive performance may occur as long-term effects of treatment, especially with higher doses of radiation. Some studies have found lower behavioral and social competence in treated

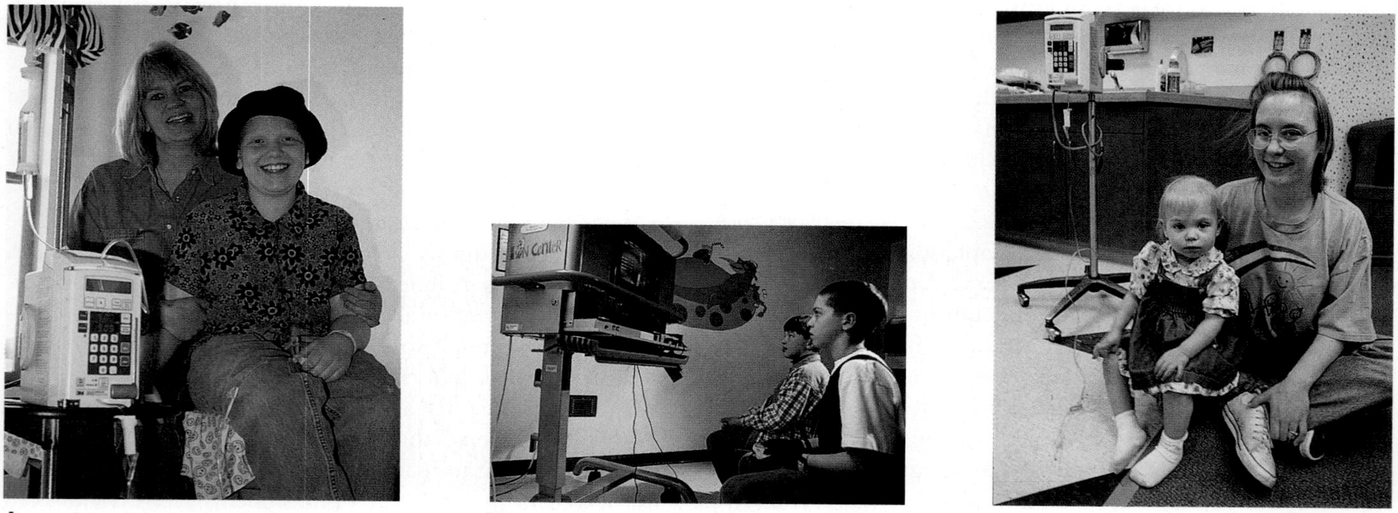

A B C

● **Figure 52–7** Survivors of childhood cancer. ***A,*** Nicole, 11 years old, is undergoing chemotherapy for Ewing's sarcoma. Her mother emphasizes, "It's our faith that has gotten us through this. The hardest part is how busy you are coming to treatments all the time. Nicole's younger brother sometimes feels neglected." ***B,*** According to Jesse, who is 10 years old and waiting for a bone marrow transplant, "The thing that has helped me the most [in dealing with acute lymphoblastic leukemia] is all the mail I got from my friends." His mother adds, "We're just really positive and think that everything will turn out all right." ***C,*** Cassie, 19 months old, has been diagnosed with neuroblastoma. At this age, it is hard for her to understand what is happening to her. Her mother has stayed with her each time she has come to the hospital, which has helped Cassie adjust to therapy. Her caregivers are confident that she will respond well to her treatment.

children and higher rates of post-traumatic stress syndrome (Rourke, Hobbie, Schwartz, et al., 2007). Secondary cancers, most commonly solid tumors, occur in some survivors. **Secondary cancers** are also called second malignant neoplasm (SMN). They occur subsequent to the primary cancer and treatment but are of a different histologic type. Other chronic conditions, such as heart failure, congestive heart failure, cognitive dysfunction, and reproductive problems are more common in cancer survivors who are adults than in the general population (Twombly, 2007).

Chemotherapy can cause a wide variety of effects, both during its administration and for years afterward. (See "Clinical Manifestations: Common Side Effects of Chemotherapy.") Cardiomyopathy can occur with some drugs, especially the anthracyclines. Temporary or permanent pulmonary toxicity and renal complications can develop. Neurologic effects of some drugs can lead to hearing loss (e.g., cisplatin and ifosfamide), cataracts, and paraplegia (e.g., intrathecal methotrexate for leukemia). Learning disabilities and change in intelligence quotient (IQ) occur in some children. Infertility may result (Nelson & Meeske, 2005). Although radiation is responsible for most secondary tumors, some chemotherapy drugs have also been implicated.

The diagnosis and stress of treatment, along with the risk of recurrence, are significant stressors for the child with cancer. Families may find it difficult to obtain full insurance coverage for the child who has had a prior cancer. Employment can be a potential problem for cancer survivors if employers have concerns about the earlier cancer diagnosis. Most people with cancer report fear of recurrence of the disease, which is a stressor. Depression, suicidal thoughts, and concerns about appearance may be more common in survivors of childhood cancer, although this finding is not consistent among all studies (Zebrack, Zevon, Turk, et al., 2006). Conversely, hopefulness and the sense of having an added purpose in life can be positive outcomes for many cancer survivors. Some meet with others who have a recent diagnosis, or work on fund-raising events that financially support cancer research.

Nurses are involved with families when a diagnosis of cancer is made, during the therapy process, and in the years that follow. For a child who survives cancer, ongoing care is essential. Evaluate the child regularly with thorough physical, psychosocial, developmental, and cognitive assessments (Houldin, Curtiss, & Haylock, 2006). Carefully monitor all body systems (e.g., cardiovascular; respiratory; musculoskeletal; eye, ear, nose, and throat; genitourinary). Record height and weight and general growth patterns. Ask about the child's interactions with peers and performance at school. Children who have received cranial radiation and intrathecal chemotherapy need regular scholastic evaluations. Impaired neurocognitive performance may occur as long-term effects of treatment, and appropriate interventions should be planned in these cases. Be alert for signs and symptoms that could indicate a secondary tumor. Ask the parents about insurance coverage and other financial difficulties during ongoing care.

Plan care to assist the family to manage any long-term effects of cancer treatment. This may involve physical rehabilitation, support related to visual impairment, or treatment for cardiac or musculoskeletal abnormalities. Provide resources for information and support. Facilitate periodic evaluations in a healthcare agency so that serious outcomes of treatment can be identified early.

The accompanying Nursing Care Plans include several diagnoses that may be appropriate for the child with cancer who is receiving care in the hospital or at home. Among the many other diagnoses that may be appropriate for a child with cancer are the following:

- *Diarrhea* related to radiation therapy and toxins
- *Impaired Urinary Elimination* related to chemotherapy
- *Impaired Oral Mucous Membrane* related to chemotherapy and radiation therapy
- *Impaired Skin Integrity* related to altered nutritional state, effects of medication, radiation, and immobilization
- *Ineffective Individual Coping* related to situational crisis of chronic and acute illness
- *Risk for Caregiver Role Strain* related to anxiety and disruption in family roles and patterns
- *Disturbed Sleep Pattern* related to biochemical agents, anxiety, and unfamiliar surroundings
- *Deficient Diversional Activity* related to frequent lengthy treatments
- *Disturbed Body Image* related to chronic illness and treatments
- *Deficient Knowledge (Child or Parents)* related to lack of exposure to disease or treatments
- *Anticipatory Grieving* related to actual or potential loss

PLANNING AND IMPLEMENTATION

The nursing care of children newly diagnosed with cancer and their families includes immediate physiologic and psychologic support, along with anticipatory guidance about imminent and future medical interventions. Assist and support the family in making decisions about types of treatment that are appropriate for their child.

Nursing care of the hospitalized child with cancer and the child receiving ongoing therapy at home is summarized in the accompanying Nursing Care Plans. These care plans are designed for the child who has progressed beyond cancer diagnosis and is receiving chemotherapy.

Physiologic care of the hospitalized child focuses on providing support during treatment. This includes ensuring optimal nutritional intake, administering medications, managing the multiple side effects of chemotherapy and radiation, ensuring adequate hydration, preventing infection, and managing pain during diagnostic procedures and treatment.

ENSURE OPTIMAL NUTRITIONAL INTAKE

The high metabolic rate of cancer growth depletes the child's nutritional stores. In addition, the catabolic effect of chemotherapy and radiation on normal cells necessitates additional cellular replacement. The child needs increased nutritional intake at a time when nausea and vomiting are occurring as drug side effects, and when decreased activity, treatment protocols, and general health status result in diminished appetite. This often leads to extreme concern on the part of parents, and they may focus excessive attention on the child's intake.

Administer antiemetic drugs to lessen nausea from chemotherapy. Integrate feeding methods and foods that the family and the child find most helpful for ensuring adequate intake. Allow the family to bring the child's favorite foods to the hospital. Ask the family what treatments they use to decrease the child's nausea and vomiting. Perform 24-hour dietary recalls to assess the child's intake, and evaluate height and weight regularly. Special nutritional products may be given orally, nasogastric or nasoduodenal tube feedings may be given, or total parenteral nutrition may be necessary.

Teaching Highlights

NUTRITION AND THE CHILD WITH CANCER

Because of the effects of cancer and chemotherapy or other treatment, the child often has a poor appetite. Mucosal sores lead to difficulty chewing and swallowing. Parents can enhance the nutritional intake of the child in a variety of ways:

- Provide frequent small feedings rather than three meals daily.
- Integrate the child's favorite foods and the cultural foods common to the family into daily menus.
- Have nutritious snacks available for times when the child feels like eating.
- Sprinkle dried milk on top of cereals and other foods.
- Smooth, soft foods are usually preferred. Avoid acidic or spicy foods. Milkshakes with added peanut butter, puddings, and soft casseroles may be well tolerated. Try a variety of liquid protein-calorie supplements to find those the child likes.
- Avoid making food an area for disagreement. Do not force foods but rather make them readily available.
- If the child is vomiting due to therapy, do not encourage food at that time. The child may develop food aversions to foods that are vomited.
- Administer antiemetics as ordered during therapy since they can prevent nausea and vomiting.
- Report weight loss and increased fatigue.
- Bring the child in for scheduled health visits so growth, development, and effects of therapy can be monitored.
- Some children need a temporary feeding tube to ensure adequate nutrition. Feedings at night can often increase intake and promote health. Occasionally a central line is inserted to provide total parenteral nutrition.
- Supplements and tube feedings will usually be covered by insurance if the provider writes an order for them.

ADMINISTER MEDICATIONS

An important intervention of the oncology nurse is administering medications safely. Most chemotherapeutic drugs are prescribed and calculated as dose per meter squared (dose/m^2), with m^2 calculated from the child's height and weight. (See Clinical Skills Manual **SKILLS**.)

A number of chemotherapeutic drugs are commonly used in combinations. These drugs are prepared with special techniques under laminar flow devices to minimize potential toxic effects on healthcare providers. Gloves and other hazardous drug protocols are used. Care must be taken to avoid **extravasation** of intravenous drugs (leakage into the soft tissue around the infusion site), as permanent tissue damage can result. The Occupational Safety and Health Administration (OSHA) publishes an instruction manual entitled *Controlling Occupational Exposure to Hazardous Drugs* that outlines general guidelines, protective equipment, and procedures.

In addition to chemotherapy drugs, the nurse administers other medications, such as antiemetics to control nausea, vitamin supplements, and antibiotics. Antiemetics such as ondansetron are given prophylactically when a cancer agent is administered that has known emetic effects. Ask parents about complementary therapy and medications they are obtaining from other sources and using at home. All medications must be safely administered and the child should be monitored for side effects. **Polypharmacy** (the use of several drugs at one time to treat multiple health conditions) can lead to multiple side effects and can challenge the body's ability to metabolize and excrete drugs.

Some children receive fluids and medications at home via central lines, or by intramuscular or subcutaneous injection. Consider referral to home healthcare infusion agencies for monitoring of these treatments and provision of supplies for home use.

MANAGE TREATMENT OF SIDE EFFECTS

All cancer treatments affect some normal body cells as well as cancer cells, causing a wide variety of side effects. Know all side effects of specific drugs administered and monitor for them. A frequent occurrence is **myelosuppression**, or suppression of blood cell production in the bone marrow. Be alert for signs of a decreased white blood cell count, such as infections. **Neutropenia** is present when the ANC is less than 500 cells/mm^3 or if between 500 and 1000 cells/mm^3 when chemotherapy is being given and falling levels are anticipated. At these levels, children will be given a broad-spectrum antibiotic; granulocyte colony-stimulating factor (G-CSF) may be given (see Table 52–3). Take the child's temperature, isolate the child from others with infections, and perform serum laboratory studies as ordered. Although elevated temperature generally indicates infection, in a child with immunosuppression the temperature may be low even in overwhelming infection. A colony-stimulating factor for white cell production may be administered, if necessary. A treatment known as *leucovorin rescue* is used in conjunction with high-dose methotrexate chemotherapy. Leucovorin (citrovorum factor) is a form of folic acid that helps to protect normal cells from the

Nursing Care Plan

HOSPITAL CARE OF THE CHILD WITH CANCER

INTERVENTION	RATIONALE	EXPECTED OUTCOME
1. Nursing Diagnosis: Pain related to tissue injury		
NIC Priority Intervention: **Pain management:** Alleviation or reduction in pain to a level of comfort acceptable to patient		**NOC Suggested Outcome:** **Comfort level:** Feelings of physical and psychologic ease
Goal: The child will report reduced pain that is manageable.		
■ Give analgesics as ordered. ■ Teach relaxation techniques, deep breathing, and distraction. ■ Insert pain management techniques appropriate for developmental age (see Chapter 42 ∞).	■ Adequate medications can reduce pain. ■ Nonpharmacologic methods work with the medication to reduce pain. ■ Developmental level determines the pain assessment method that should be used, as well as the most appropriate intervention methods, from rocking, to distraction, to providing information.	The child experiences pain reduced to the level that allows the child to interact appropriately and gain rest.
2. Nursing Diagnosis: Imbalanced Nutrition: Less than Body Requirements related to inability to ingest or digest food or absorb nutrients		
NIC Priority Intervention: **Nutrition management:** Assistance with and provision of a balanced dietary intake		**NOC Suggested Outcome:** **Nutritional status:** Extent to which nutrients are available to meet metabolic needs
Goal: The child will maintain adequate nutritional intake. The child will experience reduced effects of chemotherapy (i.e., nausea and vomiting).		
■ Offer small feedings. Encourage favorite foods. Refer to dietitian for special meals. Weigh daily. ■ Teach the child distraction and relaxation techniques. Give antiemetics according to orders.	■ Measures can increase caloric intake. Taste changes and mouth sores alter desire for food. ■ Pharmacologic and nonpharmacologic methods are effective in helping to reduce nausea.	The child maintains admission weight or pre-illness weight. The child has minimal side effects of nausea and vomiting.
3. Nursing Diagnosis: Fluid Volume Excess or Deficient related to medications		
NIC Priority Intervention: **Fluid management:** Promotion of fluid balance and prevention of complications resulting from abnormal fluid levels		**NOC Suggested Outcome:** **Fluid balance:** Balance of water in the intracellular and extracellular compartments of the body
Goal: The child will be adequately hydrated.		
■ Record all intake and output. Monitor intravenous rate and solution as appropriate. Monitor output from urine and other output routes such as vomiting or diarrhea.	■ Some drugs (e.g., cyclophosphamide) necessitate a high level of fluid intake to prevent complications. Careful balance of intake and monitoring of output are required.	The child demonstrates adequate hydration. Mucous membranes are hydrated.
■ Test specific gravity of urine daily.	■ Renal function may be affected by chemotherapy.	Specific gravity remains within normal range.
4. Nursing Diagnosis: Risk for Infection related to immunosuppression, invasive procedures, malnutrition, or pharmaceutical agents		
NOC Suggested Outcome: **Infection protection:** Prevention and early detection of infection in patient at risk		**NOC Suggested Outcome:** **Risk control:** Actions to eliminate or reduce health threats

(continued)

Nursing Care Plan—continued

HOSPITAL CARE OF THE CHILD WITH CANCER

INTERVENTION	RATIONALE	EXPECTED OUTCOME
Goal: The child will remain free of infection.		
■ Wash hands often. Maintain in isolation if needed. Transmission-based precautions may be needed to safeguard child.	■ Hand hygiene is effective to reduce organisms. Transmission-based precautions may be needed to safeguard child.	The child remains infection-free. The child with an infection is effectively treated.
■ Monitor temperature. Use a non-invasive method such as tympanic; report method used when recording temperature. Report elevation to physician.	■ Elevated temperature is a sign of infection. Children with oral or intestinal mucositis should not have temperature taken in these mucous cavities since it may cause increased irritation.	
Goal: The child will return to normal, uninfected state.		
■ Administer intravenous antibiotics as ordered. Monitor temperature. Use cooling mattress as ordered. Report elevations over 38°C (101°F) to physician.	■ Multiple antibiotics are needed to deal with bacterial and fungal infections during neutropenia. Blood cultures may be taken to identify organism.	
5. Nursing Diagnosis: Ineffective Individual Coping related to situational crisis		
NIC Priority Intervention: **Coping enhancement:** Assisting a patient to adapt to stressors that interfere with meeting life demands and roles		**NOC Suggested Outcome:** **Coping:** Actions to manage stressors that tax an individual's resources
Goal: The child will demonstrate normal adaptive coping methods.		
■ Encourage drawings and other therapeutic play for expression of feelings. Allow for expression of angry feelings, such as hitting dolls and throwing sponge balls. Discuss how to behave during treatments.	■ Expression of feelings helps identify avoidance coping for further intervention. Play is a normal way for child to express self and ideas. Misinterpretations can be corrected. Knowledge of appropriate and helpful behaviors supports self-esteem.	The child continues to use usual coping strategies expected for developmental stage.

destructive action of methotrexate. It is started within 24 hours of methotrexate administration and is given along with hydration therapy. Usual administration is every 6 hours for 72 hours or until serum methotrexate is at the desired level.

Protect the child from bruises and be alert for hemorrhage or signs of bleeding such as petechiae or the presence of blood in vomit and urine. These are all effects of thrombocytopenia, or decreased platelets. When thrombocytopenia occurs, minimize needle sticks and other intrusive procedures. Be ready to deal with nosebleeds and watch for bleeding gums. Report any bleeding episodes to the oncology specialist. Be sure parents know that the child should avoid contact sports or other rough activities and that any healthcare provider, such as a dentist, should be informed of the child's treatment and condition. Infusions to increase platelets are sometimes administered.

Inadequate red blood cell production can result in anemia. Encourage the child to eat iron-rich foods, and administer nutritional supplements as needed. Blood transfusions are sometimes needed to treat severe anemia.

Chemotherapy affects all rapidly growing cells in the body, but especially those of the mucous membranes. Provide good oral hygiene with a soft toothbrush, foam wand, or water irrigation device. Report oral breakdown promptly. See "Teaching Highlights: Oral Care" for common techniques to manage oral hygiene. Be alert for blood in vomit and stool or dark colored stools, all of which can indicate bleeding in the gastrointestinal tract. Blood in the urine may also occur. Know all side effects of specific drugs administered and monitor for them. Some side effects are late and may be seen after therapy is completed. Emphasize importance of all follow-up visits scheduled in the future for monitoring of late effects.

Radiation can cause burns to the skin. Examine the skin daily during hospitalization or weekly when making home visits. Leave the marks on the skin that outline the radiation target area.

Evidence in Action

Oral mucositis or oral ulcers are a frequent side effect of cancer treatment and are difficult to treat. They impair the child's ability to eat and cause serious discomfort. Several studies have tested the effectiveness of a variety of treatments for mucositis, including allopurinol mouth rinse, aloe vera, antibiotic paste, ice chips, and a variety of medicinal and herbal products. Many studies have found benefit for prevention or reduction in ulcers, but no clear evidence suggests that one product is better than another. Types of cancer and treatment protocols may respond differently to various ulcer interventions (Putwatana, Sanmanowong, Oonprasertpong et al., 2009; Worthington, Clardson, & Eden, 2007). Nurses can ask families what they are using, can suggest comfort measures, and evaluate the outcome in order to suggest alternative treatments if needed.

Avoid use of lotions, powders, and soaps on the target skin area. Some children may need to be anesthetized to ensure correct positioning for radiation; postanesthesia care will then be needed.

ENSURE ADEQUATE HYDRATION

Hydration management can be a challenge as the child may not be thirsty but is excreting large numbers of cell fragments and other substances as a result of treatment. Offer frequent small amounts of fluid. Include frozen ice pops or other fluid-containing foods such as Jell-O. Measure intake and output. To ensure adequate excretion, a number of chemotherapy drugs are given with intravenous fluids. It is important to administer fluids as ordered and ensure that the recommended urinary output excretion rate is maintained after drug administration.

PREVENT AND TREAT INFECTION

Children with cancer have an altered immune system, both from the disease and from the effects of immunosuppressant drugs, and must be kept away from persons with known infections. Teach parents to avoid taking the child to places that attract large gatherings of people, such as department stores, once the child returns home. Teach administration of any drugs being used to prevent infection such as pentamidine or sulfa preparations for pneumocystis pneumonia prophylaxis. Emphasize the need to report any exposure to contagious diseases, especially chickenpox. Some drugs may mask signs of infection, so be alert for any signs of mild infection. Fever, malaise, and mild respiratory infection must all be reported promptly (see "Teaching Highlights: Reportable Events for Children Receiving Chemotherapy"). Keep the child's immunization record so immunizations that have not been given yet can be administered in regular clinic visits after therapy is complete, using Centers for Disease Control and Prevention (CDC) recommendations for timing after treatment. Follow recommendations for the immunization of children with cancer as published by the CDC and the American Academy of Pediatrics. Usually, no immunizations are given to the child until 6 months after completing chemotherapy.

Teaching Highlights

ORAL CARE

Since cancer treatment and poor nutritional status can adversely affect the oral status of children, families need help to plan and carry out prophylactic and treatment measures. Children continue to lose teeth, have new teeth erupt, and require nutrients to help in building teeth not yet erupted, even during cancer treatment. Some suggestions are:

- Provide a visit to the dentist early in treatment for assessment, treatment of dental disease, and establishment of a prevention plan.
- Brush teeth twice daily with a soft bristle brush and rinse with water.
- When granulocyte counts fall below 500/mm^3 or platelets fall below 40,000/mm^3, toothettes or gauze can be used to clean the teeth. Avoiding brushes will help to prevent bleeding and infection.
- Toothpaste can be used unless it causes discomfort.
- Medications may be used to prevent infection. They may include antibacterial mouthwash, nystatin, or fluconazole. Continue oral fluoride if it is not present in the drinking water.
- If bleeding, infection, or other oral care needs emerge, consult with the dentist and pediatric oncologist to develop a treatment plan.

Management of infections is critical. Children are often hospitalized and central lines are used for antibiotic administration. Blood cultures and cultures of infected body parts help to establish the causative organisms. Due to lowered immune status, unusual agents are sometimes identified. Administer medication treatment on time and as ordered. Ensure standard precautions and transmission-based precautions are followed. Temperature, vital signs, and assessment of all body systems is performed at admission and at least every 4 hours.

MANAGE PAIN

The child with cancer may experience pain from the disease itself and from the medical interventions, such as lumbar puncture, bone marrow aspiration, and frequent intravenous infusions and blood draws. Use all possible pain management techniques to keep the child comfortable, as this encourages cooperation throughout the long treatment period. Whenever possible, include the parents in comforting the child after painful procedures. (See Chapter 42 for suggestions on methods of pain management.) (See "Complementary Care: Pain Management.")

Nurses must examine research on effective pain management for children and integrate findings into practice. See the Companion Website for relevant links.

Sedation for diagnostic and therapeutic procedures (see Chapter 42) may be used for pain management. Administer sedation as ordered for young children who are undergoing

Clinical Manifestations

COMMON SIDE EFFECTS OF CHEMOTHERAPY

SIDE EFFECT	CLINICAL MANIFESTATIONS	CLINICAL THERAPY
Bone marrow suppression	Evidence of suppression usually appears 7–10 days after administration of chemotherapy; recovery is usually complete within 3–4 weeks.	Blood transfusions are administered when anemia is severe (Hgb less than 7 g/dL) or platelets are very low. Some institutions use a low-microbial diet to decrease the possibility that infectious organisms will colonize the intestine. Septra is used for *Pneumocystis carinii* pneumonia prophylaxis; nystatin and oral vancomycin for antifungal and antibacterial prophylaxis. Instruct the family and child about the importance of protecting the body from bruising during periods of mild to moderate thrombocytopenia (platelet count, 5,000–20,000/mm^3). Careful hand hygiene is essential. Encourage use of masks if family or staff have nasopharyngeal infections.
Nausea and vomiting	Symptoms may occur immediately or 5–6 hours after administration of chemotherapy and may last 48 hours.	Antiemetics, such as Zofran, Kytril, Reglan, and Benadryl, are used to treat this side effect. Teach relaxation techniques, hypnosis, and systematic desensitization (a hypnotic process that progressively reduces reactions to objects that cause strong emotional or physical responses) to help to decrease the child's symptoms. Encourage mild exercise and change of diet (eating only easily digestible foods) 12 hours before chemotherapy.
Anorexia and weight loss	May occur at any time	Hyperalimentation is necessary if dietary changes are unsuccessful in halting the child's weight loss. Pay careful attention to changes in taste that affect food preferences. Referral to a dietician may be helpful to achieve successful modification of the child's diet.
Oral ulcers	The oral mucositis resulting from chemotherapy usually occurs within 3–4 days and is often a contributing factor in anorexia.	Antifungal agents, such as nystatin or clotrimazole, lessen the possibility of candidal infection. Promote good oral hygiene, use soft foam wand or water irrigation to clean teeth; commercial mouthwashes are not recommended because they contain alcohol and increase drying of the oral cavity; specially formulated pharmacological mouthwash may promote comfort.
Constipation	Can occur at any time in treatment but becomes more common as therapy progresses and dietary intake and physical activity decrease.	Stool softeners and laxatives are used to treat this side effect (e.g. Miralax). Advise parents to increase fluids and fibrous foods in the child's diet.
Pain	Pain can occur at any time and is best understood by subjective explanations of the child.	Acetaminophen, morphine, steroids, nonsteroidal anti-inflammatory drugs, and antidepressants may be used to manage pain. Careful pain assessment is important; the location of the pain may provide a clue to its cause, for example, metastasis to the skull, infiltration of joints, or damage to soft tissue; pain associated with chemotherapy may also be related to oral mucositis, myalgia, or tumor embolization; painful polyneuropathy can follow treatment with vincristine or cisplatin. Acetaminophen for pain can mask the presence of fever, which signals infection; careful and complete physical assessment is needed to identify infection. Pharmacologic, nonhypnotic (deep breathing, self-control), and hypnotic methods of pain control may be used; the nonpharmacologic methods often prove helpful to children with pain from multiple etiologies.

Teaching Highlights

REPORTABLE EVENTS FOR CHILDREN RECEIVING CHEMOTHERAPY

Parents require verbal and written instructions about signs and symptoms to report to the child's oncologist while the child is receiving chemotherapy. Have parents report the following events to the child's oncologist if they occur while the child is receiving chemotherapy:

- Temperature above 38°C (101°F)
- Any bleeding, such as nosebleeds, blood in stool or urine, petechiae, bruising
- Pain or discomfort with urination or defecation
- Sores in the mouth
- Vomiting or diarrhea
- Persistent pain anywhere, including headache
- Signs of infection, such as cough, fever, runny nose, tugging at ears
- Signs of infection in central lines, such as redness, drainage, or tenderness
- Exposure to communicable diseases, especially varicella (chickenpox)

Parents should also inform dentists and other healthcare providers that the child is receiving chemotherapy prior to procedures. Prophylactic antibiotics should be given before and after dental care.

Adapted from Bindler, R. M., & Howry, L. B. (2005). *Pediatric drug guide.* Upper Saddle River, NJ: Prentice Hall Health.

Complementary Care

PAIN MANAGEMENT

Children have many painful and invasive procedures during cancer treatment. In addition to use of medication, they will be helped by a variety of other pain management techniques. These include the following:

- Parental presence during procedures as support persons, if they wish to be present.
- Use of distraction and relaxation. Either a parent or healthcare provider can work with the child and integrate techniques, such as singing, counting, telling stories, and blowing bubbles. Children and teens can be taught to visualize positive scenes, use rhythmic breathing, or listen to music (Tsao & Zeltzer, 2005).
- Hypnosis has been used successfully to manage both pain and nausea/vomiting during cancer treatment with children from 5 to 18 years (Richardson, Smith, McCall, et al., 2006).

lumbar punctures, radiation, and other procedures, and monitor them after the procedure. Coordinate other painful or intrusive tests so they can be done while the child is sedated for radiation.

Topical anesthetics such as eutectic mixture of local anesthetic (EMLA) cream may be used to numb the skin before an intravenous start, lumbar puncture, or bone marrow aspiration. Do not use EMLA on infants who are a gestational age of less than 37 weeks, who are under 20 kg, or who are under 12 months receiving treatment with methemoglobin-inducing agents. For all infants, be certain that parents realize the importance of limiting the area and duration as ordered and to keep the cream in a safe place to avoid ingestion by any children. Another measure that can be effective for local anesthetic delivery is iontophoresis. A low-voltage electrical current is applied to intact skin in the area needing anesthesia. The current forces drug molecules (commonly lidocaine hydrochloride and epinephrine) across the stratum corneum. The local anesthetic is effective in approximately 10–15 minutes and has been tested for safety in children as young as 5 years of age (Pasero, 2006).

Some fast-acting sprays are available for even more minor anesthesia. Intradermal application of anesthesia with lidocaine is generally used for more painful and invasive procedures such

as central line insertion. They may be combined with sedation to help the child relax. Follow sedation monitoring protocols (see Clinical Skills Manual SKILLS).

PROVIDE PSYCHOSOCIAL SUPPORT

A diagnosis of cancer brings with it many emotions for the family. Initially parents experience shock and anger. They need basic information about the disease and the purpose of the tests that will be performed. Instructions often need to be repeated as parents may not process information the first time it is presented due to their increased stress levels. Help the parents plan how and when to tell the child the diagnosis. What the child needs to know is based on his or her developmental level and understanding.

Once the family has progressed from their initial state of shock about the diagnosis, they need to learn more about the disease. They may be interested in the pathophysiology, treatment, and expected outcome or the prognosis. Clarify their understanding of these areas and ask what questions they have. Provide verbal explanations and written material. Parents may talk with friends, purchase books, or search the Internet for information. Find out where they are getting information and provide additional resources when appropriate. Correct misconceptions and misinformation.

The family needs many strategies to deal with the challenge of long-term treatment for cancer. As the child experiences remissions and exacerbations or complications, the family feels alternately hopeful and discouraged. Identify the family's support systems and intervene as needed to enhance these systems. Facilitate contact with extended family members who might be of help, religious or spiritual connections, social service agencies, and other resources such as Internet and parent support groups. For parents who are concerned about job obligations and financial concerns, help them identify sources of financial assistance, respite from child care, and ways to take time for themselves.

Evidence-Based Nursing

CANCER AND STRESS

Clinical Question

The family of a child with cancer experiences profound stress, and each member of the family needs to adjust his or her role. The needs of family members are often overlooked as the ill child becomes the center of treatment and attention. Family members often provide care for the child, which can be emotionally and physically draining, and can deplete family financial resources.

Evidence

Major changes in the family were identified by a research study that interviewed family members when a child was diagnosed with leukemia (McGrath, Paton, & Huff, 2005). They included:

- Relocation to be closer to the treatment center
- Interruption of normal activities of daily life for family members
- Placing life "on hold" and deferring usual activities, such as classes and vacations
- Readjustment to home when the child improved and the family resumed usual living patterns
- Concerns related to school and employment for family members
- Financial difficulties

In another study, parents in 86 families that had a child with cancer were found to focus on the needs of the 159 well siblings in those families. About 50% of the parents stated that they anticipated that the well siblings would manifest some problems because of the diagnosis of cancer. Parents frequently observed depression or withdrawal among the siblings, and believed that they had received inadequate information about how to support and help the siblings. Difficulty in scheduling times for the sibling to come to the treatment center and learn more about the cancer treatment was noted. A weekend intervention program for siblings was instituted to offer activities and counseling designed to support siblings. The peer support of meeting with others was helpful to the children (Ballard, 2004).

Best Practice

Both parents and siblings expressed a need for information about the condition and treatment of the child with cancer. Nurses should provide information at each health encounter and frequently ask what questions the family members have. Ask about siblings and include them in visits when possible. Plan peer support group sessions for the siblings so they can discuss their experiences and feelings with other siblings. In addition to information, support is vital. Ask who the parents and siblings have told about the ill child. Who can they turn to when they want to talk? Who can the parents call upon for help at home? Who can the siblings invite to school performances and other events if the parents are unable to attend?

Critical Thinking

Consider the opening scenario that describes Rasheed, a 12-year-old who has leukemia, and his family. What information do his parents need? How can you best support him and his family?

See MyNursingKit for possible responses.

Consider the impact on siblings when a child is being treated for cancer. They may alternately resent and feel guilty for the sibling's illness. They may not understand the treatments or disease. School progress may be slowed and teachers may not be aware of the sibling's stress. (See "Evidence-Based Nursing: Cancer and Stress.")

The child undergoing treatment for cancer needs support appropriate to his or her developmental stage and cognitive level. (See Chapters 33 and 41 ∞ for developmental levels and effective support strategies for children of different ages.) Younger children primarily need support during painful procedures and separation from parents. Older children need intervention strategies to help work through feelings about treatments (Figure 52–8 ●). A major developmental task of adolescence is to attain independence and control, but cancer often interferes with adolescents' ability to achieve this task. Therefore, plan nursing strategies that empower adolescents as much as possible. Introduce them to other teens with similar diagnoses and allow them to make decisions and choices independent of parents when possible. An adolescent can decide which type of medication port would be best (e.g., an implantable port under the skin or a venous access device with tubing outside the body). Making this choice enables the teen to feel more in control of the disease and treatment.

Talk with the child's teachers before the return to school after treatment to explain the child's condition. Ask them to notify

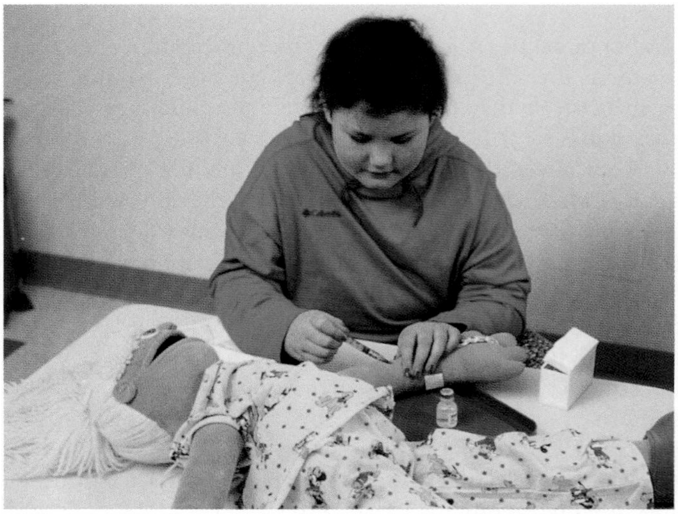

● **Figure 52–8** Play therapy. A child in a pediatric oncology clinic giving injections to a doll. This type of play therapy helps the child deal with fear, thus lowering her stress level.

the family immediately of diseases or infections in other children so the child with cancer treatment who is immunocompromised can be kept home. Arrange for tutors if necessary to assist the child with school work during hospitalization and home care. Explore the option of summer camp for children with cancer. The Make-A-Wish Foundation strives to make dreams come true for ill children by sponsoring them for a desired activity or outing. Refer the child to this foundation if appropriate. See the Companion Website for links, as well as other resources.

The siblings of a child who has cancer may grieve over the ill brother or sister and may feel sad and depressed. Inquire about what they know about the child's condition, and their reactions or behavior changes. Ask the parents if the siblings are demonstrating symptoms such as depression, behavioral changes, or decrease in school performance and suggest interventions as appropriate. Find out who is caring for siblings and whether their teachers have been informed about the family situation. Invite them to play therapy sessions and recreational activities with the ill child. They may benefit from speaking with a school counselor or can be referred to a support group for siblings of children with cancer. Some cancer summer camps welcome siblings as well as children with cancer.

Chapter 43∞ offers strategies to help the family of a child with cancer cope with the stressor of a life-threatening illness. For some types of cancer, the child may experience a remission with treatment, but a recurrence of disease later as cancer cells grow again. The family may become angry or depressed about the relapse. Repeated treatments challenge the family's support systems. Waiting for the outcome of diagnostic tests can be an especially challenging time. Provide information as soon as possible. If the child's illness progresses, refer the family to hospice to help them care for the terminally ill child and work through the grieving process. Explore cancer support groups and information to share this information with families.

DISCHARGE PLANNING AND HOME CARE TEACHING

Preparation for home care centers on creating a normal environment while supporting the child's physiologic and psychosocial responses to the cancer and treatments. Education is the primary focus of discharge planning. Teach the parents how to ensure adequate nutritional intake, to be alert for signs of infection, to protect the child from exposure to communicable diseases during times of neutropenia, to administer medications at home, and to handle vomiting and pain. Help the parents and child deal with any obstacles to normal development and functioning. Teach the parents and family about symptoms that need to be treated immediately.

Home management of a vascular access device or central line, such as a Broviac catheter, initially challenges parents (Figure 52–9 ●). An implanted port may be used; it allows the child freedom to swim and engage in other activities. Parents will need information about whatever device the child has received. Demonstrate details about cleaning the site, instilling heparin in the line or reservoir, and other needed care. After teaching the parents, observe them performing the procedure before the child is discharged.

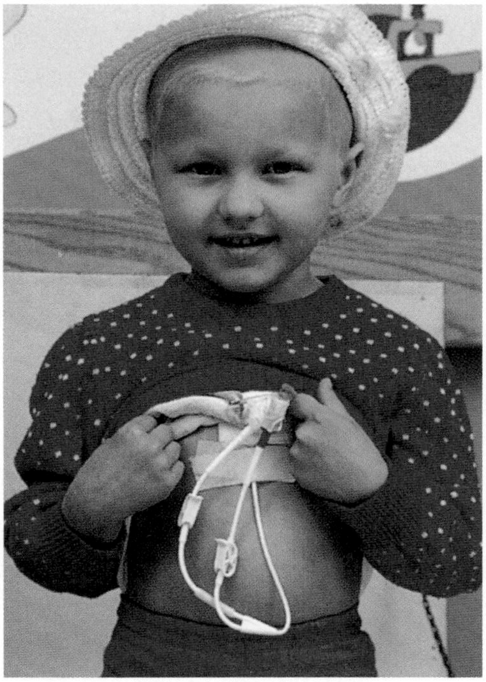

● **Figure 52–9** Comfort and convenience. A vascular access device allows chemotherapeutic agents to be administered without the need for repeated "sticks" to the child.

Emphasize the need for the child and family to have fun and be as normal as possible. Play distracts the child and is essential in reducing fears. Children, parents, and siblings often benefit from participation in cancer support groups and cancer summer camps. These activities create additional support systems, build the child's self-esteem, and enhance coping skills through role modeling. (See "Teaching Highlights: Cancer Therapy.")

Make home visits to evaluate the family's strengths and needs in the home setting. Be sure that the family has adequate support from hospice and other end-of-life services when a child's condition is terminal.

Most children are treated for cancer over a period of 2 to 3 years. Since normal developmental stages progress during this time, health promotion and health maintenance visits should still occur. Some usual care may have to be altered, but many of the same developmental concerns of all children should be addressed. Help parents to view the child as a "normal" child who is ill for a period of time, but still needs to have limits set on behavior, to develop healthy lifestyles, and to have environmental stimulation to learn to talk, read, or perform motor and cognitive tasks.

EVALUATION

Expected outcomes of nursing care for the child with cancer relate to the specific disease, treatments, and responses. Some examples of outcomes include the following:

- Adequate intake to promote normal growth
- Hydration that supports body processes and ensures drug and cancer cell product elimination

Nursing Care Plan

HOME CARE OF THE CHILD WITH CANCER

INTERVENTION	RATIONALE	EXPECTED OUTCOME
1. Nursing Diagnosis: Ineffective Management of Therapeutic Regimen related to complex therapy		
NIC Priority Intervention: **Family involvement:** Facilitating family participation in the emotional and physical care of the child		**NOC Suggested Outcome:** **Care management:** Family ability to manage complex therapy
Goal: The child will comply with oral medication regimen.		
■ Educate parents and child about the importance of taking medication as prescribed.	■ Understanding can assist parents and child in placing importance on medication intake.	The child takes all medications according to prescription.
■ Set up calendar with dates, times, and medications clearly labeled.	■ Visual reminders can help them recall instructions.	
■ Reward the child for taking medications.	■ Reinforcing desired behaviors through rewards is effective with children.	
2. Nursing Diagnosis: Delayed Growth and Development related to serious illness		
NIC Priority Intervention: **Developmental enhancement:** Facilitating patient's caregivers to promote optimal growth and development of child		**NOC Suggested Outcome:** **Child growth and development:** Normal increase in body size and developmental skills
Goal: The child will demonstrate normal physical, emotional, and cognitive development.		
■ Encourage play appropriate to age.	■ Normal activities support self-esteem and self-knowledge.	The child continues to develop physically, emotionally, and cognitively at a normal pace.
■ Encourage the child to attend school when able to do so. Arrange for tutors at home when unable to attend.	■ School is the work of the child and promotes cognitive and social growth.	
■ Encourage seeing peers when unable to attend school.	■ Peer contacts help the child in normal developmental tasks.	
■ Work with teachers to support reentry to school. Use puppets, videotape, and discussion with classmates.	■ Classmates need to understand what has happened to their friend without asking the child directly.	
3. Nursing Diagnosis: Fatigue related to disease state		
NIC Priority Intervention: **Energy management:** Regulating energy use to prevent fatigue and optimize function		**NOC Suggested Outcome:** **Energy conservation:** Extent of management of energy to initiate and sustain activity
Goal: The child will maintain energy levels necessary for normal activities.		
■ Problem-solve ways to save energy for play and school.	■ The child and parents are assisted to see school and play as important.	The child plans use of time effectively to maintain energy for school and play.
■ Plan with child for quiet activities during low-energy times.	■ The child is empowered to select and plan own activities.	The child conserves energy during times of increased fatigue.

THE CHILD RECEIVING CANCER TREATMENT

Cancer treatment often extends for several years, so the child needs to continue health promotion and health maintenance visits.

Growth and Development Surveillance

- The child is assessed for height, weight, and body mass index. This provides information about growth patterns, which may be altered by cancer treatment. If indicated, 24-hour diet recalls and other nutritional assessments are performed.
- Teaching is provided about age-appropriate foods. Since appetite may be impaired during periods of treatment, the child may be lacking fruits, vegetables, or other foods, as well as the nutrients they include. Encourage parents to be sure the child has a well-balanced diet during periods of remission.
- Perform developmental screening of young children. Provide suggestions for parents about the stimulation that is appropriate for the child's age. Include quiet activities that can be used when the child is fatigued or receiving therapy. These might include reading books, listening to tapes and music, and working on a computer. Have the parent plan for these activities on days that the child goes for chemotherapy or other treatment.
- Ask about the school-age child's progress in school. Performance may be altered due to neurologic effects of treatment as well as missing school. Plan for the family to partner with the school personnel for provision of tutors, computer programs, or other needed assistance.
- Encourage continued social contact with peers when blood counts are adequate to prevent infection.

Physical Assessment and Screening

- Careful physical assessments are performed to identify any abnormalities that may result from cancer or its treatment. Cardiopulmonary and neuromuscular assessments are particularly important. Vision and hearing should be assessed prior to treatment and periodically throughout. Include measurements of fine and gross motor activity.

Elimination

- Toddlers may have an interruption in toilet training during periods when they do not feel well. Help parents to understand this regression and encourage them to start again when the child is feeling better.
- Some medications cause diarrhea or constipation so evaluate bowel patterns and provide guidance as needed. Skin care instruction may be needed if the child has diarrhea and is relatively immobile. Increasing fluids and fiber foods may be needed for constipation.
- Evaluate urinary output since many medications have effects on kidney function. Encourage adequate fluids for age to ensure elimination of medications.

Sleep and Fatigue

- Children undergoing treatment often have disturbed sleep patterns. Parents of young children may become exhausted working all day, getting the child to treatments, and having disturbed sleep at night. Assess both the child's sleep patterns and the family's experiences. Encourage plans for respite care to enable rest periods. Provide cots, rocking chairs, and other comfortable settings for child and family members during treatments.

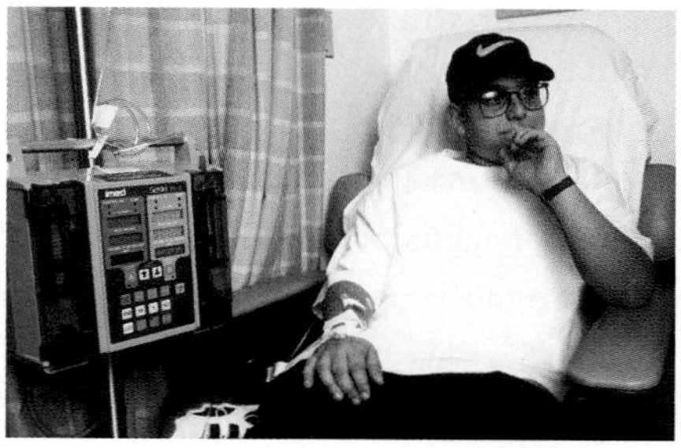

- Both child and parents may not expect or understand the profound fatigue that occurs during cancer treatment. They can be helped to plan for providing quiet times, and replenishing energy through naps, massage, relaxing baths, and spending time with family.

Physical Activity

- Since the child has periods of fatigue, patterns of physical activity may decrease. Emphasize the importance of integrating physical activity when the child feels well, since it is needed for learning gross motor skills, facilitating blood flow, improving mental status, and setting patterns for the future.

Disease and Injury Prevention Strategies

- The child with cancer has the same safety hazards as other children of the same age, and such topics as car safety seats, fire prevention, water safety, and violence prevention should be addressed.
- An important hazard for children with cancer is infection due to decreased immune response. Keep records of immunization status. Follow the recommendations of the CDC and AAP for other immunizations. Teach the hazards of large groups when the child's immune system is compromised. Teach care of central lines and other potential sources of infection. Have families report signs of infection and exposure to known illnesses promptly.

Mental and Spiritual Health

- Evaluate the child and family for signs of anxiety and depression. Ask how they are managing the cancer treatment and what poses the greatest challenges. Refer to other families with similar circumstances for support.
- Ensure that the child has contact with friends through child care, school, or via phone, letters, and computer.
- Find out the impact of the child's cancer on the parent's jobs. Ask how the siblings have been coping, what changes there are in school performance, and whether teachers and others are aware of the stress the sibling may be experiencing.

Transitional Care

- As the child's treatment ends, instruct the child's parents about needed periodic follow-up with the oncologist. Continue to perform neurological examinations and ascertain school performance. Be alert for signs of secondary tumors.
- Ask about worries regarding the future. As teens grow older, have them take over more responsibility for informing care providers of their cancer history and assist them to transition to adult healthcare providers (Florin & Hinkle 2005).

- Prompt identification and treatment to minimize treatment side effects
- Management of pain to a level of comfort satisfactory to child and family
- Family use of resources to provide necessary support during hospitalizations and treatments
- Knowledge of management of treatment regimens
- Acceptance of prognosis and support of all family members

SOLID TUMORS

BRAIN TUMORS

Central nervous system or brain tumors are the most commonly occurring solid tumors in children and the second most common malignancy, after leukemia. Each year approximately 1700 children up to 14 years, and about 2200 youth up to 20 years are diagnosed with tumors of the brain and central nervous system, accounting for one in five childhood cancers; the overall survival rate is 70% (American Cancer Society, 2005; Blaney, Kun, Hunter, et al., 2006).

Etiology and Pathophysiology

The cause of most brain tumors is unknown. About 5–10% of brain tumors are genetic in origin. Exposure to radiation is a known risk factor, such as CNS radiation used for treatment of some other cancers. There is a higher incidence in children with certain other cancers or diseases such as retinoblastoma, renal tumors, neurofibromatosis, tuberous sclerosis, or endocrine syndromes (Blaney et al., 2006).

Brain tumors in children usually occur below the roof of the cerebellum and involve the cerebellum, midbrain, and brainstem (see "Pathophysiology Illustrated: Brain Tumors"). In contrast, brain tumors in adults are usually located above the areas between the cerebrum and cerebellum.

PATHOPHYSIOLOGY ILLUSTRATED

BRAIN TUMORS

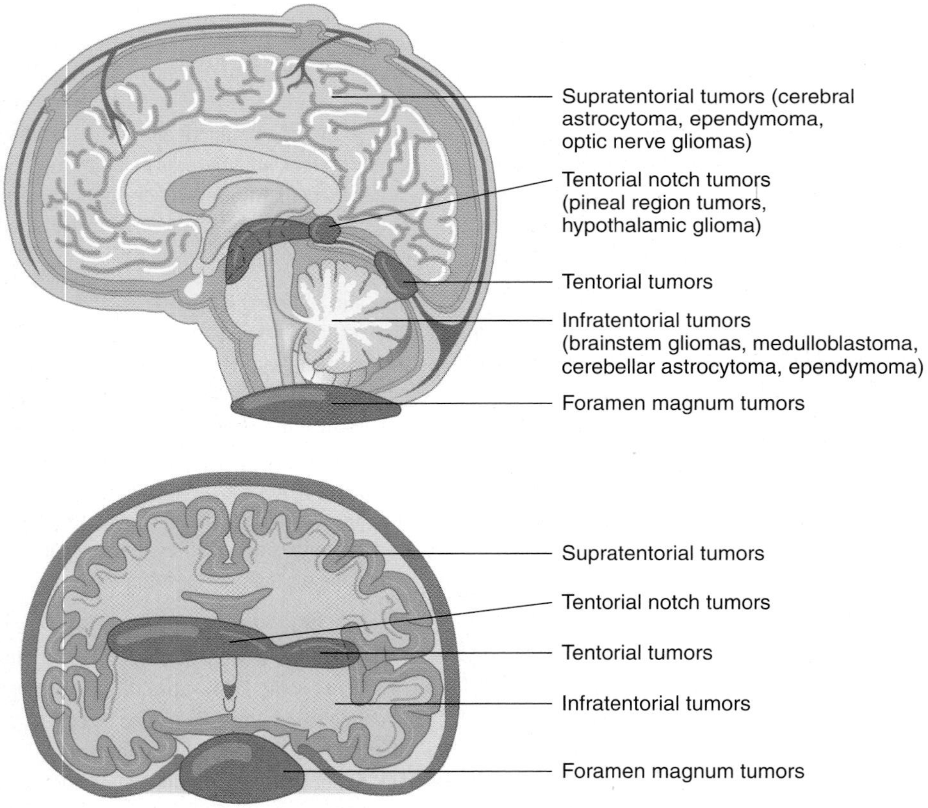

Sites of brain tumors in children. Approximately 3000 children under the age of 15 years are diagnosed annually as having tumors of the brain and central nervous system. The four most common brain tumors in children are medulloblastoma, gliomas of the cerebrum or brainstem; cerebral, cerebellar, and supratentorial astrocytoma; ependymoma (from ependymal cells lining the brain ventricles and spinal cord canal); and craniopharyngioma (Blaney et al., 2006; McKinney, 2005).

Clinical Manifestations

BRAIN TUMORS

TUMOR	ETIOLOGY	CLINICAL MANIFESTATIONS	CLINICAL THERAPY
Medulloblastoma	External layer of cerebellum	Headache, vomiting, ataxia	Surgery; chemotherapy with lomustine, vincristine, cisplatin, radiation
Astrocytomas	Glial cells, supratentorial or infratentorial	Seizures, visual disturbances, increased intracranial pressure, vomiting	Surgery; chemotherapy with vincristine, dactinomycin; radiation
Ependymoma	Fourth ventricle, posterior fossa	Hydrocephalus	Surgery, radiation
Brain stem gliomas	Pons	Cranial nerve (VI + VII) tract signs, nystagmus, ataxia, motor symptoms	Surgery, radiation

Clinical Manifestations

Children with brain tumors can manifest behavioral and nervous changes. These are often a result of increased intracranial pressure and may occur either rapidly or slowly and subtly. Some common symptoms include headache, nausea, vomiting, abnormal gait, dizziness, change in vision or hearing, fatigue, and mental status changes such as educational or behavioral problems (Wilne, Collier, Kennedy, et al., 2007; Wilne, Ferris, Nathwani, et al., 2006).

Brainstem tumors can present with weight deficits and may be mistakenly diagnosed as an eating disorder of infancy and childhood (failure to thrive). This may delay proper treatment. See "Clinical Manifestations: Brain Tumors" for common manifestations of certain types of tumors.

Medulloblastomas are brain tumors in the external layer of the cerebellum. They account for 10–20% of childhood brain tumors, and commonly occur in children 5 to 6 years of age. Astrocytomas arise from glial cells and can be either above or below the area between the cerebrum and cerebellum. They account for 40–60% of childhood brain tumors. The presenting symptoms vary depending on the location of the tumor. Endocrine, vision, and behavioral changes are all possible, as well as increased intracranial pressure and seizures. Ependymomas commonly occur in the fourth ventricle of the posterior fossa and comprise 5–10% of childhood brain tumors. Impaired growth, hydrocephalus, seizures, and cranial nerve impairments are the most common manifestations. Brain stem gliomas are located in the pons and typically spread into the surrounding tissue. They account for 15% of childhood brain tumors.

Clinical Therapy

Brain tumors are diagnosed with computed tomography (CT), magnetic resonance imaging (MRI), positron emission tomography (PET), single-photon emission computed tomography (SPECT), myelography, and angiography. Neurophysiologic tests (electroencephalography and brainstem evoked potentials) are used to assess sensory pathway integrity and disease- or drug-related sensory dysfunction. Other tests that may be performed are tumor markers and cerebrospinal fluid cytology. Lumbar puncture identifies abnormal cells in the cerebrospinal fluid. Bone marrow aspiration and bone scans identify extracranial primary neoplastic growth, since cancers in other sites can metastasize to the brain.

Treatment depends on the type of brain tumor. Surgery is common. It may be performed to obtain a biopsy specimen, to debulk (reduce the tumor by partial removal) or excise the tumor, or to treat any hydrocephalus that may be present. During surgery, radiology images allow the neurosurgeon to see computerized images of the brain while stimulating nerves to determine their functioning. These techniques provide rapid feedback to the neurosurgeon. Laser surgery, which has delicate precise control and accuracy, is used when tumors are close to sensitive neural or vascular structures.

Use of radiation after surgery and chemotherapy has improved the survival of children with medulloblastoma and ependymoma. High-dose chemotherapy is often used, and this modality has improved the survival of children with central nervous system tumors. Low-dose chemotherapy can shrink and help manage some tumors. Intrathecal administration of chemotherapy is useful in some cases. An Ommaya Reservior, a dome-shaped device with a catheter, may be surgically placed under the scalp to administer chemotherapy directly to the central nervous system.

Nursing Practices

The following drugs are used to treat brain tumors:

Cyclophosphamide	VP-16
Ifosfamide	Cisplatin
Lomustine	Carboplatin
Methotrexate	Nitrosoureas
Vincristine	Temozolomide

(Levy, 2005)

However, the blood-brain barrier reduces the effectiveness of chemotherapy for children with brain tumors. For example, when methotrexate is administered intrathecally (in the spinal canal), only a small amount crosses normal brain capillaries. Radiation is not used in children under 3 years because of resultant damage to brain cells. Hematopoietic stem cell transplantation is increasingly used. Numerous new approaches are being investigated and will be used increasingly in the years ahead. New combinations of chemotherapeutic agents, precision-guided delivery of medications and radiotherapy, gene therapy, cytokine-producing therapy to activate the immune system, and blood-brain barrier disruption are examples of emerging treatments (Khatua & Jalali, 2005).

Complications of treatment for children with brain tumors are significant. They include severe infections (associated with high-dose chemotherapy), seizure activity, sensorimotor defects, hydrocephalus, and growth problems. Care is taken to treat infections early and aggressively. If a cerebrospinal shunt is used, infection or blockage can occur (see Chapter 56 for further discussion of cerebrospinal shunts in children). Anticonvulsants are commonly given prophylactically after surgery. Endocrine problems, such as growth hormone changes, hypothyroidism, and panhypopituitarism, may occur when the tumor is in the hypothalamic-pituitary area. Treatment may also lead to impaired cognitive function and emotional or behavioral problems in some children. Memory deficits and selective attention deficits are the most common problems.

Diabetes insipidus is a special consideration in children with midline brain tumors, such as those that compress the hypothalamus, pituitary stalk, or posterior pituitary gland. Manifestations of diabetes insipidus include voiding of large amounts of dilute urine with a specific gravity of less than 1.005 to 1.010 (see Chapter 54).

Table 52–4 Physiologic Assessment of Brain Tumors

Clinical Manifestations	Assessment
Nonspecific signs: headache, morning vomiting, somnolence, irritability	Level of consciousness, pupil response, pupil shape and size
Secondary signs: disturbances of cranial nerves; other signs depend on site of tumor	All cranial nerves
Focal signs: truncal ataxia (midline brain tumors), general nystagmus, head tilting	Motor ability, head positions when watching television or looking at people (double vision, sixth cranial nerve involvement)

NURSING MANAGEMENT

NURSING ASSESSMENT AND DIAGNOSIS

The focus of physiologic assessment of the child with a brain tumor is determined by its presentation (Table 52–4). Presenting signs can be categorized as follows:

- Nonspecific signs related to increasing intracranial pressure
- Secondary signs related to displacement of intracranial structures
- Focal signs suggesting direct involvement of the brain and cranial nerves

Thorough neurologic examination before surgery is essential to provide a record of baseline functioning. The neurologic examination also allows the evaluation of the child's changing physiologic status before surgery. Ask if the child has manifested slow changes over time or has had quickly developing symptoms. Measurement of head circumference and assessment of the anterior fontanelle are necessary in children under the age of 18 months.

Perform developmental screening on young children using the Denver II or other developmental test (see Chapter 36). Ask about the child's social interactions, school performance, and any behavior changes that have occurred.

Several nursing diagnoses can be identified for the child with a brain tumor, depending on the type and location of the tumor. Some common examples follow:

- *Imbalanced Nutrition: Less than Body Requirements* related to loss of appetite
- *Impaired Physical Mobility* related to tumor pressure on coordination centers
- *Delayed Growth and Development* related to effects of disability
- *Impaired Memory* related to neurologic disturbance
- *Acute Pain* related to compression of brain tissue

PLANNING AND IMPLEMENTATION

The child with a brain tumor requires multidisciplinary care by, among others, a neurologist, neurosurgeon, pediatrician, dietitian, and social worker. Other specialists are also often needed. The nurse can act as a case manager to coordinate the complex care needed by the child.

For the nursing care of children immediately following surgery, refer to Chapter 41. In addition, close monitoring of neurologic status is needed postoperatively (refer to Chapter 56). Be especially alert for signs of increased intracranial pressure and infection. Observe for seizure activity. Administer drugs such as antibiotics and anticonvulsants as ordered.

Signs and symptoms of diabetes insipidus may occur following brain surgery (see Chapter 54 for a description of diabetes insipidus). Nursing care includes hourly measurement of intake and output, measurement of serum sodium levels every 4 to 6 hours, accurate fluid replacement, and frequent assessment of neurologic status. An indwelling urinary catheter is useful for accurate measurement of urinary output.

DISCHARGE PLANNING AND HOME CARE TEACHING

Teach the parents to watch for an increase in voiding of dilute urine. Be sure they can recognize the signs of infection and changes in the child's neurologic status. Once the child is ready for discharge, chemotherapy or radiation may begin; tell parents the reason and potential side effects of these treatments. Help the family get any special equipment they may need to care for the child at home, such as a wheelchair, bed rails, or dressings. The American Cancer Society is a potential resource for assistance with these needs. See the Companion Website for links.

Children with brain tumors, especially those who have received radiation, often have some permanent sequelae. They may have slowed development, incoordination, learning disabilities, or other effects. These sequelae are most common in children who are 3 years of age or younger at the time of radiation therapy. Perform accurate height and weight measures at each healthcare visit. Assess developmental milestones. Ask about progress in school and any special services that might be needed. Perform thorough neurologic assessments. Support the family as they learn to deal with unknown or changed expectations for the child's performance.

EVALUATION

Expected outcomes of nursing care for the child with a brain tumor depend on the site of tumor, clinical therapy, and medical outcome. Some outcomes might include the following:

- Adequate nutritional intake to support growth and prevent malnutrition
- Maintenance of a safe environment
- Physical mobility allowed by developmental level and alterations of disease
- Provision of an environment to meet normal developmental milestones within capability of the child
- Management of pain to a comfort level
- Parental understanding of the diagnosis and treatment plan

NEUROBLASTOMA

Neuroblastoma is the solid tumor most commonly occurring outside the cranium of children. It is responsible for 8–10% of childhood cancers and 15% of cancer deaths in children. The average age at onset is 2 years; it is the most common tumor in infants during the first year of life. Nearly all cases (90%) are diagnosed before 5 years of age (Ater, 2007). Prognosis varies, depending on the staging of the tumor (Table 52–5) and the age of the child, with more favorable outcomes in infants under 1 year of age and in presenting sites in the pelvis or thorax. Less favorable outcomes are associated with presence of N-myc oncogen amplification. Survival rates are 98% for stages 1 and 2, but drop to 22% for stage 4 (Kim & Chung, 2006).

Neuroblastoma is commonly a smooth, hard, nontender mass that can occur anywhere along the sympathetic nervous system chain. A frequent location is the abdomen, although other sites are the adrenal, thoracic, and cervical areas.

Table 52–5 International Neuroblastoma Staging System

Stage	Description
1	Localized tumor confined to the area of origin; complete gross excision, with or without microscopic residual disease; identifiable ipsilateral and contralateral lymph nodes negative microscopically
2A	Unilateral tumor with incomplete gross excision; identifiable ipsilateral and contralateral lymph nodes negative microscopically
2B	Unilateral tumor with complete or incomplete gross excision; with positive ipsilateral regional lymph nodes; identifiable contralateral lymph nodes negative microscopically
3	Tumor infiltrating across the midline with or without regional lymph node involvement; or unilateral tumor with contralateral regional lymph node involvement; or midline tumor with bilateral regional lymph node involvement
4	Dissemination of tumor to distant lymph nodes, bone, bone marrow, liver, and/or other organs (except as defined in stage 4S)
4S	Localized primary tumor as defined for stage 1 or 2 with dissemination limited to liver, skin, and/or bone marrow; bone marrow involvement should be minimal (less than 10% of cells); if greater it is stage 4 disease

Data from National Cancer Institute (2007b). *Neuroblastoma Treatment: Stage Information.* Retrieved from www.cancer.gov/cancertopics/pdq/treatment/neuroblastoma/HealthProfessional/page3

Etiology and Pathophysiology

Neuroblastoma originates in primitive neurocrest cells that form the adrenal medulla, paraganglia, and sympathetic nervous system of the cervical sympathetic chain and the thoracic chain. Fifty percent of neuroblastomas develop in the adrenal medulla, 30% develop in the cervical, thoracic or pelvic ganglia, and the remaining are elsewhere along the sympathetic chain (Ater, 2007). Lymph node metastasis is common because of the close proximity of the tumor origin to the lymph system drainage.

The cause of neuroblastoma is unknown. Theories center on the possible effects of environmental factors such as prenatal drug exposure from the mother and disturbed cellular nerve growth factors. A genetic defect found in many cases of neuroblastoma is a deletion of the short arm of chromosome 1 (1p del). Other abnormalities include 11q, 14q, and 17q. Oncogenes are present in neuroblastoma cells in a DNA sequence known as N-myc, located on chromosome 2. High levels of the N-myc oncogene are associated with rapid disease progression and a poorer prognosis (Ater, 2007).

Clinical Manifestations

The location of the mass determines the symptoms. A retroperitoneal mass causes altered bowel and bladder function; characteristic signs are weight loss, abdominal distention, enlarged liver, irritability, fatigue, and fever. Dyspnea or infection may occur when the tumor is mediastinal. Neck and facial edema may result from vena cava syndrome if the tumor is mediastinal and large. Intracranial lesions may be present with periorbital ecchymosis. Malaise, fever, and a limp can occur if there has been metastasis to the bone. Bone marrow disease can manifest as **pancytopenia** (abnormal depression of all cellular blood components) with neutropenia (causing infections) and anemia (causing fatigue). Metastatic spread can result in an array of symptoms affecting multiple organs.

Clinical Therapy

The International Neuroblastoma Staging System (INSS) recommends different diagnostic and laboratory evaluations for diagnosis of the primary disease and of metastases (see Table 52–5). Biopsy of the tumor is used for initial diagnosis, and metastases are diagnosed by bone marrow biopsy, radiolabeled scanning, x-ray, CT, and MRI. Vanillylmandelic acid (VMA) and homovanillic acid (HVA) levels are usually elevated in the urine and blood (see Appendix B for normal values). They are used initially to diagnose the disease and later to follow its progress. Areas of necrosis and calcification are readily identifiable with radiologic tests. These tests also help in the staging of the disease by identifying metastases. Urinary catecholamines are increased.

Routine blood cell counts are needed, including CBC with differential. The test may reveal anemia and thrombocytopenia. There is no classic WBC response, although thrombocytopenia may occur in association with disseminated intravascular coagulation. **Leukocytosis** (higher than normal leukocyte count) and **leukopenia** (lower than normal leukocyte count) have been observed with bone marrow involvement. Serum electrolytes, liver function studies, lactic dehydrogenase (LDH), coagulation studies, and urinalysis are performed. Elevations in dopamine, ferritin, NSE (an enzyme in neural tissue), LDH, and GD2 (a sugar and lipid molecule on the surface of neural cells) are seen. All of these laboratory findings are used initially to diagnose the disease and later to follow its progress. A biopsy or surgical removal of the tumor will be followed by analysis of its type and genetic abnormalities. Areas of necrosis and calcification in major organs are readily identifiable with radiologic tests and MRIs. These tests also help in the staging of the disease by identifying metastases.

The stage of the tumor determines the treatment protocol. Surgical excision of the mass is performed and may be the only treatment in low-risk stages. With higher risk, surgery is followed by chemotherapy with a combination of drugs. Radiation is often used, especially in disseminated disease or when tumors are not receptive to chemotherapy. Stem cell transplantation may be performed for advanced disease, sometimes followed by the biological modifier *cis*-retinoic acid and fenretinide (to promote apoptosis). Studies are being conducted involving GD2, natural killer cells, and other treatments, as well as gene therapy to interrupt growth of abnormal cells, antitumor vaccines, monoclobal antibodies with growth factors, and high-dose chemotherapy (Ater, 2007).

Nursing Practice

The following drugs are used to treat neuroblastoma:

Cyclophosphamide	Teniposide
Doxorubicin	Etoposide
Cisplatin	Carboplatin
Ifosfamide	

NURSING MANAGEMENT

NURSING ASSESSMENT AND DIAGNOSIS

Assess the presenting site of the tumor, such as the neck or abdomen, by observation and inspection. Palpation is contraindicated to avoid seeding tumor cells. Carefully document related functioning, such as bowel and bladder function. Take vital signs to watch for elevated temperature and vital sign changes caused by a thoracic mass. Observe gait and coordination. Take weight and height and compare to earlier percentiles for the child. Specific assessments during treatment will depend on the treatment methods used (refer to the earlier discussions of chemotherapy and radiation treatment). Psychosocial assessment and emotional assessment of the family are needed.

A variety of nursing diagnoses may be appropriate for the child with neuroblastoma, depending on the location and extent of the presenting disease. Some common diagnoses might include the following:

- *Impaired Gas Exchange* related to ventilation-perfusion imbalance
- *Impaired Physical Mobility* related to neuromuscular impairment
- *Disturbed Sensory Perception (Visual)* related to altered sensory perception
- *Pain* related to tumor pressure and injury
- *Anticipatory Grieving (Family)* related to potential loss of significant person

PLANNING AND IMPLEMENTATION

The nursing management of the child with neuroblastoma can encompass the three phases of medical treatment: chemotherapy, surgery, and radiation. Specific postsurgical care depends on the size and site of the tumor. Normal postoperative care includes providing fluid support and respiratory care and preventing infection.

Nursing care during the chemotherapy phase includes minimizing side effects, preventing infection, teaching parents about the medications their child is receiving, and monitoring physical and emotional growth and development of the young child. When radiation is part of the treatment, use common nursing measures described earlier in the chapter.

Teaching Highlights

THE CHILD WITH A NEUROBLASTOMA

Surgery Phase

- Teach the parents to observe for signs of infection at the wound site and to take the child's temperature, if necessary.
- Assist the family to provide pain management including medication administration and various comfort measures.
- Teach the parents the importance of keeping accurate records of urine output and bowel movements and to notify the healthcare provider if the child does not have a bowel movement at least every 3 days.
- Continue with progression to a regular diet.

Chemotherapy Phase

The child frequently has a central line placed early in the chemotherapy phase. The central line greatly reduces the emotional trauma associated with chemotherapy and blood tests.

- Teach the child how to help the parents with cleaning of the central line.
- Teach the child how to protect the central line.
- Teach the parents how to clean and dress the site of the central line.
- Have the parents practice central line care with a model and then on the child before discharge to increase the parents' confidence.
- Give the parents written and illustrated information about care of a central line.
- Arrange for home care dressing supplies before discharge.
- Give the parents detailed chemotherapy information.
- Teach administration of any medications that the parent will perform via central line or other routes.
- Refer the family to the American Cancer Society for coloring books for children receiving chemotherapy.

Topics for parent and family teaching and discharge planning are presented in "Teaching Highlights: The Child with a Neuroblastoma." Ongoing support and connection to resources to assist in management of the child's treatment at home will be needed. When the prognosis is poor, parents may appreciate referrals to hospice, to other parents who have experienced similar child illnesses, and to other community resources. See Chapter 41∞ for additional nursing care for the end of life.

EVALUATION

Expected outcomes of nursing care for the child with neuroblastoma include the following:

- Ventilatory exchange adequate to support daily activities
- Physical mobility to level possible considering developmental age
- Management of sensory/perceptual alterations to provide for safety and sensory input
- Management of pain to level of comfort
- Acceptance and integration of diagnosis into lives of family members

WILMS' TUMOR (NEPHROBLASTOMA)

Nephroblastoma, an intrarenal tumor of which the most common type is Wilms' tumor, is a common abdominal tumor of childhood and accounts for 6% of all childhood tumors (Dome, Perlman, Ritchey, et al., 2006). The incidence is approximately 7.6 cases per million children annually. Wilms' tumor occurs most frequently between 41 and 47 months of age, with young ages more commonly associated with bilateral disease (Dome et al., 2006; Jaffe & Huff, 2007).

Etiology and Pathophysiology

Wilms' tumor is associated with several congenital anomalies: aniridia (absence of the iris), hemihypertrophy (abnormal growth of one half of the body or a body structure), genitourinary anomalies, nevi, and hamartomas (benign, nodulelike growths). These connections suggest a genetic link; chromosome deletions at 11p13 and 11p15 (locations for WT1 and WT2 genes) have been associated with Wilms' tumor. It has a high incidence in Beckwith-Wiedemann syndrome, which is characterized by macroglossia and hypoglycemia. However, most children with Wilms' tumor have no other abnormalities. Wilms' tumor grows very quickly, doubling its size in 11 to 13 days. Such fast growth generally contributes to a large tumor by the time of diagnosis. However, chemotherapy drugs have significantly increased survival rates for children with Wilms' tumor, with 90% survival rates (Kutluk, Varan, Buyukpamukcu, et al., 2006). Tissue type is associated with outcome, with anaplastic tumors having a less favorable prognosis.

Clinical Manifestations

Wilms' tumor is usually an asymptomatic, firm, lobulated mass located to one side of the midline in the abdomen. Often a parent discovers the mass during the child's bath. Hypertension caused by increased renin activity related to renal damage is reported in 25% of cases. Hematuria or abdominal pain is sometimes present.

Clinical Therapy

The diagnosis of Wilms' tumor is based on an ultrasound study of the abdomen and an intravenous pyelogram. CT scanning or MRI of the lungs, liver, spleen, and brain may be performed to identify any metastasis. This information is used in staging the tumor (Table 52–6). A complete blood count is obtained, as well as BUN and creatinine levels. Liver function tests are performed.

Treatment is multifaceted and increasingly successful; about 90% of early stages and 70% of metastic cases have long-term survivial (Kutluk et al., 2006). Surgery is performed to remove the affected kidney, to examine the opposite kidney, and to look for other sites of metastasis. Chemotherapy or radiation therapy,

Table 52–6 National Wilms' Tumor Study Staging System

Stage	Description
I	The tumor is limited to the kidney and completely excised. The surface of the renal capsule is intact. The tumor is not ruptured before or during removal. No residual tumor is apparent beyond the margins of the excision.
II	The tumor extends beyond the kidney but is completely excised. Regional extension of the tumor is present (i.e., penetration through the outer surface of the renal capsule into the perirenal soft tissues). Vessels outside the kidney substance are infiltrated or contain tumor thrombus. Biopsy may have been performed on the tumor, or local spillage of tumor confined to the flank has occurred. No residual tumor is apparent at or beyond the margin of excision.
III	Residual nonhematogenous tumor is confined to the abdomen. Any of the following may occur: ■ Lymph nodes on biopsy are found to be involved in the hilus, the periaortic chains, or beyond. ■ Diffuse peritoneal contamination by the tumor has occurred, such as by spillage of tumor beyond the flank before or during surgery, or by tumor growth that has penetrated through the peritoneal surface. ■ Implants are found on peritoneal surfaces. ■ The tumor extends beyond the surgical margins either microscopically or grossly. ■ The tumor is not completely resectable because of local infiltration into vital structures.
IV	Hematogenous metastasis: deposits are present beyond stage III (e.g., lung, liver, bone, and/or brain).
V	Bilateral renal involvement is present at diagnosis. An attempt should be made to stage each side according to the above criteria on the basis of extent of disease before biopsy.

Data from National Cancer Institute (2007c). *Wilms' Tumor and Other Childhood Kidney Tumors: Stage Information.* Retrieved from www.cancer.gov/cancertopics/pdq/treatment/wilms/HealthProfessional/page3

alone or in combination, is sometimes used before surgery to reduce the size of the tumor. Radiation, chemotherapy, or both may also follow surgery. Children whose tumors are almost completely excised and who have a favorable prognosis do not require irradiation of the tumor bed and may receive limited chemotherapy.

Long-term complications of treatment include liver damage, portal hypertension, and mild cirrhosis, which may occur in children treated for right-sided Wilms' tumor. Radiation damage (such as thinning or weakening) of the skeleton, pelvis, and thorax has been reported. Kyphosis and scoliosis may occur from irradiation of vertebral bodies and the pelvis. Glomerular damage to the remaining kidney may also occur. Second malignancies in the original radiation field have occurred with orthovoltage radiation, but recent changes in radiation therapy have reduced this risk.

Nursing Practice

The following drugs are used to treat Wilms' tumor:

Vincristine	Doxorubicin
Actinomycin D	Cyclophosphamide

NURSING MANAGEMENT

NURSING ASSESSMENT AND DIAGNOSIS

Perform a thorough baseline assessment of the child. Do not palpate the abdomen because of the potential for spreading the cancerous cells. Monitor the child's blood pressure carefully as hypertension is a common finding that may require treatment.

Nursing diagnoses for a child with Wilms' tumor will differ depending on the phase of treatment. Some common nursing diagnoses might include the following:

- *Risk for Infection* related to inadequate defenses
- *Impaired Urinary Elimination* related to anatomic obstruction
- *Ineffective Cardiopulmonary Tissue Perfusion* related to hypertension caused by mechanical reduction of blood flow
- *Risk for Caregiver Role Strain* related to child's illness severity
- *Risk for Impaired Home Maintenance* related to child's disease

PLANNING AND IMPLEMENTATION

Nursing management can be divided into two phases: the postrenal surgery phase and the chemotherapy phase. (See Chapter 41∞ for general care of the child after surgery.) Drawings and special teaching dolls with removable kidneys can be used to teach young children about the surgery. Although chemotherapy may occur at two different times, before and after surgery, nursing management considerations remain the same.

Nursing care during the postrenal surgery phase focuses on pain management and close monitoring of fluid levels. A large incision is necessary to remove the kidney, and the resultant postoperative shift of organs and fluid in the abdominal cavity may create discomfort for the child. Frequently reposition the child and use noninvasive and pharmacologic pain interventions

Nursing Practice

If you feel a mass during palpation of a child's abdomen, stop palpating immediately and report the finding to the child's primary care practitioner. Never palpate the liver or abdomen of a child with Wilms' tumor as this could cause a piece of the tumor to dislodge. Place a sign on the child's bed and in the chart alerting health providers not to palpate the abdomen.

to improve the child's comfort. Gentle handling is important. Monitor fluids closely following surgery to prevent hypovolemia and to assess the shift of fluids out of the third space and out of the body. Assess daily weight, intake and output (I&O), and urine specific gravity. Monitor the function of the remaining kidney. Take blood pressure frequently to watch for signs of shock and to assess the functioning of the remaining kidney.

During the chemotherapy phase, monitor the child for side effects of drugs, the potential for infection from the central line site, and the function of the remaining kidney. Advise parents about home care needs, administration of medications, and monitoring for drug side effects and ongoing needs for health monitoring. A long-term complication in children who received doxorubicin treatment is congestive heart failure, so ongoing periodic healthcare evaluations are needed. Be sure care is well coordinated among all healthcare providers.

EVALUATION

Desired outcomes for nursing care of the child with nephroblastoma include balanced intake and output, normal vital signs, recovery from surgery, and successful family management of postsurgical care and ongoing treatments.

BONE TUMORS

OSTEOSARCOMA

Osteosarcoma is the most common tumor affecting the skeleton of children, with an incidence of 5.6 cases per million children. Its peak incidence is during the rapid growth years, at 13 years for girls, and 14 years for boys (Hartford, Wodowski, Rao, et al., 2006). The tumor is usually located at the metaphysis of the distal femur, proximal tibia, or proximal humerus.

Etiology and Pathophysiology

Bone tissue produced by osteosarcoma never matures into compact bone. Although the cause of osteosarcoma is unknown, radiation exposure (either environmental or treatment related) is associated with its development. Survivors of retinoblastoma have a greatly increased incidence of osteosarcoma. An abnormality of gene p53 has been noted in some cases of this cancer, leading to oncogene malformations and possibly to an absence of tumor suppressor genes (Wunder, Gokgoz, Parkes, et al., 2005).

Clinical Manifestations

The common initial symptoms are pain, swelling, and a limp. The pain can be referred to the hip or back, which can delay diagnosis. Deep bone pain causing night awakenings should be investigated (Arndt, 2007). Pulmonary metastasis occurs in 20% of cases. Other metastatic sites include kidney, adrenals, brain, and pericardium. When lung metastasis is the only site, lung resection may be successful for treatment. Disseminated metastases and bone lesions have poorer prognoses.

> **Nursing Practice**
>
> The following drugs are used to treat osteosarcoma:
>
> - Methotrexate with leucovorin rescue
> - Doxorubicin
> - Cisplatin
> - Ifosfamide with mesna

Clinical Therapy

Diagnosis is made through radiographic studies of the affected area, bone scan, CT or MRI scans of involved bone, blood test for serum alkaline phosphatase and lactic dehydrogenase (levels may be elevated), and tumor biopsy (to confirm the diagnosis). Arteriography may be performed if limb-sparing surgery is contemplated. Complete blood count, liver studies, and renal studies are performed for information about possible metastases.

Treatment involves both surgery and chemotherapy. The surgery is either a limb-salvage procedure or limb amputation. In limb-salvage procedures the tumor is removed and an internal prosthesis is inserted. A limb-salvage procedure is possible if bone growth has taken place and a neurobundle (area where several nerves converge) is not involved in the tumor. If these two criteria are not met, limb amputation is necessary. Physical rehabilitation will be needed after either amputation or limb-salvage procedure. Aggressive chemotherapy following surgery has improved the survival rate. At the time of diagnosis, most children have metastases (even though they may not be identifiable), so chemotherapy is needed. Chemotherapy is started before surgery to shrink the tumor, especially when limb-salvage surgery is planned. It is also given postoperatively to treat and prevent metastasis.

EWING'S SARCOMA

Ewing's sarcoma is a malignant, small, round cell tumor usually involving the diaphyseal (shaft) portion of the long bones. The most common sites are the femur, pelvis, tibia, fibula, ribs, humerus, scapula, and clavicle, but any bone may be involved. Ewing's sarcoma occurs in two children per million, is most common in whites and Hispanics, and is rare in black and Asian American children. The incidence is highest in children between the ages of 5 and 20 years (Khoury, 2005).

Translocations on chromosomes 11 and 22 have been identified in children with Ewing's sarcoma; these are t(11;22)(q24;q12). In addition, these tumors express a proto-oncogene, c-myc.

The symptoms are similar to those of osteosarcoma and may include pain, swelling, fever, an elevated WBC count, an elevated erythrocyte sedimentation rate, and elevated C-reactive protein. Some children present with a fracture of the affected bone. A tumor biopsy is necessary for diagnosis. Diagnostic tests are the same as those for osteosarcoma.

Initial treatment for Ewing's sarcoma is chemotherapy to reduce the tumor, followed by surgical removal of the entire bone

MyNursingKit Case Study: Teens with Ewing's Sarcoma

Nursing Practice

The following drugs are used to treat Ewing's sarcoma:

Vincristine	Doxorubicin
Cyclophosphamide	Ifosfamide
Dactinomycin	Etoposide

or intensive high-dose irradiation of the entire bone. Limb-salvage procedures are now commonly performed rather than amputation. Surgery is preferred because of the possibility of a secondary cancer from radiation. Chemotherapy is always used after initial treatment, as undetectable metastases are nearly always present.

NURSING MANAGEMENT

NURSING ASSESSMENT AND DIAGNOSIS

Carefully evaluate any child or adolescent who has a limp or complains of pain in an extremity. Confirm the onset and whether the symptoms were associated with injury. Refer for further evaluation if the discomfort persists or is not associated with injury. Physiologic assessment of the child with a bone tumor includes assessment of the site before surgery. Assess the child's pain or discomfort, mobility, and gait. Take careful vital signs, especially noting temperature and respirations. Psychologic assessments of the child and family are needed, especially if amputation is planned. Loss of a limb causes body image disturbances, particularly with school-age children and adolescents. Assess the child's understanding of the treatment and of care after surgery. Find out what support systems are available to the family.

Observe the wound postoperatively for infection and hemorrhage. Assess circulation above and below the operative site. If edema is found, elevate the limb. If a limb-salvage procedure is performed, the child's extremity will remain, but it will not function as before because muscle insertion sites and mass have been removed with the tumor during surgery. Detailed charting of the condition of the surgical site and limb function is important.

If the limb has been amputated, assess the child for the following signs indicating a disturbed body image:

- Refusal to look at or touch the altered or missing body part
- Preoccupation with loss or change
- Feelings of shame or embarrassment, either verbalized or demonstrated
- Distorted perception of normal body (easily seen in the child's drawings of the body)
- Fears of rejection or unwanted attention from others
- Overexposure or hiding of the affected body part
- Actual or perceived change in the structure and function of the body or body parts

Psychosocial assessment of the child and family is discussed in more detail earlier in the general section titled "Childhood Cancer" (see pages 1478–1480).

Nursing diagnoses for the child with a bone tumor are based on the treatment and needs of each child. The nursing diagnoses that might be appropriate include the following:

- *Risk for Infection* related to amputation or limb-salvage procedure
- *Impaired Skin Integrity* related to mechanical forces of prosthesis
- *Impaired Physical Mobility* related to musculoskeletal impairment
- *Impaired Adjustment* related to disability and lifestyle change
- *Disturbed Body Image* related to treatment and injury
- *Pain* related to physical injury of tissues

PLANNING AND IMPLEMENTATION

Care of the child after surgery involves general postoperative care (see Chapter 41∞). The child who has had an amputation has special needs regarding skin care and rehabilitation. Inspect the tissue at the surgical site, using sterile technique, and turn the child at least every 2 hours. The site needs to heal completely before chemotherapy can begin and a prosthesis can be made. Pain management is a major nursing care need. When amputation has occurred the adolescent will often experience phantom pain. This is pain that feels as if it is in the amputated extremity and is caused by trauma to the nerves in the area of the amputation. Acknowledge the pain as real since the nerve endings are intact and the patient is perceiving real discomfort. Medicate adequately and use additional pain control measures such as repositioning the limb using gentle movement, supporting the limb, and using distraction or deep breathing.

Discuss insurance and other financial arrangements with the parents, as prosthetics can be costly. Physical therapy will be needed as well. Referral to a Shriners Hospital is an option for some families.

Implement plans to help the child deal with body image disturbance. Plan for a visit from another child who is well adjusted to a prosthesis. Help the child gradually learn how to care for the stump. Slow progress may be made as the child first looks briefly, then for longer periods, and finally is willing to touch the stump. Show the child how it is possible to continue with sports such as baseball, skiing, or biking with a prosthesis. A discussion group with others can be very useful for adolescents. Plan with the child how to tell friends about the surgery and what issues he or she may face upon return to school. Make plans for elevator access if needed and emergency evacuation procedures. Some children or adolescents may need referral for counseling to assist in dealing with body image disturbance.

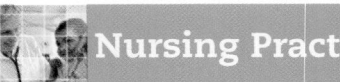

The child will receive physical rehabilitation while hospitalized and after discharge. When the child is discharged, explain to the family the importance of bringing the child for outpatient chemotherapy and physical rehabilitation visits. Special arrangements may be needed at the child's school to accommodate a wheelchair, crutches, or ambulation with a new prosthesis. Call or visit the school to see whether there are buttons to open doors, wide doorways to facilitate passage, and any limitations of the building. Contact school personnel to plan the child's return.

Follow-up care is needed to monitor for progress and to be alert for signs of metastases. Fracture may be a sign of recurrent tumor. All body systems such as lungs, heart, kidneys, and liver are monitored for signs of recurrence.

EVALUATION

Expected outcomes of nursing care for the child with a bone tumor focus on the treatments required and adaptation to changes in lifestyle. Examples include the following:

- Healed surgical site with no signs of infection
- Adaptation to changes in mobility status
- Successful adjustment to changes required in school settings
- Maintenance of healthy skin
- Positive body image
- Management of pain to comfort level
- Successful integration of continuing medical therapy

LEUKEMIA

Leukemia is among the most commonly diagnosed pediatric malignancies in children under 14 years of age. A cancer of the blood-forming organs, leukemia is characterized by a proliferation of abnormal white blood cells in the body. Several types of leukemia are differentiated, depending on the blood cells affected. The main types are acute lymphoblastic leukemia, acute nonlymphocytic leukemia (acute myelogenous leukemia), and the rare chronic leukemias of childhood.

The most common type of childhood leukemia is acute lymphoblastic leukemia (ALL), which accounts for 25% of all childhood cancer and 78% of leukemias in children. The peak age at onset is 2 to 3 years. ALL is more common in whites and in boys (American Cancer Society, 2006b). Subtypes of ALL are based on the French-American-British (FAB) system of classification. There are three types of ALL in the FAB system: L1, L2, and L3. Rasheed, who is described in the opening scenario, has ALL.

Acute nonlymphocytic leukemia (ANLL) refers to all leukemias from myeloid cells. About 17% of childhood leukemias are ANLL. ANLL is most common in children younger than 2 years of age and in adolescents. It is more common in males than females and in Asians/Pacific Islanders, Hispanics, and whites than in blacks (Brown, 2006). There are several subtypes of ANLL in the FAB classification:

M0 = acute nonlymphocytic leukemia without maturation
M1 = acute nonlymphocytic leukemia with poor maturation
M2 = acute nonlymphocytic leukemia with maturation
M3 = acute promyelocytic leukemia
M4 = acute myelomonocytic leukemia
M5 = acute monocytic leukemia
M6 = erythroleukemia
M7 = acute megakaryocytic leukemia

Developing Cultural Competence

PREVALENCE OF LEUKEMIA

Black, Hispanic, and Native American children have statistically poorer outcomes from leukemia treatment than do white and Asian children. Analysis of 5-year survival rates demonstrated poorer outcomes for black children than white children with AML (Rubnitz, Lensing, Razzouk, et al., 2007). It is unclear whether racial and ethnic groups with poorer outcomes have particular genetic characteristics placing them at risk, do not obtain treatment as soon, have more complications from the disease, enroll less often in clinical trials, or have less access to care at oncology centers. Clearly more research is needed to describe and then eliminate the racial and ethnic disparity in leukemia treatment outcomes.

Because chronic leukemias such as chronic myelocytic, chronic myelomonocytic, and chronic lymphocytic leukemia are rare in children, the following discussion will focus on ALL and ANLL.

Etiology and Pathophysiology

MyNursingKit Video: Leukemia

The causes of leukemia are not well understood. Some investigators theorize that exposure to infectious agents can predispose children to leukemia. Genetic factors are believed to play a role in some types of the disease. For instance, children with chromosomal defects such as Down syndrome, neurofibromatosis type I, Bloom syndrome, and Shwachman syndrome have an increased incidence of ALL, and chromosomal abnormalities are present in most children with ALL (Bennett & Konrokji, 2005). Children with immune deficiency states, such as ataxia-telangiectasia, congenital hypogammaglobulinemia, and Wiskott–Aldrich syndrome, have an increased risk of ALL.

Ionizing radiation exposure when in utero and chemical agents such as treatment with chemotherapy for other cancers are thought to play some role in the development of ANLL. There are several chromosomal and genetic abnormalities associated with ANLL. For example, trisomy 8 is associated with all subtypes of the disease (Jaff, Chelghoum, Elhamri, et al., 2006).

Leukemia occurs when the stem cells in the bone marrow produce immature WBCs that cannot function normally. These cells proliferate rapidly by cloning instead of normal mitosis, causing the bone marrow to fill with abnormal WBCs. The abnormal cells then spill out into the circulatory system where they steadily replace the normally functioning WBCs. As this occurs, the protective lymphocytic functions such as cellular and humeral immunity are reduced, leaving the body vulnerable to infections.

The malignant WBCs rapidly fill the bone marrow, replacing stem cells that produce erythrocytes (red blood cells) and other blood products such as platelets, thereby decreasing the amount of these products in circulation. The stem cells are replaced by leukemic clones, eventually resulting in anemia. Children with leukemia commonly experience abnormal bleeding because of the reduced amounts of platelets.

Clinical Manifestations

Children with ALL and ANLL usually have fever, pallor, overt signs of bleeding, lethargy, malaise, anorexia, and large joint or bone pain. Petechiae, frank bleeding, and joint pain are cardinal signs of bone marrow failure. Enlargement of the liver and spleen (hepatosplenomegaly) and changes in the lymph nodes (lymphadenopathy) are common. If the leukemia has infiltrated the central nervous system (entered it by means of the circulatory or lymphoid system), the child may have signs such as headache, vomiting, papilledema, and sixth cranial nerve palsy (inability to move the eye laterally). These findings are caused by the leukemic cells massing and putting pressure on nerves. The testicles, spinal cord, and bone marrow are common sites for infiltration. The leukemic cells in the testicle become a mass that causes the testicle to enlarge, often painlessly.

Clinical Therapy

Diagnosis is based initially on blood counts and bone marrow aspiration. Blood counts reveal anemia, **thrombocytopenia**, and neutropenia. Bone marrow aspiration reveals immature and abnormal lymphoblasts and hypercellular marrow and is the differential test. The percentage of blast cells in marrow is measured and 25% lymphoblasts is definitive of disease (Brown, 2006). Neutropenia, thrombocytopenia, and anemia are commonly noted. Other abnormal laboratory findings include elevated serum uric acid and elevated calcium, potassium, and phosphorus levels. New laboratory studies such as rapid flow cytometric assay are making the measurement of even very small numbers of leukemic cells possible, so that treatment can improve prognosis in children with minimal residual disease. Leukemic cells are examined and classified by FAB type, and DNA analysis may provide clues about genetic changes; all of these considerations are used to establish the protocol for treatment. Blood cells of children with ALL are B cell or T cell; these classifications are also used to establish treatment protocols.

Treatment of ALL involves radiation and chemotherapy. Radiation is used for central nervous system disease, in T cell leukemia, and for testicular involvement. Chemotherapy is organized into four phases: (1) induction, (2) consolidation, (3) delayed intensification, and (4) maintenance of remission. Additional drugs may be used for treatment of central nervous system involvement. Maintenance therapy may continue for 2 to 3 years, causing decreased resistance to infection for this prolonged period. Treatment of ANLL involves use of a wide variety of drugs during the induction and consolidation phases.

Maximum cell death occurs during the induction phase. The cells that remain after this period are more resistant to treatment. After 3 to 4 weeks, when a remission has occurred, central nervous system prophylaxis begins. Drugs are used in combination with cranial irradiation. During the consolidation phase, chemotherapy with L-asparaginase and doxorubicin is administered. Delayed intensification uses additional drugs to target the leukemic cells that have survived. Treatment during the maintenance phase is aimed at destroying the remaining leukemic cells. Combinations of active drugs are used to prevent resistance. Occasionally other drugs are added to the regimen, such as vincristine, prednisone, cyclophosphamide, intravenous methotrexate, cytosine arabinoside, or anthracyclines (See "Drug Guide" on the Companion Website).

The prognosis for children with leukemia is much improved with current therapy. However, several risk factors affect the long-term outcome. The most favorable findings are:

- Age at onset between 2 and 10 years
- Initial hemoglobin level less than 10 g/dL
- Low initial WBC count

Nursing Practice

The following drugs are used to treat acute lymphoblastic leukemia:

Induction phase

Prednisone	L-asparaginase
Vincristine	Daunorubicin
Central nervous system prophylaxis	
Intrathecal methotrexate	

Consolidation phase

L-asparaginase	Doxorubicin

Delayed intensification

Vincristine	Cyclophosphamide
Ara-C	

Maintenance phase

6-mercaptopurine or 6-thioguanine
Methotrexate

Nursing Practice

Following are the laboratory values in leukemia:

USUAL	**COMMON VALUES IN LEUKEMIA**
Leukocytes	
less than 10,000/microL	greater than 10,000/microL
Platelets	
150,000–400,000/microL	20,000–100,000/microL
Hemoglobin	
12–16 g/dL	7–11 g/dL

Nursing Practice

The following drugs are used to treat ANLL:

Induction phase

Daunorubicin	Mitoxantrone
Doxorubicin	Cytarabine

Consolidation phase

Etoposide	Teniposide

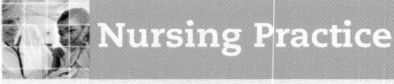

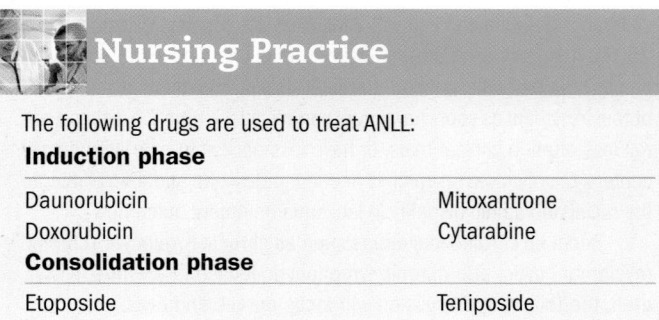

- Lack of B- or T-cell antigens
- Absence of extramedullary (outside bone marrow or spinal cord) involvement
- Rapid response to chemotherapy.

The most important factor is the initial leukocyte count. The higher the leukocyte count (over 50,000/mm³) at diagnosis, the worse the prognosis. For children in the low-risk group, the probability of prolonged survival is as high as 90%; even higher risk ALL has a 75–80% survival rate with current treatments (Pui & Evans, 2006). Infants under 12 months of age have a poor prognosis. Treatment methods and duration are adjusted for each child, depending on that child's risk factors. More aggressive treatment is undertaken for those in the higher risk groups.

Approximately 10% of children have a relapse within a year after completing treatment. Treatment for relapse consists of additional chemotherapy drugs. The prognosis is best if the relapse occurs late after the initial diagnosis and after the initial treatment is completed. Bone marrow transplantation is a treatment option for the child who has a relapse with ALL, who then achieves a second remission; the transplant is given when the child is in remission. Transplant is also used for children with ANLL; they do not need to be in remission for the transplant to be performed. Chemotherapy itself can create numerous complications, affecting all body organs. Central nervous system toxicity; damage to organs such as pituitary, liver, kidneys, heart, and lungs; and secondary malignancies sometimes occur.

NURSING MANAGEMENT

NURSING ASSESSMENT AND DIAGNOSIS

Thorough physical assessment is important to ensure prompt identification of problems without injuring the child who has deficient coagulation and immune function. Perform assessments every 8 hours or more often depending on the chemotherapy regimen. Observe carefully for bruising, other new sites of bleeding, and fever or other signs of infection. Once chemotherapy has begun, closely monitor renal functioning through specific gravity, I&O, and daily weight measurement. Monitor dietary intake, nausea, vomiting, and constipation. Observe for mucosal sores in the mouth. A central line is usually in place for intravenous infusion of medications, so carefully assess the line for proper functioning and for signs of infection. Ask the parents about any behavioral changes. Central nervous system infiltration can affect the child's level of consciousness, causing irritability, vomiting, and lethargy. However, chemotherapeutic drugs and antiemetics can also induce these nonspecific signs. Frequent venipunctures, bone marrow aspirations, and lumbar punctures require pain assessment and an evaluation of the level of knowledge and coping skills of child and family.

Leukemia causes many changes in the body, and confirmation of the disease is difficult for families to face. Among the many nursing diagnoses that might be appropriate for the child with leukemia are the following:

- *Imbalanced Nutrition: Less than Body Requirements* related to inability to ingest food
- *Risk for Infection* related to altered immune system functioning
- *Risk for Injury* related to bleeding
- *Activity Intolerance* related to generalized weakness
- *Pain* related to chemotherapy and disease process
- *Disturbed Sleep Pattern* related to chemotherapy drugs and disease process
- *Anxiety (Child and Parent)* related to change in health status
- *Risk for Caregiver Role Strain* related to length of treatment, disruptions of life patterns, and anxiety

PLANNING AND IMPLEMENTATION

Bone marrow suppression may necessitate transmission-based precautions. Instruct parents in the prevention of infection and use nursing care measures to prevent infection also. Perform careful hand hygiene; take temperature frequently; give mouth care with antibacterial mouth washes; inspect skin, mouth, rectal area, and central line site for any signs of infection. Care of mouth sores and other side effects of chemotherapy is presented in "Nursing Care Plan: Hospital Care of the Child with Cancer" earlier in this chapter.

Special attention to renal function is needed when the child receives cyclophosphamide. Gross hematuria is a side effect of this drug. Hydration with intravenous fluids to attain a specific gravity of less than 1.010 prevents or reduces the severity of hematuria. It also prepares the kidneys to manage products of tumor cell breakdown. To achieve the desired specific gravity, the child receives intravenous fluids at 1.5 times maintenance volume for at least 6 to 8 hours before and at least 1.5 hours after administration of the drug. Other chemotherapy drugs have different infusion times, while some do not require hydration prior to infusion. Check drug references carefully for recommendations with each drug. Evaluate the infusion site before and frequently during infusion. Although extravasation is not as common with central lines used in cancer treatment as in peripheral lines, it still can occur. Many chemotherapy agents are extremely toxic to tissues. In addition, lysis of the cancer cells can produce toxic side effects (see oncologic emergencies described earlier in the chapter). Careful monitoring of I&O is required to record the intravenous fluids, assess kidney functioning, and monitor excretion of by-products from destroyed tumor cells. Monitor specific gravity every 8 hours, as well as before and during administration of the drug, and when the intravenous fluids are reduced to maintenance volume levels. Daily weight measurements are important to assist in planning adequate hydration during chemotherapy, as well as to measure nutritional status.

MyNursingKit Life with Leukemia: A Teen in Transition

Drug side effects may necessitate infusion of platelets or packed red blood cells. See the Clinical Skills Manual **SKILLS** for techniques to be used in these situations.

Many children are treated in an oncology clinic, staying in the hospital only on the day of intravenous drug administration and receiving oral medications at home. The time at the

Teaching Highlights

CHILD CHEMOTHERAPY FOR LEUKEMIA

Physical Care

- Have rest periods each day.
- Avoid exposure to people with illnesses.
- Drink generous amounts of water.
- Eat a healthy diet, using frequent, small, and nutritious meals to obtain enough nutrients.
- Take medicines prescribed to decrease nausea.
- Maintain good oral hygiene with a soft toothbrush and water pick.
- Avoid sun exposure and check skin each day for any signs of bruises, pressure areas, cuts, or scratches.
- Allow time for and eat foods to promote bowel elimination.
- Promote bowel elimination through regular dietary and toileting practices.
- Report any signs of infection, changes in condition, or other concerns.

Emotional Care

- Be prepared for loss of hair with plans for hats, wigs, or other alternatives.
- Continue contact with friends via phone, Internet, and in person when possible.
- Try relaxation techniques to aid in sleep and management of treatments.
- Talk with clergy, teachers, parents, counselors, friends, or other supportive people about the experience of having leukemia.
- Keep a journal to record feelings and experiences.

(Adapt the highlights for parents when the child is too young to manage his or her own care.)

hospital is used to assess how the family is managing issues such as nutrition, sleep, medication administration, and obtaining psychosocial support. Careful teaching for the family is needed to ensure safe drug administration and identification of issues requiring further care.

Nurses play a key role in the long-term multidisciplinary treatment of children with leukemia. The impact of a diagnosis of leukemia and the long-term nature of treatment can severely stress the coping abilities of both the child and the family. Ongoing psychosocial assessment and emotional support are essential (see the general discussion of Psychosocial Assessment in the section "Childhood Cancer," pages 1478–1480). Referral to support groups and social services may be beneficial. Help the family explore alternative therapies such as relaxation, imagery, and nutritional support that may aid the child. Be alert for any interactions that could occur between alternative therapies and the medical regimen.

Thinking Critically

FAMILY SUPPORT DURING CHILDHOOD CANCER

Sam is a 4-year-old boy recently diagnosed with ALL. He has been hospitalized for initial diagnostic work and the beginning of chemotherapy. Sam lives about 70 miles from the hospital and his parents have been taking turns staying with him. He has two older siblings at home who are 6 and 9 years old. What are the most urgent needs for the parents? The siblings? What information should you collect to start a plan for psychosocial support for the family?

See MyNursingKit for possible responses.

EVALUATION

Expected outcomes for nursing care of the child with leukemia include the following:

- Prevention of infection
- Adequate hydration
- Normal urinary output
- Blood values within normal limits
- Successful family adaptation to parenting a child with chronic illness
- Adequate parental knowledge related to disease process

Complementary Care

NURSING ROLE IN CAM STUDIES

Complementary medicine practices are commonly used by families to increase children's comfort during therapeutic treatment. About one-half of families queried used some type of complementary and alternative medical (CAM) treatments for their children with cancer. Most common approaches were spiritual and mental approaches, and herbal or vitamin remedies (Martel, Bussieres, Theoret, et al., 2005). National initiatives have identified CAM treatments that should be tested for efficacy. For example, a study is being conducted to learn if tramneel-s, a compound of plant extracts, is useful in treatment of oral mucositis during cancer treatment in children (Hawks, 2006). Nurses play a major role in identifying families and children who may wish to participate in studies of cam, informing the families fully about the study, answering questions, and possibly conducting the data gathering to provide the definitive results. Additionally, nurses inquire about treatments that the family is using or those about which they need further information. Inquire about massage, vitamins, herbs, prayer, music, and other techniques. How can you phrase your questions in an open and nonthreatening manner in order to elicit the information from families?

SOFT-TISSUE TUMORS

HODGKIN DISEASE

Hodgkin disease, a disorder of the lymphoid system, usually arises in a single lymph node or an anatomic group of lymph nodes (see "Pathophysiology Illustrated: Hodgkin Disease"). Hodgkin disease is rare before 10 years of age, accounts for just 5% of cancers in children under 14 years, but 15% of cancer in youth from 15 to 19 years. The disease has a bimodal peak with higher incidence in the early 20s and after 50 years (Cairo & Bradley, 2007). Three forms of the disease exist: that in young persons under 14 years, the young adult form in persons from 15 to 34 years, and older adult form in those over 50 years. There is a slightly increased incidence in males, which is more pronounced in the disease manifested in younger children (Hudson, Onciu, & Donaldson, 2006).

Etiology and Pathophysiology

Hodgkin disease occurs in clusters and has been reported in families. This suggests a possible genetic link as well as an infectious agent (such as Epstein-Barr virus) or environmental hazard (Cairo & Bradley, 2007).

Clinical Manifestations

The main symptom of Hodgkin disease is nontender, firm lymphadenopathy, usually in the supraclavicular and cervical nodes but occasionally in the mediastinal area. A mediastinal growth can cause respiratory difficulty because of pressure on the trachea or bronchi. A characteristic large cell with multiple nuclei, called the Reed-Sternberg cell, is characteristic of Hodgkin, though the cell is found also in infectious mononucleosis and some other lymphomas. Fever, night sweats, and weight loss occur in one third of children with Hodgkin disease and are associated with a more aggressive form of the disease. The leukocyte count and erythrocyte sedimentation rate (ESR) may be elevated.

Table 52–7 Staging System for Hodgkin Disease

Stage	Description
I	Disease within a single lymph node region
IE	Disease within a single extralymphatic organ or site outside of lymphatic system (extralymphatic organ)
II	Disease within two or more lymph node regions on same side of diaphragm
IIE	Disease within extralymphatic organ, and of one or more lymph node regions on same side of diaphragm
III	Disease of lymph node regions on both sides of diaphragm; Stage III(1) indicates involvement of upper abdomen above the renal vein while Stage III(2) indicates involvement of pelvic or other lower abdomen nodes
IIIE	Disease of lymph node regions on both sides of the diaphragm with involvement of extralymphatic organ
IIIS	As in III, plus disease within spleen
IIISE	As in III, plus disease in extralymphatic organs and spleen
IV	Disseminated disease within one or more lymphatic organs with or without lymph node involvement

Data from National Cancer Institute (2008b). Stage Information for Adult Hodgkin Lymphoma. Retrieved from www.cancer.gov/cancertopics/pdq/treatment/adulthodgkins/HealthProfessional/page4

PATHOPHYSIOLOGY ILLUSTRATED

HODGKIN DISEASE

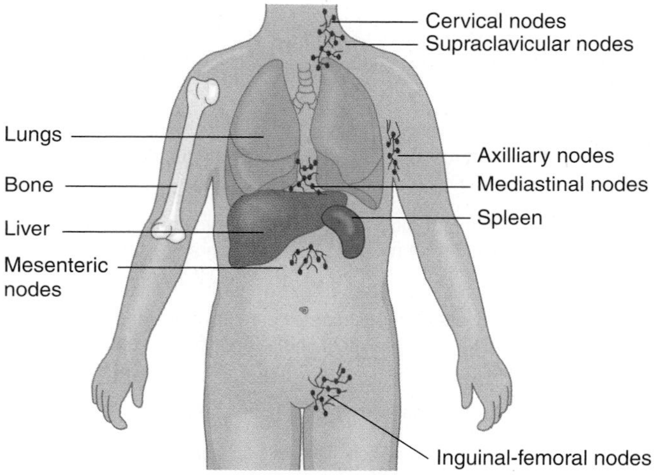

Lymph nodes and organs affected in Hodgkin disease in children.

Clinical Therapy

Diagnosis is based on lymph node biopsy; Reed-Sternberg cells are present. A staging classification is used to determine disease severity (Table 52–7). The basis for staging is data obtained from the history, physical examination, chest x-ray study (for metastasis), chest CT scan, CT or MRI scans of the retroperitoneal nodes, lymphangiogram if there is retroperitoneal involvement, laboratory studies (complete blood count, erythrocyte sedimentation rate, serum copper level, C-reactive protein, liver and renal function tests), and a radionuclide scan with gallium. Bone marrow biopsy, bone scan, or a staging laparotomy may be performed if advanced disease is suspected. Minimally invasive surgery can be used to biopsy or remove the spleen for diagnosis, avoiding the potential complications of major surgery (Hudson et al., 2006).

Chemotherapy using a four-drug combination has been found to be the most effective drug treatment. Radiation is commonly added, with low doses for children who are still growing, and larger doses for those who are physically mature or those whose disease is more advanced at diagnosis. The 5-year survival rate is approximately 85–90%, depending on the stage of the disease at diagnosis.

Nursing Practice

The following drugs are used to treat Hodgkin disease:

ABVD	Adriamycin + bleomycin + vinblastine + dacarbazine
ABVE	Adriamycin (doxorubicin) + bleomycin + vincristine + etoposide
ABVE-PC	Adriamycin (doxorubicin) + bleomycin + vincristine + etoposide + prednisone + cyclophosphamide
COPP	cyclophosphamide + Oncovin + procarbazine + prednisone
EBVP	etoposide + bleomycin + vinblastine + prednisone
MOPP	mechlorethamine + Oncovin (vincristine) + procarbazine + prednisone
OEPA	vincristine + etoposide + prednisone + Adriamycin (doxorubicin)
OPPA	Oncovin + procarbazine + prednisone + Adriamycin
VAMP	vinblastine + Adriamycin (doxorubicin) + methotrexate + prednisone
VEPA	vinblastine + etoposide + prednisone + Adriamycin (doxorubicin)

Autologous stem cell or allogeneic stem cell transplant is a treatment option in children with advanced disease or relapse.

NON-HODGKIN LYMPHOMA

There are three types of pediatric non-Hodgkin lymphoma: (1) lymphoblastic lymphoma (30% to 40%), (2) small non-cleaved cell (Burkitt) lymphoma (40% to 50%), and (3) large cell lymphoma (15%) (Mann, Attarbaschi, Steiner, et al., 2006). Lymphomas of all types are the third most common group of malignancies in children, following leukemia and brain tumors. Non-Hodgkin lymphomas are malignant tumors of lymphoreticular (internal framework of the lymph system) origin. The peak incidence for lymphomas occurs between the ages of 7 and 11 years, and they are three times more common in boys than in girls.

Lymphoblastic non-Hodgkin lymphomas are caused by T-cell abnormalities. These abnormal T cells are diffuse, highly malignant, and very aggressive and do not mature. T-cell lymphomas produced by these cells often occur in children with congenital or acquired immunodeficiency states, chronic immune stimulation, or autoimmune disease. Some lymphomas have B-cell abnormalities, most specifically Burkitt lymphoma; 8q24 chromosomal translocation may be found in these cases. Large cell lymphomas are variable in cell type affected and may also manifest chromosomal translocations (Mann et al., 2006).

The incidence of lymphomas shows geographic variability. For example, a high incidence of Burkitt lymphoma is found in equatorial Africa, where it causes 50% of childhood cancer. Incidence in Hispanic children is higher than in whites, and blacks have the lowest incidence. Males are affected more than females, and children with immune system compromise are most commonly affected. Epstein-Barr virus has been associated with Burkitt lymphoma (Cairo & Bradley, 2007).

Children with non-Hodgkin lymphoma frequently present with fever and weight loss. The lymph glands are usually enlarged or nodular, with the most frequent sites being the cervical, axillary, inguinal, and femoral nodes. However, the disease may be diffuse, without nodular glands. The anterior mediastinum is the primary site for T-cell lymphomas. Tumors that occur in this area may compress the airway (causing breathing difficulty) or superior vena cava (leading to swelling of the face, neck, or arms), and can cause pain. Jaw involvement is common in Burkitt lymphoma.

CBC is performed; additional blood tests include renal and liver function, electrolytes, uric acid, and LDH. Bone marrow aspiration and lumbar puncture are performed. Chest x-ray, bone scan, gallium scan, CT, and MRI can help to isolate affected body organs. Tissue biopsy confirms the diagnosis.

A staging system is used to describe the tumor mass and extension to other body areas (Table 52–8). Treatment is tailored to the type of cancer and its stage. Stages I and II may be treated with drugs such as vincristine, cyclophosphamide, prednisone, and methotrexate for several months. Intrathecal medication is added if head and neck cancers are present. Stages III and IV are treated with additional drugs (up to nine total) for longer periods (1 to 2 years). Radiation is uncommonly used and may be helpful to treat a tumor that is impinging on a body part. Surgery is used to biopsy the tumor mass and treat any complications caused by the cancer. HSCT is used for children with recurrent disease.

RHABDOMYOSARCOMA

Rhabdomyosarcoma is the most common soft-tissue diagnosed in children, and is especially common in children under 5 years of age. The 5-year survival rate is 64% (Punyko, Gurney, Baker,

Table 52–8 St. Jude Children's Research Hospital Staging Classification for non-Hodgkin Lymphoma

Stage	Description
I	Single tumor or node area involved; no tumor in abdomen or mediastinum
II	Single tumor with lymph node involvement; or two node areas or tumor on same side of diaphragm; or GI tumor in one site
III	Two tumors or node areas on different sides of diaphragm; or a primary mediastinal, intra-abdominal, or epidural tumor
IV	Any involvement with CNS or bone marrow metastases

Data from Hussong, M. R. (2002). Non-Hodgkin's lymphoma. In C. R. Baggott, K. P. Kelly, D. Fochtman, & G. V. Foley (Eds.), *Nursing care of children and adolescents with cancer* (3rd ed., p. 539). Philadelphia: WB Saunders.

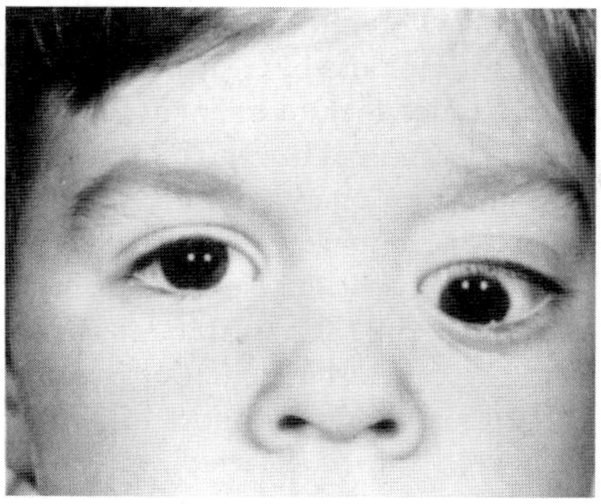

• **Figure 52–10** Rhabdomyosarcoma. Rhabdomyosarcoma is characterized by ptosis and edema.

Used with permission from Vaughn, D., Asbury, J., & Riordan-Eva, P. (1995). General ophthalmology (14th ed.). Norwalk, CT: Appleton: Lange.

Table 52–9 Classification of Rhabdomyosarcoma

Stage	Description
I	Localized tumor, completely resected disease
II	Total gross resection with regional microscopic spread
III	Locally extensive tumor with residual microscopic spread
IV	Any size primary tumor with distant metastatic disease present

Data from Wexler, L. H., Meyer, W. H., & Helman, L. J. (2006). Rhabdomyosarcoma and the undifferentiated sarcomas. In P. A. Pizzo & D. G. Poplack (Eds.). *Principles and practice of pediatric oncology* (5th ed., p. 982). Philadelphia: Lippincott Williams & Wilkins.

et al., 2006). It occurs most often in the muscles around the eyes (extraorbital), in the neck, and less commonly in the abdomen, genitourinary tract, and extremities.

The cause of rhabdomyosarcoma is unknown. However, it is more common in children with neurofibromatosis and Li-Fraumeni syndrome. Mutations in tumor suppressor gene p53 are sometimes seen. The abnormal cells arise from mesenchyme that normally grows into muscle, fat, and bone.

Tumors close to the eye produce swelling, ptosis, visual disturbances, and eye movement abnormalities (Figure 52–10 ●). When the tumor occurs in the genitourinary tract, the result can be urinary obstruction, hematuria, dysuria, vaginal discharge, and a protruding vaginal mass. Rhabdomyosarcoma occurring in the abdomen may be asymptomatic. There is rapid metastasis to the lungs, bones, bone marrow, and distant lymph nodes.

Diagnosis is confirmed by CT, MRI, PET, bone marrow aspiration, and biopsy. CBC, renal and liver studies, and urinalysis are performed. Lumbar puncture may be used in head and neck tumors. A useful biologic marker, desmin, allows differentiation of rhabdomyosarcoma from other round cell tumors. A significant number of children have metastatic disease at the time of diagnosis, so chest and lung CT scans, as well as regional lymph node biopsies are performed (Rodeberg & Paidas, 2006).

Treatment includes surgical removal of the tumor when possible. However, if the tumor involves other structures, removal may not be possible. Many children have metastasis at the time of diagnosis, so the primary tumor may not be removed. Surgery is followed by wide-field radiation and chemotherapy with a combination of drugs. Some commonly used drugs include the following:

- Vincristine
- Actinomycin
- Cyclophosphamide (VAC therapy)

Prognosis depends on the site, staging (Table 52–9), and histologic findings, with about 70% of children surviving (Rodeberg & Paidas, 2006).

RETINOBLASTOMA

Retinoblastoma is an intraocular malignancy of the retina. It may be bilateral (20% to 30%) or unilateral. In 40% of children, the disease is inherited by an autosomal dominant gene. Family history is therefore important to collect, although many cases occur with no family history of the cancer. The tumor arises from embryonic retinal cells. It may be a new mutation or may be passed on to offspring of affected individuals. The retinoblastoma gene, RB1, is on chromosome 13q14 (de Andrade, da Hora Barbosa, Vargas, et al., 2006; Herzog, 2006; Hurwitz, Shields, Shields, et al., 2006).

The first sign of retinoblastoma is a white pupil, termed leukokoria or cat's-eye reflex (Figure 52–11 ●). The red reflex is absent, asymmetric, or of a differing color in the affected eye. Other symptoms may include a fixed strabismus (a constant deviation of one eye from the other), orbital inflammation, glaucoma, and heterochromia (irises of different colors).

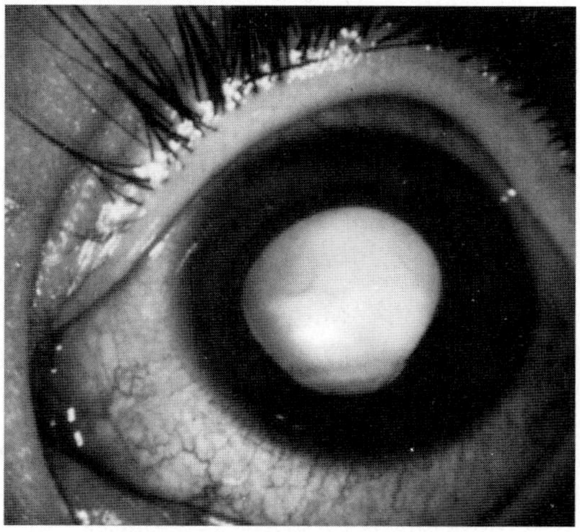

• **Figure 52–11** Retinoblastoma. Retinoblastoma is characterized by leukokoria, a white reflection in the pupil.

Used with permission from Hathaway, W. E., Hay, W. W., Jr., Grouthius, J. R., & Paisley, J. W. (1993). Current pediatric diagnosis and treatment (11th ed.). New York: McGraw-Hill Companies.

Retinoblastoma is usually diagnosed when the child is between 1 and 2 years of age. A family history should alert healthcare providers so that regular ophthalmologic examinations can be performed frequently on infants and young children in the family. The appearance of a unilateral tumor demands regular examinations of the healthy eye since bilateral disease can develop. In some children a pineal gland tumor can also develop, causing central nervous system symptoms. The overall tumor-free survival rate is 90%, 5 to 10 years after diagnosis (Kids Data, 2006).

Diagnostic tests for the cancer include full ocular examination and CT or MRI scans of the eye orbit. All children with a history of retinoblastoma in the family should be examined by an ophthalmologist after birth, at 6 weeks, every 2 to 3 months until 2 years and then every 4 months until 3 years, and then annually (de Andrade et al., 2006) to aid in early diagnosis. Tumors are classified according to a staging system, from a very small localized tumor (group I) to tumors involving more than half the retina and with seeding into the vitreous (group V).

Treatment for retinoblastoma may include removal of the eye (enucleation) when there is permanent retinal damage or failure to respond to other treatment. Other surgical treatments involve cryotherapy or photocoagulation (argon laser therapy). Radiation is nearly always used, either as the sole treatment or before surgery to shrink the tumor. Chemotherapy is sometimes used but is frequently ineffective as the drugs often fail to penetrate sufficiently into the eye. Chemotherapy drugs include carboplatin, etoposide, vincristine, and cyclosporine. Multiple therapies are more commonly used in children with bilateral retinoblastoma. Children with retinoblastoma are at increased risk of developing a secondary tumor, including another retinoblastoma or a sarcoma, most commonly osteogenic sarcoma. However, most young children who have been treated for the disease have good health and normal mental abilities several years after treatment. The most common sequela of retinoblastoma is decrease in visual acuity.

NURSING MANAGEMENT

NURSING ASSESSMENT AND DIAGNOSIS

PHYSIOLOGIC ASSESSMENT

Physiologic assessment of the child with a soft-tissue tumor, such as Hodgkin disease, non-Hodgkin lymphoma, rhabdomyosarcoma, and other lymphomas, focuses on the child's general condition. Accurate height and weight measurements are essential to provide a baseline against which to measure the child's growth during treatment, as well as for calculation of chemotherapeutic drug dosages.

Observe the area of the tumor, such as the face, neck, and abdomen, and describe any changes. Monitor respiratory status if the tumor is in the face or neck. Report any changes in respiratory pattern to the oncology specialist. Avoid palpation of any tumor site or enlarged area; injudicious palpation and manipulation of a tumor site can influence metastasis. Notify the primary healthcare provider of a change in any lymph node or any other area of the body.

Gastrointestinal and genitourinary function can be altered by the presence of a tumor and by treatment such as chemotherapy and radiation. Careful measurement of the child's intake and output is essential. Abdominal tumors may affect defecation, so charting of all bowel movements is important. Explain to the family and child why keeping accurate records is necessary.

Observe wounds closely for lack of healing as a result of chemotherapy or radiation. Examine the mouth and extremities for wounds or ulcers. Nutritional changes caused by treatment will affect the body's ability to support healthy cells and heal wounds.

A thorough eye examination is warranted for any child who has a family history of retinoblastoma or has undergone treatment for a prior tumor. Assess color and position of the iris, eye movements, cover–uncover test, and other eye tests described in Chapter 35∞. Ask whether the child has been evaluated by an ophthalmologist.

PSYCHOSOCIAL ASSESSMENT

Refer to the general discussion of psychosocial assessment under "Childhood Cancer," earlier in this chapter. Assessment of body image is needed when the child has a soft-tissue tumor affecting appearance of the head and neck.

The location and type of a soft-tissue tumor determine the specific nursing diagnoses for a particular child. Common nursing diagnoses might include the following:

- *Impaired Tissue Perfusion (Peripheral)* related to interruption of blood flow
- *Ineffective Breathing Pattern* related to effect of tumor deformity on neck or chest wall
- *Impaired Swallowing* related to tumor or treatment
- *Delayed Growth and Development* related to effects of treatment
- *Disturbed Body Image* related to illness and treatment
- *Disturbed Sensory Perception (Visual)* related to illness

PLANNING AND IMPLEMENTATION

Nursing management of children with soft-tissue tumors varies depending on the specific tumor. Children with lymphoma affecting the mediastinum may need respiratory support. Position the child so that the head is elevated. Administer chemotherapy drugs as ordered, maintaining adequate fluids to facilitate excretion of the resultant breakdown products. Monitor the central line used for chemotherapy administration, and teach parents care of the central line when the child is at home.

For the child with a rhabdomyosarcoma involving the bladder, monitor urinary output carefully. Report hematuria and painful urination. Monitor the changes that occur during therapy. For example, in children with eye tumors, observe for a decrease in ptosis, which may indicate successful treatment. Administer pain medications as needed and use distraction and other techniques to decrease the child's discomfort. Emphasize to parents the need for follow-up CT and MRI scans after completion of treatment.

When the child with retinoblastoma undergoes removal of the eye, the parents and child will need detailed instructions on postsurgical care. Demonstrate to the parents care of the socket and use of a conformer to maintain the eye socket shape. When healing is complete and the child receives a prosthetic eye, instruct parents about its insertion and care. The child can gradually be taught to take over this care when old enough. Encourage periodic healthcare visits to monitor for signs of a tumor in the other eye. Interventions to encourage normal developmental milestones are adapted if sensory alteration has resulted.

Pay attention to the body changes of the cancer and its treatment. Children and adolescents may need suggestions to deal with hair loss, disfigurement, and living with serious illness. Referral to other children and teens with similar concerns may be helpful. Parents of all children need help to encourage normal development in the child with cancer.

The child with a soft-tissue tumor often receives chemotherapy or radiation, or sometimes both modalities. Nursing management during chemotherapy and radiation is discussed earlier in this chapter in the general sections on these treatment measures (see pages 1483–1484) and in "Nursing Care Plan: Hospital Care of the Child with Cancer." Generally, the family needs help to adjust to the diagnosis of a life-threatening disease and to the care of the ill child. Refer to Chapter 40 for a description of postsurgical care. Consult Chapter 47 for strategies to assist the child and family if the child has a visual impairment resulting from a retinoblastoma. Topics for parent and family teaching and discharge planning are similar to those previously presented. Referral resources to support the families of children with these types of cancer can be found on the Companion Website.

NURSING CARE IN THE COMMUNITY

Reinforce with families the importance of long-term follow-up after treatment for a soft-tissue tumor. Increased risk for secondary cancers for 2 to 3 decades is possible, and early identification can help with prompt diagnosis (Hudson & Findlay, 2006). Partner with other healthcare providers to provide instructions to families as the child transitions from oncology treatment back to the pediatrician so they understand the importance of telling all care providers about the cancer and treatment. Establish oncology clinics to track and examine survivors. As children grow into teen and young adult years, help them to take over this important task in their care.

Some recommended annual examinations include the following:

- CBC
- Physical examination with special attention to skin, abdomen, and thyroid
- Monitoring for signs of hypo- and hyperthyroidism
- Neurologic and developmental examinations; monitoring of school performance
- First mammogram at 25 years in those with chest radiation
- Pap and pelvic examinations for teen and young adult women
- Mental status assessment

EVALUATION

The following expected outcomes of nursing care for the child with a soft-tissue tumor are examples that illustrate the varied tumor presentations:

- Successful management of treatment side effects
- Healed surgical site with no signs of infection
- Adaptation to sensory loss
- Adaptation to altered self-image
- Growth and development to maximum potential
- Anticipatory grieving by parents in cases of terminal disease

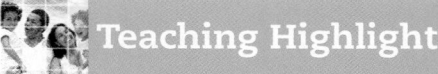

Teaching Highlights

CARE OF THE CHILD WITH A SOFT-TISSUE TUMOR

- Teach the family about the chemotherapy drugs and their side effects.
- Teach about the care of surgically placed venous access devices.
- Provide written and illustrated information about the chemotherapy protocol(s).
- Provide the family with radiation and surgery education specific to the tumor treatment.
- Refer the family to nutrition resources such as dietitians for ways to promote the child's adequate intake of food and fluid.

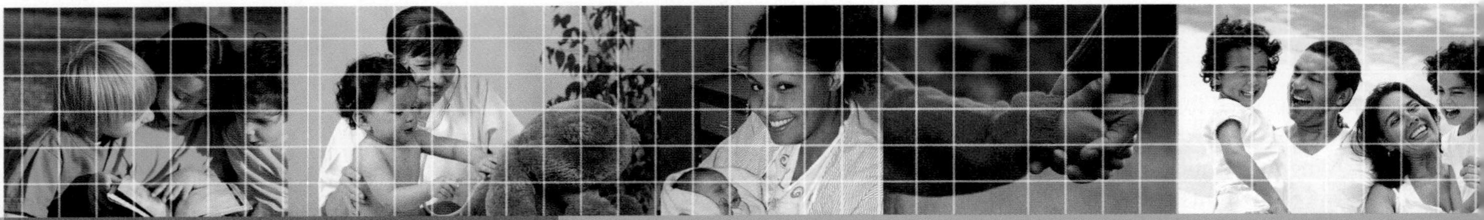

CRITICAL CONCEPT REVIEW

LEARNING OUTCOMES / CONCEPTS

52.1 Describe the incidence, known etiologies, and common clinical manifestations of cancer.

1. Incidence:
   - Approximately 11,000 children in the United States are diagnosed annually with a form of cancer.
2. Etiology:
   - External stimuli.
   - Gene abnormalities.
   - Immune system and chromosomal abnormalities.
3. Common clinical manifestations:
   - Pain.
   - Cachexia.
   - Anemia.
   - Infection.
   - Bruising.
   - Neurologic symptoms.
   - Palpable mass.

52.2 Synthesize information about diagnostic tests and clinical therapy for cancer to plan comprehensive care for children undergoing these procedures.

1. Diagnostic tests:
   - Complete blood count.
   - Bone marrow aspiration and biopsy.
   - Lumbar puncture.
   - X-ray and CT.
   - MRI.
   - Ultrasound.
   - Biopsy of tumor.
2. Clinical therapy:
   - Surgery.
   - Chemotherapy.
   - Radiation.
   - Biotherapy.
   - Bone marrow transplantation.

52.3 Integrate information about oncologic emergencies into plans for monitoring all children with cancer.

1. Closely monitor complete blood count (CBC):
   - To prevent sepsis.
   - To prevent hemorrhage.
2. Monitor intake and output closely:
   - Encourage hydration to prevent hypercalcemia.
   - Observe for signs of water intoxication.
3. Observe for behavioral changes:
   - Space-occupying lesions may cause seizures or increased ICP.

52.4 Recognize the most common solid tumors in children, describe their treatment, and plan comprehensive nursing care.

Central nervous system and brain tumors are the most common solid tumors.

1. Treatment:
   - Surgery.
   - Chemotherapy; may be delivered intrathecally.
2. Nursing care:
   - Provide and refer for psychosocial support.
   - Closely monitor neurologic status.
   - Monitor for changes in ICP, seizure activity, and other neurological indicators.
   - Observe for signs and symptoms of diabetes insipidus, and other conditions arising from the tumor and treatment.
   - Assist parents with dealing with the behavioral and educational changes that may occur with their child.

LEARNING OUTCOMES — CONCEPTS

Learning Outcomes	Concepts
52.5 Plan care for children and adolescents of all ages who have a diagnosis of leukemia.	1. Administer chemotherapy as ordered. 2. Observe for signs and symptoms of bone marrow suppression: ■ Anemia: encourage child to conserve energy. ■ Leukopenia: encourage handwashing. ■ Isolate child while counts are low; keep away from others with infection. ■ Thrombocytopenia. 3. Protect from injuries: no sports until counts increase. 4. Nutrition: frequent small feedings when dealing with nausea. 5. Monitor renal function. 6. Provide psychosocial support for child and family.
52.6 Recognize the most common soft-tissue tumors in children, describe their treatment, and plan comprehensive care.	1. The most common soft-tissue tumors: ■ Hodgkin disease. ■ Non-Hodgkin lymphoma. ■ Rhabdomyosarcoma. ■ Retinoblastoma. 2. Treatment depends upon the tumor. May require: ■ Surgery. ■ Chemotherapy. ■ Radiation.
52.7 Describe the impact of cancer survival on children and use this information to plan for ongoing physiological and psychosocial care in the children's futures.	1. Regular physical and laboratory examinations are needed. 2. Increased chance of development of other cancers due to original cancer treatment. 3. Encourage adolescents and young adults to manage their own care as much as possible. 4. Provide children, adolescents, and their families with educational and psychosocial support.

CRITICAL THINKING IN ACTION

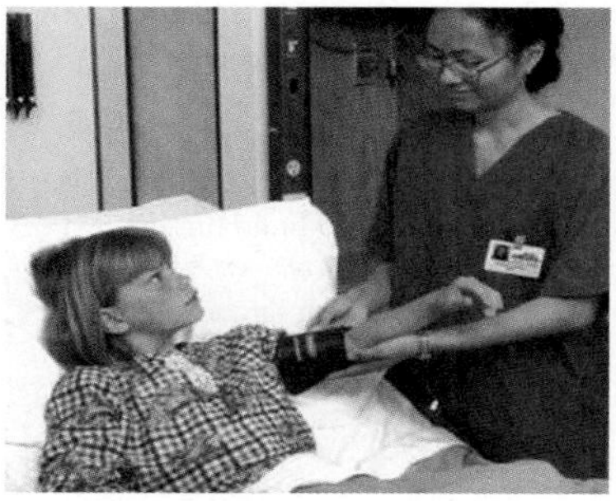

Seven-year-old Christina is brought to the hospital with an unusual rash, lethargy, and fever. Blood work is drawn, and the results are abnormal. The hematologist confirms that Christina has acute lymphoblastic leukemia (ALL), the most common childhood cancer. Her parents are in shock and disbelief about the news; she seems too young. Christina is immediately admitted to the hospital, and put on an IV with orders for more blood work.

Christina's blood work demonstrates the following: hemoglobin 9 g/dL, leukocytes 20,000/mm^3, and platelets 90,000/mm^3. Chemotherapy was initiated and precautions were taken to avoid infections. Recommendations for Christina include rest times daily, generous amounts of water, intake of healthy foods, and avoidance of sun exposure. The parents are happy when Christina comes home during the chemotherapy. The hemotologist advises them it is not uncommon to return to the hospital due to a chemotherapy complication. The parents are encouraged to remember to take care of themselves. This will help them deal with Christina's therapy more effectively.

1. What are some of the common side effects of chemotherapy?
2. Why is it important to check Christina's daily weights?
3. What symptoms should Christina's parents report to the doctor while she is on chemotherapy?
4. What are some developmentally-appropriate techniques you can encourage that will assist Christina to deal with her illness?

See MyNursingKit for possible responses.

REFERENCES

Agha, M. M., Williams, J. I., Marrett. L., To, T., Zipursky, A., & Dodds, L. (2005). Congenital abnormalities and childhood cancer. *Cancer, 106,* 1418–1419.

Alavi, S., Arzanian, M. T., Abbasian, M. R., & Ashena, Z. (2006). Tumor lysis syndrome in children with non-Hodgkin lymphoma. *Pediatric Hematology and Oncology, 23,* 65–70.

American Cancer Society. (2003). *National action plan for childhood cancer.* Retrieved from www.cancer.org

American Cancer Society. (2005). *What are the key statistics about brain and spinal cord cancers?* Retrieved from www.cancer.org/docroot/CRI

American Cancer Society. (2006a). *Cancer facts and figures.* Retrieved from www.cancer.org/docroot/STT/stt_o.asp

American Cancer Society. (2006b). *What are the key statistics about childhood leukemia?* Retrieved from www.cancer/docroot/CRI/content/

Arndt, C. A. S. (2007). Malignant tumors of bone. In R. M. Kliegman, R. E. Behrman, H. B. Jenson, & B. F. Stanton (Eds.), *Nelson textbook of pediatrics* (18th ed., pp. 2146–2149). Philadelphia: Saunders.

Ater, J. A. (2007). Neuroblastoma. In R. M. Kliegman, R. E. Behrman, H. B. Jenson, & B. F. Stanton (Eds.), *Nelson textbook of pediatrics* (18th ed., pp. 2137–2139). Philadelphia: Saunders.

Ballard, K. L. (2004). Meeting the needs of siblings of children with cancer. *Pediatric Nursing, 30,* 394–402.

Bennett, J. M., & Konrokji, R. S. (2005). The myelodysplastic syndromes: Diagnosis, molecular biology and risk assessment. *Hematology, 10* (Suppl 1), 258–269.

Bindler, R. M., & Howry, L. B. (2005). *Pediatric drug guide.* Upper Saddle River, NJ: Prentice Hall.

Bjork, M., Nordstrom, B., & Hallstrom, I. (2006). Needs of young children with cancer during their initial hospitalization: An observational study. *Journal of Pediatric Oncology Nursing, 23*(4), 210–219.

Blaney, S. M., Kun, L. E., Hunter, J., Rorke-Adams, L. B., Lau, C., Strother, D., & Pollack, I. F. (2006). Tumors of the central nervous system. In P. A. Pizzo & D. G. Poplack (Eds.), *Principles and practice of pediatric oncology* (5th ed., pp. 786–864). Philadelphia: Lippincott Williams & Wilkins.

Brody, A. C., & Simmons, L. A. (2007). Family resiliency during childhood cancer: The father's perspective. *Journal of Pediatric Oncology Nursing, 24*(3), 152–165.

Brown, P. (2006). Answers to key questions about childhood leukemias. *Contemporary Pediatrics, 23*(3), 81–84, 87, 90.

Cairo, M. S., & Bradley, M. B. (2007). Lymphoma. In R. M. Kliegman, R. E. Behrman, H. B. Jenson, & B. F. Stanton (Eds.), *Nelson textbook of pediatrics* (18th ed., pp. 2123–2127). Philadelphia: Saunders.

Da Silva, E. D., Koch Nogueira, P. C., Russo Zamataro, T. M., de Carvalho, W. B., & Petrilli, A. S. (2008). *Journal of Pediatric Hematology and Oncology, 30,* 513–518.

De Andrade, A. F., da Hora Barbosa, R., Vargas, F. R., Ferman, S., Eisenberg, A. L., Fernandes, L., & Bonvicino, C. R. (2006). *Cancer Genetics and Cytogenetics, 167,* 43–46.

Dome, J. S., Perlman, E. J., Ritchey, M. L., Coppes, M. J., Kalapurakal, J., & Grundy, P. E. (2006). Renal tumors. In P. A. Pizzo & D. G. Poplack (Eds.), *Principles and practice of pediatric oncology* (5th ed. pp. 905–932). Philadelphia: Lippincott Williams & Wilkins.

Elfenbein, G. J. (2005). Granulocyte-colony stimulating factor primed bone marrow and granulocyte-colony stimulating factor mobilized peripheral blood stem cells are equivalent for engraftment: Which to choose? *Pediatric Transplantation, 9*(Suppl 7), 37–47.

Florin, T. A., & Hinkle, A. S. (2005). A guide to caring for cancer survivors. *Contemporary Pediatrics, 22*(8), 31–48.

Hammes, B. J., Klevan, J., Kempf, M., & Williams, M. S. (2005). Pediatric advance care planning. *Journal of Palliative Medicine, 8,* 766–773.

Hartford, C. M., Wodowski, K. S., Rao, B. N., Khoury, J. D., Neel, M. D., & Daw, N. C. (2006). Osteosarcoma among children age 5 years or younger. *Journal of Pediatric Hematology and Oncology, 28,* 43–47.

Haut, C. (2005). Oncological emergencies in the pediatric intensive care unit. *AACN Clinical Issues, 16,* 232–245.

Hawks, R. (2006). Complementary and alternative medicine research initiative in the children's oncology group and the role of the pediatric oncology nurse. *Journal of Pediatric Oncology Nursing, 23,* 261–264.

Henderson, R. A., Mossman, S., Nairn, N., & Cheever, M. A. (2005). Cancer vaccines and immunotherapies: Emerging perspectives. *Vaccine, 23,* 2359–2362.

Herzog, C. E. (2007). Retinoblastoma. In R. M. Kliegman, R. E. Behrman, H. B. Jenson, & B. F. Stanton (Eds.), *Nelson textbook of pediatrics* (18th ed., pp. 2152–2152). Philadelphia: Saunders.

Himmelstein, B. P., Hilden, J. M., Boldt, A. M., & Weissman, D. (2004). Pediatric palliative care. *New England Journal of Medicine, 350,* 1752–1762.

Hon, K. L., Leung, A., Chik, K. W., Chu, C. W., Cheung, K. L., & Fok, T. F. (2005). Critical airway obstruction, superior vena cava syndrome, and spontaneous cardiac arrest in a child with acute leukemia. *Pediatric Emergency Care, 21,* 844–846.

Houldin, A., Curtiss, C. P., & Haylock, P. J. (2006). Executive summary: The state of the science on nursing approaches to managing late and long-term sequelae of cancer and cancer treatment. *American Journal of Nursing, 106*(3), 54–59.

Hudson, M. M., & Findlay, S. (2006). Health-risk behaviors and health promotion in adolescent and young adult cancer survivors. *Cancer, 107* (7 Suppl), 1695–1701.

Hudson, M. M., Onciu, M., & Donaldson, S. S. (2006). Hodgkin lymphoma. In P. A. Pizzo & D. G. Poplack (Eds.), *Principles and practice of pediatric oncology* (5th ed. pp. 695–721). Philadelphia: Lippincott Williams & Wilkins.

Hurwitz, C.A., Duncan, J. & Wolfe, J. (2004). Aring for the child with cancer at the close of life. *Journal of the American Medical Association 292,* 2141–2149.

Hurwitz, R. L., Shields, C. L., Shields, J. A., Chevez-Barrios, P., Hurwitz, J. Y., & Chintagumpala, M. M. (2006). Retinoblastoma. In P. A. Pizzo & D. G. Poplack, D. G. *Principles and practice of pediatric oncology* (5th ed. pp. 865–886). Philadelphia: Lippincott Williams & Wilkins.

Hussong, M. R. (2002). Non-Hodgkin's lymphoma. In C. R. Baggott, K. P. Kelly, D. Fochtman, & G. V. Foley (Eds.), *Nursing care of children and adolescents with cancer* (3rd ed., p. 539). Philadelphia: Saunders.

Jaff, N., Chelghoum, Y., Elhamri, M., Tigaud, I., Michallet, M., & Thomas, X. (2006). Trisomy 8 as sole anomaly or with other clonal aberrations in acute myeloid leukemia: Impact on clinical presentation and outcome. *Leukemia Research, 31,* 67–73.

Jaffe, N., & Huff, V. (2007). Neoplasms of the kidney. In R. M. Kliegman, R. E. Behrman, H. B. Jenson, & B. F. Stanton (Eds.), *Nelson textbook of pediatrics* (18th ed., pp. 2140–2143). Philadelphia: Saunders.

Kaste, S. C. (2008). Skeletal toxicities of treatment in children with cancer. *Pediatric Blood Cancer, 50* (2 suppl), 469–473, 486.

Kazak, A. E., Rourke, M. T., Alderfer, M. A., Pai, A., Reilly, A. F., & Meadows, A. T. (2007). Evidence-based assessment, intervention and psychosocial care in pediatric oncology: A blueprint for comprehensive services across treatment. *Journal of Pediatric Psychology, 32,* 1099–1110.

Kersun, L., & Elia, J. (2007). Depressive symptoms and SSRI use in pediatric oncology patients. *Pediatric Blood Cancer, 49,* 881–887.

Khatua, S., & Jalali, R. (2005). Recent advances in the treatment of childhood brain tumors. *Pediatric Hematology and Oncology, 22,* 361–371.

Khoury, J. D. (2005). Ewing sarcoma family of tumors. *Advances in Anatomy and Pathology, 12,* 212–220.

Kids Data. (2006). Net five-year cancer survival rates. Retrieved from www.kidsdata.org

Kim, S., & Chung, D. H. (2006). Pediatric solid malignancies: Neuroblastoma and Wilms' tumor. *Surgical Clinics of North America, 86,* 469–487.

Kutluk, T., Varan, A., Buyukpamukcu, N., Atahan, L., Caglar, M., Akyuz, C., & Buyukpamukcu, M. (2006). Improved survival of children with Wilms' tumor. *Journal of Pediatric Hematology and Oncology, 28,* 423–426.

Levy, A. S. (2005, July). Brain tumors in children: Evaluation and management. *Current Problems in Pediatric and Adolescent Health Care,* 230–245.

Loescher, L. J., & Merkle, C. J. (2005). The interface of genomic technologies and nursing. *Journal of Nursing Scholarship, 37,* 111–119.

Mann, G., Attarbaschi, A., Steiner, M., Simonitsch, I., Strobl, H., Urban, C., et al. (2006). Early and reliable diagnosis of non-Hodgkin lymphoma in childhood and adolescence. *Pediatric Hematology and Oncology, 23,* 167–176.

Martel, D., Bussieres, J. F., Theoret, Y., Lebel, D., Kish, S., Moghrabi, A., & Laurier, C. (2005). Use of alternative and complementary therapies in children with cancer. *Pediatric Blood and Cancer, 44*, 660–668.

McGrath, P., Paton, M. A., & Huff, N. (2005). Beginning treatment for pediatric acute myeloid leukemia: The family connection. *Issues in Comprehensive Pediatric Nursing, 28*, 97–114.

McKinney, P. A. (2005). Central nervous system tumours in children: Epidemiology and risk factors. *Bioelectromagnetics Suppl 7*, S60–S68.

National Cancer Institute (2007a). *Sun protection and cancer*. Retrieved from http://progressreport.cancer.gov/index.asp

National Cancer Institute (2007b). *Neuroblastoma treatment: Stage information.* Retrieved from www.cancer.gov/cancertopics/pdq/treatment/neuroblastoma/HealthProfessional/page3

National Cancer Institute (2007c). *Wilms' tumor and other childhood kidney tumors: Stage information.* Retrieved from www.cancer.gov/cancertopics/pdq/treatment/wilms/HealthProfessional/page3

National Cancer Institute (2008a). *A snapshot of pediatric cancers.* Retrieved from www.cancer.gov/incidence

National Cancer Institute (2008b). *Staging information of adult Hodgkin lymphoma.* Retrieved from www.cancer.gov/cancertopics/pdq/treatment/hodgkin/HealthProfessional/page4

Nelson, M. B., & Meeske, K. (2005). Recognizing health risks in childhood cancer survivors. *Journal of the American Academy of Nurse Practitioners, 17*(3), 96–103.

Packman, W., Greenhalgh, J., Chesterman, B., Shaffer, T., Fine, J., Van Zutphen, K., et al. (2005). Siblings of pediatric cancer patients: The quantitative and qualitative nature of quality of life. *Journal of Psychosocial Oncology, 23*, 87–108.

Pasero, C. (2006). Lidocaine iontophoresis for dermal procedure analgesia. *Journal of PeriAnesthesia Nursing, 21*, 48–52.

Pollack, L. A., Stewart, L., Thompson, T. D., & Li, J. (2007). Trends in childhood cancer mortality–United States, 1990–2004. *Morbidity and Mortality Weekly Report, 56*, 1257–1261.

Post-White, J., & Hawks, R. G. (2005). Complementary and alternative medicine in pediatric oncology. *Seminars in Oncology Nursing, 21*, 107–114.

Pui, C. J., & Evans, W. E. (2006). Treatment of acute lymphoblastic leukemia. *New England Journal of Medicine, 354*, 166–178.

Punyko, J. A., Gurney, J. G., Baker, K. S., Hayashi, R. J., Hudson, M. M., Liu, Y., et al. (2006). Physical impairment and social adaptation in adult survivors of childhood and adolescent rhabdomyosarcoma: A report from the Childhood Cancer Survivors Study. *Psycho-Oncology, 16*, 26–37.

Putwatana, P., Sanmanowong, P., Oonprasertpong, L., Junda, T., Pitiporn, S. & Narkwong, L. (2009). Relief of radiation-induced oral mucositis in head and neck cancer. *Cancer Nursing, 32*, 82–87.

Rheingold, S. R., & Lange, B. J. (2006). In P. A. Pizzo & D. G. Poplack (Eds.), *Principles and practice of pediatric oncology* (5th ed., pp. 1202–1230). Philadelphia: Lippincott Williams & Wilkins.

Richardson, J., Smith, J. E., McCall, G., & Pilkington, K. (2006). Hypnosis for procedure-related pain and distress in pediatric cancer patients: A systematic review of effectiveness and methodology related to hypnosis interventions. *Journal of Pain and Symptom Management, 31*, 70–84.

Rodeberg, D., & Paidas, C. (2006). Childhood rhabdomyosarcoma. *Seminars in Pediatric Surgery, 15*, 57–62.

Rollins, J. A. (2005). Tell me about it: Drawing as a communication tool for children with cancer. *Journal of Pediatric Oncology Nursing, 22*, 203–211.

Ross, J. A., Spector, L. G., Robison, L. L., & Olshan, A. F. (2005). Epidemiology of leukemia in children with Down syndrome. *Pediatric Blood Cancer, 44*, 8–12.

Rourke, M. T., Hobbie, W. L., Schwartz, L., & Kazak, A. D. (2007). Posttraumatic stress disorder (PTSD) in young adult survivors of childhood cancer. *Pediatric Blood & Cancer 49*(2), 177–182.

Rubnitz, J. E., Lensing, S., Razzouk, B. I., Pounds, S., Pui, C. H., & Ribeiro, R. C. (2007). Effect of race on outcome of white and black children with acute myeloid leukemia: The St. Jude experience. *Pediatric Blood Cancer, 48*, 10–15.

Rushton, C. H. (2005). A framework for integrated pediatric palliative care: Being with dying. *Journal of Pediatric Nursing, 20*, 311–325.

Skinner, R., Hamish, W., Wallace, B., & Levitt, G. A. (2006). Long-term follow-up of people who have survived cancer during childhood. *Lancet, 7*, 489–498.

Spinazze, S., & Schrijvers, D. (2006). Metabolic emergencies. *Critical Reviews in Oncology/Hematology, 58*, 79–89.

Stan, S. D., Kar, S., Stoner, G. D., & Singh, S. V. (2008). Bioactive food components and cancer risk reduction. *Journal of Cellular Biology 104*, 339–356.

Stanescu., L., Foarfa, C., Georgescu, A. C., & Georgescu, I. (2007). Kaposi's sarcoma associated with AIDS. *Romanian Journal of Morphology and Embryology, 48*, 181–187.

Tsao, J. C., & Zeltzer, L. K. (2005). Complementary and alternative medicine approaches for pediatric pain: A review of the state-of-the-science. *Evidence Based Complementary and Alternative Medicine, 2*, 149–159.

Twombly, R. (2007). Childhood cancer survivor study doubles to examine late effects of new treatments. *News–Journal National Cancer Institute, 99*, 1574–1576.

Wexler, L. H., Meyer, W. H., & Helman, L. J. (2006). Rhabdomyosarcoma and the undifferentiated sarcomas. In P. A. Pizzo & D. G. Poplack (Eds.), *Principles and practice of pediatric oncology* (5th ed., pp. 971–1001). Philadelphia: Lippincott Williams & Wilkins.

Wilne, S., Collier, J., Kennedy, C., Koller, K., Grundy, R., & Walker, D. (2007). Presentation of childhood CNS tumours: A systematic review and meta-analysis. *The Lancet Oncology, 8*, 685–695.

Wilne, S. H., Ferris, R. C., Nathwani, A., & Kennedy, C. R. (2006). The presenting features of brain tumors: A review of 200 cases. *Archive of Diseases in Children, 91*, 502–506.

Worthingon, H. V., Clarkson, J. E., & Eden, O. B. (2007). Interventions for preventing oral mucositis for patients with cancer receiving treatment. *Cochrane Database Systematic Review October, 17*(4), CD000978.

Wunder, J. S., Gokgoz, N., Parkes, R., Bull, S. B., Eskandarian, S., Davis, A. M., et al. (2005). TP53 mutations and outcome in osteosarcoma: A prospective, multicenter study. *Journal of Clinical Oncology, 23*, 1483–1490.

Yang, D. J., Kim, E. E., & Inoue, T. (2006). Targeted molecular imaging in oncology. *Annals of Nuclear Medicine, 20*, 1–11.

Zebrack, B. J., Zevon, M. A., Turk, N., Nagarajan, R., Whitton, J., Robison, L. L., & Zeltzer, L. K. (2007). Psychological distress in long-term survivors of solid tumors diagnosed in childhood: A report from the Childhood Cancer Survivor Study. *Pediatric Blood & Cancer 49*(1), 47–51.

EXPLORE PEARSON **mynursingkit™**

MyNursingKit is your one stop for online chapter review materials and resources. Prepare for success with additional NCLEX®-style practice questions, interactive assignments and activities, web links, animations and videos, and more!

Register your access code from the front of your book at **www.mynursingkit.com**

CHAPTER 53

The Child with Alterations in Gastrointestinal Function

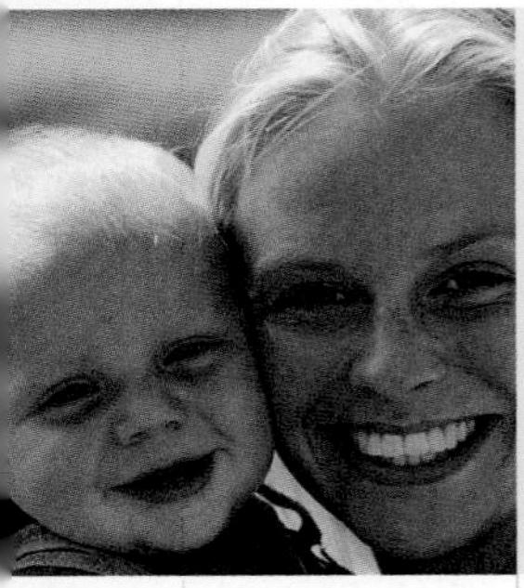

I was so worried when Jerome was born. He had no anal opening and his esophagus did not lead to his stomach. Now that he's had several surgeries, he is growing and doing pretty well, and I'm so happy to see him starting to smile. I can't wait until he is able to eat on his own instead of having tube feedings. —*Mother of Jerome, 8 months old*

LEARNING OUTCOMES

53.1 Describe the general function of the gastrointestinal system.

53.2 Discuss the pathophysiologic processes associated with specific gastrointestinal disorders in the pediatric population.

53.3 Identify signs and symptoms that may indicate a disorder of the gastrointestinal system.

53.4 Contrast nursing management and plan care for disorders of the gastrointestinal system for the child needing abdominal surgery versus the child needing nonoperative management.

53.5 Analyze developmentally appropriate approaches for nursing management of gastrointestinal disorders in the pediatric population.

53.6 Discuss nursing management of the child with an injury to the abdomen.

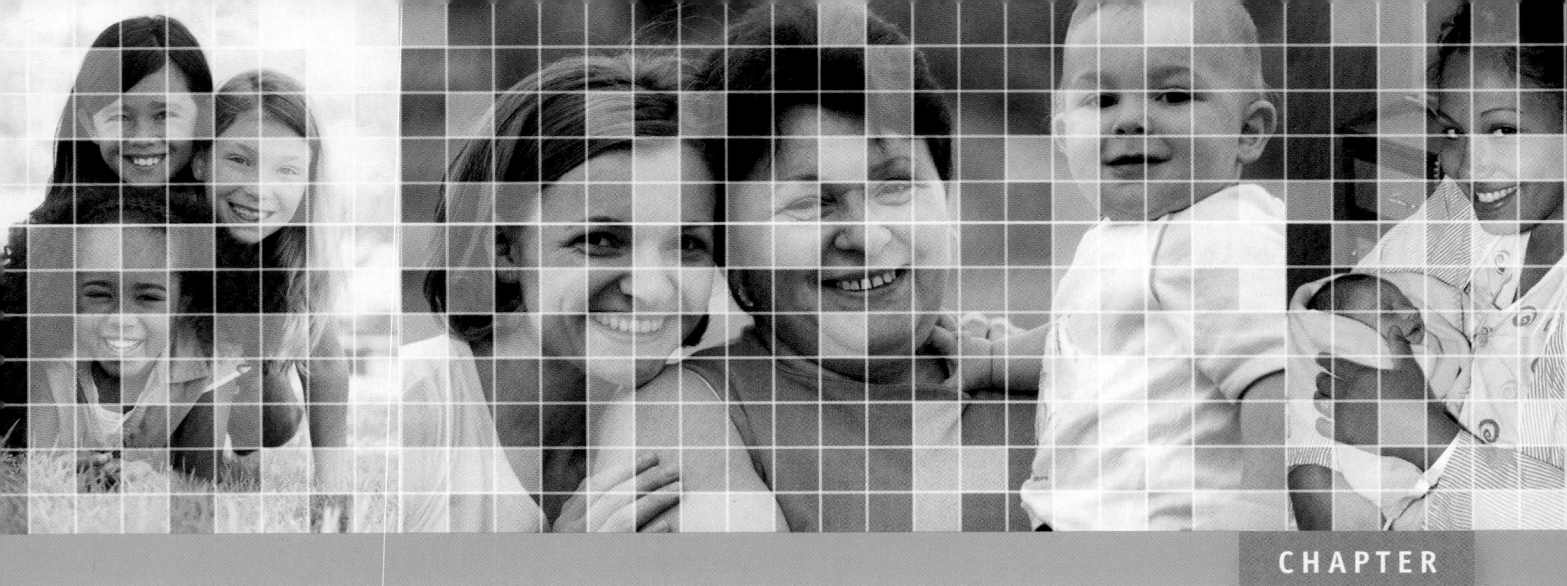

What causes structural defects of the gastrointestinal tract such as the esophageal atresia and imperforate anus experienced by Jerome? What special care do children with gastrointestinal abnormalities need to promote growth and development during treatment for anomalies? This chapter discusses the care of infants who have structural defects and those with other common disorders of gastrointestinal functioning.

Through the gastrointestinal (GI) tract, a child ingests and absorbs the foods and fluids necessary to sustain life and promote growth. Most GI disturbances produce short-term symptoms that interfere with nutrition and fluid balance only briefly. Some disorders or severe defects lead to complications that prevent optimal nutrition and adequate growth. This chapter explores some common GI disorders in children. (See Chapter 46∞ for a discussion of specific fluid imbalances that may accompany GI disorders.)

GI disorders can result from a congenital defect, acquired disease, infection, or injury. Structural problems may occur when development is altered or ceases in the first trimester of gestation. Because various parts of the GI system are developing at this point in gestation, it is not unusual for infants to have more than one structural defect of the GI system. This was the case with Jerome in the opening quote. Infections can cause an increase or decrease in motility and prevent proper absorption of nutrients. Interruption or destruction of the GI system can also result from trauma. While reading this chapter, remember that any interruption or alteration in the GI system decreases the body's ability to obtain nutrients, thus impairing growth.

ANATOMY AND PHYSIOLOGY OF PEDIATRIC DIFFERENCES

Although the fetus makes sucking and swallowing movements in utero and ingests amniotic fluid, the GI system is immature at birth. The processes of absorption and excretion do not begin until after birth because the placenta provides nutrients and removes waste. Sucking is a primitive reflex that occurs whenever the lips or cheeks are stroked. The infant does not have voluntary control over swallowing until about 6 weeks of age.

The stomach capacity of the newborn is quite small, and intestinal motility (**peristalsis**) is greater than in older children (see the nearby feature "As Children Grow"). These characteristics explain the newborn's need for small, frequent feedings and the increased frequency and liquid consistency of bowel movements. Because of the relaxed cardiac sphincter, infants frequently regurgitate small amounts of feedings.

Digestion takes place in the duodenum. Infants have a deficiency of several enzymes: amylase (which digests carbohydrates), lipase (which enhances fat absorption), and trypsin (which catabolizes protein into polypeptides and some amino acids). Enzymes are usually not present in sufficient quantities to aid digestion until 4 to 6 months of age. Thus, abdominal distention from gas is common.

Liver function is also immature. After the first few weeks of life, the liver is able to conjugate bilirubin and excrete bile. The processes of **gluconeogenesis** (formation of glycogen from noncarbohydrates), plasma protein and ketone formation, vitamin storage, and **deamination** (removal of amino group from amino compound) remain immature during the first year of life.

By the second year of life, digestive processes are fairly complete. Stomach capacity increases to accommodate a three-meals-per-day feeding schedule. At about the same time, myelination of the spinal cord becomes complete and voluntary control over excretory functions can be achieved. Around 18 months of age, the child becomes aware of soiling and may begin to have some voluntary control over excretory functions although many children are at least 2–3 years of age before continence for stool is achieved (Doughty, 2004). See Table 53–1 for guidelines for assessment of the gastrointestinal system.

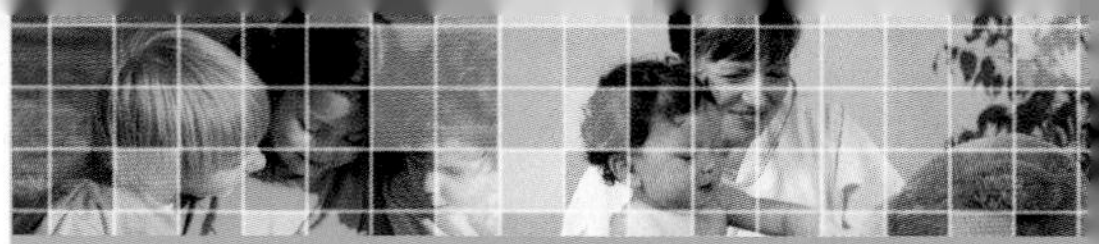

KEY TERMS

Cholestasis, 1540
Chronic vomiting, 1549
Constipation, 1532
Cyclic vomiting, 1549
Deamination, 1515
Diarrhea, 1532
Gluconeogenesis, 1515
Hernia, 1534
Occult blood, 1540
Ostomy, 1536
Peristalsis, 1515
Projectile vomiting, 1526
Stoma, 1536

MyNursingKit Animation: Digestive System

AS CHILDREN GROW

STOMACH CAPACITY

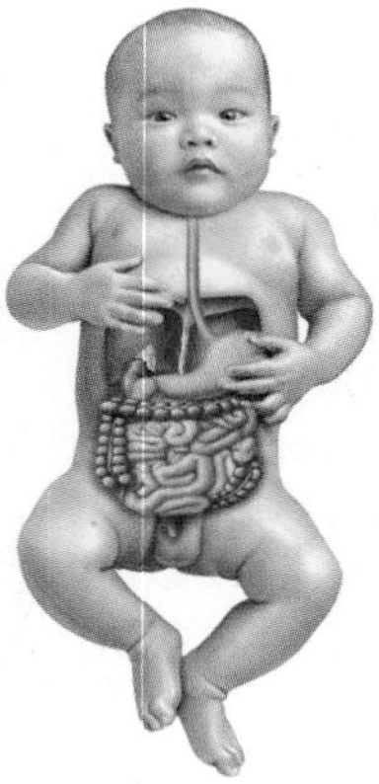

Stomach capacity throughout early childhood

Age	*Capacity (mL)*
Newborn	10 to 20
1 week	30 to 90
2 to 3 weeks	75 to 100
1 month	90 to 150
3 months	150 to 200
1 year	210 to 360
2 years	500

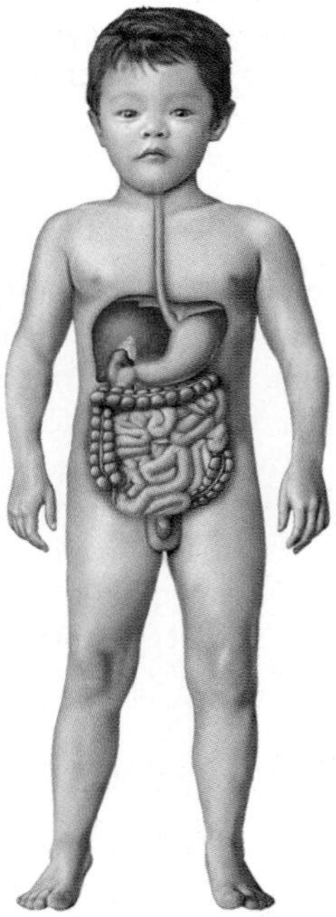

Stomach capacity increases throughout childhood.

Parents should be reminded that the young infant has a small stomach as compared to the older child or adolescent. Amounts per feeding should be determined accordingly using the guidelines seen here.

Source: From Chamley, C. A. Carson, P. Randall, D., & Sandwell. M. (2005). *Developmental anatomy and physiology of children* (p. 193). St. Louis, MO: Elsevier.

Table 53–1 Guidelines for Assessment of a Child with a Gastrointestinal Condition

Assessment Focus	Assessment Guidelines
Abdomen—Inspection	■ Observe the shape of the abdomen. ■ Note any abdominal distention. ■ Observe the umbilicus for protrusion. ■ Observe for peristaltic waves (visible rhythmic contractions of the intestinal wall smooth muscle).
Abdomen—Auscultation	■ Auscultate for bowel sounds in all four quadrants prior to palpation.
Abdomen—Palpation	■ Palpate the abdomen and note if it is soft or firm. ■ Palpate the size of the umbilical ring. ■ Does the child complain of pain or tenderness during palpation? Does the infant cry? ■ Describe any masses palpated by location, shape, size, and consistency. ■ Palpate the liver for size and tenderness. ■ Palpate the spleen for size and tenderness.
Esophagus	■ Note the presence of increased oral secretions.
Nutrition	■ Note tolerance of feedings, spitting up, emesis, and recurrent respiratory infections. ■ Observe amount, color, and frequency of emesis. ■ Note if emesis is associated with feeding and whether or not it is projectile. ■ Note amount of intake, frequency of feedings, and growth.
Stool	■ Observe color, consistency, and size of stool. Note any changes in stool patterns.
Family History	■ Ask about history of gastrointestinal illness with genetic influences such as celiac disease and inflammatory bowel disease.

STRUCTURAL DEFECTS

Structural defects can involve one or more areas of the GI tract. These defects occur when growth and development of fetal structures are interrupted during the first trimester. This can leave the structure incomplete, resulting in *atresia* (absence or closure of a normal body orifice), malposition, nonclosure, or other abnormalities.

CLEFT LIP AND CLEFT PALATE

Cleft lip and cleft palate are two distinct facial defects that can occur singly or in combination (Figure 53–1 ●). Cleft lip with or without cleft palate is the fourth most common birth defect occurring in 14 out of every 10,000 live births. The incidence of cleft palate is less common, occurring in 4 out of every 10,000 live births. Clefts are more common among Native Americans and Asians than whites, and less common in blacks (Merritt, 2005a).

Etiology and Pathophysiology

Cleft lip with or without cleft palate results when the maxillary processes fail to fuse with the elevations on the frontal prominence during the sixth week of gestation. Normally union of the upper lip is complete by the seventh week. Fusion of the secondary palate occurs between 5 and 12 weeks of gestation. Failure of the tongue to move downward at the correct time prevents the palatine processes from fusing.

The intrauterine development of the hard and soft palates is completed in the first trimester. It is during this time that other major organ systems develop. Ten percent of children with cleft lip and palate will have an associated syndrome. When cleft lip or cleft palate occurs alone, the incidence of an associated syndrome increases to 30–50%, respectively (Merritt, 2005a). There is an increased incidence in families with a prior history of cleft lip or palate. The cause is believed to be multifactorial, involving a combination of environmental and genetic influences. When fortification of cereals and breads with folate began in the United States in 1996 as a measure to decrease neural tube defects, the incidence of orofacial clefts also decreased. This may suggest a role for folate in formation of maxillary processes in the fetus (Yazdy, Honein, & Xing, 2007).

Clinical Manifestations

A cleft that involves the lip is readily apparent at birth. It may be a simple dimple in the vermilion border of the lip or a complete separation extending to the floor of the nose. The defect may be unilateral or bilateral and may occur alone or in combination with a cleft palate defect. Varying degrees of nasal deformity may also be present.

Cleft palate defects are less obvious when they occur without a cleft lip and may not be detected at birth. Clefts of the hard palate form a continuous opening between the mouth and nasal cavity and may be unilateral or bilateral, involving just the soft palate or both the soft and hard palate.

Clinical Therapy

Cleft lip and palate are usually diagnosed at birth or during the newborn assessment. Medical management requires the combined efforts of a multidisciplinary team. Because speech, hearing, and dentition may be affected, coordinated care by specialists in plastic surgery, hearing, speech, and dentistry is necessary.

The cleft lip is usually repaired by around 3 months of age (Merritt, 2005b) (Figure 53–2 ●). The lip is sutured together using either a diagonal incision or a staggered suture line (z-plasty) (Merritt, 2005b). If the defect is severe, the child may need more than one operation to achieve total repair. After surgery, soft

MyNursingKit Case Study: The Child with a Cleft Palate

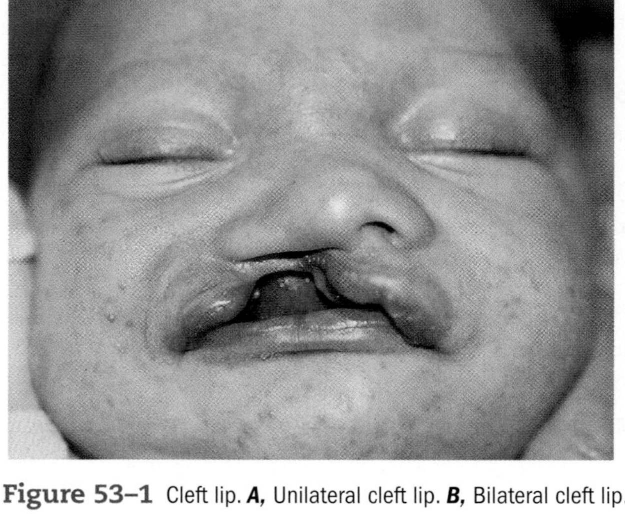

A

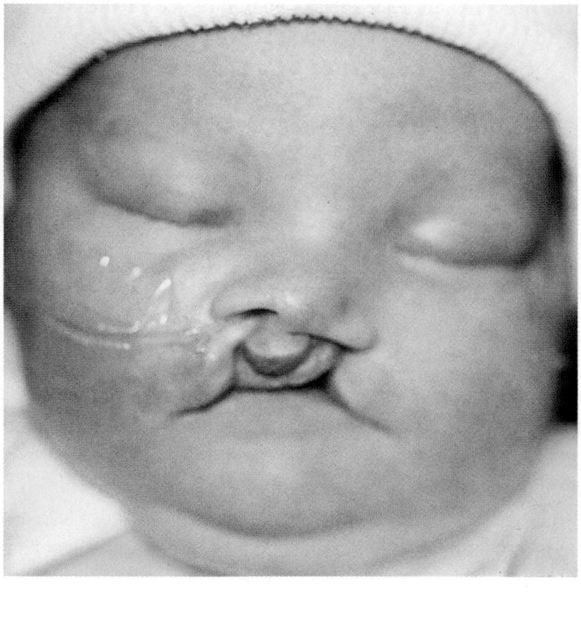

B

● **Figure 53–1** Cleft lip. ***A,*** Unilateral cleft lip. ***B,*** Bilateral cleft lip.

Courtesy of Dr. Elizabeth Peterson, Spokane, WA.

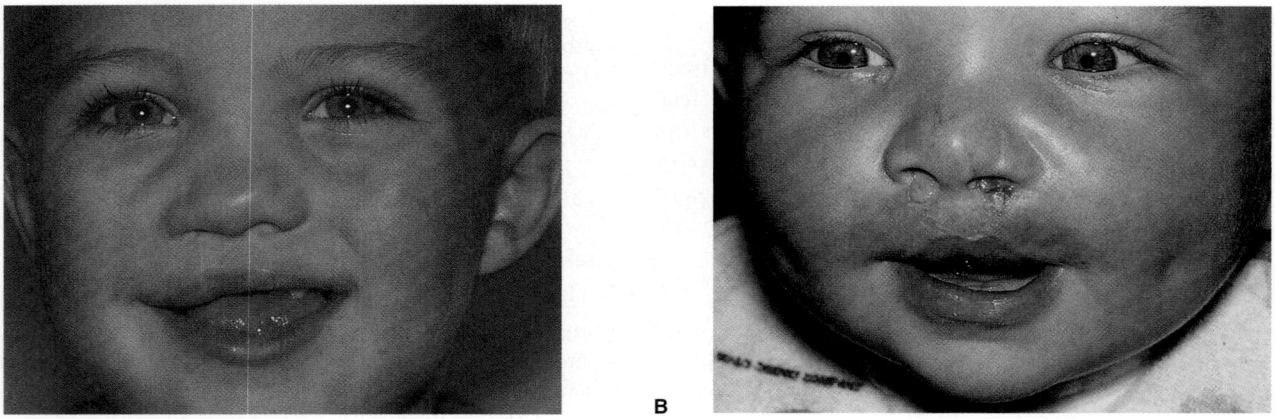

A B

● **Figure 53–2** Repaired cleft lip. ***A,*** Repaired unilateral cleft lip. ***B,*** Repaired bilateral cleft lip.

Courtesy of Dr. Elizabeth Peterson, Spokane, WA.

elbow immobilizers are used for 2 weeks to prevent the child from thumb sucking or putting their fingers in their mouth, which could disrupt the suture line (Kasten, Schmidt, Zickler, et al., 2008) (see Skill 7–6 SKILLS). The child should also receive distraction and pain medication as needed, as crying may disrupt the suture line.

Early closure of the lip enables the infant to form a better seal around the nipple for feeding. The sucking motion strengthens the muscles necessary for speech. Special feeding devices such as longer nipples with enlarged holes are available to help meet the infant's nutritional needs before surgical correction.

Timing of the cleft palate repair varies among surgeons and depends on the size and severity of the cleft. Most surgeons perform closure operations before the child reaches 18 months of age (Merritt, 2005b). This protects the formation of tooth buds and allows the infant to develop more normal speech patterns.

Infants with cleft lip and cleft palate are prone to recurrent otitis media, which can lead to hearing problems. Ear infections should be promptly evaluated by a health professional with expertise in ear care and treatment. (Refer to Chapter 48 for care of the child with chronic otitis media.) The child who has had cleft palate repair requires orthodontic care. Early visits permit assessment of tooth eruption and the need for future orthodontic work.

Developing Cultural Competence

CORRECTIVE SURGERY FOR CLEFT LIP AND PALATE

In many developing countries, infants do not have access to surgery for correction of cleft lip and palate. They may grow into childhood and adulthood with these abnormalities. Medical teams from the United States, Canada, and other countries sometimes travel to developing nations for short medical missions, performing surgery on the children and teaching local doctors surgical techniques. Are there medical missions teams from your area that perform these surgeries? What is the planning required for such trips to perform surgery safely and care for the children? What is the impact on the communities served? (WEBLINK: www.operationsmile.org)

NURSING MANAGEMENT

NURSING ASSESSMENT AND DIAGNOSIS

PHYSIOLOGIC ASSESSMENT

A cleft lip defect is observable at birth. A cleft palate defect is usually noted during the newborn assessment by palpation of the hard palate with the finger (Merritt, 2005b). A description of the location and extent of the defect helps the nurse determine the correct method of feeding. Thorough and complete physical assessment is required since additional defects are sometimes present.

PSYCHOSOCIAL ASSESSMENT

Assessment of the family's reactions is an integral part of the overall nursing assessment. Physical deformities, especially of the face, can be devastating to parents. A poorly corrected defect can lead to the development of low self-esteem in the older child. Assess the child's developmental level and social interactions with peers.

The accompanying Nursing Care Plan lists common nursing diagnoses for the infant with a cleft lip and/or palate. Other diagnoses that might be appropriate include the following:

- *Anxiety (Parent)* related to situational crisis and threat to self-concept
- *Risk for Impaired Parent/Infant Attachment* related to newborn's structural defect

- *Acute Pain* related to surgical repair of defect
- *Risk for Delayed Growth and Development* related to structural defect and altered nutritional intake

PLANNING AND IMPLEMENTATION

Nursing care involves providing emotional support, performing postsurgical care, helping parents coordinate care and maintain a healthy home environment, and making appropriate referrals. See "Nursing Care Plan: The Infant with a Cleft Lip or Palate" for a summary of nursing care.

PROVIDE EMOTIONAL SUPPORT

When a child is born with a cleft lip/cleft palate, parents may grieve the loss of the ideal child that they expected (Merritt, 2005b). Parents may need assistance to view their infant as a whole person, rather than focusing solely on the physical defect. Promote parent–infant bonding by explaining the nature of the structural defect and the procedure for correction. Interact and speak to the infant in the parents' presence and point out positive attributes such as alertness, soft skin, or active movements. Self-blame is common among parents. Parents can also be referred to the American Cleft Palate Association for information about the disorder. Pictures of children who have had repair are available at this Web site. Seeing pictures of children who have had a successful repair offers reassurance to parents (Weblink: www.cleftline.org/).

Parental anxiety is a typical response when children undergo surgery, and it is heightened when the surgery involves an infant. To minimize anxiety, give clear, concise explanations to parents. Allow sufficient time for parents to ask questions. Encourage parents to hold and cuddle the infant before surgery (Chapter 41 ∞).

PROVIDE POSTOPERATIVE CARE

Provide general postoperative care for the infant. (See "Nursing Care Plan: The Infant with a Cleft Lip or Palate" in this chapter and "Nursing Care Plan: The Child Undergoing Surgery" in Chapter 41.) Additional postoperative nursing diagnoses may include:

- Risk for infection related to location of surgical procedure
- Deficient (parent) related to lack of exposure and unfamiliarity with resources

The nurse should assess vital signs frequently and maintain the infant's airway. Intake and output should be measured. When oral fluids with clear liquids are started, they are usually given through a dropper, syringe, or special feeder. The infant should be positioned in a sitting position for the feedings to avoid aspiration. Frequent burping during feedings is also important. The infant then progresses to half-strength formula or breast milk. After each feeding, the suture line should be cleaned with water or normal saline to avoid accumulation of feedings. In addition, specific interventions are necessary to ensure healing of the suture line and include:

- Prevent the infant from rubbing the suture line on the bedding by positioning the infant in a supine or a side-lying position to avoid rubbing the suture line on the bedding.

> **Growth and Development**
>
> An infant who has had a cleft lip repair needs stimulation to provide distraction. This approach will minimize crying, which can damage the suture line. Soft, colorful toys, mobiles, and other visual objects are helpful. Music also can be used to soothe the infant. Parental presence is comforting and reassuring.

- Keep elbows in soft immobilizers.
- Maintain the suture line or Steri-Strips placed over the incision. Place antibiotic body ointment on the incision site as ordered.
- Medicate the infant as prescribed to control pain and to minimize crying and stress on the suture line.
- After cleft palate surgery, avoid the use of metal utensils or straws, which may disrupt the surgical site.

NURSING CARE IN THE COMMUNITY

Home care needs should be discussed well in advance of discharge. Discuss all aspects of the infant's care with the parents throughout hospitalization and after surgery. Involve parents in the infant's care to increase their comfort level before discharge and to promote bonding. Teach feeding techniques, how to recognize signs of infection, how to position the infant, and how to care for the suture line. Breastfeeding is usually possible with some assistance from a lactation specialist, even if the mother pumps her breasts and milk is fed by a special nurser. For infants requiring assistance to feed, several wide-based nipples, squeezable bottles, and other special bottles are available. Some infants may require a device placed in the mouth to enable them to establish suction. Management involves many different healthcare professionals. In addition to hospital, clinic, and home health nurses, members of the healthcare team often include specialists such as the plastic surgeon, orthodontist, dentist, social worker, audiologist, speech pathologist, and pediatrician (Kasten et al., 2008). The parents are the best coordinators of the child's care. Encourage them to keep a diary listing the professionals with whom they talk and the content of the discussions.

Private insurance does not always cover all the costs of care necessary for the child, therefore the financial implications of long care should be discussed with the parents by someone with expertise in this area. A social worker or financial counselor can provide information related to programs and financial assistance for which the parents and child may be eligible. Relief from financial worries enables parents to concentrate on caring for the child.

Discharge teaching related to care of the child at home is essential for the child. If the child has siblings, emphasize that they will need preparation to accept the child. Sibling rivalry can be heightened when one child receives more attention in the home. The parents should be reminded of the importance of setting limits and of spending time with each child. Determine whether additional family supports are necessary. Parents

Nursing Care Plan

THE INFANT WITH A CLEFT LIP OR PALATE

INTERVENTION	RATIONALE	EXPECTED OUTCOME
Preoperative Care		
1. Nursing Diagnosis: Risk for Aspiration (breast milk, formula, or mucus) related to anatomic defect		
NIC Priority Intervention: **Aspiration precautions:** Prevention or minimization of risk factors in the patient at risk of aspiration		**NOC Suggested Outcome:** **Respiratory Status: Ventilation** Movement of air in and out of the lungs
Goal: The infant will have no episodes of gagging or aspiration.		
■ Assess respiratory status and monitor vital signs at least every 2 hours.	■ Allows for early identification of problems.	The infant exhibits no signs of respiratory distress.
■ Keep suction equipment and bulb syringe at bedside.	■ Suctioning may be necessary to remove milk or mucus.	
■ Position upright for feedings.	■ Minimizes passage of feedings through cleft.	
■ Feed slowly and use adaptive equipment as needed.	■ Facilitates intake while minimizing risk of aspiration.	
■ Hold upright for 30 minutes after feeding.	■ Prevents aspiration of feedings.	
■ Burp frequently (after every 15–30 mL of fluid).	■ Helps to prevent regurgitation and aspiration.	
2. Nursing Diagnosis: Compromised Family Coping related to birth of a child with a defect		
NIC Priority Intervention: **Caregiver Support:** Provision of the necessary information, advocacy, and support to facilitate primary patient care by someone other than a healthcare professional		**NOC Suggested Outcome:** **Family coping:** Family actions to manage stressors that tax family resources
Goal: Parents will begin bonding process with the infant. The family's coping ability will be maximized. Parents will verbalize the nature and sequelae of the defect.		
■ Help parents to hold the infant and facilitate feeding process.	■ Contact is essential for bonding.	Parents hold, comfort, and show concern for the infant.
■ Point out positive attributes of infant (hair, eyes, alertness, etc.).	■ Helps parents see the child as a whole, rather than concentrating on the defect.	
■ Explain surgical procedure and expected outcome. Show pictures of other children's cleft lip repair.	■ Eliminating unknown factors helps to decrease anxiety.	
■ Assess parents' knowledge of the defect, their degree of anxiety and level of discomfort, and the interpersonal relationships among family members.	■ Helps to determine the appropriate timing and amount of information to be given regarding the child's defect.	The family demonstrates improved coping ability before discharge.
■ Explore the reactions of extended family members.	■ Extended family is an important source of support for most parents of a newborn. Family members can often help promote acceptance and compliance with the treatment plan.	Parents receive necessary support to care for their infant.
■ Support open visitation.	■ Allows parents to continue the bonding process.	
■ Encourage parents to participate in caretaking activities (holding, diapering, feeding).	■ Participation in infant care decreases anxiety and provides parents with a sense of purpose.	

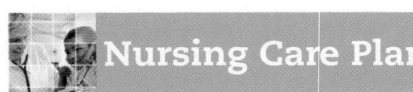

Nursing Care Plan—continued

THE INFANT WITH A CLEFT LIP OR PALATE

INTERVENTION	RATIONALE	EXPECTED OUTCOME
■ Provide information about the etiology of cleft lip and palate defects and the special needs of these infants. Encourage questions.	■ Concrete information allows parents time to understand the defect and reduces guilt.	
■ Refer to parent support groups.	■ Support groups allow parents to express their feelings and concerns, to find people with concerns similar to their own, and to seek additional information.	

3. Nursing Diagnosis: Imbalanced Nutrition: Less than Body Requirements related to the infant's inability to ingest nutrients

NIC Priority Intervention:

Nutrition management: Assistance with or provision of a balanced dietary intake of foods and fluids

NOC Suggested Outcome:

Nutrition status: Amount of food and fluid taken over a 24-hour period

Goal: The infant will gain weight steadily.

INTERVENTION	RATIONALE	EXPECTED OUTCOME
■ Assess fluid and calorie intake daily. Assess weight daily (same scale, same time, with infant completely undressed). Teach parents signs of adequate fluid intake such as frequency of wet diapers.	■ Provides an objective measurement of whether the infant is receiving sufficient caloric intake to promote growth. Using the same scale and procedure when weighing the infant provides for comparability between daily weights.	The infant maintains adequate nutritional intake and gains weight appropriately.
■ Observe for any respiratory impairment.	■ Any symptoms of respiratory compromise will interfere with the infant's ability to suck. Feedings should be initiated only if there are no signs of respiratory distress.	
■ Provide weight appropriate calories and fluid amounts. If the infant needs an increased number of calories to grow, referral to a nutritionist should be made. Formulas with higher calorie concentrations per ounce are available.	■ Provides optimal calories and fluids for growth and hydration.	
■ Facilitate breastfeeding.	■ Breast milk is recommended as the best food for an infant. The process of breastfeeding helps to promote bonding between mother and infant.	Successful breastfeeding is achieved if desired.
■ Hold the infant in an upright position.	■ Facilitates swallowing and minimizes the amount of fluid return from the nose.	
■ Give the mother information on breastfeeding the infant with a cleft lip or palate such as plugging the cleft lip and eliciting a letdown reflex before nursing.	■ Information and specific suggestions may encourage the mother to persist with breastfeeding.	
■ Contact the La Leche League for the name of a support person.	■ The La Leche League promotes breastfeeding for all infants. It can provide support people with experience who will aid the mother.	

(continued)

Nursing Care Plan—continued

THE INFANT WITH A CLEFT LIP OR PALATE

INTERVENTION	RATIONALE	EXPECTED OUTCOME
■ If the mother is unable to breastfeed (or prefers not to), initiate bottle-feeding:	■ Facilitates swallowing and minimizes the amount of fluid return from the nose.	Feeding provides necessary nutrients and is a positive experience for parents and infant.
■ Place nipple against the inside cheek toward the back of the tongue. May need to use a premature nipple (slightly longer and softer than regular nipple with a larger opening) or special cleft feeder.	■ Use of longer, softer nipples makes it easier for the infant to suck. Special cleft feeders decrease the amount of pressure in the bottle and makes the formula flow more easily.	
■ Feed small amounts slowly.	■ Small amounts and slow feeding do not tire the infant as quickly as do larger amounts given at a faster rate. They also decrease the calories used during feeding.	
■ Burp frequently, after 15–30 mL of formula has been given.	■ Frequent burping prevents the accumulation of air in the stomach, which can cause regurgitation or vomiting.	
■ Initiate nasogastric feedings if the infant is unable to ingest sufficient calories by mouth.	■ Adequate nutrition must be maintained. Use of a feeding tube allows the infant who has difficulty with oral feeding to receive adequate nutrition for growth.	

Postoperative Care

1. Nursing Diagnosis: Ineffective Breathing Pattern related to surgical correction of defect

NIC Priority Intervention:

Airway management: Facilitation of patency of air passages

NOC Suggested Outcome:

Vital signs status: Temperature, pulse, respiration, and blood pressure within expected range for the infant/child

Goal: The infant will maintain an effective breathing pattern.

INTERVENTION	RATIONALE	EXPECTED OUTCOME
■ Assess respiratory status and monitor vital signs at least every 2 hours.	■ Allows for early identification of problems.	The infant shows no signs of respiratory infection or compromise.
■ Apply a cardiorespiratory monitor.	■ Enables early detection of abnormal respirations, facilitating prompt intervention.	
■ Keep suction equipment and bulb syringe at bedside. Gently suction oropharynx and nasopharynx as needed.	■ Gentle suctioning will keep the airway clear. Suctioning that is too vigorous can irritate the mucosa.	
■ Provide cool mist for first 24 hours postoperatively if ordered.	■ Moisturizes secretions to reduce pooling in lungs. Moisturizes oral cavity.	
■ Reposition every 2 hours.	■ Ensures expansion of all lung fields.	

2. Nursing Diagnosis: Impaired Tissue Integrity related to mechanical factors

NIC Priority Intervention:

Wound care: Prevention of wound complications and promotion of wound healing

NOC Suggested Outcome:

Wound healing: The extent to which cells and tissues have regenerated following intentional closure

Goal: Lip and/or palate will heal with minimal scarring or disruption.

INTERVENTION	RATIONALE	EXPECTED OUTCOME
■ Position the infant with cleft lip repair on back.	■ Prone position could cause rubbing on suture line.	Lip/palate heals without complications.
■ Use soft elbow immobilizers. Remove every 2 hours and replace. Do not leave the infant unattended when restraints are removed.	■ Prevents the infant's hands from rubbing surgical site. Regular removal allows for skin and neurovascular checks.	

Nursing Care Plan—continued

THE INFANT WITH A CLEFT LIP OR PALATE

INTERVENTION	RATIONALE	EXPECTED OUTCOME
■ Maintain suture line or Steri-Strips placed over cleft lip repair.	■ Maintaining suture line will minimize scarring.	
■ Avoid metal utensils or straws after cleft palate repair.	■ These devices may disrupt suture line.	
■ Do not allow pacifiers.	■ Sucking can disrupt suture line.	
■ Keep the infant well medicated for pain in initial postoperative period. Have parents hold and comfort the infant.	■ Good pain management minimizes crying, which can cause stress on suture line. Increases bonding and soothes the child to decrease crying.	
■ Provide developmentally appropriate activities (i.e., mobiles, music).	■ Soothes and keeps the infant calm.	

3. Nursing Diagnosis: Imbalanced Nutrition: Less than Body Requirements related to inability to ingest nutrients

NIC Priority Intervention:

Nutrition management: Assistance with or provision of a balanced dietary intake of food and fluids

NOC Suggested Outcome:

Nutritional status: Extent to which nutrients are available to meet metabolic needs

Goal: The infant will receive adequate nutritional intake.

INTERVENTION	RATIONALE	EXPECTED OUTCOME
■ Maintain intravenous infusion as ordered.	■ Provides fluid when NPO.	The infant receives adequate nutritional intake. Infant resumes usual feeding patterns and gains weight appropriately.
■ Begin with clear liquids, then give half-strength formula or breast milk as ordered.	■ Ensures adequate fluids and nutrients.	
■ Use syringe or dropper inside of mouth.	■ Avoids suture line and resultant accumulation of formula in that area.	
■ Give high-calorie soft foods after cleft palate repair.	■ Rough foods, utensils, and straws could disrupt the surgical site.	

should be provided with information on support groups, physicians, social workers, Internet resources, and local services that can help maintain family continuity.

Discharge teaching should include ways to prevent the infant from touching the suture line such as:

- Bundling an infant in a blanket with arms tucked inside the blanket.
- Using a front-sling baby carrier to immobilize the arms. Front-sling carriers provide the additional benefits of comforting the infant through contact with the parent and of holding the infant upright, which aids in optimal positioning after feedings.

After surgical repair, parents need to be taught how to feed the infant and identify signs of complications (fever, vomiting, respiratory distress). Referral to a home healthcare agency for support may be helpful. Encourage follow-up visits with healthcare professionals (see "Health Promotion: The Child with Cleft Lip or Cleft Palate"). The child may need further evaluation of speech development, ear infections, or a recommendation for plastic surgery.

EVALUATION

Expected outcomes of nursing care are provided in the accompanying Nursing Care Plan.

ESOPHAGEAL ATRESIA AND TRACHEOESOPHAGEAL FISTULA

Esophageal atresia is a malformation that results from failure of the esophagus to develop as a continuous tube during the fourth and fifth weeks of gestation. The defect affects approximately 1 in 4000 neonates with at least 90% of those affected also having a tracheoesophageal fistula (Orenstein, Peters, Khan, et al., 2007).

Etiology and Pathophysiology

In esophageal atresia the foregut fails to lengthen, separate, and fuse into two parallel tubes (the esophagus and trachea) during fetal development. Instead the esophagus may end in a blind pouch or develop as a pouch connected to the trachea by a fistula

HEALTH PROMOTION

THE CHILD WITH CLEFT LIP OR CLEFT PALATE

The child with cleft lip or cleft palate requires close monitoring and intervention to foster growth and development. The nurse can assist the child and family to achieve healthy outcomes.

Growth and Development Surveillance

- Monitor the child's growth and developmental patterns.
- Monitor for developmental delays.
- Explain to parents that regression following surgery in the toddler or older child is normal.

Nutrition

- Refer family to sources for nipples, nursers, and other special feeding devices.
- Assist mother with learning how to express breast milk and facilitate breastfeeding.
- Teach parents to avoid foods that can pose a choking hazard to the child.
- Teach parents to feed the infant in an upright position and to burp the child frequently during feedings.

Physical Activity

- Activity for the child having surgical procedures to correct cleft palate is generally restricted for approximately 2 to 3 weeks to allow for healing.
- After healing has occurred, encourage the parents to promote the child's activities as they would any child without cleft lip or cleft palate.

Oral Health

- The child should be routinely screened for dental caries. Ask family about dental visits.
- Teach the parents to provide good dental hygiene to the child.
- Routine dental/orthodontic evaluation is necessary for the child with cleft palate.

Mental and Spiritual Health

- For uncorrected or poorly corrected cleft lip or palate, the child may experience poor self-esteem related to body image.
- Encourage family to adhere to treatment and surgical correction plan, including staged surgical corrections, dental care, and speech pathology assistance.
- Ask the family about financial ability regarding speech therapy, dental care, and other services that may be required. Financial constraints can impede compliance to recommended therapies.
- Be alert for the child who has had experiences with teasing associated with articulation or physical appearance.
- Refer parents to Web sites such as Project Smile and other resources.
- Refer the child for counseling if indicated.

Relationships

- Evaluate the parents for parent–infant bonding.
- Promote bonding by encouraging the parents to participate in the infant's care, to hold the infant, and to recognize the infant's positive attributes.

Disease Prevention Strategies

- Teach family to recognize signs and symptoms of ear or other infections and to seek immediate evaluation. Treatment of acute otitis media is necessary to prevent long-term effects of repeated infections.
- Emphasize to the parents the importance of audiology screening for children with cleft lip and palate to evaluate conductive hearing loss.

Injury Prevention Strategies (Safety)

- Assist parents to properly apply elbow restraints or to wrap child in mummy blanket to protect suture line in the postoperative period.
- Ask the parents about eating utensils the child uses.
- Teach parents to avoid straws, metal spoons, and other sharp utensils that may damage palate.

(tracheoesophageal fistula) (see "Pathophysiology Illustrated: Esophageal Atresia and Tracheoesophageal Fistula"). Esophageal atresia is often associated with a maternal history of polyhydramnios. Associated anomalies may occur, including congenital heart defects, gastrointestinal or urinary tract anomalies, and musculoskeletal abnormalities (Orenstein et al., 2007). Jerome, described at the beginning of the chapter, had esophageal atresia as well as an imperforate anus.

Clinical Manifestations

Symptoms in the newborn include excessive salivation and drooling, often accompanied by three classic signs for this defect: cyanosis, choking, coughing. Sneezing may also be manifested. During feeding, the infant returns fluid through the nose and mouth. Aspiration places the infant at risk for pneumonia. Depending on the type of defect, the infant's abdomen may be distended.

Diagnosis is usually confirmed by attempting to pass a nasogastric or orogastric tube into the stomach. In most cases the tube meets resistance and can be advanced only minimally. Radiologic examination reveals specific defects and associated anomalies. The lungs need to be examined carefully. A delay in diagnosis can be fatal because ingested fluid or secretions may enter the lungs and lead to pneumonia (Orenstein et al., 2007).

Clinical Therapy

A nasogastric tube is inserted to suction the upper pouch and intravenous antibiotics and fluids are started. Surgery is performed as soon as possible. Surgical correction may be accomplished in several stages. The first stage usually involves ligation of the fistula and insertion of a gastrostomy tube. In the second stage, the two ends of the esophagus are reconnected, if possible. When surgical closure (anastomosis) is not possible, a gastrostomy tube must remain in place for feedings. Potential postoperative complications include

PATHOPHYSIOLOGY ILLUSTRATED

ESOPHAGEAL ATRESIA AND TRACHEOESOPHAGEAL FISTULA

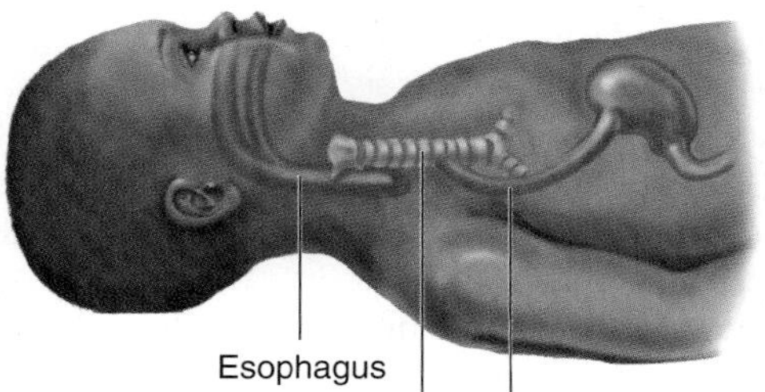

In the most common type of esophageal atresia and tracheoesophageal fistula, the upper segment of the esophagus ends in a blind pouch connected to the trachea; a fistula connects the lower segment to the trachea.

gastroesophageal reflux, aspiration, and stricture formation. The prognosis is usually good with surgery; however, some conditions are complicated, requiring repeated surgeries and long-term management. In the event that the two ends of the esophagus cannot be reconnected, colonic, jejunal, or gastric segments may be used to lengthen the esophagus (Orenstein et al., 2007).

Nursing Management

The nurse may recognize the signs and symptoms in the immediate newborn period. Assess the infant for difficulty feeding and excessive drooling and the classic signs of choking, coughing, and cyanosis. Assess for respiratory distress and assess the lung sounds carefully.

Esophageal atresia is a surgical emergency. Preoperatively the infant requires close observation and intervention to maintain a patent airway. Specific interventions include:

- Have suction readily available to remove any secretions that accumulate in the nasopharyngeal airway.
- Place the infant with the head of the bed slightly elevated to minimize aspiration of secretions into the trachea.
- Use continuous or low intermittent suction to remove secretions from the blind pouch.
- Withhold oral fluids, and provide maintenance intravenous fluids.
- Constantly monitor the infant's vital signs and overall condition.

After surgery, measure gastrostomy drainage, and administer intravenous fluids and antibiotics. Total parenteral nutrition may be needed until gastrostomy or oral feedings are tolerated. Monitoring and assessment of feeding tolerance are ongoing. Feedings are

Teaching Highlights

TEACHING THE FAMILY ABOUT GASTROSTOMY TUBE FEEDINGS

The infant or child who has difficulty swallowing, consuming oral feedings, or gaining weight may be a candidate for gastrostomy tube placement. Children with chronic conditions such as failure to thrive, cystic fibrosis, neurological impairment, or gastrointestinal anomalies may need to have a gastrostomy tube placed for long-term enteral feedings (Borkowski, 2005). Parents of children who have or will receive a gastrostomy tube need clear instructions to maximize the benefit of the device to the child. See Chapter 41 for general guidelines related to teaching plans. See also the accompanying Clinical Skills Manual, Skill 15-3 SKILLS.

General Principles

Preoperatively

- Assess the family's knowledge about gastrostomy tube placement.
- Assess the parents and extended family members' willingness to learn about care of the gastrostomy tube and enteral feedings.
- Show the family pictures or dolls with gastrostomy tubes and explain what the child's abdomen will look like in the immediate postoperative period.
- Provide the family with a booklet about gastrostomy tubes and enteral feedings.

Postoperatively

- Show the family the child's gastrostomy tube and reassess their understanding of the tube.
- When feedings are ordered, demonstrate the first feeding to the parents while explaining each step.
- Actively involve a family member in the second feeding. With subsequent feedings, have a family member demonstrate feeding to the nurse.
- Teach the family about:
  - Medication administration.
  - Daily care of the tube and the site surrounding the tube.
  - How to troubleshoot common complications.
- Provide family with phone numbers to call if needed.
- All family members that are involved in care of the child should practice feeding the child and administering medications to the child before discharge. This allows the nurse to assess for understanding of the procedure and gives the family confidence in their ability to care for the child. Some children will need bolus feedings, others may have continuous feedings via a feeding pump, and others may have bolus feedings during the day and continuous feedings at night.

Data from: Borkowski, S. (2005, May). Irritation, redness, and drainage at the site of a pediatric gastrostomy. *The Clinical Advisor, 8*(5), 90–91; Holmes, S. (2004). Enteral feeding and percutaneous endoscopic gastrostomy. *Nursing Standard, 18*(20), 41–43.

introduced slowly and in small amounts. Assess for respiratory difficulty during reintroduction of feedings. Monitor weight, growth, and developmental achievements.

The parents require emotional support throughout the infant's hospitalization. Clearly explain all procedures. Encourage parents to bond with the infant by stroking and talking to the infant. Eliciting questions and allowing parents to participate in the infant's care, especially feeding (when permitted), can facilitate bonding and help to prepare parents for care of the infant after discharge.

Once enteral feedings have been established, the infant may be discharged from the hospital with a gastrostomy tube in place. Teach the parents about gastrostomy tube care and feeding, signs of infection, and how to prevent postoperative complications.

The outcomes of nursing care will depend on the extent of the defect and correction. Examples include the following:

- Adequate intake of fluids and nutrition to promote hydration and growth
- Absence of respiratory distress
- Positive parent-infant bonding
- Healing without infection

PYLORIC STENOSIS

Pyloric stenosis is a hypertrophic obstruction of the circular muscle of the pyloric canal. Pyloric stenosis occurs in approximately 1 in 1000 live births (Vajnar, 2007). Males are affected more often than females by a 4:1 ratio (Liao, Li, Zhang, et al., 2007). There is an increased incidence in firstborn white males (Wyllie, 2007).

Etiology and Pathophysiology

The exact cause of pyloric stenosis is unknown, although frequently there is a family history of the disorder. *Hypergastrinemia* (too much gastrin in the blood) is thought to play a role in the development of pyloric stenosis. Studies have indicated a higher incidence of the disorder in infants who received prostaglandin E infusion for patent ductus arteriosis and in infants less than a month old who have received oral erythromycin. Gastroesophageal reflux is frequently also present in premature infants with pyloric stenosis, complicating the differential diagnosis (Joshi, Mahajan, & Kamat, 2006).

Hypertrophy of the circular pylorus muscle results in stenosis of the passage between the stomach and the duodenum, partially obstructing the lumen of the stomach (see "Pathophysiology Illustrated: Pyloric Stenosis"). The lumen becomes inflamed and edematous, which narrows the opening until the obstruction becomes complete. At this time vomiting becomes more forceful. As the obstruction progresses, the infant becomes dehydrated and electrolytes are depleted, resulting in metabolic imbalances.

Clinical Manifestations

Symptoms usually become evident 2 to 8 weeks after birth, although onset may vary. Most cases are diagnosed by 12 weeks of age (Vajnar, 2007). Initially the infant appears well or regurgitates slightly after feedings. The parents may describe the infant as a "good eater" who vomits occasionally. As the obstruction progresses, the vomiting becomes projectile. In **projectile vomiting**, the contents of the stomach may be ejected up to 3 feet from the

PATHOPHYSIOLOGY ILLUSTRATED

PYLORIC STENOSIS

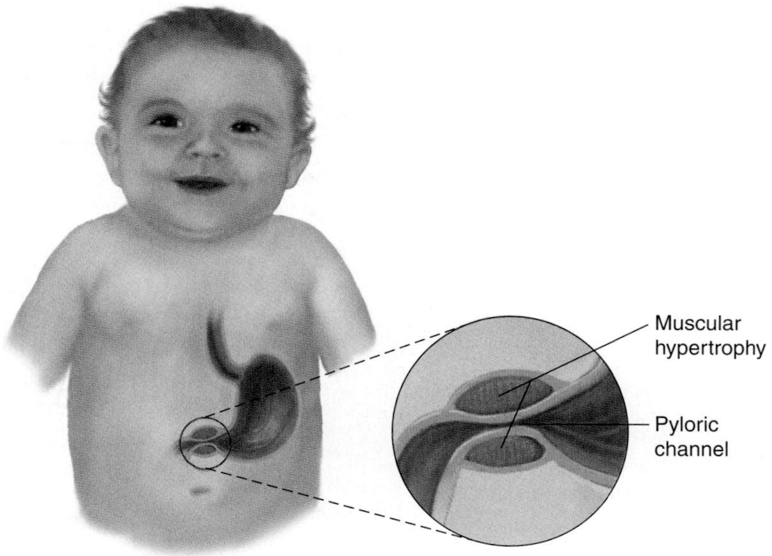

In pyloric stenosis, the hypertrophied pyloric muscle causes symptoms of projectile vomiting and visible peristalsis.

infant. The vomitus is nonbilious and may become blood tinged because of repeated irritation to the esophagus. The infant generally appears hungry, especially after emesis, irritable, fails to gain weight, and has fewer and smaller stools. Loss of gastric secretions results in dehydration and potentially metabolic alkalosis. On physical examination, visible peristaltic waves across the abdomen and an olive-sized mass in the right upper quadrant may be evident (Vajnar, 2007).

Clinical Therapy

An abdominal ultrasound to assess the diameter and length of the pyloric muscle, is usually performed to confirm the diagnosis. A thickened pylorus of greater than 4 mm in diameter and pyloric length of greater than 14 mm support a diagnosis of pyloric stenosis (Joshi et al., 2006). An upper gastrointestinal (UGI) study may be performed and reveals a narrowing of the pyloric channel, preventing the passage of the contrast medium.

Blood tests determine the degree of dehydration, electrolyte imbalance, and anemia (see Chapter 46); common findings are hypochloremia, hypokalemia, metabolic alkalosis, and hyperbilirubinemia (Vajnar, 2007). Early diagnosis will decrease the frequency with which infants present with an alteration in electrolytes.

Surgery is performed as soon as possible after the infant's fluid and electrolyte balance is restored. Open pyloromyotomy is performed through a periumbilical incision or through a small, transverse upper abdominal incision. Laparoscopic pyloromyotomy is currently used in many cases, and has been shown to be equally as successful as open pyloromyotomy (Wyllie, 2007). With both procedures, the pyloric muscle is split to allow the passage of food and fluid.

The prognosis is good. The infant is usually taking fluids within a few hours following surgery and discharged on full strength formula within 24 hours after surgery.

NURSING MANAGEMENT

NURSING ASSESSMENT AND DIAGNOSIS

Observe the infant's abdomen for the presence of peristaltic waves. Bowel sounds are hyperactive on auscultation. Auscultate before palpating the abdomen since palpation can cause a change in bowel patterns (see Chapter 35). Palpation reveals an olive-shaped mass in the right upper quadrant of the abdomen.

Assess the infant's history of vomiting, vital signs, weight, and nutritional status. Assess skin turgor, fontanels, urinary output (weigh diapers), urine specific gravity, and mucous membranes to determine whether hydration is adequate. Describe vomiting episodes and estimate emesis amount. Be alert for signs of an electrolyte imbalance, particularly low levels of serum chloride, sodium, and potassium, and an elevated pH. (See Chapter 46 for a discussion of these electrolyte imbalances.) Assess parental anxiety related to the child's condition. The child is usually hungry and tries to feed. Crying and general discomfort are frequently observed.

Among the nursing diagnoses that might be appropriate for the child with pyloric stenosis are the following:

- *Deficient Fluid Volume* related to active fluid volume loss
- *Imbalanced Nutrition: Less than Body Requirements* related to vomiting and inability to ingest nutrients
- *Sleep Pattern Disturbance* related to discomfort and hunger
- *Parental Anxiety* related to surgery
- *Pain* related to surgical incision

PLANNING AND IMPLEMENTATION

Nursing care focuses on meeting the infant's fluid and electrolyte needs, minimizing weight loss, promoting rest and comfort, preventing infection, and providing supportive care for parents.

MEET FLUID AND ELECTROLYTE NEEDS

Withhold oral feedings preoperatively because projectile vomiting will continue until the obstruction is relieved. Emphasize to the parents the importance of maintaining an NPO status preoperatively. Intravenous therapy is administered to correct fluid and electrolyte imbalances and to maintain adequate hydration. Because gastric fluid is high in potassium, hypokalemia can result (see Chapter 46 for a discussion and signs of this electrolyte imbalance). Maintain patency of nasogastric tube if one is present and measure aspirated contents. Inform parents that all diapers will be weighed to measure the infant's output of urine and stool.

MINIMIZE WEIGHT LOSS

The infant loses weight because of frequent vomiting. Monitor weight daily both preoperatively and postoperatively. Begin feedings postoperatively according to the healthcare provider's orders. Conventional feeding methods include a prolonged NPO period following pyloromyotomy, with slow, incremental increases in volume and strength of feedings once feeding has resumed. In recent years, some surgeons have implemented an earlier postoperative feeding approach.

PROMOTE REST AND COMFORT

During the preoperative period, the infant is hungry and cries often. The infant is swaddled to maintain warmth and provide comfort. Encourage the parents to hold and cuddle the infant. Provide a pacifier to meet the infant's need to suck.

Postoperatively the infant is uncomfortable due to the surgical incision. Acetaminophen or other analgesics can be administered to relieve discomfort as ordered. (See Chapter 42 for a discussion of pain management.) Instruct parents to avoid pressure on the incision. When diapering the infant, slide the diaper gently under the buttocks rather than lifting the legs. Swaddling, rocking, and use of a pacifier provide comfort to the infant.

PREVENT INFECTION

Postoperatively the incision is covered with collodion or Steri-Strips and should be kept clean and dry. Inspect the incision site for redness, swelling, or discharge. Monitor the infant's temperature every 4 hours. Auscultate the lungs to assess for any adventitious sounds.

PROVIDE SUPPORTIVE CARE

The need for hospitalization and surgery creates anxiety for parents. Encourage them to participate in the infant's care and to discuss their fears and concerns. Provide simple and clear explanations about the infant's condition and care. Advise parents that occasional vomiting after surgery may occur.

DISCHARGE PLANNING AND HOME CARE TEACHING

Instruct parents to observe the incision for redness, swelling, or discharge and to notify the physician immediately if these occur or if the infant's temperature is higher than 38.5°C (101°F). To reduce the possibility of infection, advise parents to fold the infant's diaper so that it does not touch the incision. Provide instructions about feeding to ensure the infant's intake.

EVALUATION

Expected outcomes of care include pain control, intake of recommended fluid and food with absence of vomiting, and manifestation of normal growth patterns.

GASTROESOPHAGEAL REFLUX

Gastroesophageal reflux (GER), the return of gastric contents into the esophagus, is the result of relaxation of the lower esophageal sphincter (Suwandhi, Ton, & Schwarz, 2006). GER is one of the most common gastrointestinal disorders in children, affecting approximately 50% of infants ages 0–3 months (International Pediatric Endosurgery Group [IPEG], 2008). There is a higher incidence in premature infants, and males are affected three times more often than females. Children with neurologic impairments, such as cerebral palsy, more commonly experience GER. Some "spitting up" after feedings is considered normal in newborn infants, because of the weak cardiac sphincter of the stomach. However, regurgitation that continues and increases in frequency may be caused by GER and requires further investigation.

Etiology and Pathophysiology

Gastroesophageal reflux disease (GERD) is a more serious manifestation of GER; it is a pathologic process in infants manifested by poor weight gain, recurrent vomiting, generalized irritability, refusal to feed, arching, and respiratory symptoms such as wheezing (Gold & Gremse, 2006). GERD is diagnosed in approximately one in every 300 infants (Henry, 2004). Those children most at risk include those with neurologic disorders, syndromes, trisomy 21, bronchopulmonary dysplasia, and tracheoesophageal fistula (Henry, 2004).

Clinical Manifestations

Regurgitation after feeding is the most common sign of gastroesophageal reflux in infants. The infant may spit up a small amount or may have episodes of forceful vomiting (Arguin & Swartz, 2004). Children with gastroesophageal reflux are frequently hungry and irritable. They eat often but still lose weight. They have a history of vomiting and frequent upper respiratory infections and are at risk for aspiration and episodes of apnea (Arguin & Swartz, 2004).

Diagnosis is confirmed by a thorough history of the child's feeding patterns and by diagnostic evaluation using contrast upper GI series (barium fluoroscopy), pH probe monitoring (insertion of a small catheter into the esophagus through the nose that is left in place for 18 to 24 hours to measure pH and thus determine number of reflux episodes), or nuclear medicine scintiscan (gastric emptying study) (Henry, 2004). The child should be tested for cow's milk protein allergy since there is an association between gastroesophageal reflux and cow's milk allergy. Testing includes cutaneous tests, eosinophil smears of the nasal mucosa, IgG antilactoglobulin levels, and intestinal biopsy (Arguin & Swartz, 2004).

Clinical Therapy

Treatment depends on the severity of the condition. Generally, feeding modification, thickened feeds, and positioning are effective management for milder cases. A smaller feeding volume may prove beneficial to avoid overdistention of the abdomen and subsequent reflux. The infant should be burped after every 1 to 2 ounces (Arguin & Swartz, 2004). Rice cereal is sometimes placed in the infant's bottle to thicken feedings to a consistency similar to nectar. Note that breast milk will not readily thicken with addition of cereal. Prethickened formulas are commercially available. For example, Enfamil AR contains added rice and is nutritionally balanced. These formulas can be administered without enlarging the nipple hole. Formula change to a protein hydrolysate or elemental formula, such as Pregestimil, Nutramigen, or Alimentum, may be recommended (Arguin & Swartz, 2004). Fatty foods and citrus juices are avoided.

Medications (proton pump inhibitors, antacids, and histamine antagonists) may be prescribed to reduce the amount of stomach acid and lessen the child's discomfort. See "Drug Guide: Medications Used to Treat Gastroesophageal Reflux Disease."

Treatment for severe cases of GERD may include surgery to create a valve mechanism by wrapping the greater curvature of the stomach (fundus) around the distal esophagus (fundoplication) (IPEG, 2008). A gastrostomy tube is usually inserted during

Nursing Practice

The best position in which to place the postprandial infant with GERD is the prone position with the head elevated. However, the prone position should not be used in the sleeping child due to the increased incidence of sudden infant death syndrome with this position. Caution parents to use the prone position only while the infant is awake and while being continuously observed by the parent (Arguin & Swartz, 2004). Parents are encouraged to hold their infant in an upright position for 20 to 30 minutes following feedings. Minimize seated positioning such as in an infant seat because this increases intra-abdominal pressure and promotes reflux.

Drug Guide

MEDICATIONS USED TO TREAT GASTROESOPHAGEAL REFLUX DISEASE

MEDICATION AND ACTION	NURSING IMPLICATIONS
Zantac (ranitidine) Pepcid (famotidine) Inhibition of the histamine H_2 receptor on the gastric parietal cell, thus blocking gastric acid secretion	May be administered with or without food If antacids are prescribed, administer 2 hours before or after H_2 antagonists Teach parents to avoid OTC medications without checking with healthcare provider Monitor for side effects: Bradycardia, Fatigue, Rash Constipation, Headache, Confusion Nausea, Irritability, Thrombocytopenia Dizzinesss
Prevacid (lansoprazole) Prilosec (omeprazole) These powerful inhibitors of acid secretion alleviate symptoms and help to heal esophagitis Blocks the final common pathway of acid production by inhibiting activated proton pumps in the gastric parietal cell canaliculus	Administer in the morning on an empty stomach Antacids may be administered with omeprazole Monitor for side effects: Abdominal pain, Fatigue, Nausea Diarrhea, Headache, Proteinuria Dizziness, Hematuria, Rash Teach family to inform primary healthcare provider if severe diarrhea occurs Teach family to inform primary healthcare provider if changes in urinary elimination, such as pain or discomfort associated with urination, occur.

Data from: Arguin, A. L., & Swartz, M. K. (2004). Gastroesophageal reflux in infants: A primary care perspective. *Pediatric Nursing, 30*(1), 45–51, 71. Bindler, R., & Howry, L. (2005). *Pediatric drug guide.* Upper Saddle River, NJ: Prentice Hall Health. Gold, B. D., & Gremse, D. A. (2006). Extinguishing the burn: Case Studies in pediatric reflux disease. *Self Study Supplement to Clinician Reviews.* Henry, S. M. (2004). Discerning differences: Gastroesophageal reflux and gastroesophageal reflux disease in infants. *Advances in Neonatal Care, 4*(4), 235–247.

surgery to serve as a vent for trapped gas (Henry, 2004). The gastrostomy tube may be removed after a few weeks or may be left in long term if needed for feedings.

Nursing Management

Nursing management focuses on supporting the infant's or child's nutritional intake, promoting interventions to reduce associated complications, and supporting the family.

Monitor the infant's weight daily and plot on a growth chart to note progress. Observe for any signs of respiratory distress, and keep the infant's nose and mouth clear of vomitus.

Adequate nutrition must be maintained for the child to achieve normal growth and development. Infants receiving oral feedings should be given small, frequent feedings. Elevate the head of the bed to prevent aspiration if vomiting should occur. If the child has a gastrostomy tube, it is important to maintain skin integrity around the stoma site.

Discharge planning focuses on instructing parents in how to feed and position the infant, as well as providing comfort and emotional support. Encourage parents to hold and cuddle the infant during all feedings. Providing the infant with a pacifier helps to meet nonnutritive sucking needs. Teach parents how to suction the nose and mouth if vomiting occurs.

OMPHALOCELE AND GASTROSCHISIS

Omphaloceles are congenital malformations in which intra-abdominal contents herniate through the umbilical cord (Figure 53–3 ●). An omphalocele results when the intestines fail to return to the abdomen when the abdominal wall begins to close by the 10th week of gestation. The size of the sac varies depending on the extent of the protrusion. Large defects may contain intestines, stomach, liver, and the spleen (Zimmerman, 2007). The abdominal contents are covered with peritoneum and amniotic membrane (Doughty, 2004). Rupture of the sac results in evisceration of the abdominal contents. Omphalocele with herniation of intestines into the umbilical cord occurs in 1 in 5000 births, while omphalocele with herniation of liver and intestines occurs in 1 in 10,000 births (Stoll, 2007). Thirty percent of infants with omphalocele will have an associated chromosomal anomaly and 30–50% will have congenital heart defects (Lund, Bauer, & Berrios (2007). Gastroschisis is a congenital defect of the ventral abdominal wall, characterized by herniation of abdominal viscera outside the abdominal cavity through a defect in the abdominal wall to the side (most often to the right) of the umbilicus. The most common abdominal organs involved are the small intestine and ascending colon. Unlike the omphalocele, no membrane covers the organs (Figure 53–4 ●). Gastroschisis

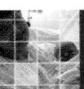

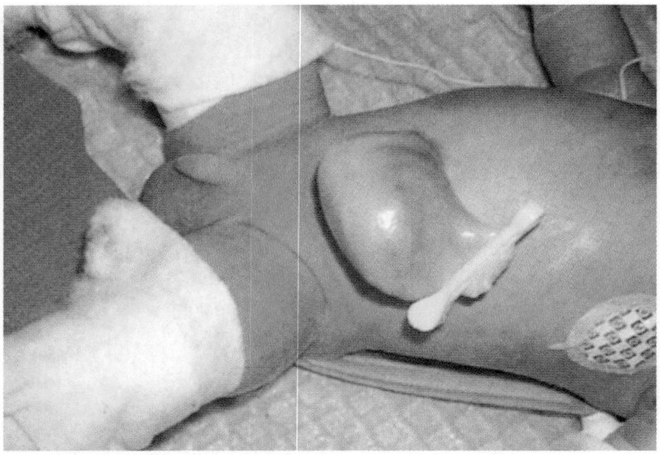

• **Figure 53–3** Omphalocele. In omphalocele, the size of the sack depends on the extent of the protrusion of abdominal contents through the umbilical cord.

Used with permission from Rudolph, A. M., Hoffman, J. I. E., & Rudolph, C. D. (Eds.). (1991). *Rudolph's pediatrics* (19th ed., p. 1040). Stamford, CT: Appleton & Lange.

occurs in approximately 1–2 in 10,000 births worldwide (Zimmerman, 2007). It is the most common abdominal wall defect in neonates (Lund et al., (2007). Gastroschisis is more common in infants of young mothers that smoke (Doughty, 2004). Approximately 10–20% of infants with gastroschisis have an associated anomaly, most often intestinal atresias. Anomalies outside of the gastrointestinal tract are uncommon in infants with gastroschisis (Lund et al., (2007). Care of the child with gastroschisis or omphalocele centers on protecting the protruding abdominal organs, correcting the defect, and preventing complications such as hypothermia, infection, and injury to involved organs.

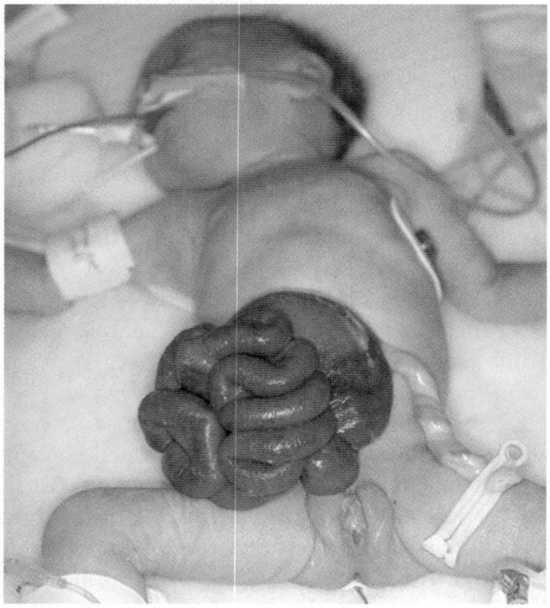

• **Figure 53–4** Gastroschisis. The newborn with gastroschisis has abdominal contents located outside the abdominal wall.

Used with permission of the authors and the University of Iowa's Virtual Hospital®, http://www.vh.org

Both gastroschisis and omphalocele are associated with elevation of maternal serum alpha-fetoprotein (MSAFP). Routine prenatal ultrasonography and determination of MSAFP levels permit early diagnosis and coordination of the team of specialists needed to manage these congenital anomalies including neonatologists and pediatric surgeons. The immediate action upon birth is to protect the sac (in omphalocele) or exposed abdominal contents (in gastroschisis) from injury by placing the infant feet first into a bowel bag that extends to the nipple line and is secured with ties. The bowel bag decreases heat loss and allows for visualization of the defect. The child with gastroschisis should first have the exposed abdominal contents covered with moist sterile gauze. The child will often be transferred to a NICU with surgical capability for this defect.

Surgical repair of omphalocele and gastroschisis may occur in one or two stages depending on the severity of the defect. For small defects one surgery may be all that is needed to repair the defect. For larger defects, the first stage of repair may involve nonoperative placement of the abdominal contents or sac into a silastic silo. Once the abdominal cavity can accommodate the intestinal contents the child will have surgery to close the abdominal wall (Lund et al., 2007; Zimmerman, 2007).

Nursing Management

Be alert for signs of associated congenital anomalies. (Refer to the discussions of tracheoesophageal fistula earlier in this chapter, of genitourinary anomalies in Chapter 54∞, and of congenital heart defects in Chapter 49∞.)

Immediately after birth, follow physician protocol for maintaining the omphalocele sac or for the exposed abdominal contents in gastroschisis as discussed previously. Monitor vital signs at least hourly, paying close attention to temperature, as the infant can lose heat through the sac. The child should be in a warmer or isolette for maintenance of temperature control. Inspect the area for signs of infection.

Because the infant is NPO preoperatively, maintain fluid and electrolyte balance with intravenous fluids. Postoperative care includes measures to control pain, prevent infection, maintain fluid and electrolyte balance, and ensure adequate nutritional intake. Attainment of bowel motility and function varies and is often delayed for weeks after surgery; parenteral nutrition for the infant is used during this period (Lund, et al, 2007).

Throughout the infant's hospitalization, parents need clear, accurate explanations about the infant's condition. To help the parents deal with the crisis of an acutely ill newborn, provide emotional support and encourage parents to express their feelings. When the child has multiple anomalies, parents need ongoing support for the lengthy treatment, numerous hospitalizations, and management of nutritional intake.

Expected outcomes of nursing care depend on the severity of the defect and its correction, but may include:

- Maintenace of fluid volume balance
- Healing without infection
- Maintenance of stable thermoregulatory function

- Effective pain management
- Parent /infant bonding and attachment demonstrated.

INTUSSUSCEPTION

Intussusception occurs when one portion of the intestine prolapses and then invaginates or telescopes into another. It is one of the most frequent causes of intestinal obstruction during infancy, second only to pyloric stenosis. Intussusception occurs at a rate of 1.5–4 per 1000 live births and is more common in males. Eighty percent of cases occur in children younger than 2 years (Fagerman & Farber, 2007).

Etiology and Pathophysiology

The etiology of intussusception is multifactorial, and direct causes cannot always be identified. While the exact cause of intussusception is unknown, it is frequently preceded by a viral infection of the gastrointestinal tract (Hackman, Newman, & Ford, 2005).

The most common site of intussusception is the ileocecal valve. Telescoping of the intestine obstructs the passage of stool. The walls of the intestine rub together, causing inflammation, edema, and decreased blood flow. This can lead to necrosis and loss of a significant portion of the intestine if not treated promptly (Fagerman & Farber, 2007) (Figure 53–5 ●).

Clinical Manifestation

The onset of intussusception is usually abrupt. A previously healthy infant or child suddenly experiences acute abdominal pain with vomiting and passage of brown stool. There may be periods of comfort between acute episodes of pain. As the condition worsens, painful episodes increase. The stools become red and resemble currant jelly because of the mix of blood and mucus (Fagerman & Farber, 2007). A palpable mass may be present in the upper right quadrant or mid-upper abdomen.

Clinical Therapy

Diagnosis is made on the basis of the history and confirmed by radiographs and ultrasound of the abdomen. A contrast enema using barium or air can be both diagnostic and therapeutic. In 70–90% of cases the hydrostatic pressure from the contrast moves the bowel back into place (Fagerman & Farber, 2007).

A nasogastric tube is inserted for gastric decompression. If reduction of the intussusception does not occur with these methods, surgical intervention to reduce the invaginated bowel and remove any necrotic tissue is necessary. Surgery is generally successful in correcting the problem; however, intussusception can recur after hydrostatic reduction or surgical correction.

Nursing Management

Nursing management focuses on maintaining or restoring fluid and electrolyte balance. Intravenous fluids are started immediately. Serum electrolyte monitoring is essential to correct imbalances.

Postoperative care focuses on monitoring for early signs of infection, managing the child's pain, and maintaining nasogastric tube patency. Assess vital signs, check for abdominal distention, and assess for return of bowel function. Feeding protocols vary among practitioners. Generally, after normal bowel function returns, clear liquid feeding or breastfeeding can resume. Feedings are then advanced to half-strength milk and other foods as the infant or child tolerates them.

Discharge usually occurs shortly after the infant or child begins taking full feedings. Instruct parents to watch for infection and to call the physician if symptoms recur, a fever develops, or appetite decreases.

Nursing Practice

The passage of a normal brown stool may indicate that an intussusception has been reduced. Report this finding to the primary care provider immediately, as the course of treatment may be altered, especially in the case of a planned surgical reduction.

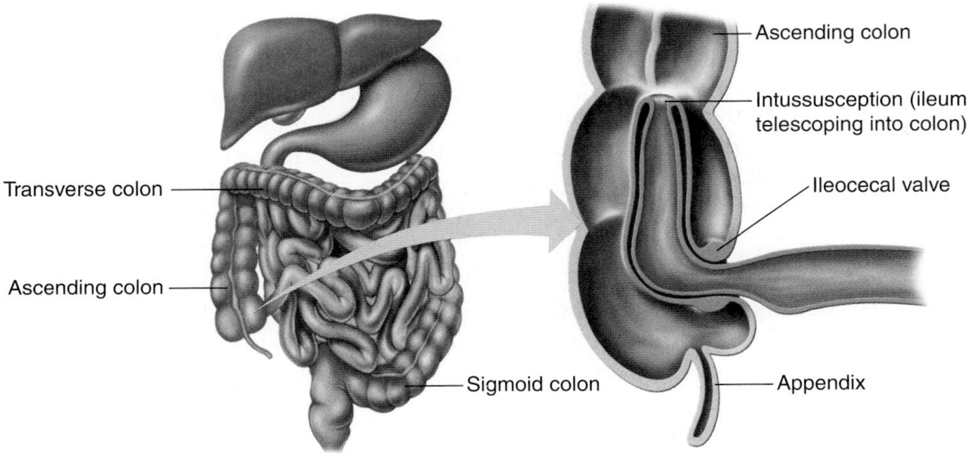

● **Figure 53–5** Intussusception. In infants, intussusception is commonly associated with viral illnesses and gastroenteritis.

Evidence in Action

Traditionally, the return of bowel sounds postoperatively has been a key indicator of the return of bowel function. Evidence-based research indicates that the best indicators of bowel function in patients undergoing abdominal surgery is passage of flatus and passage of stool (Madsen, Sebolt, Cullen, et al., 2005).

VOLVULUS

During the seventh to 12th week of gestation the small intestine undergoes rapid growth. In normal development, the intestine rotates counterclockwise as it settles into its permanent position inside the abdominal cavity. Malrotation of the intestine occurs in 1 out of 6000 live births and can lead to complications in the infant (Aiken & Oldham, 2005). If the bowel does not rotate normally during this process the child is at risk for *volvulus*, a twisting of the intestine (Doughty, 2004). Volvulus disrupts blood flow in the intestines and can lead to necrosis of the bowel, short bowel syndrome, and death. Volvulus is considered a surgical emergency (Aiken & Oldham, 2005). Early diagnosis and treatment is necessary to preserve the bowel and to save the child's life.

Symptoms of volvulus in the infant include bilious vomiting, firm abdomen with distention, irritability secondary to pain, and passage of bloody stools. Confirmation of malrotation of the intestine through upper GI series or contrast studies, supports a diagnosis of volvulus. Emergency exploratory surgery to untwist the bowel is essential (Diana-Zerpa & Shapiro-Stolar, 2007). If a portion of the bowel is necrotic, that portion of the bowel is removed. An ostomy may need to be created, depending on the amount of bowel removed (Aiken & Oldham, 2005). See the section on ostomies on page 1536. The child is at risk for developing short bowel syndrome if a significant amount of bowel is removed (see page 1554).

Nursing Management

The infant or child who presents to the emergency room with bilious vomiting and a firm and distended abdomen should be assessed quickly to determine the cause of the symptoms. Once volvulus has been diagnosed, nursing management focuses on keeping the child NPO, administering intravenous fluids, assessing of vital signs. and reporting symptoms of a worsening condition. The child who has had surgery to correct uncomplicated volvulus will need care similar to that described for the child with intussusception. If the child had necrotic bowel removed he or she may have an ostomy for a period of time.

HIRSCHSPRUNG DISEASE

Hirschsprung disease, also known as congenital aganglionic megacolon, is a congenital anomaly in which inadequate motility causes mechanical obstruction of the intestine. The disease occurs in approximately 1 in 5000 live births, and is more common in males than females. Hirschsprung disease can occur as a single anomaly or in combination with congenital heart defects and chromosomal abnormalities such as Down syndrome (Kessman, 2006).

Etiology and Pathophysiology

Hirschsprung disease is the congenital absence of ganglion cells in the wall of a variable segment of rectum and colon. It is now known that the RET protooncogene is a major gene for the disease. The absence of autonomic parasympathetic ganglion cells in the colon prevents peristalsis at that portion of the intestine, resulting in the accumulation of intestinal contents and abdominal distention. In most cases, the area lacking ganglion cells is limited to the rectosigmoid region of the colon (Kessman, 2006).

Clinical Manifestations

Clinical manifestations of Hirschsprung disease vary depending on the child's age at onset. In newborns, symptoms include failure to pass meconium within the first 48 hours after birth, abdominal distention, and bilious vomiting (Klar, 2007). If Hirschsprung disease is not treated, the condition can lead to fever, bloody **diarrhea** (frequent, watery stools), abdominal distention, and *enterocolitis* (inflammation of the intestines) (Biggs & Dery, 2006).

The older infant or child may have a history of failure to gain weight, malnutrition, chronic progressive **constipation** (difficult and infrequent defecation with passage of hard, dry stool), and recurrent fecal impaction (Kessman, 2006).The child may have a history of passage of pencil thin stools (Biggs & Dery, 2006).

Clinical Therapy

Diagnosis is made on the basis of the history, bowel patterns, anorectal manometry (reaction of the anal sphincter to distention of the rectum), radiographic contrast studies, and rectal biopsy for presence or absence of ganglion cells. The rectum is small in size on palpation and does not contain stool. Anorectal manometry demonstrates absence of relaxation of the internal sphincter, an expected response to rectal distension. Normally, distension of the rectum produces relaxation of the internal sphincter. Abdominal radiograph and contrast studies reveal a distended small bowel and proximal colon with an empty rectum. Rectal biopsy has proven to be the most reliable test for confirmation of the diagnosis; the absence of ganglionic cells and the presence of hypertrophic nerve trunks confirms the diagnosis (Kessman, 2006).

Treatment in infancy involves surgical removal of the aganglionic bowel through an endorectal pull-through procedure (Mattioli, Prato, Giunta, et al., 2008). In mild cases, in otherwise healthy infants, the affected portion of the bowel can be removed in the newborn period. In severe cases or in ill infants, a temporary colostomy is created. Timing of closure of the colostomy and reanastomosis varies among surgeons with the procedure generally being performed sometime between 2 and 6 months of age (Black, 2005; Kessman, 2006). For children not diagnosed in infancy, treatment should be implemented as soon as possible after diagnosis. Whether complete repair is possible in the first surgery, or a colostomy is required, depends on the amount of bowel affected.

The return of normal bowel function depends on the amount of bowel involved. Some fecal incontinence and constipation may persist following surgery. Enterocolitis is a serious complication that can occur before or after surgery, resulting in ischemia and ulceration of the bowel wall. Treatment includes intravenous fluids, antibiotics, and placement of a nasogastric tube for decompression of the abdomen (Kessman, 2006).

Nursing Management

Nursing assessment in the newborn period includes careful observation for the passage of meconium. Because newborns are often discharged within 24 hours of birth, tell parents to notify the physician if no stool is passed or the abdomen becomes distended. When the disease is diagnosed later in infancy or in childhood, obtain a thorough history of weight gain, nutritional intake, and bowel elimination habits.

When Hirschsprung disease is diagnosed, nursing care includes monitoring for infection, managing pain, maintaining hydration, measuring abdominal circumference to detect any distention, and providing support to the child and family. Preoperative oral intake varies depending on the surgeon; however, intake is generally restricted to clear fluids the day before surgery. Rectal irrigations may be performed to evacuate the bowel prior to surgery.

Initial postoperative nursing care is the same for any other infant or child having abdominal surgery: maintain intravenous fluids and nasogastric tube, and monitor intake and output. Administer pain medications as prescribed and assess at least every hour for evidence of pain utilizing a pain scale and documenting assessment. If a colostomy was performed, the stoma should be assessed frequently as well as the return of bowel function. See the section on ostomies on page 1536.

Children occasionally develop constipation and parents may need guidance to adapt the diet and fluid intake to manage this complication. Because some children develop malabsorption, be alert for signs of poor growth or malnutrition.

Expected outcomes of nursing care include:

- Maintenance of fluid and electrolyte balance
- Adequate nutritional intake to promote growth and development
- Adequate bowel function
- Effective pain management
- Parental coping with stress of the child's condition.

ANORECTAL MALFORMATIONS

Anorectal malformations refer to anomalies of the rectum, urinary, and reproductive system and have an incidence of 1 in 4000 births. Anorectal malformations are frequently associated with anomalies of the musculoskeletal system (Levitt & Peña, 2005). Chromosomal abnormalities such as trisomy 13, 18, or 21 may coexist, and some babies have VACTERL conditions. VACTERL refers to the presence of three or more of the following anomalies: vertebral anomalies, anal atresia, congenital heart disease, tracheoesophageal fistula, renal anomalies, and limb defects (Davies, Creighton, & Wilcox, 2004).

Nursing Practice

For the child who has had an endorectal pull-through procedure, it is very important that nothing be placed in the rectum, including thermometers and suppositories. A sign should be placed on the patient's bed to alert all staff caring for the infant. If the child requires rectal dilations, these are delayed for 3 weeks to allow for healing (Klar, 2007).

Nursing Practice

Following colostomy closure in the child who has had a colostomy for several months, the perineal area is not accustomed to contact with stool. Without meticulous skin care, breakdown is very likely. Teach parents to change diapers frequently, clean the perineal area carefully, and apply a protective barrier at each diaper change.

Etiology and Pathophysiology

The term *imperforate anus* (absence of the anal opening) is frequently used to refer to anorectal malformations and is classified according to the specific defect. Males with imperforate anus frequently have a rectourethral fistula and girls generally have a rectovestibular fistula (Levitt & Peña, 2005). Additional minor defects that may occur include anal stenosis (narrowing of the anus and imperforate anal membrane (skin covering the anal opening).

Clinical Manifestation

Imperforate anus affects males and females equally. Perineal inspection at birth reveals the absent anal opening. Failure to pass meconium within the first 24 hours of birth may be indicative of imperforate anus. Stool in the urine usually indicates the presence of a fistula between the colon and urinary tract. Cloacal malformations in females, in which the urinary tract, vagina, and rectum drain through a common channel, may occur (Levitt and Peña, 2005). Some anorectal malformations may be suspected prenatally on ultrasound, especially in the presence of associated anomalies (Levitt & Peña, 2005). Diagnosis for both defects is usually made at birth or during the newborn assessment of anorectal structures and rectal patency. Ultrasound and lower gastrointestinal radiographic studies are used to confirm the diagnosis and demonstrate the extent of the anomaly.

Clinical Therapy

Medical management depends on the extent of the malformation and presence of associated conditions. Anal stenosis may be treated with dilation alone. An imperforate anal membrane is excised surgically, followed by daily manual dilations. A single operation, anoplasty, may be used to repair rectoperineal defects (previously known as low defects). Higher defects require a three-stage procedure. A temporary colostomy in the newborn period provides for bowel decompression and for protection of the surgical site when the anomaly is repaired. Reconstructive surgery is generally performed via posterior sagittal anorectoplasty (PSARP) after 1 month of age. When the operative site has healed, approximately 2 weeks after surgery, anal dilatations are begun (Levitt & Peña, 2005). When the desired size of the anal opening has been achieved, approximately 6–8 weeks after surgery, the colostomy is closed (Levitt & Peña, 2005; Guardino, 2007).

Nursing Management

During the initial newborn assessment, the perineal area is inspected for a poorly developed anal dimple or sacral anomalies. Observation and recording of passage of meconium are essential.

Once the diagnosis has been made, intravenous fluids are initiated and a nasogastric tube is inserted to decompress the stomach. Monitor the child's intake and output, and cardiorespiratory functioning. Provide emotional support to the parents and give them information about the upcoming surgery.

Postoperative care specific to the child who has had the PSARP procedure centers on protection of the surgical site. A Foley catheter will be in place for 5 days to protect the new anal opening from urine. The colostomy that is still in place protects the surgical site from stool. Provide adequate pain management for the child. Maintain intravenous fluids until the child is able to take liquids by mouth.

Nursing care for the child who has had colostomy closure is more complex because the bowel has been manipulated during surgery. It is essential to monitor the maintenance of the nasogastric tube to low wall suction until bowel function returns. Provide intravenous fluids or total parenteral nutrition through peripheral or central venous access until the child can tolerate fluids by mouth. Monitor intake and output. The child will frequently have a Foley catheter in place for accurate measurement of urine output.

Care of the operative site may include dressing changes in addition to assessment for signs of infection. As the child begins to pass stool through the anal opening for the first time, skin breakdown is likely. Protect the perineal area with a barrier cream or paste.

Provide intravenous pain medication on a regular basis. The nurse is also responsible for administering prescribed antibiotics that protect the child from infection.

The child with associated abnormalities may need several surgeries and interventions to treat all of the conditions present. Partnering with families and the group of healthcare providers will assist in case management that facilitates the child's health and development. Health promotion and health maintenance that includes support of family members, ensuring immunizations, and monitoring developmental status are important.

Discharge planning and home care teaching. Infants are increasingly discharged shortly after birth, so parents need clear instructions about normal newborn stools and what abnormalities to report. The nurse should:

- Teach parents how to care for the ostomy site if a colostomy is performed in the newborn period (see discussion of ostomies later in this chapter).
- Reassure parents that the colostomy will be closed in the future, and help them plan for that hospitalization.
- Refer parents to ostomy support groups in the community or online.

> **Thinking Critically**
>
> **ANAL ATRESIA AND ESOPHAGEAL ATRESIA**
>
> Jerome was born with both anal atresia and esophageal atresia. He has had several surgeries, and is now 8 months old. He has a colostomy for bowel elimination and a gastrostomy tube for feedings. What assessments will you perform of the colostomy site? How can you help Jerome's parents to manage the colostomy? What developmental milestones would you expect at Jerome's age? What suggestions do you have for the family about ways to stimulate Jerome's social, physical, and cognitive skills?
>
> See MyNursingKit for possible responses.

- Discuss follow-up care and long-term management.
- Arrange follow-up visits and home care visits to evaluate the child's ostomy site and monitor growth.

After surgery to create the anal opening, teach parents how to take the infant's temperature using the axillary route (see Skill 9–13 SKILLS). Once anal dilatations have begun, the family will be taught how to perform them at home. After the final surgical procedure discuss feeding regimens and bowel habits necessary to maintain adequate nutrition for growth and development. Advise parents that children with anorectal malformations may have difficulty achieving bowel control. Patience in toilet training is important. When the child reaches an age appropriate for toilet training, encourage the family to speak with a healthcare provider to discuss the child's progress.

Expected outcomes of nursing care include:

- Effective pain management
- Healing without infection
- Maintenance of fluid and electrolyte balance
- Adequate bowel function
- Demonstration by parents of understanding of ostomy care and other treatment protocols.

HERNIAS

A **hernia** is the protrusion or projection of an organ or a part of an organ through the muscle wall of the cavity that normally contains it. This protrusion may result from the failure of normal openings to close during fetal development or from weakness in the supporting musculature. When intra-abdominal pressure increases (as when the infant cries or strains to pass stool), the weakened area separates, causing a protrusion of underlying organs. Inguinal hernias are the most common type of hernia occurring in children (see Chapter 54∞). Other hernias that occur frequently in children are diaphragmatic and umbilical.

Congenital Diaphragmatic Hernia

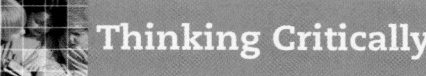

In a diaphragmatic hernia, abdominal contents protrude into the thoracic cavity through an opening in the diaphragm. Sites of herniation include the substernal space, the posterolateral region, and the esophageal hiatus. The cause is a delay or failure in closure of the pleuroperitoneal musculature. The overall incidence of diaphragmatic hernia is 1 in 3300 live births (Coha, 2007). Associated major anomalies are present in 37–47% of children with congenital diaphragmatic hernia (Colvin, Bower, Dickinson, et al., 2005).

A diaphragmatic hernia is a life-threatening condition with an overall mortality rate of 35% for infants born alive with the condition (Bagolan, Casaccia, Crescenzi, et al., 2004). Severe respiratory distress occurs shortly after birth. As the infant cries, abdominal organs extend into the thorax, decreasing the size of the thoracic cavity. The infant becomes dyspneic and cyanotic. Characteristic findings include a barrel-shaped chest and sunken abdomen.

Congenital diaphragmatic hernia may be diagnosed in utero by ultrasound. If it is not identified prenatally, the condition is first identified postnatally by physical signs and symptoms; confirmation is made by chest radiologic examination. MRI is helpful in confirming the diagnosis and in determining the position of organs in the chest and abdomen (Hedrick, Crombleholme, Flake, et al., 2004). Immediate respiratory support is essential in a NICU. Extracorporeal membrane oxygenation (ECMO) may be used to provide cardiopulmonary bypass to rest the lungs. Alternatively, inhaled nitric oxide (iNO) and high-frequency oxygen ventilation (HFVO) preoperatively may improve survival outcomes and decrease concomitant morbidity (Bagolan et al., 2004).

The infant is positioned with the head and thorax higher than the abdomen to facilitate downward movement of abdominal organs. A nasogastric tube is inserted to decompress the stomach. Ventilator support is necessary to manage respiratory compromise. Intravenous fluids are administered through an umbilical artery catheter.

Once the infant's condition is stabilized, the defect is corrected surgically. The chance for a successful repair and survival is affected by the size of the defect. Children who survive will generally continue to have health concerns and should have continued evaluation of pulmonary, nutritional and neurodevelopmental related problems (Downard, 2008).

Nursing Management

The infant with a diaphragmatic hernia is admitted to the neonatal intensive care unit (NICU) and requires continuous monitoring. Preoperative management centers on providing supportive care to the infant and parents and includes the following:

- Note the infant's vital signs every 30 minutes on the cardiorespiratory monitor.
- Observe for worsening of respiratory compromise.
- Maintain intravenous fluid administration.
- Promote decreased stimulation to keep the infant calm and thus maintain low abdominal pressure.
- Keep parents informed about the infant's condition, and provide emotional support both before and after surgery.

Postoperative care includes:

- Positioning the infant on the affected side to facilitate expansion of the lung on the unaffected side.
- Observing closely for signs of infection.
- Maintaining respiratory support.
- Carefully monitoring fluid and electrolyte balance.

Before discharge, instruct parents in wound care, prevention of infection, and feeding techniques.

Umbilical Hernia

An umbilical hernia results from a weak or imperfectly closed umbilical ring (Cilley & Shereef, 2004) (Figure 53–6 ●). Umbilical hernia is a common condition in childhood and occurs more frequently in black children and low birthweight infants (Stoll, 2007).

The hernia appears as a soft swelling covered by skin. Omentum and small intestine herniate or protrude through the opening with coughing, crying, or straining during a bowel movement. It is easily reduced by pushing the bowel back through the fibrous ring. The size of the defect is determined by measuring the diameter of the muscular ring (Stoll, 2007).

Most defects that appear prior to 6 months of age will resolve spontaneously by age 1. Surgery is indicated in cases of *strangulation* (closure of the muscular ring around a portion of the bowel, preventing it from moving back into the abdomen). Surgery is also recommended if the defect does not resolve by 3 to 4 years of age or if the defect becomes larger after 1–2 years of age (Stoll, 2007).

Nursing Management

Nursing management is generally supportive. Instruct parents not to apply tape, straps, or coins to reduce the hernia as these methods have not proven to be effective. If surgery is required, it is usually performed in a short-stay unit. Postoperatively, teach

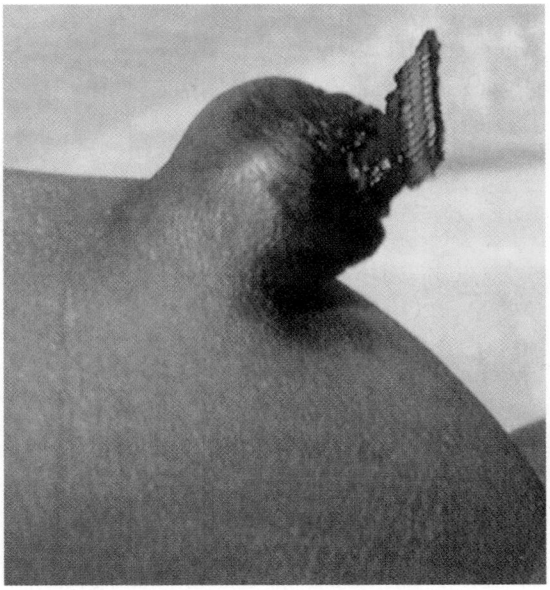

● **Figure 53–6** Umbilical hernia. The umbilical hernia of the newborn usually closes as the muscles strengthen in later infancy and childhood.

From Zitelli, B., & Davis, H. (Eds.) (2007). *Atlas of pediatric physical diagnosis.* (5th ed., p. 48). St. Louis: Mosby.

parents how to care for the surgical site, to watch for bleeding, and to recognize signs of infection. Reinforce the importance of returning for follow-up evaluation.

OSTOMIES

An intestinal **ostomy** is an opening, or **stoma**, into the small or large intestine that diverts fecal matter, providing an outlet when a distal surgical anastomosis, obstruction, or nonfunctioning structure prevents normal elimination. Depending on the integrity and function of anatomic structures, the ostomy may be temporary or permanent. Infants and small children with imperforate anus, necrotizing enterocolitis, Hirschsprung disease, or volvulus, may require a temporary or permanent colostomy or ileostomy. Ostomies may also be indicated for children with inflammatory bowel disease, intestinal tumors, or abdominal trauma.

An ostomy may be elective or considered a surgical emergency. In all cases it affects a child's lifestyle, alters body image, causes anxiety, and increases the risk for alterations in physiologic processes (electrolyte imbalance, increased nutritional requirements). For adolescents, it may also result in dependence at a time when autonomy is a major developmental need (Figure 53–7 ●).

When assessing the family and child approaching ostomy surgery, it is important to determine their ability to understand and accept the physical changes that will occur. Parents may feel guilt and anger about the need for an ostomy when the child has a genetically transmitted disease, is injured, or has developed an obstruction from necrosis of the bowel. Encourage the parents and child to express their feelings, and correct any misunderstandings. Parents and older children may be referred for counseling and to support groups to help them deal with their feelings. Adolescents often benefit from a visit with an adolescent ostomate (someone who has an ostomy) who can answer questions about living with an ostomy.

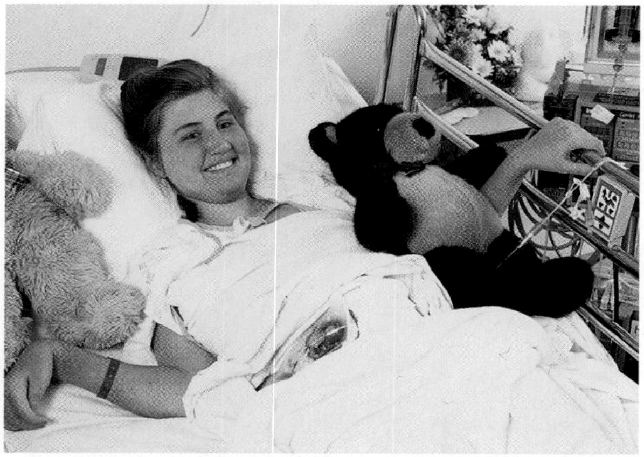

● **Figure 53–7** Adolescents with ostomies. Nursing strategies to address altered perceptions of body image and increased feelings of dependence are important when working with adolescents who have ostomies. Support groups or a visit from another teenager who has had an ostomy can facilitate positive coping, as demonstrated by this teenage girl.

Growth and Development

The preschooler has some manual dexterity and can help with some parts of the procedure for changing an ostomy appliance and cleaning the stoma. Teach the child using a doll or stuffed animal. Many school-age children are able to care for their ostomy independently. Teach them how to avoid leakage around the bag, which could be embarrassing. Adolescents are generally totally independent in their self-care of ostomies. However, they may need support to deal with the fact that they are different from their peers.

PREOPERATIVE CARE

Preoperative education focuses on educating the child and family and preparing them for postoperative management. Discuss how the ostomy pouch will look, and explain the purpose of the appliance in developmentally appropriate terms. Encourage the parents and child to touch and manipulate all equipment. Show a younger child how to place a pouch on a doll. Older children can practice placing a pouch on their skin. These measures help relieve anxiety by providing information and increasing familiarity with the appliance.

In addition to discussion of the appliance, preoperative education should include discussion of pain control and measures that will be used to prevent postoperative complications (turning, coughing, and breathing deeply). Gear the instructions to the child's developmental level. Encourage parental participation to promote compliance.

POSTOPERATIVE CARE

Postoperative care of a child with an ostomy is similar to that of any child who undergoes abdominal surgery. (See the discussion of nursing management for appendicitis later in this chapter and "Nursing Care Plan: The Child Undergoing Surgery" in Chapter 41 ∞.) Management of the stoma may be done by an "ostomy nurse" or other nurses. Major interventions involve ensuring proper function of the stoma, identifying complications, and instituting daily stoma care. Assess the stoma, quality and amount of fecal matter, skin condition, and adherence of the pouch. Evaluate for the most common complications, which are prolapse, retraction, stenosis, and skin breakdown around the stoma. Evaluate the family's understanding and their ability to care for the ostomy.

Nursing Practice

Avoid adhesive enhancers on the skin of newborns and premature infants. Their skin layers are so thin that removal of the appliance can strip off the skin. Remember also that adhesive contains latex and its frequent use is not advised due to risk of latex allergy development (see Chapter 50 ∞).

Identify and address home care needs well in advance of discharge. Instructions include skin care, care of the stoma, appliance removal and application, and frequency of appliance changes (see Skills 16–3 and 16–4 SKILLS). Begin teaching immediately after surgery with responsibility for care transferred gradually to the parents and child as they are ready. Discuss diet, activity level, hygiene, clothing, equipment, and financial considerations. Arrange for home visits to check periodically on the home management program.

Parents and children can be referred to the United Ostomy Association or a local ostomy group for information and support. Make referrals to social service, counseling, and a home health agency, if appropriate.

Expected outcomes of nursing care include successful adjustment to the ostomy, thorough evacuation of the bowel, absence of infection and other complications, intact skin, and formation of a positive self-image in the child.

PATHOPHYSIOLOGY ILLUSTRATED

APPENDICITIS

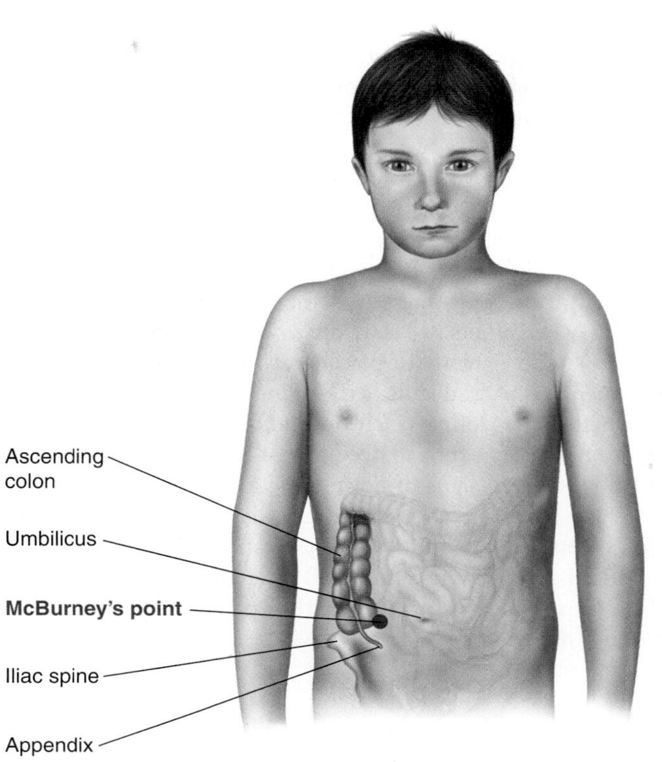

McBurney's point is the common location of pain in children and adolescents with appendicitis.

INFLAMMATORY DISORDERS

Inflammatory disorders are reactions of specific tissues of the GI tract to trauma caused by injuries, foreign bodies, chemicals, microorganisms, or surgery. These disorders may be acute or chronic and may involve various segments of the GI tract.

APPENDICITIS

Appendicitis is an inflammation of the vermiform appendix, the small sac near the end of the cecum. The condition occurs most often in adolescent boys (10 to 19 years of age). Appendicitis is the most common cause for emergency abdominal surgery in children and adolescents in the United States (Kosloske, Love, Rohrer, et al., 2004). Children account for 62,000 to 82,000 of the appendectomies performed every year in more than 250,000 Americans (Ziegler, 2004).

Etiology and Pathophysiology

Appendicitis almost always results from an obstruction in the appendiceal lumen. It can be caused by a fecalith (hard fecal mass), parasitic infestations, stenosis, hyperplasia of lymphoid tissue, or a tumor.

Continued secretion of mucus following acute obstruction of the lumen increases pressure, causing ischemia, cellular death, and ulceration. The appendix may perforate or rupture, resulting in fecal and bacterial contamination of the peritoneum. Peritonitis spreads quickly and if untreated can result in small bowel obstruction, electrolyte imbalances, septicemia, and hypovolemic shock.

Clinical Manifestations

At onset, symptoms include periumbilical cramps, abdominal tenderness, and fever. In adolescent and young adult females, symptoms must be differentiated from those associated with ovulation (mittelschmerz), ruptured ectopic pregnancy, and pelvic inflammatory disease. As the inflammation progresses, pain in the right lower abdomen becomes constant. Pain is often most intense at McBurney's point, halfway between the anterior superior iliac crest and the umbilicus (see "Pathophysiology Illustrated: Appendicitis"). In 30% of children, however, the appendix is in a different location, so the pain may occur elsewhere. Symptoms progress to include guarding, rigidity, nausea, vomiting, onset of pain before vomiting, anorexia, and rebound tenderness following palpation over the right lower quadrant. Vomiting, diarrhea, or constipation may be present.

As appendicitis progresses, the child remains motionless, usually in a side-lying position with knees flexed. Sudden relief of pain usually means that the appendix has ruptured.

Clinical Therapy

Diagnosis of appendicitis in young children can be difficult because their pain may be less localized and their symptoms more diffuse than in the older child. Continuing evaluations over several hours are often needed to establish the diagnosis.

The presence of fever and an elevated white blood cell count (above 10,000/mm^3) generally occurs in appendicitis. In addition to these symptoms, a history of mid-abdominal pain migrating to the right lower quadrant, along with rebound tenderness is highly indicative of appendicitis (Bundy, Byerly, Liles, et al., 2007). While an abdominal ultrasound can be helpful in the diagnosis of appendicitis, computed tomography (CT) is preferred and has been found to be most reliable (Jaffe & Berger, 2005; Tamburrini, Brunetti, Brown, et al., 2007).

Treatment involves immediate surgical removal (appendectomy), either through laparoscopic or open method (Vegunta, Ali, Wallace, et al., 2004). Preoperatively the child is kept NPO. Intravenous fluids, electrolytes, and antibiotics are administered. Postoperatively the child has an abdominal incision, and intravenous antibiotics are administered to prevent infection. The child with uncomplicated appendicitis will generally be discharged the next day.

If the appendix has ruptured before surgery, a drain may be placed and the wound left open. Wound irrigations may be needed to help cleanse the peritoneum. Recovery is usually complete following uncomplicated removal of the appendix.

With ruptured appendix, some surgeons prefer to close the wound, while others will leave the wound open (delayed primary closure), with or without placement of drains. If the wound is left open, it is packed with sterile saline-soaked gauze. Regardless of whether the wound is left opened or is closed, the child will have a nasogastric tube to decompress the abdomen and will remain NPO until signs of bowel function return. The child will also have a peripheral or temporary central line for administration of intravenous fluids and medications. After surgery for a ruptured appendix, the child will receive antibiotics for several days. Morphine is generally given for pain. For the child whose wound was left open, the wound will be closed under sedation in about 5 days.

NURSING MANAGEMENT

NURSING ASSESSMENT AND DIAGNOSIS

PHYSIOLOGIC ASSESSMENT

A detailed assessment of the child's pain is necessary to differentiate appendicitis from other illnesses (see Chapter 42∞). Ask the child to point to the painful area and describe the pain. Recognize that localizing the pain may be difficult for young children. Note onset, location, and intensity of pain; precipitating factors; and relief measures tried. During abdominal assessment, palpate last to avoid causing additional pain. Deep palpation of the left side of the abdomen followed by removing the hand quickly can lead to pain in the area of the appendix (rebound tenderness). However, once appendicitis is suspected or verified, avoid abdominal palpation in order to minimize pain to the child. Assess vital signs to determine baseline values, and monitor every 4 hours thereafter.

PSYCHOSOCIAL ASSESSMENT

Because appendicitis usually occurs in school-age children and adolescents, assessment of the child's coping skills is important. Adolescents, because of their preoccupation with body image, may be concerned about the surgical scar. Assess the parents' and child's anxiety about the sudden hospitalization and need for emergency surgery.

Among the nursing diagnoses that might be appropriate for the child with appendicitis are the following:

- *Acute Pain* related to inflammation and surgery
- *Risk for Deficient Fluid Volume Deficit* related to fluid volume loss and inadequate fluid volume intake
- *Anxiety/Fear* related to physical condition
- *Risk for Infection* related to bowel trauma
- *Risk for Ineffective Airway Clearance* related to retained secretions

PLANNING AND INTERVENTION

Nursing management focuses on promoting comfort, maintaining hydration, providing emotional support, supporting respiratory function, providing care of the surgical site, and monitoring for symptoms of infection.

PROMOTE COMFORT

Preoperatively, a side-lying position with knees bent is usually the most comfortable. Administer analgesics as ordered, and note relief from pain. Manage postoperative pain in a similar manner. The child should be placed in a semi-Fowler or side-lying position on the right side. If the appendix has ruptured, lying on the right side helps the peritoneal cavity drain. The child with a ruptured appendix will require intravenous pain medication frequently and prior to scheduled dressing changes if the wound was left open. The child who has an appendectomy for uncomplicated appendicitis will need oral or intravenous pain management for postoperative pain control.

MAINTAIN HYDRATION

An intravenous infusion is initiated preoperatively and continued until bowel function returns after surgery. Once bowel sounds return and after the nasogastric tube has been removed, offer water in small amounts and then other clear fluids. The child should be monitored closely to make sure he or she does not become nauseated after oral fluids are taken.

PROVIDE EMOTIONAL SUPPORT

For many children, appendicitis may be their first hospitalization and their first experience with healthcare personnel beyond their usual provider. The nurse must elicit a history, perform a physical examination, coordinate diagnostic tests, and prepare the child for surgery in a short period of time. Emotional support is essential for both child and parents. Good preoperative education can reduce anxiety. Answer any questions the child or parents may have.

SUPPORT RESPIRATORY FUNCTION

General anesthesia during surgery compromises respiratory function. It is important for the child to turn, cough, and breathe deeply to prevent atelectasis. Provide adequate analgesia and encourage the child to splint the incision area with a pillow during coughing to decrease pain. Incentive spirometry is frequently ordered for the child. Young children may be resistant to this procedure or may be too young to understand the procedure. An effective alternative approach is to give the child bubbles or a pinwheel to blow.

RECOGNIZE SYMPTOMS OF INFECTION

Assess vital signs and observe the abdominal incision every 4 hours for redness, edema, or drainage. If a drain is present, assess drainage for color, consistency, and amount. The amount of drainage from the wound should decrease gradually as the wound heals. Administer antibiotics as prescribed. The child with an open wound will require wet to dry dressing changes 2–3 times a day, depending on physician orders.

DISCHARGE PLANNING AND HOME CARE TEACHING

For children with uncomplicated appendicitis, the child is discharged once bowel function returns and he or she has a bowel movement. If the appendix was ruptured, the child will be hospitalized several days for intravenous antibiotics. Give parents instructions for home care. Teach parents to recognize the signs and symptoms of infection and to seek early treatment.

Normal activities can be resumed fairly quickly, but the child should avoid strenuous activities and contact sports in the immediate postoperative period. Parents should check with the child's physician before allowing the child to resume sports activities. Home tutoring may be needed for a short time so the child can keep up with schoolwork.

EVALUATION

Expected outcomes of nursing care include the following:

- Effective pain management
- Effective airway clearance
- Healing without development of secondary infection
- Adequate hydration achieved and maintained.

NECROTIZING ENTEROCOLITIS

Necrotizing enterocolitis (NEC) is a potentially life-threatening inflammatory disease of the intestinal tract that occurs primarily in premature infants. It affects from 4% to 13% of very low-birth-weight infants (Bell, 2005), and has an overall mortality rate of 25–30% (Tudehope, 2004). NEC is considered the most common emergency condition of the gastrointestinal tract in newborn infants (Pietz, Achanti, Lilien, et al., 2007).

The etiology of NEC is multifactorial: intestinal ischemia, bacterial or viral infection (a result of the premature infant's decreased immune response and greater risk for infection), and immaturity of the gastrointestinal mucosa (a result of the premature infant's decreased amount of gastric acid and proteolytic enzymes and underdeveloped protective intestinal mucin layer) (Kliegman & Willoughby, 2005). The disease occurs most often in the distal ileum and proximal colon (McCollough & Sharieff, 2006).

Manifestations generally occur between 3 and 14 days of age, but can occur as early as the first day of life and as late as 3 months of age. Symptoms may include poor feeding, increased gastric residuals prior to feeding, bilious emesis, abdominal distention, temperature instability, lethargy, and irritability. The infant may also have bloody stools (Kasson, 2007).

Diagnosis is made on the basis of characteristic clinical findings and the presence of free peritoneal gas, dilated bowel loops, bowel distention, and bowel wall thickening on abdominal radiographs. Stools and emesis are monitored for occult blood. Laboratory data reveal anemia, leukopenia, leukocytosis, thrombocytopenia, electrolyte imbalance, and metabolic or respiratory acidosis. Blood cultures are positive for the organism present.

Necrotizing enterocolitis requires prompt intervention. All enteral feedings are discontinued. A nasogastric or orogastric tube is inserted to prevent gastric distention, and intravenous fluids are started. Total parenteral nutrition may be initiated through a central line. Antibiotics are administered prophylactically or to treat sepsis. Radiographs of the abdomen should be performed every 6 hours to see if intestinal perforation has occurred (Kasson, 2007). Perforation or necrosis of the bowel necessitates surgical resection of the bowel. An ileostomy or colostomy may sometimes be performed. New treatments are being attempted with probiotics, live and beneficial microorganisms that promote normal gut flora. *Lactobacillus acidophilus* and *Bifidobacterium infantis* are examples of organisms that can be administered by special formula (Kliegman & Willoughby, 2005).

All cases of necrotizing enterocolitis are treated with strict enteric precautions to prevent the spread of infection to other premature infants on the unit. Early aggressive enteral formula-feedings of premature infants is avoided because of the increased incidence of the disease in these cases. Human milk has been shown to protect against the disease; thus, breastfeeding or feeding the mother's expressed milk is the feeding method of choice for premature infants.

Long-term complications of necrotizing enterocolitis include short bowel syndrome, strictures, cholestasis, impaired nutrition and growth, and delayed developmental performance.

Nursing Management

Nursing care centers on prevention and early detection of necrotizing enterocolitis to minimize bowel loss, and providing

> **Nursing Practice**
>
> The infant with NEC is at risk to develop sepsis. Signs of sepsis in the newborn or premature infant include:
>
> - Hypothermia or hyperthermia
> - Jaundice
> - Respiratory distress
> - Hepatomegaly
> - Abdominal distention
> - Anorexia
> - Vomiting
> - Lethargy
>
> Report these symptoms to the primary healthcare provider immediately.

> **Nursing Practice**
>
> **Cholestasis** is a disruption of bile flow. This is the most common problem in survivors of necrotizing enterocolitis. It is a complication of total parenteral nutrition (TPN) and commonly occurs 2 weeks after TPN therapy has been initiated. It is characterized by an elevated bilirubin (greater than 2 mg/dL), hepatomegaly, and elevated serum transaminase.

postoperative care. Observe for feeding intolerance by aspirating gastric residual (if the infant is receiving enteral feedings). Measure abdominal circumference and assess bowel sounds in the premature or high-risk infant every 4 to 8 hours. Even minimal changes in circumference can indicate necrotizing enterocolitis and should be reported to the primary care provider.

Maintaining fluid and electrolyte balance is essential. Provide comfort by holding and cuddling an infant who is NPO, and offer a pacifier to meet nonnutritive sucking needs. Careful assessment for infection and maintenance of skin integrity are essential. Feedings are gradually reestablished once bowel function returns. Administration of probiotics may be part of therapy. Offer parents emotional support, reassurance, and help in bonding with their infant. Because the symptoms of necrotizing enterocolitis do not appear until approximately 5 to 7 days after feedings begin, parents may not be prepared for the infant's decline. The recovery of a premature infant is slow and can be complicated. Give clear explanations and encourage parents to ask questions and express their fears and concerns. If the infant's condition worsens, offer the parents support (see Chapter 43).

Once the child is discharged, frequent follow-up is needed. Parents need specific education related to feedings, medications, and any other treatments prescribed. The infant requires regular and thorough physical assessments to check weight gain, assess development, and identify signs of complications. If the child had to have an ostomy created, the family must be taught ostomy care (see page 1536).

The infant requires regular and thorough physical assessments to identify any complications. Growth of the child is monitored and compared with previous findings. Developmental progress is assessed by regular administration of a developmental test such as the Denver II (see Chapter 37).

Expected outcomes of nursing care for the child with necrotizing enterocolitis include:

- Healing without infection
- Achieving and maintaining fluid and electrolyte balance
- Tissue perfusion maintained following surgical removal of necrotic bowel
- Adequate nutrition to support growth and development needs.

If the infant or child has had surgery, complete healing without infection or other complication is desired. If the infant is not successfully treated, support and comfort for the parents are necessary. When the child survives, desired long-term outcomes include normal developmental progression and nutrition to support growth.

MECKEL'S DIVERTICULUM

Meckel's diverticulum results when the omphalomesenteric duct, which connects the midgut to the yolk sac during embryonic development, fails to atrophy. Instead, an outpouching of the ileum remains, usually located near the ileocecal valve. The pouch contains gastric or pancreatic tissue, which secretes acid, causing irritation and ulceration. Meckel's diverticulum is the most common GI malformation and cause of lower GI bleeding in children; it occurs in 2% of the population. Many people are asymptomatic and do not know they have the disorder (Otten & Stoops, 2007).

Clinical manifestations usually appear by age 2. The most common sign is painless dark or bright-red rectal bleeding, which results from the obstruction or ulceration. Often blood is passed without stool. The child may have symptoms of intussusception, incarcerated hernia, volvulus, or intestinal obstruction. If untreated, diverticulitis may progress to perforation and peritonitis.

Diagnosis is based on the history. Contrast studies are usually not helpful because the diverticulum is often too small to visualize and may not fill with barium. Radionuclide imaging and scanning can usually detect the gastric tissue, confirming the diagnosis.

Treatment is surgical excision of the diverticulum and removal of any involved bowel. The prognosis is good following surgical excision.

Nursing Management

Preoperatively an intravenous infusion is initiated to correct fluid and electrolyte imbalances. Monitor intake and output. Observe for rectal bleeding, and test stools for **occult blood** (blood that is present in small quantities and is measurable only by laboratory testing). Keep the child on bed rest. Assess vital signs every 2 hours, and monitor for signs of shock. Postoperative care is similar to that for an infant or child undergoing abdominal surgery. (See the earlier discussion of postsurgical nursing management of appendicitis and "Nursing Care Plan: The Child Undergoing Surgery" in Chapter 41.)

At discharge, parents need instructions on caring for the surgical site, preventing infection, providing an adequate diet, and administering prescribed medications.

INFLAMMATORY BOWEL DISEASE

Crohn's Disease and Ulcerative Colitis

Inflammatory bowel disease encompasses two distinct chronic disorders, Crohn's disease and ulcerative colitis, that have similar symptoms and treatment. Inflammatory bowel disease differs from irritable bowel syndrome, which is discussed in the section on feeding and elimination disorders in Chapter 34.

Crohn's disease is a chronic, inflammatory process. It can occur randomly throughout the GI tract; the ileum, colon, and rectum are the most common sites. A distinct feature of Crohn's disease is the development of enteric fistulas between loops of

Clinical Manifestations

ULCERATIVE COLITIS AND CROHN'S DISEASE

	ULCERATIVE COLITIS	CROHN'S DISEASE
Type of lesions	Continuous, superficial involvement	Segmental, transmural (through the wall) involvement
Clinical manifestations		
Anal or perianal lesions	Rare	Common
Anorexia	Mild to moderate	Can be severe
Diarrhea	Often severe	Moderate
Growth retardation	Mild	Significant
Pain	Present	Common
Rectal bleeding	Present	Absent
Weight loss	Moderate	Severe
Risk of cancer	Slightly increased	Greatly increased

bowel or nearby organs. Mucosal ulcers begin in small locations, and then grow in size and depth into the mucosal wall. Submucosal inflammation can be severe. The etiology is unknown. There is strong evidence to support a genetic association. Crohn's disease is more common in whites than blacks. It is rare in the Asian and Hispanic population (Grossman & Mamula, 2007). It most often develops in adolescents and young adults. Crohn's disease has an incidence of approximately 3–4/100,000 (Hyams, 2007). The onset of Crohn's disease is subtle. Crampy abdominal pain is usually reported first, followed by diarrhea. Other symptoms include fever, anorexia, growth failure or weight loss, general malaise, and joint pain. Diagnosis is based on laboratory evaluation (anemia is common; an elevated erythrocyte sedimentation rate, hypoalbuminemia, and thrombocytosis are other possible findings), diffuse abdominal tenderness, and radiologic and biopsy examinations.

Ulcerative colitis is a chronic recurrent disease of the large intestine and rectal mucosa of unknown etiology. Inflammation is limited to the mucosa, as opposed to Crohn's disease, which extends deep into the bowel wall. Ulcerative colitis can involve the entire length of the bowel with varying degrees of inflammation, ulceration, hemorrhage, and edema. Emotional and other psychosocial factors may influence the presentation and course of the disease. It is more prevalent among persons of Jewish heritage. The disease develops before 20 years of age with peak onset at about 12 years. Ulcerative colitis develops in 15/100,000 individuals in the United States (Hyams, 2007). See the accompanying "Clinical Manifestations: Ulcerative Colitis and Crohn's Disease" feature for a comparison of the two diseases.

The first symptom of ulcerative colitis is usually diarrhea. Lower abdominal pain and cramping are present before and during a bowel movement and are relieved by the passage of stool and flatus. The stool is often mixed with blood and mucus. Weight loss or delayed growth, nutritional deficiencies, and arthralgias often occur as effects of the disease.

Diagnosis centers on evaluating the cause and identifying the extent of involved bowel and differentiating an infectious process (organisms such as *Shigella* and *Salmonella*) from ulcerative colitis. Endoscopy with biopsy is helpful to determine the extent and severity of the inflammatory process. Laboratory and bone age studies help to identify related nutritional, growth, and blood abnormalities. Common serum findings include elevated erythrocyte sedimentation rate, elevated C-reactive protein, hypoalbuminemia, thrombocytosis, and antineutrophil cytoplasmic antibodies (ANCA).

Crohn's disease and ulcerative colitis have periods of remission and exacerbation (Tanaka & Kazuma, 2005). Treatment for both diseases includes pharmacologic interventions (antibiotic, anti-inflammatory, immunosuppressive, and antidiarrheal medications), nutrition therapy, and, in severe cases, surgery. First-line pharmacologic treatment of Crohn's disease involves aminosalicylates. Sulfasalazine inhibits prostaglandin synthesis, thereby decreasing inflammation. Corticosteroids are given orally and in the form of enemas to children with more severe disease.

A nutritionist is part of the team treating the child. The goal of nutrition therapy is to provide adequate caloric intake and nutrients necessary for growth. Vitamin, iron, zinc, and folic acid supplementation is frequently required. Total parenteral nutrition (TPN) is often given to treat nutritional deficiencies and malnutrition, which accompany inflammatory bowel disease (see Skill 12–7 SKILLS). A high-protein, high-carbohydrate, low-fiber diet with normal amounts of fat is recommended.

If other treatment measures fail to reduce inflammation, surgery is generally indicated. A temporary colostomy or ileostomy is performed to allow the bowel to rest. In Crohn's disease, however, ulcerations tend to recur elsewhere in the GI tract. Biologic therapies such as infliximab (Remicade) have been effective in patients with Crohn's disease who fail to respond to other therapies. These therapies have recently been approved for use in children and are emerging as a treatment option in ulcerative colitis (Aschenbrenner, 2006; Irving & Gibson, 2007). In ulcerative colitis, removal of the diseased bowel provides a permanent cure.

Nursing Practice

The following drugs are used in the treatment of inflammatory bowel disease:

Aminosalicylates	Immunosuppressants
Sulfasalazine Mesalamine	6-Mercaptopurine (6-MP) Azathioprine Cyclosporine Methotrexate

Corticosteroids	Antibiotics
Prednisone Prednisolone Hydrocortisone enema	Metronidazole Ciprofloxacin

Biologic Therapies
Tumor necrosis factor (TNF) Infliximab (Remicade) Interleukin-10 Thalidomide

Data from: Bindler, R., & Howry, L. (2005). *Pediatric drug guide*. Upper Saddle River, NJ: Prentice Hall Health; Hyams, J. (2005). Inflammatory bowel disease. *Pediatrics in Review, 26* (9), 314–320; Irving, P. M., & Gibson, P. R. (2007). Infliximab: Getting the most for your money. *Journal of Gastroenterology and Hepatology, 22*, 1557–1565; Plante, M. L. (2004). Crohn's disease. *Advance for Nurse Practitioners* (May 2004), 28–35; Silbermintz, A., & Markowitz, J. (2006). Inflammatory bowel disease. *Pediatric Annals,* 35(4), 269–274.

Nursing Management

Nursing management occurs mainly in the community and home and focuses on helping the child and family adjust to the emotional impact of a chronic disease, administering medications and diet therapy, monitoring nutritional status, and providing appropriate referrals. Provide emotional support and counseling to help the child adjust to feeling "different" from peers. Inability to compete with peers and frequent absences from school can affect the child's self-esteem. Have the parents contact the school district to arrange for tutoring in case extended absences from school become necessary. Encourage the child who is not attending school regularly to maintain contact with friends through telephone calls, cards, and visits.

Growth and Development

Providing adequate stress reduction may be helpful in control of inflammatory bowel disease. Teach young children relaxation techniques, such as deep breathing, progressive tensing and relaxing of muscles, and visualization of favorite places. Encourage busy school-age children and teens to have quiet and restful times each day, in addition to physical activity periods.

Teaching Highlights

DIET INSTRUCTIONS FOR INFLAMMATORY BOWEL DISEASE

- Several small feedings are usually better tolerated than three meals daily.
- Limiting fiber intake can help to decrease intestine motility and inflammation. Peel fruits and avoid large quantities of whole grains and nuts.
- If the child is not eating well, offer high-calorie meals. If lactose intolerance is not a problem for the particular child, cream soups, milkshakes, puddings, and custards can be offered.
- Liquid dietary supplements may be helpful to ensure protein and caloric requirements are met.
- Watch for foods that cause intestinal problems for the individual child, and avoid them in the future.
- Avoid having mealtime become a reason for family strife. Seek help of nurses and dietitians if needed.

If the child is unable to eat or the intake of calories is insufficient to meet basic nutritional and metabolic needs, TPN is ordered (see Skill 12–7 **SKILLS**). If the child is able to eat, parents need instructions about dietary needs. Frequently measure growth and assess nutrition.

Body image is a major concern for children and adolescents with inflammatory bowel disease. Corticosteroid therapy causes growth retardation and delayed sexual maturation. Encourage the child to discuss feelings about these side effects. If a permanent colostomy or ileostomy is required, help the child and family understand the need for surgical treatment. (See the discussion of ostomies earlier in this chapter.) Introduce the child and family to other children who have stomas.

Teach parents about medication administration and diet therapy. Reinforce to both the parents and child the importance of adhering to a strict medication regimen. Emphasize that medications should be continued even when the child is asymptomatic. Discuss the side effects of the drugs and what to do if any of these symptoms occur. When the child is taking systemic corticosteroids, immunizations are generally delayed until after the medication is discontinued.

Parents need instructions for TPN if this therapy is used, as well as information about care of a central venous catheter, including dressing changes, sterile and nonsterile techniques, signs of infection, how to handle infusion pumps and tubing, and how to measure the child's intake and output. Assist parents in obtaining equipment and supplies necessary for the child's care. Have parents demonstrate their mastery of care for the central venous catheter and their understanding of TPN techniques during home visits and appointments for health care.

Refer parents to social services, the visiting nurse association, and home healthcare agencies, if they are not receiving any of these services. For information about inflammatory bowel disease, refer families to the Crohn's and Colitis Foundation.

Expected outcomes of nursing care for the child with inflammatory bowel disease include the following:

- Normal growth and development
- Ability to cope with episodes of GI distress
- Successful management of medications without demonstration of side effects
- Free from infection due to central line
- Positive body image
- Integration of stress-lowering practices into daily life.

PEPTIC ULCER

A peptic ulcer is an erosion of the mucosal tissue in the lower end of the esophagus, in the stomach (usually along the lesser curvature), or in the duodenum (gastric ulcer is the term sometimes used when the stomach mucosa is affected). Males are more likely to have peptic ulcers than females; however, peptic ulcers are much less common in children than in adults. African-American and Hispanic children are at greater risk for peptic ulcers (Shah & Carroll, 2007).

Ulcers are classified as primary or secondary, depending on their etiology. Primary peptic ulcers occur in healthy children. Secondary (stress) ulcers occur in children with a preexisting illness or injury (often a burn) and in children receiving medications such as salicylates, corticosteroids, and nonsteroidal anti-inflammatory drugs. Diet usually is not a major factor in the development of peptic ulcers in children, although caffeine and alcohol consumption in adolescents may exacerbate the disease. It is now known that many cases of ulcer, in both adults and children, are caused by *Helicobacter pylori (H. pylori),* a gram-negative rod (Vaira, Gatta, Ricci, et al., 2005). This organism is transmitted by the fecal–oral or oral–oral routes. Infections often occur in several members of a family, especially when the family's water supply is contaminated.

Clinical manifestations vary according to the age of the child and location of the ulcer. The most common symptom is abdominal pain (burning) associated with an empty stomach, which may awaken the child at night. Vomiting and pain after meals, anemia, occult blood in stools, and abdominal distention may also be present.

Diagnosis is based on the history and radiologic studies. *H. pylori* can be diagnosed by culture of the organism taken via gastroscopy, and by measuring urea in the urine and on the breath, since the organism hydrolyzes urea. The goals of medical management are to relieve discomfort and promote healing. When *H. pylori* is the causative agent, antimicrobial agents such as bismuth salts, tetracycline, and metronidazole combination are given. Other drug combinations such as antacids in liquid form (Maalox, Mylanta) and histamine antagonists (ranitidine, cimetidine, and famotidine) are also used. Antibody titers are measured several times over 6 months to evaluate the effectiveness of therapy. The prognosis is usually good with early intervention.

Nursing Management

Assess the child for abdominal pain, vomiting, and abdominal distention. Assess for family history of *H. pylori* infection. Nursing care centers on interventions to promote adequate nutritional intake, promote healing, and prevent recurrences. Provide a nutritionally sound, age-appropriate diet. Omit foods only if they exacerbate the disorder.

Antibiotics must be given as scheduled. Emphasize the importance of continuing drug therapy. The family needs encouragement to continue the medications as ordered and to return for follow-up visits. Children who attend school may prefer to take antacids in the form of tablets, which are easier to carry than liquid preparations. The appropriate form must be completed in order for the child to receive medication at school.

Parents should discuss any additional medications with the primary healthcare provider before administering to the child. Caution parents to avoid aspirin products, which irritate the gastric mucosa. If an antipyretic or pain medication is needed, acetaminophen should be given. Advise parents to read medication labels if they are unsure of product contents.

Because psychological stress can contribute to peptic ulcer disease, the parents and child should be assisted to identify sources of stress in the child's life. Assess coping mechanisms and provide referral for psychological counseling, if appropriate. Teach relaxation techniques and recommend community classes on yoga or other stress reduction.

MyNursingKit Care Plan: Managing Emesis in Pediatric Conditions

DISORDERS OF MOTILITY

Fluids are an important part of normal GI functioning. As food passes through the intestines, fluids are reabsorbed and moderately soft stool is formed and evacuated. In disorders such as diarrhea and constipation, fluid balance is altered, causing either more or less fluid to be reabsorbed. This can severely alter the characteristics of the stool. Reabsorption of too little water produces diarrhea and can lead to fluid and electrolyte alterations. Reabsorption of too much fluid can cause constipation, which if untreated can lead to bowel obstruction.

GASTROENTERITIS (ACUTE DIARRHEA)

Gastroenteritis is an inflammation of the stomach and intestines that may be accompanied by vomiting and diarrhea. Gastroenteritis can affect any part of the GI tract. It may be an acute problem, caused by viral, bacterial, or parasitic infections, or a chronic problem. Rotavirus is the leading cause of gastroenteritis in children (Hsu, Staat, Roberts, et al., 2005). Children younger than 5 years average approximately two episodes of gastroenteritis each year. Infants and small children with gastroenteritis or diarrhea can quickly become dehydrated and are at risk for hypovolemic shock if fluid and electrolyte losses are not replaced (see Chapter 46).
A significant number of infants and young children are hospitalized each year for dehydration secondary to gastroenteritis.

Etiology and Pathophysiology

Diarrhea in children is related to many different causes (Table 53–2). The specific etiology is not always identified. The common

Table 53–2 Causes of Diarrhea in Children

Etiology	Bowel Manifestations
Emotional stress (anxiety, fatigue)	Increased motility
Intestinal infection (bacteria [*E. coli, Salmonella, Shigella*], viral [human rotavirus, enteric adenovirus], fungal overgrowth)	Inflammation of mucosa; increased mucus secretion in colon
Food sensitivity (gluten, cow's milk)	Decreased digestion of food
Food intolerance (lactose, introduction of new foods, overfeeding)	Increased motility; increased mucus secretion in colon
Medications (iron, antibiotics)	Irritation and suprainfection
Colon disease (colitis, necrotizing enterocolitis, enterocolitis)	Inflammation and ulceration of intestinal walls; reduced absorption of fluid; increased intestinal motility
Surgical alterations (short bowel syndrome)	Reduced size of colon; decreased absorption surface

mechanism is a decrease in the absorptive capacity of the bowel through inflammation, decrease in surface area for absorption, or alteration of parasympathetic innervation. Children in childcare centers and those living in substandard housing with improper sanitation are at increased risk.

Clinical Manifestations

Diarrhea may be mild, moderate, or severe. In mild diarrhea, stools are slightly increased in number and have a more liquid consistency. In moderate diarrhea the child has several loose or watery stools. Other symptoms include irritability, anorexia, nausea, and vomiting. Moderate diarrhea is usually self-limiting, resolving without treatment within 1 or 2 days. In severe diarrhea, watery stools are continuous. The child exhibits symptoms of fluid and electrolyte imbalance (see Chapter 46∞), has cramping, and is extremely irritable and difficult to console.

Clinical Therapy

Diagnosis is based on the history, physical examination, and laboratory findings. Physical examination provides a guide to the severity of dehydration (see Chapter 46∞). The stool can be examined for the presence of ova, parasites, infectious organisms, viruses, fat, and undigested sugars. Laboratory evaluation of serum and urine helps identify electrolyte imbalances and other deficiencies.

Medical management depends on the severity of the diarrhea and fluid and electrolyte imbalances. The goal of treatment is to correct the fluid and electrolyte imbalances. For mild and moderate dehydration, oral rehydration therapy is the first intervention (see Chapter 46∞). This may be accomplished at home or in the short-stay observation unit in a hospital with solutions such as Pedialyte. Carbonated and very sugary beverages should not be given. Fermentation of sugar in the GI tract causes increased gas, abdominal distention, and an increased frequency of diarrhea.

For severe dehydration, rehydration is accomplished by intravenous infusion with a solution chosen to correct the specific imbalances (see Chapter 46∞ for further information about solutions to correct dehydration). As soon as possible, introduce clear liquids or breast milk and then the child progresses to his or her regular diet. Foods generally are not withheld for more than 1 to 2 days.

If the diarrhea is caused by bacteria or parasites, antimicrobial therapy may be prescribed. Antiemetics and antidiarrheals are generally not used in young children since they can mask the signs and symptoms of more serious illness (Thielman & Guerrant, 2004).

NURSING MANAGEMENT

NURSING ASSESSMENT AND DIAGNOSIS

The nurse may encounter the child and family in the emergency department, urgent care center, clinic, or office. The child may be cared for over several hours at a clinic or urgent care center so that dehydration is treated with intravenous infusion and/or oral rehydration, and then sent home with instructions for parents to care for the child. A thorough history may help in identifying the cause.

If the child is hospitalized, it is important to assess onset, frequency, color, amount, and consistency of stools. If the child is also vomiting, monitor the amount and type of vomitus. Initial and ongoing physical assessment of the child focuses on observing for signs and symptoms of dehydration, which reflect underlying fluid and electrolyte status. Evaluate urinary output and specific gravity. An accurate weight must be obtained on admission and daily thereafter. Monitor vital signs every 2 to 4 hours. A febrile child has increased water loss, contributing to the dehydration. Assess skin integrity, especially in the perineal and rectal areas, and note any breakdown or rashes.

The accompanying nursing care plan lists common nursing diagnoses for a child with gastroenteritis. The following diagnoses may also be appropriate:

- *Anxiety (Child and Parent)* related to change in health status
- *Disturbed Sleep Pattern* related to pain
- *Imbalanced Nutrition: Less than Body Requirements* related to inability to ingest sufficient nutrients

PLANNING AND IMPLEMENTATION

Nursing care focuses on providing emotional support, promoting rest and comfort, and ensuring adequate nutrition.

PROVIDE EMOTIONAL SUPPORT

The child may have been ill for several days or become suddenly ill a short time before seeking health care. The child and parents

Nursing Care Plan

THE CHILD WITH GASTROENTERITIS

INTERVENTION	RATIONALE	EXPECTED OUTCOME
1. Nursing Diagnosis: Diarrhea related to infectious process		
NIC Priority Intervention: **Diarrhea management:** Prevention and alleviation of diarrhea		**NOC Suggested Outcome:** **Fluid and electrolyte balance:** Balance of water and electrolytes in the intracellular and extracellular compartments of the body
Goal: The child's bowel function will be restored to normal.		
■ Obtain baseline vital signs and monitor every 2–4 hours.	■ Fluid and electrolyte imbalances can alter vital body functions.	The child's bowel function returns to normal.
■ Observe stools for amount, color, consistency, odor, and frequency.	■ Aids in the diagnosis and in monitoring the child's status.	
■ Test stools for occult blood.	■ Frequent defecation and some infectious organisms can cause bleeding.	
■ Monitor results of stool culture and sample for ova and parasites.	■ Rapid notification of the physician will facilitate treatment.	
■ Wash hands well before and after contact with the child.	■ Helps prevent transmission of microorganisms.	
■ Isolate the child until the cause of the diarrhea is determined.	■ Prevents exposure of other patients and staff.	
■ Assist the child with toileting and hygiene.	■ The child may be weak, incontinent, physically impaired, or anxious and require assistance to use the bathroom.	
■ Administer prescribed oral rehydration and intravenous solutions.	■ Provides necessary fluids and nutrients.	
■ Notify the physician if diarrhea persists, stool characteristics change, or other symptoms of dehydration electrolyte imbalance occur.	■ Ensures early intervention.	
2. Nursing Diagnosis: Deficient Fluid Volume related to active fluid volume loss		
NIC Priority Intervention: **Fluid monitoring:** Collection and analysis of patient data to regulate fluid balance		**NOC Suggested Outcome:** **Fluid and electrolyte balance:** Balance of water and electrolytes in the intracellular and extracellular compartments of the body
Goal: The child will remain hydrated and will begin to drink fluids within 24 hours of admission.		
■ Monitor intake and output. Document time of each voiding. Weigh all diapers.	■ Will determine if output exceeds input. Long periods of time without urine output can be an early indicator of poor renal function. A child should produce 1–2 mL of urine/kg/hr.	The child has normal fluid and electrolyte balance as indicated by laboratory evaluation and physical examination.
■ Compare admission weight to preadmission weight. Assess weight daily.	■ The degree of dehydration can be determined by the percentage of weight loss. Daily weights aid in determining progress toward rehydration.	
■ Assess level of consciousness, skin turgor, mucous membranes, skin color and temperature, capillary refill, eyes, and fontanelles every 4 hours.	■ Will determine degree of hydration and adequacy of interventions.	
■ Assess for vomiting.	■ Vomiting frequently accompanies diarrhea and contributes to the child's fluid loss.	

(continued)

Nursing Care Plan—continued

THE CHILD WITH GASTROENTERITIS

INTERVENTION	RATIONALE	EXPECTED OUTCOME
■ Provide oral fluid and electrolyte replacement solution if able to tolerate.	■ Less invasive than IV fluids. Provides for replacement of essential fluids and electrolytes.	
■ Provide and maintain IV replacement therapy, as ordered.	■ Use of IV replacement is based on the degree of dehydration, ongoing losses, insensible water losses, and electrolyte results.	

3. Nursing Diagnosis: Risk for Impaired Skin Integrity related to altered fluid status

NIC Priority Intervention: **Skin surveillance:** Collection and analysis of patient data to maintain skin integrity		**NOC Suggested Outcome:** **Tissue integrity:** Skin and mucous membranes Structural intactness and normal physiologic function of skin and mucous membranes

Goal: The child will remain free of skin breakdown and rashes.

■ Assess skin of perineum and rectum for signs of skin breakdown or irritation.	■ Early assessment and intervention can prevent worsening of the condition.	
■ Provide prevention or restorative care for infants as follows:		
Preventive Care:		
■ Change diapers every 2 hours or as needed.	■ Minimizes skin contact with chemical irritants from stool and urine.	The child's perianal and rectal tissue remains pink and intact.
■ Wash diaper area after each soiling.	■ Removes traces of stool if present.	
■ Apply A & D ointment, Aquaphor, or another barrier ointment with each diaper change.	■ Provides a barrier and protects intact or reddened skin from becoming excoriated.	
Restorative Care:		
■ Leave the buttocks open to air for a few minutes several times daily, placing absorbent pads under the infant.	■ Promotes air circulation to the area.	
■ Notify the physician if the skin is severely broken or peeling or if a rash is present.	■ Additional measures such as the use of a barrier cream or paste may be needed to ensure skin healing.	
■ For toddlers and older children: Tub bathe at least daily (if condition allows) in tepid water. Pat the area dry.	■ Helps loosen any fecal matter without scrubbing, which can cause additional irritation to the skin.	
■ Discourage the wearing of underwear if possible.	■ Allows air to circulate and prevents accumulation of moisture.	
■ Apply barrier ointment with each diaper change or as instructed.	■ Provides a barrier and protects intact or reddened skin from becoming excoriated.	

are usually anxious, so it is important to allow them to talk and ask questions. The child may require blood tests to help direct rehydration therapy. Most children are cared for at home, although care in a 24-hour monitoring unit may occur. Using therapeutic play techniques, such as allowing the child to manipulate equipment, can reduce anxiety (see Chapter 41∞).

PROMOTE REST AND COMFORT

Children with gastroenteritis may awaken frequently with periods of vomiting and diarrhea. Provide a quiet, restful environment and cluster nursing care to allow for periods of uninterrupted rest. Darken the room and keep interruptions to a minimum. To reduce the child's anxiety, encourage parents to

Nursing Practice

Hand hygiene is the most important health maintenance measure that can be taken to prevent the spread of gastroenteritis. Wash hands often and use hand hygiene products, particularly before and after care of each child. Instruct parents in the importance of and techniques for hand hygiene, especially when caring for the child with gastroenteritis. Teach children in childcare centers and school how to wash their hands effectively to prevent spread of infectious diseases.

Complementary Care

CHILDREN AND HERBAL LAXATIVES

Herbal stimulant laxatives are used by some families as complementary therapies. The following are not recommended for use in children younger than 12 years:

- Aloe
- Buckthorn bark
- Cascara sagrada bark
- Senna leaf or pod
- Coffee
- Tea
- Cola nut
- Mate
- Ma huang

Question parents about the use of complementary therapy for their child's constipation. Educate them regarding avoiding the use of any therapies that are not recommended for children.

room-in. Place the child's favorite toys and comfort objects within reach. Keep the child's mouth moistened with a wet washcloth, or an occasional ice chip. Provide skin care after each diarrheal episode to maintain skin integrity. Avoid using commercial baby wipes that contain alcohol as these irritate the skin and cause discomfort for the child.

ENSURE ADEQUATE NUTRITION

Liquids are offered throughout the illness, even if an intravenous infusion is in place. Follow guidelines for oral rehydration therapy in Chapter 46∞. Small amounts of normal diet for age are provided. Infants are breastfed or given formula. The child's diet progresses according to protocol or the child's tolerance for feedings.

DISCHARGE PLANNING AND HOME CARE TEACHING

Discharge teaching begins on arrival at the healthcare facility. Teach the parents about the symptoms of dehydration and what actions to take if diarrhea recurs. Be sure that parents understand the recommended diet progression. Emphasize the necessity of good hygiene practices to prevent the spread of microorganisms that can cause gastroenteritis. If the child attends child care, have the parent inform the care center about the infection so the staff can be alerted to watch for other cases and can take steps to prevent the spread of infection.

EVALUATION

Expected outcomes of nursing care are provided on the accompanying Nursing Care Plan.

CONSTIPATION

Constipation is a common complaint in the pediatric population and accounts for 3–5% of visits to the pediatric office (Biggs & Dery, 2006). Stools are hard but there is an absence of structural, endocrine, or metabolic conditions that cause hard stools. Constipation affects up to one third of children 6–12 years of age each year (Biggs & Dery, 2006). Constipation is more common in school-age males than females but at other ages it is more common in females. Because stool patterns vary among children, identification of an abnormal pattern is sometimes difficult. Infants usually have several bowel movements a day. For a young child, one bowel movement a day may be normal. As the child grows, however, three to four bowel movements in a week may be a normal pattern. The diagnosis of constipation must take into account the child's normal stool patterns. Constipation may be caused by an underlying disease, diet, or psychological factor. It may result from defects in filling, or more commonly emptying, of the rectum. Pathological causes of defective filling include ineffective colonic propulsive activity, caused by hypothyroidism or use of medication, and obstruction, caused by a structural anomaly (stricture or stenosis) or by an aganglionic segment (Hirschsprung disease). If the rectum fails to fill, stasis leads to excessive drying of the stools. Emptying of the rectum depends on the defecation reflex. Lesions of the spinal cord, weakness of the abdominal muscles, and local lesions blocking sphincter relaxation all may impede attempts to defecate.

Constipation during infancy is rare and is most often caused by mismanagement of diet. The transition from formula to cow's milk may cause a transient constipation because the bowel must adjust to the increased protein content of cow's milk. Constipation occurs most frequently in the toddler and preschool age groups. This increased incidence is often associated with learning to control body functions. Many children do not like the sensations of a bowel movement and may begin withholding stool, which accumulates in and dilates the rectum until the next urge to defecate. The increasingly hard and painful bowel movement reinforces the child's behavior, and a pattern develops (Biggs & Dery, 2006).

Constipation in the school-age child, older child, and adolescent is generally related to activity dietary and toileting habits. The child's diet may be lacking in fiber and contain many starchy foods such as bread and cheese (Van Orden, 2004). Constipation may occur due to limited time for toileting. The child may not take time during the day to have a bowel movement or may be hesitant to use an unfamiliar bathroom.

Diagnosis is based on a thorough history and physical examination. When digital rectal examination confirms the presence

MyNursingKit Video: Stool Toileting: Refusals and Rewards

of fecal impaction further studies are not needed (Biggs & Dery, 2006). If digital rectal examination is contraindicated or the exam does not yield any findings, abdominal radiographs may be useful in identifying fecal impaction. Refer to the section on Hirschsprung disease on page 1532 for diagnostic tests used to confirm this diagnosis. When constipation occurs along with growth failure, vomiting, or abdominal pain, further investigation is necessary to rule out other disorders. Tests may include thyroid function tests; measurements of calcium, glucose, and electrolytes; a complete blood count; and urinalysis.

Clinical Therapy

Dietary management is the treatment of choice for constipation that has no underlying pathologic cause. Constipation in young infants can usually be corrected by increasing the amount of fluids or adding 2 ounces of pear or apple juice to daily intake. Increasing physical activity and fluid intake may be effective for some children.

Removing constipating foods (e.g., bananas, rice, and cheese) from the child's diet often decreases constipation. Increasing the child's intake of high-fiber foods (e.g., whole-grain breads, raw fruits, and vegetables) and fluids also promotes bowel elimination. In older infants, increasing the intake of fluids, cereals, fruits, and vegetables in the diet should correct the problem. A single glycerin suppository or enema may be required to remove hard stool.

Encouragement from parents and relaxation of bathroom privileges at school promote regularity and return of usual bowel patterns within a short time for school age children. Children may need to get up earlier to have breakfast to allow time for toileting before going to school.

Constipation may follow surgery, especially in children who are immobilized, such as by traction or a body cast. Stool softeners and a diet high in roughage and fluids prevent and treat constipation. Many families use herbal or other plant remedies to treat constipation.

Pharmacologic management of severe constipation usually occurs in two stages. The first stage involves disimpaction followed by maintenance therapy (Biggs & Dery, 2006). The evacuation phase is the most difficult for the child and those who are managing the child's constipation.

Consider the most effective means to evacuate the stool while causing the least amount of stress and anxiety to the child. Suppositories and enemas can cause fear in children. Polyethylene glycol electrolyte solution can be administered orally or instilled via a nasogastric tube to promote stool evacuation (Biggs & Dery, 2006). More recently electrolyte-free polyethylene glycol (Miralax) has been used effectively (Kinservik & Friedhoff, 2004). Once the stool has been evacuated, a routine stimulant laxative is given to prevent reaccumulation of stool in the bowel. Behavior modification is also an important aspect of treatment for constipation. For example, establish a routine for sitting on the toilet and offer rewards for success (Croffie, 2006).

Nursing Management

Nursing care focuses on teaching parents what constitutes normal bowel patterns in children and the importance of diet in maintaining normal bowel patterns. Assess the child's diet history and obtain a description of bowel patterns from parents. Ask what the family does to treat constipation. Assessment of the child's food likes and dislikes may provide a clue as to the cause of constipation. Regular bowel habits are encouraged by placing the child on the toilet 30 minutes after a meal or around the time defecation usually occurs. Providing positive reinforcement during toilet training helps prevent a withholding pattern.

Teach parents dietary measures to promote regularity of bowel movements. Children can be given a high-fiber diet that includes fruits and vegetables. Cut-up fresh fruits, dried fruits, and fruit juice can be offered as snacks. A glycerin suppository can be used periodically. This is a natural stimulant and lubricant of the bowel. Caution parents to avoid frequent use of laxatives, stool softeners, and enemas, since overuse can cause bowel dependency. Herbal stimulant laxatives are discouraged for children younger than 12 years, whereas other intestinal motility aids are not generally harmful. Find out more about any herbs the family commonly uses. See "Complementary Care: Children and Herbal Laxatives" on page 1547.

ENCOPRESIS

Encopresis is an abnormal elimination pattern characterized by the recurrent soiling or passage of stool at inappropriate times by a child who should have achieved bowel continence. Encopresis is reported to occur in 55% of boys and 35% of girls with constipation (Biggs & Dery, 2006). Children with primary encopresis have never achieved bowel control. Children with secondary encopresis have been continent of stool for several months.

Encopresis is usually associated with voluntary or involuntary retention of stool in the lower bowel and rectum, leading to constipation, dilation of the lower bowel, and incompetence of the inner sphincter. The retention of stool is usually a result of being "too busy"; the child puts off going to the bathroom because of the inconvenience of leaving an activity. The retention of stool leads to constipation that is untreated and chronic. Loose stool leaks around the hard feces, and the child becomes unaware of a need to eliminate. Soiling may occur during the day or night. Bowel movements are irregular, painful, small, and hard. The child may be ridiculed by peers because of offensive body odor. This rejection leads to withdrawal and behavioral problems, often resulting in altered school performance and attendance. The child continues to hold stool because the passage has become painful. Parents commonly seek health care, believing that the child has diarrhea or constipation.

The underlying constipation that leads to encopresis may be caused by the stress of environmental changes (e.g., birth of a sibling, moving to a new house, attending a new school), issues of anger and control related to bowel training, diet, a full schedule of activities, or a genetic predisposition.

A thorough history, physical examination, and diagnostic studies (possibly including barium or contrast enema) are necessary to rule out organic causes and anatomic abnormalities. Information about the child's toilet training habits and parents' attitudes concerning those habits is obtained. A dietary history, including eating habits and types of foods eaten, is often helpful. Physical examination sometimes reveals a non-tender mass in the lower abdomen.

In addition to dietary management and treatment to evacuate the bowel as discussed in the preceding section, behavior modification techniques, and psychotherapy may be used. Behavior modification programs that reward and reinforce appropriate toileting habits can be successful. The child should sit on the toilet for several minutes after morning and evening meals. It takes several months for the bowel to be retrained to respond to sphincter stimulation. Psychological-based treatment that involves interactive parent and child guidance may be indicated if the child has not responded to other treatment (Reid & Bahar, 2006).

Nursing Management

Prevention of encopresis is the nursing goal. Partner with parents to teach toilet training techniques, emphasizing the child's developmental readiness. Parents are encouraged to praise the child for successes and to avoid punishment and power struggles. Encourage high-fiber diets and regular times for elimination.

Nursing care centers on educating the child and parents about the disorder and its treatment and on providing emotional support. Explain the treatment plan, including dietary changes and use of laxatives or stool softeners. Reassure the child that he or she has a healthy body and, with treatment, will achieve normal functioning. The child is monitored during clinic visits for at least 6 months to be certain new patterns have been established.

INTESTINAL PARASITIC DISORDERS

Intestinal parasitic disorders occur most frequently in tropical regions. Outbreaks take place where water is not treated, food is incorrectly prepared, or people live in crowded conditions with poor sanitation. In the United States, outbreaks of diseases caused by protozoa or helminths (worms) are increasing. Young children, especially those in day care, are most at risk of infection. Young children often lack good hygiene practices and are likely to put objects and their hands into their mouths. (See "Clinical Manifestations: Common Intestinal Parasitic Disorders.")

Another common cause of young child infection is exposure to pets and wildlife. Pets should be checked for parasites and dewormed regularly. Sandboxes should be kept covered when not in use and children should be taught good handwashing techniques after exposure to their pets (CDC, 2008a). Laboratory examination of stool specimens identifies the causative organism (protozoa, worms, larvae, or ova). Treatment usually involves an anthelmintic.

Nursing care centers on preventive teaching. Emphasize the importance of good hygiene practices, especially careful handwashing, after toileting and when handling food. Ensure the family understands proper medication administration. Instruct parents to administer prescribed medications as directed even if the child's condition seems to be improved.

FEEDING DISORDERS

Feeding problems that interfere with a child's ability to ingest or tolerate certain forms of oral intake usually become apparent during the first year of life. To prevent complications of poor nutrition, feeding methods or diet may need to be altered. The following discussion focuses on the common disorders of colic and rumination. See Chapter 34 for a discussion of food allergy and sensitivity and of feeding disorder of infancy and childhood (failure to thrive). Chapter 34 includes a discussion of the eating disorders anorexia nervosa and bulimia.

COLIC

Colic is a feeding disorder characterized by paroxysmal abdominal pain and severe crying. The crying generally lasts at least 3 hours and occurs at least 3 day per week. Crying episodes peak around 6 weeks of age and generally resolve by 3–4 months of age (Hyman, Milla, Benninga, et al., 2006).

The etiology of colic is unknown. Proposed causes include feeding too rapidly and swallowing large amounts of air.

Characteristically the infant cries loudly and continuously, often for several hours. The infant's face may become flushed. The abdomen is distended and tense. Often the infant draws up the legs and clenches the hands. Episodes occur at the same time each day, usually in the late afternoon or early evening. Crying may stop only when the child is completely exhausted or after passage of flatus or stool.

The symptoms initially may resemble intestinal obstruction or peritoneal infection. These conditions must be ruled out along with sensitivity to formula. Treatment is supportive as no general medical consensus exists on effective treatments or interventions for colic. Some healthcare providers recommend medications such as simethicone (Mylicon) drops. Some recommend formula change to a soy formula or an elemental formula such as Pregestimil (Lobo, Kotzer, Keefe, et al., 2004).

Nursing Management

Nursing care requires a thorough history of the infant's diet and daily schedule and the events surrounding episodes of colicky behavior. Assessment of the infant's feeding patterns and diet, includes type, frequency, and amount of feeding (if breastfeeding, maternal diet history), and frequency of burping. Episodes of colic for onset, duration, and characteristics of cry. Ask the parents what measures are used to relieve crying and their effectiveness.

Nursing Practice

Vomiting and feeding disorders can occur throughout childhood as well as in infancy. In older children, a pattern of **chronic vomiting** (low-grade nearly daily emesis) or **cyclic vomiting** (repeated severe vomiting of an episodic nature) can occur. These patterns differ from vomiting seen in colic or gastroesophageal reflux. Chronic vomiting is often associated with upper gastrointestinal tract diseases such as gastritis and esophagitis while cyclic vomiting is indicative of a syndrome known as abdominal migraine (Bullard & Page, 2005). Continuous vomiting of any nature should be evaluated.

Clinical Manifestations

COMMON INTESTINAL PARASITIC DISORDERS

PARASITIC INFECTION	TRANSMISSION, LIFE CYCLE, PATHOGENESIS	CLINICAL MANIFESTATIONS	CLINICAL THERAPY	COMMENTS
Giardiasis				
Organism: protozoan *Giardia lamblia* 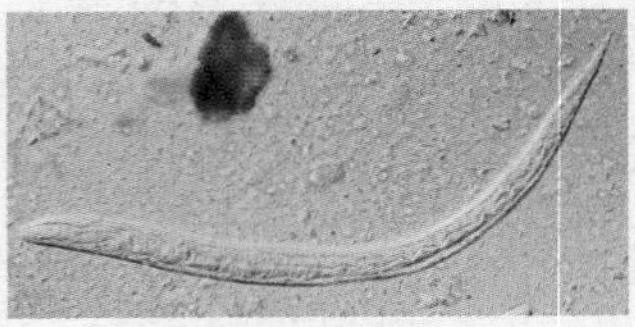 Threadworm	Transmission is through person-to-person contact, unfiltered water, improperly prepared infected food, and contact with animals. Cysts are ingested and passed into the duodenum and proximal jejunum, where they begin actively feeding. They are excreted in the stool.	May be asymptomatic. *Infants:* diarrhea, vomiting, anorexia, failure to thrive *Older children:* abdominal cramps; intermittent loose, foul-smelling, watery, pale, and greasy stools.	Available medications include furazolidone and quinacrine. Furazolidone has fewer side effects than quinacrine but is more expensive. Metronidazole is also effective but is not licensed in the United States for treatment of giardiasis.	Most common intestinal parasitic organism in the United States. Infection may resolve spontaneously in 4–6 weeks without treatment. Parents or caregivers should wear gloves when handling diapers or stool of parasite-infected infant or child.
Enterobiasis (Pinworm)				
Organism: nematode *Enterobius vermicularis* 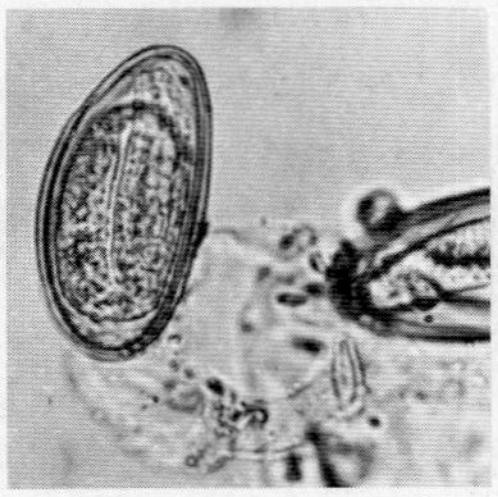 Pinworm	Transmission is from discharged eggs inhaled or carried from hand to mouth. Eggs hatch in the upper intestine and mature in 15–28 days. Larvae then migrate to the cecum. After mating, the female migrates out of the anus and lays up to 17,000 eggs. Movement of worms causes intense itching. Scratching deposits eggs on the hands and under the nails.	Intense perianal itching, irritability, restlessness, and short attention span; in females, can migrate to the vagina and urethra to cause infection. Itching intensifies at night when the female comes to the anal opening to lay eggs.	Available medications include mebendazole, pyrantel pamoate, and piperazine citrate. The child and all household members should be treated at the same time. Treatment may be repeated in 2–3 weeks.	Most common helminthic infection in United States. Transmission is increased in crowded conditions such as housing developments, schools, and childcare centers.
Ascariasis (Type of Roundworm)				
Organism: nematode *Ascaris lumbricoides* 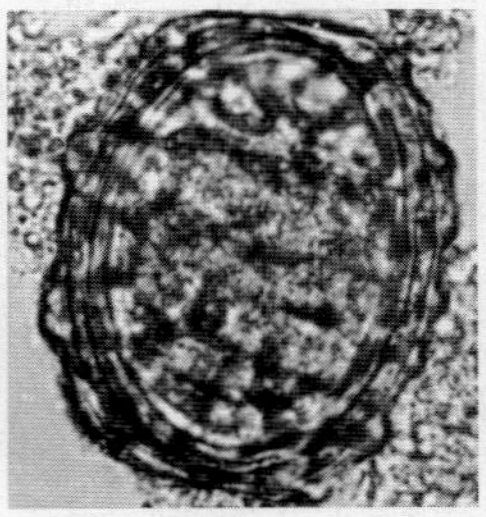 Roundworm	Transmission is from discharged eggs carried from hand to mouth. Adult lays eggs in small intestine. Eggs are excreted in stool, where they incubate for 2–3 weeks. Swallowed eggs hatch in the small intestine. Larvae may penetrate intestinal villi, entering the portal vein and liver, then moving to the lung. Larvae that ascend to upper respiratory tract are swallowed and proceed to the small intestine, where they repeat the cycle.	Mild infection may be asymptomatic. Severe infection may result in intestinal obstruction, peritonitis, obstructive jaundice, and lung involvement.	Available antihelminthic medications include mebendazole, pyrantel pamoate, or piperazine citrate. Stools should be examined 2 weeks after treatment and monthly for 3 months. Family members and contacts of the child should be treated if indicated. If the child has intestinal obstruction, treatment may include administering piperazine through a nasogastric tube and duodenal suction. Obstructing worms sometimes have to be surgically removed.	Most common in warm climates. Primarily affects children 1–4 years of age.

Clinical Manifestations—continued

COMMON INTESTINAL PARASITIC DISORDERS

PARASITIC INFECTION	TRANSMISSION, LIFE CYCLE, PATHOGENESIS	CLINICAL MANIFESTATIONS	CLINICAL THERAPY	COMMENTS
Hookworm disease				
Organism: nematode *Necator americanus* 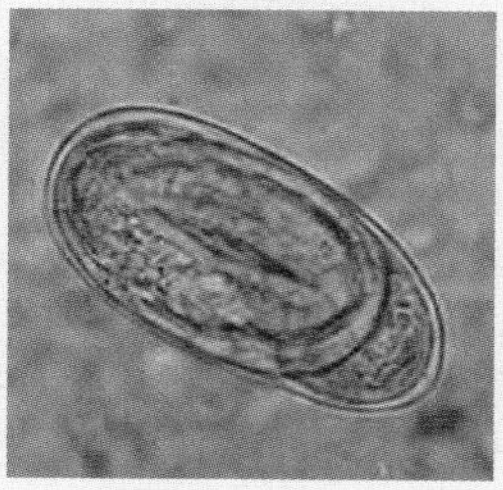 Hookworm	Transmission is through direct contact with infected soil containing larvae. Worms live in the small intestine and feed on villi, causing bleeding. Eggs are deposited in the bowel and excreted in feces. Eggs hatch in damp shaded soil. Larvae attach to and penetrate the skin, then enter the bloodstream, migrating to the lungs. Larvae then migrate to the upper respiratory passages and are swallowed.	In healthy individuals mild infection seldom causes problems. More severe infection may result in anemia and malnutrition. Presence of larvae on the skin may cause burning and itching, followed by redness and papular eruption.	Available medications include mebendazole and pyrantel pamoate. Stools should be examined 2 weeks after treatment and monthly for 3 months. Family members and contacts of the child should be treated if indicated.	Children should wear shoes when outdoors, although other unprotected areas of the skin may still come in contact with larvae.
Strongyloidiasis (Type of Roundworm)				
Organism: nematode *Strongyloides stercoralis* 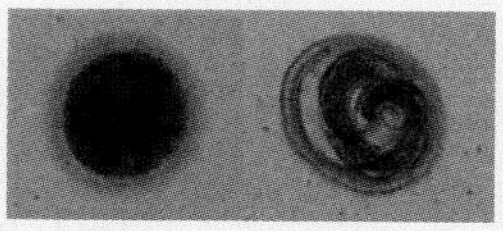 Nematode	Transmission is from the ingestion of discharged larvae in the soil. Life cycle is similar to that of the hookworm, except this roundworm does not attach to the intestinal mucosa, and feeding larvae (rather than eggs) may be deposited in the soil.	Mild infection may be asymptomatic. Severe infection may result in abdominal pain and distention, nausea, vomiting, and diarrhea. Stools may be large and pale, with mucus. Severe infection may lead to a nutritional deficiency.	Available medications include thiabendazole or mebendazole. Treatment may need to be repeated if symptoms recur after treatment. Family members and contacts of the child should be examined and treated if indicated.	Most common in older children and adolescents.
Visceral larva migrans (Toxocarlasis)				
Organism: nematode *Toxocara canis* or *T. catis*, commonly found in dogs and cats 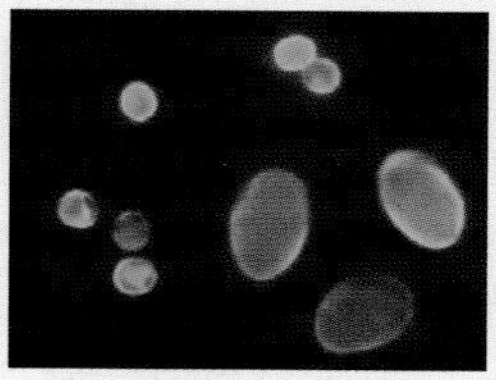 Giardia lamblia	Transmission is through the ingestion of eggs in the soil. Ingested eggs hatch in the intestine. Mobile larvae then migrate to the liver and eventually to all major organs (including the brain). Once migration is complete, they encapsulate in dense fibrous tissue.	Most cases are asymptomatic. Affected children may have a low-grade fever and recurrent upper airway diseases. Severe symptoms include hepatomegaly, pulmonary infiltration, and neurologic disturbances. In all cases there is a hypereosinophilia of the blood.	There is no specific treatment. Corticosteroids have been used in severe cases. Thiabendazole has been recommended but efficacy is not established (infection usually resolves spontaneously).	Most common in toddlers. Deworm household pets monthly if indicated. Keep children away from areas contaminated with animal droppings.

Giardia lamblia, Strongyloidiasis, Hookworm, and Toxocariasis courtesy of the Centers for Disease Control and Prevention, Atlanta, GA. Ascariasis and Enterobiasis from: Murray, D. L. (2003). Infectious diseases. In C. D. Rudolph & A. M. Rudolph (Eds.), *Rudolph's pediatrics* (21st ed., pp. 1102, 1106). New York: McGraw Hill.

Evidence-Based Nursing

REDUCING CRYING TIME IN COLIC EPISODES

Clinical Question

What interventions are needed to provide relief to the child and the family and minimize the negative impacts of the experience of having an infant with colic?

The Evidence

Approximately 15% to 25% of infants have colic during the first few months of life (Ellett, Schuff, & Davis, 2005). To determine the impact of a colicky infant on the family, a study was conducted in which parents were asked to describe their experiences of living with an infant with colic. Parents of 15 colicky infants participated in the study. Three themes emerged from this study: crying, emotions, and feelings. Half of the mothers reported that they cried with their infants. Emotions such as anger, worry, guilt, and frustration were expressed. Feelings of helplessness, hopelessness, isolation, and being unloved were expressed. The results of the study supported the need for evidence-based practice in the treatment of colic (Ellett & Swenson, 2005).

An emerging view of colic is that it is a behavioral pattern that will respond to modifications in the environment and to structured cue-based care (Keefe, Lobo, Froese-Fretz, et al., 2006). With this in mind, a study to implement the REST (Regulation, Entrainment, Structure, and Touch) program was conducted to see if the average crying time decreased in infants with colicky or unexplained crying episodes. One of the major goals of the program was to promote parent-infant bonding and to provide information and support to parents. One-hundred-and-twenty-one infants between 2 and 6 weeks of age were involved in either routine care or a home management REST program implemented by a pediatric nurse. The REST program included weekly home or clinic visits, videos, workbooks, and nursing assessments and counseling.

- *Regulation:* The focus in regulation is to avoid overstimulation and exhaustion in the young infant and to help the parents recognize when this might occur.
- *Entrainment.* The goal of entrainment is to adjust the environment depending on the infants sleep/wake cycles such as dimming the lights when the infant is asleep.
- *Structure.* Structure focuses on establishing routines for daily activities such as feeding and bathing.
- *Touch.* Touch involves different methods of tactile stimulation and various holding positions for the infant.

In addition to the guiding principles of the REST program described above, the concepts that provided guidance for parents included *reassurance, empathy, support,* and *time-out.* Results of the study showed that those infants who received REST interventions had a reduction in their crying time to 1.3 hours per day while those in the control group cried an average of 3 hours per day. At the 8-week follow-up visit, symptoms in 62% of the infants in the REST group had resolved as compared to 29% in the control group (Keefe, Barbosa, Froese-Fretz, et al., 2005; Keefe et al., 2006).

Best Practice

Open lines of communication between healthcare providers and parents are essential to minimize the trauma of having an infant with colic (Ellett & Swenson, 2005). Parents need support and a consistent approach to dealing with an infant with prolonged crying episodes. Spending time with families to implement programs such as REST not only promotes parent-infant bonding, but decreases the length of crying episodes, thereby decreasing the stress on both the infant and the parents.

Critical Thinking

How can you determine how well parents are coping with their child's colic? What are the risks to the child if the parents do not demonstrate positive coping strategies? What suggestions might you give to parents of a child with colic? What is your own view of the causes of colic and the most effective treatment plan?

See MyNursingKit for possible responses.

When possible, observe the feeding method. Parents of infants with colic are often tired and frustrated. They require frequent reassurance that they are not to blame for the infant's condition. Suggest ways of alleviating some of the infant's symptoms and discomfort. See "Evidence-Based Nursing: Reducing Crying Time in Colic Episodes."

An important consideration is the significant impact of colic on families. Colic can place extreme stress and fatigue on the family. Active support and counseling for the mother and other family members is essential to reduce the risk of abuse to the infant (Lobo et al., 2004).

RUMINATION

Rumination is a rare and serious form of chronic regurgitation of recently ingested food into the mouth, followed by rechewing and reswallowing or expulsion of the material (Hyman et al., 2006). Chewing movements and mouthing of fingers often precede or accompany regurgitation. Close observation may reveal the infant actively initiating gagging with the tongue and fingers.

Rumination is most often associated with poor maternal–infant bonding. This kind of behavior is seen in infants deprived of tactile, visual, or auditory stimuli for long periods. The infant substitutes repetitive self-stimulation for the lack of appropriate external stimulation. (See the discussion of eating disorders of infancy and childhood in Chapter 34.) Rumination can be life threatening because it can lead to weight loss, growth failure, malnutrition, and electrolyte imbalance.

Diagnostic evaluation focuses on ruling out an organic cause and determining the degree and type of nutritional deficiencies. The child should be observed ruminating to help confirm the diagnosis. Treatment involves correcting the nutritional deficits and developing normal feeding patterns. An interdisciplinary approach with medical and nursing staff and social services is often needed to help parents meet the infant's nutritional and psychologic needs (Hyman et al., 2006).

Teaching Highlights

SUGGESTIONS FOR ALLEVIATING COLIC

Provide Rhythmic Movement

Front-carrying sling carriers

Infant swing (battery-operated swing provides continuous motion)

Car ride

Ride in a stroller

Alternate Positions

Swaddle infant in a soft, stretchy blanket with knees flexed up against abdomen or with legs straight

Place infant prone on parent's arm, supporting the body with one hand under the abdomen and cradling the head in the crook of the other arm

Reduce Environmental Stimuli

Respond to crying

Provide quiet, soothing music

Prevent sudden loud noises

Avoid smoking

Provide Various Tactile Stimuli

Offer a pacifier

Provide a warm bath

Massage abdomen

Alter Intake

Feed smaller amount and burp frequently

Use a bottle with a collapsible bag to prevent sucking air

Breastfeeding mothers: eliminate milk products and spicy or gas-producing foods

Hold upright for 30 minutes after feeding

Nursing Management

Nursing care focuses on establishing a warm, caring relationship with the infant and the parents. Making eye contact with the infant, providing food regularly, and stimulating the infant through all the senses are ways to break the pattern of rumination.

Parents need to be included in the infant's care. Discuss proper nutrition and demonstrate feeding techniques and interactions that promote development. Determine the parents' support needs and make a referral to social service agencies as appropriate. A parent preoccupied with financial or other problems is less likely to attend to an infant's needs, resulting in continuation or recurrence of the pattern of rumination.

DISORDERS OF MALABSORPTION

Malabsorption occurs when a child cannot digest or absorb nutrients in the diet. Disorders of malabsorption include celiac disease, lactose intolerance, and short bowel syndrome. Cystic fibrosis, a common cause of malabsorption, is discussed in Chapter 48∞.

CELIAC DISEASE

Celiac disease, or gluten-sensitive enteropathy, is a chronic malabsorption syndrome (Nehring, 2004). Although it was previously thought to be more prevalent in European countries, recent data show that the prevalence of celiac disease in the general population of the United States is 1 in 133 people, similar to that of those countries in Europe (Hill & Hill, 2005). It is also more common among members of the same family; a genetic factor may play a role in etiology. It is estimated that 4–17% of children with Down syndrome have celiac disease (Nehring, 2004).

Celiac disease is an immunologic disorder (Zelnik, Pacht, Obeid, et al., 2004) characterized by an intolerance for gluten, a protein found in wheat, barley, rye, and oats. Inability to digest glutenin and gliadin (protein fractions) results in the accumulation of the amino acid glutamine, which is toxic to mucosal cells in the intestine. Damage to the villi ultimately impairs the absorptive process in the small intestine.

In the early stages, celiac disease affects fat absorption, resulting in excretion of large quantities of fat in the stools (steatorrhea). Stools are greasy, foul smelling, frothy, and excessive. As changes in the villi continue, the absorption of protein, carbohydrates, calcium, iron, folate, and vitamins A, D, E, K, and B_{12} becomes impaired.

Symptoms usually occur when solid foods containing gluten are introduced to the child's diet (generally between 6 months to 2 years of age), although celiac disease is sometimes first diagnosed in adulthood. The classic features of celiac disease in infancy include chronic diarrhea, growth impairment, and abdominal distention. The child also demonstrates poor appetite, lack of energy, and muscle wasting with hypotonia (Gelfond & Fasano, 2006) (Figure 53–8 ●). Atypical features are present in children diagnosed with delayed onset celiac disease around 5–7 years of age. Symptoms include nausea, vomiting, recurrent abdominal pain, and bloating. Other symptoms may include delayed growth, iron deficiency, defects in tooth enamel, and abnormal liver function tests (Gelfond & Fasano, 2006).

Diagnosis is confirmed through measurement of fecal fat content, duodenal biopsy, and improvement with removal of gluten products from the diet. Serum screening tests for IgA antiendomysial antibodies and IgA antitissue transglutaminase antibodies are commonly used in diagnosis (Murdock & Johnston, 2005).

Management of the disease is total exclusion of gluten from the diet. This gluten-free diet is a lifetime treatment. Barley, wheat, and rye are completely eliminated (Allen, 2004). Symptoms generally improve within a few days to weeks.

The intestinal villi return to normal in about 6 months. Growth should improve steadily, and height and weight should reach normal range within 1 year. Vitamin supplementation may be needed for a period of time if the child has become malnourished.

Nursing Management

Nursing care focuses on supporting the parents in maintaining a gluten-free diet for the child. Thoroughly explain the disease

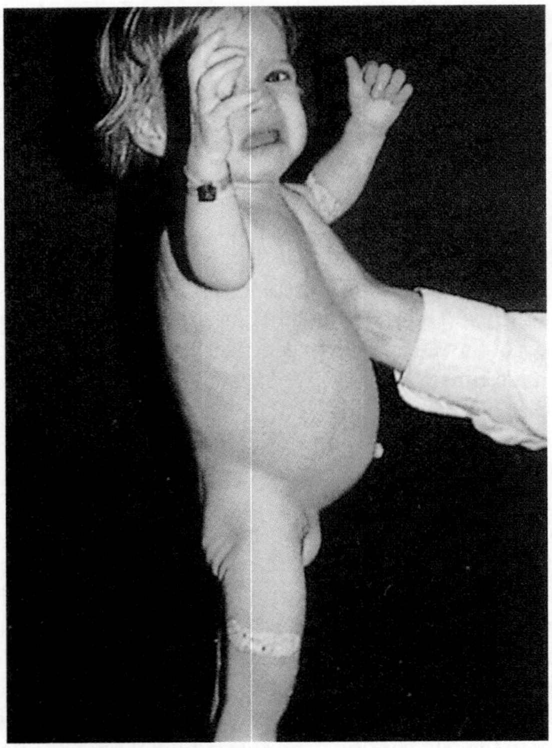

● **Figure 53–8** Celiac disease. The child with celiac disease commonly shows failure to grow and wasting of extremities. The abdomen can appear large due to intestinal bloating and malnutrition.

From Zitelli, B. J., & Davis, H. W. (Eds.). (2007). *Atlas of pediatric physical diagnosis.* (5th ed., p. 389). St. Louis: Mosby.

process to the parents. Emphasize the necessity of following a gluten-free diet. Help parents to understand that celiac disease requires lifelong dietary modifications that should not be discontinued when the child is symptom-free. Discontinuation of the diet places the child at risk for growth retardation and the development of GI cancers in adulthood. All children with celiac disease should be seen by a dietitian several times during childhood. Nutritional assessment and continued teaching to maintain a gluten-free diet take place at these visits. Dietary management is made difficult by hidden gluten in many prepared foods, such as chocolate candy, prepared meats, ice cream, soups, condiments, and food starch.

An infant or toddler's diet is easily monitored at home. When the child enters school, however, ensuring adherence to dietary restrictions becomes more difficult. In addition to easily identified gluten-based foods, such as bread, cake, doughnuts, cookies, and crackers, the child must also avoid processed foods that contain gluten as a filler. School-age children and adolescents are often tempted to eat these foods, especially when among peers. Emphasize the need for compliance while meeting the child's developmental needs.

The child's special dietary needs can place a financial burden on the family. Parents need to purchase prepared rice or corn flour products or make their own bread and bakery products. Advise parents that getting a dietary prescription enables them to deduct the cost of these ingredients and commercially prepared products as a medical expense.

Because the entire family must adapt to the diet, parents and siblings need support and management skills. For information and support, refer parents and children to several organizations, including the American Celiac Society, the Celiac Sprue Association/United States of America, and the Gluten Intolerance Group.

Expected outcomes of nursing care include the following:

- Adequate nutrition to support growth and development needs
- Growth and developmental milestones appropriate for age achieved
- Understanding of dietary restrictions and appropriate meal planning.

LACTOSE INTOLERANCE

Lactose intolerance is the inability to digest lactose, a disaccharide found in milk and other dairy products. It results from a congenital or acquired deficiency of the enzyme lactase. Congenital lactase deficiency of infancy is a rare disorder. See Chapter 34∞ for a general discussion of food intolerance. Lactose intolerance is considered a biological norm, occurring in up to 80% of African Americans, 80–100% of Native Americans, and 90–100% of Asian Americans (NDDIC, 2006).

Abdominal pain, flatulence, and diarrhea occur shortly after birth when the infant is unable to hydrolyze lactose. Diarrhea develops rapidly after the child ingests milk and milk products. Some children are able to tolerate small ingestions of lactose but have symptoms when larger amounts are consumed. Incidence of lactose intolerance increases with advancing age throughout childhood.

Diagnosis is based on a thorough history and a hydrogen breath test, which measures the amount of hydrogen left after fermentation of unabsorbed carbohydrates. Implementing a lactose-free diet for a period of time may eliminate the symptoms, thus confirming the diagnosis. Treatment for infants includes switching to lactose-free formula. For older children, eliminating lactose-containing foods is recommended. Lactase enzyme tablets can be added to milk or sprinkled on foods to aid digestion.

Nursing Management

Nursing care is primarily supportive. Carefully explain dietary modifications to parents and discuss alternative sources of calcium (see Chapter 34∞). Discuss the need for supplementation of calcium and vitamin D to prevent deficiencies. Teach families how to read food labels to find hidden sources of lactose. For example, milk solids may be found in breads, cakes, candies, salad dressings, margarine, and processed food. Suggest lactase tablets for children who want to eat some dairy products.

SHORT BOWEL SYNDROME

Short bowel syndrome is a decreased ability to digest and absorb a regular diet due to a shortened intestine. Loss of intestine may result from extensive bowel resection for treatment of necrotizing enterocolitis or from a congenital bowel anomaly such as intestinal malrotation, Hirschsprung disease, gastroschisis, or atresia (Baron & Blaber, 2005; Jackson & Buchman, 2004).

Nursing Practice

The child with short bowel syndrome will receive TPN via a central line. Meticulous care of the central line is essential to prevent a central line infection and potential septicemia (Baron & Blaber, 2005). Maintaining patency of the central line is also essential as this may be the child's only route for receiving nutrition. It is not uncommon for children with SBS to require insertion of multiple central lines over time either due to infection or to occlusion of the line, especially if they require long term TPN. This not only places a stress on the child who must undergo yet another surgical procedure, but is a stressor for the family as well.

The extent and location of the involved bowel determine the severity of the disorder. Because specific types of absorption occur primarily in certain parts of the bowel, the section lost determines which vitamins and other nutrients are inadequate. During the first 3 months after bowel resection, watery diarrhea is common. In the transition period, the remaining bowel usually increases its absorptive surface area and partially compensates for the absent intestine. At first, the infant or young child requires nutritional support to provide sufficient nutrients for growth and development. In the initial period, the child receives only TPN. Once the bowel begins to recover, in addition to TPN, feedings by mouth or by tube may be started in small amounts. Feedings by this method stimulate the bowel and prevent atrophy of the mucosa (Baron & Blaber, 2005). It is essential that the child received the appropriate nutritional components regardless of the method in which nutrition is delivered.

Nursing Management

Nursing care focuses on meeting the child's nutritional and fluid needs and teaching parents how to care for the child at home. Establishing an adequate nutritional intake and bowel pattern is a lengthy process. TPN is provided initially until a feeding regimen can be established. Oral and enteral feedings are instituted gradually to allow the bowel time to compensate. Provide support to the family and child throughout this period. Teach parents how to prepare and administer total parenteral feedings and care for the central line (see Skill 12–7 SKILLS). Once enteral or tube feedings have started, teach management of the feeding pump and care of the feeding tube. Ensure regular bowel function and maintain skin integrity. Arrange home visits to monitor the child's growth and development, care of the central line and tube-feeding site, and any side effects such as fluid and electrolyte imbalance and diarrhea.

HEPATIC DISORDERS

The liver is one of the most vital organs in the body. Its primary functions include production of blood clotting factors, fibrinogen and prothrombin; secretion of bile and *bilirubin* (yellow pigment produced from the breakdown of red blood cells); metabolism of fat, protein, and carbohydrates; detoxification of hormones, drugs, and other substances; and storage of vitamins A, D, E, and K and glycogen. Thus, any inflammatory, obstructive, or degenerative disorder that affects liver function can be life threatening. The following discussion focuses on three common liver disorders in children: biliary atresia, viral hepatitis, and cirrhosis. A discussion of hyperbilirubinemia can be found in Chapter 31.

BILIARY ATRESIA

Biliary atresia results when the extrahepatic bile ducts fail to develop or are closed (Flanigan, 2007; Bezerra, 2005). The disorder leads to cholestasis, cirrhosis, end-stage liver disease, and death by 2 years of age, if left untreated (Bezerra, 2005; Utterson, Shepherd, Sokol, et al., 2005; Weerasooriya, White, & Shepherd, 2004). It is the most common cause of pathologic jaundice in infants and is the leading indication for pediatric liver transplantation (Bezerra, 2005; Utterson et al., 2005).

Clinical Manifestations

Initially the newborn is asymptomatic. Jaundice may not be detected until 2 to 3 weeks after birth. At that point bilirubin levels increase, accompanied by abdominal distention and hepatomegaly (see Appendix B for bilirubin levels and other liver function tests). As the disease progresses, splenomegaly occurs. The infant experiences easy bruising, prolonged bleeding time, and intense itching. Stools have putty-like consistency and are white or clay colored because of the absence of bile pigments. Excretion of bilirubin and bile salts results in tea-colored urine. Failure to thrive and malnutrition occur as the destructive changes of the disease progress.

The cause of biliary atresia is unknown. Absence or blockage of the extrahepatic bile ducts results in blocked bile flow from the liver to the duodenum. This altered bile flow soon causes inflammation and fibrotic changes in the liver. In addition to blockage, the disease can also be caused by hepatocellular dysfunction. Lack of bile acids also interferes with digestion of fat and absorption of fat-soluble vitamins A, D, E, and K, resulting in steatorrhea and nutritional deficiencies. Without treatment the disease is fatal.

Clinical Therapy

Diagnosis is based on the history, physical examination, and laboratory evaluation. Laboratory findings reveal elevated bilirubin levels, elevated serum aminotransferase and alkaline phosphatase values, prolonged prothrombin time, and increased ammonia levels. Percutaneous liver biopsy suggests biliary atresia, and cholangiography and an exploratory laparatomy confirms the diagnosis (Roach & Bruny, 2008).

Treatment involves surgery to attempt correction of the obstruction (hepatoportoenterostomy) and supportive care. In the hepatoportoenterostomy (Kasai procedure), a segment of the intestine is anastomosed to the porta hepatis. The primary purpose of this procedure is to promote bile flow from the liver. Intravenous antibiotics are administered in the postoperative period to prevent cholangitis. Prophylaxis with oral antibiotics is continued for 1–2 years after surgery (Flanigan, 2007).

Additional treatment includes administration of intramuscular vitamin K prior to invasive procedures and surgery to decrease the risk of bleeding afterwards; ursodeoxycholic acid (Actigall) to promote bile flow, and vitamins A, D, E, and K to provide supplementation since absorption of these vitamins is impaired. The infant is breastfed or is given Pregestimil or Nutramigen, formulas that contain medium chain triglycerides. As the liver disease worsens the child may need cholestyramine and antihistamines to help decrease itching. Enteral feedings and TPN may be needed as well (Flanigan, 2007).

Although the Kasai procedure improves the prognosis, complications of liver disease continue to develop; liver transplantation is eventually needed. Donor shortage is the major factor limiting the use of liver transplantation (Tran, Nissen, Poordad, et al., 2004). Advances in transplantation surgery now make it possible to perform partial liver transplants from living donor resections. This enables transplantation to be performed when the child is in optimal health, rather than waiting until an appropriate-size cadaver liver is available, and allows for donations from close family members who are often good tissue matches. One-year survival rates of 85% and 86% have been reported in recent studies (Farmer, Vernick, McDiarmid, et al., 2007; D'Alessandro et al., 2007).

Nursing Management

Nursing care in the initial stages of biliary atresia is the same as that for any healthy newborn. As symptoms develop, the focus of nursing care becomes long-term management and support.

Diagnosis of this potentially fatal disorder can be devastating to parents. Provide emotional support and offer frequent explanations of tests during the initial diagnostic evaluation. As the disease progresses, the infant becomes irritable because of intense itching and the accumulation of toxins. Tepid baths may help to relieve itching and provide comfort. When drying the skin, pat the towel against the skin rather than rubbing, which promotes vasodilation and worsens the infant's itching and irritation. Promote rest by grouping nursing activities while the infant is awake. Weigh the infant daily. Administer TPN, intralipids, and fat-soluble vitamins A, D, E, and K as prescribed.

Care following a hepatoportoenterostomy is similar to that for a child undergoing abdominal surgery. (See the earlier discussion of postsurgical nursing management for appendicitis and "Nursing Care Plan: The Child Undergoing Surgery" in Chapter 41∞.) Posttransplant care includes immunosuppressant drugs and close monitoring for vascular complications. For the child who has received a transplant, teach parents how to identify signs of rejection (nausea, vomiting, fever, jaundice), as well as the administration and side effects of immunosuppressant medications.

Discharge planning focuses on teaching parents how to care for the child's skin, provide for nutritional needs, administer medications, and monitor for increasing symptoms of liver disease. Refer parents to support groups, clergy, or social services if indicated. They will need ongoing visits from a home healthcare nurse to help them manage the child's complex care. The main expected outcomes of nursing care are the parent's ability to cope with the child's health status and to provide the necessary care. The child is expected to function at maximum potential considering the extent of disease.

Expected outcomes for nursing care of the child with biliary atresia are as follows:

- Adequate nutrition to support growth and development
- Parental coping with stress of the child's condition
- Growth and developmental milestones expected for age are achieved.

VIRAL HEPATITIS

Hepatitis is an inflammation of the liver caused by a viral infection. It may be acute or chronic. Acute hepatitis is rapid in onset and if untreated may develop into chronic hepatitis. The most frequently diagnosed causative organisms are hepatitis A virus (HAV), hepatitis B virus (HBV), and hepatitis C virus (HCV). A lesser known type is hepatitis D virus (HDV). This type of hepatitis only occurs in individuals who have HBV infection (Holloway & D'Acunto, 2006). Hepatitis E (HEV) occurs primarily in developing countries and is rarely seen in the United States (CDC, 2008b). In 2006 the incidence of Hepatitis A declined to its lowest rates with only 1.2/100,000 cases reported in the United States. The incidence of hepatitis B has also decreased remarkably over the past several years to a low in 2006 of 1.6/100,000 population in the United States (Wasley, Grytdal, & Gallagher, 2008). The decline in both of these illnesses is related to routine vaccine administration, especially in children.

Etiology and Pathophysiology

Hepatitis A is highly contagious and traditionally has been called infectious hepatitis. Infection occurs primarily through the fecal–oral route. Transmission is by direct person-to-person spread or through ingestion of contaminated water or food (particularly shellfish). Hepatitis A frequently occurs in children in childcare settings where hygiene practices are poor. Food handlers can spread hepatitis A if not aware of their infection; it is a common cause of food-borne illness. Because the virus is transmitted in the early stages of the disease when individuals are often asymptomatic or only mildly ill, large numbers of people may be exposed before the diagnosis is confirmed (Table 53–3). Most children recover from hepatitis A; however, in rare instances acute liver failure may occur (Yazigi & Balistreri, 2007).

Hepatitis B, known traditionally as serum hepatitis, is a serious disease. Transmission is usually by the parenteral route through the exchange of blood or any body secretion or fluid. Other common transmission routes include sexual activity and transmission from mother to fetus in utero. Adolescents who use intravenous drugs and have unprotected sexual intercourse are at risk for contracting hepatitis B. Major sources for the spread of HBV are healthy chronic carriers. All body fluids of infected individuals are potentially contaminated with the virus.

The hepatitis C virus is transmitted primarily through blood and blood products, and blood banks now test for this virus. Infected children have commonly had repeated transfusions (as in sickle cell disease or hemophilia). Intravenous drug use, body piercing, and multiple sexual partners are also risk factors. Infected mothers may infect their children before birth or during breastfeeding. Chronic infection occurs in 70–85% of those indi-

Table 53–3 Comparison of Hepatitis Types

Type	Immunization Available	Prophylaxis	Primary Transmission	Incubation Period
Hepatitis A	Yes	Immune globulin Hepatitis A vaccine	Fecal-oral	15–19 days
Hepatitis B	Yes	Hepatitis B immune globulin Hepatitis B vaccine	Needlesticks or sharps exposure Intravenous drug use During birth Sexual activity	60–180 days
Hepatitis C	No	None	Needlesticks or sharps exposure Intravenous drug use During birth	14–160 days
Hepatitis D	No	Hepatitis B vaccine	Needlesticks or sharps exposure Intravenous drug use During birth Sexual activity	21–42 days
Hepatitis E	No	None	Fecal-oral	21–63 days

Adapted from: Centers for Disease Control and Prevention. (2008b) Viral Hepatitis. Retrieved January 10, 2009, from www.cdc.gov/hepatitis; Yazigi, N., & Balistreri, W. F. (2007) Viral hepatitis. In R. M. Kliegman, R. E. Behrman, H. B. Jenson, & B. F. Stanton (Eds.), *Nelson textbook of pediatrics* (18th ed., pp. 1680–1690). Philadelphia: Saunders.

viduals infected with hepatitis C (CDC, 2008b). Hepatitis C is now the most common blood-borne infection in the United States (Wasley et al., 2008).

Hepatitis D (delta virus) is a defective virus that can gain entry to a human only in connection with hepatitis B (CDC, 2008). Hepatitis E infection is primarily transmitted through contaminated water and is most common in developing countries. The only documented cases in the United States have been in individuals who immigrated or visited from a country where the disease is prevalent (Yazigi & Balistreri, 2007).

The liver's response to injury by the viruses that cause hepatitis is similar (see "Pathophysiology Illustrated: Viral Hepatitis"). Initially, invasion of the parenchymal cells by the virus results in local degeneration and necrosis. Subsequent infiltration of the parenchyma by lymphocytes, macrophages, plasma cells, eosinophils, and neutrophils causes inflammation that blocks biliary drainage into the intestine. Impaired bile excretion causes a buildup of bile in the blood, urine, and skin (jaundice). Structural changes in the parenchymal cells account for other altered liver functions.

Clinical Manifestations

Acute hepatitis infection is characterized by two phases, the anicteric (absence of jaundice) phase and the icteric (jaundice) phase. The anicteric phase usually lasts 5 to 7 days. Signs and symptoms include nausea, vomiting, anorexia, malaise, fatigue, right upper quadrant pain, hepatosplenomegaly, and fever. The child becomes irritable, looks ill, and requires rest. In the icteric phase, signs and symptoms include darkening of urine, clay-colored stools, and the characteristic yellowing of the skin and sclera. Many children with hepatitis do not have jaundice, leading to difficulty in disease diagnosis and management. As the jaundice worsens, the child begins to feel better. This phase lasts approximately 4 weeks. Complete recovery with return of normal liver function and laboratory values may take 1 to 3 months.

In some cases, hepatitis becomes chronic. Chronic hepatitis is described as inflammation and necrosis of the liver that lasts for 6 months or longer. A person with chronic hepatitis carries the virus, can transfer it to others, and may develop permanent liver disease (Holloway & D'Acunto, 2006).

Clinical Therapy

Diagnosis is often made on the basis of a thorough history and physical examination. A history of exposure to persons with the disease is significant. Physical examination reveals a tender, enlarged liver, abdominal pain, and flulike symptoms. Laboratory evaluation includes serologic testing (to detect the presence of antigens and antibodies to HAV, HBV, HCV, or HDV) and liver function studies (Holloway & D'Acunto, 2006).

The three goals of medical management are early detection to prevent complications, support and monitoring during the acute phase of the disease, and prevention of the spread of the disease. Early diagnosis is essential to follow the course of the illness and identify potential complications. Management includes bed rest, hydration, and adequate nutrition during the flulike phase. If prothrombin times are increased, vitamin K is administered.

The spread of viral infections can be interrupted by elimination of the virus from the infected population, institution of proper hygiene, and passive or active immunization. To date, no antiviral agent has been developed to combat the hepatitis viruses. Prevention depends on breaking the cycle of infection.

Active immunization for hepatitis A, a two-dose series, is recommended for all people at increased risk of acquiring infection, for children and for those who wish to acquire immunity to

PATHOPHYSIOLOGY ILLUSTRATED

VIRAL HEPATITIS

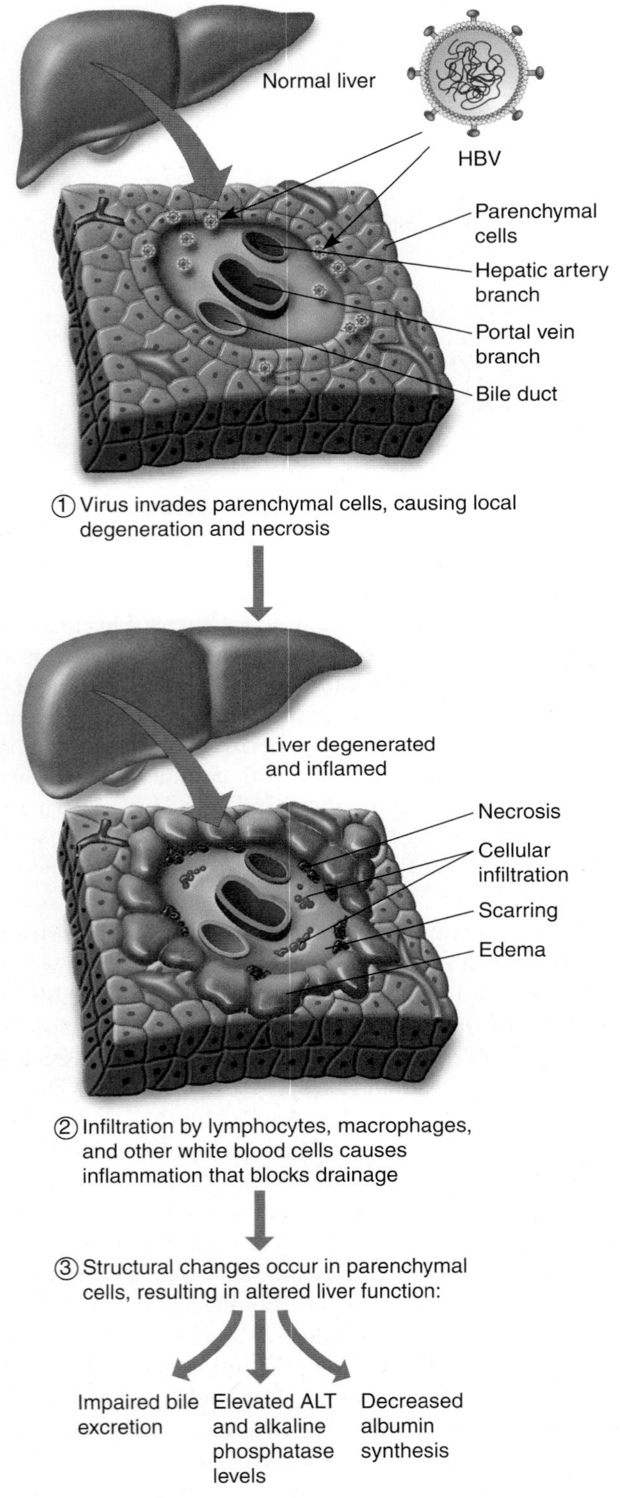
Normal liver
HBV
Parenchymal cells
Hepatic artery branch
Portal vein branch
Bile duct
① Virus invades parenchymal cells, causing local degeneration and necrosis
Liver degenerated and inflamed
Necrosis
Cellular infiltration
Scarring
Edema
② Infiltration by lymphocytes, macrophages, and other white blood cells causes inflammation that blocks drainage
③ Structural changes occur in parenchymal cells, resulting in altered liver function:
Impaired bile excretion
Elevated ALT and alkaline phosphatase levels
Decreased albumin synthesis

The hepatitis virus causes degeneration and necrosis of the liver, which results in abnormal liver function and illness.

the illness). The CDC recommends that all children receive the first hepatitis A vaccine at 1 year of age (Fiore, Wasley, & Bell, 2006). (Chapter 45 provides specific information on immunization schedules).

Passive immunity to HAV can be achieved with immune globulin from pooled human plasma. It must be administered within 2 weeks of exposure (Fiore et al., 2006). Passive immunity to HBV can be achieved with hepatitis B immune globulin (HBIG). Used for one-time exposure and for infants of infected mothers, it is given within 12 hours after birth (CDC, 2008b).

NURSING MANAGEMENT

NURSING ASSESSMENT AND DIAGNOSIS

The nurse usually encounters the child and family in an outpatient setting. In addition to observing the child for characteristic signs of hepatitis (jaundiced skin and sclera), assess for abdominal pain, anorexia, nausea and vomiting, malaise, and arthralgia. A history of the child's contacts over the past 45 days for HAV and up to 180 days for HBV is also obtained. For an infant, the hepatitis history of the mother and other family members is important.

Common nursing diagnoses for the child with acute hepatitis might include the following:

- *Risk for Imbalanced Nutrition: Less than Body Requirements* related to chronic illness
- *Fatigue* related to disease state
- *Risk for Body Image Disturbance (Older Child)* related to jaundice
- *Anxiety (Parent and Child)* related to threat to health status

PLANNING AND IMPLEMENTATION

Nursing care involves home and community considerations, as children with hepatitis are seldom admitted to the hospital. The hospitalized child is placed in isolation. Prevention of the diseases is integrated into all healthcare by discussion of immunization and universal precautions. Parents need additional detailed information about health precautions and infection control measures if hepatitis cases have occurred in the family or community. In addition, teach parents the importance of checking with health professionals before administering any medications (even nonprescription medicines), maintaining adequate nutrition, promoting rest and comfort, and providing diversional activities.

PREVENT SPREAD OF INFECTION

Teach the parents and the child infection control measures to help prevent transmission of the virus. For parents, reinforce good hygiene practices, such as washing hands before and after toileting and proper disposal of soiled diapers. Siblings of a child with hepatitis B who have not already been immunized with the hepatitis B vaccine should be vaccinated immediately. Contacts

Nursing Practice

Nurses in childcare centers can provide assessment of the center's procedures and teaching to prevent hepatitis A transmission. Help the center to set standards about:

- Hand washing after each diaper change
- Proper disposal of diapers
- Cleaning diaper-changing surfaces after each diaper change
- Enforce that food handlers never perform diaper changes
- Instructing parents to keep children at home for at least 2 weeks after a diagnosis of hepatitis A
- Informing parents of other children when there is a case of hepatitis A and teaching them the symptoms of the condition

of the child with hepatitis A should receive immune serum globulin and the first immunization in the hepatitis A series. Rifampin may be given in some cases. All health providers should receive the hepatitis B immunization series and use standard precautions at all times SKILLS.

MAINTAIN ADEQUATE NUTRITION

Initially the child is encouraged to eat favorite foods. Once the anorexia and nausea have resolved, a high-protein, high-carbohydrate, low-fat diet is recommended. Increased protein helps maintain protein stores and prevent muscle wasting. Increased carbohydrates ensure adequate caloric intake and prevent protein depletion. The use of low-fat foods lessen stomach distention. Offer the child small, frequent feedings.

PROMOTE REST AND COMFORT

Bed rest is necessary only if the child has severe fatigue and malaise. However, most children voluntarily limit their activities during the initial phase of the disease. Keep the child quiet and comfortable. Offer comfort items such as favorite toys, blankets, and pillows.

MEDICATION ADMINISTRATION

Drug metabolism is altered during hepatitis since the liver cannot detoxify medications readily. As with all liver disorders, medications need to be administered carefully and the child's condition must be monitored for possible drug side effects. Caution parents to check with health professionals before giving any nonprescription medication. For example, acetaminophen is metabolized in the liver, and liver disease can interfere with its breakdown.

PROVIDE DIVERSIONAL ACTIVITIES

Hospitalized children with hepatitis are kept in isolation. Nonhospitalized children with hepatitis do not need to be isolated, but they should be kept at home for 2 weeks following the onset of symptoms. Parents who cannot take time off from work may need to arrange home sitters to stay with the child. Offer suggestions for diversional activities during this period. Young children can be given a new toy or favorite activities. Older children and adolescents can be given board games, puzzles, books or magazines, movies, or video games. Phone calls and short visits from friends help school-age children and adolescents maintain contact with peers.

EVALUATION

Expected outcomes of nursing care for hepatitis include the following:

- Adequate nutritional intake to meet growth and development needs
- Participation in quiet, non-fatiguing activities and self-care
- Positive body image
- Parental coping with stress of the child's condition
- Reduced risk of spread of hepatitis to child's contacts.

CIRRHOSIS

Cirrhosis is a degenerative disease process that results in fibrotic changes and fatty infiltration in the liver. It can occur in children of any age as the end stage of several disorders such as hepatitis and biliary atresia (Boamah & Balistreri, 2007; A-Kader & Balistreri, 2007). The diffuse destruction and regeneration of the hepatic parenchymal cells result in an increase in fibrous connective tissue and disorganization of the liver structure. Progressive scarring that occurs in cirrhosis leads to altered blood flow to the liver, which causes further deterioration of liver function (Boamah & Balistreri, 2007).

Clinical manifestations of cirrhosis vary. Hepatomegaly may be evident on exam. Jaundice occurs as the disease progresses and is an indication of hyperbilirubinemia. Jaundice is sometimes the only sign of hepatic dysfunction so its appearance must be investigated. Pruritus is common in children with cirrhosis although it is not related to the degree of hyperbilirubinemia. Other clinical manifestations of cirrhosis in children include ascities, portal hypertension, encephalopathy and variceal hemorrhage (Boamah & Balistreri, 2007). Severe end-stage complications signaling hepatic failure can occur at any time and with little warning.

Diagnostic evaluation is based on the child's history of infection or disease with liver involvement. Physical examination may reveal jaundice, skin changes, ascites, and hemodynamic changes. Laboratory evaluation reveals abnormal liver function tests. A liver biopsy may help determine the extent of the parenchymal damage.

Medical management focuses on treating the child's symptoms and achieving optimal nutritional status and growth. See "Clinical Manifestations: Cirrhosis Complications" for a summary of treatment. Liver transplantation is the most common treatment for biliary atresia and metabolic disorders and is the only treatment for end-stage liver disease.

Nursing Management

Nursing care focuses on monitoring physiologic and psychosocial changes to identify early signs of end-stage hepatic failure. Monitor vital signs every 2 to 4 hours. Measure weight daily to assess for

Clinical Manifestations

CIRRHOSIS COMPLICATIONS

ETIOLOGY	CLINICAL MANIFESTATIONS	CLINICAL THERAPY
Fluid and electrolyte imbalance	Ascites with enlarged abdomen and potential for breathing difficulty	Restrict sodium, protein, and fluids. Administer diuretics (e.g., furosemide [Lasix]). Administer intravenous albumin.
Liver dysfunction	Hepatic encephalopathy with altered mental status potentially progressing to coma	Restrict protein. Administer lactulose to control increased ammonia levels. Administer antibiotics. Correct any imbalances that can lead to coma (fluid and electrolyte imbalance).
Esophageal varices	Hemorrhage Bloody emesis Bloody stools	Administer blood and blood products. Replace fluid and electrolytes. Administer vitamin B complex and vitamin K. Insert Sengstaken-Blakemore tube in cases of severe bleeding.

fluid retention. Close monitoring of electrolytes and liver function test results helps determine the need for fluid replacement therapy.

Careful administration of medications and monitoring for side effects are necessary because drug metabolism is altered in liver disorders. If ascites is present, provide a low-sodium, low-protein diet and restrict fluids. Remove all water pitchers, glasses, and straws to minimize the child's desire to drink.

Parents of a child with cirrhosis are coping with a life-threatening disorder, and their anxiety and stress are high. The child may be awaiting a liver transplantation that represents the only hope for recovery. Support parents and encourage them to talk about their fears and concerns (see Chapter 43). Encourage parents to participate in the child's care. Referral to a support group or counseling may be beneficial.

INJURIES TO THE GASTROINTESTINAL SYSTEM

ABDOMINAL TRAUMA

The majority of abdominal injuries are caused by blunt trauma (86%), with penetrating trauma accounting for the remainder (Pieper, 2007). Falls are the most common cause of abdominal injury in children; however, automobile accidents and pedestrian injuries are the major cause of severe blunt abdominal trauma in children (Potoka & Saladino, 2005). ATV (all-terrain vehicle) injuries are increasing in the United States as the popularity of these devices increases (Brandenberg, 2004; Aitken, Graham, Killingsworth, et al., 2004). The child may suffer severe abdominal trauma, including injury to the spleen and liver. Child abuse involving kicking or punching the abdomen is another major cause of blunt abdominal trauma. Penetrating trauma occurs due to impalement on an object, stabbing, or gunshot wounds (Potoka & Saladino, 2005). Children are more likely to have abdominal injuries because of their small pliable rib cage and less developed abdominal muscles that provide little protection for major solid organs such as the spleen, liver, and kidneys. In addition, the solid organs in children are larger in comparison than adults, exposing more surface area, making the organ more vulnerable to injury (Alterman, 2008; Saxena, 2008).

The kind of injury determines the extent of organ damage. High-velocity blunt trauma, which may occur in motor vehicle crashes, usually involves multiple organs. Solid organs such as the liver and spleen can be bruised or lacerated. The sudden increase in abdominal pressure that occurs with a lap belt injury causes hollow organs such as the stomach, intestines, and bladder to burst. Sports-related abdominal trauma is often associated with a direct blow to the abdomen, and a single organ is usually injured. Bicycle crashes can result in abdominal injury if the handlebars hit the child in the abdomen (Potoka & Saladino, 2005).

Clinical manifestations of abdominal injury include pain, abdominal distention, muscle guarding, decreased or absent bowel sounds, nausea and vomiting, hypotension, and shock. The external abdomen and back may have penetrating wounds, abrasions, bruising, or markings (e.g., tire tracks or lap belt marks) that provide a clue to injury beneath the skin surface. Ecchymosis and contusions in the lower abdominal area are classic visible signs of seatbelt trauma (Eckert, 2005). See Chapter 35 for techniques of abdominal assessment.

Suspected abdominal trauma in a child necessitates a thorough history and physical examination. The description of the event should be compared with the child's signs and symptoms. Plain abdominal radiographs may reveal air in the abdomen. An ultrasound can reveal free fluid in the abdomen. A CT scan as-

Nursing Practice

The child who is restrained in a motor vehicle with only a lap belt is at high risk for abdominal injury in a crash. As the car stops rapidly, the child's body is restrained and flexes around the lap belt. The sudden increase in abdominal pressure causes injury to hollow organs, and sometimes solid organs. Children no longer using car safety seats should sit in a booster seat so that a shoulder restraint is used in addition to the lap belt.

sesses multiple organs for injury and for the presence of free fluid in the abdomen. Serial hemoglobin and hematocrit evaluation is essential to determine hemodynamic stability. Type and cross match of blood is also necessary in case the child needs a blood transfusion. In addition, electrolytes and enzyme studies (amylase and lipase) to detect liver, spleen, and pancreas injuries are obtained (Pieper, 2007; Potoka & Saladino, 2005; Saxena, 2008).

The spleen and the liver are the organs most commonly injured in blunt abdominal trauma. Nonsurgical management is preferred. The spleen plays a major role in immune function; therefore, the organ is salvaged whenever possible to help maintain immune function. Liver lacerations are treated much like spleen lacerations as long as major vessels have not been injured. Nonsurgical management of injury to the spleen in children is successful in 90–98% of cases, while the success rate of nonsurgical management of injuries to the liver in children is 85–90% (Potoka & Saladino, 2005). Exploratory laparotomy is performed to resect hollow organ injuries or to repair liver or spleen lacerations when bleeding is not controlled.

Treatment of an abdominal, liver, or spleen injury takes place in the pediatric intensive care unit (PICU) and focuses on preventing or managing hemorrhage and monitoring for signs of shock. An intravenous infusion is initiated for fluid maintenance and to provide access for blood products. The child is kept NPO. A nasogastric tube is inserted. Blood transfusions and pharmacologic management are used to treat blood loss.

The child is maintained on strict bed rest until bleeding is controlled and the hemoglobin and hematocrit are stable. The length of time the child is hospitalized ranges from 2 to 5 days depending on the severity of the injury. The length of time for activity restrictions after discharge ranges from 3 to 6 weeks and also depends on the severity of the injury (Pieper, 2007).

Nursing Management

Nursing care includes initial and ongoing assessments of the child's condition. Initially, assess the abdomen for bruising, pain, guarding, rebound tenderness, distension, and absence of bowel sounds (Eckert, 2005). See Chapter 35 for techniques of abdominal assessment.

Nursing care includes initial and ongoing assessments of the child's condition. Monitor hematocrit and vital signs every hour as warranted to detect hypovolemia (see Chapter 26). Tachycardia and hypotension may indicate hypovolemia or internal bleeding. Strict monitoring of intake and output will give information to the child's fluid status. Monitor the respiratory status as abdominal injuries may also have thoracic involvement. The child with associated thoracic injuries may not take deep breaths if it is painful.

The child and parents are usually fearful and anxious when the child is admitted with a serious injury. If the injury was preventable, parents may have feelings of guilt or anger. Provide emotional support and avoid judgmental comments or statements that assign blame. Additional nursing care includes maintenance of the nasogastric tube, administration of antibiotics, intravenous fluids, and blood and monitoring of lab studies as appropriate. Any concerns should be reported to the physician immediately.

Once the child's condition is stabilized, the focus of nursing care shifts to preventive teaching. Parents should be taught safety measures to prevent future injuries. Discuss the use of car safety restraint devices for riding in an automobile (see Chapters 36, 37, and 38). If the child's injury was the result of a bicycle fall or crash, discuss the importance of the proper bicycle size and safety measures such as use of a helmet and proper use of hand signals. Refer to Chapter 44 for information related to injury to the GI system due to poisoning and ingestion of foreign objects.

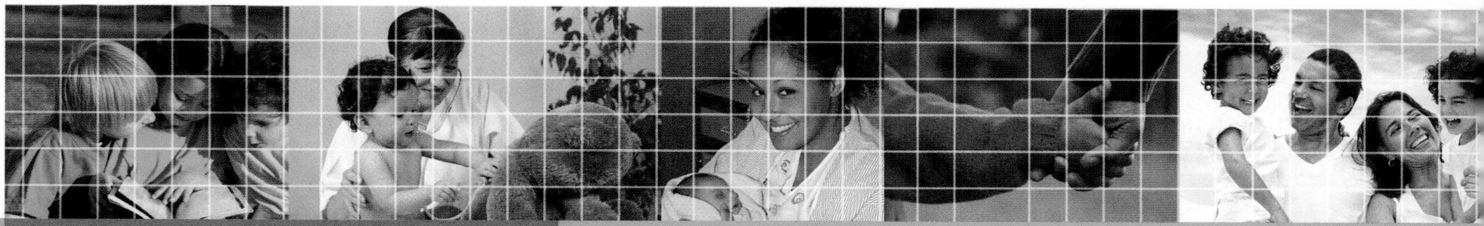

CRITICAL CONCEPT REVIEW

LEARNING OUTCOMES	CONCEPTS
53.1 Describe the general function of the gastrointestinal system.	1. Ingestion, digestion, and absorption of fluids and nutrients. 2. Metabolism of needed nutrients. 3. Excretion of waste products.

(continued)

LEARNING OUTCOMES	CONCEPTS
53.2 Discuss the pathophysiologic processes associated with specific gastrointestinal disorders in the pediatric population.	1. Structural defects: occur when growth and development of fetal structures are interrupted in the first trimester: ■ Cleft lip and palate. ■ Esophageal atresia and tracheoesophageal fistula. ■ Pyloric stenosis. 2. Gastroesophageal reflux: return of gastric contents into the esophagus caused by relaxation of the esophageal sphincter. 3. Abdominal wall defects: ■ Gastroschisis: vascular disruption of the fetal mesenteric vessels. ■ Omphalocele: intra-abdominal contents herniate through the umbilical cord. 4. Intussusception: occurs when one portion of the intestine prolapses and telescopes into another portion. 5. Volvulus: twisting of the intestine, secondary to malrotation of the bowel in utero. 6. Hirschsprung disease: congenital aganglionic megacolon. 7. Anorectal malformation: failure during fetal life for complete development of the anus and rectum. 8. Hernias: protrusion or projection of an organ through the muscle wall of the cavity that normally contains it, caused by failure to close during fetal development. ■ Diaphragmatic hernia. ■ Umbilical hernia. 9. Ostomies: May be indicated in infants and children with imperforate anus, necrotizing enterocolitis, Hirschsprung disease, volvulus, inflammatory bowel disease, intestinal tumors, or abdominal trauma. 10. Inflammatory disorders: ■ Appendicitis. ■ Necrotizing enterocolitis: caused by vascular compromise to the bowel of the newborn. ■ Meckel's diverticulum: failure of a fetal duct to atrophy. ■ Inflammatory bowel disease. ■ Peptic ulcer. 11. Motility Disorders: ■ Gastroenteritis. ■ Constipation. ■ Encopresis. 12. Intestinal Parasitic Disorders 13. Feeding Disorders: ■ Colic. ■ Rumination. 14. Disorders of Malabsorption: ■ Celiac disease. ■ Lactose intolerance. ■ Short bowel syndrome. 15. Hepatic Disorders: ■ Biliary atresia. ■ Viral Hepatitis. ■ Cirrhosis.
53.3 Identify signs and symptoms that may indicate a disorder of the gastrointestinal system.	1. Inability to gain weight or weight loss. 2. Vomiting, diarrhea, or constipation. 3. Lack of energy or lethargy. 4. Abdominal tenderness. 5. Abdominal distention.
53.4 Contrast nursing management and plan care for gastrointestinal disorders for the child needing abdominal surgery versus the child needing nonoperative management.	1. Assess abdominal girth. 2. Assess for presence of bowel sounds. 3. Begin oral feedings with frequent, small feedings of clear liquids, advance diet as tolerated. 4. Assess location and type of pain child is experiencing. 5. Determine if child is experiencing nausea or vomiting. 6. Determine stooling pattern. 7. Monitor intake and output. 8. Provide pre and postoperative care as indicated.

LEARNING OUTCOMES / CONCEPTS

53.5 Analyze developmentally appropriate approaches for nursing management of gastrointestinal disorders in the pediatric population.

1. Facilitate bottle or breastfeeding in the child with a structural defect.
2. Instruct parents in the use of thickened formula for treatment of GER and GERD.
3. Assist children with hepatitis to make appropriate food choices that are palatable and conform to the restricted diet.
4. Encourage children with ostomies to take responsibility for own care.

53.6 Discuss nursing management of the child with an injury to the abdomen.

1. Promote hemodynamic stabilization:
   - Fluid and blood replacement therapy.
   - Frequent vital sign measurement.
   - Strict measurement of intake and output.
2. Provide pre- and postoperative care.
3. Support the child and family.

CRITICAL THINKING IN ACTION

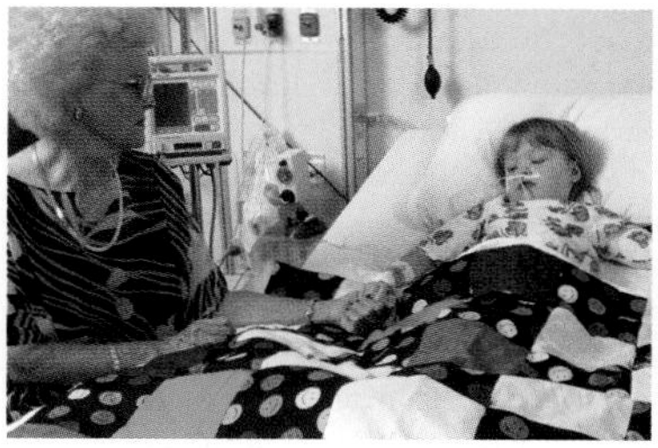

Three-year-old Jenna has just been admitted to the pediatric unit following surgery for a ruptured appendix. She complained of her stomach hurting last night, but this morning her condition was worse and she had a temperature of 102°F. Worried that this was not just a virus, Jenna's mother took her to the pediatrician. On the way to the doctor's office Jenna told her mother that her pain "just went away." While at the pediatrician's office she complained of feeling bad all over. On examination her abdomen was rigid and no bowel sounds were heard. A complete blood count revealed a white blood count (WBC) of 22,000 mm^3. The pediatrician diagnosed that Jenna had appendicitis and most likely had a ruptured appendix. He referred Jenna to the emergency department for assessment and surgical consultation. A CT scan confirmed a diagnosis of appendicitis. During surgery the appendix was found to have ruptured.

Jenna had an appendectomy and her wound was left open and packed with saline-soaked gauze. The gauze was covered with a dry dressing. Montgomery straps have been placed on Jenna's abdomen to decrease the skin irritation related to dressing changes that must be performed three times a day. Jenna has an intravenous line for fluids, pain medication, and antibiotics. She also has a nasogastric tube to suction and a Foley catheter.

Jenna's parents are anxious about the surgery and the open wound. They feel guilty that Jenna became ill so quickly and wonder if they could have done something to prevent it. This is Jenna's first hospitalization. They are worried that she will have a lot of pain and wonder how she will cope with the hospitalization.

1. What is the priority of nursing care for Jenna in the immediate postoperative period?
2. What should the nurse include when teaching Jenna's parents about the postoperative course?
3. Jenna's parents ask why she needs all of the tubes. What information should the nurse include related to the purpose of the nasogastric tube, the Foley catheter, and the central line?
4. What nursing interventions are most appropriate with a 3-year-old to decrease the risk of pulmonary complications associated with surgery?

See MyNursingKit for possible responses.

REFERENCES

Aiken, J. J., & Oldham, K. T. (2005). Malrotation. In K. W. Ashcraft, G. W. Holcomb, & J. P. Murphy (Eds.), *Pediatric surgery* (4th ed., pp. 435–447). Philadephia: Saunders.

Aitken, M. E., Graham, C. J., Killingsworth, J. B., Mullins, S. H., Parnell, D. N., & Dick, R. M. (2004). All-terrain vehicle injury in children: strategies for prevention. *British Medical Journal 10*(5), 303–307.

A-Kader, H. A., & W. F. Balistreri (2007). Cholestasis. In R. M. Kliegman, R. E. Behrman, H. B. Jenson, & B. F. Stanton (Eds.), *Nelson textbook of pediatrics* (18th ed., pp. 1168–1675). Philadelphia: Saunders.

Allen, P. L. J. (2004). Guidelines for the diagnosis and treatment of celiac disease in children. *Pediatric Nursing, 30*(6), 473–476.

Alterman, D. M. (2008). Considerations in pediatric trauma. Retrieved May 5, 2009 from http://emedicine.medscape.com/article/435031-overview

Arguin, A. L., & Swartz, M. K. (2004). Gastroesophageal reflux in infants: A primary care perspective. *Pediatric Nursing, 30*, 45–52.

Aschenbrenner, D. S. (2006). Treatment of pediatric Crohn's disease: A biologic therapy now is approved for use in children. *American Journal of Nursing, 106*(9), 30.

Bagolan, P., Casaccia, G., Crescenzi, F., Nahom, A., Trucchi, A., & Giorlandino, C. (2004). Impact of a current treatment protocol on outcome of high-risk congenital diaphragmatic hernia. *Journal of Pediatric Surgery, 39*, 313–318.

Baron, M., & Blaber, M. E. (2005). Short-bowel syndrome in children. *American Journal of Nursing, 105*(9), 72C–72H.

Bell, E. F. (2005). Preventing necrotizing enterocolitis: What works and how safe? *Pediatrics, 115*, 173–175.

Bezerra, J. A. (2005). Potential etiologies of biliary atresia. *Pediatric Transplantation, 9*, 646–651.

Biggs, W. S., & Dery, W. H, (2006). Evaluation and treatment of constipation in infants and children. *American Family Physician, 73*(3), 469–477.

Bindler, R. M., & Howry, L. B. (2005). *Pediatric drug guide*. Upper Saddle River, NJ: Prentice Hall Health.

Black, T. L. (2005). Congenital megacolon. In M. R. Dambro & J. A. Griffith (Eds.), *Griffith's*

5-minute clinical consult (13th ed., p. 260). Philadelphia: Lippincott Williams & Wilkins.

Boamah, L., & Balistreri, W. F. (2007). Manifestations of liver disease. In R. M. Kliegman, R. E. Behrman, H. B. Jenson, & B. F. Stanton (Eds.), *Nelson textbook of pediatrics* (18th ed., pp. 1661–1668). Philadelphia: Saunders.

Borkowski, S. (2005). Borkowski, S. (2005, May). Irritation, redness, and drainage at the site of a pediatric gastrostomy. *The Clinical Advisor, 8*(5) 90–91.

Brandenberg, M. A. (2004). All-terrain vehicle injuries: A growing epidemic. *Annals of Emergency Medicine, 43*(4), 536–537.

Bullard, J., & Page, N. E. (2005). Cyclic vomiting syndrome: A disease in disguise. *Journal of Pediatric Nursing, 31*, 27–29.

Bundy, D. G., Byerley, J. S., Liles, E. A., Perrin, E. M., Katznelson, J., & Rice, H. E. (2007). Does this child have appendicitis? *Journal of American Medical Association, 298*(4), 438–451.

Centers for Disease Control and Prevention. (2008a). What every pet owner should know about roundworms & hookworms. Retrieved January 10, 2009 from www.cdc.gov/healthypets/Merial_CDCBroch_rsgWEB.pdf

Centers for Disease Control and Prevention. (2008b) Viral Hepatitis. Retrieved January 10, 2009, from www.cdc.gov/hepatitis/

Cilley, R. E., & Shereef, S. (2004). Umbilical hernia repair. *Operative Techniques in General Surgery, 6*(4), 244–252.

Coha, T. (2007). Congenital lung malformations. In N. T. Browne, L. M. Flanigan, C. A. McComiskey, & P. Pieper (Eds.), *Nursing care of the pediatric surgical patient* (2nd ed., pp. 237–246). Boston: Jones & Bartlett.

Colvin, J., Bower, C., Dickinson, J., & Sokol, J. (2005). Outcomes of congenital diaphragmatic hernia: A population-based study in Western Australia. *Pediatrics, 166*(3), 356–363.

Croffie, J. M. (2006). Constipation in children. *Indian Journal of Pediatrics, 73*(8), 697–701.

Davies, M. C., Creighton, S. M., & Wilcox, D. T. (2004). Long-term outcomes of anorectal malformations. *Pediatric Surgery International, 20*, 567–572.

D'Alessandro, A. M., Knechtle, S. J., Chin, L. T., Fernandez, L. A., Yagci, G., Leverson, G., & Kalayoglu, M. (2007). Liver transplantation in pediatric patients: Twenty years of experience at the University of Wisconsin. *Pediatric Transplantation, 11*, 661–670.

Diana-Zerpa, J. A., & Shapiro-Stolar, T. J. (2007). Malrotation and Volvulus. In N. T. Browne, L. M. Flanigan, C. A. McComiskey, & P. Pieper (Eds.), *Nursing care of the pediatric surgical patient* (2nd ed., pp. 333–342). Boston: Jones & Bartlett.

Doughty, D. (2004). Structure and function of the gastrointestinal tract in infants and children. *Journal of Wound, Ostomy, and Continence Nursing, 31*, 207–212.

Downard, C. D. (2008). Congenital diaphragmatic hernia: An ongoing clinical challenge. *Current Opinion in Pediatrics, 20*(3), 300–304.

Eckert, K. (2005). Penetrating and blunt abdominal trauma. *Critical Care Nursing Quarterly, 28*, 41–59.

Ellett, M. L. C., & Swenson, M. (2005). Living with a colicky infant. *Gastroenterology Nursing, 28*(1), 19–25.

Ellett, M., Schuff, E., & Davis, J. B. (2005). Parental perceptions of the lasting effects of infant colic. *MCN: The American Journal of Maternal Child Nursing, 30*(2), 127–132.

Fagerman, L. E., & Farber, L. D. (2007). Intussusception. In N. T. Browne, L. M. Flanigan, C. A. McComiskey, & P. Pieper (Eds.), *Nursing care of the pediatric surgical patient* (2nd ed., pp. 343–348). Boston: Jones & Bartlett.

Farmer, D. G., Venick, R. S., McDiarmid, S. V., Ghobrial, R. M., Gordon, S. A., Yersiz, H., et al. (2007). Predictors of Outcomes after Pediatric Liver Transplantation: An Analysis of More Than 800 Cases Performed at a Single Institution. *Journal of the American College of Surgeons, 204*, 904–916.

Fiore, A. E., Wasley, A., & Bell, B. P. (2006). Prevention of hepatitis A through active or passive immunization. *Morbidity and Mortality Weekly Report, 55*(RR07), 1–23.

Flanigan, L. M. (2007). Biliary Atresia and Choledochal Cyst. In N. T. Browne, L. M. Flanigan, C. A. McComiskey, & P. Pieper (Eds.), *Nursing care of the pediatric surgical patient* (2nd ed., pp. 379–387). Boston: Jones & Bartlett.

Gelfond, D., & Fasano, A. (2006). Celiac disease in the pediatric population. *Pediatric Annals, 35*(4), 275–279.

Gold, B. D., & Gremse, D. A. (2006). Extinguishing the burn: Case studies in pediatric reflux disease, *Self Study Supplement to Clinician Reviews.*

Grossman, A. B., & Mamula, P. (2007). *Crohn disease.* Retrieved May 5, 2009 from http://emedicine.medscape.com/article/928288-overview

Guardino, K. O. (2007). Anorectal malformations in children. In N. T. Browne, L. M. Flanigan, C. A. McComiskey, & P. Pieper (Eds.), *Nursing care of the pediatric surgical patient* (2nd ed., pp. 301–314). Boston: Jones & Bartlett.

Hackman, D. J., Newman, K., & Ford, H. R. (2005). Pediatric surgery. In F. Brunicardi, D. K. Andersen, T. R. Billiar, D. L. Dunn, J. G. Hunter, J. B. Matthews, et al. (Eds.), *Schwartz's principles of surgery* (8th ed., pp. 1471–1517) New York: McGraw Hill.

Hedrick, H. L., Crombleholme, T. M., Flake, A. W., Nance, M. L., von Allmen, D., Howell, L. J., et al. (2004). Right congenital diaphragmatic hernia: Prenatal assessment and outcome. *Journal of Pediatric Surgery, 39*, 319–323.

Henry, S. M. (2004). Discerning differences: Gastroesophageal reflux and gastroesophageal reflux disease infants. *Advances in Neonatal Care, 4*, 235–247.

Hill, K. D., & Hill, I. D. (2005). Celiac disease: Fundamentals for pediatricians. *Contemporary Pediatrics, 22*(10), 65–77.

Holloway, M., & D'Acunto, K. (2006, June). An update on the ABC's of viral hepatitis. *The Clinical Advisor*, 26, 29–40.

Holmes, S. (2004). Enteral feeding and percutaneous endoscopic gastrostomy. *Nursing Standard, 18*(20), 41–43.

Hsu, V. P., Staat, M. A., Roberts, N., Thieman, C., Bernstein, D. L., Bresee, J., et al. (2005). Use of active surveillance to validate international classification of disease code estimates of rotavirus hospitalizations in children. *Pediatrics, 115*, 78–82.

Hyams, J. (2005). Inflammatory bowel disease. *Pediatrics in Review, 26*(9), 314–320.

Hyams, J. (2007). Inflammatory bowel disease. In R. M. Kliegman, R. E. Behrman, H. B. Jenson, & B. F. Stanton (Eds.), *Nelson textbook of pediatrics* (18th ed., pp. 1575–1585). Philadelphia: Saunders.

Hyman, P. E., Milla, P. J., Benninga, M. A., Davidson, G. P., Fleisher, D. F., & Taminiau, J. (2006). Childhood functional gastrointestinal disorders: Neonate/Toddler. *Gastroenterology*, 130(5), 1519–1526.

Irving, P. M., & Gibson, P. R. (2007). Infliximab: Getting the most for your money. *Journal of Gastroenterology and Hepatology, 22*, 1557–1565.

International Pediatric Endosurgery Group (2008). IPEG guidelines for the surgical treatment of pediatric gastroesophageal reflux disease (GERD). *Journal of Laparoendoscopic & Advanced Surgical Techniques, 18*(6), x–xiii.

Jackson, C. S., & Buchman, A. L. (2004). The nutritional management of short bowel syndrome. *Nutritional Clinical Care*, 7, 114–121.

Jaffe, B. M., & Berger, D. H. (2005). The appendix. In F. Brunicardi, D. K. Andersen, T. R. Billiar, D. L. Dunn, J. G. Hunter, J. B. Matthews, . . . S. I. Schwartz (Eds.), *Schwartz's principles of surgery*. (8th ed., pp. 1119–1137). New York: McGraw Hill.

Joshi, S., Mahajan, P., & Kamat (2006). Infantile hypertrophic pyloric stenosis. *Consultant for Pediatricians, 5*(2), 106–109.

Kasson, B. R. (2007). Necrotizing enterocolitis. In N. T. Browne, L. M. Flanigan, C. A. McComiskey, & P. Pieper (Eds.), *Nursing care of the pediatric surgical patient* (2nd ed., pp. 181–193). Boston: Jones & Bartlett.

Kasten, E. F., Schmidt, S. P., Zickler, C. R., Berner, E., Damian, L. K., Christian, G. M., et al. (2008). Team care of the patient with cleft lip and palate. *Current Problems in Pediatric and Adolescent Health, 38*, 138–158.

Keefe, M. R., Barbosa, G. A., Froese-Fretz, A., Kotzer, A. M., & Lobo, M. (2005). An intervention program for families with irritable infants. *MCN: The American Journal of Maternal Child Nursing, 30*(4), 230–236.

Keefe, M. R., Lobo, M. L., Froese-Fretz, A., Kotzer, A. M., Barbosa, G. A., & Dudley, W. N. (2006). Effectiveness of an intervention for colic. *Clinical Pediatrics, 45*, 123–133.

Kessman, J. (2006). Hirschsprung Disease: Diagnosis and management. *American Family Physician, 74*(8), 1319–1322.

Kinservik, M. A., & Friedhoff, M. M. (2004). The efficacy and safety of Polyethylene Glycol 3350 in the treatment of constipation in children. *Pediatric Nursing, 30*(3), 232–237.

Klar, M. (2007). Hirschsprung disease. In N. T. Browne, L. M. Flanigan, C. A. McComiskey, & P. Pieper, *Nursing Care of the Pediatric Surgical Patient* (2nd ed., pp. 289–300). Boston: Jones & Bartlett.

Kliegman, R. M., & Willoughby, R. E. (2005). Prevention of necrotizing enterocolitis with probiotics. *Pediatrics, 115*, 171–172.

Kosloske, A. M., Love, C. L., Rohrer, J. E., Goldthorn, J. F., & Lacey, S. R. (2004). The diagnosis of appendicitis in children: Outcomes of a strategy based on pediatric surgical evaluation. *Pediatrics, 113*, 29–34.

Levitt, M. A., & Peña, Alberto (2005). Outcomes from the correction of anorectal malformations. *Current opinion in pediatrics, 17*, 394–401.

Liao, Z., Li, Z.-S., Zhang, W.-J., Zou, D.-W., Xue, X.-C., & Zhang, X.-K. (2007). *Journal of Gastroenterology and Hepatology, 22*, 1692.

Lobo, M. L., Kotzer, A. M., Keefe, M. R., Brady, E., Deloian, B., Froese-Fretz, A., & Barbosa, G. (2004). Current beliefs and management strategies for treating infant colic. *Journal of Pediatric Health Care, 18*(3), 115–122.

Lund, C. H., Bauer, K., & Berrios, M. (2007). Gastroschisis: Incidence, complications, and clinical management in the neonatal intensive care unit. *The Journal of Perinatal & Neonatal Nursing, 21*(1), 63–68.

Madsen, D., Sebolt, T, Cullen, L., Folkedahl, B., Mueller, T., Richardson, C., & Titler, M. (2005). Listening to bowel sounds: An evidence-based practice project: Nurses find that a traditional practice isn't the best indicator of returning gastrointestinal motility in patients who've undergone abdominal surgery. *American Journal of Nursing, 105*(12), 40–49.

Mattioli, G., Prato, A. P., Giunta, C., Avanzini, S., Rocca, M. D., Montobbio, G., et al. (2008).Outcome of primary endorectal pull-through for the treatment of classic Hirschsprung disease. *Journal of Laparoendoscopic & Advanced Surgical Techniques, 18*(6), 869–874.

McCollough, M., & Sharieff, G. Q. (2006). Abdominal pain in children. *Pediatric Clinics of North America, 53*, 107–137.

Merritt, L. (2005a). Part 1. Understanding the embryology and genetics of cleft lip and palate. *Advances in Neonatal Care, 5*(2), 64–71.

Merritt, L. (2005b). Part 2. Physical assessment of the infant with cleft lip and/or palate. *Advances in Neonatal Care, 5*(3), 125–134.

Murdock, A. M., & Johnston, S. D. (2005). Diagnostic criteria for coelic disease: Time for change? *European Journal of Gastroenterology and Hepatology, 17*, 41–43.

Murray, D. L. (2003). Infectious diseases. In C. D. Rudolph & A. M. Rudolph (Eds.), *Rudolph's pediatrics* (21st ed., pp. 1102, 1106). New York: McGraw Hill.

National Digestive Diseases Information Clearinghouse: NDDIC (2006). Lactose intolerance. NIH Publication No. 06–2751. Retrieved January 10, 2009 from http://digestive.niddk.nih.gov/ddiseases/pubs/lactoseintolerance/

Nehring, W. M. (2004). Down syndrome. In P. L. Allen & J. A. Vessey (Eds.), *Primary care of the child with a chronic condition* (pp. 445–468). St. Louis: Mosby.

Orenstein, S., Peters, J., Khan, S., Youssef, N., & Hussain, S. (2007). Congenital anomalies: Esophageal atresia and tracheoesophageal fistula. In R. M. Kliegman, R. E. Behrman, H. B. Jenson, & B. F. Stanton (Eds.), *Nelson textbook of pediatrics* (18th ed., pp. 1543–1544). Philadelphia: Saunders.

Otten, M. E., & Stoops, M. M. (2007). Splenectomy, cholecystectomy, and Meckel's diverticulum. In N. T. Browne, L. M. Flanigan, C. A. McComiskey, & P. Pieper, *Nursing Care of the Pediatric Surgical Patient* (2nd ed., pp. 357–375). Boston: Jones & Bartlett.

Pieper, P. (2007). Pediatric trauma. In N. T. Browne, L. M. Flanigan, C. A. McComiskey, & P. Pieper (Eds.), *Nursing care of the pediatric surgical patient* (2nd ed., pp. 445–464). Boston: Jones & Bartlett.

Pietz, J., Achanti, B., Lilien, L., Stepka, E. C., & Mehta, S. K. (2006). Prevention of necrotizing enterocolitis in preterm infants: A 20-year experience. *Pediatrics, 119*(1), e164–e170.

Plante, M. L. (2004). Crohn's disease. *Advance for Nurse Practitioners*, (May), 28–35.

Potoka, D. A., & Saladino, R. A. (2005). Blunt abdominal trauma in the pediatric patient. *Clinical Pediatric Emergency Medicine, 6*, 23–31.

Reid, H., & Bahar, R. J. (2006). Treatment of encopresis and chronic constipation in young children: clinical results from interactive parent-child guidance. *Clinical Pediatrics, 45*(2), 157–164.

Roach, J. P., & Bruny, J. L. (2008). Advances in the treatment and understanding of biliary atresia. *Current Opinion in Pediatrics, 20*, 315–319.

Saxena, A. K. (2008). *Abdominal trauma*. Retrieved May 5, 2008 from http://emedicine.medscape.com/article/940726-overview

Shah, A., & Carroll, M. (2007). *Peptic ulcer disease*. Retrieved January 10, 2009 from http://emedicine.medscape.com/article/932308-overview

Silbermintz, A., & Markowitz, J. (2006). Inflammatory bowel disease. *Pediatric Annals, 35*(4), 269–274.

Stoll, B. J. (2007). The umbilicus. In R. M. Kliegman, R. E. Behrman, H. B. Jenson, & B. F. Stanton (Eds.), *Nelson textbook of pediatrics* (18th ed., pp. 775–777). Philadelphia: Saunders.

Suwandhi, E., Ton, M. N. & Schwarz, S. S. (2006). Gastroesophageal reflux in infancy and childhood. *Pediatric Annals, 35*(4), 259–266.

Tamburrini, S., Brunetti, A., Brown, M., Sirlin C., & Casola, G. (2007). Acute appendicitis: diagnostic value of nonenhanced CT with selective use of contrast in routine clinical settings. *European Radiology, 17*, 2055–2061.

Tanaka, M., & Kazuma, K. (2005). Ulcerative colitis: Factors affecting difficulties of life and psychological well-being of patients in remission. *Journal of Clinical Nursing, 14*, 65–73.

Thielman, N. M., & Guerrant, R. L. (2004). Acute infectious diarrhea. *New England Journal of Medicine, 350*, 38.

Tran, T. T., Nissen, N., Poordad, F. F., & Martin, P. (2004). Advances in liver transplantation: New strategies and current care expand access, enhance survival. *Postgraduate Medicine, 115*(5), 73–85.

Tudehope, D. I. (2004). The epidemiology and pathogenesis of neonatal necrotizing enterocolitus. *Journal of Paediatric Child Health, 41*, 167–168.

Utterson, E. C., Shepherd, R. W., Sokol, R. J., Bucuvalas, J., Magee, J. C., McDiarmid, S. V., & Anand, R. (2005). Biliary atresia: Clinical profiles, risk factors, and outcomes of 755 patients listed for liver transplantation. *The Journal of Pediatrics, 147*(2), 180–185.

Vaira, D., Gatta, L., Ricci, C., Tampieri, A., Cavina, M., & Bernabucci V. (2005). Symposium on peptic acid disease. Peptic ulcer and *Helicobacter pylori*: Update on testing and treatment. *Postgraduate Medicine, 117*(6), 17–22, 46.

Vajnar, J. (2007). A common cause of vomiting in infancy. *Journal of the American Academy of Physician Assistants, 20*(1), 58–59.

Van Orden, H. (2004). Constipation: An overview of treatment. *Journal of Pediatric Health Care, 18*(6), 320–322.

Vegunta, R. K., Ali, A., Wallace, L. J., Switzer, D. M., & Pearl, R. H. (2004). Laparoscopic appendectomy in children: Technically feasible and safe in all stages of acute appendicitis. *American Surgeon, 70*, 198–202.

Wasley, A., Grytdal, S., & Gallagher, K. (2008). Surveillance for acute viral hepatitis-United States, 2006. *Morbidity and Mortality Weekly Report, 57*(SS02), 1–24.

Weerasooriya, V. S., White, F. V., & Shepherd, R. W. (2004). Hepatic fibrosis and survival in biliary atresia. *The Journal of Pediatrics, 144*(1), 123–125.

Wyllie, R. (2007). Pyloric stenosis and congenital anomalies of the stomach. In R. M. Kliegman, R. E. Behrman, H. B. Jenson, & B. F. Stanton (Eds.), *Nelson textbook of pediatrics* (18th ed., pp. 1555–1558). Philadelphia: Saunders.

Yazdy, M. M., Honein, M. A., & Xing, J. (2007). Reduction in orofacial clefts following folic acid fortification of the U.S. grain supply. *Birth Defects Research (Part A), 79*(1), 16–23.

Yazigi, N., & Balistreri, W. F. (2007). Viral hepatitis. In R. M. Kliegman, R. E. Behrman, H. B. Jenson, & B. F. Stanton (Eds.), *Nelson textbook of pediatrics* (18th ed., pp. 1680–1690). Philadelphia: Saunders.

Zelnik, N., Pacht, A., Obeid, R., & Lerner, A. (2004). Range of neurological disorders in patients with celiac disease. *Pediatrics, 113*, 1672–1677.

Ziegler, M. M. (2004). The diagnosis of appendicitis: An evolving paradigm. *Pediatrics, 113*, 130–132.

Zimmerman, B. T. (2007). Abdominal wall defects. In N. T. Browne, L. M. Flanigan, C. A. McComiskey, & P. Pieper (Eds.), *Nursing care of the pediatric surgical patient* (2nd ed., pp. 261–271). Boston: Jones & Bartlett.

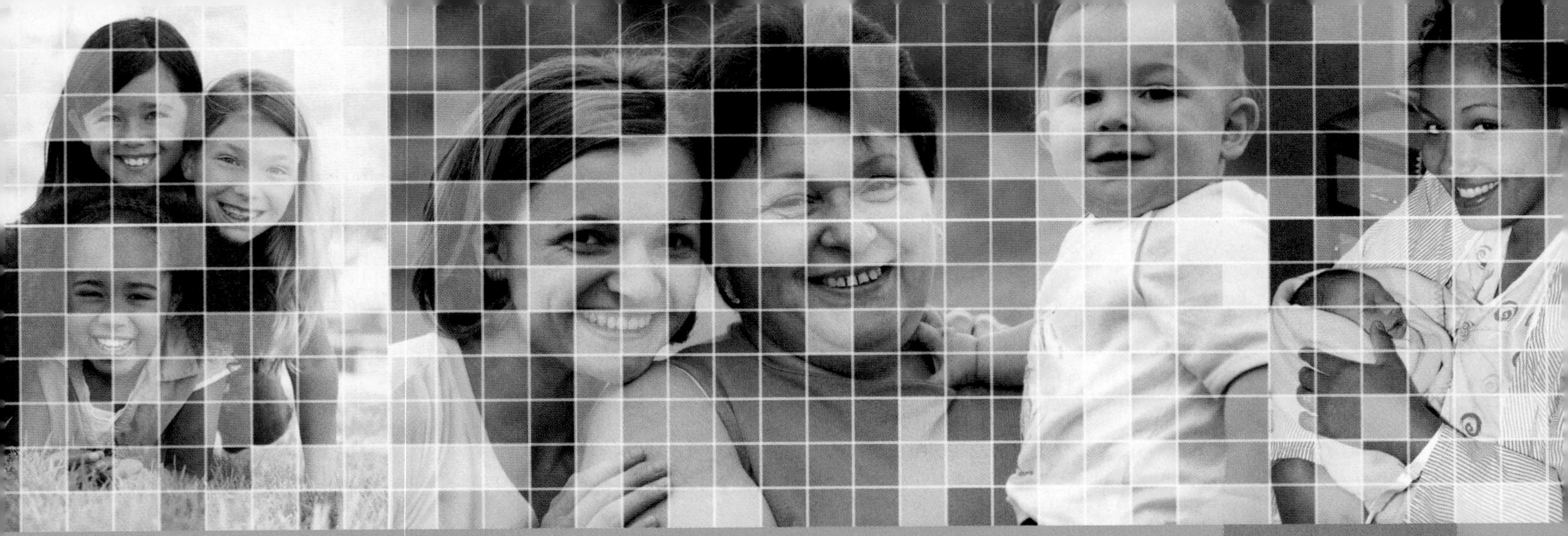

CHAPTER 54

The Child with Alterations in Genitourinary Function

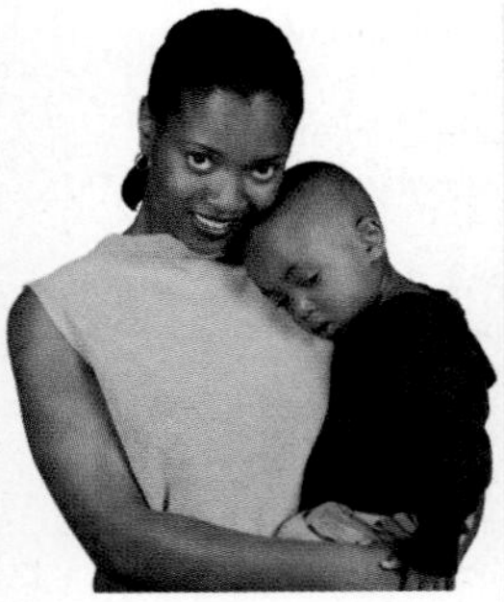

Planning Terrell's day can be a challenge, because his treatment often interferes with his activities. We all hope that Terrell receives a kidney transplant soon so his growth will improve and he will not have to miss school during treatment. —*Aunt of Terrell, 5 years old*

LEARNING OUTCOMES

54.1 Describe the pathophysiologic processes associated with genitourinary disorders in the pediatric population.

54.2 Discuss the nursing management of a child with a structural defect of the genitourinary system.

54.3 Develop a nursing care plan for the child with a urinary tract infection.

54.4 Discuss the growth and developmental issues for the child with chronic renal failure.

54.5 Summarize dietary restrictions for the child with a renal disorder.

54.6 Develop a nursing care plan for the child with acute and chronic renal failure on dialysis.

54.7 Describe psychosocial issues for the child requiring surgery on the genitourinary system.

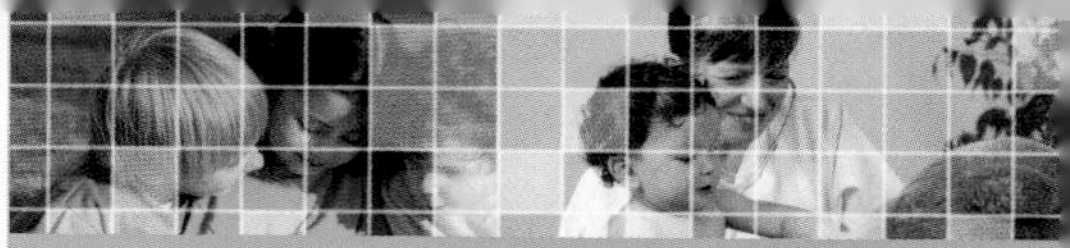

KEY TERMS

Anuria, 1586
Azotemia, 1586
Chvostek sign, 1588
Dialysate, 1594
Disequilibrium syndrome, 1597
Dysfunctional voiding, 1577
End-stage renal disease (ESRD), 1591
Enuresis, 1576
Hydronephrosis, 1571
Incarceration, 1600
Inguinal hernia, 1600
Nephrotic syndrome, 1577
Neurogenic bladder, 1573
Oliguria, 1586
Osteodystrophy, 1585
Phimosis, 1599
Pyeloplasty, 1572
Renal insufficiency, 1590
Stent, 1570
Uremia, 1586
Vesicoureteral reflux, 1573

Many infections, structural disorders, and disease processes alter genitourinary function. Because the kidneys and other urinary system organs perform several essential body functions, including removal of waste products and maintenance of fluid and electrolyte balance, disorders that affect these organs pose a significant threat to the health of children.

Although the reproductive system is functionally immature until puberty, uncorrected structural defects can have both psychologic and physiologic implications for the developing child.

ANATOMY AND PHYSIOLOGY OF PEDIATRIC DIFFERENCES

The genitourinary system is made up of the urinary and reproductive organs. The urinary system—kidneys, ureters, bladder, and urethra (Figure 54–1 ●)—excretes wastes and maintains acid–base and fluid and electrolyte balance. The reproductive system consists of internal and external organs that at maturity promote the conception and healthy development of a fetus.

URINARY SYSTEM

All of the nephrons that will make up the mature kidney are present at birth. The kidneys grow and the tubular system matures gradually during childhood, reaching full size by adolescence. Most renal growth occurs during the first 5 years of life. This increase in size is primarily a result of enlargement of the nephrons. The efficiency of the kidney also increases with age. During the first 2 years of life, the kidneys are less efficient at regulating electrolyte and acid–base balance (see Chapter 46)

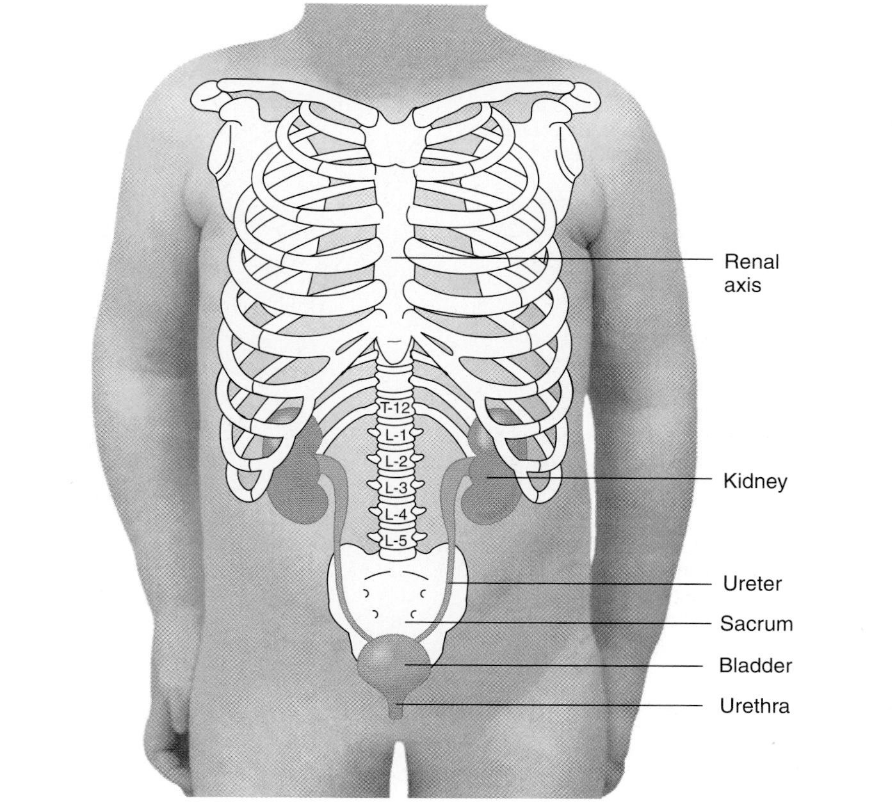

● **Figure 54–1** The urinary system: The urinary system is composed of the kidneys, ureters, bladder, and urethra. The kidneys are located between the twelfth thoracic (T12) and third lumbar (L3) vertebrae.

MyNursingKit Video: Sexually Transmitted Infections

and eliminating some drugs from the body. After the age of 2 years, the kidneys' efficiency increases markedly.

Bladder capacity increases with age from 20 to 50 mL at birth to 700 mL in adulthood. A child's bladder capacity (in ounces) can be estimated by adding 2 to the child's age (e.g., a 4-year-old has a bladder capacity of 6 ounces) (see As Children Grow). Stimulation of "stretch receptors" within the bladder wall initiates urination. Simultaneous contraction of the detrusor muscle of the bladder and relaxation of the internal and external sphincters result in emptying of the bladder. Children less than 2 years of age cannot maintain bladder control because of insufficient nerve development.

Normal renal function requires the following: unimpaired renal blood flow, adequate glomerular ultrafiltration, normal tubular function, and unobstructed urine flow.

MyNursingKit Animation: Renal Function

REPRODUCTIVE SYSTEM

The reproductive system in children is functionally immature until puberty. Throughout childhood the genitalia (with the exception of the clitoris in girls) enlarge gradually. The hormonal changes of puberty accelerate anatomic and functional development (see Chapter 35 for figures illustrating pubertal development). In girls, the mons pubis becomes more prominent and hair begins to grow. The vagina lengthens, and the epithelial layers thicken. The uterus and ovaries enlarge, and the musculature and vascularization of the uterus also increase. In boys, downy

Growth and Development

Urinary output per kilogram of body weight decreases as the child ages because the kidney becomes more efficient at concentrating urine. Expected output is as follows:

Infants	2 mL/kg/hr
Children	0.5 to 1 mL/kg/hr
Adolescents	40 to 80 mL/hr

AS CHILDREN GROW

DEVELOPMENT OF THE GENITOURINARY SYSTEM

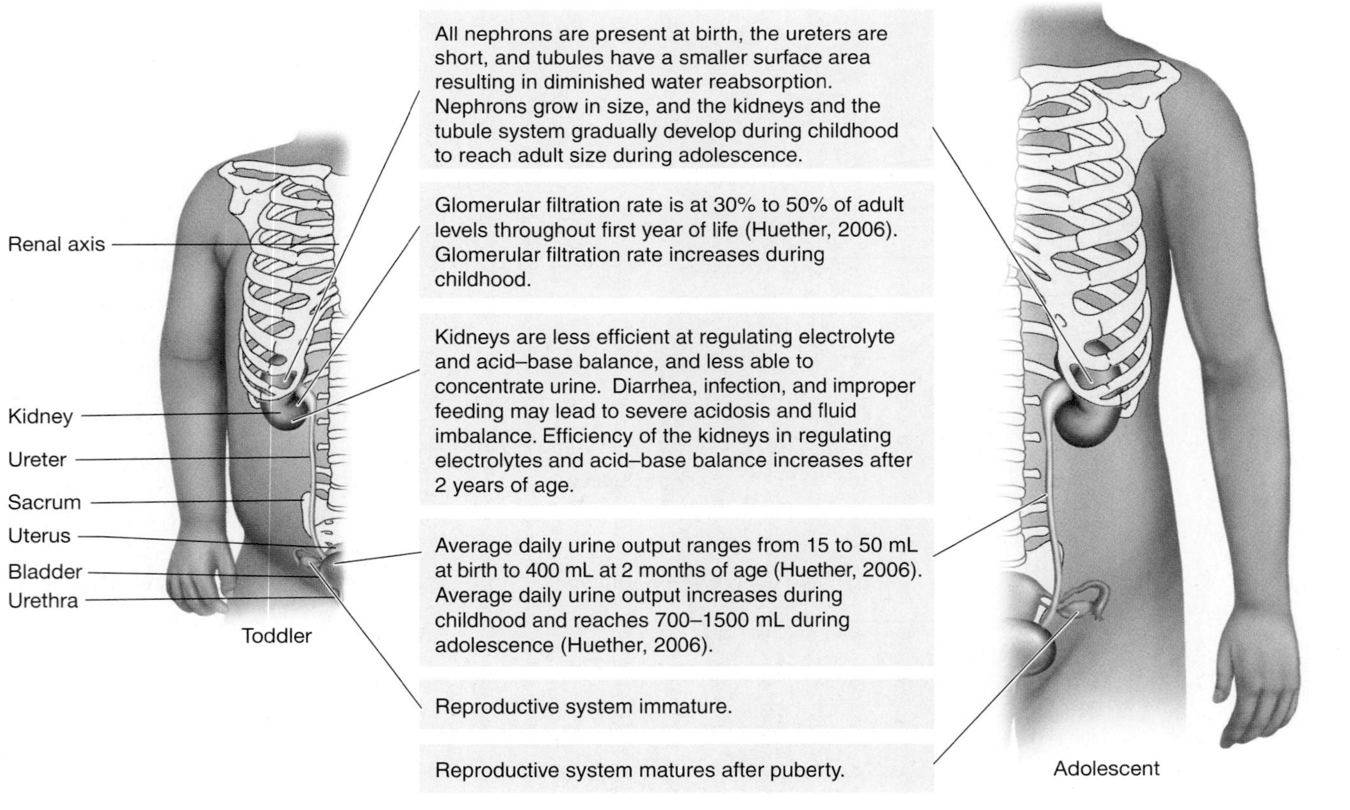

Renal axis
Kidney
Ureter
Sacrum
Uterus
Bladder
Urethra
Toddler
All nephrons are present at birth, the ureters are short, and tubules have a smaller surface area resulting in diminished water reabsorption. Nephrons grow in size, and the kidneys and the tubule system gradually develop during childhood to reach adult size during adolescence.
Glomerular filtration rate is at 30% to 50% of adult levels throughout first year of life (Huether, 2006). Glomerular filtration rate increases during childhood.
Kidneys are less efficient at regulating electrolyte and acid–base balance, and less able to concentrate urine. Diarrhea, infection, and improper feeding may lead to severe acidosis and fluid imbalance. Efficiency of the kidneys in regulating electrolytes and acid–base balance increases after 2 years of age.
Average daily urine output ranges from 15 to 50 mL at birth to 400 mL at 2 months of age (Huether, 2006). Average daily urine output increases during childhood and reaches 700–1500 mL during adolescence (Huether, 2006).
Reproductive system immature.
Reproductive system matures after puberty.
Adolescent

Data from: Huether, S. E. (2006). Alterations of renal and urinary tract function in children. In K. L. McCance, & S. E. Huether (Eds.), *Pathophysiology: The biologic basis for disease in children and adults* (5th ed., pp. 1337–1352), St. Louis: Elsevier Mosby.

hair begins to appear at the base of the penis, and the scrotum becomes increasingly pendulous as the testes enlarge. The penis increases in length and width.

STRUCTURAL DEFECTS OF THE URINARY SYSTEM

BLADDER EXSTROPHY

Bladder exstrophy is a rare congenital defect in which the posterior bladder wall extrudes through the lower abdominal wall (Figure 54–2 ●). Failure of the abdominal wall to close during fetal development results in eversion and protuberance of the bladder wall along with a wide separation of the rectus muscles and the symphysis pubis. The upper urinary tract is usually normal. The bladder mucosa appears as a mass of bright-red tissue, and urine continually leaks from the ureters onto the skin (Huether, 2006). Females have a bifid (split) clitoris. Males have a short, stubby penis, and the glans is flattened with dorsal chordee and a ventral prepuce. Epispadias and undescended testes (see pages 1570 and 1600) occur with this disorder in males. Inguinal hernias may develop in both males and females (Leung, Robson, & Wong, 2005).

The exposed bladder tissue is covered with plastic wrap until surgery is performed to keep the bladder mucosa moist (Elder, 2007). Primary closure of the bladder and abdominal wall is usually completed within 24 to 48 hours after birth. The wound and pelvis are immobilized to promote healing. An osteotomy (see Chapter 35∞) to rotate the innominate bones of the pelvis to approximate the symphysis pubis reduces tension on the closed bladder and abdominal wall to promote healing. Epispadias repair is often performed between 1 and 2 years of age or at the same times as a another surgical procedure to improve continence. Surgery to reconstruct the bladder neck and reimplant the ureters is performed when the bladder has achieved capacity of at least 80 ml (Elder, 2007). The goals of surgical reconstruction include:

- Closure of the bladder and abdominal wall
- Urinary continence, with preservation of renal function
- Creation of functional and normal-appearing genitalia, and
- Correction to promote later sexual functioning.

Some children require permanent urinary diversion because a functional bladder cannot be reconstructed.

Because the bladder epithelium is abnormal, it is prone to neoplasms. Periodic examination and cystoscopy after the age of 20 years is recommended to detect malignancies since symptoms are often ignored or ambiguous.

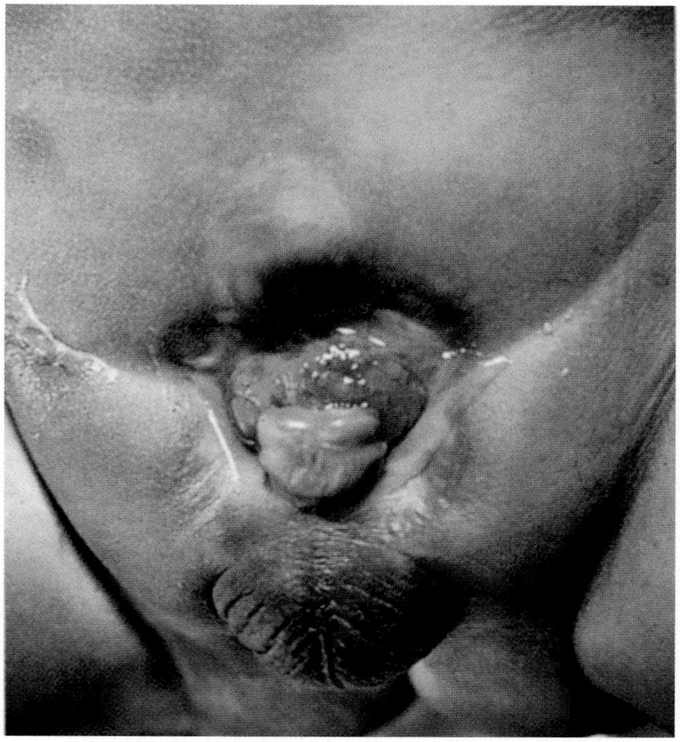

● **Figure 54–2** Bladder exstrophy. This child has bladder exstrophy, noted by extrusion of the posterior bladder wall through the lower abdominal wall.

Nursing Management

Preoperative nursing care centers on preventing infection and trauma to the exposed bladder. The bladder mucosa is protected with plastic wrap to prevent trauma and irritation and the surrounding area is cleaned daily and protected from leaking urine with a skin sealant. Saline soaked gauze may also be used to keep the area moist (Mercy & Brady-Fryer, 2004).

Postoperatively the wound and pelvis are immobilized to facilitate healing. Internal (with sutures) and external immobilization techniques are used for pelvic closure (see Chapter 58∞). Avoid abduction of the infant's legs. Nursing care includes maintaining proper alignment, monitoring peripheral circulation, and providing meticulous wound and skin care. Maintain aseptic technique for wound care and monitor for signs of infection including redness, drainage, and edema.

Monitor renal function by assessing the adequacy of urine output and blood and urine chemistries to detect signs of renal damage. Observe for any signs of obstruction in the drainage tubes such as increased intensity of bladder spasms, decreased urine output, or urine or blood draining from the urethral meatus. Promote comfort and give antibiotics as ordered.

Parents need emotional support to help them cope with the disfiguring nature of the infant's defect and the uncertainty of complete repair. To promote parent-infant bonding, encourage parents to participate in all aspects of the infant's care, including bathing, feeding, and wound care. Discharge teaching should include instructions about dressing changes and diapering and the need to immediately report any signs of infection or change in renal function. Emphasize the need for routine follow-up visits after surgery to assess urinary function and to ensure that the next stages of surgery for continence control are performed at the appropriate time in the child's development. The family should be aware that achievement of continence is more difficult in children with bladder exstrophy, and urinary diversion to achieve continence may be necessary if surgical procedures are not successful. Parents may require guidance to promote the child's self-esteem

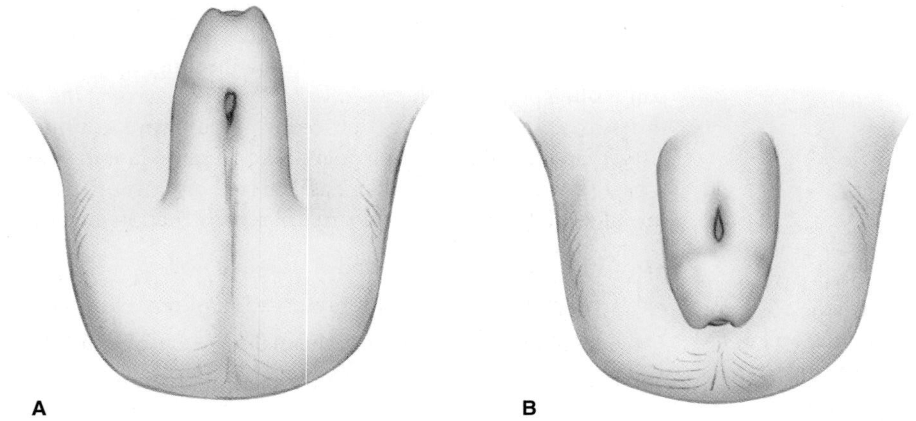

● **Figure 54–3** Hypospadias and epispadias. ***A,*** In hypospadias the urethral canal is open on the ventral surface of the penis. ***B,*** In epispadias the canal is open on the dorsal surface.

and self-confidence with sexual identity and function. Psychological counseling may be beneficial to the child during adolescence.

HYPOSPADIAS AND EPISPADIAS

Hypospadias and epispadias are congenital anomalies involving the abnormal location of the urethral meatus (Figure 54–3 ●). Both defects result when the urethral folds fail to fuse completely over the urethral groove. The reported incidence of hypospadias is 1 in 250 male births (Elder, 2007). The incidence of epispadias is 1 in 40,000 to 1 in 118,000 births. Epispadias occurs twice as often in males as females. Epispadias and exstrophy of the bladder are the same condition, but epispadias is the milder expression of the condition (Huether, 2006). See section on exstrophy of the bladder on page 1569.

In hypospadias, the urethral meatus can be located anywhere along the course of the urethra on the ventral surface of the penile shaft, from the perineum to the tip of the glans. Most cases are mild, with the meatus slightly off center from the tip of the penis; in severe cases, the meatus is located on the scrotum. Hypospadias often occurs in conjunction with congenital *chordee,* a fibrous line of tissue that results in ventral curvature of the penile shaft.

In males with epispadias, the meatal opening is located on the dorsal surface of the penile shaft. The opening may be small or a fissure may extend the entire length of the penis. Females with epispadias have a cleft of the ventral urethra that generally extends to the bladder neck (Huether, 2006). The remainder of this discussion will focus on hypospadias and males with distal epispadias as the treatment for severe epispadias in males and epispadias in females is similar to the 2nd and 3rd stages of repair of bladder exstrophy (Elder, 2007).

Diagnosis is made by prenatal ultrasound or by examination at birth. Other diagnostic studies may include urinalysis and urine culture. When the meatus is located on the perineum or scrotum, testing to rule out a chromosomal abnormality or problem in androgen metabolism is conducted (Stokowski, 2004).

The infant should not be circumcised because the foreskin tissue may be used for surgical repair (Pieretti, Pieretti, & Pieretti-Vanmarcke, 2009). The defects are corrected surgically, usually during the first year of life, to minimize psychologic effects when the child is older. Surgery is usually performed in a single operation, often as an outpatient procedure. The goals of surgical repair are (1) placement of the urethral meatus at the end of the glans penis with satisfactory caliber and configuration for a urinary stream (enabling the child to void in a standing position), (2) release of chordee to straighten the penis (enabling future sexual function), and (3) satisfactory cosmetic appearance of the penis.

A caudal nerve block is often used for postoperative pain relief. Anticholinergic medications may be prescribed to relieve bladder spasms. A urethral **stent** (a device used to maintain patency of the urethral canal) is placed to maintain patency of the new urethral canal opening.

Nursing Management

It is important to address parents' concerns at the time of birth. Preoperative teaching can relieve some of their anxiety about the future appearance and functioning of the penis.

Postoperative care focuses on protecting the surgical site from injury. The infant or child returns from surgery with the penis wrapped in a simple dressing, and a urethral stent is placed to keep the new urethral canal open. Plan care to ensure that the stent does not get removed. Refer to the hospital's policy for the appropriate use of immobilizers in this situation.

Encourage fluid intake to maintain adequate urinary output and patency of the stent. Hourly documentation of intake and output is essential to detect postoperative complications. Notify the physician if there is no urine drainage for 1 hour as this may indicate kinks in the system or obstruction. Pain may be associated with bladder spasms. Anticholinergic medications such as oxybutynin or hyoscyamine may be prescribed. Acetaminophen may also be given for pain. Antibiotics are often prescribed until the stent is out.

The child is often discharged the day of surgery. Discharge teaching should include instructions for parents about care of the reconstructed area, double-diapering to protect the stent, fluid intake, medication administration, and signs and symptoms of infection (see "Teaching Highlights: Caring for the Child after Hypospadias and Epispadias Repair" and Skill 16–2 in the Clinical Skills Manual **SKILLS**). Tell parents when the child needs to see the physician for dressing removal.

Teaching Highlights

CARING FOR THE CHILD AFTER HYPOSPADIAS AND EPISPADIAS REPAIR

- Use double-diapering to protect the stent (the small tube that drains the urine). See Skill 16–2 **SKILLS**.
- Restrict the infant or toddler from activities (e.g., playing on riding toys) that put pressure on the surgical site. Avoid holding the infant or child straddled on the hip. Limit the child's activity for 2 weeks.
- Encourage the infant or toddler to drink fluids to ensure adequate hydration. Provide fluids in a pleasant environment or using a special cup. Offer fruit juice, fruit-flavored ice pops, fruit-flavored juices, flavored ice cubes, and gelatin.
- Be sure to give the complete course of prescribed antibiotics to avoid infection.
- Watch for signs of infection: fever, swelling, redness, pain, strong-smelling urine, or change in flow of the urinary stream.
- The urine will be blood tinged for several days. Call the physician if urine is seen leaking from any area other than the penis.

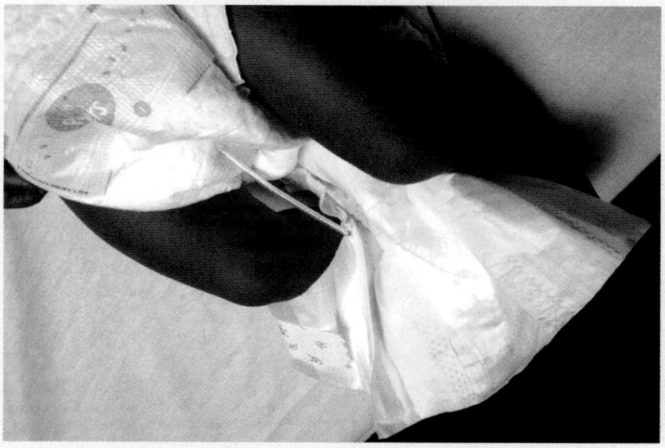

A double-diapering technique protects the urinary stent after surgery for hypospadias or epispadias repair. The inner diaper collects stool; the outer diaper, urine.

OBSTRUCTIVE UROPATHY

Obstructive uropathy refers to structural or functional abnormalities of the urinary system that interfere with urine flow. The pressure caused by urine backup compromises kidney function and often causes **hydronephrosis** (accumulation of urine in the renal pelvis as a result of obstructed outflow). Physiologic changes that may occur as a result of hydronephrosis include the following:

- Cessation of glomerular filtration when the pressure in the kidney pelvis equals the filtration pressure in the glomerular capillaries. To compensate, the blood pressure increases to increase the glomerular filtration pressure; however, increasing pressure on the glomeruli leads to cell death.
- Metabolic acidosis results when the distal nephrons' ability to secrete hydrogen ions is impaired.
- Impairment of the kidney's ability to concentrate urine results in polydipsia and polyuria.
- Obstruction results in urinary stasis, promoting bacterial growth.
- Restriction of urinary outflow causes progressive renal damage and chronic renal failure if untreated.

Obstructive uropathy may be caused by several congenital lesions such as ureteropelvic junction (UPJ) obstruction, posterior urethral valves (PUVs), and stenosis or hypoplasia of the ureterovesicular junction (see "Pathophysiology Illustrated: Obstruction Sites in the Urinary System"). The UPJ is the most common site of obstruction of the upper urinary tract in infants and children. UPJ obstruction occurs in 1 out of every 2000 live births, making it the most common cause of hydronephrosis in newborns (Small & Copel, 2004). PUVs (abnormal folds of mucosa in the male urethra) are the most common cause of anatomic bladder outlet obstruction, occurring in approximately 1 in 5000 to 8000 live male births (Small & Copel, 2004).

Clinical manifestations vary, depending on the cause and location of the obstruction (see "Clinical Manifestations: Obstructive Lesions of the Urinary System").

Clinical Manifestations

OBSTRUCTIVE LESIONS OF THE URINARY SYSTEM

OBSTRUCTIVE LESION	CLINICAL MANIFESTATIONS
Ureteropelvic junction obstruction	In infants: abdominal mass (enlarged kidney), hypertension, urinary tract infection In children: hematuria, pain, intermittent nausea and vomiting
Posterior urethral valves	In infants: abdominal mass (enlarged kidney), distended bladder, poor urinary stream, urinary tract infection, sepsis, low specific gravity, polyuria, increased creatinine level, failure to thrive In children: urinary frequency and incontinence
Ureterovesicular junction obstruction	Urinary tract infection (recurrent or chronic), hematuria, pain, abdominal mass (enlarged kidney), enuresis

PATHOPHYSIOLOGY ILLUSTRATED

OBSTRUCTION SITES IN THE URINARY SYSTEM

Obstruction may occur in either the upper or lower urinary tract. Common sites of obstruction occur at the ureteropelvic valve, the ureterovesicular junction or the posterior urethral valve. Renal failure is most likely to occur when both kidneys are affected by hydronephrosis.

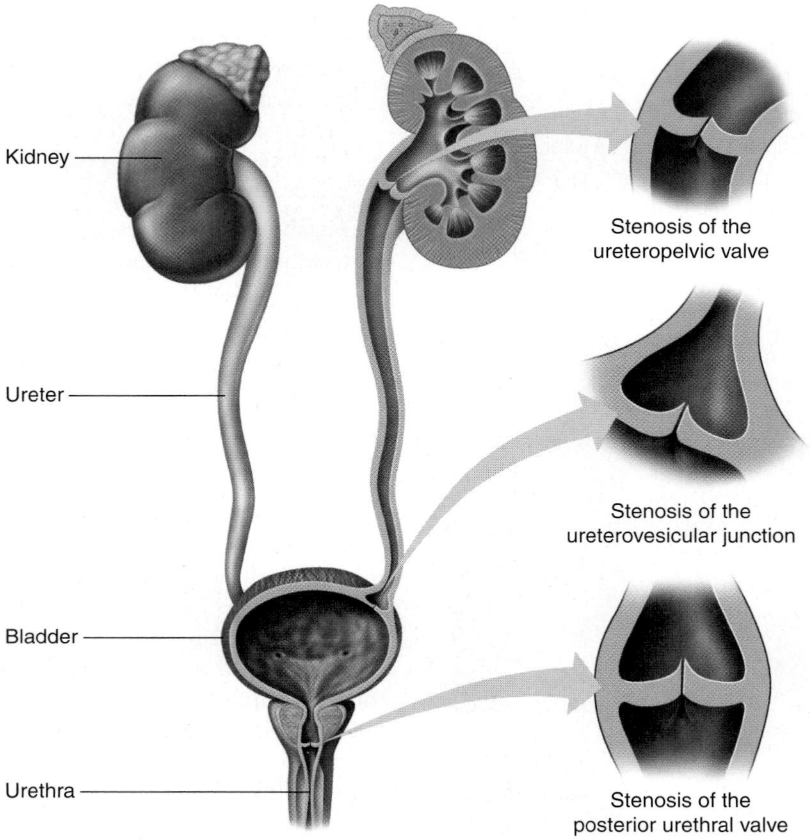

Early diagnosis and treatment prevents kidney damage and deterioration of renal function. Prenatal ultrasound may detect hydronephrosis and PUV. A diuretic enhanced radionuclide scan and voiding cystourethrogram are performed when UPJ or ureterovesicular obstruction is suspected.

The goals of surgical correction or diversion are to lower the pressure within the collecting system, which reduces renal damage, and to prevent stasis, which decreases the risk of infection. Surgical correction may necessitate **pyeloplasty** (removal of an obstructed segment of the ureter and reimplantation into the renal pelvis), valve repair or reconstruction, depending on the cause of the obstruction. Urinary incontinence resulting from sphincter weakness is a common problem after surgery.

Nursing Management

Preoperative nursing care focuses on preparing the parents and child for the procedure and addressing parents' concerns about the postsurgical outcome. Provide parents with an opportunity to discuss concerns about how the disorder will affect the child's long-term renal functioning.

Postoperative care involves monitoring vital signs and intake and output and observing for signs of urine retention, such as decreased output and bladder distention. Many children are discharged with stents or catheters. Teach parents how to change dressings, double-diaper, care for catheters, assess pain and give analgesics, and recognize signs of possible obstruction or infection. Parents should encourage the child to participate in age-appropriate activities. However, children should avoid contact sports because of their potential to injure the bladder.

PRUNE BELLY SYNDROME

Prune belly syndrome, also known as Eagle-Barrett syndrome, is a congenital defect characterized by failure of the abdominal musculature to develop. The skin covering the abdominal wall is thin and resembles a wrinkled prune. Other characteristics include urinary tract anomalies, poor ureteral peristalsis, enlarged bladder, high risk for recurrent urinary tract infection, vesicoureteral reflux, and bilateral cryptorchidism. Prune belly syndrome occurs predominantly in males (95%), with an incidence of 1 in 40,000 live births (Elder, 2007).

The etiology of prune belly syndrome is unknown; however, it is thought to be related to a fetal urinary tract obstruction or a specific injury to the mesoderm between 6 and 10 weeks of gestation. In addition to urinary tract anomalies, cardiac, pulmonary, gastrointestinal, and orthopedic anomalies also occur (Prune Belly Syndrome Network, 2008).

Diagnosis is confirmed with abdominal ultrasound. An intravenous pyelogram is useful in assessing structural defects. Abdominal wall reconstruction and correction of genitourinary defects, including orchiopexy, are performed to repair defects. The mortality rate in infants has improved significantly in the past three decades with advances in surgical techniques. Mortality in the neonatal period is related to severe pulmonary hypoplasia. Approximately 30% of children with prune belly syndrome will develop end-stage renal disease in childhood or adolescence because of inadequate renal function (Elder, 2007).

Nursing Management

Nursing management for the infant with prune belly syndrome is the same as for other defects of the genitourinary system, including preoperative and postoperative management. Additional management includes psychosocial support for the child and family related to the numerous congenital anomalies, body image concerns, and long-term consequences of the defect.

A discussion of Wilms' tumor can be found in Chapter 52∞.

URINARY TRACT INFECTION

An infection of the urinary tract may be of bacterial, viral, or fungal origin, and can occur in the lower or upper urinary tract. Cystitis is a lower urinary tract infection (UTI) that involves the urethra or bladder. Pyelonephritis is an upper UTI that involves the ureters, renal pelvis, and renal parenchyma. UTIs can be acute or chronic (the latter either recurrent or persistent).

UTIs are the second most common infection in children (Dulczak & Kirk, 2005). An estimated 7% of females and 2% of males will have a urinary tract infection (UTI) by 6 years of age (Leroy, Adamsbaum, Marc, et al., 2005). See "Growth and Development: Urinary Tract Infections."

Growth and Development

Urinary tract infections are more common in males than females during the first 3 months of life. Uncircumcised infants in this age group are 5–10 times more likely to develop a UTI than circumcised infants (Raszka & Khan, 2005). After this age, UTI is much more common in females because the shorter female urethra (2 cm [1 in.] in young girls) has closer proximity to the anus and vagina, increasing the risk of contamination by fecal bacteria.

Etiology and Pathophysiology

Many first UTIs are caused by *Escherichia coli,* a common gram-negative enteric bacterium. Other causative organisms include *Staphylococcus, Klebsiella, Proteus, Pseudomonas aeruginosa, Enterobacter,* and *Enterococcus* (Dulczak & Kirk, 2005).

Urinary stasis enhances the risk of UTI. Stasis may be caused by abnormal anatomic structures or abnormal function (e.g., **neurogenic bladder** in which an interrupted nerve supply from myelomeningocele or spinal cord trauma impairs bladder voiding function and leads to incomplete bladder emptying). Children normally void five to six times a day. Infrequent voiding, common in school-age children, results in incomplete emptying of the bladder and urinary stasis. Other factors associated with increased risk of UTI include poor hygiene, inadequate cleansing after bowel movements, an irritated perineum, uncircumcised male in the first 6 months of life, constipation, masturbation, sexual abuse, and sexual activity in adolescent females (Dulczak & Kirk, 2005). Another cause of UTI is **vesicoureteral reflux**, the backflow of urine from the bladder into the ureters during voiding. This prevents complete emptying of the bladder and creates a reservoir for bacterial growth (Huether, 2006).

The inflammatory and ischemic effects as a result of hydronephrosis or pyelonephritis can lead to renal scarring. Renal scarring has been associated with hypertension, proteinuria, and kidney failure. The risk of kidney damage increases in the following instances:

- UTI in infant less than 1 year of age
- Delay in diagnosis and effective antibacterial treatment for an upper UTI
- Anatomic obstruction or nerve supply interruption
- Recurrent episodes of upper UTIs

Clinical Manifestations

Symptoms depend on the location of the infection and the age of the child. Symptoms in the newborn period tend to be nonspecific—unexplained fever, hypothermia, failure to thrive, poor feeding, vomiting and diarrhea, strong-smelling urine, and irritability. Any child under 2 years of age with a fever of unknown origin should be tested for a UTI. Not until the toddler years are the more "classic" symptoms of lower UTI seen as listed in "Clinical Manifestations: Urinary Tract Infection." Many UTIs are asymptomatic and are discovered incidentally on routine examination.

Clinical Therapy

A urine specimen is examined for the presence of bacteria. A dipstick positive leukocyte esterase test identifies white blood cells and pyuria, and a positive nitrite dipstick detects gram negative bacteria (Raszka & Kahn, 2005). The UTI is diagnosed when a midstream clean-catch urine culture yields greater than 100,000 colony-forming units (cfu) of a single bacteria, or greater than 50,000 cfu of a single bacteria are cultured from a sterile catheterized specimen (Dulczak & Kirk, 2005). See Clinical Skills Manual for urine collection methods, Skills 10–7 through 10–12 SKILLS. Urine cultures do not distinguish between upper and lower UTIs (Raszka & Khan,

Clinical Manifestations

URINARY TRACT INFECTION

TYPE OF UTI	CLINICAL MANIFESTATIONS
Lower UTI—Cystitis	
Infants	Fever, diarrhea, vomiting, irritability, lethargy, foul-smelling diapers, poor feeding, failure to gain weight
Preschooler	Fever, hematuria, urgency, dysuria, frequency, cloudy urine, foul-smelling urine, dehydration, abdominal pain, enuresis
School-age	Dysuria, enuresis, hematuria, strong smelling urine, diarrhea, frequency or hesitancy, mood changes, abdominal pain, suprapubic or flank pain, dehydration
Upper UTI—Pyelonephritis	High fever, chills, abdominal pain, nausea, vomiting, flank pain, costovertebral angle tenderness, moderate to severe dehydration

2005). Once the presence of bacteria is confirmed, antibiotic sensitivity for the specific organisms cultured is then determined.

Radiologic studies may be performed to detect structural abnormalities and renal scarring. The most common tests performed are a renal and bladder ultrasound soon after the diagnosis of a UTI. A voiding cystourethrogram (VCUG) may be obtained to test for vesicoureteral reflux. The ultrasounds and a DMSA scan may also be used to detect pyelonephritis and renal scarring (Dulczak & Kirk, 2005).

Antibiotic therapy is begun as soon as urine samples have been collected. Generally the child receives a 7–10-day course of antibiotic matching organism sensitivity. The length of treatment may be shorter in older children. Sulfamethoxazole-trimethoprim is the preferred oral antibiotic in children over 2 months of age (Dulczak & Kirk, 2005).

Table 54–1 lists diagnostic tests commonly used to identify urinary tract conditions.

Table 54–1 Diagnostic Tests and Laboratory Procedures for the Genitourinary System

Diagnostic Procedures	Laboratory Tests
Computed tomography (CT)	Blood urea nitrogen (BUN)
Cystoscopy	Creatinine clearance
Diuretic renogram (a type of nuclear scan)	Urinalysis (UA) (Skills 10-7 to 10-12 SKILLS)
Intravenous pyelogram	Urine culture (Skill 10-10 SKILLS)
Magnetic resonance imaging (MRI)	Urine protein-to-creatinine ratio
Radionucleotide renal scan with dimercaptosuccinic acid (DMSA)	
Renal biopsy	
Renal or bladder ultrasound	
Voiding cystourethrogram (VCUG) or radionuclide cystography	

Evidence in Action

A randomized control trial of children diagnosed with pyelonephritis and mild or moderate vesicoureteral reflux (VUR) was done to evaluate the effect of prophylactic antibiotics on outcomes. The trial followed 218 children, aged 3 months to 18 years. Half of the children received antibiotics and the remainder did not. Children were seen every 3 months for the year of the study, and each had a urine culture at each visit. Results indicated that the presence of mild or moderate VUR did not increase the incidence of UTI, pyelonephritis, or renal scarring following an acute episode of pyelonephritis. The children who did not receive prophylactic antibiotics had no more infections or renal scarring than the children who did receive antibiotics (Garin, Olavarria, Nieto, et al., 2006).

Follow-up urine cultures should then be obtained according to the frequency specified by agency guidelines or physician orders. Children with pyelonephritis may have repeat urine cultures repeated monthly for 3 months, every 3 months for 6 months, and then annually. Most reinfections occur within a year, and subsequent infections may be asymptomatic. For children with vesicoureteral reflux or recurrent infections, a long-term suppressive dose of an antibiotic may be ordered for prophylaxis; however, there is limited evidence that this is effective (Raszka & Khan, 2005). Children with renal scarring should have their blood pressure monitored.

Children who appear ill and cannot tolerate oral antibiotics are often hospitalized because they need rehydration and initiation of parenteral antibiotic treatment until they are afebrile for 24 hours. Infants may develop permanent kidney damage or generalized sepsis if UTI is not treated aggressively. If a structural defect is identified, surgical correction may be necessary to prevent recurrent infections that could lead to renal damage. Children with pyelonephritis are often initially hospitalized to receive rehydration and parental antibiotics. Once the child has been afebrile for 24 hours, he or she is transitioned to oral antibiotics matching organism sensitivity for a total of 10–14 days of therapy (Dulczak & Kirk, 2005).

NURSING MANAGEMENT

NURSING ASSESSMENT AND DIAGNOSIS

PHYSIOLOGIC ASSESSMENT

Obtain a history of urinary symptoms. Assess the infant for toxic (very ill) appearance, fever, and poor feeding. Evaluate the child's oral fluid intake. Assess for quality, quantity, and frequency of voiding. Assess the infant's or child's vital signs, including blood pressure. Palpate the abdomen and suprapubic and costovertebral areas for masses, tenderness, and distention. Assess for abdominal or flank pain, frequency, urgency, and dysuria. Observe the urinary stream if possible and perform a urinalysis, including specific gravity. Proper collection of the urine specimen is essential. Obtain a clean-catch urine specimen if the child is old enough to do this. If not, get a catheterized sample (see Skill 10–10 SKILLS). An early morning urine specimen is preferred because the urine is more concentrated.

PSYCHOSOCIAL ASSESSMENT

Sexually active adolescents may deny having symptoms of a UTI because they fear disclosing their sexual activity to their parents. Careful questioning and a visit alone with the adolescent may be necessary to elicit these concerns. Be open and approachable and give the patient and family the chance to address their concerns.

Common nursing diagnoses for the child with a UTI include the following:

- *Impaired Urinary Elimination* related to recurrent urinary tract infections
- *Delayed Growth and Development* related to chronic infection and renal damage
- *Urinary Retention* related to infrequent voiding habits or vesicoureteral reflux
- *Ineffective Therapeutic Regimen Management* related to lack of knowledge of preventive UTI measures
- *Risk for deficient fluid volume* related to fever and inadequate intake

PLANNING AND IMPLEMENTATION

Nursing care for the hospitalized child with a complicated UTI centers on administering prescribed medications, promoting rehydration, assessing renal function, and teaching parents and older children how to minimize the risk of future infection.

Administer antibiotics and antipyretics as prescribed to maintain therapeutic drug levels and reduce fever. Encourage fluid intake to dilute the urine and flush the bladder. Frequent voiding minimizes urinary stasis. Document intake and output. Assess renal function by comparing the child's output to the expected urine output and weigh the child daily.

Teaching Highlights

PREVENTION OF URINARY TRACT INFECTIONS

- Teach proper perineal hygiene. Girls should always wipe the perineum from front to back after voiding.
- Encourage the child to drink plenty of fluids and avoid long periods of "holding urine."
- Caution against tight underwear; children should wear cotton rather than nylon underwear.
- Encourage the child to void more frequently and to fully empty the bladder.
- Discourage bubble baths, bath oils, and hot tubs, which can irritate the urethra.
- Encourage abstinence of sexual activity. However, if girls are sexually active, instruct them to void before and after sexual intercourse to prevent urinary stasis and flush out bacteria introduced during intercourse.

Because bladder training is such an important milestone for young children, any disorder that affects voiding may have developmental implications. A toddler who has been toilet trained may regress and require diapers temporarily as a result of UTI-related incontinence. An older child may develop enuresis after a prolonged period of being dry at night. Reassure parents that this is normal and emphasize that the child needs support. A preschooler may perceive the infection and any parental disapproval as punishment for an imagined wrong.

DISCHARGE PLANNING AND HOME CARE TEACHING

Children with UTIs are usually cared for at home. Teach parents that all doses of the antibiotic must be taken as prescribed and that they may be continued even after the infection has cleared to prevent a recurrence. Teach prevention through proper hygiene and avoidance of risk behaviors.

Give parents specific guidelines for oral fluid intake. Make sure the amount of fluids recommended for a 24-hour period equals the maintenance fluids needed plus additional fluids required because of fever and diuresis to flush out pathogens. (See Chapter 46 ∞.) Suggest that the parents avoid giving the child caffeinated and carbonated beverages as these may potentially irritate the bladder mucosa. Teach parents the signs and symptoms of recurrent infection and to seek care promptly.

The child with a neurogenic bladder requires a clean intermittent catheterization to be performed several times a day to reduce urinary stasis and the potential for UTI. While the procedure for inserting the catheter is the same as that for catheterization using sterile technique, children and families are generally taught to use clean technique (Bray & Sanders, 2007).

EVALUATION

Expected outcomes of nursing care include:

- Increased fluid intake and number of times voiding each day
- Reduced risk of recurrent UTI

DISORDERS AFFECTING URINARY ELIMINATION

ENURESIS

Enuresis is repeated involuntary voiding by a child old enough that bladder control is expected, usually about 5 to 6 years of age. (See Table 54–2 for bladder control milestones.) Enuresis can occur either at night (nocturnal), during the day (diurnal), or both night and day.

Enuresis is further categorized as primary and secondary.

- *Primary enuresis*—child has never had a dry night; attributed to maturational delay and small functional bladder; not associated with stress or psychiatric cause.
- *Secondary enuresis*—child who has been reliably dry for at least 6 months begins bedwetting; associated with stress, infections, and sleep disorders.

Primary nocturnal enuresis is the most common type of enuresis and occurs more frequently in males than females (Elder, 2007). In the United States, approximately 5 to 7 million children over 6 years of age are affected with primary nocturnal enuresis (Ward-Smith & Barry, 2006).

Enuresis may result from neurologic or congenital structural disorders, illness, preoccupation with concerns, or stress. Nocturnal enuresis occurs frequently in children whose parents have a history of bed-wetting. There is a 77% risk if both parents had enuresis, a 44% risk if one parent had enuresis (Ward-Smith & Barry, 2006).

In most children with primary enuresis, the bladder has a smaller functional capacity, and neuromuscular maturation of the inhibitory fibers is delayed. Minor abnormalities of the bladder neck and urethra are also associated with enuresis. Nocturnal enuresis is also more prevalent in children with obstructive sleep

MyNursingKit Care Plan: A School-Age Child with Enuresis

Table 54–2 Milestones in the Development of Bladder Control

Age	Developmental Milestone
1 1/2 years	Child passes urine at regular intervals.
2 years	Child announces when he or she is voiding.
2 1/2 years	Child makes known need to void; can hold urine.
3 years	Child goes to the bathroom by himself or herself; holds urge if preoccupied with play.
2 1/2–3 1/2 years	Child achieves nighttime control.
4 years	Child shows great interest in going to bathrooms when away from home (shopping centers, movies).
5 years	Child voids approximately 7 times a day; prefers privacy; is able to initiate emptying of bladder at any degree of fullness.

Growth and Development

An estimated 15% of 5 year olds experience primary nocturnal enuresis (Ward-Smith & Barry, 2006). While wetting episodes do decrease as the child gets older, an estimated 4–8% of 12 year olds and 1–3% of adolescents will continue to have nocturnal enuresis (Berry, 2006). In addition, approximately 3.8% of males and 6% of girls, seven years of age, have diurnal (daytime) enuresis (Schulman & Berry, 2007.

Nursing Practice

Questions to ask when taking an enuresis history include the following:

Family History

Is there a family history of renal or urinary structural abnormalities?

Is there a family history of bed-wetting? At what age did bed-wetting stop?

Family Management of Enuresis

How serious is the problem for the family?

What happens when the child wets? (Who gets up and changes sheets?)

How is the child treated? Is the child punished or blamed for wetting?

What remedies have been tried?

Toilet Training

When was it initiated and what method was used?

Has the child ever been dry during the day or night for an extended period?

How long was the child's longest dry period?

How often does the child void? Have a bowel movement?

Does the child have a history of constipation or encopresis?

Stressors

How is the child doing in school?

Are any new or chronic stressors present in the child's life?

How does the problem interfere with play and other activities?

Risk Factors

Diabetes—Are there any signs of polyuria or polydipsia?

Urinary tract infection—Does the child have frequency, urgency, burning on urination?

apnea syndrome (Weissbach, Leiberman, Tarasiuk, et al., 2006). Often children with nocturnal enuresis are harder to arouse and may fail to respond to full bladder signals. Some children may produce more urine and exceed the functional bladder capacity because of a lack of circadian rhythm of vasopressin that helps concentrate the urine during sleep (Mercer, 2006; Nield & Kamat, 2004). Some children with daytime enuresis may have **dysfunctional voiding**, an abnormality in the storage or emptying phase of urination (Berry, 2005).

A thorough history can help identify potential causes of enuresis. Enuretic children often have a history of constipation (Berry, 2006). Rectal pressure on the posterior bladder wall stimulates the bladder to empty. The child's lower spine is examined for fistulas, sacral dimples, or tufts of hair that could be signs of spina bifida occulta. (See Chapter 56∞.) Prolonged hospitalization, family stressors, and preoccupation with school concerns also have been associated with secondary enuresis. Laboratory evaluation includes urinalysis and urine culture. Measurement of the child's functional bladder capacity may be performed. Bladder sonography to measure residual urine after voiding and uroflow (the rate of urine flow) measurement are sometimes performed, but are not considered essential (Nield & Kamat, 2004). A multitreatment approach is usually most effective.

Fluid restriction, bladder training, and enuresis alarms are common approaches (Table 54–3). A spontaneous resolution occurs in 15% of children each year, regardless of intervention or lack of intervention (Ward-Smith & Berry, 2006). Some children with nocturnal enuresis are treated with medications. Imipramine, a tricyclic antidepressant, is often used for nocturnal enuresis. This medication requires close monitoring because of its effects on mood and sleep-arousal patterns and the associated danger of overdoses (Vemulakonda & Jones, 2006). Desmopressin has an antidiuretic effect and is given only on a nighttime basis at the beginning of treatment. Once its effectiveness has been established, it may be used as needed for times when the child is away from home for a short period (e.g., sleepovers or camp) (Berry, 2006). Oxybutynin, an anticholinergic medication, has an antispasmodic effect and is used for children with urgency or an overactive detrusor muscle (Vemulakonda & Jones, 2006). Relapse often occurs when medications are stopped.

Table 54–3 Treatment Approaches for Enuresis

Approach	Description
Fluid restriction	Fluid intake is limited in the evening and before the child goes to bed.
Bladder exercises	The child drinks a large amount and then holds urine as long as he or she can. The child practices stopping voiding midstream. Exercises should continue for at least 6 months.
Timed voiding	The child with diurnal enuresis is instructed to void every 2 hours and to use a double voiding pattern; this trains the bladder to empty completely and avoid overdistention.
Enuresis alarms	A detector strip is attached to the child's pants. The alarm sounds a buzzer that alerts the child when wetting occurs, so the child can get up and finish voiding in the bathroom. This works best for children over 7 years old, and takes 3 to 4 months for success.
Reward system	Set realistic goals for the child and reinforce dry days or nights with stars and stickers on a chart.
Medications	Imipramine, desmopressin, and oxybutynin are used as per discussion above.

Nursing Management

Teach the child and parents about the physiologic development of bladder control and causes and treatment of enuresis. Explore feelings of guilt or blame. Make sure the parents are aware that the child cannot control the wetting. Psychosocial support is an essential part of care since stress is an important cause of secondary enuresis. Provide emotional support to the parents and child, and encourage the child's participation in the treatment plan. Refer the child for counseling or therapy if appropriate.

Assess the parents' and child's motivation and readiness for interventions. The child needs to be an active participant in the treatment plan for daytime and nighttime wetting. Before parents buy an enuresis alarm, suggest they use an alarm clock in the child's room for several nights to see if the child will arouse. Find out whether the child shares a room with others who will be disturbed by the alarm. Ask if the child and parents are willing to persist with an enuresis alarm, as it may take months to work. Discuss potential strategies with the family to reduce stressors on the child or to help the child cope with the stressors. Expected outcomes of nursing care include:

- Increased number of dry nights
- Positive self-esteem

RENAL DISORDERS

NEPHROTIC SYNDROME

Nephrotic syndrome (NS) is an alteration in kidney function secondary to increased glomerular basement membrane permeability to plasma protein (see "Pathophysiology Illustrated: Nephrotic Syndrome"). Nephrotic syndrome refers not to a specific disease, but rather to a clinical state characterized by edema, massive proteinuria, hypoalbuminemia, hypoproteinemia, hyperlipidemia, and altered immunity. Congenital nephrotic (CNF) syndrome, an autosomal recessive disorder, is extremely rare. The CNF gene is localized on chromosome 19 (Huether, 2006). Primary nephrotic syndrome results from a disease that affects only the kidney, such as glomerulonephritis. Secondary nephrotic syndrome results from a systemic disease, drugs, or toxins that alter kidney function (Huether, 2006).

Approximately 85% of children with nephrotic syndrome have a type of primary disease called minimal change nephrotic

PATHOPHYSIOLOGY ILLUSTRATED

NEPHROTIC SYNDROME

Note the contrast between the normal glomerular anatomy and the changes that exist in nephrotic syndrome permitting protein to be excreted in the urine. The lower albumin blood level stimulates the liver to generate lipids and excessive clotting factors. Edema results from decreased oncotic plasma pressure, renin-angiotensin-aldosterone activation, and antidiuretic hormone secretion.

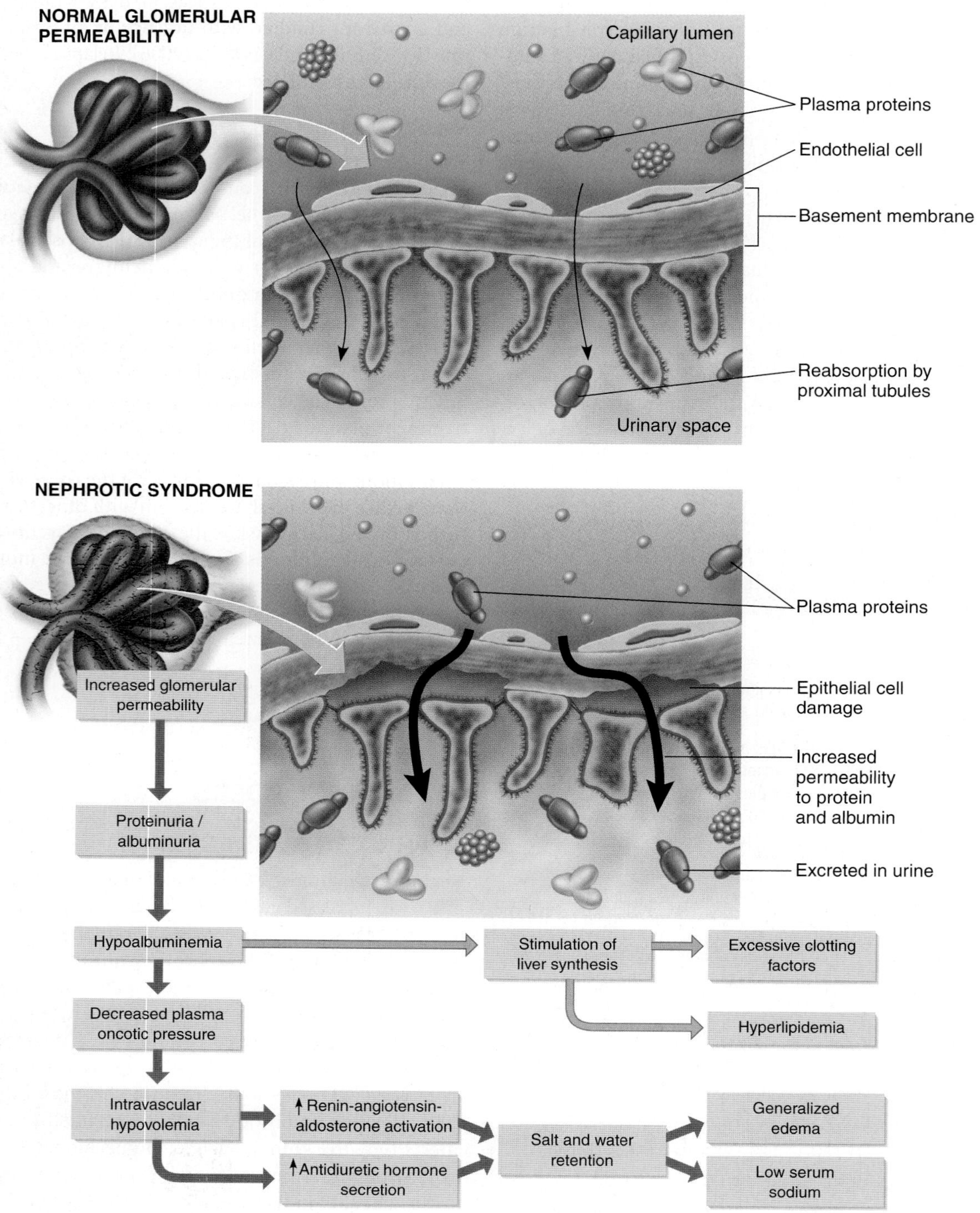

syndrome (MCNS). Ninety-five percent of these children respond to steroid therapy (Vogt & Avner, 2007a). MCNS is a common kidney disease in the pediatric population occurring in 2–16 per 100,000 children (Lahdenkari, Suvanto, Kajantie, et al., 2005) and is more common in males than females (Vogt & Avner, 2007a). MCNS derives its name from the normal or only minimally changed appearance of the glomeruli on light microscopic evaluation. Because MCNS is the most common form of nephrotic syndrome, it is the focus of the following discussion.

Etiology and Pathophysiology

The cause of primary MCNS is not clearly understood but an immune system role is suspected (Vogt & Avner, 2007a). The mechanism of increased glomerular permeability is unknown as the glomeruli appear normal; although it may be related to the loss of a negative charge in the glomerular capillary wall (Huether, 2006). In MCNS increased permeability of the glomerular membrane permits large, negatively charged molecules such as albumin to pass through the membrane and be excreted in the urine. Proteinuria results in decreased oncotic pressure and edema, because fluid remains in the interstitial spaces instead of being pulled back into the vascular compartment (Vogt & Avner, 2007a). Immunoglobulins are lost, resulting in altered immunity. Loss of protein in the urine, insufficient albumin production by the liver, and a decreased albumin concentration as a result of salt and water retention by the kidney contribute to hypoalbuminemia. Hypercoagulability occurs because of loss of antithrombin III in the urine and reduced levels of factors IX, XI, and XII. The liver, stimulated perhaps by hypoalbuminemia or decreased osmotic pressure, responds by increasing synthesis of lipoprotein, resulting in hyperlipidemia. Acute renal failure is a rare complication of MCNS, most likely resulting from changes in glomerular permeability (Walle, Mauel, Raes, et al., 2004).

Clinical Manifestations

In most children, edema develops gradually over several weeks. Children may have a history of periorbital edema on waking that resolves during the day as fluid shifts to the abdomen and lower extremities. Other signs include snug fit of clothing and shoes, pallor, hypertension, irritability, anorexia, hematuria, decreased urine output, and nonspecific malaise. The child's urine may be frothy or foamy. Parents often do not seek medical treatment until generalized edema develops on the child's extremities, abdomen, or genitals (Figure 54–4 ●). Respiratory distress from pleural effusion may occur in some cases.

Massive edema resulting in a dramatic weight gain and abdominal pain, with or without vomiting, may occur, depending on the amount of albumin lost and the amount of sodium ingested. The child becomes malnourished as a result of protein loss in the urine. The skin is pale and shiny with prominent veins, and the hair becomes more brittle. An increased risk of thrombosis is present.

Clinical Therapy

Diagnosis is based on the history, characteristic symptoms, and laboratory findings. Urinalysis as well as serum albumin, sodium, BUN, cholesterol, and electrolytes are ordered. Hypoalbuminemia of less than 25 g/L and urinary protein excretion of greater than or equal to 40 mg/m2/hour are the criteria for diagnosing nephrotic syndrome in childhood (Ruth, Kemper, Leumann, et al., 2005). Microscopic hematuria may also be present. Renal ultrasound may be performed to detect structural kidney problems. A single-needle kidney biopsy for examination of glomeruli may be performed to assess for renal failure or other disorders. Diagnostic testing for a relapse is the presence of 2+ proteinuria by dipstick testing for 3 consecutive days (Ruth et al., 2005).

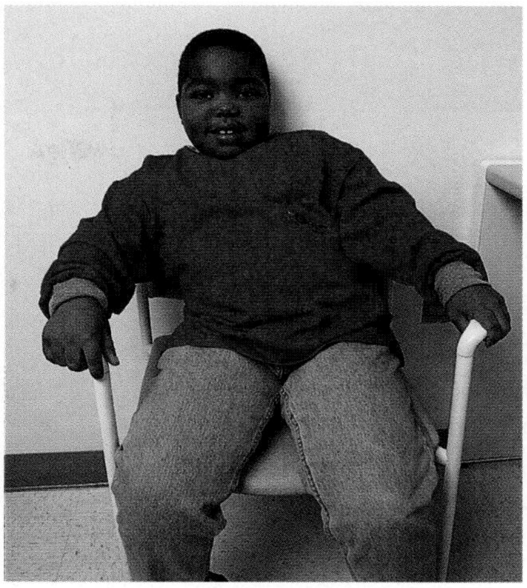

● **Figure 54–4** Generalized edema. This boy has generalized edema, a characteristic finding in nephrotic syndrome.

Children may be hospitalized when severe edema or a major infection is present, but are usually treated as outpatients. Clinical therapy focuses on decreasing proteinuria, relieving edema, managing associated symptoms, improving nutrition, and preventing infection. A corticosteroid (such as prednisone) is prescribed to decrease proteinuria. In most children, urine protein levels fall to trace or negative values within 2 to 3 weeks of the start of therapy. Children who respond successfully to therapy continue to take corticosteroids daily for 6 weeks, followed by 6 weeks of alternate-day treatment. The medication is then slowly tapered and discontinued over a 2–3 month period of time. Approximately 90% of children experience complete remission with corticosteroid therapy. Intravenous methylprednisolone may be used in children not responsive to oral steroids (Nachman, Jennette, & Falk, 2008; Vogt & Avner, 2007a). Intravenous administration of albumin followed by furosemide may occasionally be ordered in the child with massive edema who is unresponsive to fluid restriction and parenteral diuretics (Vogt & Avner, 2007a). Analgesics may be ordered for pain related to edema or flank pain from a urinary tract infection.

Relapses occur in up to 50% of children with nephrotic syndrome (Ruth, Landolt, Neuhaus, et al., 2004). Relapses may become less frequent during adolescence; however, long term studies have revealed that many adults continue to have relapses (Ruth et al., 2005).

Children who have a relapse after drug therapy is discontinued receive repeat therapy. Other medications used include diuretics, antihypertensive agents, and antibiotics. Medications such as

Drug Guide

PREDNISONE

MEDICATION AND ACTION/INDICATION	NURSING IMPLICATIONS
Prednisone Natural or synthetic, intermediate-acting glucocorticoid that has strong anti-inflammatory, immunosuppressant, and metabolic actions. Treats diseases such as renal, connective tissue, dermatologic, allergy, acute leukemia, and respiratory distress syndrome.	■ *Assess:* Obtain baseline weight and height, blood pressure, intake and output ratio and pattern. Take the blood pressure twice a day during initial stabilization period and report an ascending pattern. Obtain a fasting glucose, electrolytes, and routine laboratory studies at regular intervals. ■ *Administer:* PO: It is best to give a daily dose before 9 A.M. Alternate-day therapy is recommended to reduce growth-retarding effects. Give with food or milk to reduce gastrointestinal irritation. Tablets can be crushed and mixed with small amounts of food or fluid. Tablets are very bitter. If child is able to swallow capsules, they can be placed in a gelatin capsule. Follow with fluid of choice to cleanse child's palate. ■ *Monitor:* Carefully assess child's response to drug to determine need for dosage adjustments. Observe for side effects, especially hypocalcemia, signs of adrenal insufficiency, symptoms of infection, or worsening of condition. Monitor blood pressure and daily weights; report any sudden weight gain to the physician. With long-term usage, monitor serum electrolytes, height (to evaluate impact of medication on growth), and bone density. Encourage a well-balanced diet low in sodium, and encourage good hygiene and dental care (possible oral fungal infections). To discontinue the medication, reduce the dose gradually, especially after long-term use, so it does not cause acute life-threatening adrenal insufficiency. ■ *Patient Teaching:* Do not alter dose or stop medication abruptly as it could cause serious side effects or even death. Gradual tapering of dosage is necessary. Increasing the amount of medication will not speed the healing process. Monitor signs and symptoms of medication reactions; report signs of gastrointestinal distress, symptoms of adrenal insufficiency, or worsening of condition to physician. Obtain weekly weights; report a weight gain of 2 kg (5 lb) to physician. Stress importance of close medical supervision and follow-up. Get regular ophthalmologic examinations if on long-term therapy. Live vaccine immunizations should not be given when on high doses of corticosteroids. Inform any healthcare provider, including dentists, surgeons, or emergency care personnel, that child is on medication. Child should carry medical identification card. Observe for symptoms of infection. Do not use over-the-counter medications unless approved by the healthcare provider (Bindler & Howry, 2005).

Data from Bindler, R. M., & Howry, L. B. (2005). *Pediatric drug guide.* Upper Saddle River, NJ: Prentice Hall-Health.

MyNursingKit Care Plan: Child with Nephrotic Syndrome

cyclophosphamide, cyclosporine, tacrolimus, and mycophenolate may be used to prolong remissions in children with nephrotic syndrome who have frequent relapses (Vogt & Avner, 2007a). Since diuretics can precipitate hypovolemia, hyponatremia, and hypokalemia, electrolyte levels should be carefully monitored.

NURSING MANAGEMENT

NURSING ASSESSMENT AND DIAGNOSES

PHYSIOLOGIC ASSESSMENT

Careful assessment of the child's hydration status and edema is essential. Carefully monitor intake and output. Weigh the child daily using the same scale, and measure abdominal girth to monitor changes in edema and ascites (see Skill 9–7 SKILLS). Monitor vital signs at least every 4 hours to watch for signs of respiratory distress, hypertension, or circulatory overload. Test urine for proteinuria and specific gravity at least once each shift. In addition, assess for skin breakdown from edema, hypovolemia during periods of diuresis, indications of infection, and signs of skin breakdown.

PSYCHOSOCIAL ASSESSMENT

Children and parents are often fearful or anxious on admission. Because edema often develops gradually, parents may feel guilty if they did not seek medical attention immediately. School-age children with generalized edema are often concerned about their appearance. Careful questioning may be necessary to elicit these concerns. The child hospitalized for a recurrence of nephrotic syndrome may be frustrated or depressed. Assess individual and family coping mechanisms, support systems, and level of stress.

Common nursing diagnoses for the child with MCNS include the following:

- *Risk for Infection* related to immunosuppressive therapy
- *Risk for Impaired Skin Integrity* related to edema, lowered resistance to infection and injury, immobility, and malnutrition
- *Excess Fluid Volume* related to renal dysfunction and sodium retention
- *Imbalanced Nutrition: Less than Body Requirements* related to loss of appetite and protein loss in urine
- *Fatigue* related to fluid and electrolyte imbalance, albumin loss, altered nutrition, and renal failure
- *Deficient Diversional Activity* related to fatigue, immobility, and social isolation

PLANNING AND IMPLEMENTATION

Nursing care is mainly supportive and focuses on administering medications, preventing infection, preventing skin breakdown, meeting nutritional and fluid needs, promoting rest, and providing emotional support to the parents and child.

ADMINISTER MEDICATIONS

It is important to give prescribed medications at the scheduled times. Monitor closely for side effects of corticosteroids such as moon face, increased appetite, increased hair growth, abdominal distention, and mood swings, as well as adverse effects of corticosteroids such as hypertension, nausea, and hyperglycemia. Corticosteroids should be tapered rather than abruptly discontinued. If the child is receiving albumin intravenously, monitor closely for hypertension or signs of volume overload caused by fluid shifts. If diuretics are used, observe for shock. The child may need to have albumin infused simultaneously with diuretics.

PREVENT INFECTION

Children with MCNS are at risk for infection because of the loss of immunoglobulins in the urine and corticosteroid therapy. Implement careful hand hygiene and standard precautions. Strict aseptic technique is essential during invasive procedures. Monitor the child's white blood cell count when cytotoxic drugs are given as bone marrow suppression is a side effect. Monitor vital signs carefully to detect early signs of infection that may be masked by corticosteroid therapy. Decrease the child's social contacts during immunosuppressive treatment, and caution parents and children to avoid exposure to people with respiratory infections and communicable diseases. Emphasize the importance of avoiding shopping malls, sporting arenas, grocery stores, game stores, and other public areas where the risk of exposure to such infections is increased. Provide instructions to the parents on signs of infection, including fever and changes in behavior. Discuss with parents need for maintenance of annual recommended influenza immunizations and avoiding those who have recently been vaccinated with live viruses.

PREVENT SKIN BREAKDOWN

Meticulous skin care is essential to prevent skin breakdown and potential infection. Assess the skin repeatedly, turn the child frequently, and use therapeutic mattresses (e.g., egg crate, airflow) to help prevent skin breakdown. Keep the skin clean and dry.

MEET NUTRITIONAL AND FLUID NEEDS

Keep the child's food preferences in mind when planning menus. Encourage the child to eat by presenting attractive meals with small portions. Socialization during meals may improve the child's appetite. Fluids are not usually restricted except during severe edema.

PROMOTE REST

Provide opportunities for quiet play as tolerated, such as drawing, playing board games, listening to tapes, and watching videos/DVDs. Adjust the child's daily schedule to allow rest periods after activities. Signs of fatigue may include irritability, mood swings, or withdrawal. Tell the parents and child about the importance of rest. Limiting visitors during the acute phase of the illness may be necessary. Telephone and computer contacts may be encouraged as an alternative to visitors. To provide a sense of control, encourage the child to set his or her own limits on activity.

PROVIDE EMOTIONAL SUPPORT

Parents and children often need support to cope with this chronic disease. Thoroughly explain the child's disease and treatment regimen to parents. Parental anxiety in combination with the hospitalization may interfere with the child's independence. Help parents promote the child's independence by allowing the child to choose from the menu or to select the daily activity schedule. This gives the child some sense of control.

Children with MCNS may have a distorted body image because of sudden weight gain and edema. They may refuse to look in the mirror, refuse to participate in care, and take less interest in their appearance. Encourage children to express their feelings. Help them maintain a normal appearance by promoting normal grooming routines. Encourage children to wear their own pajamas rather than hospital gowns. Scarves or hats may be used to lessen the child's edematous appearance. Adolescents can be encouraged to write their feelings in a journal as a coping mechanism. These children may have a long-term psychosocial adjustment because of having a chronic condition with concerns about potential relapse (Ruth et al., 2004).

DISCHARGE PLANNING AND HOME CARE TEACHING

Explain the disease process, prognosis, and treatment plan to parents and school-age children. Make sure parents know how to administer medications and can identify potential side effects. Inform parents about restricting fluid intake until the edema resolves. Instruct parents about the need to monitor urine daily for protein, and have them keep a diary to record results. Monitoring the child's weight each week may help parents identify early stages of fluid retention and signs of relapse before edema occurs.

Tutoring may be required for a short period after discharge. Encourage parents to allow the child to return to normal activities once the acute episode has resolved. Emphasize the importance of avoiding contact with people with infectious diseases, because of the child's reduced immunity. Reinforce to parents that as long as the child is receiving corticosteroid therapy or shows signs of MCNS, the no-added-salt diet should be followed.

Most children do well with corticosteroid therapy; however, relapses are common. Even children with frequent relapses usually have a spontaneous resolution of MCNS before 30 years of age. Children should have periodic bone density evaluations because of the repeated steroid therapy.

EVALUATION

Expected outcomes of nursing care may include:

- Absence of infection
- Fluid, electrolyte, and acid–base balance restored and maintained
- Maintenance of skin integrity
- Nutritional requirements are met and dietary guidelines are followed

MyNursingKit Animation: Furosemide

ACUTE POSTINFECTIOUS GLOMERULONEPHRITIS

Glomerulonephritis is the most common inflammation of the glomeruli of the kidneys. In children, it is most often a response to a group A beta-hemolytic streptococcal infection of the skin or pharynx. It is also caused by other organisms, including *Staphylococcus, Pneumococcus,* and *Coxsackie* viruses. The incidence of acute postinfectious glomerulonephritis (APIGN) is highest in children between 2 and 6 years of age, and the disorder is more common in boys than in girls (Nachman et al., 2008).

Etiology and Pathophysiology

The child with APIGN usually becomes ill after contracting a nephrogenetic strain of group A beta-hemolytic streptococcal infection of the upper respiratory tract or the skin. Often the child contracts a streptococcal infection (e.g., strep throat), recovers, and then develops signs of APIGN after an interval of 10–21 days.

Glomerular damage occurs as a result of an immune complex reaction that localizes on the glomerular capillary wall. See "Pathophysiology Illustrated: Acute Postinfectious Glomerulonephritis." Antibody–antigen complexes become lodged in the glomeruli, leading to inflammation and obstruction. Capillaries in the glomeruli are obstructed by damaged tissue cells, and the glomerular filtration rate is reduced. Vascular permeability increases, allowing red blood cells and red cell casts to be excreted. Sodium and water are retained, expanding the intravascular and interstitial compartments and resulting in the characteristic finding of edema.

Clinical Manifestations

Many children are asymptomatic. In other children the onset is usually abrupt with flank or midabdominal pain, irritability, malaise, and fever. Microscopic hematuria is present in nearly all cases, and gross hematuria, resulting in tea-colored urine, is found in up to 50% of cases. Mild periorbital edema occurs early, along with dependent edema of the feet and ankles. Edema may progress in severity to cause a pulmonary effusion (dyspnea, cough, and crackles) or ascites (Gray, Huether, & Forshee, 2006). Acute hypertension may cause an encephalopathy that includes headache, nausea, vomiting, irritability, lethargy, and seizures. Oliguria may or may not be present.

Clinical Therapy

The serum BUN and creatinine concentrations are elevated. Serum protein is decreased as a result of mild or moderate proteinuria. The white blood cell count and erythrocyte sedimentation rate may be elevated. Serum lipid levels are increased in about 40% of cases. An elevated antistreptolysin O (ASO) titer reflects the presence of antibodies from a recent streptococcal respiratory infection, but the ASO level associated with a recent skin infection is low. The anti-DNAse B titer is helpful for detecting antibodies associated with recent skin infections. Up to 90% of children have reduced serum C3 as a result of the initial infection. Urinalysis reveals hematuria, proteinuria, and red and white cell casts. Anemia is common in the acute phase, usually because extracellular fluid dilutes the serum. Hemoglobin and hematocrit levels reveal anemia, which is common in the acute phase and is generally caused by dilution of the serum by the extracellular fluid. Anemia during the late phase is a result of hematuria.

Treatment focuses on relief of symptoms and supportive therapy. Bed rest is a key component of the treatment plan during the acute phase. Edema and mild to moderate hypertension should be treated with sodium restriction and a diuretic such as furosemide (Lau & Wyatt, 2005). Immediate emergency care is needed for severe hypertension with cerebral dysfunction; medication such as hydralazine or diazoxide is administered intravenously. A course of antibiotics may be given to ensure eradication of the original infectious agent.

The prognosis for over 90% of children with APIGN is good. Clinical signs, proteinuria, and hematuria resolve within several weeks. Most children recover without significant loss of renal function or recurrence of the disorder (Gray et al., 2006).

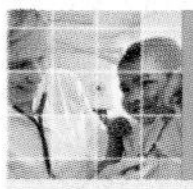

Nursing Practice

Antibiotics are *not* a treatment for acute postinfectious glomerulonephritis (APIGN). Instead, antibiotics are prescribed to treat the original infection (such as strep throat).

PATHOPHYSIOLOGY ILLUSTRATED

ACUTE POSTINFECTIOUS GLOMERULONEPHRITIS

Infection from group A beta-hemolytic streptococcus causes an immune response that causes inflammation and damage to the glomeruli. Protein and red blood cells are allowed to pass through the glomeruli. Blood flow to the glomeruli is reduced due to obstruction with damaged cells. Renal insufficiency results, leading to the retention of sodium, water, and waste.

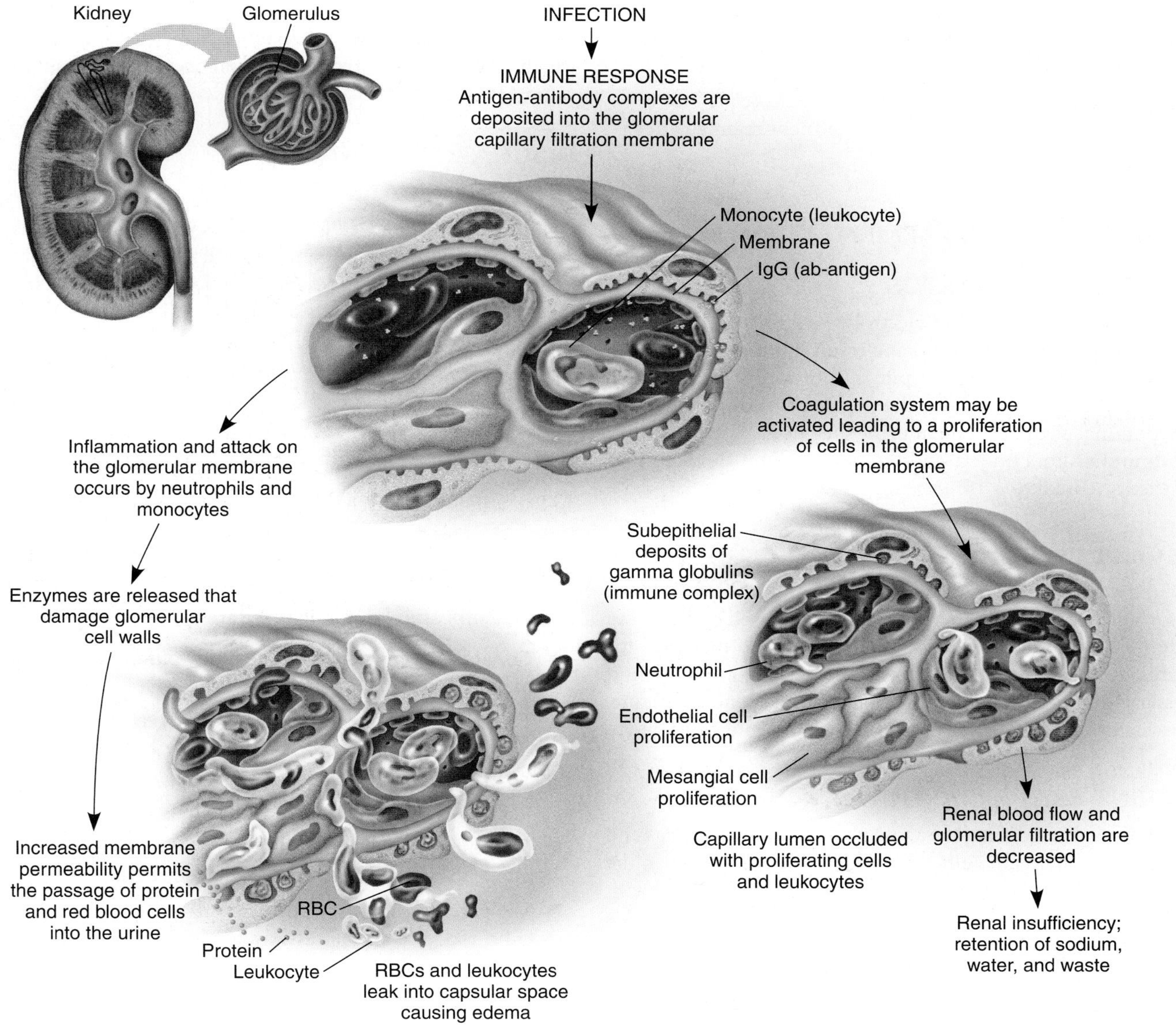
Kidney
Glomerulus
INFECTION
IMMUNE RESPONSE
Antigen-antibody complexes are deposited into the glomerular capillary filtration membrane
Monocyte (leukocyte)
Membrane
IgG (ab-antigen)
Coagulation system may be activated leading to a proliferation of cells in the glomerular membrane
Inflammation and attack on the glomerular membrane occurs by neutrophils and monocytes
Enzymes are released that damage glomerular cell walls
Subepithelial deposits of gamma globulins (immune complex)
Neutrophil
Endothelial cell proliferation
Mesangial cell proliferation
Capillary lumen occluded with proliferating cells and leukocytes
Renal blood flow and glomerular filtration are decreased
Renal insufficiency; retention of sodium, water, and waste
Increased membrane permeability permits the passage of protein and red blood cells into the urine
RBC
Protein
Leukocyte
RBCs and leukocytes leak into capsular space causing edema

NURSING MANAGEMENT

NURSING ASSESSMENT AND DIAGNOSES

As with other renal disorders, care of the child with APIGN requires careful monitoring of vital signs and fluid–electrolyte balance to evaluate renal functioning and identify complications. Frequent blood pressure monitoring is required since it can rise as high as 200/120 mm Hg. With severe hypertension, assess for signs of central nervous system problems (headache, blurred vision, vomiting, decreased level of consciousness, confusion, and convulsions). Monitor urine for proteinuria, hematuria. Record output. Assess edema, which may be periorbital or dependent and shifts as the child's position is changed. Assess for a pulmonary effusion (crackles, dyspnea, and cough).

Nursing diagnoses may include the following:

- *Excess Fluid Volume* related to decreased glomerular filtration and increased sodium retention
- *Risk for Infection* related to renal impairment and corticosteroid therapy
- *Risk for Impaired Skin Integrity* related to tissue edema
- *Imbalanced Nutrition: Less than Body Requirements* related to loss of appetite and proteinuria
- *Activity Intolerance* related to fluid and electrolyte imbalance, infectious process, and altered nutrition
- *Effective Therapeutic Regimen Management* related to child's medication schedule and treatment regimen after discharge

PLANNING AND IMPLEMENTATION

MONITOR FLUID STATUS

Monitor vital signs, fluid and electrolyte status, and intake and output. Hypovolemia can occur as a result of fluid shifting from vascular to interstitial spaces despite the outward clinical signs of excess fluid retention. Monitor the degree of ascites by measuring abdominal girth. Document urine specific gravity. Make sure parents and visitors understand the need to limit fluids to prevent excessive intake.

PREVENT INFECTION

Impaired renal function puts the child at risk for infection. Monitor for signs of infection, including fever, increased malaise, and an elevated white blood cell count. Screen family members for the presence of streptococcal infection and refer for treatment if necessary. Instruct the family in good hand hygiene technique. Limit visitors, and screen for upper respiratory infections.

PREVENT SKIN BREAKDOWN

Bed rest is required during the acute phase. Dependent areas and other pressure areas are vulnerable to skin breakdown. Turn the child frequently. Pad bony prominences or susceptible areas with sheepskin, or protect skin with a transparent dressing. Elevate lower extremities on pillows when in the dependent position or when the child is lying in bed. Make sure the child's bed is free of crumbs or sharp toys. Keep sheets tight and free of wrinkles. Maintain proper hygiene and dry skin.

MEET NUTRITIONAL NEEDS

A team approach (including the nurse, renal dietitian, parents, and child) is often needed to meet the child's nutritional needs. In most cases the child follows a "no added salt" and low-protein diet. This diet may be challenging since the child may refuse to eat foods that taste different. Anorexia presents the greatest challenge to meeting daily nutritional requirements during the acute phase of the disease. To increase the child's appetite, encourage parents to bring the child's favorite foods from home, serve foods in age-appropriate quantities, and allow the child to eat with other children or with family members.

PROVIDE EMOTIONAL SUPPORT

Parents of a child with APIGN commonly feel guilty. Parents may blame themselves for not responding more quickly to the child's initial symptoms or may believe they could have prevented the development of glomerular damage. Discuss the etiology of the disease and the child's treatment, and correct any misconceptions. Emphasize that it is not possible to predict which of the few children with streptococcal infections will develop APIGN.

DISCHARGE PLANNING AND HOME CARE TEACHING

Children are hospitalized for a few days, although it may require 3 weeks for hypertension and gross hematuria to resolve and longer for the disorder to resolve completely. Discharge planning focuses on teaching parents about the child's medication regimen, potential side effects of medications, dietary restrictions, and signs and symptoms of complications. Teach parents how to take the child's blood pressure and how to test urine for blood or protein. Emphasize that it is important to avoid exposing the child to people with upper respiratory tract infections. Advise parents to allow the child to return to his or her normal routine and activities after discharge, with periods allowed for rest.

EVALUATION

Expected outcomes of nursing care are the following:

- The child receives appropriate fluid volume each day and maintains normal urine output.
- The child develops no areas of redness, abrasions, or skin breakdown over pressure points.
- The child's temperature remains within normal limits and the child is free of secondary infection.
- The child maintains pre-illness weight and tolerates daily intake that meets nutritional requirements.
- The parents administer medications as prescribed. The child's sodium and potassium levels reflect adherence to dietary restrictions.

HEMOLYTIC-UREMIC SYNDROME

Hemolytic-uremic syndrome (HUS) is an acute renal disease. In young children it is the most common cause of acute renal failure (Huether, 2006). HUS is an important cause of chronic renal failure. It occurs most often in children under age 4 years with a peak between 1 and 2 years. The syndrome has a classic triad of signs: (1) hemolytic anemia, (2) thrombocytopenia, and (3) acute renal failure (Andersen, 2005).

Escherichia coli strain 0157:H7 produces a toxin that attaches to the glomeruli, collecting ducts, and distal tubules. The toxin damages the lining of the glomerular arterioles, causing the endothelial cells to swell and become occluded with platelets and fibrin clots. This partial occlusion damages the red blood cells, resulting in hemolytic anemia. Platelets cluster in areas of vascular endothelial damage, causing thrombocytopenia. Glomerular filtration is decreased resulting in hematuria and proteinuria. Oliguria and ARF develops in 40–50% of children with HUS. Streptococcal pneumoniae is another important organism causing HUS that is not associated with diarrhea or a gastrointestinal site of infection (Constantinescu, Bitzan, Weiss, et al., 2004).

An episode of severe gastroenteritis with bloody diarrhea, upper respiratory infection, or UTI precedes the development of HUS by 1 to 2 weeks followed by 1 to 5 days without symptoms. Signs and symptoms of HUS include hypertension, pallor, bruising, and oliguria. The child may also be irritable and have fever, anorexia, abdominal pain, vomiting, diarrhea, mild jaundice, and edema or ascites. Neurologic involvement is indicated by irritability, lethargy, and seizures (Huether, 2006).

Treatment focuses on the complications of ARF and includes fluid restrictions and a high-calorie, high-carbohydrate diet that is low in protein, sodium, potassium, and phosphorus. Enteral nutrition is sometimes needed. Medications may include calcium gluconate or calcium chloride, aluminum hydroxide gel to bind to phosphorus, Kayexalate to remove excess potassium, and antihypertensive agents. Transfusions of fresh-packed red blood cells may be ordered to treat severe anemia. Platelets are given if the child is bleeding or if surgery is needed.

Transfusions are carefully administered to prevent hypertension caused by hypervolemia. About 40% of children need dialysis and approximately 3% to 5% of those affected will die (Fiorino & Raffaelli, 2006). Peritoneal dialysis is preferred unless the child has severe colitis and abdominal tenderness. Some children may develop chronic renal failure; however, most regain normal renal function (Huether, 2006).

Nursing Management

Nursing care is the same as that for the child with acute renal failure (see page 1589). Careful monitoring of neurologic signs, laboratory values, fluid and electrolyte balance, and bleeding is essential. Monitor daily weights and assess intake and output. Assess the child for abdominal discomfort from diarrhea. Observe the child carefully for signs of progressive renal impairment. Discharge planning focuses on teaching parents about medications and dietary and fluid restrictions. Follow-up visits are necessary to evaluate the effectiveness of the treatment plan. Teach parents that HUS can be largely prevented by cooking of ground beef to 155°F throughout, meaning no more rare hamburgers. Teach them to wash hands carefully when handling raw ground meats, and to make sure utensils touching raw meat do not come into contact with cooked meats.

POLYCYSTIC KIDNEY DISEASE

Polycystic kidney disease (PKD) is a genetic disorder that has autosomal recessive and autosomal dominant forms. Liver abnormalities are associated with both forms of the disease. The incidence of the autosomal recessive form is 1 per 20,000 live births, and most are diagnosed in infancy (Asplin & Coe, 2005). The autosomal dominant form is one of the most frequently inherited diseases and is the most common inherited renal disorder with a prevalence of 1 in 800 live births in the United States (Rizk & Chapman, 2008; Watnick & Morrison, 2007). The autosomal dominant PKD results from mutations on the PKD1 locus on chromosome 16 and PKD2 on chromosome 4. The autosomal recessive gene (PKHD1) is located on chromosome 6 (National Kidney and Urologic Diseases Information Clearinghouse, 2007).

In PKD, cellular hyperplasia of the collecting ducts causes dilation of the ducts. Fluid secreted into these ducts enables cyst sacs to form. Initially, cysts are usually less than 2 mm in size and do not obstruct urinary flow. As the child grows, however, the cysts become larger and fibrosis occurs. The cysts slowly replace much of the kidney's mass and reduce kidney function. Tubular atrophy may occur in some children, whereas others have minimal changes in renal function. PKD is associated with liver abnormalities that progress in severity with age to fibrosis, portal hypertension, and biliary infection.

Newborns with autosomal recessive PKD may have enlarged kidneys, detected at birth. Those with the most severe form of the disease die shortly after birth of pulmonary hypoplasia (Asplin & Coe, 2005). Clinical manifestations in infants with autosomal recessive PKD include Potter facies (low-set ears, small jaw, and a flattened nose). Hypertension develops in early infancy and is often severe. Infants may have expected urine output or oliguria. Respiratory distress and feeding intolerance may develop from the enlarged kidneys (Davis & Avner, 2007). As uremia develops, infants and children develop renal **osteodystrophy** (a complex bone disease process of chronic kidney disease in which there is increased resorption of bone caused by chronic hyperparathyroidism) and progressive developmental delay and growth failure.

Sonogram or renal biopsy confirms the diagnosis. The disease is often diagnosed on prenatal ultrasound. Liver function tests are usually normal initially. A liver biopsy may also be performed. Other family members should be screened for subclinical cases of PKD.

Treatment is supportive. Medications such as diuretics are prescribed for hypertension. Fluid and electrolyte abnormalities are managed. Antibiotics treat urinary tract infection. Growth hormones may be used in some children to promote growth. Renal osteodystrophy is treated to suppress the parathyroid hormone. Many children develop end-stage renal disease (ESRD) by 10 years of age. Renal dialysis or a transplant prolong survival; however, liver problems may continue to complicate the child's health, even when the renal condition is well controlled. Up to 20% to 30% of children die by age 15 (Davis & Avner, 2007).

Nursing Management

Nursing care is the same as that for the child with renal insufficiency and chronic renal failure. See discussion on pages 1590 and 1592. Observe the child for signs of progressive renal impairment. Make sure the family schedules follow-up appointments to assess growth, developmental progress, and the effectiveness of the treatment plan. Family teaching for home management focuses on medications, diet adequate in protein and calories to support growth, management of acute gastrointestinal illnesses, and care for the child with progressive renal insufficiency and a liver disorder. Since the disease is inherited, the family should be referred for genetic counseling.

RENAL FAILURE

Renal failure, which may be acute or chronic, occurs when the kidney is unable to excrete wastes and concentrate urine. Acute renal failure occurs suddenly (over days or weeks) and may be reversible, whereas in chronic renal failure, kidney function diminishes gradually and permanently over months or years.

Both types of renal failure are characterized by **azotemia** (accumulation of nitrogenous wastes in the blood) and sometimes **oliguria** (reduced urine volume for age), indicating the kidney's inability to excrete metabolic waste products. Chronic renal failure eventually results in **anuria** (absence of urine output). The degree of impaired kidney function is estimated by the glomerular filtration rate (Miller & MacDonald, 2006).

ACUTE RENAL FAILURE

Acute renal failure (ARF) is a sudden loss of adequate renal function in which the kidneys are unable to clear metabolic wastes and to regulate extracellular fluid volume, sodium balance, and acid–base homeostasis. ARF is seen in 2% to 3% of children cared for in pediatric intensive care units and up to 8% of infants cared for in neonatal intensive care units (Vogt & Avner, 2007b). Potential causes include hemolytic uremic syndrome, acute glomerulonephritis, sepsis, poisoning, nephrotoxic medications, hypovolemia, obstructive uropathy, and complication of cardiac surgery. Hematologic-oncologic complications, bone marrow transplantation, and respiratory failure have become more common causes of ARF in the last few years (Bock, 2005).

Etiology and Pathophysiology

ARF may be caused by prerenal or postrenal factors as well as actual kidney damage. Prerenal ARF is a result of decreased perfusion to an otherwise normal kidney in association with a systemic condition. Hypovolemia secondary to dehydration is generally the cause; however, alterations in renal vasculature or cardiac function may also precipitate prerenal ARF. This is the most common type of ARF in infants and young children (Lum, 2007).

Primary kidney damage (intrinsic factors) may result from infection, diseases such as hemolytic uremic syndrome or acute glomerulonephritis, cortical necrosis, nephrotoxic drugs, or accidental ingestion of drugs or poisons. The structure most susceptible to damage is the kidney tubule. Injury to the tubule resulting in acute tubular necrosis is the most frequent cause of intrinsic renal failure in children (Lum, 2007). Postrenal ARF is caused by obstruction of the urinary flow from both kidneys, such as occurs in posterior urethral valves or a neurogenic bladder. Children may have oliguria, or normal or increased urine output. Renal failure without oliguria usually indicates a less severe renal injury. Children who recover from ARF may have residual kidney damage and compromised renal function.

Clinical Manifestations

Characteristically, a healthy child suddenly becomes ill with nonspecific symptoms that indicate a significant illness or injury (e.g., nausea, vomiting, lethargy, edema, gross hematuria, oliguria, and hypertension). These symptoms are a result of electrolyte imbalances, uremia, and fluid overload. The child appears pale and lethargic. See "Clinical Manifestations: Acute Versus Chronic Renal Failure" and "Clinical Manifestations: Electrolyte Imbalances in Acute and Chronic Renal Failure" for more information.

Hyperkalemia is the most life-threatening electrolyte disorder associated with ARF. Hyponatremia affects central nervous system function, resulting in symptoms that range from fatigue to seizures. Edema occurs as a result of sodium and water retention. (Refer to Chapter 43 for a discussion of these fluid and electrolyte alterations.) Children with ARF are also more susceptible to infection because of depressed immune functioning. **Uremia** occurs when there is an excess of urea and other nitrogenous waste products in the blood. Neurologic symptoms from accumulating wastes may include headache, seizures, lethargy, and confusion.

Clinical Manifestations

ACUTE VERSUS CHRONIC RENAL FAILURE

TYPE OF RENAL FAILURE	CLINICAL MANIFESTATIONS
Acute renal failure	Dark urine or gross hematuria, headache, edema, fatigue, crackles, gallop heart rhythm, hypertension, hematuria, lethargy, nausea and vomiting, oliguria Mass in flank area if a cyst, tumor, or obstructive lesion is present
Chronic renal failure	Fatigue, malaise, poor appetite, nausea and vomiting, failure to thrive or short stature Headache, decreased mental alertness or ability to concentrate Secondary enuresis, chronic anemia, hypertension, edema Fractures with minimal trauma, rickets, valgus deformity

PATHOPHYSIOLOGY ILLUSTRATED

ACUTE RENAL FAILURE

The initial kidney injury is usually associated with an acute condition such as sepsis, trauma, and hypotension, or the result of treatment for an acute condition with a nephrotoxic medication. Injury to the kidney can occur because of glomerular injury, vasoconstriction of capillaries, or tubular injury. All consequences of injury lead to decreased glomerular filtration and oliguria.

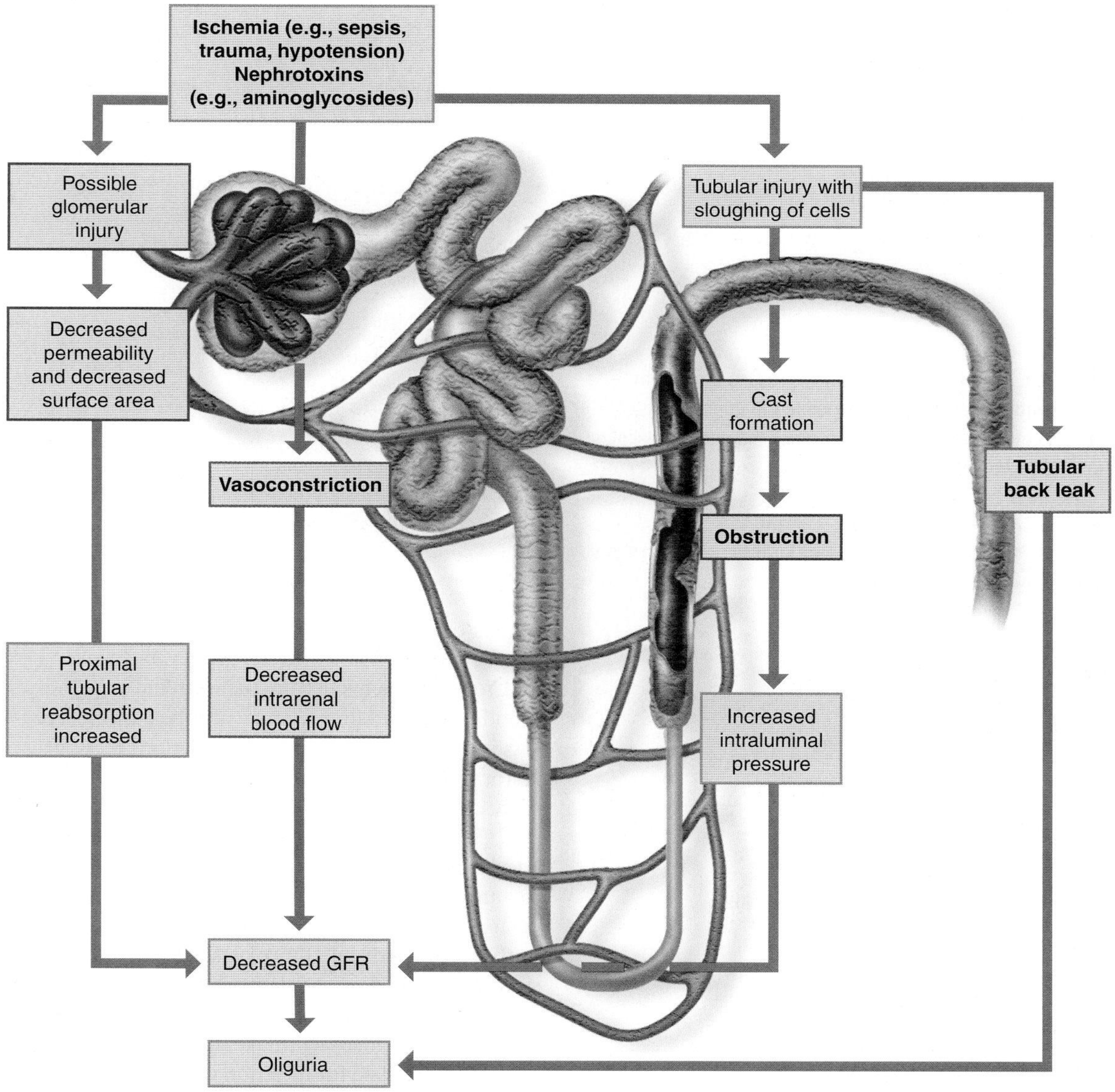

Clinical Therapy

Diagnosis of renal failure is based primarily on urinalysis and blood chemistry results, including BUN, serum creatinine, sodium, potassium, and calcium levels (Table 54–4). The kidneys are normal in size, and no signs of renal osteodystrophy are found on x-ray. Various imaging studies to assess kidney structures, renal blood flow, and renal perfusion and function may be performed to determine whether the child has ARF or chronic renal failure. A renal biopsy may be required.

Treatment depends on the underlying cause of the renal failure. The goal is to minimize or prevent permanent renal damage while maintaining fluid and electrolyte balance and managing complications. Initial emergency treatment of children with fluid depletion focuses on rapid fluid replacement of saline or lactated

Clinical Manifestations

ELECTROLYTE IMBALANCES IN ACUTE AND CHRONIC RENAL FAILURE

ELECTROLYTE IMBALANCE AND CAUSE	CLINICAL MANIFESTATIONS
Hyperkalemia	
Results from inability to adequately excrete potassium derived from diet and catabolized cells. In metabolic acidosis, potassium also moves from intracellular fluid to extracellular fluid.	■ Peaked T waves, widening of QRS waves on ECG ■ Dysrhythmias: ventricular dysrhythmias, heart block, ventricular fibrillation, cardiac arrest ■ Diarrhea ■ Muscle weakness
Hyponatremia	
In the acute oliguric phase, hyponatremia is related to the accumulation of fluid in excess of solute.	■ Change in level of consciousness ■ Muscle cramps ■ Anorexia ■ Abdominal reflexes, depressed deep tendon reflexes ■ Cheyne-Stokes respirations ■ Seizures
Hypocalcemia	
Phosphate retention (hyperphosphatemia) depresses the serum calcium ion concentration. Calcium is deposited in injured cells. Hyperkalemia and metabolic acidosis may mask the common clinical manifestations of severe hypocalcemia.	■ Muscle tingling ■ Changes in muscle tone ■ Seizures ■ Muscle cramps and twitching ■ Positive **Chvostek sign** (contraction of facial muscles after tapping facial nerve just anterior to parotid gland)

Note: See Chapter 46 for more information related to these alterations in electrolytes.

Table 54–4 Diagnostic Tests for Renal Failure

Diagnostic Tests	Findings in Renal Failure
URINALYSIS	
pH	Acidic urine
Osmolarity	Greater than 500: prerenal ARF Less than 350: intrinsic ARF
Specific gravity	High: prerenal ARF Low: intrinsic ARF Normal: postrenal ARF
Protein	Positive
SERUM CHEMISTRY*	
Potassium	Elevated
Sodium	Normal, low, or high, depends solely on the amount of water in the body
Calcium	Low
Phosphorus	High
Urea nitrogen	Increased
Creatinine	Increased
pH	Low acidic

*Please refer to Appendix B for normal values for various ages.
ARF = Acute Renal Failure

Ringer's solution at 20 mL/kg given rapidly over 5 to 10 minutes and repeated as needed to ensure renal perfusion and stabilize blood pressure. Albumin may also be administered when blood loss is the cause of circulatory depletion. If oliguria persists after restoration of adequate fluid volume, intrinsic renal damage is suspected.

Children with fluid overload, such as those with pulmonary edema, need diuretic therapy, and dialysis if they respond poorly to diuretics. Once the child is stabilized, fluid requirements are calculated to maintain zero water balance (intake should equal urine output and insensible fluid loss). All potential sources of potassium should be eliminated until hyperkalemia is controlled. Other electrolyte imbalances are treated. Nutrition must be maintained with extra carbohydrate intake during the catabolic state. Antibiotics are prescribed for infection if applicable. Nephrotoxic antibiotics should be avoided. See Drug Guide on page 1589.

Some children whose ARF is unresponsive to management require dialysis to correct severe electrolyte imbalances, manage fluid overload, and cleanse the blood of waste products. The clinical situation and age of the child determine whether hemodialysis or peritoneal dialysis is used. Refer to the "Renal Replacement Therapy" section on page 1594.

Prognosis depends on the cause of ARF. When renal failure results from drug toxicity or dehydration, the prognosis is generally good. However, ARF that results from diseases such as

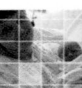

Drug Guide

MEDICATIONS USED TO TREAT COMPLICATIONS OF ACUTE RENAL FAILURE

COMPLICATION	MEDICATION / ACTION OR INDICATION	NURSING IMPLICATIONS
Hyperkalemia (> 5.8 mmol/L)	**Kayexalate** Exchanges sodium for potassium.	May require up to 4 hours to take effect.
	Calcium Gluconate 10% Counteracts potassium-induced increased myocardial irritability.	Monitor for ECG changes. Intravenous infiltration may result in tissue necrosis.
	Albuterol Beta agonist effects cause potassium to be shifted into the cells.	Give by aerosol.
Metabolic acidosis	**Sodium Bicarbonate or Sodium Citrate** Helps correct metabolic acidosis by exchanging hydrogen for potassium.	*Do not mix with calcium.* Complications include fluid overload, hypertension, and tetany.
Hypocalcemia (< 2.2 mmol/L)	**Calcium Gluconate 10%** Used in presence of tetany; provides ionized calcium to restore nervous tissue function to control serum phosphorus.	Administer slowly to prevent bradycardia. Monitor for ECG changes.
Malignant hypertension (blood pressure > 95% for age, sex, and height percentile)	**Sodium Nitroprusside, Nitroglycerin** Relaxes smooth muscle in peripheral arterioles.	Administer by continuous intravenous infusion; fall in blood pressure is seen within 10–20 minutes.

Nursing Practice

Nephrotoxic drugs include the following:

- Antimicrobials: aminoglycosides, cephalosporins, tetracycline, sulfonamides
- Radiographic contrast media with iodine (typically used for CT scans)
- Heavy metals: lead, barium, iron
- Nonsteroidal anti-inflammatory drugs: indomethacin, aspirin, ibuprofen

hemolytic-uremic syndrome or acute glomerulonephritis may be associated with residual kidney damage.

NURSING MANAGEMENT

NURSING ASSESSMENT AND DIAGNOSES

A complete history and physical examination are necessary to identify progression of symptoms and possible causes of renal failure.

PHYSIOLOGIC ASSESSMENT

Assess vital signs, level of consciousness, and other neurologic indicators to help identify clinical signs of electrolyte imbalance (see "Clinical Manifestations: Electrolyte Imbalances in Acute and Chronic Renal Failure" on page 1588). Measure the child's weight on admission to provide a baseline for evaluating changes in fluid status. Monitor urinalysis, urine culture, and blood chemistry studies. Inspect urine for color, specific gravity, amount, and odor. Cloudy urine may indicate infection; tea-colored urine suggests hematuria.

PSYCHOSOCIAL ASSESSMENT

The unexpected and acute nature of the child's hospitalization creates anxiety for both parents and child. Assess for feelings of anger, guilt, or fear associated with the hospitalization. Such feelings are likely if ARF developed as a result of dehydration, a preventable injury, or poisoning. Assess coping mechanisms, family support systems, and level of stress.

Several nursing diagnoses may apply to the child with ARF, including the following:

- *Ineffective Renal Tissue Perfusion* related to hypovolemia, sepsis, or drug toxicity
- *Excess Fluid Volume* related to renal dysfunction and sodium retention

MyNursingKit Care Plan: Child with Kidney Failure

- *Imbalanced Nutrition: Less than Body Requirements* related to anorexia, nausea, vomiting, and catabolic state
- *Risk for Infection* related to invasive procedures and monitoring equipment, and diminished immune functioning
- *Compromised Family Coping* related to sudden hospitalization and uncertain prognosis of child

PLANNING AND IMPLEMENTATION

Nursing care focuses on preventing complications, maintaining fluid balance, administering medications, meeting nutritional needs, preventing infection, and providing emotional support to the child and parents.

PREVENT COMPLICATIONS

Complications are best prevented by ensuring compliance with the treatment plan. Careful monitoring of vital signs, intake and output, serum electrolytes, and level of consciousness can alert the nurse to changes that indicate potential complications.

MAINTAIN FLUID BALANCE

Estimate the child's fluid status by daily monitoring intake and output and blood pressure two or three times daily. Also obtain a weight at least daily on the same scale at the same time of day. Monitor serum chemistry values, especially for sodium and potassium. The aim of maintaining fluid balance is to achieve a stable serum sodium concentration and a decrease in body weight by 0.5% to 1% a day.

If the child has oliguria, limit fluid intake, including parenteral nutrition, to replacement of insensible fluid loss (excreted by the lungs, skin, and gastrointestinal tract), which is about one third the daily maintenance requirements in afebrile children. If the child is febrile, fluid administration is increased by 12% for each centigrade degree of temperature elevation. The child with **renal insufficiency** (decrease in the kidney's ability to conserve sodium and concentrate urine) is at greater risk for fluid loss with illness. In cases of acute gastrointestinal illness, children are at greater risk for dehydration.

ADMINISTER MEDICATIONS

Because the kidney's ability to excrete drugs is impaired in ARF, dosages of all medications should be adjusted. The actual dosage of the drug can be reduced or the time interval between doses may be increased. Check drug levels to monitor for drug toxicity and know the signs of drug toxicity for each medication the child is receiving.

MEET NUTRITIONAL NEEDS

Children are at risk for malnutrition because of their high metabolic rate during ARF. Parenteral or enteral feeding may be used initially to minimize protein catabolism. The diet is tailored to the individual child's need for calories, carbohydrates, fats, and amino acids or protein hydrolysates. Depending on the degree of renal failure, sodium, potassium, and phosphorus may be restricted. Initiate oral feeding as soon as tolerated.

> **Developing Cultural Competence**
>
> **REDUCING SODIUM IN THE CHILD'S DIET**
>
> Special effort is often needed to reduce the sodium in the diet of an Asian child. Sauces and seasonings for foods (soy sauce, mustards, monosodium glutamate, and garlic salt) are sodium rich even though the foods seasoned (rice, vegetables, shrimp, and chicken) are low in sodium. The child may ingest up to 18 grams of sodium a day with these added sauces and seasonings; 4 grams per day is the goal. The typical Mexican diet, high in sodium and potassium (avocados, tomatoes, beans), may also require significant modification. Individualized counseling and motivation are needed to encourage families to reduce the child's sodium intake and to use spices low in sodium when preparing meals.

PREVENT INFECTION

The child with ARF is extremely susceptible to hospital-acquired infections because of altered nutritional status, compromised immunity, and numerous invasive procedures. Thorough hand hygiene and standard precautions are imperative to decrease the risk of infection. Use sterile technique for all invasive procedures and when caring for lines. Drainage from catheter sites should be cultured to check for the presence of infectious organisms. Assess vital signs and lung sounds frequently.

PROVIDE EMOTIONAL SUPPORT

The sudden onset of ARF presents parents with an unexpected threat to their child's life. Both the child and the parents experience anxiety because of the unexpected hospitalization and the uncertainty of the prognosis. Parents often feel guilty, regardless of the cause of renal failure. Guilt is intensified if the parents feel there is something they could have done to prevent the condition. Encourage parents to verbalize their fears and help them work through feelings of guilt. Explain procedures and treatment measures to decrease anxiety. Encouraging parents and older siblings to participate in the child's care can increase their sense of control.

DISCHARGE PLANNING AND HOME CARE TEACHING

Encourage parental involvement early in the child's hospitalization. Be sure parents understand the importance of administering medications correctly. Teach family members proper technique for measuring blood pressure so they can monitor the child's hypertension, if ordered. Make sure the parents can identify signs of progressive renal failure (see the following chronic renal failure discussion).

Diet counseling is a key component of discharge planning and is usually performed by a renal nutritionist. Depending on the degree of renal failure, the child's diet may include restrictions on protein, water, sodium, potassium, and phosphorus. The parents should be given written guidelines listing appropriate food choices to assist in menu planning. Ethnic and cultural preferences should be considered in listing menu options.

Continued monitoring of renal function during follow-up examinations is critical as deterioration may occur over time. Referral to support groups can be helpful for both parents and children. The National Kidney Foundation is a source of numerous publications that are helpful to the child and family.

EVALUATION

Expected outcomes of nursing care include:

- Restoration of kidney function
- Restoration and maintenance of fluid, electrolyte, and acid–base balance
- Adequate nutritional intake to promote growth and development
- Reduced risk for secondary infection

CHRONIC RENAL FAILURE

Chronic renal failure (CRF) is a progressive, irreversible reduction in kidney function. The prevalence of CRF in children is approximately 18 per 1 million (Vogt & Avner, 2007b).

Etiology and Pathophysiology

In children, CRF usually results from developmental abnormalities of the kidney or obstructed urine flow and reflux, hereditary diseases such as polycystic kidney disease, infections such as hemolytic-uremic syndrome, and glomerulonephritis (Lum, 2007).

The gradual, progressive loss of functioning nephrons ultimately results in **end-stage renal disease (ESRD)**, the most advanced form of CRF. ESRD is characterized by minimal renal function (less than 10% of normal), uremic syndrome, anemia, and abnormal blood values. In ESRD, the kidneys can no longer maintain homeostasis and the child requires dialysis.

The kidneys excrete excess acid in the body and regulate the body's fluid and electrolyte balance. Renal failure disrupts this fluid and electrolyte balance. As renal failure progresses, metabolic acidosis occurs because the kidneys cannot excrete the acids that build up in the body. Renal osteodystrophy occurs as the kidneys are unable to produce activated vitamin D and to excrete phosphorus, causing phosphorus levels to rise and serum calcium levels to fall. The parathyroid gland responds by drawing calcium and phosphorus from the bones to maintain the adequate serum calcium and phosphorus levels. Hypocalcemia may occur as the parathyroid glands become less responsive to vitamin D and lower serum calcium levels (Legg, 2005). Growth retardation is caused by disturbances in the metabolism of calcium, phosphorus, and vitamin D; decreased caloric intake; and metabolic acidosis. Healthy kidneys also produce erythropoietin (the growth factor responsible for the production and maturation of red cells); lack of erythropoietin and progressive renal disease are the underlying causes of the anemia of CRF.

Clinical Manifestations

Children with CRF frequently have no symptoms initially. Early renal failure with a glomerular filtration rate (GFR) of 50% to 75% of normal has few or no clinical signs. As progression continues, renal insufficiency occurs with polyuria as the kidneys cannot concentrate the urine. Symptoms such as pallor, headache, nausea, and fatigue become more classic as CRF progresses. Decreased mental alertness and ability to concentrate may be seen. The child may have anemia leading to tachycardia, tachypnea, and dyspnea on exertion. The child loses his or her appetite and has complications of renal impairment, including hypertension, pulmonary edema, growth retardation, osteodystrophy, delayed fine and gross motor development, and delayed sexual maturation. See the contrast with signs of acute renal failure on page 1586.

In ESRD, renal failure adversely affects all body systems. As the severity of the clinical and biochemical disturbances resulting from progressive renal deterioration increases, uremic symptoms develop. Signs and symptoms of uremic syndrome include nausea and vomiting, progressive anemia, anorexia, dyspnea, malaise, *uremic frost* (urea crystals deposited on the skin), unpleasant (uremic) breath odor, headache, progressive confusion, tremors, pulmonary edema, and congestive heart failure.

Clinical Therapy

Laboratory evaluation, including serum electrolytes, phosphate, BUN, and creatinine levels and pH, is used to confirm the diagnosis of CRF. An early morning urine sample is collected for culture, and to calculate the protein-to-creatinine ratio. The child's glomerular filtration rate is calculated from prediction equations using the serum creatinine level and the patient's height and gender. Imaging studies are performed to identify renal diseases that could be causing the renal failure. A renal biopsy may sometimes be performed.

CRF is irreversible. However, the course of the disease is variable. Some children progress quickly to renal failure, necessitating dialysis. Other children are managed with a combination of medication and diet therapy for some time before significant renal impairment occurs. Frequent modifications in the treatment plan are often necessary to address the child's changing status. Dietary management focuses on maximizing caloric intake for growth while limiting phosphorus, potassium, and sodium intake as needed to maintain electrolytes in balance (Vogt & Avner, 2007b). Adequate calcium needs to be part of the meal plan. Enteral or parenteral feedings may be required to achieve optimal protein intake, especially in children under 1 year of age. When CRF is present, extra high-quality protein such as meat, fish, poultry, milk, and eggs is needed to support growth. Optimal protein intake for children is 2.5 g/kg/day (Vogt & Avner, 2007b). Complex carbohydrates should be chosen along with vegetables and fruits that are lower in potassium. Vegetable oils, hard candy, sugar, honey, and jelly may be recommended to add calories to the child's diet. (See "Complementary Care: Avoiding Herbal Supplements in Children with CRF".)

Medications used to treat children with CRF are discussed in the Drug Guide on page 1592.

MyNursingKit Case Study: A Child with Chronic Kidney Failure

Drug Guide

MEDICATIONS COMMONLY USED BY CHILDREN WITH CHRONIC RENAL FAILURE

MEDICATION AND ACTION/INDICATION	NURSING IMPLICATIONS
Vitamin and Mineral Supplement (Nephrocaps) Adds vitamins and minerals missing from heavily restricted diet.	Only prescribed vitamins should be used; over-the-counter brands may contain elements that are harmful.
Phosphate Binding Agents: Calcium Carbonate (Tums), Calcium Acetate (PhosLo), or Sevelamer Hydrochloride (Renagel) Reduces absorption of phosphorus from the intestines.	Ensure that phosphate binding agent is aluminum-free.
Calcitriol (Rocaltrol) Replaces the calcitriol that kidneys are no longer producing to keep calcium balance normal.	Monitor serum calcium level. Ensure that calcium supplement is provided.
Epoetin Alfa (Epogen, Procrit) Stimulates bone marrow to produce red blood cells, treats anemia due to CRF.	Given by IV or subcutaneous injection. Monitor blood pressure as hypertension is an adverse effect. Monitor hematocrit and serum ferritin level according to facility guidelines.
Iron Supplementation Treats iron deficiency when epoetin alfa is prescribed.	May be administered orally or IV during hemodialysis.
Growth Hormone (rhGH) Used to stimulate growth in children with CRF.	Record accurate height measurements at regular intervals.
Antihypertensive Agents: Angiotensin-Converting Enzyme (ACE) Inhibitor (Enalapril, Lisinopril) Used with proteinuric kidney disease as it slows the progression to ESRD.	Monitor renal function and electrolyte balance.
Loop diuretics Used when volume overload is present.	

Complementary Care

AVOIDING HERBAL SUPPLEMENTS IN CHILDREN WITH CHRONIC RENAL FAILURE

Herbal supplements should not be used in children with CRF as they may contain harmful minerals, such as potassium, or they are toxic to the kidneys. The child with CRF is unable to clear waste products from the body like a healthy child. There is also the risk for interaction between the herbs and other medications taken that could place the child at risk for rejection of a transplanted kidney (National Kidney Foundation, 2009). Parents should discuss with the physician the use of any over-the-counter (OTC) or complementary therapies.

Children who progress to ESRD require renal replacement therapy. The timetable for dialysis or renal transplantation is different from that of adults; transplantation is the goal so the child has an optimal chance for a more normal childhood. Earlier initiation can prevent some complications of ESRD. In addition to the GFR, nonspecific signs such as uremic syndrome, poorly controlled hypertension, renal osteodystrophy, failure of head circumference measurement to increase normally, developmental delay, and poor growth are used in determining when to initiate therapy. (Refer to the "Renal Replacement Therapy" section in this chapter.) Infection is a common cause of hospitalization in children receiving renal replacement therapy (Chavers, Solid, Gilbertson, et al., 2007).

NURSING MANAGEMENT

NURSING ASSESSMENT AND DIAGNOSES

Nursing assessment focuses on identifying signs and symptoms of renal failure and associated complications as well as assessing the psychosocial effects of renal failure on the child and family.

PHYSIOLOGIC ASSESSMENT

The initial and ongoing assessment of the child focuses on identifying complications of renal failure. Observe for signs of hypertension, edema, poor growth and development, osteodystrophy, and anemia. Assess vital signs, particularly the blood pressure. Observe for signs of alterations in electrolyte balance (see page 1588).

PSYCHOSOCIAL ASSESSMENT

As renal disease progresses, the number of stressors on the child and family increases. Denial and disbelief are commonly the first reactions. A thorough family assessment can help to identify particular needs of the child and family (see Appendix G∞). The development of ESRD is particularly challenging during childhood and adolescence because of differences in appearance and social, psychological, and physical issues. Nonadherence to treatments can endanger the adolescent's life.

Nursing diagnoses for the child with CRF are similar to those previously listed for ARF. Additional diagnoses might include the following:

- *Delayed Growth and Development* related to decreased protein and caloric intake and loss of protein in dialysate
- *Impaired Social Interaction* related to impaired immunity and hemodialysis schedule during school hours
- *Activity Intolerance* related to anemia and fatigue
- *Ineffective Therapeutic Regimen Management* related to complexity of care plan and economic difficulties
- *Disturbed Body Image* related to short stature and visible external catheter for dialysis

PLANNING AND IMPLEMENTATION

Children with CRF are usually hospitalized for one or more of the following reasons: initial diagnostic evaluation, dialysis treatment initiation, problems with the treatment plan or infection. Nursing care for the hospitalized child with CRF focuses on monitoring for side effects of medications, preventing infection, meeting nutritional needs, and providing emotional support and anticipatory teaching.

MONITOR FOR SIDE EFFECTS OF MEDICATIONS

Assess for signs of electrolyte imbalance such as weakness, muscle cramps, dizziness, headache, and nausea and vomiting in children who are taking diuretics. Supervise the child's activities closely to prevent falls resulting from dizziness, especially at the beginning of diuretic therapy. If antihypertensive medications such as hydralazine are being administered, monitor the child's weight to detect excessive gain resulting from water and sodium retention.

PREVENT INFECTION

The child with CRF is susceptible to infections. Be alert for signs of infection, such as elevated temperature; cloudy, strong-smelling urine; dysuria; changes in respiratory pattern; or productive cough. Emphasize to the child and family the importance of good hand hygiene practices. Make sure the child receives the 23-valent pneumococcal vaccine and meningococcal vaccines in addition to usual childhood immunizations.

MEET NUTRITIONAL NEEDS

Maintaining adequate nutritional intake in a child with CRF who has dietary restrictions is challenging. Provide small, frequent feedings and present meals attractively to encourage the child to eat. A nutritionist works with the child and family to develop meal plans that meet the nutritional requirements and acknowledge the child's preferences. See Table 54–5 for foods that children with CRF should avoid.

MAINTAIN FLUID RESTRICTIONS

Plan the child's oral intake through the entire 24 hours to ensure that the child has some fluids with meals, to take medications, and when thirsty. Keep in mind that many foods have a high fluid content (gelatin, popsicles) and must be counted toward the daily fluid allowance. Use medicine cups or small cups for fluids given. Encourage parents and visitors to avoid drinking in the child's presence. Ensure that all visitors know and understand the importance of maintaining the child's fluid restriction.

PROVIDE EMOTIONAL SUPPORT

Progressive CRF requires a total lifestyle change for the child and family. The parents and child need opportunities to express and work through their feelings related to the disease, prognosis, and

Table 54–5 Nutritional Information for the Child with Kidney Disease

Children with kidney disease have restricted diets, generally low in sodium, potassium, and phosphorus. A renal dietitian works with families of children with chronic renal failure to develop meal plans that fit a restricted diet. The nurse can help families remember that certain foods must be avoided or eaten in very small quantities by reviewing this table.

High-Sodium Content Foods	High-Potassium Content Foods	High-Phosphorus Content Foods
Soups and sauces: e.g., gravy, spaghetti and tomato sauce, barbeque sauce, steak sauce *Processed lunchmeats:* e.g., bologna, ham, salami, hot dogs *Smoked meat and fish:* bacon, chipped beef, corned beef, ham, lox Sauerkraut, pickles, and other pickled foods *Seasonings:* horseradish, soy sauce, Worcestershire sauce, meat tenderizer, and monosodium glutamate (MSG)	*Fruit:* apricots, avocados, bananas, citrus fruits, fresh pears, nectarines, dates, figs, cantaloupe and other melons, prunes, and raisins *Vegetables:* celery, dried beans, lima beans, potatoes, leafy greens, spinach, tomatoes, winter squash *Whole grains:* especially those containing bran Sardines, clams Peanuts *Dairy products:* milk, ice cream, pudding, yogurt Potassium-containing salt substitutes	*Dairy products:* milk, cheese, yogurt, custard, pudding, ice cream Dried beans, peas Nuts, peanut butter Chocolate Dark cola Sausage, hot dogs

treatment restrictions. Help children express their feelings through drawings or therapeutic play.

The need for ongoing dialysis treatments and the wait for a suitable donor kidney are stressful for both parents and children. Identify effective coping methods and family support systems to promote treatment compliance. The National Kidney Foundation and local support groups for kidney disease can give the family information or additional support.

DISCHARGE PLANNING AND HOME CARE TEACHING

Parents need to understand the necessity of long-term treatments and follow-up care. Help the family develop a schedule for medication administration that fits with their routine. Emphasize the importance of consistency in administration times. Teach parents how to recognize medication side effects and complications.

Appropriate referrals are made to home care nursing agencies as indicated. Parents of children receiving peritoneal dialysis at home are taught how to perform the treatment and how to identify complications. Strict aseptic technique is necessary to prevent infection at the catheter site and peritonitis.

NURSING CARE IN THE COMMUNITY

Children with CRF require frequent outpatient visits to monitor the progression of signs and symptoms, and to evaluate the effectiveness of current treatments. The blood pressure is monitored. Blood and urine tests are performed to monitor renal function. Radiographs of the bones are often taken at 6-month intervals to assess changes caused by osteodystrophy. See "Health Promotion: The Child with Chronic Renal Failure" on page 1596.

Encourage parents to register the young child for the Early Intervention Program to promote development and interaction with other children. The dialysis schedule for school-age children should enable the child to participate in school or home tutoring should be provided.

School-age children and adolescents are often embarrassed about being seen as different from peers. Ask the child how he or she feels about the need to follow a special diet, take medications, and undergo dialysis treatments. To minimize the psychological consequences of coping with a chronic disease, encourage parents to promote the child's participation in age-appropriate activities. Attendance at school and contacts with peers promote normal growth and development. Work to promote the child's self-worth and a healthy self-esteem. Encourage adolescents to participate in a program that helps them transition to adult health services and job skill training. Begin teaching the child during early adolescence about the health condition, medications taken and their actions, how to access emergency help, and problems caused by nonadherence to treatment. As the adolescent ages, have the family begin giving more responsibility for self-care, such as making appointments for healthcare, obtaining prescription refills, and seeking out adult healthcare professionals and a dialysis program. (See "Evidence-Based Nursing: Living with End-Stage Renal Disease.") Give the parents timely information about the disease process, dialysis treatments, and issues related to renal transplantation, as the child's renal impairment progresses.

EVALUATION

Expected outcomes of nursing care include:

- Maintenance of fluid balance
- Nutritional needs with adherence to dietary restrictions
- Growth and developmental milestones are achieved.

RENAL REPLACEMENT THERAPY

Renal replacement therapy is the treatment for renal failure and includes both dialysis and renal transplantation. The preferred method of dialysis is generally dependent on the age of the child. Currently 88% of children 5 years of age and younger are treated with peritoneal dialysis, while 54% of children older than 12 years of age are treated with hemodialysis (Vogt & Avner, 2007b). The use of hemodialysis in children less than 19 years of age has increased over the past several years (Warady & Chada, 2007). Up to 87% of children with ESRD have had a kidney transplant within 5 years of diagnosis (United States Renal Data System, 2008).

Peritoneal Dialysis

In peritoneal dialysis the peritoneum of the abdomen is the membrane through which the body's waste products pass from the blood to the abdominal cavity. A catheter is inserted through the abdominal wall into the peritoneal cavity. In children receiving peritoneal dialysis for ARF, a percutaneously placed catheter can be used for a few weeks. In children with CRF, a catheter is placed surgically for long-term use. The dialysis solution (**dialysate**) that enters the abdomen typically contains dextrose that pulls body wastes and extra fluid into the abdominal cavity. These wastes and extra fluid leave the body with the drained dialysate. This method of dialysis is beneficial to small children since it allows continuous removal of fluids and waste products, decreasing the toxic effects of waste products on the child's developing body. The child can ambulate and interact with the environment. The timing of the treatment can be set to minimize the interruption of school, play, or other social events.

Two types of peritoneal dialysis are commonly used: continuous ambulatory peritoneal dialysis (CAPD) and automated peritoneal dialysis (APD). Graduated cylinders are used to monitor the volume of fluid exchanged.

- Continuous ambulatory peritoneal dialysis (CAPD) uses gravity to instill prefilled bags of dialysate into the peritoneal cavity four or five times a day. The fluid remains in the cavity for 4 to 8 hours. An attached bag is folded under the child's clothes, permitting normal activity. After the allotted time, the dialysate is drained by hanging the bag lower than the pelvis. The repeated connections and disconnections with this method are time consuming for the child and family and increase the risk of infection.

Evidence-Based Nursing

LIVING WITH END-STAGE RENAL DISEASE

Clinical Question

End-stage renal disease is a serious chronic condition that requires significant adaptations in lifestyle and complex medical treatments that take a toll on the child and family. What is the impact of the condition on children and adolescents?

The Evidence

A study of 38 children (19 with predialysis chronic renal failure [CRF] and 19 on hemodialysis) ranging in age from 9 to 15 years, found that 52% of these children had some type of psychiatric disorder. Adjustment disorders, depression, and neurocognitive disorders, respectively, were identified as the most common disorders. Of the children in the study in which a psychiatric order was identified, those on dialysis were more likely (68.4%) to have a psychiatric disorder than those with predialysis CRF (36.8%) (Bakr, Amr, Sarhan, et al., 2007).

A study of 35 adolescents, aged 13 to 18 years, with end-stage renal disease was conducted to identify strategies used to help them cope with their illness. Twenty-two hospitalized adolescents and 13 adolescents attending camp for dialysis/transplant patients served as participants for this study. A self-report tool, the A-COPE, designed to evaluate coping strategies used by adolescents, was used for this study. Listening to music was identified by a majority of the adolescents as a strategy they used most of the time to help them cope. Strategies that were used sometimes by the teens included talking with parents, use of anger and yelling to vent feelings, and trying to help others with their problems. The study also found that the older the adolescent, the less likely they were to get angry and vent their feelings. In addition, the older the adolescent, the less likely they were to use avoidance behaviors such as drugs and alcohol use to escape their problems. This could be related to the use of more coping strategies and increased independence in older adolescents (Snethen, Broome, Kelber, et al., 2004).

Best Practice

Effects of chronic illness in children and adolescents can be both physically and psychosocially overwhelming. Children and adolescents who develop end-stage renal disease are expected to develop skills to cope with the consequences of the illness. Complications and exacerbations of chronic illness directly affect the child's participation in activities with peers, making it more difficult for them to cope and develop socially (Snethen et al., 2004). It is common for children and adolescents with chronic renal disease to develop feelings of anger, fear, depression, and denial. This illness can lead not only to delays in psychomotor development but to delays in growth as well. Because of the expenses associated with this illness, parents may have difficulties providing nourishment needed to maximize growth in these children (Terrill, 2007).

Parents must modify lifestyles and their hopes and dreams for their child's future. Strategies for managing the disease differ for every family. These families view their lives and their child as different from other families because of the child's condition. Development of effective coping strategies is essential if the child is to effectively manage living with this illness. Nurses can facilitate development of these coping strategies by encouraging children and adolescents to express their feelings about the illness and the restraints it places on their lifestyle. Nurses can ensure that distraction techniques such as music are utilized for these patients to listen to when they are in the hospital or in the dialysis center receiving treatment.

Children who are having difficulty coping with their chronic illness need to be identified early so that they may receive counseling and psychiatric help if needed. Nurses can be effective in working with families by listening to the issues and offering suggestions. Often the opportunity to talk through the child's management plan will help the family consider different strategies that may be effective. The nurse may also provide linkages to community resources that may help the family.

Critical Thinking

Initiate a discussion with an older school-age child or adolescent with end-stage renal disease; listen to their description of living with the condition. Develop a nursing care plan to help the child take the next steps in self-management.

See MyNursingKit for possible responses.

- Automated peritoneal dialysis uses an automatic cycler to instill and drain the dialysate about five times over a 10-hour period, usually overnight. One additional exchange may be needed during the day. With this method the number of connections and disconnections is minimized, which reduces demands on the family as well as the risk of infection. Of the peritoneal dialysis types, this method is used most often in children (Warady & Chada, 2007). The primary complications of peritoneal dialysis are peritonitis and abdominal hernia. (See Table 54–6, "Complications of Peritoneal Dialysis.")

Nursing Practice

The predominant sign of peritonitis associated with peritoneal dialysis is cloudy dialysate. Other signs and symptoms may include fever, vomiting, diarrhea, abdominal pain, and tenderness. The nurse monitors for these symptoms and ensures that the child and family can recognize the symptoms and report them immediately.

Teach the family to perform peritoneal dialysis and to use sterile technique when performing dialysis and when doing catheter care. Peritoneal dialysis is time consuming, and family members must be committed to managing this procedure daily. Help the family develop home routines that minimize disruptions to daily family life. For additional information, refer to "Nursing Care Plan: The Child Receiving Home Peritoneal Dialysis."

HEALTH PROMOTION

THE CHILD WITH CHRONIC RENAL FAILURE

Growth and Development Surveillance

- Compare the child's height, weight, and head circumference to age-specific norms to identify growth retardation and to plot progress.
- Assess developmental progress using the Denver II or another screening tool (refer to Chapter 37∞).
- Educate parents on normal developmental milestones and measures to promote achieving those milestones.
- Assess the adolescent for signs of delayed sexual maturation and, in girls, amenorrhea.

Nutrition

- Review the dietary restrictions with the child and parents.
- Partner with the family to assist the child to make food selections and to restrict fluids and sodium as necessary, taking into account the child's likes and dislikes and cultural background. Encourage the child and family to take a list of a few favorite foods to the dietitian to see if they can be integrated into the child's meal plan.
- Make meal time pleasant and make foods taste more appealing with permitted spices.
- Discuss possible behavioral responses by older children and adolescents to dietary restrictions and limitations imposed by the treatment plan. Involve the child and adolescent in discussions about dietary restrictions, and when possible integrate their recommendations for dietary restrictions and fluid management throughout the day.
- Emphasize to the school-age child that dietary and other restrictions are not punishment.
- Use enteral feeding at night to provide the needed calories for growth.

Physical Activity

- Encourage child to participate in developmentally appropriate activities as tolerated.
- Partner with the child to establish a routine plan for physical activity as tolerated that will help promote strong bones.

Oral Health

- Promote good dentition and oral hygiene.
- Schedule regular dental visits for examination and cleaning to reduce infections.
- Partner with the family to ensure they understand the need for antibiotic prophylaxis before certain invasive procedures, including dental care.

Mental and Spiritual Health

- Ask children how they feel about the need to follow a special diet, take medications, and undergo dialysis treatments. Ask what might make it easier for them to cope with the treatments, and integrate at least one idea into the care plan.
- Encourage parents to promote their child's participation in age-appropriate activities to minimize the psychologic consequences of coping with a chronic disease.
- Adolescents often resent the dietary restrictions and ongoing dialysis treatments, which pose a threat to their independence, evolving sense of self, and their need for independence. Noncooperation, depression, and hostility are common responses.
- Assist adolescents to begin the transition to adult health services.

Relationships

- Attendance at school and contacts with peers promote normal growth and development.
- Work to promote the child's self-worth and a healthy self-esteem.
- Prepare the child for peer conflict.
- Ensure that parents understand the importance of encouraging normal socialization of their child.

Disease Prevention Strategies

- Partner with the child and family to establish plans to avoid large crowds, people with infections, or other risks that expose the child to infection.
- If possible, all immunizations should be provided before renal transplantation, as long-term immunosuppressive therapy will then be prescribed.
- Live vaccines should not be given to the child taking immunosuppressive agents.
- Encourage the family to maintain scheduled appointments for routine serum and urine diagnostic tests performed to monitor renal function.

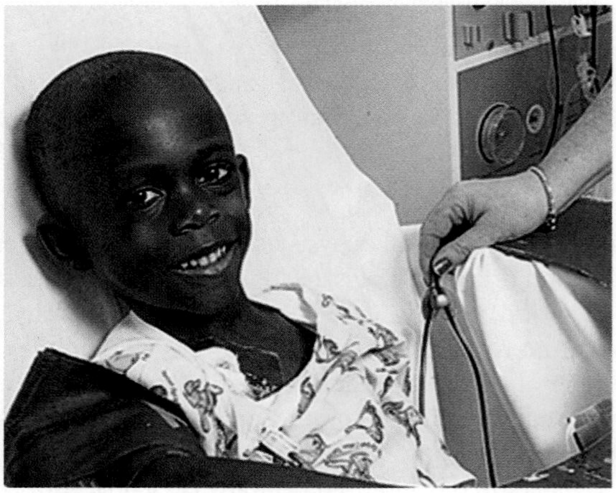

Table 54–6 Complications of Peritoneal Dialysis

Complications and Manifestations	Cause
PERITONITIS	
Cloudy dialysate, abdominal pain, tenderness, leukocytosis, fever (neonatal hypothermia), constipation	*Staphylococcus aureus, Staphylococcus epidermidis,* fungal infections, gram-negative rods (risk is proportional to duration of dialysis and inversely proportional to age)
PAIN	
During inflow	Too rapid a rate of infusion, too large a volume of dialysate, encasement of catheter in a false passage, extremes in temperature of dialysate
During outflow at end of emptying	Omentum entering catheter at end of outflow
LEAKAGE	
Fluid around catheter, edema of penis or scrotum secondary to leakage into abdominal subcutaneous tissue, fluid leakage to pleural spaces through diaphragm	Overfilling of abdomen, catheter that has migrated from peritoneal cavity
RESPIRATORY SYMPTOMS	
Shortness of breath, decreased breath sounds in lower lobes, inadequate chest expansion	Abdominal fullness that compromises diaphragm movement, hole in diaphragm allowing dialysate into chest cavity

Hemodialysis

Hemodialysis is a process in which the blood flows from the patient through a machine with a special filter that removes body wastes and extra fluids. Blood is pumped out of the body and through a dialyzer, where waste products and extra fluids diffuse out across a semipermeable membrane, before the blood is returned to the body. Dialysate is pumped in the direction opposite blood flow to promote waste extraction. Differences in osmolarity and concentration between the child's blood and the dialysate alter the intravascular electrolyte concentration and reduce the intravascular volume.

Hemodialysis is used in the critical care setting and for those children with CRF when peritoneal dialysis is not possible for technical reasons, after repeated peritonitis, or when the family is unable to provide peritoneal dialysis safely. Hemodialysis for children is offered in a special dialysis center on an outpatient basis, or it can be performed at bedside during hospitalization. Treatment is usually performed three times a week, with each session lasting approximately 3 to 4 hours.

Children over 20 kg (44 lb) often have an arteriovenous (AV) fistula (connection between an artery and a vein) created for long-term vascular access. Alternatively, a synthetic tube can be implanted under the skin creating a graft between the arterial and venous circulation to provide vascular access. Two needles are inserted into the arteriovenous fistula or the graft: one to carry blood to the dialyzer and one to return cleaned blood to the body. In emergencies and for infants, a double-lumen cannula is inserted into a large vein (e.g., the femoral, jugular, or subclavian vein) for hemodialysis.

Hemodialysis is more efficient than peritoneal dialysis but requires close monitoring for symptoms related to hypotension or rapid changes in fluid and electrolyte balance. Uncommonly, a **disequilibrium syndrome** (rapid changes in the body's water and electrolyte balance during treatment) may occur during or soon after the dialysis procedure is first initiated. Other complications include access thrombosis and infection. Heparin is used to reduce the risk of thrombosis.

Nursing management focuses on care of the child during dialysis and teaching the child and family about the administration of heparin and the control of bleeding from minor trauma.

Thinking Critically

THE CHILD ON HEMODIALYSIS

Terrell, who is now 5 years old, was born with posterior urethral valves, which caused damage to his kidneys. Despite undergoing surgery to correct the defect during infancy, his kidney function continued to deteriorate. End-stage renal disease was diagnosed 2 years ago, and dialysis treatment was initiated. Terrell requires a kidney transplant, but in the meantime he is being treated with hemodialysis. He visits the dialysis center three afternoons a week for treatments lasting approximately 3 to 4 hours. This schedule permits him to attend kindergarten classes in the morning.

At his scheduled visit to the nephrologist, Terrell has gained weight and is edematous. In talking with him, the nurse discovers that Terrell has been drinking Cokes and eating "junk food" at school. Terrell asks the nurse not to tell his mother because she will be mad, but that he just can't help eating and drinking what he isn't supposed to.

How does Terrell's growth and development level affect his adherence to the treatment regimen? What is the immediate intervention for the nurse to take with Terrell? What approach does the nurse take with discussing this nutritional issue with the family?

See MyNursingKit for possible responses.

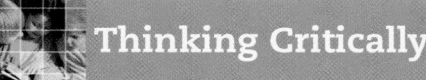

Nursing Care Plan

THE CHILD RECEIVING HOME PERITONEAL DIALYSIS

INTERVENTION	RATIONALE	EXPECTED OUTCOME
1. Nursing Diagnosis: Imbalanced Nutrition: Less than Body Requirements related to poor appetite, feeling of fullness after a small amount, and loss of protein in dialysate		
NIC Priority Intervention: **Nutrition management:** Assistance with or provision of a balanced dietary intake of foods and fluids		**NOC Suggested Outcome:** **Nutrition status:** Food and fluid intake: Amount of food and fluid taken into the body over a 24-hour period
Goal: The child will obtain adequate nutrients each day.		
■ Develop a meal plan in collaboration with a nutritionist to identify the amounts of essential nutrients needed.	■ Parents need concrete guidelines for food preparation.	The child's intake is adequate for an expected growth pattern to be maintained.
■ Provide small, frequent meals of needed nutrients.	■ The child will feel full with smaller amounts of food because of the dialysate.	
■ Make mealtimes pleasant and avoid battles over the child's intake.	■ The child will be more inclined to eat if there is less stress.	
■ Provide supplements by tube feeding if adequate oral intake is not possible.	■ Adequate nutrition is important for growth and development, and must be supported if oral intake is inadequate.	
2. Nursing Diagnosis: Risk for Infection related to daily invasive procedure		
NIC Priority Intervention: **Infection control:** Minimizing the acquisition and transmission of infectious agents		**NOC Suggested Outcome:** **Infection status:** Presence and extent of infection
Goal: The child will not develop peritonitis.		
■ Wash hands, use sterile gloves and aseptic technique for connection and disconnection of catheters.	■ Aseptic technique reduces chance of introducing bacteria into the abdomen.	The child does not develop peritonitis.
■ Perform daily catheter site care.	■ Skin around the catheter site will have fewer organisms that could potentially cause infection.	
Goal: If peritonitis occurs, it will be treated appropriately.		
■ Observe for signs of infection (fever, abdominal pain, cloudy dialysate).	■ Early identification of infection will reduce complications.	Hospitalization will not be needed for peritonitis due to early identification and prompt treatment.
■ Report signs of infection to physician immediately.	■ Rapid intervention may reduce need for hospitalization.	
3. Nursing Diagnosis: Caregiver Role Strain related to daily dialysis treatments		
NIC Priority Intervention: **Caregiver support:** Provision of necessary information, advocacy, and support to facilitate primary patient care by someone other than a healthcare professional		**NOC Suggested Outcome:** **Caregiver performance:** Direct care: Provision by family care provider of appropriate personal and health care for a family member or significant other
Goal: The family copes with daily demands for the child's dialysis treatments.		
■ Discuss the importance of daily, consistent dialysis treatments for the child's overall health status.	■ If parents understand the need for consistent dialysis treatments, they are more likely to adhere to guidelines.	The family adheres to daily dialysis treatment guidelines.

Nursing Care Plan—continued

THE CHILD RECEIVING HOME PERITONEAL DIALYSIS

INTERVENTION	RATIONALE	EXPECTED OUTCOME
■ Collaborate with the family to identify strategies that could reduce the impact of dialysis on the family's life.	■ When the family participates in planning care, adherence is more likely.	
■ Refer the family to local support groups for emotional support, treatment strategies, and respite care.	■ Support groups may help the family develop effective coping strategies.	

Nursing Practice

Monitor the child receiving hemodialysis for complications that can occur suddenly.

- Hypotension—sudden nausea and vomiting, abdominal cramping, tachycardia, and dizziness
- Rapid fluid and electrolyte exchange—muscle cramping, nausea and vomiting, and dizziness
- Dysequilibrium syndrome—restlessness, headache, nausea and vomiting, blurred vision, muscle twitching, and altered level of consciousness

Carefully monitor fluid balance in the child undergoing hemodialysis. Check vital signs and blood pressure every half hour. Monitor oral intake and urinary output every half hour when the child is on the dialysis equipment. Weigh the child before and after the dialysis to determine any fluid imbalances that require adjustment during the next hemodialysis session.

Because fluid and dietary limitations (reduced potassium, sodium, and phosphorus containing foods) are needed more often with hemodialysis than with peritoneal dialysis, make sure the family knows how to plan and provide for the child's daily nutritional needs. Review ways to reduce the risk of infection, including the daily care of the catheter site. Encourage showering rather than tub baths. Activities such as swimming may be discouraged.

Kidney Transplantation

Kidney transplantation provides the only alternative to long-term dialysis for children with ESRD. It can normalize physiology and may let children grow normally. Because of the adverse effects on growth and development resulting from the delay of transplantation, children are given some priority over adults awaiting transplantation. Blood type compatibility between the donor and recipient is essential for a transplant to be successful. A human leukocyte antigen (HLA) system match also improves survival of the graft. A living relative donor kidney has a higher survival rate than a cadaver kidney. Children and their families are carefully screened prior to transplantation in an effort to identify problems that could lead to rejection of the kidney or infection that could be life threatening if the immune system is suppressed.

After transplantation, the child must take immunosuppressive medications such as corticosteroids, azathioprine, cyclosporine, tacrolimus, and monoclonal antibodies to suppress rejection. Immunosuppression regimens use various combinations and sequences of these drugs to reduce the incidence of acute and chronic rejection. Rejection is a major cause of transplanted kidney loss (Vogler, Wang, Brink, et al., 2007). Signs of rejection include fever, increased BUN and serum creatinine levels, pain and tenderness over the abdomen, irritability, and weight gain.

Complications of immunosuppressive therapy include opportunistic infection, lymphomas and skin cancer, and hypertension. Nonadherence to therapy is the primary cause of transplanted kidney loss in 10% to 15% of pediatric kidney transplant recipients. Nonadherence is highest among families in crises without adequate support and in adolescents who refuse or forget to take their medications, have mild cognitive impairment, or depression (Feinstein, Keich, Becker-Cohen, et al., 2005). Adherence is higher in adolescents when their parents are knowledgeable and supportive, and when they promote the adolescent to become competent in self-care. Some primary kidney diseases, such as glomerulonephritis and hemolytic-uremic syndrome, can also recur in the transplanted kidney.

Nursing management includes teaching parents about the transplantation process before it occurs to help prepare them for the experience. Discuss all aspects of the child's care that will have an impact on the family's life, including follow-up appointments, medications, and general health promotion. Monitor adherence to immunosuppression treatment at each visit in an effort to identify issues early. Teach parents about the signs of acute rejection and infection, including when and how to notify the child's physician if immediate care is required.

STRUCTURAL DEFECTS OF THE REPRODUCTIVE SYSTEM

PHIMOSIS

In **phimosis**, the foreskin over the glans penis cannot be retracted. As a result of natural adhesion, phimosis is a normal finding in uncircumcised infants and young males. Circumcision, surgical removal of the foreskin, has long been a common practice performed in some countries and cultures during the newborn period. It is performed to prevent phimosis, for ease of proper male hygiene, and to prevent urinary tract infections and penile cancer. The procedure removes the skin covering the end of the penis. Circumcision is considered comparatively safe; however, complications such as damage to the urethra and disfigurement to the penis may occur. Betamethasone cream (0.05%) applied twice daily for 4–8 weeks to the outer prepuce is an effective alternative to surgery for phimosis and has few side effects. Often the child is able to achieve foreskin retraction without surgery (Steadman & Ellsworth, 2006).

MyNursingKit Video: Circumcision

CRYPTORCHIDISM

Cryptorchidism (undescended testes) occurs when one or both testes fail to descend through the inguinal canal into the scrotum. Normally, the testes descend during the seventh to ninth month of gestation.

Cryptorchidism may be the result of a testosterone deficiency, an absent or defective testis, or a structural problem such as a narrow inguinal canal, short spermatic cord, or adhesions. This disorder occurs in 3–6% of term male infants and in 20–30% of preterm infants (Morgan & McCance, 2006).

The higher temperature in the abdomen than in the scrotum results in morphologic changes to the testis that are apparent by 18 months of age. Complications of uncorrected cryptorchidism include infertility and malignancy.

Cryptorchidism is usually detected during the newborn examination when palpation of the scrotum fails to reveal one or both testes. It is not unusual for boys with cryptorchidism to have an inguinal hernia as well. In a majority of cases, the testes descend spontaneously by 3 months of age.

Although diagnosis is made on physical examination, diagnostic studies including ultrasound, CT scan, and MRI are utilized to determine the location of the testes. A diagnostic laparoscope may also be needed to locate the testis. When neither testis can be palpated, hormonal and chromosomal evaluation may be performed to detect an intersex disorder.

If the testes do not descend spontaneously, an orchiopexy is performed at 1 year of age before further damage to the testes occurs. The timing for surgery is crucial to preserve fertility and to avoid psychological effects related to fear of castration and body-image issues in older children. With an orchiopexy an incision is made at the location of the testis, either in the abdomen or in the inguinal area. Blood vessels are disentangled to allow the testis to reach into the lower scrotum. A second incision is made in the scrotum at the point where the testis is stitched to the inside wall to keep it in place. A protective sealant that peels off in 3 to 5 days is often put over the incision. If the testis is defective or undeveloped, it may be removed surgically to decrease the risk of later malignancies and a prosthesis may be placed in the scrotum. The goals of surgery are to position the testis for future accessibility to palpation, repair of any hernia, enhance the possibility of fertility, decrease the potential susceptibility for malignancy, and provide psychological benefit of a normal-appearing scrotum. The orchiopexy also makes it easier to examine the testis for tumors. It will be extremely important to have regular testicular examinations since the risk of testicular cancer is 35 to 50 times greater in men with a history of cryptorchidism (Morgan & McCance, 2006).

Nursing Management

Preoperative nursing care includes preparing the parents and child for the procedure and addressing parents' concerns about the postsurgical outcome. Orchiopexy is often performed as an outpatient procedure. If the child is hospitalized, postoperative nursing care focuses on maintaining comfort and preventing infection. Encourage bed rest, and monitor voiding. Apply ice to the surgical area, and administer prescribed analgesics to relieve pain.

Discharge instructions should include demonstration of proper incision care. The diaper area should be cleaned well with each diaper change to decrease chances of infection. Sponge bathe the child for 2 days after surgery, and then a tub bath may be given. No medicine or ointment should be placed over the incision. Teach parents to identify signs of infection such as redness, warmth, swelling, and discharge and to notify the physician if present. Ibuprofen or acetaminophen may be given for pain. Inform parents to avoid straddling the infant across the hip and to permit no strenuous activity or straddle toy riding for 2 weeks after surgery to promote healing and to prevent injury.

INGUINAL HERNIA AND HYDROCELE

An **inguinal hernia** is a painless inguinal or scrotal swelling of variable size that occurs when abdominal tissue, such as bowel, extends into the inguinal canal. An inguinal hernia is found in 3.5% to 5% of full-term infants and 9–11% of preterm infants and occurs more often in boys than girls by a 6:1 ratio (Aiken & Oldham, 2007).

A hydrocele is a fluid-filled mass in the scrotum. The condition is found in 1% to 2% of male neonates. Most hydroceles resolve spontaneously by reabsorption by one year of age (Elder, 2007).

During fetal development a peritoneal sac precedes the testicle's descent to the scrotum. The lower sac enfolds the testis to become the tunica vaginalis, and the upper sac atrophies before birth. Fluid may become trapped in the tunica vaginalis and cause the hydrocele. When the tunica vaginalis does not atrophy, an abdominal structure may move into it. Inguinal hernias are often associated with abdominal wall defects such as exstrophy of the bladder and prune belly syndrome, and are a common occurrence with undescended testes.

Diagnosis is made by physical examination at birth or in early infancy. Palpation of the scrotum reveals a round, smooth, nontender mass, which is noted with either a hernia or hydrocele. Parents may report an intermittent bulge in the groin or swelling in the scrotum. Swelling associated with a hernia may become more apparent with straining and reduced in size when quiet or asleep.

Outpatient surgery is performed as an elective procedure at an early age (usually after 3 months of age to reduce anesthesia risks) to avoid **incarceration** (hernia cannot be reduced and circulation is impaired), which is a medical emergency. A nerve block may be given in the operating room to reduce postoperative pain. The prognosis is generally excellent. Most hydroceles

Nursing Practice

Inguinal hernias can become incarcerated when a bit of bowel becomes trapped in the inguinal opening and the blood supply is constricted. The child has an acute onset of pain, abdominal distention, vomiting, and an irreducible mass. Other findings may include an edematous, erythematosus scrotum accompanied by abdominal distension, poor feeding, and bloody stools (Aiken & Oldham, 2007). Efforts are made to reduce the hernia before surgery by sedating the child and applying firm manual pressure on the affected side. If the hernia is reduced, surgery is often performed several days later. If the hernia cannot be reduced, emergency surgery is performed (Coppola, 2005).

without inguinal hernia resolve spontaneously as the fluid reabsorbs by the time an infant is 1 to 2 years of age.

Nursing care for hydroceles and inguinal hernias include assessment, explaining the disorder and its treatment, and providing preoperative and postoperative teaching, care, and support.

The incision is covered with a protective sealant rather than a dressing. Provide pain medication as ordered. Inform parents that the scrotum may be edematous and may appear bruised after surgery. Incision care involves careful cleaning of the diaper area.

TESTICULAR TORSION

Testicular torsion is an emergency condition in which the testis suddenly rotates on its spermatic cord, cutting off its blood supply. The arteries and veins in the spermatic cord become twisted and interrupt the blood supply, leading to vascular engorgement and ischemia. Testicular torsion occurs in an estimated 1 in 4000 males before 25 years of age (Ringdahl & Teague, 2006). Often the testicles are positioned horizontally in the scrotum, a congenital anomaly known as a bell clapper deformity, which predisposes the male to this condition (Eaton, Cendron, Estrado, et al., 2005).

Manifestations include severe pain and erythema in the scrotum, nausea and vomiting, abdominal pain, and scrotal swelling that is not relieved by rest or scrotal support. The testes are tender on palpation and become edematous. The cremasteric reflex is absent. Symptoms generally start when the child is sleeping or inactive, but they can occur after trauma, sexual activity, or exercise. The affected testis is positioned higher in the scrotum than the unaffected testis because of the shortened vascular pedicle. The most commonly used tests to confirm the diagnosis of testicular torsion are Doppler ultrasonography and radionuclide imaging. One of these tests may be performed to confirm the diagnosis prior to surgery if they can be performed immediately (Ringdahl & Teague, 2006).

When testicular torsion is reduced within 6 hours after onset of symptoms, there is a 90% chance of saving the testis. Manual reduction under intravenous sedation may be attempted, but emergency surgery is more common and is the only way to ensure resolution of the problem (Ringdahl & Teague, 2006). During surgery (orchiopexy), the testis is untwisted and stitched to the side of the scrotum in the correct position. The procedure is usually performed bilaterally to prevent future torsion in the other testis. If torsion was reduced manually, elective orchiopexy is recommended to prevent recurrence (Ringdahl & Teague, 2006).

Nursing management involves psychological support for the child and family related to the need for emergency surgery and concern about the child's future fertility. Reassure parents that as only one testis is usually involved, fertility should not be affected. The child often goes home within a few hours of surgery; thus the child and family need to be taught about proper care of the incision and pain management. Explain to parents that the child should not lift heavy objects for 4 weeks or participate in strenuous activity for 2 weeks after surgery to promote healing. Teach the adolescent testicular self-examination.

See Chapter 6 for information on sexually transmitted infections.

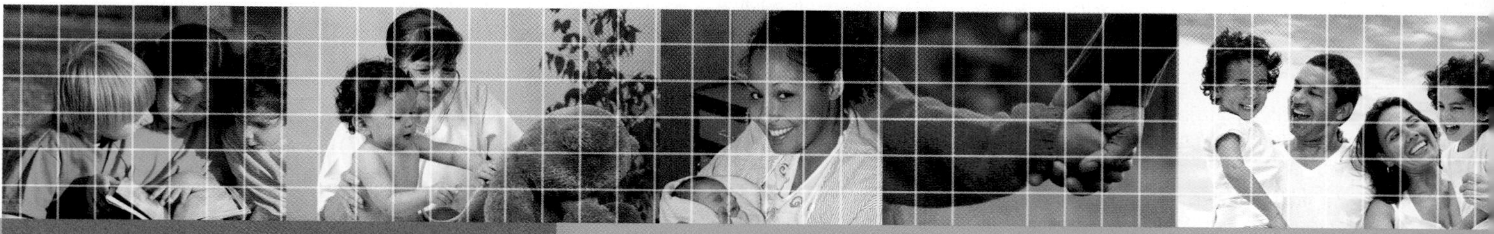

CRITICAL CONCEPT REVIEW

LEARNING OUTCOMES	CONCEPTS
54.1 Describe the pathophysiologic processes associated with genitourinary disorders in the pediatric population.	Genitourinary disorders in the pediatric population are usually caused by: 1. Incomplete organ development during fetal development. 2. Hydronephrosis. 3. Improper placement of ureters in bladder and urethra in penis. 4. Anatomic obstruction or incomplete nerve innervation. 5. Infections. 6. Genetic disorders.

(continued)

LEARNING OUTCOMES — CONCEPTS

54.2 Discuss the nursing management of a child with a structural defect of the genitourinary system.

Nursing care focuses on:
1. Preventing infection and trauma:
   - Protection of exposed surfaces prior to surgery.
   - Maintenance of proper alignment and immobility after surgery.
2. Protecting surgical site from injury.
3. Monitoring renal function:
   - Strict intake and output.
4. Providing pain management and comfort measures to infant.
5. Providing emotional support to parents:
   - Encourage parent-infant bonding.
   - Instruct in discharge care.
   - Emphasize need for follow-up care.
   - Instruct parents in signs and symptoms of complications.
6. Educating parents to care for child after surgery.

54.3 Develop a nursing care plan for the child with a urinary tract infection.

A nursing care plan for a child with a UTI includes:
1. Obtain a sterile urine specimen.
2. Begin and maintain antibiotic therapy.
3. Reinforce proper cleansing methods for girls (front to back).
4. Medicate child for fever and discomfort.
5. Reinforce need for completion of antibiotic treatment and follow-up urine specimen.

54.4 Discuss the growth and developmental issues for the child with chronic renal failure.

1. Growth retardation.
2. Decreased mental alertness and ability to concentrate.
3. Fatigue.
4. Dyspnea on exertion.
5. Delayed fine and gross motor development.
6. Delayed sexual maturation.

54.5 Summarize dietary restrictions for the child with a renal disorder.

1. Restricted fluid needs:
   - Make a visual display giving child exact amount of fluid allowed.
   - Help child choose fluids high in calories and low in sodium.
   - Separate fluids from meals.
2. Restricted dietary needs:
   - Provide small, frequent feedings in a social atmosphere.
   - Use high-calorie supplements.
   - Instruct child and family on foods to avoid that are high in sodium, potassium, and phosphorus.
   - Refer to nutritionist.

54.6 Develop a nursing care plan for the child with acute and chronic renal failure on dialysis.

Hemodialysis:
1. Weigh child before and after dialysis.
2. Monitor fluid balance during therapy.
3. Check vital signs every half hour.
4. Monitor for any signs of bleeding from dialysis catheter.
5. Monitor PO intake and urinary output every half hour.
6. Provide distractions for child during therapy.

Peritoneal dialysis:
1. Teach family to perform peritoneal dialysis using sterile technique to connect and disconnect bags of dialysate.
2. Suggest clothing to help hide dialysate bags.
3. Educate parents about signs of peritonitis.

54.7 Describe psychosocial issues for the child requiring surgery on the genitourinary system.

1. Preschool and school-age child:
   - Embarrassment due to lack of continence.
2. School-age child and adolescent:
   - Embarrassment due to need for medications and doctor's visits.
   - Development of self-esteem and self-confidence with sexual identity and function.

CRITICAL THINKING IN ACTION

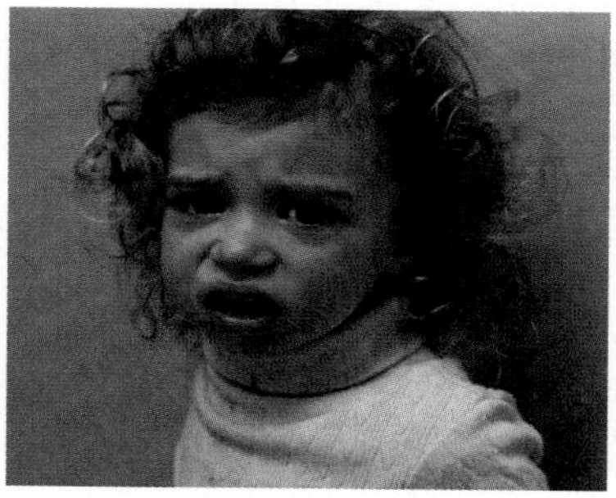

Kendra, a 2-year-old who appears ill, is brought into the urgent care center for a skin rash, fever, irritability, and edema. Her father is concerned she might also be dehydrated because she has had a decreased urine output. The doctor determines her skin rash does not blanch when pressure is applied and notes a purplish color. Last week Kendra was treated for an episode of abdominal pain, diarrhea, and vomiting. The doctor immediately admits her to the hospital and orders a urine culture, blood work, and stool tests. The stool comes back positive for the strain of *E Coli* usually found in contaminated hamburger meat. Kendra has hemolytic uremic syndrome (HUS) and is in acute renal failure (ARF). She also has a low hemoglobin, elevated BUN and creatinine, hematuria, and electrolyte imbalances.

Kendra is given medication for her electrolyte imbalances, antihypertensive medications, and is placed on a high-calorie, high-carbohydrate diet with restrictions on protein, sodium, potassium, and phosphorus. You explain to her parents the extreme importance of adhering to her dietary and fluid restrictions to help keep her electrolytes and fluid level balanced. You educate them that in some cases children with HUS need dialysis and some children have long term kidney damage. You teach them how to take her blood pressure, and how to observe for edema so that Kendra can be monitored after she goes home.

1. How is drug administration adjusted for Kendra since she has ARF? What is an important nursing role when administering various medications to her?
2. What is the reason ARF develops in HUS?
3. What is one way Kendra's condition could have been prevented?
4. Renal failure is characterized by azotemia and oliguria. Describe what these are.

See MyNursingKit for possible responses.

REFERENCES

Aiken, J. J., & Oldham, K. T. (2007). Inguinal hernias. In R. M. Kliegman, R. E. Behrman, H. B. Jenson, & B. F. Stanton (Eds.), *Nelson textbook of pediatrics* (18th ed., pp. 1644–1650). Philadelphia: Saunders.

Andersen, H. (2005). "Children on the frontline against E. coli": Typical hemolytic-uremic syndrome. *Clinical Laboratory Science, 18*(2), 90–99.

Asplin, J. R., & Coe, F. L. (2005). Tubular disorders. In D. L. Kasper, E. Braunwald, A. S. Fauci, S. L. Hauser, D. L. Longo, & J. L. Jameson (Eds.), *Harrison's principles of internal medicine* (16th ed., pp. 1694–1702). New York: McGraw-Hill.

Bakr, A., Amr, M., Sarhan, A., Hammad, A., Ragab, M., El-Refaey, A., & El-Mougy, A. (2007). Psychiatric disorders in children with chronic renal failure. *Pediatric Nephrology, 22,* 128–131.

Berry, A. (2005). Helping children with dysfunctional voiding. *Urologic Nursing, 25*(3), 193–200.

Berry, A. K. (2006). Helping children with nocturnal enuresis. *American Journal of Nursing, 106*(8), 56–63.

Bindler, R. M., &, Howry, L. B. (2005). *Pediatric drug guide.* Upper Saddle River, NJ: Prentice Hall-Health.

Bock, K. R. (2005). Renal replacement therapy in pediatric critical care medicine. *Current Opinion in Pediatrics, 17,* 368–371.

Bray & Sanders (2007). Teaching children and young people intermittent self-catheterization. *Urologic Nursing, 27*(3), 203–209, 242.

Chavers, B. M., Solid, T. A., Gilbertson, D. T., & Collins, A. J. (2007). Infection-related hospitalization rates in pediatric *versus* adult patients with end-stage renal disease in the United States. *Journal of the American Society of Nephrology, 18,* 952–959.

Constantinescu, A. R., Bitzan, M., Weiss, L. S., Christen, E., Kaplan, B. S., Cnaan, A., & Trachtman, H. (2004). Non-enteropathic hemolytic uremic syndrome: Causes and short-term course. *American Journal of Kidney Diseases, 43*(6), 976–982.

Coppola, C. P. (2005). A surgeon in your corner. *Pediatric Annals, 34*(11), 903–908.

Davis, I. D., & Avner, E. D. (2007). Conditions particularly associated with hematuria. In R. M. Kliegman, R. E. Behrman, H. B. Jenson, & B. F. Stanton (Eds.), *Nelson textbook of pediatrics* (18th ed., pp. 2168–2188). Philadelphia: Saunders.

Dulczak, S., & Kirk, J. (2005). Overview of the evaluation, diagnosis, and management of urinary tract infections in infants and children. *Urologic Nursing, 25*(3), 185–191.

Eaton, S. H., Cendron, M. A., Estrada, C. R., Bauer, S. B., Borer, J. G., Cilento, B. G., et al, (2005). Intermittent testicular torsion: Diagnostic features and management outcomes. *The Journal of Urology, 174*(4 Part 2), 1532–1535.

Elder, J. S. (2007). Urologic disorders in infants and children. In R. M. Kliegman, R. E. Behrman, H. B. Jenson, & B. F. Stanton (Eds.), *Nelson textbook of pediatrics* (18th ed., pp. 2221–2271). Philadelphia: Saunders.

Feinstein, S., Keich, R., Becker-Cohen, R., Rinat, C., Schwartz, S. B., & Frishberg, Y. (2005). Is noncompliance among adolescent renal transplant recipients inevitable? *Pediatrics, 115*(4), 969–973.

Fiorino, E. K., & Raffaelli, R. M. (2006). Hemolytic-uremic syndrome. *Pediatrics in Review, 27*(10), 398–399.

Garin, E. H., Olavarria, F., Nieto, V. G., Valenciano, B., Campos, A., & Young, L. (2006). Clinical significance of primary vesicoureteral reflux and urinary antibiotic prophylaxis after acute pyelonephritis: A multicenter, randomized controlled study. *Pediatrics, 117*(3), 626–632.

Gray, M., Huether, S. E., & Forshee, B. A. (2006). Structure and function of the renal and urologic systems. In K. L. McCance & S. E. Huether (Eds.), *Pathophysiology: The biologic basis for disease in adults and children* (5th ed., pp. 1301–1335), St. Louis: Elsevier Mosby.

Huether, S. E. (2006). Alterations of renal and urinary tract function in children. In K. L. McCance & S. E. Huether (Eds.), *Pathophysiology: The biologic basis for disease in adults and children* (5th ed., pp. 1337–1352). St. Louis: Elsevier Mosby.

Lahdenkari, A., Suvanto, M., & Kajantie, E., Koskimies, O., Kestila, M., & Jalanko, H. (2005). Clinical features and outcome of childhood minimal change nephritic syndrome: is genetics involved? *Pediatric Nephrology, 20,* 1073–1080.

Lau, K. K., & Wyatt, R. J. (2005). Glomerulonephritis. *Adolescent Medicine Clinics, 16*(1), 67–85.

Legg, V. (2005). Complications of chronic kidney disease. *American Journal of Nursing, 105*(6), 40–49.

Leroy, S., Adamsbaum, C., Marc, E., Moulin, F., Raymond, J., Gendrel, D., et al. (2005). Procalcitonin as a predictor of vesicoureteral reflux in children with a first febrile urinary tract infection. *Pediatrics, 115*(6), 706–709.

Leung, A. K. C., Robson, W. L. M., & Wong, A. L. (2005, February). What's your diagnosis? Bladder exstrophy. *Consultant for Pediatricians,* 77–80.

Lum, G. (2007). Kidney & urinary tract. In W. W. Hay, M. L. Leven, J. M. Sondheimer, & R. R. Deterding (Eds.), *Current pediatric diagnosis and treatment* (18th ed., pp. 684–707). New York: McGraw-Hill.

Mercer, R. (2006, May). Enuresis in the older child. *Nursing Spectrum,* 21.

Mercy, N., & Brady-Fryer (2004). Bladder exstrophy: A challenge for nursing care. *Journal of Wound, Ostomy & Continence Nursing, 31*(5), 293–298.

Miller, D. & MacDonald, D. (2006). Management of pediatric patients with chronic kidney disease. *Nephrology Nursing Journal, 33*(4), 415–429.

Morgan, K., & McCance, K. L. (2006). Alterations of the reproductive systems. In K. L. McCance & S. E. Huether (Eds.), Pathophysiology: The biologic basis for disease in adults and children, (5th ed., pp. 771–861). St. Louis: Elsevier Mosby.

Nachman, P. H., Jennette, J. C., & Falk, R. J. (2008). Primary glomerular disease. In B. M. Brenner (Ed.), *Brenner & Rector's the kidney* (8th ed., pp. 987–1066). Philadelphia: Saunders Elsevier.

National Kidney and Urological Diseases Information Clearinghouse. (2007). *Polycystic kidney disease* (NIH Publication No. 08-4008). Retrieved January 24, 2009 from http://kidney.niddk.nih.gov/kudiseases/pubs/pdf/PKD.pdf

National Kidney Foundation. (2009). Use of herbal supplements in chronic kidney disease. Retrieved January 24, 2009 from www.kidney.org/ATOZ/atozItem.cfm?id=123

Nield, L. S., & Kamat, D. (2004). Enuresis: How to evaluate and treat. *Clinical Pediatrics, 43,* 409–415.

Pieretti, R. V., Pieretti, A., & Pieretti-Vanmarcke, R. (2009). Circumcised hypospadias. *Pediatric Surgery International, 25,* 53–55.

Prune Belly Syndrome Network, 2008, Retrieved January 25, 2009, from http://www.prunebelly.org

Raszka, W. V., & Khan, O. (2005). Pyelonephritis. *Pediatrics in Review, 26*(10), 364–369.

Ringdahl, E., & Teague, L. (2006). Testicular Torsion. *American Family Physician, 74*(10), 1739–1743.

Rizk, D., & Chapman, A. (2008). Treatment of autosomal polycystic kidney disease (ADPKD): The new horizon for children with ADPKD. *Pediatric Nephrology, 23,* 1029–1036.

Ruth, E..M., Kemper, M. J., Leumann, E. P., Laube, G. F., & Neuhaus, T. J. (2005). Children with steroid-sensitive nephrotic syndrome come of age: Long-term outcome. *Journal of Pediatrics, 147*(2), 202–207.

Ruth, E. M., Landolt, M. A., Neuhaus, T. J., & Kemper, M. J. (2004). Health-related quality of life and psychosocial adjustment in steroid-sensitive nephrotic syndrome. *Journal of Pediatrics, 145*(6), 778–783.

Schulman, S. L., & Berry, A. K. (2007). A simple, step-wise approach to the child with daytime wetting. *Contemporary Urology, 19*(1) 19–21, 25–26, 29.

Small & Copel (2004). Practical guidelines for diagnosing and treating fetal hydronephrosis. *Contemporary OB/GYN, 49*(2) 59–77.

Snethen, J. A., Broome, M. E., Kelber, S., & Warady, B. A. (2004). Coping strategies utilized by adolescents with end-stage renal disease. *Nephrology Nursing Journal, 31*(1), 41–49.

Steadman, B., & Ellsworth, P. (2006). To circ or not to circ: Indications, risks, and alternatives to circumcision in the pediatric population with phimosis. *Urologic Nursing, 26*(3), 181–194.

Stokowski, L. A. (2004). Hypospadias in the neonate. *Advances in Neonatal Care, 4*(4), 206–215.

Terrill, C. J. (2007). Nutrition and the pediatric patient with CKD. *Nephrology Nursing Journal, 34*(1), 89–92.

United States Renal Data System. (2008). *2008 Annual data report.* Retrieved January 24, 2008, from www.usrds.org/atlas.htm

Vemulakonda, V. M., & Jones, E. A. (2006). Primer: Diagnosis and management of uncomplicated daytime wetting in children. *Nature Clinical Practice Urology, 3*(10), 551–559.

Vogler, C., Wang, Y., Brink, D., Wood, E., Belsha, C., & Walker, P. D. (2007). Renal pathology in the pediatric transplant patient. *Advances in Anatomic Pathology, 14*(3), 202–216.

Vogt, B. A., & Avner, E. D. (2007a). Conditions particularly associated with proteinuria. In R. M. Kliegman, R. E. Behrman, H. B. Jenson, & B. F. Stanton (Eds.), *Nelson textbook of pediatrics* (18th ed., pp. 2188–2195). Philadelphia: Saunders.

Vogt, B. A., & Avner, E. D. (2007b). Toxic neuropathies: Renal failure. In R. M. Kliegman, R. E. Behrman, H. B. Jenson, & B. F. Stanton (Eds.), *Nelson textbook of pediatrics* (18th ed., pp. 2204–2219). Philadelphia: Saunders.

Walle, J. V., Mauel, R., Raes, A., Vanderkerckhove, K., & Donckerwolcke, R. (2004). ARF in children with minimal change nephrotic syndrome may be related to functional changes of the glomerular basement membrane. *American Journal of Kidney Diseases, 43*(3), 399–404.

Warady, B. A., & Chada, V. (2007). Chronic kidney disease in children: The global perspective. *Pediatric Nephrology, 22*(12), 1999–2009.

Ward-Smith, P., & Barry, D. (2006). The challenge of treating enuresis. *Urologic Nursing, 26*(3), 222–224.

Watnick, S., & Morrison, G. (2007). Nephrology. In S. J. McPhee, M. A. Papadakis, & L. M. Tierny Jr. (Eds.), Current medical diagnosis and treatment (46th ed.). New York: McGraw-Hill.

Weissbach, A., Leiberman, A., Tarasiuk, A., Goldbart, A., & Tal, A. (2006). Adenotonsillectomy improves enuresis in children with obstructive sleep apnea syndrome. *Pediatric Otorhinolaryngology, 70,* 1351–1356.

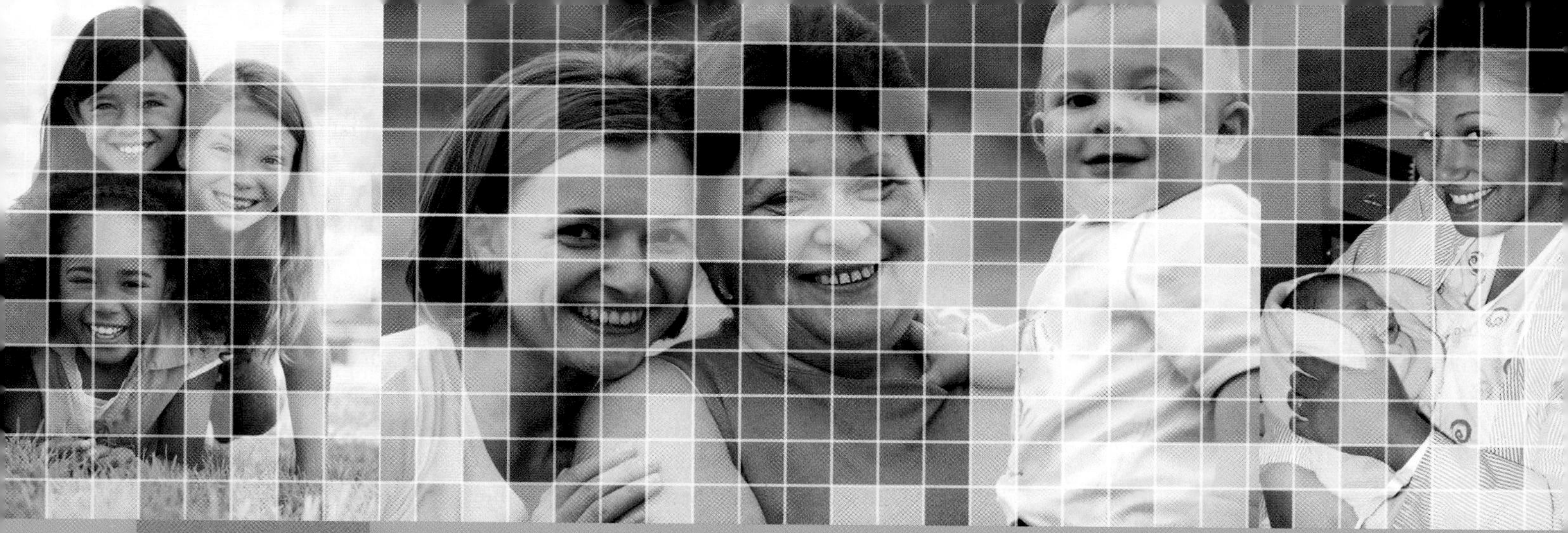

CHAPTER

55 The Child with Alterations in Endocrine Function

I am really worried about how Anthony is going to learn to manage all these aspects of diabetes care. Learning to check his blood sugar is pretty easy compared to counting calories and figuring out how much insulin to take and when to take it. I hope we have some time to get into a routine with his diabetes management before he gets sick. We have to work hard to keep the diabetes under control. —Mother of Anthony, 12 years old

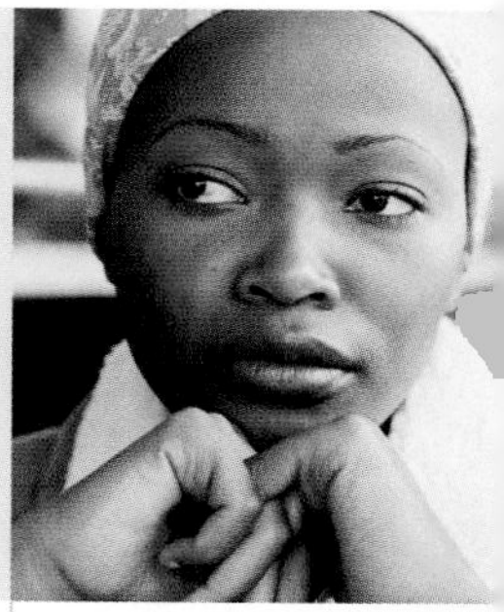

LEARNING OUTCOMES

55.1 Identify the function of important hormones of the endocrine system.
55.2 Identify signs and symptoms that may indicate a disorder of the endocrine system.
55.3 Identify all conditions for which short stature is a sign.
55.4 Develop a nursing care plan for each type of acquired metabolic disorder.
55.5 Develop a family education plan for the child that needs lifelong cortisol replacement.
55.6 Distinguish between the nursing care of the child with type 1 and type 2 diabetes.
55.7 Develop a nursing care plan for the child with an inherited metabolic disorder.

KEY TERMS

Acanthosis nigricans, 1638
Adrenarche, 1613
Bone age, 1609
Chvostek sign, 1617
Euthyroid, 1614
Glucagon, 1637
Glycosuria, 1622
Goiter, 1614
Hyperinsulinemia, 1638
Inborn errors of metabolism, 1642
Insulin deficiency, 1624
Insulin resistance, 1624
Polydipsia, 1611
Polyphagia, 1622
Polyuria, 1611
Pseudohermaphroditism, 1619
Puberty, 1608
Thelarche, 1613
Thyrotoxicosis, 1615
Virilization, 1619
Water intoxication, 1612

The endocrine system controls the cellular activity that regulates growth and body metabolism through the release of hormones. Hormones are chemical messengers secreted by various glands that exert controlling effects on the cells of the body. Overlapping with all body systems, the general functions of the endocrine system include the following:

- Differentiation of the reproductive and central nervous systems in the fetus
- Regulation of the pace of growth and development in concert with the central nervous system throughout childhood and adolescence
- Coordination of the male and female reproductive systems, enabling sexual reproduction
- Maintenance of an optimal level of hormones for body functioning
- Maintenance of homeostasis, a healthy internal environment, in the presence of a constantly changing external environment

The endocrine and nervous systems interact to regulate responses within the body and with the external environment.

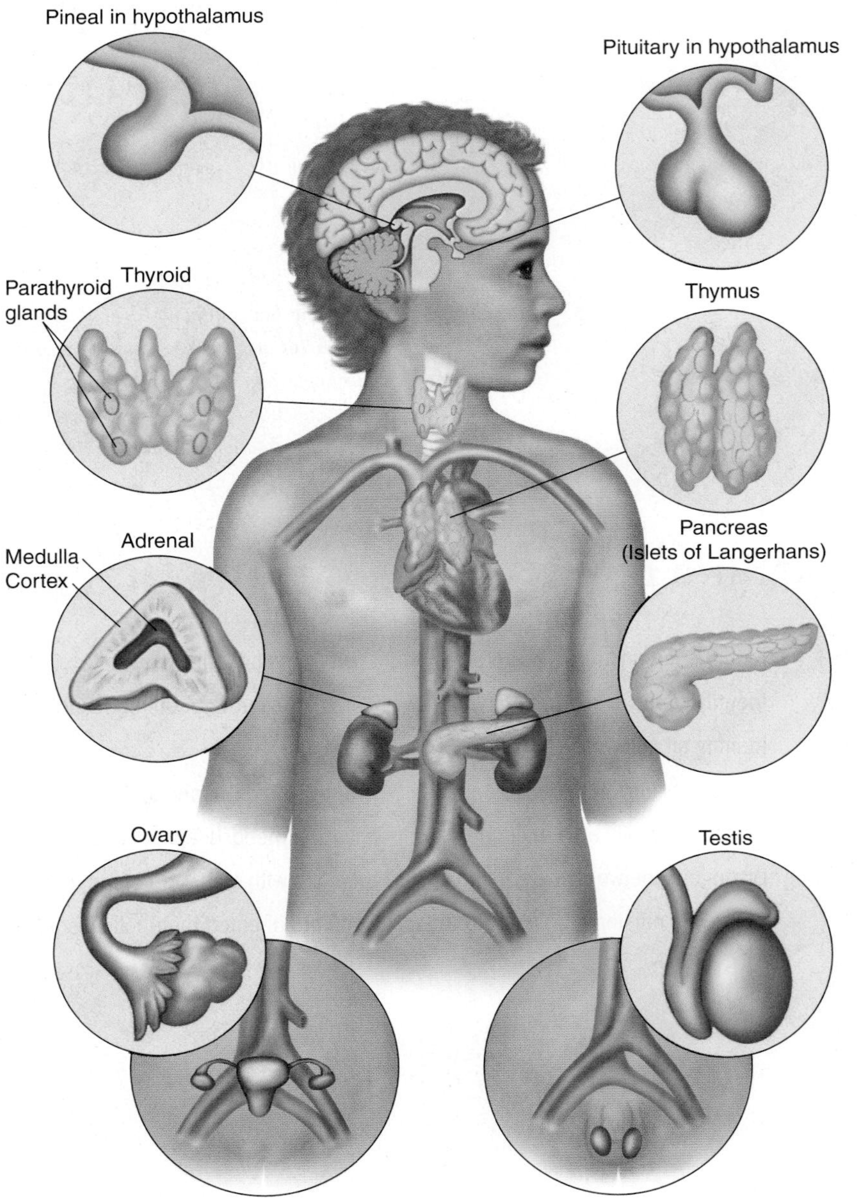

● **Figure 55–1** Major organs and glands of the endocrine system.

ANATOMY AND PHYSIOLOGY OF PEDIATRIC DIFFERENCES

The hypothalamic-pituitary axis produces several releasing and inhibiting hormones that regulate the function of many endocrine glands, including the thyroid, adrenal, and male and female reproductive glands. The hypothalamus synthesizes many hormones and the pituitary gland works by stimulating or inhibiting the release of these hormones. The pituitary gland also secretes certain hormones. Hormones originating from this axis regulate growth. Other endocrine glands include the parathyroid glands and the islets of Langerhans in the pancreas (Figure 55–1 ●). All of these glands secrete hormones into the bloodstream, which carries them to target organs or tissues. Most hormones exert their influence through interaction with receptors in the target cells of specific tissues (Table 55–1).

Hormone secretion regulation occurs through a *negative feedback* mechanism that functions to maintain an optimal internal

Table 55–1 Endocrine Glands and Their Functions

Gland/Hormone	Function
ANTERIOR PITUITARY	
Growth hormone (somatotropin)	Regulates metabolic process related to growth
Thyroid-stimulating hormone (TSH)	Stimulates thyroid hormone secretion
Adrenocorticotropic hormone (ACTH) (corticotrophin)	Stimulates secretion of glucocorticoids and androgens
Follicle-stimulating hormone (FSH) (a gonadotropin)	Stimulates secretion of estrogen; stimulates follicle maturation in ovaries. Also critical for sperm production in males.
Luteinizing hormone (LH) and interstitial cell-stimulating hormone (ICSH) (male analog) (a gonadotropin)	Stimulates secretion of androgens in males and progesterone in females
Prolactin-releasing hormone	Stimulates secretion of prolactin which stimulates the secretion of milk during lactation
Melanocyte-stimulating hormone (MSH)	Stimulates skin pigmentation
POSTERIOR PITUITARY	
Antidiuretic hormone (ADH)	Promotes water reabsorption back into blood, decreasing urine output
Oxytocin	Stimulates uterine contractions and breast milk letdown reflex
Beta endorphins	May regulate body temperature, food, and water intake
THYROID	
Thyroxine (T_4) and triiodothyronine (T_3)	Regulates metabolic rate of all cells, body heat production; protein, fat, and carbohydrate catabolism in all cells
Thyrocalcitonin	Stimulates bone ossification and development
PARATHYROID	
Parathyroid hormone	Regulates serum calcium levels and excretion of phosphorus
ADRENAL	
Aldosterone	Increases sodium ion reabsorption, and increases potassium and hydrogen ion excretion in the kidneys
Androgens	Stimulates bone development and secondary sexual characteristics
Cortisol	Stimulates anti-inflammatory reactions, protects from stress
Epinephrine	Activates sympathetic nervous system; stimulates increase in blood pressure and blood glucose levels
PANCREAS (ISLETS OF LANGERHANS)	
Insulin	Facilitates cellular glucose utilization
Glucagon	Increases blood glucose when low by stimulating glycogenolysis
Somatostatin	Inhibits insulin and glucagon secretion; may prevent excess insulin secretion
OVARIES	
Estrogen	Stimulates development of breasts and ova
Progesterone	Stimulates breast glandular development; acts to maintain pregnancy
TESTES	
Testosterone	Stimulates production of sperm, development of secondary sexual characteristics, and closure of epiphysis

environment in the body. Negative feedback occurs when an endocrine gland or secretory tissue receives a message that the target cells have received an adequate amount of hormone. In response, further secretion is inhibited. Secretion is resumed only when the secretory tissue receives another message indicating that levels of the hormone are low.

The endocrine system is responsible for sexual differentiation during fetal development and for stimulating growth and development during childhood and adolescence. This includes stimulating development of the reproductive system in both sexes.

Puberty (sexual maturation, lasting an average of 4.5 years) occurs when the gonads secrete increased amounts of the sex hormones estrogen and testosterone. At the average age of 9 years in girls and 11 years in boys, the hypothalamus produces increased amounts of gonadotropin-releasing hormone (GnRH). This hormone stimulates the anterior pituitary gland to secrete luteinizing hormone (LH) and follicle-stimulating hormone (FSH). In boys, LH stimulates testosterone production and FSH stimulates sperm production. In girls, LH and FSH stimulate development and maturation of the ova and ovulation. These hormones in turn stimulate the gonads to secrete more sex hormones, resulting in the development of primary and secondary sex characteristics (Figure 55–2 ●).

Use the Assessment Guide on page 1609 to perform a nursing assessment of the endocrine system.

DISORDERS OF PITUITARY FUNCTION

Pituitary disorders such as growth hormone deficiency, hyperpituitarism, and precocious puberty directly affect the child's growth, while diabetes insipidus and the syndrome of inappropriate antidiuretic syndrome are disorders affecting fluid balance. These disorders are discussed in the following section.

GROWTH HORMONE DEFICIENCY (HYPOPITUITARISM)

Growth hormone deficiency (GHD) is a disorder caused by decreased activity of the pituitary gland. Because most children with this disorder secrete inadequate amounts of growth hormone, the term *growth hormone deficiency* is often preferred to *hypopituitarism.* The disorder is diagnosed earlier in males than females since males are referred for evaluation of short stature (Grimberg, Kutikov, & Cucchiara, 2005).

Etiology and Pathophysiology

The release of growth hormone from the anterior pituitary gland is controlled by the hypothalamus, which secretes releasing and inhibitory factors (somatostatin). Growth hormone (GH) stimulates linear growth and bone mineral density, as well as the growth of all body tissues. Growth hormone also stimulates the synthesis of proteins in the liver, among them the somatomedins or insulin-like growth factors (IGFs), which promote glucose utilization by the cells and cell proliferation.

Infarction of the pituitary gland (related to sickle cell disease), central nervous system infection, disease, tumors of the pituitary gland or hypothalamus (primarily craniopharyngiomas and gliomas), other brain tumors, cranial irradiation, brain trauma, chemotherapy, and psychosocial deprivation may cause GHD by interfering with the production or release of growth hormone. Other major causes of short stature include familial short stature, hypothyroidism, Turner syndrome, *constitutional growth delay* (delayed pubertal hormone secretion causes a late pubertal growth spurt), chronic renal failure, Cushing syndrome, Down syndrome, inborn error of metabolism, and severe cardiac, pulmonary, immunologic, or gastrointestinal disease. Psychosocial dwarfism is a syndrome of emotional deprivation that causes suppression of pituitary hormone production, resulting in a transient growth hormone deficiency that is reversed by placing the child in a nurturing environment (Rose, Vogiatzi, & Copeland, 2005).

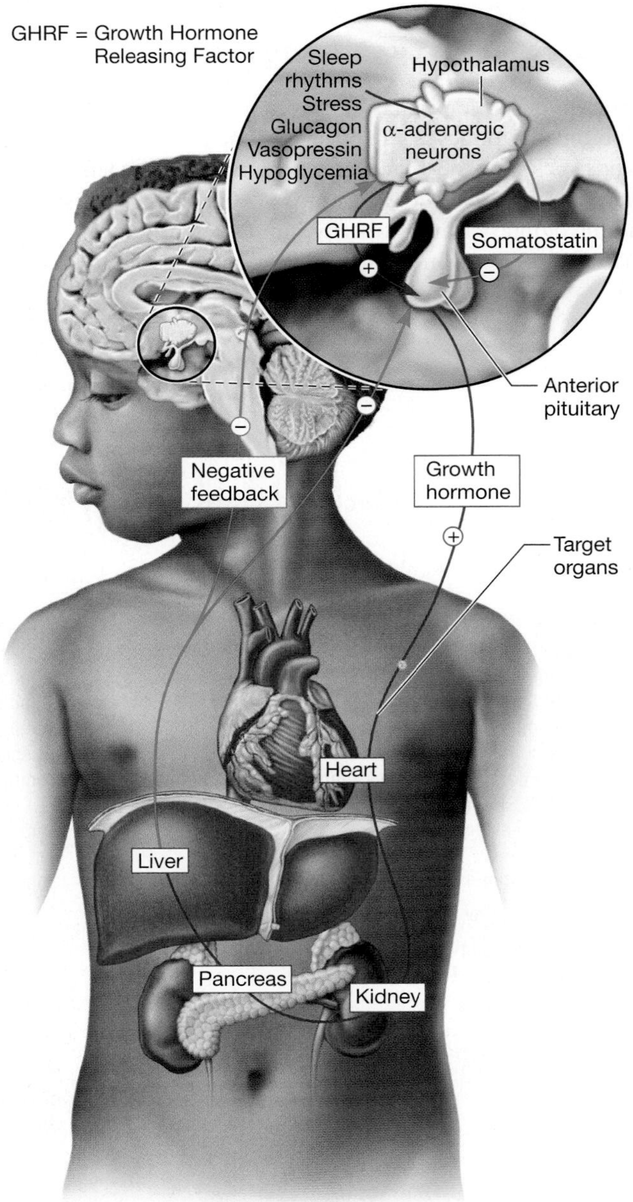

● **Figure 55–2** Feedback mechanism in hormonal stimulation of the gonads during puberty.

Assessment Guidelines

THE CHILD WITH AN ENDOCRINE CONDITION

ASSESSMENT FOCUS	ASSESSMENT GUIDELINE
Growth	■ Carefully measure weight, length, or height and plot on a growth curve. ■ Compare measurements at different ages to assess the growth pattern over time and to assess the growth velocity.
Blood pressure	■ Assess blood pressure and compare to expected norms for age. See Appendix D.
Facial characteristics	■ Inspect the face for unusual features such as a protuberant tongue, protuberant eyes, or moon face.
Neck	■ Palpate the neck for an enlarged thyroid or goiter.
Muscles	■ Assess strength and muscle tone.
Genitalia and secondary sexual characteristics	■ Assess external genitalia for signs of ambiguous genitalia, inappropriate size for age. ■ Determine the child's stage of development for each characteristic (breast and pubic hair for girls, genital and pubic hair for boys) by comparing to the images in Chapter 35 (Figures 35–29, 35–30, and 35–31). ■ Assess the sexual maturity rating with information in Chapter 35 (Figure 35–32). Compare the stage of development to the age of the boy or girl to determine early or delayed onset of puberty.
Body odor	■ Assess body odor for unusual smell (e.g., sweet, musty, cheesy, sweaty feet).
Skin	■ Assess skin color, noting areas of unusual pigmentation.
Family history	■ Assess for family history of metabolic or endocrine disorders.

Clinical Manifestations

Children with GHD have normal birth weights and lengths. By the age of 1 year, however, they are below the third percentile on the growth chart. The child characteristically grows at a rate of less than 5 cm (2 in.) per year. Other characteristic findings in infants include hypoglycemic seizures, hyponatremia, neonatal jaundice, pale optic discs, micropenis, and undescended testicles. Children with growth hormone deficiency tend to appear "cherubic" and exhibit youthful facial features, higher pitched voices, delayed dentition, "ripply" abdominal fat, decreased muscle mass, delayed skeletal maturation, and delayed sexual maturation. Slipped capital femoral epiphysis (Chapter 58) has been associated with growth hormone deficiency. Any child receiving growth hormone treatment who complains of hip pain, knee pain, or manifesting a limp must be evaluated for this disorder (Halac & Zimmerman, 2004a).

Any child whose height is 2 to 3 standard deviations below the mean height for age or whose measurement is falling off the normal growth chart should be evaluated for short stature (Table 55–2). A child whose screening tests reveal low levels of insulin-like growth factors (IGF-1) requires further evaluation by a pediatric endocrinologist. A careful history, physical examination, assessment of pubertal development and unusual facies, and radiologic studies are necessary to rule out familial short stature and constitutional growth delay, which are normal variants, and skeletal dysplasias or psychosocial short stature, which requires further evaluation.

Clinical Therapy

Radiographic imaging of the hand or wrist bone is used to evaluate the stage of bone ossification, and thus the **bone age** of the child. Using standardized norms for bone ossification, it can be

Table 55–2 Diagnostic Tests for Short Stature

Test	Purpose Related to Short Stature
IGF-1 and IGFBP-3	Screens test for growth hormone deficiency
MRI of the pituitary gland	Detects pituitary malformation or tumor
Provocative growth hormone testing	Tests for growth hormone deficiency
Bone age	Identifies other potential causes of delayed growth
Karyotype (girls)	Detects Turner syndrome (see page 1640)
Thyroid function studies	Detects hypothyroidism (see page 1613)
ACTH and cortisol levels	Detects other pituitary hormonal deficiencies
Urine creatinine, pH, specific gravity, urea nitrogen, electrolytes	Detects chronic renal failure (see Chapter 54)
Complete blood count and erythrocyte sedimentation rate	Screens for inflammatory bowel disease with anemia
Antigliadin antibodies	Screens for celiac disease

Data from: Parks, J. S., & Felner, E. I. (2007a). Hormones of the hypothalamus and pituitary. In R. M. Kliegman, R. E. Behrman, H. B. Jenson, & B. F. Stanton (Eds.), *Nelson textbook of pediatrics* (18th ed., pp. 2291–2293). Philadelphia: Saunders Elsevier; Parks, J. S., & Felner, E. I. (2007b). Hypopituitarism. In R. M. Kliegman, R. E. Behrman, H. B. Jenson, & B. F. Stanton, *Nelson textbook of pediatrics* (18th ed., pp. 2293–2299). Philadelphia: Saunders Elsevier; Grimberg, A., & DeLéon, D. D. (2005). Disorders in growth. In T. M. Moshange (Ed.), *Pediatric endocrinology: The requisites in pediatrics* (pp. 127–167). St. Louis: Elsevier Mosby.

AS CHILDREN GROW

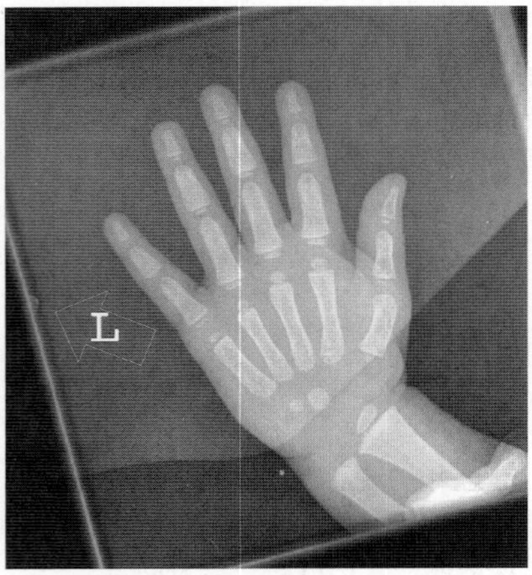

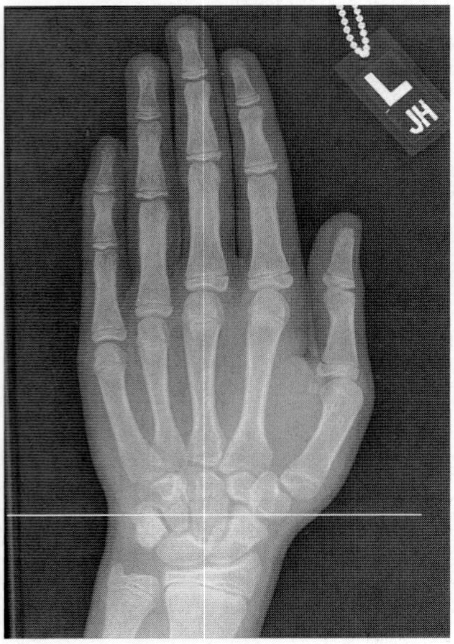

The radiograph of the hand and wrist of a 3-year-old and 13-year-old girl reveal significant differences in skeletal maturation that are closely tied to physiologic maturation. The 3-year-old has many bones in the hand and wrist that have not fully developed. The secretion of estrogen during puberty has resulted in the development and calcification of secondary ossification centers of most of the bones in the hand and wrist of the 13-year old.

Courtesy: Dorothy Bulas, M.D., Children's National Medical Center.

determined if the child's chronologic and bone ages match. Significantly delayed (less than the child's age) or advanced (greater than the child's age) bone age may be indicative of the possibility of a systemic chronic disease or hormone abnormality requiring investigation (see As Children Grow above). Provocative growth hormone testing, in which various medications (arginine, clonidine, glucagon, insulin, L-dopa) are administered to stimulate release of growth hormone, is a diagnostic test that may be used to confirm growth hormone deficiency.

For growth hormone deficiency, replacement therapy with growth hormone (GH) is administered to promote growth and development. Most indications for growth hormone replacement require daily or alternate day subcutaneous injections; however, outcomes are improved with frequent dosing (Lee & Menon, 2005).

The child usually experiences increased growth velocity for the first year of treatment, followed by a gradual decrease in growth for subsequent months or years. Growth should progress at least at the normal rate for age while maintained on growth hormone treatment. Replacement therapy is continued until either the child achieves an acceptable height or growth velocity drops to less than 2 cm (1 in.) per year. Close monitoring of growth and endocrinology visits every 3 to 4 months are needed. If growth is slower than anticipated, improper preparation and administration of growth hormone and adherence to therapy must be considered (Halac & Zimmerman, 2004a). In some cases the onset of puberty is delayed with gonadotropin-releasing hormone analogues to provide more time for growth hormone therapy to stimulate growth.

Nursing Management

Nursing care consists of monitoring growth, teaching the child and family about the disorder and its treatment, and providing emotional support. Carefully measure the child's height and weight and plot them on a growth chart (see Appendix C and Skills 9–1 to 9–7 SKILLS).

Teach the parents and child about the GH replacement therapy, preparation and administration of subcutaneous injections, rotating injection sites, potential side effects, and actions to take if noticed. Provide the parents with ideas about how to minimize the child's stress associated with daily injections. Give parents educational resources, such as information from the Magic Foundation and the Human Growth Foundation. Replacement therapy is expensive, costing $20,000 or more per year (Lee, Davis, Clark, et al., 2006) and may not be covered by insurance; therefore, parents may require financial assistance that is sometimes available from the growth hormone manufacturers.

Children with GHD, especially those whose deficiency is due to tumors and trauma from radiation or surgery, may have academic problems because of acquired learning disabilities. Before the child enters or returns to school, a comprehensive evaluation should be performed to identify potential problems.

The best results occur when treatment begins at an early age, before the psychologic effects of short stature become apparent and when attainment of near-normal height is reached. People often treat short children on the basis of their size rather than their age, and such children experience social prejudice about height. Teasing is a common problem. The teenage years may be particularly stressful because of adolescents' characteristic preoccupation with body image.

Encourage parents and teachers to treat the child in an age-appropriate manner. The child should dress in clothing that reflects chronologic age. Emphasize the child's strengths, support independence, and encourage participation in age-appropriate activities to aid in the development of a positive self-image. Suggest that the child take part in sports in which ability does not depend on size (e.g., swimming, gymnastics, wrestling, ice skating, and martial arts). Identifying positive role models, short people who accomplish their goals, also promotes a positive image. Refer the child for counseling if appropriate.

GROWTH HORMONE EXCESS (HYPERPITUITARISM)

Hyperpituitarism, a disorder in which excessive secretion of growth hormone increases the growth rate, is rare in children. If combined with precocious puberty, a tumor of the hypothalamus may be present. Affected children can grow to 7 or 8 feet in height when oversecretion occurs before closure of the epiphyseal plates. If the disorder occurs after closure of the epiphyseal plates, acromegaly occurs.

Because tall stature is valued in our society, assessment of children (particularly males) with accelerated linear growth is often delayed. Any child whose predicted height exceeds that consistent with parental height should be evaluated for possible growth problems and underlying pathologic conditions.

A complete history is obtained, and physical examination and laboratory testing are performed. Increased levels of IGF-1 establish the diagnosis of hyperpituitarism. A bone age radiologic examination is performed to determine if the epiphyseal plates have begun to fuse. Radiologic studies are used to detect a tumor. Thorough evaluation is required to differentiate hyperpituitarism from familial tall stature.

Treatment depends on the cause of the excessive growth and may involve surgical removal of a tumor or pituitary gland (hypophysectomy), radiation therapy, or radioactive implants. High doses of sex steroids are given to close the epiphyseal plates. The child may need lifelong pituitary hormone replacement following surgery.

Nursing Management

Tall stature, like short stature, can be stressful for children. Tall children are often treated as if they are older than their chronologic age. Tall adolescents may have problems with self-image, and girls in particular may worry about their appearance.

Nursing care focuses on teaching the parents and child about the disorder and its treatment, providing emotional support, and, if surgery is required, providing preoperative and postoperative teaching and care (see Chapter 40∞).

DIABETES INSIPIDUS

Two forms of diabetes insipidus occur: central (neurogenic) antidiuretic hormone (ADH) deficiency and familial nephrogenic diabetes insipidus. Both disorders involve ADH, a hormone secreted by the posterior pituitary gland. In normal circumstances, thirst is the regulator for ADH release (Kache & Ferry, 2005). The most important function of ADH is to bind to the collecting ducts of the kidney and promote reabsorption of water back into the circulation.

ADH facilitates concentration of the urine by stimulating reabsorption of water from the distal tubule of the kidney. When ADH is inadequate, the tubules do not resorb, leading to **polyuria** (passage of a large volume of urine in a given period). Therefore the body is unable to conserve water, resulting in severe dehydration.

Diabetes insipidus can occur at any age and results from inadequate production or secretion of ADH or arginine-vasopressin (central or neurogenic diabetes insipidus) or inability of the renal collecting tubules to respond to the ADH (nephrogenic diabetes insipidus). Brain tumors and their treatment are the most common cause of central DI (Kache & Ferry, 2005). Other causes of central diabetes insipidus include brain trauma, central nervous system infection, and neurosurgery. Genetic nephrogenic diabetes insipidus is not as common as the acquired type but its presentation is more severe. Transient nephrogenic diabetes insipidus may be caused by drug toxicity or an adverse drug reaction (Breault & Majzoub, 2007).

Polyuria and **polydipsia** (excessive thirst) are the cardinal signs of diabetes insipidus. Polydipsia is the body's attempt to preserve fluid balance. Additional manifestations observed in children with diabetes insipidus include hypernatremia, dilute urine, and dehydration. See "Clinical Manifestations: Diabetes Insipidus."

Clinical Manifestations

DIABETES INSIPIDUS

CAUSE	CLINICAL MANIFESTATIONS	CLINICAL THERAPY
Central Diabetes Insipidus		
ADH deficiency Familial or idiopathic	Polyuria, polydipsia Nocturia, enuresis Thirsty at night Irritable if fluids withheld Constipation, fever, dehydration	Desmopressin acetate
Nephrogenic Diabetes Insipidus		
Inherited or acquired Decreased responsiveness of kidneys to ADH	Polyuria, polydipsia Hypernatremia in neonatal period Dehydration, fever, vomiting Mental status changes	Diuretics High fluid intake Salt and protein restricted diet

Nursing Practice

During the fluid deprivation test, advise parents that the child will be frustrated and irritable from thirst. No one should drink in front of the child during the testing period. Monitor the child's vital signs, intake, and output carefully. The test is stopped if the child loses 5% of body weight and develops a fever and hypotension (Kache & Ferry, 2005).

Although the onset of symptoms is usually sudden, diagnosis is often delayed. Children who can quench their thirst may not complain to parents about symptoms. In infants, symptoms may include vomiting, polyuria, poor skin turgor, and irritability (Kache & Ferry, 2005).

In all forms of diabetes insipidus, the urine cannot be concentrated, no matter how dehydrated the child becomes. A dehydration episode usually leads to the diagnosis. Serum sodium concentration and osmolality increase rapidly to pathologic levels. Seizures may occur in response to extreme electrolyte imbalances. Often an unconscious child is admitted to the emergency department with dehydration and hypernatremia.

Urine osmolality is decreased (<300 mOsm/kg), urine specific gravity is decreased (<1.005), serum sodium is elevated, and the urine to serum osmolality ratio is less than 1 (Kache & Ferry, 2005). An MRI may be ordered to visualize the pituitary gland. Diagnosis is confirmed by measuring the plasma arginine vasopressin (AVP) level before and during a fluid deprivation test, which is usually conducted in the hospital or in a carefully controlled outpatient setting for up to 8 hours. Fluid intake is prohibited during the procedure. Weight, urine output, specific gravity, and osmolality are measured every 2 hours. The specific gravity remains low (less than 1.005) even after dehydration. A dose of aqueous vasopressin is given after several hours. A decreased urine output and increased urine concentration confirm the diagnosis of central diabetes insipidus. No response to vasopressin is seen in cases of nephrogenic diabetes insipidus.

Central ADH deficiency is treated by subcutaneous, intranasal, or oral desmopressin acetate (DDAVP). The medication educes urinary output, enabling the child to live a more normal life with a decrease in thirst, urinary output, and nocturia. The dose of DDAVP must be titered for sufficient coverage of metabolic needs while not high enough to cause water overload (Raine, Donaldson, Gregory, et al., 2006a).

Nephrogenic diabetes insipidus is treated with thiazide diuretics, which promote sodium excretion and stimulate the proximal tubule to reabsorb water. Prostaglandin inhibitors (indomethacin) may also be prescribed to have an additive effect on decreased water excretion. The child is allowed liberal fluid intake. The child's sodium and potassium levels must be carefully monitored to prevent hypernatremia and hypokalemia (Kache & Ferry, 2005; Raine et al., 2006a) (see Chapter 46).

Nursing Management

Educate parents about making fluids available to the child as needed, administering DDAVP, obtaining and recording daily weights, measuring intake and output, and recognizing signs of inadequate fluid intake (see Chapter 46). The child should consume fluids equal to the amount of output (sometimes as much as 75 mL/kg) (Ferry, 2005). Parents may need to weigh diapers to monitor urine output in infants. Cold fluids are often preferred and help relieve thirst. The child's fluid intake will need to be adjusted to prevent dehydration during an illness. Children often wake to drink fluids at night, but infants will need to have fluids provided. Many infants have coexisting brain damage and need nasogastric or gastrostomy feeding to maintain adequate hydration and nutrition. However, care should be taken to avoid the intake of excessive fluid as the child will not be able to excrete the excess water load with DDAVP treatment.

The child with chronic diabetes insipidus should always wear a medical alert identification (tag, bracelet, or necklace) to indicate the presence of the disorder. Partner with the parents and school officials to make arrangements to provide the child unrestricted access to toilet facilities and water.

SYNDROME OF INAPPROPRIATE ANTIDIURETIC HORMONE (SIADH)

Syndrome of inappropriate antidiuretic hormone (SIADH) results from an excessive amount of serum ADH. It is seen in children with central nervous system infections, brain tumors, and brain trauma; in children with pulmonary disorders such as pneumonia, asthma, or cystic fibrosis; and in children receiving positive pressure ventilation. Some medications, including diuretics and chemotherapy, have been associated with SIADH.

Failure of normal feedback mechanisms from the hypothalamus, pituitary gland, and kidney results in excessive secretion of ADH, leading to water reabsorption despite the presence of low serum osmolality. ADH secretion causes increased permeability of the distal renal tubules and collecting ducts, resulting in water reabsorption, increased intravascular volume, and decreased urine output (Ferry, 2005). Elevated ADH also causes suppression of the renin-angiotensin mechanism and sodium excretion. The outcome is **water intoxication** (an abnormal proportion of water to sodium in the extracellular fluid), hyponatremia, and cellular edema.

Signs of SIADH include elevated blood pressure, distended jugular veins, crackles in lung fields, weight gain without edema, fluid and electrolyte imbalance, and concentrated urine with decreased urine output. As serum sodium levels continue to fall, lethargy, confusion, headache, altered level of consciousness, seizures, and coma occur due to cerebral edema.

Laboratory findings include a high urine osmolality (greater than 100 mOsm/kg), elevated specific gravity (greater than 1.025), low serum osmolality (less than 260 mOsm/kg), low serum sodium (less than 125 mM), and decreased BUN (less than 22 mg/dL) (Ferry, 2005).

Fluids are restricted to prevent further dilution of the blood. Medications include diuretics, demeclocycline to block action of ADH at the renal collecting tubules, and hypertonic saline IV fluids. Oral urea has recently been evaluated for treatment with promising results (Huang, Feldman, Schwartz, et al., 2006).

Nursing Management

Nursing care focuses on maintenance of fluid and electrolyte balance and prevention of complications associated with the disorder. Monitor changes in level of consciousness, headache, and seizure activity. Monitor vital signs, intake and output, serum sodium, urine osmolality, and specific gravity. Weigh the child daily to assess for weight gain, which may indicate a sign of water intoxication. Assess nutritional intake status and appetite.

Educate the parents about the hidden sources of water and fluids in foods, avoiding excessive fluid intake, and the importance of weighing the child daily and reporting weight gain that could indicate fluid retention. Depending on the cause of the disorder, lifelong medication may be required. If the child is prescribed demeclocycline, emphasize to the family the importance of follow-up care since the drug has nephrotoxic side effects. The child should wear a medical alert identification (tag, bracelet, or necklace) identifying the disorder and treatment.

PRECOCIOUS PUBERTY

Precocious puberty is defined as the appearance of any secondary sexual characteristics before 8 years of age in girls (breast development or pubic hair) and 9 years of age in boys (pubic hair) (Pinyerd & Zipf, 2005).

Earlier than expected secretion of the normal hormones responsible for pubertal changes is not usually associated with an endocrine system abnormality (an idiopathic problem). External sources of hormones such as anabolic steroids or estrogen may be identified. Central precocious puberty or true precocious puberty occurs when the hypothalamus is activated to secrete gonadotropin-releasing hormone. Other potential causes include tumors of the ovary, adrenal gland, and pituitary gland, and a rare genetic condition known as McCune-Albright syndrome (Keefe, 2007).

Isolated signs of premature sexual development such as premature **thelarche** (breast development), premature menarche (vaginal bleeding without other signs of sexual development), and premature **adrenarche** (development of pubic and axillary sexual hair) before 8 years of age in girls and 9 years in boys often needs no treatment.

Children with precocious puberty have an advanced bone age (premature skeletal maturation) and may appear unusually tall for their age. Their growth ceases prematurely, however, as the hormones stimulate closure of the epiphyseal plates, resulting in short stature. Behavior changes may include mood swings and emotional lability.

Serum diagnostic studies include LH, FSH, testosterone, or estradiol. Provocative testing includes gonadotropin-releasing hormone (GnRH) stimulation to confirm the diagnosis. Radiologic imaging of the brain, as well as bone age, may be performed.

CNS tumors require surgery, radiation, and/or chemotherapy. Treatment may be initiated immediately to slow or stop the progression of sexual development in children below the expected age of puberty. A gonadotropin-releasing hormone analogue (GnRHa) is administered, usually leuprolide acetate (Lupron) injections once a month or nafarelin acetate (Synarel) intranasally twice a day. Treatment often continues until a more normal age for puberty is reached (e.g., 11 years in girls and 12 years in boys). Simple monitoring of growth patterns may be the only intervention for children closer to the lower than expected age for puberty to begin.

> **Developing Cultural Competence**
>
> **ONSET OF PUBERTY**
>
> Differences exist by race in the onset of puberty and secondary sexual characteristics. Black girls begin puberty one half to one year earlier than white girls (Kaplowitz, 2006).

Nursing Management

Nursing care should focus on teaching the child and parents about the condition and its treatment, promoting growth and providing emotional support. Inform the child in age-appropriate terms that the physiologic changes are normal but are occurring at an earlier than usual age. Reassure the child that friends will experience the same stages of development eventually. Emphasize to the family that the child's social, cognitive, and emotional development matches his or her age, even though the physical development is advanced.

Children with precocious puberty become self-conscious as body changes occur. Provide the child opportunities to express concerns and discuss issues related to body changes. The child may need to practice role playing as a coping mechanism to manage teasing by other children. Partner with the family to encourage dressing the child in a manner appropriate to his or her chronologic age, even though the child may look older. Provide privacy during physical examinations. Advise parents that they may need to discuss issues of sexuality with the child at an earlier age than normal. Refer the child and family for counseling if appropriate.

Teach the family proper medication administration and adherence to treatment regimen. Determine the family's ability to financially manage the cost of treatment. Assistance in covering the cost of therapy may be available through pharmaceutical companies and third-party payers.

DISORDERS OF THYROID FUNCTION

HYPOTHYROIDISM

Hypothyroidism is a disorder in which levels of active thyroid hormones are decreased. It may be congenital or acquired. Congenital hypothyroidism occurs in approximately 1 in 4000 live births and is twice as common in girls as in boys. In comparison to white infants, it is less prevalent among black infants but more prevalent in Hispanic infants (Rossi, Caplin, & Alter, 2005). It also occurs more commonly in children with Down syndrome. Acquired hypothyroidism is more common in girls than in boys.

Etiology and Pathophysiology

Thyroid hormones are important for growth and development and for metabolizing nutrients and energy. When these hormones are not available to stimulate other hormones or specific target cells, growth is delayed and mental retardation develops.

Congenital hypothyroidism is usually caused by a spontaneous gene mutation, an autosomal recessive genetic transmission of an enzyme deficiency, hypoplasia or aplasia of the thyroid gland, failure of the CNS–thyroid feedback mechanism to develop, or iodine deficiency. Mental retardation (cretinism) is irreversible if the disorder is not treated.

Acquired hypothyroidism can be idiopathic or result from autoimmune thyroiditis (Hashimoto thyroiditis), late-onset thyroid dysfunction, isolated thyroid-stimulating hormone (TSH) deficiency due to pituitary or hypothalamic dysfunction, or exposure to drugs or substances such as lithium that interfere with thyroid hormone synthesis. In the case of Hashimoto's thyroiditis, the thyroid is infiltrated by lymphocytes that cause an autoimmune reaction and an enlarged thyroid. A genetic predisposition to autoimmune thyroiditis and an autosomal dominant inheritance of thyroid antibodies has been identified (Roberts & Ladenson, 2004).

Clinical Manifestations

Infants with congenital hypothyroidism have few clinical signs of the disorder in the first weeks of life. In untreated infants the characteristic cretinoid features (thickened protuberant tongue, thick lips, and dull appearance) appear during the first few months of life. Other signs include prolonged neonatal jaundice, hypotonia, respiratory distress, bradycardia, decreased pulse pressure, hypothermia, cool extremities, mottling, pallor, umbilical hernia, a posterior fontanel larger than 1 cm in diameter, difficulty feeding, lethargy, swollen eyelids, constipation, and a hoarse cry (Palma Sisto, 2004).

Children with acquired hypothyroidism have many of the same signs as adults: decreased appetite, dry, cool skin, thinning hair or hair loss, depressed deep tendon reflexes, bradycardia, constipation, sensitivity to cold temperatures, abnormal menses, and a **goiter** (a nontender enlarged thyroid gland). Manifestations unique to children include change in past normal growth patterns with a weight increase, decreased height velocity, delayed bone and dental age, muscle hypertrophy with muscle weakness, and delayed or precocious puberty.

Clinical Therapy

Congenital hypothyroidism is usually detected during newborn screening of thyroxine (T_4) and TSH levels, which is mandatory in all U.S. states. Newborn screening has greatly reduced the morbidity of the disorder (Rossi et al., 2005). A decreased T_4, normal T_3, and elevated thyroid-stimulating hormone level indicates hypothyroidism. An elevated TSH level indicates that the disease originated in the thyroid, not the pituitary. Two tests are frequently performed so that the disorder is identified, before the newborn leaves the hospital and at the first healthcare visit at 1 to 2 weeks of age. Rapid response from the laboratory testing the samples is important to reduce the time to diagnosis and the effects of hypothyroidism on the infant's development.

If the T_4 level is below normal and the TSH level is increased, the synthetic thyroid hormone levothyroxine (Synthroid) is prescribed. The dose is increased gradually as the child grows to ensure a **euthyroid** (normal thyroid) state. A pediatric endocrinologist monitors treatment. Periodic evaluation of T_4 and TSH serum levels, bone age, and growth parameters are necessary to assess for signs of excess or inadequate thyroid hormone.

Antithyroid antibodies are measured in children with a goiter and suspected Hashimoto thyroiditis, as increased titers of antithyroglobin and antimicrosomal antibodies are often found.

To ensure an adequate growth rate and prevent mental retardation, the hormone must be taken throughout life. Children with congenital hypothyroidism that are diagnosed before 3 months of age have the best prognosis for optimal mental development. Children with acquired hypothyroidism usually have normal growth following a period of catch-up growth. Many adolescents with Hashimoto thyroiditis have a spontaneous remission.

NURSING MANAGEMENT

NURSING ASSESSMENT AND DIAGNOSIS

Routine neonatal screening is performed before discharge from the hospital and is often repeated at the infant's first health visit to evaluate levels of circulating thyroid hormones (see Skill 10–2 SKILLS).

Record the length or height and weight at each follow-up visit and plot on a growth curve. The child is assessed for signs of inadequate growth to determine if the dose of thyroid hormone needs to be adjusted and to monitor compliance with medication. Conduct developmental screening to detect delays in developmental milestones.

Among the nursing diagnoses that might be appropriate for the child with hypothyroidism are the following:

- *Imbalanced Nutrition: Less than Body Requirements* related to loss of appetite
- *Risk for Delayed Development* related to delayed initiation of thyroid replacement therapy
- *Risk for Disproportionate Growth* related to poor adherence to thyroid hormone therapy
- *Fatigue* related to inadequate dose of thyroid medication

PLANNING AND IMPLEMENTATION

Nursing care focuses on teaching the parents and child about the disorder and its treatment and monitoring the child's growth rate. Explain how to administer thyroid hormone (e.g., tablets can be crushed and mixed in a small amount of formula or applesauce as long as the child gets all of the medication). Advise parents that the child may experience temporary sleep disturbances or behavioral changes in response to therapy. Teach the parents how to assess for an increased pulse rate, which could indicate the presence of too much thyroid hormone, and advise them to report problems such as fatigue, which could indicate an improper drug dose that needs to be adjusted.

Caution parents to dress the child appropriately for the season to prevent hypothermia. Modify the child's diet by increasing the amount of fruits and bulk if constipation is a problem.

Reassure the family that the child will develop normally with hormone replacement therapy. Reinforce the importance of follow-up visits to assess growth rate and response to therapy and to regulate drug dosages as the child grows. Periodic assessments of educational achievement are needed. Even with good control, adolescents have persistent visual-spatial deficits, and memory and attention problems. Parents should be informed that therapy will be lifelong and is needed to promote the child's mental development. When the cause is genetic, make a referral for genetic counseling.

EVALUATION

Expected outcomes of nursing care of the child with hypothyroidism include the following:

- The child maintains adequate growth of height and weight, following a percentile curve throughout childhood.
- The child's diet contains adequate fruits and bulk to prevent constipation.
- The child's cognitive development is appropriate for age.

HYPERTHYROIDISM

Hyperthyroidism occurs when thyroid hormone levels are increased, resulting in excessive levels of circulating thyroid hormones. Hyperthyroidism is rare in children and adolescents occurring in only 0.02% of children, primarily in adolescents ages 11–15. The disorder is almost always due to Graves' disease (LaFranchi, 2007).

Etiology and Pathophysiology

Graves' disease is an autoimmune disorder. Immunoglobulins produced by the B lymphocytes stimulate oversecretion of thyroid hormones, resulting in the clinical symptoms. It has a high familial incidence.

Other less common causes of hyperthyroidism result from thyroiditis and thyroid hormone-producing tumors, including thyroid adenomas and carcinomas, and pituitary adenomas. Congenital hyperthyroidism can occur in infants of mothers with Graves' disease as a result of transplacental transfer of immunoglobulins.

Clinical Manifestations

Signs and symptoms are caused by hyperactivity of the sympathetic nervous system. Characteristic findings include an enlarged, nontender thyroid gland (goiter) prominent or bulging eyes (exophthalmos) (Figure 55–3 ●) eyelid lag, tachycardia, nervousness, restlessness or irritability, increased appetite with weight loss, emotional lability, heat intolerance, diaphoresis, insomnia, tremor, and muscle weakness. The thyroid gland may be slightly enlarged or grow to three to four times its normal size; feel warm, soft, and fleshy; and have an auditory bruit on auscultation. Onset is subtle, and the condition often goes unrecognized for 1 to 2 years.

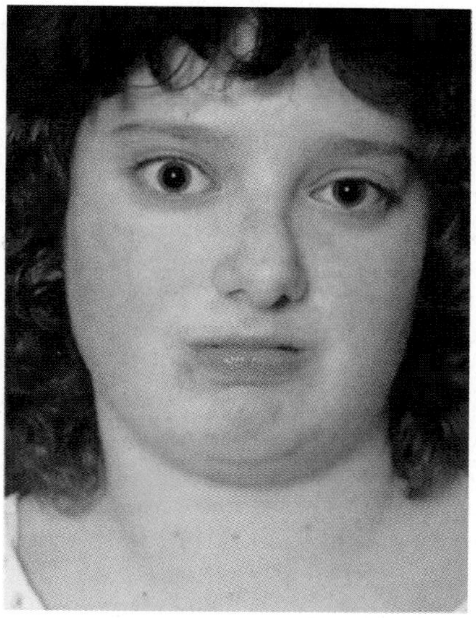

● **Figure 55–3** Exophthalmos and an enlarged thyroid in an adolescent with Graves' disease.

From Zitelli, B. J., & Davis, H. W. (Eds.). (2007). *Atlas of pediatric physical diagnosis* (5th ed., p. 357). Philadelphia: Mosby-Elsevier.

Children with Graves' disease usually have difficulty concentrating, behavioral problems and declining performance in school. They become easily frustrated in the classroom and overheated and fatigued during physical education class. Children with this disorder find it difficult to relax or sleep. These symptoms usually prompt parents to seek medical treatment for the child.

The most serious complication of hyperthyroidism is severe **thyrotoxicosis,** also called thyroid crisis or thyroid storm. It is a life-threatening emergency resulting from extreme hyperthyroidism, in which elevated circulating levels of TH result in a hypermetabolic state. The progression for thyrotoxicosis to life-threatening thyroid storm can occur. Symptoms include muscle weakness, tremor, diarrhea, excessive sweating, and palpitations and can progress to coma or cardiac failure (Amer, 2005).

Clinical Therapy

Diagnostic studies include laboratory evaluation of serum TSH, T_3 (triiodothyronine), and T_4 levels, and a thyroid scan. T_3 and T_4 levels are markedly elevated while the TSH level is decreased. Serum studies are also performed to detect thyroid autoantibodies (anti-TG and anti-TPO).

The goal of clinical therapy is to inhibit excessive secretion of thyroid hormones. Treatment may include drug therapy, radiation therapy, or surgery. Drug therapy is most often the initial treatment, but compliance is often a problem because of drug side effects. Methimazole (Tapazole) and propylthiouracil (PTU) are administered to inhibit thyroid (T_3 & T_4) secretion (Amer, 2005). PTU therapy can cause temporary side effects, including skin rashes, urticaria, and lymphadenopathy. If rash, fever, or sore throat develops, a healthcare professional should perform hematologic studies. Treatment continues for 2 years or longer until remission occurs. An estimated 25% achieve remission in 2 years, and 50% achieve it in 5 years (Amer, 2005). Symptoms usually improve within weeks of starting treatment. Adjunct therapy with beta-adrenergic blocking agents such as propranolol (Inderal) may be administered to relieve symptoms of tremors, tachycardia, lid lag, and excessive sweating (LaFranchi, 2007). Inderal may also be used during thyroid storm to prevent cardiac failure (Amer, 2005).

If medication therapy is ineffective, radiation therapy using oral radioactive iodine 1 is the next treatment choice. Current data do not indicate a relationship between radioactive iodine and cancer (Amer, 2005). Thyroidectomy (removal of most of the thyroid) provides an immediate cure and avoids radiation and possible long-term complications of radioactive iodine; however, destruction or removal of the thyroid gland often results in permanent hypothyroidism, necessitating lifelong hormone replacement therapy (Boger & Perrier, 2004). Manipulation of the parathyroid gland during surgery may result in excess release of parathyroid hormone, leading to hypercalcemia. Monitoring of serum calcium levels following a thyroidectomy is essential.

NURSING MANAGEMENT

NURSING ASSESSMENT AND DIAGNOSIS

Assess the child's vital signs, as blood pressure and pulse may be elevated. Keep a record of food intake. Accurate measurement and recording of height and weight are important to establish baselines and identify patterns of growth. Observe the child's behavior, activity, and level of fatigue.

Common nursing diagnoses for the child with hyperthyroidism include the following:

- *Ineffective Thermoregulation (Elevated)* related to illness and excessive activity of the sympathetic nervous system
- *Imbalanced Nutrition: Less than Body Requirements* related to high metabolic needs
- *Disturbed Body Image* related to changes caused by illness (prominent eyes, excessive perspiration, and tremors)
- *Fatigue* related to hypermetabolic state and sleep deprivation

PLANNING AND IMPLEMENTATION

Nursing care focuses on teaching the child and parents about the disorder and its treatment, promoting rest, providing emotional support, and, if the child needs surgery, providing preoperative and postoperative teaching and care. Promote increased caloric intake by providing five or six moderate meals per day. Encourage the child and family to express their feelings and concerns about the disorder. Pointing out even slight improvements in the child's condition increases adherence with therapy.

Children with hyperthyroidism are easily fatigued. Rest periods should be scheduled at school and home and physical activities kept to a minimum until symptoms resolve. Encourage parents to provide a cool environment and allow the child to wear fewer clothes until symptoms subside.

Children who have partial or total removal of the thyroid gland receive antithyroid drugs, such as iodine, for approximately 2 weeks before surgery to reduce the vascularity and size of the thyroid gland and to decrease the risk of thyroid storm.

Teach the child and parents about drug therapy and instruct parents to watch for side effects of antithyroid drugs, including fever, urticaria, and lymphadenopathy. Provide preoperative teaching (see Chapter 41∞). Young children in particular may be fearful about having their throat "cut."

Postoperatively, elevate the head of bed to 30 degrees to promote patent airway. A tracheostomy kit, suction supplies, and IV calcium gluconate should be immediately available for emergency treatment of hypocalcemia and respiratory distress. If thyroidectomy is performed, thyrotoxicosis does not immediately resolve because the half-life is 7 to 8 days. Antithyroid medications should be slowly tapered (Boger & Perrier, 2004).

Teach the family about the need for lifelong thyroid hormone replacement if radiation or surgery is performed. The child should wear a medical alert bracelet. Make sure the child is monitored regularly to ensure that the T_4 level is adequate to sustain growth.

EVALUATION

Expected outcomes of nursing care for the child with hyperthyroidism include the following:

- The child achieves balanced thermoregulation.
- The child participates in daily activities without experiencing fatigue.
- The child demonstrates a positive body image.

DISORDERS OF THE PARATHYROID

Children usually have four parathyroid glands located posterior to the thyroid gland. Their primary function is to work in conjunction with vitamin D to regulate total body calcium.

HYPERPARATHYROIDISM

Primary hyperparathyroidism, rare during childhood, is most often the result of a tumor (adenoma) which secretes the hormone without proper regulation (Doyle & DiGeorge, 2007). Secondary hyperparathyroidism is due to disease outside of the parathyroid gland, leading to excessive secretion of parathyroid hormone. This is commonly seen in chronic renal failure when the kidneys are unable to reabsorb calcium, causing low serum calcium levels and stimulating continual secretion of parathyroid hormone to maintain normal serum calcium levels (Molina, 2006). See Chapter 54∞.

Primary hyperparathyroidism may be asymptomatic. The most common symptoms are fatigue, exhaustion, lethargy, and constipation (Xu, 2005). There is often a delay between development of symptoms and diagnosis. Elevated serum calcium and PTH levels are diagnostic. Resection of the parathyroid is the treatment of choice in children with primary hyperparathyroidism (Kollars, Zarroug, van Heerden, et al., 2005). Treatment of secondary hyperparathyroidism focuses on prevention of hypercalcemia using vitamin D replacement and phosphorus binders.

Nursing Management

Nursing care centers on fluid management and electrolyte monitoring. In children who require surgery, assess for respiratory distress and a potential airway obstruction due to edema and a potential hematoma around the tracheal space. Monitor for signs of infection.

Following surgery, educate the child and parents to recognize signs of hypocalcemia and to provide appropriate amounts of calcium supplementation. After diagnosis or after surgical intervention, follow-up is important to monitor serum calcium and phosphorus levels to detect persistence of hyperparathyroidism.

HYPOPARATHYROIDISM

Primary hypoparathyroidism is rare, but it may result from congenital disorders (parathyroid aplasia, DiGeorge syndrome), surgical removal of the parathyroid glands, disease processes destroying the parathyroid glands (Wilson disease, hemochromatosis), or medications (e.g., aluminum, asparagine, doxorubicin, cytosine, arabinoside). Hypoparathyroidism can also be idiopathic. The primary result is hypocalcemia and hyperphosphatemia.

Infants may display hyperirritability, muscle rigidity, seizures, vomiting, abdominal distention, apneic episodes, intermittent cyanosis, or twitching. Muscle pain and cramps may progress to numbness, stiffness, and tingling of the hands and feet. A positive **Chvostek sign** (spasm of facial muscles after tapping facial nerve) reveals hyperreflexia. Life-threatening tetany and convulsions may occur with hypocalcemia (Doyle & DiGeorge, 2007).

Serum calcium and PTH levels are low and serum phosphorus is elevated. Radiographs often demonstrate increased bone density. Oral calcitriol and calcium are given for an indefinite period of time (Caplin, 2005). Foods with high phosphorus content (dairy products and eggs) are limited.

Nursing Management

Assess and stabilize the airway, breathing, and circulation. In the acute care setting, children should be placed on a cardiorespiratory monitor. Maintain seizure precautions until normal serum calcium levels are attained. Obtain intravenous access and administer calcium supplementation as ordered.

Nursing Practice

Dilute intravenous calcium per hospital protocol. Infiltration of IV calcium can cause extravasation and tissue sloughing. Always check the patency of the IV prior to administration. Monitor ECG during administration. Evaluate for hypocalcemia and hypercalcemia after administration.

Partner with the family to ensure their understanding of the need for calcium supplementation and reduced intake of phosphorus. Teach the family that periodic monitoring of calcium levels is important. Inform the family that hypoparathyroidism may require lifelong therapy.

DISORDERS OF ADRENAL FUNCTION

CUSHING DISEASE

Cushing disease, also called adrenocortical hyperfunction, is characterized by a group of symptoms resulting from excess levels of glucocorticoids (especially cortisol) in the bloodstream. It is uncommon in children and the true incidence is unknown. During infancy, most cases of endogenous Cushing disease are due to a functioning adrenocortical tumor. The tumor is usually a malignant carcinoma; however, it may be a benign adenoma (White, 2007). Other causes include hyperplasia of one or both adrenal glands and benign tumors of the adrenal glands. The increased secretion of cortisol alters metabolism.

The initial sign in most children is gradual excessive weight gain followed by growth retardation, hypertension, and mental and behavior problems. It generally takes 2 to 5 years for the child to develop the characteristic "cushingoid" appearance, which includes a moon face (chubby cheeks and a double chin) and fat pads over the shoulders and back (buffalo hump). The most common reasons for cushingoid features in children are excessive doses of corticosteroids and prolonged use of corticosteroids as treatment for other diseases. Cushingoid features may develop in a shorter time than occurs with Cushing disease. Corticosteroids suppress adrenal function when administered long term. These children may have Cushing disease. See "Clinical Manifestations: Cushing Disease."

Diagnosis is based on characteristic physical findings and laboratory values, including increased 24-hour urinary levels of free cortisol, and 17-hydroxycorticosteroid (17-OHCs); and elevated nighttime salivary cortisol level. The child has chronic hyperglycemia and an elevated glycosylated hemoglobin concentration. See Appendix B for lab values.

The adrenal suppression test using an 11 p.m. dose of dexamethasone reveals that adrenal cortisol output is not suppressed overnight as would occur normally in children. Computed tomography (CT) and magnetic resonance imaging (MRI) detect tumors in the adrenal and pituitary glands.

Surgical removal of the pituitary adenoma is the current treatment of choice when this is the cause of Cushing disease. Replacement glucocorticoid therapy may be needed for several months after surgery. Irradiation of the pituitary is performed when surgical removal of the adenoma does not substantially reduce cortisol levels. Alternatively, medications may be given for management of hypercortisolism by interrupting adrenal steroid synthesis.

Lifelong glucocorticoid and mineralocorticoid replacement is required when both adrenal glands are removed. The prognosis for children with malignant adrenal tumors is poor.

Clinical Manifestations

CUSHING DISEASE

ETIOLOGY	CLINICAL MANIFESTATIONS	NURSING MANAGEMENT
Catabolism of protein	Muscle weakness and wasting, capillary weakness and bruising, growth failure with delayed bone age, fatigue	Plan periods of rest for child Cluster nursing care Assess skin for bruising Assess and plot growth and development
Decreased absorption of calcium from the intestines	Demineralization of bones, osteoporosis	Monitor serum calcium levels
Increased appetite	Weight gain primarily on the trunk, striae on the abdomen, buttocks, thighs	Assist in meal planning Refer to nutritionist
Salt retention	Increased blood volume and hypertension	Teach family to monitor and record child's blood pressure

Nursing Management

Nursing assessment during both the pre- and postoperative phases includes monitoring the child's vital signs, fluid status, nutritional status, and weight. Additional assessment includes monitoring muscle strength and endurance during hospital play activities.

Teach the child and family about the disorder and its treatment. For children undergoing surgery, provide preoperative and postoperative teaching and care. Answer any questions the child and family may have and explain all laboratory and diagnostic tests. Explain to parents that the child's cushingoid appearance is reversible with treatment. Refer to Chapter 52 for general nursing care of the child with cancer. Provide nutritional guidance or refer the child and parents to a nutritionist to promote maintenance of an appropriate weight.

For children who need cortisol replacement therapy because both adrenal glands were surgically removed, administering the drug early in the morning or every other day causes fewer symptoms than daily administration and mimics the normal diurnal pattern of cortisol secretion. Cortisol replacement in the postoperative period must be explained carefully to parents. Hydrocortisone (Cortef, Solu-Cortef, cortisone acetate) comes in liquid, tablet, or injectable form. Parents may need to crush the tablet and mix with a small amount of applesauce, but the entire dose of medication must be taken. The oral preparations of cortisone have a bitter taste and can cause gastric irritation. Giving the dose at mealtimes and using antacids between meals helps reduce these side effects. Teach parents how and when to administer the injectable form—usually when the child is vomiting, has diarrhea, or cannot take the oral medication. Failure to give medication when the child is ill may lead to severe illness and cardiovascular collapse.

Teach parents to be alert to signs of acute adrenal insufficiency during the withdrawal of corticosteroid therapy, and to inform all healthcare providers of the child's condition and medication. The child should wear a medical alert bracelet at all times.

Teaching Highlights

HYDROCORTISONE ADMINISTRATION

Teach the family the following tips regarding hydrocortisone administration:

- Always give the medication at the times prescribed since the schedule follows the body's normal cortisol release pattern.
- Never abruptly discontinue the medication.
- If the child has vomiting or diarrhea and is unable to take the medication by mouth, administer the injections to replace oral doses as instructed and notify the physician immediately. Higher doses of hydrocortisone are needed when the child is ill.
- Always have injectable hydrocortisone available at home, at school, and everywhere the child travels. An emergency kit should be available at all times to supply cortisol to the child during acute illnesses and stressful situations. Check expiration dates frequently and maintain current medications in the emergency kit.

CONGENITAL ADRENAL HYPERPLASIA

Congenital adrenal hyperplasia (CAH), sometimes called adrenogenital syndrome, adrenocortical hyperplasia, or congenital adrenogenital hyperplasia, is an autosomal recessive disorder that causes a deficiency of one of the enzymes necessary for the synthesis of cortisol and aldosterone.

Etiology and Pathophysiology

This disorder occurs in 1 in 10,000–15,000 live births (Kwon & Tsai, 2007). This form has an autosomal recessive inheritance pattern and the defective gene CYP21 is located on the short arm of chromosome 6. About 5–8% of children have deficiency of 11 β-hydroxylase. Mutations on defective gene CPY11B1 of chromosome 8 result in inadequate cortisol and excess levels of other steroids and testosterone synthesis (Henwood & Katz, 2005). The remaining 2–5% of cases involve deficiencies of other enzymes.

Of the two classic forms of the disorder, 75% are salt-losing, caused by aldosterone deficiency and overproduction of androgen, and 25% are nonsalt-losing with **virilization** (the production of masculine secondary sexual characteristics in females). In all forms, increased secretion of ACTH occurs in response to diminished cortisol levels (Kwon & Tsai, 2007).

During fetal development the lack of cortisol triggers the pituitary to continue secretion of ACTH. This in turn stimulates overproduction of the adrenal androgens. Virilization of the female external genitalia begins in week 10 of gestation. If untreated, the overproduction of androgens results in accelerated height, early closure of the epiphyseal plates, and premature sexual development with both pubic and axillary hair.

Clinical Manifestations

Congenital adrenal hyperplasia is the most common cause of **pseudohermaphroditism** (ambiguous genitalia) in newborn girls. The female infant is born with an enlarged clitoris and partial or complete labial fusions. The vagina usually has a common opening with the urethra (Figure 55–4 ●). Severely virilized females may be mistaken for males with cryptorchidism, hypospadias, or micropenis (Chapter 54). The uterus, ovaries, and fallopian tubes are normal. The male infant may look normal at birth or may have a slightly enlarged penis and hyperpigmented scrotum. The boy may have tall stature and an adult-sized penis by school age, but the testes are appropriately sized for age. Partial enzyme deficiency produces less obvious symptoms. Precocious puberty, tall stature for age, acne, and excessive muscle development may be noted in both males and females as the child grows. Due to early epiphyseal fusion, adult stature is shorter.

Signs of adrenal insufficiency may be the first indication of the disorder. Recurrent vomiting, dehydration, metabolic acidosis, hypotension, and hypoglycemia are characteristic signs of the salt-wasting form of the disorder. Hypertension with hypokalemic alkalosis is alternately found in children with 11-hydroxylase deficiency.

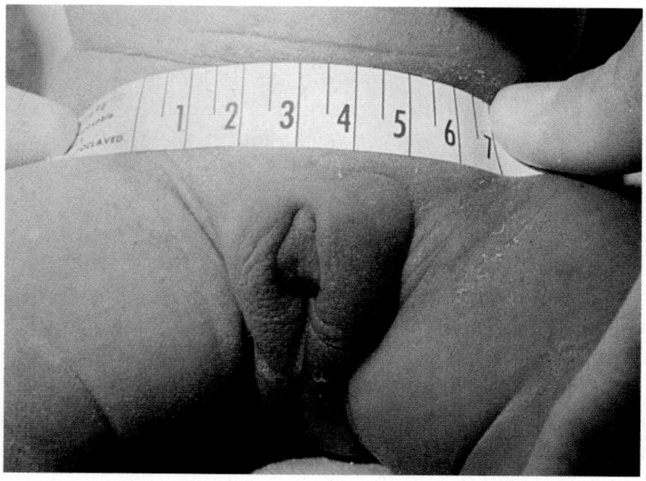

● **Figure 55–4** Newborn girl with ambiguous genitalia.
Courtesy of Patrick C. Walsh, MD.

Clinical Therapy

Diagnosis in infants and children is usually confirmed by laboratory evaluation of serum 17-hydroxyprogesterone (17-OHP) level. Routine newborn screening for congenital adrenal hyperplasia is performed in all 50 states (National Newborn Screening and Genetics Resource Center, 2009). Prenatal diagnosis is available. In instances of ambiguous genitalia, a karyotype determines the infant's gender. (See Chapter 7.) Ultrasonography may be used to visualize pelvic structures.

In the salt-wasting form of the disorder, the child may have hyponatremia, hyperkalemia, acidosis, hypoglycemia, a high urine sodium level, and low serum and urinary aldosterone levels. Serum concentrations of testosterone in girls and androstenedione in boys and girls are elevated in affected infants. Measurement of ACTH and 17-hydroxyprogesterone levels reveal high readings, while serum cortisol is inappropriately low in comparison to ACTH (White, 2007). Diagnosis may be delayed in the nonsalt-losing form until 3 to 7 years.

The goal of treatment is to suppress adrenal secretion of androgens by replacing deficient hormones. This is accomplished by the lifelong use of oral glucocorticoids (dexamethasone, prednisone, or hydrocortisone). The glucocorticoid replacement reduces secretion of ACTH, which had overstimulated the adrenal cortex. As a result, excessive adrenal androgen production is suppressed. The dose is individualized by monitoring growth parameters, bone age, and hormone levels. If the infant has the salt-wasting form of the disorder, salt is added to the infant's formula, and a mineralocorticoid (Florinef) is given to replace the missing hormone. Hormone dosage must be doubled or tripled during acute illnesses or injury and for surgery. Injectable hydrocortisone is used for severe stress. Adrenalectomy is recommended only in cases when medical therapy is ineffective (Pang, 2003).

Reconstructive surgery of the enlarged clitoris is often performed on girls during the first year of life; however, some centers support waiting until adolescence, allowing the patient to participate in the decision for surgery.

NURSING MANAGEMENT

NURSING ASSESSMENT AND DIAGNOSIS

Assess the infant and child for signs of dehydration, electrolyte imbalance, and hypovolemic shock in the salt-wasting form of the disease (see Skill 9–22 SKILLS). Monitor the airway, breathing, circulation, and responsiveness. Assess vital signs and assess peripheral perfusion (capillary refill, distal pulses, color and temperature of the extremities) frequently to detect early changes in condition such as hypovolemia.

Assess the parents' emotional response to a child with ambiguous genitalia and a chronic condition. Explore their values and beliefs regarding gender roles and sexuality while awaiting results of the karyotype.

Nursing diagnoses for the child with congenital adrenal hyperplasia might include the following:

- *Impaired Parenting* related to a child with undetermined gender identity
- *Caregiver Role Strain* related to care of a child with a chronic, potentially life-threatening condition
- *Risk for Deficient Fluid Volume* related to failure of regulatory mechanisms and excess excretion of salt by the kidneys
- *Risk for Disproportionate Growth* related to accelerated growth and premature closure of epiphyseal plates

PLANNING AND IMPLEMENTATION

Nursing care of the newborn with CAH focuses on teaching parents about the disorder and its treatment, providing emotional support, and preoperative and postoperative teaching for parents of infants undergoing reconstructive surgery. The administration of glucocorticoids and mineralocorticoids must be carefully controlled.

It is often difficult for parents to accept that their infant, whose genitalia look male, is really female. With medication and surgery, the genitalia assume a female appearance and all organs necessary for future childbearing are usually functional. Several surgeries may be performed before 2 years of age and then during adolescence to dilate the vagina. Because of the risk for adrenal insufficiency, the child will most likely be hospitalized for surgery rather than having outpatient surgery.

Nurses can assist parents in educating the child's siblings, grandparents, other family members, and childcare workers about the condition. In the newborn nursery, the infant should be referred to as "your beautiful infant," not "your son" or "your daughter," until gender identity is confirmed.

Inform parents that genetic counseling should be provided for the child during adolescence. Parents considering a future pregnancy should also be informed that prenatal testing may detect congenital adrenal hyperplasia in the fetus. Refer the family for counseling if indicated.

NURSING CARE IN THE COMMUNITY

Teach parents about the special problems that develop in the salt-wasting form of the disease during acute illness. Explain the medication regimen and help the family develop an emergency care plan. The child should wear a medical alert bracelet. Teach parents how to administer intramuscular injections of hydrocortisone. If injectable hydrocortisone is not available, the child needs urgent treatment in an emergency department. The child may become dehydrated quickly and need intravenous fluid and electrolyte replacement in addition to higher doses of hydrocortisone.

EVALUATION

Expected outcomes of nursing care for congenital adrenal hyperplasia include the following:

- Parent/newborn attachment is achieved.
- The child maintains fluid volume balance.
- The child achieves age-appropriate growth and developmental milestones.
- The parents demonstrate understanding of treatment and respond appropriately when injectable medication is needed.

ADRENAL INSUFFICIENCY (ADDISON DISEASE)

Adrenal insufficiency, also known as Addison disease, is a rare disorder in childhood characterized by a deficiency of glucocorticoids (cortisone) and mineralocorticoids (aldosterone). The lack of glucocorticoids affects the body's ability to handle stress (Gance-Cleveland, 2003). The majority of cases of Addison disease are caused by an autoimmune process. It may also be acquired after trauma, or with tuberculosis, HIV infection, meningococcemia, or fungal infections that destroy the adrenal glands.

Adrenal insufficiency usually develops slowly as the adrenal glands deteriorate. The early signs may not be noticed but include weakness with fatigue, lethargy and emotional lability, anorexia and salt craving, and poor weight gain or weight loss. Skin changes include hyperpigmentation on pressure points, lip borders, gingival margins, nipples, palms, soles, body creases, and scarred areas of the body, as well as generalized bronzing of the skin or freckling without tan lines even in winter months. Additional signs include abdominal pain, nausea and vomiting, diarrhea, and symptomatic hypoglycemia. If the child experiences a stressful period (illness, injury, or surgery), acute adrenal insufficiency may occur. Signs of an adrenal crisis include weakness, fever, abdominal pain, hypoglycemia with seizures, hypotension, dehydration, shock, and coma.

Clinical Therapy

Serum cortisol and urinary 17-hydroxycorticoid levels are measured in the early morning. Low levels of serum cortisol are associated with adrenal insufficiency. The ACTH stimulation test is used to detect adrenal gland reserve. Electrolyte values generally reveal low serum sodium, elevated serum potassium, and low fasting blood glucose levels. CT may be used to visualize the adrenal glands.

Treatment involves replacement of the deficient hormones. Oral hydrocortisone is given in the lowest therapeutic dose to control symptoms and promote normal growth. Fludrocortisone acetate (Florinef) is administered to replace the missing mineralocorticoid in children with aldosterone deficiency.

Adrenal crisis is treated by aggressive fluid resuscitation, intravenous glucose, and intravenous hydrocortisone. The precipitating illness or injury is then treated along with adequate doses of glucocorticoid, and maintenance doses of mineralocorticoid. Children will also need increased doses of steroids during periods of increased physiologic stress, such as surgical procedures, illnesses, and injuries. In these cases, the dose of hydrocortisone should be at least tripled and given three times a day for 24 hours or for as long as the stress lasts before resuming the maintenance dose (Henwood & Katz, 2005).

Nursing Management

Nursing management focuses on educating the child and parents about the disorder, providing emotional support, and caring for the child during acute episodes. See the earlier discussion of congenital adrenal hyperplasia for further detail.

PHEOCHROMOCYTOMA

Pheochromocytoma is a tumor of the adrenal gland, but it may be extra-adrenal with no anatomic connection. In most cases these tumors are benign and curable. They can occur in a familial pattern (autosomal dominant trait) with a 3:2 male to female ratio. Most tumors diagnosed in children are identified between the ages of 6 and 14 years; however, this only accounts for 10% of these tumors as most are identified during adult years (White, 2007). Pheochromocytomas may also be associated with neurofibromatosis. See Chapter 56∞.

The tumor causes an excessive release of catecholamines epinephrine and norepinephrine leading to hypertension. Clinical manifestations include labile hypertension with a systolic reading that may reach 250 mm Hg, tachycardia, arrhythmias, palpitations, profuse sweating with cool extremities, flushing, headache, abdominal pain, nausea and vomiting, weight loss, visual disturbances, weakness, polydipsia, and polyuria. The classic triad of signs includes new-onset hypertension, new or worsening diabetes mellitus, and hypertensive crisis. Because release of catecholamines (norepinephrine and epinephrine) from the tumor is not continuous, these symptoms occur intermittently. Episodes may occur daily or monthly and generally last minutes to an hour (Failor & Capell, 2003). In some cases the condition may be silent until a stressor such as surgery causes a hypertensive crisis.

Clinical Therapy

Diagnosis is based on 24-hour urine studies to detect the presence of increased urinary catecholamines and vanilmandelic (VMA) levels. Radiologic imaging with CT, PET scan, MRI, and ultrasound studies are required to locate the tumor in preparation for surgery. Most are located on the adrenal gland, but they may also be located in the chest, abdomen, pelvis, head, and neck (Karagiannis, Mikhailidis, Athyros, et al., 2007).

The treatment of choice is curative surgical removal of all identified tumors; however, the procedure is dangerous and may result in pheochromocytoma crisis. Removal of the tumor during surgery may cause a release of stored epinephrine and norepinephrine, leading to elevated blood pressure and changes in heart rate (pheochromocytoma crisis). If this occurs, alpha-adrenergic blocking agents are administered.

Alpha- and beta-adrenergic blocking agents to control hypertension, tachycardia, and catecholamine release are given for 10 to 14 days before surgery (Karagiannis et al., 2007). Plasma catecholamines are used to measure the effectiveness of the preoperative adrenergic blockade. Postoperatively, for several days, a 24-hour urine collection is measured for catecholamines to determine if all tumor sites were removed. With successful removal of all tumor sites, the prognosis is generally good. Follow-up is important to assess for recurrence.

Nursing Management

Nursing care is mainly supportive. Provide preoperative and postoperative teaching and care (see Chapter 41∞). Preoperatively, monitor vital signs and observe for signs of complications associated with pheochromocytoma crisis. Administer antihypertensives and watch for any signs of hyperglycemia (see page 1637). Postoperatively, the child may be managed initially in an intensive care unit. Monitor blood pressure and glucose levels. Hypoglycemia and hypotension may occur following the withdrawal of excessive amounts of catecholamines. Observe for changes in neurologic status, respiratory distress, and signs of shock. Lifelong follow-up care with screening for hypertension and increased urinary catecholamine levels is required as symptoms recur if the child has other tumors not yet detected that activate at a later age (White, 2007).

DISORDERS OF PANCREATIC FUNCTION

MyNursingKit Animation: Physiology of Diabetes

DIABETES MELLITUS

Diabetes mellitus, the most common metabolic disease in children, is a disorder of hyperglycemia resulting from defects in insulin secretion, insulin action, or both, leading to abnormalities in carbohydrate, protein, and fat metabolism (American Diabetes Association, 2008a). There are two main types of diabetes. Most children have immune-mediated type 1 diabetes, formerly called insulin-dependent diabetes mellitus or juvenile diabetes. However, a disturbingly large number of children are being diagnosed with type 2 diabetes, formerly called noninsulin-dependent diabetes (Alemzadeh & Wyatt, 2007).

TYPE 1 DIABETES

MyNursingKit Case Study: Diabetic Risk Factors

In the United States, approximately 1 in every 400–600 children and adolescents have type 1 diabetes (American Diabetes Association, 2008b). Peak incidence in childhood is between 7 and 15 years of age; however, type 1 diabetes can present at any age (Alemzadeh & Wyatt, 2007). Caucasians experience a higher incidence of type 1 diabetes than other racial groups. Boys and girls are equally affected.

Etiology and Pathophysiology

Type 1 diabetes results from destruction of pancreatic islet beta cells, which fail to secrete insulin. The body becomes dependent on exogenous sources of insulin. Type 1 diabetes is a multifactorial disease caused by autoimmune destruction of insulin-producing pancreatic beta cells in genetically predisposed individuals (Sepa, Wahlberg, Vaarala, et al., 2005). Type 1 diabetes has familial tendencies but does not show any specific pattern of inheritance. Inheritance of the DR3 and DR4 markers on the human leukocyte antigen (HLA) complex on chromosome 6 increases the likelihood of developing type 1 diabetes. If the child inherits one marker, the child's risk is 2 to 3 times higher. If both markers are inherited, the child's risk is 7 to 10 times higher (Alemzadeh & Wyatt, 2007). However, the child inherits a susceptibility to the disease rather than the disease itself. It is believed that an event such as a virus triggers the inflammatory process, resulting in development of islet cell serum antibodies. These antibodies can be detected in the blood years before the development of the clinical symptoms (Weinzimer & Magge, 2005).

Insulin helps transport glucose into the cells so that the body can use it as an energy source. It also prevents the outflow of glucose from the liver to the general circulation. It is hypothesized that type 1 diabetes may be caused by a genetic component, environmental influences, or an autoimmune response that damages the pancreatic beta cells (Alemzadeh & Wyatt, 2007). Environmental factors such as enteroviruses or toxins are believed to lead to an autoimmune destruction of the beta cells in the islets of Langerhans (see Pathophysiology Illustrated). Antigens are generated that lead to production of antibodies that indicate ongoing destruction of the islet cells. As the destruction continues, insulin secretion decreases.

As the secretion of insulin decreases, the blood glucose level rises and the glucose level inside the cells decreases. When the renal threshold for glucose (180 mg/dL) is exceeded, **glycosuria** (abnormal amount of glucose in the urine) occurs as a result of osmotic diuresis (Alemzadeh & Wyatt, 2007). Fluids follow the highly osmotic glucose and water is excreted in large volumes of urine (polyuria).

When glucose is unavailable to the cells for metabolism, free fatty acids provide an alternate source of energy. The liver metabolizes fatty acids at an increased rate, producing acetyl coenzyme A (CoA). The by-products of acetyl CoA metabolism (ketone bodies) accumulate in the body, resulting in a state of metabolic acidosis, or ketoacidosis. (Refer to Chapter 46 for discussion of metabolic acidosis; see page 1635 for ketoacidosis.)

Clinical Manifestations

The classic signs of type 1 diabetes are polyuria, polydipsia, and **polyphagia** (excessive appetite) with significant weight loss. See "Clinical Manifestations: Diabetes by Type." Other signs include unexplained fatigue or lethargy, headaches, stomachaches. Enuresis may also occur in a previously toilet-trained child. Adolescent girls may have vaginitis caused by *Candida,* which thrives in the hyperglycemic tissues. Symptoms develop gradually and insidiously but have usually been present less than a month when diagnosed. Approximately 30% of new onset cases of diabetes are ill with diabetic ketoacidosis (DKA), a type of metabolic acidosis (Silverstein, Klingensmith, Copeland, et al., 2005). See Nursing Practice for information about cystic fibrosis–related diabetes.

Clinical Manifestations

DIABETES BY TYPE

CAUSE	CLINICAL MANIFESTATIONS	CLINICAL THERAPY
Type 1—immune mediated, insulin deficiency due to pancreatic beta cell destruction	Polyuria, polydipsia May have polyphagia Weight loss Ketoacidosis on initial presentation in 30% to 40% of cases, at continued risk for ketoacidosis Short duration of symptoms Ketosis Initial period of decreased insulin requirement, then need insulin for survival	Blood glucose monitoring Insulin Dietary management, balancing carbohydrate intake to insulin Exercise
Type 2—insulin resistance with relative insulin secretory defect	Obese, little or no weight loss, or may have significant weight loss Acanthosis nigricans Long duration of symptoms Polyuria, polydipsia, may be mild or absent Glycosuria without ketonuria in 33% of cases on initial presentation Ketoacidosis on initial presentation in 5% to 25% of cases Lipid disorders Hypertension Androgen-mediated problems such as acne, hirsutism, menstrual disturbances, polycystic ovary disease Excessive weight gain and fatigue due to insulin resistance	Diet with decreased calories and low-fat foods Decrease sedentary activity time or increase routine physical activity Blood glucose monitoring Oral medication (metformin) to improve insulin sensitivity

PATHOPHYSIOLOGY ILLUSTRATED

MECHANISM OF DIABETES MELLITUS

Destruction of the alpha and beta cells in the islets of Langerhans produces multiple metabolic changes. Acute signs and symptoms are followed by short-term and long-term complications if the disease is not well managed.

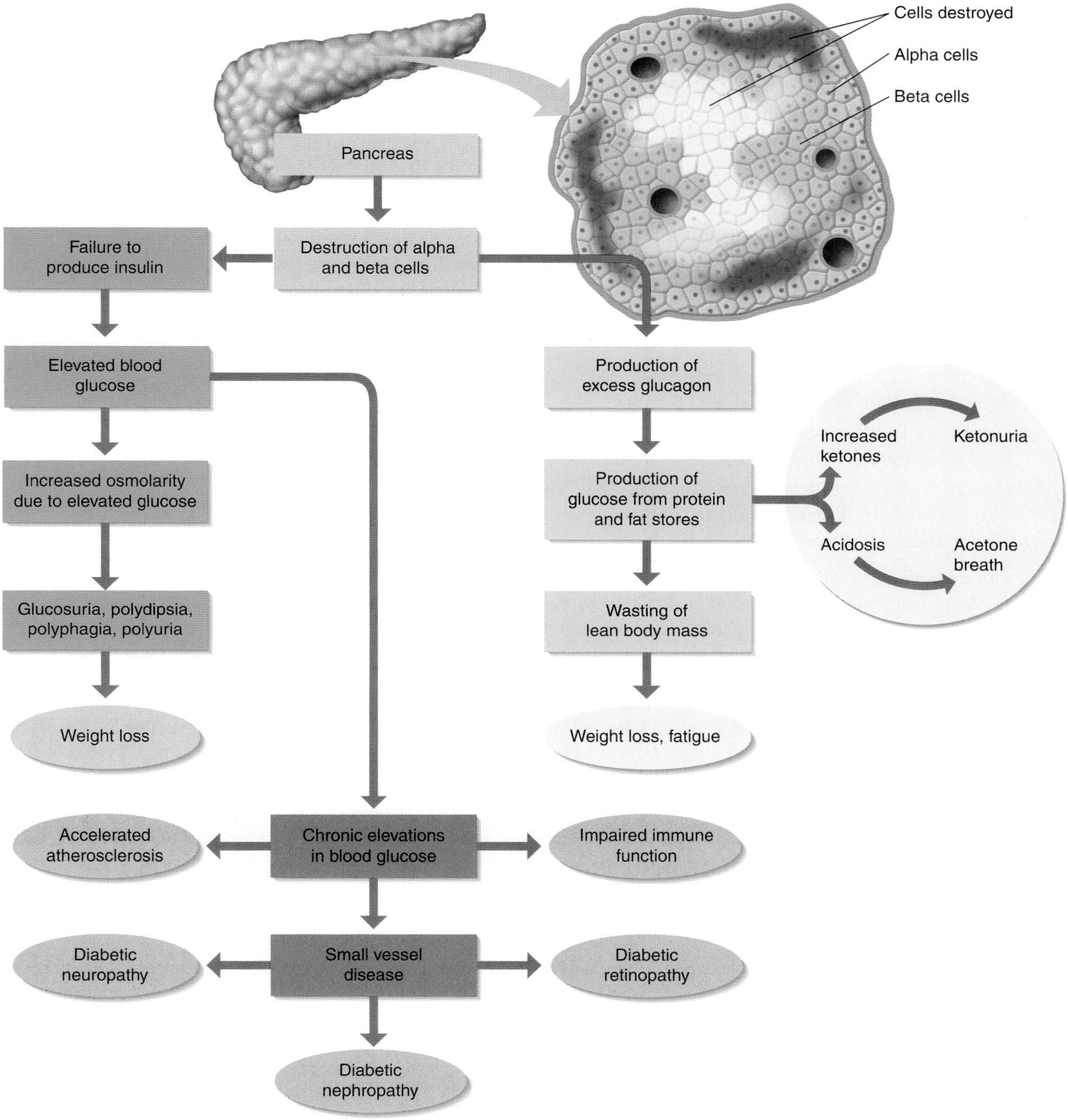

Nursing Practice

Cystic fibrosis-related diabetes (CFRD) has similar features of types 1 and 2 diabetes; however, it is considered a separate condition. In cystic fibrosis, the pancreas does not produce sufficient insulin (as in type 1 diabetes), which is referred to as **insulin deficiency**. Another mechanism of CFRD is ***insulin resistance***, an impairment in insulin receptors on cell membranes, leading to inability to transfer sufficient amounts of glucose into cells, requiring higher levels of insulin for metabolism. Insulin deficiency and insulin resistance combined in the patient with cystic fibrosis can lead to the development of diabetes more frequently in these patients than in the general population (Cystic Fibrosis Foundation, 2009).

Clinical Therapy

Diagnosis is based on the presence of classic symptoms and one of the following plasma glucose levels (American Diabetes Association, 2008a):

- Fasting plasma glucose greater than or equal to (7 mmol/L), no caloric intake for at least 8 hours
- Two-hour plasma glucose greater than or equal to (11.1 mmol/L) during an oral glucose tolerance test
- Plasma glucose concentration greater than or equal to (11.1 mmol/L) taken at any time of day regardless of time of last meal

When an asymptomatic child's screening test reveals an elevated glucose level, confirmation of a second fasting plasma glucose level should be performed. An oral glucose tolerance test is rarely required. Other laboratory tests for known autoantibodies (e.g., glutamic acid decarboxylase (GAD-65), insulin autoantibodies, and islet cell cytoplasmicautoantibodies) can indicate an autoimmune attack against the insulin-producing beta cells of the pancreas, and may be helpful in some cases to distinguish between type 1 and type 2 diabetes. Plasma c-peptide levels and fasting insulin levels will be low in type 1 diabetes (Berry, Urban, & Grey, 2006a). A careful history is necessary to rule out a stress-related illness, corticosteroid use, fracture, acute infection, cystic fibrosis, pancreatitis, or liver disease.

Nursing Practice

The American Diabetes Association considers a fasting glucose level of 100–125 mg/dL (5.6–6.9 mmol/l) to be an *impaired fasting glucose,* and a 2-hour postload glucose level of 140–199 mg/dL to be an *impaired glucose tolerance*. Individuals with impaired fasting glucose and/or impaired glucose tolerance are now referred to as having "pre-diabetes," indicating that they have a relatively high risk for development of diabetes (American Diabetes Association, 2008a).

Clinical therapy for type 1 diabetes combines insulin, nutrition management to support growth and maintain blood glucose at near-normal levels, an exercise regimen, and psychosocial support.

Insulin therapy. Multiple approaches to insulin therapy for children and adolescents are available, and an approach that works for the child and family should be selected. Children often need several daily injections of insulin before meals and at bedtime to maintain an optimal blood glucose level. See the Drug Guide for different types of insulin and action times.

The basal-bolus insulin regimen has been documented to result in stable glycemic control and less hypoglycemia in comparison to other regimens using intermediate and short acting insulin regimens (Silverstein et al., 2005). Insulin can be administered by an insulin pump or by multiple daily injections. With basal-bolus therapy, basal insulin is administered once a day using glargine, and then a bolus of rapid-acting insulin is adminis-

Drug Guide

DIABETES MELLITUS AND AVERAGE INSULIN ACTION TIMES (SUBCUTANEOUS ROUTE)

TYPE	ONSET	PEAK	DURATION	ACTION
Rapid Acting				
Insulin lispro, insulin glulisine or insulin aspart	5–10 min	0.5 to 2 hr	3–4 hr	Insulin is an endogenous hormone, secreted by the beta cells of the pancreas. It lowers the blood glucose level by stimulating glucose passage across cell membranes and uptake into the cells. It also promotes the conversion of glucose to glycogen and inhibits hepatic glucose production from glycogen.
Short Acting				
Regular	0.5–1 hr	2–5 hr	6–8 hr	
Intermediate Acting				
NPH	1–3 hr	5–8 hr	12–18 hr	
Very Long Acting				
Glargine or Detemir	1.5–4 hr	None	20–24 hr	

Adapted from: Rachmiel, M., Perlman, K., & Daneman, D. (2005). Insulin analogues in children and teens with type 1 diabetes: Advantages and caveats. *Pediatric Clinics of North America, 52*, 1651–1675.

Nursing Practice

Insulin is usually provided in prepackaged doses of 100 units/mL. Diluted insulin prepared by a pharmacist may be used for infants and toddlers who require a small insulin dosage. Insulin cartridges, disposable pens, and other devices are available, making insulin easy to carry by older children and adolescents for frequent insulin injections during the day.

tered with each meal and snack based on the carbohydrate grams consumed and the blood glucose level. This means that a child may get 6 to 7 injections a day. Stress, infection, and illness may either increase or decrease insulin needs. If basal-bolus therapy for type 1 diabetes is to be effective, the child and family need to do each of the following:

- Monitor the blood glucose four to eight times daily and once a week at midnight and 3 a.m.
- Consistently count carbohydrates consumed
- Anticipate exercise in the daily routine

Continuous subcutaneous insulin infusion (CSII) pump therapy is increasingly used by children and adolescents as the technology makes it possible to more closely match the plasma insulin levels in normal children (see Table 55–3). CSII pump therapy has been used successfully in children of all ages, including infants and toddlers. Insulin therapy can now be adjusted to the lifestyle of the child or adolescent (Weinzimer, Sikes, Steffen, et al., 2005). Advantages and disadvantages of an insulin pump are outlined in Table 55–4. CSII has been found to improve metabolic control in youth with type 1 diabetes (Doyle, Weinzimer, Steffen, et al., 2004).

The goal of insulin therapy is to maintain a range of blood glucose levels that varies by the child's age. Glycemic goals for children younger than 6 years old are generally less stringent since they lack the cognitive capacity to recognize and respond to hypoglycemic symptoms (Silverstein et al., 2005).

Insulin therapy is evaluated every 3 months with a hemoglobin A_{1c} (HbA_{1c}) level, an objective measurement of glycemic control. It represents the amount of glucose that binds to the hemoglobin molecule, predicting an index of glucose control over the prior 60–90 days. The HbA_{1c} is below 5.9% for individuals without diabetes (Howe, Jawad, Tuttle, et al., 2005) and the goal for children with diabetes is 7.5% to 8% depending on age and healthcare provider preferences. It is also important to determine if the HbA_{1c} matches recorded blood sugars.

Nutrition therapy. The goal of nutrition therapy is to provide adequate calories for the child's normal growth and development. An evaluation of the child's food intake, metabolic status, and lifestyle are necessary before establishing a nutrition plan. Daily caloric requirements are individualized for each child according

Table 55–3 Age-Based Criteria for Selecting Insulin Pump Therapy

Toddlers and Young Children	Children over 10 Years
Indications for Pump Therapy	**Disease Management Readiness**
■ Recurrent episodes of moderate and severe hypoglycemia ■ Persistent HbA_{1c} greater than or equal to 9% even with changes in insulin dosing ■ Unexplained erratic changes in blood glucose levels not resolved with insulin dosing changes ■ Recurrent diabetic ketoacidosis or severe hyperglycemia	■ 3–6 months of intensive insulin therapy, including 3 or more shots per day ■ 3–6 months of monitoring and recording blood glucose levels at least 4 times per day ■ 3–6 months of carbohydrate counting ■ Ability to give abdominal injections and no fear of needles ■ Ability to make small adjustments in treatment regimen appropriately between visits ■ Evidence of diabetes team contact in emergency situations
Parents or Caregivers Requirements for Pump Therapy	**Psychosocial Readiness**
■ Available to provide constant supervision ■ Understand pump functioning ■ Able to adjust basal and bolus doses ■ Willing to monitor blood glucose levels 4 times daily ■ Have collaborative working relationship with healthcare providers	■ Child/adolescent responsible for majority of diabetes self-care
Child Requirements for Pump Therapy	
■ Tolerate catheter and infusion set ■ Refrains from touching the catheter and pump	

Adapted from Litton, J., Rice, A., Friedman, N., Oden, J., Lee, M. M., & Freemark, M. (2002). Insulin pump therapy in toddlers and preschool children with type 1 diabetes mellitus. *Journal of Pediatrics, 141,* 490–495; Cogen, F. R., Streisand, R., & Sarin, S. (2002). Selecting children and adolescents for insulin pump therapy: Medical and behavioral considerations. *Diabetes Spectrum, 15*(2), 72–75.

Table 55–4 Advantages and Disadvantages of an External Insulin Infusion Pump

Advantages	Disadvantages
■ Delivers a continuous infusion of insulin to match the basal rate needed plus an insulin bolus at mealtime to more closely simulate normal pancreatic function ■ Helps maintain blood glucose control between meals ■ Decreases HbA_{1c} level ■ Improves glycemic control ■ Improves growth in children ■ Reduces number of injections ■ New pumps calculate bolus insulin dose to carbohydrates consumed ■ Allows child to eat with less adherence to a schedule and have more flexible lifestyle ■ Reduces number of injection sites, so variation in absorption decreases ■ Fewer incidences of diabetic ketoacidosis	■ Requires highly motivated child and supportive parents and healthcare professionals ■ Requires willingness to live connected to a device (can be disconnected for short periods by removing or clamping the catheter; however, DKA can occur within hours of interruption of insulin flow) ■ The site must be changed every 2–4 days, at least 1 inch from the last site; involves changing syringe, catheter, and skin setup ■ Infections can occur at the injection site ■ Must still monitor blood glucose levels and carbohydrates consumed ■ Weight gain is common when blood glucose control improves ■ Cost ■ Risk of DKA secondary to pump failure

Data from: Eugster, E. A., & Francis and the Lawson Wilkins Drug and Therapeutics Committee (2006). Position Statement: Continuous subcutaneous insulin infusion in very young children with type 1 diabetes. *Pediatrics, 118*(4), 1244–1249; Nimri, R., Weintrob, H. B., Ofan, R., Fayman, G., & Phillip, M. (2006). Insulin pump therapy in youth with type 1 diabetes: A retrospective paired study. *Pediatrics, 117*(6), 2126–2131; Wood, J. R., Moreland, E. C., Volkening, L. K., Svoren, B. M., Butler, D. A., & Laffel, L. M. B. (2006). Durability of insulin pump use in pediatric patients with type 1 diabetes. *Diabetes Care, 29*(11), 2355–2360.

to need. To facilitate adherence to the nutritional plan, an individualized approach with considerations of the child and family's culture, lifestyle, and financial means should be incorporated. Careful instruction by a nutritionist is essential in the management of diabetes.

Carbohydrate counting provides flexibility in meal planning and is simple for children and adolescents to use. One carbohydrate choice equals 15 grams of carbohydrates. Younger school-age children can consume two to four carbohydrate choices (one carbohydrate choice equals 15 g of carbohydrates) per meal and older children and adolescents can consume four to six per meal. Additional carbohydrate choices are necessary for more physically active children. Between-meal snacks generally consist of one to two carbohydrate choices, depending on the type of insulin used (Evert, 2004). Generally one unit of insulin covers 15 grams of carbohydrates, making insulin dosage calculation for meal coverage relatively easy. If additional carbohydrates are eaten at a meal or snack, the number of insulin units can also be adjusted providing further flexibility. A high-fiber diet is also recommended for improved control of blood glucose.

Exercise program. Physical activity is associated with increased insulin sensitivity. Regular exercise and fitness improves glucose control, reduces cardiovascular risk factors, and improves overall well-being. Blood lipid levels are also positively affected. However, the child must have an adequate caloric intake to prevent hypoglycemia. Excessive exercise associated with sports requires careful planning and management.

Some new developments for diabetes management are being evaluated. Noninvasive or continuous glucose monitoring techniques are in development and will be an important advance when integrated into insulin pumps (Weinzimer, Sikes, et al., 2005). Insulin pens that can store information regarding the amount and time of insulin doses should prove to be especially helpful to adolescents who generally do not record this type of information (Steck, Klingensmith, & Fiallo-Scharer, 2007). Pancreatic and islet transplant are not being aggressively pursued

Thinking Critically

MANAGING ADOLESCENT DIABETES

Anthony, 12 years old, has just been diagnosed with diabetes mellitus. His parents took him to their family physician after Anthony complained of being constantly thirsty and hungry for over a week. Despite this, he has lost 5 pounds. They note that he had a viral illness about 1 month ago but seemed to recover from it. His mother says that Anthony seemed lethargic for several days.

Anthony and his family must now learn to manage his diabetes using the combination of a diet, exercise, and insulin therapy. Monitoring his blood glucose level is important in determining how much insulin he will need every day. Anthony's meals and activity will need to be coordinated with the insulin doses. Anthony and his parents will need to watch closely for signs of hypoglycemia. Develop a teaching plan that includes the following information:

- What causes diabetes?
- What potential problems need prompt treatment?
- What does Anthony need to monitor for when he gets sick?
- Intensive therapy will be a goal of Anthony's treatment—how can you help Anthony and his family decide if this should be accomplished with insulin injections or an insulin pump?
- What are some strategies to help an adolescent actively participate in his disease management and maintain optimal diabetic control?

See MyNursingKit for possible responses.

until improved immunosuppression therapy regimens are available (Casu, Trucco, & Pietropaolo, 2005).

Complications of type 1 diabetes (retinopathy, heart disease, renal failure, and peripheral vascular disease) result from long-term hyperglycemic effects on the blood vessels. Without careful management, children with diabetes may develop renal failure and loss of vision in adulthood. Intensive therapy is expected to reduce the risk for or delay the development of these complications. Risk may be further reduced if the adolescent does not begin smoking and if the blood pressure is controlled.

NURSING MANAGEMENT

NURSING ASSESSMENT AND DIAGNOSIS

PHYSIOLOGIC ASSESSMENT

Children are generally admitted to the hospital at the time of diagnosis. Assess the child's physiologic status, focusing on vital signs and level of consciousness. Assess hydration by checking mucous membranes, skin turgor, and urine output. Blood initially is collected to monitor blood gases, glucose, and electrolytes. The frequency of blood collections will depend on whether or not the child is in diabetic ketoacidosis and the time of the diagnosis. Once the child is stable, assess dietary and caloric intake and the ability of the child or family to manage care.

PSYCHOSOCIAL ASSESSMENT

Parents may feel guilty at the time of diagnosis if they waited to seek care until the child began to experience symptoms of DKA. Assess coping mechanisms, family strengths and resources, ability to manage the disease, and educational needs of both the child and parents. Examples of questions to use in assessing the family's strengths and limitations in the child's disease management include:

- Do both parents or the single parent work? What hours?
- Who else is involved in the child's care?
- What is the child's usual daily schedule? Does the schedule vary on the weekend or any other days of the week?
- Does the child have health insurance? What coverage exists for diabetes education, treatment, and home management?
- Does the child have any cognitive, behavioral, motor, or visual problems coexisting with this condition?
- What other family stressors coexist with the diagnosis?

DEVELOPMENTAL ASSESSMENT

Assess the child's developmental level, particularly fine motor skills and cognitive level. The child will need to learn how to obtain and read a blood glucose sample and how to inject insulin (see Skill 10–3 SKILLS). Children can usually perform some of these tasks with supervision by 6 to 8 years of age.

Adolescents often perceive type 1 diabetes as a disability and may deny having the disease so they can be like their peers when eating and exercising. Talk with the adolescent and assess problem-solving skills associated with daily condition management, and the ability to manage special circumstances such as illness or changes in exercise. Self-management is the eventual goal, and the child's responsibilities are gradually increased.

Several diagnoses that may apply to the child newly diagnosed with type 1 diabetes are provided in the accompanying Nursing Care Plans. Additional diagnoses that may be appropriate include the following:

- *Risk for Deficient Fluid Volume* related to active fluid loss associated with hyperglycemia
- *Ineffective Breathing Pattern* related to neuromuscular dysfunction associated with metabolic acidosis
- *Ineffective Coping* related to inability to admit impact of disease on lifestyle

PLANNING AND IMPLEMENTATION

Nursing care focuses on teaching the child and parents about the disease and its management, managing dietary intake, providing emotional support, and planning strategies for daily management in the community. Refer to the accompanying Nursing Care Plans, which summarize nursing care for the child who is hospitalized with newly diagnosed type 1 diabetes, and the child who is receiving care in the community. Some hospitals have developed clinical pathways to streamline and standardize diabetes care.

PROVIDE EDUCATION

The nurse is an important member of the management team (physician, nurse, nutritionist, and social worker) and is usually responsible for educating the child and family. The majority of teaching may be performed by an advanced practice nurse or a certified diabetes nurse educator in the clinic setting, since children may be hospitalized only briefly following diagnosis.

MyNursingKit Video: Adolescent Diabetes and Quality of Life

The timing and amount of information provided are especially important in the first days following diagnosis. Both the child and parents are very tired, and they are often in a state of shock and disbelief. Information presented during this period needs to be repeated. This time should be used to assess learning needs and to answer the family's questions. Initial teaching focuses on the survival skills necessary for home management (insulin administration, blood glucose testing, record keeping, dietary management, and the recognition and treatment of both hypoglycemia and hyperglycemia) (Habich, 2006).

Explain the goals of insulin therapy. Teach the parents and child (if appropriate) how to draw up and administer insulin and perform blood glucose tests (Figure 55–5 ●). Rotating the injection sites is important to decrease the chances of *lipoatrophy,* loss of subcutaneous tissue, or hypertrophy in which collagen is replaced by fat cells (Figure 55–6 ●). The absorption rate of insulin varies by the site used. Insulin is usually absorbed most rapidly from the abdomen; however, insulin absorption is increased in the extremities with exercise. An understanding of the different types of insulin and their actions is essential.

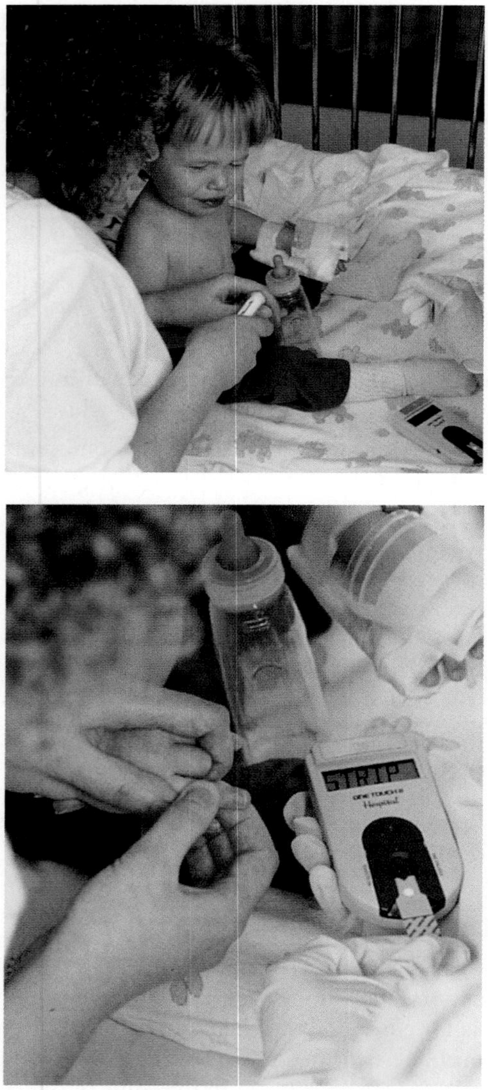

● **Figure 55–5** This mother is learning how to test her child's blood glucose level.

Once the child and parents demonstrate understanding of this information, teach guidelines for managing episodes of hyperglycemia during acute illness and using a sliding scale. A sliding scale indicates specific insulin dosages appropriate for a particular blood glucose level. The family also needs to learn "sick day" care guidelines to prevent diabetic ketoacidosis.

Teaching Highlights

CHECKING BLOOD GLUCOSE LEVELS

Caution parents to check the blood glucose level of a toddler who is extremely sleepy or irritable, as these can be signs of either hypoglycemia or hyperglycemia.

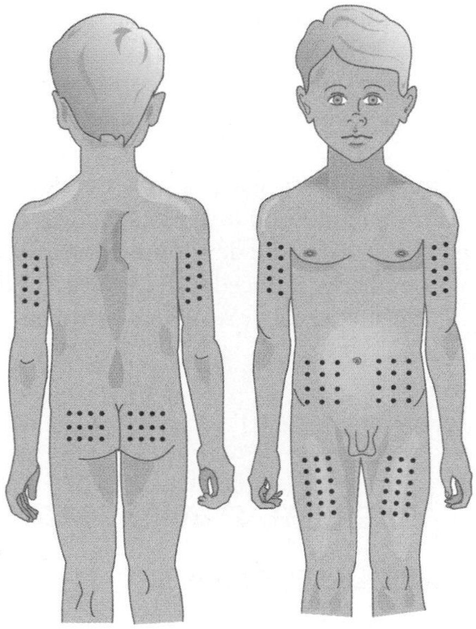

● **Figure 55–6** Insulin injection sites. Give all morning insulin in one site (e.g., arms) and all evening insulin in another (e.g., legs) because of different rates of absorption from these sites. Space injections about 1/2 inch (1.25 cm) apart.

MANAGE FOOD INTAKE

While no specific meal plan is recommended for children with diabetes, 50–55% of their calories should be carbohydrates, 15–20% of their calories protein, and 30% of their calories fat (Haller, Atkinson, & Schatz, 2005). The child needs adequate calories to reach or maintain a desirable body weight. A variety of simple and complex carbohydrates should be eaten. An increased ratio of polyunsaturated fats should be eaten to reduce serum lipid levels.

Teaching Highlights

SICK DAY GUIDELINES

When the child with diabetes is sick, parents need to be extra attentive to the child's glycemic control. The following recommendations should be followed (Boland & Grey, 2004):

- Seek medical attention for fever or other signs of infection.
- Monitor the blood glucose levels more often than routine (every 1 to 4 hours).
- Test urine ketones when the blood glucose level is greater than 200 mg/dL.
- The usual dose of insulin may be increased for high blood glucose levels.
- Do not skip doses of insulin.
- Maintain a large fluid intake (more than 8 oz hourly) even if the child cannot eat. Seek medical attention if this is not possible. Fluids should have carbohydrates to maintain the child's usual caloric intake.

Nursing Care Plan

THE CHILD HOSPITALIZED WITH NEWLY DIAGNOSED TYPE 1 DIABETES MELLITUS

INTERVENTION	RATIONALE	EXPECTED OUTCOME
1. Nursing Diagnosis: Deficient Knowledge (Survival Skills) related to lack of exposure to diabetic management in the newly diagnosed child		
NIC Priority Intervention: **Teaching, individual:** Planning, implementation, and evaluating a teaching program designed to address a patient's particular need		**NOC Suggested Outcome:** **Knowledge:** Extent of understanding conveyed about diabetic treatment regimen
Goal: The child and parents will acquire survival skills for home management.		
■ Assess the child's developmental level and select an educational approach and self-care activities to match. ■ Teach blood glucose monitoring, drawing up and injecting insulin, urine testing for ketones, record keeping, survival food guidelines, and when to call the healthcare provider. ■ Use demonstration/return demonstration until the child and family are comfortable with procedures.	■ Learning goals for the child must match knowledge and skill expectations appropriate for developmental stage. ■ Diabetic management survival skills are needed for initial home management until more extensive education can be completed that permits more independent management. ■ Return demonstration permits evaluation, positive reinforcement and guidance for modification of techniques.	The child and parents demonstrate proper technique for blood glucose monitoring, urine testing for ketones, drawing up and injecting insulin doses, survival food guidelines and record keeping.
Goal: The child and parents will recognize signs and symptoms of hypoglycemia and hyperglycemia.		
■ Teach signs and symptoms of hypoglycemic and hyperglycemic reactions. ■ Teach the child to test blood glucose when feeling different than usual, and record the reading and symptoms felt.	■ Recognition of and treatment of poor glucose control will prevent progression of symptoms. ■ Permits child to learn his/her specific symptoms of hyper- and hypoglycemia.	The child and family can describe symptoms of hypoglycemia and hyperglycemia.
2. Nursing Diagnosis: Risk for Injury (Complication) related to potential episodes of hypoglycemia and diabetic ketoacidosis		
NIC Priority Intervention: **Risk identification:** Analysis of potential risk factors, determination of health risks, and prioritization of risk reduction strategies for an individual or group.		**NOC Suggested Outcome:** **Risk control:** Actions to eliminate or reduce actual, personal, and modifiable health threats
Goal: The child will experience few episodes of hypoglycemia during hospitalization.		
■ Assess the child at least every 2 hours for signs of hypoglycemia. If signs are present, check blood glucose to verify and administer source of quick sugar. ■ When the child is NPO for a special procedure, verify with physician when food, fluids, and insulin are to be given, or if an intravenous infusion with dextrose is to be given. ■ Have glucose paste or 50% dextrose solution readily available.	■ Hypoglycemia commonly occurs during hospitalization because of change in diet, lack of food intake, or illness. ■ Giving insulin without food intake can lead to hypoglycemia. Intravenous dextrose and insulin can be used when the child must be NPO. ■ Dextrose is used for emergency intravenous treatment of severe hypoglycemia. Glucose paste is used for oral treatment.	The child and staff manage episodes of hypoglycemia without a crisis developing.
Goal: The child's condition is treated slowly to gradually reverse hyperglycemia and ketoacidosis and to prevent cerebral edema.		

(continued)

Nursing Care Plan—continued

THE CHILD HOSPITALIZED WITH NEWLY DIAGNOSED TYPE 1 DIABETES MELLITUS

INTERVENTION	RATIONALE	EXPECTED OUTCOME
■ Assess the child's mental status for improvement or deterioration.	■ Improvement in mental status may indicate successful treatment. Deterioration may indicate onset of cerebral edema.	The child's hyperglycemia and ketoacidosis resolves without additional complications.
■ Check blood glucose and urine ketones frequently to confirm reduction in blood glucose level and ketosis, and to identify the insulin dose for administration.	■ Frequent blood glucose and ketone level determination helps assess progress in treating ketoacidosis.	
■ Monitor and control IV fluid intake. Measure output.	■ The child with ketoacidosis will be dehydrated. IV fluid intake needs to be carefully controlled to prevent cerebral edema.	
■ Have insulin doses checked by a second nurse.	■ Doses are frequently small, and the possibility of error is great.	

Goal: The child and parents will demonstrate emergency management of hypoglycemia.

■ Identify sources of glucose to give in case of hypoglycemic reaction. Tell the child and parent to carry glucose tablets or paste with them at all times.	■ Access to sources of glucose and its rapid administration are important for emergency care.	The child and family can identify several glucose sources for emergencies. The child and family have a source of glucose with them at each visit.

Goal: The child and parents will demonstrate management of sick days.

■ Teach the child and family to test blood glucose and urine for ketones with acute symptoms and notify the healthcare provider.	■ When the child is ill, hyperglycemia needs special management to prevent progression to ketoacidosis.	The child's hyperglycemic episodes do not progress to ketoacidosis.

3. Nursing Diagnosis: Imbalanced Nutrition: Less than Body Requirements related to glycosuria

NIC Priority Intervention:
Nutrition management: Assistance with or provision of a balanced dietary intake of foods and fluids

NOC Suggested Outcome:
Nutritional status: Extent to which nutrients are available to meet metabolic needs

Goal: The child will eat a well-balanced diet and maintain normal height and weight proportions.

■ Encourage and serve meals and snacks with consistent carbohydrates at the same time each day.	■ Keeps blood glucose levels stable during initial disease management stages.	The child regains weight lost and demonstrates normal growth and stable blood glucose levels.
■ Provide a calorie nonrestricted diet.	■ Enables weight lost during onset of diabetes to be regained.	

Goal: The child and parents will state understanding of dietary management of diabetes mellitus.

■ Make an appointment with a nutritionist who can assess the child's favorite foods and promote their integration into the child's diet. Reinforce the dietary information taught.	■ The nutritionist can develop dietary recommendations that fit the specific needs of the child and include favorite foods, thereby increasing compliance with the diet.	The child and parents describe nutritional needs of the child and select the dietary management best suited to the family's and child's eating habits.
■ Provide sample menus and teach the use of carbohydrate counting.	■ Assists the family and adolescent with diet planning.	

Nursing Care Plan

THE CHILD WITH PREVIOUSLY DIAGNOSED TYPE 1 DIABETES BEING CARED FOR AT HOME

INTERVENTION	RATIONALE	EXPECTED OUTCOME
1. Nursing Diagnosis: Imbalanced Nutrition: Less than Body Requirements related to chronic illness (type 1 diabetes)		
NIC Priority Intervention: **Weight management:** Assistance with or provision of a balanced dietary intake of foods and fluids		**NOC Suggested Outcome:** **Nutritional status: Nutrient value:** Adequacy of nutrients taken into body
Goal: The child will eat a well-balanced diet that maintains weight proportional to height.		
■ Assess height and weight regularly and plot on growth chart. ■ Make an appointment with a nutritionist who can assess the child's favorite foods and integrate them into a food plan that controls caloric intake. Encourage the child to keep a food diary.	■ Assesses change in body mass index to identify potential weight problem early. ■ Inclusion of child's favorite foods helps child adapt to changes in the food plan.	Diet records indicate meals and snacks have the appropriate distribution of carbohydrates, protein, and fats, and daily caloric intake goals are met.
2. Nursing Diagnosis: Readiness for Enhanced Family Processes related to management of a chronic disease		
NIC Priority Intervention: **Family process maintenance:** Minimization of family process disruption effects		**NOC Suggested Outcome:** **Family functioning:** Ability of family to meet the needs of its members through developmental transitions
Goal: The child and family will manage the food plan, exercise, blood glucose monitoring, and medications regimen.		
■ Assess the family's lifestyle and attempt to fit the child's care needs into the family's schedule. ■ Discuss the family's routines for special occasions and vacations. Identify ways to modify the child's management for these occasions.	■ Fitting the care to the family's lifestyle promotes adherence with the regimen. ■ It is important for the child to participate in special events with the family and peers as a normal child to promote psychologic development.	The child and family make minimal changes in usual lifestyle while managing the type 1 diabetes.
3. Nursing Diagnosis: Ineffective Coping (Individual) related to inadequate level of confidence in ability to cope		
NIC Priority Intervention: **Coping enhancement:** Assisting a patient to adapt to perceived stressors, changes, or threats which interfere with meeting life demands and roles		**NOC Suggested Outcome:** **Coping:** Actions to manage stressors that tax an individual's resources
Goal: The child will demonstrate enhanced coping skills.		
■ Ask how the child has solved problems in the past. Review possible problems the child may encounter. Together evaluate the effectiveness of solutions. Suggest other solutions to consider.	■ Children's success in mastering maturational conflicts and daily psychosocial problems will influence their pattern of coping.	The child demonstrates enhanced coping skills and expresses positive attitude toward self. The child displays warmth and affection toward family.

(continued)

Nursing Care Plan—continued

THE CHILD WITH PREVIOUSLY DIAGNOSED TYPE 1 DIABETES BEING CARED FOR AT HOME

INTERVENTION	RATIONALE	EXPECTED OUTCOME
Goal: The child will develop positive self-esteem.		
■ Role-play ways to talk about diabetes with friends and teachers. Encourage the child to express feelings about diabetes to those he or she trusts.	■ Sharing information about the condition helps others understand changes in lifestyle needed by the child. Expressing feelings decreases anxiety.	The child demonstrates confidence in interactions with peers and maintains social network.
■ Encourage the child to attend diabetes camp.	■ Learning and support networks developed at camp can promote self-esteem.	
■ Encourage the child to continue previous social activities and hobbies.	■ Increased social interaction, especially in group sessions, improves self-esteem.	
4. Nursing Diagnosis: Health-Seeking Behaviors (Child) related to learning self-management of chronic disorder		
NIC Priority Intervention: **Self-modification assistance:** Reinforcement of self-directed change initiated by the patient to achieve personally important goals		**NOC Suggested Outcome:** **Health promotion:** Actions to sustain or increase wellness, recovery and rehabilitation
Goal: The child will develop independent ability to manage diabetes care.		
■ Allow the child to perform as many self-care procedures as possible at each developmental stage.	■ Normal growth and development are ensured if the child is encouraged to participate in care from the beginning.	The child is able to perform as many diabetic care techniques as possible for age.
■ Encourage the child to make decisions regarding care. Review decisions and discuss possible alternative solutions. Role-play possible scenarios.	■ Trust develops when children sense that their decisions are respected or at least considered by others.	
■ Encourage parents to stay involved even when the adolescent takes primary responsibility for care.	■ The child's diabetic control is likely to be better when the parents continue to show interest and supervise care.	
■ Provide 24-hour access to physician or diabetes nurse educator. Encourage the child to seek help early.	■ The child needs to overcome concerns about calling for guidance, and thus maintain better control.	

Eating at consistent intervals is important for glycemic control, whether counting carbohydrates or following a conventional meal plan (three meals a day and three snacks a day). Although the child with diabetes is not restricted from eating any food, the child and parents need to learn about the relationship between foods eaten and insulin needed. Meal plans also need to be adjusted for exercise. Non-nutritive sweeteners such as aspartame and saccharin may be used in moderation. The child and family should learn how to read food labels. The meal plan should be customized, with the assistance of a nutritionist, to the child's age, cultural and family food preferences, and activity level.

PROVIDE EMOTIONAL SUPPORT

The diagnosis of type 1 diabetes often comes as a shock to the family. If there is a familial history, parents may feel guilty about having caused the disease. The diagnosis of a chronic disease that requires daily management can be difficult to accept. Give parents information about diabetes education programs, refer them to support groups with other parents of children with diabetes, and help them to learn the role they can play in managing the disease.

Support for the child depends on age and developmental stage. Encourage the child to express feelings about the disease and its management. The adolescent may benefit from contact with other adolescents who have diabetes.

DISCHARGE PLANNING AND HOME CARE TEACHING

Home care needs should be identified and addressed before discharge. Initial survival skills described earlier are taught with the plans for ongoing outpatient education.

Make every effort to incorporate the diabetic regimen (insulin administration, food plan, blood glucose monitoring, and exercise) into the family's present lifestyle. The fewer changes the family has to make, the greater the chance of adherence.

The family and child newly diagnosed with diabetes should be made aware of the "honeymoon phase." This is a period during new-onset diabetes when the child has some residual beta-cell function, which reduces exogenous insulin requirements. The child and family may assume this is an indication that the diabetes "is better." However, the insulin requirement does eventually return. The duration of this phase varies among individuals.

Provide written materials and refer parents to books and other materials they can use in teaching the child about diabetes. The Juvenile Diabetic Research Foundation and the American Diabetes Association are good sources of information.

NURSING CARE IN THE COMMUNITY

During follow-up visits, ask the child or parents about signs indicating problems of diabetic control. Questions to ask that could help identify problems in diabetic control include:

- Is the child hungry at meals? Between meals?
- How much fluid is the child drinking?
- Has the child been going to the bathroom frequently or had episodes of bed-wetting?
- Does the child have dry skin?
- Are there sores on the feet? Do scratches or scrapes take a long time to heal?
- Has the child had any skin infections?
- Does the child have changes in mood (depression, unexplained sadness, irritability) or energy level from day to day or throughout the day?
- Have there been any changes in vision?

Record growth measurements and vital signs in the child's chart. Review the child's typical dietary intake and exercise regimens. Assess the child's sexual development using Tanner staging guidelines (see Chapter 35 ∞). Puberty may be delayed if diabetic control is inadequate. Evaluation for the potential complications of diabetes should be performed annually, including blood for lipid levels, blood pressure, liver and renal function, urine for albumin, an ophthalmologic examination for retinopathy, and a neurologic examination of the extremities for neuropathies.

Education is ongoing, especially for children who develop diabetes at a young age. As they grow and assume more responsibility for their care, they need to learn more about the pathophysiology of the disease and the rationale for its management.

The child with diabetes should be treated as any other child without a chronic condition, including limit setting and consistent discipline for unacceptable behavior. Children with type 1 diabetes may learn maladaptive behaviors, using their disease to obtain something they want. Teach parents to be alert to signs of maladaption, such as helpless, demanding, or whining behaviors, and any evidence of poor coping. Additional behaviors may include skipping blood glucose testing and losing or damaging equipment. Food may become a battleground for toddlers who are picky eaters, but must eat enough for the insulin dose. Referral for counseling may be appropriate for some families.

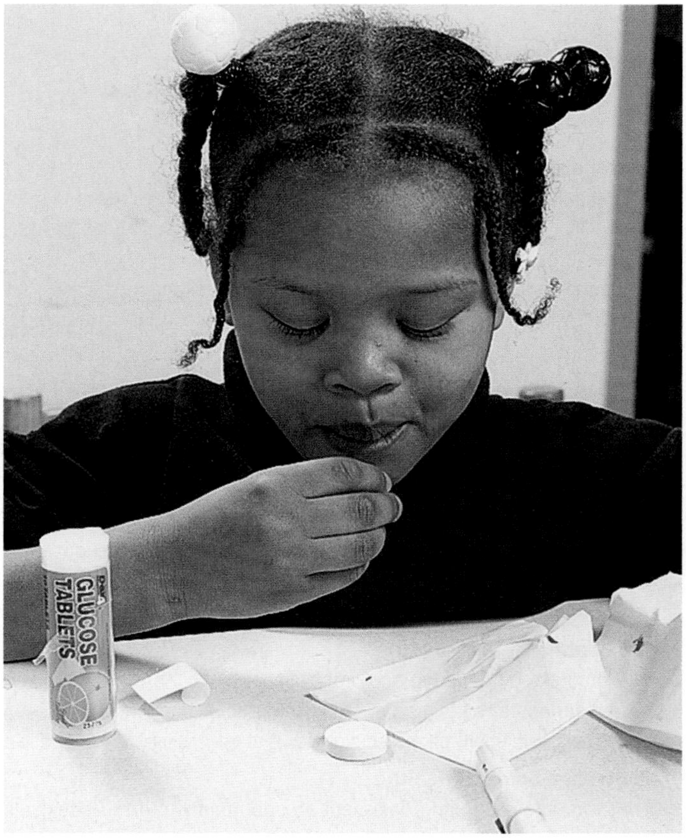

● **Figure 55–7** This girl is old enough to understand the need to take glucose tablets or another form of a rapidly absorbed sugar when her blood glucose level is low.

Continually work with the child to help him or her assume responsibility for self-care, and with parents to promote the child's self-care (Figure 55–7 ●). The child's developmental stage and cognitive level influence his or her readiness to take on responsibility for self-care. Summer camps and other programs for children with diabetes are often helpful in providing education and support.

The preschool child's need for autonomy and control can be met by allowing the child to choose snacks or to pick which finger to stick for glucose testing and by helping parents to gather necessary supplies. School-age children can learn to test blood glucose, administer insulin, and keep records. They should be taught how to select foods and portion sizes appropriate for dietary management and how to plan food intake for an exercise program. School-age children need to learn to recognize the signs of hypoglycemia and hyperglycemia, and understand the importance of carrying a rapidly absorbed sugar product.

Although adolescents understand explanations about the potential complications of diabetes, they are present-time oriented and may rebel against the daily regimen of insulin injections, the food plan, and the exercise plan. Successful self-care depends in part on the adolescent's adjustment to the chronic nature of the disease and feelings of being different from peers. Although the adolescent is able to manage self-care, the desire to be like peers may interfere with treatment adherence. Adolescents with high levels of depressive symptoms are at an increased risk

MyNursingKit Case Study: Child with Type 1 Diabetes

HEALTH PROMOTION

THE CHILD WITH DIABETES MELLITUS

Growth and Development Surveillance

- Compare the child's height, weight, and head circumference to age-specific norms to determine if growth is meeting expectations for age.
- Assess developmental progress using the Denver II or another screening tool (refer to Chapter 36). Assess school performance.
- Assess for delays in development of sexual secondary characteristics and pubertal changes.

Nutrition

- Promote adherence to nutrition guidelines by including the child's personal preferences in the food plan.

Physical Activity

- Encourage regular physical activity and educate the child to modify insulin dosage or food intake for extra physical activity periods.
- Encourage the child to participate in sports when interested and work to balance exercise, food intake, and insulin dosage.

Oral Health

- Promote good dentition and oral hygiene.
- Regular dental visits are important to reduce risk of infections.
- The child with poorly controlled diabetes is at risk of gingivitis and cavities.

Mental and Spiritual Health

- Provide the child and adolescent an opportunity to discuss feelings regarding diabetes.
- Assess the adolescent for evidence of depression.

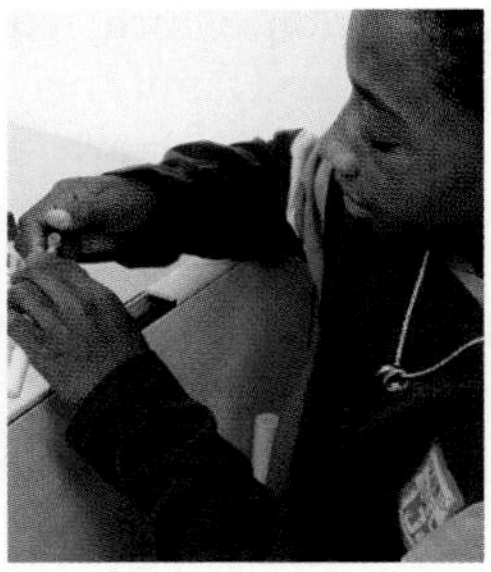

Relationships

- The child should attend school or childcare as any other child.
- Encourage the development of special friends who can be informed about the child's disorder and seek help when needed.

Disease Prevention Strategies

- Encourage family to maintain the child's active immunization status.
- Children with diabetes should receive an annual influenza vaccine.
- Refer the child for an annual ophthalmologic examination.
- Maintain appointments for regular evaluation of $HgbA_{1c}$ to monitor glycemic control.

Injury Prevention Strategies

- Encourage the child to wear a medical identification tag.
- Encourage daily inspection of feet and foot care.
- Provide the family with strategies for safe disposal of needles and syringes.

for hospitalization (Stewart, Rao, Emslie, et al., 2005). Talk with the adolescent to assess mood and to evaluate motivation to manage the meal plan, exercise regimen, blood glucose monitoring, and insulin therapy. Discuss how carbohydrate counting and insulin dose adjustment may provide the flexibility to participate in activities with peers. Collaborate with the adolescent in preparation to assume care, and assist parents in accepting the growing independence from adult supervision. A discussion of the hazards associated with having diabetes and the use of alcohol, drugs, and tobacco should occur. At every subsequent health care visit, the adolescent should be asked about alcohol intake. See "Evidence-Based Nursing: Adolescent Diabetes and Quality of Life."

The child with type 1 diabetes may develop circulatory and neurologic changes over time. Emphasize the importance of good foot care from an early age, for example, wearing clean cotton socks; changing socks and shoes when they are damp; washing, drying, and powdering feet; and keeping toenails short.

Explain to parents that the child should wear some type of medical alert identification. Help them have an individualized school health plan developed (see Chapter 40) to ensure that school administrators and teachers can identify the signs of hypoglycemia or hyperglycemia and provide emergency management.

EVALUATION

Expected outcomes of nursing care for children with type 1 diabetes can be found in the Nursing Care Plans.

Teaching Highlights

TREATING HYPOGLYCEMIC EPISODES

- If the child shows signs of hypoglycemia (pallor, sweating, tremors, dizziness, numb lips or mouth, confusion, irritability, altered mental status), test the blood glucose level.
- Assist the child to perform the test, as skills needed to get an accurate reading deteriorate with altered mental status.
- If the blood glucose reading is less than or equal to 70 mg/dL, give glucose rapidly. Use one of the following:
  - 1/2 cup orange juice
  - 3/4 cup of sugar-sweetened beverage
  - 1 small box raisins
  - 3 to 4 glucose tablets
- Wait 15 minutes and recheck the blood glucose level. Repeat the glucose if it is still less than or equal to 70 mg/dL. Recheck the blood glucose level in another 15 minutes.
- Once blood sugar has returned to at least 80 mg/dL, give a more substantial snack such as cheese and crackers if the next meal will be more than 30 minutes later or an activity or exercise is planned.
- If the child is unconscious, administer im or sq glucagon or spread glucose paste on the gums.

Evidence in Action

The dietary intake of 132 adolescents with type 1 diabetes was compared with that of 131 adolescents without diabetes. Both groups had a mean age of 12 years and were comparable by sex, race, ethnicity, and stage of pubertal development. Using a 24-hour recall method, there was no difference in the number of calories consumed by the two groups. The diet of adolescents with diabetes consumed a greater percentage (and more grams) of fat and protein and a smaller percentage of carbohydrates than adolescents without diabetes. Of concern is the greater amount of saturated fat by adolescents with diabetes that may contribute to cardiovascular disease in the future (Helgeson, Viccaro, Becker, et al., 2006).

DIABETIC KETOACIDOSIS

Potential causes of DKA include incorrect or missed insulin doses or administration just under the skin, an illness, trauma, or surgery. DKA is found in 20–40% of children with new-onset type 1 diabetes (Haley-Andrews & Mackenzie, 2005).

Insulin deficiency is accompanied by a compensatory increase in hormones (epinephrine, norepinephrine, cortisol, growth hormone, and glucagon) that are released when inadequate glucose is delivered to the cells. The muscle cells break down protein into amino acids that are then converted to glucose by the liver, leading to hyperglycemia. The adipose tissue releases fatty acids that are transformed by the liver into ketone bodies. Their accumulation leads to ketoacidosis. The hyperglycemia causes an osmotic diuresis resulting in dehydration, acidosis, and hyperosmolality. The rising ketones lead to metabolic acidosis. DKA is associated with severe metabolic, electrolyte, and fluid imbalances.

Characteristic signs of DKA include polyuria, polydipsia, weight loss, abdominal pain, nausea and vomiting, tachycardia, signs of dehydration, flushed ears and cheeks, Kussmaul respirations, acetone breath (fruity smell), altered level of consciousness, and hypotension. Hyperglycemia, glycosuria, and ketonuria are also present. In response to metabolic acidosis, children complain of abdominal or chest pain, nausea, and vomiting. The disorder may progress to electrolyte disturbances, arrhythmias, altered consciousness, pupillary changes, irregular respirations, inappropriate slowing of the heart rate and widening pulse pressure. See the table on page 1637 for clinical manifestations of hypoglycemia and hyperglycemia.

DKA is present with the following findings: blood glucose level greater than 200 mg/dL, serum ketones,

Evidence-Based Nursing

ADOLESCENT DIABETES AND QUALITY OF LIFE

Clinical Question

What factors are associated with how adolescents with diabetes view their quality of life?

The Evidence

A study involving 115 adolescents with diabetes (ages 11 to 18 years) examined their perception of parental involvement, care, and control in relation to health-related quality of life and metabolic control. Their perceptions were compared to 9345 healthy adolescents and 291 adolescents with physical disabilities. Adolescents with diabetes reported a higher level of parental control than both healthy adolescents and adolescents with disabilities, and this higher level of control was significantly associated with a lower health-related quality of life. Adolescents with diabetes reported a significantly higher health-related quality of life score when they perceived a higher degree of parental care and involvement, and a lower degree of parental control and overprotection. Their $HbA1_C$ level was not significantly related to perceptions of parental care, control, or involvement, potentially due to the challenges of maintaining metabolic control during puberty (Graue, Wentzel-Larsen, Hanestad, et al., 2005).

Another study examined responses of 39 adolescents between the ages of 13 and 17 who completed the Diabetes Quality of Life for Youths questionnaire. Of the 22 domains listed on the questionnaire, only 3 were cited as important; family, friends, and school. Functional health of the participants was perceived as similar to their peers. Seventy-four percent of the adolescents had attended a diabetes camp at least once. The study confirmed not only the importance of family to adolescents with diabetes, but the importance of peers as well, whether it be at school or summer camp (Cheung, Cureton, & Canham, 2006).

Best Practice

Developmental tasks of adolescents focus on development of self-concept and self-esteem. Adolescents with type 1 diabetes must also cope with the increasing responsibility for complex self-management, including insulin administration, blood glucose testing, exercise, and nutrition. Self-esteem and self-concept often become linked with the disease as peers react to the differences noted. Life satisfaction, perceived control, and worries associated with having diabetes are important considerations when counseling the teenager and family about the management of diabetes. Additionally, it is important to know that adolescents value parental involvement and care rather than having it be perceived as a reason for conflict. Parental involvement and supervision is important in helping adolescents transition successfully to self-management of their disease. Peers are also very important to adolescents with diabetes. Continued involvement in school activities and summer camps provide excellent avenues for friendship and promote a positive quality of life.

Critical Thinking

What questions can be used to explore an adolescent's perceptions of family involvement, care, and control? How can you address quality of life issues in adolescents with diabetes? What questions can be used to determine the adolescent's satisfaction with peer relationships?

See MyNursingKit for possible responses.

acidosis (pH less than or equal to 7.3 and bicarbonate less than 15 mEq/L), glycosuria, and ketonuria. Electrolyte disorders also occur (hyperkalemia, hyperchloremia, hyponatremia, hypophosphatemia, hypocalcemia, and hypomagnesemia). The blood urea nitrogen (BUN) and creatinine are elevated due to dehydration. Diabetic coma occurs when the serum osmolality exceeds 350 mOsm/kg. Normal serum osmolality is 275 to 295 mOsm/kg. The child with ketoacidosis is usually hospitalized. Medical management includes isotonic intravenous fluids and electrolytes for dehydration and acidosis. Short acting insulin (0.1 unit/kg per hour) is administered by continuous infusion pump to decrease the serum glucose level at a rate not to exceed 100 mg/dL/hr. Faster reduction of hyperglycemia and serum osmolality increases the risk for cerebral edema. When glucose is lowered too rapidly, water is freed and attracted to the glucose. Mannitol is kept on standby for treatment of neurologic deterioration. Bicarbonate is not routinely used for treatment of DKA as it places the child at increased risk for hypokalemia, acidosis, and cerebral edema (Glaser, 2005). As insulin is administered, potassium shifts to the cells, resulting in hypokalemia. Potassium supplementation is given only after confirmation of renal function.

Cerebral edema complicates approximately 1% of cases of DKA, and typically occurs 2 to 4 hours after treatment for DKA begins (Dunger, Sperling, Acerini, et al., 2004). Cerebral edema is the most common cause of DKA-related deaths (Glaser, 2005). See Chapter 56 for information about cerebral edema.

Nursing Management

Continuously monitor the child's vital signs, respiratory status, perfusion, and mental status. Assess for changes in neurologic status, respiratory pattern, blood pressure, and heart rate. Monitor for cardiac arrhythmias associated with hypokalemia. Assess for signs of dehydration, including dry skin and mucous membranes and depressed fontanels in infants. Monitor blood glucose levels hourly or as indicated. Frequently monitor the electrolytes and acid-base status, as well as urine glucose and ketone levels as indicated. Intake and output are monitored hourly.

Intravenous fluids are given in boluses of 10 to 20 mL/kg rapidly over 5 minutes if the child is in hypovolemic shock. Adequate fluids are given to reverse the fluid deficit. The insulin infusion must be carefully titrated to control the gradual reduction in hyperglycemia. The child is tapered off intravenous insulin and transitioned to subcutaneous insulin when clinically stable. Oral feedings are reintroduced when the child is alert and the glucose level is stabilized.

The prevention of future episodes of DKA is important. The parents and child need to learn strategies to keep hyperglycemic

MyNursingKit Animation: Responding to Hypoglycemia

Nursing Practice

Insulin binds to IV tubing. Run 50 to 100 mL run through new IV tubing to saturate all the binding sites. This ensures that the full dose of insulin reaches the child from the outset.

Teaching Highlights

RECOGNIZING SIGNS OF DKA

- Abdominal pain
- Nausea and vomiting that persists for longer than 6 hours
- More than five diarrheal stools in 1 day
- 1 or 2 day history of polyuria and polydipsia
- Has illness (e.g., viral or other) and is unable to eat
- Change in mental status
- Temperature over 102°F (38.9°C) for 12 hours
- Blood glucose 400 mg/dL on two separate readings, or > 200 mg/dL and moderate to large ketones
- Large ketones are present
- Fruity breath odor
- Evidence of a bacterial infection (e.g., fever, drainage, dysuria or other evidence of a urinary tract infection)
- Difficulty breathing
- Decreased urine output

Data from: Bismuth, E., & Laffel, L. (2007). Can we prevent diabetes ketoacidosis in children? *Pediatric Diabetes*, *8*(6), 24–33; Boland, E. A., & Grey, M. (2004). Diabetes mellitus (Types 1 and 2). In P. L. Jackson & J. A. Vessey (Eds.), *Primary care of the child with a chronic condition* (4th ed., pp. 426–444). St Louis: Mosby; Masharani, U. (2008). Diabetes mellitus and hypoglycemia. In S. J. McPhee, M. A. Papadakis, L. M. Tierney Jr., R. Gonzales, R. Zeiger (Eds.), *Current medical diagnosis and treatment 2008*. Retrieved from McGraw-Hill's Access Medicine, www.accessmedicine.com.

episodes from progressing to DKA. For example, the child's urine should be tested for ketones every 4–6 hours if the blood glucose reading is 240 mg/dL or greater or if the child is sick (American Diabetes Association, 2008c). If the child has an elevated blood glucose and moderate or large amounts of ketones, treatment with extra insulin and fluids can be initiated. Increased attention to blood glucose and urine ketone monitoring is especially important when the child has significant stressors such as an illness. It is important for the child and family to understand that insulin is required even when the child is not eating to counter the hormones secreted in response to the stressor.

HYPOGLYCEMIA

Hypoglycemia can develop within minutes in children with type 1 diabetes mellitus. The symptoms outlined in "Clinical Manifestations: Hypoglycemia and Hyperglycemia" may occur when blood glucose levels suddenly drop or fall below 70 mg/dL. Children are at risk of hypoglycemia due to their rapid growth rates and unpredictable eating habits and physical activity. Severe hypoglycemia episodes may occur at night in children who are treated with two to three injections per day. Other common causes include an error in insulin dosage, errors in injection technique, inadequate calories because of missed meals, or exercise without a

Clinical Manifestations

HYPOGLYCEMIA AND HYPERGLYCEMIA

CAUSE	CLINICAL MANIFESTATIONS	CLINICAL THERAPY
Hypoglycemia ■ Insulin dose too high for food eaten ■ Insulin injection into muscle ■ Too much exercise for insulin dose ■ Too long between meals/snacks ■ Too few carbohydrates eaten ■ Illness, stress	Rapid onset Irritability, nervousness, tremors, shaky feeling, difficulty concentrating or speaking, behavior change, confusion, repeating something over and over Unconsciousness, seizure, shallow breathing, tachycardia Pallor, sweating Moist mucous membranes, hunger Headache, dizziness, blurred vision, double vision, photophobia Numb lips or mouth	If conscious, give 15 grams of carbohydrate. Wait 15 minutes and recheck blood glucose level. Give another 15 grams of carbohydrate if 70 mg/dL or below. Recheck the blood glucose level in 15 minutes. If unconscious, give glucagon by injection.
Hyperglycemia ■ Insulin dose too low for food eaten ■ Illness or injury, stress ■ Too many carbohydrates eaten ■ Meals/snacks too close together ■ Insulin injected just under skin or injected into hypertrophied areas ■ Decreased activity	Gradual onset Lethargy, sleepiness, slowed responses, or confusion Deep, rapid breathing Flushed skin, dry skin Dry mucous membranes, thirst, hunger, dehydration Weakness, fatigue Headache, abdominal pain, nausea, vomiting Blurred vision Shock	Additional insulin given at usual injection time. Sliding scale insulin doses for specific blood glucose levels when ill or injured. Extra injections if hyperglycemia and moderate to large ketones. Increased fluids.

corresponding increase in caloric intake. Severe hypoglycemia can cause seizures.

Hypoglycemia can be diagnosed on the basis of the sudden onset of signs and symptoms. A blood glucose reading should be taken to confirm the diagnosis, since signs of hyperglycemia and hypoglycemia may be difficult to distinguish. Give glucose immediately but only in the form of a low-fat carbohydrate-containing snack or drink, sugar gel, glucose tablets, or glucose paste. If the child becomes unconscious, administer glucagon or if unavailable, administer sugar gel or glucose paste squeezed onto the gums. In the hospital setting, administer an intravenous infusion of dextrose to prevent progression of symptoms. Since the effects of dextrose and glucagon are temporary, additional snacks or a meal is provided. The child should be continually observed for several hours after treatment.

Nursing Management

Teach parents and children to recognize the signs of hypoglycemia and take appropriate action. Teach parents to give an intramuscular or subcutaneous dose of **glucagon** (a hormone produced by the pancreas that helps release stored glucose from the liver) for severe cases of hypoglycemia. Reinforce the importance of balancing dietary intake, insulin, and exercise every day. Since the effects of glucose, dextrose, and glucagon are temporary, additional snacks or a meal is provided once the child is alert. Monitor the child continually for several hours after treatment.

TYPE 2 DIABETES

Type 2 diabetes is a disease associated with insulin resistance (an alteration of the insulin receptor that signals the presence of insulin in the interior of cells). While it is sometimes connected to an insulin secretory defect in the pancreas caused by a decrease in the beta cell weight and number and insulin deficiency (Gungor & Arslanian, 2004), it is more commonly associated with decreased insulin receptors at the cellular level. Significant risk factors for type 2 diabetes includes obesity, low levels of physical activity, a diet high in fat, race, and family history of diabetes (Alemzadeh & Wyatt, 2007; Berry et al., 2006a). Several genes on chromosomes 1q, 12q, 20q, and 7q are associated with the predisposition for development of type 2 diabetes (Vivian, 2006). Most children are diagnosed between the ages of 8 and 19 years (Berry et al., 2006a).

The increasing number of children being diagnosed with type 2 diabetes has caused significant concern in the healthcare community. An estimated 8–45% of children older than 10 years of age with a new diagnosis of diabetes have type 2 (Berry, Urban, & Grey, 2006b). The true incidence in children is unknown as many children are undiagnosed.

Developing Cultural Competence

TYPE 2 DIABETES RISK

Children of African American, Native American, Hispanic, Alaska Native, and Asian/Pacific Islander origins are at greater risk for developing type 2 diabetes (Adams & Lammon, 2007; Berry et al., 2006b). Particularly affected are members of some Native American tribes that historically have had a high level of exercise and hunter-gatherer diets. In some groups, such as the Pima Indians of the Southwest, 22.3–50.9 per 1000 children are reported to have type 2 DM (Adams & Lammon, 2007).

Etiology and Pathophysiology

Type 2 diabetes is a complex metabolic disorder with insulin resistance the central abnormality. In response to increased body weight, the visceral fat produces a cytokine hormone (tumor necrosis factor) that desensitizes cellular insulin receptor to insulin. The pancreatic cells produce more insulin in an attempt to overcome the insulin resistance and facilitate glucose transfer. This results in **hyperinsulinemia** (elevated insulin levels in the blood). The child maintains a balance between hyperinsulinemia and insulin resistance and a normal glycemic state. As insulin resistance worsens, the islet of Langerhans beta cells fail in their ability to hypersecrete insulin. This leads to impaired glucose tolerance, and overt diabetes develops. The onset of puberty and increased secretion of growth hormone is believed to be a contributing factor in the development of insulin resistance (Vivian, 2006).

Clinical Manifestations

Signs and symptoms of type 2 diabetes vary upon initial presentation from those for type 1. Onset is more insidious, and symptoms of polydipsia and polyuria are absent or mild (Berry et al., 2006a). **Acanthosis nigricans,** hyperpigmentation and thickening of the skin with velvety irregularities in the skin folds of the back of the neck, medial aspect of the thighs and axillae, is a common finding and is associated with insulin resistance. The finding is present in 60–90% of children with type 2 diabetes (Adams & Lammon, 2007) (see Figure 55–8 ●). The child is usually obese with a high waist circumference. Some children (5–25%) are in ketoacidosis at the time of diagnosis (Berry et al., 2006a). Other clinical manifestations can be found on page 1622.

Clinical Therapy

Blood glucose levels of 200 mg/dL or greater without fasting, or a fasting glucose 126 mg/dL or greater are diagnostic of diabetes. Hemoglobin A_{1c} provides an indicator of the average serum glucose level for the past 60–90 days (Howe et al., 2005). Urine is tested and ketones are found in about 50% of children. Islet cell autoantibodies, fasting insulin levels, glutamic acid decarboxylase autoantibody test (GAD-65), and C-peptid levels are used to differentiate between type 1 and type 2 diabetes.

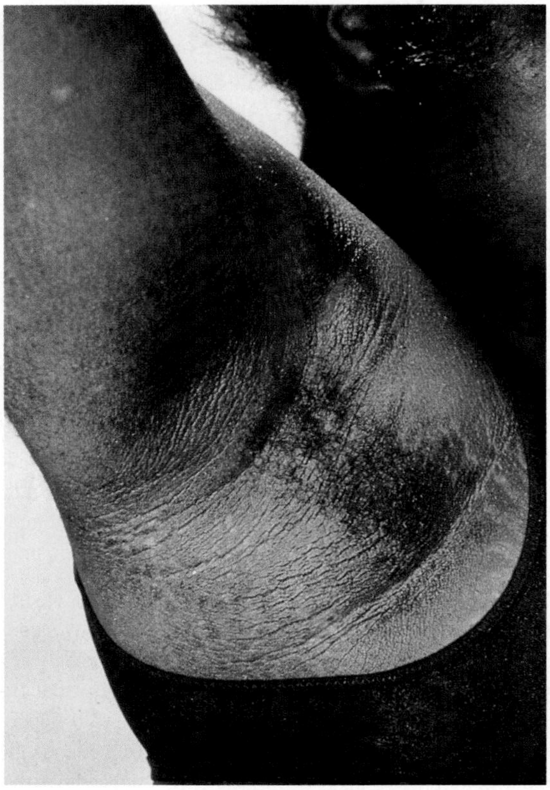

● **Figure 55–8** Acanthosis nigricans.
Courtesy of Audrey Austin, M.D., Children's National Medical Center, Washington, D.C.

The child with type 2 diabetes has normal or elevated fasting insulin C-peptid levels while these levels are normally low in the child with type 1 diabetes. Islet cell and GAD-65 autoantibodies will not be present in the child with type 2 diabetes (Berry et al., 2006a). A fasting lipid profile is obtained since dyslipidemia (primarily elevated LDL-C and triglycerides) is usually present. High blood pressure for age, gender, and height percentile is also seen (see Appendix B∞).

The multiple goals for managing the child with type 2 diabetes include the following: normalizing the blood glucose and HbA1c levels, decreasing weight, increasing exercise, normalizing lipid profile and blood pressure, and preventing complications. Nutrition education and weight loss make up the major therapy. The child needs to have gradual, sustained weight loss, metabolic control of blood glucose levels, exercise, and emotional support. If the child or adolescent presents with severe hyperglycemia or diabetic ketoacidosis, insulin will be required to gain initial glycemic control. Once metabolic control is achieved, oral medication (Metformin) is initiated as the child is weaned off of insulin. Metformin is used when diet and exercise efforts are inadequate to control hyperglycemia. Metformin improves the sensitivity of target cells to insulin, slows the gastrointestinal absorption of glucose, and reduces the hepatic and renal glucose production. It can be used when there is normal liver and kidney function and no ketosis. The dosage may be gradually increased to improve metabolic control. If additional medication is needed, sulfonylurea or meglitinides may be used; however, they are not approved for use in children in the United States due to liver toxicity (Alemzadeh & Wyatt, 2007). Insulin may only be needed for periods of increased stress, but the adolescent may ultimately require insulin for glycemic control if weight and exercise goals are not met.

NURSING MANAGEMENT

NURSING ASSESSMENT AND DIAGNOSIS

Because the child with type 2 diabetes does not often have an acute onset, assess any child with a body mass index (BMI) greater than 85th percentile for age and gender for signs of insulin resistance (acanthosis nigricans, hypertension, and dyslipidemia). Family history of diabetes in an overweight child is a reason to begin screening for the condition. Once the child has been diagnosed, monitor the child's blood glucose levels and blood pressure. Assess the child's diet and activity patterns to determine appropriate changes for disease management. Consider evaluating the siblings for diabetes. Nursing diagnoses that may apply to the child with type 2 diabetes include the following:

- *Imbalanced Nutrition: More than Body Requirements* related to obesity and ethnic and cultural norms
- *Activity Intolerance* related to sedentary lifestyle and disease state (insulin resistance)
- *Ineffective Therapeutic Regimen Management (Family and Individual)* related to family conflict over changing eating patterns
- *Situational Low Self-esteem* related to situational crisis associated with diagnosis of new-onset chronic illness

PLANNING AND IMPLEMENTATION

The child with type 2 diabetes may be hospitalized at the time of diagnosis because of ketoacidosis. However, the nurse in an inpatient setting is more likely to encounter this child when hospitalized for another condition or during visits for health care in clinics or schools. Nursing care focuses on managing the child's blood glucose levels and hypertension during the hospitalization, assessing growth and dietary intake, evaluating goals for weight loss and exercise programs, and reviewing the child's knowledge about diabetes and strategies for management at home.

NURSING CARE IN THE COMMUNITY

Since the child is initially diagnosed with type 2 diabetes and managed on an outpatient basis, nursing care focuses on teaching the child and parents about the disease and its management, managing dietary intake, providing emotional support, and planning strategies for daily management in the community.

Educate the child and family about the disease and lifestyle changes required for effective management of the condition. Focus on the need to increase activity with routine exercise of at least 30 to 60 minutes daily and by decreasing sedentary activity time, such as computer and television viewing time to no more than 2 hours daily. Customize the activity strategy for each child with motivation to develop a regular routine.

Work with the family to substitute high-calorie and high-fat foods with a meal plan sensitive to the family's resources and ethnic preferences. Suggestions include limiting fast food, and snacking on fruits and vegetables rather than foods high in fat and sugar. Assess the child's height, weight, and BMI on each visit, and plot on the appropriate growth curve for age and sex on each visit. A gradual sustained weight loss or decrease in BMI is the goal. If the child is experiencing a height-growth-height spurt, maintenance of weight rather than weight loss is the goal. Encourage the entire family to make dietary changes, especially since other family members are also at risk for the condition.

Teach the child and family to perform home blood glucose testing to monitor glycemic control. This will let the child and family know that efforts to manage the disease are successful. Take HbA_{1c} levels at each visit to determine the average blood glucose level for the past 3 months. A HbA_{1c} level of 7% or less is the goal. When dietary control and exercise are not successful in reducing blood glucose levels, teach the child and family about the prescribed oral medication.

Give the child and family opportunities to talk about the impact of the disease on their lives. Identify resources for information about strategies that have worked for other families. Identify local support groups and peer groups for the family and child. Suggest weekly activities, summer camps, and other ongoing programs to provide necessary support and motivation.

Make sure the child gets annual evaluations for potential complications of diabetes. The tests to be performed include blood for lipid levels, blood pressure, liver and renal function, urine for albumin, an eye examination for retinopathy, and a neurologic examination of the extremities for neuropathies. The child with type 2 diabetes has the same risk for developing long-term vascular complications as the child with type 1 diabetes when hyperglycemia is poorly controlled.

EVALUATION

Examples of expected outcomes of nursing care include the following:

- The child decreases sedentary activity time to less than 2 hours a day.
- The child's daily intake of fruits and vegetables increases to 5 to 8 servings daily, and total fat intake decreases to less than 30% of total calories.
- The child's body mass index slowly and consistently decreases.

DISORDERS OF GONADAL FUNCTION

GYNECOMASTIA

Gynecomastia is the presence of unilateral or bilateral enlarged breast tissue that occurs in about 65% of boys during puberty, usually at 13 to 14 years of age (Pinyerd & Zipf, 2005). It is sometimes confused with subcutaneous fat pads in obese males. Gynecomastia occurs when the ratio of estrogen to testosterone is greater than the usual male ratio. It is also associated with Klinefelter syndrome and drugs that increase the circulating concentration of prolactin such as marijuana, tricyclic antidepressants, and calcium channel blockers. The condition disappears in 1 to 2 years, and the amount of breast tissue varies among boys. If gynecomastia is severe and is causing distress to the adolescent, a referral to a plastic surgeon for possible reduction is indicated (Raine, Donaldson, Gregory, et al., 2006b).

Nursing care focuses on reassuring the boy and his parents that gynecomastia is common and transient. Because of the body image concerns common during adolescence, embarrassment is a frequent problem. Recommend clothing styles and other methods to camouflage the enlarged breasts.

AMENORRHEA

Amenorrhea, or lack of menstruation, may be primary or secondary. Criteria for primary amenorrhea include absence of menarche by age 14.5 years in association with no growth or development of secondary sexual characteristics, or absence of menses by age 16 when secondary sexual characteristics and growth are present.

Secondary amenorrhea is the cessation of menstrual periods 6 months or 3 cycles after menstruation has begun; it is characterized by an absence of spontaneous bleeding for at least 120 days. Pregnancy is the most common cause of secondary amenorrhea in adolescents. It is common for adolescents to have irregular menstrual cycles and duration of the menstrual period for 1 to 2 years after menarche. A large number of cycles are anovulatory for the first 2 years after menarche.

Primary amenorrhea is most often caused by structural defects of the reproductive system; chromosomal abnormalities (such as Turner syndrome); or hypothalamic or pituitary tumors, thyroid dysfunction, or polycystic ovary syndrome. No underlying pathologic condition is found in some adolescents. Primary or secondary amenorrhea may be found in competitive athletes.

A thorough history (including sexual activity), physical examination, and laboratory evaluation are required to determine the cause of amenorrhea. The history focuses on asking questions about recent excessive weight loss or gain; excessive physical activity or sports training; chronic illness; use of illegal drugs, birth control pills, or phenothiazines; emotional problems; and age of the mother at menarche. The physical examination focuses on evaluating the adolescent's stage of sexual development and assessing for hirsutism (see Chapter 35). A vaginal exam is performed to determine vaginal patency and if the vaginal mucosa is estrogenized. A pregnancy test is performed. Bone age and hormone levels are evaluated (estrogen, LH, FSH, and prolactin).

Treatment of amenorrhea depends on the specific cause. The most common approach is to give birth control pills containing both estrogen and progesterone. Athletic teenagers are encouraged to eat a well-balanced, high-calorie diet. Calcium supplements may be ordered. Estrogen with progesterone in low doses may be prescribed for athletes to reduce the risk for osteoporosis. Nursing management centers on patient education and emotional support. The goal is to maintain normal growth and development.

See Chapter 5 for information on dysmenorrhea.

Growth and Development

Girls competing in sports such as gymnastics, ballet, and long-distance running feel the need to maintain a low weight and specific body type. Reduced adipose tissue leads to a reduction in leptin, and subsequently a reduction in gonadotropin-releasing hormone and low serum estrogen levels (Bloomfield, 2006). Amenorrhea or oligomenorrhea and bone demineralization often result. This, in turn, may increase the girl's risk of fractures and osteoporosis in young adulthood (Landry, 2007) (See Chapter 58).

DISORDERS RELATED TO SEX CHROMOSOME ABNORMALITIES

TURNER SYNDROME

Turner syndrome is the most common sex chromosome abnormality in females. Affected girls have a missing or partial absence of one X chromosome. It occurs in approximately 1 in 2000 to 3000 live female births (Halac & Zimmerman, 2004b). Approximately 99% of fetuses with the disorder are spontaneously aborted generally during the first trimester of pregnancy (Doswell, 2006). In the absence of one X chromosome, the oocytes in the ovaries disappear and are nearly all gone by age 2 years. Other specific clinical manifestations are related to specific genes missing.

Characteristic clinical findings in the newborn include lymphedema of the hands and feet, a webbed neck, and a low hairline. During childhood, short stature becomes apparent (less than 5th percentile). During adolescence, there is a lack of breast development, pubertal delay, and amenorrhea. Other characteristic signs include cubitus valgus (increased angle at the elbow); scoliosis; broad chest with widely spaced nipples; hyperconvex fingernails; and dark and pigmented nevi (Figure 55–9 ●). Few girls have all of these features (Misra & Lee, 2005).

Growth usually proceeds at a normal rate for the first 2 to 3 years of life and then slows. Breast tissue, which begins to bud at about 10 to 12 years, fails to develop fully. Only in rare instances does a girl with Turner syndrome menstruate spontaneously or become able to conceive. Without treatment, final height is approximately 20 cm (7.8 in.) lower than the expected mean adult female height (Misra & Lee, 2005).

Among the conditions that may be associated with Turner syndrome are congenital heart defects such as coarctation of aorta or bicuspid aortic valve, hypertension, structural abnormalities of the kidney, autoimmune thyroiditis, celiac disease, hearing loss, orthodontic anomalies, strabismus, congenital hip dysplasia, and scoliosis (Morgan, 2007).

The condition is diagnosed definitively by a karyotype, which reveals the classic 45,X chromosome pattern or a combi-

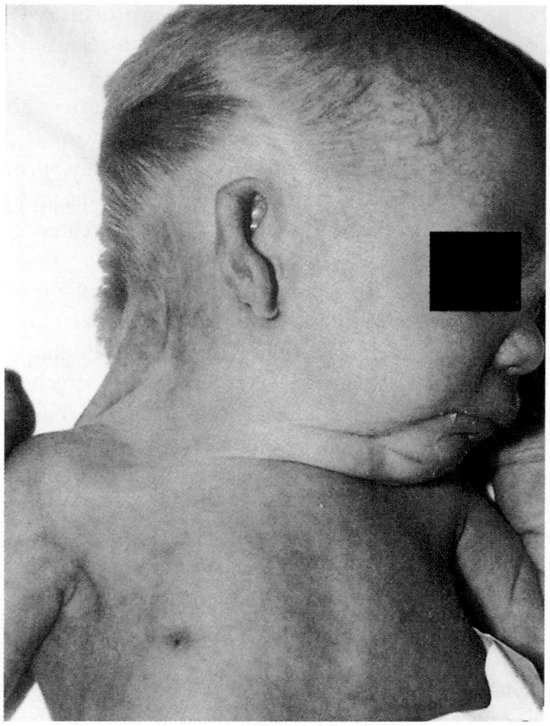

• Figure 55–9 What characteristic physical manifestations of Turner syndrome can you identify in this girl?

From Zittelli, B. J., & Davis, H. W. (Eds.). (2007). *Atlas of pediatric physical diagnosis* (5th ed., p. 14). Philadelphia: Mosby-Elsevier.

nation 45,X/46,XX pattern (Morgan, 2007). Turner syndrome may be suspected prenatally based on results of maternal serum screening and ultrasound. The diagnosis must be confirmed by chorionic villous testing or amniocentesis (Loscalzo, Bondy, & Biesecker, 2006).

Treatment involves carefully monitoring the child's growth. A growth chart made especially for girls with Turner syndrome is available from the Turner Syndrome Society. Growth hormone therapy may be prescribed to promote growth during childhood, and therapy can begin at age 2 years (Halac & Zimmerman, 2004b). Low-dose estrogen therapy is usually begun at around 12 years of age, with a gradual dosage increase to mimic natural puberty (Tyler & Edman, 2004). This treatment produces pubertal changes such as breast development and pubic hair. Progesterone is added to the estrogen therapy to initiate cyclic menstrual periods.

Nursing Management

Nursing assessment is focused on monitoring growth rates and observing for signs of cardiac, renal, gastrointestinal, vision, hearing, musculoskeletal, or thyroid dysfunction. Carefully measure the child's height and plot on the growth curve. Teach the family the correct administration of growth hormone and potential side effects.

The lack of growth and sexual development associated with Turner syndrome presents problems not only for physical growth but also for psychosocial development. The girl's perception of her body and how she differs from peers affects self-image, self-consciousness, and self-esteem. In the United States, cultural values place importance on attaining normal to tall stature. Short children tend to be treated according to their size rather than their age. Emphasis is also placed on sexual maturity. Encourage parents to treat the child by her chronologic age rather than size. The nurse can be instrumental in helping the child adapt to the condition and gain self-esteem. Be an active listener and reinforce abilities and skills that the girl exhibits. Encourage parents to provide support. Even though their intelligence is generally normal, they have a higher incidence of learning problems because of visual–spatial deficits that affect performance on mathematical and manual dexterity tasks (Tyler & Edman, 2004).

KLINEFELTER SYNDROME

Klinefelter syndrome is a genetic condition that occurs in boys who have an extra X chromosome (usually 47,XXY). It occurs in approximately 1 in 1000 live male births (Wattendorf & Muenke, 2005). It is the single most common cause of hypogonadism (decreased secretory activity of the gonad), androgen deficiency, and infertility in males.

Most infants appear normal at birth. The condition is usually diagnosed during the school-age years when the boy's behavior becomes a problem in the classroom. Boys with Klinefelter syndrome may have delayed language development and auditory processing problems that are frustrating to the child. Intelligence quotient (IQ) scores may be similar to those of siblings, but academic difficulty is common because of memory, data retrieval skills, and verbal processing problems (Misra & Lee, 2005). The onset of puberty may be delayed with an abnormal progression. Testicular size is decreased at all ages. Less facial and body hair may develop. Gynecomastia is a characteristic finding. Associated complications of Klinefelter syndrome include cardiac abnormalities, pulmonary disease, dental abnormalities, and scoliosis.

Chromosomal analysis revealing one or more extra X chromosomes confirms the diagnosis. The goal of treatment is to stimulate masculinization and the development of secondary sex characteristics when adolescence is delayed. Testosterone replacement begins when the boy is 11 or 12 years of age. A testosterone preparation is given by intramuscular injection every 3 to 4 weeks to maintain serum testosterone levels within the normal range. The dose is increased gradually until an adult dose is reached between 15 and 17 years of age; however, this does not improve fertility. Hormone treatment helps improve psychologic well-being and social functioning (Misra & Lee, 2005). It also helps to promote normal body proportions and prevent gynecomastia.

Nursing Management

Nursing care consists of educating the parents and child about the syndrome, evaluating the child's and family's coping mechanisms, assisting with school problems, and reinforcing the child's strengths. Encourage parents to channel their son's energy into areas that will provide opportunities for success and productive experiences. Emphasize the importance of rewarding the boy's successes in school, sports, or hobbies. Make genetic counseling available to adolescents, if indicated, because sexual functioning and fertility may be impaired.

INBORN ERRORS OF METABOLISM

Inborn errors of metabolism are inherited biochemical abnormalities of the urea cycle, amino acid, and organic acid metabolism. Therefore, protein, carbohydrate, fat, electrolyte, blood, and respiratory metabolism can be affected. Individually they are rare disorders; however, as a group they are a significant health problem in infancy.

The biochemical defect usually causes an abnormal chemical by-product to accumulate in the blood, urine, or tissues or results in a decreased amount of normal enzymes. Most disorders are associated with protein intolerance with symptoms developing shortly after formula or breast milk feedings begin.

Clinical manifestations usually occur within days or weeks of birth. Signs and symptoms may include lethargy and poor feeding, persistent vomiting, abnormal muscle tone and seizures, apnea and tachycardia, and an unusual urine or body odor (musty, sweet odor of maple syrup or burnt sugar, or cheesy or sweaty feet).

Newborn screening has been demonstrated to save lives and to prevent serious disability. The March of Dimes recommends that newborn screening tests for 29 disorders that have effective treatment be made available to all newborns (March of Dimes, 2006). In most states, newborn screening programs lead to the detection of several conditions before symptoms develop.

In some cases, disorders associated with inborn errors of metabolism are not detected until signs and symptoms are present. Initial laboratory tests include measurement of serum glucose, electrolytes, blood gases, and serum ammonia. Tests results make it possible to classify the disorder by the presence of hypoglycemia, metabolic acidosis, hyperammonemia, or liver dysfunction. Further diagnostic laboratory tests are then performed on newborns with positive results.

Treatment, when available, focuses on replacing or reducing the amount of the substance causing the biochemical abnormality.

Four of the more common inborn errors of metabolism—phenylketonuria, galactosemia, fatty acid oxidation defects, and maple syrup urine disease—are presented in this section. Congenital hypothyroidism and congenital adrenal hyperplasia, which are also considered inborn errors of metabolism, were discussed earlier in this chapter.

PHENYLKETONURIA

Phenylketonuria (PKU) is an autosomal recessive inherited disorder of amino acid metabolism that affects the body's use of protein. It is caused by a mutation of the phenylalanine hydroxylase gene. The incidence is greater than 1 in 25,000 live births per year in the U.S. population (March of Dimes, 2006). The defect results in an accumulation of phenylalanine in the blood or phenylalanine metabolites in the urine. If untreated, this disease leads to severe mental retardation, seizures, and death.

Children with PKU have a deficiency of the liver enzyme phenylalanine hydroxylase that normally breaks down the essential amino acid phenylalanine into tyrosine. As a result, phenylalanine accumulates in the blood, causing a musty or mousey body and urine odor, irritability, vomiting, hyperactivity, hypertonia, hyperreflexive deep tendon reflexes, seizures, and an eczema-like rash (Rezvani, 2007). Persistence of elevated phenylalanine leads to disruption of cellular processes of myelination and protein synthesis, and results in a seizure disorder and untreatable mental retardation.

Infants appear normal at birth except for lighter skin complexion than their nonaffected siblings. If diagnosis is delayed mental retardation may be severe. Microcephaly, prominent maxilla and widely spaced teeth, enamel hypoplasia, and growth retardation are other common findings in untreated children (Rezvani, 2007).

Screening for PKU is required by state law in all 50 states. For best results the newborn should have begun formula or breast milk feeding before specimen collection. Early hospital discharge places newborns at risk for false-negative screening tests if screened within 24 hours of birth. Screening needs to occur no sooner than 48 hours after birth, or the test should be repeated at 1 to 2 weeks of age. If the test shows elevated levels of plasma phenylalanine, a repeat quantitative test is performed. If the second test is positive, the family is referred to an outpatient treatment center. Serum phenylalanine should be measured periodically throughout life. Levels greater than 15 mg/dL are considered dangerous.

PKU is treated using special formulas (e.g., Lofenalac, Minafen, and Albumaid XP) and a diet low in phenylalanine to keep plasma phenylalanine levels between 2 and 6 mg/dL. The diet must also meet the child's needs for optimal growth. Breastfeeding is possible if phenylalanine levels are monitored. High-protein foods (meats and dairy products) and aspartame are avoided because they contain large amounts of phenylalanine. Elemental medical foods (modified protein hydrosylates in which the phenylalanine has been removed) are used instead. The low-phenylalanine diet should be maintained throughout life. If dietary control is lost before 6 years of age, there is a significant impact on IQ. The low phenylalanine diet is especially important for adolescent females and women prior to conception and during pregnancy to prevent congenital anomalies (low birth weight, microcephaly, mental retardation, and congenital heart defects) in the fetus (Rouse & Azen, 2004).

Nursing Management

Nursing care is mainly supportive and focuses on teaching parents about the disorder and its management. The low-phenylalanine diet is a rigid, strict diet that excludes many foods. Educate the family about sources of phenylalanine, and refer the family to a nutritionist to establish an appropriate meal plan. Parents and children need a great deal of support to promote compliance. The formula and elemental medical food costs are relatively high. The formula is usually reimbursed by insurance, but negotiations with health plans may help parents obtain some support for medical foods. The current recommendation is for all patients to remain on the phenylalanine restricted diet for life (Rezvani, 2007).

Refer parents of an affected child who are considering a future pregnancy and adolescents with the disorder for genetic counseling.

GALACTOSEMIA

Galactosemia, a disorder of carbohydrate metabolism, has an autosomal recessive inheritance pattern. It occurs in 1 in 50,000 live births (March of Dimes, 2006).

Galactosemia results from a deficiency of the liver enzyme galactose 1-phosphate uridyltransferase (GALT), one of three enzymes needed to convert galactose to glucose. The lack of enzyme leads to an accumulation of galactose metabolites in the eyes, liver, kidney, and brain, rapidly damaging the organs and causing life-threatening problems. Children become susceptible to gram-negative sepsis.

Early signs include poor sucking, failure to gain weight due to vomiting followed by diarrhea, hypoglycemia, and an enlarged liver. Later signs include mental retardation, jaundice, ascites, sepsis, lethargy, seizures, hypotonia, cataracts, and coma. Babies may die within 1 month of birth without treatment, usually due to sepsis. When diagnosis is not made at birth, damage to the liver (cirrhosis) and brain (mental retardation) become progressively more severe and irreversible.

Routine newborn screening for galactosemia is performed in all U.S. newborn screening programs (March of Dimes, 2008). (See Skill 10–2 SKILLS.) Infants who are not screened at birth are identified once they become symptomatic. The diagnosis is based on history, physical examination, and laboratory tests (galactose, AST, and ALT are abnormally high). Urine specimens are checked for reducing substances (the Clinitest is positive and the Clinistix is negative) in several specimens while the infant is receiving breast milk or formula with lactose.

Treatment involves placing infants on a lactose- or galactose-free formula (e.g., Nutramigen, a meat-based or soybean formula), which remains the child's milk substitute for life. Improvement in the infant's condition is generally seen within 24 hours. A galactose-free diet (no milk or cheese products, including foods with dry milk products) is prescribed when the infant is ready for solids. Despite compliance with the diet, complications (learning disabilities, speech defects, ovarian failure, and neurologic syndromes) develop in many children.

Nursing management focuses on educating the parents and child about the disorder and required diet, assessing coping abilities, and providing emotional support. Refer the family to a nutritionist for diet counseling. Families must learn to screen foods for added milk solids and to avoid medications, such as antibiotics, that have lactose fillers. Calcium supplementation may be needed. Advise parents that several galactose-free cheeses are sold commercially. Because the disorder is inherited, refer the family for genetic counseling.

DEFECTS IN FATTY ACID OXIDATION

Mitochondrial oxidation of fatty acids is an energy-producing pathway that becomes essential during periods of starvation, when the body fuel converts from carbohydrate to fat. Gene defects can occur in nearly every stage in the fatty acid oxidation pathway resulting in many subclasses of fatty acid oxidation defects. All of these defects are autosomal recessive traits that occur in both males and females (Stanley & Bennett, 2007).

Screening has revealed that fatty acid oxidation disorders are among the most common inborn errors of metabolism. These defects include medium-chain acyl-CoA dehydrogenase (MCAD) deficiency (most common), very long-chain acyl-CoA dehydrogenase deficiency, long-chain 3-OH acyl-CoA dehydrogenase deficiency, trifunctional protein deficiency, and carnitine uptake defect. If undiagnosed, these disorders can lead to serious complications affecting the brain and other organs. Symptoms can progress to coma and then death (March of Dimes, 2006).

The most common presentation is an acute-onset life-threatening coma and hypoglycemia induced by a period of fasting. Other manifestations often include cardiomyopathy, hepatomegaly, and muscle weakness. Infants and children can be asymptomatic except for times during fasting or stress.

Diagnosis can occur during routine newborn screening when laboratories use mass spectrometry. Most cases are identified during an acute presentation of symptoms when laboratory evaluation may include blood gases, electrolytes, hepatic profile, plasma lactate, plasma amino acids, urine organic acids, acylcamitine profile, quantitative carnitine levels and urine for ketones. Hypoglycemia is usually present and ketone levels are unusually low (Thomas & Van Hove, 2007). Liver function tests demonstrate elevated transaminases, urea, and ammonia. Plasma and tissue concentrations of total carnitine are reduced. Skin biopsies are often obtained for fibroblast analysis. Physical examination may reveal hepatomegaly due to fatty infiltration.

Treatment includes the prevention of hypoglycemia by avoiding fasting, ensuring that no more than 8–12 hours passes before food is eaten. Carnitine supplementation may be required in some disorders as it is useful in preventing low blood sugar and assists in removing metabolic waste from cells (Thomas & Van Hove, 2007).

Nursing management involves educating parents about the importance of frequent feedings and avoidance of fasting. These children should go no longer than 8 to 12 hours without food. Infants should be fed around the clock every 2 to 4 hours. If the infant or child is unable to sustain oral intake during an acute illness, he or she must be referred to the hospital for intravenous dextrose supplementation. Even simple infections such as an ear infection or influenza can become life threatening for these children. Several snack foods and meals of low-fat and high-carbohydrate foods (e.g., cereal, pasta) are recommended throughout the day. Genetic counseling should be offered to the family. If one child in the family is diagnosed with the disorder, the siblings should also be tested, even if they are asymptomatic.

MAPLE SYRUP URINE DISEASE

Maple syrup urine disease (MSUD) is a disorder of amino acid metabolism that has an autosomal recessive inheritance pattern. It is rare, occurring in approximately 1 in 180,000 newborns, but occurs as often as 1 in 176 newborns among some Pennsylvania Mennonites (Bodamer & Lee, 2008).

In MSUD, three essential amino acids (leucine, isoleucine, and valine) cannot be metabolized because of absent or defective enzyme branched chain alpha-ketoacid dehydrogenase (Simon et al., 2006). All three amino acids are essential to form normal structures such as the hair, skin, and muscle. Leucine has the potential to accumulate in the brain and cause cerebral edema, progressive neurologic impairment, and death (Bodamer & Lee, 2008).

Within 4 to 7 days of life, the newborn develops symptoms of poor appetite, lethargy, vomiting, variable muscle tone, irritability, seizures, high-pitched cry, severe ketoacidosis, and a sweet odor of maple syrup in bodily fluids. The symptoms may quickly progress to coma and death if not treated (Bodamer & Lee, 2008; March of Dimes, 2006).

Most but not all states require newborn screening for this condition. Diagnosis is made with laboratory tests of the urine for positive ketones and blood tests for elevated leucine, isoleucine, alloisoleucine (a stereoisomer of isoleucine not normally found in blood), and valine.

Treatment during the acute stage involves removal of the branched-chain amino acids and their metabolites from the tissues and body fluids. Some critically ill infants may require dialysis to remove these compounds as renal clearance is poor. Lifelong treatment includes specially designed medical formulas and foods rich in amino acids, calories, vitamins, minerals, and other nutrients as prescribed. These special medical foods have the three amino acids removed. The child needs special low-protein foods that are adequate for growth with enough calories to support twice the child's basal metabolic rate. Daily urine testing is required to determine if ketones are being excreted, an indication that the body is in a catabolic state. A liver transplant has been performed in a few affected children who were subsequently able to tolerate a normal diet (Rezvani & Rosenblatt, 2007). The long-term prognosis of affected children is guarded as severe ketoacidosis, cerebral edema, or death may occur during any stressful situation, including infection or surgery.

Nursing care includes educating the family about the disorder and special dietary requirements. The parents need to learn how to mix the child's special formula with a natural protein source, amino acid supplements, and water. The child needs formula even when ill; provide a sick day plan to prevent ketoacidosis. The child should be permitted moderate exercise only to prevent increases in leucine levels. Help families identify sources of information or support groups who can share recipes and tips for managing the child's condition.

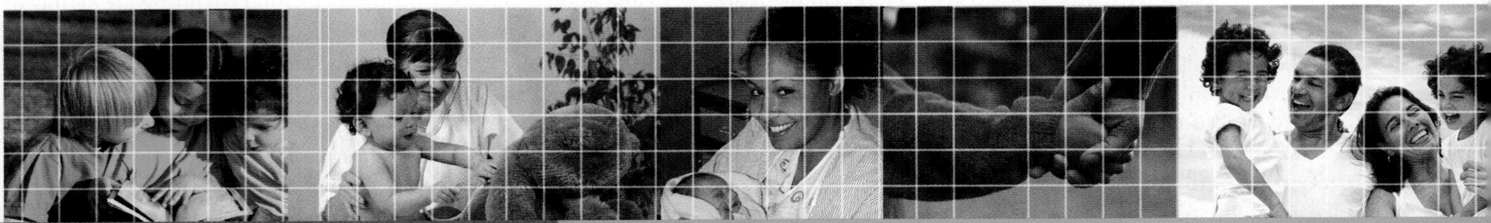

CRITICAL CONCEPT REVIEW

LEARNING OUTCOMES	CONCEPTS
55.1 Identify the function of important hormones of the endocrine system.	1. Gonadotropin-releasing hormone: ■ Stimulates anterior pituitary to produce LH and FSH. 2. Growth hormone: ■ Regulates linear bone growth and growth of all tissues. 3. Antidiuretic hormone: ■ Regulates urine concentration by the kidneys. 4. Thyroid hormone: ■ Regulates metabolism of cells and body heat production. 5. Parathyroid hormone: ■ Regulates serum calcium levels and phosphorus excretion. 6. Insulin: ■ Regulates glucose utilization by the cells.
55.2 Identify signs and symptoms that may indicate a disorder of the endocrine system.	1. Delayed or accelerated growth. 2. Impaired metabolism. 3. Mental retardation. 4. Delayed or accelerated sexual development. 5. Polyuria and polydipsia. 6. Cushingoid features.
55.3 Identify all conditions for which short stature is a sign.	1. Growth hormone deficiency. 2. Familial short stature. 3. Constitutional growth delay. 4. Hypothyroidism. 5. Precocious puberty. 6. Turner syndrome. 7. Chronic renal failure. 8. Cushing disease. 9. Inborn error of metabolism. 10. Severe cardiac, pulmonary, and GI disease.

LEARNING OUTCOMES	CONCEPTS
55.4 Develop a nursing care plan for each type of acquired metabolic disorder.	1. Diabetes insipidus: ■ Monitor intake and output and daily weight. ■ Replace fluids orally or by IV to match output. ■ Administer DDAVP as ordered. ■ Instruct child and parents in use of medication. 2. Growth hormone excess (Hyperpituitarism): ■ Teach parents and child about disorder. ■ Support a positive self-image. ■ Provide pre- and postoperative nursing care as needed. 3. SIADH: ■ Monitor fluid balance and avoid excess fluid intake. ■ Monitor for changes in behavior or level of consciousness. ■ Implement seizure precautions. ■ Monitor laboratory work for serum sodium, urine osmolality, and specific gravity. ■ Weigh child daily. 4. Precocious puberty: ■ Teach parents and child about condition and how to treat the child according to chronological age. ■ Provide emotional support. ■ Teach parents to administer medication. 5. Hyperthyroidism: ■ Carefully assess vital signs. ■ Teach parents and child about disorder. ■ Promote rest. ■ Provide increased calories in 5–6 small meals. ■ Provide a cool environment. ■ Provide pre- and postoperative care as needed. 6. Hyperparathyroidism: ■ Manage fluid and electrolytes. ■ Assess for respiratory distress and airway obstruction. ■ Monitor for signs of infection. ■ Monitor the serum calcium and phosphorus levels. ■ Provide pre- and postoperative teaching and care. ■ Teach parents and child the signs of hypocalcemia. 7. Adrenal insufficiency: ■ Educate parents and child about disorder and need for cortisol replacement. ■ Administer replacement medication. ■ Instruct parents in use of replacement cortisol. 8. Pheochromocytoma: ■ Provide pre- and postoperative teaching and care. ■ Closely monitor vital signs. ■ Administer antihypertensives as needed. ■ Postoperatively, observe for neurologic signs, respiratory distress, and signs of shock. ■ Instruct parents in need for lifelong follow-up care.
55.5 Develop a family education plan for the child that needs lifelong cortisol replacement.	1. Administer medication early in the morning: ■ May be given every other day to reduce side effects. 2. Give medication at mealtimes: ■ May use antacids between meals if medication causes GI side effects. 3. Teach parents how to inject medication: ■ Instruct in the reasons why the injectable form may be needed. 4. Assist parents to understand serious complications that can occur if medication is not given. 5. Instruct parents in signs and symptoms of acute adrenal insufficiency. 6. Instruct parents to inform all healthcare providers about the child's condition. 7. Instruct parents to have child wear a medical alert bracelet.

(continued)

LEARNING OUTCOMES — CONCEPTS

55.6 Distinguish between the nursing care of the child with type 1 and type 2 diabetes.

1. Type 1 diabetes:
   - Teach child and parents about the disease.
   - Monitor blood glucose levels frequently.
   - Administer insulin as prescribed.
   - Teach parents and the child meal planning with carbohydrate counting.
   - Teach child and parents how to administer insulin injections or teach the use of an insulin pump.
   - Encourage a balance of diet, activity, and insulin to maintain blood glucose level.
   - Provide simple sugars followed by a complex carbohydrate for symptoms of hypoglycemia.
   - Instruct child and family about symptoms of both hypo- and hyperglycemia.
   - Instruct family concerning sick day rules for the child.
2. Type 2 diabetes:
   - Monitor child's blood glucose and blood pressure.
   - Teach child and family how to check blood glucose at home.
   - Assess diet and activity pattern.
   - Administer medication to control hyperglycemia.
   - Help child and parent to plan nutritious meals that encourage weight loss.
   - Assist child to increase activity and weight loss.

55.7 Develop a nursing care plan for the child with an inherited metabolic disorder.

1. Perform newborn screening test as indicated by state law.
2. Administer special diet or medication prescribed for child.
3. Instruct parents in use of special formula and preparation of special diets.
4. Refer to a nutritional counselor.
5. Assess coping abilities of parents.
6. Support emotional status of parents.

CRITICAL THINKING IN ACTION

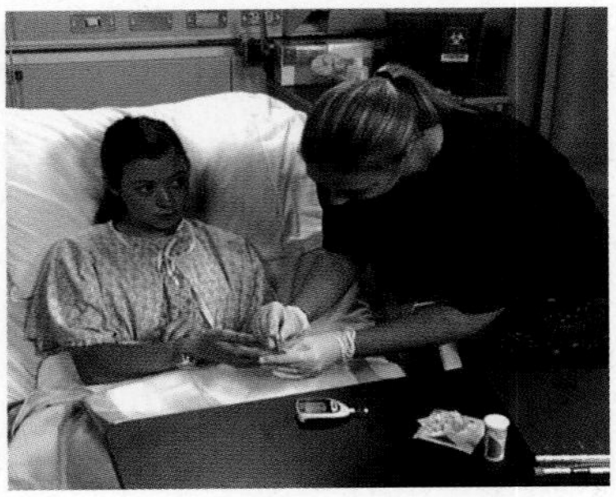

Fourteen-year-old Amanda is admitted to the hospital with newly diagnosed type 1 diabetes mellitus. She had initially been taken to her doctor's office for enuresis, polyphagia, polydipsia, and lethargy, but when assessed, her urinalysis had glucose and ketones, and she had a weight loss of 15 pounds.

Upon admission to the hospital, a full assessment is performed and the following vital signs are documented: weight 115 pounds, temperature 98.8°F, respiratory rate 40 breaths per minute, heart rate 90 beats per minute, and blood pressure 106/63. She has dry mucous membranes, but skin turgor is brisk. Blood is drawn immediately and will continue to be drawn every hour until she is stable. Amanda is able to understand the nutritional guidelines associated with type 1 diabetes and how to, under adult supervision, perform blood glucose monitoring as well as how to draw up and administer insulin. Amanda and her parents spend most of the time in the hospital learning survival skills for managing her diabetes. Daily education and monitoring will occur in the diabetes clinic until the family is confident about taking care of Amanda. Regular follow-up visits will be scheduled with the diabetes nurse educator and endocrinologist.

1. What is the blood work most likely to be done on Amanda when admitted to the hospital for type 1 diabetes?
2. How should the family be told to manage hypoglycemic episodes?
3. What should the parents be told about preventing diabetic ketoacidosis in Amanda?
4. How often should blood glucose monitoring be performed once the condition is stabilized?

See MyNursingKit for possible responses.

REFERENCES

Adams, M. H., & Lammon, C. A. B. (2007). The presence of family history and the development of Type 2 diabetes mellitus risk factors in rural children. *The Journal of School Nursing, 23*(5), 259–266.

Alemzadeh, R., & Wyatt, D. T. (2007). Diabetes mellitus in children. In R. M. Kliegman, R. E. Behrman, H. B. Jenson, & B. F. Stanton (Eds.), *Nelson textbook of pediatrics* (18th ed., pp. 2402–2431). Philadelphia: Saunders Elsevier.

Amer, K. S. (2005). Advances in assessment, diagnosis, and treatment of hyperthyroidism in children. *Journal of Pediatric Nursing, 20*(2), 119–126.

American Diabetes Association (2008a). Diagnosis and classification of diabetes mellitus. *Diabetes Care, 31*(Suppl 1), S55–S60.

American Diabetes Association. (2008b). Diabetes care in the school and day care setting. *Diabetes Care, 31*(Suppl 1), S79–S86.

American Diabetes Association (2008c). Ketoacidosis. Retrieved February 28, 2009 from www.diabetes.org/type-1-diabetes/ketoacidosis.jsp

Berry, D., Urban, A., & Grey, M. (2006a). Management of type 2 diabetes in youth (Part 2). *Journal of Pediatric Health Care, 20*(2), 88–97.

Berry, D., Urban, A., & Grey, M. (2006b). Understanding the development and prevention of type 2 diabetes in youth (Part 1*). Journal of Pediatric Health Care, 20*(1), 3–10.

Bismuth, E., & Laffel, L. (2007). Can we prevent diabetes ketoacidosis in children? *Pediatric Diabetes, 8*(6), 24–33.

Bloomfield, D. (2006). Secondary Amenorrhea. *Pediatrics in Review*, *27*(3), 113–115.

Bodamer, O. A., & Lee, B. (2008). Maple syrup urine disease. Retrieved February, 28, 2009 from http://emedicine.medscape.com/article/946234-overview

Boger, M. S., & Perrier, N. D. (2004). Advantages and disadvantages of surgical therapy and optional extent of thyroidectomy for the treatment of hyperthyroidism. *Surgical Clinics of North America, 84,* 849–874.

Boland, E. A., & Grey, M. (2004). Diabetes mellitus (Types 1 and 2). In P. L. Jackson & J. A. Vessey (Eds.), *Primary care of the child with a chronic condition* (4th ed., pp. 426–444). St Louis: Mosby.

Breault, D. T., & Majzoub, J. A. (2007). Diabetes insipidus. In R. M. Kliegman, R. E. Behrman, H. B. Jenson, & B. F. Stanton (Eds.), *Nelson textbook of pediatrics* (18th ed., pp. 2299–2301). Philadelphia: Saunders Elsevier.

Caplin, N. (2005). Calcium regulation and hypocalcemic disorders. In T. M. Moshang (Ed.), *Pediatric endocrinology: The requisites for pediatrics* (pp. 217–225). St. Louis: Elsevier Mosby.

Casu, A., Trucco, M., & Pietropaolo, M. (2005). A look at the future: Prediction, prevention, and cure including islet transplantation and stem cell therapy. *Pediatric Clinics of North America, 52,* 1779–1804.

Cheung, R., Cureton, V. Y., & Canham, D. L. (2006). Quality of life in adolescents with Type 1 diabetes who participate in diabetes camp. *Journal of School Nursing, 22,* 53–58.

Cogen, F. R., Streisand, R., & Sarin, S. (2002). Selecting children and adolescents for insulin pump therapy: Medical and behavioral considerations. *Diabetes Spectrum, 15*(2), 72–75.

Cystic Fibrosis Foundation (2009). Cystic fibrosis-related diabetes. Retrieved February 28, 2009 from www.cff.org/LivingWithCF/StayingHealthy/Diet/Diabetes/

Doswell, B. H., Visootsak, J., Brady, A. N., & Graham, J. M. (2006). Turner syndrome: An update and review for the primary physician. *Clinical Pediatrics, 45,* 301–313.

Doyle, D. A., & DiGeorge, A. M. (2007). Disorders of the parathyroid. In R. M. Kliegman, R. E. Behrman, H. B. Jenson, & B. F. Stanton, *Nelson textbook of pediatrics* (18th ed., pp. 2340–2348). Philadelphia: Saunders Elsevier.

Doyle, E. A., Weinzimer, S. A., Steffen, A. T., Ahern, J. H., Vincent, M., & Tamborlane, W. V. (2004). A randomized prospective trial comparing the efficacy of continuous subcutaneous insulin infusion with multiple daily injections using insulin glargine. *Diabetes Care, 27*(7), 1554–1558.

Dunger, D. B., Sperling, M. A., Acerini, C. L., Bohn, D. J., Daneman, D., Danne, T. P. A., et al. (2004). European Society for Paediatric Endocrinology/Lawson Wilkins Pediatric Endocrine Society consensus statement on diabetic ketoacidosis in children and adolescents. *Pediatrics, 113*(2), e133–e140.

Eugster, E. A., & Francis and the Lawson Wilkins Drug and Therapeutics Committee (2006). Position Statement: Continuous subcutaneous insulin infusion in very young children with type 1 diabetes. *Pediatrics, 118*(4), 1244–1249.

Evert, A. B. (2004). Tools and techniques for working with young people with diabetes. *Diabetes Spectrum, 17*(1), 8–14.

Failor, R. A., & Capell, P. T. (2003). Hyperaldosteronism and pheochromocytoma: New tricks and tests. *Primary Care: Clinics in Office Practice, 30*(4), 801–820viii.

Ferry, R. J. (2005). Salt wasting and the syndrome of inappropriate antidiuretic hormone. In T. M. Moshang (Ed.), Pediatric endocrinology: The requisites for pediatrics (pp. 269–274). St. Louis: Elsevier Mosby.

Gance-Cleveland, B. (2003). Adaptation to Addison's disease in a child: A case study. *Journal of Pediatric Health Care, 17*(6), 301–310.

Glaser, N. (2005). Pediatric diabetic ketoacidosis and hyperglycemic hyperosmolar state. *Pediatric Clinics of North America, 52,* 1611–1635.

Graue, M., Wentzel-Larsen, T., Hanestad, B. R., & Sovik, O. (2005). Health-related quality of life and metabolic control in adolescents with diabetes: The role of parental care, control, and involvement. *Journal of Pediatric Nursing, 20*(5), 373.

Grimberg, A., & DeLéon, D. D. (2005). Disorders in growth. In T. M. Moshang (Ed.), *Pediatric endocrinology: The requisites in pediatrics* (pp. 127–167). St. Louis: Elsevier Mosby.

Grimberg, A., Kutikov, J. K., & Cucchiara, A. J. (2005). Sex differences in patients referred for evaluation of poor growth. *Journal of Pediatrics, 146*(2), 212–216.

Gungor, N., & Arslanian, S. (2004). Progressive beta cell failure in type 2 diabetes mellitus of youth. *Journal of Pediatrics, 144*(5), 656–659.

Habich, M. (2006). Establishing a standard for pediatric inpatient diabetes education. *Pediatric Nursing, 32*(2), 113–115.

Halac, I., & Zimmerman, D. (2004a). Managing growth hormone treatment in pediatric patients. *Pediatric Annals, 33*(3), 183–190.

Halac, I., & Zimmerman, D. (2004b). Coordinating care for children with Turner syndrome. *Pediatric Annals, 33*(3), 189–196.

Haller, M. J., Atkinson, M. A., & Schatz, D. (2005). Type 1 diabetes mellitus: Etiology, presentation, and management. *Pediatric Clinics of North America, 52,* 1553–1578.

Haley-Andrews, S., & Mackenzie, J. E. (2005). Pediatric diabetic ketoacidosis: Clinical presentations and nursing considerations. *Pediatric Emergency Care, 21*(9), 624–628.

Helgeson, V. S., Viccaro, L., Becker, D., Escobar, O., & Siminerio, L. (2006). Diet of adolescents with and without diabetes. *Diabetes Care, 29*(5), 982–987.

Henwood, M. J., & Katz, L. E. L. (2005). Disorders of the adrenal gland. In T. M. Moshang (Ed.), *Pediatric endocrinology: The requisites for pediatrics* (pp. 193–213). St. Louis: Elsevier Mosby.

Howe, C. J., Jawad, A. F., Tuttle, A. K., Moser, J. T., Preis, C., Buzby, M., & Murphy, K. M. (2005). Education and telephone case management for children with type 1 diabetes: A randomized controlled trial. *Journal of Pediatric Nursing, 20*(2), 83–95.

Huang, E. A., Feldman, B. J., Schwartz, I. D., Geller, D. H., Rosenthal, S. M., & Gitelman, S. E. (2006). Oral urea for the treatment of chronic syndrome of inappropriate antidiuresis in children. *Journal of Pediatrics, 148,* 128–131.

Kache, S., & Ferry, R. J. (2005). Diabetes insipidus. In T. M. Moshang (Ed.), *Pediatric endocrinology: The requisites for pediatrics* (pp. 257–267). St. Louis: Elsevier Mosby.

Kaplowitz, P. B. (2006). Pubertal development in girls: Secular trends. *Current opinion in obstetrics and gynecology, 18*(5), 487–491.

Karagiannis, A., Mikhailidis, D. P., Athyros, V. G., & Harsoulis, F. (2007). Pheochromocytoma: An update on genetics and management. *Endocrine-Related Cancer, 14,* 935–956.

Keefe, S. (2007, Feb.). Precocious puberty. *Advance for Nurses,* 41–42.

Kollars, J., Zarroug, A. E., van Heerden, J., Lteif, A., Stavlo, P., Suarez, L. et al. (2005). Primary hyperthyroidism in pediatric patients. *Pediatrics, 115*(4), 974–980.

Kwon, K. T., & Tsai, V. W. (2007). Metabolic emergencies. *Emergency Medicine Clinics of North America, 25*(4), 1041–1060.

LaFranchi, S. (2007). Disorders of the thyroid gland. In R. M. Kliegman, R. E. Behrman, H. B. Jenson, & B. F. Stanton (Eds.), *Nelson textbook of pediatrics* (18th ed., pp. 2316–2340). Philadelphia: Saunders Elsevier.

Landry, G. L. (2007). Female athletes: Menstrual problems and the risk of osteopenia. In R. M. Kliegman, R. E. Behrman, H. B. Jenson, &

B. F. Stanton (Eds.), *Nelson textbook of pediatrics* (18th ed., p. 2865). Philadelphia: Saunders Elsevier.

Lee, J. M., & Menon, R. K. (2005). Growth hormone for short children without growth deficiency: Issues and practices. *Contemporary Pediatrics, 22*(10), 46–53.

Lee, J. M., Davis, M. M., Clark, S. J., Hofer, T. P., & Kemper, A. R. (2006). Estimated cost effectiveness of growth hormone therapy for idiopathic short stature. *Archives of Pediatric Adolescent Medicine, 160,* 263–269.

Litton, J., Rice, A., Friedman, N., Oden, J., Lee, M. M., & Freemark, M. (2002). Insulin pump therapy in toddlers and preschool children with type 1 diabetes mellitus. *Journal of Pediatrics, 141,* 490–495.

Loscalzo, M. L., Bondy, C. A., & Biesecker, B. (2006). Issues in prenatal counseling and diagnosis in Turner Syndrome. *International Congress Series, 1298,* 26–29.

March of Dimes. (2006). *Quick reference: Recommended newborn screening tests: 29 disorders.* Retrieved February 28, 2009 from http://www.marchofdimes.com/printableArticles/14332_15455.asp

March of Dimes. (2008). *Newborn screening tests.* Retrieved February 28, 2009 from http://search.marchofdimes.com

Masharani, U. (2008). Diabetes mellitus and hypoglycemia. In S. J. McPhee, M. A. Papadakis, L. M. Tierney Jr., R. Gonzales, & R. Zeiger (Eds.), *Current medical diagnosis and treatment 2008.* Retrieved February 28, 2009 from McGraw-Hill's-Access Medicine, http://www.accessmedicine.com

Misra, M., & Lee, M. M. (2005). Delayed puberty. In T. M. Moshang (Ed.), *Pediatric endocrinology: The requisites for pediatrics* (pp. 87–101). St. Louis: Elsevier Mosby.

Molina, P. E. (2006). Parathyroid gland & Ca^{2+} & Po_4^- regulation. In *Endocrine Physiology* (2nd ed.). Retrieved February 28, 2009 from McGraw-Hill's Access Medicine, www.accessmedicine.com

Morgan, T. (2007). Turner Syndrome: Diagnosis and Management. *American Family Physician, 76*(3), 406–410.

National Newborn Screening and Genetics Resource Center. (2009). *National newborn screening status report.* Retrieved February 28, 2009 from http://genes-r-us.uthscsa.edu/nbsdisorders.pdf

Nimri, R., Weintrob, H. B., Ofan, R., Fayman, G., & Phillip, M. (2006). Insulin pump therapy in youth with type 1 diabetes: A retrospective paired study. *Pediatrics, 117*(6), 2126–2131.

Palma Sisto, P. A. (2004). Endocrine disorders in the neonate. *Pediatric Clinics of North America, 51*(4), 1141–1168.

Pang, S. (2003). Newborn screening for congenital adrenal hyperplasia. *Pediatric Annals, 32*(8), 516–523.

Parks, J. S., & Felner, E. I. (2007a). Hormones of the hypothalamus and pituitary. In R. M. Kliegman, R. E. Behrman, H. B. Jenson, & B. F. Stanton (Eds.), *Nelson textbook of pediatrics* (18th ed., pp. 2291–2293). Philadelphia: Saunders Elsevier.

Parks, J. S., & Felner, E. I. (2007b). Hypopituitarism. In R. M. Kliegman, R. E. Behrman, H. B. Jenson, & B. F. Stanton (Eds.), *Nelson textbook of pediatrics* (18th ed., pp. 2293–2299). Philadelphia: Saunders Elsevier.

Pinyerd, B., & Zipf, W. B. (2005). Puberty – Timing is everything. *Journal of Pediatric Nursing, 20*(2), 75–82.

Rachmiel, M., Perlman, K., & Daneman, D. (2005). Insulin analogues in children and teens with type 1 diabetes: Advantages and caveats. *Pediatric Clinics of North America, 52,* 1651–1675.

Raine, J. E., Donaldson, M. D. C., Gregory, J. W., Savage, M. O., & Hintz, R. L. (2006a). Salt and water balance. In J. E. Raine, M. D. C. Donaldson, J. W. Gregory, M. O. Savage, & R. L. Hintz (Eds.), *Practical endocrinology and diabetes in children* (2nd ed., pp. 147–155). Malden, MA: Blackwell.

Raine, J. E., Donaldson, M. D. C., Gregory, J. W., Savage, M. O., & Hintz, R. L. (2006b). Puberty. In J. E. Raine, M. D. C. Donaldson, J. W. Gregory, M. O. Savage, & R. L. Hintz (Eds.), *Practical endocrinology and diabetes in children* (2nd ed., pp. 69–90). Malden, MA: Blackwell.

Rezvani, I. (2007). Defects in metabolism of amino acids. In R. M. Kliegman, R. E. Behrman, H. B. Jenson, & B. F. Stanton (Eds.), *Nelson textbook of pediatrics* (18th ed., pp. 529–532). Philadelphia: Saunders Elsevier.

Rezvani, I., & Rosenblatt, D. S. (2007). Valine, leucine, isoleucine and related organic acidemias. In R. M. Kliegman, R. E. Behrman, H. B. Jenson, & B. F. Stanton (Eds.), *Nelson textbook of pediatrics* (18th ed., pp 540–549). Philadelphia: Saunders Elsevier.

Roberts, C .G. P., & Ladenson, P. W. (2004). Hypothyroidism. *Lancet, 363*(9411), 793–803.

Rose, S. R., Vogiatzi, M. G., & Copeland, K. C. (2005). A general pediatric approach to evaluating a short child. *Pediatrics in Review, 26*(11), 410–419.

Rossi, W. C., Caplin, N., & Alter, C. A. (2005). Thyroid disorders in children. In T. M. Moshang (Ed.), *Pediatric endocrinology: The requisites for pediatrics* (pp. 171–190). St. Louis: Elsevier Mosby.

Rouse, B., & Azen, C. (2004). Effect of high maternal blood phenylalanine on offspring congenital anomalies and developmental outcome at ages 4 and 6 years: The importance of strict dietary control preconception and throughout pregnancy. *Journal of Pediatrics, 144,* 235–239.

Sepa, A., Wahlberg, J., Vaarala, O., Frodi, A., & Ludvigsson, J. (2005). Psychological stress may induce diabetes-related autoimmunity in infancy. *Diabetes Care, 28*(2), 290–295.

Silverstein, J., Klingensmith, G., Copeland, K., Plotnick, L., Kaufman, F., Laffel, L., et al. (2005). Care of children and adolescents with type 1 diabetes. *Diabetes Care, 28*(1), 186–212.

Simon, E., Flaschker, N., Schadewaldt, P. , Langenbeck, U., Wendel, U. (2006). Variant maple syrup urine disease (MSUD)—The entire spectrum, *Journal of Inherited Metabolic Disease,* (2006) 29: 716–724.

Stanley, C. A., & Bennett, M. J. (2007). Disorders of mitochondrial fatty acid β-oxidation. In R. M. Kliegman, R. E. Behrman, H. B. Jenson, & B. F. Stanton (Eds.), *Nelson textbook of pediatrics* (18th ed., pp. 567–573). Philadelphia: Saunders Elsevier.

Steck, A. K., Klingensmith, G. J., & Fiallo-Scharer, R. (2007). Recent advances in insulin treatment of children. *Pediatric Diabetes, 8*(Suppl 6), 49–56.

Stewart, S. M., Rao, U., Emslie, G. J., Klein, D., & White, P. C. (2005). Depressive symptoms predict hospitalization for adolescents with type 1 diabetes mellitus. *Pediatrics, 115*(5), 1315–1319.

Thomas, J. A., & Van Hove, J. L. K. (2007). Inborn errors of metabolism. In W. W. Hay, M. J. Levin, J. M. Sondheimer, & R. R. Deterding (Eds.), *Current pediatric diagnosis and treatment* (18th ed.). Access Medicine: McGraw-Hill Companies.

Tyler, C., & Edman, J. C. (2004). Down syndrome, Turner syndrome, and Klinefelter syndrome: Primary care throughout the life span. *Primary Care Clinics for Office Practitioners, 31,* 627–648.

Vivian, E. M. (2006). Type 2 diabetes in children and adolescents—The next epidemic? *Current Medical Residents Opinion, 22*(2), 297–306.

Wattendorf, D. J., & Muenke, M. (2005). Klinefelter syndrome. *American Family Physician, 72,* 2259–2262.

Weinzimer, S. A., & Magge, S. (2005). Type 1 diabetes mellitus in children. In T. M. Moshange (Ed.), *Pediatric endocrinology: The requisites for pediatrics* (pp. 3–18). St. Louis: Elsevier Mosby.

Weinzimer, S. A., Sikes, K. A., Steffen, A. T., & Tamborlane, W. V. (2005). Insulin pump treatment of childhood type 1 diabetes. *Pediatric Clinics of North America,* 52, 1677–1688.

White, P. C. (2007). Disorders of the adrenal glands. In R. M. Kliegman, R. E. Behrman, H. B. Jenson, & B. F. Stanton (Eds.), *Nelson textbook of pediatrics* (18th ed., pp. 2349–2374). Philadelphia: Saunders Elsevier.

Wood, J. R., Moreland, E. C., Volkening, L. K., Svoren, B. M., Butler, D. A., & Laffel, L. M. B. (2006). Durability of insulin pump use in pediatric patients with type 1 diabetes. *Diabetes Care, 29*(11), 2355–2360.

Xu, W. (2005). Hypercalcemic Disorders. In T. M. Moshang (Ed.), *Pediatric endocrinology: The requisites for pediatrics* (pp. 227–239). St. Louis: Elsevier Mosby.

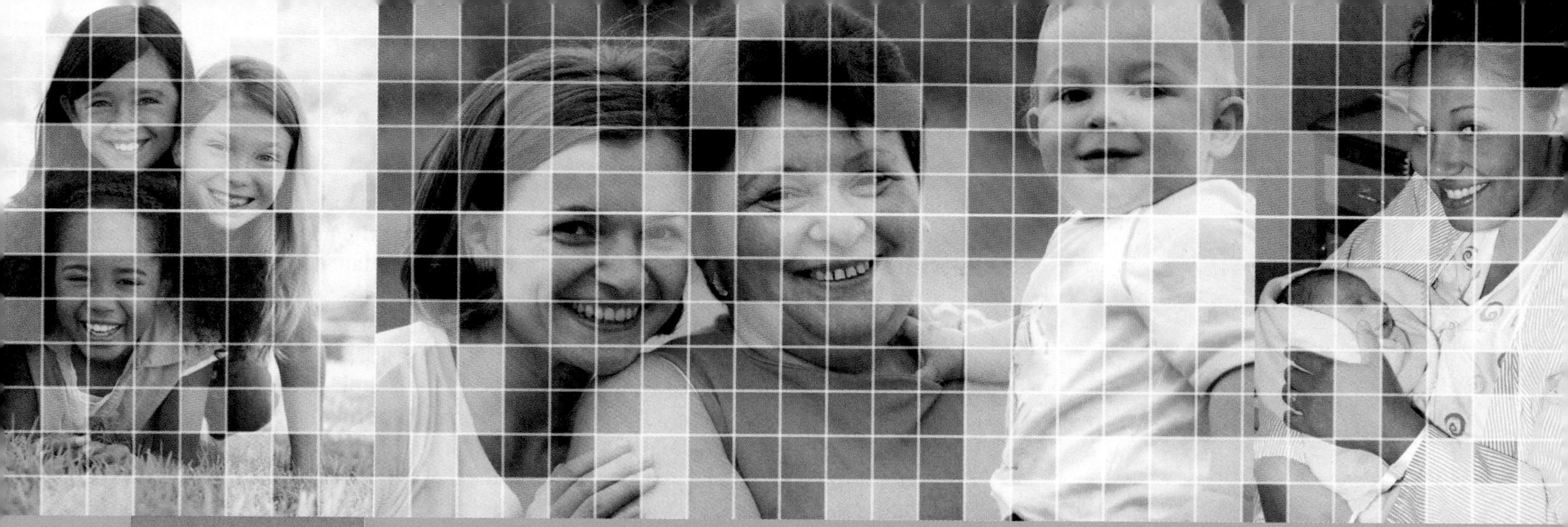

CHAPTER

56 The Child with Alterations in Neurologic Function

It's so hard to watch your child experience a brain injury and lie in a coma. All we can do is be here every day for Antwan. We keep talking to him and trying to get him to respond to us. We hope he will wake up soon. —*Mother of Antwan, 7 years old*

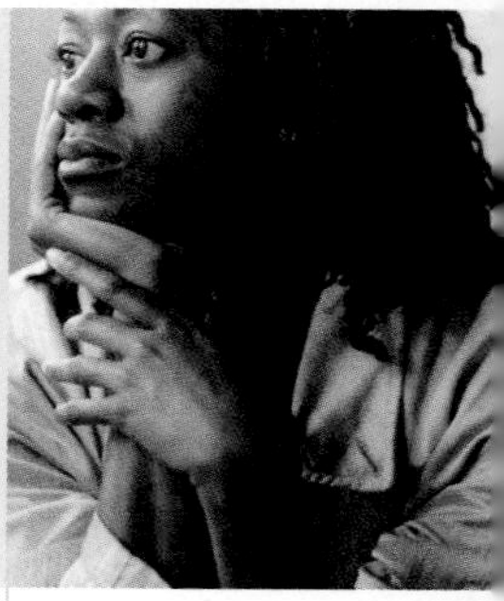

LEARNING OUTCOMES

56.1 Describe the anatomy and physiology of the neurologic system.

56.2 Describe the nursing assessment process and tools used for infants and children with altered levels of consciousness and other neurologic conditions.

56.3 Differentiate between the signs of infants and children with epilepsy and status epilepticus, and describe appropriate nursing management for each condition.

56.4 Differentiate between signs of bacterial meningitis, viral meningitis, encephalitis, and Guillain-Barré syndrome in infants and children.

56.5 Develop a nursing care plan for the infant with myelodysplasia and hydrocephalus.

56.6 Describe the focus of community-based nursing care for the child with cerebral palsy.

56.7 Distinguish among the assessment findings of the child with a mild, moderate, and severe traumatic brain injury.

56.8 Contrast the appropriate initial nursing management for mild and severe traumatic brain injury.

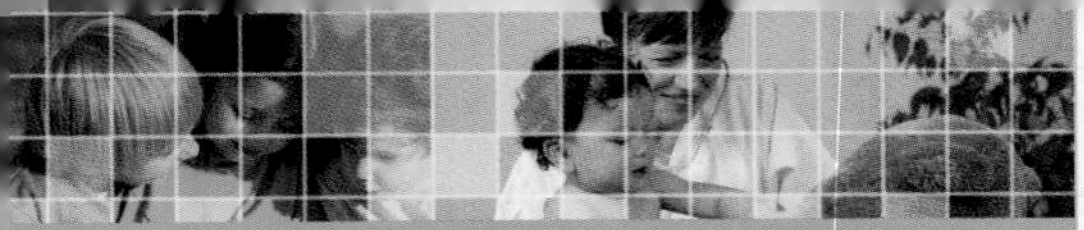

KEY TERMS

Areflexia, 1670
Assistive technology, 1687
Aura, 1656
Automatism, 1657
Autonomic dysreflexia, 1694
Cerebral edema, 1663
Cerebral perfusion pressure, 1651
Clonic, 1656
Coma, 1651
Cushing's triad, 1652
Encephalopathy, 1669
Focal, 1656
Herniation, 1652
Intracranial pressure, 1651
Intractable seizure, 1659
Level of consciousness, 1651
Microcephaly, 1671
Myelodysplasia, 1676
Neural tube defects, 1650
Nuchal rigidity, 1663
Opisthotonic position, 1663
Postictal period, 1656
Posturing, 1652
Status epilepticus, 1656
Tonic, 1656

ANATOMY AND PHYSIOLOGY OF PEDIATRIC DIFFERENCES

Knowledge of the anatomy of the nervous system makes neurologic symptoms easier to understand. The brain, spinal cord, and nerves are the major structures of the nervous system (Figure 56–1 ●). The brain controls, regulates, or coordinates many body functions, including cognition, behaviors, the senses, and motor skills. The spinal cord transmits impulses to and from the brain, conveying sensory information and relaying impulses that stimulate motor responses. Alterations in neurologic function can have widespread effects on the body's metabolism.

Central nervous system (CNS) defects account for approximately one-third of all apparent congenital malformations in live infants, and 90% of these are **neural tube defects**, anomalies of the embryonic neural tube that forms the brain and spine. CNS defects are responsible for 40% of infant deaths in the first year of life (Padgett, 2006).

At birth the nervous system is complete but immature. The infant is born with all the nerve cells he or she will have throughout life. Maturation of these nerve cells continues after birth until about 4 years of age as the number of glial cells (that build a structure around nerve cells) and dendrites (that carry nerve impulses from other nerve cells to the nerve cell body) continues to increase. Myelination, which increases the speed and accuracy of nerve impulses, is also incomplete at birth. The myelination process, which proceeds in a cephalocaudal direction, accounts for the progressive acquisition of fine and gross motor skills and coordination during early childhood.

The anatomic and physiologic differences between children and adults help explain why children and adults have different neurologic problems. See "As Children Grow: Anatomic Differences in the Structures of the Nervous System between Children and Adults."

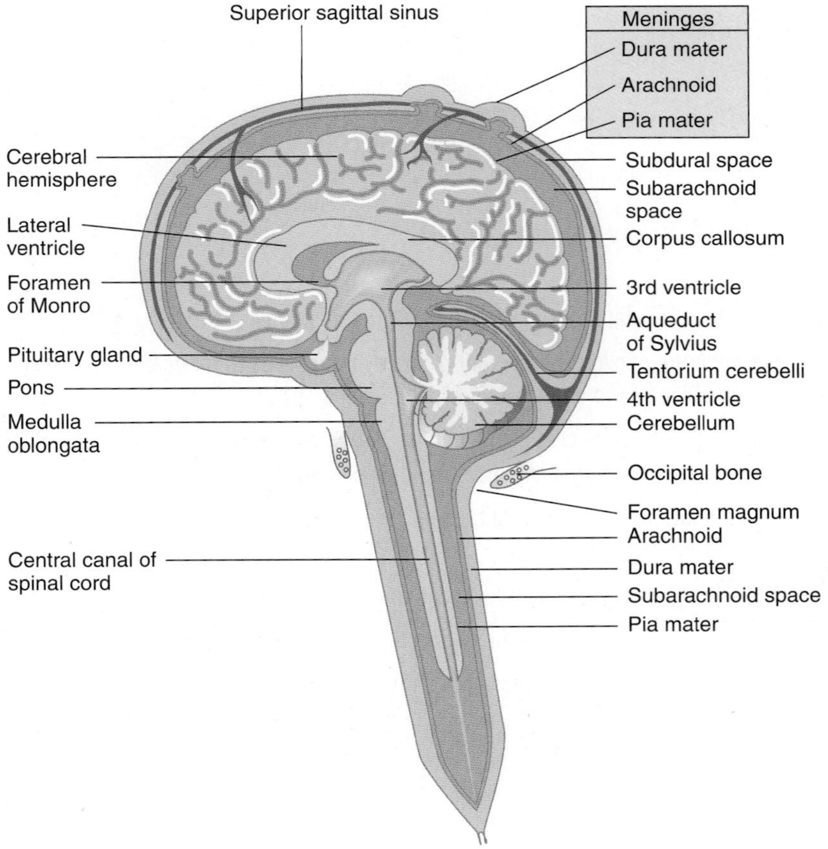

● **Figure 56–1** Transverse section of the brain and spinal cord. Knowledge of the anatomy of the brain is helpful in understanding the symptoms of neurologic dysfunction.

AS CHILDREN GROW

ANATOMIC DIFFERENCES BETWEEN CHILDREN'S AND ADULTS' NERVOUS SYSTEM STRUCTURES

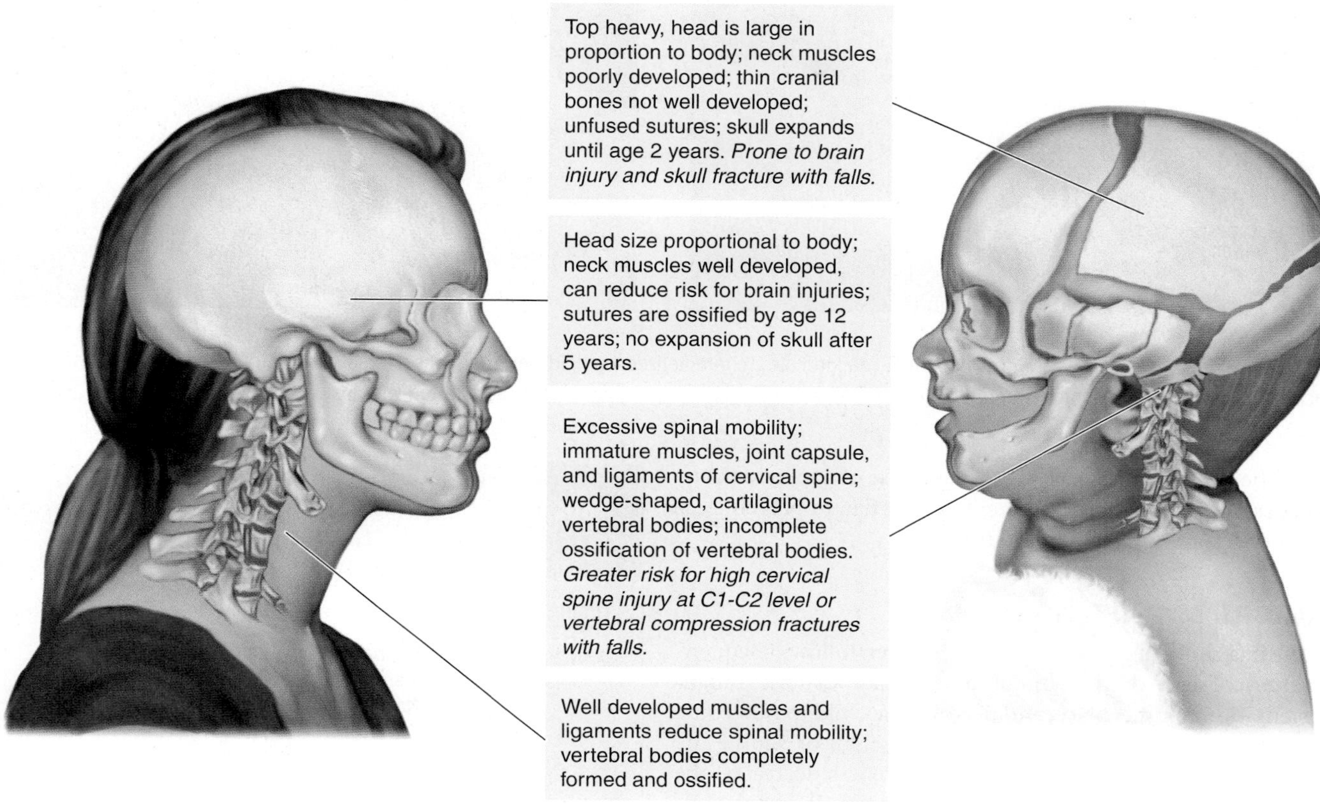

Top heavy, head is large in proportion to body; neck muscles poorly developed; thin cranial bones not well developed; unfused sutures; skull expands until age 2 years. *Prone to brain injury and skull fracture with falls.*
Head size proportional to body; neck muscles well developed, can reduce risk for brain injuries; sutures are ossified by age 12 years; no expansion of skull after 5 years.
Excessive spinal mobility; immature muscles, joint capsule, and ligaments of cervical spine; wedge-shaped, cartilaginous vertebral bodies; incomplete ossification of vertebral bodies. *Greater risk for high cervical spine injury at C1-C2 level or vertebral compression fractures with falls.*
Well developed muscles and ligaments reduce spinal mobility; vertebral bodies completely formed and ossified.

Skull and brain growth. The skull and brain grow and develop rapidly during early childhood. Infants and young children are at higher risk for injury to the brain and spinal cord because of developing anatomic structures.

ALTERED STATES OF CONSCIOUSNESS

Level of consciousness (LOC) is perhaps the most important indicator of neurologic dysfunction. *Consciousness,* the responsiveness of the mind to sensory stimuli, has two components: *alertness,* or the ability to react to stimuli, and *cognitive power,* or the ability to process the data and respond either verbally or physically. *Unconsciousness* is depressed cerebral function, or the inability of the brain to respond to stimuli. Altered levels of consciousness can be further categorized as:

- *Confusion:* disorientation to time, place, or person; loss of clear thinking. Answers to simple questions may be correct, but responses to complex ones may be inaccurate.
- *Delirium:* state characterized by disorientation, fear, irritability or agitation, and mental or motor excitement.
- *Lethargy:* profound slumber in which speech and movement are limited. The child is aroused with moderate stimulation, but falls asleep easily once stimulation is removed.
- *Stupor:* deep sleep or unresponsiveness; the child is aroused only with repeated vigorous stimulation, but returns to the unresponsive state when the stimulus is removed.
- **Coma***:* unconsciousness; cannot be aroused even by painful stimuli.

ETIOLOGY AND PATHOPHYSIOLOGY

Infection of the brain and meninges is the most common cause of an altered level of consciousness in children (Avner, 2006). Other causes include: trauma, hypoxia, poisoning, seizures, alcohol or substance abuse, endocrine or metabolic disturbances (e.g. diabetic ketoacidosis), electrolyte or acid-base imbalance, brain tumor, stroke, or a congenital structural defect. Any of these pathologic processes can cause increased **intracranial pressure** (force exerted by brain tissue, cerebrospinal fluid, and blood within the cranial vault). Decreased **cerebral perfusion pressure**, the amount of pressure needed to ensure that adequate oxygen and nutrients will be delivered to the brain, often results when the increased intracranial pressure (ICP) reduces arterial blood

MyNursingKit Animation: 3-D Brain and Brainstem

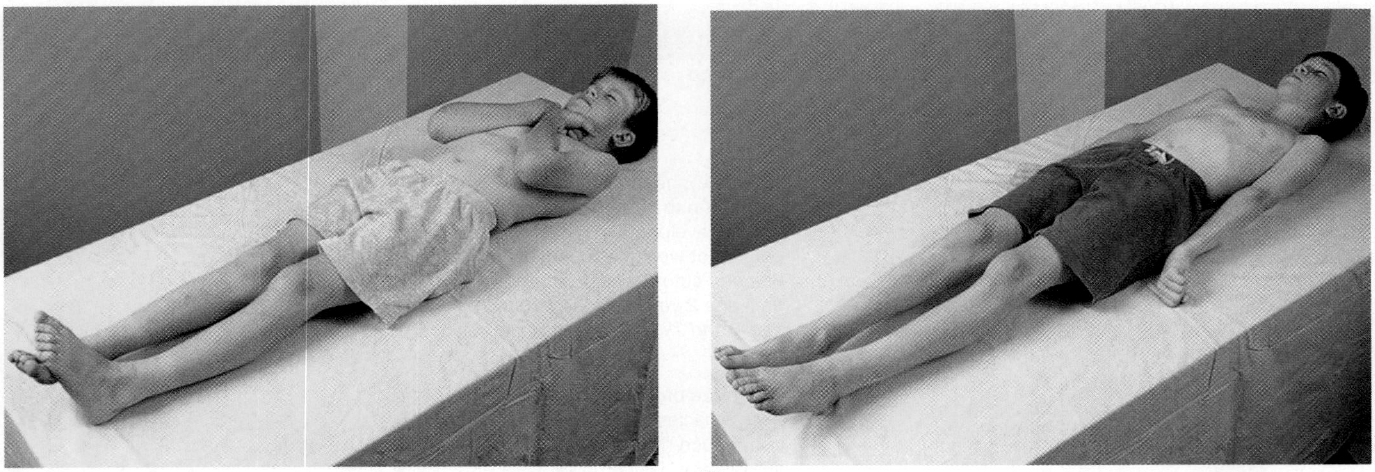

● **Figure 56–2** Posturing. ***A,*** Flexor posturing (decorticate), characterized by rigid flexion, is associated with lesions above the brainstem in the corticospinal tracts. ***B,*** Extensor posturing (decerebrate), distinguished by rigid extension, is associated with lesions of the brainstem.

flow to the brain. Rapid diagnosis of the cause of an altered consciousness and immediate treatment is essential, to prevent secondary effects of the illness or injury.

CLINICAL MANIFESTATIONS

Decline in a child's level of consciousness often follows a sequential pattern of deterioration. Initial changes may be subtle: a slight disorientation to time, place, and person. The child may become restless or fussy, and actions that normally calm or soothe the child only increase irritability. As responsiveness decreases, the child may become drowsy but still respond to loud verbal commands and withdraw from painful stimuli. Keeping the child awake is sometimes difficult. Then response to pain progresses from purposeful to nonpurposeful. The child may exhibit flexor or extensor **posturing**, the abnormal positions assumed after injury or damage to the brain (Figure 56–2 ●). Clinical manifestations of increased ICP are provided in Table 56–1.

Clinical Therapy

Clinical therapy focuses on early diagnosis of the cause of an altered consciousness and intervention to prevent further insult to the central nervous system. The Glasgow Coma Scale (GCS) is used to quantify the level of consciousness, and pediatric criteria for preverbal children are also available. See Table 56–2.

Laboratory tests include a complete blood cell count, blood chemistry, clotting factors, and blood culture; toxicology assessments of blood and urine; and urinalysis with culture. A lumbar puncture may be performed to assess the cerebrospinal fluid (CSF) for protein, glucose, blood cells, and pressure level. An electroencephalogram (EEG) identifies damaged or nonfunctioning areas of the brain. Computed tomography (CT) or magnetic resonance imaging (MRI) is used to detect any lesions, structural abnormalities, vascular malformations, or edema. Skull radiographic studies may detect fractures or bony malformations.

The child is treated with oxygen, and assisted ventilation is provided when gas exchange is inadequate. Any metabolic, acid-

Table 56–1 Signs of Increased Intracranial Pressure

Timing of Signs	Signs
Early signs	Headache Visual disturbances, diplopia Nausea and vomiting Dizziness or vertigo Slight change in vital signs Pupils not as reactive or equal Sunsetting eyes Slight change in level of consciousness, restlessness
Infant has above signs plus:	Irritability Bulging fontanelle Wide sutures, increased head circumference Dilated scalp veins High-pitched, catlike cry
Late signs	Significant decrease in level of consciousness Seizures **Cushing's triad** ■ Increased systolic blood pressure and widened pulse pressure ■ Bradycardia ■ Irregular respirations Fixed and dilated pupils, papilledema

Nursing Practice

The lumbar puncture should be postponed if any signs of increased ICP (e.g., papilledema) are present, which could place the child at risk for brain **herniation** (protrusion of brain contents into the brainstem area).

Table 56–2 Glasgow Coma Scale for Assessment of Coma in Infants and Children

Category	Score*	Preverbal Child Criteria	Older Child and Adult Criteria
Eye opening	4	Spontaneous opening	Spontaneous
	3	To loud noise	To verbal stimuli
	2	To pain	To pain
	1	No response	No response
Verbal response	5	Smiles, coos, cries to appropriate stimuli	Oriented to time, place, and person; uses appropriate words and phrases
	4	Irritable; cries	Confused
	3	Cries to pain	Inappropriate words or verbal response
	2	Moans to pain	Incomprehensible words
	1	No response	No response
Motor response	6	Spontaneous movement	Obeys commands
	5	Purposeful, localizes pain	Localizes pain
	4	Withdraws to pain	Withdraws to pain
	3	Flexor posturing	Flexor posturing
	2	Extensor posturing	Extensor posturing
	1	No response; flaccid	No response; flaccid

From Jankowitz, B. T., & Adelson, P. D. (2006). Pediatric traumatic brain injury: Past, present, and future. *Developmental Neuroscience, 28,* 264–275.

*Add the score from each category to get the total. The maximum score is 15, indicating the best level of neurologic functioning. The minimum is 3, indicating total neurologic unresponsiveness.

base, or electrolyte imbalances are corrected. Antibiotics are initiated for suspected infection.

Maintenance of the cerebral perfusion pressure is important so that adequate oxygen and nutrients are supplied to the brain. Intravenous fluids are given if the child is hypovolemic. When poor perfusion and fluid overload exist, dopamine is administered to increase cardiac output and perfusion of the brain. If the ICP is markedly increased and due to obstruction of CSF, a ventricular catheter may be inserted to drain CSF to decrease the ICP, temporarily, relieving a life-threatening condition. See page 1690 for care specific to increased ICP and traumatic brain injury.

NURSING MANAGEMENT

NURSING ASSESSMENT AND DIAGNOSIS

General guidelines for assessing the child with a neurologic condition are provided in Table 56–3.

When consciousness is altered, initially assess the child's physiologic status, focusing on the child's responsiveness to the environment or stimuli, ability to maintain the airway, vital signs, and breathing patterns. When a cough or gag reflex is present the child can protect the airway from aspiration. Assess the vital signs, respiratory effort, and color. Monitor pulse oximetry and arterial blood gas measurements. Adequate air exchange to keep oxygen and carbon dioxide levels within normal ranges and maintenance of acid-base balance are critical to reduce the risk of hypoxemia and increased ICP.

A baseline neurologic assessment should be performed, including pupils, eye movements, and motor function (see Figure 56–3 ●). Assess the cranial nerves; however, be aware that assessment and interpretation may be more challenging in the unconscious child (Table 56–4). Observe for other physiologic signs of increased ICP (Table 56–1). See Table 56–5 for a method to rapidly assess an infant's responsiveness, referred to by the acronym AVPU.

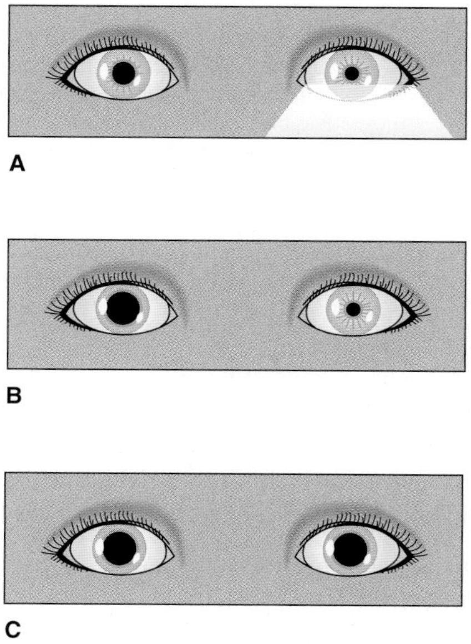

● **Figure 56–3** Pupil findings in various neurologic conditions with altered consciousness. ***A,*** A unilateral dilated and reactive pupil is associated with an intracranial mass. ***B,*** A fixed and dilated pupil may be a sign of impending brainstem herniation. ***C,*** Bilateral fixed and dilated pupils are associated with brainstem herniation from increased intracranial pressure.

Table 56–3 Guidelines for Assessment of a Child with a Neurologic Condition

Assessment Focus	Assessment Guidelines
Level of Consciousness	■ Is the infant or child lethargic or hard to arouse? ■ Is the infant or child irritable or difficult to console? ■ Use the Glasgow Coma Scale when a numerical score is important for future comparison. See Table 56–3.
Cognitive Function	■ Are the child's verbal skills appropriate for age? ■ Does the child follow directions appropriately?
Cranial Nerves	■ Assess the cranial nerves. See Table 35–17. See also Table 56–4 for methods to assess cranial nerves in the unconscious child.
Fontanelles and Sutures	■ Palpate the fontanelles and suture lines of the infant.
Pupils	■ Check the pupils for size, reaction to light, and accommodation.
Vital Signs	■ Assess the heart rate, respiratory rate, and blood pressure. ■ Monitor for late signs of increased ICP (increased systolic blood pressure, a widened pulse pressure, bradycardia, and irregular respirations).
Posture and Movement	■ Assess the infant's primitive reflexes to evaluate posture and movement. See Chapter 25∞. ■ Assess the child's strength, symmetry, coordination, and smoothness of movements during play and examination activities. Are muscle tone and strength equal bilaterally? Is any weakness present? ■ Are the child's motor skills developmentally appropriate and acquired at the appropriate age? Has the child lost a previously acquired skill? ■ Assess deep tendon reflexes. See Table 35–18.
Neck Stiffness	■ Assess for neck stiffness (nuchal rigidity). See Figure 56–6.
Pain	■ Assess level of pain when present.

A cry with a loud, energetic quality, a strong suck and suck-swallowing coordination, and appropriate primitive reflex responses for age are other signs of an infant's intact mental status.

Among the nursing diagnoses that might be appropriate for the child with an altered level of consciousness are the following:

- *Ineffective Breathing Pattern* related to neuromuscular dysfunction associated with increased intracranial pressure
- *Risk for Aspiration* related to poor control of secretions with decreased level of consciousness
- *Risk for Impaired Skin Integrity* related to agitation and skin rubbing against bedding
- *Interrupted Family Processes* related to care of a child with an acquired disability

Table 56–4 Assessment of Cranial Nerves in the Unconscious Child

Cranial Nerves	Reflex	Assessment Procedure and Normal Findings[a]
II, III	Pupillary	Shine a light source in eye. *Rapid, concentrically constricting pupils indicate intact cranial nerves, II, III.*
II, IV, VI	Oculocephalic	Perform with eyes held open (doll's eyes) and head turned from side to side. *Eyes gazing straight up or lagging slightly behind head motion indicate intact cranial nerves. Precaution:* Cervical spine injury must be ruled out before this assessment is performed.
III, VIII	Oculovestibular	Place the head in a midline and slightly elevated position. Inject ice water into ear canal. *Eyes deviating toward the irrigated ear indicate intact cranial nerves III, VIII. Precautions:* Ensure that the cervical spine is not injured and that the tympanic membranes are intact before this assessment is performed by a physician.
V, VII	Corneal	Cornea is gently swabbed with sterile cotton swab. *A blink indicates intact cranial nerves V, VII.*
IX, X	Gag	Pharynx is irritated with tongue depressor or cotton swab. *Gagging response indicates intact cranial nerves IX, X.*

[a]Italic indicates normal findings.

Table 56–5 AVPU—Infant Responsiveness Assessment*

Criterion	Description
Alert	Responsive to parents, cuddles, coos or babbles, smiles
Verbal	Responsive to verbal stimulation
Pain	Responsive to painful stimulation only
Unresponsive	No response to painful stimulation

Note: *AVPU is the acronym formed from each criterion.

PLANNING AND IMPLEMENTATION

HOSPITAL-BASED NURSING CARE

Nursing care of the child with altered consciousness or increased ICP focuses on maintaining airway patency, monitoring neurologic status, performing routine care, providing sensory stimulation, and providing emotional support to parents. Nursing care for the child with increased ICP is described on page 1691.

Make sure the child's airway is patent at all times. If the child has difficulty managing secretions or has no gag reflex, intubation or a tracheostomy is performed. Frequent suctioning may be required (see Skills 14–23 and 14-24 SKILLS). Keep suction apparatus with catheters, oxygen, resuscitation bag and mask, and extra tracheostomy tubes (if applicable) at the bedside. Pulse oximetry or arterial blood gas measurement is performed at regular intervals to ensure that gas exchange is adequate. Assisted ventilation may be required (see Skill 14–13 SKILLS).

Anticipate that seizures may occur. Raise and pad the side rails to protect the child from injury.

Perform routine nursing care. If the corneal reflex is absent, place an approved ophthalmologic ointment or artificial tears in the eyes and keep them closed with gauze and tape. Perform routine mouth care by brushing the teeth and using swabs with water.

Provide adequate nutrition. A nasogastric or gastrostomy tube may be inserted if the child remains unconscious or is not alert enough to take food by mouth (see Skill 15–2 SKILLS).

Prevent complications associated with immobility (muscle atrophy, contractures, and skin breakdown) as described in Nursing Practice. Support physical therapy efforts with extra passive range of motion exercises.

Provide sensory stimulation. Because the child with a severely altered level of consciousness may still be able to hear, talk to him or her. Listening to music or tapes of family members talking or reading can soothe the child when family members cannot be present. Encourage parents to stroke and touch the child in a soothing manner.

As the child becomes more alert, repeatedly orient the child to time, place, and person, depending on his or her age and level of understanding. Encourage parents to bring objects or toys from home to make the environment more familiar and promote a feeling of security.

Provide emotional support to the child and family. Explain the child's condition in simple terms. Encourage parents to take part in the child's care and therapy as much as possible. Give family members the opportunity to express their feelings. If the child's functioning has been permanently impaired, refer the family to the appropriate psychologic and social services. (See Chapter 43 for information about supporting families during a child's life-threatening illness.)

Nursing Practice

When caring for a child who is immobile:

- Use splints or rolls made of towels or blankets to keep the body in proper alignment.
- Perform passive or gentle range of motion exercises three or four times per day according to physician's orders.
- Maintain skin integrity.
- Change position every 2 hours.
- Place child on a special mattress designed to relieve pressure points (foam or egg-crate mattress or sheepskin covering when a special mattress is not available).
- Massage child gently using lotion.
- Place transparent dressing over skin surfaces exposed to rubbing or friction.
- Sequential compression devices may be used in some cases to prevent deep vein thrombosis.

DISCHARGE PLANNING AND HOME CARE TEACHING

The child's transition from the hospital to home, a long-term care facility, or inpatient rehabilitation center must be planned well in advance of discharge. A case manager or social worker should be identified who can help plan the child's long-term care needs, including home health nursing, adaptation of the home, and the purchase of special equipment.

NURSING CARE IN THE COMMUNITY

Home care nurses play a vital role in the care of the child with an acquired neurologic dysfunction and prolonged altered consciousness. Teach the family how to care for the child with severe neurologic dysfunction and to perform routine procedures such as maintaining the airway, skin care, feeding, positioning, exercises, and stimulation. Regular follow-up visits are needed to assess the child's progress and to modify the treatment plan.

The child should be linked with community rehabilitation services through an early intervention program or school-based program. The home health nurse or case manager should help the family have an individual education plan (IEP) developed for the child (see Chapter 40).

EVALUATION

Expected outcomes of nursing care include the following:

- The child's airway is maintained and the brain is adequately oxygenated.
- Complications of immobility are prevented.
- The family provides appropriate care to the child with prolonged altered consciousness to promote minimal long-term disabilities.

SEIZURE DISORDERS

Seizures are periods of abnormal electrical discharges in the brain that cause involuntary movement, and behavior and sensory alterations. One in 20 children will have a seizure (with or without fever) by age 18 years, but most children who have one seizure will never experience a second (Fisher, 2007).

Epilepsy is a chronic disorder characterized by recurrent, unprovoked seizures, secondary to an underlying brain abnormality.

MyNursingKit Video: Seizure Disorders

Developing Cultural Competence

SEIZURES

Seizures may have a special meaning to different cultural groups. For example, the Hmong believe the child is experiencing quag dab peg, or "the spirit catches you and you fall down." Traditional Hmong view the condition as serious, but take pride in the child who has the condition, as they have a link to the spirit world. In 1997, Anne Fadiman wrote a compelling story about the cultural conflict between a Hmong family and healthcare providers over the treatment of their daughter's seizures, *The Spirit Catches You and You Fall Down* (Spector, 2009).

Approximately 45,000 children under age 15 years develop epilepsy each year (Epilepsy Foundation, 2009). Approximately 30% of epilepsy cases occur by age 4 years (Padgett, 2006). See "Developing Cultural Competence: Seizures."

ETIOLOGY AND PATHOPHYSIOLOGY

When an excessive number of neurons in the brain become overexcited, they discharge abnormally, leading to seizures. Seizures may result from a CNS disorder or structural defect, or from a disorder that affects CNS functioning, such as brain injury, infection, electrolyte disturbance, toxins, and brain tumor. Genetic factors may predispose the child for seizures. Some seizures have no known cause. See "Clinical Manifestations: Seizures" for the etiology of various types of seizures.

Partial, or **focal**, seizures are caused by abnormal electrical activity in one brain hemisphere or a specific area of the cerebral cortex, most often the temporal, frontal, or parietal lobes. The symptoms depend on the region of the cortex affected.

Generalized seizures are the result of diffuse electrical activity that begins in both brain hemispheres simultaneously, spreading throughout the cortex into the brainstem. The child's movements and spasms are bilateral and symmetric.

Febrile seizures occur in susceptible infants and children in connection with a fever (39°C or 102°F or higher) and associated acute illness. No evidence of intracranial infection or other defined cause is present. It is believed that the sensitivity of the young child's developing brain to fever is the mechanism for the seizure. Febrile seizures commonly occur between 6 months and 5 years, with a peak incidence between 18 and 24 months of age (Blumstein & Friedman, 2007). The higher the fever, the greater the risk for a febrile seizure, especially in a child with a positive family history. Children who have one febrile seizure have a 30% to 40% greater chance of having future febrile seizures (Leung & Robson, 2007).

Status epilepticus is a condition in which a continuous seizure or recurrent seizures occur, lasting more than 20 minutes without return to baseline neurologic condition. This condition occurs in approximately 10% of children after a diagnosis of epilepsy (Goldstein, 2008). The length of a seizure, especially a generalized seizure, is important because the airway may be compromised during the tonic phase. The basal metabolic rate rises during the peak of seizure activity, increasing the demand for oxygen and glucose.

CLINICAL MANIFESTATIONS

The symptoms of a seizure depend on the type and duration of the seizure. The characteristics of the various types of partial and generalized seizures are presented in "Clinical Manifestations: Seizures."

Partial seizures often start with an **aura** (a visual, auditory, taste, or motor sensation that gives warning of an impending seizure or migraine headache) or an abrupt, unprovoked alteration in behavior. Once the pattern of an aura is recognized, the child may have time to avoid injury by getting to the floor.

Generalized tonic-clonic seizures are the most common seizure type in children (Blumstein & Friedman, 2007). The **tonic** phase is characterized by unconsciousness and continuous muscular contraction. The **clonic** phase is characterized by alternating muscular contraction and relaxation. During the **postictal period** following seizure activity, the level of consciousness is decreased. The length of the postictal period varies among children. Some children have an olfactory or visual aura. Children may have a partial seizure that progresses to a generalized seizure. During a status epilepticus the child may become pale or cyanotic as a result of hypoxia or hypoglycemia. The only evidence of seizures in neonates may be lip smacking, eye deviations, or apneic episodes (Blumstein & Friedman, 2007).

Febrile seizures involve generalized tonic-clonic movements with the eyes rolling back, generally lasting 1 to 2 minutes. A brief postictal period follows.

CLINICAL THERAPY

After the child's first seizure, a thorough history is taken from the parent, primary caretaker, or witnesses to the event. Details include the description and length of the seizure, presence or absence of an aura, and whether the child lost consciousness. This information helps to identify the type of seizure according to the International Classification of Epileptic Seizures.

Based on the physical findings and history, diagnostic tests ordered may include a complete blood cell count, blood chemistry, urine toxicology, urine culture, and lumbar puncture. A lead level and tests for inborn errors of metabolism may be considered. Radiologic tests such as CT scanning or MRI and angiography may be performed to identify a cerebral lesion or metabolic disorder in the brain. An EEG is often performed at a follow-up visit between seizures. If the child is taking any anticonvulsants, a serum drug level is checked.

Many seizures are self-limiting and require no emergency intervention. When the seizure is prolonged, emergency therapy includes airway management, supplemental oxygen, intravenous benzodiazepines, and careful monitoring of vital signs. Serum electrolytes, glucose, and blood gases may be monitored. Monitor for continued motor activity, which may be less intense after benzodiazepines are given. The postictal period ranges from 30 minutes to 2 hours. When the child's seizure does not stop as

Clinical Manifestations

SEIZURES

TYPE OF SEIZURE AND CAUSE	CLINICAL MANIFESTATIONS
PARTIAL SEIZURES	
***Simple partial seizures* (focal seizures)** Focal damage (e.g., with cerebral palsy) Tumors or lesions Arteriovenous malformation Brain abscesses	*Onset:* any age No loss of consciousness; lasts less than 30 seconds; no postseizure confusion No aura Motor responses may involve one extremity, part of extremity, or ipsilateral extremities with eyes and head turning in opposite direction Sensory responses involve paresthesias (decreased sensation or tingling); auditory, olfactory, or visual sensations; autonomic (e.g., sweating) or psychic symptoms Motor and sensory involvement may be combined and progress to generalized seizure Jacksonian march (rare in children): tonic-clonic movements start in the fingers of one hand, toes of one foot, or one side of face and spread to adjacent muscles of the affected extremity or same side of body
***Complex partial seizures* (psychomotor seizures)** Lesions, cysts, or tumors Perinatal trauma Focal sclerosis, e.g., scarring of the mediotemporal lobe from prolonged febrile seizures Vascular anomalies, e.g., arteriovenous malformations Brain trauma	*Onset:* 3 years of age to adolescence Consciousness is impaired immediately; followed by **automatisms** (unusual body movements without purpose, e.g., lip smacking, lip chewing, sucking); may have abnormal motor activity, twitching, loss of tone, tingling or numbness; may progress to involve entire brain leading to a generalized seizure Aura frequently present Abdominal pain Posturing Lasts 30 seconds up to 5 minutes, postseizure amnesia or confusion Feelings of anxiety, fear or déjà vu (sensation that event occurred before)
GENERALIZED SEIZURES	
***Tonic-clonic seizures* (grand mal seizures)** Cerebral damage from perinatal trauma, brain trauma, tumors, structural lesions, metabolic and neuromuscular degenerative disorders Genetic link Many are idiopathic	*Onset:* any age, rare before 6 months of age, strong familial incidence Abrupt onset seizure, 1–2 minute loss of consciousness, postseizure confusion (few minutes to hours) May or may not have aura Body becomes stiff and rigid (tonic phase), followed by rhythmic jerking motions (clonic phase) Drooling as secretions are not swallowed Pupils dilated; eyes roll upward or deviate to one side Abdominal or chest wall rigidity with leg, head, and neck extended, and arms flexed or contracted Cry or grunt as air is forced out when diaphragm and chest muscles contract Urinary or bowel incontinence as muscles become flaccid during clonic phase Sleepiness, difficulty in arousal; hypertension; diaphoresis; headache, nausea, vomiting; poor coordination, decreased muscle tone; confusion, amnesia; slurred speech; visual disturbances; combativeness
***Absence seizures* (petit mal, or lapse seizures)** Hyperventilation Genetic predisposition	*Onset:* age 3–12 years with remission in adolescence More prevalent in females May develop other generalized seizures Hyperventilation or flashing lights may trigger a seizure No aura; brief loss of consciousness, usually lasts 5–10 seconds, rarely exceeds 30 seconds, no postseizure confusion, lethargy, or sleepiness Frequent attacks (50–100 or more per day), may cluster, interfere with learning Child may continue simple movements such as walking or looking, but ceases activities such as reading; slight decrease or loss of muscle tone (head may droop, may drop objects) Cannot be interrupted by verbal or touch stimulation Amnesia

(continued)

Clinical Manifestations—continued

SEIZURES

TYPE OF SEIZURE AND CAUSE	CLINICAL MANIFESTATIONS
Juvenile Myoclonic Epilepsy Genetic disorder with locus on chromosome 6p and 15q14 (Padgett, 2006)	*Onset:* more prevalent in adolescents No loss of consciousness, child recovers in seconds, no postictal period Most often occur upon falling asleep or awakening Quick involuntary muscle jerks of the neck, shoulders, and arms Child usually has normal intelligence
***Infantile spasms* (myoclonic epilepsy of infancy, salaam seizures)** Tuberous sclerosis (genetic syndrome) Hypoxic-ischemic injury Inborn errors of metabolism CNS malformations	*Onset:* begin at age 4 and 8 months; resolve by 2 years May occur with altered consciousness as part of a complex partial seizure Occur in clusters, 5 to 150 per day Episodes of abrupt flexion and extension of muscle groups in the neck, trunk, and extremities, involving head nods or total body contractions (jackknife seizures); occur as infant awakens or falls asleep Eye rolling, either upward or downward Crying, pallor, or cyanosis Developmental delays Seizure activity increases in intensity and severity over time; may develop other types of epilepsy
***Lennox-Gastaut syndrome* (Akinetic or atonic seizure)** Gray matter degenerative diseases and subacute seizures Sclerosing panencephalitis Many are idiopathic	*Onset:* first seen between 1 and 5 years, predominantly in males Various types of generalized seizures, but mostly tonic-clonic, absence, and myoclonic activity; drop attack (falls to ground with sudden loss of postural tone, inability to break fall, is limp for period of time) Associated mental retardation, delayed psychomotor development, and personality disorders

expected with emergency intervention, treatment for status epilepticus is initiated (Table 56–6).

Children with febrile seizures are often not treated with an anticonvulsant at the time of the seizure because the seizure is often over before arrival at the emergency department. Acetaminophen is given to lower the temperature. Long-term antiepileptic medications are not recommended for simple febrile seizures because of their adverse effects (Leung & Robson, 2007).

Most seizure disorders are treated with antiepileptics. A single medication (monotherapy) is preferred for seizure control to minimize the side effects such as sleepiness, decreased attention and memory, behavior problems and changes in

Table 56–6 Management of Status Epilepticus and Nursing Management

Type of Care	Clinical Therapy and Nursing Management
Emergency assessment and management	■ Maintain a patent airway. Muscle rigidity may compromise the airway. Keep suction equipment at the bedside in case secretions are excessive. ■ Give supplemental oxygen as increased metabolic demands deplete oxygen stores. ■ Monitor vital signs and circulation with pulse oximeter and cardiorespiratory monitor. ■ Perform neurologic assessments every 5 to 10 minutes.
Ongoing urgent management	■ Establish an intravenous line to administer fluids or medications. ■ Assess blood glucose level; administer glucose if the child is hypoglycemic; the physical stress of the seizure may result in declining glucose levels. ■ Insert a nasogastric tube to reduce the risk for aspiration due to vomiting. ■ Protect the child from injury. ■ Manage thermoregulation.
Medications	■ Administer benzodiazepines such as diazepam, lorazepam, or midazolam. If there is no response, the dose may be repeated. Phenytoin or phenobarbital may be necessary if seizure activity continues. Cumulative doses of drugs may produce apnea, so be prepared to assist ventilations.

Nursing Practice

Children treated with antiepileptic medications should have a multivitamin with calcium to help prevent osteoporosis, and females of childbearing age taking valproate should receive folic acid supplementation (Weinstein & Gaillard, 2007). When children are treated with multiple antiepileptic medications, regular blood testing is performed to identify any developing hematologic or liver problems, and to determine if drug therapeutic ranges are maintained.

Table 56–7 Questions to Ask about Seizures

Time Period	Questions to Ask
Just before the seizure	■ What was the child doing? ■ Did the child complain of not feeling well (headache, nausea, vomiting, muscle pain, fever) or feeling "funny"? ■ Did the child suffer any trauma? Did the child get into any medications or poisons?
During the seizure	■ What movements of the arms and legs were seen? ■ On one or both sides of the body or in one extremity only? ■ Did the child exhibit any chewing or other type of automatic behavior?
	■ Were the pupils dilated or the eyes deviated to one side? ■ Did the child's color change (pale, red, blue)? ■ Was the child incontinent of urine or stool?
	■ Was the child aware of surroundings or able to respond to questions?
After the seizure	■ How long did the episode last? ■ Was the child lethargic, weak, or uncoordinated when waking up? ■ Did the child have loss of memory or confusion?

cognition. Monotherapy works for about 60% of children with new-onset epilepsy (Wolf & McGoldrick, 2006). An alternate antiepileptic may be tried if seizure control is not achieved with the first medication or when unacceptable side effects occur. Some children have refractory or **intractable seizures**, requiring multiple medications. See the Drug Guide for medications used to treat seizures. Medication dosage adjustments are often needed as the child grows.

Surgery may be performed to remove a tumor, lesion, or portion of the brain that has been identified as causing the seizures, particularly when seizures are not responsive to medication. A vagal nerve stimulator is another option for children who are unable to tolerate multiple medications and are not candidates for surgery (Saneto, Sotero de Menezes, Ojemann, et al., 2006).

A ketogenic diet (high-fat, adequate protein for growth, and very low carbohydrate) is occasionally used for children with intractable seizures. This diet is customized to help the child maintain an ideal body weight, maximize ketosis, and achieve optimal seizure control. The ketosis caused by the diet is believed to produce anticonvulsant effects, but the mechanism of action is unclear (Freeman, Kossoff, & Hartman, 2007). Family motivation must be high to maintain the rigid diet for 1 or more years because improved seizure control is directly related to diet compliance. Diet side effects include dyslipidemia, constipation, kidney stones, and slowed growth. Constipation is treated with medium chain triglycerides (MCT) oil and increased fluids. Kidney stones are treated by increasing fluids and alkalinizing the urine. About 10% to 15% of children who initiate the ketogenic diet are seizure-free after 1 year and 30% have greater than a 90% reduction in seizures, even after discontinuing the diet. Many families discontinue the diet because it is too difficult or not seen as effective (Freeman et al., 2007).

A trial of medication withdrawal is often attempted for children who have been seizure-free for at least 2 to 5 years. Approximately 70% of children remain seizure-free without medications (Wolf & McGoldrick, 2006).

NURSING MANAGEMENT

NURSING ASSESSMENT AND DIAGNOSIS

Assess and monitor the child's physiologic status. Observe the specific seizure activity, level of consciousness, vital signs, and signs of hypoxia. During the postictal period, monitor the child's vital signs, perform neurologic checks, and keep the environment safe. Once the child is stable, a more definitive assessment can be made. Level of consciousness is one of the most important indicators of neurologic function. Remember that the child's lack of response may be the result of the postictal state.

Collect and analyze historical information about the seizure activity. See Table 56–7.

Assess the family's adaptation to the seizure disorder, including how well the family is coping with the uncertainty of when the next seizure will occur.

Common nursing diagnoses for the child with a seizure disorder include the following:

- *Ineffective Breathing Pattern* related to neuromuscular dysfunction during the tonic phase of a seizure
- *Ineffective Airway Clearance* related to inability to control secretions during seizure
- *Risk for Trauma* related to seizure activity
- *Chronic Low Self-Esteem* related to refractory seizures and loss of bowel and bladder control during seizure activity
- *Anxiety* related to unpredictable nature of seizure disorder
- *Ineffective Therapeutic Regimen Management* related to poor adherence with medications

Drug Guide

MEDICATIONS USED TO TREAT SEIZURES

MEDICATION AND ACTION	NURSING MANAGEMENT
Benzodiazepines (Diazepam, Lorazepam) CNS depressant; anticonvulsant properties	■ Administer IV push medication very slowly into the IV entry site closest to the child's body. ■ Monitor for hypotension, tachycardia, and respiratory depression.
Phenobarbital Limits spread of seizure activity by increasing threshold for motor cortex stimuli	■ Administer IV push medication very slowly into the IV entry site closest to the child's body. ■ Monitor child's vital signs frequently when given IV. ■ May crush tablets and mix with food or fluid.
Phenytoin (Dilantin) Reduces voltage, frequency, and spread of electrical discharges within motor cortex to inhibit seizure activity	■ Educate family to provide an adequate intake of vitamin D, folic acid, and calcium. ■ Promote frequent dental care for gingival hyperplasia.
Carbamazepine (Tegretol) Action similar to phenytoin	■ Give with food to enhance absorption. ■ Do not administer suspension simultaneously with another liquid medication to prevent formation of a precipitate. ■ Causes photosensitivity reactions.
Valproic acid (Depacon, Depakote) Anticonvulsant, unknown mechanism of action	■ Do not use carbonated beverage to dilute syrup. Tablets and capsules should not be chewed. Give with food to decrease GI irritation. ■ Do not use drug in combination with aspirin, sedatives, and allergy medications. ■ Monitor platelet count and bleeding times.
Ethosuximide (Zarontin) Depresses motor cortex and increases CNS threshold to stimuli	■ Monitor for weight loss or anorexia. ■ Give with food if gastrointestinal upset occurs.
Felbamate (Felbatol) Blocks repetitive firing of neurons and increases seizure threshold	■ Monitor weight for gain or loss. ■ Monitor regularly for hematologic and liver problems.
Gabapentin (Neurontin) Gamma-aminobutyric acid (GABA) neurotransmitter analog	■ Monitor vision, concentration, and coordination as medication may cause impairments. ■ Do not take medication within 2 hours of an antacid.
Lamotrigine (Lamictal) Inhibits release of glutamate (neurotransmitter) in brain tissue	■ Educate family about photosensitivity side effect. ■ Monitor for adverse effects if used with valproic acid.
Tiagabine (Gabitril filmtabs) GABA inhibitor	■ Give with food. Avoid using with over-the-counter medications that cause drowsiness. ■ Monitor for signs of central nervous system depression.
Topiramate (Topamax) GABA inhibitor	■ Monitor for metabolic acidosis. ■ Increase fluid intake to reduce risk of kidney stones. ■ Monitor for adverse effect of psychomotor, speech, and language slowing.
Levetircacetam (Keppra) Anticonvulsant, unknown mechanism of action	■ Do not engage in hazardous activities such as driving any motorized vehicle (e.g., ATV or car) until effect of drug is known. ■ Do not abruptly discontinue the medication.
Oxcarbamazepine (Trileptal) May block voltage-sensitive sodium channels to stabilize hyperexcited neural membranes	■ Monitor for hyponatremia. ■ Use barrier contraception as the drug interferes with hormonal contraception methods.
Vigabatrin GABA inhibitor	■ Monitor vision, can cause blindness. ■ Not approved for use in children in the U.S.
Zonisamide (Zonegran) Facilitates dopaminergic and serotonergic neurotransmission	■ Increase fluid intake to reduce risk of kidney stones. ■ Report dizziness, excess drowsiness, lack of coordination, or double vision.

Data from Wilson, B. A., Shannon, M. T., & Shield, K. M. (2009). *Nurse's drug guide 2009*. Upper Saddle River, NJ: Prentice Hall Health; Wolf, S. M., & McGoldrick, P. E. (2006). Recognition and management of seizures. *Pediatric Annals, 35*(5), 332–344.

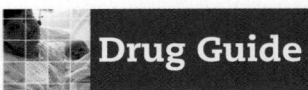

PLANNING AND IMPLEMENTATION

Nursing care focuses on maintaining airway patency, ensuring safety, administering medications, and providing emotional support. Both acute care and long-term management are involved.

MAINTAIN AIRWAY PATENCY

Place nothing in the child's mouth during a seizure; loose teeth may be knocked out and aspirated. The child is put in side-lying position for secretions to drain. Monitor the child to ensure adequate oxygenation: The child's color should be pink, the heart rate at a normal or slightly above normal rate for age, and the pulse oximetry reading (SpO_2) greater than 95%. Oxygen is usually given at SpO_2 levels below 95% (see Skill 14–1 **SKILLS**).

ENSURE SAFETY

Protect the child from self-harm during violent seizures (Figure 56–4 ●). If the child is in bed, pad the side rails to prevent injury. Children who have frequent, recurrent seizures should wear helmets to protect their heads in case they fall. All children with seizure disorders should wear some form of medical alert identification.

ADMINISTER MEDICATIONS

Take special precautions when administering intravenous medications (benzodiazepines) for the acute management of seizures. Give these medications very slowly over several minutes to minimize the risk of respiratory or circulatory collapse.

Medications for the daily management of seizures are given orally. When a child is NPO because of illness or on the day of surgery, seizure medications are usually given with a swallow of water. Obtain medication orders in these cases.

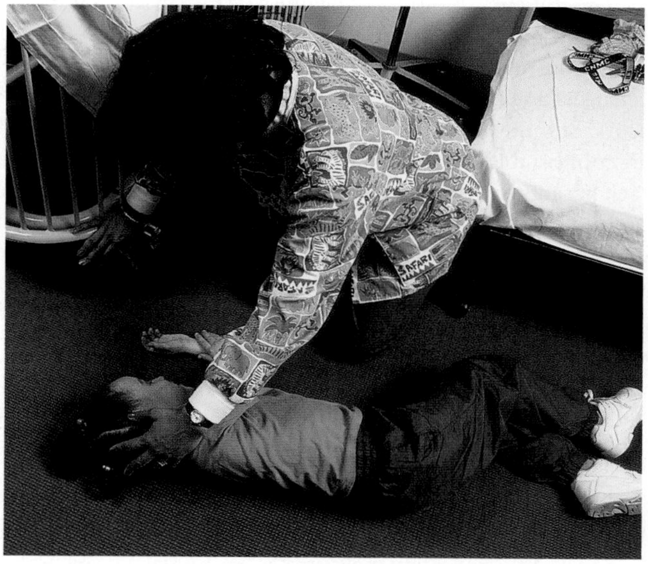

● **Figure 56–4** Safety during seizures. A child who has a seizure when standing should be gently assisted to the floor and placed in a side-lying position. Clear the area of any objects that might cause harm to the child.

> **Nursing Practice**
>
> When the child on a ketogenic diet is hospitalized, limit glucose and dextrose from all sources including IV fluids, elixirs, suspensions, and syrups. Use normal saline IV fluid. Obtain medications in pill form, crush them, and mix with an allowable food approved by the pharmacy.

PROVIDE EMOTIONAL SUPPORT

Seizures are frightening to the child and family because of the loss of control of body movements and possible loss of consciousness. Parents often feel guilty about the child's seizure disorder and need guidance to treat the child as normally as possible. Refer the child and family to support groups and counseling services if indicated. See "Evidence-Based Nursing: Supporting Children with Epilepsy and Their Parents."

DISCHARGE PLANNING AND HOME CARE TEACHING

Encourage parents to express their fears and anxieties. Answer their questions honestly, and refer them to organizations such as the Epilepsy Foundation of America, where they can get more information about the child's disorder. Be sure parents know how to administer medications and keep the child safe. Discuss with them whom to call with questions and when to return for follow-up. See MyNursingKit for Web sites with seizure information.

MyNursingKit Animation: Diazepam

NURSING CARE IN THE COMMUNITY

Educate the child and parents about medication regimens. Explain the purpose of each drug, its administration schedule, and the importance of giving all doses. Provide information about the medication side effects, and alert parents to the signs of toxic reactions. Explain the importance of follow-up visits to healthcare providers so that serum drug levels and the effectiveness of the child's medications can be monitored. Explain the use of rectal diazepam (Diastat) for acute management of a seizure when prescribed. Monitor the child's growth as a change in weight may require medication dosage adjustment to maintain seizure control. Encourage the family to schedule regular dental care for the child treated with phenytoin because of its effect on the gingiva. Ensure that information is shared directly with the older child so that he or she can begin taking more responsibility for self-care and gain a sense of self-control.

The parents of children with recurrent febrile seizures should be taught to give the proper dose of acetaminophen or ibuprofen with fever onset. Parents need to know that the fever management may not prevent a future febrile seizure. In most cases the adverse effects of antiepileptic medications for the child with febrile seizures outweigh the risk of the seizures. Reassure parents that complications from febrile seizures are rare.

Adolescent females need to be educated about the potential teratogenicity of some antiepileptics. Valproic acid and carbamazepine are associated with neural tube defects. Contraception

Evidence-Based Nursing

SUPPORTING CHILDREN WITH EPILEPSY AND THEIR PARENTS

Clinical Question

What information and support do children with epilepsy and their parents need to improve adjustment to living with epilepsy?

Evidence

One qualitative study used focus groups to identify information needs of 11 children (7 to 15 years) and 15 parents. Children reported frustration because healthcare providers talked with their parents and did not explain seizures in a way the children understood. They recognized that they were different from other children because of their diet, need to take medication at school, or limitations in some physical activities. Parents described their challenges in being their child's advocate, trying to get information about the treatment plan and expected course of the child's disorder, and wishing for coordinated care, such as a healthcare home (see Chapter 36). Parents were concerned about the different medications prescribed and became confused when medications or dosages were adjusted. Parents also worried about the physical and emotional health of their children (McNelis, Buelow, Myers, et al., 2007). A study using structured telephone interviews with parents of 224 children (4 to 14 years) having epilepsy focused on identifying family factors associated with behavior problems in children. At the onset of seizures, 32% of children had behavior problems, most commonly attention and social problems, along with anxiety and depression. Parents were interviewed about the family environment, specifically family mastery and family esteem/communication, as well as their perceived worry and need for information and support. Families with a disorganized family environment and low parent confidence in ability to discipline the child resulted in greater child behavior problems at baseline. Families were more likely to have a child with greater internalizing problems (anxiety and depression) if difficulties were found with the following tasks: family mastery, disciplining the child, encouraging child autonomy. These families also had a continuing need for information and support; and experienced greater worry 24 months after seizure onset than families whose child had less anxiety and depression. The children of families that gained confidence in child discipline over the 24-month study period had fewer internalizing problems. Some requests that parents made for support included discussions about the child's future, the child's mental health, fears about the child's seizures, and having the child talk with other children who have seizures (Austin, 2004).

Best Practice

Parents often have no prior experience with epilepsy, and studies reveal that parents and children often do not have their concerns and needs well addressed by healthcare providers. Assess for child behavior problems and parenting behaviors and provide education and support at the time of new onset seizures. Parents need guidance related to parenting their children and helping them to understand that discipline is important for all children. Referral to support groups is one way to provide ongoing support and education that can improve the child's and family's coping with a seizure disorder.

Critical Thinking

Refer to Chapters 36–38 for guidelines about child discipline methods, and develop a series of questions to identify how parents discipline their child with epilepsy. Identify some strategies to help the parent implement effective age-appropriate discipline.

See MyNursingKit for possible responses.

should be used when the adolescent is sexually active. When pregnancy is desired an alternate antiepileptic may be prescribed that reduces the risk for birth defects.

Teach families about safety guidelines for the child. Families of children with severe seizure disorders need to develop an emergency care plan so that emergency personnel know about their needs for care in advance (see Chapter 39).

Assist the family to develop an individual health plan so the child can receive medications during school hours, if necessary. Teachers and school administrators should know what to do if the child has a seizure and what information to report about the seizure. Parents may want to provide a towel and change of clothing for the child to use if incontinence occurs with the seizures.

Physical activity and exercise are important for all children. Encourage participation in sports when adequate supervision is provided. Children with well-controlled seizures may participate in most team sports, and activities such as bicycle riding. Activities such as rope climbing, rock or mountain climbing, tree climbing, snow skiing, scuba diving, and sky diving are more dangerous if seizures are not well controlled. Swimming and water sports require one-to-one supervision.

The child may be afraid of having a seizure in front of friends. Reassure the child and family that taking medications regularly should control seizures. Children need to be able to explain to peers what a seizure is and what to do if they are present when one occurs. Summer camps for children with seizures can be a safe and comfortable place for the child to enjoy outdoor activities. Teach parents to boost the child's self-image by emphasizing what the child can do, rather than focusing on contraindicated activities. Depending on state laws, most adolescents can drive after they have been seizure-free for at least 2 years.

EVALUATION

Expected outcomes of nursing management include the following:

- The child achieves good seizure control with medication, ketogenic diet, or surgical intervention.
- Injuries associated with seizures are prevented through the use of effective safety measures.
- The child's self-esteem is enhanced through participation in well-supervised sports and activities.

Teaching Highlights

SAFETY FOR THE CHILD WITH A SEIZURE DISORDER

Children with epilepsy have more injuries of all sorts, including burns and falls. Children are at increased risk for death due to drowning. Planning for safety includes the following:

- Do not leave the child alone in the bathtub.
- Children who bathe alone should use the shower.
- A buddy and lifeguard should always be present when the child swims.
- A life vest should always be worn when boating.
- A child with frequent seizures should wear a helmet to protect the head in case of a fall.
- The child should not play or stand around open flames or outdoor grills.
- The child should avoid areas where fall risks are increased.
- A form of medical identification should be worn, such as a medical alert bracelet.

INFECTIOUS DISEASES

Infections of the central nervous system need to be identified and treated rapidly because they can cause significant consequences in the developing child.

BACTERIAL MENINGITIS

Meningitis, an inflammation of the meninges, can be caused by either bacterial or viral agents. Bacterial meningitis is more virulent than viral meningitis and is sometimes fatal. Newborns and infants are at greatest risk for bacterial meningitis. Other risk factors for meningitis include immunosuppression, ventriculoperitoneal shunt, and a cochlear implant (Chàvez-Bueno & McCracken, 2005).

Etiology and Pathophysiology

Meningitis may occur secondary to other infections such as otitis media, sinusitis, pharyngitis, cellulitis, pneumonia, or septic arthritis; brain trauma; or a neurosurgical procedure. The organism causing the majority of cases in children between 2 months and 12 years of age is *Neisseria meningitides* (Prober, 2007, p. 2514). *Haemophilus influenzae* type b and *Streptococcus pneumoniae* are less common because of immunizations. Group B streptococcus and gram-negative enteric bacilli are more likely to cause meningitis in newborns (Chávez-Bueno & McCracken, 2005).

In many cases, bacteremia spreads the infectious agent to the CNS (see "Pathophysiology Illustrated: Central Nervous System Infection"), triggering an inflammatory response. White blood cells accumulate, covering the surface of the brain with a thick, white, purulent exudate. The brain then becomes hyperemic and edematous. If the infection spreads to the ventricles, the flow of cerebrospinal fluid can become obstructed and cause increased ICP and hydrocephalus. Meningitis can cause acute complications, e.g., the syndrome of inappropriate antidiuretic hormone (SIADH), and long-term morbidity.

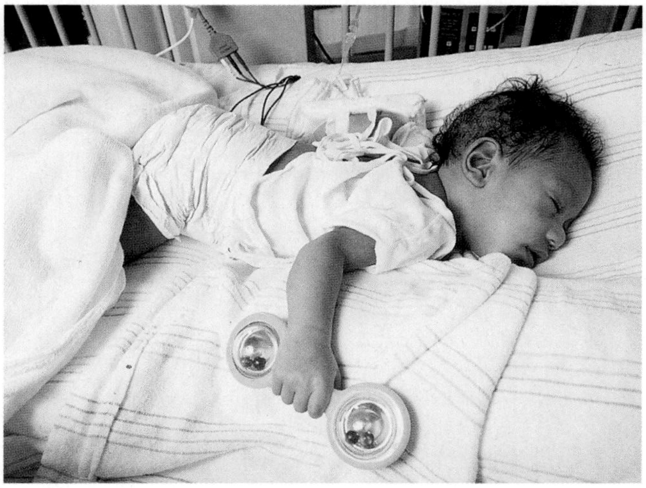

● **Figure 56–5** Bacterial meningitis. The child with bacterial meningitis assumes an opisthotonic position, with the neck and the head hyperextended, to relieve discomfort.

Clinical Manifestations

Symptoms vary by the child's age, the pathogen, and the length of the illness before diagnosis. Onset may be sudden or may develop over 1 to 2 days. Symptoms in the young infant may include fever, change in feeding pattern, vomiting, or diarrhea. The anterior fontanelle may be bulging or flat. The infant may be alert, restless, lethargic, or irritable. Rocking or cuddling, which normally calms a fussy infant, irritates the infant with meningitis.

Older children are usually febrile, have altered consciousness (e.g., confusion, delirium, lethargy, irritability), may have vomiting, and complain of muscle or joint pain. A hemorrhagic rash of petechiae that changes to purpura or large necrotic patches, may be seen in meningococcal meningitis (see Chapter 45). Other symptoms consistent with meningeal irritation may include headache (most often frontal), photophobia, back pain, and **nuchal rigidity** (resistance to neck flexion). The child is often comfortable only in an **opisthotonic position** (hyperextension of the head and neck) (Figure 56–5 ●). The child may have a positive Kernig or Brudzinski sign, or both, on examination (Figure 56–6 ●).

The condition can progress, leading to seizures, apnea, **cerebral edema** (an increase in the brain's intracellular and extracellular fluid that results from anoxia, vasodilation, or vascular stasis), increased ICP, subdural effusion, hydrocephalus, disseminated intravascular coagulation (DIC), and shock.

Clinical Therapy

Diagnosis is based on the history, clinical presentation, and laboratory findings. Laboratory tests include a complete blood count, blood cultures, serum electrolytes, blood urea nitrogen, osmolality, and clotting factors. Blood cultures usually identify the responsible organism causing meningitis. A lumbar puncture

PATHOPHYSIOLOGY ILLUSTRATED

CENTRAL NERVOUS SYSTEM INFECTION

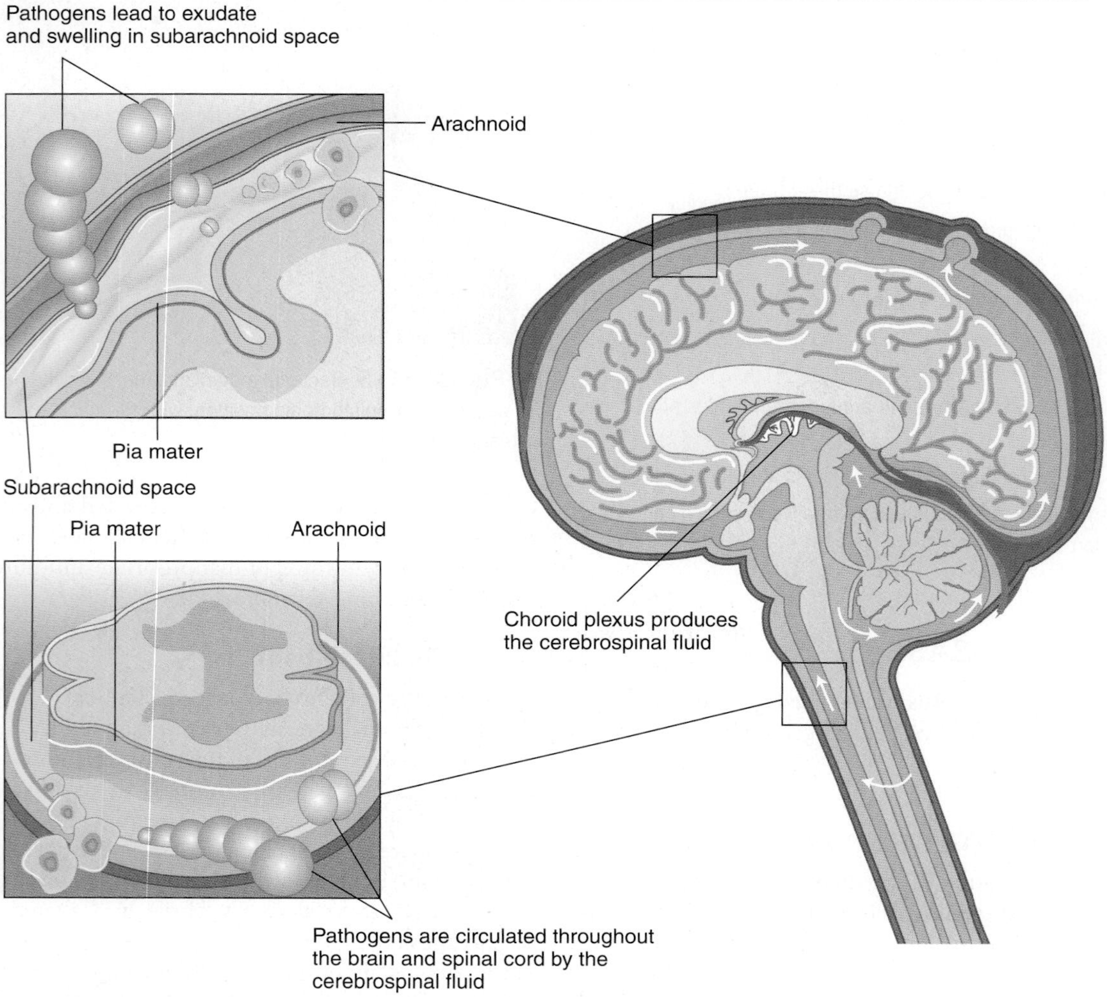
Pathogens lead to exudate and swelling in subarachnoid space
Arachnoid
Pia mater
Subarachnoid space
Pia mater
Arachnoid
Choroid plexus produces the cerebrospinal fluid
Pathogens are circulated throughout the brain and spinal cord by the cerebrospinal fluid

After bacteria reach the central nervous system, the pia mater, the arachnoid, and the cerebrospinal fluid-filled subarachnoid space become infected. The cerebrospinal fluid then circulates the pathogens throughout the brain and spinal cord.

is performed to evaluate the CSF for white blood cells, protein and glucose levels, and culture. CT scanning may be performed when increased ICP or a brain abscess is suspected.

Antibiotics are administered as soon as diagnostic tests are obtained. Antibiotics commonly used to treat bacterial meningitis include ampicillin, aminoglycosides, cefotaxime, ceftriaxone, penicillin G, and vancomycin. Antibiotics are often changed once culture and sensitivity results are known, since many organisms have resistance to certain antibiotics. These medications are administered intravenously for 7 to 21 days, depending on the organism and the child's clinical response. Corticosteroids (dexamethasone) are given as an adjunct to children over 6 weeks of age to reduce the risk of severe neurologic sequelae such as sensorineural hearing loss, especially in cases of *Hemophilus influenza* type b meningitis (Chávez-Bueno & McCracken, 2005). If increased ICP is present, medications (e.g., mannitol) may be given to reduce the pressure.

Depending on the causative organism, the disease may need to be reported to the local health department. Contacts who have not been previously immunized with the meningococcal vaccine may need to take prophylactic antibiotics, such as rifampin or ciprofloxacin.

Infants and children receive nothing by mouth and are started on IV fluids. The IV fluids are initially restricted to two-thirds maintenance as careful monitoring for increased ICP and SIADH (see Chapter 55∞) is initiated. If the child is in shock, aggressive fluid resuscitation is performed to maintain the cerebral perfusion pressure.

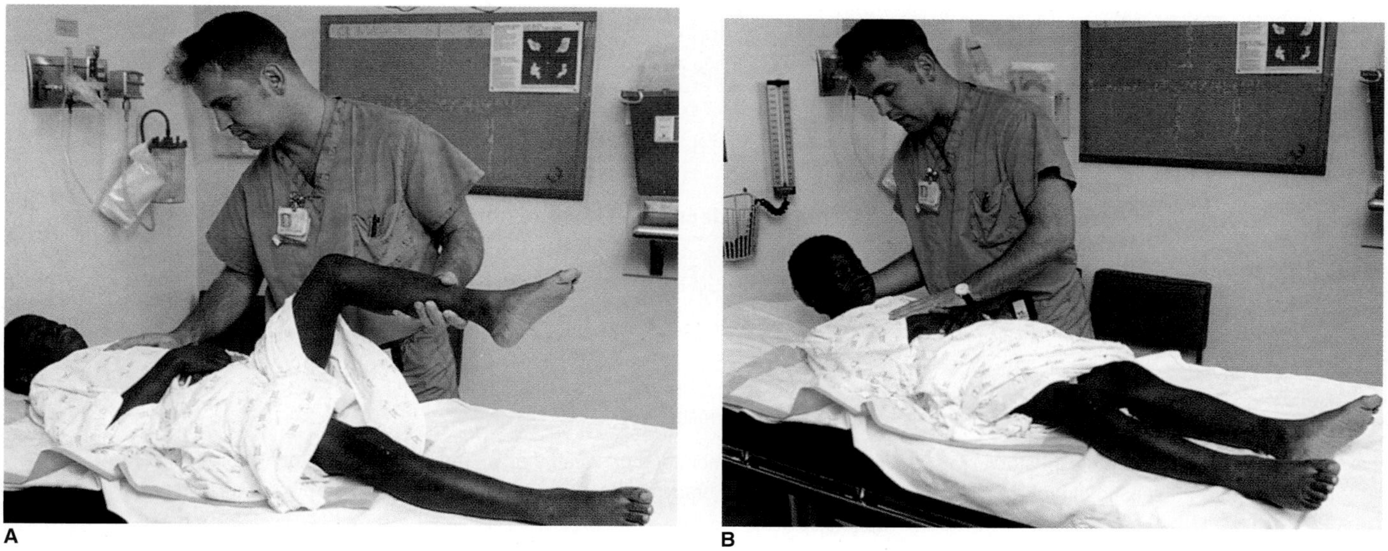

A B

● **Figure 56–6** Testing for Kernig and Brudzinski signs. ***A,*** To test for Kernig sign, raise the child's leg with the knee flexed. Then extend the child's leg at the knee. If any resistance is noted or pain is felt, the result is a positive Kernig sign. This is a common finding in meningitis. ***B,*** To test Brudzinski sign, flex the child's head while in a supine position. If this action makes the knees or hips flex involuntarily, a positive Brudzinski sign is present. This is a common finding in meningitis.

Some infants and children who have had bacterial meningitis suffer neurologic damage despite early, aggressive management. The most common sequelae involve cranial nerves, especially the eighth, resulting in hearing loss. In addition, children may develop seizures, hydrocephalus, subdural effusion, SIADH, developmental delay, learning problems, and behavior problems.

NURSING MANAGEMENT

NURSING ASSESSMENT AND DIAGNOSIS

Assess the child's physiologic status, including vital signs and level of consciousness. Measure head circumference often in hospitalized infants because of the potential for hydrocephalus. Be alert for signs of a change in the child's condition and response to treatment. Monitor the child's ability to control secretions and to drink sufficient fluids. Monitor intake and output. Assess for any sensory deficits. Identify parents' concerns about this potentially life-threatening condition.

Several nursing diagnoses that may apply to the child with bacterial meningitis appear in the accompanying Nursing Care Plan. Additional nursing diagnoses might include the following:

- *Risk for Aspiration* related to altered level of consciousness and poor secretion control
- *Risk for Deficient Fluid Volume* related to poor oral fluid intake
- *Grieving (Parent)* related to the child's life-threatening condition
- *Caregiver Role Strain* related to a hospitalized child and other family responsibilities

PLANNING AND IMPLEMENTATION

The accompanying Nursing Care Plan summarizes care for the child with bacterial meningitis. Nursing care begins with emergency treatment and continues as the child's condition stabilizes. Monitor respiratory and neurologic status, maintain hydration, administer medications, and prevent complications. Promote the child's comfort with reduced stimulation (dim lights, quiet room) and by placing in a side-lying position. Isolate the child and use standard and droplet precautions until the causative organism is identified and culture sensitivities confirm that effective treatment is being administered.

Monitor the child's response to antibiotic therapy. Observe for signs of gastrointestinal bleeding, which is a potential complication of corticosteroid use. Maintenance and replacement fluids are usually given to children with bacterial meningitis.

Respond to parents' concerns about their child's condition, explaining all measures to reduce the child's discomfort and treat the illness. Identify ways parents can help meet the child's comfort needs.

Prevention is a major role for nurses. Encourage parents to get their infants and children fully immunized with the Haemophilus influenzae, pneumococcal, and meningococcal vaccines.

Nursing Practice

Monitor the serum sodium concentration and urine specific gravity since the child is at risk for SIADH. Fluids are restricted if SIADH is suspected. Sodium chloride, potassium, and acetate or lactate are administered intravenously to balance sodium excretion.

Nursing Care Plan

THE CHILD WITH BACTERIAL MENINGITIS

INTERVENTION	RATIONALE	EXPECTED OUTCOME
1. Nursing Diagnosis: Impaired Gas Exchange related to decreased level of consciousness		
NIC Priority Intervention: **Respiratory monitoring:** Collection and analysis of patient data to ensure airway patency and adequate gas exchange		**NOC Suggested Outcome:** **Respiratory status: Ventilation:** Movement of air in and out of the lungs
Goal: The child's respiratory failure does not progress to respiratory arrest.		
■ Place the child on a cardiorespiratory monitor with a 20-second alarm.	■ The alarm on the monitor alerts staff that the child is having bradycardia or an apneic spell.	The child's respiratory failure is managed with assessment and prompt treatment.
■ Have resuscitation equipment, including oxygen, resuscitation bag with mask, and suction apparatus, at the bedside.	■ Equipment should be at the bedside in case of respiratory arrest. Bag-valve-mask ventilation is recommended because the child's respiratory secretions contain bacteria.	
■ Stimulate the child if apneic; if no response, begin manual ventilations and call for the resuscitation team.	■ Stimulation may encourage spontaneous respirations; if not, ventilation is necessary. Calling for resuscitation team ensures help in managing the child in a timely manner.	
■ Monitor heart rate and perform compressions if necessary.	■ The apneic child may have bradycardia resulting from cardiac hypoxia.	
2. Nursing Diagnosis: Risk for Injury related to infection of cerebrospinal fluid and potential sequelae		
NIC Priority Intervention: **Health screening:** Detecting health risks or problems by means of history, examination, and other procedures.		**NOC Suggested Outcome:** **Immune status:** Adequacy of natural and acquired appropriately targeted resistance to internal and external antigens
Goal: The child will suffer minimal CNS injury secondary to infection.		
■ Administer antibiotics and corticosteroids as prescribed.	■ Antibiotics help eradicate the pathogen and prevent cerebral edema. Corticosteroids diminish inflammatory response and reduce the chance of neurologic sequelae.	The child's condition improves significantly within 48–72 hours (fever decreases and no signs of neurologic sequelae are detected).
■ Note return of fever, nuchal rigidity, or irritability. Monitor vital signs, assess for signs of increased ICP. Measure head circumference once or twice daily. Note changes in responsiveness. Notify the physician immediately if any signs are detected.	■ Watching for common sequelae such as subdural effusions, hydrocephalus, or septic arthritis ensures prompt treatment.	
Goal: The child will not develop cerebral edema as a result of water retention.		
■ Monitor for SIADH and watch for signs of increased ICP.	■ SIADH can be either avoided or quickly managed if recognized early.	Cerebral edema does not develop. If SIADH or increased ICP occurs, the condition is treated promptly so effects are minimized.
■ Perform strict intake and output measurements. Determine urine specific gravity. Check electrolytes and osmolality of both serum and urine. Weigh the child daily. Restrict fluids and give sodium chloride as prescribed.	■ Low urine output with a high specific gravity is a sign of fluid retention and SIADH. The child is maintained with lower fluids and provided sodium supplements to reduce the possibility for cerebral edema.	

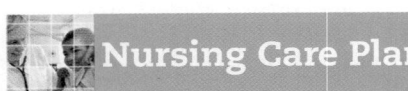

THE CHILD WITH BACTERIAL MENINGITIS

INTERVENTION	RATIONALE	EXPECTED OUTCOME
Goal: The child will be free of injury resulting from DIC.		
■ Be aware of needle sticks that continue to bleed and lesions that continue to ooze. Monitor clotting times.	■ Prompt recognition leads to management of the coagulopathy.	The child does not sustain injury from DIC.
■ Administer blood products, vitamin K, or heparin as ordered.	■ Prompt recognition allows for early initial treatment of DIC. The child may bleed to death if treatment is delayed.	
Goal: The child will be free of injury secondary to shock.		
■ Monitor vital signs, including pulse, respirations, and blood pressure. Note perfusion (capillary refill, central versus proximal pulses). Check level of consciousness. Note urine output.	■ Monitoring allows for prompt diagnosis of shock based on clinical signs.	The child recovers from shock quickly with no complications. Prompt management of shock can enhance the child's recovery, since it prevents complications associated with poor perfusion (tissue acidosis and ischemia).
■ Begin fluid resuscitation as ordered.	■ IV fluid bolus may improve perfusion.	
■ Administer inotropes if prescribed.	■ Inotropes enhance perfusion when response to fluid challenge is minimal.	
Goal: The child with any degree of hearing loss will be identified.		
■ Arrange for hearing assessment prior to discharge.	■ Hearing loss is a common complication. Early intervention is needed to promote growth and development.	The child with identified hearing loss is referred to an appropriate specialist or program for intervention.

3. Nursing Diagnosis: Acute Pain related to meningeal irritation

NIC Priority Intervention:		NOC Suggested Outcome:
Pain management: Alleviation of pain or reduction in pain to a level of comfort acceptable to patient		**Comfort level:** Feelings of physical and psychologic ease
Goal: The child will be as comfortable as possible.		
■ Assess pain with age-appropriate pain scale.	■ Pain scales provide ability to quantify pain for future comparison.	The child is calm and expresses increased comfort.
■ Minimize tactile stimulation.	■ Sensory stimulation increases discomfort.	
■ Allow the child to assume a comfortable position.	■ The child determines the most comfortable position. Opisthotonic position, with the head and neck hyperextended, may be the most comfortable.	
■ Keep the lights dim and maintain a quiet environment.	■ Dim lights reduce the discomfort from photophobia. Noise can disturb the child.	
■ Provide pain medication as prescribed.	■ Pain medication is appropriate for acute discomfort associated with illness.	

4. Nursing Diagnosis: Risk for Infection (Family and Close Contacts) related to pathogens in the cerebrospinal fluid

NIC Priority Intervention:		NOC Suggested Outcome:
Infection control: Minimizing the acquisition and transmission of infectious agents		**Infection status:** Presence and extent of infection
Goal: Caretakers or family members will have no apparent evidence of infection.		
■ Explain rationale and dose schedule for taking rifampin or ciprofloxacin.	■ Rifampin and ciprofloxacin provide prophylaxis for many bacterial pathogens responsible for meningitis.	Family members and other close contacts verbalize the schedule for rifampin or ciprofloxacin therapy.

DISCHARGE PLANNING AND HOME CARE TEACHING

Identify and address home care needs well in advance of discharge. Follow-up visits are important to monitor for complications and sequelae. Help parents deal with any physical requirements resulting from the child's illness and any emotional, social, and financial repercussions of the child's condition. Teach parents what to do if the child has a seizure.

Infants and toddlers with neurologic sequelae should be referred to an early intervention program. If the child has had a hearing loss, referral to an otolaryngologist and speech and language specialist should be made. Early identification of other neurologic sequelae, such as learning problems, should be encouraged. Children with neurologic sequelae need to have an individual education plan (IEP) developed (see Chapter 40∞), and parents may need help planning for the child's special educational needs. Refer parents to the appropriate social service agencies for support and assistance.

EVALUATION

Expected outcomes of nursing care are provided in the accompanying Nursing Care Plan.

VIRAL (ASEPTIC) MENINGITIS

Viral meningitis is an inflammatory response of the meninges characterized by an increased number of blood cells and protein in the CSF. In the United States, an enterovirus is often the cause of more than 80% of viral meningitis cases (Prober, 2007).

Generally, the child with aseptic meningitis does not appear as ill as the child with bacterial meningitis. The child may be irritable or lethargic and usually has a fever. Other symptoms include general malaise, headache, photophobia, gastrointestinal distress, upper respiratory symptoms, and a maculopapular rash. The child may also show signs of meningeal irritation such as stiff neck, back pain, and positive Kernig and Brudzinski signs (see Figure 56–6 ●). The infant may have a tense anterior fontanelle. Seizures are rare. Symptoms usually resolve spontaneously within 3 to 10 days.

The child with fever and meningeal signs is hospitalized. Blood, urine, and CSF analyses are performed. Polymerase chain reaction testing helps detect viral meningitis, often within 24 hours. Until the diagnosis of aseptic meningitis is confirmed, the child is treated aggressively for bacterial meningitis. Other treatment is supportive of symptoms.

Nursing Management

Initial nursing care focuses on providing supportive care as described for the child with bacterial meningitis. Give acetaminophen as ordered to reduce fever, headache, and muscle or joint pain. Keep the room dark and quiet (to decrease stimuli and meningeal irritation), give fluids either intravenously or orally, and promote comfort with proper positioning.

The child and family need information about the disease. Explain medical and nursing procedures in terms that the child and family can understand. Keep parents informed about the child's progress. Once the diagnosis of viral meningitis is made, immediately begin discharge planning and teaching for home care. Explain that recovery may take several weeks but that complete recovery is expected.

ENCEPHALITIS

Encephalitis is an acute CNS condition with radiographic or laboratory evidence of brain inflammation. Inflammation of the meninges is also common. Infants under age 1 year have the highest incidence (Lewis & Glaser, 2005).

Encephalitis may occur as a direct or primary infection by an organism that successfully passes through the blood-brain barrier. Viruses, bacteria, fungi, and parasites may all cause encephalitis. Herpes viruses, enteroviruses, and Epstein-Barr virus are the most common organisms (Lewis & Glaser, 2005). Postinfectious encephalitis may occur days or weeks after a measles or varicella infection. Children who survive often have significant neurologic sequelae (American Academy of Pediatrics, 2009, p. 444).

Signs and symptoms depend on the causative organism and the location of the infection within the brain. An acute onset of a febrile illness with neurologic signs is the classic manifestation. Initially the child may have a severe headache, fever, and vomiting, followed by altered consciousness or focal neurologic signs. Meningeal irritation signs such as nuchal rigidity, photophobia, and positive Kernig and Brudzinski signs are common. Other neurologic signs vary. The child may be disoriented or confused, with behavioral or personality changes. Speech disturbances; motor dysfunction such as hemiparesis, ataxia, or weakness; cranial nerve deficits; or alterations in reflex response may be present. Focal or generalized seizures may occur. The child's level of consciousness may deteriorate to coma over hours or days.

Diagnosis is based on history and laboratory findings. Information about recent immunizations, insect bites, or residence in or travel to areas where cases of encephalitis are present should be obtained (e.g., West Nile virus or eastern equine encephalitis). CSF analysis, blood serologic tests, and nasopharyngeal and stool specimens are evaluated to identify viral pathogens. Testing for virus-specific immunoglobulin M antibodies with enzyme-linked immunosorbent assay (ELISA) is performed after 5 days of acute illness. The polymerase chain reaction test is used to assay for herpes DNA in the CSF. A CT scan, MRI, and EEG may also be performed. Brain biopsy may be performed to diagnose herpes simplex and parasitic infections. Routine blood chemistry and hematology tests are often normal (Lewis & Glaser, 2005).

The child with encephalitis is at risk for seizures, respiratory failure, and increased ICP and should be cared for in an intensive care unit. Treatment is both pharmacologic and supportive. The child with a suspected bacterial infection should be treated with antibiotics until bacterial pathogens have been ruled out. Acyclovir may be used for herpes viral infections. With postinfectious encephalitis, IV immune globulin, corticosteroids, and other immune modulators are considered (Lewis & Glaser, 2005). Physical therapy may be prescribed during the acute phase.

Children with encephalitis have many permanent neurologic sequelae. Although some children recover completely, many more are left with intellectual, motor, visual, or auditory deficits. The cardiovascular system, lungs, or liver may also be affected. Generally, younger children have a more serious illness and more severe sequelae.

Nursing Management

Nursing care focuses on monitoring cardiorespiratory function, preventing complications resulting from immobility, reorienting the child, and teaching the parents about the child's condition.

Monitor the child's cardiorespiratory function. Check the child's airway and ability to handle secretions. Assess the child's color, respiratory effort, the SpO_2, and arterial blood gases. Monitor the heart rate, blood pressure, capillary refill time, and urine output.

Provide seizure precautions. Prevent complications resulting from immobility as described on page 1655. Maintain skin integrity. Proper positioning with frequent turning is important. When indicated by the physician, perform chest physiotherapy to prevent pneumonia.

Give the parents information about their child's condition and prognosis. Provide support as they cope with the child's life-threatening condition.

As the level of consciousness begins to improve, the child may at first be confused and disoriented and may have residual effects of the disease. Orient the child to the hospital environment. Have the family help to reorient the child by bringing favorite stuffed animals or music from home. Engage in therapeutic play (refer to Chapter 41∞ for techniques). Give the child age-appropriate toys to encourage a return to normal behavior.

DISCHARGE PLANNING AND HOME CARE TEACHING

Encourage parents to take an active role in the child's physical and emotional care in the hospital, and give them written instructions about home care. Encourage the parents to learn specific physical, occupational, and speech therapies so they can work with their child at home between therapy sessions. Refer parents to home care, social services, family counseling, and support groups. Plan follow-up visits so the child can be evaluated for neurologic sequelae.

REYE SYNDROME

Reye syndrome is an acute **encephalopathy**, a cerebral dysfunction caused by a toxic, injury, inflammatory, or anoxic insult that may result in permanent tissue damage, although the dysfunction may improve over time. In 1980 an association was identified between the use of aspirin for influenza or varicella and Reye syndrome. The condition is now rare since most parents give children acetaminophen or ibuprofen rather than aspirin for flulike symptoms and varicella. The mortality rate due to Reye syndrome is high.

Reye syndrome is classified as a secondary mitochondrial hepatopathy, caused by a hepatotoxic drug, toxin, metal, or metabolite caused by a poorly functioning organ. In the case of Reye syndrome, an interaction between a viral illness and aspirin occurs in a susceptible individual (Carey & Balistreri, 2007, p. 1697). The disorder is characterized by cerebral edema, hypoglycemia, and an enlarged, fatty, poorly functioning liver (due to an elevation of short chain fatty acid levels and hyperammonemia).

Reye syndrome begins with nausea and vomiting, mental status changes, seizures, and progressive unresponsiveness. The condition has five stages that indicate increasing signs of cerebral edema and neurologic dysfunction, resulting in a final stage with coma, seizures, flaccidity, loss of deep tendon reflexes, and respiratory arrest.

The diagnosis of Reye syndrome is based on an abrupt change in the child's level of consciousness and diagnostic laboratory tests that reveal no other identifiable cause of the child's coma and neurologic signs. CSF analysis usually reveals white blood cells. Radiographic imaging reveals cerebral edema. Liver enzyme and ammonia levels are elevated, blood glucose levels are below normal, and prothrombin time is prolonged. A liver biopsy is sometimes performed to confirm the diagnosis.

The child with Reye syndrome should be cared for in a pediatric intensive care unit. The goal of medical management is to provide supportive treatment and to prevent the secondary effects of cerebral edema and metabolic injury associated with the elevated short-chain fatty acids and ammonia levels. Mechanical ventilation is often needed once the child is comatose. Arterial and venous blood pressure monitoring is performed. The child is monitored for signs of increased ICP secondary to cerebral edema. Hypoglycemia is treated with IV glucose. Electrolytes, blood chemistry, and blood pH are monitored.

Nursing Management

Nursing care focuses on monitoring the child's physical status, providing emotional support, and teaching parents about disease prevention.

Check the child's respiratory and neurologic status frequently, and note any signs of improvement or deterioration. Refer to the discussion of nursing management of altered states of consciousness on page 1653 for specific nursing interventions. Look for changes in laboratory values that indicate acidosis, an elevation of ammonia levels, or hypoglycemia. Monitor the child's intake and output. Correct imbalances by administering fluids, electrolytes, or medications as ordered. Prevent complications associated with immobility.

The child who survives and is discharged is monitored to observe for sequelae. Developmental and neurologic deficits

Nursing Practice

Make sure all parents know that they should use acetaminophen or ibuprofen when the child has a viral illness such as influenza, to prevent the development of Reye syndrome. Teach parents to check all over-the-counter medicines (including homeopathic and herbal medications) for the presence of aspirin or salicylate compounds. Emphasize the importance of obtaining health care whenever a child's condition worsens at the end of a viral illness.

may occur and are more severe in children under 2 years of age. Arrange for home nursing or frequent clinic visits during the recovery period for monitoring. Inform the parents about community resources that can assist them in promoting the child's recovery.

GUILLAIN-BARRÉ SYNDROME (POSTINFECTIOUS POLYNEURITIS)

Guillain-Barré syndrome is an acute inflammatory demyelinating polyneuropathy. This condition may lead to deteriorating motor function, weakness, and paralysis that progress in an ascending pattern, as well as paresthesia and **areflexia** (no reflex response to stimulation).

Guillain-Barré syndrome is thought to be caused by an immune response to an infectious organism, usually within 1 to 3 weeks of a gastrointestinal or respiratory illness. Associated organisms are *Campylobacter jejuni*, *Helicobacter pylori*, and *Mycoplasma pneumoniae*. It has also been associated with immunizations for influenza and rabies (Sarnat, 2007). The peripheral nerve myelin is attacked by macrophages, resulting in demyelination and blocked transmission of nerve impulses to the muscles. The damaged peripheral nerves then begin to atrophy.

Infants have an onset of rapidly progressive severe hypotonia, possible respiratory distress, irritability, and feeding difficulties. Older children have rapidly progressive symmetric weakness and muscle pain with varying degrees of distal paresthesia and numbness in the legs. This ascending weakness spreads to the upper extremities, trunk, chest, neck, face, and head. Deep tendon reflexes may be diminished or absent. The child may develop acute ataxia. Difficulty swallowing and facial weakness are signs of impending respiratory failure. Respiratory effort may be inadequate for proper ventilation. Cranial nerves may be affected, causing Bell's palsy, for example. A dysfunctional autonomic nervous system may cause such symptoms as labile blood pressure and cardiac rates, postural hypotension, profound bradycardia, or asystole (Sarnat, 2007).

Diagnostic criteria of Guillain-Barré syndrome include progressive motor weakness (minimal weakness of the legs to total paralysis of all extremities), and areflexia of varying degrees. Diagnostic findings of this syndrome include a CSF protein level twice the upper limit of normal, a normal glucose level, and fewer than 10 white blood cells per cubic millimeter (Sarnat, 2007). Bacterial and viral cultures are usually negative. Electroconduction tests such as electromyography show acute muscle denervation.

Clinical therapy for Guillain-Barré syndrome is intravenous immune globulin (IVIG) for several days when the child is unable to ambulate. Guidelines for administration of IVIG can be found in Chapter 50∞. Responses to IVIG are dramatic, often within days. Physical therapy and supportive care are initiated early to promote ambulation. The condition is rarely fatal.

Nursing Management

Nursing care focuses on monitoring respiratory status, meeting nutritional needs, managing autonomic nervous system dysfunction, preventing complications associated with immobility, providing emotional support, and teaching the parents how to care for the child after discharge.

Monitor cardiorespiratory status. Place the child on a cardiorespiratory monitor for continuous assessment in the early phase of the illness. Look for such signs that may indicate the need for endotracheal intubation and mechanical ventilation (e.g., dyspnea, inability to handle secretions, inadequate respiratory effort, and color changes).

Manage autonomic nervous system dysfunction. Monitor the child's vital signs closely for episodes of tachycardia, bradycardia, and hypotension. Blood pressure fluctuations and autonomic instability are linked to asystole (Sarnat, 2007). Observe frequently for decreased responsiveness. Intervene promptly if these or other signs of autonomic nervous system dysfunction are noted.

Meet nutritional needs. Assess whether the child is having difficulty swallowing. If the child has no gag reflex, nutritional needs are maintained with intravenous supplements or nasogastric tube feedings.

Prevent complications. Prevent complications associated with immobility (see page 1655). Ensure good postural alignment, and turn the child every 2 hours. Maintaining skin integrity is also important.

Evaluate the child's muscle tone, strength, and symmetry. When the child's condition begins to improve, recovery of lost strength is the priority. Active exercise is emphasized in physical therapy. Encourage family members to participate in the child's care, especially during the recovery phase. They can help with the activities of daily living and reinforce what the child has learned in physical therapy.

Provide emotional support. Explain the progression of Guillain-Barré syndrome to the parents during the initial stages. Witnessing a rapid deterioration in their child's physical status can be frightening; therefore, preparation is essential to reduce their anxieties. Be honest when discussing recovery and prognosis for the child.

Have parents bring in favorite toys, dolls, or books to make the child feel more secure. Playing with or reading to the child can be comforting.

Discharge planning and home care teaching. Home care needs should be identified and addressed well in advance of discharge. Support the parents as they prepare for the child's return home, especially when return to full strength is expected to be slow. Provide referral to home care nurses who can manage all aspects of treatment, rehabilitation, and follow-up. Refer the parents to social workers who can help with financial arrangements and school considerations.

Nursing care in the community. Help the child to adjust to any residual effects of Guillain-Barré syndrome. Help the child practice exercises learned in physical therapy sessions, and encourage the child to perform activities of daily living, such as brushing the teeth or combing the hair. Refer the child to outpatient rehabilitation programs to promote recovery.

To promote a positive self-image, praise any effort the child makes to be self-sufficient. The child may be frustrated and angry. Allow the child to express these feelings in an appropriate way, either during play or in conversation.

HEADACHES

Up to 75% of children experience a headache by age 15 years. Migraine headaches occur in 1% of children by age 7 years, and 5% of children by age 15 years. Approximately 20% of children in the United States have chronic headaches (Rubin, Suecoff, & Knupp, 2006). Headaches may be associated with school absence, decreased extracurricular activity, and poor academic achievement.

> **Complementary Care**
>
> **TREATING HEADACHES**
>
> Self-hypnosis training can help motivated children to manage their chronic headaches. A study reviewed the outcomes of 144 children with a mean age of 11.5 years who learned to perform self-hypnosis using imagery involving favorite places. Each child selected a therapeutic hypnotic suggestion (e.g., imagining themselves to be somewhere where they had never had a headache, thinking of an elevator floor as the level of pain intensity and then pushing the elevator button to go down floor by floor until 1 or 0 is reached). The majority of children had reduced headache frequency (88%), and 26% of children became headache free after learning self-hypnosis techniques (Kohen & Zajac, 2007).

ETIOLOGY AND PATHOPHYSIOLOGY

Headaches have both benign (migraine, inflammatory, and tension) and structural causes, such as a tumor. See "Clinical Manifestations: Causes of Headaches."

- Migraine headaches may be triggered by stress; foods containing nitrates, glutamate, caffeine, tyramine, and salt; menses; oral contraceptives; fatigue; and hunger. If another family member often has similar headaches, genetic predisposition may be a factor.
- Tension headaches may be associated with stresses due to school, insecurity, or conflict in the family.
- Medication overuse (rebound) headaches are associated with the frequent use of medications for headaches, more than 2 to 3 times a week. Medications associated with this type of headache include acetaminophen, nonsteroidal anti-inflammatory drugs (NSAIDs), decongestants, triptans, opioids, benzodiazepines, and ergotamines (Gladstein & Mack, 2005).

CLINICAL MANIFESTATIONS

See the clinical manifestations table for the signs and symptoms associated with specific types of headaches.

CLINICAL THERAPY

Clinical therapy involves taking a detailed history of the headache characteristics (onset, duration, pain severity, quality, and location; aura; treatment or medications used) and associated symptoms (abdominal pain, nausea, vomiting). Assessment is focused on detecting neurologic signs such as altered consciousness, abnormal cranial nerves, papilledema, and motor or sensory deficits. Radiologic studies (CT scan or MRI) are used only in cases of abnormal neurological signs or if a structural problem is suspected. A lumbar puncture is performed if an infection or inflammatory process is suspected (Gunner & Smith, 2007).

Treatment includes relaxation techniques, analgesics, and anti-inflammatory medications. A behavior management program may help reduce common headache triggers (inadequate sleep, perimenstrual stress, and missed meals). Foods (e.g., caffeine, chocolate, processed meats, alcohol, hard cheeses, monosodium glutamate, yeast, nuts, figs, aspartame, and sauerkraut) may also be headache triggers (Rubin et al., 2006). Medications to abort migraines (e.g., sumatriptan by mouth or nasal spray) are used in children old enough to identify an aura. Some children and adolescents have prophylactic medications prescribed (e.g., propanolol, amitriptyline, valproic acid, topiramate), but side effects may outweigh the benefits (Rubin et al., 2006).

Nursing Management

Assess the child for potential neurologic signs associated with headaches. Encourage the child to keep a headache diary, writing down the events and stresses at the time of a headache to help identify patterns and potential triggers. Behavior changes that may reduce headaches include a consistent sleeping and wake-up time 7 days a week, a regular eating schedule and avoiding hunger, regular physical activity for 30 to 45 minutes at least 5 days a week, avoidance of identified food triggers, and avoidance of smoke and other strong odors (Unger, 2006).

Assist the child and family to see patterns in the headache diary and discuss potential strategies for relieving the headaches. Teach the child to take the prescribed medications at the first sign of a headache, but caution the child not to take medications in any combination for more than 2 to 3 days a week. See "Complementary Care: Treating Headaches."

See Chapter 52 for care of the child with a brain tumor.

STRUCTURAL DEFECTS

Common structural defects include microcephaly, hydrocephalus, neural tube defects, craniosynostosis, positional plagiocephaly, and neurofibromatosis.

MICROCEPHALY

Microcephaly is a small brain with a head circumference below the third percentile on growth curves (Kinsman & Johnson,

Clinical Manifestations

CAUSES OF HEADACHES

TYPE OF HEADACHE AND CAUSE	CLINICAL MANIFESTATIONS
Migraine Vascular, acute recurrent	■ Unilateral or bilateral pulsatile throbbing pain lasting for hours or days, moderate to severe pain intensity lasting for 4 to 72 hours, aggravated by routine activity ■ Nausea and vomiting ■ Photophobia and phonophobia ■ Visual or motor aura several minutes before headache starts; child may have no aura ■ Preschool-age children may have irritability, restlessness, malaise, head banging, head holding, and sensitivity to light and sound ■ Recurrent abdominal pain ■ Relief with sleep
Tension Muscular contraction, acute recurrent or chronic nonprogressive	■ Dull, achy pain of mild to moderate intensity in bilateral or frontal areas, may last for days; not aggravated by increased physical activity ■ Intermittent or constant pain with fluctuations in intensity ■ Unlikely to have nausea and vomiting ■ Sensitive to light or sound
Rebound or medication overuse Acute recurrent	■ Dull, bilateral or unilateral pain in frontal area ■ Occurs at least 2 to 4 times a week or daily ■ Can vary in character, location, and severity from time to time ■ Usually increases in frequency and severity over time, paralleling the increase in medication use ■ Recurs when medication wears off
Inflammatory Sinusitis or dental abscess, acute localized	■ Facial pain or tenderness over affected sinus ■ Dull, constant pressure ■ Severity of pain varies with head position ■ Fever
Structural Space-occupying lesion, hemorrhage, increased ICP, chronic progressive	■ Severe pain that is increasing in frequency and severity, often in occipital or frontal location; awakens child in the morning or is present on awakening; increases with coughing, sneezing, or straining ■ Vomiting that is persistent or preceded by recurrent headache ■ Abnormal neurologic signs (e.g., double vision, papilledema, strabismus, weakness, ataxia)

Data from: Fisher, P. G. (2005). Help for headaches: A strategy for your busy practice. *Contemporary Pediatrics, 22*(11), 34–40; Rubin, D. H., Suecoff, S. A., & Knupp, K. G. (2006). Headaches in children. *Pediatric Annals, 35*(5), 345–353.

2007). Causes may include chromosomal abnormalities, fetal insult, maternal infection, or an infection, metabolic disorder, or anoxia during infancy. Children with microcephaly have cognitive impairments. See Chapter 57 for more information.

HYDROCEPHALUS

Hydrocephalus is the body's response to an imbalance between the production and absorption of CSF. The condition is often congenital and associated with other CNS malformations. Hydrocephalus can develop as a complication of illness or trauma. The incidence is estimated to be 1 per 500 children (National Institute for Neurologic Disorders and Stroke, 2008). It is commonly associated with myelomeningocele, a spinal fluid–filled meningeal sac that contains a portion of the spinal cord and nerves protruding through a vertebral defect (see page 1676).

Etiology and Pathophysiology

Hydrocephalus may be either communicating or noncommunicating. In communicating hydrocephalus the CSF flows freely among normal channels and pathways, but CSF absorption in the subarachnoid space and the arachnoid villi is impaired. It may be acquired from postinfectious meningitis or from intraventricular hemorrhage in a preterm infant, or it may be caused by a congenital malformation in the subarachnoid spaces.

Noncommunicating hydrocephalus is responsible for most cases in children. It results from an obstruction in the ventricular system (e.g., infection, hemorrhage, tumor, surgery, or struc-

PATHOPHYSIOLOGY ILLUSTRATED

HYDROCEPHALUS

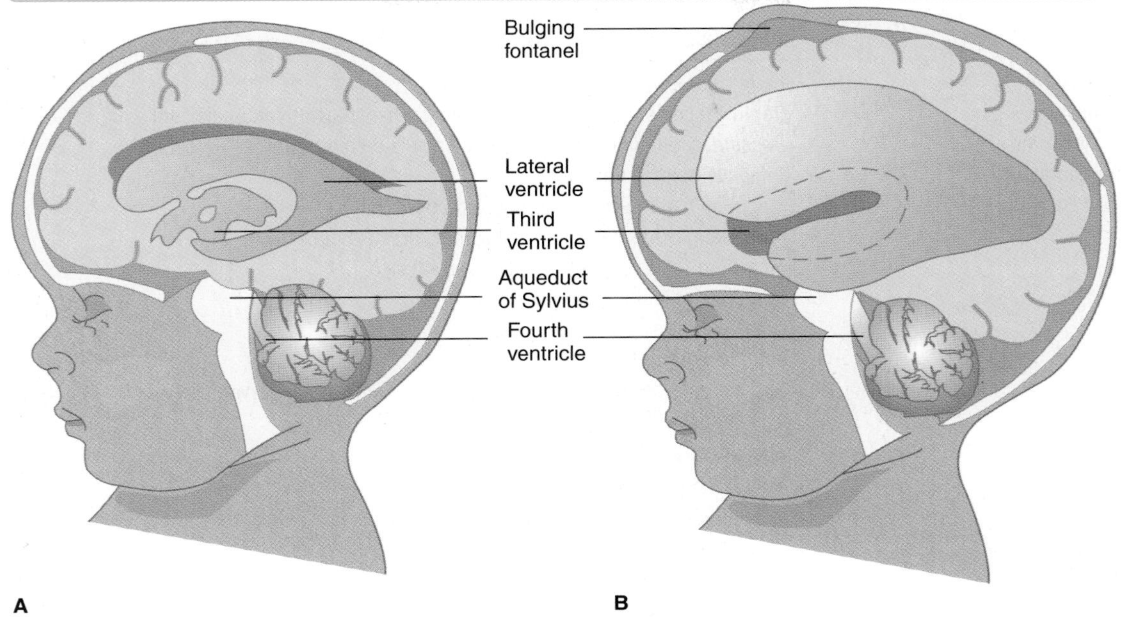

A, Normal size of ventricles. ***B,*** Enlarged ventricles, characteristic of hydrocephalus.

tural defects) that prevents CSF from entering the subarachnoid space (see "Pathophysiology Illustrated: Hydrocephalus"). Congenital structural defects include the Chiari II malformation (found in children with myelomeningocele), aqueduct of Sylvius stenosis, and the Dandy-Walker syndrome. Enlargement of one or more of the ventricles results.

The Chiari II malformation involves a downward displacement of the cerebellum, brainstem, and fourth ventricle and herniation through the foramen magnum into the cervical spaces. This displacement can cause sudden death, respiratory difficulty, swallowing difficulties, and the need for assisted ventilation. Rapid surgical decompression may be needed to reduce brainstem compression and to prevent death if the ventriculoperitoneal shunt does not resolve the problem (Warner, 2007).

Clinical Manifestations

The signs and symptoms of hydrocephalus vary with the age of the child (see "Clinical Manifestations: Hydrocephalus"). Infants have a rapidly increasing head circumference (Figure 56–7 ●). Older children show signs of increased ICP.

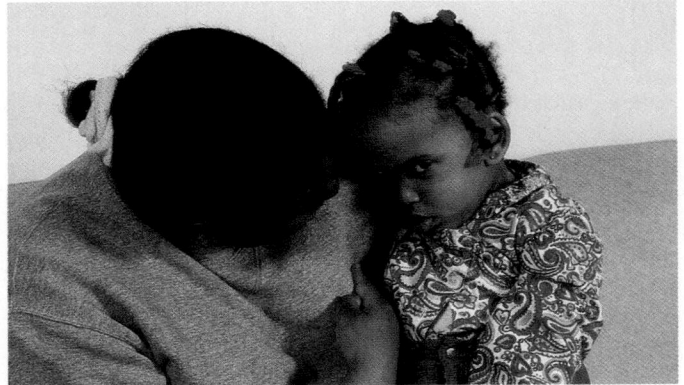

● **Figure 56–7** Hydrocephalus. In communicating hydrocephalus, an excessive amount of cerebrospinal fluid accumulates in the subarachnoid space, producing the characteristic head enlargement seen here. When observing the child with hydrocephalus, look for a downward deviation of the eyes in which the lower half of the iris is hidden by the lower eyelid (sunsetting eyes). This finding occurs in severe hydrocephalus, but is not present in this child.

Clinical Therapy

The diagnosis of hydrocephalus may be made prenatally by ultrasound or based on physical findings and neuroimaging studies after birth. Daily measurements of the head circumference are critical in any infant at risk of developing hydrocephalus. In children with closed sutures, signs of increased ICP are noted. CT and MRI imaging diagnose hydrocephalus, and in some cases reveal the anatomic cause. When the infant's fontanelle is still open, ultrasonography or echoencephalography may be used to confirm the diagnosis. CT and MRI imaging are also used to evaluate shunt failure.

Clinical therapy for hydrocephalus involves surgery to remove the obstruction (e.g., surgical removal of a tumor) or to place a shunt

Clinical Manifestations

HYDROCEPHALUS

CAUSE	CLINICAL MANIFESTATIONS
Congenital Structural Defect in Infancy Dandy-Walker syndrome Chiari II malformation Intraventricular hemorrhage	*Early signs* Rapidly increasing head circumference; tense, bulging fontanelle, split sutures *Bossing* (protrusion) of frontal area, face is disproportionate for skull size Difficulty holding head up Macewen's or "cracked-pot" sign with percussion Prominent, distended scalp veins, translucent scalp skin Increased tone or hyperreflexia, Babinski sign Irritability or lethargy, poor feeding Decline in level of consciousness *Late signs* Sunsetting eyes (sclera visible above iris), sixth cranial nerve palsy Apnea spells Shrill, high-pitched cry Difficulty swallowing or feeding; vomiting Cardiopulmonary depression (severe cases)
Acquired Hydrocephalus in Older Child after Closure of Sutures Postinfectious Tumor Hemorrhage	No head enlargement Signs of increased intracranial pressure Headache upon arising with vomiting Fussiness or irritability, sleepiness, confusion, lethargy, apathy, altered consciousness Personality change, loss of interest in daily activities Poor judgment or verbal incoherence, worsening school performance, memory loss Ataxia, spasticity, or other alterations in motor development Visual defects secondary to pressure on second, third, and sixth cranial nerves

in the ventricle to divert CSF to the peritoneal cavity, right atrium of the heart, or the pleural spaces of the lungs (Figure 56–8 ●). Shunt systems consist of four parts: a ventricular catheter, a pumping chamber or reservoir, a one-way pressure valve, and a distal catheter. Initial shunt placement is usually performed early in infancy. At this stage, adequate tubing is inserted to accommodate the child's growth and reduce the need for future surgery. Children with ventriculatrial shunts receive perioperative intravenous antibiotics to reduce the risk for infection (Chiafery, 2006).

Mechanical complications may include a blocked catheter, kinked tube, or valve breakdown. Infants or children with shunt failure show signs and symptoms of recurrent hydrocephalus and increased ICP. Shunt materials and systems continue to be refined in an attempt to reduce mechanical problems.

The most serious complication is shunt infection, most prevalent in the first 2 months after placement (Simpkins, 2005). Up to 12% of patients develop a shunt infection, and low birth weight infants have a higher risk (Chiafery, 2006). To confirm the infection, a CSF culture is obtained from the shunt reservoir located in a burr hole placed in the skull. Intravenous antibiotics are usually prescribed. The shunt is surgically removed, and an external drainage device is placed. A new shunt is inserted when the CSF cultures are sterile.

Endoscopic third ventriculoscopy (creating a CSF pathway around the obstruction) is an alternate surgical procedure for

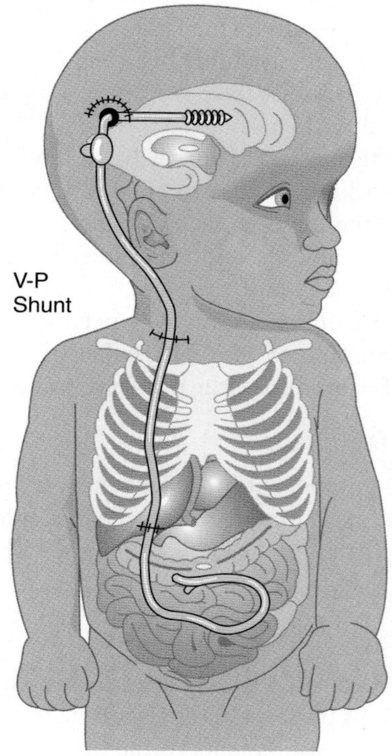

● **Figure 56–8** Ventriculoperitoneal shunt. A ventriculoperitoneal shunt, commonly used to treat children with hydrocephalus, is often placed at 3 to 4 months of age.

Nursing Practice

Some new shunt valves are programmable, enabling adjustment of pressure with the use of a magnet. Children must have these valves checked and reprogrammed to the correct pressure level after having an MRI diagnostic procedure. The valve should be checked regularly because exposure to other magnetic sources (e.g., telephone speakers and toy magnets) may affect pressure settings (Chiafery, 2006).

some patients with obstructive hydrocephalus from a tumor or aqueductal stenosis (Chiafery, 2006).

NURSING MANAGEMENT

NURSING ASSESSMENT AND DIAGNOSIS

Nurses should monitor all infants to ensure prompt identification and treatment of children with hydrocephalus. Measure the head circumference of all infants at each well-child visit and compare to prior measurements plotted on the growth curve (see Skill 9–5 SKILLS).

Assess the child with a ventriculoperitoneal shunt for signs and symptoms of shunt failure and infection. Signs of infection may include changes in responsiveness, irritability after fever is controlled, low-grade fever, malaise, headache, nausea, redness along the shunt device system, abdominal discomfort, or apnea. Measure the infant's head circumference daily and compare to prior measurements when shunt failure is suspected. Report any abnormalities to the physician immediately.

Nursing diagnoses that might be appropriate for the child with hydrocephalus include the following:

- *Risk for Infection* related to surgical procedure
- *Impaired Physical Mobility (Level 2)* related to insufficient muscle mass to lift the increased weight of head
- *Risk for Caregiver Role Strain* related to care of a child with a chronic condition or life-threatening illness
- *Risk for Delayed Development* related to repeated shunt infections and hospitalizations
- *Risk for Injury* related to potential shunt failure

PLANNING AND IMPLEMENTATION

Hospital-Based Nursing Care

Nursing care focuses on providing preoperative and postoperative care and providing emotional support.

Provide preoperative care. Position the infant carefully; do not stretch or strain the neck muscles, since they must support the large head. Holding the infant may be difficult because of the additional weight of the head. Provide good skin care. Reduce the risk for skin breakdown by placing sheepskin or a lamb's wool blanket under the head. Prevent any other complications associated with immobility (see page 1655). Attend to the child's special nutritional needs. Because the infant is prone to vomiting, frequent small feedings and frequent burping are beneficial.

Provide postoperative care. After surgery the child is usually placed in a flat position to prevent rapid CSF drainage. The head of the bed is elevated gradually over a day or two. Take vital signs every 2 to 4 hours. Monitor the child carefully for any signs of shunt malfunction, increased ICP, or infection.

Support the parents and explain the child's condition and all procedures to be performed. Encourage parents and family to help with the child's care in the hospital when appropriate. Be sympathetic and understanding, and allow parents to express their concerns. If hydrocephalus occurs during early infancy, the parents will be anxious about the impact of the chronic condition and subsequent surgical procedures. If hydrocephalus is secondary to neoplasm, however, the parents' anxieties are compounded by their child's life-threatening illness. Assure parents that most children with shunts lead normal lives, attending school and interacting with others no differently from their peers.

DISCHARGE PLANNING AND HOME CARE TEACHING

Identify and address home care needs well in advance of discharge. Parents must learn how to care for a child with a shunt. Educate parents and other family members about important signs and symptoms of shunt failure (signs of increased ICP) and infection (changes in responsiveness, irritability, malaise, headache, nausea, and low-grade fever). Provide the telephone numbers of health care providers, and reinforce the need to contact a physician immediately if a problem with the shunt is suspected. Inform parents that the child may develop a seizure disorder (or seizure characteristics may change in a child with seizures), and teach them how to care for the child if a seizure occurs. Refer families to the appropriate home care, social services, and support groups such as the Hydrocephalus Association. (See the Companion Website for links to such resources.)

NURSING CARE IN THE COMMUNITY

Infants and children need frequent monitoring to ensure proper shunt functioning. Head circumference is measured at each visit to monitor growth. Assess the child for visual problems and cognitive, speech, and motor developmental delays. Refer the child and family to an early intervention program to promote developmental progress. School-age children may need an IEP (see Chapter 40∞). See MyNursingKit for a Web site with information on hydrocephalus.

Encourage parents to promote optimal health status by providing good nutrition and reducing exposure to infections. Encourage parents to use a child care setting with a small number of children, such as family or home-based child care, to decrease exposure to infection. Encourage good hand hygiene by all caregivers.

Constipation that increases abdominal pressure may interfere with CSF drainage through the ventriculoperitoneal shunt.

Parents should monitor the child's bowel pattern and implement dietary changes and occasional laxatives to promote regular bowel movements (Chiafery, 2006).

Teach parents to protect the infant from injury. Do not place infants with poor head control and an enlarged head in forward-facing car safety seats, regardless of their age. This position increases their risk of cervical spine injury and death in a car crash. Participation in sports with a high potential for head and abdominal impact should be discouraged, although other sports should be encouraged.

EVALUATION

Expected outcomes of nursing care include the following:

- The infant develops adequate neck muscle control to interact with the environment.
- Shunt infections and malfunctions are rapidly identified by the parents, and medical attention is sought quickly.
- The child's potential for growth and development is maximized by care and a stimulating environment.

NEURAL TUBE DEFECTS

The neural tube is the tissue that ultimately develops into the CNS, including the brain and spinal cord. The incidence of neural tube defects is 0.7 to 1 per 1000 live births in the United States (Padgett, 2006). Neural tube defects include the following:

- *Anencephaly*—The brain does not develop above the brainstem.
- *Encephalocele*—A protrusion of meningeal tissue or meningeal-covered brain is observed through a defect in the skull.
- *Spina bifida occulta*—The posterior vertebral arches fail to fuse, most commonly at the fifth lumbar or first sacral vertebrae. The spinal cord and meninges lie entirely within the vertebral canal. A tuft of hair, a dermoid cyst, or hemangioma may be found over the site.
- *Spina bifida cystica*—A posterior vertebral arch defect is observed with protrusion through the bony spine.
- *Meningocele*—A spinal fluid–filled meningeal sac protrudes through a vertebral defect without abnormalities of the spinal cord. The sac may be translucent or membranous. The spinal cord and spinal root are in normal position.
- *Myelodysplasia (spina bifida or meningomyelocele)*—A spinal fluid–filled meningeal sac contains a portion of the meninges, spinal cord, or nerve roots that protrude through a vertebral defect. Fluid leakage may also occur as the lesion is poorly covered with imperfect tissue.

MyNursingKit Video: Living with Spina Bifida

MYELODYSPLASIA (SPINA BIFIDA)

Myelodysplasia (sometimes called spina bifida or meningomyelocele) refers to a malformation of the spinal cord and spinal canal. One or more defective vertebrae allow spinal cord contents to protrude. The malformation can occur anywhere along the vertebral column, but is most common at the lumbar or sacral portion of the spine.

Nursing Practice

All women of childbearing age should take 400 mcg of folic acid daily (Brand, 2006). Mandatory fortification of all enriched grain products with folate in 1998 resulted in a significant reduction in spina bifida and anencephaly (Williams, Rasmussen, Flores, et al., 2005).

This is the most common developmental disorder of the CNS. The condition occurs in about 0.4 to 1.43 per 1000 live births in the United States (Dias, 2005). The highest rates occur in Hispanics while Asians have the lowest rates (Brand, 2006). Blacks have a lower rate than whites (Dias, 2005).

Etiology and Pathophysiology

The cause of spina bifida is unknown, although environmental factors have been implicated, such as chemicals (excessive use of alcohol), medications (e.g., valproic acid and carbamazepine used for seizures, isotretinoin for acne), genetic factors, and maternal health conditions (diabetes mellitus, gestational diabetes, folic acid deficiency, and maternal obesity). The increased incidence of the condition in families points to a possible genetic influence.

Clinical Manifestations

A saclike protrusion on the infant's back indicates meningocele or myelodysplasia (Figure 56–9 ●). The clinical manifestations (paralysis, weakness, and sensory loss) depend on the location of

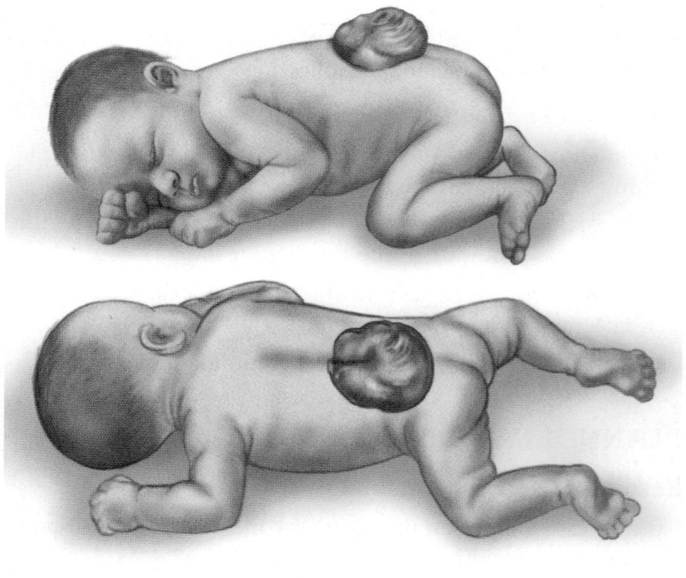

● **Figure 56–9** Lumbosacral myelomeningocele. Lumbosacral myelomeningocele is caused by a neural tube defect that results in incomplete closure of the vertebral column. As shown here, the meninges (and sometimes the spinal cord) protrude as a saclike structure. Observe for leakage of cerebrospinal fluid.

the defect. The higher the defect on the spinal cord, the greater the neurologic dysfunction:

- Thoracic or lumbar 1–2 level—paralysis of the legs; weakness and sensory loss in the trunk and lower body region.
- Lumbar 3 level—can flex hips and extend the knees; paralyzed ankles and toes.
- Lumbar 4–5 level—can flex hips and extend the knees; weak or absent ankle extension, toe flexion, and hip extension.
- Sacral level—mild weakness in ankles and toes; bladder and bowel function may be affected.

Sensory loss is more pronounced on the back of the legs, and the loss of lower extremity motor and sensory functioning may not be symmetric.

Bowel and bladder sphincters may be affected. Renal damage may result from neurologic impairment and urinary retention (neurogenic bladder). Hydrocephalus is usually present in children with a myelomeningocele defect above the sacral level because of the Chiari II malformation. The range of potential problems for the child with spina bifida is listed in "Clinical Manifestations: Myelodysplasia."

Clinical Therapy

Diagnosis is usually made by fetal ultrasound, but it is not until after birth that the lesion is examined and the neurologic status is evaluated. Radiologic imaging by ultrasonography, CT scan, MRI, and flat films of the spinal column can pinpoint the bony defect. Subsequent testing is performed to evaluate bowel and bladder function, neurologic and motor function, and cognitive function.

Surgery to close and repair the lesion usually occurs within 24 to 48 hours of the infant's birth to reduce infection. In some cases, a repair is performed on the fetus in utero.

Braces are used to support joint position and mobility. Assistive devices such as walkers, crutches, and wheelchairs are used to enhance mobility. To minimize the risk for osteoporosis, the diet should ensure adequate calcium and vitamin D, and weight-bearing activities should be encouraged. Acquired scoliosis may be a sign of a tethered cord, hydromyelia (expansion of the central canal of the spinal cord with increased CSF accumulation), or shunt failure. Surgery to address these problems may improve the scoliosis (Rowe & Jadhav, 2008).

Interventions for a neurogenic bladder are initiated early to prevent kidney damage, to maintain bladder function, and to promote urinary continence. Clean intermittent catheterization is performed on a regular schedule (every 3 to 4 hours) (see Chapter 54∞). A Mitrofanoff procedure that creates a reservoir for urine and a stoma for catheterization in the umbilicus may be performed.

Dietary fiber, stool softeners and glycerin or bisacodyl suppositories are prescribed for bowel evacuation and to promote bowel continence. Surgery to create a channel between the skin and bowel using the appendix (Malone antegrade continence enema) is often performed in older children. This procedure enables a child or adolescent to infuse an enema into the ascending and transverse colon to promote bowel evacuation (Doolin, 2006).

Prognosis depends on the type of defect, the level of the lesion, and other complicating factors. Children need multiple surgeries and invasive procedures. A team of physicians, nurses, and therapists from the neurosurgery, orthopedic, urology, and physical medicine departments work with the child and family to form a comprehensive care plan.

Clinical Manifestations

MYELODYSPLASIA

CAUSE	CLINICAL MANIFESTATIONS
Interruption of the spinal cord at site of the spinal defect	Loss of motor and sensory function of the abdomen and lower extremities, dependent on defect level Scoliosis or kyphosis Incontinence of urine or urinary retention Incontinence of feces or constipation Sensory loss around genitalia
Muscle imbalance	Hip abnormalities, hip dysplasia Foot deformities (e.g., clubfoot)
Chiari II malformation	Hydrocephalus **Infants:** Difficulty swallowing Apnea, respiratory difficulty, inspiratory stridor Weak or poor cry **Older children:** Choking, hoarseness, vocal cord paralysis Disordered breathing during sleep; breath-holding episodes Aspiration Stiffness or spasticity of arms and hands
Brain and spinal cord abnormalities	Learning problems, attention deficit disorder Problems with perceptual motor skills Memory and organization problems Problems with numerical reasoning

NURSING MANAGEMENT

HOSPITAL-BASED NURSING CARE

Nursing care focuses on providing preoperative and postoperative care, promoting mobility, and providing emotional support.

Cover the sac with a sterile saline dressing to protect its integrity, and monitor for CSF leakage and signs of infection.

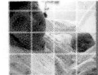

Nursing Practice

More than half of children with myelodysplasia develop a latex allergy, and the risk increases as the child ages (Liptak, 2007) (see Chapter 50). All children with latex allergy need to carry a kit with premeasured epinephrine for emergency treatment of anaphylaxis. Use nonlatex materials when providing care to the child in all settings. The Spina Bifida Association maintains an updated list of products containing latex and potential substitutes (see also Table 50–10). See MyNursingKit for links to such resources.

Maintain the newborn in a prone position with hips slightly flexed and legs abducted to minimize tension on the sac. Assess the infant's vital signs and intake and output. Evaluate the newborn for motor deficits as well as bladder and bowel involvement.

Following surgery, monitor the infant's vital signs carefully. Watch closely for symptoms of infection, especially meningitis. If a ventriculoperitoneal shunt was placed, watch for signs of hydrocephalus, increased ICP, or infection. Inspect the surgical site for CSF leakage. The infant should be placed in a prone or side-lying position for sleep until healing has occurred (despite guidelines to put infants to sleep on their backs), and then supine position for sleep may be used. Keep the diaper away from the incision site.

Begin gentle range of motion exercises as soon as possible to prevent muscle contractures and atrophy. Extreme caution should be used because these children have brittle bones that fracture easily. Splints may be used to maintain extremity alignment.

Support the parents by keeping them informed about their child's status. Allow them to express their frustrations and anger. As soon as parents are able to cope with the child's condition, encourage them to become involved in the child's care in the hospital.

The child with myelodysplasia may be hospitalized for surgery numerous times to correct deformities. Assess the child's vital signs, responsiveness, and level of pain. Because the child may have decreased pain sensation in the lower extremities, careful assessment is needed. Assess dressing sites for bleeding and drainage. Monitor the distal extremities for swelling and circulation.

DISCHARGE PLANNING AND HOME CARE TEACHING

Address home care needs well in advance of discharge. Help parents obtain special devices such as splints, wedges, and rolls, if needed, to prevent complications. Instruct parents how to position, handle, and feed the infant, and to perform range of motion exercises. Teach parents to perform intermittent clean catheterization and establish a schedule for catheterization every 3 to 4 hours. See Skill 10–10 SKILLS.

Teach parents the symptoms of increased ICP, hydrocephalus, shunt infection or malfunction, and urinary tract infection. Arrange for home care nursing or a case manager, if needed. The home care nurse reinforces the skills learned in the hospital and the case manager helps coordinate the child's care with numerous healthcare professionals. Refer parents to resource groups such as the Spina Bifida Association of America. See MyNursingKit for Web sites with information on myelodysplasia.

NURSING CARE IN THE COMMUNITY

To reduce complications and promote optimal development, children with myelodysplasia need comprehensive care planned and coordinated by a knowledgeable team of healthcare professionals. This care may be provided in partnership with the primary care physician.

At an appropriate age, teach the child to perform intermittent self-catheterization. If the child has a Mitrofanoff procedure performed, monitor for any signs that the stoma is becoming stenosed. If stenosis occurs, dilatation can be performed and prevent the need for surgical revision of the stoma (Gray, Blackinton, & White, 2006). When the child begins school, an Individualized Health Plan should be developed so the child has access to the restroom, assistance as needed for toileting, and accommodations for mobility challenges.

Good nutrition planning is important to prevent obesity and to reduce constipation and fecal impaction. Bowel training is initiated to control bowel evacuation. A diet high in fiber helps ensure adequate stool. A glycerin or bisacodyl suppository can be given to promote bowel evacuation at the appropriate time of day.

Promote safety and independent mobility with proper use of braces, walkers, crutches, canes, and in some cases custom-designed wheelchairs and car safety seats (Figure 56–10 ●). For other safety guidelines, see "Teaching Highlights: Safety for the Child with Spina Bifida."

Parents are faced with the long-term financial issues as the child regularly needs medical supplies as well as new adaptive

Nursing Practice

The child who has clean intermittent catheterization performed usually has bacteria in the urine. Unless the child is symptomatic (e.g., foul odor or discharge, a change in mood or personality, or fatigue) no treatment is usually provided (Gray et al., 2006).

Growth and Development

Treat older children according to their intellectual level, not their motor development. Encourage them to take responsibility for self-care, and recognize their need to control their body functions. Monitor adolescents for mental health problems, especially as differences from peers and challenges in lifestyle become of greater concern. Refer for counseling as needed.

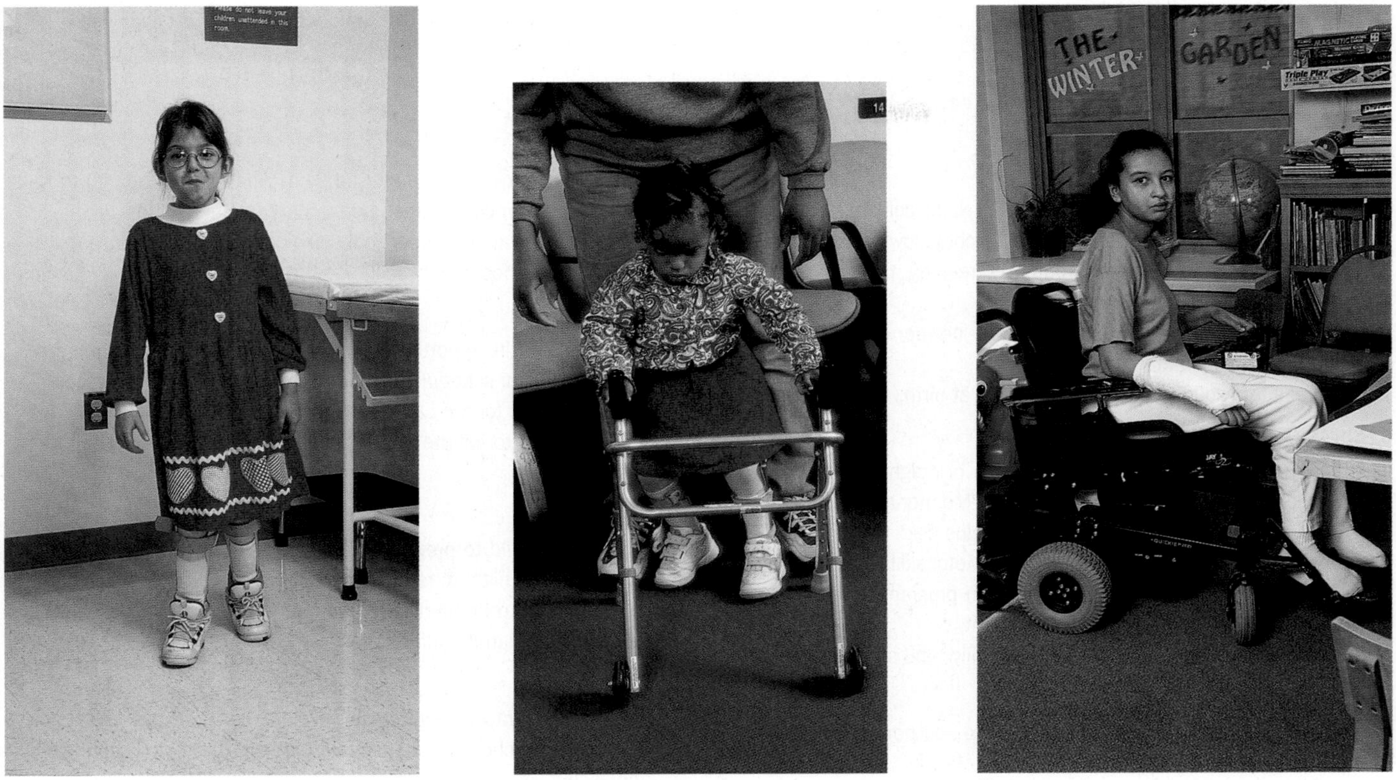

A B C

● **Figure 56–10** Promoting mobility. Help determine the best assistive device for the child to gain the most independence for mobilizing and to promote development. The child may change devices in different settings to promote optimal independence. ***A*** and ***B,*** Braces and walkers may be best for young children to promote an upright posture that encourages a normal interaction with the environment. ***C,*** A motorized wheelchair can assist the child with a significant neurologic impairment to achieve independence and mobility.

Teaching Highlights

SAFETY FOR THE CHILD WITH SPINA BIFIDA

Due to the loss of sensation in the lower extremities, injuries to the skin may not be immediately noticed by the child. Several routine actions will help reduce the risk for injury.

- Perform a daily check of all skin surfaces and pressure points associated with sitting, braces, and shoes to identify abrasions, scrapes, reddened areas, and other lesions. Stop using the braces or shoes until the skin heals or redness disappears.
- Keep all skin surfaces clean and dry. Wear socks under braces.
- Use a gel-filled cushion in the wheelchair, and teach the child to shift positions hourly to prevent pressure sores.
- Avoid burns to the lower extremities by checking the temperature of bath water and car safety seats in a hot car.
- Teach parents how to avoid the use of latex products and to inform all healthcare providers about the child's latex allergy or risk.
- Use safe ambulation techniques with walkers, canes, and crutches.

equipment as the child grows. At least 75% of children born with spina bifida survive to at least the early adult years (Nehring & Faux, 2006). Parents thus need to learn how to act as the child's case manager to promote the child's health, or to work effectively with the child's case manager. See Health Promotion and Maintenance.

CRANIOSYNOSTOSIS

Craniosynostosis is the premature closure of cranial sutures during the first 18 months of life. This condition occurs in 1 per 2100 live births, and boys are affected twice as often as girls (Padgett, 2006). Genetic syndromes (Alpert and Crouzon) account for 10% to 20% of cases (Kinsman & Johnston, 2007).

The cause of craniosynostosis is unknown. When one or more sutures closes too early, bone growth continues in a direction parallel to the suture line, leading to compensatory overgrowth at normal suture lines and classic skull deformities (Figure 56–11 ●). Sagittal synostosis (scaphocephaly) accounts for 40% to 60% of cases (Komotar, Zacharia, Ellis, et al., 2006). Bicoronal synostosis is associated with Alpert or Crouzon syndromes.

Positional *plagiocephaly* (a totally flat occiput) and *brachycephaly* are seen increasingly in healthy infants put to sleep on their backs to prevent sudden infant death syndrome. Since

HEALTH PROMOTION

THE CHILD WITH MYELODYSPLASIA

Preventive Health Care

- Provide all recommended immunizations. If the child has a seizure disorder, alert parents that seizures may occur following immunizations.
- Perform all recommended routine screening procedures (vision, hearing, hematocrit, blood pressure).
- Obtain a urinalysis with culture in the newborn period and when signs of infection are noted.
- Screen for scoliosis annually beginning at birth.

Growth and Development Surveillance

- Monitor the growth of the child (length or height, weight, head circumference) and plot on growth curves. Monitor head circumference growth carefully because of hydrocephalus risk.
- Assess developmental status regularly. Motor skills are often delayed.
- Enroll the infant in an early intervention program to assist the parents to promote the child's development.
- Promote gradual independence in mobility and self-care.

Nutrition

- Teach families appropriate caloric intake and portion control for the child at each age to reduce the risk for obesity.
- Provide guidance about increased fluids and fiber in the diet to reduce the risk for constipation and urinary tract infections.
- Alert parents that allergies to foods like bananas, avocados, papaya, kiwi, and other foods may occur.

Elimination

- Teach families the importance of performing intermittent catheterization on a regular schedule. Teach the child to perform self-catheterization and care for the catheter in preparation for school entry.
- Teach families to initiate bowel training so that a bowel regimen is established.

Sleep and Rest

- Position the child to prevent contractures. Change the child's position during the night to reduce pressure over skin surfaces.
- Teach parents to be alert for apnea spells or snoring that could be related to a Chiari II malformation.

Relationships

- Encourage interaction with peers.
- Be alert for psychosocial adjustment problems, especially during the adolescent years.

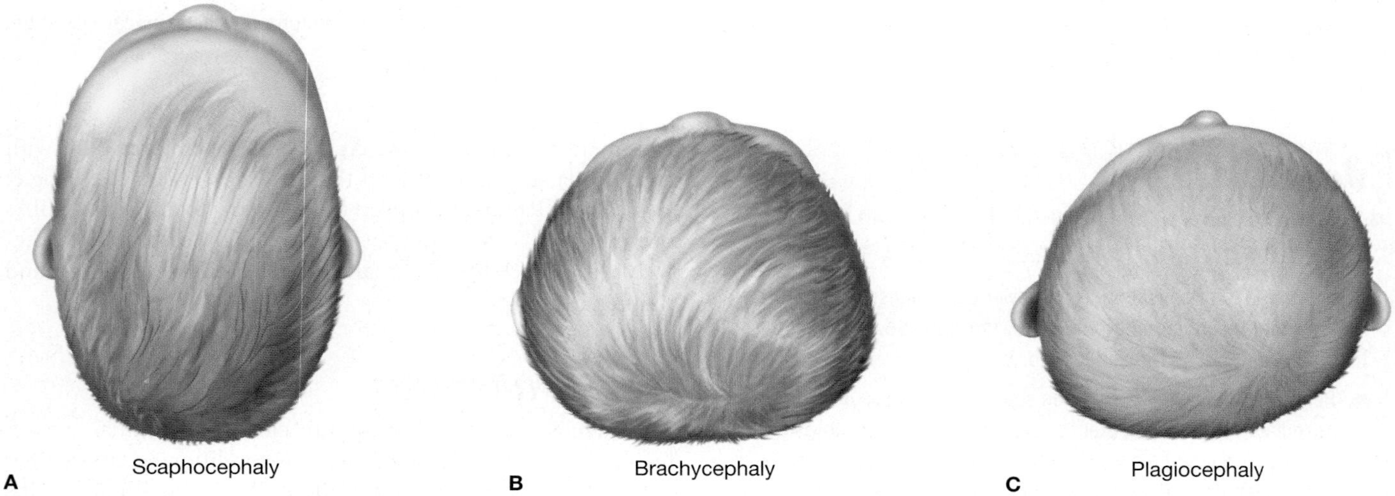

● **Figure 56–11** Craniosynostosis. In craniosynostosis, the head shape is dependent on which sutures are involved. ***A,*** Scaphocephaly, premature closure of the sagittal suture causes a long, narrow skull, flattened parietal bones with a prominent occiput, a broad forehead, and a small or absent anterior fontanel. ***B,*** Brachycephaly, premature closure of the bicoronal suture causes a head shape shortened anterior to posterior, and the occiput is flattened. ***C,*** Positional plagiocephaly is often asymmetric flattening of the occiput due to preferred sleep position when supine or due to torticollis.

the infant's sleep position does not change, the weight of the head flattens the skull. Congenital torticollis may also contribute to a position preference when supine. It is speculated that infants who develop these skull shapes do not have enough supervised tummy time that helps correct positional preference (Graham, Kreutzman, Earl, et al., 2005).

Diagnosis of craniosynostosis is made by clinical appearance and measurement of the skull with metal calipers. Skull radiographs and CT or MRI imaging confirm the diagnosis. The hands and feet should be carefully examined to detect any skeletal defect that might help identify a syndrome (Kinsman & Johnston, 2007).

Nursing Practice

Encourage parents to try to reduce the infant's preference for lying supine in one position. One strategy is to rotate the crib every day so the infant must turn his or her head in a different direction to look at who comes into the room. Rotate the arm used for formula feeding the infant. When the child is alert and can be continuously supervised, place the infant in prone position on the floor for short periods to promote neck muscle strength and interaction with nearby objects.

Reconstructive surgery of the skull, the most common form of treatment, is performed to protect brain development and vision, and to improve cosmetic appearance. Many children need multiple procedures. Children having surgery before 1 year of age have a better outcome.

Nursing Management

After surgery, keep the incision dry and intact. Observe the child for symptoms of increased ICP (see Table 56–1). A special molding helmet may be used after surgery to promote proper cranial growth. Explain to parents that surgery will improve the child's appearance. Assure them that most children with craniosynostosis are healthy, and that their brains develop normally.

In cases of severe positional plagiocephaly or brachycephaly a helmet device to correct the condition is most effective when treatment is initiated at 6 months of age when the skull bones are most malleable. The helmet is worn for 23 hours a day for 3 months. Remolding of the head shape continues naturally after that treatment period because the infant spends more time awake and upright. Younger infants may be successfully treated with positioning and physical therapy for torticollis (Graham, Gomez, Halberg, et al., 2005).

NEUROFIBROMATOSIS

Neurofibromatosis 1 (NF1), or von Recklinghausen disease, is an autosomal dominant genetic disorder in which tumors grow along nerves. One in 3500 individuals develops the disorder, and more than half of new cases result from a mutation (Hart, 2005; Theos & Korf, 2006).

The NF1 gene is located on chromosome 17. Neurofibromas develop from cells of the nerve sheath, usually along the peripheral nerves or at nerve endings. The neurofibroma may be an isolated growth, or extend along the length of a nerve and include nerve branches (plexiform neurofibroma). Dermal neurofibromas, which usually begin to appear around the time of puberty, may reside in the skin or project above the skin surface. Neurofibromas may also develop on spinal nerve roots in the central nervous system. Children with NF1 may be at risk for leukemia, rhabdomyosarcoma, and pheochromocytoma (Theos & Korf, 2006).

The disorder is characterized by six or more café-au-lait spots (darker than surrounding skin) 5 mm in diameter or larger seen at birth or by 2 years of age. The spots grow to 15 mm or larger by adulthood. Freckling in the axillary and inguinal areas is common. Multiple neurofibromas or benign tumors grow on or under the skin beginning during puberty. Pain may occur when a tumor compresses a nerve or grows in the spinal cord. Lisch nodules, tan or brown benign tumors on the iris of the eye, are characteristic. Vision deficits or blindness is found in 20% of children due to a tumor along the optic pathway. Precocious puberty or delayed puberty and menarche may occur when the optic tumor invades the hypothalamus. Other manifestations include hyperactivity, learning disabilities, speech problems, seizures, scoliosis, and thinning or bowing of the tibia.

Diagnosis is made in early childhood by the presence of characteristic physical findings (café-au-lait spots, Lisch nodules, small skin tumors), and a positive family history. Radiologic imaging (MRI of brain and radiographs of the spine and other bones) is performed when problems are detected. Ophthalmologic examinations should be performed at least annually. Clinical therapy focuses on monitoring the child for signs of problems associated with the condition. When neurofibromas are disfiguring or cause problems because of their location, surgery may be performed to remove the tumor.

Nursing Management

Nurses assess the child for signs of neurofibromatosis. Monitor the blood pressure as renal vascular stenosis or pheochromocytoma may cause hypertension. Pay attention to any mass that is rapidly enlarging or causing new pain.

Provide psychologic support to the child and family. As tumor development increases during adolescence, problems with self-image and self-esteem are common. Adolescents may fear the response of peers to the tumors and isolate themselves. Identify potential peers or refer the adolescent to a support group.

CEREBRAL PALSY

Cerebral palsy (CP) is a group of permanent disorders of movement and posture development causing activity limitation. It results from a nonprogressive disturbance that occurred in the fetal or infant brain. CP is primarily a motor disorder, but the child may also have sensory, perceptual, cognitive, communicative, and behavioral problems (Rosenbaum, Paneth, Leviton, et al., 2007). CP occurs in 1.5 to 2 cases per 1000 live births (Jones, Morgan, & Shelton, 2007a). Four types of motor dysfunction are seen with cerebral palsy—spastic, dyskinetic, ataxic, and mixed—related to the location of brain insult.

ETIOLOGY AND PATHOPHYSIOLOGY

Most CP cases are caused by brain insult (complications of prematurity, prenatal, perinatal, and genetic factors, or fetal viral infection). Injury to the immature periventricular white matter in the fetus or premature infant is thought to be the most common cause (Johnston, Ferriero, Vannucci, et al., 2005). The rate of CP increases with decreasing gestational age and in premature infants with intraventricular hemorrhage (Rais-Bahrami & Short, 2007). An estimated 6% to 7% of CP cases are associated with birth asphyxia (Nield, Nanda, Someshwar, et al., 2007). After birth, risk factors for CP include neonatal sepsis and hyperbilirubinemia, as well as CNS infection, and brain injury in children under 2 years.

CLINICAL MANIFESTATIONS

Cerebral palsy is characterized by abnormal muscle tone and lack of coordination:

- Hypotonia—floppiness, increased range of motion, diminished reflex response
- Rigidity—hypertonia with tense, tight muscles
- Spasticity—hypertonia with uncoordinated, awkward, stiff movements; scissoring or crossing of the legs; exaggerated reflex reactions; found in majority of cases
- Athetosis—constant involuntary writhing motions; more severe distally
- Ataxia—irregularity in muscle coordination or action
- Hemiplegia—involvement of one side of the body; upper extremities are more dysfunctional than lower extremities
- Diplegia—involvement of all extremities, lower extremities are more affected than upper; usually spastic
- Quadriplegia—involvement of all extremities; arms in flexion and legs in extension

Symptoms vary depending on the child's age, the area of the brain involved, and degree of brain injury. See "Clinical Manifestations: Cerebral Palsy by Type of Insult." Children with CP usually have delayed developmental milestones. Other common disabilities include mental retardation and epilepsy, as well as vision, hearing, language, cognitive, and behavior problems. Feeding and speech may be difficult because of oral motor involvement.

CLINICAL THERAPY

Diagnosis is usually based on clinical findings. CP is difficult to diagnose in the early months of life. Many children with delayed developmental milestones or neuromuscular abnormalities at 1 year of age continue to show gradual improvement in function. CP must be distinguished from other neurologic conditions, and signs may be subtle. Suspicious historical findings include a premature infant (less than 1500 g birth weight or less than 28 weeks' gestation), maternal intrauterine infection, multiple birth, or anoxic event (Pellegrino, 2007).

Ultrasonography can be used to detect fetal and neonatal abnormalities of the brain, such as intraventricular hemorrhage.

Clinical Manifestations

CEREBRAL PALSY BY TYPE OF INSULT

CLASSIFICATION AND TYPE OF INSULT	CLINICAL MANIFESTATIONS
Spastic	Persistent hypertonia, rigidity related to location of brain damage
Cerebral cortex or pyramidal tract injury 75% of cases	Exaggerated deep tendon reflexes Persistent primitive reflexes Leads to contractures and abnormal curvature of the spine
Dyskinetic	Abnormalities of muscle tone that affect the entire body
Extrapyramidal, basal ganglia injury 10% to 15% of cases	Inconsistent muscle tone, may change hour to hour or day to day, may have rigid muscle tone when awake and normal or decreased muscle tone when asleep Involuntary movements Tremors, difficulty with fine and purposeful motor movements Exaggerated posturing
Ataxic Cerebellar (extrapyramidal) injury 5% to 10% of cases	Abnormalities of voluntary movement involving balance and position of the trunk and limbs Difficulty controlling hand and arm movements during reaching (overshooting or past-pointing) Increased or decreased muscle tone Hypotonia in infancy Muscle instability and wide-based unsteady gait
Mixed	No dominant motor pattern
Injuries to multiple areas	Unique compensatory movements and posture to maintain control over specific neuromotor deficits Combination of characteristics from other types

Neuromotor tests are used to evaluate the presence of normal movement patterns, absence of primitive reflexes, and abnormal tone. Once CP is suspected, CT and MRI imaging provide information about anatomic structures and help identify the cause of CP. Positron emission tomography (PET) or single photon emission computed tomography (SPECT) may provide information about brain metabolic functioning (Pellegrino, 2007).

Clinical therapy focuses on helping the child develop to a maximum level of independence. Referrals are made for physical, occupational, and speech therapy, as well as special education to improve motor function and ability. Braces and splints, serial casting, and positioning devices (prone wedges, standers, and side-lyers) are used to promote range of motion, skeletal alignment, stability, control of involuntary movements, and prevent contractures.

Surgical interventions may be required to improve function by balancing muscle power and stabilizing uncontrollable joints, e.g., an Achilles tendon lengthening to increase the ankle range of motion or releasing the hamstrings to correct knee flexion contractures. A dorsal rhizotomy may be performed for spastic diplegia to cut the afferent fibers that contribute to spasticity; however, some muscle weakness may result from the procedure (Pelligrino, 2007).

Medications are given to control seizures, to control spasms (skeletal muscle relaxants, baclofen, and benzodiazepines), and to minimize gastrointestinal side effects (cimetidine or ranitidine). Benzodiazopines affect brain control of muscle tone to help control spasticity. Dantrolene is a calcium channel blocker that inhibits muscle contraction. Baclofen is administered orally or by intrathecal pump to decrease spasticity. See Figure 56–12 ●. Botulinum toxin injection into specific muscles is a relatively new therapy that helps to temporarily control spasticity.

The prognosis for infants and children with CP depends on the level of motor disability and on the presence of intellectual, visual, or hearing deficits. Early intervention programs can help improve performance. Many children with hemiplegia or ataxia show some improvement with maturation and are able to ambulate. Others need assistance with mobility and activities of daily living.

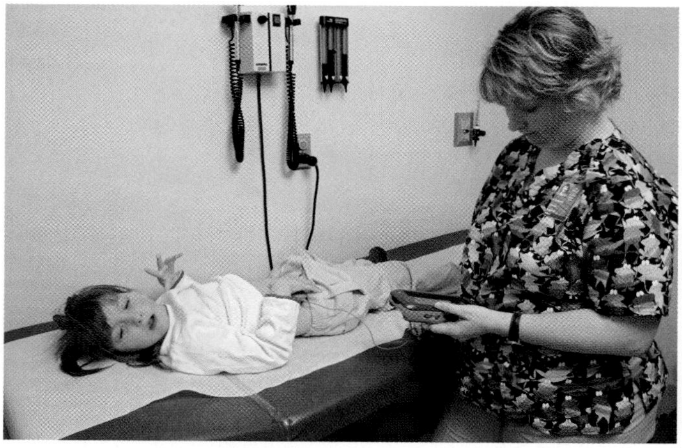

● **Figure 56–12** Baclofen by intrathecal pump. A child having a baclofen pump filled.

NURSING MANAGEMENT

NURSING ASSESSMENT AND DIAGNOSIS

Be alert for children whose histories indicate an increased risk for CP. Assess all children at each healthcare visit for developmental delays. Note any orthopedic, visual, auditory, or intellectual deficits. When an infant's primitive reflexes persist beyond the normal age refer for further evaluation (see Chapter 28∞). Identify infants who appear to have an abnormal muscle tone or abnormal posture (head lag beyond 6 months of age, arched back, poor trunk control and balance, toe walking or scissoring) (Jones et al., 2007a). Asymmetric or abnormal crawling by using 2 or 3 extremities and hand dominance prior to 18 months of age indicates a motor problem. A simple screening test involves placing a clean cloth on the infant's face. Infants normally use two hands to remove it, but the infant at risk for CP uses one hand or does not remove the cloth. Record dietary intake as well as height and weight percentiles for children suspected to have or diagnosed with the condition.

Nursing diagnoses for the child with CP often vary by the type of CP, the child's symptoms and age, and the family situation. The "Nursing Care Plan: The Child with Cerebral Palsy" includes several nursing diagnoses. Additional nursing diagnoses might include the following:

- *Risk for Constipation* related to low intake of fiber and fluids and insufficient physical activity
- *Impaired Tissue Integrity* related to decreased physical mobility and limited self-care ability
- *Impaired Verbal Communication* related to hearing and/or speech impairment
- *Chronic Pain* related to spasticity and stretching exercises to prevent contractures
- *Delayed Growth and Development* related to lack of muscle strength or limited social interaction

PLANNING AND IMPLEMENTATION

The accompanying Nursing Care Plan summarizes care for the child with CP. Since the condition varies in severity and manifestations, interventions need to be customized to the child and family. Nursing care focuses on providing adequate nutrition, maintaining skin integrity, promoting physical mobility, promoting safety, promoting growth and development, teaching parents how to care for the child, and providing emotional support.

PROVIDE ADEQUATE NUTRITION

Children with CP require high-calorie diets because of feeding difficulties associated with spasticity. Many children have difficulty chewing and swallowing. Give the child small amounts of soft foods at a time. Utensils with large, padded handles may be easier for the child to use. Make sure the child gets adequate fluids as the child may not be able to communicate thirst. Children with severe CP may need a gastrostomy tube to obtain adequate nutrition. Adequate fiber is needed to prevent constipation, and

(continues on page 1686)

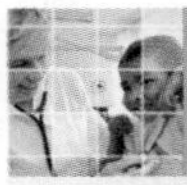

Nursing Care Plan

THE CHILD WITH CEREBRAL PALSY

INTERVENTION	RATIONALE	EXPECTED OUTCOME
1. Nursing Diagnosis: Impaired Physical Mobility related to decreased muscle strength and control		
NIC Priority Intervention:		**NOC Suggested Outcome:**
Exercise therapy, joint mobility: Use of active and passive body movement to maintain joint flexibility		**Joint movement—active:** Range of motion of joints with self-initiated movement
Goal: The child will attain maximum physical abilities possible.		
■ Perform development assessment and record age of milestones achieved (e.g., reaching for objects, sitting).	■ Delayed development milestones are common with CP. As one milestone is achieved, interventions are revised to focus on the next skill.	The child reaches maximum physical mobility and all developmental milestones.
■ Plan activities to use gross and fine motor skills (e.g., holding eating utensils, toys positioned to encourage reaching).	■ Many activities of daily living and play activities promote physical development.	
■ Allow time for the child to complete activities.	■ The child may perform tasks more slowly than most children.	
■ Perform range of motion exercises every 4 hours for the child unable to move body parts. Position the child to promote tendon stretching (e.g., foot plantar flexion, legs extended at the knees and hips).	■ Exercises and positioning promote mobility and increased circulation, and decreases the risk of contractures.	
■ Arrange for and encourage parents to keep appointments with a rehabilitation therapist.	■ A regular and frequently reevaluated rehabilitation program assists in promoting development.	
■ Teach the family to maintain appropriate brace wear.	■ Adaptive devices are often necessary to maximize physical mobility.	
2. Nursing Diagnosis: Disturbed Sensory Perception (Visual or Auditory) related to cerebral damage		
NIC Priority Intervention:		**NOC Suggested Outcome:**
Communication enhancement: Visual deficit: Assistance with accepting or learning alternative methods for living with diminished vision		**Sensory function: Vision:** Extent to which visual images are sensed, with and without assistive devices
Goal: The child will receive and benefit from varied forms of sensory and perceptual input.		
■ Facilitate vision examinations by specialist. Promote the use of glasses or contact lens and encourage recommended return visits to specialists.	■ Corrective lenses enhance sensory input. Regular vision assessment may identify lens prescription changes.	The child receives adequate visual sensory/perceptual input to maximize developmental outcome.
3. Nursing Diagnosis: Imbalanced Nutrition: Less than Body Requirements related to difficulty in chewing and swallowing and high metabolic needs		
NIC Priority Intervention:		**NOC Suggested Outcome:**
Nutrition management: Assistance with or provision of a balanced dietary intake of foods and fluids		**Nutritional status: Nutrient intake:** Adequacy of nutrients taken into body
Goal: The child will receive nutrients needed for normal growth.		

Nursing Care Plan—continued

THE CHILD WITH CEREBRAL PALSY

INTERVENTION	RATIONALE	EXPECTED OUTCOME
■ Monitor height and weight and plot on a growth grid. Perform hydration status assessment.	■ Insufficient intake can lead to impaired growth and dehydration.	The child shows normal growth patterns for height, weight, and other physical parameters.
■ Teach the family techniques to promote caloric and nutrient intake: ■ Position the child upright for feedings. ■ Place foods far back in the mouth to overcome tongue thrust. ■ Use soft and blended foods. ■ Allow extra time for chewing and swallowing. ■ Obtain adaptive handles for utensils and encourage self-feeding skills.	■ Special techniques can facilitate food intake. Adaptive handles may help the child better manage feeding self.	
■ Perform frequent respiratory assessment. Teach the family the preceding techniques to prevent aspiration. Teach care of gastrostomy and tube-feeding technique as appropriate.	■ Aspiration pneumonia is a risk for the child with poor swallowing. Special feeding techniques or tube feeding may be needed.	

4. Nursing Diagnosis: Ineffective Therapeutic Regimen Management (family) related to excessive demands made on the family for the child's complex care needs

NIC Priority Intervention:

Family mobilization: Utilization of family strengths to influence patient's health in a positive direction

NOC Suggested Outcome:

Family functioning: Ability of the family to meet the needs of its members through developmental transitions

Goal: The family will adapt to growth and development needs of the child with CP.

INTERVENTION	RATIONALE	EXPECTED OUTCOME
■ Allow chances for parents to verbalize the impact of CP on the family. Provide referral to other parents and support groups.	■ The family needs to explore the emotional and social impact of the child's care so they can integrate and grow from the experience.	The child demonstrates appropriate growth and developmental progress. The family successfully supports all of its members.
■ Explore community services for rehabilitation, respite care, child care, early intervention program, and refer family as appropriate.	■ Diverse services are available and will be needed due to the multiple impacts of CP on the child.	
■ During home and office visits, review the child's achievements and praise the family for care provided.	■ The child's achievements are positive reinforcement of the family's efforts.	
■ Teach the family skills needed to manage the child's care (e.g., medication administration, muscle stretching, seizure management).	■ Complex skills must be learned before they can be performed efficiently.	
■ Teach case management techniques.	■ The child requires care by many specialists, and many parents become case managers to coordinate care.	
■ Involve siblings in the care for the child with CP. Review with parents the needs of all children in the family.	■ Siblings of the child with CP may feel left out because of the care provided. Special efforts help to meet the developmental needs of all family members.	

(continued)

Nursing Care Plan—continued

THE CHILD WITH CEREBRAL PALSY

INTERVENTION	RATIONALE	EXPECTED OUTCOME
5. Nursing Diagnosis: Deficient Diversional Activity (child) related to poor social skills		
NIC Priority Intervention: **Recreation therapy:** Purposeful use of recreation to promote relaxation and enhancement of social skills		**NOC Suggested Outcome:** **Play participation:** Use of activities as needed for enjoyment, entertainment, and development by children
Goal: The child will engage in activities that maximize growth and development.		
■ Refer the family to an early intervention program. Encourage contact with other children. When hospitalized, place the child in a room with other children whenever possible.	■ The child needs a variety of activities and contact with other children and adults to maximize development.	The child engages in activities to maximize development.
■ Work with the school to develop an individualized education plan that encourages interaction with peers and a variety of activities that support development.	■ The education system is obligated to work with families to provide methods to enhance learning, including social interactions.	
■ Investigate recreational programs for children with disabilities and share information with the parents.	■ Recreational programs for children with disabilities may promote social experiences and physical activity.	

some children need a bowel management program to treat chronic constipation.

MAINTAIN SKIN INTEGRITY

Protect bony prominences from skin breakdown. Monitor splints and braces for proper fit and the skin under them for redness. If the skin is red or broken, the braces or splints should be removed and not worn until the skin is healed.

Proper body alignment should be maintained at all times. Support the child with pillows, towels, and bolsters whether the child is in bed or in a chair. Support the head and body of a floppy infant. A spastic child with scissored, extended legs or a child with athetosis who writhes constantly is difficult to carry and transport.

PROMOTE PHYSICAL MOBILITY

Range of motion exercises are essential to maintain joint flexibility and to prevent contractures. Consult with the physical therapists who work with the child and assist with recommended exercises. Refer parents to the appropriate resources for help getting adaptive devices (Figure 56–13 ●). Teach parents to position the child to foster flexion rather than extension so that the child can more easily interact with the environment (for example, by bringing objects closer to the face). Encourage parents to bring in the child's *adaptive appliances* (braces, positioning devices) for use during the hospitalization; however, secure them as the family may have difficulty replacing them if lost.

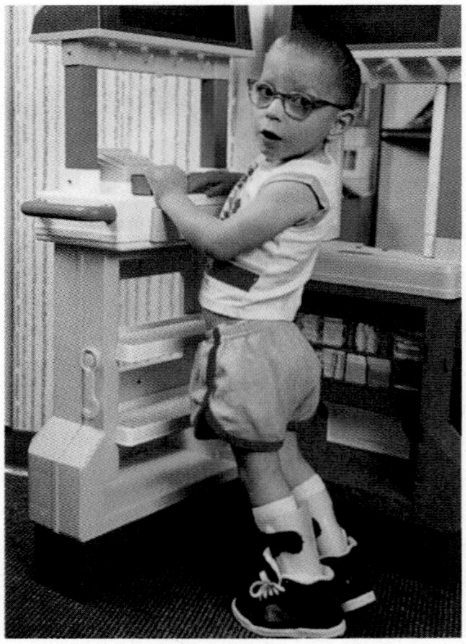

● **Figure 56–13** Cerebral palsy. This child has glasses for vision impairment. The lower leg braces are used for abnormal muscle tone that may cause deformities.

PROMOTE SAFETY

Safety belts should be used for children in strollers and wheelchairs (see Skills 8–1 to 8–3 SKILLS). Determine if an adaptive car safety seat is needed so the child can be safely transported. A

Complementary Care

TECHNIQUES FOR THE CHILD WITH CEREBRAL PALSY

The child with CP may benefit from massage therapy or hippotherapy (horse riding). Riding a horse benefits the child's body posture and promotes balance and muscle functioning (Jones, Morgan, & Shelton, 2007b).

child with chronic seizures should wear a helmet to protect against further injury.

PROMOTE GROWTH AND DEVELOPMENT

Remember that many children with CP are physically but not intellectually disabled. Use terminology appropriate for the child's developmental level. Help the child develop a positive self-image to ensure emotional health and social growth. Children with a hearing impairment may need referral to learn American Sign Language or other communication methods. Provide audio and visual activities for the child who is quadriplegic.

Adaptive and assistive technology may be needed to promote mobility and communication. **Assistive technology** is any item, equipment, or product customized for use to promote the functional capabilities and independence of an individual with disabilities. Examples include computers, adaptive utensils, and customized wheelchairs.

FOSTER PARENTAL KNOWLEDGE

Teach parents about the disorder and arrange sessions to teach them about all of the child's special needs. Teach administration, desired effects, and side effects of medications prescribed for seizures. Make sure parents are aware of the need for dental care for children because of the enamel defects and malocclusion that commonly occur in children with CP, and the gum hyperplasia that occurs when taking some antiepileptics.

PROVIDE EMOTIONAL SUPPORT

Listen to the parents' concerns and encourage them to express their feelings and ask questions. Explain what they can expect from future treatment. Work with other healthcare professionals to help families adjust to this chronic disease. Refer parents to individual and family counseling if appropriate.

NURSING CARE IN THE COMMUNITY

Children with CP need continuous support in the community. A case manager such as the parent or nurse is often needed to coordinate care. Parents may need financial assistance to provide the care that the child needs and to obtain appliances such as braces, wheelchairs, or adaptive utensils. Children need new adaptive devices, ongoing developmental assessment and care planning, and possibly surgery as they grow. Although the brain lesion does not change, it manifests differently as the child grows. For example, once the child begins to walk, the extensor tone may cause Achilles cord tightening. Braces may decrease deformities, but surgery may eventually be needed. Technology offers many new strategies to promote communication and self-care by these children. See MyNursingKit for Web sites with information on cerebral palsy.

Monitor the child's growth. If the child is unable to ambulate, use a scale that accommodates a wheelchair when weighing. Height measurements may be inaccurate and tools to assess ulnar length may be more accurate for a height measurement (Jones et al., 2007b). Schedule regular vision and hearing screening during health promotion visits, and give immunizations according to the recommended schedule. Educate parents about the possible risk for a seizure associated with the vaccines.

Early intervention programs can help parents learn to meet their child's special needs and obtain physical, occupational, and speech therapy. The child often needs an IEP to maximize learning potential (see Chapter 40). The nurse can help parents meet the needs of the child with CP in preschool, school, and health care settings. The nurse also makes referrals as appropriate to support groups and organizations such as the United Cerebral Palsy Association and Shriners Hospitals. Recreational activities may be identified through the National Association of Sports for Cerebral Palsy. An individualized transition plan should be developed during adolescence to assist the family and adolescent with CP with plans for adult living. Vocational training options can be explored. See Chapter 40.

EVALUATION

Expected outcomes of nursing care for the child with CP are provided on the Nursing Care Plan. For information on Neonatal Substance Abuse, see Chapter 31.

INJURIES OF THE NEUROLOGIC SYSTEM

Injuries to the brain and spinal cord are major causes of disability in previously healthy children. Drowning is another cause of brain injury in children.

TRAUMATIC BRAIN INJURY

A traumatic brain injury (TBI) is a blunt force or penetrating injury to the head that disrupts normal brain functioning, such as a loss of consciousness. Nearly 475,000 children under age 15 years experience a TBI annually, with 435,000 requiring an emergency department visit, 37,000 requiring hospitalization, and 2685 dying (Centers for Disease Control and Prevention, 2006). Children are at greatest risk when under 5 years or during adolescence. TBI is commonly associated with bicycling, sports, and playground activites.

Children under age 2 years have a higher risk for intracranial injury after TBI. Infants have thinner and more pliable skulls, putting them at even greater risk for skull fractures and intracranial injury (Atabaki, 2007).

Etiology and Pathophysiology

The injury impact transfers energy through the skull and meninges to the brain. Primary injury occurs at the time of the

MyNursingKit Animation: Coup-Contrecoup Injury

PATHOPHYSIOLOGY ILLUSTRATED

BRAIN INJURY

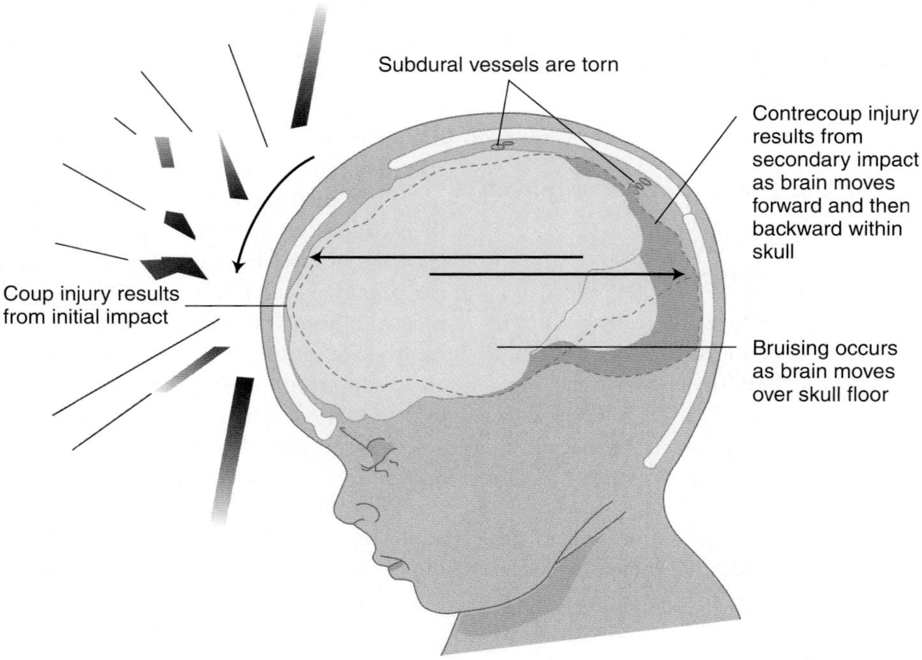
Subdural vessels are torn
Contrecoup injury results from secondary impact as brain moves forward and then backward within skull
Coup injury results from initial impact
Bruising occurs as brain moves over skull floor

Brain injury can result from a direct blow to the head (coup injury) or the acceleration-deceleration movement of the brain (contrecoup injury). Movement of the brain in the skull tears nerves, fibers, and blood vessels causing altered level of consciousness. Scalp injuries, skull fractures, contusions, and hematomas of brain tissue may also occur.

insult when the initial cellular damage takes place. See "Pathophysiology Illustrated: Brain Injury" for an explanation of the primary injury. The secondary injury is a biochemical and cellular response to the primary injury. Cerebral edema begins immediately and increases for the next 72 hours (Marcoux, 2005). Increased ICP and cerebral ischemia worsen the brain injury. The inflammatory response also damages brain cells by increasing the permeability of the blood-brain barrier.

Clinical Manifestations

TBI signs and symptoms in children depend on the pathologic features and severity of the injury. The child with a mild TBI (concussion) may remain conscious or have brief loss of consciousness (seconds to a few minutes). The child with a moderate TBI loses consciousness for 5 to 10 minutes. Following mild or moderate TBI, children may have amnesia about the event, headache, nausea, and vomiting. See "Clinical Manifestations: Traumatic Brain Injury by Severity."

Unconsciousness may result from increased ICP, edema, hemorrhage, or parenchymal damage to the cortex in both cerebral hemispheres or the brainstem. See "Clinical Manifestations: Intracranial Hematomas." Posttraumatic seizures are common. Children with inflicted TBI are more likely to have retinal hemorrhages, skull fractures, and rib and long bone fractures (Frasier, 2008).

Growth and Development

Mechanisms of injury are related to developmental stages and exposures, such as the following (Keenan & Bratton, 2006):

- Infants—shaken baby syndrome, child abuse, falls, and motor vehicle crashes
- Toddlers and preschoolers—falls down stairs, out a window, or from climbing; motor vehicle-related injuries as passengers or pedestrians
- School-age children—motor vehicle crashes, either as passengers or pedestrians, bicycle crash, roller-blading, scooter, or skateboard mishaps
- Adolescents—motor vehicle crashes; often alcohol or drugs are involved, struck by an object, sports-related injuries, and firearm injuries

Changes in respiratory effort or periods of apnea can occur secondary to shock, injury to the spinal cord above C4, or damage to or pressure on the medulla. Heart rate and blood pressure are indices of brainstem function. Tachycardia can be a sign of blood loss, shock, hypoxia, anxiety, or pain. Cushing's triad, associated with increased ICP or compromised blood flow to the brainstem, is characterized by hypertension,

Clinical Manifestations

TRAUMATIC BRAIN INJURY BY SEVERITY

TYPE OF BRAIN INJURY	CLINICAL MANIFESTATIONS
Concussion or mild brain injury	Low-grade headache that will not go away Slowness in thinking, acting, speaking, reading Memory problems Loss of balance, unsteady walking Difficulty paying attention or concentrating, change in performance at school Feeling tired all the time, change in sleeping pattern, lack of motivation or interest in favorite toys Change in eating patterns Increased sensitivity to lights, sounds, distractions; easily irritated
Moderate brain injury	Glasgow Coma Scale score of 9–12 Posttraumatic amnesia for 1–24 hours Loss of consciousness
Severe brain injury	Glasgow Coma Scale score of 8 or less Posttraumatic amnesia greater than 24 hours Coma Increased intracranial pressure

Clinical Manifestations

INTRACRANIAL HEMATOMAS

TYPE OF HEMATOMA	CLINICAL MANIFESTATIONS
SUBDURAL HEMATOMA	
Results from severe brain trauma, including shaken child syndrome More common in infants less than age 1 year Inertial forces cause laceration of the bridging veins; a venous hematoma forms beneath the dura and presses directly on brain	■ Symptoms may occur 48–72 hours after the injury ■ Change in level of consciousness (confusion, agitation, or lethargy) ■ Nausea or vomiting ■ Headache ■ Retinal hemorrhages in both eyes ■ Pupil on side of injury may be fixed and dilated ■ Seizures
EPIDURAL HEMATOMA	
Rare in children, especially those less than 4 years of age Results from blunt trauma (most often falls), assaults, or baseball to temporal area; may have linear skull fracture Arterial or venous bleeding occurs between the skull and the dura	■ Minimal or absent symptoms from initial impact ■ Delayed onset followed by rapid deterioration in mental status and signs of increased ICP ■ Headache or full fontanelle ■ Paresis of cranial nerves III and VI ■ Papilledema ■ Fixed and dilated pupil
INTRACEREBRAL HEMATOMA	
Result of deep contusion or intracerebral laceration (secondary to foreign body, bony penetration, or impalement) Causes diffuse bleeding in parenchyma; there may be a hematoma with associated small areas of bleeding	■ Symptoms depend upon the size and location of the hematoma; may change if size increases due to uncontrolled bleeding ■ Altered consciousness

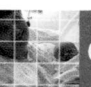

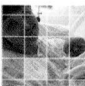

Nursing Practice

Any infant who arrives in the emergency department with seizures, failure to thrive, respiratory irregularities, or coma should be evaluated for child abuse (shaken child syndrome). Lethargy and vomiting may be additional signs. Because an infant has a large head and relatively weak neck muscles, a frustrated adult can cause acceleration and deceleration injuries to the head by shaking the infant.

increased systolic pressure with wide pulse pressure, bradycardia, and irregular respirations. Refer to the earlier discussion of altered states of consciousness for more information about increased ICP.

Reflexes may be hyporesponsive, hyperresponsive, or nonexistent. The child may assume a flexor, extensor, areflexic, or flaccid posture (see Figure 56–2).

Clinical Therapy

The severity of a brain injury is diagnosed from the history, physical examination, pediatric Glasgow Coma Scale, and diagnostic tests. Important historical information includes the mechanism of injury, the child's initial and current responses, any loss of consciousness, and the child's memory of the event.

Laboratory tests include a complete blood cell count, blood chemistry, toxicology screening, and urinalysis. Skull and spinal radiographs detect fractures of the skull and cervical vertebrae. A CT scan detects fractures, intracranial hemorrhage, swelling, and diffuse axonal injury. An MRI scan is used during recovery to determine the extent of brain damage. PET scans measure the blood flow in the brain. A fracture indicates a more serious injury. Many children with brain injuries have multiple other injuries. All children with a TBI should be evaluated for a potential cervical spine injury.

The initial management of a child with a brain injury is based on the child's physiologic status (see page 1692 for mild TBI or concussion). The airway must be clear and stable, and hypoxia must be prevented. Hypoxia and hypercapnia cause vasodilation and increased ICP. Mechanical ventilation with 100% oxygen at the child's normal respiratory rate is used in the first 24 hours after injury to maintain oxygenation levels. (see Skill 14–14 SKILLS). Paralytic agents may be administered to eliminate the child's resistance to mechanical ventilation and lower the ICP (Mansfield, 2007).

Nursing Practice

In the child with moderate head injury, the oxygen saturation should remain over 95%. For the severely injured child who is intubated, monitor arterial blood gas results. The PaO_2 of 70–100 mm Hg indicates satisfactory management of oxygenation.

Increased intracranial pressure. If increased ICP occurs and is not relieved, brain shifting begins in the cranium, a precursor of herniation. Invasive ICP monitoring (catheter into the ventricle or a bolt into the subarachnoid space) may be initiated in the child with severe TBI. Increased ICP must be controlled, and the goal is to maintain the ICP to less than 20 mm Hg (Marcoux, 2005). Mannitol or a continuous infusion of hypertonic saline (3%) may be used to decrease ICP. Pain and sedation management promote comfort and help control the ICP. Corticosteroids are not recommended for reducing ICP.

Invasive procedures may be used to reduce ICP. Burr holes or more extensive surgery may be performed to evacuate a lesion or hematoma. A ventricular catheter may be placed to drain CSF and to monitor pressure. The child may be placed in a chemically induced coma to reduce brain activity during this acute care phase. Hypothermia is sometimes used to treat coma associated with TBI (Haque, LaTour, & Zaritsky, 2006).

Intracranial hematomas are space-occupying lesions that expand rapidly or slowly, depending on whether they are arterial or venous in origin. Some lesions require immediate surgical evacuation to minimize the secondary effects of the injury.

If there is no cervical spine injury, the head of the bed is elevated up to 30 degrees. The child's head is kept in the midline to promote venous (jugular) drainage. Hip flexion is avoided. Normothermia is maintained. The environment is kept as quiet as possible. A urinary catheter is inserted to monitor output, and electrolytes should be checked frequently. Enteral nutrition support should be started within 72 hours using a postpyloric feeding tube to reduce the risk for aspiration.

Rehabilitation. Aggressive support continues until the child regains consciousness and rehabilitation can be initiated. Physical therapists, occupational therapists, speech-language specialists, and social workers all play vital roles. Moderate and severe TBI may result in a permanent disability, such as epilepsy, motor and cognitive impairments, learning problems, hearing and vision impairment, communication problems, and behavioral or emotional problems. Difficulties with learning skills are common, such as short-term memory, problem solving, sequencing, concrete thinking, and visual-spatial organization. No new learning can occur before short-term memory returns (Blackman, 2005). Reliable predictions of outcome in the child who has suffered a severe brain injury cannot be made until 6 to 12 months postinjury during which most recovery occurs.

Evidence in Action

Beliefs that young age and brain development are protective and allow more recovery after TBI are changing. In children with severe TBI it has been found that less-well-established skills are more likely to be disrupted than well-established skills. Functional recovery may be limited to the younger child's fewer well-established skills (Kirkwood, Yeates, & Wilson, 2006).

NURSING MANAGEMENT

NURSING ASSESSMENT AND DIAGNOSIS

Assess the child's neurologic status and pediatric Glasgow Coma Scale frequently, compare to prior evaluations, and note improvement, stability, or deterioration. Assess the cranial nerves and pupils for size and reactivity. Monitor vital signs and behavior carefully, noting any signs that might indicate increased ICP (see Table 56–1). See Table 56–3 for neurologic evaluation guidelines. See altered states of consciousness on page 1651. Changes in these signs may indicate hypoxia, decreased perfusion, shock, or increased ICP (see Skill 9–17 SKILLS). When the child has a decreased level of consciousness shortly after a brain injury, consider if a posttraumatic seizure occurred and if the child could still be in the postictal state. The cause of any deterioration must be quickly determined and appropriate interventions taken.

Observe for physiologic and behavioral signs of pain. Assume that the child with increased ICP is in pain, even when unresponsive.

Examples of nursing diagnoses appropriate for the child with TBI include the following:

- *Ineffective Cerebral Tissue Perfusion* related to hypoventilation, hypovolemia, and/or reduction of arterial blood flow to the brain due to increased ICP
- *Risk for Aspiration* related to decreased level of consciousness and loss of protective reflexes
- *Risk for Imbalanced Fluid Volume* related to therapies for reducing ICP
- *Compromised Family Coping* related to life-threatening injury to child

PLANNING AND IMPLEMENTATION

HOSPITAL-BASED NURSING CARE

The child with a severe TBI is initially cared for in the pediatric intensive care unit. Nursing care focuses on maintaining cerebral perfusion pressure and minimizing increased ICP, preventing complications, and providing emotional support.

Maintain cardiopulmonary function. In the moderately injured child, observe breathing patterns and check color, neurologic signs, and level of consciousness. The oxygen saturation should remain over 95%. Report any sign of decreased oxygenation or signs and symptoms of increased ICP to the physician immediately (see Table 56–1). Keep suction equipment at the bedside in case aspiration occurs.

Reduce physiologic stresses on the body that could increase ICP. The nurse should minimize unpleasant stimuli when possible, keep the environment quiet, and avoid jarring the bed. Pain management and temperature control are important. Position the child to avoid excessive flexion of the hips and neck that could slow venous circulation. Monitor the effect of nursing procedures on level of ICP and determine if clustering procedures is better than spreading procedures over time. Encourage parents to talk to the child and provide comforting touch.

Administer medications as prescribed. Provide oral care to keep mucous membranes moist and intact. Pad and cushion bony prominences, provide skin care, and change the child's position frequently. The eyes should be protected from corneal irritation with ophthalmic ointment and patching. Enteral feeding may be used initially, slowly progressing to oral foods as tolerated. Fluids are given to meet daily fluid requirements, or to maintain the child's blood pressure within normal ranges for age. Stool softeners and suppositories should be used as needed to prevent constipation. The side rails of the bed should be padded to protect the child if a seizure occurs.

Promote recovery and prevent physical deformities. Perform passive range of motion exercises to prevent contractures. Splints may be used to position extremities in functional positions. Work with physical, occupational, and speech therapists to reinforce exercises and help teach parents the techniques so they can work with the child in the hospital and at home. Provide stimulation and promote general awareness when the child is ready, based on the child's age and ability by using toys, books, music, or games.

Provide emotional support to the family in collaboration with the social workers, physicians, psychologists, rehabilitation therapists, and members of the clergy caring for the child and family. All can help the family adjust to having a child with a new disability.

Sometimes despite all efforts, the child dies due to the consequences of the brain injury. Provide support for the family while brain death testing is perfomed. See Chapter 43 for information to support the family when termination of life support and organ donation are discussed.

Thinking Critically

THE CHILD WITH SEVERE BRAIN INJURY

Antwan, 7 years old, was injured when he was struck by a car and thrown several feet. He was unconscious upon admission to the emergency department and showed some signs of increased ICP (dilated and fixed pupils). He was treated for shock, and his neurologic status and vital signs were frequently assessed. Antwan was found to have sustained several contusions of the brain, but no skull fracture. He was intubated and medicated to manage the increased ICP.

Antwan's ICP has now stabilized, but he has not totally regained consciousness. He is restless and agitated, and unable to follow directions. His parents stay at his bedside and provide auditory and tactile stimulation, hoping he will eventually respond. Physical therapy has been initiated to prevent contractures and to maintain function. Long-term rehabilitation will be needed to help Antwan and his family achieve the best outcome possible after this injury.

What is the role of the nurse in acute care of the child with a severe brain injury? What support does the family need to contribute to the child's care? How would you work with other healthcare professionals to coordinate care during the acute care phase? How would you help plan the long-term care for a child such as Antwan?

See MyNursingKit for possible responses.

DISCHARGE PLANNING AND HOME CARE TEACHING

Home care needs should be identified and addressed well in advance of discharge. Children with serious TBIs benefit from inpatient or outpatient rehabilitation to promote optimal achievement of function. A case manager is often needed to coordinate services and resources during rehabilitation. Social services intervention may be needed when brain injury results from child abuse.

Give parents information about caring for children with mild or moderate TBIs at home and possible behaviors to expect from the child. For children with disabilities, determine what adaptations and assistive technology are needed in the home to care for the child, such as a wheelchair, a walker, braces, or a special bed. Social work and home health agencies can often help the parents make special arrangements.

NURSING CARE IN THE COMMUNITY

Home care nursing may be important for the child with an acquired neurologic dysfunction and prolonged altered consciousness. The home care nurse may assume case management responsibilities for the child and make sure the environment is safe. The nurse can teach the family to meet the child's needs, monitor the intake of fluids and foods, position the child, provide skin care, and perform range of motion exercises to reduce contractures. Regular follow-up visits are needed to assess the child's recovery and to modify the treatment plan.

Even though the child may look normal within days of a brain injury, parents and teachers need to be aware that brain healing takes up to 6 weeks. Typical behaviors during this healing period may include any of the following: tiring easily, memory loss or forgetfulness, easy distractibility, difficulty concentrating, difficulty following directions, irritability or short temper, and needing help starting and finishing tasks. Return the child to a full school schedule gradually to prevent fatigue and frustration. Educational assessment should be initiated if recovery takes longer than 6 weeks.

Children with moderate brain injuries often have long-term problems with attention, problem solving, speed of information processing, and behavior problems (e.g., impulsivity, irritability, apathy, aggression, and social withdrawal). Neuropsychologic testing is needed to identify subtle learning disabilities that are not usually revealed on standardized school achievement tests.

The child or adolescent facing long-term rehabilitation needs support to adjust to the disability and to find the strength to maximize his or her abilities. Identify recreational opportunities for the child with disabilities to promote exercise and self-esteem. The adolescent may need to gain vocational skills and learn to live independently. Refer parents to the Brain Injury Association for further information. (See MyNursingKit for Web links to such resources.)

Prevention of brain injury is another important role of the nurse. Encourage parents to obtain protective helmets and require children to use them for bicycling and skateboarding. Parents should be encouraged to wear a helmet themselves as role models. Encourage parents to monitor playgrounds for appropriate use of wood chips or cushioning tiles to reduce the severity of injuries associated with falls.

EVALUATION

Examples of expected outcomes of nursing care for the family and child with TBI include the following:

- Cerebral perfusion pressure is maintained at an adequate rate to sustain oxygenation of the brain.
- Muscle function is maintained and physical deformities are prevented with range of motion exercises and splinting during the recovery stages of the brain injury.
- Parents are supported through the child's acute recovery phase and learn to provide care the child will need at home.
- The child's school performance is monitored and appropriate educational resources are provided to support the child's learning.

SPECIFIC HEAD INJURIES

Some specific head injuries occur simultaneously with TBI that have specific care needs in addition to that provided for TBI. Recognition of these additional injuries is important to promote the child's recovery.

Scalp Injuries

Injuries to the scalp, which can be caused by falls, blunt trauma, or penetration of a foreign body, are usually benign. Although bleeding may be extensive, hypovolemia or shock is uncommon unless the patient is an infant.

Lacerations should be irrigated with copious amounts of sterile normal saline solution and inspected for bony fragments or depressions, CSF leakage with a dural tear, or debris. If the injury is simple, the laceration can be sutured and the child discharged from the emergency department. If not, a neurosurgeon should be consulted.

Concussion

A concussion is a mild TBI that results from a direct blow to the head, face, or neck that causes an alteration in mental status (e.g., amnesia, dizziness, memory or orientation impairment, unsteady gait), but not necessarily loss of consciousness (Kirkwood, Yeates, & Wilson, 2006). The signs are caused by stretching, compression, or shearing of nerve fibers as the brain moves within the skull, disrupting brain chemicals responsible for brain functioning (Adirim, 2007). The injury is metabolic rather than gross structural damage or focal injury. A simple concussion progressively resolves without complications over 7 to 10 days. A complex concussion is associated with persistent recurrence of symptoms with exertion, seizures, loss of consciousness longer than 1 minute, or prolonged cognitive impairment (McCrory, Johnston, Meeuwisse, et al., 2005). See "Clinical Manifestations: Concussion Severity Level."

Pediatric concussive syndrome, a complex concussion, is thought to be caused by an injury to the brainstem and occurs in children less than age 3 years. Toddlers seem stunned at the time of

Clinical Manifestations

CONCUSSION SEVERITY LEVEL

SEVERITY	CLINICAL MANIFESTATIONS
Grade 1	Transient confusion, no loss of consciousness, no posttraumatic amnesia, mental status abnormalities last less than 15 minutes
Grade 2	Transient confusion with posttraumatic amnesia, no loss of consciousness, mental status abnormalities last 15 minutes or longer
Grade 3	Any loss of consciousness, seconds or minutes

MyNursingKit Case Study: Post-Concussion Return to Competitive Play

injury, but have no loss of consciousness. Later these children become pale, clammy, and lethargic, and they may vomit. These children may be placed in a short-stay unit for observation and usually recover within 24 hours. Postconcussive cognitive deficits do not become apparent until at least 24 hours after injury (Adirim, 2007).

No standard practice exists for evaluation of children with mild TBI or concussion (Adirim, 2007). Brain imaging studies are usually normal, and may not be ordered. Treatment is supportive. Children are observed in the emergency department for several hours before being sent home with instructions to the parents to watch them closely for decreased responsiveness. The child who is unconscious for more than 5 minutes or has amnesia of the event may be admitted to the hospital or be observed in a short-stay unit to rule out other injury. Symptoms from postconcussive syndrome usually disappear within several weeks but may last up to 6 months. Tell parents and teachers to expect the child to have altered behavior, and encourage them to help the child who is aware of differences to maintain self-esteem.

Children who have had one brain injury are at greater risk for a subsequent brain injury (Swaine, Tremblay, Platt, et al., 2007). Young athletes suffering a second concussion before complete recovery from the first may develop *second impact syndrome.* This syndrome results in acute brain swelling, neurologic or cognitive deficits, and sometimes death from the cumulative effect of these concussions. Recommendations should be followed for the management of sports-related concussions to reduce the risk of disability and death. Removal from sports participation ranges from 7 days to the entire season, depending on the severity of concussion and neurologic symptoms. The athlete should be allowed to return to full game play only when symptom-free after a gradual increase in activities (Kirkwood et al., 2006).

Skull Fractures

A fracture to any of the eight cranial bones requires considerable force. Any area of the skull with swelling or a hematoma should be evaluated for possible fracture. Diagnosis is made by visual inspection, palpation, radiologic study, or CT scan. Treatment should always include neurosurgical consultation.

Management of skull fractures depends on the type and extent of the injury (Table 56–8).

Penetrating Injuries

Gunshot wounds to the head can damage tissue, bone, and blood vessels. Low-velocity bullets enter and ricochet within the cranial vault, destroying brain tissue and blood vessels. The child's level of consciousness quickly deteriorates because of the edema surrounding the penetration tract. High-velocity bullets cause immediate, severe damage on impact.

CT scans evaluate gunshot trauma and pinpoint the location of bullet and bone fragments as well as parenchymal damage. Surgery is performed to debride the tract, evacuate any hematomas, and remove accessible bone or bullet particles. Children with gunshot wounds to the head have a high mortality. Those who survive may suffer multiple focal deficits and seizures.

Impalement injuries may occur in children in association with darts, dog bites, or other sharp objects. All objects must be left in place and removed in the operating room by a neurosurgeon. The child with an impalement injury is at high risk for focal injury and infection. After surgery, children are managed as with other postoperative brain injuries, with attention focused on level of consciousness, management of increased ICP, and infection control.

SPINAL CORD INJURY

The incidence of spinal cord injury in children is estimated to be 2 cases per 100,000 children (Vitale, Goss, Matsumoto, et al., 2006). Children account for about 2% to 5% of all spinal cord injuries, and half of these injuries occur in the cervical area (Hayes & Arriola, 2005). Motor vehicle crashes account for 55% of cases, either pedestrian, passenger, driver, or bicycle-vehicular related (Vitale et al., 2006). Other causes in toddlers and young children include falls and child abuse. Recreation or sports-related trauma accounts for more injuries as children grow older. Penetrating injuries such as stabbing and gunshot wounds are becoming more prevalent.

The mechanism of injury and direction of forces determines the type of lesion that occurs (Figure 56–14 ●). Hyperflexion injuries (e.g., bending around a safety seatbelt) produce tears or avulsions and fractures of vertebral bodies, as well as subluxation and dislocation. Rotation may cause joint dislocations or unstable spinal fractures. Hyperextension may result in the so-called hangman's fracture, ligament tears, avulsion fractures of vertebral

Table 56–8 Skull Fractures

Injury	Diagnosis and Clinical Therapy
Linear Fracture	
Results from impact to large area of the skull. Usually no symptoms. May have overlying hematoma or soft-tissue swelling. Such fractures in newborns may result from pressure from forceps or from maternal pelvic bones.	If fracture is on temporal bone or crosses sagittal suture line, a CT scan is performed to detect potential epidural hematoma. Consider the possibility of an inflicted injury. No treatment is commonly needed.
Depressed Fracture	
Break in skull itself or an area shattered into many fragments. Pieces of bone may be depressed into brain tissue with hematoma forming on top. This type of fracture in a newborn may be the result of a forceps injury.	Plain radiographic film or CT scan. Surgery to elevate bone fragments when depression is greater than 5 mm. Tetanus prophylaxis is given as needed. Many are associated with intracranial injury and posttraumatic epilepsy.
Compound Fracture	
Combination of a full-thickness scalp laceration and depressed skull fracture with the bone exposed, considered penetrating fractures if the dura is torn.	Visual diagnosis along with radiographic studies. Surgical debridement, a search for foreign bodies, and copious irrigation are performed. Parenteral antibiotics and tetanus prophylaxis are provided as needed.
Basilar Fracture	
Fracture at the base of the skull that may involve the frontal, ethmoid, sphenoid, temporal, or occipital bones. A dural tear may be present.	Diagnosis is confirmed by signs of blood behind the tympanic membranes, CSF leakage from the nose or ears, periorbital ecchymosis (raccoon eyes), or bruising of the mastoid (Battle sign). Radiographic imaging locates the fracture site. Antibiotics may be prescribed. Surgical repair of the site of the CSF leak is performed if it persists after 7–10 days. Cranial nerve injuries may occur (e.g., hearing loss, facial nerve palsy).

Data from Dias, M. S. (2004). Traumatic brain injury and spinal cord injury. *Pediatric Clinics of North America, 51,* 271–303.

Growth and Development

The vertebrae are incompletely ossified in children under 9 years. The facet joints are more shallow and horizontal. The young child's head is relatively large compared to the strength of the neck muscles. Atlanto-occipital dislocation (C1 to C3 level) occurs more frequently in infants and young children because of the horizontal articulation between the occiput and the top cervical vertebra. The ligaments supporting this spinal cord are more elastic and allow for more stretching between the vertebrae, but the spinal cord does not stretch (McCall, Fassett, & Brockmeyer, 2006). Injuries are more likely to occur at the C4 to C6 level in children over age 9 years.

bodies, as well as central or posterior spinal cord syndrome. Compression injuries cause anterior cord syndrome, occlusion of the anterior spinal artery resulting in loss of motor function, and pain and temperature sensation below the level of the injury. Touch, pressure, position and vibratory sensations remain intact (Boss, 2006).

Children are prone to specific kinds of spinal cord injuries because of the mobility and flexibility of their spinal column, especially in the upper cervical region (C1 to C4).

Table 56–9 describes the spinal cord injuries most common in children. Spinal cord injuries are classified as complete or incomplete. Complete lesions are irreversible and involve a loss of sensory, motor, and autonomic function below the level of the injury. Incomplete lesions involve varying degrees of sensory, motor, and autonomic function below the level of injury. Hypotension, loss of bladder and bowel control, and loss of environmental thermoregulatory function are associated with autonomic dysfunction. The higher the level of spinal cord injury, the more severe the neurologic damage.

At the time of injury, the child is flaccid and areflexic below the lesion. The child who experiences spinal shock has flaccidity and loss of reflexes, but some return of function occurs within the first 72 hours of injury. As neurologic recovery begins, spinal reflex activity returns and increasing spasticity is seen below the level of the lesion.

The child can experience neurogenic shock in which there is loss of vasomotor tone and sympathetic innervations of the heart, resulting in hypotension, bradycardia, and peripheral vasodilation (a form of distributive shock). See Chapter 49 ∞. Priapism may be seen. Respiratory compromise may be present due to paralysis of the diaphragm.

Nursing Practice

Autonomic dysreflexia is a medical emergency in which overactivity of the autonomic nervous system causes an abrupt onset of hypertension, bradycardia, severe headaches, pallor below and flushing above the level of the spinal cord lesion, and seizures. This response can be triggered by a full bladder.

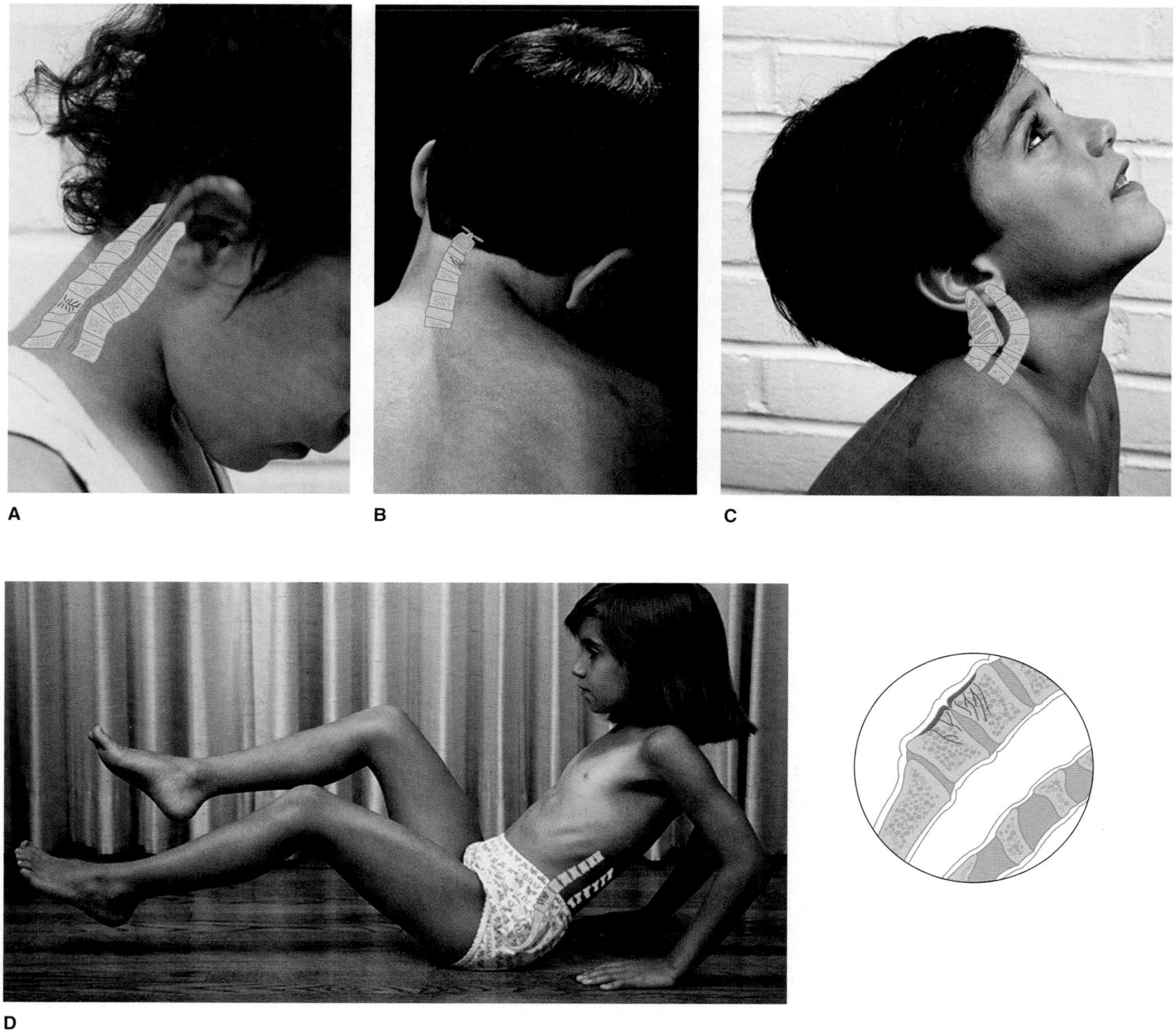

● **Figure 56–14** Mechanics of injury to the spinal cord. ***A,*** Hyperflexion. ***B,*** Lateral flexion. ***C,*** Hyperextension. ***D,*** Compression.

Diagnosis is made by observation, neurologic examination, and radiologic studies of the cervical, thoracic, and lumbosacral spine to determine if a vertebral fracture or compression on the spinal cord is present. The child's immobilized position is unchanged until a radiologist has declared the spine uninjured. In addition, CT scanning, MRI, fluoroscopy, or myelography may be performed. More than 20% of children have spinal cord injury without radiographic abnormality (SCIWORA) because initial films or CT scans show no bony deformity. The child under 8 years has a more tenuous spinal cord blood supply and greater elasticity of the vertebral column, so the initial radiological films and CT scan show no bony injury (McCall et al., 2006). If profound or progressive paralysis occurs immediately or within 48 hours, an MRI can detect the injury to ligaments and soft tissues.

Spinal injuries are managed aggressively as the spinal injury extends upward 1 to 2 levels during the immediate hours and days after the injury (Hayes & Arriola, 2005). The child with a spinal cord injury may be placed in external immobilization with a halo device. Surgery to reduce and internally fixate the fracture is performed for unstable fractures, dislocations, and progressive deformity. Decompression of the spinal cord and nerve roots may be performed if transaction is not complete.

To decrease neurologic sequelae in children with motor deficits, a high-dose methylprednisolone continuous infusion is administered over 24 to 48 hours. Administration must be started within 8 hours of the injury (Mendelson & Fallat, 2007). Gastrointestinal prophylaxis is started to reduce the risk for an ulcer. Atropine and norepinephrine may be given to manage spinal shock.

Complications of spinal cord injury include:

- Impaired respiratory function due to a paralyzed diaphragm or diminished vital capacity.

Table 56–9 Spinal Cord Injuries in Children

Spine Region	Injury Characteristics
Cervical	■ Site of 60% of spinal injuries in children under 10 years ■ Injury above C3 segment causes respiratory arrest and death without ventilatory support; many of these injuries are fatal ■ Diaphragm function is present when injury is at C5 level ■ Quadriplegia, some function of upper extremities when injury is at C6–C7 level ■ Loss of sphincter function ■ Sensory level lost below the sternum
Thoracic	■ Site of 20% of spinal injuries usually between 8 and 14 years ■ Full control of upper extremities including hands ■ Poor trunk balance
Thoracolumbar	■ Full control of muscles in abdomen and upper back ■ Good trunk balance
Lumbar	■ Most injuries occur at the L2–L4 level; often results when children 4 to 8 years are restrained with a lap belt only during a frontal motor vehicle crash (Elliott, Arbogast, & Durbin, 2006). ■ Below L3 may have functioning of muscles in upper leg ■ Loss of ankle and foot control

- Scoliosis if injury occurs before the skeleton is mature.
- Hip instability due to poor acetabular development.
- Pathologic fractures of the long bones due to immobilization hypercalcemia.
- Pressure sores.
- Deep vein thrombosis.
- Autonomic dysreflexia.

An interdisciplinary approach is required to manage the rehabilitation and long-term care needs of the child and family.

NURSING MANAGEMENT

HOSPITAL-BASED NURSING CARE

Nursing care focuses on monitoring vital signs, meeting nutritional needs, maintaining skin integrity, promoting independent functioning, providing emotional support, and promoting rehabilitation.

Be alert for any changes in vital signs, especially those that may signify increased respiratory difficulty or neurogenic shock (hypotension, bradycardia, and peripheral vasodilation), increased ICP (see Table 56–1), or autonomic dysreflexia. Monitor intake and output. Monitor bladder and bowel function. Assess the skin for integrity.

With higher cervical injuries, assess the cranial nerves as they may be affected by swelling around the spinal cord. Note the return of reflexes and change from flaccid tone to spasticity. Identify any changes in level of sensation or motor function. Carefully check the immobilizing device to ensure that the spine stays stable.

Ensure adequate nutrition. A child with complete paralysis may require a gastrostomy tube. When the child begins to eat, feed soft foods slowly as the child may have some swallowing difficulties.

Prevent skin breakdown. See Chapter 58∞. Observe surgical sites for signs of infection or inflammation. Provide regular traction pin site care according to institutional guidelines.

Promote independent functioning by reinforcing the exercises and skills learned in physical and occupational therapy. Use supports, boots, footboards, splints, and braces as recommended by the therapists to prevent contractures (Figure 56–15 ●). If hand mobility is limited, explore options for independence. Encourage the child to be as independent as possible in a wheelchair. An important mobility goal is to achieve wheelchair transfer and to perform self-care. Identify adaptive equipment that makes these goals possible.

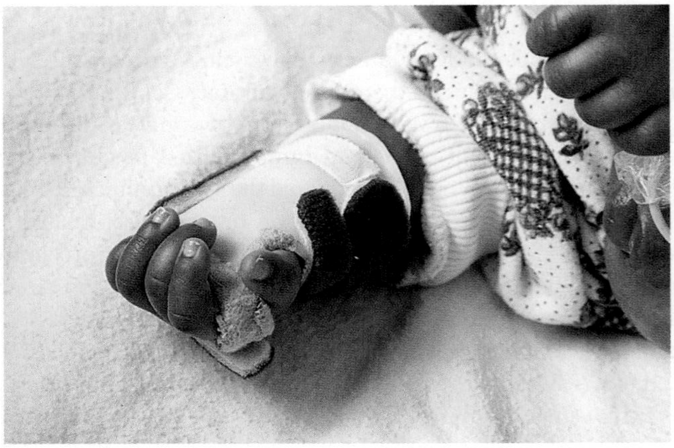

● **Figure 56–15** Preventing contractures. Splints are often used to prevent contractures, thus maintaining optimal functioning of the child's hands or feet.

Achieving bowel and bladder control may be difficult. Intermittent catheterizations may be necessary if urinary retention occurs (see Skill 10–10 SKILLS). Anticipate that constipation will occur and initiate bowel training with a diet high in fiber and the use of stool softeners.

Therapeutic play appropriate for the child's developmental level is an important part of the healing process. Provide as many normal activities for the child as possible, but do not give the child tasks that he or she will have difficulty completing. Child life teachers or tutors can help the child keep up with schoolwork.

Television, DVDs, computer games, Internet connections, and music can offer diversion for prolonged hospitalization. Children with paraplegia can learn to use their arms and hands to play interactive games. Devices can also be adapted so that the child can play computer games or manipulate the television or radio.

Support the child emotionally. Encourage the child to meet small, short-term goals, including those that involve self-care. Encourage the child to express fears and frustrations.

Be compassionate and understanding. Encourage siblings to visit, answer their questions honestly, and help them to discuss their feelings. Involve the parents and siblings in the child's care as much as possible. When appropriate, encourage them to help with activities of daily living.

DISCHARGE PLANNING AND HOME CARE TEACHING

Many children are discharged to inpatient rehabilitation facilities. Assist with arrangements for the transfer. Work closely with the child, parents, and other members of the healthcare team concerning placement. Home care needs, reintegration into educational programs, and safety issues should be identified and addressed well in advance of discharge from the rehabilitation facility. Refer families to social services, family counseling, and support groups if indicated. See MyNursingKit for Web links to resources about spinal cord injury.

HYPOXIC-ISCHEMIC BRAIN INJURY (DROWNING)

Drowning is defined as the process resulting in primary respiratory impairment from submersion/immersion in a liquid medium. Children between 1 and 4 years and males 15 to 24 years have the highest risk for drowning (Meyer, Theodorou, & Berg, 2006). Drowning is a leading cause of injury-related deaths in children.

Infants most commonly drown in the bathtub (78%). Children 1 to 4 years more frequently drown in artificial pools (56%) and bodies of fresh water. Hot tubs, toilets, and large water-filled buckets are other drowning mechanisms for this age group. Older children and adolescents frequently drown in natural bodies of fresh water (63%) (Zuckerbraun & Saladino, 2005). Children with seizure disorders are at higher risk for drowning. Adolescent drowning is often related to risk-taking behaviors and illicit substance use.

A child can drown in as little water as it takes to cover the nose and mouth. The events preceding drowning follow a sequential pattern. The child trapped in water panics, struggles, tries to move using swimming motions, and holds his or her breath. The child aspirates a small amount of water from the oropharynx, causing a laryngospasm that lasts no more than 2 minutes and hypoxia. Because of increasing panic and hypoxia, the child swallows more liquid. As the laryngospasm passes, the child breathes water into the lungs. The child may also vomit and aspirate stomach contents. Aspirated water damages the lung surfactant and impairs alveolar gas exchange. As the arterial oxygen saturation falls, cardiac output decreases, and hypoxia, hypercarbia, and respiratory acidosis develop (Zuckerbraun & Saladino, 2005). Hypothermia may result because the child's body cools faster in water than in air, and systemic perfusion decreases as a result. See Chapter 58∞. With increasing hypoxia, the cardiac muscle becomes impaired and ultimately the heart stops.

Anoxia is the major insult associated with drowning. Anoxia leads to cerebral edema and increased ICP, and secondary cerebral injuries. Little can be done to resuscitate the brain, but with aggressive cardiopulmonary resuscitation, more severely brain-injured children survive in a permanent vegetative state. Approximately 10% of drowning victims have severe neurologic impairment (Burford, Ryan, Stone, et al., 2005).

The child who has been immersed exhibits a wide variety of signs and symptoms depending on the length of time underwater, the temperature of the water, the response to the episode, and the initial treatment performed at the scene. The child may be apneic and pulseless. Signs and symptoms in the rescued child may be decreased level of consciousness ranging from stupor to total unresponsiveness, apnea or irregular respirations, gastric distention, and seizures. Children submerged for short periods (5 to 10 minutes) have few symptoms and often recover without neurologic impairment. The child with a submersion of 25 minutes or longer will likely die or have severe neurologic impairment, except in some rare cases of submersion in icy water (Meyer et al., 2005).

Immediate cardiopulmonary resuscitation (CPR) performed at the scene is associated with the best outcomes. Initial emergency treatment is 100% oxygen and rewarming. The airway may be secured with an endotracheal tube. Emergency personnel with a defibrillator should assess the heart rhythm and defibrillate if ventricular fibrillation is present. The child should be transported to the hospital even if the child begins breathing spontaneously.

All submersion victims should be admitted to the hospital for at least 24 hours or observed in a short-stay observation unit for several hours, even when asymptomatic. Many life-threatening complications, including respiratory distress and cerebral edema, may not become evident for at least 12 hours after the incident.

The child may need mechanical ventilation to keep the alveoli open, to promote adequate oxygenation, and to prevent respiratory acidosis. After hypovolemia is corrected, fluids may be restricted and diuretics may be used to help reduce cerebral edema. Vasopressor medication may be used to maintain a normal blood pressure. Predictors of good outcome are spontaneous purposeful movements and normal brainstem function in the first 24 hours after submersion (Meyer et al., 2006).

Nursing Management

Nursing care of the child who survives a submersion incident focuses on monitoring the child's neurologic and cardiopulmonary status and providing emotional support to the family.

Assess the child's responsiveness, spontaneous respiratory efforts, oxygenation, and vital signs. Perform frequent neurologic status assessments. Attach a cardiorespiratory monitor and pulse oximeter for continuous assessment information about the child's oxygenation status.

Implement the nursing interventions for a child with altered states of consciousness as described on page 1653. If cerebral edema develops, implement nursing interventions as described on page 1691.

Provide emotional support to the family. Be nonjudgmental and provide a forum for parents to express their feelings. Reassure parents who exhibit guilt reactions that their child is receiving all possible medical treatment. Parents may be faced with an unknown prognosis. Encourage them to seek assistance from social workers, members of the clergy, close friends, and relatives. Arrange for appropriate referrals. If the child's prognosis is poor, an ethical consult may be offered to educate the family about options for decision making regarding sustaining or terminating life support. See Chapter 43.

Identify and address home care needs well in advance of discharge. Assist with arrangements for the child with minor deficits. Assign a case manager to the child with significant neurologic impairments so that long-term care options can be explored. Inpatient or outpatient rehabilitation options should be matched to the child's needs and family resources.

Drowning can be prevented by education, legislation, and changes in the environment. Pool owners should erect climb-proof 5-foot fences around all four sides of the pool. If fencing is on 3 sides, the house door to the pool area should be kept locked and have an alarm. Local ordinances may require such fences. Adolescents should learn the dangers of mixing alcohol or drugs and swimming. Five- and 10-gallon buckets should be kept empty when not in use. Emphasize the importance of closely supervising children when near or in the water, whether at pools, at the beach, or in the bathtub.

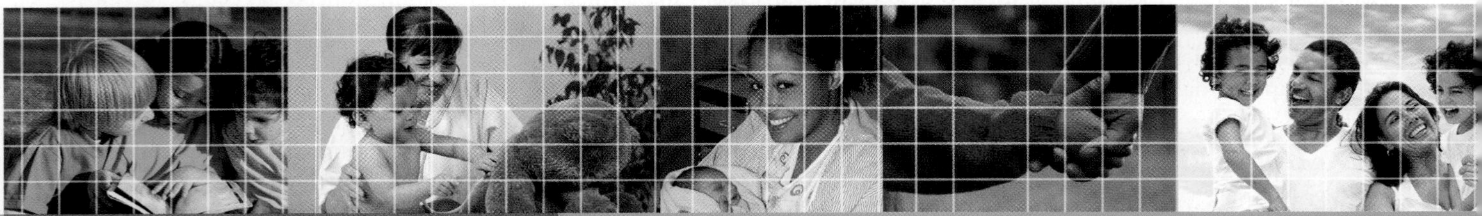

CRITICAL CONCEPT REVIEW

LEARNING OUTCOMES	CONCEPTS
56.1 Describe the anatomy and physiology of the neurologic system.	The major structures of the neurologic system are: 1. Brain. 2. Spinal cord: transmits impulses to and from the brain, conveying sensory information and relaying impulses that stimulate motor responses. 3. Nerves: the infant is born with all the nerve cells he or she will have throughout life. Maturation of these nerves continue until age 4. Myelination proceeds in a cephalocaudal direction.
56.2 Describe the nursing assessment process and tools used for infants and children with altered levels of consciousness and other neurologic conditions.	1. Infants and children with altered levels of consciousness should be monitored for: ■ Responsiveness to environmental and sensory stimuli. ■ Pupil size and reactivity. ■ Movement of extremities. ■ Ability to maintain an airway. ■ Changes in vital signs. ■ Changes in breathing patterns. ■ Status of the cranial nerves. ■ Orientation and cognitive functioning. 2. Nurses should use the Glasgow Coma Scale as well as cardiorespiratory monitors and pulse oximetry to monitor the child.
56.3 Differentiate between the signs of infants and children with epilepsy and status epilepticus, and describe appropriate nursing management for each condition.	1. Epilepsy: ■ Clinical manifestations depend upon type of seizure. ■ Lasts from 5 seconds to 1–2 minutes, depending upon type of seizure. ■ Signs range from momentary lapse of attention to unconsciousness with repetitive muscular contraction and relaxation. ■ Decreased level of consciousness during postictal period.

LEARNING OUTCOMES	CONCEPTS
	2. Nursing management of epilepsy: ■ Administer medications as ordered. ■ Protect child from injury. ■ Instruct parents concerning importance of giving medications as prescribed to maintain blood levels of medications. ■ Instruct parents in management of seizures and when to call for emergency assistance. 3. Status epilepticus: ■ Continuous seizure that lasts longer than 20 minutes. ■ Series of seizures during which consciousness is not regained. 4. Nursing management of status epilepticus: ■ Maintain the airway of the child. ■ Establish IV access. ■ Monitor vital signs and oxygen saturation with pulse oximetry. ■ Administer medications as prescribed. ■ Monitor for respiratory depression and apnea due to cumulative doses of medications.
56.4 Differentiate among signs of bacterial meningitis, viral meningitis, encephalitis, and Guillain-Barré syndrome in infants and children.	1. Bacterial meningitis: ■ Fever. ■ Lethargic and irritable. ■ Change in feeding, vomiting, and diarrhea. ■ Hemorrhagic rash (meningococcal meningitis). ■ Nuchal rigidity, positive Kernig and Brudzinski signs, opisthotonic position. ■ Headache, back pain, photophobia. 2. Viral meningitis: ■ Child appears less ill than child with bacterial meningitis. ■ Fever. ■ Irritable and lethargic. ■ General malaise, headache, photophobia. ■ Upper respiratory symptoms. ■ Positive Kernig and Brudzinski signs, stiff neck. 3. Encephalitis: ■ Fever. ■ Severe headache. ■ Altered mental status. ■ Speech disturbance. ■ Motor dysfunction. 4. Guillain-Barré syndrome: ■ Rapidly progressive severe hypotonia (infants). ■ Rapidly progressive ascending symmetric weakness and muscle pain (children). ■ Absent or diminished deep tendon reflexes. ■ Difficulty swallowing and facial weakness. ■ Respiratory effort inadequate for ventilation.
56.5 Develop a nursing care plan for the infant with myelodysplasia and hydrocephalus.	1. Myelodysplasia: ■ Keep newborn in prone position. ■ Cover defect with sterile, saline dressing. ■ Monitor for signs of infection. ■ After surgery, monitor for wound healing and CSF leakage. ■ Measure head circumference daily. ■ Assess intake and output. ■ Avoid the use of latex products. ■ Assess neurologic status of the extremities. ■ Perform range of motion exercises and promote positioning for function. 2. Hydrocephalus: ■ Measure head circumference daily. ■ Observe for signs and symptoms of increased ICP. ■ Assess level of responsiveness. ■ Observe surgical site for signs of wound healing. ■ Position infant to aid in drainage of CSF.

(continued)

LEARNING OUTCOMES / CONCEPTS

56.6 Describe the focus of community-based nursing care for the child with cerebral palsy.

1. The nurse in the community assists in:
   - Care planning and coordination of multiple healthcare services and referring the family to community resources.
   - Providing health promotion care to the child. Supporting family with ways to promote growth and development.
   - Providing information to schools and other community agencies to meet the needs of the child.
   - Assuring access to adaptive equipment or assistive technology needed.
   - Planning the transition from adolescence to adulthood.

56.7 Distinguish among the assessment findings of the child with a mild, moderate, and severe traumatic brain injury.

1. Mild brain injury:
   - No loss (or very brief loss) of consciousness.
   - Possible amnesia of event.
   - Mild headache unrelieved by medication.
   - Easily irritated.
   - Slowed thinking, acting, speaking.
   - Difficulty paying attention or concentrating.
2. Moderate brain injury:
   - Loss of consciousness.
   - Headache.
   - Nausea and vomiting.
   - Amnesia.
   - Glasgow Coma Score of 9–12.
3. Severe brain injury:
   - Prolonged period of unconsciousness.
   - Signs of increased ICP.
   - Glasgow Coma Score of 8 or less.
   - Amnesia lasting longer than 24 hours.

56.8 Contrast the appropriate initial nursing management for mild and severe traumatic brain injury.

Nursing management of traumatic brain injury is as follows:

1. Mild injury:
   - Observe for changing levels of consciousness.
   - Instruct parents concerning signs and symptoms of increased ICP indicating need to return for immediate care.
   - Educate parents about behavior changes to expect and rest needed during the child's recovery.
2. Severe injury:
   - Assess airway, breathing, and circulation. Be prepared to assist ventilations.
   - Assess neurologic status and vital signs frequently. Monitor for increased ICP.
   - Elevate head of bed if there is no neck injury.
   - Administer medications and IV fluids as ordered.
   - Keep environment quiet.
   - Provide nutrition, with enteral feeding if child is unable to eat.
   - Provide oral care and promote skin integrity.
   - Prevent physical deformities.

CRITICAL THINKING IN ACTION

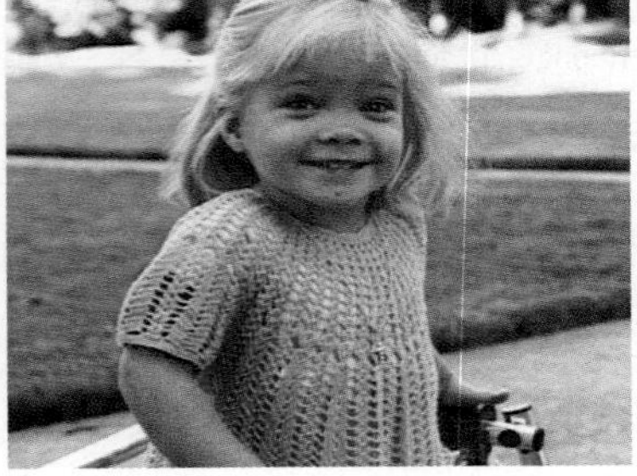

Abigail, a 3-year-old with myelodysplasia, is seen every few months with her parents in the multidisciplinary spina bifida clinic where you work. Her lesion is at the L3 level, so she can flex her hips and extend her knees, but her ankles and toes are paralyzed. She also has a ventriculoperitoneal shunt for hydrocephalus. She uses lower leg braces and a walker to mobilize and has minimal sensation in her lower legs and feet. Her bladder and bowel sphincters are also affected, so Abigail and her parents have worked hard to establish bowel control with a high-fiber diet and by establishing specific times for bowel evacuation. Abigail's parents learned to perform intermittent catheterization for bladder control to reduce the risk for kidney damage.

Her health history reveals she has experienced a case of otitis media since her last visit and responded well to antibiotics. Her legs are well protected by stockings to reduce rubbing by her braces. Her gait is becoming steadier with the walker, and her parents are encouraging exercise of her arms and upper trunk with swimming. You encourage Abigail's parents to promote her cognitive development with age-appropriate games and interaction with siblings.

1. What are the safety issues to discuss with Abigail's parents about spina bifida?
2. Describe spina bifida.
3. Identify important health promotion issues to discuss with Abigail's parents.
4. Describe the relationship between hydrocephalus and spina bifida.

See MyNursingKit for possible responses.

REFERENCES

Adirim, T. A. (2007). Concussions in sports and recreation. *Clinical Pediatric Emergency Medicine, 8*, 2–6.

American Academy of Pediatrics Committee on Infectious Disease. (2009). *Red book: Report of the committee on infectious disease* (28th ed.). Elk Grove Village, IL: Author.

Atabaki, S. M. (2007). Pediatric head injury. *Pediatrics in Review, 28*(6), 215–223.

Austin, J. K. (2004). Behavioral issues involving children and adolescents with epilepsy and the impact of their families: recent research data. *Epilepsy and Behavior, 5* (Suppl 3), S33–41.

Avner, J. R. (2006). Altered states of consciousness, *Pediatrics in Review, 27*(9), 331–337.

Blackman, J. A. (2005). Severe brain injury: Helping patient and family on the long road back. *Contemporary Pediatrics, 22*(1), 63–78.

Blumstein, M. D., & Friedman, M. J. (2007). Childhood seizures. *Emergency Clinics of North America, 25*, 1061–1086.

Boss, B. J. (2006). Alterations in neurologic function. In K. L. McCance & S. E. Huether (Eds.), *Pathophysiology: The biologic basis for disease in adults and children* (5th ed., pp. 547–603). St. Louis: Mosby.

Brand, M. C. (2006). Part 2: Examining the newborn with an open spinal dysraphism. *Advances in Neonatal Care, 6*(4), 181–196.

Burford, A. E., Ryan, L. M., Stone, B. J., Hirshon, J. M., & Klein, B. L. (2005). Drowning and near drowning in children and adolescents. *Pediatric Emergency Care, 21*(9), 610–616.

Carey, R. G., & Balistreri, W. F. (2007). Mitochondrial hepatopathies. In R. M. Kliegman, R. E. Behrman, H. B. Jenson, B. F. Stanton (Eds.), *Nelson textbook of pediatrics* (18th ed., pp. 1696–1698). Philadelphia: Elsevier Saunders.

Centers for Disease Control and Prevention. (2006). *What is traumatic brain injury?* Retrieved February 5, 2009, from http://www.cdc.gov/ncipc/tbi/TBI.htm

Chávez-Bueno, S., & McCracken, G. H. (2005). Bacterial meningitis in children. *Pediatric Clinics of North America, 52*, 795–810.

Chiafery, M. (2006). Care and management of the child with shunted hydrocephalus. *Pediatric Nursing, 32*(3), 222–225.

Dias, M. S. (2004). Traumatic brain injury and spinal cord injury. *Pediatric Clinics of North America, 51*, 271–303.

Dias, M. S. (2005). Neurosurgical management of myelomeningocele (spina bifida). *Pediatrics in Review, 26*(2), 50–59.

Doolin, E. (2006). Bowel management for patients with myelodysplasia. *Surgical Clinics of North America*, 86, 505–514.

Elliott, M. R., Arbogast, K. A., & Durbin, D. R. (2006). A latent class analysis of injury patterns among rear-seated, seat-belted children. *Journal of Trauma Injury, Infection, and Critical Care, 61*(5), 1244–1248.

Epilepsy Foundation. (2009). *Epilepsy and seizure statistics.* Retrieved January 28, 2009 from http://www.epilepsyfoundation.org/about/statistics.cfm

Fadiman, A. (1997). *The spirit catches you and you fall down.* New York: Farrar, Strauss, Giroux.

Fisher, P. G. (2005). Help for headaches: A strategy for your busy practice. *Contemporary Pediatrics, 22*(11), 34–40.

Fisher, P. G. (2007). First and second seizure: What to know and do. *Contemporary Pediatrics, 24*(4), 80–89.

Frasier, L. D. (2008). Abusive head trauma in infants and young children: A unique contributor to developmental disabilities. *Pediatric Clinics of North America, 55*(6), 1269–1285.

Freeman, J. M., Kossoff, E. H., & Hartman, A. L. (2007). The ketogenic diet: One decade later. *Pediatrics, 119*(3), 535–543.

Gladstein, J., & Mack, K. J. (2005). Chronic daily headaches in adolescents. *Pediatric Annals, 34*(6), 472–479.

Goldstein, J. (2008). Status epilepticus in the pediatric emergency department. *Clinical Pediatric Emergency Medicine, 9*, 96–100.

Graham, J. M., Gomez, M., Halberg, A., Earl, D. L., Kreutzman, J. T., Cui, J., & Guo, X. (2005). Management of deformational plagiocephaly: Repositioning versus orthotic therapy. *Journal of Pediatrics, 146*(2), 258–262.

Graham, J. M., Kreutzman, J., Earl, D., Halberg, A., Samayoa, C., & Guo, X. (2005). Deformational brachycephaly in supine-sleeping infants. *Journal of Pediatrics, 146*(2), 253–257.

Gray, E. H., Blackinton, J., & White, G. M. (2006). Stoma care in the school setting. *Journal of School Nursing, 22*(2), 74–80.

Gunner, K. B., & Smith, H. D. (2007). Practice guideline for diagnosis and management of migraine headaches in children and adolescents: Part one. *Journal of Pediatric Health Care, 21*(5), 327–332.

Haque, I. U., LaTour, M. C., & Zaritsky, A. L. (2006). Pediatric critical care community survey of knowledge and attitudes toward therapeutic hypothermia in comatose children after cardiac arrest. *Pediatric Critical Care Medicine, 7*, 7–14.

Hart, L. (2005). Primary care for patients with neurofibromatosis 1. *The Nurse Practitioner, 30*(6), 38–43.

Hayes, J. S., & Arriola, T. (2005). Pediatric spinal injuries. *Pediatric Nursing, 31*(6), 464–467.

Jankowitz, B. T., & Adelson, P. D. (2006). Pediatric traumatic brain injury: Past, present, and future. *Developmental Neuroscience, 28*, 264–275.

Johnston, M. V., Ferriero, D. M., Vannucci, S. J., & Hagberg, H. (2005). Models of cerebral palsy: Which ones are best? *Journal of Child Neurology, 20*(12), 984–987.

Jones, M. W., Morgan, E., Shelton, J. E. (2007a). Cerebral palsy: Introduction and diagnosis (Part 1). *Journal of Pediatric Health Care, 21*(3), 146–152.

Jones, M. W., Morgan, E., & Shelton, J. E. (2007b). Primary care of the child with cerebral palsy: A review of systems (Part II). *Journal of Pediatric Health Care, 21*(4), 226–237.

Keenan, H. T., & Bratton, S. L. (2006). Epidemiology and outcomes of pediatric traumatic brain injury. *Developmental Neuroscience, 28*, 256–263.

Kinsman, S. L., & Johnson, M. V. (2007). Congenital anomalies of the central nervous system. In R. M. Kliegman, R. E. Behrman, H. B. Jenson, B. F. Stanton (Eds.), *Nelson textbook of pediatrics* (18th ed., pp. 2443–2456). Philadelphia: Elsevier Saunders.

Kirkwood, M. W., Yeates, K. O., & Wilson, P. E. (2006). Pediatric sports-related concussion: A review of the clinical management of an oft-neglected population. *Pediatrics, 117*(4), 1359–1371.

Knapp, J. M. (2005). Hyperosmolar therapy in the treatment of severe head injury in children: Mannitol and hypertonic saline. *AACN Clinical Issues, 16*(2), 199–211.

Kohen, D. P., & Zajac, R. (2007). Self-hypnosis training for headaches in children and adolescents. *Journal of Pediatrics, 150*, 635–639.

Komotar, R. J., Zacharia, B. E., Ellis, J. A., Feldstein, N. A., & Anderson, R. C. E. (2006). Pitfalls for the pediatrician: Positional molding or craniosynostosis? *Pediatric Annals, 35*(5), 365–375.

Leung, A. K. C., & Robson, W. L. M. (2007). Febrile seizures. *Journal of Pediatric Health Care, 21*(4), 250–255.

Lewis, P., & Glaser, C. A. (2005). Encephalitis. *Pediatrics in Review, 26*(10), 353–362.

Liptak, G. S. (2007). Neural tube defects. In M. L. Batshaw (Ed.), *Children with disabilities* (6th ed., pp. 419–438). Baltimore: Paul H. Brooks.

Mansfield, R. T. (2007). Severe traumatic brain injury. *Clinical Pediatric Emergency Medicine, 8*, 156–164.

Marcoux, K. K. (2005). Management of increased intracranial pressure in the critically ill child with an acute neurologic injury. *AACN Clinical Issues, 16*(2), 212–231.

McCall, T., Fassett, D., & Brockmeyer, D. (2006). Cervical spine trauma in children: A review. *Neurosurgical Focus, 20*(2), E5.

McCrory, P., Johnston, K., Meeuwisse, W., Aubry, M., Cantu, R., Dvorak, J., et al. (2005). Summary and agreement statement of the 2nd international conference on concussion in sport, Prague 2004. *British Journal of Sports Medicine, 39*, 196–204.

McNelis, A., Buelow, J., Myers, J., & Johnson, E. A. (2007). Concerns and needs of children with epilepsy and their parents. *Clinical Nurse Specialist, 21*(4), 195–202.

Mendelson, K. G., & Fallat, M. E. (2007). Pediatric injuries: Prevention to resolution. *Surgical Clinics of North America, 87*, 207–228.

Meyer, R. J., Theodorou, A. A., & Berg, R. A. (2006). Childhood drowning. *Pediatrics in Review, 27*(5), 163–168.

National Institute for Neurologic Disorders and Stroke. (2008). Hydrocephalus fact sheet. Retrieved February 8, 2009 from http://www.ninds.nih.gov/disorders/hydrocephalus/detail_hydrocephalus.htm

Nehring, W. M., & Faux, S. A. (2006). Transitional and health issues of adults with neural tube defects. *Journal of Nursing Scholarship, 38*(1), 63–70.

Nield, L. S., Nanda, S., Someshwar, J., Dalcanto, F. C., Someshwar, S., Collins, J. J., & Jaynes, M. (2007, June). Cerebral palsy: A multisystem review. *Consultant for Pediatricians, 6*(6), 337–343.

Padgett, K. (2006). Alterations in neurologic function in children. In K. L. McCance & S. E. Huether (Eds.), *Pathophysiology: The biologic basis for disease in adults and children* (5th ed., pp. 623–654). St. Louis: Mosby.

Pellegrino, L. (2007). Cerebral palsy. In M. L. Batshaw, L. Pellegrino, & N. J. Roizen (Eds.), *Children with disabilities* (6th ed., pp. 387–408). Baltimore: Paul H. Brooks.

Prober, C. G. (2007). Central nervous system infections. In R. M. Kliegman, R. E. Behrman, H. B. Jenson, & B. F. Stanton (Eds.), *Nelson textbook of pediatrics* (18th ed., pp. 2512–2524). Philadelphia: Elsevier Saunders.

Rais-Bahrami, K., & Short, B. L. (2007). Premature and small-for-dates infants. In M. L. Batshaw, L. Pellegrino, & N. J. Roizen (Eds.), *Children with disabilities* (6th ed., pp. 107–122). Baltimore: Paul H. Brooks.

Rosenbaum, P., Paneth, N., Leviton, A., Goldstein, M., Bax, M., et al. (2007). A report: The definition and classification of cerebral palsy, April 2006. *Developmental Medicine and Child Neurology, 49*, 8–14.

Rowe, D. E., & Jadhav, A. L. (2008). Care of the adolescent with spina bifida. *Pediatric Clinics of North America, 55*, 1359–1374.

Rubin, D. H., Suecoff, S. A., & Knupp, K. G. (2006). Headaches in children. *Pediatric Annals, 35*(5), 345–353.

Saneto, R. P., Sotero de Menezes, M. A., Ojemann, J. G., Bournival, B. D., Murphy, P. J., Cook, W. B., et al. (2006). Vagus nerve stimulation for intractable seizures in children. *Pediatric Neurology, 35*, 323–326.

Sarnat, H. B. (2007). Neuromuscular disorders. In R. M. Kliegman, R. E. Behrman, H. B. Jenson, B. F. Stanton (Eds.), *Nelson textbook of pediatrics* (18th ed., pp. 2531–2567). Philadelphia: Elsevier Saunders.

Simpkins, C. J. (2005). Ventriculoperitoneal shunt infections in patients with hydrocephalus. *Pediatric Nursing, 31*(6), 457–462.

Spector, R. E. (2009). *Cultural diversity in health and illness* (7th ed., pp. 3–4). Upper Saddle River, NJ: Pearson.

Swaine, B. R., Tremblay, C., Platt, R. W., Grimard, G. Zhang, X., & Pleiss, I. B. (2007). Previous head injury is a risk factor for subsequent head injury in children: A longitudinal cohort study. *Pediatrics, 119*(4), 749–758.

Theos, A., & Korf, B. R. (2006). Pathophysiology of neurofibromatosis type 1. *Annals of Internal Medicine, 144*(11), 842–849.

Unger, J. (2006, September). Pediatric migraine: Clinical pearls in diagnosis and therapy. *Consultant for Pediatricians, 5*(9), 545–551.

Vitale, M. G., Goss, J. M., Matsumoto, H., & Roye, D. P. (2006). Epidemiology of pediatric spinal cord injury in the United States, Years 1997 and 2000. *Journal of Pediatric Orthopedics, 26*(6), 745–749.

Warner, W. C. (2007). Myelomeningocele. In S. T. Canale & J. H. Beaty (Eds.), *Campbell's operative orthopedics* (11th ed., pp. 1450–1474), Philadelphia: Mosby Elsevier.

Weinstein, S. L., & Gaillard, W. D. (2007). Epilepsy. In M. L. Barshaw, L. Pellegrino, & N. J. Roizen (Eds.), *Children with disabilities* (6th ed., pp. 439–460). Baltimore: Paul H. Brooks.

Williams, L. J., Rasmussen, S. A., Flores, A., Kirby, R. S., & Edmonds, L. D. (2005). Decline in the prevalence of spina bifida and anencephaly by race/ethnicity: 1995–2002. *Pediatrics, 116*(3), 580–586.

Wilson, B. A., Shannon, M. T., & Shield, K. M. (2009). *Nurse's drug guide 2009.* Upper Saddle River, NJ: Prentice Hall Health.

Wolf, S. M., & McGoldrick, P. E. (2006). Recognition and management of pediatric seizures. *Pediatric Annals, 35*(5), 332–344.

Zuckerbraun, N. S., & Saladino, R. A. (2005). Pediatric drowning: Current management strategies for immediate care. *Clinical Pediatric Emergency Medicine, 6*, 49–56.

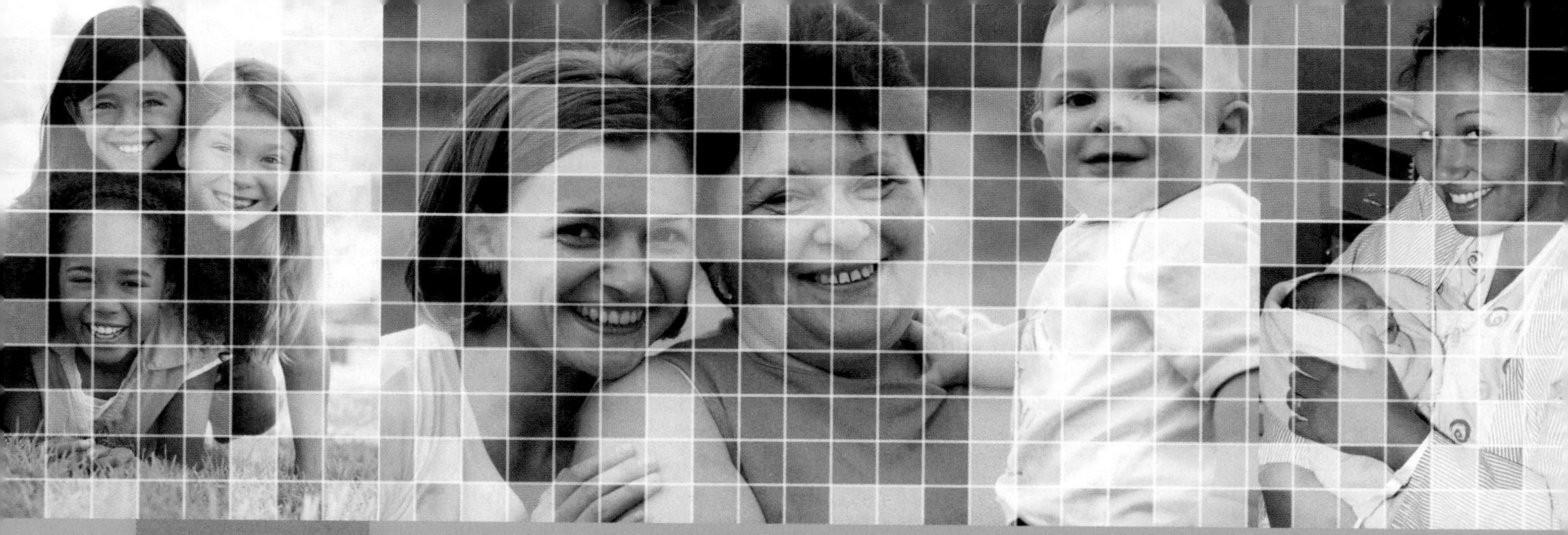

CHAPTER

57 The Child with Alterations in Mental Health and Cognitive Function

We've been so worried about Cassandra. After being in the car crash, she has become so frightened of everything. She wakes up at night screaming and has lost interest in school and friends. We hope that her work with the therapist will help to decrease her fears and get her involved in all of her activities again. —*Mother of Cassandra, 9 years old*

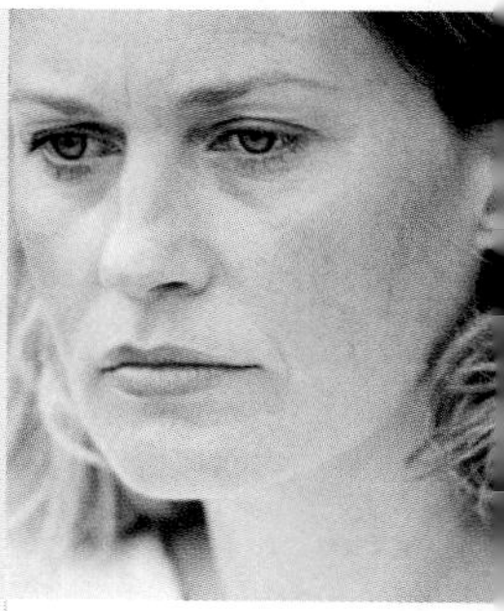

LEARNING OUTCOMES

57.1 Define mental health and describe major mental health alterations in childhood.

57.2 Discuss the clinical manifestations of the major mental health alterations of childhood and adolescence.

57.3 Plan for the nursing management of children and adolescents with mental health alterations in the hospital and community settings.

57.4 Describe characteristics of common cognitive alterations of childhood.

57.5 Plan nursing management for children with cognitive alterations.

57.6 Establish and evaluate expected outcomes of care for the child with a cognitive alteration.

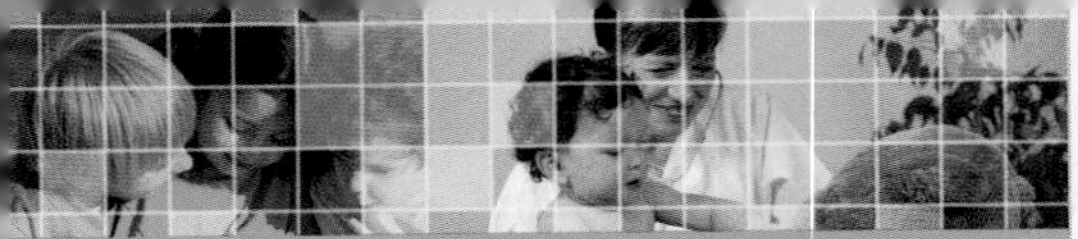

KEY TERMS

Adaptive functioning, 1731
Affect, 1729
Agoraphobia, 1724
Behavior modification, 1706
Cognition, 1704
Cognitive therapy, 1705
Developmental disability, 1731
Echolalia, 1710
Evidence-based practice, 1705
Intellectual disability, 1731
Mental health, 1704
Pervasive developmental disorders, 1709
Play therapy, 1706
Stereotypy, 1710

This chapter will provide the knowledge and tools needed to provide appropriate care for children with alterations in mental health and cognition. Mental health care is provided by psychiatric–mental health specialists, so the nurse's role often centers on identification, support of the therapy, teaching, and referral. Cognitive conditions are commonly managed by the family and the school personnel. The nurse also forms partnerships with families and school personnel to plan and evaluate care for the child with cognitive conditions such as intellectual disability (mental retardation). A thorough knowledge of development is a prerequisite to understanding both mental health alterations and cognitive conditions since developmental status is often altered in both mental health and cognitive conditions. Review Chapter 33 as needed to understand the relationships of development to the conditions described in the present chapter.

Some cognitive/mental health conditions in children originate from a genetic or physiologic cause. Examples include intellectual disability and childhood schizophrenia. The environments in which children live also influence their characteristics and contribute to dysfunctions such as anxiety, depression, and posttraumatic stress disorder.

Most mental health and cognitive conditions are treated in community settings, and nurses in these settings play an active role in the treatment and support of the child and family. Nurses may function as case managers, assisting a family to deal with all areas of the child's care. Occasionally a child is hospitalized for treatment of a significant mental health alteration, or a child hospitalized for another health problem requires continued mental health services.

MENTAL HEALTH ALTERATIONS OF CHILDREN AND ADOLESCENTS

Mental health is foundational to a sense of personal well-being. It involves successful engagement in activities and relationships and the ability to adapt and cope with change. **Cognition** refers to the change in thought, intelligence, and language that occurs over time as brain maturation and life experiences interact to mutually influence child performance (Santrock, 2007).

Approximately 25% of children, or 15 million, in the United States suffer from mental illness that is severe enough to impair functioning at home or school, and only 30% of those children receive any mental health services. Overall, about one in four or five children and adolescents has a mental health disorder, 1 in 10 has a disorder that profoundly interferes with daily functioning, and 1/2 of adult mental health disorders begin in childhood (National Institute for Health Care Management Foundation, 2008). Less than 35% of children with mental health alterations receive mental health services to treat their impairment (Mark & Buck, 2006; Stein, Zitner, & Jensen, 2006). Further, some of the services received are not comprehensive or multidisciplinary, leading to unmet mental health needs.

From the ages of 10 to 21 years, mental health issues are among the top two leading causes of hospitalization in all age groups (see Chapter 1). This high rate of hospitalization suggests that children are not receiving clinical therapy early, when outpatient care is appropriate and prognosis is best. The Surgeon General led an initiative to examine mental health in the United States and identified a series of goals and steps toward improving mental health care for children (U.S. Department of Health and Human Services, 2004). In order to confront this childhood mental health crisis, the Surgeon General's agenda includes promoting mental health as an essential part of child health, integrating mental health services into all health services provided to children, engaging families and youth in planning for mental health care, and developing and enhancing the infrastructure to support child and youth mental health services (Chambers, Ringeisen, & Hickman, 2005; U.S. Department of Health and Human Services, 2004). See Table 57–1 for a list of the goals established in the Surgeon General's report.

Table 57–1 Goals of the Surgeon General's National Action Agenda for Children's Mental Health

1. Promote public awareness of children's mental health issues and reduce stigma associated with mental illness.
2. Continue to develop, disseminate, and implement scientifically proven prevention and treatment services in the field of children's mental health.
3. Improve the assessment and recognition of mental health needs in children.
4. Eliminate racial/ethnic and socioeconomic disparities in access to mental health care.
5. Improve the infrastructure for children's mental health services, including support for scientifically proven interventions across professions.
6. Increase access to and coordination of quality mental healthcare services.
7. Train frontline providers to recognize and manage mental health issues, and educate mental health providers in scientifically proven prevention and treatment services.
8. Monitor the access to and coordination of quality mental health care services.

Note: From U.S. Department of Health and Human Services (2004). Report on the surgeon general's conference on children's mental health: A national action agenda. Washington, DC: Author.

Nurses have been leaders in the field of pediatric mental health care. An initiative known as KySS (Keep Your children/yourself Safe and Secure) was launched by nurses in 2001 and was the subject of a summit for health professional collaboration in 2003. The goals of the summit included identifying assessment, implementation, and dissemination strategies for promoting the mental health of children and teens in primary care and alternative care settings, and reviewing evidence-based practice to make recommendations for interventions and needed research areas (Melnyk & Moldenhauer, 2006; National Association of Pediatric Nurse Practitioners, 2007).

During all health visits, mental health screening should be integrated into care so that alterations can be identified. See Chapters 36–38 for specific questions to ask during health promotion and health maintenance visits. When a potential mental health condition exists, the child receives further assessment from a mental health specialist. A resource commonly used is the *Diagnostic and Statistical Manual,* which lists diagnostic criteria for known mental health conditions. The current edition is the DSM-IV-TR (American Psychiatric Association, 2000), and its criteria for several conditions are listed throughout this chapter.

CLINICAL THERAPY

Diagnosis of mental health conditions involves careful physical and psychological assessment. Studies such as magnetic resonance imaging (MRI), radiograph, electroencephalogram, and toxicology screening may be useful. Mental health is linked to development so developmental screening tests are administered. Mental health status can influence activity level, physiologic parameters, and risk for certain conditions. Therefore, height and weight, review of systems, vital signs, and medication/substance use history are important to perform. Family interactions, stressors, and methods of coping are assessed.

The primary treatment goal for children and adolescents with psychosocial disorders is to assist the child and family to achieve and maintain an optimal level of functioning through interventions designed to reduce the impact of stressors. Therapeutic interventions and communication are based on the principle that feelings motivate behaviors. Parents and others close to the child often fall into the habit of reacting to the child's behaviors rather than trying to find out what feelings may be precipitating the undesirable actions. While behaviors may be considered in treatment, feelings and life experiences are often explored to provide insight and to lead to behavior change. Medication may be used to enhance and support other therapy, or may be the major therapeutic measure.

When possible, mental health interventions should be founded on **evidence-based practice**, or a body of scientific knowledge. While the research basis for care in all areas of pediatric health is generally scant, there is even less scientific basis to support interventions in mental health services because of a lack of pediatric mental health research. Nurses must seek to apply evidence-based practice to enhance mental health care when possible, and to participate in research and outcomes measurement so that additional strong evidence can be gathered on the best approaches to care (Dulcan, 2005; Hoagwood & Burns, 2005).

Treatment Modes

Three basic treatment modes are used: individual, family, and group therapy. The choice of treatment mode must take into account the child's age and developmental stage. Most therapists use several intervention strategies simultaneously. Different strategies are more or less effective and appropriate for children and adolescents in various stages of development. A thorough understanding of developmental needs, expectations, and abilities is therefore essential for mental health professionals.

Individual therapy. Individual therapy involves only the child and the therapist. Treatment of specific emotional problems or disorders may involve various techniques such as play therapy, psychodrama, art therapy, and **cognitive therapy** (a technique used to help a person recognize automatic negative thinking). Individual therapy may be short term (four to six sessions) or long term (lasting for several years).

Family therapy. Family therapy involves the exploration of a particular emotional problem and its manifestations among the family members. Family therapy is based on the idea that the emotional symptoms or problems of an individual are an expression of emotional symptoms or problems in the family. The focus is on the relationships among the family members, not the psychologic conflict within each individual member.

Group therapy. Group therapy involves an ongoing or limited number of sessions in which several individuals participate. The emphasis is on the interpersonal styles of relating to one another in the group. Group therapy is particularly effective with adolescents because of the importance of the peer group at this age. An advantage of group therapy is that stimuli and feedback come from multiple sources (the group members) instead of just one person (the therapist).

Therapeutic Strategies

Play therapy. Play is often called the language or work of the child. From a developmental perspective, children progressively learn to express feelings and needs through action, fantasy, and finally language. The special quality of play buffers children against the pressures and demands of daily life. Play helps children master developmental stages by strengthening physical and neurologic processes. Play also assists in cognitive learning, setting the stage for problem solving and creativity.

Play therapy is a technique that reveals problems on a fantasy level through the use of toys, dolls, clay, art, and other creative objects. It is often used with preschool and school-age children who are experiencing anxiety, stress, and other specific nonpsychotic mental disorders. Play therapy encourages the child to act out feelings such as anger, hostility, sadness, and fear. It also gives the therapist a chance to help the child understand, on a conscious or unconscious level, his or her own responses and behavior in a safe, supportive environment. This type of therapy was used for Cassandra, described in the opening quotation, who needed to gain some control over a frightening environment by acting out fears and trying solutions during play with a therapist. Play therapy is different from therapeutic play, which may be used with hospitalized children (see Chapter 41∞). Only a specialist is qualified to provide play therapy for mental health disorders.

Art therapy. Children who may be apprehensive about playing can sometimes be encouraged to participate in art therapy, using brief drawing exercises. This technique is appropriate for children of all ages, including adolescents. The drawings can help the therapist gain information about the child, the family, and the interactions between the child and family. However, children's drawings should never be the only basis for a definitive diagnosis.

When used in conjunction with a thorough history and appropriate psychologic testing information, art therapy can guide the child's treatment. These drawing exercises provide an opportunity to help in the healing process. The therapist can assist the child to release feelings of anger, pain, or fear onto paper, where they can be examined objectively. (Figures 57–1 ● to 57–4 ● present several examples of this technique.)

Cognitive and behavioral therapy (CBT). Cognitive therapy teaches thinking patterns to change reactions to situations that cause anxiety or other undesirable conditions. The child is taught how his or her brain and body are working; this understanding assists the child in having control over the experience.

Behavior modification is a therapeutic technique that uses stimulus and response conditioning to alter inappropriate behaviors. It reinforces desirable behaviors, helping the child to replace maladaptive behaviors with more appropriate ones. This technique is based on the assumption that any learned behavior can be unlearned. Thus, if parents, nurses, teachers, and other adults consistently reinforce desirable behaviors, the child will eventually alter or discontinue undesirable behaviors.

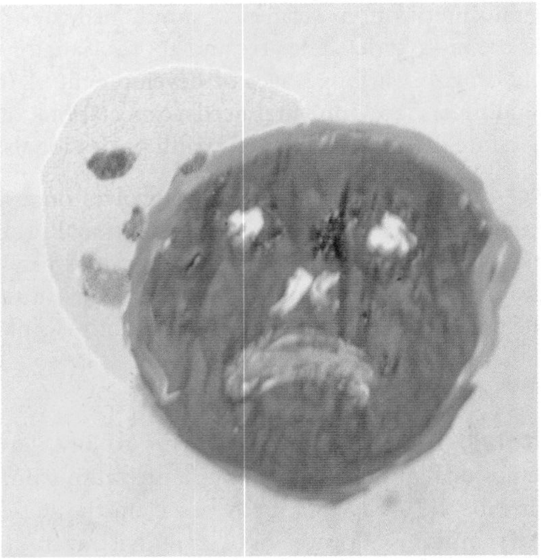

● **Figure 57–1** "Me." Drawn by a 14-year-old girl with major depression, anxiety, and school phobia who had experienced multiple losses over several years. Her mother had severe chronic lung problems and diabetes, and the girl had stopped attending school for fear that something would happen to her mother. This drawing represents the girl's obvious feelings of sadness and depression but also indicates a glimmer of hope (represented by the yellow mask coming from behind the dark mask of depression).

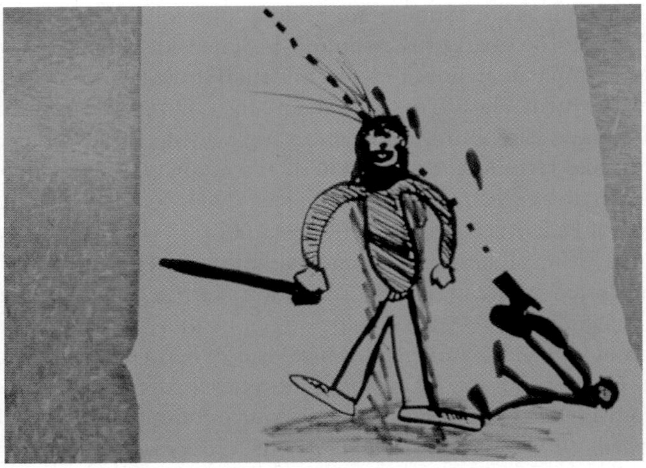

● **Figure 57–2** "Self-Portrait." Drawn by a 15-year-old boy who was admitted through the emergency department after a failed suicide attempt by hanging. He had a psychiatric diagnosis of depression and polysubstance abuse (including inhalants and alcohol) and insisted that he was a member of a satanic cult in his hometown. Most of his drawings depicted a preoccupation with violence and suicide. The boy said that he always felt a "darkness" like a shadow that followed him around and wanted him dead. His family history was significant for depression and suicide on both his mother's and his father's side. His father also had a lengthy history of polysubstance abuse and alcoholism. The boy was discharged to a long-term residential treatment facility for adolescents.

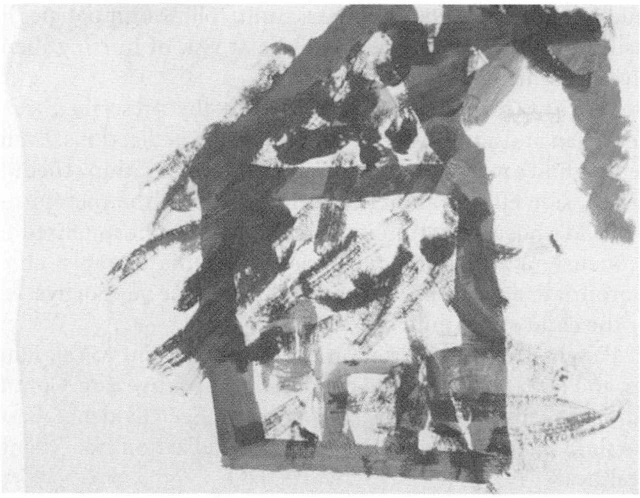

● **Figure 57–3** "An Activity." Drawn by an 8-year-old boy who was initially admitted to the medical-surgical floor of a pediatric hospital for dehydration resulting from vomiting and diarrhea. Psychiatric evaluation was ordered for extreme anxiety. These drawings, completed during the initial interview, led to further investigation, which revealed that the child had started a house fire in which his grandmother (his primary caretaker at the time) was killed. The family's home and all their belongings were lost. No one had known that the child had set the fire. Further sessions indicated that he had been setting neighborhood garage fires and watching them burn from a distance.

Behavior modification may include (1) removing the child from the home to a more structured environment, such as a hospital, for a brief time, and (2) teaching the parents, teachers, and other appropriate adults to be agents of behavioral change. Several ongoing sessions may be required with the adults involved, using role play and other techniques. Consistency is the most important principle in the success of behavior modification.

A combination of cognitive and behavioral therapy (CBT) is useful in treating many mental health conditions in children.

Visualization and guided imagery. The techniques of visualization and guided imagery begin with specific directions for progressive relaxation according to the child's ability. This form of therapy uses the child's own imagination and positive thinking to reduce stress and anxiety, decrease the experience of pain or discomfort, and promote healing. The techniques are especially useful for managing anxiety disorders and chronic pain. It is not easy for every child to use his or her imagination in this way, so the technique may not work or be appropriate for everyone.

Hypnosis. Hypnosis involves varying degrees of suggestibility and deep relaxation effects. This technique is useful for children and adolescents because they can usually be hypnotized more easily than adults. Hypnosis is especially helpful in treating physical symptoms with a psychologic component, anxiety, and phobias. It is also useful in managing severe physical symptoms or discomfort (pain or nausea) associated with a physiologic disorder or its treatment (e.g., cancer or juvenile rheumatoid arthritis).

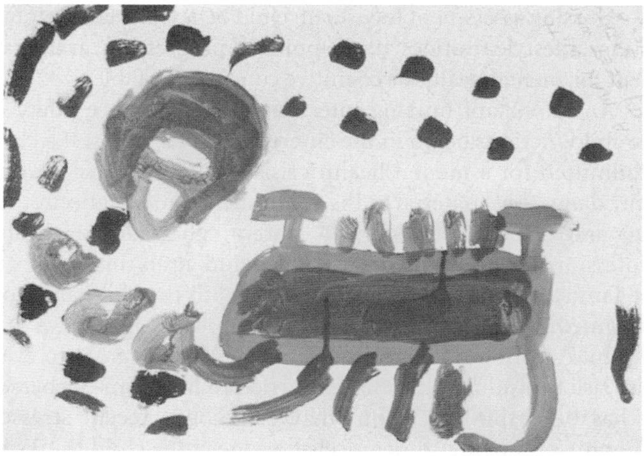

● **Figure 57–4** "A Family Activity." By the same boy who drew Figure 57–3. This drawing depicts a recurring incident of physical and emotional abuse by his mother's live-in boyfriend. It shows the family bathtub with feces and blood smeared on the floors and walls. The boy reported that when either he or his 3-year-old brother had a toileting accident the boyfriend would make them go into the bathroom and stand in the bathtub while he smeared the feces on the walls. He would then hit the children and make them clean up the mess. The boy had previously been removed from the mother's custody for neglect. He was transferred from the medical-surgical area to the inpatient children's psychiatric unit, where he received a diagnosis of depression, overanxious disorder, and child abuse (physical and emotional). Charges were filed against the mother's boyfriend and custody of both children was temporarily revoked.

Nursing Management

Ongoing assessment of all children and their families for mental health risk should be performed from the beginning of life and throughout childhood and adolescence (National Association of Pediatric Nurse Practitioners, 2007). When a potential mental health condition exists, the child should receive further assessment from a mental health specialist. Many mental health disorders are managed effectively with therapy, medication, or both on an outpatient basis, while some necessitate admission to an inpatient psychiatric setting. Therefore the nurse may encounter the child with a mental health disorder in a variety of community settings or during hospitalization for a concurrent physiologic problem.

Developing Cultural Competence

SPIRITUAL BELIEFS AND MENTAL HEALTH

In many cultures, care of the "spirit" is believed necessary to promote mental health. An identity with one's community and spiritual wholeness is promoted by storytelling, singing, rites of passage, and use of certain objects such as bags of herbs. Use of healers, family and community support, relaxation or meditation, exorcism, or other procedure may be used by families. Ask what the family believes about mental health, and integrate safe and culturally acceptable practices into the plan of care to enhance the child's mental health.

Nursing assessment focuses on child behaviors, family interactions, lifestyle routines, developmental progression, and treatment for mental health or cognitive conditions (Table 57–2).

An important nursing intervention is to ensure safety of the child. Actions begin in the emergency department if a child is admitted for a mental health crisis. Remove or lock potentially dangerous material in the room such as medications, tubing, and sharps containers. A parent, guardian, or health professional should remain with the child at all times. Inform the family member of the need to stay with the child and how to immediately notify the nurse if the adult needs to leave or if the child's condition changes. Part of the initial care is to evaluate risk by asking if the child has tried to hurt him- or herself or has been thinking about that. Ask about recent stresses, thoughts of hurting someone else, and why the child thinks he or she has been brought to the emergency department. If the child is admitted to the psychiatric unit, follow unit policies for ensuring safety for children who are at risk of hurting themselves or others.

Nursing care includes carrying out the prescribed treatment plan and administering psychotropic medications. Evaluate the child's medication regimen for administration schedule, dosage, side effects, and effectiveness. Inform the therapist of the child's hospitalization if the child has been hospitalized for a concurrent condition, and consult with the therapist about appropriate approaches for the child. Provide supportive care for the child and family.

Psychiatric hospitalization is a stressful event for all families, and both the family and child need supportive care. Continuation of family involvement is critical. (See "Evidence-Based Nursing: Family Needs During Hospitalization for Mental Healthcare.")

Table 57–2 Assessment Guidelines for the Child with an Alteration in Mental Health or Cognition

Assessment Focus	Assessment Guidelines
History	■ Describe prenatal care and problems. Was there any trauma at birth? ■ Is there a diagnosed mental health disorder in the child or other family members? ■ Is there a history of any neurological injuries or diseases? ■ What medications is the child taking?
Growth	■ Is growth progressing along the same channel or growth percentile? ■ Is head circumference within normal limits?
Development	■ Perform regular developmental screening to identify any variations from expected developmental milestones. Further testing is required if screening suggests any abnormalities. ■ What is the progression of skills reported by the family? ■ Are there any unusual capabilities or deficits? ■ Inquire about progression in school and extracurricular activities.
Social skills	■ Describe the relationship between the child and significant adults. Is close attachment evident? Are there signs of attachment disorders such as lack of eye contact, smiles, or response to others in the environment? ■ Describe the school-age child's daily schedule, including family and peer activities. Does the child have friends and engage in several activities with them on a regular basis? Does the child generally interact well with others? Has the child recently had a change in school performance? ■ Have the teen describe daily activities and friends. Is there a combination of peer and family influence on personal decision making?
Affect	■ Describe facial expression and response to nurse. ■ Observe body size, position, and posture. ■ Are interaction behaviors typical for the setting and age of the child? ■ Does the child display interest in surroundings? ■ Is the child dressed in an appropriate manner? Does the child establish eye contact?
Appearance	■ Is the child's clothing appropriate for age, setting, and developmental level?
Behaviors	■ Describe level of consciousness and interaction with surroundings. ■ Inquire about recent reported changes in behavior (e.g., sleep, eating patterns, communication with others, school performance, friendships, risky activities). ■ Are problem behaviors identified by the child or parent? ■ Are there particular events that were associated with problem behaviors?
Life events	■ Has the child or family experienced recent stress or trauma? ■ Have there been any changes in family structure? ■ Evaluate chronic health conditions in family members.

Evidence-Based Nursing

FAMILY NEEDS DURING HOSPITALIZATION FOR MENTAL HEALTH CARE

Clinical Question

Hospitalization for mental health care is always a stressful event. Families frequently do not understand treatment procedures or the child's condition and diagnosis. Treatment may last for several days to months, causing disruption in family roles and routines. Family stresses must be understood so that the nurse can adequately support both the child and the family.

Evidence

Recognizing that mental health hospitalizations are often brief, a nurse researcher applied information about parental needs to plan social support for families. The nurse researcher conducted a pilot study with families of children hospitalized for psychiatric illness. Themes that emerged during the interviews were analyzed and categorized into three categories of social support.

The first was a need for *information.* Parents often did not receive information about admission and unit procedures. Many felt that the physicians and other therapists were hard to reach and did not provide adequate information about the child's condition and treatment. Parents identified a need to have access to hospital records and the child's diagnosis. Such information was viewed as important to link to outpatient facilities where the child was also treated.

The second set of needs was for *instrumental support.* These items included reasonably priced lodging near the hospital, ready access to the hospitalized child, assistance with providing physical care for the hospitalized child, and improved physical environment of the hospital unit and rooms. Some parents voiced a lack of mental health services in their own communities, resulting in lack of care both before and after hospitalization.

The third need was for *emotional support.* Parents often felt isolated and did not know where to turn. They suggested that staff could provide additional emotional support, and that having a parent to call who had similar experiences would have been helpful.

As a strategy to meet the identified needs of children and families receiving mental health care, an internet discussion board was used to identify parental concern about the child's illness, developmental concerns, and parental support and well-being (Scharer, 2005a). Based on this work and that of other researchers, it is suggested that nurses who work in areas with information systems can offer regular electronic discussions with families. While ethical concerns mandate careful security guidelines, technology offers one approach and can provide valuable support for families (Scharer, 2005b).

Best Practice

The nurse in a mental health facility is in a unique position to offer support to the family of the child or adolescent. Information about the unit can be provided by videotape, tour, and written materials. Daily updates on the child's condition and treatment plan are needed. Families must be viewed as partners in the treatment, along with the child and health professionals. Provide an opportunity for parents to ask questions and be sure they understand the diagnosis and treatment.

Consider visiting hours and access to children. If they are limited to certain times, explain the reason to parents. Provide access to Ronald McDonald House or other low-cost facilities if the parent is from out of town. Provide assistance and instruction with any physical care the child needs. Consider changes that can be made to make the unit more welcoming and pleasant, such as color of walls, presence of posters and brochures, and general cleanliness.

Facilitate parent-to-parent communication. Ask parents each day about how they feel and what can be done for them. Use empathy and interest to convey support.

Critical Thinking

Why do you think that families find psychiatric facilities frightening or strange? How can you explain the need to remove items with which children could injure themselves or others? What questions will you ask early in the hospitalization to learn about facilities that are present in the home community that can be used for referral upon discharge? How could you locate available treatment options for a family from a community some distance from the hospital? How could support of the family influence the care and condition of their child or adolescent?

See MyNursingKit for possible responses.

The nurse frequently is the liaison between the family and the therapist in making follow-up arrangements at the time of discharge. Be aware of the meaning of mental illness in various cultural groups and the treatments that may be commonly used. Integrate these complementary therapies into the care plan whenever safe. Families must feel that their responses and approaches to the child with a mental disorder are not judged by health professionals.

The nurse in the community assesses how a child with a mental health disorder is functioning in each microsystem, such as home, day care, school, and with friends. Assess risk and protective factors of the child and family (see Chapter 33∞). Evaluate involvement in therapy sessions and ability to manage prescribed pharmacologic interventions.

DEVELOPMENTAL AND BEHAVIORAL DISORDERS

PERVASIVE DEVELOPMENTAL DISORDERS (AUTISTIC SPECTRUM DISORDERS)

It is estimated that 12% to 16% of children have a developmental or behavioral disorder. One of the most common sets of disorders is pervasive developmental disorders. **Pervasive developmental disorders (PDDs)** begin in early childhood and are characterized by impaired social interactions and communication, with restricted interests, activities, and behaviors (Centers for Disease Control and Prevention, 2006a). PDDs are called autistic spectrum disorders (ASDs), and include autistic disorder (the most common type), Rett syndrome, Asperger syndrome, childhood disintegrative disorder, and pervasive developmental disorder not otherwise specified. About 5.7 to 6.6 children in 1000 have autistic spectrum disorder, with about half of the cases consisting of autistic disorder (commonly called simply *autism*). While incidence varies geographically, about one in 150 children has autism (Centers for Disease Control and Prevention, 2007a; Schieve, Rice, Boyle, et al., 2006). This incidence represents an increase from formerly described levels. Before 1985, about 0.4 to 0.5 children in 1000 were diagnosed with autistic disorder; it is unclear whether there is a true increase in cases or simply improved techniques in making the diagnosis, as well as an enlarged diagnostic category that includes more children (Johnson, Myers, and the Council on Children with Disabilities, 2007). The disorder is more common in males than females, peak age at diagnosis is 6–11 years, but symptoms often begin by 18–24 months of age (Johnson et al., 2007).

ETIOLOGY AND PATHOPHYSIOLOGY

The etiology of autistic spectrum disorders is unknown. Genetic transmission, immune responses, and neuroanatomy are all being investigated as causes Neurotransmitters such as dopamine, serotonin, and opioids are abnormal in some children and are a focus of research. Brain size and head circumference may be enlarged in the young child with the disorder, so malfunction of the cortex and connectivity among brain regions may be abnormal (DiCicco-Bloom, Lord, Zwaigenbaum, et al., 2006; Williams & Minshew, 2007). Fetal alcohol syndrome, fragile X syndrome, phenylketonuria, Down syndrome, and tuberous sclerosis are all associated with a higher than normal incidence of autism (Johnson et al., 2007). Advanced parental age, rubella infection in pregnancy, and teratogens have been associated with ASDs. Despite concern expressed in earlier medical and lay press, there has been no demonstrated relationship of measles-mumps-rubella vaccine, nor thimerosol (mercury-based preservative in some vaccines) with the incidence of ASDs (see Chapter 45 for further information on immunizations) (D'Souza, Fombonne, & Ward, 2006; Katz, 2006; Richler, Luyster, Risi, et al., 2006).

CLINICAL MANIFESTATIONS

The essential features of the disorder typically become apparent by the time a child is 3 years of age. They involve impairments in the following three areas:

- Social interactions
- Communication
- Adapting to new situations
- Attention span and organizing responses to situations (Volkmar, Wiesner, & Westphal, 2006).

Children with autism are unable to relate to people as is normal for young children, or to respond to social and emotional cues. In addition, they engage in **stereotypy**, or rigid, repetitive, and machinelike movement with obsessive behavior (see Figure 57–5 ●).

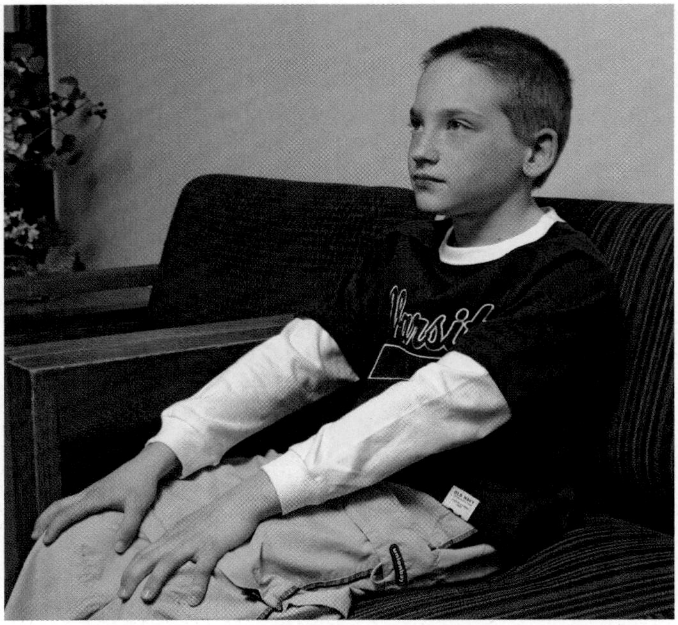

● **Figure 57–5** Stereotypy. This child with autism sits stiffly in the chair and engages in rhythmic rocking behavior. He has a disengaged look and does not readily interact with other children or adults who are in his environment.

Characteristically these repetitive behaviors in affected children include head banging, twirling in circles, biting themselves, and flapping their hands or arms. Frequently a child's behavior is self-stimulating or self-destructive. Responses to sensory stimuli are frequently abnormal and include an extreme aversion to touch, loud noises, and bright lights. Emotional lability is common.

Communication difficulties or delays in speech and language are common, and are often the first symptoms that lead to diagnosis. Abnormal communication patterns include both verbal and nonverbal communication. Absence of babbling and other communication by 1 year, absence of two-word phrases by 2 years, and deterioration of previous language skills are characteristic (Johnson et al., 2007). Children with autism may eventually learn to talk, in some cases well, but their speech is likely to show certain abnormalities: use of *you* in place of *I;* **echolalia** (a compulsive parroting of what is heard); repeating questions rather than answering them; and fascination with rhythmic, repetitive songs, and verses.

Behaviors of children with autism show several differences from others. They do not commonly explore objects but display stereotypy. They may line up objects, play with the same objects over and over, and have certain rituals that must be performed. They often become upset if these normal routines are disrupted. Rituals may involve eating only certain types or colors of foods or eating in specific patterns. Children may manifest disturbances in the rate or sequence of development. They are frequently cognitively impaired but can demonstrate a wide range of intellectual ability and functioning. Cognitive impairment may manifest early in life as slow developmental progression, particularly in social skills. Some children are impaired in particular areas of development, whereas others are above normal. About 25% have reduced head size at birth, followed by excessive

Clinical Manifestations

AUTISTIC SPECTRUM DISORDERS (PERVASIVE DEVELOPMENTAL DISORDERS)

DISORDER	CLINICAL MANIFESTATIONS	CLINICAL THERAPY
Autistic disorder	Impaired social, communicative, and behavioral development, usually noted in first year of life.	Early intervention is key to maximal performance. Interventions focus on improving behaviors and communication skills, providing physical and occupational therapy, structuring play interactions with other children, and educating parents about the child's needs.
Asperger syndrome	Impaired social interactions with normal language development for age; pitch, tone, and other speech characteristics may be abnormal. Verbal skills involving spelling and vocabulary are high but concept formation, language flexibility, and comprehension are low. Intellectual functioning may be at a high level, particularly in certain areas, while social skills are limited.	Social interactions are focus of therapy.
Rett disorder	Early development appears normal and symptoms emerge at 6–18 months. Ataxia, handwringing, intermittent hyperventilation, dementia, and growth retardation show progressive increase. Appears only in females as an X-linked dominant disorder; mutations occur in the gene MeCP2, affecting methyl-CpG-binding protein 2, which is important in brain development.	Early intervention in areas of abnormal behaviors.
Childhood disintegrative disorder	First 2–5 years of development appear normal followed by deterioration in many areas of functioning. Behaviors finally stabilize at some point without further deterioration.	Focus on areas of developmental function that show abnormality. Individualized education plans are needed in school to deal with communication, play, physical therapy, and teaching management skills to parents. Regression in toileting and other skills may occur.
Pervasive developmental disorder not otherwise specified	Severe social impairment without meeting DSM criteria for other types of autistic spectrum disorder.	Behavioral therapy focuses on building social skills.

growth of the head at 1 to 2 months and 6 to 14 months of age (Dementieva, Vance, Donnelly, et al., 2005).

The specific differences in clinical manifestations of the types of autistic spectrum disorder are listed in "Clinical Manifestations: Autistic Spectrum Disorders (Pervasive Developmental Disorders")).

CLINICAL THERAPY

The first step in identifying children at risk of ASD is surveillance at each healthcare visit. Since diagnosis and treatment have often been delayed, the American Academy of Pediatrics has now identified a multistage process for surveillance and screening:

1. Perform surveillance at early healthcare visits to identify if a sibling has ASD, parents or other caregivers are concerned about the developmental progression of the child, or the provider notes abnormalities in child behavior.
2. The healthcare provider determines if the child appears to be at risk for ASD.
3. The healthcare provider evaluates the risks. If risk exists, the provider administers an age-appropriate and ASD-specific screening tool.
4. If no risk exists, an ASD-specific tool is administered at the 18- and 24-month visits.
5. Select appropriate screening tool for age and risk profile of the child.
6. If screening is negative for a child with some risk, provide information to parents and evaluate again in one month. If screening is positive, refer for comprehensive ASD evaluation, including audiology, and begin early intervention programs (Johnson et al., 2007).

Several screening tests are available for use in health maintenance visits if autistic disorder is suspected. Additional testing is

Table 57–3 DSM-IV-TR Diagnostic Criteria for Autistic Disorder

A. A total of six or more items from 1, 2, and 3, with at least two from 1, and one each from 2 and 3:
   1. Qualitative impairment in social interaction, as manifested by at least two of the following:
      a. Marked impairment in the use of multiple nonverbal behaviors such as eye-to-eye gaze, facial expression, body posture, and gestures to regulate social interaction
      b. Failure to develop peer relationships appropriate to developmental level
      c. A lack of spontaneous seeking to share enjoyment, interests, or achievements with other people
      d. Lack of social or emotional reciprocity
   2. Qualitative impairments in communication as manifested by at least one of the following:
      a. Delay in, or total lack of, the development of spoken language (not accompanied by an attempt to compensate through alternative modes of communication such as gesture or mime)
      b. In individuals with adequate speech, marked impairment in the ability to initiate or sustain a conversation with others
      c. Stereotyped and repetitive use of language or idiosyncratic language
      d. Lack of varied, spontaneous make-believe play or social imitative play appropriate to developmental level
   3. Restricted repetitive and stereotyped patterns of behavior, interests, and activities, as manifested by at least one of the following:
      a. Encompassing preoccupation with one or more stereotyped and restricted patterns of interest that is abnormal either in intensity or in focus
      b. Apparently inflexible adherence to specific, nonfunctional routines or rituals
      c. Stereotyped and repetitive motor mannerisms (e.g., hand or finger flapping or twisting, or complex whole-body movements)
      d. Persistent preoccupation with parts of objects

B. Delays or abnormal functioning in at least one of the following areas, with onset prior to age 3 years: (1) social interaction, (2) language as used in social communication, or (3) symbolic or imaginative play.

C. The disturbance is not better accounted for by Rett Syndrome or Childhood Disintegrative Disorder.

performed to rule out other causes of the child's behavior. Tests may include neuroimaging (CT scan or MRI), lead screening, metabolic studies, DNA analysis, and electroencephalogram. See Chapters 35 and 56 for further descriptions related to neurological system assessment. Diagnosis is based on the presence of specific criteria, as described in the American Psychiatric Association's *Diagnostic and Statistical Manual of Mental Disorders,* 4th edition (DSM-IV), outlined in Table 57–3.

Early intervention helps maximize the child's potential by improving developmental skills and decreasing severity of symptoms, as well as establishing helpful support for parents (Giarelli, Souders, Pinto-Martin, et al., 2005; Rogers & Vismara, 2008). Treatment focuses on behavior management to reward appropriate behaviors, foster positive or adaptive coping skills, and facilitate effective communication. Speech therapy is an essential part of treatment (Weber & Newmark, 2007). The goals of treatment are to reduce rigidity or stereotypy and other maladaptive behaviors. Often the child must be physically restrained from aggressive or self-destructive behaviors. Some parents choose to use complementary therapies (see "Complementary Care: Autism").

The overall prognosis for autistic children to become functioning members of society varies. Successful adjustment is more

Complementary Care

AUTISM

Some parents who have a child with autism choose to use complementary therapy in an attempt to help the child. A popular treatment approach includes dietary therapy with vitamin A, vitamin C, vitamin B_6, magnesium, omega-3 fatty acids, probiotics, zinc, or use of gluten-free or casein-free diets. Parents may also try drug therapy including secretin, a pancreatic gastrointestinal peptide, and Pepcid or other antacids. Some parents believe that detoxification by limiting intake of certain dietary components, or using Epsom salt baths can be helpful (Hyman & Levy, 2005; Levy & Hyman, 2005). Music therapy has been used to improve social interaction, and massage to enhance response to touch and communication (Gold, Wigram, & Elefant, 2006; Cullen-Powell, Barlow, & Cushway, 2005). Additional therapies include homeopathy, craniosacral therapy, Reiki, hyperbaric chambers, and biofeedback (Weber & Newmark, 2007). Chelation therapy is not approved but has been used by some physicians and families as a treatment for autism. The rationale is that autism is related to a collection of heavy metals such as mercury in the body. Chelation is a treatment with serious potential side effects (see Chapter 44 for further information about chelation for treatment of lead poisoning). The report of a death of a young boy being treated for autism with chelation reinforces the danger of using untested therapies (Beauchamp, Willis, Betz, et al., 2006).

Nurses can help parents to evaluate studies on CAM and encourage them to initiate only one treatment at a time to measure effectiveness. Ask about therapies being used and discuss safeguards to avoid any undesired side effects. Read about new studies on complementary therapies and evaluate the rationale, efficacy, side effects, and other pertinent findings in order to bring current information to families.

likely for children with higher IQs, adequate speech, and access to specialized programs.

NURSING MANAGEMENT

NURSING ASSESSMENT AND DIAGNOSIS

The nurse may encounter the child with autism during routine well child visits, or when parents seek care for a suspected hearing impairment, speech difficulty, or developmental delay. Early and frequent developmental screening of all children can help in referral for thorough assessment and identification of cases. Be alert to parental observations that the baby or young child does not look at them or provides other developmental or behavioral cues (Beauchesne & Kelley, 2004). Parents may report abnormal interaction such as lack of eye contact, disinterest in cuddling, minimal facial responsiveness, and failure to talk. Be alert for the "red flags": no babbling or communication gestures by 12 months, no single word by 16 months, no spontaneous two-word phrases by 24 months, loss of language or social skills previously achieved (Johnson et al., 2007).

Assessment at every healthcare visit focuses on language development, response to others, and hearing acuity (see Chapters 33 and 35∞). Specialized screening tests for autism may be administered.

When a child with a diagnosis of autistic disorder is hospitalized for a concurrent problem, obtain a history from the parents about the child's routines, rituals, and likes and dislikes, as well as ways to promote interaction and cooperation. Autistic children may carry a special toy or object that they play with during times of stress. Ask parents about these objects and their use.

Ask about the child's behaviors and observe them on admission. Obtain a history of acute and chronic illnesses and injuries. Ask about eating patterns and food restrictions. Inquire about complementary and alternative medicine treatments in a nonjudgmental and supportive manner.

Nursing diagnoses must be tailored to fit the individual needs of the child. Examples of nursing diagnoses that might be appropriate for autistic children include the following:

- *Impaired Verbal Communication* related to psychological condition
- *Impaired Social Interaction* related to developmental disability
- *Disturbed Thought Processes* related to mental disorder
- *Risk for Injury* related to cognitive impairment
- *Risk for Caregiver Role Strain* related to chronicity and demands of child's condition
- *Disabled Family Coping: Compromised* related to having a child with prolonged disability

PLANNING AND IMPLEMENTATION

Nursing care focuses on stabilizing environmental stimuli, providing supportive care, enhancing communication, maintaining a safe environment, giving the parents anticipatory guidance, and providing emotional support.

STABILIZE ENVIRONMENTAL STIMULI

Autistic children interpret and respond to the environment differently from other individuals. Sounds that are not distressing to the average person may be interpreted by autistic children as louder, more frightening, and overwhelming. The child needs to be oriented to new settings such as a classroom or the hospital room and may adjust best to a small classroom or a hospital room with only one other child. Encourage parents to bring the child's favorite objects from home, and try to keep these objects in the same places, because the child does not cope well with changes in the environment.

PROVIDE SUPPORTIVE CARE

Developing a trusting relationship with the autistic child is often difficult. Adjust communication techniques and teaching to the child's developmental level. Ask parents about the child's usual home routines, and maintain these routines as much as possible when the child is out of the home. Because self-care abilities are often limited, the child may need help meeting basic needs. School programs and individualized education plans (IEPs) (see Chapter 39∞) can help the child learn self-care skills. When possible, schedule daily care and routine procedures at consistent times to maintain predictability. Encourage parents to remain with the hospitalized child and to participate in daily care planning. Parents are integral parts of the treatment team when the child's learning goals are established in early intervention or school programs. Identify rituals for naptime and bedtime, and maintain them to promote rest and sleep. Establish patterns that help the child eat nutritious foods at mealtimes.

ENHANCE COMMUNICATION

Since children with autism have impaired communication, nursing care focuses on using and improving communication with the child. Speech is used when possible; short, direct sentences are usually most effective. When the child responds well to visual cues, pictures, computers, and other visual aids may form an important part of interactions. Some children use sign language.

MAINTAIN A SAFE ENVIRONMENT

Monitor autistic children at all times, including bathtime and bedtime. Close supervision is needed to ensure that the child does not obtain any harmful objects or engage in dangerous behaviors. Bicycle helmets and mittens are sometimes used to protect autistic children so that they can safely participate in activities.

PROVIDE ANTICIPATORY GUIDANCE

Approximately half of all children with autistic disorder require lifelong supervision and support. This is especially true if the disorder is accompanied by intellectual disability (mental retardation). Some children may grow up to lead independent lives, although they will have social limitations with impaired interpersonal relationships. Encourage parents to promote the child's development through behavior modification and specialized educational programs. The overall goal is to provide the child with the guidance, education, and support necessary for optimal functioning.

NURSING CARE IN THE COMMUNITY

Families need a great deal of support to cope with the challenges of caring for the autistic child. Help the family identify resources for child care, such as special toddler programs, preschools, and parent support groups (Luther, Canham, & Cureton, 2005). The child will need an individualized education and health plan; the school nurse is instrumental in team management to establish these plans (Lobar, Fritts, Arbide, et al., 2008). The parent or primary caretaker often has a hard time getting respite care and may need assistance to find suitable resources. Siblings of the autistic child may need help explaining the disorder to their friends or teachers. Family support programs are available in some states to provide assistance to parents.

Offer the family genetic counseling. Parents need information on the need for immunizations since they may have heard about a potential connection between immunization and the disorder. Encourage parents to have the child immunized on the recommended schedule. Parents may have questions about where to find information on complementary and alternative therapies.

Local support groups for parents of autistic children are available in most areas. Parents can also be referred to the Autism Society of America, the American Academy of Pediatrics and the Centers for Disease Control and Prevention for information. (See the Companion Website for links to such resources.)

EVALUATION

Expected outcomes of nursing care for the child with autism include the following:

- Management of behavioral symptoms
- Maximization of self-care
- Maintenance of safe environment
- Consistent developmental progression
- Successful communication strategies

ATTENTION DEFICIT DISORDER AND ATTENTION DEFICIT HYPERACTIVITY DISORDER

MyNursingKit Video: ADD/ADHD

Attention deficit disorder (ADD) is a variation in central nervous system processing characterized by developmentally inappropriate behaviors involving inattention. When hyperactivity and impulsivity accompany inattention, the disorder is called attention deficit hyperactivity disorder (ADHD). The latter is the more common condition and affects from 6% to 9% of all school-age children (Froelich, Lanphear, Epstein, et al., 2007; Wolraich, Wibbelsman, Brown, et al., 2005). Boys are affected almost 4 times as often as girls. It is also known to affect adolescents and adults, and those with the disorder often continue to manifest at least some of the symptoms as they grow into adulthood. Hyperactivity and impulsivity may improve as the child nears adulthood, with inattentiveness the most persistent characteristic (Reiff, 2006).

ETIOLOGY AND PATHOPHYSIOLOGY

Although a variety of physical and neurologic disorders are associated with ADHD, children with identifiable causes represent a small proportion of this population. Examples of known associations include exposure to high levels of lead or mercury in childhood and prenatal exposure to alcohol or tobacco smoke. Other prenatal factors associated with a higher incidence of ADHD include preterm labor, impaired placenta functioning, and impaired oxygenation. Seizures and serious head injury are other potential associations. Genetic factors may be important, as well as family dynamics and environmental characteristics. Although ADHD occurs more commonly within families (25% have a first-degree relative with the disorder), a single gene has not been located and a specific mechanism of genetic transmission is not known. It is believed that a genetic predisposition interacts with the child's environment, so that both factors contribute to the appearance of the condition. Family stress, poverty, and poor nutrition may also be contributing factors. Daily television exposure at ages 1 to 3 years is associated with attentional symptoms of the condition at 7 years (Christakis, Zimmerman, DiGiuseppe, et al., 2004). It is likely that there are many types of attention deficit, resulting from several different mechanisms that involve interaction of genetic, biological, and environmental risk factors.

The pathophysiology of ADD/ADHD is not totally known. However, some children exhibit a deficit in the catecholamines dopamine and norepinephrine, lowering the threshold for stimuli input. The disorder is marked by brain maturation delay in the area of self-regulation. Increased input from stimuli and decreased self-regulation cause the hallmark inability to inhibit stimuli and motor activity. Slow brain maturity, as much as three years, has now been demonstrated on imaging studies. The cortex was particularly affected and may explain the school and concentration difficulty associated with the disorder (National Institutes of Health, 2007).

CLINICAL MANIFESTATIONS

Children with ADD and ADHD have problems related to decreased attention span, impulsiveness, or increased motor activity. Symptoms can range from mild to severe. The disorders often coexist with various developmental learning disabilities. The child has difficulty completing tasks, fidgets constantly, is frequently loud, and interrupts others. Sleep disturbances are common. Because of these behaviors, the child often has difficulty developing and maintaining social relationships and may be shunned or teased by other children. This only increases the anxiety of the already compromised child, whose behavior is set on a downward-spiraling course.

Typically, girls with ADHD show less aggression and impulsiveness than boys, but far more anxiety, mood swings, social withdrawal, rejection, and cognitive and language problems. Girls tend to be older at the time of diagnosis. Children are frequently diagnosed with the disorder soon after beginning school, with its demands for attentive behavior.

CLINICAL THERAPY

Children are usually brought for evaluation when behaviors escalate to the point of interfering with the daily functioning of teachers or parents. When children have learning disabilities or anxiety disorders, the problem is commonly misdiagnosed as ADHD if full and accurate evaluation of the child's symptoms is not performed. Obtaining an accurate diagnosis by a pediatric mental health specialist is vital (Brown, Amler, Freeman, et al., 2005; Wolraich et al., 2005). Specific diagnostic criteria must be applied to all children with the potential diagnosis (see DSM-IV criteria in Table 57–4). The diagnosis of ADD is often difficult because of the absence of hyperactivity behaviors. Behaviors both at home and school or childcare must be evaluated, because abnormal patterns in two settings are needed for diagnosis. A variety of tests are available for use by the trained professional in establishing the diagnosis.

Diagnosis begins with a careful history of the child, including family history, birth history, growth and developmental milestones, behaviors such as sleep and eating patterns, progression and patterns in school, social and environmental conditions, and reports from parents and teachers. A physical examination should be performed to rule out neurologic diseases and other health problems. The mental health specialist then performs testing of the child and administers questionnaires to the parent and teacher. It is important to identify other conditions that may either mimic ADD/ADHD or exist in conjunction with the disorders. These might include depression, anxiety, learning disorder, conduct disorder, or oppositional defiant disorder.

Treatment is established to meet the desired behavioral outcomes, and includes a combination of approaches, such as environmental changes, behavior therapy, and pharmacotherapy (Brown et al., 2005). It is expected that treatment will be long term.

Children often benefit from environmental changes. Decreasing stimulation—for example, by turning off television, keeping the environment quiet, and maintaining an orderly and clutter-free desk or study area without distraction—may help the child to stay focused on the task at hand. Another relatively simple change is appropriate classroom placement, preferably in a small class with a teacher who can provide close supervision and

Table 57–4 DSM-IV-TR Diagnostic Criteria for Attention Deficit Hyperactivity Disorder

A. Either 1 or 2:
   1. *Inattention:* Six (or more) of the following symptoms of inattention have persisted for at least 6 months to a degree that is maladaptive and inconsistent with developmental level:
      a. Often fails to give close attention to details or makes careless mistakes in schoolwork, work, and other activities
      b. Often has difficulty sustaining attention in tasks or play activities
      c. Often does not seem to listen when spoken to directly
      d. Often does not follow through on instructions and fails to finish schoolwork, chores, or duties in the workplace (not due to oppositional behavior or failure to understand instructions)
      e. Often has difficulty organizing tasks and activities
      f. Often avoids, dislikes, or is reluctant to engage in tasks that require sustained mental effort (such as schoolwork or homework)
      g. Often loses things necessary for tasks or activities (e.g., toys, school assignments, pencils, books, or tools)
      h. Is often easily distracted by extraneous stimuli
      i. Is often forgetful in daily activities
   2. *Hyperactivity-impulsivity:* Six (or more) of the following symptoms of hyperactivity-impulsivity have persisted for at least 6 months to a degree that is maladaptive and inconsistent with developmental level:

      Hyperactivity

      a. Often fidgets with hands or feet or squirms in seat
      b. Often leaves seat in classroom or in other situations in which remaining seated is expected
      c. Often runs about or climbs excessively in situations in which it is inappropriate (in adolescents or adults, may be limited to subjective feelings of restlessness)
      d. Often has difficulty playing or engaging in leisure activities quietly
      e. Is often "on the go" or often acts as if "driven by a motor"
      f. Often talks excessively

      Impulsivity

      g. Often blurts out answers before questions have been completed
      h. Often has difficulty awaiting turn
      i. Often interrupts or intrudes on others (e.g., butts into conversations or games)

B. Some hyperactive-impulsive or inattentive symptoms that caused impairment were present before age 7 years.
C. Some impairment from the symptoms is present in two or more settings (e.g., at school [or work] and at home).
D. There must be clear evidence of clinically significant impairment in social, academic, or occupational functioning.
E. The symptoms do not occur exclusively during the course of a Pervasive Developmental Disorder, Schizophrenia, or other Psychotic Disorder and are not better accounted for by another mental disorder (e.g., Mood Disorder, Anxiety Disorder, Dissociative Disorder, or a Personality Disorder).

Complementary Care

ALTERNATIVE TREATMENTS FOR ADHD

In addition to drug therapy, a variety of other treatments have been attempted for ADHD and are commonly used by families. Chiropractic manipulation, biofeedback, visual or auditory therapy, and dietary interventions are examples of complementary or alternative therapies. Some dietary interventions include elimination of dietary components, such as highly processed foods, sugar, aspartame, or yeast. Other therapies include supplements, such as iron, magnesium, zinc, and vitamin B_6. Herbs such as Pycnogenol, melatonin, and *Ginkgo biloba* are sometimes used. Essential fatty acids (EFAs) have been used for ADHD treatment, specifically omega-3 and omega-6 fatty acids. Because the body does not manufacture EFAs, they must be obtained from the diet. Sources of omega-3 and omega-6 fatty acids include evening primrose oil, flaxseed oil, borage oil, and oils from coldwater fish such as cod and salmon. Ask parents about alternative therapies used, investigate what is known about them, and share this information with parents (Rojas & Chan, 2005).

a structured daily routine. Consistent limits and expectations should be set for the child. Children living in chaotic homes and communities may function better if the environment can be simplified. When aggressive behaviors occur, therapeutic approaches such as play and group therapy may be useful.

Behavior therapy involves rewarding the child for desired behaviors and applying consequences for undesirable behaviors. Children may be rewarded by praise or earn points toward a movie or other desired outing for staying seated during meals or quietly listening in a classroom.

Children with moderate to severe ADHD are treated with pharmacotherapy. Methylphenidate (Ritalin, Concerta) is most often prescribed, with alternatives of dextroamphetamine (Dexedrine or Adderall) and the nonstimulant medication Atomoxetine. A skin patch that releases medication over a 9-hour period is now available, facilitating ease of administration (Anderson & Scott, 2006). Usually a favorable response (a decrease in impulsive behaviors and an increase in the ability to sit still and attend to an activity for at least 15 minutes) is seen in the first 10 days of treatment and frequently with the first few doses. New guidelines have been issued to recommend thorough evaluation of children before stimulant or other medication is prescribed, in order to rule out any cardiac condition that could be affected by medication use. Guidelines include:

- Patient and family history of conditions associated with sudden cardiac death
- All medications and health supplements
- Physical examination, especially of the cardiovascular system
- Electrocardiogram
- Pediatric cardiology consult if any abnormalities are identified (Vetter, Elia, Erickson, et al., 2008).

Although ADHD was once thought to be a disorder of childhood that gradually improved with age, it is now believed that symptoms continue into adulthood and that careful management in childhood helps lessen problems of social functioning later in life.

NURSING MANAGEMENT

NURSING ASSESSMENT AND DIAGNOSIS

The nurse often encounters the family who is concerned about the child's behavior before a diagnosis has been made. Ask about family and birth history and have the parents describe the child's behaviors. Perform developmental testing and look specifically for attention span and physical activity. Refer the family to their pediatric healthcare home for further assessment, and then to a mental healthcare specialist who is experienced in diagnosing ADHD. Schedule a visit for complete patient and family history, physical examination, and electrocardiogram before medication is begun (Vetter et al., 2008).

Nurses may encounter the child with ADHD in the hospital when parents bring the child for treatment of an injury (e.g., fracture) or other problem. Explore the parent's report of the child's attention span in detail. Usually within a few minutes in an unstructured setting or waiting area, the child with ADHD becomes restless and searches for distraction. Gather information about the child's activity level and impulsiveness. Be alert for information that reveals a serious problem, such as hurting animals or other children. Find out about distractibility, attention deficit in activities of daily living, characteristic ways of reacting, and the extent of impulsiveness when the child is receiving medication. Find out how the family manages at home. Ask about a family history of the disorder, as that is a common finding among children with ADHD.

Examples of nursing diagnoses that might be appropriate for a child with ADHD include the following:

- *Impaired Verbal Communication* related to altered perceptions
- *Impaired Social Interaction* related to chronic episodes of impulsive behavior
- *Chronic Low Self-esteem* related to behaviors associated with ADD/ADHD
- *Risk for Injury* related to high level of impulsiveness and excitability
- *Risk for Caregiver Role Strain* related to management of child with unpredictable moods and high energy

PLANNING AND IMPLEMENTATION

Prevention can focus on discouraging regular television exposure for young children from 1 to 3 years and encouraging daily vigorous physical activity for all children. Nursing care of the hospitalized child with ADD/ADHD focuses on administering medications, managing the child's environment, implementing behavioral management plans, providing emotional support to

Drug Guide

METHYLPHENIDATE HYDROCHLORIDE (RITALIN)

Overview of Action

Methylphenidate hydrochloride (Ritalin) is a derivative of piperidine, which acts like an amphetamine. It causes CNS and respiratory stimulation and has some sympathomimetic activity. It may work by enhancing catecholamine effects in the reticular activating system, thereby affecting the cortex to improve attention span and task performance. It may also prevent flooding of sensory impulses into the cortex so that they enter in a more integrated manner. It is used to treat children with attention deficit hyperactivity disorder and adults with narcolepsy.

Routes, Dosage, Frequency

PO: For children 6 years or older: 2.5 to 5 mg before breakfast and lunch initially, increased in 2.5- to 5-mg increments weekly as needed or 0.25 mg/kg/day in 2 doses initially, increased by doubling weekly as needed; not to exceed 2 mg/kg/day or 60 mg/day. A sustained-release form is available so that children can take one pill in the morning and do not have to take more at school in the middle of the day; this can be used after the child is stabilized on the proper dose. The preparation called Concerta is dosed at 18 mg each morning, increased at weekly intervals as needed, with a maximum dose not to exceed 54 mg/day.

A skin patch (Daytrana) is now available also.

Side Effects: Insomnia, nervousness and agitation, palpitations, changes in blood pressure and pulse, blurred vision, anorexia and weight loss, hepatotoxicity, dermatitis

Contraindications: Tic syndromes, allergy to the drug, children under 6 years; do not give within 14 days of any MAO inhibitors

Nursing Implications

Measure height and weight and plot on growth grid. Take baseline vital signs. Do CBC and platelet count. Take history of previous drug therapy and reactions.

- *Administer:* Schedule II drug under Federal Controlled Substance Act. Do not give tablets late in afternoon or evening because doing so may interrupt sleep. Extended-release tablets are given once daily in early morning and should not be crushed or chewed.
- *Monitor:* Patient is seen in office for regular visits, when vital signs, height, weight, cardiac exam, and CBC and platelet counts are performed. Observe for signs of bleeding and bruising. Question parents and teachers about child's behavior and ability to concentrate and perform tasks. If drug is to be effective, behavior change occurs within 1 month. Some drug-free holidays are recommended; monitor for behavior changes at these times. Supervise drug withdrawal carefully after prolonged use since severe depression and psychotic behavior have occurred.
- *Patient Teaching:* Take drug as directed. Do not withdraw quickly; tapering is recommended under supervision of prescriber. Measure child's weight weekly and report weight loss. Report signs of bleeding, fever, sore throat, or bruising. Report changes in child's ability to concentrate and general behavior. Store the medication out of reach of children. If the drug is taken during school hours, work with personnel to plan for safe administration.

Data from Bindler, R. M., & Howry, L. B. (2005). Pediatric drug guide with nursing implications. *Upper Saddle River, NJ: Prentice Hall-Health.*

the child and family, promoting self-esteem, and ensuring ongoing care.

ADMINISTER MEDICATIONS

Stimulant and nonstimulant medications increase the child's attention span and decrease distractibility. Be alert for the common side effects of these medications, including anorexia, insomnia, and tachycardia. Administering medication early in the day helps to alleviate insomnia. Anorexia can be managed by giving medication at mealtimes. Baseline cardiac examinations are needed, as well as periodic reevaluation. Careful monitoring of weight, height, and blood pressure is necessary. Instruct families about the abuse potential of stimulant drugs and teach them to keep the medications locked and to administer them only as directed.

MINIMIZE ENVIRONMENTAL DISTRACTIONS

The child may need an environment with minimal distractions. When hospitalized, this may mean a room with only one other child. Keep potentially harmful equipment out of reach. Monitor and limit television and video game time. Use shades to darken the room at nap- or bedtime, and minimize noise. Teach parents to minimize distractions at home during periods when the child needs to concentrate; for example, when doing schoolwork. Visits to areas such as shopping malls and playgrounds may need to be limited. Plenty of daily exercise and minimal use of television and video games may help the child concentrate when needed for school and other tasks.

IMPLEMENT BEHAVIORAL MANAGEMENT PLANS

Behavior modification programs can help reduce specific impulsive behaviors. An example is setting up a reward program for the child who has taken medication as ordered or completed a homework assignment. The rewards may be daily as well as weekly or monthly, depending on the child's age. For example, one completed homework assignment might be rewarded with 30 minutes of basketball or a bike ride; assignments completed for a week might be rewarded with an activity of the child's choice on the weekend.

If punishment is necessary, the behavior should be corrected while simultaneously supporting the child as a person. Punishment is generally withdrawal of a privilege, and should follow the offense quickly, as the child may not otherwise connect the punishment with the behavior.

Nursing Practice

Many families who have a child with ADHD or another mental health disorder are embarrassed and feel shame because of the diagnosis. This may be especially true in certain cultures, such as some Asian groups, and in highly structured and highly achieving families. When taking histories from family members, it is best to be sensitive to the stigma some may feel. Ask questions in a private setting and ask about the family's feelings about a mental health disorder. Provide information in a nonjudgmental manner and if appropriate provide support from other families with similar experiences.

PROVIDE EMOTIONAL SUPPORT

Children with ADD or ADHD offer a special challenge to parents, teachers, and healthcare providers. Parents must cope simultaneously with managing the difficult needs and demands of a hard-to-handle child, obtaining appropriate evaluation and treatment, and understanding and accepting the diagnosis, even when the child exhibits different behaviors with different people. Family support is essential. Educate both the parents and the child about the importance of appropriate expectations and consequences of behaviors. Teach skills that will help as the child grows older: making lists of tasks to accomplish; having routines for eating, sleeping, recreation, and school work; minimizing stimuli in the environment when completing work; and asking teachers and friends to identify when behavior is inappropriate.

PROMOTE SELF-ESTEEM

Help the child understand the disorder at an appropriate developmental level, and facilitate a trusting relationship with healthcare providers. Assist the child with social skills through role-play, playing in small groups, and modeling. Promote the child's self-esteem by pointing out the positive aspects of behavior and treating instances of negative behavior as learning opportunities. Help the child to develop ego strengths (the consciousness to be able to screen outside stimuli and control internal demands), which will result in better impulse control and thus increase self-esteem over time. Encourage skills at which the child excels and consider offering support groups for children in school (Barber, Grubbs, & Cottrell, 2005).

NURSING CARE IN THE COMMUNITY

Most children with ADD or ADHD are hospitalized only when needing care for another condition. Parents need support to understand the diagnosis and to learn how to manage the child. Emphasize the importance of a stable environment, at home as well as at school. At home the child may have difficulty staying on task. Parents need to consider age and developmental appropriateness of tasks, give clear and simple instructions, and provide frequent reminders to ensure completion. Routines in the evening can promote good sleep patterns.

The nurse can serve as a liaison to teachers and school personnel, or as the case manager for the child. An individualized education plan may be needed (see Chapter 39), with clear expected outcomes stated for the child's behaviors. Special classrooms or periods of instruction free from the distractions of the entire class may enable the child to improve school performance. Parents may have difficulty understanding the need for these approaches because the child often tests with above-average intelligence. Reinforce the importance of providing a structured environment free from unnecessary external stimuli. Be sure that parents understand behavioral approaches that will help the child, how to administer prescribed medications, and the importance of returning for healthcare visits to monitor for side effects. Medication should be locked safely away at home to keep it away from other children and prevent illegal use of this controlled substance. An individual school health plan may be needed for medication management.

Parents may have heard about ADHD in the media and often have many questions about its cause and management. Providing information about complementary and alternative treatments is a nursing role.

As the child grows older, explain the disorder and teach about techniques that will assist in dealing with problems. Assist in planning for quiet environment during work. Encourage children with attention deficits to write down instructions from teachers and to use checklists to help them accomplish specific tasks.

EVALUATION

Expected outcomes of nursing care for the child with ADD or ADHD include the following:

- Understanding of disorder by parents and child
- Management of medication administration
- Increase in attentiveness and decrease in hyperactivity, impulsivity, and sleep disturbances
- Formation of positive self-image in the child
- Educational performance to maximum potential

MOOD DISORDERS

DEPRESSION

Depression is psychological distress that can range from mild to severe. Only in recent years has depression in children been recognized as a clinical condition. Many children referred to child guidance centers and mental health professionals because of behavioral difficulties or poor achievement actually suffer from depression. The incidence of major depression is estimated to be about 0.3% in preschoolers, 2% in prepubertal children, and about 5% to 10% in adolescents (Dopheide, 2006). Males and females are equally affected until adolescence, when the incidence in girls rapidly increases. A history of substance abuse and anxiety disorder increases risk and cultural variations in rates exist (Dopheide, 2006).

Developing Cultural Competence

DEPRESSION RATES

Ethnic/racial differences in depression rates exist, with 29% of American Indian youth, 22% of Hispanic youth, 18% of White Americans, 17% of Asian Americans, and 15% of African American youth displaying signs of depression (Dopheide, 2006). It is unclear if genetics, environment, or cultural issues influence the differences in prevalence; perhaps all of those factors play a role.

Growth and Development

Symptoms of depression in children vary according to their developmental levels. Infants may fail to eat and grow; toddlers can show regressive behaviors in toileting and other activities; preschoolers have less symbolic and other play activities, may be irritable and lack confidence; school children may show a decrease in academic performance, increased or decreased activity, somatic complaints, and loss of friends; and adolescents can have a wide array of symptoms such as anxiety, decreased social contact, poor school performance, lack of prior involvement in activities, poor self-care, difficulty with parents and teachers, or focus on violence (Dopheide, 2006; Luby, Heffelfinger, Koenig-McNaught, et al., 2004; Pruett & Luby, 2004).

ETIOLOGY AND PATHOPHYSIOLOGY

Many theories have been proposed to explain the cause of depression in children and adolescents. Depression may be biologic in origin or a result of learned helplessness, cognitive distortion, social skills deficit, or family dysfunction. The physiologic theory focuses on monoamine neurotransmission. These amines include indolamine, serotonin, norepinephrine, and dopamine, and decreases are sometimes found in depression. Magnetic resonance imaging has identified brain changes in individuals who are depressed, suggesting a biological basis (Dopheide, 2006).

Parental depression is a strong predictor of childhood depression. Abuse and neglect, family conflict, parental death, and low socioeconomic status predispose children to depression. Other psychiatric diagnoses are common in children with depression; these include conditions such as ADHD, anxiety disorder, bipolar disease, or substance abuse (Richardson & Katzenellenbogen, 2005).

CLINICAL MANIFESTATIONS

Characteristic findings of major depression in children and adolescents include declining school performance; withdrawal from social activities; sleep disturbance (either too much or too little); appetite disturbance (too much or too little); multiple somatic complaints, especially headaches and stomachaches; decreased energy; difficulty concentrating and making decisions; low self-esteem; and feelings of hopelessness. There is much variation among children in the symptoms displayed, and they often have some but not all of the major criteria. Symptoms vary according to children's developmental levels.

CLINICAL THERAPY

Initial assessment is performed by a child psychologist or child psychiatrist. A variety of scales and techniques are used; examples of useful tools are the Children's Depression Inventory, the Revised Children's Manifest Anxiety Scale, and Beck Depressive Inventory. The child is tested for other mental health problems since comorbidities (combination with other disorders) are common.

Treatment may include psychotherapy in combination with psychotropic medication. Often a combination of individual, family, and group therapy provides the greatest benefits for young children and adolescents. Involving parents, other family members, school personnel, and friends in the treatment plan is essential. Group therapy is often effective for adolescents. Cognitive behavioral therapy (CBT) may be used with adolescents, and play therapy with younger children (see discussion of play therapy earlier in this chapter). CBT focuses on thoughts and behaviors, leading to understanding of negative thoughts, and increasing activities that provide pleasure (Cheung, Zuckerbrot, Jensen, et al., 2008; Zuckerbrot, Cheung, Jensen, et al., 2007). Supportive interactions with healthcare providers and active problem solving are approaches that improve outcomes in adolescents (Stein et al., 2006). Healthcare providers should educate families about depression and counsel as needed. Confidentiality should be ensured. Refer to community resources as needed. Ensure a plan for safety of the adolescent.

Antidepressant medications, most commonly the selective serotonin reuptake inhibitors (SSRIs), imipramine (Tofranil),

Nursing Practice

Serotonin syndrome, the serious and life-threatening side effect of SSRIs, is caused by overstimulation of serotonin receptors. It is characterized by agitation, muscle twitching, gastric upset, chills, fever, confusion, and dizziness. It is more likely to develop when the child or adolescent is also taking St. John's wort, other antidepressants, alcohol, diet pills, or drugs such as ecstasy and LSD (Hu, Yang, Ho, et al., 2005). Be certain to ask questions in a nonjudgmental way about intake of any alternative therapies, other medications, or substance use to identify those most at risk.

Sudden cardiac death has occurred in several children on tricyclic antidepressants (TCAs). Because of this risk, serum levels should be monitored and electrocardiograms (ECGs) performed. Specific ECG changes along with a resting heart rate above 100, systolic blood pressure above 130 mm Hg, and diastolic blood pressure above 85 mm Hg necessitate immediate report to the prescriber. A narrow margin exists between the therapeutic and lethal dose in children. Additionally, TCAs have not shown efficacy in treating depression in children, so the risk outweighs benefit (Hirsch & Carlson, 2007).

Nursing Practice

There have been reports of increased suicidal ideation and other behavioral changes in children and adolescents taking antidepressant medications. In both the United States and Canada, the medications are now accompanied by clear warnings for use in these age groups. In particular, paroxetine (Paxil) has been implicated in suicidal thoughts and should not be used in children (Pruett & Luby, 2004). Agencies in both countries have alerted healthcare providers and families of the risks, but leave decisions about medications to the prescribers and families, since the risk of depressive illness in itself carries a risk of harm to the individual.

In the U.S., the Food and Drug Administration recommends that a Patient Medication Guide (MedGuide) be provided to each patient explaining the risks of the drug and precautions to take. In addition, the following information should be in a boxed warning on the drug labels (called a "Black Box" warning):

- Antidepressants increase the risk of suicidal thinking and behavior in children and adolescents with major depressive disorder and other psychiatric disorders.
- Anyone considering the use of an antidepressant in a child or adolescent for any clinical use must balance the risk of increased suicidality with the clinical need.
- Patients who begin medication therapy should be observed closely for clinical worsening, suicidality, or unusual changes in behavior.
- Families and caregivers should be advised to closely observe the patient and to communicate with the prescriber.
- A statement regarding whether the particular drug is approved for any pediatric indication and if so, which one(s).

Note: The only antidepressant approved to treat major depressive disorder in pediatric patients is fluoxetine HCL (Prozac). Drugs approved for obsessive-compulsive disorder (see discussion later in this chapter) in pediatrics include fluoxetine HCL (Prozac), sertraline HCL (Zoloft), fluvoxamine maleate (Luvox), and clomipramine HCL (Anafranil).

In Canada, a Therapeutic Products Directorate has been issued by Health Canada. It notes that SSRIs and other new antidepressants in patients under 18 years may be associated with behavioral and emotional changes, including severe agitation-type adverse events coupled with self-harm or harm to others. The agitation-type events include akathisia, agitation, disinhibition, emotional lability, hostility, aggression, depersonalization, often within several weeks of starting treatment.

Nurses must reinforce this important teaching for all families when the child or adolescent receives medication, and emphasize the importance of follow-up visits and prompt reporting of any changes in the child/adolescent behavior. Recommended follow-up is for weekly face-to-face contact with the patient and family for the first four weeks of treatment, followed by biweekly visits for four weeks, and contact at 12 weeks to monitor response (Hamrin & Scahill, 2005).

Data from U.S. Food and Drug Administration (2004). FDA Public Health Advisory, October 15, 2004. Antidepressant use in children, adolescents, and adults. Accessed from http://www.fda.gov/Drugs/DrugSafety/InformationbyDrugClass/UCM096273

MyNursingKit Case Study: Calculate SSRI Dosage

desipramine (Norpramin), and amitriptyline (Elavil), may be prescribed. The only antidepressant approved to treat major depressive disorders in pediatric patients is fluoxetine HCl (Prozac), but clinicians use others when the child does not respond to Prozac.

NURSING MANAGEMENT

NURSING ASSESSMENT AND DIAGNOSIS

Take a thorough history and physical examination, including observation of behavior, at the time of admission. Assess the child for common risk factors for depression (Table 57–5).

Several nursing diagnoses that might be appropriate for the child or adolescent hospitalized with depression are included in the accompanying Nursing Care Plan. Other diagnoses might include the following:

- *Imbalanced Nutrition: More than Body Requirements* related to eating in response to internal cues other than hunger
- *Powerlessness* related to sense of helplessness
- *Chronic Low Self-esteem* related to negative self-evaluation

PLANNING AND IMPLEMENTATION

Nursing care of the child or adolescent hospitalized for depression includes administering medications and other therapy, and providing supportive care. Monitor vital signs of youth receiving antidepressant medications. Watch for common side effects of the agent(s) used. Carefully monitor for serious side effects of TCAs or SSRIs and be aware that lower doses are used at initiation, with doses increasing slowly to the desired level. Frequent face-to-face follow-up visits are needed. When dosages are altered, behavior and ideation changes must be closely monitored. Monitor cardiovascular status, including hypertension and tachycardia, observe motor movement, and record dietary intake. Help parents to evaluate inpatient settings to be certain the care provided will best meet the needs of the child or adolescent. Refer to "Nursing Care Plan: The Child or Adolescent Hospitalized with Depression" for specific nursing interventions.

DISCHARGE PLANNING AND HOME CARE TEACHING

When the child has been hospitalized and is returning home, teach parents to recognize signs and symptoms of worsening depression. Also teach them dosages and side effects of any prescribed medications. Refer the family to appropriate healthcare professionals and to support groups for family members dealing with depression.

Table 57–5 Risk Factors for Child and Adolescent Depression

Child	Family	School and Social Situations
■ Frequent feelings of sadness, sleep problems, loss of interest in activities ■ Increase in risk taking and impulsivity ■ Previous suicide attempt ■ Alcohol or substance abuse ■ Diagnosed psychotic disorder ■ Chronic illness and frequent hospitalization	■ Parental neglect, abuse, or loss ■ Dysfunctional family relationships ■ Family history of depression, suicide, substance abuse, alcoholism, other psychopathology	■ Academic pressures and underachievement ■ Stressful social relationships ■ Declining participation in social events

Teaching Highlights

SELECTING RESIDENTIAL AND INPATIENT CARE FOR THE CHILD WITH MENTAL ILLNESS

Families need guidelines to help them evaluate inpatient facilities when a child with a mental disorder must be placed in an institution. You can refer them to the National Alliance for the Mentally Ill Web site. Provide questions for the families to ask:

- What is the staff-to-youth ratio?
- What are the guidelines for chemical and physical restraint?
- Are children isolated when behaviors are inappropriate?
- Are children constantly monitored visually when in restraint or when potentially dangerous to self or others?
- Does the child have a full physical and psychologic evaluation by a specialist within 24 hours of entry to the facility?
- What professionals review the plan of care and how often?
- Who can the family speak to for regular updates on the child?
- How often can the family visit?
- What services will be covered by insurance?
- What subjective feelings do the family members have as they visit the unit and facility?
- What services will be offered on an ongoing basis upon discharge?

NURSING CARE IN THE COMMUNITY

Most children with depression are cared for in the community. Maintain regular contact with the family through their health-care visits to outpatient agencies and by making home visits. Monitor the child's affect, activity, and food intake. School teachers and counselors often are aware of the child's ability to perform in the school setting. Have the family schedule after-school care so young children are not left at home alone for extended periods. Assist the family in finding support for financial and emotional needs related to managing the child's depression. Major expected outcomes for nursing care of the child with depression are found on the accompanying Nursing Care Plan.

BIPOLAR DISORDER (MANIC DEPRESSION)

Bipolar disorder is a mental illness in which extreme changes in affect and energy are manifested. Moods most often alter between mania (high energy and euphoria) and depression. Children often present with irritability or hyperactivity. About 1% of children and adults have bipolar illness, with a high rate of onset from 15 to 19 years (Lansford, 2005). The disorder has been diagnosed in children as young as preschool age (Apps, Winkler, & Jandrisevits, 2008. There is a high rate of attempted suicide in those with bipolar disease, as well as co-occurrence with other disorders such as ADHD, anxiety, and substance abuse, all of which complicates diagnosis (Kowatch, Fristad, Birmaher, et al., 2005).

Bipolar disorder is classified into four types. They include:

- Bipolar I—includes a severe manic episode that requires hospitalization or causes functional impairment in life
- Bipolar II—at least one episode of mild to moderate mania (hypomania) and one of depression
- Cyclothymic disorder—manifests as multiple mild manic and depressive episodes
- Bipolar not otherwise specified—rapid mood fluctuations, mania without depressive episodes, or chronic depression with hypomania episodes (Roberts, 2007).

When parents or close relatives are affected, the child is more likely to have the disorder. Thus, a genetic etiology is probable. It is believed that genetics and environment interact to create the condition in youth. Brain imaging shows abnormalities of the frontal and prefrontal cortex, the hippocampus, the basal ganglia, and the left amygdala, which is the center for experiencing fear (Schapiro, 2005).

The manic phase of bipolar illness is characterized by hyperactivity and high energy, irritability, aggression, and sometimes hallucinations. In the depressive phase, the child is sad, has alterations in sleep and eating patterns, and is socially withdrawn, similar to any depressive illness. Mania may be the persistent symptom in children, or rapid cycles of mania and depression can occur throughout the day (Lansford, 2005).

Diagnosis and treatment of bipolar disorder should be performed by mental health specialists. Use of alcohol or illegal

Nursing Care Plan

THE CHILD OR ADOLESCENT HOSPITALIZED WITH DEPRESSION

INTERVENTION	RATIONALE	EXPECTED OUTCOME
1. Nursing Diagnosis: Hopelessness related to long-term stress		
NIC Priority Intervention: **Hope instillation:** Facilitation of the development of a positive outlook		**NOC Suggested Outcome:** **Hope:** Presence of internal state of optimism that is personally satisfying and life supporting
Goal: The child or adolescent will discuss feelings of hopelessness.		
■ Encourage open expression of feelings. Explore hopeless, sad, or lonely feelings. Point out the connection between feelings and behavior. Assess the child or adolescent to identify the precipitating event when feelings of sadness arose. Maintain an accepting and nonjudgmental attitude regarding any feelings expressed by the child.	■ Expressing feelings may help to relieve sadness, loneliness, despair, and hopelessness.	By discharge, the child or adolescent expresses an interest in the future.
■ Encourage the child or adolescent to take part in self-care and unit activities. Use routines to establish feelings of control.	■ An active role in self-care and treatment helps the child or adolescent to feel more in control.	
■ Medicate as ordered and document results.	■ Antidepressants modify mood to a more hopeful outlook.	
2. Nursing Diagnosis: Ineffective Individual Coping related to inadequate social support or disturbance in pattern of appraisal of threat		
NIC Priority Intervention: **Coping enhancement:** Assisting a patient to adapt to perceived stressors, changes, or threats that interfere with meeting life demands and roles		**NOC Suggested Outcome:** **Coping:** Actions to manage stressors that tax an individual's resources
Goal: The child or adolescent will use effective coping skills.		
■ Teach positive, effective coping strategies such as guided imagery and relaxation. Assist the child or adolescent to focus on strengths rather than weaknesses.	■ Therapeutic techniques can help the child or adolescent to replace negative thoughts and images with more positive and effective beliefs and images. These interventions foster resilience.	The child or adolescent verbalizes and demonstrates ability to cope appropriately for his or her age.
■ Assist the child or adolescent to identify friends, family members, and others who are positive and supportive.	■ Helps the child or adolescent to become aware that people can be caring and supportive (thus validating self-esteem).	
3. Nursing Diagnosis: Impaired Social Interaction related to self-concept disturbance		
NIC Priority Intervention: **Socialization enhancement:** Facilitation of ability to interact with others		**NOC Suggested Outcome:** **Social interaction skills:** An individual's use of effective interaction behaviors
Goal: The child or adolescent will participate in and initiate activities and conversation.		

Nursing Care Plan—continued

THE CHILD OR ADOLESCENT HOSPITALIZED WITH DEPRESSION

INTERVENTION	RATIONALE	EXPECTED OUTCOME
■ Assist the child or adolescent to identify topics and activities of interest.	■ The more the child or adolescent focuses on areas of interest, the less he or she will focus on internal anxiety and depression.	By discharge, the child or adolescent initiates conversation and activities with staff and peers.
■ Encourage interaction with peers and staff.	■ Each positive interaction reinforces feelings of success. Each success reinforces the desire for future social interaction.	
■ Facilitate visits from family and friends.	■ Reinforces positive and rewarding relationships.	
■ Provide guidance to family regarding interaction that promotes self-esteem.	■ The family's existing interaction style is often negative.	

4. Nursing Diagnosis: Imbalanced Nutrition: Less than Body Requirements related to loss of appetite secondary to depression

NIC Priority Intervention:

Nutrition management: Assistance with or provision of a balanced dietary intake of foods and fluids

NOC Suggested Outcome:

Nutritional status: Amount of food and fluid taken into the body over a 24-hour period

Goal: The child's or adolescent's daily intake will be adequate to maintain optimal nutritional status.

INTERVENTION	RATIONALE	EXPECTED OUTCOME
■ Offer nutritious finger foods, sandwiches, and high-calorie liquid supplements frequently throughout the day.	■ Convenient easy-to-eat foods encourage the child or adolescent to eat and maintain nutritional status.	The child or adolescent's daily intake will be adequate to maintain optimal nutritional status by discharge.
■ Offer easy-to-carry drinks that are high in vitamins, minerals, and calories.	■ These are a convenient method for meeting hydration and electrolyte needs.	
■ Encourage daily vigorous physical activity of at least 30 minutes.	■ Physical activity stimulates appetite.	

drugs should be ruled out as a cause of symptoms, even in children. Since the manic phase is often manifested by hyperactivity, the child may incorrectly be treated with stimulants (see treatment of ADHD earlier in this chapter), and the disease can be worsened. Irritability, elation, labile moods, and sleep disturbance are commonly seen in children (Apps et al., 2008; DelBello, Adler, & Strakowski, 2006; Kowatch et al., 2005).

The treatment of bipolar disease involves a variety of drugs used to stabilize mood. Lithium, valproate, divalproex, carbamazepine, olanzapine, oxcarbazepine, lamotregine, quetiapine, and risperidone are examples of drugs used. Only lithium is approved by the FDA for use in those from 12 to 18 years (Apps et al., 2008). However, clinicians prescribe other drugs with careful monitoring performed. Early treatment is key to preventing chronic, serious mental illness (Ferguson-Noyes, 2005; Kowatch et al., 2005). Individual and family education and therapy can be helpful.

Nurses are instrumental in identifying children with the disorder, providing information to families, and monitoring the drugs and psychotherapy for the child. Nurses should observe for side effects to the specific drug regimen used and assist parents to find resources for healthcare since medications and other treatments may be costly. Parents and children need information about the disorder since it may recur several times during the child's life. Nurses can assist the child to find social events and groups that build a sense of self-esteem.

ANXIETY AND RELATED DISORDERS

A large group of anxiety disorders can affect youth as well as adults. Some of the more common types seen in children and adolescents are described in the following sections, with detailed nursing management described for posttraumatic stress disorder.

GENERALIZED ANXIETY DISORDER

Anxiety is a subjective feeling of uncertainty and helplessness, usually accompanied by central nervous system (CNS) signs, including restlessness, trembling, perspiration, and rapid pulse. Anxiety is second only to substance abuse (see Chapter 44∞) in incidence for mental disorders and is a common mental disorder among children. From 3% to 12% of chidren experience generalized anxiety disorder, with 8 to 19 years of age the most frequent time for its emergence (Hudson, Deveny, & Taylor, 2005).

Anxiety disorders are strongly linked to familial and genetic factors. They may coexist with other mental health disorders, or children sometimes have more than one type of anxiety (Shear, Jin, Ruscio, et al., 2006). Diagnosis is performed by a mental health specialist, and treatment is usually cognitive behavioral therapy (CBT) and may involve medication. CBT can include child or family interventions that focus on relaxation, recognition of feelings, and self-talking. Medications that have been reported to be successful in children include sertraline and fluvoxamine (Hudson et al., 2005).

SEPARATION ANXIETY DISORDER

Separation anxiety disorder is characterized by an extreme state of uneasiness when in unfamiliar surroundings and often by refusal to visit friends' homes or attend school for at least 2 weeks. It is the most common type of anxiety disorder manifested by children (Cartwright-Hatton, McNicol, & Doubleday, 2006). Approximately 75% of children with separation anxiety disorder refuse to attend school (see "School Phobia," to follow). Many children worry about losing a parent or significant other. This disorder occurs in approximately 4% to 5% of children and in twice as many girls as boys (Shear et al., 2006). The peak age for occurrence is 7 to 9 years. It may come and go and may be acute in onset (preceded by a traumatic event) or slow to develop over time (Hanna, Fischer, & Fluent, 2006).

Children with separation anxiety disorder tend to be perfectionistic, overly compliant, and eager to please. They appear to cling to the parent or caretaker. They may use physical complaints such as headaches, abdominal pain, nausea, and vomiting in an attempt to avoid being away from the parent. Depression frequently accompanies separation anxiety disorder. The resulting avoidant behaviors can interfere with personal growth and development, academic achievement, and social functioning.

Diagnosis is made by a mental health specialist. Treatment includes CBT with both child and parents. Parents learn about the disorder and how to structure the setting so that the child is expected to attend school. Consistency in expectations is needed since if the child is permitted to stay home some days or has missed school and other activities for longer periods, treatment is more difficult. The child learns what situations cause anxiety and how to manage the situations and feelings elicited. Both parents and child work out the expectations for behavior for the child with the mental health therapist; school personnel are included in the treatment plan. Medication has occasionally been used but only if CBT is not helpful (Jurbergs & Ledley, 2005). The SSRI fluoxetine has been used with a dose of 10–20 mg/day for children and adolescents; the dose may be increased as needed at weekly intervals to a maximum of 60 mg/day (Bindler & Howry, 2005).

Growth and Development

The separation anxiety commonly experienced by a 2-year-old differs from the psychiatric disorder in age appropriateness, duration, and severity. Separation anxiety disorder affects children of preschool age or older, lasts for at least 2 weeks, and is characterized by excessive anxiety. In contrast, the separation anxiety experienced by the 2-year-old involves a single episode of separation from a familiar caretaker and is a characteristic response in toddlers.

PANIC DISORDER

Panic disorder is the presence of recurrent, unexpected panic attacks. Panic attacks are periods of intense fear and discomfort in the absence of real danger. The risk of panic disorder ranges from 0.4% in adolescent boys, to 0.7% in adolescent girls, and 1.5% in adults. Predictive factors for panic attacks in adolescence include a history of separation anxiety disorder earlier in life, history of parental panic attacks, and history of parental chronic illness (Hayward, Wilson, Lagle, et al., 2004).

Examples of the physical symptoms experienced are palpitations, sweating, chills, hot flashes, shaking, shortness of breath, choking, chest pain, nausea, and dizziness. The person describes feelings of danger or doom. Some people may have accompanying agoraphobia. **Agoraphobia** is an anxiety of being in places or situations from which escape may be difficult or embarrassing, or in which help may not be available. The attacks may be continuous or episodic, but generally are chronic.

Diagnosis is made by a mental health specialist. Similar to anxiety, treatment may involve individual and family therapy, with use of medication in some cases. Nurses can help identify the disorder, refer for evaluation, and provide care in the community so that the child attends therapy sessions and takes medication as ordered.

OBSESSIVE-COMPULSIVE DISORDER

People with obsessive-compulsive disorder (OCD) may be mildly or severely affected. From 1% to 4% of children are affected, and about 80% of adults with OCD had the condition in childhood (Lewin, Storch, Adkins, et al., 2005). Affected children have recurrent obsessive thoughts, commonly about contamination, harm, sex, or moral concerns. These obsessions are handled through a series of compulsive behaviors that interfere with daily life. Examples of behaviors are excessive handwashing, counting objects, and hoarding substances. These practices may take one hour or more of time each day. Children with OCD differ from adults in several ways. They have more aggressive obsessions, such as fears of catastrophe, more commonly hoard objects, and are more likely to have religious obsessions. The presence of additional mental health disorders is common (Lewin et al., 2005).

Nursing Practice

Pediatric autoimmune neuropsychiatric disorders (PANDAS) are characterized by obsessive-compulsive and/or tic disorder, childhood onset, association with Group A beta hemolytic streptococcal infection, and neurological abnormalities. It is believed that in certain children, the strep infection leads to a neural autoimmune response, resulting in the psychiatric disorder. Research continues to identify possible mechanisms, results, and treatments for this cause of OCD (Gabbay, Coffey, Babb, et al., 2008; Mell, Davis, & Owens, 2005).

The basal ganglia of the brain are affected and a genetic link is observed. A neurochemical cause may be related to abnormal serotonin metabolism. MRI changes in the globus pallidus and anterior cingulated gyrus of the brain have been noted (Lewin et al., 2005). Poststreptococcal autoimmune disorder may be a cause in some cases.

Diagnosis is made by a mental health specialist. Treatment may involve CBT, where the feared occurrence is presented and the person learns that no harm will occur. Involvement of the family in treatment is important so that members learn how to handle the child's ritualistic behaviors. Medications, such as clomipramine and the SSRIs, are effective in most children and adolescents. Nurses can identify cases and refer for mental health evaluation, and provide teaching and support for families.

SCHOOL PHOBIA (SOCIAL PHOBIA)

School phobia (also called *social phobia, school avoidance,* or *school refusal*) is a persistent, irrational, or excessive fear of negative evaluation or embarrassment in social situations and therefore of attending school. The child may fear being harmed or losing control. Social and school phobia occur in children as young as 5 years of age, often presents at 11 or 12 years, but can occur in children up to 16 years (Ginsburg & Grover, 2005).

Children with social phobia may fear asking for directions, ordering food at a restaurant, and speaking in the classroom. They commonly report that teachers and peers "pick on" them. Somatic complaints are similar to those in children with separation anxiety disorder. Characteristically, symptoms are present only on school days and not on weekends or holidays. The social withdrawal that occurs in this disorder further impairs the child since social interactions are needed for normal developmental progression.

Diagnosis is made by a mental health specialist. Treatment includes the family and child, and establishes firm limits for behavioral expectations and consequences. CBT is used, commonly 12- to 16-week group sessions with other youth, and additional sessions involving the family (Ginsburg & Grover, 2005). SSRI medications may sometimes be needed to lessen anxiety in social situations.

CONVERSION REACTION

Conversion reaction is a disorder in which a disturbance or loss of sensory, motor, or other physical functions suggests neurologic or other somatic disease. The disturbance or loss cannot be explained by any known pathophysiologic mechanism. Instead, psychologic factors are involved. About 3% of the population experiences conversion reactions at some time. Adolescence and early adulthood are common times for the onset to occur, with onset rare before 10 years or after 35 years (Powsner & Dufel, 2006).

Conversion reactions develop in response to a catastrophic event such as threat, loss, or harm. Clinical manifestations include altered sensations such as blindness or deafness; paralysis or ataxia, including inability to stand or walk and loss of ability to speak (aphonia); involuntary movements, such as pseudoepileptic convulsions; and constant complaints of pain with no physical basis (psychogenic pain). Children under 10 years usually present with gait abnormalities or seizures. The onset of conversion symptoms is usually dramatic and sudden. Symptoms often appear to be neurologic, but on careful examination obvious discrepancies are found. The person is usually calm about the symptoms even though they are serious. Often the child or family members appear indifferent or unconcerned over what healthcare providers consider an overwhelming physical disability. Other psychiatric conditions may coexist with conversion reaction (Haugaard, 2004).

Children suspected of having a conversion reaction require a complete physical and neurologic evaluation to rule out any possible physiologic basis for the symptoms. Individual and family therapy is usually necessary to identify the source of the psychologic conflict, pain, or need resulting in the conversion symptoms. Pharmacologic approaches may also be used (Diseth & Christie, 2005).

POSTTRAUMATIC STRESS DISORDER

MyNursingKit Critical Thinking: Females and PTSD

Acute stress disorder can occur after any life-threatening event and is manifested in the first month after exposure to the event. Symptoms include repeatedly reliving the traumatic experience, anxiety, and increased arousal. Similarly, *posttraumatic stress disorder* (PTSD) victims have experienced or witnessed a life-threatening event; however, the symptoms of distress continue for more than 1 month and cause impairment in functioning. Estimates of the incidence of PTSD are hard to obtain. It is assumed that about 40% of youth have an episode of trauma that could lead to PTSD and that 6% have symptoms of the disorder (Caffo & Belaise, 2003). While 20% of children may experience PTSD after traumatic events, the prevalence rises to 90% when the trauma is severe (Centers for Disease Control and Prevention, 2006b).

Examples of events associated with posttraumatic stress include sexual or other child abuse, rape, car crash, fire, witnessing violence, and having experience in war (Kaminer, Seedat, & Stein, 2005; Schafer, Barkmann, Riedesser, et al., 2006). The events that occurred in the United States on September 11, 2001, are causes of posttraumatic stress in children who either had a family member involved, lived near the events, or in some other way were profoundly affected. Cassandra, described in the opening quotation of this chapter, was experiencing posttraumatic stress disorder (PTSD) resulting from a frightening car crash as

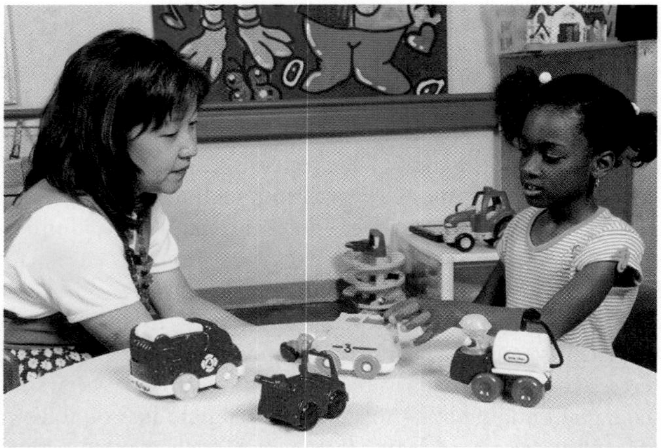

● **Figure 57–6** Play therapy. The psychologist uses play therapy to help Cassandra reenact her car crash. This helps her gain some control over the event so that it is not so frightening.

she was driven to school. She was too young to describe her feelings verbally to her mother or school personnel; however, she manifested the sleep abnormalities and other complaints common in the disorder (Figure 57–6 ●).

The disorder involves both a traumatic event and the child's reaction to this event. It is believed that brain changes occur in trauma, leading to neurobiologic alterations that cause dysfunction of memory. Overreactivity of the amygdala, underreactivity of the prefrontal cortex, and increased dopamine in the medial prefronal cortex are observed (Brown, 2005). Female gender, having other psychiatric disorders, a family history of psychiatric illness, and severe or lengthy trauma are all risk factors.

The child with PTSD has feelings of fear, terror, and helplessness, and may relive the event frequently in thought and nightmares. The child may become emotionally numb in a subconscious attempt to protect the self, but may have a persistently increased state of arousal. The child exhibits a state of hypervigilance and an exaggerated startle response, such as to touch or loud noises. The child with PTSD is often irritable, and has sleep problems and inattentiveness. The person feels detached from others and alone. Immediately after the event, the child may appear to have adapted and functions normally. However, after several weeks or even months, the symptoms of the disorder begin to appear.

The diagnosis is made by a mental health specialist; a variety of instruments assist in screening for the disorder. Counseling by a mental health specialist is the main therapy for PTSD. Cassandra saw a clinical psychologist who used play therapy to help her communicate her fears related to a car crash. CBT is the treatment of choice, with both the child and family members included. Young children show significant improvement in symptoms after a course of CBT (Scheeringa, Salloum, Arnberger, et al., 2007; Smith, Yule, Perrin, et al., 2007). A variety of antidepressants and SSRIs are used for pharmacologic treatment.

Nursing Management

Nurses often help identify PTSD victims so that care can be obtained. Ask about traumatic events in the past and how the child reacted. Inquire about recent changes in the child's behavior. Include school attendance, complaints of physical illness, sleep patterns, and rituals in behavior. A family history of mental disorders may be useful. Youth who run away from home and present at homeless shelters are often suffering from PTSD. Assessment for the condition should be part of initial history (Thompson, Maccio, Desselle, et al., 2007).

Nursing care for anxiety disorders focuses on behavioral and cognitive therapies to enhance coping skills. Mental health nurses may conduct group therapy sessions (Figure 57–7 ●). Group sessions for children often provide a forum for discussion of fears, an opportunity to enhance skills of working together, and an opportunity to learn coping skills. Being a member of a group with other children experiencing anxiety or trauma can remove the stigma and allow the child the freedom to explore the behavior and its causes. Several of the techniques described in the chapter, such as drawing pictures and discussing them or telling stories, are used by mental health nurses in child therapy groups.

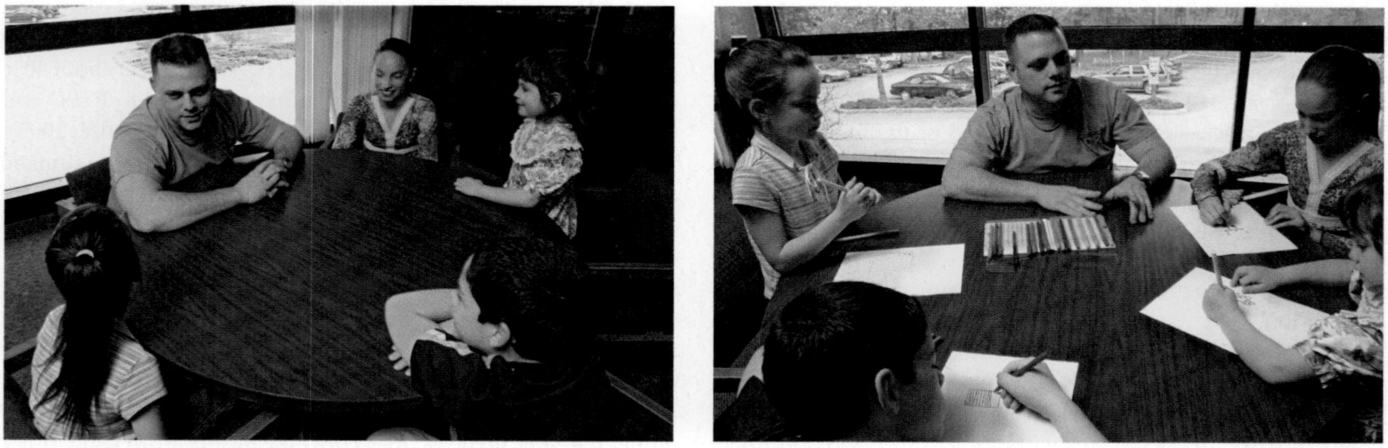

● **Figure 57–7** Group therapy for children. This nurse conducts a group therapy session for children who have experienced traumatic events and have resulting anxiety disorders. He is clearly engaged, has a positive rapport, and fosters exchanges among the children. Games and drawing are frequent techniques used in the group.

Teaching Highlights

TALKING WITH CHILDREN ABOUT TRAUMATIC EVENTS

Whether a child or adolescent experiences trauma from a car crash, abuse, or environmental event, parents can help to decrease the effects of the stress and prevent the appearance of PTSD. Some suggestions for parents include:

- Be sure children feel free to ask parents, teachers, or others about the events and their feelings.
- Assure children that their feelings are normal and may return over time.
- Be honest and open in responses, without overloading children with more details than they need.
- Be prepared to repeat answers and discuss the same topics many times.
- Get help from counselors who can suggest how to talk with the child.
- Use communication methods appropriate at various ages, such as reading books, doing art projects, or drawing.
- Show children that they are loved by spending time and planning activities with them.
- Limit the television and other media time where the child is exposed to violence and traumatic events.
- Restore a sense of normal routines into the child's life.
- Be alert for increasing signs of distress and seek care from a professional if they occur.

Children need to learn relaxation techniques and nurses may teach such techniques or recommend that the child consider participation in yoga or guided imagery classes. Inquire about alternative therapies that the child and family are using or have an interest in beginning, and refer as needed. Parents or other significant people should be included in the treatment program. Nurses often teach them basic information about the child's diagnosis and therapy. They should be in at least some therapy sessions with the child. Provide the family with resources that will assist with relief from worry about the child, guilt about causing an accident that triggered the child's symptoms, or other feelings related to the diagnosis.

Insurance companies may provide limited payment for mental health services. Help the family to see the importance of recommended therapy and assist them to find resources for care if needed. School personnel may need to know about the child's treatment. Partner with the families to provide needed information. Some schools have counselors that can be instrumental in carrying out treatment plans at school and acting as a resource in that setting. School personnel may be asked to provide feedback about the child's attendance, performance, and social skills as a measure of the success of therapy, and the community or school nurse can relay this information.

Thinking Critically

POSTTRAUMATIC STRESS DISORDER

Cassandra is a 9-year-old girl who has recently become fearful about attending school and has awakened crying at night. She is in the third grade at a school she has attended for 2 years. A few weeks ago, she was in a car crash as her mother drove her to school. She received only minor injuries and returned to school the next day. However, her mother believes that Cassandra's behavior has been worsening since the car crash. She spoke with the school nurse, who is aware of no trauma at school, but did learn from the teacher that Cassandra has not been paying attention in class recently. Cassandra cannot explain why she does not want to go to school, only that her stomach aches or some other part of her body hurts.

Cassandra visited her pediatrician, who ruled out any physical cause for her complaints, and referred her to a child psychologist. The psychologist has scheduled several sessions with Cassandra to help her learn to verbalize her fears and learn strategies to deal with them. She uses dolls in an attempt to help Cassandra act out her fears and gain some understanding. The psychologist communicates Cassandra's progress to you, the school nurse.

- How can you ensure Cassandra's attendance at school?
- What does the teacher need to know to support Cassandra in the classroom?
- What is your role as liaison between the psychologist, family, and school personnel?
- Parents often feel guilty when a child experiences a mental health disorder. What type of information and support do Cassandra's parents need?

See MyNursingKit for possible responses.

Nurses often administer medications to children being treated for PTSD and other mental health concerns. Be alert for side effects and ensure the family knows how to safely administer the drugs. They should be kept locked securely. Have the child return for follow-up as needed since some medications may take several weeks to achieve effects, and close monitoring is essential. The child should have a medication alert tag for drugs being taken.

OTHER DISORDERS

SUICIDE

Suicide is the third leading cause of death in adolescents between 15 and 19 years of age. The suicide rate decreased in individuals from 10 to 24 years during 1990–2003. However, since then suicide rates have increased, with about 7.32 per 100,000 (Centers for Disease Control and Prevention, 2007c). Suicide accounts for about 12% of deaths in teens and about 4500 deaths annually in the United States. About 9.7% of teens report at least one suicide attempt, and 29.9% have suicidal ideation at some time (Evans, Hawton, Rodham, et al., 2005; Shaw, Fernandez, & Rao, 2005).

Developing Cultural Competence

SUICIDE AND ETHNICITY

Some ethnic groups have a high rate of suicide. For example, Native Americans and Alaskan Natives have a rate of suicide at 1.5 times the national average; suicide is the second leading cause of death in these ethnic groups (Centers for Disease Control and Prevention, 2007b). The historic pain experienced by this ethnic group and lack of opportunities for many youth may be some of the reasons for a high suicide rate. Hispanic females have a higher rate of suicide than other gender and ethnic groups. White males have traditionally had highest rates of suicide, but recently blacks have had greatly increasing numbers of suicides (Centers for Disease Control and Prevention, 2004; Centers for Disease Control and Prevention, 2006b). *Healthy People 2010* goals focus on eliminating such health disparities by finding the causes, setting up prevention programs, and providing more support and opportunities for native populations.

Males die as a result of suicide four times more often than females. This statistic is reversed for suicide attempts, perhaps because boys use lethal methods such as guns, hanging, and jumping more often than girls, who use drug overdose and wrist cutting (Evans et al., 2005). It is not unusual for healthcare professionals and parents to label suicide attempts by children and adolescents "accidents." Up to half of childhood suicides may be recorded as accidents; suicide data for children under age 10 years are not maintained. Adults may have difficulty believing that young children, in particular, would have any reason to want to end their lives. Because of this, many children brought to the emergency department with indications of a suicide attempt are often classified as unintentional injury victims and released without arrangements for appropriate follow-up care. Accurate identification and treatment are needed for youth at risk of suicide (Pompili, Mancinelli, Girardi, et al., 2005).

Many risk factors for suicide exist in children and adolescents, while some protective factors are influential as well (Table 57–6). The most common precursor to adolescent suicide is depression (see earlier discussion). Common signs or symptoms of an underlying depression that could lead to suicide include boredom, restlessness, problems with concentration, irritability, lethargy, intentional misbehavior, preoccupation with one's own body or health, and excessive dependence on or isolation from others (especially adults or caregivers).

The child or adolescent at high risk for suicide may be admitted to a mental health unit for care or cared for in a community mental health facility. Treatment may include individual, group, or family therapy. Negotiating a "no suicide" contract is one method that may be used with a suicidal youth. In the contract, the child agrees not to attempt suicide during a specified time period. When a suicide attempt is made, the child or adolescent may be hospitalized for 24 hours, kept in a short-term monitoring unit, or sent home under close observation to ensure adequate assessment and monitoring. It is important to provide crisis intervention at the time of suicide attempt to minimize the opportunity for repeat attempts and begin a therapeutic treatment plan.

Table 57–6 Risk and Protective Factors for Suicide in Children and Adolescents

Risk Factors	Protective Factors
History of previous attempted suicide	Emotional well-being
Friend committed or attempted suicide	Satisfactory school performance
School problems or changes in grades	Participation in sports or other group events
Pregnancy	Weight satisfaction
Drug use or abuse	Parent/family connectedness
Problems with a romantic relationship	Frequent discussions of important issues with family
Minority sexual practice	School connectedness
Loneliness, withdrawal	Safe school
Feelings of anxiety	Safe neighborhood
History of chronic family problems	Caring adult presence at school or elsewhere
Chronic illness	Availability of school counseling
Physical, emotional, or sexual abuse	School policies to limit and cope with fighting, bullying
History of suicide in a family member	
History of depression	
Chronic low self-esteem	
Change in behavior	
Change in weight	
Giving away special possessions	
Access to firearms and ammunition	

Nursing Management

The major nursing role is in prevention of suicide. All children and adolescents in health promotion visits and emergency rooms should be evaluated for risk. Health promotion visits are an opportunity to be alert for children with depression (see previous discussion), substance abuse, recent stresses, and changes in behavior. Inquire about sleep patterns, feelings of sadness, and use of alcohol and other substances. Gather a family history of mental health disorders, suicide attempts, and stresses. Ask about how often the youth talks with or has meals with the family. Be aware of the risk of self-inflicted strangulation.

Recall that all youth who receive medications for treatment of depression should be carefully monitored, especially in the first several weeks in order to identify those who may develop suicide ideation and risk. While antidepressants have demonstrated efficacy for treating depression in youth, there is a twofold increased risk of suicidal ideation or behaviors in children and adolescents treated with these drugs (Bridge, Iyengar, Salary, et al., 2007).

Most suicides are committed with firearms that are usually obtained from the home (Roche, Giner, & Zalsman, 2005). Determine at each healthcare visit if the family has firearms. Teach them to keep the guns unloaded, with ammunition and firearms locked in separate locations. Be sure that children and adolescents do not have access to the keys for the locked firearms. Never underestimate the resourcefulness or abilities of a suicidal child or adolescent, regardless of age, IQ, or physical abilities.

Education in all school settings is appropriate to teach children about resources that can help them if they need it and to identify peers at risk. Mental health services of all types should be available and embedded in schools since that is the setting where youth spend much of their time (U.S. Department of Health and Human Services, 2006). Be alert for children and adolescents at risk for suicide in any setting. Assess children and adolescents in schools, outpatient settings, and emergency departments for the possibility of suicidal behavior. Report threats of suicide and depressive behavior. When a child or adolescent persists in threatening suicide after establishment of a "no suicide" contract, hospitalization is necessary to ensure safety. Recognize that when a child or adolescent has committed suicide, friends of the victim may be at increased risk. Teach students to report to teachers, nurses, or counselors about friends who have threatened suicide or seem depressed or display behaviors different from usual. Nurses often plan with mental health specialists to implement suicide prevention programs in schools and communities. Provide supportive services to family and friends whenever suicide occurs. Consult Web sites and refer parents as appropriate. The Suicide Prevention Resource Center has helpful regional offices to facilitate networks at national, state, territorial, community, and tribal levels.

Nursing care during hospitalization for suicide centers on taking appropriate precautions to ensure the child's safety. Monitor both the child and the hospital environment for any object that could be used for self-harm. Remove all potentially harmful objects, such as shoestrings, belts, pantyhose, and hair ribbons. Keep all personal care items (including toothbrush and shampoo) locked at the nursing station and monitor them constantly when used by the child.

Children or adolescents considered at high risk for suicidal behaviors are attended by a nursing staff member at all times, including while using the bathroom and sleeping. It may be necessary for the child to dress in a plain hospital gown, be kept in a visually monitored seclusion room, or (if seriously impaired and self-abusive) be medicated for restraint for a period of time. Restraints are used only when ordered by the physician and interdisciplinary team caring for the youth. Physical restraint is only a short-term approach to provide immediate safety if necessary. Chemical (medication) restraint may be needed to prevent self-injury by the suicidal person. See "Teaching Highlights: Selecting Residential and Inpatient Care for the Mentally Ill Child" on page 1721 for information to help families consider when choosing care for their suicidal child.

Hospitalization continues as long as the child's behavior is self-destructive. Children are referred for intensive individual and family therapy. Encourage parents to keep follow-up clinic appointments, to watch for self-destructive behaviors, and to administer any prescribed medications according to the treatment schedule. Arrange home visits and other community resources for families.

TIC DISORDERS AND TOURETTE SYNDROME

Tics are sudden, rapid, recurrent, nonrhythmic, and brief motor movements or vocalizations. They may involve movement of the head or upper body, blinking of eyes, or a variety of verbal noises. They may be worse during periods of stress or tiredness. Many children have mild motor tics at some time that gradually disappear with no intervention. When the tics are severe or last over one year, they are considered chronic and may require attention from a mental health provider.

Severe motor tics accompanied by verbal utterances are known as Tourette syndrome. The syndrome is often accompanied by other diagnoses such as attention deficit and learning disabilities. Children with Tourette syndrome may exhibit coprolalia, the involuntary utterance of obscenities, profanities and racial slurs, or copropraxia, the involuntary use of obscene gestures (Schapiro, 2004).

Tic disorders are characterized by disruptions in the levels of dopamine, serotonin, and other neurotransmitter and neuropeptide levels. Nursing care involves supporting parents and encouraging normal developmental progression for the child. Nurses should carefully monitor symptoms after medication is begun, minimize stress, and teach relaxation techniques.

SCHIZOPHRENIA

Schizophrenia is a psychotic disorder that is relatively rare in young children and adolescents, occurring in 1 in 10,000 children. The prevalence increases after puberty, most commonly manifesting from 15 to 20 years of age, and reaches adult levels by late adolescence (Remschmidt & Theisen, 2005).

The cause of schizophrenia is unknown, but genetic predisposition or neurointegration deficits are suspected (Remschmidt & Theisen, 2005). The brain is altered in the disease, with progressively enlarged ventricles and nervous system arousal. Impaired glucose metabolism is often present. Onset is usually slow with increasing intensity. Most often the child demonstrates restlessness, poor appetite, and social withdrawal over several weeks to months. Behavioral problems, slowed development, and minor neurologic symptoms may occur.

The clinical manifestations of schizophrenia are the same in children as in adults. Characteristic behaviors include social withdrawal, impaired social relationships, flat **affect** (outward appearance of feeling or emotion), regression, loose associations (thought characterized by speech in which ideas shift from one subject to another that is unrelated), poor judgment and problem solving, anxiety, delusions, and hallucinations. Motor abnormalities may include rocking and arm flapping.

During adolescence, acute schizophrenia can occur suddenly while the teenager is making plans to leave home and family to attend college, marry, or work in another area. Onset of symptoms may be triggered by an important loss (death of a significant other, parent, child, or friend).

Prompt diagnosis can lead to early treatment and more positive outcomes. Clinical therapy for childhood schizophrenia is multifaceted, including individual psychotherapy, family therapy, and various psychotropic medications (antipsychotics such as haloperidol [Haldol], antianxiety agents such as lorazepam [Ativan], antidepressants such as imipramine [Tofranil], and newer antipsychotics such as clozapine, olanzapine, and risperidone) (Remschmidt & Theisen, 2005). Drugs are only moderately effective at controlling hallucinations and delusions. Responses vary considerably, and children may have different responses than adults. Side effects determine what drugs are used and for how long. Antipsychotic medication is continued for at least 4 to 6 weeks before effectiveness can be determined. Medications often must be continued for several months or years after recovery from an acute schizophrenic episode, although medication-free trials may be tried in children who have not shown symptoms for 6 to 12 months.

Episodes of acute schizophrenia may require inpatient hospitalization on a psychiatric unit for thorough diagnosis and beginning management. Treatment may include an intensive school-based program in a structured, supervised setting with specially trained professionals. The goal of initial treatment is to reduce or control schizophrenic episodes and provide a safe, structured environment for the child or adolescent, enabling the child to live each day at an optimal level of functioning. Outpatient care is provided in the community following initial diagnosis and establishment of a treatment regimen.

Most children require long-term treatment, including intermittent periods of hospitalization. Children or adolescents whose symptoms are difficult to control and who present a safety risk to themselves or others may require long-term residential treatment. Earlier age at diagnosis and delay in treatment lead to poorer prognosis.

Nursing Management

The nurse may encounter the child or adolescent with schizophrenia during hospitalization for an acute episode, for treatment of another problem, or while working with the individual in the community. Nursing care centers on providing for physical safety and psychologic care, and normal growth and development for the child.

Family education and involvement in the treatment plan are essential. Teach the family to monitor the child's symptoms and progression. Educating the child and parents about the risk of recurrence and methods to alleviate side effects of prescribed medications may increase compliance with the treatment plan. Assess the child for common medication side effects. For example, when excess weight is a potential side effect, frequent growth measurements are made. Neurologic assessment and laboratory studies may be needed with some medications. Help the family establish educational plans and integration within the school system. Communicate with school personnel to ensure understanding of the child's condition and ongoing management of the individualized education plan.

COGNITIVE ALTERATIONS

A wide array of cognitive conditions occur in childhood. Some are mild and not diagnosed until a child has difficulty in school, while others may be associated with physical signs that are visible at birth. Two common conditions, learning disabilities and intellectual disabilities (mental retardation), are discussed in this section.

LEARNING DISABILITIES

Learning disabilities are a common problem of young children, affecting about 5% of school children. They involve neurologic conditions in which the brain cannot receive or process information in the normal manner. Often the impairment is only in one or two types of learning, making diagnosis difficult. Common types of learning disorders are listed in "Clinical Manifestations: Various Learning Disabilities."

Children may have difficulty in processing visual information, which may be manifested in reading, writing, and mathematics performance. Others may have more difficulty with oral information, leading to problems in language development and reading (Kelly & Aylward, 2005).

The causes of learning disorders are complex. Sometimes they are related to low birth weight or problems during the perinatal period. There may be a genetic component since their occurrence is more common when other family members are affected.

Learning disabilities should be diagnosed by a learning specialist such as a psychologist with special training. A series of cognitive and developmental tests are commonly used; magnetic resonance imaging (MRI) is sometimes used. Treatments involve learning how to compensate for the difficulties by using capabilities that are intact. Some children need to have all material written for them, and others need to have verbal presentations. Specific learning goals are established with the assistance of learning specialists. Children with learning disabilities should have individualized education plans (IEPs) established with realistic goals for school performance (see Chapter 39 for further information about IEPs ∞).

Nurses play a major role in identifying children with learning disabilities. The nurse may be in contact with families during health promotion visits or in other settings when parents relay concern about the child's performance or difficulty in some aspect of school. Nurses should assess the child for the following developmental milestones, which can indicate learning disability:

- Lack of ability to phrase sentences together by 2 1/2 years
- Inability to use speech that is understandable at least 50% of the time by 3 years
- Inability to ties shoes, button, hop, or cut with scissors by kindergarten
- Inability to sit for a short story by 3 to 5 years (Kelly & Aylward, 2005).

When a child may have a learning disability, the nurse should refer the family to the school or other testing resource. The nurse should partner with the family to plan for the child's learning needs, help the family to work closely with the child, suggest pro-

Clinical Manifestations

EXAMPLES OF LEARNING DISABILITIES

DISORDER	CLINICAL MANIFESTATIONS
Dyslexia	Difficulty with writing, reading, spelling
Dyscalculia	Mathematics and computation problems
Dysgraphia	Difficulty with writing, spelling, and composition
Dyspraxia	Problems with manual dexterity and coordination

viding a setting at home to maximize potential for learning, and offer suggestions for building healthy self-esteem in the child. The nurse should assist the family to work with the school to establish annual goals for the child. Most children with learning disabilities can learn to perform well in their areas of strength and compensate for areas of difficulty. Early intervention is key to success and building a positive self-image regarding abilities.

INTELLECTUAL DISABILITY (MENTAL RETARDATION)

Intellectual disability is now the preferred term for what was previously called mental retardation. **Intellectual disability** is defined as significant limitation in intellectual functioning and adaptive behavior. It is manifested in differences in conceptual, social, and practical adaptive skills, beginning before the age of 18 years (American Association of Intellectual and Developmental Disabilities, 2008). Later events that lead to limitations in function are commonly referred to as brain injury. Intellectual functioning is generally characterized by an IQ below 70 to 75, and there are significant impairments in **adaptive functioning** (the ability to meet the standards expected for a cultural group). The child with intellectual disability has adaptive deficits in at least two areas such as communication, self-care, home living, social/interpersonal skills, use of community resources, self-direction, functional academic skills, work, leisure, health, or safety. A low IQ score by itself does not necessarily correlate with an impaired ability to carry out adaptive skills. The child should be evaluated within the contexts of the individual cultural and community environment. The IQ score and the level of adaptive skills together determine the degree of severity of intellectual disability.

Intellectual disability is one type of **developmental disability,** any of a variety of chronic conditions that are characterized by mental or physical impairments. Other examples include pervasive developmental disorder, cerebral palsy, and sensory loss. A developmental disability begins through the age of 21 years, and lasts throughout life (Bhasin, Brocksen, Avchen, et al., 2006).

ETIOLOGY AND PATHOPHYSIOLOGY

Intellectual disability occurs in 12 per 1000 children, a decrease from 15.5 per 1000 one decade ago (Bhasin et al., 2006). Its causes can be grouped into three general categories: prenatal errors in the development of the central nervous system, prenatal or postnatal changes in the person's biologic environment, and external forces leading to central nervous system damage. In each instance, the precipitating factor changes the form, function, and adaptation of the central nervous system. Table 57–7 provides examples of common conditions associated with intellectual disability.

Three conditions from prenatal life that are associated with intellectual disability are Down syndrome, fragile X syndrome, and fetal alcohol syndrome. In the United States, about 1 in 800 to 1000 infants, or 5500 infants each year, are born with Down syndrome (Centers for Disease Control and Prevention, 2006a; van Riper, 2007). The syndrome is caused by an extra chromosome; the child has 47 rather than 46 chromosomes (see discussion of genetic transmission in Chapter 3 ∞). The most common chromosome affected is 21 so that the child often has "trisomy 21," or three instead of two copies of number 21 chromosome. In addition to intellectual disability and physical signs, the child with Down syndrome is at higher risk of developing some other conditions such as cardiac defects, hearing loss, gastrointestinal problems, orthodontic conditions, thyroid disease, dermatologic conditions, and leukemia (Van Cleve, Cannon, & Cohen, 2006).

Table 57–7 Common Conditions Associated with Intellectual Disability

Prenatal Conditions	Biologic Environment	External Forces
Down syndrome Fragile X syndrome Fetal alcohol syndrome Maternal infection (e.g., rubella, cytomegalovirus)	Inborn errors of metabolism (e.g., phenylketonuria, hypothyroidism)	Traumatic brain injury (e.g., accident) Poison ingestion (acute or chronic) Hypoxia/anoxic insult Infection (e.g., meningitis) Environmental deprivation

MyNursingKit Video: Down Syndrome

Fragile X syndrome is caused by a single recessive gene abnormality on the X chromosome. A permutation to the X chromosome may occur in males or females. When a father or mother passes the faulty X chromosome to a daughter, it may remain as a permutation or may change into a true mutation. The daughter has two X chromosomes and therefore does not manifest this recessive disorder. However, she can pass the mutated X chromosome to her son who becomes affected with fragile X. The mutation of fragile X is on gene FMRP-1, which instructs cells to make a protein necessary for normal brain development. The faulty gene creates a deficiency in the FMRI protein that leads to brain changes. The condition is often associated with other conditions such as SDHD, anxiety, and autism (Hagerman, 2006).

Fetal alcohol syndrome (FAS) is caused by the effect of ethyl alcohol on the developing fetus. The term *fetal alcohol spectrum disorder* (FASD) describes the wide range of effects from the condition, which can range from FAS to a milder condition called fetal alcohol effects (FAE) (Caley, Shipkey, Winkelman, et al., 2006). Alcohol ingestion by the pregnant woman can influence development of many body organs, and effects can range from

Developing Cultural Competence

FETAL ALCOHOL SYNDROME

Fetal alcohol syndrome is more common in groups with higher intake of alcohol. Since some Native-American tribes have a high rate of alcoholism, the federal government and some tribes have joined together to lower that risk among this ethnic group. On some reservations, such as the Yakama Nation in Washington State, alcoholic beverages are not sold and educational programs are in place.

mild to severe. Despite many years of public health education, alcohol use remains a leading cause of intellectual disability. From 0.3 to 1.5 per 1000 births are affected by fetal alcohol syndrome (Centers for Disease Control and Prevention, 2006a).

For a discussion of phenylketonuria and hypothyroidism, two common biochemical causes of intellectual disability, see Chapter 55. Other causes involve traumatic brain injury and infections of the central nervous system (see Chapter 56). Intellectual disability is more common in children born prematurely.

CLINICAL MANIFESTATIONS

Mild intellectual disability was originally described as an intelligence quotient (IQ) between 50 and 70, moderate disability with IQ of 35 to 50, severe disability with IQ 20 to 35, and profound disability below 20. Although an IQ below 70 is generally considered indicative of intellectual disability, the functional assessment of the child is now considered a more accurate identification of children's performance and needs. Children who are intellectually disabled manifest delays in all areas of development, including motor movement, language, and adaptive behavior. They usually achieve developmental milestones more slowly than the average child. These developmental delays may be the first indication to parents and care providers of the child's condition.

Intellectual disability is sometimes accompanied by sensory impairment, speech problems, motor and orthopedic disabilities, and seizure disorders. Of children with the disability, 10% to 30% manifest one of these other disorders. Table 57–8 lists several physical characteristics associated with Down syndrome, fragile X syndrome, and fetal alcohol syndrome.

CLINICAL THERAPY

Intellectual disability is diagnosed and initial treatment is planned in a multistep process, and by involving a multidisciplinary team. Team members may include a developmental specialist, physician, geneticist, nurse, teacher, language therapist, occupational therapist, and physical rehabilitation specialist. See Table 57–9 for a description of the DSM-IV-TR diagnostic criteria for intellectual disability. Diagnosis begins with a comprehensive history and evaluation of the child's physical characteristics, developmental level, and intellectual and adaptive functioning. Laboratory tests such as chromosome analysis, blood enzyme levels, lead levels, or cranial imaging provide valuable information in some circumstances. A three-generation family history is performed (Moeschler, Shevell, and the American Academy of Pediatrics, 2006).

Developmental screening using a test such as the Denver II (see Chapter 36) can help identify children at risk. Tests of intellectual and adaptive functioning are performed when disability is suspected. A neurologic examination may indicate asymmetry of movement or strength, irritability or lethargy, or abnormal pitch to an infant's cry. Because intellectual disability may be accompanied by physical abnormalities, it is important to observe the child for facial symmetry, distance between the eyes, level of the ears, hair growth, and palmar creases. These abnormalities may be clues to other health problems.

Based on the results of the evaluation, a multidisciplinary team plans the support needed to maximize the child's potential for development. Management focuses on early intervention to

Table 57–8 Characteristics Associated with Three Common Types of Intellectual Disability

Syndrome	Characteristics
Down Syndrome (see Figures 35-8 and 35-38B)	Small head (microcephaly) Flattened forehead Wide, short neck Epicanthal eye folds White spots on eye iris (Brushfield spots) Congenital cataracts Flat nose Small, low-set ears Protruding tongue Short broad hands Simian line on palm Wide space between first and second toes Hearing loss Increased incidence of diabetes, congenital heart defect, and leukemia Hypotonia
Fragile X Syndrome	Long face Prominent jaw Large ears Frequent otitis media Large testicles Epicanthal eye folds Strabismus High arched palate Scoliosis
Fetal Alcohol Syndrome (see Figure 33-4)	Flat midface Low nasal bridge Long philtrum with narrow upper lip Short upturned nose Poor coordination Failure to thrive Skeletal and joint abnormalities Hearing loss

Table 57–9 DSM-IV-TR Diagnostic Criteria for Intellectual Disability

A. Significantly subaverage intellectual functioning: an IQ of approximately 70 or below on an individually administered IQ test (for infants, a clinical judgment of significantly subaverage intellectual functioning)
B. Concurrent deficits or impairments in present adaptive functioning (i.e., the person's effectiveness in meeting the standards expected for his or her age by his or her cultural group) in at least two of the following areas: communication, self-care, home living, social/interpersonal skills, use of community resources, self-direction, functional academic skills, work, leisure, health, and safety
C. The onset is before age 18 years

improve the degree of adaptive functioning. Associated physical, emotional, and behavioral problems are treated simultaneously. Depending on the child's condition, special education programs and physical or occupational therapy may be necessary (Figure 57–8 ●). The Education for All Handicapped Children Act, PL 94-142, provides free appropriate education to all handicapped children between 2 and 21 years of age. Amendments to this act in 1986 (PL 99-457) encouraged states to provide early intervention services for infants and toddlers with developmental delay conditions through federal funding.

The child may require supportive care and assistance with activities of daily living. The plans for intervention need to change as the child grows and the family situation alters. Classes and special services are needed for youth and families when the adolescent with intellectual disability transitions into young adulthood.

NURSING MANAGEMENT

NURSING ASSESSMENT AND DIAGNOSIS

Nurses can help to identify children with intellectual disability through history taking, observation, and developmental screening during early childhood. The history should provide information about the mental and adaptive functioning of birth parents and other family members, as intellectual disability may cluster in some families, and conditions such as fragile X syndrome are genetic in origin. The pregnancy and birth history can provide important information about the mother's alcohol and drug use during pregnancy. Be alert for a history of difficult pregnancy and problems during birth. Prematurity places the child at risk of below normal cognitive development. Frequent developmental testing during early childhood is needed for infants born prematurely. When genetic conditions in the family predispose family members to intellectual disability, assess the child carefully. Children from deprived environments or those at risk because of environmental factors such as lead poisoning (see Chapter 44∞) are more likely to manifest intellectual disability.

Many children with intellectual disability are not diagnosed until they reach school age, particularly if the condition is mild. Early intervention, however, can help to enhance the child's functioning later. During home visits, during clinic appointments, in childcare centers, and during hospitalization, be alert for signs such as developmental delays, multiple (more than three) physical anomalies associated with a specific condition (see Table 57–8), or neurologic alterations. Developmental assessment should be part of each healthcare visit; see Chapters 36 to 38∞ for developmental surveillance recommended at each age.

Once the diagnosis of intellectual disability has been made, assess the adaptive functioning of the child and family. Perform a functional assessment of the child, including toileting, dressing, and feeding skills. Assess the child's language, sensory, and psychomotor functioning. Assess the home and community for safety hazards. Observe how the family is managing with the child. Ask about family activities that include the child, community and school attitudes and support, and care management as well as planning for the future. Assess the availability of services such as groups for parents and special education opportunities for children. Evaluate the coping skills of family members.

A B

● **Figure 57–8** Physical therapy. Physical therapy is an important component of medical management for many children who are intellectually disabled. ***A,*** This girl, who is severely intellectually disabled and uses a wheelchair, is being positioned in a mobile prone stander, which enables her to interact in a different manner with her therapists and the environment. ***B,*** Physical therapists also provide outpatient care in the community to children with varying degrees of disability.

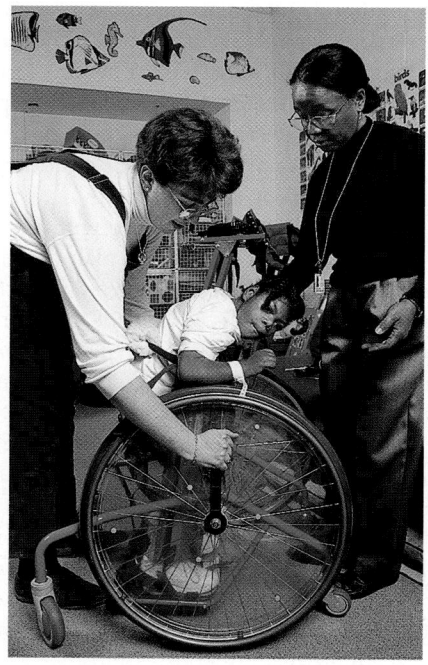

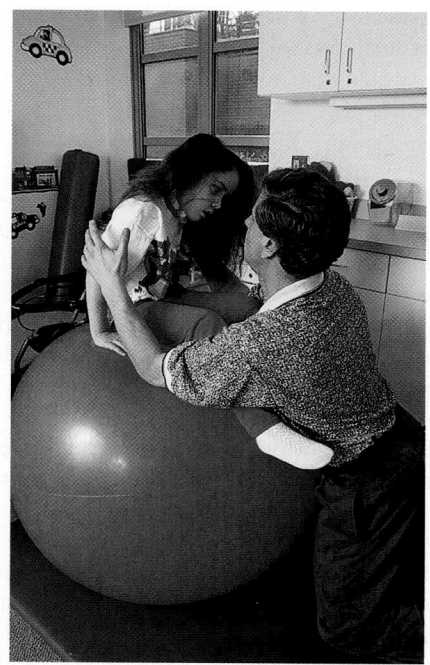

Several nursing diagnoses may be appropriate for the child with intellectual disability, depending on the degree, cause, and outcome of the child's condition. Some of these diagnoses relate to impairments in adaptive functioning; others relate to the impact on the family. Examples include the following:

- *Delayed Growth and Development* related to neonatal disease or condition
- *Imbalanced Nutrition: Less than Body Requirements* related to inability to ingest sufficient food
- *Self-care Deficit: Dressing, Toileting, Bathing* related to developmental disability
- *Impaired Verbal Communication* related to developmental disability
- *Risk for Injury* related to lack of understanding of environmental hazards
- *Compromised Family Coping* related to the child's developmental variations

PLANNING AND IMPLEMENTATION

Nearly all children with intellectual disability are cared for in the community. However, they may have conditions that require periodic hospitalization or frequent healthcare visits. Nursing care focuses on providing emotional support and information to family members, assisting the child with adaptive functioning, and fostering parental management of the child's activities. Whenever possible, the nurse uses preventive teaching to lower the risk of disabilty. For example, nurses can integrate teaching into care for all women about the importance of avoiding all alcohol during any times when they might become pregnant. This helps prevent fetal alcohol syndrome, especially in early pregnancy when women may not know they are pregnant.

PROVIDE EMOTIONAL SUPPORT AND INFORMATION

Family members need empathy and support both at the time of diagnosis and in the ensuing years. Parents may be in an acute or chronic state of grief over the loss of the healthy child. Encourage them to verbalize their feelings. Introducing them to parents of other intellectual disabled children may help and support them as they learn how to manage the child's needs. Discuss the availability of respite care to provide parents with a break from caretaking. Other family members such as grandparents and siblings may also feel grief or guilt and should be given an opportunity to talk about their feelings.

Parents need honest information and answers to their questions about the child's condition. Reinforce information provided by genetic counselors and other healthcare professionals. Parents need to know about community resources designed to assist children with intellectual disability. The Education for All Handicapped Children Act, PL 94-142, provides free appropriate education to all handicapped children between 2 and 21 years of age. States and local communities may provide early intervention services for infants and toddlers with disabilities. Examples of programs include the Zero to Three project early intervention programs, special education preschools and schools, county health services, and respite care, among others. Ask parents if they have questions about individualized education plans and refer them to Internet sources if that may be helpful. Review federal and state laws and services that might be helpful to the family, and help them interpret information they find to analyze its strengths and limitations.

MyNursingKit Help Families Evaluate Internet Information

MAINTAIN A SAFE ENVIRONMENT

The child with intellectual disability requires close supervision because he or she may not understand common hazards. Ensure safety in the hospital. Assist parents to provide safety at home and school, and teach the child necessary skills such as pedestrian safety. Consider both physical and emotional safety. The child may be indiscriminately trusting and sometimes is at risk for physical or sexual abuse.

PROVIDE ASSISTANCE WITH ADAPTIVE FUNCTIONING

Encourage parents' efforts to maximize the child's areas of strength and identify needs related to adaptive behaviors. Refer them to resources to help with the child's impaired areas of adaptive functioning, such as communication, self-care, or social skills. During hospitalization, support parents' efforts to maintain the child's skills in toileting, dressing, and self-care by planning interventions to use the skills being taught at home.

NURSING CARE IN THE COMMUNITY

The child with intellectual disability needs ongoing care throughout childhood; interventions must be adapted as the child develops and the family's needs evolve. Parents often act as case managers for the child's care. Assist parents as necessary to acquire the skills required to coordinate the child's plan of care. Evaluate the child's needs regularly and help parents with the treatment plan as necessary. Provision of education including services such as physical or speech therapy is a primary goal (Johnson & Walker, 2006). Most children with intellectual disability have an individualized education plan designed to meet their specific learning needs. Parents, nurses, and others such as teachers and language therapists are part of the team that establishes the child's individualized education plan. Promote optimal development and socialization. As the child reaches adolescence, education is directed toward a vocation, issues of sexuality, and the goal of independent living, when appropriate. Transition classes for adolescents with intellectual disability can teach self-care skills that may enable some to live in group homes or other community settings. Parents need help planning for the child's future and their own retirement.

Specific guidelines for care are available for the child with Down syndrome. These guidelines suggest times for evaluation of hearing, growth, cardiac function, and other areas designed for early identification and treatment of associated disorders (Van Cleve & Cohen, 2006). There are growth grids for children with Down syndrome, and specific topics to suggest for anticipatory guidance during healthcare visits.

EVALUATION

The expected outcomes of nursing care depend on the child's needs and developmental level. Early in the diagnostic phase, desired outcomes may involve the family's understanding of the diagnosis and the child's special needs. Later outcomes may focus on the child's communication of self-help skills. Outcomes related to cognitive performance and adaptive skills may be developed during childhood. Successful transition into adulthood at the maximal level of function is the ultimate desired outcome.

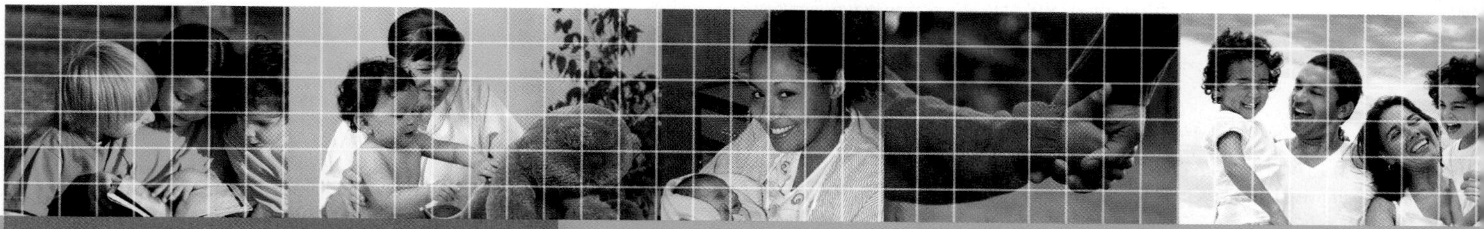

CRITICAL CONCEPT REVIEW

LEARNING OUTCOMES	CONCEPTS
57.1 Define mental health and describe major mental health alterations in childhood.	1. Mental health: ■ Successful engagement in activities and relationships and the ability to adapt to and cope with change. 2. Pervasive developmental disorders (autistic spectrum disorders): ■ Impaired social interactions and communication with restricted interests, activities, and behaviors. 3. Attention deficit and attention deficit hyperactivity disorder: ■ Characterized by developmentally inappropriate behaviors involving attention. 4. Mood disorders: ■ Depression. ■ Bipolar disorder. 5. Anxiety disorders: ■ Group of disorders characterized by feelings of worry and uncertainty. 6. Tic disorders and Tourette syndrome. 7. Schizophrenia.
57.2 Discuss the clinical manifestations of the major mental health alterations of childhood and adolescence.	1. Pervasive development disorders: ■ Impaired social interaction and communication. ■ Restricted interests, social activities, and behaviors. 2. ADD and ADHD: ■ Decreased attention span. ■ Impulsiveness. ■ Increased motor activity. 3. Mood disorders: ■ Sadness. ■ Declining school performance. ■ Appetite and sleep disturbances. ■ Somatic complaints. ■ Extreme changes in affect and energy. 4. Anxiety disorders: ■ Restlessness. ■ Poor concentration. ■ Irritability. ■ Sleep disturbances. ■ Uneasiness in unfamiliar surroundings. 5. Tic disorders and Tourette syndrome: ■ Sudden, rapid recurrent, nonrhythmic, and brief motor movements and vocalizations. 6. Schizophrenia: ■ Social withdrawal. ■ Impaired social relationships. ■ Flat affect. ■ Regression. ■ Hallucinations.

(continued)

LEARNING OUTCOMES	CONCEPTS
57.3 Plan for the nursing management of children and adolescents with mental health alterations in the hospital and community settings.	Hospital: 1. Assess child's current level of mental health functioning. 2. Continue prescribed treatments and medications. 3. Ensure child has no access to potentially dangerous materials and has adequate supervision. 4. Assess child's potential for self-harm. Community settings: 1. Conduct ongoing assessment and evaluation of the child's mental health functioning. 2. Provide individual and group therapy sessions. 3. Refer families to mental health resources and support groups.
57.4 Describe characteristics of common cognitive alterations of childhood.	1. Learning disabilities: ■ Difficulty processing information by reading, writing, and math. Difficulty understanding oral information. Usually have normal IQ. 2. Down syndrome: ■ Hypotonia. ■ Epicanthal eye folds. ■ Simian crease on palm. ■ Flat nose. ■ Wide, short neck. ■ Intellectual disability (mental retardation). 3. Fragile X syndrome: ■ Long face with prominent jaw and large ears. ■ Strabismus. ■ Aggressive behaviors. ■ Intellectual disability. 4. Fetal alcohol syndrome: ■ Failure to thrive. ■ Flat midface with low nasal bridge. ■ Poor coordination. ■ Poor impulse control. ■ Low normal IQ to intellectual disability.
57.5 Plan nursing management for children with cognitive alterations.	1. Assess for signs and symptoms of developmental delay. 2. Refer child for early intervention programs. 3. Refer parents to support groups. 4. Assist parents to obtain needed adaptive equipment. 5. Refer parents to programs that provide respite care. 6. When child is hospitalized, maintain home routine as much as possible.
57.6 Establish and evaluate expected outcomes of care for the child with a cognitive alteration.	Expected outcomes include: 1. The family will understand the child's diagnosis and the specific physical and developmental needs of the child. 2. The child will develop self-care skills appropriate to his or her developmental level. 3. The family will be able to access the necessary community and educational resources. Evaluations include: 1. The family's ability to function and care for the child's needs. 2. The child's ability to perform self-help skills. 3. The family's ability to cope with changing needs of the child.

CRITICAL THINKING IN ACTION

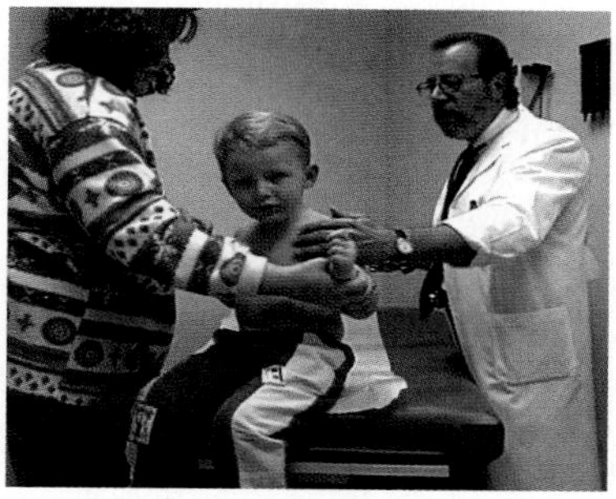

Cooper, a 5-year-old child with autism, comes into the office for his annual checkup and school immunizations of diphtheria tetanus acellular pertussis (DTaP), inactivated polio vaccine (IPV), and measles-mumps-rubella (MMR). He is very combative and it takes four people to help hold him and administer the vaccines. He will be attending a special school for children with autism and similar disorders. Diagnosed at 3 years old, he has never been in the hospital or had surgery. It is extremely difficult to examine him as he does not like to be touched. During prior visits in the office, Cooper has stood facing the wall and twisting his hands. He continues to be combative for most of the exam, even with the use of decreased stimuli, communication, and slow movements, but you are able to assess that his blood pressure is 95/53. He is in the 50th percentile for both height and weight and his temperature is 99°F.

You give Cooper's mother information about local support groups for children with autism and about local psychiatrists who can treat autism with types of medication to help control aggressive behavior. You also supply her with contact information for counselors in the area to help her deal with her own stress. She is appreciative of your help and support and looks forward to being able to send Cooper to school.

1. The mother has questions about the MMR vaccine and whether it causes autism. What can you tell her about that? Would you administer the vaccine today?
2. What can you tell the mother about safety issues with Cooper?
3. How can you enhance communication with Cooper when he comes into the office?

See MyNursingKit for possible responses.

REFERENCES

American Association on Intellectual and Developmental Disabilities. (2008). Frequently asked questions on intellectual disability and the AAIDD definition. Retrieved from www.aamr.org/content_185.cfm

American Psychiatric Association. (2000). *Diagnostic* and *statistical manual of mental disorders* (4th ed., text revision). Washington, DC: American Psychiatric Association.

Anderson, V. R., & Scott, L. J. (2006). Methylphenidate transdermal system: In attention-deficit hyperactivity disorder in children. *Drugs, 66,* 1117–1126.

Apps, J., Winkler, J., & Jandrisevits, M. D. (2008). Bipolar disorders: Symptoms and treatment in children and adolescents. *Pediatric Nursing, 34,* 84–88.

Barber, S., Grubbs, L., & Cottrell, B. (2005). Self-perception in children with attention deficit/hyperactivity disorder. *Journal of Pediatric Nursing, 20,* 235–245.

Beauchamp, R. A., Willis, T. M., Betz, T. G., Villanacci, J., Rozin, L., Brown, M.J., et al. (2006). Deaths associated with hypocalcemia from chelation therapy—Texas, Pennsylvania, and Oregon, 2003–2005. *Morbidity and Mortality Weekly Report, 55,* 204–207.

Beauchesne, M. A., & Kelley, B. R. (2004). Evidence to support parental concerns as an early indicator of autism in children. *Pediatric Nursing, 30,* 57–67.

Bhasin, T. K., Brocksen, S., Avchen, R. N., & Braun, K. V. (2006). Prevalence of four developmental disabilities among children aged 8 years—Metropolitan Atlanta developmental disabilities surveillance program, 1996 and 2000. *Morbidity and Mortality Weekly Report, 55,* SS-1, 1–9.

Bindler, R., & Howry, L. (2005). *Pediatric Drug Guide.* Upper Saddle River, NJ: Prentice Hall Health.

Bridge, J. A., Iyengar, S., Salary, C. B., Barbe, R. P., Birmaher, B., Pincus, H. A., et al. (2007). Clinical response and risk for reported suicidal ideation and suicide attempts in pediatric antidepressant treatment. *JAMA, 297,* 1683–1696.

Brown, E. J. (2005). Clinical characteristics and efficacious treatment of posttraumatic stress disorder in children and adolescents. *Pediatric Annals, 34,* 139–146.

Brown, R. T., Amler, R. W., Freeman, W. S., Perrin, J. M., Stein, M. T., Feldman, H., et al. and Committee and Quality Improvement Subcommittee on Attention—Deficit/Hyperactivity Disorder (2005). Treatment of hyperactivity disorder: Overview of the evidence. *Pediatrics, 115,* e749–e757.

Caffo, E., & Belaise, C. (2003). Psychological aspects of traumatic injury in children and adolescents. *Child and Adolescent Psychiatric Clinics of North America, 12,* 493–535.

Caley, L. M., Shipkey, N., Winkelman, T., Dunlap, C., & Rivera, S. (2006). Evidence-based review of nursing interventions to prevent secondary disabilities in fetal alcohol spectrum disorder. *Pediatric Nursing, 32,* 155–162.

Cartwright-Hatton, S., McNicol, K., & Doubleday, E. (2006). Anxiety in a neglected population: Prevalence of anxiety disorders in pre-adolescent children. *Clinical Psychology Review, 26,* 817–833.

Centers for Disease Control and Prevention. (2004). Suicide: Fact sheet. Retrieved from www.cdc.gov/ncipc/factsheets/suifacts.htm

Centers for Disease Control and Prevention. (2006a). Improved national prevalence estimates for 18 selected major birth defects—United States, 1999–2001. *Morbidity and Mortality Weekly Report, 54,* 1301–1305.

Centers for Disease Control and Prevention (2006b). Youth risk behavior surveillance—United States, 2005. *Morbidity and Mortality Weekly Report 55*(SS-5), 1–112.

Centers for Disease Control and Prevention (2007a). Prevalence of autism spectrum Disorders—Autism and developmental disorders monitoring network. *Morbidity and Mortality Weekly Report, 56*(SS-1), 1–40.

Centers for Disease Control and Prevention (2007b). *Suicide.* Atlanta: Author.

Centers for Disease Control and Prevention (2007c). Suicide trends among youths and young adults aged 10–24 years—United States, 1990–2004. *Morbidity and Mortality Weekly Report, 56,* 905–908.

Chambers, D. A., Ringeisen, J., & Hickman, E. E. (2005). Federal, state, and foundation initiatives around evidence-based practices for child and adolescent mental health. *Child and Adolescent Psychiatric Clinics of North America 14,* 307–327.

Cheung, A. H., Zuckerbrot, R. A., Jensen, P. S., Ghalib, K., Laraque, D., Stein, R. E. L., and the GLAD-PC Steering Group (2008). Guidelines for adolescent depression in primary care (GLAD-PC): II. Treatment and ongoing management. *Pediatrics, 120,* e1313–1326.

Christakis, D. A., Zimmerman, F. J., DiGiuseppe, D. L., & McCarty, C. A. (2004). Early television exposure and subsequent attentional problems in children. *Pediatrics, 113,* 708–713.

Cullen-Powell, L. A., Barlow, J. H., & Cushway, D. (2005). Exploring a massage intervention for parents and their children with autism: The implications for bonding and attachment. *Journal of Child Health Care, 9,* 245–255.

DelBello, M. P., Adler, C. M., & Strakowski, S. M. (2006). The neurophysiology of childhood and adolescent bipolar disorder. *CNS Spectrum, 11,* 298–311.

Dementieva Y. A., Vance, D. D., Donnelly, S. L., Elston, L. A., Wolpert, C. M., Ravan, S.A., et al.

(2005). Accelerated head growth in early development of individuals with autism. *Pediatric Neurology, 32,* 102–108.

DiCicco-Bloom, E., Lord, C., Zwaigenbaum, L., Courchesne, E., Dager, S. R., Schmitz, C., et al. (2006). The developmental neurobiology of autism spectrum disorder. *Journal of Neuroscience, 26,* 6897–6906.

Diseth, T. H., & Christie, H. J. (2005). Trauma-related dissociative (conversion) disorders in children and adolescents—an overview of assessment tools and treatment principles. *Nordic Journal of Psychiatry, 59,* 278–292.

Dopheide, J. A. (2006). Recognizing and treating depression in children and adolescents. *American Journal of Health-Systems Pharmacy, 63,* 233–243.

D'Souza, Y., Fombonne, E., & Ward, B. J. (2006). No evidence of persisting measles virus in peripheral blood mononuclear cells from children with autism spectrum disorder. *Pediatrics, 118,* 1664–1675.

Dulcan, M. K. (2005). Practitioner perspectives on evidence-based practice. *Child and Adolescent Psychiatric Clinics of North America, 14,* 225–240.

Evans, E., Hawton, K., Rodham, K., & Deeks, J. (2005). The prevalence of suicidal phenomena in adolescents: A systematic review of population-based studies. *Suicide and Life Threatening Behaviors, 35,* 239–250.

Faedda, G. L., Baldessarini, R. J., Glovinsky, I. P., & Austin, N. B. (2004). Pediatric bipolar disorder: Phenomenology and course of illness. *Bipolar Disorders, 6,* 305–313.

Ferguson-Noyes, N. (2005). Bipolar disorder in children. *Advance for Nurse Practitioners, 13*(3), 35–42.

Froehlich, T. E., Lanphear, B. P., Epstein, J. N., Barbaresi, W. J., Katusic, S. K., & Kahn, R. S. (2007). Prevalence, recognition, and treatment of attention-deficit/hyperactivity disorder in a national sample of US children. *Archives of Pediatric and Adolescent Medicine 161,* 857–864.

Gabbay, V., Coffey, B. J., Babb, J. S., Meyer, L., Wachtel, C., Anam, S., & Rabinovitz, B. (2008). Pediatric autoimmune neuropsychiatric disorders associated with streptococcus: Comparison of diagnosis and treatment in the community and at a specialty unit. *Pediatrics, 122,* 273–278.

Giarelli, E., Souders, M., Pinto-Martin, J., Bloch, J., & Levy, S. E. (2005). Intervention pilot for parents of children with autistic spectrum disorder. *Pediatric Nursing, 31,* 389–399.

Ginsburg, G. S., & Grover, R. L. (2005). Assessing and treating social phobia in children and adolescents. *Pediatric Annals, 34,* 119–127.

Gold, C., Wigram, T., & Elefant, C. (2006). Music therapy for autistic spectrum disorder. *Cochrane Database Systematic Review, 19*(2), CD004381.

Hagerman, R. J. (2006). Lessons from fragile X regarding neurobiology, autism, and neurodegeneration. *Journal of Developmental and Behavioral Pediatrics, 27,* 63–74.

Hamrin, V., & Scahill, L. (2005). Selective serotonin reuptake inhibitors for children and adolescents with major depression: Current controversies and recommendations. *Issues in Mental Health Nursing, 26,* 433–450.

Hanna, G. L., Fischer, D. J., & Fluent, T. E. (2006). Separation anxiety disorder and school refusal in children and adolescents. *Pediatrics in Review, 27,* 56–62.

Haugaard, J. J. (2004). Recognizing and treating uncommon behavioral and emotional disorders in children and adolescents who have been severely maltreated: Somatization and other somatoform disorders. *Child Maltreatment, 9,* 169–176.

Hayward, C., Wilson, K. A., Lagle, K., Killen, J. D., & Taylor, B. (2004). Parent-reported predictors of adolescent panic attacks. *Journal of the American Academy of Child and Adolescent Psychiatry, 43,* 613–620.

Hirsch, A. J., & Carlson, J. S. (2007). Prescription practices and empirical efficacy of psychopharmacologic treatments for pediatric major depressive disorder. *Journal of Child and Adolescent Psychiatric Nursing, 20,* 222–233.

Hoagwood, K. E., & Burns, B. J. (2005). Evidence-based practice, part II: Effecting change. *Child and Adolescent Psychiatric Clinics of North America, 14,* xv–xvii.

Hu, Z., Yang, X., Ho, P. C., Chan, S. Y., Heng, P. W., Chan, E., et al. (2005). Herb-drug interactions. *A Literature Review Drugs, 65,* 1239–1282.

Hudson, J. L., Deveney, C., & Taylor, L. (2005). Nature, assessment, and treatment of generalized anxiety disorder in children. *Pediatric Annals, 34,* 97–106.

Hyman, S. L., & Levy, S. E. (2005). Introduction: novel therapies in developmental disabilities—Hope, reason, and evidence. *Mental Retardation and Developmental Disabilities Research Review, 11,* 107–109.

Johnson, C. P., Myers, S. M., and the Council on Children with Disabilities (2007). Identification and evaluation of children with autism spectrum disorders. *Pediatrics, 120,* 1183–1215.

Johnson, C. P., & Walker, W. O. (2006). Mental retardation: Management and prognosis. *Pediatrics in Review, 27,* 249–255.

Jurbergs, N., & Ledley, D. R. (2005). Separation anxiety disorder. *Pediatric Annals, 34,* 108–115.

Kaminer, D., Seedat, S., & Stein, D. J. (2005). Post-traumatic stress disorder in children. *World Psychiatry, 4,* 121–125.

Katz, S. L. (2006). Has the measles-mumps-rubella vaccine been fully exonerated? *Pediatrics, 118,* 1744–1745.

Kelly, D. P., & Aylward, G. P. (2005). Identifying school performance problems in the pediatric office. *Pediatric Annals, 34,* 288–298.

Kowatch, R., Fristad, M., Birmaher, B., Wagner, K. D., Findling, R. L., Hellander, M., and the Child Psychiatric Workgroup on Bipolar Disorder. (2005). Treatment guidelines for children and adolescents with bipolar disorder. *Journal of American Academy of Child and Adolescent Psychiatry, 44,* 236–239.

Lansford, A. H. (2005). The importance of recognizing a child with bipolar disorder. *Contemporary Pediatrics, 22*(2), 69–78.

Levy, S. E., & Hyman, S. L. (2005). Novel treatments for autistic spectrum disorders. *Mental Retardation and Developmental Disabilities Research Review, 11,* 131–142.

Lewin, A. B., Storch, E. A., Adkins, J., Murphy, T. K., & Geffken, G. R. (2005). Current directions in pediatric obsessive-compulsive disorder. *Pediatric Annals, 34,* 128–134.

Lobar, S. L., Fritts, M. K., Arbide, Z., & Russell, D. (2008). The role of the nurse practitioner in an Individualized Education Plan and coordination of care for the child with Asperger's syndrome. *Journal of Pediatric Health Care, 22,* 111–119.

Luby, J. L., Heffelfinger, A., Koenig-McNaught, A. L., Brown, K., & Spitznagel, E. (2004). The Preschool Feelings Checklist: A brief and sensitive screening measure for depression in young children. *Journal of the American Academy of Child and Adolescent Psychiatry, 43,* 708–717.

Luther, E. H., Canham, D. L., & Cureton, V. Y. (2005). Coping and social support for parents of children with autism. *Journal of School Nursing, 21,* 40–47.

Mark, T. L., & Buck, J. A. (2006). Characteristics of U.S. youths with serious emotional disturbance: Data from the National Health Interview Survey. *Psychiatric Services, 57,* 1573–1578.

Mell, L. K., Davis, R. L., & Owens, D. (2005). Association between streptococcal infection and obsessive-compulsive disorder, Tourette's syndrome, and tic disorder. *Pediatrics, 116,* 56–60.

Melnyk, B. M., & Moldenhauer, Z. (2006). *The KySS guide to child and adolescent mental health screening, early intervention and health promotion.* Cherry Hill, NJ: NAPNAP.

Moeschler, J. B., Shevell, M., and the American Academy of Pediatrics Committee on Genetics. (2006). Clinical genetic evaluation of the child with mental retardation or developmental delays. *Pediatrics, 117,* 2304–2316.

National Association of Pediatric Nurse Practitioners. (2007). NAPNAP position statement on integration of mental health care in pediatric primary care settings. *Journal of Pediatric Health Care, 21,* 19A–30A.

National Institute for Health Care Management Foundation. (2008). *Pediatric Mental Health Care.* Retrieved from http://nihcm.org/page/pediatric_mental_health

National Institutes of Health (2007). *Brain matures a few years late in ADHD, but follows normal pattern.* News Release. Retrieved from www.nih.gov/news/pr/nov2007/nimh-12.htm

Pompili, M., Mancinelli, I., Girardi, P., Ruberto, A., & Tatarelli, R. (2005). Childhood suicide: A major issue in pediatric health care. *Issues in Comprehensive Pediatric Nursing, 28,* 63–68.

Powsner, S., & Dufel, S. (2006). Conversion disorder. Retrieved from www.emedicine.com/EMERG/topic_112.htm

Pruett, J. R., & Luby, J. L. (2004). Recent advances in prepubertal mood disorders: Phenomenology and treatment. *Current Opinion in Psychiatry, 17,* 31–36.

Reiff, M. I. (2006). ADHD: A guide to assessment and diagnosis. *Psychiatric Times 5*(8), 104. Retrieved from www.psychiatric_times.com/topic/ADHD

Remschmidt, J., & Theisen, F. M. (2005). Schizophrenia and related disorders in children and adolescents. *Journal of Neural Transmission, 69,* 121–124.

Richardson, L. P., & Katzenellenbogen, R. (2005). Childhood and adolescent depression: The role of primary care providers in diagnosis and treatment. *Current Problems in Pediatric and Adolescent Health Care, 35,* 6–24.

Richler, J., Luyster, R., Risi, S., Hsu, W. L. Dawson, G., Bernier, R., et al. (2006). Is there a "regressive phenotype" of autism spectrum disorder associated with the measles-mumps-rubella vaccine? A CPEA Study. *Journal of Autism and Developmental Disorders, 36, 299–316.*

Roberts, M. (2007). The many faces and facets of BP. Retrieved from www.nami.org/Content/Contentgroups/bp_and_Schizophrenia_Digest/The_Many_Faces_and_Facets_of_BP.htm

Roche, A. M., Giner, L., & Zalsman, G. (2005). Suicide in early childhood: A brief review. *International Journal of Adolescent Medical Health, 17,* 221–224.

Rogers, S. J., & Vismara, L. A. (2008). Evidence-based comprehensive treatments for early autism. *Journal of Clinical Child and Adolescent Psychology, 37,* 8–38.

Rojas, N. L., & Chan, E. (2005). Old and new controversies in the alternative treatment of attention-deficit hyperactvitiy disorder. *Mental Retardation and Developmental Disability Research Review, 11,* 116–130.

Santrock, J. W. (2007). *Children* (9th ed.). Boston: McGraw-Hill.

Schafer, I., Barkmann, C., Riedesser, P., & Schulte-Markwort, M. (2006). Posttraumatic syndromes in children and adolescents after road traffic accidents—a prospective cohort study. *Psychopathology, 39,* 159–164.

Schapiro, N. A. (2004). Tourette's syndrome and obsessive-compulsive disorder. In P. J. Allen & J. A. Vessey (Eds.), *Primary care of the child with a chronic condition.* St. Louis: Mosby.

Schapiro, N. A. (2005). Bipolar disorders in children and adolescents. *Journal of Pediatric Health Care, 19,* 131–141.

Scharer, K. (2005a). An internet discussion board for parents of mentally ill young children. *Journal of Child and Adolescent Psychiatric Nursing 18,* 17–35.

Scharer, K. (2005b). Internet social support for parents: The state of science. *Journal of Child and Adolescent Psychiatric Nursing 18,* 26–35.

Scheeringa, M. S., Salloum, A., Arnberger, R. A., Weems, C. F., Amaya-Jackson, L., & Cohen, J. A. (2007). Feasibility and effectiveness of cognitive-behavioral therapy for posttraumatic stress disorder in preschool children: Two case reports. *Journal of Traumatic Stress, 20,* 631–636.

Schieve, L. A., Rice, C., Boyle, C., Visser, S. M., & Blumberg, S. J. (2006). Mental health in the United States: Parental report of diagnosed autism in children age 4–17 years—United States, 2003–2004. *Morbidity and Mortality Weekly Report, 55,* 481–487.

Shaw, D., Fernandes, J. R., & Rao, C. (2005). Suicide in children and adolescents: A 10-year retrospective review. *American Journal of Forensic Medicine and Pathology, 26,* 309–315.

Shear, K., Jin, R., Ruscio, A. M., Walters, E. E., & Kessler, R. C. (2006). Prevalence and correlates of estimated *DSM-IV* child and adult separation anxiety disorder in the National Comorbidity Survey Replication. *American Journal of Psychiatry, 163,* 1074–1083.

Smith, P., Yule, W., Perrin, S., Tranah, T., Dalfleish, T., & Clark, D. M. (2007). Cognitive-behavioral therapy for PTSD in children and adolescents: A preliminary randomized controlled trial. *Journal of the American Academy of Child and Adolescent Psychiatry, 46,* 1051–1061.

Stein, R. E. K., Zitner, L. E., & Jensen, P. S. (2006). Interventions for adolescent depression in primary care. *Pediatrics, 118,* 669–682.

Thompson, S. J., Maccio, E. M., Desselle, S. K., & Zittel-Palamara, K. (2007). Predictors of posttraumatic stress symptoms among runaway youth utilizing two service sectors. *Journal of Traumatic Stress, 20,* 553–563.

U.S. Department of Health and Human Services. (2004). *Report of the surgeon general's conference on children's mental health: A national action agenda.* Washington, DC: U.S. Department of Health and Human Services.

U.S. Department of Health and Human Services. (2006). *The current status of mental health in schools: A policy and practice analysis.* Washington, DC: Author.

U.S. Food and Drug Administration (2004). FDA launches a multi-pronged strategy to strengthen safeguards for children treated with antidepressant medications. Retrieved from www.Fda.gov/bbs/topics/news/2004/NEW01129.html

Van Cleve, S. N., Cannon, S., & Cohen, W. I. (2006). Part II: Clinical practice guidelines for adolescents and young adults with Down syndrome: 12 to 21 years. *Journal of Pediatric Health Care, 20,* 198–205.

Van Cleve, S. N., & Cohen, W. I. (2006). Part I: Clinical practice guidelines for children with Down syndrome from birth to 12 years. *Journal of Pediatric Health Care, 20,* 47–54.

Van Riper, M. (2007). Families of children with Down syndrome: Responding to "a change of plans" with resilience. *Journal of Pediatric Nursing, 22,* 116–127.

Vetter, V. L., Elia, J., Erickson, C., Berger, S., Blum, N., Uzark, K., & Webb, C. L. (2008). Cardiovascular monitoring of children and adolescents with heart disease receiving stimulant drugs: A scientific statement from the American Heart Association Council on Cardiovascular Disease in the Young Congenital Cardiac Defects Committee and the Council on Cardiovascular Nursing. *Circulation, 117,* 2407–2423.

Volkmar, F. R., Wiesner, L. A., & Westphal, A. (2006). Healthcare issues for children on the autism spectrum. *Current Opinions in Psychiatry, 19,* 361–366.

Weber, W., & Newmark, S. (2007). Complementary and alternative medical therapies for attention-deficit/hyperactivity disorder and autism. *Pediatric Clinics of North America, 54,* 983–1006.

Williams, D. L., & Minshew, N. J. (2007). Understanding autism and related disorders: What has imaging taught us? *Neuroimaging Clinics of North America, 17,* 495–509.

Wolraich, M. L., Wibbelsman, C. J., Brown, T. E., Evans, S. W., Gotlieb, E. M., Knight, J. R., et al. (2005). Attention-deficit/hyperactivity disorder among adolescents: A review of the diagnosis, treatment, and clinical implications. *Pediatrics, 115,* 1734–1746.

Zuckerbrot, R. A., Cheung, A. H., Jensen, P. S., Stein, R. E. K., Laraque, D., and the GLAD-PC Steering Group 2007). Guidelines for adolescent depression in primary care (GLAD-PC): I. Identification, assessment, and initial management. *Pediatrics, 119,* 101–108.

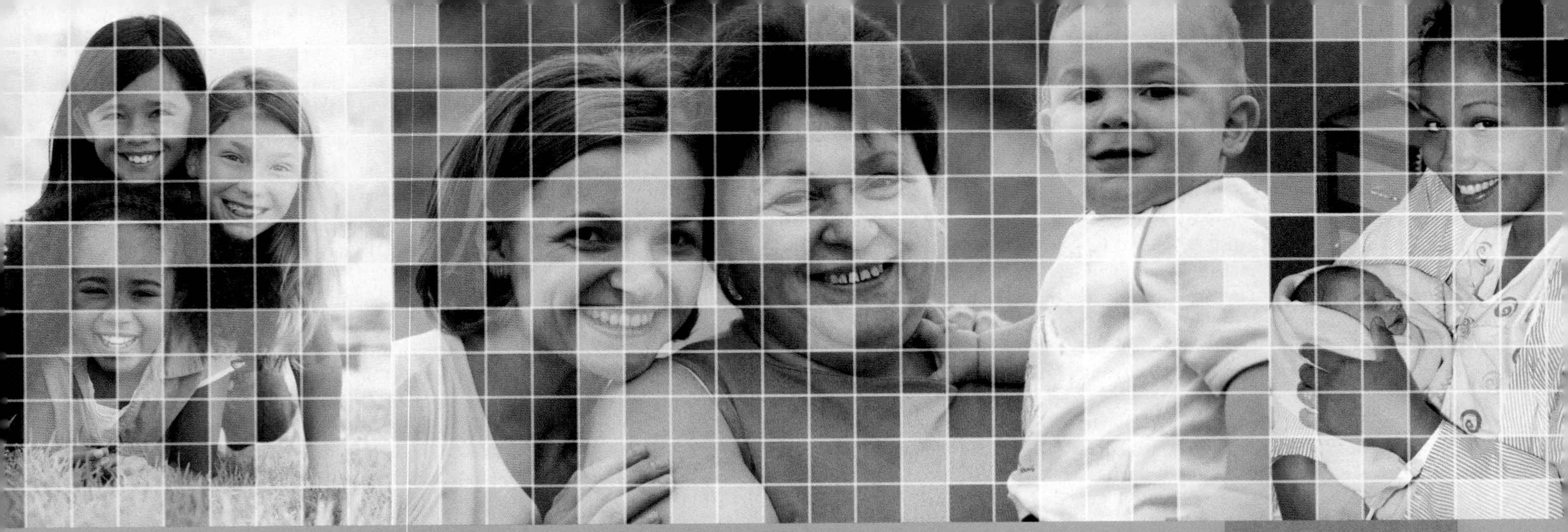

CHAPTER

The Child with Alterations in Musculoskeletal Function

58

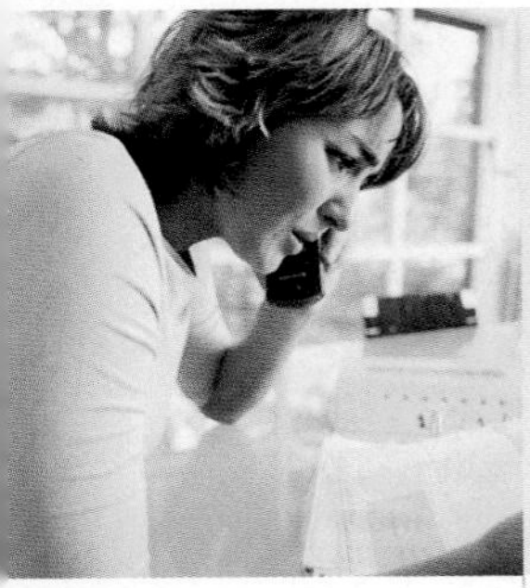

When I got the call that Douglass was in the emergency room I was so scared. I guess we're lucky it was just a broken leg. I don't know what to do now, though—he broke his leg on a friend's trampoline. Should he go back to his friend's house? Should I tell him not to use the trampoline? It's hard to decide. And I never had a cast. What do you need to do with it?
—Mother of Douglass, 12 years old

LEARNING OUTCOMES

58.1 Describe pediatric variations in the musculoskeletal system.

58.2 Plan nursing care for children with structural deformities of the foot, hip, and spine.

58.3 Recognize signs and symptoms of infectious musculoskeletal disorders and refer for appropriate care.

58.4 Partner with families to plan care for children with musculoskeletal conditions that are chronic or require long-term care.

58.5 Plan nursing interventions to promote safety and developmental progression in children who require braces, casts, traction, and surgery.

58.6 Provide nursing care for fractures, including teaching for injury prevention and nursing implementations for the child who has sustained a fracture.

The musculoskeletal system helps the body protect its vital organs, support weight, control motion, store minerals, and supply red blood cells. Bones provide a rigid framework for the body, muscles provide for active movement, and tendons and ligaments hold the bones and muscles together. Alterations in musculoskeletal functioning, therefore, can have a significant impact on a child's growth and development.

What concerns do parents and children have when a child has musculoskeletal conditions? Will the child need any special adaptations in the home and school? Can musculoskeletal injuries be prevented? The information in this chapter will answer these questions, and enable nurses to provide effective care for children who have musculoskeletal disorders.

Musculoskeletal disorders may be congenital, such as clubfoot, or acquired, such as osteomyelitis. They may require short- or long-term management, and may be treated on an outpatient basis or require hospitalization. Many musculoskeletal disorders require surgical correction, casting, or braces.

Figure 58–1 ● reviews several terms that will be used throughout this chapter in describing the positioning of a child's limbs. See the Assessment Guide for assessment guidelines for the child with alterations in musculoskeletal function.

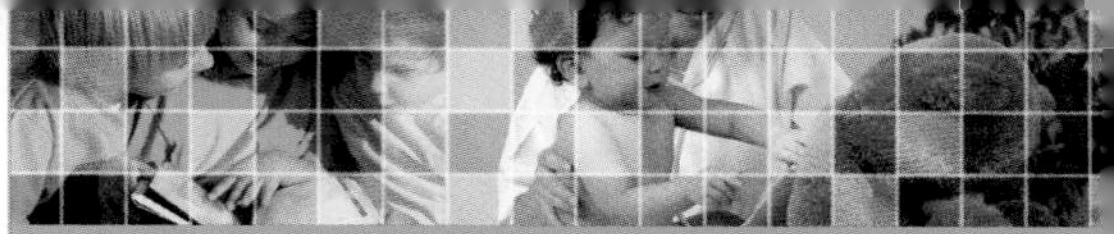

KEY TERMS

compartment syndrome, 1775
chondrolysis, 1754
dislocation, 1748
dwarfism, 1764
dysplasia, 1748
equinus, 1744
ossification, 1741
osteotomy, 1748
pseudohypertrophy, 1767
sprain, 1743
subluxation, 1748
varus, 1744

ANATOMY AND PHYSIOLOGY OF PEDIATRIC DIFFERENCES

BONES

The bones of children and those of adults differ in several ways. Although primary centers of **ossification** (bone formation) are nearly complete at birth, a fibrous membrane still exists between the cranial bones (fontanelles) (see "As Children Grow: Sutures" in Chapter 35). The posterior fontanelle closes between 2 and 3 months of age. The anterior fontanelle does not close until approximately 18 months of age, allowing for growth of the brain and skull (Chamley, Carson, Randall, et al., 2005). In addition, the ends of the long bones (epiphyses) remain cartilaginous (Figure 58–2 ●). Long-bone growth continues until approximately age 20 years, when skeletal maturation is complete.

Secondary ossification occurs as the long bones grow. Cartilage cells at the epiphyses are replaced by osteoblasts (immature bone cells), resulting in the deposition of calcium. Calcium intake during childhood and adolescence is essential to provide adequate bone density that will prevent osteoporosis and fractures in adulthood. See Chapter 34 for a discussion of inadequate calcium intake during school age and adolescence.

The long bones of children are porous and less dense than those of adults. For this reason, children's bones can bend, buckle, or break as a result of a simple fall. Children and adolescents may suffer injuries to the musculoskeletal system from falls, car crashes, and sports. Fractures are one type of common injury. Because growth takes place at the epiphyseal plates, injuries to this portion of a long bone are of particular concern in young children.

In addition to the structural differences between the bones of children and adults, there are also functional differences in the skeletal system of children (see "As Children Grow: Children Are Not Just Small Adults" in Chapter 35). Before birth the thoracic and sacral regions of the spine are convex curves. As the infant learns to hold up the head, the cervical region becomes concave. When the child learns to stand, the lumbar region also becomes concave. Failure of the spine to assume these final curves results in an abnormal curvature of the spine (kyphosis or lordosis). The rapid bone growth of childhood facilitates healing after fractures, but may also lead to "growing pains," as muscles are pulled when bones grow quickly.

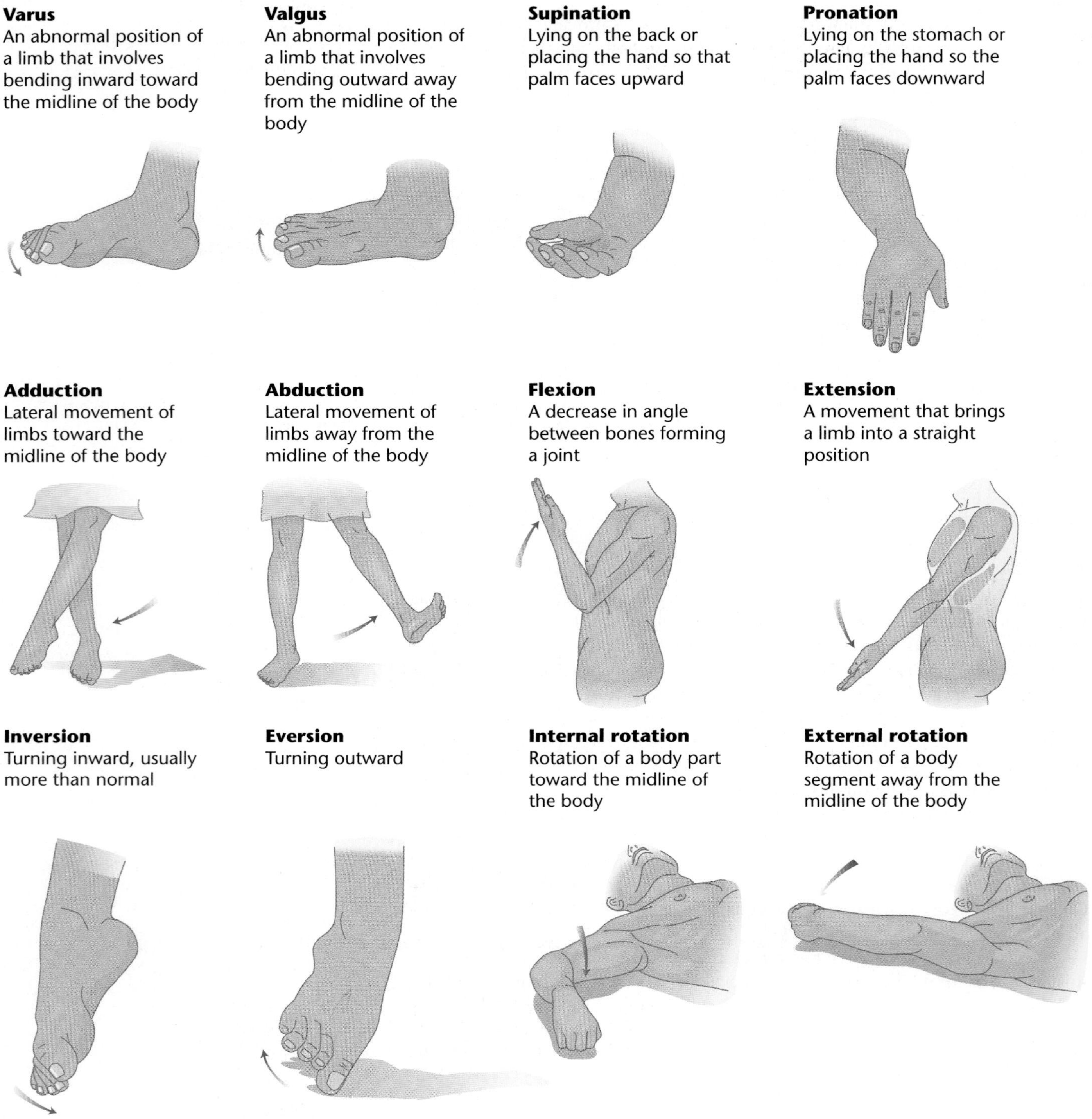

Varus
An abnormal position of a limb that involves bending inward toward the midline of the body
Valgus
An abnormal position of a limb that involves bending outward away from the midline of the body
Supination
Lying on the back or placing the hand so that palm faces upward
Pronation
Lying on the stomach or placing the hand so the palm faces downward
Adduction
Lateral movement of limbs toward the midline of the body
Abduction
Lateral movement of limbs away from the midline of the body
Flexion
A decrease in angle between bones forming a joint
Extension
A movement that brings a limb into a straight position
Inversion
Turning inward, usually more than normal
Eversion
Turning outward
Internal rotation
Rotation of a body part toward the midline of the body
External rotation
Rotation of a body segment away from the midline of the body

● **Figure 58–1** Musculoskeletal positions and joint motions.

Assessment Guide

THE CHILD WITH A MUSCULOSKELETAL SYSTEM ALTERATION

ASSESSMENT FOCUS	ASSESSMENT GUIDELINES
Muscles	■ Is muscle mass symmetrical? ■ Do fine and gross motor movements correspond to developmental expectations? ■ Can you identify any abnormal signs such as asymmetry of movement, tenderness, masses, weakness, hypotonia, hypertonia? ■ Can the school-age child get up from a lying or sitting position in the usual manner? ■ Can you describe the child's usual daily physical activity? ■ Has there been a loss of ability to perform developmental milestones?
Joints	■ Are movements smooth and symmetrical? ■ Are there any signs of tenderness, decreased range of motion, inflammation, crepitus/grinding, or masses? ■ Do the hips of newborns and infants manifest symmetrical full range of motion? ■ Were there recent events of trauma such as in sports or a fall?
Bones	■ Are there any masses noted? ■ Are arms and legs the same length? ■ Is there a recent decrease or change in mobility, such as limping? ■ Are bones in alignment, or are abnormalities noted such as bowlegs or knock-knees? ■ Upon spinal screening, is the spine properly aligned (see screening procedure within this chapter)? ■ In what sports does the child participate? Is recommended protective gear worn?
Tendons and ligaments	■ Do all joints move through full range of motion? ■ Is there any pain upon joint motion or palpation? ■ Are there feelings of grinding or crepitus as the joint moves? ■ Has there been a recent sports or other injury? ■ In what sports does the child participate?
Family history	■ Is there a family history of disorders of the muscular or skeletal systems?

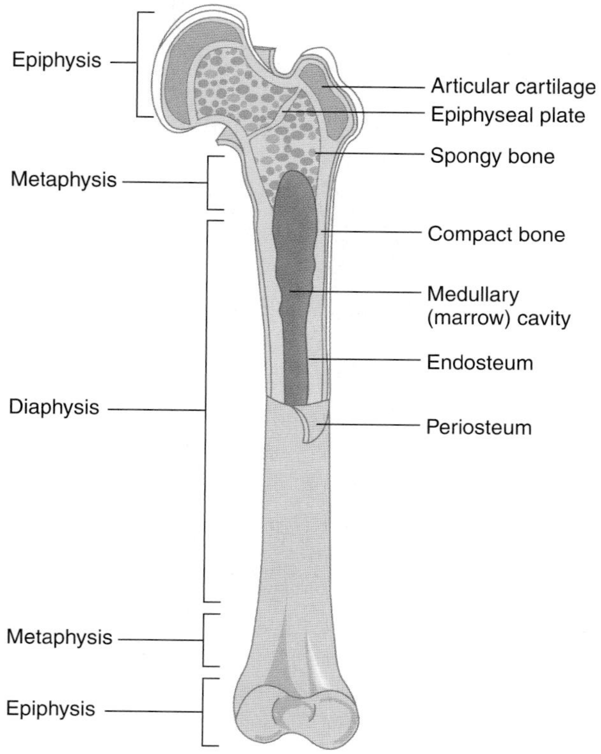

● **Figure 58–2** The parts of long bones.

MUSCLES, TENDONS, AND LIGAMENTS

The muscular system, unlike the skeletal system, is almost completely formed at birth. As a child grows, muscles do not increase in number, but rather in length and circumference. Until puberty, both ligaments and tendons are stronger than bone. When these structural differences are not recognized, a childhood fracture is sometimes mistaken for a **sprain**. A sprain is a tearing of ligaments, the structural support connecting bones, usually caused when a joint is twisted or otherwise traumatized. Tendons, which connect bones to muscles, grow in length and fibrous tissue as mechanical pressure is placed on them.

MyNursingKit Muscle Physiology Animation

DISORDERS OF THE FEET AND LEGS

METATARSUS ADDUCTUS

Metatarsus adductus, the most common congenital foot deformity, is characterized by an inward turning of the forefoot at the tarsometatarsal joints (Figure 58–3 ●). Often referred to as "intoeing," metatarsus adductus affects male and female infants equally and occurs in approximately 1 in 1000 births, with more common incidence among siblings, twins, and multiple births (Hart, Grottkau, Rebello, et al., 2005; Wan, 2006). It occurs more often in certain neurological conditions such as cerebral palsy (Rethlefsen, Healy, Wren, et al., 2006). This condition is most likely caused by

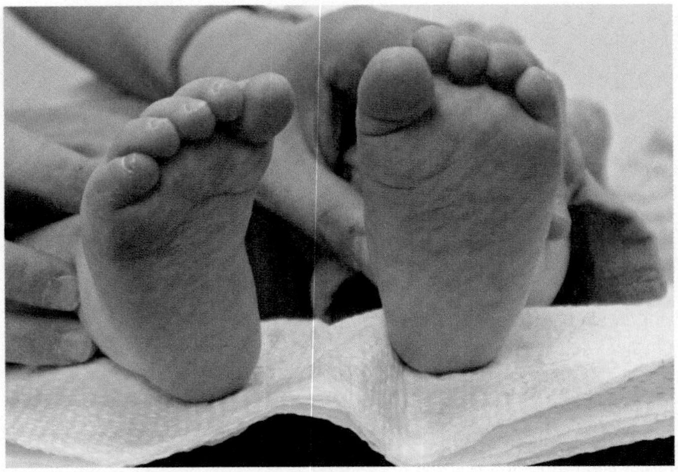

● **Figure 58–3** Metatarsus adductus. This disorder is characterized by convexity (curvature) of the lateral border of the foot. The child's right foot demonstrates the disorder. Note that the forefoot turns inward and appears out of alignment with the remainder of the foot.

both intrauterine positioning and genetic factors. Metatarsus adductus is differentiated from other causes of intoeing, such as internal tibial torsion (more common in children 12 to 18 months and learning to walk), and femoral anteversion (seen more often in preschool-age children).

Treatment depends on the degree of foot flexibility. If the foot can be readily maneuvered past the neutral position, simple exercises may correct the problem. Most cases resolve spontaneously by the time the infant is about 3 months of age. Serial casting is the treatment of choice for curvature angles greater than 15 degrees, or in cases that do not improve. The infant's feet are placed in a position as close to neutral as possible and are held secure with casts. Casts are changed weekly until the desired correction is achieved. Braces and orthopedic shoes may also be used to maintain correction after casting.

Nursing Management

Reassure parents that the child's condition can be corrected. If the child's deformity is mild, teach parents simple stretching exercises to perform at each diaper change. The foot is held securely by the heel, and the forefoot is moved outward from the body with the other hand. The position is maintained for 5 seconds, and repeated 5 times at each diaper change. If casting is necessary, provide cast care as outlined in Table 58–1 and teach parents how to care for the child in a cast at home. If metatarsus adductus persists into childhood without correction, the challenge is to find shoes that accommodate the unusual shape of the foot.

CLUBFOOT

Clubfoot is a congenital abnormality in which the foot is twisted out of its normal position. It occurs in approximately 1 to 2 in 1000 births, affects boys nearly twice as often as girls, and is bilateral in about half of affected infants (Hart et al., 2005).

Etiology and Pathophysiology

The exact cause of clubfoot is unknown; however, several possible etiologies have been proposed. Some authorities believe abnormal intrauterine positioning causes the deformity. Others suspect neuromuscular or vascular problems as causes. Yet other experts believe there is a genetic component, either at the chromosomal level or by the arrest of normal fetal development. Uterine positioning and biochemical causes are also cited as possible causes (Faulks & Luther, 2005). A positive family history increases the chance of the deformity, with an occurrence rate 17 times higher in families with affected members than in the general population (Morcuende, 2006). The incidence varies among ethnic groups; it is least common in Asian populations and most common in Polynesian groups (Faulks & Luther, 2005).

Clinical Manifestations

A clubfoot (talipes equinovarus) involves three areas of deformity: The midfoot is directed downward (**equinus**), the hindfoot turns inward (**varus**), and the forefoot curls toward the heel (adduction) and turns upward in partial supination. Muscles, tendons, and bones are all involved in the abnormality, and it cannot be corrected by exercise. Most children have this combination of findings. The foot is small with a shortened Achilles' tendon. Muscles in the lower leg are atrophied, but leg lengths are generally normal (see "Pathophysiology Illustrated: Clubfoot").

PATHOPHYSIOLOGY ILLUSTRATED

CLUBFOOT

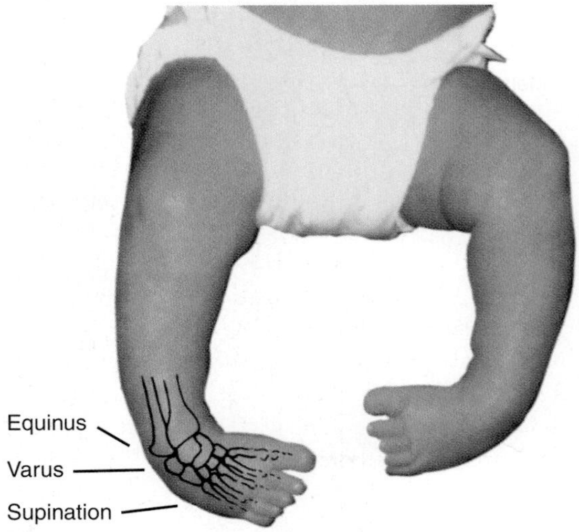

Bilateral clubfoot deformity. Parents of a child with clubfoot will have many questions. Can the condition be treated? Will the child be able to walk normally after surgery? Will they need help caring for the infant? How much will surgery and other care cost? Will any subsequent children have a clubfoot?

Table 58–1 Nursing Care of the Child in a Cast

- A plaster cast takes anywhere from 24 to 48 hours to dry. When handling the wet cast, be gentle and use the palms of your hands, as fingertips can indent plaster and create pressure areas.
- After the cast is applied, elevate the extremity on a pillow above the level of the heart. Elevation helps reduce swelling and increases venous return.
- If the cast is applied after surgery, there may be drainage or bleeding through the cast material. Circle the stain and note the date and time on the cast to provide a way to assess the amount of fluid lost.
- Assess the distal pulses, and check the fingers and toes for color, warmth, capillary refill, and edema. Assess sensation as well as movement. Any deviation from normal may indicate nerve damage or decreased blood supply.
- During the first 24 hours, check the casted extremity every 15–30 minutes for 2 hours, then every 1–2 hours thereafter. The skin should be warm. It should blanch when slight pressure is applied and then return to its normal color within 3 seconds (**A**). For the next 2 days, assess the casted extremity at least every 4 hours.

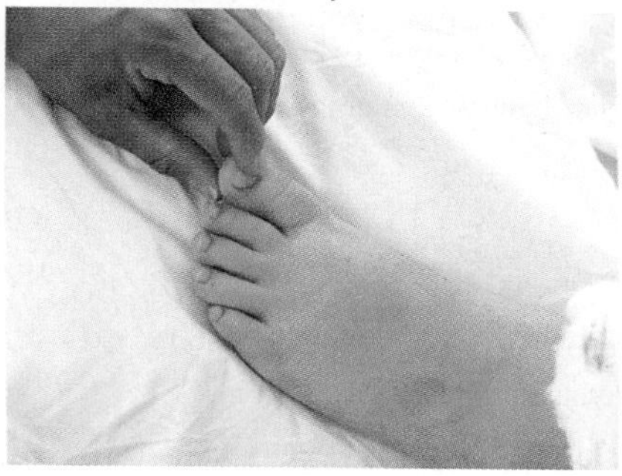

A

- Check the edges of the cast for roughness or crumbling. If necessary, pull the inner stockinette over the edge of the cast and tape in place.
- The rough edges of the cast may also be alleviated by "petaling." This is done by securing tape or padding to the inside of the cast and pulling it over the edge, covering the jagged or broken pieces of plaster, and securing it to the outer surface of the cast **(B, C, D)**. Moleskin may be used on the cast as well.
- Keep the cast as clean and dry as possible. Cover the cast with a plastic bag or plastic wrap when the child bathes or showers.
- The skin under the cast may itch; however, do not use powders or lotions near the edges or under the cast as they can cause skin irritation.
- Be sure that children do not put small objects between the casts and their extremities; that can cause skin irritation as well as neurovascular compromise.

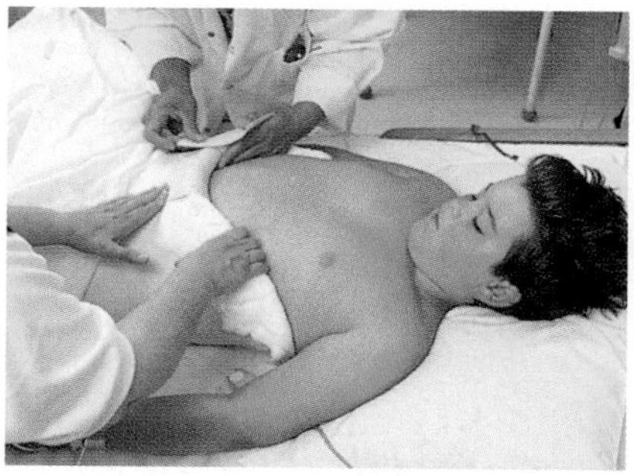

B

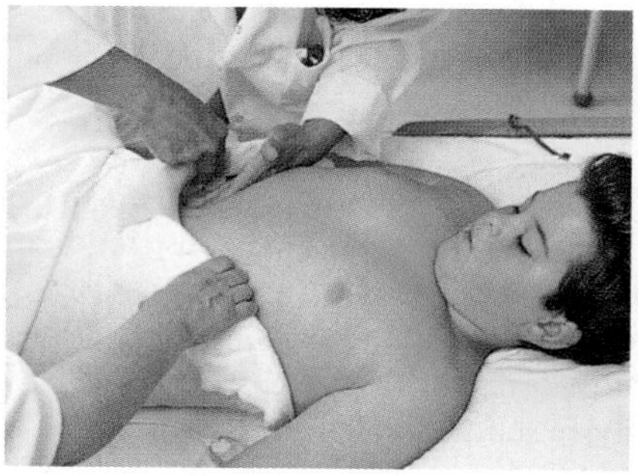

C

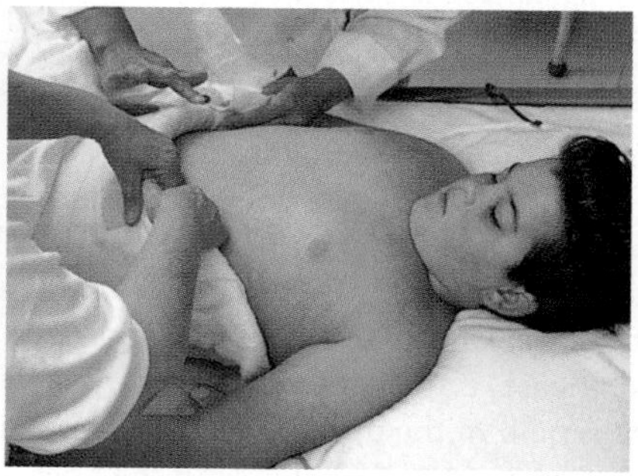

D

Clinical Therapy

Diagnosis is made at birth on the basis of visual inspection. Radiographs are used to confirm the severity of the condition.

Early treatment is essential to achieve successful correction and reduce the chance of complications. Serial casting is the treatment of choice. Casting should begin as soon as possible after birth. Timing is critical because the short bones of the foot, which are primarily cartilaginous at birth, begin to ossify shortly thereafter. The foot is manipulated to achieve maximum correction first of the varus deformity and then of the equinus deformity. A long leg cast holds the foot in the desired position (Figure 58–4 ●). The cast is changed every 1 to 2 weeks. This regimen of manipulation and casting continues for approximately 8 to 12 weeks until maximum correction is achieved. If the deformity has been corrected, the child may begin wearing a splint or reverse cast (shaped so that the foot turns outward away from the body instead of the normal inward turn) corrective shoes to maintain the correction (Morcuende, 2006). If the deformity has not been corrected, surgery is required. Casting holds the foot in position until surgery is performed.

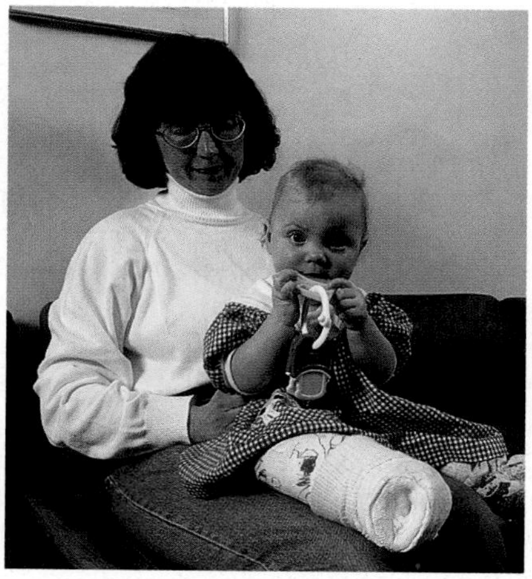

● **Figure 58–4** Long leg cast. This girl has a long leg cast, which was applied after surgery to correct her clubfoot deformity.

Teaching Highlights

CARE OF THE CHILD WITH A CAST

Skin Care

- Check the skin around the cast edges for irritation, rubbing, or blistering. The skin should be clean and dry.
- You may cleanse the skin just under the cast edges and between the toes or fingers with a cotton-tipped applicator and rubbing alcohol. Avoid using lotions, oils, and powders near the cast as they may cause caking.
- Avoid poking sharp objects down inside the cast as this may result in sores.

Cast Care

- Keep the cast dry. Protect plaster with a cast shoe, thick sock, or sling.
- Allow a new, wet cast to air-dry for 24 hours. Raise it on pillows just above heart level to prevent swelling.
- You may walk on a leg cast only if your physician has given you permission to do so.

Be Alert for Possible Complications

- Toes or fingers should be pink, not blue or white.
- Skin should be warm and the tips of the toes should blanch when pinched.

Notify Your Healthcare Provider If Any of the Following Occurs

- Unusual odor beneath the cast
- Burning, tingling, or numbness in the casted arm or leg
- Drainage through the cast
- Swelling or inability to move the fingers or toes
- Slippage of the cast
- Cast cracked, soft, or loose
- Sudden unexplained fever
- Unusual fussiness or irritability in an infant or child
- Fingers or toes that are blue or white
- Pain that is not relieved by any comfort measures (e.g., repositioning or pain medication)

Courtesy of Shriners Hospital for Children, Spokane, WA.

The age at which a child undergoes clubfoot surgery varies among surgeons. However, most children have surgery between 3 and 12 months of age. The one-stage posteromedial release procedure, which involves realignment of the bones of the foot and release of the constricting soft tissue, is most common. The foot is held in the proper position by one or more stainless steel pins. A cast is then applied with the knee flexed to prevent damage to the pin and to discourage weight bearing. Casting continues for 6 to 12 weeks. The child may then need to wear a brace or corrective shoes, depending on the severity of the deformity and the surgeon's preference.

More severe cases or those not corrected in infancy may require more than one surgery to correct the foot.

NURSING MANAGEMENT

NURSING ASSESSMENT AND DIAGNOSIS

Nursing assessment, which begins at birth and continues throughout the child's subsequent outpatient casting visits and hospitalization for surgery, includes taking a genetic and birth history, performing a physical examination (including position and appearance of the foot), and assessing the child's motor development and family's coping mechanisms. Because parents will need to bring the child for frequent cast changes, assess access to transportation and other arrangements needed for these visits.

Among the nursing diagnoses that might apply to the child with a clubfoot deformity are the following:

- *Impaired Physical Mobility* related to prescribed movement restriction of cast
- *Risk for Impaired Skin Integrity* related to cast
- *Altered Parenting* related to birth of a child with a physical defect
- *Health-Seeking Behaviors (Parental)* related to lack of information about deformity, treatment, and home care

PLANNING AND IMPLEMENTATION

Nursing management involves providing emotional support, educating the family about home care of the child in a cast and the importance of keeping appointments at the outpatient facility for cast changes, preparing the family for the child's hospitalization if surgery is to occur, and providing postsurgical care.

PROVIDE EMOTIONAL SUPPORT

Clubfoot affects both the child and the family. The child's foot deformity is upsetting to parents, and they need emotional support to allay their fears. Helping parents understand the condition and its treatment is essential.

Promote bonding by encouraging parents to hold and cuddle the child and to take an active role in the child's care. Explain that, with treatment, the child is expected to grow and develop normally.

PROVIDE CAST AND BRACE CARE

Routine cast care is outlined in Table 58–1 and is important to ensure skin and neurovascular integrity. After serial casting is

Teaching Highlights

GUIDELINES FOR BRACE WEAR

- Braces should be as comfortable as possible and the child should have adequate mobility while wearing the brace.
- Begin wearing the brace for periods of 1 to 2 hours and then progress to 2 to 4 hours.
- Check the skin at 1- to 2-hour intervals initially, then lengthening to every 4 hours once skin has been clear for several days. If redness is apparent, leave the brace off and allow the skin to clear. If breakdown has occurred, the brace cannot be replaced until healing is complete. (See Chapter 59 for a discussion of pressure ulcers.)
- Always have the child wear a clean white sock, T-shirt, or other thin white liner beneath the brace. Be sure the liner is wrinkle-free under the brace. Avoid using powders or lotions that can cause skin to break down. Toughen any sensitive areas using alcohol wipes 3–4 times daily.
- Reapply the brace when the skin returns to its normal color.
- Return to the physician or orthotic specialist if discomfort or red areas persist or if the brace needs adjustment or repair or is outgrown.
- Check the brace daily for rough edges.

complete, or after surgery, the child may progress to wearing a brace or special shoe for 6 to 12 months. Braces should fit snugly but should not interfere with neurovascular function. Before the child begins to wear a brace, check the skin for any areas of redness or breakdown. Give parents guidelines for brace wear. Emphasize that proper skin care is essential. If skin redness develops, arrange to have the fit of the brace evaluated and modified if necessary.

PROVIDE POSTSURGICAL CARE

Routine postoperative care after surgical correction includes neurovascular status checks every 2 hours for the first 24 hours and observing for any swelling around the cast edges (see Table 58–1). Apply ice bags to the foot, and keep the ankle and foot elevated on a pillow for 24 hours. This promotes healing and helps with venous return. Check for drainage or bleeding. Administer pain medication routinely for 24 to 48 hours. Popliteal or epidural blocks may be placed during surgery and used in the immediate postsurgical period for pain control. Monitor these blocks for effectiveness and any undesired effects (see Chapter 42 for detailed instructions on pain management).

DISCHARGE PLANNING AND HOME CARE TEACHING

Give parents written instructions for care of the child with a cast (see page 1746). In addition, assist them in the following ways:

- Demonstrate the use of a sponge bath to protect the cast from water breakdown. Have parents contact the healthcare provider if the cast gets wet with water or urine.
- Discuss options for clothing that accommodate a cast, for example, one-piece snap suits or sweatpants.
- Discuss potential safety hazards that may result from awkward positioning. Be sure the child is properly situated in a car safety seat for the trip home.
- Provide resources for strollers and other equipment that will support the cast so it does not hang down during the baby's activities.
- Suggest that parents try to place toys within the child's reach, since the movements of a child in a cast may be slowed.

EVALUATION

Expected outcomes of nursing care include maintenance of skin integrity, recovery without complications after surgery, normal developmental progression of the child, and demonstrated parental knowledge of care of braces or casts, as needed.

GENU VARUM AND GENU VALGUM

Genu varum (bowlegs) is a deformity in which the knees are widely separated while the ankles are close together and the lower legs are turned inward (varus). In genu valgum (knock-knees), the knees are close together and the lower legs are directed outward (valgus) (Figure 58–5 ●). Chapter 35 discusses the assessment of bowlegs and knock-knees in children.

At certain stages of a child's development, the appearance of bowlegs or knock-knees is normal. Until 2 to 3 years of age, the knees are normally bowed, showing varus alignment, and by 4 to 5 years, some knock-knee or valgus alignment is common. However, the

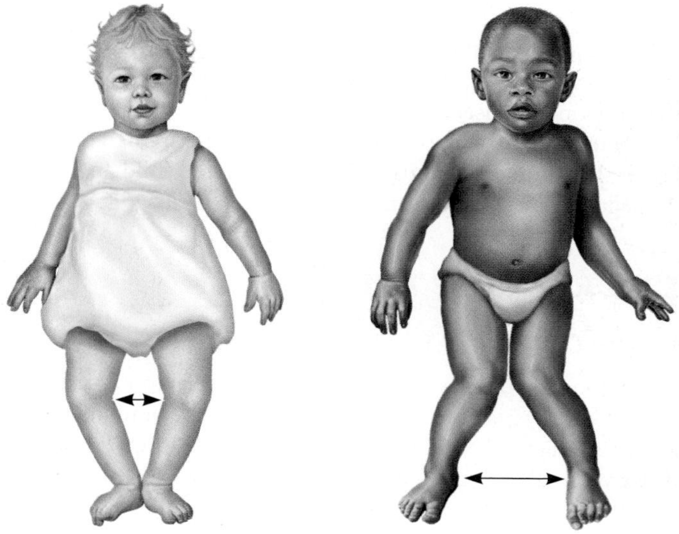

A B

● **Figure 58–5** Genu varum and genu valgum. ***A,*** Genu varum, or bowlegs. The legs are bowed so that the knees are far apart as the child stands. ***B,*** Genu valgum, or knock-knees. Note that the ankles are far apart when the knees are together.

MyNursingKit Care Plan: Home Care of the Infant in a Spica Cast persistence of knock-knees beyond the age of 4 to 5 years necessitates further evaluation. The most common pathologic causes of bowed legs are Blount disease and rickets (see Chapter 34∞). Blount disease is characterized by abnormal growth on the medial side of the proximal tibia, which causes an increasing varus deformity. It is believed to be due to increasing compression forces across the medial knee and is more common in overweight, black, and female children (Hosalkar, Gholve, & Wells, 2007). Rickets is a result of inadequate bone mineralization, usually caused by a deficiency of calcium, vitamin D, or both. Since the bones are decalcified or softened, long bones such as those in the legs may bend into a bowed position. Occasionally rickets is congenital and is caused by an x-linked autosomal dominant or recessive gene with the chromosomal location Xp22.31-p21.3. It results in an enzyme deficiency of alkaline phosphatase, which in turn leads to excessive inhibitors of bone mineralization. This type of rickets is rare and is called familial hypophosphatemic rickets (FHR).

Measurements, radiographs, arthrography (joint radiograph), magnetic resonance imaging (MRI), and computed tomography (CT) imaging may be used for accurate diagnosis. Braces are often used to correct mild deformities that could worsen as the child grows. Braces for bowlegs are worn at night; those for knock-knees both day and night. Duration of brace wear is determined by the severity of the deformity, which is usually evaluated by radiographs. If the deformity continues to worsen, surgery is necessary. Surgery is common in treatment of Blount disease. An **osteotomy** (cutting of the bone) is performed and the tibiofemoral angle surgically corrected. The child is then placed in a cast for approximately 6 to 10 weeks, or until completely healed. When dietary rickets is the cause of varus deformity, supplementation with calcium and vitamin D is needed. FHR is treated with calcium and phosphorus in 5 to 6 daily doses.

Nursing Management

Reassure parents that bowlegs and knock-knees are usually a normal part of a child's growth and development. These conditions often resolve on their own and need no treatment other than continued observation.

Nursing care focuses on educating the parents and child about the condition and its treatment. Give the child and family guidelines for brace wear and maintenance (see page 1747).

DISORDERS OF THE HIP

DEVELOPMENTAL DYSPLASIA OF THE HIP

Developmental dysplasia of the hip (DDH) refers to a variety of conditions in which the femoral head and the acetabulum are improperly aligned. These conditions include hip instability, **dislocation** (displacement of the bone from its normal articulation with the joint), **subluxation** (in this instance, a partial dislocation), and acetabular **dysplasia** (abnormal cellular or structural development leading to instability) (Shipman, Helfand, Nygren, et al., 2006). In the past, DDH was referred to as congenital dislocated hip (CDH). The revised name of the disorder emphasizes that many cases of dislocation, subluxation, and dysplasia occur well after the neonatal period and involve more than a simple dislocation.

One in 100 newborns has hip instability, while dislocation occurs in 1.5 to 20 in 1000 births, depending on the studies examined. The condition affects girls four times as often as boys. It is unilateral in 80% of affected children, and the left hip is affected three times as often as the right (Shipman et al., 2006).

Etiology and Pathophysiology

Although the exact cause of DDH is unknown, genetic factors appear to play a role. DDH is 20 to 50 times more common in first-degree relatives of an infant with the condition than in the general population. If one child of a set of identical twins has DDH, the other twin is affected 30% to 40% of the time. Some types of DDH are linked to early gestational events at 12 and 18 weeks' gestation, as the lower limbs rotate and surrounding muscles develop. On the other hand, milder cases may be influenced by mechanical forces in the last month of pregnancy such as breech position or fetal size, and can occur after birth as the hip assumes an extended rather than flexed posture (Cady, 2006). The left hip is involved more often than the right hip as a result of intrauterine positioning of the left side of the fetus against the mother's sacrum. Maternal estrogen may cause laxity of the hip joint and capsule, leading to joint instability, especially in females who respond to these estrogen levels. DDH is more common in infants born in the breech position. Cultural factors may also be associated with DDH. (See "Developing Cultural Competence: Developmental Dysplasia of the Hip.")

Clinical Manifestations

Common signs and symptoms of DDH include limited abduction of the affected hip, asymmetry of the gluteal and thigh fat folds, and telescoping or pistoning of the thigh (Figure 58–6 ●). The older child with untreated DDH walks with a significant limp, which results from telescoping of the femoral head into the pelvis. The longer the disorder goes untreated, the more pronounced the clinical manifestations become, and the worse the prognosis.

Clinical Therapy

From 60% to 80% of hip abnormalities noted in infants resolve by 2 months of age, so practitioners use care and caution in diagnosing DDH. However only 15–25% of infants have known risk fac-

Developing Cultural Competence

DEVELOPMENTAL DYSPLASIA OF THE HIP

Infants who are positioned on cradleboards or traditionally swaddled, as in some Native American cultures, have a high incidence of developmental dysplasia of the hip (DDH). Eastern European children, who are commonly swaddled also have a high incidence; in both of these cases the legs are maintained in an adducted position. The condition occurs less commonly in infants carried on the mothers' hips since the infants' legs are maintained in the abducted position. The disorder is rarely seen in Chinese and African children (hip carrying is common in these groups) (Hosalkar, Horn, Friedman, et al., 2007).

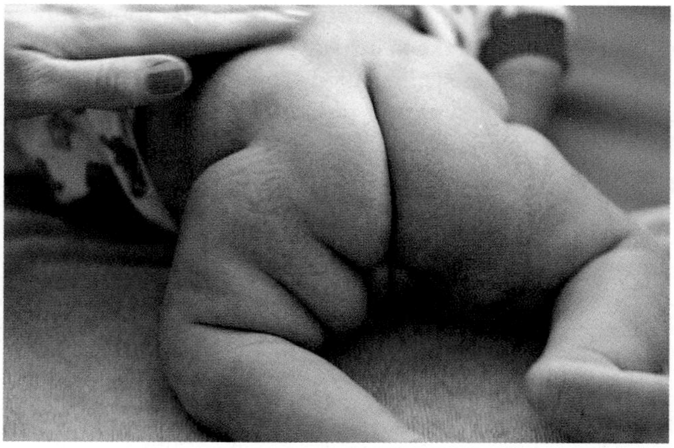

● **Figure 58–6** Common signs of developmental dysplasia of the hip (DDH). The asymmetry of the gluteal and thigh fat folds is easy to see in this child with DDH.

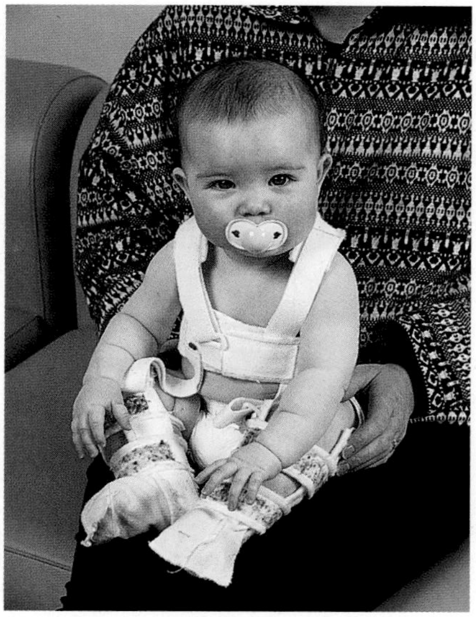

● **Figure 58–7** Pavlik harness for DDH. The most common treatment for DDH in a child under 3 months is a Pavlik harness. A shirt should be worn under the harness to prevent skin irritation. (It was omitted for clarity in this photograph.)

tors for the disorder. Therefore, the American Academy of Pediatrics and the Pediatric Orthopaedic Society of North America recommend that all infants and young children should be screened for DDH until walking is well established at about 1 year of age (Schwend, Schoenecker, Richards, et al., 2007; U.S. Preventive Services Task Force, 2006a; U.S. Preventive Services Task Force, 2006b). Physical examination reveals Allis' sign (one knee lower than the other when the knees are flexed) and positive Ortolani and Barlow maneuvers in babies under 8 to 12 weeks. Refer to Chapter 35∞ for a discussion of the assessment of hip dysplasia in newborns and infants. Radiographs are generally not reliable until approximately 4 months of age because the pelvis in a newborn is still primarily cartilaginous. Before 4 months of age, ultrasonography may be useful for diagnosis. Family history of DDH and a female in the breech position necessitate careful evaluation (U.S. Department of Health and Human Services, 2006; Schwend et al., 2007).

Treatment plans vary according to the child's age. For infants younger than 3 months, the Pavlik harness is the most commonly used method for hip reduction (Figure 58–7 ●). The Pavlik harness is a dynamic splint—a splint that allows movement. It ensures hip flexion and abduction and does not allow hip extension or adduction. For infants older than 6 months of age, surgery with closed reduction is performed (positioning of the head of the femur into the acetabulum without an incision of the skin) followed by the application of a spica cast (Figure 58–8 ●). In children over 18 months of age, open or closed reduction surgery and casting are usually necessary and bracing may also be required.

Early screening, detection, and treatment enable most affected children to attain normal hip function. Late diagnosis has lowered prognosis for full function.

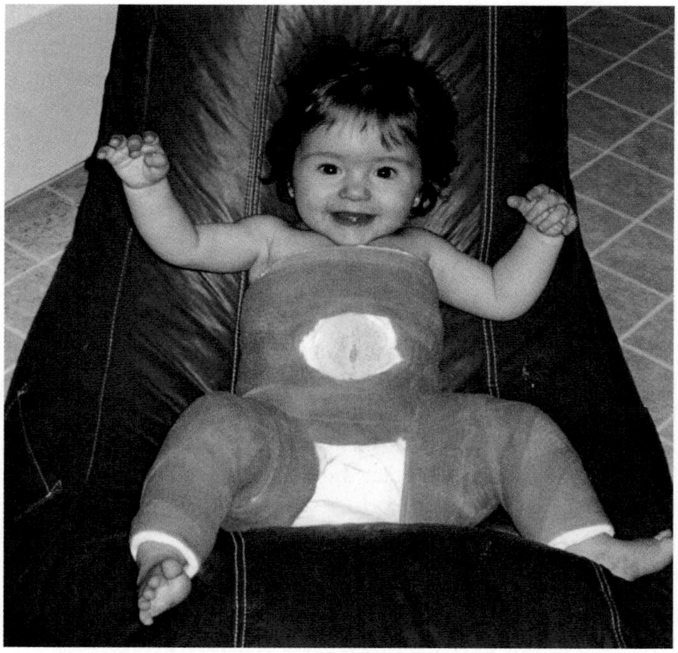

● **Figure 58–8** Spica cast. Surgery followed by spica cast application is commonly used in treatment of DDH.

NURSING MANAGEMENT

NURSING ASSESSMENT AND DIAGNOSIS

Assessment for DDH begins at birth and continues through all health promotion visits during the first two years of life. The family history or birth data may indicate a high-risk infant. Instructions for performing the physical examination to assess the infant for DDH are provided in Chapter 35∞. Once treatment begins, assessments are performed based on risks of the treatment. Assess the skin of the child in traction or a cast every few minutes in the immediate postoperative period, progressing to once or twice daily at home. Include respiratory and circulatory assessments when the child is immobilized. Ongoing assessment of the child's growth and development is needed. Weigh the child in a cast once the cast is dry so a baseline casted weight can be used for comparison while the cast remains in place.

Several nursing diagnoses that may apply to the child with DDH include the following:

- *Impaired Physical Mobility* related to prescribed movement restriction (Pavlik harness, traction, spica cast, brace)
- *Risk for Impaired Skin Integrity* related to irritation from harness straps or skin traction
- *Risk for Altered Urinary Elimination or Constipation* related to immobility caused by treatment
- *Risk for Impaired Nutrition* related to decreased appetite
- *Risk for Delayed Growth and Development* related to limited mobility and potential decreased exposure to stimulation
- *Health-Seeking Behaviors (Parental)* related to lack of information about disease process and treatment

PLANNING AND IMPLEMENTATION

The infant with DDH is often cared for at home and in outpatient facilities. If surgery is performed, the child is hospitalized for surgery and the immediate postoperative period. Nursing care varies according to the medical treatment and the child's age. Management includes maintaining traction, if ordered; providing cast care; preventing complications resulting from immobility; promoting normal growth and development; and teaching parents how to care for a child in a cast, traction, or a Pavlik harness at home. Because treatment may interfere with the child's normal movement, the treatment plan should take into consideration the age and developmental stage of the child.

PROVIDE CAST CARE

The principles of routine cast care presented in Table 58–1 apply to the care of spica casts. Special techniques should be used to help keep the cast clean and dry in children who are not toilet trained. Female and male urinals can be used for older children. Use a plastic lining to protect the cast edges during elimination for older children and use a small disposable diaper to cover the perineum in babies, tucking edges beneath the cast. Be sure to change the diaper frequently to prevent soiling of the cast.

PREVENT COMPLICATIONS RESULTING FROM IMMOBILITY

Immobilization from traction or a cast can cause alterations in physiologic functioning. To prevent complications:

- Assess breathing patterns and lung sounds frequently for congestion or respiratory compromise.
- Perform skin and neurovascular assessments approximately every 2 hours.
- Use adequate padding and skin wrapping to avoid placing pressure on the popliteal space. Such pressure could lead to nerve damage.
- For the child in a cast, change the child's position every 2 to 3 hours while awake to help avoid areas of pressure and promote increased circulation. The child can be placed either prone or supine or positioned on the floor and supported with pillows.
- Help prevent skin irritation and breakdown in the child with a cast. Use moleskin to protect from rough edges. Place tape around the perineal opening of the cast to prevent soiling.
- Increase fluids and fiber in the child's diet, as a change in bowel or bladder status is commonly associated with immobility.
- If permitted by physician orders, release the child from traction for meals and daily care. The time out of traction should not exceed 1 hour per day. Encourage parents to hold and cuddle the child at this time to promote comfort and bonding.

PROMOTE NORMAL GROWTH AND DEVELOPMENT

Engage the child in activities that stimulate the upper extremities and all five senses. Provide stimulating toys such as stacking blocks, brightly colored mobiles, soft balls, or musical toys. Position toys within the child's reach and interact with the child as much as possible.

DISCHARGE PLANNING AND HOME CARE TEACHING

Teach parents how to care for a child in traction or a spica cast at home. Family members' active participation in the child's daily care during hospitalization gradually increases their confidence in their ability to provide care once home. Identify and address home care needs well in advance of discharge. Before discharge, be sure the parents have:

- Information about general cast care (see page 1746), positioning, bathing, toileting, and age-appropriate diversional activities. Include body mechanics for the adults moving the child.
- Knowledge of the importance of performing neurovascular checks and reporting any abnormalities immediately. Teach them circulation, motion, and sensitivity checks.
- The parents should understand that the bar between the legs on the cast is not to be used for holding or turning the child. The bar is used to position the legs at the proper distance; using it to lift can cause the cast to fracture, weaken, or disintegrate.
- Information on feeding the child.
- Safety teaching to minimize chance of injury to a casted child.
- Instruction about types of toys that are age-appropriate and measures to prevent them from being placed into the cast (a tee-shirt should be placed over the cast, covering its edges).

- Appropriate referrals for periodic assessment by a visiting nurse or home health nurse.
- Family resources to care for the child.

Before discharge, have parents demonstrate how to dress and feed a child in a spica cast. Ensure that safe travel arrangements have been made for the day of discharge. Help parents get an appropriate car safety seat in advance of discharge. Encourage parents to let the child interact with other children at home, and to provide the child in a cast with similar opportunities for play and social activities.

NURSING CARE IN THE COMMUNITY

Have parents of an infant in a Pavlik harness demonstrate proper application of the harness and care of the infant in the harness. Teach family members about daily care (bathing, dressing, and feeding) of the infant. Ideally, the harness is worn 23 hours per day and is removed only for skin checks and bathing. The hips and buttocks should be supported carefully when the infant is out of the harness. Demonstrate how to feed the infant in an upright position to maintain abduction and how to change a diaper without removing the harness. Double-diapering may be recommended to support the hips.

Teaching Highlights

GUIDELINES FOR PAVLIK HARNESS APPLICATION

1. Position the chest halter at nipple line and fasten with Velcro.
2. Position the legs and feet in the stirrups, being sure the hips are flexed and abducted. Fasten with Velcro.
3. Connect the chest halter and leg straps in front.
4. Connect the chest halter and leg straps in back.

All the straps are marked at the first fitting with indelible ink so they can be reattached easily after the harness is rinsed and dried.

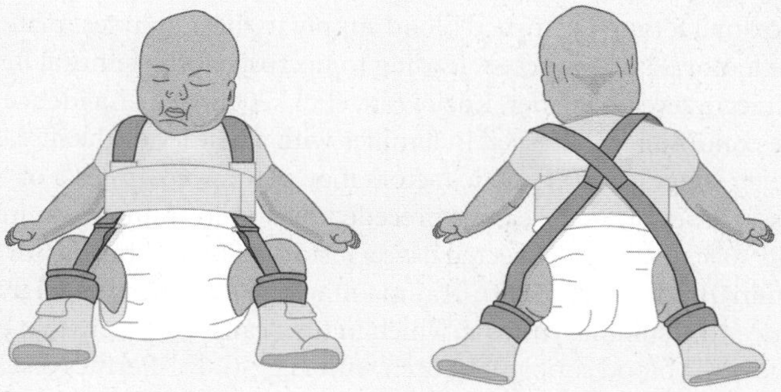

Teaching Highlights

TRANSPORTING THE CHILD WITH ORTHOPEDIC DEVICES

The American Academy of Pediatrics has established guidelines for transporting children with special healthcare needs.

- Riding in the rear seat is preferable.
- If the front seat must be used, the front passenger airbag should be disconnected. The National Highway and Traffic Safety Administration provides information and assistance (1-888-327-4236 or www.nhtsa.dot.gov).
- Use only car seat transport systems approved for use with special needs children.
- Install and use seats as instructed. Never alter a car safety seat to transport a child.
- Move a child from a wheelchair or other special device to the vehicle safety seat whenever this is reasonable.
- Pieces of medical equipment required during transportation (such as monitors or oxygen) or that are being transported with the child (such as wheelchair or walker) should be secured to the floor of the vehicle.
- If the child is transported by school bus, follow state and federal recommendations for school bus transportation of children with special needs.
- Keep a cellular phone and emergency equipment in the vehicle.

Data adapted from American Academy of Pediatrics, Committee on Injury and Poison Prevention. (1999 and 2006). Children with Special Health Care Needs. Retrieved from www.aap.org/healthtopics/shpecialneeds.cfm; Parenting Corner: Questions and Answers: Transporting Children with Special Health Care Needs. Retrieved from www.aap.org/publiced/BR_SpNeedsCarSeats.htm

Instruct the parents of an infant with a harness or a child in a cast to look for any reddened or irritated areas near the harness or cast edges and to check toes frequently for proper circulation. Frequent repositioning reduces the risk of pressure sores or circulatory compromise. The infant should wear an undershirt and socks under the harness to prevent rubbing of the skin.

Safety precautions are important as the child will not have normal mobility. Parents will need to use a specially designed car seat that accommodates the child with abducted hips. Strollers and cribs should provide sufficient room to protect the legs from injury and to prevent hip adduction.

EVALUATION

Expected outcomes for nursing care of the child with developmental dysplasia of the hip include the following:

- Maintenance of skin integrity
- Absence of complications due to immobility
- Knowledge by parents about the condition, treatment, and necessary home care
- Maintenance of a safe environment for the child
- Eventual attainment of normal mobility

LEGG-CALVÉ-PERTHES DISEASE

Legg-Calvé-Perthes disease (or simply Perthes Disease) is a self-limiting condition in which there is avascular necrosis of the femoral head. The disease occurs in approximately 1 in 12,000 children and affects boys four times more often than girls. It usually occurs between the ages of 2 and 12 years, with an average age of 7 years at onset. The disease is bilateral in 20% of cases (Hosalkar et al., 2007).

Etiology and Pathophysiology

The necrosis associated with Legg-Calvé-Perthes disease results from an interruption of the blood supply to the femoral epiphysis. How and why this occurs is not completely understood, but several predisposing factors have been identified. A coagulation system disorder causes repeated vascular interruptions to the proximal femur. Disturbed blood supply to the epiphyseal plate of the femoral bone is noted, leading to necrosis of the femoral head (Grzegorzewski, Synder, Kozlowski, et al., 2006). The incidence of the condition is increased in families with a history of the disease, which suggests that genetic factors may play a role. In 17% of the cases, onset of the disease is preceded by a mild traumatic injury, and 10% of children affected have a history of breech birth (Burns, Dunn, Brady, et al., 2009). Trauma may cause a subchondral fracture and resultant synovitis, which in turn causes pressure that occludes the blood supply. Children with Legg-Calvé-Perthes disease often have delayed skeletal maturation, increased thyroid levels, and low somatomedin C (insulin-like growth factor). It is more common in those with low birth weight, increased parental age, and exposure to environmental tobacco smoke.

Clinical Manifestations

Legg-Calvé-Perthes disease progresses through four distinct stages after the original insult (usually unidentified) occurs, over a period of 1 to 4 years. Early symptoms of Perthes disease include a mild pain in the hip or anterior thigh and a limp, which are aggravated by increased activity and relieved by rest. The child favors the affected hip and limits hip movement to avoid discomfort. (See "Clinical Manifestations: Legg-Calvé-Perthes Disease.")

As the disease progresses, range of motion becomes limited and weakness and muscle wasting develop. The affected thigh is 2 to 3 cm smaller than the unaffected thigh. Prolonged hip irritability may produce muscle spasms and increased pain. This period of the disease varies from 1 to 4 years. Gradually, revascularization begins and pain decreases.

Developing Cultural Competence

LEGG-CALVÉ-PERTHES DISEASE

Legg-Calvé-Perthes disease is most common among white, Chinese, and Japanese children. It is less common among blacks and Native Americans. This suggests a genetic link to the disease, as does the more frequent occurrence in certain families. However, the cause of the disease is not known so the reason for ethnic variation in incidence is not certain (Hosalkar et al., 2007).

Clinical Manifestations

LEGG-CALVÉ-PERTHES DISEASE

STAGE	CLINICAL MANIFESTATIONS
Prenecrosis	An insult causes loss of blood supply to the femoral head.
I–Necrosis	Avascular stage (3-6 months); the child is asymptomatic, bone radiographs are normal, and the head of the femur is structurally intact but avascular.
II–Revascularization	Period of 1-4 years characterized by pain and limitation of movement. Bone radiographs show new bone deposition and dead bone resorption. Fracture and deformity of the head of the femur can occur.
III–Bone healing	Reossification takes place; pain decreases.
IV–Remodeling	The disease process is over, pain is absent, and improvement in joint function occurs.

Clinical Therapy

Because the child's initial symptoms are so mild, parents often do not seek medical attention until symptoms have been present for several months. Diagnosis is made using standard anteroposterior and frog-leg radiographs. However, radiographs taken early in the course of the disease may be normal or show vague widening of the cartilage space. Bone scans and MRI may show the disease process earlier than radiographs. Laboratory studies of the blood, such as white blood cell count, help to rule out inflammatory synovitis of the hip. Protein C, protein S, and APC-R (resistance to activated protein C) may sometimes be performed to evaluate if a coagulation abnormality is present (Burns et al., 2009).

Medical management and prognosis depend on the degree of femoral involvement. Early detection is important. The desired outcome is a pain-free hip that functions properly. To promote healing and prevent deformity, the femoral head must be contained within the hip socket until ossification is complete. This can happen only if the hips remain in an abducted position. At the beginning of treatment, traction can be used to maintain the hips in an abducted and internally rotated position. Once abduction is accomplished, treatment consists of Petrie (leg abduction) casting, or surgical soft-tissue releases such as adductor tenotomy, followed by bracing. Toronto (Figure 58–9 ●) and Scottish-Rite braces are most commonly used. Prognosis is good if the femoral head can be contained long enough for proper healing to occur. Severe disease may be treated by surgery to release adductor muscles, treat the acetabulum or femur, and restore range of motion. Children with untreated disease or those diagnosed late in the disease process occasionally develop osteoarthritis, leg length discrepancy, or hip dysfunction later in life (Herring, Kim, & Browne, 2005).

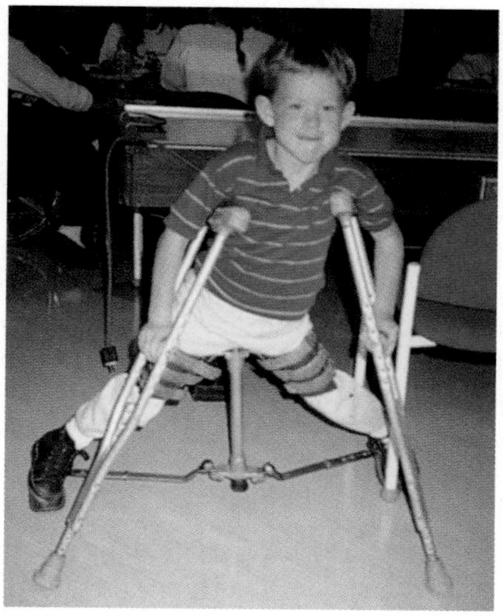

● **Figure 58–9** Toronto brace. Although the Toronto brace may seem formidable for a child to wear, you can see by this photograph that, as usual, children adapt quite well to it.

NURSING MANAGEMENT

NURSING ASSESSMENT AND DIAGNOSIS

Suspect Legg-Calvé-Perthes disease in any child, especially a boy 2 to 12 years of age, who complains of hip discomfort accompanied by a limp. The school nurse may be the first person to observe the child with symptoms of Legg-Calvé-Perthes disease. The child may complain of pain and have to rest during physical education classes. Refer the child to the healthcare provider immediately. Question the child who has an apparent limp about pain, and assess the child's range of motion. Ask if the child injured the hip at some time in the past.

Nursing diagnoses, which center on altered activities and compliance, might include the following:

- *Impaired Physical Mobility* related to restriction of brace or cast
- *Risk for Injury* related to potential complications resulting from noncompliance with the treatment regimen
- *Impaired Adjustment* related to duration of treatment and non-adherence to recommended therapy
- *Deficient Diversional Activity* related to forced inactivity
- *Potential Disturbed Body Image* related to brace

PLANNING AND IMPLEMENTATION

Children with Legg-Calvé-Perthes disease often receive all of their treatment at home. Helping the child and family comply with the prescribed treatment plan may be challenging, because children develop the disease at an age when they are usually very active. The child, who may have little pain, often finds immobilization difficult.

Growth and Development

Legg-Calvé-Perthes disease primarily affects boys with an average age of 7 years. These school-age children are industrious and independent. Suggest activities that redirect energy and promote normal development. These may include horseback riding, which promotes hip abduction; swimming to increase mobility; handcrafts to promote fine motor skills; and computer activities to stimulate cognitive development.

PROMOTE NORMAL GROWTH AND DEVELOPMENT

Give parents suggestions to help redirect the child's energy within the limitations in mobility imposed by treatment. A return to school promotes a feeling of normality. Coordinate the return to school by facilitating the child's use of an elevator or ramp as needed in that setting. Partner with the family to provide instruction for school personnel and other children to foster understanding of the child's condition and treatment. Activities that involve peers also help the child achieve developmental milestones. Help the child adjust to wearing a brace.

NURSING CARE IN THE COMMUNITY

Both the child and the family should be aware that treatment generally takes more than 2 years. Emphasize the importance of following the treatment plan to ensure adequate hip containment and proper healing. Teach the family how to care for a child in traction and how to check the child's skin for breakdown (see Table 58–6 later in this chapter). Follow-up visits should be arranged at regular intervals, in addition to home care visits during the period of traction.

EVALUATION

Expected outcomes of nursing care are elimination of hip pain and discomfort, normal development during the period of immobilization, absence of complications, and parent and child knowledge of the treatment regimen.

SLIPPED CAPITAL FEMORAL EPIPHYSIS

Slipped capital femoral epiphysis (SCFE) occurs when the femoral head is displaced from the femoral neck. This condition is seen in 10/100,000 adolescents, commonly in the prepubertal growth spurt, between the ages of 12 to 15 years in boys and 10 to 13 years in girls. Boys are more often affected than girls. Black children are affected more often than other ethnic groups, as are children who are overweight, those with sports injuries or other trauma, a history of radiation therapy, or endocrine disease (Manoff, Banffy, & Winell, 2005).

Evidence in Action

Obesity is a known risk factor for SCFE. Increasing rates of obesity among children contributes to an increasing risk for the disorder. Research continues to demonstrate a relationship between body mass index (BMI) and SCFE. In one study of over 100 youth from 8 to 18 years, over 81% had a BMI above the 95th percentile for their age and gender (Manoff et al., 2005). Another study examined factors associated with bilateral SCFE; about 20% of children with SCFE eventually develop the condition in both hips. In a study of 54 children with unilateral disease, 16 (30%) developed bilateral disease. Those progressing to the bilateral condition had significantly higher BMI percentiles (Bhatia, Pirpiris, & Otsuka, 2006). Nurses are well-positioned to work with children and families to teach weight reduction strategies and to share information about the numerous health risks associated with elevated BMI.

Etiology and Pathophysiology

The cause of SCFE is unknown. Predisposing factors include obesity, a recent growth spurt, and endocrine disorders such as hypothyroidism and hypogonadism.

Slippage of the femoral head occurs at the proximal epiphyseal plate, and the femur displaces from the epiphysis (see "Pathophysiology Illustrated: Slipped Epiphysis"). Slippage is usually gradual (chronic), but may also result from acute trauma. The synovial membrane becomes inflamed, edematous, and painful. If untreated, callous formation occurs, resulting in a deformed hip with limited range of motion.

PATHOPHYSIOLOGY ILLUSTRATED

SLIPPED EPIPHYSIS

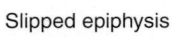

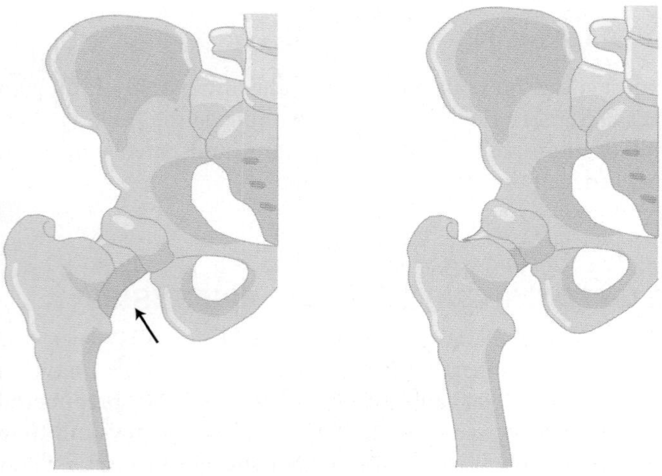

In slipped capital femoral epiphysis, the femoral head is displaced from the femoral neck at the proximal epiphyseal plate.

Clinical Manifestations

Symptoms include limp; knee, thigh, groin or hip pain; and loss of hip motion. Out-toeing, decreased internal rotation, and external rotation with flexion of the leg are symptomatic (Katz, 2006). The condition is categorized as acute (sudden onset with less than 3 weeks' duration), chronic (longer than 3 weeks' duration), or acute-on-chronic (an additional slippage in a child with a chronic condition), depending on the onset and severity of symptoms. The child with an acute slip has sudden, severe pain and cannot bear weight. An acute slip may be associated with traumatic injury. The youth may be able to walk (stable), or unable to bear weight (unstable) (Aronsson, Loder, Breur, et al., 2006).

Clinical Therapy

A complete history provides information about risk factors and the development of the condition. Radiographs confirm the diagnosis. A bone scan, ultrasound, CT, and MRI may also be performed.

The goal of medical management is to stabilize the femoral head while keeping displacement to a minimum and retaining as much hip function as possible. Surgical treatment is usually necessary; this involves fixation of the epiphysis with screws or pins. If the condition is stable, a single screw into the hip in an outpatient procedure is sufficient for stabilization; if unstable, surgery may involve two or three pins placed through the physis into the epiphysis to stabilize the femoral head (Aronsson et al., 2006). Medical treatment, which is occasionally used, includes a regimen of no weight bearing, bed rest, a spica cast, and Buck or Russell traction (see Table 58–5 later in this chapter).

Prognosis is related to the severity of the deformity and the occurrence of complications, such as avascular necrosis of the femoral head or **chondrolysis** (the breaking down and absorption of cartilage).

NURSING MANAGEMENT

NURSING ASSESSMENT AND DIAGNOSIS

The child usually presents with hip pain or referred pain to the groin, thigh, or knee, and limited mobility. A thorough history is needed to assess for injury as a cause. Assess the child's range of motion, pain, and limp, if apparent. Refer the child for treatment immediately if SCFE is suspected. This condition is considered to be an emergency, and it is essential that the child be treated immediately to keep weight off the affected joint (Katz, 2006).

Among the nursing diagnoses that may apply to the child with SCFE are the following:

- *Impaired Physical Mobility* related to treatment
- *Pain* related to hip injury
- *Risk for Disturbed Body Image* related to treatment
- *Risk for Delayed Growth and Development* related to mobility restrictions
- *Risk for Imbalanced Nutrition: More than Body Requirements* related to immobility

- *Ineffective Tissue Perfusion: Peripheral* related to traction, casting, and other treatments
- *Health-Seeking Behaviors (Child and Parental)* related to disease process and treatment

PLANNING AND IMPLEMENTATION

Nursing management involves caring for the child in traction or after surgery, administering medications and other pain-control interventions, maintaining mobility within the limits imposed by treatment, providing adequate nutrition, educating the child and family about the disorder, providing emotional support, and promoting compliance with the treatment plan.

ENCOURAGE APPROPRIATE NUTRITIONAL INTAKE AND PHYSICAL ACTIVITY

A growing adolescent needs increased amounts of proteins, carbohydrates, and calcium to promote skeletal healing. Provide written instructions about nutritional requirements to promote bone healing and maintain an ideal body weight. If a child is overweight, encourage weight loss by decreasing the percentage of fat and sugar in the diet and by increasing physical activity that is safe to do. Weight loss decreases pressure on the femoral epiphysis and can also lead to a more positive self-image. Incorporate upper body exercises into treatment, both to assist in weight control and to build muscle. A few visits to physical therapy may facilitate a program of upper body exercise and teach safe ways of increasing the total amount of physical activity.

PROVIDE EMOTIONAL SUPPORT

Because the onset of SCFE is usually unexpected, the child and family may find themselves facing surgery with little warning. Explain the treatment plan simply and thoroughly. Reassure the child and family that with proper compliance, treatment should be successful.

DISCHARGE PLANNING AND HOME CARE TEACHING

Help the family plan for the child's return to school. If attendance is not possible for a time due to traction or surgery, arrange for tutors and computer communication with school as needed. Follow-up visits are necessary until the child's epiphyseal plates close. It is not uncommon for SCFE to occur in the other hip. Make sure the child and family are aware of symptoms such as decreased range of motion or pain that could indicate onset of the disorder in the other hip. Tell parents to contact their healthcare provider immediately if these symptoms occur.

EVALUATION

Expected outcomes of nursing care for the child with slipped capital femoral epiphysis include maintenance of normal weight and recommended nutritional intake, absence of complications of immobility, successful adaptation to school following treatment, and family recognition of the need for ongoing monitoring for complications.

DISORDERS OF THE SPINE

SCOLIOSIS

Scoliosis is a lateral S- or C-shaped curvature of the spine that is often associated with a rotational deformity of the spine and ribs. Many people exhibit some degree of spinal curvature; curvatures of more than 10 degrees are considered abnormal. Curves are either idiopathic or compensatory, the latter occurring as the spine curves to compensate for a structural deformity such as leg length discrepancy. Idiopathic scoliosis occurs most often in girls, especially during the growth spurt between the ages of 10 and 13 years. From 1% to 3% of adolescents manifest with idiopathic scoliosis of greater than 10 degrees (Hart & Grottkau, 2006; Mooney, Mayer, & Woodbridge, 2007). Early onset of idiopathic scoliosis occurs before 10 years of age and comprises 15% of cases (Spiegel, Hosalkar, & Dormans, 2007).

Etiology and Pathophysiology

The cause of scoliosis is complex. Structural scoliosis may be congenital, idiopathic, or acquired (associated with neuromuscular disorders such as muscular dystrophy or myelodysplasia, or secondary to spinal cord injuries).

In idiopathic structural scoliosis (the most common type), the spine for unknown reasons begins to curve laterally, with vertebral rotation. The most common curve is a right thoracic and left lumbar deformity. As the curve progresses, structural changes occur. The ribs on the concave side (inside of the curve) are forced closer together, while the ribs on the convex side separate widely, causing narrowing of the thoracic cage and formation of the rib hump. The lateral curvature affects the vertebral structure. Disk spaces are narrowed on the concave side and spread wider on the convex side, resulting in an asymmetric vertebral canal (Figure 58–10 ●).

Scoliosis can also occur in congenital diseases involving the spinal structure and in the musculoskeletal changes seen in conditions such as myelomeningocele, cerebral palsy (see Chapter 56∞), or muscular dystrophy. It can also be acquired after injury to the spinal cord.

Clinical Manifestations

The classic signs of scoliosis include truncal asymmetry, uneven shoulder and hip height, a one-sided rib hump, and a prominent scapula. The child does not complain of pain or discomfort.

Clinical Therapy

Generally, observation and radiographic examination are used to diagnose scoliosis. Additional diagnostic studies include MRI, CT, and bone scanning, which are used occasionally to assess the degree of curvature. The goal of medical management is to limit or stop progression of the curvature.

Early detection is essential to successful treatment. Adequate treatment and follow-up maximize the child's chances for proper

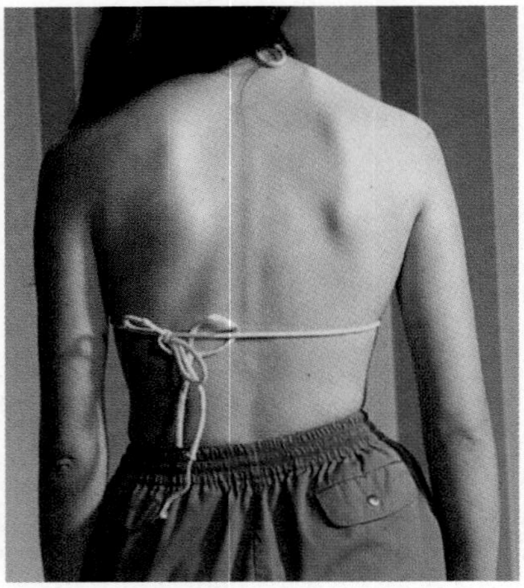

• **Figure 58–10** Clues for early detection of scoliosis. A child may have varying degrees of scoliosis. For mild forms, treatment will focus on strengthening and stretching. Moderate forms will require bracing. Severe forms may necessitate surgery and fusion. Clothes that fit at an angle, such as this teenage girl's shorts, and anatomic asymmetry of the back provide clues for early detection.

spinal alignment. The treatment regimen chosen depends on the degree and progression of the curvature and the reaction of the child and family to medical management.

Treatment of children with mild scoliosis (curvatures of 10 to 20 degrees) consists of exercises to improve posture and muscle tone and to maintain, or possibly increase, flexibility of the spine. Emphasis is placed on building strength toward the outside of the curve while stretching the inside of the curve. These exercises are not a cure, however, and the child should be evaluated by a physician at 3-month intervals, with radiographic evaluation every 6 months.

Medical management of moderate scoliosis (curvatures of 20 to 40 degrees) includes bracing with a Boston brace. The goal of wearing a brace is to maintain the existing spinal curvature with no increase. Brace wear begins immediately after diagnosis. To achieve maximum effectiveness, the brace should be worn 23 hours per day. Brace treatment is lengthy and requires a high degree of compliance, which can be difficult for adolescents, for whom body image or sports involvement is often important.

Children with severe scoliosis (curvatures of 40 degrees or more) require surgery, which involves spinal fusion. The majority of spinal fusions are performed using instrumentation of the spinal cord. Examples of surgical approaches include Luque wires, Coutrel-Dubosset (CD) instrumentation, Texas Scottish Rite Hospital system, and Moss-Miami system (Lonstein, 2006). These treatments stabilize the spine well during surgery, may be accompanied by bone grafting to the spine, and require no long-term therapy. Following surgery with wires or instrumentation, the child is on bed rest during a recovery period and then is generally fitted with anteroposterior plastic shells (also called thoracolumbar sacral orthotics) that are worn for several months to provide stability for the spine. The wires will remain in the back permanently.

NURSING MANAGEMENT

NURSING ASSESSMENT AND DIAGNOSIS

School nurses often screen children for scoliosis, generally in the fifth and seventh grades. Several states mandate this screening, but it is not universal in all states (U.S. Preventive Services Task Force, 2006b). When abnormalities are noted, refer the child to an orthopedic center for further evaluation. Children should be examined every 6 to 9 months thereafter. If scoliosis is detected, the child's brothers and sisters should be examined and observed closely. Scoliosis screening involves visual observations of the following.

From the front:

- Is the head midline?
- Are the shoulders at the same height?
- Is there the same amount of space between the arms and body on each side?

From the back:

- Is the head midline?
- Are the shoulders at the same height?
- Are the scapulae equally prominent and at the same height?
- Is the spine straight?
- Is there the same amount of space between the arms and body on each side?
- Are the hips at the same height?

With the adolescent holding hands together and bent over slightly:

- Are the scapula humps even?

With the adolescent holding hands together and bent over toward the floor:

- Are the flank humps even?
- Is the spine straight?
- Is there a marked roundness when viewed from the side? (evidence of kyphosis)

Once scoliosis has been identified, the focus becomes education and follow-up. Any child with scoliosis should have a comprehensive neurologic, cardiac, and respiratory examination, since the rib cage deformity can influence the functioning of these systems.

The following nursing diagnoses may apply to the child with scoliosis. See additional nursing diagnoses in the nursing care plan.

- *Risk for Impaired Adjustment* to the exercise program related to duration and intensity of exercise
- *Impaired Physical Mobility* related to brace or movement restrictions and pain following surgery
- *Risk for Impaired Skin Integrity* related to brace
- *Health-Seeking Behaviors (Child and Parental)* related to unfamiliarity with disease process

- *Disturbed Body Image* related to deformity and brace wear
- *Risk for Deficient Knowledge (child and parent)* related to lack of information about home care following surgery

Common nursing diagnoses for the child having surgery can be found in the accompanying Nursing Care Plan.

PLANNING AND IMPLEMENTATION

An important aspect of nursing care is patient education. Patient adherence with prescribed measures is critical to the success of treatment. Children and their families need to understand the condition and the stages of treatment, particularly true for adolescents undergoing treatment for scoliosis.

Children or adolescents facing surgery require education, reassurance, and support. Teach about pain control and the patient-controlled analgesia (PCA) pump. Often the child donates some of his or her own blood prior to surgery, and the family may also donate so blood transfused in surgery is the child's or a family member's. Teach the child the safety that this ensures. The adolescent will benefit from learning about deep breathing, positioning, surgical incision, and all other aspects of postoperative care. The Nursing Care Plan summarizes nursing care for the child undergoing surgery for scoliosis.

PROMOTE ACCEPTANCE OF THE TREATMENT PLAN

Provide instructions about exercises that will help to decrease the severity of the spinal curvature, and obtain baseline exercise levels (Mooney et al., 2007). Demonstrate the exercises, and explain their purpose (i.e., to strengthen back muscles). Help the child adjust to wearing a brace. Adolescents, in particular, may be reluctant to wear an external device such as a brace. To promote a sense of control, allow the adolescent to choose when to exercise and when to be out of the brace, within the treatment guidelines. Provide reassurance and encouragement and promote interaction with peers. Suggest that the adolescent work with a peer support person who is being treated for scoliosis or has had the condition in the past. Provide information about fashionable clothing that can be worn with the brace and facilitate visits to department stores that will help the teen shop for clothing.

DISCHARGE PLANNING AND HOME CARE TEACHING

Identify and address home care needs well in advance of discharge after spinal surgery. The child will need to adapt to a new set of body mechanics. Show the child how to do simple tasks without bending or twisting the torso. Have the child demonstrate the ability to perform activities of daily living before discharge from the hospital. Partner with physical therapy/rehabilitation personnel to plan for the youth's needs related to safe and effective movement with the brace.

Activities for the child who has had spinal surgery are commonly limited for a period of time. The child can usually walk and perform physical activity such as gentle swimming, but lifting heavy loads, bending or twisting at the waist, or engaging in activities such as skiing, rollerblading, bicycle riding, and many other sports may not be allowed. Restrictions usually should be followed for 6 to 8 months, depending on the type of surgery and the surgeon. Emphasize to both the child and the family the importance of compliance. Give written discharge instructions to the child and family. Follow-up visits are important. The child should be examined 4 to 6 weeks after discharge, then every 3 to 4 months for 1 year, and every 1 to 2 years thereafter. The metal hardware in the back necessitates that after surgery the teen must carry a written physician explanation since the hardware will set off metal detectors at airports.

Several organizations provide information and assistance to families of children with scoliosis. Make referrals as appropriate.

Thinking Critically

ADOLESCENT SELF-IMAGE AND BRACES

In a study that used interviews to learn about feelings related to brace wear among youth with scoliosis, the youth expressed feelings of stress, anger, denial, and shame. They reported receiving support from family and friends but did not receive adequate support from healthcare professionals (Sapountzi-Krepia, Psychogiou, Peterson, et al., 2006). The findings that adolescents are concerned with body image is not surprising, considering that adolescence is a developmental stage that focuses on appearance and fitting in with others. It is surprising that this is not acknowledged and discussed sufficiently during healthcare visits. Health professionals should realize that wearing a brace can be difficult for adolescents and provide a chance for youth to discuss how they feel about the diagnosis and treatment. Consider interventions that aid in improving body image. For example, some department stores sponsor fashion shows for adolescents with scoliosis who must wear braces. Children with braces model and demonstrate how popular clothing can be worn to disguise the wearing of the brace. These events can have a positive impact on the self-esteem of adolescents who participate in and view the shows.

See MyNursingKit for possible responses.

EVALUATION

Expected outcomes of nursing care for the child with scoliosis treated by brace are maintenance of intact skin and compliance with prescribed therapy. Expected outcomes after surgical correction are listed on the accompanying Nursing Care Plan.

MyNursingKit Musculoskeletal Resources

TORTICOLLIS, KYPHOSIS, AND LORDOSIS

Torticollis is tilt of the head caused by rotation of the cervical spine. The cause is generally an injury sustained to the sternocleidomastoid muscle at the time of birth or to a cervical spine abnormality. Stretching exercises or surgical lengthening of the sternocleidomastoid muscle are usual treatments. Occasionally the cause of torticollis is visual impairment, leading to constant turning in one direction to see with the better eye.

Nursing Care Plan

THE CHILD UNDERGOING SURGERY FOR SCOLIOSIS

1. Nursing Diagnosis: Deficient Knowledge (Child and Parents) related to lack of information about surgery

NIC Priority Intervention:

Teaching disease process and preoperative: Assisting the patient to understand information and mentally prepare for surgery and postoperative recovery

NOC Suggested Outcome:

Knowledge: Extent of understanding conveyed about scoliosis treatment

Goal: The child and parents will verbalize understanding of the disease, its treatment, and the surgical procedure.

INTERVENTION	RATIONALE	EXPECTED OUTCOME
■ Teach the child and family about the course of the disease, its signs and symptoms, and treatment. Provide appropriate handouts. Encourage the child and parents to ask questions.	■ Understanding and involvement increase motivation and compliance while reducing fear.	The child and family accurately verbalize knowledge about the disease and its treatment. The child and family ask appropriate questions about postoperative care.
■ Begin preoperative teaching at the time of admission. Orient the child to hospital and postoperative procedures. Before surgery, have the child demonstrate log-rolling, range of motion exercises, and the use of an incentive spirometer. Discuss pain management.	■ Preoperative teaching and familiarity with hospital procedures reduce the stress related to surgery and postoperative complications.	

2. Nursing Diagnosis: Ineffective Breathing Pattern related to hypoventilation syndrome

NIC Priority Intervention:

Airway management and respiratory monitoring: Facilitation of patency of air passages and analysis of patient data

NOC Suggested Outcome:

Respiratory status ventilation: Movement of air in and out of the lungs

Goal: The child will show no signs of respiratory compromise.

INTERVENTION	RATIONALE	EXPECTED OUTCOME
■ Monitor respiratory status, especially after the administration of analgesics. Apply pulse oximeter.	■ Evaluation of the child's respiratory condition anticipates and avoids complications. Analgesics such as morphine may increase or potentiate respiratory compromise.	The child has normal respiratory patterns.
■ Administer oxygen if ordered.	■ Oxygen increases peripheral oxygen saturation to 95–100%.	
■ Have the child use an incentive spirometer.	■ Spirometry increases lung expansion and aeration of the alveoli.	
■ Monitor intake and output.	■ Good hydration promotes loose secretions and helps prevent infection.	
■ Reposition the child at least every 2 hours.	■ Repositioning ensures inflation of the lung fields.	

3. Nursing Diagnosis: Risk for Injury related to neurovascular deficit secondary to instrumentation

NIC Priority Intervention:

Injury prevention: Instituting special precautions with patient at risk

NOC Suggested Outcome:

Risk control: Actions to eliminate or reduce modifiable health risks

Nursing Care Plan—continued

THE CHILD UNDERGOING SURGERY FOR SCOLIOSIS

Goal: The child's neurovascular system will remain intact as evidenced by circulation, sensation, and motor checks. The child will feel no numbness or tingling.

INTERVENTION	RATIONALE	EXPECTED OUTCOME
■ Monitor the child's color, circulation, capillary refill, warmth, sensation, and motion in all extremities. Perform neurovascular checks every 2 hours for the first 24 hours and then every 4 hours for the next 48 hours. Record presence of pedal and distal tibial pulses every hour for 48 hours. Report changes and abnormal findings immediately.	■ When the spinal column is manipulated during surgery, altered neurovascular status, thrombosis formation, and paralysis are possible complications. Postoperative risks include loss of bowel or bladder control, weakness or paralysis, and impaired vision or sensation.	The child exhibits only temporary alteration (pale skin, faint pulse, and edema occur but they resolve within the initial postoperative phase). The child returns to the preoperative baseline state by discharge.
■ Have the child wear antiembolism stockings until ambulatory. The stockings may be removed for 1 hour 2–3 times daily.	■ Antiembolism stockings prevent blood clots and promote venous return. Thrombus formation is a postoperative risk.	
■ Check for any pain, swelling, or a positive Homans' sign (pain in the calf of the leg when the toes are dorsiflexed). Record any evidence of edema.	■ Swelling may indicate a tight dressing and tissue damage. A positive Homans' sign and pain may indicate thrombus formation.	
■ Monitor input and output.	■ Abnormalities may indicate a fluid shift problem.	
■ Encourage and assist the child with range of motion exercises, both passive and active.	■ Activity promotes mobility and reduces risk of thrombus formation.	

4. Nursing Diagnosis: Pain related to spinal fusion with instrumentation

NIC Priority Intervention:

Pain management: Alleviation of pain or a reduction of pain to a level of comfort acceptable to the patient

NOC Suggested Outcome:

Pain level: Amount of reported or demonstrated pain

Goal: The child will verbalize an adequate level of comfort or show absence of pain behavior within 1 hour of a specific nursing intervention.

INTERVENTION	RATIONALE	EXPECTED OUTCOME
■ Assess the level of pain and initiate pain management strategies as soon as possible. Use patient-controlled analgesia if ordered.	■ Adequate pain management allows for faster healing and a more cooperative patient. Patient-controlled analgesics may be effective.	The child experiences pain relief early in the postoperative period.
■ Administer pain medication around-the-clock to help ensure pain relief, especially during the first 48 hours. Monitor epidural blocks and patient-controlled analgesia or other methods used for pain control.	■ Medicating around-the-clock helps to maintain comfort. Monitoring ensures patient safety.	
■ Use nonpharmacologic pain management techniques, such as imagery, relaxation, touch, music, application of heat and cold, and reduced environmental stimulation to supplement medications (see Chapter 42 ∞).	■ Alternative treatments also interrupt the pain stimulus and provide relief. Nonpharmacologic methods can be an effective adjunct to pain management.	
■ Document pain assessment interventions and the child's reactions.	■ Proper documentation guides the selection of the most effective means of pain control.	
■ Reassure the child that some discomfort is expected and that a variety of measures can be tried to reduce discomfort.	■ Realistic expectations decrease anxiety and give the child a sense of control.	

Clinical Manifestations

KYPHOSIS AND LORDOSIS

CONDITION	CLINICAL MANIFESTATIONS	DIAGNOSTIC TESTS AND CLINICAL THERAPY	NURSING MANAGEMENT
KYPHOSIS Excessive convex curvature of the cervical thoracic spine	Visible hunchback or rounded shoulders; shortness of breath or fatigue; abdominal creases and tight hamstrings in severe cases	*Diagnostic tests:* Spinal curvature is assessed by having the child bend 90 degrees at the waist and looking at the scapular area from side. Diagnosis is confirmed by radiograph. *Clinical therapy:* Exercises are prescribed for mild condition; bracing is commonly used; surgery is performed in severe cases.	Provide support. Encourage exercises and diligent brace wear. Help the child to deal with the psychologic stress of altered body image.
LORDOSIS Excessive concave curvature of the lumbar spine with an angle of more than 60 degrees; most common in prepubescent girls and African Americans	Presence of swayback; prominent buttocks; hip flexion contractures; tight hamstrings	Diagnostic tests: Spinal curvature is assessed by looking at the standing child from the side. Lumbar lordosis is confirmed by visualizing the spine on standing, lateral radiograph. Clinical therapy: Treatment focuses on exercises and postural awareness. Bracing and surgery are rarely prescribed.	Provide support. Reassure the child and family that the condition is often outgrown as the child matures. Encourage physical conditioning exercises and follow-up examinations on a yearly basis.

Growth and Development

Postural lordosis is a characteristic finding in toddlers but should disappear by the school-age years.

Kyphosis (hunchback) and lordosis (swayback) are two other types of spinal curvature that may occur in children. Clinical therapy depends on the cause and degree of the curvature, and the age of the child at onset. Nurses can perform thorough musculoskeletal assessments of children (see Chapter 35∞) and refer any children with abnormalities for further evaluation. (See "Clinical Manifestations: Kyphosis and Lordosis.")

ADDITIONAL DISORDERS OF THE BONES AND JOINTS

OSTEOPOROSIS AND OSTEOPENIA

Osteoporosis, a condition in which there is decreased density and mass of bone, promotes the risk of fractures and is commonly associated with aging. However, children can have osteoporosis (also known as metabolic bone disease or a bone mineral density more than 2.5 standard deviations below the norm) related to imbalanced nutrition or other pathologic conditions. Osteoporosis is preceded by osteopenia or low bone mass, which is between 1 and 2.5 standard deviations below the norm (Bowman & Russell, 2006).

Etiology and Pathophysiology

Very-low-birth-weight infants who are premature often have osteopenia of prematurity because much of bone mass is usually acquired in the latter weeks of pregnancy. In addition, they may have other health problems after birth and be unable to ingest enough nutrients to meet metabolic needs for bone growth. Premature infants are often less active than others, which decreases the amount of mechanical loading on their bones, a factor known to increase bone resorption and decrease bone mass (Eliakim & Nemet, 2005).

A group of children who may show signs of osteoporosis are those who have decreased mechanical loading. Children with spina bifida or cerebral palsy, conditions that interfere with ambulation, have limited pressure on bones and resultant lowered bone mass in affected extremities and spine. Some other conditions are associated with lower bone mass, including Turner syndrome, growth hormone deficiency, osteogenesis imperfecta, juvenile rheumatoid arthritis, and diabetes. Children who are

PATHOPHYSIOLOGY ILLUSTRATED

EFFECTS OF IMMOBILITY

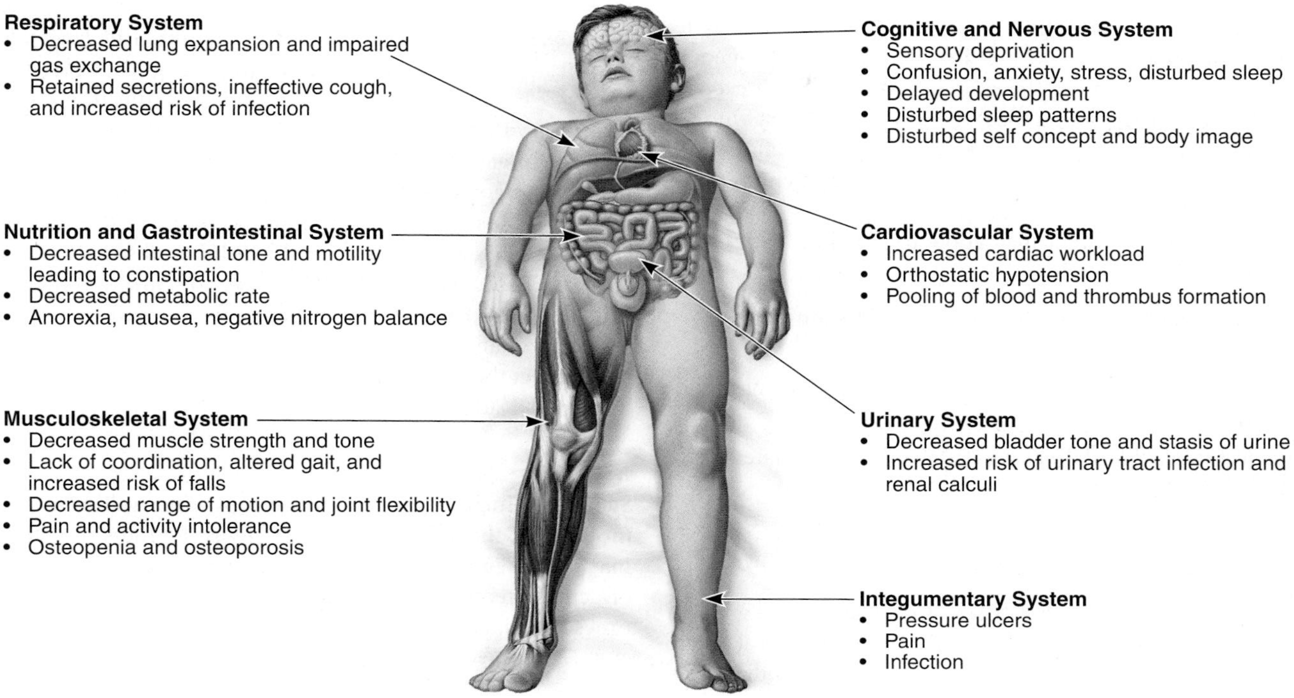
Respiratory System
• Decreased lung expansion and impaired gas exchange
• Retained secretions, ineffective cough, and increased risk of infection
Nutrition and Gastrointestinal System
• Decreased intestinal tone and motility leading to constipation
• Decreased metabolic rate
• Anorexia, nausea, negative nitrogen balance
Musculoskeletal System
• Decreased muscle strength and tone
• Lack of coordination, altered gait, and increased risk of falls
• Decreased range of motion and joint flexibility
• Pain and activity intolerance
• Osteopenia and osteoporosis
Cognitive and Nervous System
• Sensory deprivation
• Confusion, anxiety, stress, disturbed sleep
• Delayed development
• Disturbed sleep patterns
• Disturbed self concept and body image
Cardiovascular System
• Increased cardiac workload
• Orthostatic hypotension
• Pooling of blood and thrombus formation
Urinary System
• Decreased bladder tone and stasis of urine
• Increased risk of urinary tract infection and renal calculi
Integumentary System
• Pressure ulcers
• Pain
• Infection

treated for disorders or injuries with casting and bracing are also at high risk of osteoporosis due to immobilization.

Lastly, adolescence is a period when adequate intakes of calcium and vitamin D are needed to maximize bone formation and prevent osteoporosis later in life. Adolescents, particularly females, often do not meet the recommended daily allowance (RDA) for these nutrients and are at risk for osteoporosis even though it may not be manifested for years. Other lifestyle patterns of youth that decrease bone formation are smoking, alcohol use, excessive soda intake, and keeping weight at a very low level. Those with anorexia nervosa are clearly at risk for osteoporosis.

Clinical Manifestations

Osteoporosis is a silent disease, as is its precursor osteopenia; those who have the disorders are often without signs or symptoms for years. It may become apparent when a baby or child has a fracture and radiologic studies make the problem evident.

Clinical Therapy

Bone mineral content and density are measured by single-photon absorptiometry (SPA), dual-photon absorptiometry (DPA), and dual-energy x-ray absorptiometry (DEXA). Although uncommonly used, serum studies such as bone-specific alkaline phosphatase, phosphorus, and type-I collagen can be used to measure osteoblastic and osteoclastic activity. Over 90% of the body's calcium is stored in bone so serum calcium is not reflective of bone density.

Premature newborns at risk of osteopenia of prematurity need collaborative management by neonatologists, neonatal nutritionists, and neonatal nurses. Breast milk is enhanced by adding special fortifiers; premature formula should be used rather than regular baby formula. When babies need enteral or parenteral feedings, calcium-to-phosphorus ratios are carefully balanced to enhance osteoblastic activity. Extremity range of motion for very-low-birth-weight newborns can decrease bone loss in the period after birth. Up to eight weeks of assisted range of motion exercise decreases loss of bone strength and enhances bone health in low-birth-weight premature infants (Litmanovitz, Dolfin, Amon, et al., 2007).

For older children at risk of developing osteoporosis, calcium and vitamin D intake is encouraged and oral supplements may be given. Standing therapy for those who are nonambulatory can provide mechanical weight and enhance bone density (Caulton, Ward, Alsop, et al., 2004). When a cast or other immobilizing device is removed from a child, a program of gradually increasing exercise in collaboration with physical rehabilitation professionals promotes bone strengthening and lowered risk for fractures or related sequelae.

NURSING MANAGEMENT

NURSING ASSESSMENT AND DIAGNOSIS

Nurses identify newborns, children, and adolescents at risk of developing low bone mass and density. This is accomplished by identifying diseases putting the child at risk. Ask about exercise and activity patterns, and physical therapy for children who are nonambulatory. Dietary intake is measured periodically for all youth at health promotion visits, and RDAs for calcium, phosphorus, and vitamin D are compared to intake.

Nursing diagnoses that may apply to the child with osteoporosis include the following:

- *Imbalanced Nutrition* related to inability to consume essential nutrients
- *Risk for Injury to Bones* related to decreased bone mass and density
- *Ineffective Health Maintenance* related to inadequate dietary intake

PLANNING AND IMPLEMENTATION

Perform a dietary analysis of children at risk (see Chapter 34 for detailed methods for diet assessment). Refer children at risk to nutritionists and physicians for further education and diagnosis. Suggest referrals to physical rehabilitation to recommend weight-bearing exercise. Administer nutritional supplements when prescribed, and teach families how to give these medications. Partner with families to provide therapy that stimulates weight bearing for nonambulatory children. Teach parents how to recognize fractures in children who may not have normal sensation and are unable to report them. Edema, unusual shape of a limb, fussiness of the child, and falls should be reported promptly.

When osteoporosis is due to immobility, many other symptoms occur as well. Be alert for these problems and integrate physical activity into care as much as possible to minimize their effects.

EVALUATION

Expected outcomes of nursing care for the child with a potential for osteoporosis include adequate intake of recommended amounts of nutrients, absence of fractures, and normal findings on studies of bone mineral content and density.

OSTEOMYELITIS

Osteomyelitis is an infection of the bone, most often one of the long bones of the lower extremity. It may be acute or chronic and may spread into surrounding tissues. Although osteomyelitis may occur at any age, it is most common in children between the ages of 1 and 12 years. Boys are affected two to three times as often as girls, primarily because they have a greater incidence of trauma. Overall incidence is 1 in 5000 youth (Kocher, Lee, & Dolan, 2006).

Etiology and Pathophysiology

Osteomyelitis is caused by a microorganism, usually bacterial but possibly viral or fungal. *Staphylococcus aureus* is the most common causative pathogen, followed by *Escherichia coli,* group B streptococci, *Streptococcus aureus, Streptococcus pyogenes, Pseudomonas aeruginosa* (in foot puncture), and *Haemophilus influenzae; Kingella kingae* is increasingly diagnosed (Frank, Mahoney, & Eppes, 2005). Common sources of infection are upper respiratory infection, trauma to the bone, and surgery.

The infecting organism spreads through the bloodstream or through a penetrating injury to the bone, where it becomes established. Most infections in children begin in the metaphysis (see Figure 58–2), which has a sluggish blood supply (Bautista, Gholve, & Dormans, 2006). Eventually the infection may penetrate the bone cortex and periosteum. Inflammation and abscess formation can interrupt the blood supply to the underlying bone, affect the surrounding soft tissue, and, if the infection is left untreated, lead to necrosis.

Clinical Manifestations

Symptoms include pain and tenderness with swelling, decreased mobility of the infected joint, and fever. Redness over the area may occur. The child may refuse to walk or may limp. The onset of acute osteomyelitis is generally rapid and is therefore sometimes misdiagnosed as a sports injury (Kaplan, 2005; Kocher et al., 2006).

Clinical Therapy

A history suggestive of osteomyelitis includes an upper respiratory infection or blunt trauma followed by pain at the area of a growth plate. Laboratory evaluation shows leukocytosis and an elevated erythrocyte sedimentation rate (ESR) and C-reactive protein (Gutierrez, 2005). The degree of ESR elevation is directly related to the severity of the infection. Radiographs and bone scans may identify the area of involvement. A needle aspiration of the site or a blood culture can confirm the diagnosis and provide a culture of the causative organism. Other studies may include ELISA for Lyme antibody titer, antistreptolysin-O for recent streptococcus infections, or PPD for exposure to tuberculosis (Bautista et al., 2006).

Medical management begins with the intravenous administration of a broad-spectrum antibiotic, even before culture results are available. Since *S. aureus* is a common cause of infection, the antibiotic should be effective against this organism. Treatment is influenced by the possibility of methicillin-resistant *S. aureus* (MRSA), so beginning antibiotics are usually

Growth and Development

Osteomyelitis in a newborn is of great concern, as before 18 months of age the blood vessels cross the growth plates. This creates a higher risk of epiphyseal involvement with resultant limb length discrepancy.

vancomycin or clindamycin, drugs effective against MRSA (see Chapter 45∞). Once the culture results are obtained, the antibiotic may be altered. Oral antibiotics are given once an adequate response has occurred. However, extended intravenous home therapy may be used. Antibiotic therapy continues for about 3 to 6 weeks. The cause of infection is not always identified from culture so ESR and C-protein are followed carefully in these cases to identify if treatment is successful. When an adequate response is not obtained within 2 to 3 days, the area may be aspirated again, or surgically drained. Intravenous fluids may be administered to ensure adequate hydration. In children with extensive orthopedic surgery, or in those with immunosuppression, a short course of prophylactic antibiotic may be administered after surgery.

Prompt diagnosis and treatment usually completely resolve the infection. The prognosis is related to the initiation of therapy—the earlier treatment begins, the better the outcome. Long-term unfavorable outcomes include disruption of the growth plate, which can interrupt growth, and damage to the joints from septic arthritis.

NURSING MANAGEMENT

NURSING ASSESSMENT AND DIAGNOSIS

A thorough history, including information about the onset of symptoms and a history of recent infections or puncture wounds, is essential. Ask about immunization status, especially tetanus vaccine. Assess the affected area for signs of redness, swelling, pain, and decreased range of motion. Measure vital signs; increased temperature and pulse in particular may provide clues about worsening infection. When osteomyelitis is possible, all cultures of blood or wound must be taken before antibiotic therapy is started.

Among the nursing diagnoses that may apply to the child with osteomyelitis are the following:

- *Acute Pain* related to biologic injury
- *Impaired Physical Mobility* related to discomfort
- *Risk for Infection (Sepsis)* related to spread of infection
- *Risk for Imbalanced Nutrition: Less than Body Requirements* related to loss of appetite
- *Health-Seeking Behaviors (Child and Parental)* related to lack of information about disease process

PLANNING AND IMPLEMENTATION

Nursing management focuses on administering antibiotics, protecting the child from spread of the infection, and encouraging a well-balanced diet. Use standard precautions, with transmission-based precautions for any drainage from the site of infection.

OBTAIN CULTURES AND BLOOD WORK

Blood cultures and cultures of any open wound must be performed before the first dose of antibiotic when osteomyelitis is suspected. Obtain continuing blood samples as needed to monitor ESR and C-reactive protein. See Skill 10–5 SKILLS.

ADMINISTER FLUIDS AND MEDICATIONS

Administer intravenous fluids as ordered to maintain the child's hydration status. Antibiotics are administered intravenously, at first, then orally. Monitor the intravenous site and provide care for the central line, if one is used. See Skill 12–5 SKILLS.

In the early stages of the infection, analgesics are prescribed to relieve the associated pain and joint tenderness.

PROTECT FROM THE SPREAD OF INFECTION

Strict aseptic technique and transmission-based precautions should be used during all dressing changes. Children and family members should avoid direct contact with any dressings or drainage. Teach good hygiene practices, including hand hygiene, to maintain infection control. Take vital signs and evaluate the child frequently for symptoms indicating the spread of infection (e.g., increasing pain, difficulty breathing, increased pulse rate, fever).

ENCOURAGE A WELL-BALANCED DIET

Educate both the child and the parents about healthy dietary choices that promote healing. A high-protein diet and extra vitamin C will contribute to this process. Encourage increased fluid intake to provide adequate hydration and circulation.

DISCHARGE PLANNING AND HOME CARE TEACHING

Emphasize the importance of completing the full course of antibiotic therapy, especially for children who have had an abscess or lesion surgically drained. Some children may be discharged on intravenous antibiotics if the family is willing to learn the procedure for medication administration and care of the central line. Several sessions of demonstration and return demonstration are needed to ensure safe administration. If the family is unable to perform antibiotic therapy, a home infusion company may be available to come to the home and administer the medication. Explain that failure to follow the prescribed antibiotic therapy may result in chronic infection. Emphasize the importance of returning for blood analysis to monitor progression of healing.

Consider the child's age and developmental level and partner with the family to plan quiet activities and access to school work. Provide suggestions for the family if the child will be immobilized at home.

EVALUATION

Expected outcomes of nursing care for the child with osteomyelitis include the following:

- Absence of signs of infection or sepsis
- Completion of prescribed course of antibiotics
- Prevention of infection in contacts
- Adequate intake of fluids and nutrients
- Absence of pain
- Return to normal activities of daily living

Nursing Practice

If the child needs to remain home for a period of time during treatment for osteomyelitis, help the family plan for completion of school tasks.

- Contact the school and ask that work be sent home.
- Arrange for a tutor if needed.
- Facilitate computer communication between child, teacher, and other students.
- Help the family plan for help at home to monitor the child when the family needs to be at work or performing other tasks.
- Refer families to financial resources as appropriate for the services the child needs.
- Suggest activities that the child can do at home that foster developmental progress.

SKELETAL TUBERCULOSIS AND SEPTIC ARTHRITIS

Skeletal tuberculosis (Figure 58–11 ●) and septic arthritis are two infections that, although infrequent, may affect children and adolescents. See "Clinical Manifestations: Skeletal Tuberculosis and Septic Arthritis" for diagnostic tests and medical and nursing management for these infections.

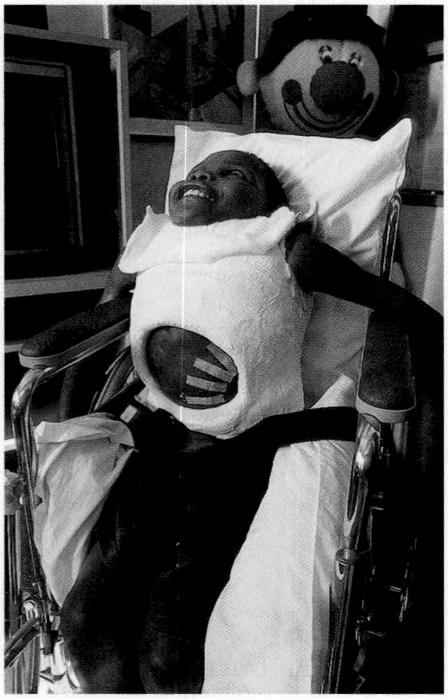

● **Figure 58–11** Risser cast. This boy from Kenya had surgery to correct severe kyphosis and scoliosis, caused by tuberculosis of the spine. A Risser cast has been applied to maintain stability of the spine and thoracic cage during healing. Notice the area cut out of the cast to allow for auscultation of the abdomen, as well as to facilitate the child's comfort and adequate intake of food.

ACHONDROPLASIA

Dwarfism is a genetic condition usually resulting in an adult height of 58 inches or less. The most common cause of dwarfism is achondroplasia, which causes short arms and legs. The torso and head are approximately normal size, but decreased growth of long bones causes short stature. This is known as disproportionate short stature. Achondroplasia is caused by an abnormal gene of chromosome 4 and occurs in 1 in 26,000 births (March of Dimes, 2007). The gene is coded to produce proteins called fibroblast growth factor receptors. When fewer receptors are produced, the cells cannot respond normally to signals from growth factors. Achondroplasia may occur as a new genetic mutation with no previous family history or can occur when one or both parents are also dwarfs. There are other less common forms of dwarfism with about 200 identified types.

Children with achondroplasia have short legs and arms, short fingers with a separation between middle and ring fingers, and a large, prominent forehead. Hydrocephalus sometimes occurs in children with achondroplasia (see Chapter 56 for a description of hydrocephalus). Most children with the disorder inherit the gene from one parent. Since only one faulty gene must be present for manifestation of the disorder, it is a dominant characteristic. When a child inherits two copies of the gene from two affected parents, a fatal form of achondroplasia occurs, which is characterized by a small thorax, respiratory failure, and death in infancy.

Children with the disorder are diagnosed prenatally, at birth or shortly after. When there is a family history, genetic testing before or after birth identifies the presence of the faulty gene. Characteristics common in the growth disorder include frequent otitis media, dental malocclusion, short fingers, bowing of legs, marked lordosis, and sleep apnea. The child may be slow at meeting gross motor developmental milestones (Trotter, Hall, & the Committee on Genetics, 2005).

There is no treatment for the disorder at this time. Gene therapy and human growth hormone therapy are being explored as possible future treatments. Some children and adults with dwarfism have undergone limb-lengthening procedures such as that described later in this chapter (see page 1776). Other orthopedic intervention may be needed to treat back pain or bone problems. For those children who develop hydrocephalus, insertion of a shunt to divert excess fluid may be needed. Treatment of conditions such as otitis media and malocclusion of teeth is provided.

Nursing Management

Nurses play an important role in helping families when a child is diagnosed with achondroplasia. If a parent is a dwarf or there is a positive family history of dwarfism, genetic counseling should be offered prenatally. Explain findings of testing and provide assistance with decision making about pregnancy if needed. Nurses assist parents who have a child with achondroplasia to adjust to the diagnosis, particularly if the parents have had no previous experience with the condition. They may feel guilt and anxiety; contact with other families who have children with achondroplasia can be a supportive intervention.

Nurses help the child with achondroplasia to develop a positive self-concept during childhood. Many resources, such as the

Clinical Manifestations

SKELETAL TUBERCULOSIS AND SEPTIC ARTHRITIS

CONDITION	CLINICAL MANIFESTATIONS	DIAGNOSTIC TESTS AND CLINICAL THERAPY	NURSING MANAGEMENT
SKELETAL TUBERCULOSIS Rare microbacterial infection that can be very destructive. The spine is the most frequent site of infection (Pott's disease), with joints and other sites sometimes affected.	Depending on the site, pain, limp, severe muscle spasms, kyphosis, muscle atrophy, "doughy" swelling of joints, decreased joint motion, changes in reflexes, low-grade fever	*Diagnostic tests:* Diagnostic studies include tuberculosis skin test, complete blood count, synovial fluid analysis, and radiographs of affected limb or joint. *Clinical therapy:* Antibiotic therapy (using a combination of drugs) for 6–9 months is the treatment of choice. The affected site is immobilized. Disease may become resistant to these drugs, and additional drug therapy may be necessary.	Educate the child and family about the disorder and stress the importance of complying with long-term antibiotic therapy. Test all members of the family for tuberculosis. Report the disease to the local health department. Facilitate the immobilization and physical therapy of the child at home.
SEPTIC ARTHRITIS Joint infection of the synovial space most often caused by Haemophilus influenzae, Staphylococcus, and Streptococcus. The most common site of infection is the knee, followed by the hip, ankle, and elbow.	Fever, pain and local inflammation, joint tenderness, swelling, loss of spontaneous movement	Diagnostic tests: CBC with differential, ESR, blood cultures. Diagnosis is made based on joint aspiration findings. Results are commonly 100,000 WBCs and 75% neutrophils, ESR .44 mm/h. Radiographic changes may not be evident until later in the disease process. Clinical therapy: This is a medical emergency requiring prompt treatment to avoid permanent disability. Treatment involves joint aspiration, open drainage, and irrigation, followed by intravenous antibiotic therapy for 3–4 weeks and then oral antibiotics. If the full course of antibiotic treatment is not completed, the child risks recurrent infection and further degeneration of the infected joint.	Educate the child and family about the disorder and emphasize the importance of proper antibiotic therapy. Carefully position the painful joint. Administer antibiotics as prescribed. Use transmission-based precautions. Encourage fluids to ensure adequate hydration. Support and rest the joint; provide activities that do not require joint movement.

Little People of America Web site, provide suggestions about how to foster a positive self-concept, adjust the home to facilitate the dwarf, and assist the child with adjustments in school settings. Partner with school nurses or counselors to ensure the child's successful inclusion in all school facilities and an individualized education plan. While some families decide to explore limb-lengthening procedures, most organizations state that focus should be placed on development of a healthy self-image rather than encouraging limb lengthening.

Nurses provide careful assessments of children throughout childhood. Head circumference is especially important in early childhood to identify hydrocephalus if it should occur. Carefully evaluate growth with specialized growth grids for achondroplasia (Trotter at al., 2005), evaluate dental health at each visit, and perform developmental assessment with special emphasis on gross motor skills. Suggest activities such as swimming and biking that provide activity with little stress on bones. Assist the family by providing resources that assist with planning for car safety seats, methods of adjusting the home, and partnering with the school to provide a supportive atmosphere for the child. Some helpful organizations include Little People of America, Dwarf Athletic Association of America, Human Growth Foundation, Magic Foundation for Children's Growth and Related Adult Disorders, and March of Dimes. Refer for care for otitis media and provide postoperative care if ear tubes are inserted (see Chapter 47). Refer to dentists and orthodontists and encourage regular dental care.

MARFAN SYNDROME

Marfan syndrome is another example of a condition inherited in an autosomal dominant manner. About 1 in 5000 children are affected with the syndrome, which manifests with several conditions of connective tissue (Ha, Seo, Lee, et al., 2007; von Kodolitsch & Robinson, 2007). The most common problems are cardiac (mitral valve prolapse, aortic regurgitation, abnormal aortic root dimensions), skeletal (pectus excavatum, long arms and digits, scoliosis, elongated head, high arched palate), ocular (lens subluxation), and respiratory (pneumothorax) (Mayo Clinic, 2007). The woman with Marfan syndrome has an increased risk of complications during pregnancy, primarily due to the extra requirements placed on the heart. The average age for diagnosis is 3 years, with a heart murmur the usual finding. Careful assessment identifies additional characteristics of the condition along with a positive family history.

Diagnosis is made after a complete family history, a detailed physical examination, an eye examination, a thorough heart examination, radiographs of the chest, and MRI or CT.

There is no treatment for the syndrome, which causes abnormal formation of fibrillin matrix in connective tissue. However, early diagnosis can be successful in treating the cardiac abnormalities with medication or surgery to prevent dissection of the aorta, the major cause of death. Diagnosis in children is often difficult because many features of Marfan syndrome are not apparent until adolescence (Mayo Clinic, 2007). Surgery may be needed to correct scoliosis, pectus excavatum, or pneumothorax. Careful monitoring throughout life is needed to prevent and treat abnormalities associated with the disorder.

Nursing Management

Nursing management of Marfan syndrome begins with identification of infants and children with symptoms of the disorder. Once diagnosed, collaboration with a cardiologist, ophthalmologist, and orthopedist is needed throughout the child's life. The child may require surgery for one or more conditions, can require antibiotics during elective procedures or dental care if the mitral valve is affected, and needs echocardiogram and other cardiac studies regularly. The nurse may need to explain the disorder to the family and provide referrals for genetic counseling. The child needs support during childhood to learn about the disorder and to manage the medication and monitoring required.

> **Thinking Critically**
>
> **AUTOSOMAL DOMINANT DISORDERS**
>
> Both achondroplasia and Marfan syndrome are autosomal dominant disorders. Does this mean that the child needs one or two genes to manifest the disorders? If one parent has the disorder, what is the chance that a pregnancy will result in an affected child? Will there ever be a carrier who does not manifest the disease? See Chapter 3 for further information about autosomal dominant inheritance.
>
> See MyNursingKit for possible responses.

OSTEOGENESIS IMPERFECTA

Osteogenesis imperfecta, also known as brittle bone disease, is a connective tissue disorder that primarily affects the bones. Children with this condition have fragile bones that are more likely to fracture. The major type of osteogenesis imperfecta occurs in 1 in 30,000 live births and affects boys and girls equally.

The underlying disorder is a biochemical defect in the production of collagen. The disease is genetically transmitted, generally in an autosomal dominant inheritance pattern, although some types are transmitted in a recessive pattern. The most common types are caused by mutations on the COL1A 1 or COL1A 2 genes on chromosomes 17 and 7 respectively (Online Mendelian Inheritance in Man, 2008).

Clinical manifestations include multiple and frequent fractures; blue sclerae; thin, soft skin; altered joint flexibility; short stature; enlargement of the anterior fontanelle; weak muscles; soft, pliable, brittle bones; and short stature. Conductive hearing loss can occur by adolescence or young adulthood (Devogelaer & Coppin, 2006).

The disease is classified into four types (Martin & Shapiro, 2007). In type I disease, the most common form, children have fragile bones, blue sclerae, weakened tooth dentin, and possible hearing loss that manifests in adolescence. In type II disease, the ribs and skeleton are extensively involved; most children with this form of the disease die in utero or shortly after birth. Type III disease is identified in the newborn period or in infancy when the child sustains numerous fractures and manifests blue sclerae. Severe bone fragility and kyphoscoliosis are observed. Type IV disease is characterized by fractures without other symptoms of the disease. Bowing of the legs and other structural deformities can occur; however, the incidence of fractures decreases beginning in puberty.

Improved knowledge about the genetic transmission of this disease means that some cases of osteogenesis imperfecta can be identified before birth using ultrasound or collagen analysis of chorionic villus cells. In many cases, however, diagnosis of osteogenesis imperfecta is made only when the child has a delay in walking or sustains a fracture. Radiographic evaluation may detect old as well as new fractures. This may lead to an erroneous diagnosis of child abuse. Tests such as DEXA can be used to measure bone density. Serum alkaline phosphatase may be elevated; other measures of bone metabolism such as serum osteocalcin, procollagen 1 C-terminal peptide, collagen 1 teleopeptide, and urine deoxypyridinoline may be performed occasionally to measure effects of medication.

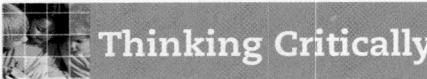

There is no cure for osteogenesis imperfecta. Medical management consists primarily of fracture care and prevention of deformities. The goal is to maximize the child's independence and mobility while minimizing the risk of fractures. Treatment includes physical therapy; casting, bracing, or splinting; surgical stabilization; nutritional management with high vitamin D and calcium; and bisphosphonate medication. Hematologic stem cell transplant has been used successfully in some children with severe osteogenesis imperfecta and is under further research (Lee & Hui, 2006).

Nursing Management

Nursing care is primarily supportive and focuses on educating the parents and child about the disease and its treatment. The family may have been suspected of child abuse before the disease was diagnosed; explain the similar presenting symptoms of these cases. Ask about favorite activities of the child since these will need to be integrated into plans for physical activity and developmental progression. Perform careful growth measurements and developmental screening.

To prevent fractures, children with osteogenesis imperfecta must be handled gently. Support the trunk and extremities using a blanket whenever moving the child. Tasks such as bathing and diapering may cause fractures and should be performed carefully. Never pull the legs upward during diaper changes, but slip a hand gently under the hips to raise them.

Children commonly have several fractures during childhood. The period of immobility and casting causes further bone breakdown due to decreased weight bearing, further increasing the chance of fracture. The child should have a well-balanced diet with additional vitamin C, vitamin D, and calcium to encourage healing and bone growth. Calories should be limited to maintain weight at recommended levels since immobility can lead to overweight and the child is generally short for his or her age. Partner with parents if the child is receiving experimental bisphosphonate medication so that doses are properly administered and serum/urine samples are obtained for monitoring.

When the child needs a fracture stabilized in surgery, or is having rods inserted to strengthen bones, surgical care management is important. Assess the child's vital signs and growth measurements. Obtain accurate weight before surgery and again after with the cast in place. Administer fluids and use pain control techniques such as medication and other comfort measures. Be alert for signs of infection such as osteomyelitis, or respiratory or urinary tract infection. Begin fluids and perform dietary teaching before discharge to promote intake that fosters healing. Follow activity orders precisely to minimize safety hazards for the child. Partner with physical and occupational therapists to plan for the child's return to home and school, and to ensure the family can perform range of motion exercises and other therapies. Ensure that the family has an approved car safety seat to transport the child.

Emphasize the importance of maintaining normal patterns of growth and development. Help toddlers explore and interact safely in their environment. Socialization is essential during the school-age and adolescent years. Encourage exercise, such as swimming, to improve muscle tone and prevent obesity. Adaptive equipment and motorized wheelchairs promote independent functioning. Maintenance of function can depend on proper rehabilitation services. Arrange and manage such services for the family.

The Osteogenesis Imperfecta Foundation provides information about the disease and can put families in touch with others who have the disease. See My Nursing Kit for links to these resources. Parents should receive genetic counseling. For parents who have a child with type II or III osteogenesis imperfecta, the terminal nature of the condition necessitates psychologic support, linkage to potential resources, and assistance with managing other tasks of family life (see Chapter 43 for management of end-of-life care). The siblings and extended family will need support to understand the disease and deal with their feelings and the affected child.

Expected outcomes include minimal fractures with optimal healing, normal range of motion, maintenance of a healthy diet and recommended weight, achievement of developmental milestones, family support, and adequate resources to provide necessary treatments for the child.

MUSCULAR DYSTROPHIES

The muscular dystrophies are a group of inherited diseases characterized by muscle fiber degeneration and muscle wasting. These disorders can begin early or late in life, and onset can be at birth or gradual. They are all terminal disorders but the progression can vary from a few to many years.

Many types of muscular dystrophies affect children and adults. The most common form of childhood muscular dystrophy is Duchenne muscular dystrophy (pseudohypertrophic), which occurs in 2.2 to 5.5 of 10,000 live male births (Kemper & Wake, 2007). **Pseudohypertrophy** refers to enlargement of the muscles as a result of their infiltration with fatty tissue. The gene for Duchenne muscular dystrophy was identified in 1987; it is carried in the Xp21.2 region of the chromosome and is either absent or deleted in affected children. This area codes for a protein called dystrophin, which is needed as a muscle membrane stabilizer. In the absence of dystrophin, a cascade of cellular events occurs, leading to necrosis in the fibers and their replacement by connective tissue. Since this is an X-linked disorder, it is seen only in males. There is similar incidence in various ethnic groups.

Becker muscular dystrophy is also X-linked and affects 1 in 30,000 males (American Academy of Pediatrics, Section on Cardiology and Cardiac Surgery, 2005). Although the gene mutation is similar to Duchenne, it is milder in form. Other rare muscular dystrophies manifest in infancy, later childhood, or adolescence. There are a variety of genetic mutations ranging from X-linked to autosomal.

Children with muscular dystrophy have generalized muscle weakness. They compensate for weak lower extremities by using the upper extremity muscles to raise themselves to a standing position (Gowers' maneuver) (Figure 58–12 ●). (See "Clinical Manifestations: Muscular Dystrophies of Childhood.")

Diagnosis and classification are most often based on clinical signs and the pattern of muscle involvement. Biochemical examinations such as serum enzyme assay, muscle biopsy, and electromyography confirm the diagnosis. Serum creatine kinase (CK) is elevated early in the disease. Muscle biopsy can measure dystrophin, the muscle protein that is deficient in muscular dystrophy. Genetic testing establishes the specific abnormality and type of disease present. Testing of newborns may be offered to families who have one child with the disease since this helps some

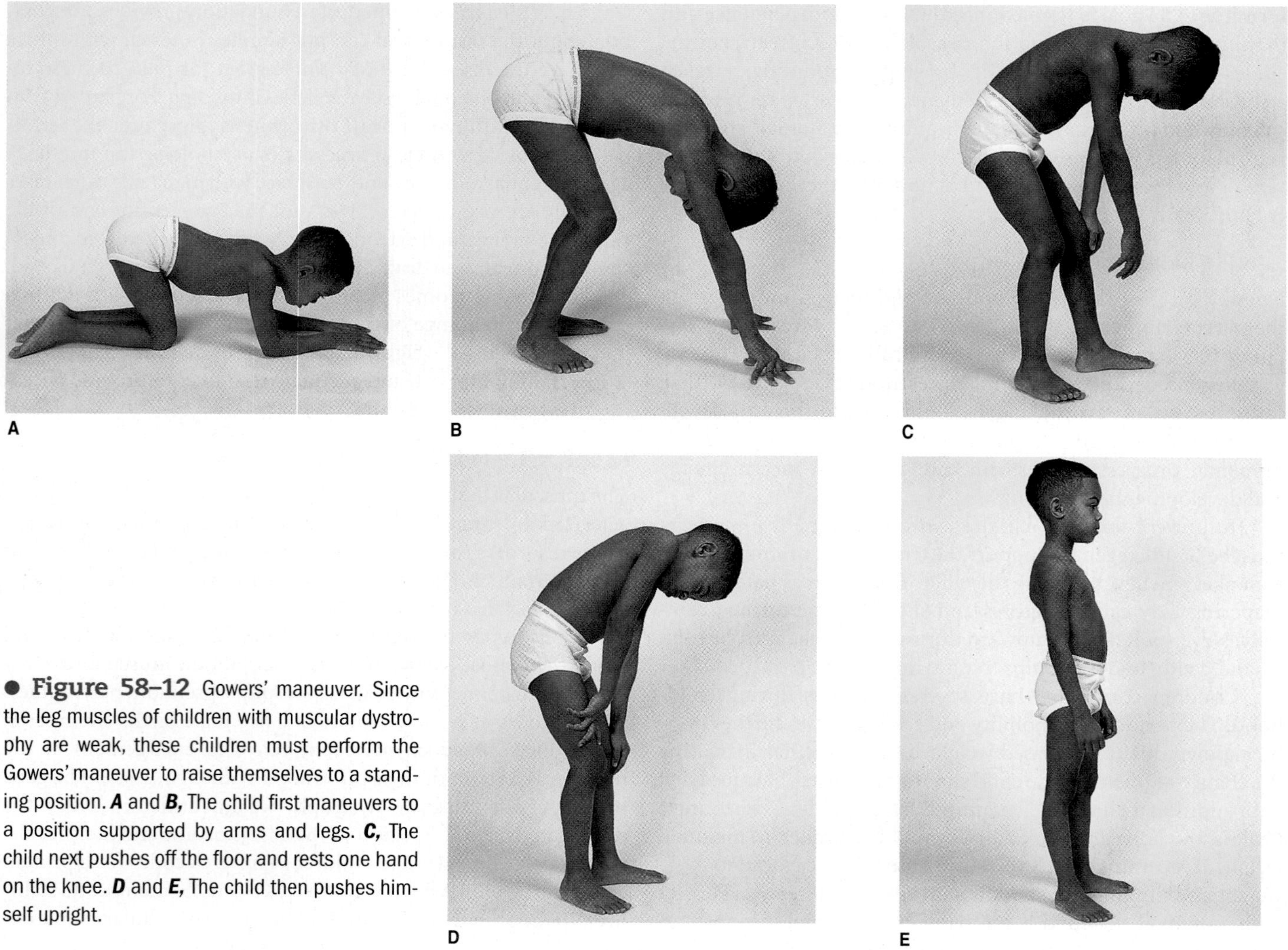

● **Figure 58–12** Gowers' maneuver. Since the leg muscles of children with muscular dystrophy are weak, these children must perform the Gowers' maneuver to raise themselves to a standing position. ***A*** and ***B,*** The child first maneuvers to a position supported by arms and legs. ***C,*** The child next pushes off the floor and rests one hand on the knee. ***D*** and ***E,*** The child then pushes himself upright.

families to adapt and prepare for the care the child will need. Respiratory function is measured periodically with pulmonary function tests and overnight pulse oximetry (Beck, Weinberg, Hamnegard, et al., 2006).

There is no effective treatment for childhood muscular dystrophy. Research is being directed at several techniques to repair mutations by gene therapy, override the genetic error in order to produce dystrophin and apply stem cell therapy (Kuehn, 2007; Lee & Hui, 2006). The steroids prednisone and deflazacort may preserve muscle function, preserving walking for a longer period. Rehabilitative therapy is needed to maximize independence and physical activity and to decrease hazards of immobility. Children and families can benefit from mental health support due to the progressive and terminal nature of the disease.

Progressive weakness and muscle deformity result in chronic disability (Figure 58–13 ●). Respiratory infections are vigorously

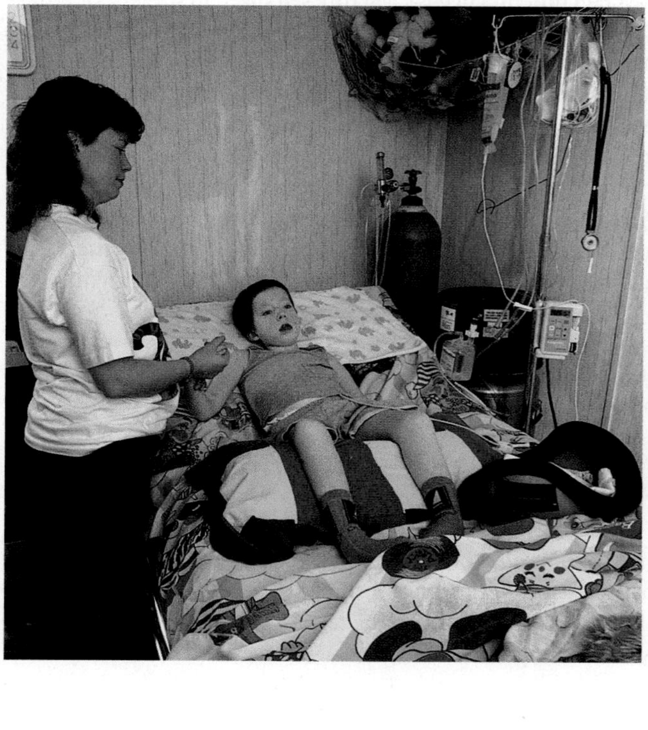

● **Figure 58–13** Muscular dystrophy. This young boy with muscular dystrophy needs to receive tube feedings and home nursing care. He attends school when possible and is able to use an adapted computer.

Clinical Manifestations

MUSCULAR DYSTROPHIES OF CHILDHOOD

TYPE OF DYSTROPHY	CLINICAL MANIFESTATIONS	CLINICAL THERAPY
DUCHENNE MUSCULAR DYSTROPHY		
X-linked recessive disorder seen in boys (on Xp21 gene); however, 30–50% of affected children have no family history Onset: within the first 3–4 years of life	Delayed walking; frequent falls; easily tired when walking, running, or climbing stairs; toe walking, hypertrophied calves; waddling gait; lordosis; positive Gowers' maneuver; mental retardation frequently seen	Supportive care; physical therapy and braces to help maintain mobility and prevent contractures Most children are wheelchair bound by 12 years of age; death usually occurs during adolescence from respiratory or cardiac failure
BECKER MUSCULAR DYSTROPHY		
X-linked recessive disorder Onset: usually after 5 years	Symptoms are similar to those of Duchenne muscular dystrophy, but milder and delayed; child is mobile until late teens; normal intelligence; congestive heart failure; contractures	Supportive care, same as for Duchenne muscular dystrophy Slow progression; death usually occurs from the third to the fifth decade of life
FACIOSCAPULOHUMERAL MUSCULAR DYSTROPHY		
Autosomal dominant disorder (on 4q35 chromosome) Onset: later childhood and adolescence	Face, shoulder girdle, lower limbs affected; unable to raise arms over head; lordosis; cannot close eyes, whistle, smile, or drink from a straw because of inability to move face; characteristic appearance includes facial weakness, winging of the scapula, thin arms, well-developed forearms	Physical therapy Slow progression; confined to wheelchair as older adult, but usually attains normal life span
EMERY-DREIFUSS MUSCULAR DYSTROPHY		
X-linked recessive disorder (on Xq28 gene) Onset: childhood	Early onset of contractures followed by weakness; Achilles' tendon, elbow, and spine affected; muscle weakness in upper body follows, with lower body weakness occurring later; cardiac conduction defect may occur	Physical therapy Surgery Pacemaker insertion
CONGENITAL MUSCULAR DYSTROPHIES		
Autosomal recessive group of disorders Onset: present at birth	Muscle weaknesses present at birth; motor development delay; contractures and joint deformities; hypotonia	Correction of skeletal deformity (orthosis or surgery) Usually nonprogressive

treated with deep breathing, coughing, nebulizer treatments, and antibiotics. Comprehensive and regular cardiac evaluations are recommended (American Academy of Pediatrics, 2005). The team approach to managing the child with muscular dystrophy ensures a comprehensive management plan. Team members should include physicians (pediatrician, orthopedic surgeon, neurologist), nurses, physical and occupational therapists, a nutritionist, psychologist or mental health therapist, and a social worker.

Nursing Management

Nursing care focuses on promoting independence and mobility and providing psychosocial support that helps the child and family deal with this progressive, incapacitating disease. Nearly all body systems become involved in the disease, and emotional care is important as well for child and family.

Monitor cardiac and respiratory functioning frequently. Assess urinary function and frequency of bowel movements. Periodically measure strength and range of motion. Assess mobility via ambulation or assisted device. Perform periodic developmental and nutritional assessments. Meet with teachers to evaluate the child's learning needs and functional level in the classroom. Evaluate the family's risk and protective factors for dealing with this chronic and fatal disorder.

Administer oxygen or respiratory therapy as ordered. Encourage the child to be independent for as long as possible. Concentrate on what the child can accomplish, and do not ask the child to complete tasks that may prove frustrating. Encourage parents to establish an individualized education plan with the school system. Reading books to the child, listening to tapes, and watching television offer the child stimulation

HEALTH PROMOTION

THE CHILD WITH MUSCULAR DYSTROPHY

The child with muscular dystrophy needs close monitoring and intervention to foster growth and development in spite of a chronic and terminal disease. The nurse in health promotion can assist the child and family in many ways.

Growth and Development Surveillance

- Perform developmental screening of the young child.
- Refer to early intervention programs that establish educational plans to foster development.
- Provide resources and ideas for the parents based on the child's status rather than expected age norms.
- Measure growth at each healthcare visit and plot on growth grids. Be alert for the child who is gaining weight due to decreased activity in order to avoid overweight.
- Ensure visits with specialists in respiratory medicine and cardiology as recommended.

Nutrition

- Perform 24-hour analysis and evaluate for all essential nutrients. Base the analysis on the child's height and weight rather than chronological age.
- Ask about appetite and food likes and dislikes.
- Encourage adequate fluid, whole grains, fruits, and vegetables to maintain bowel function.
- For the infant with muscular dystrophy, evaluate intake carefully; gavage feeding or nutritional supplementation such as with high-calorie formula may be needed.

Physical Activity

- Carefully monitor physical ability at each visit. Observe for decreases in movement, difficulty ambulating, or a history of falls.
- Partner with physical therapists to ensure range of motion and proper positioning of extremities.
- Explore activities that the child can do as mobility decreases. Swimming and upper body exercise may be good options.
- If the child is using a wheelchair, evaluate fit, safety, and ability to move the chair by arm controls.
- Physical activity should be regular and daily. Ensure that the family has resources to accomplish this need.

Activities of Daily Living

- Partner with occupational therapy to evaluate the child's ability to feed, bathe, dress, and provide own oral care. Provide adaptive devices as needed.
- Encourage the family to provide time for the child to perform own self-care as much as possible.
- Make a home visit or discuss with the family adaptations that could make it easier for the child to be independent in activities of daily living. Low drawers for clothing, or open shelves that do not require pulling out to get items are examples of important adaptations.

Mental and Spiritual Health

- Inquire about the child's general mood.
- Ask the parents what is best and worst about their lives at this time. Use the information to establish a list of their meaningful activities and to identify the areas most in need of support.
- Ask about sources of support such as a group for parents of a child with muscular dystrophy, family participation in faith-based activity, and extended family or neighbors.
- Be alert for signs of depression in child or family (see Chapter 57).

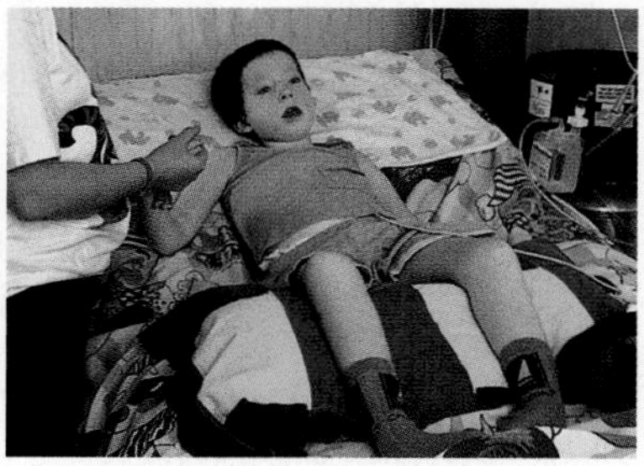

- Assist the family to establish activities to increase self-esteem in the youth. The youth should be able to make choices appropriate for developmental age.
- If the child was diagnosed at a younger age, ask what the parents have now told him or her about the disease. Provide support and role-playing opportunities for parents who wish to tell the child about the terminal nature of the disorder.
- Refer for services such as genetic counseling, grief counseling, or other supportive interventions.

Relationships

- Ask about siblings and their relationship with the child with muscular dystrophy.
- Inquire about the child's participation in early intervention or school programs, and community groups. Refer the family to resources that encourage the child's interactions with peers. This is particularly important for teens.
- Ask the parents if and how often they are able to spend time with other adults.

Disease Prevention Strategies

- Immunize the child at recommended times. If the child is ill and immunization is delayed, be sure to call the family back promptly to reschedule administration of vaccines so that infectious diseases can be avoided. Annual influenza vaccine is needed. If the child is treated with steroids for the disease, follow recommendations for immunization of children on steroids.
- Teach the family to avoid crowds and known infectious persons. The child may need to be out of school for a few days or weeks if there is an influenza or other disease outbreak in the school population.
- Teach the family signs of infection, especially of the respiratory tract. Have them report these symptoms promptly.
- Monitor effects of antibiotics when administered for infection.
- Encourage daily activities that encourage deep breathing. Swimming, blowing into an incentive spirometer, or playing with a pinwheel are examples.

Injury Prevention Strategies

- Inquire about whether the family has an emergency evacuation plan for the child in case of house fire or other emergency. Assist them to develop a plan.
- If the child is using oxygen, teach about fire safety.
- When mechanical ventilation is used at home, help the family establish emergency backup systems for power outage, such as portable generators.
- Assist the family to learn proper body mechanics to safely transfer and provide care for the child.

Complementary Care

MUSCULAR DYSTROPHY

Many families who have a child with muscular dystrophy will use different types of complementary care. The nurse always assesses for such approaches, provides information as needed by the family, makes recommendations for complementary therapies that may be helpful, and cautions against those that could be harmful due to interactions with medications or other problems. A common complementary care used for muscular dystrophy is dietary enhancement. This enhancement includes giving vitamins A, C, E, D, and B-complex; minerals such as calcium, magnesium, zinc, and selenium; probiotic supplement; omega-3 fatty acids; herbal remedies such as green and rhodioloa rosea teas; muscular and immunologic enzymes such as coenzyme Q10, N-acetyl cysteine, acetyl-L-carnitine, creatine, L-theanine; and melatonin to promote sleep. Massage is often used to assist with reduction of muscle spasms (University of Maryland Medical Center, 2007).

during hospitalization. Exercise as tolerated contributes to muscle strength. Physical therapy helps the child ambulate and prevents joint contractures. It is important to provide good back support and posture by keeping the child's body in alignment when confined to a wheelchair.

Parents may feel guilty and hopeless. Encourage parents to express their feelings. Genetic counseling is recommended for the entire family, and it is especially important to identify female relatives who are carriers of one of the X-linked disorders. Siblings may feel neglected because their brother or sister is receiving so much attention. They may be concerned that they will develop the disease, and in some families, this indeed occurs. Encourage the parents to spend individual time with each child and to involve siblings in the child's care.

Refer family members to resource and support groups such as the Muscular Dystrophy Association. The Companion Website contains such resources. Provide ongoing support during hospitalizations, management of home care, and the child's changes in condition.

INJURIES TO THE MUSCULOSKELETAL SYSTEM

Musculoskeletal injuries are classified according to the mechanism, the location, and the force of the injury. Strains, sprains, dislocations, and fractures are the most common musculoskeletal injuries in children; athletic participation and injuries from car crashes are frequent causes. Distinguishing among these injuries is often difficult. See "Clinical Manifestations: Strains, Sprains, and Dislocations." See Evidence-Based Nursing for a discussion of backpack use by children. A detailed discussion of fractures follows.

Evidence-Based Nursing

DO HEAVY BACKPACKS CAUSE BACK PAIN?

Clinical Question

Many children wear backpacks that are heavy and are carried for large parts of the day. Low back, neck, and shoulder pain seem to be increasing in children (Shilt & Barnett, 2007), and a possible connection with backpacks has been suggested.

Evidence

Several studies have now investigated the relationships between backpack use and complaints of pain. In one study of over 500 youth, student backpacks were weighed and the student was also weighed. The students were then interviewed about back pain incidence. Pain was reported more often by females (57.8%) than males (38.9%). Backpack weight was higher (11.8% of body weight) for those reporting pain than backpack weight (10% of body weight) for those not reporting pain (Moore, White, & Moore, 2007). In another study of 1263 adolescents, back pain was also more common among females, and it was associated with assymetrical carrying of backpacks. The researchers found that such asymmetry caused shifts of upper trunk and shoulders, leading to cervical lordosis (Korovessis, Koureas, Zacharatos, et al., 2005). Another study found that female pain reports were associated with lower body mass index in the females. The researchers suggest further studies to include separate populations of males and females, quantification of time spent carrying backpacks, and whether stairs are climbed with packs in place (Navuluri & Navuluri, 2006).

Best Practice

A clear association between backpack use and weight and complaints of pain appears to be evident, especially among females. Therefore, nurses should ask about backpack use at health promotion visits and advise on how to wear them. The American Academy of Pediatrics and North American Spine Society list recommendations for backpack use:

- Have wide, padded shoulder straps and wear the pack on both shoulders, close to the body.
- Use a padded back and waist strap.
- Be sure the backpack is lightweight (no more than 10%–15% of the youth's weight) or consider a rolling pack if it is heavy.
- Practice back strengthening exercises and learn to bend at the knees when lifting objects.

Critical Thinking

How will you partner with youth who are in sports after school to plan how to carry school items and sports gear safely? What exercises can you plan to help strengthen the back and thighs for carrying a pack? What children are most at risk for back pain from heavy backpacks (consider gender and weight)?

See MyNursingKit for possible responses.

Clinical Manifestations

STRAINS, SPRAINS, AND DISLOCATIONS

CONDITION	CLINICAL MANIFESTATIONS	CLINICAL THERAPY
STRAIN		
■ Stretching or tearing of either a muscle or a tendon, usually from overuse (example: back strain resulting from improper or overly heavy lifting).	■ Vary according to the type and severity of the strain. Pain can be acute or chronic.	■ Rest and support of the injured part until the muscle or tendon heals and normal activity can occur.
SPRAIN		
■ Stretching or tearing of a ligament, usually caused by falls, sports injuries, or motor vehicle crashes. For example, an anterior cruciate ligament (ACL) tear is a severe sprain requiring reconstruction.	■ Edema, joint immobility, and pain.	■ For the first 24–36 hours: **R**est **I**ce **C**ompression **E**levation ■ After the first 24–36 hours, mobility is gradually increased.
DISLOCATION		
■ Complete displacement of an articular joint surface, usually associated with falls, sports injuries, or motor vehicle crashes. Although almost any joint may be dislocated, most dislocations occur in the shoulder, knee, and hip.	■ Pain and tenderness, swelling and obvious deformity, and instability of the joint.	■ Varies according to the site and severity of the injury, and consists of: Shoulder: Open or closed reduction followed by the application of a sling. Knee: Closed reduction with gentle traction, then immobilization with a splint. Hip (posterior): Immediate closed reduction or possibly open reduction, traction, or hip spica cast. Hip (anterior): Immediate closed reduction, extension traction, and hip spica cast.

MyNursingKit Case Study: Fracture Assessment

FRACTURES

A fracture is a break in a bone that occurs when more stress is placed on the bone than the bone can withstand. Fractures may occur at any age; they are frequent in children because their bones are less dense and more porous than those of adults (see "Pathophysiology Illustrated: Classification and Types of Fractures").

Etiology and Pathophysiology

Fractures in children may result from direct trauma to a bone (falls, sports injuries, abuse, motor vehicle crashes) or bone diseases that result in weakening of the bone (osteogenesis imperfecta). Children with osteoporosis or osteopenia are more prone to fractures (see description of these conditions earlier in the chapter). Trauma may be caused by an acute injury, by direct and forceful impact, or by overuse such as in chronic and repetitive activities. Child abuse is a cause of fracture and should be suspected when the type of fracture is uncommon for a given age (see Chapter 44∞).

Clinical Manifestations

Signs and symptoms of fractures vary depending on the location, type, and nature of the causative injury. Fractures are generally characterized by pain, abnormal positioning, edema, immobility or decreased range of motion, ecchymosis, guarding, and crepitus. Childhood fractures most often involve the clavicle, tibia, ulna, and femur, with distal forearm fractures the most common type (Carson, Woolridge, Colletti, et al., 2006). Douglass, described in the opening vignette, had a fracture of his tibia. Fractures to the pelvis

Growth and Development

Stress fractures are becoming more common in adolescents and are most common in those who limit their intake of calories and calcium in an attempt to remain lean for sports such as distance running or gymnastics. These fractures may present with chronic pain that changes in intensity. Be alert to this possibility when teenagers' diets and athletic activities place them at risk. The risk of bone fractures is significantly increased with high cola consumption and television viewing time and with lower levels of physical activity and lower milk intake (Manias, McCabe, & Bishop, 2006). Teach healthy diet and activity patterns to youth and their families to decrease these health risks.

PATHOPHYSIOLOGY ILLUSTRATED

CLASSIFICATION AND TYPES OF FRACTURES

CLASSIFICATION

Complete (transverse) fracture

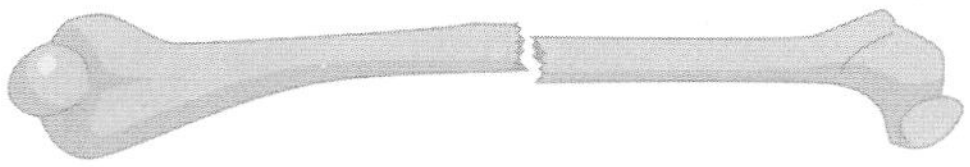

Break across entire section of a bone at a right angle to the bone shaft resulting in two or more fragments

Open fracture

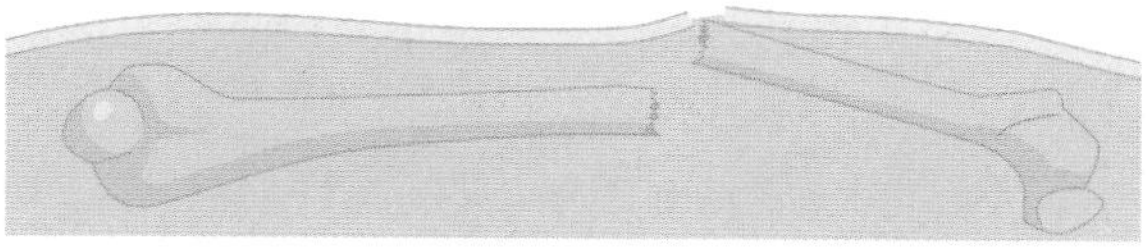

Broken bone protrudes through the skin leaving a path to the fracture site; high risk of infection exists

Greenstick fracture

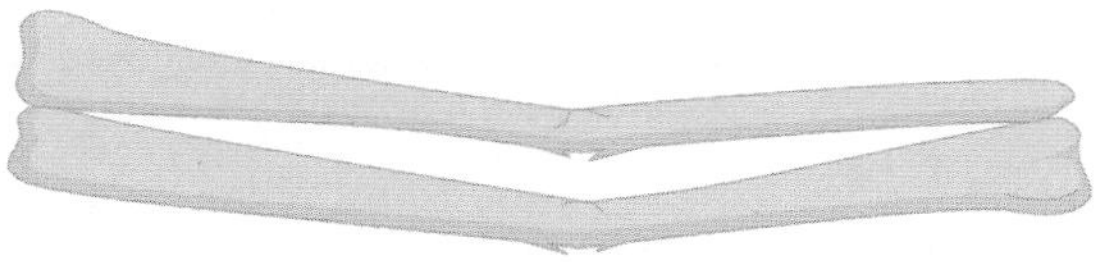

Caused by compression force; often seen in young children

TYPE

Spiral fracture

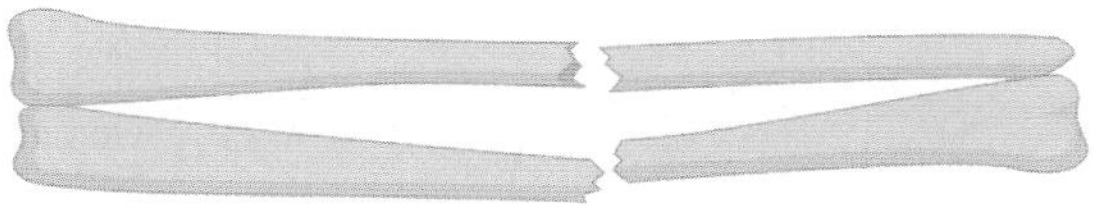

Associated with twisting force; fracture coils around the bone

Closed fracture

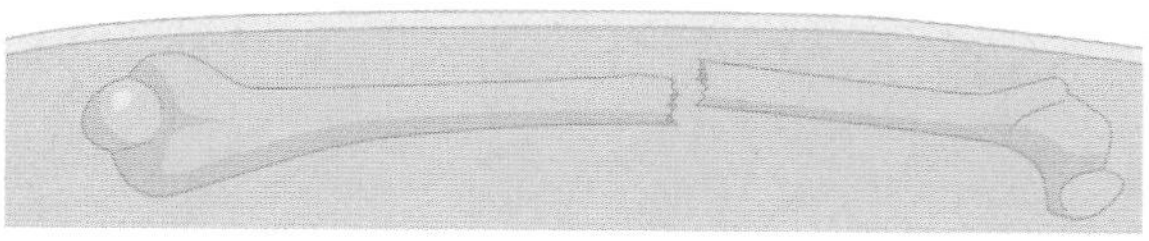

Broken bone does not protrude through the skin

Comminuted fracture

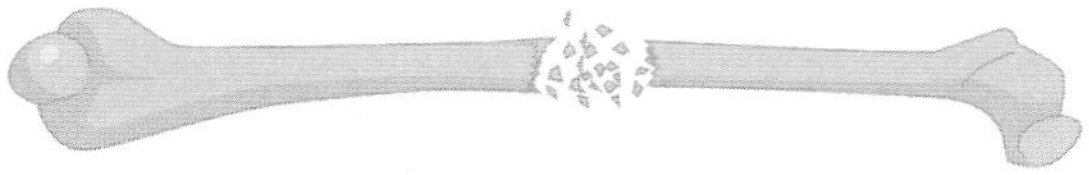

Associated with high-impact forces; bone breaks into three or more segments

Additional types of fractures include: incomplete, in which the break occurs in only one side of the cortex; oblique, in which the fracture slants across the long axis of the bone; compression, in which two bones are jammed together (usually occurs in spinal area); and compacted, in which one bone fragment is wedged into another.

are often associated with motor vehicle crashes. Epiphyseal injuries are dangerous in children as they can interfere with bone growth at the site. These injuries are described using the Salter-Harris classification system (Figure 58–14 ●).

Clinical Therapy

Emergency care focuses on accurate diagnosis, pain management, and establishment of a treatment plan. Radiographs are useful for determining the exact location and type of the fracture. Medical management consists of two basic steps: (1) reduction to realign displaced or fragmented bones, and (2) immobilization so that healing can take place.

Immobilization is needed for bone healing A closed reduction aligns the bone by manual manipulation or traction. Sedation and additional pain management techniques will be used during closed reduction. An open reduction requires surgical alignment of the bone, often using pins, plates, wires, or screws. For open fractures, surgery must also be performed for debridement, to remove dead tissue and clean the wound. Casting is the most common external method of immobilization. Casts may be placed on extremities (short or long leg or arm cast), the upper body to immobilize the spine, or from chest to legs to stabilize pelvis or hips (spica cast). Leg casts may be walking or nonwalking casts. Cast material is either plaster or a synthetic fabric. Other external methods of stabilization include traction and splinting (see Table 58–3 later in this chapter for types of traction). Pins may be inserted to stabilize the fracture, and can be used with or without casts or traction. A child with multiple fractures following a car crash or other trauma may need a combination of treatments.

Immobilization is essential for the bone-healing process. Healing of fractures is influenced by factors including age, size of the involved bone, and fracture site. Fractures heal more quickly in children than in adults. If a fracture is properly

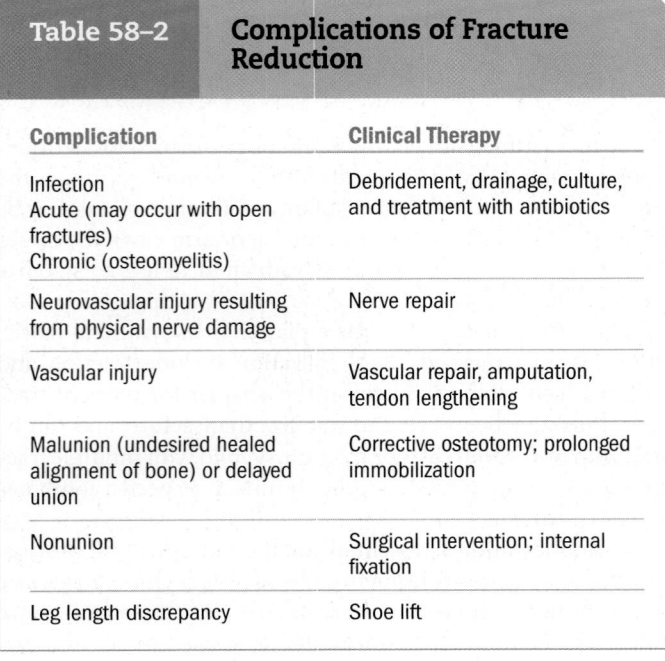

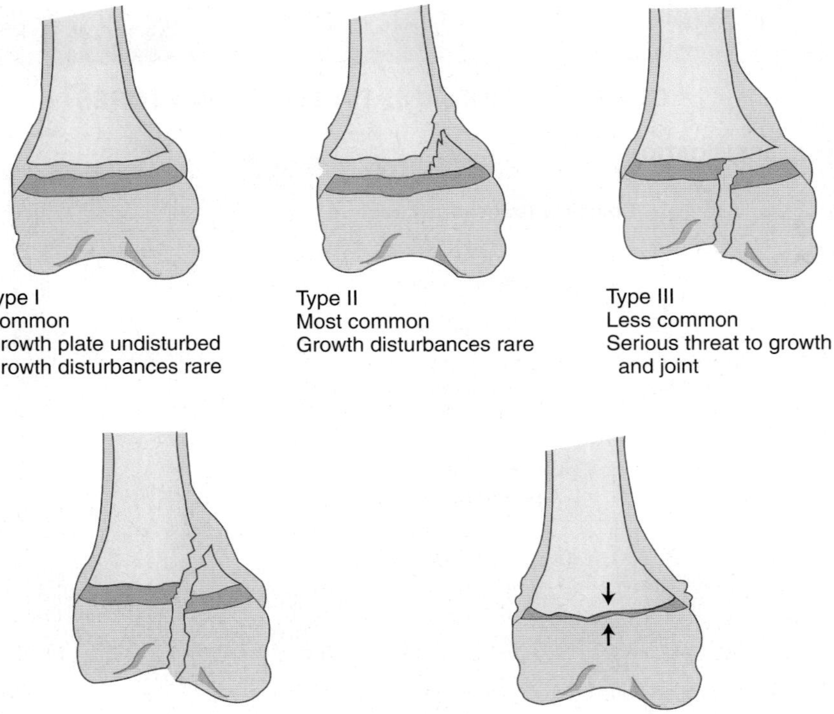
Type I
Common
Growth plate undisturbed
Growth disturbances rare
Type II
Most common
Growth disturbances rare
Type III
Less common
Serious threat to growth and joint
Type IV
Serious threat to growth
Type V
Rare
Crush injury causes cell death in growth plate, resulting in arrested growth and limited bone length
If growth plate is partially destroyed, angular deformities may result

● **Figure 58–14** Salter-Harris classification system. The Salter-Harris classification system is based on the angle of the fracture in relation to the epiphysis.

reduced, complications should be minimal (Table 58–2). Fractures involving the epiphyseal growth plate must be treated properly to minimize the chance for limb length discrepancy, joint incongruity, and angular deformities.

Table 58–2 Complications of Fracture Reduction

Complication	Clinical Therapy
Infection Acute (may occur with open fractures) Chronic (osteomyelitis)	Debridement, drainage, culture, and treatment with antibiotics
Neurovascular injury resulting from physical nerve damage	Nerve repair
Vascular injury	Vascular repair, amputation, tendon lengthening
Malunion (undesired healed alignment of bone) or delayed union	Corrective osteotomy; prolonged immobilization
Nonunion	Surgical intervention; internal fixation
Leg length discrepancy	Shoe lift

NURSING MANAGEMENT

NURSING ASSESSMENT AND DIAGNOSIS

When dealing with an injured child, be alert to the signs and symptoms of fractures before moving the child. When in doubt about the type of injury, apply a splint to immobilize the joints above and below the injury. Try to identify the cause of the injury by asking the child, parents, or other family members what happened. Evaluate pain, edema, and any abnormal positioning of the injured area. When a child is admitted to the emergency department or hospital, nursing assessment includes the extent of the injury, the degree of pain, and the child's vital signs (respiratory status, pulse, and blood pressure). Monitor all systems since infection, fat emboli, and other problems can emerge during the treatment period.

Several nursing diagnoses may apply to the child with a fracture. They include the following:

- *Pain* related to injury
- *Risk for Impaired Skin Integrity* related to treatment
- *Risk for Infection* related to open fracture or trauma
- *Impaired Physical Mobility* related to treatment
- *Health-Seeking Behaviors* related to lack of information about treatment and expected outcome

PLANNING AND IMPLEMENTATION

Nurses may be in community settings when children experience a fracture and may need to provide emergency care and arrange for transport. Inform emergency personnel of the assessment data to provide for safe care. In addition, be aware that repeated fractures in the same child can be a sign of other healthcare conditions. Young children may have osteogenesis imperfecta, an older child may be experimenting with risky behavior, and child abuse may have occurred if there are several fractures in various states of healing or if the parental explanation does not match the clinical presentation. Nursing care focuses on care of the child before and after fracture reduction, encouraging mobility as ordered, maintaining skin integrity, preventing infection, and teaching the parents and child how to care for the fracture. If sedation or pain blocks are used, nursing care for these procedures is needed. See Skill 13–4 **SKILLS**. When caring for a child who has undergone fracture reduction, it is important to know the signs of complications. Notify the physician immediately if these signs occur. The major serious complication is **compartment syndrome**, or a condition of increased pressure in a limited space such as the soft tissue of an extremity, which compromises circulation and nervous innervation. (See "Clinical Manifestations: Compartment Syndrome.")

MAINTAIN PROPER ALIGNMENT

Immobilization maintains proper alignment of the fracture. Casts and traction are methods used for immobilizing an injured child. Cast care guidelines are included in Table 58–1, earlier in this chapter.

Different types of traction are used, depending on the location and type of fracture (Table 58–3). Nursing care for the child in traction is described in Table 58–4.

MONITOR NEUROVASCULAR STATUS

Neurovascular assessment is used for early detection of compartment syndrome. Compartment syndrome may occur with a crush injury or when a fracture is reduced. The swelling of inflammation reduces blood flow to the affected area, and casting causes further constriction of blood flow. Douglass, who was described in the chapter opener quote, had a splint applied for several days, with casting later, to allow swelling to decrease and to minimize risk for compartment syndrome. Monitor the child's sensation to touch, temperature, movement, strength of the pulse, and capillary refill time in the extremity distal to the injury. Monitor every 15 minutes after the cast is applied for at least 2 hours and then every 1 to 2 hours, depending on the facility's policy and the child's condition. Keep the cast elevated above heart level to minimize edema. Report symptoms of compartment syndrome immediately as permanent damage to nerves and circulatory system can occur.

PROMOTE MOBILITY

The amount of mobility the child is allowed is ordered by the physician; restrictions depend on the extent and site of the fracture. Fractures of the hip or pelvis may involve body casts; wheeled carts make mobility possible. Children with leg fractures can sometimes bear weight on the cast, but if they cannot, they move around with crutches, walkers, or wheelchairs. See Skill 17–7 **SKILLS**.

> **Clinical Manifestations**
>
> **COMPARTMENT SYNDROME**
>
> Clinical manifestations begin about 30 minutes after tissue ischemia starts. Major manifestations are:
>
> - Paresthesia (tingling, burning, loss of 2-point discrimination)
> - Pain (unrelieved by medication, characterized by crying in the young child)
> - Pressure (skin is tense, cast appears tight)
> - Pallor* (pale, gray or white skin tone)
> - Paralysis* (weakness or inability to move extremity)
> - Pulselessness* (weak or absent pulse)
>
> * = late sign
>
> Check extremities for:
>
> - Color
> - Temperature
> - Capillary refill
> - Peripheral pulses
> - Edema
> - Sensation
> - Motor ability
> - Pain
>
> Document results and report changes or abnormal results immediately. Changes are a medical emergency (Grottkau, Epps, & DiScala, 2005).

DISCHARGE PLANNING AND HOME CARE TEACHING

Most fractures can be easily managed at home. Activities are generally limited for approximately 8 weeks. Teach the parents and child cast care, activity restrictions, and how to identify problems that should be reported (see page 1746). Help parents to identify any modifications that may be needed at home and school. The child who has to manage steps at home or school may need special training with crutches or a temporary ramp. Refer parents to home health nurses or home teaching services if indicated. Provide pertinent teaching to prevent future injuries. Reinforce the need for protective gear for many sports (see Chapter 44).

EVALUATION

Desired outcomes for treatment of injuries is proper healing of the body parts affected, return to usual strength and range of motion, and no impairment of musculoskeletal development.

SPORTS INJURIES

Sports injuries are the most common type of injury in youth from 13 to 19 years. Football, cycling, and basketball are the sports most commonly associated with injury (Simon, Bublitz, & Hambidge, 2006). Fractures, described earlier, are common sports injuries of young athletes, and may be treated on an outpatient basis or may require surgery and hospitalization (Deakin, Crosby & Moran et al.,

Table 58–3 Types of Traction

Skin Traction
Pull is applied to the skin surface, which puts traction directly on the bones and muscles. Traction is attached to the skin with adhesive materials or straps, or foam boots, belts, or halters.

Dunlop Traction (can be either skeletal or skin)
Used for fracture of the humerus. The flexed arm is suspended horizontally with straps placed on both the upper and lower portions for pull from both sides.

Skeletal Traction
Pull is directly applied to the bone by pins, wires, tongs, or other apparatus that have been surgically placed through the distal end of the bone.

Skeletal Cervical Traction
Used for cervical spine injuries to reduce fractures and dislocations. Crutchfield, Gardner-Wells, or Vinke tongs are placed in the skull with bur holes. Weights are attached to the apparatus with a rope and pulley system to the hyperextended head.

Halo Traction
Used to immobilize the head and neck after cervical injury or dislocation. Also used for positioning and immobilization after cervical injury.

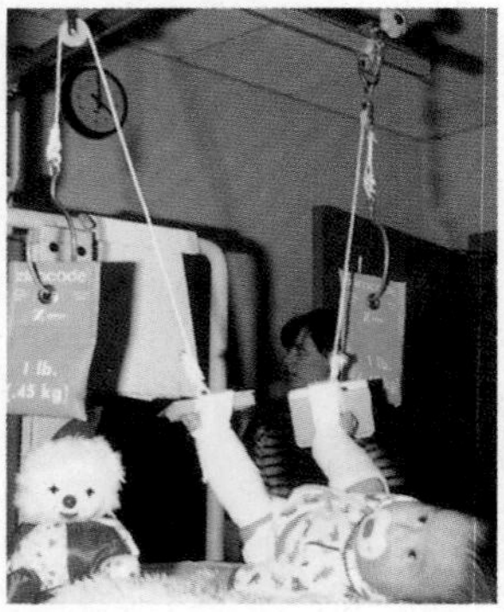

A

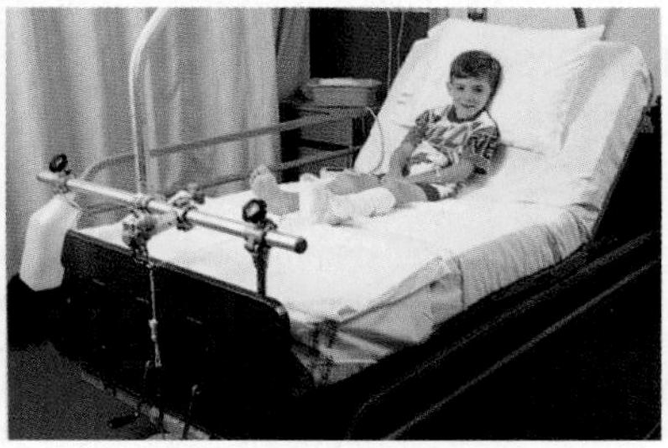
B

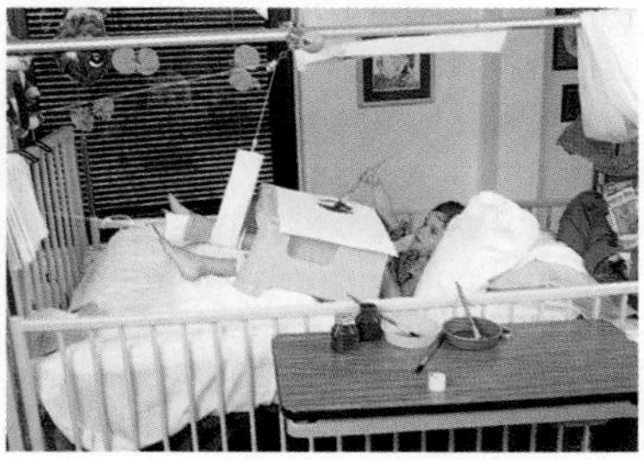
C

Bryant Traction (A)
Used specifically for the child under 3 years of age and weighing less than 35 pounds (17.5 kg), who has developmental dysplasia of the hip or a fractured femur. This bilateral traction is applied to the child's legs and kept in place by wrapping the legs from foot to thigh with elastic bandages. The hips are flexed at a 90-degree angle, with knees extended. This position is maintained by attaching the traction appliance to weights and pulleys suspended above the crib. The buttocks do not rest on the mattress, but are slightly elevated off the bed.

Buck Traction (B)
Used for knee immobilization; to correct contractures or deformities; or for short-term immobilization of a fracture. It keeps the leg in an extended position, without hip flexion. Traction is applied to the extremity in one direction (straight line) with a single pulley system.

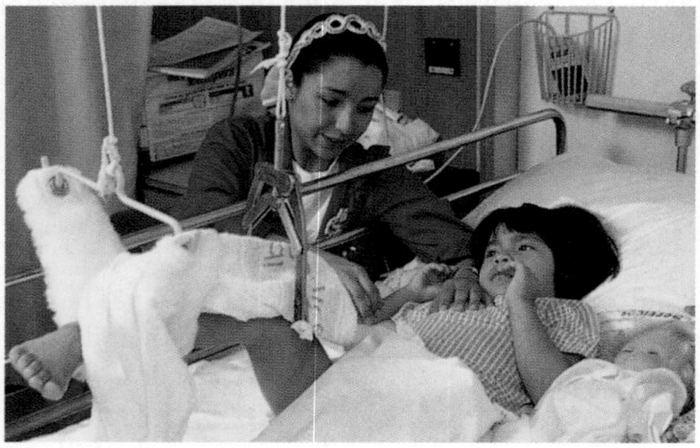
D

90–90 Traction (D)
Used for fractures of the femur or tibia. A skeletal pin or wire is surgically placed through the distal part of the femur, while the lower part of the extremity is in a boot cast. Traction ropes and pulleys are applied at the pin site and on the boot cast to maintain the flexion of both the hip and knee at 90 degrees. This traction can also be used for treatment of an upper extremity fracture.

Russell Traction (C)
Used for fractures of the femur and lower leg. Traction is placed on the lower leg while the knee is suspended in a padded sling. The slightly flexed hips and knees are immobilized. One force is applied by a double pulley to the foot and another force is applied upward using a sling under the knee and an overhead pulley.

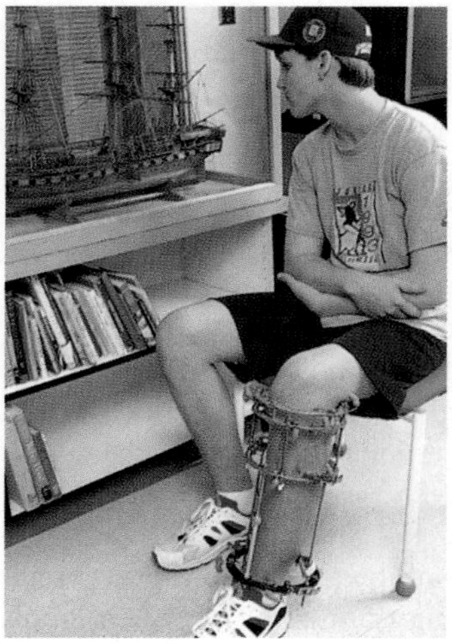
E

External Fixators (E)
These devices can be used in the treatment of simple fractures, both open and closed; complex fractures with extensive soft tissue involvement; correction of bony or soft tissue deformities; pseudoarthroses; and limb length discrepancy. They are attached to the extremity by percutaneous transfixing of pins or wires to the bone. When used to lengthen an extremity, the device can be "distracted" or turned as ordered by the surgeon for a very small amount several times daily. This separates the bone and allows new growth, gradually lengthening the extremity.

Table 58–4 Care of the Child with Traction or External Fixator

1. Assess the child in traction by first checking the equipment. Make sure that the equipment is in the proper position. Observe both the body appliance and the attached weights and pulleys. Make certain that the child's body is in proper alignment.
2. Assess the skin under the straps and pin insertion sites for any signs of redness, edema, or skin breakdown.
3. Assess the extremity by checking neurovascular status frequently (check warmth, color, distal pulses, capillary refill time, movement, sensation).
4. Provide pin care when ordered using sterile technique. Clean the area surrounding the pin with cotton-tipped applicators saturated with normal saline or half-strength hydrogen peroxide. Clean the area again with sterile water or more saline. Apply an antibacterial ointment, if ordered, using another cotton-tipped applicator.
5. When external skin traction is used, perform skin care every 4 hours when the traction device is removed.
6. Place a sheepskin pad under the child's extremity if prescriptions permit.

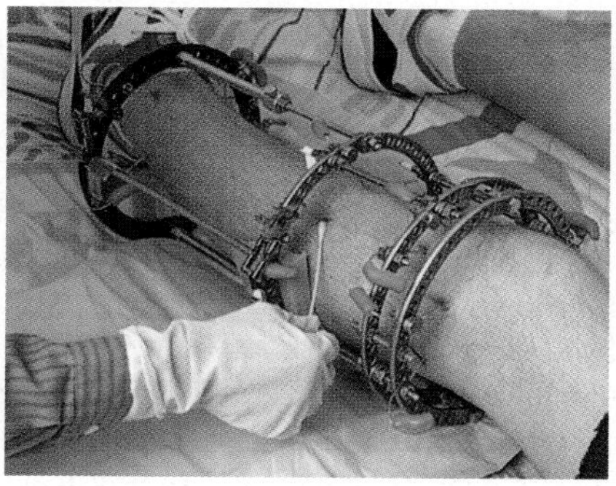

2007). Douglass, in the opening scenario, is a good example of a youth with this type of injury. However, a variety of other injuries that affect the musculoskeletal system are common in sports; strains and sprains are examples. Children and adolescents have characteristics that put them at risk for injury. These include:

- Vulnerability of growth plates to injury, especially the distal tibia and fibula.
- Increased joint mobility from lax tendons and ligaments, leading to injury of the knee, ankle, and hip.
- More porous bones, leading to fractures and to more common injury to underlying organs.
- Lack of experience in the sport and inadequate training.
- Lack of acceptance of protective gear.
- Impatience with taking the time to heal after injury.
- Vulnerability to spinal injury related to high impact sports and recreation such as diving in unsupervised locations.

Common sports injuries are listed in Table 58–5. Treatments for sprains, strains, dislocations, and fractures are described in the preceding sections. Head and neck injuries are discussed in Chapter 56 and dental emergencies in Chapter 47. General approaches to minimize and treat injuries for youth athletes follow.

Athletes can benefit from teaching that enhances performance of their sports and also minimizes chance of injury. They should receive instruction in correct techniques from a person qualified to coach and supervise children. Nurses should encourage youths to gradually increase time and intensity at a sport, rather than immediately playing a new sport for long periods of time. Parents should be encouraged to inquire about the coach's experience and also verify that the coaching staff is prepared in emergency care.

The nurse should be alert for sports injuries during contacts with children and adolescents in health promotion visits. The nurse should ask about sports participation for all youths, but especially when there are complaints of sore muscles, edema of body parts, and bruises. Neurovascular assessment of extremities, including color, temperature, capillary refill time, edema, pulses, sensation, and pain, should be performed. Questions should be phrased so that sports such as skateboarding or snowboarding, which might not be performed under supervision or in organized sports programs, can be identified. Youths might not consider these "sports."

Teach the importance of warming up for 10 to 15 minutes before participation and cooling down for a corresponding period at the end of activity. Encourage wearing recommended safety gear for the sport, including equipment such as a well-fitted protective helmet, face masks, eye protection, mouth guards, elbow and wrist guards, gloves, knee pads, and shin pads. Parents may need assistance to learn about the recommended equipment and resources

Table 58–5 Common Sports Injuries

Sport	Type of Injuries
Baseball/Basketball	■ Hand and finger fractures and sprains ■ Contusions and sprains of upper or lower extremities; wrists, elbows, knees, and ankles are common sites ■ Injury to body parts when hit by a ball, (e.g., broken teeth, face, head, eye, and chest injuries)
Football	■ Head and neck injury such as skull or cervical vertebrae fracture ■ Pulled muscles or dislocations in shoulders and legs
Gymnastics	■ Wrist and elbow fractures and strains ■ Tendonitis in elbows and ankles/legs
Hockey (ice and inline)	■ Dental injury ■ Leg fractures ■ Head and neck injuries
Soccer	■ Head and neck injury ■ Strains and fractures of legs
Wrestling	■ Fractures and dislocations of upper and lower extremities

for purchase. Frequent updates are needed as the child grows. The child should be taught not to ignore pain.

Injuries such as muscle strains should be treated promptly. They involve several steps:

- Resting the injury for 24 to 48 hours, applying ice for 20 minutes 4 times daily, compression with an elastic wrap to provide comfort and decrease edema, and elevating the part affected above heart level
- Gradually increasing motion to the part
- Adding flexibility and resistance or strengthening exercises
- Returning gradually to the sport, usually in 2 to 3 weeks after injury

The nurse should partner with the child, family, and other health professionals to plan for activity whenever an injury has occurred. Praise the family and youth for physical activity, an important part of a healthy lifestyle. Provide community resources to foster sports participation.

AMPUTATIONS

Amputation—the complete absence of a body extremity—can be either congenital or acquired. Approximately two thirds of amputations in children are congenital and one third are acquired. Congenital amputations can be caused by constrictive amniotic bands, drugs, or irradiation. Acquired amputations are generally associated with trauma or the result of a disease or disorder. Children are prone to such injuries because of small extremities and limited skeletal mass. Lawn mower injury, exercise equipment, and car crashes are common causes and the peak age for occurrence is 1 year (Hostetler, Schwartz, Shields, et al., 2005). Most common traumatic amputations involve fingers or toes but hands and limbs are also at risk.

The child with an absent limb should be fitted with a prosthesis as soon as feasible. This fosters a positive body image, independence, and self-confidence, and also ensures that motor skills develop as normally as possible. The prosthetic device should be reevaluated as the child progresses physically and developmentally. Children with traumatic amputations may need frequent stump reconstructions because as children grow, so do their bones, and the skin tends to adhere to the bone. Bone may need to be cut and soft tissue added to keep the stump rounded. Joint fusions or stump lengthenings may also be needed to allow the effective use of a prosthesis. Several prosthetic revisions will be needed as the child grows and develops.

Nursing Management

Nursing care focuses on providing emotional support regarding altered body image, managing pain, maintaining skin integrity, and encouraging maximal independent functioning.

Recovering from the loss of a limb is one of the most difficult challenges facing a child. Emphasize what the child can do rather than what he or she cannot do. Good listening skills are important.

The child who has had surgery or a traumatic injury experiences pain. Many techniques discussed in Chapter 42 are useful interventions. After surgery, an epidural may be the treatment of choice. Oral analgesics are used during the period of adaptation to a prosthesis if the stump is tender. Children may have "phantom" limb pain in the lost extremity although this phenomenon is less common in children than in adults (Wilkins, McGrath, Finley, et al., 2004).

The child usually begins wearing the prosthetic device for 1- to 2-hour intervals. Check the skin for any redness or breakdown. If redness or breakdown develops, leave the prosthesis off and allow the skin to clear before reapplying. Have the prosthesis adjusted if necessary, and increase wearing time as tolerated by the child.

Children with amputated limbs quickly learn how to accommodate to the prosthetic device. Use physical therapy programs specifically designed to help the child perform activities of daily living.

Thinking Critically

THE CHILD WEARING A CAST

Douglass was admitted to the clinic today for application of a short leg cast. He broke his leg nearly a week ago when he was on a trampoline with three friends, trying to see who could jump the highest. Douglass slipped and his leg hit the frame on the side. His friends helped him off the trampoline and found someone to transport Douglass to the emergency department. They then reached his mother by phone, who rushed to the hospital when she heard the news.

His mother states that he is now 12 years old and in middle school. He has been going to a friend's house nearly every day after school and spending time on activities such as the trampoline and rollerblading, as well as watching television and playing video games. She felt this was safer than him being at home alone during her work hours, but is now starting to wonder about whether to allow Douglass to engage in activities with his friend.

A splint has provided support for several days and has allowed the swelling to decrease before today's cast application. Douglass has been non-weight bearing on his leg and has been using crutches. He returned to school yesterday for part of the day and found it was hard to get to all of his classes.

- What concerns will Douglass have once his cast is in place?
- What teaching should you provide to help him keep the cast intact and to ensure his safety?
- What signs or symptoms might indicate infection or loss of circulation and need to be reported immediately?
- Will any special adaptations be needed in his home and school?
- Is there any way his injury could have been avoided? What teaching does he need now to avoid further injuries?

See MyNursingKit for possible responses.

DISCHARGE PLANNING AND HOME CARE TEACHING

Answer any questions the family has about how to care for the prosthetic device and how to perform skin checks. Encourage parents to allow the child to participate in physically and emotionally challenging peer activities. Sporting activities that enable the child to participate using modified equipment are a good way to build self-confidence and motivation. For example, ski centers may offer programs that teach children with physical disabilities how to ski, or the Paralympics may be motivating for some children. Assess the need for counseling and offer referrals as appropriate.

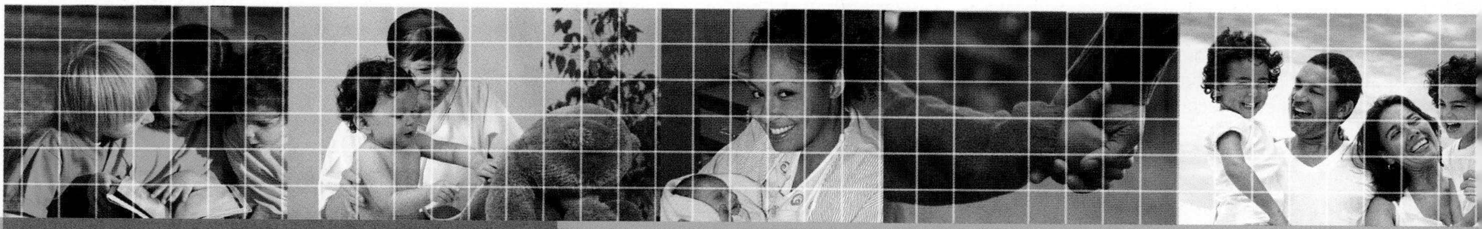

CRITICAL CONCEPT REVIEW

LEARNING OUTCOMES → CONCEPTS

58.1 Describe pediatric variations in the musculoskeletal system.

1. A fibrous membrane exists between the cranial bones to allow for skull growth.
2. Ends of the long bones remain cartilaginous.
3. Long bones are porous and less dense.
4. Bones can bend, buckle, or break due to a simple fall.
5. Muscles increase only in length and circumference.

58.2 Plan nursing care for children with structural deformities of the foot, hip, and spine.

1. Foot:
   - Instruct parents in simple stretching exercises.
   - Provide cast care and instruct parents in cast care.
2. Hip:
   - Provide frequent assessment of the skin and neurovascular status of the affected leg or legs after surgery, or if placed in cast or harness.
   - Maintain traction, if ordered.
   - Increase fluids and fiber in the child's diet.
   - Instruct parents in the use of the Pavlik harness and have them return demonstration of application.
3. Spine:
   - Support self-image if placed in brace.
   - Instruct in exercises to strengthen muscles of spine.
   - Monitor respiratory and circulatory status after fusion surgery.
   - Provide adequate pain medication and instruct in use of PCA.
   - Instruct family in use of brace postoperatively.

58.3 Recognize signs and symptoms of infectious musculoskeletal disorders and refer for appropriate care.

1. Signs and symptoms of infection include:
   - Pain and tenderness with swelling of affected extremity.
   - Decreased mobility of infected joint.
   - Fever.
   - Redness over the area.

58.4 Partner with families to plan care for children with musculoskeletal conditions that are chronic or require long-term care.

1. Help child establish a positive self-image.
2. Assist parents in locating support groups.
3. Provide resources to assist with safety issues such as car seats and home adjustments.
4. Instruct parents in identifying signs and symptoms of complications.
5. Assist parents in dealing with changing condition of the child (for example, with muscular dystrophy).
6. Collaborate with multiple providers who care for child.

(continued)

LEARNING OUTCOMES / CONCEPTS

Learning Outcomes	Concepts
58.5 Plan nursing interventions to promote safety and developmental progression in children who require braces, casts, traction, and surgery.	1. Position child on side (casts and braces), or with head slightly elevated for feeding. 2. Provide age-appropriate toys. 3. Monitor neurovascular and skin status. 4. Promote mobility as allowed. 5. Instruct parents in cast and brace care.
58.6 Provide nursing care for fractures, including teaching for injury prevention and nursing implementations for the child who has sustained a fracture.	1. Immobilize site of fracture until casted or surgically corrected. 2. Keep extremity elevated. 3. Use palms to handle cast until dry. 4. Monitor neurovascular status of the extremity frequently. 5. Provide pain medication as needed. Injury prevention instruction should include: 1. Warm-up before beginning exercise. 2. Use protective equipment. 3. Treat sprains and strains promptly.

CRITICAL THINKING IN ACTION

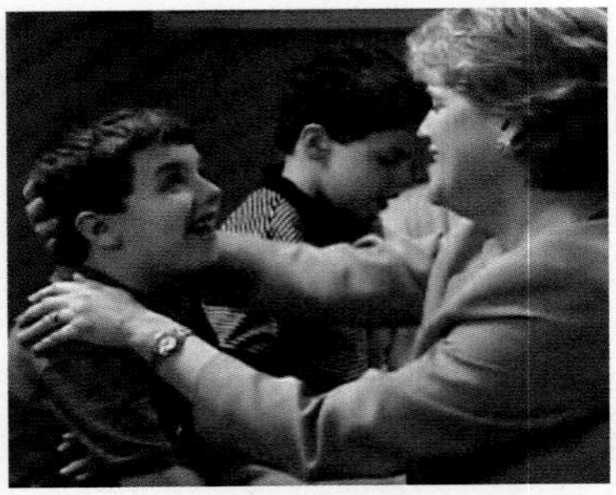

Peter, now 7 years old, was diagnosed at 5 years with Duchenne muscular dystrophy. His parents are well-informed about the disease since they had an older son who died of the disorder at 19 years. At the present time he walks on his toes but is able to ambulate well with leg braces. Today Peter is visiting the specialty clinic for children with muscular dystrophies. His braces will be checked for fit and performance, physical therapy will be performed, and he will attend a group session with other school-age children. During these visits, the parents also meet in a support group with other families and receive instruction and resources to help them with Peter's health management. As a nurse in the clinic you perform a physical and mental assessment on Peter. All findings are within normal limits, although he has had some constipation and several upper respiratory infections. You learn that he has an individualized education plan (IEP) in place at school that allows for periods of rest and physical therapy; the parents report that he is at grade level and excels at computer skills.

1. What are the main roles of the nurse working with Peter in the specialty clinic?
2. Children with muscular dystrophy often get to a standing position by mainly using arm muscles. What is the name of the maneuver?
3. What are some of the tests performed to see if a child has muscular dystrophy, and what are the expected results?
4. Who can Peter expect to meet with on the days he goes to the specialty clinic for muscular dystrophy?

See MyNursingKit for possible responses.

REFERENCES

American Academy of Pediatrics (1999 and 2006). Children with special health care needs. Retrieved from www.aap.org/healthtopics/specialneeds.cfm

American Academy of Pediatrics, Section on Cardiology and Cardiac Surgery (2005). Cardiac health supervision for individuals affected with Duchenne or Becker muscular dystrophy. *Pediatrics, 116*, 1569–1573.

Aronsson, D. D., Loder, R. T., Breur, G. J., & Weinstein, S. L. (2006). Slipped capital femoral epiphysis: Current concepts. *Journal of the American Academy of Orthopedic Surgeons, 14*, 666–679.

Bachrach, L. K. (2007). Consensus and controversy regarding osteoporosis in the pediatric population. *Endocrine Practice, 13*, 513–520.

Bautista, S. R., Gholve, P., & Dormans, J. P. (2006). Pediatric musculoskeletal infections: Advances in diagnosis and management. *Consultant for Pediatricians August*, 481–494.

Beck, J., Weinberg, J., Hamnegard, C. H., Spahija, J., Olofson, J., Grimby, G. Y., & Sindery, C. (2006). Diaphragmatic function in advanced Duchenne muscular dystrophy. *Neuromuscular Disorders, 16*, 161–167.

Bhatia, N. N., Pirpiris, M., & Otsuka, M. Y. (2006). Body mass index in patients with slipped capital femoral epiphysis. *Journal of Pediatric Orthopaedics, 26*, 197–199.

Bowman, B. A., & Russell, R. M. (Eds.). (2006). *Present knowledge of nutrition* (9th ed.). Washington, DC: International Life Sciences Institute.

Burns, C. E., Dunn, A. M., Brady, M. A., Starr, N. B., & Blosser, C. G. (2009). *Pediatric primary care* (4th ed.). Philadelphia: Elsevier Saunders.

Cady, R. B. (2006). Developmental dysplasia of the hip: Definition, recognition, and prevention of late sequelae. *Pediatric Annals, 35*, 92–101.

Carson, S., Woolridge, D. P., Colletti, J., & Kilgore, D. (2006). Pediatric upper extremity injuries. *Pediatric Clinics of North America, 53*, 41–67.

Caulton, J. M., Ward, K. A., Alsop, C. W., Dunn, G., Adams, J. E., & Mughal, M. Z. (2004). A randomized controlled trial of standing programme on bone mineral density in non-ambulant children with cerebral palsy. *Archives of Disease in Childhood, 89*, 131–135.

Chamley, C. A., Carson, P., Randall, D., & Sandwell, M. (2005). *Developmental anatomy and physiology of children.* St. Louis: Elsevier.

Deakin, D. E., Crosby, J. M., Moran, C. G., & Chell, J. (2007). Childhood fractures requiring inpatient management. *Injury, 38*, 1241–1246.

Devogelaer, J. P., & Coppin, C. (2006). Osteogenesis imperfecta: Current treatment options and future prospects. *Treatments in Endocrinology, 5*, 229–242.

Eliakim, A., & Nemet, D. (2005). Osteopenia of prematurity—The role of exercise in prevention and treatment. *Pediatric Endocrinology Review, 2*, 675–682.

Faulks, S., & Luther, B. (2005). Changing paradigm for the treatment of clubfeet. *Orthopaedic Nursing, 24*, 25–30.

Frank, G., Mahoney, H. M., & Eppes, S. C. (2005). Musculoskeletal infections in children. *Pediatric Clinics of North America, 52,* 1083–1106.

Grottkau, B. E., Epps, H. R., & DiScala, C. (2005). Compartment syndrome in children and adolescents. *Journal of Pediatric Surgery, 40,* 678–682.

Grzegorzewski, A., Synder, M., Kozkkowski, P., Szymczak, W., & Bowen, R. J. (2006). The role of the acetabulum in Perthes Disease. *Journal of Pediatric Orthopaedics, 26,* 316–321.

Gutierrez, K. (2005). Bone and joint infections in children. *Pediatric Clinics of North America, 52,* 779–794.

Ha, H. I., Seo, J. B., Lee, S. H., Kang, J. W., Goo, H. W., Lim, T. H., & Shin, M. J. (2007). Imaging of Marfan syndrome: Multisystemic manifestations. *Radiographics, 27,* 989–1004.

Hart, E. S., & Grottkau, B. E. (2006). *The Clinical Advisor, February,* 43–47.

Hart, E. S., Grottkau, B. E., Rebello, G. N., & Albright, M. B. (2005). The newborn foot: Diagnosis and management of common conditions. *Orthopedic Nursing, 24,* 313–321.

Herring, J. A., Kim, H. T., & Browne, R. (2005). Legg-Calve-Perthes disease. *Journal of Bone and Joint Surgery,* 86-A, 2121–2134.

Hosalkar, H. S., Gholve, P. A., & Wells, L. (2007). Torsional and angular deformities. In R. M. Kliegman, R. E. Behrman, H. B. Jenson, & B. F. Stanton (Eds.), *Nelson textbook of pediatrics* (18th ed., pp. 2784–2790). Philadelphia: Saunders Elsevier.

Hosalkar, H. S., Horn, B. D., Friedman, J. E., & Dormans, J. P. (2007). The hip. In R. M. Kliegman, R. E. Behrman, H. B. Jenson, & B. F. Stanton (Eds.), *Nelson textbook of pediatrics* (18th ed., pp. 2800–2811). Philadelphia: Saunders Elsevier.

Hostetler, S. G., Schwartz, L., Shields, B. J., Xiang, H., & Smith, G. A. (2005). Characteristic of pediatric traumatic amputations treated in hospital emergency departments: United States, 1990–2002. *Pediatrics, 116,* e667–e674.

Kaplan, S. L. (2005). Osteomyelitis in children. *Infectious Disease Clinics of North America, 19,* 787–797.

Katz, D. A. (2006). Slipped capital femoral epiphysis: The importance of early diagnosis. *Pediatric Annals 35,* 102–111.

Kemper, A. R., & Wake, M. A. (2007). Duchenne muscular dystrophy: Issues in expanding newborn screening. *Current Opinion in Pediatrics, 19,* 700–704.

Kocher, M. S., Lee, B., Dolan, M., Weinberg, J., & Shulman, S. T. (2006). Pediatric orthopedic infections: Early detection and treatment. *Pediatric Annals, 35,* 112–122.

Korovessis, P., Koureas, G., Zacharatos, S. & Papazisis, Z. (2005). Backpacks, back pain, sagittal spinal curves and trunk alignment in adolescents. *Spine, 30,* 247–255.

Kuehn, B. M. (2007). Studies point way to new therapeutic prospects for muscular dystrophy. *JAMA, 298,* 1385–1386.

Lee, E. H., & Hui, J. H. (2006). The potential of stem cells in orthopaedic surgery. *Journal of Bone and Joint Surgery, 88,* 841–851.

Litmanovitz, I., Dolfin, T., Arnon, S., Regev, R. H., Nemet, D., & Eliakim, A. (2007). Assisted exercise and bone strength in preterm infants. *Calcified Tissue International, 80,* 39–43.

Lonstein, J. E. (2006). Scoliosis: Surgical versus nonsurgical treatment. *Clinical Orthopaedics and Related Research, 443,* 248–259.

Manias, K., McCabe, D., & Bishop, N. (2006). Fractures and recurrent fractures in children: varying effects of environment factors as well as bone size and mass. *Bone, 39,* 652–657.

Manoff, E. M., Banffy, M. B., & Winell, J. J. (2005). Relationship between body mass index and slipped capital femoral epiphysis. *Journal of Pediatric Orthopedics, 25,* 744–746.

March of Dimes. (2007). *Achondroplasia.* Retrieved from www.marchofdimes.com/

Martin, E., & Shapiro, J. R. (2007). Osteogenesis imperfecta: Epidemiology and pathophysiology. *Current Osteoporosis Reports, 5*(3), 91–97.

Mayo Clinic (2007). Marfan Syndrome. Retrieved from www.mayoclinic.com/health/marfan-syndrome/DS00540/DSECTION=6

Mooney, V., Mayer, J., & Woodbridge, D. (2007). Adolescent scoliosis: Exercise therapy may help correct the condition. *Consultant for Pediatricians, September,* 509–515.

Moore, M. J., White, G. L., & Moore, D. L. (2007). Association of relative backpack weight with reported pain, pain sites, medical utilization, and lost school time in children and adolescents. *Journal of School Health, 77,* 232–239.

Morcuende, J. A. (2006). Congenital idiopathic clubfoot: Prevention of late deformity and disability by conservative treatment with the Ponseti technique. *Pediatric Annals, 35,* 128–136.

Navuluri, N., & Navuluri, R. G. (2006). Study on the relationship between backpack use and back and neck pain among adolescents. *Nursing and Health Sciences, 8,* 208–215.

Online Mendelian Inheritance in Man (2008). Osteogenesis Imperfecta. Retrieved from www.ncbi.nlm.nih.gov/entrez/dispomin/cgi?id=166200

Rethlefsen, S. A., Healy, B. S., Wren, T. A. L., Skaggs, D. L., & Kay, R. M. (2006). Causes of intoeing gait in children with cerebral palsy. *Journal of Bone & Joint Surgery, 88,* 2175–2180.

Sapountzi-Krepia, D., Psychogiou, M., Peterson, D., Zafari, B., Iordanopoulou, E., Michailidou, F., & Christodoulou, A. (2006). The experience of brace treatment in children/adolescents with scoliosis. *Scoliosis, 22,* 8.

Schwend, R. M., Schoenecker, P., Richards, B. S., Flynn, J. M., & Vitale, J. (2007). Screening the newborn for developmental dysplasia of the hip. *Journal of Pediatric Orthopaedics, 27,* 607–610.

Shilt, J. S., & Barnett, T. M. (2007). Back pain in children: Keys to evaluation and treatment. *Consultant for Pediatricians, May,* 281–290.

Shipman, S., Helfand, M., Nygren, P., & Bougatsos, C. (2006). Screening for developmental dysplasia of the hip. Evidence synthesis 42. *Agency for Healthcare Research and Quality,* 1–98.

Simon, T. D., Bublitz, C., & Hambidge, S. J. (2006). Emergency department visits among pediatric patients for sports-related injury: Basic epidemiology and impact of race-ethnicity and insurance status. *Pediatric Emergency Care, 22,* 309–315.

Spiegel, D. A., Hosalkar, H. S., & Dormans, J. P. (2007). The spine. In R. M. Kliegman, R. E. Behrman, H. B. Jenson, & B. F. Stanton (Eds.), *Nelson textbook of pediatrics* (18th ed., pp. 2811–2822). Philadelphia: Saunders Elsevier.

Trotter, T. L., Hall, J. G., and the Committee on Genetics (2005). Health supervision for children with achondroplasia. *Pediatrics, 116,* 771–783.

Unal, E., Abaci, A., Bober, E., & Buyukgebiz, A. (2006). Efficacy and safety of oral alendronate treatment in children and adolescents with osteoporosis. *Journal of Pediatric Endocrinology and Metabolism, 19,* 523–528.

University of Maryland Medical Center. (2007). Muscular dystrophy. Retrieved from www.umm.edu/altmed/ConsConditions/MuscularDystrophycc.html

U.S. Department of Health and Human Services. (2006). Screening for developmental dysplasia of the hip: Recommendation statement. Agency for Healthcare Quality and Research. AHRQ Publication #05(06)-0585-A.

U.S. Preventive Services Task Force. (2006a). Screening for developmental dysplasia of the hip: Recommendation statement. *American Family Physician, 73,* 1192–1198.

U.S. Preventive Services Task Force (2006b). The Guide to clinical preventive services. Agency for Healthcare Research and Quality. Available at www.preventiveservices.ahrq.gov

Von Kodolitsch, Y., & Robinson, P. N. (2007). Marfan syndrome: An update of genetics, medical and surgical treatment. *Heart, 93,* 755–760.

Wan, S. C. (2006). Metatarsus adductus and skewfoot deformity. *Clinics in Podiatric Medicine and Surgery, 23,* 23–40.

Wilkins, K. L., McGrath, P. J., Finley, G. A., & Katz, J. (2004). Prospective diary study of nonpainful and painful phantom sensations in a preselected sample of child and adolescent amputees reporting phantom limbs. *Clinical Journal of Pain, 20,* 293–301.

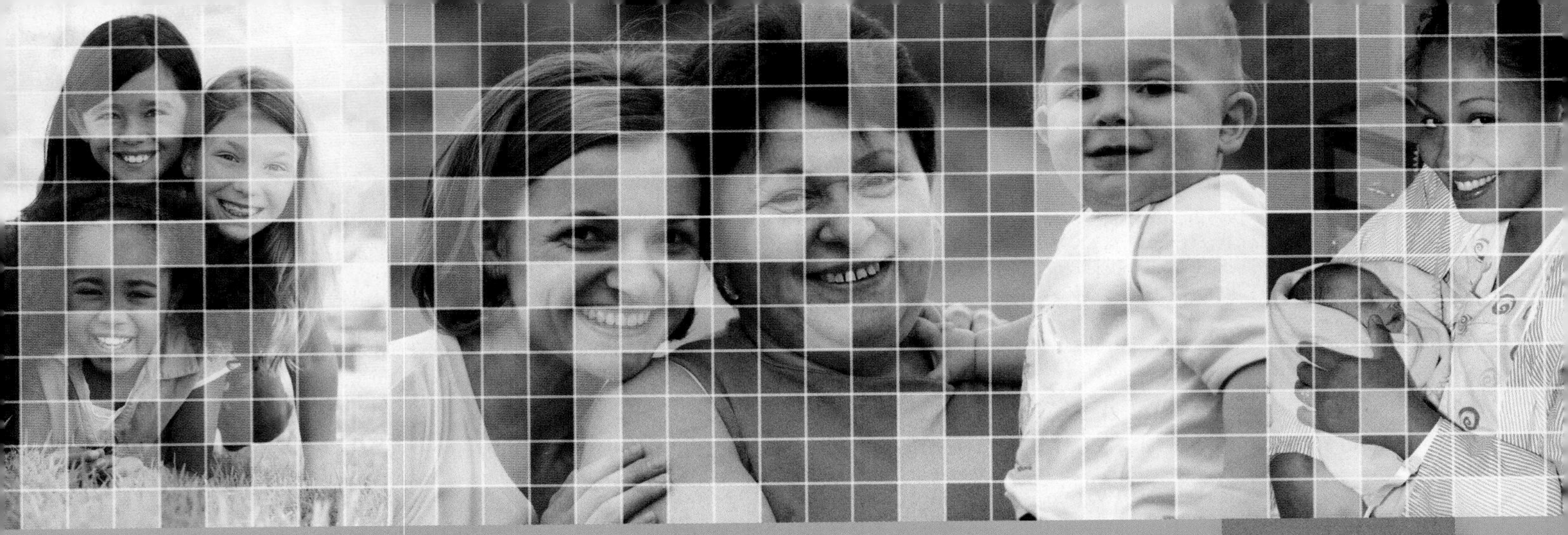

CHAPTER 59

The Child with Alterations in Skin Integrity

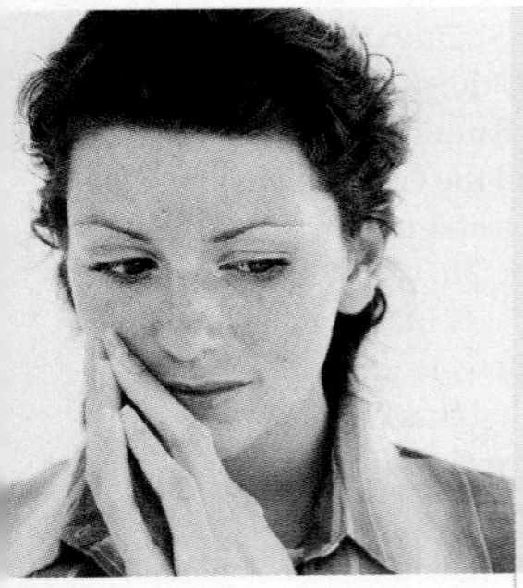

I didn't know that hot coffee could cause such a bad injury. I am worried about the scars Shanelle might have over her chest from this scald burn. —Mother of Shanelle, 1 year old

LEARNING OUTCOMES

59.1 Identify the characteristics of different skin lesions by their cause, including those caused by irritants, drug reactions, mites, infection, and injury.

59.2 Describe the stages of wound healing.

59.3 Describe a nursing care plan for a child with acute skin disorders, including dermatitis, infectious disorders, and infestations.

59.4 Plan the nursing care for the child with a chronic skin condition.

59.5 Develop an education plan for adolescents with acne to promote self-care.

59.6 Describe the process to measure the extent of burns and burn severity in children.

59.7 Develop a nursing care plan for the child with a full-thickness burn injury.

59.8 Identify preventive strategies to reduce the risk of injury from burns, hypothermia, bites and stings.

The skin is the largest organ in the body and performs several essential functions. The skin protects underlying tissues from invasion by microorganisms and from trauma. The nerves in the skin enable the perception of touch, pain, heat, and cold. The body regulates its temperature by dilating or constricting blood vessels and sweat glands that act under the control of the central nervous system. The skin also supplements the body's intake of vitamin D by synthesizing this vitamin from ultraviolet light. The sweat glands secrete a solution of water, electrolytes, and urea, thus helping to rid the body of toxins.

ANATOMY AND PHYSIOLOGY OF PEDIATRIC DIFFERENCES

The skin has three distinct layers: the epidermis, the dermis, and the subcutaneous fatty layer that separates the skin from the underlying tissue (Figure 59–1 ●). The epidermis is the thin, outermost layer of skin that grows rapidly and contains the melanocytes that synthesize and secrete melanin when the skin is exposed to ultraviolet light. Within the dermis are nerves, muscles, connective tissue, hair follicles, sebaceous and sweat glands, lymph channels, and blood vessels. The subcutaneous layer contains the hair, sebaceous glands, eccrine and apocrine sweat glands, and a layer of fat to help insulate the body from cold temperatures.

The infant's skin is thin, with little underlying subcutaneous fat. Because of this the infant loses heat more rapidly, has greater difficulty regulating body temperature,

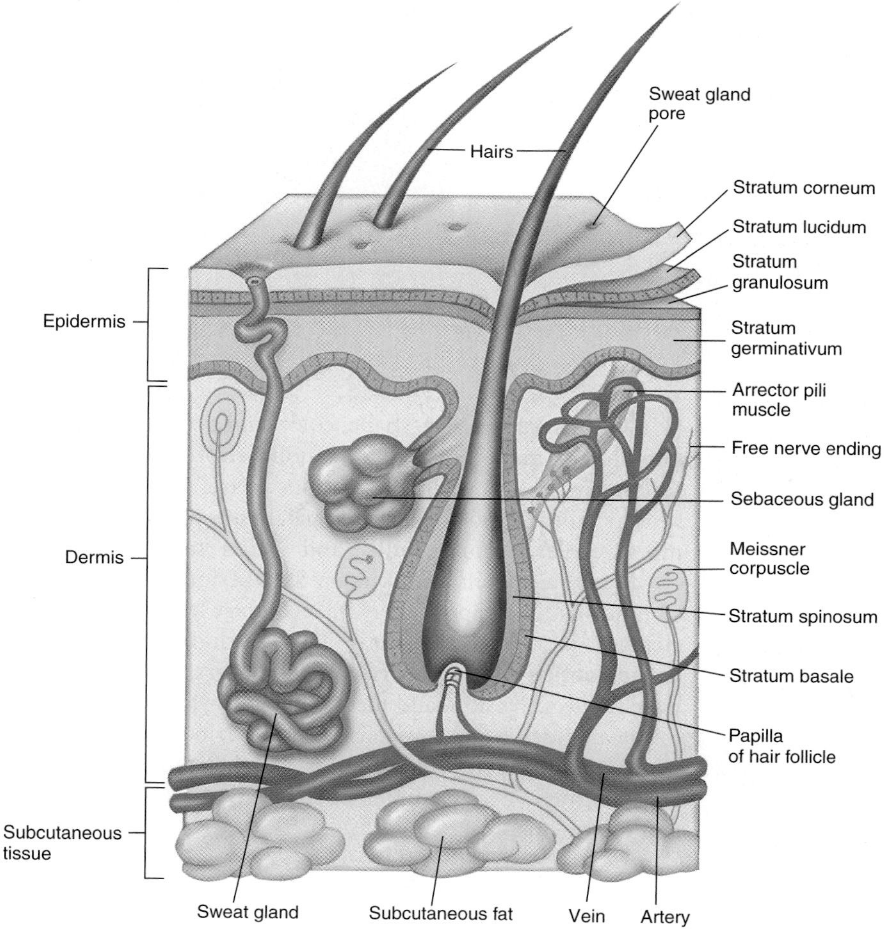

● **Figure 59–1** Layers of the skin with accessory structures.

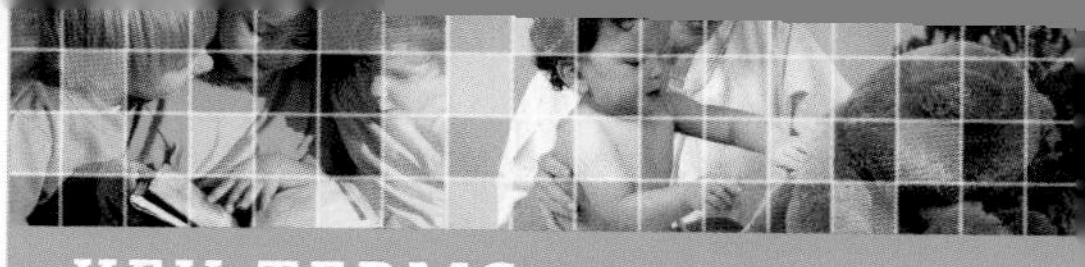

KEY TERMS

Allograft, 1812
Atopy, 1796
Autografting, 1812
Circumferential, 1810
Comedone, 1798
Cryotherapy, 1791
Debridement, 1785
Dermatophytoses, 1792
Epithelialization, 1785
Eschar, 1810
Escharotomy, 1810
Intertriginous, 1788
Involution, 1805
Keloid, 1785
Kerion, 1793
Lichenification, 1784
Phototoxic, 1800
Telangiectasia, 1806
Xerosis, 1795

MyNursingKit Animation: Layers of the Skin

AS CHILDREN GROW

INTEGUMENTARY SYSTEM CHANGES

The structures of the skin mature during childhood, reaching adult function at puberty.

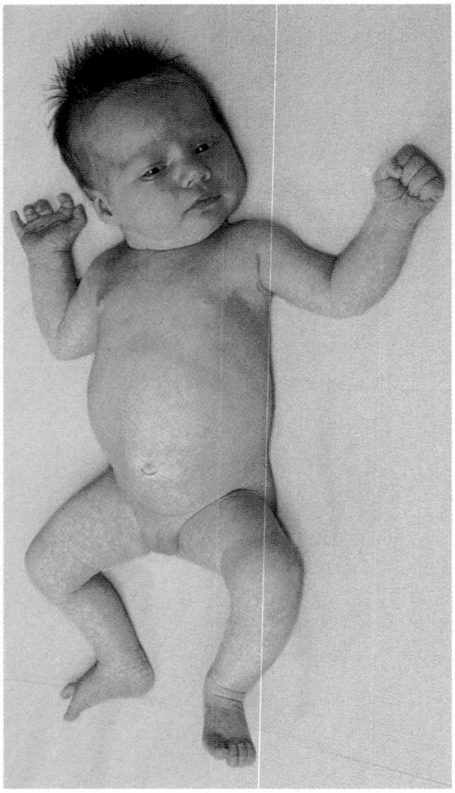

Newborns
Skin is very thin
Epidermis is loosely bound to the dermis, friction can cause separation of the layers with blistering
Eccrine sweat glands function, produce sweat in response to heat and emotional stimuli
Apocrine sweat glands are small and nonfunctional
Less melanin is present at birth so skin is lighter colored

Adolescents
Skin thickens
Epidermis and dermis are tightly bound, increasing resistance to infection and irritation
Eccrine sweat glands achieve full function, after puberty males sweat more than females
Apocrine sweat glands mature during puberty
Melanin is at adult levels, determining skin color and serving as a shield against ultraviolet radiation

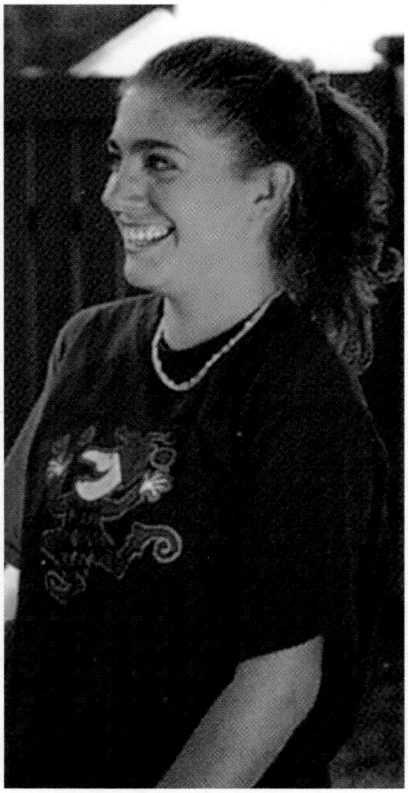

and becomes more easily chilled than an older child or an adult. The thinner skin also leads to increased absorption of harmful chemical substances and topical medications. The infant's skin contains more water than an adult's and has loosely attached cells. As the infant grows, the skin toughens and becomes less hydrated, making it less susceptible to bacteria. See changes in skin characteristics in "As Children Grow: Integumentary System Changes."

MyNursingKit Animation: Integumentary Repair

Sebaceous glands function at birth, although somewhat immaturely. They vary in size and appear all over the body except on the hands and soles of the feet. Sebum, a lipid substance produced and secreted into the hair follicle or directly onto the skin, lubricates the skin and hair.

Eccrine glands, located in the dermis, open onto the skin surface. They secrete an odorless, watery fluid, primarily in response to emotional stress. They also respond to changes in body temperature. As body temperature increases, the glands increase production of sweat; its evaporation cools the body. All eccrine sweat glands are present and functional at birth.

Apocrine glands, located mainly in the axillary and genital areas, do not function until puberty.

SKIN LESIONS

Skin lesions vary in size, shape, color, and texture characteristics. The two major types of skin lesions are primary lesions and secondary lesions. Primary lesions arise from previously healthy skin and include macules, patches, papules, nodules, tumors, vesicles, pustules, bullae, and wheals (see "Pathophysiology Illustrated: Common Primary Skin Lesions and Associated Conditions" in Chapter 35∞). Secondary lesions result from changes in primary lesions. They include crusts, scales, **lichenification** (thickening of the skin), scars, keloids, excoriation, fissures, erosion, and ulcers (Table 59–1). It is important for the nurse to be able to identify and describe the primary and secondary skin lesions and understand their underlying cause and treatment. See "Complementary Care: Oils, Gels, Creams, and Ointments."

WOUND HEALING

Wound healing occurs in three overlapping phases: inflammation, proliferation, and remodeling or maturation (see "Patho-

Table 59–1 Common Secondary Skin Lesions and Associated Conditions

Lesion Name	Description	Example
Burrow	A narrow, raised irregular channel caused by a parasite	Scabies
Comedone	A plug of sebaceous and keratin material in a hair follicle	Acne
Crust	Dried residue of serum, pus, or blood	Impetigo
Erosion	Loss of superficial epidermis; moist but does not bleed	Ruptured chickenpox vesicle
Excoriation	Abrasion or scratch mark	Scratched insect bite
Fissure	Linear crack in skin	Tinea pedis (athlete's foot)
Keloid	Overdevelopment or hypertrophy of scar that extends beyond wound edges and above skin line due to excess collagen	Healed skin area following traumatic injury
Lichenification	Thickening of skin with increased visibility of normal skin furrows	Eczema (atopic dermatitis)
Scale	Thin flake of exfoliated epidermis	Dandruff, psoriasis
Scar	Replacement of destroyed tissue with fibrous tissue	Healed surgical incision
Telangiectasia	Dilated, superficial blood vessels	Birthmark
Ulcer	Deeper loss of skin surface; bleeding or scarring may ensue	Chancre

Complementary Care

OILS, GELS, CREAMS, AND OINTMENTS

Some skin conditions have complementary therapies for which scientific studies have demonstrated a benefit. Evening primrose oil given orally is used for atopic eczema. Aloe vera gel used topically is effective for superficial burns and abrasions. Chamomile topical cream or ointment is effective for skin inflammation (National Center for Complementary and Alternative Medicine, 2006).

physiology Illustrated: Phases of Wound Healing") (Sagerman, 2005; Trask, Rote, & Huether, 2006).

Inflammation, the initial response at the injury site, is the phase that prepares the injury site for the repair process. Vasodilation, which occurs shortly after injury, allows leukocytes to travel to the injury site, where they ingest bacteria and debris. The blood coagulates as platelets, red blood cells, and fibrin gather to form a clot. This seals the wound, preventing bacterial invasion and joining the wound edges.

Reconstruction, or **epithelialization** (the process by which epithelial cells grow into the wound from surrounding healthy tissue), is the second phase in which capillaries bud to reestablish the blood flow. Natural **debridement** (enzyme action to clean the lesion and dissolve the clot or scab) also occurs. The wound contracts as the wound edges grow toward each other. Fibroblasts multiply, producing collagen and shiny, red granulation tissue to fill the wound to skin level. A fine layer of epithelial cells forms over the site.

Maturation or remodeling, the third phase, involves continued collagen production for scar production. The scar gradually strengthens and devascularizes, eventually achieving about 80% of the tissue's preinjury strength (Frask, Rote, & Huether, 2006).

Formation of a **keloid**, a scar that extends beyond the original boundaries of the wound, occurs because of an imbalance between collagen synthesis and collagen breakdown. The cause is unknown, but there is a familial tendency. A hypertrophic scar is raised but stays within the original boundaries of the wound.

DERMATITIS

Many skin inflammations occur in early childhood. Most are easily treated and have no long-term consequences. Dermatitis is a condition in which skin changes occur in response to external stimuli. The four most common types of dermatitis in infants, children, and adolescents are contact dermatitis, diaper dermatitis, seborrheic dermatitis, and atopic eczema (atopic dermatitis). See page 1795 for atopic eczema. These skin disorders may cause some emotional problems for the family and child, since they can see the skin condition. Reassure them that the child is not infectious.

CONTACT DERMATITIS

Contact dermatitis is an inflammation of the skin that occurs in response to direct contact with an allergen or irritant.

When contact dermatitis is caused by an external irritant, an inflammatory response occurs, but there is no immune response. Common irritants include soaps, detergents, fabric softeners, bleaches, lotions, urine, and stool. An irritant can affect the skin any time there is adequate concentration and contact duration. Sweating and friction enhance the absorption of the allergen or irritant.

Phytodermatitis can result when the child has contact with a chemical found in citrus fruits, celery, parsley, fig leaves, or ragweed that sensitizes the skin to sunlight. Following sun exposure the child develops erythema and blistering at the site of the contact that then becomes hyperpigmented. The hyperpigmentation fades over 2 to 3 months (Khachemoune, Khechmoune, & Blanc, 2006).

PATHOPHYSIOLOGY ILLUSTRATED

PHASES OF WOUND HEALING

Wound healing occurs in three overlapping phases.

Inflammation (3–5 days)

Clot formation that seals the wound with fibrin and trapped cells and platelets

Increased blood flow to area carrying exudate with phagocytes and lymphocytes to the site

Increased capillary permeability, causing swelling

Dilute toxic products released by dying cells

Phagocytosis

Inflammation

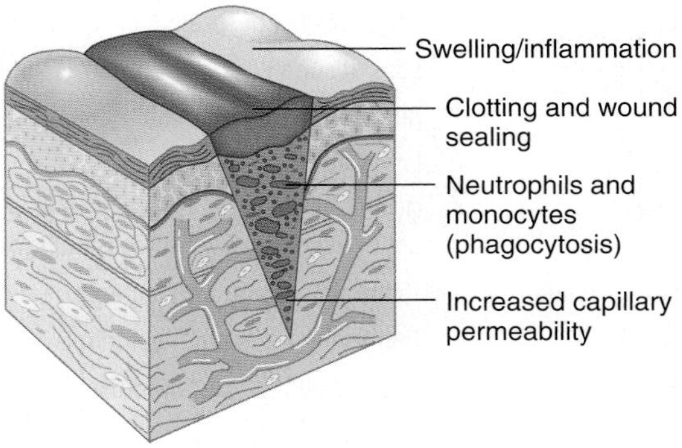

Reconstruction (4 days to 2 weeks)

Debridement or cleanup of the site, fibrinolytic enzymes dissolve the fibrin clots

Regeneration of destroyed cells if injury is minor

Collagen production for scar formation occurs when tissue is too injured to regenerate

Epithelialization with granulation tissue that includes capillary budding and becomes scar tissue

Wound contraction, inward movement of the wound edge

Reconstruction

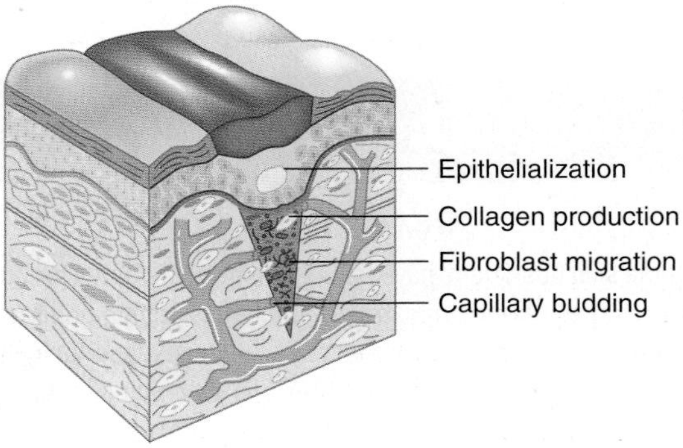

Maturation (Months to 2 Years)

Remodeling of the site as scar tissue forms

Scar formation and strengthening

Capillary disappearance from scar tissue

Maturation

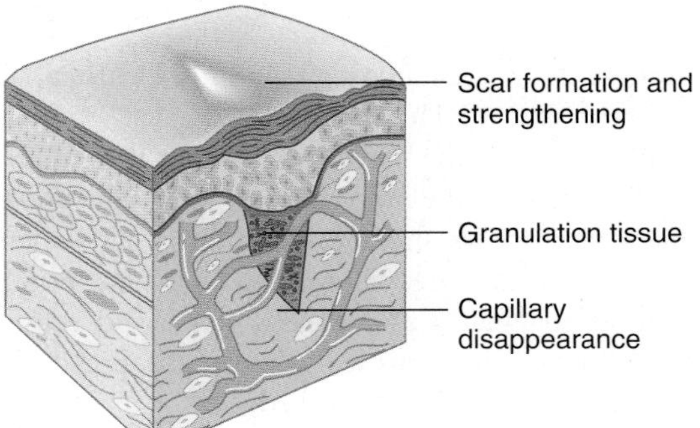

Data from Nicol, N. H., Huether, S. E., & Weber, R. (2006). Structure, function, and disorders of the integument. In K. L. McCance & S. E. Huether (Eds.), *Pathophysiology: The basis for disease in adults and children* (5th ed., pp. 1573–1607). St. Louis, MO: Elsevier Mosby.

Allergic contact dermatitis is a delayed hypersensitivity reaction. An antigen is absorbed from the skin surface during the initial sensitization phase, and an immune memory is created. Generally, repeated exposures or a long-term exposure is required to cause the immune response and the dermatitis. See Chapter 50 to review the immune response to allergens. Common allergens include poison ivy, poison oak, lanolin, neomycin, rubber, chemicals in shoe leather, nickel, fragrances, and latex. Children may have both irritant and allergic reactions to latex, found in many types of hospital equipment and supplies, and products in the home.

Table 59–2 Distribution of Lesions by Type of Allergen

Distribution of Lesion	Allergen
Face, eyelids	Cosmetics, skin care products, nail cosmetics
Earlobes, neck	Nickel, fragrances
Lips, mouth	Oral hygiene products, gum, lipstick
Dorsal aspects of toes and feet	Rubber or leather chemical in shoes
Trunk	Snaps on pants, moisturizers, cleansers, sunscreens

Adapted from Timm-Knudson, V. L., Johnson, J. S., Ortiz, K. J., & Yiannias, J. A. (2006). Allergic contact dermatitis to preservatives. *Dermatologic Nursing, 18*(2), 130–136.

Teaching Highlights

EXPOSURE TO POISON IVY OR POISON OAK

- The rash is caused by contact with the urushiol oil from the sap of the plants, either directly or indirectly, such as on another person, animal or clothing. Avoid hugging a pet exposed to poison ivy until after it has been bathed. Once the rash develops it is not contagious.
- React quickly after contact. Wash exposed areas with Zanfel® (a product that removes urushiol that has bonded with the skin) or with soap and lukewarm water within 10 minutes if possible, making sure to scrub under the nails.
- Do not rub fingers exposed to poison ivy against broken skin or in eyes.
- Launder clothing worn during exposure, and wash hands after handling exposed clothing.
- Wear vinyl gloves to handle plants (cloth and rubber gloves allow sap to penetrate).
- Search the yard and remove all plants. Do not burn plants removed. A person with a sensitivity may inhale the smoke and develop airway inflammation.
- For children with sensitivity to poison ivy, an over-the-counter barrier cream such as IvyBlock® can help prevent skin penetration of plant oil.

Allergic contact dermatitis is characterized by erythema, edema, pruritus, vesicles, or bullae that rupture, ooze, and crust. The rash is usually limited to the area of contact. Symptoms of allergic contact dermatitis can develop several hours to 3 days after exposure when the immune response has been activated (see Table 59–2). The rash takes 2 to 4 weeks to resolve naturally without treatment (Amer & Fischer, 2006). In contrast, irritant contact dermatitis is a discrete area of redness that corresponds to the exposure location. The rash usually develops within a few hours of contact, peaks within 24 hours, and quickly resolves with removal of the irritant. Reactions to irritants include painful erythema, edema, vesiculation, skin dryness, scaling, fissuring, and necrosis.

The distribution of lesions provides clues about the source and identity of the allergen or irritant. Treatment involves removing the offending agent (e.g., clothes, plant, soap). Calamine lotion can be applied to the affected skin. Cool compresses with aluminum acetate (e.g., Burow's solution) promote drying. Wet dressings and colloidal oatmeal soaks relieve itching. Antihistamines may be given for a sedative effect when the child is too irritable to sleep. Acute allergic contact dermatitis is managed with medium potency topical corticosteroids when less than 10% of the body surface area is affected, but the medication should not be applied to open lesions. The topical corticosteroids are applied to the affected area twice a day for 2 to 3 weeks. Stopping the treatment too soon can cause rebound dermatitis. Reactions to poison ivy or other allergens covering more than 10% of the body surface area require treatment with oral corticosteroids for 7 to 14 days and a tapered dose for 7 to 10 additional days.

Nursing Management

Patient education for home care management focuses on care of the skin and prevention of future exposures. Teach parents how to apply topical corticosteroids and to keep using the ointment for 2 to 3 weeks even when the skin shows signs of healing. When oatmeal soaks are used, caution parents that the tub will be slippery, and teach them to pat the child dry to leave the oatmeal film in place. Wet dressings may be soothing and help loosen crusts. Burow's or Domeboro solution applied to blistered or oozing lesions for 20 minutes daily helps dry lesions (Allen, 2004). Familiarize parents with the symptoms of infection in the affected area (i.e., increased redness, oozing, fever) and tell them when to return for follow-up care.

Teach parents to avoid exposure to allergens or irritants. Advise parents to wash all clothes before the first wearing and to rinse clothes an extra time to remove all the soap. Mild soap should be used to clean the skin. Place a barrier between the irritant (e.g., metal, shoe leather) and the skin. If a nickel allergy exists, avoid use of nickel jewelry and belt buckles.

DIAPER DERMATITIS

Diaper dermatitis, a common cause of irritant contact dermatitis, occurs in approximately one third of young children, usually in a mild form. It is most common in infants from 9 to 12 months of age (Alberta, Sweeney, & Wiss, 2005). Diaper dermatitis is a primary reaction to urine, feces, moisture, or friction. Urine and feces interact with the skin to cause dermatitis. The urine increases the wetness and pH of the skin, increasing abrasion and its permeability to irritants and microbes. Fecal enzymes are activated by the alkalinity of the urine and cause skin irritation. Urine breaks down to ammonia, also a skin irritant.

Infection with *Candida albicans* is a common complication of diaper dermatitis or antibiotic therapy for another condition. It is frequently the underlying cause of severe diaper rash. Diaper candidiasis often occurs simultaneously with oral candidiasis (see page 1792).

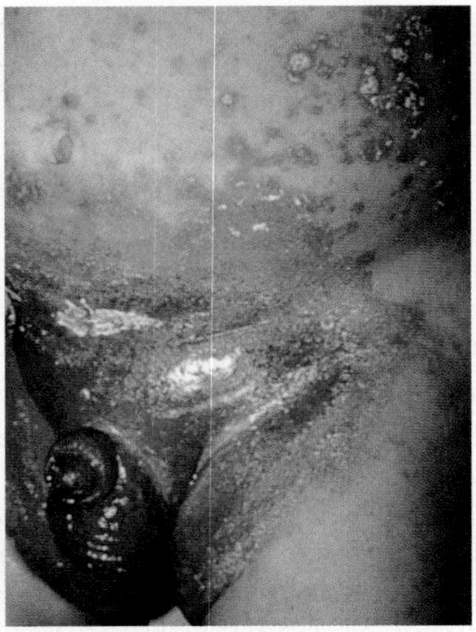

• **Figure 59–2** Diaper dermatitis. Note the skinfold that is free of inflammation.

Courtesy of the Centers for Disease Control, Atlanta, GA.

The rash is characterized by glazed red plaques over skin in contact with the diaper. Usually the perineum, genitals, and buttocks are affected, and the skinfolds are spared. In severe cases, the infant develops a rash that is fiery red, raised, and confluent (Figure 59–2 ●). Pustules with tenderness can also be present. When a *Candida albicans* infection occurs, the rash has bright-red scaly plaques with sharp margins in the skinfolds. Small papules and pustules may be seen, along with satellite lesions.

Mild diaper dermatitis is treated with a water-impermeable barrier or protective sealant such as zinc oxide, Aquaphor, Desitin, or Balmex after every diaper change. In some cases a combination product (e.g., karaya powder, Stomahesive Protective powder) may be effective. An antifungal topical medication (e.g., nystatin) is applied to the skin before the barrier product when *Candida albicans* is present, and continued for 3 days after the rash clears (Nield & Kamat, 2006). Diaper dermatitis with severe inflammation is rarely treated with a low-potency hydrocortisone cream applied once or twice daily for no more than 3 days. Occlusion in the diaper area increases corticosteroid systemic absorption, so its use for diaper dermatitis is very limited (Borkowski, 2004).

Nursing Management

MyNursingKit Care Plan: Atopic Dermatitis

Diaper dermatitis can be a major source of stress for parents who must deal with a child in constant discomfort. Instruct parents to change the diaper as soon as the infant is wet, or at least every 2 hours during the day and once during the night.

Encourage parents to use superabsorbent disposable diapers, which tend to reduce the frequency and severity of diaper dermatitis. When wet, these diapers form a gel that keeps the skin drier than cloth diapers; however, diapers should still be changed every 2 to 3 hours. Tell parents to avoid using tight diapers and waterproof pants. A & D ointment, zinc oxide, and other barrier products can be used to protect the skin from urine and stool. Mineral oil may be helpful in removing pastes so fresh medication can be applied.

Advise parents to wash the perianal area with warm water or a waterless cleanser (Aquanil HC lotion or Cetaphil) after a bowel movement. Most soaps remove lipids, making the skin more permeable to irritants (Borkowski, 2004). Advise parents to use soft paper towels with water or babywipes without alcohol at other times. Talcum powder is abrasive and offers no protection (Atherton, 2004).

Exposing the diaper area to air helps aid healing; for example, parents could allow the child to go without a diaper while lying on an absorbent pad or cloth. Watch for signs of infection since the skin is damaged and can allow infectious organisms to grow. The child should return for further care if the skin condition has not improved within a week.

SEBORRHEIC DERMATITIS

Seborrheic dermatitis is a recurrent inflammatory skin condition thought to be caused by an overgrowth of a yeast, *Malassezia furfur* (formerly *Pityrosporum ovale*). The condition is thought to be influenced by hormones. The rash is found over the areas of the body where the sebaceous glands are most plentiful: scalp (cradle cap), forehead, and postauricular and periorbital areas. It may also occur on the skin of the eyelids, inguinal area, or nasolabial folds. The condition is frequently seen in infants up to 3 months of age and in adolescents.

Common symptoms are pruritus and a mildly erythematous, adherent, waxy scaling of the scalp (or "dandruff"). Yellow-red patches with greasy scaling may be present, typically on the scalp and nasolabial folds on the face, behind the ears, on the upper chest, and sometimes on the **intertriginous** (skin folds of the neck, axillae, antecubital fossa) areas (Figure 59–3 ●). Itching is less intense than with atopic eczema.

Prevention for young infants consists of daily shampooing with baby shampoo. Once seborrhea develops, an emollient (e.g., white petroleum or baby oil) is left on the scalp for about 20 minutes to soften the crusts after shampooing. The scales are removed by brushing with the fingertips or a soft toothbrush. The hair is then shampooed again and rinsed thoroughly. A tar-containing

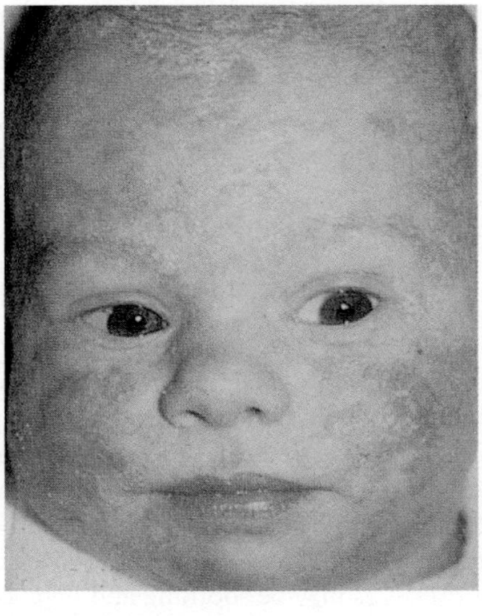

• **Figure 59–3** Seborrheic dermatitis.

shampoo may be used in infants if baby shampoo is not effective (O'Connor, McLaughlin, & Ham, 2008). Lesions on the body can be treated with shampoos containing selenium sulfide or salicylic acid. Use baby shampoo to wash lesions on the eyelids and eyelashes. Treatments are continued for several days after the lesions disappear. Topical corticosteroids are used to treat seborrhea that is not on the scalp, but avoid its use around the eyes.

Nursing Management

Teach new parents to wash the infant's hair regularly with each bath. Reassure parents that gentle cleansing will not harm the infant's "soft spot." Demonstrate bathing to show them the proper technique, if necessary. Follow-up is seldom necessary, as the condition resolves with treatment. Advise adolescents that emotional distress may trigger future flare-ups and to initiate treatment promptly when symptoms begin.

BACTERIAL INFECTIONS

IMPETIGO

Impetigo, the most common bacterial skin condition, is a highly contagious, superficial (epidermal) infection caused by streptococci, staphylococci, or both. The most common sites are the face, around the mouth, the hands, the neck, and the extremities.

Minor skin injuries, insect bites, and dermatitis provide the portal for the infectious agent. Group A *beta-hemolytic streptococcus* and *Staphylococcus aureus* are usually responsible. *Staphylococcus aureus* colonizes on the skin and mucous membranes, particularly in the nose and throat. This infection occurs more commonly in children who are in close physical contact with others, such as in childcare settings, or who have poor hygiene.

Impetigo lesions begin as a papule that turns into a vesicle at the injury site. The vesicle ruptures and forms an erosion, and serous fluid forms the characteristic honey-colored crusts. Pruritis and regional lymphadenopathy may be present. The rash may spread to the face and extremities by self-inoculation (Figure 59–4 ●). In bullous impetigo, vesicles stimulated by a toxin enlarge and coalesce to form bullae with sharp margins and no surrounding erythema. A thin honey-colored crust forms when the bullae rupture. When the crust is removed, a moist, erythematous lesion with a collar of skin around the erosion is seen. These lesions occur more commonly in moist skinfold areas. Impetigo is diagnosed by appearance or lesions, or a Gram stain and bacterial culture.

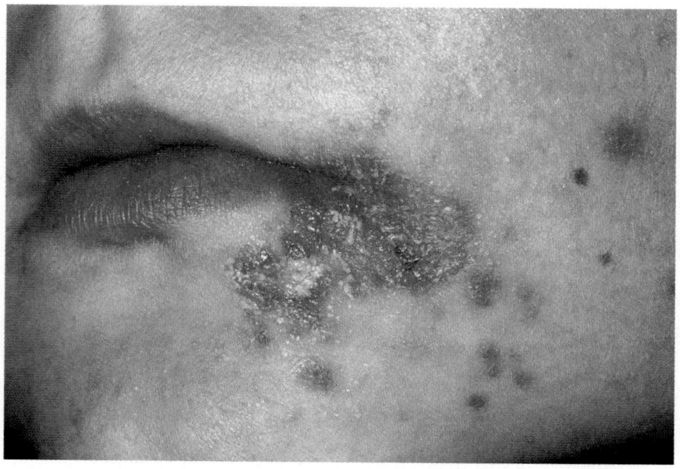

● **Figure 59–4** Impetigo. Note the honey-colored crusts over the lesion.

> **Nursing Practice**
>
> If the child has a history of recurrent impetigo, investigate whether a caregiver or family member is a nasal carrier of *Staphylococcus aureus*. The carrier can be effectively treated with topical mupirocin ointment applied to the nares twice daily for 5 days (McLeod, 2004).

Methicillin-resistant *Staphylococcus aureus* (MRSA) is becoming more common and identifying the appropriate antibiotic to which it is sensitive is important when initial treatment response is poor. Local treatment involves removal of the crusts and application of a topical antibiotic. Crusts are soaked in warm water and gently scrubbed off with an antiseptic soap. Mupirocin, a topical bactericidal ointment, is applied 3 times a day for 5 to 7 days. Alternatively, retapamulin 1% ointment (Altabax) is applied twice a day for 5 days (Bell, 2007). If there is no response to topical antibiotics, a culture and systemic antibiotic may be needed. The infection is communicable for 24 hours after antibiotic ointment treatment is begun.

Some cases of postinfectious streptococcal glomerulonephritis have occurred following impetigo caused by specific strains of group A *beta-hemolytic streptococcus*, as an immune response to the infection (see Chapter 54). Prompt treatment of impetigo does not decrease its incidence (Popovich & McAlhany, 2007).

Nursing Management

Advise parents that they must continue topical or oral medications for the full number of days prescribed. Inform the parents to observe all close contacts and family members for lesions. Caution them that an infected child should not share towels or toiletries with others and to wash separately with detergent and hot water all linens and clothing used by the child. Keep fingernails short and clean to prevent spreading infection by scratching. Inform the childcare center about the infection, so staff can sanitize toys and surfaces.

Increased cases of MRSA have been reported among athletes in high school, particularly when skin trauma occurs or when items are shared. Educate parents, adolescents, coaches, and teachers about the importance of a regular schedule for cleaning equipment and taking showers with soap and water after all practice sessions. Discourage athletes from sharing of towels and clothing. Cover wounds to reduce exposure to other athletes. Skin infections that worsen rather than heal with regular topical antibiotics should be seen by a healthcare provider.

FOLLICULITIS

Folliculitis is a superficial inflammation of the pilosebaceous follicle caused by infection, trauma, or irritation. The causative organism is usually *Staphylococcus aureus*. The condition is common in children and teenagers because of increased sweat production. Folliculitis may be associated with *Pseudomonas aeruginosa* exposure in a poorly chlorinated pool or hot tub.

Symptoms include pain or pruritus, localized swelling, and the formation of tiny dome-shaped, yellowish pustules and red papules at follicular openings with surrounding erythema. Individual lesions may become deeper and form an abscess (furuncle). Lesions are usually seen in clusters on the face, scalp, trunk, and extremities. Some children have fever, aching, and flulike symptoms. If associated with *Pseudomonas* exposure in a pool or hot tub, lesions may develop on areas covered by bathing suits.

Treatment of inflamed follicles consists of washing the affected area with a topical antibiotic cleanser (e.g., chlorhexidine) and water. A benzoyl peroxide gel or wash or another drying agent will also help clear the infection. Ruptured lesions heal with hyperpigmentation and no scarring. Complications are rare. If lesions do not resolve within a week, the child may need systemic antibiotics (e.g., ciprofloxacin). If a furuncle develops, incision and drainage may be needed.

Nursing Management

Nursing management focuses on educating the parents and child about prevention. Advise children to shower daily and shortly after exercise, to cleanse with an antibacterial soap, and to wear loose cotton clothing. Talk with parents about the importance of maintaining the correct pH level and chlorine concentration in swimming pools and hot tubs. Bathing suits of affected children should be laundered and well dried before the next use.

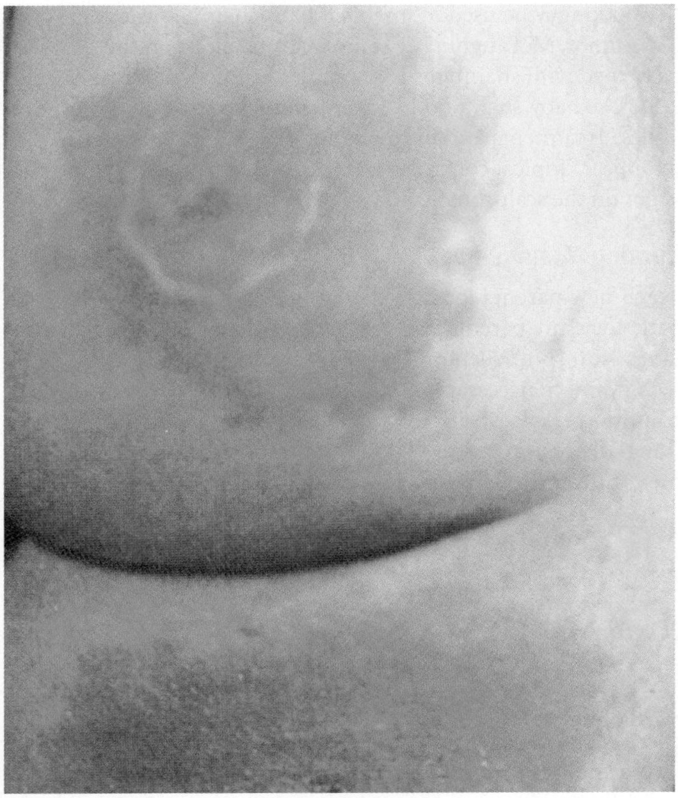

● **Figure 59–5** Characteristic appearance of cellulitis.

Used with permission from Ben-Amitai, D., & Ashkenazi, S. (1993). Common bacterial skin infections in children. *Pediatric Annals, 22*(4), 226. Photograph courtesy of Dr. Aryeh Metzker.

CELLULITIS

Cellulitis is an acute inflammation of the dermis and underlying connective tissue characterized by red or lilac, tender, warm, edematous skin. The condition usually occurs on the face and extremities as a result of trauma or a compromised skin barrier.

Etiology and Pathophysiology

The child may have a history of trauma, impetigo, folliculitis, or recent otitis media. Common causative organisms are *Staphylococcus aureus*, *Streptococcus pyogenes*, and *Streptococcus pneumoniae*. The condition may also result from a nearby abscess or sinusitis. Onset is usually rapid.

Clinical Manifestations

Children with cellulitis have a rapid onset and they appear ill. Classic signs and symptoms include erythema, edema of the face or infected limb, and warmth and tenderness around the infected site (Figure 59–5 ●). The border is often indistinct because the infection is deep in the tissue. Other symptoms include fever, chills, malaise, and enlargement and tenderness of regional lymph nodes. Lymphangitis may be present. In some cases, a rapidly progressive lesion may result in septicemia.

Clinical Therapy

Blood studies may show an increase in white blood cells. Cultures are taken by needle aspiration to identify the causative organisms. Blood cultures and a lumbar puncture are performed if the child has a toxic (very ill) appearance (see Skill 10–5 SKILLS).

If the face is involved, intravenous antibiotic therapy is administered to avoid serious complications. Children with severe cases or a large affected surface area are treated with systemic antibiotics and analgesics in the hospital to prevent sepsis. Children with cellulitis on the trunk, limbs, or perianal area may be treated on an outpatient basis with oral antibiotics. Recovery begins within 48 hours, but therapy should continue for at least 10 days (Morelli, 2007b). See Chapter 47 for treatment of periorbital cellulitis.

NURSING MANAGEMENT

NURSING ASSESSMENT AND DIAGNOSIS

Assessment centers on recognition of infection, documentation of location and related symptoms, and monitoring of vital signs.

Nursing diagnoses that may be appropriate for the child with cellulitis include the following:

- *Impaired Skin Integrity* related to mechanical factors (injury, the inflammatory process, and presence of infection)

- *Acute Pain* related to swelling and inflammation of the skin
- *Interrupted Family Processes* related to home care needs of child with acute illness

PLANNING AND IMPLEMENTATION

Because of the risk of sepsis, cellulitis is managed carefully. Administer prescribed oral or IV antibiotics as scheduled. Supportive care includes warm compresses to the affected area four times daily, elevation of the affected limb, and bed rest. Outpatient follow-up is crucial to ensure response to therapy.

Advise parents about possible complications, such as abscess formation. Instruct parents of children treated at home to contact their healthcare provider if the child has any of the following signs:

- Spread of the infected area in the 24- to 48-hour period after the start of treatment
- Temperature over 38.3°C (101°F)
- Increased lethargy

Reinforce to parents the importance of compliance with the treatment regimen and the seriousness of the possible complications.

EVALUATION

Expected outcomes of nursing care include pain control, adherence with administration of antibiotics, and resolution of the infection without progression to systemic infection.

VIRAL INFECTIOUS DISORDERS

MOLLUSCUM CONTAGIOSUM

Molluscum contagiosum is a skin infection caused by a poxvirus. It is transmitted by direct contact, by contact with contaminated objects, or by sexual contact. Multiple pearl-like flesh-colored smooth papules are about 2 mm to 5 mm in size. The lesion has a central depression, and a plug of cheesy material can be expressed when punctured. Lesions may appear anywhere on the body, but tend to be seen more commonly on the face, trunk, and extremities. Adolescents may have lesions on the genital mucous membranes. Children generally have up to 20 lesions that appear singly or in groups. Children with impaired immunity or atopic eczema may have a more severe infection with hundreds of lesions (Silverberg, 2007). Each lesion lasts for up to 6 months, but new lesions may appear over 2 to 4 years.

Clinical therapy focuses on symptom care in most cases because aggressive treatments often leave scars or cause pigment change in children with darker skin. Pruritus can be managed with emollients, topical corticosteroids, or oral antihistamines. Aggressive treatment options include application of Cantharidin (a vesicant or blistering agent), liquid nitrogen, or curettage by a dermatologist. Secondary infections are a potential complication.

Nursing Management

Nursing education focuses on reducing disease transmission. Infected children should avoid public swimming pools, hot tubs, and other joint bathing as the virus is more easily transmitted when the skin is wet. Transmission of the virus among household members is high. Towels and sponges should not be shared. The skin should be washed daily with gentle fragrance-free cleansers, followed by application of a hypoallergenic moisturizer or emollient to the entire skin surface. Teach parents to recognize potential secondary infections.

When intervention such as curettage or **cryotherapy** (application of a freezing agent) is performed, ensure that a topical anesthetic is used to minimize pain. Inform the child about what will happen, and provide distraction during the procedure to reduce anxiety.

WARTS (PAPILLOMAVIRUS)

Several types of human papillomavirus infect epithelial cells and cause warts. Various types of warts are found in children: common warts that appear on any skin surface and plantar warts found on the feet. The human papillomavirus is commonly transmitted by direct skin-to-skin contact or mucous membrane contact. The virus also survives on various surfaces, and transmission can occur with contact, such as plantar warts from locker room floors. The incubation period may be 2 to 6 months; however, a latency period may exist in some cases. Children with immune compromise are more susceptible and often have numerous warts.

Common warts appear as skin-colored, rough, scaly papules and nodules on exposed skin surfaces. Individual and multiple warts may be seen, or large plaques may form if autoinoculation occurs. Warts usually cause no pain or itching unless on skin surface areas that become irritated. Plantar warts appear as papules and plaques on the bottom of feet that grow inward and cause pain. Small black dots result from thrombosed vessels on the surface of the warts caused by weight bearing.

No intervention may be recommended as warts often resolve spontaneously over a couple of years. Application of duct tape that is changed every 1 to 3 days over a couple of months is often effective and painless (Smolinski & Yan, 2005). If warts cause pain or a social stigma, clinical therapy may be initiated. Treatment may involve cryotherapy, application of caustic substances or peeling agents, electrocautery, and laser therapy. Treatment is not always successful and may result in scarring.

Nursing Management

Educate the parents and child about how warts are spread by picking at it or chewing on it. Teach parents about the application of peeling agents and caustic substances, or duct tape when prescribed for home use. If the reaction to the substance is painful, encourage the parents to reduce the frequency of the treatment until the pain subsides and then to resume the original treatment schedule. Successful treatment may take several months, and parents may need encouragement to continue the therapy and remain optimistic.

Other viral skin conditions are described in Chapter 45∞.

FUNGAL INFECTIONS

ORAL CANDIDAL INFECTION (THRUSH)

Thrush is a fungal infection, usually caused by *Candida albicans,* that occurs as an acute condition in a child who regularly uses a corticosteroid inhaler or has received antibiotics that disturbed the normal flora and allowed fungal growth. It may occur as a chronic condition in young children who have an immune disorder. See Chapter 32∞ for newborn oral candidal infection.

Oral thrush is characterized by white patches that look like coagulated milk on the oral mucosa and may bleed when removed (Figure 59–6 ●). To distinguish between the two, teach parents that attempts at gentle removal of patches are unsuccessful, whereas actual milk residue can be removed with gentle swabbing. The infant may refuse to nurse or feed because of discomfort and pain. The infant may also have diaper dermatitis. Fever is usually not present.

Treatment involves oral nystatin suspension or clotrimazole, which is applied to the mouth and tongue after feedings. Fluconazole or itraconazole may be used for immunocompromised patients with oropharyngeal candidiasis. If infection is severe, occurs in the esophagus, or invades other body systems, oral fluconazole or intravenous amphotericin B may be prescribed for a minimum of 21 days.

Nursing Management

Teach parents to give the medication by swabbing the suspension on the buccal mucosa and tongue surfaces, allowing the infant to swallow the remaining suspension. Older children should be told to swish the solution around in the mouth before swallowing it.

To help prevent a reinfection, educate parents to use good hand hygiene and to sterilize bottle nipples and pacifiers. Teach parents and older children with asthma to rinse the mouth well with water after using a corticosteroid inhaler. If a spacer is used, it should also be rinsed with water after use. A commercial antiseptic spray may be used on toys that cannot be autoclaved, but follow directions carefully so the child does not ingest any harmful residue.

DERMATOPHYTOSES (RINGWORM)

Dermatophytoses are fungal infections that affect the skin, hair, or nails. Children of all ages may be affected. The most common infections are tinea capitis, tinea corporis, tinea cruris, and tinea pedis. See "Clinical Manifestations: Tinea Infections." Dermatophytoses may be spread from another person, an animal, or by contact with a contaminated object.

Diagnosis is confirmed through microscopic examination of the hair and scalp scrapings using a potassium hydroxide (KOH) wet mount to reveal rows and chains of spores within the hair shaft. A fungal culture can also be taken from a scalp lesion by rubbing a cotton-tipped applicator across the scalp or body lesion. A Wood's lamp is also useful in identifying some forms of tinea. For example, microsporum infection fluoresces a brilliant green under ultraviolet light. However, the most common causes of tinea (e.g., *Trichophyton tonsurans*) do not fluoresce (American Academy of Pediatrics, 2009, p. 662). See the Clinical Manifestations table for clinical therapy.

Nursing Management

All members of the family and household pets should be assessed for fungal lesions. Since person-to-person transmission is common, family members should avoid sharing hair accessories, brushes, and hats. In some cases, a family member may be an asymptomatic carrier, so all family members should be treated. Teach parents and older children or teenagers that

> **Nursing Practice**
>
> Some children treated for tinea capitis will develop an "id" reaction, an extensive, itchy rash on the trunk, extremities, and face similar to atopic eczema. This is a hypersensitivity reaction to the fungus antigen, not an allergic reaction to the oral medication (Shy, 2007). A systemic antihistamine may be given for itching. Antifungal therapy is continued to resolve the infection.

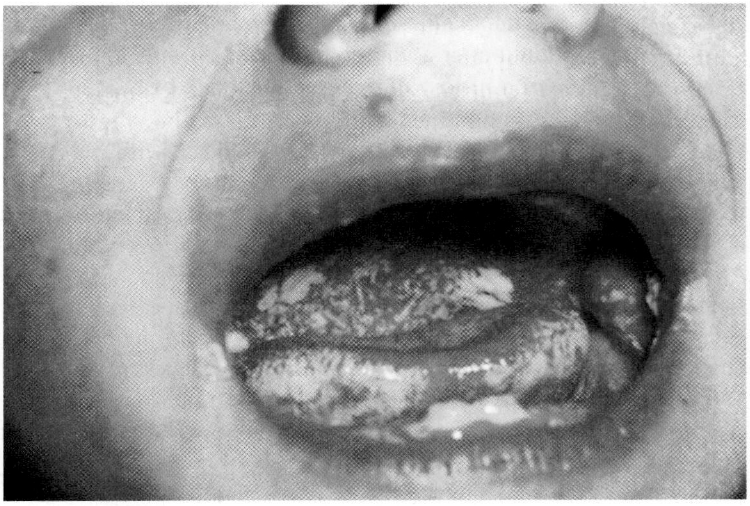

● **Figure 59–6** Oral thrush. Thrush is an acute pseudomembranous form of candidiasis. It is a common fungal infection in infants and children.

Used with permission from Zitelli, B. J., & Davis, H. W. (Eds.). (1997). *Atlas of pediatric physical diagnosis* (3rd ed., p. 104, Fig. 4–50a). St. Louis, MO: Mosby.

Clinical Manifestations

TINEA INFECTIONS

INFECTION SITE AND CLINICAL MANIFESTATIONS	CLINICAL THERAPY
TINEA CAPITIS (SCALP) Scaly pustular bald areas with indistinct margins; may appear as seborrhea, with yellow, greasy scales; erythema or lesion lighter than skin color Broken hairs; dotted stubbed appearance where weakened hair has broken off Mild itching **Kerion**—large purulent tender boggy mass on scalp with drainage	Griseofulvin orally for 8–12 weeks, OR Terbinafine orally for 6 weeks in children over age 4 years. Selenium sulfide shampoo 2–3 times weekly leaving the shampoo on the scalp for 10 minutes before rinsing. Encourage family members to use the shampoo 2–3 times a week to reduce the number of fungus spores in the household. Oral antifungal agents for kerions, but oral corticosteroids may also be prescribed (American Academy of Pediatrics, 2009, p. 662).
TINEA CORPORIS (TRUNK) Pink, scaly circular patch with an expanding border, may be scaly or erythematous throughout; slightly raised borders with a clearing center Usually acquired from contact with infected human, cat, dog, or horse (Monroe, 2005)	Topical cream (e.g., clotrimazole, miconazole, ketoconazole, naftifine, terbinafine) twice a day for 4 weeks. Do not use a topical corticosteroid to prevent a persistent or recurrent infection. Selenium sulfide shampoo 2–3 times a week on the child's body to help reduce the number of spores. Family members may also use the shampoo. An oral antifungal agent for extensive lesions or when no response to topical therapy.
TINEA CRURIS ("JOCK ITCH") Scaly, erythematous annular lesions; may have elevated lesions, papules, or vesicles May spread to abdomen, buttocks, and upper thighs, usually spares the penis and scrotum	Topical antifungal agent such as imidazole for 2 weeks or butenafine, naftifine, or terbinafine for 1 week. Wash body area with selenium sulfide shampoo. Decrease moisture and occlusion in area.
TINEA PEDIS ("ATHLETE'S FOOT") Vesicles or erosions on instep or between toes (fissures, red scaly); dry scaly patches or plaques with erythema on plantar and lateral surfaces of foot Peeling maceration and fissures in lateral toe web spaces indicates secondary bacterial involvement Pruritus	Broad-spectrum topical antifungal agent with antibacterial properties, e.g., econazole or ciclopirox. Allow feet to air dry. Use 100% cotton socks, change twice daily; put socks on before other clothing to reduce transmission of fungus.

fungi are found in soil and animals and are transmitted through direct contact.

Advise parents to give oral griseofulvin with fatty foods such as whole milk or peanut butter to enhance absorption. To prevent recurrence of the infection, the medications must be used for the entire prescribed period, even if the lesions are gone. Advise parents about the possibility of the "id" reaction so they will continue to give the medication.

For children with tinea cruris, encourage loose-fitting undergarments to promote dryness. With tinea pedis, feet should be kept clean and dry and nails clipped short. Encourage the use of 100% cotton socks that wick moisture away from the skin. Encourage children to wear shower shoes in public showers and locker rooms.

Parents of children with tinea capitis should be told that hair regrowth is slow and may take 6 to 12 months. In rare cases hair loss is permanent, which can be particularly stressful for older children or adolescents. Provide emotional support.

DRUG REACTIONS

Adverse reactions to over-the-counter or prescription medications are relatively common. Children with drug allergies usually have reactions after ingestion (e.g., aspirin, antibiotics, sedatives), injection (e.g., penicillin), or direct skin contact with medications. Drug sensitivities may result from variations in an individual's ability to tolerate a particular drug or concentration of a drug or from allergic responses. (See Chapter 50 for a description of allergic reactions.)

Reactions may occur after 1 or 2 doses when the child has previously taken the drug, but it may take up to 7 days for sensitivity to occur to a drug not previously administered. The most common reactions in children are erythematous macules and papules or urticaria, which may be pruritic. Drugs most likely to cause maculopapular eruptions, urticaria, and pruritus include the following: sulfonamides, anticonvulsants, antibiotics (penicillins, cephalosporins, erythromycin,

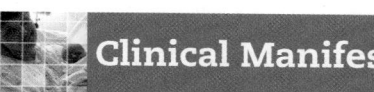

Clinical Manifestations

DRUG REACTIONS

TYPE OF REACTION	CLINICAL MANIFESTATIONS
ALLERGIC DRUG REACTION Most commonly caused by sulfonamides, tetracyclines, NSAIDs, oral contraceptives, barbiturates, and phenolphthalein.	Erythematous, pruritic macules and papules; urticaria that moves from one body part to another. A fixed drug reaction (lesion occurs in same site as earlier drug reaction) is unusual; may commonly involve the face, genitals, sacrum; may heal with hyperpigmentation.
ERYTHEMA MULTIFORME MINOR Hypersensitivity reaction to anticonvulsants, penicillins, salicylates, sulfa antibiotics, barbiturates, and phenytoin; infectious agents (e.g., herpes simplex virus).	Skin lesions may be preceded by fever, malaise, and upper respiratory symptoms. Widespread pruritic macules progress to target lesions (papules, vesicles, or bullae in a pale ring with an erythematous border), and then to plaques. May progress to blisters and bullous lesions. Lesions common on palms and soles, elbows, extensor surface of forearms and legs; few mucosal lesions.
STEVENS-JOHNSON SYNDROME (SJS) AND TOXIC EPIDERMAL NECROLYSIS (TEN) Potentially life-threatening hypersensitivity reaction or autoimmune response to penicillins, sulfonamides, anticonvulsants, NSAIDs, or reaction to infectious disease such as *Mycoplasma pneumoniae*. Believed to be forms of the same disease and the most severe form of erythema multiforme.	Prodromal infection for 1–7 days with cough, coryza, sore throat, fever, malaise, headache, muscle aches, joint pain. Vomiting and diarrhea may be seen. Widespread blistering, erosions, and ulcerations of mucous membranes followed by crusting and conjunctivitis; precedes skin rash by 1 to 2 days. Target lesions, bullae, and erosions (similar to partial thickness burns) may spread to cover up to 10% of the skin surface in SJS, 10% to 30% in overlapping SJS and TEN, and more than 30% in TEN; full thickness epidermis peels off in sheets easily with light pressure. Corneal blistering can lead to scarring and blindness. Respiratory and gastrointestinal tracts may have mucosal sloughing. Causes hypopigmentation in children with dark skin, but hyperpigmentation in children with white skin. Hyperpigmentation fades over time. Signs of sepsis.

Data from Nicol, N. H., Huether, S. E., & Weber, R. (2006). Structure, function, and disorders of the integument. In K. L. McCance & S. E. Huether, *Pathophysiology: The biologic basis for disease in adults and children* (5th ed., pp. 1589–1590), St. Louis: Elsevier Mosby; Aber, C., Connelly, E. A., & Schachner, L. A. (2007). Fever and rash in a child: When to worry? *Pediatric Annals, 36*(1), 30–38; Morelli, J. G. (2007c). Vesiculobullous disorders. In R. M. Kliegman, R. E. Behrman, H. B. Jensen, & B. F. Stanton, *Nelson Textbook of Pediatrics* (18th ed., 2685–2693), St. Louis: Elsevier Mosby; Schmidt, C. E. (2003). A 12-month-old girl with maculopapular lesions and lower extremity edema. *Journal of Emergency Nursing, 29*(3), 204–207.

vancomycin), and nonsteroidal anti-inflammatory drugs (NSAIDS). Be alert to the possibility of serious drug reactions that may become a medical emergency. See "Clinical Manifestations: Drug Reactions."

The treatment of choice for most drug sensitivity reactions is discontinuation of the causative drug. In rare cases, a drug may be continued with careful monitoring when the child has a sensitivity reaction because it is the best treatment choice. Supportive measures should be taken to decrease the intensity of the reaction. An antihistamine may be used to block the release of histamine, which causes the rash. Topical corticosteroids, cool compresses, and baths may also be prescribed for pruritus. For some severe drug reactions, the child must be hospitalized and treated on a burn unit.

Nursing Management

Teach parents to be alert for the signs of drug sensitivity reactions. Obtain a careful history of the child's past reactions to medications before starting new therapies. If a reaction occurs,

Nursing Practice

Children with a true drug allergy (having a past serious systemic reaction) should never be treated with that drug again. Prominently mark the child's records so that all allergies are easily identified. The child should wear a medical alert bracelet.

discontinue the medication until the physician is notified. See nursing care of the burned child on page 1812 for the care of damaged skin due to severe drug reactions.

CHRONIC SKIN CONDITIONS

ATOPIC ECZEMA

Atopic eczema (atopic dermatitis) is a chronic, relapsing, superficial inflammatory skin disorder characterized by intense pruritus (Figure 59–7 ●). The condition affects approximately 17% of infants, children, and adolescents (Tofte, 2007). Up to 65% of children who develop the condition do so during the first year of life, and 90% develop it by 5 years of age (Schachner, Lamerson, Sheehan, et al., 2005). Atopic eczema is a risk factor for development of asthma and allergic rhinitis (Simpson & Hanifin, 2006).

Etiology and Pathophysiology

The etiology of eczema is unknown, but the immune system plays a role, along with a complex interaction of genetic predisposition, environmental exposure, infectious agents, defects in the skin barrier function, and immunologic responses (Akdis, Akdis, Bieber, et al., 2006). Two forms of eczema have been identified: an allergic form (70% to 85% of children) and a nonallergic form (15% to 30% of children) (Peterson & Chan, 2006). Most affected children have T-cell activation and increased IgE levels. The allergic form begins in early childhood and the nonallergic form onset is at a later age (Peterson & Chan, 2006). Triggers of atopic eczema include stress, temperature and humidity changes, allergens (foods before age 3 years and inhalants at later ages), and irritants (e.g., soaps, detergents, abrasive clothing) (Akdis et al., 2006).

Children with eczema have **xerosis**, generally dry skin that is more likely to crack and fissure. The lipid barrier function of the skin is impaired, leading to increased water loss from the epidermis and decreased elasticity. When the skin is chronically dry, irritants have a greater chance to penetrate, and the child is more susceptible to infection.

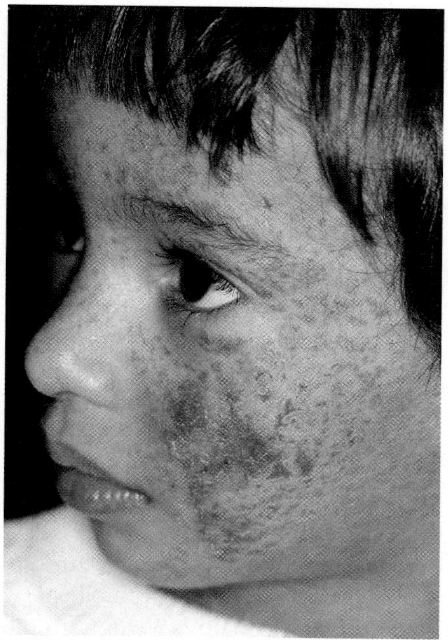

● **Figure 59–7** Chronic eczema.

Clinical Manifestations

Acute eczema is characterized by patches with vesicles, exudate, and crusts. Subacute eczema is characterized by scaling with erythema and excoriation. Some patches may weep. Chronic eczema characteristics include darkened thickened skin with prominent skin lines (lichenification), excoriation, dryness, and scaling. Inflammation usually occurs on the face, neck and extensor surfaces in infants and children. Skinfolds such as the antecubital and popliteal areas are often affected. The itching interferes with sleep and causes irritability. The child moves so much because of the itching discomfort that a perception of hyperactivity may occur. Erythema and warmth may indicate a secondary bacterial infection. See "Clinical Manifestations: Eczema" for the three phases of eczema.

Clinical Manifestations

ECZEMA

ECZEMA TYPE	CLINICAL MANIFESTATIONS
Infantile - 2 months to 2 years	Papulovesicular, and erythematous lesions on face, neck, scalp, and extensor surfaces of extremities; not in diaper area Some patches may weep or have exudate Intensely pruritic; child wiggles to rub and scratch areas out of reach
Childhood - 2 years to puberty	Erythematous, papular, well-circumscribed lesions; pruritus, but less weeping and exudates More thickened, lichenified, and excoriated lesions on flexor and extensor surfaces of extremities, hands, feet, and in neck, perioral, periorbital, and retroauricular folds Dry skin; once toilet trained, buttocks are affected
Adolescent - puberty and onward	Much the same as childhood eczema but generalized form is less acute Localized areas affected may include eyelids, where earlobe touches the face, fingertips, toes, nipple, and the vulvar area plus sites affected in childhood phase

Source: Data from Peterson, J. D., & Chan, L. S. (2006). A comprehensive management guide for atopic dermatitis. *Dermatology Nursing, 18*(6), 531–542.

Clinical Therapy

Eczema is distinguished from other forms of dermatitis by its history and clinical manifestations. No laboratory tests are diagnostic. Diagnostic criteria for eczema include an itching skin condition with three of these factors (Ong & Boguniewicz, 2007):

- History of flexural dermatitis (flexion surfaces of knees, ankles, neck, or cheeks) if less than 4 years old
- History of **atopy**, asthma, or hay fever in a child, or in a first-degree relative if less than 4 years old
- History of dry skin in past year
- Skin rash occurring before 2 years of age
- Visible flexural dermatitis; dermatitis on cheeks, forehead, and outer limbs if less than 4 years old

As there is no cure, the goals of treatment are to hydrate and lubricate the skin, reduce pruritus, minimize inflammatory changes, and try to determine what triggers flare-ups. The skin is lubricated by applying occlusive topical emollients within 3 minutes of leaving the water after bathing. This traps moisture in the skin and promotes flexibility of the skin without cracking. Moisturizing ointments and creams should be applied 3 to 4 times a day, or whenever the skin feels dry.

Topical corticosteroids reduce inflammation and achieve quick control. Ointments are preferred over creams because of their occlusive effect, which ensures a stronger barrier and absorption into the skin. Many different preparations and seven categories of corticosteroid strength exist. Corticosteroids are used twice daily for 2 weeks and must be applied before the skin moisturizer is used. Newer corticosteroid ointments such as fluticasone propionate and mometasone furoate are effective for once-daily use (Dohil & Eichenfield, 2005). Lower potency ointments are used for thinner skin areas, such as the face, diaper area, and skin folds. A higher potency ointment is used for flare-ups. When the inflammation resolves, topical corticosteroids are tapered in frequency of application and potency and then discontinued. Topical steroids are not used on healthy skin to reduce the risk for steroid side effects. Oral corticosteroids may be used for an acute exacerbation; however, there is often a rebound effect (the rash returns after the medication is discontinued). Complementary therapy may also be beneficial. (See "Complementary Therapy: Chamomile.")

Topical antibiotics are used to treat excoriated, open lesions and those that appear infected. Oral antibiotics such as cephalosporin for 5 days may be used to treat superinfections. In some cases a longer course of an antibiotic is needed for chronic recurrent infections (Tofte, 2007). Superinfections with herpes simplex may be treated with acyclovir.

Immunomodulator ointments such as tacrolimus and pimecrolimus are increasingly used as a second-line treatment for some children. However, the medication expense may be too much for some families. The medication has been approved by the U.S. Food and Drug Administration (FDA) for children over 2 years of age, for short-term or intermittent treatment, who are not responsive to conventional therapy. Recent warnings of increased risk for lymphoma and skin cancer associated with duration of use may be of concern to parents (FDA, 2005). Advocates of these medications contrast the adverse effects of long term corticosteroid use and emphasize that all treatments have risks (Tharp, 2005).

Antihistamine agents such as diphenhydramine (Benadryl) or hydroxyzine (Vistaril and Atarax) have a limited effect on itching, but the sedative effect may help promote sleep. Because tolerance to the sedating effects of these medications occurs, their use should be limited to 2 to 7 nights during a flare-up, when scratching interferes with sleep (Kelsay, 2006). Methods to reduce pruritus include aggressively treating flare-ups and environmental controls, such as humidification in the winter and air conditioning in the summer. A humidifier counteracts dryness of the surrounding air, minimizing loss of skin moisture. Air conditioning limits unnecessary sweating that can exacerbate inflamed areas.

The relationship between food allergies and eczema continues to be discussed. An evidence-based review of food allergy and eczema concluded that the avoidance of foods, except perhaps eggs, does not have therapeutic value (Simpson & Hanifin, 2006). Dietary restrictions should not be implemented unless the child has a diagnosis of food hypersensitivity (Akdis et al., 2006). A food elimination test (withholding cow's milk, wheat, eggs, soy products, citrus, and peanuts) may be suggested to see if improvements in the skin condition occur. See Chapter 50 for more information on food allergies.

Complementary Care

CHAMOMILE

Chamomile applied topically to the lesions of atopic eczema has been the focus of a couple of small European studies, and some positive effects have been noted. However, studies with more patients are needed to confirm the benefit of chamomile for atopic eczema. It is important to note that chamomile can cause adverse effects when the individual is allergic to plants in the aster family (ragweed, aster, and chrysanthemums), leading to contact dermatitis (Gardiner, 2007).

Nursing Practice

The potency or strength of a topical corticosteroid is based on whether it is fluorinated and contains other ingredients. Do not rely on the percentage listed on the medication label to inform you about the medication's potency. Refer to a drug manual to identify the potency classification of prescribed topical corticosteroids. Topical corticosteroids bought over-the-counter are low strength.

Avoid the use of fluorinated corticosteroids on the face, genitalia, and skin folds where absorption of the medication is increased because of the thinness of the skin. Occlusive dressings, such as may occur with a tight-fitting diaper, further increase the potential absorption. The lowest concentration of topical corticosteroids should also be used in these areas. Posterior cataracts and glaucoma are a potential adverse effect of topical corticosteroid use around the eyes. Other adverse effects may include skin atrophy due to decreased collagen synthesis and striae after 3 to 4 weeks of therapy.

NURSING MANAGEMENT

NURSING ASSESSMENT AND DIAGNOSIS

Take a thorough history, including any family history of allergy, environmental or dietary factors, past exacerbations, and what makes the eczema flare up. Note distribution and type of lesions, presence of weeping, or signs of infection.

Identify the impact that the skin disorder is having on the child and family. Do the child, siblings, or other family members have disturbed sleep? Is the child's self-esteem disturbed? What other stresses has the child's skin disorder placed on the family? Does the family have concerns about medication use?

Common nursing diagnoses that may be appropriate for the child with eczema include the following:

- *Impaired Tissue Integrity* related to chemical irritants and mechanical factors (abrasive clothing)
- *Insomnia* related to prolonged physical discomfort (itching)
- *Risk for Infection* related to breaks in skin barrier
- *Chronic Low Self-Esteem* related to peer reaction to visible skin lesions
- *Ineffective Therapeutic Regimen Management (Families)* related to excessive demands made on the family to keep the condition under control

PLANNING AND IMPLEMENTATION

Nursing management focuses on education and emotional support. Eczema can be controlled, but there is no cure. Advise parents that the lesions are not contagious and will not usually result in scarring. Help parents and adolescents deal with the frustration of the acute flare-ups of the condition by reinforcing that remissions do occur with good home care.

Bathing once a day is important to hydrate the skin and to allow topical corticosteroids to penetrate the skin. Salt or baking soda added to the bath water may help if water stings the child's open lesions. See "Teaching Highlights: Atopic Eczema Skin Care."

The child, parents, and siblings may be tired because of lost sleep when the child scratches during the night during a flare-up. School performance may be affected if the child has sleep deprivation or if the child has physical discomfort that interferes with learning. If an oral antihistamine has been ordered, make sure the parents understand when to give the medication to maximize its effectiveness to produce a full night of sleep.

Eczema produces visible changes that can affect a child's self-confidence and self-esteem. Identify activities that the child can participate in to improve self-esteem. Because humidity and sweating can make eczema worse, encourage the child to shower after a sporting event or strenuous activity. Needed medications and emollients can then be applied in the order described in the accompanying Teaching Highlights box.

Provide encouragement and positive reinforcement for improvements in the child's skin during healthcare visits. Eczema that is difficult to manage is more stressful and has a more profound effect on the child's and family's quality of life. The use of immunomodulators in children with moderate or severe eczema significantly improves the quality of life in children and adults as measured by daily activities, feelings, relationships, and sleep (Schachner et al., 2005).

When eczema is under control, educate parents about the food elimination diet if a food allergy is suspected (see Chapter 50 ∞).

Teaching Highlights

ATOPIC ECZEMA SKIN CARE

- Help the parents select an unscented emollient ointment or cream (Eucerin, Aveeno, Vanicream, Cetaphil, SBR Lipocream, or white petroleum) that fits into the family's budget. White petroleum is inexpensive, safe, and easily applied. Lotions have a high water and alcohol content that will further dry the skin (Tofte, 2007).
- Help ensure that parents receive adequate amounts of topical corticosteroids for effective treatment. It takes about 6 g to cover the entire body of a 6-month-old infant, so a 12 g tube of corticosteroid ointment is enough for only 1 day, and 84 g are needed for an entire week. Similarly, it takes 10 g to cover the entire body of a 2 year old, 13 g for a 5 year old, and 18 g for a 10 year old (Findlay, 2007). Fortunately most children do not have atopic eczema over the entire body, and the ointment is used only where there is inflammation.
- For immunomodulators, a pea-size amount should cover a 2-in. circle.
- Let the child soak in warm water for up to 20 minutes once or twice a day. Use mild, unscented soap only on dirty areas. Rinse well. Immediately apply the emollient to wet skin, within 3 minutes of leaving the water, covering the entire body.
- When the child has a flare, bathe the child twice a day and apply the topical medications on affected areas. Emollients are applied on top of medications, as well as over the rest of the body.
- In areas with low humidity, apply emollients to the skin more frequently. Corticosteroids should be applied no more than twice a day.
- Encourage the child to wear loose cotton clothing rather than wool or other irritating fabrics.
- Keep the child's fingernails trimmed and use clean cotton gloves or socks over the infant's or child's hands to decrease scratching and reduce the chance of secondary infection.
- Emphasize the importance of following the treatment plan to promote healing of existing lesions and to reduce the risk of secondary infections.

Thinking Critically

THE CHILD WITH ATOPIC ECZEMA

Noah, 15 months of age, has had atopic eczema since 6 months of age. Today he has skin lesions on his face, neck, elbows, and knees. The patches on his elbows and knees are weeping, and he is very uncomfortable because of the itching. His mother has worked hard to treat his eczema, but is very frustrated at this latest flare-up, and she has run out of the corticosteroid ointment. Noah visited his grandmother a few days ago, and she gave him some strawberries to eat. Noah has had skin reactions to certain foods in the past, but never strawberries. Noah's mother cannot think of any other food that could be causing this flare-up.

When talking with Noah's mother, the nurse recommends the following daily skin care routine. Noah is bathed each evening with warm water, and a small amount of soap is used on his legs if they are dirty. She puts the corticosteroid ointment over skin lesions and then white petroleum over his entire body.

- What signs of infection should the nurse and mother be observing for?
- What information can you provide to Noah's mother regarding the role of food allergies in causing atopic eczema?
- Contrast the treatment of acute flare-ups with daily maintenance care for atopic eczema.
- What information can you provide to help control Noah's itching and scratching?

See MyNursingKit for possible responses.

Inform them that increased itching within hours of eating a food may be associated with an eczema flare-up. Once a specific food allergy, such as eggs, has been identified, refer the parents to a nutritionist for counseling about alternative food options that will fulfill daily nutritional requirements. Food allergies can change and new food sensitivities may develop. A food connected with eczema may sometimes be safely eaten later in life. Refer the family to the Food Allergy Network. (See the MyNursingKit for links to such resources.)

EVALUATION

Expected outcomes of nursing care include the following:

- Control of the child's eczema is maintained and no infection occurs.
- Parents identify triggers of the child's eczema and avoid or eliminate them.
- The child's sleep is minimally disturbed by itching.

ACNE

Acne is a chronic inflammatory disorder of the pilosebaceous hair follicles on the face and trunk. It is the most common skin disorder in the pediatric population, affecting 85% of the population aged 12 to 25 years (Nicol & Huether, 2006). Acne is found in all ethnic groups, and occurs equally in males and females. Severe acne is more common in males.

Etiology and Pathophysiology

Keratin and sebum usually flow to the skin surface. Androgens, released as puberty begins, trigger the sebaceous glands to increase the production of sebum. When the extra sebum mixes with the keratinocytes and causes them to clump together, the pilosebaceous follicular canal becomes obstructed by **comedones** (whiteheads and blackheads). The sebum behind the comedone is an ideal environment for the anaerobic *Propionibacterium acnes*, and this bacterium metabolizes the sebum causing an inflammatory rather than infectious reaction (Zaenglein & Thiboutot, 2006). When the inflammatory reaction is close to the surface, a papule or pustule develops. If the inflammatory reaction is deeper, a larger papule or nodule develops. Extensive rupture and inflammation leads to cysts that can result in scars. Familial trends have been recognized, but a pattern of inheritance has not been identified.

Acne may occur in neonates in response to maternal androgen hormones, and it resolves spontaneously in a few months. Drugs such as anabolic steroids, corticosteroids, phenytoin, lithium, and isoniazid are reported to cause acne (Morelli, 2007a). Friction of the skin from hairbands, helmets, and hats, as well as oil-based cosmetics can also trigger acne.

Clinical Manifestations

Comedones are initial skin lesions. Closed comedones are whiteheads or flesh-colored papules with tiny follicular openings. Open comedones are blackheads in which the follicular plug has enlarged and dilated the follicular opening. As inflammation occurs, papules and pustules develop (Figure 59–8 ●). Nodules are larger areas of inflammation that may involve more than one hair follicle. Cysts are compressible nodules without overlying inflam-

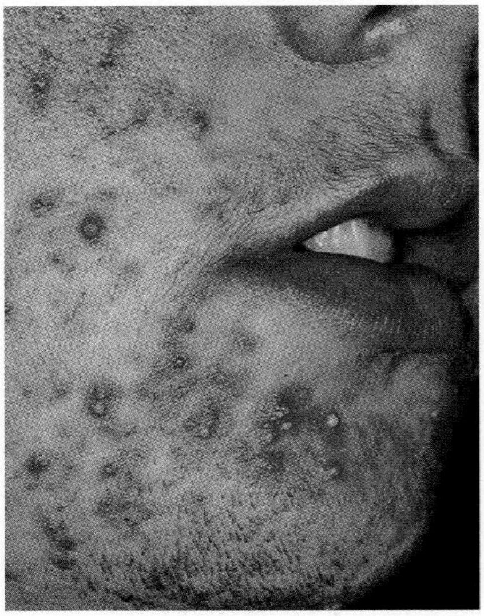

● **Figure 59–8** Pustular acne. Acne can have a significant effect on an adolescent's self-esteem.

Used with permission from Habif, T. P. (1990). *Clinical dermatology: A color guide to diagnosis and therapy* (2nd ed., p. 113). St. Louis, MO: Mosby-Year Book.

mation. Scars form when the surrounding dermis is damaged and may be pitted, atrophic, or hypertrophic (keloid). Lesions occur most often on the face, upper chest, shoulders, and back.

Clinical Therapy

Diagnosis is based upon the examination of the skin. Treatment is customized to the predominant type of lesion present and severity of the lesions. The goal of treatment is to suppress lesions until the condition is outgrown, thus preventing infection and scarring, and minimizing psychologic distress (see the accompanying Drug Guide). Acne will recur gradually if the treatment is stopped, so maintenance therapy is recommended once acne is controlled (Zaenglein & Thiboutot, 2006).

Skin irritation related to topical preparations may occur in adolescents with sensitive skin. Using a lower-concentration product and removing it after a few hours may reduce the initial irritation. With continued use the skin adapts, permitting the product concentration to be changed. Creams are used when skin is more sensitive, while gels are used when skin is more oily. (See the accompanying boxes, "Developing Cultural Competence: Acne Lesions in Individuals with Dark Skin"; and "Complementary Care: Light Treatment.")

Isotretinoin (Accutane) is reserved for severe acne that is not responsive to other therapies. A 5-month course of treatment is given. Because the medication causes sebaceous gland atrophy,

Developing Cultural Competence

ACNE LESIONS IN INDIVIDUALS WITH DARK SKIN

Inflammatory acne in adolescents with darker skin color is associated with a hyperpigmented macule. Extra pigment gets deposited in the areas of inflammation. This color change can last for 4 months or longer, but hyperpigmentation may be permanent when scars form. Azelaic acid has a mild bleaching action that helps with postinflammatory pigment changes that occur in individuals with darker skin (Keri, 2006).

Sunscreen (SPF 30 or higher and noncomedonic) should be used, and may help reduce the postinflammatory discoloration that develops in patients with dark skin (Silverberg, Silverberg, & Silverberg, 2005).

Drug Guide

ACNE

MEDICATION AND ACTION	NURSING MANAGEMENT
Topical retinoids (Tretinoin (Retin-A), Adalpalene, Tazarotene) Inhibits formation of initial comedones, regulates follicular keratinocyte shedding, has anti-inflammatory properties	Use lower concentrations initially as skin irritation is common. Divide and spread a pea-sized amount over the entire face. Do not use as spot therapy. Apply at night as drug stability is affected by light.
Benzoyl peroxide For mild or moderate papulopustular acne Topical antimicrobial with bacteriocidal action	A lower strength may be used initially if skin irritation occurs. Apply in the morning.
Antibiotics (tetracyclines and macrolides) Topical for mild inflammatory acne; oral for moderate to severe inflammatory acne Antimicrobial action, reduces resident skin bacteria	Combined with topical retinoid and benzoyl peroxide to reduce antibiotic resistance. Takes 6 to 8 weeks to see improvement, antibiotic is changed if no response. Discontinued once inflammatory lesions are under good control.
Isotretinoin (Accutane) For severe nodular acne, especially when resistant to other treatment Causes sebaceous gland atrophy and decreases sebum production; reverses effect of androgens on sebaceous glands Represses inflammatory response and comedone production	Requires informed consent. Females need 2 negative pregnancy tests before beginning the medication and a monthly pregnancy test before each prescription refill. Females must use contraception, beginning 1 month prior to treatment, during treatment, and for 1 month after completing treatment due to teratogenic effects of the drug. Take medication with food to increase oral absorption. Monthly monitoring of cholesterol, triglycerides, and liver function is performed.
Oral contraceptives For persistent inflammatory papules and nodules Suppresses gonadotropin secretion and reduces ovarian androgen production	Teach adolescent the correct administration schedule.

Data from Zaenglein, A. L., & Thiboutot, D. M. (2006). Expert committee recommendations for acne management. *Pediatrics, 118*(3), 1188–1199; Kaymak, Y., & Ilter, N. (2006). The results and side effects of systemic isotretinoin treatment in 100 patients with acne vulgaris. *Dermatology Nursing, 18*(6), 576–580.

MyNursingKit Adolescents and Acne Management

Complementary Care

LIGHT THERAPY

Daily treatment with mixed blue and red light for several weeks is an alternate treatment for mild to moderate acne on the face. The bacteria *P. acnes* has porphyrins that fluoresce, and these porphyrins become excited by the wavelength of the blue light and kill the bacteria. Red light has an anti-inflammatory effect. Studies have reported improvement for many patients with acne with light therapy, laser therapy, and most recently with photodynamic therapy preceded by application of methyl aminolevulinic acid (Nestor, 2007).

the improvement in acne is permanent in 70% to 75% of those treated. Recent studies, conducted after a link between taking the medication and an increased risk for suicide became suspected, have found no such association (Hull, Derm, & D'Arcy, 2005). See the Drug Guide for important care guidelines.

NURSING MANAGEMENT

NURSING ASSESSMENT AND DIAGNOSIS

Physical assessment should include documentation regarding distribution, type, and severity of acne lesions. Assess the adolescent's and parents' knowledge about the cause and treatment of acne. Also explore the amount of emotional distress the acne is causing the adolescent.

The "Nursing Care Plan: The Adolescent with Acne" lists common nursing diagnoses and summarized nursing care.

PLANNING AND IMPLEMENTATION

Nursing management focuses on educating the adolescent and parents about acne and its treatment. Encourage good hand hygiene before touching affected areas. Educate them that picking and squeezing lesions may increase the inflammation that occurs with the rupture of lesions below the skin surface. Additional nursing education focuses on avoiding any cleansing products with a greasy base, shampooing the hair regularly, and treating seborrheic dermatitis that can accompany acne. Correct misconceptions about dietary causes. Although no food has been found to cause acne or an increase in severity of lesions, good nutrition is important.

Topical medications should be spread in a thin film over the skin, according to directions. Emphasize that treatment is often long term. Inform the adolescent that treatment may seem to worsen the acne as the comedones are being pushed out, and this is a sign that the medication is working. Significant improvement may not be seen until at least 6 to 12 weeks after beginning treatment, and flare-ups are expected despite treatment. Both increased sweating and emotional stress can contribute to flare-ups.

Caution patients using tretinoin that this medication is **phototoxic** (a rapid nonimmunologic reaction of the skin when exposed to sunlight), resulting in sunburn with even minimal exposure. Teach correct procedures for taking other prescribed drugs, such as tetracycline and isotretinoin (Accutane), and discuss possible side effects. Emphasize the importance of return visits to the adolescent's healthcare provider to monitor medication side effects.

Psychologic support is an important aspect of care. Because adolescents are preoccupied with their body image and peer relationships, they often find having acne embarrassing. Encourage them to express their feelings and refer for counseling, if necessary.

EVALUATION

Expected outcomes of nursing care can be found in "Nursing Care Plan: The Adolescent with Acne."

PSORIASIS

Psoriasis is a chronic, pruritic, papulosquamous skin condition with an onset most commonly between 15 and 35 years of age, although it can occur during infancy. Males, females, and all races are affected equally (Sullivan-Whalen & Gilleaudeau, 2007). A multifactorial inheritance pattern is suspected, and a positive family history of psoriasis is often present.

Psoriasis is a T-cell mediated autoimmune disease. Inflammatory cytokines from activated T-cells are responsible for the skin changes (Nicol, Huether, & Weber, 2006). The dermis and epidermis become thickened and an excessive proliferation of keratinocytes occurs. Because cells proliferate so rapidly, the keratinocytes do not mature.

The typical psoriatic lesion is a thick, silvery scaly erythematous plaque with an irregular border, surrounded by normal skin. Pruritus is often present. These lesions commonly are found on the scalp, elbows, knees, umbilicus, and genitals. Lesions also often appear at the site of trauma. Small points of bleeding may be noted when a scale is removed. Psoriasis may be triggered in children, particularly guttate type, by a streptococcal infection (Wong & Rogers, 2006). Guttate psoriasis is characterized by an eruption of small round or oval papules on the trunk, face, and extremities. Nails may also be affected. The child may have remissions and exacerbations that occur throughout life.

Diagnosis is based on skin lesion characteristics or microscopic examination. Treatment includes topical steroids and topical vitamin D. A tar shampoo may be used to clear scales in the scalp prior to topical steroid application. Ultraviolet B phototherapy is used for children who do not respond to topical therapy. Systemic therapy with drugs such as methotrexate, oral retinoids, and cyclosporine are reserved for children with severe psoriasis.

Nursing Management

The child's skin should be assessed for extent of lesions and response to therapy. Spend time talking with the child and family to learn how the condition affects them. Educate them about the condition and reasonable expectations related to treatment. Families need to understand that lesions are not contagious, and

Nursing Care Plan

THE ADOLESCENT WITH ACNE

INTERVENTION	RATIONALE	EXPECTED OUTCOME
1. Nursing Diagnosis: Effective, Individual Therapeutic Regimen Management related to daily hygiene and skin care		
NIC Priority Intervention: Health education: Developing and providing instruction and learning experiences to facilitate voluntary adaptation of behavior conducive to health in individuals, families, groups, or communities		**NOC Suggested Outcome:** Symptom control behavior: Personal actions to minimize perceived adverse changes in physical and emotional functioning
Goal: The adolescent will verbalize proper hygiene, nutrition, and treatment of acne.		
■ Teach good skin care: ■ Wash skin with mild soap and water twice a day. ■ Do not use astringents or abrasive cleansers. ■ Wash hands frequently, especially after eating greasy foods. ■ Apply topical retinoid 20 minutes after washing and drying face.	■ Good hygiene and appropriate skin care reduces irritation, surface oils and bacteria, which intensify inflammatory reactions. Astringents and aftershave may contain alcohol and further dry the skin.	The adolescent exhibits good hygiene habits and nutrition.
■ Praise good habits.	■ Positive reinforcement encourages continued effort.	
■ Advise the adolescent to wash hair with antiseborrheic shampoo, avoid oil-based cosmetics, pomades or petroleum-based hair products.	■ Seborrhea frequently accompanies acne. Oil-based products can obstruct sebaceous glands, exacerbating acne.	
■ Encourage a balanced diet, adequate fluids, exercise, and adequate rest.	■ Adequate nutrients, water, and exercise promote healthy skin.	
Goal: The adolescent will verbalize understanding of treatment regimen.		
■ Educate the adolescent about medications (action, side effects, dosage, method of application).	■ Proper application of medication enhances healing of lesions.	The adolescent implements the treatment regimen as outlined, resulting in a noticeable reduction in lesions.
■ Encourage application of tretinoin at night. Encourage use of noncomedonic sunscreens of at least SPF 30 during the day.	■ Nighttime application helps reduce sensitivity to sun and sunscreen helps to avoid sunburn.	
■ Educate the adolescent about time needed for a therapeutic response and importance of adhering to daily regimen.	■ Up to 3 months may be needed for significant improvement. The adolescent needs a reason to continue with the care plan.	
■ Encourage continuation of daily therapies even when acne has improved significantly.	■ Acne will return if treatment stops.	
2. Nursing Diagnosis: Disturbed Body Image related to biophysical factors (visible facial lesions)		
NIC Priority Intervention: **Self-esteem enhancement:** Assisting a patient to increase his or her personal judgment of self-worth		**NOC Suggested Outcome:** **Self-esteem:** Personal judgment of self-worth
Goal: The adolescent will demonstrate increased self-confidence and self-esteem.		

(continued)

Nursing Care Plan—continued

THE ADOLESCENT WITH ACNE

INTERVENTION	RATIONALE	EXPECTED OUTCOME
■ Establish a rapport with the adolescent.	■ A trusting relationship promotes verbalization of concerns and fears.	The adolescent freely discusses concerns and fears.
■ Provide education about the condition and therapy modalities.	■ Providing information better enables the adolescent to take control of the condition.	The adolescent demonstrates active involvement in own care.
■ Encourage the adolescent to be responsible for treatment and follow-up, and give positive reinforcement.	■ Responsibility reinforces sense of self-esteem.	The adolescent shows increased confidence, as demonstrated by involvement in extracurricular activities.
■ Encourage the adolescent to become involved with school activities and peers.	■ Involvement in activities helps enhance self-esteem and allows the adolescent to explore new experiences and friendships.	

periods of remissions and flare-ups are common. Actively involve the family and child in decision making regarding the treatment plan. Parents and adolescents need education to appropriately apply topical medications.

Children and adolescents may have feelings of embarrassment, anger, and frustration related to their visible skin lesions. Psoriasis may impact their daily lives causing problems at school, with personal relationships, and with social acceptance. Children may anticipate rejection and withdraw from social interactions. Children and adolescents may withdraw from physical activities that require them to expose affected skin areas, such as swimming. The mental health of adolescents should be monitored to identify psychological distress, depression, or substance abuse. The National Psoriasis Foundation provides supportive information and local or Internet support group contacts. Peers may help the child learn how to handle social situations. See the Companion Website for these resources.

EPIDERMOLYSIS BULLOSA

Epidermolysis bullosa (EBS) is a rare and severe chronic blistering skin disorder that is associated with minor trauma. The most common variants are inherited in an autosomal dominant pattern while other variants are inherited in an autosomal recessive pattern. (See Chapter 7∞.) The incidence in the United States is estimated to be 2 per million live births (Schachner, Feiner, & Camisulli, 2005).

The classifications for this disorder are distinguished by the inheritance pattern and skin layer where the split or blistering occurs (within epidermis, at the junction between the epidermis and dermis, or within the dermis). The most common form (EBS Weber-Cockayne) has blistering that is limited to the hands and feet. Blistering due to friction can occur on any skin surface area with the EBS Koebner form. The most severe form of EBS has a high mortality rate, and it is associated with blisters that develop in the mouth and the respiratory and gastrointestinal tracts. In some forms the blistering lessens in severity with age.

Children with EBS have extremely fragile skin, and blisters form with minor trauma, friction, or heat applied to the skin. In severe forms, the blistering can be extensive and damage to the skin is apparent. Fingers and toes may fuse leading to malformations. Children experience pain with blisters and may have difficulty walking when feet are affected.

Diagnosis can be made prenatally by amniocentesis or chorionic villus sampling or by skin lesion biopsy of the skin lesions (Podraza & Miller, 2007). The condition is managed by prevention of new blisters, wound care, good nutrition, and minimizing the risk for infection. In the more common form of the disorder, blisters generally heal without scarring, and the condition may gradually improve with age. Open wounds increase the risk of infection so wound care is important. Blisters are pricked on two sides with a sterile needle each day and drained so that they do not extend. The blister roof is not removed as it acts as a natural biological dressing. Antibiotic ointments are applied to wounds, and changed monthly to reduce the risk for bacterial resistance. Wounds are covered, and care is taken to avoid placing adhesives directly on the skin. These infants need additional protein and calories, similar to children with burns, because of the chronic wound healing.

Nursing Management

Teach the family to provide daily wound care at home. Wound care can be quite time consuming, so help the parents select the best time to do routine dressing changes. Determine if financial support is needed to ensure that parents have the dressing supplies needed to effectively manage the child's wounds. Provide parents with guidance on all aspects of dressing changes.

- Gather all supplies and have an assistant present. Ask the assistant to gently hold the child's extremities to prevent movement of the extremity during blister lancing and dressing changes. Holding or grabbing the extremity too tightly can cause friction injury.

- Use soft music and distraction to help calm the infant.
- Soak off dressings that are stuck to the skin.
- Inspect the skin each day for signs of infection. Encourage parents to remove dressings from one location at a time as exposure to the air may be painful for the infant.
- Use nonadherent dressings that can absorb the blister fluid to help prevent dressings from sticking to the skin. Place a bulky cover over the dressing to protect the skin and promote healing. Wrap fingers and toes separately so they do not fuse together with healing.

Help the parents to identify ways to protect the skin but still permit the child to interact with other children and have opportunities for development. Dress the child in soft cotton clothing that covers the skin, placing rough seams that can irritate the skin on the outside. Foam padding can be sewn into clothing over the knees and elbows for the infant who is crawling or walking. Shoes without seams on the inside should be worn with seamless cotton socks. Cotton socks can be used to mitten the infant's hands during sleep. The child should also avoid sun exposure and to stay where temperatures are cool (Schachner et al., 2005).

Protein is lost with blisters and chronic wound healing requires extra calories. Promote good nutrition with adequate calories and high protein to meet the child's growth and healing requirements. In infants, blistering in the mouth may interfere with feeding. A soft nipple with a larger hole may be easier for the infant to use. Vaseline on the lips may help reduce trauma to the mouth. Food temperature should be cool or room temperature and nonacidic to prevent injury to the gastrointestinal tract. In some cases a gastrostomy tube is inserted for nutritional supplementation. Regularly measure height and weight and plot measurements on a growth curve to monitor growth and to identify growth deficiencies early.

Help parents and the child manage the psychological impact of this disfiguring disorder and the inability to fully participate in all activities. An Individual Health Plan with educational accommodations will be necessary. Because the hands and feet are often involved, writing and test taking may be challenging. Mobility and walking throughout the school may also be a problem. Information needs to be provided to classroom teachers and classmates to help minimize injury.

INFESTATIONS

PEDICULOSIS CAPITIS (LICE)

Pediculosis capitis is a lice infestation of the hair and scalp. Infestation occurs among children of all socioeconomic levels, and it is most common in children ages 4 to 11 years (Sladden & Johnston, 2005). Parents or teachers may be the first to notice lice, or healthcare providers may spot them during routine examination (see Chapter 35). Outbreaks occur periodically among preschool and school-age children, particularly those in child care and elementary school.

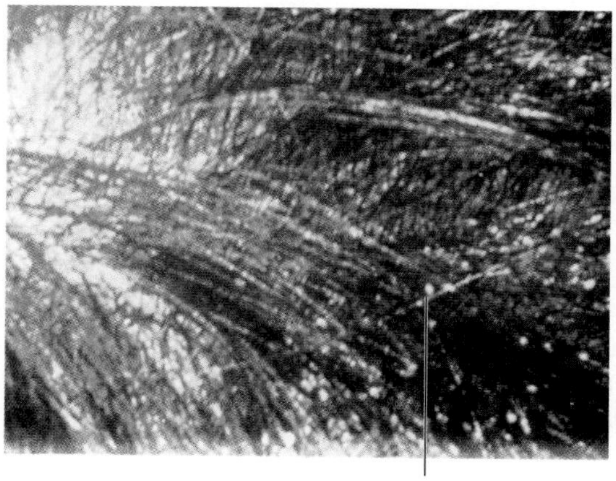

● **Figure 59–9** Lice. Note the presence of lice nits adhering to hair shafts.

Courtesy of Centers for Disease Control.

Head lice live and reproduce only on humans and are transmitted by direct hair-to-hair contact or indirect contact such as sharing of hair accessories, hats, towels, and bedding. Lice are wingless insects about the size of a sesame seed. They move quickly away from light and are not often seen. Lice do not fly or jump, but they can crawl quickly.

The female louse lays her eggs (nits) on the hair shaft, close to the scalp (Figure 59–9 ●). Nits look like silvery white, yellow, or darker 1-mm teardrops adhering to one side of the hair shaft. The incubation period for eggs to hatch is 8 to 10 days. Lice feed on human blood several times a day.

Clinical manifestations include intense pruritus and complaints of "dandruff" that sticks to the hair (actually the nits) and "bugs" in the hair. Secondary effects of scratching include inflammation, pustules, and bacterial infection. Nits are found most commonly behind the ears and at the base of the head. Posterior cervical nodes are frequently palpable.

Treatment involves a pediculicide shampoo, such as pyrethrin within an enzymatic lice egg remover, or an ovicidal rinse, such as permethrin (Nix). Permethrin cream rinse is applied to dry hair and left in place for 10 minutes, before rinsing. The hair is towel-dried, and the nits are removed with a fine-toothed comb. A second treatment is needed in 7 to 10 days as the neurotoxin is not effective on nits. Permethrin resistance has been reported, but a 5% concentration is effective. See the Drug Guide

Nursing Practice

Lindane must be used with caution because of neurotoxicity and potential to cause seizures. It should only be used when other approved treatments are not tolerated or have failed. It should not be used in infants because they may absorb too much of the pesticide through their thin skin (FDA, 2007). It is also contraindicated in children with seizure disorders or hypersensitivity to the product (Leung, Fong, & Pinto-Rojas, 2005).

Drug Guide

TREATMENT FOR HEAD LICE

NAME OF MEDICATION/PREPARATION	NURSING MANAGEMENT
Insecticide-Free	
Lice B Gone Lice Away Enzyme Shampoo Hair Clean 1-2-3 LiceFreee!	Apply all products to *dry hair*.
Cetaphil cleanser	Apply lotion to wet scalp and dry it with a hair dryer to shrink wrap and suffocate lice (Pearlman, 2004).
Oil, petroleum jelly, mayonnaise	Cover with shower cap overnight.
Distilled white vinegar or formic acid	Used as a rinse to loosen nits after use of pediculicide.
First-Line Pesticide Treatment	
Permethrin 1% Crème Rinse–Nix Pyrethrin shampoo (0.33%) or Piperonyl butoxide–Rid, A-200, Bayer, and generic brands	Should be applied to *dry hair and scalp*. Massage into the hair one section at a time. Wet hair dilutes the product and may contribute to treatment failure. Permethrin is approved for children 2 months and older.
Second-Line Pesticide Treatment	
Malathion 0.5%–Ovide lotion Lindane 1% or "lindano"–Kwell, limited effectiveness as a result of resistance; central nervous system toxicity	Apply to *dry scalp and hair* until soaked and allowed to dry naturally. Leave on for 8–12 hours. Do not expose the child treated with malathion to electric heat sources or flames as it is flammable.
Non-FDA Approved	
Trimethoprim/sulfamethoxazole Ivermectin–antiparasitic	Drug in bloodstream is ingested by louse, destroys bacterial flora in louse intestine. Trimethoprim/sulfamethazole is reserved for cases resistant to pediculicides (Leung et al., 2005). Medications do not treat the nits.

Complementary Care

HOT-AIR TREATMENT FOR LICE

Hot air with high volume and a comb-like device at the end of the hose has been found to be effective in the treatment of lice. While the hot air is blowing, the hair is slowly combed, taking about 30 minutes to treat the entire scalp. The mortality rate for eggs and lice was nearly 100% without the use of any medications. The specially developed hot air machine, not currently on the market, could potentially be available for use in schools and other healthcare setting (Goates, Atkin, Wilding, et al., 2006).

for products used to treat lice. See "Complementary Care: Hot-Air Treatment for Lice" for one new therapy being investigated.

Nursing Management

Carefully assess children who have been exposed to head lice using a bright light and magnifying glass to look for lice and nits along the hair shaft close to the scalp. To avoid potential reinfestation of other children, change gloves frequently when assessing several children in a classroom setting.

Infestation with lice can be upsetting for both the child and family. Emphasize to the family that anyone can get lice. Thorough interventions and education are essential for effective treatment. All family members and contacts of the child should be examined for infestation and treated as necessary. Tell parents that children infested with lice should not return to child care or school until after the first pediculicide treatment is completed. Teach the child not to share clothing, headwear, or combs.

Explain to parents that the shampoo and rinses prescribed are pesticides and must be used for the time specified and as directed. An extra bottle of shampoo may be needed if the child has extra long hair. Keep these products out of the eyes and mouth of the child during their use as they will irritate mucous membranes.

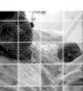

To remove nits, use a small-toothed comb, tweezers, and a basin filled with water or isopropyl alcohol to dip and clean the comb and tweezers. Comb 1-inch sections from the scalp outward and pin these out of the way when done. Nits adhere to the hair shaft and must be manually pulled down the shaft with the comb, tweezers, or fingernails. All nits should be removed. Have blunt-nosed scissors available to cut a hair shaft below the level of the nit when the nit cannot be removed. Put the child under a bright light and use distractions such as a video to keep the child entertained during the procedure. Check the hair every 2 to 3 days and remove any lice or nits seen. An alternative therapy for boys is to cut off the hair in a close buzz cut. A shorter hair cut for girls may help with nit removal.

Although lice can survive for only about 3 days away from a human host, shed nits may hatch 8 to 10 days later. For this reason, the child's bedding, towels, and clothing should be changed daily, laundered in hot water with detergent, and dried in a hot dryer for 20 minutes. Nonessential bedding and clothing can be stored in a tightly sealed bag for 2 to 3 weeks and then washed. Hair accessories, brushes, and combs should be discarded or soaked in hot soapy water (54.4°C [130°F]) for 10 minutes. Vacuum furniture and carpets and treat them with a hot iron when possible. It is not recommended that the family use an insecticide in the home to kill the lice on carpets, furniture, and other items with which young children and pets come into contact. Seal toys and other personal items that cannot be washed or dry-cleaned in a plastic bag for 2 weeks.

SCABIES

Scabies is a highly contagious infestation caused by the mite *Sarcoptes scabiei*. It is spread by skin-to-skin and sexual contact. Transmission within a household is common. Children of all ages and both sexes can be affected. Because the mite usually takes at least 45 minutes to burrow into the skin, transient contact is unlikely to cause infestation.

The female mite burrows into the outer layer of the epidermis (stratum corneum) to lay her eggs, leaving a trail of debris and feces under the skin. The larvae hatch in approximately 2 to 4 days and proceed toward the surface of the skin. The cycle is repeated 14 to 17 days later. A delayed type IV hypersensitivity reaction to the mites, debris, and feces occurs within 2 to 4 weeks of infestation, causing irritation and intense pruritus; however, response to reinfestation can occur within 48 hours (Sladden & Johnston, 2005). Nodules develop as a granulomatous response to the dead mites' antigen and feces and can persist for weeks after effective treatment.

Symptoms include a rash with various types of lesions, severe pruritus that worsens at night, and restlessness. Lesions are usually located in the webs of the fingers, in the intergluteal folds, around the axillae, or on the palms, wrists, head, neck, legs, buttocks, chest, abdomen, and waist. In children under age 2 years, the head, neck, face, palms, and soles of the feet can be affected. Lesions may appear as linear, threadlike, grayish burrows 1 to 10 cm in length, which may end in a pinpoint vesicle. The child's scratching and secondary infection may obliterate the burrow lesions.

Diagnosis is confirmed by microscopic examination of scrapings from a burrow, which reveals actively moving mites, fecal pellets, eggs, or nits. Treatment involves application of a scabicide, such as 5% permethrin lotion, over the entire body with special attention to the hands, fingers, feet, toes, and skin under the nails. The scabicide should be applied to the face, neck, ears, and scalp, avoiding the eyes and mucous membranes. Application of 5% permethrin lotion or malathion is preceded by a warm soap-and-water bath. When the skin is cool and dry apply the lotion. The lotion is left in place for 8 to 12 hours (6 hours for infants under 1 month of age), before washing off (Idriss & Khachemoune, 2006). A second treatment is used one week later. Topical and oral ivermectin is a new antiparasitic product with FDA approval for children weighing more than 15 kg, but it is used when other treatments are unsuccessful. All members of the household and child-care contacts should be treated at the same time, even if they have no symptoms.

Itching may persist for 1 to 2 weeks after treatment. An oral antihistamine (e.g., Benadryl, Atarax) may be prescribed to help relieve itching. Antibiotics may be needed when a secondary infection occurs.

Nursing Management

Advise parents that scabies is transmitted by close contact and is very contagious. All clothing, bedding, and pillowcases used by the child should be changed daily, washed with hot water, and ironed before reuse. Nonwashable toys and other items should be sealed in plastic bags for 5 to 7 days.

Educate the parents about the proper application of the scabicide. The child should have the scabicide reapplied to the hands if hands are washed or the child sucks the fingers or thumb. Socks over the hands of young children may reduce the chance of the child ingesting scabicide.

All household members should be treated simultaneously. Individuals who are not infected should avoid touching the affected child until after treatment is completed. If contact is made, they should wash their hands well. Inform the parents about signs of secondary infections and that itching and nodules may persist for weeks after effective treatment. Encourage the use of emollients as the treatment dries the skin.

Scabies, like pediculosis, can be embarrassing or upsetting for the child and family. Educate the child and parents about the condition, its spread, and treatment measures to prevent recurrence.

VASCULAR TUMORS (HEMANGIOMAS)

Vascular tumors or hemangiomas occur in 1% to 3% of all newborns; however, by the age of 1 year, approximately 10% of infants are affected. An increased incidence has been noted in females, preterm, and low birth weight infants who are fair-skinned (Haggstrom, Drolet, Baselga, et al., 2007). The risk for a hemangioma is greater in children of women who had chorionic villus sampling during pregnancy (Christinson-Lagay & Fishman, 2006).

Hemangiomas may initially arise from embolized placental tissue or a mutation that arrests vascular differentiation, perhaps one reason for their rapid growth in the first few months of life (Miller & Frieden, 2005). Vascular tumors are neoplasms of endothelial cells and increased numbers of small blood vessels that undergo rapid growth and proliferation during the first 6 to 10 months of life and may lead to ulceration. The proliferation phase is followed by a slow **involution** (process of decreasing in size) that is completed in 95% of children by adolescence (Cohen, 2004). Hemangiomas may be superficial (located in the epidermis), deep (located in the dermis or subcutaneous tissue), or mixed superficial and deep. When multiple hemangiomas are found, some may be in major organs, such as the liver. Complications caused by the rapid growth and pressure against or obstruction of vital structures (e.g., airway, eye, or ear canal) may occur.

Infantile hemangiomas begin as barely visible **telangiectasias** (dilated superficial blood vessels) or red macules that begin to grow rapidly and become bright red and compressible. Superficial hemangiomas are bright-red vascular cutaneous plaques that resemble strawberries. Deep hemangiomas appear as bluish tumors covered with normal-appearing epidermis. Mixed hemangiomas have features of both superficial and deep tumors. The lesions, appearing any place on the body, are minimally compressible and have no bruit or thrill. As the vascular tumor involutes, signs of tissue atrophy, wrinkles, telangiectasias, and hypopigmentation may be noted.

Initial diagnosis is by physical examination and monitoring the growth of the vascular tumor. When a vital organ could become obstructed or a large facial hemangioma is present, ultrasound, computed tomography, or magnetic resonance imaging may be performed.

Simple hemangiomas are monitored and receive no treatment. Hemangiomas in problem areas may be treated with high doses of systemic corticosteroids during the proliferation phase to slow growth (Cohen, 2004). Pulsed dye laser treatment at 2 to 3 week intervals is used for superficial hemangiomas during the proliferation phase. The hemangioma may darken for 1 to 2 weeks as purpura results from the extravasation of red blood cells when blood vessels rupture (Jones, 2007). The darkness will fade to red, and eventual lightening of the treated skin surface occurs. Surgical removal of an ulcerated hemangioma may be considered if the scarring outcome would be acceptable (Christinson-Lagay & Fishman, 2006).

Nursing Management

Assess the distribution of the hemangioma and consider the potential for complications as it goes through a rapid growth stage. Monitor the child for signs of any complications, such as ulceration or stridor that could be associated with compression on the airway. Assess the parents' response to the infant's appearance and how they are managing interactions with friends and family about the infant's changing appearance. Take photos of the infant at each visit so that parents have a record of improvements once therapy is initiated.

Teach the parents about the type of vascular lesion and potential treatment options. When corticosteroids are prescribed, teach the parents about administration, the need to take the full course as prescribed, and potential side effects. Inform parents about the possible ulceration of a rapidly growing hemangioma, what signs to expect, and how to protect the ulcerated skin until the infant is seen by the physician.

Talk with parents about comments made about the infant's appearance and provide some possible responses that parents can make. To promote attachment, help the parents see the infant's positive characteristics, such as responsiveness and smiling. Show photos of other children with similar lesions who have completed therapy to show that improvements in appearance are gradual, but possible.

Prepare parents for the changes in the child's appearance with pulsed-dye laser therapy. Some swelling may occur after the treatment, so the application of ice packs for 10 minutes every hour during the first day may help. Teach parents to protect the skin surface from trauma after pulsed dye laser treatments and to keep the infant's nails short to prevent scratching. Cleanse the area treated with water and pat it dry. Inform parents to avoid sun exposure for several weeks after the treatments, and to use sunscreen in the future.

INJURIES TO THE SKIN

PRESSURE ULCERS

More and more children with disabilities are cared for in hospital, community, and home care settings. Many are at risk for skin breakdown and pressure ulcers. Children at greatest risk are those with limited mobility, the inability to change positions, sensory deficits, or incontinence. Children also at risk include those with high activity, such as occurs when the skin rubs against bedding (Table 59–3). A reported rate in pediatric critical care settings was 27%, while other hospital settings may have a rate of 1% to 13% (Noonan, Quigley, & Curley, 2006).

Soft tissues and capillary beds can be compressed between a bony prominence and an external surface. Tissue ischemia occurs when high pressure is maintained over a short period of time or low pressure is maintained over a prolonged time (Butler, 2006). The cells are deprived of oxygen and nutrients, and metabolic waste products accumulate, resulting in hypoxia and soft tissue injury. Without appropriate intervention, the injury progresses rapidly and a pressure ulcer forms. See Figure 59–10 ● for clinical manifestations of four common stages of pressure ulcers. With unstageable pressure ulcers, the base of a full-thickness lesion wound bed is covered with exudate or eschar. A sixth classification is a suspected deep tissue injury, in which a purple or maroon localized area of discolored intact skin or blood-filled blister exists due to damage to the underlying soft tissue from pressure or a shear injury (National Pressure Ulcer Advisory Panel, 2007).

The Braden Q Scale (for children under age 5 years) and the Braden scale can be used to assess the child's risk for pressure ulcers. Initial treatment for early stages of skin damage involves removing pressure from the affected site until the skin has healed. Children who use leg braces for alignment and mobility are of-

Table 59–3 Sites and Potential Causes of Pressure Ulcers

Sites	Potential Causes
Occipital region of scalp	Inability to lift head
Sacrum and buttocks	Confinement to bed or wheelchair
Legs and feet	Orthotics, leg braces, casts
Spine and neck	Scoliosis brace
Knees, elbows, heels of feet	Rubbing against bed sheet
Sternum, iliac crest	Prone positioning for mechanical ventilation

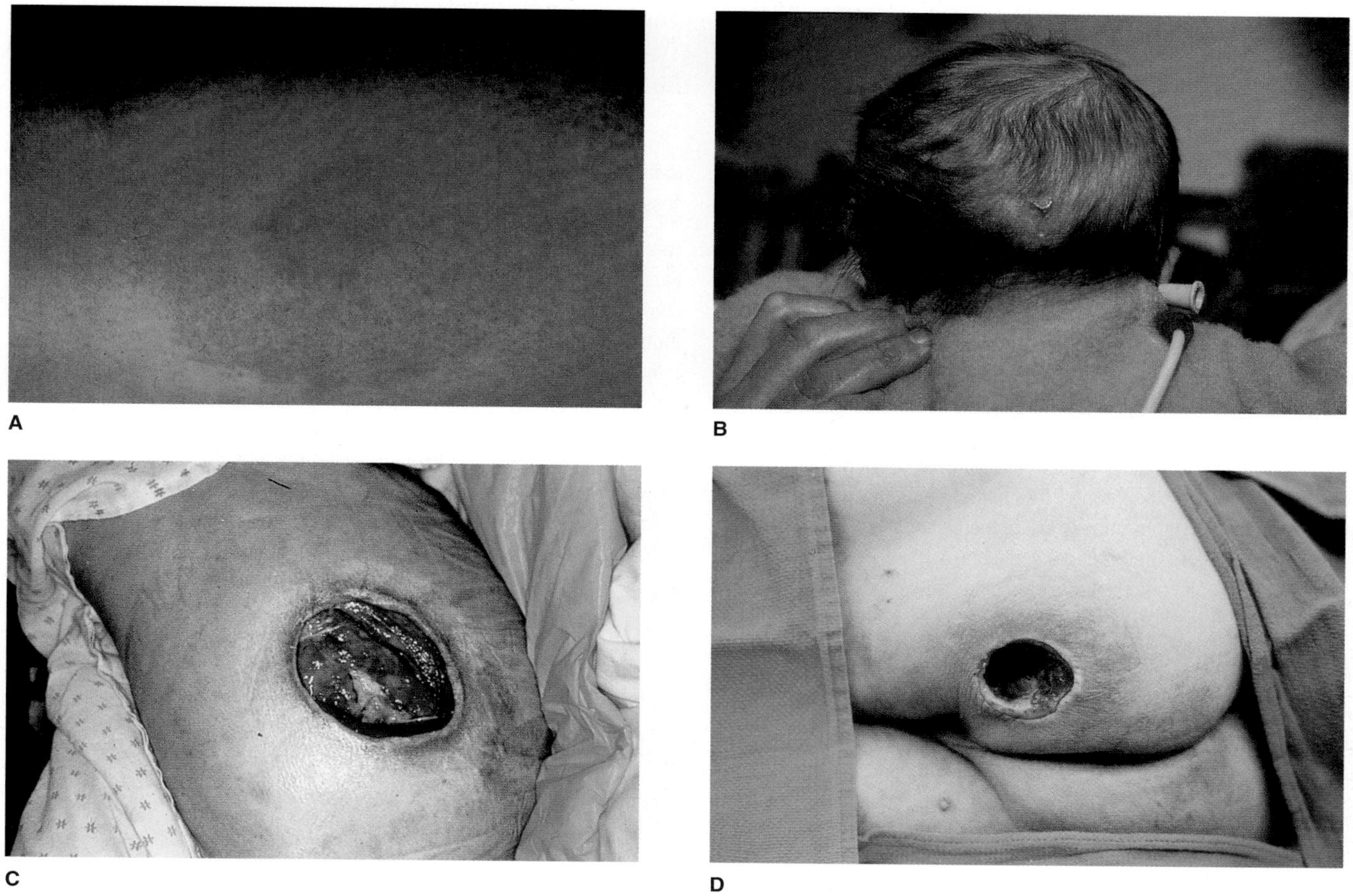

● **Figure 59–10** The Stages of Ulcer Formation. ***A,*** Stage 1, an area of redness does not go away within 30 minutes of removing the pressure or skin irritant. Children with dark skin may have persistent red, blue, or purple discoloration. ***B,*** Stage 2, the skin looks rubbed or raw like a blister or abrasion, a partial-thickness injury with damage through epidermis, dermis, or both. ***C,*** Stage 3, an ulcer forms as the subcutaneous tissue is exposed, a full thickness injury. ***D,*** Stage 4, the ulcer deepens and extends to muscle, bone, or supporting tissues.

Courtesy of Sandra Quigley, Children's Hospital, Boston, MA.

ten put in wheelchairs. Children who use wheelchairs are often put on bed rest on a pressure-reducing surface. Frequent repositioning is needed. A transparent film may be applied to affected red skin to minimize friction. Pressure ulcers are treated with dressings, such as hydrocolloids, gels or hydrogels, and calcium alginates that do not adhere to the wound.

Nursing Management

Carefully inspect the dependent skin surfaces of all infants and children confined to bed at least three times in each 24-hour period. Evaluate the risk for skin damage based on factors that can contribute to skin breakdown. Identify the size (length, width, and depth) and character of the skin lesion. Note any signs of infection, the appearance of wound edges, type of tissue at the wound base, and drainage. Describe any drainage amount, color, and type.

Develop protocols for pressure ulcer prevention so that children at high risk are identified and have appropriate interventions initiated (e.g., increased ambulation, frequent position changes, pressure-reducing surfaces, and moisture barriers). If the child is incontinent, change the diaper frequently to keep the skin clean and dry. Ensure an adequate intake of fluids, proteins, and vitamins to keep the skin healthy. (See "Evidence-Based Nursing: Pressure Ulcers in Children.")

Moist wounds heal more rapidly than dry wounds because cell migration across the moist wound bed more effectively fights infection and removes cellular debris (Butler, 2006). Provide wound care and dressing changes according to agency guidelines. These guidelines may include saline irrigation, debridement, and a dressing appropriate for the wound condition (see Skill 17–1 SKILLS). Gauze wraps to hold the dressing in place help prevent skin damage caused by adhesives.

Teach parents of children with braces to inspect the skin under the braces every day for irritation (redness or blisters). Help the child to use a mirror with a long handle to inspect skin on the bottom and sides of the feet, behind the knees, and on the lower legs. Check all edges of the braces for roughness or breakage that can pinch or scrape the skin. If any skin irritation is seen and redness does not go away within 30 minutes, do not put the brace back on until the skin heals. Inform the child's physician so that treatment can be started immediately. To reduce irritation, have the child wear cotton socks under the braces and make sure the shoes are large enough to accommodate the brace, socks, and the

Evidence-Based Nursing

PRESSURE ULCERS IN CHILDREN

Clinical Question

What information about the prevalence of pressure ulcers and factors that increase the child's risk for development of pressure ulcers is important for nursing management of children at risk?

Evidence

Investigators identified a pressure ulcer prevalence of 13% in 97 hospitalized children after inspecting the skin of all children during an 8-hour period. Children less than age 1 year had the highest rate, and sites of skin breakdown were the ears, occiput, nose, and heels. Approximately 75% of pressure ulcers were Stage 1 (Groeneveld, Anderson, Allen, et al., 2004). An audit of skin integrity among 252 child patients in a large children's hospital found that approximately 6% of the children were at high risk for a pressure ulcer using the Braden Q scale and 1.6% had a pressure ulcer. Thirteen children had a pressure-related skin injury associated with pulse oximetry or other medical devices such as a leg cast, and an intravenous catheter hub (Noonan et al., 2006). Pilot testing of a simplified scale (Starkid Skin Scale) for skin integrity assessment was conducted in a large pediatric hospital. The prevalence of skin breakdown was 23% (80 of 347 children), and approximately 75% were described as Stage 1. Common skin breakdown sites were the buttocks, perineum, and occiput. Children with skin breakdown were more likely to be younger, smaller, have more medical devices, more episodes of diarrhea, and a lower score on the assessment scale (Suddaby, Barnett, & Facteau, 2005).

Best Practices

Factors that increase a child's risk for development of pressure ulcers include the following: friction from casts and orthotic devices, excessive motion, inability to move independently, diminished or no sensation, moisture on the skin from soiling, sedation and care in a critical care unit with medical devices, and preterm or sick newborns. Knowledge of these risk factors can be used to develop guidelines for prevention of pressure ulcers, such as a turning schedule; careful inspection of skin under braces, orthotics, and medical devices; frequently relocating pulse oximetry sensors; and positioning and taping endotracheal, tracheostomy, and nasogastric tubes to reduce pressure against the skin.

Critical Thinking in Action

Use the Braden scale or Braden Q scale (for children under 5 years) to assess the risk of a child with an acute illness and one with a chronic illness for pressure ulcers. Then perform a complete assessment of these children to identify any skin breakdown. Develop a nursing care plan for the high risk child to prevent and treat skin breakdown.

See MyNursingKit for possible responses.

foot. Advise parents to return to a prosthetist regularly for brace refitting as the child grows.

Children who use a wheelchair are at risk for skin breakdown on the buttocks and lower back from the pressure of sitting for hours. A wheelchair cushion can distribute and shift the child's weight when sitting in the chair. Teach the child to change position frequently by doing wheelchair push-ups or by shifting the weight (leaning to the side or forward) for several minutes every 10 to 15 minutes. Make sure the child wears a safety belt when sitting in the wheelchair. Teach school personnel about the child's recommended protocol so they can provide opportunities in school to change positions and reinforce the routine.

BURNS

Burns are among the top five leading causes of injury and death in children between 1 and 14 years of age (National Center for Health Statistics, National Vital Statistics System, 2007). Daily in the United States 435 children ages 0 to 19 are treated in emergency departments for burn-related injuries, and two children die as a result of being burned (Centers for Disease Control and Prevention, 2008). Males are at greater risk for burn injury and mortality.

The four main types of burns are thermal, chemical, electrical, and radioactive. Thermal burns, the most common in children, result from flames, scalds (such as coffee or grease), or contact with hot objects (such as a wood stove or curling iron). Chemical burns occur when children touch or ingest caustic agents. Electrical burns are caused by direct or alternating current in electrical wires, appliances, or high-voltage wires. Radiation burns result from exposure to radioactive substances or sunlight. About 10% to 25% of all burns in children result from child abuse, and are most common under age 3 years (Horner, 2005). See Chapter 44 ∞ for a description of child abuse.

Etiology and Pathophysiology

Children at different developmental stages are at risk for different types of burns.

- Infants are most often injured by thermal burns (scalding liquids, house fires) (Figure 59–11 ●).
- Toddlers are at risk for thermal burns (pulling hot liquids or grease onto themselves), electrical burns (biting electrical cords) (Figure 59–12 ●), contact burns, and chemical burns (ingesting cleaning agents and other substances) associated with exploring the environment.
- Preschool-age children are most often injured by scalding or contact with hot appliances (curling irons, ovens).
- School-age children are at risk for thermal burns (playing with matches, fireworks), electrical burns (climbing high-voltage towers, climbing trees, and contact with electrical wires), and chemical burns (combustion experiments).
- Adolescents also experience thermal, chemical, and electrical burns, as well as radiation burns associated with sunbathing.

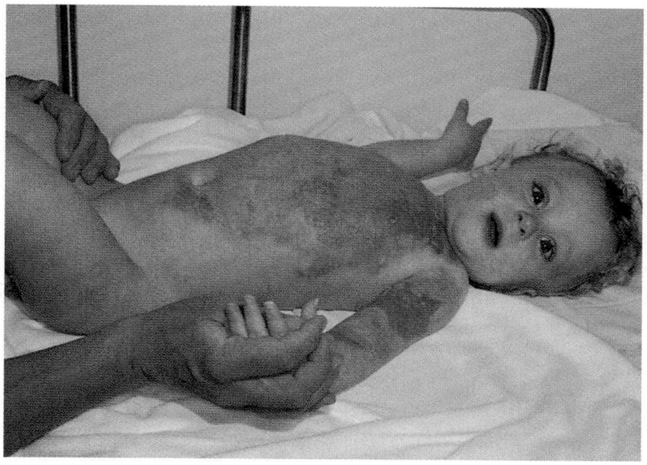

● **Figure 59–11** Thermal burns. Also known as scalds, thermal burns are the most common burn injury in infancy.

Immediately after the burn, intense vasoconstriction occurs in response to substances released by the injured cells. Ischemia resulting from vasoconstriction may increase the depth of the burn injury. Vasoactive hormones are then released, which increases capillary permeability. This permits fluid and plasma to shift into the interstitial spaces, causing edema and decreased circulating volume in the blood vessels. Capillary integrity is not restored for 18 to 36 hours after the burn injury. The child loses increased water and heat through the injured epidermis. The child's metabolic rate and need for calories increase in the attempt to maintain body temperature and begin healing. The depth of the burn depends upon the temperature and duration of the heat application, and on the ability of tissues to dissipate the transferred energy.

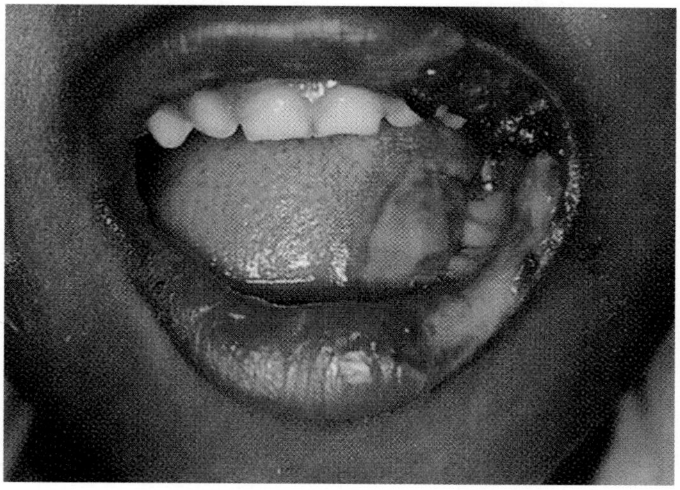

● **Figure 59–12** Electrical burn caused by biting on electrical cord. The burn is caused when the current arcs through the lips, often causing a full-thickness injury through the mucosa, muscle, nerves, and blood vessels. The labial artery may be injured and cause significant bleeding once the eschar falls off after 2 to 3 weeks.

Courtesy Dr. Lezley McIveen, Department of Dentistry, Children's National Medical Center, Washington, DC.

Nursing Practice

A full-thickness burn can occur in adults after immersion for only 5 seconds in water with a temperature of 60°C (140°F). The amount of time for a burn to occur increases to 5 minutes when water temperature is 48°C (120°F). Coffee and other hot beverages are often served at temperatures between 71° to 82°C (160° to 180°F) (Grant, 2004).

Clinical Manifestations

Burns are classified by the depth of their penetration into the layers of the skin. Burn depth may be defined as partial thickness or full thickness. Partial-thickness burns, in which the injured tissue can regenerate and heal, may be either first- or second-degree. Full-thickness burns, in which the injured tissue cannot regenerate, are also known as third-degree burns. See "Pathophysiology Illustrated: Classification of Burns by Depth" for clinical manifestations by burn depth.

Signs of infection include purulent drainage, swelling, erythema, discoloration of wound margins, and pain in the uninjured skin around the wound (Sheridan, 2005a).

Clinical Therapy

Assessment of burn severity. Burn severity is determined by the depth of the burn injury, percentage of body surface area (BSA) affected, and involvement of specific body parts. A Lund and Browder chart with BSA distributions for various body parts at different ages is used to calculate the area affected by the burn injury (Figure 59–13 ●). The palm of a child's hand (without fingers and thumb) is 1% of his or her body surface area and can be used to make a quick estimate of the burn size. Reassessment of the extent of burn injury is performed 24 to 48 hours after the injury. Criteria for major burns that should be cared for in a specialized burn center include (Reed & Pomerantz, 2005):

- A partial-thickness burn greater than 10% BSA in a child under 10 years; greater than 20% in an older child
- Burns involving the hands, face, feet, genitalia, perineum, and major joints
- Full-thickness burns greater than 5% BSA
- Electrical burns, including lightning injury
- Inhalation injury

Initial treatment. The first step is to ensure that the child has an airway, is breathing, and has a pulse. Then stop the burning process by removing jewelry and clothing. Moist soaks or ice (if a small surface area is affected) is used to stop the burning process and to relieve pain. A tetanus vaccine booster is given if more than 5 years have passed since the last vaccine, or when the child has not completed the full vaccine series.

Treatment of major burns. The goals of treatment include decreasing burn fluid losses, preventing infection, controlling pain, promoting nutrition, and salvaging all viable tissue. Fluid replacement is necessary to maintain the cardiovascular and renal systems. Fluid shifts from the vasculature to the interstitial spaces (third spacing) soon after the burn and can cause hypovolemic shock. Fluid replacement for the first 24 hours after the injury is based on a fluid volume formula calculated from the child's body weight, affected BSA, and normal maintenance needs (e.g., the Parkland and Galveston formulas):

- Parkland Formula: 4 mL × body weight (kg) × percentage of total body surface area burned = total 24 hour fluid requirement in mL. Maintenance fluids must be added to the amount of fluid calculated with this formula.
- Carvajal or Galveston Formula: 5,000 mL/m^2 burned area + 2,000 mL/m^2 of total body surface area = total 24 hour fluid requirement in mL.

Lactated Ringer's or normal saline solution is the preferred IV fluid. Half of the total volume calculated for the 24-hour period is infused over the first 8 hours, starting at the time of the burn rather than arrival time in the emergency department. The remainder is distributed evenly over the next 16 hours. Vascular integrity is usually restored after the first 24 hours and the fluid volume administered is reduced. Efforts are focused on maintaining the child's temperature because heat is lost rapidly through burned skin.

Fever is a normal, expected outcome of any significant burn injury, but in some cases it may also be a sign of infection. Treatment may include analgesics, ice packs, cooling blankets, or cool hydrotherapy sessions. Infection is a frequent complication. Wounds are cultured to identify specific organisms for antibiotic therapy rather than routinely giving prophylactic antibiotic treatment (Sheridan, 2005b).

Continuous enteral feedings are often begun within 6 hours of the burn injury to support the child's increased nutritional requirements for additional protein, vitamins, and minerals. These nutrients are needed for the significantly increased metabolic rate and to support healing and the body's stress response to injury (Klein & Herndon, 2004).

Aggressive pain management with intravenous opioids is needed around the clock and for all procedures. The burns cause a significant emotional distress that increases the perception of pain. See Chapter 42∞ for pain management information. Cimetidine or other H_2 blockers may be ordered to prevent a burn stress ulcer.

Special consideration is needed when burns involve certain areas of the body:

- Deep partial-thickness and full-thickness burns develop **eschar** (the tough leathery scab that forms over severely burned areas) with no elasticity. When the burn is **circumferential** (surrounds the chest or an extremity), blood flow can become restricted as a result of edema, leading to tissue hypoxia. An **escharotomy** (incision into the constricting tissue) may be necessary to restore peripheral circulation.
- Facial burns usually cause significant edema. Care must be taken to ensure airway patency. An ophthalmologist should assess burns to the eye and prescribe treatment. If the lips are burned, an infant may be unable to suck.
- Burns of the hands require careful management to maintain function. Special splinting and physical therapy are usually necessary.

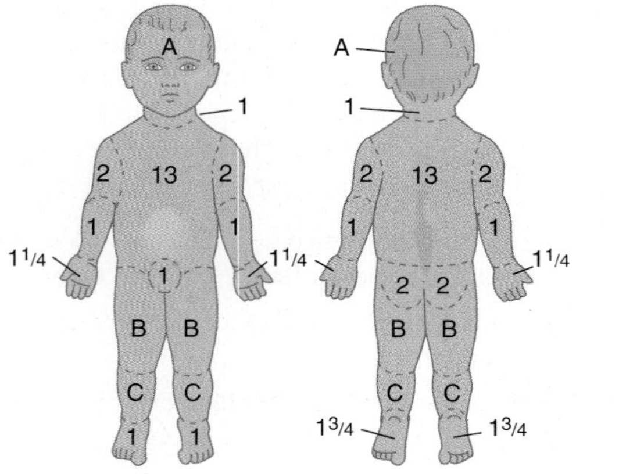

Relative Percentages of Areas Affected by Growth

	Age in years					
Area	0	1	5	10	11	Adult
A = 1/2 of head	9 1/2	8 1/2	6 1/2	5 1/2	4 1/2	3 1/2
B = 1/2 of one thigh	2 3/4	3 1/4	4	4 1/2	4 1/2	4 3/4
C = 1/2 of one lower leg	2 1/2	2 1/2	2 3/4	3	3 1/4	3 1/2

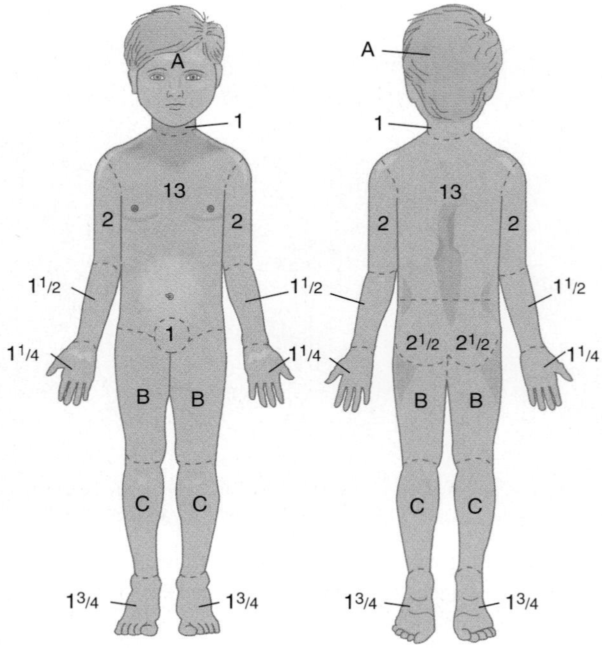

● **Figure 59–13** Lund and Browder chart with BSA distributions. This chart is used for determining percentage of body surface areas in pediatric burn injuries.

Adapted with permission from Artz, C. P., & Moncrief, J. A. (1969). *The treatment of burns* (2nd ed.). Philadelphia: Saunders.

PATHOPHYSIOLOGY ILLUSTRATED

CLASSIFICATION OF BURNS BY DEPTH

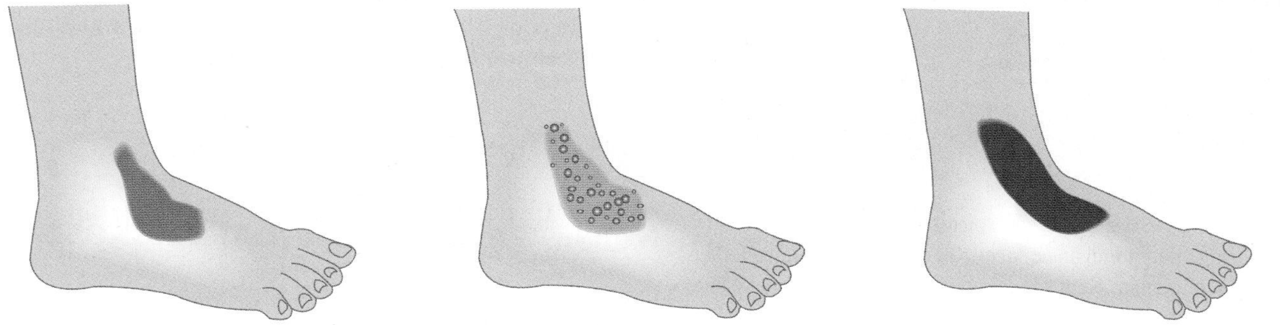

SUPERFICIAL PARTIAL THICKNESS (FIRST DEGREE)	PARTIAL THICKNESS (SECOND DEGREE)	FULL THICKNESS (THIRD DEGREE)
Damages only outer layer of skin; burn is painful and red; heals in a few days (e.g., sunburn)	Involves epidermis and upper layers of dermis; may have sparing of sweat glands and sebaceous glands; heals in 10–14 days	Involves all of epidermis and dermis; may also involve underlying tissue; nerve endings usually destroyed; requires skin grafting
Erythema, blanches on pressure, no bullae, peeling after a few days due to premature cell death	Blisters or bullae, erythema, blanches on pressure, pain and sensitivity to cold air, minimal scar formation	Skin may appear brown, black, deep cherry red, white to gray, waxy or translucent; usually no pain, injured area may appear sunken

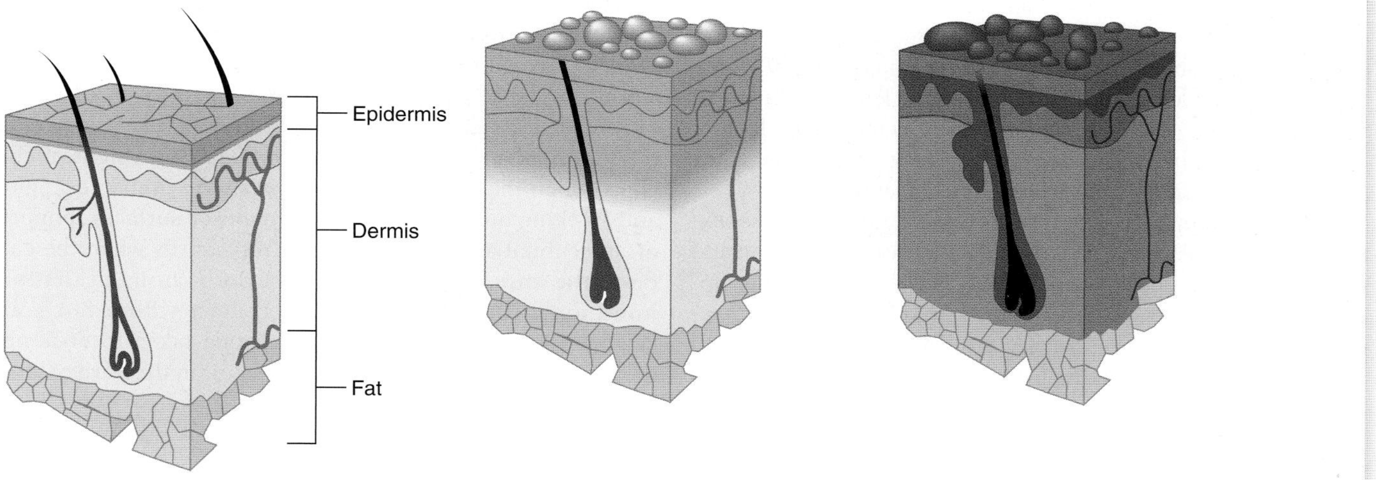

- Perineal burns are at higher risk for infection because of frequent contamination with urine and stool. Frequent dressing changes are required. A urinary catheter is usually inserted but is removed once hydration status is stable, to minimize the risk of urinary tract infection.

Wound management. Burn wound care has several goals: (1) to remove necrotic tissue and speed wound debridement, (2) to maintain moist wound conditions and adequate circulation, (3) to conserve body heat and fluids, (4) to protect from infection, and (5) to control scarring and prevent scar contracture. Several treatment regimens are used to achieve these goals.

When the burn is extensive, the entire body is bathed to initiate debridement. Sedation and anesthesiology support may be ordered for pain management during debridement. Intact blisters provide a natural, pain-free, sterile dressing. However, some healthcare providers break blisters open, believing that the fluid provides a medium for bacterial infection. The tissues should be carefully cut away when the wound is being prepared for skin grafting.

Various options are used for wound management after debridement. Traditional burn care for a partial-thickness injury involves the application of antibacterial agents, such as silver sulfadiazine (Silvadene), mafenide acetate (Sulfamylon),

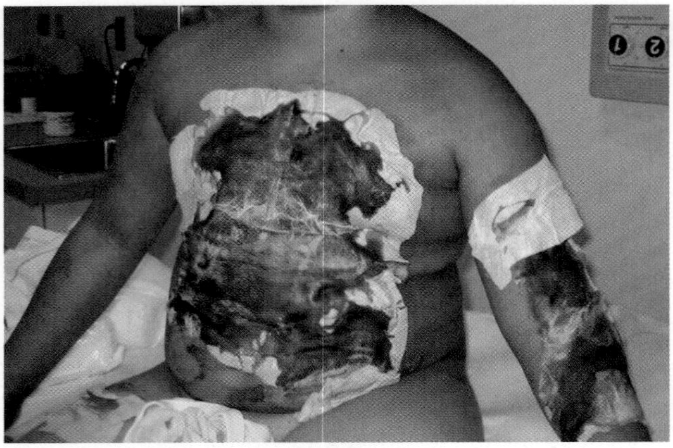

● **Figure 59–14** Silver-based antimicrobial dressing. This child's scald burn is being treated with an Aquacel AG® dressing, one of the newer silver-embedded dressings. Note the absorbed exudate that is visible through the burn dressing.

Courtesy of Martin Eichelberger, MD, and Lisa Ring, RN, PNP, Children's National Medical Center, Washington, DC.

or bacitracin after initial cleansing. Dressings are added to cover the burned area and are changed once or twice daily. (See Skill 17–2 SKILLS).

Newer silver-based antimicrobial dressings (e.g., Aquacel, Acticoat) have been developed that provide a sustained-release delivery of silver and also absorb exudate from the wound (Figure 59–14 ●). Dressings can be left in place for many days (Duffy, McLaughlin, Eichelberger, et al., 2006). When the dressing is removed, a layer of eschar may also be debrided. These dressing changes are often painful, so pain management is needed. See Chapter 42.

Hydrotherapy (whirlpool) baths may be given to cleanse extensive wounds before debridement, to increase vasodilation and circulation, and to speed healing. The water loosens exudate, topical medications, and dead tissue, and it may help soak off dressings that adhere to the skin. Gentle washing is necessary to protect new epithelial cells. Superficial second-degree burns reepithelialize within 3 weeks.

Skin grafting is necessary with any deep second- or third-degree burn. Often a temporary skin substitute or **allograft** (cadaver skin from a skin bank) is used to cover a second-degree burn until healing occurs or until **autografting** (use of healthy skin taken from a nonburned area of the child's body) can be performed. The graft is placed after the wound is debrided in the operating room to reveal healthy, bleeding tissue. The allograft forms a protective barrier over the wound surface to decrease infection risk and to protect against fluid loss. An autograft is permanent. The donor site (where the autograft was harvested) is a new wound, causing pain and requiring close monitoring for signs of infection. Various temporary skin substitutes, such as Integra or Biobrane may be applied to the debrided skin to form a protective barrier over the wound surface. This covering is effective in decreasing infection and pain, protecting against fluid loss, and promoting revascularization until autografting is performed.

During the rehabilitation stage, pressure garments, also known as Jobst garments, are used to reduce development of hypertrophic scarring and contractures. Such garments are worn 23 hours a day for 6 to 8 months to shorten the time of scar maturation and to reduce the thickness of the scars.

Severe morbidity is likely to occur with major burns. Significant scarring may occur regardless of autografting and the use of pressure garments. Contractures and loss of function are also possible. Children with major burns require comprehensive follow-up, sometimes involving repeated hospitalizations for surgery to release burn contractures or perform new grafting, or cosmetic surgery for scar revision.

NURSING MANAGEMENT

NURSING ASSESSMENT AND DIAGNOSIS

Emergency assessment first focuses on the potential for life-threatening injuries that need immediate care. Assessment of the airway is necessary, especially when there are signs of smoke inhalation or burns to the face and neck. Other potential injuries are important to identify when the mechanism of injury also includes a fall or explosion. Identify signs of respiratory distress and any potential bleeding source. A weak, thready pulse, tachycardia, and pallor are important signs of early shock that may provide clues to an internal injury.

Obtain information about the type of burn (e.g., thermal, electrical, chemical) and a complete history. If a burn injury was preventable, parents may be emotionally stressed by feelings of guilt. Take care to avoid sounding accusatory when questioning parents about the injury. Be alert to signs of child abuse when the history does not match the injury (e.g., glove and stocking burns, burns that spare flexor surfaces [popliteal or antecubital areas are protected from burns when the child flexes the knees or elbows], contact burns from cigarettes or irons, and zebra burn lines from contact with a hot grate) (Figure 59–15 ●). Photographs are often taken to document these injuries. Child neglect can be a factor in the burn of an inadequately supervised child.

Assess the extent of burn injury (BSA and depth). Frequently monitor the vital signs and pain control. Monitor the child's circulatory and respiratory status to identify signs of hypovolemia in the first 24 hours or fluid overload as capillary integrity is restored. A head-to-toe assessment is performed at the beginning of every shift, followed by system-specific assessments, depending on clinical findings and changes in the child's status. A urinary catheter may be inserted to enable close monitoring of urine output (see Skill 16–1 SKILLS). Weigh the child daily, as the increased metabolic rate may result in weight loss if nutritional intake is inadequate. Be alert to signs of infection such as purulent drainage and edematous, red, or discolored wound margins.

Assess the child's concerns over appearance and the stress of hospitalization. Determine if the child has memories or nightmares about the burn and arrange psychologic support as needed. Identify any family stressors that might need to be addressed during the child's care.

MyNursingKit Nursing in Action: Topical Medication: Burn Wound Care

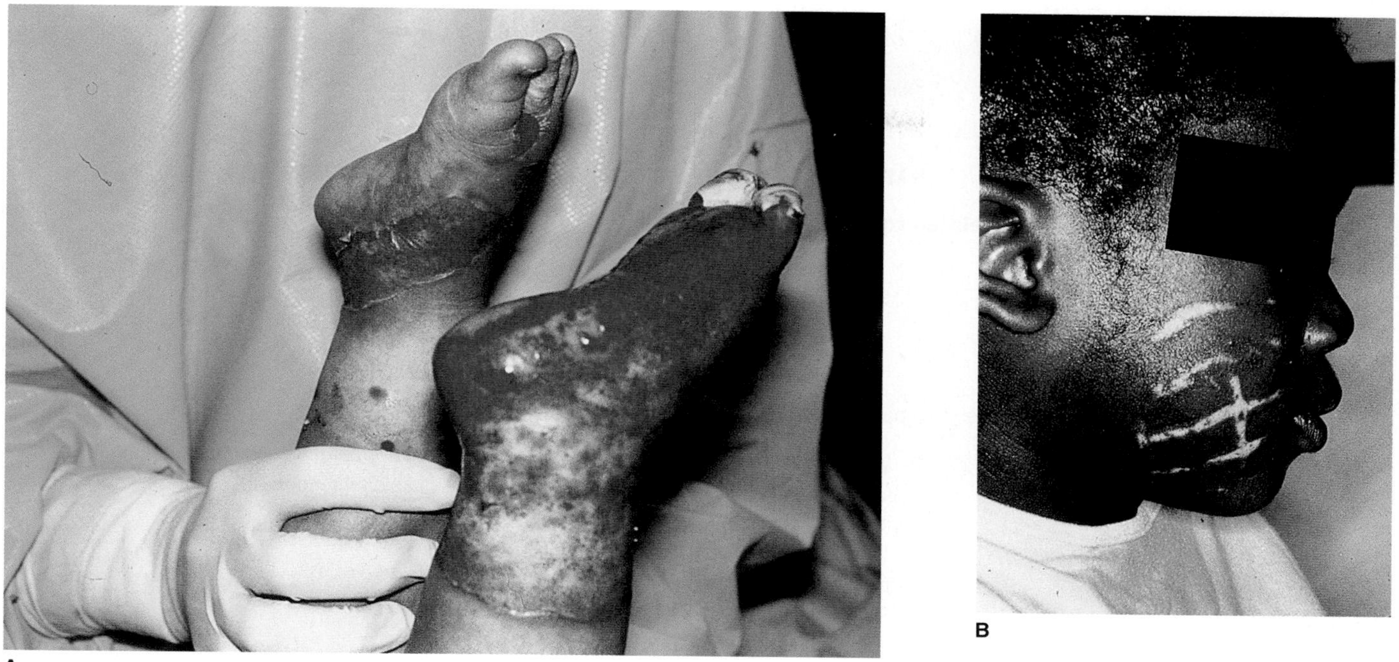

A B

● **Figure 59–15** Burn injuries associated with child abuse. ***A,*** Burns of the hands or feet that are distributed like gloves or stockings. ***B,*** Zebra burns from a grate.

Used with permission from American Academy of Pediatrics, Elk Grove Village, IL, and the Kempe Children's Center, Denver, CO.

Nursing Practice

If a burn is circumferential, assess for an increase in cyanosis, deep tissue pain, and capillary refill time, and a decreased pulse distal to the burn. If these signs are detected, notify the physician immediately.

Common nursing diagnoses for the child with a major burn injury are included in the accompanying Nursing Care Plan. Additional nursing diagnoses for the child with a major burn might include the following:

- *Hyperthermia* related to increased metabolic rate and trauma
- *Disturbed Body Image* related to burn injury
- *Anxiety* related to situational crisis and threat of death or disfigurement

PLANNING AND IMPLEMENTATION

Care of the burned child involves various treatments designed to promote healing and prevent complications. These include dressing changes, hydrotherapy, antibiotic therapy, fluid and nutrition management, analgesic support, physical therapy, play therapy, and possible skin grafting.

To reduce the stress on the child, begin pain management as soon as possible for the initial debridement. Continue effective pain management around the clock with intravenous opioids (see Chapter 42). Elevated body temperature from the burn may cause discomfort. Promote the child's comfort while keeping burns covered to reduce pain. Keep the room temperature at a comfortable level. Change bed linens as needed when the child perspires heavily.

Soak charred clothing off with sterile saline and clip any hair within 2 inches of the burn to keep it out of the burn site. Cleanse the burn with mild soap and water and remove any foreign matter. If a chemical is the burning agent, remove the clothing and wash with plenty of water. Elevate burned extremities.

A semipermeable wound membrane may be applied to clean superficial partial-thickness burns. These membranes protect the burned tissues from trauma, prevent fluid loss, create a moist environment for healing, and provide a physical barrier to bacteria. Monitor the burn under the semipermeable membrane for infection, which could potentially cause sepsis or a deepening burn wound (Sheridan, 2005a). When the burn heals, the wound membrane loosens, permitting it to be trimmed.

Allografts or autografts may be put in place in the operating room after debridement to prepare the burned tissue for the graft. Following the grafting process, wet dressings with antibiotic solution are used for several days, commonly followed by other dry dressings with antibiotics. Splints may be required to promote healing when the skin over a joint is burned. The child may be kept on bed rest for several days following an autograft to protect the graft until it has a vascular supply. Donor sites are treated as separate wounds.

Fluids should be administered at the rate prescribed for resuscitation for the first 24 hours, and then adjusted as prescribed. Enteral feeding may be needed initially by the child with extensive

(continues on page 1816)

Nursing Care Plan

THE CHILD WITH A MAJOR BURN INJURY

INTERVENTION	RATIONALE	EXPECTED OUTCOME
1. Nursing Diagnosis: Acute Pain related to physical injury agents		
NIC Priority Intervention: **Pain management:** Alleviation of pain or a reduction in pain to a level of comfort that is acceptable to the patient		**NOC Suggested Outcome:** **Comfort level:** Feelings of physical and psychologic ease
Goal: The child will verbalize adequate relief from pain and will be able to perform activities of daily living (ADLs).		
■ Assess the level of pain frequently using pain scales (see Chapter 42).	■ Provides objective pain measurement. Changes in pain location and intensity may indicate complications.	The child verbalizes adequate relief from pain and is able to perform ADLs.
■ Cover burns as much as possible.	■ Temperature change or air movement causes pain.	
■ Change the child's position frequently. Perform range of motion exercises.	■ Reduces joint stiffness and prevents contractures and increases comfort.	
■ Provide diversional activities.	■ Helps lessen focus on pain.	
■ Promote uninterrupted sleep with use of medications.	■ Sleep deprivation can increase pain perception.	
■ Use analgesics and sedation (as appropriate) before all dressing changes and burn care.	■ Helps to reduce pain and decreases anxiety for subsequent dressing changes.	
2. Nursing Diagnosis: Risk for Infection related to trauma and destruction of skin barrier		
NIC Priority Intervention: **Infection protection:** Prevention and early detection of infection in a patient at risk		**NOC Suggested Outcome:** **Risk control:** Actions to eliminate or reduce actual, personal, and modifiable health threats
Goal: The child will be free of infection during healing process.		
■ Take vital signs frequently.	■ Increased temperature is an early sign of infection, but it is also a common response to burn injury.	The child either stays free of secondary infection, or has infection diagnosed and treated early.
■ Use standard precautions (gown, gloves, mask) when wounds of a major burn are exposed. Do not allow visitors who have an infectious disease.	■ Reduces risk of wound contamination.	
■ Clip hair around burns.	■ Hair harbors bacteria and can irritate the wound.	
■ Keep burn dressing clean and intact.	■ Helps reduce the number of bacteria introduced to the burned site.	
■ Do not place the IV in any burned area.	■ Reduces risk of wound contamination.	
■ Administer oral or IV antibiotics for diagnosed infections as prescribed.	■ Antibiotics administered as prescribed help to clear the infection quickly.	
3. Nursing Diagnosis: Risk for Imbalanced Fluid Volume related to loss of fluids through wounds and to subsequent excess fluid intake		
NIC Priority Intervention: **Fluid management:** Promotion of fluid balance and prevention of complications resulting from abnormal or undesired fluid levels		**NOC Suggested Outcome:** **Fluid balance:** Balance of water in the intracellular and extracellular compartments of the body

Nursing Care Plan—continued

THE CHILD WITH A MAJOR BURN INJURY

INTERVENTION	RATIONALE	EXPECTED OUTCOME
Goal: The child will maintain adequate urine output.		
■ Monitor vital signs, central venous pressure, capillary refill time, pulses.	■ The child is initially at risk for hypovolemic shock and needs fluid resuscitation (see Chapter 49 ∞).	The child maintains normal urine output and burn site edema is not excessive.
■ Administer IV and oral fluids as ordered.	■ Careful calculation of fluid needs and ensuring proper intake helps keep the child properly hydrated.	
■ Estimate insensible fluid losses.	■ Losses are increased during the first 72 hours after burn injury. Plasma is lost through burn because of capillary damage.	
■ Monitor intake and output.	■ The child is at risk for fluid overload during hydration, and for edema in the burned tissues.	
■ Weigh child daily using the same scale and amount of clothing.	■ Significant weight loss or gain can help determine fluid imbalances.	
■ Insert urinary catheter if prescribed.	■ Helps maintain accurate output measurement during critical care stage.	
■ Monitor for hyponatremia and hypercalcemia (see Chapter 46 ∞).	■ Sodium is lost with burn fluid and potassium is lost from damaged cells, causing electrolyte imbalances.	

4. Nursing Diagnosis: Ineffective Peripheral Tissue Perfusion related to mechanical reduction of venous and/or arterial blood flow (edema) of circumferential burns

NIC Priority Intervention: **Circulatory care:** Promotion of arterial and venous circulation		**NOC Suggested Outcome:** **Tissue perfusion (peripheral):** Extent to which blood flows through the small vessels of the extremities and maintains tissue function
Goal: The child will maintain adequate perfusion in burned extremities.		
■ Elevate extremities. Check distal pulse hourly. Notify the physician of decreased or absent pulses.	■ Elevation helps to reduce dependent edema by promoting venous return. Dependent edema can constrict peripheral circulation.	The child has no episodes of poor perfusion in the burned extremity.
■ Assess the eschar and edema of the extremity.	■ Eschar can constrict peripheral circulation in edematous extremity.	

5. Nursing Diagnosis: Impaired Physical Mobility related to joint stiffness due to burns

NIC Priority Intervention: **Exercise therapy, joint mobility:** Use of active or passive body movement to maintain or restore joint flexibility		**NOC Suggested Outcome:** **Joint movement (active):** Range of motion of joints with self-initiated movement
Goal: The child will maintain maximum range of motion.		
■ Arrange physical and occupational therapy twice daily for stretching and range of motion exercises. Splint as ordered.	■ Positioning in alignment and range of motion exercises help to prevent contractures.	The child maintains maximum range of motion without contractures.
■ Encourage activities to promote range of motion (toss a bean bag, mimic animal movements).	■ Fun activities help the child with diversion and provide movement.	

(continued)

Nursing Care Plan—continued

THE CHILD WITH A MAJOR BURN INJURY

INTERVENTION	RATIONALE	EXPECTED OUTCOME
6. Nursing Diagnosis: Imbalanced Nutrition: Less than Body Requirements related to high metabolic needs		
NIC Priority Intervention: **Nutrition management:** Assistance with or provision of balanced dietary intake of foods and fluids		**NOC Suggested Outcome:** **Nutritional status:** Extent to which nutrients are available to meet metabolic needs
Goal: The child will maintain weight and demonstrate adequate serum albumin and hydration.		
■ Provide an opportunity to choose meals. Offer a variety of high protein and high calorie foods. Provide snacks.	■ Encourages intake. General malaise and anorexia lead to poor healing.	The child maintains weight, adequate hydration, normal serum albumin.
■ Encourage the child to have meals with other children.	■ Socialization improves intake.	
■ Provide a multivitamin supplement.	■ Vitamin C aids zinc absorption; zinc aids in healing.	
■ Provide enteral feedings as needed.	■ A child with a burn greater than 10% of BSA cannot usually meet nutrition requirements without assistance.	
■ Weigh the child daily.	■ Provides objective evaluation.	

burns until the child is able to eat adequate amounts. Once the child is able to eat, provide a diet high in protein and calories in small frequent feedings. Identify food items that the child likes, and encourage the family to bring in food that the child may prefer to eat.

PREVENT COMPLICATIONS

Severe complications of burns include infections, pneumonia, and renal failure, as well as possible irreversible loss of function of the burned area. The healthcare team's goal is to prevent complications. Parents need to be involved in their child's care and to learn how to change dressings, assess for infection and dehydration, and perform range of motion exercises to aid in the child's recovery.

PROVIDE EMOTIONAL SUPPORT

Children with burns have received a profound insult to their body and their self-image. Fear and anxiety about disfigurement and scarring are common, especially among adolescents. The shock and pain of the injury cause increased stress, as do the unfamiliar surroundings and presence of healthcare providers.

Psychologic support is essential to the child's recovery. Continuity of care providers is important in developing a trusting relationship with the child and family. Encourage the child and parents to voice concerns, and show understanding and support for their concerns. Social workers, chaplains, and child life specialists are all trained to help the child and family deal with the stressors of recovery. Make appropriate referrals to ensure that the child and family receive necessary services.

Evidence in Action

A study of 52 children between 12 and 48 months of age admitted to a burn hospital evaluated for evidence of an acute stress response within 1 month of the burn injury. An acute stress response was found in 29% of these children. Symptoms of these children included reliving the injury, hyperarousal, and avoidance (detachment or emotionally numb). Risk factors associated with the child's acute stress response included size of the burn, pulse rate, pain, and parents' stress symptoms. The child's pain was related to the parents' acute stress response (Stoddard, Saxe, Ronfeldt, et al., 2006).

Play therapy is encouraged for children, even if they can only observe initially. Play therapy serves several purposes for the child with a major burn:

- It provides an outlet for frustration, independence, and creativity.
- It promotes activities that challenge range of motion.
- It normalizes the child's daily routine.
- It encourages the child, who sees the progress other children make day by day.

Families are at risk for emotional stress. Forewarn them about the expected edema and the changes in the child's body. Parents often feel guilty and responsible for the child's injury. Help parents focus on recovery rather than past actions. Fear usually results from lack of knowledge about the severity of the burn and the child's status, especially in the early stages of burn care and admission to the hospital ICU. Include the family in the child's care whenever possible. The family needs information and frequent updates. This promotes trust between the family and the healthcare team.

DISCHARGE PLANNING AND HOME CARE TEACHING

Identify and address home care needs well in advance of discharge. Discharge planning may include instructing parents in nutrition and diet needs, safety in the home, protection of the burned area, wound care, signs of infection and actions to take, use of pressure garments, and range of motion exercises to prevent contractures.

Provide support and encouragement to parents as they learn how to care for the burned child. Many burn centers use silver-embedded burn dressings to reduce the frequency of dressing changes needed. Many burn centers perform the dressing changes in a clinic setting because parents find it so difficult to change the dressings knowing that they will inflict pain on their child. If parents do choose to perform dressing changes, provide pain medication and guidelines for how far in advance of the dressing change the medication should be given. Specific guidelines for dressing changes should be outlined so that parents and healthcare team members have the same focus. Parents should first observe care being performed and then provide repeat demonstrations until competent.

NURSING CARE IN THE COMMUNITY

Care of the child with a burn requires long-term therapy and rehabilitation. Long-term care commonly occurs in the home, with frequent visits to healthcare professionals. In some cases, children regularly return to the hospital clinic for dressing changes. Children with extensive burns or with burns in locations where scarring may limit function must often wear a pressure (Jobst) garment, and sometimes a face mask if the face was burned. The garment is removed only for bathing and laundering. The pressure garment may present a threat to the child's body image, but it is an important way to decrease scarring. Help families understand the need for the special garments and masks, and how to clean and care for them. Moisturizing creams can be used after burns heal to relieve drying. The healed skin is highly sensitive to sunburn, so cover the area or use a sunscreen. The sunscreen will also help prevent hyperpigmentation after burn healing.

Continued physical therapy and occupational therapy are often needed to increase strength and dexterity in performing self-care skills and to prevent contractures. Emphasis is placed on returning to normal activities of daily living as soon as possible, such as returning to school. Some children have home tutors or computer connections to school for a time to ensure opportunities for learning while decreasing their risk of exposure to infection.

School reentry is often a traumatic experience, especially for older children and adolescents, because of the fear of rejection, decreased self-esteem, and impaired body image. The child's primary nurse, social worker, and child life specialist may visit the school of a child with a burn injury before the child returns to school—bringing photographs of the child, pressure garments, or other items—to inform classmates and allow them to explore their feelings about the child's burn injury. Some communities may offer support groups for families and children with burn injuries. Referral to these groups may be beneficial.

A major role of nurses in the community is prevention. Provide burn prevention information to parents at each health promotion visit. Become involved with a Safe Kids coalition or with local firefighters to help educate families and caregivers about ways to prevent scald burns and house fires. Examples of prevention messages include the following:

- Appropriate temperature settings for hot water heaters
- Keeping the handles of pots on the stove turned toward the wall and dishes with hot liquids out of the toddler's reach
- Keeping infants and toddlers off the lap when drinking hot beverages or eating soup
- Keeping matches, lighters, and flammable materials away from children
- Installing smoke detectors and replacing the batteries annually

MANAGEMENT OF MINOR BURNS

Many children with minor burns are cared for at home after an initial visit to the emergency department or urgent care clinic. Discuss home remedies for minor burn care (see "Developing Cultural Competence: Litargirio Use"). For superficial burns covering a small area, use moist soaks to stop the burning process and to relieve pain. Any open blisters are debrided, and a thin layer of antibiotic medication is applied over the burn. Do not place this medication close to the eyes or mouth. Bacitracin is often used for burns on the face. The burn is then covered with one or two layers of gauze. Acetaminophen with codeine may be prescribed for burn dressing changes at home. Burn dressings should be changed twice daily. This involves cleaning the burn and reapplying antibiotic cream. See "Teaching Highlights: Caring for Minor Burns."

MyNursingKit Scald Burn Reduction in Children

Teaching Highlights

CARING FOR MINOR BURNS

- Place burn under cool, running water to stop the burning process and to help reduce pain.
- Do not use ice, as it can cause more damage to the injured skin.
- Remove all clothing and jewelry from the burned area.
- Apply a topical antibiotic such as bacitracin to the burned area and cover the area with a couple of layers of gauze. Keep the area clean and dry. Clean and change the dressing twice daily.
- Monitor for signs of infection, such as odor, increased drainage, and increasing redness of the skin around the burn. Contact the healthcare provider if infection is suspected.

Developing Cultural Competence

LITARGIRIO USE

When taking a history about methods used to treat minor burns in children, inquire about the use of "litargirio." This is a traditional remedy used for burn and wound healing and as a deodorant and foot fungicide in the Dominican Republic. The powder is sold in small packets at specialty stores that cater to Spanish-speaking populations. It contains up to 79% lead and can cause lead toxicity in children (FDA, 2003).

EVALUATION

Examples of expected outcomes of nursing management are included in the nursing care plan. Some additional outcomes include the following:

- The child expresses and shows signs of reduced anxiety.
- Effective pain management is provided for dressing changes.

SUNBURN

Sunburn is a burn injury to the outer layer of skin caused by excess ultraviolet light exposure, or sun exposure after taking phototoxic drugs (acne medication, sulfonamides, tetracycline, nonsteroidal anti-inflammatory drugs, and birth control pills) (Boe & Tillotson, 2006). Young children have less melanin to protect their skin against harmful ultraviolet rays. It is estimated that 80% of a person's lifetime exposure to sunburns occurs before 18 years of age, and much of this sun exposure occurs between peak sun hours of 10 a.m. and 4 p.m. (Boe & Tillotson, 2006). Melanoma is the most common cancer in individuals less than 30 years of age, and the rate of melanoma is increasing rapidly in children and adolescents (Oliveria, Saraiya, Geller, et al., 2006). Avoiding sunburn during childhood is believed to be more important than protecting skin during adulthood.

Erythema and skin tenderness usually develop between 30 minutes and 4 hours after exposure to sunlight. Increased vasodilation and vascular permeability result in the extravasation of fluid to the tissues and white blood cell migration to the damaged skin. The erythema peaks at 24 hours. Prolonged exposure can result in edema, vesiculation, bullae, or ulceration. Systemic complaints include malaise, poor sleep due to skin tenderness, fatigue, headaches, and chilling resulting from rapid heat loss.

Nursing Practice

Behaviors and skin characteristics that increase the risk for pediatric melanoma include blue eyes, freckling, fair skin with an inability to tan, blond or red hair, family history of melanoma, intermittent intense sun exposure (e.g., blistering sunburns before 20 years of age), frequent sun exposure without use of sunscreen, melanocytic nevi, and immunosuppression (Muhrer, 2009).

Treatment is generally supportive. Pain can be relieved by cool compresses followed by application of a low-potency topical corticosteroid (on unblistered skin). Children with severe sunburn may need nonsteroidal anti-inflammatory drugs (NSAIDs) for pain relief and to reduce inflammation. See Chapter 42 for information on NSAIDs.

Nursing Management

Educate parents and children about preventing sunburn, especially if the child is taking a phototoxic medication. Advise them that repeated sunburns may lead to permanent skin damage, skin cancer, cataracts, and premature aging of the skin. Recommend to parents that children use sunscreens, use a sun block such as zinc oxide, wear protective clothing, and limit the amount of time they spend in the sun. Children should also wear sunglasses with 99% ultraviolet blockage. See "Teaching Highlights: Preventing Sunburn."

HYPOTHERMIA

Hypothermia is a condition in which the core body temperature falls below 35°C (95°F). This occurs when the heat produced by the body is less than the heat lost. Hypothermia is a life-threatening emergency that can occur in any season and any geographic location. Infants and young children are at risk because of immature temperature regulatory mechanisms, thinner skin, limited subcutaneous fat, and high skin surface area to body mass ratio. Adoles-

Teaching Highlights

PREVENTING SUNBURN

- Keep children out of direct sunlight as much as possible, especially between 10 a.m. and 2 p.m. Encourage children to play in the shade. A child can still be burned on a cloudy day, since up to 80% of ultraviolet rays can penetrate the cloud cover.
- Be aware that water, concrete, and sand reflect sunlight and increase exposure up to 90% by reflecting up to 85% of the ultraviolet rays.
- Minimize sun exposure by wearing a hat with a 3-inch brim, closely woven cotton long-sleeved clothing and pants, and wraparound UV blocking sunglasses. Wear a T-shirt while swimming.
- Use sunscreen with 15 or higher SPF. For optimal protection, apply as thickly as directed to all exposed areas 30–45 minutes before sun exposure. Reapply every 2 hours, or sooner if swimming, toweling off, or perspiring heavily.
- Use a waterproof sunscreen when swimming for protection in water that lasts 60–80 minutes. Reapply as needed. Avoid placing it near the eyes as it causes a chemical burn and pain. Call the poison control center immediately for guidance.
- Use UV blocking agents such as zinc oxide or titanium oxide for infants under 6 months of age as infants may absorb sunscreen chemical through their skin.

cents are at risk because of risk-taking behaviors such as drug and alcohol use and engaging in remote outdoor activities without proper equipment.

Primary hypothermia results from environmental exposure. As with newborns, heat is lost through radiation, conduction, convection, and evaporation. As the core body temperature falls, the body tries to conserve body heat and to rewarm the blood by vasoconstriction (to shunt blood to the body core) and increasing muscle tone and shivering. Hypothermia leads to increased blood viscosity, slows blood through the capillaries, and facilitates blood coagulation.

Symptoms of mild hypothermia include slurred speech, poor coordination, poor judgment and inappropriate behavior, shivering, and muscle stiffness. Symptoms of moderate hypothermia include depressed respirations, slow pulse, low blood pressure, pale or cyanotic color, shivering, and dilated pupils. Lethargy, mental impairment, irrational thinking, hallucinations, and coma develop as the central nervous system becomes depressed. Profound hypothermia (body temperature below 28°C [84°F]) is characterized by apnea, no shivering, low blood pressure, ventricular fibrillation, dilated and unresponsive pupils, and coma.

Clinical therapy focuses on resuscitation, if necessary, and gradual core body rewarming. The child who has profound hypothermia should receive cardiopulmonary resuscitation until the body temperature returns to normal because the hypothermia may have preserved vital organs. Aggressive techniques for rewarming may include humidified, warm oxygen, warmed intravenous fluids, warm packs to the core circulation areas (axillae, groin, and neck), and peritoneal lavage and dialysis. Hypoglycemia is a common complication and is treated with IV glucose.

For mild hypothermia (temperature above 35°C [95°F]), external heat lamps, immersion in warm water, and an electric blanket are used.

Nursing Management

Monitor vital signs and urine output during rewarming. Prevention is geared toward educating parents to layer children's clothing in cold climates, recognize signs of hypothermia, decrease time of exposure to cold, and know how to treat mild hypothermia. Teach school-age children and adolescents who go on camping and hunting trips how to recognize and manage hypothermia in themselves and others. Teach preventive techniques such as avoiding riding snowmobiles or walking on ice that is not known to be deep enough to support the weight.

If a child becomes hypothermic during an outing such as a camping trip, a warm person should get into a sleeping bag (or under the blankets) next to the child after any wet or heavy clothing is removed. This action will warm the child and prevent further heat loss. First aid for hypothermia includes moving the child to a dry area and removing any wet clothing. Replace with warm, dry clothing, and encourage the child to drink a warm, high-calorie liquid, if able.

FROSTBITE

Frostbite is a cold injury that results from overexposure of the water in skin cells to temperatures low enough to cause crystal formation. Frostbite develops in tissues exposed to temperatures below freezing for more than an hour when environmental protection is inadequate. Areas of the body at high risk for frostbite include the hands, feet, cheeks, nose, and ears. Ice crystallizes in the tissues, resulting in dehydration of the cells and ischemic damage. Frostbite can also occur if a chemical cold pack used for first aid is left in contact with the skin for an extended period.

Clinical manifestations depend on the severity and depth of the cellular damage (Nicol, Huether, & Weber, 2006):

- Superficial skin affected—numb, central white area surrounded by redness and edema, no blistering.
- Full-thickness skin affected—erythema, vesicle formation with clear or pink fluid, surrounded by edema and redness.
- Full-thickness and subcutaneous skin affected—local edema, grayish blue discoloration, hemorrhagic vesicles, tissue necrosis.
- Deeper cold injury—deep cyanosis, no vesicles or local edema, necrosis of subcutaneous tissue or deeper, possibly involving the muscles or tendons.

The skin at first appears pale and is numb. Rapid rewarming causes a flush and the sensation of tingling, burning, or prickling in the affected area. The erythema and mild swelling develop into bullae. The extent of injury is not initially apparent.

If frostbite is suspected, get the child to a warmer environment, loosen all constricting clothing, and remove any wet clothes. Because the frostbitten area is numb, extreme caution is needed to protect it from any trauma. Rewarming is done slowly to decrease the chance of cellular damage. The affected part is immersed for 10 to 15 minutes in water warmed to between 38°C and 40°C (100.4°F and 104°F). Analgesics are prescribed because thawing causes severe pain. The affected skin is gently cleaned with saline and covered with sterile dressings. Wound care may be similar to that provided to a child with burns. Whirlpool and physical therapy treatment are important to improve circulation and maintain function. Amputation may be needed when circulation is not restored.

Nursing Management

As with hypothermia, the goal of management is prevention. Teach parents to layer children's clothing for warmth and to pack extra blankets and clothing if cold temperatures are expected during outdoor activities. Teach adolescents how to avoid frostbite during hunting and other cold weather expeditions. Wet clothing should be changed quickly.

Early care is instrumental in minimizing permanent injury. Severe frostbite requires hospitalization, fluid management, dressing changes, and careful attention to diet. Provide emotional support to the child and family while they wait to learn the full extent of injury and disability.

MyNursingKit Dog Bite Reduction

BITES

Animal Bites

Approximately 42% of nonfatal dog bites treated in emergency departments (150,000 visits) in the United States occur among children under 14 years of age, and the injury rates are highest among male children ages 5 to 9 years (Howell & Powell, 2007). In many cases the dog is known by the child, and most bites occur in the home or a familiar place. Bites are often associated with the child's inappropriate behavior, such as teasing, rough play, or interfering with feeding or care of puppies. Other animals that may bite include cats, birds, turtles, and wild animals such as bats, squirrels, and raccoons.

Assessment includes noting the location and number of puncture wounds, abrasions, lacerations, and crushing injuries; redness or swelling at entry sites; redness extending out from site (possible cellulitis); and any drainage related to the bite. Dog bites tend to be crushing, rather than clean, sharp lacerations. Cat bites tend to be puncture wounds. Damage to nerves, muscles, tendons, and vascular structures is identified. Head and neck bites require radiographic examination to rule out any associated injury, such as trauma to the airway or a depressed skull fracture.

Initial treatment involves irrigation of the wound, removal of devitalized tissue, and application of a clean dressing. Sedation and pain management may be needed for some children. Small wounds may be closed with adhesive strips rather than suturing because of the potential for infection. Wounds that are several hours old are often left open. Severe bites sometimes require surgical closure or reconstruction. Wounds over joints should be immobilized and elevated. Puncture wounds should *not* be irrigated or sutured. The major complication of bites is infection, such as cellulitis. Cat bites can result in septic arthritis and osteomyelitis if a bone or joint is punctured. Antibiotics and early treatment can greatly decrease these complications.

Dog bites should be reported to animal control, and the dog should be confined and observed for 10 days for signs of rabies. Cat bites are also dangerous as they are less commonly immunized against rabies. Human rabies immune globulin (HRIG) or human diploid cell rabies vaccine (HDCV) should be given to all children bitten by wild animals in which rabies cannot be excluded, as well as to children bitten by domestic animals (cats and dogs) suspected or proven to be rabid. See Chapter 45 for a description of rabies treatment.

Nursing Management

If a child is bitten by an animal, obtain information about the extent of the injury, circumstances surrounding the attack, present location of the animal, and attempts to assess the animal's health.

To decrease infection, the wound is gently washed with antibacterial soap and water. The wound (unless it is a puncture wound) is then irrigated with large quantities of sterile saline or lactated Ringer's solution. A 19-gauge needle on a 60-mL syringe may be used to provide high pressure irrigation. After dead tissue is debrided, apply a clean dressing and elevate the affected body part to reduce bleeding. Check the child's immunization record to determine whether a tetanus booster is necessary. Teach parents how to care for the wound and signs of infection that indicate a need to return for care.

Prevention of animal bites is another important nursing role (see "Teaching Highlights: Preventing Animal Bites").

Teaching Highlights

PREVENTING ANIMAL BITES

General guidelines for pets in the home

- Never leave a young child alone with an animal.
- Do not buy or adopt a pet unless you are confident of your child's ability to respect it.
- Spay or neuter the pet to reduce aggression.
- If an animal (wild or unknown) is sick or acting strangely, notify the health department.

Teach children the following rules

- Avoid all unfamiliar animals and report them to a parent.
- Avoid contact with all wild animals.
- Do not touch an animal when it is eating, sleeping, or nursing.
- Never overexcite an animal, even in play. Do not roughhouse or play games that stimulate aggressive behavior.
- Never tease or throw objects at an animal.
- Never put your face close to an animal. Seek permission before hugging or petting an animal.
- If approached by a dog, stay calm, stand still, talk softly, and back away slowly until the dog loses interest; do not run.
- If attacked, pretend to be a tree or a log and protect the face. If knocked down, curl into a ball and protect the face and neck.

Human Bites

Human bites are more common than most people realize. They usually occur in toddlers and young children. Adolescents may also receive human bites during altercations. The skin may be broken, with erythema, abrasion, bruising, or laceration. Because the mouth harbors many bacteria, infection is fairly common. Assess the risk for hepatitis B and HIV infection; however, saliva is believed to inhibit the transmission of HIV infection (Conlon, 2007). Initial treatment includes irrigating with sterile saline and debridement. Antibiotics may be prescribed to prevent systemic complications. Parents should be instructed about how to care for the wound and to observe for infection.

Insect Bites and Stings

Insect bites and stings occur frequently in children and usually are not a cause for concern. Exceptions include bites or stings by insects that carry parasites or communicable diseases (ticks, mosquitos), those of a venomous nature (spiders), and those that produce an allergic reaction. About 3% of the population is sensitized to *Hymenoptera* (bee, wasps, fire ants) stings and have a generalized response (Steen, Carbonaro, & Schwartz, 2004); see "Clinical Manifestations: Insect Bites and Stings." For a discussion of communicable diseases carried by ticks and mosquitoes (e.g., Lyme disease and Rocky Mountain spotted fever) see Chapter 45.

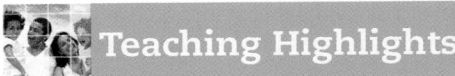

Clinical Manifestations

INSECT BITES AND STINGS

TYPE OF BITE AND CLINICAL MANIFESTATIONS	CLINICAL THERAPY
MOSQUITOES AND FLEAS Local inflammation results from injected foreign protein or chemicals. ■ Local reactions: discrete, red papules and edema at the bite site with itching, burning, pain, and hives; minimal discomfort; pruritic wheals and bullae tend to develop with repeat exposure. ■ Systemic reactions: wheezing, urticaria; laryngeal edema; shock	Local reactions: ■ Cold compresses or ice applied to the site ■ Antihistamine medication Systemic reactions need emergency medical treatment.
BEE OR WASP STING Venoms contain enzymes that affect vascular tone and permeability. ■ Local reaction: mild, local pain; erythema and edema ■ Systemic reaction: generalized urticaria, flushing, angioedema, pruritus; wheezing; anaphylaxis is rare.	Local reactions: ■ Remove stinger as soon as possible ■ Cold compresses and elevate extremity ■ A dash of meat tenderizer (papain powder) and a drop of water massaged into the skin for 5 minutes relieves the pain. ■ Antihistamine medication Systemic reactions are treated with glucocorticoids and antihistamines or epinephrine. Desensitization for severe reactions
FIRE ANTS Venom is hemolytic and neurotoxic, causing a histaminelike response. ■ Local reaction: a black center at the point of the bite, or trail of lesions across skin; initial wheal becomes a vesicle in a few hours; in 24 hours the fluid is cloudy, and the vesicle has a red halo; pruritus, erythema, edema, induration ■ Systemic and anaphylactic reactions can occur.	Local reactions: ■ Ice or cold compresses ■ Antihistamine medication ■ Elevate extremity Systemic reactions—same as bees and wasps
BLACK WIDOW SPIDER Venom is neurotoxic. ■ Local reaction: stinging sensation at time of bite; localized edema and erythema, two fang marks, petechiae branching from site ■ Systemic reaction in 1–3 hours, symptoms peak in 3–12 hours, diminish in 72 hours; muscle rigidity of torso and abdomen, priapism, muscle cramps near the bite; malaise, sweating, nausea, vomiting, dizziness, restlessness, insomnia, and diaphoresis; hypertension and arrhythmias; oliguria	Ice Diazepam and opioids Antihistamine medication Hydrocortisone may decrease the inflammatory response. Antivenom IV is used in severe reactions after negative skin test for hypersensitivity to horse serum.
BROWN RECLUSE SPIDER Venom contains proteolytic enzymes and sphingomyelinase D, a cytotoxic factor. ■ Local reaction: itching, pain, and erythema at bite site in first 6–12 hours; evolves to purple bull's-eye lesion that signals beginning of necrosis; reddish blisters; a white ring is surrounded by an irregular erythematous ring (Zeglin, 2005). ■ Systemic reaction: severe progressive reactions may occur in 12–72 hours; fever, chills, restlessness, malaise, joint pain, and nausea and vomiting	Ice Cleanse the wound and good wound care Analgesics Oral anti-inflammatory agent Antibiotics for secondary infection Excision and skin grafting in cases of severe necrosis

Nursing Management

The goal of nursing care is prevention. Become familiar with the harmful insects in your area, so you can identify them and recognize their effects. Children should be taught to avoid spiders and other biting or stinging insects. Many commercial repellents (OFF, Cutter's, Deep Woods OFF) are available. Most products contain DEET (diethyltoluamide) and are effective against many insects, including mosquitoes, fleas, ticks, and chiggers. However, DEET does not repel stinging insects. Teach children to stay calm when a bee or wasp approaches and to slowly walk away without swatting.

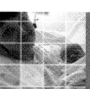

Warn parents against using heavily perfumed shampoos, powders, soaps, or lotions, or dressing children in bright-colored or floral print clothing when outdoors, as these may attract insects. Avoid eating sweet foods and beverages outdoors as these will attract bees and wasps. Bees and wasps may crawl into a canned beverage and not be seen. Pour beverages into a cup rather than drinking from a can to prevent stings to the mouth and lips.

Household pets may be a source of fleas or ticks. Encourage frequent inspection of pets and preventive treatments against fleas and ticks before pets are allowed prolonged contact with children.

When a systemic reaction to Hymenoptera has occurred, the child should wear a medical alert identification and carry an emergency kit with epinephrine. See Chapter 50∞. Teach parents and school personnel how to administer epinephrine. Desensitization injections may be given.

Snake Bites

Venomous snakes are found in most areas of the country. During warm months, snakes are active and likely to bite if disturbed. Fortunately, many bites are dry, delivering no venom. Fatalities are rare.

Rattlesnake, copperhead, and cottonmouth venom is composed of enzymes and toxins that cause hemolysis and tissue necrosis (Singletary, Rochman, Bodmer, et al., 2005). Coral snake venom causes neuromuscular paralysis. The amount and toxicity of the venom injected has an impact on the consequences of the snakebite. Because children usually receive a higher amount of venom relative to body mass, their response maybe greater than an adult's.

Puncture marks, white wheal, and burning sensation appear at the site of the bite. Erythema, bruising, and edema rapidly develop and extend from the site for up to 24 hours. Systemic signs include dizziness, tachycardia, nausea, vomiting, diarrhea, sweating, and chills. Signs of a severe response may include hypotension, altered consciousness, and bleeding from multiple sites (disseminated intravascular coagulation), pulmonary edema, and renal failure.

Clinical therapy involves immobilization of the extremity and a cold compress to slow the spread of the venom. Laboratory studies include complete blood count, platelet count, coagulation studies, electrolytes, and renal function. Attempts to identify the snake causing the bite should be made to determine if it is venomous. The poison control center is contacted to obtain treatment guidelines. Specific antivenom is usually administered within 4 to 6 hours. CroFab®, a newer antivenom used for cottonmouth, copperhead, and rattlesnake bites, is available, but limited data on use in children exist (Schmidt, 2005). Because antivenom contains a hyperimmune horse serum product, anaphylaxis or delayed serum sickness may develop. A skin test may be performed first to detect hypersensitivity. Antihistamines are often given in anticipation of a hypersensitivity reaction. Pain medication may be provided. A tetanus booster is given if vaccination status is unknown or the tetanus series is incomplete.

Nursing Management

Nursing care involves assessing the child for initial and progressive signs of envenomation. First aid involves immobilizing the extremity, keeping it in a dependent position to slow the spread of venom, and cold compresses. Rings or constricting items should be quickly removed from the injured extremity. Monitor the distal extremity's color, pulse, and sensation, and measure the circumference of the extremity every 20 to 30 minutes to track progression in swelling and response to treatment. Provide skin care for the swollen and tense skin to prevent abrasions and to prevent additional injury.

Help the child identify the snake from pictures of snakes common to the area; however, some venomous snakes are kept as exotic pets.

The child receiving antivenom may be cared for in the critical care unit. The antivenom is diluted in saline and slowly administered intravenously as ordered. Administer the antihistamines after tests for sensitivity to horse serum are completed. Have resuscitation equipment on hand in preparation for an anaphylactic reaction. Help locate additional antivenom if the hospital does not have an adequate supply.

Provide emotional support to the child and family. Teach children and their families to avoid future snakebites.

CONTUSIONS

Contusions are soft-tissue injuries that have a variety of causes. Often it is difficult to assess whether an injury has caused underlying tissue damage. An injury does not have to break the skin to result in internal damage. Radiographic examination may be necessary to rule out broken bones or further tissue damage. Signs and symptoms that indicate a need for treatment include swelling that does not subside within 72 hours, intense pain, inability to move the injured part, and infection. Elevate the injured extremity and apply ice as soon as possible after injury. This can reduce inflammation and swelling in the area.

FOREIGN BODIES

Many skin injuries result from penetration of foreign particles. Common substances include gravel from abrasions, bee stingers, and splinters. Treatment of superficial foreign bodies involves irrigating the wound to try to forcibly dislodge the debris. A deeply embedded foreign body is best removed under medical supervision to avoid permanent injury or scarring.

LACERATIONS

Lacerations are cuts or tears to the skin. In many cases the cut is minor and can be managed at home with gentle cleansing, antibiotic ointment, and a bandage. More extensive lacerations and those on the face or over joints often need suturing to promote healing and reduce scarring. Laceration repair is performed after wound cleansing and appropriate local analgesia to control pain. Sutures or dermal adhesive may be used. Sutures are usually removed about 7 days later.

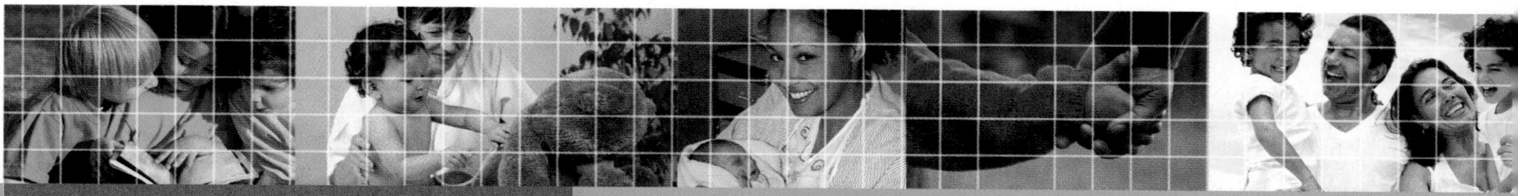

CRITICAL CONCEPT REVIEW

LEARNING OUTCOMES / CONCEPTS

59.1 Identify the characteristics of different skin lesions by their cause, including those caused by irritants, infections, drug reactions, mites, infection, and injury.

1. Irritant skin lesions:
   - Pruritic papulovesicular lesions.
   - Erythematous.
   - Well circumscribed.
2. Infection:
   - Localized swelling and erythema.
   - Papular and vesicular lesions that rupture, leaving an erosion and serous fluid crusts.
3. Drug reactions:
   - Erythematous macules and papules.
   - Pruritus and urticaria.
4. Mites:
   - Intense pruritus.
   - Papular, pustular, vesicular, and nodular lesions.
   - Linear threadlike grayish burrows.
5. Injuries:
   - Pressure ulcers: reddened area progressing to skin breakdown and erosion.
   - Burn (partial thickness): erythema, blistering, and pain.
   - Animal bites: usually cause crush or puncture wounds.

59.2 Describe the stages of wound healing.

1. Inflammation (3–5 days):
   - Clot formation to seal the wound.
   - Vasodilation allows white blood cells to reach the injured tissue for phagocytosis.
   - Swelling.
2. Reconstruction/epithelialization (4 days to 2 weeks):
   - Regeneration of destroyed cells.
   - Clot dissolves and wound edges grow together.
   - Collagen and granulation tissue are produced.
3. Maturation (months–2 years):
   - Scar formation and strengthening.

59.3 Describe a nursing care plan for a child with acute skin disorders, including dermatitis, infectious disorders, and infestations.

1. Eliminate possible allergens from the child's environment.
2. Cleanse skin as ordered.
3. Apply appropriate topical medications.
4. Keep child's fingernails short to prevent damage from scratching.
5. Provide medications to decrease itching.
6. Provide cool soaks to reduce itching.
7. Treat infestation sites of body with appropriate medication.
8. Treat all clothing, linens, and toys that have been in contact with the child with infestation.

59.4 Plan the nursing care for the child with a chronic skin condition.

1. Provide guidelines for bathing and moisturizing the skin.
2. Teach appropriate application of topical medications.
3. Identify potential for food allergies as a trigger for skin flare-ups.
4. Help family deal with frustrations of acute flare-ups, and provide emotional support.
5. Identify strategies to promote the child's self-esteem.

(continued)

LEARNING OUTCOMES	CONCEPTS
59.5 Develop an education plan for adolescents with acne to promote self-care.	1. Inform parents and adolescents that acne does not have a dietary cause. 2. Inform adolescents that excessive perspiration and emotional stress may increase the number of acne lesions. 3. Instruct the adolescent in a recommended skin cleansing routine. 4. Teach the adolescent and parents about oral and topical medication administration, including side effects. 5. Caution the adolescent that some acne medications increase the skin's sensitivity to the sun and the importance of using sunscreen. 6. Emphasize the importance of returning to the healthcare provider for scheduled follow-up appointments.
59.6 Describe the process to measure the extent of burns and burn severity in children.	1. Assessment of burn severity includes: ■ Depth of the burn injury. ■ Percentage of body surface area affected using the Lund and Browder chart for age of child. ■ Involvement of specific body parts. 2. Burns to the hands, feet, face, or perineal area are treated as major injuries due to the potential for impairment in function and cosmetic appearance.
59.7 Develop a nursing care plan for the child with a full-thickness burn injury.	1. Maintain adequate fluid volume: ■ Monitor vital signs. ■ Administer volume-expanding IV fluids as ordered. ■ Monitor intake and output. 2. Observe for any respiratory difficulties. 3. Provide enteral nutrition or a high-protein and high-calorie diet. 4. Provide adequate pain management. 5. Promote functional use of joints and extremities. 6. Maintain sterile technique when changing dressings. 7. Assist child in the use of guided imagery and distraction during dressing changes. 8. Provide psychological support to the child and family.
59.8 Identify preventive strategies to reduce the risk of injury from burns, hypothermia, bites, and stings.	1. Burns ■ Lower the temperature settings for hot water heaters. ■ Keep pot handles on the stove turned toward the wall and keep dishes with hot liquids out of a toddler's reach. ■ Keep infants and toddlers off the lap when drinking hot beverages or eating soup. ■ Keep matches, lighters, and flammable materials away from children. ■ Install smoke detectors and replace the batteries annually. 2. Hypothermia ■ Layer children's clothing for warmth. ■ Pack extra blankets and clothing if cold temperatures are expected during outdoor activities. ■ Change wet clothing quickly. 3. Bites and Stings ■ Avoid contact with unknown animals and wild animals. ■ Do not play with animals while they are eating, sleeping, or nursing. ■ Do not tease or overexcite an animal. ■ Parents should apply appropriate commercial insect repellent to exposed skin and clothes of children. ■ Instruct children to stay calm when near stinging insects. ■ Wear light-colored clothes and avoid eating sweetened foods and beverages when outside. ■ Inspect and treat pets for fleas and ticks.

CRITICAL THINKING IN ACTION

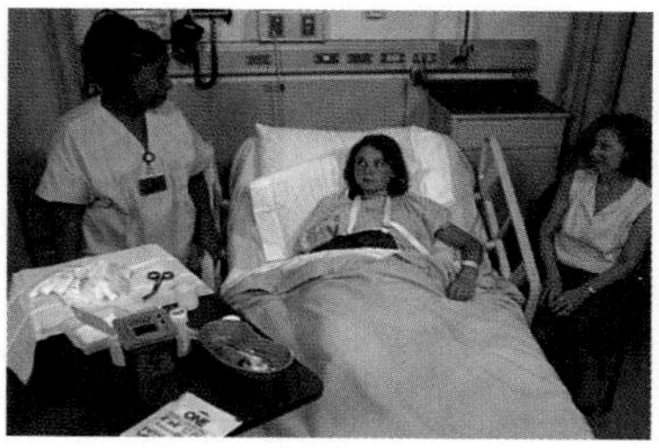

Twelve-year-old Rebecca is admitted to the burn unit after being scalded after spilling boiling spaghetti water on her chest, abdomen, and legs when attempting to carry the pot to the sink. The burn is classified as a partial-thickness burn covering 12% of her body surface area (BSA) and full-thickness burn covering 3% of BSA. IV fluids are started in the emergency department and a continuous infusion of morphine is given for pain. Her temperature is 101°F. The initial debridement of the burns is performed in the operating room so that Rebecca is anesthetized and does not feel pain from the procedure. A silver-embedded dressing is applied to her partial thickness burns, and an allograft is placed over the full thickness injury. Following debridement, Rebecca is put on a high-calorie, high-protein diet to help meet her increased nutritional requirements. Her parents are encouraged to bring in foods Rebecca enjoys to encourage her to eat. Wound care around the allograft is performed twice a day, and all burn sites are inspected for signs of infection. The dressing over the partial thickness burns is replaced every 3 days. Pain medication for wound care is provided through the IV. After several days, Rebecca is scheduled for an autograft for the full thickness injury. Rebecca's nutritional intake and urine output are carefully monitored while she is hospitalized. Physical therapy is initiated to maintain range of motion and to prevent contractures.

The nurse talks with Rebecca and her family about what to expect as the burns heal. Education of the family includes signs and symptoms of infection and the care of the graft donor site and the graft site. After a few days in the hospital, Rebecca is discharged with daily follow-up in the burn clinic for wound care.

1. What is the most likely type of initial IV fluid started on Rebecca in the emergency department and hospital? Why?
2. Why is it important to monitor Rebecca's urine output?
3. What are the advantages of the type of dressing used for Rebecca's partial thickness burns?
4. What regular assessments of Rebecca's burn sites should be performed?
5. What are some high-protein, high-calorie foods that might appeal to Rebecca?

See MyNursingKit for possible responses.

REFERENCES

Aber, C., Connelly, E. A., & Schachner, L. A. (2007). Fever and rash in a child: When to worry? *Pediatric Annals, 36*(1), 30–38.

Akdis, C. A., Akdis, M., Bieber, T., Bindslev-Jensen, C., Boguniewicz, M., Eigenmann, P., et al. (2006). Diagnosis and treatment of atopic dermatitis in children and adults: European Academy of Allergology and Clinical Immunology/American Academy of Allergy, Asthma and Immunology/PRACTALL consensus report. *Journal of Allergy and Clinical Immunology, 118*(1), 152–169.

Alberta, L., Sweeney, S. M., & Wiss, K. (2005). Diaper dye dermatitis. *Pediatrics, 116*(3), e450–e452.

Allen, P. L. J. (2004). Leaves of three, let them be: If it were only that easy! *Pediatric Nursing, 30*(2), 129–135.

Amer, A., & Fischer, H. (2006). Linear rash leaves your patient itching. *Contemporary Pediatrics, 23*(10), 20, 23.

American Academy of Pediatrics Committee on Infectious Disease. (2009). *Red book, report of the Committee on Infectious Disease* (28th ed). Elk Grove Village, IL: Author.

Atherton, D. J. (2004). A review of the pathophysiology, prevention, and treatment of irritant diaper dermatitis. *Current Medical Research and Opinion, 20*(5), 645–649.

Bell, E. A. (2007). New topical offers a choice in impetigo treatment. *Infectious Diseases in Children, 20*(10), 12.

Boe, K., & Tillotson, E. A. (2006). Encouraging sun safety for children and adolescents. *Journal of School Nursing, 22*(3), 136–141.

Borkowski, S. (2004). Diaper rash care and management. *Pediatric Nursing, 30*(6), 467–470.

Butler, C. T. (2006). Pediatric skin care: Guidelines for assessment, prevention, and treatment. *Pediatric Nursing, 32*(5), 443–450.

Centers for Disease Control and Prevention. (2008). Protect the ones you love: Burns. Retrieved June 10, 2009 from http://www.cdc.gov/SafeChild/Burns/default.htm

Christinson-Lagay, E. R., & Fishman, S. J. (2006). Vascular anomalies. *Surgical Clinics of North America, 86*, 393–425.

Cohen, B. A. (2004). Another baby and another cutaneous lesion—and more on efficient recognition and management. *Contemporary Pediatrics, 21*(10), 39–57.

Conlon, H. A. (2007). Human bites in the classroom: Incidence, treatment, and complications. *Journal of School Nursing, 23*(4), 197–201.

Dohil, M. A., & Eichenfield, L. F. (2005). A treatment approach for atopic dermatitis. *Pediatric Annals, 34*(3), 201–210.

Duffy, B. J., McLaughlin, P. M., & Eichelberger, M. R. (2006). Assessment, triage, and early management of burns in children. *Clinical Pediatric Emergency Medicine, 7*, 82–93.

Findlay, J. (2007). Treating atopic dermatitis. *Contemporary Pediatrics, 24*(6 Suppl.), 4–12.

Food and Drug Administration. (2003). *FDA warns consumers about use of Litargirio - Traditional remedy that contains dangerous levels of lead.* Retrieved February 21, 2009, from http://www.fda.gov/bbs/topics/ANSWERS/2003/ANS01253.html

Food and Drug Administration. (2005). *FDA public health advisory: Elidel (pimecrolimus) and Protopic (tacrolimus) ointment.* Retrieved April 3, 2005, from http://www.fda.gov/cder/drug/advisory/elidel_protopic.htm

Food and Drug Administration. (2007). *Lindane shampoo and lindane lotion: Questions and answers.* Retrieved February 19, 2009, from http://www.fda.gov/cder/drug/infopage/lindane/lindaneQA.htm

Gardiner, P. (2007). Complementary, holistic, and integrative medicine: Chamomile. *Pediatrics in Review, 28*(4), e16–e18.

Goates, B. M., Atkin, S. J., Wilding, K. G., Birch, K. G., Cottam, M. R., Bush, S. E., & Clayton, D. H., (2006). An effective nonchemical treatment for head lice: A lot of hot air. *Pediatrics, 118*(5), 1962–1970.

Grant, E. J. (2004). Burn prevention. *Critical Care Nursing Clinics of North America, 16*, 127–138.

Groeneveld, A., Anderson, M., Allen, S., Bressmer, S., Golberg, M., et al. (2004). The prevalence of pressure ulcers in a tertiary care pediatric and adult hospital. *Journal of Wound Ostomy Care Management, 31*(3), 108–120.

Haggstrom, A. N., Drolet, B. A., Baselga, E., Chamlin, S. L., Garzon, M. C., Horii, K. A., et al., (2007). Prospective study of infantile hemangiomas: Demographic, prenatal, and perinatal characteristics. *Journal of Pediatrics, 150*(3), 291–294.

Horner, G. (2005). Physical abuse: Recognition and reporting. *Journal of Pediatric Health Care, 19*(1), 4–11.

Howell, J. F., & Powell, S. T. (2007). Companion animals and human health risk: Animal bites and rabies. *Topics in Advanced Practice Nursing eJournal, 7*(2).

Hull, P. R., Derm, F. F., & D'Arcy, C. (2005). Acne, depression, and suicide. *Dermatology Clinics, 23*, 665–674.

Idriss, N., & Khachemoune, A. (2006). Scabies. *Dermatology Nursing, 18*(6), 588, 616.
Jones, H. (2007). Nurse-administered laser in dermatology. *Nursing Clinics of North America, 42*, 393–406.
Kaymak, Y., & Ilter, N. (2006). The results and side effects of systemic isotretinoin treatment in 100 patients with acne vulgaris. *Dermatology Nursing, 18*(6), 576–580.
Kelsay, K. (2006). Management of sleep disturbance associated with atopic dermatitis. *Journal of Allergy and Clinical Immunology, 118*(1), 198–201.
Keri, J. E. (2006). Acne: Improving skin and self-esteem. *Pediatric Annals, 35*(3), 174–179.
Khachemoune, A., Khechmoune, K., & Blanc, D. (2006). Assessing phytophotodermatitis: Boy with erythema and blisters on both hands. *Dermatology Nursing, 18*(2), 153–154.
Klein, G. L., & Herndon, D. N. (2004). Burns. *Pediatrics in Review, 25*(12), 411–416.
Leung, A. K. C., Fong, J. H. S., & Pinto-Rojas, A. (2005). Pediculosis capitus. *Journal of Pediatric Health Care, 19*(6), 369–378.
McLeod, R. P. (2004). Lungs, bumps, and things that go itch in your office! *Journal of School Nursing, 20*(6), 361–362.
Miller, T., & Frieden, I. J. (2005). Hemangiomas: New insights and classification. *Pediatric Annals, 34*(3), 179–187.
Monroe, J. R. (2005). All that is round is not fungal. *Clinician Reviews, 15*(2), 46–53.
Morelli, J. G. (2007a). Acne. In R. M. Kliegman, R. E. Behrman, H. B. Jensen, & B. F. Stanton (Eds.), *Nelson Textbook of Pediatrics* (18th ed., 2759–2764), Philadelphia: Elsevier Saunders.
Morelli, J. G. (2007b). Cutaneous bacterial infections. In R. M. Kliegman, R. E. Behrman, H. B. Jensen, & B. F. Stanton (Eds.), *Nelson Textbook of Pediatrics* (18th ed., 2759–2764), Philadelphia: Elsevier Saunders.
Morelli, J. G. (2007c). Vesiculobullous disorders. In R. M. Kliegman, R. E. Behrman, H. B. Jensen, & B. F. Stanton (Eds.), *Nelson Textbook of Pediatrics* (18th ed., 2685–2693), Philadelphia: Elsevier Saunders.
Muhrer, J. C. (2009). Melanoma: Current incidence, diagnosis, and preventive strategies. *Journal for Nurse Practitioners, 5*(1), 35–41.
National Center for Complementary and Alternative Medicine. (2006). *Herbs at a glance*. Retrieved February 16, 2009, from http://nccam.nih.gov/health
National Center for Health Statistics, National Vital Statistics System. (2007). *Injury deaths and rates for children and teenagers by age, external cause, and intent, 2004*. Retrieved February, 19, 2009 from http://webapppa.cdc.gov/sasweb/ncicp/leadcause10.htm
National Pressure Ulcer Advisory Panel. (2007). *Updated staging system*. Retrieved June 7, 2009 from http://www.npuap.org/pr2.htm
Nestor, M. S. (2007). The use of photodynamic therapy for treatment of acne vulgaris. *Dermatologic Clinics, 25*, 47–57.
Nicol, N. H., & Huether, S. E. (2006). Alterations of the integument in children. In K. L. McCance & S. E. Huether, *Pathophysiology: The biologic basis for disease in adults and children* (5th ed., pp. 1609–1623). St. Louis: Elsevier Mosby.
Nicol, N. H., Huether, S. E., & Weber, R. (2006). Structure, function, and disorders of the integument. In K. L. McCance & S. E. Huether (Eds.), *Pathophysiology: The basis for disease in adults and children* (5th ed., pp. 1573–1607). St. Louis: Elsevier Mosby.
Nield, L. S., & Kamat, D. M. (2006). Diaper dermatitis: From "A" to "Pee." *Consultant for Pediatricians, 5*(6), 373–380.
Noonan, C., Quigley, S., & Curley, M. A. Q. (2006). Skin integrity in hospitalized infants and children: A prevalence survey. *Journal of Pediatric Nursing, 21*(6), 445–453.
O'Connor, N. R., McLaughlin, M. R., & Ham, P. (2008). Newborn skin: Part 1. Common rashes. *American Family Physician, 77*(1), 47–52.
Oliveria, S. A., Saraiya, M., Geller, A. C., Heneghan, M. K., & Jorgensen, C. (2006). Sun exposure and risk of melanoma. *Archives of Disease in Childhood, 91,* 131–138.
Ong, P. Y., & Boguniewicz, M. (2007). Atopic dermatitis and contact dermatitis in the emergency department. *Clinical Pediatric Emergency Medicine, 8*, 81–86.
Pearlman, D. L. (2004). A simple treatment for head lice. Dry-on suffocation based pediculicide. *Pediatrics, 114*, 275–279.
Peterson, J. D., & Chan, L. S. (2006). A comprehensive management guide for atopic dermatitis. *Dermatologic Nursing, 18*(6), 531–542.
Podraza, J., & Miller, R. (2007). What's your diagnosis? *Consultant for Pediatricians, 6*(9), 517–521.
Popovich, D., & McAlhany, A. (2007). Accurately diagnosing commonly misdiagnosed circular rashes. *Pediatric Nursing, 33*(4), 315–320.
Reed, J. L., & Pomerantz, W. J. (2005). Emergency management of pediatric burns. *Pediatric Emergency Care, 21*(2), 118–129.
Sagerman, P. J. (2005). Wounds. *Pediatrics in Review, 26*(2), 43–48.
Schachner, L., Feiner, A., & Camisulli, S. (2005). Epidermolysis bullosa: Management principles for the neonate, infant, and young child. *Dermatology Nursing, 17*(1), 56–59.
Schachner, L. A., Lamerson, C., Sheehan, M. P., Boguniewicz, M., Mosser, J., Raimer, S., et al. (2005). Tacrolimus ointment 0.03% is safe and effective for the treatment of mild to moderate atopic dermatitis in pediatric patients: Results from a randomized, double-blind, vehicle controlled study. *Pediatrics, 116*(3), e334–e342.
Schmidt, C. E. (2003). A 12-month-old girl with maculopapular lesions and lower extremity edema. *Journal of Emergency Nursing, 29*(3), 204–207.
Schmidt, J. M. (2005). Antivenom therapy for snakebites in children: Is there evidence? *Current Opinion in Pediatrics, 17*, 234–238.
Sheridan, R. L. (2005a). Outpatient burn care in the emergency department. *Pediatric Emergency Care, 21*(7), 449–456.
Sheridan, R. L. (2005b). Sepsis in pediatric burn patients. *Pediatric Critical Care Medicine, 6*(3, Suppl.), S112–S119.
Shy, R. (2007). Tinea corporis and tinea capitis. *Pediatrics in Review, 28*(5), 164–174.
Silverberg, N. B. (2007). A practical approach to molluscum contagiosum, Part 1. *Contemporary Pediatrics, 24*(8), 73–81.
Silverberg, N. P., Silverberg, J. I., & Silverberg, A. I. (2005). Eradicating acne vulgaris of puberty: What makes for optimal therapy? *Contemporary Pediatrics, 22*(10 suppl), 12–22.
Simpson, E. L., & Hanifin, J. M. (2006). Atopic dermatitis. *Medical Clinics of North America, 90*, 149–167.
Singletary, E. M., Rochman, A. S., Bodmer, J. C. A., & Holstege, C. P. (2005). Envenomations. *Medical Clinics of North America, 89*, 1195–1224.
Sladden, M. J., & Johnston, G. A. (2005, May 21). Clinical review: More common skin infections in children. *British Medical Journal, 330*, 1194–1198.
Smolinski, K. N., & Yan, A. C. (2005). How and when to treat molluscum contagiosum and warts in children. *Pediatric Annals, 34*(3), 211–221.
Steen, C. J., Carbonaro, P. A., & Schwartz, R. A. (2004). Arthropods in dermatology. *Journal of American Academy of Dermatology, 50*, 819–942.
Stoddard, F. J., Saxe, G., Ronfeldt, H., Drake, J. E., Burns, J., Edgren, C., & Sheridan, R. (2006). Acute stress symptoms in young children with burns. *Journal of American Academy of Child and Adolescent Psychiatry, 45*(1), 87–93.
Suddaby, E. C., Barnett, S., & Facteau, L. (2005). Skin breakdown in acute care pediatrics. *Pediatric Nursing, 31*(2), 132–138, 148.
Sullivan-Whalen, M., & Gilleaudeau, P. (2007). Psoriasis: Hope for the future. *Nursing Clinics of North America, 42*, 467–484.
Tharp, M. D. (2005). A multifaceted approach to the treatment of atopic dermatitis. *Medscape Dermatology, 6* (1). Retrieved July 5, 2005, from http://www.medscape.com/viewarticle/506964.
Timm-Knudson, V. L., Johnson, J. S., Ortiz, K. J., & Yiannias, J. A. (2006). Allergic contact dermatitis to preservatives. *Dermatologic Nursing, 18*(2), 130–136.
Tofte, S. (2007). Atopic dermatitis. *Nursing Clinics of North America, 42*, 407–419.
Trask, B. C., Rote, N. S., & Huether, S. E. (2006). Innate immunity: Inflammation. In K. L. McCance & S. E. Huether (Eds.), *Pathophysiology: The biologic basis for disease in adults and children* (5th ed., pp. 175–209). St. Louis: Elsevier Mosby.
Wong, L., & Rogers, M. (2006). Psoriasis: Varied presentations, individualized treatment. *Contemporary Pediatrics, 23*(1), 33–39.
Zaenglein, A. L., & Thiboutot, D. M. (2006). Expert committee recommendations for acne management. *Pediatrics, 118*(3), 1188–1199.
Zeglin, D. (2005). Brown recluse spider bites. *American Journal of Nursing, 105*(2), 64–68.

PEARSON
EXPLORE mynursingkit™

MyNursingKit is your one stop for online chapter review materials and resources. Prepare for success with additional NCLEX®-style practice questions, interactive assignments and activities, web links, animations and videos, and more!

Register your access code from the front of your book at
www.mynursingkit.com

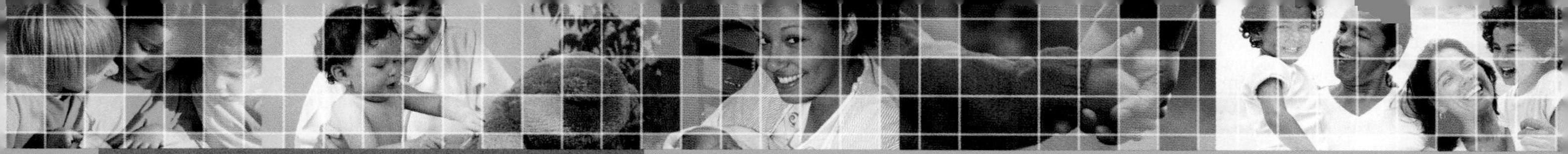

APPENDIX A

SELECTED MATERNAL-NEWBORN LABORATORY VALUES

Normal Maternal Laboratory Values

Test	Nonpregnant Values	Pregnant Values
Hematocrit	37% to 47%	32% to 42%
Hemoglobin	12 to 16 g/dL**	10 to 14 g/dL**
Platelets	150,000 to 350,000/mm^3	Significant increase 3 to 5 days after birth (predisposes to thrombosis)
Partial thromboplastin time (PTT)	12 to 14 seconds	Slight decrease in pregnancy and again in labor (placental site clotting)
Fibrinogen	250 mg/dL	400 mg/dL
Serum glucose		
Fasting	70 to 80 mg/dL	65 mg/dL
2-hour postprandial	60 to 110 mg/dL	Less than 140 mg/dL
Total protein	6.7 to 8.3 g/dL	5.5 to 7.5 g/dL
White blood cell total	4500 to 10,000/mm^3	5000 to 15,000/mm^3
Polymorphonuclear cells	54% to 62%	60% to 85%
Lymphocytes	38% to 46%	15% to 40%

**At sea level

Normal Term Neonatal Cord Blood Laboratory Values

Test	Normal Values
Hematocrit	43% to 63%*
Hemoglobin	14 to 20 g/dL
Platelets	150,000 to 350,000/mm^3
Reticulocyte	3% to 7%
White blood cell total	10,000 to 30,000/mm^3
White blood cell differential	
Polymorphonuclear (segs)	40% to 80%
Lymphocytes	20% to 40%
Monocytes	3% to 10%
Serum glucose	45 to 96 mg/dL*
Serum electrolytes	
Sodium	126 to 144 mEq/L*
Potassium	5.6 to 12.0 mEq/L*
Chloride	100 to 121 mEq/L*
Carbon dioxide	13 to 29 mmol/L
Bicarbonate	18 to 23 mEq/L
Calcium	8.2 to 11.1 mg/dL
Total protein	4.8 to 7.3 g/dL

Note: Adapted from Fanaroff, A. A., & Martin, R. J. (Eds.). (2006). *Neonatal-perinatal medicine* (8th ed.). Philadelphia: Mosby.

*All laboratory values are approximate. Consult your local laboratory for guidelines as to normal values.

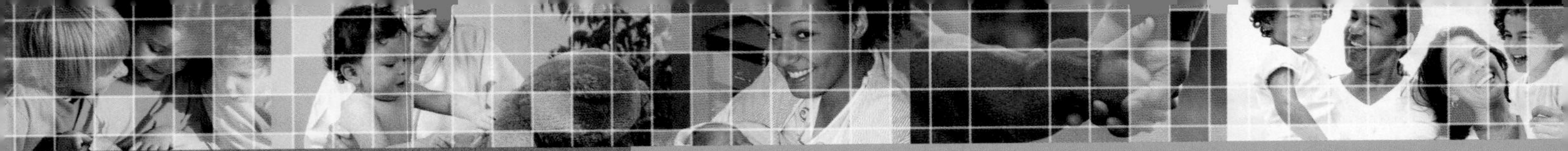

APPENDIX B

SELECTED PEDIATRIC LABORATORY VALUES

All laboratory value intervals listed are approximate. Consult your local laboratory for guidelines as to normal values for the specific testing procedures used.

NORMAL BLOOD CHEMISTRY VALUE INTERVALS

Albumin (S)[1]

1 month–1 year: 2.8–4.8 g/dL
1–18 years: 3.2–4.7 g/dL

Alkaline Phosphatase (S)[1]

Age	Male Units/L	Female Units/L
1-30 days	75-316	48-406
1-3 years	104-345	108-317
4-6 years	93-309	96-297
7-9 years	86-315	69-325
10-12 years	42-362	51-332
13-15 years	74-390	50-162
16-18 years	52-171	47-119

Alpha-fetoprotein (AFP) (S)[1]

Newborn: 50–100,000 ng/mL
1–3 mo: 40–1000 ng/mL

Bilirubin (S)[1]

Conjugated Newborn: Less than 0.6 mg/dL
Total Birth–5 days: Less than 11.7 mg/dL

Blood Gases

Carbon Dioxide, Partial Pressure (P_{CO_2}) (B)[1]

Infant: 27–41 mmHg (3.6–5.5 kPa)
Children: 32–48 mmHg (4.3–6.4 kPa)

Oxygen, Partial Pressure (P_{O_2}) (B)[1]
Less than 1 day: 83–108 mmHg (11–14.4 kPa)

Bicarbonate, Actual (P)[3]
22–29 mmol/L

pH (B)[1]

0–6 months: 7.18–7.51
6–12 months: 7.27–7.49

Base Excess (B)[1]

Infant: –7 to –1 mmol/L
Child: –4 to +2 mmol/L
Thereafter: –3 to +3 mmol/L

Oxygen Saturation (B)[1]

Newborns: 85–90%
Thereafter: 95–99%

Cholesterol (S)[2]

Total Cholesterol

Borderline: 170–199 mg/dL
Elevated: Greater than 200 mg/dL

High-Density Lipoprotein
Less than 35 mg/dL

Low-Density Lipoprotein

Borderline: 110–129 mg/dL
Elevated: 130 mg/dL and higher

Triglycerides
Less than 150 mg/dL

Coagulation Values[4]

Fibrinogen: 175–400 mg/dL
Partial thromboplastin time, activated (aPTT): 22–34 seconds
Prothrombin time (PT): 11–15 seconds
Thrombin time: 14–16 seconds

C-Reactive Protein (CRP) (P, S)[1]

0.68–8.2 mg/L

Creatinine (S, P)[1]

1–7 days: 0.7–1.2 mg/dL (0.06–0.11 micromol/L)
7 days–1 yr: 0.2–0.5 mg/dL (0.02–0.04 micromol/L)
1–9 years: 0.2–0.8 mg/dL (0.02–0.07 micromol/L)
10–18 years: 0.5–1.1 mg/dL (0.04–0.1 micromol/L)

Electrolytes[1]

Calcium (S, P)

Newborn: 7.9–10.7 mg/dL
Thereafter: 8.7–10.7 mg/dL

Chloride (S, P)

96–110 mmol/L

Glucose (S, P)

70–126 mg/dL (3.9–7 mmol/L)

Magnesium (P, S)

1.6–2.4 mg/dL (0.66–0.99 mmol/L)

Osmolality (S)

280–300 mOsm/kg

Phosphorus, Inorganic (S, P)

2.5–6.5 mg/dL (0.81–2.1 mmol/L)

Potassium (S, P)

3.3–4.6 mmol/L

Sodium (P, S)

134–143 mmol/L

Urea Nitrogen (S, P)

1–13 years: 5–17 mg/dL (1.8–6 mmol/L)
14–19 years: 8–21 mg/dL (2.9–7.5 mmol/L)

Hematology Values (B)

Values for children 2 to 12 years

Hematocrit (HCT)[1]

31.7–39.8%

Hemoglobin (HGB)[1]

10.2–13.4 g/dL

Mean Corpuscular Hemoglobin (MCH)[1]

23.7–29.5 picograms

Mean Corpuscular Hemoglobin Concentration (MCHC)[1]

31.8–34.9%

Mean Corpuscular Volume (MCV)[1]

71.3–87.6 mm^3

Red Blood Cell (RBC)[1]

3.89–5.03 × 10^{12}/L

White Blood Cell (WBC)[1]

4.86–1140 × 10^9/L

Differential[1]

Neutrophils	34.3-76.9%
Eosinophils	0-4.8%
Basophils	0-1%
Lymphocytes	1-50.6%
Atypical Lymphocytes	2-4%
Monocytes	3.5-13.9%

Platelet Count[3]

150–400 × 10^9/L

Reticulocyte Count[1]

0.8–2.8%

Erythrocyte Sedimentation Rate (Micro)[4]

1–13 mm/hr

Hemoglobin A_{1c} (B)[1]

Normal: 4–7%

Hemoglobin F(B)[4]

0–2% Fetal hemoglobin

Growth Hormone (P, S)[1]

0 to 6.9 years: Less than 13.7 mcg/L
7 to 10.9 years: Less than 16.5 mcg/L
11 to 14.9 years: Less than 14.5 mcg/L
15 to 18.9 years: Less than 13.5 mcg/L

Iron-Related Values

Ferritin (P, S)[1]

1–5 years: 6–24 ng/mL
6–9 years: 10–55 ng/mL
10–19 years: Males 23–70 ng/mL, Females 6–40 ng/mL

Iron (S, P)[1]
5–11 am: 20–105 mcg/dL (3.6–18.8 micromol/L)

Iron-Binding Capacity (S, P)[1]

1–5 years: 268–441 mcg/dL (48–79 micromol/L)
6–9 years: 240–508 mcg/dL (43–91 micromol/L)
10–19 years: 290–570 mcg/dL (52–102 micromol/L)

Lead (B)[3]

Less than 10 mcg/dL (0.48 mmol/L)

Phenylalanine (P)[3]

Less than 2 mg/dL (0.04–0.21 micromol/L)

Thyroid Hormones

Thyroid-Stimulating Hormone (TSH) (P, S)[1]

Age	Males	Females
1-30 days	0.52-16 mUnit/mL	0.72-13.1 mUnit/mL
1 month-5 years	0.55-7.1 mUnit/mL	0.46-8.1 mUnit/mL
6-18 years	0.37-6 mUnit/mL	0.36-5.8 mUnit/mL

Thyroxine (T_4) (S, P)[1]

1–3 days: 8–20 mcg/dL
Under 1 year: 5–15 mcg/dL
Over 1 year: 4.5–11 mcg/dL

Thyroxine, "Free" (Free T_4) (S, P)[1]

1–3 days: 2–5 ng/mL
3–30 days: 0.9–2.2 ng/mL
Thereafter: 0.8–2 ng/mL

Thyroxine-Binding Globulin (TBG) (P)[1]

0–6 years: 16.2–33.8 mg/L
7–12 years: 15–29.2 mg/L
13–18 years: 13.4–28.7 mg/L

Triiodothyronine (T_3) (S)[1]

0–11 years: 90–260 ng/dL
12–18 years: 100–210 ng/dL

NORMAL VALUE RANGES: URINE

Albumin[4]

Less than 1 mg/dL

Catecholamines (Norepinephrine, Epinephrine)[1]

Values in mmol/mol creatinine

Age	Norepinephrine	Epinephrine
<1 year	0.017-0.207	0-0.232
1-4 years	0.017-0.194	0-0.051
4-10 years	0.018-0.072	0.003-0.057
10-18 years	0.003-0.07	0.001-0.027

Creatinine[1]

3–8 years: 0.11–0.68 g/24 hr
9–12 years: 0.17–1.41 g/24 hr
13–17 years: 0.29–1.87 g/24 hr
Adults: 0.63–2.5 g/24 hr

Osmolality[4]

500–800 mOsm/kg water
Should be higher than serum osmolality

Protein[4]

Less than 150 mg/24 hr

Specific Gravity

1.01–1.03

NORMAL VALUE RANGES: SWEAT

Electrolytes[1]

Sodium and chloride: under 40 mmol/L

NORMAL VALUE RANGES: CEREBROSPINAL FLUID

Protein[1]

Under 1 month: 15–153 mg/dL
Over 1 month: 15–48 mg/dL

Glucose[1]

All ages: 41–84 mg/dL (60–80% of blood glucose)

[1]Adapted from: Soldin, S. J., Brugnara, C., & Wong, E. C. (2007). *Pediatric reference ranges* (6th ed.). Washington, DC: AACC Press.

[2]Data from: Daniels, S. R., Greer, F. R., and the Committee on Nutrition. (2008). Lipid screening and cardiovascular health in childhood. *Pediatrics, 122*(1), 198–208.

[3]Data from: Kliegman, R. M., Behrman, R. E., Jenson, H. B., & Stanton, B. F. (2007). *Nelson textbook of pediatrics* (18th ed.). Philadelphia: Saunders Elsevier.

[4]Data from Corbett, J. V. (2008). *Laboratory tests and diagnostic procedures with nursing diagnoses* (7th ed.). Upper Saddle River, NJ: Pearson Prentice Hall.

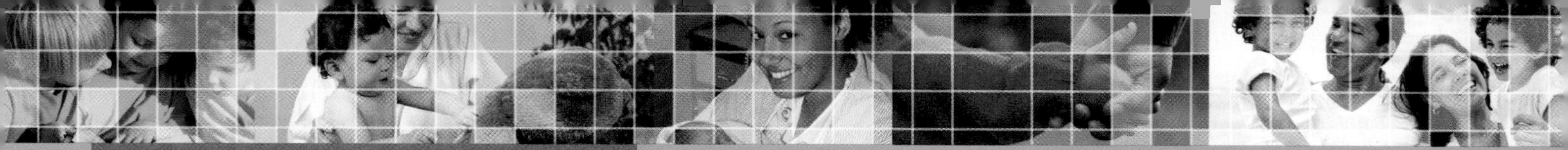

APPENDIX C

GROWTH CHARTS

● **Figure C–1**

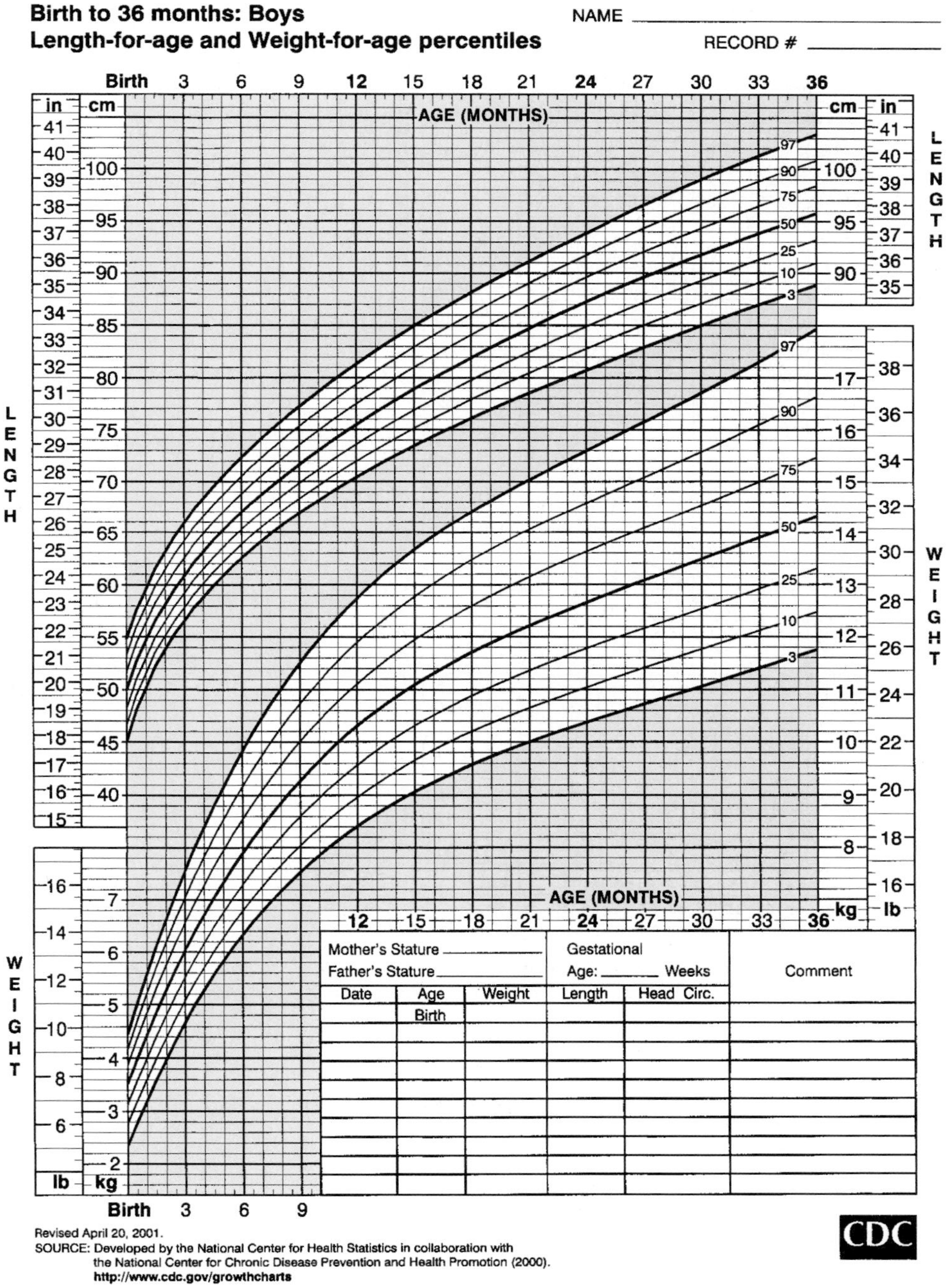

Physical growth percentiles for length and weight—boys: birth to 36 months.

From CDC, 2001. www.cdc.gov/growthcharts

• Figure C–2

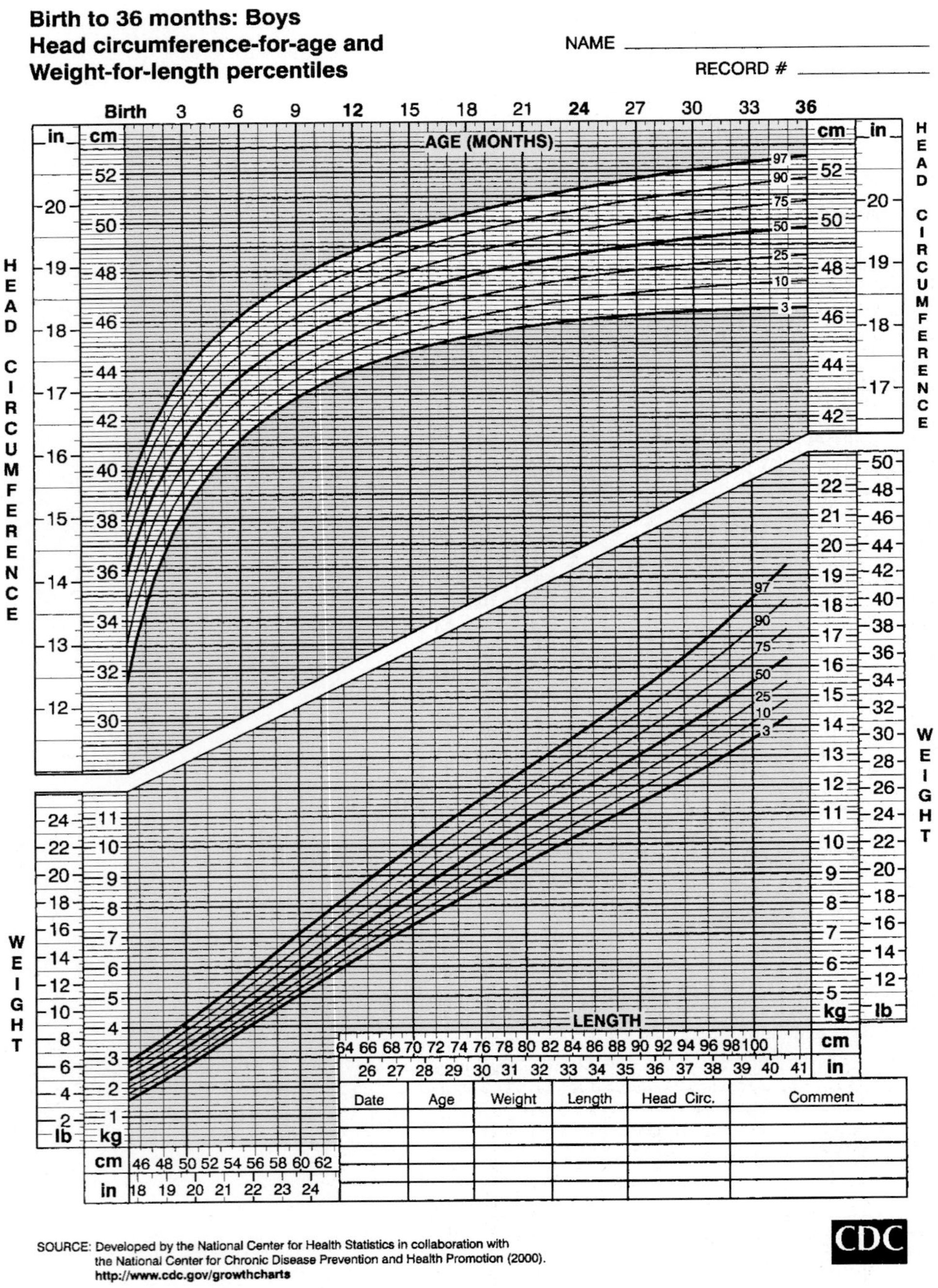

Physical growth percentiles for head circumference, weight for length—boys: birth to 36 months.

From CDC, 2001. www.cdc.gov/growthcharts

● **Figure C–3**

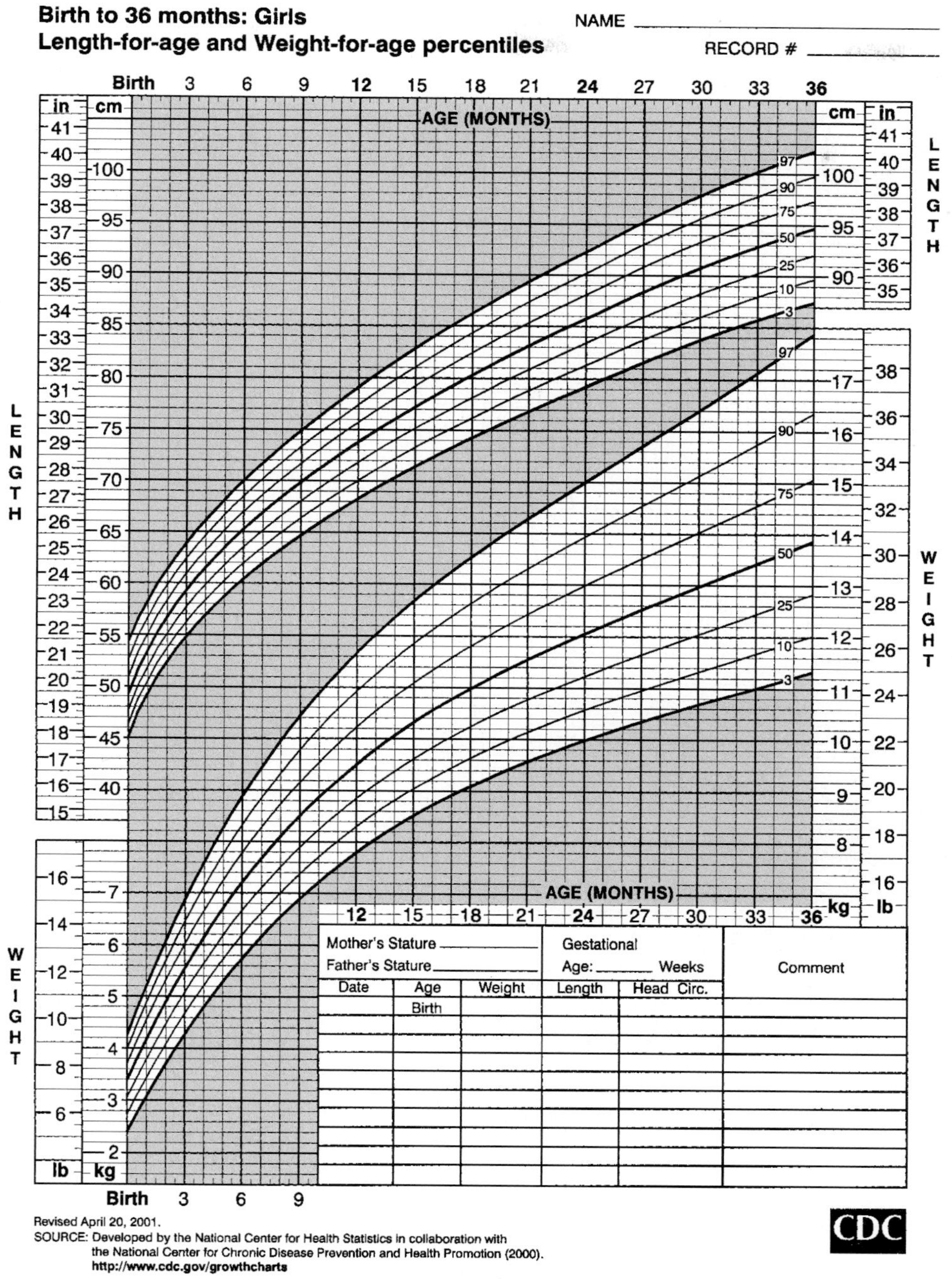

Physical growth percentiles for length and weight—girls: birth to 36 months.

From CDC, 2001. www.cdc.gov/growthcharts

● **Figure C–4**

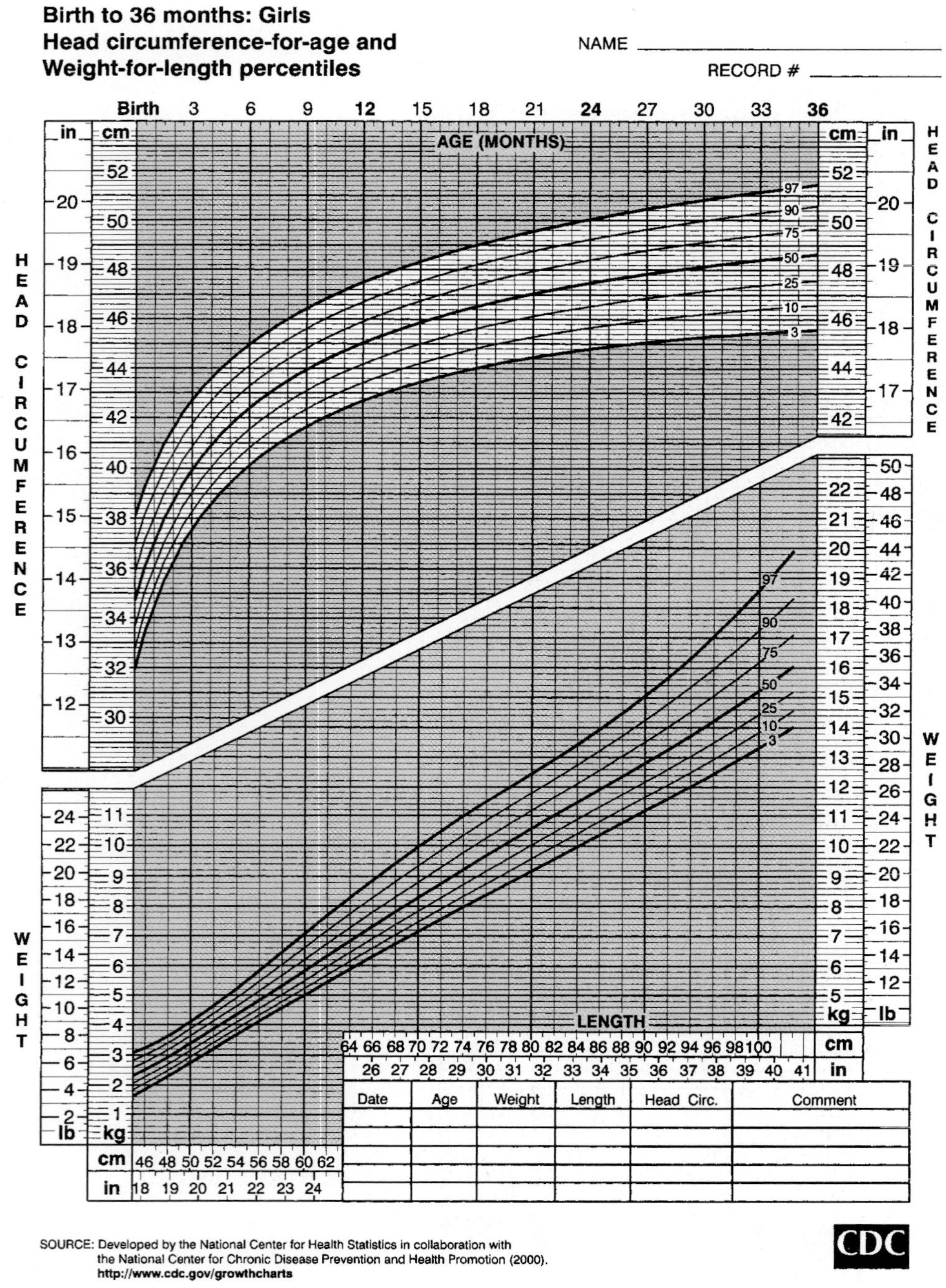

Physical growth percentiles for head circumference, weight for length—girls: birth to 36 months.

From CDC, 2001. www.cdc.gov/growthcharts

• **Figure C–5**

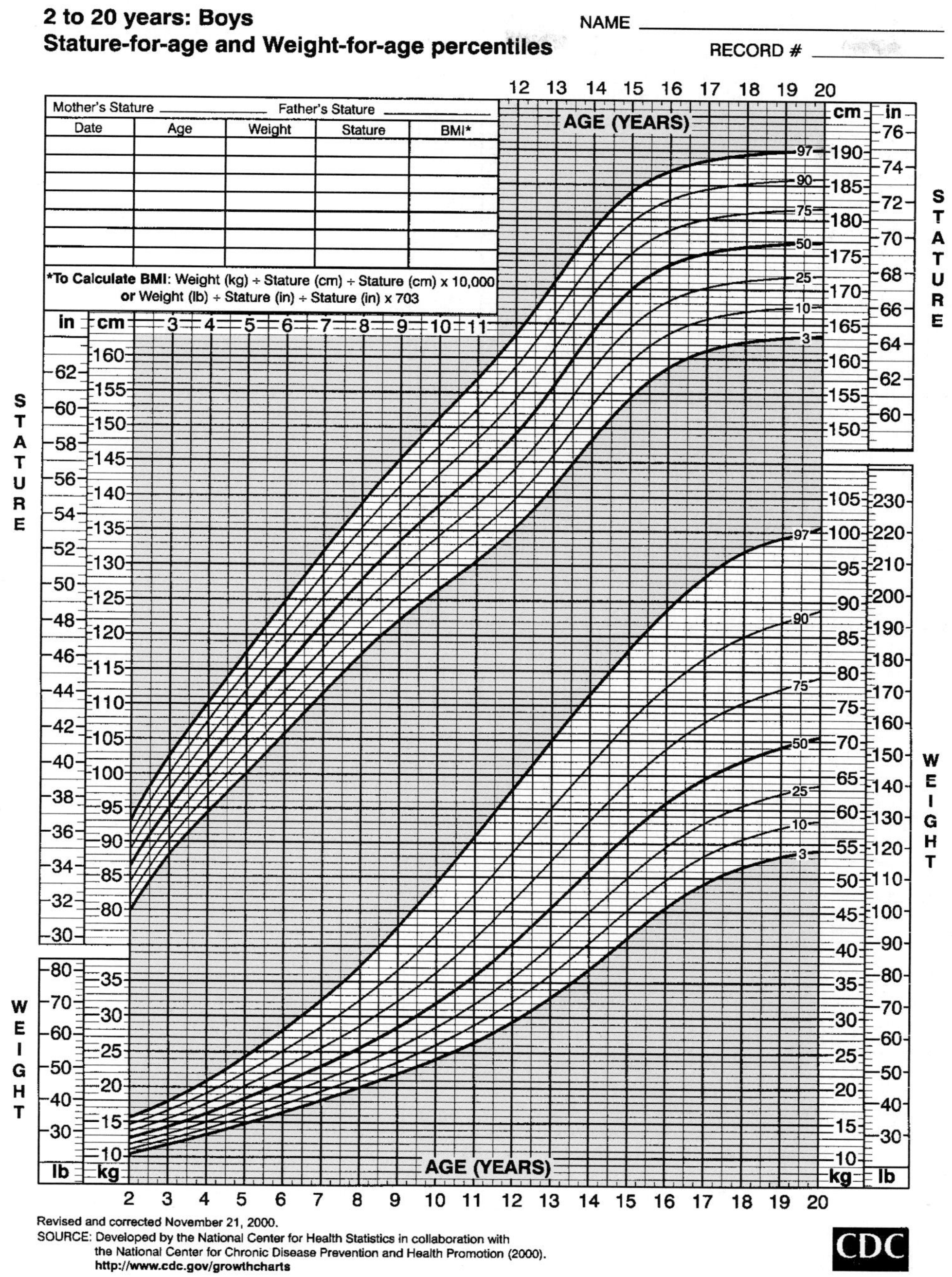

Physical growth percentiles for stature and weight according to age—boys: 2 to 20 years.

From CDC, 2001. www.cdc.gov/growthcharts

• Figure C–6

2 to 20 years: Boys
Body mass index-for-age percentiles

NAME ______________________

RECORD # ____________

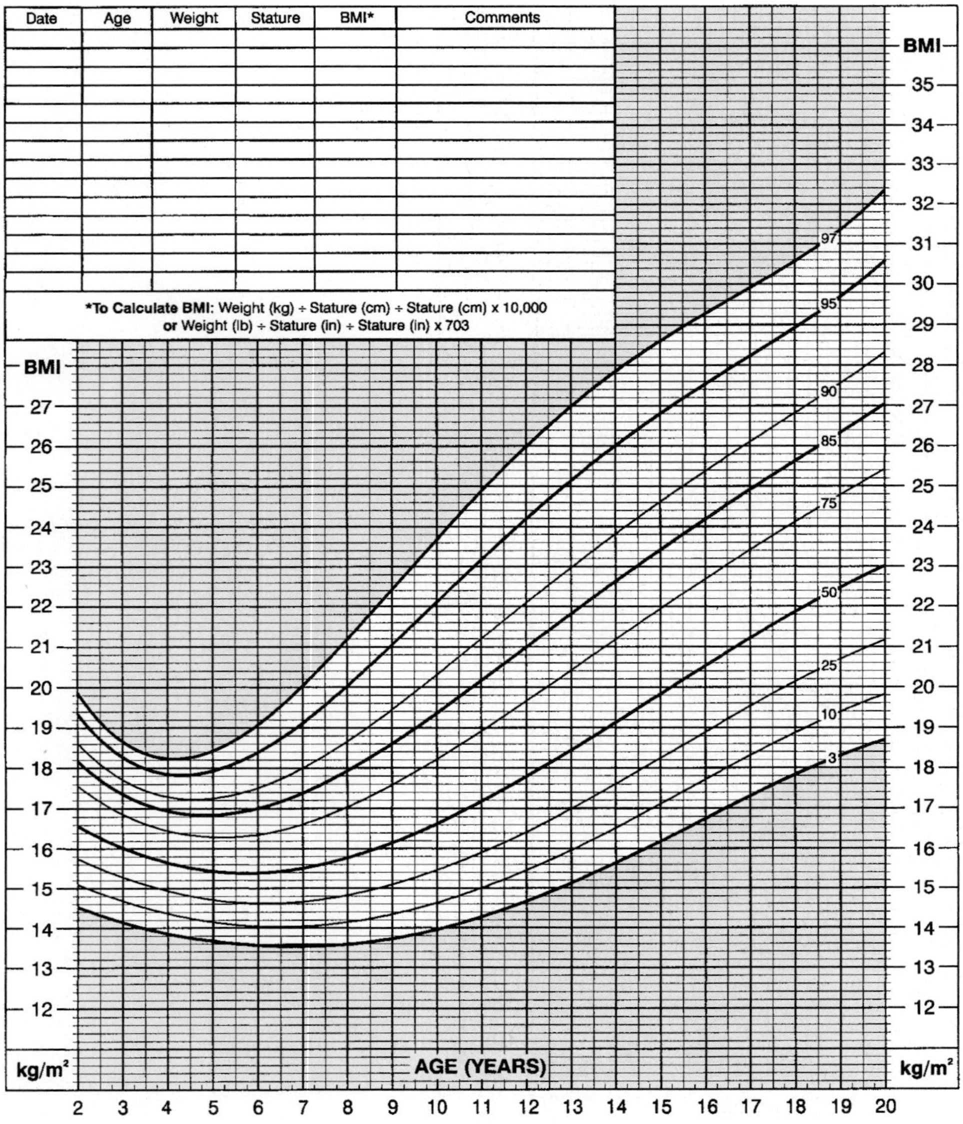

SOURCE: Developed by the National Center for Health Statistics in collaboration with the National Center for Chronic Disease Prevention and Health Promotion (2000). http://www.cdc.gov/growthcharts

CDC

Physical growth percentiles for body mass index according to age—boys: 2 to 20 years.

From CDC, 2001. www.cdc.gov/growthcharts

● **Figure C–7**

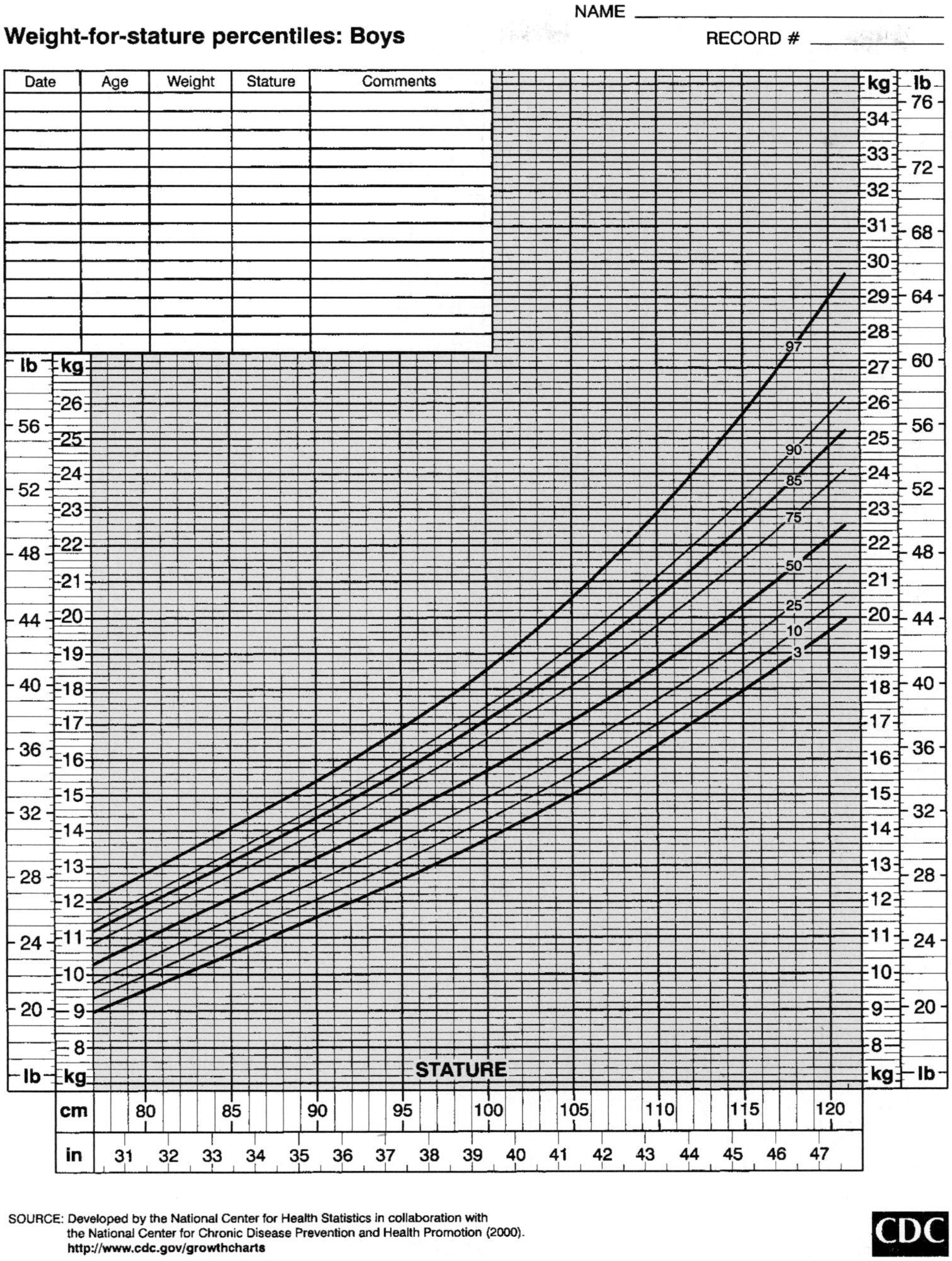

Physical growth percentiles for weight for stature—boys: 2 to 20 years.

From CDC, 2001. www.cdc.gov/growthcharts

● **Figure C–8**

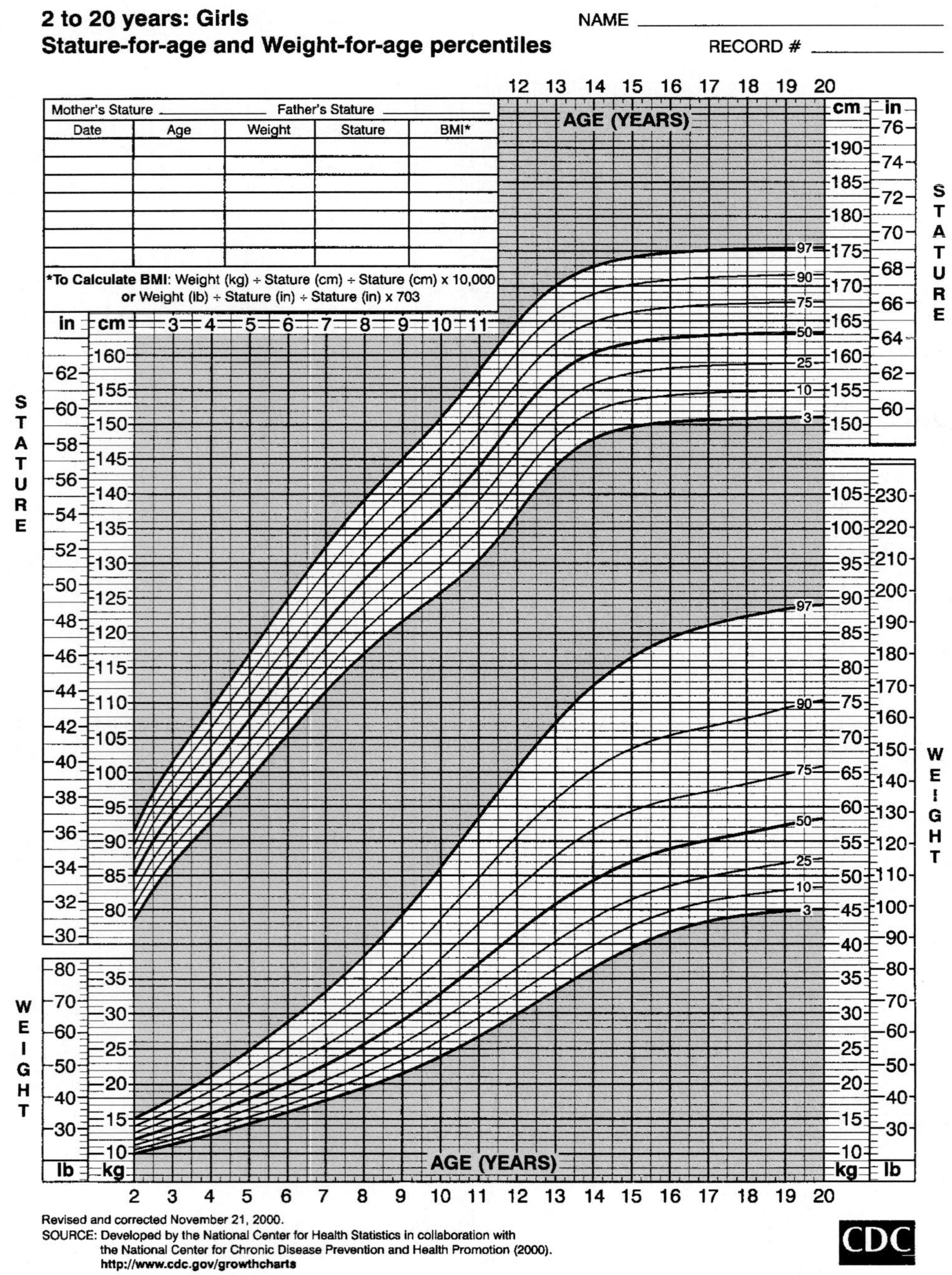

Physical growth percentiles for stature and weight according to age—girls: 2 to 20 years.

From CDC, 2001. www.cdc.gov/growthcharts

● **Figure C–9**

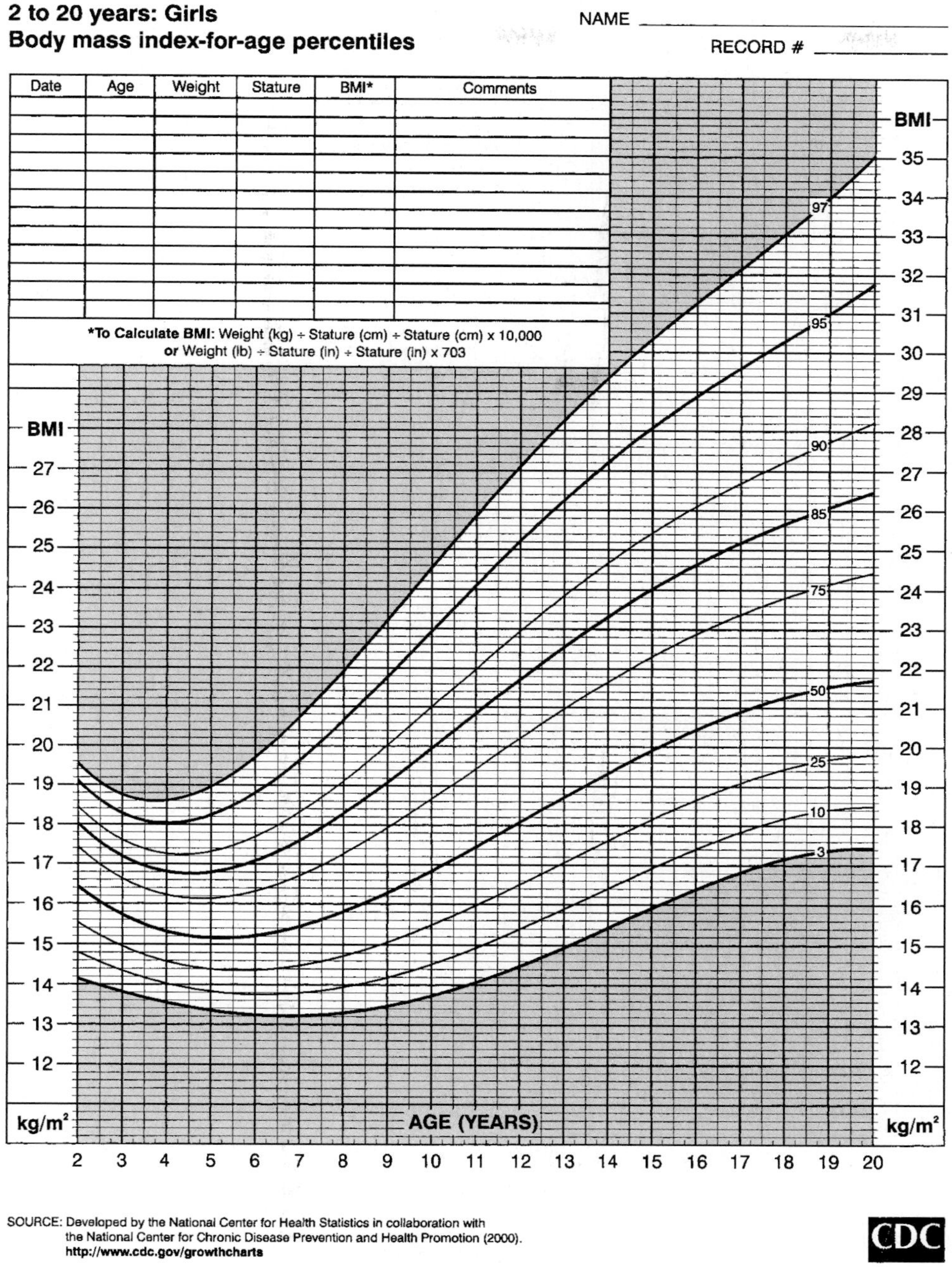

Physical growth percentiles for body mass index according to age—girls: 2 to 20 years.

From CDC, 2001. www.cdc.gov/growthcharts

● **Figure C–10**

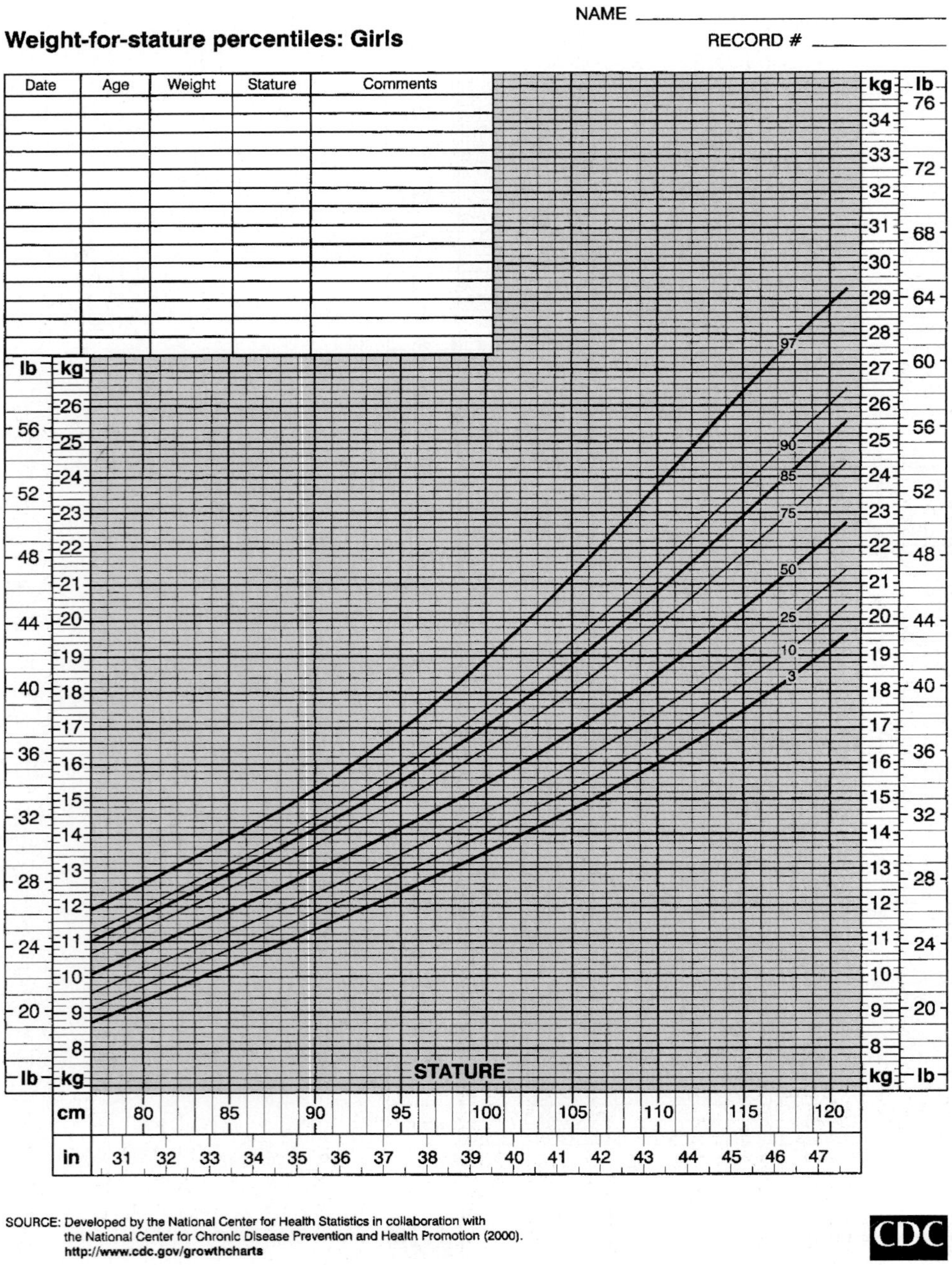

Physical growth percentiles for weight for stature–girls: 2 to 20 years.

From CDC, 2001. www.cdc.gov/growthcharts

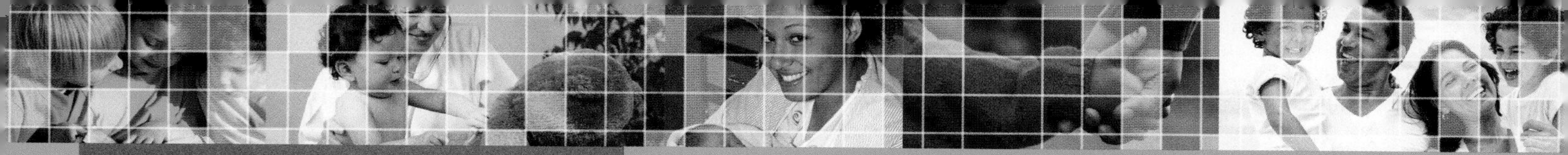

APPENDIX D

PEDIATRIC BLOOD PRESSURE TABLES

Table D–1 Blood Pressure Levels for Boys by Age and Height Percentile

Use the child's height percentile for the age and sex from the standard growth charts found in Appendix A. A blood pressure value at the 50th percentile for the child's age, sex, and height percentile is considered the midpoint of the normal range. A reading above the 95th percentile indicates hypertension.

		SYSTOLIC BP (mmHG)							DIASTOLIC BP (mmHG)						
		PERCENTILE OF HEIGHT							PERCENTILE OF HEIGHT						
Age (Year)	BP Percentile	5th	10th	25th	50th	75th	90th	95th	5th	10th	25th	50th	75th	90th	95th
1	50th	80	81	83	85	87	88	89	34	35	36	37	38	39	39
	95th	98	99	101	103	104	106	106	54	54	55	56	57	58	58
2	50th	84	85	87	88	90	92	92	39	40	41	42	43	44	44
	95th	101	102	104	106	108	109	110	59	59	60	61	62	63	63
3	50th	86	87	89	91	93	94	95	44	44	45	46	47	48	48
	95th	104	105	107	109	110	112	113	63	63	64	65	66	67	67
4	50th	88	89	91	93	95	96	97	47	48	49	50	51	51	52
	95th	106	107	109	111	112	114	115	66	67	68	69	70	71	71
5	50th	90	91	93	95	96	98	98	50	51	52	53	54	55	55
	95th	108	109	110	112	114	115	116	69	70	71	72	73	74	74
6	50th	91	92	94	96	98	99	100	53	53	54	55	56	57	57
	95th	109	110	112	114	115	117	117	72	72	73	74	75	76	76
7	50th	92	94	95	97	99	100	101	55	55	56	57	58	59	59
	95th	110	111	113	115	117	118	119	74	74	75	76	77	78	78
8	50th	94	95	97	99	100	102	102	56	57	58	59	60	60	61
	95th	111	112	114	116	118	119	120	75	76	77	78	79	79	80
9	50th	95	96	98	100	102	103	104	57	58	59	60	61	61	62
	95th	113	114	116	118	119	121	121	76	77	78	79	80	81	81
10	50th	97	98	100	102	103	105	106	58	59	60	61	61	62	63
	95th	115	116	117	119	121	122	123	77	78	79	80	81	81	82
11	50th	99	100	102	104	105	107	107	59	59	60	61	62	63	63
	95th	117	118	119	121	123	124	125	78	78	79	80	81	82	82
12	50th	101	102	104	106	108	109	110	59	60	61	62	63	63	64
	95th	119	120	122	123	125	127	127	78	79	80	81	82	82	83
13	50th	104	105	106	108	110	111	112	60	60	61	62	63	64	64
	95th	121	122	124	126	128	129	130	79	79	80	81	82	83	83
14	50th	106	107	109	111	113	114	115	60	61	62	63	64	65	65
	95th	124	125	127	128	130	132	132	80	80	81	82	83	84	84
15	50th	109	110	112	113	115	117	117	61	62	63	64	65	66	66
	95th	126	127	129	131	133	134	135	81	81	82	83	84	85	85
16	50th	111	112	114	116	118	119	120	63	63	64	65	66	67	67
	95th	129	130	132	134	135	137	137	82	83	83	84	85	86	87
17	50th	114	115	116	118	120	121	122	65	66	66	67	68	69	70
	95th	131	132	134	136	138	139	140	84	85	86	87	87	88	89

Source: National Heart, Lung, and Blood Institute. (2004). Blood pressure tables for children and adolescents from the fourth report on the diagnosis, evaluation, and treatment of high blood pressure in children and adolescents. www.nhlbi.nih.gov/guidelines/hypertension/child_tbl.htm, accessed 6/11/2004.

BP, blood pressure

*The 90th percentile is 1.28 SD, the 95th percentile is 1.645 SD, and the 99th percentile is 2.326 SD over the mean.

Table D-2 Blood Pressure Levels for Girls by Age and Height Percentile

Use the child's height percentile for the age and sex from the standard growth charts found in Appendix A. A blood pressure value at 50th percentile for the child's age, sex, and height percentile is considered the midpoint of the normal range. A reading above the 95th percentile indicates hypertension.

		SYSTOLIC BP (mmHG)							DIASTOLIC BP (mmHG)						
		PERCENTILE OF HEIGHT							PERCENTILE OF HEIGHT						
Age (Year)	**BP Percentile**	**5th**	**10th**	**25th**	**50th**	**75th**	**90th**	**95th**	**5th**	**10th**	**25th**	**50th**	**75th**	**90th**	**95th**
1	50th	83	84	85	86	88	89	90	38	39	39	40	41	41	42
	95th	100	101	102	104	105	106	107	56	57	57	58	59	59	60
2	50th	85	85	87	88	89	91	91	43	44	44	45	46	46	47
	95th	102	103	104	105	107	108	109	61	62	62	63	64	65	65
3	50th	86	87	88	89	91	92	93	47	48	48	49	50	50	51
	95th	104	104	105	107	108	109	110	65	66	66	67	68	68	69
4	50th	88	88	90	91	92	94	94	50	50	51	52	52	53	54
	95th	105	106	107	108	110	111	112	68	68	69	70	71	71	72
5	50th	89	90	91	93	94	95	96	52	53	53	54	55	55	56
	95th	107	107	108	110	111	112	113	70	71	71	72	73	73	74
6	50th	91	92	93	94	96	97	98	54	54	55	56	56	57	58
	95th	108	109	110	111	113	114	115	72	72	73	74	74	75	76
7	50th	93	93	95	96	97	99	99	55	56	56	57	58	58	59
	95th	110	111	112	113	115	116	116	73	74	74	75	76	76	77
8	50th	95	95	96	98	99	100	101	57	57	57	58	59	60	60
	95th	112	112	114	115	116	118	118	75	75	75	76	77	78	78
9	50th	96	97	98	100	101	102	103	58	58	58	59	60	61	61
	95th	114	114	115	117	118	119	120	76	76	76	77	78	79	79
10	50th	98	99	100	102	103	104	105	59	59	59	60	61	62	62
	95th	116	116	117	119	120	121	122	77	77	77	78	79	80	80
11	50th	100	101	102	103	105	106	107	60	60	60	61	62	63	63
	95th	118	118	119	121	122	123	124	78	78	78	79	80	81	81
12	50th	102	103	104	105	107	108	109	61	61	61	62	63	64	64
	95th	119	120	121	123	124	125	126	79	79	79	80	81	82	82
13	50th	104	105	106	107	109	110	110	62	62	62	63	64	65	65
	95th	121	122	123	124	126	127	128	80	80	80	81	82	83	83
14	50th	106	106	107	109	110	111	112	63	63	63	64	65	66	66
	95th	123	123	125	126	127	129	129	81	81	81	82	83	84	84
15	50th	107	108	109	110	111	113	113	64	64	64	65	66	67	67
	95th	124	125	126	127	129	130	131	82	82	82	83	84	85	85
16	50th	108	108	110	111	112	114	114	64	64	65	66	66	67	68
	95th	125	126	127	128	130	131	132	82	82	83	84	85	85	86
17	50th	108	109	110	111	113	114	115	64	65	65	66	67	67	68
	95th	125	126	127	129	130	131	132	82	83	83	84	85	85	86

BP, blood pressure

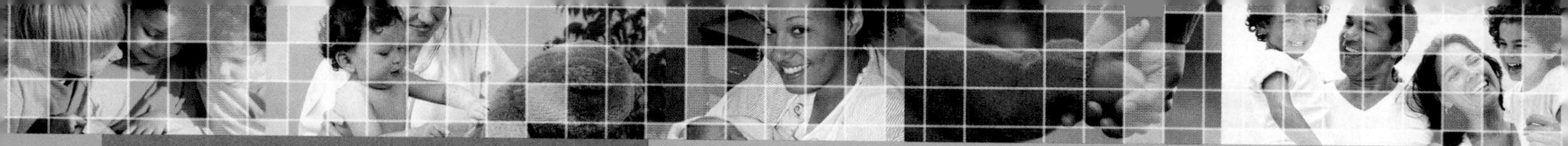

APPENDIX E

CONVERSIONS AND EQUIVALENTS

Temperature Conversion

(Fahrenheit temperature − 32) × 5/9 = Centigrade temperature

(Centigrade temperature × 9/5) + 32 = Fahrenheit temperature

Selected Conversion to Metric Measures

Known Value	Multiply By	To Find
inches	2.54	centimeters
ounces	28	grams
pounds	454	grams
pounds	0.45	kilogram

Selected Conversion from Metric Measures

Known Value	Multiply By	To Find
centimeters	0.4	inches
grams	0.035	ounces
grams	0.0022	pounds
kilograms	2.2	pounds

Conversion of Pounds and Ounces to Grams

POUNDS \ OUNCES	0	1	2	3	4	5	6	7	8	9	10	11	12	13	14	15
0	–	28	57	85	113	142	170	198	227	255	283	312	340	369	397	425
1	454	482	510	539	567	595	624	652	680	709	737	765	794	822	850	879
2	907	936	964	992	1021	1049	1077	1106	1134	1162	1191	1219	1247	1276	1304	1332
3	1361	1389	1417	1446	1474	1503	1531	1559	1588	1616	1644	1673	1701	1729	1758	1786
4	1814	1843	1871	1899	1928	1956	1984	2013	2041	2070	2098	2126	2155	2183	2211	2240
5	2268	2296	2325	2353	2381	2410	2438	2466	2495	2523	2551	2580	2608	2637	2665	2693
6	2722	2750	2778	2807	2835	2863	2892	2920	2948	2977	3005	3033	3062	3090	3118	3147
7	3175	3203	3232	3260	3289	3317	3345	3374	3402	3430	3459	3487	3515	3544	3572	3600
8	3629	3657	3685	3714	3742	3770	3799	3827	3856	3884	3912	3941	3969	3997	4026	4054
9	4082	4111	4139	4167	4196	4224	4252	4281	4309	4337	4366	4394	4423	4451	4479	4508
10	4536	4564	4593	4621	4649	4678	4706	4734	4763	4791	4819	4848	4876	4904	4933	4961
11	4990	5018	5046	5075	5103	5131	5160	5188	5216	5245	5273	5301	5330	5358	5386	5415
12	5443	5471	5500	5528	5557	5585	5613	5642	5670	5698	5727	5755	5783	5812	5840	5868
13	5897	5925	5953	5982	6010	6038	6067	6095	6123	6152	6180	6209	6237	6265	6294	6322
14	6350	6379	6407	6435	6464	6492	6520	6549	6577	6605	6634	6662	6690	6719	6747	6776
15	6804	6832	6860	6889	6917	6945	6973	7002	7030	7059	7087	7115	7144	7172	7201	7228
16	7257	7286	7313	7342	7371	7399	7427	7456	7484	7512	7541	7569	7597	7626	7654	7682
17	7711	7739	7768	7796	7824	7853	7881	7909	7938	7966	7994	8023	8051	8079	8108	8136
18	8165	8192	8221	8249	8278	8306	8335	8363	8391	8420	8448	8476	8504	8533	8561	8590
19	8618	8646	8675	8703	8731	8760	8788	8816	8845	8873	8902	8930	8958	8987	9015	9043
20	9072	9100	9128	9157	9185	9213	9242	9270	9298	9327	9355	9383	9412	9440	9469	9497
21	9525	9554	9582	9610	9639	9667	9695	9724	9752	9780	9809	9837	9865	9894	9922	9950
22	9979	10007	10036	10064	10092	10120	10149	10177	10206	10234	10262	10291	10319	10347	10376	10404

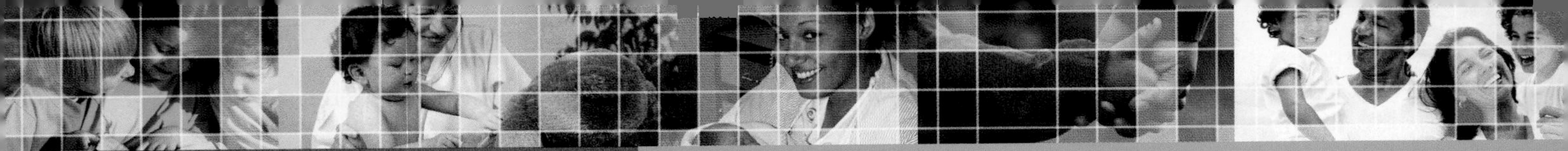

APPENDIX F

ACTIONS AND EFFECTS OF SELECTED DRUGS DURING BREASTFEEDING*

ANTICOAGULANTS

Coumarin derivatives (warfarin, dicumarol): Relatively safe to use; only small amount in breast milk; check PTT
Heparin and derivatives (Lovenox): Does not cross into breast milk; check PTT

ANTICONVULSANTS

Phenytoin (Dilantin), phenobarbital: Generally considered safe; if high doses of phenobarbital are ingested, may cause drowsiness; short-acting phenobarbiturates (secobarbital) preferred, because they appear in lower concentration in milk
Magnesium sulfate: Lactogenesis may be delayed

ANTIDEPRESSANTS

SSRI class:

Fluoxetine (Prozac), fluvoxamine: Effect on newborn unknown but may be of concern
Tricyclic antidepressants: (Doxepin) sedation, potential respiratory arrest in infant

ANTIHISTAMINES

Diphenhydramine (Benadryl), Claritin, Allegra: May cause decreased milk supply; infant may become drowsy or irritable
Clemastine (Tavist): Counterindicated.

ANTIHYPERTENSIVES

β adrenergic blockers:

Atenolol, acebutolol: Cyanosis, bradycardia, hypotension
Tenormin: Hypotension, bradycardia

ANTIMETABOLITES/ANTINEOPLASTICS

Unknown, probably long-term anti-DNA effect on the infant; potentially very toxic

ANTIMICROBIALS

Aminoglycosides: May cause ototoxicity or nephrotoxicity if given for more than 2 weeks
Ampicillin: Skin rash, candidiasis; diarrhea
Azithromycin: No risk to newborn
Chloramphenicol (rarely used): Possible bone marrow suppression; too low a dose for Gray syndrome; refusal of breast
Erythromycin: Accumulates in breast milk, idiopathic hypertrophic pyloric stenosis
Methacycline: Possible inhibition of bone growth; may cause discoloration of the teeth; use should be avoided
Metronidazole (Flagyl): Possible neurologic disorders or blood dyscrasias; delay breastfeeding for 12 hours after dose
Penicillin: Possible allergic response; candidiasis
Quinolones (synthetic antibiotics): Can cause arthropathies
Sulfonamides: May cause hyperbilirubinemia; use contraindicated until infant over 1 week old
Tetracycline: Long-term use and large doses should be avoided; may cause tooth staining or inhibition of bone growth

ANTITHYROIDS

Thiouracil: Contraindicated during lactation; may cause goiter or agranulocytosis
Propylthiouracil: Safe; monitor infant thyroid function

BARBITURATES

Phenothiazines: May produce sedation

BRONCHODILATORS

Aminophylline: May cause insomnia or irritability in the infant
Leukotriene inhibitors (Zyflo, Accolate): Potential tumorigenicity

CAFFEINE

Excessive consumption may cause jitteriness or wakefulness

CARDIOVASCULAR

Amiodarone: Transient bradycardia, IUGR; contains iodine-potential for thyroid gland problems
Clonidine (Catapres): May reduce milk volume
Methyldopa: May increase milk volume; monitor for hypotension for 48 hrs after birth
Propranolol (Inderal): May cause hypoglycemia; possibility of other blocking effects, especially if infant has renal or liver dysfunction

Quinidine: May cause arrhythmias in infant
Reserpine (Serpasil): Nasal stuffiness, lethargy, or diarrhea in infant

CORTICOSTEROIDS

Adrenal suppression may occur with long-term administration of doses greater than 20 mg/day

DIURETICS

Furosemide (Lasix): Not excreted in breast milk
Thiazide diuretics (Esidrix, HydroDIURIL Oretic): Safe but can cause dehydration, reduce milk production

HEAVY METALS

Gold: Potentially toxic; gold salts—compatible with breastfeeding
Lead: Excreted in breast milk; high maternal levels can affect neuropsychologic development
Mercury: Excreted in the milk and hazardous to infant

HORMONES

Androgens: Suppress lactation
Thyroid hormones: May mask hypothyroidism

LAXATIVES

Peri-Colace, Dulcolax: Relatively safe
Milk of magnesia, Metamucil: Relatively safe

NARCOTIC ANALGESICS

Codeine: Accumulation may lead to neonatal depression
Meperidine: Avoid use. May lead to neonatal depression
Morphine: Long-term use may cause newborn addiction

NONNARCOTIC ANALGESICS, NSAIDs

Acetaminophen (Tylenol): Relatively safe for short-term analgesia
Ibuprofen (Motrin): Safe
Propoxyphene (Darvon): May cause sleepiness and poor breastfeeding in infant
Salicylates (aspirin): Safe after first week of life; monitor PTT

ORAL CONTRACEPTIVES

Combined estrogen/progestin pills: Significantly decrease milk supply; may alter milk composition; may cause gynecomastia in male infants
Progestin only (DMPA, Norplant): Safe if started after lactation is established

RADIOACTIVE MATERIALS FOR TESTING

Gallium citrate (67G): Insignificant amount excreted in breast milk; no breastfeeding for 2 weeks
Iodine: Contraindicated; may affect infant's thyroid gland
^{125}I: Discontinue breastfeeding for 24 hours
^{131}I: Breastfeeding should be discontinued until excretion is no longer significant; may be resumed after 10 days
Technetium-99m: Discontinue breastfeeding for 24 hours (half-life = 6 hours)

SEDATIVES/TRANQUILIZERS

Diazepam (Valium): May accumulate to high levels; may increase neonatal jaundice; may cause lethargy, weight loss, and poor suck
Lithium: Contraindicated; may cause neonatal flaccidity, hypotonia; may affect thyroid and cardiac arrhythmia

SMOKING CESSATION

Nicotine patch (NicoDerm, Nicotrol): Irritability, abnormal sleep patterns, poor feeding
Bupropion (Zyban, Wellbutrin): No effect on breastfeeding

SUBSTANCE ABUSE

Alcohol: Potential motor developmental delay; mild sedative effect
Amphetamines: Controversial; may cause irritability, poor sleeping pattern
Cocaine, crack: Extreme irritability, tachycardia, vomiting, apnea
Marijuana: Drowsiness
Heroin: Tremors, restlessness, vomiting, poor feeding
Nicotine (smoking): Shock, vomiting, diarrhea, decreased milk production

*Based on data from Riordan, J., & Auerbach, K. J. (2005). *Breastfeeding and human lactation* (3rd ed., pp. 146–166). Boston: Jones & Bartlett; Briggs, G. G., Freeman, R. K., & Yaffe, S. J. (2005). *Drugs in pregnancy and lactation* (7th ed.). Baltimore: Williams & Wilkins; Hale, T. (2006). *Medications and mothers' milk* (12th ed.). Amarillo, TX: Pharmasoft Publishing; Committee on Drugs, American Academy of Pediatrics. (2001). The transfer of drugs and other chemicals into human milk. *Pediatrics, 108*(3), 776.

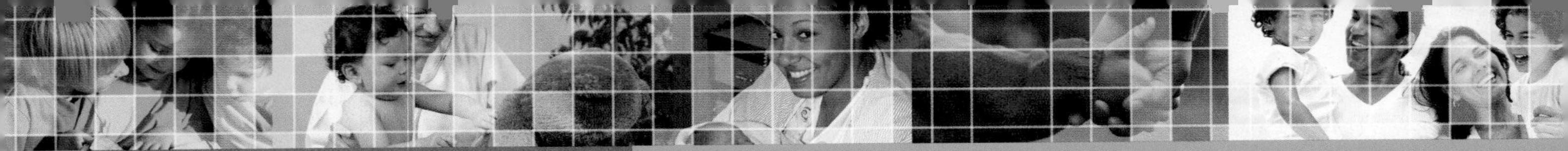

APPENDIX G

THE FRIEDMAN FAMILY ASSESSMENT MODEL (SHORT FORM)

The following form is shortened for ease in assessing a family. If you are not sure what data should be covered in each of the assessment areas below, please refer to the original reference where more detailed questions/areas are presented.

Before using the following guidelines in completing family assessments, note that not all areas included below will be germane for each of the families visited. The guidelines are comprehensive and allow depth when probing is necessary. Do not feel that every subarea needs to be covered when the broad area of inquiry poses no problems to the family or concern to the health worker. Second, by virtue of the interdependence of the family system, one will find unavoidable redundancy. The assessor should try not to repeat data, but to refer the reader back to sections where this information has already been described.

IDENTIFYING DATA

1. Family Name
2. Address and Phone
3. Family Composition: The Family Genogram
4. Type of Family Form
5. Cultural (Ethnic) Background
6. Religious Identification
7. Social Class Status
8. Social Class Mobility

DEVELOPMENTAL STAGE AND HISTORY OF FAMILY

9. Family's Present Developmental Stage
10. Extent of Family Developmental Tasks Fulfillment
11. Nuclear Family History
12. History of Family of Origin of Both Parents

ENVIRONMENTAL DATA

13. Characteristics of Home
14. Characteristics of Neighborhood and Larger Community
15. Family's Geographical Mobility
16. Family's Associations and Transactions with Community

FAMILY STRUCTURE

17. Communication Patterns
    - Extent of Functional and Dysfunctional Communication (types of recurring patterns)
    - Extent of Emotional (Affective) Messages and How Expressed
    - Characteristics of Communication within Family Subsystems
    - Extent of Congruent and Incongruent Messages
    - Types of Dysfunctional Communication Processes Seen in Family
    - Areas of Closed Communication
    - Familial and Contextual Variables Affecting Communication
18. Power Structure
    - Power Outcomes
    - Decision-Making Process
    - Power Bases
    - Variables Affecting Family Power
    - Overall Family System and Subsystem Power (Family Power Continuum Placement)
19. Role Structure
    - Formal Role Structure
    - Informal Role Structure
    - Analysis of Role Models (optional)
    - Variables Affecting Role Structure
20. Family Values
    - Compare the family to American core values or family's reference group values and/or identify important family values and their importance (priority) in family.
    - Congruence between the Family's Values and the Family's Reference Group or Wider Community
    - Disparity in Value Systems
    - Presence of Value Conflicts in Family
    - Effect of the Above Values and Value Conflicts on Health Status of Family

FAMILY FUNCTIONS

21. Affective Function
    - Mutual Nurturance, Closeness, and Identification
    - Separateness and Connectedness
    - Family's Need–Response Patterns
22. Socialization Function
    - Family Childrearing Practices
    - Adaptability of Childrearing Practices for Family Form and Family's Situation
    - Who Is (Are) Socializing Agent(s) for Child(ren)?
    - Value of Children in Family
    - Cultural Beliefs That Influence Family's Childrearing Patterns
    - Social Class Influence on Childrearing Patterns
    - Estimation about Whether Family Is at Risk for Childrearing Problems and if so, Indication of High-Risk Factors
    - Adequacy of Home Environment for Children's Needs to Play
23. Health Care Function
    - Family's Health Beliefs, Values, and Behavior
    - Family's Definitions of Health–Illness and Its Level of Knowledge
    - Family's Perceived Health Status and Illness Susceptibility
    - Family's Dietary Practices
    - Adequacy of Family Diet (recommended 3-day food history record)
    - Function of Mealtimes and Attitudes toward Food and Mealtimes
    - Shopping (and its planning) Practices.
    - Person(s) Responsible for Planning, Shopping, and Preparation of Meals
    - Sleep and Rest Habits
    - Physical Activity and Recreation Practices
    - Family's Therapeutic and Recreational Drug, Alcohol, and Tobacco Practices
    - Family's Role in Self-care Practices
    - Medically Based Preventive Measures (physicals, eye and hearing tests, immunizations, dental care)

Complementary and Alternative Therapies
Family Health History (both general and specific diseases—environmentally and genetically related)
Health Care Services Received
Feelings and Perceptions Regarding Health Services
Emergency Health Services
Source of Payments for Health and Other Services
Logistics of Receiving Care

FAMILY STRESS, COPING, AND ADAPTATION

24. Family Stressors, Strengths, and Perceptions
    Stressors Family Is Experiencing
    Strengths That Counterbalance Stressors
    Family's Definition of the Situation
25. Family Coping Strategies
    How the Family Is Reacting to the Stressors
    Extent of Family's Use of Internal Coping Strategies (past/present)
    Extent of Family's Use of External Coping Strategies (past/present)
    Dysfunctional Coping Strategies Utilized (past/present; extent of use)
26. Family Adaptation
    Overall Family Adaptation
    Estimation of Whether Family Is in Crisis
27. Tracking Stressors, Coping, and Adaptation Over Time

Used with permission from Friedman, M. M., Bowden, V. R., & Jones, E. G. (2003). *Family nursing: Research, theory, and practice* (5th ed.). Upper Saddle River, NJ: Prentice Hall.

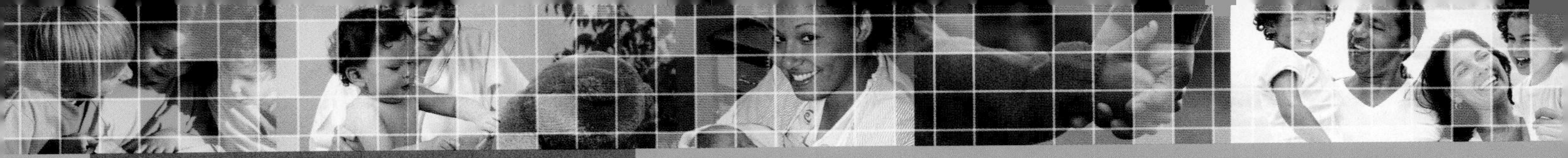

APPENDIX H

Table H–1 Dietary Reference Intakes (DRI's) for Nonpregnant Females and for Pregnant and Lactating Females

	Age	Vitamin A (mcg/d)	Vitamin D (mcg/d)	Vitamin E (mg/d α-tocopherol)	Vitamin K (mcg/d)	Vitamin C (mg/d)	Thiamine (mg/d)	Riboflavin (mg/d)
Females	9–13 y	600	5*	11	60*	45	0.9	0.9
	14–18 y	700	5*	15	75*	65	1.0	1.0
	19–30 y	700	5*	15	90*	75	1.1	1.1
	31–50 y	700	5*	15	90*	75	1.1	1.1
	50–70 y	700	10*	15	90*	75	1.1	1.1
	> 70 y	700	15*	15	90*	75	1.1	1.1
Pregnancy	≤ 18 y	750	5*	15	75*	80	1.4	1.4
	19–30 y	770	5*	15	90*	85	1.4	1.4
	31–50 y	770	5*	15	90*	85	1.4	1.4
Lactation	≤ 18 y	1200	5*	19	75*	115	1.4	1.6
	19–30 y	1300	5*	19	90*	120	1.4	1.6
	31–50 y	1300	5*	19	90*	120	1.4	1.6

Source: All data is from the Institute of Medicine (1997–2001). Dietary reference intakes. Washington, D.C. National Academy Press. Also available at http://www.nap.edu

*Values are adequate intakes (AIs) rather than recommended dietary allowances (RDAs). All other values on chart are RDAs.

Table H–2 Dietary Reference Intakes for Infants, Children, and Adolescents

	Age	Vitamin A (mcg/d)	Vitamin D (mcg/d)	Vitamin E (mg/d α-tocopherol)	Vitamin K (mcg/d)	Vitamin C (mg/d)	Thiamin (mg/d)	Riboflavin (mg/d)
Infants	0–6 months	400*	5*	4*	2.0*	40*	0.2*	0.3*
	7–12 months	500*	5*	5*	2.5*	50*	0.3*	0.4*
Children	1–3 years	300	5*	6	30*	15	0.5	0.5
	4–8 years	400	5*	7	55*	25	0.6	0.6
Males	9–13 years	600	5*	11	60*	45	0.9	0.9
	14–18 years	900	5*	15	75*	75	1.2	1.3
Females	9–13 years	600	5*	11	60*	45	0.9	0.9
	14–18 years	700	5*	15	75*	65	1.0	1.0

*Values are Adequate Intakes (AI) rather than Recommended Dietary Allowances (RDAs). All other values on chart are RDAs. See Chapter 34 for a discussion of nutrient requirements.

Note: Data from Otten, J. J., Hellwig, J. P., & Meyers, L. D. (Eds.). (2006). *Dietary reference intakes: The essential guide to nutrient requirements.* Washington, DC: The National Academies Press.

Niacin (mg/d)	Vitamin B_6 (mg/d)	Folate (µg/d)	Vitamin B_{12} (mcg/d)	Calcium (mg/d)	Phosphorus (mg/d)	Magnesium (mg/d)	Iron (mg/d)	Zinc (mg/d)	Iodine (mcg/d)	Selenium (mcg/d)
12	1.0	300	1.8	1300*	1250	240	8	8	120	40
14	1.2	400	2.4	1300*	1250	360	15	9	150	55
14	1.3	400	2.4	1000*	700	310	18	8	150	55
14	1.3	400	2.4	1000*	700	320	18	8	150	55
14	1.5	400	2.4	1200*	700	320	8	8	150	55
14	1.5	400	2.4	1200*	700	320	8	8	150	55
18	1.9	600	2.6	1300*	1250	400	27	12	220	60
18	1.9	600	2.6	1000*	700	350	27	11	220	60
18	1.9	600	2.6	1000*	700	360	27	11	220	60
17	2.0	500	2.8	1300*	1250	360	10	13	290	70
17	2.0	500	2.8	1000*	700	310	9	12	290	70
17	2.0	500	2.8	1000*	700	320	9	12	290	70

Niacin (mg/d)	Vitamin B_6 (mg/d)	Folate (mcg/d)	Vitamin B_{12} (mcg/d)	Calcium (mg/d)	Phosphorus (mg/d)	Magnesium (mg/d)	Iron (mg/d)	Zinc (mg/d)	Iodine (mcg/d)	Selenium (mcg/d)
~0.2*	0.1*	65*	0.4*	210*	100*	30*	0.27*	2.0*	110*	15*
~0.4*	0.3*	80*	0.5*	270*	275*	75*	11	3	130*	20*
6	0.5	150	0.9	500*	460	80	7	3	90	20
8	0.6	200	1.2	800*	500	130	10	5	90	30
12	1.0	300	1.8	1300*	1250	240	8	8	120	40
16	1.3	400	2.4	1300*	1250	240	11	11	150	55
12	1.0	300	1.8	1300*	1250	410	8	8	120	40
14	1.2	400	2.4	1300*	1250	360	15	9	150	55

Table H-3 Recommended Dietary Allowances

	Age	Protein	Carbohydrate	Polyunsaturated Fatty Acids n-6	Polyunsaturated Fatty Acids n-3	Total Fat	Fiber
Infants	0–6 months	9.1 g/d or 1.52 g/kg/d*	60 g/d*	4.4 g/d	0.5 g/d	31 g/d	NE
	7–12 months	1.5 g/kg/d	95 g/d*	4.6 g/d	0.5 g/d	30 g/d	NE
Children	1–3 years	1.1 g/kg/d or 13 g/d	130 g/d	7 g/d (linoleic)	0.7 g/d (α-linolenic)	NE	19 g/d
	4–8 years	0.95 g/kg/d or 19 g/d	130 g/d	10 g/d (linoleic)	0.9 g/d (α-linolenic)	NE	25 g/d
Males	9–13 years	0.95 g/kg/d or 34 g/d	130 g/d	12 g/d (linoleic)	1.2 g/d (α-linolenic)	NE	31 g/d
	14–18 years	0.85 g/kg/d or 52 g/d	130 g/d	16 g/d (linoleic)	1.6 g/d (α-linolenic)	NE	38 g/d
Females	9–13 years	0.95 g/kg/d or 34 g/d	130 g/d	10 g/d (linoleic)	1.0 g/d (α-linolenic)	NE	26 g/d
	14–18 years	0.85 g/kg/d or 46 g/d	130 g/d	11 g/d (linoleic)	1.1 g/d (α-linolenic)	NE	26 g/d

*Values are Adequate Intakes (AIs) rather than Recommended Dietary Allowances (RDAs). All other values on charts are RDAs.

NE = not established. All data from Institute of Medicine. (2002). Dietary Reference Intakes. Washington DC: National Academy Press. www.nap.edu/iom

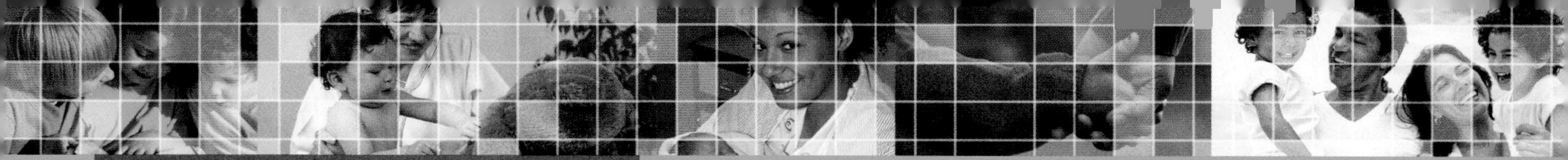

APPENDIX I

WEST NOMOGRAM-BODY SURFACE AREA

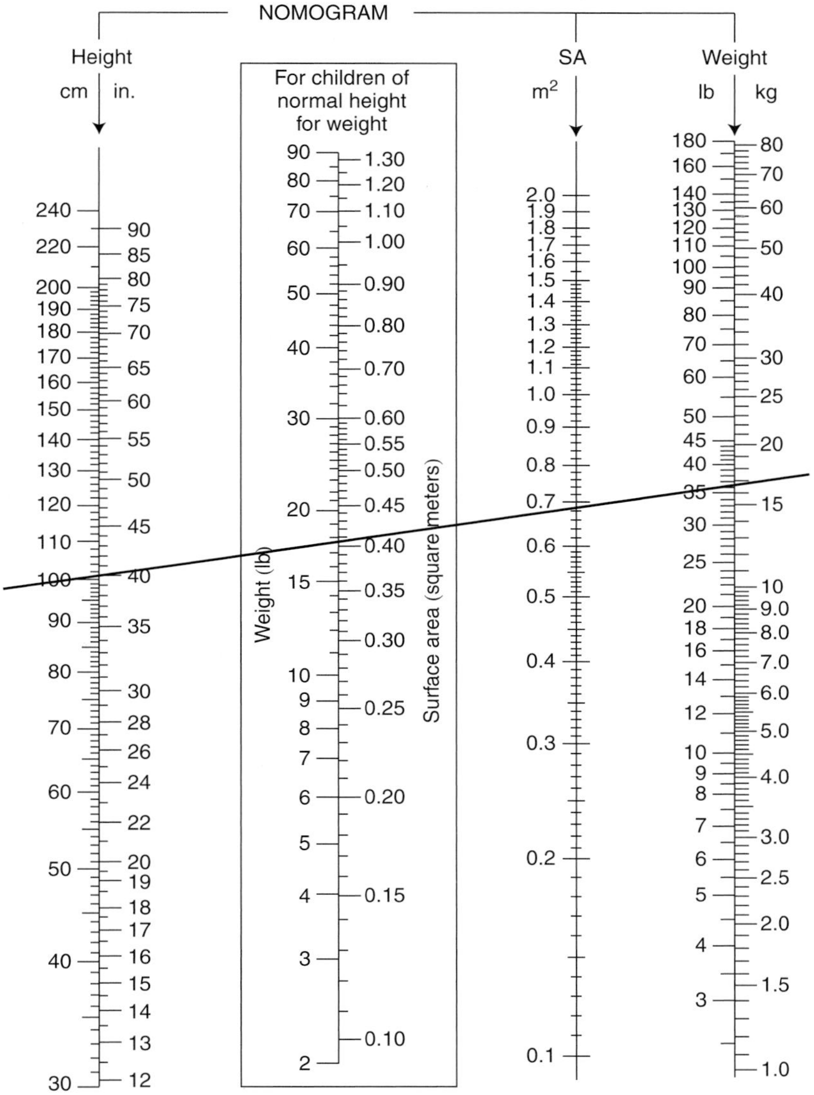

● Figure App-I–1

The proportion between height and weight in children is different from the proportion in adults. These differences are most manifest in newborns, infants, and young children. Therefore, dosages of drugs that have been established for adults cannot simply be reduced, and correspondingly be safe for young children. Weight is used as a better method of calculating drug dosage in children and is used when medications have a dose of drug recommended in mg/kg.

However, weight alone is not always accurate as a method of calculating a drug dosage for a child. Another more accurate method is that of body surface area (BSA). BSA is a relationship of height to weight and is measured in squared meters. BSA increases about 7 times from birth to adulthood, and is a good reflection of many physiologic processes significant in metabolizing, transporting, and eliminating drugs, such as metabolic rate, extracellular fluid and total fluid volumes, cardiac output, and glomerular filtration rate. BSA is calculated by the formula:

$$\text{Surface area } (\text{m}^2) = \sqrt{\frac{\text{height (cm)} \times \text{weight (kg)}}{3600}}$$

Rather than calculating the BSA by this method, a graph can be used. See the nomogram here to demonstrate that method. To calculate a child's BSA, draw a straight line from the height (in the left column) to the weight (in the right column). The point at which the line intersects the surface area (SA) column is the BSA (measured in squared meters [m^2]). If the child is of normal height-weight proportions, the BSA can be calculated from the weight alone (in the enclosed area). In the example shown here, the child's height and weight percentiles varied, so it is most accurate to use the SA line. The child's SA (or BSA) is 0.48 m^2.

Medications that are prescribed using the BSA system will be dosed in mg/m^2. For example, an initial lowest recommended dosage of cyclophosphamide for children is 60 mg/m^2. The child who has a BSA of 0.48 m^2, as in the example here, should receive 60 times 0.48, or 28.8 mg of the drug.

Nomogram modified from data of G. L. Briars & B. J. Bailey, from Robertson, J., & Shilkofshi, N. (Eds.). (2005). This article was published in *The Harriet Lane Handbook*, 2005, p. 599, Robertson et al.

GLOSSARY

A

Abdominal effleurage A light stroking movement made over the abdominal wall with the fingertips.

Abortion Loss of pregnancy before the fetus is viable outside the uterus; miscarriage.

Abruptio placentae Partial or total premature separation of a normally implanted placenta.

Acanthosis nigricans Hyperpigmentation and thickening of the skin associated with chronic hyperinsulinemia.

Accelerations Periodic increases in the baseline fetal heart rate.

Accommodation The process of changing one's cognitive structures to include data from recent experiences.

Acculturation The process by which people adapt to a new cultural norm.

Acellular pertussis vaccine A vaccine that uses pertussis proteins rather than the whole cell to stimulate active immunity.

Acidemia Decreased blood pH.

Acidosis Condition caused by excess acid in the blood.

Acquired immunity Humoral (antibody-mediated) and cell-mediated immunity that is not fully developed until a child is about 6 years of age.

Acquired immunodeficiency syndrome (AIDS) An immunological disorder caused by infection with the human immunodeficiency virus (HIV) and characterized by increasing susceptibility to opportunistic infections and rare cancers.

Acrocyanosis Cyanosis of the extremities.

Acrosomal reaction Breakdown of the hyaluronic acid in the corona radiata by enzymes from the heads of sperm; allows one spermatozoon to penetrate the ovum zona pellucida.

Active acquired immunity Formation of antibodies by the pregnant woman in response to illness or immunization.

Active alert (state) The awake state in which the newborn's eyes are open and motor activity is quite intense, with thrusting movements of the extremities.

Active immunity Stimulation of antibody production without causing clinical disease.

Acute pain Sudden pain of short duration, associated with a tissue-damaging stimulus.

Adaptation phase Period during a crisis when the child and family meet the challenge and use resources effectively.

Adaptive functioning The ability of an individual to meet the standards expected for his or her age by his or her cultural group.

Adjustment phase Period just after a family is confronted by a crisis, characterized by disorganization and unsuccessful attempts to deal with the problem.

Adrenarche The development of pubic and axillary sexual hair.

Advance directives A patient's living will or appointed durable power of attorney for healthcare decisions.

Adventitious Breath sounds that are not normally heard, such as crackles and rhonchi.

Affect Outward manifestation of feeling or emotion; the tone of a person's reaction or response to people or events.

Afterpains Cramplike pains due to contractions of the uterus that occur after childbirth. They are more common in multiparas, tend to be most severe during nursing, and last 2 to 3 days.

Agoraphobia Anxiety of being in places or situations from which escape may be difficult or embarrassing, or in which help may not be available.

Air hunger The most severe form of dyspnea, when a person or child looks panicked, gasps for breath, and sits upright.

Airway remodeling A thickening of the sub-basement membrane, subepithelial fibrosis, airway smooth muscle hypertrophy and hyperplasia, blood vessel proliferation and dilation, and mucous gland hyperplasia and hypersecretion. Decreased airway elasticity and decreased lung function result.

Airway resistance The effort or force needed to move oxygen through the trachea to the lungs.

Alkalemia Increased blood pH.

Alkalosis Condition caused by too little acid in the blood.

Allergen An antigen capable of inducing hypersensitivity.

Allergy An abnormal or altered reaction to an antigen.

Allograft The use of cadaver skin from a skin bank in skin grafting; an allograft is used to cover a second-degree burn until healing occurs.

Alternative therapy Usually considered a substance or procedure that has not undergone rigorous scientific testing in this country, although it might have been thoroughly tested in other countries.

Alveolar hypoventilation The condition in which the volume of air entering the alveoli during gas exchange is inadequate to meet the body's metabolic needs.

Amenorrhea Suppression or absence of menstruation.

Amniocentesis Removal of amniotic fluid by insertion of a needle into the amniotic sac; amniotic fluid is used to assess fetal health or maturity.

Amnion The inner of the two membranes that form the sac containing the fetus and the amniotic fluid.

Amniotic fluid The liquid surrounding the fetus in utero. It absorbs shocks, permits fetal movement, and prevents heat loss.

Amniotic fluid embolism Amniotic fluid that has leaked into the chorionic plate and entered the maternal circulation.

Amniotomy The artificial rupturing of the amniotic membrane.

Ampulla The outer two-thirds of the fallopian tube; fertilization of the ovum by a spermatozoon usually occurs here.

Analgesic potentiators A group of tranquilizers that potentiate the effects of narcotic analgesics without increasing unwanted side effects.

Anemia Reduction in the number of red blood cells, the quantity of hemoglobin, and the volume of packed red cells per 100 mL of blood to below-normal levels.

Animal-assisted therapy A form of therapy used in hospitals and units in which specially trained animals (commonly dogs) provide diversion, distraction, comfort, and relaxation during health care.

Antepartum Time between conception and the onset of labor; usually used to describe the period during which a woman is pregnant.

Anthropometric measurements The term used to refer to growth assessment of various parts of the body.

Antibodies Proteins capable of responding to specific infectious agents.

Anticipatory guidance The process of understanding upcoming developmental needs and then teaching caretakers to meet those needs.

Antigen A foreign substance that triggers an immune system response.

Anxiolysis Minimal sedation by medication in which cognitive and motor functions may be impaired.

Apgar score A scoring system used to evaluate newborns at 1 minute and 5 minutes after birth. The total score is achieved by assessing five signs: heart rate, respiratory effort, muscle tone, reflex irritability, and color. Each of the signs is assigned a score of 0, 1, or 2. The highest possible score is 10.

Apical impulse Also called the point of maximum intensity, is located where the left ventricle taps the chest wall during contraction. The apical impulse is usually seen in thin children.

Apnea Cessation of respiration lasting longer than 20 seconds.

Apoptosis Programmed cell death. When the cell "realizes" something is wrong and destroys itself.

Areflexia A lack of reflex response to verbal, sensory, or pain stimulation.

Areola Pigmented ring surrounding the nipple of the breast.

Arrhythmias Abnormal rhythms or dysrhythmias.

Artificial rupture of membranes (AROM) A procedure in which the amniotic membranes are ruptured by a certified nurse-midwife or physician, using an instrument called an amniohook. Also known as *amniotomy*.

Asplenia An absent or dysfunctional spleen.

Assimilation The process of incorporating new experiences into an individual's cognitive awareness.

Assisted reproductive technology (ART) The term used to describe highly technologic approaches used to produce pregnancy. In vitro fertilization and embryo transfer (IVF-ET) is an example of ART.

Assistive technology The process of incorporating new experiences into one's cognitive awareness.

Associative play A type of play that emerges in preschool years when children interact with one another, engaging in similar activities and participating in groups.

Atopy A hereditary allergic tendency.

Audiography A test used to assess hearing in which sounds of various pitches and intensity are presented to children through earphones.

Aura A visual, auditory, taste, or motor sensation that gives warning of an impending seizure or migraine headache.

Auscultation The technique of listening to sounds produced by the airway, lungs, stomach, heart, and blood vessels to identify their characteristics. Auscultation is usually performed with the stethoscope to enhance the sounds heard.

Autografting Use of healthy skin taken from a nonburned area of the child's body.

Automatism Unusual body movements without purpose, e.g., lip smacking, lip chewing, sucking.

Autonomic dysreflexia Condition in which hypertension, bradycardia, severe headaches, pallor below and flushing above the level of the spinal cord lesion, and seizures occurs due to an impaired autonomic nervous system, triggered by simultaneous sympathetic and parasympathetic activity.

Autosomes Chromosomes that are not a sex chromosome.

Azotemia Accumulation of nitrogenous wastes in the blood.

B

Bag of waters (BOW) The membrane containing the amniotic fluid and the fetus.

Ballottement A technique of palpation to detect or examine a floating object in the body. In obstetrics, the fetus, when pushed, floats away and then returns to touch the examiner's fingers.

Barlow's maneuver Test designed to detect subluxation or dislocation of the hip. A dysplastic joint will be felt to be dislocated as the femur leaves the acetabulum.

Basal body temperature (BBT) The lowest waking temperature.

Baseline rate The average fetal heart rate observed during a 10-minute period of monitoring.

Baseline variability A measure of the interplay (the push-pull effect) between the sympathetic and parasympathetic nervous systems over a 10-minute period.

Becoming a mother (BAM) Alternative term for *maternal role attainment* (MRA). The transition process of becoming a mother that changes throughout the maternal-child relationship.

Behavior modification A technique used to reinforce desirable behaviors, helping the child to replace maladaptive behaviors with more appropriate ones.

Benign Describing a growth that does not endanger life or health.

Bilirubin encephalopathy The yellow staining and degenerative lesions in basal ganglia associated with high levels of unconjugated bilirubin in infants. Also known as *kernicterus*.

Binge eating A compulsion to consume large quantities of food in a short period of time.

Binocularity Ability of the eyes to function together.

Biophysical profile (BPP) Assessment of five variables in the fetus that help to evaluate fetal risk: breathing movement, body movement, tone, amniotic fluid volume, and fetal heart rate reactivity.

Biotherapy Use of biologic response modifiers to treat cancer.

Birth preference plan A written list of preferences of the prospective parents that identifies aspects of the childbearing experience that are most important to them. Used as a tool for communication among the expectant parents, the healthcare provider, and the healthcare professionals at the birth setting, the written plan identifies options that are available as well as those that are not.

Birth rate Number of live births per 1000 population.

Birthing room In hospitals or birthing centers, single rooms where the woman and her partner or other family members will stay for the labor, birth, recovery, and possibly the postpartum period. Also called *labor, delivery, recovery,* and *postpartum rooms* or *single-room maternity care.*

Bisexual An adjective used to describe or refer to a person who is attracted to both men and women.

Blastocyst The inner solid mass of cells within the morula.

Bloody show Pink-tinged mucous secretions resulting from rupture of small capillaries as the cervix effaces and dilates.

Body fluid Body water that has substances (solutes) dissolved in it.

Body image The idea that one forms about one's body.

Body mass index (BMI) A calculation (kilograms of weight/m^2 of height) used to determine the proportion between a child's height and weight.

Boggy uterus (uterine atony) A term used to describe the uterine fundus when it is not firmly contracted after the birth of the baby and in the early postpartum period; excessive bleeding occurs from the placental site, and maternal hemorrhage may occur.

Bone age A radiographic image of the bones of the wrist used to evaluate the stage of bone ossification.

Brain death The irreversible cessation of all functions of the brain, including the cerebral cortex and brainstem.

Braxton Hicks contractions Intermittent painless contractions of the uterus that may occur every 10 to 20 minutes. They occur more frequently toward the end of pregnancy and are sometimes mistaken for true labor signs.

Brazelton Neonatal Behavioral Assessment Scale A brief examination used to identify the infant's behavioral states and responses.

Breast self-examination (BSE) A manual examination conducted monthly by a woman to evaluate her own breasts for signs of masses, changes, nipple discharge, or evidence of abnormalities.

Breasts Mammary glands.

Breech presentation A birth in which the buttocks and/or feet are the presenting part rather than the head.

Broad ligament A ligament that keeps the uterus centrally placed and provides stability within the pelvic cavity. It is a double layer that is continuous with the abdominal peritoneum. The broad ligament covers the uterus anteriorly and posteriorly and extends outward from the uterus to enfold the fallopian tubes.

Bronchophony Change in vocal resonance in the presence of a lung consolidation, in which there is increased intensity and clarity of sounds while the words remain indistinct.

Brown adipose tissue (BAT) Fat deposits in neonates that provide greater heat-generating activity than ordinary fat. Found around the kidneys, adrenals, and neck; between the scapulas; and behind the sternum. Also called *brown fat.*

Buffer Related acid-base pair that gives up or takes up hydrogen ions as needed to prevent large changes in the pH of a solution.

Bullying Repeatedly aggressive behavior intended to cause physical or emotional harm that exists in a relationship with an imbalance of power.

C

Calorie Amount of heat required to raise the temperature of 1 kg of water 1 degree centigrade.

Capacitation Removal of the plasma membrane overlying the spermatozoa's acrosomal area with the loss of seminal plasma proteins and the glycoprotein coat. If the glycoprotein coat is not removed, the sperm will not be able to penetrate the ovum.

Caput succedaneum Swelling or edema occurring in or under the fetal scalp during labor.

Carcinogens Chemicals or processes that, when combined with genetic traits and in interaction with one another, cause cancer.

Cardiac output Volume of blood ejected from the left ventricle each minute.

Cardinal ligaments The chief uterine supports, the cardinal ligaments suspend the uterus from the side walls of the true pelvis. Also known as *Mackenrodt's* or *transverse cervical ligaments,* they arise from the sides of the pelvic walls and attach to the cervix in the upper vagina. They prevent uterine prolapse and support the upper vagina.

Cardinal movements The positional changes of the fetus as it moves through the birth canal during labor and birth. The positional changes are descent, flexion, internal rotation, extension, restitution, and external rotation.

Cardiopulmonary adaptation Adaptation of the neonate's cardiovascular and respiratory systems to life outside the womb.

Care coordination The process of planning and integrating healthcare services among providers in an effort to achieve and promote good health in the child.

Caregiver burden The unrelenting pressure and anxiety related to providing daily care to a child with disabilities while meeting other family obligations.

Case management A process of coordinating the delivery of healthcare services in a manner that focuses on both quality and cost outcomes.

Case manager Person who coordinates health care to prevent gaps or overlaps.

Cephalocaudal development The process by which development proceeds from the head downward through the body and toward the feet.

Cephalohematoma Subcutaneous swelling containing blood found on the head of an infant several days after birth; it usually disappears within a few weeks to 2 months.

Cephalopelvic disproportion (CPD) A condition in which the fetal head is of such a shape or size, or in such a position, that it cannot pass through the maternal pelvis.

Cerebral edema Increase in intracellular and extracellular fluid in the brain that results from anoxia, vasodilation, or vascular stasis.

Cerebral perfusion pressure Amount of pressure needed to ensure that adequate oxygen and nutrients will be delivered to the brain.

Certified nurse-midwife (CNM) An RN who has received special training and education in the care of the family during childbearing and the prenatal, labor and birth, and postpartal periods. After a period of formal education, the nurse-midwife takes a certification test to become a CNM.

Cervical cap A cup-shaped device placed over the cervix to prevent pregnancy.

Cervical ripening Softening of the cervix; occurs normally as a physiologic process prior to labor or is stimulated to occur through the process of induction of labor.

Cervix The "neck" between the external os and the body of the uterus. The lower end of the cervix extends into the vagina.

Cesarean birth Birth of fetus accomplished by performing a surgical incision through the maternal abdomen and uterus.

Chadwick's sign An objective change or probable sign of pregnancy, is a blue-purple discoloration of the cervix caused by increased vascularization of the uterus during pregnancy.

Chelation A reaction in which an organic compound, containing carbonyl (CO) and hydroxyl (OH) groups coordinates with a metal to form a firmly bound ring-like structure.

Chemical conjunctivitis Irritation of the mucous membrane lining of the eyelid; may be due to instillation of silver nitrate ophthalmic drops.

Chemotherapy Treatment to combat cancer that involves drugs taken orally, intravenously, intrathecally, or by injection, which kill both normal and cancerous cells.

Child life specialist Trained professional who plans therapeutic activities for hospitalized children.

Child sexual abuse The exploitation of a child for the sexual gratification of an adult.

Children with special healthcare needs (CSHCN) Children who have or are at increased risk for a chronic physical, developmental, behavioral, or emotional condition and who also require health and related services of a type or amount beyond that required by children generally.

Chlamydial infection A sexually transmitted infection caused by *Chlamydia trachomatis.*

Chloasma (melasma gravidarum) Brownish pigmentation over the bridge of the nose and the cheeks during pregnancy and in some women who are taking oral contraceptives. Also called *mask of pregnancy*.

Cholestasis Disruption of bile flow.

Chondrolysis The breaking down and absorption of cartilage.

Chorion The fetal membrane closest to the intrauterine wall that gives rise to the placenta and continues as the outer membrane surrounding the amnion.

Chorionic villus sampling (CVS) Procedure in which a specimen of the chorionic villi is obtained from the edge of the developing placenta at about 8 weeks' gestation. The sample can be used for chromosomal, enzyme, and DNA tests.

Chromosomes The threadlike structures within the nucleus of a cell that carry the genes.

Chronic condition A health condition that lasts or is expected to last 3 months or more.

Chronic pain Persistent pain lasting longer than 6 months, generally associated with a prolonged disease process.

Chronic vomiting Low-grade nearly daily emesis.

Chvostek sign A spasm of facial muscles after tapping facial nerve. A positive Chvostek sign reveals hyperreflexia. It is used to assess for hypoparathyroidism.

Circumcision Surgical removal of the prepuce (foreskin) of the penis.

Circumferential Injury completely surrounding the thorax or an extremity.

Cleavage Rapid mitotic division of the zygote; cells produced are called *blastomeres*.

Clinical practice guidelines Outlines detailing specific medical and nursing assessments and interventions during specific time intervals for a specific condition. This guideline is often adopted in an institution for all healthcare providers to follow so that quality of care is increased and costs of care are minimized.

Clonic Alternating muscular contraction and relaxation; often used to describe seizure activity.

Cognition The change in thought, intelligence, and language that occurs from the mutual interaction of brain maturation with life experiences.

Cognitive therapy A therapeutic approach that attempts to help the person recognize automatic thought patterns that lead to unpleasant feelings.

Coitus interruptus Method of contraception in which the male withdraws his penis from the vagina prior to ejaculation.

Cold stress Excessive heat loss resulting in compensatory mechanisms (increased respirations and nonshivering thermogenesis) to maintain core body temperature.

Coloboma A keyhole-shaped pupil caused by a notch in the iris.

Colostrum Secretion from the breast before the onset of true lactation; contains mainly serum and white blood corpuscles. It has a high protein content, provides some immune properties, and cleanses the neonate's intestinal tract of mucus and meconium.

Colposcopy The use of an instrument inserted into the vagina to examine the cervical and vaginal tissues by means of a magnifying lens.

Coma State of unconsciousness in which the child cannot be aroused, even with powerful stimuli.

Combined oral contraceptives (COCs) Commonly called *birth control pills* or "the pill." A form of contraception that uses a combination of a synthetic estrogen and a progestin.

Comedone A plug of sebaceous and keratin material in a hair follicle; commonly known as "whiteheads" and "blackheads."

Communicable disease An illness that is transmitted directly or indirectly from one person to another.

Compartment syndrome A condition of increased pressure in a limited space that compromises circulation and tissue function.

Complementary therapy May be defined as an adjunct to conventional medical treatment that has been through rigorous scientific testing, which shows that it has some reliability.

Compliance Approaches to health care that are usually not part of conventional western medicine; sometimes called *alternative therapy*.

Condom A rubber sheath that covers the penis to prevent conception or disease.

Conduction Loss of heat to a cooler surface by direct skin contact.

Conductive hearing loss Hearing loss caused by inadequate conduction of sound from the outer to the middle ear.

Condylomata acuminata A common sexually transmitted infection caused by the human papillomavirus (HPV). The infection is called *condylomata acuminata*. Also known as *venereal warts.*

Conjugate vera The true conjugate, which extends from the middle of the sacral promontory to the middle of the pubic crest.

Conjugated forms Forms of a vaccine against childhood diseases in the United States in which an altered organism is joined with another substance to increase the immune response.

Conservation The knowledge that matter is not changed when its form is altered.

Constipation Difficult and infrequent defecation with passage of hard, dry stool.

Continuous epidural infusion (CEI) Postcesarean pain control technique in which the epidural catheter is left in place and medication is continually administered via an electric pump.

Contraction stress test (CST) A method of assessing the reaction of the fetus to the stress of uterine contractions. This test may be utilized when contractions are occurring spontaneously or when contractions are artificially induced by oxytocin challenge test (OCT) or breast self-stimulation test (BSST).

Convection Loss of heat from the warm body surface to cooler air currents.

Cooperative play A type of play that emerges in school years when children join into groups to achieve a goal or play a game.

Coping The cognitive and behavioral responses that manage specific internal and external demands exceeding a person's resources, enabling the person to solve problems and to respond emotionally.

Cornua The elongated portion of the uterus where the fallopian tubes enter.

Cor pulmonale Obstruction of pulmonary blood flow that leads to right ventricular hypertrophy and heart failure.

Corpus The upper two-thirds of the uterus.

Corpus luteum A small yellow body that develops within a ruptured ovarian follicle; it secretes progesterone in the second half of the menstrual cycle and atrophies about 3 days before the beginning of menstrual flow. If pregnancy occurs, the corpus luteum continues to produce progesterone until the placenta takes over this function.

Cosleeping Practice whereby children and parents regularly sleep together in an adult bed.

Cotyledon One of the rounded portions into which the placenta's uterine surface is divided, consisting of a mass of villi, fetal vessels, and an intervillous space.

Couplet care A form of health care that is focused on keeping the mother and baby together as much as the mother desires. Also known as *mother-baby care,* this type of care provides increased opportunities for parent-child interaction because the newborn shares the mother's room and they are cared for together. Mother-baby care enables the mother to have time to bond with her baby and learn to care for her or him in a supportive environment.

Couvade In some cultures, the male's observance of certain rituals and taboos to signify the transition to fatherhood.

Crepitus A crinkly sensation palpated on the chest surface caused by air escaping into the subcutaneous tissues.

Crowning Appearance of the presenting fetal part at the vaginal orifice during labor.

Cryotherapy The use of cold or cold agents to treat specific injuries or conditions. Often used for treating warts and other skin conditions.

Cultural competence Refers to the skills and knowledge necessary to appreciate, understand, and work with individuals from different cultures.

Culture Defined as the beliefs, values, attitudes, and practices that are accepted by a population, community, or an individual.

Cushing's triad Reflex response associated with increased intracranial pressure or compromised blood flow to the brainstem; characterized by hypertension, increased systolic pressure with wide pulse pressure, bradycardia, and irregular respirations.

Cyberbullying A situation in which a child or adolescent is targeted by another via Internet posting or other digital technology, and threatened, tormented, harassed, humiliated, or embarrassed.

Cyclic vomiting Repeated severe vomiting of an episodic nature.

Cystocele The downward displacement of the bladder, which appears as a bulge in the anterior vaginal wall.

D

Date rape A form of acquaintance rape that occurs between a dating couple.

Deamination Removal of an amino group from an amino compound.

Death anxiety A feeling of apprehension or fear of death.

Death imagery Any reference to death or death-related topics, such as going away, separation, funerals, and dying, given in response to a picture or story that would not usually stimulate other children to discuss death-related topics.

Debridement Enzyme action to clean a lesion and dissolve fibrin clots or scabs; or removal of dead tissue to speed the healing process.

Decelerations Periodic decreases in the baseline fetal heart rate.

Decibels Units used to measure the loudness of sounds.

Decidua basalis The part of the decidua that unites with the chorion to form the placenta. It is shed in lochial discharge after childbirth.

Decidua capsularis The part of the decidua surrounding the chorionic sac.

Decidua vera (parietalis) Nonplacental decidua lining the uterus.

Deciduous teeth Primary set of 20 teeth that are complete by about 2 years and will be lost during childhood, beginning at about 6 years.

Deep sedation A controlled state of depressed consciousness or unconsciousness in which the child may experience partial or complete loss of protective reflexes.

Deep sleep State of sleep in which the infant will be nearly still except for occasional startles, twitches, and sucking.

Defense mechanism Technique used by the ego to unconsciously change reality, thereby protecting itself from excessive anxiety.

Dehydration The state of body water deficit.

Depo-Provera A long-acting, injectable progestin contraceptive.

Dermatophytoses Fungal infections that affect primarily the skin but may affect the hair and nails.

Desaturated blood Blood with a lower than normal oxygen level resulting when a heart defect causes oxygenated and unoxygenated blood to mix.

Development An increase in capability or function.

Developmental delay A delay in mastering functions, such as motor coordination and behavioral skills.

Developmental disability Any of a variety of chronic conditions that are characterized by mental or physical impairments. Intellectual disability, pervasive developmental disorder, cerebral palsy, and sensory loss are examples of developmental disabilities.

Developmental surveillance A flexible, continuous process of skilled observations that also provides data about the child's capabilities, allows for early identification of any neurologic problems, and helps to verify that the home environment is stimulating.

Diagonal conjugate An anteroposterior diameter that extends from the subpubic angle to the middle of the sacral promontory and is typically 12.5 cm. One of three diameters that are used to assess the size and shape of the pelvic inlet.

Dialysate The solution used in dialysis.

Diaphragm A flexible disk that covers the cervix to prevent pregnancy.

Diarrhea Frequent passage of abnormally watery stool.

Diastasis recti abdominis Separation of the recti abdominis muscles along the median line. In women, it is seen with repeated childbirths or multiple gestations. In the newborn, it is usually caused by incomplete development.

Dietary Reference Intakes (DRIs) A set of nutrient values that can be used to assess and plan intake for individuals of different ages.

Digitalization Process of giving a higher than normal dose of digoxin initially to speed response to the drug.

Diploid number of chromosomes Containing a set of maternal and a set of paternal chromosomes; in humans, the diploid number of chromosomes is 46.

Direct transmission The passage of an infectious disease through physical contact between the source of the pathogen and a new host.

Disability Impairment in one or more of five categories of function—cognition, communication, motor abilities, social abilities, or patterns of interactions.

Disaster A serious and massive event that impacts many people and is beyond the community's ability to manage.

Disaster preparedness Planning and coordinated response readiness by a community to meet the personal safety, healthcare, emotional, and environmental needs of children and their families in the event of a natural or manmade disaster.

Dislocation Displacement of a bone from its normal articulation with a joint.

Distraction The ability to focus attention on something other than pain, such as an activity, music, or a story.

Domestic violence Defined as the collective methods used to exert power and control by one individual over another in an adult intimate relationship. Forms of abuse typically fall into three categories: psychological abuse, physical abuse, and sexual abuse.

Doula A supportive companion who accompanies a laboring woman to provide emotional, physical, and informational support and acts as an advocate for the woman and her family.

Dramatic play A type of play in which a child acts out the drama of daily life.

Drowsy A subcategory of the alert state of infants. Aspects of the drowsy state include open or closed eyes, fluttering eyelids, semidozing appearance, and slow, regular movements of the extremities. Mild startles may be noted from time to time.

Dubowitz tool A scoring tool to estimate gestational age of the newborn by maturity rating. It can be used from birth to 5 days of life.

Ductus arteriosus A communication channel between the main pulmonary artery and the aorta of the fetus. It is obliterated after birth by rising PO2 and changes in intravascular pressure in the presence of normal pulmonary functioning. It normally becomes a ligament after birth but sometimes remains patent (patent ductus arteriosus, a treatable condition).

Ductus venosus A fetal blood vessel that carries oxygenated blood between the umbilical vein and the inferior vena cava, bypassing the liver; it becomes a ligament after birth.

Duration The time length of each contraction, measured from the beginning of the increment to the completion of the decrement.

Dwarfism A genetic condition usually resulting in an adult height of 58 inches or less. The most common cause of dwarfism is achondroplasia, which causes short arms and legs. The torso and head are approximately normal size, but decreased growth of long bones causes short stature.

Dysmenorrhea Painful menstruation.

Dyspareunia Painful intercourse.

Dysphagia Difficulty in swallowing.

Dysphonia Muffled, hoarse, or absent voice sounds.

Dysplasia Abnormal development resulting in altered size, shape, and cell organization.

Dyspnea Shortness of breath; difficulty in breathing.

Dystocia Difficult labor due to mechanical factors produced by the fetus or the maternal pelvis or due to inadequate uterine or other muscular activity.

E

Early adolescence Refers to adolescents who are age 14 and under.

Early childhood caries (ECC) The presence of one or more decayed, lost, or filled tooth surfaces in primary teeth from birth to 71 months of age; frequently caused by drinking from a bottle or nursing for prolonged periods, especially when sleeping; previously referred to as *nursing bottle mouth syndrome* and *baby bottle tooth decay*.

Early deceleration A periodic decrease in fetal heart rate from the normal baseline.

Early intervention Special services provided by state or local education programs for infants and toddlers up to age 3 years who have developmental delay or are at risk for developmental delay in the hopes that these children will have a lowered total cost of educational services.

Early (primary) postpartal hemorrhage A loss of blood of greater than 500 mL following birth. The hemorrhage is classified as early if it occurs within the first 24 hours and late if it occurs after the first 24 hours.

Ecchymosis A bruise.

Echolalia A compulsive parroting of what is heard.

Eclampsia Defined as the occurrence of either seizure or coma associated with pregnancy and not caused by other neurologic disease.

Ecologic theory A theory of development that emphasizes the importance of interactions between the developing child and the settings in which the child lives.

Ectoderm Outer layer of cells in the developing embryo that gives rise to the skin, nails, and hair.

Ectopic pregnancy (EP) Implantation of the fertilized ovum outside the uterine cavity; common sites are the abdomen, fallopian tubes, and ovaries. Also called *oocyesis*.

Effacement Thinning and shortening of the cervix that occurs late in pregnancy or during labor.

Egophony A change in vocal resonance in the presence of a lung consolidation condition in which the transmission of the "eee" sound becomes a nasal "ay" sound.

Electroanalgesia A method of delivering electrical stimulation to the skin, to compete with pain stimuli for transmission to the spinal cord; also known as *transcutaneous electrical nerve stimulation* (TENS).

Electrolytes Charged particles (ions) dissolved in body fluid.

Electronic fetal monitoring (EFM) A method of placing a fetal monitor on the fetus in order to obtain a continuous tracing of the FHR, which allows many characteristics of the fetal heart rate to be observed and evaluated.

Emancipated minors Minors who are legally considered to have assumed the rights of an adult. An adolescent may be considered emancipated if he or she is self-supporting and living away from home, married, pregnant, a parent, or in the military.

Embryo The early stage of development of the young of any organism. In humans the embryonic period is from about 2 to 8 weeks' gestation and is characterized by cellular differentiation and predominantly hyperplastic growth.

Embryonic membranes The amnion and chorion.

Emergency contraception Commonly called "Plan B," or the "morning after pill" a progestin-only approach (levonorgestrel) that is used within 72 hours of unprotected intercourse to eliminate the possibility of pregnancy.

Emergency preparedness Readiness to manage a healthcare emergency that involves planning, equipment and supplies for responses, and provider training and guidelines for action when an emergency occurs.

Emotional abuse Shaming, ridiculing, embarrassing, or insulting a child.

Emotional neglect A caretaker's inability to meet the psychosocial needs of a child.

En face An assumed position in which one person looks at another and maintains his or her face in the same vertical plane as that of the other.

Encephalopathy Cerebral dysfunction resulting from an insult (toxin, injury, inflammation, or anoxic event) of limited duration; the tissue damage is often permanent, but the dysfunction may improve over time.

Endoderm The inner layer of cells in the developing embryo that give rise to internal organs such as the intestines.

Endogenous pyrogenes Pyrogens released in response to an invasive organism that travel through the circulatory system to the hypothalamus, where they trigger the production of prostaglandins.

Endometrial biopsy Procedure provides information about the effects of progesterone produced by the corpus luteum after ovulation and endometrial receptivity.

Endometriosis Ectopic endometrium located outside the uterus in the pelvic cavity. Symptoms may include pelvic pain or pressure, dysmenorrhea, dyspareunia, abnormal bleeding from the uterus or rectum, and sterility.

Endometritis (metritis) An inflammation of the endometrium portion of the uterine lining.

Endometrium The mucous membrane that lines the inner surface of the uterus.

End-stage renal disease (ESRD) Irreversible kidney failure.

Engagement The entrance of the fetal presenting part into the superior pelvic strait and the beginning of the descent through the pelvic canal.

Engrossment Characteristic sense of absorption, preoccupation, and interest in the infant demonstrated by fathers during early contact with their infants.

Enteral therapy Nutrition introduced through the intestinal tract, including oral or tube feedings.

Enuresis Involuntary micturition by a child who has reached the age at which bladder control is expected.

Epidural block Regional anesthesia effective through the first and second stages of labor.

Episiotomy Incision of the perineum to facilitate birth and to avoid laceration of the perineum.

Epithelialization The process by which epithelial cells grow into the wound from surrounding healthy tissue.

Epstein's pearls Small, white blebs found along the gum margins and at the junction of the hard and soft palates; commonly seen in the newborn as a normal manifestation.

Equianalgesic dose The amount of a drug, whether administered orally or parenterally, needed to produce the same analgesic effect.

Equinus A condition that limits dorsiflexion to less than normal; usually associated with clubfoot.

Erb-Duchenne paralysis (Erb's palsy) Paralysis of the arm and chest wall as a result of a birth injury to the brachial plexus or a subsequent injury to the fifth and sixth cervical nerves.

Ergogenic aids Products that enhance physical performance.

Erythema toxicum Innocuous pink papular rash of unknown cause with superimposed vesicles; it appears within 24 to 48 hours after birth and resolves spontaneously within a few days.

Erythroblastosis fetalis Hemolytic disease of the newborn characterized by anemia, jaundice, enlargement of the liver and spleen, and generalized edema. Caused by isoimmunization due to Rh incompatibility or ABO incompatibility.

Erythropoiesis Formation of red blood cells.

Eschar Slough or layer of dead skin or tissue.

Escharotomy Incision into constricting dead tissue of a burn injury to restore peripheral circulation.

Estimated date of birth (EDB) During a pregnancy, the approximate date when childbirth will occur; the "due date."

Estrogens The hormones estradiol and estrone, produced by the ovary.

Ethnicity A social identity that is associated with shared beliefs, behaviors, and patterns.

Ethnocentrism An individual's belief that the values and practices of his or her own culture are the best ones.

Euthyroid Normal thyroid state.

Evaporation Loss of heat incurred when water on the skin surface is converted to a vapor.

Evidence-based practice An approach to problem solving and decision making that is based on the consideration of data from research, statistical analysis, quality measures, risk management measurements, and other sources of reliable information.

Expressive jargon Use of unintelligible words with normal speech intonations as if truly communicating in words; common in toddlerhood.

External cephalic version (ECV) Procedure involving external manipulation of the maternal abdomen to change the presentation of the fetus from breech to cephalic.

Extracellular fluid The fluid in the body that is outside the cells.

Extravasation Damage that occurs when a chemotherapeutic drug leaks into the soft tissue surrounding the infusion site.

F

Fallopian tubes Tubes that extend from the lateral angle of the uterus and terminate near the ovary; they serve as a passageway for the ovum from the ovary to the uterus and for the spermatozoa from the uterus toward the ovary. Also called *oviducts* and *uterine tubes.*

False pelvis The portion above the pelvic brim, or linea terminalis, that serves to support the weight of the enlarged pregnant uterus and direct the presenting fetal part into the true pelvis below.

Family Refers to two or more persons who are joined together by bonds of sharing and emotional closeness and who identify themselves as being part of a family.

Family crisis An event occurring when a family encounters problems that for a time seem insurmountable and with which the family is unable to cope in its usual ways.

Family resilience The family's capacity to demonstrate a positive response to an adverse situation and to emerge from the situation feeling strengthened, more resourceful, and more confident.

Family strengths Relationships and processes that support and protect families and family members during times of adversity and change.

Family-centered care A philosophy of care that integrates the family's values and potential contributions in the plans for and provision of care to the child.

Female reproductive cycle (FRC) The monthly rhythmic changes in sexually mature women.

Ferning capacity Formation of a palm-leaf pattern by the crystallization of cervical mucus as it dries at mid-menstrual cycle. Helpful in determining time of ovulation. Observed via microscopic examination of a thin layer of cervical mucus on a glass slide. This pattern is also observed when amniotic fluid is allowed to air dry on a slide and is a useful and quick test to determine whether amniotic membranes have ruptured.

Fertility awareness-based methods Also known as *natural family planning,* are based on an understanding of the changes that occur throughout a woman's ovulatory cycle. All these methods require periods of abstinence and recording of certain events throughout the cycle; cooperation of the partners is important.

Fertilization Impregnation of an ovum by a spermatozoon; conception.

Fetal alcohol spectrum disorder (FASD) An umbrella term that includes all categories of prenatal alcohol exposure, including fetal alcohol syndrome (FAS). It is not meant to be used as a clinical diagnosis.

Fetal alcohol syndrome (FAS) Syndrome caused by maternal alcohol ingestion and characterized by microcephaly, intrauterine growth restriction, short palpebral fissures, and maxillary hypoplasia.

Fetal attitude Relationship of the fetal parts to one another. Normal fetal attitude is one of moderate flexion of the arms onto the chest and flexion of the legs onto the abdomen.

Fetal blood sampling A procedure to collect a small amount of blood from the umbilical cord or fetus during pregnancy to diagnose, treat, and monitor various fetal problems.

Fetal bradycardia Fetal heart rate less than 110 bpm during a 10-minute period or longer.

Fetal lie Relationship of the cephalocaudal axis (spinal column) of the fetus to the cephalocaudal axis (spinal column) of the woman. The fetus may be in a longitudinal or transverse lie.

Fetal movement record (FMR) A method for tracking fetal activity taught to pregnant women.

Fetal position Relationship of the landmark on the presenting fetal part to the front, sides, or back of the maternal pelvis.

Fetal presentation The fetal body part that enters the maternal pelvis first. The three possible presentations are cephalic, shoulder, and breech.

Fetal tachycardia Sustained fetal heart rate of 161 bpm or higher.

Fetus The child in utero from about the seventh to ninth week of gestation until birth.

Fibrocystic breast changes Benign breast changes characterized by bilateral, cyclic breast pain and breast nodularities that may be unilateral or bilateral, and often in the upper outer quadrants of the breasts.

Filtration Movement into or out of capillaries as the net result of several opposing forces.

Fimbria The funnel-like structure at the abdominal opening of the uterine tube that has many fingerlike projections (fimbriae) reaching out to the ovary.

First-trimester combined screening A comprehensive screening testing that includes the nuchal translucency testing and serum screening for pregnancy-associated plasma protein-A (PAPP-A) and free beta human chorionic gonadotropin (BHCG) to determine whether a fetus is at risk for the genetic anomalies of trisomies 13, 18, and 21.

Focal Specific area of the brain; often used to describe seizures or neurologic deficits.

Folic acid A member of the vitamin B complex, required for amino acid metabolism, DNA synthesis, and production of red blood cells.

Follicle-stimulating hormone (FSH) Hormone produced by the anterior pituitary during the first half of the menstrual cycle, stimulating development of the graafian follicle.

Fontanelles In the fetus, unossified space, or soft spots, consisting of a strong band of connective tissue lying between the cranial bones of the skull.

Food allergy An IgE-mediated reaction to a given food that is potentially systemic, characteristically rapid in onset, and may be manifested as swelling of the lips, mouth, uvula or glottis, generalized urticaria, and, in severe reactions, anaphylaxis.

Food insecurity An inability or uncertainty that one will be able to acquire or consume adequate quality or quantity of foods in socially acceptable ways.

Food intolerance An abnormal physiologic response (flatulence, sweating, hives, indigestion) to a food that is not immunoglobulin E (IgE)-mediated.

Food jags Eating only a few foods for several days or weeks.

Food security Access at all times to enough nourishment for an active, healthy life.

Foramen ovale Special opening between the atria of the fetal heart. Normally, the opening closes shortly after birth; if it remains open, it can be repaired surgically.

Forceps-assisted birth A birth in which a set of instruments, known as *forceps,* are applied to the presenting part of the fetus to provide traction or to enable the fetal head to be rotated to an occiput-anterior position. Forceps-assisted birth is also known as *instrumental delivery, operative delivery,* or *operative vaginal delivery*.

Forceps marks Reddened areas over the cheeks and jaws caused by application of forceps. The red areas usually disappear within 1 or 2 days.

Foremilk Breast milk obtained at the beginning of the breastfeeding episode.

Frequency The time between the beginning of one contraction and the beginning of the next contraction.

Fundus The upper portion of the uterus between the fallopian tubes.

Funic presentation The condition in which the umbilical cord is interposed between the cervix and the presenting part. It can be located by clinical evaluation or by ultrasound.

G

Gamete intrafallopian transfer (GIFT) procedure Retrieval of oocytes by laparoscopy; immediately combining oocytes with washed, motile sperm in a catheter; and placement of the gametes into the fimbriated end of the fallopian tube.

Gametes Female or male germ cells; contain a haploid number of chromosomes.

Gametogenesis The process by which germ cells are produced.

Gay An adjective used to describe or refer to a homosexual male.

General anesthesia A state of induced unconsciousness that may be achieved through intravenous injection, inhalation of anesthetic agents, or a combination of both methods.

Genotype The genetic composition of an individual.

Gestation The number of weeks of pregnancy since the first day of the last menstrual period.

Gestational age assessment tools Systems used to evaluate the newborn's external physical characteristics and neurologic and/or neuromuscular development to accurately determine gestational age. These replace or supplement the traditional calculation from the woman's last menstrual period.

Gestational diabetes mellitus (GDM) A form of diabetes of variable severity with onset or first recognition during pregnancy.

Gestational trophoblastic disease (GTD) Disorder classified into two types: benign (hydatidiform mole) and malignant.

Glucagon A hormone produced by the pancreas that helps release stored glucose from the liver.

Gluconeogenesis Formation of glycogen from noncarbohydrate sources such as protein or fat.

Glycosuria Abnormal amount of glucose in the urine.

Goiter Enlargement of the thyroid gland.

Gonadotropin-releasing hormone (GnRH) A hormone secreted by the hypothalamus that stimulates the anterior pituitary to secrete FSH and LH.

Goodell's sign Softening of the cervix that occurs during the second month of pregnancy.

Graafian follicles The ovarian cyst containing the ripe ovum; it secretes estrogens.

Graft-versus-host disease A series of immunologic responses mounted by the host of a transplanted organ with the purpose of destroying the transplant cells.

Grasping reflex Normal newborn reflex elicited by stimulating the palm with a finger or object, resulting in newborn firmly holding on to the finger or object.

Gravida A pregnant woman.

Growth An increase in physical size.

H

Habituation Infant's ability to diminish innate responses to specific repeated stimuli.

Haploid number of chromosomes Half the diploid number of chromosomes. In humans there are 23 chromosomes, the haploid number, in each germ cell.

Harlequin sign A rare color change that occurs between the longitudinal halves of the newborn's body, such that the dependent half is noticeably pinker than the superior half when the newborn is placed on one side; it is of no pathologic significance.

Hazing An activity that is forced upon an individual, which causes humiliation and is required for membership in an organization or group. It can sometimes be harmful.

Health A state of complete physical, mental, and social well-being and not merely the absence of disease and infirmity.

Health maintenance (health protection) Activities that preserve an individual's present state of health and prevent disease or injury occurrence.

Health promotion Activities that increase well-being, enhance wellness or health, and lead to actualization of positive health potential; strategies that seek to foster conditions to allow populations to be healthy and to make healthy choices.

Health supervision The process of health promotion services, growth and development monitoring, and disease and injury prevention throughout the child's life.

Heaving Lifting of the chest wall during contraction.

Hegar's sign A softening of the lower uterine segment found upon palpation in the second or third month of pregnancy.

HELLP syndrome A cluster of changes including hemolysis, elevated liver enzymes, and low platelet count; sometimes associated with severe preeclampsia.

Hemarthrosis Bleeding into joint spaces.

Hematopoiesis Blood cell production.

Hemodynamics Pressures generated by blood and passage of blood through the heart and pulmonary system.

Hemoglobinopathy Disease characterized by abnormal hemoglobin.

Hemolytic disease of the newborn Hyperbilirubinemia secondary to Rh incompatibility.

Hemosiderosis Increased storage of iron in body tissues; associated with diseases involving the destruction of red blood cells.

Herd immunity Immunization of healthy children so that pathogens do not have hosts to reproduce and survive, indirectly protecting unimmunized infants.

Hernia Protrusion or projection of a body part or structure through the muscle wall of the cavity that normally contains it.

Herniation Protrusion of brain contents through the cranial vault at the base of the skull.

Hindmilk Breast milk released after initial letdown reflex; high in fat content.

Homosexuality Sexual attraction to people of the same sex.

Hormone replacement therapy (HRT) Administration of hormones, usually estrogen and a progestin, to alleviate the symptoms of menopause.

Hospice care A philosophy of care that focuses on helping persons with short life expectancies to live their remaining lives to the fullest—without pain and with choices and dignity.

Huhner test A test performed 1 or 2 days before the expected date of ovulation that evaluates the cervical mucus, the number of active sperm in the cervical mucus, and the length of sperm survival (in hours) after intercourse. Also called the *postcoital test.*

Human chorionic gonadotropin (hCG) A hormone produced by the chorionic villi and found in the urine of pregnant women. Also called *prolan.*

Human immunodeficiency virus (HIV) A virus that causes a progressive disease that ultimately results in the development of acquired immunodeficiency syndrome (AIDS).

Hydatidiform mole Degenerative process in chorionic villi, giving rise to multiple cysts and rapid growth of the uterus, with hemorrhage.

Hydramnios An excess of amniotic fluid, leading to overdistension of the uterus. Frequently seen in diabetic pregnant women, even if there is no coexisting fetal anomaly. Also called *polyhydramnios.*

Hydronephrosis Collection of urine in the renal pelvis as a result of obstructed outflow.

Hydrops fetalis Hemolytic disease of the newborn characterized by anemia, jaundice, enlargement of the liver and spleen, and generalized edema. Caused by isoimmunization due to Rh incompatibility or ABO incompatibility. See *Erythroblastosis fetalis.*

Hyperbilirubinemia Excessive amount of bilirubin in the blood; indicative of hemolytic processes due to blood incompatibility, intrauterine infection, septicemia, neonatal renal infection, and other disorders.

Hypercapnia Greater than normal amounts of carbon dioxide in the blood.

Hyperemesis gravidarum Excessive vomiting during pregnancy, leading to dehydration and starvation.

Hyperinsulinemia Elevated insulin levels in the blood.

Hypersensitivity response An overreaction of the immune system, responsible for allergic reactions.

Hypersplenism A syndrome characterized by splenomegaly and blood cell deficiencies.

Hypertelorism Widely spaced eyes.

Hypertonic dehydration (or hypernatremic dehydration) Sodium loss that is proportionately greater than water loss.

Hypertonic saline A solution that is more concentrated than body fluid. Used to rapidly increase body fluid concentration, but it must be monitored carefully because it can easily cause rebound hypernatremia.

Hypoglycemia Abnormally low level of sugar in the blood.

Hypotonic dehydration (or hyponatremic dehydration) Fluid loss characterized by a proportionately greater loss of sodium than water.

Hypotonic fluid Fluid that is more dilute than normal body fluid.

Hypoxemia Lower than normal amounts of oxygen in the blood.

Hypoxia Lower than normal amounts of oxygen in the tissues.

Hysterectomy Surgical removal of the uterus.

Hysterosalpingography (HSG) Testing by instillation of radiopaque substance into the uterine cavity to visualize the uterus and fallopian tubes.

I

Immunodeficiency A state of the immune system in which it cannot cope effectively with foreign antigens.

Immunoglobulin A protein that functions as an antibody. Immunoglobulins are responsible for humoral immunity.

In vitro fertilization (IVF) Procedure during which oocytes are removed from the ovary, mixed with spermatozoa, fertilized, and incubated in a glass petri dish; then up to four viable embryos are placed in the woman's uterus.

Inborn errors of metabolism Hereditary deficiencies of a specific enzyme needed for normal metabolism of specific chemicals.

Incarceration Occurs when the presence of intestine in the groin causes constriction of the blood supply to the scrotal sac, leading to intestinal strangulation and testicular ischemia.

Incest Sexual activity between family members close enough that marriage between them would be legally or culturally prohibited.

Incompetent cervix The premature dilatation of the cervix, usually in the second trimester of pregnancy.

Incubation period The time interval between infection exposure and development of symptoms.

Indirect transmission The passage of an infectious disease involving survival of pathogens outside humans before they invade a new host.

Individualized approach An assessment approach that involves measuring individual children seen in a clinic, to share results with the family, and address appropriate teaching about weight control and nutritious intake.

Individualized education plan (IEP) Formulation of a specific learning approach for a child with a physical or mental handicap, following thorough assessment of the child's capabilities and areas of need.

Individualized family service plan (IFSP) A form of education planning/intervention that is developed for early intervention with infants with special healthcare needs and their families. The IFSP contains information about the services required to support a child's development and enhance the family's capacity to facilitate the child's development. The family and education service providers work as a team to plan, implement, and evaluate services specific to the family's unique concerns, priorities, and resources.

Individualized health plan A formal mechanism to ensure that the child's health needs are managed in the school setting.

Individualized transition plan A plan that focuses on assisting the individual in moving successfully from school into the community.

Infant mortality rate Number of deaths of infants under 1 year of age per 1000 live births in a given population per year.

Infant of a diabetic mother (IDM) At-risk infant born to a woman previously diagnosed as diabetic or who develops symptoms of diabetes during pregnancy.

Infant of a substance-abusing mother (ISAM) Formerly called *infant of an addicted mother.* An infant who is born to a mother who abuses or is addicted to drugs or alcohol.

Infectious disease Illness, caused by a microorganism, that is commonly communicated from one host (human or otherwise) to another.

Infertility Diminished ability to conceive.

Informed consent A legal concept that protects a person's rights to autonomy and self-determination by specifying that no action may be taken without that person's prior understanding and freely given consent.

Infundibulopelvic ligament The ligament that suspends and supports the ovaries. It arises from the outer third of the broad ligament and contains the ovarian vessels and nerves.

Insensible water loss Water loss not directly measurable or observable, such as through skin and respirations.

Inspection The technique of purposeful observation by carefully looking at the characteristics of the child's physical features and behaviors. Physical feature characteristics include size, shape, color, movement, position, and location.

Insulin deficiency A condition in which the pancreas does not produce sufficient insulin (as in type 1 diabetes).

Insulin resistance An alteration of the insulin receptor that signals the presence of insulin in the interior of cells.

Intellectual disability Significant limitation in intellectual functioning and adaptive behavior, manifested by differences in conceptual, social, and practical adaptive skills, beginning before the age of 18 years.

Intensity The strength of a uterine contraction during acme.

Interstitial fluid That portion of the extracellular fluid that is between the cells and outside the blood and lymphatic vessels.

Intertriginous (areas) Skin folds of the neck, axillae, and antecubital fossa.

Intimate partner violence A pattern of coercive behavior and methods used to exert power and control by one individual over another in an adult domestic or intimate relationship. Also known as *domestic violence.*

Intracellular fluid The fluid in the body that is inside the cells.

Intracranial pressure Force exerted by brain tissue, cerebrospinal fluid, and blood within the cranial vault.

Intractable seizure Seizures that continue to occur even with optimal medical management.

Intrapartum The time from the onset of true labor until the birth of the infant and delivery of the placenta.

Intrathecal A method of drug or medication delivery in which the drug is introduced into the spinal canal.

Intrauterine device (IUD) Small metal or plastic form that is placed in the uterus to prevent implantation of a fertilized ovum.

Intrauterine drug-exposed infants Infants whose mothers used marijuana, alcohol, nicotine or illicit drugs while pregnant.

Intrauterine fetal surgery Surgery performed on a fetus to correct anatomic lesions that are not compatible with life if left untreated.

Intrauterine growth restriction (IUGR) Fetal undergrowth due to any etiology, such as intrauterine infection, deficient nutrient supply, or congenital malformation. A term used to describe fetuses falling below the 10th percentile in ultrasonic estimation of weight at a given gestational age. Formerly called *intrauterine growth retardation.*

Intrauterine pressure catheter A catheter that can be placed through the cervix into the uterus to measure uterine pressure during labor. Some types of catheters may be inserted for the purpose of infusing warmed saline to add additional intrauterine fluid when oligohydramnios is present.

Intrauterine resuscitation Corrective measures used to optimize the oxygen exchange within the maternal-fetal circulation.

Intravascular fluid That portion of the extracellular fluid that is in the blood vessels.

Involution Rolling or turning inward; the reduction in size of the uterus following childbirth.

Ischial spines Prominences that arise near the junction of the ilium and ischium and jut into the pelvic cavity; used as a reference point during labor to evaluate the descent of the fetal head into the birth canal.

Isotonic dehydration (or isonatremic dehydration) Fluid loss that is not balanced by intake; the loss of water and sodium are in proportion.

Isotonic fluid Fluid that has the same osmolality as normal body fluid.

Isthmus The straight, narrow part of the fallopian tube with a thick muscular wall and an opening (lumen) 2–3 mm in diameter; the site of tubal ligation. Also, a constriction in the uterus that is located above the cervix and below the corpus.

J

Jaundice Yellow pigmentation of body tissues caused by the presence of bile pigments. See also *Physiologic jaundice.*

K

Karyotype The set of chromosomes arranged in a standard order.

Kegel exercises Perineal muscle tightening that strengthens the pubococcygeus muscle and increases its tone.

Keloid Overdevelopment or hypertrophy of scar that extends beyond wound edges and above skin line due to excess collagen.

Kerion A large tender boggy mass on scalp with drainage associated with tinea capitis.

Kernicterus The yellow staining and degenerative lesions in basal ganglia associated with high levels of unconjugated bilirubin in infants. Also known as *bilirubin encephalopathy.*

Killed virus vaccine A vaccine that contains a killed microorganism that is still capable of inducing the human body to produce antibodies to the disease.

Kilocalorie Equivalent to 1000 calories, it is the unit used to express the energy value of food.

Kinesthesia The sense of one's body position and movement.

Kussmaul respirations Increased rate and depth of respirations (hyperventilation).

L

La Leche League International A nonprofit organization that promotes breastfeeding and provides information on and assistance with breastfeeding.

Labor induction The stimulation of uterine contractions before the spontaneous onset of labor, with or without ruptured fetal membranes, for the purpose of accomplishing birth.

Lactase deficiency (lactose intolerance) A condition characterized by difficulty digesting milk and dairy products, results from an inadequate amount of the enzyme lactase, which breaks down the milk sugar lactose into smaller digestible substances.

Lacto-ovo-vegetarians Vegetarians who include milk, dairy products, and eggs in their diets and occasionally fish, poultry, and liver.

Lactovegetarians Vegetarians who include dairy products but no eggs in their diets.

Lamellar body count (LBC) A fetal test to predict or establish the presence of fetal lung maturity.

Lanugo Fine, downy hair found on all body parts of the fetus, with the exception of the palms of the hands and the soles of the feet, after 20 weeks' gestation.

Laparoscopy Procedure that enables direct visualization of pelvic organs.

Large for gestational age (LGA) Excessive growth of a fetus in relation to the gestational time period.

Laryngospasm Spasmodic vibrations of the larynx, which create sudden, violent, unpredictable, involuntary contraction of airway muscles.

Late adolescence Refers to adolescents who are ages 18 to 19 years.

Late deceleration Symmetrical decrease in fetal heart rate beginning at or after the peak of the contraction and returning to baseline only after the contraction has ended, indicating possible uteroplacental insufficiency and potential that the fetus is not receiving adequate oxygenation.

Late (secondary) postpartal hemorrhage A loss of blood of greater than 500 mL following birth. The hemorrhage is classified as late if it occurs from 24 hours to 6 weeks after birth.

Late preterm infant Infants born between 34 and 37 weeks. These infants are at a greater risk for increases in mortality and morbidity because they are physically not mature and are more prone to have physiological and metabolic complications.

Lecithin/sphingomyelin ratio (L/S ratio) Lecithin and sphingomyelin are phospholipid components of surfactant; their ratio changes during gestation. When the L/S ratio reaches 2:1, the fetal lungs are thought to be mature and the fetus will have a low risk of respiratory distress syndrome (RDS) if born at that time.

Leopold's maneuvers A series of four maneuvers designed to provide a systematic approach whereby the examiner may determine fetal presentation and position.

Lesbian An adjective used to describe or refer to a homosexual woman.

Let-down reflex Pattern of stimulation, hormone release, and resulting muscle contraction that forces milk into the lactiferous ducts, making it available to the infant. Also called *milk ejection reflex.*

Leukocytosis A higher than normal leukocyte count.

Leukopenia A lower than normal white blood cell count.

Leukorrhea Mucous discharge from the vagina or cervical canal that may be normal or pathologic, as in the presence of infection.

Level of consciousness General description of cognitive, sensory, and motor response to stimuli.

Lichenification Thickening of the skin.

Life-threatening condition A condition in which considerable likelihood of death may occur even though treatment may prolong the child's life or the child may have a complete recovery from the illness or injury.

Light sleep State that makes up the highest proportion of newborn sleep and precedes awakening; characterized by some body movements, rapid eye movements (REM), and brief fussing or crying.

Lightening Moving of the fetus and uterus downward into the pelvic cavity.

Linea nigra The line of darker pigmentation extending from the umbilicus to the pubis noted in some women during the later months of pregnancy.

Live virus vaccine A vaccine that contains the microorganism in a live but attenuated, or weakened, form.

Local infiltration anesthesia Anesthesia accomplished by injecting an anesthetic agent into the intracutaneous, subcutaneous, and intramuscular areas of the perineum. Generally used at the time of birth, both in preparation for an episiotomy if one is needed and for the episiotomy repair.

Lochia Maternal discharge of blood, mucus, and tissue from the uterus; may last for several weeks after birth.

Lochia alba White vaginal discharge that follows lochia serosa and that lasts from about the 10th to the 21st day after birth.

Lochia rubra Red, blood-tinged vaginal discharge that occurs following birth and lasts 2 to 4 days.

Lochia serosa Pink, serous, and blood-tinged vaginal discharge that follows lochia rubra and lasts until the 7th to 10th day after birth.

Luteinizing hormone (LH) Anterior pituitary hormone responsible for stimulating ovulation and for development of the corpus luteum.

M

Macronutrients The major building blocks of the body: carbohydrates, protein, and fat.

Macrosomia A condition seen in neonates of large body size and high birth weight (more than 4000–4500 grams [8 lb/13 oz – 9 lb/4 oz]), such as those born of prediabetic and diabetic mothers.

Malignant The progressive growth of a tumor that will, if not checked by treatment, result in death.

Malpresentations Presentations of the fetus into the birth canal that are not "normal"—that is, brow, face, shoulder, or breech presentation.

Mammogram A soft tissue radiograph of the breast without the injection of a contrast medium.

Mastitis Inflammation of the breast.

Maternal-child nursing Care of women during pregnancy, birth, and postpartum, as well as the care of infants, children, and adolescents.

Maternal mortality rate The number of maternal deaths from any cause during the pregnancy cycle per 100,000 live births.

Mature milk Breast milk that contains 10% solids for energy and growth.

Mature minors Adolescents of 14 and 15 years of age who are able to understand treatment risks and who in some states can consent to or refuse treatment.

McDonald's sign A probable sign of pregnancy characterized by an ease in flexing the body of the uterus against the cervix.

Meconium Dark green or black material present in the large intestine of a full-term infant; the first stools passed by the newborn.

Meconium aspiration syndrome (MAS) Respiratory disease of term, postterm, and SGA newborns caused by inhalation of meconium or meconium-stained amniotic fluid into the lungs; characterized by mild to severe respiratory distress, hyperexpansion of the chest, hyperinflated alveoli, and secondary atelectasis.

Medically fragile Children who need skilled nursing care with or without medical equipment to support vital functions.

Meiosis The process of cell division that occurs in the maturation of sperm and ova that decreases their number of chromosomes by one-half.

Melanin Skin pigment.

Mendelian (single-gene) inheritance A major category of inheritance whereby a trait is determined by a pair of genes on homologous chromosomes. Also called single *gene inheritance.*

Menopause The permanent cessation of menses.

Menorrhagia Increased menstrual bleeding.

Mental health Foundational to a sense of personal well-being, it involves successful engagement in activities and relationships and the ability to adapt and cope with change.

Mesoderm The intermediate layer of germ cells in the embryo that gives rise to connective tissue, bone marrow, muscles, blood, lymphoid tissue, and epithelial tissue.

Metastasis The spread of cancer cells to other sites in the body.

Microcephaly A small brain with a head circumference below the third percentile on growth curves.

Micronutrients Substances needed in small quantities for healthy body functioning; vitamins and minerals are micronutrients.

Middle adolescence Refers to adolescents who are ages 15 to 17 years.

Milia Tiny white papules appearing on the face of a neonate as a result of unopened sebaceous glands; they disappear spontaneously within a few weeks.

Miscarriage Abortion that occurs naturally. Also called *miscarriage.*

Mitosis Process of cell division whereby both daughter cells have the same number and pattern of chromosomes as the original cell.

Mixed hearing loss Hearing loss having a combination of conductive and sensorineural causes.

Modeling Exhibiting appropriate behavior for someone else.

Moderate sedation A lower sedative dose that enables the child to maintain protective reflexes, independently and continuously maintain a patent airway, and make an appropriate response to physical stimuli or verbal command.

Molding Shaping of the fetal head by overlapping of the cranial bones to facilitate movement through the birth canal during labor.

Mongolian spots Macular areas of bluish black or gray-blue pigmentation on the dorsal area and the buttocks that are common in newborns of Asian, Hispanic, and African descent and other dark-skin races. They gradually fade during the first or second year of life.

Monosomies Genetic condition that occurs when a normal gamete unites with a gamete that is missing a chromosome.

Morning sickness A term that refers to the nausea and vomiting that a woman may experience in early pregnancy. This lay term is sometimes used because these symptoms frequently occur in the early part of the day and disappear within a few hours.

Moro reflex Flexion of the newborn's thighs and knees accompanied by fingers that fan, then clench, as the arms are simultaneously thrown out and then brought together, as though embracing something. This reflex can be elicited by startling the newborn with a sudden noise or movement. Also called the *startle reflex.*

Morula Developmental stage of the fertilized ovum in which there is a solid mass of cells.

Mosaicism Condition of an individual who has at least two cell lines with differing karyotypes.

Mother-baby care A type of family health care that is focused on keeping the mother and baby together as much as the mother desires. Also known as *couplet care,* it provides increased opportunities for parent-child interaction because the newborn shares the mother's room and they are cared for together. Mother-baby care enables the mother to have time to bond with her baby and learn to care for her or him in a supportive environment.

Mottling Discoloration of the skin in irregular areas; may be seen with chilling, poor perfusion, or hypoxia.

Mucous plug A collection of thick mucus that blocks the cervical canal during pregnancy. Also called *operculum.*

Multigravida Woman who has been pregnant more than once.

Multipara Woman who has had more than one pregnancy in which the fetus was viable.

Myelinization Establishment of the myelin or fatty sheath on nerve fibers.

Myelodysplasia Any malformation of the spinal cord and spinal canal.

Myelosuppression A decreased production of blood cells in the bone marrow.

Myometrium Uterine muscular structure.

Myringotomy A procedure whereby an incision is made in the tympanic membrane to drain fluid.

N

Nadir The lowest point.

Nägele's rule A method of determining the estimated date of birth (EDB): after obtaining the first day of the last menstrual period, subtract 3 months and add 7 days.

Nasal flaring A sign of respiratory distress; an effort the child makes to widen the airway.

Natural immunity The defenses present at birth, such as intact skin, body pH, natural antibodies from the mother, and inflammatory and phagocytic properties.

Nature The genetic or hereditary capability of an individual.

Neonatal mortality risk The infant's chance of death within the newborn period—that is, within the first 28 days of life.

Neonatal transition The first few hours of life, in which the newborn stabilizes its respiratory and circulatory functions.

Neoplasms Cancerous growths.

Neurogenic bladder The result of urinary tract obstruction related to an interrupted nerve supply to the bladder.

Neuropathic pain A form of chronic pain, initiated or caused by a primary lesion or dysfunction of the nervous system.

Neutral thermal environment (NTE) An environment that provides for minimal heat loss or expenditure.

Neutropenia A low neutrophil count.

Nevus flammeus (port-wine stain) Large port-wine stain.

Nevus vasculosus (strawberry mark) Strawberry mark: raised, clearly delineated, dark-red, rough-surfaced birthmark commonly found in the head region.

New Ballard Score A postnatal gestational age assessment tool that is used within 12 hours of birth.

Newborn screening tests Tests that detect inborn errors of metabolism that, if left untreated, cause mental retardation and physical handicaps.

Nidation Implantation of a fertilized ovum in the endometrium.

Nightmares Frightening dreams that awaken the child, who is often crying and upset.

Night terrors (or sleep terrors) A situation in which the child cries out and appears frightened while sleeping, but in contrast to nightmares, the child having a night terror is not fully awake and may appear disoriented.

Nipple A protrusion about 0.5 to 1.3 cm in diameter in the center of each mature breast.

Nonmendelian (multifactorial) inheritance The occurrence of congenital disorders that result from an interaction of multiple genetic and environmental factors.

Nonsteroidal antiinflammatory drugs (NSAIDs) Drugs, used for the treatment of pain.

Nonstress test (NST) An assessment method by which the reaction (or response) of the fetal heart rate to fetal movement is evaluated.

Nosocomial infection An infection acquired in a health care agency, not present at the time of entrance to the agency.

Nuchal translucency testing A genetic screening test that uses ultrasound to scan the translucent or clear area on the back of the fetal neck, measuring the diameter of the area. Fetuses that have a nuchal translucency measurement of greater than 3 mm are at risk for trisomies 13, 18, and 21 and the mother should be offered an amniocentesis.

Nulligravida A woman who has never been pregnant.

Nullipara A woman who has not delivered a viable fetus.

Nurse researcher A nurse with an advanced doctoral degree (typically a Ph.D.) who assumes a leadership role in generating new research.

Nurture The effects of environment on an individual's performance.

Nutrition Taking in food and assimilating it metabolically for use by the body.

O

Object permanence The knowledge that an object or person continues to exist when not seen, heard, or felt.

Obstetric conjugate Distance from the middle of the sacral promontory to an area approximately 1 cm below the pubic crest.

Occult blood Blood that is present in minute quantities and can be seen only on microscopic examination or through chemical testing.

Oligohydramnios Decreased amount of amniotic fluid, which may indicate a fetal urinary tract defect.

Oliguria Diminished urine output (less than 0.5–1 mL/kg/hr).

Oncogene A portion of the DNA that is altered and, when duplicated, causes uncontrolled cellular division.

Oncotic pressure The part of the blood osmotic pressure that is due to plasma proteins; also called *blood colloid osmotic pressure.*

Opioids Synthetic narcotic drugs used for the treatment of pain.

Opisthotonos Rigid hyperextension of the entire body.

Opportunistic infection An infection that is often caused by normally nonpathogenic organisms in persons who lack normal immunity.

Orientation Infant's ability to respond to auditory and visual stimuli in the environment.

Ortolani's maneuver A manual procedure performed to rule out the possibility of developmental dysplastic hip.

Osmolality The amount of concentration of a fluid; technically, the number of moles of particles per kilogram of water in the solution.

Osmosis Movement of water across a semipermeable membrane into an area of higher particle concentration.

Ossification Formation of bone from fibrous tissue or cartilage.

Osteodystrophy Defective mineralization of bone caused by renal failure and chronic hyperphosphatemia.

Osteoporosis A condition, more common in postmenopausal women, that is characterized by decreased bone strength related to diminished bone density and bone quality. Thought to be associated with lowered estrogen and androgen levels, osteoporosis puts an individual at increased risk for fractures of the hip, forearm, and vertebrae.

Osteotomy Surgical cutting of bone.

Ostomy An artificial abdominal opening into the urinary or gastrointestinal canal that provides an outlet for the diversion of urine or fecal matter.

Outcome expectancy What the person expects to get from performing a certain behavior.

Ovarian ligaments Ligaments that anchor the lower pole of the ovary to the cornua of the uterus. They are surrounded by muscle fibers that allow the ligaments to contract.

Ovaries The pair of almond-shaped female reproductive organs that contain the ova. The two structures lie just below the pelvic brim. One ovary is located on each side of the pelvic cavity.

Ovulation Normal process of discharging a mature ovum from an ovary approximately 14 days prior to the onset of menses.

Oxytocin Hormone normally produced by the posterior pituitary, responsible for stimulation of uterine contractions and the release of milk into the lactiferous ducts.

P

Pain An unpleasant sensory and emotional experience associated with actual or potential tissue damage. Pain exists when the patient says it does.

Palliative care Active and compassionate therapies intended to comfort and support those with short life expectancies.

Palliative procedure Intervention used to preserve life in children with a potentially fatal or lethal condition.

Palpation The technique of touch to identify characteristics of the skin, internal organs, and masses. Characteristics include texture, moistness, tenderness, temperature, position, shape, consistency, and mobility of masses and organs.

Pancytopenia A decreased number of blood cell components.

Para A woman who has borne offspring who reached the age of viability.

Paradox breathing Severe respiratory distress in which the chest falls and the abdomen rises on inspiration.

Parallel play A type of play that emerges in toddlerhood when children play side by side with similar or different toys, demonstrating little or no social interaction.

Parenteral Nutrition introduced outside of the intestinal tract, usually by the intravenous route.

Parent-newborn attachment Close affectional ties that develop between parent and child. See also *Attachment.*

Partnership A relationship in which participants join together to ensure healthcare delivery in a way that recognizes the critical role and contribution of each partner in promoting health, preventing illness, and managing healthcare conditions.

Passive acquired immunity Transfer of antibodies (IgG) from the mother to the fetus in utero.

Passive immunity Immunity produced through introduction of specific antibodies to the disease, which are usually obtained from the blood or serum of immune persons and animals. Does not confer lasting immunity.

Patient-controlled analgesia (PCA) A method of pain control where anesthesia, usually morphine or meperidine, is initially administered by the anesthesiologist and subsequent doses are self-administered by pushing a button controlled by a special IV pump system.

Pediatric healthcare home The site of comprehensive, continuous, culturally sensitive, coordinated, and compassionate healthcare by a pediatric healthcare professional focused on the overall well-being of children and families.

Pedigree Graphic representation of a family tree.

Pelvic cavity The lower portion of the abdominopelvic cavity that contains the urinary bladder, the rectum, and internal parts of the reproductive system. The pelvic cavity is divided into the false pelvis and the true pelvis.

Pelvic cellulitis (parametritis) Inflammation of the parametrial layer of the uterus.

Pelvic diaphragm Part of the pelvic floor composed of deep fascia and the levator ani and the coccygeal muscles.

Pelvic inflammatory disease (PID) An infection of the fallopian tubes that may or may not be accompanied by a pelvic abscess; may cause infertility secondary to tubal damage.

Pelvic inlet Upper border of the true pelvis.

Pelvic outlet Lower border of the true pelvis.

Pelvic tilt Also called *pelvic rocking;* exercise designed to reduce back strain and strengthen abdominal muscle tone.

Percussion The technique of striking the surface of the body, either directly or indirectly, to set up vibrations that reveal the density of underlying tissues and borders of internal organs.

Perimenopause Refers to the period of time prior to menopause during which the woman moves from normal ovulatory cycles to cessation of menses.

Perimetrium The outermost layer of the corpus of the uterus. Also known as the *serosal layer.*

Perinatal loss Death of a fetus or infant from the time of conception through the end of the newborn period 28 days after birth.

Perineal body Wedge-shaped mass of fibromuscular tissue found between the lower part of the vagina and the anal canal.

Periodic breathing Sporadic episodes of apnea, not associated with cyanosis, that last for about 10 seconds and commonly occur in preterm infants.

Periods of reactivity Predictable patterns of neonate behavior during the first several hours after birth.

Peristalsis A progressive, wavelike muscular movement that occurs involuntarily throughout the gastrointestinal tract.

Peritonitis Infection involving the peritoneal cavity.

Persistent occiput posterior position (POP position) Malposition of the fetus in which the fetal occiput is posterior in the maternal pelvis.

Pervasive developmental disorders Conditions that begin in early childhood and are characterized by impaired social interactions and communication, with restricted interests, activities, and behaviors.

Petechiae Pinpoint red lesions.

pH Negative logarithm of the hydrogen ion concentration; used to monitor the acidity of body fluid.

Phenotype The whole physical, biochemical, and physiologic makeup of an individual as determined both genetically and environmentally.

Phosphatidylglycerol (PG) A phospholipid in surfactant that appears when fetal lung maturity has been attained, at about 35 weeks' gestation. Because PG is not present in blood or vaginal fluids, its presence is reliable in predicting fetal lung maturity.

Phototherapy The treatment of jaundice by exposure to light.

Phototoxic A rapid nonimmunologic reaction of the skin when exposed to sunlight.

Physical abuse The deliberate maltreatment of another individual that inflicts pain or injury and may result in permanent or temporary disfigurement or even death.

Physical dependence The physiologic adaptation to an analgesic or sedative drug at the peripheral and central neurons.

Physical neglect The deliberate withholding of or failure to provide the necessary and available resources to a child.

Physiologic anemia of infancy A harmless condition in which the hemoglobin level drops in the first 6 to 12 weeks after birth, then reverts to normal levels.

Physiologic anemia of pregnancy Apparent anemia that results because during pregnancy the plasma volume increases more than the erythrocytes increase.

Physiologic anorexia A decrease in appetite manifested when the extremely high metabolic demands of infancy slow to keep pace with the more moderate growth rate of toddlerhood.

Physiologic jaundice A harmless condition caused by the normal reduction of red blood cells, occurring 48 or more hours after birth, peaking at the 5th to 7th day, and disappearing between the 7th and 10th day.

Pica The eating of substances not ordinarily considered edible or to have nutritive value.

Pitting edema A "pit" or concave indentation that remains after an edematous area is pressed downward by the examiner's fingers.

Placenta Specialized disk-shaped organ that connects the fetus to the uterine wall for gas and nutrient exchange. Also called *afterbirth.*

Placenta previa Abnormal implantation of the placenta in the lower uterine segment. Classification of type is based on proximity to the cervical os: total—completely covers the os; partial—covers a portion of the os; marginal—is in close proximity to the os.

Play therapy A therapeutic intervention often used with preschool and school-aged children. The child reveals conflicts, wishes, and fears on an unconscious level while playing with dolls, toys, clay, and other objects.

Podalic version Type of version used to turn a second twin during a vaginal birth.

Polycystic ovarian syndrome (PCOS) A complex endocrine disorder of ovarian dysfunction that is evidenced by amenorrhea or oligomenorrhea and clinical signs of androgen excess (typically hirsutism, acne) in the absence of other conditions that might have these same signs and symptoms.

Polycythemia An abnormal increase in the number of total red blood cells in the body's circulation.

Polydipsia Excessive thirst.

Polyphagia Excessive or voracious eating.

Polypharmacy A term used to describe the act of taking multiple drugs to treat symptoms, when the etiology of the symptoms is actually a side effect from one or more prescribed medications.

Polysomnography A sleep study that simultaneously records the brain activity, eye movement, and respiration.

Polyuria Passage of a large volume of urine in a given period.

Population-based approach Health assessment and intervention performed with a group of children.

Postcoital test A test performed 1 or 2 days before the expected date of ovulation that evaluates the cervical mucus, the number of active sperm in the cervical mucus, and the length of sperm survival (in hours) after intercourse. Also called the *Huhner test.*

Postconception age periods Period of time in embryonic/fetal development calculated from the time of fertilization of the ovum.

Postictal period Period after seizure activity during which the level of consciousness is decreased.

Postmaturity See *Postterm newborn.*

Postpartal home care Focused more on assessment, teaching, facilitating learning, and counseling than on physical care.

Postpartum Describing the period after giving birth.

Postpartum blues (adjustment reaction with depressed mood) A maternal adjustment reaction occurring in the first few postpartal days, characterized by mild depression, tearfulness, anxiety, headache, and irritability.

Postpartum major mood disorder (postpartum depression) Depression that the mother experiences after birth of a child. The periods of greatest risk occur around the fourth week, just before the initiation of menses, and upon weaning.

Postpartum psychosis Psychosis that the mother experiences after birth of a child. Usually becomes evident within the first 1 to 3 months postpartum. Considered an emergency because of the risk of suicide and/or infanticide.

Postterm labor Labor that occurs after 42 weeks' gestation.

Postterm newborn Any infant born after 42 weeks' gestation.

Posturing Abnormal position assumed after injury or damage to the brain that may be seen as extreme flexion or extension of the limbs.

Precipitous birth Labor lasting less than 3 hours.

Precipitous labor Unduly rapid progression of labor.

Preeclampsia Toxemia of pregnancy, characterized by hypertension, albuminuria, and edema. See also *Eclampsia*.

Preload Volume of blood in the ventricle at the end of diastole that stretches the heart muscle before contraction.

Premature rupture of membranes (PROM) Rupture may be PROM (premature), SROM (spontaneous), or AROM (artificial). Some clinicians may use the abbreviation RBOW (rupture of bag of waters).

Premenstrual syndrome (PMS) Cluster of symptoms experienced by some women, typically occurring from a few days up to 2 weeks prior to the onset of menses.

Prenatal education Programs offered to expectant families, adolescents, women, or partners to provide education regarding the pregnancy, labor, and birth experience.

Presenting part The fetal part present in or on the cervical os.

Preterm infant Any infant born before 38 weeks' gestation.

Preterm labor (PTL) Labor occurring between 20 and 38 weeks of pregnancy. Also called *premature labor*.

Primary immune response The process in which B lymphocytes produce antibodies specific to a particular antigen on first exposure.

Primary immunodeficiency Congenital immunodeficiency.

Primigravida A woman who is pregnant for the first time.

Primipara A woman who has given birth to her first child (past the point of viability), whether or not that child is living or was alive at birth.

Probiotics Live microorganisms thought to provide a health benefit.

Prodrome The phase of early manifestations of the infection until the development of the overt clinical syndrome.

Progesterone A hormone produced by the corpus luteum, adrenal cortex, and placenta whose function is to stimulate proliferation of the endometrium to facilitate growth of the embryo.

Projectile vomiting Vomiting in which the stomach contents are ejected with great force.

Prolactin A hormone secreted by the anterior pituitary that stimulates and sustains lactation in mammals.

Prolapsed umbilical cord Umbilical cord that becomes trapped in the vagina before the fetus is born.

Prolonged (postterm) pregnancy A pregnancy that extends more than 294 days or 42 weeks past the first day of the last menstrual period (LMP). Distinct from *postdate* pregnancy, in which the pregnancy has gone beyond the estimated date of birth (EDB) at 40 weeks.

Prostaglandins (PGs) Complex lipid compounds synthesized by many cells in the body.

Prostration Extreme exhaustion.

Protective factors Characteristics of a child and family that provide strength and assistance in dealing with a crisis.

Protocol A plan of action for chemotherapy that is based on the type of cancer, its stage, and the particular cell type.

Proto-oncogene A gene that regulates cellular growth and development but can become an oncogene, capable of causing cancerous growth.

Proximodistal development The process by which development proceeds from the center of the body outward to the extremities.

Pseudohermaphroditism Ambiguous development of the external genitalia.

Pseudohypertrophy Enlargement of the muscles as a result of infiltration by fatty tissue.

Pseudomenstruation In female infants, in the first weeks of life, a vaginal discharge composed of thick, whitish mucus that can become tinged with blood; caused by the withdrawal of maternal hormones.

Ptyalism Excessive salivation.

Puberty The developmental period between childhood and attainment of adult sexual characteristics and functioning.

Pubis Pertaining to the pubes or pubic area.

Pudendal block Injection of an anesthetizing agent at the pudendal nerve to produce numbness of the external genitals and the lower one-third of the vagina, to facilitate childbirth and permit episiotomy if necessary.

Puerperal infection Infection of the reproductive tract associated with childbirth and occurs any time up to 6 weeks postpartum.

Puerperal morbidity A maternal temperature of 38 degrees C (100.4 degrees F) or higher on any 2 of the first 10 postpartal days, excluding the first 24 hours. The temperature is to be taken by mouth at least four times per day.

Puerperium The period after completion of the third stage of labor until involution of the uterus is complete, usually 6 weeks.

Purpura Bleeding into the tissues, particularly beneath the skin and mucous membranes, causing lesions that vary from red to purple.

Pyeloplasty Removal of an obstructed segment of the ureter and reimplantation into the renal pelvis.

Q

Quadruple screen Prenatal test of amniotic fluid or blood that assesses for appropriate levels of alpha-fetoprotein (AFP), human chorionic gonadotropin (hCG), unconjugated estriol (UE3), and the substance dimeric inhibin-A. It is used to screen for Down syndrome (trisomy 21), trisomy 18, and neural tube defects (NTDs). A more sensitive and accurate detector of trisomy 21 than the triple screen.

Quickening The first fetal movements felt by the pregnant woman, usually between 16 and 18 weeks' gestation.

Quiet alert (state) An alert state characterized by a brightening of the eyes and face. Infants are most attentive to their environment in this state and provide positive feedback to caregivers.

R

Race A group of people who share biologic similarities such as skin color, bone structure, and genetic traits. Examples of races include white (sometimes called Caucasian or European American), black (sometimes called African American in the United States), Hispanic, Natives (such as Native Americans, Alaskan Native, Hawaiian Native, and First Nation people of Canada), and Asian.

Radiation Heat loss incurred when heat transfers to cooler surfaces and objects not in direct contact with the body.

Radioallergosorbent test (RAST) A technique in which radioimmunoassay is used to measure the presence in the blood of IgE antibodies to certain antigens.

Radiofrequency ablation The use of radio energy to destroy a very small section of the myocardium through which an accessory conduction pathway passes.

Rape Sexual activity, often intercourse, against the will of the victim.

Reciprocity An interactional cycle that occurs simultaneously between mother and infant. It involves mutual cuing behaviors, expectancy, rhythmicity, and synchrony.

Recombinant form An organism has been genetically altered for use in vaccines.

Rectocele A condition that results when the posterior vaginal wall is weakened. The anterior wall of the rectum can then sag forward, ballooning into the vagina, pushing the weakened posterior wall of the vagina in front of it.

Regional analgesia The temporary and reversible loss of sensation produced by injecting an anesthetic agent (called a local anesthetic) into an area that will bring the agent into direct contact with nervous tissue.

Regional anesthesia Injection of local anesthetic agents so that they come into direct contact with nervous tissue.

Regression Return to an earlier behavior. A defense mechanism often displayed by children with life-threatening or mortal illness, regression is a common reaction to stress.

Rehabilitation Assisting a child with physical or mental challenges to reach his or her fullest potential through therapy and education that considers the physiologic, psychologic, and environmental strengths and limitations of the child.

Renal insufficiency Any degree of renal failure in which the kidneys' ability to conserve sodium and concentrate the urine decreases.

Repression Involuntary forgetting. A defense mechanism often displayed by children with life-threatening or mortal illness.

Resilience The ability to function with healthy responses, even with significant stress and adversity.

Resiliency theory An assessment theory that holds that all individuals experience crises that lead to adaptation and development of inner strengths and the ability to handle future crises.

Respiratory distress syndrome (RDS) Respiratory disease of the newborn characterized by interference with ventilation at the alveolar level, thought to be caused by the presence of fibrinoid deposits lining the alveolar ducts. Formerly called *hyaline membrane disease.*

Respite care Short-term home care to relieve the primary caregiver and allow time away from home.

Retained placenta Retention of the placenta beyond 30 minutes after birth.

Retractions A visible drawing in of the skin of the neck and chest, which occurs on inhalation in infants and young children in respiratory distress.

Rh immune globulin (RhoGAM) An anti-Rh (D) gamma globulin given after delivery to an Rh-negative mother of an Rh-positive fetus or child. Prevents the development of permanent active immunity to the Rh antigen.

Risk factors Any findings that suggest the pregnancy may have a negative outcome, for either the woman or her unborn child.

Rooming-in Practice in which parents stay in the child's hospital room and care for the child.

Rooting reflex An infant's tendency to turn the head and open the lips to suck when one side of the mouth or cheek is touched.

Round ligaments Ligaments that arise from the sides of the uterus near the fallopian tube insertions. They extend outward between the folds of the broad ligament, passing through the inguinal ring and canals and eventually fusing with the connective tissue of the labia majora.

S

Sacral promontory A projection into the pelvic cavity on the anterior upper portion of the sacrum; serves as an obstetric guide in determining pelvic measurements.

Saline A mixture of salt and water; normal saline refers to the mixture of salt and water in equal concentration in body fluids.

Screening Procedures used to detect the presence of a health condition before symptoms are apparent.

Secondary cancers Cancers (most commonly solid tumors) that appear subsequent to the primary cancer and treatment but are of a different histologic type. Also called *second malignant neoplasms* (SMN).

Secondary immune response The body's response to an antigen at any time other than the initial exposure.

Secondary immunodeficiency Acquired immunodeficiency.

Self-concept Evaluation of the self in certain specific areas, such as those related to academic achievement, athletic ability, physical appearance, and social interactions.

Self-efficacy A person's belief that he or she can change behavior to produce a desired outcome.

Self-esteem The feelings and beliefs of children about their competence and worth as individuals, ability to meet challenges, and to learn lessons from success and failure.

Self-quieting ability Infant's ability to use personal resources to quiet and console him- or herself.

Self-regulation The infant's ability to maintain state and self-console, for example by sucking his fingers to stay calm instead of crying.

Sensible water loss Water loss that is measurable and observable, such as urine and drainage from tubes.

Sensorineural hearing loss Hearing loss caused by damage to the inner ear structures or the auditory nerve.

Separation anxiety Distress behaviors observed in young children separated from familiar caregivers.

Sepsis neonatorum Infections experienced by a neonate during the first month of life.

Sexual assault Involuntary sexual contact with another person.

Sexuality A person's view of him- or herself as a sexual being.

Sexually transmitted infection (STI) Refers to an infection ordinarily transmitted by direct sexual contact with an infected individual. Also called *sexually transmitted disease.*

Shaken baby injuries A collection of symptoms that are caused by vigorously shaking an infant. Shaking can cause brain hemorrhage, spinal cord injury, retinal hemorrhage or detachment, long-term developmental problems, mental retardation, or even death.

Shaman In the Native American culture, a man or woman who enters an altered state of consciousness, at will, to contact and utilize another type of reality to acquire knowledge and power and to help other people.

Shock An acute, complex state of circulatory dysfunction resulting in failure to deliver sufficient oxygen and other nutrients to meet cell and tissue demands.

Shunt Movement of blood between heart chambers through an abnormal anatomic or surgically created opening.

Skin turgor Elasticity of skin; provides information on hydration status.

Sleep hygiene Behaviors that foster a regular and sufficient sleep pattern and daytime alertness.

Small for gestational age (SGA) Inadequate weight or growth for gestational age; birth weight below the 10th percentile.

Solitary play When infants play by themselves.

Spermatogenesis The process by which mature spermatozoa are formed, during which the number of chromosomes is halved.

Spermicides A variety of creams, foams, jellies, and suppositories that, when inserted into the vagina prior to intercourse, destroy sperm or neutralize any vaginal secretions and thereby immobilize sperm.

Spinal block Injection of a local anesthetic agent directly into the spinal fluid in the spinal canal to provide anesthesia for vaginal and cesarean births.

Spinnbarkeit The elasticity of the cervical mucus that is present at ovulation.

Spiritual dimension Belief in a connection with a greater power that guides a person to strive for inspiration, respect, meaning, and purpose in life.

Spiritual health The ability to develop a spiritual nature, including awareness of a life purpose and fulfillment.

Spirituality A belief in a transcendent power pertaining to the spirit or soul.

Spontaneous rupture of membranes (SROM) The breaking of the "water" or membranes marked by the expulsion of amniotic fluid from the vagina.

Sprain A tearing of ligaments usually caused when a joint is twisted or otherwise traumatized.

Station Relationship of the presenting fetal part to an imaginary line drawn between the pelvic ischial spines.

Status epilepticus A continuous seizure or recurrent seizures that last for more than 20 minutes without return to baseline.

Stenosis Narrowing of a valve or below the valve, or in the blood vessel.

Stent A device used to maintain patency of the urethral canal after surgery.

Stereotyping The assumption that all members of a culture, ethnic, or racial group are alike and share the same attitudes and beliefs.

Stereotypy Repetitive, obsessive, machine-like movements, commonly seen in autistic or schizophrenic children.

Sterilization An inclusive term that refers to surgical procedures that permanently prevent pregnancy. In the man, sterilization is achieved through a procedure called vasectomy. In the female, sterilization is done by tubal ligation.

Stillbirth The delivery of a dead infant.

Stoma An opening, commonly in the abdominal wall, to provide for drainage from the intestinal or urinary systems.

Stranger anxiety Wariness of strange people and places, often shown by infants between 6 and 18 months of age.

Striae Stretch marks; shiny reddish lines that appear on the abdomen, breasts, thighs, and buttocks of pregnant women as a result of stretching the skin.

Stridor An abnormal, high-pitched musical respiratory sound caused when air moves through a narrowed larynx or trachea.

Subconjunctival hemorrhage Hemorrhage on the sclera of a newborn's eye, usually caused by changes in vascular tension during birth.

Subdermal implants A subdermal progestin contraceptive that is implanted in a woman's arm and provides contraceptive protection for up to 5 years.

Subfertility A couple who have difficulty conceiving because both partners have reduced fertility.

Subinvolution Failure of a part to return to its normal size after functional enlargement, such as failure of the uterus to return to normal size after pregnancy.

Subluxation Partial or complete dislocation of a joint.

Sucking reflex Normal newborn reflex elicited by inserting a finger or nipple in the newborn's mouth, resulting in forceful, rhythmic sucking.

Supine hypotensive syndrome (vena caval syndrome, aortocaval compression) Also called *vena caval syndrome* or *aortocaval compression,* refers to a condition that can develop during pregnancy when the enlarging uterus puts pressure on the vena cava when the woman is supine. This pressure interferes with returning blood flow and produces a marked decrease in blood pressure with accompanying dizziness, pallor, and clamminess, which can be corrected by having the woman lie on her left side.

Support systems The extended network of family, friends, and religious and community contacts that provide nurturance, emotional support, and direct assistance to parents.

Surfactant A surface-active mixture of lipoproteins secreted in the alveoli and air passages that reduces surface tension of pulmonary fluids and contributes to the elasticity of pulmonary tissue.

Sutures Fibrous connections of opposed joint surfaces, as in the skull.

Symphysis pubis A firm joint between the two pelvic bones.

Syncope Transient loss of consciousness and muscle tone.

T

Taboo Describing behaviors or things that are avoided due to cultural customs and beliefs.

Tachypnea An abnormally rapid rate of respiration.

Tactile fremitus Producing vibrations by either crying or talking that can be palpated on the chest.

Technology-assisted State of depending on a medical device that is required to sustain life (mechanical ventilators, intravenous nutrition or drugs, tracheostomy, suctioning, oxygen, or nutritional support with tube feedings).

Telangiectasia Permanent dilation of superficial capillaries and venules.

Telangiectatic nevi (stork bites) Small clusters of pink-red spots appearing on the nape of the neck and around the eyes of infants; localized areas of capillary dilatation.

Teratogens Nongenetic factors that can produce malformations of the fetus.

Term The normal duration of pregnancy.

Testosterone The male hormone; responsible for the development of secondary male characteristics.

Thelarche Breast development.

Therapeutic insemination A procedure to produce a pregnancy in which sperm obtained from a woman's husband or from a donor is deposited in the woman's vagina. Process by which semen is deposited at the cervical os or in the uterus by mechanical means.

Therapeutic play Planned play techniques that provide an opportunity for children to deal with their fears and concerns related to illness or hospitalization.

Thrombocytopenia A low platelet count.

Thrombophlebitis Inflammation of a vein wall, resulting in thrombus.

Thrush A fungal infection of the oral mucous membranes caused by Candida albicans. Most often seen in infants; characterized by white plaques in the mouth.

Thyrotoxicosis A condition that can occur when thyroid hormone is suddenly released into the bloodstream during surgery. The child experiences fever, diaphoresis, and tachycardia, progressing to shock and, if untreated, death.

Tinnitus Ringing in the ears.

Tocolysis Use of medications to arrest preterm labor.

Tolerance Adaptation to an opioid dosage that results in a shorter duration of drug effectiveness over time.

Tonic Continuous muscular contraction; often used to describe seizure activity.

Tonic neck reflex Postural reflex seen in the newborn. When the supine infant's head is turned to one side, the arm and leg on that side extend while the extremities on the opposite side flex. Also called the *fencing position.*

Total parenteral nutrition A feeding regimen accomplished entirely by intravenous injection or other nongastrointestinal route.

Total serum bilirubin Sum of conjugated (direct) and unconjugated (indirect) bilirubin.

Toxic appearance Lethargy, poor perfusion, hypoventilation or hyperventilation, and cyanosis.

Toxic shock syndrome (TSS) Infection caused by *Staphylococcus aureus*, found primarily in women of reproductive age.

Toxicants Harmful natural or synthetic chemicals not metabolically produced by an organism.

Toxins Harmful or poisonous chemicals produced by metabolism or an organism (e.g., ricin).

Toxoid A toxin that has been treated (by heat or chemical) to weaken its toxic effects but retain its antigenicity.

Transgendered An adjective used to describe or refer to someone who feels compelled to (and does) dress and act like a member of the opposite sex.

Transitional milk Breast milk produced from the end of colostrum production until about 2 weeks postpartum.

Transplacental immunity Passive immunity that is transferred from mother to infant.

Transvaginal ultrasound A follicular monitoring test that is used in women undergoing induction cycles, for timing ovulation for insemination and intercourse, for retrieving oocytes for in vitro fertilization, and for monitoring early pregnancy.

Transverse diameter The largest diameter of the pelvic inlet; helps determine the shape of the inlet.

Treatment room In a hospital or medical center, a room designated for performing treatments such as intravenous starts, blood drawing, and lumbar punctures to promote the child's sense of security that his or her own room is a "safe" and relatively pain-free site.

Trigger A stimulus that initiates an asthmatic episode; a substance or condition, including exercise, infection, allergy, irritants, weather, or emotions.

Tripod position Sitting forward with arms on knees for support and extending the neck.

Trisomies The presence of three homologous chromosomes rather than the normal two.

Trophoblast The outer layer of the blastoderm that will eventually establish the nutrient relationship with the uterine endometrium.

True pelvis The portion that lies below the linea terminalis, made up of the inlet, cavity, and outlet.

Trunk incurvation (Galant reflex) Reflex resulting from the stroking of the spine which causes the pelvis to turn to the stimulated side.

Tubal embryo transfer (TET) Procedure in which eggs are retrieved and incubated with the man's sperm then transferred back into the women's body at the embryo stage.

Tubal ligation Sterilization of a woman accomplished by transecting or occluding the fallopian tubes.

Tummy time Prone positioning while awake. Important for all babies because it assists them with learning developmentally appropriate skills; builds muscle strength for their shoulders, neck, and back; and prevents SIDS.

Tumor suppressor genes Genetic material that controls the growth of cells, decreasing the effects of oncogenes.

Tympanogram A graph showing the ability of the middle ear to transmit sound energy; measured by inserting an airtight probe into the external ear entrance and emitting a tone.

Tympanometry A hearing evaluation test that measures middle ear pressure and tympanic membrane movement.

Tympanostomy tubes Pressure-equalizing tubes inserted to drain fluid from the middle ear.

U

Ultrasound High-frequency sound waves that may be directed, through the use of a transducer, into the maternal abdomen. The ultrasonic sound waves reflected by the underlying structures of varying densities allow identification of various maternal and fetal tissues, bones, and fluids.

Umbilical cord The structure connecting the placenta to the umbilicus of the fetus and through which nutrients from the woman are exchanged for wastes from the fetus.

Umbilical velocimetry A noninvasive ultrasound test that measures blood flow changes that occur in maternal and fetal circulation in order to assess placental function.

Uremia Toxicity resulting from the buildup of urea and nitrogenous waste in the blood.

Urinary tract infection (UTI) Significant bacteriuria in the presence of symptoms.

Uterus The hollow muscular organ in which the fertilized ovum is implanted and in which the developing fetus is nourished until birth.

Uterine atony Relaxation of uterine muscle tone following birth.

Uterosacral ligaments Ligaments that provide support for the uterus and cervix at the level of the ischial spines. They arise on each side of the pelvis from the posterior wall of the uterus and sweep back around the rectum to insert on the sides of the first and second sacral vertebrae.

V

Vacuum-assisted birth An obstetric procedure used to assist in the birth of a fetus by applying suction to the fetal head with a soft suction cup attached to a suction bottle (pump) by tubing and placing the device against the occiput of the fetal head.

Vagina The musculomembranous tube or passageway located between the external genitals and the uterus of a woman.

Vaginal birth after cesarean (VBAC) Practice of permitting a trial of labor and possible vaginal birth for women following a previous cesarean birth for nonrecurring causes such as fetal distress or placenta previa.

Variable decelerations Periodic change in fetal heart rate caused by umbilical cord compression; decelerations vary in onset, occurrence, and waveform.

Varus A condition in which the hindfoot turns inward; usually associated with clubfoot.

Vasectomy Surgical removal of a portion of the vas deferens (ductus deferens) to produce infertility.

Vaso-occlusion Blockage of a blood vessel.

Vegans Strict vegetarians who eat absolutely no animal products.

Vegetarian One who eats no poultry, meat, or fish.

Vernix caseosa A protective, cheeselike, whitish substance made up of sebum and desquamated epithelial cells that is present on the fetal skin.

Vertical transmission The passage of disease from the mother to the fetus during the period of pregnancy.

Vesicoureteral reflux The backflow of urine from the bladder into the ureters during voiding.

Violence Threatened or actual use of physical force that leads to potential or actual physical or emotional trauma.

Virilization The production of masculine secondary sexual characteristics in females.

Vision A complex process of acquiring meaning from what is seen, involving the eye, brain, and related neurologic and physiologic structures.

Visual acuity Measurement of the ability to discriminate a letter or other object to test sight.

Vulva The external structure of the female genitals, lying below the mons veneris.

W

Water intoxication An abnormal proportion of water to sodium in the extracellular fluid.

Wharton's jelly Yellow-white gelatinous material surrounding the vessels of the umbilical cord.

Whispered pectoriloquy Change in vocal resonance when syllables are heard distinctly as a whisper.

Withdrawal The physical signs and symptoms that occur when a sedative or pain drug is suddenly stopped in a patient who is physically tolerant.

X

Xerosis Generally dry skin that is more likely to crack and fissure.

Z

Zygote A fertilized egg.

Zygote intrafallopian transfer (ZIFT) Retrieval of oocytes under ultrasound guidance, followed by in vitro fertilization and laparoscopic replacement of fertilized eggs into the fimbriated end of the fallopian tube.

INDEX

Page numbers followed by f indicate figures and those followed by t indicate tables or boxes.

A

B

C

D

E

F

G

H

I

J

K

L

M

N

O

Q

R

S

T

U

V

W

X

Y

Z

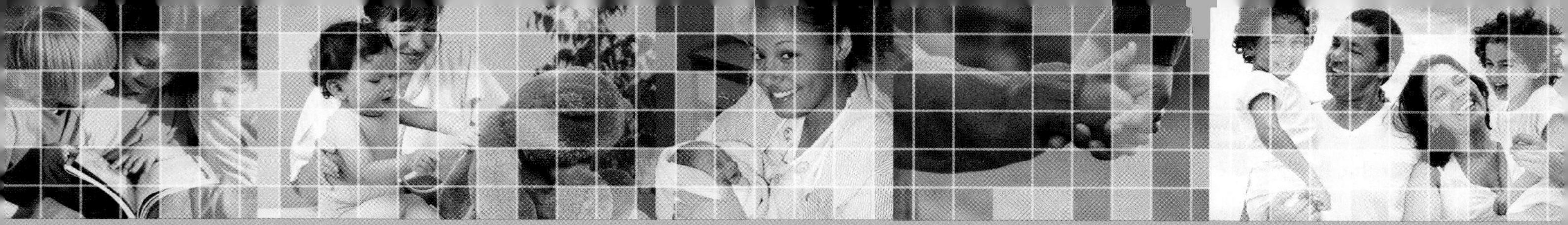

Special Features

DEVELOPING CULTURAL COMPETENCE

DRUG GUIDE

EVIDENCE-BASED NURSING

HEALTH PROMOTION

NURSING CARE PLAN

PATHOPHYSIOLOGY ILLUSTRATED

TEACHING HIGHLIGHTS

THINKING CRITICALLY